Contents

SECTION I. REPRODUCTIVE BASICS

SECTION II. NORMAL OBSTETRICS

SECTION III. PREGNANCY AT RISK

SECTION IV. GENERAL GYNECOLOGY

Authors

Paola Aghajanian, MD
Resident Physician, Department of Obstetrics and
  Gynecology, UCLA Medical Center, Los
  Angeles, California
Gestational Trophoblastic Diseases

Steven W. Ainbinder, MD
Obstetrics and Gynecology Medical Consultant,
  Los Angeles, California
Sexually Transmitted Diseases & Pelvic Infections

Mohammed W. Akhter, MD
Fellow, Division of Cardiovascular Medicine,
  Department of Internal Medicine, University of
  Southern California, Los Angeles, California
Cardiac Disorders in Pregnancy

D. Ellene Andrew, MD
Chief Resident, Department of Obstetrics and
  Gynecology, Tufts University School of Medicine
  and New England Medical Center, Boston,
  Massachusetts
Hirsutism

Dennis R. Anti, Esquire
Partner, Morrison Mahoney LLP, Springfield,
  Massachusetts
The Borderland Between Law & Medicine

Carol L. Archie, MD
Associate Professor of Obstetrics and Gynecology,
  David Geffen School of Medicine at UCLA, Los
  Angeles, California
The Course and Conduct of Normal Labor & Delivery

Christina Arnett, MD
Department of Obstetrics and Gynecology,
  University of Southern California, Los Angeles,
  California
Hematologic Disorders in Pregnancy

Michael P. Aronson, MD, FACOG, FACS
Director of Women's Health Services, University of
  Massachusetts Memorial Medical Center,
  Worcester, Massachusetts
*Intraoperative & Postoperative Complications of
  Gynecologic Surgery*

Vicki V. Baker, MD
Professor, Obstetrics and Gynecology, Wayne State
  University, Detroit, Michigan
*Premalignant & Malignant Disorders of the Ovaries
  & Oviducts*

David L. Barclay, MD
Professor/Director Gynecologic Oncology,
  Department of Obstetrics and Gynecology, Texas
  Tech University Health Sciences Center,
  Amarillo, Texas
*Benign Disorders of the Vulva & Vagina;
  Premalignant & Malignant Disorders of the Vulva
  & Vagina*

Joseph D. Bast, PhD
Professor, Anatomy and Cell Biology, University of
  Kansas Medical Center, Kansas City, Kansas
*Embryology of the Urogenital System & Congenital
  Abnormalities of the Female Genital Tract*

Heather Beattie, RN, JD
Partner, Morrison Mahoney LLP, Springfield,
  Massachusetts
The Borderland Between Law & Medicine

Avi Ben-Shushan, MD
Department of Obstetrics and Gynecology,
  Hadassah University Hospital, Ein Kerem,
  Jerusalem, Israel
Benign Disorders of the Uterine Cervix

Helene B. Bernstein, MD
Assistant Professor, Department of Obstetrics and
  Gynecology, Division of Maternal Fetal
  Medicine, David Geffen School of Medicine at
  UCLA, Los Angeles, California
Normal Pregnancy & Prenatal Care

Narender N. Bhatia, MD
Chief of Urogynecology, Director of Fellowship in
  Female Pelvic Medicine and Reconstructive
  Surgery, Professor-in-Residence of Obstetrics and
  Gynecology, David Geffen School of Medicine at
  UCLA, Los Angeles, California
Urinary Incontinence

Muriel Boreham, MD
Clinical Instructor, Department of Obstetrics and
  Gynecology, Baylor University Medical Center,
  Dallas, Texas
Perioperative Considerations in Gynecology

Kathleen M. Brennan, MD
Resident Physician, Department of Obstetrics and
  Gynecology, The David Geffen School of
  Medicine at UCLA, Los Angeles, California
*Premalignant & Malignant Disorders of the Ovaries
  & Oviducts*

Ronald T. Burkman, MD
Chair, Department of Obstetrics and Gynecology,
  Baystate Medical Center, Springfield,
  Massachusetts
Contraception & Family Planning

Melissa C. Bush, MD
Assistant Clinical Professor, Department of
  Obstetrics and Gynecology, University of
  California, Irvine, Orange, California
Multiple Pregnancy

Wendy Y. Chang, MD
Assistant Clinical Professor of Obstetrics and
  Gynecology, The David Geffen School of
  Medicine at UCLA, Los Angeles, California
Amenorrhea

David Chelmow
Department of Obstetrics and Gynecology, Tufts
  New England Medical Center, Boston,
  Massachusetts
*Intraoperative & Postoperative Complications of
  Gynecologic Surgery*

Caroline M. Colin, MD
Senior Resident, Department of Obstetrics and
  Gynecology, University of California, Los
  Angeles, Los Angeles, California
*Complications of Menstruation; Abnormal Uterine
  Bleeding*

Joseph V. Collea, MD
Vice Chairman, Professor and Director, Division of
  Maternal-Fetal Medicine, Department of
  Obstetrics and Gynecology, Georgetown
  University Hospital, Washington, DC
Malpresentation & Cord Prolapse

Dipika Dandade, MD
Associate Physician, Obstetrics and Gynecology,
  Southern California Kaiser Permanente, Baldwin
  Park, Baldwin Park, California
Therapeutic Gynecologic Procedures

Alan H. DeCherney, MD
Chief, Reproductive Biology and Medicine Branch,
  National Institute of Child Health and Human
  Development, National Institutes of Health,
  Bethesda, Maryland
*Amenorrhea; Assisted Reproductive Technologies: In
  Vitro Fertilization & Related Techniques;
  Endometriosis; Infertility; The Role of Imaging
  Techniques in Gynecology; Sexually Transmitted
  Diseases & Pelvic Infections*

Catherine M. DeUgarte, MD
Staff Physician, Reproductive Endocrinology,
  Obstetrics and Gynecology, Henry Ford
  Hospital, Troy, Michigan
*Assisted Reproductive Technologies: In Vitro
  Fertilization & Related Techniques; Embryology of
  the Urogenital System & Congenital Abnormalities
  of the Female Genital Tract*

Oliver Dorigo, MD, PhD
Assistant Professor, Division of Gynecologic
  Oncology, Department of Obstetrics and
  Gynecology, The David Geffen School of
  Medicine at UCLA, Los Angeles, California
*Premalignant & Malignant Disorders of the Ovaries
  & Oviducts; Premalignant & Malignant Disorders
  of the Uterine Corpus; Radiation Therapy &
  Chemotherapy for Gynecologic Cancers*

Peter Drewes, MD, FACOG
Assistant Instructor, University of Texas
  Southwestern Medical Center at Dallas, Dallas,
  Texas
Perioperative Considerations in Gynecology

Jamie S. Drinville, MD
Chief Resident, Department of Obstetrics and
  Gynecology, The David Geffen School of
  Medicine at UCLA, Los Angeles, California
Benign Disorders of the Uterine Corpus

Adelina M. Emmi, MD
Medical Director, Reproductive Laboratories of
  Augusta, Augusta, Georgia
Hirsutism

Niloofar Eskandari, MD
Staff Physician, Department of Obstetrics and
Gynecology, Southern California Kaiser
Permanente, Baldwin Park, Baldwin Park,
California
Infertility

James E. Fanale, MD
Associate Professor of Medicine, University of
Massachusetts Medical School, Worcester,
Massachusetts
The Borderland Between Law & Medicine

Carol L. Gagliardi, MD
Assistant Professor, Department of Obstetrics and
Gynecology, Mount Sinai School of Medicine,
Jersey City Medical Center Program, Jersey City,
New Jersey
Hirsutism

William F. Ganong, MD
Lange Professor of Physiology Emeritus, University of
California, San Francisco, San Francisco, California
Physiology of Reproduction in Women

Sara H. Garmel, MD
Adjunct Clinical Assistant Professor, Department
of Obstetrics and Gynecology, University of
Michigan Medical School, Ann Arbor, Michigan
Early Pregnancy Risks

Shahin Ghadir, MD
Reproductive Endocrinologist and Infertility
Specialist, Department of Obstetrics and
Gynecology, The David Geffen School of
Medicine at UCLA and Cedars-Sinai Medical
Center, Los Angeles, California
Infertility

Ronald C. Gibbs, MD
E. Stewart Taylor Chair in Obstetrics and
Gynecology and Professor and Chairman,
Department of Obstetrics and Gynecology,
University of Colorado Health Sciences Center,
Denver, Colorado
Antimicrobial Chemotherapy

Johanna Weiss Goldberg, MD
Clinical Instructor, Department of Obstetrics and
Gynecology, Joan and Sanford I. Weill Medical
College, Cornell University, New York, New York
Critical Care Obstetrics

Annekathryn Goodman, MD
Associate Professor in Obstetrics, Gynecology,
Reproductive Biology, Harvard Medical School,
Boston, Massachusetts
*Premalignant & Malignant Disorders of the Uterine
Corpus*

T. Murphy Goodwin, MD
Chief, Division of Maternal-Fetal Medicine,
Department of Obstetrics and Gynecology,
University of Southern California, Los Angeles,
California
*Nervous System & Autoimmune Disorders in Pregnancy;
Renal/Urinary Tract, Gastrointestinal, &
Dermatologic Disorders in Pregnancy*

Robert A. Graebe, MD
Chairman and Program Director, Director of
Reproductive Endocrinology, Department of
Obstetrics and Gynecology, Monmouth Medical
Center, Long Branch, New Jersey
The Role of Imaging Techniques in Gynecology

Jeffrey S. Greenspoon, MD
Maternal-Fetal Medicine Specialist, Olive-View
UCLA Medical Center, Los Angeles, California
*Diabetes Mellitus & Pregnancy; Renal/Urinary
Tract, Gastrointestinal, & Dermatologic
Disorders in Pregnancy; Hematologic Disorders in
Pregnancy*

Cristiane Guberman, MD
Resident, Obstetrics and Gynecology, University
of Southern California, Los Angeles,
California
*Renal/Urinary Tract, Gastrointestinal, &
Dermatologic Disorders in Pregnancy*

Marsha K. Guess, MD
Fellow, Division of Urogynecology and
Reconstructive Surgery, Albert Einstein College
of Medicine, Montefiore Medical Center, Bronx,
New York
Hirsutism

Alexandra Haessler, MD
Fellow, Female Pelvic Medicine and Reconstructive
Surgery, Harbor-UCLA Medical Center, Los
Angeles, California
Psychological Aspects of Obstetrics & Gynecology

Vivian P. Halfin, MD
Associate Clinical Professor of Psychiatry and
   Obstetrics and Gynecology, Tufts University
   School of Medicine, Boston, Massachusetts
Domestic Violence & Sexual Assault

Afshan B. Hameed, MD, FACC
Assistant Clinical Professor, Division of Maternal
   Fetal Medicine, Department of Obstetrics and
   Gynecology, University of California, Irvine,
   Orange, California
Cardiac Disorders in Pregnancy

Kathleen Harney, MD
Chief, Department of Obstetrics and Gynecology,
   Cambridge Health Alliance, Cambridge,
   Massachusetts
The Breast

Christine H. Holschneider, MD
Assistant Professor, Obstetrics and Gynecology,
   The David Geffen School of Medicine at UCLA,
   Los Angeles, California
*Premalignant & Malignant Disorders of the Uterine
   Cervix; Surgical Diseases & Disorders in Pregnancy*

Andy Huang, MD
Fellow, Reproductive Endocrinology and Infertility,
   Department of Obstetrics and Gynecology, The
   David Geffen School of Medicine at UCLA, Los
   Angeles, California
*Genetic Disorders & Sex Chromosome Abnormalities,
   The Role of Imaging Techniques in Gynecology*

Marc H. Incerpi, MD
Associate Professor, Division of Maternal-Fetal
   Medicine, Department of Obstetrics and
   Gynecology, University of Southern California
   Keck School of Medicine, Los Angeles, California
Operative Delivery

Carla Janzen, MD
Clinical Instructor, Department of Obstetrics and
   Gynecology, The David Geffen School of
   Medicine at UCLA, Los Angeles, California
*Diabetes Mellitus & Pregnancy; Essentials of Normal
   Newborn Assessment & Care*

Howard L. Judd, MD
Professor, Department of Obstetrics and
   Gynecology, David Geffen School of Medicine at
   UCLA, Los Angeles, California
Menopause & Postmenopause

Daniel A. Kahn, MD, PhD
Chief Resident Physician, Department of
   Obstetrics and Gynecology, David Geffen School
   of Medicine at UCLA, Los Angeles, California
Maternal Physiology During Pregnancy

Laura A. Kalayjian, MD
Assistant Professor of Neurology, Co-director,
   Comprehensive Epilepsy Center, University of
   Southern California Keck School of Medicine,
   Los Angeles, California
Nervous System & Autoimmune Disorders in Pregnancy

Charles Kawada, MD
Department of Obstetrics, Gynecology, and
   Reproductive Biology, Harvard Medical School,
   Cambridge, Massachusetts
*Gynecologic History, Examination & Diagnostic
   Procedures*

Karen Kish, MD
Private Practice, Austin, TX
Malpresentation & Cord Prolapse

Robert A. Knuppel, MD, MPH, MBA, FACOG
Chief Medical Officer, Winhealthcare, Rye Brook,
   New York
*Maternal-Placental Fetal Unit; Fetal & Early
   Neonatal Physiology*

Anna Kogan, MD
Resident, Department of Obstetrics and
   Gynecology, David Geffen School of Medicine at
   UCLA, Los Angeles, California
Benign Disorders of the Uterine Cervix

Brian J. Koos, MD, PhD
Professor, Obstetrics and Gynecology, The David
   Geffen School of Medicine at UCLA, Los
   Angeles, California
Maternal Physiology during Pregnancy

Kermit E. Krantz, MD, LittD
Professor and Chairman Emeritus, Professor of
   Anatomy Emeritus, University of Kansas School
   of Medicine, Kansas City, Kansas
Anatomy of the Female Reproductive System

Ashim Kumar, MD
Fertility and Surgical Associates of California,
   Thousand Oaks, California
Infertility

Melanie Landay, MD
Resident Physician, Department of Obstetrics and Gynecology, UCLA Medical Center, Los Angeles, California
Premalignant & Malignant Disorders of the Vulva & Vagina

Kim Lipscomb
Department of Obstetrics and Gynecology, David Geffen School of Medicine at UCLA, Los Angeles, California
The Normal Puerperium

Jessica S. Lu, MPH
Medical Student, UCLA, Los Angeles, California
Domestic Violence & Sexual Assault

Michael C. Lu, MD, MPH
Assistant Professor, Department of Obstetrics and Gynecology, David Geffen School of Medicine at UCLA, Los Angeles, California
Domestic Violence & Sexual Assault

Somjate Manipalviratn, MD
Fellow in Reproductive Endocrinology and Infertility, Department of Obstetrics and Gynecology, University of California Los Angeles, Los Angeles, California
Genetic Disorders & Sex Chromosome Abnormalities

Fariborz Mazdisnian, MD
Physician-In-Charge, Palmdale Medical Office, Southern California Permanente Medical Group, Palmdale, California
Benign Disorders of the Vulva & Vagina; Complications of Menstruation; Abnormal Uterine Bleeding

John S. McDonald, MD
Professor and Chairman, Department of Anesthesiology; Professor, Obstetrics and Gynecology; Harbor-UCLA Medical Center, Torrance, California
Obstetric Analgesia & Anesthesia

Shobha H. Mehta, MD
Maternal-Fetal Medicine Fellow, Department of Obstetrics and Gynecology, Wayne State University/Hutzel Women's Hospital, Detroit, Michigan
Methods of Assessment for Pregnancy at Risk

Sandaz Memarzadeh, MD
Clinical Instructor, Division of Gynecologic Oncology, Department of Obstetrics and Gynecology, David Geffen School of Medicine at UCLA, Los Angeles, California
Benign Disorders of the Uterine Corpus; Premalignant & Malignant Disorders of the Vulva & Vagina

David A. Miller, MD
Associate Professor, Division of Maternal-Fetal Medicine, University of Southern California Keck School of Medicine, Los Angeles, California
Hypertension in Pregnancy

Martin N. Montoro, MD
Professor of Clinical Medicine and Obstetrics and Gynecology, University of Southern California Keck School of Medicine, Women's and Children's Hospital, Los Angeles, California
Pulmonary Disorders in Pregnancy; Thyroid & Other Endocrine Disorders during Pregnancy

David Muram, MD
Professor Emeritus, Department of Obstetrics and Gynecology, University of Tennessee, Memphis, Tennessee
Pediatric & Adolescent Gynecology

Kenneth N. Muse, MD, MPH
Associate Professor, Department of Obstetrics and Gynecology, University of Kentucky, Lexington, Kentucky
Endometriosis

Lauren Nathan, MD
Associate Professor, Department of Obstetrics and Gynecology, The David Geffen School of Medicine at UCLA, Los Angeles, California
Menopause & Postmenopause

Mikio Nihira MD, MPH
Associate Professor of Obstetrics and Gynecology, Division of Female Pelvic Medicine and Reconstructive Surgery, University of Oklahoma Health Sciences Center, Oklahoma City, Oklahoma
Perioperative Considerations in Gynecology

Miles J. Novy, MD
Professor of Obstetrics and Gynecology, Oregon Health and Science University, Beaverton, Oregon
The Normal Puerperium

John P. O'Grady, MD
Professor, Department of Obstetrics and
Gynecology, Tufts University School of
Medicine, Boston, Massachusetts
The Borderland Between Law & Medicine

Sue M. Palmer, MD, PA
Department of Obstetrics and Gynecology,
University of Texas, Houston, Texas
Diabetes Mellitus & Pregnancy

Sujatha Pathi, MD
Resident, Department of Obstetrics and
Gynecology, The David Geffen School of
Medicine at UCLA, Los Angeles, California
*Radiation Therapy & Chemotherapy for Gynecologic
Cancers*

Alan S. Penzias, MD
Surgical Director, Boston IVF, Boston,
Massachusetts
*Assisted Reproductive Technologies: In Vitro
Fertilization & Related Techniques*

Martin L. Pernoll, MD
Executive Dean, Kansas University School of
Medicine, Kansas City, Kansas
*Benign Disorders of the Uterine Cervix; Late
Pregnancy Complications; Multiple Pregnancy*

Matthew M. Poggi, MD
Assistant Professor of Radiology and Radiological
Sciences, Uniformed Services University of the
Health Sciences, Bethesda, Maryland
The Breast

Sarah H. Poggi, MD
Perinatologist, Inova Alexandria Hospital
Alexandria, Virginia
Postpartum Hemorrhage & the Abnormal Puerperium

Karen Purcell, MD, PhD
Clinical Instructor, Department of Obstetrics,
Gynecology, and Infertility, University of
California, San Francisco, San Francisco, California
Benign Disorders of the Ovaries & Oviducts

Elisabeth L. Raab, MD
Neonatologist, Children's Hospital, Los Angeles,
Los Angeles, California
*Essentials of Normal Newborn Assessment & Care;
Neonatal Resuscitation & Care of the Newborn at Risk*

Jeannine Rahimian, MD
Assistant Clinical Faculty, University of California,
Los Angeles, Los Angeles, California
Disproportionate Fetal Growth

Susan M. Ramin, MD
Professor and Director, Division of Maternal-Fetal
Medicine, Department of Obstetrics, Gynecology
and Reproductive Sciences, The University of
Texas Medical School at Houston, Houston, Texas
Sexually Transmitted Diseases & Pelvic Infections

Ashley S. Roman, MD, MPH
Assistant Professor, Department of Obstetrics and
Gynecology, New York University School of
Medicine, New York, New York
Late Pregnancy Complications

Miriam B. Rosenthal, MD
Associate Professor Emerita, Psychiatry and
Obstetrics and Gynecology, Case Western
Reserve School of Medicine, Cleveland, Ohio
Psychological Aspects of Obstetrics & Gynecology

Susan Sarajari, MD, PhD
Fellow, Division of Reproductive Endocrinology
and Infertility, Department of Obstetrics and
Gynecology, UCLA Medical Center and
Cedars-Sinai Medical Center, Los Angeles,
California
*Endometriosis; The Role of Imaging Techniques in
Gynecology*

Wendy A. Satmary, MD, FACOG
Obstetrics and Gynecology, Kaiser Permanente
Medical Center, Woodland Hills, California
*Premalignant & Malignant Disorders of the Vulva &
Vagina*

Jennifer Scearce, MD
Department of Obstetrics and Gynecology,
University of Southern California Keck School of
Medicine, Los Angeles, California
Third-Trimester Vaginal Bleeding

Asher Shushan, MD
Department of Obstetrics and Gynecology,
Hadassah University Hospital, Ein Kerem,
Jerusalem, Israel
*Complications of Menstruation; Abnormal Uterine
Bleeding*

Donna M. Smith, MD
Associate Professor, Department of Obstetrics and Gynecology, Loyola University Medical Center, Maywood, Illinois
Premalignant & Malignant Disorders of the Vulva & Vagina

Ramada S. Smith, MD
Director, Gaston Perinatal Center, Gaston Memorial Hospital, Gastonia, North Carolina
Critical Care Obstetrics

Robert J. Sokol, MD
Distinguished Professor and Director, C.S. Mott Center for Human Growth and Development, Department of Obstetrics and Gynecology, Wayne State University School of Medicine, Detroit, Michigan
Methods of Assessment for Pregnancy at Risk

Kari Sproul, MD
Resident, Department of Obstetrics and Gynecology, The David Geffen School of Medicine at UCLA, Los Angeles, California
Approach to the Patient

Stacy L. Strehlow, MD
Fellow, Maternal-Fetal Medicine, University of Southern California Women's and Children's Hospital, Los Angeles, California
Complications of Labor & Delivery; Diabetes Mellitus & Pregnancy

Christopher M. Tarnay, MD
Associate Clinical Professor, Division of Female Pelvic Medicine and Reconstructive Pelvic Surgery, Department of Obstetrics and Gynecology, The Olive View-UCLA Medical Center and The David Geffen School of Medicine at UCLA, Los Angeles, California
Pelvic Organ Prolapse; Urinary Incontinence

Bradley Trivax, MD
Fellow, Department of Reproductive Endocrinology and Infertility, UCLA Medical Center, Los Angeles, California
Genetic Disorders & Sex Chromosome Abnormalities

Mor Tzadik, MD
Department of Obstetrics and Gynecology, The David Geffen School of Medicine at UCLA, Los Angeles, California
Benign Disorders of the Ovaries & Oviducts

Peter S. Uzelac, MD
Assistant Professor, Department of Obstetrics and Gynecology, University of Southern California Keck School of Medicine, Los Angeles, California
Complications of Labor & Delivery; Early Pregnancy Risks; Third-Trimester Vaginal Bleeding

Michael W. Varner, MD
Professor, Department of Obstetrics and Gynecology, University of Utah Health Sciences Center, Salt Lake City, Utah
Disproportionate Fetal Growth

Milena Weinstein, MD
Fellow of Urogynecology and Pelvic Reconstructive Medicine, Reproductive Medicine Department, University of California, San Diego, San Diego, California
Neonatal Resuscitation & Care of the Newborn at Risk; Normal Pregnancy & Prenatal Care

James M. Wheeler, MD, MPH, JD
Center for Women's Healthcare, Houston, Texas
Benign Disorders of the Ovaries & Oviducts; Therapeutic Gynecologic Procedures

Cecilia K. Wieslander, MD
Assistant Instructor, Division of Urogynecology/ Reconstructive Pelvic Surgery, Department of Obstetrics and Gynecology, University of Texas Southwestern Medical Center, Dallas, Texas
Therapeutic Gynecologic Procedures

Uchechi Wosu, MD
Department of Obstetrics and Gynecology, University of Massachusetts Memorial Hospital, Worcester, Massachusetts
Intraoperative & Postoperative Complications of Gynecologic Surgery

Ralph Yarnell, MD
Associate Professor, Department of Anesthesiology, University of Vermont, Burlington, Vermont
Obstetric Analgesia & Anesthesia

Preface

As in the previous editions, this text is a single-source reference for practitioners in both the inpatient and outpatient setting focusing on the practical aspects of clinical diagnosis and patient management.

Contained within the text is a thorough review of all of obstetrics and gynecology, including medical advances up to the time of publication. More than 1000 diseases and disorders are included.

A continued emphasis on disease prevention and evidence-based medicine remains paramount. In addition to diagnosis and treatment of disease, pathophysiology is a major area of focus. The concise format facilitates quick access.

A new and improved layout will certainly be appreciated, with more than 500 anatomic drawings, imaging studies, and diagrams as part of the basic text.

Medical students will find *CDTOG* to be an authoritative introduction to the specialty and an excellent source for reference and review. House officers will welcome the concise practical information for commonly encountered health problems. Practicing obstetricians and gynecologists, family physicians, internists, nurse practitioners nurse midwives, physician assistants, and other healthcare providers whose practice includes women's health can use the book to answer questions that arise in the daily practice of obstetrics and gynecology.

Medicine, including OB/GYN, is undergoing rapid change and every attempt has been made to keep the Lange Series current. A great deal of effort has gone into checking the sources to make sure that this book presents standards of care and acceptable modes of treatment and diagnosis.

Just as the preface has been updated, modified, and modernized from the ninth edition, so has what lies between the covers of the tenth edition of *Current Diagnosis & Treatment Obstetrics & Gynecology*.

Alan H. DeCherney, MD
Lauren Nathan, MD
T. Murphy Goodwin, MD
Neri Laufer, MD

SECTION I
Reproductive Basics

Approach to the Patient

Kari Sproul, MD

An effective relationship between health care provider and patient is based on the knowledge and skill that qualify the provider for adequate communication between the individuals and for an appreciation of the ethical standards that govern the conduct of the participants in the relationship.

THE KNOWLEDGE BASE

The health care of women encompasses all aspects of medical science and therapeutics. Physicians in the practice of obstetrics and gynecology are called upon as consultants. In addition, they frequently act as primary care providers for their patients. The special medical needs and concerns of women vary with the patient's age, reproductive status, and desire to reproduce. Certainly the diagnostic possibilities and the choice of diagnostic or therapeutic intervention will be influenced by the possibility of, or desire for, pregnancy or, in some cases, by the patient's hormonal profile. In addition, the gynecologic or obstetric assessment must include an evaluation of the patient's general health status and should be placed in the context of the psychologic, social, cultural, and emotional status of the patient. In this day of e-medicine and evidence-based medicine, the patient's and physician's knowledge base will be dependent on information that is retrieved online. It will become the job of the physician to use the most up-to-date evidence for medical decision making and to assist the patient in deciphering what Internet information is true or false.

History

To offer each woman optimal care, the information obtained at each visit should be as complete as possible. Whether the contact is a routine visit or is occasioned by a particular problem or complaint, the woman should be encouraged to view the visit as an opportunity to participate in improving her health. The clinical database should include general information about the patient and her goals in seeking care. The history of the present problem, past medical history, family history, medications used, allergies, social history, and review of systems should be concise but thorough. Portions of the history provided by questionnaires or by other members of the health care team should be reviewed with the patient, in part to verify the information but also to begin assessing the patient's personality and to determine her attitude toward the health care system. The developmental history, menstrual history, sexual history, and obstetric history obviously assume central importance for the gynecologic or obstetric visit. In addition, the habit of systematically categorizing the nature of complaints such as pain, abnormal bleeding, or vaginal discharge will usually narrow the differential diagnoses. For example, the categorization of a complaint of pain should include its character, location, onset, radiation, intensity, events associated, and palliative and provocative factors. Such thoroughness will permit assessment of change as well as determination of the appropriate mode of investigation or therapy.

The initial contact with the patient, made while she is fully clothed and comfortable, may help in decreasing her anxiety about the physical examination. Concerns about the examination may be elicited, and a history of previous unfortunate experiences may alert the examiner to the need for extra attention, time, and gentleness.

Physical Examination

The second component of the patient assessment, the physical examination, should also be directed toward evaluation of the total patient. The patient again should be encouraged to view the examination as a positive opportunity to gain information about her body, and she should be offered feedback regarding the general physical examination and any significant findings. The examination should always include a discussion of any concerns expressed by the patient. The breast examination provides a good opportunity to reinforce the practice of breast self-examination. The pelvic examination is usually an occasion of heightened anxiety for the patient, and every effort should be made to make the experience a positive one. Starting from the beginning, with the correct positioning of the patient, the physician should give the patient as much control over the process as possible, by asking if she is ready, asking for feedback on whether the examination is painful, and seeking her cooperation in relaxation and muscle control. Information about each step of the examination can be provided so that the patient is involved and appropriately aware of the value of each maneuver.

Inspection of the external genitalia is followed by the gentle insertion of an appropriately sized, warmed metal speculum or a plastic vaginal speculum with a small amount of water-soluble gel lubricant on the outer inferior blade, to permit examination of the vagina and the cervix. For patients with pain or increased anxiety, their cooperation must be continually reinforced by slow, gentle placement of the instrument, maintaining downward pressure against the relaxed perineal body and away from the urethral and anterior vaginal areas. Some women may wish to watch, using a mirror, as the genitalia are inspected and may gain confidence from visualizing the cervix and vagina. The Papanicolaou (Pap) smear may be uncomfortable for some women, so patients should be alerted when the test is being done. The bimanual examination should also be explained to the patient. When the uterus is anteflexed, the woman may want to appreciate the size and location of her uterus by feeling it with the guidance of the examiner. The rectovaginal and rectal examinations, if performed while the patient relaxes her anal sphincter, provide additional information and can be another source of reassurance for the normal patient or a means of diagnosis for the patient with disease. If an ultrasound is indicated as part of the gynecologic or obstetric examination, additional patient participation in the evaluation can be obtained by providing explanations of the visualized anatomy.

Implications of Technology

The scientific knowledge base for obstetric and gynecologic care has grown in parallel with general medical advances. In some cases this proliferation of information and technology has profoundly altered the relationship between health care providers and their patients. For example, the change from an intuitive management of labor and delivery to active monitoring and subsequent interpretation of data has provided a more rational basis for decision making. This change of management style has also created a potential for conflict or confusion in the relationship between patient and physician. In seeking to obtain additional information, the physician can be perceived to be intervening unnecessarily. More than ever before, issues of consumerism and participation in decision making require an understanding of the expectations of each individual woman. Whether a woman perceives herself as a "client" or as a "patient," and the degree to which this perception coincides with the views of her physician, may alter her acceptance of recommendations for care. Women are turning to the Internet for health information, and the quality of this information is an important factor in determining whether it will have a negative or positive impact on their health care experience. The fact that several options are available in the management of many obstetric or gynecologic situations may further complicate the relationship. However, this situation provides an opportunity to allow the patient to participate actively in choosing the best therapy for her particular circumstance.

COMMUNICATION

If the first foundation of a strong therapeutic relationship is knowledge, the second is communication. The ability to establish trust, to obtain and deliver complete and accurate information, and to ensure compliance with recommendations depends in large measure on the health care provider's communication skills. In some individuals these skills are innate, but for most the ability to become an effective communicator in a variety of settings requires an active process of learning and a willingness to be evaluated by peers. The information communicated in each encounter, whether by written material, face-to-face discussion, telephone contact, or e-mail, extends beyond the factual content provided to include a demonstration of the provider's willingness to be available to answer questions and to encourage patient involvement in decision making.

One common barrier from the patient's perspective is that medical information is communicated via medical jargon to the layperson. This medical jargon is often spoken in a hurried fashion, and the listener is not given the opportunity to ask questions for clarification. The patient may also find it difficult to voice her concerns within the traditional doctor–patient relationship. She may be embarrassed to reveal intimate details about her personal life to a provider who does not take the time to show interest in her story. By not allowing the patient to express her fears, concerns, or questions, the provider can miss valuable clues to diagnosis and formulation of a treatment plan. Also, with the rapidly growing proportion of minority groups within the United States (U.S.) population, the physician is faced with barriers such as foreign languages and the use of translators.

Solutions to these communication barriers can be found by educating patients and providers. The physician should provide a comfortable environment, encourage the patient to ask questions, listen carefully to both her story and the way she tells it, explore with her the goals and expectations she has about the treatment, and have interpreter services available for patients in need. Videotaped interviews as well as more structured teaching programs in medical schools are very effective means of educating providers about these skills. The patient should be asked to repeat instructions, and written material should be provided whenever possible. For her part the patient can be asked to take notes and keep a diary for review at subsequent visits.

To enhance women's health and to decrease the discontinuation of hormones taken to prevent unintended pregnancy, clinicians need to focus on communication and counseling issues. In doing so, physicians can provide patients with the knowledge of benefits of hormone therapy, dispel fears about contraceptives, and promote the health benefits in an effort to increase adherence and continuance of hormonal contraceptives. For the health care practitioner, the counterbalance of a litigious society that may hold the physician responsible for treatment outcome places a high premium on documentation and scientific justification for each intervention or nonintervention and can place the physician in an adversarial position with respect to the patient's desires. The obligation to inform the patient, to obtain surgical informed consent, or to advise about choices regarding pregnancy outcome is becoming in some instances a matter of law rather than established medical practice. These legislative initiatives, while offensive to many, are signals that the public feels it requires protection from manipulation at the hands of those who have the power of knowledge and training not available to the layperson. Regardless of the validity of this perception, it can only be countered by efforts to establish and maintain the trust of each individual with whom the physician has a medical relationship. This trust is rooted in the physician's medical knowledge and is maintained by conscientious structured lifetime learning, the frank assessment and acknowledgment of areas of ignorance, and the willingness to discuss with the patient what is known and what is uncertain.

ETHICS

If the bricks of the foundation of the relationship between physician and patient are knowledge and communication, then the mortar that forms the basis for trust is the integrity and ethical behavior of all participants in the relationship. Ethical dilemmas in obstetrics and gynecology are receiving increasing recognition, particularly as they deal with the provocative issues surrounding the beginnings of life and the control of individual patients over their own treatment plans, including their route of delivery (vaginal versus elective cesarean section). Ethical dilemmas only arise when there are conflicting obligations, rights, or claims. Because the delivery of health care involves multiple participants, a consensus of values often must be sought when the patient is cared for by a team, even when significant pluralism of views might be represented. To minimize potential ethical conflicts, to anticipate potential areas of difficulty, and to achieve consistency in behavior, individuals may avail themselves of a number of resources for ethical decision making. In addition to the growing literature in the field, many hospitals and practice settings have formal consultation services for resolution of ethical dilemmas. Before seeking an external framework, however, the practitioner should be aware of his or her own values and understand the basis of these values. The values of the medical profession and of the institutions in which the physician practices, as formulated by codes and standards but also as expressed indirectly through past actions, usually are helpful in providing a decision-making framework. Finally, a familiarity with ethical theories may permit decision making that achieves an acceptable consensus in the face of conflicting values. Discussions based on consideration of the ethical principles of patient autonomy (respect for persons), beneficence (doing good), nonmalfeasance (refraining from doing harm), and justice (consideration of resources and fairness of opportunity) will prevent capricious and arbitrary decisions.

The principle of autonomy, or respect for each individual person, may form the underlying basis for resolving many ethical questions and will determine appropriate attitudes toward confidentiality, privacy, right to information, and the ultimate primacy of the patient in making treatment decisions. Because caring for women necessarily involves information regarding sensitive and intimate relationships and activities, as well as access to a woman's thoughts, feelings, and emotions, full disclosure of such information by the patient places a burden of trust on the health care provider to protect the rights and privacy of each patient. The relationship established at an initial gynecologic visit between a young adolescent and the physician may potentially extend throughout the patient's adult life and include major life events such as education about reproductive health, assistance in family planning and childbearing, and preservation of physical fitness and well-being through the postmenopausal years. To successfully establish such an enduring clinical relationship requires a sensitivity to the changing goals and needs of the individual patient. Offering care to some patients or providing some types of services may not be comfortable for all practitioners. For example, establishing a rapport with an adolescent seeking birth control or providing health care to a lesbian may require a nonjudgmental approach when interviewing the patient and a balanced consideration of lifestyle options. Recognition of these special needs has led to a compartmentalization of health care in some regions such that specialty practices or clinics directed toward adolescent health care, family planning, fertility, oncology, and menopausal care are frequently available. These resources can best be utilized by referral, with guidance from the primary care provider, so that appropriate use of such resources can be an integral part of the general health care of each woman. In addition, we can integrate these multiple disciplines in a deliberate effort to expand the concept of women's health beyond its traditional focus on reproductive health to more fully evaluate and care for the female patient.

REFERENCES

ACOG Committee Opinion: The ethics of decision making. Obstet Gynecol 2003;102:1101.

American College of Physicians: Racial and ethnic disparities in health care. Ann Intern Med 2004;141:226.

Amies AM: The effect of vaginal speculum lubrication on the rate of unsatisfactory cervical cytology diagnosis. Obstet Gynecol 2002;100:889.

Bickley L: *Bates' Guide to Physical Examination and History Taking*, 7th ed. Lippincott Williams & Wilkins, 1999.

Kassirer JP: Patients, physicians and the Internet. Health Affairs 2000;19:115.

La Valleur J, Wysocki S: Selection of oral contraceptives or hormone replacement therapy: Patient communication and counseling issues. Am J Obstet Gynecol 2001;185(2 Suppl):S57.

Minkoff H: Ethical dimensions of primary elective cesarean delivery. Obstet Gynecol 2004;103:387.

Murray E: The impact of health information on the internet on health care and the physician-patient relationship: National U.S. survey among 1,050 U.S. physicians. J Med Internet Res 2003;6:17.

Teutsch C: Patient-doctor communication. Med Clin North Am 2003;87:1115.

Anatomy of the Female Reproductive System

2

Kermit E. Krantz, MD, LittD

ABDOMINAL WALL

Topographic Anatomy

The anterior abdominal wall is divided into sections for descriptive purposes and to allow the physician to outline relationships of the viscera in the abdominal cavity. The centerpoint of reference is the sternoxiphoid process, which is in the same plane as the tenth thoracic vertebra. The upper 2 sections are formed by the subcostal angle; the lower extends from the lower ribs to the crest of the ilium and forward to the anterior superior iliac spines. The base is formed by the inguinal ligaments and the symphysis pubica.

The viscera are located by dividing the anterolateral abdominal wall into regions. One line is placed from the level of each ninth costal cartilage to the iliac crests. Two other lines are drawn from the middle of the inguinal ligaments to the cartilage of the eighth rib. The 9 regions formed (Fig 2–1) are the epigastric, umbilical, hypogastric, and right and left hypochondriac, lumbar, and ilioinguinal.

Within the right hypochondriac zone are the right lobe of the liver, the gallbladder at the anterior inferior angle, part of the right kidney deep within the region, and, occasionally, the right colic flexure.

The epigastric zone contains the left lobe of the liver and part of the right lobe, the stomach, the proximal duodenum, the pancreas, the suprarenal glands, and the upper poles of both kidneys (Fig 2–2).

The left hypochondriac region marks the situation of the spleen, the fundus of the stomach, the apex of the liver, and the left colic flexure.

Within the right lumbar region are the ascending colon, coils of intestine, and, frequently, the inferior border of the lateral portion of the right kidney.

The central umbilical region contains the transverse colon, the stomach, the greater omentum, the small intestine, the second and third portions of the duodenum, the head of the pancreas, and parts of the medial aspects of the kidneys.

Located in the left lumbar region are the descending colon, the left kidney, and small intestine. Within the limits of the right ilioinguinal region are the cecum and appendix, part of the ascending colon, small intestine, and, occasionally, the right border of the greater omentum.

The hypogastric region includes the greater omentum, loops of small intestine, the pelvic colon, and often part of the transverse colon.

The left ilioinguinal region encloses the sigmoid colon, part of the descending colon, loops of small intestine, and left border of the greater omentum.

There is considerable variation in the position and size of individual organs due to differences in body size and conformation. Throughout life, variations in the positions of organs are dependent not only on gravity but also on the movements of the hollow viscera, which induce further changes in shape when filling and emptying. The need to recognize the relationships of the viscera to the abdominal regions becomes most apparent when taking into account the distortion that occurs during pregnancy. For example, the appendix lies in the right ilioinguinal region (right lower quadrant) until the 12th week of gestation. At 16 weeks, it is at the level of the right iliac crest. At 20 weeks, it is at the level of the umbilicus, where it will remain until after delivery. Because of this displacement, the symptoms of appendicitis will be different during the 3 trimesters. Similarly, displacement will also affect problems involving the bowel.

Skin, Subcutaneous Tissue, & Fascia

The abdominal skin is smooth, fine, and very elastic. It is loosely attached to underlying structures except at the umbilicus, where it is firmly adherent. Beneath the skin is the superficial fascia (tela subcutanea) (Fig 2–3). This fatty protective fascia covers the entire abdomen. Below the navel, it consists principally of 2 layers: Camper's fascia, the more superficial layer containing most of the fat; and Scarpa's fascia (deep fascia), the fibroelastic membrane firmly attached to midline aponeuroses and to the fascia lata.

Arteries

The anterior cutaneous branches of the superficial arteries are grouped with the anterior cutaneous nerves

5

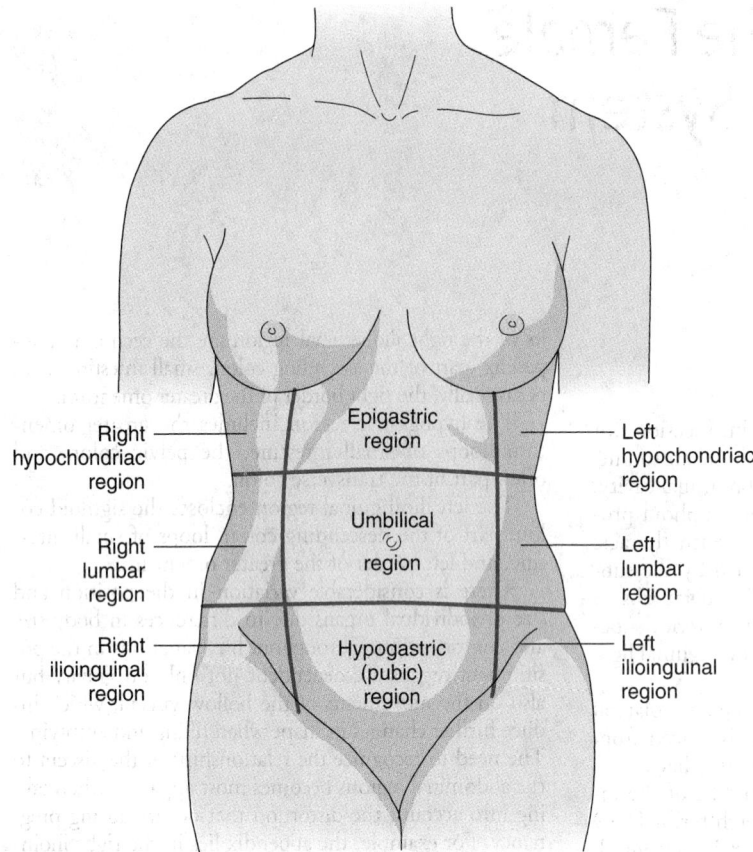

Right
hypochondriac
region

Epigastric
region

Left
hypochondriac
region

Right
lumbar
region

Umbilical
region

Left
lumbar
region

Right
ilioinguinal
region

Hypogastric
(pubic)
region

Left
ilioinguinal
region

Figure 2–1. Regions of the abdomen.

(Fig 2–4). The lateral cutaneous branches stem from the lower aortic intercostal arteries and the subcostal arteries. The femoral artery supplies both the superficial epigastric and the superficial circumflex iliac arteries. From its origin beneath the fascia lata at approximately 1.2 cm beyond the inguinal ligament, the superficial epigastric artery passes immediately through the fascia lata or through the fossa ovalis. From there, it courses upward, primarily within Camper's fascia, in a slightly medial direction anterior to the external oblique muscle almost as far as the umbilicus, giving off small branches to the inguinal lymph nodes and to the skin and superficial fascia. It ends in numerous small twigs that anastomose with the cutaneous branches from the inferior epigastric and internal mammary arteries. Arising either in common with the superficial epigastric artery or as a separate branch from the femoral artery, the superficial circumflex iliac artery passes laterally over the iliacus. Perforating the fascia lata slightly to the lateral aspect of the fossa ovalis, it then runs parallel to the inguinal ligament almost to the crest of the ilium, where it terminates in branches

within Scarpa's fascia that anastomose with the deep circumflex iliac artery. In its course, branches supply the iliacus and sartorius muscles, the inguinal lymph nodes, and the superficial fascia and skin.

Veins

The superficial veins are more numerous than the arteries and form more extensive networks. Above the umbilicus, blood returns through the anterior cutaneous and the paired thoracoepigastric veins, the superficial epigastric veins, and the superficial circumflex iliac veins in the tela subcutanea. A cruciate anastomosis exists, therefore, between the femoral and axillary veins.

Lymphatics

The lymphatic drainage of the lower abdominal wall (Fig 2–5) is primarily to the superficial inguinal nodes, 10–20 in number, which lie in the area of the inguinal ligament. These nodes may be identified by dividing the area into quadrants by intersecting horizontal and

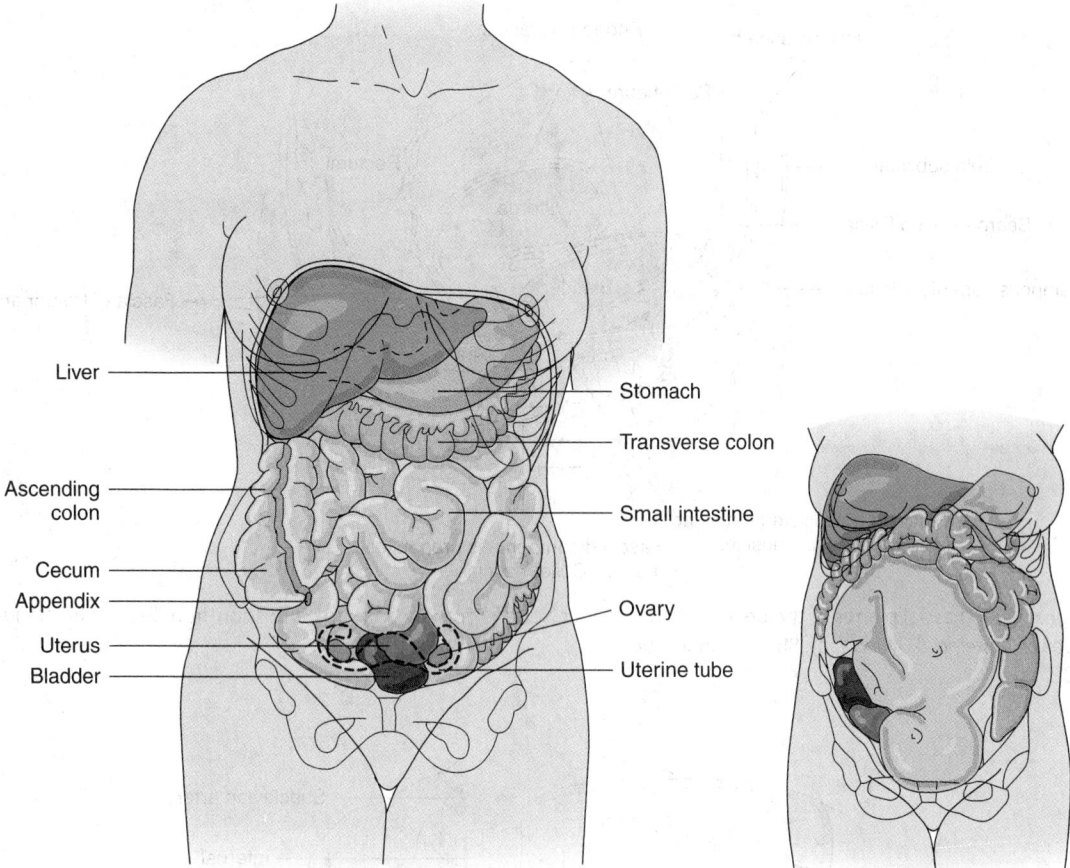

Figure 2–2. Abdominal viscera in situ. Inset shows projection of fetus in situ.

vertical lines that meet at the saphenofemoral junction. The lateral abdominal wall drainage follows the superficial circumflex iliac vein and drains to the lymph nodes in the upper lateral quadrant of the superficial inguinal nodes. The drainage of the medial aspect follows the superficial epigastric vein primarily to the lymph nodes in the upper medial quadrant of the superficial inguinal nodes. Of major clinical importance are the frequent anastomoses between the lymph vessels of the right and left sides of the abdomen.

Abdominal Muscles & Fascia

The muscular wall that supports the abdominal viscera (Fig 2–6) is composed of 4 pairs of muscles and their aponeuroses. The 3 paired lateral muscles are the external oblique, the internal oblique, and the transversus. Their aponeuroses interdigitate at the midline to connect opposing lateral muscles, forming a thickened band at this juncture, the linea alba, which extends from the xiphoid process to the pubic symphysis. Anteriorly, a pair of muscles—the rectus abdominis, with the paired pyramidalis muscles at its inferior border with its sheath—constitute the abdominal wall.

A. EXTERNAL OBLIQUE MUSCLE

The external oblique muscle consists of 8 pointed digitations attached to the lower 8 ribs. The lowest fibers insert into the anterior half of the iliac crest and the inguinal ligament. At the linea alba, the muscle aponeurosis interdigitates with that of the opposite side and fuses with the underlying internal oblique.

B. INTERNAL OBLIQUE MUSCLE

The internal oblique muscle arises from thoracolumbar fascia, the crest of the ilium, and the inguinal ligament. Going in the opposite oblique direction, the muscle inserts into the lower 3 costal cartilages and into the linea alba on either side of the rectus abdominis. The apo-

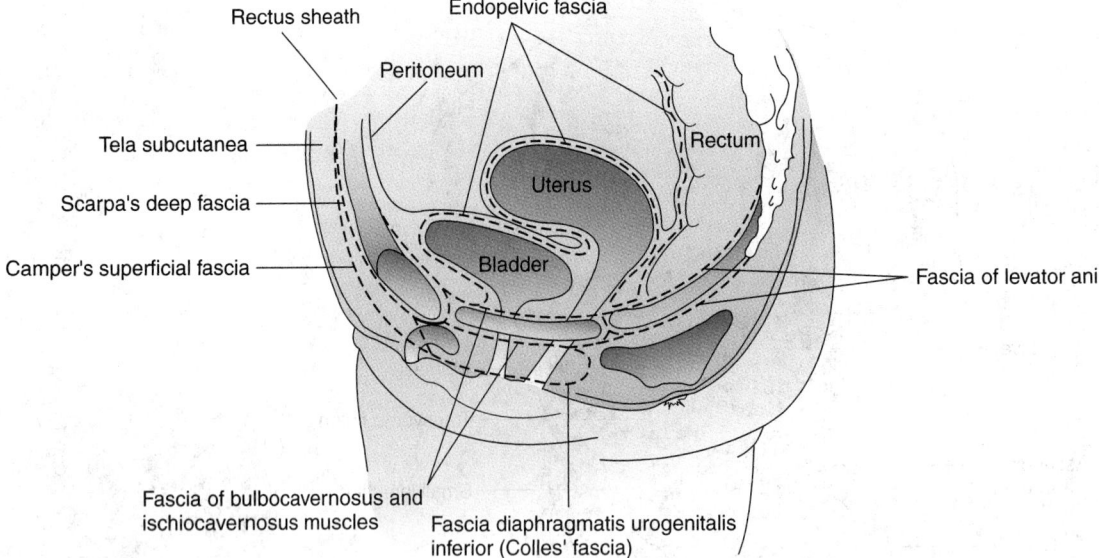

Figure 2–3. Fascial planes of the pelvis. (Modified after Netter. Reproduced, with permission, from Benson RC: *Handbook of Obstetrics & Gynecology*, 8th ed. Lange, 1983.)

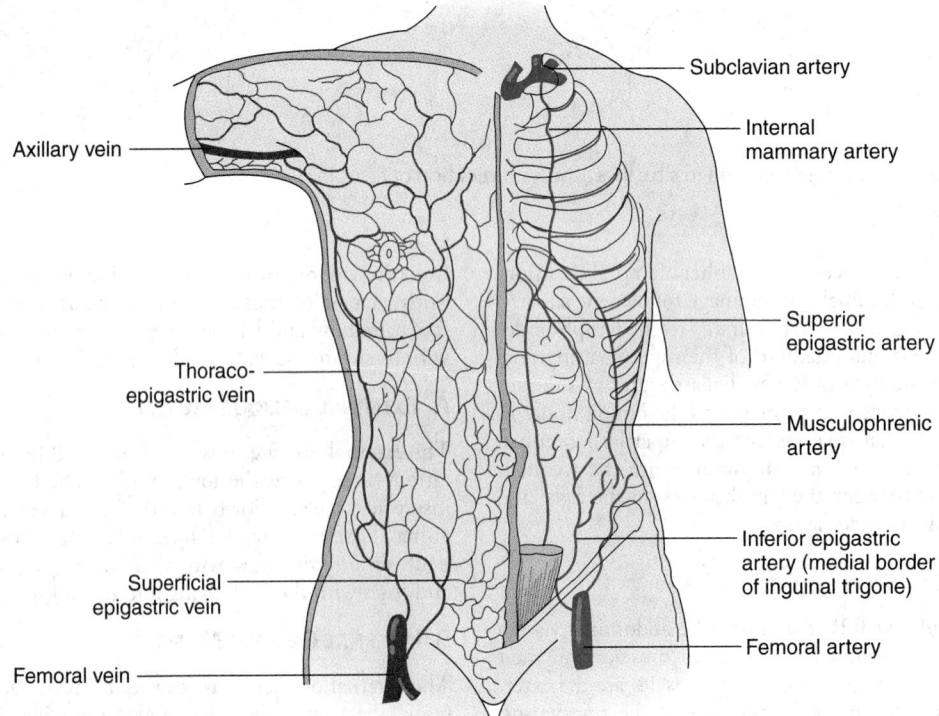

Figure 2–4. Superficial veins and arteries of abdomen.

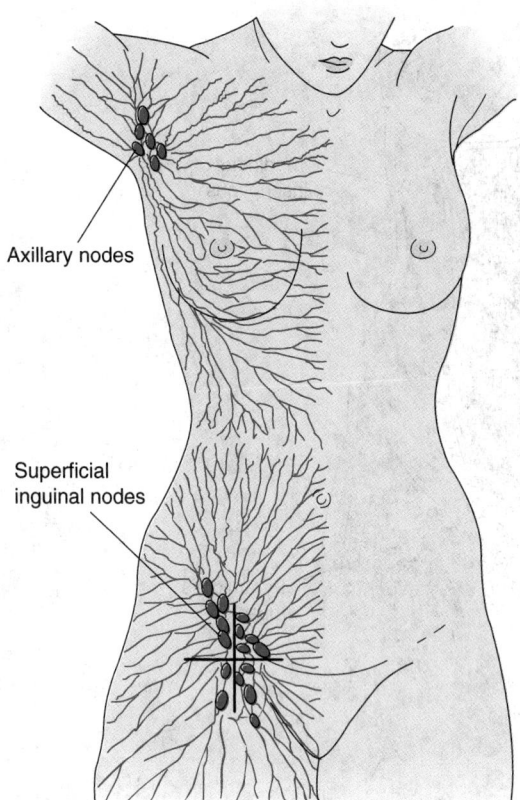

Axillary nodes

Superficial inguinal nodes

Figure 2–5. Lymphatics of abdominal wall. Only one side is shown, but contralateral drainage occurs, ie, crosses midline to the opposite side.

neurosis helps to form the rectus sheath both anteriorly and posteriorly. The posterior layer extends from the rectus muscle rib insertions to below the umbilicus.

C. TRANSVERSUS MUSCLE

The transversus muscle, the fibers of which run transversely and arise from the inner surfaces of the lower 6 costal cartilages, the thoracolumbar fascia, the iliac crest, and the inguinal ligament, lies beneath the internal oblique. By inserting into the linea alba, the aponeurosis of the transversus fuses to form the posterior layer of the posterior rectus sheath. The termination of this layer is called the arcuate line, and below it lie transversalis fascia, properitoneal fat, and peritoneum. Inferiorly, the thin aponeurosis of the transversus abdominis becomes part of the anterior rectus sheath.

D. RECTUS MUSCLES

The rectus muscles are straplike and extend from the thorax to the pubis. They are divided by the linea alba and

outlined laterally by the linea semilunaris. Three tendinous intersections cross the upper part of each rectus muscle, and a fourth may also be present below the umbilicus. The pyramidalis muscle, a vestigial muscle, is situated anterior to the lowermost part of the rectus muscle. It arises from and inserts into the pubic periosteum.

Beneath the superficial fascia and overlying the muscles is the thin, semitransparent deep fascia. Its extensions enter and divide the lateral muscles into coarse bundles.

Abdominal incisions are shown in Fig 2–7. The position of the muscles influences the type of incision to be made. The aim is to adequately expose the operative field, avoiding damage to parietal structures, blood vessels, and nerves. The incision should be placed so as to create minimal tension on the lines of closure.

Abdominal Nerves

The lower 6 thoracic nerves align with the ribs and give off lateral cutaneous branches (Fig 2–8). The intercostal nerves pass deep to the upturned rib cartilages and enter the abdominal wall. The main trunks of these nerves run forward between the internal oblique and the transversus. The nerves then enter the rectus sheaths and the rectus muscles, and the terminating branches emerge as anterior cutaneous nerves. The iliohypogastric nerve springs from the first lumbar nerve after the latter has been joined by the communicating branch from the last (12th) thoracic nerve. It pierces the lateral border of the psoas and crosses anterior to the quadratus lumborum muscle but posterior to the kidney and colon. At the lateral border of the quadratus lumborum, it pierces the aponeurosis of origin of the transversus abdominis and enters the areolar tissue between the transversus and the internal oblique muscle. Here, it frequently communicates with the last thoracic and with the ilioinguinal nerve, which also originates from the first lumbar and last thoracic nerves. The iliohypogastric divides into 2 branches. The iliac branch pierces the internal and external oblique muscles, emerging through the latter above the iliac crest and supplying the integument of the upper and lateral part of the thigh. The hypogastric branch, as it passes forward and downward, gives branches to both the transversus abdominis and internal oblique. It communicates with the ilioinguinal nerve and pierces the internal oblique muscle near the anterior superior spine. The hypogastric branch proceeds medially beneath the external oblique aponeurosis and pierces it just above the subcutaneous inguinal ring to supply the skin and symphysis pubica.

Abdominal Arteries

A. ARTERIES OF THE UPPER ABDOMEN

The lower 5 intercostal arteries and the subcostal artery accompany the thoracic nerves. Their finer, terminal

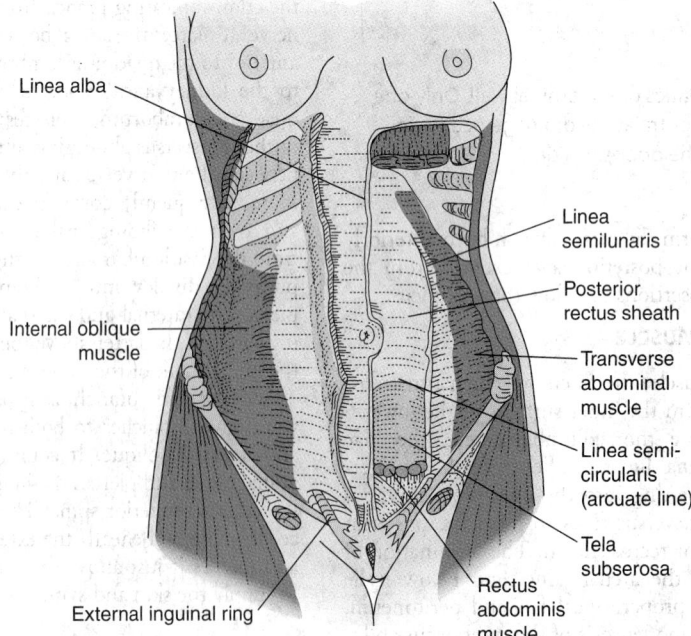

Figure 2–6. Musculature of abdominal wall.

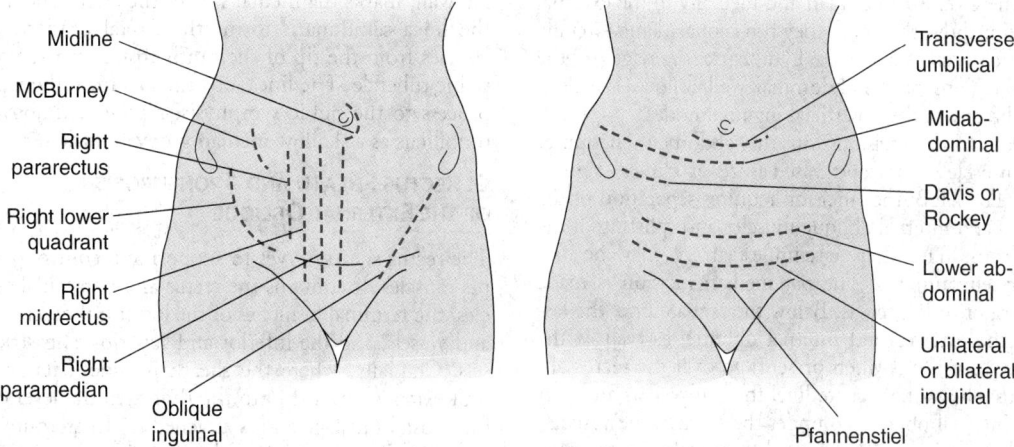

Figure 2–7. Abdominal incisions. Transverse incisions are those in which rectus muscles are cut. A Cherney incision is one in which the rectus is taken off the pubic bone and then sewed back; the pyramidalis muscle is left on pubic tubercles.

branches enter the rectus sheath to anastomose with the superior and inferior epigastric arteries. The superior epigastric artery is the direct downward prolongation of the internal mammary artery. This artery descends between

Figure 2–8. Cutaneous innervation of the abdominal wall.

the posterior surface of the rectus muscle and its sheath to form an anastomosis with the inferior epigastric artery upon the muscle. The inferior epigastric artery, a branch of the external iliac artery, usually arises just above the inguinal ligament and passes on the medial side of the round ligament to the abdominal inguinal ring. From there, it ascends in a slightly medial direction, passing above and lateral to the subcutaneous inguinal ring, which lies between the fascia transversalis and the peritoneum. Piercing the fascia transversalis, it passes in front of the linea semicircularis, turns upward between the rectus and its sheath, enters the substance of the rectus muscle, and meets the superior epigastric artery. The superior epigastric supplies the upper central abdominal wall, the inferior supplies the lower central part of the anterior abdominal wall, and the deep circumflex supplies the lower lateral part of the abdominal wall.

B. ARTERIES OF THE LOWER ABDOMEN

The deep circumflex iliac artery is also a branch of the external iliac artery, arising from its side either opposite the epigastric artery or slightly below the origin of that vessel. It courses laterally behind the inguinal ligament lying between the fascia transversalis and the peritoneum. The deep circumflex artery perforates the transversus near the anterior superior spine of the ilium and continues between the transversus and internal oblique along and slightly above the crest of the ilium, finally running posteriorly to anastomose with the iliolumbar artery. A branch of the deep circumflex iliac artery is important to the surgeon because it forms anastomoses with branches of the inferior epigastric. The deep veins correspond in name with the arteries they accompany. Below the umbilicus, these veins run caudad and medially to the external iliac vein; above that level, they run cephalad and laterally into the intercostal veins. Lymphatic drainage in the deeper regions of the abdominal wall follows the deep veins directly to the superficial inguinal nodes.

The various incisions on the abdomen encounter some muscle planes and vasculature of clinical significance. The McBurney incision requires separation of the external and internal oblique muscles and splitting of the transversus. The deep circumflex artery may be frequently encountered. The paramedian incision is made in the right or left rectus. Below the arcuate line, the fascia of the external and internal oblique, as well as the transversus muscles when present, go over the rectus abdominis; above the arcuate line, the transversus and part of the internal oblique go under the rectus. The vasculature is primarily perforators and frequently the thoracoabdominal vein. Inferiorly, the superficial epigastric may be encountered. In the Pfannenstiel incision, the fascia of the external and internal oblique go over the rectus muscle as well as the transversus muscle when present. After the fascia over the rectus is incised, the muscles can be separated. The superficial epigastric artery and vein are encountered in Camper's fascia. Laterally, the superficial and deep circumflex iliac arteries may be at the margin of the incision. Lying under the transversus muscle and entering the rectus approximately halfway to the umbilicus is the inferior epigastric artery.

In the transverse incision, the arcuate line may be encountered. As the rectus muscle is incised, the inferior epigastric within the muscle and its anastomosis with the thoracoabdominal artery must be recognized.

In the Cherney incision, care should be taken to avoid the inferior epigastric artery, which is the primary blood supply to the rectus abdominis.

Special Structures

There are several special anatomic structures in the abdominal wall, including the umbilicus, linea alba, linea semilunaris, and rectus sheath.

A. UMBILICUS

The umbilicus is situated opposite the disk between the third and fourth lumbar vertebrae, approximately 2 cm below the midpoint of a line drawn from the sternoxiphoid process to the top of the pubic symphysis. The umbilicus is a dense, wrinkled mass of fibrous tissue enclosed by and fused with a ring of circular aponeurotic fibers in the linea alba. Normally, it is the strongest part of the abdominal wall.

B. LINEA ALBA

The linea alba, a fibrous band formed by the fusion of the aponeuroses of the muscles of the anterior abdominal wall, marks the medial side of the rectus abdominis; the linea semilunaris forms the lateral border, which courses from the tip of the ninth costal cartilage to the pubic tubercle. The linea alba extends from the xiphoid process to the pubic symphysis, represented above the umbilicus as a shallow median groove on the surface.

C. RECTUS SHEATH AND APONEUROSIS OF THE EXTERNAL OBLIQUE

The rectus sheath serves to support and control the rectus muscles. It contains the rectus and pyramidalis muscles, the terminal branches of the lower 6 thoracic nerves and vessels, and the inferior and superior epigastric vessels. Cranially, where the sheath is widest, its anterior wall extends upward onto the thorax to the level of the fifth costal cartilage and is attached to the sternum. The deeper wall is attached to the xiphoid process and the lower borders of the seventh to ninth costal cartilages and does not extend upward onto the anterior thorax. Caudally, where the sheath narrows considerably, the anterior wall is attached to the crest and the symphysis pubica. Above the costal margin on the anterior chest wall, there is no complete rectus sheath (Fig 2–9). Instead, the rectus muscle is covered only by the aponeurosis of the external oblique. In the region of the abdomen, the upper two-thirds of the internal oblique aponeurosis splits at the lateral border of the rectus muscle into anterior and posterior lamellas. The anterior lamella passes in front of the external oblique and blends with the external oblique aponeurosis. The posterior wall of the sheath is formed by the posterior lamella and the aponeurosis of the transversus muscle. The anterior and posterior sheath join at the midline. The lower third of the internal oblique aponeurosis is undivided. Together with the aponeuroses of the external oblique and transversus muscles, it forms the anterior wall of the sheath. The posterior wall is occupied by transversalis fascia, which is spread over the interior surfaces of both the rectus and the transversus muscles, separating them from peritoneum and extending to the inguinal and lacunar ligaments. The transition from aponeurosis to fascia usually is fairly sharp, marked by a curved line called the arcuate line.

D. FUNCTION OF ABDOMINAL MUSCLES

In general, the functions of the abdominal muscles are 3-fold: (1) support and compression of the abdominal viscera by the external oblique, internal oblique, and transversus muscles; (2) depression of the thorax in conjunction with the diaphragm by the rectus abdominis, external oblique, internal oblique, and transversus muscles, as evident in respiration, coughing, vomiting, defecation, and parturition; and (3) assistance in bending movements of the trunk through flexion of the vertebral column by the rectus abdominis, external oblique,

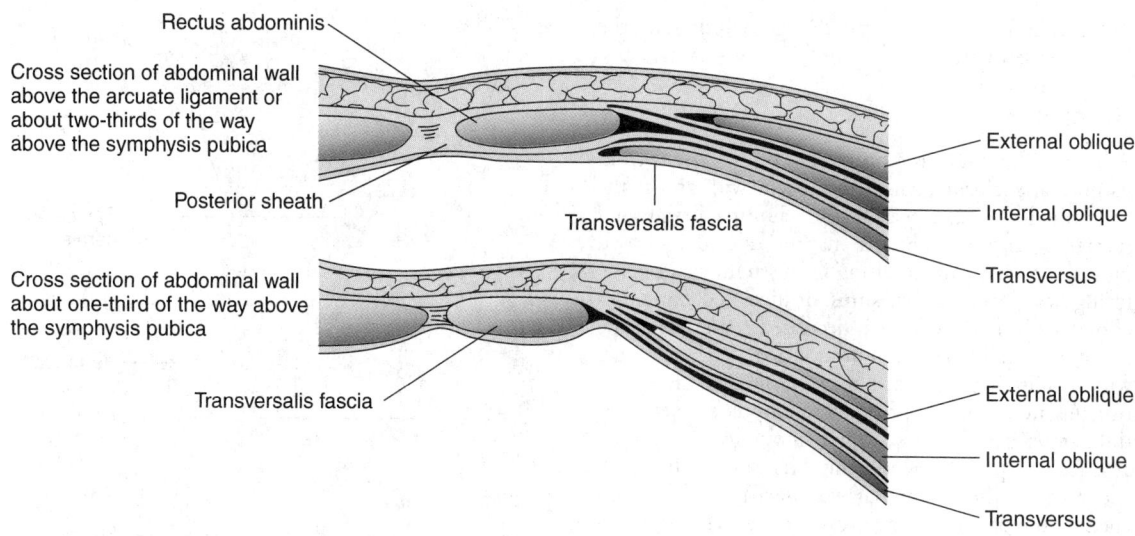

Figure 2–9. Formation of rectus sheath.

and internal oblique muscles. There is partial assistance in rotation of the thorax and upper abdomen to the same side when the pelvis is fixed by the internal oblique and by the external oblique to the opposite side. In addition, the upper external oblique serves as a fixation muscle in abduction of the upper limb of the same side and adduction of the upper limb of the opposite side. The pyramidalis muscle secures the linea alba in the median line.

Variations of Abdominal Muscles

Variations have been noted in all of the abdominal muscles.

A. Rectus Muscle

The rectus abdominis muscle may differ in the number of its tendinous inscriptions and the extent of its thoracic attachment. Aponeurotic slips or slips of muscle on the upper part of the thorax are remnants of a more primitive state in which the muscle extended to the neck. Absence of part or all of the muscle has been noted. The pyramidalis muscle may be missing, only slightly developed, double, or may extend upward to the umbilicus.

B. External Oblique Muscle

The external oblique muscle varies in the extent of its origin from the ribs. Broad fascicles may be separated by loose tissue from the main belly of the muscle, either on its deep or on its superficial surface. The supracostalis anterior is a rare fascicle occasionally found on the upper portion of the thoracic wall. Transverse tendinous inscriptions may also be found.

C. Internal Oblique Muscle

The internal oblique deviates at times, both in its attachments and in the extent of development of the fleshy part of the muscle. Occasionally, tendinous inscriptions are present, or the posterior division forms an extra muscle 7–7.5 cm wide and separated from the internal oblique by a branch of the iliohypogastric nerve and a branch of the deep circumflex iliac artery.

D. Transversus Muscle

The transversus muscle fluctuates widely in the extent of its development but is rarely absent. Rarely, it extends as far inferiorly as the ligamentum teres uteri (round ligament), and infrequently it is situated superior to the anterior superior spine. However, it generally occupies an intermediate position.

E. Other Variations

Several small muscles may be present.

1. The pubotransversalis muscle may extend from the superior ramus of the pubis to the transversalis fascia near the abdominal ring.
2. The puboperitonealis muscle may pass from the pubic crest to the transversus near the umbilicus.
3. The posterior rectus abdominis (tensor laminae posterioris vaginae musculi recti abdominis) may spread from the inguinal ligament to the rectus sheath on the deep surface of the rectus muscle near the umbilicus.
4. The tensor transversalis (tensor laminae posterioris vaginae musculi recti et fasciae transversalis abdominis) has appeared from the transversalis

fascia near the abdominal inguinal ring to the linea semicircularis.

Hernias

A hernia (Fig 2–10) is a protrusion of any viscus from its normal enclosure, which may occur with any of the abdominal viscera, especially the jejunum, ileum, and greater omentum. A hernia may be due to increased pressure, such as that resulting from strenuous exercise, lifting heavy weights, tenesmus, or increased expiratory efforts, or it may result from decreased resistance of the abdominal wall (congenital or acquired), such as occurs with debilitating illness or old age, prolonged distention from ascites, tumors, pregnancy, corpulence, emaciation, injuries (including surgical incisions), congenital absence, or poor development. Hernias are likely to occur where the abdominal wall is structurally weakened by the passage of large vessels or nerves and developmental peculiarities. Ventral hernias occur through the linea semilunaris or the linea alba. Umbilical hernias occur more frequently and can be 1 of 3 types.

During early fetal development, portions of the mesentery and a loop of the intestine pass through the opening to occupy a part of the body cavity (the umbilical coelom) situated in the umbilical cord. Normally, the mesentery and intestine later return to the abdominal cavity. If they fail to do so, a congenital umbilical hernia results. Infantile umbilical hernias occur if the component parts fail to fuse completely in early postnatal stages. The unyielding nature of the fibrous tissue forming the margin of the ring predisposes to strangulation. Adult umbilical hernias occur frequently in females. When the hernia comes through the ring itself, it is always at the upper part.

INGUINAL REGION

The inguinal region of the abdominal wall is bounded by the rectus abdominis muscle medially, the line connecting the anterior superior iliac spines superiorly, and the inguinal ligament inferiorly. The region contains 8 layers of abdominal wall. These layers, from the most superficial inward, are (1) the skin, (2) the tela subcutanea, (3) the aponeurosis of the external oblique muscle, (4) the internal oblique muscle, (5) the transversus abdominis muscle (below the free border, the layer is incomplete), (6) the transversalis fascia, (7) the subperitoneal fat and connective tissue, and (8) the peritoneum. The tela subcutanea consists of the superficial fatty Camper's fascia, which is continuous with the tela subcutanea of the whole body, and the deeper membranous Scarpa's fascia, which covers the lower third of the abdominal wall and the medial side of the groin, both joining below the inguinal ligament to form the fascia lata of the thigh.

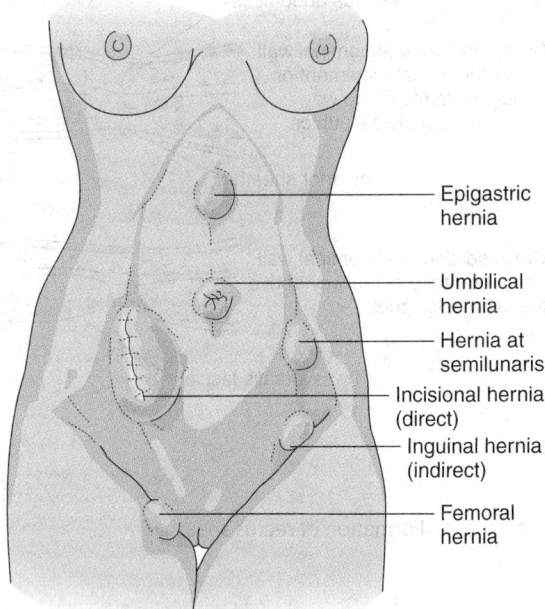

- Epigastric hernia
- Umbilical hernia
- Hernia at semilunaris
- Incisional hernia (direct)
- Inguinal hernia (indirect)
- Femoral hernia

Figure 2–10. Hernia sites.

Subcutaneous Inguinal Ring

A triangular evagination of the external oblique aponeurosis, the subcutaneous inguinal ring (external abdominal ring), is bounded by an aponeurosis at its edges and by the inguinal ligament inferiorly. The superior or medial crus is smaller and attaches to the symphysis pubica. The inferior or lateral crus is stronger and blends with the inguinal ligament as it passes to the pubic tubercle. The sharp margins of the ring are attributed to a sudden thinning of the aponeurosis. In the female, the ligamentum teres uteri (round ligament) passes through this ring. The subcutaneous inguinal ring is much smaller in the female than in the male, and the abdominal wall is relatively stronger in this region.

Ligaments, Aponeuroses, & Fossae

The inguinal ligament itself forms the inferior thickened border of the external oblique aponeurosis, extending from the anterior superior iliac spine to the pubic tubercle. Along its inferior border, it becomes continuous with the fascia lata of the thigh. From the medial portion of the inguinal ligament, a triangular band of fibers attaches separately to the pecten ossis pubis. This band is known as the lacunar (Gimbernat's) ligament. The reflex inguinal ligament (ligament of Colles or triangular fascia) is represented by a small band of fibers, often poorly developed, and derived from the superior crus of the subcutaneous inguinal ring and the lower part of the linea alba. These fibers cross to the opposite side to attach to the pecten ossis pubis. The falx inguinalis or conjoined tendon is formed by the aponeurosis of the transversus abdominis and internal oblique muscles. These fibers arise from the inguinal ligament and arch downward and forward to insert on the pubic crest and pecten ossis pubis, behind the inguinal and lacunar ligaments. The interfoveolar ligament is composed partly of fibrous bands from the aponeurosis of the transversalis muscle of the same and opposite sides. Curving medial to and below the internal abdominal ring, they attach to the lacunar ligament and pectineal fascia.

Abdominal Inguinal Ring

The abdominal inguinal ring (internal abdominal ring) is the rounded mouth of a funnel-shaped expansion of transversalis fascia that lies approximately 2 cm above the inguinal ligament and midway between the anterior superior iliac spine and the symphysis pubica. Medially, it is bounded by the inferior epigastric vessels; the external iliac artery is situated below. The abdominal inguinal ring represents the area where the round ligament emerges from the abdomen. The triangular area medial to the inferior epigastric artery, bounded by the inguinal ligament below and the lateral border of the rectus sheath, is known as the trigonum inguinale (Hesselbach's triangle), the site of congenital direct hernias.

Inguinal Canal

The inguinal canal in the female is not well demarcated, but it normally gives passage to the round ligament of the uterus, a vein, an artery from the uterus that forms a cruciate anastomosis with the labial arteries, and extraperitoneal fat. The fetal ovary, like the testis, is an abdominal organ and possesses a gubernaculum that extends from its lower pole downward and forward to a point corresponding to the abdominal inguinal ring, through which it continues into the labia majora. The processus vaginalis is an evagination of peritoneum at the level of the abdominal inguinal ring occurring during the third fetal month. In the male, the processus vaginalis descends with the testis. The processus vaginalis of the female is rudimentary, but occasionally a small diverticulum of peritoneum is found passing partway through the inguinal region; this diverticulum is termed the processus vaginalis peritonei (canal of Nuck). Instead of descending, as does the testis, the ovary moves medially, where it becomes adjacent to the uterus. The intra-abdominal portion of the gubernaculum ovarii becomes attached to the lateral border of the developing uterus, evolving as the ligament of the ovary and the round ligament of the uterus. The extra-abdominal portion of the round ligament of the uterus becomes attenuated in the adult and may appear as a small fibrous band. The inguinal canal is an intermuscular passageway that extends from the abdominal ring downward, medially, and somewhat forward to the subcutaneous inguinal ring (about 3–4 cm). The canal is roughly triangular in shape, and its boundaries are largely artificial. The lacunar and inguinal ligaments form the base of the canal. The anterior or superficial wall is formed by the external oblique aponeurosis, and the lowermost fibers of the internal oblique muscle add additional strength in its lateral part. The posterior or deep wall of the canal is formed by transversalis fascia throughout and is strengthened medially by the falx inguinalis.

Abdominal Fossae

The abdominal fossae in the inguinal region consist of the foveae inguinalis lateralis and medialis. The fovea inguinalis lateralis lies lateral to a slight fold, the plica epigastrica, formed by the inferior epigastric vessels, and just medial to the abdominal inguinal ring, which slants medially and upward toward the rectus muscle. From the lateral margin of the tendinous insertion of the rectus muscle, upward toward the umbilicus, and over the obliterated artery extends a more accentuated fold, the plica umbilicalis lateralis. The fovea inguinalis medialis lies between the plica epigastrica and the plica umbilicalis lateralis, the bottom of the fossa facing the trigonum inguinale (Hesselbach's triangle). This region is strengthened by the interfoveolar ligament at the medial side of the abdominal inguinal ring and the conjoined tendon lateral to the rectus muscle; however, these bands vary in width and thus are supportive.

Ligaments & Spaces

The inguinal ligament forms the roof of a large osseoligamentous space leading from the iliac fossa to the thigh. The floor of this space is formed by the superior ramus of the pubis medially and by the body of the ilium laterally. The iliopectineal ligament extends from the inguinal ligament to the iliopectineal eminence, dividing this area into 2 parts. The lateral, larger division is called the muscular lacuna and is almost completely filled by the iliopsoas muscle, along with the femoral nerve medially and the lateral femoral cutaneous nerves laterally. The medial, smaller division is known as the vascular lacuna and is traversed by the external iliac (femoral) artery, vein, and lymphatic vessels, which do not completely fill the space. The anterior border of the vascular lacuna is formed by the inguinal ligament and the transversalis fascia. The posterior boundary is formed by the ligamentum pubicum superius (Cooper's ligament), a thickening of fascia along the public pecten where the pectineal fascia and iliopectineal ligament meet. The transversalis fascia and iliac fascia are extended with the vessels, forming a funnel-shaped fibrous investment, the femoral sheath. The sheath is divided into 3 compartments: (1) the lateral compartment, containing the femoral artery; (2) the intermediate compartment, containing the femoral vein; and (3) the medial compartment or canal, containing a lymph node (nodi lymphatici inguinales profundi [node of Rosenmüller or Cloquet]) and the lymphatic vessels that drain most of the leg, groin, and perineum. The femoral canal also contains areolar tissue, which frequently condenses to form the "femoral septum." Because of the greater spread of the pelvis in the female, the muscular and vascular lacunae are relatively large spaces. The upper or abdominal opening of the femoral canal is known as the femoral ring and is covered by the parietal peritoneum.

Arteries

In front of the femoral ring, the arterial branches of the external iliac artery are the inferior epigastric and the deep circumflex iliac. The inferior epigastric artery arises from the anterior surface of the external iliac, passing forward and upward on the anterior abdominal wall between peritoneum and transversalis fascia. It pierces the fascia just below the arcuate line, entering the rectus abdominis muscle or coursing along its inferior surface to anastomose with the superior epigastric from the internal thoracic. The inferior epigastric artery forms the lateral boundary of the trigonum inguinale (Hesselbach's triangle). At its origin, it frequently gives off a branch to the inguinal canal, as well as a branch to the pubis (pubic artery), which anastomoses with twigs of the obturator artery. The pubic branch of the inferior epigastric often becomes the obturator artery. The deep circumflex iliac artery arises laterally and traverses the iliopsoas to the anterior superior iliac spine, where it pierces the transversus muscle to course between the transversus and the internal oblique, sending perforators to the surface. It often has anastomoses with penetrating branches of the inferior epigastric via its perforators through the rectus abdominis. The veins follow a similar course.

As the external iliac artery passes through the femoral canal, which underlies the inguinal ligament, it courses medial to the femoral vein and nerve, resting in what is termed the femoral triangle (Scarpa's triangle). The femoral sheath is a downward continuation of the inguinal ligament anterior to the femoral vessel and nerve.

The branches of the femoral artery supplying the groin are (1) the superficial epigastric, (2) the superficial circumflex iliac, (3) the superficial external pudendal, and (4) the deep external pudendal. The superficial epigastric artery passes upward through the femoral sheath over the inguinal ligament, to rest in Camper's fascia on the lower abdomen. The superficial circumflex iliac artery arises adjacent to the superior epigastric, piercing the fascia lata and running parallel to the inguinal ligament as far as the iliac crest. It then divides into branches that supply the integument of the groin, the superficial fascia, and the lymph glands, anastomosing with the deep circumflex iliac, the superior gluteal, and the lateral femoral circumflex arteries. The superficial external pudendal artery arises from the medial side of the femoral artery, close to the preceding vessels. It pierces the femoral sheath and fascia cribrosa, coursing medially across the round ligament to the integument on the lower part of the abdomen and the labium majus, anastomosing with the internal pudendal. The deep external pudendal artery passes medially across the pectineus and adductor longus muscles, supplying the integument of the labium majus and forming, together with the external pudendal artery, a rete with the labial arteries.

PUDENDUM

The vulva consists of the mons pubis, the labia majora, the labia minora, the clitoris, and the glandular structures that open into the vestibulum vaginae (Fig 2–11). The size, shape, and coloration of the various structures, as well as the hair distribution, vary among individuals and racial groups. Normal pubic hair in the female is distributed in an inverted triangle, with the base centered over the mons pubis. Nevertheless, in approximately 25% of normal women, hair may extend upward along the linea alba. The type of hair is dependent, in part, on the pigmentation of the individual. It varies from heavy, coarse, crinkly hair in black women to sparse, fairly fine, lanugo-type hair in Asian women. The length and size of the various structures of the vulva are influenced by the pelvic architecture, as is the position of the external genitalia in the perineal area. The external genitalia of the female have their exact counterparts in the male.

Labia Majora

A. Superficial Anatomy

The labia majora are comprised of 2 rounded mounds of tissue, originating in the mons pubis and terminating in the perineum. They form the lateral boundaries of the vulva and are approximately 7–9 cm long and 2–4 cm wide, varying in size with height, weight, race, age, parity, and pelvic architecture. Ontogenetically, these permanent folds of skin are homologous to the scrotum of the male. Hair is distributed over their surfaces, extending superiorly in the area of the mons pubis from

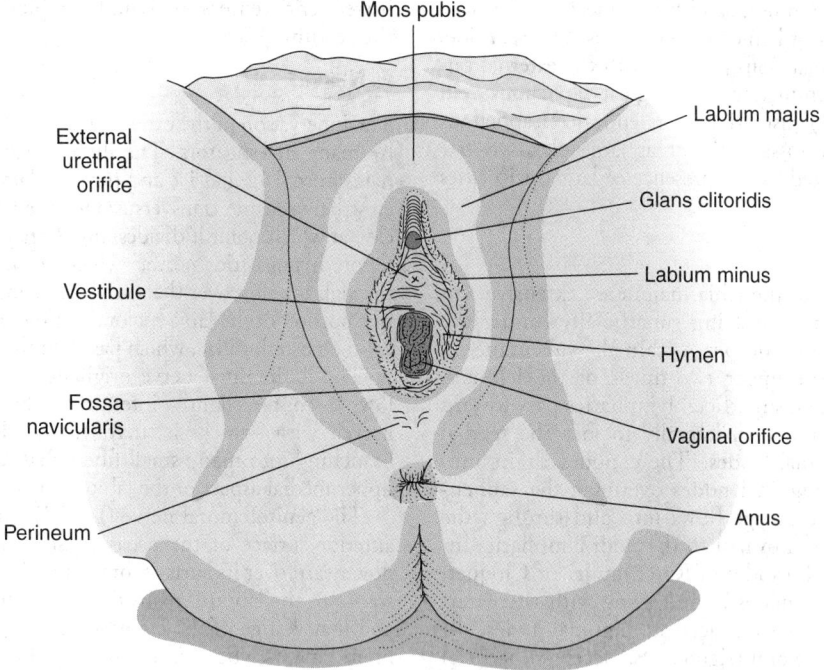

Figure 2–11. External genitalia of adult female (parous).

one side to the other. The lateral surfaces are adjacent to the medial surface of the thigh, forming a deep groove when the legs are together. The medial surfaces of the labia majora may oppose each other directly or may be separated by protrusion of the labia minora. The cleft that is formed by this opposition anteriorly is termed the anterior commissure. Posteriorly, the cleft is less clearly defined and termed the posterior commissure. The middle portion of the cleft between the 2 labia is the rima pudendi.

B. Deep Structures

Underlying the skin is a thin, poorly developed muscle layer called the tunica dartos labialis, the fibers of which course, for the most part, at right angles to the wrinkles of the surface, forming a crisscross pattern. Deep to the dartos layer is a thin layer of fascia, most readily recognizable in the old or the young because of the large amount of adipose and areolar tissue. Numerous sweat glands are found in the labia majora, with the greater number on the medial aspect. In the deeper substance of the labia majora are longitudinal bands of muscle that are continuous with the ligamentum teres uteri (round ligament) as it emerges from the inguinal canal. Occasionally, a persistent processus vaginalis peritonei (canal of Nuck) may be seen in the upper region of the labia. In most women, it has been impossible to differ-entiate the presence of the cremaster muscle beyond its area of origin.

C. Arteries

The arterial supply into the labia majora comes from the internal and external pudendals, with extensive anastomoses. Within the labia majora is a circular arterial pattern originating inferiorly from a branch of the perineal artery, from the external pudendal artery in the anterior lateral aspect, and from a small artery of the ligamentum teres uteri superiorly. The inferior branch from the perineal artery, which originates from the internal pudendal as it emerges from the canalis pudendalis (Alcock's canal), forms the base of the rete with the external pudendal arteries. These arise from the medial side of the femoral and, occasionally, from the deep arteries just beneath the femoral ring, coursing medially over the pectineus and adductor muscles, to which they supply branches. They terminate in a circular rete within the labium majus, penetrating the fascia lata adjacent to the fossa ovalis and passing over the round ligament to send a branch to the clitoris.

D. Veins

The venous drainage is extensive and forms a plexus with numerous anastomoses. In addition, the veins communicate with the dorsal vein of the clitoris, the veins of the labia minora, and the perineal veins, as well as with the inferior hemorrhoidal plexus. On each side, the posterior labial veins connect with the external pudendal vein, terminating in the great saphenous vein (saphena magna) just prior to its entrance (saphenous opening) in the fossa ovalis. This large plexus is frequently manifested by the presence of large varicosities during pregnancy.

E. LYMPHATICS

The lymphatics of the labia majora are extensive and utilize 2 systems, one lying superficially (under the skin) and the other deeper, within the subcutaneous tissues. From the upper two-thirds of the left and right labia majora, superficial lymphatics pass toward the symphysis and turn laterally to join the medial superficial inguinal nodes. These nodes drain into the superficial inguinal nodes overlying the saphenous fossa. The drainage flows into and through the femoral ring (fossa ovalis) to the nodi lymphatici inguinales profundi (nodes of Rosenmüller or Cloquet; deep subinguinal nodes), connecting with the external iliac chain. The superficial subinguinal nodes, situated over the femoral trigone, also accept superficial drainage from the lower extremity and the gluteal region. This drainage may include afferent lymphatics from the perineum. In the region of the symphysis pubica, the lymphatics anastomose in a plexus between the right and left nodes. Therefore, any lesion involving the labia majora allows direct involvement of the lymphatic structures of the contralateral inguinal area. The lower part of the labium majus has superficial and deep drainage that is shared with the perineal area. The drainage passes, in part, through afferent lymphatics to superficial subinguinal nodes; from the posterior medial aspects of the labia majora,

it frequently enters the lymphatic plexus surrounding the rectum.

F. NERVES

The innervation of the external genitalia has been studied by many investigators. The iliohypogastric nerve originates from T12 and L1 and traverses laterally to the iliac crest between the transversus and internal oblique muscles, at which point it divides into 2 branches: (1) the anterior hypogastric nerve, which descends anteriorly through the skin over the symphysis, supplying the superior portion of the labia majora and the mons pubis; and (2) the posterior iliac, which passes to the gluteal area.

The ilioinguinal nerve originates from L1 and follows a course slightly inferior to the iliohypogastric nerve, with which it may frequently anastomose, branching into many small fibers that terminate in the upper medial aspect of the labium majus.

The genitofemoral nerve (L1–L2) emerges from the anterior surface of the psoas muscle to run obliquely downward over its surface, branching in the deeper substance of the labium majus to supply the dartos muscle and that vestige of the cremaster present within the labium majus. Its lumboinguinal branch continues downward onto the upper part of the thigh.

From the sacral plexus, the posterior femoral cutaneous nerve, originating from the posterior divisions of S1 and S2 and the anterior divisions of S2 and S3, divides into several rami that, in part, are called the perineal branches. They supply the medial aspect of the thigh and the labia majora. These branches of the posterior femoral cutaneous nerve are derived from the sacral plexus. The pudendal nerve, composed primarily of S2, S3, and S4, often with a fascicle of S1, sends a small number of fibers to the medial aspect of the labia majora. The pattern of nerve endings is illustrated in Table 2–1.

Table 2–1. Quantitative distribution of nerve endings in selected regions of the female genitalia.

	Touch			Pressure	Pain	Other Types	
	Meissner Corpuscles[1]	Merkel Tactile Disks[1]	Peri-trichous Endings	Vater-Pacini Corpuscles[2]	Free Nerve Endings	Ruffini Corpuscles[2]	Dogiel and Krause Corpuscles[3]
Mons pubis	++++	++++	++++	+++	+++	++++	+
Labia majora	+++	++++	++++	+++	+++	+++	+
Clitoris	+	+	0	++++	+++	+++	+++
Labia minora	+	+	0	+	+	+	+++
Hymenal ring	0	+	0	0	+++	0	0
Vagina	0	0	0	0	+ Occasionally	0	0

[1]Also called corpuscula tactus.
[2]Also called corpuscula lamellosa.
[3]Also called corpuscula bulboidea.

Figure 2–12. Arteries and nerves of perineum.

Labia Minora

A. SUPERFICIAL ANATOMY

The labia minora are 2 folds of skin that lie within the rima pudendi and measure approximately 5 cm in length and 0.5–1 cm in thickness. The width varies according to age and parity, measuring 2–3 cm at its narrowest diameter to 5–6 cm at it widest, with multiple corrugations over the surface. The labia minora begin at the base of the clitoris, where fusion of the labia is continuous with the prepuce, extending posteriorly and medially to the labia majora at the posterior commissure. On their medial aspects superiorly beneath the clitoris, they unite to form the frenulum adjacent to the urethra and vagina, terminating along the hymen on the right and left sides of the fossa navicularis and ending posteriorly in the frenulum of the labia pudendi, just superior to the posterior commissure. A deep cleft is formed on the lateral surface between the labium majus and the labium minus. The skin on the labia minora is smooth and pigmented. The color and distention vary, depending on the level of sexual excitement and the pigmentation of the individual. The glands of the labia are homologous to the glandulae preputiales (glands of Littre) of the penile portion of the male urethra.

B. ARTERIES

The main source of arterial supply (Fig 2–12) occurs through anastomoses from the superficial perineal artery, branching from the dorsal artery of the clitoris, and from the medial aspect of the rete of the labia majora. Similarly, the venous pattern and plexus are extensive.

C. VEINS

The venous drainage is to the medial vessels of the perineal and vaginal veins, directly to the veins of the labia majora, to the inferior hemorrhoidals posteriorly, and to the clitoral veins superiorly.

D. LYMPHATICS

The lymphatics medially may join those of the lower third of the vagina superiorly and the labia majora laterally, passing to the superficial subinguinal nodes and to the deep subinguinal nodes. In the midline, the lymphatic drainage coincides with that of the clitoris, communicating with that of the labia majora to drain to the opposite side.

E. NERVES

The innervation of the labia minora originates, in part, from fibers that supply the labia majora and from branches of the pudendal nerve as it emerges from the canalis pudendalis (Alcock's canal) (Fig 2–12). These branches originate from the perineal nerve. The labia minora and the vestibule area are homologous to the skin of the male urethra and penis. The short membranous portion, approximately 0.5 cm of the male urethra, is homologous to the midportion of the vestibule of the female.

Clitoris

A. SUPERFICIAL ANATOMY

The clitoris is the homologue of the dorsal part of the penis and consists of 2 small erectile cavernous bodies, terminating in a rudimentary glans clitoridis. The erectile body, the corpus clitoridis, consists of the 2 crura clitoridis and the glans clitoridis, with overlying skin and prepuce, a miniature homologue of the glans penis. The crura extend outward bilaterally to their position in the anterior portion of the vulva. The cavernous tissue, homologous to the corpus spongiosum penis of the male, appears in the vascular pattern of the labia minora in the female. At the lower border of the pubic arch, a small triangular fibrous band extends onto the clitoris (suspensory ligament) to separate the 2 crura, which turn inward, downward, and laterally at this point, close to the inferior rami of the pubic symphysis. The crura lie inferior to the ischiocavernosus muscles and bodies. The glans is situated superiorly at the fused termination of the crura. It is composed of erectile tissue and contains an integument, hoodlike in shape, termed the prepuce. On its ventral surface, there is a frenulum clitoridis, the fused junction of the labia minora.

B. ARTERIES

The blood supply to the clitoris is from its dorsal artery, a terminal branch of the internal pudendal artery, which is the terminal division of the posterior portion of the internal iliac (hypogastric) artery. As it enters the clitoris, it divides into 2 branches, the deep and dorsal arteries. Just before entering the clitoris itself, a small branch passes posteriorly to supply the area of the external urethral meatus.

C. VEINS

The venous drainage of the clitoris begins in a rich plexus around the corona of the glans, running along the anterior surface to join the deep vein and continuing downward to join the pudendal plexus from the labia minora, labia majora, and perineum, forming the pudendal vein.

D. LYMPHATICS

The lymphatic drainage of the clitoris coincides primarily with that of the labia minora, the right and left sides having access to contralateral nodes in the superficial inguinal chain. In addition, its extensive network provides further access downward and posteriorly to the external urethral meatus toward the anterior portion of the vestibule.

E. NERVES

The innervation of the clitoris is through the terminal branch of the pudendal nerve, which originates from the sacral plexus as previously discussed. It lies on the lateral side of the dorsal artery and terminates in branches within the glans, corona, and prepuce. The nerve endings in the clitoris vary from a total absence within the glans to a rich supply primarily located within the prepuce (Table 2–1). A total absence of endings within the clitoris itself takes on clinical significance when one considers the emphasis placed on the clitoris in discussing problems of sexual gratification in women.

Vestibule

A. SUPERFICIAL ANATOMY

The area of the vestibule is bordered by the labia minora laterally, by the frenulum labiorum pudendi (or posterior commissure) posteriorly, and by the urethra and clitoris anteriorly. Inferiorly, it is bordered by the hymenal ring. The opening of the vagina or junction of the vagina with the vestibule is limited by a membrane stretching from the posterior and lateral sides to the inferior surface of the external urethral orifice. This membrane is termed the hymen. Its shape and openings vary and depend on age, parity, and sexual experience. The form of the opening may be infantile, annular, semilunar, cribriform, septate, or vertical; the hymen may even be imperforate. In parous women and in the postcoital state, the tags of the hymenal integument are termed carunculae myrtiformes. The external urethral orifice, which is approximately 2–3 cm posterior to the clitoris, on a slightly elevated and irregular surface with depressed areas on the sides, may appear to be stellate or crescentic in shape. It is characterized by many small mucosal folds around its opening. Bilaterally and on the surface are the orifices of the paraurethral and periurethral glands (ductus paraurethrales [ducts of Skene and Astruc]). At approximately the 5 and 7 o'clock positions, just external to the hymenal rings, are 2 small papular elevations that represent the orifices of the ducts of the glandulae vestibulares majores or larger vestibular glands (Bartholin) of the female (bulbourethral gland of the male). The fossa navicularis lies between the frenulum labiorum pudendi and the hymenal ring. The skin surrounding the vestibule is stratified squamous in type, with a paucity of rete pegs and papillae.

B. ARTERIES

The blood supply to the vestibule is an extensive capillary plexus that has anastomoses with the superficial transverse perineal artery. A branch comes directly from the pudendal anastomosis with the inferior hemorrhoidal artery in the region of the fossa navicularis. The blood supply of the urethra anteriorly, a branch of the dorsal artery of the clitoris and the azygos artery of the anterior vaginal wall, also contributes.

C. VEINS

Venous drainage is extensive, involving the same areas described for the arterial network.

D. LYMPHATICS

The lymphatic drainage has a distinct pattern. The anterior portion, including that of the external urethral meatus, drains upward and outward with that of the labia minora and the clitoris. The portion next to the urethral meatus may join that of the anterior urethra, which empties into the vestibular plexus to terminate in the superficial inguinal nodes, the superficial subinguinal nodes, the deep subinguinal nodes, and the external iliac chain. The lymphatics of the fossa navicularis and the hymen may join those of the posterior vaginal wall, intertwining with the intercalated lymph nodes along the rectum, which follow the inferior hemorrhoidal arteries. This pattern becomes significant with cancer. Drainage occurs through the pudendal and the hemorrhoidal chain and through the vestibular plexus onto the inguinal region.

E. NERVES

The innervation of the vestibular area is primarily from the sacral plexus through the perineal nerve. The absence of the usual modalities of touch is noteworthy. The vestibular portion of the hymenal ring contains an abundance of free nerve endings (pain).

Vestibular Glands

The glandulae vestibulares majores (larger vestibular glands or Bartholin glands) have a duct measuring approximately 5 mm in diameter. The gland itself lies just inferior and lateral to the bulbocavernosus muscle. The gland is tubular and alveolar in character, with a thin capsule and connective tissue septa dividing it into lobules in which occasional smooth muscle fibers are found. The epithelium is cuboid to columnar and pale in color, with the cytoplasm containing mucigen droplets and colloid spherules with acidophilic inclusions. The epithelium of the duct is simple in type, and its orifice is stratified squamous like the vestibule. The secretion is a clear, viscid, and stringy mucoid substance with an alkaline pH. Secretion is active during sexual activity. Nonetheless, after about age 30, the glands undergo involution and become atrophic and shrunken.

The arterial supply to the greater vestibular gland comes from a small branch of the artery on the bulbocavernosus muscle, penetrating deep into its substance. Venous drainage coincides with the drainage of the bulbocavernosus body. The lymphatics drain directly into the lymphatics of the vestibular plexus, having access to the posterior vaginal wall along the inferior hemorrhoidal channels. They also drain via the perineum into the inguinal area. Most of this minor drainage is along the pudendal vessels in the canalis pudendalis and explains, in part, the difficulty in dealing with cancer involving the gland.

The greater vestibular gland is homologous to the bulbourethral gland (also known as Cowper's glands, Duverney's glands, Tiedemann's glands, or the Bartholin glands of the male). The innervation of the greater vestibular gland is from a small branch of the perineal nerve, which penetrates directly into its substance.

Muscles of External Genitalia

The muscles (Fig 2–13) of the external genitalia and cavernous bodies in the female are homologous to those of the male, although they are less well developed.

A. BULBOCAVERNOSUS MUSCLE

The bulbocavernosus muscle and deeper bulbus vestibuli or cavernous tissue arise in the midline from the posterior part of the central tendon of the perineum, where each opposes the fibers from the opposite side. Each ascends around the vagina, enveloping the bulbus vestibuli (the corpus cavernosum bodies of the male) to terminate in 3 heads: (1) the fibrous tissue dorsal to the clitoris, (2) the tunica fibrosa of the corpus cavernosa overlying the crura of the clitoris, and (3) decussating fibers that join those of the ischiocavernosus to form the striated sphincter of the urethra at the junction of its middle and lower thirds. The blood supply is derived from the perineal branch of the internal pudendal artery as it arises in the anterior part of the ischiorectal fossa. Deep to the fascia diaphragmatis urogenitalis inferior (Colles' fascia) and crossing between the ischiocavernosus and bulbocavernosus muscles, the pudendal artery sends 1–2 branches directly into the bulbocavernosus muscle and vestibular body, continuing anteriorly to terminate in the dorsal artery of the clitoris. The venous drainage accompanies the pudendal plexus. In addition, it passes posteriorly with the inferior hemorrhoidal veins and laterally with the perineal vein, a branch of the internal pudendal vein. The lymphatics run primarily with those of the vestibular plexus, with drainage inferiorly toward the intercalated nodes of the rectum and anteriorly and laterally with the labia minora and majora to the superficial inguinal nodes. Con-

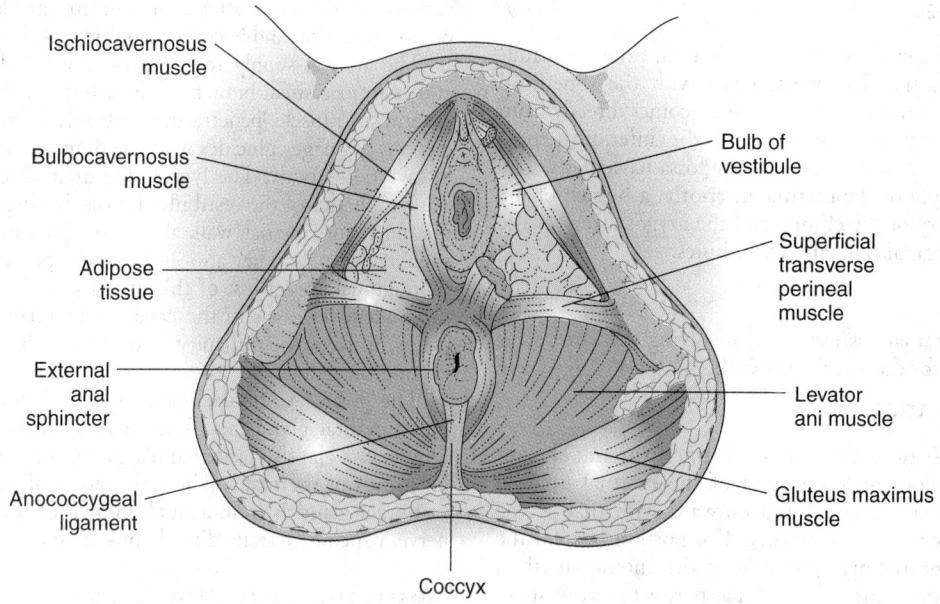

Figure 2–13. Pelvic musculature (inferior view).

tralateral drainage in the upper portion of the muscle and body is evident.

B. Ischiocavernosus Muscle

The ischiocavernosus muscle and its attendant cavernous tissue arise from the ischial tuberosity and inferior ramus to the ischium. It envelops the crus of its cavernous tissue in a thin layer of muscle ascending toward and over the medial and inferior surfaces of the symphysis pubica to terminate in the anterior surface of the symphysis at the base of the clitoris. It then sends decussating fibers to the region of the upper and middle thirds of the urethra, forming the greater part of the organ's voluntary sphincter. The blood supply is through perforating branches from the perineal artery as it ascends between the bulbocavernosus and ischiocavernosus muscles to terminate as the dorsal artery of the clitoris. The innervation stems from an ischiocavernosus branch of the perineal division of the pudendal nerve.

C. Transversus Muscle

The transversus perinei superficialis muscle arises from the inferior ramus of the ischium and from the ischial tuberosity. The fibers of the muscle extend across the perineum and are inserted into its central tendon, meeting those from the opposite side. Frequently, the muscle fibers from the bulbocavernosus, the puborectalis, the superficial transverse perinei, and occasionally the external anal sphincter will interdigitate. The blood supply is from a perforating branch of the perineal divi-

sion of the internal pudendal artery, and the nerve supply is from the perineal division of the pudendal nerve.

D. Sensory Corpuscles

In the cavernous substances of both the bulbocavernosus and ischiocavernosus muscles, Vater-Pacini corpuscles (corpuscula lamellosa) and Dogiel and Krause corpuscles (corpuscula bulboidea) are present.

E. Inferior Layer of Urogenital Diaphragm

The inferior layer of urogenital diaphragm is a potential space depending upon the size and development of the musculature, the parity of the female, and the pelvic architecture. It contains loose areolar connective tissue interspersed with fat. The bulbocavernosus muscles, with the support of the superficial transverse perinei muscles and the puborectalis muscles, act as a point of fixation on each side for support of the vulva, the external genitalia, and the vagina.

F. Surgical Considerations

A midline perineotomy is most effective to minimize trauma to vital supports of the vulva, bulbocavernosus, and superficial transverse perinei muscles. Overdistention of the vagina caused by the presenting part and body of the infant forms a temporary sacculation. If distention occurs too rapidly or if dilatation is beyond the resilient capacity of the vagina, rupture of the vaginal musculature may occur, often demonstrated by a cuneiform groove on the anterior wall and a tonguelike protrusion on the posterior wall of the vagina. Therefore, return of the vagina and vulva to the nonpregnant state is dependent upon the tonus of the muscle and the degree of distention of the vagina during parturition.

BONY PELVIS

The pelvis (Fig 2–14) is a basin-shaped ring of bones that marks the distal margin of the trunk. The pelvis rests upon the lower extremities and supports the spinal column. It is composed of 2 innominate bones, one on each side, joined anteriorly and articulated with the sacrum posteriorly. The 2 major pelvic divisions are the pelvis major (upper or false pelvis) and the pelvis minor (lower or true pelvis). The pelvis major consists primarily of the space superior to the iliopectineal line, including the 2 iliac fossae and the region between them. The pelvis minor, located below the iliopectineal line, is bounded anteriorly by the pubic bones, posteriorly by the sacrum and coccyx, and laterally by the ischium and a small segment of the ilium.

Innominate Bone

The innominate bone is composed of 3 parts: ilium, ischium, and pubis.

A. ILIUM

The ilium consists of a bladelike upper part or ala (wing) and a thicker, lower part called the body. The body forms the upper portion of the acetabulum and unites with the bodies of the ischium and pubis. The medial surface of the ilium presents as a large concave area: the anterior portion is the iliac fossa; the smaller posterior portion is composed of a rough upper part, the iliac tuberosity; and the lower part contains a large surface for articulation with the sacrum. At the inferior medial margin of the iliac fossa, a rounded ridge, the arcuate line, ends anteriorly in the iliopectineal eminence. Posteriorly, the arcuate line is continuous with the anterior margin of the ala of the sacrum across the anterior aspect of the sacroiliac joint. Anteriorly, it is continuous with the ridge or pecten on the superior ramus of the pubis. The lateral surface or dorsum of the ilium is traversed by 3 ridges: the posterior, anterior, and inferior gluteal lines. The superior border is called the crest, and at its 2 extremities are the anterior and posterior superior iliac spines. The principal feature of the anterior border of the ilium is the heavy anterior inferior iliac spine. Important aspects of the posterior border are the posterior superior and the inferior iliac spines and, below the latter, the greater sciatic notch, the inferior part of which is bounded by the ischium. The inferior border of the ilium participates in the formation of the acetabulum.

The main vasculature (Fig 2–15) of the innominate bone appears where the bone is thickest. Blood is supplied to the inner surface of the ilium through twigs of the iliolumbar, deep circumflex iliac, and obturator arteries by foramens on the crest, in the iliac fossa, and below the terminal line near the greater sciatic notch. The outer surface of the ilium is supplied mainly below the inferior gluteal line through nutrient vessels derived from the gluteal arteries. The inferior branch of the deep part of the superior gluteal artery forms the external nutrient artery of the ilium and continues in its course to anastomose with the lateral circumflex artery. Upon leaving the pelvis below the piriform muscle, it divides into a number of branches, a group of which passes to the hip joint.

B. ISCHIUM

The ischium is composed of a body, superior and inferior rami, and a tuberosity. The body is the heaviest part of the bone and is joined with the bodies of the ilium and pubis to form the acetabulum. It presents 3 surfaces. (1) The smooth internal surface is continuous above with the body of the ilium and below with the inner surface of the superior ramus of the ischium. Together, these parts form the posterior portion of the lateral wall of the pelvis minor. (2) The external surface of the ischium is the portion that enters into the formation of the acetabulum. (3) The posterior surface is the area between the acetabular rim and the posterior border. It is convex and is separated from the ischial tuberosity by a wide groove. The posterior border, with the ilium, forms the bony margin of the greater sciatic notch. The superior ramus of the ischium descends from the body of the bone to join the inferior ramus at an angle of approximately 90 degrees. The large ischial tuberosity and its inferior portion are situated on the convexity of this angle. The inferior portion of the tuberosity forms the point of support in the sitting position. The posterior surface is divided into 2 areas by an oblique line. The lesser sciatic notch occupies the posterior border of the superior ramus between the spine and the tuberosity. The inferior ramus, as it is traced forward, joins the inferior ramus of the pubis to form the arcus pubis (ischiopubic arch).

The ischium is supplied with blood from the obturator medial and lateral circumflex arteries. The largest vessels are situated between the acetabulum and the sciatic tubercle.

C. PUBIS

The pubis is composed of a body and 2 rami, superior and inferior. The body contributes to the formation of the acetabulum, joining with the body of the ilium at the iliopectineal eminence and with the body of the is-

Figure 2–14. The bony pelvis. (Reproduced, with permission, from Benson RC: *Handbook of Obstetrics & Gynecology,* 8th ed. Lange, 1983.)

ANTERIOR VIEW

Anterior longitudinal ligament

Iliolumbar ligament

Iliofemoral ligament

Anterior sacroiliac ligament

Obturator membrane

INFERIOR VIEW

Dorsal sacrococcygeal ligament

Sacrospinous ligament

Arcuate pubic ligament

Inguinal ligament

Sacrotuberous ligament

POSTERIOR VIEW

Iliolumbar ligament

Short posterior sacroiliac ligament

Long posterior sacroiliac ligament

Ilioischial ligament

Dorsal sacrococcygeal ligament

Interspinal ligament

Iliofemoral ligament

Sacrotuberous ligament

SUPERIOR VIEW

Iliolumbar ligament

Sacrospinous ligament

Iliofemoral ligament

Anterior longitudinal ligament

Anterior sacroiliac ligament

Arcuate pubic ligament

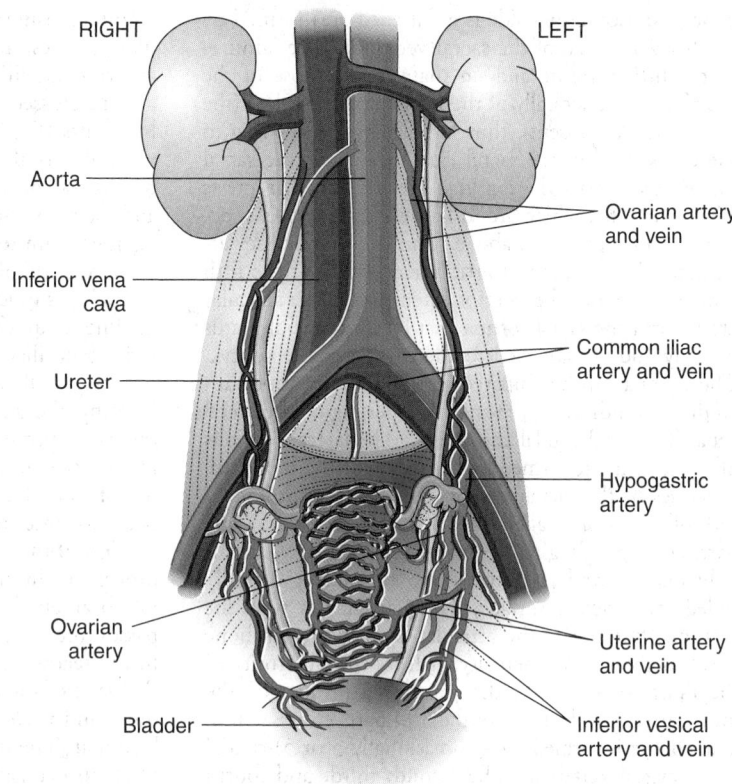

RIGHT   LEFT

Aorta

Ovarian artery and vein

Inferior vena cava

Common iliac artery and vein

Ureter

Hypogastric artery

Ovarian artery

Uterine artery and vein

Bladder

Inferior vesical artery and vein

Figure 2–15. Blood supply to pelvis.

chium in the region of the acetabular notch. The superior ramus passes medially and forward from the body to meet the corresponding ramus of the opposite side at the symphysis pubica. The medial or fore portion of the superior ramus is broad and flattened anteroposteriorly. Formerly called "the body," it presents an outer and an inner surface, the symphyseal area, and an upper border or "crest." Approximately 2 cm from the medial edge of the ramus and in line with the upper border is the prominent pubic tubercle, an important landmark. Below the crest is the anterior surface and the posterior or deep surface. The medial portion of the superior ramus is continuous below with the inferior ramus, and the lateral part presents a wide, smooth area anterosuperiorly, behind which is an irregular ridge, the pecten ossis pubis. The pecten pubis forms the anterior part of the linea terminalis. In front of and below the pectineal area is the obturator crest, passing from the tubercle to the acetabular notch. On the inferior aspect of the superior ramus is the obturator sulcus. The inferior ramus is continuous with the superior ramus and passes downward and backward to join the inferior ramus of the ischium, forming the "ischiopubic arch." The pubis receives blood from the pubic branches of the obturator artery

and from branches of the medial and lateral circumflex arteries.

Sacrum

The sacrum is formed in the adult by the union of 5 or 6 sacral vertebrae; occasionally, the fifth lumbar vertebra is partly fused with it. The process of union is known as "sacralization" in the vertebral column. The sacrum constitutes the base of the vertebral column. As a single bone, it is considered to have a base, an apex, 2 surfaces (pelvic and dorsal), and 2 lateral portions. The base faces upward and is composed principally of a central part, formed by the upper surface of the body of the first sacral vertebra, and 2 lateral areas of alae. The body articulates by means of a fibrocartilage disk with the body of the fifth lumbar vertebra. The alae represent the heavy transverse processes of the first sacral vertebra that articulate with the 2 iliac bones. The anterior margin of the body is called the promontory and forms the sacrovertebral angle with the fifth lumbar vertebra. The rounded anterior margin of each ala constitutes the posterior part (pars sacralis) of the linea terminalis. The pelvic surface of the sacrum is rough and convex. In the midline is the median sacral crest (fused spinal processes), and on either side is a flattened area formed by the fused laminae of the sacral vertebrae. The laminae of the fifth vertebra and, in many cases, those of the fourth and occasionally of the third are incomplete (the spines also are absent), thus leaving a wide opening to the dorsal wall of the sacral canal known as the sacral hiatus. Lateral to the laminae are the articular crests (right and left), which are in line with the paired superior articular processes above. The lateral processes articulate with the inferior articular processes of the fifth lumbar vertebra. The inferior extensions of the articular crests form the sacral cornua that bind the sacral hiatus laterally and are attached to the cornua of the coccyx. The cornua can be palpated in life and are important landmarks indicating the inferior opening of the sacral canal (for sacral-caudal anesthesia). The lateral portions of the sacrum are formed by the fusion of the transverse processes of the sacral vertebrae. They form dorsally a line of elevations called the lateral sacral crests. The parts corresponding to the first 3 vertebrae are particularly massive and present a large area facing laterally called the articular surface, which articulates with the sacrum. Posterior to the articular area, the rough bone is called the sacral tuberosity. It faces the tuberosity of the ilium. The apex is the small area formed by the lower surface of the body of the fifth part of the sacrum. The coccyx is formed by 4 (occasionally 3 or 5) caudal or coccygeal vertebrae. The second, third, and fourth parts are frequently fused into a single bone that articulates with the first by means of a fibrocartilage. The entire coccyx may become ossified and fused with the sacrum (the sacrococcygeal joint).

The sacrum receives its blood supply from the middle sacral artery, which extends from the bifurcation of the aorta to the tip of the coccyx, and from the lateral sacral arteries that branch either as a single artery that immediately divides or as 2 distinct vessels from the hypogastric artery. The lowest lumbar branch of the middle sacral artery ramifies over the lateral parts of the sacrum, passing back between the last vertebra and the sacrum to anastomose with the lumbar arteries above and the superior gluteal artery below. The lateral sacral branches (usually 4) anastomose anteriorly to the coccyx with branches of the inferior lateral sacral artery that branch from the hypogastric artery. They give off small spinal branches that pass through the sacral foramens and supply the sacral canal and posterior portion of the sacrum.

Sacroiliac Joint

The sacroiliac joint is a diarthrodial joint with irregular surfaces. The articular surfaces are covered with a layer of cartilage, and the cavity of the joint is a narrow cleft. The cartilage on the sacrum is hyaline in its deeper parts but much thicker than that on the ilium.

A joint capsule is attached to the margins of the articular surfaces, and the bones are held together by the anterior sacroiliac, long and short posterior sacroiliac, and interosseous ligaments. In addition, there are 3 ligaments (Fig 2–16), classed as belonging to the pelvic girdle itself, which also serve as accessory ligaments to the sacroiliac joint: the iliolumbar, sacrotuberous, and sacrospinous ligaments. The anterior sacroiliac ligaments unite the base and the lateral part of the sacrum to the ilium, blending with the periosteum of the pelvic surface and, on the ilium, reaching the arcuate line to attach in the paraglenoid grooves. The posterior sacroiliac ligament is extremely strong and consists essentially of 2 sets of fibers, deep and superficial, forming the short and long posterior sacroiliac ligaments, respectively. The short posterior sacroiliac ligament passes inferiorly and medially from the tuberosity of the ilium, behind the articular surface and posterior interior iliac spine, to the back of the lateral portion of the sacrum and to the upper sacral articular process, including the area between it and the first sacral foramen. The long posterior sacroiliac ligament passes inferiorly from the posterior superior iliac spine to the second, third, and fourth articular tubercles on the back of the sacrum. It partly covers the short ligament and is continuous below with the sacrotuberous ligament. The interosseous ligaments are the strongest of all and consist of fibers of different lengths passing in various directions between the 2 bones. They extend from the rough surface of the sacral tuberosity to the corresponding surface on the lateral aspect of the sacrum, above and behind the articular surface.

Ligaments

The sacrotuberous ligament, in common with the long posterior sacroiliac ligament, is attached above to the crest of the ilium and posterior iliac spine and to the posterior aspect of the lower 3 sacral vertebrae. Below, it is attached chiefly to the medial border of the ischial tuberosity. Some of the fibers at the other end extend forward along the inner surface of the ischial ramus, forming the falciform process. Other posterior fibers continue into the tendons of the hamstrings.

The sacrospinous ligament is triangular and thin, extending from the lateral border of the sacrum and coccyx to the spine of the ischium. It passes medially (deep) to the sacrotuberous ligament and is partly blended with it along the lateral border of the sacrum.

The iliolumbar ligament connects the fourth and fifth lumbar vertebrae with the iliac crest. It originates from the transverse process of the fifth lumbar vertebra, where it is closely woven with the sacrolumbar ligament. Some of its fibers spread downward onto the body of the fifth vertebra and others ascend to the disk above. It is attached to the inner lip of the crest of the

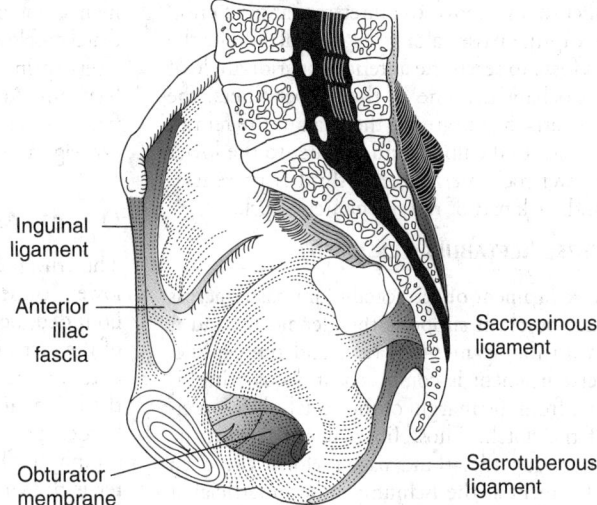

Figure 2–16. Ligaments of the pelvis.

ilium for approximately 5 cm. The sacrolumbar ligament is generally inseparable from the iliolumbar ligament and is regarded as part of it.

Pubic Symphysis

The pubic symphysis is a synarthrodial joint of the symphyseal surfaces of the pubic bones. The ligaments associated with it are (1) the interpubic fibrocartilage, (2) the superior pubic ligament, (3) the anterior pubic ligament, and (4) the arcuate ligament. The interpubic fibrocartilage is thicker in front than behind and projects beyond the edges of the bones, especially on the posterior aspect, blending intimately with the ligaments at its margins. Sometimes it is woven throughout, but often the interpubic fibrocartilage presents an elongated, narrow fissure with fluid in the interspace, partially dividing the cartilage into 2 plates. The interpubic cartilage is intimately adherent to the layer of hyaline cartilage that covers the symphyseal surface of each pubic bone. The superior pubic ligament extends laterally along the crest of the pubis on each side to the pubic tubercle, blending in the middle line with the interpubic cartilage. The thick and strong anterior pubic ligament is closely connected with the fascial covering of the muscles arising from the conjoined rami of the pubis. It consists of several strata of thick, decussating fibers of different degrees of obliquity, the superficial being the most oblique and extending lowest over the joint. The arcuate ligament is a thick band of closely connected fibers that fills the angle between the pubic rami to form a smooth, rounded top to the pubic arch. Both on the anterior and posterior aspects of the joint, the ligament gives off decussating fibers that, interlacing with one another, strengthen the joint.

Hip Joint

The hip joint is a typical example of a ball-and-socket joint, the round head of the femur received by the deep cavity of the acetabulum and glenoid lip. Both articular surfaces are coated with cartilage. The portion covering the head of the femur is thicker above, where it bears the weight of the body, and thins out to a mere edge below. The pit in the femoral head receives the ligamentum teres, the only part uncoated by cartilage. The cartilage is horseshoe-shaped on the acetabulum and, corresponding to the lunate surface, thicker above than below. The ligaments are the articular capsule, transverse acetabular ligament, iliofemoral ligament, ischiocapsular ligament and zona orbicularis, pubocapsular ligament, and ligamentum teres.

A. ARTICULAR CAPSULE

The articular capsule is one of the strongest ligaments in the body. It is attached superiorly to the base of the anterior inferior iliac spine at the pelvis, posteriorly to a point a few millimeters from the acetabular rim, and inferiorly to the upper edge of the groove between the acetabulum and tuberosity of the ischium. Anteriorly, it is secured to the pubis near the obturator groove, to the iliopectineal eminence, and posteriorly to the base of the inferior iliac spine. At the femur, the articular capsule is fixed to the anterior portion of the superior border of the greater trochanter and to the cervical tubercle. The capsule runs down the intertrochanteric line as far as the medial aspect of the femur, where it is on a level with the inferior part of the lesser trochanter. It then runs superiorly and posteriorly along an oblique line, just in front of and above the lesser trochanter, and continues along the back of the neck of the femur nearly parallel to and above the intertrochanteric crest. Finally, the capsule passes along the medial side of the trochanteric fossa to reach the anterior superior angle of the greater trochanter. Some of the deeper fibers, the retinacula, are attached nearer to the head of the femur. One corresponds to the upper and another to the lower part of the intertrochanteric line; a third is present at the upper and back part of the trochanteric neck.

B. TRANSVERSE ACETABULAR LIGAMENT

The transverse ligament of the acetabulum passes across the acetabular notch. It supports the glenoid lip and is connected with the ligamentum teres and the capsule. The transverse ligament is composed of decussating fibers that arise from the margin of the acetabulum on either side of the notch. Those fibers coming from the pubis are more superficial and pass to form the deep part of the ligament at the ischium; those superficial at the ischium are deep at the pubis.

C. ILIOFEMORAL LIGAMENT

The iliofemoral ligament is located at the front of the articular capsule and is triangular. Its apex is attached to a curved line on the ilium immediately below and behind the anterior inferior spine; its base is fixed beneath the anterior edge of the greater trochanter and to the intertrochanteric line. The upper fibers are almost straight whereas the medial fibers are oblique, giving the appearance of an inverted Y.

D. ISCHIOCAPSULAR LIGAMENT

The ischiocapsular ligament, on the posterior surface of the articular capsule, is attached to the body of the ischium along the upper border of the notch. Above the notch, the ligament is secured to the ischial margin of the acetabulum. The upper fibers incline superiorly and laterally and are fixed to the greater trochanter. The other fibers curve more and more upward as they pass laterally to their insertion at the inner side of the trochanteric fossa. The deeper fibers take a circular course and form a ring at the back and lower parts of the capsule, where the longitudinal fibers are deficient. This ring, the zona orbicularis, embraces the neck of the femur.

E. PUBOCAPSULAR LIGAMENT

The pubocapsular ligament is fixed proximally to the obturator crest and to the anterior border of the iliopectineal eminence, reaching as far down as the pubic end of the acetabular notch. Below, the fibers reach to the neck of the femur and are fixed above and behind the lowermost fibers of the iliofemoral band, blending with it.

F. LIGAMENTUM TERES

The ligamentum teres femoris extends from the acetabular fossa to the head of the femur. It has 2 bony attachments, one on either side of the acetabular notch immediately below the articular cartilage, with intermediate fibers springing from the lower surface of the transverse ligament. At the femur, the ligamentum teres femoris is fixed to the anterior part of the fovea capitis and to the cartilage around the margin of the depression.

Outlets of the True Pelvis

The true pelvis is said to have an upper "inlet" and a lower "outlet." The pelvic inlet to the pelvis minor is bounded, beginning posteriorly, by (1) the promontory of the sacrum; (2) the linea terminalis, composed of the anterior margin of the ala sacralis, the arcuate line of the ilium, and the pecten ossis pubis; and (3) the upper border or crest of the pubis, ending medially at the symphysis. The conjugate or the anteroposterior diameter is drawn from the center of the promontory to the symphysis pubica, with 2 conjugates recognized: (1) the true conjugate, measured from the promontory to the top of the symphysis; and (2) the diagonal conjugate, measured from the promontory to the bottom of the symphysis. The transverse diameter is measured through the greatest width of the pelvic inlet. The oblique diameter runs from the sacroiliac joint of one side to the iliopectineal eminence of the other. The pelvic outlet, which faces downward and slightly backward, is very irregular. Beginning anteriorly, it is bounded by (1) the arcuate ligament of the pubis (in the midline), (2) the ischiopubic arch, (3) the ischial tuberosity, (4) the sacrotuberous ligament, and (5) the coccyx (in midline). Its anteroposterior diameter is drawn from the lower border of the symphysis pubica to the tip of the coccyx. The transverse diameter passes between the medial surfaces of the ischial tuberosities.

Musculature Attachments

A. ILIUM

The crest of the ilium gives attachment to the external oblique, internal oblique, transversus (anterior two-thirds), latissimus dorsi and quadratus lumborum (posteriorly), sacrospinalis (internal lip, posteriorly), and tensor fasciae latae and sartorius muscles (anterior superior iliac spine) (Fig 2–17). The posterior superior spine of the ilium gives attachment to the multifidus muscle. The rectus femoris muscle is attached to the anterior inferior iliac spine. The iliacus muscle originates on the iliac fossa. Between the anterior inferior iliac spine and the iliopectineal eminence is a broad groove for the tendon of the iliopsoas muscle. A small portion of the gluteus maximus muscle originates between the posterior gluteus line and the crest. The surface of bone between the anterior gluteal line and the crest gives origin to the gluteus medius muscle. The

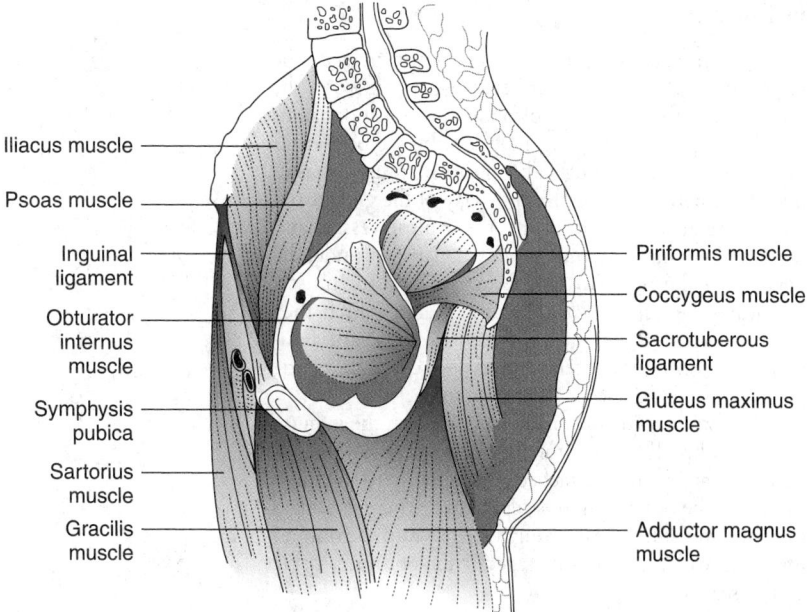

Iliacus muscle

Psoas muscle

Inguinal ligament

Obturator internus muscle

Symphysis pubica

Sartorius muscle

Gracilis muscle

Piriformis muscle

Coccygeus muscle

Sacrotuberous ligament

Gluteus maximus muscle

Adductor magnus muscle

Figure 2–17. Pelvic muscles.

gluteus minimus muscle has its origin between the anterior and inferior gluteal lines.

B. Ischium

The body and superior ramus of the ischium give rise to the obturator internus muscle on the internal surface. The ischial spine provides, at its root, attachments for the coccygeus and levator ani muscles on its internal surface and for the gemellus superior muscle externally. The outer surface of the ramus is the origin of the adductor magnus and obturator externus muscles. The transversus perinei muscle is attached to the lower border of the ischium. The ischial tuberosity gives rise on its posterior surface to the semimembranosus muscles, the common tendon of the biceps, and semitendinosus muscles and on its inferior surface to the adductor magnus muscle. The superior border is the site of origin of the inferior gemellus and the outer border of the quadratus femoris muscle. The superior ramus of the pubis gives origin to the adductor longus and obturator externus muscles on its anterior surface and to the levator ani and obturator internus muscles. The superior border provides attachment for the rectus abdominis and pyramidalis muscles. The pectineal surface gives origin at its posterior portion to the pectineus muscle. The posterior surface of the superior ramus is the point of attachment of a few fascicles of the obturator internus muscle. The anterior surface of the inferior ramus attaches to the abductor brevis, adductor magnus, and obturator externus muscles, and

its posterior surface attaches to the sphincter urogenitalis and the obturator internus.

C. Sacrum

The pelvic surface of the sacrum is the origin of the piriform muscle. The lateral part of the fifth sacral vertebra is the point of insertion of the sacrospinalis and gluteus maximus muscles. The ala is attached to fibers of the iliacus muscle.

D. Coccyx

The dorsal surface of the coccyx is attached to the gluteus maximus muscle and the sphincter ani externus muscle. The lateral margins receive parts of the coccygeus and of the iliococcygeus muscles.

E. Greater Trochanter

The lateral surface of the greater trochanter of the femur receives the insertion of the gluteus medius muscle. The medial surface of the greater trochanter receives the tendon of the obturator externus in the trochanteric fossa, along with the obturator internus and the 2 gemelli. The superior border provides insertion for the piriformis and, with the anterior border, receives the gluteus minimus. The quadratus femoris attaches to the tubercle of the quadratus. The inferior border gives origin to the vastus lateralis muscle. The lesser trochanter attaches to the iliopsoas muscle at its summit. Fascicles of the iliacus extend beyond the trochanter and are inserted into the surface of the shaft.

Foramens

Several foramens are present in the bony pelvis. The sacrospinous ligament separates the greater from the lesser sciatic foramen. These foramens are subdivisions of a large space intervening between the sacrotuberous ligament and the femur. The piriform muscle passes out of the pelvis into the thigh by way of the greater sciatic foramen, accompanied by the gluteal vessels and nerves. The internal pudendal vessels, the pudendal nerve, and the nerve to the obturator internus muscle also leave the pelvis by this foramen, after which they enter the perineal region through the lesser sciatic foramen. The obturator internus muscle passes out of the pelvis by way of the lesser sciatic foramen.

The obturator foramen is situated between the ischium and the pubis. The obturator membrane occupies the obturator foramen and is attached continuously to the inner surface of the bony margin except above, where it bridges the obturator sulcus, converting the latter into the obturator canal, which provides passage for the obturator nerve and vessels.

On either side of the central part of the pelvic surface of the sacrum are 4 anterior sacral foramens that transmit the first 4 sacral nerves. Corresponding to these on the dorsal surface are the 4 posterior sacral foramens for transmission of the small posterior rami of the first 4 sacral nerves.

Types of Pelves

Evaluation of the pelvis is best achieved by using the criteria set by Caldwell and Moloy, which are predicated upon 4 basic types of pelves: (1) the gynecoid type (from Greek *gyne* woman); (2) the android type (from Greek *aner* man); (3) the anthropoid type (from Greek *anthropos* human); and (4) the platypelloid type (from Greek *platys* broad and *pella* bowl) (Fig 2–18).

A. GYNECOID

In pure form, the gynecoid pelvis provides a rounded, slightly ovoid, or elliptical inlet with a well-rounded forepelvis (anterior segment). This type of pelvis has a well-rounded, spacious posterior segment, an adequate sacrosciatic notch, a hollow sacrum with a somewhat backward sacral inclination, and a Norman-type arch of the pubic rami. The gynecoid pelvis has straight side walls and wide interspinous and intertuberous diameters. The bones are primarily of medium weight and structure.

B. ANDROID

The android pelvis has a wedge-shaped inlet, a narrow forepelvis, a flat posterior segment, and a narrow sacrosciatic notch, with the sacrum inclining forward. The side walls converge, and the bones are medium to heavy in structure.

Figure 2–18. Types of pelves. White lines in the diagrams at right (after Steele) show the greatest diameters of the pelves at left. (Reproduced, with permission, from Benson RC: *Handbook of Obstetrics & Gynecology,* 8th ed. Lange, 1983.)

C. ANTHROPOID

The anthropoid pelvis is characterized by a long, narrow, oval inlet; an extended and narrow anterior and posterior segment; a wide sacrosciatic notch; and a long, narrow sacrum, often with 6 sacral segments. The subpubic arch may be an angled Gothic type or rounded Norman type. Straight side walls are characteristic of the anthropoid pelvis, whose interspinous and intertuberous diameters are less than those of the average gynecoid pelvis. A medium bone structure is usual.

D. PLATYPELLOID

The platypelloid pelvis has a distinct oval inlet with a very wide, rounded retropubic angle and a wider, flat posterior segment. The sacrosciatic notch is narrow and has a nor-

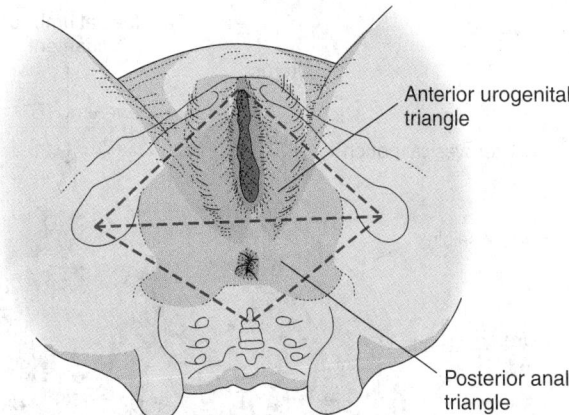

Anterior urogenital triangle

Posterior anal triangle

Figure 2–19. Urogenital and anal triangles.

mal sacral inclination, although it is often short. The sub-pubic arch is very wide and the side walls are straight, with wide interspinous and intertuberous diameters.

The pelvis in any individual case may be one of the 4 "pure" types or a combination of mixed types. When one discusses the intermediate pelvic forms, the posterior segment with its characteristics generally is described first and the anterior segment with its characteristics next, eg, anthropoid-gynecoid, android-anthropoid, or platypelloid-gynecoid. Obviously, it is impossible to have a platypelloid-anthropoid pelvis or a platypelloid-android pelvis.

Pelvic Relationships

Several important relationships should be remembered, beginning with those at the inlet of the pelvis. The transverse diameter of the inlet is the widest diameter, where bone is present for a circumference of 360 degrees. This diameter stretches from pectineal line to pectineal line and denotes the separation of the posterior and anterior segments of the pelvis. In classic pelves (gynecoid), a vertical plane dropped from the transverse diameter of the inlet passes through the level of the interspinous diameter at the ischial spine. These relationships may not hold true, however, in combination or intermediate (mixed type) pelves. The anterior transverse diameter of the inlet reaches from pectineal prominence to pectineal prominence; a vertical plane dropped from the anterior transverse passes through the ischial tuberosities. For good function of the pelvis, the anterior transverse diameter should never be more than 2 cm longer than the transverse diameter (Fig 2–19).

A. OBSTETRIC CONJUGATE

The obstetric conjugate differs from both the diagonal conjugate and the true conjugate. It is represented by a line drawn from the posterior superior portion of the

pubic symphysis (where bone exists for a circumference of 360 degrees) toward intersection with the sacrum. This point need not be at the promontory of the sacrum. The obstetric conjugate is divided into 2 segments: (1) the anterior sagittal, originating at the intersection of the obstetric conjugate with the transverse diameter of the inlet and terminating at the symphysis pubica; and (2) the posterior sagittal, originating at the transverse diameter of the inlet to the point of intersection with the sacrum.

B. INTERSPINOUS DIAMETER

A most significant diameter in the midpelvis is the interspinous diameter. It is represented by a plane passing from ischial spine to ischial spine. The posterior sagittal diameter of the midpelvis is a bisecting line drawn at a right angle from the middle of the interspinous diameter, in the same plane, to a point of intersection with the sacrum. This is the point of greatest importance in the midpelvis. It is sometimes said that the posterior sagittal diameter should be drawn from the posterior segment of the intersecting line of the interspinous diameter, in a plane from the inferior surface of the symphysis, through the interspinous diameter to the sacrum. However, this configuration often places the posterior sagittal diameter lower in the pelvis than the interspinous diameter. It is the interspinous diameter, together with the posterior sagittal diameter of the midpelvis, that determines whether or not there is adequate room for descent and extension of the head during labor.

C. INTERTUBEROUS DIAMETER

The intertuberous diameter of the outlet will reflect the length of the anterior transverse diameter of the inlet, ie, the former cannot be larger than the latter if convergent or straight side walls are present. Therefore, the intertuberous diameter determines the space available in the anterior segment of the pelvis at the inlet, and, simi-

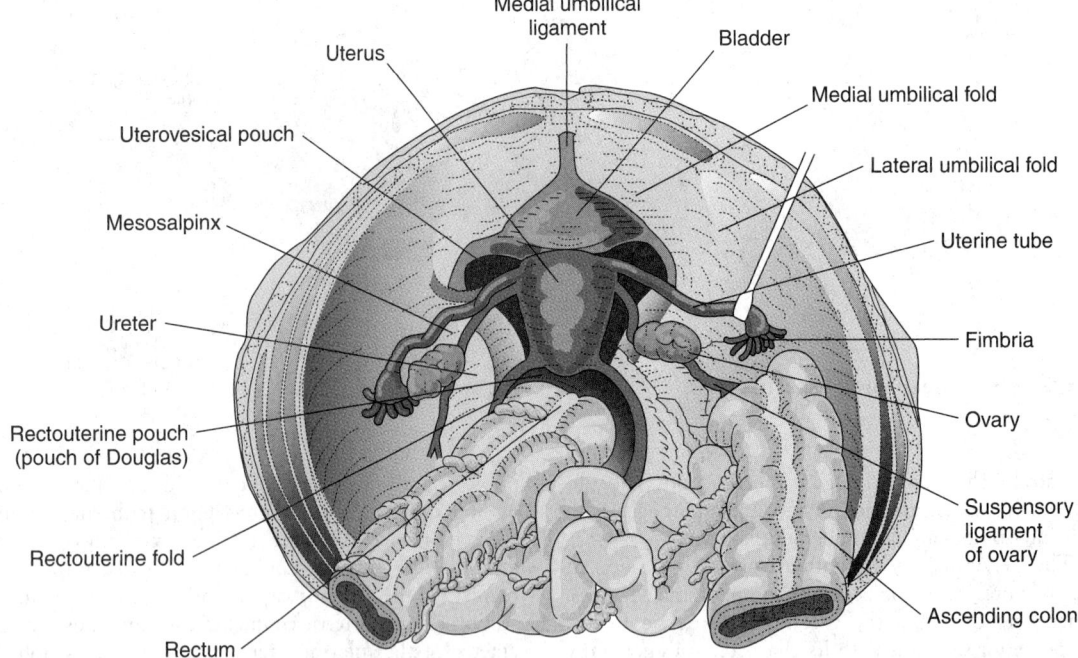

Medial umbilical
ligament

Bladder

Uterus

Medial umbilical fold

Uterovesical pouch

Lateral umbilical fold

Mesosalpinx

Uterine tube

Ureter

Fimbria

Rectouterine pouch
(pouch of Douglas)

Ovary

Suspensory
ligament
of ovary

Rectouterine fold

Ascending colon

Rectum

Figure 2–20. Female pelvic contents from above.

larly, the degree of convergence influences the length of the biparietal diameter at the outlet.

D. POSTERIOR SAGITTAL DIAMETER

The posterior sagittal diameter of the outlet is an intersecting line drawn from the middle of the intertuberous diameter to the sacrococcygeal junction and reflects the inclination of the sacrum toward the outlet for accommodation of the head at delivery. It should be noted that intricate measurements of the pelvis are significant only at minimal levels. Evaluation of the pelvis for a given pregnancy, size of the fetus for a given pelvis, and conduct of labor engagement are far more important.

CONTENTS OF THE PELVIC CAVITY

The organs that occupy the female pelvis (Figs 2–20 to 2–22) are the bladder, the ureters, the urethra, the uterus, the uterine (fallopian) tubes or oviducts, the ovaries, the vagina, and the rectum.* With the exception of the inferior portion of the rectum and most of the vagina, all lie immediately beneath the peritoneum. The uterus, uterine tubes, and ovaries are almost completely covered with peritoneum and are suspended in peritoneal ligaments. The remainder are partially covered. These organs do not

completely fill the cavity; the remaining space is occupied by ileum and sigmoid colon.

1. Bladder

The urinary bladder is a muscular, hollow organ that lies posterior to the pubic bones and anterior to the uterus and broad ligament. Its form, size, and position vary with the amount of urine it contains. When empty, it takes the form of a somewhat rounded pyramid, having a base, a vertex (or apex), a superior surface, and a convex inferior surface that may be divided by a median ridge into 2 inferolateral surfaces.

Relationships

The superior surface of the bladder is covered with peritoneum that is continuous with the medial umbilical fold, forming the paravesical fossae laterally. Posteriorly, the peritoneum passes onto the uterus at the junction of the cervix and corpus, continuing upward on the anterior surface to form the vesicouterine pouch. When the bladder is empty, the normal uterus rests upon its superior surface. When the bladder is distended, coils of intestine may lie upon its superior surface. The base of the bladder rests below the peritoneum and is adjacent to the cervix and the anterior fornix of the vagina. It is separated from these structures by areolar tissue containing plexiform veins. The

---

* The rectum is not described in this chapter.

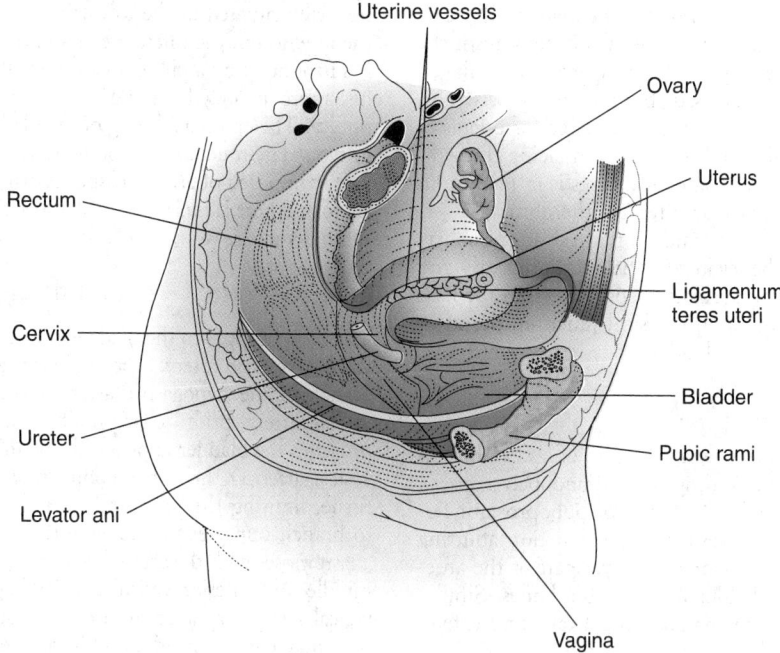

Figure 2–21. Pelvic viscera (sagittal view).

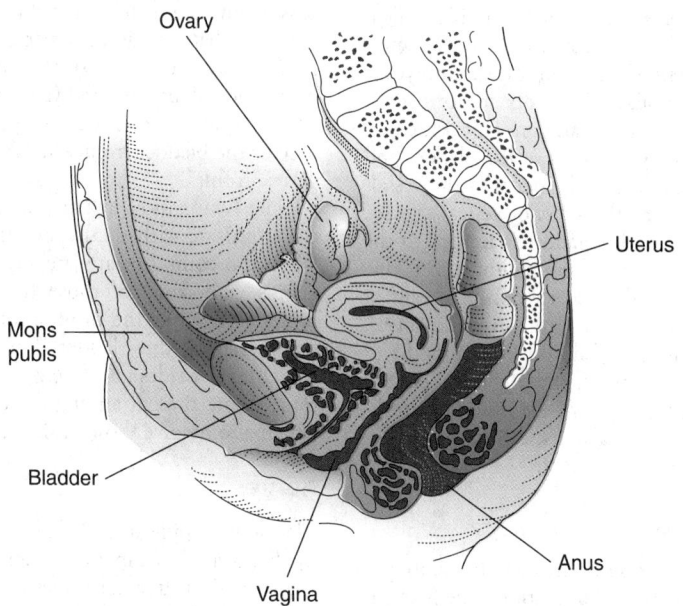

Figure 2–22. Pelvic organs (midsagittal view). (Reproduced, with permission, from Benson RC: *Handbook of Obstetrics & Gynecology,* 8th ed. Lange, 1983.)

area over the vagina is extended as the bladder fills. The inferolateral surfaces are separated from the wall of the pelvis by the potential prevesical space, containing a small amount of areolar tissue but no large vessels. This surface is nonperitoneal and thus suitable for operative procedures. Posterolateral to the region facing the symphysis, each of the inferolateral surfaces is in relation to the fascia of the obturator internus, the obturator vessels and nerve, the obliterated umbilical artery above, and the fascia of the levator ani below. Posteriorly and medially, the inferior surface is separated from the base by an area called the urethrovesical junction, the most stationary portion of the bladder.

Fascia, Ligaments, & Muscle

The bladder is enclosed by a thin layer of fascia, the vesical sheath. Two thickenings of the endopelvic fascia, the medial and lateral pubovesical or puboprostatic ligaments, extend at the vesicourethral junction abutting the levator ani muscle from the lower part of the anterior aspect of the bladder to the pubic bones. Similar fascial thickenings, the lateral true ligaments, extend from the sides of the lower part of the bladder to the lateral walls of the pelvis. Posteriorly, the vesicourethral junction of the bladder lies directly against the anterior wall of the vagina.

A fibrous band, the urachus or medial umbilical ligament, extends from the apex of the bladder to the umbilicus. This band represents the remains of the embryonic allantois. The lateral umbilical ligaments are formed by the obliterated umbilical arteries and are represented by fibrous cords passing along the sides of the bladder and ascending toward the umbilicus. Frequently, the vessels will be patent, thus forming the superior vesical arteries. The peritoneal covering of the bladder is limited to the upper surface. The reflections of the peritoneum to the anterior abdominal wall and the corresponding walls of the pelvis are sometimes described as the superior, lateral, and posterior false ligaments. The muscle (smooth) of the bladder is represented by an interdigitated pattern continuous with and contiguous to the inner longitudinal and anterior circumferential muscles of the urethra. No distinct muscle layers are apparent.

Mucous Membrane

The mucous membrane is rose-colored and lies in irregular folds that become effaced by distention. The 3 angles of the vesical trigone are represented by the orifices of the 2 ureters and the internal urethral orifice. This area is redder in color and free from plication. It is bordered posteriorly by the plica interureterica, a curved transverse ridge extending between the orifices of the ureters. A median longitudinal elevation, the uvula vesicae, extends toward the urethral orifice. The internal urethral orifice is normally situated at the lowest point of the bladder, at the junction of the inferolateral and posterior surfaces. It is surrounded by a circular elevation, the urethral annulus, approximately level with the center of the symphysis pubica. The epithelial lining of the bladder is transitional in type. The mucous membrane rests on the submucous coat, composed of areolar tissue superficial to the muscular coat. There is no evidence of a specific smooth muscle sphincter in the vesical neck.

Arteries, Veins, & Lymphatics

The blood supply to the bladder comes from branches of the hypogastric artery. The umbilical artery, a terminal branch of the hypogastric artery, gives off the superior vesical artery prior to its obliterated portion. It approaches the bladder (along with the middle and inferior vesical arteries) through a condensation of fatty areolar tissue, limiting the prevesical "space" posterosuperiorly, to branch out over the upper surface of the bladder. It anastomoses with the arteries of the opposite side and the middle and inferior vesical arteries below. The middle vesical artery may arise from one of the superior vessels, or it may come from the umbilical artery, supplying the sides and base of the bladder. The inferior vesical artery usually arises directly from the hypogastric artery—in common with or as a branch of the uterine artery—and passes downward and medially, where it divides into branches that supply the lower part of the bladder. The fundus may also receive small branches from the middle hemorrhoidal, uterine, and vaginal arteries.

The veins form an extensive plexus at the sides and base of the bladder from which stems pass to the hypogastric trunk.

The lymphatics, in part, accompany the veins and communicate with the hypogastric nodes (Table 2–2). They also communicate laterally with the external iliac glands, and some of those from the fundus pass to nodes situated at the promontory of the sacrum. The lymphatics of the bladder dome are separate on the right and left sides and rarely cross; but extensive anastomoses are present among the lymphatics of the base, which also involve those of the cervix.

Nerves

The nerve supply to the bladder is derived partly from the hypogastric sympathetic plexus and partly from the second and third sacral nerves (the nervi erigentes).

2. Ureters

Relationships

The ureter is a slightly flattened tube that extends from the termination of the renal pelvis to the lower outer corner of the base of the bladder, a distance of 26–28 cm. It

Table 2-2. Lymphatics of the female pelvis.

A. Superficial Lymphatics:

Skin of abdomen (lateral) ——————— Superficial nodes

⎫ Frequent anastomoses

Skin of abdomen (medial) ——————— Superficial circumflex vein and nodes

Thigh (medial) and perineal skin ——————— Superficial epigastric vein and nodes ——— Frequently cross to contralateral side

Thigh (lateral)

B. Deep Lymphatics:

Clitoral plexus

Lymphatics through labia majora

Superior vestibular plexus ——— To respective superficial inguinal nodes (10–20 along inguinal ligament) (under internal oblique fascia)

Superior network of fourchette

Abdomen ——— Saphenous fossa ——— Femoral nodes (3–4); nodes in deep inguinal ring (nodi lymphatici inguinales profundi [nodes of Rosenmüller or Cloquet]) ——— External iliac chain

Inner rectum ——— Superficial subinguinal nodes (3–4)

Lateral thigh

(continued)

Table 2–2. Lymphatics of the female pelvis. (continued)

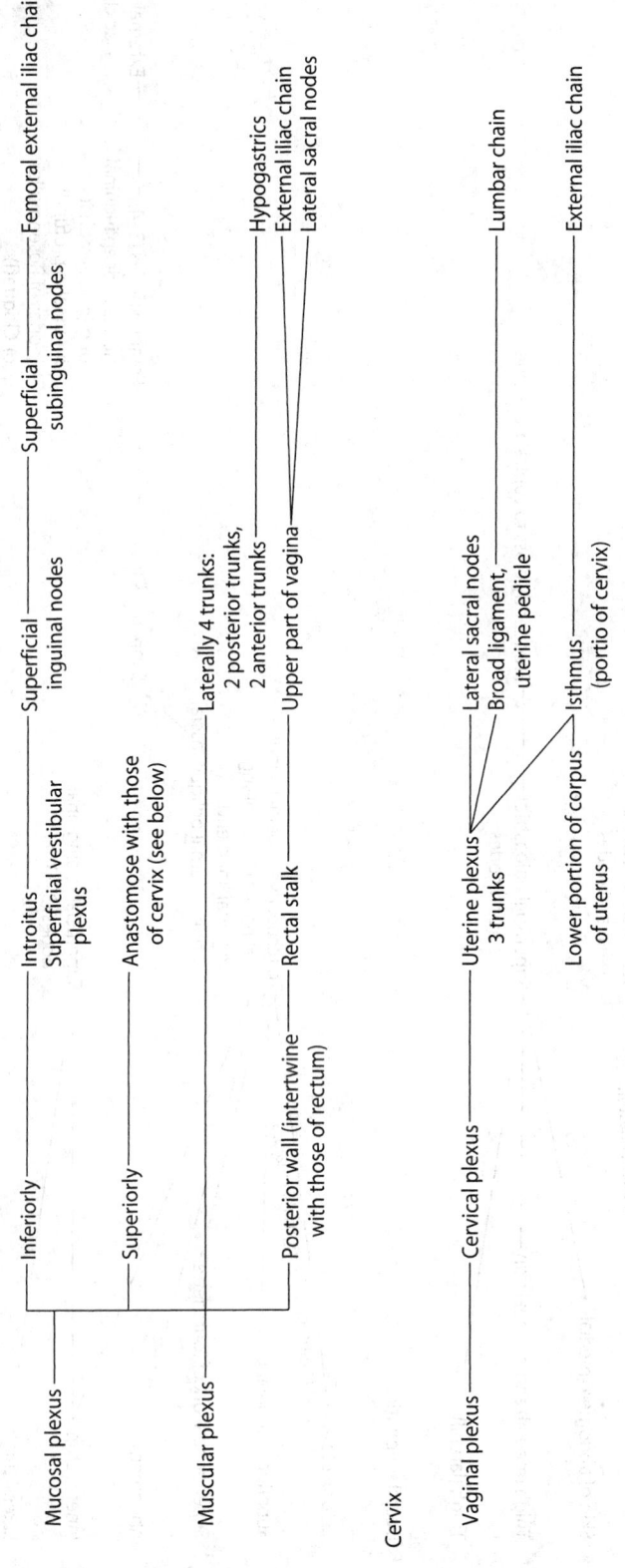

Vagina

Mucosal plexus —— Inferiorly —— Introitus —— Superficial —— Femoral external iliac chain
                                Superficial vestibular   inguinal nodes   Superficial
                                plexus   subinguinal nodes

              —— Superiorly —— Anastomose with those
                                of cervix (see below)

Muscular plexus —— Laterally 4 trunks:
                    2 posterior trunks,
                    2 anterior trunks

                 —— Upper part of vagina —— Hypogastrics
                                            External iliac chain
                                            Lateral sacral nodes

                 —— Posterior wall (intertwine —— Rectal stalk
                     with those of rectum)

Cervix

Vaginal plexus —— Cervical plexus —— Uterine plexus —— Lateral sacral nodes —— Lumbar chain
                                      3 trunks   Broad ligament,
                                                          uterine pedicle

                 —— Lower portion of corpus —— Isthmus —— External iliac chain
                     of uterus   (portio of cervix)

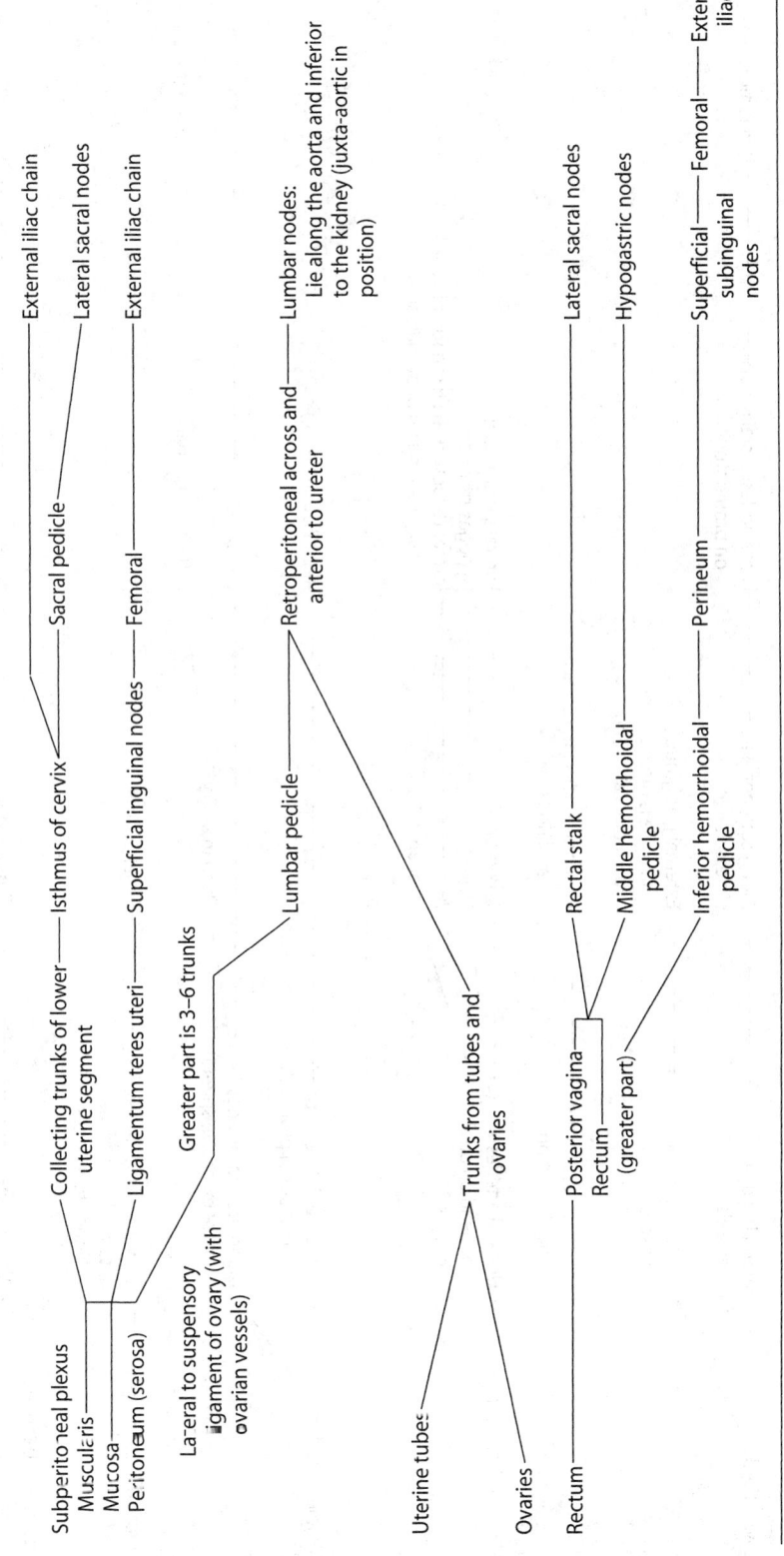

Uterus

Subperitoneal plexus
Muscularis
Mucosa
Peritoneum (serosa)

Collecting trunks of lower uterine segment —— Isthmus of cervix —— Sacral pedicle —— Lateral sacral nodes
—— External iliac chain

Ligamentum teres uteri —— Superficial inguinal nodes —— Femoral —— External iliac chain

Greater part is 3–6 trunks

Lateral to suspensory ligament of ovary (with ovarian vessels)

Lumbar pedicle —— Retroperitoneal across and anterior to ureter —— Lumbar nodes:
Lie along the aorta and inferior to the kidney (juxta-aortic in position)

Uterine tubes

Ovaries

Trunks from tubes and ovaries

Rectum

Posterior vagina
Rectum (greater part) —— Rectal stalk —— Lateral sacral nodes

Middle hemorrhoidal pedicle —— Hypogastric nodes

Inferior hemorrhoidal pedicle —— Perineum —— Superficial subinguinal nodes —— Femoral —— External iliac chain

(continued)

Table 2-2. Lymphatics of the female pelvis. (continued)

Ureters

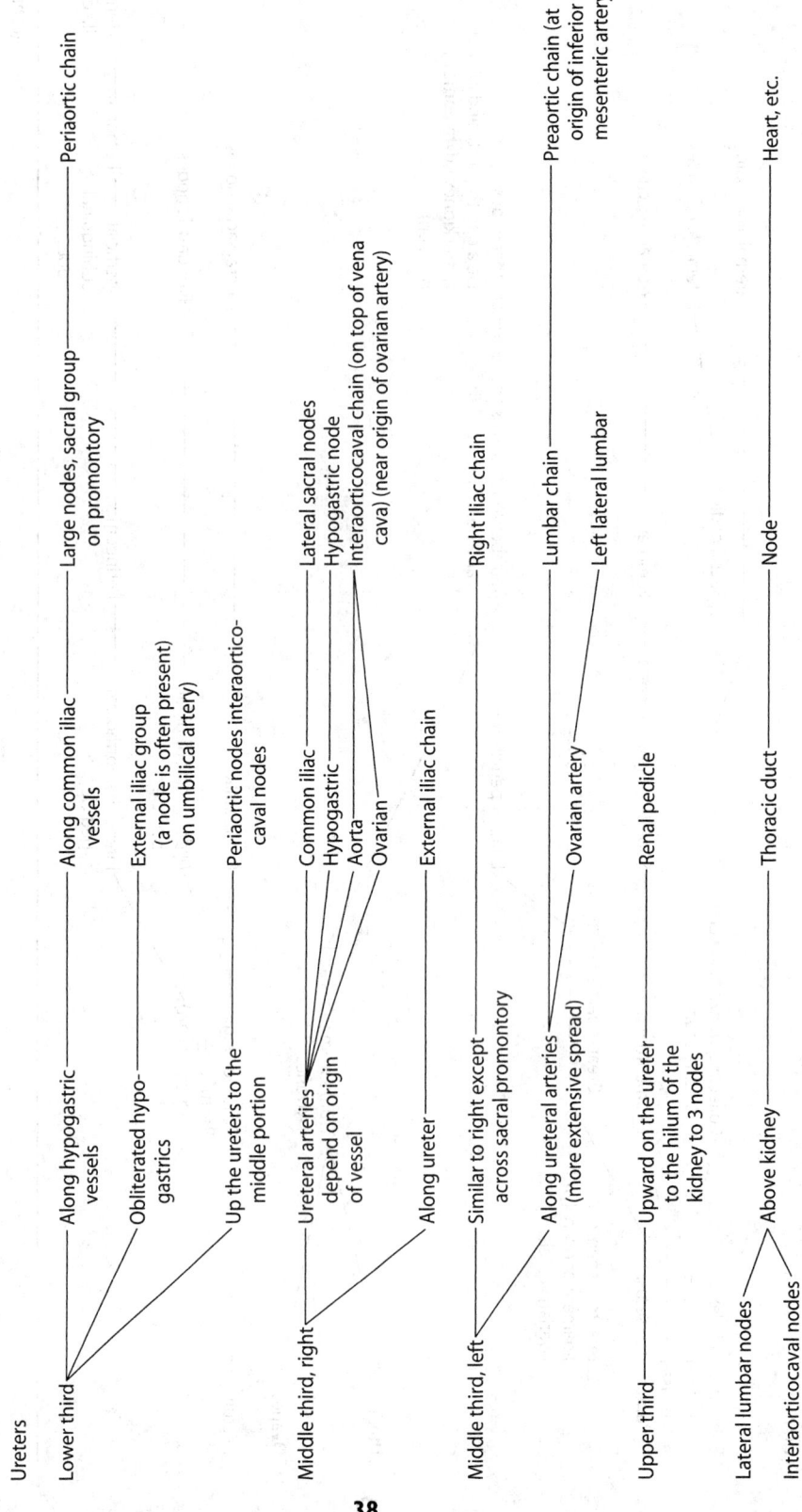

Table 2-2. Lymphatics of the female pelvis. (continued)

Ureters

Lower third ———— Along hypogastric vessels ———— Along common iliac vessels ———— Large nodes, sacral group on promontory ———— Periaortic chain

Lower third ———— Obliterated hypogastrics ———— External iliac group (a node is often present) on umbilical artery

Lower third ———— Up the ureters to the middle portion ———— Periaortic nodes interaortico-caval nodes

Middle third, right ———— Ureteral arteries depend on origin of vessel ———— Common iliac ———— Lateral sacral nodes
Hypogastric ———— Hypogastric node
Aorta ———— Interaorticocaval chain (on top of vena cava) (near origin of ovarian artery)
Ovarian

Middle third, right ———— Along ureter ———— External iliac chain

Middle third, left ———— Similar to right except across sacral promontory ———— Right iliac chain

Middle third, left ———— Along ureteral arteries (more extensive spread) ———— Ovarian artery ———— Lumbar chain ———— Preaortic chain (at origin of inferior mesenteric artery)
Left lateral lumbar

Upper third ———— Upward on the ureter to the hilum of the kidney to 3 nodes ———— Renal pedicle

Lateral lumbar nodes ———— Above kidney ———— Thoracic duct ———— Node ———— Heart, etc.
Interaorticocaval nodes

Urethra

Anterior urethra —— Vestibular plexus —— Superficial inguinal nodes —— Superficial subinguinal nodes —— Femoral —— External iliac chain

Posterior urethra

1. Anterior superior part —— Trunks —— Interior bladder wall —— Lateral inferior border of umbilical artery —— Middle chain, external iliacs

2. Anterolateral —— Trunks —— Lateral bladder wall ——┬—— Internal chain, external iliac group at the obturator nerve (obturator node)
                                                       └—— Hypogastrics at bifurcation of external and internal iliacs

    Posteriorly along internal pudendal artery

Ischiorectal fossa —— Canalis pudendalis (Alcock's canal) —— 3 nodes —— Greater sciatic foramen —— Along inferior gluteal artery —— Onto obturator artery —— Lateral sacral nodes, hypogastric nodes

3. Posterior aspect

Urethrovaginal septum —— Cervix —— Uterine plexus —— Over ureter —— Lower uterine pedicle —— Middle chain, external iliac nodes, hypogastric nodes

Bladder

Right and left sides remain separate

1. Anterior bladder wall —— (Laterally along umbilical ligaments) —— Along umbilical ligaments —— One trunk near ureter —— Nodes of posterior abdominal group

2. Posterior bladder wall ——————————————————————— (Frequent anastomoses between cervix, vagina, and fundus; large vessels upper third, medium middle third, small lower third)

is partly abdominal and partly pelvic and lies entirely behind the peritoneum. Its diameter varies from 4–6 mm, depending on distention, and its size is uniform except for 3 slightly constricted portions. The first of these constrictions is found at the junction of the ureter with the renal pelvis and is known as the upper isthmus. The second constriction—the lower isthmus—is at the point where the ureter crosses the brim of the pelvis minor. The third (intramural) constriction is at the terminal part of the ureter as it passes through the bladder wall. The pelvic portion of the ureter begins as the ureter crosses the pelvic brim beneath the ovarian vessels and near the bifurcation of the common iliac artery. It conforms to the curvature of the lateral pelvic wall, inclining slightly laterally and posteriorly until it reaches the pelvic floor. The ureter then bends anteriorly and medially at about the level of the ischial spine to reach the bladder. In its upper portion, it is related posteriorly to the sacroiliac articulation; then, lying upon the obturator internus muscle and fascia, it crosses the root of the umbilical artery, the obturator vessels, and the obturator nerve. In its anterior relationship, the ureter emerges from behind the ovary and under its vessels to pass behind the uterine and superior and middle vesical arteries. Coursing anteriorly, it comes into close relation with the lateral fornix of the vagina, passing 8–12 mm from the cervix and vaginal wall before reaching the bladder. When the ureters reach the bladder, they are about 5 cm apart. They pass through the bladder wall on an oblique course (about 2 cm long) and in an anteromedial and downward direction. The ureters open into the bladder by 2 slitlike apertures, the urethral orifices, about 2.5 cm apart when the bladder is empty.

Wall of Ureter

The wall of the ureter is approximately 3 mm thick and is composed of 3 coats: connective tissue, muscle, and mucous membrane. The muscular coat has an external circular and an internal longitudinal layer throughout its course and an external longitudinal layer in its lower third. The mucous membrane is longitudinally plicated and covered by transitional epithelium. The intermittent peristaltic action of the ureteral musculature propels urine into the bladder in jets. The oblique passage of the ureter through the bladder wall tends to constitute a valvular arrangement, but no true valve is present. The circular fibers of the intramural portion of the ureter possess a sphincterlike action. Still, under some conditions of overdistention of the bladder, urine may be forced back into the ureter.

Arteries, Veins, & Lymphatics

The pelvic portion of the ureter receives its blood supply from a direct branch of the hypogastric artery, anastomosing superiorly in its adventitia with branches from the iliolumbar and inferiorly with branches from the inferior vesical and middle hemorrhoidal arteries. Lymphatic drainage passes along the hypogastric vessels to the hypogastric and external iliac nodes, continuing up the ureters to their middle portion where drainage is directed to the periaortic and interaorticocaval nodes (Table 2–2).

Nerves

The nerve supply is provided by the renal, ovarian, and hypogastric plexuses. The spinal level of the afferents is approximately the same as the kidney (T12, L1, L2). The lower third of the ureter receives sensory fibers and postganglionic parasympathetic fibers from the Frankenhäuser plexus and sympathetic fibers through this plexus as it supplies the base of the bladder. These fibers ascend the lower third of the ureter, accompanying the arterial supply. The middle segment appears to receive postganglions of sympathetic and parasympathetic fibers through and from the middle hypogastric plexus. The upper third is supplied by the same innervation as the kidney.

3. Urethra

Relationships

The female urethra is a canal 2.5–5.25 cm long. It extends downward and forward in a curve from the neck of the bladder (internal urethral orifice), which lies nearly opposite the symphysis pubica. Its termination, the external urethral orifice, is situated inferiorly and posteriorly from the lower border of the symphysis. Posteriorly, it is closely applied to the anterior wall of the vagina, especially in the lower two-thirds, where it actually is integrated with the wall, forming the urethral carina. Anteriorly, the upper end is separated from the prevesical "space" by the pubovesical (puboprostatic) ligaments, abutting against the levator ani and vagina and extending upward onto the pubic rami.

Anatomy of Walls

The walls of the urethra are very distensible, composed of spongy fibromuscular tissue containing cavernous veins and lined by submucous and mucous coats. The mucosa contains numerous longitudinal lines when undistended, the most prominent of which is located on the posterior wall and termed the crista urethralis. Also, there are numerous small glands (the homologue of the male prostate, paraurethral and periurethral glands of Astruc, ducts of Skene) that open into the urethra. The largest of these, the paraurethral glands of Skene, may open via a pair of ducts beside the external urethral orifice in the vestibule. The epithelium begins as transitional at the upper end and becomes squamous in the lower part. External to the urethral lumen is a smooth muscle coat composed of an outer circular layer and an inner longitudinal layer in the lower two-thirds. In the upper third, the muscle bundles of the layers interdigitate in a basket-like weave to become continuous with and contiguous to those of the bladder. The entire urethral circular smooth muscle acts as the involuntary sphincter. In the region of the juncture of the middle and lower thirds of the urethra, decussating fibers (striated in type) form the middle heads of the bulbocavernosus and ischiocavernosus muscles and encircle the urethra to form the sphincter urethrae (voluntary sphincter).

Arteries & Veins

The arterial supply is intimately involved with that of the anterior vaginal wall, with cruciate anastomoses to the bladder. On each side of the vagina are the vaginal arteries, originating in part from the coronary artery of the cervix, the inferior vesical artery, or a direct branch of the uterine artery. In the midline of the anterior vaginal wall is the azygos artery, originating from the coronary or circular artery of the cervix. Approximately 5 branches traverse the anterior vaginal wall from the lateral vaginal arteries to the azygos in the midline, with small sprigs supplying the urethra. A rich anastomosis with the introitus involves the clitoral artery (urethral branches) as the artery divides into the dorsal and superficial arteries of the clitoris, a terminal branch of the internal pudendal artery. The venous drainage follows the arterial pattern, although it is less well defined. In the upper portion of the vagina, it forms an extensive network called the plexus of Santorini (Table 2–3).

Lymphatics

The lymphatics are richly developed (Fig 2–23). Those of the anterior urethra drain to the vestibular plexus, the superficial inguinal nodes, the superficial subinguinal nodes, and the femoral and external iliac chain. The lymphatic drainage of the posterior urethra can be divided into 3 aspects: the anterior superior, anterolateral, and posterior. The anterior superior portion drains to the anterior bladder wall and up the lateral inferior border of the umbilical artery to the middle chain of the external iliacs. The anterolateral portion drains in several directions. Part extends to the lateral bladder wall and onto the internal chain of the external iliacs at the obturator nerve or to the hypogastrics at the bifurcation of the external and internal iliacs. Another part drains into the ischiorectal fossa and through the canalis pudendalis (Alcock's canal), following the inferior gluteal artery and obturator artery to the lateral sacral and hypogastric nodes. The posterior aspect of the drainage is into the urethrovaginal septum, onto the cervix and the uterine plexus, over the ureter, and along the umbilical ligaments to the middle chain of the external iliacs or to the lower uterine pedicle and the hypogastrics.

Nerves

The nerve supply is parasympathetic, sympathetic, and spinal. The parasympathetic and sympathetic nerves are derived from the hypogastric plexus; the spinal supply is via the pudendal nerve.

4. Uterus

Anatomy

The uterus is a pear-shaped, thick-walled, muscular organ, situated between the base of the bladder and the rectum. Covered on each side by the 2 layers of the broad ligament, it communicates above with the uterine tubes and below with the vagina. It is divided into 2 main portions, the larger portion or body above and the smaller cervix below, connected by a transverse constriction, the isthmus. The body is flattened so that the side-to-side dimension is greater than the anteroposterior dimension and larger in women who have borne children. The anterior or vesical surface is almost flat; the posterior surface is convex. The uterine tubes join the uterus at the superior (lateral) angles. The round portion that extends above the plane passing through the points of attachment of the 2 tubes is termed the fundus. This portion is the region of greatest breadth. The cavity of the body, when viewed from the front or back, is roughly triangular with the base up. The communication of the cavity below with the cavity of the cervix corresponds in position to the isthmus and forms the internal orifice (internal os uteri). The cervix is somewhat barrel-shaped, its lower end joining the vagina at an angle varying from 45–90 degrees. It projects into the vagina and is divided into a supravaginal and a vaginal portion by the line of attachment. About one-fourth of the anterior surface and half of the posterior surface of the cervix belong to the vaginal portion. At the extremity of the vaginal portion is the opening leading to the vagina, the external orifice (external os uteri), which is round or oval before parturition but takes the form of a transverse slit in women who have borne children. It is bounded by anterior and posterior labia. The cavity of the cervix is fusiform in shape, with longitudinal folds or furrows, and extends from the internal to the external orifice.

The size of the uterus varies, under normal conditions, at different ages and in different physiologic states. In the adult woman who has never borne children, it is approximately 7–8 cm long and 4–5 cm at its widest point. In the prepubertal period, it is consider-

Table 2–3. Arterial supply to the female pelvis.

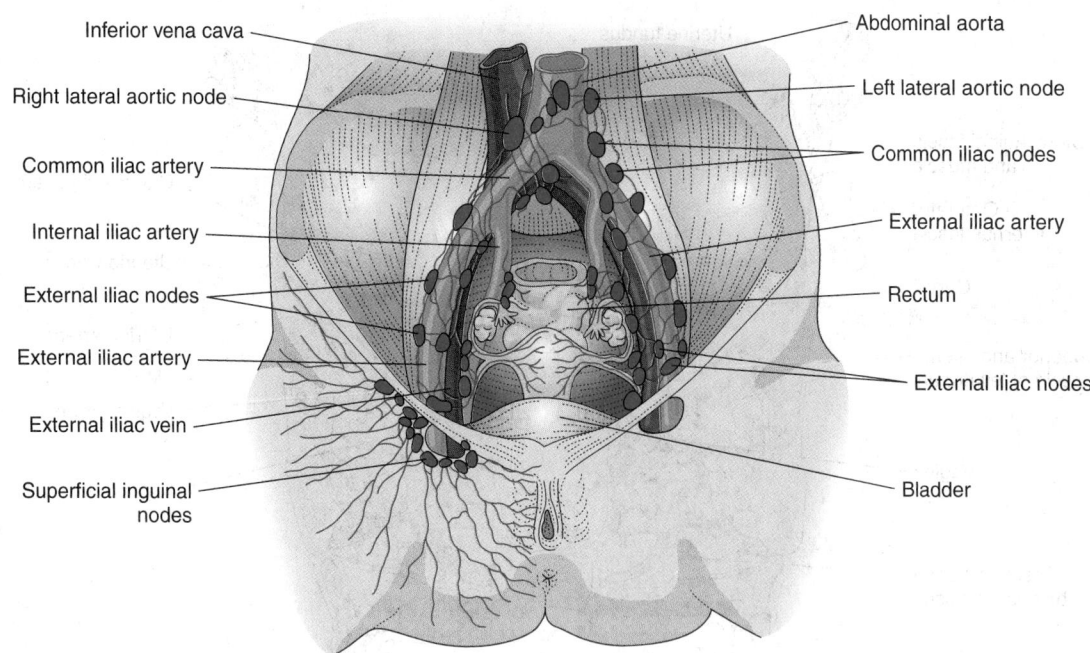

Figure 2–23. Lymphatic drainage of pelvis.

ably smaller. In women who have borne children, it is larger. Its shape, size, and characteristics in the pregnant state become considerably modified depending on the stage of gestation.

Position & Axis Direction

The direction of the axis of the uterus varies greatly. Normally, the uterus forms a sharp angle with the vagina so that its anterior surface lies on the upper surface of the bladder and the body is in a horizontal plane when the woman is standing erect. There is a bend in the area of the isthmus, at which the cervix then faces downward. This position is the normal anteversion or angulation of the uterus, although it may be placed backward (retroversion), without angulation (military position), or to one side (lateral version). The forward flexion at the isthmus is referred to as anteflexion, or there may be a corresponding retroflexion or lateral flexion. There is no sharp line between the normal and pathologic state of anterior angulation.

Relationships

Anteriorly, the body of the uterus rests upon the upper and posterior surfaces of the bladder, separated by the uterovesical pouch of the peritoneum. The whole of the anterior wall of the cervix is below the floor of this pouch, and it is separated from the base of the bladder

only by connective tissue. Posteriorly, the peritoneal covering extends down as far as the uppermost portion of the vagina; therefore, the entire posterior surface of the uterus is covered by peritoneum, and the convex posterior wall is separated from the rectum by the rectouterine pouch (cul-de-sac or pouch of Douglas). Coils of intestine may rest upon the posterior surface of the body of the uterus and may be present in the rectouterine pouch. Laterally, the uterus is related to the various structures contained within the broad ligament: the uterine tubes, the round ligament and the ligament of the ovary, the uterine artery and veins, and the ureter. The relationships of the ureters and the uterine arteries are very important surgically. The ureters, as they pass to the bladder, run parallel with the cervix for a distance of 8–12 mm. The uterine artery crosses the ureter anterosuperiorly near the cervix, about 1.5 cm from the lateral fornix of the vagina. In effect, the ureter passes under the uterine artery "as water flows under a bridge."

Ligaments

Although the cervix of the uterus is fixed, the body is free to rise and fall with the filling and emptying of the bladder. The so-called ligaments supporting the uterus consist of the uterosacral ligaments, the transverse ligaments of the cervix (cardinal ligaments, cardinal supports, ligamentum transversum colli, ligaments of

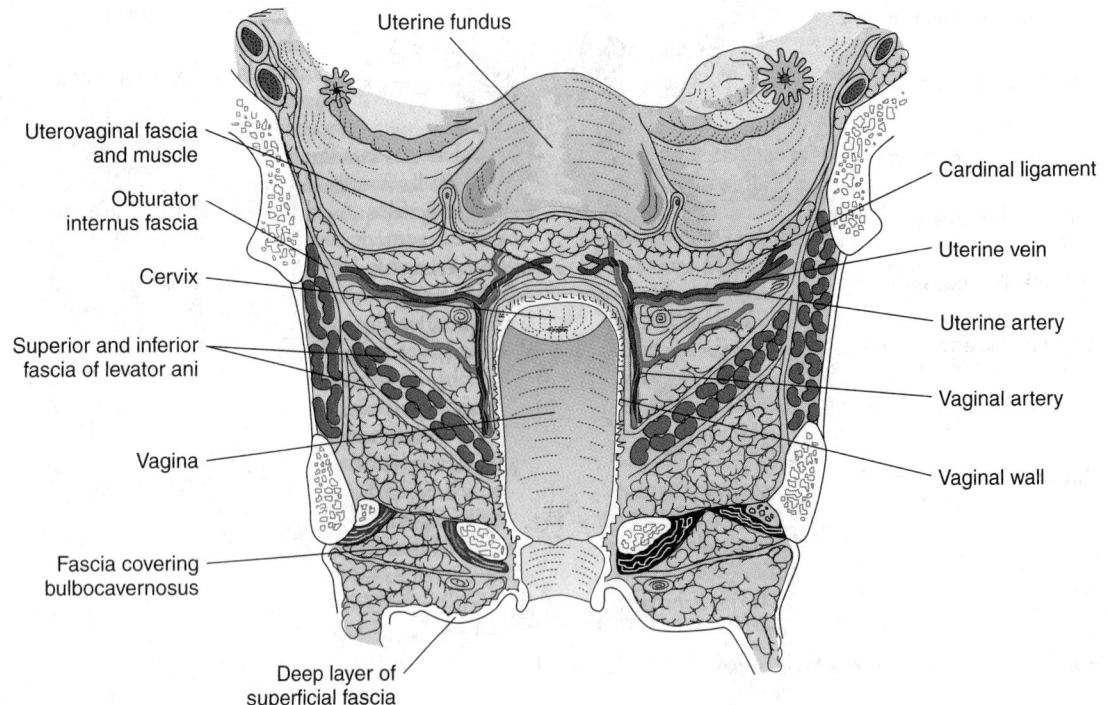

Uterine fundus

Uterovaginal fascia and muscle

Obturator internus fascia

Cervix

Superior and inferior fascia of levator ani

Vagina

Fascia covering bulbocavernosus

Deep layer of superficial fascia

Cardinal ligament

Uterine vein

Uterine artery

Vaginal artery

Vaginal wall

Figure 2–24. Ligamentous and fascial support of pelvic viscera. (Redrawn from original drawings by Frank H. Netter, MD, that first appeared in *Ciba Clinical Symposia,* Copyright ©1950. Ciba Pharmaceutical Co. Reproduced with permission.)

Mackenrodt), the round ligaments, and the broad ligaments (Fig 2–24). The cervix is embedded in tissue called the parametrium, containing various amounts of smooth muscle. There are 2 pairs of structures continuous with the parametrium and with the wall of the cervix: the uterosacral ligaments and the transverse (cardinal) ligament of the neck, the latter of which is the chief means of support and suspends the uterus from the lateral walls of the pelvis minor. The uterosacral ligaments are, in fact, the inferior posterior folds of peritoneum from the broad ligament. They consist primarily of nerve bundles from the inferior hypogastric plexus and contain preganglionic and postganglionic fibers and C fibers of the sympathetic lumbar segments, parasympathetic in part from sacral components and in part from sensory or C fibers of the spinal segments.

The cardinal ligaments are composed of longitudinal smooth muscle fibers originating superiorly from the uterus and inferiorly from the vagina, fanning out toward the fascia visceralis to form, with the internal os of the cervix, the primary support of the uterus. There is a natural defect in the muscle at its sides (hilum of the uterus) and at the cervical isthmus (internal os), where the vasculature and nerve supply enter the uterus. The round ligaments of the uterus, although forming no real support, may assist in maintaining the

body of the uterus in its typical position over the bladder. They consist of fibrous cords containing smooth muscle (longitudinal) from the outer layer of the corpus. From a point of attachment to the uterus immediately below that of the ovarian ligament, each round ligament extends downward, laterally, and forward between the 2 layers of the mesometrium, toward the abdominal inguinal ring that it traverses and the inguinal canal, to terminate in a fanlike manner in the labia majora and become continuous with connective tissue. The round ligament is the gubernaculum (ligamentum teres uteri), vestigial in the female. It is accompanied by a funicular branch of the ovarian artery, by a branch from the ovarian venous plexus, and, in the lower part of its course, by a branch from the inferior epigastric artery, over which it passes as it enters the inguinal ring. Through the inguinal canal, it is accompanied by the ilioinguinal nerve and the external spermatic branch of the genitofemoral nerve.

The broad ligament, consisting of a transverse fold of peritoneum that arises from the floor of the pelvis between the rectum and the bladder, provides minimal support. In addition to the static support of these ligaments, the pelvic diaphragm (levator ani) provides an indirect and dynamic support. These muscles do not actually come in contact with the uterus, but they aid in supporting the vagina and maintain the entire pelvic floor in resisting downward pressure. The effectiveness of these muscles depends on an intact perineum (perineal body, bulbocavernosus muscle and body), for if it is lacerated or weakened the ligaments will gradually stretch and the uterus will descend. The uterus and its components and the vagina are, in fact, one continuous unit.

Layers of Uterine Wall

The wall of the uterus is very thick and consists of 3 layers: serous, muscular, and mucous. The serous layer (perimetrium) is simply the peritoneal covering. It is thin and firmly adherent over the fundus and most of the body, then thickens posteriorly and becomes separated from the muscle by the parametrium. The muscular layer (myometrium) is extremely thick and continuous with that of the tubes and vagina. It also extends into the ovarian and round ligaments, into the cardinal ligaments at the cervix, and minimally into the uterosacral ligaments. Two principal layers of the muscular coat can be distinguished: (1) the outer layer, which is weaker and composed of longitudinal fibers; and (2) a stronger inner layer, the fibers of which are interlaced and run in various directions, having intermingled within them large venous plexuses. The muscle layer hypertrophies with the internal os to form a sphincter. The cervix, from the internal os distally, progressively loses its smooth muscle, finally to be entirely devoid of smooth muscle and elastic in its distal half. It is, in fact, the "dead-end tendon" of the uterus, at which point, during the active component of labor, both the uterus and the vagina direct their efforts. The mucous layer (endometrium) is soft and spongy, composed of tissue resembling embryonic connective tissue. The surface consists of a single layer of ciliated columnar epithelium. The tissue is rather delicate and friable and contains many tubular glands that open into the cavity of the uterus.

Arteries

The blood supply to the uterus is from the uterine and ovarian arteries. As a terminal branch of the hypogastric artery, the uterine artery runs downward and medially to cross the ureter near the cervix. It then ascends along the lateral border of the uterus in a tortuous course through the parametrium, giving off lateral branches to both uterine surfaces. Above, it anastomoses to join with the ovarian artery in the mesometrium, which creates the main accessory source of blood. The uterine arteries within the uterus form a series of arches over the fundus, creating cruciate anastomoses with the opposite side. Branches of the arcuate arteries (radial) penetrate the myometrium at right angles to terminate in the

basilar arterioles for the basilar portion of the endometrium and in the spinal arteries of the endometrium. The spinal arteries are tortuous in structure, not because of endometrial growth but because, ontogenically, an organ carries its arterial supply with it as it changes size and position. Therefore, the spiral arteries are able to maintain adequate arterial flow to the placenta while it is attached within the uterus. On the other hand, the veins of the endometrium are a series of small sinusoids that connect to the larger sinusoids of the myometrium, the latter coalescing into the larger veins of the uterine complex. It is useful here to note the significance of the muscular role of the uterus in helping to control venous bleeding during parturition.

The arterial supply to the cervix is primarily through the cervical branches of the right and left uterine arteries, which form a rete around the cervix (coronary artery), creating the azygos artery in the midline anteriorly and posteriorly. Anastomoses between this artery and the vaginal artery on both sides afford cruciate flow on the anterior wall, whereas on the posterior wall of the vagina, anastomoses occur with the right and left middle hemorrhoidal arteries as they supply the wall and the rectum.

Veins

The veins form a plexus and drain through the uterine vein to the hypogastric vein. There are connections with the ovarian veins and the inferior epigastric by way of the vein accompanying the round ligament.

Lymphatics

Lymphatic drainage involves several chains of lymph nodes (Table 2–2). From the subperitoneal plexus, the collecting trunks of the lower uterine segment may drain by way of the cervix to the external iliac chain or by way of the isthmus to the lateral sacral nodes. Drainage along the round ligament progresses to the superficial inguinal nodes, then to the femoral, and finally to the external iliac chain. Drainage laterally to the suspensory ligament of the ovary involves the lumbar pedicle and progresses in a retroperitoneal manner across and anteriorly to the ureter, to the lumbar nodes (interaorticocaval) that lie along the aorta, and inferiorly to the kidney.

Nerves

The pelvic autonomic system can be divided into the superior hypogastric plexus (the presacral plexus and the uterinus magnus), the middle hypogastric plexus, and the inferior hypogastric plexus. The superior hypogastric plexus begins just below the inferior mesenteric artery. It is composed of 1–3 intercommunicating nerve bundles connected with the inferior mesenteric ganglia, but no ganglia are an integral part of the plexus. The intermesenteric nerves receive branches from the lumbar sympathetic ganglia.

A. Superior Hypogastric Plexus

The superior hypogastric plexus continues into the midhypogastric plexus. The presacral nerves spread out into a latticework at the level of the first sacral vertebra, with connecting rami to the last of the lumbar ganglia. The greater part of the superior midhypogastric plexus may be found to the left of the midline.

B. Inferior Hypogastric Plexus

At the first sacral vertebra, this plexus divides into several branches that go to the right and left sides of the pelvis. These branches form the beginning of the right and left inferior hypogastric plexus. The inferior hypogastric plexus, which is the divided continuation of the midhypogastric plexus, the superior hypogastric plexus, the presacral nerve, and the uterinus magnus, is composed of several parallel nerves on each side. This group of nerves descends within the pelvis in a position posterior to the common iliac artery and anterior to the sacral plexus, curves laterally, and finally enters the sacrouterine fold or ligaments. The medial section of the primary division of the sacral nerves sends fibers (nervi erigentes) that enter the pelvic plexus in the sacrouterine folds. The plexus now appears to contain both sympathetic (inferior hypogastric plexus) and parasympathetic (nervi erigentes) components.

C. Nervi Erigentes

The sensory components, which are mostly visceral, are found in the nervi erigentes; however, if one takes into account the amount of spinal anesthetic necessary to eliminate uterine sensation, one must assume that there are a number of sensory fibers in the sympathetic component.

D. Common Iliac Nerves

The common iliac nerves originate separately from the superior hypogastric plexus and descend on the surface of the artery and vein, one part going through the femoral ring and the remainder following the internal iliac, finally rejoining the pelvic plexus.

E. Hypogastric Ganglion

On either side of the uterus, in the base of the broad ligament, is the large plexus described by Lee and Frankenhäuser, the so-called hypogastric ganglion. The plexus actually consists of ganglia and nerve ramifications of various sizes, as well as branches of the combined inferior hypogastric plexus and the nervi erigentes. It lies parallel to the lateral pelvic wall, its lateral surface superficial to the internal iliac and its branches;

the ureter occupies a position superficial to the plexus. The middle vesical artery perforates and supplies the plexus, its medial branches supplying the rectal stalk. The greater part of the plexus terminates in large branches that enter the uterus in the region of the internal os, while another smaller component of the plexus supplies the vagina and the bladder. The branches of the plexus that supply the uterus enter the isthmus primarily through the sacrouterine fold or ligament. In the isthmus, just outside the entrance to the uterus, ascending rami pass out into the broad ligament to enter the body of the uterus at higher levels—besides supplying the uterine tubes. A part of the inferior hypogastric plexus may pass directly to the uterus without involvement in the pelvic plexus.

Ganglia are in close proximity to the uterine arteries and the ureters, in the adventitia of the bladder and vagina, and in the vesicovaginal septum. The nerve bundles entering the ganglia contain both myelinated and unmyelinated elements. Corpuscula lamellosa (Vater-Pacini corpuscles) may be found within the tissues and are often observed within nerve bundles, especially within those in the lower divisions of the plexus. Both myelinated and unmyelinated nerves are present within the uterus. The nerves enter along the blood vessels, the richest supply lying in the isthmic portion of the uterus. The fibers following the blood vessels gradually diminish in number in the direction of the fundus, where the sparsest distribution occurs. The fibers run parallel to the muscle bundles, and the nerves frequently branch to form a syncytium before terminating on the sarcoplasm as small free nerve endings.

Sensory Corpuscles

Vater-Pacini corpuscles (corpuscula lamellosa) are present outside the uterus. Dogiel and Krause corpuscles (corpuscula bulboidea) appear in the region of the endocervix. They may also be found in the broad ligament along with Vater-Pacini corpuscles and at the juncture of the uterine arteries with the uterus. These corpuscles may act to modulate the stretch response that reflexively stimulates uterine contractions during labor.

The innervation of the cervix shows occasional free endings entering papillae of the stratified squamous epithelium of the pars vaginalis. The endocervix contains a rich plexus of free endings that is most pronounced in the region of the internal os. The endocervix and the isthmic portion of the uterus in the nonpregnant state both contain the highest number of nerves and blood vessels of any part of the uterus. The presence here of a lamellar type of corpuscle has already been noted.

Nerves pass through the myometrium and enter the endometrium. A plexus with penetrating fibers involving the submucosal region is present in the basal third of the endometrium, with branches terminating in the stroma, in the basilar arterioles, and at the origin of the spiral arterioles. The outer two-thirds of the endometrium is devoid of nerves.

5. Uterine (Fallopian) Tubes (Oviducts)

Anatomy

The uterine tubes serve to convey the ova to the uterus. They extend from the superior angles of the uterus to the region of the ovaries, running in the superior border of the broad ligament (mesosalpinx). The course of each tube is nearly horizontal at first and slightly backward. Upon reaching the lower (uterine) pole of the ovary, the tube turns upward, parallel with the anterior (mesovarian) border, then arches backward over the upper pole and descends posteriorly to terminate in contact with the medial surface. Each tube is 7–14 cm long and may be divided into 3 parts: isthmus, ampulla, and infundibulum. The isthmus is the narrow and nearly straight portion immediately adjoining the uterus. It has a rather long intramural course, and its opening into the uterus, the uterine ostium, is approximately 1 mm in diameter. Following the isthmus is the wider, more tortuous ampulla. It terminates in a funnel-like dilatation, the infundibulum. The margins of the infundibulum are fringed by numerous diverging processes, the fimbriae, the longest of which, the fimbria ovarica, is attached to the ovary. The funnel-shaped mouth of the infundibulum, the abdominal ostium, is about 3 mm in diameter and actually leads into the peritoneal cavity, although it probably is closely applied to the surface of the ovary during ovulation.

Layers of Wall

The wall of the tube has 4 coats: serous (peritoneal), subserous or adventitial (fibrous and vascular), muscular, and mucous. Each tube is enclosed within a peritoneal covering except along a small strip on its lower surface, where the mesosalpinx is attached. At the margins of the infundibulum and the fimbriae, this peritoneal covering becomes directly continuous with the mucous membrane lining the interior of the tube. The subserous tissue is lax in the immediate vicinity of the tube. The blood and nerve supply is found within this layer. The muscular coat has an outer longitudinal and an inner circular layer of smooth muscle fibers, more prominent and continuous with that of the uterus at the uterine end of the tube. The mucous coat is ciliated columnar epithelium with coarse longitudinal folds, simple in the region of the isthmus but becoming higher and more complex in the ampulla. The epithelial lining extends outward into the fimbriae. The ciliary motion is directed toward the uterus.

Ligament

The infundibulum is suspended from the pelvic brim by the infundibulopelvic ligament (suspensory ligament of the ovary). This portion of the tube may adjoin the tip of the appendix and fuse with it.

Arteries & Veins

The blood supply to the tubes is derived from the ovarian and uterine arteries. The tubal branch of the uterine artery courses along the lower surface of the uterine tube as far as the fimbriated extremity and may also send a branch to the ligamentum teres. The ovarian branch of the uterine artery runs along the attached border of the ovary and gives off a tubal branch. Both branches form cruciate anastomoses in the mesosalpinx. The veins accompany the arteries.

Lymphatics

The lymphatic drainage occurs through trunks running retroperitoneally across and anterior to the ureter, into the lumbar nodes along the aorta, and inferior to the kidney.

Nerves

The nerve supply is derived from the pelvic plexuses (parasympathetic and sympathetic) and from the ovarian plexus. The nerves of the ampulla are given off from the branches passing to the ovary, whereas those of the isthmus come from the uterine branches. The nerve fibers enter the muscularis of the tube through the mesosalpinx to form a reticular network of free endings among the smooth muscle cells.

6. Ovaries

Anatomy

The ovaries are paired organs situated close to the wall on either side of the pelvis minor, a little below the brim. Each measures 2.5–5 cm in length, 1.5–3 cm in breadth, and 0.7–1.5 cm in width, weighing about 4–8 g. The ovary has 2 surfaces, medial and lateral; 2 borders, anterior or mesovarian and posterior or free; and 2 poles, upper or tubal and lower or uterine. When the uterus and adnexa are in the normal position, the long axis of the ovary is nearly vertical, but it bends somewhat medially and forward at the lower end so that the lower pole tends to point toward the uterus. The medial surface is rounded and, posteriorly, may have numerous scars or elevations that mark the position of developing follicles and sites of ruptured ones.

Relationships

The upper portion of this surface is overhung by the fimbriated end of the uterine tube, and the remainder lies in relation to coils of intestine. The lateral surface is similar in shape and faces the pelvic wall, where it forms a distinct depression, the fossa ovarica. This fossa is lined by peritoneum and is bounded above by the external iliac vessels and below by the obturator vessels and nerve; its posterior boundary is formed by the ureter and uterine artery and vein, and the pelvic attachment of the broad ligament is located anteriorly. The mesovarian or anterior border is fairly straight and provides attachment for the mesovarium, a peritoneal fold by which the ovary is attached to the posterosuperior layer of the broad ligament. Because the vessels, nerves, and lymphatics enter the ovary through this border, it is referred to as the hilum of the ovary. Anterior to the hilum are embryonic remnants of the male and female germ cell ducts. The posterior or free border is more convex and broader and is directed freely into the rectouterine pouch. The upper or tubal pole is large and rounded. It is overhung closely by the infundibulum of the uterine tube and is connected with the pelvic brim by the suspensory ligament of the ovary, a peritoneal fold. The lower or uterine pole is smaller and directed toward the uterus. It serves as the attachment of the ligament of the ovary proper.

Mesovarium

The ovary is suspended by means of the mesovarium, the suspensory ligament of the ovary, and the ovarian ligament. The mesovarium consists of 2 layers of peritoneum, continuous with both the epithelial coat of the ovary and the posterosuperior layer of the broad ligament. It is short and wide and contains branches of the ovarian and uterine arteries, with plexuses of nerves, the pampiniform plexus of veins, and the lateral end of the ovarian ligament. The suspensory ligament of the ovary is a triangular fold of peritoneum and is actually the upper lateral corner of the broad ligament, which becomes confluent with the parietal peritoneum at the pelvic brim. It attaches to the mesovarium as well as to the peritoneal coat of the infundibulum medially, thus suspending both the ovary and the tube. It contains the ovarian artery, veins, and nerves after they pass over the pelvic brim and before they enter the mesovarium. The ovarian ligament is a band of connective tissue, with numerous small muscle fibers, that lies between the 2 layers of the broad ligament on the boundary line between the mesosalpinx and the mesometrium, connecting the lower (uterine) pole of the ovary with the lateral wall of the uterus. It is attached just below the uterine tube and above the attachment of the round ligament of the uterus and is continuous with the latter.

Structure of Ovary

The ovary is covered by cuboid or low columnar epithelium and consists of a cortex and a medulla. The medulla is made up of connective tissue fibers, smooth muscle cells, and numerous blood vessels, nerves, lymphatic vessels, and supporting tissue. The cortex is composed of a fine areolar stroma, with many vessels and scattered follicles of epithelial cells within which are the definitive ova (oocytes) in various stages of maturity. The more mature follicles enlarge and project onto the free surface of the ovary, where they are visible to the naked eye. They are called graafian follicles. When fully mature, the follicle bursts, releasing the ovum and becoming transformed into a corpus luteum. The corpus luteum, in turn, is later replaced by scar tissue, forming a corpus albicans.

Arteries

The ovarian artery is the chief source of blood for the ovary. Though both arteries may originate as branches of the abdominal aorta, the left frequently originates from the left renal artery; the right, less frequently. The vessels diverge from each other as they descend. Upon reaching the level of the common iliac artery, they turn medially over that vessel and ureter to descend tortuously into the pelvis on each side between the folds of the suspensory ligament of the ovary into the mesovarium. An additional blood supply is formed from anastomosis with the ovarian branch of the uterine artery, which courses along the attached border of the ovary. Blood vessels that enter the hilum send out capillary branches centrifugally.

The veins follow the course of the arteries and, as they emerge from the hilum, form a well-developed plexus (the pampiniform plexus) between the layers of the mesovarium. Smooth muscle fibers occur in the meshes of the plexus, giving the whole structure the appearance of erectile tissue.

Lymphatics

Lymphatic channels drain retroperitoneally, together with those of the tubes and part of those from the uterus, to the lumbar nodes along the aorta inferior to the kidney. The distribution of lymph channels in the ovary is so extensive that it suggests the system may also provide additional fluid to the ovary during periods of preovulatory follicular swelling.

Nerves

The nerve supply of the ovaries arises from the lumbosacral sympathetic chain and passes to the gonad along with the ovarian artery.

7. Vagina

The vagina is a strong canal of muscle approximately 7.5 cm long that extends from the uterus to the vestibule of the external genitalia, where it opens to the exterior. Its long axis is almost parallel with that of the lower part of the sacrum, and it meets the cervix of the uterus at an angle of 45–90 degrees. Because the cervix of the uterus projects into the upper portion, the anterior wall of the vagina is 1.5–2 cm shorter than the posterior wall. The circular cul-de-sac formed around the cervix is known as the fornix and is divided into 4 regions: the anterior fornix, the posterior fornix, and 2 lateral fornices. Toward its lower end, the vagina pierces the urogenital diaphragm and is surrounded by the 2 bulbocavernosus muscles and bodies, which act as a sphincter (sphincter vaginae). In the virginal state, an incomplete fold of highly vascular tissue and mucous membrane, the hymen, partially closes the external orifice.

Relationships

Anteriorly, the vagina is in close relationship to the bladder, ureters, and urethra in succession. The posterior fornix is covered by the peritoneum of the rectovaginal pouch, which may contain coils of intestine. Below the pouch, the vagina rests almost directly on the rectum, separated from it by a thin layer of areolar connective tissue. Toward the lower end of the vagina, the rectum turns back sharply, and the distance between the vagina and rectum greatly increases. This space, filled with muscle fibers, connective tissue, and fat, is known as the perineal body. The lateral fornix lies just under the root of the broad ligament and is approximately 1 cm from the point where the uterine artery crosses the ureter. The remaining lateral vaginal wall is related to the edges of the anterior portion of the levator ani. The vagina is supported at the introitus by the bulbocavernosus muscles and bodies, in the lower third by the levator ani (puborectalis), and superiorly by the transverse (cardinal) ligaments of the uterus. The ductus epoophori longitudinalis (duct of Gartner), the remains of the lower portion of the wolffian duct (mesonephric duct), may often be found on the sides of the vagina as a minute tube or fibrous cord. These vestigial structures often become cystic and appear as translucent areas.

Wall Structure

The vaginal wall is composed of a mucosal layer and a muscular layer. The smooth muscle fibers are indistinctly arranged in 3 layers: an outer longitudinal layer, circumferential layer, and a poorly differentiated inner longitudinal layer. In the lower third, the circumferential fibers envelop the urethra. The submucous area is abundantly supplied with a dense plexus of veins and lymphatics. The mucous layer shows many transverse and oblique rugae, which project inward to such an extent that the lumen in transverse section resembles an H-shaped slit. On the anterior and posterior walls, these ridges are more prominent, and the anterior column forms the urethral carina at its lower end, where the urethra slightly invaginates the anterior wall of the vagina. The mucosa of the vagina is lined throughout by stratified squamous epithelium. Even though the vagina has no true glands, there is a secretion present. It consists of cervical mucus, desquamated epithelium, and, with sexual stimulation, a direct transudate.

Arteries & Veins

The chief blood supply to the vagina is through the vaginal branch of the uterine artery. After forming the coronary or circular artery of the cervix, it passes medially, behind the ureter, to send 5 main branches onto the anterior wall to the midline. These branches anastomose with the azygos artery (originating midline from the coronary artery of the cervix) and continue downward to supply the anterior vaginal wall and the lower two-thirds of the urethra. The uterine artery eventually anastomoses to the urethral branch of the clitoral artery. The posterior vaginal wall is supplied by branches of the middle and inferior hemorrhoidal arteries, traversing toward the midline to join the azygos artery from the coronary artery of the cervix. These branches then anastomose on the perineum to the superficial and deep transverse perineal arteries.

The veins follow the course of the arteries.

Lymphatics

The lymphatics are numerous mucosal plexuses, anastomosing with the deeper muscular plexuses (Table 2–2). The superior group of lymphatics joins those of the cervix and may follow the uterine artery to terminate in the external iliac nodes or form anastomoses with the uterine plexus. The middle group of lymphatics, which drain the greater part of the vagina, appears to follow the vaginal arteries to the hypogastric channels. In addition, there are lymph nodes in the rectovaginal septum that are primarily responsible for drainage of the rectum and part of the posterior vaginal wall. The inferior group of lymphatics forms frequent anastomoses between the right and left sides and either courses upward to anastomose with the middle group or enters the vulva and drains to the inguinal nodes.

Nerves

The innervation of the vagina contains both sympathetic and parasympathetic fibers. Only occasional free nerve endings are seen in the mucosa; no other types of nerve endings are noted.

STRUCTURES LINING THE PELVIS

The walls of the pelvis minor are made up of the following layers: (1) the peritoneum, (2) the subperitoneal or extraperitoneal fibroareolar layer, (3) the fascial layer, (4) the muscular layer, and (5) the osseoligamentous layer (not further discussed). The anatomy of the floor of the pelvis is comparable to that of the walls except for the absence of an osseoligamentous layer.

1. Peritoneum

The peritoneum presents several distinct transverse folds that form corresponding fossae on each side. The most anterior is a variable fold, the transverse vesical, extending from the bladder laterally to the pelvic wall. It is not the superficial covering of any definitive structure. Behind it lies the broad ligament, which partially covers and aids in the support of the uterus and adnexa.

Ligaments

The broad ligament extends from the lateral border on either side of the uterus to the floor and side walls of the pelvis. It is composed of 2 layers, anterior and posterior, the anterior facing downward and the posterior facing upward, conforming to the position of the uterus. The inferior or "attached" border of the broad ligament is continuous with the parietal peritoneum on the floor and on the side walls of the pelvis. Along this border, the posterior layer continues laterally and posteriorly in an arc to the region of the sacrum, forming the uterosacral fold. Another fold—the rectouterine fold—frequently passes from the posterior surface of the cervix to the rectum in the midline. The anterior layer of the broad ligament is continuous laterally along the inferior border with the peritoneum of the paravesical fossae and continuous medially with peritoneum on the upper surface of the bladder. Both layers of the attached border continue up the side walls of the pelvis to join with a triangular fold of peritoneum, reaching to the brim of the pelvis to form the suspensory ligament of the ovary or infundibular ligament. This ligament contains the ovarian vessels and nerves. The medial border of the broad ligament on either side is continuous with the peritoneal covering on both uterine surfaces. The 2 layers of the ligament separate to partially contain the uterus, and the superior or "free" border, which is laterally continuous with the suspensory ligament of the ovary, envelops the uterine tube.

The broad ligament can be divided into regions as follows: (1) a larger portion, the mesometrium, which is associated especially with the lateral border of the uterus; (2) the mesovarium, the fold that springs from the posterior layer of the ovary; and (3) the thin portion, the mesosalpinx, which is associated with the uterine tube in the region of the free border. The superior lateral corner of the broad ligament has been referred to as the suspensory ligament of the ovary, or infundibulopelvic ligament, because it suspends the infundibulum as well as the ovary.

Fossae & Spaces

Corresponding to the peritoneal folds are the peritoneal fossae. The prevesical or retropubic space is a potential space that is crossed by the transverse vesical fold. It is situated in front of the bladder and behind the pubis. When the bladder is displaced posteriorly, it becomes an actual space, anteriorly continuous from side to side and posteriorly limited by a condensation of fatty areolar tissue extending from the base of the bladder to the side wall of the pelvis. The vesicouterine pouch is a narrow cul-de-sac between the anterior surface of the body of the uterus and the upper surface of the bladder when the uterus is in normal anteflexed position. In the bottom of this pouch, the peritoneum is reflected from the bladder onto the uterus at the junction of the cervix and corpus. Therefore, the anterior surface of the cervix is below the level of the peritoneum and is connected with the base of the bladder by condensed areolar tissue. The peritoneum on the posterior surface of the body of the uterus extends downward onto the cervix and onto the posterior fornix of the vagina. It is then reflected onto the anterior surface of the rectum to form a narrow cul-de-sac continuous with the pararectal fossa of either side. The entire space, bounded anteriorly by the cervix and by the fornix in the midline, the uterosacral folds laterally, and the rectum posteriorly, is the rectouterine pouch or cul-de-sac (pouch of Douglas).

2. Subperitoneal & Fascial Layers

The subperitoneal layer consists of loose, fatty areolar tissue underlying the peritoneum. External to the subperitoneal layer, a layer of fascia lines the wall of the pelvis, covering the muscles and, where these are lacking, blending with the periosteum of the pelvic bones. This layer is known as the parietal pelvic fascia and is subdivided into the obturator fascia, the fascia of the urogenital diaphragm, and the fascia of the piriformis. The obturator fascia is of considerable thickness and covers the obturator internus muscle. Traced forward, it partially blends with the periosteum of the pubic bone and assists in the formation of the obturator canal. Traced upward, it is continuous at the arcuate line with the iliac fascia. Inferiorly, it extends nearly to the margin of the ischiopubic arch, where it is attached to the bone. In this lower region, it also becomes continuous with a double-layered triangular sheet of fascia, the fasciae of the urogenital diaphragm, passing across the anterior part of the pelvic outlet. A much thinner portion of the parietal pelvic fascia covers the piriform and coccygeus muscles in the posterior pelvic wall. Medially, the piriformis fascia blends with the periosteum of the sacrum around the margins of the anterior sacral foramens and covers the roots and first branches of the sacral plexus. Visceral pelvic fascia denotes the fascia in the bottom of the pelvic bowl, which invests the pelvic organs and forms a number of supports that suspend the organs from the pelvic walls. These supports arise in common from the obturator part of the parietal fascia, along or near the arcus tendineus. This arc or line extends from a point near the lower part of the symphysis pubica to the root of the spine of the ischium. From this common origin, the fascia spreads inward and backward, dividing into a number of parts classified as either investing (endopelvic) fascia or suspensory and diaphragmatic fascia.

3. Muscular Layer

The muscles of the greater pelvis are the psoas major and iliacus. Those of the lesser pelvis are the piriformis, obturator internus, coccygeus, and levator ani; they do not form a continuous layer.

Greater Pelvis

A. PSOAS MAJOR

The fusiform psoas major muscle originates from the 12th thoracic to the fifth lumbar vertebrae. Parallel fiber bundles descend nearly vertically along the side of the vertebral bodies and extend along the border of the minor pelvis, beneath the inguinal ligament, and on toward insertion in the thigh. The medial border inserts into the lesser trochanter, whereas the lateral border shares its tendon with the iliacus muscle. Together with the iliacus, it is the most powerful flexor of the thigh, acting as a lateral rotator of the femur when the foot is off the ground and free and as a medial rotator when the foot is on the ground and the tibia is fixed. The psoas component flexes the spine and the pelvis and abducts the lumbar region of the spine. The psoas, having longer fibers than the iliacus, gives a quicker but weaker pull.

B. ILIACUS

The fan-shaped iliacus muscle originates from the iliac crest, the iliolumbar ligament, the greater part of the iliac fossa, the anterior sacroiliac ligaments, and frequently the ala of the sacrum. It also originates from the ventral border of the ilium between the 2 anterior spines. It is inserted in a penniform manner on the lateral surface of the tendon that emerges from the psoas above the inguinal ligament and directly on the femur immediately distal to the lesser trochanter. The lateral portion of the muscle arising from the ventral border of the ilium is adherent to the direct tendon of the rectus femoris and the capsule of the hip joint.

Lesser Pelvis

A. PIRIFORMIS

The piriformis has its origin from the lateral part of the ventral surface of the second, third, and fourth sacral vertebrae, from the posterior border of the greater sciatic notch, and from the deep surface of the sacrotuberous ligament near the sacrum. The fiber bundles pass through the greater sciatic foramen to insert upon the anterior and inner portion of the upper border of the greater trochanter. The piriformis acts as an abductor, lateral rotator, and weak extensor of the thigh.

B. OBTURATOR INTERNUS

The obturator internus arises from the pelvic surface of the pubic rami near the obturator foramen, the pelvic surface of the ischium between the foramen and the greater sciatic notch, the deep surface of the obturator internus fascia, the fibrous arch that bounds the canal for the obturator vessels and nerves, and the pelvic surface of the obturator membrane. The fiber bundles converge toward the lesser sciatic notch, where they curve laterally to insert into the trochanteric fossa of the femur. The obturator internus is a powerful lateral rotator of the thigh. When the thigh is bent at a right angle, the muscle serves as an abductor and extensor.

C. COCCYGEUS

The coccygeus muscle runs from the ischial spine and the neighboring margin of the greater sciatic notch to the fourth and fifth sacral vertebrae and the coccyx. A large part of the muscle is aponeurotic. It supports the pelvic and abdominal viscera and possibly flexes and abducts the coccyx.

D. LEVATOR ANI

The levator ani muscle forms the floor of the pelvis and the roof of the perineum. It is divisible into 3 portions: (1) the iliococcygeus, (2) the pubococcygeus, and (3) the puborectalis.

1. Iliococcygeus—The iliococcygeus arises from the arcus tendineus, which extends from the ischial spine to the superior ramus of the pubis near the obturator canal and for a variable distance downward below the obturator canal. Its insertion is into the lateral aspect of the coccyx and the raphe that extends from the tip of the coccyx to the rectum. Many fiber bundles cross the median line.

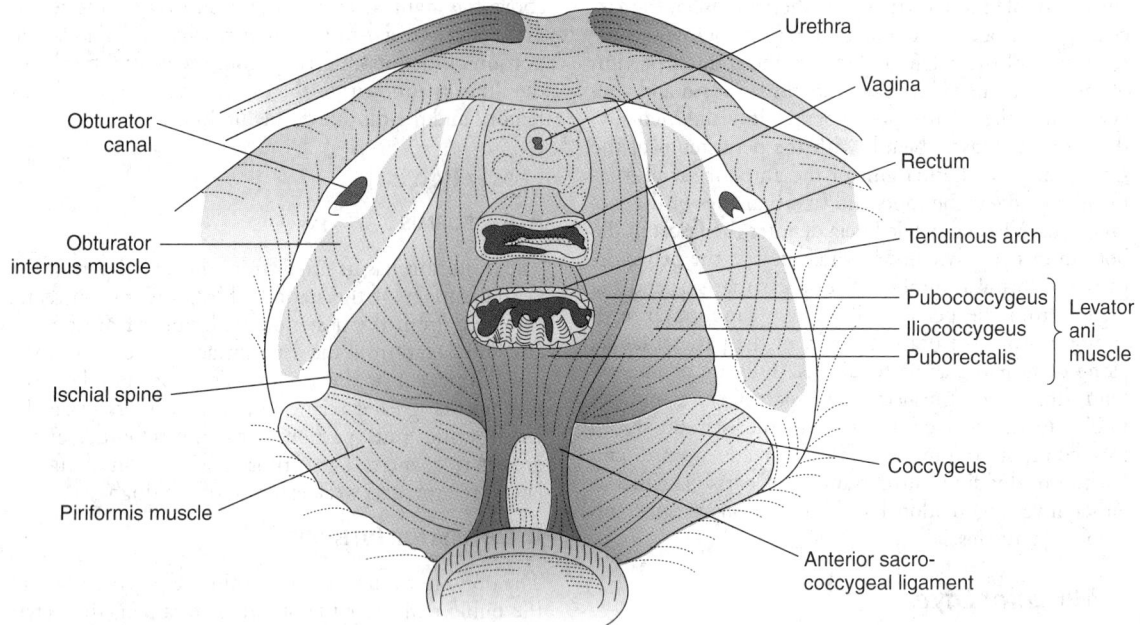

Obturator canal

Obturator internus muscle

Ischial spine

Piriformis muscle

Urethra

Vagina

Rectum

Tendinous arch

Pubococcygeus ⎫
Iliococcygeus ⎬ Levator ani muscle
Puborectalis ⎭

Coccygeus

Anterior sacro-coccygeal ligament

Figure 2–25. Pelvic diaphragm from above.

2. Pubococcygeus—The pubococcygeus arises from the inner surface of the os pubis, the lower margin of the symphysis pubica to the obturator canal, and the arcus tendineus as far backward as the origin of the iliococcygeus. It passes backward, downward, and medially past the urogenital organs and the rectum, inserting into the anterior sacrococcygeal ligament, the deep part of the anococcygeal raphe, and each side of the rectum. The pubococcygeus lies to some extent on the pelvic surface of the insertion of the iliococcygeus.

3. Puborectalis—The puborectalis arises from the body and descending ramus of the pubis beneath the origin of the pubococcygeus, the neighboring part of the obturator fascia, and the fascia covering the pelvic surface of the urogenital diaphragm. Many of the fiber bundles interdigitate with those of the opposite side, and they form a thick band on each side of the rectum behind which those of each side are inserted into the anococcygeal raphe.

The levator ani serves to slightly flex the coccyx, raise the anus, and constrict the rectum and vagina. It resists the downward pressure that the thoracoabdominal diaphragm exerts on the viscera during inspiration.

Pelvic Diaphragm

The pelvic diaphragm (Fig 2–25) extends from the upper part of the pelvic surface of the pubis and ischium to the rectum, which passes through it. The pelvic diaphragm is formed by the levator ani and coccygeus muscles and covering fasciae. The diaphragmatic fasciae cloaking the levator ani arise from the parietal pelvic fascia (obturator fascia), the muscular layer lying between the fasciae. As viewed from above, the superior fascia is the best developed and is reflected onto the rectum, forming the "rectal sheath." The coccygeus muscle forms the deeper portion of the posterolateral wall of the ischiorectal fossa, helping to bound the pelvic outlet. The diaphragm presents a hiatus anteriorly, occupied by the vagina and urethra. The pelvic diaphragm is the main support of the pelvic floor; it suspends the rectum and indirectly supports the uterus.

Arteries & Veins

The blood supply to the muscles lining the pelvis is primarily from branches of the hypogastric artery, accompanied by contributions from the external iliac artery. The iliolumbar branch of the hypogastric artery runs upward and laterally beneath the common iliac artery, then beneath the psoas muscle to the superior aperture of the pelvis minor, where it divides into iliac and lumbar branches. The iliac supplies both the iliacus and psoas muscles. It passes laterally beneath the psoas and the femoral nerve and, perforating the iliacus, ramifies in the iliac fossa between the muscle and the bone. It supplies a nutrient artery to the bone and then divides into several branches that can be traced as follows: (1) upward toward the sacroiliac synchondrosis to anastomose with the last lumbar artery, (2) laterally toward the crest of the ilium to anastomose with the lateral circumflex and gluteal arteries, and (3) medially toward the pelvis minor to anastomose with the deep circumflex iliac from the external iliac. The lumbar branch ascends beneath the psoas and supplies that muscle along with the quadratus lumborum. It then anastomoses with the last lumbar artery.

Another branch of the hypogastric artery, the lateral sacral artery, may be represented as 2 distinct vessels. It passes medially in front of the sacrum and turns downward to run parallel with the sympathetic trunk. Crossing the slips of origin of the piriform muscle, it sends branches to that muscle. On reaching the coccyx, it anastomoses in front of the bone with the middle sacral artery and with the inferior lateral sacral artery of the opposite side. The obturator artery usually arises from the hypogastric, but occasionally it may stem from the inferior epigastric or directly from the external iliac artery. It runs forward and downward slightly below the brim of the pelvis, lying between the peritoneum and endopelvic fascia. Passing through the obturator canal, it emerges and divides into anterior and posterior branches that curve around the margin of the obturator foramen beneath the obturator externus muscle.

When the obturator artery arises from the inferior epigastric or external iliac artery, its proximal relationships are profoundly altered, the vessel coursing near the femoral ring where it may be endangered during operative procedures. The anterior branch of the obturator artery runs around the medial margin of the obturator foramen and anastomoses with both its posterior branch and the medial circumflex artery. It supplies branches to the obturator muscles. The internal pudendal artery is a terminal branch of the hypogastric artery that arises opposite the piriform muscle and accompanies the inferior gluteal artery downward to the lower border of the greater sciatic foramen. It leaves the pelvis between the piriform and coccygeus muscles, passing over the ischial spine to enter the ischiorectal fossa through the small sciatic foramen. Then, running forward through the canalis pudendalis (Alcock's canal) in the obturator fascia, it terminates by dividing into the perineal artery and the artery of the clitoris.

Within the pelvis, the artery lies anterior to the piriform muscle and the sacral plexus of nerves, lateral to the inferior gluteal artery. Among the small branches that it sends to the gluteal region are those that accompany the nerve to the obturator internus. Another of its branches, the inferior hemorrhoidal artery, arises at the posterior part of the ischiorectal fossa. Upon perforating the obturator fascia, it immediately breaks up into several branches. Some of them run medially toward the rectum to supply the levator ani muscle. The superior gluteal artery originates as a short trunk from the

lateral and back part of the hypogastric artery, associated in origin with the iliolumbar and lateral sacral and sometimes with the inferior gluteal or with the inferior gluteal and the internal pudendal. It leaves the pelvis through the greater sciatic foramen above the piriform muscle, beneath its vein and in front of the superior gluteal nerve. Under cover of the gluteus maximus muscle, it breaks into a superficial and a deep division.

The deep portion further divides into superior and inferior branches. The inferior branch passes forward between the gluteus medius and minimus toward the greater trochanter, where it anastomoses with the ascending branch of the lateral circumflex. It supplies branches to the obturator internus, the piriformis, the levator ani, and the coccygeus muscles and to the hip joint. The deep circumflex iliac artery arises from the side of the external iliac artery either opposite the epigastric or a little below the origin of that vessel. It courses laterally behind the inguinal ligament, lying between the fascia transversalis and the peritoneum or in a fibrous canal formed by the union of the fascia transversalis with the iliac fascia. It sends off branches that supply the psoas and iliacus muscles, as well as a cutaneous branch that anastomoses with the superior gluteal artery.

PLACENTA*

At term, the normal placenta is a blue-red, rounded, flattened, meaty discoid organ 15–20 cm in diameter and 2–4 cm thick. It weighs 400–600 g, or about one-sixth the normal weight of the newborn. The umbilical cord arises from almost any point on the fetal surface of the placenta, seemingly at random. The fetal membranes arise from the placenta at its margin. In multiple pregnancy, one or more placentas may be present depending upon the number of ova implanted and the type of segmentation that occurs. The placenta is derived from both maternal and fetal tissue. At term, about four-fifths of the placenta is of fetal origin.

The maternal portion of the placenta amounts to less than one-fifth of the total placenta by weight. It is composed of compressed sheets of decidua basalis, remnants of blood vessels, and, at the margin, spongy decidua. Irregular grooves or clefts divide the placenta into cotyledons. The maternal surface is torn from the uterine wall at birth and as a result is rough, red, and spongy.

The fetal portion of the placenta is composed of numerous functional units called villi. These are branched terminals of the fetal circulation and provide for transfer of metabolic products. The villous surface, which is exposed to maternal blood, may be as much as 12 m² (130 square feet). The fetal capillary system within the villi is

---

* This section is contributed by Robert C. Goodlin, MD.

almost 50 km (27 miles) long. Most villi are free within the intervillous spaces, but an occasional anchor villus attaches the placenta to the decidua basalis. The fetal surface of the placenta is covered by amniotic membrane and is smooth and shiny. The umbilical cord vessels course over the fetal surface before entering the placenta.

Placental Types

A. CIRCUMVALLATE (CIRCUMMARGINATE) PLACENTAS

In about 1% of cases, the delivered placenta shows a small central chorionic plate surrounded by a thick whitish ring that is composed of a double fold of amnion and chorion with fibrin and degenerated decidua in between. This circumvallate placenta may predispose to premature marginal separation and second-trimester antepartum bleeding (Fig 2–26). This uncommon extrachorial placenta is of uncertain origin. It is associated with increased rates of slight to moderate antepartal bleeding, early delivery, and perinatal death. Older multiparas are more prone to its development. Low-birth-weight infants and extrachorial placentas seem related.

B. SUCCENTURIATE LOBE

Occasionally there may be an accessory cotyledon, or succenturiate lobe, with vascular connections to the main body of the placenta. A succenturiate lobe may not always deliver with the parent placenta during the third stage of labor. This leads to postpartal hemorrhage. If a careful examination of the delivered membranes reveals torn vessels, immediate manual exploration of the uterus is indicated for removal of an accessory lobe (Fig 2–27).

C. BIPARTITE PLACENTA

A bipartite placenta is an uncommon variety. The placenta is divided into 2 separate lobes but united by primary ves-

Figure 2–27. Succenturiate placenta.

sels and membranes. Retention of one lobe after birth will cause hemorrhagic and septic complications. Examine the vasculature and note the completeness of membranes of a small placenta for evidence of a missing lobe, and recover the adherent portion without delay (Fig 2–28).

D. MARGINAL INSERTION OF CORD (BATTLEDORE PLACENTA)

The umbilical cord may be found inserted into the chorionic plate at almost any point, but when it inserts at the margin it is sometimes called a battledore placenta (Fig 2–29).

E. PLACENTA MEMBRANACEA

This type of placenta is one in which the decidua capsularis is so well vascularized that the chorion laeve does not atrophy and villi are maintained. Hence, the entire fetal envelope is functioning placenta.

F. PLACENTA ACCRETA

In rare cases, the placenta is abnormally adherent to the myometrium, presumably because it developed where there was a deficiency of decidua. Predisposing factors include placenta previa in one-third of cases, previous cesarean in one-fourth, a prior dilatation and curettage

Figure 2–26. Marked circumvallate or extrachorial placenta.

Figure 2–28. Bipartite placenta.

Figure 2–29. Marginal insertion of battledore placenta.

(D&C) in one-fourth, and grand multiparity. The adherence may be partial or total. Rarely, the placenta may invade the myometrium deeply (placenta increta) or even perforate the uterus (placenta percreta). When attempts are made to remove a placenta accreta manually, hemorrhage may be severe. The treatment is hysterectomy.

G. PLACENTA PREVIA

This abnormality is discussed in Chapter 20.

H. MULTIPLE PREGNANCY PLACENTA

In fraternal twins, the placentas may be 2 distinct entities or fused. There are 2 distinct chorions and amnions. In the case of identical twins, the picture may be more confusing. Depending upon the time of division of the fertilized ovum, the position of the placentas and

number of membranes will vary. If the division occurs soon after fertilization, 2 distinct placentas and sets of membranes are the result. From that point on, many variations (eg, monochorionic monoamniotic fused placentas and, possibly, interchange of blood supply) may occur. Further variations may be noted when triplets or more are derived from one ovum. When the presence of identical twins is suspected, it is always wise to clamp the cord on the placental side at the time it is clamped on the infant to minimize the chance of exsanguination of the uterine twin.

REFERENCES

Caldwell WE, Moloy HC: Anatomical variations in the female pelvis. Am J Obstet Gynecol 1933;26:479.

Clemente C: *Gray's Anatomy of the Human Body,* 30th ed. Lippincott Williams & Wilkins, 1985.

Donnelly JE: *Living Anatomy,* 2nd ed. Human Kinetics, 1990.

Goscicka D, Murawski E: Tendinous intersections of the rectus abdominis muscle in human fetuses. Folia Morphol (Warsz) 1980;39:427.

Harrison RJ, Navarainam V (editors): *Progress in Anatomy.* Vol. 3. Cambridge University Press, 1984.

Junqueira LC, Carneiro J, Kelley RO: *Basic Histology,* 9th ed. McGraw-Hill, 1998.

Moore KL: *Clinically Oriented Anatomy,* 4th ed. Lippincott Williams & Wilkins, 1999.

Netter FH et al: *The Ciba Collection of Medical Illustrations.* Vol. 2: Reproductive System. Novartis Medical Education, 1986.

Schlossberg L, Zuidema GD (editors): *The Johns Hopkins Atlas of Human Functional Anatomy,* 4th ed. Johns Hopkins University Press, 1997.

Wilson DB, Wilson WJ: *Human Anatomy,* 2nd ed. Oxford University Press, 1983.

The Role of Imaging Techniques in Gynecology

3

Susan Sarajari, MD, PhD, Andy Huang, MD, Alan H. DeCherney, MD, & Robert A. Graebe, MD

CASE REPORT

C.O. is a 29-year-old white woman who presented with a history of infertility for several years, followed by a history of recurrent pregnancy losses.

Her past medical and surgical histories were negative. Gynecologically, she was remarkable in that she reported severe dysmenorrhea for several years that was relieved by nonsteroidal anti-inflammatory drugs. Her gynecologist found a low luteal phase progesterone level and treated her with 50 mg of clomiphene citrate on days 5–9 of the cycle.

She responded well to the medication, with a subsequent conception. The pregnancy resulted in a spontaneous abortion 5 weeks later. No dilatation and curettage (D&C) was required, and the patient recovered well. She still was unable to conceive on her own and was again given clomiphene citrate therapy. Again, she conceived and had a spontaneous abortion—this time at 7 weeks' gestation. No D&C was performed.

The patient was evaluated for recurrent pregnancy losses. Karyotype was normal for both partners. Hormonal evaluation was normal with the exception of a low midluteal phase progesterone level. Immunologic and infectious screening failed to reveal a cause for the recurrent losses. The hysterosalpingogram (HSG) demonstrated a midline filling defect similar to that shown in Figure 3–1.

The patient was informed of the results and the potential for future miscarriages. The need for further evaluation and possible repair performed hysteroscopically or abdominally, together with its risks and benefits, was carefully explained to the patient. She elected to try clomiphene citrate therapy one more time and hoped to avoid surgery.

At 8 weeks' gestation, vaginal ultrasonography (US) revealed positive fetal cardiac activity in an ovulation induced by clomiphene citrate. While still taking micronized progesterone 100 mg 3 times daily, she was referred to her gynecologist for routine obstetric care.

At 12 weeks' gestation, the patient had an incomplete abortion that required a D&C. She recovered uneventfully and later returned to the office for further evaluation and treatment.

Several months were allowed to lapse before a hysteroscopy/laparoscopy was performed, which revealed a broad-based intrauterine septum and stage I endometriosis. To evaluate the depth and width of the septum, a LaparoScan (EndoMedix, Irvine, CA) laparoscopic 7.5-Hz probe was used during the procedure. The septum was removed with a hysteroscopic resectoscope loop on a 40-W setting. After the resection, the ultrasonic probe was again used to measure the thickness of the myometrium and to verify the resection of the septum. A 30-mL 18F Foley catheter with the distal tip resected was placed in the fundus and inflated. The patient was discharged and placed on therapy consisting of a broad-spectrum antibiotic and conjugated estrogen 2.5 mg daily.

DISCUSSION

The new millennium saw a proliferation of imaging techniques used in medical practice. Research into the development, refinement, and application of imaging in gynecology is apparent in the literature.

The HSG has been considered the gold standard for imaging the uterine corpus for benign disorders (submucous myomas, submucous polyps, localization of tubal occlusion, and evaluation of müllerian fusion defects) and malignant disease (endometrial carcinoma).

In the case reported, the standard scout film was obtained, and the cervix was prepared after the following were assured: position of the uterus, absence of pelvic tenderness, and negative pregnancy test. The water-soluble contrast medium was injected into the uterine cavity, and oblique and anteroposterior films were obtained. These films showed a midline uterine filling defect of the type usually seen with septate or bicornuate uteri.

US performed on this patient during her pregnancies failed to show the filling defect. If suspected, the septum might have been encountered by more careful scanning. The scans of the last pregnancy revealed

Figure 3–1. Müllerian anomaly as demonstrated by hysterosalpingogram. (Reproduced, with permission, from Doyle MB: Magnetic resonance imaging in müllerian fusion defects. J Reprod Med 1992;37:33.)

only an eccentrically placed pregnancy that might have been seen ultrasonographically even in normally structured uteri. Although not helpful at this point, ultrasonographic examination of the uterus between conceptions might have been helpful if used with a distending medium. This is especially useful in patients allergic to iodine contrast medium (Table 3–1). This technique of ultrasonic HSG is performed by occluding the cervix with a uterine injector and distending the uterus. The method can demonstrate the separate cavities as well as the possible difference between the septate and the bicornuate uterus while demonstrating tubal patency. The technique was adopted for this patient during her uterine septum resection, with the addition of ultrasonic contrast between the endometrial cavity and septum and the myometrium. Readers are referred to the many fine texts on diagnostic pelvic ultrasound for instruction and further discussion of these techniques. The development of "sonicated" contrast solutions may add greatly to the usefulness of US.

Using 2 video cameras (1 for the resectoscope and the other for the laparoscope and the LaparoScan laparoscopic ultrasound probe), all aspects of the surgery were evaluated. This setup allowed the operating surgeon adequate visualization of the uterine cavity during the resection and enabled other personnel in the operating room to follow the progress of surgery. The laparoscopic video allowed for careful monitoring of the uterine surface and assured the surgeon that there would be less likelihood of a uterine perforation, a complication that could result in bowel injury.

The laparoscopic ultrasound probe with a picture within a picture was useful because it allowed visualization of the 2 separate cavities and measurement of the length and width of the septum. It also enabled the operator to demonstrate the complete removal of the septum (Fig 3–2).

IMAGING OF THE UTERUS & CERVIX

Plain radiographs are rarely the test of choice for identifying gynecologic pathology, but they can be used to detect calcified leiomyomas as well as an intrauterine device (IUD). Such films can help determine if an IUD has been expelled from the uterine cavity or has penetrated the uterine wall and migrated to an ectopic location.

Pelvic US plays a significant role in the diagnosis of uterine leiomyomas (submucosal, intramural, and subserosal) and polyps. Occasionally, the detection and localization of myomas, assessment of size, and their differential diagnosis are difficult. In these circumstances it is sometimes useful to perform magnetic resonance imaging (MRI) of the pelvis. MRI produces images with excellent soft-tissue resolution. MRI can be used for evaluation of congenital abnormalities of the uterus, leiomyomas, adenomyosis, gestational trophoblastic disease, and endometrial carcinoma diagnosis and staging. MRI can accurately measure the volume of the myoma, which aids in determining whether medical management of myomas has resulted in shrinkage or whether conservatively treated myomas are growing. Malignant degeneration of myomas visualized by MRI as described by some authors allows for early and appropriate intervention.

Table 3–1. Indications for saline infusion sonohysterosalpingogram.

Abnormal x-ray hysterosalpingogram
Abnormal uterine bleeding
Allergies to iodine dyes
Amenorrhea
Infertility

Figure 3–2. Uterine septum. **A:** Laparoscopic view showing a broad uterine fundus. **B:** Laparoscopic probe on the fundus of the uterus showing the depth and width of the septum. **C:** Hysteroscopic view showing the resection of the uterine septum. **D:** Laparoscopic probe on the fundus of the uterus showing the resected septum. (Note the echogenicity of the debris in the fundus.)

MRI can effectively discern between the septate and the bicornuate uterus, thus avoiding the more costly laparoscopy. MRI may provide a clear anatomic picture of complicated müllerian fusion defects (didelphys with transverse vaginal septum or noncommunicating uterine segment) and allow for proper planning of surgical repair. If pelvic MRI had been performed on the patient in the opening case report, the image probably would have appeared the same as the MRI shown in Figure 3–3. (See review of MRI findings of müllerian fusion defects in Table 3–2.)

Currently, histopathologic evaluation of colposcopic biopsies is required to diagnose cervical cancer and its precursor lesions. However, the technique is expensive and often requires a waiting period before histopathologic results are available and necessary treatment can be scheduled. Several new imaging techniques that evaluate the cervical epithelium are under investigation. Optical techniques, such as elastic backscattering and fluorescence and Raman spectroscopies, have been used to noninvasively examine tissue morphology and the biochemical composition of the cervix. Optical coherence tomography (OCT) is a noninvasive imaging technique that uses coherent light to form images of subsurface tissue structures with 10- to 20-μm resolution and up to 1-mm depth. A study by Zuluaga et al showed that simple quantitative analysis of images obtained with an OCT system can be used for noninvasive evaluation of normal and abnormal cervical tissue in vivo. Optical coherence tomographic imaging could have broad applications for screening and detection of cervical malignancies and their precursors. It also may aid in surgical planning by allowing surgeons to identify margins in vivo without obtaining frozen sections.

Figure 3–3. Complete uterine septum extending to the cervix. (Reproduced, with permission, from Doyle MB: Magnetic resonance imaging in müllerian fusion defects. J Reprod Med 1992;37:33.)

IMAGING OF THE ENDOMETRIUM

Pelvic ultrasound has been used to evaluate the uterine cavity, and endometrial thickness has been used as a marker for endometrial pathology. The following guidelines should be used to obtain interobserver consistency in the evaluation of the endometrium. Obtain measurements from the midfundal region in the sagittal plane. Obtain the maximal double-thickness dimension, remembering to exclude the hypoechoic area between the myometrium and the endometrium. Any fluid between the anterior and posterior walls should be subtracted from the total measurement. Endometrial thickness ranges from 4–8 mm during the follicular phase. The uterine lining ranges from 7–14 mm during the luteal phase and has a uniform echogenic appearance.

Premenopausal women should be evaluated during the early follicular phase, immediately following the menses when the endometrium has a uniform linear appearance.

Menopausal women usually have an endometrial stripe less than 4 mm. Menopausal women on hormone replacement therapy (HRT) may have an endometrial thickness exceeding 8 mm and a small amount of fluid (< 1 mm).

Table 3–2. Types of müllerian anomalies and associated MRI findings.

Class and Type	No.	Finding
I: Segmental agenesis/hypoplasia	7 (24%)	Agenesis: no identifiable organ or small amorphous tissue remnant. Hypoplasia: uterus small for patient's age, maintains adult body/cervix ratio of 2:1, reduced intercornual distance (< 2 cm), low signal intensity on T_2-weighted images with poor zonal differentiation, endometrial/myometrial width reduced
A. Vaginal	0	
B. Cervical	0	
C. Fundal	0	
D. Tubal	0	
E. Combined	7	
II: Unicornuate uterus	5 (17%)	Banana-shaped uterus, normal width of endometrium and myometrium, endometrial/myometrial ratio preserved
A1. Rudimentary horn with endometrium		
(A) Communicating with main uterine cavity	0	
(B) Not communicating with main uterine cavity	1	
A2. Rudimentary horn without endometrium	1	
B. No rudimentary horn	3	
III: Didelphys	5 (17%)	Double, separate uterus, cervix and upper vagina; each uterine cavity of normal volume; endometrium and myometrium of normal width; endometrial/myometrial ratio normal
IV: Bicornuate uterus	10 (34%)	Uterine fundus concave or flattened outward, two horns visible with increased intercornual distance (> 4 cm), high-signal-intensity septum myometrium on T_2-weighted images at level of fundus; high-signal-intensity myometrium (7 patients) or low-signal-intensity fibrous tissue at level of lower uterine segment (3 patients)
A. Complete	3	
B. Partial	3	
C. Arcuate	4	
V: Septate	2 (7%)	Uterine fundus convex outward, normal intercornual distance (2–4 cm), each uterine cavity reduced in volume, endometrial/myometrial width and ratio normal, low-signal-intensity septum on T_1- and T_2-weighted images
A. Complete	1	
B. Incomplete	1	

Because of rounding, the percentages do not add up to 100.
Reproduced, with permission, from Doyle MB: Magnetic resonance imaging in müllerian fusion defects. J Reprod Med 1992;37:33.

Figure 3–4. Proposed algorithm for evaluating women with abnormal vaginal bleeding. (Reproduced, with permission, from Davidson KG et al: Ultrasonographic evaluation of the endometrium in postmenopausal vaginal bleeding. Radiol Clin North Am 2003;41:769.)

Approximately one-fifth of patients with abnormal uterine bleeding have submucous myomas and/or polyps. These lesions may be detected by irregularities in the endometrial stripe or by saline infusion sonohysterography (SIS), a technique that involves saline infusion to distend the uterine cavity. Using SIS, a polyp appears as a smoothly marginated focal lesion that protrudes into the endometrial cavity. A study comparing transvaginal sonography and SIS for detection of endometrial polyps found SIS had significantly greater sensitivity (93% versus 65%) and specificity (94% versus 76%) than transvaginal sonography alone.

The sensitivity and specificity rates of ultrasound in detecting endometrial pathology reportedly increase when color flow and power Doppler imaging are used. However, tissue sampling would be required to make a definitive diagnosis and to rule out malignancy in any patient not on HRT with a hyperechogenic endometrial stripe greater than 4 mm.

Three-dimensional ultrasonography (3-D US) has been studied for evaluation of the endometrium. The ability of 3-D US to produce coronal images of the cornua may increase slightly the sensitivity of SIS for detecting lesions in this location that otherwise might be difficult to evaluate. Endometrial abnormalities that can be seen in women with congenital malformations of the uterus may be imaged to greater advantage with 3-D US techniques. Three-dimensional ultrasonography has also been demonstrated to be a valid measurement technique for assessing volume. However, hysteroscopy likely will become the new gold standard for evaluating the endometrium because of the ability of hysteroscopy to visualize directly the endometrium and perform biopsies as indicated. The technique may become more cost-effective as use of office hysteroscopy becomes more widespread. Evaluation of the endometrium using transvaginal sonography as the initial screening tool, followed by endometrial biopsy or possibly hysteroscopy, is likely to become the standard of care (Fig 3–4).

OVARIAN TUMOR ULTRASOUND-DOPPLER CLASSIFICATION
Circle all characteristics seen and add numbers in parentheses for a score.

Patient name _____ Date _____ Institution _____

	FLUID			INTERNAL BORDERS		SIZE
UNILOCULAR	Clear	(0)		Smooth	(0)	
	Internal echoes	(1)		Irregular	(2)	
MULTILOCULAR	Clear	(1)		Smooth	(1)	
	Internal echoes	(1)		Irregular	(2)	
CYSTIC-SOLID	Clear	(1)		Smooth	(1)	
	Internal echoes	(2)		Irregular	(2)	

PAPILLARY PROJECTIONS	Suspicious	(1)		Definite	(2)
SOLID	Homogenous	(1)		Echogenic	(2)
PERITONEAL FLUID	Absent	(0)		Present	(1)
LATERALITY	Unilateral	(0)		Bilateral	(1)

ULTRASOUND SCORE

≤2 Benign
3–4 Questionable
>4 Suspicious

Figure 3–5. Scoring system used to evaluate the morphology of adnexal tumor. RI, resistance index. (Reproduced, with permission, from Kurjak A et al: Transvaginal ultrasound, color flow, and Doppler waveform of the postmenopausal adnexal mass. Obstet Gynecol 1992;80:917.)

COLOR DOPPLER		**RI (resistance index)**	
No vessels seen	(0)		(0)
Regular separate vessels	(1)	>0.40	(1)
Randomly dispersed vessels	(2)	<0.41	(2)

If suspected corpus luteum, repeat in next menstrual cycle in proliferative phase.

COLOR DOPPLER SCORE

≤2 Benign
3–4 Questionable

IMAGING OF THE OVARIES

Approximately 12,000 women in the United States die annually of ovarian cancer. Unfortunately, the ability of the pelvic examination to detect early ovarian malignancy is poor. Cancer antigen (CA)-125 monoclonal marker for ovarian cancer also is a poor predictor of early cases.

The flat plate of the abdomen may still be useful in the diagnosis of dermoid cysts of the ovary, which are identified by the presence of calcified teeth. However, cystic and solid structures of the ovary now are better evaluated by transabdominal ultrasonography, transvaginal ultrasonography (TVUS), computed tomography (CT), and MRI.

US is frequently used in the evaluation of ovarian pathology. TVUS combined with color flow and Doppler can be used for evaluation of blood flow to the adnexal structures and for diagnosis of ovarian torsion.

Venous and lymphatic flow is occluded in early torsion, but arterial flow may be present. Arterial flow ceases completely later in the torsion. Torsion is diagnosed by Doppler study showing no venous or arterial flow, but a study showing arterial blood flow does not necessarily rule out the diagnosis.

In an attempt to discriminate between malignant and benign adnexal masses, morphologic criteria have been assigned to increase suspicion concerning ultrasound findings when ovarian cancer is suspected. Cysts larger than 4 cm, solid and cystic components, septa, and papillary nodules have all been described (Fig 3–5). In addition, Doppler flow studies have been used to distinguish between benign and malignant masses (Table 3–3).

CT may be useful for preoperative staging of ovarian cancer or for planning second-look procedures. CT may be useful for biopsy and drainage in patients with benign-appearing adnexal masses (ovarian cysts or

Table 3–3. Histology and blood flow characteristics.

Histology	N	Flow Detected	RI
Malignant			
Papillary adeno-carcinoma	13	12	0.39 ± 0.04
Serous cystadeno-carcinoma	3	3	0.30 ± 0.04
Endometrioid adeno-carcinoma	4	4	0.38 ± 0.02
Metastatic carcinoma	7	7	0.37 ± 0.07
Theca-granulosa cell	2	1	0.37
Total	29	27	0.37 ± 0.08
Benign			
Simple cyst	25	5	0.75 ± 0.17
Papillary serous cyst	4	1	0.6
Mucinous cyst	5	3	0.62 ± 0.09
Inflammatory mass	2	1	0.62
Parasitic cyst	1	0	0
Fibroma	4	3	0.56 ± 0.03
Thecoma	2	2	0.60
Cystadenofibroma	1	1	0.56
Endometrioma	4	1	0.56
Cystic teratoma	1	1	0.36
Pseudo- and parovarian cyst	4	0	0
Brenner tumor	1	1	0.50
Total	54	19	0.62 ± 0.11[1]

Data are presented as N or mean ± SD.
[1]$P < .001$.
RI, resistance index.
Reproduced, with permission, from Kurjak A et al: Transvaginal ultrasound, color flow, and Doppler waveform of the post-menopausal adnexal mass. Obstet Gynecol 1992;80:917.

tubo-ovarian abscesses). Contraindications to needle biopsy and drainage include lack of a safe unobstructed path for the needle, bleeding disorders, and lack of a motivated patient. Three-dimensional ultrasonography can be useful in the evaluation of gynecologic diseases. It can reconstruct any plane of interest and is particularly valuable in visualizing abnormalities in the coronal plane. In addition, 3-D US is better able to measure volumes than is 2-dimensional ultrasonography and therefore is helpful when evaluating patients with conditions ranging from fibroids to infertility. CT can be used in conjunction with pelvic US to diagnose and manage several conditions, such as pelvic inflammatory disease, adnexal torsion, ovarian vein thrombosis, and hemorrhagic ovarian cysts. In addition, MRI has been shown to be particularly useful in the evaluation of ovarian vein thrombosis.

IMAGING OF THE FALLOPIAN TUBES

Endoscopic techniques provide the best direct evaluation of the patency and architecture of the fallopian tubes. HSG provides the best indirect evaluation of tubal function. HSG allows demonstration of tubal patency and visualization of tubal rugations while avoiding the more costly laparoscopic surgery. Some disadvantages of HSG are pelvic infection, dye allergies, failure to detect adnexal adhesions, and false-positive results for tubal occlusion. Hysterosalpingo-contrast sonography and MRI are alternatives to laparoscopy, as women with normal findings probably have a normal pelvis. For example, transvaginal sonography may detect dilated fallopian tubes and tubo-ovarian complexes. (See the sections on pelvic inflammatory disease and tubo-ovarian abscess in Chapter 41 for more on the radiographic diagnosis and management of these conditions.)

IMAGING IN ECTOPIC PREGNANCY

Adnexal sonography is a valuable tool in assessing women with suspected ectopic pregnancy (Table 3–4). When human chorionic gonadotropin (hCG) levels reach 6500 mIU/mL, most normal intrauterine pregnancies can be detected as a gestational sac by transabdominal US. However, the sonographic appearance of a pseudogestational sac should not be confused with the gestational sac. In the latter, a double-ring sign resulting from the decidua parietalis is seen abutting the decidua capsularis.

TVUS, on the other hand, has the advantage of earlier and better localization of the pregnancy, with less pelvic

Table 3–4. Criteria for diagnosis of ectopic pregnancy.

Criteria	Sensitivity (%)	Specificity (%)
Extrauterine gestational sac with yolk sac or embryo	8–34	100
Adnexal ring	40–68	100
Complex adnexal mass separate from ovary	89–100	92–99
Any fluid	46–75	69–83
Moderate to large amount of free fluid	29–63	21–96
Echogenic fluid	56	96
Decidual cyst	21	92

Reproduced, with permission, from Harrison BE et al: Imaging modalities in obstetrics and gynecology. Emerg Med Clin North Am 2003;21:711.

discomfort because the bladder is not painfully distended. An hCG level of 1000–2000 mIU/mL is the discriminatory zone in which an intrauterine pregnancy can be detected by TVUS. The double-ring sign and/or the yolk sac must be identified to ensure that the pregnancy is intrauterine. When an intrauterine pregnancy is not visualized on TVUS and the hCG level exceeds 1000–2000 mIU/mL, then suspicion for an ectopic pregnancy should be high. Also, multiple gestations may take several more days to be identified, and heterotopic pregnancies are encountered more frequently in patients using assisted reproductive techniques. Transvaginal sonography may also detect dilated fallopian tubes and tubo-ovarian complexes.

CONCLUSION

The imaging techniques prevalent today have proved to be valuable tools in the diagnosis and early treatment of benign and malignant gynecologic disorders. To provide the patient with the highest level of medical care, the contemporary practicing gynecologist must constantly keep abreast of the new developments and applications of diagnostic imaging.

No matter what technology is used today and in the future, the goal will always be the same: to provide quick, low-risk, accurate diagnosis of gynecologic conditions while keeping in mind the cost-effectiveness of the care delivered.

REFERENCES

Davidson KG et al: Ultrasonographic evaluation of the endometrium in postmenopausal vaginal bleeding. Radiol Clin North Am 2003;41:769.

Doyle MB: Magnetic resonance imaging in müllerian fusion defects. J Reprod Med 1992;37:33.

Fielding JR: MR imaging of the female pelvis. Radiol Clin North Am 2003;41:179.

Harrison BP et al: Imaging modalities in obstetrics and gynecology. Emerg Med Clin North Am 2003;21:711.

Krampl E et al: Transvaginal ultrasonography, sonohysterography and operative hysteroscopy for the evaluation of abnormal uterine bleeding. Acta Obstet Gynecol Scand 2001;80:616.

Kurjak A et al: Transvaginal ultrasound, color flow, and Doppler waveform of the postmenopausal adnexal mass. Obstet Gynecol 1992;80:917.

Laing FC: Gynecologic ultrasound. Radiol Clin North Am 2001;39:523.

Moore C et al: Ultrasound in pregnancy. Emerg Med Clin North Am 2004;22:697.

Soper JT: Radiographic imaging in gynecologic oncology. Clin Obstet Gynecol 2001;44:485.

Thurmond AS: Imaging of female infertility. Radiol Clin North Am 2003;41:757.

Vitiello D et al. Diagnostic imaging of myomas. Obstet Gynecol Clin 2006;33:85.

Zuluaga AF et al: Optical coherence tomography: A pilot study of a new imaging technique for noninvasive examination of cervical tissue. Am J Obstet Gynecol 2005;193:83.

Embryology of the Urogenital System & Congenital Anomalies of the Female Genital Tract

4

Catherine M. DeUgarte, MD, & Joseph D. Bast, PhD

In the urogenital system, knowledge of the embryology is crucial in understanding the functions and interconnections between the reproductive and urologic systems. The adult genital and urinary systems are distinct in both function and anatomy, with the exception of the male urethra, where the two systems are interconnected. During development, these two systems are closely associated. The initial developmental overlap of these systems occurs 4–12 weeks after fertilization. The complexity of developmental events in these systems is evident by the incomplete separation of the 2 systems found in some congenital anomalies. For the sake of clarity, this chapter describes the embryology of each system separately, rather than following a strict developmental chronology.

In view of the complexity and duration of differentiation and development of the genital and urinary systems, it is not surprising that the incidence of malformations involving these systems is one of the highest (10%) of all body systems. Etiologies of congenital malformations are sometimes categorized on the basis of genetic, environmental, or genetic-plus-environmental (so-called polyfactorial inheritance) factors. Known genetic and inheritance factors reputedly account for about 20% of anomalies detected at birth, aberration of chromosomes for nearly 5%, and environmental factors for nearly 10%. The significance of these statistics must be viewed against reports that (1) an estimated one-third to one-half of human zygotes are lost during the first week of gestation and (2) the cause of possibly 70% of human anomalies is unknown. Even so, congenital malformations remain a matter of concern because they are detected in nearly 3% of infants, and 20% of perinatal deaths are purportedly due to congenital anomalies.

The inherent pattern of normal development of the genital system can be viewed as one directed toward somatic "femaleness," unless development is directed by factors for "maleness." The presence and expression of a Y chromosome (and its testis-determining genes) in a normal 46,XY karyotype of somatic cells directs differentiation toward a testis, and normal development of the testis

makes available hormones for the selection and differentiation of the genital ducts. When male hormones are present, the mesonephric (wolffian) system persists; when male hormones are not present, the "female" paramesonephric (müllerian) ducts persist. Normal feminization or masculinization of the external genitalia is also a result of the respective timely absence or presence of androgen.

An infant usually is reared as female or male according to the appearance of the external genitalia. However, genital sex is not always immediately discernible, and the choice of sex of rearing can be an anxiety-provoking consideration. Unfortunately, even when genital sex is apparent, later clinical presentation may unmask disorders of sexual differentiation that can lead to problems in psychological adjustment. Whether a somatic disorder is detected at birth or later, investigative backtracking through the developmental process is necessary for proper diagnosis and treatment.

OVERVIEW OF THE FIRST FOUR WEEKS OF DEVELOPMENT*

Transformation of the bilaminar embryonic disk into a trilaminar disk composed of **ectoderm, mesoderm,** and **endoderm** (the 3 embryonic germ layers) occurs during the third week by a process called **gastrulation** (Fig 4–1). During this process, a specialized thickening of epiblast, the **primitive streak,** elongates through the midline of the disk. Some epiblastic cells become **mesoblastic cells,** which migrate peripherally between the epiblast and hypoblast, forming a middle layer of **embryonic mesoderm.** Other mesoblastic cells migrate into the hypoblastic layer and form **embryonic endoderm,** which displaces the hypoblastic cells. The remaining overlying epiblast becomes the **embryonic ectoderm.**

---

*Embryonic or fetal ages given in this chapter are relative to the time of fertilization and should be considered estimates rather than absolutes.

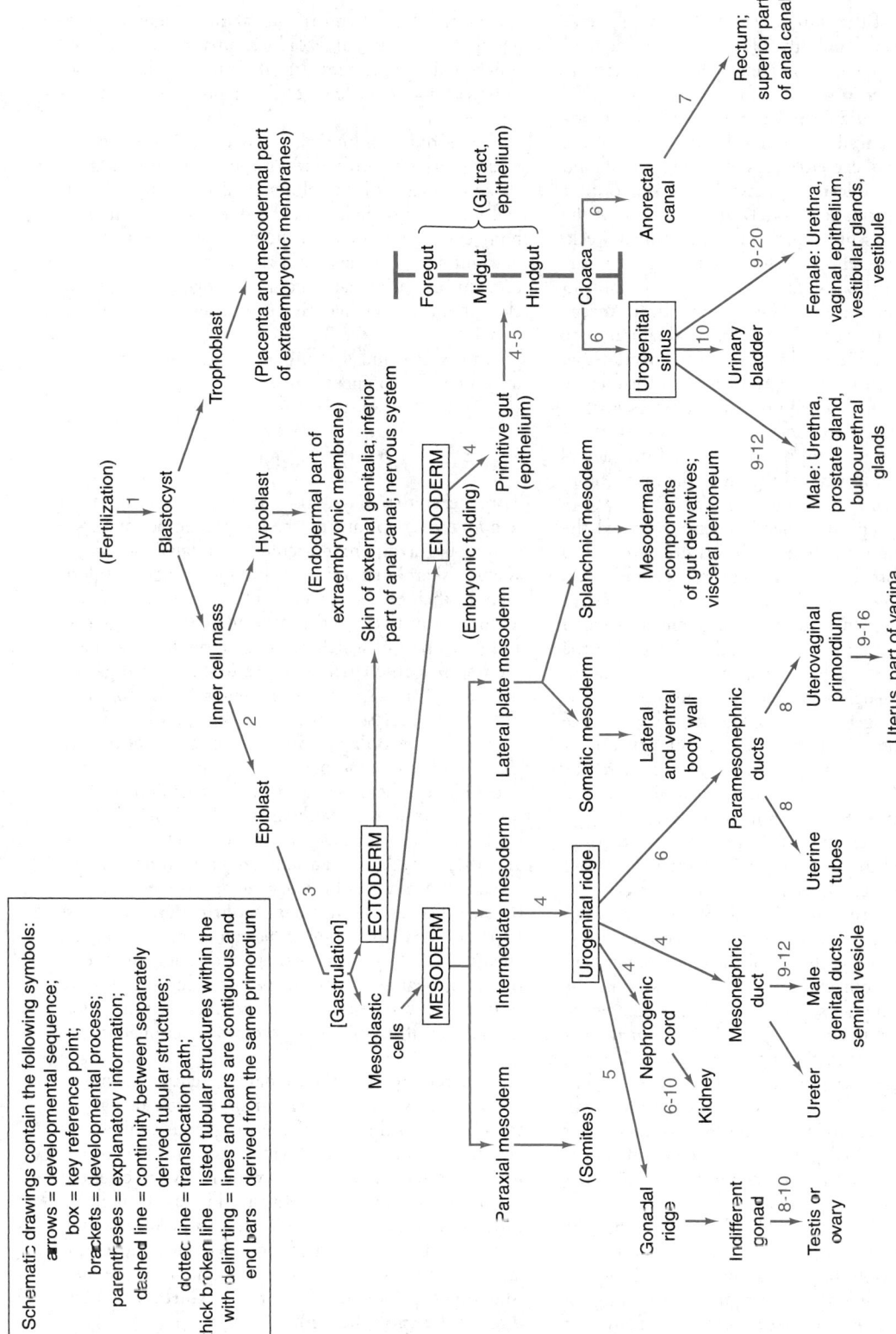

Schematic drawings contain the following symbols:
 arrows = developmental sequence;
   box = key reference point;
 brackets = developmental process;
parentheses = explanatory information;
dashed line = continuity between separately
              derived tubular structures;
 dottec line = translocation path;
thick broken line = listed tubular structures within the
with delimiting = lines and bars are contiguous and
 end bars = derived from the same primordium

Figure 4–1. Schematic overview of embryonic development of progenitory urinary and genital tissues and structures considered to be derivatives of embryonic ectoderm, mesoderm, or endoderm. Numbers indicate the weeks after fertilization when the indicated developmental change occurs.

By the end of the third week, 3 clusters of mesoderm are organized on both sides of the midline neural tube. From medial to lateral, these clusters are **paraxial mesoderm,** which forms much of the axial skeleton; **intermediate mesoderm,** which is the origin of the **urogenital ridge** and, hence, much of the reproductive and excretory systems (Fig 4–2); and **lateral plate mesoderm,** which splits and takes part in body cavity formation. Rarely, degeneration of the primitive streak is incomplete after the fourth week, and presumptive remnants form a teratoma in the sacrococcygeal region of the fetus (more common in females than in males). The **intermediate mesoderm** is located between the paraxial and lateral plate mesoderm and is the origin of the **urogenital ridge** and, hence, much of the reproductive and excretory systems (Fig 4–2). The primitive streak regresses after the fourth week. Rarely, degeneration of the streak is incomplete, and presumptive remnants form a teratoma in the sacrococcygeal region of the fetus (more common in females than in males).

Weeks 4 through 8 of development are called the **embryonic period** (the **fetal period** is from week 9 to term) because formation of all major internal and external structures, including the 2 primary forerunners of the urogenital system (urogenital ridge and urogenital sinus), begins during this time. During this period the embryo is most likely to develop major congenital or acquired morphologic anomalies in response to the effects of various agents. During the fourth week, the shape of the embryo changes from that of a trilaminar disk to that of a crescentic cylinder. The change results from "folding," or flexion, of the embryonic disk in a ventral direction through both its transverse and longitudinal planes. Flexion occurs as midline structures (neural tube and somites) develop and grow at a faster pace than more lateral tissues (ectoderm, 2 layers of lateral plate mesoderm enclosing the coelom between them, and endoderm). Thus, during transverse folding, the lateral tissues on each side of the embryo curl ventromedially and join the respective tissues from the other side, creating a midline ventral tube (the endoderm-lined **primitive gut**), a mesoderm-lined coelomic cavity (the **primitive abdominopelvic cavity**), and the incomplete ventral and lateral body wall. Concurrent longitudinal flexion ventrally of the caudal region of the disk establishes the pouchlike distal end, or **cloaca,** of the primitive gut as well as the distal attachment of the cloaca to the yolk sac through the allantois of the sac (Fig 4–3).

A noteworthy point (see The Gonads) is that the primordial germ cells of the later-developing gonad initially are found close to the allantois and later migrate to the gonadal primordia. Subsequent partitioning of the cloaca during the sixth week results in formation of the anorectal canal and the **urogenital sinus,** the progenitor of the urinary bladder, urethra, vagina, and other genital structures (Fig 4–1 and Table 4–1; see Subdivision of the Cloaca & Formation of the Urogenital Sinus).

Embryonic folding also moves the intermediate mesoderm—the forerunner of the **urogenital ridge**—to its characteristic developmental locations as bilateral longitudinal bulges in the dorsal wall of the new body cavity and lateral to the dorsal mesentery of the new gut tube. By the end of the fourth week of development, the principal structures (urogenital ridge and cloaca) and tissues that give rise to the urogenital system are present.

Tables 4–1 and 4–2 provide a general overview of urogenital development.

THE URINARY SYSTEM

Three excretory "systems" form successively, with temporal overlap, during the embryonic period. Each system has a different excretory "organ," but the 3 systems share anatomic continuity through development of their excretory ducts. The 3 systems are mesodermal derivatives of the urogenital ridge (Figs 4–2 and 4–3), part of which becomes a longitudinal mass, the **nephrogenic cord.** The **pronephros,** or organ of the first system, exists rudimentarily, is nonfunctional, and regresses during the fourth week. However, the developing pronephric ducts continue to grow and become the mesonephric ducts of the subsequent kidney, the **mesonephros.** The paired mesonephroi exist during 4–8 weeks as simplified morphologic versions of the third, or permanent, set of kidneys, and they may have transient excretory function. Although the mesonephroi degenerate, some of its tubules, called **epigenital mesonephric tubules,** persist to participate in formation of the gonad and male ductuli efferentes (Fig 4–4). The permanent kidney, the **metanephros,** begins to form in response to an inductive influence of a diverticulum of the mesonephric ducts during the fifth week and becomes functional at 10–13 weeks.

Differentiation of the caudal segment of the mesonephric ducts results in (1) incorporation of part of the ducts into the wall of the urogenital sinus (early vesicular trigone, see following text), and (2) formation of a ductal diverticulum, which plays an essential role in formation of the definitive kidney. If male sex differentiation occurs, the major portion of each duct becomes the epididymis, ductus deferens, and ejaculatory duct. Only small vestigial remnants of the duct sometimes persist in the female (**Gartner's duct; duct of the epoophoron**).

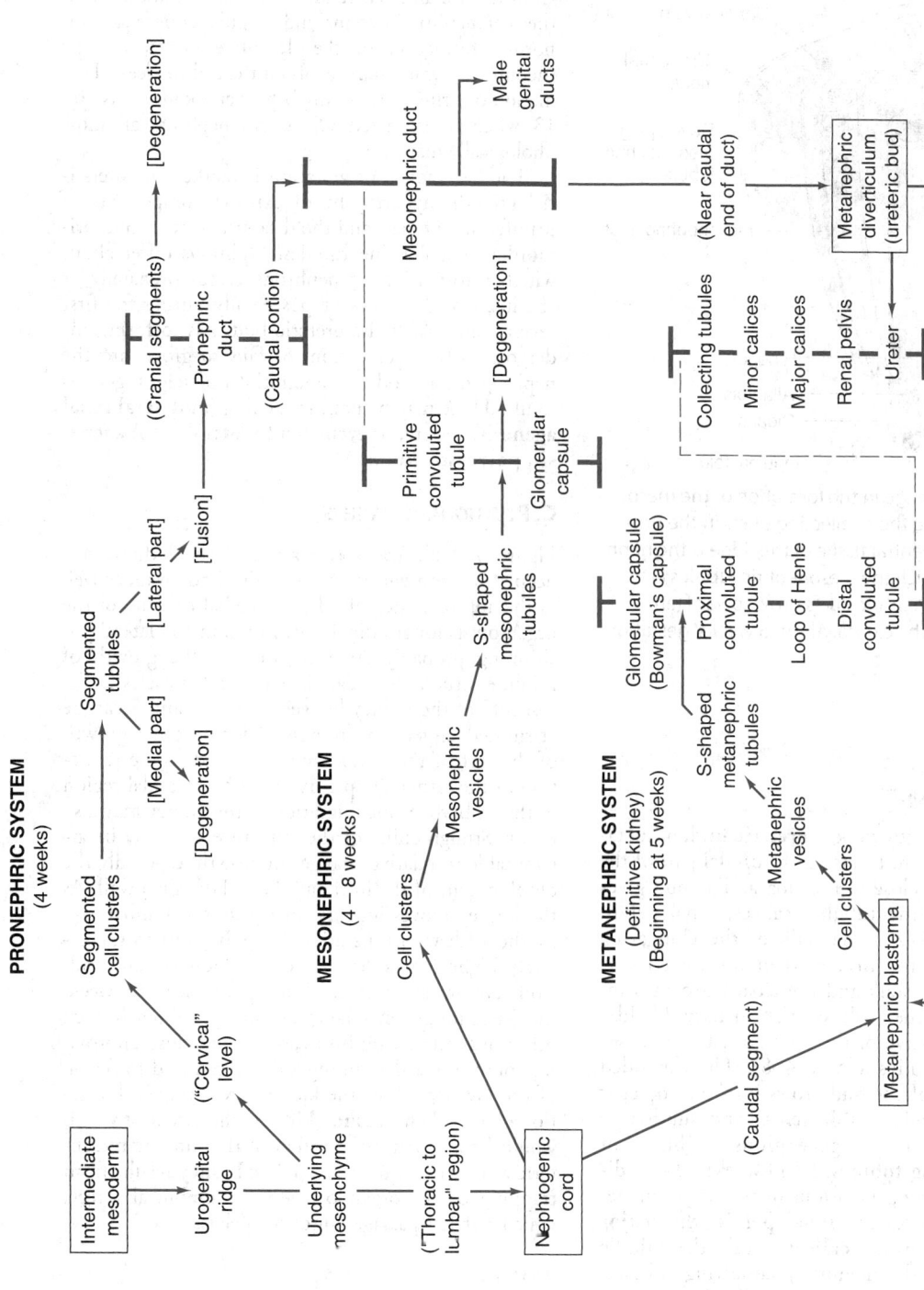

Figure 4–2. Schematic drawing of formation of the definitive kidney and its collecting ducts. The pronephric duct is probably the only structure that participates in all 3 urinary systems, as its caudal portion continues to grow and is called the mesonephric duct when the mesonephric system develops. (Explanatory symbols are given in Fig 4–1.)

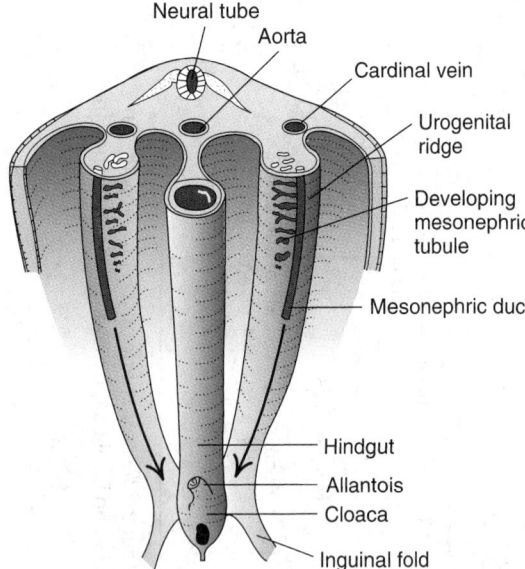

Neural tube
Aorta
Cardinal vein
Urogenital ridge
Developing mesonephric tubule
Mesonephric duct
Hindgut
Allantois
Cloaca
Inguinal fold

Figure 4–3. Early stage in the formation of the meso-nephric kidneys and their collecting ducts in the uro-genital ridge. The central tissue of the ridge is the neph-rogenic cord, in which the mesonephric tubules are forming. The mesonephric ducts grow toward (arrows) and will open into the cloaca. About 5 weeks' gestation.

Metanephros (Definitive Kidney)

A. COLLECTING DUCTS

By the end of the fifth week, a **ureteric bud,** or meta-nephric diverticulum, forms on the caudal part of the mesonephric duct close to the cloaca. The bud gives rise to the collecting tubules, calices, renal pelvis, and ureter (Fig 4–2). The stalk of the elongating bud will become the **ureter** when the ductal segment between the stalk and the cloaca becomes incorporated into the wall of the urinary bladder (which is a derivative of the partitioned cloaca, see text that follows; Figs 4–5 to 4–8). The expanded tip, or **ampulla,** of the bud grows into the adjacent metanephric mesoderm (**blastema**) and subdivides successively into 12–15 generations of buds, or eventual **collecting tubules.** From weeks 10–14, dilatation of the early generations of tubular branches successively produces the **renal pelvis,** the **major calices,** and the **minor calices,** while the middle generations form the medullary collecting tubules. The last several generations of collecting tubules grow centrifugally into the cortical region of the kidney between weeks 24 and 36.

B. NEPHRONS

Continued maintenance of the intimate relationship of the metanephric blastema and ampulla is necessary for normal formation of the definitive excretory units (nephrons), which starts at about the eighth week. Formation of urine purportedly begins at about weeks 10–13, when an estimated 20% of the nephrons are morphologically mature.

The last month of gestation is marked by interstitial growth, hypertrophy of existing components of uriniferous tubules, and the disappearance of bud primordia for collecting tubules. Opinions differ about whether formation of nephrons ceases prenatally at about 28 or 32 weeks or postnatally during the first several months. If the ureteric bud fails to form, undergoes early degeneration, or fails to grow into the nephrogenic mesoderm, aberrations of nephrogenesis result. These may be nonthreatening (**unilateral renal agenesis**), severe, or even fatal (**bilateral renal agenesis, polycystic kidney**).

C. POSITIONAL CHANGES

Figure 4–9 illustrates relocation of the kidney to a deeper position within the posterior body wall, as well as the approximately 90-degree medial rotation of the organ on its longitudinal axis. Rotation and lateral positioning probably are facilitated by the growth of midline structures (axial skeleton and muscles). The "ascent" of the kidney between weeks 5 and 8 can be attributed largely to differential longitudinal growth of the rest of the lumbosacral area and to the reduction of the rather sharp curvature of the caudal region of the embryo. Some migration of the kidney may also occur. Straightening of the curvature also may be attributable to relative changes in growth, especially the development of the infraumbilical abdominal wall. As the kidney moves into its final position (lumbar 1–3 by the 12th week), its arterial supply shifts to successively higher aortic levels. Ectopic kidneys can result from abnormal "ascent." During the seventh week, the "ascending" metanephroi closely approach each other near the aortic bifurcation. The close approximation of the 2 developing kidneys can lead to fusion of the lower poles of the kidneys, resulting in formation of a single **horseshoe kidney,** the ascent of which would be arrested by the stem of the interior mesenteric artery. Infrequently, a **pelvic kidney** results from trapping of the organ beneath the umbilical artery, which restricts passage out of the pelvis.

THE GENITAL SYSTEM

Sexual differentiation of the genital system occurs in a basically sequential order: genetic, gonadal, ductal,

Table 4–1. Adult derivatives and vestigial remains of embryonic urogenital structures.

Embryonic Structure	Male	Female
Indifferent gonad 　Cortex 　Medulla	*Testis* 　*Seminiferous tubules* 　*Rete testis*	*Ovary* 　*Ovarian follicles* 　*Medulla* 　*Rete ovarii*
Gubernaculum	Gubernaculum testis	*Ovarian ligament* *Round ligament of uterus*
Mesonephric tubules	*Ductus efferentes* Paradidymis	Epoophoron Paroophoron
Mesonephric duct	Appendix of epididymis *Ductus epididymidis* *Ductus deferens* *Ureter, pelvis, calices, and collecting tubules* *Ejaculatory duct and seminal vesicle*	Appendix vesiculosa Duct of epoophoron Duct of Gartner *Ureter, pelvis, calices, and collecting tubules*
Paramesonephric duct	Appendix of testis	Hydatid (of Morgagni) *Uterine tube* *Uterus* *Vagina (fibromuscular wall)*
Urogenital sinus	*Urinary bladder* *Urethra* (except glandular portion) Prostatic utricle *Prostate gland* *Bulbourethral glands*	*Urinary bladder* *Urethra* *Vagina* *Urethral and paraurethral glands* *Greater vestibular glands*
Müllerian tubercle	Seminal colliculus	Hymen
Genital tubercle	*Penis* 　*Glans penis* 　*Corpora cavernosa penis* 　*Corpus spongiosum*	*Clitoris* 　*Glans clitoridis* 　*Corpora cavernosa clitoridis* 　*Bulb of the vestibule*
Urogenital folds	*Ventral aspect of penis*	*Labia minora*
Labioscrotal swellings	*Scrotum*	*Labia majora*

Functional derivatives are in italics.
Modified and reproduced, with permission, from Moore KL, Persaud TVN: *The Developing Human: Clinically Oriented Embryology*, 5th ed. Saunders, 1993.

and genital. **Genetic sex** is determined at fertilization by the complement of sex chromosomes (ie, XY specifies a genotypic male and XX a female). However, early morphologic indications of the sex of the developing embryo do not appear until about the eighth or ninth week after conception. Thus, there is a so-called **indifferent stage,** when morphologic identity of sex is not clear or when preferential differentiation for one sex has not been imposed on the sexless primordia. This is characteristic of early developmental stages for the gonads, genital ducts, and external genitalia. When the influence of genetic sex has been expressed on the indifferent gonad, **gonadal sex** is established. The **SRY** (**sex-determining region of the Y chromo-**

some) gene in the short arm of the Y chromosome of normal genetic males is considered the best candidate for the gene encoding for the **testis-determining factor** (**TDF**). TDF initiates a chain of events that results in differentiation of the gonad into a testis with its subsequent production of antimüllerian hormone and testosterone, which influences development of somatic "maleness" (see Testis). Normal genetic females do not have the SRY gene, and the early undifferentiated medullary region of their presumptive gonad does not produce the TDF (see Ovary).

The testis and ovary are derived from the same primordial tissue, but histologically visible differentiation toward a testis occurs sooner than that toward an ovary.

Table 4–2. Developmental chronology of the human urogenital system.

Age in Weeks[1]	Size (C–R) in mm	Urogenital System
2.5	1.5	Allantois present.
3.5	2.5	All pronephric tubules formed. Pronephric duct growing caudad as a blind tube. Cloaca and cloacal membrane present.
4	5	Primordial germ cells near allantois. Pronephros degenerated. Pronephric (mesonephric) duct reaches cloaca. Mesonephric tubules differentiating rapidly. Metanephric bud pushes into secretory primordium.
5	8	Mesonephros reaches its caudal limit. Ureteric and pelvic primordia distinct.
6	12	Cloaca subdividing into urogenital sinus and anorectal canal. Sexless gonad and genital tubercle prominent. Paramesonephric duct appearing. Metanephric collecting tubules begin branching.
7	17	Mesonephros at peak of differentiation. Urogenital sinus separated from anorectal canal (cloaca subdivided). Urogenital and anal membranes rupturing.
8	23	Earliest metanephric secretory tubules differentiating. Testis (8 weeks) and ovary (9–10 weeks) identifiable as such. Paramesonephric ducts, nearing urogenital sinus, are ready to unite a uterovaginal primordium. Genital ligaments indicated.
10	40	Kidney able to excrete urine. Bladder expands as sac. Genital duct of opposite sex degenerating. Bulbourethral and vestibular glands appearing. Vaginal bulbs forming.
12	56	Kidney in lumbar location. Early ovarian folliculogenesis begins. Uterine horns absorbed. External genitalia attain distinctive features. Mesonephros and rete tubules complete male duct. Prostate and seminal vesicle appearing. Hollow viscera gaining muscular walls.
16	112	Testis at deep inguinal ring. Uterus and vagina recognizable as such. Mesonephros involuted.
20–38 (5–9 months)	160–350	Female urogenital sinus becoming a shallow vestibule (5 months). Vagina regains lumen (5 months). Uterine glands begin to appear (5 months). Scrotum solid until sacs and testes descend (7–8 months). Kidney tubules cease forming at birth.

[1]After fertilization.
C–R, crown–rump length.
Modified and reproduced, with permission, from Arey LB: *Developmental Anatomy,* 7th ed. Saunders, 1965.

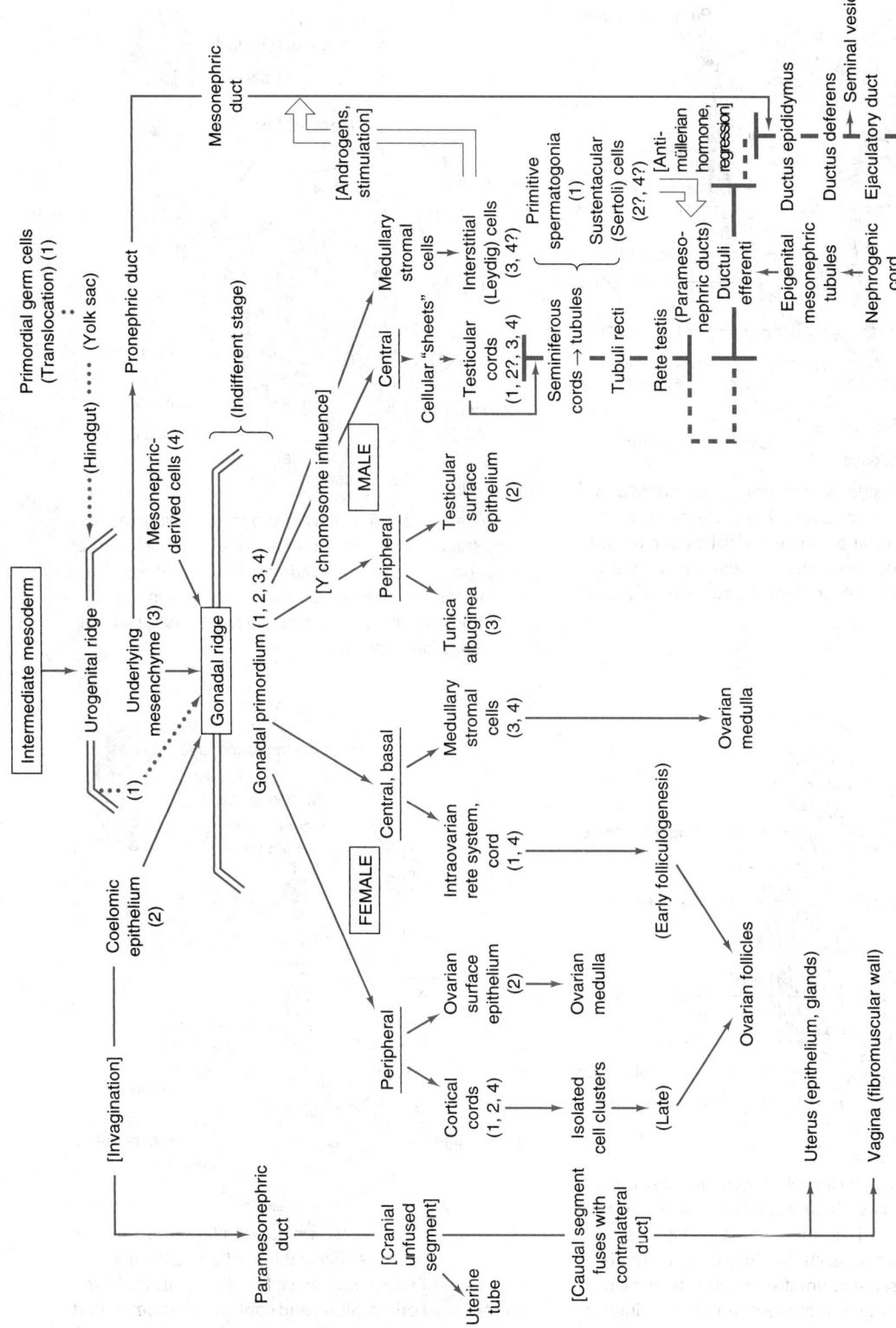

Figure 4-4. Schematic drawing of the formation of the gonads and genital ducts.

71

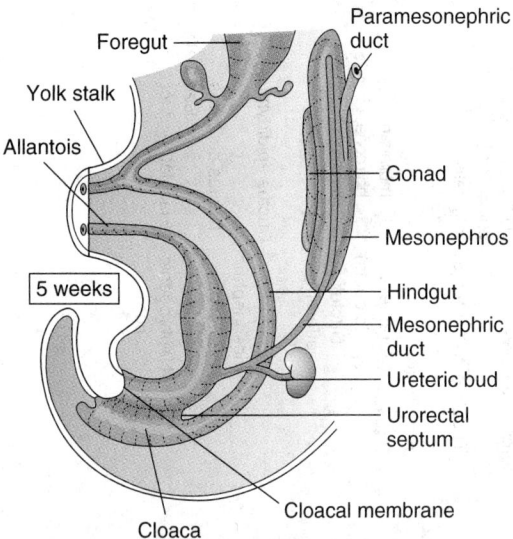

Figure 4–5. Left-side view of urogenital system and cloacal region prior to subdivision of cloaca by urorectal septum (Tourneux and Rathke folds). Position of future paramesonephric duct is shown (begins in the sixth week). Gonad is in the indifferent stage (sexually undifferentiated).

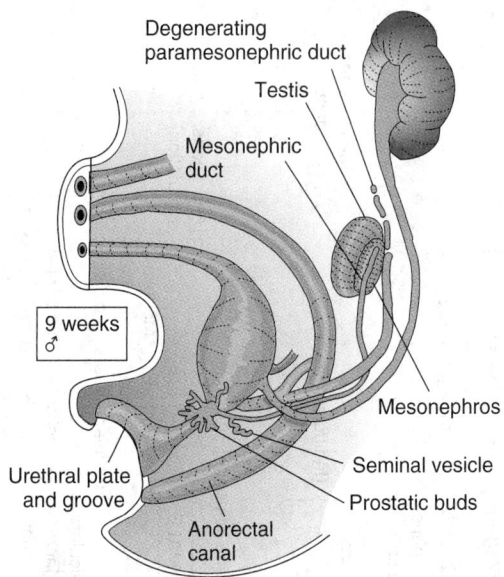

Figure 4–7. Left-side view of urogenital system at an early stage of male sexual differentiation. Phallic part of urogenital sinus is proliferating anteriorly to form the urethral plate and groove. Seminal vesicles and prostatic buds are shown at a more advanced stage (about 12 weeks) for emphasis.

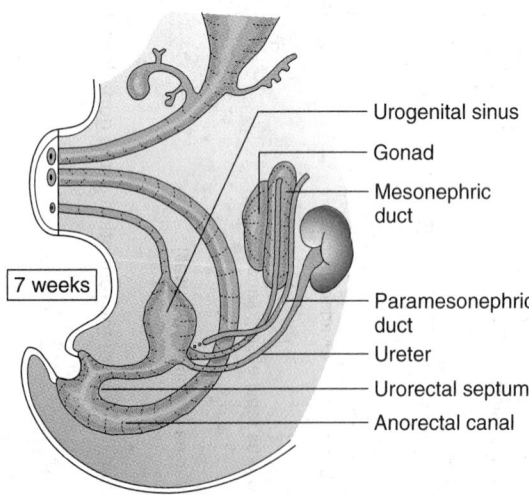

Figure 4–6. Left-side view of urogenital system. Urorectal septum nearly subdivides the cloaca into the urogenital sinus and the anorectal canal. Paramesonephric ducts do not reach the sinus until the ninth week. Gonad is sexually undifferentiated. Note incorporation of caudal segment of mesonephric duct into urogenital sinus (compare with Fig 4–5).

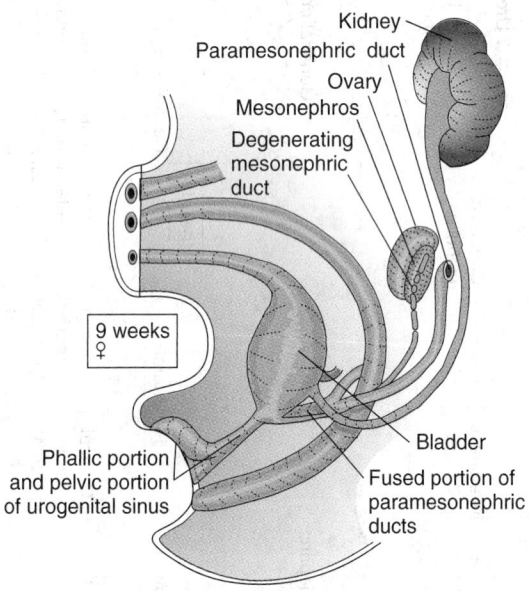

Figure 4–8. Left-side view of urogenital system at an early stage of female sexual differentiation. Paramesonephric (müllerian) ducts have fused caudally (to form uterovaginal primordium) and contacted the pelvic part of the urogenital sinus.

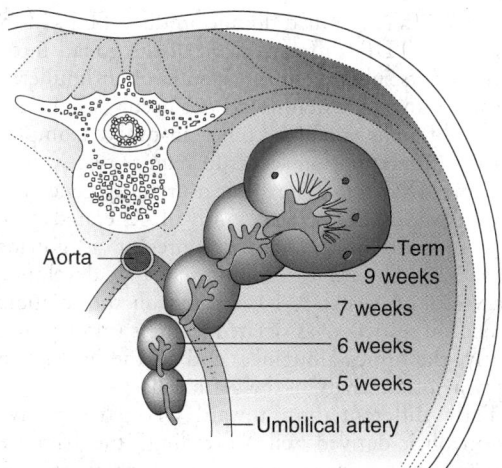

Figure 4–9. Positional changes of the definitive kidney at 5 different stages but projected on one cross-sectional plane.

An "ovary" is first recognized by the absence of testicular histogenesis (eg, thick tunica albuginea) or by the presence of germ cells entering meiotic prophase between the 8th and about the 11th week. The different primordia for male and female genital ducts exist in each embryo during overlapping periods, but establishment of male or female **ductal sex** depends on the presence or absence, respectively, of testicular products and the sensitivity of tissues to these products. The 2 primary testicular products are androgenic steroids (**testosterone** and nonsteroidal **antimüllerian hormone**) (see Testis). Stimulation by testosterone influences the persistence and differentiation of the "male" mesonephric ducts (**wolffian ducts**), whereas antimüllerian hormone influences regression of the "female" paramesonephric ducts (**müllerian ducts**). Absence of these hormones in a nonaberrant condition specifies persistence of müllerian ducts and regression of wolffian ducts, ie, initiation of development of the uterus and uterine tubes. **Genital sex** (external genitalia) subsequently develops according to the absence or presence of androgen. Thus, *the inherent pattern of differentiation of the genital system can be viewed as one directed toward somatic "femaleness" unless the system is dominated by certain factors for "maleness" (eg, gene expression of the Y chromosome, androgenic steroids, and antimüllerian hormone).*

THE GONADS

Indifferent (Sexless) Stage

Gonadogenesis temporally overlaps metanephrogenesis and interacts with tissues of the mesonephric system.

Formation of the gonad is summarized schematically in Fig 4–4.

Around the fifth week, the midportion of each urogenital ridge thickens as cellular condensation forms the **gonadal ridge.** For the next 2 weeks, this ridge is an undifferentiated cell mass, lacking either testicular or ovarian morphology. As shown in Fig 4–4, the cell mass consists of (1) **primordial germ cells,** which translocate into the ridge, and a mixture of **somatic cells** derived by (2) proliferation of the **coelomic epithelial cells,** (3) condensation of the **underlying mesenchyme** of part of the urogenital ridge, and (4) ingrowth of **mesonephric-derived cells.**

The end of the gonadal indifferent stage in the male is near the middle of the seventh week, when a basal lamina delineates the coelomic epithelium and the developing tunica albuginea separates the coelomic epithelium from the developing testicular cords. The indifferent stage in the female ends around the ninth week, when the first oogonia enter meiotic prophase.

Primordial germ cells, presumptive progenitors of the gametes, become evident in the late third to early fourth week in the dorsocaudal wall of the yolk sac and the mesenchyme around the allantois. The **allantois** is a caudal diverticulum of the yolk sac that extends distally into the primitive umbilical stalk and, after embryonic flexion, is adjacent proximally to the cloacal hindgut. The primordial germ cells are translocated from the allantoic region (about the middle of the fourth week) to the urogenital ridge (between the middle of the fifth week and late in the sixth week). It is not known whether primordial germ cells must be present in the gonadal ridge for full differentiation of the gonad to occur. The initial stages of somatic development appear to occur independently of the germ cells. Later endocrine activity in the testis, but not in the ovary, is known to occur in the absence of germ cells. The germ cells appear to have some influence on gonadal differentiation at certain stages of development.

Testis

During early differentiation of the testis, there are condensations of germ cells and somatic cells, which have been described as platelike groups, or sheets. These groups are at first distributed throughout the gonad and then become more organized as primitive **testicular cords.** The cords begin to form centrally and are arranged somewhat perpendicular to the long axis of the gonad. In response to TDF, these cords differentiate into Sertoli cells. The first characteristic feature of male gonadal sex differentiation is evident around week 8, when the **tunica albuginea** begins to form in the mesenchymal tissue underlying the coelomic epithelium. Eventually, this thickened layer of tissue causes the developing testicular cords to be separated from the surface epithelium and placed deeper in the central region of the gonad. The surface epithelium re-forms a basal lamina and later thins to a mesothelial covering of the gonad. The testicular cords coil peripherally and thicken as their cellular organization becomes more distinct. A basal lamina eventually develops in the testicular cords, although it is not known if the somatic cells, germ cells, or both are primary contributors to the lamina.

Throughout gonadal differentiation, the developing testicular cords appear to maintain a close relationship to the basal area of the mesonephric-derived cell mass. An interconnected network of cords, **rete cords,** develops in this cell mass and gives rise to the **rete testis.** The rete testis joins centrally with neighboring epigenital mesonephric tubules, which become the **efferent ductules** linking the rete testis with the epididymis, a derivative of the mesonephric duct. With gradual enlargement of the testis and regression of the mesonephros, a cleft forms between the 2 organs, slowly creating the mesentery of the testis, the **mesorchium.**

The differentiating testicular cords are made up of primordial germ cells (primitive spermatogonia) and somatic "supporting" cells (**sustentacular cells,** or **Sertoli cells**). Some precocious meiotic activity has been observed in the fetal testis. Meiosis in the germ cells usually does not begin until puberty; the cause of this delay is unknown. Besides serving as "supporting cells" for the primitive spermatogonia, Sertoli cells also produce the glycoprotein **antimüllerian hormone** (also called **müllerian-inhibiting substance**). Antimüllerian hormone causes regression of the paramesonephric (müllerian) ducts, apparently during a very discrete period of ductal sensitivity in male fetuses. At puberty, the seminiferous cords mature to become the seminiferous tubules, and the Sertoli cells and spermatogonia mature.

Shortly after the testicular cords form, the steroid-producing **interstitial (Leydig) cells** of the extracordal compartment of the testis differentiate from stromal mesenchymal cells, probably due to antimüllerian hormone. Mesonephric-derived cells may also be a primordial source of Leydig cells. Steroidogenic activity of Leydig cells begins near the tenth week. High levels of testosterone are produced during the period of differentiation of external genitalia (weeks 11–12) and maintained through weeks 16–18. Steroid levels then rise or fall somewhat in accordance with changes in the concentration of Leydig cells. Both the number of cells and the levels of testosterone decrease around the fifth month.

Ovary

A. DEVELOPMENT

In the normal absence of the Y chromosome or the sex-determining region of the Y chromosome (SRY gene; see The Genital System), the somatic sex cords of the indifferent gonad do not produce TDF. In the absence of TDF, differentiation of the gonad into a testis and its subsequent production of antimüllerian hormone and testosterone do not occur (see Testis). The indifferent gonad becomes an ovary. Complete ovarian differentiation seems to require two X chromosomes (XO females exhibit ovarian dysgenesis, in which ovaries have precociously degenerated germ cells and no follicles and are present as gonadal "streaks"). The first recognition of a developing ovary around weeks 9–10 is based on the temporal absence of testicular-associated features (most prominently, the tunica albuginea) and on the presence of early meiotic activity in the germ cells.

Early differentiation toward an ovary involves mesonephric-derived cells "invading" the basal region (adjacent to mesonephros) and central region of the gonad (central and basal regions represent the primitive "medullary" region of the gonad). At the same time, clusters of germ cells are displaced somewhat peripherally into the "cortical" region of the gonad. Some of the central mesonephric cells give rise to the rete system that subsequently forms a network of cords (**intraovarian rete cords**) extending to the primitive cortical area. As these cords extend peripherally between germ clusters, several epithelial cell proliferations extend centrally, and some mixing of these somatic cells apparently takes place around the germ cell clusters. These early cordlike structures are more irregularly distributed than early cords in the testis and not distinctly outlined. The cords open into clusters of germ cells, but all germ cells are not confined to cords. The first oogonia that begin meiosis are located in the innermost part of the cortex and are the first germ cells to contact the intraovarian rete cords.

Folliculogenesis begins in the innermost part of the cortex when the central somatic cells of the cord contact and surround the germ cells while an intact basal lamina is laid down. These somatic cells are morphologically similar to the mesonephric cells that form the intraovarian rete cords associated with the oocytes and apparently differentiate into the presumptive granulosa cells of the early follicle. Folliculogenesis continues peripherally. Between weeks 12 and 20 of gestation, proliferative activity causes the surface epithelium to become a thickened, irregular multilayer of cells. In the absence of a basal lamina, the cells and apparent epithelial cell cords mix with underlying tissues. These latter cortical cords often retain a connection to and appear similar to the surface epithelium. The epithelial cells of these cords probably differentiate into granulosa cells and contribute to folliculogenesis, although this occurs after the process is well under way in the central region of the gonad. Follicles fail to form in the absence of oocytes or with precocious loss of germ cells, and oocytes not encompassed by follicular cells degenerate.

Stromal mesenchymal cells, connective tissue, and somatic cells of cords not participating in folliculogenesis form the **ovarian medulla** in the late fetal ovary. Individual **primordial follicles** containing diplotene oocytes populate the inner and outer cortex of this ovary. The rete ovarii may persist, along with a few vestiges of mesonephric tubules, as the vestigial epoophoron near the adult ovary. Finally, similar to the testicular mesorchium, the **mesovarium** eventually forms as a gonadal mesentery between the ovary and old urogenital ridge. Postnatally, the epithelial surface of the ovary consists of a single layer of cells continuous with peritoneal mesothelium at the ovarian hilum. A thin, fibrous connective tissue, the tunica albuginea, forms beneath the surface epithelium and separates it from the cortical follicles.

B. ANOMALIES OF THE OVARIES

Anomalies of the ovaries encompass a broad range of developmental errors from complete absence of the ovaries to supernumerary ovaries. The many variations of gonadal disorders usually are subcategorized within classifications of disorders of sex determination. Unfortunately, there is little consensus for a major classification, although most include pathogenetic consideration. Extensive summaries of the different classifications are offered in the references to this chapter.

Congenital absence of the ovary (no gonadal remnants found) is very rare. Two types have been considered, agenesis and agonadism. By definition, **agenesis** implies that the primordial gonad did not form in the urogenital ridge, whereas **agonadism** indicates the absence of gonads that may have formed initially and subsequently degenerated. It can be difficult to distinguish one type from the other on a practical basis. For example, a patient with female genital ducts and external genitalia and a 46,XY karyotype could represent either gonadal agenesis or agonadism. In the latter condition, the gonad may form but undergo early degeneration and resorption before any virilizing expression is made. *Whenever congenital absence of the ovaries is suspected, careful examination of the karyotype, the external genitalia, and the genital ducts must be performed.*

Descriptions of agonadism usually have indicated that the external genitalia are abnormal (variable degree of fusion of labioscrotal swellings) and that either very rudimentary ductal derivatives are present or there are no genital ducts. The cause of agonadism is unknown, although several explanations have been suggested, such as (1) failure of the primordial gonad to form, along with abnormal formation of ductal an-

lagen, and (2) partial differentiation and then regression and absorption of testes (accounting for suppression of müllerian ducts but lack of stimulation of mesonephric, or wolffian, ducts). Explanations that include teratogenic effects or genetic defects are more likely candidates in view of the associated incidence of nonsexual somatic anomalies with the disorder. The **streak gonad** is a product of primordial gonadal formation and subsequent failure of differentiation, which can occur at various stages. The gonad usually appears as a fibrouslike cord of mixed elements (lacking germ cells) located parallel to a uterine tube. Streak gonads are characteristic of **gonadal dysgenesis** and a 45,XO karyotype (**Turner's syndrome;** distinctions are drawn between Turner's syndrome and **Turner's stigmata** when consideration is given to the various associated somatic anomalies of gonadal dysgenesis). However, streak gonads may be consequent to genetic mutation or hereditary disease other than the anomalous karyotype.

Ectopic ovarian tissue occasionally can be found as **accessory ovarian tissue** or as **supernumerary ovaries.** The former may be a product of disaggregation of the embryonic ovary, and the latter may arise from the urogenital ridge as independent primordia.

SUBDIVISION OF THE CLOACA & FORMATION OF THE UROGENITAL SINUS

The endodermally lined urogenital sinus is derived by partitioning of the endodermal cloaca. It is the precursor of the urinary bladder in both sexes and the urinary and genital structures specific to each sex (Fig 4–1). The cloaca is a pouchlike enlargement of the caudal end of the hindgut and is formed by the process of "folding" of the caudal region of the embryonic disk between 4 and 5 weeks' gestation (see Overview of the First Four Weeks of Development; Figs 4–1 and 4–3). During the "tail-fold" process, the posteriorly placed allantois, or allantoic diverticulum of the yolk sac, becomes an anterior extension of the cloaca (Figs 4–3 and 4–5). Soon after the cloaca forms, it receives posterolaterally the caudal ends of the paired mesonephric ducts and hence becomes a junctional cistern for the allantois, the hindgut, and the ducts. A **cloacal membrane,** composed of ectoderm and endoderm, is the caudal limit of the primitive gut and temporarily separates the cloacal cavity from the extraembryonic confines of the amniotic cavity (Fig 4–5).

Between weeks 5 and 7, 3 wedges of splanchnic mesoderm, collectively called the **urorectal septum,** proliferate in the coronal plane in the caudal region of the embryo to eventually subdivide the cloaca (Figs 4–5 to 4–8). The superior wedge, called the **Tourneux**

fold, is in the angle between the allantois and the primitive hindgut, and it proliferates caudally into the superior end of the cloaca (Fig 4–5). The other 2 mesodermal wedges, called the **Rathke folds,** proliferate in the right and left walls of the cloaca. Beginning adjacent to the cloacal membrane, these laterally placed folds grow toward each other and the Tourneux fold. With fusion of the 3 folds creating a urorectal septum, the once single chamber is subdivided into the primitive **urogenital sinus** (ventrally) and the **anorectal canal** of the hindgut (dorsally; Figs 4–6 to 4–8). The mesonephric ducts and allantois then open into the sinus. The uterovaginal primordium of the fused paramesonephric ducts will contact the sinusal wall between the mesonephric ducts early in the ninth week of development. However, it can be noted that the junctional point of fusion of the cloacal membrane and urorectal septum forms the **primitive perineum** (later differentiation creates the so-called perineal body of tissue) and sub-

divides the cloacal membrane into the **urogenital membrane** (anteriorly) and the **anal membrane** (posteriorly; Figs 4–5, 4–8, 4–10, and 4–20).

THE GENITAL DUCTS
Indifferent (Sexless) Stage

Two pairs of genital ducts are initially present in both sexes: (1) the **mesonephric (wolffian) ducts,** which give rise to the male ducts and a derivative, the seminal vesicles; and (2) the **paramesonephric (müllerian) ducts,** which form the oviducts, uterus, and part of the vagina. When the adult structures are described as derivatives of embryonic ducts, this refers to the epithelial lining of the structures. Muscle and connective tissues of the differentiating structures originate from splanchnic mesoderm and mesenchyme adjacent to ducts. Mesonephric ducts are originally the excretory ducts of the mesonephric

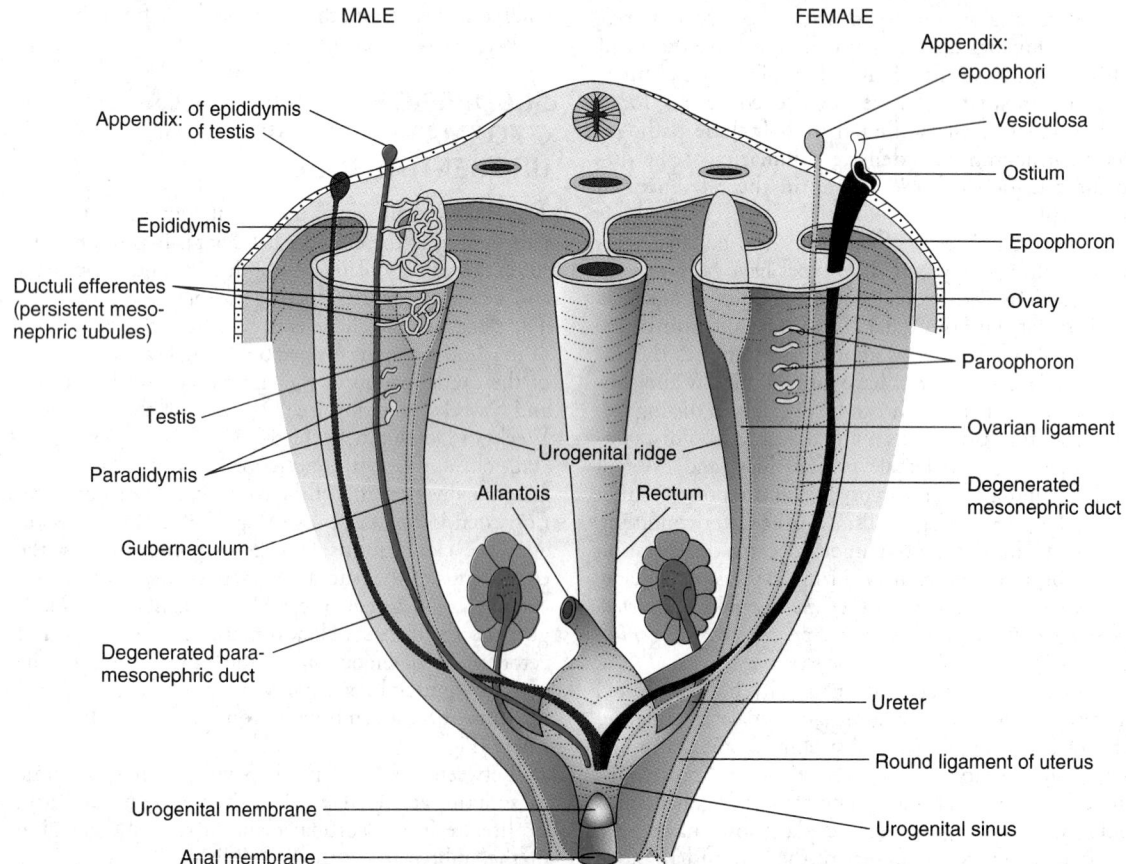

Figure 4–10. Diagrammatic comparison between male and female differentiation of internal genitalia.

"kidneys" (see previous text), and they develop early in the embryonic period, about 2 weeks before development of paramesonephric ducts (weeks 6–10). The 2 pairs of genital ducts share a close anatomic relationship in their bilateral course through the urogenital ridge. At their caudal limit, both sets contact the part of the cloaca that is later separated as the urogenital sinus (Figs 4–5, 4–6, and 4–10). *Determination of the ductal sex of the embryo (ie, which pair of ducts will continue differentiation rather than undergo regression) is established initially by the gonadal sex and later by the continuing influence of hormones.*

Formation of each paramesonephric duct begins early in the sixth week as an invagination of coelomic epithelium in the lateral wall of the cranial end of the urogenital ridge and adjacent to each mesonephric duct. The free edges of the invaginated epithelium join to form the duct except at the site of origin, which persists as a funnel-shaped opening, the future **ostium of the oviduct.** At first, each paramesonephric duct grows caudally through the mesenchyme of the urogenital ridge and laterally parallel to a mesonephric duct. More inferiorly, the paramesonephric duct has a caudomedial course, passing ventral to the mesonephric duct. As it follows the ventromedial bend of the caudal portion of the urogenital ridge, the paramesonephric duct then lies medial to the mesonephric duct, and its caudal tip lies in close apposition to its counterpart from the opposite side (Fig 4–10). At approximately the eighth week, the caudal segments of the right and left ducts fuse medially and their lumens coalesce to form a single cavity. This conjoined portion of the Y-shaped paramesonephric ducts becomes the uterovaginal primordium, or canal.

Male: Genital Ducts

A. MESONEPHRIC DUCTS

The mesonephric ducts persist in the male and, under the stimulatory influence of testosterone, differentiate into the internal genital ducts (epididymis, ductus deferens, and ejaculatory ducts). Near the cranial end of the duct, some of the mesonephric tubules (epigenital mesonephric tubules) of the mesonephric kidney persist lateral to the developing testis. These tubules form a connecting link, the **ductuli efferentes,** between the duct and the rete testis (Fig 4–10). The cranial portion of each duct becomes the convoluted **ductus epididymis.** The **ductus deferens** forms when smooth muscle from adjacent splanchnic mesoderm is added to the central segment of the mesonephric duct. The seminal vesicle develops as a lateral bud from each mesonephric duct just distal to the junction of the duct and the urogenital sinus (Fig 4–7). The terminal segment of the duct between the sinus and seminal vesicle forms the

ejaculatory duct, which becomes encased by the developing prostate gland early in the 12th week (see Differentiation of the Urogenital Sinus). A vestigial remnant of the duct may persist cranially near the head of the epididymis as the **appendix epididymis,** whereas remnants of mesonephric tubules near the inferior pole of the testis and tail of the epididymis may persist as the **paradidymis** (Fig 4–10).

B. PARAMESONEPHRIC DUCTS

The paramesonephric ducts begin to undergo morphologic regression centrally (and progress cranially and caudally) about the time they meet the urogenital sinus caudally (approximately the start of the ninth week). Regression is effected by nonsteroidal antimüllerian hormone produced by the differentiating Sertoli cells slightly before androgen is produced by the Leydig cells (see Testis). Antimüllerian hormone is produced from the time of early testicular differentiation until birth (ie, not only during the period of regression of the paramesonephric duct). However, ductal sensitivity to antimüllerian hormone in the male seems to exist for only a short "critical" time preceding the first signs of ductal regression. Vestigial remnants of the cranial end of the ducts may persist as the **appendix testis** on the superior pole of the testis (Fig 4–10). Caudally, a ductal remnant is considered to be part of the prostatic utricle of the seminal colliculus in the prostatic urethra.

C. RELOCATION OF THE TESTES AND DUCTS

Around weeks 5–6, a bandlike condensation of mesenchymal tissue in the urogenital ridge forms near the caudal end of the mesonephros. Distally, this gubernacular precursor tissue grows into the area of the undifferentiated tissue of the anterior abdominal wall and toward the genital swellings. Proximally, the **gubernaculum** contacts the mesonephric duct when the mesonephros regresses and the gonad begins to form. By the start of the fetal period, the mesonephric duct begins differentiation and the gubernaculum adheres indirectly to the testis via the duct, which lies in the mesorchium of the testis. The external genitalia differentiate over the seventh to about the 19th week. By the 12th week, the testis is near the deep inguinal ring, and the gubernaculum is virtually at the inferior pole of the testis, proximally, and in the mesenchyme of the scrotal swellings, distally.

Although the testis in early development is near the last thoracic segment, it is still close to the area of the developing deep inguinal ring. With rapid growth of the lumbar region and "ascent" of the metanephric kidney, the testis remains relatively immobilized by the gubernaculum, although there is the appearance of a lengthy transabdominal "descent" from an upper abdominal position. The testis descends through the in-

Figure 4–11. Female genital tract. Gubernacular derivatives and mesonephric vestiges are shown.

guinal canal around the 28th week and into the scrotum about the 32nd week. Testicular blood vessels form when the testis is located on the dorsal body wall and retain their origin during the transabdominal and pelvic descent of the testis. The mesonephric duct follows the descent of the testis and hence passes anterior to the ureter, which follows the retroperitoneal ascent of the kidney (Fig 4–10).

Female: Uterus and Uterine Tubes

A. MESONEPHRIC DUCTS

Virtually all portions of these paired ducts degenerate in the female embryo, with the exception of the most caudal segment between the ureteric bud and the cloaca, which is later incorporated into the posterior wall of the urogenital sinus (Figs 4–5 and 4–6) as the **trigone of the urinary bladder.** Regression begins just after gonadal sex differentiation and is finished near the onset of the third trimester. Cystlike or tubular vestiges of mesonephric duct (Fig 4–11) may persist to variable degrees parallel with the vagina and uterus (**Gartner's cysts**). Other mesonephric remnants of the duct or tubules may persist in the broad ligament (**epoophoron**).

B. PARAMESONEPHRIC DUCTS

Differentiation of müllerian ducts in female embryos produces the uterine tubes, uterus, and probably the fibromuscular wall of the vagina. In contrast to the ductal/gonadal relationship in the male, ductal differentiation in the female does not require the presence of ovaries. Formation of the bilateral paramesonephric ducts during the second half of the embryonic period has been described [see Indifferent (Sexless) Stage]. By the onset of the fetal period, the 2 ducts are joined caudally in the midline, and the fused segment of the new Y-shaped ductal structure is the **uterovaginal primordium** (Fig 4–8). The nonfused cranial part of each

paramesonephric duct gives rise to the **uterine tubes** (oviducts), and the distal end of this segment remains open and will form the **ostium of the oviduct.**

Early in the ninth week, the uterovaginal primordium contacts medially the dorsal wall of the urogenital sinus. This places the primordium at a median position between the bilateral openings of the mesonephric ducts, which joined the dorsal wall during the fifth week before subdivision of the urogenital sinus from the cloaca occurred (Figs 4–8 and 4–9). A ventral protrusion of the dorsal wall of the urogenital sinus forms at the area of contact of the uterovaginal primordium with the wall and between the openings of the mesonephric ducts. In reference to its location, this protrusion is called the **sinusal tubercle (sinus tubercle, paramesonephric tubercle, müllerian tubercle).** This tubercle may consist of several types of epithelia derived from the different ducts as well as from the wall of the sinus.

Shortly after the sinusal tubercle forms, midline fusion of the middle and caudal portions of the paramesonephric ducts is complete, and the vertical septum (apposed walls of the fused ducts) within the newly established uterovaginal primordium degenerates, creating a single cavity or canal (Fig 4–12). The solid tip of this primordium continues to grow caudally, while a mesen-

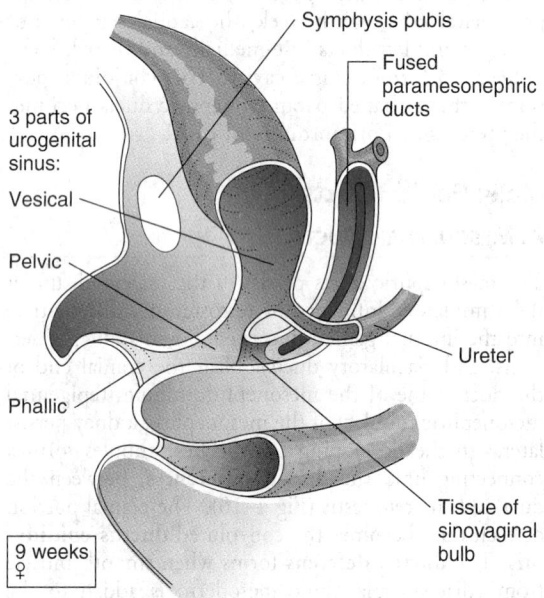

Figure 4–12. Sagittal cutaway view of female urogenital sinus and uterovaginal primordium (fused paramesonephric ducts). Sinovaginal bulbs form in the tenth week.

chymal thickening gradually surrounds the cervical region of the uterovaginal primordium. The primordium gives rise to the fundus, body, and isthmus of the uterus, specifically the endometrial epithelium and glands of the uterus. The endometrial stroma and smooth muscle of the myometrium are derived from adjacent splanchnic mesenchyme. The epithelium of the cervix forms from the lower aspect of the primordium. Development of the various components of the uterus covers the 3 trimesters of gestation. The basic structure is generated during the latter part of the first trimester. The initial formation of glands and muscular layer occurs near midgestation, whereas mucinous cells in the cervix appear during the third trimester.

The formation of the vagina is discussed in Differentiation of the Urogenital Sinus, even though the question of whether the vaginal epithelium is a sinusal or paramesonephric derivative (or both) has not been resolved. The fibromuscular wall of the vagina is generally considered to be derived from the uterovaginal primordium (Fig 4–13).

C. RELOCATION OF THE OVARIES AND FORMATION OF LIGAMENTS

Transabdominal "descent" of the ovary, unlike that of the testis, is restricted to a relatively short distance, presumably (at least partly) because of attachment of the gubernaculum to the paramesonephric duct. Hence, relocation of the ovary appears to involve both (1) a passive rotatory movement of the ovary as its mesentery is drawn by the twist of the developing ductal mesenteries and (2) extensive growth of the lumbosacral region of the fetus. The ovarian vessels (like the testicular vessels) originate or drain near the point of development of the gonad, the arteries from the aorta just inferior to the renal arteries and the veins to the left renal vein or to the vena cava from the right gonad.

Initial positioning of the ovary on the anteromedial aspect of the urogenital ridge is depicted in Fig 4–10, as is the relationship of the paramesonephric duct lateral to the degenerating mesonephros, the ovary, and the urogenital mesentery. The urogenital mesentery between the ridge and the dorsal body wall represents the first mesenteric support for structures developing in the ridge.

Alterations within the urogenital ridge eventually result in formation of contiguous double-layered mesenteries supporting the ovary and segments of the paramesonephric ducts. Enlargement of the ovary and degeneration of the adjacent mesonephric tissue bring previously separated layers of coelomic mesothelium into near apposition, establishing the mesentery of the ovary, the **mesovarium.** Likewise, mesonephric degeneration along the region of differentiation of the unfused cranial segment of the paramesonephric ducts establishes the **mesosalpinx.** Caudally, growth and fusion ventromedially of these bilateral ducts "sweep" the once medially attached mesenteries of the ducts toward the midline. These bilateral mesenteries merge over the fused uterovaginal primordium and extend laterally to the pelvic wall to form a continuous double-layered "drape," the **mesometrium of the broad ligament,** between the upper portion of the primordium and the posterolateral body wall. This central expanse of mesentery creates the rectouterine and vesicouterine pouches. The midline caudal fusion of the ducts also alters the previous longitudinal orientation of the upper free segments of the ducts (the oviducts) to a near transverse orientation. During this alteration, the attached mesovarium is drawn from a medial relationship into a posterior relationship with the paramesonephric mesentery of the mesosalpinx and the mesometrium.

The **suspensory ligament of the ovary,** through which the ovarian vessels, nerves, and lymphatics traverse, forms when cranial degeneration of the mesonephric tissue and regression of the urogenital ridge adjacent to the ovary reduce these tissues to a peritoneal fold.

The **round ligament of the uterus** and the **proper ovarian ligament** are both derivatives of the **gubernaculum,** which originates as a mesenchymal condensation at the caudal end of the mesonephros and extends over the initially short distance to the anterior abdominal wall (see Relocation of the Testes and Ducts). As the gonad enlarges and the mesonephric tissue degenerates, the cranial attachment of the gubernaculum appears to "shift" to the inferior aspect of the ovary. Distally, growth of the fibrous gubernaculum continues into the inguinal region. However, the midportion of the gubernaculum becomes attached, inexplicably, to the paramesonephric duct at the uterotubal junction. Formation of the uterovaginal primordium by caudal fusion of the paramesonephric ducts apparently carries the attached gubernaculum medially within the cover of the encompassing mesentery of the structures (ie, the parts of the developing broad ligament). This fibrous band of connective tissue eventually becomes 2 ligaments.

Cranially, the band is the proper ligament of the ovary, extending between the inferior pole of the ovary and the lateral wall of the uterus just inferior to the oviduct. Caudally, it continues as the uterine round ligament from a point just inferior to the proper ovarian ligament and extending through the inguinal canal to the labium majus.

D. ANOMALIES OF THE UTERINE TUBES (OVIDUCTS, FALLOPIAN TUBES)

The uterine tubes are derivatives of the cranial segments of the paramesonephric (müllerian) ducts, which differ-

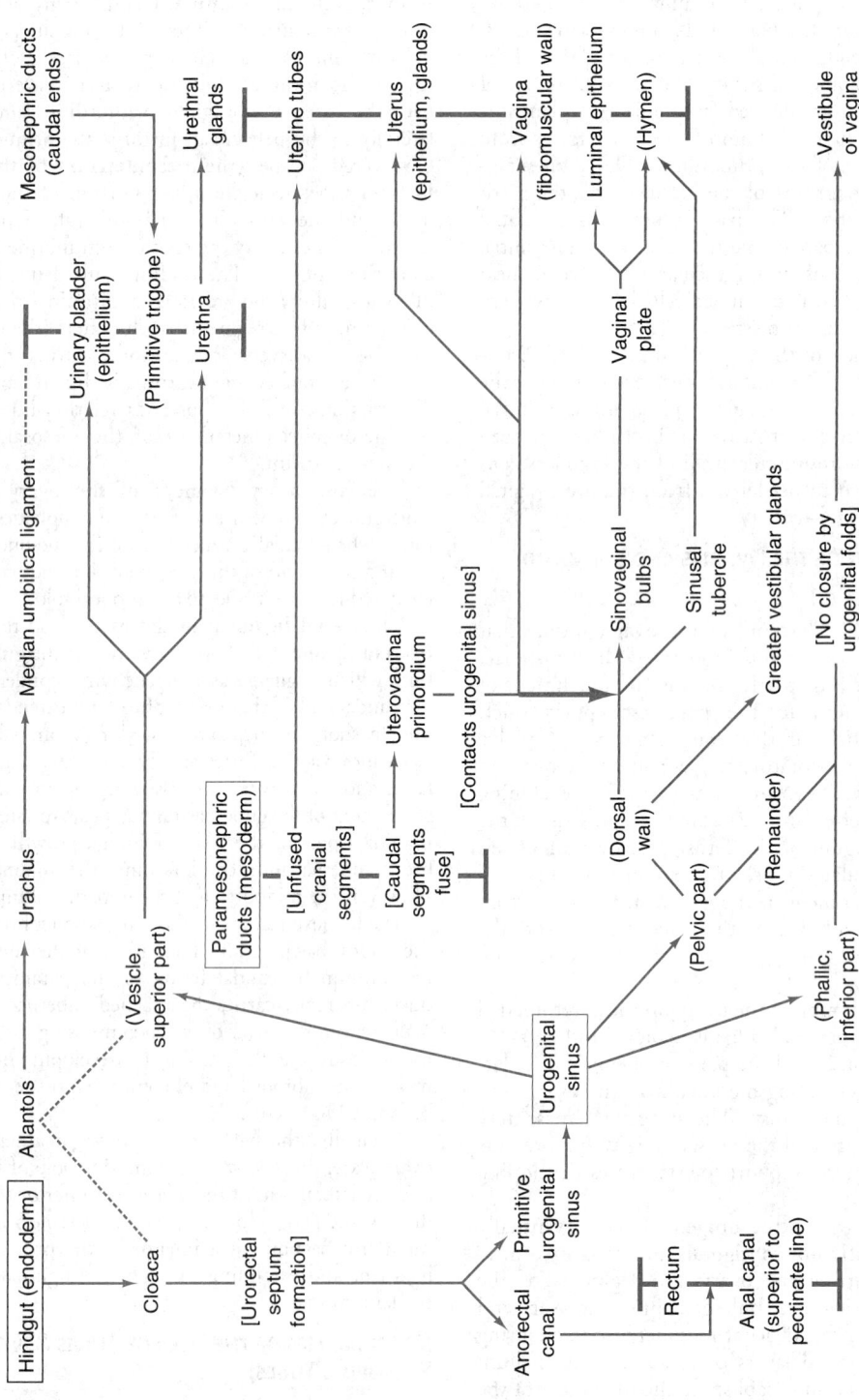

Figure 4–13. Schematic drawing of differentiation of urogenital sinus and paramesonephric ducts in the female; formation of urinary bladder, urethra, uterine tubes, uterus, and vagina. (Explanatory symbols are given in Fig 4–1.)

entiate in the urogenital ridge between the sixth and ninth weeks (Fig 4–10). Ductal formation begins with invagination of the coelomic epithelium in the lateral coelomic bay. The initial depression remains open to proliferate and differentiate into the ostium (Fig 4–10). Variable degrees of **duplication of the ostium** sometimes occur; in such cases, the leading edges of the initial ductal groove presumably did not fuse completely or anomalous proliferation of epithelium around the opening occurred.

Absence of a uterine tube is very rare when otherwise normal ductal and genital derivatives are present. This anomaly has been associated with (1) ipsilateral absence of an ovary and (2) ipsilateral unicornuate uterus (and probable anomalous broad ligament). Bilateral absence of the uterine tubes is most frequently associated with lack of formation of the uterus and anomalies of the external genitalia. Interestingly, absence of the derivatives of the lower part of the müllerian ducts with persistence of the uterine tubes occurs more frequently than the reverse condition. This might be expected, as the müllerian ducts form in a craniocaudal direction.

Partial absence of a uterine tube (middle or caudal segment) also has been reported. The cause of partial absence is unknown, although several theories have been advanced. One theory holds that when the unilateral anomaly coincides with ipsilateral ovarian absence, a "vascular accident" might occur following differentiation of the ducts and ovaries. Obviously, various factors resulting in somewhat localized atresia could be proposed. From a different perspective, bilateral absence of the uterine tubes as an associated disorder in a female external phenotype is characteristic of **testicular feminization syndrome** (nonpersistence of the rest of the paramesonephric ducts, anomalous external genitalia, hypoplastic male genital ducts, and testicular differentiation with usual ectopic location).

E. ANOMALIES OF THE UTERUS

The epithelium of the uterus and cervix and the fibromuscular wall of the vagina are derived from the paramesonephric (müllerian) ducts, the caudal ends of which fuse medially to form the uterovaginal primordium. Most of the primordium gives rise to the uterus (Fig 4–13). Subsequently, the caudal tip of the primordium contacts the pelvic part of the urogenital sinus, and the interaction of the sinus (sinovaginal bulbs) and primordium leads to differentiation of the vagina. Various steps in this sequential process can go awry, such as (1) complete or partial failure of one or both ducts to form (agenesis), (2) lack of or incomplete fusion of the caudal segments of the paired ducts (abnormal uterovaginal primordium), or (3) fail-

ure of development *after* successful formation (aplasia or hypoplasia). Many types of anomalies may occur because of the number of sites for potential error, the complex interactions necessary for the development of the müllerian derivatives, and the duration of the complete process.

Complete **agenesis of the uterus** is very rare, and associated vaginal anomalies are usually expected. Also, a high incidence of associated structural or positional abnormalities of the kidney has been reported; there has been speculation that the initial error in severe cases may be in the development of the urinary system and then in the formation of the paramesonephric ducts.

Aplasia of the paramesonephric ducts (**müllerian aplasia**) is more common than agenesis and could occur after formation and interaction of the primordium with the urogenital sinus. A rudimentary uterus or a vestigial uterus (ie, varying degrees of fibromuscular tissue present) is most frequently accompanied by partial or complete absence of the vagina. As in uterine agenesis, ectopic kidney or absence of a kidney is frequently associated with uterine aplasia (in about 40% of cases). **Uterine hypoplasia** variably yields a rudimentary or infantile uterus and is associated with normal or abnormal uterine tubes and ovaries. Unilateral agenesis or aplasia of the ducts gives rise to **uterus unicornis,** whereas unilateral hypoplasia may result in a rudimentary horn that may or may not be contiguous with the lumen of the "normal" horn (**uterus bicornis unicollis** with one unconnected rudimentary horn; Fig 4–14). The status of the rudimentary horn must be considered for potential hematometra, or blood in the uterus that cannot exit, at puberty.

Anomalous **unification** caudally of the paramesonephric ducts results in many uterine malformations (Fig 4–14). The incidence of defective fusion is estimated to be 0.1–3% of females. Furthermore, faulty unification of the ducts has been cited as the primary error responsible for most anomalies of the female genital tract. Partial or complete retention of the apposed walls of the paired ducts can produce slight (**uterus subseptus unicollis**) to complete (**uterus bicornis septus**) septal defects in the uterus. Complete failure of unification of the paramesonephric ducts can result in a double uterus (**uterus didelphys**) with either a single or double vagina.

F. ANOMALIES OF THE CERVIX

Because the cervix forms as an integral part of the uterus, cervical anomalies are often the same as uterine anomalies. Thus, absence or hypoplasia of the cervix is rarely found with a normal uterovaginal tract. The cervix appears as a fibrous juncture between the uterine corpus and the vagina.

Uterus subseptus
unicollis

Uterus septus
duplex

Uterus septus
duplex with
double vagina

Herniated level
of cervix

Uterus bicornis
unicollis

Uterus didelphys with
double vagina

Uterus bicornis
septus

Uterus bicornis unicollis
with one unconnected
rudimentary horn

Uterus unicornis

Uterus acollis with
absence of vagina

Uterus communicans septus,
cervix septa, vagina septa*

Uterus communicans bicornis,
cervix duplex, vagina septa
unilateralis atretica*

Uterus communicans bicornis,
cervix duplex, vagina septa*

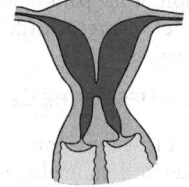

Uterus communicans septus,
cervix duplex, vagina septa*

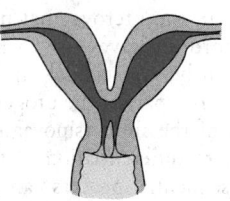

Uterus communicans bicornis,
cervix septa, vagina simplex*

Figure 4–14. **Uterine anomalies.** (*Redrawn and reproduced, with permission, from Toaff R: A major genital malformation: Communicating uteri. Obstet Gynecol 1974;43:221.)

DIFFERENTIATION OF THE UROGENITAL SINUS

Until differentiation of the genital ducts begins, the urogenital sinus appears similar in both sexes during the middle and late embryonic period. For purposes of describing the origin of sinusal derivatives, the sinus can be divided into 3 parts: (1) the **vesical part,** or the large dilated segment superior to the entrance of the mesonephric ducts; (2) the **pelvic part,** or the narrowed tubular segment between the level of the mesonephric ducts and the inferior segment; and (3) the **phallic part,** often referred to as the definitive urogenital sinus (the anteroposteriorly elongated, transversely flattened inferiormost segment) (Fig 4–8). The **urogenital membrane** temporarily closes the inferior limit of the phallic part. The superior limit of the vesical part becomes delimited by conversion of the once tubular allantois to a thick fibrous cord, the **urachus,** by about 12 weeks. After differentiation of the vesical part of the sinus to form the epithelium of the **urinary bladder,** the urachus maintains its continuity between the apex of the bladder and the umbilical cord and is identified postnatally as the **median umbilical ligament.** Various anomalies of urachal formation can present as **urachal fistula, cyst,** or **sinus,** depending on the degree of patency that persists during obliteration of the allantois.

In both sexes, the caudal segments of each mesonephric duct between the urogenital sinus and the level of the ureter of the differentiating metanephric diverticulum (or ureteric bud) become incorporated into the posterocaudal wall of the vesical part (ie, urinary bladder) of the sinus (Figs 4–5 and 4–6). As the dorsal wall of the bladder grows and "absorbs" these caudal segments, the ureters are gradually "drawn" closer to the bladder and eventually open directly and separately into it, dorsolateral to the mesonephric ducts (Figs 4–6 and 4–7). The mesodermal segment of mesonephric duct incorporated into the bladder defines the epithelium of the **trigone of the bladder,** although this mesodermal epithelium is secondarily replaced by the endodermal epithelium of the sinusal bladder. After formation of the trigone, the remainder of each mesonephric duct (ie, the portion that was cranial to the metanephric diverticulum) is joined to the superior end of the pelvic part of the urogenital sinus. Thereafter, the ducts either degenerate (in females) or undergo differentiation (in males).

Male: Urinary Bladder and Urethra (Fig 4–15)

The urogenital sinus gives rise to the endodermal epithelium of the **urinary bladder,** the prostatic and membranous urethra, and most of the spongy (penile) urethra (except the glandular urethra). Outgrowths from its derivatives produce epithelial parts of the prostate and bul-

bourethral glands (Fig 4–15). The **prostatic urethra** receives the ejaculatory ducts (derived from the mesonephric ducts) and arises from 2 parts of the urogenital sinus. The portion of this urethral segment superior to the ejaculatory ducts originates from the inferiormost area of the vesical part of the sinus. The lower portion of the prostatic urethra is derived from the pelvic part of the sinus near the entrance of the ducts and including the region of the sinusal tubercle—the latter apparently forming the seminal colliculus. Early in the 12th week, endodermal outgrowths of the prostatic urethra form the prostatic anlage, the **prostatic buds,** from which the glandular epithelium of the **prostate** will arise. Differentiation of splanchnic mesoderm contributes other components to the gland (smooth muscle and connective tissue), as is the case for mesodermal parts of the urinary bladder. The pelvic part of the sinus also gives rise to the epithelium of the **membranous urethra,** which later yields endodermal buds for the **bulbourethral glands.** The phallic, or inferior, part of the urogenital sinus proliferates anteriorly as the external genitalia form (during weeks 9–12) and results in incorporation of this phallic part as the endodermal epithelium of the **spongy (penile) urethra** (the distal glandular urethra is derived from ectoderm.

Female: Urinary Bladder, Urethra, and Vagina

A. DEVELOPMENT

Differentiation of the female sinus is schematically presented in Fig 4–13 and illustrated in Figs 4–8, 4–12, 4–16, and 4–17. In contrast to sinusal differentiation in the male, the vesical part of the female urogenital sinus forms the epithelium of the **urinary bladder** and entire **urethra.** Derivatives of the pelvic part of the sinus include the epithelium of the **vagina,** the **greater vestibular glands,** and the **hymen.** Controversy exists about how the vagina is formed, mainly because of a lack of consensus about the origin and degree of inclusion of its precursor tissues (mesodermal paramesonephric duct, endodermal urogenital sinus, or even mesonephric duct). The most common theory is that 2 endodermal outgrowths, the **sinovaginal bulbs,** of the dorsal wall of the pelvic part of the urogenital sinus form bilateral to and join with the caudal tip of the uterovaginal primordium (fused paramesonephric ducts) in the area of the sinusal tubercle (Fig 4–12). This cellular mass at the end of the primordium occludes the inferior aspect of the canal, creating an endodermal **vaginal plate** within the mesodermal wall of the uterovaginal primordium. Eventually, the vaginal segment grows, approaching the vestibule of the vagina. The process of growth has been described either as "downgrowth" of the vaginal segment away from the uterine canal and along the urogenital sinus or, more commonly, as "upgrowth" of the segment away from the

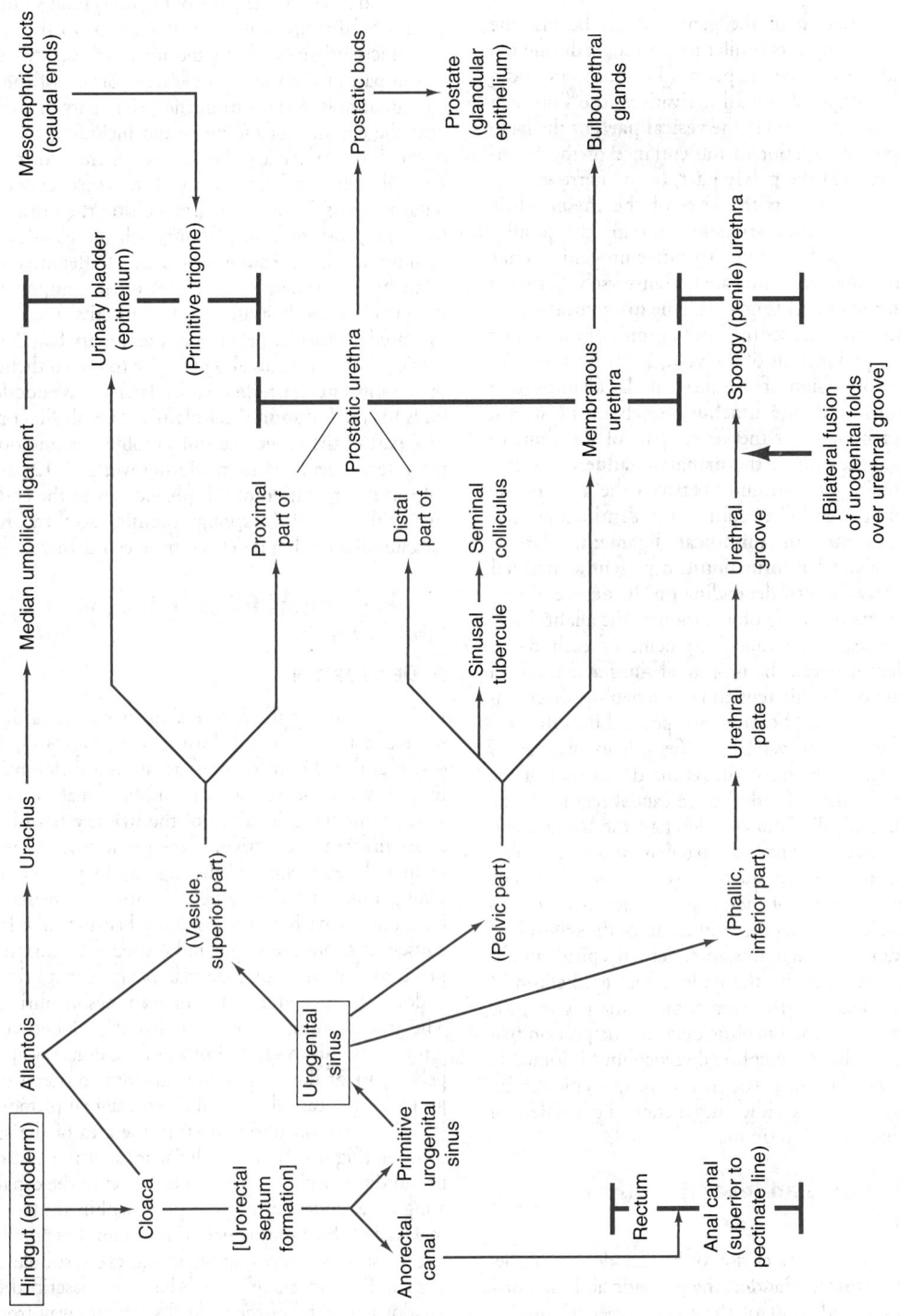

Figure 4-15. Schematic drawing of male differentiation of the urogenital sinus; formation of urinary bladder and urethra. (Explanatory symbols are given in Fig 4-1.)

84

sinus and toward the uterovaginal canal. In either case, the vaginal segment is extended between the paramesonephric-derived cervix and the sinus-derived vestibule (Figs 4–12, 4–16, and 4–17). Near the fifth month, the breakdown of cells centrally in the vaginal plate creates the vaginal lumen, which is delimited peripherally by the remaining cells of the plate as the epithelial lining of the vagina. The solid vaginal fornices become hollow soon after canalization of the vaginal lumen is complete. The upper one-third to four-fifths of the vaginal epithelium has been proposed to arise from the uterovaginal primordium, whereas the lower two-thirds to one-fifth has been proposed as a contribution from the sinovaginal bulbs.

The fibromuscular wall of the vagina is derived from the uterovaginal primordium. The cavities of the vagina and urogenital sinus are temporarily separated by the thin **hymen,** which probably is a mixture of tissue derived from the vaginal plate and the remains of the sinusal tubercle. With concurrent differentiation of female external genitalia, inferior closure of the sinus does not occur during the 12th week of development, as it does in the male. Instead, the remainder of the pelvic part and all of the inferior phallic part of the urogenital sinus expand to form the **vestibule of the vagina.** Presumably, the junctional zone of pigmentation on the labia minora represents the distinction between endodermal derivation from the urogenital sinus (medially) and ectodermal skin (laterally).

B. ANOMALIES OF THE VAGINA

The vagina is derived from interaction between the uterovaginal primordium and the pelvic part of the uro-

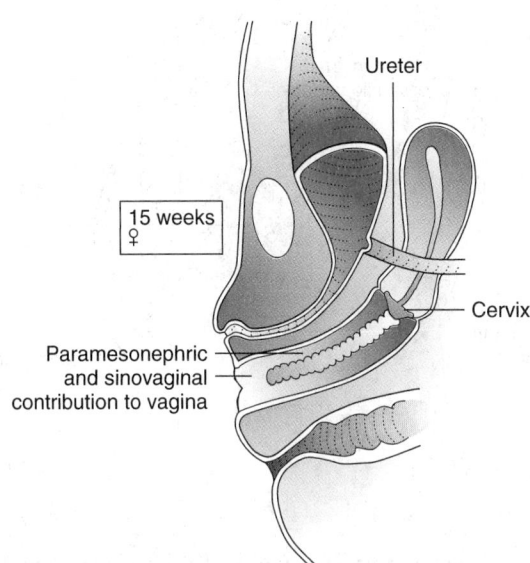

Figure 4–17. Sagittal cutaway view of differentiated urogenital sinus and precanalization stage of vaginal development. The drawing depicts one of several theories about the relative contributions of paramesonephric ducts and sinovaginal bulbs to the vagina.

genital sinus (Fig 4–13; see Development). The causes of vaginal anomalies are difficult to assess because integration of the uterovaginal primordium and the urogenital sinus in the *normal* differentiation of the vagina remains a controversial subject. Furthermore, an accurate breakdown of causes of certain anomalous vaginal presentations, as with many anomalies of the external genitalia, would have to include potential moderating factors of endocrine and genetic origin as well.

The incidence of absence of the vagina due to suspected **vaginal agenesis** is about 0.025%. Agenesis may be due to failure of the uterovaginal primordium to contact the urogenital sinus. The uterus is usually absent (Fig 4–18). Ovarian agenesis is not usually associated with vaginal agenesis. The presence of greater vestibular glands has been reported with presumed vaginal agenesis; their presence emphasizes the complexity of differentiation of the urogenital sinus.

Vaginal atresia, on the other hand, is considered when the lower portion of the vagina consists merely of fibrous tissue while the contiguous superior structures (the uterus, in particular) are well differentiated (perhaps because the primary defect is in the sinusal contribution to the vagina). In **müllerian aplasia** almost all of the vagina and most of the

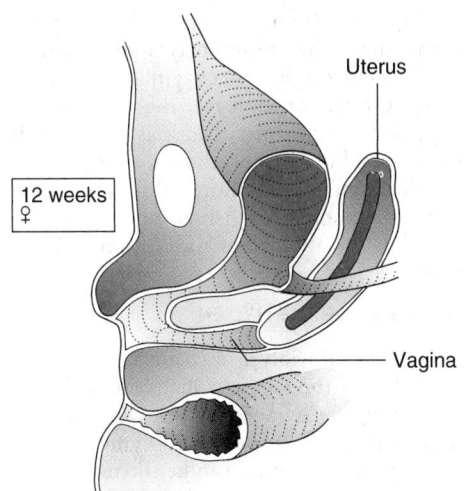

Figure 4–16. Sagittal cutaway view of developing vagina and urethra.

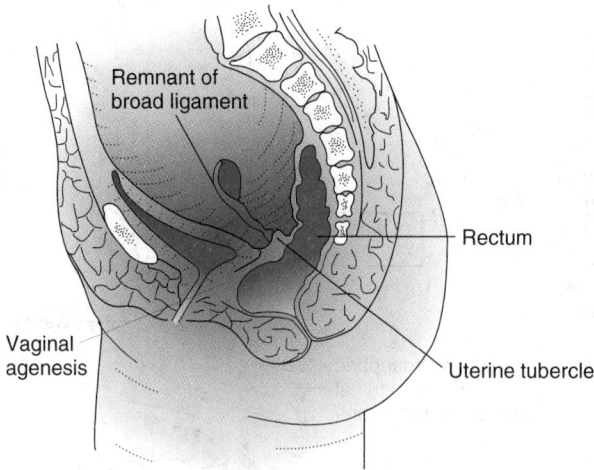

Remnant of
broad ligament

Rectum

Vaginal
agenesis

Uterine tubercle

Figure 4–18. Midsagittal view of vaginal agenesis and uterine agenesis with normal ovaries and oviducts. (Reproduced, with permission, from Ingram JM: The Ingram technique for the management of vaginal agenesis and stenosis. The Pelvic Surgeon 1981;2:1.)

uterus are absent (Rokitansky-Küster-Hauser syndrome, with a rudimentary uterus of bilateral, solid muscular tissue, was considered virtually the same as this aplasia). Most women with absence of the vagina (and normal external genitalia) are considered to have müllerian aplasia rather than vaginal atresia.

Other somatic anomalies are sometimes associated with müllerian aplasia, suggesting multiple malformation syndrome. Associated vertebral anomalies are much more prevalent than middle ear anomalies, eg, müllerian aplasia associated with **Klippel-Feil syndrome** (fused cervical vertebrae) is more common than müllerian aplasia associated with Klippel-Feil syndrome plus middle ear anomalies ("conductive deafness"). **Winter's syndrome,** which is thought to be autosomal recessive, is evidenced by middle ear anomalies (somewhat similar to those in the triad above), renal agenesis or hypoplasia, and vaginal atresia (rather than aplasia of the paramesonephric ducts). **Dysgenesis** (partial absence) of the vagina and **hypoplasia** (reduced caliber of the lumen) have also been described.

Transverse vaginal septa (Fig 4–19) are probably not the result of vaginal atresia but rather of incomplete canalization of the vaginal plate or discrete fusion of sinusal and primordial (ductal) derivatives. Alternative explanations are likely because the histologic composition of septa is not consistent. A rare genetic linkage has been demonstrated. A single septum or multiple septa can be present, and the location may vary in upper or lower segments of the lumen. **Longitudinal vaginal septa** can also occur. A variety of explanations have been advanced, including true duplication of vaginal primordial tissue, anomalous differentiation of the uterovaginal primordium, abnormal variation of the caudal fusion of the

müllerian ducts, persistence of vaginal plate epithelium, and anomalous mesodermal proliferation. Septa may be imperforate or perforated. A transverse septum creates the potential for various occlusive manifestations (eg, hydrometrocolpos, hematometra, or hematocolpos, depending on the composition and location of the trapped fluid.

Abnormalities of the vagina are often associated with anomalies of the urinary system and the rectum because differentiation of the urogenital sinus is involved in formation of the bladder and urethra as well as the vagina and vestibule. Furthermore, if partitioning of the cloaca into the sinus and anorectal canal is faulty, then associated rectal defects can occur. Compound anomalies may affect the urinary tract or rectum. The urethra may open into the vaginal wall; even a single vesicovaginal cavity has been described. On the other hand, the vagina can open into a persistent urogenital sinus, as in certain forms of female pseudohermaphroditism. Associated rectal abnormalities include vaginorectal fistula, vulvovaginal anus, rectosigmoidal fistula, and vaginosigmoidal cloaca in the absence of the rectum (see Cloacal Dysgenesis).

C. ANOMALIES OF THE HYMEN

The hymen is probably a mixture of tissue derived from remains of the sinusal tubercle and the vaginal plate. Usually, the hymen is patent, or perforate, by puberty, although an **imperforate hymen** is not rare. The imperforate condition can be the result of a congenital error of lack of central degeneration or the result of inflammatory occlusion after perforation. Obstruction of menstrual flow at puberty may be the first sign (Fig 4–19).

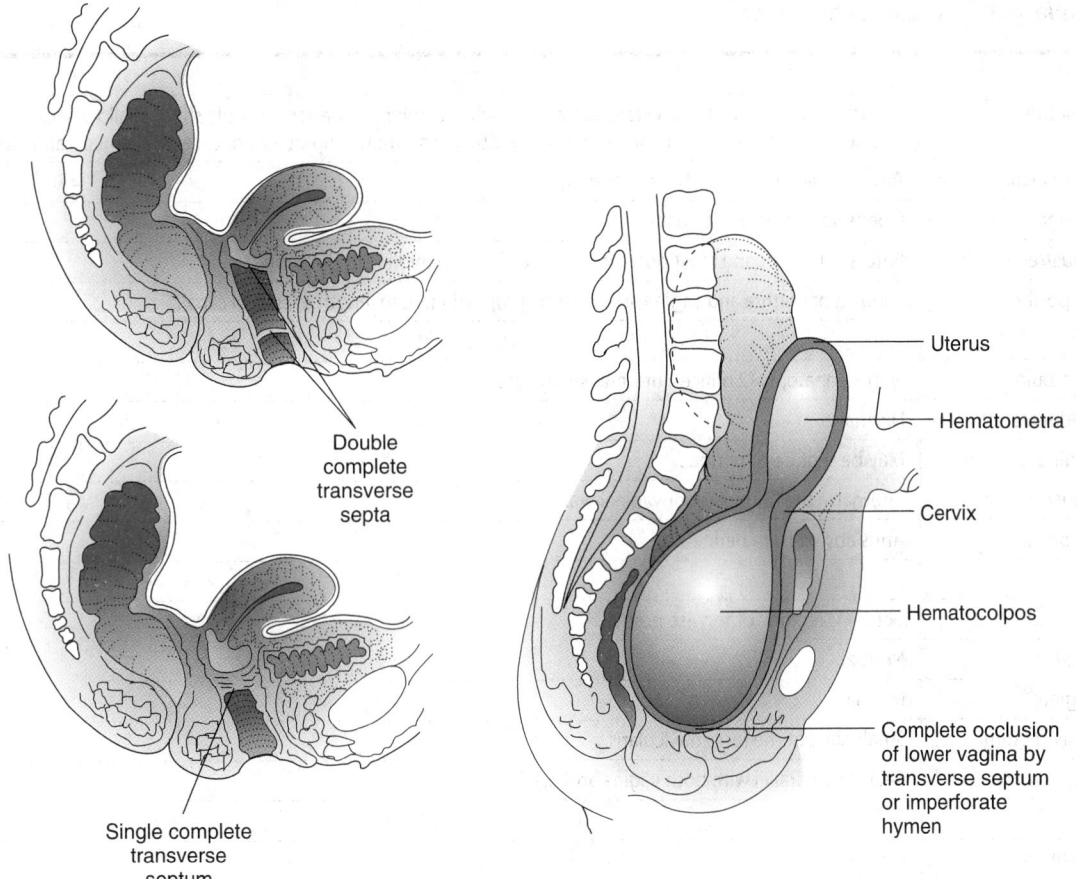

Double
complete
transverse
septa

Single complete
transverse
septum

Uterus

Hematometra

Cervix

Hematocolpos

Complete occlusion
of lower vagina by
transverse septum
or imperforate
hymen

Figure 4–19. Transverse vaginal septa.

D. CLOACAL DYSGENESIS (INCLUDING PERSISTENCE OF THE UROGENITAL SINUS)

Anomalous partitioning of the cloaca by abnormal development of the urorectal septum is rare, at least based on reported cases in the literature. As anticipated from a developmental standpoint, the incidence of associated genitourinary anomalies is high. Five types of cloacal or anorectal malformations are summarized in Table 4–3.

Rectocloacal fistula with a persistent cloaca provides a common canal or outlet for the urinary, genital, and intestinal tracts. The distinction between a canal and an outlet is one of depth (deep versus very shallow, respectively) of the persistent lower portion of the cloaca and, thus, the length of the individual urethral and vaginal canals emptying into the cloaca. The inverse relationship between depth (or length) of the cloaca and length of the vaginal and urethral canals is probably a reflection of the time when arrest of formation of the urorectal septum occurs. Although the bladder, the vagina, and the rectum

can empty into a common cloaca as just described, other unusual variations of persistent cloaca can also occur.

For example, the vagina and rectum develop, but the urinary bladder does not develop as a separate entity from the cloaca. Instead, the vagina and rectum open separately into a "urinary bladder," which has ureters entering posterolaterally to the vagina (vaginal orifice is in the "anatomic trigone" of the bladderlike structure). The external orifice from the base of this cloacal "bladder" is a single narrow canal. One explanation for this variant might be that arrest of formation of the urorectal septum occurs much earlier than does the separate development of distal portions of the 3 tracts (urethra, vagina, and anorectum) to a more advanced (but still incomplete) stage before urorectal septal formation ceases. The anomaly is probably rare.

With a **rectovaginal fistula,** the vestibule may appear anatomically normal, but the anus does not appear in the perineum. The defect probably results from anorectal agenesis due to incomplete subdivision of the cloaca (sim-

Table 4–3. Cloacal malformations.

Rectocloacal Fistula	
Vestibule	Deformed; flanked by labia; clitoris in front, fourchette behind; anterior vestibule short, shallow, and moist; single external orifice in posterior half of vestibule (common conduit for urine, cervical mucus, and feces).
Bladder/urethra	Anterior; directed cranially and ventrally.
Vagina	Opens into the vault of cloaca.
Anus/rectum	Enters at highest and most posterior point; orifice is in midline and stenotic.
Disposition	Lengths of urethra and vagina are inversely proportionate to length of cloacal canal.
Rectovaginal Fistula	
Vestibule	Normal anatomy (2 orifices: urethral & vaginal).
Bladder/urethra	Normal.
Vagina	May be septate or normal.
Anus/rectum	Internal in the midposterior vaginal wall.
Disposition	Anus absent from perineum.
Rectovestibular Fistula	
Vestibule	Contains rectum, otherwise normal.
Urethra	Normal.
Vagina	Normal.
Anus/rectum	Small, sited at the fossa navicularis.
Disposition	Rectum is parallel with both vagina and urethra.
Covered Anus	
Vestibule	Normal.
Urethra	Normal.
Vagina	(Probably normal.)
Anus	At any point between the normal site and the fourchette; anocutaneous; anovulvar.
Disposition	Genital folds are abnormally fused anterior and posterior to common orifice and give rise to hypertrophied perineal raphe.
Ectopic Anus	
Vestibule	Normal.
Urethra	Normal.
Vagina	Normal.
Anus	Anterior to the normal site; normal function.
Disposition	Fault lies in the development of the perineum.

Modified and reproduced, with permission, from Okonkwo JEN, Crocker KM: Cloacal dysgenesis. Obstet Gynecol 1977; 50:97.

ilar agenesis in the male could result in a rectourethral fistula). The development of the anterior aspect of the vagina completes the separation of the urethra from the vagina, so there is not a persistent urogenital sinus. **Anorectal agenesis** is reputedly the most common type of anorectal malformation, and usually a fistula occurs. Rectovaginal, anovestibular (or rectovestibular; Table 4–3), and anoperineal fistulas account for most anorectal malformations.

In the absence of the anorectal defect (normal anal presentation) but presence of a **persistent urogenital sinus** with a single external orifice, various irregularities of the urethra and genitalia can appear. The relative positions of urethral and vaginal orifices in the sinus can even change as the child grows. In the discussion of anomalies of the labia majora, there may be a persistent urogenital sinus in female pseudohermaphroditism due to congenital adrenal hyperplasia. The vagina opens into the persisting pelvic part of the sinus, which extends with the phallic part of the sinus to the external surface at the urogenital opening. The sinus can be deep and narrow in the neonate, approximating the size of a urethra, or it can be relatively shallow.

Urinary tract disorders associated with persistent urogenital sinus include duplication of the ureters, unilateral ureteral and renal agenesis or atresia, and lack of or abnormal ascent of the kidneys. Variations in the anomalies of derivatives of the urogenital sinus appear to be related in part to the time of arrest of normal differentiation and development of the urogenital sinus, as well as to the impact of other factors associated with abnormal sexual differentiation, such as the variable degrees of response to adrenal androgen in congenital adrenal hyperplasia.

THE EXTERNAL GENITALIA

Undifferentiated Stage

The external genitalia begin to form early in the embryonic period, shortly after development of the cloaca. The progenitory tissues of the genitalia are common to both sexes, and the early stage of development is virtually the same in females and males. Although differentiation of the genitalia can begin around the onset of the fetal period if testicular differentiation is initiated, definitive genital sex is usually not clearly apparent until the 12th week. Formation of external genitalia in the male involves the influence of androgen on the interaction of subepidermal mesoderm with the inferior parts of the endodermal urogenital sinus. In the female, this androgenic influence is absent.

The external genitalia form within the initially compact area bounded by the umbilical cord (anteriorly), the developing limb buds (laterally), the embryonic tail (posteriorly), and the cloacal membrane (centrally).

Two of the primordia for the genitalia first appear bilaterally adjacent to the cloacal membrane (a medial pair of cloacal folds and a lateral pair of genital [labioscrotal] swellings). The **cloacal folds** are longitudinal proliferations of caudal mesenchyme located between the ectodermal epidermis and the underlying endoderm of the phallic part of the urogenital sinus. Proliferation and bilateral anterior fusion of these folds create the **genital tubercle,** which protrudes near the anterior edge of the cloacal membrane by the sixth week (Figs 4–20 to 4–22). Extension of the tubercle forms the phallus, which at this stage is the same size in both sexes.

By the seventh week, the urorectal septum subdivides the bilayered (ectoderm and endoderm) cloacal membrane into the **urogenital membrane** (anteriorly) and the **anal membrane** (posteriorly). The area of fusion of the urorectal septum and the cloacal membrane becomes the **primitive perineum,** or **perineal body.** With formation of the perineum, the cloacal folds are divided transversely as **urogenital folds** adjacent to the urogenital membrane and **anal folds** around the anal membrane. As the mesoderm within the urogenital folds thickens and elongates between the perineum and the phallus, the urogenital membrane sinks deeper into the fissure between the folds. Within a week, this membrane ruptures, forming the **urogenital orifice** and, thus, opening the urogenital sinus to the exterior. Similar thickening of the anal folds creates a deep anal pit, in which the anal membrane breaks down to establish the **anal orifice** of the anal canal (Figs 4–20 and 4–21).

Subsequent masculinization or feminization of the external genitalia is a consequence of the respective presence or absence of androgen and the androgenic sensitivity or insensitivity of the tissues. The significance of both of these factors (availability of hormone and sensitivity of target tissue) is exemplified by the rare condition (about 1 in 50,000 "females") of **testicular feminization,** wherein testes are present (usually ectopic) and produce testosterone and antimüllerian hormone. The antimüllerian hormone suppresses formation of the uterus and uterine tubes (from the paramesonephric ducts), whereas testosterone supports male differentiation of the mesonephric ducts to form the epididymis and ductus deferens. The anomalous feminization of the external genitalia is considered to be due to androgenic insensitivity of the precursor tissues consequent to an abnormal androgen receptor or postreceptor mechanism set by genetic inheritance.

Male

Early masculinization of the undifferentiated or indifferent genitalia takes place during the first 3 weeks of the fetal period (weeks 9–12) and is caused by androgenic stimulation. The phallus and urogenital

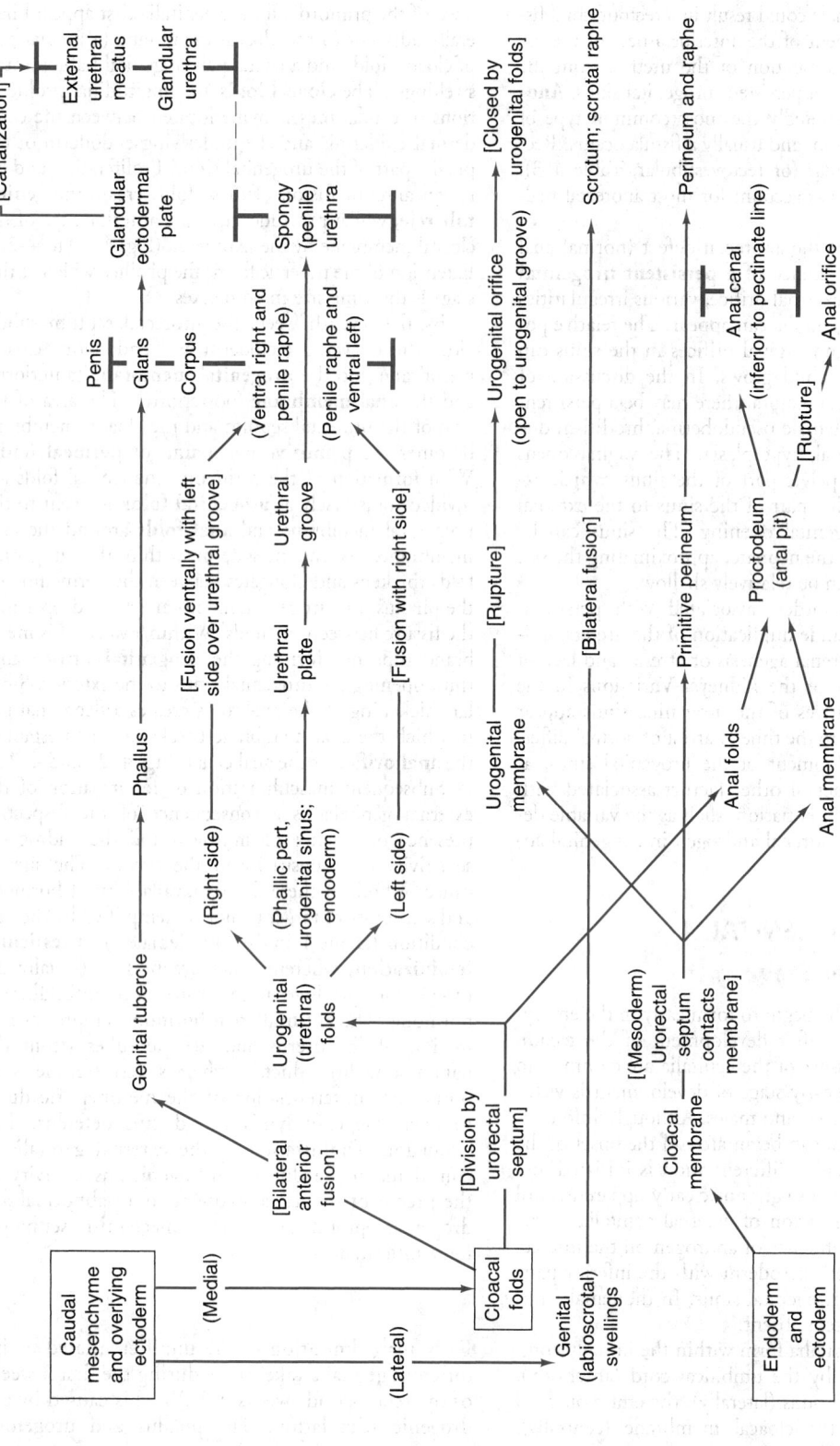

Figure 4–20. Schematic drawing of formation of male external genitalia. (Explanatory symbols are given in Fig 4–1.)

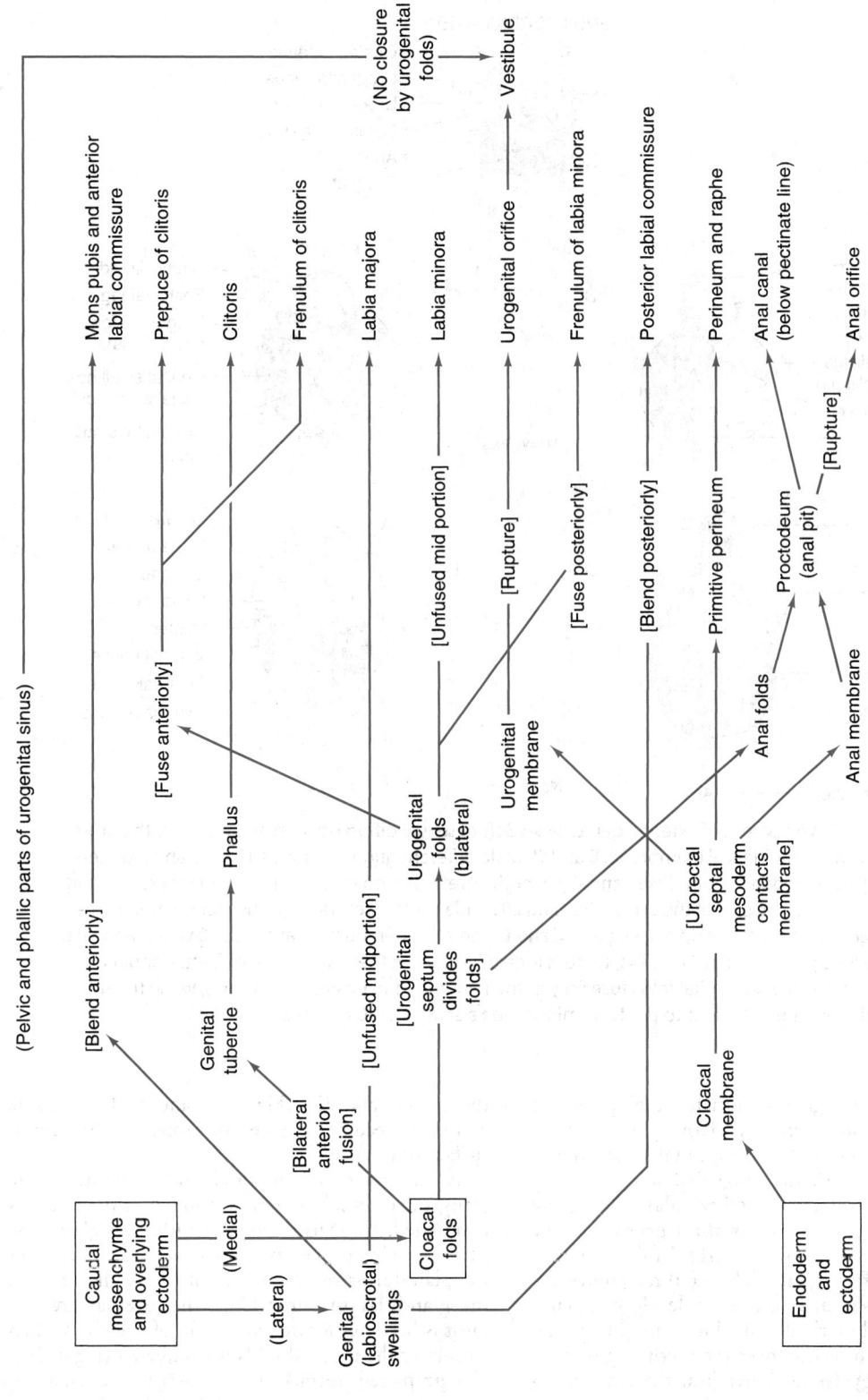

Figure 4–21. Schematic drawing of formation of female external genitalia. (Explanatory symbols are given in Fig 4–1.)

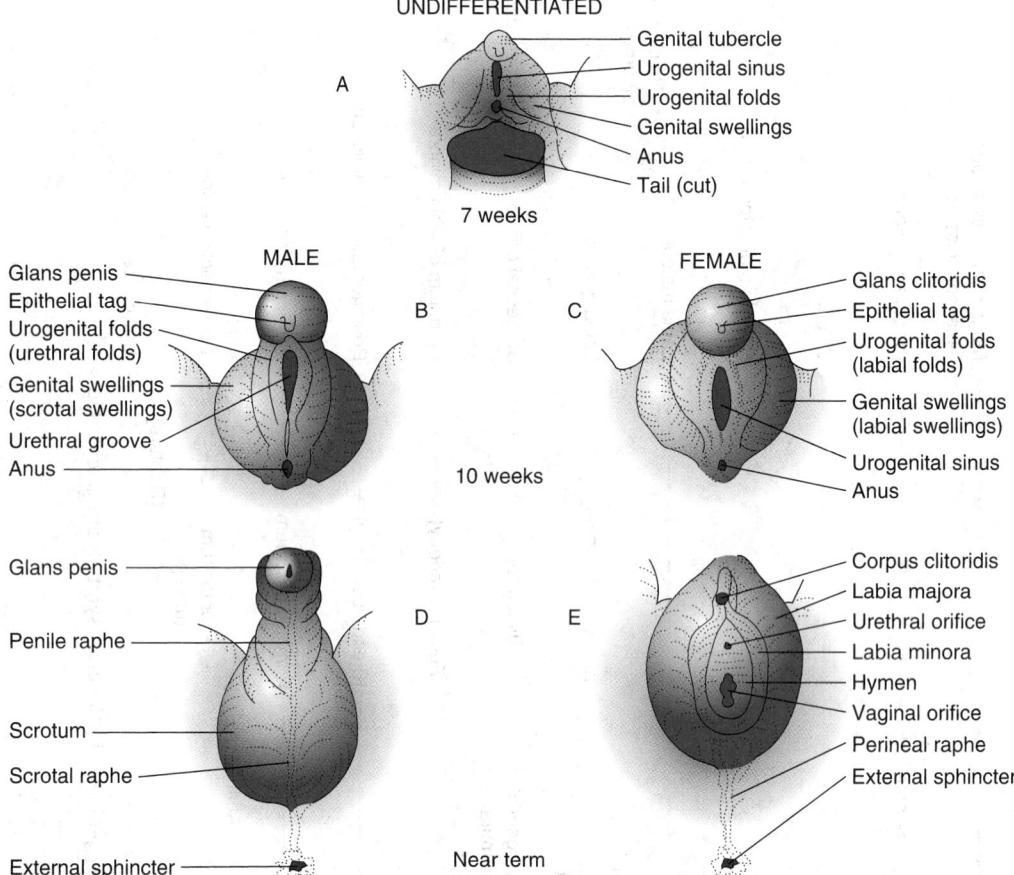

UNDIFFERENTIATED

A

Genital tubercle
Urogenital sinus
Urogenital folds
Genital swellings
Anus
Tail (cut)

7 weeks

MALE

B

Glans penis
Epithelial tag
Urogenital folds
(urethral folds)
Genital swellings
(scrotal swellings)
Urethral groove
Anus

FEMALE

C

Glans clitoridis
Epithelial tag
Urogenital folds
(labial folds)
Genital swellings
(labial swellings)
Urogenital sinus
Anus

10 weeks

D

Glans penis
Penile raphe
Scrotum
Scrotal raphe
External sphincter

E

Corpus clitoridis
Labia majora
Urethral orifice
Labia minora
Hymen
Vaginal orifice
Perineal raphe
External sphincter

Near term

Figure 4–22. Development of external genitalia. **A:** Before sexual differentiation and just after the urorectal septum divides the cloacal membrane. **B** and **D:** Male differentiation at about 10 weeks and near term, respectively. The urogenital folds fuse ventrally over the urethral groove to form the spongy urethra and close the inferior phallic part of the urogenital sinus. The glandular urethra forms by canalization of invaginated ectoderm from the tip of the glans. **C** and **E:** Female differentiation at about 10 weeks and near term, respectively. Until about 12 weeks, there is little difference in the appearance of female and male external genitalia. The urogenital folds fuse only at their anterior and posterior extremes, while the unfused remainder differentiates into the labia minor. (See also Figs 4–20 and 4–21.)

folds gradually elongate to initiate development of the **penis.** The subjacent endodermal lining of the inferior part (phallic) of the urogenital sinus extends anteriorly along with the urogenital folds, creating an endodermal plate, the **urethral plate.** The plate deepens into a groove, the **urethral groove,** as the urogenital folds (now called **urethral folds**) thicken on each side of the plate. The urethral groove extends into the ventral aspect of the developing penis, and the bilateral urethral folds slowly fuse in a posterior to anterior direction over the urethral groove to form the **spongy (penile) urethra,** thereby closing

the urogenital orifice (Figs 4–15 and 4–20). The line of fusion becomes the **penile raphe** on the ventral surface of the penis.

As closure of the urethral folds approaches the glans, the external urethral opening on this surface is eliminated. Concurrently, an **ectodermal glandular plate** invaginates the tip of the penis. Canalization of the plate forms the distal end of the penile urethra, the **glandular urethra.** Thus, the external urethral meatus becomes located at the tip of the glans when closure of the urethral folds is completed (Fig 4–20). The **prepuce** is formed slightly later by a circular invagination of ectoderm at the tip of the **glans penis.** This cylindric ectodermal plate then cleaves to leave a double-layered fold of skin extending over the glans.

While the cloacal folds and phallic urogenital sinus were differentiating into the penis and the urethra, the **genital** (**labioscrotal**) swellings of the undifferentiated stage were enlarging lateral to the cloacal folds. Medial growth and fusion of the scrotal swellings to form the **scrotum** and **scrotal raphe** around the 12th week virtually complete the differentiation of the male external genitalia (Figs 4–20 and 4–22).

Female

A. DEVELOPMENT OF EXTERNAL GENITALIA

Feminization of the external genitalia proceeds in the absence of androgenic stimulation (or nonresponsiveness of the tissue). The 2 primary distinctions in the general process of feminization versus masculinization are (1) the lack of continued growth of the phallus and (2) the near absence of fusion of the urogenital folds and the labioscrotal swellings. Female derivatives of the indifferent sexual primordia for the external genitalia are virtually homologous counterparts of the male derivatives. Formation of the female genitalia is schematically presented in Fig 4–21.

The growth of the phallus slows relative to that of the urogenital folds and labioscrotal swellings and becomes the diminutive **clitoris.** The anterior extreme of the urogenital folds fuses superior and inferior to the clitoris, forming the **prepuce** and **frenulum of the clitoris,** respectively. The midportions of these folds do not fuse but give rise to the **labia minora.** Lack of closure of the folds leaves the urogenital orifice patent and results in formation of the **vestibule of the vagina** from the inferior portion of the pelvic part and the phallic part of the urogenital sinus at about the fifth month (Fig 4–21). Derivatives of the vesical part of the sinus (the **urethra**) and the superior portion of the pelvic part of the sinus (**vagina** and **greater vestibular glands**) then open separately into the vestibule. The **frenulum of the labia minora** is formed by fusion of the posterior ends of the urogenital folds. The mesoderm of the labioscrotal swellings proliferates beneath the ectoderm and remains virtually unfused to create the **labia majora** lateral to the labia minora. The swellings blend together anteriorly to form the **anterior labial commissure** and the tissue of the **mons pubis,** while the swellings posteriorly less clearly define a **posterior labial commissure.** The distal fibers of the round ligament of the uterus project into the tissue of the labia majora.

B. ANOMALIES OF THE LABIA MINORA

In otherwise normal females, 2 somewhat common anomalies occur—labial fusion and labial hypertrophy. True labial fusion as an early developmental defect in the normally unfused midportions of the urogenital folds is purportedly less frequent than "fusion" due to inflammatory-type reactions. **Labial hypertrophy** can be unilateral or bilateral and may require surgical correction in extreme cases.

C. ANOMALIES OF THE LABIA MAJORA

The labia majora are derived from the bilateral genital (labioscrotal) swellings, which appear early in the embryonic period and remain unfused centrally during subsequent sex differentiation in the fetal period. Anomalous conditions include **hypoplastic** and **hypertrophic labia** as well as different gradations of fusion of the labia majora. Abnormal fusion (masculinization) of labioscrotal swellings in genetic females is most commonly associated with ambiguous genitalia of female pseudohermaphroditism consequent to **congenital adrenal hyperplasia** (**adrenogenital syndrome**). Over 90% of females with congenital adrenal hyperplasia have a steroid 21-hydroxylase deficiency (autosomal recessive), resulting in excess adrenal androgen production. This enzyme deficiency has been reported to be "the most common cause of ambiguous genitalia in genetic females." Associated anomalies include clitoral hypertrophy and persistent urogenital sinus. Formation of a penile urethra is extremely rare.

D. ANOMALIES OF THE CLITORIS

Clitoral agenesis is extremely rare and is due to lack of formation of the genital tubercle during the sixth week. Absence of the clitoris could also result from **atresia** of the genital tubercle. The tubercle forms by fusion of the anterior segments of the cloacal folds. Very rarely, these anterior segments fail to fuse, and a **bifid clitoris** forms. This anomaly also occurs when unification of the anterior parts of the folds is restricted by exstrophy of the cloaca or bladder. Duplication of the genital tubercle with consequent formation of a **double clitoris** is equally rare. **Clitoral hypertrophy** alone is not common but may be associated with various intersex disorders.

E. ANOMALIES OF THE PERINEUM

The primitive perineum originates at the area of contact of the mesodermal urorectal septum and the endodermal dorsal surface of the cloacal membrane (at 7 weeks). During normal differentiation of the external genitalia in the fetal period, the primitive perineum maintains the separation of the urogenital folds and ruptured urogenital membrane from the anal folds and ruptured anal membrane, and later develops the perineal body. Malformations of the perineum are rare and usually associated with malformations of cloacal or anorectal development consequent to abnormal development of the urorectal septum. Imperforate anus has an incidence of about 0.02%. The simplest form (rare) is a thin membrane over the anal canal (the anal membrane failed to rupture at the end of the embryonic period). Anal stenosis can arise by posterior deviation of the urorectal septum as the septum approaches the cloacal membrane, causing the anal membrane to be smaller (with a relatively increased anogenital distance through the perineum). Anal agenesis with a fistula detected as an ectopic anus is considered to be a urorectal septal defect. The incidence of agenesis with a fistula is only slightly less than that without a fistula. In females, the fistula commonly may be located in the perineum (perineal fistula) or may open into the posterior aspect of the vestibule of the vagina (anovestibular fistula; see Cloacal Dysgenesis).

REFERENCES

Cadeddu JA, Watumull L, Corwin TS: Laparoscopic gonadectomy and excision of müllerian remnant in an adult intersex patient. Urology 2001;57:554.

Cho S, Moore SP, Fangman T: One hundred three consecutive patients with anorectal malformations and their associated anomalies. Arch Pediatr Adolesc Med 2001;155:587.

Cook CL, Siow Y, Taylor S: Serum müllerian-inhibiting substance levels during normal menstrual cycles. Fertil Steril 2000;73:859.

Di Lorenzo C: Pediatric anorectal disorders. Gastroenterol Clin North Am 2001;30:269.

Drews U: Local mechanisms in sex-specific morphogenesis. Cytogenet Cell Genet 2000;91:72.

Edmonds DK: Congenital malformations of the genital tract. Obstet Gynecol Clin North Am 2000;27:49.

Folch M, Pigem I, Konje JC: Müllerian agenesis: Etiology, diagnosis, and management. Obstet Gynecol Surv 2000;55:644.

Hiort O: Neonatal endocrinology of abnormal male sexual differentiation: Molecular aspects. Horm Res 2000;53(Suppl)1:38.

Larsen WJ: Development of the urogenital system. In: Larsen WJ et al (editors): *Human Embryology.* Churchill Livingstone, 2001, p. 235.

Malik E et al: Reproductive outcome of 32 patients with primary or secondary infertility and uterine pathology. Arch Gynecol Obstet 2000;264:24.

Mittwoch U: Genetics of sex determination: Exceptions that prove the rule. Mol Genet Metab 2000;71:405.

Nef S, Parada LF: Hormones in male sexual development. Genes Dev 2000;14:3075.

Ostrer H: Sexual differentiation. Semin Reprod Med 2000;18:41.

Resendes BL, Sohn SH, Stelling JR: Role for anti-müllerian hormone in congenital absence of the uterus and vagina. Am J Med Genet 2001;98:129.

Salas-Cortes L et al: SRY protein is expressed in ovotestis and streak gonads from human sex reversal. Cytogenet Cell Genet 2000;91:212.

Shimanda K, Hosokawa S, Matsumoto F: Urological management of cloacal anomalies. Int J Urol 2001;8:282.

Vendeland LL, Shehadeh L: Incidental finding of an accessory ovary in a 16 year old at laparoscopy. A case report. J Reprod Med 2000;45:435.

Genetic Disorders & Sex Chromosome Abnormalities

5

Somjate Manipalviratn, MD, Bradley Trivax, MD, & Andy Huang, MD,

■ GENETIC DISORDERS

MENDELIAN LAWS OF INHERITANCE

1. Types of Inheritance
Autosomal Dominant

In autosomal dominant inheritance, it is assumed that a mutation has occurred in 1 gene of an allelic pair and that the presence of this new gene produces enough of the changed protein to give a different phenotypic effect. Environment must also be considered because the effect may vary under different environmental conditions. The following are characteristic of autosomal dominant inheritance:

1. The trait appears with equal frequency in both sexes.
2. For inheritance to take place, at least 1 parent must have the trait unless a new mutation has just occurred.
3. When a homozygous individual is mated to a normal individual, all offspring will carry the trait. When a heterozygous individual is mated to a normal individual, 50% of the offspring will show the trait.
4. If the trait is rare, most persons demonstrating it will be heterozygous (Table 5–1).

Autosomal Recessive

The mutant gene will not be capable of producing a new characteristic in the heterozygous state in this circumstance under customary environmental conditions—ie, with 50% of the genetic material producing the new protein, the phenotypic effect will not be different from that of the normal trait. When the environment is manipulated, the recessive trait occasionally becomes dominant. The characteristics of this form of inheritance are as follows:

1. The characteristic will occur with equal frequency in both sexes.

2. For the characteristic to be present, both parents must be carriers of the recessive trait.
3. If both parents are homozygous for the recessive trait, all offspring will have it.
4. If both parents are heterozygous for the recessive trait, 25% of the offspring will have it.
5. In pedigrees showing frequent occurrence of individuals with rare recessive characteristics, consanguinity is often present (Table 5–2).

X-Linked Recessive

This condition occurs when a gene on the X chromosome undergoes mutation and the new protein formed as a result of this mutation is incapable of producing a change in phenotype characteristic in the heterozygous state. Because the male has only 1 X chromosome, the presence of this mutant will allow for expression should it occur in the male. The following are characteristic of this form of inheritance:

1. The condition occurs more commonly in males than in females.
2. If both parents are normal and an affected male is produced, it must be assumed that the mother is a carrier of the trait.
3. If the father is affected and an affected male is produced, the mother must be at least heterozygous for the trait.
4. A female with the trait may be produced in 1 of 2 ways. (A) She may inherit a recessive gene from both her mother and her father; this suggests that the father is affected and the mother is heterozygous. (B) She may inherit a recessive gene from 1 of her parents and may express the recessive characteristic as a function of the Lyon hypothesis; this assumes that all females are mosaics for their functioning X chromosome. It is theorized that this occurs because at about the time of implantation, each cell in the developing female embryo selects 1 X chromosome as its functioning X and that all progeny cells thereafter use this X chromosome as their functioning X chromosome. The other X

95

Table 5–1. Examples of autosomal dominant conditions and traits.

Achondroplasia
Acoustic neuroma
Aniridia
Cataracts, cortical and nuclear
Chin fissure
Color blindness, yellow-blue
Craniofacial dysostosis
Deafness (several forms)
Dupuytren's contracture
Ehlers-Danlos syndrome
Facial palsy, congenital
Huntington's chorea
Hyperchondroplasia
Intestinal polyposis
Keloid formation
Lipomas, familial
Marfan's syndrome
Mitral valve prolapse
Muscular dystrophy
Neurofibromatosis (Recklinghausen's disease)
Night blindness
Pectus excavatum
Adult polycystic renal disease
Tuberous sclerosis
Von Willebrand's disease
Wolff-Parkinson-White syndrome (some cases)

chromosome becomes inactive. Because this selection is done on a random basis, it is conceivable that some females will be produced who will be using primarily the X chromosome bearing the recessive gene. Thus, a genotypically heterozygous individual may demonstrate a recessive characteristic phenotypically on this basis (Table 5–3).

X-Linked Dominant

In this situation, the mutation will produce a protein that, when present in the heterozygous state, is sufficient to cause a change in characteristic. The following are characteristic of this type of inheritance:

1. The characteristic occurs with the same frequency in males and females.
2. An affected male mated to a normal female will produce the characteristic in 50% of the offspring.
3. An affected homozygous female mated to a normal male will produce the affected characteristic in all offspring.
4. A heterozygous female mated to a normal male will produce the characteristic in 50% of the offspring.

5. Occasional heterozygous females may not show the dominant trait on the basis of the Lyon hypothesis (Table 5–4).

2. Applications of Mendelian Laws

Identification of Carriers

When a recessive characteristic is present in a population, carriers may be identified in a variety of ways. If the gene is responsible for the production of a protein (eg, an enzyme), the carrier often possesses 50% of the amount of the substance present in homozygous normal persons. Such a circumstance is found in galactosemia, where the carriers will have approximately half

Table 5–2. Examples of autosomal recessive conditions and traits.

Acid maltase deficiency
Albinism
Alkaptonuria
Argininemia
Ataxia-telangiectasia
Bloom's syndrome
Cerebrohepatorenal syndrome
Chloride diarrhea, congenital
Chondrodystrophia myotonia
Color blindness, total
Coronary artery calcinosis
Cystic fibrosis
Cystinosis
Cystinuria
Deafness (several types)
Dubowitz's syndrome
Dysautonomia
Fructose-1,6-diphosphatase deficiency
Galactosemia
Gaucher's disease
Glaucoma, congenital
Histidinemia
Homocystinuria
Laron's dwarfism
Maple syrup urine disease
Mucolipidosis I, II, III
Mucopolysaccharidosis I-H, I-S, III, IV, VI, VII
Muscular dystrophy, autosomal recessive type
Niemann-Pick disease
Phenylketonuria
Sickle cell anemia
17α-Hydroxylase deficiency
18-Hydroxylase deficiency
21-Hydroxylase deficiency
Tay-Sachs disease
Wilson's disease
Xeroderma pigmentosum

as much galactose-1-phosphate uridyltransferase activity in red cells as do noncarrier normal individuals.

At times, the level of the affected enzyme may be only slightly below normal, and a challenge with the substance to be acted upon may be required before the carrier can be identified. An example is seen in carriers of phenylketonuria, in whom the deficiency in phenylalanine hydroxylase is in the liver cells, and serum levels may not be much lower than normal. Nonetheless, when the individual is given an oral loading dose of phenylalanine, plasma phenylalanine levels may remain high because the enzyme is not present in sufficient quantities to act upon this substance properly.

In still other situations where the 2 alleles produce different proteins that can be measured, a carrier state will have 50% of the normal protein and 50% of the other protein. Such a situation is seen in sickle cell trait, where 1 gene is producing hemoglobin A and the other hemoglobin S. Thus, the individual has half the amount of hemoglobin A as a normal person and half the hemoglobin S of a person with sickle cell anemia. An interesting but important problem involves the detection of carriers of cystic fibrosis. This is the most common autosomal recessive disease in Caucasian populations of European background, occurring in 1 in 2500 births in such populations but found in the carrier state in 1 in 25 Americans. By 1990, over 230 alleles of the single gene responsible have been discovered. The gene is known as the cystic fibrosis transmembrane conductance regulator (CFTR), and the most common mutation, delta F508, accounts for about 70% of all mutations, with 5 specific point mutations accounting for over 85% of cases. Because so many alleles are

Table 5–3. Examples of X-linked recessive conditions and traits.

Androgen insensitivity syndrome (complete and incomplete)
Color blindness, red-green
Diabetes insipidus (most cases)
Fabry's disease
Glucose-6-phosphate dehydrogenase deficiency
Gonadal dysgenesis (XY type)
Gout (certain types)
Hemophilia A (factor VIII deficiency)
Hemophilia B (factor IX deficiency)
Hypothyroidism, X-linked infantile
Hypophosphatemia
Immunodeficiency, X-linked
Lesch Nyhan syndrome
Mucopolysaccharidosis II
Muscular dystrophy, adult and childhood types
Otopalatodigital syndrome
Reifenstein's syndrome

Table 5–4. Examples of X-linked dominant conditions and traits.

Acro-osteolysis, dominant type
Cervico-oculo-acoustic syndrome
Hyperammonemia
Orofaciodigital syndrome I

present, population screening poses logistical problems that have yet to be worked out. Most programs screen for the most common mutations using DNA replication and amplification studies.

3. Polygenic Inheritance

Polygenic inheritance is defined as the inheritance of a single phenotypic feature as a result of the effects of many genes. Most physical features in humans are determined by polygenic inheritance. Many common malformations are determined in this way also. For example, cleft palate with or without cleft lip, clubfoot, anencephaly, meningomyelocele, dislocation of the hip, and pyloric stenosis each occur with a frequency of 0.5–2 per 1000 in white populations. Altogether, these anomalies account for slightly less than half of single primary defects noted in early infancy. They are present in siblings of affected infants—when both parents are normal—at a rate of 2–5%. They are also found more commonly among relatives than in the general population. The increase in incidence is not environmentally induced because the frequency of such abnormalities in monozygotic twins is 4–8 times that of dizygotic twins and other siblings. The higher incidence in monozygotic twins is called concordance.

Sex also plays a role. Certain conditions appear to be transmitted by polygenic inheritance and are passed on more frequently by the mother who is affected than by the father who is affected. Cleft lip occurs in 6% of the offspring of women with cleft lip, as opposed to 2.8% of offspring of men with cleft lip.

Many racial variations in diseases are believed to be transmitted by polygenic inheritance, making racial background a determinant of how prone an individual will be to a particular defect. In addition, as a general rule, the more severe a defect, the more likely it is to occur in subsequent siblings. Thus, siblings of children with bilateral cleft lip are more likely to have the defect than are those of children with unilateral cleft lip.

Environment undoubtedly plays a role in polygenic inheritance, because seasonal variations alter some defects and their occurrence rate from country to country in similar populations.

EPIGENETIC

Epigenetic is the regulation of gene expression not encoded in the nucleotide sequence of the gene. Gene expression can either be turned on or off by DNA methylation or histone modification (methylation, acetylation, phosphorylation, ubiquitination, or ADP-ribosylation). Epigenetic can subsequently be inherited by its descendants.

Genomic Imprinting

Genomic imprinting is an epigenetic process by which the male and female genomes are differently expressed. The imprinting mark on genes is either by DNA methylation or histone modification. The imprinting patterns are different according to the parental origin of the genes. Genomic imprints are erased in primordial germ cells and re-established again during gametogenesis. The imprinting process is completed by the time of round spermatids formation in males and at ovulation of metaphase-II oocytes in females. The imprinted genes survive the global waves of DNA demethylation and remethylation during early embryonic development. In normal children, 1 set of chromosomes is derived from the father and the other from the mother. If both sets of chromosomes are from only 1 parent, the imprinted gene expression will be unbalanced. Prader-Willi syndrome and Angelman syndrome are examples of imprinting disorders. In Prader-Willi syndrome, both 15q13 regions are from the father, whereas in Angelman syndrome both 15q13 regions are from the mother.

CYTOGENETICS

1. Identification of Chromosomes

In 1960, 1963, 1965, and 1971, international meetings were held in Denver, London, Chicago, and Paris, respectively, for the purpose of standardizing the nomenclature of human chromosomes. These meetings resulted in a decision that all autosomal pairs should be numbered in order of decreasing size from 1 to 22. Autosomes are divided into groups based on their morphology, and these groups are labeled by the letters A–G. Thus, the A group is comprised of pairs 1–3; the B group, pairs 4 and 5; the C group, pairs 6–12; the D group, pairs 13–15; the E group, pairs 16–18; the F group, pairs 19 and 20; and the G group, pairs 21 and 22. The sex chromosomes are labeled X and Y, the X chromosome being similar in size and morphology to the number 7 pair and thus frequently included in the C group (C-X) and the Y chromosome being similar in morphology and size to the G group (G-Y) (Fig 5–1).

The short arm of a chromosome is labeled p and the long arm q. If a translocation occurs in which the short arm of a chromosome is added to another chromosome,

it is written p+. If the short arm is lost, it is p–. The same can be said for the long arm (q+ and q–).

It has been impossible to separate several chromosome pairs from one another on a strictly morphologic basis because the morphologic variations have been too slight. However, there are other means of identifying each chromosome pair in the karyotype. The first of these is the incorporation of ^{3}H-thymidine, known as the autoradiographic technique. This procedure involves the incorporation of radioactive thymidine into growing cells in tissue culture just before they are harvested. Cells that are actively undergoing DNA replication will pick up the radioactive thymidine, and the chromosomes will demonstrate areas of activity. Each chromosome will incorporate thymidine in a different pattern, and several chromosomes can therefore be identified by their labeling pattern. Nonetheless, with this method it is not possible to identify each chromosome, although it is possible to identify chromosomes involved in pathologic conditions, eg, D_1 trisomy and Down syndrome.

Innovative staining techniques have made it possible to identify individual chromosomes in the karyotype and to identify small anomalies that might have evaded the observer using older methods. These involve identification of chromosome banding by a variety of staining techniques, at times with predigestion with proteolytic agents. Some of the more commonly used techniques are the following:

Q banding: Fixed chromosome spreads are stained without any pretreatment using quinacrine mustard, quinacrine, or other fluorescent dyes and observed with a fluorescence microscope.

G banding: Preparations are incubated in a variety of saline solutions using any 1 of several pretreatments and stained with Giemsa's stain.

R banding: Preparations are incubated in buffer solutions at high temperatures or at special pH and stained with Giemsa's stain. This process yields the reverse bands of G banding (Fig 5–1).

C banding: Preparations are either heated in saline to temperatures just below boiling or treated with certain alkali solutions and then stained with Giemsa's stain. This process causes prominent bands to develop in the region of the centromeres.

2. Cell Division

Each body cell goes through successive stages in its life cycle. As a landmark, cell division can be considered as the beginning of a cycle. Following this, the first phase, which is quite long but depends on how rapidly the particular cell is multiplying, is called the G_1 stage. During this stage, the cell is primarily concerned with carrying out its function. Following this, the S stage, or

Figure 5–1. Karyotype of a normal male demonstrating R banding.

period of DNA synthesis, takes place. Next there is a somewhat shorter stage, the G₂ stage, during which time DNA synthesis is completed and chromosome replication begins. Following this comes the M stage, when cell division occurs.

Somatic cells undergo division by a process known as **mitosis** (Fig 5–2). This is divided into 4 periods. The first is **prophase,** during which the chromosome filaments shorten, thicken, and become visible. At this time they can be seen to be composed of 2 long parallel spiral strands lying adjacent to one another and containing a small clear structure known as the **centromere.** As prophase continues, the strands continue to unwind and may be recognized as chromatids. At the end of prophase, the nuclear membrane disappears and **metaphase** begins. This stage is heralded by the formation of a spindle and the lining up of the chromosomes in pairs on the spindle. Following this, **anaphase** occurs, at which time the centromere divides and each daughter chromatid goes to 1 of the poles of the spindle. **Telophase** then ensues, at which time the spindle breaks and cell cytoplasm divides. A nuclear membrane now forms, and mitosis is complete. Each daughter cell

has received chromosome material equal in amount and identical to that of the parent cell. Because each cell contains 2 chromosomes of each pair and a total of 46 chromosomes, a cell is considered to be **diploid.** Occasionally, an error takes place on the spindle, and instead of chromosomes dividing, with identical chromatids going to each daughter cell, an extra chromatid goes to 1 daughter cell and the other lacks that particular member. After completion of cell division, this leads to a trisomic state (an extra dose of that chromosome) in 1 daughter cell and a monosomic state (a missing dose of the chromosome) in the other daughter cell. Any chromosome in the karyotype may be involved in such a process, which is known as mitotic nondisjunction. If these cells thrive and produce their own progeny, a new cell line is established within the individual. The individual then has more than 1 cell line and is known as a **mosaic.** A variety of combinations and permutations have occurred in humans.

Germ cells undergo division for the production of eggs and sperm by a process known as **meiosis.** In the female it is known as oogenesis and in the male as spermatogenesis. The process that produces the egg and the

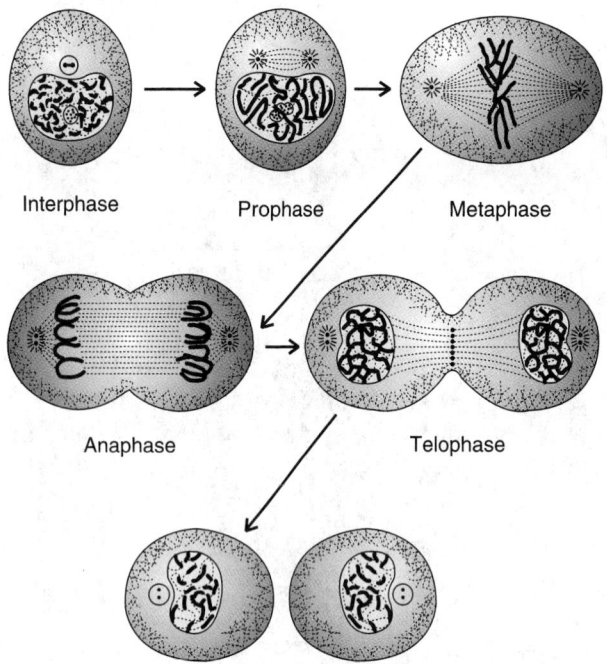

Interphase   Prophase   Metaphase

Anaphase   Telophase

Daughter cells at interphase

Figure 5–2. Mitosis of a somatic cell.

sperm for fertilization essentially reduces the chromosome number from 46 to 23 and changes the normal diploid cell to an aneuploid cell, ie, a cell that has only 1 member of each chromosome pair. Following fertilization and the fusion of the 2 pronuclei, the diploid status is reestablished.

Meiosis can be divided into several stages (Fig 5–3). The first is **prophase I.** Early prophase is known as the **leptotene stage,** during which chromatin condenses and becomes visible as a single elongated threadlike structure. This is followed by the **zygotene stage,** when the single threadlike chromosomes migrate toward the equatorial plate of the nucleus. At this stage, homologous chromosomes become arranged close to one another to form **bivalents** that exchange materials at several points known as **synapses.** In this way, genetic material located on 1 member of a pair is exchanged with similar material located on the other member of a pair. Next comes the **pachytene stage** in which the chromosomes contract to become shorter and thicker. During this stage, each chromosome splits longitudinally into 2 chromatids united at the centromere. Thus, the bivalent becomes a structure composed of 4 closely opposed chromatids known as a **tetrad.** The human cell in the pachytene stage demonstrates 23 tetrads. This stage is followed by the **diplotene stage,** in which the chromosomes of the bivalent are held together only at certain points called bridges or chiasms. It is at these points that crossover takes place. The sister chro-

matids are joined at the centromere so that crossover can only take place between chromatids of homologous chromosomes and not between identical sister chromatids. In the case of males, the X and Y chromosomes are not involved in crossover. This stage is followed by the last stage of prophase, known as **diakinesis.** Here the bivalents contract, and the chiasms move toward the end of the chromosome. The homologs pull apart, and the nuclear membrane disappears. This is the end of prophase I.

Metaphase I follows. At this time, the bivalents are now highly contracted and align themselves along the equatorial plate of the cell. Paternal and maternal chromosomes line up at random. This stage is then followed by **anaphase I** and **telophase I,** which are quite similar to the corresponding events in mitosis. However, the difference is that in meiosis the homologous chromosome of the bivalent pair separates and not the sister chromatids. The homologous bivalents pull apart, 1 going to each pole of the spindle, following which 2 daughter cells are formed at telophase I.

Metaphase, anaphase, and telophase of meiosis II take place next. A new spindle forms in metaphase, the chromosomes align along the equatorial plate, and, as anaphase occurs, the chromatids pull apart, 1 each going to a daughter cell. This represents a true division of the centromere. Telophase then supervenes, with reconstitution of the nuclear membrane and final cell division. At the end, a haploid number of chromosomes is present in each daughter

FIRST MEIOTIC DIVISION

Prophase

Leptotene Zygotene Pachytene Diplotene Diakinesis

Metaphase I Anaphase I Telophase I

SECOND MEIOTIC DIVISION

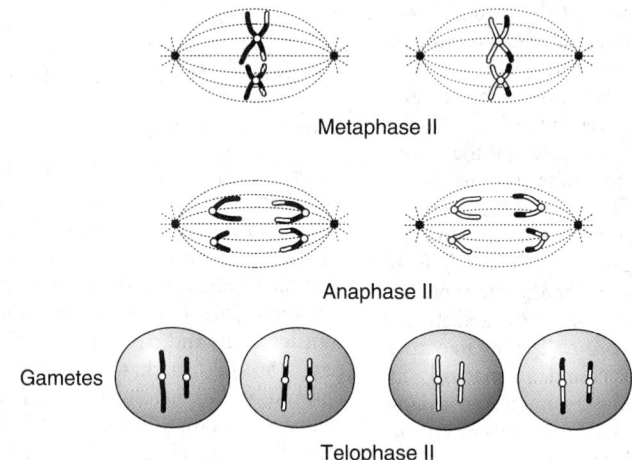

Metaphase II

Anaphase II

Gametes

Telophase II

Figure 5–3. Meiosis in the human.

cell (Fig 5–3). In the case of spermatogenesis, both daughter cells are similar, forming 2 separate sperms. In the case of oogenesis, only 1 egg is produced, the nuclear material of the other daughter cell being present and intact but with very little cytoplasm, this being known as the **polar body.** A polar body is formed at the end of meiosis I and the end of meiosis II. Thus, each spermatogonium produces 4 sperms at the end of meiosis, whereas each oogonium produces 1 egg and 2 polar bodies.

Nondisjunction may also occur in meiosis. When it does, both members of the chromosome pair go to 1 daughter cell and none to the other. If the daughter cell that receives the entire pair is the egg, and fertilization ensues, a triple dose of the chromosome, or trisomy, will oc-

cur. If the daughter cell receiving no members of the pair is fertilized, a monosomic state will result. In the case of autosomes, this is lethal, and a very early abortion will follow. In the case of the sex chromosome, the condition may not be lethal, and examples of both trisomy and monosomy have been seen in humans. Any chromosome pair may be involved in trisomic or monosomic conditions.

3. Abnormalities in Chromosome Morphology & Number

As has been stated, nondisjunction may give rise to conditions of trisomy. In these cases, the morphology of the chromosome is not affected, but the chromosome number is. Be this as it may, breaks and rearrangements in chromosomes may have a variety of results. If 2 chromosomes undergo breaks and exchange chromatin material between them, the outcome is 2 morphologically new chromosomes known as **translocations.** If a break in a chromosome takes place and the fragment is lost, **deletion** has occurred. If the deletion is such that the cell cannot survive, the condition may be lethal. Nonetheless, several examples of deleted chromosomes in individuals who have survived have been identified. If a break takes place at either end of a chromosome and the chromosome heals by having the 2 ends fuse together, a ring chromosome is formed. Examples of these have been seen clinically in all of the chromosomes of the karyotype, and generally they exhibit a variety of phenotypic abnormalities.

At times a chromosome will divide by a horizontal rather than longitudinal split of the centromere. This leaves each daughter cell with a double dose of 1 of the arms of the chromosome. Thus, 1 daughter cell receives both long arms and the other both short arms of the chromosome. Such a chromosome is referred to as an **isochromosome,** the individual being essentially trisomic for 1 arm and monosomic for the other arm of the chromosome. Examples of this abnormality have been seen in humans.

Another anomaly that has been recognized is the occurrence of 2 breaks within the chromosome and rotation of the center fragment 180 degrees. Thus, the realignment allows for a change in morphology of the chromosome although the original number of genes is preserved. This is called an **inversion.** At meiosis, however, the chromosome has difficulty in undergoing chiasm formation, and abnormal rearrangements of this chromosome, leading to partial duplications and partial losses of chromatin material, do take place. This situation may lead to several bizarre anomalies. If the centromere is involved in the inversion, the condition is called a **pericentric inversion.**

Breaks occasionally occur in 2 chromosomes, and a portion of 1 broken chromosome is inserted into the body of another, leading to a grossly abnormal chromosome. This is known as an **insertion** and generally leads to gross anomalies at meiosis.

4. Methods of Study

Sex Chromatin (X-Chromatin) Body (Barr Body)

The X-chromatin body was first seen in the nucleus of the nerve cell of a female cat in 1949 by Barr and Bertram. It has been found to be the constricted, nonfunctioning X chromosome. As a general rule, only 1 X chromosome functions in a cell at a given time. All other X chromosomes present in a cell may be seen as X-chromatin bodies in a resting nucleus. Thus, if one knows the number of X chromosomes, one can antici-

pate that the number of Barr bodies will be 1 less. If one counts the number of Barr bodies, the number of X chromosomes can be determined by adding 1.

Drumsticks on Polymorphonuclear Leukocytes

Small outpouchings of the lobes of nuclei in polymorphonuclear leukocytes of females have been demonstrated to be the X-chromatin body in this particular cell. Hence, leukocyte preparations may be used to detect X-chromatin bodies in much the same way as buccal cells are used.

Chromosome Count

In the karyotypic analysis of a patient, it is the usual practice to count 20–50 chromosome spreads for chromosome number. The purpose of this practice is to determine whether mosaicism exists because if a mosaic pattern does exist, there will be at least 2 cell lines of different counts. Photographs are made of representative spreads, and karyotypes are constructed so that the morphology of each chromosome can be studied.

Banding Techniques

As previously described, it is possible after appropriate pretreatment to stain metaphase spreads with special stains and construct a karyotype that demonstrates the banding patterns of each chromosome. In this way, it is possible to identify with certainty every chromosome in the karyotype. This is of value with problems such as translocations and trisomic conditions. Another use depends on the fact that most of the long arm of the Y chromosome is heterochromic and stains deeply with fluorescent stains. Thus, the Y chromosome can be identified at a glance, even in the resting nucleus.

APPLIED GENETICS & TERATOLOGY

1. Chromosomes & Spontaneous Abortion

An entirely new approach to reproductive biology problems became available with the advent of tissue culture and cytologic techniques that made it possible to culture cells from any tissue of the body and produce karyotypes that could be analyzed. In the early 1960s, investigators in a number of laboratories began to study chromosomes of spontaneous abortions and demonstrated that the earlier the spontaneous abortion occurred, the more likely it was due to a chromosomal abnormality. It is now known that in spontaneous abortions occurring in the first 8 weeks, the fetuses have about a 50% incidence of chromosome anomalies.

Of abortuses that are abnormal, approximately one-half are trisomic, suggesting an error of meiotic nondisjunction. One-third of abortuses with trisomy have trisomy 16.

Although this abnormality does not occur in liveborn infants, it apparently is a frequent problem in abortuses. The karyotype 45,X occurs in nearly one-fourth of chromosomally abnormal abortuses. This karyotype occurs about 24 times more frequently in abortuses than in liveborn infants, a fact that emphasizes its lethal nature. Over 15% of chromosomally abnormal abortuses have polyploidy (triploidy or tetraploidy). These lethal conditions are seen only in abortuses except in extremely rare circumstances and are due to a variety of accidents, including double fertilization and a number of meiotic errors. Finally, a small number of chromosomally abnormal abortuses have unbalanced translocations and other anomalies.

Recurrent Pregnancy Loss

Couples who experience habitual abortion constitute about 0.5% of the population. The condition is defined as 2 or more spontaneous abortions. Several investigators have studied groups of these couples using banding techniques and have found that 10–25% of them have a chromosome anomaly in either the male or female partner. Those seen are 47,XXX, 47,XYY, and a variety of balanced translocation carriers. Those with sex chromosome abnormalities frequently demonstrate other nondisjunctional events. Chromosome anomalies are thus a major cause of habitual abortion, and the incorporation of genetic evaluation into such a work-up is potentially fruitful.

Lippman-Hand and Bekemans reviewed the world literature and studied the incidence of balanced translocation carriers among 177 couples who had 2 or more spontaneous abortions. These studies suggest that in 2–3% of couples experiencing early fetal loss, 1 partner will have balanced translocations. This percentage is not markedly increased when more than 2 abortions occur. Females had a somewhat higher incidence of balanced translocations than did males.

2. Chromosomal Disorders

This section is devoted to a brief discussion of various autosomal abnormalities. Table 5–5 summarizes some of the autosomal abnormalities that have been diagnosed. They are represented as syndromes, together with some of the signs typical of these conditions. In general, autosomal monosomy is so lethal that total loss of a chromosome is rarely seen in an individual born alive. Only a few cases of monosomy 21–22 have been reported to date, which attests to the rarity of this disorder. Trisomy may occur with any chromosome. The 3 most common trisomic conditions seen in living individuals are trisomies 13, 18, and 21. Trisomy of various C group chromosomes has been reported sporadically. The most frequently reported is trisomy 8. Generally, trisomy of other chromosomes must be assumed to be lethal, because they occur only in abortuses,

not in living individuals. To date, trisomy of every autosome except chromosome 1 has been seen in abortuses.

Translocations can occur between any 2 chromosomes of the karyotype, and a variety of phenotypic expressions may be seen after mediocre arrangements. Three different translocation patterns have been identified in Down syndrome: 15/21, 21/21, and 21/22.

Deletions may also occur with respect to any chromosome in the karyotype and may be brought about by a translocation followed by a rearrangement in meiosis, which leads to the loss of chromatin material, or by a simple loss of the chromatin material following a chromosome break. Some of the more commonly seen deletion patterns are listed in Table 5–5.

The most frequent abnormality related to a chromosome abnormality is Down syndrome. Down syndrome serves as an interesting model for the discussion of autosomal diseases. The 21 trisomy type is the most common form and is responsible for approximately 95% of Down syndrome patients. There is a positive correlation between the frequency of Down syndrome and maternal age. Babies with Down syndrome are more often born to teenage mothers and even more frequently to mothers over 35. Although the reason for these findings is not entirely clear, it may be that, in older women at least, the egg has been present in prophase of the first meiotic division from the time of fetal life and that as the egg ages there is a greater tendency for nondisjunction to occur, leading to trisomy. A second theory is that coital habits are more erratic in both the very young and the older mothers, and this may lead to an increased incidence of fertilization of older eggs. This theory maintains that these eggs may be more likely to suffer nondisjunction or to accept abnormal sperm. Be this as it may, the incidence of Down syndrome in the general population is approximately 1 in 600 deliveries and at age 40 approximately 1 in 100 deliveries. At age 45, the incidence is approximately 1 in 40 deliveries (Table 5–6). The other 5% of Down syndrome patients are the result of translocations, the most common being the 15/21 translocation, but examples of 21/21 and 21/22 have been noted. In the case of 15/21, the chance of recurrence in a later pregnancy is theoretically 25%. In practice, a rate of 10% is observed if the mother is the carrier. When the father is the carrier, the odds are less because there may be a selection not favoring the sperm carrying both the 15/21 translocation and the normal 21 chromosome. In the case of 21/21 translocation, there is no chance for formation of a normal child because the carrier will contribute either both 21s or no 21 and, following fertilization, will produce either a monosomic 21 or trisomic 21. With regard to 21/22 translocation, the chance of producing a baby with Down syndrome is 1 in 2.

In general, other trisomic states occur with greater frequency in older women, and the larger the chromo-

Table 5–5. Autosomal disorders.

Type	Synonym	Signs
Monosomy		
Monosomy 21–22		Moderate mental retardation, antimongoloid slant of eyes, flared nostrils, small mouth, low-set ears, spade hands.
Trisomy		
Trisomy 13	Trisomy D: the "D₁" syndrome	Severe mental retardation, congenital heart disease (77%), polydactyly, cerebral malformations (especially aplasia of olfactory bulbs), eye defects, low-set ears, cleft lip and palate, low birth weight. Characteristic dermatoglyphic pattern.
Trisomy 18	Trisomy E: the "E" syndrome, Edward's syndrome	Severe mental retardation, long narrow skull with prominent occiput, congenital heart disease, flexion deformities of fingers, narrow palpebral fissures, low-set ears, harelip and cleft palate. Characteristic dermatoglyphics, low birth weight.
Trisomy 21	Down syndrome	Mental retardation, brachycephaly, prominent epicanthal folds. Brushfield spots, poor nasal bridge development, congenital heart disease, hypotonia, hypermobility of joints, characteristic dermatoglyphics.
Translocations		
15/21	Down syndrome	Same as trisomy 21.
21/21	Down syndrome	Same as trisomy 21.
21/22	Down syndrome	Same as trisomy 21.
Deletions		
Short arm chromosome 4(4p–)	Wolf's syndrome	Severe growth and mental retardation, midline scalp defects, seizures, deformed iris, beak nose, hypospadias.
Short arm chromosome 5(5p–)	Cri-du-chat syndrome	Microcephaly, catlike cry, hypertelorism with epicanthus, low-set ears, micrognathism, abnormal dermatoglyphics, low birth weight.
Long arm chromosome 13(13q–)	. . .	Microcephaly, psychomotor retardation, eye and ear defects, hypoplastic or absent thumbs.
Short arm chromosome 18(18p–)	. . .	Severe mental retardation, hypertelorism, low-set ears, flexion deformities of hands.
Long arm chromosome 18(18q–)	. . .	Severe mental retardation, microcephaly, hypotonia, congenital heart disease; marked dimples at elbows, shoulders, and knees.
Long arm chromosome 21(21q–)	. . .	Associated with chronic myelogenous leukemia.

some involved, the more severe the syndrome. Because trisomy 21 involves the smallest of the chromosomes, the phenotypic problems of Down syndrome are the least severe, and a moderate life expectancy may be anticipated. Even these individuals will be grossly abnormal, however, because of mental retardation and defects in other organ systems. The average life expectancy of patients with Down syndrome is much lower than for the general population.

3. Prenatal Diagnosis

Currently the most common use for applied genetics in obstetrics and gynecology is in prenatal counsel-

Table 5–6. Estimates of rates per thousand of chromosome abnormalities in live births by single-year interval.

Maternal Age	Down Syndrome	Edward's Syndrome (Trisomy 18)	Patau's Syndrome (Trisomy 13)	XXY	XYY	Turner's Syndrome Genotype	Other Clinically Significant Abnormality[1]	Total[2]
< 15	1.0[3]	< 0.1[3]	< 0.1–0.1	0.4	0.5	< 0.1	0.2	2.2
15	1.0[3]	< 0.1[3]	< 0.1–0.1	0.4	0.5	< 0.1	0.2	2.2
16	0.9[3]	< 0.1[3]	< 0.1–0.1	0.4	0.5	< 0.1	0.2	2.1
17	0.8[3]	< 0.1[3]	< 0.1–0.1	0.4	0.5	< 0.1	0.2	2.0
18	0.7[3]	< 0.1[3]	< 0.1–0.1	0.4	0.5	< 0.1	0.2	1.9
19	0.6[3]	< 0.1[3]	< 0.1–0.1	0.4	0.5	< 0.1	0.2	1.8
20	0.5–0.7	< 0.1–0.1	< 0.1–0.1	0.4	0.5	< 0.1	0.2	1.9
21	0.5–0.7	< 0.1–0.1	< 0.1–0.1	0.4	0.5	< 0.1	0.2	1.9
22	0.6–0.8	< 0.1–0.1	< 0.1–0.1	0.4	0.5	< 0.1	0.2	2.0
23	0.6–0.8	< 0.1–0.1	< 0.1–0.1	0.4	0.5	< 0.1	0.2	2.0
24	0.7–0.9	0.1–0.1	< 0.1–0.1	0.4	0.5	< 0.1	0.2	2.1
25	0.7–0.9	0.1–0.1	< 0.1–0.1	0.4	0.5	< 0.1	0.2	2.1
26	0.7–1.0	0.1–0.1	< 0.1–0.1	0.4	0.5	< 0.1	0.2	2.1
27	0.8–1.0	0.1–0.2	< 0.1–0.1	0.4	0.5	< 0.1	0.2	2.2
28	0.8–1.1	0.1–0.2	< 0.1–0.2	0.4	0.5	< 0.1	0.2	2.3
29	0.8–1.2	0.1–0.2	< 0.1–0.2	0.5	0.5	< 0.1	0.2	2.4
30	0.9–1.2	0.1–0.2	< 0.1–0.2	0.5	0.5	< 0.1	0.2	2.6
31	0.9–1.3	0.1–0.2	< 0.1–0.2	0.5	0.5	< 0.1	0.2	2.6
32	1.1–1.5	0.1–0.2	0.1–0.2	0.6	0.5	< 0.1	0.2	3.1
33	1.4–1.9	0.1–0.3	0.1–0.2	0.7	0.5	< 0.1	0.2	3.5
34	1.9–2.4	0.2–0.4	0.1–0.3	0.7	0.5	< 0.1	0.2	4.1
35	2.5–3.9	0.3–0.5	0.2–0.3	0.9	0.5	< 0.1	0.3	5.6
36	3.2–5.0	0.3–0.6	0.2–0.4	1.0	0.5	< 0.1	0.3	6.7
37	4.1–6.4	0.4–0.7	0.2–0.5	1.1	0.5	< 0.1	0.3	8.1
38	5.2–8.1	0.5–0.9	0.3–0.7	1.3	0.5	< 0.1	0.3	9.5
39	6.6–10.5	0.7–1.2	0.4–0.8	1.5	0.5	< 0.1	0.3	12.4
40	8.5–13.7	0.9–1.6	0.5–1.1	1.8	0.5	< 0.1	0.3	15.8
41	10.8–17.9	1.1–2.1	0.6–1.4	2.2	0.5	< 0.1	0.3	20.5
42	13.8–23.4	1.4–2.7	0.7–1.8	2.7	0.5	< 0.1	0.3	25.5
43	17.6–30.6	1.8–3.5	0.9–2.4	3.3	0.5	< 0.1	0.3	32.6
44	22.5–40.0	2.3–4.6	1.2–3.1	4.1	0.5	< 0.1	0.3	41.8
45	28.7–52.3	2.9–6.0	1.5–4.1	5.1	0.5	< 0.1	0.3	53.7
46	36.6–68.3	3.7–7.9	1.9–5.3	6.4	0.5	< 0.1	0.3	68.9
47	46.6–89.3	4.7–10.3	2.4–6.9	8.2	0.5	< 0.1	0.3	89.1
48	59.5–116.8	6.0–13.5	3.0–9.0	10.6	0.5	< 0.1	0.3	15.0
49	75.8–152.7	7.6–17.6	3.8–11.8	13.8	0.5	< 0.1	0.3	49.3

[1]XXX is excluded.
[2]Calculation of the total at each age assumes rate for autosomal aneuploidies is at the midpoints of the ranges given.
[3]No range may be constructed for those under 20 years by the same methods as for those 20 and over.
Reproduced with permission, from Hook EB: Rates of chromosome abnormalities at different maternal ages. *Obstet Gynecol* 1981;58:282.

ing, screening, and diagnosis. Prenatal diagnosis first came into use in 1977 with the discovery of the significance of serum α-fetoprotein (AFP). The United Kingdom Collaboration Study found that elevated AFP in maternal serum drawn between 16 and 18 weeks of gestation correlated with an increased incidence of neural tube defects (NTDs). Since that time, much research effort has been aimed at perfecting the technique. We now can screen not only for NTDs but also for trisomy 21 and trisomy 18. In addition, cystic fibrosis, sickle cell disease, and Huntington's disease, as well as many inborn errors of metabolism and other genetic disorders, can now be identified prenatally.

Neural Tube Disease

Most neural tube diseases, eg, anencephaly, spina bifida, and meningomyelocele, are associated with a multifactorial inheritance pattern. The frequency of their occurrence varies in different populations (eg, rates as high as 10 per 1000 births in Ireland and as low as 0.8 per 1000 births in the western United States). Ninety percent are index cases, ie, they occur spontaneously without previous occurrence in a family. In general, if a couple has a child with such an anomaly, the chance of producing another affected child is 2–5%. If they have had 2 such children, the risk can be as high as 10%. However, other diagnostic possibilities involving different modes of inheritance should be considered. Siblings also run greater risks of having affected children, with the highest risk being to female offspring of sisters and the lowest to male offspring of brothers. Maternal serum screening is now available to all mothers between 16 and 20 weeks of gestation. If an elevation of 2.5 or more standard deviations above the mean is noted, amniocentesis for AFP should be done along with a careful ultrasound study of the fetus for structural anomalies. Evidence for an NTD noted on ultrasound and suspected by amniotic fluid AFP elevation of 3.0 or more standard deviations indicates a diagnosis of an NTD and allows for appropriate counseling and decision making for the parents.

Maternal serum AFP screening detects about 85% of all open NTDs, thus allowing detection of 80% of all open NTDs and 90% of all anencephalic infants. Serum AFP screening does not detect skin-covered lesions or the closed form of NTDs. Thus, most encephaloceles may be missed.

Approximately 5–5.5% of women screened will have abnormally elevated values (≥ 2.5 times the mean). Most of these will be false-positive results (a repeat test should determine this) due to inaccurate dating of gestational age, multiple gestation, fetal demise or dying fetus, or a host of other structural abnormalities. In most cases, repeat AFP testing and ultrasound examination will identify the problem. If the serum AFP level remains elevated and ultrasound examination does not yield a specific diagnosis, amniotic fluid AFP levels should be measured as well as amniotic fluid acetylcholinesterase levels. Further testing and counseling may be necessary before a final diagnosis can be made. When the correct gestational age is used, the false-positive rate for second-trimester maternal screening is 3–4%.

Chromosomal Abnormalities

In 1984, maternal serum AFP levels were found to be lower in patients who delivered infants with Down syndrome. Using the AFP value with maternal age, 25–30% of fetuses with Down syndrome were detected prenatally. In 1988, 2 additional tests were added to the maternal AFP: human chorionic gonadotropin (hCG) and unconjugated estriol (uE$_3$). Using the "triple screen" a 60% detection rate for Down syndrome was accomplished. In addition, the use of uE$_3$ allowed for detection of trisomy 18.

Fetuses with Down syndrome have low maternal AFP, low uE$_3$, and high hCG. Fetuses with trisomy 18 have low values across all of the serum markers. The false-positive rate for women less than 35 years of age is 5%. Above this age cutoff the false-positive rate is increased. The definitive diagnosis of a chromosomal abnormality must be confirmed with a fetal karyotype.

The risk of fetal trisomies increases with increasing maternal age. At age 35 the risk of a trisomy is approximately 1 in 200. At age 40 the risk is 1 in 20 (Table 5–6). Prior to the discovery of serum markers, advanced maternal age was used to guide which women received fetal karyotyping. Trisomies, however, are not the only abnormality increased in this population of women. Sex chromosome aneuploidies (47,XXY and 47,XXX) also occur at an increased rate in women 35 years of age and older. Despite the advances in serum screening, fetal karyotyping continues to be the gold standard for prenatal testing in this group of women. The use of maternal serum screening in this subset of women is hindered by a high false-positive rate, less than 100% detection rate for trisomy 18 and 21, and the lack of ability to screen for the sex chromosome aneuploidies.

Cystic Fibrosis

Cystic fibrosis affects 1 in 3300 individuals of European descent in the United States. The carrier frequency is 1 in 29 for North Americans of European descent and Ashkenazi Jewish descent and 1 in 60 for African Americans. A deletion of phenylalanine at position 508 of the CFTR gene on chromosome 7 leads to the disease. All individuals with a family history of cystic fibrosis or a high carrier frequency should be offered carrier testing. For couples who are both carriers of the defective allele, fetal testing may be provided.

Future Advances in Prenatal Screening

In the detection of certain trisomies, the triple-marker screen provides better sensitivity than any single marker alone. Nonetheless, the detection rate for trisomy 18 and trisomy 21 still remains quite low. According to the Serum Urine and Ultrasound Screening Study (SURUSS), integration of nuchal translucency measurement and pregnancy-associated plasma protein-A (PAPP-A) in the first trimester improves screening. This information in conjunction with early second-trimester measurement of AFP, uE$_3$, free β-hCG (or total hCG), and inhibin-A with maternal age provides the most effective method for screening of Down Syndrome, with an 85% detection rate and 0.9% falsepositive rate. As the field of prenatal diagnostics continues to evolve, higher detection rates with lower false-positive rates can be expected. With continued research and advancing technology, prenatal screening may move into the first trimester. It may involve new markers (proform of eosinophil major basic protein [proMBP], nasal bone) and may even involve markers taken in both the first and second trimesters.

Fetal Karyotyping

A. AMNIOCENTESIS

Amniocentesis for prenatal diagnosis of genetic diseases is an extremely useful tool in the following circumstances or classes of patients:

1. Maternal age 35 years or above
2. Previous chromosomally abnormal child
3. Three or more spontaneous abortions
4. Patient or husband with chromosome anomaly
5. Family history of chromosome anomaly
6. Possible female carrier of X-linked disease
7. Metabolic disease risk (because of previous experience or family history)
8. NTD risk (because of previous experience or family history)
9. Positive second-trimester maternal serum screen

Currently, so many metabolic diseases can be diagnosed prenatally by amniocentesis that when the history elicits the possible presence of a metabolic disease, it is prudent to check with a major center to ascertain the availability of a diagnostic method.

Amniocentesis generally is carried out at 15 to 17 weeks of gestation but can be offered earlier (12–14 weeks). The underlying risk of amniocentesis when performed at 15 weeks of gestation and beyond is increased risk of miscarriage. This risk is estimated at 1 in 200 (0.5%), which is approximately the risk of Down syndrome in a 35-year-old woman. When amniocentesis is performed prior to 15 weeks the miscarriage rate is slightly increased. Table 5–7 lists some of the conditions that now can be diagnosed prenatally by biochemical means.

B. CHORIONIC VILLUS SAMPLING

Chorionic villus sampling (CVS) is a technique used in the first trimester to obtain villi for cytogenetic testing. Most commonly, it is performed transcervically; however, transabdominal routes may also be attempted. The value of CVS is that it can be performed earlier in the pregnancy, and thus the decision of pregnancy termination can be made earlier. The downfall of CVS, however, is a slightly higher

Table 5–7. Examples of hereditary diseases diagnosable prenatally.

Lipidoses: Gaucher's, Tay-Sachs, Fabry's, etc.
Mucopolysaccharidoses: Hurler's, Hunter's, etc.
Aminoacidurias: Cystinosis, homocystinuria, maple syrup urine disease, etc.
Diseases of carbohydrate metabolism: Glucose-6-phosphate dehydrogenase deficiency, glycogen storage disease, etc.
Miscellaneous: Adrenogenital syndrome, Lesch-Nyhan syndrome, sickle cell disease, cystic fibrosis, Huntington's disease, etc.

---

miscarriage rate of 1–5% and an association with distal limb defects. These risks appear to be dependent on operator experience, and lower numbers have been reported when CVS is performed between 10 and 12 weeks of gestation.

Karyotyping & Fluorescence In Situ Hybridization Analysis

Once the fetal cells are obtained they must be processed. Formal karyotyping should be performed on all specimens. This involves culturing the cells, replication, and eventually karyotyping. The entire process often takes 10–14 days until the final report becomes available. Fortunately, a quicker analysis can be obtained for some of the most common chromosomal anomalies.

The fluorescence in situ hybridization (FISH) study is a rapid assay for the detection of specific chromosomal aneuploidies using fluorescent-labeled DNA probes. Currently, probes exist for chromosomes 13, 18, 21, and 22, as well as the X and Y sex chromosomes among others. The average time to obtain a result is 24 hours. However, certain chromosomal probes may return as quickly as 4 hours. The more rapid turnaround time can be attained because the probes are mixed with uncultured amniocytes obtained from amniotic fluid or cells from CVS. If a patient is late in gestation or if the ultrasound is highly suggestive of a certain chromosomal composite, FISH analysis may be an appropriate study. With the development of multicolor FISH, all human chromosomes are painted in 24 different colors, allowing identification of chromosome rearrangement.

Single Gene Defects

If 1 parent is affected and the condition is caused by an autosomal dominant disorder, the chances are 1 in 2 that a child will be affected. If both parents are carriers of an autosomal recessive condition, the chances are 1 in 4 that the child will be affected and 1 in 2 that the child will be a carrier. Carrier status of both parents can be assumed if an affected child has been produced or if a carrier testing program is available and such testing determines that both parents are carriers. Tay-Sachs disease and sickle cell disease detection programs are examples of the latter possibility.

When carrier testing is available and the couple is at risk, as with Tay-Sachs disease in Jewish couples and sickle cell disease in blacks, the physician should order these carrier tests before pregnancy is undertaken, or immediately if the patient is already pregnant. When parents are carriers and pregnancy has been diagnosed, prenatal diagnostic testing is indicated if a test is available. If a physician does not know whether or not a test exists or how to obtain the test, the local genetic counseling program, local chapter of the National Foundation/March of Dimes, or state health department should be called for consultation. These sources may be able to inform the physician about new research that may have produced a prenatal test. A new test may be likely because this area of research is very dynamic. If genetic counseling services are readily available, patients with specific problems should be referred to those agencies for consultation. It is impossible for a physician to keep track of all of the current developments in the myriad conditions caused by single gene defects.

X-linked traits are frequently amenable to prenatal diagnostic testing. When such tests are not available, the couple has the option of testing for the sex of the fetus. If a fetus is noted to be a female, the odds are overwhelming that it will not be affected, although a carrier state may be present. If the fetus is a male, the chances are 1 in 2 that it will be affected. With this information, the couple can decide whether or not to continue the pregnancy in the case of a male fetus. Again, checking with genetic counseling agencies may reveal a prenatal diagnostic test that has only recently been described or information such as gene linkage studies that may apply in the individual case.

All options should be presented in a nonjudgmental fashion with no attempt to persuade, based on the best information available at the time. The couple should be encouraged to decide on a course of action that suits their particular needs. If the decision is appropriate, it should be supported by the physician and the genetic counselor. Very rarely, the patient will make a decision the physician regards as unwise or unrealistic. Such a decision may be based on superstition, religious or mystical beliefs, simple

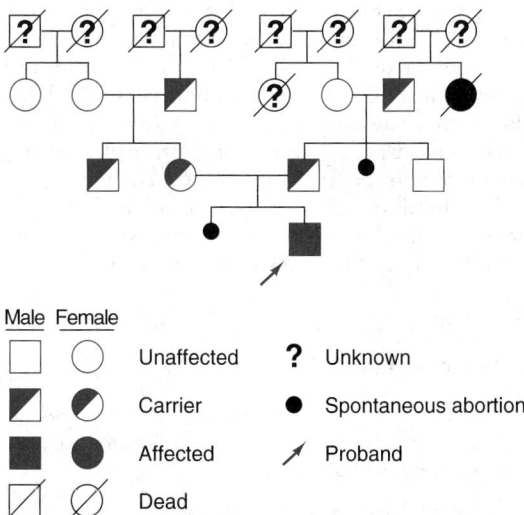

Male Female

☐	◯	Unaffected	?	Unknown
◨	◑	Carrier	●	Spontaneous abortion
■	●	Affected	↗	Proband
▱	∅	Dead		

Figure 5–4. Pedigree showing unaffected offspring, carrier offspring, and affected offspring in a family with an autosomal recessive trait (sickle cell anemia).

naivete, or even personality disorder. The physician should make every attempt to clarify the issues for the patient. Rarely, other resources such as family members or spiritual leaders may be consulted in strict confidence. The physician and the genetic counselor must clearly set forth the circumstances of the problem in the record, in case the patient undertakes a course of action that ends in tragedy and perhaps attempts to blame the professional counselors for not preventing it.

Genetic Counseling

Genetic counseling involves interaction between the physician, the family, and the genetic counselor. It is the physician's responsibility to utilize the services of the genetic consultant in the best interest of the patient. The genetic counselor will take a formal family history and construct a family tree (Fig 5–4). The assessment of the underlying general population risk of a disease and the specific family risk should be provided. When a specific diagnosis is known in the proband and the relatives are dead or otherwise not available, the counselor may ask to see photographs, which may show characteristics of the suspected condition. In many cases, when the pedigree is constructed, the inheritance pattern can be determined. If this can be done, the relative risks that future progeny will be affected can be estimated. This pedigree information is also useful in discussing the case with a genetic counselor.

■ GYNECOLOGIC CORRELATES

THE CHROMOSOMAL BASIS OF SEX DETERMINATION

Syngamy

The sex of the fetus normally is determined at fertilization. The cells of normal females contain 2 X chromosomes; those of normal males contain 1 X and 1 Y. During meiotic reduction, half of the male gametes receive a Y chromosome and the other half an X chromosome. Because the female has 2 X chromosomes, all female gametes contain an X chromosome. If a Y-bearing gamete fertilizes an ovum, the fetus is male; conversely, if an X-bearing gamete fertilizes an ovum, the fetus is female.

Arithmetically, the situation described previously should yield a male/female sex ratio of 100—the sex ratio being defined as 100 times the number of males divided by the number of females. However, for many years, the male/female sex ratio of the newborns in the white population has been approximately 105. Apparently the sex ratio at fertilization is even higher than at birth; most data on the sex of abortuses indicate a preponderance of males.

Abnormalities of Meiosis and Mitosis

The discussion in this section is limited to anomalies of meiosis and mitosis that result in some abnormality in the sex chromosome complement of the embryo.

Chromosome studies in connection with various clinical conditions suggest that errors in meiosis and mitosis do indeed occur. These errors result in any of the following principal effects: (1)an extra sex chromosome, (2) an absent sex chromosome, (3) 2 cell lines having different sex chromosomes and arising by mosaicism, (4) 2 cell lines having different sex chromosomes and arising by chimerism, (5) a structurally abnormal sex chromosome, and (6) a sex chromosome complement inconsistent with the phenotype.

By and large, an extra or a missing sex chromosome arises as the result of an error of disjunction in meiosis I or II in either the male or the female. In meiosis I, this means that instead of each of the paired homologous sex chromosomes going to the appropriate daughter cell, both go to 1 cell, leaving that cell with an extra sex chromosome and the daughter cell with none. Failure of disjunction in meiosis II simply means that the centromere fails to divide normally.

A variation of this process, known as anaphase lag, occurs when 1 of the chromosomes is delayed in arriving at the daughter cell and thus is lost. Theoretically, chromosomes may be lost by failure of association in prophase and by failure of replication, but these possibilities have not been demonstrated.

Persons who have been found to have 2 cell lines apparently have experienced problems in mitosis in the very early stage of embryogenesis. Thus, if there is nondisjunction or anaphase lag in an early (first, second, or immediately subsequent) cell division in the embryo, mosaicism may be said to exist. In this condition, there are 2 cell lines; 1 has a normal number of sex chromosomes, and the other is deficient in a sex chromosome or has an extra number of sex chromosomes. A similar situation exists in chimerism, except that there may be a difference in the sex chromosome: 1 may be an X and 1 may be a Y. This apparently arises by dispermy, by the fertilization of a double oocyte, or by the fusion, very early in embryogenesis, of 2 separately fertilized oocytes. Each of these conditions has been produced experimentally in animals.

Structural abnormalities of the sex chromosomes—deletion of the long or short arm or the formation of an isochromosome (2 short arms or 2 long arms)—result from injury to the chromosomes during meiosis. How such injuries occur is not known, but the results are noted more commonly in sex chromosomes than in autosomes—perhaps because serious injury to an autosome is much more likely to be lethal than injury to an X chromosome, and surviving injured X chromosomes would therefore be more common.

The situation in which there is a sex chromosome complement with an inappropriate genotype arises in special circumstances of true hermaphroditism and XX males (see later sections).

The X Chromosome in Humans

At about day 16 of embryonic life, there appears on the undersurface of the nuclear membrane of the somatic cells of human females a structure 1 μm in diameter known as the X-chromatin body. There is genetic as well as cytogenetic evidence that this is 1 of the X chromosomes (the only chromosome visible by ordinary light microscopy during interphase). In a sense, therefore, all females are hemizygous with respect to the X chromosome. However, there are genetic reasons for believing that the X chromosome is not entirely inactivated during the process of formation of the X-chromatin body. In normal females, inactivation of the X chromosome during interphase and its representation as the X-chromatin body are known as the Lyon phenomenon (for Mary Lyon, a British geneticist). This phenomenon may involve, at random, either the maternal or the paternal X chromosome. Furthermore, once the particular chromosome has been selected early in embryogenesis, it is always the same X chromosome that is inactivated in the progeny of that particular cell. Geneticists have found that the ratio of maternal to paternal X chromosomes inactivated is approximately 1:1.

The germ cells of an ovary are an exception to the X inactivation concept in that X inactivation does not characterize the meiotic process. Apparently, meiosis is impossible without 2 genetically active X chromosomes. Although random structural damage to 1 of the X chromosomes seems to cause meiotic arrest, oocyte loss, and therefore failure of ovarian development, an especially critical area necessary for oocyte development has been identified on the long arm of the X. This essential area involves almost all of the long arm and has been specifically located from Xq13 to Xq26. If this area is broken in 1 of the X chromosomes as in a deletion or translocation, oocyte development does not occur. However, a few exceptions to this rule have been described.

It is a curious biologic phenomenon that if 1 of the X chromosomes is abnormal, it is always this chromosome that is genetically inactivated and becomes the X-chromatin body, regardless of whether it is maternal or paternal in origin. Although this general rule seems to be an exception to the randomness of X inactivation, this is more apparent than real. Presumably, random inactivation does occur, but the disadvantaged cells—ie, those left with a damaged active X—do not survive. Consequently, the embryo develops only with cells with a normal active X chromosome (X-chromatin body) (Fig 5–5).

If there are more than 2 X chromosomes, all X chromosomes except 1 are genetically inactivated and become X-chromatin bodies; thus, in this case, the number of X-chromatin bodies will be equal to the number of X chromosomes minus 1. This type of inactivation applies to X chromosomes even when a Y chromosome is present, eg, in Klinefelter's syndrome.

Although the X chromosomes are primarily concerned with the determination of femininity, there is abundant genetic evidence that loci having to do with traits other than sex determination are present on the X chromosome. Thus, in the catalog of genetic disorders given in the 10th edition of *Mendelian Inheritance in Man,* 320 traits are listed as more or less definitely X-linked. Substantial evidence for X linkage has been found for about 160 of these traits; the rest are only suspected of having this relationship. Hemophilia, color blindness, childhood muscular dystrophy (Duchenne's dystrophy), Lesch-Nyhan syndrome, and glucose-6-phosphate dehydrogenase deficiency are among the better known conditions controlled by loci on the X chromosome. These entities probably arise from the expression of a recessive gene due to its hemizygous situation in males.

X-linked dominant traits are infrequent in humans. Vitamin D–resistant rickets is an example.

At least 1 disorder can be classified somewhere between a structural anomaly of the X chromosome and a single gene mutation. X-linked mental retardation in males is associated with a fragile site at q26, but a special culture medium is required for its demonstration. Furthermore, it has been shown that heterozygote female carriers for this fragile site have low IQ test scores.

The Y Chromosome in Humans

Just as the X chromosome is the only chromosome visible by ordinary light microscopy during interphase, the Y chromosome is the only chromosome visible in interphase, after exposure to quinacrine compounds, by fluorescence microscopy. This is a very useful diagnostic method.

In contrast to the X chromosome, few traits have been traced to the Y chromosome except those having to do with testicular formation and those at the very tip of the short arm, homologous with those at the tip of the short arm of the X. Possession of the Y chromosome alone, ie, without an X chromosome, apparently is lethal, because such a case has never been described.

Present on the Y chromosome is an area that produces a factor which allows for testicular development. This factor is termed testis-determining factor (TDF). Without the presence of TDF normal female anatomy will develop. When TDF is present, testicular development occurs with subsequent differentia-

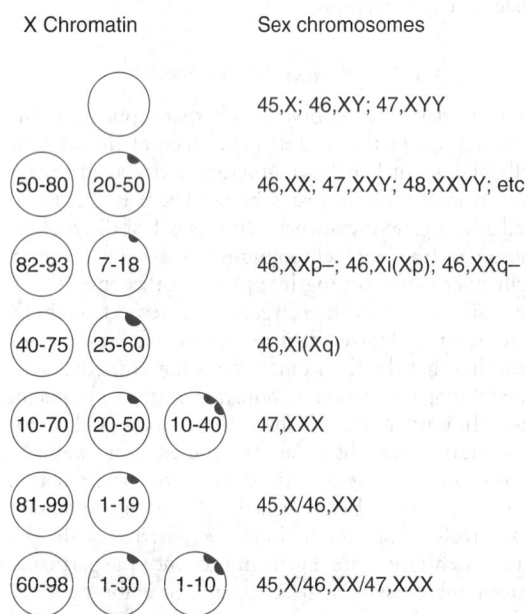

X Chromatin			Sex chromosomes
			45,X; 46,XY; 47,XYY
50-80	20-50		46,XX; 47,XXY; 48,XXYY; etc.
82-93	7-18		46,XXp–; 46,Xi(Xp); 46,XXq–
40-75	25-60		46,Xi(Xq)
10-70	20-50	10-40	47,XXX
81-99	1-19		45,X/46,XX
60-98	1-30	1-10	45,X/46,XX/47,XXX

Figure 5–5. Relation of X-chromatin body to the possible sex chromosome components.

tion of Sertoli cells. The Sertoli cells in turn produce a second factor central to male differentiation, müllerian-inhibiting factor (MIF), also termed antimüllerian factor (AMF). The presence of MIF causes the regression of the müllerian ducts and thereby allows for the development of normal internal male anatomy.

ABNORMAL DEVELOPMENT

1. Ovarian Agenesis–Dysgenesis

In 1938, Turner described 7 girls 15–23 years of age with sexual infantilism, webbing of the neck, cubitus valgus, and retardation of growth. A survey of the literature indicates that "Turner's syndrome" means different things to different writers. After the later discovery that ovarian streaks are characteristically associated with the clinical entity described by Turner, "ovarian agenesis" became a synonym for Turner's syndrome. After discovery of the absence of the X-chromatin body in such patients, the term ovarian agenesis gave way to "gonadal dysgenesis," "gonadal agenesis," or "gonadal aplasia."

Meanwhile, some patients with the genital characteristics mentioned previously were shown to have a normally positive X-chromatin count. Furthermore, a variety of sex chromosome complements have been found in connection with streak gonads. As if these contradictions were not perplexing enough, it has been noted that streaks are by no means confined to patients with Turner's original tetrad of infantilism, webbing of the neck, cubitus valgus, and retardation of growth but may be present in girls with sexual infantilism only. Since Turner's original description, a host of additional somatic anomalies (varying in frequency) have been associated with his original clinical picture; these include shield chest, overweight, high palate, micrognathia, epicanthal folds, low-set ears, hypoplasia of nails, osteoporosis, pigmented moles, hypertension, lymphedema, cutis laxa, keloids, coarctation of the aorta, mental retardation, intestinal telangiectasia, and deafness.

For our purposes, the eponym Turner's syndrome will be used to indicate sexual infantilism with ovarian streaks, short stature, and 2 or more of the somatic anomalies mentioned earlier. In this context, terms such as ovarian agenesis, gonadal agenesis, and gonadal dysgenesis lose their clinical significance and become merely descriptions of the gonadal development of the person. At least 21 sex chromosome complements have been associated with streak gonads (Fig 5–6), but only about 9 sex chromosome complements have been associated with Turner's syndrome. However, approximately two-thirds of patients with Turner's syndrome have a 45,X chromosome complement, whereas only one-fourth of patients without Turner's syndrome but with streak ovaries have a 45,X chromosome complement.

```
45,X
46,XX
46,XY
46,XXp–
46,XXq–
46,Xi(Xp)
46,Xi(Xq)
46,XXq–?
45,X/46,XX
45,X/46,XY
45,X/46,Xi(Xq)
45,X/46,XXp–
45,X/46,XXq–
45,X/46,XXq–?
45,X/46,XX        ⎫
45,X/46,Xi(Xq)    ⎭
45,X/46,XX/47,XXX       ⎫
45,X/47,XXX            ⎭
45,X/46,XX/47,XXX            ⎫
45,X/46,Xi(Xq)/47,XXX       ⎭
45,X/46,XXr(X)
45,X/46,XX/46,XXr(X)
45,X/46,XXr(X)/47,XXr(X)r(X)
45,X/46,XX/47,XXX       ⎫
45,X/46,XXq–            ⎭
```

Figure 5–6. The 21 sex chromosome complements that have been found in patients with streak gonads.

Karyotype–phenotype correlations in the syndromes associated with ovarian agenesis are not completely satisfactory. Nonetheless, if gonadal development is considered as 1 problem and if the somatic difficulties associated with these syndromes are considered as a separate problem, one can make certain correlations.

With respect to failure of gonadal development, it is important to recall that diploid germ cells require 2 normal active X chromosomes. This is in contrast to the somatic cells, where only 1 sex chromosome is thought to be genetically active, at least after day 16 of embryonic life in the human, when the X-chromatin body first appears in the somatic cells. It is also important to recall that in 45,X persons no oocytes persist, and streak gonads are the rule. From these facts, it can be inferred that failure of gonadal development is not the result of a specific sex chromosome defect but rather of the absence of 2 X chromosomes with the necessary critical zones.

Karyotype–phenotype correlations with respect to somatic abnormalities are even sketchier than the correlations with regard to gonadal development. However, good evidence shows that monosomy for the short arm of the X chromosome is related to somatic difficulties, although some patients with long-arm deletions have somatic abnormalities.

History of Gonadal Agenesis

The histologic findings in these abnormal ovaries in patients with gonadal streaks are essentially the same regardless of the patient's cytogenetic background (Fig 5–7).

Fibrous tissue is the major component of the streak. It is indistinguishable microscopically from that of the normal ovarian stroma. The so-called germinal epithelium, on the surface of the structure, is a layer of low cuboid cells; this layer appears to be completely inactive.

Tubules of the ovarian rete are invariably found in sections taken from about the midportion of the streak.

In all patients who have reached the age of normal puberty, hilar cells are also demonstrated. The number of hilar cells varies among patients. In those with some enlargement of the clitoris, hilar cells are present in large numbers. These developments may be causally related. Nevertheless, hilar cells are also found in many normal ovaries. The origin of hilar cells is not precisely known, but they are associated with development of the medullary portion of the gonad. Their presence lends further support to the concept that in ovarian agenesis the gonad develops along normal lines until just before the expected appearance of early oocytes. In all cases in which sections of the broad ligament have been available for study, it has been possible to identify the mesonephric duct and tubules—broad ligament structures found in normal females.

Clinical Findings

A. SYMPTOMS AND SIGNS

1. In newborn infants—The newborn with streak ovaries often shows edema of the hands and feet. Histologically, this edema is associated with large dilated vascular spaces. With such findings, it is obviously desirable to obtain a karyotype. However, some children with streak ovaries—particularly those who have few or no somatic abnormalities—cannot be recognized at birth.

2. In adolescents—The arresting and characteristic clinical finding in many of these patients is their short stature. Typical patients seldom attain a height of 1.5 m (5 ft) (Fig 5–8). In addition, sexual infantilism is a striking finding. As mentioned earlier, a variety of somatic abnormalities may be present; by definition, if 2 or more of these are noted, the patient may be considered to have Turner's syndrome. Most of these patients have only 1 normal X chromosome, and two-thirds of them have no other sex chromosome. Patients of normal height without somatic abnormalities may also have gonadal streaks. Under these circumstances, there is likely to be a cell line with 2 normal sex chromosomes but often a second line with a single X. The internal findings are exactly the same as in patients with classic Turner's syndrome, however.

B. LABORATORY FINDINGS

An important finding in patients of any age—but especially after expected puberty, ie, about 12 years—is elevation of total gonadotropin production. From a practical point of view, ovarian failure in patients over age 15 cannot be considered a diagnostic possibility unless the serum follicle-stimulating hormone level is more than 50 mIU/mL and luteinizing hormone level is more than 90 mIU/mL.

Nongonadal endocrine functions are normal. Urinary excretion of estrogens is low, and the maturation index and other vaginal smear indices are shifted well to the left.

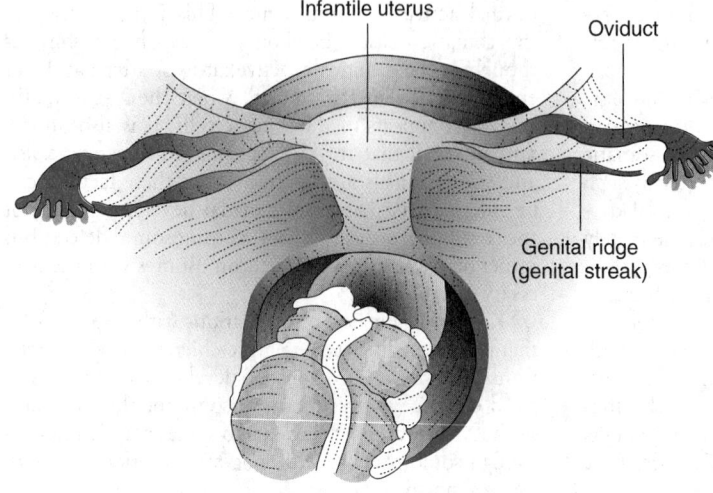

Infantile uterus
Oviduct
Genital ridge (genital streak)

Figure 5–7. Gonadal streaks in a patient with the phenotype of Turner's syndrome. (Redrawn and reproduced, with permission, from Jones HW Jr, Scott WW: *Hermaphroditism, Genital Anomalies and Related Endocrine Disorders,* 2nd ed. Williams & Wilkins, 1971.)

Figure 5–8. Patient with Turner's syndrome. (Reproduced, with permission, from Jones HW Jr, Scott WW: *Hermaphroditism, Genital Anomalies and Related Endocrine Disorders,* 2nd ed. Williams & Wilkins, 1971.)

Treatment

Substitution therapy with estrogen is necessary for development of secondary characteristics.

Therapy with growth hormone will increase height. Whether ultimate height will be greater than it otherwise would be is uncertain, but current evidence suggests that it will be.

The incidence of malignant degeneration is increased in the gonadal streaks of patients with a Y chromosome, as compared with normal males. Surgical removal of streaks from all patients with a Y chromosome is recommended.

2. True Hermaphroditism

By classic definition, true hermaphroditism exists when both ovarian and testicular tissue can be demonstrated in 1 patient. In humans, the Y chromosome carries genetic material that normally is responsible for testicular development; this material is active even when multiple X chromosomes are present. Thus, in Klinefelter's syndrome, a testis develops with up to 4 Xs and only 1 Y. Conversely (with rare exceptions), a testis has not been observed to develop in the absence of the Y chromosome. The exceptions are found in true hermaphrodites and XX males, in whom testicular tissue has developed in association with an XX sex chromosome complement.

Clinical Findings

A. SYMPTOMS AND SIGNS

No exclusive features clinically distinguish true hermaphroditism from other forms of intersexuality. Hence, the diagnosis must be entertained in an infant with any form of intersexuality, except only those with a continuing virilizing influence, eg, congenital adrenal hyperplasia. Firm diagnosis is possible after the onset of puberty, when certain clinical features become evident, but the diagnosis can and should be made in infancy.

In the past, most true hermaphrodites have been reared as males because they have rather masculine-appearing external genitalia (Fig 5–9). Nevertheless, with early diagnosis, most should be reared as females.

Almost all true hermaphrodites develop female-type breasts. This helps to distinguish male hermaphroditism from true hermaphroditism, because few male hermaphrodites other than those with familial feminizing hermaphroditism develop large breasts.

Many true hermaphrodites menstruate. The presence or absence of menstruation is partially determined by the development of the uterus; many true hermaphrodites have rudimentary or no development of the müllerian ducts (Fig 5–10).

A few patients who had a uterus and menstruated after removal of testicular tissue have become pregnant and delivered normal children.

Figure 5–9. External genitalia of a patient with true hermaphroditism. (Reproduced, with permission, from Jones HW Jr, Scott WW: *Hermaphroditism, Genital Anomalies and Related Endocrine Disorders,* 2nd ed. Williams & Wilkins, 1971.)

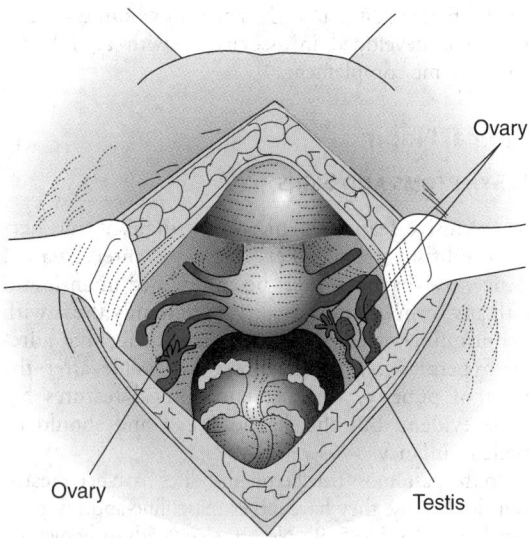

Figure 5–10. Internal genitalia of a patient with true hermaphroditism. (Reproduced, with permission, from Jones HW Jr, Scott WW: *Hermaphroditism, Genital Anomalies and Related Endocrine Disorders,* 2nd ed. Williams & Wilkins, 1971.)

B. SEX CHROMOSOME COMPLEMENTS

Most true hermaphrodites have X-chromatin bodies and karyotypes that are indistinguishable from those of normal females. In contrast to these, a few patients who cannot be distinguished clinically from other true hermaphrodites have been reported to have a variety of other karyotypes—eg, several chimeric persons with karyotypes of 46,XX/46,XY have been identified.

In true hermaphrodites, the testis is competent in its müllerian-suppressive functions, but an ovotestis may behave as an ovary insofar as its müllerian-suppressive function is concerned. The true hermaphroditic testis or ovotestis is as competent to masculinize the external genitalia as is the testis of a patient with the virilizing type of male hermaphroditism. This is unrelated to karyotype.

Deletion mapping by DNA hybridization has shown that most (but not all) XX true hermaphrodites have Y-specific sequences. Abnormal crossover of a portion of the Y chromosome to the X in meiosis may explain some cases. This latter is further supported by the finding of a positive H-Y antigen assay in some patients with 46,XX true hermaphroditism.

In general, the clinical picture of true hermaphroditism is not compatible with the clinical picture in other kinds of gross chromosomal anomalies. For example, very few true hermaphrodites have associated somatic anomalies, and mental retardation almost never occurs.

Treatment

The principles of treatment of true hermaphroditism do not differ from those of the treatment of hermaphroditism in general. Therapy can be summarized by stating that surgical removal of contradictory organs is indicated, and the external genitalia should be reconstructed in keeping with the sex of rearing. The special problem in this group is how to establish with certainty the character of the gonad. This is particularly difficult in the presence of an ovotestis, because its recognition by gross characteristics is notoriously inaccurate, and one must not remove too much of the gonad for study. In some instances the gonadal tissue of 1 sex is completely embedded within a gonadal structure primarily of the opposite sex.

3. Klinefelter's Syndrome

This condition, first described in 1942 by Klinefelter, Reifenstein, and Albright, occurs only in apparent males. As originally described, it is characterized by small testes, azoospermia, gynecomastia, relatively normal external genitalia, and otherwise average somatic development. High levels of gonadotropin in urine or serum are characteristic.

Clinical Findings

A. SYMPTOMS AND SIGNS

By definition, this syndrome applies only to persons reared as males. The disease is not recognizable before puberty except by routine screening of newborn infants. Most patients come under observation at 16–40 years of age.

Somatic development during infancy and childhood may be normal. Growth and muscular development may also be within normal limits. Most patients have a normal general appearance and no complaints referable to this abnormality, which is often discovered during the course of a routine physical examination or an infertility study.

In the original publication by Klinefelter and co-workers, gynecomastia was considered an essential part of the syndrome. Since then, however, cases without gynecomastia have been reported.

The external genitalia are perfectly formed and in most patients are quite well developed. Erection and intercourse usually are satisfactory.

There is no history of delayed descent of the testes in typical cases, and the testes are in the scrotum. Neither is there any history of testicular trauma or disease. Although a history of mumps orchitis is occasionally elicited, this disease has not been correlated with the syndrome. However the testes are often very small in contrast to the rest of the genitalia (about 1.5×1.5 cm).

Psychological symptoms are often present. Most studies of this syndrome have been performed in psychiatric institutions. The seriousness of the psychological disturbance seems to be partly related to the number of extra X chromosomes—eg, it is estimated that about one-fourth of XXY patients have some degree of mental retardation.

B. LABORATORY FINDINGS

One of the extremely important clinical features of Klinefelter's syndrome is the excessive amount of pituitary gonadotropin found in either urine or serum assay.

The urinary excretion of neutral 17-ketosteroids varies from relatively normal to definitely subnormal levels. There is a rough correlation between the degree of hypoleydigism as judged clinically and a low 17-ketosteroid excretion rate.

C. HISTOLOGIC AND CYTOGENETIC FINDINGS

Klinefelter's syndrome may be regarded as a form of primary testicular failure.

Several authors have classified a variety of forms of testicular atrophy as subtypes of Klinefelter's syndrome. Be this as it may, Klinefelter believed that only those patients who have a chromosomal abnormality could be said to have this syndrome. Microscopic examination of the adult testis shows that the seminiferous tubules lack epithelium and are shrunken and hyalinized. They contain large amounts of elastic fibers, and Leydig cells are present in large numbers.

Males with positive X-chromatin bodies are likely to have Klinefelter's syndrome. The nuclear sex anomaly reflects a basic genetic abnormality in sex chromosome constitution. All cases studied have had at least 2 X chromosomes and 1 Y chromosome. The most common abnormality in the sex chromosome constitution is XXY, but the literature also records XXXY, XXYY, XXXXY, and XXXYY, and mosaics of XX/XXY, XY/XXY, XY/XXXY, and XXXY/XXXXY. In all examples except the XX/XXY mosaic, a Y chromosome is present in all cells. From these patterns, it is obvious that the Y chromosome has a very strong testis-forming impulse, which can operate in spite of the presence of as many as 4 X chromosomes.

Thus, patients with Klinefelter's syndrome will have not only a positive X-chromatin body but also a positive Y-chromatin body.

The abnormal sex chromosome constitution causes differentiation of an abnormal testis, leading to testicular failure in adulthood. At birth or before puberty, such testes show a marked deficiency or absence of germinal cells.

By means of nursery screening, the frequency of males with positive X-chromatin bodies has been estimated to be 2.65 per 1000 live male births.

Treatment

There is no treatment for the 2 principal complaints of these patients: infertility and gynecomastia. No pituitary preparation has been effective in the regeneration of the hyalinized tubular epithelium or the stimulation of gametogenesis. Furthermore, no hormone regimen is effective in treating the breast hypertrophy. When the breasts are a formidable psychological problem, surgical removal may be a satisfactory procedure. In patients who have clinical symptoms of hypoleydigism, substitution therapy with testosterone is an important physiologic and psychological aid. Donor sperm may be offered for treatment of infertility.

4. Double-X Males

A few cases of adult males with a slightly hypoplastic penis and very small testes but no other indication of abnormal sexual development have been reported. These males are sterile. Unlike those with Klinefelter's syndrome, they do not have abnormal breast development. They are clinically very similar to patients with Del Castillo's syndrome (testicular dysgenesis). Nevertheless, the XX males have a positive sex chromatin and a normal female karyotype. These may be extreme examples of the sex reversal that usually is partial in true hermaphroditism.

5. Multiple-X Syndromes

The finding of more than 1 X-chromatin body in a cell indicates the presence of more than 2 X chromosomes in that particular cell. In many patients, such a finding is associated with mosaicism, and the clinical picture is controlled by this fact—eg, if 1 of the strains of the mosaicism is 45,X, gonadal agenesis is likely to occur. There also are persons who do not seem to have mosaicism but do have an abnormal number of X chromosomes in all cells. In such persons, the most common complement is XXX (triplo-X syndrome), but XXXX (tetra-X syndrome) and XXXXX (penta-X syndrome) have been reported.

An additional X chromosome does not seem to have a consistent effect on sexual differentiation. The body proportions of these persons are normal, and the external genitalia are normally female. A number of such persons have been examined at laparotomy, and no consistent abnormality of the ovary has been found. In a few cases, the number of follicles appeared to be reduced, and in at least 1 case the ovaries were very small and the ovarian stroma poorly differentiated. About 20% of postpubertal patients with the triplo-X syndrome report various degrees of amenorrhea or some irregularity in menstruation. For the most part, however, these patients have a normal menstrual history and are of proved fertility.

Almost all patients known to have multiple-X syndromes have some degree of mental retardation. A few have mongoloid features. (The mothers of these patients tended to be older than the mothers of normal children, as is true with Down syndrome.) Perhaps these findings are in part circumstantial, as most of these patients were discovered during surveys in mental institutions. The important clinical point is that mentally retarded infants should have chromosomal study.

Uniformly, the offspring of triplo-X mothers have been normal. This is surprising, because theoretically in such cases meiosis should produce equal numbers of ova containing 1 or 2 X chromosomes, and fertilization of the abnormal XX ova should give rise to XXX and XXY individuals. Nevertheless, the triplo-X condition seems selective for normal ova and zygotes.

The diagnosis of this syndrome is made by identifying a high percentage of cells with double X-chromatin bodies in the buccal smear and by finding 47 chromosomes with a karyotype showing an extra X chromosome in all cells cultured from the peripheral blood. It should be noted that in the examination of the buccal smear, some cells have a single X-chromatin body. Hence, based on the chromatin examination, one might suspect XX/XXX mosaicism. Actually, in triplo-X patients, only a single type of cell can be demonstrated in cultures of cells from the peripheral blood. The absence of the second X-chromatin body in some of the somatic cells may result from the time of examination of the cell (during interphase) and from the spatial orientation, which could have prevented visualization of the 2 X-chromatin bodies (adjacent to the nuclear membrane). In this syndrome, the number of cells containing either 1 or 2 X-chromatin bodies is very high—at least 60–80%, as compared with an upper limit of about 40% in normal females.

6. Female Hermaphroditism due to Congenital Adrenal Hyperplasia

ESSENTIALS OF DIAGNOSIS

- *Female pseudohermaphroditism, ambiguous genitalia with clitoral hypertrophy, and, occasionally, persistent urogenital sinus.*
- *Early appearance of sexual hair; hirsutism, dwarfism.*
- *Urinary 17-ketosteroids elevated; pregnanetriol may be increased.*
- *Elevated serum 17-hydroxyprogesterone level.*
- *Occasionally associated with water and electrolyte imbalance—particularly in the neonatal period.*

General Considerations

Female hermaphroditism due to congenital adrenal hyperplasia is a clearly delineated clinical syndrome. The syndrome has been better understood since the discovery that cortisone may successfully arrest virilization. The problem usually is due to a deficiency of a gene required for 21-hydroxylation in the biosynthesis of cortisol.

If the diagnosis is not made in infancy, an unfortunate series of events ensues. Because the adrenals secrete an abnormally large amount of virilizing steroid even during embryonic life, these infants are born with abnormal genitalia (Fig 5–11). In extreme cases, there is fusion of the scrotolabial folds and, in rare instances, even formation of a penile urethra. The clitoris is greatly enlarged so that it may be mistaken for a penis (Fig 5–12). No gonads are palpable within the fused scrotolabial folds, and their absence has sometimes given rise to the mistaken impression

Figure 5–11. External genitalia of a female patient with congenital virilizing adrenal hyperplasia. Compare with Fig 5–12. (Reproduced, with permission, from Jones HW Jr, Scott WW: *Hermaphroditism, Genital Anomalies and Related Endocrine Disorders,* 2nd ed. Williams & Wilkins, 1971.)

Figure 5–12. External genitalia of a female patient with congenital virilizing adrenal hyperplasia. This is a more severe deformity than that shown in Fig 5–11.

of male cryptorchidism. Usually, there is a single urinary meatus at the base of the phallus, and the vagina enters the persistent urogenital sinus as noted in Figure 5–13.

During infancy, provided there are no serious electrolyte disturbances, these children grow more rapidly than normal. For a time, they greatly exceed the average in both height and weight. Unfortunately, epiphyseal closure occurs by about age 10, and as a result these people are much shorter than normal as adults (Fig 5–14).

The process of virilization begins at an early age. Pubic hair may appear as early as age 2 years but usually somewhat later. This is followed by growth of axillary hair and finally by the appearance of body hair and a beard, which may be so thick as to require daily shaving. Acne may develop early. Puberty never ensues. There is no breast development. Menstruation does not occur. During the entire process, serum adrenal androgens and 17-hydroxyprogesterone levels are abnormally high.

Although our principal concern here is with this abnormality in females, it must be mentioned that adrenal hyperplasia of the adrenogenital type may also occur in males, in whom it is called macrogenitosomia precox. Sexual development progresses rapidly, and the sex organs attain adult size at an early age. Just as in the female, sexual hair and acne develop unusually early, and the voice becomes deep. The testes are usually in the scrotum; however, in early childhood they remain small and immature, although the genitalia are of adult dimensions. In adulthood, the testes usually enlarge and spermatogenesis occurs, allowing impregnation rates similar to those of a control population. Somatic development in the male corresponds to that of the female; as a child, the male exceeds the average in height and strength, but (if untreated) as an adult he is stocky, muscular, and well below average height.

Both the male and the female with this disorder—but especially the male—may have the complicating

problem of electrolyte imbalance. In infancy, it is manifested by vomiting, progressive weight loss, and dehydration and may be fatal unless recognized promptly. The characteristic findings are an exceedingly low serum sodium level, low CO_2-combining power level, and high potassium level. The condition is sometimes misdiagnosed as congenital pyloric stenosis.

A few of these patients have a deficiency in 11-hydroxylation that is associated with hypertension in addition to virilization.

Adrenal Histology

The adrenal changes center on a reticular hyperplasia, which becomes more marked as the patient grows older. In some instances, he glomerulosa may participate in the hyperplasia, but the fasciculata is greatly diminished in amount or entirely absent. Lipid studies show absence of fascicular and glomterular lipid but an abnormally strong lipid reaction in the reticularis (Fig 5–15).

Ovarian Histology

The ovarian changes can be summarized by stating that in infants, children, and teenagers, there is normal follicular development to the antrum stage but no evidence of ovulation. With increasing age, less and less follicular activity occurs, andprimordial follicles disappear. This disappearance must not be complete, however, because cortisone therapy, even in adults, usually results in ovulatory menstruation after 4–6 months of treatment.

Developmental Anomalies of the Genital Tubercle & Urogenital Sinus Derivatives

The phallus is composed of 2 lateral corpora cavernosa, but the corpus spongiosum is normally absent. The external urinary meatus is most often located at the base of the phallus (Fig 5–11). An occasional case may be seen in which the urethra does extend to the end of the clitoris (Fig 5–12). The glans penis and the prepuce are present and indistinguishable from these structures in the male. The scrotolabial folds are characteristically fused in the midline, giving a scrotumlike appearance with a median perineal raphe; however, they seldom enlarge to normal scrotal size. No gonads are palpable within the scrotolabial folds. When the anomaly is not severe (eg, in patients with postnatal virilization), fusion of the scrotolabial folds is not complete, and by gentle retraction it is often possible to locate not only the normally located external urinary meatus but also the orifice of the vagina.

An occasional patient has no communication between the urogenital sinus and the vagina. In no case does the vagina communicate with that portion of

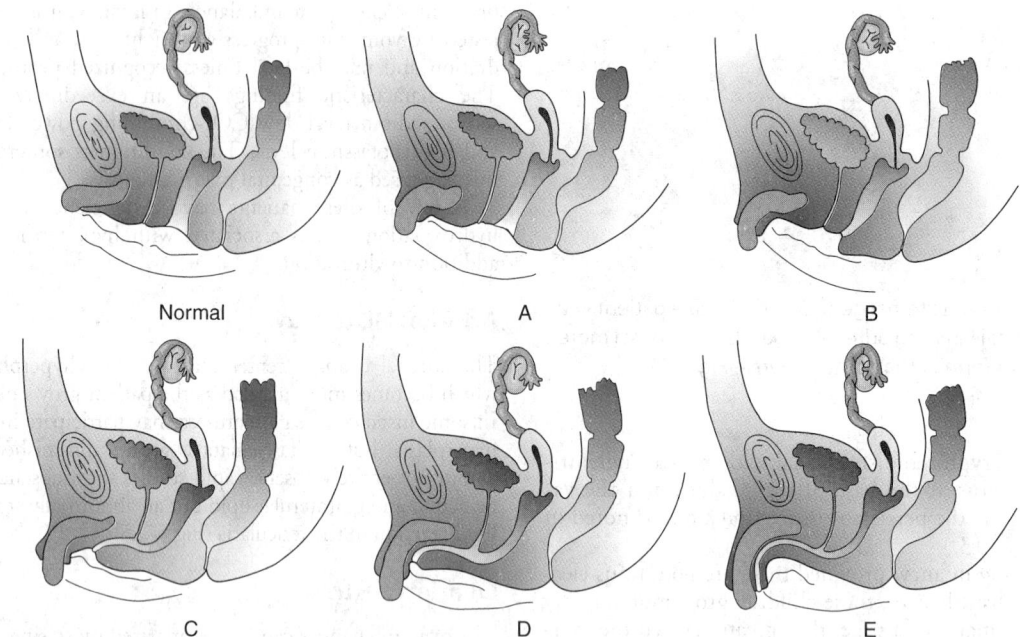

Figure 5–13. Sagittal view of genital deformities of increasing severity **(A–E)** in congenital virilizing adrenal hyperplasia. (Redrawn and reproduced, with permission, from Verkauf BS, Jones HW Jr: Masculinization of the female genitalia in congenital adrenal hyperplasia. South Med J 1970;63:634.)

the urogenital sinus that gives rise to the female urethra or the prostatic urethra. Instead, the vaginal communication is via caudal urogenital sinus derivatives; thus, fortunately, the sphincter mechanism is not involved, and the anomalous communication is with that portion of the sinus that develops as the vaginal vestibule in the female and the membranous urethra in the male. From the gynecologist's point of view, it is much more meaningful to say that the vagina and (female) urethra enter a persistent urogenital sinus than to say that the vagina enters the (membranous [male]) urethra. This conclusion casts some doubt on the embryologic significance of the prostatic utricle, which is commonly said to represent the homologue of the vagina in the normal male.

Hormone Changes

Important and specific endocrine changes occur in congenital adrenal hyperplasia of the adrenogenital type. The ultimate diagnosis depends on demonstration of these abnormalities.

A. URINARY ESTROGENS

The progressive virilization of female hermaphrodites caused by adrenal hyperplasia would suggest that estrogen secretion in these patients is low, and this hypothesis is further supported by the atrophic condition of both the ovarian follicular apparatus and the estrogen target organs. Actually, the determination of urinary estrogens, both fluorometrically and biologically, indicates that it is elevated.

B. SERUM STEROIDS

The development of satisfactory radioimmunoassay techniques for measuring steroids in blood serum has resulted in an increased tendency to measure serum steroids rather than urinary metabolites in diagnosing the condition and monitoring therapy. Serum steroid profiles of many patients with this disorder show that numerous defects in the biosynthesis of cortisol may occur. The most common defect is at the 21-hydroxylase step. Less frequent defects are at the 11-hydroxylase step and the 3β-ol-dehydrogenase step. Rarely, the defect is at the 17-hydroxylase step. In the most common form of the disorder—21-hydroxylase deficiency—the serum 17-hydroxyprogesterone level and, to a lesser extent, the serum progesterone level are elevated. This is easily understandable when it is recalled that 17-hydroxyprogesterone is the substrate for the 21-hydroxylation step (Fig 5–16). Likewise, in the other enzyme defects, the levels of serum steroid substrates are greatly elevated.

Figure 5–14. Untreated adult with virilizing adrenal hyperplasia. Note the short stature and the relative shortness of the limbs. (Reproduced, with permission, from Jones HW Jr, Scott WW: *Hermaphroditism, Genital Anomalies and Related Endocrine Disorders,* 2nd ed. Williams & Wilkins, 1971.)

Pathogenesis of Virilizing Adrenal Hyperplasia

The basic defects in congenital virilizing adrenal hyperplasia are 1 or more enzyme deficiencies in the biosynthesis of cortisol (Fig 5–16). With the reduced production of cortisol, normal feedback to the hypothalamus fails, with the result that increased amounts of adrenocorticotropic hormone (ACTH) are produced. This excess production of ACTH stimulates the deficient adrenal gland to produce relatively normal amounts of cortisol—but also stimulates production of abnormally large amounts of estrogen and androgens by the zona reticularis. In this overproduction, a biologic preponderance of androgens causes virilization. These abnormal sex steroids suppress the gonadotropins so that untreated patients never reach puberty and do not menstruate.

Therefore, the treatment of this disorder consists in part of the administration of sufficient exogenous cortisol to suppress ACTH production to normal levels. This in turn should reduce overstimulation of the adre-

nal so that the adrenal will cease to produce abnormally large amounts of estrogen and androgen. The gonadotropins generally return to normal levels, with consequent feminization of the patient and achievement of menstruation.

The pathogenesis of the salt-losing type of adrenal hyperplasia involves a deficiency in aldosterone production.

Diagnosis

Hermaphroditism due to congenital adrenal hyperplasia must be suspected in any infant born with ambiguous or abnormal external genitalia. It is exceedingly important that the diagnosis be made at a very early age if undesirable disturbances of metabolism are to be prevented.

All patients with ambiguous external genitalia should have an appraisal of their chromosomal characteristics. In all instances of female pseudohermaphroditism due to congenital hyperplasia, the chromosomal composition is that of a normal female. A pelvic ultrasound in the newborn to determine he presence of a uterus is very helpful and, if positive, strongly suggests a female infant.

The critical determinations are those of the urinary 17-ketosteroid and serum 17-hydroxyprogesterone le-

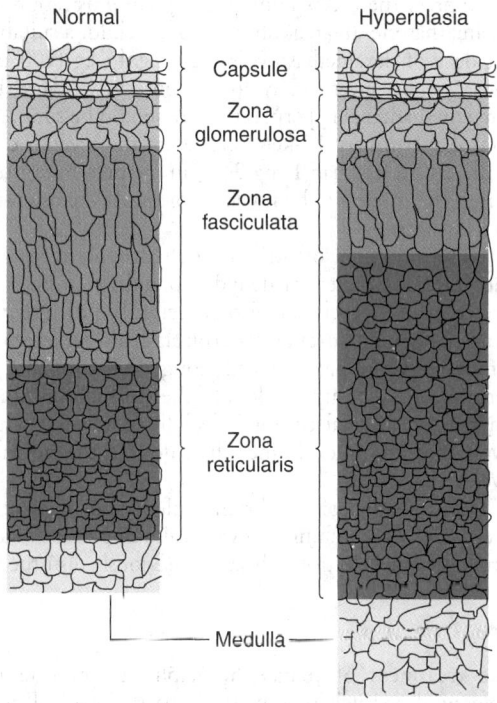

Figure 5–15. Normal adrenal architecture and adrenal histology in congenital virilizing adrenal hyperplasia. Note the great relative increase in the zona reticularis.

Figure 5–16. Enzymatic steps in cortisol synthesis. Localization of defects in congenital adrenal hyperplasia.

vels. If these are elevated, the diagnosis must be either congenital adrenal hyperplasia or tumor. In the newborn, the latter is very rare, but in older children and adults with elevated 17-ketosteroids the possibility of tumor must be considered. One of the most satisfactory methods of making this different diagnosis is to attempt to suppress the excess androgens by administration of dexamethasone. In an adult or an older child, a suitable test dose of dexamethasone is 1.25 mg/45 kg (100 lb) body weight, given orally for 7 consecutive days. In congenital adrenal hyperplasia, there should be suppression of the urinary 17-ketosteroids on the seventh day of the test to less than 1 mg/24 h; in the presence of tumor, either there will be no effect or the 17-ketosteroid levels will rise.

Determination of urinary dehydroepiandrosterone (DHEA) or serum dehydroepiandrosterone sulfate (DHEAS) levels can also be helpful in differentiating congenital adrenal hyperplasia from an adrenal tumor. Levels in patients with congenital adrenal hyperplasia may be up to double the normal amount, whereas an adrenal tumor is usually associated with levels that are much higher than double the normal level.

Determination of the serum sodium and potassium levels and CO_2-combining power is also important to ascertain whether electrolyte balance is seriously disturbed.

Treatment

The treatment of female hermaphroditism due to congenital adrenal hyperplasia is partly medical and partly surgical. Originally, cortisone was administered; today, it is known that various cortisone derivatives are at least as effective. It is most satisfactory to begin treatment with relatively large doses of hydrocortisone divided in 3 doses orally for 7–10 days to obtain rapid suppression of adrenal activity. In young infants, the initial dose is about 25 mg/d; in older patients, 100 mg/d. After the output of 17-ketosteroids has decreased to a lower level, the dose should be reduced to the minimum amount required to maintain adequate suppression. This requires repeated measurements of plasma 17α-hydroxyprogesterone in order to individualize the dose.

It has been found that even with suppression of the urinary 17-ketosteroids to normal levels, the more sensitive serum 17-hydroxyprogesterone level may still be elevated. It seems difficult and perhaps undesirable to suppress the serum 17-hydroxyprogesterone values to normal because to do so may require doses of hydrocortisone that tend to cause cushingoid symptoms.

In the treatment of newborns with congenital adrenal hyperplasia who have a defect of electrolyte regulation, it is usually necessary to administer sodium chloride in amounts of 4–6 g/d, either orally or parenterally, in addition to cortisone. Furthermore, fludrocortisone acetate usually is required initially. The dose is entirely dependent on the levels of the serum electrolytes, which must be followed serially, but it is generally 0.05–0.1 mg/d.

In addition to he hormone treatment of this disorder, surgical correction of the external genitalia is usually necessary.

During acute illness or other stress, as well as during and after an operation, additional hydrocortisone is indicated to avoid the adrenal insufficiency of stress. Doubling the maintenance dose is usually adequate in such circumstances.

7. Female Hermaphroditism without Progressive Masculinization

Females with no adrenal abnormality may have fetal masculinization of the external genitalia with the same anatomic findings as in patients with congenital virilizing adrenal hyperplasia. Unlike patients with adrenogenital syndrome, patients without adrenal abnormality do not have elevated levels of serum steroids or urinary 17-ketosteroids, nor do they show precocious sexual development or the metabolic difficulties associated with adrenal hyperplasia as they grow older. At onset of puberty, normal feminization with menstruation and ovulation may be expected.

The diagnosis of female hermaphroditism not due to adrenal abnormality depends on the demonstration of a 46,XX karyotype and the finding of normal levels of serum steroids or normal levels of 17-ketosteroids in the urine. If fusion of the scrotolabial folds is complete, it is necessary to determine the exact relationship of the urogenital sinus to the urethra and vagina and to demonstrate the presence of a uterus by rectal examination or ultrasonography or endoscopic observation of the cervix. When there is a high degree of masculinization, the differential diagnosis between this condition and true hermaphroditism may be very difficult; an exploratory laparotomy may be required in some cases.

Classification

Patients with this problem may be seen because of a variety of conditions.

1. Exogenous androgen:
   a. Maternal ingestion of androgen
   b. Maternal androgenic tumor
   c. Luteoma of pregnancy
   d. Adrenal androgenic tumor
2. Idiopathic: No identifiable cause.
3. Special or nonspecific: The same as condition 2 except that it is associated with various somatic anomalies and with mental retardation.
4. Familial: A very rare anomaly.

8. Male Hermaphroditism

Persons with abnormal or ectopic testes may have external genitalia so ambiguous at birth that the true sex is not identifiable (Fig 5–17). At puberty, these persons tend to become masculinized or feminized depending on factors to be discussed. Thus, the adult habitus of these persons may be typically male, ie, without breasts, or typically female, with good breast development. In some instances, the external genitalia may be indistinguishable from those of a normal female; in others, the clitoris may be enlarged; and in still other instances there may be fusion of the labia in the midline, resulting in what seems to be a hypospa-

Figure 5–17. External genitalia in male hermaphroditism. (Reproduced, with permission, from Jones HW Jr, Scott WW: *Hermaphroditism, Genital Anomalies and Related Endocrine Disorders,* 2nd ed. Williams & Wilkins, 1971.)

diac male. A deep or shallow vagina may be present. A cervix, a uterus, and uterine tubes may be developed to varying degrees; however, müllerian structures are often absent. Mesonephric structures may be grossly or microscopically visible. Body hair may be either typically feminine in its distribution and quantity or masculine in distribution and of sufficient quantity as to require plucking or shaving if the person is reared as a female. In a special group, axillary and pubic hair is congenitally absent. Although there is a well-developed uterus in some instances, all patients so far reported have been amenorrheic—in spite of the interesting theoretic possibility of uterine bleeding from endometrium stimulated by estrogen of testicular origin. There is no evidence of adrenal malfunction. In the feminized group, and less frequently in the nonfeminized group, there is a strong familial history of the disorder. Male hermaphrodites reared as females may marry and be well adjusted to their sex role. Others, especially when there has been equivocation regarding sex of rearing in infancy, may be less than attractive as women because of indecisive therapy. Psychiatric studies indicate that the best emotional adjustment comes from directing endocrine, surgical, and psychiatric measures toward improving the person's basic characteristics. Fortunately, this is consonant with the surgical and endocrine possibilities for those reared as females, because current operative techniques can produce more satisfactory feminine than masculine external genitalia. Furthermore, the testes of male hermaphrodites are nonfunctional as far as spermatogene-

Figure 5–18. External genitalia in male hermaphroditism. (Reproduced, with permission, from Jones HW Jr, Scott WW: *Hermaphroditism, Genital Anomalies and Related Endocrine Disorders,* 2nd ed. Williams & Wilkins, 1971.)

sis is concerned. Only about one-third of male hermaphrodites are suitable for rearing as males.

Classification

Since about 1970, considerable progress has been made in identifying specific metabolic defects that are

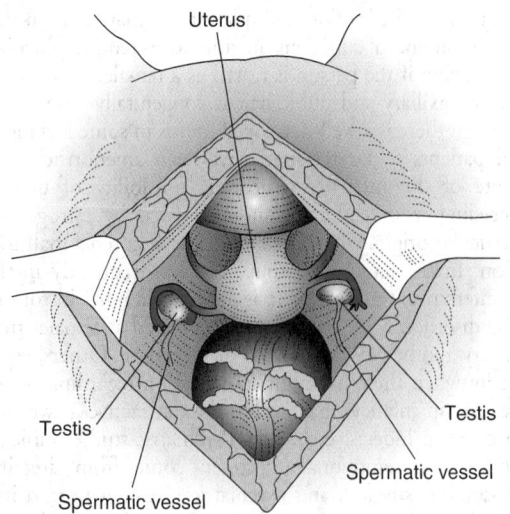

Figure 5–19. Internal genitalia of the patient whose external genitalia are shown in Fig 5–18. (Reproduced, with permission, from Jones HW Jr, Scott WW: *Hermaphroditism, Genital Anomalies and Related Endocrine Disorders,* 2nd ed. Williams & Wilkins, 1971.)

etiologically important for the various forms of male hermaphroditism. Details are beyond the scope of this text. Nevertheless, it is important to point out that all cases of male hermaphroditism have a defect in either the biologic action of testosterone or the MIF of the testis. Furthermore, it now seems apparent that nearly all—if not all—of these defects have a genetic or cytogenetic background. The causes and pathogenetic mechanisms of these defects may vary, but the final common pathway is 1 of the 2 problems just mentioned; in the adult a study of the serum gonadotropins and serum steroids, including the intermediate metabolites of testosterone, can often pinpoint a defect in the biosynthesis of testosterone. In other cases, the end-organ action of testosterone may be defective. In children, the defect is sometimes more difficult to determine before gonadotropin levels rise at puberty, but one may suspect a problem by observing abnormally high levels of steroids that act as substrates in the metabolism of testosterone. A working classification of male hermaphroditism is as follows:

I. Male hermaphroditism due to a central nervous system defect
   A. Abnormal pituitary gonadotropin secretion
   B. No gonadotropin secretion
II. Male hermaphroditism due to a primary gonadal defect
   A. Identifiable defect in biosynthesis of testosterone
      1. Pregnenolone synthesis defect (lipoid adrenal hyperplasia)
      2. 3β-Hydroxysteroid dehydrogenase deficiency
      3. 17α-Hydroxylase deficiency
      4. 17,20-Desmolase deficiency
      5. 17β-Ketosteroid reductase deficiency
   B. Unidentified defect in androgen effect
   C. Defect in duct regression (Figs 5–18 and 5–19)
   D. Familial gonadal destruction
   E. Leydig cell agenesis
   F. Bilateral testicular dysgenesis
III. Male hermaphroditism due to peripheral endorgan defect
   A. Androgen insensitivity syndrome (Fig 5–20)
      1. Androgen-binding protein deficiency
      2. Unknown deficiency
   B. 5α-Reductase deficiency
   C. Unidentified abnormality of peripheral androgen effect
IV. Male hermaphroditism due to Y chromosome defect
   A. Y chromosome mosaicism (asymmetric gonadal differentiation) (Fig 5–21)
   B. Structurally abnormal Y chromosome
   C. No identifiable Y chromosome

Figure 5–20. Androgen insensitivity syndrome.

9. Differential Diagnosis in Infants with Ambiguous Genitalia

Accurate differential diagnosis is possible in most patients with ambiguous genitalia (Table 5–8). This requires a complex history of the mother's medication use, a complex sex chromosome study, rectal examination for the presence or absence of a uterus, measurement of serum steroid levels, pelvic ultrasonography, and information about other congenital anomalies. The following disorders, however, do not yield to differentiation by the parameters given in Table 5–8: (1) idiopathic masculinization, (2) the "special" forms of female hermaphroditism, (3) 46,XX true hermaphroditism, and, occasionally, (4) the precise type of male hermaphroditism. For these differentiations, laparotomy may be necessary for diagnosis and for therapy.

10. Treatment of Hermaphroditism

The sex of rearing is much more important than the obvious morphologic signs (external genitalia, hormone dominance, gonadal structure) in forming the gender role. Furthermore, serious psychological consequences may result from changing the sex of rearing after infancy. Therefore, it is seldom proper to advise a change of sex after infancy to conform to the gonadal structure of the external genitalia. Instead, the physician should exert efforts to complete the adjustment of the person to the sex role already assigned. Fortunately, most aberrations of sexual development are discovered in the newborn period or in infancy, when reassignment of sex causes few problems.

Regardless of the time of treatment (and the earlier the better), the surgeon should reconstruct the external genitalia to correspond to the sex of rearing. Any contradictory sex structures that may function to the patient's disadvantage in the future should be eradicated. Specifically, testes should always be removed from male hermaphrodites reared as females, regardless of hormone production. In cases of testicular feminization, orchiectomy is warranted because a variety of tumors may develop in these abnormal testes if they are retained, but the orchiectomy may be delayed until after puberty in this variety of hermaphroditism.

In virilized female hermaphroditism due to adrenal hyperplasia, suppression of adrenal androgen production by the use of cortisone from an early age will result in completely female development. It is no longer necessary to explore the abdomen and the internal genitalia

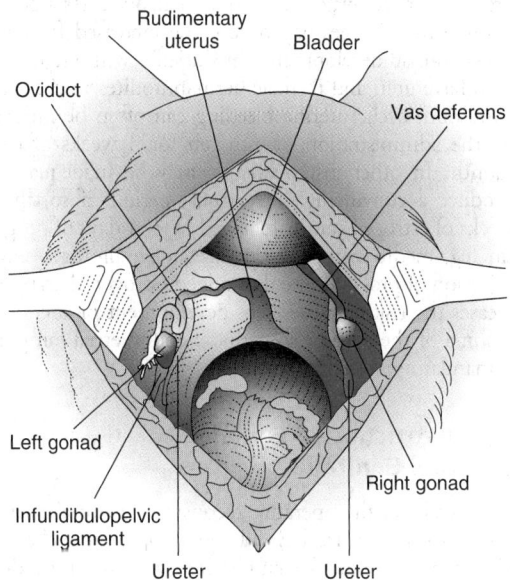

Figure 5–21. Internal genitalia in asymmetric gonadal differentiation. (Reproduced, with permission, from Jones HW Jr, Scott WW: *Hermaphroditism, Genital Anomalies and Related Endocrine Disorders,* 2nd ed. Williams & Wilkins, 1971.)

Table 5–8. Differential diagnosis of ambiguous external genitalia.

Diagnosis	Karyotype	History	Uterus	Anomalies	17-KS	Sex Chromosomes
Adrenal hyperplasia	46,XX	+	+	–	E	XX
Maternal androgen	46,XX	+	+	–	N	XX
Idiopathic masculinization	46,XX	–	+	–	N	XX
Special or nonspecific	46,XX	–	+	–	N	XX
Female familial	46,XX	+	+	+	N	XX
True hermaphroditism	46,XX; 46,XY; etc	–	+ or –	–	N	XX or other
Male hermaphroditism	46,XY	+	+ or –	–	N	XY or other
Streak gonad	45,X; 46,XX; 46,XY; etc	–	+	+ or –	N	XO or other

+, positive, –, negative, N, normal, E, elevated; 17-KS, 17-ketosteroid level.

in this well-delineated syndrome. The surgical effort should be confined to reconstruction of the external genitalia along female lines.

Patients with streak gonads or Turner's syndrome, who are invariably reared as females, should be given exogenous estrogen when puberty is expected. Those hermaphrodites reared as females who will not become feminized also require estrogen to promote the development of the female habitus, including the breasts. In patients with a well-developed system, cyclic uterine withdrawal bleeding can be produced even though reproduction is impossible. Estrogen should be started at about age 12 and may be given as conjugated estrogens, 1.5 mg/d orally (or its equivalent). In some patients, after a period of time this dosage may have to be increased for additional breast development. In patients without ovaries who have uteri and in male hermaphrodites in the same condition, cyclic uterine bleeding can often be induced by the administration of estrogen for 3 weeks of each month. In other instances, this may be inadequate to produce a convincing "menstrual" period; if so, the 3 weeks of estrogen can be followed by 3–4 days of progestin (eg, medroxyprogesterone acetate) orally or a single injection of progesterone. Prolonged estrogen therapy increases the risk of subsequent development of adenocarcinoma of the corpus, so periodic endometrial sampling is mandatory in such patients.

Reconstruction of Female External Genitalia

The details of the operative reconstruction of abnormal external genitalia are beyond the scope of this chapter. However, it should be emphasized that the procedure should be carried out at the earliest age possible so as to enhance the desired psychological, social, and sexual orientation of the patient and to facilitate adjustment by the parents. Sometimes the reconstruction can be done during the neonatal period. In any case, operation should not be delayed beyond the first several months of life. From a technical point of view, early operation is possible in all but the most exceptional circumstances.

REFERENCES

Antonarakis SE et al: Prenatal diagnosis of haemophilia A by factor VIII gene analysis. Lancet 1985;1:1407.

Botto L et al: Neural tube defects. N Engl J Med 1999;341:1509.

Eiben B et al: Rapid prenatal diagnosis of aneuploidies in uncultured amniocytes by fluorescence in situ hybridization. Fetal Diagn Ther 1999;14:193.

Eiben B, Glaubitz R: First-trimester screening: an overview. J Histochem Cytochem 2005;53:281.

Feunteun J et al: A breast-ovarian cancer susceptibility gene maps to chromosome 17q21. Am J Hum Genet 1993;52:736.

Golbus MS et al: Prenatal genetic diagnosis in 3000 amniocenteses. N Engl J Med 1979;300:157.

Hook EB: Rates of chromosome abnormalities at different maternal ages. Obstet Gynecol 1981;58:282.

Horsthemke B, Ludwig M: Assisted reproduction: the epigenetic perspective. Hum Reprod Update 2005;11:473.

Jones HW Jr, Ferguson-Smith MA, Heller RH: Pathologic and cytogenetic findings in true hermaphroditism: Report of six cases and review of 23 cases from the literature. Obstet Gynecol 1965;25:435.

Kajii T et al: Anatomic and chromosomal anomalies in 639 spontaneous abortuses. Hum Genet 1980;55:87.

Klinefelter HF Jr, Reifenstein EC Jr, Albright F: Syndrome characterized by gynecomastia, aspermatogenesis without aleydigism and increased excretion of follicle-stimulating hormone. J Clin Endocrinol 1942;2:615.

Langer S et al: Multicolor chromosome painting in diagnostic and research application. Chromosome Res 2004;12:15.

Lidsky AS, Guttler F, Woo SLC: Prenatal diagnosis of classic phenylketonuria by DNA analysis. Lancet 1985;1:549.

Lippman-Hand A, Bekemans M: Balanced translocations among couples with two or more spontaneous abortions: Are males and females equally likely to be carriers? Hum Genet 1983;68:252.

McKusick VA: Mendelian Inheritance in Man, 10th ed. Johns Hopkins University Press, 1992.

Menutti MT et al: An evaluation of cytogenetic analysis as a primary tool in the assessment of recurrent pregnancy wastage. Obstet Gynecol 1978;52:308.

Page DC et al: The sex determining region of the human Y chromosome encodes a finger protein. Cell 1987;51:1091.

Park IJ, Aimakhu VE, Jones HW Jr: An etiologic and pathogenetic classification of male hermaphroditism. Am J Obstet Gynecol 1975;123:505.

Raskin S et al: Cystic fibrosis genotyping by direct PCR analysis of Guthrie blood spots. PCR Methods Appl 1992;2:154.

Rode L et al: Combined first- and second-trimester screening for Down syndrome: An evaluation of proMBP as a marker. Prenat Diagn 2003;23:593.

Rose NC et al: Maternal serum alpha-fetoprotein screening for chromosomal abnormalities: a prospective study in women aged 35 and older. Am J Obstet Gynecol 1999;170:1073.

Salozhin SV, Prokhorchuk EB, Georgiev GP: Methylation of DNA: One of the major epigenetic markers. Biochemistry (Mosc) 2005;70:525.

Sant-Cassia LJ, Cooke P: Chromosomal analysis of couples with repeated spontaneous abortions. Br J Obstet Gynaecol 1981;88:52.

Simpson E et al: Separation of the genetic loci for the H-Y antigen and for testis determination on human Y chromosome. Nature 1987;326:876.

Stoll CG et al: Interchromosomal effect in balanced translocation. Birth Defects 1978;14:393.

Tiepalo L, Zuffardi O: Location of factors controlling spermatogenesis in the nonfluorescent portion of the human Y chromosome long arm. Hum Genet 1976;34:119.

Turner G et al: Heterozygous expression of X-linked mental retardation and X-chromosome marker fra(X)(q27). N Engl J Med 1980;303:662.

Turner HH: A syndrome of infantilism, congenital webbed neck, and cubitus valgus. Endocrinology 1938;23:566.

Wald NJ et al: Maternal serum screening for Down's syndrome in early pregnancy. Br Med J 1988;297:883.

Wald NJ et al: SURUSS in perspective. Semin Perinatol 2005;29:225.

Physiology of Reproduction in Women*

6

William F. Ganong, MD

This chapter is concerned with the function of the female reproductive system from birth through puberty and adulthood to the menopause.

After birth, the gonads are quiescent until they are activated by gonadotropins from the pituitary to bring about the final maturation of the reproductive system. This period of final maturation is known as **adolescence.** It is often called **puberty,** although strictly defined, puberty is the period when the endocrine and gametogenic functions of the gonads first develop to the point where reproduction is possible. In girls, the first event is **thelarche,** the development of breasts, followed by **pubarche,** the development of axillary and pubic hair, and then **menarche,** the first menstrual period. The initial periods are generally anovulatory, and regular ovulation begins about 1 year later. In contrast to the situation in adulthood, removal of the gonads during the period from soon after birth to puberty causes little or no increase in gonadotropin secretion, so gonadotropin secretion is not being held in check by the gonadal hormones. In children between the ages of 7 and 10, a slow increase in estrogen and androgen secretion precedes the more rapid rise in the early teens (Fig 6–1).

PUBERTY

The age at the time of puberty is variable; in Europe and the United States, it has been declining at the rate of 1–3 months per decade for more than 175 years. In the United States in recent years, puberty has generally been occurring between the ages of 8 and 13 in girls and 9 and 14 in boys.

Another event that occurs in humans at the time of puberty is an increase in the secretion of adrenal androgens (Fig 6–2). The onset of this increase is called **adrenarche.** It occurs at age 8–10 years in girls and 10–12 years in boys. Dehydroepiandrosterone (DHEA) values peak at about 25 years of age and are slightly higher in boys. They then decline slowly to low values after the age of 60.

The increase in adrenal androgen secretion at adrenarche occurs without any changes in the secretion of cortisol or adrenocorticotropic hormone (ACTH). Adrenarche is probably due to a rise in the lyase activity of a 17α-hydroxylase. Thereafter, there is a gradual decline in this activity as plasma adrenal androgen secretion declines to low levels in old age.

The adrenal androgens contribute significantly to the growth of axillary and pubic hair. The breasts develop under the influence of the ovarian hormones estradiol and progesterone, with estradiol primarily responsible for the growth of ducts and progesterone primarily responsible for the growth of lobules and alveoli. The sequence of changes that occur at puberty in girls is summarized in Fig 6–3.

Control of the Onset of Puberty

A neural mechanism is responsible for the onset of puberty. In children, the gonads can be stimulated by gonadotropins, the pituitary contains gonadotropins, and the hypothalamus contains gonadotropin-releasing hormone (GnRH). However, the gonadotropins are not secreted. In immature monkeys, normal menstrual cycles can be brought on by pulsatile injection of GnRH, and the cycles persist as long as the pulsatile injection is continued. In addition, GnRH is secreted in a pulsatile fashion in adults. Thus, it seems clear that during the period from birth to puberty, a neural mechanism is operating to prevent the normal pulsatile release of GnRH. The nature of the mechanism inhibiting the GnRH pulse generator is unknown.

Relation to Leptin

It has been argued for some time that normally a critical body weight must be reached for puberty to occur. Thus, for example, young women who engage in strenuous athletics lose weight and stop menstruating. So do girls with anorexia nervosa. If these girls start to eat and gain weight, they menstruate again, ie, they "go back through

---

This chapter is based in large part on Chapter 23 in Ganong WF: *Review of Medical Physiology,* 22nd ed. McGraw-Hill, 2005.

Figure 6–1. Changes in plasma hormone concentrations during puberty in boys (**top**) and girls (**bottom**). Stage 1 of puberty is preadolescence in both sexes. In boys, stage 2 is characterized by beginning enlargement of the testes, stage 3 by penile enlargement, stage 4 by growth of the glans penis, and stage 5 by adult genitalia. The stages of puberty in girls are summarized in Fig 6–3. (Reproduced, with permission, from Grumbach MM: Onset of puberty. In: Berenberg SR [editor]: *Puberty: Biologic and Psychosocial Components.* HE Stenfoert Kroese BV, 1975.)

puberty." It now appears that leptin, the satiety-producing hormone secreted by fat cells, may be the link between body weight and puberty. Obese ob/ob mice that cannot make leptin are infertile, and their fertility is restored by injections of leptin. Leptin treatment also induces precocious puberty in immature female mice. However, how leptin fits into the overall control of puberty remains to be determined.

Sexual Precocity

The major causes of precocious sexual development in humans are listed in Table 6–1. Early develop-

ment of secondary sexual characteristics without gametogenesis is caused by abnormal exposure of immature males to androgen or of females to estrogen. This syndrome should be called **precocious pseudopuberty** to distinguish it from true precocious puberty due to an early but otherwise normal pubertal pattern of gonadotropin secretion from the pituitary (Fig 6–4).

In 1 large series of cases, precocious puberty was the most frequent endocrine symptom of hypothalamic disease. It is interesting that in experimental animals and humans, lesions of the ventral hypothalamus near the infundibulum cause precocious puberty. The effect of the lesions may be due to interruption of neural pathways that produce inhibition of the GnRH pulse generator. Pineal tumors are sometimes associated with precocious puberty, but there is evidence that these tumors are associated with precocious puberty only when there is secondary damage to the hypothalamus. Precocity due to this and other forms of hypothalamic damage probably occurs with equal frequency in both sexes, although the constitutional form of precocious puberty is more common in girls. In addition, it has now been proved that precocious gametogenesis and steroidogenesis can occur without the pubertal pattern of gonadotropin secretion (gonadotropin-independent precocity). At least in some cases of this condition, the sensitivity of luteinizing hormone (LH) receptors to

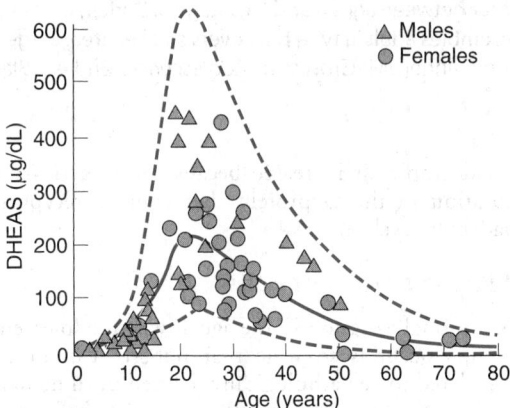

Figure 6–2. Change in serum dehydroepiandrosterone sulfate (DHEAS) with age. The middle line is the mean, and the dashed lines identify ±1.96 standard deviations. (Reproduced, with permission, from Smith MR et al: A radioimmunoassay for the estimation of serum dehydroepiandrosterone sulfate in normal and pathological sera. Clin Chim Acta 1975;65:5.)

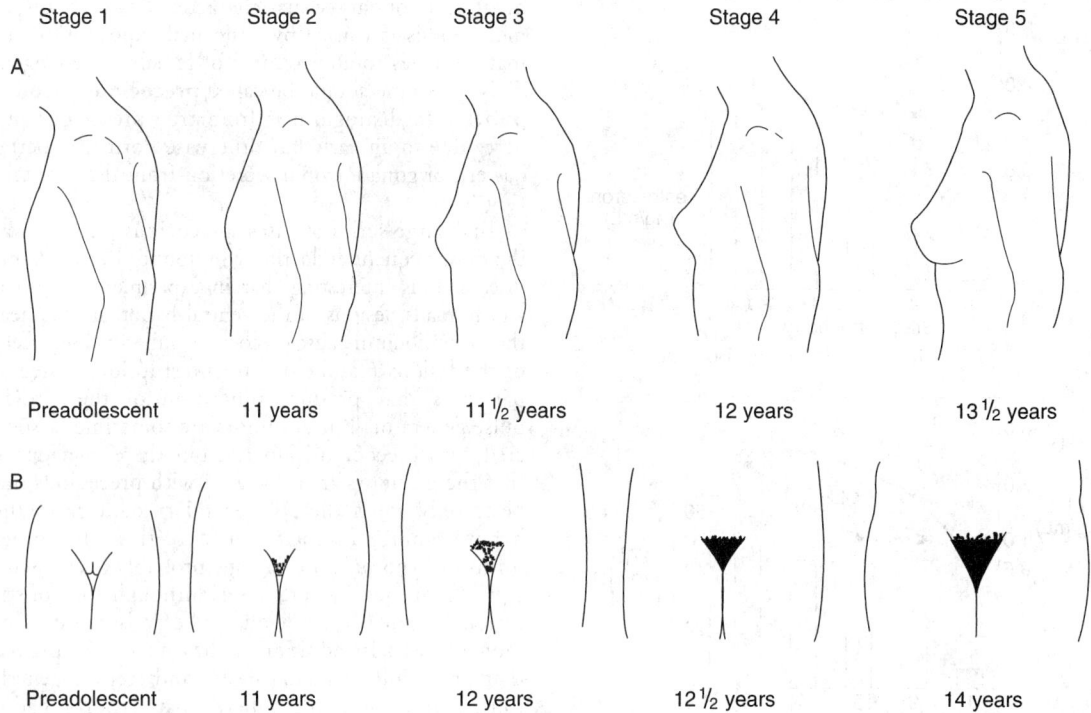

Stage 1   Stage 2   Stage 3   Stage 4   Stage 5

A

Preadolescent   11 years   11 ½ years   12 years   13 ½ years

B

Preadolescent   11 years   12 years   12 ½ years   14 years

Figure 6–3. Sequence of events at adolescence in girls. **A:** Stage 1: Preadolescent; elevation of breast papillae only. Stage 2: Breast bud stage (may occur between ages 8 and 13); elevation of breasts and papillae as small mounds, with enlargement of areolar diameter. Stage 3: enlargement and elevation of breasts and areolas with no separation of contours. Stage 4: Areolas and papillae project from breast to form a secondary mound. Stage 5: Mature; projection of papillae only, with recession of areolas into general contour of breast. **B:** Stage 1: Preadolescent; no pubic hair. Stage 2: Sparse growth along labia of long, slightly pigmented, downy hair that is straight or slightly curled (may occur between ages 8 and 14). Stage 3: Darker, coarser, more curled hair growing sparsely over pubic area. Stage 4: Resembles adult in type but covers smaller area. Stage 5: Adult in quantity and type. (Redrawn, with permission, from Tanner JM: *Growth at Adolescence,* 2nd ed. Blackwell, 1962.)

gonadotropins is increased because of an activating mutation in the G protein that couples receptors toadenylyl cyclase.

Delayed or Absent Puberty

The normal variation in the age at which adolescent changes occur is so wide that puberty cannot be considered to be pathologically delayed until menarche has failed to occur by the age of 17. Failure of maturation due to panhypopituitarism is associated with dwarfing and evidence of other endocrine abnormalities. Patients with the XO chromosomal pattern and gonadal dysgenesis are also dwarfed. In some individuals, puberty is delayed and menarche does not occur (primary amenorrhea), even though the gonads are present and other endocrine functions are normal.

REPRODUCTIVE FUNCTION AFTER SEXUAL MATURITY

Menstrual Cycle

The anatomy of the reproductive system of adult women is described in Chapter 2. Unlike the reproductive system of men, this system shows regular cyclic changes that teleologically may be regarded as periodic preparation for fertilization and pregnancy. In primates, the cycle is a **menstrual cycle,** and its most conspicuous feature is the periodic vaginal bleeding that occurs with shedding of the uterine mucosa (**menstruation**). The length of the cycle is notoriously variable, but the average figure is 28 days from the start of 1 menstrual period to the start of the next. By common usage, the days of the cycle are identified by number, starting with the first day of menstruation.

Table 6–1. Classification of the causes of precocious sexual development in humans

---

True precocious puberty
  Constitutional
  Cerebral: Disorders involving posterior hypothalamus
    Tumors
    Infections
    Developmental abnormalities
  Gonadotropin-independent precocity
Precocious pseudopuberty
(no spermatogenesis or ovarian development)
  Adrenal
    Congenital virilizing adrenal hyperplasia (without
      treatment in males; following cortisone treatment in
      females)
    Androgen-secreting tumors (in males)
    Estrogen-secreting tumors (in females)
  Gonadal
    Interstitial cell tumors of testis
    Granulosa cell tumors of ovary
  Miscellaneous

Reproduced, with permission, from Ganong WF: *Review of Medical Physiology*, 22nd ed. McGraw-Hill, 2005.

Ovarian Cycle

From the time of birth, there are many **primordial follicles** under the ovarian capsule. Each contains an immature ovum (Fig 6–5). At the start of each cycle, several of these follicles enlarge and a cavity forms around the ovum (antrum formation). This cavity is filled with follicular fluid. In humans, 1 of the follicles in 1 ovary starts to grow rapidly on about the sixth day and becomes the **dominant follicle.** The others regress, forming **atretic follicles.** It is not known how 1 follicle is singled out for development during this **follicular phase** of the menstrual cycle, but it seems to be related to the ability of the follicle to secrete the estrogen inside it that is needed for final maturation. When women are given highly purified human pituitary gonadotropin preparations by injection, many follicles develop simultaneously.

The structure of a mature ovarian follicle (**graafian follicle**) is shown in Fig 6–5. The cells of the **theca interna** of the follicle are the primary source of circulating estrogens. The follicular fluid has a high estrogen content, and much of this estrogen comes from the **granulosa cells.**

At about the 14th day of the cycle, the distended follicle ruptures, and the ovum is extruded into the abdominal cavity. This is the process of **ovulation.** The ovum is picked up by the fimbriated ends of the uterine tubes (oviducts) and transported to the uterus. Unless fertiliza-

tion occurs, the ovum degenerates or is passed on through the uterus and out the vagina.

The follicle that ruptures at the time of ovulation promptly fills with blood, forming what is sometimes called a **corpus hemorrhagicum.** Minor bleeding from the follicle into the abdominal cavity may cause peritoneal irritation and fleeting lower abdominal pain ("mittelschmerz"). The granulosa and theca cells of the follicle lining promptly begin to proliferate, and the clotted blood is rapidly replaced with yellowish, lipid-rich **luteal cells,** forming the **corpus luteum.** This is the **luteal phase** of the menstrual cycle, during which the luteal cells secrete estrogens and progesterone. Growth of the corpus luteum depends on its developing an adequate blood supply, and there is evidence that vascular endothelial growth factor (VEGF) is essential for this process. If pregnancy occurs, the corpus luteum persists, and there are usually no more menstrual periods until after delivery. If there is no pregnancy, the corpus luteum begins to degenerate about 4 days before the next menses (day 24 of the cy-

Figure 6–4. Constitutional precocious puberty in a 3½-year-old girl. The patient developed pubic hair and started to menstruate at the age of 17 months. (Reproduced, with permission, from Jolly H: *Sexual Precocity.* Thomas, 1955.)

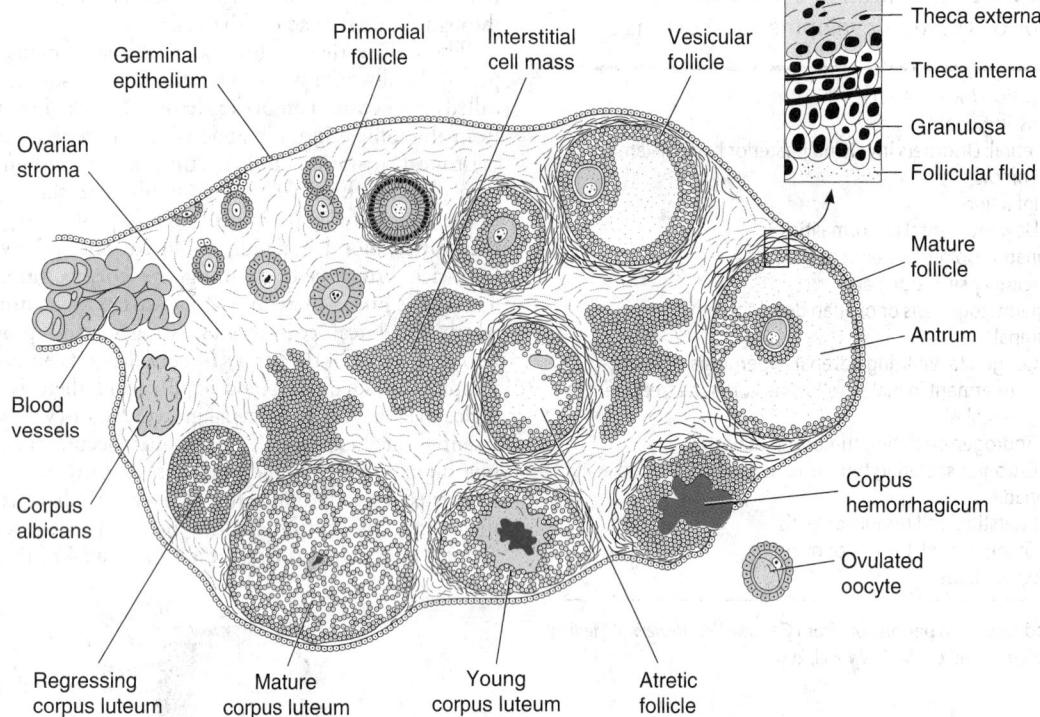

Figure 6–5. Diagram of a mammalian ovary, showing the sequential development of a follicle, formation of a corpus luteum, and, in the center, follicular atresia. A section of the wall of a mature follicle is enlarged at the upper right. The interstitial cell mass is not prominent in primates. (After Patten B, Eakin RM. Reproduced, with permission, from Gorbman A, Bern H: *Textbook of Comparative Endocrinology.* Wiley, 1962.)

cle) and is eventually replaced by fibrous tissue, forming a **corpus albicans.**

In humans, no new ova are formed after birth. During fetal development, the ovaries contain over 7 million germ cells; however, many undergo involution before birth, and others are lost after birth. At the time of birth, there are approximately 2 million primordial follicles containing ova, but approximately 50% of these are atretic. The million or so ova that are normal undergo the first part of the first meiotic division at about this time and enter a stage of arrest in prophase in which those that survive persist until adulthood. Atresia continues during development, and the number of ova in both the ovaries at the time of puberty is less than 300,000 (Fig 6–6). Normally, only 1 of these ova per cycle (or about 500 in the course of a normal reproductive life) is stimulated to mature; the remainder degenerate. Just before ovulation, the first meiotic division is completed. One of the daughter cells, the **secondary oocyte,** receives most of the cytoplasm, while the other, the **first polar body,** fragments and disappears. The secondary oocyte immediately begins the second meiotic division, but this division stops at metaphase and is completed only when a sperm penetrates the oocyte. At that time, the **second polar body** is cast off, and the fertilized ovum proceeds to form a new individual. The arrest in metaphase is due, at least in some species, to formation in the ovum of the protein **pp39^{mos},** which is encoded by the *c-mos* proto-oncogene. When fertilization occurs, the pp39^{mos} is destroyed within 30 minutes by **calpain,** a calcium-dependent cysteine protease.

Uterine Cycle

The events that occur in the uterus during the menstrual cycle terminate in the menstrual flow. By the end of each menstrual period, all but the deep layer of the endometrium has sloughed. Under the influence of estrogens from the developing follicles, the endometrium regenerates from the deep layer and increases rapidly in thickness during the period from the fifth to 16th days of the menstrual cycle. As the thickness increases, the uterine glands are drawn out so that they lengthen (Fig 6–7), but they do not become convoluted or secrete to any degree. These endometrial changes are called proliferative, and this part of the menstrual cycle is some-

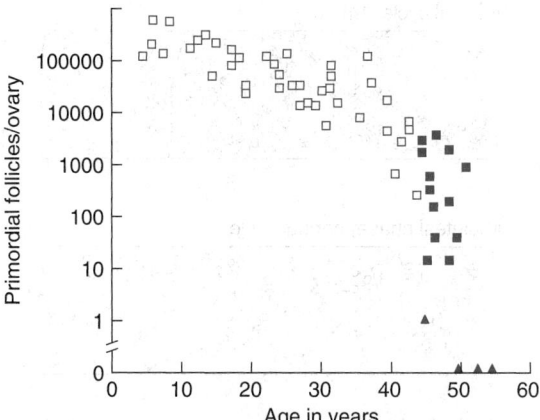

Figure 6-6. Number of primordial follicles per ovary in women at various ages. □, premenopausal women (regular menses); ■, perimenopausal women (irregular menses for at least 1 year); ▲, postmenopausal women (no menses for at least 1 year). Note that the vertical scale is a log scale and that the values are from 1 rather than 2 ovaries. (Redrawn by Wise PM and reproduced, with permission, from Richardson SJ, Senikas V, Nelson JF: Follicular depletion during the menopausal transition: evidence for accelerated loss and ultimate exhaustion. J Clin Endocrinol Metab 1987;65:1231.)

times called the **proliferative phase.** It is also called the preovulatory or follicular phase of the cycle. After ovulation, the endometrium becomes more highly vascularized and slightly edematous under the influence of estrogen and progesterone from the corpus luteum. The glands become coiled and tortuous (Fig 6–7), and they begin to secrete a clear fluid. Consequently, this phase of the cycle is called the **secretory** or **luteal phase.** Late in the luteal phase, the endometrium, like the anterior pituitary, produces prolactin, but the function of this endometrial prolactin is unknown.

The endometrium is supplied by 2 types of arteries. The superficial two-thirds of the endometrium that is shed during menstruation, the stratum functionale, is supplied by long, coiled spiral arteries, whereas the deep layer, the stratum basale, which is not shed, is supplied by short, straight basilar arteries.

When the corpus luteum regresses, hormonal support for the endometrium is withdrawn. The endometrium becomes thinner, which adds to the coiling of the spiral arteries. Foci of necrosis appear in the endometrium, and these coalesce. There is, in addition, necrosis of the walls of the spiral arteries, leading to spotty hemorrhages that become confluent and produce the menstrual flow.

Vasospasm occurs and probably is produced by locally released prostaglandins. There are large quantities of prostaglandins in the secretory endometrium and in menstrual blood, and infusions of prostaglandin F_{2a} (PGF_{2a}) produce endometrial necrosis and bleeding. One theory of the onset of menstruation holds that in necrotic endometrial cells, lysosomal membranes break down with the release of enzymes that foster the formation of prostaglandins from cellular phospholipids.

From the point of view of endometrial function, the proliferative phase of the menstrual cycle represents the restoration of epithelium from the preceding menstruation, and the secretory phase represents the preparation of the uterus for implantation of the fertilized ovum. The length of the secretory phase is remarkably constant, at about 14 days, and the variations seen in the length of the menstrual cycle are mostly due to variations in the length of the proliferative phase. When fertilization fails to occur during the secretory phase, the endometrium is shed, and a new cycle starts.

Figure 6-7. Changes in the endometrium during the menstrual cycle. (Reproduced, with permission, from Ganong WF: *Review of Medical Physiology,* 22nd ed. McGraw-Hill, 2005.)

Normal Menstruation

Menstrual blood is predominantly arterial, with only 25% of the blood being of venous origin. It contains tissue debris, prostaglandins, and relatively large amounts of fibrinolysin from the endometrial tissue. The fibrinolysin lyses clots, so menstrual blood does not normally contain clots unless the flow is excessive.

The usual duration of the menstrual cycle is 3–5 days, but flows as short as 1 day and as long as 8 days can occur in normal women. The average amount of blood lost is 30 mL but normally may range from slight spotting to 80 mL. Loss of more than 80 mL is abnormal. Obviously, the amount of flow can be affected by various factors, including thickness of the endometrium and medications and diseases that affect the clotting mechanism. After menstruation, the endometrium regenerates from the stratum basale.

Anovulatory Cycles

In some instances, ovulation fails to occur during the menstrual cycle. Such anovulatory cycles are common for the first 12–18 months after menarche and again before the onset of menopause. When ovulation does not occur, no corpus luteum is formed, and the effects of progesterone on the endometrium are absent. Estrogens continue to cause growth, however, and the proliferative endometrium becomes thick enough to break down and begin to slough. The time it takes for bleeding to occur is variable, but it usually occurs less than 28 days from the last menstrual period. The flow is also variable and ranges from scanty to relatively profuse.

Cyclic Changes in the Uterine Cervix

Although it is contiguous with the body of the uterus, the cervix of the uterus is different in a number of ways. The mucosa of the uterine cervix does not undergo cyclic desquamation, but there are regular changes in the cervical mucus. Estrogen makes the mucus thinner and more alkaline, changes that promote the survival and transport of sperms. Progesterone makes it thick, tenacious, and cellular. The mucus is thinnest at the time of ovulation, and its elasticity, or **spinnbarkeit,** increases so that by midcycle, a drop can be stretched into a long, thin thread that may be 8–12 cm or more in length. In addition, it dries in an arborizing, fernlike pattern when a thin layer is spread on a slide (Fig 6–8). After ovulation and during pregnancy, it becomes thick and fails to form the fern pattern.

Vaginal Cycle

Under the influence of estrogens, the vaginal epithelium becomes cornified, and cornified epithelial cells can be identified in the vaginal smear. Under the influence of progesterone, a thick mucus is secreted, and the

Normal cycle, 14th day

Midluteal phase, normal cycle

Anovulatory cycle with estrogen present

Figure 6–8. Patterns formed when cervical mucus is smeared on a slide, permitted to dry, and examined under the microscope. Progesterone makes the mucus thick and cellular. In the smear from a patient who failed to ovulate (**bottom**), there is no progesterone to inhibit the estrogen-induced fern pattern. (Reproduced, with permission, from Ganong WF: *Review of Medical Physiology,* 22nd ed. McGraw-Hill, 2005.)

epithelium proliferates and becomes infiltrated with leukocytes. The cyclic changes in the vaginal smear in rats are particularly well known. The changes in humans and other species are similar but unfortunately not so clear-cut. However, the increase in cornified epithelial cells is apparent when a vaginal smear from an adult woman in the follicular phase of the menstrual cycle is compared, for example, with a smear taken from a prepubescent female (Fig 6–9).

Cyclic Changes in the Breasts

Although lactation normally does not occur until the end of pregnancy, there are cyclic changes in the breasts during the menstrual cycle. Estrogens cause proliferation of mammary ducts, whereas progesterone causes growth of lobules and alveoli (see Actions of Progesterone). The breast swelling, tenderness, and pain experienced by many women during the 10 days preceding menstruation probably are due to distention of the ducts, hyperemia, and edema of the interstitial tissue of the breasts. All of these changes regress, along with the symptoms, during menstruation.

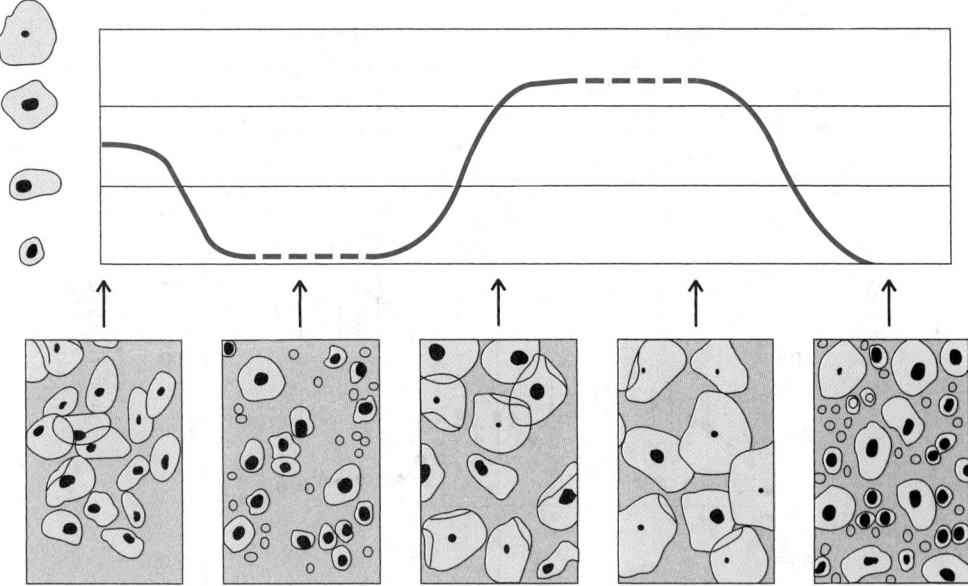

Figure 6–9. Vaginal cytologic picture in various stages of life. **Top:** Graphic representation of the maturation of vaginal epithelium. **Bottom:** Left to right: Epithelial maturation at birth; atrophic cell picture in childhood; beginning of estrogenic influence in puberty; complete maturation in the reproductive period; regression in old age.

Cyclic Changes in Other Body Functions

In addition to cyclic breast swelling and tenderness, there is usually a small increase in body temperature during the luteal phase of the menstrual cycle. This change in body temperature (see Indicators of Ovulation) probably is due to the thermogenic effect of progesterone.

Changes During Sexual Intercourse

During sexual excitation, the vaginal walls become moist as a result of transudation of fluid through the mucus membrane. A lubricating mucus is secreted by the vestibular glands. The upper part of the vagina is sensitive to stretch, while tactile stimulation from the labia minora and clitoris adds to the sexual excitement. The stimuli are reinforced by tactile stimuli from the breasts and, as in men, by visual, auditory, and olfactory stimuli; eventually, the crescendo or climax known as orgasm may be reached. During orgasm, there are autonomically mediated rhythmic contractions of the vaginal wall. Impulses also travel via the pudendal nerves and produce rhythmic contractions of the bulbocavernosus and ischiocavernosus muscles. The vaginal contractions may aid in the transport of spermatozoa but are not essential for it, as fertilization of the ovum is not dependent on orgasm.

Indicators of Ovulation

Knowing when during the menstrual cycle ovulation occurs is important in increasing fertility or, conversely, in contraception. A convenient but retrospective indicator of the time of ovulation is a rise in the basal body temperature (Fig 6–10). Accurate temperatures can be obtained by using a thermometer that is able to measure temperature precisely between 96 and 100 °F. The woman should take her temperature orally, vaginally, or rectally in the morning before getting out of bed. The cause of the temperature change at the time of ovulation is unknown but probably is due to the increase in progesterone secretion, as progesterone is thermogenic. A rise in urinary LH occurs during the rise in circulating LH that causes ovulation, and this increase can be measured as another indicator of ovulation. Kits using dipsticks or simple color tests for detection of urinary LH are available for home use.

Ovulation normally occurs about 9 hours after the peak of the LH surge at midcycle (Fig 6–10). The ovum lives approximately 72 hours after it is extruded from the follicle but probably is fertilizable for less than half this time. In a study of the relationship of isolated intercourse to pregnancy, 36% of women had a detected pregnancy following intercourse on the day of ovulation, but with intercourse on days after ovulation, the percentage was zero. Isolated intercourse on the first

Figure 6–10. Basal body temperature and plasma hormone concentrations (mean ± standard error) during the normal human menstrual cycle. Values are aligned with respect to the day of the midcycle LH peak. (Reproduced, with permission, from Ganong WF: *Review of Medical Physiology*, 22nd ed. McGraw-Hill, 2005.)

and second days before ovulation led to pregnancy in about 36% of the women. A few pregnancies resulted from isolated intercourse on day 3, 4, or 5 before ovulation, although the percentage was much lower, ie, 8% on day 5 before ovulation. Thus, some sperms can survive in the female genital tract and produce fertilization for up to 120 hours before ovulation, but the most fertile period is clearly the 48 hours before ovulation.

However, for those interested in the "rhythm method" of contraception, it should be noted that there are rare but documented cases in the literature of pregnancy resulting from isolated coitus on every day of the cycle.

OVARIAN HORMONES

Chemistry, Biosynthesis, & Metabolism of Estrogens

The naturally occurring estrogens are **17β-estradiol, estrone,** and **estriol** (Fig 6–11). They are C_{18} steroids, ie, they do not have an angular methyl group attached to the 10 position or a Δ^4-3-keto configuration in the A ring. They are secreted primarily by the granulosa and the thecal cells of the ovarian follicles, the corpus luteum, and the placenta. The biosynthetic pathway involves their formation from androgens. They are also formed by aromatization of androstenedione in the circulation. Aromatase (CYP19) is the enzyme that catalyzes the conversion of androstenedione to estrone (Fig 6–11). It also catalyzes the conversion of testosterone to estradiol.

Theca interna cells have many LH receptors, and LH acts on them via cyclic adenosine 3′,5′-monophosphate (cAMP) to increase conversion of cholesterol to androstenedione. Some of the androstenedione is converted to estradiol, which enters the circulation. The theca interna cells also supply androstenedione to the granulosa cells. The granulosa cells only make estradiol when provided with androgens (Fig 6–12), and they secrete the estradiol that they produce into the follicular fluid. They have many follicle-stimulating hormone (FSH) receptors, and FSH facilitates the secretion of estradiol by acting via cyclic AMP to increase the aromatase activity in these cells. Mature granulosa cells also acquire LH receptors, and LH stimulates estradiol production.

The stromal tissue of the ovary also has the potential to produce androgens and estrogens. However, it probably does so in insignificant amounts in normal premenopausal women. 17β-Estradiol, the major secreted estrogen, is in equilibrium in the circulation with estrone. Estrone is further metabolized to **estriol** (Fig 6–11), probably mainly in the liver. Estradiol is the most potent estrogen of the three, and estriol is the least potent.

Figure 6–11. Biosynthesis and metabolism of estrogens. (Reproduced, with permission, from Ganong WF: *Review of Medical Physiology,* 22nd ed. McGraw-Hill, 2005.)

CIRCULATION THECA INTERNA CELLS GRANULOSA CELLS ANTRUM

Figure 6–12. Interactions between theca and granulosa cells in estradiol synthesis and secretion. (Reproduced, with permission, from Ganong WF: *Review of Medical Physiology,* 22nd ed. McGraw-Hill, 2005.)

Two percent of the circulating estradiol is free. The remainder is bound to protein: 60% to albumin and 38% to the same gonadal steroid-binding globulin (GBG) that binds testosterone (Table 6–2).

In the liver, estrogens are oxidized or converted to glucuronide and sulfate conjugates. Appreciable amounts are secreted in the bile and reabsorbed in the bloodstream (enterohepatic circulation). There are at least 10 different metabolites of estradiol in human urine.

Secretion of Estrogens

The concentration of estradiol in plasma during the menstrual cycle is shown in Fig 6–10. Almost all of the estrogen comes from the ovary. There are 2 peaks of secretion: 1 just before ovulation and 1 during the midluteal phase. The estradiol secretion rate is 36 μg/d (133 nmol/d) in the early follicular phase, 380 μg/d just before ovulation, and 250 μg/d during the midluteal phase (Table 6–3). After menopause, estrogen secretion declines to low levels. For comparison, the estradiol production rate in men is about 50 μg/d (184 nmol/d).

Table 6–2. Distribution of gonadal steroids and cortisol in plasma.

Steroid	% Free	% Bound to		
		CBG	GBG	Albumin
Testosterone	2	0	65	33
Androstenedione	7	0	8	85
Estradiol	2	0	38	60
Progesterone	2	18	0	80
Cortisol	4	90	0	6

CBG, corticosteroid-binding globulin; GBG, gonadal steroid–binding globulin.
Courtesy of S Munroe.

Effects on Female Genitalia

Estrogens facilitate the growth of the ovarian follicles and increase the motility of the uterine tubes. Their role in the cyclic changes in the endometrium, cervix, and vagina is discussed above. They increase uterine blood flow and have important effects on the smooth muscle of the uterus. In immature and ovariectomized females, the uterus is small and the myometrium atrophic and inactive. Estrogens increase the amount of uterine muscle and its content of contractile proteins. Under the influence of estrogens, the myometrium becomes more active and excitable, and action potentials in the individual muscle fibers are increased. The "estrogen-dominated" uterus is also more sensitive to oxytocin.

Prolonged treatment with estrogens causes endometrial hypertrophy. When estrogen therapy is discontinued, there is some sloughing and **withdrawal bleeding.** Some "breakthrough" bleeding may also occur during prolonged treatment with estrogens.

Effects on Endocrine Organs

Estrogens decrease FSH secretion. In some circumstances, estrogens inhibit LH secretion (negative feedback); in others, they increase LH secretion (positive feedback). Estrogens also increase the size of the pituitary. Women are sometimes given large doses of estrogens for 4–6 days to prevent conception during the fertile period (postcoital or "morning-after" contraception). In this instance, pregnancy probably is prevented by interference with implantation of the fertilized ovum rather than by changes in gonadotropin secretion.

Estrogens cause increased secretion of angiotensinogen and thyroid-binding globulin. They exert an important protein anabolic effect in chickens and cattle, possibly by stimulating the secretion of androgens from the adrenal; estrogens have been used commercially to increase the weight of domestic animals. They cause epiphyseal closure in humans.

Table 6–3. Twenty-four–hour production rates of sex steroids in women at different stages of the menstrual cycle.

Sex Steroids	Early Follicular	Preovulatory	Midluteal
Progesterone (mg)	1.0	4.0	25.0
17-Hydroxyprogesterone (mg)	0.5	4.0	4.0
Dehydroepiandrosterone (mg)	7.0	7.0	7.0
Androstenedione (mg)	2.6	4.7	3.4
Testosterone (μg)	144.0	171.0	126.0
Estrone (μg)	50.0	350.0	250.0
Estradiol (μg)	36.0	380.0	250.0

Modified and reproduced, with permission, from Yen SSC, Jaffe RB: *Reproductive Endocrinology,* 3rd ed. Saunders, 1991.

Effects on the Central Nervous System

Estrogens are responsible for estrus behavior in animals, and they may increase libido in humans. They apparently exert this action by a direct effect on certain neurons in the hypothalamus (Fig 6–13).

Estrogens increase the proliferation of dendrites on neurons and the number of synaptic knobs in rats. In humans, they have been reported to slow the progression of Alzheimer's disease, but this role of estrogens remains controversial.

Effects on the Breasts

Estrogens produce duct growth in the breasts and are largely responsible for breast enlargement at puberty in girls. Breast enlargement that occurs when estrogen-containing skin creams are applied locally is due primarily to systemic absorption of the estrogen, although a slight local effect is also produced. Estrogens are responsible for the pigmentation of the areolas. Pigmentation usually becomes more intense during the first pregnancy than it does at puberty.

Effects on Female Secondary Sex Characteristics

The body changes that develop in girls at puberty—in addition to enlargement of the breasts, uterus, and vagina—are due in part to estrogens, which are the "feminizing hormones," and in part simply to the absence of testicular androgens. Women have narrow shoulders and broad hips, thighs that converge, and arms that diverge (wide **carrying angle**). This body configuration, plus the female distribution of fat in the breasts and buttocks, is also seen in castrated males. In women, the larynx retains its prepubertal proportions and the voice is high-pitched. There is less body hair and more scalp hair, and the pubic hair generally has a characteristic flattop pattern (**female escutcheon**). Growth of pubic and axillary hair in the female is due primarily to androgens rather than estrogens, although estrogen treatment may cause some hair growth. The androgens are produced by the adrenal cortex and, to a lesser extent, by the ovaries.

Other Actions of Estrogens

Normal women retain salt and water and gain weight just before menstruation. Estrogens can cause some degree of salt and water retention. However, aldosterone secretion is slightly elevated in the luteal phase, and this also contributes to premenstrual fluid retention.

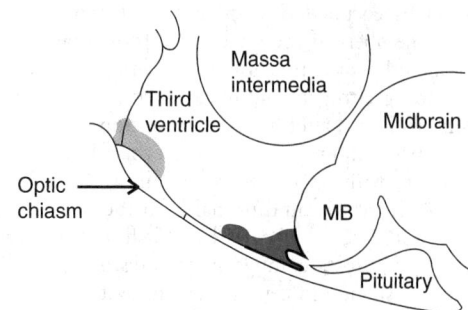

Figure 6–13. Loci where implantations of estrogen in the hypothalamus affect ovarian weight and sexual behavior in rats, projected on a sagittal section of the hypothalamus. The implants that stimulate sex behavior are located in the suprachiasmatic area above the optic chiasm, whereas ovarian atrophy is produced by implants in the arcuate nucleus and surrounding ventral hypothalamus just above the pituitary stalk. MB, mamillary body. (Reproduced, with permission, from Ganong WF: *Review of Medical Physiology,* 22nd ed. McGraw-Hill, 2005.)

Estrogens make sebaceous gland secretions more fluid and thus counter the effect of testosterone and inhibit formation of **comedones** ("blackheads") and acne. The liver palms, spider angiomas, and slight breast enlargement seen in advanced liver disease are due to increased circulating estrogens. The increase appears to be due to decreased hepatic metabolism of androstenedione, making more of this androgen available for conversion to estrogens.

Estrogens have a significant plasma cholesterol-lowering action. They produce vasodilation and inhibit vascular smooth muscle proliferation, possibly by increasing the local production of nitric oxide (NO). Estrogen has also been shown to prevent expression of factors important in the initiation of atherosclerosis. These actions may account for the low incidence of myocardial infarction and other complications of atherosclerotic-vascular disease in premenopausal women. There is considerable evidence that small doses of estrogen may reduce the incidence of cardiovascular disease after menopause. However, some recently published data do not support this conclusion, and additional research is needed. Large doses of oral estrogens also promote thrombosis, apparently because they reach the liver in high concentrations in the portal blood and alter hepatic production of clotting factors.

Mechanism of Action

The 2 principal types of nuclear estrogen receptors are estrogen receptor-α (ER-α), which is encoded by a gene on chromosome 6, and estrogen receptor-β (ER-β), which is encoded by a gene on chromosome 14. Both are members of the nuclear receptor superfamily, which includes receptors for many different steroids. After binding estrogen, the nuclear receptors dimerize and bind to DNA, altering its transcription (Fig 6–14). Some tissues contain 1 type or the other, but there is also overlap, with some tissues containing both ER-α and ER-β. ER-α is found primarily in the uterus, kidneys, liver, and heart, whereas ER-β is found primarily in the ovaries, prostate, lungs, gastrointestinal tract, hemopoietic system, and central nervous system. The receptors also form heterodimers, with ER-α binding to ER-β. Male and female mice in which the gene for ER-α has been knocked out are sterile, develop osteoporosis, and continue to grow because their epiphyses do not close. ER-β female knockouts are infertile, but ER-β male knockouts are fertile even though they have hyperplastic prostates and loss of fat. Thus, the actions of the estrogen receptors are complex, multiple, and varied. However, this is not surprising because it is now known that both receptors exist in various isoforms and, like thyroid receptors, can bind to various activating and stimulating factors.

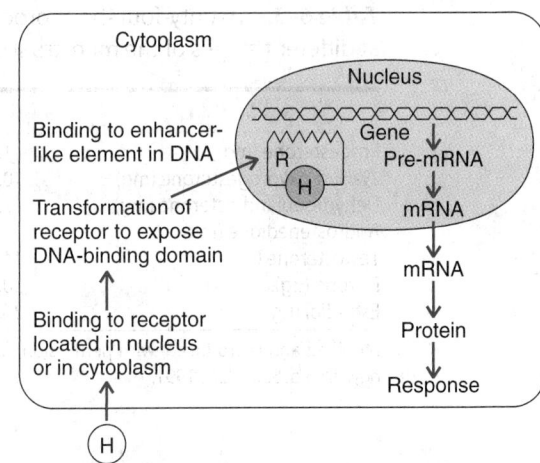

Figure 6–14. Mechanism of action of steroid hormones. The estrogen, progestin, androgen, glucocorticoid, mineralocorticoid, and 1,25-dihydroxycholecalciferol receptors have different molecular weights, but all have a ligand-binding domain and a DNA-binding domain that is exposed when the ligand binds. The receptor–hormone complex then binds to DNA, producing increased or decreased transcription. H, hormone; R, receptor. (Reproduced, with permission, from Ganong WF: *Review of Medical Physiology,* 22nd ed. McGraw-Hill, 2005.)

Most of the actions of estrogens are genomic, ie, mediated by actions on the nucleus. However, some effects are so rapid that it is difficult to believe they are mediated via increased expression of mRNAs. These include effects on neuronal discharge in the brain and possibly feedback effects on gonadotropin secretion. Their existence has led to the hypothesis that, in addition to genomic actions, there are nongenomic effects of estrogens that are presumably mediated by membrane receptors. Similar rapid effects of progesterone, testosterone, and aldosterone may also be produced by membrane receptors.

Synthetic Estrogen

The ethinyl derivative of estradiol (Fig 6–15) is a potent estrogen. Unlike naturally occurring estrogens, it is relatively active when given orally because it has an ethinyl group in position 17, which makes it resistant to hepatic metabolism. Naturally occurring hormones have low activity when given orally because the portal venous drainage of the intestine carries them to the liver, where they are largely inactivated before they can reach the general circulation. Some nonsteroidal substances and a few compounds found in plants have estrogenic activity.

Ethinyl estradiol

Diethylstilbestrol

Figure 6–15. Synthetic estrogens. (Reproduced, with permission, from Ganong WF: *Review of Medical Physiology,* 22nd ed. McGraw-Hill, 2005.)

Plant estrogens rarely affect humans but may cause undesirable effects in farm animals. Diethylstilbestrol (Fig 6–15) and a number of related compounds are strongly estrogenic, possibly because they are converted to steroidlike ring structures in the body.

Estradiol reduces the hot flashes and other symptoms of the menopause, and it prevents the development of osteoporosis. It may reduce the initiation and progression of atherosclerosis and the incidence of heart attack. However, it also stimulates the growth of the endometrium and the breast, and it can lead to cancer of the uterus and probably of the breast. Therefore, there has been an active search for "tailor-made" estrogens that have the bone and cardiovascular effects of estradiol but lack its growth-stimulating effects on the uterus and the breast. Two compounds, **tamoxifen** and **raloxifene,** show promise in this regard. Neither combats the symptoms of the menopause, but both have the bone-preserving effects of estradiol. They may also have cardioprotective effects, but the clinical relevance of these effects has not been established. In addition, tamoxifen does not stimulate the breast, and raloxifene does not stimulate the breast or uterus. The clinical uses of these 2 drugs are discussed elsewhere in this book.

Chemistry, Biosynthesis, & Metabolism of Progesterone

Progesterone (Fig 6–16) is a C_{21} steroid secreted in large amounts by the corpus luteum and the placenta. It is an important intermediate in steroid biosynthesis in all tissues that secrete steroid hormones, and small amounts enter the circulation from the testes and adrenal cortex. The 20α- and 20β-hydroxy derivatives of progesterone are formed in the corpus luteum. About 2% of the progesterone in the circulation is free (Table 6–2), whereas 80% is bound to albumin and 18% is bound to corticosteroid-binding globulin. Progesterone has a short half-life and is converted in the liver to pregnanediol, which is conjugated to glucuronic acid and excreted in the urine (Fig 6–16).

Secretion of Progesterone

The plasma progesterone level in women during the follicular phase of the menstrual cycle is approximately 0.9 ng/mL (3 nmol/L), whereas the level in men is ap-

Sodium pregnanediol-20-glucuronide

Figure 6–16. Biosynthesis of progesterone and major pathway for its metabolism. Other metabolites are also formed. (Reproduced, with permission, from Ganong WF: *Review of Medical Physiology,* 22nd ed. McGraw-Hill, 2005.)

proximately 0.3 ng/mL (1 nmol/L). The difference is due to secretion of small amounts of progesterone by cells in the ovarian follicle. During the luteal phase, the large amounts secreted by the corpus luteum cause ovarian secretion to increase about 20-fold. The result is an increase in plasma progesterone to a peak value of approximately 18 ng/mL (60 nmol/L) (Fig 6–10).

The stimulating effect of LH on progesterone secretion by the corpus luteum is due to activation of adenylyl cyclase and involves a subsequent step that is dependent on protein synthesis.

Actions of Progesterone

The principal target organs of progesterone are the uterus, the breasts, and the brain. Progesterone is responsible for the progestational changes in the endometrium and the cyclic changes in the cervix and vagina described above. It has antiestrogenic effects on the myometrial cells, decreasing their excitability, their sensitivity to oxytocin, and their spontaneous electrical activity, while increasing their membrane potential. It decreases the number of estrogen receptors in the endometrium and increases the rate of conversion of 17β-estradiol to less active estrogens.

In the breast, progesterone stimulates the development of lobules and alveoli. It induces differentiation of estrogen-prepared ductal tissue and supports the secretory function of the breast during lactation.

The feedback effects of progesterone are complex and are exerted at both the hypothalamic and the pituitary level. Large doses of progesterone inhibit LH secretion and potentiate the inhibitory effects of estrogens, preventing ovulation.

Progesterone is thermogenic and probably is responsible for the rise in basal body temperature at the time of ovulation (Fig 6–10). Progesterone stimulates respiration, and the fact that alveolar PCO_2 in women during the luteal phase of the menstrual cycle is lower than that in men is attributed to the action of secreted progesterone. In pregnancy, alveolar PCO_2 falls as progesterone secretion rises.

Large doses of progesterone produce natriuresis, probably by blocking the action of aldosterone on the kidney. The hormone does not have a significant anabolic effect.

Mechanism of Action

The effects of progesterone, like those of other steroids, are brought about by an action on DNA to initiate synthesis of new mRNA. The progesterone receptor is bound to a heat shock protein in the absence of the steroid, and progesterone binding releases the heat shock protein, exposing the DNA-binding domain of the receptor. The synthetic steroid **mifepristone (RU-486)** binds to the receptor but does not release the heat shock protein, and it blocks the binding of progeste-

rone. As the maintenance of early pregnancy depends on the stimulatory effect of progesterone on endometrial growth and its inhibition of uterine contractility, mifepristone causes abortion. In some countries, mifepristone combined with a prostaglandin is used to produce elective abortions.

Two isoforms of the progesterone receptor are produced by differential processing from a single gene. Progesterone receptor A (PR_A) is a truncated form that when activated is capable of inhibiting some of the actions of progesterone receptor B (PR_B). However, the physiologic significance of the existence of the 2 isoforms remains to be determined.

Substances that mimic the action of progesterone are sometimes called **progestational agents, gestagens,** or **progestins.** They are used along with synthetic estrogens as oral contraceptive agents.

RELAXIN

Relaxin is a polypeptide hormone that is secreted by the corpus luteum in women and by the prostate in men. During pregnancy, it relaxes the pubic symphysis and other pelvic joints and softens and dilates the uterine cervix during pregnancy. Thus, it facilitates delivery. It also inhibits uterine contractions and may play a role in the development of the mammary glands. In nonpregnant women, relaxin is found in the corpus luteum and the endometrium during the secretory but not the proliferative phase of the menstrual cycle. Its function in nonpregnant women is unknown.

In most species, there is only 1 relaxin gene, but in humans there are 2 genes on chromosome 9 that code for 2 structurally different polypeptides with relaxin activity. However, only 1 of these genes is active in the ovary and the prostate. The structure of the polypeptide produced in these 2 tissues is shown in Fig 6–17.

INHIBINS AND ACTIVINS

Polypeptides called **inhibins** that inhibit FSH secretion were first isolated from testes but soon were discovered to also be produced by the ovaries. There are 2 inhibins, and they are formed from 3 polypeptide subunits: a glycosylated α subunit with a molecular weight of 18,000, and 2 nonglycosylated β subunits, $β_A$ and $β_B$, each with a molecular weight of 14,000. The subunits are formed from precursor proteins (Fig 6–18). The α subunit combines with $β_A$ to form a heterodimer and with $β_B$ to form another heterodimer, with the subunits linked by disulfide bonds. Both $αβ_A$ (inhibin A) and $αβ_B$ (inhibin B) inhibit FSH secretion by a direct action on the pituitary, although it now appears that inhibin B is the FSH-regulating hormone in adults. Inhibins are produced by Sertoli cells in males and by granulosa cells in females.

Figure 6–17. Structure of human luteal and prostatic relaxin. Note the A and B chains are connected by disulfide bridges. Pca, pyroglutamic acid residue at N-terminal of A chain. (Modified and reproduced, with permission, from Winslow JW et al: Human seminal relaxin is a product of the same gene as human luteal relaxin. Endocrinology 1992;130:2660.)

The heterodimer $\beta_A\beta_B$ and the homodimers $\beta_A\beta_A$ and $\beta_B\beta_B$ stimulate rather than inhibit FSH secretion and consequently are called **activins.** Their function in reproduction is unsettled. However, the inhibins and activins are members of the transforming growth factor-β superfamily of dimeric growth factors that also includes the müllerian inhibitory substance (MIS) that is important in embryonic development of the gonads. Two **activin receptors** have been cloned, and both appear to be serine kinases. Inhibins and activins are found not only in the gonads but also in the brain and many other tissues. In the bone marrow, activins are involved in the development of white blood cells. In embryonic life, activins are involved in the formation of mesoderm. All mice in which a targeted deletion of the α-inhibin gene was produced initially grew in a normal fashion but then developed gonadal stromal tumors, so the α-inhibin gene is a tumor suppressor gene.

In plasma, α_2-macroglobulin binds activins and inhibins. In tissues, activins bind to a family of 4 glycoproteins called **follistatins.** Binding of the activins inactivates their biologic activity, but the relation of follistatins to inhibin and their physiologic function are unsettled.

PITUITARY HORMONES

Ovarian secretion depends on the action of hormones secreted by the anterior pituitary gland. The anterior pituitary gland secretes 6 established hormones: ACTH, growth hormone, thyroid-stimulating hormone (TSH), FSH, LH, and prolactin (Fig 6–19). It also secretes 1 putative hormone: β-lipotropic hormone (β-LPH).

GONADOTROPINS

The gonadotropins FSH and LH act in concert to regulate the cyclic secretion of the ovarian hormones. They are glycoproteins made up of α and β subunits. The α subunits have the same amino acid composition as the α subunits in the glycoproteins TSH and human chorionic gonadotropin (hCG); the specificity of these 4 glycoprotein hormones is imparted by the different structures of their β subunits. The carbohydrates in the gonadotropin molecules increase the potency of the hormones by markedly slowing their metabolism. The half-life of human FSH is about 170 minutes; the half-life of LH is about 60 minutes.

The receptors for FSH and LH are serpentine receptors coupled to adenylyl cyclase through G_S. In addition, each has an extended, glycosylated extracellular domain.

Hypothalamic Hormones

Secretion of the anterior pituitary hormones is regulated by the hypothalamic hypophysiotropic hormones. These substances are produced by neurons and enter the portal hypophysial vessels (Fig 6–20), a special group of blood vessels that transmit substances directly from the hypothalamus to the anterior pituitary gland. The actions of these hormones are summarized in Fig 6–21. The structures of 6 established hypophysiotropic hormones are known (Fig 6–22). No single prolactin-releasing hormone has been isolated and identified. However, several polypeptides that are found in the hypothalamus can increase prolactin secretion, and 1 or more of these may stimulate prolactin secretion under physiologic conditions.

Figure 6–18. Inhibin precursor proteins and the various inhibins and activins that are formed from them. SS, disulfide bonds. (Reproduced, with permission, from Ganong WF: *Review of Medical Physiology,* 22nd ed. McGraw-Hill, 2005.)

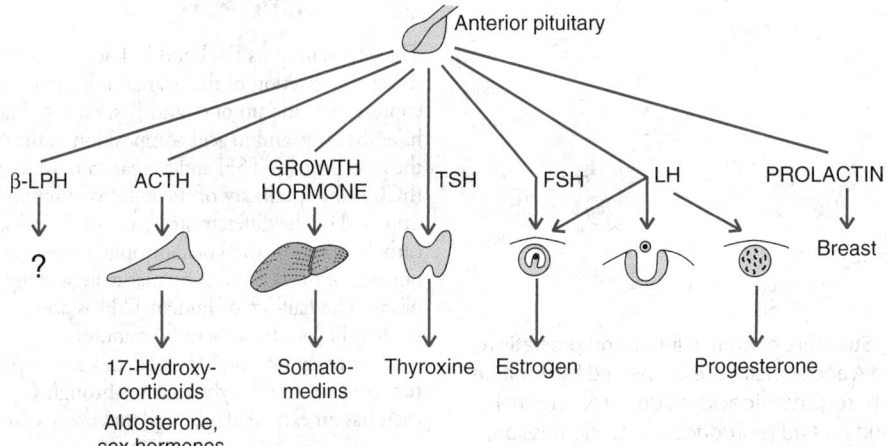

Figure 6–19. Anterior pituitary hormones. In women, FSH and LH act in sequence on the ovary to produce growth of the ovarian follicle, which secretes estrogen, then ovulation, followed by formation and maintenance of the corpus luteum, which secretes estrogen and progesterone. In men, FSH and LH control the functions of the testes. Prolactin stimulates lactation. β-LPH, β-lipotropic hormone; ACTH, adrenocorticotropic hormone; TSH, thyroid-stimulating hormone; FSH, follicle-stimulating hormone; LH, luteinizing hormone. (Reproduced, with permission, from Ganong WF: *Review of Medical Physiology*, 22nd ed. McGraw-Hill, 2005.)

The posterior pituitary differs from the anterior pituitary in that its hormones oxytocin and arginine vasopressin are secreted by neurons directly into the systemic circulation. These hormones are produced in the cell bodies of neurons located in the supraoptic and paraventricular nuclei of the hypothalamus and transported down the axons of these neurons to their endings in the posterior lobe of the pituitary. The hormones are released from the endings into the circulation when action potentials pass down the axons and reach the endings. The structures of the hormones are shown in Fig 6–23.

CONTROL OF OVARIAN FUNCTION

FSH from the pituitary is responsible for early maturation of the ovarian follicles, and FSH and LH together are responsible for final follicle maturation. A burst of LH secretion (Fig 6–10) triggers ovulation and the initial formation of the corpus luteum. There is also a smaller midcycle burst of FSH secretion, the significance of which is uncertain. LH stimulates the secretion of estrogen and progesterone from the corpus luteum.

Hypothalamic Components

The hypothalamus occupies a key role in the control of gonadotropin secretion. Hypothalamic control is exerted by GnRH secreted into the portal hypophysial vessels. GnRH stimulates the secretion of FSH as well as LH, and it is unlikely that there is an additional separate follicle-stimulating hormone–releasing hormone (FRH).

GnRH is normally secreted in episodic bursts (**circhoral secretion**). These bursts are essential for normal secretion of gonadotropins, which are also exerted in an episodic fashion (Fig 6–24). If GnRH is administered by constant infusion, the number of GnRH receptors in the anterior pituitary decreases (**downregulation**), and LH secretion falls to low levels. However, if GnRH is administered episodically at a rate of 1 pulse per hour, LH secretion is stimulated. This is true even when endogenous GnRH secretion has been prevented by a lesion of the ventral hypothalamus.

It is now clear not only that episodic secretion of GnRH is a general phenomenon but that fluctuations in the frequency and amplitude of the GnRH bursts are important in generating the other hormonal changes that are responsible for the menstrual cycle. Frequency is increased by estrogens and decreased by progesterone and testosterone. The frequency increases late in the follicular phase of the cycle, culminating in the LH surge. During the secretory phase, the frequency decreases as a result of the action of progesterone, but when estrogen and progesterone secretion decrease at the end of the cycle, frequency once again increases.

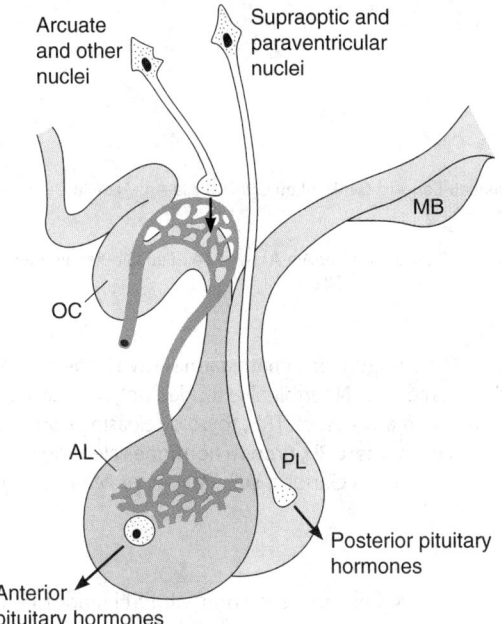

Figure 6–20. Secretion of hypothalamic hormones. The hormones of the posterior lobe (PL) are released into the general circulation from the endings of supraoptic and paraventricular neurons, whereas hypophysiotrophic hormones are secreted into the portal hypophysial circulation from the endings of arcuate and other hypothalamic neurons. AL, anterior lobe; MB, mamillary bodies; OC, optic chiasm. (Reproduced, with permission, from Ganong WF: *Review of Medical Physiology*, 22nd ed. McGraw-Hill, 2005).

At the time of the midcycle LH surge, the sensitivity of the gonadotropes to GnRH is greatly increased because of their exposure to GnRH pulses of the frequency that exist at this time. This self-priming effect of GnRH is important in producing a maximum LH response.

The nature and the exact location of the GnRH pulse generator in the hypothalamus are still unsettled. However, it is known in a general way that norepinephrine and possibly epinephrine in the hypothalamus increase GnRH pulse frequencies. Conversely, opioid peptides such as the enkephalins and β-endorphin reduce the frequency of GnRH pulses.

The downregulation of pituitary receptors and the consequent decrease in LH secretion produced by constantly elevated levels of GnRH has led to the use of long-acting GnRH agonists to inhibit LH secretion in precocious puberty and cancer of theprostate.

Feedback Effects

Changes in plasma levels of LH, FSH, sex steroids, and inhibin B during the menstrual cycle are shown in Fig 6–10, and their feedback relations are diagrammed in Fig 6–25. At the start of the follicular phase, the inhibin B level is low and the FSH level is modestly elevated, fostering follicular growth. LH secretion is held in check by the negative feedback effect of the rising plasma estrogen level. At 36–48 hours before ovulation, the estrogen feedback effect becomes positive, which initiates the burst of LH secretion (LH surge) that produces ovulation. Ovulation occurs about 9 hours after the LH peak. FSH secretion also peaks, despite a small rise in inhibin B level, probably because of the strong stimulation of gonadotropes by GnRH. During the luteal phase, se-

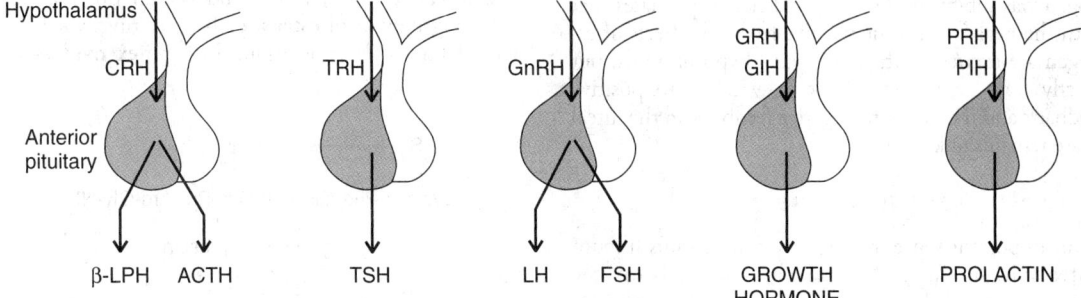

Figure 6–21. Effects of hypophysiotropic hormones on the secretion of anterior pituitary hormones. β-LPH, β-lipotropic hormone; ACTH, adrenocorticotropic hormone; CRH, corticotropin-releasing hormone; TRH, thyroid-releasing hormone; TSH, thyroid-stimulating hormone; GnRH, gonadotropin-releasing hormone; FSH, follicle-stimulating hormone; LH, luteinizing hormone; GRH, growth hormone-releasing hormone; GIH, growth-inhibiting hormone; PRH, prolactin-releasing hormone; PIH, prolactin-inhibiting hormone. (Reproduced, with permission, from Ganong WF: *Review of Medical Physiology*, 22nd ed. McGraw-Hill, 2005.)

TRH	(pyro)Glu-His-Pro-NH$_2$
GnRH	(pyro)Glu-His-Trp-Ser-Tyr-Gly-Leu-Arg-Pro-Gly-NH$_2$
Somatostatin	Ala-Gly-Cys-Lys-Asn-Phe-Phe-Trp-Lys-Thr-Phe-Thr-Ser-Cys
CRH	Ser-Glu-Glu-Pro-Pro-Ile-Ser-Leu-Asp-Leu-Thr-Phe-His-Leu-Leu-Arg-Glu-Val-Leu-Glu-Met-Ala-Arg-Ala-Glu-Gln-Leu-Ala-Gln-Gln-Ala-His-Ser-Asn-Arg-Lys-Leu-Met-Glu-Ile-Ile-NH$_2$
GRH	Tyr-Ala-Asp-Ala-Ile-Phe-Thr-Asn-Ser-Tyr-Arg-Lys-Val-Leu-Gly-Gln-Leu-Ser-Ala-Arg-Lys-Leu-Leu-Gln-Asp-Ile-Met-Ser-Arg-Gln-Gln-Gly-Glu-Ser-Asn-Gln-Glu-Arg-Gly-Ala-Arg-Ala-Arg-Leu-NH$_2$
PIH	Dopamine

Figure 6–22. Structures of hypophysiotropic hormones in humans. The structure of somatostatin shown is the tetradecapeptide (somatostatin 14). In addition, preprosomatostatin is the source of an N-terminal extended polypeptide containing 28 amino acid residues (somatostatin 28). Both forms are found in many tissues. TRH, thyroid-releasing hormone; GnRH, gonadotropin-releasing hormone; CRH, corticotropin-releasing hormone; GRH, growth hormone-releasing hormone; PIH, prolactin-inhibiting hormone. (Reproduced, with permission, from Ganong WF: *Review of Medical Physiology,* 22nd ed. McGraw-Hill, 2005.)

cretion of LH and FSH is low because of the elevated levels of estrogen, progesterone, and inhibin B.

It should be emphasized that a moderate, constant level of circulating estrogen exerts a negative feedback effect on LH secretion, whereas an elevated estrogen level exerts a positive feedback effect and stimulates LH secretion. It has been demonstrated in monkeys that there is also a minimum time that estrogen levels must be elevated to produce positive feedback. When the circulating estrogen level was increased about 300% for 24 hours, only negative feedback was seen; but when it was increased about 300% for 36 hours or more, a brief decline in secretion was followed by a burst of LH secretion that resembled the midcycle surge. When circulating levels of progesterone were high, the positive feedback effect of estrogen was inhibited. There is evidence in primates that both the negative and the positive feedback effects of estrogen are exerted in the mediobasal hypothalamus, but exactly how negative feedback is switched to positive feedback and then back to negative feedback in the luteal phase remains unknown.

Control of Menstrual Cycle

In an important sense, regression of the corpus luteum (**luteolysis**) starting 3–4 days before menses is the key to the menstrual cycle. PGF$_{2a}$ appears to be a physiologic luteolysin, but this prostaglandin is only active when endothelial cells producing endothelin-1 (ET-1) are present. Therefore, it appears that at least in some species luteolysis is produced by the combined action of PGF$_{2a}$ and ET-1. In some domestic animals, oxytocin secreted by the corpus luteum appears to exert a local luteolytic effect, possibly by causing the release of prostaglandins. Once luteolysis begins, estrogen and proges-

terone levels fall, and secretion of FSH and LH increases. A new crop of follicles develops, and then a single dominant follicle matures as a result of the action of FSH and LH. Near midcycle, there is a rise in estrogen secretion from the follicle. This rise augments the responsiveness of the pituitary to GnRH and triggers a burst of LH secretion. The resulting ovulation is followed by formation of a corpus luteum. There is a drop in estrogen secretion, but progesterone and estrogen levels then rise together, along with inhibin B. The elevated levels inhibit FSH and LH secretion for a while, but luteolysis again occurs and a new cycle starts.

Reflex Ovulation

Female cats, rabbits, mink, and certain other animals have long periods of **estrus,** or heat, during which they ovulate only after copulation. Such **reflex ovulation** is

Cys-Tyr-Phe-Gln-Asn-Cys-Pro-Arg-Gly-NH$_2$

Arginine vasopressin

Cys-Tyr-Ile-Gln-Asn-Cys-Pro-Leu-Gly-NH$_2$

Oxytocin

Figure 6–23. Structures of arginine vasopressin and oxytocin. (Reproduced, with permission, from Ganong WF: *Review of Medical Physiology,* 22nd ed. McGraw-Hill, 2005.)

Figure 6–24. Profertility and antifertility actions of GnRH and its agonists. The normal secretion of GnRH is pulsatile, occurring at 30- to 60-minute intervals. This mode, which can be mimicked by timed injections, produces circhoral peaks of LH and FSH secretion and promotes fertility. If GnRH is administered by continuous infusion or if 1 of its long-acting synthetic agonists is injected, there is initial stimulation of the pituitary receptors. However, this stimulation lasts for only a few days and is followed by receptor downregulation with inhibition of gonadotropin secretion (antifertility effect). (Reproduced, with permission, from Conn PM, Crowley WF Jr: Gonadotropin-releasing hormone and its analogues. N Engl J Med 1991;324:93.)

brought about by afferent impulses from the genitalia and the eyes, ears, and nose that converge on the ventral hypothalamus and provoke an ovulation-inducing release of LH from the pituitary. In species such as rats, monkeys, and humans, ovulation is a spontaneous periodic phenomenon, but afferent impulses converging on the hypothalamus can also exert effects. Ovulation can be delayed for 24 hours in rats by administering pentobarbital or other neurally active drugs 12 hours before the expected time of follicle rupture. In women, menstrual cycles may be markedly influenced by emotional stimuli.

Contraception

Methods commonly used to prevent conception, along with their failure rates, are listed in Table 6–4. Contraception is considered in detail in Chapter 36. It is briefly reviewed here because the techniques used are excellent examples of the practical application of the physiologic principles discussed in this chapter.

Among the most extensively used contraceptives are estrogens and/or progestins in varying doses and combinations. They interfere with gonadotrophic secretion or, in some cases, inhibit the union of sperms with ova.

Once conception has occurred, abortion can be produced by progesterone antagonists such as mifepristone.

Implantation of foreign bodies in the uterus causes changes in the duration of the sexual cycle in a number of mammalian species. In humans, such foreign bodies do not alter the menstrual cycle, but they act as effective contraceptive devices. Intrauterine implantation of pieces of metal or plastic (**intrauterine devices [IUDs]**) has been used in programs aimed at controlling population growth. Although their mechanism of action is still unsettled, they seem in general to prevent sperms from fertilizing ova.

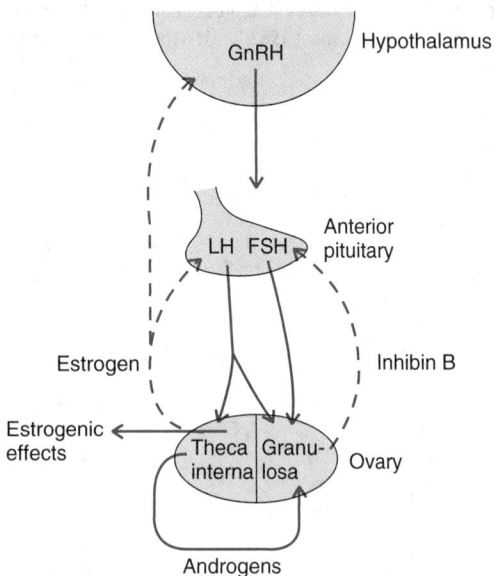

Figure 6–25. Feedback regulation of ovarian function. The cells of the theca interna provide androgens to the granulosa cells, and the thecal cells produce the circulating estrogens, which inhibit the secretion of LH, GnRH, and FSH. Inhibin B from the granulosa cells also inhibits FSH secretion. LH regulates thecal cells, whereas the granulosa cells are regulated by both LH and FSH. The dashed arrows indicate inhibition, and the solid arrows indicate stimulation. GnRH, gonadotropin-releasing hormone; LH, luteinizing hormone; FSH, follicle-stimulating hormone. (Reproduced, with permission, from Ganong WF: *Review of Medical Physiology*, 22nd ed. McGraw-Hill, 2005.)

Table 6–4. Relative effectiveness of frequently used contraceptive methods.

Method	Failures per 100 Women–Years
Vasectomy	0.02
Tubal ligation and similar procedures	0.13
Oral contraceptive	
> 50 μg estrogen and progestin	0.32
< 50 μg estrogen and progestin	0.27
Progestin only	1.2
IUD	
Copper 7	1.5
Loop D	1.3
Diaphragm	1.9
Condom	3.6
Withdrawal	6.7
Spermicide	11.9
Rhythm	15.5

Data from Vessey M, Lawless M, Yeates D: Efficacy of different contraceptive methods. Lancet 1982;1:841. Reproduced with permission.

Implants made up primarily of progestins are now being increasingly used in some parts of the world. The implants are inserted under the skin and can prevent pregnancy for up to 5 years. They often produce amenorrhea but otherwise appear to be well tolerated.

PROLACTIN

Chemistry of Prolactin

Prolactin is another anterior pituitary hormone that has important functions in reproduction and pregnancy. The human prolactin molecule contains 199 amino acid residues and 3 disulfide bridges (Fig 6–26) and has considerable structural similarity to human growth hormone and human chorionic somatomammotropin (hCS). The half-life of prolactin, like that of growth hormone, is about 20 minutes. Structurally similar prolactins are secreted by the endometrium and by the placenta.

Receptors

The human prolactin receptor resembles the growth hormone receptor and is 1 of the superfamily of receptors that includes the growth hormone receptor and receptors for many cytokines and hematopoietic growth factors. It dimerizes and activates the JAK-STAT and other intracellular enzyme cascades.

Figure 6–26. Structure of human prolactin. (Reproduced, with permission, from Bondy PK, Rosenberg LE: *Metabolic Control and Disease,* 8th ed. Saunders, 1980.)

Actions

Prolactin causes milk secretion from the breast after estrogen and progesterone priming. Its effect on the breast is increased production of casein and lactalbumin. However, the action of the hormone is not exerted on the cell nucleus and is prevented by inhibitors of microtubules. Prolactin also inhibits the effects of gonadotropins, possibly by an action at the level of the ovary. Consequently, it is a "natural contraceptive" that spaces pregnancies by preventing ovulation in lactating women. The function of prolactin in normal males is unsettled, but excess prolactin secreted by tumors causes impotence. An action of prolactin that has been used as the basis for bioassay of this hormone is stimulation of the growth and "secretion" of the crop sacs in pigeons and other birds. The paired crop sacs are outpouchings of the esophagus that form, by desquamation of their inner cell layers, a nutritious material ("milk") that the birds feed to their young. However, prolactin, FSH, and LH are now regularly measured by radioimmunoassay.

Regulation of Prolactin Secretion

The normal plasma prolactin concentration is approximately 5 ng/mL in men and 8 ng/mL in women. Secretion is tonically inhibited by the hypothalamus, and section of the pituitary stalk leads to an increase in circulating prolactin. Thus, the effect of the hypothalamic prolactin-inhibiting hormone (PIH) dopamine is greater than the effect of the putative prolactin-releasing hormone. In humans, prolactin secretion is increased by exercise, surgical and psychological stresses, and stimulation of the nipple (Table 6–5). The plasma prolactin level rises during sleep, the rise starting after the onset of sleep and persisting throughout the sleep period. Secretion is increased during pregnancy, reaching a peak at the time of parturition. After delivery, the plasma concentration falls to nonpregnant levels in about 8 days. Suckling produces a prompt increase in secretion, but the magnitude of this rise gradually declines after a woman has been nursing for more than 3 months.

L-Dopa decreases prolactin secretion by increasing the formation of dopamine, and bromocriptine and other dopamine agonists inhibit secretion because they stimulate dopamine receptors. Chlorpromazine and related drugs that block dopamine receptors increase prolactin secretion. Thyroid-releasing hormone (TRH) stimulates the secretion of prolactin in addition to TSH, and there are additional prolactin-releasing polypeptides in hypothalamic tissue. Estrogens produce a slowly developing increase in prolactin secretion as a result of a direct action on the lactotropes.

It has now been established that prolactin facilitates the secretion of dopamine in the median eminence.

Table 6–5. Factors affecting the secretion of human prolactin and growth hormone.

Factor	Prolactin	Growth Hormone
Sleep	I+	I+
Nursing	I++	N
Breast stimulation in nonlactating women	I	N
Stress	I+	I+
Hypoglycemia	I	I+
Strenuous exercise	I	I
Sexual intercourse in women	I	N
Pregnancy	I++	N
Estrogens	I	I
Hypothyroidism	I	N
TRH	I+	N
Phenothiazines, butyrophenones	I+	N
Opiates	I	I
Glucose	N	D
Somatostatin	N	D+
L–Dopa	D+	I+
Apomorphine	D+	I+
Bromocriptine and related ergot derivatives	D+	I

I, moderate increase; I+, marked increase; I++, very marked increase; N, no change; D, moderate decrease; D+, marked decrease.

(Modified from Frantz and reproduced, with permission, from Ganong WF: *Review of Medical Physiology*, 22nd ed, McGraw–Hill, 2005.)

Thus, prolactin acts in the hypothalamus in a negative feedback fashion to inhibit its own secretion.

Hyperprolactinemia

Up to 70% of patients with chromophobe adenomas of the anterior pituitary have elevated plasma prolactin levels. In some instances the elevation may be due to damage to the pituitary stalk, but in most cases the tumor cells are actually secreting the hormone. The hyperprolactinemia may cause galactorrhea, but in many individuals there are no demonstrable abnormalities. Indeed, most women with galactorrhea have normal prolactin levels; definite elevations are found in less than one-third of patients with this condition.

Another interesting observation is that 15–20% of women with secondary amenorrhea have elevated prolactin levels, and when prolactin secretion is reduced, normal menstrual cycles and fertility return. It appears that the prolactin may produce amenorrhea by blocking the action of gonadotropins on the ovaries, but definitive proof of this hypothesis must await further research. The hypogonadism produced by prolactinomas is associated with osteoporosis due to estrogen deficiency.

Hyperprolactinemia in men is associated with impotence and hypogonadism that disappear when prolactin secretion is reduced.

MENOPAUSE

The human ovary gradually becomes unresponsive to gonadotropins with advancing age and its function declines so that sexual cycles and menstruation disappear (menopause). This unresponsiveness is associated with and probably caused by a decline in the number of primordial follicles (Fig 6–6). The ovaries no longer secrete progesterone and 17β-estradiol in appreciable quantities. Estrone is formed by aromatization of androstenedione in fat and other tissues, but the amounts are normally small. The uterus and vagina gradually become atrophic. As the negative feedback effect of the estrogens and progesterone is reduced, secretion of FSH and LH is increased, and plasma FSH and LH rise to high levels. Old female mice and rats have long periods of diestrus and increased levels of gonadotropin secretion, but a clear-cut "menopause" has apparently not been described in experimental animals.

In women, the menses usually become irregular and cease between the ages of 45 and 55. The average age at onset of the menopause has increased since the turn of the century and is currently about 52 years.

Sensations of warmth spreading from the trunk to the face ("hot flushes," also called hot flashes), night sweats, and various psychic symptoms are common after ovarian function has ceased. Hot flushes are said to occur in 75% of menopausal women and may last as long as 40 years. They are prevented by administration of estrogen. They are not peculiar to the menopause; they also occur in premenopausal women and men whose gonads are removed surgically or destroyed by disease. Their cause is unknown. However, it has been demonstrated that they coincide with surges of LH secretion. LH is secreted in episodic bursts at intervals of 30–60 minutes or more (circhoral secretion), and in the absence of gonadal hormones, these bursts are large. Each hot flush begins with the start of a burst. However, LH itself is not responsible for the symptoms, as they can continue after removal of the pituitary. Instead, it appears that some event in the hypothalamus initiates both the release of LH and the episode of flushing. The menopause and the clinical management of patients with menopausal symptoms are discussed in more detail in Chapter 59.

REFERENCES

Chabbert Buffet N et al: Regulation of the human menstrual cycle. Front Neuroendocrinol 1998;19:151.

Ganong WF: *Review of Medical Physiology,* 22nd ed. McGraw-Hill, 2005.

Kelley PA et al: Implications of multiple phenotypes observed in prolactin receptor knockout mice. Front Neuroendocrinol 2001;22:140.

Knobil E, Neill JD (editors): *The Physiology of Reproduction,* 2nd ed, 2 vols. Raven Press, 1994.

Larsen PR et al: *William's Textbook of Endocrinology,* 10th ed. Saunders, 2003.

Mather JP, Moore A, Li R-H: Activins, inhibins, and follistatins: Further thoughts on a growing family of regulators. Proc Soc Exp Biol Med 1997;215:209.

Mathews J. Gustattson J-A: Estrogen signaling: A subtle balance between ER and ER. Mol Interv 2003; 3:281

Mendelsohn ME, Karas RH: The protective effects of estrogen on the cardiovascular system. N Engl J Med 1999;340:1801.

Ness RB et al: Oral contraceptives, other methods of contraception and risk reduction for ovarian cancer. Epidemiology 2001;12:307.

Palment NR, Boepple PA: Variation in the onset of puberty: Clinical spectrum and genetic investigation. J Clin Endocrinol Metab 2001;86:2364.

Reyelli A, Massobrio M, Tesarik J: Nongenomic actions of steroid hormones in reproductive tissues. Endocrinol Rev 1998;19:3.

Yen SSC, Jaffe RB, Barbieri RL (editors): *Reproductive Endocrinology: Physiology, Pathophysiology, and Clinical Management,* 4th ed. Saunders, 1999.

Maternal Physiology During Pregnancy

Daniel A. Kahn, MD, PhD, & Brian J. Koos, MD, PhD

Pregnancy involves a number changes in anatomy, physiology, and biochemistry, which can challenge maternal reserves. A basic knowledge of these adaptations is critical for understanding normal laboratory measurements, knowing the drugs likely to require dose adjustments, and recognizing women who are predisposed to medical complications during pregnancy.

CARDIOVASCULAR SYSTEM

Anatomic Changes

With uterine enlargement and diaphragmatic elevation, the heart rotates on its long axis in a left-upward displacement. As a result of these changes, the apical beat (point of maximum intensity) shifts laterally. Overall, the heart size increases by about 12%, which results from both an increase in myocardial mass and intracardiac volume (approximately 80 mL). Vascular changes include hypertrophy of smooth muscle and a reduction in collagen content.

Blood Volume

Blood volume expansion begins early in the first trimester, increases rapidly in the second trimester, and plateaus at about the 30th week (Fig 7–1). The approximately 50% elevation in plasma volume, which accounts for most of the increment, results from a cascade of effects triggered by pregnancy hormones. For example, increased estrogen production by the placenta stimulates the renin-angiotensin system, which, in turn, leads to higher circulating levels of aldosterone. Aldosterone promotes renal Na^+ reabsorption and water retention. Progesterone also participates in plasma volume expansion through a poorly understood mechanism; increased venous capacitance is another important factor. Human chorionic somatomammotropin, progesterone, and perhaps other hormones promote erythropoiesis, resulting in the about a 30% increase in red cell mass.

The magnitude of the increase in blood volume varies according to the size of the woman, the number of prior pregnancies, and the number of fetuses she is carrying. This hypervolemia of pregnancy compensates for maternal blood loss at delivery, which averages 500–600 mL for vaginal and 1000 mL for cesarean delivery.

Cardiac Output

Cardiac output increases approximately 40% during pregnancy, with maximum values achieved at 20–24 weeks' gestation. This rise in cardiac output is thought to result from the hormonal changes of pregnancy as well as the arteriovenous-shunt effect of uteroplacental circulation.

Stroke volume increases 25–30% during pregnancy, reaching peak values at 12–24 weeks' gestation (Fig 7–2). Thus, elevations in cardiac output after 20 weeks of gestation depend critically on the rise in heart rate. Maximum cardiac output is associated with a 24% increase in stroke volume and a 15% rise in heart rate. Cardiac output increases in labor in association with painful contractions, which increase venous return and activate the sympathetic nervous system. Cardiac output is further increased, albeit transiently, at delivery.

Stroke volume is sensitive to maternal position. In lateral recumbency, stroke volume remains roughly the same from 20 weeks' gestation until term, but in the supine position stroke volume decreases after 20 weeks and can even fall to nonpregnant levels by 40 weeks' gestation.

The resting maternal heart rate, which progressively increases over the course of gestation, averages at term about 15 beats/min more than the nonpregnant rate (Fig 7–2). Of course, exercise, emotional stress, heat, drugs, and other factors can further increase heart rate.

Multiple gestations have even more profound effects on the maternal cardiovascular system. In twin pregnancies, cardiac output is about 20% greater than for singletons, because of greater stroke volume (15%) and heart rate (3.5%). Other differences include greater left ventricular end-diastolic dimensions and muscle mass.

Cardiac output is generally resistant to postural stress. For example, the fall in cardiac output that develops immediately after standing does not occur in the middle of the third trimester, although some reduction can occur earlier in pregnancy. In the third trimester, the supine

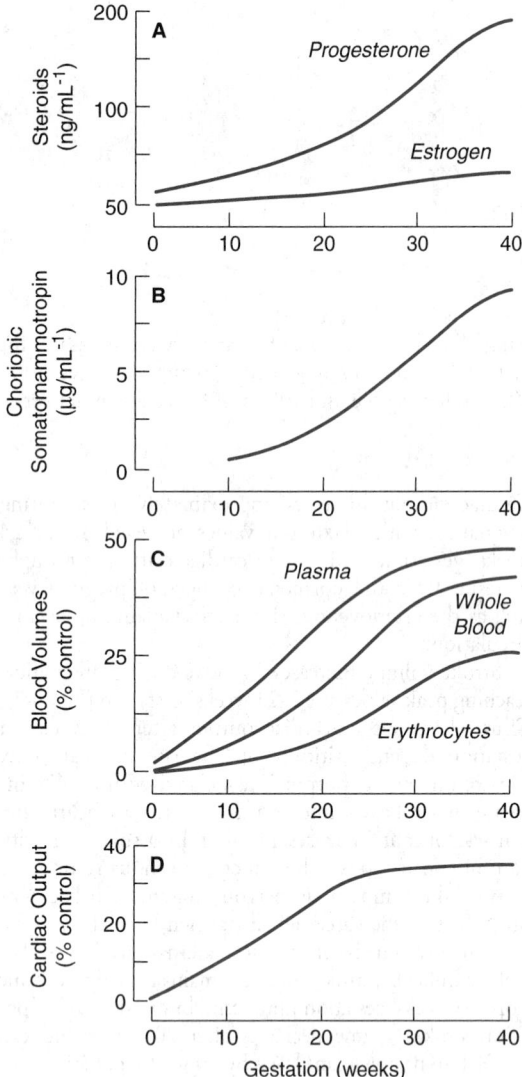

Figure 7–1. Increases in maternal hormones (**A**, **B**), blood volume (**C**), and cardiac output (**D**) over gestation. % control represents the increment relative to nonpregnant values. (Modified from Longo LD: Maternal blood volume and cardiac output during pregnancy: A hypothesis of endocrinologic control. Am J Physiol 1983;245:R720.)

tance in venous collaterals. Shifting the gravida to a right or left lateral recumbent position will alleviate caval compression, increase blood return to the heart, and restore cardiac output and arterial pressure.

Blood Pressure

Systemic arterial pressure declines slightly during pregnancy, reaching a nadir at 24–28 weeks of gestation. Pulse pressure widens because the fall is greater for diastolic than for systolic pressures (Fig 7–3). Systolic and diastolic pressures (and mean arterial pressure) increase to prepregnancy levels by about 36 weeks.

Venous pressure progressively increases in the lower extremities, particularly when the patient is supine, sitting, or standing. The rise in venous pressure, which can cause edema and varicosities, results from compression of the inferior vena cava by the gravid uterus and possibly from the pressure of the fetal presenting part on the common iliac veins. Lying in lateral recumbency minimizes changes in venous pressure. As expected, venous pressure in the lower extremities falls immediately after delivery. Venous pressure in the upper extremities is unchanged by pregnancy.

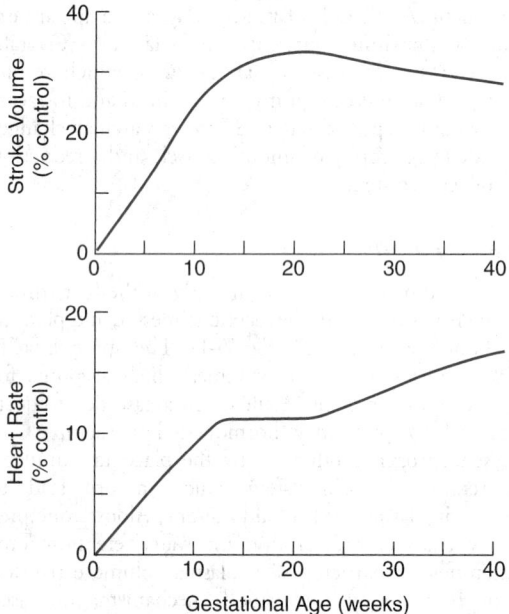

Figure 7–2. Increases in maternal stroke volume and heart rate. The % control represents increment relative to measurements in patients who are not pregnant. (Reproduced, with permission, from Koos BJ: Management of uncorrected, palliated, and repaired cyanotic congenital heart disease in pregnancy. Prog Ped Cardiol 2004;19:250.)

position can reduce cardiac output and arterial pressure caused by compression of the vena cava by the gravid uterus with an associated reduction in venous return to the heart. About 8% of gravidas will develop supine hypotensive syndrome, characterized by hypotension, bradycardia, and syncope. These women are particularly sensitive to caval compression because of reduced capaci-

Peripheral Vascular Resistance

Vascular resistance decreases in the first trimester, reaching a nadir of about 34% below nonpregnancy levels by 14 to 0 weeks of gestation with a slight increase toward term (Fig 7–3). The hormonal changes of pregnancy likely trigger this fall in vascular resistance by enhancing local vasodilators, such as nitric oxide, prostacyclin, and possibly adenosine. Delivery is associated with nearly a 40% fall in peripheral vascular resistance, although mean arterial pressure is generally maintained because of the associated rise in cardiac output.

Blood Flow Distribution

Blood flow to the uterus increases in a gestational age-dependent manner. Uterine blood flow can be as high as 800 mL/min, which is about 4 times the nonpregnant value. The increased flow during pregnancy results from the relatively low resistance in the uteroplacental circulation.

Renal blood flow increases approximately 400 mL/min above nonpregnant levels, and blood flow to the breasts increases approximately 200 mL/min. Blood flow to the skin also increases, particularly in the hands and feet. The increased skin blood flow helps dissipate heat produced by metabolism in the mother and fetus.

In absolute terms, blood flow increases to the uterus, kidneys, skin, breast, and possibly other maternal organs; the total augmented organ flow reflects virtually the entire increment in maternal cardiac output. However, when expressed as a percentage of cardiac output, blood flow in some of these organs may not be elevated compared to the nonpregnant state.

Strenuous exercise, which diverts blood flow to large muscles, has the potential to decrease uteroplacental perfusion and thus O_2 delivery to the fetus. Women who are already adapted to an exercise routine can generally continue the program in pregnancy; however, pregnant women should discuss their exercise plans with the physician managing the pregnancy.

Heart Murmurs and Rhythm

The physiologic changes of pregnancy alter several clinical findings. For example, systolic ejection murmurs, which result from increased cardiac output and decreased blood viscosity, can be detected in 90% or more gravidas. Thus, caution should be exercised in interpreting systolic murmurs in pregnant women.

The first heart sound may be split, with increased loudness of both portions, and the third heart sound may also be louder. Continuous murmurs or bruits may be heard at the left sternal edge, which arise from the internal thoracic (mammary) artery.

Pregnancy decreases the threshold for reentrant supraventricular tachycardia. Normal pregnancy can also be

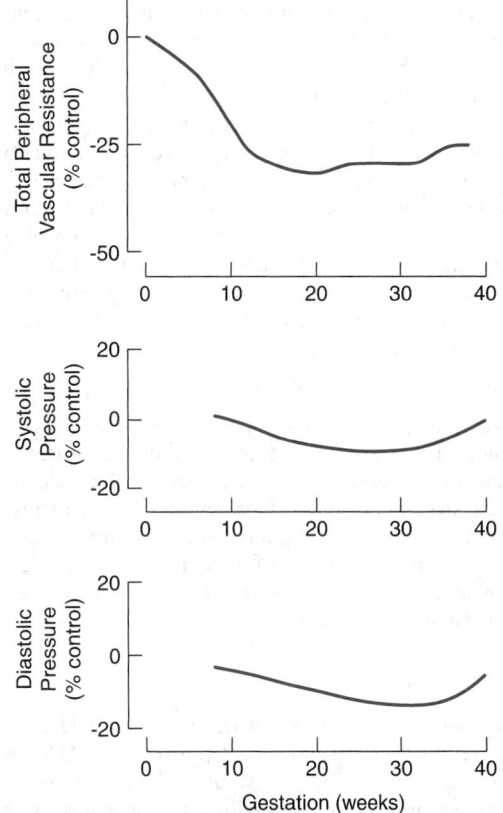

Figure 7–3. Changes in maternal peripheral vascular resistance and arterial pressures over gestation. Pressures were measured in the left lateral recumbent position. The % control represents the relative change from nonpregnant values. (Modified from Thornburg KL et al: Hemodynamic changes in pregnancy. Semin Perinatol 2000;24:11; Wilson M et al: Blood pressure, the renin-aldosterone system and sex steroids throughout normal pregnancy. Am J Med 1980;68:97.)

accompanied by sinus tachycardia, sinus bradycardia, and isolated atrial and ventricular premature contractions.

Electrocardiographic changes can include a 15- to 20-degree shift to the left in the electrical axis. Changes in ventricular repolarization can result in ST segment depression or T-wave flattening. However, pregnancy does not alter the amplitude and duration of the P wave, QRS complex, or T wave.

PULMONARY SYSTEM

Anatomic Changes

Pregnancy alters the circulation of a number of tissues involved in respiration. For example, capillary dilatation leads to engorgement of the nasopharynx, larynx, trachea, and bronchi. Prominent pulmonary vascular markings observed on x-ray are consistent with increased pulmonary blood volume.

As the uterus enlarges, the diaphragm is elevated by as much as 4 cm. The rib cage is displaced upward, increasing the angle of the ribs with the spine. These changes increase the lower thoracic diameter by about 2 cm and the thoracic circumference by up to 6 cm. Elevation of the diaphragm does not impair its function. Abdominal muscles have less tone and activity during pregnancy, causing respiration to be more diaphragm dependent.

Lung Volumes and Capacities

Several lung volumes and capacities are altered by pregnancy (Table 7–1). Dead space volume increases because of relaxation of the musculature of conducting airways. Tidal volume and inspiratory capacity increase. Elevation of the diaphragm is associated with reduction in total lung capacity and functional residual capacity. The latter involves a decrease in both expiratory reserve and residual volumes.

Respiration

Pregnancy has little affect on respiratory rate. Thus, the increase in minute ventilation (approximately 50%) results from the rise in tidal volume. This increment in minute ventilation is disproportionately greater than the rise (approximately 20%) in total oxygen consumption in maternal muscle tissues (cardiac, respiratory, uterine, skeletal) and in the products of the fetal genome (placenta, fetus), as shown in Figure 7–4. This hyperventilation, which decreases maternal arterial PCO_2 to about 27–32 mm Hg, results in a mild respiratory alkalosis (blood pH of 7.4–7.5). The hyperventilation and hyperdynamic circulation slightly increase arterial PO_2.

Increased levels of progesterone appear to have a critical role in the hyperventilation of pregnancy, which develops early in the first trimester. As in the luteal phase of the menstrual cycle of nonpregnant women, the increased ventilation appears to be caused by the action of progesterone on central neurons involved in respiratory regulation. The overall respiratory effect appears to be a decrease in the threshold and an increase in the sensitivity of central chemoreflex responses to CO_2. Maternal hyperventilation may be protective in that that it prevents the fetus from being exposed to high CO_2 tensions, which might adversely affect the development of respiratory control and other critical regulatory mechanisms.

Functional measurement of ventilation can also change according to posture and duration of pregnancy. For example, the peak expiratory rate, which declines throughout gestation in the sitting and stand-

Table 7–1. Effects of pregnancy on lung volumes and capacities.

	Definition	Change
I. Volumes		
Tidal	Volume inspired and expired with each normal respiratory cycle	↑ 35–50%
Inspiratory reserve	Maximum volume that can be inspired over normal end-tidal inspiration	↓
Expiratory reserve	Maximum volume that can be expired from resting end-tidal expiration	↓ 20%
Residual	Volume remaining in the lungs following maximum expiration	↓ 20%
II. Capacities		
Total lung	Total volume at the end of maximum inspiration	↓ 5%
Vital	Maximum volume expired after maximum inspiration	→
Inspiratory	Maximum volume inspired from end-tidal expiration	↑ 5–10%
Functional	Volume at end-tidal expiration that mixes with tidal air upon inspiration	↓ 20%

ing positions, is particularly compromised in the supine position.

RENAL SYSTEM

Anatomic Changes

During pregnancy, the length of the kidneys increases by 1–1.5 cm, with a proportional increase in weight. The renal calyces and pelves are dilated in pregnancy, with the volume of the renal pelvis increased up to 6-fold compared to the nonpregnant value of 10 mL. The ureters are dilated above the brim of the bony pelvis, with more prominent effects on the right. The ureters elongate, widen, and become more curved. The entire dilated collecting system may contain up to 200 mL of urine, which predisposes to ascending urinary infections. Urinary tract dilatation disappears in virtually all women by postpartum day 4.

Figure 7-4. Components of increased oxygen consumption during pregnancy. (Reproduced, with permission, from Hytten FE, Leitch I: *The Physiology of Human Pregnancy.* Blackwell, 1964.)

Several factors likely contribute to the hydronephrosis and hydroureter of pregnancy: (1) Pregnancy hormones (eg, progesterone) may cause hypotonia of ureteral smooth muscle. Against this possibility is the observation that high progesterone levels in nonpregnant women do not cause hydroureter. (2) Enlargement of the ovarian vein complex in the infundibulopelvic ligament may compress the ureter at the brim of the bony pelvis. (3) Hyperplasia of smooth muscle in the distal one-third of the ureter may cause reduction in luminal size, leading to dilatation in the upper two-thirds. (4) The sigmoid colon and dextrorotation of the uterus likely reduce compression (and dilatation) of the left ureter relative to the right.

Renal Function

Renal plasma flow increases 50–85% above nonpregnant values during the first half of pregnancy, with a modest decrease in later gestation. The changes in renal plasma flow reflect decreases in renal vascular resistance, which achieves lowest values by the end of the first trimester. Elevated renal perfusion is the principal factor involved in rise in glomerular filtration rate (GFR), which is increased by approximately 25% in the second week after conception. GFR reaches a peak increment of 40–65% by the end of the first trimester and remains high until term (Fig 7–5). The fraction of renal plasma flow that passes through the glomerular membrane (filtration fraction) decreases during the first 20 weeks of gestation, which subsequently rises toward term.

Hormones involved in these changes in renal vascular resistance may include progesterone and relaxin (via up-regulation of vascular matrix metalloproteinase-2). Agents elaborated by the endothelium, such as endothelin (ET) (via activation of ET_B receptor subtype) and nitric oxide

(via increased cyclic guanosine –3',5'-monophosphate), are likely to be critically involved in the reduction of renal vascular resistance. An additional factor is the increased cardiac output, which permits increased renal perfusion without depriving other organs of blood flow.

Urinary flow and sodium excretion rates in late pregnancy are increased 2-fold in lateral recumbency compared to the supine position. Thus, measurements of urinary function must take into account maternal posture. Collection periods should be at least 12–24 hours to allow for errors caused by the large urinary dead space. However, reasonable estimates of urinary excretion of a particular substance over shorter time periods generally can be calculated by referencing the level to the creatinine concentration in the same sample of urine (substance/creatinine ratio) with the assumption that a pregnant woman excretes 1 g of creatinine per day. Creatinine production (0.7-1.0 g/day) by skeletal muscle is virtually unchanged by pregnancy.

Figure 7-5. Increases in glomerular filtration over gestation as reflected by changes in inulin and endogenous creatinine clearances. The % control represents relative change from postpartum values. (Data from Davison JM, Hytten FE: Glomerular filtration during and after pregnancy. *J Obstet Gynaecol Br Commonw* 1974;81:558.)

Up to 80% of the glomerular filtrate is reabsorbed by the proximal tubules, a process that is independent of hormonal control. Aldosterone regulates sodium reabsorption in the distal tubules, while arginine vasopressin activity, which regulates free water clearance, determines the ultimate urine concentration. Pregnancy is associated with increased circulating concentrations of aldosterone. Even though the GFR increases dramatically during gestation, the volume of urine excreted per day is unchanged.

Renal clearance of creatinine increases as the GFR rises, with maximum clearances approximately 50% more than nonpregnant levels. The creatinine clearance decreases somewhat after about 30 weeks of gestation. The rise in GFR lowers mean serum creatinine concentrations (pregnant, 0.46 ± 0.13 mg/100 mL; nonpregnant, 0.67 ± 0.14 mg/100 mL) and blood urea nitrogen (pregnant, 8.17 ± 1.5 mg/100 mL; nonpregnant, 13 ± 3 mg/100 mL) concentrations.

Increased GFR with saturation of tubular resorption capacity for filtered glucose can result in glucosuria. In fact, more than 50% of women have glucosuria sometime during pregnancy. Increased urinary glucose levels contribute to increased susceptibility of pregnant women to urinary tract infection.

Urinary protein loss normally does not exceed 300 mg over 24 hours, which is similar to the nonpregnant state. Thus, proteinuria of more than 300 mg over 24 hours suggests a renal disorder.

Renin activity increases early in the first trimester, and continues to rise until term. This enzyme is critically involved in the conversion of angiotensinogen to angiotensin I, which subsequently forms the potent vasoconstrictor angiotensin II. Angiotensin II levels also increase in pregnancy, but the vasoconstriction and hypertension that might be expected do not occur. In fact, normal pregnant women are very resistant to the pressor effects of elevated levels of angiotensin II and other vasopressors; this effect is likely mediated by increased vascular synthesis of nitric oxide and other vasodilators.

Angiotensin II is also a potent stimulus for adrenocortical secretion of aldosterone, which, in conjunction with arginine vasopressin, promotes salt and water retention in pregnancy. The net effect is a decrease in plasma sodium concentrations by approximately 5 mEq/L and a fall in plasma osmolality by nearly 10 mOsm/kg. These effects on electrolyte homeostasis likely involve a resetting of the pituitary osmostat. In pregnancy, the increased pituitary secretion of vasopressin is largely balanced by placental production of vasopressinase. Pregnant women who are unable to sufficiently augment vasopressin secretion can develop a diabetes insipidus–like condition characterized by massive diuresis and profound hypernatremia. Cases have been described with maternal sodium levels reaching 170 mEq/L.

Bladder

As the uterus enlarges, the urinary bladder is displaced upward and flattened in the anteroposterior diameter. One of the earliest symptoms of pregnancy is increased urinary frequency, which may be related to pregnancy hormones. In later gestation, mechanical effects of the enlarged uterus may contribute to the increased frequency. Bladder vascularity increases and muscle tone decreases, which increases bladder capacity up to 1500 mL.

GASTROINTESTINAL SYSTEM

Anatomic Changes

As the uterus grows, the stomach is pushed upward and the large and small bowels extend into more rostrolateral regions. The appendix is displaced superiorly in the right flank area. These organs return to their normal positions in the early puerperium.

Oral Cavity

Salivation appears to increase although this may be caused in part by swallowing difficulty associated with nausea. Pregnancy does not predispose to tooth decay or to mobilization of bone calcium.

The gums may become hypertrophic and hyperemic; often, they are so spongy and friable that they bleed easily. This may be caused by increased systemic estrogen because similar problems sometimes occur with the use of oral contraceptives.

Esophagus and Stomach

Reflux symptoms (heartburn) affect 30–80% of pregnant women. Gastric production of hydrochloric acid is variable and sometimes exaggerated but more commonly reduced. Pregnancy is associated with greater production of gastrin, which increases stomach volume and acidity of gastric secretions. Gastric production of mucus also may be increased. Esophageal peristalsis is decreased. Most women first report symptoms of reflux in the first trimester (52% vs 24% in the second trimester vs 8.8% in the third trimester), although the symptoms can become more severe with advanced gestation.

The underlying predisposition to reflux in pregnancy is related to hormone-mediated relaxation of the lower esophageal sphincter (Fig 7–6). With advancing gestation, the lower esophageal sphincter has decreased pressure as well as blunted responses to sphincter stimulation. Thus, decreased motility, increased acidity of gastric secretions, and reduced function of the lower esophageal sphincter contribute to the increased gastric reflux. The increased prevalence of gastric reflux and delayed gastric emptying of solid food make the gravida

Figure 7–6. Lower esophageal sphincter pressures for 3 periods of pregnancy and the postpartum state. The shaded area represents the normal range in nonpregnant women. The horizontal bars show the mean ± SE for measurements in 4 women. The rectangles show the mean ± SE for each gestational age. (Modified from Van Theil DH, Gravaler JS, Joshi SN et al: Heartburn in pregnancy. Gastroenterology 1977;72:666.)

more vulnerable to regurgitation and aspiration with anesthesia. The rate of gastric emptying of solid foods is slowed in pregnancy, but the rate for liquids remains generally the same as in the nonpregnant state.

Intestines

Intestinal transit times are decreased in the second and third trimesters (Fig 7–7), whereas first trimester and postpartum transit times are similar. Transit times return to normal within 2 to 4 days postpartum.

The reduced gastrointestinal motility during pregnancy has been thought to be caused by increased circulating concentrations of progesterone. However, experimental evidence suggests that elevated estrogen concentrations are critically involved through an enhancement of nitric oxide release from the nonadrenergic, noncholinergic nerves that modulate gastrointestinal motility. Other factors may also be involved.

The slow transit time of food through the gastrointestinal tract potentially enhances water absorption, predisposing to constipation. However, diet and cultural expectations may be more important factors in this disorder.

Gallbladder

The emptying of the gallbladder is slowed in pregnancy and often incomplete. When visualized at cesarean delivery, the gallbladder commonly appears dilated and atonic. Bile stasis of pregnancy increases the risk for gallstone formation, although the chemical composition of bile is not appreciably altered.

Liver

Liver morphology does not change in normal pregnancy. Plasma albumin levels are reduced to a greater extent than the slight decrease in plasma globulins. This fall in the albumin/globulin ratio mimics liver disease in nonpregnant individuals. Serum alkaline phosphatase activity can double as the result of alkaline phosphatase isozymes produced by the placenta.

HEMATOLOGIC SYSTEM

Red Blood Cells

The red cell mass expands by about 33%, or by approximately 450 mL of erythrocytes for the average pregnant woman (Fig 7–1). The increase is greater with iron supplementation. The greater increase in plasma volume accounts for the anemia of pregnancy. For example, maternal hemoglobin levels average 10.9 ± 0.8 (SD) g/dL in the second trimester and 12.4 ± 1.0 g/dL at term.

Iron

The enhanced erythropoiesis of pregnancy increases utilization of iron, which can reach 6 to 7 mg per day in the latter half of pregnancy. Many women begin preg-

Figure 7–7. Small-bowel transit times measured by the lactulose hydrogen breath method in a single woman in the third trimester and postpartum. Hydrogen concentrations in maternal breath were determined after administration of a lactulose meal. Hydrogen is released when bacteria in the colon break down lactulose. (Modified from Wald A, Van Thiel DH, Hoeschstetter L et al: Effect of pregnancy on gastrointestinal transit. Dig Dis Sci 1982;27:1015.)

nancy in an iron-deficient state, making them vulnerable to iron deficiency anemia. Thus, supplemental iron is commonly given to pregnant women. Because the placenta actively transports iron from the mother to the fetus, the fetus generally is not anemic even when the mother is severely iron deficient.

White Blood Cells

The total blood leukocyte count increases during normal pregnancy from a prepregnancy level of 4,300–4,500/μL to 5000–12,000/μL in the last trimester, although counts as high as 16,000/μL have been observed in the last trimester. Counts in the 20,000–25,000/μL range can occur during labor. The cause of the rise in the leukocyte count, which primarily involves the polymorphonuclear forms, has not been established.

Polymorphonuclear leukocyte chemotaxis may be impaired in pregnancy, which appears to be a cell-associated defect. Reduced polymorphonuclear leukocyte adherence has been reported in the third trimester. These observations may predispose pregnant women to infection. Basophil counts decrease slightly as pregnancy advances. Eosinophil counts, although variable, remain largely unchanged.

Platelets

Some studies have reported increased production of platelets (thrombocytopoiesis) during pregnancy that is accompanied by progressive platelet consumption. Platelet counts fall below 150,000/μL in 6% of gravidas in the third trimester. This *pregnancy-associated thrombocytopenia*, which appears to be caused by increased peripheral consumption, resolves with delivery and is of no pathologic significance. Levels of prostacyclin (PGI$_2$), a platelet aggregation inhibitor, and thromboxane A$_2$, an inducer of platelet aggregation and a vasoconstrictor, increase during pregnancy.

Clotting Factors

Circulating levels of several coagulation factors increase in pregnancy. Fibrinogen (factor I) and factor VIII levels increase markedly, whereas factors VII, IX, X, and XII increase to a lesser extent.

Plasma fibrinogen concentrations begin to increase from nonpregnant levels (1.5–4.5 g/L) during the third month of pregnancy and progressively rise by nearly 2-fold by late pregnancy (4–6.5 g/L). The high estrogen levels of pregnancy may be involved in the increased fibrinogen synthesis by the liver.

Prothrombin (factor II) is only nominally affected by pregnancy. Factor V concentrations are mildly increased. Factor XI decreases slightly toward the end of pregnancy, and factor XIII (fibrin-stabilizing factor) is appreciably reduced, up to 50% at term. The free form

of protein S declines in the first and second trimesters and remains low for the rest of gestation.

Fibrinolytic activity is depressed during pregnancy through a poorly understood mechanism. Plasminogen concentrations increase concomitantly with fibrinogen, but there is still a net procoagulant effect of pregnancy.

Coagulation and fibrinolytic systems undergo major alterations during pregnancy. Understanding these physiologic changes is critical for the management of some of the more serious pregnancy disorders, including hemorrhage and thromboembolic disease.

SKIN

Anatomic Changes

Hyperpigmentation is one of the well-recognized skin changes of pregnancy, which is manifested in the linea nigra and melasma, the *mask of pregnancy*. The latter, which is exacerbated by sun exposure, develops in up to 70% of pregnancies and is characterized by an uneven darkening of the skin in the centrofacial-malar area. The hyperpigmentation is probably because of the elevated concentrations of melanocyte-stimulating hormone and/or estrogen and progesterone effects on the skin. Similar hyperpigmentation of the face can be seen in nonpregnant women who are taking oral contraceptives.

Striae gravidarum consist of bands or lines of thickened, hyperemic skin. These "stretch marks" begin to appear in the second trimester on the abdomen, breasts, thighs, and buttocks. Decreased collagen adhesiveness and increased ground substance formation are characteristically seen in this skin condition. A genetic predisposition appears to be involved because not every gravida develops these skin changes. Effective treatment (preventive or therapeutic) has yet to be found.

Other common cutaneous changes include spider angiomas, palmar erythema, and cutis marmorata (mottled appearance of skin secondary to vasomotor instability). The development or worsening of varicosities accompanies nearly 40% of pregnancies. Compression of the vena cava by the gravid uterus increases venous pressures in the lower extremities, which dilates veins in the legs, anus (hemorrhoids), and vulva.

The nails and hair also undergo changes. Nails become brittle and can show horizontal grooves (Beau's lines). Thickening of the hair during pregnancy is caused by an increased number of follicles in anagen (growth) phase, and generalized hirsutism can worsen in women who already have hair that is thick or has a male pattern of distribution. The thickening of the hair ends 1 to 5 months postpartum with the onset of the telogen (resting) phase, which results in excessive shedding and thinning of hair. Normal hair growth returns within 12 months.

Table 7–2. Estimate of extracellular and intracelluar water added during pregnancy.

	Total Water (mL)	Extracellular (mL)	Intracellular (mL)
Fetus	2343	1360	983
Placenta	540	260	280
Amniotic fluid	792	792	...
Uterus	743	490	253
Mammary glands	304	148	156
Plasma	920	920	...
Red cells	163	...	163
Extracellular, extra-vascular water	1195	1195	...
Total	7000	5165	1835

Reproduced, with permission, from Hytten FE, Leitch I: *The Physiology of Human Pregnancy.* Blackwell, 1964.

METABOLISM

Pregnancy increases nutritional requirements, and several maternal alterations occur to meet this demand. Pregnant women tend to rest more often, which conserves energy and thereby enhances fetal nutrition. The maternal appetite and food intake usually increase, although some have a decreased appetite or experience nausea and vomiting (see Chapter 9). In rare instances, women with pica may crave substances such as clay, cornstarch, soap, or even coal.

Pregnancy is associated with profound changes in structure and metabolism. The most obvious physical changes are weight gain and altered body shape. Weight gain results not only from the uterus and its contents, but also from increased breast tissue, blood volume, and water volume (about 6.8 L) in the form of extravascular

and extracellular fluid (Table 7–2). Deposition of fat and protein and increased cellular water are added to maternal stores. The average weight gain during pregnancy is 12.5 kg (27.5 lb). Distribution of weight gain over gestation is shown in Figure 7–8.

Protein accretion accounts for about 1 kg of maternal weight gain, which is evenly divided between the mother (uterine contractile protein, breast glandular tissue, plasma protein, and hemoglobin) and the fetoplacental unit.

Total body fat increases during pregnancy, but the amount varies with the total weight gain. During the second half of pregnancy, plasma lipids increase (plasma cholesterol increases 50%, plasma triglyceride concentration may triple), but triglycerides, cholesterol, and lipoproteins decrease soon after delivery. The ratio of low-density lipoproteins (LDLs) to high-density lipoproteins (HDLs) increases during pregnancy. It has been suggested that most fat is stored centrally during midpregnancy and that as the fetus extracts more nutrition in the latter months, fat storage decreases.

Metabolism of carbohydrates and insulin during pregnancy is discussed in Chapter 18. Pregnancy is associated with insulin resistance, which can lead to hyperglycemia (gestational diabetes) in susceptible women. This metabolic disorder usually disappears after delivery, but may arise later in life as type II diabetes.

REFERENCES

Abram SR, et al. Role of neuronal nitric oxide synthase in mediating renal hemodynamic changes during pregnancy. Am J Physiol Regul Integr Comp Physiol 2001;281:Rl390.

Bamber JH, Dresner M. Aortocaval compression in pregnancy: The effect of changing the degree and direction of lateral tilt on maternal cardiac output. Anesth Analg 2003;97:256.

Barankin B, et al. The skin in pregnancy. J Cutan Med Surg 2002; 6:236.

Baron TH, et al. Gastrointestinal motility disorders during pregnancy. Ann Intern Med 1993;118:366.

Bremme KA. Haemostatic changes in pregnancy. Best Pract Res Clin Haematol 2003;16:153.

Bridges EJ, et al. Hemodynamic monitoring in high-risk obstetrics patients, I. Expected hemodynamic changes in pregnancy. Crit Care Nurse 2003;23:53.

Carbillon L, et al. Pregnancy, vascular tone, and maternal hemodynamics: A crucial adaptation. Obstet Gynecol Surv 2000;55:574.

Conrad KP. Mechanisms of renal vasodilation and hyperfiltration during pregnancy. J Soc Gynecol Investig 2004; 11:438-48.

Del Bene R, et al. Cardiovascular function in pregnancy: Effects of posture. Br J Obstet Gynaecol 2001;108:344.

Desai DK, et al. Echocardiographic assessment of cardiovascular hemodynamics in normal pregnancy. Obstet Gynecol 2004; 104(1):20.

Domali E, Messinis IE. Leptin in pregnancy. J Matern Fetal Neonatal Med 2002;12:222.

Figure 7–8. Components of weight gain during pregnancy. (Reproduced, with permission, from Hytten FE, Leitch I: *The Physiology of Human Pregnancy.* Blackwell, 1964.)

Granger JP. Maternal and fetal adaptations during pregnancy: Lessons in regulatory and integrative physiology. Am J Physiol Regul Integr Comp Physiol 2002;283:Rl289.

Graves CR. Acute pulmonary complications during pregnancy. Clin Obstet Gynecol 2002;45:369.

Harirah HM, et al. Effect of gestational age and position on peak expiratory flow rate: A longitudinal study. Obstet Gynecol 2005;105(2):372.

Jankowski M, et al. Pregnancy alters nitric oxide synthase and natriuretic peptide systems in the rat left ventricle. J Endocrinol 2005;184:209.

Jensen D, et al. Effects of human pregnancy on the ventilatory chemoreflex response to carbon dioxide. Am J Physiol Regul Integr Comp Physiol 2005;288:R1369.

Kametas NA, et al. Maternal cardiac function in twin pregnancy. Obstet Gynecol 2003;102:806.

Karabulut N, et al. Renal vein Doppler ultrasound of maternal kidneys in normal second and third trimester pregnancy. Br J Radiol 2003;76:444.

Lindheimer MD. Polyuria and pregnancy: Its cause, its danger. Obstet Gynecol 2005;105:1171.

Poppas A, et al. Serial assessment of the cardiovascular system in normal pregnancy. Role of arterial compliance and pulsatile arterial load. Circulation 1997;95:2407.

Puskar D, et al. Symptomatic physiologic hydronephrosis in pregnancy: Incidence, complications and treatment. Eur Urol 2001;39:260.

Spaanderman ME, et al. Cardiac output increases independently of basal metabolic rate in early human pregnancy. Am J Physiol Heart Circ Physiol 2000;278:H1585.

Stachenfeld NS, et al. Progesterone increases plasma volume independent of estradiol. J Appl Physiol 2005;98:1991.

Stein AD, et al. Measuring energy expenditure in habitually active and sedentary pregnant women. Med Sci Sports Exerc 2003;35:1441.

Tihtonen K, et al. Maternal hemodynamics during cesarean delivery assessed by whole-body impedance cardiography. Acta Obstet Gynecol Scand 2005;84:355.

Varga I, et al. Analysis of maternal circulation and renal function in physiologic pregnancies; parallel examinations of the changes in the cardiac output and the glomerular filtration rate. J Matern Fetal Med 2000;9:97.

Maternal-Placental-Fetal Unit; Fetal & Early Neonatal Physiology

8

Robert A. Knuppel, MD, MPH, MBA

Fetal genetics, physiology, anatomy, and biochemistry can now be studied with ultrasonography, fetoscopy, chorionic villus sampling, amniocentesis, and fetal cord and scalp blood sampling. Embryology and fetoplacental physiology must now be considered when providing direct patient care. Currently, some medical centers measure fetal pulse oximetry, fetal electroencephalograms, and fetal heart rate monitoring to make sure the fetus is not hypoxic or asphixic. As the technology improves, we are reaching further into the early perinatal period to determine abnormal physiology and growth.

■ THE PLACENTA

A **placenta** may be defined as any intimate apposition or fusion of fetal organs to maternal tissues for physiologic exchange. The basic parenchyma of all placentas is the **trophoblast;** when this becomes a membrane penetrated by fetal **mesoderm,** it is called the **chorion.**

In the evolution of viviparous species, the yolk sac presumably is the most archaic type of placentation, having developed from the egg-laying ancestors of mammals. In higher mammals, the **allantoic sac** fuses with the chorion, forming the chorioallantoic placenta, which has mesodermal vascular villi. When the trophoblast actually invades the maternal endometrium (which in pregnancy is largely composed of decidua), a deciduate placenta results. In humans, maternal blood comes into direct contact with the fetal trophoblast. Thus, the human placenta may be described as a discoid, deciduate, hemochorial chorioallantoic placenta.

DEVELOPMENT OF THE PLACENTA

Soon after ovulation, the endometrium develops its typical secretory pattern under the influence of progesterone from the corpus luteum. The peak of development occurs at about 1 week after ovulation, coinciding with the expected time for implantation of a fertilized ovum.

Pregnancy occurs when healthy spermatozoa in adequate numbers penetrate receptive cervical mucus, ascend through a patent uterotubal tract, and fertilize a healthy ovum within about 24 hours following ovulation. The spermatozoa that penetrate favorable mucus travel through the uterine cavity and the uterine tubes at a rate of about 6 mm/min. During this transit, an enzymatic change occurs that renders the spermatozoa capable of fertilizing the ovum. This process is called **capacitation.** The cellular union between the sperm and the egg is referred to as **syngamy.** The tip of the sperm head (**acrosome**) loses its cell membrane and probably releases a lytic enzyme that facilitates penetration of the zona pellucida surrounding the ovum. Once the sperm head containing all of the paternal genetic material enters the cytoplasm of the ovum, a **zona reaction** occurs that prevents the entrance of a second sperm. The first cleavage occurs during the next 36 hours. As the conceptus continues to divide and grow, the peristaltic activity of the uterine tube slowly transports it to the uterus, a journey that requires 6–7 days. Concomitantly, a series of divisions creates a hollow ball, the **blastocyst,** which then implants within the endometrium. Most cells in the wall of the blastocyst are trophoblastic; only a few are destined to become the embryo. This evolution of our understanding of conception is critical to the success of artificial reproductive technology, the treatment of infertility, and the emergence of preimplantation genetic diagnoses as acceptable medical procedures.

Within a few hours after implantation, the trophoblast invades the endometrium and begins to produce **human chorionic gonadotropin (hCG),** which is thought to be important in converting the normal corpus luteum into the corpus luteum of pregnancy. As the cytotrophoblasts (**Langhans' cells**) divide and proliferate, they form transitional cells that are ultrastructurally more mature and a likely source of hCG. Next, these transitional cells fuse, lose their individual membranes, and form the multinucleated **syncytiotrophoblast.** Mitotic division then ceases. Thus, the syncytial layer becomes the front line of the invading fetal tissue. Maternal capillaries and venules are tapped by the invading fetal tissue to cause extravasation of maternal blood and the formation of small lakes (lacunae), the forerunners of the intervillous space. These lacunae fill with maternal blood by reflux from previously tapped veins. An occasional maternal artery then opens, and a sluggish circulation is established (hematotropic phase of the embryo).

The lacunar system is separated by trabeculae, many of which develop buds or extensions. Within these branching projections, the cytotrophoblast forms a mesenchymal core.

The proliferating trophoblast cells then branch to form secondary and tertiary villi. The **mesoblast,** or central stromal core, also formed from the original trophoblast, invades these columns to form a supportive structure within which capillaries are formed. The **embryonic body stalk** (later to become the umbilical cord) invades this stromal core to establish the fetoplacental circulation. If this last step does not occur, the embryo will die. Sensitive tests for hCG suggest that at this stage, more embryos die than live.

Where the placenta is attached, the branching villi resemble a leafy tree (the **chorion frondosum**), whereas the portion of the placenta covering the expanding conceptus is smoother (**chorion laeve**). When the latter is finally pushed against the opposite wall of the uterus, the villi atrophy, leaving the amnion and chorion to form the 2-layered sac of fetal membranes (Fig 8–1).

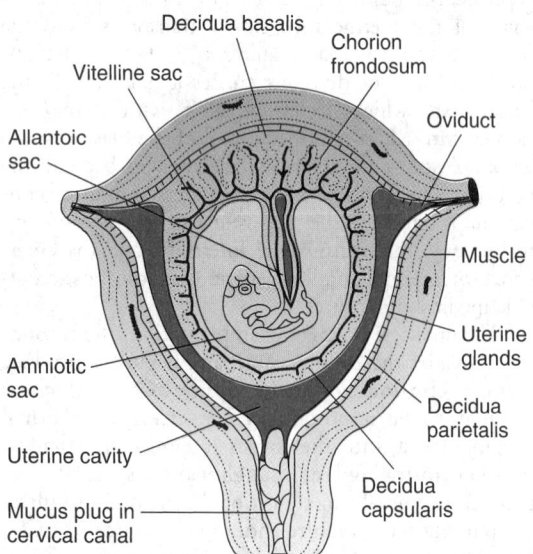

Figure 8–1. Relationships of structures in the uterus at the end of the seventh week of pregnancy. (Reproduced, with permission, from Benson RC: *Handbook of Obstetrics & Gynecology,* 8th ed. Lange, 1983.)

Around 40 days after conception, the trophoblast has invaded approximately 40–60 spiral arterioles, of which 12–15 may be called major arteries. The pulsatile arterial pressure of blood that spurts from each of these major vessels pushes the chorionic plate away from the decidua to form 12–15 "tents," or maternal **cotyledons.** The remaining 24–45 tapped arterioles form minor vascular units that become crowded between the larger units. As the chorionic plate is pushed away from the basal plate, the anchoring villi pull the maternal basal plate up into septa (columns of fibrous tissue that virtually surround the major cotyledons). Thus, at the center of each maternal vascular unit there is 1 artery that terminates in a thin-walled sac, but there are numerous maternal veins that open through the basal plate at random. The human placenta has no peripheral venous collecting system. Within each maternal vascular unit is the fetal vascular "tree," with the tertiary free-floating villi (the major area for physiologic exchange) acting as thousands of baffles that disperse the maternal bloodstream in many directions. A cross-sectional diagram of the mature placenta is shown in Fig 8–2.

Table 8–1 summarizes the major morphologic-functional correlations that take place during placental development.

FUNCTIONS OF THE MATERNAL-PLACENTAL-FETAL UNIT

The placenta is a complex organ of internal secretion, releasing numerous hormones and enzymes into the maternal bloodstream. In addition, it serves as the organ of transport for all fetal nutrients and metabolic products as well as for the exchange of oxygen and CO_2. Although fetal in origin, the placenta depends almost entirely on maternal blood for its nourishment.

The arterial pressure of maternal blood (60–70 mm Hg) causes it to pulsate toward the chorionic plate into the low-pressure (20 mm Hg) intervillous space. Venous blood in the placenta tends to flow along the basal plate and out through the venules directly into maternal veins. The pressure gradient within the fetal circulation changes slowly with the mother's posture, fetal movements, and physical stress. The pressure within the placental intervillous space is about 10 mm Hg when the pregnant woman is lying down. After a few minutes of standing, this pressure exceeds 30 mm Hg. In comparison, the fetal capillary pressure is 20–40 mm Hg.

Clinically, placental perfusion can be altered by many physiologic changes in the mother or fetus. When a precipitous fall in maternal blood pressure occurs, increased plasma volume improves placental perfusion. Increasing the maternal volume with saline infusion increases the fetal oxygen saturation. An increased rate of rhythmic uterine contractions benefits placental perfusion, but te-

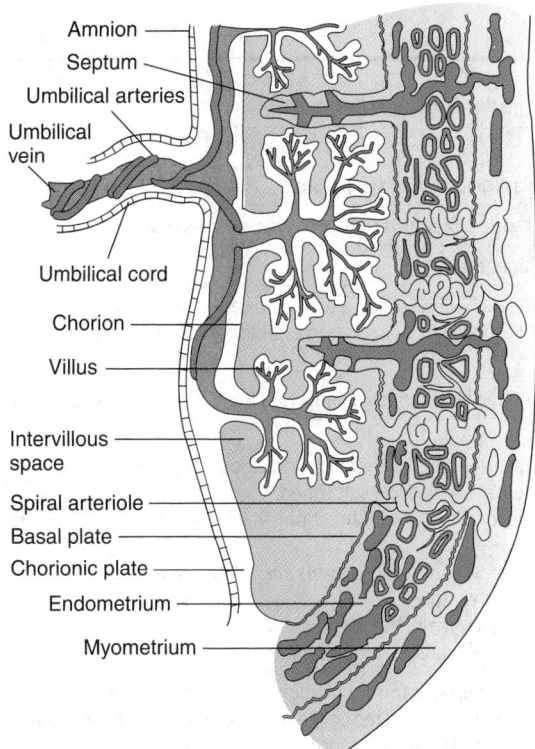

Amnion
Septum
Umbilical arteries
Umbilical vein
Umbilical cord
Chorion
Villus
Intervillous space
Spiral arteriole
Basal plate
Chorionic plate
Endometrium
Myometrium

Figure 8–2. Schematic cross section of the circulation of the mature placenta. (Reproduced, with permission, from Benson RC: *Handbook of Obstetrics & Gynecology,* 8th ed. Lange, 1983.)

tanic labor contractions are detrimental to placental and fetal circulation as they do not allow a resting period in which normal flow resumes to the fetus. An increased fetal heart rate tends to expand the villi during systole, but this is a minor aid in circulatory transfer.

Circulatory Function

A. UTEROPLACENTAL CIRCULATION

The magnitude of the uteroplacental circulation is difficult to measure in humans. The consensus is that total uterine blood flow near term is 500–700 mL/min. Not all of this blood traverses the intervillous space. It is generally assumed that about 85% of the uterine blood flow goes to the cotyledons and the rest to the myometrium and endometrium. One may assume that blood flow in the placenta is 400–500 mL/min in a patient near term who is lying quietly on her side and is not in labor.

As the placenta matures, thrombosis decreases the number of arterial openings into the basal plate. At term, the ratio of veins to arteries is 2:1 (approximately the ratio found in other mature organs).

Near their entry into the intervillous spaces, the terminal maternal arterioles lose their elastic reticulum. Because the distal portions of these vessels are lost with the placenta, bleeding from their source can be controlled only by uterine contraction. Thus, uterine atony causes postpartum hemorrhage.

B. PLASMA VOLUME EXPANSION AND SPIRAL ARTERY CHANGES

Structural alterations occur in the human uterine spiral arteries found in the decidual part of the placental bed. As a consequence of the action of cytotrophoblast on the spiral artery vessel wall, the normal musculoelastic tissue is replaced by a mixture of fibrinoid and fibrous tissue. The small spiral arteries are converted to large tortuous channels, creating low-resistance channels or arteriovenous shunts.

In dogs, when a surgically created arteriovenous shunt is opened, a marked increase in plasma volume, cardiac output, and retention of sodium soon appears. An apparent anemia occurs, as the red blood cell mass is slower to expand. The reverse happens when the shunt is closed. This situation is similar to that of early normal pregnancy, when there is an early increase in plasma volume and resulting physiologic anemia as the red blood cell mass slowly expands. Immediately after delivery, with closure of the placental shunt, diuresis and natriuresis occur. When the spiral arteries fail to undergo these physiologic changes, fetal growth retardation often occurs with preeclampsia. Campbell and colleagues (1983) and more recently Voigt and Becker (1992) used gated, pulsed Doppler ultrasound to study the uterine arcuate arteries serving the spiral arteries and placenta in pregnant women. Among the patients who showed evidence of failure of the spiral arteries to dilate and increased vascular resistance, subsequently a high frequency of proteinuric hypertension, poor fetal growth, and fetal hypoxia occurred. Voigt and Becker (1992) also noted that Doppler ultrasound profiles correlated well with the histologic findings on subsequent biopsy of the placental bed.

Fleischer and colleagues (1986) reported that normal pregnancy is associated with a uterine artery Doppler velocimetry systolic/diastolic ratio of less than 2:6. With a higher ratio and a notch in the waveform, the pregnancy is usually complicated by stillbirth, premature birth, intrauterine growth retardation, or preeclampsia.

Wells and coworkers (1984) demonstrated that decidual spiral arteries that have been attacked by the cytotrophoblast have a fibrinoid matrix that develops amniotic antigens, apparently to maintain the structural integrity of the vessel wall. Thus, there are histologic and immu-

Table 8–1. Development of the human placenta.[1]

Days After Ovulation	Important Morphologic-Functional Correlations
6–7	Implantation of blastocyst.
7–8	Trophoblast proliferation and invasion. Cytotrophoblast gives rise to syncytium.
9–11	Lacunar period. Endometrial venules and capillaries tapped. Sluggish circulation of maternal blood.
13–18	Primary and secondary villi form; body stalk and amnion form.
18–21	Tertiary villi, 2–3 mm long, 0.4 mm thick. Mesoblast invades villi, forming a core. Capillaries form in situ and tap umbilical vessels, which spread through blastoderm. Fetoplacental circulation established. Sluggish lacunar circulation.
21–40	Chorion frondosum; multiple anchored villi, which form free villi shaped like "inverted trees." Chorionic plate forms.
40–50	Cotyledon formation: (1) Cavitation. Trophoblast invasion opens 40–60 spiral arterioles. Further invasion stops. Spurts of arterial blood form localized hollows in chorion frondosum. Maternal circulation established. (2) Crowning and extension. Cavitation causes concentric orientation of anchoring villi around each arterial spurt, separating chorionic plate from basal plate. (3) Completion. Main supplying fetal vessels for groups of second-order vessels are pulled from the chorioallantoic mesenchyme to form first-order vessels of fetal cotyledons. (4) About 150 rudimentary cotyledons with anchoring villi remain, but without cavitation and crowning ("tent formation"). Sluggish, low-pressure (5–8 mm Hg) flow of maternal blood around them.
80–225	Continued growth of definitive placenta. Ten to 12 large cotyledons form, with high maternal blood pressures (40–60 mm Hg) in the central intervillous spaces; 40–50 small to medium–sized cotyledons and about 150 rudimentary ones are delineated. Basal plate pulled up between major cotyledons by anchoring villi to form septa.
225–267 (term)	Cellular proliferation ceases, but cellular hypertrophy continues.

[1]Adapted from Reynolds SRM: Formation of fetal cotyledons in the hemichorial placenta. Am J Obstet Gynecol 1966;94:425. (Reproduced, with permission, from Page EW, Villee CA, Villee DB: *Human Reproduction.* Saunders, 1976.)

nologic explanations for the presence or absence of the marked increase in uterine blood flow and plasma volume expansion seen in human pregnancies.

Goodlin and associates (1984) believed that failure of the spiral arteries to dilate and adequately expand plasma volume evokes increased maternal venous reactivity and multiple organ dysfunction. This disorder probably cannot be corrected by medical therapy, but therapy may modify secondary effects. Delivery may be the correct medical decision if the intrauterine environment is determined to be irreversibly detrimental to the fetus. The exact primary cause(s) remain unknown, thus extraction from the environment into the neonatal nursery may be justified.

C. FETOPLACENTAL CIRCULATION

At term, a normal fetus has a total umbilical blood flow of 350–400 mL/min. Thus, the maternoplacental and fetoplacental flows have a similar order of magnitude.

The villous system is best compared with an inverted tree. The branches pass obliquely downward and out-

ward within the intervillous spaces. This arrangement probably permits preferential currents or gradients of flow and undoubtedly encourages intervillous fibrin deposition, commonly seen in the mature placenta.

Cotyledons (subdivisions of the placenta) can be identified early in placentation. Although they are separated by the placental septa, some communication occurs via the subchorionic lake in the roof of the intervillous spaces.

Before labor, placental filling occurs whenever the uterus contracts (*Braxton Hicks contractions*). At these times, the maternal venous exits are closed but the thicker-walled arteries are only slightly narrowed. When the uterus relaxes, blood drains out through the maternal veins. Hence, blood is not squeezed out of the placental lake with each contraction, nor does it enter the placental lake in appreciably greater amounts during relaxation.

During the height of an average first-stage contraction, most of the cotyledons are devoid of any flow and the remainder are only partially filled. Thus, intermittently—for periods of up to a minute—maternoplacental flow virtually ceases. Therefore, it should be evident that any extended prolongation of the contractile phase, as in uterine tetany, could lead to fetal hypoxia.

Maternal Circulation

Aortocaval compression is a common cause of abnormal fetal heart rate during labor. In the third trimester, the contracting uterus obstructs its own blood supply to the level of L3–4 (**Poseiro effect**) when the mother is supine. This obstruction is completely relieved by turning the patient on her side. Although only about 30% of pregnant women will demonstrate aortocaval compression when supine, women in labor (particularly after epidural anesthesia) should not be maintained in a supine position and should be placed on their left side.

In all supine pregnant women at term, obstruction of the inferior vena cava by uterine pressure is relatively complete. However, only about 10% have inadequate collateral circulation (intervertebral venous plexus, lumbar venous plexus, abdominal wall superficial and deep veins, hemorrhoidal plates, vertebral azygous and portal system) and develop **maternal supine hypotension syndrome.** This syndrome is characterized by decreased cardiac output, bradycardia, and hypotension. Relief is obtained when the woman is placed in the lateral position. Most pregnant women near term sleep on their sides instinctively to avoid such problems.

Uterine blood flow and placental perfusion values are directly correlated with the pregnancy-related increase in maternal plasma volume. Relative maternal hypovolemia is found in association with many complications of pregnancy, including preeclampsia, small-for-gestational age (SGA) fetus, premature labor, and various fetal anomalies.

Endocrine Function

A. SECRETIONS OF THE MATERNAL-PLACENTAL-FETAL UNIT

The placenta and the maternal-placental-fetal unit produce increasing amounts of steroids late in the first trimester. Of greatest importance are the steroids required in fetal development from 7 weeks' gestation through parturition. Immediately following conception and until 12–13 weeks' gestation, the principal source of circulating gestational steroids (progesterone is the major one) is the corpus luteum of pregnancy.

After 42 days, the placenta assumes an increasingly important role in the production of several steroid hormones. Steroid production by the embryo occurs even before implantation is detectable in utero. Before implantation, production of progesterone by the embryo may assist ovum transport.

Once implantation occurs, trophoblastic hCG and other pregnancy-related peptides are secreted. A more sophisticated array of fetoplacental steroids is produced during organogenesis and with the development of a functioning hypothalamic-pituitary-adrenal axis. Adrenohypophyseal basophilic cells first appear at about 8 weeks in the development of the fetus and indicate the presence of significant quantities of adrenocorticotropic hormone (ACTH). The first adrenal primordial structures are identified at approximately 4 weeks, and the fetal adrenal cortex develops in concert with the adenohypophysis.

The fetus and the placenta acting in concert are the principal sources of steroid hormones controlling intrauterine growth, maturation of vital organs, and parturition. The fetal adrenal cortex is much larger than its adult counterpart. From midtrimester until term, the large inner mass of the fetal adrenal gland (80% of the adrenal tissue) is known as the **fetal zone.** This tissue is supported by factors unique to the fetal status and regresses rapidly after birth. The outer zone ultimately becomes the bulk of the postnatal and adult cortex.

The trophoblastic mass increases exponentially through the seventh week, after which time the growth velocity gradually increases to an asymptote close to term. The fetal zone and placenta exchange steroid precursors to make possible the full complement of fetoplacental steroids. Formation and regulation of steroid hormones also take place within the fetus itself.

In addition to the steroids, another group of placental hormones unique to pregnancy are the polypeptide hormones, each of which has an analogue in the pituitary. These placental protein hormones include hCG and human chorionic somatomammotropin. The existence of placental human chorionic corticotropin also has been suggested.

A summary of the hormones produced by the maternal-placental-fetal unit is shown in Table 8–2.

B. PLACENTAL SECRETIONS

1. Human chorionic gonadotropin—hCG was the first of the placental protein hormones to be described. Its molecular weight is 36,000–40,000 Da. It is a glycoprotein that has biologic and immunologic similarities to the luteinizing hormone (LH) from the pituitary. Recent evidence suggests that hCG is produced by the syncytiotrophoblast of the placenta. hCG is elaborated by all types of trophoblastic tissue, including that of hydatidiform moles, chorioadenoma destruens, and choriocarcinoma. As with all glycoprotein hormones (LH, follicle-stimulating hormone [FSH], thyroid-stimulating hormone [TSH]), hCG is composed of 2 subunits, alpha and beta. The alpha subunit is common to all glycoproteins, and the beta subunit confers unique specificity to the hormone. Typically,

Table 8–2. Summary of maternal-placental-fetal endocrine-paracrine functions.

Peptides of exclusively placental origin
    Human chorionic gonadotropin (hCG)
    Human chorionic somatomammotropin (hCS)
    Human chorionic corticotropin (hCC)
    Pregnancy-associated plasma proteins (PAPP)
        PAPP-A
        PAPP-B
        PAPP-C
        PAPP-D (hCS)
    Pregnancy-associated β_1 macroglobulin (β_1 PAM)
    Pregnancy-associated α_2 macroglobulin (α_2 PAM)
    Pregnancy-associated major basic protein (pMBP)
    Placental proteins (PP) 1 through 21
    Placental membrane proteins (MP) 1 through 7.
        MP1 also known as placental alkaline phosphatase
        (PLAP)
    Hypothalamic-like hormone (β-endorphin, ACTH-like)
Steroid of mainly placental origin
    Progesterone
Hormones of maternal-placental-fetal origin
    Estrone
    Estradiol 50% from maternal androgens
Hormone of placental-fetal origin
    Estriol
Hormone of corpus luteum of pregnancy
    Relaxin
Fetal hormones
    Thyroid hormone
    Fetal adrenal zone hormones
    α-Melanocyte-stimulating hormone
    Corticotropin intermediate lobe peptide (CLIP)
    Anterior pituitary hormone
    Adrenocorticotropic hormone (ACTH)
    Tropic hormones for fetal zone of placenta
    β-Endorphin
    β-Lipotropin

neither subunit is active by itself; only the intact molecule exerts hormonal effects.

Antibodies have been developed to the beta subunit of hCG. This specific reaction allows for differentiation of hCG from pituitary LH. hCG is detectable 9 days after the midcycle LH peak, which occurs 8 days after ovulation and only 1 day after implantation. This measurement is useful because it can detect pregnancy in all patients on day 11 after fertilization. Concentrations of hCG rise exponentially until 9–10 weeks' gestation, with a doubling time of 1.3–2 days.

Concentrations peak at 60–90 days' gestation. Afterward, hCG levels decrease to a plateau that is maintained until delivery. The half-life of hCG is approximately 32–37 hours, in contrast to that of most protein and steroid hormones, which have half-lives measured in minutes. Structural characteristics of the hCG molecule allow it to interact with the human TSH receptor in activation of the membrane adenylate cyclase that regulates thyroid cell function. The finding of hCG-specific adenylate stimulation in the placenta may mean that hCG provides "order regulation" within the cell of the trophoblast.

2. Human chorionic somatomammotropin—Human chorionic somatomammotropin (hCS) is a protein hormone with immunologic and biologic similarities to the pituitary growth hormone. It has also been designated **human placental lactogen (hPL)** and is synthesized in the syncytiotrophoblastic layer of the placenta. It can be found in maternal serum and urine in both normal and molar pregnancies. However, it disappears so rapidly from serum and urine after delivery of the placenta or evacuation of the uterus that it cannot be detected in the serum after the first postpartum day. The somatotropic activity of hCS is 3%, which is less than that of human growth hormone (hGH). In vitro, hCS stimulates thymidine incorporation into DNA and enhances the action of hGH and insulin. It is present in microgram-per-milliliter quantities in early pregnancy, but its concentration increases as pregnancy progresses, with peak levels reached during the last 4 weeks. Prolonged fasting at midgestation and insulin-induced hypoglycemia are reported to raise hCS concentrations. Amniotic instillation of prostaglandin PGF_2 causes a marked reduction in hCS levels. hCS may exert its major metabolic effect on the mother to ensure that the nutritional demands of the fetus are met.

It has been suggested that hCS is the "growth hormone" of pregnancy. The in vivo effects of hCS owing to its growth hormonelike and anti-insulin characteristics result in impaired glucose uptake and stimulation of free fatty acid release, with resultant decrease in insulin effect. The maternal metabolism appears to be directed toward mobilization of maternal sources to furnish substrate for the fetus.

3. Human chorionic corticotropin—Human chorionic corticotropin (hCC) is another pituitary-like hormone. The physiologic role of hCC and its regulation are unknown.

4. Placental proteins—A number of proteins thought to be specific to the pregnant state have been isolated. The most commonly known are the 4 pregnancy-associated plasma proteins (PAPPs) designated as PAPP-A, PAPP-B, PAPP-C, and PAPP-D. PAPP-D is the hormone hCS (described earlier). All these proteins are produced by the placenta and/or decidua. The physiologic role of these proteins, except for PAPP-D, are at present unclear. Numerous investigators have postulated various functions ranging from facilitating fetal "allograft" survival and the regulation of coagulation and complement cascades to the maintenance of the placenta and the regulation of carbohydrate metabolism in pregnancy. A host of other pregnancy-specific and pregnancy-associated proteins have since been isolated. The greatest challenge, however, lies in the identification of their function. Such knowledge will provide important insights into placental function and hopefully allow us to understand more completely the pregnant state.

C. Fetoplacental Secretions

The placenta may be an incomplete steroid-producing organ that must rely on precursors reaching it from the fetal and maternal circulations (an integrated maternal-placental-fetal unit). The adult steroid-producing glands can form progestins, androgens, and estrogens, but this is not true of the placenta. Estrogen production by the placenta is dependent on precursors reaching it from both the fetal and maternal compartments. Placental progesterone formation is accomplished in large part from circulating maternal cholesterol.

In the placenta, cholesterol is converted to pregnenolone and then rapidly and efficiently to progesterone. Production of progesterone approximates 250 mg/d by the end of pregnancy, at which time circulating levels are on the order of 130 mg/mL. To form estrogens, the placenta, which has an active aromatizing capacity, uses circulating androgens obtained primarily from the fetus but also from the mother. The major androgenic precursor is **dehydroepiandrosterone sulfate (DHEA-S)**. This compound comes from the fetal adrenal gland. Because the placenta has an abundance of sulfatase (sulfate-cleaving) enzyme, DHEA-S is converted to free unconjugated DHEA when it reaches the placenta, then to androstenedione, testosterone, and finally estrone and 17β-estradiol.

The major estrogen formed in pregnancy is estriol. Ninety percent of the estrogen in the urine of pregnant women is estriol. It is excreted into the urine as sulfate and glucuronide conjugates. Excretion rates increase with advancing gestation, ranging from approximately 2 mg/24 h at 16 weeks to 35–40 mg/24 h at term. Estriol is formed during pregnancy by a unique biosynthetic process that demonstrates the interdependence of the fetus, placenta, and mother. DHEA-S is quantitatively the major steroid produced by the fetal adrenal gland, with most of it being produced in the fetal zone. When DHEA-S of the fetus or mother reaches the placenta, estrone and estradiol are formed. However, little of either is converted to estriol by the placenta; instead, some of the DHEA-S undergoes 16α-hydroxylation, primarily in the fetal liver. When the 16-hydroxydehydroepiandrosterone sulfate (16-OHDHEA-S) reaches the placenta, the placental sulfatase enzyme acts to cleave the sulfate side chain, and the unconjugated 16-OHDHEA-S is aromatized to form estriol. The estriol is then secreted into the maternal circulation. When it reaches the maternal liver, it is conjugated to estriol sulfate and estriol glucosiduronate in a mixed conjugate. These forms are excreted into the maternal urine.

Circulating progesterone and estriol are thought to be important during pregnancy because they are present in such large amounts. Progesterone may play a role in maintaining the myometrium in a state of relative quiescence during much of pregnancy. A high local (intrauterine) concentration of progesterone may block cellular immune responses to foreign antigens. Progesterone appears to be essential for maintaining pregnancy in almost all mammals examined. This suggests that progesterone may be instrumental in conferring immunologic privilege to the uterus.

The functional role of estriol in pregnancy is the subject of wide speculation. It appears to be effective in increasing uteroplacental blood flow, as it has a relatively weak estrogenic effect on other organ systems. Indeed, estrogens may exert their effect on blood flow via prostaglandin stimulation.

Placental Transport

The placenta has a high rate of metabolism, with consumption of oxygen and glucose occurring at a faster rate than in the fetus. Presumably, this high metabolism requirement is caused by multiple transport and biosynthesis activities.

The primary function of the placenta is the transport of oxygen and nutrients to the fetus and the reverse transfer of CO_2, urea, and other catabolites back to the mother. In general, those compounds that are essential for the minute-by-minute homeostasis of the fetus (eg, oxygen, CO_2, water, sodium) are transported very rapidly by diffusion. Compounds required for the synthesis of new tissues (eg, amino acids, enzyme cofactors such as vitamins) are transported by an active process. Substances such as certain maternal hormones, which may modify fetal growth and are at the upper limits of admissible molecular size, may diffuse very slowly, whereas proteins such as IgG immunoglobulins probably reach the fetus by the process of pinocytosis. This transfer takes place by at least 5 mechanisms: simple diffusion, facilitated diffusion, active transport, pinocytosis, and leakage.

A. Mechanisms of Transport

1. Simple diffusion—Simple diffusion is the method by which gases and other simple molecules cross the placenta. The rate of transport depends on the chemical gradient, the diffusion constant of the compound in question, and the total area of the placenta available for transfer (Fick's law). The chemical gradient (ie, the differences in concentration in fetal and maternal plasma) is in turn affected by the rates of flow of uteroplacental and umbilical blood. Simple diffusion is also the method of transfer for exogenous compounds such as drugs.

2. Facilitated diffusion—The prime example of a substance transported by facilitated diffusion is glucose, the major source of energy for the fetus. The transfer of glucose from mother to fetus occurs more rapidly than can be accounted for by Fick's equation. Presumably, a carrier system operates *with* the chemical gradient (as opposed to active transport, which operates *against* the gradient) and may become saturated at high glucose concentrations. In the steady state, the glucose concentration in fetal plasma is about two-thirds that of the maternal concentration, reflecting the rapid rate of fetal utilization. Substances of low molecular weight, minimal electric charge, and high lipid solubility diffuse across the placenta with ease.

3. Active transport—When compounds such as the essential amino acids and water-soluble vitamins are found in higher concentration in fetal blood than in maternal blood, and when this difference cannot be accounted for by differential protein-binding effects, the presumption is that the placenta concentrates the materials during passage by an active transport system. This has been proved in the case of selected amino acids in human subjects by observing that the natural L forms are transferred with greater rapidity than the unnatural D forms, which are simply optical isomers of identical molecular size. Thus, the selective transport of specific essential nutrients is accomplished by enzymatic mechanisms.

4. Pinocytosis—Electron microscopy has shown pseudopodial projections of the syncytiotrophoblastic layer that reach out to surround minute amounts of maternal plasma. These particles are carried across the cell virtually intact to be released on the other side, whereupon they promptly gain access to the fetal circulation. Certain other proteins (eg, foreign antigens) may be immunologically rejected. This process may work both to and from the fetus, but the selectivity of the process has not been determined. Complex proteins, small amounts of fat, some immunoglobulins, and even viruses may traverse the placenta in this way. For the passage of complex proteins, highly selective processes involving special receptors are involved. For example, maternal antibodies of the IgG class are freely transferred, whereas other antibodies are not.

5. Leakage—Gross breaks in the placental membrane may occur, allowing the passage of intact cells. Despite the fact that the hydrostatic pressure gradient is normally from fetus to mother, tagged red cells and white cells have been found to travel in either direction. Such breaks probably occur most often during labor or with placental disruption (abruptio placentae, placenta previa, or trauma), cesarean section, or intrauterine fetal death. It is at these times that fetal red cells can most often be demonstrated in the maternal circulation. This is the mechanism by which the mother may become sensitized to fetal red cell antigens such as the D (Rh) antigen.

B. PLACENTAL TRANSPORT OF DRUGS

The placental membranes are often referred to as a "barrier" to fetal transfer, but there are few substances (eg, drugs) that will not cross the membranes at all. A few compounds, such as heparin and insulin, are of sufficiently large molecular size or charge that minimal transfer occurs. This lack of transfer is almost unique among drugs. Most medications are transferred from the maternal to the fetal circulation by simple diffusion, the rate of which is determined by the respective gradients of the drugs.

These diffusion gradients are influenced in turn by a number of serum factors, including the degree of drug-protein binding (such as sex hormone binding globulin). Because serum albumin concentration is considerably lower during pregnancy, drugs that bind almost exclusively to plasma albumin (eg, warfarin, salicylates) may have relatively higher unbound concentrations and, therefore, an effectively higher placental gradient. By contrast, a compound such as carbon monoxide may attach itself so strongly to the increased total hemoglobin that there will be little left in the plasma for transport.

The placenta also acts as a lipoidal resistance factor to the transfer of water-soluble foreign organic chemicals; as a result, chemicals and drugs that are readily soluble in lipids are transferred much more easily across the placental barrier than are water-soluble drugs or molecules. Ionized drug molecules are highly water soluble and are therefore poorly transmitted across the placenta. Because ionization of chemicals depends in part on their pH-pK relationships, multiple factors determine this "simple diffusion" of drugs across the placenta. *Obviously, drug transfer is not simple, and one must assume that some amount of almost any drug will cross the placenta.*

C. PLACENTAL TRANSFER OF HEAT

The core temperature of the human fetus is only about 0.5 °C above that of the maternal colon (core temperature) and about 0.2 °C above that of the amniotic fluid. There is a further temperature gradient of approximately 0.1 °C between the amniotic fluid and the uterine wall. Given these low fetomaternal temperature gradients, it appears that virtually all fetal heat loss is from the umbilical flow through the placenta, as the thermal diffusion capacity of the placental villous surface is considerably greater than that of the fetal body surface.

ANATOMIC DISORDERS OF THE PLACENTA

Observation of structural alterations within the placenta may indicate fetal and maternal disease that otherwise might go undetected.

Twin-Twin Transfusion Syndrome

Nearly all monochorionic twin placentas show an anastomosis between the vessels of the 2 umbilical circulations. These usually involve the major branches of the arteries and veins in the placental surface. Artery-to-artery communications are by far the most common, but the less frequent venovenous anastomosis may also occur. Of great pathologic significance are deep arteriovenous communications between the 2 circulations. This occurs when there are shared lobules supplied by an umbilical arterial branch from one fetus and drained by an umbilical vein branch of the other fetus. Fortunately, one-way flow to the shared lobule may be compensated for by reverse flow through a superficial arterioarterial or venovenous anastomosis, if they coexist.

Twin-twin transfusion syndrome (TTS) is believed to arise when shared lobules causing blood flow from one twin to the other are not compensated for by the presence of superficial anastomosis or by shared lobules causing flow in the opposite direction. This syndrome occurs in 15–30% of cases of monochorial placentation and is defined, at birth, in terms of a difference in cord hemoglobin between the pair of greater than 5 g/dL. The twin receiving the transfusion is plethoric and polycythemic and may show cardiomegaly. The donor twin is pale and anemic and may have organ weights similar to those seen in the intrauterine malnutrition form of SGA. Criteria for TTS diagnosed in utero differ substantially, but the underlying mechanism is the same.

The exchange of blood flow in multiple gestations is very important, as the death of one may affect the neurologic function of the living either because the shared blood flow allows thrombi to invade the affected twin or because the surviving twin bleeds into the dead twin. Treatment of TTS in utero via fetoscopic laser ablation of the communicating vessels is now feasible.

Placental Infarction

A placental infarct is an area of ischemic necrosis of placental villi resulting from obstruction of blood flow through the spiral arteries as a result of thrombosis. The lesions have a lobular distribution. However, the spiral arteries are not true end arteries, and if there is adequate flow through the arteries supplying adjacent lobules, sufficient circulation will be maintained to prevent necrosis. Thus, ischemic necrosis of one placental lobule probably indicates not only that the spiral artery supplying the infarcted lobule is thrombosed but that flow through adjacent spiral arteries is severely impaired. Placental infarction may serve as a mechanism allowing the fetus to redistribute blood flow to those placental lobules that are adequately supplied by the maternal circulation. The infarct is usually extensive before the fetus is physiologically impaired.

Chorioangioma of the Placenta

A benign neoplasm composed of fetoplacental capillaries may occur within the placenta. It is grossly visible as a purple-red, apparently encapsulated mass, variable in size, and occasionally multicentered. Placental hemangioma, or "chorioangioma," may be linked with maternal, fetal, and neonatal complications. Many placental tumors are accompanied by hydramnios, and some have been associated with preeclampsia-eclampsia. The developing fetus may be subjected to hypoxia, resulting in low birth weight, because blood within the tumor fails to reach the placental villi (and become oxygenated). The tumor may act as an arteriovenous shunt requiring increased fetal cardiac output, with resulting cardiomegaly. Fetal hydrops may occur, as may hypoalbuminemia and a microangiopathic type of hemolytic anemia. Neonatal thrombocytopenia has been associated with disseminated intravascular coagulation secondary to the liberation of thromboplastic substances.

Amniotic Bands

Close inspection of the fetal membranes, particularly near the umbilical cord insertion, may reveal band or stringlike membrane segments that are easily lifted above the placental surface. Such amniotic bands appear to be the result of a tear in the amnion early in pregnancy. They may cause constriction of the developing limbs or other fetal parts. Amputation has been known to result. Syndactyly, clubfoot, and fusion deformities of the cranium and face may also be explained in certain instances on the basis of amniotic bands. Myometrial bands also have been found within the intrauterine cavity but do not appear to place the same amount of tension on fetal anatomy as do amniotic bands.

Amnion Nodosum

Examination of the fetal surface of the placental peripheral membranes after delivery may disclose small elevated nodules several millimeters in diameter. Microscopic examination of these nodules may reveal areas of ulceration of amniotic epithelium covered with deposits of celluloid debris probably representing vernix caseosa.

These nodules reflect severe oligohydramnios regardless of cause. They frequently occur in association with underlying congenital anomalies of the fetal genitourinary system. With this information, one is alerted to the possibility that Potter's syndrome or a variant with pulmonary hypoplasia may affect the infant.

Chronic Intrauterine Infection

Chronic intrauterine infection may have a deleterious effect on organogenesis and interfere with organ development. Infections such as toxoplasmosis, rubella, cytomegalovirus, herpes, and syphilis are seen most frequently. Only in the past 2 decades has chronic inflammation within placental villi been recognized and linked with intrauterine infection. Such inflammatory foci have an incidence of approximately 20% in referral institutions. Usually, no causative organism is found, and the term **chronic villitis of unknown etiology** is used. This is an inflammatory lesion that focuses on placental villi. It has a significant correlation with unexplained stillbirth and a considerable association with fetal morbidity and SGA newborns. An increased risk of recurrence with associated adverse pregnancy outcome is suggested.

The placenta should be sent to the pathology laboratory for examination in the following cases: (1) perinatal death; (2) malformation, edema, or anemia; (3) extremes of amniotic fluid volume; (4) extreme SGA; (5) unexpected severe birth asphyxia; (6) preterm birth; (7) multiple gestation; (8) abnormal placenta; and (9) perinatal infection.

Placental Pathology

Any infant born with a complication may benefit from histologic evaluation of the placenta and umbilical cord. Histopathologic features of a placenta with uteroplacental insufficiency include nonmarginal infarcts, shrunken placental villi, increased syncytial knots, increased perivillous fibrin, and multifocal and diffuse fibrin deposition. Similarly, if the ratio of nucleated red blood cells to leukocytes exceeds 2:3, this indicates fetal hypoxic stress. Chorangiosis is a pathologic change that indicates long-standing placental hypoperfusion or low-grade tissue hypoxia.

The presence of meconium and its location can also give insight into the possible time of the presumed insult. Under gross observation, meconium will stain the placenta and cord after just 3 hours of exposure. Stained infant fingernails indicate meconium exposure for at least 6 hours. Stained vernix equates with exposure of meconium for 15 hours or longer.

Microscopic evaluation also sheds light on the timing of the release of meconium. Meconium-laden macrophages at the chorionic surface of the placenta can be seen when meconium has been present for 2–3 hours. When these macrophages are found deep within the extraplacental membranes, meconium has been present for at least 6–12 hours.

Lastly, when evaluation of the umbilical cord demonstrates necrobiotic and necrotic arterial media with surrounding meconium-laden macrophages, the release of meconium occurred more than 48 hours before delivery.

Abnormalities of Placental Implantation

Normally the placenta selects a location on the endometrium that benefits the growing fetus. However, there are numerous instances when the placental implantation site is not beneficial.

Placenta previa, or the implantation of the placenta over the cervical os, is the most common. The incidence at 12 weeks' gestation is about 6% because of the advancement of transvaginal imaging (Taipale et al., 1997). Fortunately, most cases of placenta previa resolve by the time of delivery (reported incidence of 5/1,000 births in Ananth et al., 2001). A marginal placenta previa occurs when the edge of the placenta lies within 2–3 cm of the cervical os; the prevalence ranges from 10–45% when the less accurate abdominal ultrasonogram is used.

Associated consequences of these abnormal placentation sites include increased risk for bleeding, both for the mother and the fetus; increased need for cesarean delivery; and possible risk of placenta accreta and increta or percreta, abruption, and growth restriction. Once the placental edge moves beyond 2–3 cm from the cervical os, these risks are minimized.

Placenta accreta is the most dangerous consequence of placenta previa. It involves abnormal trophoblastic invasion beyond the Nitabuch's layer. Placenta increta is the term used to describe invasion into the myometrium. Placenta percreta describes invasion through the serosa with possible invasion into surrounding tissues such as the bladder. Placenta accreta is associated with life-threatening postpartum hemorrhage and increased need for immediate hysterectomy.

The risk factors for placenta previa and placenta accreta are similar. Advanced maternal age, increased parity, and prior uterine surgery are common risk factors for both entities. The strongest correlation appears to exist with prior uterine surgeries. The prevalence of placenta previa after one prior cesarean delivery reaches 0.65% versus 0.26% in the unscarred uterus. However, after 4 or more cesarean deliveries the prevalence reaches 10%. Similarly, the frequency of accreta in the presence of placenta previa increases as the number of uterine surgeries increases. In patients with one prior uterine surgery, accreta occurs in 24% of placenta previas, whereas after 4 or more surgeries the frequency of placenta accreta may be as high as 67%.

Placenta accreta may be suspected with certain ultrasound findings such as loss of the hypoechoic retroplacental myometrial zone, thinning or disruption of the hyperechoic uterine serosa-bladder interface or with visualization of an exophytic mass. In all cases of placenta previa, and especially if placenta accreta is suspected, the patient must be counseled that hysterectomy may be needed to control excessive bleeding after delivery. Blood products must be available before delivery of the infant to ensure prompt replacement.

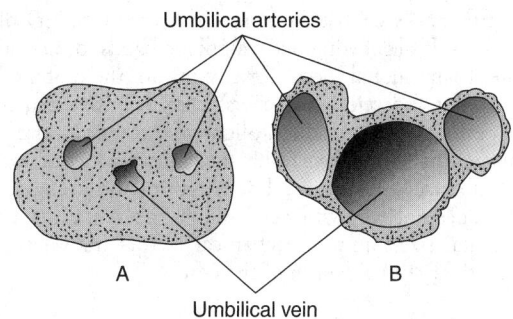

Figure 8–3. Drawings of cross-sections of umbilical cord (**A**) after blood vessels are empty and (**B**) while they are filled, as in utero. The central vein and 2 arteries occupy most of the space. (Based on photography by SRM Reynolds.)

■ THE UMBILICAL CORD

Development

In the early stages, the embryo has a thick embryonic stalk containing 2 umbilical arteries, 1 large umbilical vein, the allantois, and the primary mesoderm. The arteries carry blood from the embryo to the chorionic villi, and the umbilical vein returns blood to the embryo. The umbilical vein and 2 arteries twist around one another.

In the fifth week of gestation, the amnion expands to fill the entire extraembryonic coelom. This process forces the yolk sac against the embryonic stalk and covers the entire contents with a tube of amniotic ectoderm, forming the umbilical cord. The cord is narrower in diameter than the embryonic stalk and rapidly increases in length. The connective tissue of the umbilical cord is called **Wharton's jelly** and is derived from the primary mesoderm. The umbilical cord can be found in loops around the baby's neck in approximately 23% of normal spontaneous vertex deliveries.

At birth, the mature cord is about 50–60 cm in length and 12 mm in diameter. A long cord is defined as more than 100 cm, and a short cord as less than 30 cm. There may be as many as 40 spiral twists in the cord, as well as false knots and true knots. When umbilical blood flow is interrupted at birth, the intra-abdominal sections of the umbilical arteries and vein gradually become fibrous cords. The course of the umbilical vein is discernible in the adult as a fibrous cord from the umbilicus to the liver (ligamentum teres) contained within the falciform ligament. The umbilical arteries are retained proximally as the internal iliac arteries and give off the superior vesicle arteries and the medial umbilical ligaments within the medial umbilical folds to the umbilicus. When the umbilical cord is cut and the end examined at the time of delivery, the vessels ordinarily are collapsed (Fig 8–3A), but if a segment of cord is fixed while the vessels are distended, the characteristic appearance is as shown in Fig 8–3B.

Analysis of the Umbilical Cord in Fetal Abnormalities

A segment of umbilical cord should be kept available as a source of umbilical cord blood for blood gas measurements at the time of delivery. Cord blood gases are a more objective measure of oxygenation than Apgar scores, especially in dark-skinned babies.

The umbilical cord has recently become a means of evaluating the fetus in utero. Umbilical cord sampling under ultrasonographic guidance has opened new vistas in perinatal physiology, teratology, genetics, and therapeutic endeavors to correct Rh isoimmunization.

ABNORMALITIES OF THE UMBILICAL CORD

Velamentous Insertion

In velamentous insertion, the umbilical vessels divide to course through the membranes before reaching the chorionic plate. Velamentous insertion occurs in about 1% of placentas. When these vessels present themselves ahead of the fetus (vasa previa), they may rupture during labor or before to cause fetal exsanguination. When painless vaginal bleeding occurs, the blood may be tested to determine if it is of fetal origin (Apt test). In practical terms, a high index of suspicion for vasa previa is needed because the time to fetal collapse with bleeding from vasa previa is often too rapid to allow test interpretation.

Short Umbilical Cord

It appears from indirect evidence in the human fetus that the length of the umbilical cord at term is determined by the amount of amniotic fluid present during the first and second trimesters and by the mobility of the fetus. If oligohydramnios, amniotic bands, or limitation of fetal motion occur for any reason, the umbilical cord will not develop to an average length. Amniocentesis performed to produce oligohydramnios in pregnant rats at 14–16 days results in significant reduction of umbilical cord length. The length of the umbilical cord does not vary with fetal weight, presentation, or placental size. Simple mechanical factors may determine the eventual length of the cord.

Knots in the Umbilical Cord

True knots occur in the cord in 1% of deliveries, leading to a perinatal loss of 6.1% in such cases. False knots are developmental variations with no clinical importance.

Loops of the Umbilical Cord

Twisting of the cord about the fetus may be the reason for excessive cord length. One loop of cord is present about the neck in 21% of deliveries, 2 loops in 2.5%, and 3 loops in 0.2%. When 3 loops are present, the cord is usually longer than 70 cm. One study of 1000 consecutive deliveries found 1 or more loops of cord around the neck in approximately 24% of cases. Single or multiple loops of umbilical cord around the neck caused no fetal morbidity or mortality in that series, but Naeye's report (1987) illustrates that cord entanglement may be an important cause of stillbirth.

Torsion of the Umbilical Cord

Torsion of the cord occurs counterclockwise in most cases. If twisting is extreme, fetal asphyxia may result.

Single Artery

A 2-vessel cord (absence of one umbilical artery) occurs about once in 500 deliveries (6% of twins). The cause may be aplasia or atrophy of the missing vessel. The anomaly is more common in blacks than whites but equally frequent in primiparas and multiparas. In older studies, about 30% of these infants were found to have structural defects. Because many associated anomalies are detected on ultrasound antenatally, the main clinical question at present is the association of the apparently isolated single umbilical artery (SUA) and fetal anomalies. In this setting the risk of anomalies is much lower, but the finding should still prompt a careful search. There is also a strong association between fetal structural anomalies and placental vascular occlusion or thrombosis. Perinatal examination for such vascular defects should be routine.

■ THE FETUS

The human fetus is born about 40 weeks after the first day of the last menstrual period (LMP). The **gestational age** is measured from the first day of the LMP, although obviously conception can not occur until 2 weeks after the beginning of this calculation. The 9.5 calendar months are divided into trimesters for convenient classification of certain obstetric events. The term fetus is born 9.5 lunar cycles (29.53 days each) after conception, and the postconceptional age in weeks is used to denote the stage of development of the embryo.

Because of the error in estimating the date of conception from the LMP, early ultrasound using the crown rump length measurement is widely used in clinical practice to correct and confirm the gestational age.

GROWTH & DEVELOPMENT

During the first 8 weeks, the term **embryo** is used to denote the developing organism because it is during this time that all the major organs are formed (Table 8–3). After the eighth week, the word **fetus** is proper; this is a period when further growth and organ maturation occur. The loss of a fetus weighing less than 500 g (about 22 weeks' gestational age) is called a **spontaneous abortion.** A fetus weighing 500–1000 g (22–28 weeks) is called **immature.** From 28–36 weeks, it is referred to as **premature.** A **term fetus** is arbitrarily defined as one that has attained 37 weeks' gestational age. An alternative means of describing the premature fetus is widely used in clinical practice: 500–750 g, extremely low birth weight; 750–1500 g, very low birth weight; 1500–2500, low birth weight. The growth of the fetus may be conveniently described in units of 4 weeks' gestational age, beginning with the first day of the LMP:

8 weeks: The embryo is 2.1–2.5 cm long and weighs 1 g, and the head makes up almost half the bulk. The hepatic lobes may be recognized. Red blood cells are forming in the yolk sac and liver and contain hemoglobin. The kidneys are beginning to form.

16 weeks: The length is 14–17 cm and the weight about 100 g. The sex is discernible. Hemoglobin F is present, and formation of hemoglobin A begins.

20 weeks: The weight is about 300 g. Movements may have been perceived by the mother for 2–3 weeks. The uterine fundus is near the level of the umbilicus.

24 weeks: The weight is 600 g. Some fat is beginning to be deposited beneath the wrinkled skin. Viability is reached by the 24th week with approximately 50% survival.

28 weeks: The weight is about 1050 g and the length

about 37 cm. The lungs are now capable of breathing, but the surfactant content is low; survival is 90%.

32 weeks: The weight is about 1700 g and the length about 42 cm. If born at this stage, 99% of infants survive.

36 weeks: The weight is about 2500 g and the length about 47 cm. The skin has lost its wrinkled appearance.

40 weeks: The term fetus averages 50 cm in length and 3200–3500 g in weight. The head has a maximal transverse (biparietal) diameter of 9.5 cm, and when the neck is well flexed, the diameter from the brow to a point beneath the occiput (suboccipitobregmatic) is also 9.5 cm. The average fetus, therefore, requires cervical dilatation of almost 10 cm before it can descend into the vagina.

FETAL & EARLY NEONATAL PHYSIOLOGY

During the past 2 decades, improved neonatal care has led to increased survival rates for very low–birth-weight infants, even those as young as 23–24 weeks. Obviously, an understanding of fetal and early neonatal physiology is critical in the appropriate management of these babies.

Hematology

The fetal circulation is established at about 25 postconceptional days. At that time, the major sources of red blood cells are blood islands in the body stalk. By 10 weeks, the liver assumes the major role in erythropoiesis, but the spleen and bone marrow gradually take over this function. At term, the bone marrow is the source of at least 90% of the red cells. The hormone erythropoietin is produced in considerable quantities by 32 weeks, but levels fall almost to zero during the first week after birth, unless the infant is anemic, in which case the values are higher.

Erythrocytes are the first blood cells produced by the fetus and have a life span of 120 days. The earliest erythrocytes are megaloblastic and circulate as nucleated cells. Mean red cell values change as the fetus grows (Table 8–4).

After the first week of life, erythrocyte concentrations begin to decline gradually, reaching zero by 6–12 weeks after birth. The hemoglobin concentration decreases to about 10 g/dL and by term to as low as 7–8 g/dL (**physiologic anemia of the newborn**).

The synthesis of **hemoglobin** occurs in the proerythroblast, normoblast, and reticulocyte, but not in the mature red blood cell. Types of fetal hemoglobin present before 12 weeks are Gower I and II and Portland I. There are at least 7 types of hemoglobin chains. The synthesis of each chain is under the genetic control of a separate structural gene locus. The complete amino acid sequences of the 7 normal globin

Figure 8–4. Hemoglobin chains.

chains have been determined. A functional hemoglobin molecule is a tetramer composed of 4 globin chains and 4 heme groups. From the eighth week of gestation to term, **hemoglobin F** is the major hemoglobin in the fetus, but a small amount of hemoglobin A can also be detected. The ratio of beta to gamma synthesis remains approximately 1:10 during this period and until term (Fig 8–4). Around the time of birth, the ratio changes because of the gradually decreased synthesis of gamma chains and increased synthesis of beta chains (Table 8–5).

Fortuitously, blood in the fetus has a 50% higher hemoglobin concentration than in the adult and a greater oxygen affinity than maternal blood. Even though fetal oxygen tension is less, fetal blood carries an amount of oxygen comparable to that in maternal blood. The resistance of hemoglobin F to acid digestion makes it possible to demonstrate hemoglobin F–containing cells in the maternal circulation (**Kleihauer-Betke test**).

The higher affinity of hemoglobin F for oxygen is accentuated by **2,3-diphosphoglycerate** (**2,3-DPG**), which is present in adult red cells. Fetal and maternal blood have different oxygen saturation curves, mostly because 2, 3-DPG competes with oxygen for binding sites on adult cells.

Immunology

There are 3 basic types of leukocytes found in the blood: **granulocytes, monocytes,** and **lymphocytes.** The granular acidic leukocytes are subdivided into 3 types, based on the sustaining characteristics of the acidic plasma granules and their function—eosinophilic, basophilic, and neutrophilic granulocytes. A functional difference also exists among the lymphocytes, which are divided into 2 broad groups designated as **T cells** and **B cells.** The functions of monocytes vary greatly during maturation or with environmental influences; thus, it is not currently possible to divide them into distinct subgroups. Although all these cells are gen-

Table 8–3. Embryonic and fetal growth and development.

Fertilization Age (weeks)	Crown-Rump Length	Crown-Heel Length	Weight	Gross Appearance	Internal Development
Embryonic stage					
1	0.5 mm	0.5 mm	?	Minute clone free in uterus.	Early morula. No organ differentiation.
2	2 mm	2 mm	?	Ovoid vesicle superficially buried in endometrium.	External trophoblast. Flat embryonic disk forming 2 inner vesicles (amnio-ectomesodermal and endodermal).
3	3 mm	3 mm	?	Early dorsal concavity changes to convexity; head, tail folds form; neural grooves close partially.	Optic vesicles appear. Double heart recognized. Fourteen mesodermal somites present.
4	4 mm	4 mm	0.4 g	Head is at right angle to body; limb rudiments obvious, tail prominent.	Vitelline duct only communication between umbilical vesicle and intestines. Initial stage of most organs has begun.
8	3 cm	3.5 cm	2 g	Eyes, ears, nose, mouth recognizable; digits formed, tail almost gone.	Sensory organ development well along. Ossification beginning in occiput, mandible, and humerus (diaphysis). Small intestines coil within umbilical cord. Pleural pericardial cavities forming. Gonadal development advanced without differentiation.
Fetal stage					
12	8 cm	11.5 cm	19 g	Skin pink, delicate; resembles a human being, but head is disproportionately large.	Brain configuration roughly complete. Internal sex organs now specific. Uterus no longer bicornuate. Blood forming in marrow. Upper cervical to lower sacral arches and bodies ossify.
16	13.5 cm	19 cm	100 g	Scalp hair appears. Fetus active. Arm-leg ratio now proportionate. Sex determination possible.	External sex organs grossly formed. Myelination. Heart muscle well developed. Lobulated kidneys in final situation. Meconium in bowel. Vagina and anus open. Ischium ossified.
20	18.5 cm	22 cm	300 g	Legs lengthen appreciably. Distance from umbilicus to pubis increases.	Sternum ossifies.
24	23 cm	32 cm	600 g	Skin reddish and wrinkled. Slight subcuticular fat. Vernix. Primitive respiratory-like movements.	Os pubis (horizontal ramus) ossifies.
28	27 cm	36 cm	1100 g	Skin less wrinkled; more fat. Nails appear. If delivered may survive with optimal care.	Testes at internal inguinal ring or below. Talus ossifies.
32	31 cm	41 cm	1800 g	Fetal weight increased proportionately more than length.	Middle fourth phalanges ossify.

(continued)

Table 8–3. Embryonic and fetal growth and development. (continued)

Fertilization Age (weeks)	Crown-Rump Length	Crown-Heel Length	Weight	Gross Appearance	Internal Development
36	34 cm	46 cm	2200 g	Skin pale, body rounded. Lanugo disappearing. Hair fuzzy or wooly. Ear lobes soft with little cartilage. Umbilicus in center of body. Testes in inguinal canals; scrotum small with few rugae. Few sole creases.	Distal femoral ossification centers present.
40	40 cm	52 cm	3200+ g	Skin smooth and pink. Copious vernix. Moderate to profuse silky hair. Lanugo hair on shoulders and upper back. Ear lobes stiffened by thick cartilage. Nasal and alar cartilages distinguishable. Nails extend over tips of digits. Testes in full, pendulous, rugous scrotum (or labia majora) well developed. Creases cover sole.	Proximal tibial ossification centers present. Cuboid, tibia (proximal epiphysis) ossify.

erally regarded as white blood cells, they should be viewed as cell types that merely use the blood as a means of transportation from sites of production to sites of function. Both the sites of production and (for the most part) sites of function are extravascular. The fetus presents with relative leukocytosis, the white count being 15,000–20,000/dL at term.

Circulating white cells constitute the first line of defense against pathogenic bacteria, as outlined in Table 8–6. Leukocytes appear in the fetal circulation after 2 months' gestation. The prothymocytes migrate from the fetal liver or bone marrow to enter the embryonic thymus at approximately 8 weeks' gestation. Soon after, the splenic anlage begins to mature. Both produce lymphocytes, a major source of the antibodies that constitute the second line of defense against harmful foreign antigens. Both antibody-mediated immunity and cell-mediated immunity depend on the activity of small lymphocytes derived from bone marrow precursors. The stem cells, which during the early embryonic stage originate in the yolk sac, in later stages of development in the liver, and in adults in the bone marrow, differentiate to form 2 distinct lymphocyte populations. One group is **thymus-derived (T lymphocytes)** and the other is **bone marrow-derived (B lymphocytes)**. T lymphocytes can be detected in the thymus after 11 weeks' gestation; they appear in the peripheral blood, spleen, and lymph nodes by 16–18 weeks, and by 30–32 weeks the fetus has a near-adult number of circulating T lymphocytes.

The life span of lymphocytes is not uniform. Recent studies suggest that B- and T-cell populations contain similar proportions of long- and short-lived lymphocytes. The T lymphocytes constitute 65–85% of the lymphocytes present in the thoracic duct, blood, and lymph nodes. The long-lived lymphocytes represent the major portion (90%) of the thoracic duct cells, whereas the short-lived lymphocytes are located mainly in the thymus, spleen, and bone marrow. The T cells are effector cells in delayed sensitivity reactions and elimination of foreign tissues. They also play an important role in the expression of some humoral immune responses. The T cells can release a variety of nonspecific chemical mediators called **lymphokines** (eg, **interferon, transfer factor, mitogenic factor, migration** and **inhibition factors**, and **cytotoxic** and **growth inhibitory factors**).

B lymphocytes originate in the bone marrow of most mammals. B cells seem to be more sessile than T cells. B cells are found primarily in the perilymphoid organs, lymph nodes, and thymic-independent areas around germinal centers. They are also present in very small amounts in the peripheral blood. They seem to be short-lived. B cells differentiate into **plasma cells,** which are ultimately responsible for the synthesis and secretion of all forms of antibody and all circulating immunoglobulins. The average life span of plasma cells is 0.5–2 days.

Immunoglobulins (Ig) are serum globulins with antibody activity as their primary property. The 5 classes of Ig have been designated IgG, IgM, IgA, IgD, and IgE. In the human newborn, plasma cells are absent from the bone marrow and the lamina propria of

Table 8–4. Mean red cell values during gestation.

Age (weeks)	Hemoglobin (g/dL)	Hematocrit (%)	Red Blood Cells (10^6/μL)	Mean Corpuscle Volume (μm³/L)
12	8–10	33	1.5	180
16	10	35	2	140
20	11	37	2.5	135
24	14	40	3.5	123
28	14.5	45	4	120
34	15	47	4.4	118

Reproduced, with permission, from Oskl FA, Naiman JL: *Hematologic Problems in the Newborn,* 3rd ed, Saunders, 1982.

the ileum and appendix. They appear only 4–6 weeks after birth. However, beginning at 20 weeks' gestation, the fetal spleen synthesizes IgG and IgM but not IgA or IgD (Fig 8–5).

IgG is normally produced only in trace amounts prenatally, with its full synthesis beginning 3–4 weeks after birth. **IgM** is also found in small amounts in the fetus, primarily in the circulation but not diffused into extravascular spaces. They are synthesized in lymphocytoid plasma cells and reticular cells of the spleen and lymph nodes. Fetal production of IgG and IgM is low, however, in comparison with adult production. The fetal spleen synthesizes relatively more IgM than IgG. IgM is the first class to appear in the circulation after initial immunization and is the predominant class produced by infants in the neonatal period. At birth, the plasma level of IgM is about 5% of the normal adult level, with most, if not all, of this antibody being of fetal origin. Within 2–5 days after birth, the rate of IgM synthesis increases rapidly. IgM, unlike IgG, does not cross the human placenta, and the half-life of IgM is 5 days.

This comparison between IgG and IgM is important in determining possible intrauterine infection. The fetal IgG serum concentration at term equals the maternal concentration because IgG crosses the placenta. IgG constitutes 90% of all serum antibodies in the fetus because of the maternal contribution. IgM is predominantly of fetal origin and, therefore, is used to determine whether fetal infection is present, but there are many false-positive and false-negative results. After birth, the IgG half-life in the newborn circulation is 3–4 weeks. IgE does not cross the placenta, and cord levels are only 10% of maternal levels.

The fetus and newborn are not as well equipped immunologically as the adult to combat infection. The primary deficiency is both cellular and humoral. T lymphocytes do not respond to specific antigens, and B lymphocytes do not develop into plasma cells. This results in IgG levels that are below maternal levels until late in the third trimester, and complement and properdin proteins, which are necessary for opsonization of bacteria, are consistently reduced.

IgA production does not begin until several weeks after birth. Because IgA is produced in response to the antigens of enteric organisms, the newborn is particularly susceptible to intestinal infections.

The response of the fetus to antigens of maternal origin depends on the level of immunologic competence achieved by the fetus. During the first trimester, for example, rubella virus elicits no response from the embryo, whose tissues are therefore subject to damage.

Endocrinology

The thyroid is the first endocrine gland to develop in the fetus. As early as the fourth postconceptional week, the thyroid can synthesize thyroxine. The **pancreas** develops early as an outgrowth of the duodenal endoderm, and as early as 12 weeks' gestation, **insulin** may be extracted from the B cells of the pancreas. Maternal insulin is not transferred to the fetus in physiologic quantities, so the fetus must supply whatever is needed for metabolizing glucose. Insulin is thus the primary hormone regulating the rate of fetal growth. The beta cells of the normal fetal pancreas respond poorly to hyperglycemia unless the stimulus is repeated many times (eg, diabetes in the mother may cause hyperplasia of fetal beta cells so that larger quantities of insulin will be produced). This may be why some infants of diabetic mothers grow to an excessive size or show evidence of hyperinsulinism immediately after birth.

All the tropic hormones synthesized by the **anterior pituitary gland** are present in the fetus, although

Mean Corpuscle Hemoglobin (pg)	Mean Corpuscle Hemoglobin Concentration (g/dL)	Nucleated Red Blood Cells (% or red blood cells)	Reticulocytes (%)	Diameter (μm)
60	34	5–8	40	10.5
45	33	2–4	10–25	9.5
44	33	1	10–20	9
38	31	1	5–10	8.8
40	31	0.5	5–10	8.7
38	32	0.2	3–10	8.5

the precise role of these protein hormones in fetal growth and metabolism is not well understood. **ACTH** plays a vital role, however, in stimulating growth of the adrenal cortex because the tropic hormones are too large for placental transfer from the mother in significant quantities.

The fetal **adrenal cortex** consists mainly of a fetal zone that disappears about 6 months after birth. The cortex is an active endocrine organ that produces large quantities of steroid hormones. There is evidence that the steadily increasing activity of the fetal zone triggers the sequence of events that leads to the initiation of labor. Atrophy of the fetal adrenal gland (as in anencephalic fetuses) may result in marked prolongation of pregnancy. The fetal adrenal cortex is larger in premature infants, when the cause of labor is unknown, than when the pregnancy is terminated by placental abruption or by elective

Table 8–5. Embryonic, fetal, and adult hemoglobin concentrations.

Hemoglobin	Globin Polypeptides	Percent in Cord Blood
Embryo		
Gower I	Zeta-2, epsilon-2	—
Gower II	Alpha-2, epsilon-2	—
Portland I	Zeta-2, gamma-2	—
Portland II	Zeta-4	—
Fetus		
Bart's	Gamma-4	< 1
Hemoglobin F	Alpha-2f, gamma-2	60–85
Adult		
Hemoglobin A	Alpha-2, beta-2	15–40
Hemoglobin A$_2$	Alpha-2, delta-2	< 1

induction of labor. The fetal adrenal gland is an important source of catecholamines, which will respond to stress placed on the fetal myocardium. There is a preferential blood flow to the fetal adrenal in acidosis, unlike the adult response to acidosis.

CIRCULATORY FUNCTION IN THE FETUS & NEWBORN

The abrupt transition from intrauterine life to independent existence necessitates circulatory adaptations in the newborn. These include diversion of blood flow through the lungs, closure of the ductus arteriosus and foramen ovale, and obliteration of the ductus venosus and umbilical vessels.

Infant circulation has 3 phases: (1) the intrauterine phase, in which the fetus depends on the placenta; (2) the transition phase, which begins immediately after delivery with the infant's first breath; and (3) the adult phase, which is normally completed during the first few months of life.

Intrauterine Phase

The umbilical vein carries oxygenated blood from the placenta to the fetus (Figs 8–6 and 8–7). In the abdomen, the vein branches and enters the liver; a small branch bypasses the liver as the ductus venosus to enter the inferior vena cava directly.

Almost all the blood from the superior vena cava is directed through the tricuspid valve into the right ventricle, which ejects into the pulmonary trunk. Most of this relatively deoxygenated blood then passes directly through the ductus arteriosus to the descending aorta and on to the placenta. Blood from the inferior vena cava, which includes the oxygenated umbilical venous blood, largely passes directly through the foramen ovale into the left atrium and left ventricle to be ejected into the ascending aorta. The left ventricle ejects about one-third of the com-

Table 8–6. Defense mechanisms against infectious pathogens.

	Humoral Defense	**Cellular Defense**
General	Complement system Properdin system	Granulocytes Monocytes Reticuloendothelial system
Immune	Immunoglobulins	Lymphocytes

bined ventricular output of the fetus. Most of the left ventricular output passes to the fetal head, whereas the right ventricle, with blood of lower oxygen content, ejects mainly into the descending aorta. The aortic oxygen saturation difference is related not only to superior and inferior vena caval flow patterns but also to flow of the umbilical venous blood as it enters the inferior vena cava. The well-oxygenated blood preferentially passes to the cerebral and coronary circulations. This system preferentially supplies better-oxygenated blood (saturation 65%) to the heart and brain, whereas the less well-oxygenated (postductal saturation 60%) blood supplies the less vital structures including the abdomen and the lower extremities. Both ventricles pump in parallel, unlike the situation in adults.

The fetal cardiovascular responses to stress represent a complex interplay between state of arousal,

changes in blood gases, hydrogen ion concentration, reflex effects initiated by chemoreceptor or baroreceptor stimulation, and hormonal levels.

Superficially, the fetal hypoxemic-asphyxial response is much like the response in an adult when diving into water—they both involve selective vasoconstriction and the baroreceptor reflex, a primitive reflex involving changes in heart rate, arterial and venous dilatation, and cardiac performance. This reflex is evoked by changes in mean blood pressure and is modified by blood gas levels. The ability of some mammals to remain submerged for long periods of time remained a mystery until it was recognized that there is a "heart-brain" preparation through selective vasoconstriction.

In diving mammals, lactic acid is washed out of hypoperfused tissues after relief of the vasoconstriction. The same process occurs with the hypoxic fetus, producing a brief period of acidemia after birth or after oxygenation. While selective vasoconstriction provides a "heart-brain" preparation, at the same time it disturbs the flow of oxygenated blood to other essential organs.

A depressed central nervous system often produces a relatively constant heart rate with lack of beat-to-beat variability. Fetal beat-to-beat variability is mediated through autonomic stimulation resulting from the push-and-pull nature of the parasympathetic systems. Such central nervous system activity reflects general

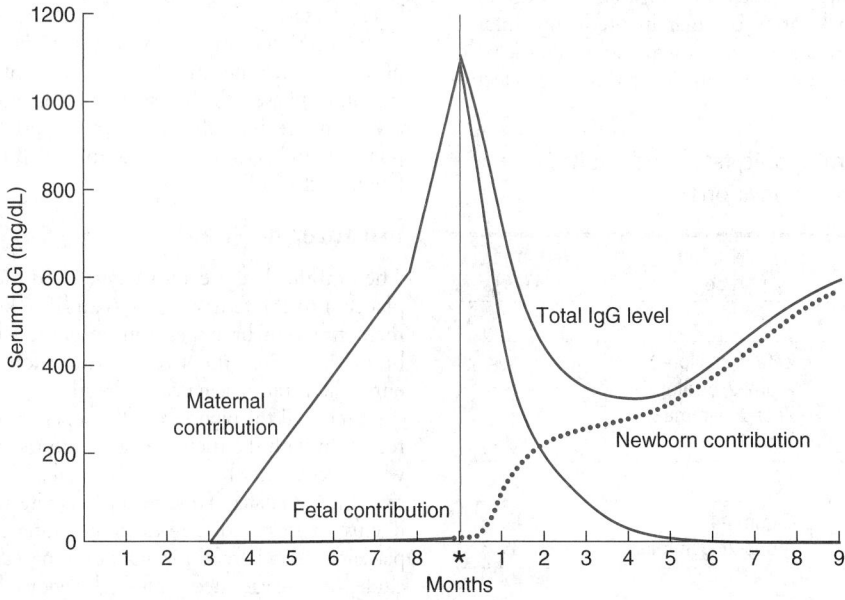

Figure 8–5. Development of IgG levels with age. Relationship of development of normal serum levels of IgG during fetal and newborn stages, and maternal contribution. (Modified from Allan-smith M et al: The development of immunoglobulin levels in man. J Pediatr 1968;72:289.)

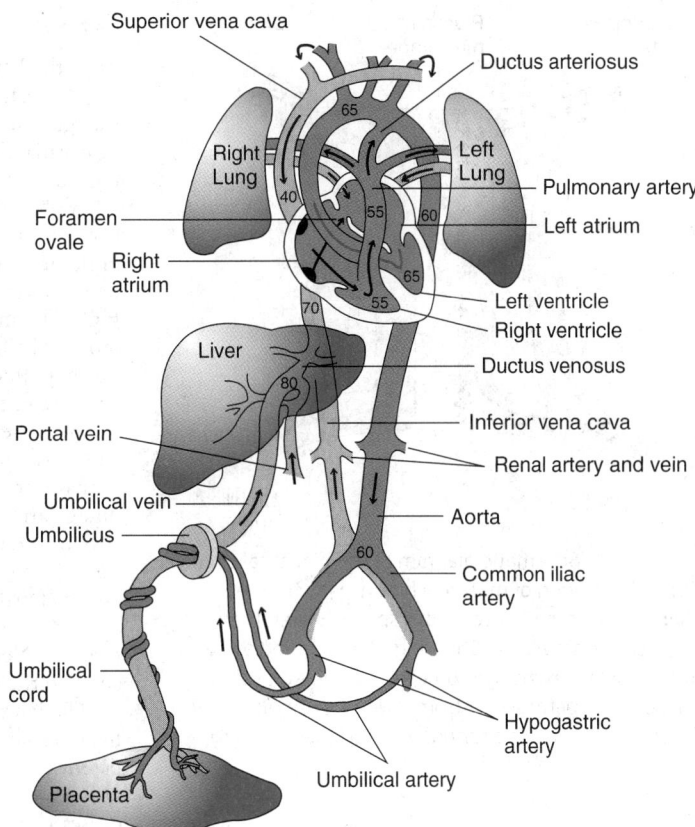

Figure 8–6. The fetal circulation. Numbers represent approximate values of the percentage of oxygen saturation of the blood in utero. (Reproduced, with permission, from Parer JT: *Handbook of Fetal Heart Rate Monitoring.* WB Saunders, 1983.)

fetal arousal levels and is decreased when the fetus is immature, asleep, drugged, or asphyxiated. Lack of fetal heart rate variability plus other signs of fetal stress can be an ominous sign. The central nervous system and cardiovascular system respond differently to hypoxia according to gestational age.

The umbilical vessels are relatively nonreactive, but the systemic and pulmonary circulations respond, when stressed, with vasoconstriction. The fetal pulmonary circulation receives a small portion (8–10%) of the fetal cardiac output, and therefore it does not play a central role in the fetal cardiovascular hypoxia response. Changes in fetal arterial pressure tend to be buffered by fetal umbilical-placental circulation. Likewise, the decrease in fetal cardiac output seen during bradycardia is modified by the redistribution of cardiac output to vital organs such as the brain, heart, placenta, and adrenal gland, so that the baroreceptor reflex may not be as effective during fetal life. The response of the fetus to hypoxia is even more complex, with chemoreceptor reflex stimulation from the aortic receptors, baroreceptor reflexes, and direct myocardial depression. Fetal tachycardia may result from

sympathetic nervous stimulation and circulating catecholamines. Because the capacity to respond to any one of these different stimuli varies with gestational age, arousal levels, general health, and the presence of drugs and hormones, there are no universal, precise fetal heart rate responses to distress.

When placental transfer of oxygen is inadequate, anaerobic glycolysis leads to the accumulation of excessive amounts of lactic acid in the fetus. There is then an associated accumulation of CO_2 and hydrogen ion (H^+), which results in decreased fetal pH. Although the maternal and fetal H^+ values maintain a relatively constant gradient, differences in the bicarbonate levels allow variation in fetal pH. Thus, determination of fetal scalp or cord blood gases can be useful in assessing fetal well-being. During fetal distress (seriously altered homeostasis), fetal blood levels of prostaglandins, catecholamines, steroids, endorphins, and pituitary hormones are often elevated (Table 8–7).

When the fetus shows signs of distress during labor, placental transfer can be improved by use of several maneuvers. First, a vaginal examination should be performed, and if prolapse of the umbilical cord has oc-

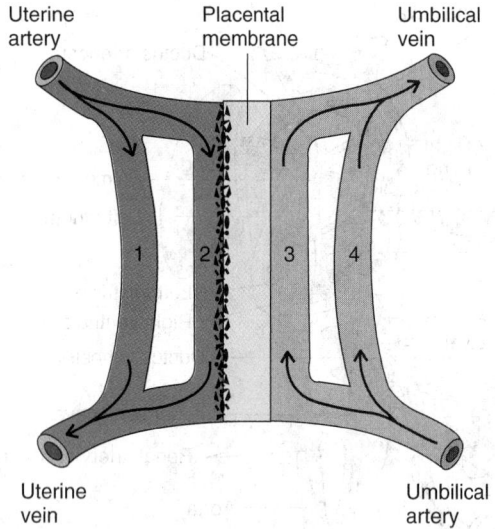

Figure 8–7. Schematic diagram of the placental circulation. (1) Shunting of maternal blood away from exchange surfaces. (2) Intervillous space. (3) Fetal capillaries of chorionic villi. (4) Shunting of fetal blood away from capillary exchange surfaces. (Modified and reproduced, with permission, from Parer JT: *Handbook of Fetal Heart Rate Monitoring.* WB Saunders, 1983.)

curred, compression of the cord should be relieved immediately by lifting the presenting fetal part off the cord. The second maneuver is to roll the mother from one side to the other to check for maternal aortocaval compression. Third, it may be helpful to administer oxygen to the mother; however, this only slightly increases the oxygen content of the uterine arterial blood because the arterial hemoglobin is already nearly saturated. Fourth, discontinuing oxytocin and possibly administering a tocolytic agent may inhibit uterine activity. The fifth maneuver is to rapidly administer 1 L of intravenous fluids to acutely expand the maternal plasma volume; a colloid solution such as 5% albumin is preferred, but a balanced salt solution is acceptable and usually more readily available.

Blood from the umbilical vein reflects uteroplacental status and is influenced by maternal and placental problems. Blood from the umbilical arteries, on the other hand, reflects uteroplacental status plus fetal status. The umbilical artery should be sampled shortly after birth with a needle inserted into the cord or one can use the placenta for both venous and arterial samples (the arteries run over the veins). Most newborns have umbilical venous and arterial blood gas samples accurately reflect the fetal status. Fetal blood samples are more accurate than Apgar scores in determining fetal status (Pomerance, 2004).

Transition Phase

At birth, 2 events occur that alter the fetal hemodynamics: (1) ligation of the umbilical cord causes an abrupt though transient rise in arterial pressure, and (2) a rise in plasma CO_2 and a fall in blood PO_2 help to initiate regular breathing.

With the first few breaths, the intrathoracic pressure of the newborn remains low (–40 to –50 mm Hg); after distention of the airways, however, the pressure rises to the normal adult level (–7 to –8 mm Hg). The initially high vascular resistance of the pulmonary bed is probably reduced by 75–80%. Pressure in the pulmonary artery falls by at least 50%, whereas pressure in the left atrium doubles.

In the fetus, the high resistance of the pulmonary bed causes most of the deoxygenated blood in the pulmonary artery to enter the descending aorta via the ductus arteriosus. At birth, expansion of the lungs occurs in the newborn, and most of the blood from the right ventricle then enters the lungs via the pulmonary artery. Furthermore, increased systemic arterial pressure reverses the flow of blood through the ductus arteriosus. Neonatal blood flows from the high-pressure aorta to the low-pressure pulmonary artery.

The increased pressure in the left atrium would normally result in backflow into the right heart through a patent foramen ovale. However, the anatomic configuration of the foramen is such that the increased pressure causes closure of the foramen by a valvelike fold situated in the wall of the left atrium.

Table 8–7. Average "normal" fetal scalp[1] and cord acid-base values.[2]

	Before Labor	Second Stage of Labor
Scalp		
pH	7.37	7.3
CO_2 pressure (mm Hg)	38	43
Bicarbonate (mmol/L)	21	21
Base excess (mmol/L)	–3	–5
	Umbilical Vein	**Umbilical Artery**
Cord		
pH	7.32	7.26
PO_2	38.9	17.7
PCO_2	37.1	40
Base deficit	6.8	6.7

[1]Population unrelated to cord sample population.
[2]Related to babies 28–43 weeks with Apgar scores greater than 7 at 1.5 minutes.

The neonatal circulation is complete with closure of the ductus arteriosus and foramen ovale, but adjustments continue for 1–2 months, until the adult phase begins.

Adult Phase

The ductus arteriosus usually is obliterated in the early postnatal period, probably by reflex action secondary to elevated oxygen tension and the interaction of prostaglandins. If the ductus remains open, a systolic crescendo murmur that diminishes during diastole (**"machinery murmur"**) is often heard over the second left interspace.

Obliteration of the foramen ovale is usually complete in 6–8 weeks, with fusion of its valve to the left interatrial septum. The foramen may remain patent in some individuals, however, with few or no symptoms. The obliterated ductus venosus from the liver to the vena cava becomes the ligamentum venosum. The occluded umbilical vein becomes the ligamentum teres of the liver.

The hemodynamics of the normal adult differ from those of the fetus in the following respects: (1) venous and arterial blood no longer mix in the atria; (2) the vena cava carries only deoxygenated blood into the right atrium, where it goes to the right ventricle and then is pumped into the pulmonary arteries and finally to the pulmonary capillary bed; and (3) the pulmonary veins deliver oxygenated blood to the left heart for distribution to the rest of the body via the aorta.

RESPIRATORY FUNCTION IN THE FETUS & NEWBORN

Gas exchange in the fetus occurs in the placenta. Transfer of gases is proportionate to the difference in partial pressure of each gas and surface area and inversely proportionate to membrane thickness. Thus, the placenta can be viewed as the fetal "lungs in utero."

Until about 12 weeks, placental permeability is low because of the small surface area of the placental "lake" and the early relative thickness of the trophoblastic membrane. From 12–32 weeks, the membrane thins and the surface area steadily increases. However, placental oxygen utilization makes accurate quantitation of oxygen transfer difficult.

The PO_2 of fetal blood is less than that of maternal blood. Although not compatible with extrauterine life, the PO_2 is adequate for the fetus, as there is a higher concentration of hemoglobin in fetal blood, much of which is hemoglobin F. Hemoglobin F has a much greater affinity for oxygen than adult hemoglobin A, resulting in greater fetal oxygen saturation. However, the enhanced ability of the fetus to deliver oxygen to the peripheral tissues seems primarily dependent on a car-

diac output that is 2.5–3 times greater than in the adult.

Both the PCO_2 and the CO_2 contents of fetal blood are slightly greater than levels in the mother's blood. As a result, CO_2 diffuses from fetus to mother for elimination.

The central and motor pathways of the fetal respiratory system are active, and respiration at birth is the culmination of in utero processes. Two main types of fetal breathing movements are recognized. One is a paradoxic irregular sequence, in which the abdominal wall moves outward as the chest wall moves inward. The other is a regular gentle movement, in which the chest and abdominal wall move outward and inward together. Fetal respiratory activity permits neuromuscular and skeletal maturation as well as development of the respiratory epithelium. As term approaches, the fetal diaphragm is usually active only during fetal rapid eye movement (REM) sleep. Without such activity, the lungs would be hypoplastic and inadequate for gas exchange. Curiously, the alveolar membrane does excrete chloride into tracheal fluid and perhaps absorbs nutrients from amniotic fluid. Consequently, it has been proposed that, like the fish gill, the fetal alveolar membrane functions as an organ of osmoregulation. In sheep, prolactin acts on both the fetal lung and amniotic membrane in facilitating sodium transport, and this may be a mechanism of control of fetal blood volume.

Hypoxia or maternal cigarette smoking reduces fetal breathing movements, whereas hyperglycemia increases fetal breathing movements. In general, these movements are governed by the same central nervous system patterns that control changes in fetal heart rate and body movements. The greatest clinical accuracy in the biophysical identification of the abnormal fetus is achieved when multiple variables are considered (eg, fetal breathing, general movements, heart rate patterns, and response to stimuli). In both sheep and humans, fetal breathing movements diminish or cease 24–36 hours before the onset of true labor. In preterm labor with intact membranes, the presence of fetal breathing movements may indicate that pregnancy will continue, while fetal apnea may indicate early delivery.

The first breath of the newborn normally occurs within the first 10 seconds after delivery. The first breath usually is a gasp, the result of central nervous system reaction to sudden pressure, temperature change, and other external stimuli. With the first breath, the slight increase in PO_2 may activate chemoreceptors to send impulses to the central nervous system respiratory center and then to the respiratory musculature. As a result, a rhythmic but rapid breathing sequence occurs, which persists into the neonatal period. The amniotic fluid usually drains from the respiratory tract or is absorbed. If meconium is present, it may be aspirated; if it is not cleared shortly after birth, it will migrate peripherally as continued respiration is established. Complete or partial obstruction of the respiratory tract or chemical pneumonitis may result.

Contrary to popular belief, the fetal lungs are not highly plastic. As development progresses, tissue elastin probably falls as the density of tissue to potential air space decreases. At the same time, liquid and future air space is enriched with phospholipid surfactants secreted by maturing type 2 saccular alveolar cells. When air breathing begins at birth, dispersion of air into the surfactant-rich liquid of the mature lungs results in formation of stable alveoli. Overall, a mature volume-pressure relationship is developed, characterized by relatively low opening pressures, high maximal volume, wide hysteresis, and retention of large volumes at end deflation or expiration.

With the onset of breathing, pulmonary vascular resistance is reduced and the capillaries fill with blood. Normally, the foramen ovale closes and pulmonary circulation is established.

Surfactant-poor lungs do not have the capacity to produce alveolar stability. As a consequence, initial aeration requires greater opening pressure, achieves a smaller maximal volume, and results in little hysteresis and gas retention during deflation. This is the underlying pathophysiologic mechanism of neonatal respiratory distress syndrome.

GASTROINTESTINAL FUNCTION IN THE FETUS & NEWBORN

The gastrointestinal tract is not truly functional until after birth, because the placenta is the organ of alimentation during fetal life. Nevertheless, when contrast medium is injected into the amniotic fluid as early as the fourth month of gestation, it may be promptly observed within the stomach and small intestine.

The full development of proteolytic activity does not develop until after birth, but the fetal gastrointestinal tract is quite capable of absorbing amino acids, glucose, and other soluble nutrients.

Meconium is produced during late pregnancy, but the amount is small. Passage of meconium in utero probably occurs with asphyxia, which increases intestinal peristalsis and relaxation of the anal sphincter. Passage of meconium is also seen in increasing frequency as the fetus reaches term and moves beyond term. Meconium is rarely seen in fetuses before 36 weeks. Between 36 and 42 weeks, meconium may be found in 25% of births. After 42 weeks meconium may be seen in 50% of all deliveries. In many circumstances, the passage of meconium may simply represent a mature gastrointestinal tract and not be an indicator of an acute hypoxic event.

Intrahepatic erythropoiesis begins during the eighth week in the embryo, and the liver is well developed histologically by midpregnancy. During fetal life, the liver acts as a storage depot for glycogen and iron. Reasonably complete liver function is not achieved until well after the neonatal period has passed. Liver deficiencies at birth are many, including reduced hepatic production of fibrinogen and coagulation factors II, VII, IX, XI, and XII.

Vitamin K stored in the liver is deficient at birth because its formation depends on bacteria in the intestine. These deficiencies predispose the newborn to hemorrhage during the first few days of life.

The formation of glucose from amino acids (gluconeogenesis) in the liver and adequate storage of glucose are not well established in the newborn. Moreover, levels of carbohydrate-regulating hormones such as cortisol, epinephrine, and glucagon may be initially insufficient. As a consequence, neonatal hypoglycemia is common after stressful stimuli such as exposure to cold or malnutrition.

Glucuronidation is limited during the early neonatal period, with the result that bilirubin is not readily conjugated for excretion as bile. After physiologic hemolysis of excess red blood cells in the first week of life or with pathologic hemolysis in isoimmunized newborns, jaundice occurs. If marked hyperbilirubinemia develops, kernicterus may ensue.

Metabolism of drugs by the liver is poor in the newborn period (eg, sulfonamides and chloramphenicol). Moreover, numerous inborn errors of metabolism (eg, galactosemia) may be diagnosed soon after birth. Neonatal liver function gradually improves, assuming proper food, freedom from infection, and a favorable environment.

Secretory and absorptive functions are accelerated after delivery. Most digestive enzymes are present, but the gastric contents are neutral at birth, although acidity soon develops. The initial neutrality may briefly delay the growth in the bowel of bacteria necessary for the formation of vitamin K in the intestine. The newborn can assimilate simple solutions and breast milk immediately after birth but cannot digest cow's milk as well until the second or third day after elimination of excessive gastric mucus. Slow progress of milk through the stomach and upper intestine is usual during the early neonatal period.

Normally, some air enters the stomach during feedings. Pocketing of air in the upper curvature of the stomach occurs when the newborn is lying flat. Hence, turning the infant and "burping" with the infant upright are necessary.

Large bowel peristalsis promptly increases after delivery, and 1–6 stools per day are passed. Absence of stool within 48 hours after birth is indicative of intestinal obstruction or imperforate anus.

RENAL FUNCTION IN THE FETUS & NEWBORN

During uterine growth and development, the placenta serves as the major regulator of fluid and electrolyte balance. The kidneys are unnecessary for fetal growth and development, as demonstrated by the rare neonate born with renal agenesis. Hence, the placenta and maternal lungs and kidneys normally maintain fetal fluid and electrolyte balance. When the connection between fetal circulation and the placenta is interrupted during delivery, the kidneys are called on to assume the homeostatic functional demands of extrauterine life.

The placenta (the major homeostatic organ) receives 40–65% of the fetal cardiac output. Renal blood flow in fetal lambs is constant when expressed per gram of renal tissue, and renal vascular resistance is maintained at a constant value. Following birth, renal blood flow increases significantly and renal vascular resistance decreases by about 25%. However, renal blood flow is low and vascular resistance high when compared with adult levels.

The high neonatal vascular resistance may be attributable to increased renal adrenergic activity in the newborn. The neonatal renal vasculature is sensitive to catecholamines, and the kidneys have a high density of high-affinity alpha-adrenoceptors. At birth, a greater percentage of blood perfuses the deeper cortical nephrons. With maturation, the rise in blood flow to the outer cortical region increases faster than the rise to the inner cortex.

The **glomerular filtration rate** (**GFR**) in fetal animals, particularly lambs, increases proportionally with growth of the kidney (GFR expressed per gram of kidney weight) and rises significantly after birth. Renal blood flow has a similar pattern. During the first 24 hours of life, measurements of the GFR reflect the status of renal function during intrauterine life; at least 24 hours are needed for the GFR to adapt to the extrauterine environment. The GFR and renal blood flow follow a similar postnatal pattern, with values more than doubling during the first 2 weeks of life. This is also true in preterm neonates, although values start at lower levels.

Preterm infants have a negative sodium balance during the first 1–3 weeks of life. The mechanism for sodium wasting in premature infants probably involves proximal and distal tubule function. Preterm infants have a lower rate of sodium resorption in the proximal tubule than term infants. Newborns also have a limited ability to excrete a salt load when compared with adults. The functional tubular immaturity of the kidney in newborns is also demonstrated by increased renal excretion of glucose and amino acids and by decreased ability to concentrate, dilute, and acidify the urine. A normal serum bicarbonate level for a preterm infant may be as low as 14–16 mmol/L, but this level increases to 21 mmol/L during the first week of life (the value is similar in term newborns). Thus, newborn infants have a limited ability to excrete an acid load as well as a lower renal threshold

for bicarbonate. Preterm infants do not concentrate urine as well as term infants. Most infants do not concentrate urine as well as adults until 6–12 months of age. Maximal urine osmolality in preterm newborns is 500–600 mOsm/kg water; in term infants, maximum osmolality is 500–700 mOsm/kg water.

Formation of urine is thought to begin at 9–12 weeks' gestation. By 32 weeks, fetal production of urine approaches 12 mL/h, and by term, 28 mL/h. From midgestation, urine is the major component of amniotic fluid. As mentioned before, the relative amounts of amniotic fluid can provide information on the status of fetal renal function. Oligohydramnios may be associated with renal hypoplasia, dysplasia, or obstructive uropathy. A normal amount of amniotic fluid indicates that there is some function in at least one kidney. Moreover, oligohydramnios is a most clinically useful determinant of hypoxia and asphyxia as used in the Biophysical Profile and the Modified Biophysical Profile. A profound decrease in amniotic fluid may indicate chronic hypoxia and decreased urinary output in the stressed state.

Ninety-three percent of all infants, either term or preterm, will void within the first 24 hours of life; 99% will void within 48 hours. Inadequate urine formation by the neonate can be associated with intravascular volume depletion, hypoxia, congenital nephrotic syndrome, tubular necrosis, renal agenesis, bilateral renal arterial or venous thrombosis, or obstructive uropathy. Normal infants may have transient glycosuria or proteinuria and a urine pH of 6.0–7.0.

Ultrasonography allows diagnosis of hydronephrosis prenatally and has stimulated research into therapeutic use of antenatal urinary aspiration or diversion techniques.

CENTRAL NERVOUS SYSTEM FUNCTION IN THE FETUS & NEWBORN

It has been known for at least a century that the fetus is capable of sustained motor activity well before quickening. Through the eighth week of gestation, nearly 95% of responses are contralateral. Ipsilateral responses (torso stimulus) begin to appear with much greater frequency during the ninth week. By 12–13 weeks, local reflexes have almost completely replaced the total pattern of response. Recent ultrasonographic evaluations have followed motor activity in utero and all confirm a transition from simple whole body movements to complex motor responses. Thus, the sensation of fetal movement is an increasing part of sensory input to the brainstem.

The cortex begins to develop during the eighth week. The neural maturational events that have been evaluated emphasize 2 transitional periods: (1) a possible consolidation of brainstem influence over motor activity and sensory input near the end of the first trimester, and

(2) establishment of the sensory input channel to the neothalamocortical connection around midgestation. However, it is apparent that the brainstem is only partially developed and functional at term.

The functional development of the human central nervous system is too complex to summarize. Nevertheless, a few clinical correlates must be mentioned. An individual's development neither begins nor ends at birth. Abnormal neuronal migrations in the developing human brain are generally early gestational events induced by genetic factors, teratogens, or infections. Although the major neuronal migrations have formed the cortical plate by 16 weeks' gestation, late migrations from the germinal matrix into the cerebral cortex continue until 5 months postnatally. The external granular layer of the cerebellar cortex continues to migrate until age 1 year. Thus, ample opportunity exists for disturbances of these migratory processes in the postnatal period. Moreover, myelination is only rudimentary in the cerebral cortex of term infants. Axons of the large pyramidal cells of the motor cortex are myelinated only as far cortically as the cerebral peduncles of the midbrain, as demonstrated by light microscopy, and pyramidal tract axons in the medulla oblongata have only 1 or 2 turns of myelin, as seen on electron microscopy.

Neurologic development not only implies acquisition of perceptual, motor, linguistic, and intellectual skills, but also signifies progressive organization of the anatomic and physiologic substrates of those achievements. Formation of the nervous system begins with the embryonic neural plate and terminates with completion of the final myelination cycle in the brain (ie, the frontal temporal association bundle at age 32–34 years). It is obvious that there are many things that can interrupt the normal migration, such as a premature infant who suffers a subependymal hemorrhage affecting the radial glial process that is guiding a neuron to the surface. The neuron may retract from the cortical surface after its cell origin is destroyed. The maturation is in situ, but the migrating neuron is unable to establish the intended synaptic relations with the cortex. Perhaps the faulty synaptic circuitry of this "incidental finding" at autopsy contributes to the development of an epileptic focus. Another mechanism of prenatal or postnatal cerebral dysgenesis involves toxins that destroy the cytoskeletal elements of glial and nerve cells (eg, methylmercury poisoning). Methylmercury chloride abruptly arrests the active movement of migrating neurons in vitro, causing damage to the neural membrane of the growth zone, interferes with DNA synthesis, and ultimately compromises cytoskeletal proteins.

Psychiatrists and psychologists have long recognized in utero modifying influences, and Freud stated that "each individual ego is endowed from the beginning with its own peculiar disposition and tendencies." For example, maternal anxiety levels do affect fetal development, and intrauterine stimuli determine, to a degree, the maturation of nerve cells and structural patterns of the developing brain. Maternal emotional stress can have immediate and long-term effects on fetal development, but it is unclear whether these effects are predictable.

Between 10 and 20 weeks' gestational age, the fetus displays several basic motor patterns that are later integrated into specific actions. The first jerky patterns of the second trimester become the functional movement patterns that allow the fetus to move about in utero. After midpregnancy, these motor patterns mature in a manner similar to the mature repertoire of the newborn. Clues to future central nervous system development may be found in the study of these various fetal motor patterns, and failure to progress at various stages seems to indicate subsequent cerebral dysfunction. Real-time ultrasonic examination of such fetal motor patterns may lead to improved care in high-risk situations.

The fetus demonstrates various sleep-wake patterns throughout its development in utero. During most of its antenatal life, fetal electrocortical activity is of low voltage, associated with REMs, slow heart rate, and fetal breathing activity. In the third trimester, high-voltage activity is associated with more-lively activity. Finally, near term, the fetus appears to be awake at least 30% of the time. These fetal states may be discerned by ultrasonic study of eye movements, which may be altered by drugs or maternal anxiety levels. These, in turn, affect fetal heart rate responses to stress.

The term fetus has high **endorphin** levels that may modify the behavioral state, including heart rate responses. Endorphin levels may be responsible for the primary apnea of the newborn and for the lack of heart rate reactivity in otherwise normal intrapartum fetuses. The fetus probably suffers pain, as does any other individual, and high endorphin levels may limit pain and other effects of stress. The near-term fetus, then, has nearly all the neurologic attributes of the newborn infant.

▮ INTRAUTERINE NUTRITION

Maternal diet among mammals is incredibly varied. For instance, the female black bear hibernates during her pregnancy, but she supplies metabolites to her fetus while neither eating nor drinking. In contrast, the pregnant guinea pig eats continuously. Obviously, forced fasting may have different effects on these different species during pregnancy. As shown in Fig 8–8, many maternal and placental modifications of nutrients occur before the nutrients reach the fetus. The mother and the placenta have first priority in use of these nutrients. Although vitamin

Figure 8–8. Schematic diagram showing the pathway of nutrients in the mother as they are broken down into different concentrations in the maternal portal vein and, finally, the umbilical vein. (Modified and reproduced, with permission, from Battaglia FC: The comparative physiology of fetal nutrition. Am J Obstet Gynecol 1984;148:850.)

B accumulates in greater concentrations in fetal blood than in maternal blood, the placental release of most vitamins to the fetus seems to depend on the degree of saturation of the vitamin reserve in the placenta. Because these nutrient-modifying factors differ markedly in different species, it is hazardous to interpolate data from laboratory animals to humans. The human newborn is 16% fat. Normally, the human fetus has a large accumulation of high-calorie fat, which during the last few weeks of gestation represents more than 80% of the fetal caloric accretion. There are 2 components of fetal caloric intake: the building-block, or accretion, component and the growth, or heat production, component. Starvation and protein-turnover studies suggest that the fetus uses calories primarily for maintenance rather than growth.

In pregnant sheep at term (pregnancy in sheep and humans is comparable in terms of relative fetal/maternal weights), one-third of the maternal glucose is used by the uterus; of this amount, two-thirds is consumed by the uteroplacental tissue and only one-third by the fetus. In sheep, the placenta rather than the fetus is clearly the primary intrauterine glucose consumer. This large glucose uptake by the placenta is partially explained by its high rate of lactate production. Laboratory studies have shown that when the human fetus is well oxygenated, the umbilical arterial lactate concentration and the umbilical arteriovenous difference are positive, indicating that lactate is also an important nutrient for the human fetus.

Ammonia is another compound produced in large quantities by the placenta and, like lactate, is released into the umbilical circulation. In humans, ketones and free fatty acids play a large role in fetal nutrition. The fetus actively synthesizes fatty acids in the liver, brain, and lung, which have special requirements for myelin and surfactant. Although fatty acids can be transported across the placenta, their oxidation does not seem to add much to the total energy economy of the fetus. The fetus regularly uses protein for oxidative metabolism. The metabolism of the human brain is very active during the perinatal period, and the brain is an obligatory consumer of glucose. Ketone bodies may partially replace glucose during periods of hypoglycemia and may also be a source of carbon for central nervous system lipids and proteins.

The placenta transports more water than any other substance. Because maternal hydrostatic and serum colloid osmotic pressures vary significantly during a normal day, unknown placental mechanisms protect the fetus against rapid shifts of water, which could cause either hydrops or dehydration. It may be that placental water transport is a passive process resulting from active solute transfer, as in the intestine.

The most widely recognized fetal hormone known to modify the rate of fetal growth is insulin. Fetuses with anomalies that preclude the availability of fetal growth hormone, thyroxine, adrenocortical steroids, or sex steroids achieve normal birth weights. Inasmuch as maternal insulin is not transferred to the fetus in physiologic quantities, the fetal pancreas must supply sufficient insulin for the oxidation of glucose. Under the stimulus of recurring hyperglycemia—as with maternal diabetes mellitus—the B cells of the fetal pancreas may become hyperplastic and secrete larger quantities of insulin.

■ THE AMNIOTIC FLUID

There is a vital need for a nonrestricting intrauterine environment, which develops before the fetus. This environment can only be ensured if it is part of the development of the fetus. Every fetus is surrounded by a protective cushion of amniotic fluid, whether the fetus develops inside the mother as a viviparous species or in an egg. In the first half of pregnancy, amniotic fluid volume appears to increase in association with growth of the fetus, and the correlation between fetal weight and amniotic fluid is very close. The serum osmolality and sodium, urea, and creatinine content of maternal serum and amniotic fluid are not significantly different. This suggests that amniotic fluid is an ultrafiltrate of maternal serum. Ultrasonographic evaluation during the first half of pregnancy reveals that the fetus does empty its bladder during the first half of gestation.

The average volume of amniotic fluid at term is 800 mL, and the sodium concentration is fairly constant. The volume and sodium concentration remain the same despite the fact that a normal fetus will swallow some of the fluid and will also contribute urine, which concentrates sodium. Analysis of amniotic fluid provides unique information about the fetus. In the first half of pregnancy, amniotic fluid appears to maintain the extracellular fluid chemistry of the fetus. In the second half, amniotic fluid reflects the development of renal function and, by virtue of the cells it sheds, the morphologic development of skin and mucous membranes. Amniotic fluid has a low specific gravity (1.008)

and a pH of 7.2. Pathways of solute and water exchange in amniotic fluid are shown in Fig 8–9.

In the past decade, morphologic chromosomal abnormalities and more than 100 inborn errors of metabolism have been identified. The amniotic fluid collects cells shed from the skin, amnion, and gastrointestinal and genitourinary tracts. In amniotic fluid obtained by amniocentesis at about 16 weeks, 30–80% of these cells are usually alive. Recent cytotechnologic advances may allow karyotyping from amniotic fluid as early as 11 weeks of gestation. The total number of cells increases with the length of gestation, but the proportion of viable cells does not increase, and at about 24 weeks, only 10–15% of the total number of cells are viable. The live cells are induced to adhere to the bottom of a tissue culture vessel after 3–4 days in culture, and they develop either an epithelial or fibroblastic morphology. The cells eventually form a monolayer, and when introduced into a suitable culture medium (containing nutrients and supplied with serum) are induced to divide. The dividing cells are arrested at metaphase with colchicine to prevent formation of the mitotic spindle. The advantage of this method is that a number of slides can be prepared, so that specific stain methods can be used and the chromosome preparation can be banded satisfactorily.

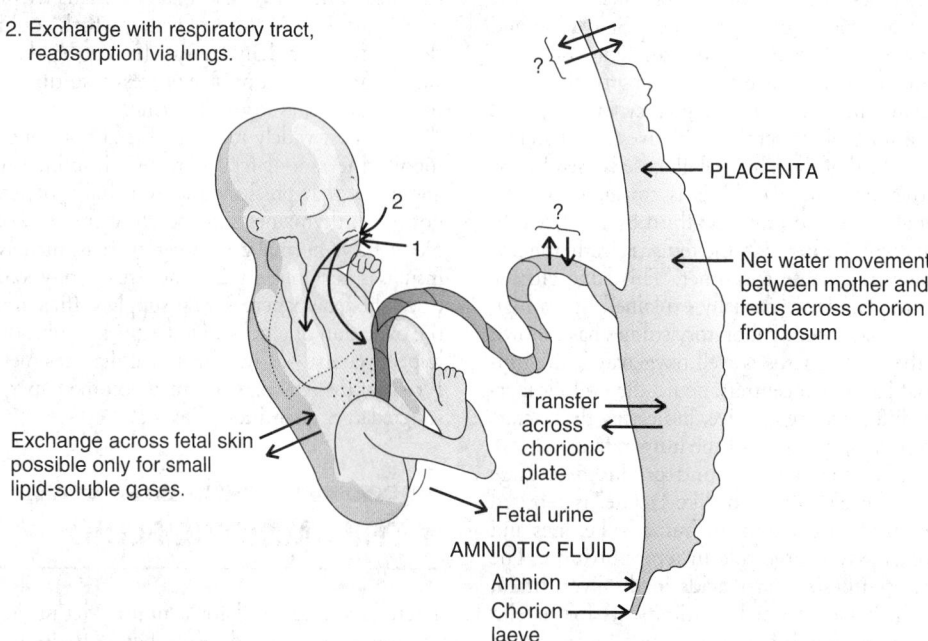

1. Fetal swallowing and reabsorption by intestine.

2. Exchange with respiratory tract, reabsorption via lungs.

PLACENTA

Net water movement between mother and fetus across chorion frondosum

Transfer across chorionic plate

Fetal urine

Exchange across fetal skin possible only for small lipid-soluble gases.

AMNIOTIC FLUID

Amnion

Chorion laeve

Figure 8–9. Solute and water exchange in amniotic fluid.

There is no simple or accurate method currently available to measure amniotic fluid volume. **Oligohydramnios** often indicates the presence of some abnormality. Polyhydramnios may occur in normal pregnancy but is also often associated with some abnormality of mother or fetus.

Oligohydramnios may be more objectively determined by identification of the largest pocket of fluid measuring less than 2 cm × 2 cm or the total of 4 quadrants less than 5 cm. However, this definition is associated with many false-positive and false-negative readings.

Oligohydramnios is associated with an SGA fetus, renal tract abnormalities such as renal agenesis, and urinary tract dysplasia. The clinical manifestation of oligohydramnios is a direct result of the impairment of urine flow to the amniotic fluid in the late part of the first half of pregnancy or during the second and third trimesters.

Amniotic fluid inhibits bacterial growth; the phosphate to zinc ratio is a predictor of inhibitory activity. In cases of intra-amniotic fluid infection, "inorganic phosphorus" levels in amniotic fluid are often elevated.

Amniotic Fluid Markers

Alpha-fetoprotein (AFP) is of fetal origin, and concentrations in amniotic fluid and maternal serum are of value in prenatal diagnosis of neural tube defects and other fetal malformations. Fetal serum contains AFP in a concentration 150 times that of maternal serum. High levels of maternal serum AFP are associated with an elevated level of amniotic fluid protein and subsequent findings of open neural tube defects.

In neural tube defects where there is an open lesion (even when covered with a membrane) in the spinal canal, fetal cerebrospinal fluid passes into the amniotic fluid. A suitable neural marker to determine whether cerebrospinal fluid is leaking into the amniotic fluid would be a protein of molecular size so large that it would not normally be excreted in the urine. The enzyme acetylcholinesterase has a molecular weight on the order of 300,000. Acetylcholinesterase levels in amniotic fluid appear to be more specific than the AFP test in predicting neural tube defects.

The clinical importance of low levels of AFP in maternal serum has also been recognized. Low levels of AFP in conjunction with estriol and comparatively high levels of hCG (roughly twice normal for given gestational age) have been shown to be predictive for Down syndrome. As an illustration, if one assumes a base rate of diagnostic amniocentesis of 5% (the approximate proportion of pregnancies occurring beyond age 35), the likelihood of detecting Down syndrome using only maternal age as a risk factor would be only 30%. However, if amniocentesis were to be performed on the basis of age, AFP, estriol, and hCG levels, the yield would rise to almost 60%. Down syndrome is the most common congenital cause of severe mental retardation, occurring with an incidence of about

1.3 per 1000 live births. Advanced maternal age is the most common consideration in selecting women for diagnostic amniocentesis. This policy derives from the fact that the risk of Down syndrome rises with advancing maternal age. The greatly improved detection rate (Fig 8–10) afforded by combining serum screening and age as screening criteria is fast establishing this method as the screening test of choice in many centers throughout the world.

Some proteins enter the amniotic fluid by transudation of placental components, but they also enter from other sources, including maternal uterine decidua; fetal skin; amnion; chorion; the umbilical cord; amniotic fluid cells; fetal urine; meconium; and fetal nasopharyngeal, oral, and lacrimal secretions. It is assumed that the relative contribution of these tissues will change during pregnancy. The major proportion of soluble proteins in amniotic fluid between 10 weeks' gestation and term is thought to be (1) of serum type and (2) of maternal origin entering the fluid by diffusing through the chorion. The observed concentration gradient for AFP between fetal serum and amniotic fluid should not be taken to imply that the presence of α-fetoprotein (AFP) in amniotic fluid is explained largely by permeation. Indeed, the concentration of AFP in fetal urine during the second trimester is comparable with levels of AFP in amniotic fluid at this time.

The amniotic fluid serves a number of important functions besides being a valuable source for analysis of fetal tissues and fluids. It cushions the fetus against severe injury; provides a medium in which the fetus can move easily; may be a source of fetal nutrients; and, in early

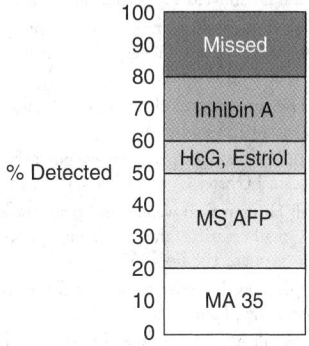

Figure 8–10. Maternal age 35 (MA 35) identifies about 20% of Down syndrome pregnancies. Low alpha fetoprotein (AFP) brings the total to about 50%. Double or triple screening (for HcG or estriol) raises that number to about 60% of the total and quadruple screening (including inhibin A) brings that number of identified cases to 80%, which is over half of those occurring in women under age 35. MS = maternal serum.

pregnancy, is essential for fetal lung development. The amniotic fluid is continuously exchanged at a rapid rate. Indeed, it is possible, at least on a temporary basis, to increase amniotic fluid volume by rapid expansion of maternal plasma volume with an intravenous infusion of colloid fluid such as 5% albumin. After 34–36 weeks, determination of amniotic fluid volume becomes even more complicated because the larger fetus swallows more fluid, upsetting the relationship between fetal size and fluid volume. After 38 weeks, both amniotic fluid and maternal plasma volume decrease. These relative decreases are even more apparent in postmature pregnancy.

Studies have shown that the fetus near term drinks 400–500 mL of amniotic fluid per day; this is about the same as the amount of milk consumed by a newborn infant. To maintain a reasonable stability of volume, the fetus must excrete about the same volume of urine into the amniotic fluid each day.

During late pregnancy, the amniotic fluid contains increasing quantities of particulate material, including desquamated cells of fetal origin; lanugo and scalp hairs; vernix caseosa; a few leukocytes; and small quantities of albumin, urates, and other organic and inorganic salts. The calcium content of amniotic fluid is low (5.5 mg/dL), but the electrolyte concentration is otherwise equivalent to that of maternal plasma. As mentioned previously, meconium is ordinarily absent but is excreted by the fetus in response to vagal activity.

REFERENCES

Altshuler G: Role of the placenta in perinatal pathology revisited. Pediatr Pathol Lab Med 1996;16:207.

Ananth CV et al: Relationship among placenta previa, fetal growth restriction, and preterm delivery: A population-based study. Obstet Gynecol 2001;98:299.

Battaglia FC: The comparative physiology of fetal nutrition. Am J Obstet Gynecol 1984;148:850.

Bonds DR et al: Fetal weight/placental weight ratio and perinatal outcome. Am J Obstet Gynecol 1984;149:195.

Bonds DR et al: Human fetal weight and placental weight growth curves: A mathematical analysis from a population at sea level. Biol Neonate 1984;45:261.

Campbell S et al: New Doppler technique for assessing uteroplacental blood flow. Lancet 1983;1:675.

Castle BM, Turnbull AC: The presence or absence of fetal breathing movements predicts the outcome of preterm labour. Lancet 1983;2:471.

Crane J et al: Neonatal outcomes with placenta previa. Obstet Gynecol 1999;93:541.

Dawes GS: The central control of fetal breathing and skeletal muscle movements. J Physiol 1984;346:1.

Farmakides G et al: Prenatal surveillance using nonstress testing and Doppler velocimetry. Obstet Gynecol 1988;71:184.

Finberg HJ et al: Placenta accreta: Prospective sonographic diagnosis in patients with placenta previa and prior cesarean section. J Ultrasound Med 1992;11:333.

Fisher DJ: Oxygenation and metabolism in the developing heart. Semin Perinatol 1984;8:217.

Fleischer A et al: Uterine artery Doppler velocimetry in pregnant women with hypertension. Am J Obstet Gynecol 1986;154:806.

Fritz MA, Guo SM: Doubling time of human chorionic gonadotrophin (hCG) in normal early pregnancy: Relationship to hCG concentration and gestational age. Fertil Steril 1987; 47:584.

Goldenberg RL, Huddleston JF, Nelson KG: Apgar scores and umbilical arterial pH in preterm newborn infants. Am J Obstet Gynecol 1984;149:651.

Goodlin RC: Expanded toxemia syndrome or gestosis. Am J Obstet Gynecol 1986;154:1227.

Goodlin RC, Anderson JC, Gallagher TF: Relationship between amniotic fluid volume and maternal plasma volume expansion. Am J Obstet Gynecol 1984;146:505.

Harris R, Andrews T: Prenatal screening for Down's syndrome. Arch Dis Child 1988;63:705.

Hustin J, Foidart JM, Lambote R: Maternal vascular lesions in preeclampsia and intrauterine growth retardation. Placenta 1983;4:489.

Jaffe RB: Fetoplacental endocrine and metabolic physiology. Clin Perinatol 1983;10:669.

Juchau MR, Faustman-Watts E: Pharmacokinetic considerations in the maternal-placental-fetal unit. Clin Obstet Gynecol 1983; 26:379.

Kaapa P: Prostanoids in neonatology. Ann Clin Res 1984; 16:330.

Longo LD: Maternal blood volume and cardiac output during pregnancy: A hypothesis of endocrinologic control. Am J Physiol 1983;245(5-Part 1):R720.

Miller PW et al: Dating the time interval from meconium passage to birth. Obstet Gynecol 1985;66:459.

Naeye RL: Functionally important disorders of the placenta, umbilical cord, and fetal membranes. Hum Pathol 1987;18: 680.

Rosenfeld CR: Consideration of the uteroplacental circulation in intrauterine growth. Semin Perinatol 1984;8:42.

Reed KL: Fetal pulmonary artery and aorta: Two-dimensional Doppler echocardiography. Obstet Gynecol 1987;69:175.

Sarnat HB: Disturbances of late neuronal migrations in the perinatal period. Am J Dis Child 1987;141:969.

Scarpelli EM: Perinatal lung mechanics and the first breath. Lung 1984;162:61.

Silverman F et al: The Apgar score: Is it enough? Obstet Gynecol 1985;66:331.

Suidan JS, Wasserman JF, Young BK: Placental contribution to lactate production by the human fetoplacental unit. Am J Perinatol 1984;1:306.

Taipale P et al: Diagnosis of placenta previa by transvaginal sonographic screening at 12–16 weeks in a nonselected population: Obstet and Gynecol 1997;89:364.

Voigt HJ, Becker V: Doppler flow measurements and histomorphology of the placental bed in uteroplacental insufficiency. J Perinat Med 1992;20:139.

Wasmoen TL: Placental proteins. In: Polin RA, Fox WW (editors): *Fetal and Neonatal Physiology.* WB Saunders, 1992.

Wells M et al: Spiral (uteroplacental) arteries of the human placental bed show the presence of amniotic basement membrane antigens. Am J Obstet Gynecol 1984;150:973.

SECTION II
Normal Obstetrics

Normal Pregnancy & Prenatal Care | 9

Helene B. Bernstein, MD, PhD, & Milena Weinstein, MD

■ NORMAL PREGNANCY

Pregnancy (gestation) is the maternal condition of having a developing fetus in the body. The human conceptus from fertilization through the eighth week of pregnancy is termed an **embryo;** from the eighth week until delivery, it is a **fetus.** For obstetric purposes, the duration of pregnancy is based on **gestational age:** the estimated age of the fetus is calculated from the first day of the last (normal) menstrual period (LMP), assuming a 28-day cycle. Gestational age is expressed in completed weeks. This is in contrast to **developmental age (fetal age)**, which is the age of the offspring calculated from the time of implantation.

The term **gravid** means pregnant, and **gravidity** is the total number of pregnancies (normal or abnormal). **Parity** is the state of having given birth to an infant or infants weighing 500 g or more, alive or dead. In the absence of known weight, an estimated duration of gestation of 20 completed weeks or more (calculated from the first day of the LMP) may be used. From a practical clinical viewpoint, a fetus is considered viable when it has reached a gestational age of 23–24 weeks and a weight of 500–600 g or more. However, only very rarely will a fetus of 20–23 weeks weighing 500 g or less survive, even with optimal care. With regard to parity, a multiple birth is a single parous experience.

Live Birth

Live birth is the complete expulsion or extraction of a product of conception from the mother, regardless of

the duration of pregnancy, which, after such separation, breathes or shows other evidence of life (e.g., beating of the heart, pulsation of the umbilical cord, or definite movements of the involuntary muscles) whether or not the cord has been cut or the placenta detached. An **infant** is a live-born individual from the moment of birth until the completion of 1 year of life.

In the most recent nomenclature, a **preterm infant** is defined as one born prior to the 37th week of gestation (259 days). Unfortunately, for purposes of evaluating statistical data, this definition does not specify that there are great differences among fetuses in this group. Therefore, it is useful to preserve the classification by weight or duration of gestation still used by many (Fig 9–1). Using the latter system, an **abortion** is the expulsion or extraction of all (complete) or any part (incomplete) of the placenta or membranes, without an identifiable fetus or with a fetus (alive or dead) weighing less than 500 g. In the absence of known weight, an estimated duration of gestation of under 20 completed weeks (139 days) calculated from the first day of the LMP may be used.

An **immature infant** weighs 500–1000 g and has completed 20 to less than 28 weeks of gestation. A **premature infant** is one with a birthweight of 1000–2500 g and a duration of gestation of 28 to less than 37 weeks. A **low-birthweight infant** is any live-born infant weighing 2500 g or less at birth. An **undergrown** or **small-forgestational age infant** is one who is significantly undersized (< 2 SD) for the period of gestation. A **mature infant** is a live-born infant who has completed 37 weeks of gestation (and usually weighs more than 2500 g). A **postmature infant** is one who has completed 42 weeks

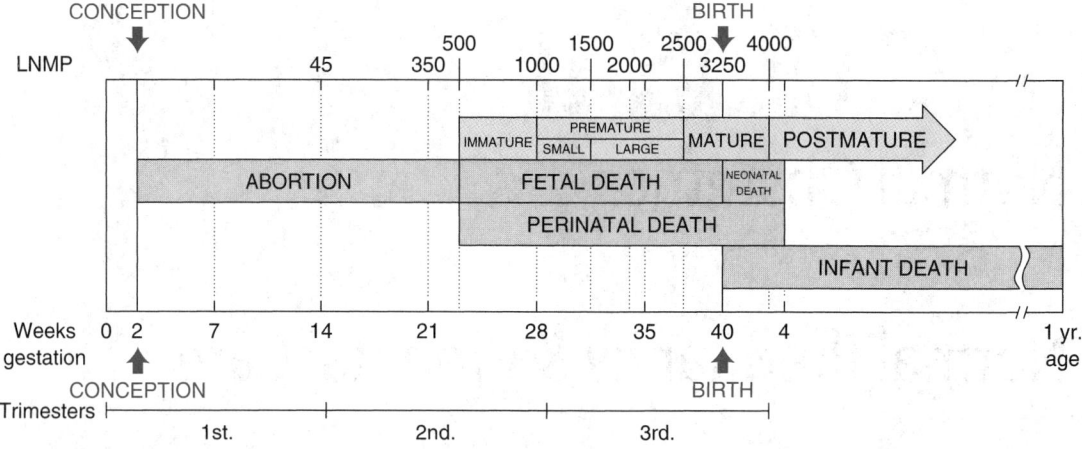

Figure 9–1. Graphic display of perinatal nomenclature.

or more of gestation. The **postmaturity syndrome** is characterized by prolonged gestation, sometimes an excessive-size fetus (see Large-for-Gestational-Age Pregnancy in Chapter 16), and diminished placental capacity for sufficient exchange, associated with cutaneous and nutritional changes in the newborn infant.

Significantly increased morbidity and mortality rates may be associated with the relative dystocia created by the large fetus. Approximately 10% of newborn infants weigh more than 4000 g and 1.5% of infants weigh in excess of 4500 g. With better nutrition and heavier infants, there has not been a commensurate increase in maternal pelvic dimensions. Excessive fetal size should be suspected in women who have previously delivered a large baby and in those with diabetes mellitus.

Predicting the end of pregnancy constitutes a major problem of perinatal care. The factors that lead to the initiation of labor and the subsequent termination of pregnancy remain unknown. This is the case for both preterm and postterm deliveries. A prolonged pregnancy (postterm) has traditionally been defined as gestation that has advanced 2 weeks past the due date (294 days). Because the perinatal mortality rate increases dramatically as gestation advances past the due date and because the cesarean rate is not increased with induction at 41 weeks, it is now common practice to offer induction of labor to all women at 7 days past the due date.

Birth Rate & Fertility Rate

Birth rate is commonly expressed in terms of the number of live births per 1000 population. The **fertility rate** is expressed as the number of live births per 1000 women ages 15–44 years and is thus a more sensitive measure of the reproductive activity of a given population. There were an estimated 4,115,590 live births in the United

States in 2004. The birth rate is currently 14.0 per 1000 total population, which is slightly increased compared to its nadir of 13.9 in 2002. The general fertility rate is currently 66.3 births per 1000 women aged 15–44. Indeed, the fertility rate appears to have peaked in 1990 at 71.1, after having been 67.1 in 1988.*

Neonatal Interval

The **neonatal interval** is from birth until 28 days of life. During this interval, the infant is referred to as a newborn. The interval may be divided into 3 periods:

Neonatal period I: birth through 23 hours, 59 minutes.

Neonatal period II: 24 hours of life through 6 days, 23 hours, 59 minutes.

Neonatal period III: seventh day of life through 27 days, 23 hours, 59 minutes.

Perinatal Period

The **perinatal period** is the time from 28 weeks of completed gestation to the first 7 days of life, spanning the fetal and early neonatal interval.

Perinatal Mortality Rates

Jeopardy to life is greatest during the perinatal period than at any subsequent time. Current data indicate that

---

* These data are provisional and are from *National Vital Statistics Report* v54 #8, the preeminent source of data concerning births, marriages, divorces, and deaths. It is available on a monthly basis from the National Center for Health Statistics (Centers for Disease Control, Public Health Service), U.S. Department of Health and Human Services.

the number of lives lost during the 5-month period from the 20th week of gestation to the 7th day after birth is almost equal to the number lost during the next 40 years of life. One half of these deaths occur *in utero*. In addition, 70% of deaths occurring in the first year of life will occur in the first 28 days of life (the neonatal period). Thus if one adds the neonatal loss rate to the fetal loss rate, it is the period of greatest threat to life for a given interval. There are gender and racial differences in mortality rates; the pertinent data are available through the *Monthly Vital Statistics Report.*

There are many causes of death during the perinatal period. The relative importance of each can only be assessed in the context of overall mortality rates and appraisal of those factors that present the greatest hazard to the fetus and infant.

DIAGNOSIS

The diagnosis of pregnancy is usually made on the basis of a history of amenorrhea and a positive pregnancy test. Nausea and breast tenderness are also often present. It may be crucial to diagnose pregnancy before the first missed menstrual period to prevent exposure of the fetus to hazardous substances (e.g., x-rays, teratogenic drugs), to manage ectopic or nonviable pregnancies, and to provide better health care for the mother.

The manifestations of pregnancy are classified into three groups: presumptive, probable, and positive.

Presumptive Manifestations

A. SYMPTOMS

1. Amenorrhea—Cessation of menses is caused by increasing estrogen and progesterone levels produced by the corpus luteum. Thus, amenorrhea is a fairly reliable sign of conception in women with regular menstrual cycles. In women with irregular cycles, amenorrhea is not a reliable sign. Delayed menses may also be caused by other factors such as emotional tension, chronic disease, opioid and dopaminergic medications, endocrine disorders, and certain genitourinary tumors. Spotting caused by bleeding at the implantation site may occur from the time of implantation (about 6 days after fertilization) until 29–35 days after the LMP in many women. Some women have unexplained cyclic bleeding throughout pregnancy.

2. Nausea and vomiting—This common symptom occurs in approximately 50% of pregnancies and is most marked at 2–12 weeks' gestation. It is usually most severe in the morning but can occur at any time and may be precipitated by cooking odors and pungent smells. Extreme nausea and vomiting may be a sign of multiple gestation or molar pregnancy. Protracted vomiting associated with dehydration and ketonuria (**hyperemesis**

gravidarum) may require hospitalization and relief of symptoms with antiemetic therapy.

Treatment for uncomplicated nausea consists of light, dry foods, small, frequent meals, and emotional support. Some improvement can be seen with the addition of high-dose vitamin B$_6$ therapy and the preconceptional use of prenatal vitamins. Antiemetic medications and alternative therapies, such as acupressure or ginger, are used for women whose symptoms interfere with daily life. The nausea is probably related to rapidly rising serum levels of human chorionic gonadotropin (hCG), although the mechanism is not understood.

3. Breasts—

a. Mastodynia—Mastodynia, or **breast tenderness,** may range from tingling to frank pain caused by hormonal responses of the mammary ducts and alveolar system. Circulatory increases result in breast engorgement and venous prominence. Similar tenderness may occur just before menses.

b. Enlargement of circumlacteal sebaceous glands of the areola (Montgomery's tubercles)—Enlargement of these glands occurs at 6–8 weeks' gestation and is a result of hormonal stimulation.

c. Colostrum secretion—Colostrum secretion may begin after 16 weeks' gestation.

d. Secondary breasts—Secondary breasts may become more prominent both in size and in coloration. These occur along the nipple line. Hypertrophy of axillary breast tissue often causes a symptomatic lump in the axilla.

4. Quickening—The first perception of fetal movement occurs at 18–20 weeks in primigravidas and at 14–16 weeks in multigravidas. Intestinal peristalsis may be mistaken for fetal movement; therefore, perceived fetal movement alone is not a reliable symptom of pregnancy, although it may be useful in determining the duration of pregnancy.

5. Urinary tract—

a. Bladder irritability, frequency, and nocturia—These conditions occur because of increased bladder circulation and pressure from the enlarging uterus.

b. Urinary tract infection—Urinary tract infection must always be ruled out because pregnant women are more likely than nonpregnant women to have significant bacteriuria which may be asymptomatic (7% versus 3%). Asymptomatic bacteriuria can also lead to pyelonephritis, which is associated with miscarriage, preterm birth, and intrauterine fetal demise.

B. SIGNS

1. Increased basal body temperature—Persistent elevation of basal body temperature over a 3-week period usually indicates pregnancy if temperatures have been carefully charted.

2. Skin—

a. Chloasma—Chloasma, or the **mask of pregnancy,** is darkening of the skin over the forehead, bridge of the nose, or cheekbones and is most marked in those with dark complexions. It usually occurs after 16 weeks' gestation and is intensified by exposure to sunlight.

b. Linea nigra—Linea nigra is darkening of the nipples and lower midline of the abdomen from the umbilicus to the pubis (darkening of the linea alba). The basis of these changes is stimulation of the melanophores by an increase in melanocyte-stimulating hormone.

c. Stretch marks—Stretch marks, or striae of the breast and abdomen, are caused by separation of the underlying collagen tissue and appear as irregular scars. This is probably an adrenocorticosteroid response. These marks generally appear later in pregnancy when the skin is under greater tension.

d. Spider telangiectases—Spider telangiectases are common skin lesions that result from high levels of circulating estrogen. These vascular stellate marks blanch when compressed. Palmar erythema is often an associated sign. Both of these signs are also seen in patients with liver failure.

Probable Manifestations

A. Symptoms

Symptoms are the same as those discussed under Presumptive Manifestations, above.

B. Signs

1. Pelvic organs—Many changes in the pelvic organs are perceivable to the experienced physician, including the following.

a. Chadwick's sign—Congestion of the pelvic vasculature causes bluish or purplish discoloration of the vagina and cervix.

b. Leukorrhea—An increase in vaginal discharge consisting of epithelial cells and cervical mucus is due to hormone stimulation. Cervical mucus that has been spread on a glass slide and allowed to dry no longer forms a fernlike pattern but has a granular appearance.

c. Hegar's sign—This is widening of the softened area of the isthmus, resulting in compressibility of the isthmus on bimanual examination. This occurs by 6–8 weeks.

d. Bones and ligaments of pelvis—The bony and ligamentous structures of the pelvis also change during pregnancy. There is slight but definite relaxation of the joints. Relaxation is most pronounced at the pubic symphysis, which may separate to an astonishing degree.

2. Abdominal enlargement—There is progressive abdominal enlargement from 7–28 weeks. At 16–22 weeks, growth may appear more rapid as the uterus rises out of the pelvis and into the abdomen (Fig 9–2).

3. Uterine contractions—As the uterus enlarges, it becomes globular and often rotates to the right. Painless uterine contractions (**Braxton Hicks contractions**) are felt as tightening or pressure. They usually begin at about 28 weeks' gestation and increase in regularity. These contractions usually disappear with walking or exercise, whereas true labor contractions become more intense.

Figure 9–2. Height of fundus at various times during pregnancy.

Figure 9–3. Regression of hCG following delivery, assuming a 1.5-day half-life.

Positive Manifestations

The various signs and symptoms of pregnancy are often reliable, but none is diagnostic. A positive diagnosis must be made on objective findings, many of which are not produced until after the first trimester. However, more methods are becoming available to diagnose pregnancy at an early stage.

A. FETAL HEART TONES (FHTS)

It is possible to detect FHT by hand held Doppler as early as 10 weeks' gestation. The normal fetal heart rate is 120–160 beats per minute. It may be detected by fetoscope by 18–20 weeks' gestation, although this device is rarely used at present.

B. PALPATION OF FETUS

After 22 weeks, the fetal outline can be palpated through the maternal abdominal wall. Fetal movements may be palpated after 18 weeks. This may be more easily accomplished by a vaginal examination.

C. ULTRASOUND EXAMINATION OF FETUS

Sonography is one of the most useful technical aids in diagnosing and monitoring pregnancy. Cardiac activity is discernible at 5–6 weeks, limb buds at 7–8 weeks, and finger and limb movements at 9–10 weeks. At the end of the embryonic period (10 weeks by LMP), the embryo has a human appearance. Fetal well-being can be monitored by ultrasound as the pregnancy progresses.

Pregnancy Tests

Sensitive, early pregnancy tests measure changes in levels of hCG. There is less cross-reaction with luteinizing hormone (LH), follicle stimulating hormone (FSH), and thyrotropin, which all share a common α subunit with hCG, when the β subunit of hCG is measured. hCG is produced by the syncytiotrophoblast 8 days after fertilization and may be detected in the maternal serum after implantation occurs, 8–11 days after conception. hCG levels peak at approximately 10–12 weeks of gestation. Levels gradually decrease in the second and third trimesters and increase slightly after 34 weeks. The half-life of hCG is 1.5 days (Fig 9–3). After termination of pregnancy, levels drop exponentially. Normally, serum and urine hCG levels return to nonpregnant values (< 5 mIU/mL) 21–24 days after delivery.

A. URINE PREGNANCY TEST

This is the most common method used to confirm pregnancy. Using antibodies, the test identifies the β subunit of hCG, minimizing cross-reaction with similarly structured hormones. The test is affordable, reliable and fast (1–5 minutes to obtain results) tool to diagnose pregnancy in the office. The urine pregnancy test is qualitative—positive or negative, based on color change, with the level of hCG detection ranging between 5 and 50 mIU/mL, depending on the kit used.

B. HOME PREGNANCY TESTS

hCG is detected in a first-voided morning urine sample. A positive test is indicated by a color change or confirmation mark in the test well. Because the accuracy of the home pregnancy test depends on technique and interpretation, it should always be repeated in the office.

C. SERUM PREGNANCY TEST

hCG can be detected in the serum as early as a week after conception. The serum pregnancy test can be quantitative or qualitative with a threshold as low as 2–4 mIU/mL, depending on the technique used. The serum pregnancy test is a reliable method to diagnose an early pregnancy;

it is widely used in the evaluation of threatened abortion, ectopic pregnancy, and other conditions.

CALCULATION OF GESTATIONAL AGE & ESTIMATED DATE OF DELIVERY

After the diagnosis of pregnancy is made, it is imperative to determine the duration of pregnancy and the estimated date of confinement (EDC).

Calculation of Gestational Age

A. Pregnancy Calendar or Calculator

Normally, human pregnancy lasts 280 days or 40 weeks (9 calendar months or 10 lunar months) from the last normal menstrual period (LNMP). This may also be calculated as 266 days or 38 weeks from the last ovulation in a normal 28-day cycle. The easiest method of determining gestational age is with a pregnancy calendar or calculator. The estimated date of delivery (EDD) can be determined mathematically using Nägele's rule: subtract 3 months from the month of the LNMP, and add 7 to the first day of the LNMP. Example: With an LNMP of July 14, the EDC is April 21.

B. Clinical Parameters of Gestational Age

1. Ultrasonography—Ultrasonography is now the most widely used technique for determination of gestational age. Fetal crown to rump length can be measured at 5–13 weeks and is the most accurate means to determine gestational age. Beyond 13 weeks, measurement of fetal biparietal diameter is used in conjunction with the femur length and abdominal circumference to assess gestational age and/or interval fetal growth. Beyond 30 weeks, the accuracy of gestational age assessment by ultrasound is much less.

Ultrasound is used to measure fetal growth parameters, to estimate fetal weight, to access fetal anatomy, and to measure amniotic fluid volume. Fetal well-being can also be evaluated by measuring biophysical characteristics.

2. Uterine size—An early first-trimester examination usually correlates well with the estimated gestational age. The uterus is palpable just at the pubic symphysis at 8 weeks. At 12 weeks, the uterus becomes an abdominal organ and at 16 weeks is usually at the midpoint between the pubic symphysis and the umbilicus. The uterus is palpable at 20 weeks at the umbilicus. Fundal height (determined by measuring the distance in centimeters from the pubic symphysis to the curvature of the fundus) correlates roughly with the estimated gestational age at 26–34 weeks (Fig 9–2). After 36 weeks, the fundal height may decrease as the fetal head descends into the pelvis.

3. Quickening—The first fetal movement is usually appreciated at 17 weeks in the average multipara and at 18 weeks in the average primipara.

4. Fetal heart tones—FHTs may be heard by fetoscope at 20 weeks, whereas Doppler ultrasound usually detects heart rates by 10 weeks.

DIAGNOSIS OF PREGNANCY AT TERM

A **term fetus** has reached a stage of development that will allow the best chance for extrauterine survival (37–41 weeks). Whether a fetus has reached this stage can be determined by the methods outlined above for ascertaining fetal age and EDD.

At term, a fetus usually weighs more than 2500 g. Depending on maternal factors such as obesity and diabetes, amniotic fluid volume, and genetic and racial factors, the baby may be larger or smaller than expected; therefore, the clinician must rely on objective data to determine fetal maturity.

Amniotic Fluid Analysis

The most accurate test of fetal maturity is analysis of amniotic fluid obtained by amniocentesis. This is discussed in Chapter 13.

Ultrasonography

Early ultrasound examination is the most accurate means of determining gestational age and indirectly confirming maturity. Because of the variation in late-pregnancy ultrasound parameters, they are not helpful in confirming maturity.

DIAGNOSIS OF FETAL DEATH

The accepted method of diagnosing pregnancy failure early is ultrasound.

Early in pregnancy, failure to visualize a fetal pole with cardiac activity at the appropriate gestational age suggests fetal death. Serial measurements of serum β-hCG may be helpful when the ultrasound findings are equivocal.

In late pregnancy, the first sign of fetal death is usually absence of fetal movement noted by the mother. This is followed by absence of FHTs. Real-time ultrasonography is virtually 100% accurate in determining the absence of fetal heart motion.

Hypofibrinogenemia may rarely develop 4–5 weeks after fetal death as thromboplastic substances are released from the degenerating products of conception. Coagulation studies should be started 2 weeks after intrauterine death, and delivery should be attempted by 4 weeks or if serum fibrinogen falls below 200 mg/mL. This is only clinically applicable in the case of death of one of twins; otherwise, the singleton demise would be delivered promptly.

PRENATAL CARE

Prenatal care as we know it today is a relatively new development in medicine. It originated in Boston in the first decade of the 20th century. Before that time, the patient who thought she was pregnant may have visited a physician for confirmation but did not visit again until delivery was imminent. The nurses of the Instructive Nursing Association in Boston, thinking they might contribute to the health of pregnant mothers, began making house calls on all mothers registered for delivery at the Boston Lying-In Hospital. These visits were so successful that the principle behind them was gradually accepted by physicians, and our present system of prenatal care, which stresses prevention, evolved.

Pregnancy is a normal physiologic event that is complicated by pathologic processes dangerous to the health of the mother and fetus in only 5–20% of cases. The physician who undertakes care of pregnant patients must be familiar with the normal changes that occur during pregnancy, so that significant abnormalities can be recognized and their effects minimized.

Prenatal care should have as a principal aim the identification and special treatment of the high-risk patient—the one whose pregnancy, because of some factor in her medical history or an issue that develops during pregnancy, is likely to have a poor outcome.

The purpose of prenatal care is to ensure, as much as possible, an uncomplicated pregnancy and the delivery of a live, healthy infant. There is evidence that mothers and offspring who receive prenatal care have a lower risk of complications. There is also evidence that the mother's emotional state during pregnancy may have a direct effect on fetal outcome. In one study, it was reported that anxiety in labor is positively correlated with plasma epinephrine levels, which, in turn, seem to result in abnormal fetal heart rate patterns and low Apgar scores. Similarly, another study, which measured anxiety in women in the third trimester, noted that in newborns of anxious women, the 5-minute Apgar score was significantly lower.

Ideally, a woman planning to have a child should have a medical evaluation before she becomes pregnant. This allows the physician to establish by history, physical examination, and laboratory studies the patient's overall fitness for undertaking pregnancy. This is the ideal time to stress the dangers of cigarette smoking, alcohol and drug use, and exposure to teratogens. Instruction on proper diet and exercise habits can also be

given. Vitamins, especially folic acid, taken 3 months before conception may be beneficial (decreasing the incidence of open neural tube defects). Unfortunately, most patients do not seek preconceptional care, and the initial prenatal visit is scheduled well after pregnancy is under way.

Common reasons why pregnant women may not receive adequate prenatal care are inability to pay for health care, fear of or lack of confidence in health care professionals, lack of self-esteem, delays in suspecting pregnancy or in reporting pregnancy to others, different individual or cultural perceptions of the importance of prenatal care, adverse initial feelings about being pregnant, and religious or cultural prohibitions. These factors should be screened for and addressed.

INITIAL OFFICE VISIT

The purpose of the first visit to the physician is to identify all risk factors involving the mother and fetus. Once identified, high-risk pregnancies require individualized specialized care. The diagnosis of pregnancy is made on the basis of physical signs and symptoms and the results of laboratory tests discussed earlier in this chapter.

History

A. PRESENT PREGNANCY

The interview should begin with a full discussion of the symptoms. The patient should have time to express her ideas on childbearing and parenting and to discuss the effect of pregnancy on her life situation.

The patient with regular menses may be able to accurately calculate the EDC using the first day of the LMP and Nägele's rule (see above). The EDC may also be determined if the patient knows the probable date of conception.

B. PREVIOUS PREGNANCY

Outcomes of all prior pregnancies provide important clues to potential problems in the current gestation. The following information should be obtained: length of gestation, birthweight, fetal outcome, length of labor, fetal presentation, type of delivery, and complications (prenatal, during labor, postpartum). If a cesarean section was performed, an operative report details the type of uterine incision and allows the physician to estimate the patient's subsequent risk for uterine scar dehiscence.

C. MEDICAL HISTORY

Many medical disorders are exacerbated by pregnancy. Many cardiovascular, gastrointestinal, and endocrine disorders require careful evaluation and counseling concerning possible deleterious effects on the mother. A history of previous blood transfusion may suggest the rare possibility of associated hemolytic disease of the newborn because of maternal antibodies from a minor blood group mismatch. Knowledge of drug sensitivities is also important.

A history of maternal infections during pregnancy should be obtained. If possible, current infections should be treated to prevent hazardous fetal effects. Review of the patient's knowledge about avoiding infectious and teratogenic risks (see Chapter 14) is prudent.

The prenatal history should include important social aspects, such as the number of sexual partners, the history of sexually transmitted diseases, and possible contact with intravenous drug users. Human immunodeficiency virus (HIV) testing should be offered to all patients.

D. SURGICAL HISTORY

Of special importance is a history of previous gynecologic surgery. Prior uterine surgery may necessitate cesarean delivery. A history of multiple induced abortions or midtrimester losses may suggest an incompetent cervix. Patients with previous cesarean deliveries may be candidates for vaginal delivery if they are adequately counseled and meet established guidelines.

E. FAMILY HISTORY

A family history of diabetes mellitus should alert the physician to possible gestational diabetes, especially if the patient has a history of large or anomalous babies or previous stillbirths. Glucose tolerance testing must be done to determine current endocrine function.

Awareness of familial disorders is also important in pregnancy management. Thus, a brief three-generation pedigree is useful. Antenatal screening tests are available for many hereditary diseases.

A history of twinning is important, because dizygotic twinning (polyovulation) may be a maternally inherited trait.

Physical Examination

A. GENERAL EXAMINATION

A complete physical examination must be performed on every new patient. In a young, healthy woman, this may be the first complete examination she has ever had.

B. PELVIC EXAMINATION

The pelvic examination is of special importance to the obstetrician.

1. Pelvic soft tissue—Any pelvic mass should be described accurately and evaluated by ultrasonography.

2. Bony pelvis—The pelvic configuration should be appraised to determine which patients are more likely to develop cephalopelvic disproportion in labor. Pelvimetry has been largely replaced, however, by clinical trial of the pelvis ("trial of labor").

a. Pelvic inlet—Although the transverse diameter of the inlet cannot be measured clinically, the anteroposterior diameter or diagonal conjugate usually can be estimated. For this measurement, the middle finger of the examining hand reaches for the promontory of the sacrum, and the tissue between the examiner's index finger and thumb is pushed against the pubic symphysis while the point of pressure is noted (Fig 9-4). The distance between the tip of the examining finger and this point of pressure measures the **diagonal conjugate** of the inlet. Subtracting 1.5 cm from the diagonal conjugate gives a satisfactory estimate of the **true conjugate** (conjugata vera), or the true anterior diameter of the pelvic inlet.

b. Midpelvis—Precise clinical measurement of the diameter of the midpelvic space is not feasible. With some experience, however, the physician can estimate this distance by noting the prominence and relative closeness of the ischial spines. If the walls of the pelvis seem to converge; if the curve of the sacrum is straightened or shallow; or if the sacrosciatic notches are unusually narrow, doubt about the adequacy of the midpelvis is justified.

c. Pelvic outlet—For clinical purposes, the outlet can be adequately estimated by physical examination. The shape of the outlet can be determined by palpating the pubic rami from the symphysis to the ischial tuberosities and noting the angle of the rami. A subpubic angle of less than 90 degrees suggests inadequacy of the outlet. A prominent or angulated coccyx diminishes the anteroposterior diameter of the pelvic outlet.

On rare occasions, extreme abnormality of the pelvis precludes vaginal delivery. In most cases, below average clinical measurements alert the obstetrician to the possibility of fetopelvic disproportion, and therefore dystocia. However, an adequate trial of labor is usually the final determinant of true adequacy of the bony pelvis.

d. Cervical length—Assessment should be made by bimanual examination of the cervical length and dilation. Average cervical length is 3–4 cm. A nulliparous woman or one who has never given birth vaginally will have a closed os. In women with prior preterm birth, transvaginal ultrasonographic evaluation of cervical length is replacing digital exam; a scan in the midtrimester (18–20 weeks) and further serial examinations can be predictive of preterm delivery.

Figure 9–4. Measurement of the diagonal conjugate (DC) (conjugata diagonalis, CD). (Reproduced, with permission, from Benson RC: Handbook of Obstetrics & Gynecology, 8th ed. Norwalk, CT: Lange, 1983.)

Laboratory Tests

The following laboratory assessments should be performed as early as possible in pregnancy and some of these repeated at least once between 24 and 36 weeks' gestation.

A. Blood Screening

At the first visit, the following is obtained: hematocrit, hemoglobin, white blood cell count and differential, blood type group, Rh factor, and antibodies to blood group antigens; also needed are a serologic test for syphilis (Venereal Disease Research Laboratory [VDRL] or rapid plasma reagent [RPR] test), rubella, hepatitis B, and HIV. At-risk individuals may need testing for toxoplasmosis. Women with prior gestational diabetes should be given early 1-hour postglucose testing. The glucose level is checked after ingestion of 50 g of glucose. In a woman with no increased risk, this is done at 24–28 weeks' gestation. If the test is abnormal, a 3-hour glucose tolerance test is obtained (fasting glucose level, followed by glucose levels 1, 2, and 3 hours after a 100-g glucose load). Hematocrit should be repeated in the third trimester.

Maternal serum testing for hCG, unconjugated estriol, and α-fetoprotein (AFP) and inhibin (the quad screen) should be offered between 15 and 20 weeks' gestation (ideally at 16–18 weeks) to screen for open neural tube defects and chromosomal abnormalities, primarily trisomies 21 and 18.

To allow earlier detection of certain chromosomal abnormalities, first trimester screening using a combination of maternal serum analytes (pregnancy-associated plasma protein A [PAPP-A] and free β-hCG) and ultrasound measurement of fetal nuchal translucency is becoming more widely available.

B. Genetics Testing

Genetic studies should be offered to women older than age 35 and to those with abnormal pedigrees or other risk factors for inherited diseases. Chorionic villus sampling (CVS) is done at 10–14 weeks' gestation by either a transabdominal or transcervical technique. Amniocentesis is usually offered at 16–20 weeks' gestation. With ultrasound guidance, the complication rate of either of these procedures is well below 1%.

C. Urine Testing

Perform urinalysis and screening tests (eg, dipstick nitrite testing) or culture for urinary tract infection. If the bacteria count is over 10^5/mL on a voided sample or if bacteria are noted on a catheterized specimen, perform antibiotic sensitivity testing. Testing for urinary protein, glucose, and ketones should be done at each prenatal visit. Proteinuria of more than 300 mg/24 h ($\geq$ 2+ on standard dipstick testing) may indicate renal dysfunction, or, if associated with relative hypertension, the onset or progression of preeclampsia. The presence of glucosuria signifies that the delivery of glucose to the kidneys exceeds renal resorptive capacity. This is not important if blood levels are normal, but elevated blood levels indicate carbohydrate intolerance. During pregnancy, the presence of ketones in the urine usually indicates inadequate intake of carbohydrates but not fetal jeopardy or maternal diabetes. The diet should be evaluated in this case to make certain that carbohydrate intake is adequate.

D. PAPANICOLAOU SMEAR

Papanicolaou smears are performed unless recent results are available. Some obstetricians routinely screen for gonorrhea and chlamydia; others reserve this for high-risk patients. Microscopic examination of vaginal secretions is performed if indicated.

E. GROUP B STREPTOCOCCUS

The current recommendations are to perform routine screening for group B streptococcus between 35 and 37 weeks' gestation. The rationale is that if the mother is positive, she should be treated (penicillin is the drug of choice) at the time of admission in labor, thus decreasing the risk of group B streptococcal sepsis in the newborn.

F. TUBERCULIN SKIN TEST

A tuberculin skin test (**purified protein derivative [PPD]**) is appropriate for high-risk patients.

SUBSEQUENT VISITS

The standard schedule for prenatal office visits is 0–32 weeks' gestation: once every 4 weeks; 32–36 weeks' gestation: once every 2 weeks; and 36 weeks' gestation to delivery: once each week. At each visit, weight gain, blood pressure, fundal height, and findings on abdominal examination by Leopold's maneuvers should be recorded. Additionally, FHTs should be documented and urine should be checked for glucose and protein. These findings should be reviewed and compared with those of previous examinations.

MATERNAL WELL-BEING AS A SIGN OF FETAL WELL-BEING

In modern obstetric practice, fetal well-being has been determined mainly by direct monitoring and testing, but it is important not to overlook the status of the mother when determining fetal well-being. Maternal health is obviously crucial to fetal development and must be continuously assessed during pregnancy.

Maternal Height & Weight

Maternal height and prepregnancy weight along with the rate and amount of weight gain during pregnancy are important in fetal development. Women who are underweight or of short stature tend to have smaller babies, and are at risk for low birthweight and preterm delivery. A teenage mother is compromised if her diet is inadequate to meet her own growth requirements and those of her fetus. In such circumstances, women less than 157 cm (5 ft) tall, especially those weighing less than 45 kg (100 lb), should be encouraged to gain at least a minimum of 11–12 kg (25 lb), if not more.

Inadequate progressive weight gain may reflect nutritional deficit, maternal illness, or a hormonal milieu that does not promote proper volume expansion and anabolic state. Often, this is associated with poor fundal growth and a small fetus and placenta, suggesting fetal growth retardation. Weight gain and fundal height should be closely monitored during pregnancy.

Blood Pressure

Blood pressure levels may provide a clue to subtle circulatory compromise. Normally, the mean arterial pressure drops somewhat from prepregnancy or early pregnancy values during the middle trimester. It is important to note this decline so that it does not mask a subsequent rise in blood pressure that may signal the onset of hypertension. In the third trimester, blood pressure recordings taken in the supine position may be higher than those taken in the recumbent or seated position; this also may indicate the onset of hypertension. Normal patients may have a significant drop in blood pressure in the supine position (supine hypotensive syndrome), which is corrected when the patient is in the left lateral position.

Fundal Height

Fundal height should be measured and recorded at each visit after 20 weeks' gestation. Measurements should be made with a centimeter tape (**McDonald's technique**) from the pubic symphysis to the top of the uterine mass over the curvilinear abdominal surface. Progress is especially important in the third trimester, when fetal growth retardation is most easily determined.

Fetal Heart Tones

FHTs can usually be heard by 10–12 postmenstrual weeks using a hand-held Doppler device. This may be helpful when gestational age is in doubt or in the presence of threatened abortion or other abnormal observations in the late first trimester. Attention should be paid both to rate and rhythm and to any accelerations, decelerations, or irregularities. Significant abnormalities may be further assessed by ultrasonography, fetal echocardiography, or electronic fetal heart rate monitoring, depending on gestational age.

Edema

At each prenatal visit, abnormal or potentially abnormal findings should be noted, and a careful record should be made of any unusual events that have occurred since the last visit. Transient episodes of general edema or swelling should be noted. Lower-extremity edema in late pregnancy is a natural consequence of hydrostatic changes in lower body circulation.

Edema of the upper body (eg, face and hands), especially in association with relative or absolute increases in blood pressure, may be the first sign of preeclampsia. A moderate rise in blood pressure without excessive fluid retention may suggest a predisposition to chronic hypertension.

Fetal Size & Position

Manual assessment of fetal size and position is always indicated after about 26 weeks' gestation. The fetus may assume a number of positions before late gestation, but persistence of an abnormal lie into late pregnancy suggests abnormal placentation, uterine anomalies, or other problems that should be investigated by ultrasound. If an abnormal lie persists, consider external version after 37 weeks' gestation. Suspected abnormal fetal size should also be investigated; a difference between gestational age and fetal heart size by 2 cm or more should prompt consideration of ultrasound evaluation.

PREPARATION FOR LABOR

As term approaches, the patient must be instructed on the physiologic changes associated with labor. She is usually admitted to the hospital when contractions occur at 5- to 10-minute intervals. She should be told to seek medical advice for any of the following danger signals: (a) rupture of membranes, (b) vaginal bleeding, (c) decreased fetal movement, (d) evidence of preeclampsia (eg, marked swelling of the hands and face, blurring of vision, headache, epigastric pain, convulsions), (e) chills or fever, (f) severe or unusual abdominal or back pain, or (g) any other severe medical problems.

NUTRITION IN PREGNANCY

The mother's nutrition from the moment of conception is an important factor in the development of the infant's metabolic pathways and future well-being. The pregnant woman should be encouraged to eat a balanced diet and should be made aware of special needs for iron, folic acid, calcium, and zinc.

The average woman weighing 58 kg (127 lb) has a normal dietary intake of 2300 kcal/d. An additional 300

kcal/d is needed during pregnancy and an additional 500 kcal/d is needed during breastfeeding (Table 9–1). Consumption of fewer calories could result in inadequate intake of essential nutrients.

WEIGHT GAIN

The American College of Obstetricians and Gynecologists along with the Institute of Medicine (IOM) recommend a weight gain of 11.5–16 kg (25–35 lb) during singleton pregnancy. Underweight women may need to gain more, whereas obese women should gain only 7–11.5 kg (15–25 lb). Heavier women and those with excessive weight gain during pregnancy are likely to have macrosomic infants. Inadequate weight gain is associated with small-for-gestational age (SGA) infant.

The fetus accounts for about one-third of the normal weight gain (3500 g); the placenta, amniotic fluid, and uterus for 650–900 g; interstitial fluid and blood volume for 1200–1800 g each; and breast enlargement for 400 g. The remaining 1640 g or more is largely maternal fat.

NUTRITIONAL REQUIREMENTS

A. PROTEIN

Protein needs in the second half of pregnancy are 1 g/kg plus 20 g/d (approximately 80 g/d for the average woman). Protein intake is essential for embryonic development.

B. CALCIUM

Calcium intake should be increased to 1.5 g/d in the later months and during lactation. If calcium intake is inadequate, fetal needs will be met through demineralization of the maternal skeleton. Maternal calcium stores may be further drained during lactation.

C. IRON

To avoid iron-deficiency anemia, the IOM recommends supplementing the diet of every pregnant woman with 30 mg/d of elemental iron during the second and third trimester. If iron-deficiency anemia is diagnosed, the therapeutic doses of elemental iron prescribed range between 60 and 120 mg/d.

D. VITAMINS AND MINERALS

Vitamin and mineral preparations are commonly given but should not be substituted for adequate food intake. Folic acid has been shown to effectively reduce the risk of neural tube defects (NTDs). A daily 4-mg dose is recommended for patients who have had a previous pregnancy affected by NTDs. It should begin more than 1 month prior to pregnancy (preferably 3 months) and continued

Table 9–1. Recommended daily dietary allowances for nonpregnant, pregnant, and lactating women.

	Nonpregnant Women (years)				Pregnant Women	Lactating Women
	15–18	19–24	25–50	50+		
Energy (kcal)	2100	2100	2100	2000	+300	+500
Protein (g)	48	46	46	46	+30	+20
Fat-soluble vitamins						
Vitamin A (RE)/(IU)	800	800	800	800	800	1300
Vitamin D (IU)	400	400	200	200	400	400
Vitamin E (IU)	8	8	8	8	10	12
Water-soluble vitamins						
Vitamin C (mg)	60	60	60	60	70	95
Folate (µg)	180	180	180	180	400	280
Niacin (mg)	15	15	15	13	17	20
Riboflavin (mg)	1.3	1.3	1.3	1.2	1.6	1.8
Thiamine (mg)	1.1	1.1	1.1	1.0	1.5	1.6
Vitamin B_6 (mg)	1.5	1.6	1.6	1.6	2.2	2.1
Vitamin B_{12} (µg)	2	2	2	2	2.2	2.6
Minerals						
Calcium (mg)	1300	1000	1000	1200	1000	1000
Iodine (µg)	150	150	150	150	175	200
Iron (mg)	15	15	15	10	30	15
Magnesium (mg)	300	280	280	280	300	355
Phosphorus (mg)	1200	800	800	800	1200	1200
Zinc (mg)	12	12	12	12	15	19

through the first 6–12 weeks of pregnancy. Studies show this amount reduces the risk of recurrence by 70%. For all other women, a daily intake of at least 0.4 mg taken before conception and through the first 6 weeks of pregnancy is recommended. Patients with insulin-dependent diabetes mellitus and those with seizure disorders treated by valproic acid and carbamazepine are also at greater risk for neural tube defects and these women should ingest at least 1 mg/d of folic acid. Vitamin B_{12} supplements are also desirable for vegetarian patients and those with known megaloblastic anemia.

Salt Restriction

Moderate amounts of foods containing sodium are not harmful during normal pregnancy. In fact, sodium restriction may be potentially dangerous. There is no evidence that rapid weight gain in preeclampsia can be controlled with sodium restriction.

COMMON COMPLAINTS DURING PREGNANCY

Most of the minor complaints during pregnancy can be minimized with patient education and prompt treatment.

Ptyalism

Excessive salivation (sialism, ptyalism) is an infrequent but troublesome complaint of pregnant women. The cause is unknown but it is strongly associated with severe nausea and vomiting of pregnancy.

Pica

Pica (cissa) is the ingestion of substances that have no value as food or are unwholesome. Common examples are clay and laundry starch. Pica is harmful because it interferes with good nutrition by substituting nonnutritious bulk for nutritionally important foods. The necessity for good nutrition must be explained to these patients.

Frequency of Urination

Urinary frequency is a common complaint throughout pregnancy. Vascular engorgement of the pelvis and hormonal changes are responsible for altered bladder function. Late in pregnancy, when pressure on the bladder by the enlarging uterus and the fetal presenting part decreases bladder capacity, urination becomes even more frequent.

Dysuria or hematuria may be signs that infection has developed; diagnostic and therapeutic measures are needed.

Sexually Transmitted Diseases (STDs)

A. SYPHILIS

Syphilis screening tests such as the VDRL slide test and the RPR tests are sensitive, but not specific, for syphilis infection and may remain positive even after disease treatment. They are used to screen for syphilis infections secondary to their cost-effectiveness. Treponemal antibody tests are used to confirm syphilis infection in patients with a positive VDRL or RPR. Penicillin remains the treatment of choice in pregnancy, secondary to its ability to cross the placenta and treat the fetus, with treatment protocols correlating with disease severity. Erythromycin or ceftriaxone are treatment alternatives for the pregnant patient, but because of treatment failures, penicillin desensitization is recommended. Monthly serologic tests are followed to assess treatment response.

B. CHLAMYDIA

The most effective screening consists of DNA probe analysis for this infection. Treatment usually consists of 7 days of erythromycin or one dose of azithromycin in the pregnant woman. Amoxicillin is used for patients with intolerance to erythromycin base or ethylsuccinate.

C. GONORRHEA

Gonorrhea is best detected by cervical culture or DNA probe. Because many strains are penicillin-resistant, ceftriaxone is the drug of choice. Amoxicillin is used for nonresistant strains and spectinomycin is recommended for the penicillin-allergic patient.

D. HERPES SIMPLEX VIRUS

Tissue culture is the best confirmation of herpes infection. Topical acyclovir may improve symptoms. Oral acyclovir may be used for recurrent outbreaks and should be considered after 36 weeks for prophylaxis against outbreaks at the time of delivery. Cultures are recommended when a lesion is suspected. If no lesions are found, vaginal delivery is safe. Cesarean delivery is the route of choice for patients with active lesions at the time of delivery or with prodromal symptoms at the time of delivery secondary to the high rate of morbidity and mortality associated with neonatal herpes infection.

E. HIV

The standard approach to HIV testing in prenatal care includes testing via ELISA (enzyme-linked immunosorbent assay) followed by confirmatory Western blot or immunofluorescence assay (IFA) for ELISA positive specimens. The Centers for Disease Control and Prevention (CDC) recommends that women who have not had prenatal HIV testing be offered rapid HIV testing at delivery to initiate prophylaxis of neonate in the event that the mother is HIV seropositive. The goal of prenatal care for HIV-positive pregnant women focuses on appropriately treating maternal disease and minimizing vertical transmission of HIV, which correlates with the concentration of virus in maternal plasma (viral load). Management of an HIV-infected pregnant woman involves serial measurements of viral load and CD4 T-cell count. The pharmacotherapy varies, but usually consists of regimen of highly active anti-retroviral therapy (HAART) and intrapartum infusion of azidothymidine (AZT). Cesarean delivery is recommended only for patients with high viral load (> 1000 copies/mL); otherwise mode of delivery is dictated by obstetric indications.

Other Infections

A. TRICHOMONIASIS

Trichomonas vaginalis can be found in 20–30% of pregnant patients, but only 5–10% complain of leukorrhea or irritation. This flagellated, pear-shaped, motile organism can be seen under magnification when the vaginal discharge is diluted with warm normal saline solution and examined microscopically. Suspect trichomoniasis when the discharge is fetid, foamy, or greenish, or when there are reddish ("strawberry") petechiae on the mucous membranes of the cervix or vagina.

Treatment is discussed in Chapter 41.

B. CANDIDIASIS

Candida albicans can be cultured from the vagina in many pregnant women, but symptoms occur in less than 50%. When symptoms do occur, they consist of severe vaginal burning and itching and a profuse, caseous, white discharge. Marked inflammation of the vagina and introitus may be noted. The symptoms are likely to be aggravated by intercourse, and the male partner not infrequently develops mild irritation of the penis. Topical miconazole nitrate or nystatin suppositories are the preferred treatment during pregnancy. Oral fluconazole should be avoided for the uncomplicated vaginal infection. The infection often flares up during pregnancy, in which case retreatment is necessary.

C. BACTERIAL VAGINOSIS (BV)

This is a change in the vaginal bacterial milieu characterized by a diminution in lactobacilli and overgrowth of other species. The pH is decreased. The presence of BV is associated with a 2-fold increased risk of preterm birth in general. Many authorities advocate screening for BV and treating it in women at high risk for preterm birth.

Varicose Veins

Varicosities may develop in the legs or in the vulva. A family history of varicosities is often present. Pressure by the enlarging uterus on the venous return from the legs is a major factor in the development of varicosities. The physician should warn the patient early in pregnancy of the need for elastic stockings and elevation of the legs if varices develop. Specific therapy (injection or surgical correction) usually is contraindicated during pregnancy. Superficial varicosities may rarely signal deeper venous disease. These patients should be examined carefully for signs of deep vein thrombosis.

Joint Pain, Backache, & Pelvic Pressure

Although the main bony components of the pelvis consist of 3 separate bones, the symphysial and sacro-iliac articulations permit practically no motion in the nonpregnant state. In pregnancy, however, endocrine relaxation of these joints permits some movement. The pregnant patient may develop an unstable pelvis, which produces pain. A tight girdle or a belt worn about the hips, together with frequent bed rest, may relieve the pain; however, hospitalization is sometimes necessary.

Improvement in posture often relieves backache. The increasingly protuberant abdomen causes the patient to throw her shoulders back to maintain her balance; this causes her to thrust her head forward to remain erect. Thus, she increases the curvature of both the lumbar spine and the cervicothoracic spine. A maternity girdle to support the abdominal protuberance and shoes with 2-inch heels, which tend to keep the shoulders forward, may reduce the lumbar lordosis and thus relieve backache. Local heat and back rubs may relax the muscles and ease discomfort. Exercises to strengthen the back are most rewarding.

Leg Cramps

The cause of leg cramps in pregnancy is unknown but may be the result of a reduced level of diffusible serum calcium or elevation of serum phosphorus. Treatment for this includes curtailment of phosphate intake (less milk and nutritional supplements containing calcium phosphate) and an increase of calcium intake (without phosphorus) in the form of calcium carbonate or calcium lactate tablets. Alternatively, a randomized trial showed that magnesium citrate, 300 mg/d, reduces leg cramps. Symptomatic treatment consists of leg massage, gentle flexing of the feet, and local heat. Tell the patient to avoid pointing toes when she stretches her legs (eg, on awakening in the morning) as this triggers a gastrocnemius cramp. She should also practice "leading with the heel" in walking.

Breast Soreness

Physiologic breast engorgement may cause discomfort, especially during early and late pregnancy. A well-fitting brassiere worn 24 hours a day affords relief. Ice bags are temporarily effective. Hormone therapy is of no value.

Discomfort in the Hands

Acrodysesthesia of the hands consists of periodic numbness and tingling of the fingers (the feet are never involved). It affects at least 5% of pregnant women. In some cases it is thought to be a brachial plexus traction syndrome caused by drooping of the shoulders during pregnancy; carpal tunnel syndrome is a common cause of a similar symptom complex. The discomfort is most common at night and early in the morning. It may progress to partial anesthesia and impairment of manual proprioception. The condition is apparently not serious, but it may persist after delivery as a consequence of lifting and carrying the baby.

Other Common Complaints

See Chapters 7 and 25 for discussions of other common complaints during pregnancy, including abdominal pain, nausea and vomiting, syncope and faintness, heartburn, constipation, hemorrhoids, genital tract complications, headache, and carpal tunnel syndrome.

DRUGS, CIGARETTE SMOKING, & ALCOHOL DURING PREGNANCY

Drugs

Teratogenicity has been established for only a few drugs. The U.S. Food and Drug Administration (FDA) proposed a classification system for drugs in pregnancy and lactation that uses available data to address relative safety of administering medications to pregnant women. The physician should have good reason for prescribing any drug early in pregnancy, or indeed during the last half of the menstrual cycle, when any fertile, sexually active woman might become pregnant.

Little is known about the effects of marijuana on the fetus, but major deleterious consequences have not been reported. Heroin and methadone, on the other hand, are associated with major problems in the neonate, especially potentially fatal withdrawal symptoms.

Cigarette Smoking

An increased incidence of low-birth-weight infants has been ascribed to heavy cigarette smoking by pregnant women. Smoking during pregnancy is associated with increased risk of intrauterine growth restriction, placenta previa, placenta accreta, preterm birth, low birth weight, and perinatal mortality. Pregnant women should be encouraged not to smoke, and can be offered pharmaceutical agents to assist with smoking cessation. If cessation is not possible, reducing the number of cigarettes smoked per day is encouraged.

Alcoholic Beverages

In the past, it was thought that moderate ingestion of alcohol caused no deleterious effects on the uterus or fetus despite the easy passage of alcohol across the placenta. Instances of newborns showing alcoholic withdrawal symptoms have been reported, but usually these infants were born to chronic alcoholics who drank heavily during pregnancy. However, the precise level of alcohol consumption during pregnancy that causes adverse fetal effects has not been established. Moreover, the chronic alcoholic may suffer from malnutrition, to the extent that the craving for alcohol exceeds the desire for food.

A **fetal alcohol syndrome** (**FAS**) following maternal ethanol ingestion has been described, with an incidence varying from 1 in 1500 to 1 in 600 live births. The rate of reported cases identified among newborns in the United States during 1979–1992 increased approximately 4-fold. The major features include growth retardation, characteristic facial dysmorphology (including microcephaly and microphthalmia), central nervous system deficiencies, and other abnormalities.

There is no exact dose–response relationship between the amount of alcohol consumed during the prenatal period and the extent of damage caused by alcohol in the infant. Infants whose mothers consume alcohol during pregnancy can have fetal alcohol effects (FAEs), alcohol-related birth defects (ARBDs), FAS, or be normal. The term *fetal alcohol spectrum disorder* has been coined to describe the broad range of adverse sequelae in alcohol exposed offspring.

Pregnant women should be encouraged to avoid alcohol intake completely during pregnancy. If this is not possible, the intake should be reduced to a minimum.

OTHER MATTERS OF CONCERN DURING PREGNANCY

Intercourse

There has always been a suspicion that intercourse may be responsible for early abortion. Few adverse consequences can be attributed directly to intercourse during pregnancy. Naturally, if cramps or spotting follow coitus, it should be proscribed for the time being. Coitus late in pregnancy may initiate labor, perhaps because of an orgasm that causes a uterine contraction reflex. Pelvic rest should be considered for patients who have had a previ-

ous premature delivery or are currently experiencing uterine bleeding.

Bathing

Bath water does not enter the vagina. Even swimming is not contraindicated during normal pregnancy. Diving should be avoided because of possible trauma. A woman in the last trimester of pregnancy may have impaired balance. For this reason, she should be cautioned about slipping and falling in the tub or shower.

Douching

Douching, which is seldom necessary, may be harmful during pregnancy.

Dental Care

There may be generalized gum hypertrophy and bleeding during pregnancy. Interdental papillae (epulis) may also form in the upper gingivae, and these rarely resorb and must be excised. Normal dental procedures under local anesthesia (ie, drilling and filling) may be carried out at any time during gestation. Lengthy procedures should be postponed until the second trimester. Antibiotics are given for dental abscesses and in cases of rheumatic heart disease and mitral valve prolapse. Periodontal disease has been associated with an increased risk of preterm birth but there have been no trials of treatment during pregnancy.

Immunization

Killed virus, toxoid, or recombinant vaccines may be safely administered during pregnancy, and patients should be vaccinated appropriately for both maternal and fetal benefit. The American College of Obstetricians and Gynecologists recommends that all women who are pregnant in the second or third trimester during the flu season (October to March) should receive the influenza vaccination. Diphtheria and tetanus toxoid may be administered in pregnancy if a woman has not received a booster in 10 years, or if no primary series had been received. The hepatitis B vaccine series and killed polio vaccine may be given during pregnancy to women at risk. Live, attenuated vaccines, including those for varicella, measles, mumps, polio, and rubella, should be given 3 months prior to pregnancy or immediately postpartum. These vaccines are contraindicated in pregnancy secondary to the potential of fetal infection. Viral shedding occurs in children receiving vaccination, but they do not transmit the virus; consequently, vaccination may be safely given to the children of pregnant women. Secondary prophylaxis with specific immune globulin is recommended for pregnant women exposed to measles, hepatitis A, hepatitis B, tetanus, chickenpox, or rabies.

Clothing

Loose-fitting conventional clothing often suffices until late in pregnancy, although maternity garments may be used as desired. A well-fitted brassiere is essential. A maternity girdle is rarely prescribed except for the relief of back pain or for abdominal weakness. Panty girdles and garters should be avoided because they interfere with circulation in the legs. Well-fitted shoes with heels of medium height are best in pregnancy.

Exercise

Exercise in moderation is acceptable during pregnancy, but the patient should also rest an hour or two during the day. Those activities with high risk of falling or for abdominal trauma (eg, horseback riding, downhill skiing) and undue physical stress should be avoided. Aerobic and exercise classes have to be designed for pregnancy. Target heart rates are adjusted for age and weight, and routines are aimed to protect joints and promote flexibility.

Employment

Women who have sedentary jobs may continue to work throughout the pregnancy. Employment that requires physical exertion calls for a careful evaluation by the obstetrician and an occupational medical practitioner. It is unwise to adopt rigid policies regarding work during pregnancy—each patient has a different level of capability, level of prepregnancy conditioning, exercise tolerance, and physique.

Substantial physical effort increases maternal oxygen consumption and places an increased demand on cardiac reserve that may result in decreased uterine blood flow. There are no studies as yet that prove this theory beyond doubt, but a conservative approach to the problem is recommended.

Travel

Travel (by automobile, train, or plane) does not adversely affect a pregnancy, but separation from the physician may be of concern. For this reason, instruct patients with a history of spontaneous abortion and those who have experienced vaginal bleeding in the course of the present pregnancy to avoid travel to distant places.

REFERENCES

Abrams B, Altman SL, Pickett KE: Pregnancy weight gain: still controversial. Am J Clin Nutr 2000;71(Suppl):1233S.

ACOG Committee Opinion No. 267: Exercise during pregnancy and the postpartum period. American College of Obstetricians and Gynecologists. Obstet Gynecol 2002;99:171.

ACOG Committee Opinion No. 282: Immunization during pregnancy. American College of Obstetricians and Gynecologists. Obstet Gynecol 2003;101:207.

American College of Obstetricians and Gynecologists: Fetal macrosomia. ACOG Practice Bulletin No. 22, November 2000.

American College of Obstetricians and Gynecologists: Prenatal diagnosis of fetal chromosomal abnormalities. ACOG Practice Bulletin No. 27, May 2001.

American College of Obstetricians and Gynecologists: Scheduled cesarean delivery and the prevention of vertical transmission of HIV infection. ACOG Committee Opinion No. 234, May 2000.

American College of Obstetricians and Gynecologists: Smoking cessation during pregnancy. ACOG Educational Bulletin No. 260, September 2000.

Brown ZA et al: Effect of serologic status and cesarean delivery on transmission rates of herpes simplex virus from mother to infant. JAMA 2003;289:203.

Centers for Disease Control and Prevention: Early-onset group B streptococcal disease—United States, 1998–1999. MMWR Morb Mortal Wkly Rep 2000;49:793.

Centers for Disease Control and Prevention: HIV/AIDS update: A glance at the HIV epidemic. Available at: http://www.cdc.gov/nchstp/od/news/At-a-Glance.pdf. Retrieved June 22, 2004.

Centers for Disease Control and Prevention: Update: Trends in fetal alcohol syndrome—United States, 1979–1993. MMWR Morb Mortal Wkly Rep 1995;44:13.

Koren G et al: Fetal alcohol spectrum disorder. CMAJ 2003;169:1181.

Martin JA et al: Births: Final Data for 2002. Natl Vital Stat Rep 2003;52:10.

Owen J et al: Mid-trimester endovaginal sonography in women at high risk for spontaneous preterm birth. JAMA 2001;286:1340.

Raman S, Samuel D, Suresh K: A comparative study of X-ray pelvimetry and CT pelvimetry. Aust N Z J Obstet Gynaecol 1991;31(3):217.

Spencer K et al: One-stop clinic for assessment of risk for fetal anomalies: A report of the first year of a prospective screening for chromosomal anomalies in the first trimester. Br J Obstet Gynaecol 2000;107:1271.

Watts DH et al: A double-blind, randomized, placebo-controlled trial of acyclovir in late pregnancy for the reduction of herpes simplex virus shedding and cesarean delivery. Am J Obstet Gynecol 2003;188:836.

Wijnberger LD et al: The accuracy of lamellar body count and lecithin/sphingomyelin ratio in the prediction of: neonatal respiratory distress syndrome: A meta-analysis. BJOG 2001;108583.

Wilcox AJ et al: Natural limits of pregnancy testing in relation to the expected menstrual period. JAMA 2001;286(14):1759.

The Course & Conduct of Normal Labor & Delivery

Carol L. Archie

Labor is a sequence of uterine contractions that results in effacement and dilatation of the cervix and voluntary bearing-down efforts leading to the expulsion per vagina of the products of conception. Delivery is the mode of expulsion of the fetus and placenta. Labor and delivery is a normal physiologic process that most women experience without complications. The goal of the management of this process is to foster a safe birth for mothers and their newborns. Additionally, the staff should attempt to make the patient and her support person(s) feel welcome, comfortable, and informed throughout the labor and delivery process. Physical contact between the newborn and the parents in the delivery room should be encouraged. Every effort should be made to foster family interaction and to support the desire of the family to be together. The role of the obstetrician/midwife and the labor and delivery staff is to anticipate and manage complications that may occur that could harm the mother or the fetus. When a decision is made to intervene, it must be considered carefully, because each intervention carries both potential benefits and potential risks. The best management in the majority of cases may be close observation and, when necessary, cautious intervention.

PHYSIOLOGIC PREPARATION FOR LABOR

Prior to the onset of true labor, several preparatory physiologic changes commonly occur. The settling of the fetal head into the brim of the pelvis, known as **lightening,** usually occurs 2 or more weeks before labor in first pregnancies. In women who have had a previous delivery, lightening often does not occur until early labor. Clinically, the mother may notice a flattening of the upper abdomen and increased pressure in the pelvis. This descent of the fetus is often accompanied by a decrease in discomfort associated with crowding of the abdominal organs under the diaphragm (eg, heartburn, shortness of breath), and an increase in pelvic discomfort and frequency of urination.

During the last 4–8 weeks of pregnancy irregular, generally painless uterine contractions occur with slowly increasing frequency. These contractions, known as **Braxton Hicks contractions,** may occur more frequently, sometimes every 10–20 minutes, and with greater intensity during the last weeks of pregnancy. When these contractions occur early in the third trimester, they must be distinguished from true preterm labor. Later, they are a common cause of "false labor," which is distinguished by the lack of cervical change in response to the contractions.

During the course of several days to several weeks before the onset of true labor, the cervix begins to soften, efface, and dilate. In many cases, when labor starts, the cervix is already dilated 1–3 cm in diameter. This is usually more pronounced in the multiparous patient, the cervix being relatively more firm and closed in nulliparous women. With cervical effacement, the mucus plug within the cervical canal may be released. When this occurs, the onset of labor is sometimes marked by the passage of a small amount of blood-tinged mucus from the vagina known as **bloody show.**

In true labor, the woman is usually aware of her contractions during the first stage. The intensity of pain depends on the fetal/pelvic relationships, the quality and strength of uterine contractions, and the emotional and physical status of the patient. Few women experience no discomfort during the first stage of labor. Some women describe slight low back pain that radiates around to the lower abdomen. Each contraction starts with a gradual build-up of intensity, and dissipation of discomfort promptly follows the climax. Normally, the contraction will be at its height well before discomfort is reported. Dilatation of the lower birth canal and distention of the perineum during the second stage of labor will almost always cause discomfort.

CHARACTERISTICS OF NORMAL LABOR

Normal labor is a continuous process that has been divided into three stages for purposes of study, with the first stage further subdivided into two phases, the latent phase and the active phase. The first stage of labor is the interval between the onset of labor and full cervical dilatation. The second stage is the interval between full cervical dilatation and delivery of the infant. The third stage of labor is the period between the delivery of the infant and the delivery of the placenta.

In his classic studies of labor in 1967, Friedman presented data describing the process of spontaneous labor over time. The duration of the first stage of labor in primipara patients is noted to range from 6–18 hours, while in multiparous patients the range is reported to be 2–10 hours. The lower limit of normal for the rate of cervical dilatation during the active phase is 1.2 cm per hour in first pregnancies and 1.5 cm per hour in subsequent pregnancies. The duration of the second stage in the primipara is 30 minutes to 3 hours, and is 5–30 minutes for multiparas. For both, the duration of the third stage was reported to be 0–30 minutes for all pregnancies. These data, while extremely helpful as guidelines, should not be used as strict deadlines that trigger interventions if not met. Even if a numerical (statistical) approach is used to define "abnormal," the cutoff figure would not be the average range, but the 5th percentile numbers (eg, 25.8 hours for the first stage of labor in a primipara). The course that is more appropriate is to consider the overall clinical presentation and use the progress of labor to estimate the likelihood that successful vaginal delivery will occur.

Evaluation of Labor Progress

The first stage of labor is evaluated by the rate of change of cervical effacement, cervical dilatation, and descent of the fetal head. The frequency and duration of uterine contractions alone is not an adequate measure of labor progress. The second stage of labor begins after full cervical dilatation. The progress of this stage is measured by the descent, flexion, and rotation of the presenting part.

■ CLINICAL MANAGEMENT OF NORMAL LABOR

Women most likely to have a normal labor and delivery have had adequate prenatal care without significant maternal or fetal complications and are at 36 weeks' gestation or beyond. Whenever a pregnant woman is evaluated for labor, the following factors should be assessed and recorded:

- Time of onset and frequency of contractions, status of membranes, any history of bleeding, and any fetal movement.

- History of allergies, use of medication, and time, amount, and content of last oral intake.
- Prenatal records with special attention to prenatal laboratory results that impact intrapartum and immediate postpartum management (eg, human immunodeficiency virus [HIV] and hepatitis B status).
- Maternal vital signs, urinary protein and glucose, and uterine contraction pattern.
- Fetal heart rate, presentation, and clinical estimated fetal weight.
- Status of the membranes, cervical dilatation and effacement (unless contraindicated, eg, by placenta previa), and station of the presenting part.

If no complications are detected during the initial assessment and the patient is found to be in prodromal labor, admission for labor and delivery may be deferred. When a patient is admitted, a hematocrit or hemoglobin measurement should be obtained and a blood clot should be obtained in the event that a cross-match is needed. A blood group, Rh type, and antibody screen should also be done.

The First Stage of Labor

In the first stage of normal labor, the pregnant woman may be allowed to ambulate or sit in a comfortable chair as desired. When the patient is lying in bed, the supine position should be discouraged. Patients in active labor should avoid ingestion of anything except sips of clear liquids, ice chips, or preparations for moistening the mouth and lips. When significant amounts of fluids and calories are required because of long labor, they should be given intravenously.

Maternal pulse and blood pressure should be recorded at least every 2–4 hours in normal labor, and more frequently if indicated. Maternal fluid balance (ie, urine output and intravenous and oral intake) should be monitored and both dehydration and fluid overload should be avoided.

Management of discomfort and pain during labor and delivery is a necessary part of good obstetric practice. A patient's request is sufficient justification for providing pain relief during labor. Specific analgesic and anesthetic techniques are discussed in Chapter 29. Some patients tolerate the pain of labor by using techniques learned in childbirth preparation programs. Common methods of preparation include Lamaze, Bradley, Read, hypnotherapy, and prenatal yoga. While specific techniques vary, these classes usually teach relief of pain through the application of principles of education, emotional support, touch, relaxation, paced breathing, and mental focus. The staff at the bedside should be knowledgeable about these pain-management techniques and should be supportive of the patient's decision to use them. When such methods fail to provide adequate pain relief, some patients will ask for medical assistance and such requests should be respected. Indeed, the use of appropriate medical analgesic techniques should be explained to the patient and her labor partner and their use encouraged where medically indicated.

Reassurance of fetal well-being is sought through fetal monitoring. In patients with no significant obstetric risk factors, the fetal heart rate should be auscultated or the electronic monitor tracing should be evaluated at least every 30 minutes in the active phase of the first stage of labor, and at least every 15 minutes in the second stage of labor. In patients with obstetric risk factors, the fetal heart rate should be evaluated every 15 minutes during the active phase of the first stage of labor, and at least every 5 minutes during the second stage.

Uterine contractions should be monitored by palpation every 30 minutes to assess their frequency, duration, and intensity. For at-risk pregnancies, uterine contractions should be monitored continuously along with the fetal heart rate. This can be achieved by using either an external tocodynamometer or an internal pressure catheter in the amniotic cavity. The latter method is particularly useful when abnormal progression of labor is suspected or when the patient requires oxytocin for augmentation of labor.

The progress of labor is monitored by examination of the cervix. During the latent phase, especially when the membranes are ruptured, vaginal examinations should be done sparingly to decrease the risk of an intrauterine infection. In the active phase the cervix should be assessed approximately every 2 hours. The cervical effacement and dilatation, and the station and position of the fetal head should be recorded (Fig 10–1). Additional examinations to determine if full dilation has occurred may be required if the patient reports the urge to push, or to search for prolapse of the umbilical cord or perform fetal scalp stimulation if a significant fetal heart rate deceleration is detected.

The therapeutic rupture of fetal membranes (amniotomy) has been largely discredited as a means of induction when used alone. Moreover, artificial rupture of the membranes increases the risk of chorioamnionitis and the need for antibiotics (especially if labor is prolonged), as well as the risk of cord prolapse if the presenting part is not engaged. Amniotomy may, however, provide information on the volume of amniotic fluid and the presence of meconium. In addition, rupture of the membranes may cause an increase in uterine contractility. Amniotomy should not be performed routinely. It should be used when internal fetal or uterine monitoring is required, and may be helpful when enhancement of uterine contractility in the active phase of labor is indicated. Care should be taken to palpate for the umbilical cord and to avoid dislodging the fetal head. The fetal heart rate should be recorded before, during, and immediately after the procedure.

Figure 10–1. Stations of the fetal head. (Reproduced, with permission, from Benson RC: Handbook of Obstetrics & Gynecology, 8th ed. Lange, 1983.)

Second Stage of Labor

At the beginning of the second stage of labor the mother usually feels a desire to bear down with each contraction. This abdominal pressure, together with the force of the uterine contractions, expels the fetus. During the second stage of labor the descent of the fetal head is measured to assess the progress of labor. The descent of the fetus is evaluated by measuring the relationship of the bony portion of the fetal head to the level of the maternal ischial spines (station) (Fig 10–1). When the bony portion of the fetal head is at the level of the ischial spines, the station is "0." The ACOG (American College of Obstetricians and Gynecologists)-endorsed method for describing station is to estimate the number of centimeters from the ischial spines, but some practitioners find it useful to refer to station in estimated thirds of the maternal pelvis. An approximate correlation of these two methods would be: 2 cm = +1, 4 cm = +2, and 6 cm = +3.

The second stage generally takes from 30 minutes to 3 hours in primigravid women and from 5–30 minutes in multigravid women. The median duration is 50 minutes in a primipara and 20 minutes in a multipara. These times may vary depending on the pushing efforts of the mother, the quality of the uterine contractions, and the type of analgesia.

Mechanism of Labor

The mechanism of labor in the vertex position consists of engagement of the presenting part, flexion, descent, internal rotation, extension, external rotation, and expulsion (Table 10–1). The progress of labor is dictated by the pelvic dimensions and configuration, the size of

Table 10–1. Mechanisms of labor: vertex presentation.

Engagement	Flexion	Descent	Internal Rotation	Extension	External Rotation (Restitution)
Generally occurs in late pregnancy or at onset of labor. Mode of entry into superior strait depends on pelvic configuration.	Good flexion is noted in most cases. Flexion aids engagement and descent. (Extension occurs in brow and face presentations.)	Depends on pelvic architecture and cephalopelvic relationships. Descent is usually slowly progressive.	Takes place during descent. After engagement, vertex usually rotates to the transverse. It must next rotate to the anterior or posterior to pass the ischial spines, whereupon, when the vertex reaches the perineum, rotation from a posterior to an anterior position generally follows.	Follows distention of the perineum by the vertex. Head concomitantly stems beneath the symphysis. Extension is complete with delivery of the head.	Following delivery, head normally rotates to the position it originally occupied at engagement. Next, the shoulders descend (in a path similar to that traced by the head). They rotate anteroposteriorly for delivery. Then the head swings back to its position at birth. The body of the baby is then delivered.

the fetus, and the strength of the contractions. In essence, delivery proceeds along the line of least resistance, that is, by adaptation of the smallest achievable diameters of the presenting part to the most favorable dimensions and contours of the birth canal.

The sequence of events in vertex presentation is as follows:

A. ENGAGEMENT

This usually occurs late in pregnancy in the primigravida, commonly in the last 2 weeks. In the multiparous patient, engagement usually occurs with the onset of labor. The head enters the superior strait in the occiput transverse position in 70% of women with a gynecoid pelvis (Figs 10–2 and 10–3).

B. FLEXION

In most cases, flexion is essential for both engagement and descent. This will vary, of course, if the head is small in relation to the pelvis or if the pelvis is unusually large. When the head is improperly fixed—or if there is significant narrowing of the pelvic strait (as in the platypelloid type of pelvis)—there may be some degree of deflexion if not actual extension. Such is the case with a brow (deflexion) or face (extension) presentation.

C. DESCENT

Descent is gradually progressive and is affected by the forces of labor and thinning of the lower uterine segment. Other factors also play a part (eg, pelvic configuration and the size and position of the presenting part). The greater the pelvic resistance or the poorer the con-

tractions, the slower the descent. Descent continues progressively until the fetus is delivered; the other movements are superimposed on it (Fig 10–4).

D. INTERNAL ROTATION

With the descent of the head into the midpelvis, rotation occurs so that the sagittal suture occupies the anteroposterior diameter of the pelvis. Internal rotation normally begins with the presenting part at the level of the ischial spines. The levator ani muscles form a V-shaped sling that tends to rotate the vertex anteriorly. In cases of occipitoanterior vertex, the head has to rotate 45 degrees, and in occipitoposterior vertex, 135 degrees, to pass beneath the pubic arch (Fig 10–5).

E. EXTENSION

Because the vaginal outlet is directed upward and forward, extension must occur before the head can pass through it. As the head continues its descent, there is a bulging of the perineum followed by crowning. Crowning occurs when the largest diameter of the fetal head is encircled by the vulvar ring (Fig 10–6). At this time, spontaneous delivery is imminent and careful management by the practitioner with controlled efforts of the mother will minimize perineal trauma. Routine episiotomy is unnecessary, and is associated with increased maternal blood loss, increased risk of disruption of the anal sphincter (third-degree extension) and rectal mucosa (fourth-degree extension), as well as delay in the patient's resumption of sexual activity. Further extension follows extrusion of the head beyond the introitus. Once the head is delivered, the airway is cleared of

Gynecoid	Android	Platypelloid (flat)	Anthropoid

Figure 10–2. Flexions of the fetal head in the 4 major pelvic types. (Reproduced, with permission, from Danforth DN, Ellis AH: Midforceps delivery: A vanishing art? Am J Obstet Gynecol 1963;86:29.)

blood and amniotic fluid using a bulb suction device. The oral cavity is cleared initially, followed by clearing of the nares.

After the airway is cleared, an index finger is used to check whether the umbilical cord encircles the neck. If so, the cord can usually be slipped over the infant's head. If the cord is too tight, it can be cut between two clamps.

F. EXTERNAL ROTATION

External rotation (restitution) follows delivery of the head when it rotates to the position it occupied at en-

gagement. Following this, the shoulders descend in a path similar to that traced by the head. The anterior shoulder rotates internally about 45 degrees to come under the pubic arch for delivery (Fig 10–7). As this occurs, the head swings back to its position at birth. Delivery of the anterior shoulder is aided by gentle downward traction on the externally rotated head (Fig 10–8). The posterior shoulder is then delivered by gentle upward traction on the head (Fig 10–9). The brachial plexus may be injured if excessive force is used. Following these maneuvers, the body, legs,

Figure 10–3. Left occipitoanterior engagement.

Figure 10–4. Descent in left occipitoanterior position.

Figure 10–5. Anterior rotation of head.

Figure 10–7. External rotation of the head.

and feet are delivered with gentle traction on the shoulders.

After delivery, blood will be infused from the placenta into the newborn if the baby is held below the mother's introitus. Delayed cord clamping can result in neonatal hyperbilirubinemia as additional blood is transferred to the newborn infant. Generally, a vigorous newborn can be delivered directly from the introitus to the abdomen and waiting arms of a healthy, alert mother. Placing the child skin to skin (abdomen to abdomen) results in optimum warmth for the newborn. Then the cord, which has been doubly clamped may then be cut between the clamps, by either the practitioner, the mother, or her partner.

Third Stage of Labor

Immediately after the baby is delivered, the cervix and vagina should be inspected for actively bleeding lacerations and surgical repair should be performed as needed. Repair of vaginal lacerations should be performed using absorbable suture material, either 2-0 or 3-0. The inspec-

tion and repair of the cervix, vagina, and perineum is often easier prior to the separation of the placenta before uterine bleeding obscures visualization.

Separation of the placenta generally occurs within 2–10 minutes of the end of the second stage, but it may take 30 minutes or more to spontaneously separate. Signs of placental separation are: (a) a fresh show of blood from vagina, (b) the umbilical cord lengthens outside the vagina, (c) the fundus of the uterus rises up, and (d) the uterus becomes firm and globular. When these signs appear, it is safe to place traction on the cord. The gentle traction, with or without counterpressure between the symphysis and fundus to prevent descent of the uterus, allows delivery of the placenta.

After the delivery of the placenta, attention is turned to prevention of excessive postpartum bleeding. Uterine contractions which reduce this bleeding may be en-

Figure 10–6. Extension of the head.

Figure 10–8. Delivery of anterior shoulder.

Figure 10–9. Delivery of posterior shoulder.

hanced with uterine massage and/or the infusion of a dilute solution of oxytocin. The placenta should be examined to ensure complete removal and to detect placental abnormalities.

Puerperium

The puerperium consists of the period following the delivery of the baby and placenta to approximately 6 weeks postpartum. The immediate postpartum period (within the first hour of delivery) is a critical time for both maternal and neonatal physiologic and emotional adjustment. During that hour, the maternal blood pressure, pulse rate, and uterine blood loss must be monitored closely. It is during this time that most postpartum hemorrhage usually occurs, largely as a result of uterine relaxation, retained placental fragments, or unrepaired lacerations. Occult bleeding (eg, vaginal wall hematoma formation) may manifest as increasing pelvic pain.

At the same time, maternal bonding to the newborn is evolving, and ideally breastfeeding is initiated. Early initiation of breastfeeding is beneficial to the health of both the mother and the newborn. Both benefit because babies are extremely alert and programmed to latch onto the breast during this period. Mother–infant pairs that begin breastfeeding early are most able to continue breastfeeding for longer periods of time. For the mother, nursing accelerates the involution of the uterus, thereby reducing blood loss by increasing uterine contractions. For the newborn, there are important immunologic advantages. For example, various maternal antibodies are present in breast milk, which provide the newborn with passive immunity against certain infections. Also immunoglobulin (Ig) A, a secretory immunoglobulin present in significant amounts in breast milk, protects the infant's gut by preventing attachment of harmful bacteria to cells of the gut mucosal surface. It is also believed that maternal lymphocytes pass through the infant's gut wall and initiate immunologic processes that are not yet fully understood. In addition to the immunologic benefits, breast milk is the ideal nutritional source for the newborn. Moreover it is inexpensive and is usually in good supply. Given all the advantages (the above is only a partial list of the benefits), encouraging successful breastfeeding is an important health goal.

Induction and Augmentation of Labor

Induction of labor is the process of initiating labor by artificial means; augmentation is the artificial stimulation of labor that has begun spontaneously. Labor induction should be performed only after appropriate assessment of the mother and fetus. Additionally, the risks, benefits, and alternatives to induction in each case must be evaluated and explained to the patient. In the absence of medical indications for induction, fetal maturity must be confirmed by either exact pregnancy dating, first trimester ultrasound measurements, and/or amniotic fluid analysis. Evaluation of the cervical status in terms of effacement and softening is important in predicting success of induction and is highly recommended before any elective induction (Table 10–2). Generally, induction should be done in response to specific indications.

A. Indications

The following are common indications for induction of labor:

1. Maternal—Preeclampsia, diabetes mellitus, heart disease, and history of fast labors.

2. Fetal/maternal—Prolonged pregnancy, Rh incompatibility, fetal abnormality, chorioamnionitis, premature rupture of membranes, placental insufficiency, suspected intrauterine growth restriction.

Table 10–2. Bishop method of pelvic scoring for elective induction of labor.

Examination	Points		
	1	2	3
Cervical dilatation (cm)	1–2	3 4	5–6
Cervical effacement (%)	40–50	60–70	80
Station of presenting part	−1, −2	0	+1, +2
Consistency of cervix	Medium	Soft	...
Position of cervix	Middle	Anterior	...

Modified and reproduced, with permission, from Bishop EH: Pelvic scoring for elective induction. Obstet Gynecol 1964;24:66. Elective induction of labor may be performed safely when pelvic score is 9 or more.

B. Contraindications

Absolute contraindications to induction of labor include contracted pelvis; placenta previa; uterine scar because of previous classical cesarean section, myomectomy entering the endometrium, hysterotomy, or unification surgery; and transverse lie.

Labor induction should be carried out with caution in the following situations: breech presentation, oligohydramnios, multiple gestation, grand multiparity, previous cesarean section with transverse scar, prematurity, suspected fetal macrosomia.

Complications of Induction of Labor

A. For the Mother

In many cases, induction of labor exposes the mother to more distress and discomfort than judicious delay and subsequent vaginal or cesarean delivery. The following hazards must be kept in mind: (a) failure of induction with increased risk of cesarean delivery; (b) uterine inertia and prolonged labor; (c) tumultuous labor and tetanic contractions of the uterus, causing premature separation of the placenta, rupture of the uterus, and laceration of the cervix; (d) intrauterine infection; and (e) postpartum hemorrhage.

B. For the Fetus

An induced delivery exposes the infant to the risk of prematurity if the estimated date of conception has been inaccurately calculated. Precipitous delivery may result in physical injury. Prolapse of the cord may follow amniotomy. Injudicious administration of oxytocin or inadequate observation during induction could lead to fetal heart rate abnormalities or delivery of a baby with poor Apgar scores.

Methods of Cervical Ripening

Cervical ripening prior to induction of labor could facilitate the onset and progression of labor and increase the chance of vaginal delivery, particularly in primigravid patients.

A. Prostaglandin

Two forms of prostaglandins are commonly used for cervical ripening prior to induction at term: misoprostol (PGE_1) and dinoprostone (PGE_2) Although only dinoprostone, commercially available as prostaglandin gel, is currently Food and Drug Administration (FDA)-approved for this use, off-label use of misoprostol for cervical ripening is widely practiced. Indeed, although both misoprostol and dinoprostone applied locally intravaginally can provide significant improvement in the Bishop score, a meta-analysis of randomized, controlled trials focusing on cervical ripening and induction of labor found the time to delivery was shorter and the rate of cesarean delivery was lower in the misoprostol group.

Dinoprostone comes prepackaged in a single-dose syringe containing 0.5 mg of PGE_2 in 2.5 mL of a viscous gel of colloidal silicon dioxide in triacetin. The syringe is attached to a soft-plastic catheter for intracervical administration, and the catheter is shielded to help prevent application above the internal cervical os. Misoprostol is manufactured in 100-μg unscored and 200-μg scored tablets that can be administered orally, vaginally, and rectally. PGE_2 should not be used in patients with a history of asthma, glaucoma, or myocardial infarction. Unexplained vaginal bleeding, chorioamnionitis, ruptured membranes, and previous cesarean section are relative contraindications to the use of prostaglandins for cervical ripening.

For cervical ripening and induction at term, misoprostol is given vaginally at a dose of 25 μg every 4–6 hours. With dinoprostone, usually 12 hours should be allowed for cervical ripening, after which oxytocin induction should be started. PGE_1 and PGE_2 have similar side-effect and risk profiles, including fetal heart rate deceleration, fetal distress, emergency cesarean section, uterine hypertonicity, nausea, vomiting, fever, and peripartum infection. However, a current literature review does not indicate any significant differences in reported side effects between control and treatment groups with prostaglandin cervical ripening.

B. Relaxin

Relaxin is a polypeptide hormone that is produced in the human corpus luteum, decidua, and chorion. Purified protein relaxin, 2 mg in tylose gel, given vaginally or intracervically is noted to induce cervical ripening in 80% of cases and labor in about one-third of patients over a 12-hour period.

C. Balloon Catheter

A Foley catheter with a 25- to 50-mL balloon is passed into the endocervix above the internal os using tissue forceps. The balloon is then inflated with sterile saline, and the catheter is withdrawn gently to the level of internal cervical os. This method should induce cervical ripening over 8–12 hours. The cervix will be dilated 2–3 cm when the balloon falls out, which will make amniotomy possible, but effacement may be unchanged.

D. Hygroscopic Dilators

Laminaria tents are made from desiccated stems of the cold-water seaweed *Laminaria digitata* or *L. japonica.* When placed in the endocervix for 6–12 hours, the laminaria increases in diameter 3- to 4-fold by extracting water from cervical tissues, gradually swelling and expanding the cervical canal. Synthetic dilators like lamicel, a polyvinyl alcohol polymer sponge impregnated with 450 mg of magnesium sulfate, and dilapan, which is made from a stable nontoxic hydrophilic polymer of polyacrylonitrile, are also noted to be highly effective in mechanical cervical dilation.

Induction of Labor

A. OXYTOCIN

Intravenous administration of a very dilute solution of oxytocin is the most effective medical means of inducing labor. Oxytocin exaggerates the inherent rhythmic pattern of uterine motility, which often becomes clinically evident during the last trimester and increases as term is approached.

The dosage must be individualized. The administration of oxytocin is determined with a biologic assay: the smallest possible effective dose must be determined for each patient and then used to initiate and maintain labor. Constant observation by qualified attendants is required when this method is used.

In most cases it is sufficient to add 1 mL of oxytocin (10 units oxytocin to 1 L of 5% dextrose in water [1 mU/mL]). One acceptable oxytocin infusion regimen is to begin induction or augmentation at 1 mU/min, preferably with an infusion pump or other accurate delivery system, and increase oxytocin in 2-mU increments at 15-minute intervals.

When contractions of 50–60 mm Hg (per the internal monitor pressure) or lasting 40–60 seconds (per the external monitor) occur at 2.5- to 4-minute intervals, the oxytocin dose should be increased no further. Oxytocin infusion is discontinued whenever hyperstimulation or fetal distress is identified, but can be restarted when reassuring fetal heart rate and uterine activity patterns are restored.

B. AMNIOTOMY

Early and variable decelerations of the fetal heart rate are noted to be relatively common with amniotomy. Nonetheless, amniotomy may be an effective way to induce labor in carefully selected cases with high Bishop scores. Release of amniotic fluid shortens the muscle bundles of the myometrium; the strength and duration of the contractions are thereby increased and a more rapid contraction sequence follows. The membranes should be ruptured with an amniohook. Make no effort to strip the membranes, and do not displace the head upward to drain off amniotic fluid. Because amniotomy has not been proven effective in augmenting labor uniformly, it is recommended that the active phase of labor be entered prior to performing amniotomy for augmentation. Amniotomy in selected cases, while slightly increasing the risk of infectious morbidity, could shorten the course of labor without increasing or reducing the incidence of operative delivery.

REFERENCES

Bernal AL: Overview of current research in parturition. Exp Physiol 2000;86:213.

Eason E et al: Preventing perineal trauma during childbirth: A systematic review. Obstet Gynecol 2000;95:464.

El-Turkey M, Grant JM: Sweeping of the membrane is an effective method of induction of labor in prolonged pregnancy: A report of a randomized trial. Br J Obstet Gynaecol 1992;99:455.

Forman A et al: Evidence for a local effect of intracervical prostaglandin E_2. Am J Obstet Gynecol 1982;143:756.

Fraser WD, Sokol R: Amniotomy and maternal position in labor. Clin Obstet Gynecol 1992;35:535.

Goldberg AB, Greenberg BS, Darney PD: Misoprostol and pregnancy. N Engl J Med 2001;344:1.

Harbort GM Jr: Assessment of uterine contractility and activity. Clin Obstet Gynecol 1992;35:546.

Kazzi GM, Bottoms SF, Rosen MG: Efficacy and safety of *Laminaria digitata* for preinduction ripening of the cervix. Obstet Gynecol 1982;60:440.

Klein MC et al: Relationship of episiotomy to perineal trauma and morbidity, sexual dysfunction, and pelvic floor relaxation. Am J Obstet Gynecol 1994;171:591.

Laifer SA: Oral intake during labor. Clin Consult Obstet Gynecol 1992;4:206.

Lange AP et al: Prelabor evaluation of inducibility. Obstet Gynecol 1982;60:137.

Martin JN Jr, Morrison JC, Wiser WL: Vaginal birth after cesarean section: The demise of routine repeat abdominal delivery. Obstet Gynecol Clin North Am 1988;15:719.

McColgin SW et al: Stripping membranes at term: Can it safely reduce the incidence of postterm pregnancy? Obstet Gynecol 1990;76:678.

Owen J, Hauth JC: Oxytocin for the induction or augmentation of labor. Clin Obstet Gynecol 1992;35:464.

Renfrew MJ et al: Practices that minimize trauma to the genital tract in childbirth: A systematic review of the literature. Birth 1998;25:143.

Sheiner E et al: The impact of early amniotomy on mode of delivery and pregnancy outcome. Arch Gynecol Obstet 2000;264:63.

Essentials of Normal Newborn Assessment and Care

Elisabeth L. Raab, MD

A full-term newborn is a baby born at 37 weeks' or more gestation. Term newborns are evaluated in the delivery room immediately following birth to assure that they do not require respiratory or circulatory support, have no birth-related trauma or congenital anomalies requiring immediate intervention and are transitioning as expected to extrauterine life. Approximately 97% of newborns are healthy and are transferred to the normal newborn nursery after birth. In the nursery, newborns receive a thorough evaluation to determine maturity, evaluate growth and development and identify those with signs of acute illness or underlying congenital disease.

DELIVERY ROOM MANAGEMENT

At every delivery there should be at least one person whose primary responsibility is attending to the newborn. Although approximately 90% of the time no resuscitation will be required, the attendant must be able to recognize signs of distress in a newborn and carry out a skilled resuscitation.

After the umbilical cord is cut, newborns should be placed in a warm environment. They may be placed on the mother's chest, skin-to-skin, or they may be brought to a radiant warmer. Early skin-to-skin contact increases the likelihood and duration of breastfeeding, decreases infant crying, and positively impacts early signs of bonding, and is therefore encouraged when possible. However, it should only be done when the newborn is vigorous and there are no risk factors that increase the likelihood that resuscitation will be required. The infant is dried with prewarmed towels to prevent heat loss and the airway is positioned and cleared to ensure patency. The airway is cleared by suctioning the mouth and nares with a bulb syringe or a suction catheter connected to mechanical suction. If the newborn is well-appearing and not at increased risk, the airway can be cleared simply by wiping the mouth and nose with a towel.

During this initial postpartum period the newborn's respiratory effort, heart rate, color, and activity are evaluated to determine the need for intervention. If drying and suctioning do not provide adequate stimulus, it is appropriate to flick the soles or rub the back to stimulate breathing. It is important to note the presence of meconium in the amniotic fluid or on the newborn's skin. All newborns born with meconium-stained amniotic fluid should have the oropharynx suctioned by the obstetrician upon delivery of the head. If a newborn is in distress or has depressed respiratory effort and there is evidence that meconium was passed in utero, the appropriate intervention is to intubate and suction the trachea before stimulating the baby in any way. Meconium can block the airway, preventing the newborn lungs from filling with oxygen, a vital step in normal transitioning. An active, crying, well-appearing newborn does not require endotracheal intubation, regardless of the presence of meconium staining or the thickness of the meconium.

If the newborn remains apneic despite drying, suctioning, and stimulation, or if there are signs of distress such as grunting, central cyanosis, or bradycardia, resuscitation should quickly be initiated. The initial step in neonatal resuscitation is to provide positive pressure ventilation (PPV) and the decision to initiate PPV should ideally be made within the first 30 seconds after birth.

THE ASSIGNMENT OF APGAR SCORES

The Apgar score was introduced by Virginia Apgar in 1952 to quantitatively evaluate the newborn's condition after birth (Table 11–1). Scores between 0 and 2 in each of 5 different categories are assigned at 1 and 5 minutes of life. The score reflects the cardiorespiratory and neurologic status at those time points. If the score is less than 7 at 5 minutes, scores should be assigned every 5 minutes until the baby has a score of 7 or greater or has reached 20 minutes of life. The Apgar score is not what determines the need for resuscitation. Although scores are based on the same elements used to evaluate the newborn's status, the assessment of the need for intervention with PPV should already have been made by the time the 1-minute Apgar score is assigned. Studies do not show a correlation between a low 1-minute Apgar score and outcome. However, the change between the scores at 1 and

Table 11–1. Apgar scoring.

Signs	Points Scored		
	0	1	2
Heartbeats per minute	Absent	Slow (< 100)	Over 100
Respiratory effort	Absent	Slow, irregular	Good, crying
Muscle tone	Limp	Some flexion of extremities	Active motion
Reflex irritability	No response	Grimace	Cry or cough
Color	Blue or pale	Body pink, extremities blue	Completely pink

5 minutes is a meaningful measure of the effectiveness of the resuscitation efforts and a 5-minute score of 0–3 is associated with increased mortality in both preterm and full-term infants. It is important to know that factors such as prematurity, maternal medications and congenital disease can adversely impact scores.

THE IMPORTANCE OF THE PRENATAL AND INTRAPARTUM HISTORY

Knowledge of the prenatal and intrapartum history is essential for adequate care of the newborn. The history should be reviewed before delivery (if possible) as it may alter care in the immediate postpartum period. For example, information about the use of certain anesthetic drugs during labor and delivery alerts those attending the delivery to the possibility of newborn respiratory depression and allows them to anticipate a role for the use of naloxone in the resuscitation. Other important pieces of information are the presence of chronic disease in the mother (such as diabetes mellitus, Grave's disease, or systemic lupus erythematosus), maternal illicit or prescription drug use, prenatal ultrasound findings, maternal screening laboratory test results, and the presence of risk factors for neonatal infection. All of these will impact how the newborn is monitored during the nursery admission and in the first few weeks of life, and adequate care is not possible without them.

INITIAL EXAM

Although a complete and detailed physical exam is delayed until the newborn is admitted to the nursery and has had time to transition to extrauterine life, a brief examination should be done shortly after delivery to rule out any problems that require immediate attention.

Airway

The airway should be evaluated for patency. A suction catheter may be passed through each naris if needed to remove secretions from the nasopharynx or if there is concern about the possibility of choanal atresia, but is not necessary if adequate clearance of secretions is achieved with a bulb syringe and the newborn is breathing comfortably. Although a suction catheter is an effective means of removing secretions, it should be used cautiously as it can induce bradycardia and cause trauma and edema to the mucous membranes.

Chest

The chest should be examined to determine the adequacy of the respiratory effort. One should assess chest wall movement, respiratory rate and breathing pattern and look for signs of distress such as retractions. Crackles are often audible initially, but should clear over time as fetal lung fluid is being resorbed and the lungs inflate with air. Decreased breath sounds may result from pneumothorax, atelectasis, and consolidation as a result of pneumonia or effusions. The presence of asymmetric breath sounds should be noted as they may alert the examiner to the presence of an intrathoracic mass. Heart rate and rhythm should be evaluated and the presence or absence of a murmur noted. The heart rate should be greater than 100 beats per minute.

Abdomen

The abdomen should be soft and nondistended. A distended, firm abdomen may indicate a bowel obstruction, pneumoperitoneum, or intra-abdominal mass. A scaphoid abdomen, when accompanied by respiratory distress, should raise the examiner's suspicion of a diaphragmatic hernia. The umbilical stump should be examined and the number of blood vessels noted. A single umbilical artery may be a clue to the presence of other anomalies, renal anomalies in particular.

Skin

The skin color should be evaluated. Although acrocyanosis, bluish discoloration of the hands and feet, may be seen in well newborns, central cyanosis of the trunk is not normal for longer than a few seconds after birth and is a sign that the newborn is not receiving sufficient oxygen. Cyanosis and pallor can result from a wide variety of causes such as sepsis, anemia, respiratory insufficiency with or without abnormally elevated cardiac vascular resistance, congenital heart disease, and hypoxic–ischemic injury with cardiac dysfunction; the pre- and intrapartum history is often useful in determining the etiology. A cyanotic infant with a normal heart rate and respiratory effort may be given free-flow 100% oxygen by face mask or tubing held close to the nose and should be observed for improvement in skin coloring. If the skin does not become pink, the patient may require positive pressure ventilation to achieve improved oxygenation.

Genitalia

It is important to closely evaluate the genitalia prior to pronouncing the sex of the newborn. If there is ambiguity of the genitalia the situation must be explained to the parents and a full evaluation, including karyotyping and consultation with a pediatric endocrinologist and urologist, should be done prior to gender assignment.

General

Alertness, activity, tone and movement of the extremities should be noted. The face and extremities should be evaluated for evidence of congenital anomalies or birth trauma. The most common birth-related injuries are nerve injuries (facial and brachial nerve palsies) and fractures (primarily clavicular). Unilateral peripheral facial nerve palsy should be suspected when the newborn has normal movement of the forehead, but difficulty closing the eye and flattening of the nasolabial folds on the affected side and an asymmetric facial expression with crying (the unaffected side will go down). Peripheral facial nerve injury is thought to result from compression of the nerve against the sacrum during delivery and is not associated with the use of forceps in delivery. The risk of brachial plexus injury is increased when there is shoulder dystocia or the baby is large for gestational age (LGA). Erb's palsy (C5-C6 injury) manifests as an inability to externally rotate or abduct the shoulder; the affected arm is held adducted and internally rotated and is extended and pronated at the elbow ("waiter-tip" position). If the C5-T1 nerve roots are all affected, the function of the hand will be affected as well.

CARE AND OBSERVATION IN THE FIRST FEW HOURS OF LIFE

A single 1 mg intramuscular injection of vitamin K is recommended for all newborns to prevent bleeding as a result of vitamin K deficiency. Vitamin K prophylaxis has been standard of care since 1961, when it was first recommended by the American Academy of Pediatrics (AAP). Standard newborn care also includes applying either 0.5% erythromycin ointment, 1% silver nitrate solution, or 1% tetracycline ointment to the infant's eyes shortly after birth to prevent infectious neonatal conjunctivitis.

The well newborn may remain with the mother after birth and attempt an initial feed. There should be continued intermittent assessment to assure that there is no cardiorespiratory distress, temperature instability, altered level of activity, or other signs of distress. It is important that caregivers are aware that babies that require resuscitation after birth are at increased risk of difficulties with transitioning and must be monitored closely.

NEWBORN NURSERY CARE

Vital Signs

Vital signs should be recorded by the nursing staff for all newborns admitted to the nursery. Body temperature is typically measured in the axilla. Fever, defined as a temperature greater than 38.0° Celsius, is often caused by excessive environmental heat or overbundling when it occurs shortly after birth. Hypothermia may result if newborns are left in the delivery room unbundled and off the radiant warmer. A newborn with hypothermia or hyperthermia whose temperature fails to normalize in response to appropriate environmental measures should be evaluated for possible sepsis and central nervous system pathology.

A normal respiratory rate for a newborn is typically between 40 and 60 breaths per minute. A normal heart rate for a newborn is generally 100–160 bpm, but varies considerably with sleep and activity level. If measured, pulse oximetry should be > 95% in the term baby. Blood pressure varies with gestation and birth weight. There is still debate about what constitutes an abnormal blood pressure in a neonate, but hypotension in the first 12–24 hours of life is typically defined as a mean blood pressure less than the gestational age. Hypertension in the full-term newborn is defined as a systolic blood pressure greater than 90 mm Hg and diastolic blood pressure greater than 60 mm Hg and a mean blood pressure > 70 mm Hg. Blood pressures should be measured in all 4 extremities if there is any suspicion of cardiac disease. Coarctation of the aorta is characterized by elevated blood pressure in the upper extremities and decreased pressure in the lower extremities.

Growth and Development

Weight, length, and head circumference should be measured and plotted on curves to assess intrauterine growth (Fig 11–1). Newborns that are small for gestational age (SGA), historically defined as less than the 10th percentile on the growth curve, may warrant evaluation for congenital infections, chromosomal syndromes or other causes if there is no identifiable cause for the growth retardation, such as multiple pregnancy or preeclampsia or other evidence of placental insufficiency. Infants that are SGA or large for gestational age (LGA) should be treated similarly to the infants of diabetic mothers, and should be monitored for hypoglycemia in the first few hours of life.

Although gestational age is usually estimated prior to delivery by prenatal ultrasounds (preferably early on in the pregnancy) or the mother's last menstrual period, information is sometimes unavailable or inaccurate and maturity should be reassessed postnatally. There are measures, such as Ballard's modified version of the Dubowitz exam (Table 11–2), which incorporate multiple elements of the physical exam and may be useful at 12–24 hours of life to help determine gestational age.

Physical Exam

A physician should perform a complete physical exam of the newborn within the first 24 hours of life.

A. SKIN

As on the initial brief examination, the color of the skin should be evaluated and the presence of cyanosis, pallor, or jaundice noted. The healthy newborn should be pink. Postterm infants often have dry, cracked skin. Clinical jaundice is rare in the first 24 hours of life and should trigger an evaluation. Plethora, often seen in infants of diabetic mothers, may indicate significant polycythemia. Practice varies, but most neonatologists consider a hematocrit greater than 70% in an asymptomatic newborn and 65% in a symptomatic newborn grounds for a partial exchange transfusion. Symptoms of hyperviscosity include hypoxia, hypoglycemia, increased work of breathing, and seizures. Neurologic sequelae can be serious.

Petechiae are often present over the face and upper torso, particularly when a nuchal cord is present. When present below the nipple line, petechiae should raise concern about the possibility of sepsis or platelet dysfunction. Bruising occurs frequently, especially with breech presentation, but should be noted as it may lead to excessive hemolysis and hyperbilirubinemia when extensive. Mongolian spots are dark purple-blue hyperpigmented areas usually over the back and buttocks that look like bruising, but are clusters of melanocytes deep within the dermis. They are present in a majority of black and Asian newborns and fade over time. Dermal sinuses, dimples, and cysts should be noted; they may indicate underlying defects or pose a risk for infection.

The most common newborn rash is erythema toxicum, which presents at 24–48 hours of life in almost half of all newborns as erythematous papular-pustular lesions that tend to spare the palms and soles. Other

Figure 11–1. Classification of newborns based on gestational age plotted against head circumference, length, and weight. AGA, appropriate for gestational age; LGA, large for gestational age; SGA, small for gestational age.

Table 11–2. Newborn maturity rating and classification.

	0	1	2	3	4	5
Neuromuscular maturity						
Posture						
Square window (wrist)	90°	60°	45°	30°	0°	
Arm recoil	180°		100°–180°	90°–100°	< 90°	
Popliteal angle	180°	160°	130°	110°	90°	< 90°
Scarf sign						
Heel to ear						
Physical maturity						
Skin	Gelatinous, red, transparent	Smooth, pink; visible veins	Superficial peeling and/or rash; few veins	Cracking, pale area; rare veins	Parchment, deep cracking; no vessels	Leathery, cracked, wrinkled
Lanugo	None	Abundant	Thinning	Bald areas	Mostly bald	
Plantar creases	No crease	Faint red marks	Anterior transverse crease only	Creases anterior two-thirds	Creases cover entire sole	
Breast	Barely perceptible	Flat areola; no bud	Stippled areola; bud, 1–2 mm	Raised areola; bud, 3–4 mm	Full areola; bud, 5–10 mm	
Ear	Pinna flat; stays folded	Slightly curved pinna; soft; slow recoil	Well-curved pinna; soft; ready recoil	Formed and firm; instant recoil	Thick cartilage; ear stiff	
Genitalia (male)	Scrotum empty; no rugae		Testes descending; few rugae	Testes down; good rugae	Testes pendulous; deep rugae	
Genitalia (female)	Prominent clitoris and labia minora		Majora and minora equally prominent	Majora large; minora small	Clitoris and minora completely covered	

The following information should be recorded: Birth date and Apgar score at 1 and 5 minutes. Two separate examinations should be made within the first 24 hours to determine the estimated gestational age according to maturity rating. Each examination and the age of the infant at each examination should be noted.

Maturity rating:

Score	5	10	15	20	25	30	35	40	45	50
Weeks	26	28	30	32	34	36	38	40	42	44

frequently seen benign rashes include milia, small white papules typically around the nares, and transient neonatal pustular melanosis, small vesicles or pustules present at birth that leave pigmented macules surrounded by scale when they disappear.

Hemangiomas and vascular malformations may be present at birth. Hemangiomas are benign tumors of vascular endothelium and are often not present at birth, but may be noted soon after. They eventually involute without therapy, but only after an initial period of growth, usually of 6–12 months. If present near the eyes or airways they may require early intervention to prevent visual or airway compromise. In contrast, vascular malformations such as port-wine stains and salmon patches are always present at birth. Developmental anomalies composed of one or more types of vessels typically grow as the child grows and do not resolve spontaneously.

B. HEAD, FACE, AND NECK

The head should be evaluated for any asymmetry. The sutures lines may be open or slightly overriding, but premature fusion requires intervention as it presents a constraint to brain growth. The anterior fontanelle should be soft, not tense or bulging, when the newborn is calm. It is typically 1–4 cm in size, and may be enlarged with hypothyroidism or increased intracranial pressure. The posterior fontanelle is typically <1 cm and may not be palpable.

Scalp edema (caput succedaneum) can most easily be differentiated from a cephalohematoma (a localized collection of blood under the dura mater) by noting whether or not the swelling crosses suture lines; cephalohematoma is typically confined by suture lines. A cephalohematoma should raise awareness of the possible development of hyperbilirubinemia as the collection of blood is broken down and resorbed. Skull fractures can occur and the skull should be palpated carefully.

The face should be evaluated for dysmorphic features, malformations, and asymmetries. Micrognathia may cause significant airway compromise in the neonate and is associated with various syndromes. The palate should be palpated to ensure that it is not high-arched or clefted. A naris is patent if there is air movement through it (demonstrated by holding cotton in front of it) when the mouth and other naris are closed. Subconjunctival hemorrhages are a common finding as a result of the birth process. An absent red reflex should prompt an immediate ophthalmologic evaluation to rule out a congenital cataract, retinoblastoma, or glaucoma. Pupils should be equal and reactive. Abnormalities of the positioning or formation of the eyes, nose, or ears may suggest specific syndromes or chromosomal defects. Although preauricular tags and pits have been associated with renal malformations, there is no current evidence to suggest that their presence, when an isolated finding, is sufficient to warrant a renal ultrasound. The neck should be examined for masses, cysts, and webbing. The clavicles should be palpated for crepitus, swelling, and tenderness, which would suggest an underlying fracture. Although not usually detected until several weeks of age, torticollis may occur as a result of ischemia within, or hemorrhage into, the sternocleidomastoid muscle at birth. It manifests as a head tilt with or without a fibrous mass palpable in the muscle. Surgery is rarely necessary; the overwhelming majority of cases are managed with a home stretching regimen or physical therapy.

C. CHEST

The chest should be evaluated for deformities such as widely spaced or accessory nipples and pectus excavatum. Breast buds may be present in both sexes and are normal, a product of exposure to circulating maternal hormones in utero.

The respiratory effort and rate should be evaluated, looking for signs of respiratory distress. Early on, tachypnea may be the only sign of pathologic processes as varied as pneumonia, amniotic fluid and/or meconium aspiration syndrome, sepsis, or congenital heart disease (CHD). Breath sounds are auscultated, paying attention to the quality of the breath sounds, the air entry, and any asymmetry that is present across the lung fields. Asymmetry of the breath sounds may indicate an area of consolidation from atelectasis or infection, a pneumothorax, effusion, or mass. Upper airway sounds, such as congestion or stridor, are often mistaken for abnormal breath sounds on exam. The listener can usually distinguish noises of upper airway origin from those of intrathoracic origin by listening for the presence of the sounds over the patient's neck. Respiratory distress or an abnormal lung exam should be evaluated with a chest radiograph. In an emergency situation where a pneumothorax is suspected, a transilluminator may be used. Transillumination is increased over the side of a pneumothorax, but it is sometimes difficult to assess accurately and should be confirmed by chest radiograph when possible prior to needle aspiration or chest tube placement.

A hyperdynamic precordium may indicate underlying heart disease with volume overload to one or both ventricles. The heart is auscultated to evaluate the heart rate and rhythm and characterize the heart sounds. A split-second heart sound can assure the examiner that both the aortic and pulmonary valves are present. A murmur should be described by where it is heard, what it sounds like, if it occurs in systole or diastole, and how loud it is. Murmurs are often audible in the newborn and are frequently innocent. Innocent murmurs are often attributed to a closing ductus arteriosus or foramen ovale, but the most commonly heard innocent murmur in the neonate is produced by peripheral pulmonic stenosis (PPS). PPS murmurs occur during systole and are best heard over the back or axillae.

Murmurs may or may not be present in newborns with CHD. Ventricular septal defects, the most common form of CHD, have a characteristic harsh, systolic murmur associated with them. However, the pressures in the newborn pulmonary system are still high (roughly equal to systemic pressures) and thus there is usually no flow gradient across a large ventricular defect to produce a murmur in the first few days of life. Complex CHD typically presents as cyanosis, tachypnea, or shock, and will rarely present as an asymptomatic murmur. Signs may develop quickly with closure of the ductus arteriosus if the lesion has ductal-dependent pulmonary or systemic flow. The initial steps in evaluating a stable patient for suspected CHD include 4-extremity blood pressure measurements, measurement of pre- and postductal saturations, electrocardiogram, chest radiography, and a hyperoxia test. The diagnosis of CHD is usually established by echocardiogram.

D. ABDOMEN

The examiner should listen for bowel sounds and palpate the abdomen for masses, organomegaly, or abnormal musculature. The liver is easily palpable in the newborn and the inferior edge is usually 1–2 cm below the right costal margin. It is often possible to palpate the kidneys and spleen. Absence of the abdominal musculature may be associated with significant urinary tract abnormalities. The umbilical stump should be assessed for redness or induration to suggest infection. Umbilical hernias are common and typically require no intervention in infancy. Omphalocele and gastroschisis are major abdominal wall defects and require emergent surgical evaluation. Omphalocele is a > 4-cm midline abdominal wall defect. Bowel, and often liver, herniate through the defect, and the umbilicus is typically on the anterior aspect of the omphalocele. Unless ruptured, an omphalocele is covered by a membrane, unlike a gastroschisis. The defect in gastroschisis is typically to the right of the umbilicus on the abdominal wall. The entire bowel may be externalized, but the liver typically remains internal. Bowel atresias may be present in gastroschisis. Omphalocele is more frequently associated with other congenital anomalies whereas gastroschisis occurs more commonly in intrauterine growth restriction (IUGR) and with young maternal age.

E. GENITALIA

The penile length and clitoral size should be inspected to rule out ambiguous genitalia. The labia majora should cover the labia minora and clitoris in a term female. White mucouslike discharge from the vagina is often present and is physiologic.

The scrotum should be evaluated for hernias or masses and descent of the testicles. Transillumination of the scrotum will help to distinguish a hydrocele from an inguinal hernia. The position of the urethral meatus is important to note, as the presence of hypospadias should preclude routine circumcision so as to allow for optimal surgical correction of the hypospadias.

F. ANUS

The rectum should be evaluated for patency and position. An anteriorly displaced rectum may be associated with a rectogenital fistula.

G. MUSCULOSKELETAL SYSTEM

The extremities, spine, and hips are examined for signs of fracture, malformation, or deformation. Range of motion of the joints is assessed. Arthrogryposis, contractures of the joints, may be seen with neuromuscular disease or oligohydramnios as a result of decreased or limited movement in utero. Abnormalities of the extremities, such as polydactyly or syndactyly, are seen in different chromosomal abnormalities and syndromes, and may help in making the diagnosis. Particular attention should be paid to the examination of the hips (despite the fact that a dislocation may not be detectable in the first weeks of life) because developmental dysplasia of the hip (DDH) can cause permanent damage if left undetected throughout the first year of life. Either the Barlow or Ortolani test may be used to determine whether a dislocation is present. The Barlow test involves positioning the patient on the back, bringing the knees together at midline, and then pushing down and out on the upper inner thighs. The Ortolani test involves pushing downward on the femurs while abducting the hips. With both maneuvers the dislocation is detected as a clunk as the femoral head is dislocated from the acetabulum (posteriorly with the Barlow, laterally with the Ortolani). Asymmetry of the gluteal folds and skin creases of the legs is another clue to the presence of DDH.

H. NEUROLOGIC SYSTEM

Observing the activity level, alertness and positioning of the newborn provides a tremendous amount of information about the overall state of health. A healthy, full-term newborn at rest should lie with the extremities flexed. Decreased tone may be a sign of neuro-muscular or systemic illness such as sepsis. There should be spontaneous intermittent movement of all 4 limbs and the baby should be alert during at least portions of the examination. Pupil size and symmetry should be noted. Primitive reflexes such as the Moro, grasp, suck, and tonic neck reflex should all be present at birth. To elicit the Moro reflex, the newborn is supported with a hand under the back and then rapidly dropped a few centimeters back toward the examination bed. The full Moro reflex consists of extension and then flexion and adduction of the arms ("embrace"), opening of the eyes, and a cry. Reflexes are elicited by tapping a finger over the appropriate tendon. Significant clonus may be a sign of central nervous system injury. A sacral dimple or tuft of hair over the sacral spine may indicate spina bifida occulta and should be evaluated with a spinal ultrasound; if the findings of the ultrasound are equivocal, a magnetic resonance imaging (MRI) scan should be done at approximately 3 months of age.

FEEDING

The benefits of breastfeeding on everything from the strength of the immune system to developmental outcomes and IQ have been well documented. The caloric value of human milk is clearly superior to formula and it is the most easily digested form of infant nutrition. Mothers should be counseled prenatally about the benefits of breastfeeding and encouraged by their obstetric caregivers to consider breastfeeding. Contraindications to breastfeeding include human immunodeficiency virus (HIV) infection, active tuberculosis infection and the use of certain medications. Maternal hepatitis C virus (HCV) infection is not a contraindication to breastfeeding. Transmission of HCV via breastmilk is not documented in the absence of coexisting maternal infection with HIV. Nevertheless, infected mothers should be informed that transmission via breastmilk is theoretically possible.

Breastfeeding may be difficult and frustrating for new mothers. It is important that the newborn nursery staff work to provide mothers with the support and knowledge they need to make breastfeeding a positive experience. It is also important that mothers of newborns who require bottle supplementation (such as a dehydrated, jaundiced infant) are reassured that their efforts at breastfeeding will not be derailed by exposure to the bottle during a limited, medically necessary period, and that breastfeeding can still ultimately succeed.

Regardless of the overwhelming literature to support the value of breastmilk, many mothers in the United States choose to bottle-feed their children. Selection of the formula given to the newborn is often based on what formula is available in the nursery or by the mother's preference. Standard-term infant formula contains iron supplementation and provides 20 kcal/oz. No one formula is better than another for healthy term infants. Mothers with a family history of lactose intolerance sometimes request soy formula and standard soy formula will provide adequate nutrition for growth and development. Formulas such as Alimentum and Nutramigen are available for infants with more significant protein allergy. Premature infant formulas contain 24 kcal/oz and provide higher amounts of protein, medium-chain triglycerides, and vitamins and minerals (such as calcium and phosphorous) than standard formulas. The AAP currently recommends formula for the first year of life.

VOIDING AND STOOLING

Voiding should be monitored closely in the nursery. Changes in the baby's weight and the frequency of urination can be used to assess the hydration status and adequacy of intake in a breastfeeding baby. The time of the first void of urine and stool should be documented. Failure to void in the first 24 hours of life should prompt an evaluation for renal function and hydration status. Failure to pass stool in the first 48 hours of life should prompt an evaluation for possible bowel obstruction; 94% of normal term newborns will pass meconium in the first 24 hours of life. Obstruction can result from conditions such as bowel atresia or stenosis, Hirschsprung disease, and meconium ileus.

NEWBORN SCREENING AND PROPHYLAXIS

The initial newborn exam may be normal despite the presence of serious occult illness. Signs of complex congenital heart disease, sepsis, gastrointestinal obstruction, significant jaundice, inborn errors of metabolism, and other illnesses may not be present until the second or third day of life at the earliest: shortly before, and at times after, the baby's discharge. Screening is done in the hopes of detecting disease before a patient becomes symptomatic. Screening is usually reserved for processes that have a worse prognosis if not detected early and for which we have effective therapy. The maternal medical history, the obstetric and perinatal history, and state laws determine what screening is done on any given baby.

Standard newborn screening tests screen for the following:

1. Phenylketonuria by Guthrie test for phenylalanine level.
2. Congenital hypothyroidism by thyroid function testing.

3. Congenital syphilis by either rapid plasma reagent (RPR) or Venereal Disease Research Laboratory (VDRL) test (whichever test was performed on the mother).
4. ABO incompatibility using infant blood type and direct Coombs' test (standard if mother has O blood type, done at many institutions for all newborns).
5. Hearing loss (evaluated by auditory brainstem response or otoacoustic emissions).

In most states, standard screening also includes testing for sickle cell anemia, galactosemia, congenital adrenal hyperplasia and a small number of less common diseases. Some states are now doing expanded newborn screens by tandem mass spectrometry, a method that can screen for a large number of metabolic diseases from a single blood sample.

Additional targeted screening often includes evaluation for infection, illicit drug exposure, hyperbilirubinemia and hypoglycemia when there are risk factors that increase the yield of the testing. A history of rupture of amniotic membranes for greater than 18 hours prior to delivery, maternal intrapartum fever, chorioamnionitis and a positive maternal group B streptococcus culture without adequate treatment prior to delivery are all risk factors for newborn sepsis. A history of any of these risk factors warrants a screening evaluation of the asymptomatic newborn for laboratory evidence of infection. Screening is routinely done for hypoglycemia in infants of diabetic mothers as well as for SGA and LGA babies. At many institutions, infants of diabetic mothers are screened for polycythemia as well.

Information about maternal hepatitis B, HIV, herpes simplex virus (HSV), chlamydia, and syphilis status is essential to newborn care. Adequate prophylaxis for hepatitis B can prevent transmission in 95% of infants born to hepatitis B surface antigen-positive (HBsAg+) mothers. A baby born to a mother who is HBsAg+ should receive the hepatitis B vaccine and hepatitis B immune globulin (HBIg) within the first 12 hours of life in order to prevent hepatitis B virus (HBV) transmission. If the mother's status is unknown, the newborn should receive the vaccine within 12 hours of birth and every effort should be made to determine the mother's status. If the baby weighs more than 2 kg, HBIg can be given as late as 7 days of life if maternal status is positive or still unknown and still provide effective postexposure prophylaxis. However, a baby who weighs <2 kg at birth should receive HBIg by 12 hours of postnatal life to receive adequate prophylaxis. Appropriate screening and treatment for infants born to mothers with a history of infection with HIV, chlamydia, HSV, or syphilis are detailed in the AAP's *Red Book*.

CIRCUMCISION

Routine circumcision is not currently recommended by the AAP. Although there is evidence that supports some medical benefits of circumcision (such as decreased incidence of urinary tract infections during infancy, sexually transmitted disease, and penile cancer), the data is insufficient for the AAP to recommend the procedure for all newborn males given concerns about the impossibility of informed consent in an infant and evidence of the pain and stress caused by the procedure. Parents should be provided with unbiased information about the procedure and the decision to proceed should be left to them. If circumcision is performed, analgesia, either topical or by nerve block, should be given.

DISCHARGE PLANNING

The physician should complete another thorough examination on the day of discharge to reevaluate the overall health of the newborn. Anticipatory guidance should be given to parents to help them care for their newborns and recognize signs of illness and distress. Safety issues, such as the use of car seats, should be addressed. Parents should be alerted to problems such as fever, lethargy, and poor feeding that should prompt them to see a physician. They should be taught about expected newborn behavior, adequate feeding, monitoring of voiding and stooling, and umbilical cord care.

Anticipatory guidance is particularly important now that hospital stays after delivery are often only 36–48 hours. Criteria for newborn discharge at less than 48 hours of life are outlined in a 2004 AAP policy statement. Newborns discharged before 48 hours of life must be examined by a health care professional within 48 hours of the discharge. The plan for the newborn's first visit to the physician and any necessary follow-up laboratory testing or nursing visits to the home should be clearly established at the time of discharge and parents should be able to demonstrate skill and comfort with feeding and tending to the baby's basic needs.

REFERENCES

American Academy of Pediatrics: AAP 2003 Red Book: Report of the Committee on Infectious Diseases, 26th ed. American Academy of Pediatrics, 2003.
American Academy of Pediatrics, Committee on Fetus and Newborn: Controversies concerning vitamin K and the newborn policy statement. Pediatrics 2003;112(1):191.

American Academy of Pediatrics, Committee on Fetus and New-born: Hospital stay for healthy term newborns policy statement. Pediatrics 2004;113(5):1434.

American Academy of Pediatrics, Committee on Fetus and New-born and American College of Obstetricians and Gynecologists, Committee on Obstetric Practice: Use and abuse of the apgar score. Pediatrics 1996;98(1):141.

American Academy of Pediatrics, Task Force on Circumcision: Circumcision policy statement. Pediatrics 1999;103(3):686.

American Academy of Pediatrics and American Heart Association: Textbook of Neonatal Resuscitation, 4th ed. American Academy of Pediatrics, 2000.

Casey BM, McIntire DD, Leveno KJ: The continuing value of the Apgar score for the assessment of newborn infants. N Engl J Med 2001;344(7):467.

Swenson D, Sherman JO, Fisher JH: Diagnosis of congenital megacolon: An analysis of 501 patients. J Pediatr Surg 1973;8(5):587.

The Normal Puerperium

Kim Lipscomb, MD, & Miles J. Novy, MD

The puerperium, or postpartum period, generally lasts 6–12 weeks and is the period of adjustment after delivery when the anatomic and physiologic changes of pregnancy are reversed, and the body returns to the normal nonpregnant state. The postpartum period has been arbitrarily divided into the immediate puerperium—the first 24 hours after parturition—when acute postanesthetic or postdelivery complications may occur; the early puerperium, which extends until the first week postpartum; and the remote puerperium, which includes the period of time required for involution of the genital organs and return of menses, usually by 6 weeks in nonlactating women, and the return of normal cardiovascular and psychological function, which may require months.

ANATOMIC & PHYSIOLOGIC CHANGES DURING THE PUERPERIUM

Uterine Involution

The uterus increases markedly in size and weight during pregnancy (about 10 times the nonpregnant weight, reaching a crude weight of 1000 g) but involutes rapidly after delivery to the nonpregnant weight of 50 to 100 g. The gross anatomic and histologic characteristics of this process have been studied through autopsy, hysterectomy, and endometrial specimens. In addition, the decrease in size of the uterus and cervix has been demonstrated by magnetic resonance imaging, sonography, and computed tomography.

Immediately following delivery, the uterus weighs about 1 kg, and its size approximates that of a 20-week pregnancy (at the level of the umbilicus). At the end of the first postpartum week, it normally will have decreased to the size of a 12-week gestation and is just palpable at the symphysis pubis (Fig 12–1). Ultrasonography can be used to measure length and width of the uterine cavity. During the first week, there is a 31% decrease in uterine area; during the second and third weeks, a 48% decrease; and subsequently, an 18% decrease. The observed changes in uterine area are mainly due to changes in uterine length, as the transverse diameter remains relatively constant during the puerperium.

Myometrial contractions or **afterpains** assist in involution. These contractions occur during the first 2–3 days of the puerperium and produce more discomfort in multiparas than in primiparas. Such pains are accentuated during nursing as a result of oxytocin release from the posterior pituitary. During the first 12 hours postpartum, uterine contractions are regular, strong, and coordinated (Fig 12–2). The intensity, frequency, and regularity of contractions decrease after the first postpartum day as involutional changes proceed. Uterine involution is nearly complete by 6 weeks, at which time the organ weighs less than 100 g. The increase in the amount of connective tissue and elastin in the myometrium and blood vessels and the increase in numbers of cells are permanent to some degree, so the uterus is slightly larger following pregnancy.

Changes in the Placental Implantation Site

Following delivery of the placenta, there is immediate contraction of the placental site to a size less than half the diameter of the original placenta. This contraction, as well as arterial smooth muscle contractions, leads to hemostasis. Involution occurs by means of the extension and downgrowth of marginal endometrium and by endometrial regeneration from the glands and stroma in the decidua basalis.

By day 16, placental site, endometrial, and superficial myometrial infiltrates of granulocytes and mononuclear cells are seen. Regeneration of endometrial glands and endometrial stroma has also begun. Endometrial regeneration at the placental site is not complete until 6 weeks postpartum. In the disorder termed **subinvolution of the placental site,** complete obliteration of the vessels in the placental site fails to occur. Patients with this condition have persistent lochia and are subject to brisk hemorrhagic episodes. This condition usually can be treated with uterotonics. In the rare event uterine curettage is performed, partly obliterated hyalinized vessels can be seen on the histologic specimen.

Normal postpartum discharge begins as **lochia rubra,** containing blood, shreds of tissue, and decidua. The amount of discharge rapidly tapers and changes to a reddish-brown color over the next 3–4 days. It is termed **lochia serosa** when it becomes serous to mucopurulent, paler, and often malodorous. During the second or third postpartum week, the lochia becomes thicker, mucoid, and yellowish-white (**lochia alba**), coincident with a pre-

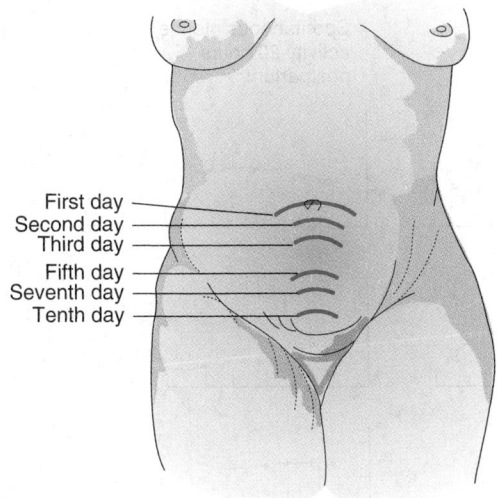

First day
Second day
Third day
Fifth day
Seventh day
Tenth day

Figure 12–1. Involutional changes in the height of the fundus and the size of the uterus during the first 10 days postpartum.

dominance of leukocytes and degenerated decidual cells. Typically during the fifth or sixth week postpartum, the lochial secretions cease as healing nears completion.

Changes in the Cervix, Vagina, & Muscular Walls of the Pelvic Organs

The cervix gradually closes during the puerperium; at the end of the first week, it is little more than 1 cm dilated. The external os is converted into a transverse slit, thus distinguishing the parous woman who delivered vaginally from the nulliparous woman or from one who delivered by cesarean section. Colposcopic examination soon after delivery may reveal ulceration, ecchymosis, and laceration. Complete healing and reepithelialization occur 6–12 weeks later. Stromal edema and round cell infiltration and the endocervical glandular hyperplasia of pregnancy may persist for up to 3 months. Cervical lacerations heal in most uncomplicated cases, but the continuity of the cervix may not be restored, so the site of the tear may remain as a scarred notch.

After vaginal delivery, the overdistended and smooth-walled vagina gradually returns to its antepartum condition by about the third week. Thickening of the mucosa, cervical mucus production, and other estrogenic changes may be delayed in a lactating woman. The torn hymen heals in the form of fibrosed nodules of mucosa, the **carunculae myrtiformes.**

Two weeks after delivery, the fallopian tube reflects a hypoestrogenic state marked by atrophy of the epithelium. Fallopian tubes removed between postpartum

days 5 and 15 demonstrate acute inflammatory changes that have not been correlated with subsequent puerperal fever or salpingitis. Normal changes in the pelvis after uncomplicated term vaginal delivery include widening of the symphysis and sacroiliac joints and occasionally gas in these joints. Gas is often seen by ultrasonography in the endometrial cavity after uncomplicated vaginal delivery and does not necessarily indicate the presence of endometritis.

Ovulation occurs as early as 27 days after delivery, with a mean time of 70–75 days in nonlactating women and 6 months in lactating women. In lactating women the duration of anovulation ultimately depends on the frequency of breastfeeding, duration of each feed, and proportion of supplementary feeds. Ovulation suppression is due to high prolactin levels, which remain elevated until approximately 3 weeks after delivery in nonlactating women and 6 weeks in lactating women. However, estrogen levels fall immediately after delivery in all mothers and remain suppressed in lactating mothers. Menstruation returns as soon as 7 weeks in 70% and by 12 weeks in all nonlactating mothers, and as late as 36 months in 70% of breastfeeding mothers.

The voluntary muscles of the pelvic floor and the pelvic supports gradually regain their tone during the puerperium. Tearing or overstretching of the musculature or fascia at the time of delivery predisposes to genital hernias. Overdistention of the abdominal wall during pregnancy may result in rupture of the elastic fibers of the cutis, persistent striae, and diastasis of the rectus muscles. Involution of the abdominal musculature may require 6–7 weeks, and vigorous exercise is not recommended until after that time.

Urinary System

In the immediate postpartum period, the bladder mucosa is edematous as a result of labor and delivery. In addition, bladder capacity is increased. Overdistention and incomplete emptying of the bladder with the presence of residual urine are therefore common problems. The diminished postpartum bladder function appears to be unaffected by infant weight and episiotomy but perhaps is transiently diminished by epidural anesthesia and prolonged labor. Nearly 50% of patients have a mild proteinuria for 1–2 days after delivery. Ultrasonographic examination demonstrates resolution of collecting system dilatation by 6 weeks postpartum in most women. Urinary stasis, however, may persist in more than 50% of women at 12 weeks postpartum. The incidence of urinary tract infection is generally higher in women with persistent dilatation. Significant renal enlargement may persist for many weeks postpartum.

Pregnancy is accompanied by an estimated increase of about 50% in the glomerular filtration rate. These values return to normal or less than normal during the

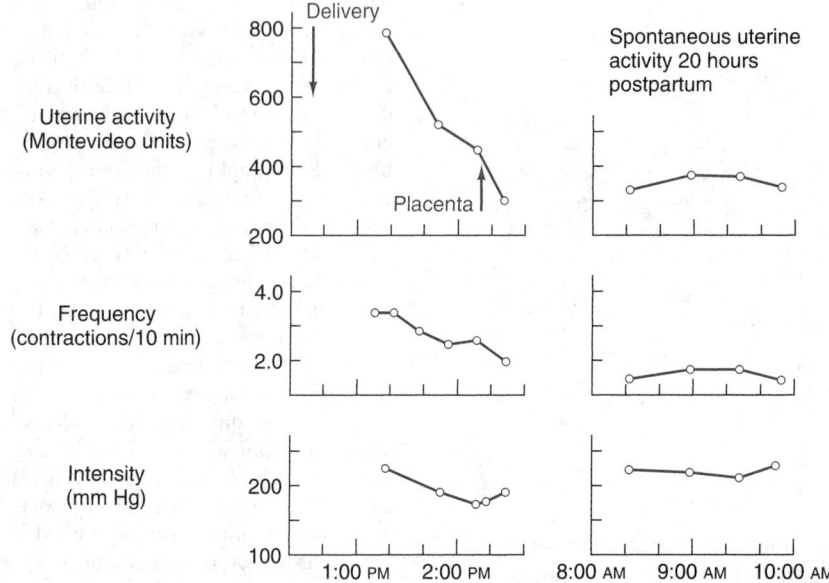

Figure 12–2. Uterine activity during the immediate puerperium (**left**) and at 20 hours postpartum (**right**).

eighth week of the puerperium. Endogenous creatinine clearance similarly returns to normal by 8 weeks. Renal plasma flow, which increased during pregnancy by 25% in the first trimester, falls in the third trimester and continues to fall to below normal levels for up to 24 months. Normal levels return slowly over 50–60 weeks. The glucosuria induced by pregnancy disappears. The blood urea nitrogen rises during the puerperium; at the end of the first week postpartum, values of 20 mg/dL are reached, compared with 15 mg/dL in the late third trimester.

Fluid Balance & Electrolytes

An average decrease in maternal weight of 10–13 lb occurs intrapartum and immediately postpartum due to the loss of amniotic fluid and blood as well as delivery of the infant and placenta. The average patient may lose an additional 4 kg (9 lb) during the puerperium and over the next 6 months as a result of excretion of the fluids and electrolytes accumulated during pregnancy. Contrary to widespread belief, breastfeeding has minimal effects on hastening weight loss postpartum.

There is an average net fluid loss of at least 2 L during the first week postpartum and an additional loss of approximately 1.5 L during the next 5 weeks. The water loss in the first week postpartum represents a loss of extracellular fluid. A negative balance must be expected of slightly more than 100 mEq of chloride per kilogram of body weight lost in the early puerperium. This negative balance probably is attributable to the discharge of maternal extracellular fluid. The puerperal losses of salt and water are generally larger in women with preeclampsia–eclampsia.

The changes occurring in serum electrolytes during the puerperium indicate a general increase in the numbers of cations and anions compared with antepartum values. Although total exchangeable sodium decreases during the puerperium, the relative decrease in body water exceeds the sodium loss. The diminished aldosterone antagonism due to falling plasma progesterone concentrations may partially explain the rapid rise in serum sodium. Cellular breakdown due to tissue involution may contribute to the rise in plasma potassium concentration noted postpartum. The mean increase in cations, chiefly sodium, amounts to 4.7 mEq/L, with an equal increase in anions. Consequently, the plasma osmolality rises by 7 mOsm/L at the end of the first week postpartum. In keeping with the chloride shift, there is a tendency for the serum chloride concentration to decrease slightly postpartum as serum bicarbonate concentration increases.

Metabolic & Chemical Changes

Total fatty acids and nonesterified fatty acids return to nonpregnant levels on about the second day of the puerperium. Both cholesterol and triglyceride concentrations decrease significantly within 24 hours after delivery, and this change is reflected in all lipoprotein fractions. Plasma triglycerides continue to fall and approach nonpregnant values 6–7 weeks postpartum. By comparison, the decrease in plasma cholesterol levels is slower; low-density lipoprotein (LDL) cholesterol remains above nonpregnant levels for at least 7 weeks postpartum. Lactation does not influence lipid levels, but, in contrast to pregnancy, the postpartum hyperlipidemia is sensitive to dietary manipulation.

During the early puerperium, blood glucose concentrations (both fasting and postprandial) tend to fall below the values seen during pregnancy and delivery. This fall is most marked on the second and third postpartum days. Accordingly, the insulin requirements of diabetic patients are lower. Reliable indications of the insulin sensitivity and the blood glucose concentrations characteristic of the nonpregnant state can be demonstrated only after the first week postpartum. Thus, a glucose tolerance test performed in the early puerperium may be interpreted erroneously if nonpuerperal standards are applied to the results.

The concentration of free plasma amino acids increases postpartum. Normal nonpregnant values are regained rapidly on the second or third postpartum day and are presumably a result of reduced utilization and an elevation in the renal threshold.

Cardiovascular Changes

A. Blood Coagulation

The production of both prostacyclin (prostaglandin I_2 [PGI_2]), an inhibitor of platelet aggregation, and thromboxane A_2, an inducer of platelet aggregation and a vasoconstrictor, is increased during pregnancy and the puerperium. Possibly, the balance between thromboxane A_2 and PGI_2 is shifted to the side of thromboxane A_2 dominance during the puerperium because platelet reactivity is increased at this time. Rapid and dramatic changes in the coagulation and fibrinolytic systems occur after delivery (Table 12–1). A decrease in the fibrinogen concentration begins to decrease during labor and reaches its lowest point during the first day postpartum. Thereafter, rising plasma fibrinogen levels reach prelabor values by the third or fifth day of the puerperium. This secondary peak in fibrinogen activity is maintained until the second postpartum week, after which the level of activity slowly returns to normal nonpregnant levels during the following 7–10 days. A similar pattern occurs with respect to factor VIII and plasminogen. Circulating levels of antithrombin III are decreased in the third trimester of pregnancy. Patients with a congenital deficiency of antithrombin III (an endogenous inhibitor of factor X) have recurrent venous thromboembolic disease, and a low level of this factor has been associated with a hypercoagulable state.

Table 12–1. Changes in blood coagulation and fibrinolysis during the puerperium.

	Time Postpartum				
	1 Hour	**1 Day**	**3–5 Days**	**1st Week**	**2nd Week**
Platelet count	↓	↑	↑↑	↑↑	↑
Platelet adhesiveness	↑	↑↑	↑↑↑	↑	0
Fibrinogen	↓	↓	↑	0	↓
Factor V		↑	↑↑	↑	0
Factor VIII	↓	↓	↑		
Factors II, VII, X		↓	↓	↓↓	↓↓
Plasminogen	↓	↓↓	0	↓	↓
Plasminogen activator	↑↑↑	↑↑	0		
Fibrinolytic activity	↑	↑↑	↑↑	↑	
Fibrin split products	↑	↑↑	↑↑		

The arrows indicate the direction and relative magnitude of change compared with the late third trimester or antepartum values. Zero indicates a return to antepartum but not necessarily nonpregnant values.
Prepared from data from Manning FA et al: Am J Obstet Gynecol 1971;110:900, Bonnar J et al: Br Med J 1970;2:200; Ygg J: Am J Obstet Gynecol 1969;104:2; and Shaper AG et al: J Obstet Gynaecol Br Commonw 1968;75:433.

The fibrinolytic activity of maternal plasma is greatly reduced during the last months of pregnancy but increases rapidly after delivery. In the first few hours postpartum, an increase in tissue plasminogen activator (t-PA) develops, together with a slight prolongation of the thrombin time, a decrease in plasminogen activator inhibitors, and a significant increase in fibrin split products. Protein C is an important coagulation inhibitor that requires the nonenzymatic cofactor protein S (which exists as a free protein and as a complex) for its activity. The level of protein S, both total and free, increases on the first day after delivery and gradually returns to normal levels after the first week postpartum.

According to current concepts, the fibrinolytic system is in dynamic equilibrium with the factors that promote coagulation. Thus, after delivery, the increased plasma fibrinolytic activity coupled with the consumption of several clotting factors suggests a large deposition of fibrin in the placental bed. Because of the continued release of fibrin breakdown products from the placental site, the concentration of fibrin split products continues to rise even after spontaneous plasma fibrinolytic activity decreases. Increased levels of soluble fibrin monomer complexes are observed during the early puerperium compared with levels at 3 months postpartum.

The increased concentration of clotting factors normally seen during pregnancy can be viewed as teleologically important in providing a reserve to compensate for the rapid consumption of these factors during delivery and in promoting hemostasis after parturition. Nonetheless, extensive activation of clotting factors, together with immobility, sepsis, or trauma during delivery, may set the stage for later thromboembolic complications (see Chapter 26). The secondary increase in fibrinogen, factor VIII, or platelets (which remain well above nonpregnant values in the first week postpartum) also predisposes to thrombosis during the puerperium. The abrupt return of normal fibrinolytic activity after delivery may be a protective mechanism to combat this hazard. A small percentage of puerperal women who show a diminished ability to activate the fibrinolytic system appears to be at high risk for the development of postpartum thromboembolic complications.

B. Blood Volume Changes

The total blood volume normally decreases from the antepartum value of 5–6 L to the nonpregnant value of 4 L by the third week after delivery. One-third of this reduction occurs during delivery and soon afterward, and a similar amount is lost by the end of the first postpartum week. Additional variation occurs with lactation. The hypervolemia of pregnancy may be viewed as a protective mechanism that allows most women to tolerate considerable loss of blood during parturition. The quantity of blood lost during delivery generally determines the blood volume and hematocrit during the puerperium. Normal vaginal delivery of a single fetus entails an average blood loss of about 400 mL, whereas cesarean section leads to a blood loss of nearly 1 L. If total hysterectomy is performed in addition to cesarean section delivery, the mean blood loss increases to approximately 1500 mL. Delivery of twins and triplets entails blood losses similar to those of operative delivery, but a compensatory increase in maternal plasma volume and red blood cell mass is observed during multiple pregnancy.

Dramatic and rapid readjustments occur in the maternal vasculature after delivery so that the response to blood loss during the early puerperium is different from that occurring in the nonpregnant woman. Delivery leads to obliteration of the low-resistance uteroplacental circulation and results in a 10–15% re-

duction in the size of the maternal vascular bed. Loss of placental endocrine function also removes a stimulus to vasodilatation.

A declining blood volume with a rise in hematocrit is usually seen 3–7 days after vaginal delivery (Fig 12–3). In contrast, serial studies of patients after cesarean section indicate a more rapid decline in blood volume and hematocrit and a tendency for the hematocrit to stabilize or even decline in the early puerperium. Hemoconcentration occurs if the loss of red cells is less than the reduction in vascular capacity. Hemodilution takes place in patients who lose 20% or more of their circulating blood volume at delivery. In patients with preeclampsia–eclampsia, resolution of peripheral vasoconstriction and mobilization of excess extracellular fluid may lead to significant expansion of vascular volume by the third postpartum day. Plasma atrial natriuretic peptide levels nearly double during the first days postpartum in response to atrial stretch caused by blood volume expansion and may have relevance for postpartum natriuresis and diuresis. Occasionally, a patient sustains minimal blood loss at delivery. In such a patient, marked hemoconcentration may occur in the puerperium, especially if there has been a preexisting polycythemia or a considerable increase in the red cell mass during pregnancy.

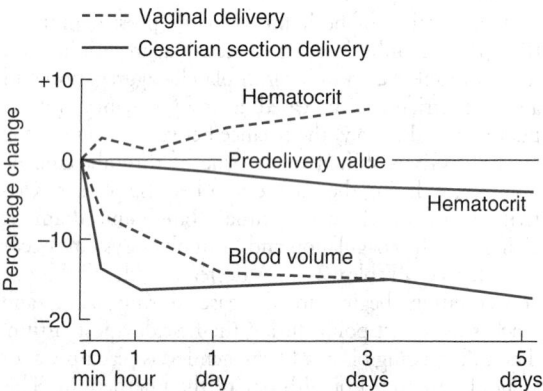

Figure 12–3. Postpartum changes in hematocrit and blood volume in patients delivered vaginally and by cesarean section. Values are expressed as the percentage change from the predelivery hematocrit or blood volume. (Based upon data from Ueland K et al: Maternal cardiovascular dynamics. 1. Cesarean section under subarachnoid block anesthesia. Am J Obstet Gynecol 1968;100:42; and Ueland K, Hansen J: Maternal cardiovascular dynamics. 3. Labor and delivery under local and caudal analgesia. Am J Obstet Gynecol 1969;103: 8.)

C. HEMATOPOIESIS

The red cell mass increases by about 30% during pregnancy, whereas the average red cell loss at delivery is approximately 14%. Thus, the mean postpartum red cell mass level should be about 15% above nonpregnant values. The sudden loss of blood at delivery, however, leads to a rapid and short-lived reticulocytosis (with a peak on the fourth postpartum day) and moderately elevated erythropoietin levels during the first week postpartum.

The bone marrow in pregnancy and in the early puerperium is hyperactive and capable of delivering a large number of young cells to the peripheral blood. Prolactin may play a minor role in bone marrow stimulation.

A striking leukocytosis occurs during labor and extends into the early puerperium. In the immediate puerperium, the white blood cell count may be as high as 25,000/mL, with an increased percentage of granulocytes. The stimulus for this leukocytosis is not known, but it probably represents a release of sequestered cells in response to the stress of labor.

The serum iron level is decreased and the plasma iron turnover is increased between the third and fifth days of the puerperium. Normal values are regained by the second week postpartum. The shorter duration of ferrokinetic changes in puerperal women compared with the duration of changes in nonpregnant women who have had phlebotomy is due to the increased erythroid marrow activity and the circulatory changes described above.

Most women who sustain an average blood loss at delivery and who received iron supplementation during pregnancy show a relative erythrocytosis during the second week postpartum. Because there is no evidence of increased red cell destruction during the puerperium, any red cells gained during pregnancy will disappear gradually according to their normal life span. A moderate excess of red blood cells after delivery, therefore, may lead to an increase in iron stores. Iron supplementation is not necessary for normal postpartum women if the hematocrit or hemoglobin concentration 5–7 days after delivery is equal to or greater than a normal predelivery value. In the late puerperium, there is a gradual decrease in the red cell mass to nonpregnant levels as the rate of erythropoiesis returns to normal.

D. HEMODYNAMIC CHANGES

The hemodynamic adjustments in the puerperium depend largely on the conduct of labor and delivery, eg, maternal position, method of delivery, mode of anesthesia or analgesia, and blood loss. Cardiac output increases progressively during labor in patients who have received only local anesthesia. The increase in cardiac output peaks immediately after delivery, at which time it is approximately 80% above the prelabor value. During a uterine contraction there is a rise in central venous pressure, arterial pressure, and stroke volume—and, in the absence of pain and anxiety, a reflex decrease in the pulse rate. These changes are magnified in the supine position. Only minimal changes occur in the lateral recumbent position because of unimpaired venous return and absence of aortoiliac compression by the contracting uterus (Poseiro effect). Epidural anesthesia modifies the progressive rise in cardiac output during labor and reduces the absolute increase observed immediately after delivery, probably by limiting pain and anxiety.

Although major hemodynamic readjustments occur during the period immediately following delivery, there is a return to nonpregnant conditions in the early puerperium. A trend for normal women to increase their blood pressure slightly in the first 5 days postpartum reflects an increased uterine vascular resistance and a temporary surplus in plasma volume. A small percentage will have diastolic blood pressures of 100 mm Hg. Cardiac output (measured by Doppler and cross-sectional echocardiography) declines 28% within 2 weeks postpartum from peak values observed at 38 weeks' gestation. This change is associated with a 20% reduction in stroke volume and a smaller decrease in myocardial contractility indices. Postpartum resolution of pregnancy-induced ventricular hypertrophy takes longer than the functional postpartum changes (Fig 12–4). In fact, limited data support a slow return of cardiac hemodynamics to prepregnancy levels over a 1-year period. There are no hemodynamic differences between lactating and nonlactating mothers.

Respiratory Changes

The pulmonary functions that change most rapidly are those influenced by alterations in abdominal contents and thoracic cage capacity. Lung volume changes in the puerperium are compared with those occurring during pregnancy in Figure 12–5. The residual volume increases, but the vital capacity and inspiratory capacities decrease. The maximum breathing capacity is also reduced after delivery. An increase in resting ventilation and oxygen consumption and a less efficient response to exercise may persist during the early postpartum weeks. Comparisons of aerobic capacity prior to pregnancy and again postpartum indicate that lack of activity and weight gain contribute to a generalized detraining effect 4–8 weeks postpartum.

Changes in acid base status generally parallel changes in respiratory function. The state of pregnancy is characterized by respiratory alkalosis and compensated metabolic acidosis, whereas labor represents a transitional period. A significant hypocapnia (< 30 mm Hg), a rise in blood lactate, and a fall in pH are first noted at the end of the first stage of labor and extend into the puerperium. Within a few days, a rise toward the normal nonpregnant values of P_{CO_2} (35–40 mm Hg) occurs. Progesterone influences the rate of ventilation by means of a central effect, and rapidly decreasing levels of this hormone are largely responsible for the increased P_{CO_2} seen in the first week postpartum. An increase in base

excess and plasma bicarbonate accompanies the relative postpartum hypercapnia. A gradual increase in pH and base excess occurs until normal levels are reached at about 3 weeks postpartum.

The resting arterial P_{O_2} and oxygen saturation during pregnancy are higher than those in nonpregnant women. During labor, the oxygen saturation may be depressed, especially in the supine position, probably as a result of a decrease in cardiac output and a relative increase in the amount of intrapulmonary shunting. However, a rise in the arterial oxygen saturation to 95% is noted during the first postpartum day. An apparent oxygen debt incurred during labor extends into the immediate puerperium and appears to depend on the length and severity of the second stage of labor. Many investigators have commented on the continued elevation of the basal metabolic rate for a period of 7–14 days following delivery. The increased resting oxygen consumption in the early puer-

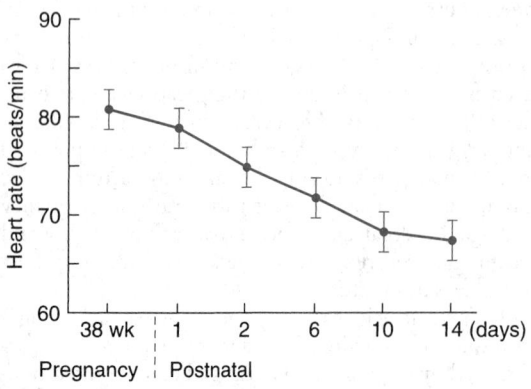

Figure 12–4. Changes in cardiac output, stroke volume, and heart rate during the puerperium after normal delivery. (Reproduced, with permission, from Hunter S, Robson SC: Adaptation of the maternal heart in pregnancy. Br Heart J 1992;68:540.)

Figure 12–5. Alterations in lung volumes during pregnancy and 1 week and 6 months postpartum. (Modified, with permission, from Cugell DW et al: Pulmonary function in pregnancy. Am Rev Tuberc 1953;67:568.)

perium has been attributed to mild anemia, lactation, and psychologic factors.

Pituitary–Ovarian Relationships

The plasma levels of placental hormones decline rapidly following delivery. Human placental lactogen has a half-life of 20 minutes and reaches undetectable levels in maternal plasma during the first day after delivery. Human chorionic gonadotropin (hCG) has a mean half-life of about 9 hours. The concentration of hCG in maternal plasma falls below 1000 mU/mL within 48–96 hours postpartum and falls below 100 mU/mL by the seventh day. Follicular phase levels of immunoreactive luteinizing hormone (LH)-hCG are reached during the second postpartum week. Highly specific and sensitive radioimmunoassays for the subunit of hCG indicate virtual disappearance of hCG from maternal plasma between the 11th and 16th days following normal delivery. The regressive pattern of hCG activity is slower after first-trimester abortion than it is after term delivery and even more prolonged in patients who have undergone suction curettage for molar pregnancy.

Within 3 hours after removal of the placenta, the plasma concentration of 17b-estradiol falls to 10% of the antepartum value. The lowest levels are reached by the seventh postpartum day (Fig 12–6). Plasma estrogens do not reach follicular phase levels (> 50 pg/mL) until 19–21 days postpartum in nonlactating women. The return to normal plasma levels of estrogens is delayed in lactating women. Lactating women who resume spontaneous menses achieve follicular phase estradiol levels (> 50 pg/mL) during the first 60–80 days postpartum. Lactating amenorrheic persons are markedly hypoestrogenic (plasma estradiol < 10 pg/mL) during the first 180 days postpartum. The onset of breast engorgement on days 3–4 of the puerperium coincides with a significant fall in estrogen levels and supports the view that high estrogen levels suppress lactation.

The metabolic clearance rate of progesterone is high, and, as with estradiol, the half-life is calculated in minutes. By the third day of the puerperium, the plasma progesterone concentrations are below luteal phase levels (< 1 ng/mL).

Prolactin levels in maternal blood rise throughout pregnancy to reach concentrations of 200 ng/mL or more. After delivery, prolactin declines in erratic fashion over a period of 2 weeks to the nongravid range in nonlactating women (Fig 12–6). In women who are breastfeeding, basal concentrations of prolactin remain above the nongravid range and increase dramatically in response to suckling. As lactation progresses, the amount of prolactin released with each suckling episode declines. If breastfeeding occurs only 1–3 times each day, serum prolactin levels return to normal basal values within 6 months postpartum; if suckling takes place

more than 6 times each day, high basal concentrations of prolactin will persist for more than 1 year. The diurnal rhythm of peripheral prolactin concentrations (a daytime nadir followed by a nighttime peak) is abolished during late pregnancy but is re-established within 1 week postpartum in non-nursing women.

Serum follicle-stimulating hormone (FSH) and LH concentrations are very low in all women during the first 10–12 days postpartum, whether or not they lactate. The levels increase over the following days and reach follicular phase concentrations during the third week postpartum (Fig 12–6). At this time, marked LH pulse amplification occurs during sleep but disappears as normal ovulatory cycles are established. In this respect, the transition from postpartum amenorrhea to cyclic ovulation is reminiscent of puberty, when gonadotropin secretion increases during sleep. There is a preferential release of FSH over LH postpartum during spontaneous recovery or after stimulation by exogenous gonadotropin-releasing hormone (GnRH). In the early puerperium, the pituitary is relatively refractory to GnRH, but 4–8 weeks postpartum the response to GnRH is exaggerated. The low levels of FSH and LH postpartum are most likely related to insufficient endogenous GnRH secretion during pregnancy and the early puerperium, resulting in depletion of pituitary gonadotropin stores. The high estrogen and progesterone milieu of late pregnancy is associated with increased endogenous opioid activity, which may be responsible for suppression of GnRH activity in the puerperium. Resumption of FSH and LH secretion can be accelerated by administering a long-acting GnRH agonist during the first 10 days postpartum.

The frequency with which menstruation is reestablished in the puerperium in lactating and nonlactating women is shown in Figure 12–7. The first menses after delivery usually follows an anovulatory cycle or one associated with inadequate corpus luteum function. The ovary may be somewhat refractory to exogenous gonadotropin stimulation during the puerperium in both lactating and nonlactating women. When prolactin is suppressed with bromocriptine, postpartum ovarian refractoriness to gonadotropin stimulation persists, suggesting that hyperprolactinemia plays only a partial role in the diminished gonadal response. Lactation is characterized by an increased sensitivity to the negative feedback effects and a decreased sensitivity to the positive feedback effects of estrogens on gonadotropin secretion.

Because ovarian activity normally resumes upon weaning, either the suckling stimulus itself or the raised level of prolactin is responsible for suppression of pulsatile gonadotropin secretion. Hyperprolactinemia may not entirely account for the inhibition of gonadotropin secretion during lactation, as bromocriptine treatment abolishes the hyperprolactinemia of suckling but not

Figure 12–6. Serum concentrations of prolactin, FSH, LH, estradiol, and progesterone in a lactating and nonlactating woman during the puerperium. The hatched bars for the prolactin data represent the normal nongravid range. To convert the FSH and LH to milli-international units per milliliter, divide the FSH values by 2 and multiply the LH values by 4.5. FSH, follicle-stimulating hormone; LH, luteinizing hormone. (Reproduced, with permission, from Reyes FI, Winter JS, Faiman C: Pituitary-ovarian interrelationships during the puerperium. Am J Obstet Gynecol 1972;114:589.)

the inhibition of gonadotropin secretion. Sensory inputs associated with suckling (if sufficiently intense), as well as oxytocin and endogenous opioids that are released during suckling, may affect the hypothalamic control of gonadotropin secretion, possibly by inhibiting the pulsatile secretion of GnRH. It appears that by 8 weeks after delivery, while ovarian activity still remains suppressed in fully breastfeeding women, pulsatile secretion of LH has resumed at a low and variable frequency in most women. However, the presence or absence of GnRH or LH pulses at 8 weeks does not predict the time of resumption of ovarian activity.

The time of appearance of the first ovulation is variable, but it is delayed by breastfeeding. Approximately 10–15% of non-nursing mothers ovulate by the time of the 6-week postpartum examination, and approximately

30% ovulate within 90 days postpartum. An abnormally short luteal phase is noted in 35% of first ovulatory cycles. The earliest reported time of ovulation as determined by endometrial biopsy is 33 days postpartum. Patients who have had a first-trimester abortion or ectopic pregnancy generally ovulate sooner after termination of pregnancy (as early as 14 days) than do women who deliver at term. Moreover, the majority of these women do ovulate before the first episode of postabortal bleeding—in contrast to women who have had a term pregnancy.

Endometrial biopsies in lactating women do not show a secretory pattern before the seventh postpartum week. Provided that nursing is in progress and that menstruation has not returned, ovulation before the tenth week postpartum is rare. In well-nourished women who breastfed for an extended period of time,

Figure 12–7. Frequency at which menstruation is re-established in the puerperium in lactating and nonlactating multiparous women. (Adapted, with permission, from Sherman A: *Reproductive Physiology of the Post-partum Period.* Livingstone, 1966.)

less than 20% had ovulated by 6 months postpartum. Much of the variability in the resumption of menstruation and ovulation observed in lactating women may be due to individual differences in the strength of the suckling stimulus and to partial weaning (formula supplementation). This emphasizes the fact that suckling is not a reliable form of birth control. Because the period of lactational infertility is relatively short in Western societies, some form of contraception must be used if pregnancy is to be prevented. Among women who have unprotected intercourse only during lactational amenorrhea but adopt other contraceptive measures when they resume menstruation, only 2% will become pregnant during the first 6 months of amenorrhea. In underdeveloped countries, lactational amenorrhea and infertility may persist for 1–2 years owing to frequent suckling and poor maternal nutrition. When maternal dietary intake is improved, menstruation resumes at least 6 months earlier.

Other Endocrine Changes

Progressive enlargement of the pituitary gland occurs during pregnancy, with a 30–100% increase in weight achieved at term. Magnetic resonance imaging shows a linear gain in pituitary gland height of about 0.08 mm/wk during pregnancy. An additional increase in size occurs during the first week postpartum. Beyond the first week postpartum, however, the pituitary gland returns rapidly to its normal size in both lactating and nonlactating women.

The physiologic hypertrophy of the pituitary gland is associated with an increase in the number of pituitary lactotroph cells at the expense of the somatotropic cell types. Thus, growth hormone secretion is depressed during the second half of pregnancy and the early puerperium. Because levels of circulating insulinlike growth factor (IGF)-1 increase throughout pregnancy, a placental growth hormone has been postulated and recently identified. Maternal levels of IGF-1 correlate highly with this distinct placental growth hormone variant but not with placental lactogen during pregnancy and in the immediate puerperium.

Late pregnancy and the early puerperium are also characterized by pituitary somatotroph hyporesponsiveness to growth hormone-releasing hormone and to insulin stimulation. Whatever the inhibitory mechanism may be (possibly increased somatostatin secretion), it persists during the early postpartum period.

The rapid disappearance of placental lactogen and the low levels of growth hormone after delivery lead to a relative deficiency of anti-insulin factors in the early puerperium. It is not surprising, therefore, that low fasting plasma glucose levels are noted at this time and that the insulin requirements of diabetic patients usually drop after delivery. Glucose tolerance tests performed in women with gestational diabetes demonstrate that only 30% have abnormal test results 3–5 days after delivery and 20% have abnormal glucose tolerance at 6 weeks postpartum. When the relative hyperinsulinism and hypoglycemia of pregnancy return to the nonpregnant range at 6–8 weeks postpartum, a paradoxical decline in fasting glucagon levels is found. Because the early puerperium represents a transitional period in carbohydrate metabolism, the results of glucose tolerance tests may be difficult to interpret.

Evaluation of thyroid function is also difficult in the period immediately after birth because of rapid fluctuations in many indices. Characteristically, the plasma thyroxine level and other indices of thyroid function are highest at delivery and in the first 12 hours thereafter. A decrease to antepartum values is seen on the third or fourth day after delivery. Reduced available estrogens postpartum lead to a subsequent decrease in circulating thyroxine-binding globulin and a gradual diminution in bound thyroid hormones in serum. Serum concentrations of thyroid-stimulating hormone (TSH) are not significantly different postpartum from those of the pregnant or nonpregnant state. Administration of thyroid-releasing hormone (TRH) in the puerperium results in a normal increase in both TSH and prolactin, and the response is similar in lactating and nonlactating patients. Because pregnancy is associated with some immunosuppressive effects, hyperthyroidism or hypothyroidism may recur postpartum in autoimmune thyroid disease. Failure of lactation and prolonged disability may be the result of hypothyroidism postpartum. In Sheehan's syndrome of pituitary infarction, postpartum cachexia and myxedema are seen secondary to anterior hypophyseal insufficiency.

Maternal concentrations of total and unbound (free) plasma cortisol, adrenocorticotropic hormone (ACTH), immunoreactive corticotropin-releasing hormone (CRH), and β-endorphin rise progressively during pregnancy and increase further during labor. Plasma 17-hydroxycorticosteroid levels increase from a concentration of 4–14 μg/dL at 40 weeks' gestation. A 2- to 3-fold increase is seen during labor. ACTH, CRH, and β-endorphin decrease rapidly after delivery and return to nonpregnant levels within 24 hours. Prelabor cortisol values are regained on the first day postpartum, but a return to normal, nonpregnant cortisol and 17-hydroxycorticosteroid levels is not reached until the end of the first week postpartum.

Much of the rise in total cortisol (but not in the unbound fraction) can be explained by the parallel increase in corticosteroid-binding globulin (CBG) during pregnancy. Displacement of cortisol from CBG by high concentrations of progesterone cannot account for the increased free cortisol levels because saliva progesterone levels (a measure of the unbound hormone) do not fluctuate, whereas a normal diurnal rhythm of saliva cortisol is maintained during pregnancy and postpartum. An extrapituitary source of ACTH, a progesterone-modulated decrease in the hypothalamic–pituitary sensitivity to glucocorticoid feedback inhibition, and an extrahypothalamic (eg, placental) source of CRH have been suggested as explanations for elevated plasma ACTH levels and the inability of dexamethasone to completely suppress ACTH in pregnant women.

In the third trimester, the placenta produces large amounts of CRH, which is released into the maternal circulation and may contribute to the hypercortisolemia of pregnancy. Present evidence suggests that it stimulates the maternal pituitary to produce ACTH while desensitizing the pituitary to further acute stimulation with CRH. Maternal hypothalamic control of ACTH production is retained (perhaps mediated by vasopressin secretion); this permits a normal response to stress and a persistent diurnal rhythm.

Overall, it is most likely that under the influence of rising estrogens and progesterone, there is a resetting of the hypothalamic–pituitary sensitivity to cortisol feedback during pregnancy, which persists for several days postpartum. Several studies have suggested a relationship between peripartum alterations in maternal levels of cortisol and β-endorphin and the development of postnatal mood disturbances.

The excretion of urinary 17-ketosteroids is elevated in late pregnancy as a result of an increase in androgenic precursors from the fetoplacental unit and the ovary. An additional increase of 50% in excretion occurs during labor. Excretion of 17-ketosteroids returns to antepartum levels on the first day after delivery and to the nonpregnant range by the end of the first week. The mean levels of testosterone during the third trimester of pregnancy range from 3 to 7 times the mean values for nonpregnant women. The elevated levels of testosterone decrease after parturition parallel with the gradual fall in sex hormone-binding globulin (SHBG). Androstenedione, which is poorly bound to SHBG, falls rapidly to nonpregnant values by the third day postpartum. Conversely, the postpartum plasma concentration of dehydroepiandrosterone sulfate (DHEAS) remains lower than that of nonpregnant women, because its metabolic clearance rate continues to be elevated in the early puerperium. Persistently elevated levels of 17-ketosteroids or androgens during the puerperium are an indication for investigation of ovarian abnormalities. Plasma renin and angiotensin II levels fall during the first 2 hours postpartum to levels within the normal nonpregnant range. This suggests that an extrarenal source of renin has been lost with the expulsion of the fetus and placenta.

There is little direct information about the puerperal changes in numerous other hormones, including aldosterone, parathyroid hormone, and calcitonin. More research should be done on these important endocrine relationships in the puerperium.

CONDUCT AND MANAGEMENT OF THE PUERPERIUM

Most patients will benefit from 2–4 days of hospitalization after delivery. Only 3% of women with a vaginal delivery and 9% of women having a cesarean section have a childbirth-related complication requiring prolonged postpartum hospitalization or readmission. Although a significant amount of symptomatic morbidity may exist postpartum (painful perineum, breastfeeding difficulties, urinary infections, urinary and fecal incontinence, and headache), most women can return home safely 2 days after normal vaginal delivery if proper education and instructions are given, if confidence exists with infant care and feeding, and if adequate support exists at home. Earlier discharge is acceptable in select mothers and infants who have had uncomplicated labors and deliveries. Discharge criteria should be met and follow-up care provided. Optimal care includes home nursing visits through the fourth postpartum day. Disadvantages of early discharge are the increased risks of rehospitalization of some neonates for hyperbilirubinemia and neonatal infection (eg, from group B streptococci).

Activities & Rest

The policy of early ambulation after delivery benefits the patient. Early ambulation provides a sense of well-being, hastens involution of the uterus, improves uterine drainage, and lessens the incidence of postpartum thrombophlebitis. If the delivery has been uncomplicated, the patient may be out of bed as soon as tolerated. Early ambulation does not mean immediate return to normal activity or work. Commonly mothers complain of lethargy and fatigue. Therefore, rest is essential after delivery, and the demands on the mother should be limited to allow for adequate relaxation and adjustment to her new responsibilities. It is helpful to set aside a few hours each day for rest periods. Many mothers do not sleep well for several nights after delivery, and it is surprising how much of the day is occupied with the care of the newborn.

In uncomplicated deliveries, more vigorous activity, climbing stairs, lifting of heavy objects, riding in or driving a car, and performing muscle toning exercises may be resumed without delay. Specific recommendations should be individualized. Current American College of Obstetricians and Gynecologists committee opinions support gradual resumption of exercise routines as soon as medically and physically safe, as detraining may have occurred during pregnancy. No known maternal complications are associated with resumption of exercise, even in women who choose to resume an exercise routine within days. Exercise postpartum does not compromise lactation or neonatal weight gain. It may be beneficial in decreasing anxiety levels and decreasing the incidence of postpartum depression.

Sexual Activity during the Postpartum Period

Establishment of normal prepregnancy sexual response patterns is delayed after delivery. However, it is safe to resume sexual activity when the woman's perineum is comfortable and bleeding is diminished. Although the median time for resumption of intercourse after delivery is 6 weeks and the normal sexual response returns at 12 weeks, sexual desire and activity vary tremendously among women. Most women report low or absent sexual desire during the early puerperium and ascribe this to fatigue, weakness, pain on intromission, irritative vaginal discharge, or fear of injury. Nearly 50% report a return of sexual desire within 2–3 weeks postpartum. In spite of minimal desire in a substantial proportion of women, nearly all resume sexual intercourse by 6–8 weeks after delivery. Roughly 20% of women have no desire for sexual activity at 3 months from delivery, and an additional 21% lose the desire completely or develop an aversion. The variation in desire depends on the site and state of perineal or vaginal healing, return of libido,

and vaginal atrophy resulting from breastfeeding. Lactating women, however, generally report higher sexual interest than do bottle-feeding mothers.

Sexual counseling is indicated before the mother is discharged from the hospital. A discussion of the normal fluctuations of sexual interest during the puerperium is appropriate, as are suggestions for noncoital sexual options that enhance the expression of mutual pleasure and affection. The importance of sleep and rest and of the partner's emotional and physical support are emphasized. If milk ejection during sexual relations is a concern, nursing the baby prior to sexual intimacy can help. Sexual relations can generally be resumed by the third week postpartum, if desired. A water-soluble lubricant or vaginal estrogen cream is especially helpful in lactating amenorrheic mothers in whom vaginal atrophy occurs, usually because of low circulating estrogen levels. Patients should be informed that roughly 50% of women engaging in sexual intercourse by 6 weeks will experience dyspareunia, which may last for 1 year. Dyspareunia also occurs in women with cesarean sections and in women using oral contraceptives who are not breastfeeding.

Diet

A regular diet is permissible as soon as the patient regains her appetite and is free from the effects of analgesics and anesthetics. Protein foods, fruits, vegetables, milk products, and a high fluid intake are recommended, especially for nursing mothers. However, even lactating women probably require no more than 2600–2800 kcal/d. It may be advisable to continue the daily vitamin–mineral supplement during the early puerperium. Following cesarean section, there is no evidence to support compromise of safety or comfort from the introduction of solid food early and allowing the patient to decide when to eat postoperatively. In fact, early feeding as tolerated by the patient has been shown to be safe and to facilitate a more rapid return to normal diet and bowel function.

Care of the Bladder

Most women empty the bladder during labor or have been catheterized at delivery. Even so, serious bladder distention may develop within 12 hours. A long and difficult labor or a forceps delivery may traumatize the base of the bladder and interfere with normal voiding. In some cases, overdistention of the bladder may be related to pain or spinal anesthesia. The marked polyuria noted for the first few days postpartum causes the bladder to fill in a relatively short time. Hence, obstetric patients require catheterization more frequently than most surgical patients. The patient should be catheterized every 6 hours after delivery if she is unable to void or empty her bladder completely. Intermittent catheterization is preferable to an indwelling catheter because the incidence of urinary tract infection is lower. However, if the bladder fills to more than 1000 mL, 1–2 days of decompression by a retention catheter usually is required to establish voiding without significant residual urine.

The incidence of true asymptomatic bacteriuria is approximately 5% in the early puerperium. Postpartum patients with a history of previous urinary tract infection, conduction anesthesia, and catheterization during delivery and operative delivery should have a bacterial culture of a midstream urine specimen. In cases of confirmed bacteriuria, antibiotic treatment should be given; otherwise, bacteriuria will persist in nearly 30% of patients. Three days of therapy is sufficient and avoids prolonged antibiotic exposure to the lactating mother.

Bowel Function

Pregnancy itself is associated with increased gastric emptying, but gastrointestinal motility is commonly delayed after labor and delivery. The mild ileus that follows delivery, together with perineal discomfort and postpartum fluid loss by other routes, predisposes to constipation during the puerperium. Obstruction of the colon by a retroverted uterus is a rare complication during the puerperium. If an enema was given before delivery, the patient is unlikely to have a bowel movement for 1–2 days after childbirth. Milk of magnesia, 15–20 mL orally on the evening of the second postpartum day, usually stimulates a bowel movement by the next morning. If not, a rectal suppository, such as bisacodyl or a small tap water or oil retention enema, may be given. Less bowel stimulation will be needed if the diet contains sufficient roughage. Stool softeners, such as dioctyl sodium sulfosuccinate, may ease the discomfort of early bowel movements. Hemorrhoidal discomfort is a common complaint postpartum and usually responds to conservative treatment with compresses, suppositories containing corticosteroids, local anesthetic sprays or emollients, and sitz baths. Surgical treatment of hemorrhoids postpartum is rarely necessary unless thrombosis is extensive.

Operative vaginal delivery and lacerations involving the anal sphincter increase a woman's risk for anal incontinence. However, 5% of pregnant women overall have some degree of anal incontinence at 3 months postpartum. Complaints of fecal incontinence are often delayed because of embarrassment. Most cases are transient; however, cases persisting beyond 6 months require investigation and probable treatment.

Bathing

As soon as the patient is ambulatory, she may take a shower. Sitz or tub baths probably are safe if performed in a clean environment, because bath water will not gain access to the vagina unless it is directly introduced. Most patients prefer showers to tub baths because of the profuse flow of lochia immediately postpartum. However, sitz baths may be beneficial for perineal pain relief. Vaginal douching is contraindicated in the early puerperium. Tampons may be used whenever the patient is comfortable. However, use should be limited to daylight hours to prevent long hours of use or inadvertent tampon loss.

Care of the Perineum

Postpartum perineal care, even in the patient with an uncomplicated and satisfactorily repaired episiotomy or laceration, usually requires no more than routine cleansing with a bath or shower and analgesia.

Immediately after delivery, cold compresses (usually ice) applied to the perineum decrease traumatic edema and discomfort. The perineal area should be gently cleansed with plain soap at least once or twice per day and after voiding or defecation. If the perineum is kept clean, healing should occur rapidly. Cold or iced sitz baths, rather than hot sitz baths, may provide additional perineal pain relief for some patients. The patient should be put in a lukewarm tub to which ice cubes are added for 20–30 minutes. The cold promotes pain relief by decreasing the excitability of nerve endings, decreased nerve conduction, and local vasoconstriction, which reduces edema, inhibits hematoma formation, and decreases muscle irritability and spasm. Episiotomy pain is easily controlled with nonsteroidal anti-inflammatory agents, which appear to be superior to acetaminophen or propoxyphene.

An episiotomy or repaired lacerations should be inspected daily. A patient with mediolateral episiotomy, a third- or fourth-degree laceration or extension, or extensive bruising or edema may experience severe perineal pain. In the case of persistent or unusual pain, a vaginal and/or rectal examination should be performed to identify a hematoma, perineal infection, or potentially fatal conditions, such as angioedema, necrotizing fasciitis, or perineal cellulitis. Episiotomy wounds rarely become infected, which is remarkable considering the difficulty of preventing contamination of the perineal area. In the event of sepsis, local heat and irrigation should cause the infection to subside. Appropriate antibiotics may be indicated if an immediate response to these measures is not observed. In rare instances, the wound should be opened widely and sutures removed for adequate drainage.

Uterotonic Agents

Prophylactic administration of oxytocin after the second stage of labor and/or after placental delivery is beneficial in preventing postpartum hemorrhage and the need for therapeutic uterotonics. The routine use of ergot preparations or prostaglandins may be as effective as oxytocin but has significantly more side effects. There appear to be no data supporting the prophylactic use of oxytocic agents beyond the immediate puerperium. These agents should be limited to patients with specific indications, such as postpartum hemorrhage or uterine atony.

Emotional Reactions

Several basic emotional responses occur in almost every woman who has given birth to a normal baby. A woman's first emotion is usually one of extreme relief, followed by a sense of happiness and gratitude that the new baby has arrived safely. A regular pattern of behavior occurs in the human mother immediately after birth of the infant. Touching, holding, and grooming of the infant under normal conditions rapidly strengthen maternal ties of affection. However, not all mothers react in this way, and some may even feel detached from the new baby. These reactions range from the common, physiologic, relatively mild and transient "maternity blues," which affect some 50–70% of postpartum women, to more severe reactions including depression and rare puerperal psychosis.

Postpartum blues or maternity blues occurs in up to 70% of postpartum women and appear to be a normal psychological adjustment or response. It is generally characterized by tearfulness, anxiety, irritation, and restlessness. This symptomatology can be quite diverse and may include depression, feelings of inadequacy, elation, mood swings, confusion, difficulty concentrating, headache, forgetfulness, insomnia, depersonalization, and negative feelings toward the baby. These transient symptoms usually occur within the first few days after delivery and cease by postpartum day 10, although bouts of weeping may occur for weeks after delivery. The blues are self-limiting, but the distress can be diminished by physical comfort and reassurance. Evidence suggests that rooming-in during the hospital stay reduces maternal anxiety and results in more successful breastfeeding.

Prematurity or illness of the newborn delays early intimate maternal–infant contact and may have an adverse effect on the rapid and complete development of normal mothering responses. Stressful factors during the puerperium (eg, marital infidelity or loss of friends as a result of the necessary confinement and preoccupation with the new baby) may leave the mother feeling unsupported and may interfere with the formation of a maternal bond with the infant.

When a baby dies or is born with a congenital defect, the obstetrician should tell the mother and father about the problem together, if possible. The baby's normal, healthy features and potential for improvement

should be emphasized, and positive statements should be made about the present availability of corrective treatment and the promises of ongoing research. In the event of a perinatal loss, parents should be assisted in the grieving process. They should be encouraged to see and touch the baby at birth or later, even if maceration or anomalies are present. Mementos such as footprints, locks of hair, or a photograph can be a solace to the parents after the infant has been buried. During the puerperium, the obstetrician has an important opportunity to help the mother whose infant has died work through her period of mourning or discouragement and to assess abnormal reactions of grief that suggest a need for psychiatric assistance. Pathologic grief is characterized by the inability to work through the sense of loss within 3–4 months, with subsequent feelings of low self-esteem.

Postpartum Immunization

A. PREVENTION OF RH ISOIMMUNIZATION

The postpartum injection of Rh_o (D) immunoglobulin* will prevent sensitization in the Rh-negative woman who has had fetal-to-maternal transfusion of Rh-positive fetal red cells. The risk of maternal sensitization rises with the volume of fetal transplacental hemorrhage. The usual amount of fetal blood that enters the maternal circulation is less than 0.5 mL. The usual dose of 300 μg of Rh_o (D) immunoglobulin is in excess of the dose generally required, because 25 mg of RhoGAM per milliliter of fetal red cells is sufficient to prevent maternal immunization. If neonatal anemia or other clinical symptoms suggest the occurrence of a large transplacental hemorrhage, the amount of fetal blood in the maternal circulation can be estimated by the Kleihauer-Betke smear and the amounts of RhoGAM to be administered adjusted accordingly. A dose of 10 mL per estimated milliliter of whole fetal blood should be administered. An alternative to the acid elution smear is the Du test, which will detect 20 mL or more of Rh-positive fetal blood in the maternal circulation.

Rh_o (D) immunoglobulin is administered after abortion without qualifications or after delivery to women who meet all of the following criteria: (1) The mother must be Rh_o (D)-negative without Rh antibodies; (2) the baby must be Rh_o (D)- or Du-positive; and (3) the cord blood must be Coombs-negative. If these criteria are met, a 1:1000 dilution of Rh_o (D) immunoglobulin is cross-matched to the mother's red cells to ensure compatibility, and 1 mL (300 μg) is given intramuscularly to the mother within 72 hours after delivery. If the 72-hour interval has been exceeded, it is advisable to give the immunoglobulin rather than withhold it because it may still protect against sensitization 14–28 days after delivery, and the time required to mount a response

*Trade names include Gamulin Rh, HypRh$_o$-D, and RhoGAM.

varies among cases. The 72-hour time limit for administration of Rh immune globulin was a study limitation in a study in which patients in prison were allowed to be visited only every 3 days; thus, the use of Rh immunoglobulin past the 3-day interval was never studied. Rh_o (D) immunoglobulin should also be given after delivery or abortion when serologic tests of maternal sensitization to the Rh factor are questionable.

The average risk of maternal sensitization after abortion is approximately half the risk incurred by full-term pregnancy and delivery; the latter has been estimated at 11%. Even though mothers have received Rh_o (D) immunoglobulin, they should be screened with each subsequent pregnancy because postpartum prophylaxis failures still exist. Failures are related to inadequate Rh_o (D) immunoglobulin administration postpartum, an undetected very low titer in the previous pregnancy, and inexcusable oversights. Routine use of postpartum screening protocols to identify excess fetomaternal hemorrhage and strict adherence to recommended protocols for the management of unsensitized Rh-negative women will prevent most of these postpartum sensitizations.

B. RUBELLA VACCINATION

A significant number of women of childbearing age have never had rubella. When tested by the hemagglutination inhibition method, 10–20% of women are seronegative (titer of 1:8 or less). Women who are susceptible to rubella can be vaccinated safely and effectively with a live attenuated rubella virus vaccine (RA 27/3 strain) during the immediate puerperium. It is more immunogenic than earlier forms of the vaccine and is available in monovalent, bivalent (measles-rubella [MR]), and trivalent (measles-mumps-rubella [MMR]) forms. Seroconversion occurs in approximately 95% of women vaccinated postpartum The puerperium is an ideal time for vaccination because there is no risk of inadvertently vaccinating a pregnant woman. Breastfeeding mothers are not excluded from immunization. There is concern, however, that 75% of such women may shed rubella virus in the breast milk, and a persistent rubella carrier state with periodic viral reactivation may rarely occur in the child. The neonate's exposure to the virus in breast milk is not associated with an alteration of responses to subsequent immunization. Women who receive rubella vaccinations are not contagious and cannot transmit infection to other susceptible children or adults. In addition, the serologic response against rubella is satisfactory when given concomitantly with other immunoglobulins such as Rh-immunoglobulin. However, blood transfusions can prevent the success of rubella vaccination if it is performed soon after the transfusion.

Vaccinated patients should be informed that transient side effects can result from rubella vaccination.

Mild symptoms such as low-grade fever and malaise may occur in less than 25% of patients, arthralgias and rash in less than 10%, and, rarely, overt arthritis may develop. Among adult women there is a 10–15% incidence of acute polyarthritis following immunization. Although the Centers for Disease Control and Prevention (CDC) registry of approximately 400 women receiving rubella vaccination within 3 months of conception reports no cases of congenital rubella, the recommendation that secure contraception be used for 3 months after vaccination remains. Rubella virus was, however, isolated from some women who received the vaccination during early pregnancy and elected to terminate. The theoretical maximum theoretical risk of congenital rubella resulting from vaccination during early pregnancy is 1–2%.

Contraception & Sterilization

The immediate puerperium has long been recognized as a convenient time for the discussion of family planning, although these discussions ideally should begin during prenatal care. Pregnancy prevention and birth control decisions should be made prior to discharge with a qualified nurse, physician, or physician's assistant, or with the aid of educational tools. Anovulation infertility lasts only 5 weeks in nonlactating women and greater than 8 weeks in fully lactating women. The lactational pregnancy rate is approximately 1% at 1 year postpartum.

Tubal sterilization is the most common method of contraception used in the United States. It is the procedure of choice for women desiring permanent sterilization. It can be performed easily at the time of cesarean section, 24–48 hours after an uncomplicated vaginal delivery, or immediately postpartum in uncomplicated patients with a labor epidural in place, without prolonging hospitalization or significantly increasing morbidity. Sterilization is not recommended in young women of low parity or when the neonatal outcome is in doubt and survival of the infant is not assured. Postponing tubal sterilization 6–8 weeks postpartum is desirable for many couples, as it allows time to ensure that the infant is healthy, to fully understand the implications of permanent sterilization, and, according to the United States Collaborative Review on Sterilization, to decrease feelings of guilt and regret.

Appropriate counseling regarding risks of failure, permanence of the procedure, the medical risks, and the potential psychosocial reactions to the procedure should be discussed with the patient. Patient ambivalence at the last minute is not unusual, in which case it is advisable to defer the procedure until after the puerperium. The 10-year failure rate of postpartum sterilization is less than 1%, with rate variations dependent on the type of sterilization procedure performed. The risks of postpartum or interval tubal ligation are infrequent, and deaths from the procedure occur in 2–12 per 100,000 cases. Long-term complications, such as the posttubal syndrome (irregular menses and increased menstrual pain) have been reported in some 10–15% of women; however, well-controlled prospective studies have failed to confirm that these symptoms occur more frequently with sterilization than in controls. A major anesthetic should be initiated only after careful evaluation by the anesthesia service because the parturient may have an increased risk of regurgitation and aspiration of gastric contents. Postpartum laparoscopic sterilization has not gained popularity because of increased pelvic vascularity, the large size of the uterus, and the risk of visceral injury.

Natural family planning as contraception may begin after normal menses resumes. Breastfeeding with no supplementation will provide 98% contraceptive protection for up to 6 months. When menses returns, natural family planning may begin. This method, which has pregnancy rates comparable to barrier methods, utilizes detection of the periovulation period by evaluating cervical mucous changes and/or basal body temperature changes. These techniques are often misrepresented by providers who have limited understanding of their use and success in pregnancy prevention.

Use of spermicides, a condom, or both may be prescribed until the postpartum examination; these methods carry a failure rate of 1.6–21 per 100 woman-years. Fitting of a diaphragm is not practical until involution of the reproductive organs has taken place and may be more difficult in lactating women with vaginal dryness. It should always be used in conjunction with a spermicidal lubricant containing nonoxynol-9. The failure rate for the diaphragm varies from 2.4–19.6 per 100 woman-years, with the lowest failure rates (comparable to the intrauterine device [IUD]) occurring in women who are older, motivated, experienced, or familiar with the technique.

In patients who are not breastfeeding, combination oral contraceptive agents can be taken as early as 2–3 weeks postpartum. These agents should not be given sooner than this period in view of the hypercoagulable state postpartum. The combined estrogen–progestin preparations, which contain 35 μg or less of estrogen and varying amounts of progestin, are associated with pregnancy rates of less than 0.5 per 100 woman-years. In addition, these low-estrogen compounds used in nonsmokers have fewer cardiovascular complications. Lactating women should be given progestin-only oral contraceptives (norethindrone 0.35 mg/d) because they do not suppress lactation and may enhance it.

Intramuscular injection of a long-acting progestin such as depot medroxyprogesterone acetate (Depo-Provera®), 150 mg given every 3 months, provides effective contraception (> 99% contraceptive efficacy) for the lactating woman without provoking maternal thromboembolism or decreasing milk yield. However, concerns related to prolonged amenorrhea, the inconvenience of unpredictable and irregular bleeding, as well as reversible bone density reduction and lipid metabolism changes, limit the usefulness of this method.

Levonorgestrel implants placed after establishment of lactation (immediately postpartum or by 6 weeks) provide acceptable contraception with no effect on lactation or infant growth. They have gained little favor, probably because of irregular bleeding, high cost, and difficulty in insertion and removal.

Insertion of an IUD (copper-containing TCu 380 Ag® and ParaGard T380A®, progesterone-releasing Progestasert®, or levonorgestrel-releasing Mirena®) is highly effective in preventing pregnancy (< 2–3 pregnancies per 100 woman-years) and is not considered an abortifacient. Ideally, an IUD should be placed at the first postpartum visit; however, it may be placed as early as immediately postpartum. In this latter case, the incidence of expulsion is high. The main side effects include syncope from vagal response to insertion, pelvic infection (relative risk 1.7–9.3), uterine perforation (0–8 per 1000), and abnormal uterine bleeding. The risk of ectopic pregnancy is higher among women using Progestasert compared to women not using contraception. The risk of uterine perforation during IUD insertion is higher in lactating women, probably because of the accelerated rate of uterine involution. However, the risk of expulsion is not increased. Uterine perforation is highest when insertion is performed in the first 1–8 weeks following delivery.

Discharge Examination & Instructions

Before the patient's hospital discharge, the breasts and abdomen should be examined. The degree of uterine involution and tenderness should be noted. The calves and thighs should be palpated to rule out thrombophlebitis. The characteristics of the lochia are important and should be observed. The episiotomy wound should be inspected to see whether it is healing satisfactorily. A blood sample should be obtained for hematocrit or hemoglobin determination. Unless the patient has an unusual pelvic complaint, there is little need to perform a vaginal examination. The obstetrician should be certain that the patient is voiding normally, has normal bowel function, and is physically able to assume her new responsibilities at home.

The patient will require some advice on what she is allowed to do when she arrives home. Hygiene is essentially the same as practiced in the hospital, with a premium on cleanliness. Upon discharge from the hospital, the patient should be instructed to rest for at least 2 hours during the day, and her usual household activities should be curtailed. Activities, exercise, and return to work will be individualized. Accepted disability following delivery is 6 weeks. Various forms of social support are critical for mothers, especially those employed outside the home: available, high-quality day care; parental leave for both mothers and fathers; and support provided by the workplace such as flexible hours, the opportunity to breastfeed, on-site day care, and care for sick children. The patient who has had frequent prenatal visits to her obstetrician may feel cut off from the doctor during the interval between discharge and the first postpartum visit. She will feel reassured in this period if she receives thoughtful advice on what she is allowed to do and what she can expect when she arrives home. She should be instructed to take her temperature at home twice daily and to notify the physician or nurse in the event of fever, vaginal bleeding, or back pain. At the time of discharge, the patient should be informed that she will note persistent but decreasing amounts of vaginal lochia for about 3 weeks and possibly for a short period during the fourth or fifth week after delivery.

Postpartum Examination

At the postpartum visit—4–6 weeks after discharge from hospital—the patient's weight and blood pressure should be recorded. Most patients retain about 60% of any weight in excess of 11 kg (24 lb) that was gained during pregnancy. A suitable diet may be prescribed if the patient has not returned to her approximate prepregnancy weight. If the patient was anemic upon discharge from the hospital or has been bleeding during the puerperium, a complete blood count should be determined. Persistence of uterine bleeding demands investigation and definitive treatment.

The breasts should be examined, and the adequacy of support, abnormalities of the nipples or lactation, and the presence of any masses should be noted. The patient should be instructed concerning self-examination of the breasts. A complete rectovaginal evaluation is required.

Nursing mothers may show a hypoestrogenic condition of the vaginal epithelium. Prescription of a vaginal estrogen cream to be applied at bedtime should relieve local dryness and coital discomfort without the side effects of systemic estrogen therapy. The cervix should be inspected and a Papanicolaou (Pap) smear obtained. Women whose prenatal smears are normal are still at risk for an abnormal Pap smear at their postpartum visit.

The episiotomy incision and repaired lacerations must be examined and the adequacy of pelvic and perineal support noted. Bimanual examination of the uterus and adnexa is indicated. At the time of the postpartum examination, most patients have some degree of retrodisplacement of the uterus, but this may soon correct itself.

Asymptomatic retroposition of the uterus is not regarded as an abnormal condition. If pain, abnormal bleeding, or other symptoms are present, a vaginal pessary may be inserted as a trial procedure to encourage anteversion of the fundus. However, pessary support for long periods of time is not recommended. In the absence of pelvic disease, uterine retrodisplacement rarely, if ever, requires surgical correction. If marked uterine descensus is noted or if the patient develops stress incontinence, symptomatic cystocele, or rectocele, surgical correction should be considered if childbearing has been completed. Hysterectomy or vaginal repair is best postponed for at least 3 months after delivery to allow maximal restoration of the pelvic supporting structures.

The patient may resume full activity or employment if her course to this point has been uneventful. Once again, the patient should be advised regarding family planning and contraceptive practices. The postnatal visit is an important opportunity to consider general disorders such as backache and depression and to discuss infant feeding and immunization. The rapport established between the obstetrician and the patient during the prenatal and postpartum periods provides a unique opportunity to establish a preventive health program in subsequent years.

■ LACTATION PHYSIOLOGY

PHYSIOLOGY

The mammary glands are modified exocrine glands that undergo dramatic anatomic and physiologic changes during pregnancy and in the immediate puerperium. Their role is to provide nourishment for the newborn and to transfer antibodies from mother to infant.

During the first half of pregnancy, proliferation of alveolar epithelial cells, formation of new ducts, and development of lobular architecture occur. Later in pregnancy, proliferation declines, and the epithelium differentiates for secretory activity. At the end of gestation, each breast will have gained approximately 400 g. Factors contributing to increase in mammary size include hypertrophy of blood vessels, myoepithelial cells, and connective tissue; deposition of fat; and retention of water and electrolytes. Blood flow is almost double that of the nonpregnant state.

The mammary gland has been called the mirror of the endocrine system, because lactation depends on a delicate balance of several hormones. An intact hypothalamic–pituitary axis is essential to the initiation and maintenance of lactation. Lactation can be divided into 3 stages: (1) mammogenesis, or mammary growth and development; (2) lactogenesis, or initiation of milk secretion; and (3) galactopoiesis, or maintenance of established milk secretion (Table 12–2). Estrogen is responsible for the growth of ductular tissue and alveolar budding, whereas progesterone is required for optimal maturation of the alveolar glands. Glandular stem cells undergo differentiation into secretory and myoepithelial cells under the influence of prolactin, growth hormone, insulin, cortisol, and an epithelial growth factor. Although alveolar secretory cells actively synthesize milk fat and proteins from midpregnancy onward, only small amounts are released into the lumen. However, lactation is possible if pregnancy is interrupted during the second trimester.

Prolactin is an necessary hormone for milk production, but lactogenesis also requires a low-estrogen environment. Although prolactin levels continue to rise as pregnancy advances, placental sex steroids block prolactin-induced secretory activity of the glandular epithelium. It appears that sex steroids and prolactin are synergistic in mammogenesis but antagonistic in galactopoiesis. Therefore, lactation is not initiated until plasma estrogens, progesterone, and human placental lactogen (hPL) levels fall after delivery. Progesterone inhibits the biosynthesis of lactose and α-lactalbumin; estrogens directly antagonize the lactogenic effect of prolactin on the mammary gland by inhibiting α-lactalbumin production. hPL may also exert a prolactin-antagonist effect through competitive binding to alveolar prolactin receptors.

The maintenance of established milk secretion requires periodic suckling and the actual emptying of ducts and alveoli. Growth hormone, cortisol, thyroxine, and insulin exert a permissive effect. Prolactin is required for galactopoiesis, but high basal levels are not mandatory, because prolactin concentrations in the nursing mother decline gradually during the late puerperium and approach that of the nonpregnant state. However, if a woman does not suckle her baby, her serum prolactin concentration will return to nonpregnant values within 2–3 weeks. If the mother suckles twins simultaneously, the prolactin response is about double that when 1 baby is fed at a time, illustrating an apparent synergism between the number of nipples stimulated and the frequency of suckling. The mechanism by which suckling stimulates prolactin release probably involves the inhibition of dopamine, which is thought to be the hypothalamic prolactin-inhibiting factor.

Nipple stimulation by suckling or other physical stimuli evokes a reflex release of oxytocin from the neurohypophysis. Because retrograde blood flow can be demonstrated within the pituitary stalk, oxytocin may reach the adenohypophysis in very high concentrations and affect pituitary release of prolactin independently of any effect on dopamine. The release of oxytocin is mediated by afferent fibers of the fourth to sixth intercostal nerves via the dorsal roots of the spinal cord to the midbrain.

The paraventricular and supraoptic neurons of the hypothalamus make up the final afferent pathway of the milk ejection reflex. The central nervous system can modulate the release of oxytocin by either stimulating or inhibiting the hypothalamus to increase or decrease prolactin-inhibiting factor (dopamine) and thus the release of oxytocin from the posterior pituitary. Thus, positive senses related to nursing, crying of an infant, positive attitudes in pregnancy and toward breastfeeding can improve milk yield and the ultimate success of breastfeeding. Likewise, the expectation of nursing is sufficient to release oxytocin prior to milk let-down but is not effective in releasing prolactin in the absence of suckling. Contrarily, negative stimuli, such as pain, stress, fear, anxiety, insecurity, or negative attitudes, may inhibit the let-down reflex. Oxytocin levels may rise during orgasm, and sexual stimuli may trigger milk ejection.

SYNTHESIS OF HUMAN MILK

Prolactin ultimately promotes milk production by inducing the synthesis of mRNAs for the production of milk enzymes and milk proteins at the membrane of mammary epithelial cells (alveolar cells). Milk synthesis and secretion are then initiated via four major transcellular and paracellular pathways. The substrates for milk production are primarily derived from the maternal gut or produced in the maternal liver. The availability of these substrates is aided by a 20–40% increased blood flow to the mammary gland, gastrointestinal tract, and liver, as well as increased cardiac output during breastfeeding. The principal carbohydrate in human milk is lactose.

Table 12–2. Multihormonal interaction in mammary growth and lactation.

Mammogenesis	Lactogenesis	Galactopoiesis
Estrogens	Prolactin	↓Gonadal hormones
Progesterone	↓Estrogens	Suckling (oxytocin, prolactin)
Prolactin	↓Progesterone	Growth hormone
Growth hormone	↓hPL(?)	Glucocorticoids
Glucocorticoids	Glucocorticoids	Insulin
Epithelial growth factor	Insulin	Thyroxine and parathyroid hormone

Arrows signify that lower than normal levels of the hormone are necessary for the effect to occur.

Glucose metabolism is a key function in human milk production, because lactose is derived from glucose and galactose; the latter originates from glucose-6-phosphate. A specific protein, α-lactalbumin, catalyzes lactose synthesis. This rate-limiting enzyme is inhibited by gonadal hormones during pregnancy. Prolactin and insulin, which enhance the uptake of glucose by mammary cells, also stimulate the formation of triglycerides. Fat synthesis takes place in the endoplasmic reticulum. Most proteins are synthesized de novo in the secretory cells from essential and nonessential plasma amino acids. The formation of milk protein and mammary enzymes is induced by prolactin and enhanced by cortisol and insulin.

Mature human milk contains 7% carbohydrate as lactose, 3–5% fat, 0.9% protein, and 0.2% mineral constituents expressed as ash. Its energy content is 60–75 kcal/dL. About 25% of the total nitrogen of human milk represents nonprotein compounds, eg, urea, uric acid, creatinine, and free amino acids. The principal proteins of human milk are casein, α-lactalbumin, lactoferrin, immunoglobulin (Ig) A, lysozyme, and albumin. Milk also contains a variety of enzymes that may contribute to the infant's digestion of breast milk, eg, amylase, catalase, peroxidase, lipase, xanthine oxidase, and alkaline and acid phosphatase. The fatty acid composition of human milk is rich in palmitic and oleic acids and varies somewhat with the diet. The major ions and mineral constituents of human milk are Na^+, K^+, Ca^{2+}, Mg^{2+}, Cl^-, phosphorus, sulfate, and citrate. Calcium concentrations vary from 25–35 mg/dL and phosphorus concentrations from 13–16 mg/dL. Iron, copper, zinc, and trace metal contents vary considerably. All the vitamins except vitamin K are found in human milk in nutritionally adequate amounts. The composition of breast milk is not greatly affected by race, age, parity, normal diet variations, moderate postpartum dieting, weight loss, or aerobic exercise. Volume and caloric density may be reduced in extreme scenarios, such as developing countries where starvation or daily caloric intake is less than 1600 kcal/d. In addition, milk composition does not differ between the 2 breasts unless 1 breast is infected. However, the volume and concentration of constituents varies during the day. The volume per feed increases in the late afternoon and evening. Nitrogen peaks in the late afternoon. Fat concentrations peak in the morning and are lowest at night. Lactose levels remain fairly constant.

Colostrum, the premilk secretion, is a yellowish alkaline secretion that may be present in the last months of pregnancy and for the first 2–3 days after delivery. It has a higher specific gravity (1.040–1.060); a higher protein, vitamin A, immunoglobulin, and sodium and chloride content; and a lower carbohydrate, potassium, and fat content than mature breast milk. Colostrum has a normal laxative action and is an ideal natural starter food.

Ions and water pass the membrane of the alveolar cell in both directions. Human milk differs from the milk of many other species by having a lower concentration of monovalent ions and a higher concentration of lactose. The aqueous phase of milk is isosmotic with plasma; thus, the higher the lactose, the lower the ion concentration. The ratio of potassium/sodium is 3:1 in both milk and mammary intracellular fluid. Because milk contains about 87% water and lactose is the major osmotically active solute, it follows that milk yield is largely determined by lactose production.

IMMUNOLOGIC SIGNIFICANCE OF HUMAN MILK

The neonate's secretory immune system and cellular responses are immature. In particular, the IgM and IgA responses are poor and cellular immunity is impaired for several months. Maternal transfer of immunoglobulins through breast milk provides support for the infant's developing immune system and thereby enhances neonatal defense against infection. All classes of immunoglobulins are found in milk, but IgA constitutes 90% of immunoglobulins in human colostrum and milk. The output of immunoglobulins by the breast is maximal in the first week of life and declines thereafter as the production of milk-specific proteins increases. Lacteal antibodies against enteric bacteria and their antigenic products are largely of the IgA class. IgG and IgA lacteal antibodies provide short-term systemic and long-term enteric humoral immunity to the breastfed neonate. IgA antipoliomyelitis virus activity present in breastfed infants indicates that at least some transfer of milk antibodies into serum does occur. However, maternal lacteal antibodies are absorbed systemically by human infants for only a very short time after birth. Long-term protection against pathogenic enteric bacteria is provided by the adsorption of lacteal IgA to the intestinal mucosa. In addition to providing passive immunity, there is evidence that lacteal immunoglobulins can modulate the immunocompetence of the neonate, but the exact mechanisms have not been described. For instance, the secretion of IgA into the saliva of breastfed infants is enhanced in comparison with bottle-fed controls.

Breast milk is highly anti-infective, containing more than 4000 cells/mm^3, the majority of which are leukocytes. The total cell count is even higher in colostrum. In human milk, the leukocytes are predominantly mononuclear cells and macrophages. Both T and B lymphocytes are present. During maternal infection, antigen-specific lymphocytes can migrate to the breast mucosa or produce immunoglobulins, both of which are key in the fight against infection. Fully functional immunoglobulins are present, primarily as IgA, IgG, and IgM. Polymeric secretory IgA is easily transported across the mucous membrane of the breast, blocking the mucosal receptors of infectious agents.

Elements in breast milk other than immunoglobulins and cells have prophylactic value against infections. The marked difference between the intestinal flora of breastfed and bottle-fed infants is due to a dialyzable nitrogen-containing carbohydrate (bifidus factor) that supports the growth of *Lactobacillus bifidus* in breastfed infants. The stool of bottle-fed infants is more alkaline and contains predominantly coliform organisms and *Bacteroides* spp. *L bifidus* inhibits the growth of *Shigella* spp, *Escherichia coli,* and yeast. Human milk also contains a nonspecific antimicrobial factor, lysozyme (a thermostable, acid-stable enzyme that cleaves the peptidoglycans of bacteria), and a "resistance factor," which protect the infant against staphylococcal infection. Lactoferrin, an iron chelator, exerts a strong bacteriostatic effect on staphylococci and *E coli* by depriving the organisms of iron. Both C3 and C4 components of complement and antitoxins for neutralizing *Vibrio cholerae* are found in human milk. Unsaturated vitamin B_{12}–binding protein in milk renders the vitamin unavailable for utilization by *E coli* and *Bacteroides*. Finally, interferon in milk may provide yet another nonspecific antiinfection factor.

Human milk may also have prophylactic value in childhood food allergies. During the neonatal period, permeability of the small intestine to macromolecules is increased. Secretory IgA in colostrum and breast milk reduces the absorption of foreign macromolecules until the endogenous IgA secretory capacity of the newborn intestinal lamina propria and lymph nodes develops at 2–3 months of age. Protein of cow's milk can be highly allergenic in the infant predisposed by heredity. The introduction of cow's milk–free formulas has considerably reduced the incidence of milk allergy. Thus, comparative studies on the incidence of allergy, bacterial and viral infections, severe diarrhea, necrotizing enterocolitis, tuberculosis, and neonatal meningitis in breastfed and bottle-fed infants support the concept that breast milk fulfills a protective function.

ADVANTAGES & DISADVANTAGES OF BREASTFEEDING

For the Mother

A. ADVANTAGES

Breastfeeding is convenient, economical, and emotionally satisfying to most women. It helps to contract the uterus and accelerates the process of uterine involution in the postpartum period, including decreased maternal blood loss. It promotes mother–infant bonding and self-confidence and improves maternal tolerance to stress through an oxytocin-associated antifight/fight response. Maternal gastrointestinal motility and absorption are enhanced. Ovulatory cycles are delayed with nonsupplemented breastfeeding. According to epidemiologic studies, breastfeeding may help to protect against premenopausal cancer and ovarian cancer.

B. DISADVANTAGES

Regular nursing restricts activities and may be perceived by some mothers as an inconvenience. Twins can be nursed successfully, but few women are prepared for the first weeks of almost continual feeding. Cesarean section may necessitate modifications of early breastfeeding routines. Difficulties such as nipple tenderness and mastitis may develop. Compared with nonlactating women, breastfeeding women have a significant decrease (mean 6.5%) in bone mineral content at 6 months postpartum, but there is "catch-up" remineralization after weaning.

Breastfeeding by a hypoparathyroid mother is undesirable, because adequate calcium supplementation to replace losses in breast milk is difficult in these patients. Furthermore, large amounts of 25-hydroxyvitamin D_3 appear in the milk of mothers receiving therapy for hypoparathyroidism. There are few absolute contraindications to breastfeeding (see Disadvantages and Contraindications for the Infant).

Many women with breast implants breastfeed successfully, but reduction mammoplasty involving nipple autotransplantation severs the lactiferous ducts and precludes nursing. Several situations may arise in which a case-by-case assessment will be needed to determine the impact of breastfeeding: environmental exposures, hepatitis C, illicit drugs, metabolic disorders, use of pharmaceutical drugs, and tobacco and alcohol consumption.

For the Infant

A. ADVANTAGES

Breast milk is digestible, of ideal composition, available at the right temperature and the right time, and free of bacterial contamination. Infants of breastfed mothers have a decreased incidence of all of the following: diarrhea, lower respiratory tract infection, otitis media, pneumonia, urinary tract infections, necrotizing enterocolitis, invasive bacterial infection, and sudden infant death. Breastfed infants may have a decreased risk of developing insulin-dependent diabetes, Crohn's disease, ulcerative colitis, lymphoma, and allergic diseases later in life. Breastfed infants are less likely to become obese as neonates and adolescents. Suckling promotes infant–mother bonding. Cognitive development and intelligence may be improved.

B. DISADVANTAGES AND CONTRAINDICATIONS

Absolute contraindications to breastfeeding are use of street drugs or excess alcohol; human T-cell leukemia virus type 1; breast cancer; active herpes simplex infection of the breast; active pulmonary tuberculosis in the mother; galactosemia in the infant; and maternal intake of cancer chemotherapeutic agents or certain other drugs. Table 12–3 lists some of the medications that are contraindicated during breastfeeding. Additional medications are not recommended during breastfeeding. Therefore, specific precautions for individual medications should be reviewed when prescribing drugs to lactating women. Human immunodeficiency virus (HIV) infection in the United States is also a contraindication to breastfeeding. Breastfeeding has been recognized as a mode of HIV transmission. Breastfeeding might pose an additional risk (about 15%) for an infant above that already present at birth because the mother had HIV. The risk of HIV transmission through breast milk is substantially higher among women who become infected during the postpartum lactation period. Most mothers in developed countries who know of their seropositivity choose not to breastfeed; in underdeveloped countries where lactation is critical to infant survival, HIV-infected mothers may choose to breastfeed their infants.

Breastfeeding does not protect against the deleterious effects of congenital hypothyroidism. The milk of a nursing mother with cystic fibrosis is high in sodium and places the infant at risk for hypernatremia. A woman with clinically infectious varicella should be isolated from the infant and should neither breastfeed nor bottle-feed. Once the infant has received varicella zoster immune globulin and there are no skin lesions on the mother's breast, she may provide expressed milk for her infant. A small number of otherwise healthy breastfed infants develop unconjugated hyperbilirubinemia (sometimes exceeding 20 mg/dL) during the first few weeks of life because of the higher-than-normal glucuronyl transferase inhibitory activity of the breast milk. The inhibitor may be a pregnanediol, although increased milk lipase activity and free fatty acids are likely the critical factors.

Breastfeeding is not usually possible for weak, ill, or very premature infants or for infants with cleft palate, choanal atresia, or phenylketonuria. It is common practice in many nurseries to feed premature infants human milk collected fresh from their mothers or processed from donors. The effects of processing and storage on the persistence of viral agents are not well studied. Cytomegalovirus transmission through breast milk has been documented and may pose a significant

Table 12–3. Medications contraindicated during breastfeeding.

Medication	Reason
Bromocriptine	Suppresses lactation; may be hazardous to the mother
Cocaine	Cocaine intoxication
Cyclophosphamide	Possible immune suppression; unknown effect on growth or association with carcinogenesis; neutropenia
Cyclosporine	Possible immune suppression; unknown effect on growth or association with carcinogenesis
Doxorubicin[1]	Possible immune suppression; unknown effect on growth or association with carcinogenesis
Ergotamine	Vomiting, diarrhea, convulsions (at doses used in migraine medications)
Lithium	One third to one half of therapeutic blood concentration in infants
Methotrexate	Possible immune suppression; unknown effect on growth or association with carcinogenesis; neutropenia
Phencyclidine	Potent hallucinogen
Phenindione	Anticoagulant; increased prothrombin and partial thromboplastin time in one infant; not used in United States
Radioactive iodine and other radiolabeled elements	Contraindications to breastfeeding for various periods

[1]Medication is concentrated in human milk.
American Academy of Pediatrics, American College of Obstetricians and Gynecologists. Guidelines for perinatal care, 4th ed. Elk Grove Village, Illinois: AAP; Washington, DC: ACOG, 1997.

hazard for preterm infants. It is recommended that seronegative preterm infants receive milk from seronegative donors only. Because maternal antibodies are present in breast milk, an otherwise healthy term infant may do better if breastfed.

PRINCIPLES & TECHNIQUES OF BREASTFEEDING

In the absence of anatomic or medical complications, the timing of the first feeding and the frequency and duration of subsequent feedings largely determine the outcome of breastfeeding. Infants and mothers who are able to initiate breastfeeding within 1–2 hours of delivery are more successful than those whose initial interactions are delayed for several hours. Lactation is established most successfully if the baby remains with the mother and she can feed on demand for adequate intervals throughout the first 24-hour period. The initial feeding should last 5 minutes at each breast in order to condition the let-down reflex. At first, the frequency of feedings may be very irregular (8–10 times per day), but after 1–2 weeks a fairly regular 4- to 6-hour pattern will emerge.

When the milk "comes in" abruptly on the third or fourth postpartum day, there is an initial period of discomfort caused by vascular engorgement and edema of the breasts. The baby does not nurse so much by developing intermittent negative pressure as by a rhythmic grasping of the areola; the infant "works" the milk into its mouth. Little force is required in nursing because the breast reservoirs can be emptied and refilled without suction. Nursing mothers notice a sensation of drawing and tightening within the breast at the beginning of suckling after the initial breast engorgement disappears. They are thus conscious of the milk ejection reflex, which may even cause milk to spurt or run out.

Some women expend a great deal of emotion on the subject of breastfeeding, and a few are almost overwhelmed by fear of being unable to care for their babies in this way. If attendants are sympathetic and patient, however, a woman who wants to nurse usually can do so. Attendants must be certain that the baby "latches" on (actually over) the nipple and the areola so as to feed properly without causing pain for the mother (Fig 12–8).

The baby should nurse at both breasts at each feeding, because overfilling of the breasts is the main deterrent to the maintenance of milk secretion. Nursing at only 1 breast at each feeding inhibits the reflex that is provoked simultaneously in both breasts. Thus, nursing at alternate breasts from 1 feeding to the next may increase discomfort due to engorgement and reduce milk output. It is helpful for the mother to be taught to empty the breasts after each feeding; a sleepy baby may not have accomplished this. The use of supplementary formula or other food during the first 6–8 weeks of breastfeeding can interfere with lactation and should be avoided except when absolutely necessary. The introduction of an artificial nipple, which requires a different sucking mechanism, will weaken the sucking reflex required for breastfeeding. Some groups, such as the La Leche League, recommend that other fluids be given by spoon or dropper rather than by bottle.

In preparing to nurse, the mother should (1) wash her hands with soap and water, (2) clean her nipples and breasts with water, and (3) assume a comfortable position, preferably in a rocking or upright chair with the infant and mother chest-to-chest. If the mother is unable to sit up to nurse her baby because of painful perineal sutures, she may feel more comfortable lying on her side. An alternative position is the football hold. A woman with large pendulous breasts may find it difficult to manage both the breasts and the baby. If the baby lies on a pillow, the mother will have both hands free to guide the nipple.

Each baby nurses differently; however, the following procedure is generally successful:

1. Allow the normal newborn to nurse at each breast on demand or approximately every 3–4 hours, for 5 minutes per breast per feeding the first day. Over the next few days, gradually increase feeding time to initiate the let-down reflex, but do not exceed 10–15 minutes per breast. Suckling for longer than 15 minutes may cause maceration and cracking of the nipples and thus lead to mastitis.
2. Stimulating the cheek or lateral angle of the baby's mouth should precipitate a reflex turn to the nipple and opening of the mouth. The infant is brought firmly to the breast, and the nipple and areola are placed into the mouth as far as the nipple–areola line. Slight negative pressure holds the teat in place, and milk is obtained with a peristaltic motion of the tongue. Compressing the periareolar area and expressing a small amount of colostrum or milk for the baby to taste may stimulate the baby to nurse.
3. Try to keep the baby awake by moving or patting, but do not snap its feet, work its jaw, push its head, or press its cheeks.
4. Before removing the infant from the breast, gently open its mouth by lifting the outer border of the upper lip to break the suction.

After nursing, gently wipe the nipples with water and dry them.

MILK YIELD

The prodigious energy requirements for lactation are met by mobilization of elements from maternal tissues and from dietary intake. Physiologic fat stores laid down during pregnancy are mobilized during lactation, and the return to prepregnancy weight and figure is promoted. A variety of studies suggest that a lactating woman should increase her normal daily food intake by 600 kcal/d, but intakes of 2000–2300 calories are sufficient for lactating women. The recommended daily dietary increases for lactation are 20 g of protein; a 20% increase in all vitamins and minerals except folic acid, which should be increased by 50%; and a 33% increase

Figure 12–8. Mechanism of suckling in the neonate. **A:** Tongue moves forward to draw nipple in as glottis still permits breathing. **B:** Tongue moves along nipple, pressing it against the palate with the glottis closed. Ductules under the areola are compressed, and milk flow begins. The cheeks fill the mouth and provide negative pressure.

in calcium, phosphorus, and magnesium. There is no evidence that increasing fluid intake will increase milk volume. Fluid restriction also has little effect because urine output will diminish in preference to milk output.

With nursing, average milk production on the second postpartum day is about 120 mL. The amount increases to about 180 mL on the third postpartum day and to as much as 240 mL on the fourth day. In time, milk production reaches about 300 mL/d.

A good rule of thumb for the calculation of milk production for a given day in the week after delivery is to multiply the number of the postpartum day by 60. This gives the approximate number of milliliters of milk secreted in that 24-hour period.

If all goes well, sustained production of milk will be achieved by most patients after 10–14 days. A yield of 120–180 mL per feeding is common by the end of the second week. When free secretion has been established, marked increases are possible; a wet nurse can often suckle 3 babies successfully for weeks.

Early diminution of milk production often is due to failure to empty the breasts because of weak efforts by the baby or ineffectual nursing procedures; emotional problems, such as aversion to nursing; or medical complications, such as mastitis, debilitating systemic disease, or Sheehan's syndrome. Late diminution of milk production results from too generous complementary feedings of formula, emotional or other illness, and pregnancy.

Adequate rest is essential for successful lactation. Sometimes it is difficult to ensure an adequate milk yield if the mother is working outside the home. If it is not possible to rearrange the nursing schedule to fit the work schedule or vice versa, it may be necessary to empty the breasts manually or by pump. Milk output can be estimated by weighing the infant before and after feeding. If there has been a bowel movement during feeding, the baby should be weighed before the diaper is changed.

It may be necessary to substitute bottle-feeding for breastfeeding if the mother's supply continues to be inadequate (less than 50% of the infant's needs) after 3 weeks of effort, if nipple or breast lesions are severe enough to prevent pumping, or if the mother is either pregnant or severely (physically or mentally) ill. Nourishment from the inadequately lactating breast can be augmented with the Lact-Aide Nursing Trainer, a device that provides a supplemental source of milk via a plastic capillary tube placed beside the breast and suckled simultaneously with the nipple. Disposable plastic bags serve as reservoirs, and the supplemental milk is warmed by hanging the bag next to the mother. The Lact-Aide supplementer has also been used to help nurse premature infants and to re-establish lactation after untimely weaning due to illness. The long-term success of breastfeeding is increased by a structured home support system of postnatal visits by allied health personnel or experienced volunteers.

DISORDERS OF LACTATION

Painful Nipples

Tenderness of the nipples, a common symptom during the first days of breastfeeding, generally begins when the baby starts to suck. As soon as milk begins to flow, nipple sensitivity usually subsides. If maternal tissues are unusually tender, dry heat may help between feedings. Nipple shields should be used only as a last resort because they interfere with normal sucking. Glass or plastic shields with rubber nursing nipples are preferable to shields made entirely of rubber.

Nipple fissures cause severe pain and prevent normal let-down of milk. Local infection around the fissure can lead to mastitis. The application of vitamin A and D ointment or hydrous lanolin, which do not have to be removed, is often effective. To speed healing, the following steps are recommended. Apply dry heat for 20 minutes 4 times per day with a 60-watt bulb held 18 inches away from the nipple. Conduct prefeeding manual expression. Begin nursing on the side opposite the fissure with the other breast exposed to air to allow the initial let-down to occur atraumatically. Apply expressed breast milk to nipples and let it dry in between feedings. If necessary, use a nipple shield while nursing, and take ibuprofen or acetaminophen with or without codeine just after nursing. On rare occasions, it may be necessary to stop nursing temporarily on the affected side and to empty the breast either manually or by gentle pumping.

A cause of chronic severe sore nipples without remarkable physical findings is candidal infection. Prompt relief is provided by topical nystatin cream. Thrush or candidal diaper rash or maternal candidal vaginitis must be treated as well.

Engorgement

Engorgement of the breasts occurs in the first week postpartum and is due to vascular congestion and accumulation of milk. Vascularity and swelling increase on the second day after delivery; the areola or breast may become engorged. Prepartum breast massage and around-the-clock demand feedings help to prevent engorgement in these patients. When the areola is engorged, the nipple is occluded and proper grasping of the areola by the infant is not possible. With moderately severe engorgement, the breasts become firm and warm, and the lobules may be palpable as tender, irregular masses. Considerable discomfort and often a slight fever can be expected.

Mild cases may be relieved by acetaminophen or other analgesics, cool compresses, and partial expression of the milk before nursing. In severe cases, the patient should empty the breasts manually or with an electric pump.

Mastitis

Mastitis occurs most frequently in primiparous nursing patients and usually is caused by coagulase-positive *Staphylococcus aureus*. High fever should never be ascribed to simple breast engorgement alone. Inflammation of the breast seldom begins before the fifth day postpartum. Most frequently, symptoms of a painful erythematous lobule in an outer quadrant of the breast are noted during the second or third week of the puerperium. Inflammation may occur with weaning when the flow of milk is disrupted, or the nursing mother may acquire the infection during her hospital stay and then transmit it to the infant. Demonstration of antibody-coated bacteria in the milk indicates the presence of infectious mastitis. Many infants harbor an infection and, in turn, infect the mother's breast during nursing. Neonatal streptococcal infection should be suspected if mastitis is recurrent or bilateral.

Infection may be limited to the subareolar region but more frequently involves an obstructed lactiferous duct and the surrounding breast parenchyma. If cellulitis is not properly treated, a breast abscess may develop. When only mastitis is present, it is best to prevent milk stasis by continuing breastfeeding or by using a breast pump. Apply local heat, provide a well-fitted brassiere, and institute appropriate antibiotic treatment. Cephalosporins, methicillin sodium, and dicloxacillin sodium are the antibiotics of choice to combat penicillinase-producing bacteria.

Pitting edema over the inflamed area and some degree of fluctuation are evidence of abscess formation. It is necessary to incise and open loculated areas and provide wide drainage. Unlike the case with mastitis, continuing breastfeeding is not recommended in the presence of a breast abscess.

Miscellaneous Complications

A galactocele, or milk-retention cyst, is caused by blockage of a milk duct. It usually will resolve with warm compresses and continuation of breastfeeding. Sometimes the infant will reject 1 or both breasts. Strong foods such as beans, cabbage, turnips, broccoli, onions, garlic, and rhubarb may cause aversion to milk or neonatal colic. A common cause of nursing problems is maternal fatigue.

INHIBITION & SUPPRESSION OF LACTATION

Despite a recent upsurge in breastfeeding in Western countries, many women will not or cannot breastfeed, and others will fail in the attempt. Lactation inhibition is desirable in the event of fetal or neonatal death as well.

The oldest and simplest method of suppressing lactation is to stop nursing, to avoid nipple stimulation, to refrain from expressing or pumping the milk, and to wear a supportive bra. Analgesics are also helpful. Patients will complain of breast engorgement (45%), pain (45%), and leaking breasts (55%). Although the breasts will become considerably engorged and the patient may experience discomfort, the collection of milk in the duct system will suppress its production, and resorption will occur. After approximately 2–3 days, engorgement will begin to recede, and the patient will be comfortable again. Medical suppression of lactation with estrogens or bromocriptine is no longer recommended.

REFERENCES

Anatomy & Physiology of the Puerperium

Allolio B et al: Diurnal salivary cortisol patterns during pregnancy and after delivery: Relationship to plasma corticotrophin-releasing-hormone. Clin Endocrinol 1990;33:279.

Bacigalupo G et al: Quantitative relationships between pain intensities during labor and beta-endorphin and cortisol concentrations in plasma: Decline of the hormone concentrations in the early postpartum period. J Perinat Med 1990;18:289.

Battin DA et al: Effect of suckling on serum prolactin, luteinizing hormone, follicle-stimulating hormone, and estradiol during prolonged lactation. Obstet Gynecol 1985;65:785.

Bremme K et al: Enhanced thrombin generation and fibrinolytic activity in normal pregnancy and the puerperium. Obstet Gynecol 1992;80:132.

Brewer MM, Bates RM, Vannoy LP: Postpartum changes in maternal weight and body fat deposits in lactating versus nonlactating women. Am J Clin Nutr 1989;49:259.

Clapp JF III, Capeless E: Cardiovascular function before, during, and after the first and subsequent pregnancies. Am J Cardiol 1997;80:1469.

Coppleson M, Reid BL: A colposcopic study of the cervix during pregnancy and the puerperium. J Obstet Gynaecol Br Commonw 1966;73:575.

Crowell DT: Weight change in the postpartum period: A review of the literature. J Nurse Midwifery 1995;40:418.

Dawood MY et al: Oxytocin release and plasma anterior pituitary and gonadal hormones in women during lactation. J Clin Endocrinol Metab 1981;52:678.

DeAlvarez RR: Renal glomerulotubular mechanisms during normal pregnancy. Am J Obstet Gynecol 1958;75:931.

De Leo V et al: Control of growth hormone secretion during the postpartum period. Gynecol Obstet Invest 1992;33:31.

DeSantis M, Cavaliere AF, Straface G, Caruso A: Rubella infection in pregnancy. Reprod Toxicol 2006;21:390.

Elster AD et al: Size and shape of the pituitary gland during pregnancy and postpartum: Measurement with MR imaging. Radiology 1991;181:531.

Gray RH et al: Risk of ovulation during lactation. Lancet 1990;335:25.

Hatjis CG et al: Atrial natriuretic factor concentrations during pregnancy and in the postpartum period. Am J Perinatol 1992;9:275.

Hellgren M: Hemostasis during normal pregnancy and puerperium. Semin Thromb Hemost 2003;29:125.

Hornnes PJ, Kuhl C: Plasma insulin and glucagon responses to isoglycemic stimulation in normal pregnancy and postpartum. Obstet Gynecol 1980;55:425.

Kerr-Wilson RHJ et al: Effect of labor on the postpartum bladder. Obstet Gynecol 1984;64:115.

Kremer JAM et al: Pulsatile secretion of luteinizing hormone and prolactin in lactating and nonlactating women and the response to naltrexone. J Clin Endocrinol Metab 1991;72:294.

Lavery JP, Shaw LA: Sonography of the puerperal uterus. J Ultrasound 1989;8:481.

Lewis PR et al: The resumption of ovulation and menstruation in a well-nourished population of women breastfeeding for an extended period of time. Fertil Steril 1991;55:529.

Liu JH, Park KH: Gonadotropin and prolactin secretion increases during sleep during the puerperium in nonlactating women. J Clin Endocrinol Metab 1988;66:839.

Oats JN, Beisher NA: The persistence of abnormal glucose tolerance after delivery. Obstet Gynecol 1990;75:397.

Oppenheimer LW et al: The duration of lochia. Br J Obstet Gynaecol 1986;93:754.

Reader D, Franz MJ: Lactation, diabetes and nutrition recommendations. Curr Diab Rep 2004;4:370.

Robson SC et al: Hemodynamic changes during the puerperium: A Doppler and M-mode echocardiographic study. Br J Obstet Gynaecol 1987;94:1028.

Scholl TO et al: Gestational weight gain, pregnancy outcome, and postpartum weight retention. Obstet Gynecol 1995;86:423.

Sheehan KL, Yen SSC: Activation of pituitary gonadotropic function by an agonist of luteinizing hormone-releasing factor in the puerperium. Am J Obstet Gynecol 1979;135:755.

Smith R, Thomson M: Neuroendocrinology of the hypothalamo-pituitary-adrenal axis in pregnancy and the puerperium. Baillieres Clin Endocrinol Metab 1991;5:167.

South-Paul JE, Rajagopal KR, Tenholder MF: Exercise responses prior to pregnancy and in the postpartum state. Med Sci Sports Exerc 1992;24:410.

Tay CCK, Glasier AF, McNeilly AS: The 24 h pattern of pulsatile luteinizing hormone, follicle stimulating hormone and prolactin release during the first 8 weeks of lactational amenorrhoea in breastfeeding women. Hum Reprod 1992;7:951.

Ueland K: Maternal cardiovascular dynamics. VIII. Intrapartum blood volume changes. Am J Obstet Gynecol 1976;126:671.

Visness CM, Kennedy KI, Ramos R: The duration and character of postpartum bleeding among breast-feeding women. Obstet Gynecol 1997;89:159.

Walters BNJ et al: Blood pressure in the puerperium. Clin Sci 1986;71:589.

Wilms AB et al: Anatomic changes in the pelvis after an uncomplicated vaginal delivery: evaluation with serial MRI imaging. Radiology 1995;195:91.

Ylikorkala O, Viinikka L: Thromboxane A$_2$ in pregnancy and puerperium. Br Med J 1980;281:1601.

Conduct of the Puerperium

American College of Obstetricians and Gynecologists: Exercise during pregnancy and the postpartum period. ACOG Committee Opinion No. 267, January 2002.

American College of Obstetricians and Gynecologists: *Prevention of RhD Alloimmunization.* ACOG Practice Bulletin No. 4. American College of Obstetricians and Gynecologists, 1999.

Aranda C et al: Laparoscopic sterilization immediately after term delivery: preliminary report. J Reprod Med 1963;14:171.

Baskett TF, Parsons ML, Peddle LJ: The experience and effectiveness of the Nova Scotia Rh Program, 1964–84. Can Med Assoc J 1986;134:1259.

Black NA et al: Postpartum rubella immunization: A controlled trial of two vaccines. Lancet 1983;2:990.

Bledin KD, Brice B: Psychological conditions in pregnancy and the puerperium and their relevance to postpartum sterilization: A review. Bull WHO 1983;61:533.

Bowman JM: Controversies in Rh prophylaxis. Who needs Rh immune globulin and when should it be used? Am J Obstet Gynecol 1985;151:289.

Britton JR, Britton HL, Gronwaldt V: Early perinatal hospital discharge and parenting during infancy. Pediatrics 1999;104:1070.

Brumfield CG: Early postpartum discharge. Clin Obstet Gynecol 1998;41:611.

Burrows WR, Gingo AJ Jr, Rose SM: Safety and efficacy of early postoperative solid food consumption after cesarean section. J Reprod Med 1995;40:463.

Chaliha C et al: Antenatal prediction of postpartum fecal incontinence. Obstet Gynecol 1999;94:689.

Chi IC, Gates D, Thapa S: Performing tubal sterilizations during women's postpartum hospitalization: A review of the United States and international experiences. Obstet Gynecol Surv 1992;47:71.

Darney PD: Hormonal implants: Contraception for a new century. Am J Obstet Gynecol 1994;170:1536.

De Santis M, Cavaliere AF, Satraface G, Caruso A. Rubella infection in Pregnancy. Reprod Toxicol 2006;21:390.

Freda VJ et al: Prevention of Rh hemolytic disease: Ten years' clinical experience with Rh-immunoglobulin. N Engl J Med 1975;292:1014.

Glass M, Rosenthal AH: Cervical changes in pregnancy, labor and puerperium. Am J Obstet Gynecol 1950;60:353.

Glazener CMA: Sexual function after childbirth: Women's experiences, persistent morbidity and lack of professional recognition. Br J Obstet Gynaecol 1997;104:330.

Goetsch MF : Postpartum dyspareunia. An unexplored problem. J Reprod Med 1999;44:963.

Hale RW, Milne L: The elite athlete and exercise in pregnancy. Semin Perinatol 1996;20:277.

Hebert PR et al: Serious maternal morbidity after childbirth: prolonged hospital stays and readmissions. Obstet Gynecol 1999;94:942.

Hillis SD et al: Poststerilization regret: Findings from the United States Collaborative Review of Sterilization. Obstet Gynecol 1999;93:889.

Hume AL, Hijab JC: Oral contraceptives in the immediate postpartum period. J Fam Pract 1991;32:423.

Kazzi A et al: Effectiveness of the lactational amenorrhea method in Pakistan. Fertil Steril 1995;64:717.

Kennedy K, Visness C: Contraceptive efficacy of lactational amenorrhea. Lancet 1992;339:227.

Kennedy KI, Sort RV, Tully MR: Premature introduction of progestin-only contraceptive methods during lactation. Contraception 1997;55:347.

Koetsawang S: The effects of contraceptive methods on the quality and quantity of breast milk. Int J Gynaecol Obstet 1987;25(Suppl):115.

Koltyn KF, Schultes SS: Psychological effects of an aerobic exercise session and a rest session following pregnancy. J Sports Med Phys Fitness 1997;37:287.

Liu LI et al: The safety of early newborn discharge: The Washington state experience. JAMA 1997;278:293.

Mandl KD et al: Maternal and infant health: effects of moderate reductions in postpartum length of stay. Arch Pediatr Adolesc Med 1997;151:915.

McCrory MA et al: Randomized trial of the short-term effects of dieting compared with dieting plus aerobic exercise on lactation performance. Am J Clin Nutr 1999;69:959.

O'Hanley K, Huber DH: Postpartum IUDs: Keys for success. Contraception 1992;45:351.

Perez A, Labbok M, Queenan J: Clinical study of the lactational amenorrhea method for family planning. Lancet 1992; 339: 968.

Ryding E-L: Sexuality during and after pregnancy. Acta Obstet Gynecol Scand 1984;63:679.

Schanler RJ, Hurst NM, Lau C: The use of human milk and breastfeeding in premature infants. Clin Perinatol 1999;26:379.

Soriano D, Dulitzki M, Keidar N: Early oral feeding after cesarean delivery. Obstet Gynecol 1996;87:1006.

Stanford JB, Thurnau PB, Lemaire JC: Physician's knowledge and practices regarding natural family planning. Obstet Gynecol 1999;94:672.

Vessey M et al: Tubal sterilization: Findings in a large prospective study. Br J Obstet Gynaecol 1983;90:203.

Vessey M, Wiggins P: Use-effectiveness of the diaphragm in a selected family planning clinic population in the United Kingdom. Contraception 1974;9:15.

Windle ML, Booker LA, Rayburn WF: Postpartum pain after vaginal delivery: A review of comparative analgesic trials. J Reprod Med 1989;34:891.

Lactation

American Academy of Pediatrics Committee on Pediatric AIDS: Human milk, breastfeeding, and transmission of human immunodeficiency virus in the United States (RE9542). Pediatrics 2003;112:1196.

American Academy of Pediatrics Policy Statement: Breastfeeding and the use of human milk. Pediatrics 2005;115:496.

American College of Obstetricians and Gynecologists: *Breastfeeding: Maternal and Infant Aspects.* ACOG Educational Bulletin No. 258. American College of Obstetricians and Gynecologists, 2000.

Briggs GG, Freeman RK, Yaffe SJ (editors): *Drugs in Pregnancy and Lactation,* 7th ed. Lippincott Williams & Wilkins, 2005.

Dunn DT et al: Risk of human immunodeficiency virus type 1 transmission through breast-feeding. Lancet 1992;340:585.

Dusdieker LB et al: Effect of supplemental fluids on human milk production. J Pediatr 1985;106:207.

Fowler MG, Bertolli J, Nieburg P: When is breast-feeding not best? The dilemma facing HIV-infected women in resource-poor settings. JAMA 1999;282:781.

Garofalo RP, Goldman AS: Expression of functional immunomodulatory and anti-inflammatory factors in human milk. Clin Perinatol 1999;26:361.

Hayslip CC et al: The effects of lactation on bone mineral content in healthy postpartum women. Obstet Gynecol 1989;73:588.

Labbok MH: Health sequela of breastfeeding for the mother. Clin Perinatol 1999;26:491.

Lawrence RA: A review of the medical benefits and contraindications to breastfeeding in the United States. Maternal and Child Health Technical Information Bulletin. National Center for Education in Maternal and Child Health, 1997, p. 3.

Losh M et al: Impact of attitudes on maternal decisions regarding infant feeding. J Pediatr 1996;126:507.

Neville MC: Physiology of lactation. Clin Perinatol 1999;26:251.

Specker B, Tsang R, Ho M: Changes in calcium homeostasis over the first year postpartum: Effect of lactation and weaning. Obstet Gynecol 1991;78:56.

Van de Perre P et al: Postnatal transmission of HIV type 1 from mother to infant. N Engl J Med 1991;325:593.

West CP: The acceptability of a progestin-only contraceptive during breast-feeding. Contraception 1983;27:563.

Ziegler JB: Breast feeding and HIV. Lancet 1993;342:1437.

Zinaman M et al: Acute prolactin and oxytocin response and milk yield to infant suckling and artificial methods of expression in lactating women. Pediatrics 1992;89:437.

SECTION III
Pregnancy Risk

Methods of Assessment for Pregnancy at Risk

13

Shobha H. Mehta, MD, & Robert J. Sokol, MD

 ESSENTIALS OF DIAGNOSIS

- *A careful history to reveal specific risk factors.*
- *A maternal physical examination organized to identify or exclude risk factors.*
- *Routine maternal laboratory screening for common disorders.*
- *Special maternal laboratory evaluations for disorders suggested by any evaluative process.*
- *Comprehensive fetal assessment by an assortment of techniques over the entire course of the pregnancy.*

OVERVIEW

High-risk pregnancy is broadly defined as one in which the mother, fetus, or newborn is, or may possibly be, at increased risk of morbidity or mortality before, during, or after delivery. Factors that may lead to this increased risk include maternal health, obstetric abnormalities, and fetal disease. Table 13–1 provides an overview of some major categories that comprise a high-risk pregnancy.

The purpose of this chapter is to outline basic and essential aspects of diagnostic modalities available for determination of pregnancies at risk that can be used in practice in a rational manner.

The incidence of high-risk pregnancy varies according to the criteria used to define it. A great many factors are involved, and the effects of any given factor differ from patient to patient. Outcomes can include mortality of the mother and/or the fetus/neonate. Leading causes of maternal death include thromboembolic disease, hypertensive disease, hemorrhage, infection, and ectopic pregnancy. The leading causes of infant mortality (death from birth to 1 year of age) are congenital malformations and prematurity-related conditions. Although there is legal variation by jurisdiction in the United States, a perinatal death is one that occurs at any time after 22 weeks' gestation (or above 500 g if gestational age is not known) through 28 days after delivery. The perinatal mortality rate is the sum of fetal (stillbirths) and neonatal deaths. Preterm birth is the leading cause of perinatal morbidity and neonatal mortality.

In assessing pregnancies to determine risk, several key concepts may offer tremendous insight. Human reproduction is a complex social, biochemical, and physiologic process that is not as successful as once thought. Approximately half of all conceptions are lost before pregnancy is even recognized. Another 15–20% are lost in the first trimester. Of this latter group, more than half have abnormal karyotypes and defy current methodologies for prevention of loss. However, many other causes of reproductive loss are amenable to diagnosis and treatment. In this chapter we discuss the indications and justifications for antepartum care and intrapartum management.

Table 13–1. Risk factors related to specific pregnancy problems.

Preterm labor
- Age below 16 or over 35 years
- Low socioeconomic status
- Maternal weight below 50 kg (110 lb)
- Poor nutrition
- Previous preterm birth
- Incomplete cervix
- Uterine anomalies
- Smoking
- Drug addiction and alcohol abuse
- Pyelonephritis, pneumonia
- Multiple gestation
- Anemia
- Abnormal fetal presentation
- Preterm rupture of membranes
- Placental abnormalities
- Infection

Polyhydramnios
- Diabetes mellitus
- Multiple gestation
- Fetal congenital abnormalities
- Isoimmunization (Rh or ABO)
- Nonimmune hydrops
- Abnormal fetal presentation

Intrauterine growth restriction (IUGR)
- Multiple gestation
- Poor nutrition
- Maternal cyanotic heart disease
- Chronic hypertension
- Pregnancy-induced hypertension
- Recurrent antepartum hemorrhage
- Smoking
- Maternal diabetes with vasculopathy
- Fetal infections
- Fetal cardiovascular anomalies
- Drug addiction and alcohol abuse
- Fetal congenital anomalies
- Hemoglobinopathies

Oligohydramnios
- Renal agenesis (Potter's syndrome)
- Prolonged rupture of membranes
- Intrauterine growth restriction
- Intrauterine fetal demise

Postterm pregnancy
- Anencephaly
- Placental sulfatase deficiency
- Perinatal hypoxia, acidosis
- Placental insufficiency

Chromosomal abnormalities
- Maternal age 35 years or more at delivery
- Balanced translocation (maternal and paternal)

Preconceptional Care

Preconceptional evaluation and counseling of women of reproductive age has gained increasing acceptance as an important component of women's health. Care given in family planning and gynecology centers provides an opportunity that is rarely seen in the prenatal visits. This valuable opportunity to maximize maternal and fetal health benefits before conception should be taken advantage of. Issues of potential consequence to a pregnancy, such as medical problems, lifestyle (including substance abuse, weight, and exercise), or genetic issues should be investigated and interventions devised prior to pregnancy. Specific recommendations include folic acid for the prevention of fetal neural tube defects (0.4 mg/d), strict blood sugar control in diabetic women, and general management of any medical problems in the mother.

PRENATAL PERIOD

Initial Screening

The initial prenatal visit is important in evaluation and assessment of risk during the pregnancy and should take place as early in the pregnancy as possible, preferably in the first trimester. Information of vital importance includes maternal medical and obstetric history, physical examination, and key laboratory findings.

A. MATERNAL AGE

Extremes of maternal age increase risks of maternal or fetal morbidity and mortality. Adolescents are at increased risk for preeclampsia–eclampsia, intrauterine growth restriction (IUGR), and maternal malnutrition.

Women 35 years of age or older at the time of delivery are at higher risk for pregnancy-induced hypertension, diabetes, and obesity, as well as other medical conditions. Chromosomal abnormalities are also more common in infants born to older women. An increased risk of cesarean section, preeclampsia, and placenta previa is noted in women with advanced maternal age.

B. MODALITY OF CONCEPTION

It is important to differentiate spontaneous pregnancy from that resulting from assisted reproductive technologies (ART). Use of ART increases the risks of multiple gestation, preterm delivery, and low birth weight.

C. PAST MEDICAL HISTORY

Many medical disorders can complicate the pregnancy course for the mother and thus the fetus. It is important that these diseases and their severity be addressed before conception if possible. During pregnancy the patient may require aggressive management and additional visits and testing to follow the course of the disease, in addition to possible consultation or management of a high-risk specialist. Table 13–2 lists the most important disorders that may complicate pregnancy.

D. Family History

A detailed family history is helpful in determining any increased risk of heritable disease states (eg, Tay-Sachs, cystic fibrosis, sickle cell disease) that may affect the mother or fetus during the pregnancy or the fetus following delivery.

E. Ethnic Background

Population screening for certain inheritable genetic diseases is not cost effective because of the relative rarity of those genes in the general population. However, many genetic diseases affect certain ethnicities in disproportionate amounts, allowing cost-effective screening of those particular groups. Table 13–3 lists several common inheritable genetic diseases for which screening is possible. It includes the group at risk as well as the method of screening.

F. Past Obstetric History

1. Recurrent abortion—A diagnosis of recurrent abortion can be made after 3 or more consecutive spontaneous losses of a previable fetus. Recurrent abortion is best investigated before another pregnancy occurs. If the patient is currently pregnant, however, as much of the work-up as possible should be performed.

- Karyotype of abortus specimen
- Parental karyotype
- Survey for cervical and uterine anomalies
- Connective tissue disease work-up
- Screening for hormonal abnormalities (ie, hypothyroidism)
- Acquired and inherited thrombophilias
- Infectious disease evaluation of the genital tract

2. Previous stillbirth or neonatal death—A history of previous stillbirth or neonatal death should trigger an immediate investigation as to the conditions or circumstances surrounding the event. If the demise was the result of a nonrecurring event, such as cord prolapse or traumatic injury, then the present pregnancy has a risk approaching a background risk. However, stillbirth or neonatal death may suggest a cytogenetic abnormality, structural malformation syndrome, fetomaternal hemorrhage, or thrombophilia (fetal or maternal), requiring a work-up similar to that just listed.

3. Previous preterm delivery—A history of preterm birth confers an increased risk of early delivery in subsequent pregnancies. Furthermore, the risk of a subsequent preterm birth increases as the number of prior preterm births increases, and the risk decreases with each birth that is not preterm. The recurrence risk also rises as the gesta-

Table 13–2. Some diseases and disorders complicating pregnancy.

Chronic hypertension
Renal disease
Diabetes mellitus
Heart disease
Previous endocrine ablation (eg, thyroidectomy)
Maternal cancer
Sickle cell trait and disease
Substance use or abuse
Pulmonary disease (eg, tuberculosis, sarcoidosis, asthma)
Thyroid disorders
Gastrointestinal and liver disease
Epilepsy
Blood disorders (eg, anemia, coagulopathy)
Others, including previous pelvic injury or disease producing pelvic deformity, connective tissue disorders, mental retardation, psychiatric disease

tional age of the previous preterm delivery decreases. Despite intense investigation, the incidence of preterm delivery has slightly increased in the United States, due in large measure to medical intervention producing indicated preterm deliveries. Eighty-five percent of preterm deliveries occur between 32 and 36 weeks, and they carry minimal fetal or neonatal morbidity. The remaining 15% of preterm deliveries, however, account for nearly all of the perinatal morbidity and mortality. Common causes of perinatal morbidity in premature infants include respiratory distress syndrome, intraventricular hemorrhage, bronchopulmonary dysplasia, necrotizing enterocolitis, sepsis, apnea, retinopathy of prematurity, and hyperbilirubinemia. Preterm deliveries can be divided into 2 types: spontaneous and indicated, with indicated preterm deliveries caused by medical or obstetric disorders that place the mother and/or fetus at risk. The clinical risk factors most often associated with spontaneous preterm birth include history of previous preterm birth, genital tract infection, nonwhite race, multiple gestation, bleeding in the second trimester, and low prepregnancy weight. Recent multicenter trials have shown that progesterone in the form of 17α-hydroxyprogesterone, given as weekly injections of 250 mg beginning in the second trimester, can decrease the risk of preterm delivery in patients with a history of prior spontaneous preterm delivery.

4. Rh isoimmunization or ABO incompatibility—All pregnant patients should undergo an antibody screen at the first prenatal visit. Those patients who are RhD-negative with no evidence of anti-D alloimmunization should receive Rh_o (D) immunoglobulin (RhoGAM) 300 μg at 28 weeks of gestation. In patients who are Rh sensitized, the patient can be followed by maternal titers and/or amniocentesis for fetal blood typing, followed by

Table 13–3. Common inheritable genetic diseases.

Disease	Population at Increased Risk	Method of Testing
Alpha thalassemia	Chinese, Southeast Asian, African	CBC
		Hemoglobin electrophoresis
Beta thalassemia	Chinese, Southeast Asians, Mediterraneans, Pakistanis, Bangladeshis, Middle Easterners, African	CBC
		Hemoglobin electrophoresis
Bloom's syndrome	Ashkenazi Jews	Mutation analysis
Canavan's disease	Ashkenazi Jews	Mutation analysis
Cystic fibrosis	North American Caucasians of European ancestry, Ashkenazi Jews	Mutation analysis
Familial dysautonomia	Ashkenazi Jews	Mutation analysis
Fanconi's anemia	Ashkenazi Jews	Mutation analysis
Gaucher's disease	Ashkenazi Jews	Mutation analysis
Niemann-Pick disease	Ashkenazi Jews	Mutation analysis
Sickle cell disease and other structural hemoglobinopathies	African-Americans, Africans, Hispanics, Mediterranean, Middle Easterners, Caribbean Indians	CBC
		Hemoglobin electrophoresis
Tay-Sachs	Ashkenazi Jews, French Canadians, Cajuns	Enzyme and mutation analysis

either serial amniocentesis for ΔOD_{450} or serial middle cerebral artery velocity measurements, as well as fetal blood sampling via cordocentesis.

5. Previous preeclampsia–eclampsia—Previous preeclampsia–eclampsia increases the risk for hypertension in the current pregnancy, especially if underlying chronic hypertension or renal disease is present.

6. Previous infant with genetic disorder or congenital anomaly—A woman with a previous history of a fetus with a chromosomal abnormality is a frequent indication of cytogenetic testing, although this may be proceeded by first- or second-trimester screening and anatomy ultrasound (US). The rate of recurrence depends on the abnormality.

7. Teratogen exposure—A teratogen is any substance, agent, or environmental factor that has an adverse effect on the developing fetus. Whereas malformations caused by teratogen exposure are relatively rare, knowledge of exposure can aid in the diagnosis and management.

   a. Drugs—Alcohol, antiseizure medications (phenytoin, valproic acid, etc), lithium, mercury, thalidomide, diethylstilbestrol (DES), warfarin (Coumadin), isotretinoin, etc.

   b. Infectious agents—Cytomegalovirus, *Listeria,* rubella, toxoplasmosis, varicella, *Mycoplasma,* etc.

   c. Radiation—It is believed that medical diagnostic radiation delivering less than 0.05 Gy (5 rad) to the fetus has no teratogenic risk.

Physical Examination

Physical examination is important not only during the initial visit but also throughout the pregnancy. Vital sign ab-

normalities can lead to the diagnosis of many key obstetric complications. Fever, defined as a temperature of 100.4°F or greater, can be a sign of chorioamnionitis. Signs or symptoms of chorioamnionitis should be assessed, and, if chorioamnionitis is suspected, amniocentesis for microscopy and culture should be considered. Depending on clinical correlation, delivery may be necessary. Maternal tachycardia can be a sign of infection, anemia, or both. Isolated mild tachycardia (> 100 bpm) should be evaluated and followed up, as should maternal tachyarrhythmias. Maternal heart rate is noted to increase normally in pregnancy, however. The normal pattern of maternal blood pressure readings is a decrease from baseline during the first trimester, reaching its nadir in the second trimester, and slightly rising in the third trimester, although not as high as the baseline levels. Repeated blood pressure readings of 140/90 mm Hg taken 6 hours apart should be considered evidence of pregnancy-induced hypertension. Increases in systolic and diastolic blood pressure, although no longer a part of the definition, may also be an indication of development of pregnancy-induced hypertension. The rest of the physical examination should be performed during the initial visit and focused examination during each visit. Fundal height measurements and fetal heart tone checks should also be performed.

Urinalysis

At the first prenatal visit, a clean-catch urine culture and sensitivity should be performed. Any growth should be treated with the appropriate antibiotics. At all subsequent visits, urine dipstick testing to screen for protein, glucose, leukocyte esterase, blood, or any combination of markers is useful in identifying patients with a change in baseline urinary composition.

Screening Tests

Screening tests during the initial visit include testing for rubella, rapid plasma reagin, hepatitis B, blood type, human immunodeficiency virus, gonorrhea, and *Chlamydia*, and Pap smear.

ANTEPARTUM MANAGEMENT

Genetic Testing

A. FIRST-TRIMESTER SCREENING

Nuchal translucency, measured between 11(0/7) and 13(6/7) weeks, combined with free β-human chorionic gonadotropin (β-hCG) and pregnancy-associated plasma protein-A levels, has been found to have 87.0% sensitivity for detection of trisomy 21 with a 5% false positive rate. In the absence of chromosomal abnormalities, an increased nuchal translucency is associated with an increased risk of structural cardiac abnormalities and skeletal dysplasias, etc. Further US findings in the first trimester, including absence of nasal bone and abnormal ductus venosus Doppler findings, may further improve the detection rate for aneuploidy but require a high level of sonographic skill.

Maternal Serum Analyte Testing

Frequently known as the "triple screen," this test includes maternal serum α-fetoprotein (MSAFP), β-hCG, and estriol. In some institutions, only the MSAFP is used, whereas in other institutions a fourth test for inhibin is included, making it a "quad test." The usefulness of this screen is its ability to identify pregnancies at increased risk for open neural tube defects, as well as for certain chromosomal abnormalities, especially trisomy 21 (70% sensitivity for Down syndrome detection). This test is effective at 15–22 weeks' gestation and therefore can identify an at-risk pregnancy in time to pursue more definitive diagnosis, if desired. It is important to note, however, that the triple screen is not a definitive test, and that many positive screens have yielded normal fetuses and many abnormal fetuses have had normal screens.

Syndromic Testing

Screening for sickle cell disease should be offered to individuals of African and African American descent and those from the Mediterranean basin, the Middle East, and India. Hemoglobin electrophoresis is the definitive test to determine the carrier status of sickle cell disease.

The decision on who to offer cystic fibrosis testing to remains controversial, as the sensitivity of the testing depends on the ethnicity of the parents, with the highest pick-up rate in those with the highest risk—Caucasian and Ashkenazi Jewish descent. Current guidelines recommend offering testing to all groups but counseling lower-risk groups of the limitations of the testing.

The current standard of care is to offer carrier testing for Tay-Sachs disease and Canavan's disease to those of Ashkenazi Jewish descent.

Preterm Labor Detection

Many patients present throughout pregnancy with signs and symptoms of preterm labor, specifically uterine contractions. Although the cost of missing true preterm labor is high, many patients are not in true labor, and the financial cost of aggressive management of these patients is also high. Two screening tests have aided in the management of these patients: cervical length measurement and fetal fibronectin. A preterm birth is very unlikely (97–99%) when the cervical length is 30 mm (before 34–35 weeks) or when the fetal fibronectin is negative (within 14 days).

Diabetes Screening/Gestational Diabetes

Although recent consensus groups have recommended screening for gestational diabetes based on risk factors, many studies have shown this to be inadequate for detecting patients with gestational screening versus universal screening.

Routine screening consists of performing a glucose challenge test between 24 and 28 weeks. The test consists of a 50-g oral glucose load with a plasma glucose level drawn exactly 1 hour after. If the value is 140 mg/dL or over, a more specific glucose tolerance test (GTT) should be performed (the cutoff may be lowered to 130 mg/dL to improve sensitivity). The GTT involves obtaining a fasting plasma glucose level, giving a 100-g oral glucose load, then drawing plasma levels at 1 hour, 2 hours, and 3 hours after the glucose load. A test is considered positive for gestational diabetes if 2 of the 4 values are elevated. The thresholds proposed by Carpenter and Coustan are currently favored (fasting > 95 mg/dL, 1 hour > 180 mg/dL, 2 hour > 155 mg/dL, 3 hour > 140 mg/dL).

Group B Streptococcus

Group B streptococcus (GBS) asymptomatically colonizes between 10% and 30% of pregnant women, but perinatal transmission can result in a severe and potentially fatal neonatal infection. Recent changes to the protocol for GBS testing emphasize the importance of culture screening and treatment over risk factor-based screening. For this reason, patients should be screened with a rectovaginal culture at 35–37 weeks. If the culture is positive, patients should be treated with intrapartum antibiotics. Intrapartum antibiotic prophylaxis has been shown to decrease the risk of perinatal GBS transmission. If the culture result is unknown, patients should be treated if in preterm labor, with rupture of membranes greater than or equal to 18 hours, or maternal fever greater than 100.4°F during labor. All patients with GBS bacteriuria during the pregnancy or previous neonate with GBS sepsis should be treated with intrapartum antibiotics.

FETAL ASSESSMENT

Performed during all trimesters, the techniques used are diverse, and the information obtained varies according to the quality of imaging, depth of investigation, and gestational age of pregnancy.

Ultrasound

US has evolved continuously over the last 30 years, with better equipment produced each year. Real-time sonography allows a 2-dimensional (2-D) image to demonstrate fetal anatomy, as well as characteristics such as fetal weight, movement, volume of amniotic fluid, and structural anomalies such as myomas or placenta previa that may affect the pregnancy. Three-dimensional sonography allows volume to be ascertained, creating a 3-D–appearing image on the 2-D screen, which assists in identifying certain anatomic anomalies. Most recently, 4-D machines have been developed, which produce a 3-D image in real time. As the machines become more technically advanced and the computers that run them become faster, the images obtained will continue to improve and push the boundaries of sonographic prenatal diagnosis.

Diagnostic ultrasonography is widely used in the assessment of the pregnancy and the fetus. However, it is not the standard of care, nor is it recommended by the American College of Obstetricians and Gynecologists (ACOG) for every pregnancy. The indications for ultrasonography are multiple and diverse, and the type and timing of the examination varies depending on the information being sought.

A **standard** US examination should provide information such as fetal number, presentation, documentation of fetal viability, assessment of gestational age, amniotic fluid volume, placental location, fetal biometry, and an anatomic survey. A **limited** US examination is a goal-directed search for a suspected problem or finding. A limited US can be used for guidance during procedures such as amniocentesis or external cephalic version, assessment of fetal well-being, or documentation of presentation or placental location intrapartum. A **specialized** US examination is performed when an anomaly is suspected based on history, biochemical abnormalities, or results of either the limited or standard scan. Other specialized examinations include fetal Dop-

pler, biophysical profile (BPP), fetal echocardiogram, or additional biometric studies.

US evaluation of fetal anatomy may detect major structural anomalies. Gross malformations such as anencephaly and hydrocephaly are commonly diagnosed and rarely missed; however, more subtle anomalies such as facial clefts, diaphragmatic hernias, and neural tube defects are more commonly reported to have been missed by US. The basic fetal anatomy survey should include visualization of the cerebral ventricles, 4-chamber view of the heart, and examination of the spine, stomach, urinary bladder, umbilical cord insertion site, and renal region. Any indication of an anomaly should be followed by a more comprehensive sonogram. Typically, the fetal anatomic survey is performed at 17–20 weeks; however, there is controversy regarding the potential benefits of an earlier sonogram at 14–16 weeks using the transvaginal probe. The earlier scan allows earlier detection of anomalies that are almost always present by the second trimester, as well as allowing greater detailed viewing of the fetal anatomy by using the higher-resolution vaginal transducers.

Aneuploidy Screening

Multiple sonographic findings associated with markers for aneuploidy have been identified. The presence of single or multiple markers adjusts the patient's age-related risk of aneuploidy based on the particular markers present. Such sonographic findings include, but are not limited to:

- Echogenic intracardiac focus
- Choroid plexus cysts
- Pyelectasis
- Echogenic bowel
- Short femur
- Hypomineralization of the fifth digit of the fetal hand

Amniocentesis

Amniocentesis is now almost always performed under the guidance of ultrasonography. A needle is inserted transcutaneously through the abdominal wall into the amniotic cavity, and fluid is removed. There are many uses for this amniotic fluid. In the early second trimester, these include AFP evaluation for neural tube defect assessment and the most common indication of cytogenetic analysis. In this case, amniocentesis is often performed between 15 and 20 weeks' gestation, and fetal cells from the amniotic fluid are obtained. Risks associated with the procedure are considered to be very low, with the risk of abortion as a result of amniocentesis considered to be between 1 in 200 to 1 in 450 amniocenteses.

Amniocentesis also provides a useful tool later in pregnancy, at low risk, for diagnosis of intra-amniotic inflammation and infection as a risk factor for preterm labor and adverse outcome, as well as documentation of fetal lung maturity.

Chorionic Villus Sampling

Chorionic villus sampling (CVS) is an alternative to amniocentesis. It is performed between 10 and 12 weeks' gestation and can be performed either transcervically or transabdominally. CVS is also performed under sonographic guidance, with the passing of a sterile catheter or needle into the placental site. Chorionic villi are aspirated and undergo cytogenetic analysis. The benefit of CVS over amniocentesis is its availability earlier in pregnancy; however, the rate of abortion is higher—as high as 1%. One disadvantage of CVS is that, unlike amniocentesis, it does not allow diagnosis of neural tube defects.

Fetal Blood Sampling

Also referred to as cordocentesis or percutaneous umbilical blood sampling (PUBS), fetal blood sampling is an option for chromosomal or metabolic analysis of the fetus. Benefits of the procedure include a rapid result turnaround and the ability to perform the procedure in the second and third trimesters. Intravascular access to the fetus is useful for assessment and treatment of certain fetal conditions such as Rh sensitization and alloimmune thrombocytopenia. However, there is a higher risk of fetal death compared to the other methods. Fetal loss rates are approximately 2% but can vary depending on the fetal condition involved.

ANTEPARTUM FETAL TESTING

Fetal Movement Assessment

A decrease in maternal perception of fetal movement can precede fetal death, sometimes by several days. Perception of 10 distinct movements in a period of up to 2 hours is considered reassuring; if less, patients are often advised to undergo further testing.

Nonstress Test

Fetal movements associated with accelerations of fetal heart rate (FHR) provide reassurance that the fetus is not acidotic or neurologically depressed. A reactive and therefore reassuring nonstress test (NST) is defined as 2 or more FHR accelerations, at least 15 bpm above the baseline and lasting at least 15 seconds within a 20 minute period. Vibroacoustic stimulation can elicit FHR accelerations that can reduce overall testing time without compromising detection of an acidotic fetus. In the case of a nonreassuring NST, further evaluation or delivery depend on the clinical context. In a patient at term, delivery is warranted. Pregnancy remote from term poses a more challenging dilemma to the clinician. If resuscitative efforts are not successful in restoring reactivity to the NST, ancillary tests or testing techniques may prove useful in avoiding a premature iatrogenic delivery for nonreassuring FHR patterns, as the false-positive rate may be as high as 50–60%.

Biophysical Profile

The BPP is composed of 5 components: NST, fetal breathing movements (30 seconds or more in 30 minutes), fetal movement (3 or more in 30 minutes), fetal tone (extension/flexion of an extremity), and amniotic fluid volume (vertical pocket of 2 cm or more). Each component is worth 2 points; a score of 8 or 10 is normal, 6 is equivocal, and 4 or less is abnormal.

Modified Biophysical Profile

Modified BPP combines NST, a short-term indicator of fetal acid–base status, with amniotic fluid index (AFI), a long-term indicator of placental function. AFI is measured by dividing the uterus into 4 equal quadrants and measuring the largest vertical pocket in each quadrant; the results are then summed and expressed in millimeters. The modified BPP has become a primary mode of antepartum fetal surveillance; a nonreactive NST or an AFI less than 50 mm (oligohydramnios) requires further intervention.

Contraction Stress Test

The contraction stress test (CST) is based on the response of HFR to uterine contractions, with the premise that fetal oxygenation will be worsened. This results in late decelerations in an already suboptimally oxygenated fetus. The test requires 3 contractions in 10 minutes, a positive or abnormal test when late decelerations occur with more than half of the contractions, suspicious with any late decelerations, and negative with no late decelerations. Contraindications to CST include any contraindications to labor, such as placenta previa or prior classic cesarian section. This test is now rarely used.

Growth Ultrasound

Growth US studies, performed every 3–4 weeks, are useful for assessment of fetuses that may be at risk for growth restriction secondary to medical conditions of pregnancy or fetal abnormalities.

Doppler Studies

Fetal Doppler studies initially were used to assess the placenta by evaluation of umbilical artery outflow. They have since evolved to a more comprehensive multivessel evaluation of fetal status. Doppler studies can be used to assess a compromised fetus (particularly the growth-restricted fetus) and may function as a diagnostic tool that alerts the clinician to the need for further intervention, including BPP, continuous fetal monitoring, or possibly delivery.

Fetal Maturity Tests

A. INDICATIONS FOR ASSESSING FETAL LUNG MATURITY

ACOG has recommended that fetal pulmonary maturity should be confirmed before elective delivery at less than 39 weeks' gestation unless fetal maturity can be inferred from any of these criteria: fetal heart tones have been documented for 20 weeks by nonelectronic fetoscope or for 30 weeks by Doppler; 36 weeks have elapsed since a serum or urine hCG-based pregnancy test was reported to be positive; US measurement of crown–rump length at 6–11 weeks of gestation or measurements at 12–20 weeks support a gestational age equal to or greater than 39 weeks.

1. Lecithin/sphingomyelin ratio— The lecithin/sphingomyelin (L/S) ratio for assessment of fetal pulmonary maturity was first introduced by Gluck and colleagues in 1971. The test depends upon outward flow of pulmonary secretions from the lungs into the amniotic fluid, thereby changing the phospholipid composition of the latter and permitting measurement of the L/S ratio in a sample of amniotic fluid. In the absence of complications, the ratio of these 2 components reaches 2.0 at about 35 weeks. The presence of blood or meconium may interfere with test interpretation.

2. Phosphatidylglycerol—Phosphatidylglycerol (PG) is a minor constituent of surfactant. It begins to increase appreciably in amniotic fluid several weeks after the rise in lecithin. Its presence is more indicative of fetal lung maturity because PG enhances the spread of phospholipids on the alveoli. However, it is not commonly used at present because of a high false-negative rate.

3. Fluorescence polarization— The fluorescence polarization test, currently the most widely used test, uses polarized light to quantitate the competitive binding of a probe to both albumin and surfactant in amniotic fluid; thus, it is a true direct measurement of surfactant concentration. It reflects the ratio of surfactant to albumin and is measured by an automatic analyzer, such as the TDx-FLM. An elevated ratio has been correlated with the presence of fetal lung maturity; the threshold for maturity is 55 mg of surfactant per gram of albumin.

Table 13–4 lists all fetal maturity tests available, discriminating levels, and specific characteristics of the tests.

INTRAPARTUM MANAGEMENT

Fetal Heart Rate Monitoring

Use of electronic fetal monitoring (EFM) has been increasing over the last several decades, up to 85% in 2002. No randomized controlled trials have compared the benefits of EFM versus no form of monitoring during labor. Randomized clinical trials comparing EFM with intermittent auscultation showed an increase in cesarian section rate, cesarian section rate for fetal distress, and operative vaginal delivery rate, with no reduction in overall perinatal mortality but possibly a decrease in perinatal mortality from fetal hypoxia. Given these findings, ACOG has stated that either EFM or intermittent auscultation is acceptable, given that guidelines for intermittent auscultation are met. Intermittent auscultation may not be acceptable in high-risk patients, however.

Despite its widespread use, EFM suffers from poor interobserver and intraobserver reliability, uncertain efficacy, and a high false-positive rate. To improve consistency, the National Institute of Child Health and

Table 13–4. Fetal maturity tests.

Test	Positive Discriminating Value	Positive Predictive Value	Relative Cost	Pros and Cons
L/S ratio	> 2.0	95–100%	High	Large laboratory variation
PG	"Present"	95–100%	High	Not affected by blood, meconium; can use vaginal pooled sample
FSI	> 47	95%	Low	Affected by blood, meconium silicone tubes
TDx-FLM	> 55	96–100%	Moderate	Minimal inter/intra-assay variability; simple test
Optical density	OD 0.15	98%	Low	Simple technique
Lamellar body counts	30–40,000	97–98%	Low	Still investigational

Human Development (NICHD) Planning Workshop proposed definitions for intrapartum FHR tracing.

Fetal Heart Rate

The baseline is the mean FHR rounded to increments of 5 bpm, at least 2 minutes in any 10-minute segment. Normal baseline is between 110 and 160 bpm. Baseline FHR below 110 is defined as *bradycardia*; above 160 is defined as *tachycardia*. Either bradycardia (particularly when the new baseline is below 80 bpm) or tachycardia (particularly when associated with a decrease in variability or repetitive late or severe variable decelerations) suggests a nonreassuring fetal status. *Accelerations* (at 32 weeks or greater) are defined as elevations above the baseline of 15 bpm lasting 15 seconds or longer; less than 32 weeks it is defined by elevations of 10 bpm lasting at least 10 seconds. Two or more accelerations in a 20-minute interval are reassuring; this defines reactivity in an NST. *Variability* is defined by fluctuations in the FHR of 2 cycles per minute or greater and can range from absent to marked. Decelerations are categorized as early, late, and variable. *Early decelerations* generally mirror contractions in timing and shape and are generally not ominous, often representing head compression. *Late decelerations* are smooth falls in the FHR beginning after the contraction has started and ending after the contraction has ended. They are associated with fetal hypoxemia and a potential for perinatal morbidity and mortality. *Variable decelerations* are abrupt in decline and return to baseline, vary in timing with the contraction, and usually represent cord compression. These are most ominous when repetitive and severe (below 60 bpm). A *prolonged deceleration* is a decrease of 15 bpm below the baseline lasting between 2 and 10 minutes.

Ancillary Tests

A. FETAL SCALP BLOOD SAMPLING

In the presence of a nonreassuring FHR pattern, a scalp blood sample for determination of pH or lactate can be considered. Although the specificity is high (normal values rule out asphyxia), the sensitivity and positive predictive value of a low scalp pH in identifying a newborn with hypoxic–ischemic encephalopathy is low. For these reasons, in addition to the technical skill and expense of the procedure, fetal scalp pH is no longer used in many institutions.

B. VIBROACOUSTIC STIMULATION/SCALP STIMULATION

The presence of an acceleration after a vaginal examination in which the examiner stimulates the fetal vertex with the examining finger or after vibroacoustic stimulation (as described above) confirms the absence of acidosis (pH > 7.2). Some clinicians prefer these methods over fetal scalp blood sampling because they are less invasive.

C. FETAL PULSE OXIMETRY

Fetal pulse oximetry, the measure of the fetus' oxygenation during labor, was developed with the goal of improving the specificity of FHR monitoring and decreasing the number of cesarean sections secondary to nonreassuring fetal status. It is performed using a sensor placed transcervically, resting against the fetal cheek. Normal oxygenation is 35–65%, and a metabolic acidosis does not develop until the oxygen saturation falls below 30% for at least 10–15 minutes. One randomized controlled trial showed that although fetal pulse oximetry did decrease the number of cesarean sections for nonreassuring fetal status, it was associated with an increased number of cesarian sections for dystocia and thus no difference overall in the rate of operative deliveries. Further studies suggest that nonreassuring fetal status may be a marker for later dystocia in labor, leading to the outcomes seen. The role of fetal pulse oximetry in practice is not yet defined.

CONCLUSION

Assessing pregnancy to determine risk, as well as careful monitoring of pregnancies with a recognized risk, begins early in the gestation. Preconceptual counseling of patients with known medical or genetic disorders helps to optimize outcomes. Early and frequent prenatal care allows the care provider to screen his or her patient population to identify pregnancies at risk and act accordingly. Additionally, pregnancies identified as complicated by 1 or more issues can be followed by assortments of maternal and fetal surveillance techniques to maximize therapeutic treatment.

As technology advances and our ability to both diagnose and treat improve, the methods for assessment and care of the pregnancy at risk will be a constantly changing field.

REFERENCES

American College of Obstetricians and Gynecologists: *Antepartum Fetal Surveillance.* ACOG Practice Bulletin No. 9. American College of Obstetricians and Gynecologists, 1999.

American College of Obstetricians and Gynecologists: *Assessment of Fetal Lung Maturity.* ACOG Practice Bulletin No. 230. American College of Obstetricians and Gynecologists, 1996.

American College of Obstetricians and Gynecologists: *Gestational Diabetes.* ACOG Practice Bulletin No. 30. American College of Obstetricians and Gynecologists, 2001.

American College of Obstetricians and Gynecologists: *Prenatal Diagnosis of Fetal Chromosomal Abnormalities.* ACOG Practice Bulletin No. 97. American College of Obstetricians and Gynecologists, 2001.

American College of Obstetricians and Gynecologists: *Prevention of Early-Onset Group B Streptococcal Disease in Newborns.* ACOG Committee Opinion No. 279. American College of Obstetricians and Gynecologists, 2002.

American College of Obstetricians and Gynecologists: *Ultrasonography in Pregnancy.* ACOG Practice Bulletin No. 58. American College of Obstetricians and Gynecologists, 2004.

American Institute of Ultrasound in Medicine: AIUM practice guideline for the performance of an antepartum obstetric ultrasound examination. J Ultrasound Med 2003;22:1116.

Baschat AA: Integrated fetal testing in growth restriction: Combining multivessel Doppler and biophysical parameters. Ultrasound Obstet Gynecol 2003;21:1.

Cunningham FG et al: Intrapartum assessment. In: Cunningham FG et al. (editors): *Williams Obstetrics.* Appleton & Lange, 2005, p. 457.

Electronic fetal heart rate monitoring: Research guidelines for interpretation. National Institute of Child Health and Human Development Research Planning Workshop. Am J Obstet Gynecol 1997;177:1385.

Gabbe SG, Graves CR: Management of diabetes mellitus complicating pregnancy. Obstet Gynecol 2003;102:857.

Garite TJ et al: A multicenter controlled trial of fetal pulse oximetry in the intrapartum management of nonreassuring fetal heart rate patterns. Am J Obstet Gynecol 2000;183:1049.

Gillen-Goldstein J et al: Prediction of respiratory distress syndrome from amniotic fluid surfactant measures: The NACB Fetal Lung Maturity Project [abstract]. J Soc Gynecol Invest 2001;716:257.

Gluck L et al: Diagnosis of the respiratory distress syndrome by amniocentesis. Am J Obstet Gynecol 1971;109:440.

Iams JD: Prediction and early detection of preterm labor. Obstet Gynecol 2003;101:402.

Iams JD, Resnik R: Preterm labor and delivery. In: Creasy RK, Resnik R (editors): *Maternal-Fetal Medicine: Principles and Practice.* WB Saunders, 2004, p. 624.

Jenkins TM, Wapner RJ: Prenatal diagnosis of congenital disorders. In: Creasy RK, Resnik R (editors): *Maternal-Fetal Medicine: Principles and Practice.* WB Saunders, 2004, p. 239, 250.

Jobe AH: Fetal lung development, tests for maturation, induction of maturation and treatment. In: Creasy RK, Resnik R (editors): *Maternal-Fetal Medicine.* WB Saunders, 1999, p. 417.

Kruger K et al: Predictive value of fetal scalp blood lactate concentration and pH as markers of neurologic disability. Am J Obstet Gynecol 1999;181:1072.

Low JA, Victory R, Derrick EJ: Predictive value of electronic fetal monitoring for intrapartum fetal asphyxia with metabolic acidosis. Obstet Gynecol 1999;93:285.

Mercer BM, Macpherson CA, Goldenberg RL, et al: Are women with recurrent spontaneous preterm births different from those without such history? Am J Obstet Gynecol 2006;194:1176.

Mari G et al: Noninvasive diagnosis by Doppler ultrasonography of fetal anemia due to maternal red cell alloimmunization. Collaborative group for Doppler assessment of the blood velocity in anemic fetuses. N Engl J Med 2000;342:9.

Meis PJ et al: Prevention of recurrent preterm delivery by 17 alpha-hydroxyprogesterone caproate. N Engl J Med 2003;348:24.

Mires G, Williams F, Howie P: Randomised controlled trial of cardiotocography versus Doppler auscultation of fetal heart at admission in labour in low risk obstetric population. BMJ 2001;322:1457.

National Center for Health Statistics: *Preterm Birth, 1988–1998.* March of Dimes Perinatal Data Center, 2000.

Nicolaides KH: Nuchal translucency and other first-trimester sonographic markers of chromosomal abnormalities. Am J Obstet Gynecol 2004;191:45.

Porreco RP et al: Dystocia in nulliparous patients monitored with fetal pulse oximetry. Am J Obstet Gynecol 2004;190:113.

Schieve LA et al: Perinatal outcome among singleton infants conceived through assisted reproductive technology in the United States. Obstet Gynecol 2004;103:1144.

Sonek JD, Cicero S, Neiger R, et al: Nasal bone assessment in prenatal screening for Trisomy 21. Am J Obstet Gynecol 2006 (Epub ahead of print).

Yoon BH et al: Clinical significance of intra-amniotic inflammation in patients with preterm labor and intact membranes. Am J Obstet Gynecol 2001;185:1130.

Early Pregnancy Risks

Peter S. Uzelac, MD, & Sara H. Garmel, MD

SPONTANEOUS ABORTION

 ESSENTIALS OF DIAGNOSIS

- *Suprapubic pain, uterine cramping, and/or back pain.*
- *Vaginal bleeding.*
- *Cervical dilatation.*
- *Extrusion of products of conception.*
- *Disappearance of symptoms and signs of pregnancy.*
- *Quantitative β-human chorionic gonadotropin that is not properly increasing.*
- *Abnormal ultrasound findings (eg, empty gestational sac, fetal disorganization, lack of fetal growth).*

General Considerations

Spontaneous abortion is the most common complication of pregnancy and is defined as the passing of a pregnancy prior to completion of the 20th gestational week. It implies delivery of all or any part of the products of conception, with or without a fetus weighing less than 500 g. **Threatened abortion** is bleeding of intrauterine origin occurring before the 20th completed week, with or without uterine contractions, without dilatation of the cervix, and without expulsion of the products of conception. **Complete abortion** is the expulsion of all of the products of conception before the 20th completed week of gestation, whereas **incomplete abortion** is the expulsion of some, but not all, of the products of conception. **Inevitable abortion** refers to bleeding of intrauterine origin before the 20th completed week, with dilatation of the cervix without expulsion of the products of conception. In **missed abortion,** the embryo or fetus dies, but the products of conception are retained in utero. In **septic abortion,** infection of the uterus and sometimes surrounding structures occur.

Incidence

Although the true incidence of spontaneous abortion is unknown, approximately 15% of clinically evident pregnancies and 60% of chemically evident pregnancies end in spontaneous abortion. Eighty percent of spontaneous abortions occur prior to 12 weeks' gestation.

The incidence of abortion is influenced by the age of the mother and by a number of pregnancy-related factors, including a history of a previous full-term normal pregnancy, the number of previous spontaneous abortions, a previous stillbirth, and a previous infant born with malformations or known genetic defects. Additionally, parental influences, including balanced translocation carriers and medical complications, may influence the rate of spontaneous abortion.

Etiology

An abnormal karyotype is present in approximately 50% of spontaneous abortions occurring during the first trimester. The incidence decreases to 20–30% in second-trimester losses and to 5–10% in third-trimester losses. As discussed in the next section, the first-trimester losses are typically autosomal trisomies or monosomy X, whereas later losses reflect chromosomal abnormalities seen in neonates.

Other suspected causes of spontaneous abortion account for a smaller percentage of losses and include infection, anatomic defects, endocrine factors, immunologic factors, and maternal systemic diseases. In a significant percentage of spontaneous abortions, the etiology is unknown.

A. MORPHOLOGIC AND GENETIC ABNORMALITIES

Aneuploidy (an abnormal chromosomal number) is the most common genetic abnormality, accounting for at least 50% of early spontaneous abortions. Monosomy X or Turner's syndrome is the single most common aneuploidy, comprising approximately 20% of these gestations. As a group, the autosomal trisomies account for over half of aneuploid losses, with trisomy 16 being the most common. Autosomal trisomies have been noted for every chromosome except chromosome number 1.

Polyploidy, usually in the form of triploidy, is found in approximately 20% of all miscarriages. Polyploid conceptions typically result in empty sacs or blighted ova but occasionally can lead to partial hydatidiform moles.

The remaining half of early abortuses appear to have normal chromosomal complements. Of these, 20% have other genetic abnormalities that may account for the loss. Mendelian or polygenic factors resulting in anatomic defects may play a role. These factors tend to be more common in later fetal losses.

B. MATERNAL FACTORS

1. Systemic disease

a. Maternal infections—Organisms such as *Treponema pallidum, Chlamydia trachomatis, Neisseria gonorrhoeae, Streptococcus agalactiae,* herpes simplex virus, cytomegalovirus, and *Listeria monocytogenes* have been implicated in spontaneous abortion. Although these agents have been identified in early losses, a causal relationship has not been established.

b. Other diseases—Endocrine disorders such as hyperthyroidism and poorly controlled diabetes mellitus; cardiovascular disorders, such as hypertensive or renal disease; and connective tissue disease, such as systemic lupus erythematosus, may be associated with spontaneous abortion.

2. Uterine defects—Congenital anomalies that distort or reduce the size of the uterine cavity, such as unicornuate, bicornuate, or septate uterus, carry a 25–50% risk of miscarriage. A diethylstilbestrol (DES)-related anomaly, such as a T-shaped or hypoplastic uterus, also carries an increased risk of miscarriage. Acquired anomalies, particularly submucous or intramural myomas, have been associated with spontaneous abortions as well.

Previous scarring of the uterine cavity following dilatation and curettage (D&C; Asherman's syndrome), myomectomy, or unification procedures has been implicated in spontaneous miscarriage, as has anatomic or functional incompetence of the uterine cervix.

3. Immunologic disorders—Blood group incompatibility due to ABO, Rh, Kell, or other less common antigens has been associated with spontaneous abortions. Furthermore, similar maternal and paternal human leukocyte antigen (HLA) status may enhance the possibility of abortion by causing insufficient maternal immunologic recognition of the fetus.

4. Malnutrition—Severe malnutrition has been implicated in spontaneous losses.

5. Emotional disturbances—Emotional causes of abortion are speculative. No valid evidence supports the concept that abortion may be induced by fright, grief, anger, or anxiety.

C. TOXIC FACTORS

Agents such as radiation, antineoplastic drugs, anesthetic gases, alcohol, and nicotine have been shown to be embryotoxic. Other agents such as lead, ethylene oxide, and formaldehyde have also been implicated.

D. TRAUMA

Direct trauma, such as injury to the uterus from a gunshot wound, or indirect trauma, such as surgical removal of an ovary containing the corpus luteum of pregnancy, may result in spontaneous abortion.

Pathology

In spontaneous abortion, hemorrhage into the decidua basalis often occurs. Necrosis and inflammation appear in the area of implantation. The pregnancy becomes partially or entirely detached. Uterine contractions and dilatation of the cervix result in expulsion of most or all of the products of conception.

Clinical Findings

A. THREATENED ABORTION

At least 20–30% of pregnant women have some first-trimester bleeding. In most cases, this is thought to represent an implantation bleed. The cervix remains closed, and slight bleeding with or without cramping may be noted.

B. INEVITABLE ABORTION

Abdominal or back pain and bleeding with an open cervix indicate impending abortion. Abortion is inevitable when cervical effacement, cervical dilatation, and/or rupture of the membranes is noted.

C. INCOMPLETE ABORTION (FIG 14–1)

In incomplete abortion the products of conception have partially passed from the uterine cavity. In gestations of less than 10 weeks' duration, the fetus and placenta are usually passed together. After 10 weeks, they may be passed separately, with a portion of the products retained in the uterine cavity. Cramps are usually present. Bleeding generally is persistent and is often severe.

D. COMPLETE ABORTION (FIG 14–2)

Complete abortion is identified by passage of the entire conceptus. Slight bleeding may continue for a short time, although pain usually ceases after pregnancy has traversed the cervix.

E. MISSED ABORTION

Missed abortion implies that the pregnancy has been retained following death of the fetus. Why the pregnancy is not expelled is not known. It is possible that normal progestogen production by the placenta continues while estrogen levels fall, which may reduce uterine contractility.

Figure 14–1. Incomplete abortion. **Right:** Product of incomplete abortion. (Reproduced, with permission, from Benson RC: *Handbook of Obstetrics & Gynecology,* 8th ed. Lange, 1983.)

F. BLIGHTED OVUM

Blighted ovum or anembryonic pregnancy represents a failed development of the embryo so that only a gestational sac, with or without a yolk sac, is present. An alternative hypothesis proposes that the fetal pole has been resorbed prior to ultrasound diagnosis.

Laboratory Findings

A. COMPLETE BLOOD COUNT

If significant bleeding has occurred, the patient will be anemic. Both the white blood cell count and the sedimentation rate may be elevated even without the presence of infection.

B. PREGNANCY TESTS

Falling or abnormally rising plasma levels of β-human chorionic gonadotropin (hCG) are diagnostic of an abnormal pregnancy, either a blighted ovum, spontaneous abortion, or ectopic pregnancy.

Ultrasonography

Transvaginal ultrasound is helpful in documenting intrauterine pregnancies as early as 4–5 weeks' gestation. Fetal heart motion should be seen in embryos > 5 mm from crown to rump or in embryos at least 5–6 weeks' gestation. Ultrasound is useful in determining which pregnancies are viable and which are most likely to miscarry.

In threatened abortion, ultrasound will reveal a normal gestational sac and viable embryo. However, a large or irregular sac, an eccentric fetal pole, the presence of a large (> 25% of sac size) retrochorionic bleed, and/or a slow fetal heart rate (< 85 bpm) carry a poor prognosis. Miscarriage becomes increasingly less likely the further the gestation progresses. If a viable fetus of 6 weeks or less is seen on ultrasound, the risk of miscarriage is approximately 15–30%. The risk decreases to 5–10% at 7–9 weeks' gestation and to less than 5% after 9 weeks' gestation.

In incomplete abortion, the gestational sac usually is deflated, and irregular, echogenic material representing placental tissue is seen in the uterine cavity. In complete abortion, the endometrium appears closely apposed, with no visible products of conception.

An embryo or fetus without heart motion is consistent with a missed abortion, whereas an abnormal gestational sac, without a yolk sac or embryo, is consistent with a blighted ovum (Figs 14–3 to 14–6). Most pregnancies are lost weeks before mothers complain of signs or symptoms.

Ectopic pregnancy may cause similar symptoms of miscarriage, namely, menstrual abnormality and abdominal or pelvic pain. An adnexal mass may or may not be present. Ultrasound can virtually exclude an ectopic pregnancy by documenting an intrauterine pregnancy, as the chance of a simultaneous intrauterine and extrauterine pregnancy (heterotopic pregnancy) is exceedingly rare in spontaneous pregnancies, occurring in only 1 in 15,000–40,000 pregnancies.

Hydatidiform mole usually ends in abortion before the fifth month. Theca lutein cysts, when present, cause bilateral ovarian enlargement; the uterus may be unusually large. Bloody discharge may contain hydropic villi.

Figure 14–2. Complete abortion. **Right:** Product of complete abortion. (Reproduced, with permission, from Benson RC: *Handbook of Obstetrics & Gynecology,* 8th ed. Lange, 1983.)

Figure 14–3. Intrauterine pregnancy at 8 weeks' gestation, demonstrating embryo (E) and yolk sac (Ys).

Figure 14–5. Empty gestational sac, consistent with a blighted ovum.

Other entities that may be confused with abortion include cervical infection, extruding pedunculated myoma, and cervical neoplasia. However, the pregnancy test will be negative unless a pregnancy coexists.

Complications

Severe or persistent hemorrhage during or following abortion may be life threatening. The more advanced the gestation, the greater the likelihood of excessive blood loss. Sepsis develops most frequently after self-induced abortion. Infection, intrauterine synechia, and

infertility are other complications of abortion. Perforation of the uterine wall may occur during D&C because of the soft and vaguely outlined uterine wall and may be accompanied by injury to the bowel and bladder, hemorrhage, infection, and fistula formation.

Multiple pregnancy with the loss of 1 fetus and retention of another ("vanishing twin") not only is possible but has been well documented in 20% of early pregnancies closely monitored by ultrasound. Usually the fetus is simply resorbed, but the loss of 1 fetus in multiple gestation may be accompanied by cramping or vaginal bleeding.

Figure 14–4. Embryonic demise at 8 weeks' gestation, with irregular gestational sac.

Figure 14–6. Empty uterus (U) with an adnexal mass (A) suspicious for an ectopic pregnancy. β-hCG at the time of transabdominal ultrasound was just over 100 mIU/mL.

Even with very early miscarriage, a loss can have a significant effect on the family. The fact that most of these losses are unexpected intensifies this grief. Each person responds differently to his or her tragedy. It is the health care worker's responsibility to help parents mourn by acknowledging their loss and identifying potential support systems.

Prevention

Some losses can be prevented by early obstetric care, with adequate treatment of maternal disorders such as diabetes and hypertension, and by protection of pregnant women from environmental hazards and exposure to infectious diseases.

Treatment of Abortions

Successful management of spontaneous abortion depends upon early diagnosis. Every patient should receive a general physical examination, and a complete history should be taken. Laboratory studies should include a complete blood count, blood typing, and cervical cultures to determine pathogens in case of infection.

If the diagnosis of threatened abortion is made, bed rest and pelvic rest typically are recommended, although neither has been shown to be helpful in preventing subsequent miscarriage. Prognosis is good when bleeding and/or cramping resolve.

If the diagnosis of inevitable or incomplete abortion is made, evacuation of the uterus by a surgical method should be considered. Significant bleeding or retained products usually require a D&C; however, cases in which blood loss is minimal can be observed for spontaneous completion. A type and cross-match for possible blood transfusion and determination of Rh status should be obtained. The prognosis for the mother is excellent if the retained tissue is promptly and completely evacuated.

If the diagnosis of complete abortion is made, the patient should be observed for further bleeding. The products of conception should be examined. As with inevitable and incomplete abortion, the prognosis for the mother is excellent.

If abortion has occurred after the first trimester, hospitalization should be considered. Oxytocics are helpful in contracting the uterus, limiting blood loss, and aiding in expulsion of clots and tissue. Ergot preparations, which contract the cervix and the uterus, may also be given if needed. As with a first-trimester loss, a D&C may be necessary if significant bleeding persists or if products of conception are retained.

Treatment of Complications

Uterine perforation may be manifested by signs of intraperitoneal bleeding, rupture of the bowel or bladder, or peritonitis. Oftentimes, there are no clinical signs and no sequelae. When uterine perforation is suspected, however, laparoscopy and/or laparotomy are indicated to determine the extent of laceration or bowel injury.

RECURRENT ABORTION

General Considerations

Recurrent abortion in its broadest definition is defined as 2 to 3 or more consecutive pregnancy losses before 20 weeks of gestation, each with a fetus weighing less than 500 g. Approximately 1% of women are habitual aborters. Prognosis for a successful subsequent pregnancy is correlated with the number of previous abortions. The risk of having a spontaneous abortion for the first time is about 15%, and this risk is at least doubled in women experiencing recurrent abortion (Table 14–1).

Other factors with prognostic implications include maternal age and abortus karyotype. The former is directly correlated with the risk of abortion. A normal karyotype carries a higher recurrence risk than does an abnormal karyotype, as this subset presumably is susceptible to maternal etiologies.

Table 14–1. Probability of spontaneous abortion.

Type of Study	Number of Previous Abortions			
	0	1	2	3+
Retrospective studies				
Stevenson et al (1959)		16.3	19.2	26.2
Warburton and Fraser (1964)	12.3	26.2	32.2	30.2
Leridon (1976)	15.2	22.0	35.3	
Poland et al (1977)		19.0	35.0	47.0
Naylor and Warburton (1978)	11.0	20.3	29.2	37.0
Cohort studies				
Shapiro et al (1970)	10.9	18.0		
Awan (1974)	10.4	22.1	27.4	
Prospective studies				
Boué at al (1975)		13.8		
Harger et al (1983)			17.4	29.2
Fitzsimmons et al (1983)			31.3	45.7
Regan (1988)	5.6	11.5	29.4	36.4

Percentage of women aborting in relation to number of previous abortions.

Reproduced, with permission, from Regan L: Prospective study of spontaneous abortion. In: Beard RW, Sharp F (editors). *Early Pregnancy Loss: Mechanisms and Treatment.* Royal College of Obstetricians and Gynaecologists, 1988.

Despite some controversy regarding the evaluation and management of recurrent abortion, the prognosis following repeated losses is good, with most couples having an approximately 60% chance of a viable pregnancy.

Etiology & Treatment

Chromosomal abnormalities, uterine malformations, and antiphospholipid syndrome are the three generally accepted etiologies of recurrent miscarriages. Currently evidence is insufficient to support routine evaluation of other causes, including hormonal abnormalities, infection, systemic disease, environmental agents, and alloimmune factors. Table 14–2 summarizes a diagnostic work-up and possible therapies for recurrent abortion.

A. GENETIC ERRORS

Genetic errors associated with recurrent abortion include parental structural chromosome abnormalities and recurrent aneuploidy. Balanced rearrangements of parental chromosomes are found in approximately 2–5% of couples with repetitive abortions. Of these, balanced translocations are the most common. In couples who have a normal chromosome analysis, recurrent fetal aneuploidy has been proposed as a distinct etiology.

A careful reproductive history and pedigree should be taken for both partners, and karyotype screening should be performed. Couples with a history of other reproductive problems, such as stillbirth or congenital anomalies, are more likely to be affected by a balanced structural chromosome abnormality. If the defect is paternal, artificial insemination by a donor is available. For a maternal defect, a donor egg may be fertilized by the husband's sperm. Preimplantation diagnosis is also an option.

B. UTERINE ABNORMALITIES

Anatomic abnormalities were the first described causes of habitual abortion and account for up to 15% of recurrent pregnancy losses. Defects include congenital uterine anomalies, cervical incompetence, submucous leiomyomas, abnormalities due to DES exposure in utero, and Asherman's syndrome. A major difficulty in counseling affected couples is that approximately 50% of women with uterine defects have no reproductive problem. Septate uteri account for the vast majority of patients with uterine malformations and recurrent pregnancy loss. Unicornuate and bicornuate uteri are less commonly associated. Submucous leiomyomas are responsible for a much smaller percentage of repeated losses. Generally, losses from anatomic abnormalities occur in the second trimester. Interference with implantation, lack of an adequate blood supply, and growth restriction are possible mechanisms for recurrent loss.

Diagnosis of uterine anatomic abnormalities usually is accomplished by hysterosalpingography or hysteroscopy. Treatment is primarily surgical, with reported success rates of 70–85% after surgical correction.

Table 14–2. Diagnosis and treatment of recurrent abortion.

Cause	Diagnosis	Treatment
Genetic error	Obtain a 3-generation pedigree and karyotype of both parents and any previously aborted material.	Artificial insemination by donor, embryo transfer, preimplantation diagnosis, or prenatal testing on subsequent conceptions
Anatomic abnormalities of reproductive tract	Perform hysterosalpingogram or hysteroscopy.	Uterine operation: hysteroscopic resection, myomectomy. Cervical cerclage (abdominal or vaginal), reconstruction of cervical isthmus.
Hormonal abnormalities	Perform laboratory studies for T_4 and TSH, serum progesterone or endometrial biopsy during luteal phase, and consider glucose tolerance test.	Thyroid replacement, progesterone or clomiphene citrate, diabetic diet and/or insulin, as indicated.
Infection	Obtain cervical cultures for *Chlamydia* and gonorrhea, and consider cultures for *Mycoplasma* and *Ureaplasma*.	Appropriate antibiotics.
Autoimmune disease	Evaluate blood pressure and kidney function, check for lupus anticoagulant and anticardiolipin antibody.	Low-dose aspirin and heparin.
Exogenous agents	Patient history and/or drug screen.	Discourage smoking, alcohol, and recreational drug use.
Immunologic factors	Testing not readily available.	Treatment under investigation.

Cervical incompetence may be due to congenital abnormalities (eg, DES exposure), trauma from a vigorous D&C or cone biopsy, and/or possibly hormonal influences. It classically presents in mid-second or early third trimester with rapid, painless cervical dilatation. If other causes of recurrent losses are excluded and the presumed etiology is incompetent cervix, a cervical cerclage is recommended between 12 and 14 weeks' gestation. Success rates with cerclage are 85–90%. Complications include risks from anesthesia, bleeding, infection, rupture of membranes, and miscarriage. Contraindications to cerclage placement include bleeding of unknown etiology, infection, labor, ruptured membranes, and congenital anomalies.

C. HORMONAL CAUSES

Possible hormonal causes of habitual abortion include hypothyroidism and hyperthyroidism, progesterone insufficiency, and uncontrolled diabetes mellitus.

Progesterone deficiency or luteal phase defect (LPD) is a controversial etiology of habitual abortion. A defective endometrium resulting in faulty implantation is the proposed mechanism. Inadequate hormonal support of the embryo may also be involved. The diagnosis usually is made by luteal phase endometrial biopsies, which attempt to identify a lag in endometrial development when compared to menstrual age. Critics of the diagnosis of LPD note intraobserver and interobserver variations in biopsy results, the presence of LPD in normal women, and the inconsistent occurrence in women affected by LPD. Furthermore, controlled studies demonstrating an improvement in pregnancy outcome with progesterone treatment are lacking. For these reasons, many experts are skeptical about the importance of LPD as an etiology of recurrent pregnancy loss.

D. INFECTION

Infectious agents that have been implicated in repetitive losses include *Mycoplasma hominis, Ureaplasma urealyticum, Toxoplasma gondii, C trachomatis, T pallidum, Borrelia burgdorferi, N gonorrhoeae, S agalactiae, L monocytogenes,* herpes simplex, and cytomegalovirus. Although these agents have been identified in early losses, a causal relationship has not been demonstrated.

E. SYSTEMIC DISEASE

Systemic causes of recurrent abortion include uncontrolled diabetes, uncontrolled thyroid disease, and collagen vascular disease. The incidence of systemic disease as a cause of habitual abortion is unknown but probably is low. Furthermore, in patients without risk factors, asymptomatic disease is an unlikely culprit, precluding routine screening. Therapy involves treatment of the specific disease.

F. IMMUNOLOGIC FACTORS

Antiphospholipid antibodies (lupus anticoagulant and anticardiolipin antibodies) may damage platelets and vascular endothelium, resulting in thrombosis. This may account for the relationship to miscarriage when found in combination with clinical features of antiphospholipid syndrome. Low-dose aspirin and/or heparin are beneficial in this situation.

Compared to women who carry a pregnancy to term, women who are habitual aborters share more HLAs with their partners and have blunted responses to paternal antigen with lower levels of blocking antibodies or antileukocytotoxic antibodies. The maternal immunologic response may not be as effective in protecting the pregnancy, resulting in pregnancy loss.

Diagnostic tests for immunologic abnormalities are available in few centers. The efficacy of leukocyte immunotherapy is unknown, and treatment such as paternal leukocyte immunization is still experimental.

In up to 50% of women with recurrent abortion, a definitive cause may not be found. However, although the loss rate may be higher than that in the general population, the majority of these women will have a successful pregnancy in their reproductive lifetime.

SEPTIC ABORTION

General Considerations

Septic abortion is manifested by fever, malodorous vaginal discharge, pelvic and abdominal pain, and cervical motion tenderness. Peritonitis and sepsis may be seen. Trauma to the cervix or upper vagina may be recognized if there has been a criminal abortion.

A complete blood count, urinalysis, endometrial cultures, blood cultures, chest x-ray, and abdominal x-ray to rule out uterine perforation should be obtained. Ultrasound may be helpful in ruling out retained products of conception.

Treatment

Treatment of septic abortion involves hospitalization and intravenous antibiotic therapy. Selection of antibiotic agents should provide for both anaerobic and aerobic coverage. A D&C should be performed, and a hysterectomy may be necessary if the infection does not respond to treatment.

ECTOPIC PREGNANCY

In ectopic pregnancy, a fertilized ovum implants in an area other than the endometrial lining of the uterus (Fig 14–7). More than 95% of extrauterine pregnancies occur in the fallopian tube.

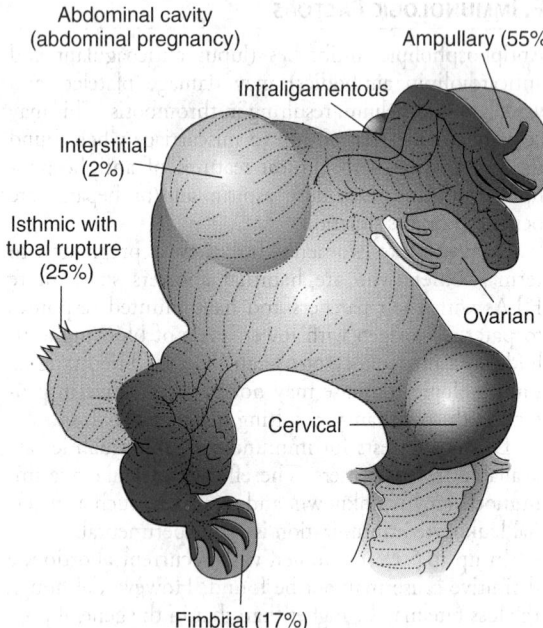

Abdominal cavity
(abdominal pregnancy)

Ampullary (55%)

Intraligamentous

Interstitial
(2%)

Isthmic with
tubal rupture
(25%)

Ovarian

Cervical

Fimbrial (17%)

Figure 14–7. Sites of ectopic pregnancies. (Adapted, with permission, from Benson RC: *Handbook of Obstetrics & Gynecology,* 8th ed. Lange, 1983.)

The incidence of ectopic pregnancy has increased from 4.5 in 1000 in 1970 to 19.7 in 1000 in 1992. This may be due, at least in part, to a higher incidence of salpingitis, an increase in ovulation induction and assisted reproductive technology, and more tubal sterilizations.

Ectopic pregnancy is a significant cause of maternal morbidity and mortality, as well as fetal loss. It is the leading cause of pregnancy-related death in the first trimester and accounts for 9% of all pregnancy-related deaths. The development of sensitive β-hCG assays, along with the increasing use of ultrasound and laparoscopy, has allowed for earlier diagnosis of ectopic pregnancy. This has resulted in a decrease in both maternal morbidity and mortality.

Classification & Incidence

Ectopic pregnancy can be classified as follows (Fig 14–7).

1. Tubal (> 95%)—Includes ampullary (55%), isthmic (25%), fimbrial (17%), and interstitial (2%).

2. Other (< 5%)—Includes cervical, ovarian, and abdominal (primary abdominal pregnancies have been reported, but most abdominal pregnancies are secondary pregnancies, from tubal abortion or rupture and subsequent implantation in the bowel, omentum, or mesentery). Cesarean delivery scar pregnancy is becom-

ing an increasingly recognized clinical entity, with its incidence presumably paralleling a rise in cesarean section rates.

3. Intraligamentous

4. Heterotopic pregnancy—An ectopic pregnancy occurs in combination with an intrauterine pregnancy in 1 in 15,000–40,000 spontaneous pregnancies and in up to 1% of patients undergoing in vitro fertilization.

5. Bilateral ectopic—These pregnancies have occasionally been reported.

Etiology

The etiology of ectopic pregnancy is not well understood. However, several risk factors have been found to be associated with ectopic pregnancy (Table 14–3).

A. TUBAL FACTORS

Ectopic pregnancy is 5–10 times more common in women who have had salpingitis. In women with ectopic pregnancies, up to 50% will have had salpingitis previously, and in most of these patients, the uninvolved tube is also abnormal. Other tubal factors that interfere with the progress of the fertilized ovum include adherent folds of tubal lumen due to salpingitis isthmica nodosa, developmental abnormalities of the tube or abnormal tubal anatomy due to DES exposure in utero, previous tubal surgery including tubal ligation with a 16–50% ectopic pregnancy rate if pregnancy oc-

Table 14–3. Risk factors for ectopic pregnancy.

Risk Factor	Odds Ratio[1]
High risk	
Tubal surgery	21.0
Sterilization	9.3
Previous ectopic pregnancy	8.3
In utero exposure to diethylstilbestrol	5.6
Use of IUD	4.2–45.0
Documented tubal pathology	3.8–21.0
Moderate risk	
Infertility	2.5–21.0
Previous genital infections	2.5–3.7
Multiple sexual partners	2.1
Slight risk	
Previous pelvic/abdominal surgery	0.9–3.8
Cigarette smoking	2.3–2.5
Vaginal douching	1.1–3.1
Early age at first intercourse (< 18 years)	1.6

[1]Single values indicate common odds ratio from homogeneous studies; point estimates indicate range of values from heterogeneous studies. Reproduced, with permission, from Pisarska MD, Carson SA, Buster JE: Ectopic pregnancy. Lancet 1998;351:1115.

curs after tubal ligation, conservative treatment of an unruptured ectopic with a recurrent ectopic rate of 4–16%, and tubal anastomosis with a 4% ectopic rate. Adhesions from infection or previous abdominal surgery, endometriosis, and even leiomyomas have been associated with ectopic pregnancy. Most of these abnormalities are bilateral and irreversible.

B. Zygote Abnormalities

A variety of zygote abnormalities have been reported in ectopic pregnancy, including chromosomal abnormalities, gross malformations, and neural tube defects. In theory, these abnormal pre-embryos are more likely to result in abnormal or ectopic implantation.

C. Ovarian Factors

Ovarian factors that may result in the development of an ectopic pregnancy are fertilization of an unextruded ovum, transmigration of the ovum into the contralateral tube with subsequent delayed and faulty implantation, and postmidcycle ovulation and fertilization.

D. Exogenous Hormones

Abnormal hormonal stimulation and/or exogenous hormones may play a role in ectopic gestation. For example, 4–6% of pregnancies occurring in women taking progestin-only oral contraceptives are ectopic. This may be due to progesterone's smooth muscle relaxant effects and subsequent "ovum trapping." Patients with DES exposure are also at risk, as are patients undergoing ovulation induction.

E. Other Factors

Intrauterine device (IUD) users are at risk for ectopic pregnancy if pregnancy occurs, although the risk of ectopic pregnancy is still lower than if no contraceptive method is used. Whether the IUD prevents intrauterine but not ectopic pregnancy or whether an associated salpingitis is responsible for this increased risk is unclear. Smoking and increasing age are also associated with ectopic pregnancy. Multiple previous elective abortions are also believed to be a risk factor for ectopic pregnancy, as postabortal infection may lead to salpingitis.

Time of Rupture

Rupture usually is spontaneous. Isthmic pregnancies tend to rupture earliest, at 6 to 8 weeks' gestation, because of the small diameter of this portion of the tube. Ampullary pregnancies rupture later, generally at 8–12 weeks. Interstitial pregnancies are the last to rupture, usually at 12–16 weeks, as the myometrium allows more room to grow than the tubal wall. Interstitial rupture is quite dangerous because its proximity to uterine and ovarian vessels can result in massive hemorrhage.

After rupture, the conceptus may be resorbed or remain as a mass in the abdominal cavity or cul-de-sac. Rarely, if not damaged during rupture, it may implant elsewhere in the abdominal cavity and continue to grow.

Clinical Findings

No specific symptoms or signs are pathognomonic for ectopic pregnancy, and many disorders can present similarly. Normal pregnancy, threatened or incomplete abortion, rupture of an ovarian cyst, ovarian torsion, gastroenteritis, and appendicitis can all be confused with ectopic pregnancy. Because early diagnosis is crucial, a high index of suspicion should be maintained when any pregnant woman in the first trimester presents with bleeding and/or abdominal pain. Fifteen to twenty percent of ectopic gestations will present as surgical emergencies.

A. Symptoms

The following symptoms may assist in the diagnosis of ectopic pregnancy.

1. Pain—Pelvic or abdominal pain is present in close to 100% of cases. Pain can be unilateral or bilateral, localized or generalized. The presence of subdiaphragmatic or shoulder pain is more variable, depending on the amount of intra-abdominal bleeding.

2. Bleeding—Abnormal uterine bleeding, usually spotting, occurs in roughly 75% of cases and represents decidual sloughing. A decidua cast is passed in 5–10% of ectopic pregnancies and may be mistaken for products of conception.

3. Amenorrhea—Secondary amenorrhea is variable. Approximately half of women with ectopic pregnancies have some spotting at the time of their expected menses and thus do not realize they are pregnant.

4. Syncope—Dizziness, lightheadedness, and/or syncope is present in one-third to one-half of cases and represent advanced stages of intra-abdominal bleeding.

B. Signs

On examination, the following signs are important in the diagnosis of ectopic gestation.

1. Tenderness—Diffuse or localized abdominal tenderness is present in over 80% of ectopic pregnancies. Adnexal and/or cervical motion tenderness is present in over 75% of cases.

2. Adnexal mass—A unilateral adnexal mass is palpated in one-third to one-half of patients. Occasionally, a cul-de-sac mass is present. The patient's discomfort may preclude an adequate examination, and effort should be made to avoid an iatrogenic tubal rupture from an overzealous assessment.

3. Uterine changes—The uterus may undergo typical changes of pregnancy, including softening and a slight increase in size.

4. Hemodynamic instability—Vital signs will reflect hemodynamic status of patients with tubal rupture and massive intra-abdominal hemorrhage.

Laboratory Findings

Hematocrit: The hematocrit will vary depending on the patient population and the degree, if any, of intra-abdominal bleeding.

β-hCG: The qualitative serum or urine β-hCG assay is positive in virtually 100% of ectopic pregnancies. The value of this test is limited, however, because a positive result does not help to elicit the location of the pregnancy. More helpful is a quantitative β-hCG value that, in conjunction with transvaginal ultrasound, can usually make the diagnosis. In an unclear clinical picture, serial titers can be followed that, in the face of a normal pregnancy, should double every 2 days. Two-thirds of ectopic pregnancies have abnormally rising values, whereas the remaining third show a normal progression.

Special Examinations

Several special procedures are helpful in diagnosing ectopic pregnancy.

1. Ultrasound—Ultrasound is useful in evaluating patients at risk for ectopic pregnancy, namely, by documenting the presence or absence of an intrauterine pregnancy. β-hCG titers and ultrasound complement each another in detecting ectopic pregnancy and have led to earlier detection with a subsequent decrease in adverse outcome. By correlating β-hCG titers with ultrasound findings, an ectopic pregnancy often can be differentiated from an intrauterine pregnancy. Furthermore, ultrasound can help distinguish a normal intrauterine pregnancy from a blighted ovum, incomplete abortion, or complete abortion.

A normal intrauterine sac appears regular and well defined on ultrasound. It has been described as a "double ring," which represents the decidual lining and the amniotic sac. In ectopic pregnancy, ultrasound may reveal only a thickened, decidualized endometrium. With more advanced ectopics, decidual sloughing with resultant intracavitary fluid or blood may create a so-called "pseudogestational sac," a small and irregular structure that may be confused with an intrauterine gestation.

An intrauterine sac should be visible by transvaginal ultrasound when the β-hCG level is approximately 1000 mIU/mL and by transabdominal ultrasound approximately 1 week later, when the β-hCG level is 1800–3600 mIU/mL. Thus, when an empty uterine cavity is seen with a β-hCG titer above this threshold, an ectopic pregnancy is more likely.

The presence of an adnexal mass with an empty uterus raises the suspicion for an ectopic pregnancy, especially if the β-hCG titers are above the discriminatory zone. Although direct visualization of an adnexal gestational sac along with a yolk sac or embryo secures the diagnosis, it is more likely to detect a "tubal ring" or complex mass adjacent to, but separate from, both the uterus and ovary. If rupture has occurred, a dilated fallopian tube with fluid in the cul-de-sac may be visualized. Ultrasound is increasingly being relied upon to differentiate several less common types of ectopic pregnancies. Both interstitial tubal and cesarean section scar pregnancies can masquerade as intrauterine gestations because of their proximity to the intrauterine cavity.

The most likely alternative diagnosis to an adnexal mass in early pregnancy is a corpus luteum cyst, which can rupture and bleed, thus contributing to a highly confusing clinical picture.

2. Laparoscopy—The need for laparoscopy in the diagnosis of ectopic pregnancy has declined with the increasing use of ultrasound. However, it still is useful in certain situations where a definitive diagnosis is difficult, especially in the case of a desired, potentially viable intrauterine pregnancy when a D&C is contraindicated. Laparoscopy may also be used as definitive management in early ectopic gestation.

3. D&C—D&C may confirm or exclude intrauterine pregnancy in the case of an undesired pregnancy. D&C may interrupt an intrauterine gestation and should not be performed if the pregnancy is desired, unless the β-hCG titers have plateaued or fallen and the pregnancy is definitely abnormal. When chorionic villi are recovered, the diagnosis of an intrauterine pregnancy is confirmed. On the other hand, if only decidua is obtained on D&C, ectopic pregnancy is highly likely.

4. Laparotomy—Laparotomy is indicated when the presumptive diagnosis of ectopic pregnancy in an unstable patient necessitates immediate surgery, or when definitive therapy is not possible by medical management or laparoscopy.

5. Culdocentesis—Culdocentesis, the transvaginal passage of a needle into the posterior cul-de-sac in order to determine whether free blood is present in the abdomen (Fig 14–8), has largely been replaced by transvaginal ultrasound.

6. Magnetic resonance imaging—Magnetic resonance imaging is a useful adjunct to ultrasound in cases where an unusual ectopic location is suspected. An accurate diagnosis of cervical, cesarean scar, or interstitial

Figure 14–8. Culdocentesis.

pregnancy urges conservative intervention with methotrexate (MTX) in order to avoid the potentially catastrophic hemorrhage associated with surgical management of these sites.

Pathology

In tubal ectopic pregnancy, implantation typically occurs in the wall of the tube, in the connective tissue beneath the serosa. There may be little or no decidual reaction and minimal defense against the permeating trophoblast. The trophoblast invades blood vessels, causing local hemorrhage. A hematoma in the subserosal space enlarges as pregnancy progresses. Progressive distention of the tube eventually leads to rupture.

Vaginal bleeding is of uterine origin and is caused by endometrial involution and decidual sloughing. Atypical changes in the endometrium may be suggestive of ectopic pregnancy. The Arias-Stella reaction consists of hyperchromatic, hypertrophic, irregularly shaped nuclei, and foamy, vacuolated cytoplasm. These changes can be seen in normal pregnancy and in miscarriage and therefore are not diagnostic of ectopic pregnancy.

Occasionally, endometrial tissue may be passed as a so-called decidual cast. Superficial secretory endometrium usually is present, but no trophoblastic cells are seen.

Prevention

Prevention of sexually transmitted disease, with early and vigorous treatment of cases that do occur, may avoid tubal damage with subsequent ectopic pregnancy. Other risk factors for ectopic pregnancy are more difficult to control. Early diagnosis of unruptured tubal pregnancy by maintaining a high index of suspicion and liberal use of β-hCG titers, ultrasound, and lap-

aroscopy will minimize potential problems of hemorrhage, infertility, and extensive surgery.

Treatment

A. EXPECTANT MANAGEMENT

Because many ectopic pregnancies resolve spontaneously, it may be reasonable to manage an asymptomatic, compliant patient expectantly if β-hCG titers are low (< 200 mIU/mL) or decreasing, and the risk of rupture is low.

B. MEDICAL MANAGEMENT

MTX, a folinic acid antagonist, has been shown to destroy proliferating trophoblast and may be effective in the medical management of small, unruptured ectopic pregnancies in asymptomatic women. Exclusion criteria include a patient who is noncompliant or has completed childbearing, peptic ulcer disease, immunodeficiency, pulmonary disease, liver disease, renal disease, blood dyscrasias, hemodynamic instability, free fluid in the cul-de-sac plus pelvic pain, or known sensitivity to MTX. Relative contraindications include an adnexal mass ≥ 3.5 cm or an extrauterine gestation with fetal heart motion, because of the higher failure rate. In select cases, approximately 90% of ectopics resolve, taking on average just under 1 month. Protocols vary from single to multiple injections, typically given systemically. The dose of MTX depends on the patient's body surface area, and nomograms are available for determining the correct dose. Follow-up β-hCG levels, along with a complete blood count, serum creatinine, and serum aspartate transaminase, are obtained for comparison with baseline values. β-hCG levels should decrease by at least 15% between days 4 and 7 after MTX administration. Failure of MTX therapy is suggested by a persistent rise or plateau in β-hCG titer and can be managed by a second dose of MTX or surgery. A recurrent episode of abdominal pain or enlargement of the adnexal mass during the first week of therapy may be part of a normal response to successful MTX treatment. Vigilant observation should be the rule, and follow-up ultrasound should be used liberally. Persistent and worsening pain in conjunction with a hemoperitoneum on ultrasound, and/or hemodynamic instability, mandates immediate surgical intervention.

Available studies comparing MTX to traditional surgical management report similar subsequent tubal patency and fertility rates. Arguments against its use include its toxicity, namely, marrow suppression, dermatitis, and stomatitis, as well as potential for treatment failure and tubal rupture.

Chronic ectopics, with decreasing but persistent β-hCG titers, pose a management dilemma. Some will resolve on their own, whereas others will require surgery. Unfortunately, at present it is impossible to predict which patients will fail expectant management.

C. Surgical Treatment

Once the mainstay of therapy for ectopic pregnancy, surgery is now mainly reserved for patients with contraindications to medical management. The extent of surgery depends on the degree of damage to the uterus and adnexa. Preservation of the ovary should be attempted if feasible. Conservative surgery (ie, preservation of the fallopian tube) may be indicated in the hemodynamically stable patient with an ampullary pregnancy who wishes to preserve fertility.

A linear salpingostomy may be performed with a small (< 3 cm), intact ampullary pregnancy. The linear incision is allowed to heal by secondary intention, minimizing recurrent ectopics as compared to salpingotomy. Both methods yield similar subsequent pregnancy rates of 40–90%.

Depending on operator skill and comfort level, both of these procedures can be performed through the laparoscope, assuming the pregnancy is < 3 cm, unruptured, and easily accessible. With both salpingostomy and salpingotomy, a β-hCG titer should be obtained weekly after surgery to ensure adequate removal of trophoblast and rule out a persistent ectopic. In stable patients, laparoscopy is preferred over laparotomy because of the associated reduction in morbidity and cost.

"Milking" the pregnancy out of the distal end of the tube is often tempting but has been associated with persistent trophoblast and need for re-exploration, as well as increased risks of recurrent ectopic pregnancy.

With an isthmic ectopic pregnancy, segmental resection with subsequent anastomosis (usually at a later date) is typically recommended. As opposed to ampullary ectopics, the muscularis is well developed, forcing the pregnancy to grow in the lumen. More conservative treatment, such as salpingostomy or salpingotomy, would likely cause scarring and compromise of the lumen. Furthermore, a tubal fistula may result if the tube were allowed to heal by secondary intention.

With fimbrial pregnancy, products of conception are often visible at the most distal end of the tube, which may be "plucked out." As with ampullary ectopics, "milking" should be avoided.

Interstitial pregnancies pose a high surgical risk with the potential for massive intra-abdominal bleeding. Most cases are managed with a cornual wedge resection, uterine reconstruction, and, sometimes, salpingectomy on the affected side. If extensive tissue damage is present or if the patient is unstable, a hysterectomy may be needed. Likewise, cervical ectopics may be associated with massive vaginal bleeding with the potential for hysterectomy. Attempts at medical management with MTX should be considered for both.

Ovarian pregnancy requires oophorectomy and sometimes salpingectomy on the affected side. Abdominal pregnancy involves delivery of the fetus (sometimes at term) with ligation of the umbilical cord close to the placenta. The placenta is usually left in place to avoid hemorrhage following removal.

D. Emergency Treatment

Immediate surgery is indicated when the diagnosis of ectopic pregnancy with hemorrhage is made. Blood products should be available because transfusion is often necessary. There is no place for conservative therapy in a hemodynamically unstable patient.

Rh_o (D) immunoglobulin should be given to any Rh-negative mother with the diagnosis of ectopic pregnancy because sensitization may occur.

EXPOSURE TO FETOTOXIC AGENTS

Many variations occur in the complex process of human development. Although population heterogeneity is based on such events, some deviations from the usual developmental process result in aberrations of normal structure and function. These adverse alterations have been scrutinized in an effort to determine their cause. The clinician investigating the effects of exposure to fetotoxic agents must consider whether the patient is known to have reproductive risks, whether the patient has been exposed to fetotoxic agents during pregnancy, and whether structural or functional abnormalities are likely to develop in the fetus.

Many harmful agents are responsible for altering the biologic process of human development (eg, radiation, viruses, medications, and drugs). Aberrations that result from fetal exposure to harmful agents is especially tragic because such exposure often is preventable. However, even the most careful investigation will fail to reveal the cause in the majority of developmental handicaps.

Approximately 3–5% of newborns in the United States have abnormalities at birth that are serious enough to require some form of treatment. Moreover, full recognition of malformations, anomalies, or defects may take years. Thus, estimates that as much as 10% of the total population suffers from some structural or functional developmental disability do not appear unreasonable.

Evaluation

The timing of exposure is crucial, as fetal organs or structures are most vulnerable to adverse influences during organogenesis. Table 14–4 lists some of the potential adverse effects related to the timing of fetotoxic exposure. The route of exposure, the length of exposure, and the total dose received during exposure may also influence the outcome of the pregnancy.

Evaluation of studies of potential toxic exposures is difficult because of the large number of possible fetotoxic agents and interactive effects of certain agents, the retrospective nature of most studies, the difficulty evaluating damage, the presence or absence of influences that may alter the effects of an agent, and the presence or absence of certain genotypes that might alter an individual's susceptibility. Therefore, specific criteria for recognizing teratogens in humans have been defined (Table 14–5). Table 14–6 summarizes the known mechanisms of abnormal development and outlines a working hypothesis of the pathogenesis, common pathways, and final manifestations of abnormal development.

Table 14–4. Potential adverse effects of fetotoxic exposure at selected stages of development.

Week Since Ovulation	Potential Adverse Effect
1–8	Miscarriage, structural malformations
9–40	Central nervous system abnormalities, growth restrictions, neurobehavioral abnormalities, reproductive effects

Table 14–5. Criteria used to recognize teratogens in humans.

Abrupt increase in the incidence of a particular defect or association of defects
Known environmental change coincident with this increase.
Known exposure to the environmental change early in pregnancy, yielding characteristically affected infants.
Absence of other factors common to all pregnancies, yielding infants with the characteristic defects.

Counseling of parents should include review of the exposure history and discussion of the particular agent involved, as well as possible sequelae. In some cases, intervention may be possible. In other cases, if an abnormal pregnancy is found, the parents may elect to abort an affected fetus. Effective counseling should provide the best information available to assist the parents in what is always a very difficult decision.

Table 14–6. General principles of teratology.

Mechanisms	Mutation Chromosome disruption Mitotic interference Altered nucleic acid integrity or function Precursor or substrate deprivation Altered energy sources Changed membrane characteristics Altered osmolar balance Enzyme inhibition
Pathogenesis	Excessive or reduced cell interactions Failed cell interactions Reproduced biosynthesis Impeded morphogenetic movement Mechanical disruption of tissues
Common pathways	Too few cells or cell products to affect localized morphogenesis or functional maturation Other imbalances in growth and differentiation
Final defects	Malformation Growth retardation Functional disorder Death

Table 14–7. Teratogenicity drug labeling now required by the FDA.[1]

Category A: Well-controlled human studies have not disclosed any fetal risk.

Category B: Animal studies have not disclosed any fetal risk; or have suggested some risk not confirmed in controlled studies in women; or no adequate studies in women are available.

Category C: Animal studies have revealed adverse fetal effects; no adequate controlled studies in women are available.

Category D: Some fetal risk, but benefits may outweigh risk (eg, life-threatening illness, no safer effective drug).

Category X: Fetal abnormalities in animal and human studies; risk not outweighed by benefit. *Contraindicated in pregnancy.*

---

[1]The FDA has established 5 categories of drugs based on their potential for causing birth defects in infants born to women who use them during pregnancy. By law, the label must provide available information on teratogenicity.

The United States Food and Drug Administration (FDA) standards for drug labeling with regard to teratogenicity are listed in Table 14–7.

REFERENCES

American College of Obstetricians and Gynecologists: *Early Pregnancy Loss.* ACOG Technical Bulletin No. 212. American College of Obstetricians and Gynecologists, 1995.

American College of Obstetricians and Gynecologists: *Medical Management of Tubal Pregnancy.* ACOG Practice Bulletin No. 3. American College of Obstetricians and Gynecologists, 1998.

American College of Obstetricians and Gynecologists: *Management of Recurrent Early Pregnancy Loss.* ACOG Practice Bulletin No. 24. American College of Obstetricians and Gynecologists, 2001.

Centers for Disease Control and Prevention: Current Trends Ectopic Pregnancy—United States, 1990–1992. MMWR Morb Mortal Wkly Rep 1995;44:46.

Levine D: Ectopic pregnancy. In: Callen PW (editor): *Ultrasonography in Obstetrics and Gynecology,* 4th ed. Saunders, 2000.

Nanda K, Peloggia A, Grimes D, Lopez L, Nanda G: Expectant care versus surgical treatment for miscarriage. *Cochrane Database Syst Rev* 2006;Apr19:CD003518.

Pisarska MD, Carson SA, Buster JE: Ectopic pregnancy. Lancet 1998;351:1115.

Regan L: Prospective study of spontaneous abortion. In: Beard RW, Sharp F (editors): *Early Pregnancy Loss: Mechanisms and Treatment.* Royal College of Obstetricians and Gynaecologists, 1988.

Seeber BE, Barnhart KT: Suspected ectopic pregnancy. *Obstet Gynecol* 2006;107:399.

Tulandi T: New protocols for ectopic pregnancy. Contemp Obstet Gynecol 1999;44:42.

Yao M, Tulandi T: Current status of surgical and nonsurgical management of ectopic pregnancy. Fertil Steril 1997;67:421.

Late Pregnancy Complications

15

Ashley S. Roman, MD, MPH, & Martin L. Pernoll, MD

PRETERM LABOR

ESSENTIALS OF DIAGNOSIS

- *Estimated gestational age of greater than 20 weeks and less than 37 weeks.*
- *Regular uterine contractions at frequent intervals.*
- *Documented cervical change or appreciable cervical dilatation or effacement (at least 2 cm dilated without previous examination).*

General Considerations

Labor is the process of coordinated uterine contractions leading to progressive cervical effacement and dilatation by which the fetus and placenta are expelled. Preterm labor is defined as labor occurring after 20 weeks' but before 37 weeks' gestation. Although there is no strict definition in the literature regarding the amount of uterine contractions required for preterm labor, there is consensus that contractions need to be regular and at frequent intervals. Generally, more than 4 contractions per hour are needed to cause cervical change. The uterine contractions need not be painful to cause cervical change and may manifest themselves as abdominal tightening, lower back pain, or pelvic pressure. In addition, there must be demonstrated cervical effacement or dilatation to meet a diagnosis of preterm labor.

It is important to distinguish preterm labor from other similar clinical entities such as cervical incompetence (cervical change in the absence of uterine contractions) and preterm uterine contractions (regular contractions in the absence of cervical change) because the treatment for these situations differs. Cervical incompetence may require cerclage placement, and preterm uterine contractions without cervical change is generally a self-limited phenomenon that resolves spontaneously and requires no intervention. If ruptured membranes accompany preterm labor, these cases are classified as preterm premature rupture of membranes (for discussion of diagnosis see Premature Rupture of Membranes).

Preterm birth complicates 10–15% of all pregnancies. It is the number 1 cause of neonatal morbidity and mortality and causes 75% of neonatal deaths that are not due to congenital anomalies.

Thirteen percent of all infants are classified as low birth weight (< 2500 g). Three percent of these are mature low-birth-weight infants and about 10% are truly premature. The latter group accounts for nearly two-thirds of infant deaths (approximately 25,000 annually in the United States). Approximately 30% of premature births are due to miscalculation of gestational age or to medical intervention required by the mother or fetus.

The care of premature (birth weight 1000–2500 g) and immature (birth weight < 1000 g) infants is costly. Compared with term infants, those born prematurely suffer greatly increased morbidity and mortality (eg, functional disorders, abnormalities of growth and development). Thus, every effort is made to prevent or inhibit premature labor. If preterm labor cannot be inhibited or is best allowed to continue, it should be conducted with the least possible trauma to the mother and infant.

Pathogenesis

Many obstetric, medical, and anatomic disorders are associated with preterm labor. Some of the risk factors are listed in Table 15–1. Detailed discussions of these conditions are given in other chapters. The cause of preterm labor in 50% of pregnancies, however, is idiopathic. Although several prospective risk-scoring tools are in use, they have not been convincingly demonstrated to be of value.

Clinical Findings

A. SYMPTOMS AND SIGNS

1. Uterine contractions—Regular uterine contractions at frequent intervals as documented by tocometer or uterine palpation, generally more than 2 in one-half hour.

Table 15–1. Risk factors associated with preterm labor.

Obstetric complications
  In previous or current pregnancy
    Severe hypertensive state of pregnancy
    Anatomic disorders of the placenta (eg, abruptio placen-
      tae, placenta previa, circumvallate placenta)
    Placental insufficiency
    Premature rupture of membranes
    Polyhydramnios or oligohydramnios
  Previous premature or low-birth-weight infant
  Low socioeconomic status
  Maternal age < 18 years or > 40 years
  Low prepregnancy weight
  Non-Caucasian race
  Multiple pregnancy
  Short interval between pregnancies (< 3 months)
  Inadequate or excessive weight gain during pregnancy
  Previous abortion
  Previous laceration of cervix or uterus
Medical complications
  Pulmonary or systemic hypertension
  Renal disease
  Heart disease
  Infection: pyelonephritis, acute systemic infection, urinary
    tract infection, genital tract infection (eg, gonorrhea,
    herpes simplex, mycoplasmosis), fetotoxic infection (eg,
    cytomegalovirus infection, toxoplasmosis, listeriosis),
    maternal systemic infection (eg, pneumonia, influenza,
    malaria), maternal intra-abdominal sepsis (eg, appendici-
    tis, cholecystitis, diverticulitis)
  Heavy cigarette smoking
  Alcoholism or drug addiction
  Severe anemia
  Malnutrition or obesity
  Leaking benign cystic teratoma
  Perforated gastric or duodenal ulcer
  Adnexal torsion
  Maternal trauma or burns
Surgical complications
  Any intra-abdominal procedure
  Conization of cervix
  Previous incision in uterus or cervix (eg, cesarean delivery)
Genital tract anomalies
  Bicornuate, subseptate, or unicornuate uterus
  Congenital cervical incompetency

2. Dilatation and effacement of cervix—Documented cervical change in dilatation or effacement of at least 1 cm or a cervix that is well effaced and dilated (at least 2 cm) on admission is considered diagnostic.

3. Vaginal bleeding—Many patients present with bloody mucous vaginal discharge or "bloody show." More significant vaginal bleeding should be evaluated for abruptio placentae or placenta previa.

B. EVALUATION

Evaluation should include determination of the following:

1. Gestational age—Gestational age must be between 20 and 37 weeks' estimated gestational age (EGA), which should be calculated based upon the patient's last menstrual period (LMP) or date of conception, if known, or the previous sonographic estimation if these dates are uncertain.

2. Fetal weight—Care must be taken to determine fetal size by ultrasonography.

3. Presenting part—The presenting part must be noted because abnormal presentation is more common in earlier stages of gestation.

4. Fetal monitoring—Continuous fetal monitoring should be performed to ascertain fetal well-being.

C. LABORATORY STUDIES

1. Complete blood count with differential.
2. Urine obtained by catheter for urinalysis, culture, and sensitivity testing.
3. Ultrasound examination for fetal size, position, and placental location.
4. Amniocentesis may be useful to ascertain fetal lung maturity in instances where EGA is uncertain, the size of the fetus is in conflict with the estimated date of conception (EDC) (too small, suggesting intrauterine growth restriction, IUGR, or too large, suggesting more advanced EGA), or the fetus is more than 34 weeks' EGA. Specifically, the amniotic fluid can be tested for lecithin/sphingomyelin (L/S) ratio, the presence of phosphatidylglycerol, fluorescence polarization assay, or lamellar body count. Amniocentesis should also be performed in instances where chorioamnionitis is suspected; the fluid should be tested for Gram's stain, bacterial culture, glucose levels, cell count, and, if available, interleukin-6 level.
5. Speculum examination should be performed. Cervical cultures should be sent for gonorrhea and chlamydia. A wet mount should be performed to look for signs of bacterial vaginosis. Group B streptococcus (GBS) cultures should be taken from the vaginal and rectal mucosa.
6. Hematologic work-up in cases associated with vaginal bleeding (see Chapter 20).
7. Fetal fibronectin enzyme immunoassay kits have been approved by the Food and Drug Administration (FDA) as a means to assess the risk of preterm birth in patients with preterm labor. A cervical swab is taken to look for fetal fibronectin. A negative test is effective at ruling out imminent delivery (within 2 weeks). A positive test result, however, is less sensitive at predicting preterm birth.

Treatment

Decisions regarding management are made based on EGA, estimated weight of the fetus, and existence of contraindications to suppressing preterm labor. Table 15–2 lists factors indicating that preterm labor should be allowed to continue. Once the patient is determined to not have any of these contraindications, the management of preterm labor depends on fetal age and size. Generally, management falls into 1 of 2 categories: expectant management (observation) or intervention. In pregnancies between 24 and 34 weeks' EGA or estimated fetal weight (EFW) between 600 and 2500 g, intervention with corticosteroids has been shown to be of benefit in reducing fetal morbidity and mortality rates. Although the efficacy of tocolysis has been much debated, it is generally accepted that a delay in delivery of 48 hours may be achieved at a minimum. Because this window can be used for corticosteroid administration, tocolysis is favored in many centers.

Extremes of preterm gestational age pose special problems. Fetuses of very preterm pregnancies (20–23 weeks EGA or EFW less than 550g) are generally not considered to be viable. If these pregnancies can be continued for several more weeks, the fetuses will become viable but have a high risk for significant morbidity if they are born in this periviable period and survive. Furthermore, intervention carries significant risks to the mother, including the risks of prolonged bed rest and side effects of tocolysis. Given these risks, expectant management is an acceptable and, in certain instances, preferable alternative to intervention. Mothers who

Table 15–2. Some cases in which preterm labor should not be suppressed.

Maternal factors
   Severe hypertensive disease (eg, acute exacerbation of chronic hypertension, eclampsia, severe preeclampsia)
   Pulmonary or cardiac disease (eg, pulmonary edema, adult respiratory distress syndrome, valvular disease, tachyarrhythmias)
   Advanced cervical dilatation (> 4 cm)
   Maternal hemorrhage (eg, abruptio placentae, placenta previa, disseminated intravascular coagulation)
Fetal factors
   Fetal death or lethal anomaly
   Fetal distress
   Intrauterine infection (chorioamnionitis)
   Therapy adversely affecting the fetus (eg, fetal distress due to attempted suppression of labor)
   Estimated fetal weight ≥ 2500 g
   Erythroblastosis fetalis
   Severe intrauterine growth retardation

---

choose intervention as opposed to expectant management should be extensively counseled by a multidisciplinary team, including the neonatologist, obstetrician, and social worker.

Conversely, once a pregnancy has continued beyond 34–37 weeks' EGA or EFW greater than 2500 g, the fetal survival rate is within 1% of the survival rate at 37 weeks. Fetal morbidity is less severe and is rarely a cause of long-term sequelae. Furthermore, corticosteroids have not been shown to be of benefit in fetuses of this age or size. Therefore, expectant management is usually the recommended course of action. Several factors should be considered when deciding between intervention and expectant management, including the certainty of the patient's dates, EFW, presence of maternal problems that could delay fetal lung maturity such as diabetes mellitus, and family history of late-onset respiratory distress syndrome (RDS).

There are other cases in which maternal or fetal factors indicate that preterm labor should be allowed to continue regardless of gestational age. Table 15–2 lists cases in detail.

The following is a protocol for management of pregnancies with preterm labor between 24 and 34 weeks' gestation or EFW 600–2500 g.

A. BED REST

Bed rest should be instituted immediately upon presentation. It is common practice for patients to receive hydration as well, although randomized trials have not shown a specific benefit.

The risk of preterm birth can be assessed using fibronectin and transvaginal scanning of the cervix. A negative fibronectin and a long cervix (> 1.5 cm) are strong negative predictors of imminent preterm birth. Decisions about tocolysis and administration of corticosteroids can be based in part on whether these tests indicate a low or high risk of preterm birth.

B. CORTICOSTEROIDS

The administration of corticosteroids to accelerate fetal lung maturity has become the standard of care in the United States for all women at risk of preterm delivery between 24 and 34 weeks' EGA. It has been shown to decrease the incidence of neonatal respiratory distress, intraventricular hemorrhage, and neonatal mortality. Steroids can be given according to 1 of 2 protocols: (1) betamethasone 12 mg IM every 24 hours for a total of 2 doses; or (2) dexamethasone 6 mg IM every 12 hours for a total of 4 doses.

The optimal benefits of antenatal corticosteroids are seen 24 hours after administration, peak at 48 hours, and continue for at least 7 days. If therapy for preterm labor is successful and the pregnancy continues beyond 1 week, there appears to be no added benefit with repeated courses of corticosteroids. In fact, multiple courses may be associated with growth abnormalities and delayed psychomotor development in the infant. In terms of safety of a single course of antenatal steroids, there does not appear to be an increased risk of infection or suppression of the fetal adrenal glands with steroid administration, and long-term follow-up of fetuses who received antenatal steroids shows no sequelae that can be attributed directly to steroid administration.

C. TOCOLYSIS

If the patient continues to contract and falls into a high-risk group based on a history of preterm birth, positive fibronectin, short cervix on transvaginal sonography (TVS), or changing dilatation on cervical examination, tocolytic therapy may be initiated. When using tocolysis to treat preterm labor, it is important to keep the following goals in mind. The short-term goal is to continue the pregnancy for 48 hours after steroid administration, after which the maximum effect of the steroids can be achieved. The long-term goal is to continue the pregnancy beyond 34–36 weeks (depending on the institution), at which point fetal morbidity and mortality are dramatically reduced and tocolysis can be discontinued.

Tocolytic therapy should be considered in the patient with cervical dilatation less than 5 cm. Successful tocolysis is generally considered fewer than 4–6 uterine contractions per hour without further cervical change.

The beta-mimetics and magnesium sulfate are the most commonly used tocolytic agents. The decision to use a specific tocolytic should be carefully considered because of contraindications and side effects associated with each agent (Table 15–3).

Table 15–3. Side effects and complications of common tocolytics.

Tocolytic	Maternal Effects	Fetal/Neonatal Effects
Beta–mimetics (ritodrine, terbutaline)	Pulmonary edema Hypotension Tachycardia Nausea/vomiting Hyperglycemia Hypokalemia Cardiac arrhythmias	Tachycardia Hyperglycemia Hypoglycemia Ileus Possible increased risk for intraventricular hemorrhage
Magnesium sulfate	Flushing Nausea/vomiting Headache Generalized muscle weakness Shortness of breath Diplopia Pulmonary edema Chest pain Hypotension Tetany Respiratory depression	Lethargy Hypotonia Respiratory depression
Indomethacin	Gastrointestinal effects: Nausea/vomiting, heartburn, bleeding Coagulation disturbances Thrombocytopenia Renal failure Hepatitis Elevated blood pressure in hypertensive patients	Renal dysfunction Oligohydramnios Pulmonary hypertension Postpartum patent ductus arteriosus Premature constriction of ductus arteriosus in utero Increased risk for necrotizing enterocolitis and intraventricular hemorrhage
Nifedipine	Hypotension Tachycardia Headache Flushing Dizziness Nausea/vomiting	Tachycardia Hypotension

1. Beta-mimetic adrenergic agents—Beta-mimetic adrenergic agents act directly on beta receptors (β_2) to relax the uterus. Their use is limited by dose-related cardiovascular side effects, including pulmonary edema, adult RDS, elevated systolic blood pressure and reduced diastolic blood pressure, and both maternal and fetal tachycardia. Other dose-related effects are decreased serum potassium level and increased blood glucose and plasma insulin levels and lactic acidosis. Maternal medical contraindications to the use of β-adrenergic agents include cardiac disease, hyperthyroidism, uncontrolled hypertension or pulmonary hypertension, asthma requiring sympathomimetic drugs or corticosteroids for relief, uncontrolled diabetes, and chronic hepatic or renal disease. Commonly observed effects during intravenous administration are palpitations, tremors, nervousness, and restlessness. Beta-mimetics in common use are ritodrine and terbutaline. Because of the side effects, beta-mimetic tocolysis in the United States is now limited almost exclusively to subcutaneous intermittent injections as a method of temporizing and triaging patients prior to definitive therapy with other agents.

    a. Terbutaline—Although not approved by the FDA, terbutaline has been studied in the United States and is used widely as a tocolytic agent. In tocolysis it is administered via subcutaneous boluses, subcutaneous pump, by mouth, or, less commonly, by intravenous bolus. The most common regimen is subcutaneous injection of 0.25 mg every 3–4 hours for 12 hours.

2. Magnesium sulfate—Although its exact mechanism of action is unknown, magnesium sulfate appears to inhibit calcium uptake into smooth muscle cells, reducing uterine contractility. The efficacy of magnesium is debated, but several small studies have shown an effect comparable to that of beta-mimetics. Magnesium sulfate is better tolerated than the beta-mimetics and, as a result, has become the first-line agent for tocolysis in many institutions in the United States. A protocol for use of magnesium sulfate is given in Table 15–4. Magnesium sulfate may appear less likely to cause serious side effects than the beta-mimetics, but its therapeutic range is close to the range at which it will cause respiratory and cardiac depression. Therefore, patients receiving magnesium sulfate should be monitored closely for signs of toxicity, with frequent checks of deep tendon reflexes, pulmonary examinations, and strict calculations of the patient's fluid balance. These effects may be reversed by calcium gluconate (10 mL of a 10% solution given intravenously), and this antidote should be kept at the bedside when magnesium sulfate is used.

3. Calcium channel blockers—Calcium channel blockers such as nifedipine work as tocolytics by inhibiting calcium uptake into uterine smooth muscle cells via voltage-dependent channels, thereby reducing uterine contractility. Several studies have shown nifedipine to be equally or more efficacious than beta-mimetics in preterm labor. Other advantages are its low incidence of maternal side effects and ease of administration. Nifedipine can be given by mouth. A common regimen for tocolysis is nifedipine 20 mg by mouth, then 10–20 mg by mouth every 6 hours until contractions diminish sufficiently.

4. Prostaglandin synthase inhibitors—Prostaglandin synthase inhibitors such as indomethacin have been shown to be as effective as ritodrine for tocolysis, but their use has been limited by potentially serious fetal effects. Indomethacin works as a tocolytic by inhibiting prostaglandin synthesis, an important mediator in uterine smooth muscle contractility. The advantages of indomethacin are its ease of administration (it can be given by rectum or by mouth) and its potent tocolytic activity. However, it has been associated with oligohydramnios and premature closure of the ductus arteriosus. In preterm infants delivered prior to 30 weeks' EGA, some studies have demonstrated an increased risk of intracranial hemorrhage, necrotizing enterocolitis, and patent ductus arteriosus after birth. A common regimen for to-

Table 15–4. Protocol for use of magnesium sulfate in suppression of preterm labor.

Criteria for admission to protocol
    Preterm labor has been confirmed.
    Gestational age of 20–34 weeks has been confirmed.
    Examinations and tests have ruled out any cases of maternal or fetal diseases or disorders in which it would be best to allow labor to continue.
    Any specific contraindications to magnesium sulfate therapy have been ruled out.
Protocol
    Begin intravenous infusion of magnesium sulfate, 4 g (40 mL of 10% solution). The rate of infusion should be slow enough to prevent flushing or vomiting. Then, continuous infusion of magnesium sulfate should be started at 2 g/h (magnesium sulfate 10% solution, 200 mL, in 5% dextrose, 800 mL, at a rate of 100 mL/h). This infusion can be titrated up by increments of 0.5 g/h to a maximum of 4.0 g/h until adequate tocolysis is achieved (< 4–6 uterine contractions per hour). Infusion should be continued until labor subsides or progresses to an irreversible stage (cervical dilatation of 5 cm).
    Reduce the rate of infusion if magnesium toxicity is observed.
Protocol for recurrent preterm labor
    If contraindications recur after discontinuation of the infusion, the procedure may be repeated.

colysis is indomethacin 100 mg per rectum loading dose (or 50 mg by mouth), then 25–50 mg by mouth or rectum every 4–6 hours. Ultrasound should be performed every 48–72 hours to check for oligohydramnios. Because of the potentially serious fetal effects, many centers limit its use to infants less than 32 weeks' EGA and its duration of use to less than 48 hours.

5. Treatment with multiple tocolytics—All tocolytics have significant failure rates; therefore, if 1 tocolytic appears to be failing, that agent should be stopped and another agent should be tried. The use of multiple tocolytics at the same time appears to have an additive tocolytic effect but also appears to increase the risk of serious side effects. For example, magnesium sulfate used in combination with nifedipine theoretically can cause serious maternal hypotension. Likewise, magnesium sulfate supplemented by 1–2 doses of subcutaneous terbutaline can be safe and effective, but sustained treatment with the 2 can increase the patient's risk of pulmonary edema. It should be remembered that the patient who is difficult to tocolyze may have an unrecognized chorioamnionitis or placental abruption, conditions that may be contraindications to use of any tocolysis at all.

6. Results of tocolytic therapy—With all tocolytics, a point may be reached where further therapy is not indicated. This may be due to adverse maternal or fetal response to the progress of labor. Thus, if cervical dilatation reaches 5 cm, the treatment should be considered a failure and abandoned. Conversely, if labor resumes after a period of quiescence, treatment should be carefully considered because the recrudescence of contractions may be a sign of intrauterine infection. In some cases, therapy may be reinstituted using the same or a different drug.

D. ANTIBIOTICS

Antibiotic therapy as a treatment of preterm labor and a means of prolonging pregnancy has been studied and, for the most part, has shown no benefit in delaying preterm birth in this population of patients. Patients with preterm labor should be started on antibiotics for prevention of neonatal GBS infection if the patient's GBS status is positive or unknown. Penicillin or ampicillin is used as first-line agents; cefazolin, clindamycin, erythromycin, or vancomycin can be used if the patient is allergic to penicillin. If the patient is successfully tocolyzed and there is no sign of imminent delivery, GBS prophylaxis can be discontinued.

Conduct of Labor & Delivery

Premature infants less than 34 weeks should be delivered in a hospital equipped for neonatal intensive care whenever possible, because transfer following birth is more hazardous. Premature breech infants weighing less than 2000 g are generally delivered by cesarean section. Although the route of delivery for very-low-birth-weight infants has been hotly debated, there is no conclusive evidence of a benefit to routine cesarean delivery. A generous episiotomy should be considered to further reduce the risk of injury.

If cesarean delivery is indicated, the decision to operate is based on maturity of the fetus and prognosis for survival. In borderline cases (23–24 weeks' gestation and 500–600 g EFW), the wishes of the parents with regard to intervention assume an important place. When performing a cesarean delivery, it is important to ascertain that the uterine incision is adequate for extraction of the fetus without delay or unnecessary trauma. This often requires a vertical incision when the lower uterine segment is incompletely developed. Trauma to the newborn may be minimized by en caul delivery.

When birth follows the unsuccessful use of parenteral tocolytic agents, keep in mind the potential residual adverse effects of these drugs. β-Adrenergic agents may cause neonatal hypotension, hypoglycemia, hypocalcemia, and ileus. Magnesium sulfate may be responsible for respiratory and cardiac depression.

Cord pH & Blood Gases

Apgar scores are often low in low-birth-weight babies. This finding does not indicate asphyxia or compromised status but merely reflects the immaturity of the physiologic systems. Therefore, it is crucial to obtain cord pH and blood gas measurements for premature (and other high-risk) infants in order to document the status at birth. Cord pH and blood gas measurements may also be helpful in reconstructing intrapartum events, clarifying resuscitative measures, and determining the need for more intensive neonatal care.

Prognosis

Excellent neonatal care in the delivery room and nursery will do much to ensure a good prognosis for the preterm infant (see Chapter 32). Lower-birth-weight babies have a lesser chance of survival and a greater chance of permanent sequelae in direct relationship to size. Making generalizations regarding survival rates and sequelae is difficult because of the many causes of preterm delivery, the different levels of perinatal care, and the institutional differences in reported series. However, general figures for survival and morbidity have been reported and are helpful in counseling patients (Table 15–5).

Table 15–5. Approximate neonatal survival of preterm infants.[1]

Gestation Age (weeks)	Birth Weight (g)	Survivors (%)	Intact[2] Survivors (%)
24–25	500–750	60	35
25–27	751–1000	75	60
28–29	1000–1250	90	80
30–31	1251–1500	96	90
32–33	1500–1750	99	98
>34	1751–2000	100	99

[1]Delivered in a tertiary care center.
[2]Intact defined as not blind, deaf, retarded, or with cerebral palsy.

PREMATURE RUPTURE OF MEMBRANES

ESSENTIALS OF DIAGNOSIS

- *History of a gush of fluid from the vagina or watery vaginal discharge.*
- *Demonstration of amniotic fluid leakage from the cervix.*

General Considerations

Rupture of the membranes may occur at any time during pregnancy. It becomes a problem if the fetus is preterm (preterm premature rupture of membranes [PROM]) or, in the case of a term fetus, if the period of time between rupture of the membranes and the onset of labor is prolonged. If 24 hours elapse between rupture of the membranes and the onset of labor, the problem is one of prolonged PROM.

The exact cause of rupture is not known, although many conditions are associated with PROM (Table 15–6). PROM occurs in approximately 10.7% of all pregnancies. In approximately 94% of cases, the fetus is mature (approximately 20% of these are cases of prolonged rupture). Premature fetuses (1000–2500 g) account for about 5% of the total number (about 50% of cases are prolonged), whereas immature fetuses (< 1000 g) account for less than 0.5% (about 75% of cases are prolonged).

Pathology & Pathophysiology

PROM is an important cause of preterm labor, prolapse of the cord, placental abruption, and intrauterine infection. Chorioamnionitis is an important sequela of PROM and may precede endomyometritis or puerperal sepsis.

In extremely prolonged rupture of the membranes, the fetus may have an appearance similar to that of Potter's syndrome (ie, flattened facial features, wrinkling of the skin). If rupture of membranes occurs early in pregnancy at less than 26 weeks' EGA, it can cause pulmonary hypoplasia and limb positioning defects in the newborn.

Clinical Findings

A. Symptoms

The diagnostic evaluation must be efficient and impeccably conducted to minimize the number of vaginal examinations and the risk of chorioamnionitis. Symptoms are the key to diagnosis; the patient usually reports a sudden gush of fluid or continued leakage. Additional symptoms that may be useful include the color and consistency of the fluid and the presence of flecks of vernix or meconium, reduced size of the uterus, and increased prominence of the fetus to palpation.

B. Sterile Speculum Examination

A most important step in accurate diagnosis is examination with a sterile speculum. This examination is the key to differentiating PROM from hydrorrhea gravidarum, vaginitis, increased vaginal secretions, and urinary incontinence. The examiner should look for the 3 hallmark confirmatory findings associated with PROM:

1. Pooling—the collection of amniotic fluid in the posterior fornix.
2. Nitrazine test—a sterile cotton-tipped swab should be used to collect fluid from the posterior fornix and apply it to Nitrazine (phenaphthazine) paper. In the presence of amniotic fluid, the Nitrazine paper turns blue, demonstrating an alkaline pH (7.0–7.25).
3. Ferning—Fluid from the posterior fornix is placed on a slide and allowed to air-dry. Amniotic fluid will form a fernlike pattern of crystallization.

Table 15–6. Diseases and disorders associated with premature rupture of the membranes.

Maternal infection (eg, urinary tract infection, lower genital tract infection, sexually transmitted diseases)
Intrauterine infection
Cervical incompetency
Multiple previous pregnancies
Hydramnios
Nutritional deficit
Decreased tensile strength of membranes
Familial history of premature rupture of membranes

Together, these 3 findings confirm ruptured membranes, although several factors may produce false-positive results. Alkaline pH on Nitrazine test can also be caused by vaginal infections or the presence of blood or semen in the sample. Cervical mucus can cause ferning, but usually patchy and less extensive than with PROM. During the speculum examination, the patient's cervix should be visually inspected to determine the degree of dilatation and effacement and the presence of cord prolapse. If vaginal pool is significant, the pool can be collected and sent for fetal lung maturity determination if the gestational age is greater than 32 weeks. Cervical secretions should also be sent for culture, and a wet mount should be performed.

If no free fluid is found, a dry pad should be placed under the patient's perineum and observed for leakage. Other confirmatory tests for PROM include observed loss of fluid from the cervical os when the patient coughs or performs a Valsalva maneuver during speculum examination and oligohydramnios on ultrasound examination. If the examiner still cannot confirm rupture of membranes and the patient's history is highly suspicious for PROM, it may be necessary to perform amniocentesis and inject a dilute solution of Evans blue or indigo carmine dye. This is done following removal of amniotic fluid for physiologic maturity testing, analysis for white blood cells or bacteria, and possible culture and sensitivity testing. After 15–30 minutes, examination of the patient's perineal pad will reveal blue dye if the membranes are ruptured.

C. Physical Examination

Once PROM is confirmed, a careful physical examination is necessary to search for other signs of infection. Given the risk of infection, there is no indication for digital cervical examination if the patient is in early labor. The sterile speculum examination is sufficient to distinguish between early and advanced labor.

D. Laboratory Studies

Initial laboratory studies should include a complete blood count with differential. In preterm pregnancies, evaluation should also include urine collected by catheterization for urinalysis, culture, and sensitivity testing; ultrasound examination for fetal size and amniotic fluid index; and amniocentesis in some cases to determine fetal lung maturity and the presence of infection.

E. Chorioamnionitis

In all cases of chorioamnionitis, it is safer for the fetus to be delivered than to be retained in utero. The most common organisms causing chorioamnionitis are those that ascend from the vagina (eg, *Escherichia coli*, *Bacteroides*, GBS, group D streptococcus, and other anaerobes). The most reliable signs of infection include

the following: (1) Fever—the temperature should be checked every 4 hours. (2) Maternal leukocytosis—a daily leukocyte count and differential can be obtained. An increase in the white blood cell count or neutrophil count may indicate the presence of intra-amniotic infection. (3) Uterine tenderness—check every 4 hours. (4) Tachycardia—either maternal pulse > 100 bpm or fetal heart rate > 160 bpm—is suspicious. (5) Foul-smelling amniotic fluid.

A number of confounding factors may complicate the diagnosis of chorioamnionitis. For example, corticosteroid administration may cause mild leukocytosis (increase of 20–25%), and labor is associated with leukocytosis. If the diagnosis of chorioamnionitis is equivocal, amniocentesis can be performed to evaluate for evidence of infection as described earlier in this chapter.

Treatment

The management of PROM depends on several factors, including gestational age and the presence or absence of chorioamnionitis.

A. Chorioamnionitis

If chorioamnionitis is present in the patient with PROM, the patient should be actively delivered *regardless of gestational age.* Broad-spectrum antibiotics should be started to treat the chorioamnionitis. If the patient is not in labor, labor should be induced to expedite delivery.

B. Term Pregnancy without Chorioamnionitis

The term pregnancy (EGA greater than 37 weeks) with PROM in the absence of infection can be managed expectantly or actively. Expectant management entails nonintervention while waiting for the patient to go into labor spontaneously, whereas active management entails induction of labor with an agent such as oxytocin (Pitocin). Nonintervention is an acceptable initial course of treatment, but if the patient does not go into labor within 6–12 hours after PROM, labor should be induced to minimize the risk of infection.

C. Preterm Pregnancy without Chorioamnionitis

The principles of managing the preterm PROM patient are similar to those for managing the preterm labor patient. The key difference is the much increased risk of developing chorioamnionitis associated with preterm PROM. Pregnancies beyond 34 weeks' EGA can be managed as a term pregnancy because there is no evidence that antibiotics, corticosteroids, or tocolytics improve outcome in these patients. These patients can be managed expectantly as long as they show no signs of chorioamnionitis.

Rupture of membranes prior to viability can be managed by active termination of pregnancy because of the poor prognosis. Nevertheless, many case series have documented substantial survival rates (15–50%) with PROM at 18–22 weeks. Although many patients may be unwilling to accept the risk of chorioamnionitis (30%) and even sepsis, they should be informed of the option of expectant management with antibiotic therapy.

For pregnancies with PROM between 24 and 32 weeks' EGA, several interventions have been shown to prolong pregnancy and improve outcome. After chorioamnionitis has been ruled out and a specimen of amniotic fluid from vaginal pool collection or amniocentesis sent for determination of fetal lung maturity, management should consist of the following interventions.

1. Antibiotics—Over the past decade, antibiotics have emerged as an important treatment for preterm PROM. In contrast to preterm labor where antibiotics have shown no benefit in prolonging pregnancy, antibiotics appear to be effective in prolonging the latency period from rupture of membranes to delivery in patients with preterm PROM. They have also been shown to decrease the infection rate in these patients. A number of well-designed studies have shown improved neonatal outcomes with antibiotics alone and with antibiotics combined with corticosteroid therapy. Table 15–7 provides 1 recommended protocol for antibiotic use in preterm PROM.

2. Corticosteroids—The National Institutes of Health (NIH) consensus development panel recommends the use of steroids in PROM patients prior to 32 weeks' EGA in the absence of intra-amniotic infection. In this patient population, corticosteroids have been shown to decrease the rate of RDS, necrotizing enterocolitis, and intraventricular hemorrhage.

Table 15–7. Antibiotic therapy for preterm premature rupture of membranes.

Once preterm PROM is confirmed, start:
Ampicillin 2 g IV every 6 hours
    plus
Erythromycin 250 mg IV every 6 hours
After 48 hours, if the patient is still undelivered, this regimen should be changed to:
Amoxicillin 250 mg by mouth every 8 hours
    plus
Erythromycin 333 mg by mouth every 8 hours
These antibiotics should be continued for 7 days if the patient remains undelivered. Women with GBS-positive cultures should receive prophylaxis intrapartum.

From Mercer BM et al: Antibiotic therapy for reduction of infant morbidity after preterm premature rupture of the membranes. JAMA 1997;278:989.

3. Tocolytics—The role of tocolytics in the preterm PROM patient is controversial. No study has shown that tocolytics alone improve fetal outcome. In general, the use of tocolytics in the preterm PROM patient should be limited to 48 hours' duration, to permit administration of corticosteroids and antibiotics.

If after starting these interventions the fetal lung profile returns as mature, the tocolytics should be abandoned and delivery considered. Again, if at any time the patient shows signs of chorioamnionitis, she should be delivered.

D. ROLE OF OUTPATIENT MANAGEMENT

In rare selected cases, patients who remain undelivered may be candidates for outpatient management. If leakage of fluid stops, the amniotic fluid volume normalizes, and the patient remains afebrile without evidence of increasing uterine irritability, she can be discharged home. These patients should be monitored very closely on an outpatient basis. They must be reliable and compliant with follow-up appointments. They also must take their temperature 4 times per day and be counseled on the warning signs of chorioamnionitis. These patients should also be monitored with frequent biophysical profiles; some sources recommend daily testing.

PROLONGED PREGNANCY

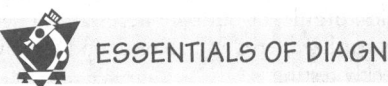 ESSENTIALS OF DIAGNOSIS

- *Confirmation of gestational age greater than 42 completed weeks.*

General Considerations

Prolonged pregnancy is defined as pregnancy that has reached 42 weeks of completed gestation from the first day of the LMP or 40 weeks' gestation from the time of conception. Most fetuses will show effects of impaired nutritional supply (weight loss, reduced subcutaneous tissue, scaling, parchmentlike skin). This condition is referred to as dysmaturity. The most common cause of prolonged pregnancy is incorrect dating due to variable length of the menstrual cycle. This has been reduced in recent years with widespread use of first-trimester ultrasound for dating. The cause of most cases of true prolonged pregnancy remains unknown. Experiments of nature, such as anencephalic fetuses and those with placental sulfatase deficiency, suggest that changes in placental steroid metabolism due to fetal hormonal signaling play a central role in the timing of delivery. At least 3% of infants are born after 42 completed weeks' gestation (in some series, as many as 12%). Because of the potential risks of dysmaturity, these infants deserve particular attention.

The maternal risks usually relate to extraordinary fetal size (ie, dysfunctional labor, arrested progress of labor, fetopelvic disproportion). Extraordinary fetal size may result in birth injury (eg, shoulder dystocia). Placental insufficiency is thought to be associated with aging of the placenta and is the basis for another group of fetal problems. Oligohydramnios, which is more common in postterm gestation, may lead to cord compromise.

Complications resulting from prolonged pregnancy result in a sharp rise in perinatal mortality and morbidity rates (2–3 times those of infants born at 37–42 weeks). Complications in the survivors increase the chance of neurologic sequelae.

Diagnosis

The diagnosis of prolonged pregnancy is made by confirmation of the gestational age by referring to records of early pregnancy tests and ultrasound examinations, the exact time of conception (if known), and clinical parameters (eg, LMP, quickening, detection of fetal heart tones).

To adequately assess the risk of fetal compromise, the following is a useful protocol for pregnancies beyond 41 weeks' gestation:

1. Perform nonstress testing 2 times weekly. (Some authorities believe that contraction stress testing, a biophysical profile, or both are necessary to detect the jeopardized fetus and recommend weekly or semiweekly testing.)
2. Perform ultrasonic monitoring at least twice weekly to assess amniotic fluid volume (biophysical profiles may be obtained at the same time).
3. Have the mother count fetal movements each day.

Treatment

The principal risk of labor induction has been thought to be an increased rate of cesarean birth. It has now been conclusively demonstrated, however, that induction of labor at 41 weeks does not increase the cesarean rate compared to expectant management with antepartum testing. Therefore, many authorities offer induction of labor at 41 completed weeks, reserving expectant management for those patients who refuse induction. If the choice is to continue the pregnancy, it may be advisable to have the patient monitor fetal activity. The following precautions should be taken:

1. Decreased fetal movement warrants an immediate biophysical profile evaluation.
2. Abnormalities in the nonstress test mandate induction or a backup test such as the full biophysical profile.

3. An abnormal contraction stress test, decreased amniotic fluid volume, abnormal biophysical profile, or other signs of fetal require delivery.
4. A large or compromised fetus may require cesarean delivery (see discussion of macrosomia in Chapter 16)
5. In the absence of fetopelvic disproportion or fetal distress, labor can be induced. Fetal monitoring should be continuous.

Rh ISOIMMUNIZATION & OTHER BLOOD GROUP INCOMPATIBILITIES

 ESSENTIALS OF DIAGNOSIS

- *Maternal Rh-negativity and presence of antibody on indirect Coombs' test.*
- *Rh or other antibody titer posing fetal risk.*
- *May have a previous infant with hemolytic disease of the newborn.*
- *Postnatal fetal cord blood findings of Rh-positivity and anemia (hemoglobin < 10 g).*

General Considerations

A fetus receives half of its genetic components from its mother and half from its father; therefore, the fetus may have different blood groups than those of its mother. Some blood groups may act as antigens in individuals not possessing those blood groups. The antigens reside on red blood cells. If enough fetal cells cross into the maternal blood, a maternal antibody response may be provoked. If these maternal antibodies cross the placenta, they then can enter the fetal circulation and destroy the fetal erythrocytes, causing hemolytic anemia. This leads to fetal responses to meet the challenge of enhanced blood cell breakdown. These changes in the fetus and newborn are called erythroblastosis fetalis. Several blood groups are capable of producing fetal risk, but those in the Rh group have caused the overwhelming majority of cases of erythroblastosis fetalis, so the Rh group is used as the example.

The Rh blood group is the most complex human blood group. The Rh antigens are grouped in 3 pairs: Dd, Cc, and Ee. The major antigen in this group, Rh_o (D), or Rh factor, is of particular concern. A woman who is lacking the Rh factor (Rh-negative) may carry an Rh-positive fetus. If fetal red blood cells pass into the mother's circulation in sufficient numbers, maternal antibodies to the Rh-positive antigen may develop and cross the placenta, causing hemolysis of fetal blood cells

(Fig 15–1). Hemolytic disease of the newborn may occur, and severe disease may cause fetal death.

In standard testing when the father is Rh-positive, 2 possibilities exist: he is either homozygous or heterozygous. Forty-five percent of Rh-positive persons are homozygous for D and 55% are heterozygous. If the father is homozygous, all of his children will be Rh-positive; if he is heterozygous, his children will have a 50% chance of being Rh-positive. By way of contrast, the Rh-negative individual is always homozygous.

Incidence

Basque populations have the highest incidence of Rh-negativity (30–35%). Caucasian populations in general have a higher incidence than other ethnic groups (15–16%). Blacks in the United States have a rate of 8%, African blacks 4%, Indoeurasians 2%, and North American Indians 1%.

In mothers who do not receive prophylaxis with Rh immunoglobulin, the overall risk of isoimmunization for an Rh-positive ABO-compatible infant with an Rh-negative mother is about 16%. Of these, 1.5–2% of reactions will occur antepartum and 7% within 6 months of delivery; the remainder (7%) manifest early in the second pregnancy, most likely as the result of an amnestic response. ABO incompatibility between an Rh-positive fetus and an Rh-negative mother provides some protection against Rh isoimmunization; in these cases the overall incidence is 1.5–2%. In mothers who receive prophylaxis with Rh immunoglobulin, the risk of isoimmunization is reduced to 0.2%.

Pathogenesis

A. MATERNAL RH ISOIMMUNIZATION

Rh antigens are lipoproteins that are confined to the red cell membrane. Isoimmunization may occur by 2 mechanisms: (1) following incompatible blood transfusion or (2) following fetomaternal hemorrhage between a mother and an incompatible fetus. Fetomaternal hemorrhage may occur during pregnancy or at delivery. With no apparent predisposing factors, fetal red cells have been detected in maternal blood in 6.7% of women during the first trimester, 15.9% during the second trimester, and 28.9% during the third trimester. Predispositions to fetomaternal hemorrhage include spontaneous or induced abortion, amniocentesis, chorionic villus sampling, abdominal trauma (eg, due to motor vehicle accidents or external version), placenta previa, abruptio placentae, fetal death, multiple pregnancy, manual removal of the placenta, and cesarean section.

Although the exact number of Rh-positive cells necessary to cause isoimmunization of the Rh-negative pregnant woman is unknown, as little as 0.1 mL of Rh-positive cells can cause sensitization. Even with delivery, this amount occurs in less than half of cases.

Fortunately, there are other mitigating factors to Rh isoimmunization. A very important factor is that about 30% of Rh-negative persons never become sensitized (nonresponders) when given Rh-positive blood. ABO incompatibility also confers a protective effect (see Incidence).

The initial maternal immune response to Rh sensitization is low levels of immunoglobulin (Ig) M. Within 6 weeks to 6 months, IgG antibodies become detectable. In contrast to IgM, IgG is capable of crossing the placenta and destroying fetal Rh-positive cells.

B. OTHER BLOOD GROUP ISOIMMUNIZATION

Of the other blood groups that may evoke an immunoglobulin capable of crossing the placenta (often called atypical or irregular immunizing antibodies), those that may cause severe fetal hemolysis (listed in descending order of occurrence) are Kell, Duffy, Kidd, MNSs, and Diego. P, Lutheran, and Xg groups may also cause fetal hemolysis, but it usually is less severe.

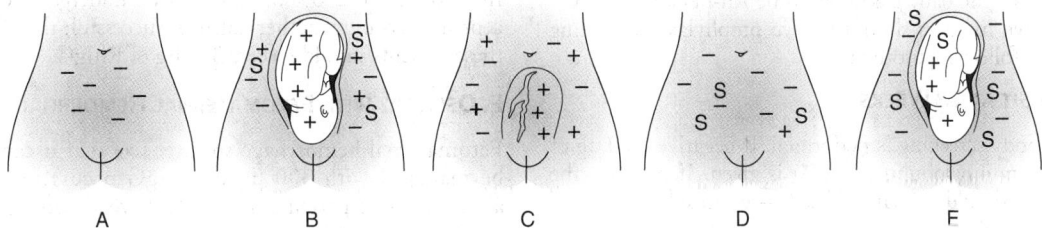

Figure 15–1. **A:** Rh-negative woman before pregnancy. **B:** Pregnancy occurs. The fetus is Rh-positive. **C:** Separation of the placenta. **D:** Following delivery, Rh isoimmunization occurs in the mother, and she develops antibodies (S) to the Rh-positive antigen. **E:** The next pregnancy with an Rh-positive fetus. Maternal antibodies cross the placenta, enter the fetal bloodstream, and attach to Rh-positive red cells, causing hemolysis.

C. FETAL EFFECTS

Hemolytic disease of the newborn occurs when the maternal antibodies cross the placenta and destroy the Rh-positive fetal red blood cells. Fetal anemia results, stimulating extramedullary erythropoietic sites to produce high levels of nucleated red cell elements. Immature erythrocytes are present in the fetal blood because of poor maturation control. Hemolysis produces heme, which is converted to bilirubin; both of these substances are neurotoxic. However, while the fetus is in utero, heme and bilirubin are effectively removed by the placenta and metabolized by the mother.

When fetal red blood cell destruction far exceeds production and severe anemia occurs, erythroblastosis fetalis may result. This is characterized by extramedullary hematopoiesis, heart failure, edema, ascites, and pericardial effusion. Tissue hypoxia and acidosis may result. Normal hepatic architecture and function may be disturbed by extensive liver erythropoiesis, which may lead to decreased protein production, portal hypertension, and ascites.

D. NEONATAL EFFECTS

In the immediate neonatal interval, the primary problem may relate to anemia and the sequelae mentioned above. However, hyperbilirubinemia may also pose an immediate risk and certainly poses a risk as further red cell breakdown occurs. The immature (and often compromised) liver, with its low levels of glucuronyl transferase, is unable to conjugate the large amounts of bilirubin. This results in a high serum bilirubin level, with resultant kernicterus (bilirubin deposition in the basal ganglia).

Management of the Unsensitized Rh-Negative Pregnancy

A. PREPREGNANCY OR FIRST PRENATAL VISIT

On the first prenatal visit, all pregnant women should be screened for the ABO blood group and the Rh group, including Du. They should also undergo antibody screening (indirect Coombs' test). Unless the father of the baby is known to be Rh-negative, all Rh-negative mothers should receive prophylaxis according to the following protocol.

B. VISIT AT 28 WEEKS

Antibody screening is performed. If negative, 300 μg of Rh immunoglobulin (RhIgG) is given. If positive, the patient should be managed as Rh-sensitized.

C. VISIT AT 35 WEEKS

Antibody screening is repeated. If negative, the patient is merely observed. If screening is positive, the patient is managed as Rh-sensitized.

D. POSTPARTUM

If the infant is Rh-positive or Du-positive, 300 μg of RhIgG is administered to the mother (provided maternal antibody screening is negative). Although RhIgG should generally be given within 72 hours after delivery, it has been shown to be effective in preventing isoimmunization if given up to 28 days after delivery. If the antibody screen is positive, the patient is managed as if she will be Rh-sensitized during the next pregnancy.

E. SPECIAL FETOMATERNAL RISK STATES

Several circumstances that may occur during pregnancy mandate administration of RhIgG to the unsensitized patient outside the management protocol described.

1. Abortion—Sensitization will occur in 2% of spontaneous abortions and 4–5% of induced abortions. In the first trimester, because of the small amount of fetal blood, 50 μg of RhIgG apparently is sufficient to prevent sensitization. However, because the cost of RhIgG has dropped, a full 300-μg dose is usually given. The same dose is recommended for exposure after the first trimester. The risk of Rh isoimmunization after threatened abortion is less well understood, but many experts agree that RhIgG should also be given to these patients.

2. Amniocentesis, chorionic villus sampling, and cord blood sampling—If the placenta is traversed by the needle, there is up to an 11% chance of sensitization. Therefore, administration of 300 μg of RhIgG is recommended when these procedures are performed in the unsensitized patient.

3. Antepartum hemorrhage—In cases of placenta previa or abruptio placentae, administration of 300 μg of RhIgG is recommended. If the pregnancy is carried more than 12 weeks from the time of RhIgG administration, a repeat prophylactic dose is recommended.

4. External cephalic version—Fetomaternal hemorrhage occurs in 2–6% of patients who undergo external cephalic version, whether failed or successful; therefore, these patients should receive 300 μg of RhIgG.

F. DELIVERY WITH FETOMATERNAL HEMORRHAGE

Fetomaternal hemorrhage so extensive that it cannot be managed with 300 μg of RhIgG occurs in only about 0.4% of patients. If the sensitive screening test is positive for persistent antibody after RhIgG administration, the amount of hemorrhage is quantitated by the Kleihauer-Bethke test and additional doses of RhIgG given according to the amount of excess hemorrhage.

Evaluation of the Pregnancy with Isoimmunization

Evaluation of the pregnancy complicated by isoimmunization is guided by 2 factors: whether the patient has a history of an affected fetus in a previous pregnancy (ie, fetus with severe anemia or hydrops) and maternal antibody titers.

A. No History of Previous Fetus Affected by Rh Isoimmunization

Once the antibody screen is positive for isoimmunization, these patients should be followed by antibody titers at intake, 20 weeks' EGA, and then every 4 weeks. As long as antibody titers remain below the critical titer (<1:32 in our laboratory, but each laboratory must establish its own norms), there is no indication for further intervention. Once antibody titers reach 1:32, amniocentesis should be performed because a titer of 1:32 places the fetus at significant risk for demise before 37 weeks. An alternative to serial amniocentesis in patients with abnormal antibody titers or a history of a prior affected fetus is assessment of blood flow in the fetal middle cerebral artery (MCA) by Doppler. Ultrasound is performed to identify the circle of Willis, and blood flow in the proximal third of the MCA can be estimated using Doppler. High peak velocity blood flow in this area (> 1.5 multiples of the median) correlates well with severe fetal anemia. This test can be performed at 2-week intervals in these patients, so more invasive diagnostic interventions can be avoided until evidence of severe anemia is observed.

B. History of a Prior Fetus Affected by Rh Isoimmunization

Antibody titers need not be followed in these pregnancies because amniocentesis is indicated by the history of prior affected fetus. Amniocentesis should be performed 4–8 weeks earlier than the gestational age in the previous pregnancy when Rh-associated morbidity was first identified. Amniocentesis, when determined to be necessary, should be performed under ultrasound guidance to minimize the risk of transplacental hemorrhage.

The amniotic fluid is analyzed by spectrophotometry. The optical density of the fluid at a wavelength of 450 nm is plotted on a semilogarithmic scale versus gestational age. The amniotic fluid concentration of bilirubin in the unsensitized patient gradually decreases as pregnancy progresses. Thus, the severity of fetal affliction may be approximated and this information used as a guide for further studies and treatment. The alternative of MCA Doppler peak velocity assessment is now more widely used.

In addition to MCA Doppler, ultrasound plays an important role in evaluating the isoimmunized patient for hydrops. Ultrasound can be used to evaluate fetal heart size and amniotic fluid index and to detect edema, pericardial effusion, and ascites. Serial ultra-sounds can document the progression or reversal of disease.

Management of the Pregnancy with Isoimmunization

Management of these patients is dictated by amniocentesis or MCA Doppler results (Fig 15–2).

A. Mildly Affected Fetus

The fetus that falls into zone 1 on the Liley curve or has normal MCA Doppler studies is considered to unaffected or mildly affected. Testing should be repeated every 2–3 weeks, and delivery should be near term and after the fetus has achieved pulmonary maturity.

B. Moderately Affected Fetus

The fetus that falls into zone 2 or has MCA Doppler studies nearing 1.5 multiples of the median (Fig 15–2) should be tested more frequently, every 1–2 weeks. Delivery may be required prior to term, and the fetus is delivered as soon as pulmonary maturity is reached. In some cases, enhancement of pulmonary maturity by use of corticosteroids may be necessary.

C. Severely Affected Fetus

The severely affected fetus falls into zone 3 on the Liley curve, has MCA Doppler studies > 1.5 multiples of the median, or has frank evidence of hydrops (eg, ascites, pleural or pericardial effusion, subcutaneous edema). Intervention usually is needed to allow the fetus to reach a gestational age at which delivery and neonatal risks are fewer than the risks of in utero therapy.

If the fetus is preterm, cordocentesis or percutaneous umbilical cord blood sampling (PUBS) is recommended at this stage to directly assess the fetal hematocrit. Once severe anemia is confirmed, intrauterine transfusion can be performed directly into the umbilical vein. The transfusion is performed using O-negative, cytomegalovirus-negative, washed, leukocyte-depleted, irradiated packed red cells. The intraperitoneal technique was used in years past but has largely been replaced by intravascular fetal transfusion secondary to its more predictable absorption.

After transfusion, repeat transfusions or delivery usually will be necessary as production of fetal blood markedly decreases or ceases. Timing of these transfusions may be assisted by ultrasonic determination of MCA Doppler studies. Delivery should take place when the fetus has documented pulmonary maturity

ABO HEMOLYTIC DISEASE

ABO hemolytic disease is much milder than the isoimmunization evoked by Rh₀ and the other antigens. The reason for this difference is poorly understood, because

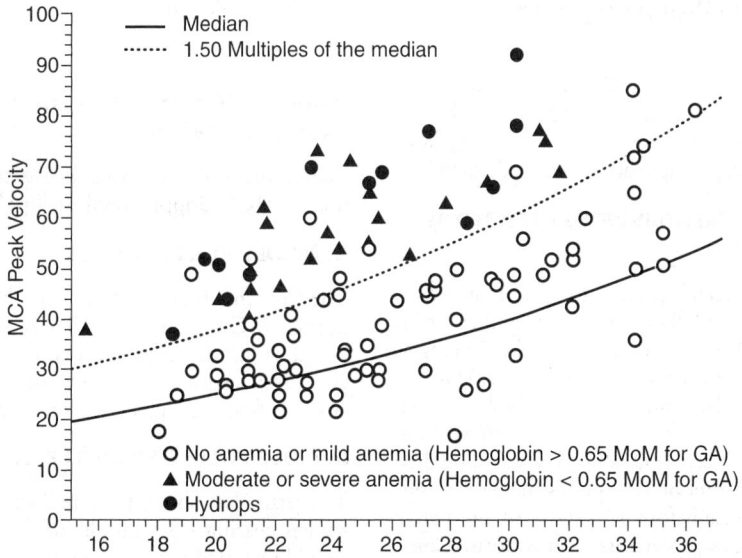

Figure 15–2. Peak velocity of systolic blood flow in the middle cerebral artery in 111 fetuses at risk for anemia due to maternal red-cell alloimmunization.
(From Mari G et al: Noninvasive diagnosis by Doppler ultrasonography of fetal anemia due to maternal red-cell alloimmunization. Collaborative Group for Doppler Assessment of the Blood Velocity in Anemic Fetuses. N Engl J Med 2000;342:9.)

both IgG and IgM are produced antenatally. Although 20–25% of pregnancies have potential maternal–infant ABO incompatibility, a recognizable process in the neonate occurs in only 10% of those cases. Those affected are almost always group A (especially A1) or B infants of group O mothers. The neonatal direct Coombs' test may be positive or negative, and maternal antibodies are also variable.

In Rh isoimmunization, only 1–2% of cases occur in the first-born infant, whereas 40–50% of ABO incompatibilities occur in the first-born infant. Serious fetal sequelae (eg, stillbirth, hydrops) almost never occur, and severe fetal anemia is rare.

ABO hemolytic disease is primarily manifest following birth, with early neonatal onset of jaundice (at < 24 hours) and variable elevation of the indirect bilirubin level. Management of ABO incompatibility relates to bilirubin surveillance and phototherapy (required in 10% of cases). The infants may have hepatosplenomegaly. Exchange transfusion is necessary in only 1% of cases, and the incidence of late anemia is rare. Sequelae such as kernicterus almost never occur.

REFERENCES

American College of Obstetricians and Gynecologists: *Premature Rupture of Membranes.* ACOG Practice Bulletin No. 1. American College of Obstetricians and Gynecologists, 1998.

American College of Obstetricians and Gynecologists: *Prevention of Rh D Alloimmunization.* ACOG Practice Bulletin No. 4. American College of Obstetricians and Gynecologists, 1999.

American College of Obstetricians and Gynecologists: *Assessment of Risk Factors for Preterm Birth. Clinical Management Guidelines for Obstetrician-Gynecologists.* ACOG Practice Bulletin No. 31. American College of Obstetricians and Gynecologists, 2001.

American College of Obstetricians and Gynecologists: *Antenatal Corticosteroid Therapy for Fetal Maturation.* ACOG Committee Opinion No. 273. American College of Obstetricians and Gynecologists, 2002.

Elimian A et al: Effectiveness of multidose antenatal steroids. Obstet Gynecol 2000;95:34.

Guinn DA et al: Single vs weekly courses of antenatal corticosteroids for women at risk of preterm delivery: A randomized controlled trial. JAMA 2001;286:1581.

How HY et al: Preterm premature rupture of membranes: aggressive tocolysis versus expectant management. J Matern Fetal Med 1998;7:8.

Huang WL et al: Effect of corticosteroids on brain growth in fetal sheep. Obstet Gynecol 1999;94:213.

Kay HH et al: Antenatal steroid treatment and adverse fetal effects: What is the evidence? J Soc Gynecol Investig 2000;7:269.

Kenyon SL et al: Broad-spectrum antibiotics for preterm, prelabour rupture of fetal membranes: The ORACLE I randomised trial. Lancet 2001;357:979.

Kenyon SL et al: Broad-spectrum antibiotics for spontaneous preterm labour: The ORACLE II randomised trial. Lancet 2001;357:989.

Macones GA et al: Predicting delivery within 48 hours in women treated with parenteral tocolysis. Obstet Gynecol 1999; 93:432.

Mari G et al: Noninvasive diagnosis by Doppler ultrasonography of fetal anemia due to maternal red-cell alloimmunization. Collaborative Group for Doppler Assessment of the Blood Velocity in Anemic Fetuses. N Engl J Med 2000;342:9.

Mercer MD et al: Antibiotic therapy for reduction of infant morbidity after preterm premature rupture of the membranes: A randomized controlled trial. JAMA 1997;278:989.

Saade GR: Noninvasive testing for fetal anemia. N Engl J Med 2000;342:52.

Schaap AH et al. Effects of antenatal corticosteroid administration on mortality and long-term morbidity in early preterm, growth-restricted infants. Obstet Gynecol 2001;97:954.

Seaward PG et al: International multicentre term prelabor rupture of membranes study: evaluation of predictors of clinical chorioamnionitis and postpartum fever in patients with prelabor rupture of membranes at term. Am J Obstet Gynecol 1997;177:1024.

Disproportionate Fetal Growth

Jeannine Rahimian, MD, MBA, & Michael W. Varner, MD

Weight at delivery once was considered evidence of prematurity (birthweight < 2500 g) or postmaturity (macrosomia; birthweight > 4500 g). These criteria later were revised upon the realization that abnormal growth was reflected in factors other than birthweight. Normative standards such as birthweight, length, and head circumference (HC) according to gestational age were developed. Abnormal fetal growth now is defined according to percentiles: infants ≤ 10th percentile are classified as having intrauterine growth restriction (IUGR) and those ≥ 90th percentile are classified as large for gestational age (LGA). Standards also vary among different populations.

Both IUGR and LGA fetuses have increased risk for perinatal morbidity and mortality (Tables 16–1 and 16–2). The pathogenesis, differential diagnosis, and treatment are different for the two extremes of growth.

INTRAUTERINE GROWTH RESTRICTED PREGNANCY

Terminology

Many terms have been used to describe fetuses with disproportionately small growth. These include small for gestational age (SGA), IUGR, and fetal growth restriction (FGR). Most often, SGA refers to the infant, whereas IUGR refers to the fetus. *Intrauterine growth restriction* is defined as estimated fetal weight (EFW) at or below the 10th percentile for gestational age. By definition, 10% of infants in any population will be at or below the 10th percentile. Approximately 70% of fetuses with EFW below the 10th percentile are simply constitutionally small, thus the term IUGR is inaccurate for many fetuses. Distinguishing between normal and pathologic growth can be difficult. Some nonpathologic factors that affect fetal birthweight are maternal height, paternal height, parity, ethnicity, and fetal sex.

Pathophysiology

Compared with an average-for-gestational-age (AGA) fetus, the IUGR fetus has altered body composition (including decreased body fat, total protein, whole body DNA and RNA, glycogen, and free fatty acids), altered distribution of weight among organs, and altered body proportions. Approximately 20% of IUGR infants are symmetrically small, with a relatively proportionate decrease in many organ weights. Eighty percent are asymmetrically small, with relative sparing of brain weight, especially when compared with that of the liver or thymus.

In asymmetric IUGR infants, brain weight is decreased only slightly compared with that of AGA controls, primarily as a result of decreased brain cell size and not to decreased brain cell numbers. Cerebral abnormalities include decreased myelination, decreased utilization of metabolic substrates other than glucose, and altered protein synthesis. In experimental animals, these changes are more likely to produce adverse effects in the brainstem and cerebellum. This differential sparing is particularly prominent when deprivation occurs in the latter half of pregnancy. Deprivation early in pregnancy is associated with less cerebral sparing and diffusely slowed brain growth.

Symmetric IUGR infants have proportionately small brains, usually because of a decreased number of brain cells. Although this may be the result of early, severe nutritional deprivation, the cause is more often a genetic disorder, infection, or other problem. Usually the thymus is small, with an average decrease of 25%. This decrease may explain in part the decreased cellular immunity seen in IUGR infants.

The liver is frequently affected, at least partly because of diminished glycogen deposition. The liver also may have functional (metabolic) abnormalities, as manifested by abnormal cord blood and neonatal serum chemistries. Such abnormalities often reflect the underlying cause of decreased size.

Blood flow to the lungs may be decreased, lessening the pulmonary contribution to amniotic fluid volume. This may be partly responsible for the often-encountered oligohydramnios. Decreased pulmonary blood flow may also be associated with accelerated functional pulmonary maturity.

Renal blood flow frequently is reduced in asymmetric IUGR pregnancies. The resultant diminished glomerular filtration rate may further contribute to oligohydramnios.

Differential Diagnosis

A classification of IUGR pregnancy delineated by cause is given in Table 16–3. Any inference of suboptimal

Table 16–1. Some complications associated with IUGR pregnancy.

Maternal Complications
Complications due to underlying disease, preeclampsia, premature labor, cesarean delivery
Fetal Complications
Stillbirth, hypoxia and acidosis, malformations
Neonatal Complications
Hypoglycemia, hypocalcemia, hypoxia and acidosis, hypothermia, meconium aspiration syndrome, polycythemia, congenital malformations, sudden infant death syndrome
Long-Term Complications
Lower IQ, learning and behavior problems, major neurologic handicaps (seizure disorders, cerebral palsy, mental retardation), hypertension

growth requires, by definition, serial observations. It cannot be emphasized too strongly that a pregnancy cannot be described as IUGR unless the gestational age is known with certainty.

Numerous authors have differentiated between symmetric and asymmetric IUGR pregnancy in terms of cause and prognosis. *Symmetric IUGR* refers to infants in which all organs are decreased proportionally. Symmetric IUGR infants are more likely to have an endogenous defect that results in impairment of early fetal cellular hyperplasia. *Asymmetric IUGR* refers to infants in which all organs are decreased disproportionately (abdominal circumference is affected to a greater degree than is HC). Asymmetric IUGR more likely is caused by intrauterine deprivation that results in redistribution of flow to the brain and heart at the expense of less important organs, such as the liver and kidneys. Although this classification is helpful in establishing a differential diagnosis and framework for discussion, it is not sufficiently precise to serve as a basis for decisions regarding intervention or viability.

Table 16–2. Some complications of LGA pregnancy.

Maternal Complications
Cesarean section, postpartum hemorrhage, shoulder dystocia, perineal trauma, operative vaginal delivery
Fetal Complications
Stillbirth, anomalies, shoulder dystocia
Neonatal Complications
Low Apgar score, hypoglycemia, birth injury, hypocalcemia, polycythemia, jaundice, feeding difficulties
Long-Term Complications
Obesity, type 2 diabetes, neurologic or behavioral problems

Table 16–3. Pathogenic classification of IUGR pregnancy.

A. Fetoplacental Causes
Genetic disorders
Autosomal: trisomy 13, 18, 21; ring chromosomes; chromosomal deletions; partial trisomies
Sex chromosomes: Turner's syndrome, multiple chromosomes (XXX, XYY)
Neural tube defects
Skeletal dysplasias: achondroplasia, chondrodystrophies, osteogenesis imperfecta
Abdominal wall defects
Other rare syndromes
Congenital infection
Viral: cytomegalovirus, rubella, herpes, varicella-zoster
Protozoan: toxoplasmosis, malaria
Bacterial: listeriosis
Placental disorders: placenta previa, placental infarction, chorionic villitis, chronic partial separation, placental malformations (circumvallate placenta, battledore placenta, placental hemangioma, twin-twin transfusion syndrome)
Multiple gestation
B. Maternal Factors
Coexistent maternal disease: hypertension, anemia (hemoglobinopathy, decreased normal hemoglobin [especially < 12 g/dL]), renal disease (hypertension, protein loss), malnutrition (inflammatory bowel disease [ulcerative colitis, regional enteritis], pancreatitis, intestinal parasites), cyanotic cardiopulmonary disease
Substance abuse/drugs: alcohol, cigarette smoking, cocaine, heroin, warfarin, folic acid antagonists (methotrexate, aminopterin), anticonvulsants
Small maternal stature

A. FETOPLACENTAL CAUSES

1. Congenital abnormalities—Genetic disorders account for approximately one-third of IUGR infants. Data from the Metropolitan Atlanta Congenital Defects Program suggest that 38% of chromosomally abnormal infants are IUGR and that the risk of an IUGR infant having a major congenital anomaly is 8–19%. An infant with an autosomal trisomy is more likely to be IUGR. The most common trisomy is **trisomy 21 (Down syndrome)**, with an incidence of 1.6 per 1000 live births. At term, such infants weigh an average of 350 g less than comparable normal infants and are 4 times more likely to be IUGR. This decrease is most apparent in the last 6 weeks of pregnancy. A similar decrease in birthweight occurs in translocation Down syndrome, whereas mosaic Down syndrome is associated with an intermediate decrease in birthweight.

The second most common autosomal trisomy is **trisomy 18** (**Edwards' syndrome**), which occurs in 1 in 6000–8000 live births. Eighty-four percent of these infants are IUGR. Ultrasound evaluation may reveal associated anomalies. The condition is associated with an increased likelihood of breech presentation, polyhydramnios, fetal neural tube defects, and visceral anomalies. The average birthweight of infants with trisomy 18 is almost 1000 g less than that of controls. In contrast to the placental weight in infants with trisomies 13 and 21, the placental weight in infants with trisomy 18 also is markedly reduced.

Trisomy 13 occurs in 1 in 5000–10,000 live births. More than 50% of affected infants have IUGR. Birthweights average 700–800 g less than those of controls.

Other more rare autosomal chromosome abnormalities, such as ring chromosomes, deletions, and partial trisomies, are associated with an increased likelihood of IUGR. Sex chromosome abnormalities may be associated with lower birthweight. Extra X chromosomes (> 2) are associated with a 200-g to 300-g decrease in birthweight for each extra X. **Turner's syndrome** is associated with an average birthweight of approximately 400 g below average. Fetuses with mosaic Turner's syndrome are intermediately affected.

Growth impairment as a result of fetal chromosome abnormalities usually occurs earlier than impairment caused by placental abnormalities. However, there is considerable clinical overlap, so gestational age at the time of diagnosis is not always of clinical value.

Fetuses with neural tube defects frequently are IUGR, weighing approximately 250 g less than controls. Anencephalic fetuses are IUGR, even considering the absent brain and skull, with average third-trimester birthweights of approximately 1000 g less than matched controls. Certain dysmorphic syndromes are associated with an increased incidence of IUGR fetuses. **Achondroplasia** may be associated with low birthweight if either parent is affected but usually is associated with normal birthweight if a spontaneous mutation is the cause. **Osteogenesis imperfecta** consists of a spectrum of diseases, all of which result in IUGR fetuses.

Infants born with abdominal wall defects are characteristically IUGR, particularly those with **gastroschisis**.

Other autosomal recessive syndromes associated with IUGR include **Smith-Lemli-Opitz syndrome, Meckel's syndrome, Robert's syndrome, Donohue's syndrome,** and **Seckel's syndrome.** These conditions are rare and are most likely to be diagnosed antepartum in families with a previously affected child. Infants with renal anomalies such as renal agenesis (**Potter's syndrome**) or complete urinary tract outflow obstruction often have IUGR.

Other congenital anomalies associated with an increased incidence of IUGR outcome are **duodenal atresia** and **pancreatic agenesis**.

2. Congenital infections—Chronic intrauterine infection is responsible for 5–10% of IUGR pregnancies (Table 16–3). The most commonly identified pathogen is cytomegalovirus (CMV). Although CMV can be isolated from 0.5–2% of all newborns in the United States, clinically obvious infection at the time of birth affects only 0.2–2 in 1000 live births. Active fetoplacental infection is characterized by cytolysis, followed by secondary inflammation, fibrosis, and calcification. Only infants with clinically apparent infection at birth are likely to be IUGR. Signs of congenital infection are nonspecific but include central nervous system involvement (eg, microcephaly), chorioretinitis, intracranial (periventricular) calcifications, pneumonitis, hepatosplenomegaly, and thrombocytopenia.

Congenital rubella infection increases the risk of IUGR. Infection in the first trimester results in the most severely affected fetuses, primarily as a result of microvascular endothelial damage. Such infants are likely to have structural cardiovascular and central nervous system defects such as microcephaly, deafness, glaucoma, and cataracts.

Other viruses implicated in causing IUGR are herpesvirus, varicella-zoster virus, influenza virus, and poliovirus, but the number of such cases is small. As expected by virtue of their chronic, indolent nature, protozoan infections are associated with IUGR. The most common protozoan, *Toxoplasma gondii,* usually is acquired by ingestion of raw meat. Only women with a primary infection are at risk for having an affected infant. The average incidence is 1 in 1000 live births in the United States, but the incidence varies widely among locations and social populations. Approximately 20% of newborns with congenital toxoplasmosis will have IUGR. Malaria is another protozoan infection associated with IUGR.

Although bacterial infections occur commonly in pregnancy and frequently are implicated in premature delivery, they are not commonly associated with IUGR. Chronic infection from *Listeria monocytogenes* is an exception. Infants usually are critically ill at the time of delivery and often have encephalitis, pneumonitis, myocarditis, hepatosplenomegaly, jaundice, and petechiae.

3. Placental factors—The placenta plays an important role in normal fetal growth. Placental weight has shown to be less in IUGR infants than in AGA infants irrespective of birthweight, suggesting that appropriate fetal growth may depend on the size or weight of the placenta. Several placental abnormalities are associated with an increased likelihood of an IUGR fetus. **Placenta previa** is associated with an increased incidence of IUGR, probably because of the unfavorable site of placental implantation. Complete placenta previa is associated with a higher incidence of IUGR than is partial placenta previa. Decreased functional exchange area as a result of **placental infarction** also is associated with an increased incidence of IUGR fetuses. **Premature placental separation** may occur at any time during pregnancy, with variable effects. When not associated with fetal death or premature labor, premature placental separation may increase the risk of IUGR. Malformations of the placenta or umbilical cord, such as **single umbilical artery (UA), velamentous umbilical cord insertion, circumvallate placenta, placental hemangioma, battledore placenta,** and **twin-twin transfusion syndrome,** also are associated with an increased risk of IUGR. **Chronic villitis,** chronic inflammation of placental villi, is seen with increased frequency when the placentas of IUGR pregnancies are examined histologically. Finally, **uterine anomalies** may result in impaired fetal growth, primarily because of the likelihood of suboptimal uterine blood flow.

4. Multiple gestation—Multiple gestation has long been associated with premature delivery. However, it also is associated with a 20–30% increased incidence of IUGR fetuses, possibly as a result of placental insufficiency, twin-twin transfusion syndrome, or anomalies. Serial ultrasound estimates of fetal weights should be considered in a multiple gestation pregnancy.

B. Maternal Factors

Numerous maternal diseases are associated with suboptimal fetal growth. Any woman who has borne 1 IUGR infant is at increased risk for recurrence, with a 2-fold and 4-fold increased risk for IUGR birth after 1 or 2 IUGR births, respectively.

1. Hypertension—Hypertension is the most common maternal complication causing IUGR. Systemic hypertension results in decreased blood flow through the spiral arterioles and decreased delivery of oxygen and nutrients to the placenta and fetus. Hypertension may be associated with placental infarction.

2. Drugs—Both social drugs and prescribed medications can affect fetal growth. **Alcohol** use has long been known to be associated with impaired fetal growth. Virtually all infants with fetal alcohol syndrome exhibit signs of growth restriction.

Cigarette smoking is much more common among women of childbearing age in the United States than is alcoholism. Smoking causes one-third of IUGR cases and is the single most preventable cause of IUGR pregnancy in the United States today. Women who smoke have a 3-fold to 4-fold increase in IUGR infants. Birthweight is reduced by approximately 200 g, with the amount of growth restriction proportional to the number of cigarettes smoked per day. Women who quit smoking at 7 months' gestation have newborns with higher mean birthweights than do women who smoke throughout the entire pregnancy. Women who stop smoking before 16 weeks' gestation are not at increased risk for having an IUGR infant.

Heroin and cocaine addicts have an increased incidence of IUGR infants, but confounding variables make determination of a direct cause-and-effect relationship difficult. Methadone use has not been shown to be associated with an increased incidence of IUGR.

Pharmacologic agents have been associated with an increased incidence of IUGR, primarily as a result of teratogenic effects. Warfarin has been associated with an increased incidence of IUGR fetuses, primarily as a result of the sequelae of intrauterine hemorrhage. Folic acid antagonists are associated with an increased risk of spontaneous abortion stillbirth, severe malformations, and IUGR infants.

IUGR fetuses are more common with maternally administered immunosuppressive drugs (eg, cyclosporine, azathioprine, corticosteroids), but when controlled for the underlying maternal disease, the medications per se probably have little effect on fetal growth.

3. Malnutrition and malabsorption—Poor maternal weight gain is associated with an increased risk of having an IUGR infant. Studies of infants borne by women who were pregnant during the Siege of Leningrad during World War II showed that daily intake must be reduced to less than 1500 kcal/d before a measurable effect on birthweight becomes evident. Maternal **malabsorption** may predispose to IUGR pregnancy. The most common clinical situations are inflammatory bowel disease (ulcerative colitis or regional enteritis), pancreatitis, and intestinal parasites.

4. Vascular disease—Diseases that affect maternal microvascular perfusion can be associated with IUGR. These include collagen vascular disease, insulin-dependent diabetes mellitus associated with microvasculopathy, and preeclampsia.

5. Maternal features—A small woman may have a smaller-than-normal infant because of reduced uterine growth potential. These mothers and infants are completely normal and healthy, but they are small because of genetic variation. The infants are described by the ponderal index (PI), which is calculated using the following formula:

$$PI = Birthweight \times 1000/(crown-heel\ length)^3$$

Asymmetric IUGR infants will have a low ponderal index (ie, they will be long, lightweight infants), whereas small normal infants will have a normal ponderal index. (A normal index at 28 weeks is 1.8. This value increases by 0.2 every 4 weeks to reach 2.4 at 40 weeks.)

Maternal parity exerts a modest effect on birthweight. First-born infants tend to be smaller and more often categorized as IUGR. This effect decreases with successive deliveries and is not seen beyond the third birth.

6. Sex of fetus—At term, female fetuses are an average 5% (150 g) smaller and 2% (1 cm) shorter than male fetuses. Referring to separate norms for male and female fetuses may increase the power of biometry in assessing IUGR.

Antenatal Diagnosis

In any pregnancy at risk for IUGR outcome, baseline studies should be obtained early in gestation. Careful attention should always be given to gestational dating (menstrual history, serial examinations, biochemical pregnancy testing, quickening, ultrasound). An IUGR outcome also may develop in pregnancies without identified risk factors. Careful attention to fundal height measurements is associated with a diagnostic sensitivity of 46–86%.

Ultrasound examination early in pregnancy is accurate in establishing the estimated date of confinement (EDC) and may sometimes identify genetic or congenital causes of IUGR pregnancy. Serial ultrasound examinations are important in documenting growth and excluding anomalies. Antenatal diagnosis of IUGR is not precise given that EFW cannot be measured directly and must be calculated from a combination of directly measured parameters. Overall prediction of weight via birthweight formulas can have a 10–20% error rate. Selection of the most useful biometric parameter depends on the timing of measurements. The crown–rump length is the best parameter for early dating of pregnancy. The biparietal diameter (BPD) and HC are most accurate in the second trimester, with a margin of error of 7–11 days for BPD and 3–5 days for HC. Head circumference is more useful in establishing gestational age in the third trimester because BPD loses its accuracy secondary to variations in shape. Abdominal circumference measurements are less accurate than BPD, HC, and femur length but is the most useful measurement for evaluating fetal growth. The fetal abdominal circumference reflects the volume of fetal subcutaneous fat and the size of the liver, which in turn correlates with the degree of fetal nutrition. Acidemia and hypoxemia are more common when the abdominal circumference is below the 5th percentile for gestational age.

The femur length is not helpful for identifying IUGR but can identify skeletal dysplasia. Because the definition of IUGR ultimately depends on birthweight and gestational age criteria, formulas that optimally predict birthweight in a given population will be the most important contributor to ultrasonographic criteria.

Fetuses from different populations show different growth patterns. The growth curves developed by Battaglia and Lubchenco in the 1960s do not reflect the variation in birthweight for various ethnic populations. The growth curves used today also do not reflect the median birthweight increase over the last 3 decades. Racial and ethnic anthropometric variations may suggest a need for specific charts for different communities. Ultrasound evaluation should also be used to identify the development of oligohydramnios in fetuses at risk for, or diagnosed with, IUGR. Decreased amniotic fluid volume is clinically associated with IUGR and may be the earliest sign detected on ultrasound. This finding is thought to result from decreased perfusion of the fetal kidneys, which leads to decreased urine production. Oligohydramnios is present in the majority of IUGR infants, but the presence of a normal amniotic fluid index (AFI) should not preclude the diagnosis of IUGR.

In fetuses with known IUGR, UA Doppler velocimetry can estimate the likelihood of adverse perinatal outcome and may be useful in determining the intensity of fetal surveillance. Placental circulatory insufficiency is associated with increased placental resistance, which causes a fall in umbilical flow and therefore hypoxia. During the compensated stage, diastolic flow in the UA is reduced or absent. Retrograde diastolic flow in the UA is a sign that severe hypoxemia and acidemia are present. Although the use of UA Doppler studies for general population screening remains unproven, Doppler studies can be helpful in following already identified IUGR fetuses. Doppler flow studies help in reducing interventions and improving overall fetal outcome in IUGR pregnancies. A recent study showed that of fetuses with suspected IUGR evaluated by Doppler studies, none of those with normal Doppler flow measurements (UA systolic/diastolic [S/D] ratio) were delivered with metabolic acidemia. This finding suggests that intense antenatal surveillance may be unnecessary in a fetus with a normal UA S/D ratio and normal AFI.

Abnormal UA flow is associated with a higher risk for fetal growth restriction and an increased likelihood of requiring cesarean or operative delivery. In fetuses with suspected IUGR, abnormal middle cerebral artery (MCA) and UA S/D ratios are strongly associated with low gestational age at delivery, low birthweight, and low UA pH. Also, mean birthweight, interval to delivery, need for emergent delivery, and occurrence of fetal distress all are related to the severity of abnormal Doppler findings after correction for gestational age. Abnormal Doppler cerebroplacental ratio (MCA pulsatile index divided by UA pulsatile index) also has been associated with a statistically significant increase in perinatal morbidity and mortality. Respiratory distress syndrome and intracranial hemorrhage are not associated with abnormal Doppler studies.

In addition to the UA and MCA, the descending aorta has altered perfusion in fetuses with growth restriction. The redistribution of systemic blood flow in order to maintain perfusion to the brain at the expense of abdominal organs is believed to result in increased vascular resistance in the perfusion area of the descending aorta and decreased vascular resistance in the cerebrum. An elevated pulsatility index of the descending aorta is associated with both IUGR and adverse outcomes, such as necrotizing enterocolitis, fetal distress, and perinatal mortality. Absent end-diastolic flow of the descending aorta is associated with a higher rate of cesarean delivery and perinatal mortality.

Elevated maternal serum α-fetoprotein (MSAFP) levels predict increased risk for IUGR outcome, regardless of maternal weight. Elevated MSAFP levels also predict an increased risk for other obstetric problems, including preeclampsia, placental abruption, preterm labor, and stillbirth.

In some centers, fetal blood sampling has been advocated for severe fetal growth restriction. Although this procedure can provide useful information on fetal karyotype, acid–base balance, fetal metabolism, and possible fetal infection, it is associated with much increased morbidity and mortality in the presence of IUGR. With advances in molecular diagnosis of amniotic fluid, most diagnostic information can be obtained rapidly by amniocentesis. If clinically indicated, studies should be performed to exclude infection. Initially this process usually involves determining maternal immune status (immunoglobulin [Ig] M antibodies against cytomegalovirus, rubella virus, and *T gondii*). If these levels are suggestive of recent infection, direct assessment of the amniotic fluid by polymerase chain reaction and culture may be required. A careful targeted ultrasound examination should be performed to determine the degree of fetal involvement, particularly of the central nervous system.

Complications

Numerous maternal and perinatal complications occur more frequently in IUGR pregnancy (Table 16–1). Underlying maternal disease is more likely to be present (Table 16–3), and these women require more intensive prenatal care. Premature labor or preeclampsia is more common. IUGR fetuses at any gestational age are less likely to tolerate labor well, and the need for operative delivery is increased.

Perinatal morbidity and mortality are significantly increased in low-birthweight infants, with an inverse relationship between neonatal weight and perinatal mortality. At any given gestational age, IUGR neonates have a higher mortality than do AGA neonates. However, at any given birthweight, outcomes are similar for IUGR and AGA neonates. Perinatal morbidity and mortality are especially increased in infants born at term with birthweights at or below the 3rd percentile. Increased risk of mortality is affected by the primary

etiology of growth restriction and may be modified by the severity and progression of maternal factors (eg, hypertension control). With the advent of fetal surveillance, perinatal mortality rate has decreased to 2–3 times that of the AGA population. The past decade has witnessed increased attention to minimizing the perinatal complications of surviving IUGR neonates. With continued improvements in antenatal surveillance and neonatal care, the perinatal mortality rate for IUGR pregnancies in most centers now is 1.5–2 times that of the AGA population. Unfortunately, this rate likely will not reach that of the AGA population in the near future because of the persistent occurrence of lethal anomalies and severe congenital infections.

IUGR fetuses are at risk for in utero complications, including hypoxia and metabolic acidosis, which may occur at any time but are likely to occur during labor. Up to 50% of growth-restricted fetuses exhibit abnormal fetal heart rate patterns, most often variable decelerations. Hypoxia is the result of increasing fetal oxygen requirements during pregnancy, with a rapid increase during the third trimester. If the fetus receives inadequate oxygen, hypoxia and subsequent metabolic acidosis will ensue. If undetected or untreated, this condition will lead to decreased glycogen and fat stores, ischemic end-organ damage, meconium-stained amniotic fluid, and oligohydramnios, eventually resulting in vital organ damage and intrauterine death.

IUGR infants are at increased risk for neonatal complications, including meconium aspiration syndrome, low Apgar scores, UA pH < 7.0, need for intubation in the delivery room, seizures, sepsis, polycythemia, hypoglycemia, hypocalcemia, temperature instability, apneic episodes, and neonatal death. All IUGR infants require a thorough evaluation for congenital anomalies.

Prevention

Because many causes of IUGR are nonpreventable, few interventions have proved effective for prevention. Interventions that have shown benefit include smoking cessation, antimalarial chemoprophylaxis, and balanced protein and energy supplementation. Smoking is the single most common preventable cause of IUGR in infants born in the United States. As discussed in Maternal Factors, women who quit smoking at 7 months' gestation have newborns with higher mean birthweights than do women who smoke throughout the pregnancy. Women who quit smoking before 16 weeks' gestation are not at any increased risk for an IUGR infant. Limited data suggest that **balanced nutritional supplementation** improves mean birthweight. As expected, such supplementation more likely will benefit those with poor nutrition or adolescent pregnancies. Pregnant women should avoid close contact with individuals known to be infected or colonized with rubella virus or cytomegalovirus. Nonpregnant women of reproductive age should be tested for immunity to rubella virus and, if susceptible, should be immunized. Currently no vaccine exists for cytomegalovirus.

Women of childbearing age should be tested for immunity to *T gondii* if this protozoan infection is clinically suspected. If the woman is immune, her risk of having an affected infant is remote. However, if she is susceptible, she should be cautioned to avoid cat feces and uncooked meat. If the screening IgM for toxoplasma is positive, no action should be taken based on this result without confirmation by a regional reference laboratory with expertise in toxoplasma testing.

Therapeutic medications are not a major cause of IUGR pregnancy, but benefits and risks should be weighed whenever medications are prescribed. Any woman of childbearing age should be questioned about the possibility of pregnancy before receiving therapeutic or diagnostic radiation to the pelvis.

Placental factors causing IUGR pregnancies are not generally preventable. It has been postulated that low-dose aspirin and dipyridamole may increase prostacyclin production in certain patients and thus prevent idiopathic uteroplacental insufficiency. The role of these agents in preventing IUGR resulting from placental insufficiency in at-risk populations is unclear at this time.

Preventive measures for the maternal diseases listed in Table 16–3 are beyond the scope of this chapter. Treatment of many of these conditions may decrease the likelihood of IUGR pregnancy. Treatment of hypertension has a positive effect on birthweight, at least in the third trimester. However, strict bed rest and hospitalization do not seem to have any beneficial effects for patients with a history of hypertension. Although a complex issue, protein supplements for patients with significant proteinuria may increase the amount of protein available for placental transfer. Correction of maternal anemia (of whatever cause) improves oxygen delivery to the fetus, thus improving fetal growth. However, routine supplements, such as with iron, have not been shown to be associated with any altered clinical outcomes.

Treatment of malabsorption syndrome (of whatever cause) can be expected to improve nutrient absorption and subsequent nutrient transfer to the fetus. Inflammatory bowel disease should be treated if required, but if possible, pregnancy should be deferred until the disease has been quiescent for approximately 6 months. Intestinal parasites should be appropriately treated and negative cultures confirmed prior to pregnancy.

Treatment

Treatment of IUGR pregnancy presupposes an accurate diagnosis. Even with the history, physical examination, and ultrasound examination, diagnosis remains difficult, and some IUGR pregnancies will not be detected.

All pregnant women should discontinue cigarette smoking as well as use of alcohol and all recreational drugs. Cessation should be accomplished before conception to allow time for clearance of toxins, particularly if the woman previously had an IUGR infant. Although bed rest often is recommended, no evidence shows that bed rest results in improved outcome or increased fetal birthweight for fetuses with suspected IUGR. The increased uterine blood flow that occurs when the patient is in the lateral recumbent position theoretically may result in some benefit for fetuses with asymmetric IUGR. However, a paucity of data support this theory.

Because IUGR fetuses are at risk for antepartum or intrapartum compromise, they should be followed carefully. The best method for monitoring a fetus with suspected IUGR is not established. Because the diagnosis of IUGR most often is made relatively late in pregnancy, patients are seen every 1 to 2 weeks. In addition to fetal kick counts, antepartum testing with nonstress test and assessment of amniotic fluid volume are performed once or twice weekly in conjunction with UA Doppler velocimetry. The significance of abnormal UA Doppler results can be clarified by investigations of middle cerebral circulation and Doppler studies of venous structures, including the ductus venosus. If a nonstress test is nonreactive or if variable or spontaneous decelerations are seen, further assessment of fetal well-being is indicated with either a contraction stress test or a fetal biophysical profile. Because the contraction stress test is more cumbersome to perform and difficult to interpret, it has largely been replaced by the biophysical profile as a backup test.

Ultrasound examinations to assess adequacy of fetal growth should be performed at least every 3–4 weeks. Measurements should include BPD, HC, abdominal circumference, and femur length, especially in patients in whom an asymmetric IUGR fetus is suspected. Probably the most sensitive index of an asymmetric IUGR fetus is the abdominal circumference. The femur length/abdominal circumference ratio is a gestational age-independent ratio (normal 0.20–0.24). Asymmetric IUGR fetuses generally have a ratio > 0.24.

In selected cases, amniocentesis may be indicated for determination of fetal pulmonary maturity with an uncertain EDC, for assessment of fetal karyotype, or for diagnosis of fetal infection.

Every IUGR pregnancy must be individually assessed for the optimal time of delivery (ie, the point at which the baby will do as well or better outside the uterus than inside). This would be whenever surveillance indicates fetal maturity, fetal compromise, or gestational age of 38 weeks (beyond which time there is no advantage to an IUGR fetus remaining in utero). Data are conflicting as to whether IUGR accelerates pulmonary maturity. Therefore, the current recommendation is to administer gluco-corticoids to women likely to deliver before 34 weeks, as would be done with any other pregnancy.

IUGR pregnancies are at increased risk for intrapartum problems, so whenever possible delivery should take place in a center where appropriate obstetric care, anesthesia, and neonatal care are readily available. Cesarean delivery may be necessary, and the presence of meconium-stained amniotic fluid or a compromised infant should be anticipated.

The mode of delivery must be individualized. Cesarean section delivery is often indicated, especially when fetal monitoring reveals fetal compromise, malpresentation, or situations where traumatic vaginal delivery might be expected.

Continuous electronic fetal heart rate monitoring should be performed during labor in all cases, even if recent antepartum testing has been reassuring. Arteriovenous cord blood gas determinations also are useful; as many as 50% of IUGR infants have some degree of metabolic acidosis. Minimization of anesthesia is generally preferable, but controlled epidural anesthesia usually is safe. Maternal hypotension or hypovolemia must be avoided.

Prognosis

IUGR pregnancy per se is not considered life-threatening for the mother. However, increased maternal morbidity and mortality may result from an underlying condition (eg, hypertension or renal disease). Most women who deliver IUGR infants can be expected to have long-term prognoses equivalent to those of women delivering AGA infants. Infants with a low birthweight have a relatively high morbidity and mortality. Studies have shown that the rate of neonatal death, Apgar score at 5 minutes < 3, UA pH < 7.0, seizures during the first day of life, and incidence of intubation are significantly increased when the fetus is at or below the 3rd percentile for birthweight.

As for long term-prognosis, reports of national survey data show that IUGR infants appear to catch up in weight in the first 6 months of life. However, IUGR infants tend to remain physically small and are shorter, lighter, and have smaller HCs than do AGA infants.

Taken as a group, IUGR infants have more neurologic and intellectual deficits than do their AGA peers. IUGR infants have lower IQs as well as a higher incidence of learning and behavioral problems. Major neurologic handicaps, such as severe mental retardation, cerebral palsy, and seizures, are more common in IUGR infants. The incidence of sudden infant death syndrome (SIDS) is increased in IUGR infants, who account for 30% of all SIDS cases. Adults who were IUGR at birth are at higher risk for developing ischemic heart disease and related disorders, including hypertension, stroke, diabetes, and hypercholesterolemia.

LARGE-FOR-GESTATIONAL-AGE PREGNANCY

Terminology

Although LGA pregnancy is defined according to the same concept as IUGR pregnancy (LGA = heaviest 10% of newborns), LGA pregnancy has received substantially less attention. *Large for gestational age* is defined as above the 90th percentile of weight for any specific gestational age. **Macrosomia** generally refers to fetuses with an EFW of at least 4500 g. The risk of morbidity is greater for infants born weighing between 4000 and 4500 g compared to the average population. However, the risk of infant morbidity is substantially increased at birthweights greater than 4500 g. Although there are numerous reports and studies regarding macrosomia, few data regarding large for gestational age as defined here are available. Therefore, this section concentrates on fetal macrosomia, with additional comments regarding LGA pregnancies.

Pathophysiology

Numerous endocrinologic changes occur during pregnancy to ensure an adequate fetal glucose supply. In the second half of pregnancy, increased concentrations of human placental lactogen, free and total cortisol, and prolactin combine to produce modest maternal insulin resistance, which is countered by postprandial hyperinsulinemia. In those who are unable to mount this hyperinsulinemic response, relative hyperglycemia may develop (ie, gestational diabetes). Because glucose crosses the placenta by facilitated diffusion, fetal hyperglycemia ensues. This in turn produces fetal hyperinsulinemia with resultant intracellular transfer of glucose, leading to fetal macrosomia.

Differential Diagnosis

Factors that predispose to LGA pregnancy are listed in Table 16–4. As with IUGR pregnancy, diagnosis of LGA pregnancy depends on knowing with certainty the gestational age of the fetus.

Table 16–4. Factors that may predispose to fetal macrosomia or LGA pregnancy.

Maternal factors
  Diabetes (gestational, chemical, or insulin-dependent), obesity, postdatism, multiparity, advanced age, previous LGA infant, large stature
Fetal Factors
  Genetic or congenital disorders, male gender

A. MATERNAL DIABETES

Maternal diabetes, whether gestational, chemical, or insulin dependent, is the condition classically associated with fetal macrosomia. The "Pedersen hypothesis" was long assumed to account for fetal macrosomia, that is, the condition was the result of inadequate management of diabetes during pregnancy. Initial reports suggested that careful control of blood glucose level in insulin-dependent diabetic women would prevent fetal macrosomia, but recent studies have suggested that the problem is not so simple and that the incidence may correlate better with cord blood concentrations of maternally acquired anti-insulin IgG antibodies and/or increased serum levels of free fatty acids, triglycerides, and the amino acids alanine, serine, and isoleucine. Cord serum epidermal growth factor concentrations also have been found to be higher than normal in pregnancies complicated by prepregnancy diabetes and gestational diabetes.

A significant correlation exists between plasma leptin levels and neonatal birthweight, which suggests that leptin levels are directly related to the quantity of body fat tissue in fetal macrosomia.

B. MATERNAL OBESITY

Maternal obesity is associated with a 3- to 4-fold increased likelihood of fetal macrosomia. This situation may result in part from associated gestational or chemical diabetes, although these disorders are not present in most obese women who deliver macrosomic babies. One study showed a significantly higher rate of cesarean delivery for obese mothers, even after comorbidities such as diabetes were excluded.

C. POSTDATISM

Prolonged pregnancy is more likely to result in a macrosomic fetus, presumably because of continued delivery of nutrients and oxygen to the fetus. Placental sulfatase deficiency or congenital adrenal hypoplasia are rare causes of postdatism.

D. GENETIC AND CONGENITAL DISORDERS

Several genetic and congenital syndromes are associated with an increased incidence of macrosomia. **Beckwith-Wiedemann syndrome** is frequently associated with fetal macrosomia, usually because of pancreatic islet cell hyperplasia (nesidioblastosis). Affected infants usually have hypoglycemia, macroglossia, and omphalocele. They also may have intestinal malrotation or visceromegaly. Although usually a sporadic event, other inheritance patterns have been suggested in a few families. Other rare syndromes include **Weaver's syndrome, Sotos' syndrome, Nevo's syndrome, Ruvalcaba-Myhre syndrome,** and **Marshall's syndrome. Carpenter's syn-**drome and the **fragile X syndrome** may be associated with an increased incidence of LGA infants.

E. CONSTITUTIONALLY LARGE FETUS

Fetuses who are suspected of being large for gestational age may simply be large secondary to constitutional factors. **Large maternal stature** should be considered as contributing to macrosomia because birthweight tends to correlate more closely with maternal height than maternal weight. **Male gender fetuses** are more likely to be considered LGA because male fetuses are an average of 150 g heavier than appropriately matched female fetuses at each gestational week during late pregnancy. Series addressing fetal macrosomia generally report an increased incidence of male fetuses, usually approximately 60–65%. One recent study showed that male fetuses were twice as likely to be diagnosed with macrosomia as compared with female fetuses.

Complications

Macrosomic pregnancies are at increased risk for many complications (Table 16–2). Macrosomic pregnancies are more likely to require cesarean delivery, usually because of failure to progress. In particular, primigravidas delivering a macrosomic infant are at increased risk for complications such as prolonged labor, postpartum hemorrhage, operative vaginal delivery, and emergency cesarean section as compared to delivering a normal weight infant. Primigravidas also have a higher risk of prolonged labor, operative delivery, and emergency cesarean sections compared with multiparous women delivering a macrosomic infant. Fetal distress, as determined by electronic fetal monitoring, is not more common in macrosomic pregnancies.

Shoulder dystocia occurs in 5–24% of vaginally delivered macrosomic fetuses. The incidence of shoulder dystocia correlates not only with progressive fetal weight but also with increasing chest circumference to HC. Shoulder dystocia of macrosomic infants also is related to maternal stature, but the associate is not as clear. From 10–15% of infants with shoulder dystocia experience brachial plexus injury; facial nerve injury and fractures of the humerus or clavicle also may be seen. The risk of brachial plexus injury in macrosomic infants delivered vaginally is 0.3–4%. Brachial plexus injury with shoulder dystocia is approximately 7% in infants whose birthweights exceed 4000 g but is 14% for mothers with gestational diabetes. The doubled risk may be secondary to increased abdominal obesity in diabetic mothers. In diabetic patients, a correlation exists between the level of fetal truncal asymmetry (abdominal circumference/biparietal diameter ratio) as measured by ultrasound and the incidence and severity of shoulder dystocia. In addition to macrosomia, risk factors for shoulder dystocia include previous shoulder dystocia and maternal diabetes (3- to 4-fold increase compared to nondiabetic mothers). Lesser risk factors that are mediated through fetal size include previous delivery of a large fetus and excessive maternal weight gain during pregnancy. The risk of shoulder dystocia is similar in primigravidas and multigravidas delivering macrosomic infants. Perineal trauma is more likely with a macrosomic pregnancy and is related to an increased incidence of shoulder dystocia and operative vaginal delivery. Vaginal delivery of a macrosomic infant increases by 5-fold the risk of third- or fourth-degree laceration.

Although gestational diabetes and postdatism predispose to fetal macrosomia, no evidence indicates that fetal macrosomia or an LGA fetus predisposes to gestational diabetes or postdatism.

The incidence of stillbirth remains higher in macrosomic fetuses than in controls of average weight. This problem has persisted even with the availability of fetal monitoring and presumably reflects the increased incidence of maternal diabetes and postdatism. Stillbirths are known to be increased in nonanomalous diabetic mothers, but the cause is not understood. Additionally, excessive prepregnancy weight is an independent risk factor for unexplained death. In fact, large for gestational age is statistically associated with unexplained fetal death even after controlling for maternal age, diabetes, and hypertension.

Many of the neonatal complications of fetal macrosomia are the result of underlying maternal diabetes or birth trauma and include low Apgar scores, hypoglycemia, hypocalcemia, polycythemia, jaundice, and feeding difficulties. Large-for-gestational-age infants have significantly higher absolute nucleated red blood cell counts, lymphocyte counts, and packed cell volumes. These hematologic abnormalities are the same for all LGA infants regardless of whether they are infants of nondiabetic mothers, insulin-dependent diabetic mothers, or non–insulin-dependent gestational diabetics. This situation is believed to reflect a compensatory increase in erythropoiesis as a result of chronic intrauterine hypoxia resulting from increased placental oxygen consumption and decreased fetal oxygen delivery.

LGA infants of diabetic mothers have an increased incidence of cardiac septal hypertrophy.

Prevention

Prevention of macrosomia and ensuing complications requires early detection of risk factors. Risk factors for having a macrosomic infant include multiparity, advanced maternal age, and previous delivery of a macrosomic infant. When controlled for gestational age and fetal gender, the average birthweight with successive pregnancies

increases by 80–120 g up to the fifth pregnancy. Multiparity is also associated with other risk factors (eg, obesity, diabetes) and therefore may be a confounding variable. Advanced maternal age also contributes to increased birthweight. However, as with multiparity, it is also associated with obesity and diabetes.

Patients with the risk factors noted in Table 16–4 should be evaluated for possible fetal macrosomia with an ultrasound estimate of fetal size and weight. EFW by ultrasound is not very accurate. More than 30 different formulas for EFW calculation have been proposed, attesting to the inadequacy of each individual method. No single formula has been consistently better than the others. Even in skillful hands, the error of fetal weight estimates by ultrasound is 10–20%. One review of ultrasonographic diagnosis of macrosomia shows sensitivity ranging from 24–88% and specificity from 60–98%. The margin of error in estimating fetal weight means that the EFW by ultrasound must be at least 4750 g in order to predict a birthweight of 4000 g with a confidence interval of 90%. The best single measurement in evaluating macrosomia in diabetic mothers is abdominal circumference. An initial abdominal circumference above the 70th percentile is significantly associated with subsequent delivery of an LGA infant. Fetal body composition and fetal shoulder width cannot be accurately assessed by ultrasound.

Adequate control of maternal glucose levels is thought to prevent the development of macrosomia in gestational diabetics, although neonatal complications despite excellent metabolic control have been reported. Prepregnancy weight and degree of weight gain are strong indicators for macrosomia regardless of glycemic control. However, the rates of macrosomia and complications are reduced overall when postprandial levels are monitored. Studies have shown that the risk of macrosomia is reduced to near normal in diabetic women who monitor 1-hour postprandial glucose levels and that 1-hour postprandial glucose levels are directly related to fetal abdominal circumference values. One study showed that when postprandial glucose levels were kept below 104 mg/dL, macrosomia rates of diabetic women were similar to those of nondiabetics. Furthermore, high carbohydrate intake is associated with a decreased incidence of newborn macrosomia. Essential management principles in known diabetics includes nutrition and exercise counseling beginning in the preconception period. Furthermore, euglycemia is crucial in the first trimester, a period when insulin requirements are frequently less than prepregnancy, and intake can be altered by nausea and vomiting. Insulin adjustments are frequently necessary.

Infants of women who participate in regular aerobic exercise programs have lower average birthweights compared with infants in the general population but no demonstrable adverse effects. To date, no studies have evaluated the potential efficacy of exercise programs as a means of decreasing birthweight in women at risk for LGA pregnancy.

Treatment

Although widely recommended, labor induction in at-risk pregnancy for reducing the incidence of fetal macrosomia and intrapartum complications remains an unproven hypothesis. Intrapartum treatment considerations center on the increased likelihood of traumatic vaginal delivery.

Several published reviews of fetal macrosomia suggest routine cesarean delivery for fetuses with estimated weights of 5000 g or more (or estimated weights ≥ 4500 g in diabetic pregnancies). This suggestion is based in part on the data given in Table 16–2 and in part on anthropometric studies suggesting that very macrosomic fetuses have bisacromial circumferences in excess of HCs. Because of current limitations in the sensitivity and specificity of ultrasound-derived fetal weight calculations, decisions regarding scheduled abdominal delivery must be partially based on clinical grounds. Such considerations are particularly warranted in women who are obese or are diabetic or in postdate pregnancies. Maternal age and maternal preference also should be considered when deciding on delivery method. Vacuum-assisted vaginal delivery increases the risk of shoulder dystocia. If the estimate of fetal weight is greater than 4000 g, the vacuum should be avoided if the second stage is prolonged, and in general the vacuum should be used with caution. Some physicians have adopted the practice of discussing the option of vaginal delivery versus cesarean delivery if the EFW is greater than 4500 g in nondiabetic women or greater than 4000–4250 g in diabetic women. No firm data indicate that this practice offers greater benefit in preventing complications such as shoulder dystocia than risks associated with many unnecessary cesarean births. Because of these factors, women at risk for macrosomic or LGA babies should deliver in facilities where adequate obstetric care, pediatric care, and anesthesia are available. Large-bore intravenous access must be established, and blood must be available. Delivery should occur in a setting where immediate operation can be accomplished. In many situations, delivery should occur in a delivery room.

Prognosis

Any woman who delivers an LGA baby should be informed that the risk of her having another LGA baby is increased by 2.5- to 4-fold. Such women should be screened for previously undiagnosed chemical or insulin-dependent diabetes and, even if screening is nega-

tive, should be followed carefully in any subsequent pregnancy to rule out gestational diabetes.

Obese women should be strongly encouraged to lose weight prior to becoming pregnant. Any woman who has delivered an LGA infant should be encouraged to seek early care for any subsequent pregnancy, if for no other reason than early confirmation of the EDC, which can minimize the likelihood of subsequent postdatism. Women who deliver an LGA infant with an underlying genetic or congenital disorder should receive genetic counseling regarding recurrence risks and the feasibility of antepartum diagnosis.

In addition to the many neonatal complications previously noted, infants of mothers with gestational or chemical diabetes are at increased risk for subsequent obesity, type 2 diabetes, or both. Infants who suffer from neonatal complications are at increased risk for subsequent neurologic or behavioral problems.

FUTURE DIAGNOSIS OF IUGR & LGA PREGNANCIES

Although much more is known about the risks of IUGR than of LGA pregnancy, both are known to be associated with increased risks of in utero, intrapartum, neonatal, and long-term compromise. The ability to diagnose and optimally manage these pregnancies remains poor. Further effort must be directed toward precise diagnosis at a point in the pregnancy when intervention can still be effective.

REFERENCES

Terminology

American College of Obstetricians and Gynecologists: *Clinical Management Guidelines for Obstetrician-Gynecologists.* ACOG Practice Bulletin No. 12. American College of Obstetricians and Gynecologists, 2000.

Chatfield J: Practice guidelines. ACOG issues guidelines on fetal macrosomia. Am Fam Physician 2001;64:169.

Degani S: Fetal biometry: Clinical, pathological, and technical considerations. Obstet Gynecol Surv 2001;56:159.

Jovanovic L: What is so bad about a big baby? Diabetes Care 2001;24;1317.

Differential Diagnosis

American College of Obstetricians and Gynecologists: *Clinical Management Guidelines for Obstetrician-Gynecologists.* ACOG Practice Bulletin No. 12. American College of Obstetricians and Gynecologists, 2000.

Clausson B et al: Perinatal outcome in SGA births defined by customized versus population-based birthweight standards. Br J Obstet Gynaecol 2001;108:830.

Degani S: Fetal biometry: Clinical, pathological, and technical considerations. Obstet Gynecol Surv 2001;56:159.

Heinonen S et al: Weights of placentae from small-for-gestational age infants revisited. Placenta 2001;22:399.

Loukavaara M et al: Diabetic pregnancy associated with increased epidermal growth factor in cord serum at term. Obstet Gynecol 2004;103:240.

Sheiner E et al: Gender does matter in perinatal medicine. Fetal Diagn Ther 2004;19:366.

Sheiner E et al: Maternal obesity as an independent risk factor for caesarean delivery. Pediatr Perinat Epidemiol 2004;18:196.

Wiznitzer A et al: Cord leptin level and fetal macrosomia. Obstet Gynecol 2000;96:707.

Antenatal Diagnosis

Aardema M et al: Uterine artery Doppler flow and uteroplacental vascular pathology in normal pregnancy and pregnancies complicated by preeclampsia and small for gestational age fetuses. Placenta 2001;22:405.

American College of Obstetricians and Gynecologists: *Clinical Management Guidelines for Obstetrician-gynecologists.* ACOG Practice Bulletin No. 12. American College of Obstetricians and Gynecologists, 2000.

Baschat A et al: Umbilical artery Doppler screening for detection of the small fetus in need of antepartum surveillance. Am J Obstet Gynecol 2000;182:154.

Benson CB et al: Doppler criteria for intrauterine growth retardation: Predictive values. J Ultrasound Med 1988;7:655.

Bush K et al: The utility of umbilical artery Doppler investigation in women with the HELLP (hemolysis, elevated liver enzymes, and low platelets) syndrome. Am J Obstet Gynecol 2001;184:1087.

Degani S: Fetal biometry: Clinical, pathological, and technical considerations. Obstet Gynecol Surv 2001;56:159.

Fouron J et al: Correlation between prenatal velocity waveforms in the aortic isthmus and neurodevelopmental outcome between the ages of 2 and 4 years. Am J Obstet Gynecol 2001;184:630.

Goffinet F et al: Screening with a uterine Doppler in low risk pregnancy women followed by low dose aspirin in women with abnormal results: A multicenter randomized control trial. Br J Obstet Gynaecol 2001;108:510.

Mandruzzano G et al: Antepartal assessment of IUGR fetuses. J Perinatal Med 2001;29:227.

Maruyama K et al: Superior mesenteric artery blood flow velocity in small for gestational age infants of very low birth weight during the early neonatal period. J Perinat Med 2001;29:64.

Park Y et al: Clinical significance of early diastolic notch depth: Uterine artery Doppler velocimetry in the third trimester. Am J Obstet Gynecol 2000;182:1204.

Sterne G et al: Abnormal fetal cerebral and umbilical Doppler measurements in fetuses with intrauterine growth restriction predicts the severity of perinatal morbidity. J Clin Ultrasound 2001;29:146.

Complications

Bloomgarden Z: American Diabetes Association 60th Scientific Sessions, 2000: Diabetes and pregnancy. Diabetes Care 2000;23:1699.

Cundy T et al: Perinatal mortality in type 2 diabetes mellitus. Obstet Gynecol Surv 2000;55:538.

Dollberg S et al: Normoblasts in large for gestational age infants. Arch Dis Child Fetal Neonatal Ed 2000;83:148.

Gupta N et al: The incidence, risk factors and obstetric outcome in primigravid women sustaining anal sphincter tears. Acta Obstet Gynecol Scand 2003;82:736.

Lim J et al: Delivery of macrosomic babies: management and outcomes of 330 cases. J Obstet Gynecol 2002;22:370.

Lindley A et al: Maternal cigarette smoking during pregnancy and infant ponderal index at birth in the Swedish Medical Birth Register. Am J Public Health 2000;90:420.

Mocanu E et al: Obstetric and neonatal outcome of babies weighing more than 4.5 kg: An analysis by parity. Eur J Obstet Gynecol 2000;92:229.

Nassar A et al: Fetal macrosomia (>4500g): Perinatal outcome of 231 cases according to mode of delivery. J Perinat 2003;23:136.

Raio L et al: Perinatal outcome of fetuses with a birth weight greater than 4500 g: An analysis of 3356 cases. Eur J Obstet Gynecol Reprod Biol 2003;109:160.

Schwartz R et al: What is the significance of macrosomia? Diabetes Care 1999;22:1201.

Vela-Huerta M: Asymmetrical septal hypertrophy in newborn infants of diabetic mothers. Am J Perinatol 2000;17:89.

Prevention

Ben-Haroush A: Fetal weight estimation in diabetic pregnancies and suspected fetal macrosomia. J Perinat Med 2004;32:113.

Bloomgarden Z: American Diabetes Association 60th Scientific Sessions, 2000: Diabetes and pregnancy. Diabetes Care 2000;23:1699.

Gulmezoglu M et al: Effectiveness of interventions to prevent or treat impaired fetal growth. Obstet Gynecol Surv 1999;54:58.

Holcomb W: Parity and maternal age affect excess fetal growth contrariwise in diabetes. Am J Obstet Gynecol 2000;182:83.

Jovanovic L: What is so bad about a big baby? Diabetes Care 2001;24:1317.

Kjos S: Prediction of large for gestational age infants in gestational diabetes with moderate fasting hyperglycemia. Am J Obstet Gynecol 2000;182:79.

Lindley A et al: Maternal cigarette smoking during pregnancy and infant ponderal index at birth in the Swedish Medical Birth Register. Am J Public Health 2000;90:420.

Romon M et al: Higher carbohydrate intake is associated with decreased incidence of newborn macrosomia in women with gestational diabetes. J Am Diet Assoc 2001;101:897.

Schwartz R et al: What is the significance of macrosomia? Diabetes Care 1999;22:1201.

Treatment

Chatfield J: Practice Guidelines. American College of Obstetricians and Gynecologists issues guidelines on fetal macrosomia. Am Fam Physician 2001;64:169.

Degani S: Fetal biometry: Clinical, pathological, and technical considerations. Obstet Gynecol Surv 2001;56:159.

Gulmezoglu M et al: Effectiveness of interventions to prevent or treat impaired fetal growth. Obstet Gynecol Surv 1999;54:58.

Owen P et al: Interval between fetal measurements in predicting growth restriction. Obstet Gynecol 2001;97:499.

Parretti E et al: Third-trimester maternal glucose levels from diurnal profiles in nondiabetic pregnancies: Correlation with sonographic parameters of fetal growth. Diabetes Care 2001;24:1319.

Sheiner E et al: Failed vacuum extraction: Maternal risk factors and pregnancy outcome. Am J Obstet Gynecol 2001;184:165.

Prognosis

Barker DJP: Fetal growth and adult disease. Br J Obstet Gynaecol 1992;99:275.

Bloomgarden Z: American Diabetes Association 60th Scientific Sessions, 2000: Diabetes and pregnancy. Diabetes Care 2000;23:1699.

Bos AF et al: Intrauterine growth retardation, general movements, and neurodevelopmental outcome: A review. Dev Med Child Neurol 2001;43:61.

Georgieff MK: Intrauterine growth retardation and subsequent somatic growth and neurodevelopment. J Pediatr 1998;133:3.

Hediger M et al: Growth and fatness at three to six years of age of children born small- or large-for-gestational age. Pediatrics 1999;104:555.

Hediger ML et al: Growth of infants and young children born small or large for gestational age: Findings from the Third National Health and Nutrition Examination Survey. Arch Pediatr Adolesc Med 1998;152:1225.

Leitner Y et al: Six-year follow-up of children with intrauterine growth retardation: Long-term prospective study. J Child Neurol 2000;15:781.

McIntire D et al: Birth weight in relation to morbidity and mortality among newborn infants. N Engl J Med 1999; 340:1234.

Weinerroither H et al: Intrauterine blood flow and long-term intellectual, neurologic and social development. Obstet Gynecol 2001;91:449.

Multiple Pregnancy

Melissa C. Bush, MD, & Martin L. Pernoll, MD

Monozygotic twins ("identical twins") result from the division of a single fertilized ovum. Monozygotic twinning occurs in approximately 2.3–4 of 1000 pregnancies in all races. The rate is remarkably constant and is not influenced by heredity, mother's age, or other factors. Dizygotic twins ("fraternal twins") are produced from separately fertilized ova. Slightly more than 30% of twins are monozygotic; nearly 70% are dizygotic. Although monozygosity is random (ie, it does not fit any discernible genetic pattern), dizygosity has hereditary determinants.

In North America, spontaneous dizygotic twinning occurs in approximately 1 in 83 conceptions and triplets in approximately 1 in 8000 conceptions. A traditional approximation of the incidence of multiple pregnancies is as follows:

Twins	1:80
Triplets	$1:80^2 = 1:6400$
Quadruplets (etc.)	$1:80^3 = 1:512,000$

The incidence of twin and higher-order multiple gestations has increased significantly over the past 15 years primarily because of the availability and increased use of ovulation-inducing drugs and assisted reproductive technology (ART). Multiple gestations now compose 3% of all pregnancies, and twins compose 25–30% of deliveries resulting from ART. Significant maternal and neonatal effects result from this increase in multiple births. The financial costs are staggering, with combined costs of ART plus pregnancy care and delivery averaging $39,249.

Maternal morbidity and mortality rates are much higher in multiple pregnancy than in singleton pregnancy because of preterm labor, hemorrhage, and pregnancy-induced hypertension. Approximately two-thirds of twin pregnancies end in a single birth; the other embryo is lost from bleeding, is absorbed within the first 10 weeks of pregnancy, or becomes mummified (fetus papyraceous). Moreover, the perinatal mortality rate of twins is 3–4 times higher—and for triplets much higher still—than in singleton pregnancies as a result of chromosomal abnormalities, prematurity, anomalies, hypoxia, and trauma. This is particularly true of monozygotic twins.

Pathogenesis

A. MONOZYGOTIC MULTIPLE GESTATION

Monozygotic twins, which result from the fertilization of a single ovum by a single sperm, are always of the same sex. However, the twins may develop differently depending on the time of preimplantation division. Normally, monozygotic twins share the same physical characteristics (skin, hair and eye color, body build) and the same genetic features (blood characteristics: ABO, M, N, haptoglobin, serum group; histocompatible genes; skin grafting possible), and they are often mirror images of one another (one left-handed, the other right-handed, etc.). However, their fingerprints differ.

The paradox of "identical" twins is that they may be the antithesis of identical. The very earliest splits are sometimes accompanied by a simultaneous chromosomal error, resulting in heterokaryotypic monozygotes, 1 with Down syndrome and the other normal.

Monozygotic triplets result from repeated twinning (also called *supertwinning*) of a single ovum. Trizygotic triplets develop by individual fertilization of 3 simultaneously expelled ova. Triplets also may be produced by the twinning of 2 ova and the elimination of 1 of the 4 resulting embryos. Similarly, quadruplets may be monozygotic, paired dizygotic, or quadrizygotic (ie, they may arise from 1–4 ova).

B. DIZYGOTIC MULTIPLE GESTATION

Dizygotic twins are the product of 2 ova and 2 sperm. The 2 ova are released from separate follicles (or, very rarely, from the same follicle) at approximately the same time. Dizygotic (fraternal) twins may be of the same or different sexes. They bear only the resemblance of brothers or sisters and may or may not have the same blood type. Significant differences usually can be identified over time.

Approximately 75% of dizygotic twins are the same sex. Both twins are males in approximately 45% of cases (a lesser preponderance of males in twins than in singletons) and both females in approximately 30%.

Many factors influence dizygotic twinning. Race is a factor, with multiple pregnancy most common in blacks, least common in Asians, and of intermediate occurrence in whites. The incidence of spontaneous dizygotic twinning varies from 1.3 in 1000 in Japan to 49 in 1000 in western Nigeria. The rate in the United States is approximately 12 in 1000.

Dizygotic multiple pregnancy tends to be recurrent. Women who have borne dizygotic twins have a 10-fold increased chance of subsequent multiple pregnancy. Dizygotic twinning probably is inherited via the female descendants of mothers of twins; the father's genetic contribution plays little or no part. White women who are dizygotic twins or who are siblings of dizygotic twin mothers have a higher twinning rate among their offspring than do women in the general population.

Parity does not influence the incidence of dizygotic twinning but aging does, with the rate of dizygotic twinning peaking between 35 and 40 years of age and then declining sharply. In women who are twins or daughters of twins, the twinning rate peaks at approximately age 35 years, at which time it plateaus until almost age 45 years and then declines. Black women, whether or not they are twins or siblings of twins, have a prolonged period of dizygotic twinning from 35–45 years of age.

Women of increased height and weight have a higher incidence of twinning, but the rate does not vary among social classes. Blood groups O and A are more prevalent in white mothers of twins than in the general population, for unknown reasons.

High fertility (polyovulation) is associated with multiple pregnancy. Excessive production of pituitary gonadotropins, relatively high frequency of coitus, and inability of 1 graafian follicle to inhibit others have been postulated as reasons for a higher incidence of dizygotic twinning. Undernutrition appears to be a negative factor. Women who conceive late in an ovulatory cycle have a greater chance of multiple pregnancy, perhaps because of ovular "overripeness."

Dizygotic twinning is more common among women who become pregnant soon after cessation of long-term oral contraception. This may be a reflection of high "rebound" gonadotropin secretion. Induction of ovulation in previously infertile patients has resulted in many multiple pregnancies—even the gestation of septuplets and octuplets. The estrogen analogue clomiphene citrate increases the incidence of dizygotic pregnancy to approximately 5–10%.

Clinically zygosity cannot be ascertained prenatally, so chorionicity seen on ultrasound is a useful marker.

C. OTHER FORMS OF MULTIPLE GESTATION

Other kinds of twinning are theoretically possible in humans. Dispermic mosaicism may result from fertilization of 2 ova that were not independently released but have instead developed from the same oocyte. Another possibility is the fertilization of 1 ovum by 2 sperms. Twinning of discordant twins may be ex-

plained by meiotic abnormalities, including polar body twinning, delayed implantation of the embryo, retarded or arrested intrauterine development, or superfetation.

Superfecundation is the fertilization of 2 ova, released at approximately the same time, by sperm released at intercourse on 2 different occasions. The rare cases in which the fetuses are of disparate size or skin color and have blood groups corresponding to those of the mother's 2 male partners lend credence to (but do not conclusively validate) this possibility.

Superfetation is the fertilization of 2 ova released in different menstrual cycles. This is virtually impossible in humans because the initial corpus luteum of pregnancy would have to be suppressed to allow for a second ovulation approximately 1 month later.

Pathologic Factors Associated with Twinning

Although the blood volume is increased in multiple pregnancy, maternal anemia often develops because of greater demand for iron by the fetuses. However, prior anemia, poor diet, and malabsorption may precede or compound iron deficiency during multiple pregnancy. Respiratory tidal volume is increased, but the woman pregnant with twins often is "breathless" (possibly because of increased progesterone levels).

Marked uterine distention and increased pressure on the adjacent viscera and pelvic vasculature are typical of multiple pregnancy. Lutein cysts and even ascites are the result of abnormally high levels of chorionic gonadotropin in occasional multiple pregnancies. Placenta previa develops more frequently because of the large size of the placenta or placentas.

The maternal cardiovascular, respiratory, gastrointestinal, renal, and musculoskeletal systems are especially subject to stress in multiple pregnancy, combined with greater maternal–fetal nutritional requirements. Multiple pregnancy is classified as high risk because of the increased incidence of maternal anemia, urinary tract infection, preeclampsia–eclampsia, hemorrhage (before, during, and after delivery), and uterine atony.

A. PLACENTAL AND CORD

The placenta and membranes of monozygotic twins may vary considerably (Fig 17–1), depending on the time of initial division of the embryonic disk. Variations are noted here.

1. Division prior to the morula stage and differentiation of the trophoblast (day 3) results in separate or fused placentas, 2 chorions, and 2 amnions. (This process grossly resembles dizygotic twinning and accounts for almost one-third of monozygotic twinning.) This is clinically relevant as dichorionic twins have a much lower rate of complications.

Figure 17–1. Placental variations in twinning. (Reproduced, with permission, from Benson RC: *Handbook of Obstetrics & Gynecology*, 8th ed. Lange, 1983.)

2. Division after differentiation of the trophoblast but before formation of the amnion (days 4–8) yields a single placenta, a common chorion, and 2 amnions. (This accounts for about two-thirds of monozygotic twinning.)

3. Division after differentiation of the amnion (days 8–13) results in a single placenta, 1 (common) chorion, and 1 (common) amnion. This is rare.

4. Division later than day 15 may result in incomplete twinning. Just prior to that time (days 13–15), division may result in conjoined twins.

At delivery, the membranous T-shaped septum or dividing membrane of the placenta between the twins must be inspected and sectioned for evidence of the probable type of twinning (Fig 17–2). Monozygotic twins most commonly have a transparent (< 2 mm) septum made up of 2 amniotic membranes only (no chorion and no decidua). Dizygotic twins almost always have an opaque (thick) septum made up of 2 chorions, 2 amnions, and intervening decidua.

A monochorionic placenta can be identified by stripping away the amnion or amnions to reveal a single chorion over a common placenta. In virtually every case of monochorionic placenta, vascular communications between the 2 parts of the placenta can be identified by careful dissection or injection. In contrast, dichorionic placentas (of dizygotic twinning) only rarely have an anastomosis between the fetal blood vessels.

Placental and membrane examination is a certain indicator of zygosity in twins with monochorionic placentas because these are always monozygotic. Overall, approximately 1% of twins are monoamniotic, and these too are monozygotic. Determination of zygosity is clinically significant in case intertwin organ transplantation is needed later in life, as well as for assessing obstetric risks. Monozygotic twins can rarely be discordant for phenotypic sex when 1 twin is phenotypically female as a result of Turner's syndrome (45,XO) and its sibling is male (46,XY).

Monochorionic placentation is associated with more disease processes as a result of placental vascular problems. Inequities of the placental circulation in 1 area (marginal insertion, partial infarction, or thinning) may lead to growth discordance between the twins. Because of vascular anastomoses in monochorionic placentation, multifetal reduction can only be performed with dichorionic placentation.

The most serious problem with monochorionic placentas is local shunting of blood—also called **twin-twin transfusion syndrome.** This occurs because of vascular anastomoses to each twin that are established early in embryonic life. The possible communications are artery to artery, vein to vein, and combinations of these. Artery-to-vein communication is by far the most seri-

Figure 17–2. Amniotic membranes of twins. (Reproduced, with permission, from Benson RC: *Handbook of Obstetrics & Gynecology*, 8th ed. Lange, 1983.)

ous; it is most likely to cause twin-twin transfusion. In uncompensated cases, the twins, although genetically identical, differ greatly in size and appearance. The recipient twin is plethoric, edematous, and hypertensive. Ascites and kernicterus are likely. The heart, liver, and kidneys are enlarged (glomerulotubular hypertrophy). Hydramnios follows fetal polyuria. Although ruddy and apparently healthy, the recipient twin with hypervolemia may die of heart failure during the first 24 hours after birth. The donor twin is small, pallid, and dehydrated (from growth restriction, malnutrition, and hypovolemia). Oligohydramnios may be present. Severe anemia, due to chronic blood loss to the other twin, may lead to hydrops and heart failure.

Various modes of treatment have been advocated for twin transfusion syndrome, including amnioreduction, amniotic septotomy, and laser ablation of communicating vessels. In a recent randomized trial, laser ablation has been shown to be the superior treatment, although access to the procedure is limited because experience with the technique is not broadly available.

Both twins are threatened by prolapse of the cord. The second twin may be harmed by premature separation of the placenta, hypoxia, constriction ring dystocia, operative manipulation, or prolonged anesthesia.

Velamentous insertion of the cord occurs in approximately 7% of twins but in only 1% of singletons. There is a corresponding increase in the potentially catastrophic vasa previa. The incidence of 2-vessel cord (single umbilical artery) is 4–5 times higher in monozygotic twins than in singletons.

Monochorionic, monoamniotic twins (1:100 sets of twins) have a < 90% likelihood of both surviving because of cord entanglement that compromises fetoplacental blood flow. Some authors advocate planned cesarean delivery at 32–34 weeks in an attempt to prevent in utero demise due to cord accidents, as well as continuous external fetal monitoring from approximately 27 weeks until delivery.

B. FETAL

Earlier and more precise sonography has revealed the incidence of multiple gestation is 3.29–5.39% before 12 weeks. However, in > 20% of such cases, 1 or more of the pregnancies spontaneously disappears ("vanishing twin"). Although this event may be associated with vaginal bleeding, the prognosis remains good for the remaining twin.

Major malformations are present in approximately 2% of twin infants, compared with 1% of singletons, whereas minor malformations are found in 4% of twins compared with approximately 2.5% in singletons. Monozygotic twins are at higher risk than dizygotic twins.

Conjoined or Siamese twins result from incomplete segmentation of a single fertilized ovum between the 13th and 14th days; if cleavage is further postponed,

incomplete twinning (2 heads, 1 body) may occur. Lesser abnormalities are also noted, but they occur without regard to specific organ systems. Conjoined twins are described by site of union: pygopagus (at the sacrum), thoracopagus (at the chest), craniopagus (at the heads), and omphalopagus (at the abdominal wall). Curiously, conjoined twins usually are female. Numerous conjoined twins have survived separation.

Each twin and its placenta generally weigh less than the newborn and placenta of a singleton pregnancy after the 30th week, but near term the aggregate weight may approach twice that of a singleton. In general, the larger the number of fetuses, the greater the degree of growth restriction. Interestingly, multifetal reduction of triplets to twins before 12 weeks results in a growth pattern typical of twins rather than triplets, who are growth restricted compared with twins. Thus the number of fetuses residing in the uterus later in pregnancy, and not their embryonic potential, seems to govern growth. Normal-weight twins that differ considerably in birthweight commonly have diamniotic-dichorionic placentas. This suggests independent intrauterine growth of co-twins. The converse is true of twins with fused diamniotic-dichorionic placentas. Low-birth-weight monochorionic twins are the rule rather than the exception. Low birthweight in the various types of multiple pregnancy probably is evidence of growth restriction due to inadequate nutrition. This is at least partially responsible for the much higher early neonatal mortality rate of newborns from multiple births.

Prematurity is the major reason for the increased risk of neonatal death and morbidity in twins. Growth restriction, competition for nutrition, cord compression and entanglement, and operative delivery also are responsible for a significant part of the perinatal mortality rate in multiple pregnancy.

In growth-restricted human fetuses, the brain and heart seem to be relatively less affected than the liver or peripheral musculature. Because placental growth and function are limited, hormone alterations may develop to trigger early labor. Moreover, restricted fetal growth has a small but lasting effect on postnatal physical development.

In late pregnancy, the fetus is jeopardized by the frequency of premature delivery, abnormal presentation and position, and hydramnios.

A fetus acardiacus is a parasitic monozygotic fetus without a heart. It is thought to develop from reversed circulation, perfused by 1 arterial-arterial and 1 venous-venous anastomosis. This represents twin reversed arterial perfusion (TRAP) syndrome. The otherwise normal donor twin is at risk for cardiac hypertrophy and failure and has a 35% mortality. Various methods of cord occlusion can be accomplished by in utero therapy.

Fetus papyraceous is a small, blighted, mummified fetus usually discovered at the delivery of a well-developed newborn. This occurs in 1 in 17,000–20,000 pregnancies. The cause is thought to be death of 1 twin, amniotic fluid loss, or reabsorption and compression of the dead fetus by the surviving twin.

Clinical Findings

With the ready availability of ultrasound, twin gestations are not commonly undiagnosed before labor and delivery. Early diagnosis facilitates appropriate prenatal care.

A. SYMPTOMS AND SIGNS

All of the common annoyances of pregnancy are more troublesome in multiple pregnancy. The effects of multiple pregnancy on the patient include earlier and more severe pressure in the pelvis, nausea, backache, varicosities, constipation, hemorrhoids, abdominal distention, and difficulty in breathing. A "large pregnancy" may be indicative of twinning (distended uterus). Fetal activity is greater and more persistent in twinning than in singleton pregnancy.

Considering the possibility of multiple pregnancy is essential to early diagnosis. In most clinical settings, the diagnosis of twins is made by routine ultrasound examination. If routine ultrasound is not performed, the following signs should alert the physician to the possibility or definite presence of multiple pregnancy:

1. Uterus larger than expected (> 4 cm) for dates.
2. Excessive maternal weight gain that is not explained by edema or obesity.
3. Polyhydramnios, manifested by uterine size out of proportion to the calculated duration of gestation, is almost 10 times more common in multiple pregnancy.
4. Outline or ballottement of more than 1 fetus.
5. Multiplicity of small parts.
6. Simultaneous recording of different fetal heart rates, each asynchronous with the mother's pulse and with each other and varying by at least 8 bpm. (The fetal heart rate may be accelerated by pressure or displacement.)

Some of the common complications in early pregnancy may also occur as a result of multiple gestation. For example, maternal bleeding in the first trimester can indicate threatened or spontaneous abortion; however, the dead fetus may be 1 of twins, as demonstrated by real-time ultrasonography (1 anechoic or hypoechoic amniotic sac and 1 normal sac). In the second and third trimesters, the demise of 1 fetus in a multiple gestation may trigger disseminated intravascular coagulation ("dead fetus syndrome"), just as a singleton intrauterine demise might. This complication is very rarely seen and generally becomes a problem only 3 weeks or more after fetal demise.

B. LABORATORY FINDINGS

The majority of multiple pregnancies are currently identified by ultrasound or by maternal serum screening. Indeed, identification of multiple gestation is so important for the institution of appropriate care that many authorities recommend routine ultrasonic scanning at 18–20 weeks. First-trimester ultrasonography is even more helpful for determining chorionicity.

The hematocrit and hemoglobin values and the red cell count usually are considerably reduced, in direct relationship to the increased blood volume. Indeed, maternal hypochromic normocytic anemia occurs so frequently in multiple pregnancy that it has been suggested that all patients with the process be suspected of having a multiple gestation. Fetal demand for iron increases beyond the mother's ability to assimilate iron in the second trimester.

Glucose tolerance tests demonstrate that both gestational diabetes mellitus and gestational hypoglycemia are much higher in multiple gestation compared with findings in singleton pregnancy. Glucose screening is the standard of care in multiple pregnancy.

C. PRENATAL DIAGNOSIS

The usual indications for prenatal diagnosis and counseling in a singleton pregnancy also apply to twin and higher-order gestations. Because the incidence of twin gestation increases with maternal age, women with multiple gestations are often candidates for prenatal genetic diagnosis. As the risk of aneuploidy is increased, some centers offer invasive testing to all patients carrying multiple gestation who will be older than 33 years at delivery. Genetic counseling should make clear to the patient the need to obtain a sample from each fetus, the risk of a chromosomal abnormality, potential complications of the procedure, the possibility of discordant results, and the ethical and technical concerns when 1 fetus is found to be abnormal.

In twin pregnancies not accompanied by neural tube defects, the median maternal serum α-fetoprotein level will be 2.5 that of the median level for singleton pregnancies at 14–20 weeks' gestation. The levels in triplets and quadruplets are 3 and 4 times as high, respectively. A value > 4.5 times the median is considered abnormal and requires a targeted ultrasound and possible amniocentesis for determination of amniotic fluid α-fetoprotein and acetylcholinesterase levels. Serum screening is less effective in multiple pregnancy, with triple screening detecting only 47% of Down syndrome pregnancies. Nuchal translucency screening with first-trimester serum markers can detect approximately 70% of Down syndrome fetuses in twin pregnancies.

Both amniocentesis and chorionic villus sampling (CVS) can be performed in women with multiple gestation in experienced centers. Documentation of the location of the fetuses and the membrane separating the sacs is important in case of discordance for aneuploidy. Selective termination of an aneuploid fetus can be performed via ultrasound-guided intracardiac injection of potassium chloride. The pregnancy then can continue carrying the normal twin only. Multifetal reduction may be performed to decrease the risk of serious perinatal morbidity and mortality associated with preterm delivery by reducing the number of fetuses from 3 or more to twins.

D. ULTRASOUND FINDINGS

Ultrasonography is the preferred imaging modality for diagnosis of multiple gestation and is potentially able to differentiate multiple gestation as early as 4 weeks (by intravaginal probe). Dichorionicity is suggested by fetuses of different genders, separate placentas, a thick (> 2 mm) dividing membrane, or a "twin peak sign" in which the membrane inserts into 2 fused placentas. In the absence of these findings, monochorionicity is likely. A first-trimester scan is highly recommended because definitive diagnosis of chorionicity may not be possible with second- and third-trimester scans.

Both twins present as vertex in almost 50% of cases. Twin A will be vertex and twin B will be breech in slightly > 33% of cases (Fig 17–3). Both fetuses will be breech presentations in 10% of cases, and almost that many will be single (or double) transverse presentations. Approximately 70% of first twins present by the vertex. Breech presentation occurs in slightly > 25%. Overall, nonvertex presentation occurs 10 times more often in multiple pregnancy than in singleton pregnancy.

Differential Diagnosis

Multiple pregnancy must be distinguished from the following conditions.

A. SINGLETON PREGNANCY

Inaccurate dates may give a false impression of the duration of the pregnancy, and the fetus may be larger than expected.

B. POLYHYDRAMNIOS

Either single or multiple pregnancy may be associated with excessive accumulation of fluid.

C. HYDATIDIFORM MOLE

Although usually easily distinguished from multiple gestation, this complication must be considered in diagnosis early in pregnancy.

D. ABDOMINAL TUMORS COMPLICATING PREGNANCY

Fibroid tumors of the uterus, when present in great numbers, are readily identified. Ovarian tumors are generally

***Figure 17–3.* Left:** Both twins presenting by the vertex. **Right:** One vertex and one breech presentation. (Reproduced, with permission, from Benson RC: *Handbook of Obstetrics & Gynecology*, 8th ed. Lange, 1983.)

single, discrete, and harder to diagnose. A distended bladder or full rectum may elevate the pregnant uterus.

E. COMPLICATED TWIN PREGNANCY

If 1 dizygotic twin dies early in pregnancy and the other lives, the dead fetus may become flattened and mummified (fetus papyraceous; see section on Pathologic Factors Associated with Twinning, B. Fetal). Its portion of a fused placenta will be pale and atrophic, but remnants of 2 sacs and 2 cords may be found. If 1 twin dies in late pregnancy, considerable enlargement of the uterus persists, although the findings on palpation may be unusual and only 1 fetal heartbeat will be heard. Ultrasonography can confirm the diagnosis.

Prevention

A. MULTIPLE PREGNANCY

Although ovulation induction agents result in fewer multiple pregnancies when used by experts, even in the best of hands some multiple pregnancies inevitably will occur. For example, clomiphene citrate induction of multiple ovulation increases the rate of dizygotic pregnancy to 5–10%.

With many forms of ART (eg, ovulation induction, in vitro fertilization), iatrogenic multiple pregnancies regularly occur in which the number of fetuses is so great that they may preclude any being carried to the point of viability. When this occurs, many authorities recommend multifetal pregnancy reduction by transabdominal intracardiac potassium injection. Efforts are underway to recommend limiting the number of embryos transferred; legislation to this effect has been enacted in the United Kingdom.

B. COMPLICATIONS OF MULTIPLE PREGNANCY

To prevent the complications of multiple pregnancy, it is imperative to make the diagnosis as early in pregnancy as possible. Later in pregnancy, ultrasonography is useful for monitoring the growth of the fetuses and for detecting gross anomalies. Routine growth scans on twins are recommended every 4 weeks in the third trimester or more frequently if growth restriction is detected. Recall that the risk of fetal anomalies in twins is approximately 3 times that in singleton pregnancy.

Enhanced antenatal care assists in improving outcome. The most commonly used techniques are iron and calcium supplementation, vitamin and folic acid administration (in an attempt to prevent anemia), a high-protein diet, and more weight gain than usual (ideal weight for height plus 35–45 lb). Supplementation with magnesium, zinc, as well essential fatty acids also have been recommended.

Insufficient evidence is available to suggest a policy of routine hospitalization for bed rest in multiple pregnancy because no reduction in the risk of preterm birth or perinatal death is observed. There is also no evidence that prophylactic cerclage improves outcome. More frequent antenatal visits are scheduled, and several authorities recommend closely following cervical length by ultrasound. Rescue cerclage can be offered for a short cervix (< 1.5 cm) or a large funnel of membranes prior to 24 weeks. Early and prompt therapy for any complications (eg, vaginal infections, preeclampsia–eclampsia) should be instituted, bearing in mind that preeclampsia–eclampsia is a common complication of multiple pregnancy.

Tocolytic drugs may suppress premature labor and extend gestation by 48 hours so that the effects of steroids can be realized. There is no evidence that long-term oral or intravenous tocolysis improves outcome. Most authorities recommend starting with intravenous magnesium sulfate. If terbutaline is used, very close monitoring for pulmonary edema must be maintained, because this complication is much more likely with administration of β-mimetic agents in multiple gestation. Also, because indomethacin may influence fetal ductal constriction, it should not be used after 32 weeks' gestation. Fetal fibronectin can be helpful, particularly when negative, to determine how aggressively to administer tocolytics.

In cases of antepartum bleeding or hydramnios, try to delay the delivery until each twin weighs at least 2000 g or until fetal lung maturity can be documented, usually after 34 weeks' gestation.

All patients with multiple pregnancy should be delivered in a well-equipped hospital by an experienced physician who has adequate assistance. It is desirable to

have a pediatrician (or neonatologist) in attendance. Delivery must be done in the operating room in case an emergent cesarean section is needed for twin B. An early epidural is recommended; in case of emergent cesarean section, anesthesia is already established and general anesthesia can usually be avoided. Prematurity, trauma of manipulative delivery, and associated asphyxia are the major preventable causes of morbidity and mortality in twins, especially the second twin.

Treatment

A. LABOR AND DELIVERY

Admit the patient to the hospital at the first sign of labor or if leakage of amniotic fluid or significant bleeding occurs. An ultrasound evaluation should be performed to ascertain the presentation of each fetus and its estimated fetal weight. Routine, continuous electronic fetal heart rate monitoring is recommended. Labor should be conducted so that immediate cesarean section can be performed if required. A pediatric team for each infant plus obstetric and anesthesiologic attendants should be present. Insert an intravenous line and send a specimen of blood for typing, antibody screening, and complete blood count.

If either twin shows signs of persistent compromise, proceed promptly to cesarean delivery. Other indications for primary cesarean section include (but are not limited to) compound or monoamniotic twins and probable twin-twin transfusion syndrome (gross disparity in fetal size) and placenta previa. In the United States, all triplets warrant cesarean delivery.

In a woman with a previous lower-segment cesarean scar, limited literature suggests that delivery of twins does not mandate a repeat cesarean section in the absence of other complications. Concomitant with increasing rates of elective and nonelective cesarean section, cesarean delivery by patient request is becoming more common. In addition, less resident training in vaginal breech delivery can decrease a clinician's comfort with breech extraction of a second twin.

Management of twins that are candidates for vaginal delivery may proceed as outlined in the following. Intrapartum twin presentations may be classified (1) twin A and twin B vertex (slightly > 40% of all twins), (2) twin A vertex and twin B nonvertex (almost 40%), or (3) twin A nonvertex and twin B vertex, breech, or transverse (approximately 20%).

The current intrapartum management of twins is as follows. For vertex-vertex presentations in labor (category 1), vaginal delivery of both twins may be chosen in the absence of standard indications for cesarean section delivery. Of course, if either twin develops fetal distress, cesarean delivery should be performed. Category 2 twins, each weighing more than 2000 g, can usually be managed successfully by vaginal delivery of both. This is generally accomplished by total breech extraction of twin B immediately after the delivery of twin A. External cephalic version of twin B has also been described. When either twin A or both twins are nonvertex (category 3), primary cesarean section should be performed. This is also sometimes recommended in cases of nonvertex twin B where the estimated fetal weight is much greater than that of twin A. The ultrasound machine should be present in the operating room to confirm the presentation of twin B after the delivery of twin A.

Difficult forceps operation or rapid extraction should be avoided, but forceps to protect the aftercoming premature head may be useful. The umbilical cord should be clamped promptly to prevent the second twin of a monozygotic twin pregnancy from exsanguinating into the first born.

Perform a vaginal examination immediately after delivery of twin A to note the presentation of the second twin, the presence of a second sac, an occult cord prolapse, or cord entanglement.

Cut the cord as far outside the vagina as possible so that it can hang loose to permit vaginal examination or manipulation. This eliminates inadvertent cord traction on the placenta. Tag and label the cords (twin A and twin B) so that they can be associated with the proper placenta or placentas.

Use external version whenever possible for conversion of twin B from breech to vertex. Cautious rupture of the second sac will allow slow loss of fluid while twin B's vertex is being gently guided into the inlet. The amount of time between delivery of twin A and twin B is still a matter of controversy. If electronic fetal monitoring suggests fetal well-being, delivery of twin B within 30 minutes is not necessary.

One twin may obstruct the delivery of both fetuses in locked twins. In this circumstance, twin A is always a breech and twin B is a vertex presentation. The heads become impacted in the pelvis. Locked twins can be avoided by cesarean delivery in all cases in which twin A is not vertex. However, if the obstetrician is presented with a case of locked twins (Fig 17–4), having an assistant support the twin already partially delivered as a breech while pushing both heads upward out of the pelvis with rotation of both fetuses may accomplish delivery of the first twin. This process may require deep anesthesia. If this cannot be done, cesarean with abdominal delivery of both fetuses may be the safest route. An alternative procedure while cesarean preparations are underway is to elevate the partially delivered twin, establish an airway, and protect the cord.

Postpartum hemorrhage is common in multiple pregnancy. Increased intravenous oxytocin, elevation, and light massage of the fundus and an intravenous ergot or prostaglandin product (only after the last fetus

Figure 17–4. Locked twins. (Reproduced, with permission, from Benson RC: *Handbook of Obstetrics & Gynecology,* 4th ed. Lange, 1971.)

is delivered) may be required. After delivery, if separation of the placenta is delayed or bleeding is brisk, manual extraction of the placenta may be necessary. Send the placenta, cord, and membranes to the pathology laboratory to assist in determining whether the fetuses are monozygotic or dizygotic.

Preeclampsia–eclampsia and premature labor and delivery are managed as outlined in Chapters 15 and 19.

Complications

A. MATERNAL

The incidence of spontaneous abortion of at least 1 of several fetuses is increased in multiple pregnancy. Stillbirth occurs twice as often among twins as among singleton pregnancies. Premature labor and delivery as well as premature rupture of the membranes are also greatly increased. The average gestational age at delivery is 36–37 weeks for twins, 33 weeks for triplets, and 31 weeks for quadruplets. Efforts to reduce the incidence of prematurity thus far have been largely unsuccessful.

Placenta previa may be responsible for antepartum bleeding, malpresentation, or unengagement of the first fetus. A large placenta (or placentas) and possibly fundal scarring or tumor may lead to low implantation of the placenta. Premature separation of the placenta may occur antepartum, perhaps in association with preeclampsia–eclampsia or rupture of membranes of twin A and the initiation of strong uterine contractions, or after the delivery of the first twin. Careless traction on the first cord may encourage early partial separation of the placenta.

Hypochromic normocytic anemia is 2–3 times more common in multiple pregnancy than in singleton pregnancy. Urinary tract infection is at least twice as frequent in multiple pregnancy as in singleton pregnancy because of increased ureteral dilatation secondary to a higher serum progesterone level and greater uterine pressure on the ureters. Preeclampsia–eclampsia occurs approximately 3 times more often in multiple pregnancy than in singleton pregnancy.

A thinned uterine wall, secondary to unusually large uterine contents, is associated with hypotonic uterine contractions and a longer latent stage of labor. However, prolonged labor is uncommon in multiple pregnancy because rupture of the membranes generally is followed by improvements in the uterine contraction pattern. Uterine atony often is accompanied by excessive loss of blood postpartum owing to inability of the overdistended uterus to contract well and remain contracted after delivery.

When 2 separate placentas are present, 1 of them may deliver immediately after the first twin. Although the second twin may not be compromised, it is best to proceed with its delivery, both for its protection and to conserve maternal blood.

Operative intervention is more likely in multiple pregnancy because of increased obstetric problems such as malpresentation, prolapsed cord, and fetal distress.

B. FETAL

Fetal death is approximately 3 times more common in multiple pregnancy than in singleton pregnancy. Death may be the result of developmental anomalies, cord compression, or placental disorders. The greatest hazard from cord compression is cord entanglement of monozygotic twins with only 1 amniotic sac. Developmental anomalies and polyhydramnios are common in monozygotic twins.

Almost twice as many monozygotic as dizygotic twins die in the perinatal period. Attrition is even greater for triplets, quadruplets, and higher-order pregnancies. Even so, preterm delivery and intrapartum complications are the most common causes of fetal loss in multiple pregnancy. All too frequently preterm delivery is occasioned by premature rupture of the membranes, which occurs in approximately 25% of twin, 50% of triplet, and 75% of quadruplet pregnancies.

Abnormal and breech presentation, circulatory interference by 1 fetus with the other, and operative delivery all increase fetal loss. Prolapse of the cord occurs 5 times more often in multiple pregnancy than in singleton pregnancy. Premature separation of the placenta before delivery of the second twin may cause death of the second twin by hypoxia.

Neonatal outcome is very much dependent on gestational age at delivery. In general, morbidity and mortality rates are similar for twins and singletons of equivalent gestational ages. Many outcome data are stratified according to birthweight. Therefore, the slowing of growth in the third trimester can give twin fetuses the advantage of increased gestational age for weight. Advances in neonatal intensive care have made survival possible even at 23 weeks' gestation, although usually with considerable morbidity, including but not limited to intraventricular hemorrhage, chronic lung disease, and necrotizing enterocolitis. Because intact survival is much more likely after 34 weeks, prolonging gestation at least to this point when possible is desirable. The adage "1 day in utero saves 2 days in intensive care" applies to the economic as well as the emotional costs of caring for premature infants.

It is imperative that an experienced physician be present for resuscitation and stabilization of each infant born premature. Antenatal diagnosis of multiple gestation facilitates delivery at an appropriate center. Delivery before week 36 is twice as frequent in twin pregnancies as in singleton pregnancies. Intracranial injury is more common in premature infants, even those delivered spontaneously. An increased risk of cerebral palsy is found in twins, especially very low-birthweight babies, and in liveborn co-twins of fetuses who died in utero.

Treatment of twin-twin transfusion syndrome in utero remains experimental. After delivery, therapy includes replacing blood in the donor twin to correct fluid and electrolyte imbalance. In the recipient twin, phlebotomy is necessary until normal venous pressure is restored. Often, other therapy for cardiac failure (eg, digitalis) is necessary.

Prognosis

The U.S. maternal mortality rate for multiple pregnancy is only slightly higher than for singleton pregnancy. A history of previous dizygotic twins increases the likelihood of subsequent multiple pregnancy 10-fold. Hemorrhage is approximately 5 times as frequent in multiple pregnancies as in single pregnancies. The probability of abnormal presentation and of operative delivery and its complications is increased in multiple pregnancy. Premature rupture of the membranes and premature labor, often with a long prodromal phase, are common occurrences in multiple pregnancy. A gravida with a multiple pregnancy has approximately 5 times the likelihood of having a morbid (febrile, complicated) course as an average patient of the same parity with a single fetus.

Hydramnios is 5 times more frequent in multiple pregnancies as in singleton pregnancies, principally because of fetal abnormality. Perinatal mortality and morbidity rates are increased in multiple pregnancy, mainly because of preterm delivery and its complications (eg, trauma or asphyxia).

Almost 50% of twins weigh < 2500 g, but the majority of these twins are of 36 weeks' gestational age or more. Directly or indirectly, multiple pregnancies are responsible for approximately 15% of premature births and approximately 9% of perinatal deaths, a rate 7 times that of single births. Approximately 55% of twins are premature; 80% of perinatal deaths occur in those born before 31 weeks' gestation, and 93% of deaths are in those with birthweight < 1500 g. The incidence of intrauterine growth restriction is increased in multiple gestation, and multiple gestations account for 17% of infants with intrauterine growth restriction. Congenital malformations and abnormal presentation are more serious in monozygous twins. Preeclampsia–eclampsia, diabetes mellitus, and other disorders may further jeopardize the fetuses.

Efforts to reduce the incidence of prematurity have not met with much success in singletons or in multiple gestations. In order to maximize fetal growth, good nutrition, frequent rest periods, and cessation of smoking are encouraged. Approximately 90% of twins born at greater than 28 weeks survive.

Recent studies have found that neonatal morbidity is reduced when delivery occurs at approximately 38 weeks, so routine induction at that time is recommended.

The comparative occurrence of perinatal death (per 1000) for single and multiple pregnancy are as follows: singletons, 39; twins, 152; triplets, 309; and quadruplets, 509. The rates are proportionately higher for higher-order pregnancies.

Central nervous system disease and respiratory disease are frequently diagnosed in the surviving second twin.

Discordance noted at birth is associated with a slower weight gain during extrauterine life. A twin whose birthweight is < 20% that of its partner will not gain as rapidly and may never catch up with the other twin with regard to weight and height. The IQ of the larger monozygotic twin is likely to be higher than that of the smaller twin if the weight difference is > 300 g at birth. The female twin of a female–male pair who survives cross-transfusion is not sterile (in contrast to the situation encountered in the bovine freemartin).

Concordance of placental examination, clinical comparisons, and hematologic and serologic tests provides presumptive evidence of monozygotic twinning. The total probability of diagnosis of zygosity is > 95% using ABO, MNSs, Rh, Kell, Kidd, Duffy, and Lewis A and B antigens, and approaches 100% using chromosomal analysis.

In comprehensive perinatal care centers, morbidity and mortality rates decrease greatly. In a report of triplets receiving optimal care, the mean weight at delivery was 1779 g, and the incidence of neonatal mortality was only 23 in 1000. First twins have an approximately 3% greater chance of survival than do second twins.

REFERENCES

American College of Obstetricians and Gynecologists: *Multiple Gestation: Complicated Twin, Triplet and Higher-Order Multifetal Pregnancy.* ACOG Practice Bulletin No. 56. American College of Obstetricians and Gynecologists, 2004.

Blickstein I: Growth aberration in multiple pregnancy. Obstet Gynecol Clin North Am 2005;32:39.

Bush MC, Malone FD: Down syndrome screening in twins. Clin Perinatol 2005;32:373.

Cleary-Goldman J, D'Alton M: Management of single fetal demise in a multiple gestation. Obstet Gynecol Surv 2004;59:285.

Crowther CA: Hospitalization and bed rest for multiple pregnancy (Cochrane Review). Cochrane Database Sys Rev 2001;(1):CD000110.

Dodd JM, Crowther CA: Elective delivery of women with a twin pregnancy from 37 weeks' gestation. Cochrane Database Syst Rev 2003;(1):CD003582.

Evans MI et al: Update on selective reduction. Prenat Diagn 2005;9:807.

Harkness UF, Crombleholme TM: Twin-twin transfusion syndrome: Where do we go from here? Semin Perinatol 2005;29:296.

Healy AJ, Gaddipati S: Intrapartum management of twins: Truths and controversies. Clin Perinatol 2005;32:455.

Heyborne KD et al; Obstetrix/Pediatrix Research Study Group: Improved perinatal survival of monoamniotic twins with intensive inpatient monitoring. Am J Obstet Gynecol 2005;192:96.

Hogle KL et al: Cesarean delivery for twins: A systematic review and meta-analysis. Am J Obstet Gynecol 2003;188:220.

Lewi L et al: Pregnancy and infant outcome of 80 consecutive cord coagulations in complicated monochorionic multiple pregnancies. Am J Obstet Gynecol 2006;194:782.

Luke B: Nutrition and multiple gestation. Semin Perinatol 2005;29:349.

Nakhuda GS, Sauer MV: Addressing the growing problem of multiple gestations created by assisted reproductive therapies. Semin Perinatol 2005;29:355.

Oleszczuk JJ, Keith LG, Oleszczuk AK: The paradox of old maternal age in multiple pregnancies. Obstet Gynecol Clin North Am 2005;32:69.

Rochon M, Stone J: Invasive procedures in multiple gestations. Curr Opin Obstet Gynecol 2003;15:167.

Rustico MA et al: Managing twins discordant for fetal anomaly. Prenat Diagn 2005;25:766.

Shetty A, Smith AP: The sonographic diagnosis of chorionicity. Prenat Diagn 2005;25:735.

Spadola AC, Simpson LL: Selective termination procedures in monochorionic pregnancies. Semin Perinatol 2005;29:330.

Sperling L et al: How to identify twins at low risk of spontaneous preterm delivery. Ultrasound Obstet Gynecol 2005;26138.

Diabetes Mellitus & Pregnancy 18

Stacy L. Strehlow, MD, Jeffrey S. Greenspoon, MD, Carla Janzen, MD, & Sue M. Palmer, MD

Diabetes mellitus is the most common medical complication of pregnancy. The Centers for Disease Control and Prevention estimated that 20.8 million persons in the United States had diabetes in 2005. Minority groups are disproportionately affected. Diabetes is undiagnosed in nearly one-third of adults with the condition.

Preexisting (type 1 or type 2) diabetes mellitus affects approximately 1–3 per 1000 pregnancies. Although preconception care and glycemic control are advised, pregnancy will be the first time many women present for medical care. Gestational diabetes mellitus (GDM) is defined as any degree of glucose intolerance with first recognition during pregnancy. GDM complicates approximately 4% of pregnancies. Women with GDM have an approximately 50% risk of developing type 2 diabetes over the next 10 years. Pregnancy affords a unique opportunity to diagnose or possibly prevent diabetes among women at risk to develop type 2 diabetes later in life.

Diabetes during pregnancy poses significant risks to the mother and fetus. With poorly controlled diabetes, spontaneous abortion risk is high, and the rate of major congenital anomalies is 6–12% among women with pregestational diabetes. Diabetic ketoacidosis (DKA) is an immediate threat to maternal and fetal life. Fetal death occurs in approximately 10% of pregnant patients with DKA, which is an improvement from rates of 30–50% in the recent past. GDM increases the risk of fetal macrosomia, which is associated with secondary complications such as operative delivery, shoulder dystocia, and birth trauma. There is an increase in neonatal complications, such as hypoglycemia, respiratory distress syndrome (RDS), hypocalcemia, and hyperbilirubinemia.

Before the introduction of insulin in 1922, diabetic patients often died during the course of their pregnancy. Just 20 years ago, delivery of an unexplained stillbirth from a mother with type 1 diabetes was not uncommon. Today this tragedy is rare, with a reduction in perinatal mortality rate to less than 5%. When diabetic patients receive preconception care, including medical nutrition therapy and insulin therapy as needed to achieve near-normal glycemic goals as well as antepartum fetal surveillance, morbidity and mortality approach that of women with uncomplicated pregnancies. Two decades ago, most diabetics required prolonged hospitalization, but today few require more than a brief hospital stay. This is partly due to the accessibility of self-monitoring of blood glucose level with its concomitant effect on glycemic control.

Currently, the priorities for diabetes care providers are first to identify and control diabetes prior to conception and second to appropriately screen and treat even mild gestational diabetes during pregnancy.

Pathophysiology: Metabolism in Normal & Diabetic Pregnancy

Insulin is an anabolic hormone with essential roles in carbohydrate, fat, and protein metabolism. It promotes the uptake of glucose, storage of glucose as glycogen, lipogenesis, and uptake and utilization of amino acids. The lack of insulin results in hyperglycemia and lipolysis. Elevation of free fatty acids leads to an increase in the formation of ketone bodies, acetoacetate and β-hydroxybutyrate. When blood glucose levels exceed the renal threshold for absorption of filtered glucose, glycosuria occurs and causes an osmotic diuresis with dehydration and electrolyte losses.

Insulin sensitivity decreases as gestation advances in all pregnant women, mainly due to anti-insulin signals produced by the placenta. In the first trimester, increasing maternal estrogen and progesterone levels are associated with a decrease in fasting glucose levels, which reach a nadir by the 12th week. The decrease averages 15 mg/dL; thus, fasting values of 70–80 mg/dL are common by the 10th week of pregnancy.

In the second trimester, as the placenta increases secretion of anti-insulin hormones, higher fasting and postprandial glucose levels occur that facilitate transfer of glucose from mother to fetus. Glucose transfer occurs via a carrier-mediated active transport system that becomes saturated at 250 mg/dL. Fetal glucose levels are 80% of maternal levels. In contrast, maternal amino acid levels are lowered due to active placental transfer to the fetus. Lipid metabolism in the second trimester shows continued storage until midgestation, then enhanced mobilization (lipolysis) as fetal fuel demands increase.

Human placental lactogen (hPL) is the hormone mainly responsible for insulin resistance and lipolysis. hPL also decreases the hunger sensation and diverts maternal carbohydrate metabolism to fat metabolism in the third trimester. hPL is similar in structure to growth hormone and acts by reducing the insulin affinity to insulin receptors. The net effect is to favor placental transfer of glucose to the fetus and to reduce the maternal use of glucose. The hPL levels rise steadily during the first and second trimesters, with a plateau in the late third trimester.

Cortisol levels rise during pregnancy and stimulate endogenous glucose production and glycogen storage and decrease glucose utilization. The "dawn phenomenon" (elevated fasting glucose to facilitate brain metabolism) is marked in normal pregnancies and enhanced even more in women with polycystic ovarian syndrome (PCOS) who conceive. Therefore, pregestational and early pregnancy screening for prediabetes and diabetes are advised for women with PCOS.

Prolactin levels are increased 5- to 10-fold during pregnancy and may impact carbohydrate metabolism. Thus, women with hyperprolactinemia also should undergo early glucose screening.

Fetal Effects

Elevated glucose levels are toxic to the developing fetus, producing an increase in miscarriages and major malformations in direct proportion to the glucose level. These birth defects (Table 18–1) are fatal or seriously deleterious to quality of life and are preventable by preconceptional glucose control. Because malformations occur within the first 8 weeks of gestation, when most women are just beginning prenatal care, preconceptional care is essential for women with diabetes. The hemoglobin A_{1c} level, which reflects the blood glucose concentration over the previous 2 months, can predict the risk for malformations when measured in the first trimester (Table 18–2).

The fetus continues to experience the effects of hyperglycemia beyond the period of organogenesis. Whereas glucose crosses the placenta, insulin does not, leading to increased fetal production of insulin to compensate for its hyperglycemic environment. Higher insulin levels promote increased fetal somatic growth, leading not only to macrosomia and central fat deposition but also to enlargement of internal organs such as the heart.

Diagnostic Criteria for Diabetes Mellitus Prior to Pregnancy

The 3 ways of diagnosing preexisting diabetes mellitus are as follows:

1. Symptoms of diabetes plus random plasma glucose concentration equal to or greater than 200 mg/dL. The classic symptoms of diabetes include polyuria, polydipsia, and unexplained weight loss.

2. Fasting plasma glucose (FPG) equal to or greater than 126 mg/dL. Fasting is defined as no caloric intake for at least 8 hours.

3. Two-hour postload glucose level equal to or greater than 200 mg/dL during an oral glucose tolerance test (OGTT). The test uses a glucose load containing the equivalent of 75 g anhydrous glucose dissolved in water.

In the absence of unequivocal hyperglycemia, these criteria should be confirmed by repeat testing on a different day. The third measure (OGTT) is not recommended for routine clinical use in nonpregnant adults.

Diagnostic Criteria for Gestational Diabetes Mellitus

Risk assessment for GDM is performed at the first prenatal visit in all women who do not already have diagnosed diabetes. Women with risk factors should be screened as soon as feasible. Risk factors include obesity (nonpregnant body mass index ≥ 30), prior history of GDM, heavy glycosuria (> 2+), unexplained stillbirth, prior infant with major malformation, and family history of diabetes in a first-degree relative. If results of testing do not demonstrate diabetes, these

Table 18–1. Some congenital anomalies of infants of diabetic mothers.

Cardiac	Atrial septal defects
	Ventricular septal defects
	Transposition of the great vessels
	Coarctation of the aorta
	Tetralogy of Fallot
	Truncus arteriosus
	Dextrocardia
	Cardiomegaly
Central nervous system	Neural tube defects
	Anencephaly
	Holoprosencephaly
Renal	Hydronephrosis
	Renal agenesis
	Ureteral duplication
Gastrointestinal	Duodenal atresia
	Anorectal atresia
	Omphalocele
Spinal	Caudal regression syndrome, sacral agenesis

Reprinted with permission from Reece EA, Hobbins JC: Diabetes embryopathy, pathogenesis, prenatal diagnosis and prevention. Obstet Gynecol Surv 1986;41:325.

Table 18–2. Relationship between initial pregnancy value of glycosylated hemoglobin and rate of major fetal congenital malformations.

Initial Maternal Hemoglobin A$_{1c}$ Level	Major Congenital Malformations (%)
≤7.9	3.2
8.9–9.9	8.1
≥ 10	23.5

women should be retested between 24 and 28 weeks' gestation. All women of ordinary or high risk should be screened between 24 and 28 weeks' gestation. In the United States, a 2-step approach usually is taken. The first step is a screening test consisting of a 50-g oral glucose challenge test (GCT). Plasma or serum glucose level is measured 1 hour later. The GCT can be performed at any time of day and without regard to time of prior meal. The sensitivity and specificity of the test are related to the cutoff value designated to be an "abnormal" result. A cutoff value of 140 mg/dL has a sensitivity of approximately 80% and results in progression to definitive testing in 14% of patients; a cutoff value of 130 mg/dL has a sensitivity of 90% and results in definitive testing in 24% of patients. Either cutoff value is acceptable. If the GCT result is 180 mg/dL or more, then the FPG should be obtained the next day, before the 3-hour, 100-g OGTT because many of these women can be diagnosed by FPG alone if the FPG is 95 or more.

Screening can be omitted for the small group of women with low risk. The low-risk group comprises women who fulfill all of the following criteria: age less than 25 years, normal body weight, no family history (first-degree relatives) of diabetes, no history of abnormal glucose metabolism or poor obstetric outcome, and not a member of an ethnic/racial group with a high prevalence of diabetes (eg, Hispanic American, Native American, Asian American, African American, Pacific Islander). The American Diabetes Association (ADA) diagnoses GDM based on 2 abnormal results on the 3-hour, 100-g OGTT or on the 2-hour, 75-g OGTT (Table 18–3).

There is increasing evidence that 1 abnormal value is sufficient to adversely affect the fetus; some physicians now use a single abnormal value to initiate treatment. Outside the United States, a 1-step approach using a 75-g oral glucose load is widely used.

During the antenatal period, clinical findings that suggest maternal hyperglycemia, such as fetal weight 70% or greater for gestational age or polyhydramnios (amniotic fluid index ≥ 24 cm) should prompt reevaluation for GDM.

■ PREGESTATIONAL DIABETES

TYPE 1 DIABETES (INSULIN-DEPENDENT)

Type 1 diabetes mellitus (T1DM) results from beta cell destruction, usually leading to absolute insulin deficiency. Onset often occurs in the young. T1DM may appear in older persons and may rarely present during pregnancy. Profound thirst, increased urination, and weight loss or even overt ketoacidosis are the usual symptoms prompting medical evaluation.

T1DM has multiple identified genetic predispositions. Susceptibility to T1DM is increased by a gene or genes located near or within the human leukocyte antigen (HLA) locus on the short arm of chromosome 6 (6p). The risk to offspring of developing T1DM with an affected sibling is 5% if 1 haplotype is shared, 13% for 2 haplotypes, and 2% if no haplotypes are shared. If both parents are affected, the risk of T1DM is 33%. The incidence of type 1 diabetes is 0.1–0.4% (1–4 per 1000) in the general population.

TYPE 2 DIABETES (NONINSULIN DEPENDENT)

Type 2 diabetes mellitus (T2DM) is characterized by insufficient insulin receptors to effect proper glucose control after insulin is released (insulin resistance). Women with T2DM typically have a body habitus consisting of increased abdominal girth, often described as an "apple shape."

T2DM is a multifactorial illness that is influenced by heredity, environment, and lifestyle choices. Although several genes have been associated with T2DM, progression to frank disease can be modified by factors such as diet and exercise. With T2DM, the risk of diabetes in a first-degree relative is almost 15%, and ap-

Table 18–3. Diagnostic criteria for gestational diabetes mellitus.

	100-g Glucose Load (mg/dL)	75-g Glucose Load (mg/dL)
Fasting	95	95
1 hour	180	180
2 hour	155	155
3 hour	140	—

Diagnosis based on ≥ 2 values above listed cutoff values.

proximately 30% more will have impaired glucose tolerance. If both parents have T2DM, the incidence of diabetes in the offspring is 60–75%, although lifestyle modification can decrease the risk.

GESTATIONAL DIABETES

GDM is defined as any degree of glucose intolerance with onset or first recognition during pregnancy. In the majority of GDM cases, glucose levels return to normal after delivery. The risk of recurrence in future pregnancies is at least 60%. The definition applies regardless of which therapies—insulin, diet, activity, or oral hypoglycemics—are used during pregnancy. Clinically unrecognized glucose intolerance may have antedated, or begun concomitantly with, the pregnancy.

Significance

Normal growth and maturation of the fetus are closely associated with the normal delivery of maternal nutrients, especially glucose. The duration and degree of hyperglycemia are directly related to excessive growth, especially in the third trimester. There is an increase in miscarriages, congenital malformations, preterm birth, pyelonephritis, preeclampsia, in utero meconium, fetal heart rate abnormalities, cesarean deliveries, and stillbirths.

Incidence & Etiology

The incidence of gestational diabetes ranges from 1% in rural areas with a predominantly white population to 12% in racially heterogeneous urban regions. However, the increasing prevalence of obesity, metabolic syndrome, and prediabetes make it likely that the incidence of gestational diabetes also will increase.

Pathophysiology

GDM is pathophysiologically similar to T2DM. Women most likely to develop GDM are those who are overweight, with a body habitus often described as an "apple shape." hPL increases insulin resistance and increases in direct relation to the length of gestation. Normally, insulin release by pancreatic beta cells is increased in an attempt to maintain glucose homeostasis. Women with GDM continue to demonstrate postpartum defects in insulin action. These defects include the regulations of glucose clearance, glucose production, and plasma free fatty acid concentrations, together with defects in pancreatic beta-cell function, which precede the development of T2DM.

APPROACH TO DIABETES IN PREGNANCY

Prevention of hyperglycemia through rigorous control of blood glucose level is the mainstay of treatment in the pregnant woman with pregestational diabetes. This is best accomplished by careful preconceptional counseling and achievement of normal hemoglobin A_{1c} levels before pregnancy in pregestational diabetics, frequent (usually 4–5 times per day) home glucose level monitoring, adjustment of diet, and regular exercise.

Nonweight-bearing or low-impact exercise can be initiated or continued. Even short episodes of exercise will sensitize the patient's response to insulin for approximately 24 hours. All care providers should stress the importance of diet. Soluble fiber provides satiety and improves both the number of insulin receptors and their sensitivity. Carbohydrate restriction improves glycemic control and may enable a patient to achieve her glycemic goals using diet and activity. Calories are prescribed at 25–35 kcal/kg of actual body weight, generally 1800–2400 kcal/day. The diet should be 40–50% carbohydrate, 30–40% fat, and 20% protein. Morbidly obese women may have a lower metabolism rate; therefore, begin low and increase calories as needed. When postprandial values exceed the targets, review all recent food intake to adjust food choice, preparation, and portion size.

Self-monitoring of fasting, 1- or 2-hour postprandial, and nighttime blood glucose levels using a glucose meter provides instant feedback to assess the patient's diet and behavior. When the glycemic goals are met, the feedback is a powerful motivator. Diet and/or activity errors are identified and corrected as needed. Optimal glucose levels during pregnancy are fasting levels of 70–95 mg/dL and 1-hour postprandial values less than 140 mg/dL or 2-hour postprandial values less than 120 mg/dL.

A minimum of 2 visits to a dietitian improves education and active participation regarding diet. Food records are useful. The dietitian reviews content and calories and suggests how to include favorite ethnic foods to improve compliance. Other family members should be encouraged to participate in the dietary education because their understanding and support increase the chance for a successful diet. Often, the other family members will benefit from the healthful diet changes. Additional follow-up visits between patient and dietitian are important when glycemic goals are not reached, weight change is too great or too small, or the patient is having difficulty maintaining the diet.

Insulin therapy is added when necessary to achieve goals. The addition of insulin should not be presented or perceived as a failure or a punishment. Insulin is simply the next rational step to achieving worthwhile glycemic goals.

Patient resistance should be addressed with support, reassurance, and education by diabetes health provider team members. There are different approaches to introducing insulin, but the plan should be as simple as possible.

Subcutaneous insulin pumps may be considered in highly motivated patients and should not be discontinued in women who began the pump prior to conception. Use of subcutaneous pumps during pregnancy has been associated with better control of hyperglycemia and increased patient satisfaction.

When pharmacologic therapy is required during pregnancy, insulin has long been the treatment of choice. However, recent evidence suggests that glyburide or metformin are safe and effective alternatives. Until further research is done, treatment with oral hypoglycemics should be limited and individualized.

ANTEPARTUM CARE

Care of the insulin-dependent pregestational diabetic must be intensive. The initial evaluation of a patient, ideally done prior to conception, includes assessment of other end-organ damage. A comprehensive eye examination for retinopathy should be performed annually. When a patient is already pregnant at time of presentation, the rapid introduction of tight glycemic control may worsen retinopathy. Thus, gradually achievement of euglycemia is best accomplished before conception. If needed, laser therapy can be performed during pregnancy. Renal function is assessed with a serum creatinine level and a 24-hour urine collection or urinary albumin/creatinine ratio to measure protein excretion. In patients with T1DM, thyroid function should be evaluated because of increased rates of thyroid disease. Electrocardiography can be performed on patients older than 30 years or who have disease duration of more than 5 years. Prenatal vitamins should be started with supplementation of at least 0.4 mg of folate daily.

Gestational age should be confirmed with a first-trimester ultrasound examination. In all pregestational diabetics, a fetal ultrasound for anatomy, including the heart, should be completed at 18–20 weeks. Additional tests to screen for anomalies should be offered, if available, such as first-trimester nuchal translucency and serum screening and/or second-trimester triple or quadruple screening.

Women with diabetes have triple the rate of asymptomatic bacteriuria compared to other pregnant women. A urine culture is obtained at the initial visit. After administration of a complete course of appropriate antibiotic treatment, a repeat culture (test of cure) is performed to confirm cure. The development of edema, including carpal tunnel syndrome, is monitored because of the increased risk of preeclampsia in patients with diabetes.

Evaluation of maternal glycemic control by self-monitoring of blood glucose level and of fetal growth and development by ultrasound are essential. Excellent glycemic control in a nonsmoking woman without end-organ disease from the diabetes increases the chance for a more normal outcome. Patients with poor glycemic control, often suggested by fetal macrosomia or polyhydramnios, are at increased risk for poor pregnancy outcome. Surveillance for fetal well-being often begins at 32 weeks' gestation in patients with end-organ disease using a twice-weekly nonstress test (NST) or the modified biophysical profile (BPP) done twice weekly by measuring the fetal heart rate and the amniotic fluid volume. A weekly BPP is similarly useful. Women without end-organ disease who require insulin often begin fetal monitoring at 32–34 weeks. Women with diet-controlled gestational diabetes usually begin testing at 36–40 weeks until delivered.

Maternal fetal movement monitoring ("kick counts") using a count to 10 or similar method is recommended for all pregnant women, including those with diabetes, to reduce the stillbirth rate.

When fetal assessment is not reassuring, the mature fetus should be delivered. In such cases near term, amniocentesis to obtain amniotic fluid for pulmonary maturity may be helpful. If the fetus is mature, delivery may proceed. If the fetus is immature, then a decision must be made in which the risk of fetal jeopardy is balanced against the risks of preterm birth. Participation of the patient, her partner, and the neonatology and perinatology departments may facilitate a plan. Assessment of fetal lung maturity is recommended for elective delivery at less than 38 weeks' gestation or when maternal glycemic control has been inadequate and there is risk of delay in fetal lung maturity.

Preterm labor is more frequent among patients with diabetes. The main goal of tocolysis is to delay delivery so that glucocorticoid therapy to accelerate fetal lung maturation can be administered over 48 hours. Magnesium sulfate tocolysis is widely used. Nifedipine is a reasonable alternative. β-Adrenergic mimetics such as terbutaline should be avoided if possible because these drugs may cause severe hyperglycemia and, rarely, ketoacidosis. Because glucocorticoids also cause hyperglycemia, a continuous intravenous infusion of insulin often is necessary to maintain normal glucose levels.

Many obstetricians induce the patient if she reaches 39 weeks' gestation. One prospective randomized controlled study demonstrated that patients requiring insulin for GDM or class B diabetes benefited from induction of labor at 38.5–39 weeks' gestation compared to expectant care. These pregnancies had excellent dates and good glycemic control. Lung maturity was not assessed, but RDS was not a complication. Patients with poor glycemic control may be evaluated for delivery at 38 weeks, although demonstrating fetal lung maturity in these cases is prudent. Patients with pregestational diabetes and vascular complications often require induction at or near term if preeclampsia, fetal growth restriction, or fetal heart rate abnormalities occur. The practice of offering cesarean delivery to prevent traumatic birth injury at a given estimated fetal weight (EFW) is controversial. Although a clear benefit outweighing the risk has not been firmly established, some practitioners have adopted a threshold EFW above which they counsel patients about the risks of vaginal delivery and offer cesarean delivery.

SEVERE HYPERGLYCEMIA & KETOACIDOSIS

During pregnancy, severe hyperglycemia and ketoacidosis are treated exactly the same as in the nonpregnant state. Insulin therapy, careful monitoring of potassium level, and fluid replacement are crucial for maternal survival. Fetal heart rate monitoring often demonstrates recurrent late decelerations, but these improve as maternal ketoacidosis is corrected.

INTRAPARTUM MANAGEMENT

Glucose infusion is provided to all patients in labor as 5% dextrose in lactated Ringer's solution or a similar crystalloid. The rate usually is 125 mL/h (providing 6.25 g of glucose per hour) unless the patient requires more. Intravenous fluid bolus prior to conduction anesthesia should not contain glucose. A bedside glucose monitor can be used to monitor glucose levels every 2–4 hours in early labor and every 1–2 hours in active labor. Patients requiring insulin may receive a continuous infusion of regular insulin, often prepared as 25 U in 250 mL saline (0.1 unit/mL) according to the institution's protocol for intravenous insulin. Most patients require approximately 0.5–2.0 U/h, although rates are adjusted based on the capillary glucose level.

Cervical ripening for induction of labor, if indicated, is conducted in the same manner as for nondiabetic parturients. Continuous electronic fetal monitoring is used. In diabetic pregnancies, the fetus's ability to tolerate the stress of labor may be limited. Fetal heart rate abnormalities should be evaluated with acoustic or scalp stimulation or fetal oxygen saturation monitoring. If fetal well-being cannot be demonstrated, expeditious delivery, often by cesarean section, is indicated. If fetal macrosomia is suspected, operative vaginal delivery should be considered with great caution, if at all. The infant of the diabetic is at increased risk for shoulder dystocia, and this should be anticipated with adequate personnel, obstetric anesthesia, and neonatal resuscitation available at delivery.

If a repeat cesarean delivery or other elective surgery is planned, the patient can take her evening insulin doses on the preceding night, but she cannot take the morning dose. The morning of surgery, glucose level is monitored and basal insulin needs usually are treated with continuous intravenous insulin to maintain a glucose between 70 and 120 mg/dL.

POSTPARTUM CARE

Postpartum, the patient should start back on an ADA diet as soon as clinically indicated. The dose of insulin should be reduced because insulin sensitivity increases markedly postpartum. The general rule is two-thirds of the prepregnancy dose or one-half of the present dose. If the patient underwent surgery, a sliding scale may be implemented until oral intake can be established. The glucose levels should be kept below 140–150 mg/dL to assist the patient in healing. Breastfeeding is encouraged, and snacks can be used to decrease the risk of hypoglycemia.

If hypoglycemic agents are necessary postpartum, insulin is continued for those women who are breastfeeding, whereas oral agents can be used in the non–breastfeeding mothers. Postpartum weight loss is encouraged. All patients with a history of diabetes or with risk factors should be re-evaluated prior to the next planned pregnancy.

CONTRACEPTION

Contraceptive options for diabetic women without vascular complications are the same as for nondiabetic women. In women with an increased risk for embolism, hormonal contraception containing estrogen is not recommended, but progesterone-only methods, including the levonorgestrel intrauterine system, can be offered. Permanent sterilization should be made available to women with diabetes who have completed childbearing.

NEONATAL COMPLICATIONS

Hyperglycemia at the time of conception results in enhanced rates of spontaneous abortion and major congenital malformations. Hyperglycemia in later pregnancy increases the risks for macrosomia, hypocalcemia, polycythemia, respiratory difficulties, cardiomyopathy, and congestive heart failure. Macrosomia is associated with increased risk for fetal intolerance to continued intrauterine existence and the stress of labor and of birth trauma. RDS and transient tachypnea are more common in infants of women with poorly controlled diabetics. Excellent antepartum glycemic control eliminates any delay in fetal lung maturity. Maternal hyperglycemia causes excess glycogen deposition and hypertrophy of the fetal heart muscle, which may cause fetal cardiomyopathy and congestive heart failure.

Table 18–4. Diagnostic criteria for diabetes and prediabetes in the nonpregnant state.

Diabetes	Prediabetes with Impaired Fasting Glucose (mg/dL)	Prediabetes with Impaired Glucose Tolerance (mg/dL)	Normal (mg/dL)
FPG ≥ 126	126 ≥ FPG ≥ 100		FPG < 100
2-hour OGTT ≥ 200		2-hour OGTT ≥ 140 and < 200	2-hour OGTT < 140

FPG, fasting plasma glucose; OGTT, oral glucose tolerance test with 75 g of glucose.

The fetus responds to maternal hyperglycemia with pancreatic hyperplasia and increased basal insulin secretion, which are associated with a lifetime increased risk of diabetes. Mothers with diabetes during pregnancy have offspring with higher rates of diabetes at age 20–24 years than do women who develop diabetes after the pregnancy (45% vs 8.6%). This observation suggests that the hyperglycemia during pregnancy had an effect beyond the mother's genetic tendency.

PROGRESSION FROM GDM TO T2DM

Women diagnosed with GDM are at increased risk to develop diabetes (in nearly all cases type 2) in the future. They have a 50–60% risk of developing diabetes within 10–15 years. Lifestyle modification may delay or entirely prevent the onset of diabetes in adults with impaired glucose tolerance.

All patients with GDM should have a 2-hour, 75-g OGTT approximately 6 weeks postpartum. Those with normal glucose tolerance should be reassessed every 3 years. Those with prediabetes should be re-evaluated annually (Table 18–4).

If the patient is breastfeeding, the same calorie ADA diet is continued postpartum. All women should be encouraged to eliminate or reduce any other risk factors (in addition to glucose intolerance) for cardiovascular disease. In practice, this means referral to programs, as needed, to cease smoking and to avoid environmental smoke; to engage in regular physical activity; to consume an appropriate diet; to achieve and maintain a normal weight; and to be treated for individual cardiovascular disease risk factors.

REFERENCES

American College of Obstetricians and Gynecologists: *Gestational Diabetes.* ACOG Practice Bulletin No. 30. American College of Obstetricians and Gynecologists, 2001.

American College of Obstetricians and Gynecologists: *Pregestational Diabetes Mellitus.* ACOG Practice Bulletin No. 60. American College of Obstetricians and Gynecologists, 2005.

American Diabetes Association: Diagnosis and classification of diabetes mellitus. Diabetes Care 2006;29:S43.

American Diabetes Association: Preconception care of women with diabetes. Diabetes Care 2004;27(Suppl 1):S76.

Boulot P et al; Diabetes and Pregnancy Group, France: French multicentric survey of outcome of pregnancy in women with pregestational diabetes. Diabetes Care 2003;26:2990.

Clausen TD et al: Poor pregnancy outcome in women with type 2 diabetes. Diabetes Care 2005;28:323.

Crowther CA et al; Australian Carbohydrate Intolerance Study in Pregnant Women (ACHOIS) Trial Group: Effects of treatment of gestational diabetes mellitus on pregnancy outcomes. N Engl J Med 2005;352:2477.

Dang K, Homko C, Reece EA: Factors associated with fetal macrosomia in offspring of gestational diabetic women. J Matern Fetal Med 2000;9:114.

Engelgau MM et al: The evolving diabetes burden in the United States. Ann Intern Med 2004;140:945.

Jimenez-Moleon JJ et al: Prevalence of gestational diabetes mellitus: Variations related to screening strategy used. Eur J Endocrinol 2002;146:831.

Jovanovic L, Nakai Y: Successful pregnancy in women with type 1 diabetes: From preconception through postpartum care. Endocrinol Metab Clin North Am 2006;35:79.

Kamalakannan D et al: Diabetic ketoacidosis in pregnancy. Postgrad Med J 2003;79:454.

Kim C et al; TRIAD Study Group: Preconception care in managed care: The Translating Research Into Action for Diabetes study. Am J Obstet Gynecol 2005;192:227.

Langer O et al: A comparison of glyburide and insulin in women with gestational diabetes mellitus. N Engl J Med 2000;343:1134.

Lusignan S et al: Trends in the prevalence and management of diagnosed type 2 diabetes 1994-2001 in England and Wales. BMC Fam Pract 2005;6:13.

Ray JG, O'Brien TE, Chan WS: Preconception care and the risk of congenital anomalies in the offspring of women with diabetes mellitus: A meta-analysis. QJM 2001;94:435.

Reece EA, Hobbins JC: Diabetic embryopathy: Pathogenesis, prenatal diagnosis and prevention. Obstet Gynecol Surv 1986;41:325.

Rendell M: Dietary treatment of diabetes mellitus. N Engl J Med 2000;342:1440.

Schaefer-Graf UM et al: Patterns of congenital anomalies and relationship to initial maternal fasting glucose levels in pregnancies complicated by type 2 and gestational diabetes. Am J Obstet Gynecol 2000;182:313.

Strehlow SL, Mestman JH: Prevention of T2DM in women with a previous history of GDM. Curr Diab Rep 2005;5:272.

Hypertension in Pregnancy

David A. Miller, MD

INTRODUCTION

Hypertension is a common medical disorder that affects 20–30% of adults in the United States and complicates as many as 5–8% of all pregnancies. Hypertensive disorders of pregnancy rank among the leading causes of maternal morbidity and mortality. Approximately 15% of maternal deaths are attributable to hypertension, making it the second leading cause of maternal mortality in the United States. Severe hypertension increases the mother's risk of heart attack, cardiac failure, cerebral vascular accidents, and renal failure. The fetus and neonate also are at increased risk from complications such as poor placental transfer of oxygen, fetal growth restriction, preterm birth, placental abruption, stillbirth, and neonatal death.

Hypertension is defined as a sustained blood pressure higher than 140/90 mm Hg. In the nonpregnant patient, essential hypertension accounts for more than 90% of cases; however, many other conditions must be considered (Table 19–1). In the pregnant patient, hypertension may be attributable to any of the conditions summarized in Table 19–1. In addition, a unique form of hypertension, "preeclampsia," occurs only during pregnancy. Preeclampsia is characterized by the onset of hypertension and proteinuria, usually during the third trimester of pregnancy. The National High Blood Pressure Education Program Working Group recently stated that edema occurs too frequently in normal pregnant women to be a useful marker in the diagnosis of preeclampsia. Therefore, edema is no longer recommended as a diagnostic criterion for preeclampsia. Management of preeclampsia differs from the management of other forms of hypertension during pregnancy. Therefore, it is important to distinguish preeclampsia from other forms of hypertension that may complicate pregnancy.

Classification of hypertension during pregnancy can be viewed as a continuum. On one end of the spectrum is the patient with hypertension that was present before pregnancy (or was recognized during the first half of pregnancy), does not worsen appreciably during pregnancy, and persists after delivery. This condition would be classified as *chronic hypertension.* On the other end of the spectrum is the patient with no evidence of chronic hypertension who experiences the abrupt onset of hypertension and proteinuria late in pregnancy followed by complete resolution postpartum. In this case, the hypertension observed during pregnancy may be the result of factors related entirely to pregnancy and *not* to an underlying medical cause. This condition would be classified as *preeclampsia.* Between these 2 extremes are cases in which varying degrees of preeclampsia are superimposed upon varying degrees of chronic hypertension. These broad categories have some value in estimating risk. Isolated mild to moderate chronic hypertension may have little effect on pregnancy outcome. On the other hand, severe hypertension of any cause may increase the risk to mother and fetus. The highest risks are associated with preeclampsia or eclampsia. The classification system of hypertension in pregnancy proposed by the National High Blood Pressure Education Program Working Group is summarized in Table 19–2.

CHRONIC HYPERTENSION

Chronic hypertension complicates as many as 5% of pregnancies. It is characterized by a history of high blood pressure before pregnancy, elevation of blood pressure during the first half of pregnancy, or high blood pressure that lasts for longer than 12 weeks after delivery. The search for an underlying cause should include a complete history and physical examination, taking into account the normal changes that accompany pregnancy. During normal pregnancy, maternal blood volume increases by 40% to 60%. Cardiac output and renal blood flow increase significantly. Blood pressure normally decreases throughout the first half of pregnancy under the influence of progesterone, reaching a nadir in midpregnancy and returning to prepregnancy levels by the end of the third trimester.

In women with hypertension, underlying disorders must be excluded (Table 19–1). Blood pressure should be measured in both arms with the patient in a sitting position and the arm at the level of the heart, and multiple measurements should be obtained on different occasions. If possible, measurements should be obtained outside of the office setting. The fifth Korotkoff sound should be used to determine diastolic pressure. Auscul-

Table 19–1. Causes of chronic hypertension.

Idiopathic
  Essential hypertension
Vascular disorders
  Renovascular hypertension
  Aortic coarctation
Endocrine disorders
  Diabetes mellitus
  Hyperthyroidism
  Pheochromocytoma
  Primary hyperaldosteronism
  Hyperparathyroidism
  Cushing's syndrome
Renal disorders
  Diabetic nephropathy
  Chronic renal failure
  Acute renal failure
  Tubular necrosis
  Cortical necrosis
  Pyelonephritis
  Chronic glomerulonephritis
  Nephrotic syndrome
  Polycystic kidney
Connective tissue disorders
  Systemic lupus erythematosus

tation of the flanks may reveal a renal artery bruit. Funduscopic examination may reveal typical findings associated with long-standing hypertension or possibly diabetes. An enlarged thyroid gland may indicate thyroid disease. Absent peripheral pulses suggest coarctation of the aorta. Heart, skin, and joints should be evaluated thoroughly. After evaluating the possible causes of chronic hypertension, further assessment is directed at end-organs and systems most likely to be affected by hypertension, including the eyes, heart, kidneys, uteroplacental circulation, and the fetus.

Laboratory tests include a complete blood count, glucose screen, electrolyte panel, serum creatinine, urinalysis, and urine culture. In some cases, additional tests may be needed. In patients with possible renal disease (serum creatinine $\geq$ 0.8 mg/dL, urine protein > 1+ on dipstick), a 24-hour urine collection for creatinine clearance and total protein will provide baseline information that may be helpful in diagnosing the onset of preeclampsia later in pregnancy. Diabetes should be excluded. Antinuclear antibody may help confirm a diagnosis of collagen vascular disease. A suppressed thyroid-stimulating hormone level suggests hyperthyroidism. Rarely, elevated urinary catecholamine levels may point to pheochromocytoma. An electrocardiogram may reveal left ventricular hypertrophy in the patient with long-standing hyper-

tension. Chest radiography with abdominal shielding may reveal cardiomegaly.

Fetal Assessment in Chronic Hypertension

Pregnancies complicated by chronic hypertension, regardless of the cause, are at increased risk for poor fetal growth. An initial ultrasound examination should be performed as early as possible to confirm the due date and to ensure that no obvious fetal anomalies are present. Thereafter, fetal growth may be assessed by ultrasound as needed, usually no more frequently than every 2–4 weeks. Antepartum fetal monitoring usually is started by 32–34 weeks. If the nonstress test is used as the method of surveillance, it should be accompanied by assessment of amniotic fluid volume. Doppler velocimetry of the umbilical, uterine, and middle cerebral arteries are helpful in optimizing the timing of delivery, particularly in cases of suspected fetal growth restriction.

Management of Mild Chronic Hypertension

In pregnant women with mild hypertension and no evidence of renal disease, serious medical complications are rare. Moreover, there is no consensus that antihypertensive medication can reduce the risk of fetal death, growth restriction, placental abruption, preeclampsia, or eclampsia in these women. Therefore, antihypertensive medication is not usually necessary. Avoidance of alcohol and tobacco is encouraged. Sodium restriction may be considered (2–3 g/d). Rigorous activity should be avoided, as should weight reduction. Despite the lack of evidence supporting the benefit of antihypertensive therapy in women with blood pressure < 180/110 mm Hg, many clinicians are reluctant to withhold medication when the blood pressure remains $\geq$ 150/100 mm Hg despite lifestyle modifications. A practical management algorithm using a blood pressure of 150/100 mm Hg as the threshold for initiation of antihypertensive therapy in women without evidence of end-organ involvement and 140/90 mm Hg as the threshold in women with evidence of renal involvement is summarized in Figure 19–1. Prenatal visits are scheduled every 2–4 weeks until 34–36 weeks, and weekly thereafter. At each visit, blood pressure, urine protein, and fundal height are evaluated. Patients are questioned regarding signs and symptoms of preeclampsia, including headache, abdominal pain, blurred vision, scotomata, rapid weight gain, or marked swelling of the hands and/or face. Antepartum fetal monitoring usually is started around 32–34 weeks, and, in most cases, delivery is accomplished by 39–40 weeks' gestation.

Table 19–2. Classification of hypertension in pregnancy.

Definition of hypertension

Mild: Systolic blood pressure ≥ 140 mm Hg
Diastolic blood pressure ≥ 90 mm Hg
Severe: Systolic blood pressure ≥ 180 mm Hg
Diastolic blood pressure ≥ 110 mm Hg

Chronic hypertension
Hypertension with onset before pregnancy or before 20th week gestation
Use of antihypertensive medications before pregnancy
Persistence of hypertension beyond 12 weeks postpartum

Preeclampsia
Hypertension that occurs after 20 weeks of gestation in a woman with previously normal blood pressure. Systolic blood pressure ≥ 140 mm Hg or diastolic blood pressure ≥ 90 mm Hg on two occasions at least 6 hours apart
Proteinuria, defined as urinary excretion of ≥ 0.3 g protein in a 24-hour urine specimen. This finding usually correlates with a finding of 1+ or greater on dipstick
Note edema is no longer a diagnostic criterion
Note a systolic rise of 30 mm Hg or a diastolic rise of 15 mm Hg is no longer a diagnostic criterion

Eclampsia
New-onset grand mal seizures in a woman with preeclampsia that cannot be attributed to other causes

Superimposed preeclampsia–eclampsia
Preeclampsia or eclampsia that occurs in a woman with a pre-existing chronic hypertension

Gestational hypertension
Hypertension detected for the first time after midpregnancy
Distinguished from preeclampsia by the absence of proteinuria
Working diagnosis only during pregnancy

Transient hypertension of pregnancy
Gestational hypertension that resolves by 12 weeks postpartum
If proteinuria develops in a patient with gestational hypertension, the diagnosis is preeclampsia
If gestational hypertension does not resolve by 12 weeks postpartum, the diagnosis is chronic hypertension

---

Management of Severe Chronic Hypertension

Women with sustained blood pressure ≥ 180/110 mm Hg or those with evidence of renal disease may be at higher risk for serious complications, such as heart attack, stroke, or progression of renal disease, and are candidates for antihypertensive medication. As summarized in Figure 19–1, many clinicians would use a lower threshold of 150/100 mm Hg for instituting antihypertensive therapy during pregnancy.

Frequent prenatal visits may be needed to check the effectiveness of the medication. Fetal growth, blood pressure, and proteinuria are assessed at each visit, and evidence of superimposed preeclampsia is aggressively sought. Management of preeclampsia is described later in this chapter. In women with evidence of renal disease, some clinicians measure creatinine clearance and 24-hour urinary protein excretion each trimester. Sonographic assessment of fetal growth is performed every 2–4 weeks, antepartum testing is initiated by 32–34 weeks, and delivery is accomplished after 38 weeks or when fetal lung maturity is demonstrated. In some cases, hypertension worsens significantly during pregnancy without the development of overt preeclampsia. If exacerbation of chronic hypertension necessitates preterm delivery, corticosteroids should be considered in attempt to accelerate fetal maturity.

Antihypertensive Therapy in Chronic Hypertension

Several choices for initial antihypertensive therapy during pregnancy are available. Methyldopa has been studied extensively and is recommended by many as the first-line antihypertensive agent in pregnancy. It is a centrally acting α-adrenergic agonist that appears to inhibit vasoconstricting impulses from the medullary vasoregulatory center. The total daily dosage of 500 mg to 2 g is administered in 2–4 divided doses. Peak

Figure 19–1. Management algorithm for severe chronic hypertension in pregnancy.

plasma levels occur 2–3 hours after administration, and the maximum effect occurs 4–6 hours after an oral dose. The agent is excreted primarily by the kidney. Sedation and postural hypotension are the most common side effects. A positive direct Coombs' test may be seen, usually after 6–12 months of therapy. Hemolytic anemia may occur in these patients and is an indication to stop the medication. Fever, liver function abnormalities, granulocytopenia, and thrombocytopenia are rare side effects.

Labetalol is an α_1-adrenergic blocker and a nonselective β-adrenergic blocker. The β-blockade/α-blockade ratio is 7:1. A large body of clinical evidence suggests that use of labetalol is safe during pregnancy. It appears to lack teratogenicity and crosses the placenta in small amounts. One randomized study showed no advantages of labetalol over methyldopa. Another study reported a higher incidence of small for gestational age (SGA) newborns in patients treated with labetalol. The usual starting dose is 100 mg BID, and the dose can be increased weekly to a maximum of 2400 mg daily. Titration increments should not exceed 200 mg BID.

Nifedipine is a calcium channel blocker that has been used during pregnancy for tocolysis and treatment of hypertension. Several reports suggest that nifedipine use is safe during pregnancy; however, the cumulative experience with this agent is not as extensive as with methyldopa and labetalol. When nifedipine is used for treatment of chronic hypertension during pregnancy, the long-acting formulation (Procardia XL, Adalat CC) may improve patient compliance. The principal benefit of this agent is once-daily dosing. The usual starting dose is 30 mg daily. If necessary, the dose may be increased to 60–90 mg daily. The neuromuscular-blocking action of magnesium may be potentiated by simultaneous calcium channel blockade; therefore, nifedipine should be used with caution in patients receiving magnesium sulfate. The sublingual route of administration is associated with unpredictable blood levels and should be avoided.

Other antihypertensive medications used in pregnancy include atenolol, metoprolol, prazosin, minoxidil, hydralazine, thiazide diuretics, and clonidine. Published experience with these agents is limited, and they should not supplant methyldopa, labetalol, or nifedipine as first-line agents in pregnancy.

Use of angiotensin-converting enzyme inhibitors (enalapril, captopril) during pregnancy is associated fetal hypocalvaria, renal defects, anuria, and fetal and neonatal death. These agents are contraindicated in pregnancy. With few exceptions, diuretics (furosemide, hydrochlorothiazide) should be avoided during pregnancy. Fetal bradycardia, growth retardation, and neonatal hypoglycemia have been reported in patients treated with blockers.

Prognosis

Pregnancy outcome usually is good in patients with mild chronic hypertension and no other serious medical conditions. Fetal growth restriction, superimposed preeclampsia, placental abruption, and preterm delivery are the most common complications. The outlook is less favorable in women with severe hypertension early in pregnancy and in those with evidence of end-organ compromise, such as renal insufficiency and/or cardiovascular disease. By necessity, management is individualized. Close monitoring for development of fetal growth restriction and superimposed preeclampsia is indicated.

PREECLAMPSIA

Preeclampsia complicates 5–7% of all pregnancies. The classic diagnostic triad included hypertension, proteinuria, and edema. Recently, the National High Blood Pressure Education Working Group recommended eliminating edema as a diagnostic criterion because it is too frequent an observation during normal pregnancy to be useful in diagnosing preeclampsia. Preeclampsia occurs with increased frequency among young, nulliparous women. However, the frequency distribution is bimodal, with a second peak occurring in multiparous women greater than 35 years of age. Among daughters of preeclamptic women, the risk of preeclampsia is significantly higher than the population risk. Other predisposing factors for preeclampsia are listed in Table 19–3.

Normal pregnancy is associated with decreased maternal sensitivity to endogenous vasopressors. Apparent early in gestation, this effect leads to expansion of the maternal intravascular space and a decline in blood pressure throughout the first half of pregnancy, with a nadir at midgestation. Thereafter, continued expansion of intravascular volume leads to a gradual rise in the blood pressure to prepregnancy levels by term. Women destined to develop preeclampsia do not exhibit normal refractoriness to endogenous vasopressors. As a result, normal expansion of the intravascular space does not occur, and the normal decline

Table 19–3. Risk factors for preeclampsia.

Age < 20 years or > 35 years
Nulliparity
Multiple gestation
Hydatidiform mole
Diabetes mellitus
Thyroid disease
Chronic hypertension
Renal disease
Collagen vascular disease
Antiphospholipid syndrome
Family history of preeclampsia

in blood pressure during the first half of pregnancy may be absent or attenuated. Despite normal to elevated blood pressure, intravascular volume is reduced. In addition to the classic findings of hypertension and proteinuria, women with preeclampsia may complain of scotomata, blurred vision, or pain in the epigastrium or right upper quadrant. Examination often reveals brisk patellar reflexes and clonus. Laboratory abnormalities include elevated levels of hematocrit, lactate dehydrogenase, serum transaminases and uric acid, and thrombocytopenia. Although biochemical evidence of disseminated intravascular coagulation (DIC) may be detected with increased fibrin degradation products, hypofibrinogenemia and prolongation of the prothrombin time and activated partial thromboplastin time usually are seen only in cases complicated by abruption or multiple organ failure.

Pathophysiology

A. Brain

Pathologic findings in preeclampsia-induced cerebral injury include fibrinoid necrosis, thrombosis, microinfarcts, and petechial hemorrhages, primarily in the cerebral cortex. Cerebral edema may be observed. Head computed tomographic findings include focal white matter hypodensities in the posterior cerebral hemispheres, temporal lobes, and brainstem, possibly reflecting petechial hemorrhage with resultant local edema. Magnetic resonance imaging may reveal occipital and parietal abnormalities in the watershed distribution of the major cerebral arteries, as well as lesions in the brainstem and basal ganglia. Subarachnoid or intraventricular hemorrhage may occur in severe cases.

B. Heart

Preeclampsia is characterized by the absence of normal intravascular volume expansion, a reduction in normal circulating blood volume, and a loss of normal refractoriness to endogenous vasopressors, including angiotensin II. Invasive hemodynamic monitoring in preeclamptic patients has yielded conflicting information. Depending upon disease severity, effects of previous therapy, and other factors, preeclampsia has been described variously as a state of abnormally high cardiac output and low systemic vascular resistance, a state of abnormally low cardiac output and high systemic vascular resistance, or a state of high cardiac output and high systemic vascular resistance. These divergent observations underscore the complexity of the disorder.

C. Lungs

Alterations in colloid oncotic pressure, capillary endothelial integrity, and intravascular hydrostatic pressure in preeclampsia predispose to noncardiogenic pulmonary edema. In women with preeclampsia superimposed on chronic hypertension, preexisting hypertensive cardiac disease may exacerbate the situation, superimposing cardiogenic pulmonary edema on noncardiogenic, preeclampsia-related pulmonary edema. Excessive administration of intravenous (IV) fluid and postpartum mobilization of accumulated extravascular fluid also increase the risk of pulmonary edema. In eclampsia, pulmonary injury may result from aspiration of gastric contents, leading to pneumonia, pneumonitis, or adult respiratory distress syndrome.

D. Liver

Histologic lesions in the liver are characterized by sinusoidal fibrin deposition in the periportal areas with surrounding hemorrhage and portal capillary thrombi. Centrilobular necrosis may result from reduced perfusion. Inflammation is not characteristic. Subcapsular hematomas may develop. In severe cases involving hepatocellular necrosis and DIC, intrahepatic hematomas may progress to liver rupture. Right upper quadrant pain or epigastric pain are classic symptoms attributed to stretching of Glisson's capsule. Elevation of serum transaminases is a hallmark of HELLP (hemolysis, elevated liver enzymes, and low platelets) syndrome.

E. Kidneys

Distinct histologic changes have been described in the kidneys of women with preeclampsia. The classic renal lesion of preeclampsia, "glomeruloendotheliosis," is characterized by swelling and enlargement of glomerular capillary endothelial cells, leading to narrowing of the capillary lumen. There is an increased amount of cytoplasm containing lipid-filled vacuoles. Mesangial cells may be swollen as well. Immunoglobulins, complement, fibrin, and fibrin degradation products have been observed in the glomeruli, but their presence is variable.

F. Eyes

Retinal vasospasm, retinal edema, serous retinal detachment, and cortical blindness may occur in the setting of preeclampsia. Blindness is uncommon and usually transient, resolving within hours to days of delivery.

Etiology

The etiology of preeclampsia is not known; however, a growing body of evidence suggests that maternal vascular endothelial injury plays a central role in the disorder. Some reports suggest that endothelial damage in preeclampsia results in decreased endothelial production of prostaglandin I_2 (prostacyclin), a potent vasodilator and inhibitor of platelet aggregation. Endothelial cell injury exposes subendothelial collagen and can trigger platelet aggregation, activation, and release of platelet-derived thromboxane A_2 (TXA_2), a potent vasoconstrictor and stimulator of platelet aggregation. Decreased prostacyclin production by dysfunctional endothelial cells and increased TXA_2 release by activated platelets and trophoblast may be responsible for reversal of the normal ratio of prostacyclin and TXA_2 observed in preeclampsia. The predominance of TXA_2 may contribute to the vasoconstriction and hypertension that are central features of the disorder. Elevated intravascular pressure combined with damaged vascular endothelium results in movement of fluid from the intravascular to the extravascular spaces, leading to edema in the brain, retinae, lungs, liver, and subcutaneous tissues. Hypertension and glomerular endothelial damage lead to proteinuria. The resultant decrease in intravascular colloid oncotic pressure contributes to further loss of intravascular fluid. Hemoconcentration is reflected in a rising hematocrit. Consumption of platelets and activation of the clotting cascade at the sites of endothelial damage may lead to thrombocytopenia and DIC. Soluble fibrin monomers produced by the coagulation cascade may precipitate in the microvasculature, leading to microangiopathic hemolysis and elevation of the serum lactate dehydrogenase level. Cerebral edema, vasoconstriction, and capillary endothelial damage may lead to hyperreflexia, clonus, convulsions, or hemorrhage. Hepatic edema and/or ischemia may lead to hepatocellular injury and elevation of serum transaminases and lactate dehydrogenase levels. The right upper quadrant or epigastric pain observed in severe preeclampsia is thought to be caused by stretching of Glisson's capsule by hepatic edema or hemorrhage. Intravascular fluid loss across damaged capillary endothelium in the lungs may result in pulmonary edema. In the retinae, vasoconstriction and/or edema may lead to visual disturbances, retinal detachment, or blindness. Movement of fluid from the intravascular space into the subcutaneous tissues produces the characteristic nondependent edema of preeclampsia.

Endothelial damage appears to be capable of triggering a cascade of events culminating in the multiorgan system dysfunction observed in preeclampsia. However, the mechanism of endothelial injury remains speculative. In one theory, decreased placental oxygenation triggers the placenta to release an unknown factor into the maternal circulation. This circulating factor is capable of damaging or altering the function of maternal endothelial cells and triggering the cascade of events described. In support of this theory, cultured trophoblasts exposed to a hypoxic environment release a variety of potentially vasoactive factors, including thromboxane, interleukin-1, and tumor necrosis factor. Moreover, serum from preeclamptic women, when applied to human endothelial cell cultures,

alters the release of a variety of procoagulant, vasoactive, and mitogenic factors, including endothelin, nitric oxide, and prostacyclin. Serum from the same woman 6 weeks after delivery does not produce this effect. Likewise, serum from a nonpreeclamptic woman at the same gestational age fails to trigger these endothelial changes. In many cases, reduced placental oxygenation may be explained by maternal vasculopathy (chronic hypertension, renal disease, collagen vascular disease) and in others by abnormal placental mass (multiple gestation, diabetes, hydatidiform mole). In another subset of patients, reduced placental oxygenation late in pregnancy may be the result of abnormal endovascular trophoblast invasion early in pregnancy. In the first trimester of a normal pregnancy, proliferating trophoblast invades the decidual segments of the maternal spiral arteries, replacing endothelium and destroying the medial elastic and muscular tissue of the arterial wall. The arterial wall is replaced by fibrinoid material. During the second trimester, a second wave of endovascular trophoblastic invasion extends down the lumen of the spiral arteries deeper in the myometrium. The endothelium and musculoelastic architecture of the spiral arteries are destroyed, resulting in dilated, thin-walled, funnel-shaped vessels that are passive conduits of the increased uteroplacental blood flow of pregnancy. In some women destined to develop preeclampsia, the first wave of endovascular trophoblastic invasion may be incomplete, and the second wave does not occur. As a result, the deeper segments of the spiral arteries are not remodeled but instead retain their musculoelastic architecture and their ability to respond to endogenous vasoconstrictors, reducing maternal perfusion of the placenta and predisposing to relative placental hypoxia later in pregnancy. In addition, myometrial portions of the spiral arteries exhibit a unique abnormality characterized by vessel wall damage, fibrinoid necrosis, lipid deposition, and macrophage and mononuclear cell infiltration of vessel walls and surrounding tissues. These changes, histologically similar to those observed in atherosclerosis, are referred to as acute atherosis and may lead to vascular lumen obliteration and placental infarction. Importantly, these changes are attributed to abnormal endovascular trophoblastic invasion during the second trimester of pregnancy, predisposing the fetus to suboptimal placental perfusion early in gestation. Interestingly, the clinical manifestations are observed most often in the third trimester, possibly due to increasing fetal and placental oxygen demands with advancing gestation.

The reason that endovascular trophoblastic invasion progresses normally in most pregnancies but abnormally in others is unclear. One theory maintains that maternal antibodies directed against paternal antigens on invading trophoblasts are necessary to shield those antigens from recognition by decidual natural killer cells, protecting the invading trophoblast from attack and rejection by the cellular arm of the maternal immune system. Supporting this theory is the observation that preeclampsia appears to be associated with primipaternity and the presumed lack of previous maternal exposure and sensitization to paternal trophoblast antigens in a previous pregnancy. Additional support for this theory is provided by the observation that preeclampsia is more common among women using barrier contraception than among those using nonbarrier forms of contraception prior to pregnancy. This suggests that maternal exposure (and presumably sensitization) to paternal antigens on sperm is protective against preeclampsia. The observed inverse relationship between duration of cohabitation before pregnancy and the incidence of preeclampsia provides further evidence that maternal sensitization to paternal antigens is protective against preeclampsia. The interplay between immunology and genetics is underscored by the observation that preeclampsia may be more common in pregnancies in which the father was the product of a preeclamptic pregnancy. Applied to the theory under discussion, this suggests that some genetically determined paternal antigens are less antigenic than others and therefore less likely to provoke an antibody response in an exposed mother, decreasing maternal production of "blocking" antibodies and increasing the likelihood of abnormal placental invasion and preeclampsia. Alternatively, paternally inherited genes may code for altered fetal production of insulinlike growth factor-2, an insulin homologue related to placental invasion. Other genes that may be inherited from the father and play a role in the development of preeclampsia include genes coding for angiotensinogen, methylenetetrahydrofolate reductase, and the factor V Leiden mutation.

Some studies have demonstrated that invading trophoblastic cells in normal pregnancy undergo an "antigenic shift" to resemble vascular endothelial antigens, masking them from recognition and rejection by decidual natural killer cells. Invading trophoblasts in preeclamptic pregnancies may fail to make this antigenic shift, exposing them to recognition by natural killer cells and halting normal invasion.

Recent work has demonstrated that soluble fms-like tyrosine kinase-1 (sFlt-1) is increased in the placenta and serum of women with preeclampsia. This protein adheres to placental growth factor and vascular endothelial growth factor (VEGF), preventing their interaction with endothelial receptors and causing endothelial dysfunction. Interrupted angiogenesis may contribute to faulty placental invasion early in pregnancy and subsequent risk for placental hypoxia–ischemia and preeclampsia. Unbound placental growth factor and VEGF have been found in decreased concentration during and even before the development of clinical preeclampsia.

Genetic, immunologic, and other factors govern the complex interaction between the maternal host and the invading trophoblast. Detailed discussion of these and other possible etiologies of the entity of preeclampsia are beyond the scope of this chapter. Regardless of the etiology, thorough familiarity with the clinical aspects of the disorder can help guide thoughtful and coherent management.

Management

In the management of preeclampsia, with few exceptions, maternal interests are best served by immediate delivery. However, this approach may not be in the best interest of the fetus. In the case of extreme prematurity, for example, the fetus may benefit from a period of expectant management during which corticosteroids are administered to accelerate fetal maturation. The decision to proceed with immediate delivery versus expectant management is based upon several factors, including disease severity, fetal maturity, maternal and fetal condition, and cervical status. For the purposes of management, preeclampsia may be classified as mild or severe, as outlined in Table 19–4.

A. MILD PREECLAMPSIA

Women with mild preeclampsia are hospitalized for further evaluation and, if indicated, delivery. If mild preeclampsia is confirmed and the gestational age is 40 weeks or greater, delivery is indicated. At gestational ages of 37–40 weeks, cervical status is assessed and, if favorable, induction is initiated. If the cervical status is unfavorable, preinduction cervical ripening agents are used as needed. Occasionally, women with very unfavorable cervical examinations between 37 and 40 weeks may be managed expectantly for a limited time with bed rest, antepartum fetal surveillance, and close monitoring of maternal condition, including blood pressure measurement every 4–6 hours and daily assessment of patellar reflexes, weight gain, proteinuria, and symptoms. A complete blood count and levels of serum transaminases, lactate dehydrogenase, and uric acid should be checked weekly to twice weekly. Delivery is indicated if the cervical status becomes favorable, antepartum testing is abnormal, the gestational age reaches 40 weeks, or evidence of worsening preeclampsia is seen. If expectant management is undertaken after 37 weeks, the patient should understand that the only known benefit is a possible reduction in the rate of cesarean birth.

Women with mild preeclampsia before 37 weeks are managed expectantly with bed rest, twice-weekly antepartum testing, and maternal evaluation as described. Corticosteroids are administered if the gestational age is less than 34 weeks; amniocentesis is performed as needed to assess fetal pulmonary maturity. When extended expectant management is undertaken, fetal growth is assessed with ultrasound every 3–4 weeks. Occasionally, outpatient management is reasonable in carefully selected, reliable, asymptomatic patients with minimal pro-

Table 19-4. Classification of preeclampsia.

Mild Preeclampsia	Severe Preeclampsia
Blood pressure ≥ 140/90 mm Hg but < 160/110 mm Hg on two occasions at least 6 hours apart while the patient is on bed rest	Blood pressure ≥ 160 mm Hg systolic or ≥ 110 mm Hg diastolic on two occasions at least 6 hours apart while the patient is on bed rest
Proteinuria ≥ 300 mg/24 h but < 5 g/24 h	Proteinuria of 5 g or higher in 24-hour urine specimen or 3+ or greater on two random urine samples collected at least 4 hours apart
Asymptomatic	Oliguria < 500 mL in 24 hours
	Cerebral or visual disturbances
	Pulmonary edema or cyanosis
	Epigastrica or right upper quadrant pain
	Impaired liver function
	Thrombocytopenia
	Fetal growth restriction

teinuria and normal laboratory test results. This approach includes bed rest at home, daily fetal movement counts, twice-weekly antepartum testing, serial evaluation of fetal growth, and frequent assessment, often by a visiting nurse, of blood pressure, proteinuria, weight gain, patellar reflexes, and symptoms. Any evidence of disease progression constitutes an indication for hospitalization and consideration of delivery. Regardless of severity, all women with preeclampsia at the University of Southern California receive prophylactic intrapartum magnesium sulfate to prevent convulsions. The benefit of prophylactic magnesium sulfate in preventing convulsions in patients with mild preeclampsia has not been demonstrated conclusively in the literature.

B. SEVERE PREECLAMPSIA

Severe preeclampsia mandates hospitalization. Delivery is indicated if the gestational age is 34 weeks or greater, fetal pulmonary is confirmed, or evidence of deteriorating maternal or fetal status is seen. Acute blood pressure control may be achieved with hydralazine, labetalol, or nifedipine. The goal of antihypertensive therapy is to achieve a systolic blood pressure < 160 mm Hg and a diastolic blood pressure < 105 mm Hg. Overly aggressive control of the blood pressure may compromise maternal perfusion of the intervillous space and adversely impact fetal oxygenation. Hydralazine is a peripheral vasodilator that can be given in doses of 5–10 mg IV. The onset of action is 10–20 minutes, and the dose can be repeated in 20–30 minutes if necessary. Labetalol can be administered in doses of 5–20 mg by slow IV push. The dose can be repeated in 10–20 minutes. Nifedipine is a calcium channel blocker that can be used in doses of 5–10 mg orally. The sublingual route of administration should not be used. The dose can be repeated in 20–30 minutes, as needed.

Management of severe preeclampsia before 34 weeks is controversial. In some institutions, delivery is accomplished regardless of fetal maturity. At the University of Southern California, delivery often is delayed for a limited period of time to permit the administration of corticosteroids. Magnesium sulfate is initiated, fetal status is monitored continuously, and antihypertensive agents are used as needed to maintain a systolic blood pressure < 160 mm Hg and a diastolic blood pressure < 105 mm Hg. Between 33 and 35 weeks, consideration should be given to amniocentesis for pulmonary maturity studies. If mature, immediate delivery is indicated. If immature, corticosteroids are administered and, if possible, delivery is delayed 24–48 hours. Between 24 and 32 weeks, antihypertensive therapy is instituted as indicated, corticosteroids are administered, and extensive maternal counseling is undertaken to clarify the risks and benefits of pregnancy prolongation. Neonatology consultation is helpful to delineate the neonatal risks specific to gestational age and estimated fetal weight. The duration of expectant management is determined on an individual basis, taking into account maternal wishes, estimated fetal weight, gestational age, and maternal and fetal status. Expectant management is contraindicated in the presence of fetal compromise, uncontrollable hypertension, eclampsia, DIC, HELLP syndrome, cerebral edema, pulmonary edema, or evidence of cerebral or hepatic hemorrhage. When severe preeclampsia is diagnosed before 24 weeks of gestation, the likelihood of a favorable outcome is low. Thorough counseling should address realistically the risks and anticipated benefits of expectant management and should include the option of pregnancy termination. If an appropriately informed patient declines the option of pregnancy termination, expectant management should proceed as outlined above.

C. INTRAPARTUM MANAGEMENT OF PREECLAMPSIA

In women with preeclampsia without contraindications to labor, vaginal delivery is the preferred approach. Cervical ripening agents and oxytocin are used as needed. During labor, magnesium sulfate is administered for seizure prophylaxis as an IV loading dose of 4–6 g over 20–60 minutes, followed by a maintenance dose of 1–2 g/h. Urine output and serum creatinine level are monitored, and the magnesium dose is adjusted accordingly to prevent hypermagnesemia. Patellar reflexes and respiratory rate should be assessed frequently. In the presence of patellar reflexes, serum magnesium levels usually are unnecessary. Therapeutic magnesium levels range from 4–8 mg/dL. Loss of patellar reflexes is observed at magnesium levels of 10 mg/dL or higher, respiratory paralysis may occur at levels of 15 mg/dL or above, and cardiac arrest is possible with levels in excess of 25 mg/dL. Calcium gluconate (10 mL of 10% solution) should be available in the event of hypermagnesemia. To avoid pulmonary edema, total IV fluids should not exceed 100 mL/h. Pain control is achieved with regional anesthesia or with intramuscular or IV narcotic analgesics. Invasive hemodynamic monitoring is reserved for refractory pulmonary edema, adult respiratory distress syndrome, or oliguria unresponsive to fluid challenge. If cesarean section is required, platelets should be available for possible transfusion for patients with platelet counts < 50,000/mm^3. Use of other blood products is guided by clinical and laboratory findings.

Eclampsia

The estimated incidence of eclampsia is 1–3 in 1000 preeclamptic patients. Leveno reported no seizures among 1049 preeclamptic women receiving magnesium sulfate prophylaxis. Nonetheless, tonic–clonic convulsions may occur despite magnesium sulfate therapy. In most cases seizures are self-limited, lasting 1–2 minutes. The first priorities are to ensure that the airway is clear and to prevent injury and aspiration of gastric contents. Diazepam or lorazepam should be used only if seizures are sustained. Nearly all tonic–clonic seizures are accompanied by a prolonged fetal heart rate deceleration that resolves after the seizure has ended. If possible, a 10- to 20-minute period of in utero resuscitation should be permitted prior to delivery. Convulsions alone do not constitute an indication for cesarean section. However, if vaginal birth is not possible within a reasonable period of time, cesarean delivery is performed in most cases.

HELLP Syndrome

The HELLP syndrome is a variant of preeclampsia that is characterized by *h*emolysis, *e*levated *l*iver enzymes, and *l*ow *p*latelets. It complicates 10% of cases of severe preeclampsia and up to 50% of cases of eclampsia. Right upper quadrant pain, nausea, vomiting, and malaise are common. Hypertension and proteinuria are variable. The hallmark of the disorder is microangiopathic hemolysis leading to elevation of serum lactate dehydrogenase level and fragmented red blood cells on peripheral smear. Transaminase levels are elevated, thrombocytopenia is present, and DIC may be evident. Management is similar to that of severe preeclampsia. Recent reports suggest that dexamethasone may hasten the improvement of HELLP syndrome following delivery. Dexamethasone is administered IV in 4 doses of 10 mg, 10 mg, 5 mg, and 5 mg at 12-hour intervals or in doses of 10 mg IV at 12-hour intervals until improvement. In another protocol, dexamethasone is administered in doses of 10 mg IV every 6 hours for 2 doses, followed by 6 mg every 6 hours for 2–4 doses. If elevated transaminase levels or thrombocytopenia persist beyond the fourth postpartum day, alternative explanations should be considered, including thrombotic thrombocytopenic purpura, hemolytic uremic syndrome, acute fatty liver of pregnancy, viral- or drug-induced hepatitis, and systemic lupus erythematosus.

Prevention of Preeclampsia

The observed alteration in the ratio of vasoconstrictive and vasodilatory prostaglandins in preeclampsia led investigators to study the effectiveness of prostaglandin synthesis inhibitors in preventing the disorder. Several small trials of low-dose aspirin reported significant reductions in the incidence of preeclampsia in high-risk populations. However, in 1994 the Collaborative Low-Dose Aspirin Study in Pregnancy (CLASP) Collaborative Group reported a large randomized trial comparing low-dose aspirin to placebo in more than 9300 high-risk patients. Low-dose aspirin did not reduce the incidence of preeclampsia in this high-risk population. Hauth reported a significant reduction in preeclampsia among low-risk women treated with low-dose aspirin. However, a larger trial by Sibai reported no benefit. Reviewing all the conflicting evidence, investigators for the Cochrane Collaboration concluded there may be a small to moderate benefit of low-dose aspirin in preventing preeclampsia. Because the risks of the regimen are few, some physicians may reasonably choose to use it.

Calcium is essential in the synthesis of nitric oxide, a potent vasodilator believed to contribute to the maintenance of reduced vascular tone in pregnancy. Although several small studies suggested a possible benefit of calcium supplementation in preventing preeclampsia, a large trial by Levine that included more than 4400 women reported no benefit.

CONCLUSION

Hypertensive disorders of pregnancy remain among the most common causes of adverse maternal and perinatal outcome. These disorders can be regarded as a spectrum of disease, ranging from isolated chronic hypertension to pure preeclampsia–eclampsia. Isolated mild or moderate chronic hypertension appears to have little effect on pregnancy outcome. Morbidity and mortality are highest among patients with severe preeclampsia or eclampsia.

Appropriate management of newly diagnosed chronic hypertension entails a thorough search for an underlying cause. Use of antihypertensive medications are reserved for women with severe chronic hypertension. Close maternal and fetal surveillance is necessary, and a high index of suspicion must be maintained for the development of superimposed preeclampsia.

The management of preeclampsia is influenced by many factors, including disease severity, gestational age, and fetal condition. Optimal management requires an appreciation of the complexity of the disease process and familiarity with its manifestations in multiple organ systems. Maternal and fetal risks and benefits must be assessed thoroughly. Individualized treatment plans should be formulated and discussed with the patient, and she should be encouraged to participate in major decisions regarding her care. In atypical cases, alternative diagnoses must be considered.

REFERENCES

American College of Obstetricians and Gynecologists: Chronic hypertension in pregnancy. ACOG Practice Bulletin No. 29. Obstet Gynecol 2001;98:177.

American College of Obstetricians and Gynecologists: Diagnosis and management of preeclampsia and eclampsia. ACOG Practice Bulletin No. 33. Obstet Gynecol 2002;99:159.

Chambers JC et al: Association of maternal endothelial dysfunction with preeclampsia. JAMA 2001;285:1607.

CLASP: A randomised trial of low-dose aspirin for the prevention and treatment of pre-eclampsia among 9364 pregnant women. CLASP (Collaborative Low-dose Aspirin Study in Pregnancy) Collaborative Group. Lancet 1994;343:619.

Duley L: Pre-eclampsia and hypertension. Clin Evid 2002;7:1296.

Duley L, Gulmezoglu AM, Henderson-Smart DJ: Magnesium sulphate and other anticonvulsants for women with pre-eclampsia. Cochrane Database Syst Rev 2003;(2):CD000025.

Duley L et al: Antiplatelet agents for preventing pre-eclampsia and its complications. Cochrane Database Syst Rev 2004;(1):CD004659.

Esplin MS et al: Paternal and maternal components of the predisposition to preeclampsia. N Engl J Med 2001;344:867.

Isler CM et al: A prospective, randomized trial comparing the efficacy of dexamethasone and betamethasone for the treatment of antepartum HELLP (hemolysis, elevated liver enzymes, and low platelet count) syndrome. Am J Obstet Gynecol 2001;184:1332.

Lain KY, Roberts JM: Contemporary concepts in the pathogenesis and management of preeclampsia. JAMA 2002;287:3183.

Levine RJ et al: Trial of calcium to prevent preeclampsia. N Engl J Med 1997;337:69.

Levine RJ et al: Circulating angiogenic factors and the risk of preeclampsia. N Engl J Med 2004;350:672.

O'Brien JM, Milligan DA, Barton JR: Impact of high-dose corticosteroid therapy for patients with HELLP (hemolysis, elevated liver enzymes, and low platelet count) syndrome. Am J Obstet Gynecol 2000;183:921.

Report of the National High Blood Pressure Education Program Working Group on High Blood Pressure in Pregnancy. Am J Obstet Gynecol 2000;183:S1.

Sibai BM: Prevention of preeclampsia: A big disappointment. Am J Obstet Gynecol 1998;179:1275.

Sibai BM et al: Risk factors associated with preeclampsia in healthy nulliparous women. The Calcium for Preeclampsia Prevention (CPEP) Study Group. Am J Obstet Gynecol 1997;177:1003.

Taylor RN: Review: Immunobiology of preeclampsia. Am J Reprod Immunol 1997;37:79.

Third-Trimester Vaginal Bleeding

20

Jennifer Scearce, MD, & Peter S. Uzelac, MD

Third-trimester hemorrhage continues to be one of the most ominous complications of pregnancy. Bleeding in late pregnancy is common and requires medical evaluation in 5–10% of pregnancies. The seriousness and frequency of obstetric hemorrhage make third-trimester hemorrhage one of the 3 leading causes of maternal death and a major cause of perinatal morbidity and mortality in the United States. Fortunately, most patients have only slight blood loss. However, even minor bleeding may be caused by a life-threatening disorder.

Differentiation must be made between obstetric causes of bleeding (usually more hazardous) and nonobstetric causes (usually less hazardous) (Table 20–1). Nonobstetric causes usually result in relatively little blood loss and little threat to mother or fetus. An exception is invasive carcinoma of the cervix. Obstetric causes are of more concern. Most serious hemorrhages (2–3% of pregnancies) result in loss of more than 800 mL of blood and are due to premature separation of the placenta or placenta previa. Less common but still dangerous causes of bleeding are circumvallate placenta, abnormalities of the blood clotting mechanism, and uterine rupture. Bleeding from the peripheral portion of the intervillous space, or marginal sinus rupture, is a diagnosis of exclusion. Extrusion of cervical mucus ("bloody show") is the most common cause of bleeding in late pregnancy. Although blood loss in this setting occasionally is heavy, medical intervention almost never is necessary.

Although almost all of the blood loss from placental accidents is maternal, some fetal loss is possible, particularly if the substance of the placenta is traumatized. Bleeding from vasa praevia is the only cause of pure fetal hemorrhage but fortunately is rare. If fetal bleeding is suspected, the presence of fetal hemoglobin can be confirmed by elution or electrophoretic techniques.

This chapter focuses on 3 major causes of hemorrhage: premature separation of the placenta, placenta previa, and uterine rupture. Circumvallate placenta and marginal sinus rupture (usually self-limited) are considered variants of premature separation of the placenta.

INITIAL EVALUATION

Principles of Management

Two principles in the investigation of third-trimester hemorrhage must be followed. (1) Any woman experiencing vaginal bleeding in late pregnancy must be evaluated in a hospital capable of dealing with maternal hemorrhage and a compromised perinate. (2) A vaginal or rectal examination must not be performed until placenta previa has been ruled out. Vaginal or rectal examination is extremely hazardous because of the possibility of provoking an uncontrollable, catastrophic hemorrhage.

Life-Threatening Hemorrhage Associated with Hypovolemic Shock

Early recognition of hypovolemia is essential. Signs and symptoms of hypovolemic shock include pallor, clammy skin, syncope, thirst, dyspnea, restlessness, agitation, anxiety, confusion, falling blood pressure, tachycardia, thready pulse, and oliguria. Abnormalities in the fetal heart tracing (decelerations of change in baseline) occur as the mother decompensates (Table 20–2).

Most healthy gravidas remain hemodynamically stable until they lose approximately 1500 mL (25%) of their blood volume. If adequate treatment is not provided, the patient will rapidly decompensate.

In the unstable patient, the standard ABCDs of resuscitation should be initiated. Guarantee a patent airway. Place the patient in Trendelenburg position with a left tilt, which will maximize venous return by preventing the gravid uterus from compressing the inferior vena cava. Two large-bore (16-gauge or larger) intravenous catheters should be placed and fluid replacement with crystalloid or colloid volume expanders initiated. In this case, the "D" in the ABCDs represents continuous electronic fetal monitoring while the mother is being stabilized.

A. Blood Transfusion

The initial hematocrit may be deceptively normal until equilibration is reached in a patient with rapid blood loss hemoconcentration. Therefore, the clinical evaluation

Table 20–1. Common causes of third-trimester bleeding.

Obstetric Causes	Nonobstetric Causes
Bloody show	Cervical cancer or dysplasia
Placenta previa	Cervicitis[1]
Abruptio placentae	Cervical polyps
Vasa previa	Cervical eversion
Disseminated intravascular coagulopathy (DIC)	Vaginal laceration
	Vaginitis
Uterine rupture	
Marginal sinus bleed[2]	

[1]Due to trichomoniasis, *Chlamydia trachomatis, Neisseria gonorrhoeae,* herpes simplex virus, etc.
[2]Marginal sinus bleed is a form of abruptio placentae.

should be the primary guide in managing the patient with hemorrhage.

When clinically indicated, whole blood or packed red blood cells (PRBCs) should be administered rapidly. When packed cells are used, it is important to be aware of the potential for dilution coagulopathy. After 4 units of PRBCs are transfused, a coagulation panel in addition to calcium and potassium levels should be obtained and electrolytes replenished if needed. If fluid overload is a concern, such as in the preeclamptic patient, cryoprecipitate can be used in place of fresh-frozen plasma. Invasive hemodynamic monitoring may be necessary in extraordinary cases.

B. VASOACTIVE DRUGS

Vasoactive drugs should be used only when specific pharmacologic effects are desired (eg, to increase myocardial contractility), when volume expanders are not available, or when volume expansion and other measures are ineffective. Even in these cases, efficacy may be questioned; these agents should be used only when their benefit clearly outweighs their potential risks. Delivery will have been accomplished prior to use of these agents in almost all cases. The most commonly used agent is dopamine (a mixed α- and β-adrenergic stimulant), 200 mg in 500 mL sodium chloride intravenously, starting at 2–5 μg/kg/min and increasing gradually by 5–10 μg/kg/min to 20–50 μg/kg/min. Other agents that might be given by experienced personnel include levarterenol bitartrate, isoproterenol, metaraminol bitartrate, and phenylephrine. Intra-arterial blood pressure monitoring usually is required when these medications are given.

Nonemergency Bleeding

A. HISTORY AND ABDOMINAL EXAMINATION

Once the patient is evaluated and found to be hemodynamically stable, the cause of bleeding must be quickly identified. After a brief history is obtained, the patient's abdomen should be examined and a bedside ultrasound performed to evaluate the location of the placenta and the fetal status.

Table 20–2. Clinical picture in hemorrhagic shock and expected response to volume replacement.

Clinical Sign	Primary Shock		Secondary Shock
	Early	Late	
Mental state	Alert and anxious	Confused	Coma
General appearance	Normal and warm	Pale and cold	Cyanotic and cold
Blood pressure	Slightly hypotensive	Moderately hypotensive	Markedly hypotensive
Respiratory system	Slight tachypnea	Tachypnea	Tachypnea and cyanosis
Urinary output	30 to 60 mL/h	< 30 mL/h	Anuria
	(0.5–1.0 mL/kg/h)	(<0.5 mL/kg/h)	
Effect of volume challenge on			
Blood pressure	Increased	Slightly increased	No response
Urinary output	Increased	Slightly increased	No response

If ultrasound is not immediately available, fetal heart tones should be obtained and the fundal height marked on the abdomen with a ballpoint or other indelible pen. This aids in determining gestational age and later aids in ascertaining if the uterus is rapidly expanding from concealed hemorrhage due to abruptio placentae. Leopold's maneuvers assist in determination of fetal size, presentation, position, and engagement. It is crucial to determine whether the presenting part is well engaged in the pelvis. When there is engagement, total placenta previa is unlikely. Palpation for uterine contractions, tone, and tenderness should be conducted. Hemodynamic status can change after initial assessment and therefore should be continuously re-evaluated.

B. LABORATORY EVALUATION

Laboratory evaluation should include blood type and cross-match for 2–6 units, depending on the hemodynamic status, as well as a complete blood count with platelets and baseline coagulation status (prothrombin time and partial thromboplastin time). D-Dimer or fibrin split products are useful when abruptio placentae is suspected. These are the most sensitive tests to confirm coagulopathy; however, they are qualitative studies and provide little information about the severity of abruption.

C. VAGINAL EXAMINATION

Once placenta previa has been ruled out, both a speculum and a manual vaginal examination should be performed to evaluate for the presence of either a nonobstetric etiology or labor. When other causes have been excluded, placental abruption (including marginal sinus bleed) becomes the assumed diagnosis.

D. ULTRASOUND EXAMINATION

Ultrasound is the most accurate way to confirm a diagnosis of placenta previa. A translabial or transvaginal study can be safely performed if the diagnosis is unclear from a transabdominal scan. Transvaginal ultrasound is the most accurate means to evaluate for placenta previa and has been demonstrated to be safe in experienced hands. The addition of color flow Doppler to real-time ultrasound increases the sensitivity. Ultrasound has limited sensitivity in diagnosing a retroplacental clot (caused by abruption), even in experienced hands. However, it occasionally is useful for diagnosis of a concealed hemorrhage.

Ultrasound evaluation should be performed in the labor and delivery suite if possible. Fetal heart rate (FHR) monitoring should continue at regular intervals throughout the study. Assessment of amniotic fluid volume and confirmation of fetal age should be obtained at the time of ultrasound study.

E. MANAGEMENT OF BLEEDING

At this point, findings regarding the status of the mother, fetus, and placenta and evaluation of labor should be combined to provide a diagnosis and to plan the course of management. The 3 general management options are immediate delivery, continued labor, and expectant management, depending on the diagnosis.

If the fetus is immature, the patient should be treated expectantly unless additional complications (eg, continuing bleeding, evidence of fetal compromise, labor, or spontaneous rupture of the membranes) appear. In approximately 90% of cases, third-trimester bleeding subsides within 24 hours. If placental studies signify a high placental implantation and bleeding stops, repeat vaginal examination is indicated prior to patient discharge to exclude nonobstetric causes of bleeding (Fig 20–1).

Nonobstetric causes of bleeding in late pregnancy usually result only in spotting that does not increase with activity. There are no uterine contractions, and the definitive diagnosis usually is made by speculum examination, Papanicolaou smear, culture, or colposcopy. Only advanced cancer is associated with a poor maternal prognosis. Vaginal lacerations and varices may require repair but have a good prognosis. Most infections causing bleeding clear readily when treated with appropriate agents. Benign neoplasias and eversions require simple treatment and have a good prognosis.

PREMATURE SEPARATION OF THE PLACENTA (ABRUPTIO PLACENTAE, MARGINAL SINUS BLEED)

 ESSENTIALS OF DIAGNOSIS

- *Unremitting abdominal (uterine) or back pain.*
- *Irritable, tender, and often hypertonic uterus.*
- *Visible or concealed hemorrhage.*
- *Evidence of fetal distress may or may not be present, depending on the severity of the process.*

General Considerations

Premature separation of the placenta is defined as separation from the site of uterine implantation before delivery of the fetus (approximately 1 in 77–89 deliveries). The severe form (resulting in fetal death) has an incidence of approximately 1 in 500–750 deliveries. Two principal forms of premature separation of the pla-

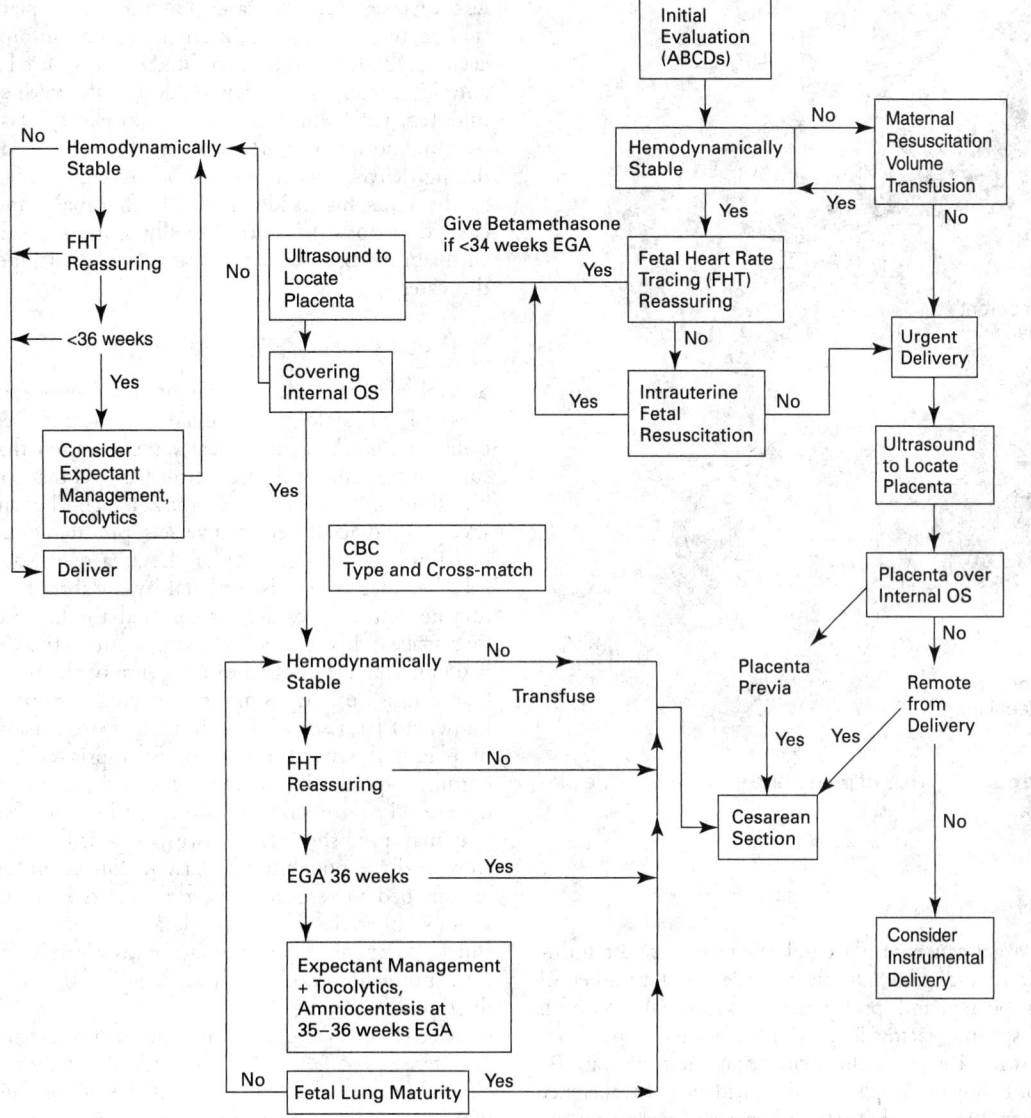

Figure 20–1. Algorithm for evaluating third-trimester vaginal bleeding.

centa can be recognized, depending on whether the resulting hemorrhage is external or concealed (Fig 20–2). In the **concealed form** (20%), the hemorrhage is confined within the uterine cavity, detachment of the placenta may be complete, and the complications often are severe. Approximately 10% of abruptions are associated with clinically significant coagulopathies (disseminated intravascular coagulation [DIC]), but 40% of those severe enough to cause fetal death are associated with coagulopathy. In the **external form** (80%), the blood drains through the cervix, placental detachment is more likely to be incomplete, and the compli-

cations are fewer and less severe. Occasionally, the placental detachment involves only the margin or placental rim. Here, the most important complication is the possibility of premature labor.

Approximately 30% of cases of third-trimester bleeding are due to placental separation, with the initial hemorrhage usually encountered after the 26th week. Placental separation in early pregnancy cannot be distinguished from other causes of abortion. Approximately 50% of separations occur before the onset of labor, and 10–15% are not diagnosed before the second stage of labor.

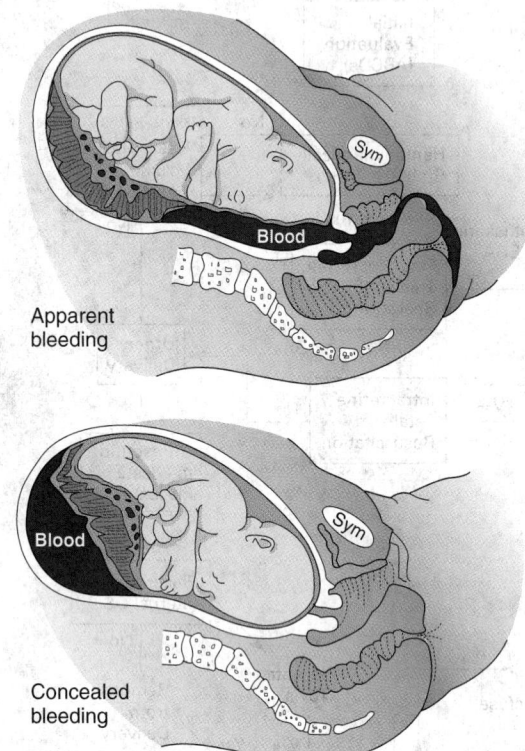

Apparent
bleeding

Blood

Sym

Blood

Sym

Concealed
bleeding

Figure 20–2. Types of premature separation of the placenta.

Etiology

The exact causes of placental separation are often difficult to ascertain, although there are a number of predisposing and precipitating factors. A common predisposing factor is previous placental separation. Following 1 episode, the incidence of recurrence is 10–17%. Following 2 episodes, the incidence of recurrence exceeds 20%. The hypertensive states of pregnancy are associated with 2.5–17.9% incidence of placental separation. In abruptio placentae extensive enough to cause fetal death, approximately 50% of cases are associated with hypertensive states of pregnancy. Approximately half of these cases have chronic hypertension and half pregnancy-induced hypertension. Other predisposing factors include advanced maternal age, multiparity, uterine distention (eg, multiple gestation, hydramnios), vascular disease (eg, diabetes mellitus, systemic lupus erythematosus), thrombophilias, uterine anomalies or tumors (eg, leiomyoma), cigarette smoking, alcohol consumption (> 14 drinks per week), cocaine use, and possibly maternal type O blood.

Precipitating causes of premature separation of the placenta, although more direct and definable, are no less diverse. All are rare. Circumvallate placenta, trauma (eg, external or internal version, automobile accident, abdominal trauma directly transmitted to an anterior placenta), sudden reduction in uterine volume (eg, rapid amniotic fluid loss, delivery of a first twin), abnormally short cord (usually only a problem during delivery, when traction is exerted on the cord as the fetus moves down the birth canal), and increased venous pressure (usually only problematic with abrupt or extreme alterations) are included in this category.

Pathophysiology & Pathology

Several mechanisms are thought to be important in the pathophysiology of premature placental separation. One mechanism is local vascular injury that results in vascular rupture into the decidua basalis, bleeding, and hematoma formation. The hematoma shears off adjacent denuded vessels, producing further bleeding and enlargement of the area of separation. Another mechanism is initiated by an abrupt rise in uterine venous pressure transmitted to the intervillous space. This results in engorgement of the venous bed and separation of all or a portion of the placenta. Conditions predisposing to vascular injury and known to be associated with an increased incidence of placental separation are preeclampsia–eclampsia, chronic hypertension, diabetes mellitus, chronic renal disease, cigarette smoking, and cocaine use. Factors that may predispose to a disturbed vascular equilibrium and the possibility of passive congestion of the venous bed in response to an abrupt rise in uterine venous pressure are vasodilatation secondary to shock, compensatory hypertension as a result of aortic compression, and paralytic vasodilatation of conduction anesthesia.

Mechanical factors causing premature separation are rare (1–5%). They include transabdominal trauma, sudden decompression of the uterus, such as with the delivery of a first twin or rupture of the membranes in hydramnios, or traction on a short umbilical cord.

Another possible mechanism is initiation of the coagulation cascade. This may occur, for example, with trauma causing release of tissue thromboplastin. These activated coagulation factors in turn may act to initiate clot formation in the relative hemodynamic stasis occurring in the placental pool.

Anatomically, placental abruption may occur by hemorrhage into the decidual basalis, which splits, leaving a thin layer adjacent to the myometrium. This decidual hematoma leads to separation, compression, and further bleeding. Alternatively, a spiral artery may rupture, creating a retroplacental hematoma. In either case, bleeding occurs, a clot forms, and the placental surface can no longer provide metabolic exchange between mother and fetus.

The clot depresses the adjacent placenta. Nonclotted blood courses from the site of injury. In concealed hemorrhage, this effusion may be totally retained behind the placental margins, behind the membrane attachment to the uterine wall, or behind a closely applied fetal presenting part. The blood may rupture through the membranes or placenta and gain access to the amniotic fluid (and vice versa). The tissue disruption by bleeding may allow maternofetal hemorrhage, fetomaternal hemorrhage, maternal bleeding into the amniotic fluid, or amniotic fluid embolus, depending on the areas disrupted and their relative pressure differences.

Concealed hemorrhage is more likely to be associated with complete placental detachment. If the placental margins remain adherent, central placental separation may result in hemorrhage that infiltrates the uterine wall. Uterine tetany may follow. Occasionally, extensive intramyometrial bleeding results in uteroplacental apoplexy—so-called **Couvelaire uterus,** a purplish and copper-colored, ecchymotic, indurated organ that may lose its contractile force because of disruption of the muscle bundles.

In the more severe cases of separation, there may be a clinically significant amount of DIC associated with depletion of fibrinogen and platelets as well as other clotting factors. The mother may then develop a hemorrhagic diathesis that is manifested by widespread petechiae, active bleeding, hypovolemic shock, and failure of the normal clotting mechanism. In addition, fibrin deposits in small capillaries (along with the hypoxic vascular damage of shock) can result in potentially lethal complications, including acute cor pulmonale, renal cortical and tubular necrosis, and anterior pituitary infarction (Sheehan's syndrome).

The likelihood of fetal hypoxia and fetal death depends on the amount and duration of placental separation and, in severe cases, the loss of a significant amount of fetal blood.

Clinical Findings

A. SYMPTOMS AND SIGNS

In general, the clinical findings correspond to the degree of separation. Approximately 30% of separations are small, produce few or no symptoms, and usually are not noted until the placenta is inspected. Larger separations are accompanied by abdominal pain and uterine irritability. Hemorrhage may be visible or concealed. If the process is extensive, evidence of fetal distress, uterine tetany, DIC, or hypovolemic shock may be seen. Increased uterine tonus and frequency of contractions may provide early clues of abruption.

Approximately 80% of patients will present with vaginal bleeding, and two-thirds will have uterine tenderness and abdominal or back pain. One-third will have abnormal contractions; about half of these will have high-frequency contractions and half hypertonus. More than 20% of patients with abruptio placentae will be diagnosed erroneously as having idiopathic premature labor. Fetal distress will be present in more than 50% of cases, and 15% will present with fetal demise.

If placental separation is marginal, there will be only minimal irritability and no uterine tenderness or fetal distress. There may be a limited amount of external bleeding (50–150 mL), either bright or dark red depending on the rapidity of its appearance.

B. LABORATORY AND IMAGING FINDINGS

The degree of anemia probably will be considerably less than would seem to be justified by the amount of blood loss because changes in hemoglobin and hematocrit are delayed during acute blood loss until secondary hemodilution has occurred. A peripheral blood smear may show a reduced platelet count; the presence of schistocytes, suggesting intravascular coagulation; and fibrinogen depletion with release of fibrin split products. If serial laboratory determinations of fibrinogen levels are not available, the clot observation test, a simple but invaluable bedside procedure, can be performed. A venous blood sample is drawn every hour, placed in a clean test tube, and observed for clot formation and clot lysis. Failure of clot formation within 5–10 minutes or dissolution of a formed clot when the tube is gently shaken is proof of a clotting deficiency that almost surely is due principally to a lack of fibrinogen and platelets.

More sophisticated studies should be available on an emergency basis in most hospitals. The following tests will assist in determining coagulation status: prothrombin time and partial thromboplastin time, platelet count, fibrinogen, and fibrin split products.

Ultrasonography may be considered in the diagnosis of placental abruption but often is inconclusive. Possible findings include hyperechoic foci posterior to the placenta suggestive of a collection of fresh blood or a hypoechoic area suggestive of a formed clot. Lack of findings does not provide reassurance, and use of ultrasound should not be substituted for clinical judgment, especially in the face of a concerning clinical situation.

Treatment

A. EXPECTANT THERAPY

Expectant management of suspected placental abruption is the exception, not the rule. This management pathway should be attempted only with careful observation of the patient and a clear clinical picture. In general, expectant management may be appropriate when the mother is stable, the fetus is immature, and the fetal heart tracing is reassuring. The patient should be observed in the labor and delivery suite for 24–48 hours to ensure that further placental separation is not occurring. Continuous fetal and uterine monitoring should be maintained. Changes in fetal status may be the earliest indication of an expanding abruption.

In retrospective studies of women with placental abruption, tocolytic use was associated with increasing gestational age at delivery. Tocolytic use did not increase the incidence of hemorrhage, fetal distress, or stillbirth. Currently no prospective trials addressing the efficacy of tocolytic therapy in preventing an abruption from expanding have been reported.

Once the patient is stable, the decision to manage the patient as an outpatient should be tailored to the clinical situation. If outpatient surveillance is selected, the fetus should be followed closely with nonstress testing.

B. Emergency Measures

Most cases of placental abruption are diagnosed as an acute event (upon presentation to labor and delivery or during the intrapartum period), making immediate intervention necessary. If the patient exhibits clinical findings that become progressively more severe or if a major placental separation is suspected as manifested by hemorrhage, uterine spasm, or fetal distress, an acute emergency exists.

Blood should be drawn for laboratory studies and at least 4 units of PRBCs typed and crossed. Two large-bore intravenous catheters should be placed and crystalloid administered.

C. Vaginal Delivery

An attempt at vaginal delivery is indicated if the degree of separation appears to be limited and if the continuous FHR tracing is reassuring. When placental separation is extensive but the fetus is dead or of dubious viability, vaginal delivery is indicated. The exception to vaginal delivery is the patient in whom hemorrhage is uncontrollable and operative delivery is necessary to save the life of the fetus or mother.

Induction of labor with an oxytocin infusion should be instituted if active labor does not begin shortly after amniotomy. In practice, augmentation often is not needed because usually the uterus is already excessively irritable. If the uterus is extremely spastic, uterine contractions cannot be clearly identified unless an internal monitor is used, and the progress of labor must be judged by observing cervical dilatation. Pudendal block anesthesia is recommended. Conduction anesthesia is to be avoided in the face of significant hemorrhage because profound, persistent hypotension may result.

However, in the volume-repleted patient in early labor, a preemptive epidural should be considered because rapid deterioration of maternal or fetal status can occur as labor progresses.

D. Cesarean Section

The indications for cesarean section are both fetal and maternal. Abdominal delivery should be selected whenever delivery is not imminent for a fetus with a reasonable chance of survival who exhibits persistent evidence of distress. Cesarean section also is indicated if the fetus is in good condition but the situation is not favorable for rapid delivery in the face of progressive or severe placental separation. This includes most nulliparous patients with less than 3–4 cm of cervical dilatation. Maternal indications for cesarean section are uncontrollable hemorrhage from a contracting uterus, rapidly expanding uterus with concealed hemorrhage (with or without a live fetus) when delivery is not imminent, uterine apoplexy as manifested by hemorrhage with secondary relaxation of a previously spastic uterus, or refractory uterus with delivery necessary (20%).

Complications

A. Disseminated Intravascular Coagulation

Placental abruption can lead to initiation of the coagulation cascade by release of tissue thromboplastin into the maternal circulation. Consumption of coagulation factors and platelets is followed by coagulopathic hemorrhage. A cycle ensues as further bleeding worsens the depletion of coagulation factors. Continuous monitoring for evidence of a clotting deficiency is mandatory from the time the diagnosis of placental abruption is considered well into the postpartum period. Treatment will depend not only on the demonstration of hematologic deficiencies but also on the amount of active bleeding and the anticipated route of delivery.

1. **Fresh whole blood**—Fresh whole blood is generally reserved for massive hemorrhage (more than 5–6 L blood loss in a 24-hour period). Each unit has a volume of 500 cc and contains red blood cells, white blood cells, coagulation factors, and other plasma proteins. Like PRBCs, 1 unit can be expected to raise the hematocrit by 3%.

2. **Packed red blood cells**—PRBCs are satisfactory for immediate replacement of blood loss, but they do not contain clotting factors. Each unit has a volume of 250 cc. Because the amount of white blood cells and plasma proteins is less than in whole blood, the chance of transfusion reaction is decreased.

3. **Fresh-frozen plasma**—Fresh-frozen plasma is a preparation of unconcentrated clotting factors without platelets. Each unit has a volume of 250 cc and can be expected to raise any clotting factor concentration by 2–3%. Fibrinogen concentration is raised by 10 mg% per unit. Fresh-frozen plasma usually is given in increments of 2 units.

4. **Cryoprecipitate packs**—Cryoprecipitate is prepared as a concentrate of fresh-frozen plasma and contains all the necessary labile coagulation factors. Because each unit contains a volume of only 40 cc, it is useful in avoiding fluid overload when treating hypofibrinogenemia.

5. **Platelets**—During active bleeding, transfusion of platelets often is the best practical means of counteracting a clotting deficiency. Each unit of platelets has a volume of 40–50 cc and can be expected to raise the platelet count by 10,000. Transfusions are customarily ordered as a minimum of 6–8 units.

6. **Heparin**—Prophylactic administration of heparin to block conversion of prothrombin to thrombin (and thereby reduce the consumption of coagulation factors) has been used successfully in the management of DIC associated with fetal death ("dead fetus syndrome"). With prompt diagnosis of fetal death and uterine evacuation, this syndrome is rarely seen. There is no role for heparin in treatment of DIC related to abruption.

7. **Preparation for surgery**—If cesarean section is indicated, preparation for surgery must be completed quickly. Two to 4 units of PRBCs should be secured from the moment the diagnosis is entertained. Fresh-frozen plasma can be ordered as indicated by coagulation studies. Empiric treatment of a clotting disorder may be necessary if intraoperative findings suggest abnormal coagulation and confirmatory laboratory results are not readily available. In cases of uncontrollable hemorrhage, despite maximal attempts to correct coagulopathy, alternatives include whole pelvis embolization, intrauterine balloon tamponade, and abdominal packing. Rarely, hysterectomy is necessary to control bleeding, even in the presence of some degree of coagulopathy.

B. Renal Cortical and Tubular Necrosis

The possibility of renal cortical or tubular necrosis must be considered if oliguria persists after an adequate blood volume has been restored. An attempt should be made to improve renal circulation and promote diuresis by increasing fluid volume (with the aid of monitoring). If oliguria or anuria persists, renal necrosis is probable, and fluid intake and output must be carefully monitored. Continuing impairment of renal function may require peritoneal dialysis or hemodialysis.

C. Uterine Atony

Extensive infiltration of the myometrial wall with blood may result in loss of myometrial contractility. If, as a result, bleeding from the placental bed is not controlled, hysterectomy may be necessary. If future childbearing is an important consideration, bilateral ligation of the ascending branches of the uterine arteries should be accomplished before resorting to hysterectomy. Not only will blood flow be reduced, but the relative ischemia produced may result in a satisfactory contraction of the damaged uterus. If ligation of the uterine vessels proves ineffective, bilateral ligation of the hypogastric arteries, reducing arterial pressure within the uterus to venous levels, may effect hemostasis. Following ligation of either the uterine or hypogastric arteries, collateral circulation should be adequate to preserve uterine function, including subsequent pregnancies.

A relatively new approach to uterine atony is the B-Lynch suture. This technique involves mechanical involution of an atonic uterus with chromic suture, mimicking the hemostasis obtained with bimanual compression. The B-Lynch technique is quick, easy to learn, and safe, providing a useful alternative to performing a hysterectomy.

Prognosis

External or concealed bleeding, excessive blood loss, shock, nulliparity, a closed cervix, absence of labor, and delayed diagnosis and treatment are unfavorable prognostic factors. Maternal mortality rates ranging from 0.5–5% are currently reported from various parts of the world. Most women die of hemorrhage (immediate or delayed) or cardiac or renal failure. A high degree of suspicion, early diagnosis, and definitive therapy should reduce the maternal mortality rate to 0.5–1%.

The perinatal mortality rate reported with abruption overall is approximately 5%. With severe abruption, the rate is much higher. In approximately 15% of cases, no fetal heartbeat can be heard on admission to the hospital, and in another 50% an abnormal FHR pattern is noted early. In cases in which transfusion of the mother is urgently required, the fetal mortality rate probably will be at least 50%. Liveborn infants have a high rate of morbidity resulting from predelivery hypoxia, birth trauma, and the hazards of prematurity (40–50%).

PLACENTA PREVIA

ESSENTIALS OF DIAGNOSIS

- *Spotting during first and second trimesters.*
- *Sudden, painless, profuse bleeding in third trimester.*
- *Initial cramping in 10% of cases.*

General Considerations

In placenta previa, the placenta is implanted in the lower uterine segment within the zone of effacement and dilatation of the cervix, constituting an obstruction to descent of the presenting part (Fig 20–3). Placenta previa is encountered in approximately 1 in 200 births, but only 20% are complete (placenta over the entire cervix). Approximately 90% of patients will be parous. Among grand multiparas the incidence may be as high as 1 in 20.

Etiology

The incidence of placenta previa is increased by multiparity, advancing age, and previous cesarean delivery. Thus, possible etiologic factors include scarred or poorly vascularized endometrium in the corpus, a large placenta, and abnormal forms of placentation such as succenturiate lobe. The incidence of placenta previa is slightly higher in multiple gestation. A cesarean section scar triples the incidence of placenta previa. Another contributory factor is an increased average surface area of a placenta implanted in the lower uterine segment, possibly because these tissues are less well suited for nidation.

Bleeding in placenta previa may be due to any of the following causes: (1) mechanical separation of the placenta from its implantation site, either during the formation of the lower uterine segment or during effacement and dilatation of the cervix in labor, or as a result of intravaginal manipulation; (2) placentitis; or (3) rupture of poorly supported venous lakes in the decidua basalis that have become engorged with venous blood.

Classification

1. *Complete placenta previa:* The placenta completely covers the internal cervical os.

Figure 20–3. **A:** Marginal placenta previa. **B:** Partial placenta previa. **C:** Complete placenta previa.

2. *Marginal placenta previa:* The placenta is implanted at the margin of the internal cervical os, within 2 cm. If the placenta is seen to be more than 2 cm from the internal os, the rate of antepartum or intrapartum hemorrhage is not increased.

Diagnosis

Every patient suspected of placenta previa should be hospitalized, and cross-matched blood should be at hand. To avoid provoking hemorrhage, both vaginal and rectal examination should not be performed.

A. SYMPTOMS AND SIGNS

Painless hemorrhage is the cardinal sign of placenta previa. Although spotting may occur during the first and second trimesters of pregnancy, the first episode of hemorrhage usually begins after the 28th week and is characteristically described as sudden, painless, and profuse. With the initial bleeding episode, clothing or bedding may be soaked by an impressive amount of bright red, clotted blood, but the blood loss usually is not extensive, seldom produces shock, and almost never is fatal. In approximately 10% of cases there is some initial pain, probably because of coexisting placental separation and localized uterine contractions. Spontaneous labor can be expected over the next few days in 25% of patients. In a small minority of cases, bleeding is less dramatic or does not begin until after spontaneous rupture of the membranes or the onset of labor. A few nulliparous patients even reach term without bleeding, possibly because the placenta has been protected by an uneffaced cervix.

The uterus usually is soft, relaxed, and nontender. A high presenting part cannot be pressed into the pelvic inlet. The infant will present in an oblique or transverse lie in approximately 15% of cases. FHR abnormalities are unlikely unless there are complications such as hypovolemic shock, placental separation, or a cord accident.

B. ULTRASONOGRAPHY (FIG 20–4)

Bedside transabdominal ultrasonography can definitively identify 95% of placenta previas. Transvaginal or transperineal studies can make the diagnosis in virtually every case. This approach is particularly helpful with the posterior placenta previa.

During the middle of the second trimester, the placenta is observed by ultrasound to cover the internal cervical os in approximately 30% of cases. With development of the lower uterine segment, almost all of these low implantations will be carried to a higher station. An early ultrasonic diagnosis of placenta previa requires the confirmation of an additional study before definitive action is taken.

Figure 20–4. Total placenta previa at 18 weeks' gestation. Placenta (PLAC) completely overlies the cervical os. (Courtesy of Dr. Rigoberto Santos.) (From Cunningham FG, Leveno KJ, Bloom SL, et al: Williams Obstetrics, 22nd ed. New York: McGraw-Hill, 2005.)

Differential Diagnosis

Placental causes of bleeding other than placenta previa include partial premature separation of the normally implanted placenta or circumvallate placenta.

Treatment

The treatment depends on the amount of uterine bleeding; the duration of pregnancy and viability of the fetus; the degree of placenta previa; the presentation, position, and station of the fetus; the gravidity and parity of the patient; the status of the cervix; and whether or not labor has begun. The patient must be admitted to the hospital to establish the diagnosis and ideally should remain in the hospital once the diagnosis is made. Blood should be readily available for transfusion.

A. EXPECTANT THERAPY

The initial hemorrhage of placenta previa may occur before pulmonary maturity is established. In such cases, fetal survival can often be enhanced by expectant therapy. Early in pregnancy, transfusions to replace blood loss and the use of tocolytic agents to prevent premature labor are indicated to prolong pregnancy to at least 32–34 weeks. After 34 weeks, the benefits of further maturation must be weighed against the risk of major hemorrhage. The possibility that repeated small hemorrhages may be accompanied by intrauterine growth retardation also must be considered. Approximately 75% of cases of placenta previa are now delivered between 36 and 40 weeks.

In selecting the optimum time for delivery, tests of fetal lung maturation, including assessment of amniotic fluid surfactants and ultrasonic growth measurements, are valuable adjuvants.

If the patient is between 24 and 34 weeks' gestational age, a single course of betamethasone (2 doses of 12 mg intramuscularly separated by 24 hours) or dexamethasone (4 doses of 6 mg intravenously or intramuscularly separated by 12 hours) should be given to promote fetal lung maturity. Repeat courses of steroids are not necessary and usually are considered only for patients who initially present and receive treatment with steroids at less than 24 weeks.

Because of the costs of hospitalization, patients with a presumptive diagnosis of placenta previa are sometimes sent home on strict bed rest after their condition has become stable under ideal, controlled circumstances. Such a policy is always a calculated risk in view of the unpredictability of further hemorrhage, but the practice has been studied and is an acceptable alternative.

B. DELIVERY

1. Cesarean section—Cesarean section is the delivery method of choice with placenta previa. Cesarean section has proved to be the most important factor in lowering maternal and perinatal mortality rates (more so than blood transfusion or better neonatal care).

If possible, hypovolemic shock should be corrected by administration of intravenous fluids and blood before the operation is started. Not only will the mother be better protected, but an at-risk fetus will recover more quickly in utero than if born while the mother is still in shock.

The choice of anesthesia depends on current and anticipated blood loss. A combination of rapid induction, endotracheal intubation, succinylcholine, and nitrous oxide is a suitable method for proceeding in the presence of active bleeding.

The choice of operative technique is of importance because of the placental location and the development of the lower uterine segment. If the incision passes through the site of placental implantation, there is a strong possibility that the fetus will lose a significant amount of blood—even enough to require subsequent transfusion. With posterior implantation of the placenta, a low-transverse incision may be best if the lower uterine segment is well developed. Otherwise, a classic incision may be required to secure sufficient room and to avoid incision through the placenta. Preparations should be made for care and resuscitation of the infant if it becomes necessary. In addition, the possibility of blood loss should be monitored in the newborn if the placenta has been incised.

In a small percentage of cases, hemostasis in the placental bed is unsatisfactory because of the poor contractility of the lower uterine segment. Mattress sutures or packing may be required in addition to the usual oxytocin, prostaglandins, and methylergonovine. If placenta previa accreta is found, hemostasis may necessitate a total hysterectomy. Puerperal infection and anemia are the most likely postoperative complications.

2. Vaginal delivery—Vaginal delivery usually is reserved for patients with a marginal implantation and a cephalic presentation. If vaginal delivery is elected, the membranes should be artificially ruptured prior to any attempt to stimulate labor (oxytocin given before amniotomy likely will cause further bleeding). Tamponade of the presenting part against the placental edge usually reduces bleeding as labor progresses.

Because of the possibility of fetal hypoxemia due to either placental separation or a cord accident (as a result of either prolapse or compression of low insertion of the cord by the descending presenting part), continuous fetal monitoring must be used. If FHR abnormalities develop, a rapid cesarean section should be performed unless vaginal delivery is imminent.

Deliver the patient in the easiest and most expeditious manner as soon as the cervix is fully dilated and the presenting part is on the perineum. For this purpose, a vacuum extractor is particularly valuable because it expedites delivery without risking rupture of the lower uterine segment.

Complications

A. MATERNAL

Maternal hemorrhage, shock, and death may follow severe antepartum bleeding resulting from placenta previa. Death may occur as a result of intrapartum and postpartum bleeding, operative trauma, infection, or embolism.

Premature separation of a portion of a placenta previa occurs in virtually every case and causes excessive external bleeding without pain; however, complete or wide separation of the placenta before full dilatation of the cervix is uncommon.

Placenta previa accreta is a serious abnormality in which the sparse endometrium and the myometrium of the lower uterine segment are penetrated by the trophoblast in a manner similar to placenta accreta higher in the uterus. In patients with 1 prior cesarean section, the rate of accreta in the presence of previa is 20–25% and rises to 50% with 2 or more prior cesarean sections.

B. FETAL

Prematurity (gestational age < 36 weeks) accounts for 60% of perinatal deaths due to placenta previa. The fetus may die as a result of decreased oxygen delivery intrapartum or birth injury. Fetal hemorrhage due to tearing of the placenta occurs with vaginal manipulation and especially upon entry into the uterine cavity as cesarean section is done for placenta previa. About half of these cesarean babies lose some blood. Fetal blood loss is directly proportional to the time that elapses between lacerating the cotyledon and clamping the cord.

Prognosis

A. MATERNAL

With rapid recourse to cesarean section, use of banked blood, and expertly administered anesthesia, the overall maternal mortality has fallen to less than 1 in 1000.

B. FETAL

The perinatal mortality rate associated with placenta previa has declined to approximately 1%. Although premature labor, placental separation, cord accidents, and uncontrollable hemorrhage cannot be avoided, the mortality rate can be greatly reduced if ideal obstetric and newborn care is given.

RUPTURE OF THE UTERUS

ESSENTIALS OF DIAGNOSIS

- *Fetal heart rate abnormalities.*
- *Increased suprapubic pain and tenderness with labor.*
- *Sudden cessation of uterine contractions with a "tearing" sensation.*
- *Vaginal bleeding (or bloody urine).*
- *Recession of the fetal presenting part.*

General Considerations

Rupture of the pregnant uterus is a potential obstetric catastrophe and a major cause of maternal death. The incidence of uterine rupture is 0.8% for women with a prior low-transverse uterine scar and 4–8% for women with a prior classic scar. Complete rupture includes the entire thickness of the uterine wall and, in most cases, the overlying serosal peritoneum (broad ligament) (Fig 20–5). *Occult* or *incomplete rupture* is a term usually reserved for dehiscence of a uterine incision from previous surgery, in which the visceral peritoneum remains intact. Such defects usually are asymptomatic unless converted to complete rupture during the course of pregnancy or labor.

Risk factors for uterine rupture include history of hysterotomy (cesarean section, myomectomy, metroplasty, cornual resection), trauma (motor vehicle accident, rotational forceps, extension of a cervical lacera-

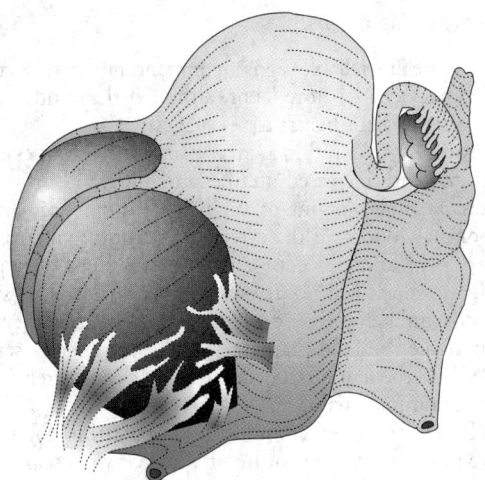

Figure 20–5. Rupture of the lower uterine segment into the broad ligament.

tion), uterine overdistention (hydramnios, multiple gestation, macrosomia), uterine anomalies, placenta percreta, and choriocarcinoma.

Ruptures usually occur during the course of labor. One notable exception is scars from a classic cesarean section (or hysterotomy), one-third of which rupture during the third trimester before term and before the onset of labor. Other causes of rupture without labor are placenta percreta, invasive mole, choriocarcinoma, and cornual pregnancy.

Complete ruptures can be classified as traumatic or spontaneous. Traumatic ruptures occur most commonly as a result of motor vehicle accidents, improper administration of an oxytocic agent, or an inept attempt at operative vaginal delivery. Breech extraction through an incompletely dilated cervix is the type of operative vaginal delivery most likely to produce uterine rupture. Other maneuvers that impose risk of rupture are internal podalic version and extraction, difficult forceps, destructive operations, and cephalic replacement to relieve shoulder dystocia. Neglected obstructed labor may be responsible for rupture of the uterus. Causes of obstructed labor include contracted pelvis, fetal macrosomia, brow or face presentation, hydrocephalus, or tumors involving the birth canal. The vast majority of uterine ruptures are associated with prior uterine surgery. Previous uterine surgery includes both classic and low cervical section, intramural or submucous myomectomy, resection of the uterine cornu, metroplasty, and trachelectomy. Other operative procedures that may have damaged the uterus are vigorous curettage, induced abortion, and manual removal of the placenta.

Clinical Findings

There are no reliable signs of impending uterine rupture that occurs before labor, although the sudden appearance of gross hematuria is suggestive.

Rupture may produce local pain and tenderness associated with increased uterine irritability and, in some cases, a small amount of vaginal bleeding. Premature labor may follow. As the extent of the rupture increases, more pain, more bleeding, and perhaps signs of hypovolemic shock will occur. Exsanguination prior to surgery is unlikely because of the reduced vascularity of scar tissue, but the placenta may be completely separated and the fetus extruded partially or completely into the abdominal cavity.

By far the most common clinical setting for rupture of the uterus is rupture of a low cervical scar; this almost always occurs during active labor. Clearly identifiable signs and symptoms may be lacking. However 78–90% of patients have FHR abnormalities as the first sign of rupture. Although it is possible that labor will progress to the vaginal birth of an unaffected infant, rupture may lacerate a uterine artery, producing exsanguination, or the fetus may be extruded into the abdominal cavity. If a defect is palpated in the lower uterine segment following vaginal delivery, laparotomy may be necessary to assess the damage. Laparotomy is mandatory if continuing hemorrhage is present. If such a defect is palpated in a stable patient who does not require exploration, a subsequent trial of labor is contraindicated.

Although much less common than FHR abnormalities, other findings of spontaneous rupture during labor are suprapubic pain and tenderness, cessation of uterine contractions, disappearance of fetal heart tones, recession of the presenting part, and vaginal hemorrhage—followed by the signs and symptoms of hypovolemic shock and hemoperitoneum. Ultrasound examination might confirm an abnormal fetal position or extension of the fetal extremities. Hemoperitoneum can sometimes be seen on ultrasound.

The clinical picture depends on the extent of rupture. Unfortunately, valuable time is often lost because the rupture was not diagnosed at the time of initial examination. Whenever a newly delivered patient exhibits persistent bleeding or shock, the uterus must be carefully reexamined for signs of a rupture that may have been difficult to palpate because of the soft, irregular tissue surfaces.

Whenever an operative delivery is performed—especially if the history includes events or problems that increase the likelihood of uterine rupture—the initial examination of the uterus and birth canal must be diligent. A dehiscence of the lower uterine segment contained only by a layer of visceral peritoneum is not an uncommon finding at time of repeat cesarean section.

Treatment

Treatment is dictated by clinical scenario and can range from simply repairing the defect and obtaining hemostasis to removing the entire uterus. If hysterectomy is deemed necessary, either total hysterectomy or the subtotal operation can be performed, depending on the site of rupture and the patient's condition. The most difficult cases are lateral ruptures involving the lower uterine segment and a uterine artery with hemorrhage and hematoma formation obscuring the operative field. Care must be taken to avoid ureteral damage by blind suturing at the base of the broad ligament. If there is a question of ureteral occlusion by a suture, it is best to perform cystotomy to observe the bilateral appearance of an intravenously injected dye such as indigo carmine. If doubt still exists, a retrograde ureteral catheter can be passed upward through the cystotomy wound.

If childbearing is important and the risks—both short and long term—are acceptable to the patient, rupture repair can be attempted. Many ruptures can be repaired. Successful pregnancies have been reported following uterine repair; however, the risk of rupture in a subsequent pregnancy is at least as high as the risk with a prior classic cesarean section. Occult ruptures of the lower uterine segment encountered at repeat section can be treated by freshening the wound edges and secondary repair, but the newly repaired incision is at increased risk for rupture, and a subsequent trial of labor is contraindicated.

Prevention

Most causes of uterine rupture can be avoided by carefully selecting patients for trial of labor. Thorough and well-documented informed consent that includes mention of fetal or maternal death is needed. The ideal candidate will have a single prior low-transverse cesarean for a nonrepetitive indication (eg, breech), will have a prior vaginal delivery, will present in active labor, and will not require augmentation during labor. The further the characteristics diverge from those of this ideal patient, the greater the chance of a failed trial of labor and complications including uterine rupture. Continuous FHR monitoring by fetal scalp electrode as soon as feasible is the best means of detecting evolving rupture during labor. Two-layer closure of the uterine incision and increasing interval between pregnancies appears to decrease the risk of subsequent rupture of the low-transverse scar.

Complications

The complications of ruptured uterus are hemorrhage, shock, postoperative infection, bladder or ureteral damage, thrombophlebitis, amniotic fluid embolus, DIC, pituitary failure, and death.

Prognosis

The maternal mortality rate is 4.2%. The perinatal mortality rate is approximately 46%.

REFERENCES

Ananth CV, Getahun D, Peltier MR, Smulian JC: Placental abruption in term and preterm gestations: Evidence for heterogeneity in clinical pathways. Obstet Gynecol 2006;107:785.

Ananth CV, Smulian JC, Vintzileos AM: The association of placenta previa with history of cesarean delivery and abortion: A metaanalysis. Am J Obstet Gynecol 1997;177:1071.

Besinger RE: The effect of tocolytic use in the management of symptomatic placenta previa. Am J Obstet Gynecol 1995;172:1770.

Bhide A, Thilaganathan B: Recent advances in the management of placenta previa. Curr Opin Obstet Gynecol 2004;16:447.

Cho JH, Jun HS, Lee CN: Hemostatic suturing technique for uterine bleeding during cesarean delivery. Obstet Gynecol 2000;96:129.

Claydon CS, Greenspoon JS: Emergency management of third trimester vaginal bleeding. Postgrad Obstet Gynecol 2001;21:8.

Landon MB, et al. The MFMU Cesarean Registry: Factors affecting the success of trial of labor after previous cesarean delivery. Am J Obstet Gynecol 2005;193:1016.

McGee S, Abernethy WB III, Simel DL: Is this patient hypovolemic? JAMA 1999;281:1022.

Miller DA et al: Intrapartum rupture of the unscarred uterus. Obstet Gynecol 1997;89:671.

Miller DA, Chollet JA, Goodwin TM: Clinical risk factors for placenta previa-placenta accreta. Am J Obstet Gynecol 1997;177:210.

Miller DA, Diaz FG, Paul RH: Vaginal birth after cesarean: a 10-year experience. Obstet Gynecol 1994;84:255.

Rasmussen S et al: Perinatal mortality and case fatality after placental abruption in Norway 1967–1991. Acta Obstet Gynecol Scand 1996;75:229.

Rasmussen S et al: The occurrence of placental abruption in Norway 1967–1991. Acta Obstet Gynecol Scand 1996;75:222.

Sholl JS: Abruptio placentae: Clinical management on nonacute cases. Am J Obstet Gynecol 1987;156:40.

Spinillo A et al: Early morbidity and neurodevelopmental outcome in low-birthweight infants born after third trimester bleeding. Am J Perinatol 1994;11:85.

Towers CV, Pircon RA, Heppard M: Is tocolysis safe in the management of third-trimester bleeding? Am J Obstet Gynecol 1999;180(6 Pt 1):1572.

Wing DA, Paul RH, Millar LK: Management of the symptomatic placenta previa: A randomized, controlled trial of inpatient versus outpatient expectant management. Am J Obstet Gynecol 1996;175:806.

Malpresentation & Cord Prolapse

Karen Kish, MD, & Joseph V. Collea, MD

■ BREECH PRESENTATION

Breech presentation, which complicates 3–4% of all pregnancies, occurs when the fetal pelvis or lower extremities engage the maternal pelvic inlet. Three types of breech are distinguished, according to fetal **attitude** (Fig 21–1). In **frank breech,** the hips are flexed with extended knees bilaterally. In **complete breech,** both hips and knees are flexed. In **footling breech,** 1 (single footling breech) or both (double footling breech) legs are extended below the level of the buttocks.

In singleton breech presentations in which the infant weighs less than 2500 g, 40% are frank breech, 10% complete breech, and 50% footling breech. With birth weights of more than 2500 g, 65% are frank breech, 10% complete breech, and 25% footling breech. The incidences of singleton breech presentations by birth weight and gestational age are listed in Table 21–1.

Fetal **position** in breech presentation is determined by using the fetal sacrum as the point of reference to the maternal pelvis. This is true for frank, complete, and footling breeches. Eight possible positions are recognized: sacrum anterior (SA), sacrum posterior (SP), left sacrum transverse (LST), right sacrum transverse (RST), left sacrum anterior (LSA), left sacrum posterior (LSP), right sacrum anterior (RSA), and right sacrum posterior (RSP). The **station** of the breech presenting part is the location of the fetal sacrum with regard to the maternal ischial spines.

Causes

Before 28 weeks, the fetus is small enough in relation to intrauterine volume to rotate from cephalic to breech presentation and back again with relative ease. As gestational age and fetal weight increase, the relative decrease in intrauterine volume makes such changes more difficult. In most cases, the fetus spontaneously assumes the cephalic presentation to better accommodate the bulkier breech pole in the roomier fundal portion of the uterus.

Breech presentation occurs when spontaneous version to cephalic presentation is prevented as term approaches or if labor and delivery occur prematurely before cephalic version has taken place. Some causes include oligohydramnios, hydramnios, uterine anomalies such as bicornuate or septate uterus, pelvic tumors obstructing the birth canal, abnormal placentation, advanced multiparity, and a contracted maternal pelvis.

In multiple gestations, each fetus may prevent the other from turning, with a 25% incidence of breech in the first twin, nearly 50% for the second twin, and higher percentages with additional fetuses. Additionally, 6% of breech presentations are found to have congenital malformations, which include congenital hip dislocation, hydrocephalus, anencephalus, familial dysautonomia, spina bifida, meningomyelocele, and chromosomal trisomies 13, 18, and 21. Thus, those conditions that alter fetal muscular tone and mobility increase the likelihood of breech presentation.

Diagnosis

A. Palpation and Ballottement

Performance of Leopold's maneuvers and ballottement of the uterus may confirm breech presentation. The softer, more ill-defined breech may be felt in the lower uterine segment above the pelvic inlet. Diagnostic error is common, however, if these maneuvers alone are used to determine presentation.

B. Pelvic Examination

During vaginal examination, the round, firm, smooth head in cephalic presentation can easily be distinguished from the soft, irregular breech presentation if the presenting part is palpable. However, if no presenting part is discernible, further studies are necessary (ie, ultrasound).

C. Radiographic Studies

X-ray studies will differentiate breech from cephalic presentations and help determine the type of breech by locating the position of the lower extremities. X-ray studies can reveal multiple gestation and skeletal defects. Fetal attitude may be seen, but fetal size cannot readily be determined by x-ray film. Because of the risks of radiation exposure to the fetus with this technique, ultrasonography is now used instead of radiography to determine fetal presentation or malformations.

Single footling breech

Frank breech

Complete breech

Figure 21–1. Types of breech presentations. (Reproduced, with permission, from Pernoll ML: *Benson and Pernoll's Handbook of Obstetrics and Gynecology,* 10th ed. McGraw-Hill, 2001.)

D. ULTRASOUND

Ultrasonographic scanning by an experienced examiner will document fetal presentation, attitude, and size; multiple gestation; location of the placenta; and amniotic fluid volume. Ultrasound also will reveal skeletal and soft-tissue malformations of the fetus.

Management

A. ANTEPARTUM MANAGEMENT

Following confirmation of breech presentation, the mother must be closely followed to evaluate for spontaneous version to cephalic presentation. If breech presentation persists beyond 36 weeks, external cephalic version should be considered (see below).

In women considering a vaginal breech delivery, radiographic pelvimetry using x-ray, computed tomogra-

phy, or magnetic resonance imaging should be performed to rule out women with a borderline or contracted pelvis. Attempts at vaginal delivery with an inadequate pelvis are associated with a high rate of difficulty and significant trauma to mother and fetus. Difficult vaginal delivery may still occur in women with adequate pelvic measurements.

B. MANAGEMENT DURING LABOR

1. Examination—Patients with singleton breech presentations are admitted to the hospital with the onset of labor or when spontaneous rupture of membranes occurs because of the increased risk of umbilical cord complications. Upon admission, a repeat ultrasound is obtained to confirm the type of breech presentation and to ascertain head flexion. The fetus is again screened for lethal congenital malformations, such as anencephaly, which would preclude cesarean delivery for fetal indications. A thorough history is taken, and a physical examination is performed to evaluate the status of mother and fetus. Based on these findings, a decision must be made regarding the route of delivery (see below).

2. Electronic fetal monitoring—Continuous electronic fetal heart rate monitoring is essential during labor. If a fetal electrocardiographic electrode is needed, care should be taken to avoid injury to the fetal anus, perineum, and genitalia when attaching the electrode to the breech presenting part. An intrauterine pressure catheter can be used to assess the frequency, strength, and duration of uterine contractions. With the catheter in place, fetal distress or dysfunctional labor can easily be identified and the decision to proceed with a cesarean section made expeditiously to optimize fetal outcome.

3. Oxytocin—The use of oxytocin in the management of breech labor is controversial. Although some obstetricians condemn its use, others use oxytocin with benefit and without complications. Generally, oxytocin

Table 21–1. Incidence of singleton breech presentations by birthweight and gestational age.

Birthweight (g)	Gestational Age (weeks)	Incidence (%)
1000	28	35
1000–1499	28–32	25
1500–1999	32–34	20
2000–2499	34–36	8
2500	36	2–3
All weights		3–4

Table 21–2. Criteria for vaginal or cesarean delivery in breech presentation.

Vaginal Delivery	Cesarean Delivery
Frank breech presentation	**Estimated fetal weight of 3500 g or more, or less than 1500 g.**
Gestational age of 34 weeks or more.	**Contracted or borderline maternal pelvic measurements.**
Estimated fetal weight of 2000–3500 g.	Deflexed or hyperextended fetal head.
Flexed fetal head.	Prolonged rupture of membranes.
Adequate maternal pelvis as determined by x-ray pelvimetry (pelvic inlet with transverse diameter of 11.5 cm and anteroposterior diameter of 10.5 cm; midpelvis with transverse diameter of 10 cm and anteroposterior diameter of 11.5 cm).	Unengaged presenting part.
	Dysfunctional labor.
	Elderly primigravida.
	Mother with infertility problems or poor obstetric history.
No maternal or fetal indications for cesarean section.	Premature fetus (gestational age of 25–34 weeks).
Previable fetus (gestational age < 25 weeks and weight < 700 g).	Most cases of complete or footling breech over 25 weeks' gestation without detectable lethal congenital malformations (to prevent umbilical cord prolapse).
Documented lethal fetal congenital anomalies.	
Presentation of mother in advanced labor with no fetal or maternal distress, even if cesarean delivery was originally planned (a carefully performed, controlled vaginal delivery is safer in such cases than is a hastily executed cesarean section).	Fetus with variable heart rate decelerations on electronic monitoring
	Footling presentation

should be administered only if uterine contractions are insufficient to sustain normal progress in labor. Continuous fetal and uterine monitoring should be used whenever oxytocin is administered.

C. DELIVERY

The decision regarding route of delivery must be made carefully on an individual basis. Criteria for vaginal or cesarean delivery are outlined in Table 21–2.

Prior to 1975, virtually all viable singleton breech presentations were delivered vaginally. Cesarean section was reserved for specific fetal indications, such as unremitting distress or prolapsed umbilical cord, or maternal indications, such as placenta previa, abruptio placentae, or failure of progress in labor. However, breech infants delivered vaginally had a 5-fold higher mortality rate in comparison to cephalic presentations.

Recent studies have shown that planned cesarean delivery decreases perinatal and neonatal morbidity and mortality, with no difference in maternal morbidity and mortality versus planned vaginal breech delivery. Thus, cesarean delivery has now become much more common in breech presentation. Only obstetricians skilled in breech techniques should attempt any breech delivery, whether vaginal or cesarean. Nevertheless, broader familiarity with the technique is needed because unanticipated vaginal breech delivery is still encountered.

1. Cesarean delivery—The type of incision chosen is extremely important. If the lower uterine segment is well developed, as is usually the case in women at term in labor, a transverse "lower segment" incision is adequate for easy delivery. In premature gestations, in an unlabored uterus, or in many cases of malpresentation, the lower uterine segment may be quite narrow, and a low vertical incision is almost always required for atraumatic delivery.

2. Vaginal delivery—Obstetricians who contemplate performing a vaginal breech delivery should be experienced in the maneuver and should be assisted by 3 physicians: (1) an experienced obstetrician who will assist with delivery; (2) a pediatrician capable of providing total resuscitation of the newborn; and (3) an anesthesiologist, to ensure that the mother is comfortable and cooperative during labor and delivery. The type of anesthesia required depends on the type of breech delivery. Multiparous women undergoing spontaneous breech delivery may require no anesthesia or only intravenous analgesia for pain relief during labor and a pudendal anesthetic during delivery. Epidural anesthesia may also be administered during labor or in anticipation of partial breech extraction, including application of Piper forceps to the aftercoming head. In emergency circumstances, complete relaxation of the perineum and uterus is essential for a successful outcome. This is accomplished by immediate induction of inhalation anesthesia or by administration of intravenous nitroglycerin.

a. Spontaneous vaginal delivery—During spontaneous delivery of an infant in the frank breech position, delivery occurs without assistance, and no obstetric maneuvers are applied to the body. The fetus negotiates the maternal pelvis as outlined below, while the operator simply supports the body as it delivers.

Engagement occurs when the bitrochanteric diameter of the fetus has passed the plane of the pelvic inlet. As the fetus descends into the pelvis (Fig 21–2),

Figure 21–2. Mechanism of labor in breech delivery. **A:** Mechanism of breech delivery. Right sacrum transverse (RST) at the onset of labor; engagement of the buttocks usually occurs in the oblique or transverse diameter of the pelvic brim. **B:** Early second stage. The buttocks have reached the pelvic floor, and internal rotation has occurred so that the bitrochanteric diameter lies in the anteroposterior (AP) diameter of the pelvic outlet. **C:** Late second stage. The anterior buttock appears at the vulva by lateral flexion of the trunk around the pubic symphysis. The shoulders have not yet engaged in the pelvis. **D:** The buttocks have been delivered, and the shoulders are adjusting to engage in the transverse diameter of the brim. This movement causes external rotation of the delivered buttocks so that the fetal back becomes uppermost. **E:** The shoulders have reached the pelvic floor and have undergone internal rotation so that the bisacromial diameter lies in the AP diameter of the pelvic outlet. Simultaneously, the buttocks rotate anteriorly through 90 degrees. This is called **restitution.** The head is engaging in the pelvic brim, and the sagittal suture is lying in the transverse diameter of the brim. **F:** The anterior shoulder is born from behind the pubic symphysis by lateral flexion of the delivered trunk.

the buttocks reach the levator ani muscles of the maternal pelvis. At this point, internal rotation occurs, whereby the anterior hip rotates beneath the pubic symphysis, resulting in a sacrum transverse position. The bitrochanteric diameter of the fetal pelvis is now in an anteroposterior position within the maternal pelvis. The breech then presents at the pelvic outlet and, upon emerging, rotates from sacrum transverse to sacrum anterior. Crowning occurs when the bitrochanteric diameter passes under the pubic symphysis. As this occurs, the shoulders enter the pelvic inlet with the bisacromial diameter in the transverse position. As descent occurs, the bisacromial diameter rotates to an oblique or anteroposterior diameter, until the anterior shoulder rests beneath the pubic symphysis. Delivery of the anterior shoulder occurs as it slips beneath the pubic symphysis. Upward flexion of the body allows for easy delivery of the posterior shoulder over the perineum.

As the shoulders descend, the head engages the pelvic inlet in a transverse or oblique position. Rotation of the head to the occiput anterior position occurs as it enters the midpelvis. The occiput then slips beneath the pubic symphysis, and the remainder of the head is delivered by flexion as the chin, mouth, nose, and forehead slip over the maternal perineum.

As delivery of the breech occurs, increasingly larger diameters (bitrochanteric, bisacromial, biparietal) of the body enter the pelvis, whereas in cephalic presentation, the largest diameter (biparietal diameter) enters the pelvis first. Particularly in preterm labors, the head is considerably larger than the body and provides a better "dilating wedge" as it passes through the cervix and into the pelvis. The smaller bitrochanteric and bisacromial diameters may descend into the pelvis through a partially dilated cervix, but the larger biparietal diameter may be trapped. Delivery in these cases is described in the following.

b. Partial breech extraction—Partial breech extraction (assisted breech extraction) is used when the operator discerns that spontaneous delivery will not occur or that expeditious delivery is indicated for fetal or maternal reasons. The body is allowed to deliver spontaneously up to the level of the umbilicus. The operator then assists in delivery of the legs, shoulders, arms, and head.

As the umbilicus appears at the maternal perineum, the operator places a finger medial to 1 thigh and then the other thigh, pressing laterally as the fetal pelvis is rotated away from that side by an assistant. Thus, the thigh is externally rotated at the hip and results in flexion of the knee and delivery of one, then the other, leg. The fetal trunk is then wrapped in a towel to support the body. When both scapulae are visible, the body is rotated counterclockwise. The operator locates the right

Figure 21–3. Assisted delivery of the shoulders. **A:** Shoulders engaged, posterior (left) shoulder at lower level in pelvis than anterior shoulder. **B:** Rotation of trunk causing posterior shoulder to rotate to anterior and slip beneath the pubic symphysis.

humerus and laterally sweeps the arm across the chest and out the perineum (Fig 21–3). In a similar fashion, the body is rotated clockwise to deliver the left arm. The head then spontaneously delivers by gently lifting the body upward and applying fundal pressure to maintain flexion of the fetal head (Fig 21–4). During partial breech extraction, the anterior shoulder may be difficult to deliver if it is impacted behind the pubic symphysis. In this event, the body is gently lifted upward toward the pubic symphysis, and the operator inserts 1 hand along the hollow of the maternal pelvis and identifies the posterior humerus of the fetus. By gentle downward traction on the humerus, the posterior arm can be easily delivered, thus allowing for easier delivery of the anterior shoulder and arm.

The operator may elect to manually assist in delivery of the head by performing the **Mauriceau-Smellie-Veit**

Figure 21–4. Maneuver for delivery of the head. The fingers of the left hand are inserted into the infant's mouth or over the infant's mandible; the right hand exerts pressure on the head from above. (Modified and reproduced, with permission, from Pernoll ML: *Benson and Pernoll's Handbook of Obstetrics and Gynecology,* 10th ed. McGraw-Hill, 2001.)

maneuver (Fig 21–5). In this procedure, the index and middle fingers of 1 of the operator's hands are applied over the maxilla as the body rests on the palm and forearm of the operator. Two fingers of the operator's other hand are applied on either side of the neck with gentle downward traction. At the same time, the body is ele-

Figure 21–5. Mauriceau-Smellie-Veit maneuver for delivery of the head. The fingers of the left hand are inserted into the infant's mouth or over the infant's mandible; the fingers of the right hand curve over the shoulders. An assistant exerts suprapubic pressure on the head. (Reproduced, with permission, from Pernoll ML: *Benson and Pernoll's Handbook of Obstetrics and Gynecology,* 10th ed. McGraw-Hill, 2001.)

vated toward the pubic symphysis, allowing for controlled delivery of the mouth, nose, and brow over the perineum. Likewise, Piper forceps may be used electively or when the Mauriceau-Smellie-Veit maneuver fails to deliver the aftercoming head. Piper forceps may only be used when the cervix is completely dilated and the head is engaged in the pelvis. Ideally, the head is in a direct occiput anterior position, but a left or right occiput anterior position is acceptable. Piper forceps should not be attempted in the occiput transverse positions because this may result in significant fetal and maternal injury. An assistant supports and slightly elevates the fetal trunk while the operator places each forceps blade alongside the fetal parietal bones (Fig 21–6). After proper placement is confirmed, the forceps are locked, and gentle traction is applied to flex and deliver the head over the perineum. A midline episiotomy is often indicated to allow for easier application of the forceps and for delivery.

If, after delivery of the body, the spine remains in the posterior position and rotation is unsuccessful, extraction of the head in a persistent occiput posterior position may be accomplished by the **modified Prague maneuver.** One hand of the operator supports the shoulders from below, while the other hand gently elevates the body upward toward the maternal abdomen. This action flexes the head within the birth canal and results in delivery of the occiput over the perineum.

In premature breech presentations, the incompletely dilated cervix may allow delivery to the smaller body, but the relatively larger aftercoming head may be en-

Figure 21–6. Application of Piper forceps, using towel sling support. The forceps are introduced from below, left blade first, aiming directly at intended positions on sides of the head. (Reproduced, with permission, from Pernoll ML: *Benson and Pernoll's Handbook of Obstetrics and Gynecology,* 10th ed. McGraw-Hill, 2001.)

A   B

Figure 21–7. Extraction of breech. **A:** Abduction of thigh and pressure in popliteal fossa cause the knee to flex and become accessible. **B:** Delivery of leg by traction on the foot.

trapped. Prompt delivery is mandatory because severe asphyxia leading to death may rapidly ensue. Gentle downward traction on the shoulders combined with fundal pressure applied by an assistant may effect delivery. If this fails, the anesthesiologist should administer nitroglycerin or inhalation anesthesia to obtain complete relaxation of the lower uterine segment and pelvic floor with reattempt at delivery.

If delivery is still not accomplished, **Dührssen's incisions** must be considered to preserve fetal life. Incisions are made in the posterior cervix at the 6 o'clock position to loosen the entrapped head. Occasionally, additional incisions are necessary at the 2 and 10 o'clock positions. Dührssen's incisions invariably release the fetal head, but the maternal consequences may be severe with resultant hemorrhage. Thus, this procedure should be performed only in an emergent situation. Prevention of head entrapment can be accomplished by delivering viable premature breech gestations by cesarean section.

c. Total breech extraction—In total breech extraction (Fig 21–7), the entire body is manually delivered. This procedure is used only occasionally when fetal distress is encountered and an expeditious delivery is

indicated, and under certain conditions in the setting of delivery of a second twin in a nonvertex position following successful vaginal delivery of a first twin. Total breech extraction has been virtually replaced by cesarean delivery in modern obstetrics.

For complete or footling presentation, total breech extraction is accomplished by initially grasping both feet and applying gentle downward pressure until the buttocks are delivered (Fig 21–8). A generous midline or mediolateral episiotomy is then performed. The operator gently grasps the fetal pelvis, with both thumbs placed directly on either side of the sacrum. The spine is rotated, if necessary, until it rests under the pubic symphysis. Gentle, firm downward pressure is applied to the body until both scapulas are visible. The shoulders, arms, and head are delivered as in partial breech extraction.

If the fetus is in frank breech presentation, the index finger of the right hand must initially be placed into the anterior groin of the fetus and gentle downward pressure applied (Fig 21–9). As the fetus descends further into the birth canal, the left index finger is inserted into the posterior groin, and additional gentle downward traction is applied, until the buttocks are delivered through the vaginal introitus (Fig

Figure 21–8. Extraction of breech. **A:** Buttocks brought to hollow of sacrum. **B:** Traction on anterior leg causes buttocks to advance and rotate into direct AP diameter of pelvis. Continued downward traction causes the back to rotate anteriorly. **C:** Further downward traction causes the shoulders to engage in the transverse diameter of the inlet.

21–10). The fetus is gently rotated until the spine rests directly under the pubic symphysis. To deliver the extended legs from the birth canal, the operator places the index finger in the popliteal fossa of 1 leg and applies pressure upward and outward, causing the knee to flex. As the knee flexes, the foot is often seen or easily palpated. The lower leg is grasped firmly and gently delivered, and the opposite leg is then delivered. The rest of the body is extracted as previously described for footling presentation.

Complications of Breech Delivery

A. BIRTH ANOXIA

Umbilical cord compression and prolapse may be associated with breech delivery, particularly in complete (5%) and footling (15%) presentations. This is due to the inability of the presenting part to fill the maternal pelvis, either because of prematurity or poor application of the presenting part to the cervix so that the umbilical cord is allowed to prolapse below the level of the breech (see below). Frank breech presentation offers a contoured presenting part, which is better accommodated to the maternal pelvis and is usually well applied to the cervix. The incidence of cord prolapse in frank breech is only 0.5% (the same as for cephalic presentations).

Figure 21–9. Delivery of breech with 1 finger in the groin. The wrist is supported with the other hand. When the posterior groin is accessible, the index finger of the other hand is placed in the groin to complete delivery of the breech.

Figure 21–10. Flexion and abduction of the thigh to deliver extended leg.

Compression of the prolapsed cord may occur during uterine contractions, causing moderate to severe variable decelerations in the fetal heart rate and leading to fetal anoxia or death. Continuous electronic monitoring is mandatory during labor in these cases to detect ominous decelerations. If they occur, immediate cesarean delivery must be performed.

B. Birth Injury

The incidence of birth trauma during vaginal breech delivery is 6.7%, 13 times that of cephalic presentations (0.51%). Only high forceps and internal version and extraction procedures have higher rates of birth injury than do vaginal breech deliveries. The types of perinatal injuries reported in breech delivery include tears in the tentorium cerebellum, cephalohematomas, disruption of the spinal cord, brachial palsy, fracture of long bones, and rupture of the sternocleidomastoid muscles. Vaginal breech delivery is the main cause of injuries to the fetal adrenal glands, liver, anus, genitalia, spine, hip joint, sciatic nerve, and musculature of the arms, legs, and back.

Factors contributing to difficult vaginal breech delivery include a partially dilated cervix, unilateral or bilateral nuchal arms, and deflexion of the head. The type of procedure used may affect the neonatal outcome.

1. Partially dilated cervix—Delivery of a breech fetus may progress even though the cervix is only partially dilated because the bitrochanteric and bisacromial diameters are smaller than the biparietal diameter. This is true especially in prematurity. The hips and shoulders may negotiate the cervix, but the aftercoming head becomes entrapped, resulting in difficult delivery and birth injury.

2. Nuchal arms—During partial breech extraction and more often in total breech extraction, excessive downward traction on the body results in a single or double nuchal arm. This occurs because of the rapid descent of the body, leading to extension of 1 or both arms, which become lodged behind the neck. When delivery of the shoulder is difficult to accomplish, a nuchal arm should be suspected. To dislodge the arm, the operator rotates the body 180 degrees to bring the elbow toward the face. The humerus can then be identified and delivered by gentle downward traction. In cases of double nuchal arm, the fetus is rotated counterclockwise to dislodge and deliver the right arm and rotated clockwise to deliver the left arm. If this action is unsuccessful, the operator must insert a finger into the pelvis, identify the humerus, and possibly extract the arm, resulting in fracture of the humerus or clavicle. Nuchal arms cause a delay in delivery and increase the incidence of birth asphyxia.

3. Deflexion of the head—*Hyperextension of the head* is defined as deflexion or extension of the head posteriorly beyond the longitudinal axis of the fetus (5% of all breech deliveries). Causes of hyperextension include neck cysts, spasm of the neck musculature, and uterine anomalies, but over 75% have no known cause. Although deflexion may be documented by ultrasonographic or x-ray studies weeks before delivery, there is little apparent risk to the fetus until vaginal delivery is attempted. At that time, deflexion causes impaction of the occipital portion of the head behind the pubic symphysis, which may lead to fractures of the cervical vertebrae, lacerations of the spinal cord, epidural and medullary hemorrhages, and perinatal death. If head deflexion is diagnosed prior to delivery, cesarean section should be performed to avert injury. Cesarean section cannot prevent injuries such as minor meningeal hemorrhage or dislocation of the cervical vertebrae, which may develop in utero secondary to longstanding head deflexion.

4. Type of delivery—More complex delivery procedures have a higher rate of birth trauma. Whereas few infants are injured during spontaneous breech births, as many as 6% are injured during partial breech extraction and 20% during total breech extraction. Injuries associated with total breech extraction usually are extensive and severe, and this procedure should never be attempted unless fetal survival is in jeopardy and cesarean section cannot be immediately performed.

An additional important factor in breech injury and perinatal outcome is the experience of the operator. Inexperience may lead to hasty performance of obstetric maneuvers. Delay in delivery may result in birth asphyxia due to umbilical cord compression, but haste in the management of breech delivery results in application of excessive pressure on the fetal body, causing soft-tissue damage and fracture of long bones. Too-rapid extraction of the body from the birth canal causes the arms to extend above the head, resulting in unilateral or bilateral nuchal arms and difficult delivery of the aftercoming head. All breech deliveries hould be performed slowly and methodically by experienced obstetricians who execute the maneuvers with gentleness and skill—not speed.

Prognosis

The incidence of cesarean section for breech delivery has been steadily increasing, from approximately 30% in 1970 to 85% in 1999. A recent review of breech deliveries in California revealed an 88% cesarean section rate, with more vaginal deliveries performed in public teaching hospitals and far fewer in private facilities. A decreased number of practitioners currently are skilled in vaginal breech delivery, and although academic faculty support its teaching, there are insufficient numbers of vaginal breech deliveries to properly teach this procedure at most institutions. It should be noted that cesarean section for the immature or malformed fetus does not improve chances for perinatal survival; vaginal delivery should be performed in these cases.

The Term Breech Trial Collaborative Group recently conducted a randomized controlled trial to compare planned cesarean section with vaginal birth for selected breech presentation pregnancies. They found that fetuses of women who underwent planned cesarean sections were less likely to die or to experience poor outcomes in the immediate neonatal period than were fetuses of women who underwent vaginal birth. There was no difference in the 2 groups in terms of maternal mortality or serious morbidity. They concluded that a policy of planned cesarean section will result in 7 cesarean births to avoid 1 infant death or serious morbidity. Because of the results of this trial, the American College of Obstetricians and Gynecologists recommends planned cesarean delivery for persistent breech presentations at term.

■ VERSION

Version is a procedure used to turn the fetal presenting part from breech to cephalic presentation (cephalic version) or from cephalic to breech presentation (podalic version). Because cephalic version is performed by manipulating the fetus through the abdominal wall, the maneuver is known as **external cephalic version.** Podalic version is performed by means of internal maneuvers and is known as **internal podalic version.** External cephalic version is regaining popularity, whereas internal podalic version is rarely used.

EXTERNAL CEPHALIC VERSION

External cephalic version is used in the management of singleton breech presentations or in a nonvertex second twin. In carefully selected patients, it is safe for both mother and fetus. The goal is to increase the proportion of vertex presentations near term, thus increasing the chance for a vaginal delivery. In the past, external cephalic version was performed earlier in gestation but was accompanied by high reversion rates, making additional procedures necessary. Now it is performed in patients who have completed 36 weeks of gestation so that the risk of spontaneous reversion is decreased, and, if complications arise, delivery of a term infant can be accomplished. Current success rates for external cephalic version range from 35–85% (mean 60%).

Indications

Patients with unengaged singleton breech presentations of at least 36 weeks' gestation are candidates for external cephalic version. The procedure is more successful in multigravidas and those with a transverse or oblique lie. Use of fetal heart rate monitoring and real-time ultrasonography are essential to document fetal well-being during the procedure. The use of tocolytics in external cephalic version is controversial. Recent evidence indicates that tocolytics offer an advantage in nulliparous women, but reports on which type of tocolytic confers the highest success rate are conflicting. Thus, these agents should be used at the discretion of the physician. Additionally, evidence regarding the use of regional anesthesia is inconsistent. Recent randomized controlled trials have shown an increased success rate in those with epidural anesthesia. However, the ultimate decision should be based on physician experience.

Contraindications

Contraindications to external cephalic version include engagement of the presenting part in the pelvis, marked oligohydramnios, placenta previa, uterine anomalies, presence of nuchal cord, multiple gestation, premature rupture of membranes, previous uterine surgery (including myomectomy or metroplasty), and suspected or documented congenital malformations or abnormalities (including intrauterine growth retardation).

Complications

Complications are rare, occurring in only 1–2% of all external cephalic versions. Complications include placental abruption, uterine rupture, rupture of membranes with resultant umbilical cord prolapse, amniotic fluid embolism, preterm labor, fetal distress, fetomaternal hemorrhage, and fetal demise. Thus, given the potential for catastrophic outcome, this procedure should be performed in a facility where immediate access to cesarean delivery is available. Patients require extensive counseling regarding the version procedure, with disclosure of all risks, benefits, and alternatives so that an informed medicolegal decision can be made.

A. FETAL HEART RATE ABNORMALITIES

Fetal heart rate abnormalities can be readily documented during external cephalic version by intermittent electronic fetal monitoring (EFM) or ultrasonographic surveillance. Fetal bradycardia occurs in 20% of cases, but normal cardiac activity usually will return if the procedure is stopped for a short time. If significant unremitting fetal cardiac alterations occur, the attempt at version should be discontinued and preparation for cesarean delivery undertaken immediately.

B. FETOMATERNAL TRANSPLACENTAL HEMORRHAGE

Fetomaternal (transplacental) hemorrhage (FMH) may occur during version and has been reported to occur in 6–28% of patients undergoing external cephalic version, although the amount of hemorrhage rarely results in clinically significant anemia. The **Kleihauer-Betke acid elution test** should be performed if this condition is suspected. In cases of an Rh-negative–unsensitized woman, Rh immune globulin should be administered after external cephalic version to cover the calculated amount of FMH.

Technique

External cephalic version is performed as follows:

1. Obtain informed consent from the patient.
2. Perform an ultrasound examination to verify presentation and to rule out fetal or uterine abnormalities.
3. Perform a nonstress test. Results must be reactive.
4. If desired, administer a tocolytic to prevent contractions or irritability.
5. Administer anesthesia if desired.
6. Perform external cephalic version. Place both hands on the patient's abdomen, and perform a forward roll by lifting the breech upward while placing pressure on the head downward toward the pelvis. If this maneuver is unsuccessful, a backward roll can be attempted.
7. Fetal well-being should be monitored intermittently with Doppler or real-time ultrasound scanning. The procedure should be abandoned in case of any significant fetal distress or patient discomfort, or if multiple attempts are unsuccessful.
8. Following the procedure, external fetal heart rate monitoring should be continued for 1 hour to ensure stability. If the patient is Rh-negative, administer anti-D immune globulin.
9. If the patient is stable, she can be sent home to await the onset of spontaneous labor if the version is successful. If unsuccessful, the patient can be scheduled for an elective cesarean section or a trial of labor with a breech vaginal delivery planned if the mother is a good candidate.

INTERNAL PODALIC VERSION

Internal podalic version is now rarely used because of the high fetal and maternal morbidity and mortality associated with the procedure. It is occasionally performed as a life-saving procedure or in cases of a noncephalic second twin (see Chapter 17 for delivery of a second twin).

Indications

Internal podalic version is the only alternative to cesarean section for rapid delivery of the second twin in a noncephalic presentation if external cephalic version fails. Thus, when cesarean section is unavailable or when a life-threatening condition arises (maternal hemorrhage due to premature placental separation, fetal distress, prolapsed umbilical cord), internal version may be required.

A life-threatening condition is the only indication for internal podalic version. The cervix must be completely dilated, and the membranes must be intact. A skilled operator is crucial for safe performance of this procedure. In several French studies, internal podalic version was found to be a reliable and effective technique with excellent long-term maternal and fetal prognoses.

Contraindications

Internal podalic version is contraindicated in cases in which the membranes are ruptured or oligohydramnios is present, precluding easy version. This procedure should not be performed through a partially dilated cervix or if the uterus is firmly contracted down on the fetal body. However, recent studies have indicated that intravenous nitroglycerin can be used to provide transient uterine relaxation without affecting maternal or fetal outcome.

Complications

Internal podalic version is associated with considerable risk of traumatic injury to both fetus and mother. Prior to 1950, when this procedure was performed much more frequently than it is today, associated uterine rupture and hemorrhage caused 5% of all maternal deaths. Perinatal mortality rates were 5–25% (primarily due to traumatic intracerebral hemorrhage and birth asphyxia). Considerable birth trauma, including long bone fractures, dislocations, epiphyseal separations, and central nervous system deficits, was also linked to this procedure. For these reasons, internal podalic version has been abandoned with rare exceptions in favor of cesarean section.

Technique

Internal podalic version is performed as follows:

1. Establish an intravenous line for administration of parenteral fluids, including blood. Cross-matched blood should be available in the hospital blood bank.
2. Administer anesthesia to achieve relaxation of the uterus.
3. Place the patient in the dorsolithotomy position. Insert a hand through the fully dilated cervix along the fetal body until both feet are identified, and apply traction to bring the feet into the pelvis and out the introitus. Then, grasp both feet firmly. Perform an amniotomy. Apply dorsal traction on both lower extremities until both feet are delivered through the vagina. Then, perform a total breech extraction for delivery of the body (Fig 21–11).

■ COMPOUND PRESENTATION

Compound presentation is prolapse of a fetal extremity alongside the presenting part. Prolapse of the hand in cephalic presentation is most common, followed by prolapse of an upper extremity in breech presentation. Prolapse of a lower extremity in cephalic presentation is relatively rare. Compound presentations are uncommon, occurring in only 1 in 1000 pregnancies.

Causes

Obstetric factors that prevent descent of the presenting part into the pelvic inlet predispose to prolapse of an extremity alongside the presenting part (ie, prematurity, cephalopelvic disproportion, multiple gestation, grand multiparity, and hydramnios). Prematurity occurs in over 50% of compound presentations. In twin gestations, over 90% of compound presentations are associated with the second twin.

Because of poor application of the presenting part to the cervix found in compound presentations, umbilical cord prolapse is common (occurring in 11–20% of cases) and is a major contributor to fetal loss during labor.

Diagnosis

The diagnosis of compound presentation is made by palpation of a fetal extremity adjacent to the presenting part on vaginal examination. The diagnosis is usually made during labor; as the cervix dilates, the prolapsed extremity is more easily palpated alongside the vertex or breech. Compound presentation may be suspected if poor progress in labor is noted, particularly when the presenting part fails to engage during the active phase. If the diagnosis of compound presentation is suspected but uncertain, ultrasound can be used to locate the position of the extremities and search for malformations.

Management

Management of compound presentation depends on gestational age and type of presentation. Given that 50% of compound presentations are associated with prematurity, viability of the fetus should be documented prior to delivery. If the fetus is considered nonviable, labor should be permitted and vaginal delivery anticipated. The small size of the fetus makes dystocia or difficult vaginal delivery uncommon.

Labor can be allowed and vaginal delivery anticipated in viable cephalic presentations with a prolapsed hand. These cases generally pose no difficulty in labor or delivery because the hand moves upward into the lower uterine segment as the vertex descends into the birth canal.

Umbilical cord prolapse is a risk in all cases of compound presentation, and continuous fetal heart rate monitoring should be performed to detect fetal distress or changes in the fetal heart rate. Umbilical cord complications should be managed by immediate cesarean delivery (see below).

Prognosis

Compound presentations have been associated historically with perinatal mortality rates ranging from 9–19%. Contributing factor are prematurity, prolapsed umbilical cord, and traumatic vaginal delivery.

■ SHOULDER DYSTOCIA

Shoulder dystocia is defined as an inability to deliver the shoulders after the head has delivered. Characteristically, after the head is delivered, the chin presses tightly against the perineum as the anterior shoulder becomes impacted behind the pubic symphysis. This condition is an acute obstetric emergency requiring prompt, skill-

Figure 21–11. Internal podalic version and extraction. **A:** Feet are grasped. **B:** Baby is turned; hand on abdomen pushes head toward uterine fundus. **C:** Feet are extracted. **D:** Torso is delivered. From this point onward, procedure is the same as for uncomplicated breech delivery.

ful management in order to prevent significant fetal damage or death. The incidence of shoulder dystocia ranges from 0.15–1.7% of all vaginal deliveries.

Risk Factors

Primary risk factors that can influence clinical management are fetal macrosomia, gestational or overt diabetes mellitus, a history of shoulder dystocia in a prior birth, a prolonged second stage of labor, and instrumental delivery, particularly a midpelvic delivery. Other risk factors, such as a history of a macrosomic infant, maternal obesity, multiparity, and postterm pregnancy, are mediated through the primary risk factors. However, most women who experience shoulder dystocia have no combination of risk factors that allows clinically useful identification.

Complications

Birth injuries related to shoulder dystocia include fracture of the humerus or clavicle and injury to the brachial plexus (**Erb's palsy**). Fractures of the humerus and clavicle generally heal without incident, and most injuries to the brachial plexus resolve with minimal or no neurologic deficit detectable during the neonatal period. However, 10–15% cases of Erb's palsies do not resolve. Studies attempting to distinguish the clinical course of patients with permanent injuries from those with transient injuries have found no clinically distinct characteristics. Maternal complications of shoulder dystocia include postpartum hemorrhage and lacerations involving the cervix, vagina, and perineum.

Prevention

Efforts at prevention focus on patients with the clinically important risk factors: history of shoulder dystocia, macrosomia by estimated fetal weight (EFW), diabetes, prolonged second stage of labor, and instrumental delivery. Although no study has shown conclusively that offering a cesarean birth in the presence of various combinations of these risk factors is advisable from a risk–benefit analysis, most practitioners apply some or all of these in an attempt to reduce the risk of shoulder dystocia. An example of 1 approach follows.

1. Prior shoulder dystocia: Offer cesarean.
2. Prior brachial plexus injury: Strongly suggest cesarean.
3. Nondiabetic with macrosomia by EFW (varying thresholds applied between 4500g and 5000g): Offer cesarean.
4. Diabetic with macrosomia (varying thresholds applied between 4000g and 4500g): Offer cesarean.
5. Macrosomia by EFW: Avoid instrumental delivery.

Management

Shoulder dystocia should be anticipated given any indications of macrosomia. The diagnosis is confirmed when gentle downward pressure on the head fails to deliver the anterior shoulder from behind the pubic symphysis. At this point, the fetus is at risk for asphyxiation as the fetus cannot expand its chest to breathe, and umbilical cord circulation is compressed within the birth canal. Confronted with this terrifying dilemma, the inexperienced operator often continues to apply downward pressure on the head in a vain attempt to deliver the anterior shoulder. Such action should be avoided, not only because it is ineffective but also because it can potentially damage the brachial plexus and result in permanent Erb's palsy. A number of maneuvers designed to alleviate shoulder dystocia without increasing traction have been described. No specific sequence of these maneuvers has be shown to be superior to any other, but a commonsense approach based on ease of performance and limitations of risk can be described. Initially, the operator places a hand in the birth canal to assess the posterior outlet. If inadequate, an episiotomy or a proctoepisiotomy is performed. At the same time, assistants including a pediatrician and an anesthesiologist are summoned to aid in the delivery.

The **McRoberts' maneuver** should be used initially because it is simple and resolves shoulder dystocia in 42% of cases. The maternal legs are hyperflexed onto the maternal abdomen, resulting in flattening of the sacrum and cephalad rotation of the symphysis pubis. If the shoulders remain undelivered, suprapubic pressure is applied by an assistant to dislodge the anterior shoulder while gentle downward pressure on the head is applied. Suprapubic pressure and/or proctoepisiotomy increases success rates to between 54 and 58%. If these attempts are unsuccessful, the examiner can attempt to rotate the fetal shoulders into the oblique position by placing 2 fingers against the posterior shoulder and pushing it around toward the fetal chest (**Rubin maneuver**) or pushing the posterior shoulder around toward the fetal back (**Wood's maneuver**) in a corkscrew fashion.

If the maneuvers to this point fail, delivery of the posterior arm (Barnum maneuver) is indicated. The obstetrician's hand is inserted posteriorly into the hollow of the maternal sacrum, and the posterior arm of the fetus is identified. Gentle pressure by the examiner's forefinger on the fetal antecubital fossa will cause flexion of the arm. As the arm flexes across the chest, the forearm is gently grasped, and the hand and forearm are gently delivered from the birth canal. If not, the trunk can be rotated to bring the free arm anteriorly, resulting in delivery. Deliberate fracture of the clavicle also can be performed, preferably in a direction away from the fetal lungs. This action diminishes the size of the shoulder girdle and should facilitate delivery.

Finally, if all previous techniques fail, a **Zavanelli maneuver** can be performed in which the fetal head is replaced in anticipation of a cesarean delivery. A subcutaneous symphysiotomy also can be performed to allow disimpaction of the fetal shoulders. Both of these procedures can be very difficult, are associated with high maternal and fetal morbidity, and should be performed only when other conventional maneuvers have failed.

■ UMBILICAL CORD PROLAPSE

Umbilical cord prolapse is defined as descent of the umbilical cord into the lower uterine segment, where it may lie adjacent to the presenting part (occult cord prolapse) or below the presenting part (overt cord prolapse) (Fig 21–12). In occult prolapse, the umbilical cord cannot be palpated during pelvic examination, whereas in funic presentation, which is characterized by prolapse of the umbilical cord below the level of the presenting part before the rupture of membranes occurs, the cord often can be easily palpated through the membranes. Overt cord prolapse is associated with rupture of the membranes and displacement of the umbilical cord into the vagina, often through the introitus.

Prolapse of the umbilical cord to a level at or below the presenting part exposes the cord to intermittent compression between the presenting part and the pelvic inlet, cervix, or vaginal canal. Compression of the umbilical cord compromises fetal circulation and, depending on the duration and intensity of compression, may lead to fetal hypoxia, brain damage, and death. In overt cord prolapse, exposure of the umbilical cord to air causes irritation and cooling of the cord, resulting in further vasospasm of the cord vessels.

The incidence of overt umbilical cord prolapse in cephalic presentations is 0.5%, frank breech 0.5%, complete breech 5%, footling breech 15%, and transverse lie 20%. The incidence of occult prolapse is unknown because it can be detected only by fetal heart rate changes characteristic of umbilical cord compression. However, some degree of occult prolapse appears to be common, given that as many as 50% of monitored labors demonstrate fetal heart rate changes compatible with umbilical cord compression. In most cases, the compression is transient and can be rectified simply by changing the patient's position.

Whether occult or overt, umbilical cord prolapse is associated with significant rates of perinatal morbidity and mortality because of intermittent compression of blood flow and resultant fetal hypoxia. The perinatal mortality rate associated with all cases of overt umbilical cord prolapse approaches 20%. Prematurity, itself a contributor to the incidence of umbilical cord prolapse, accounts for a considerable portion of this perinatal loss.

Causes

Any obstetric condition that predisposes to poor application of the fetal presenting part to the cervix can result in prolapse of the umbilical cord. Cord prolapse

Occult prolapse   Funic presentation   Overt prolapse

Figure 21–12. Types of prolapsed cords.

is associated with prematurity (< 34 weeks' gestation), abnormal presentations (breech, brow, compound, face, transverse), occiput posterior positions of the head, pelvic tumors, multiparity, placenta previa, low-lying placenta, and cephalopelvic disproportion. In addition, cord prolapse is possible with hydramnios, multiple gestation, or premature rupture of the membranes occurring before engagement of the presenting part. A recent study revealed that obstetric intervention contributes to nearly half of cases of umbilical cord prolapse. Examples cited include amniotomy, scalp electrode application, intrauterine pressure catheter insertion, attempted external cephalic version, and expectant management of preterm premature rupture of membranes.

Clinical Findings

A. OVERT CORD PROLAPSE

Overt cord prolapse can be diagnosed simply by visualizing the cord protruding from the introitus or by palpating loops of cord in the vaginal canal.

B. FUNIC PRESENTATION

The diagnosis of funic presentation is made by pelvic examination if loops of cord are palpated through the membranes. Antepartum detection of funic presentation is discussed below.

C. OCCULT PROLAPSE

Occult prolapse is rarely palpated during pelvic examination. This condition can be inferred only if fetal heart rate changes (variable decelerations, bradycardia, or both)

associated with intermittent compression of the umbilical cord are detected during monitoring.

D. FETUS

The fetus in good condition whose well-being is jeopardized by umbilical cord compression may exhibit violent activity readily apparent to the patient and the obstetrician. Variable fetal heart rate decelerations will occur during uterine contractions, with prompt return of the heart rate to normal as each contraction subsides. If cord compression is complete and prolonged, fetal bradycardia occurs. Persistent, severe, variable decelerations and bradycardia lead to development of hypoxia, metabolic acidosis, and eventual damage or death. As the fetal status deteriorates, activity lessens and eventually ceases. Meconium staining of the amniotic fluid may be noted at the time of membrane rupture.

Complications

A. MATERNAL

Cesarean section is a major operative procedure with known anesthetic, hemorrhagic, and operative complications. These risks must be weighed against the real risk to the fetus of continued hypoxia if labor were to continue.

Maternal risks encountered at vaginal delivery include laceration of the cervix, vagina, or perineum resulting from a hastily performed delivery.

B. NEONATAL

The neonate at delivery may be hypoxic, acidotic, or moribund. A pediatric team should be present to effect immediate resuscitation of the newborn.

Prevention

Patients at risk for umbilical cord prolapse should be treated as high-risk patients. Patients with malpresentations or poorly applied cephalic presentations should be considered for ultrasonographic examination at the onset of labor to determine fetal lie and cord position within the uterine cavity. Because most prolapses occur during labor as the cervix dilates, patients at risk for cord prolapse should be continuously monitored to detect abnormalities of the fetal heart rate. Artificial rupture of membranes should be avoided until the presenting part is well applied to the cervix. At the time of spontaneous membrane rupture, a prompt, careful pelvic examination should be performed to rule out cord prolapse. Should amniotomy be required and the presenting part remains unengaged, careful needling of the membranes and slow release of the amniotic fluid can be performed until the presenting part settles against the cervix.

Management

A. OVERT CORD PROLAPSE

The diagnosis of overt cord prolapse demands immediate action to preserve the life of the fetus. An immediate pelvic examination should be performed to determine cervical effacement and dilatation, station of the presenting part, and strength and frequency of pulsations within the cord vessels. If the fetus is viable, the patient should be placed in the knee–chest position, and the examiner should apply continuous upward pressure against the presenting part to lift and maintain the fetus away from the prolapsed cord until preparations for cesarean delivery are complete. Alternatively, 400–700 mL of saline can be instilled into the bladder in order to elevate the presenting part. Oxygen should be given to the mother until the anesthesiologist is prepared to administer a rapid-acting inhalation anesthetic for delivery. Successful reduction of the prolapsed umbilical cord has been described, but such an attempt may worsen fetal heart rate changes and should not delay preparation for cesarean delivery. Abdominal delivery should be accomplished as rapidly as possible through a generous midline abdominal incision, and a pediatric team should be on standby in the event immediate resuscitation of the newborn is necessary.

B. OCCULT CORD PROLAPSE

If cord compression patterns (variable decelerations) of the fetal heart rate are recognized during labor, an immediate pelvic examination should be performed to rule out overt cord prolapse. If occult cord prolapse is suspected, the patient should be placed in the lateral Sims or Trendelenburg position in an attempt to alleviate cord compression. If the fetal heart rate returns to normal, labor can be allowed to continue, provided no further fetal insult occurs. Oxygen should be administered to the mother, and the fetal heart rate should be continuously monitored electronically. Amnioinfusion can be performed via an intrauterine pressure catheter in order to instill fluid within the uterine cavity and possibly decrease the incidence of variable decelerations. If the cord compression pattern persists or recurs to the point of fetal jeopardy (moderate to severe variable decelerations or bradycardia), a rapid cesarean section should be accomplished.

C. FUNIC PRESENTATION

The patient at term with funic presentation should be delivered by cesarean section prior to membrane rupture. However, there is no consensus on management if the fetus is premature. The most conservative approach is to hospitalize the patient on bed rest in the Sims or Trendelenburg position in an attempt to reposition the cord within the uterine cavity. Serial ultrasonographic examinations should be performed to ascertain cord position, presentation, and gestational age.

D. ROUTE OF DELIVERY

Vaginal delivery can be successfully accomplished in cases of overt or occult cord prolapse if, at the time of prolapse, the cervix is fully dilated, cephalopelvic disproportion is not anticipated, and an experienced physician determines that delivery is imminent. Internal podalic version, midforceps rotation, or any other operative technique is generally more hazardous to mother and fetus in this situation than is a judiciously performed cesarean delivery. Cesarean delivery is the preferred route of delivery in most cases. Vaginal delivery is the route of choice for the previable or dead fetus.

Prognosis

A. MATERNAL

Maternal complications include those related to anesthesia, blood loss, and infection following cesarean section or operative vaginal delivery. Maternal recovery is generally complete.

B. NEONATAL

Although the prognosis for intrapartum cord prolapse is greatly improved, fetal mortality and morbidity rates still can be high, depending on the degree and duration of umbilical cord compression occurring before the diagnosis is made and neonatal resuscitation is started. If the diagnosis is made early and the duration of complete cord occlusion is less than 5 minutes, the prognosis is good. Gestational age and trauma at delivery also affect the final neonatal outcome. If complete cord occlusion has occurred for longer than 5 minutes or if intermittent partial cord occlusion has occurred over a prolonged period of time, fetal damage or death may occur.

REFERENCES

Breech Presentation

Alarab M et al: Singleton vaginal breech delivery at term: Still a safe option. Obstet Gynecol 2004;103:407.

American College of Obstetrics and Gynecology: *Mode of Term Singleton Breech Delivery.* ACOG Committee Opinion No. 265. American College of Obstetrics and Gynecology, 2001.

Belfrage P et al: The term breech presentation. A retrospective study with regard to the planned mode of delivery. Acta Obstet Gynecol Scand 2002;81:544.

Caukwell S et al: Women's attitudes towards management of breech presentation at term. J Obstet Gynaecol 2002;22:486.

Demol S et al: Breech presentation is a risk factor for intrapartum and neonatal death in preterm delivery. Eur J Obstet Gynecol Reprod Biol 2000;93:47.

Dunn PM: Erich Bracht (1882–1969) of Berlin and his "breech" manoeuvre. Arch Dis Child Fetal Neonatal Ed 2003;88:F76.

Gilbert WM et al: Vaginal versus cesarean delivery for breech presentation in California: A population-based study. Obstet Gynecol 2003;102:911.

Gregory KD et al: Variation in vaginal breech delivery rates by hospital type. Obstet Gynecol 2000;97:385.

Hannah M et al: Planned cesarean section versus planned vaginal birth for breech presentation at term: A randomized multicentre trial. Lancet 2000;356:1375.

Hofmeyer GJ, Hannah ME: Planned cesarean section for term breech delivery. Cochrane Database Syst Rev 2003;(3):CD000166.

Lavin JP Jr et al: Teaching vaginal breech delivery and external cephalic version. A survey of faculty attitudes. J Reprod Med 2000;45:808.

Munstedt K et al: Term breech and long-term morbidity—Cesarean section versus vaginal breech delivery. Eur J Obstet Gynecol Reprod Biol 2001;96:163.

Sanchez-Ramos L et al: Route of breech delivery and maternal and neonatal outcomes. Int J Gynaecol Obstet 2001;73:7.

Su M et al: Factors associated with adverse perinatal outcome in the Term Breech Trial. Am J Obstet Gynecol 2003;189:740.

Tunde-Byass MO et al: Breech vaginal delivery at or near term. Semin Perinatol 2003;27:34.

Winn HN et al: Intrapartum management of nonvertex second born twins: A critical analysis. Am J Obstet Gynecol 2001;185:1204.

Version

American College of Obstetricians and Gynecologists: *External Cephalic Version.* ACOG Practice Bulletin No. 13. American College of Obstetricians and Gynecologists, 2000.

Andarsio F, Feng TI: External cephalic version. Nitroglycerin versus terbutaline (abst). Am J Obstet Gynecol 2000;182:S161.

Ben-Haroush A et al: Mode of delivery following successful external cephalic version. Am J Perinatol 2002;19:355.

Chauhan AR et al: Is internal podalic version a lost art? Optimum mode of delivery in transverse lie. J Postgrad Med 2001;47:15.

Collaris RJ et al: External cephalic version: a safe procedure? A systemic review of version-related risks. Acta Obstet Gynecol Scand 2004;83:511.

Ezra Y et al: Significance of success rate of external cephalic versions and vaginal breech deliveries in counseling women with breech presentation at term. Eur J Obstet Gynecol Reprod Biol 2000;90:63.

Hofmeyer GJ: Interventions to help external cephalic version for breech presentation at term. Cochrane Database Syst Rev 2004;(1):CD000184.

Hutton EK et al: External cephalic version beginning at 34 weeks versus 37 weeks gestation. A randomized multicenter trial. Am J Obstet Gynecol 2003;189:245.

Hutton EK et al: Use of external cephalic version for breech pregnancy and mode of delivery for breech and twin pregnancy. A survey of Canadian practitioners. J Obstet Gynaecol Can 2002;24:804.

Mancuso KM et al: Epidural anesthesia for cephalic version: a randomized trial. Obstet Gynecol 2000;95:648.

Skupski DW et al: External cephalic version: An approach with few complications. Gynecol Obstet Invest 2003;56:83.

Compound Presentation

Goplerud J, Eastman NJ: Compound presentation: Survey of 65 cases. Obstet Gynecol 1953;1:59.

Weissberg SM, O'Leary JA: Compound presentation of the fetus. Obstet Gynecol 1973;41:60.

Shoulder Dystocia

Alhadi M et al: Shoulder dystocia. Risk factors and maternal and perinatal outcome. J Obstet Gynaecol 2001;21:352.

American College of Obstetricians and Gynecologists: *Shoulder Dystocia.* ACOG Practice Bulletin No. 40. American College of Obstetricians and Gynecologists, 2002.

Beall MH et al: Clavicular fracture in labor: risk factors and associated morbidity. J Perinatol 2001;21:513.

Buhimschi CS et al: Use of McRoberts' position during delivery and increase in pushing efficiency. Lancet 2001;358:470.

Christoffersson M et al: Shoulder dystocia and brachial plexus injury: A population-based study. Gynecol Obstet Invest 2002;53:42.

Gherman RB et al: A comparison of shoulder dystocia-associated transient and permanent brachial plexus palsies. Obstet Gynecol 2003;102:544.

Ginsberg NA, Moisidis C: How to predict recurrent shoulder dystocia. Am J Obstet Gynecol 2001;184:1427.

Keenan J et al: The Zavanelli maneuver in two cases of shoulder dystocia. J Matern Fetal Neonatal Med 2003;13:135.

Lam MH et al: Reappraisal of neonatal clavicular fracture. Relationship between infant size and risk factors. J Reprod Med 2002;47:903.

Lam MH et al: Relationship between infant size and neonatal morbidity. Obstet Gynecol 2002;100:115.

Poggi SH et al: Prioritizing posterior arm delivery during severe shoulder dystocia. Obstet Gynecol 2003;101:1068.

Robinson H et al: Is maternal obesity a predictor of shoulder dystocia? Obstet Gynecol 2003;101:24.

Rubin A: Management of shoulder dystocia. JAMA 1964;189:835.

Woods CE: A principle of physics is applicable to shoulder delivery. Am J Obstet Gynecol 1943;45:796.

Wykes CB et al: Symphysiotomy: a lifesaving procedure. BJOG 2003;110:219

Umbilical Cord Prolapse

Ezra Y et al: Does cord presentation on ultrasound predict cord prolapse? Gynecol Obstet Invest 2003;56:6.

Faiz SA et al: Results of delivery in umbilical cord prolapse. Saudi Med J 2003;24:757.

Kahana B et al: Umbilical cord prolapse and perinatal outcomes. Int J Gynaecol Obstet 2004;84:127.

Katz Z, Lancet M, Borenstein R: Management of labor with umbilical cord prolapse. Am J Obstet Gynecol 1982;142:239.

Qureshi NS et al: Umbilical cord prolapse. Int J Gynaecol Obstet 2004;86:29.

Uygur D et al: Risk factors and infant outcomes associated with umbilical cord prolapse. Int J Gynaecol Obstet 2002;78:127.

Cardiac Disorders in Pregnancy

Afshan B. Hameed, MD, & Mohammed W. Akhter, MD

CARDIOVASCULAR CHANGES IN NORMAL PREGNANCY

Hemodynamic changes during pregnancy are meant to increase blood flow to the fetoplacental unit. These changes create hemodynamic burden on the maternal heart and may cause symptoms and signs similar to those of heart disease. It is important to be familiar with these cardiovascular adaptations, as women with preexisting cardiovascular disease may exhibit marked clinical deterioration during the course of pregnancy.

Blood volume begins to rise as early as 6 weeks' gestation and continues to increase until midpregnancy. The hormonally mediated increase in plasma volume is disproportionately higher than the red cell mass and, therefore, results in the "physiologic anemia of pregnancy." On average, hematocrit level is reduced to 30–38% by week 30. Increases in blood volume and heart rate result in increased cardiac output. Cardiac output peaks during the second trimester and then remains constant until term. Myocardial contractility improves, left atrial and left ventricular chamber sizes increase, and peripheral vascular resistance falls (as a result of progesterone, circulating prostaglandins, atrial natriuretic peptides, endothelial nitric oxide, and the low-resistance vascular bed of the placenta). The net effect of these changes is an approximately 50% increase in cardiac output.

The overall increment in heart rate by the third trimester averages 10 to 20 bpm. The systemic arterial pressure falls during the first trimester, remains stable during the second trimester, and returns to pregestational levels before term. The reduction in diastolic pressure is more than the reduction in systolic pressure, leading to widening of the pulse pressure. Supine hypotensive or uterocaval syndrome occurs in 0.5–11% of pregnancies and is related to acute occlusion of the inferior vena cava by the gravid uterus in the supine position; and it is characterized by significant decreases in blood pressure and heart rate. This contrasts with the tachycardia seen with hypotension in the nonpregnant state. Patients usually complain of lightheadedness, nausea, dizziness, and syncope in extreme cases. Symptoms are alleviated by changing to a left lateral recumbent position.

Some hemodynamic changes, especially the increases in cardiac output during labor and delivery, are related to the fear, anxiety, and pain experienced by the patient at this stage. Uterine contractions displace 300 to 500 mL of blood with each contraction, augmenting cardiac output by 20%. Oxygen consumption increases 3-fold. The changes in cardiac output are less pronounced if the patient is in the supine position and receives adequate analgesia.

Immediately after delivery, relief of caval compression coupled with autotransfusion from the contracting uterus produces a further increase in cardiac output. This can cause acute decompensation in the immediate postpartum period. Most of the hemodynamic changes revert to prepregnancy levels by 2 weeks postpartum.

HEART DISEASE

Heart disease is quickly becoming one of the leading causes of maternal death. It complicates approximately 1% of all pregnancies. Pregnant patients with significant symptoms on exertion, such as patients in New York Heart Association (NYHA) functional classes III and IV (Table 22A–1), have high event rates and succumb to complications of heart disease, such as heart failure, arrhythmias, and stroke. Patients with stenotic lesions (eg, mitral or aortic stenosis) and minimal baseline symptoms (NYHA class I or II) may deteriorate rapidly. Some other diseases associated with the highest risk of maternal mortality include Eisenmenger's syndrome, primary pulmonary hypertension, fragile aortas as in Marfan's syndrome, left-sided obstructive lesions, and already dilated poorly functioning left ventricles (Table 22A–2).

Women of childbearing age are as susceptible to myocarditis, pericarditis, or infective endocarditis as is the general population. Healthy, pregnant women can develop many cardiovascular complications, such as varicose veins, preeclampsia, pulmonary emboli, amniotic fluid emboli, disseminated intravascular coagulation, and shock due to hemorrhage or aortic dissection.

As a result of successful pediatric surgical correction of congenital anomalies, many children are reaching adulthood and subsequently becoming pregnant. Pregnant women with congenital heart disease now outnumber

Table 22A–1. New York Heart Association functional classification of heart disease.

Class I	No signs or symptoms (chest pain or shortness of breath)
Class II	No symptoms at rest, slight limitation with mild to moderate activity (walking > 2 blocks)
Class III	No symptoms at rest, marked limitation with less than ordinary activity (walking < 2 blocks)
Class IV	Symptoms at rest

those with rheumatic heart disease in most developing countries. It is important to recognize, however, that subtle clinical clues, such as shortness of breath, may be the only manifestation of conditions such as mitral stenosis or pulmonary hypertension related to rheumatic heart disease. Acquired conditions such as ischemic heart disease are not uncommon today as women are delaying childbearing to the third and fourth decades of life. As the general population becomes more susceptible to diabetes mellitus, morbid obesity, and hypertension, more frequent encounters with ischemic heart disease in pregnant patients are expected.

CARDIOVASCULAR EVALUATION DURING PREGNANCY

Most women with heart disease have successful pregnancies, but complacency in the diagnosis and management of pregnant patients can have dire consequences for both the mother and the fetus. Therefore it is essential to evaluate every pregnant woman with heart disease for her risk of adverse outcomes during pregnancy, labor, delivery, and postpartum. In general, all such women should be referred to a specialist center where their care can be managed jointly by an obstetrician, cardiologist, clinical geneticist, and neonatologist. Ideally, patients with heart disease should consult their physicians prior to their becoming pregnant. Preconception counseling allows for optimal timing for conception, completion of all diagnostic procedures beforehand (especially those involving harmful radiation exposure), discontinuation of teratogenic drugs, and scheduling of corrective/palliative surgery before pregnancy.

The initial evaluation should include a careful medical history, comprehensive physical examination, and noninvasive laboratory testing. Common findings in normal pregnancy are listed in Table 22A–3.

Medical History

Most patients admit to reduced exercise tolerance and easy fatigability. This condition is related to both the weight gained during gestation and the physiologic anemia of pregnancy. Syncopal episodes or lightheadedness occur as a result of mechanical compression of the gravid uterus on the inferior vena cava leading to poor venous return to the heart, especially in the third trimester. Other frequent complaints include hyperventilation and orthopnea (from mechanical pressure of the enlarged uterus on the diaphragm). Palpitations are common and probably are related to the hyperdynamic circulation of pregnancy rather than arrhythmias in most cases.

In patients with an established history of heart disease, it is important to inquire about their functional capacity, prevalence of other associated symptoms, therapeutic regimens, prior diagnostic tests (eg, echocardiogram, exercise testing, and cardiac catheterization), and history of corrective or palliative surgery. In patients with no known heart disease, it is essential to ask about a history of rheumatic heart disease, episodes of cyanosis at birth or early childhood, presence of rheumatologic disorders (eg, systemic lupus erythematosus), episodes of arrhythmias, occurrence of exertional syncope or chest pain, and persistence of lower-extremity edema. In addition, ask about a family history of congenital heart disease, premature coronary artery disease, or sudden death in family members. Signs and symptoms of cardiovascular disease are listed in Table 22A–4.

Physical Examination

Hyperventilation is a common phenomenon in pregnancy likely related to the effect of progesterone on the respiratory center. It is important to differentiate hyperventilation from dyspnea, which is a common finding in congestive heart failure. Bibasilar crackles are commonly heard in normal pregnancy that result from atelectasis that develops from basal compression of the

Table 22A–2. High-risk pregnancy in women with heart disease.

Etiology	Disease
Pump failure	Severe cardiomyopathy
Symptomatic valve narrowing	Mitral stenosis, aortic stenosis, pulmonary stenosis
Cyanotic heart disease	Tetralogy of Fallot, transposition of great arteries
Aortic rupture	Marfan's syndrome with dilated aorta
Artificial prosthesis	Mechanical heart valves
Elevated pulmonary artery pressures	Eisenmenger's syndrome, primary pulmonary hypertension, pulmonary vascular disease

Table 22A–3. Common findings in normal pregnancy.

Symptoms	Fatigue, decreased exercise capacity
	Lightheadedness, syncope
	Palpitations
	Dyspnea, orthopnea
Physical examination	Distended neck veins
	Increased intensity of S_1, exaggerated splitting
	Exaggerated splitting of S_2
	Midsystolic, soft, ejection-type murmurs (lower left sternal border or over the pulmonary area)
	Third heart sound
	Continuous murmurs (cervical venous hum, mammary soufflé)
	Brisk, diffused, displaced left ventricular impulse
	Palpable right ventricular impulse
Electrocardiogram	QRS axis deviation
	Small Q and inverted P in lead III (abolished by inspiration)
	Sinus tachycardia, higher incidence of arrhythmias
Chest radiograph	Horizontal position of heart
	Increased lung markings
Doppler and echocardiography	Slightly increased systolic and diastolic left ventricular dimensions
	Moderate increase in size of right atrium, right ventricle, and left atrium
	Functional pulmonary, tricuspid and mitral regurgitation

lungs due to uterine enlargement and the subsequent increase in intra-abdominal pressure.

The left ventricular impulse is easily palpated, is brisk, and is nonsustained. The peripheral pulse often is collapsing in character and can be confused with the findings in aortic regurgitation. The jugular veins present a more distended pulse, with prominent *a* and *v* peaks with rapid *x* and *y* descents. A significant number of pregnant women have leg edema. It develops as a result of a fall in colloid oncotic pressure of the plasma with a concomitant increase in femoral venous pressure as a result of poor venous return.

The physical examination should focus on facial, digital, or skeletal abnormalities that suggest the presence of congenital anomalies. One should observe for clubbing, cyanosis, or pallor. Inspection of the chest can rule out pectus excavatum deformity, precordial bulge, or presence of right or left ventricular heave. The first heart sound usually is widely split (which can be misinterpreted as a fourth heart sound). A loud first heart sound suggests mitral stenosis, whereas a low-intensity first heart sound indicates first-degree heart block. A widely split second heart sound can be interpreted as an atrial septal defect, whereas a paradoxically split sound occurs in severe left ventricular hypertrophy or left bundle branch block. A third heart sound is normal in pregnancy. A fourth heart sound, ejection click, opening snap, or mid to late systolic click suggests heart disease. Innocent systolic murmurs can be heard in most pregnant women and can result from the hyperkinetic circulation of pregnancy. These murmurs are midsystolic and are heard best at the lower left sternal border and over the pulmonic area. Continuous benign murmurs, such as the cervical venous hum and mammary soufflé, also result from increased flow secondary to the hemodynamic changes of pregnancy. The venous hum is best heard over the right supraclavicular fossa, and the mammary soufflé is best auscultated over the breast in late gestation. Diastolic murmurs heard during pregnancy require further investigation by echocardiography and Doppler ultrasound.

Laboratory Examinations

A. ELECTROCARDIOGRAPHY

The QRS axis in normal pregnancy usually is within normal limits but can shift to the extreme right or left of that range. A small Q wave and an inverted P wave in lead III are abolished by deep inspiration. Greater R-wave amplitude can be seen in leads V_1 and V_2. The incidences of sinus tachycardia and premature atrial/ventricular beats as well as the susceptibility to paroxysmal supraventricular and ventricular arrhythmias are increased.

B. CHEST RADIOGRAPH

The radiation exposure from a routine chest radiograph is minimal; however, chest x-ray films still should not be taken casually in pregnancy because of the potential biologic adverse effects of radiation exposure irrespective of the dose used. When chest films are taken, the pelvic area should be shielded with protective lead material. The findings on chest films can mimic abnormal disease conditions. Straightening of the left heart border due to enlargement of the main pulmonary artery can be seen. The heart is more horizontally located, and the lung markings are more prominent due to redistribution secondary to increased pulmonary venous pressure.

C. ECHOCARDIOGRAPHY

Small pericardial effusions are seen in normal pregnant women late in pregnancy. Dilation of mitral, tricuspid, and pulmonary annuli and enlargement of all the cardiac chambers are seen. Mild physiologic regurgitation of these valves is observed. Transthoracic echocardiography can be used safely on both the

Table 22A–4. Signs and symptoms indicative of significant cardiovascular disease.

Symptoms	Progressively worsening shortness of breath
	Cough with frothy pink sputum
	Paroxysmal nocturnal dyspnea
	Chest pain with exertion
	Syncope preceded by palpitations or exertion
	Hemoptysis
Physical examination	Abnormal venous pulsations
	Rarely audible S_1
	Single S_2 or paradoxically split S_2
	Loud systolic murmurs, any diastolic murmur
	Ejection clicks, late systolic clicks, opening snaps
	Friction rub
	Sustained right or left ventricular heave
	Cyanosis or clubbing
Electrocardiogram	Significant arrhythmias
	Heart blocks
Chest radiograph	Cardiomegaly
	Pulmonary edema

mother and the fetus to rule out congenital heart disease, ventricular dilatation, and aortic root disease. Doppler ultrasound can evaluate the significance of valvular lesions, estimate pulmonary pressures, and rule out intracardiac shunts. Transesophageal echocardiography can improve visualization of posteriorly situated cardiac structures, such as the left atrium and mitral valve.

D. EXERCISE STRESS TESTING

Stress testing usually is indicated for preconception work-up for estimation of myocardial reserve to determine if a woman can safely carry a pregnancy to term. Some low-level exercise protocols have been developed for implementation during pregnancy to evaluate for ischemic heart disease. These protocols allow the heart rate to go up to only 70% of age-predicted heart rate along with concomitant fetal monitoring.

E. CARDIAC CATHETERIZATION

Pulmonary artery catheterization without fluoroscopy, at the bedside, is a relatively safe procedure and allows for hemodynamic monitoring during labor and delivery in patients with significant heart disease. Left or right heart catheterization under fluoroscopy should be undertaken only when absolutely essential (eg, for

percutaneous coronary intervention or balloon valvuloplasty). Every effort should be taken to shield the abdominal and pelvic areas and to avoid direct irradiation of the fetus.

VALVULAR HEART DISEASE

1. Mitral Stenosis

Mitral stenosis is the most common valvular lesion seen in pregnancy. It may be congenital or may be caused by rheumatic heart disease, Libman-Sacks endocarditis in lupus, and Lutembacher's syndrome (mitral stenosis in association with an atrial septal defect). Rheumatic heart disease develops after a group A β-hemolytic streptococcal infection of the upper airway. Even though its incidence in developing countries has declined as a result of the prevalent use of antibiotics, rheumatic valvular disease still afflicts a large majority of women of childbearing age in Asia, Central America, and South America. Major Jones criteria for diagnosing rheumatic heart disease include prior evidence of a group A streptococcal infection (elevated antistreptolysin titer, positive throat culture), carditis, polyarthritis, chorea, subcutaneous nodules, and erythema marginatum. Minor criteria consist of fevers, arthralgias, elevated sedimentation rate, and first-degree heart block.

Pregnancy-related complications of mitral stenosis are mostly related to narrowing of the mitral valve in the setting of increasing heart rate and stroke volume. As left atrial pressure rises, the patient begins to develop symptoms of dyspnea, decreased exercise capacity, orthopnea, paroxysmal nocturnal dyspnea, and pulmonary edema. Eventually left atrial outflow obstruction leads to severe pulmonary venous congestion, resulting in pulmonary hypertension and right ventricular failure. Patients can have frank hemoptysis, and the low cardiac output can cause symptoms of dizziness and even syncope. The augmented atrial pressures, increasing atrial irritability, and presence of increasing sympathetic tone predispose the patient to development of atrial fibrillation. This new-onset atrial fibrillation can precipitate acute decompensation of heart disease even in the setting of mild to moderate mitral stenosis due to acceleration of ventricular rate that results in unfavorable hemodynamics.

The normal hemodynamic changes of pregnancy place patients with mitral stenosis at special risk for developing pulmonary congestion. The increased heart rate with consequent shortening of the diastolic filling period, augmented cardiac output and blood volume, and increased pulmonary venous pressure all contribute to raising left atrial pressure. The increased atrial irritability and increased sympathetic tone predispose to atrial fibrillation. The pregnant cardiac patient also is at risk for developing thromboembolic complications because of the hypercoagulable state of the blood during pregnancy as well as venous stasis in the legs. The risk of developing heart failure increases progressively throughout pregnancy and increases further during labor and delivery and immediately postpartum. Symptoms can be aggravated by associated anemia, thyrotoxicosis, fever, respiratory infections, and tachycardia resulting from anxiety, stress, and unusual physical exertion, as well as a hot, humid environment. The risk of infective endocarditis remains throughout pregnancy, delivery, and early puerperium.

Labor imposes an additional load, and congestive failure may develop for the first time during labor in a previously well-controlled patient with mitral stenosis. The overall mortality rate in women with rheumatic mitral valve disease is 1% overall and reaches 3–4% in women with class III and IV severity.

Clinical Findings

The symptoms of mitral valve disease are similar to those of pulmonary venous congestion: dyspnea on exertion and later at rest, right ventricular failure, atrial arrhythmias, and occasionally hemoptysis. The characteristic findings on physical examination include a right ventricular lift, a loud first heart sound (S_1), an accentuated pulmonic component of the second heart sound (P_2), an opening snap, and a low-frequency diastolic rumble at the apex with presystolic accentuation (if the patient is in sinus rhythm). The murmur is best heard with the bell of the stethescope in the left lateral decubitus position. The electrocardiogram often is normal but may indicate left atrial enlargement, right-axis deviation, or even right ventricular hypertrophy. The echocardiogram is particularly useful for defining the anatomy of the valvular and intravalvular structures, quantifying the degree of stenosis and associated regurgitation, and identifying the presence of abnormalities in other valves and pulmonary hypertension.

Treatment

The goals of treatment for the patient with mitral stenosis is to prevent/treat tachycardia and atrial fibrillation, prevent fluid overload, and prevent unnecessary increases in oxygen demands that may occur with anxiety or physical activity. Digitalis, quinidine, occasionally β-adrenergic blocking agents, sodium restriction, and diuretics may be necessary to treat congestive failure and atrial arrhythmias. Patients with chronic atrial fibrillation should be anticoagulated with subcutaneous heparin. Anemia, intercurrent infection, and thyrotoxicosis should be corrected. Large fluctuations in hemodynamics due to venous pooling in the legs should be prevented by the use of elastic support hose, especially late in pregnancy.

Medical management remains the first-line therapy in patients with mitral stenosis. In patients with severe mitral stenosis, mitral valvotomy may be performed for symptom relief before they become pregnant. Closed surgical mitral commissurotomy is an option during pregnancy. Balloon valvuloplasty has become a preferred, less invasive procedure, especially for patients with a noncalcified, pliable valve. Occasionally mitral valve placement is necessary as an emergency procedure during pregnancy, for instance, in a patient with prior valve replacement whose valve becomes obstructed by pannus or thrombus. Recent reports indicate a lower mortality rate for both mother and fetus with cardiopulmonary bypass. However, open heart surgery should be deferred until after the pregnancy if possible.

Patients who have a prosthetic valve require anticoagulation and should be switched from warfarin (Coumadin) to heparin during the pregnancy. The teratogenic and fetotoxic effects of warfarin and the risks of bleeding for the mother and fetus during labor and delivery must be balanced against the risks of thromboembolic episodes, especially in patients with earlier-model prosthetic valves. The use of tissue valves obviates the need for anticoagulants, but the life span of bioprosthetic valves is only 8–10 years, and anticoagulation is still required if the patient is in atrial fibrillation.

Patients with mitral stenosis should be delivered vaginally at term unless cesarean section in indicated for obstetric reasons. Narcotic-epidural anesthesia without epinephrine is the preferred option for delivery. Other considerations include maintenance of meticulous fluid balance, oxygen administration, and left lateral decubitus position during labor. The second stage of labor may be shortened with use of outlet forceps. Careful hemodynamic monitoring during labor and delivery is indicated in patients with compromised circulation. Postpartum uterotonics should be given cautiously and blood loss carefully monitored. Redistribution of fluid from the interstitial to the intravascular space immediately postpartum can precipitate pulmonary edema in compromised patients.

2. Mitral Regurgitation

Patients with isolated or predominant mitral regurgitation tolerate the physiologic consequences of pregnancy better than do patients with predominant mitral stenosis. The fall in systemic vascular resistance decreases left ventricular afterload and actually reduces the regurgitant fraction, thus reducing the risk of pulmonary congestion. The risks of atrial fibrillation and endocarditis, however, are no less in patients with predominant mitral insufficiency. Although mitral regurgitation frequently is the result of rheumatic disease, other causes include genetic defects in collagen synthesis (as occur in Marfan's syndrome and Ehlers-Danlos syndrome) or following endocarditis of a previously abnormal valve, late complication of mitral valve prolapse, or papillary muscle infarction or rupture. The characteristic finding on physical examination is a long systolic murmur that ends with the second heart sound and is best heard at the apex with radiation into the axilla. An associated third heart sound is often present, and an opening snap may be present with associated mitral valve stenosis.

3. Rheumatic Disease in Other Valves

The aortic, pulmonary, and tricuspid valves may be involved by the rheumatic process, usually in association with mitral valve disease. Involvement of multiple valves compounds the problems of management in these patients. Patients with aortic or pulmonary stenosis have a fixed ventricular outflow obstruction. The gradient across the valve increases with progressive increase in cardiac output during pregnancy, leading to increased systolic pressure load on the ventricle. Although left ventricular failure is rare, postexertional syncope and angina due to inadequate cardiac output reserve may develop for the first time during pregnancy, especially in the last trimester, when venous return may be abruptly reduced due to compression of the inferior vena cava by the uterus. Patients with severe aortic stenosis should be advised to undergo surgical correction before they become pregnant. Because patients with high-grade aortic stenosis are unable to maintain normal cardiac output, hypotension, hypertension, and increased cardiac work must be prevented by restricting physical activity and carefully replacing intrapartum blood loss.

Patients with aortic insufficiency (eg, those with mitral regurgitation) tolerate pregnancy well because the fall in peripheral resistances favors blood flow and decreases the regurgitant fraction. The risk of endocarditis is present in both stenotic and insufficient valves regardless of severity, and antibiotic prophylaxis during delivery is recommended. Patients with elevated left ventricular end-diastolic pressure, however, are more likely to develop left ventricular failure during pregnancy.

Corrective surgical procedures for rheumatic valve disease include balloon valvuloplasty, surgical commissurotomy, and valve replacement. Two types of valves are available for valve replacement. Tissue valves do not require systemic anticoagulation but tend to deteriorate in 8–10 years. Prosthetic valves, such as the tilting disk or caged ball valves, may last 20 years or longer but always require anticoagulation, complicating the management of pregnancy.

4. Peripartum Cardiomyopathy

Peripartum cardiomyopathy occurs in 1 in 1500 to 1 in 15,000 pregnancies. It is a dilated cardiomyopathy of an unknown cause. Patients usually present with symptoms of congestive heart failure late in pregnancy or in the early postpartum period. Treatment includes bed rest, fluid and salt restrictions, diuretics, vasodilators, digitalis, and β blockers. In addition, prophylactic anticoagulation during pregnancy and full anticoagulation for 1–2 weeks after delivery is recommended. Cardiac function normalizes within 6 months of delivery in approximately half of patients with peripartum cardiomyopathy. Because these patients are at risk for developing heart failure and death in subsequent pregnancy, they should be counseled against future pregnancies.

SUMMARY

Most pregnant patients with cardiac disease have successful outcomes with meticulous follow-up. Valvular stenotic lesions pose a high risk to the mother and the fetus, whereas regurgitant lesions are tolerated well by pregnant women. Extremely high-risk patients should be advised against pregnancy and be offered termination if they become pregnant.

REFERENCES

Abbas AE, Lester SJ, Connolly H: Pregnancy and the cardiovascular system. Int J Cardiol 2005;98:179.

Bonow RO et al: ACC/AHA Guidelines for the Management of Patients with Valvular Heart Disease. Executive Summary. A report of the American College of Cardiology/American Heart Association Task Force on Practice Guidelines (Committee on Management of Patients with Valvular Heart Disease). J Heart Valve Dis 1998;7:672.

Campuzano K et al: Bacterial endocarditis complicating pregnancy: case report and systematic review of the literature. Arch Gynecol Obstet 2003;268:251.

de Souza JA et al: Percutaneous balloon mitral valvuloplasty in comparison with open mitral valve commissurotomy for mitral stenosis during pregnancy. J Am Coll Cardiol 2001;37: 900.

Elkayam U et al: Maternal and fetal outcomes of subsequent pregnancies in women with peripartum cardiomyopathy. N Engl J Med 2001;344:1567.

Elkayam U, Bitar F: Valvular heart disease and pregnancy: part II: prosthetic valves. J Am Coll Cardiol 2005;46:403.

Elkayam U, Bitar F: Valvular heart disease and pregnancy: part I: native valves. J Am Coll Cardiol 2005;46:223.

Hameed A et al: The effect of valvular heart disease on maternal and fetal outcome of pregnancy. J Am Coll Cardiol 2001; 37:893.

Hung L, Rahimtoola SH: Prosthetic heart valves and pregnancy. Circulation 2003;107:1240.

Reimold SC, Rutherford JD: Clinical practice. Valvular heart disease in pregnancy. N Engl J Med 2003;349:52.

Siu SC et al: Prospective multicenter study of pregnancy outcomes in women with heart disease. Circulation 2001;104: 515.

Sutton SW et al: Cardiopulmonary bypass and mitral valve replacement during pregnancy. Perfusion 2005;20:359.

Pulmonary Disorders in Pregnancy 22B

Martin N. Montoro, MD

ASPIRATION PNEUMONITIS

Pregnant women are at increased risk for aspiration of gastric contents as a result of elevated intra-abdominal pressure, decreased gastroesophageal sphincter tone, delayed gastric emptying, and diminished laryngeal reflexes. Aspiration may be the result of passive regurgitation or active vomiting. Aspiration has been reported to account for 30–50% of maternal deaths related to anesthetic complications. Superimposed bacterial infection following aspiration may occur after 24–72 hours, with mortality rates even higher in these cases. The main determinants of outcome are related to the acidity (pH ≤ 2.5) and the volume (≥ 25 mL) of the aspirate and the presence or absence of solid particles in the aspirate.

Clinical Findings

The pathologic mechanism and clinical manifestations depend on the volume and composition of the aspirate. Small volumes of a very acidic aspirate will be highly toxic, whereas relatively large volumes of a buffered aspirate can be tolerated. Aspiration of large, solid particulate matter may occlude portions of the larger bronchi, resulting in hypoxia, pulmonary hypertension, and even death. With smaller particles, bronchial obstruction occurs more distally, resulting in atelectasis, hypoxia, and inflammation of the bronchial mucosal and respiratory distress. Symptoms immediately after aspiration include dyspnea, bronchospasm, cyanosis, tachycardia, and even respiratory arrest. The patient will be hypoxic, hypercapnic, and acidotic. The chest x-ray film may reveal interstitial pulmonary edema.

Prevention

Given the high rate of maternal death associated with aspiration pneumonitis, every effort should be made to prevent this catastrophic condition. General anesthesia is the main risk factor associated with aspiration, and expert airway management during induction and intubation is extremely important.

Oral intake during labor must be avoided. Women undergoing elective cesarean delivery must not be given anything by mouth for at least 6–8 hours prior to the procedure. All anesthetized obstetric patients should be intubated. Laryngeal reflexes will generally prevent aspiration while patients are awake, but the reflexes will be altered in patients who are given excessive sedation, in patients who are under anesthesia, or in patients with seizures. Pain, anxiety, narcotics, and labor itself may cause delayed gastric emptying and increased intragastric pressure. Lowering the volume of gastric contents to < 25 mL and raising the gastric pH to > 2.5 will reduce the risk of pulmonary injury if aspiration occurs. Clear, nonparticulate systemic alkalizers (eg, sodium citrate-Bacitra, or Alka-Seltzer) must be used instead of particulate oral antacids (eg, magnesium trisilicate, Maalox, Riopan). Thirty milliliters of a clear antacid should be routinely given to all women 30 minutes prior to induction of anesthesia.

Gastric acidity may be reduced by histamine-2 (H_2) receptor blockers. Cimetidine and ranitidine have been reported to be safe for use during pregnancy. Metoclopramide may increase lower esophageal sphincter tone and enhance gastric emptying. However, antacids are preferred, particularly in emergency situations, because they are reliable and fast acting. H_2 blockers and metoclopramide are not recommended for routine use.

Treatment

If aspiration occurs during anesthesia, immediate intubation and suction should be performed, followed by ventilation and adequate oxygenation. Positive end-expiratory pressure may help to better expand areas of fluid-filled collapsed lung. Bronchoscopic suction should be performed as soon as possible if the aspirate contains solid particles. A chest x-ray film should be taken and serial blood gas determinations made. These patients should be managed in the intensive care unit.

If the gastric fluid pH is > 3.0 and the patient appears to be well oxygenated, she can be followed closely with periodic chest x-ray films and blood gas determinations. Use of corticosteroids is not universally agreed upon. Antibiotics should not be given empirically; they should be administered only when clinical evidence and cultures indicate the presence of a superimposed bacterial infection.

ASTHMA DURING PREGNANCY

Frequency

The general prevalence of asthma appears to be increasing. Recent studies report that asthma occurs in 9% of the general U.S. population and in 3.7–8.4% of pregnant women. Therefore, asthma has become one of the most common medical illnesses complicating pregnancy. The most recent government-compiled statistics in 2003 reveal that 20.3 million persons in the United States have asthma; 9 million of these persons are younger than 18 years. There were 1.8 million emergency room visits, half a million hospitalizations, and 5000 deaths in 2003, half of which occurred in those younger than 18 years. The increased prevalence is reported worldwide, particularly in urban areas, and is generally attributed to industrial pollution. However, marked geographic variations occur, and the extent to which genetic predisposition plays a role is under active investigation.

Effect of Asthma on Pregnancy

Childhood-onset asthma affects males more often than females. In contrast, adult-onset asthma reportedly occurs more frequently in women than in men. Overall, the prevalence and severity of asthma are consistently reported to be greater in women than in men. Women also are reported to require more frequent emergency room visits and more hospitalizations. Therefore, sex hormones are believed to play a role in the differences observed in the occurrence of asthma, although the exact mechanisms are not completely elucidated. Asthma shows variations during the menstrual cycle, with premenstrual exacerbation more often reported. Reports on asthma during the menopause are more conflicting, with some studies noting improvement but others reporting more episodes of bronchospasm after 6 months of hormone replacement therapy.

No consistent effect (either worsening or improvement) during pregnancy has been observed, although one-third of women with more severe disease reportedly became worse late in the second trimester or during the third trimester. Others speculate that pregnancy does not have an effect on asthma and that the variations observed are simply part of the natural history of the disease. The responses in subsequent pregnancies are more consistent and tend to be similar to those that occurred during the first pregnancy.

Potential maternal complications include hyperemesis gravidarum, pneumonia (women with asthma account for > 60% of pneumonia cases in pregnancy), preeclampsia, vaginal bleeding, more complicated labors, and more cesarean deliveries. Fetal complications can include intrauterine growth restriction, preterm birth, low birthweight, neonatal hypoxia, and increased overall perinatal mortality. Women with severe asthma are at the highest risk. However, patients are at little or no increased risk when the disease is effectively treated and controlled.

Classification

Asthma currently is classified according to severity as (1) mild intermittent, (2) mild persistent, (3) moderate persistent, and (4) severe persistent. In mild intermittent asthma, symptoms do not occur more often than twice per week, and nocturnal symptoms do not occur more often than twice per month. The peak expiratory flow (PEF) or the forced expiratory volume in 1 second (FEV_1) is > 80% of normal, with a variability < 20%. In mild persistent asthma, symptoms occur more often than twice per week but not daily, and nocturnal symptoms occur more often than twice per month. The PEF or FEV_1 still is at least 80% of normal, but the variability is greater at 20–30%. In moderate persistent asthma, symptoms occur daily, and nocturnal symptoms occur more than once per week. The PEF or FEV_1 is < 80% but > 60% of normal, with variability > 30%. In severe persistent asthma, daytime symptoms occur continually, and nocturnal attacks occur frequently. The PEF or FEV_1 is < 60% of normal, with variability > 30%.

Diagnosis

The diagnosis of asthma usually is made on clinical grounds and rarely is difficult if an adequate history and physical examination are obtained. Most patients are diagnosed before pregnancy and already are receiving treatment. Symptoms suggestive of asthma include cough, dyspnea, chest tightness, and wheezing, particularly when episodes occur episodically. Pulmonary function studies are useful to confirm the diagnosis and should be part of the initial investigations. The FEV_1/ FVC (forced vital capacity) ratio will be < 70%, and the airway obstruction can be reversed by administration of a short-acting β_2-agonist preparation. Rarely, bronchospasm is caused by a condition other than asthma. These conditions include acute left ventricular heart failure (also called *cardiac asthma*), pulmonary embolism, exacerbation of chronic bronchitis, carcinoid tumors, upper airway obstruction (laryngeal edema, foreign body), gastroesophageal reflux, and cough caused by some medications.

Common triggers of asthma include upper respiratory infections (more commonly viral); administration of blockers, aspirin, or nonsteroidal anti-inflammatory drugs; sulfites and other food preservatives; allergens such as pollen, animal dander, mites, or molds; smoking; (environmental asthma); gastric reflux; and exercise or other causes of hyperventilation. Both cigarette smoking and other major environmental pollutants are specifically associated with fetal damage.

Treatment

A. GENERAL MEASURES

The main goal of therapy is to maintain normal or near-normal maternal pulmonary function to allow adequate fetal oxygenation, prevent exacerbations, and allow the patient to maintain her usual activities. In general, pregnant women are receptive to educational interventions that will improve their asthma management, and the benefits are likely to continue after delivery. A good example is learning the proper use of portable peak flow meters to objectively evaluate asthma severity because clinical symptoms and the patient's own perception of the severity of asthma often are inaccurate. The PEF rate correlates well with FEV_1 and allows the detection of worsening at an early stage before serious symptoms appear and the evaluation of response to treatment while the patient is still at home. Avoidance of potential asthma triggers also is extremely important. The general principles of management for pregnant asthmatic women are similar to those for nonpregnant patients and include removing pets if necessary, encasing mattresses and pillows in airtight covers, carefully washing the bedding, keeping ambient humidity < 50%, avoid vacuuming (or at least wear a mask), using air conditioning and air filters, avoiding outdoor activities when allergens and air pollution levels are high, and avoiding nonallergen irritants, such as strong odors, food additives, aspirin, β blockers, and particularly tobacco smoke. Several recent studies have shown that these measures not only are beneficial but are cost-effective as well.

Patients undergoing immunotherapy may continue doing so during pregnancy but without any further dose increase. Starting immunotherapy de novo during pregnancy is not recommended because uterine contractions are likely to develop if anaphylaxis occurs.

Influenza vaccination is currently recommended for all pregnant women during the flu season. This recommendation is of the utmost importance for pregnant women with asthma. Asthma sufferers also should receive the pneumococcal vaccine but preferably prior to pregnancy.

Treating rhinitis and sinusitis, which often are associated with asthma and may trigger exacerbations, is important. Treatment of rhinitis includes reducing exposure to antigens (environmental control); intranasal cromolyn sodium, antihistamines (tripelennamine or chlorpheniramine), and intranasal steroids are very beneficial. For treatment of sinusitis, amoxicillin (erythromycin if allergic to penicillin), oxymetazoline (nasal spray or drops), and pseudoephedrine are more often used.

B. PHARMACOLOGIC THERAPY

Many women have the impression that most, if not all, medications might be harmful to the fetus. However, they should be informed that the risk of uncontrolled asthma is far worse than any of the potential side effects of the most common medications used to treat asthma. Most women with asthma can be managed effectively during pregnancy, and complications are generally confined to patients with uncontrolled asthma.

1. Mild intermittent asthma—These patients do not need daily medications. When symptoms occur, 2–4 puffs of a short-acting $β_2$ agonist can be used as needed. More data are available for use of albuterol than for any other $β_2$ agonist during pregnancy, and no harm to the fetus has been observed to date. These women may still experience severe exacerbations, which may be separated by long asymptomatic periods, and a short course of systemic corticosteroids may be needed.

2. Mild persistent asthma—The preferred therapy for this group of patients is a low-dose inhaled corticosteroid. More experience is available for budesonide use in pregnancy, and the published data regarding its safety and lack of risk for congenital anomalies are reassuring. Less experience is reported with beclomethasone, but the published data also are reassuring. Inhaled corticosteroids suppress and may even prevent airway inflammation, which plays a critical role in the pathogenesis of asthma and may decrease airway responsiveness as well. Because they may decrease and sometimes even obviate the need for systemic steroids, their use is now recommended at earlier stages of asthma. However, the full benefits may not be seen for 2–4 weeks, so they are not recommended as part of the treatment of acute attacks. Use of a mouth spacer to minimize systemic absorption is strongly recommended. Inhaled corticosteroids are likewise beneficial for rhinitis (2 sprays in each nostril twice daily).

Alternative, but not preferred, therapies for this group include inhaled cromolyn sodium, leukotriene receptor antagonists, or sustained-release theophylline. Cromolyn sodium is also anti-inflammatory drug, but its efficacy is less predictable than that of the inhaled corticosteroids, and the benefits may not be seen for 4–6 weeks. Nevertheless, cromolyn sodium seems to be free of side effects for mother or fetus. Few data on the use of leukotriene receptor modifiers during pregnancy are available, but they are reported to be safe in animals. The extensive experience with theophylline during pregnancy indicates theophylline is safe for the fetus except when maternal levels exceed 12 μg/mL. In these cases, the fetus or newborn may develop jitteriness, tachycardia, and vomiting.

3. Moderate persistent asthma—The preferred treatment is a combination of a low-dose or medium-dose inhaled corticosteroid and a long-acting β_2 agonist. Alternative therapies (but again not preferred) include a low-dose or medium-dose inhaled corticosteroid and either theophylline or a leukotriene receptor antagonist. However, given the scarcity of data on human pregnancy, the use of leukotriene receptor modifiers is reserved for patients who showed a very good response before pregnancy but are not responding well to other medications while pregnant.

4. Severe persistent asthma—The preferred treatment is a high-dose inhaled corticosteroid and a long-acting inhaled β_2 agonist as well as (if needed) a systemic corticosteroid, such as 2 mg/kg/d of prednisone or equivalent steroid not to exceed 60 mg/d, with an attempt to taper to the minimal effective dose. An alternative, but not preferred, treatment includes a high-dose inhaled corticosteroid and sustained-release theophylline (keeping maternal systemic levels at 5–12 µg/mL for the reasons explained above).

Systemic corticosteroids are used when any of the other drug combinations cannot control the asthma. They usually are given first as a short, rapidly tapering course (eg, 40–60 mg/d of prednisone or equivalent steroid for 1 week, tapering off during the second week). If these courses fail to effectively control symptoms for < 2–3 weeks, long-term systemic corticosteroid treatment may be needed. In these cases, the lowest effective dose or alternate-day therapy, if possible, should be used. Potential maternal side effects include impaired glucose tolerance or frank diabetes mellitus, preeclampsia, intrauterine growth restriction, and premature delivery. With prolonged use (1–2 months), maternal adrenal insufficiency may occur, and adequate coverage during periods of stress (including labor and delivery) is mandatory. Use during the first trimester is associated with a higher risk for facial clefts (lip and palate). Pregnant women with asthma who are steroid dependent should be managed by an internist/pulmonologist who is experienced in the treatment of asthma during pregnancy.

C. OTHER ASTHMA MEDICATIONS

Nonselective β agonists such as epinephrine and isoproterenol are sometimes given subcutaneously during acute asthma attacks. Epinephrine use during pregnancy should be avoided because epinephrine causes vasoconstriction and reduces fetal oxygenation. It is teratogenic in animals as well as in humans. Isoproterenol also is teratogenic in animals. Because many other alternative therapies are available, isoproterenol use in humans is best avoided. Iodine-containing medications should be avoided during pregnancy because the fetus may be at risk for developing a goiter, which

may become very large and cause airway obstruction and even asphyxia. Nedocromil sodium is similar to cromolyn sodium. No reports on humans are available, but nedocromil sodium has not been observed to be teratogenic in animal experiments. Anticholinergic medications such as atropine (which block bronchoconstriction by inhaled irritants) may accelerate the fetal heart rate and inhibit breathing. Ipratropium has not been reported to be teratogenic in animals, but data on humans are lacking. Glycopyrrolate has been used safely in humans near term, and no defects have been reported in animal experiments.

1. Acute asthmatic attack—During acute exacerbations, dyspnea, cough, wheezing, and chest tightness increase and expiratory flow decreases. A few, well-educated patients with a relatively mild attacks might be managed at home taking advantage of the judicious use of peak flow measurements. However, any serious exacerbation most likely will require hospitalization. Great care should be exercised to maintain a maternal PO_2 > 70 mm Hg and O_2 saturation > 95%. A maternal PO_2 < 60 mm Hg will result in marked fetal hypoxia.

General measures include reassuring the patient and avoiding sedatives, which may depress respiration. Oxygen can be administered by mask or nasal catheter with the goal of maintaining PO_2 > 70 mm Hg and O_2 saturation > 90% to ensure adequate fetal oxygenation at all times. A few patients may require endotracheal intubation and mechanical ventilation to maintain an adequate oxygen supply. Blood gas determinations are necessary for this purpose. A chest x-ray film should be part of the initial evaluation. Antibiotics are given only if evidence of bacterial infection is present. Some pregnant women receiving large amounts of intravenous fluids, β_2 agonists, and corticosteroids reportedly develop pulmonary edema, so this risk should be considered under these circumstances.

Initial pharmacologic treatment includes an inhaled β_2 agonist administered by a metered-dose inhaler, 2–4 puffs every 20 minutes to a maximum of 3 doses or less if side effects appear. A subcutaneous β_2 agonist (eg, terbutaline 0.25 mg) is also given and can be repeated once 20 minutes later. Systemic corticosteroids are recommended early in the course of treatment of acute exacerbations. The most frequently used corticosteroid is methylprednisolone intravenously at an initial dose of 1–2 mg/kg/d. At present, intravenous theophylline is used much less frequently for acute exacerbations because of the early use of corticosteroids. When necessary, the recommended initial loading dose is 5–6 mg/kg given intravenously over 20–30 minutes. The loading dose is not given if the patient was receiving adequate oral doses prior to the acute attack, or only half the loading dose is given if the patient was receiving theophylline but only intermittently. Maintenance doses are 0.7 mg/kg/h. Serum levels should be monitored to avoid maternal levels in excess of 12 μg/mL.

After admission to the hospital, administration of β$_2$ agonists is continued by nebulized aerosol every 4–6 hours; administration of intravenous corticosteroids also is continued (eg, methylprednisolone 0.5–1 mg/kg twice daily). If theophylline was started, it is continued per the maintenance dose protocol, with careful monitoring of maternal serum levels to avoid fetal toxicity. As the patient improves, the β$_2$-agonist aerosols are continued (2 puffs every 4–6 hours), and at this point the inhaled steroids (high dose, per the protocol for the severe persistent asthma) are resumed or the therapy initiated if the patient was not receiving them prior to the acute attack. If the clinical improvement continues, the systemic steroids can be switched to the oral route (eg, prednisone 0.5 mg/kg/d, with gradual tapering attempted while maximizing inhaled steroid treatment). If theophylline was being given, it also should be changed to the oral route (6 mg/kg), with close monitoring of maternal serum levels.

Management during Labor and Delivery

The medications that were being administered prior to the onset of labor should be continued during labor. Adequate control should be maintained because labor has been reported to trigger an acute attack in approximately 10% of women with asthma. Peak expiratory flow measurements should be obtained at regular intervals to monitor pulmonary status closely. Adequate hydration should be maintained and pain relief provided as necessary. Fentanyl is considered a good analgesic choice for these patients. Analgesics and/or narcotics, which can cause histamine release, should be avoided because of the possibility of respiratory depression and bronchospasm. Continuous O$_2$ monitoring is mandatory to ensure that O$_2$ saturation is > 95% at all times.

Medications to avoid include prostaglandin F$_2$ because it may cause bronchospasm. Prostaglandin E$_2$, either gel or suppository, is safe for women with asthma and can be used if necessary from the obstetric standpoint. Oxytocin is safe and considered the medication of choice for induction.

Epidural anesthesia is preferred because it reduces O$_2$ consumption and minute ventilation. General anesthesia may trigger an attack, but the risk may be reduced by pretreatment with atropine (see above for potential fetal effects) and glycopyrrolate, which have a bronchodilatory effect. A low concentration of halogenated anesthetic may provide bronchodilation as well. For induction, ketamine is preferred. An anesthesiologist experienced in the care of pregnant women should be consulted ahead of time when anticipating anesthesia needs.

Ergot derivatives should be avoided because they may precipitate bronchospasm. If postpartum hemorrhage occurs, oxytocin is the best choice. If a prostaglandin is needed, then prostaglandin E$_2$ is preferred. Aspirin and nonsteroidal anti-inflammatory drugs (eg, indomethacin) may trigger severe bronchospasm as well as ocular, nasal, dermal and gastrointestinal inflammation in 3–8% of asthmatic patients and are best avoided. Magnesium is safe for asthma but with careful monitoring to avoid respiratory depression.

Fetal Monitoring

An ultrasound examination in early pregnancy is useful to confirm dating and to provide a baseline to evaluate future growth assessment. Serial ultrasounds are recommended for women with moderate and severe asthma because they are the most at risk for fetal growth restriction. No specific guidelines have been issued for antepartum fetal surveillance other than very general recommendations such as "when needed in the third trimester to assure fetal well being" and "daily recording of fetal movements is encouraged." Many institutions offer fetal surveillance starting at 32–34 weeks to patients with moderate and severe asthma and at any time during the third trimester when an exacerbation occurs. There is unanimous agreement that all patients with asthma should undergo continuous fetal monitoring during labor and delivery.

Breastfeeding

Inhaled β$_2$ agonists, cromolyn sodium, steroids (inhaled), and ipratropium are safe while breastfeeding. Systemic (oral or parenterally administered) steroids may enter into breast milk but only in small amounts if the total daily dosage contains less than 40 mg of prednisone (or equivalent steroid).

TUBERCULOSIS

Tuberculosis was one the leading causes of death in the United States for many years until the introduction of effective therapy in the early 1950s. Since then, the number of reported cases declined steadily until recently, when the number of cases has increased. This situation is attributed to increased immigration from countries with a high tuberculosis prevalence and particularly to the human immunodeficiency virus (HIV)/acquired immunodeficiency syndrome (AIDS) epidemic.

Tuberculosis in adults is mainly (> 95%) a disease of the pulmonary parenchyma caused by *Mycobacterium tuberculosis,* a nonmotile, acid-fast aerobic rod. Transmission usually occurs by inhalation of droplets produced by infected individuals when coughing. The droplets can remain suspended in the air for prolonged periods (several hours). The persons most at risk for becoming infected are family members and other close contacts, such as coworkers and roommates (elderly residents and employees in long-term care facilities, correctional institutions), homeless individuals, and intravenous drug users. After the initial inhalation, the bacilli multiply in the alveoli and subsequently spread to the regional lymph nodes and to other organs such as the upper lung regions, kidneys, bones, central nervous system (CNS), and, rarely, during pregnancy, to the placenta. In most people, the infection is contained by cell-mediated immunity, which develops 2–10 weeks after exposure when the infected sites are walled off by granulomatous inflammation and the tuberculin tests then becomes reactive. At this stage, these persons are not infectious and are asymptomatic except for the positive tuberculin skin test. After the initial exposure, the risk of developing active disease during the following 2–5 years is generally given as 5–15%, but the risk later falls to very low levels < 1–2%. However, active disease may ensue if a person is unable to contain the infection when first exposed or if the person subsequently becomes immunocompromised and the infection is reactivated at a time remote from the initial exposure.

Clinical Findings

Most cases of tuberculosis can be diagnosed on the basis of a history of cough, weight loss, positive tuberculin skin test, and chest x-ray film.

A. Symptoms and Signs

Typical symptoms include cough, weight loss, fatigue, night sweats, and anorexia. However, some patients may have very few symptoms.

Laboratory Findings

The definitive diagnosis is made after positive identification of the bacilli by Ziehl-Neelsen staining and a positive culture.

A. Tuberculin Skin Test

The tuberculin skin test is the most important screening test for tuberculosis. It should be performed early in pregnancy, especially in high-risk populations. An induration of 5 mm or greater is considered positive in individuals with HIV infection, in close contacts of persons with active, infectious tuberculosis, in persons with typical x-ray findings who were never previously treated, and in intravenous drug users. An induration of 10 mm or more is considered positive in persons who have risk factors other than HIV, such as diabetes

mellitus, silicosis, chronic use of corticosteroids or other immunosuppressive drugs, cancer (solid tumors as well as leukemias and lymphomas), chronic renal insufficiency, gastrectomy or intestinal bypass, or malabsorption and chronic malnutrition with body weight 10% or less below the ideal.

B. Chest X-Ray Film

With the abdomen shielded and preferably after the first trimester, a chest x-ray film should be taken in patients in whom skin testing is positive after an earlier negative test and in patients with a suggestive history or physical examination even though skin testing is negative.

C. Congenital Tuberculosis

Congenital tuberculosis is rare. The criteria for diagnosis include positive bacteriologic studies, primary disease complex in the liver, disease occurring within the first few days of life, and exclusion of extrauterine infection. The most common signs are nonspecific and include fever, failure to thrive, lymphadenopathy, hepatomegaly, and splenomegaly. The disease usually is miliary or disseminated. An early diagnosis is necessary for effective treatment.

Treatment

A. Medical Therapy

Untreated tuberculosis is far riskier to the mother and fetus than any of the potential medications necessary to treat active disease. A preventive course of isoniazid (isonicotinic acid hydrazide [INH]) is generally recommended for those with a positive skin test and no evidence of active disease if they are at risk for developing active tuberculosis. However, such preventive therapy is withheld in those older than 35 years and during pregnancy and early postpartum because of an increased risk for INH-related hepatitis. In those at high risk (particularly in cases of HIV/AIDS), preventive INH treatment is initiated as soon as evidence of tuberculosis infection (but no active disease) is documented. The recommended dose of INH is 300 mg/d for 9 months as well as pyridoxine (vitamin B_6) to prevent INH-related neuropathy. Periodic evaluation of liver function is recommended to detect hepatotoxicity early if it occurs. Most studies have shown no teratogenic effects of INH.

Active tuberculosis should be treated as soon as the diagnosis is made. Most treatment programs consist of a 3-drug regimen, usually INH 5 mg/kg/d (total 300 mg/d), and ethambutol 15 mg/kg/d, and rifampin 10 mg/kg/d (maximum 600 mg/d) for 8 weeks and the INH and rifampin to complete 9 months. Pyridoxine should be given along with INH. Local public health departments should be consulted to obtain data about drug resistance. These three medications cross the placenta, but no adverse fetal side effects have been reported to date. Pyrazinamide has been used in addition to the three medications mentioned in areas of highly drug-resistant tuberculosis but is not recommended during pregnancy because of limited safety data. Because of the risk for fetal (and maternal) ototoxicity, streptomycin, kanamycin, and capreomycin should not be used. Isoniazid has many therapeutic advantages (eg, high efficacy, patient acceptability, and low cost) and appears to be the safest drug for use during pregnancy. The major side effects of INH are hepatitis, hypersensitivity reactions, peripheral neuropathy, and gastrointestinal distress. A baseline liver function test should be obtained and then repeated periodically. *Pyridoxine 50 mg/d should be administered to prevent INH-induced neuritis due to vitamin B6 deficiency.* Optic neuritis is a rare complication reported with ethambutol use. Rifampin may cause hepatitis, hypersensitivity reactions, occasional hematologic toxicity, flulike syndrome, abdominal pain, acute renal failure, and thrombocytopenia. Rifampin may increase the metabolic rate of oral contraceptives through activation of the hepatic P450 enzyme system, so an alternative form of contraception may be necessary after delivery in these patients while they are taking rifampin.

Obstetric Management

Routine antepartum obstetric management includes adequate rest and nutrition, family support, correction of anemia if present, and regular follow-up visits.

Immediate neonatal contact is allowed if the mother has received treatment for inactive disease and no evidence of reactivation is present. In patients with inactive disease in whom prophylactic INH was not given or those with active disease in whom adequate treatment was given, early neonatal contact may be allowed, provided the mother is reliable in continuing therapy. A mother with active disease should receive at least 3 weeks of treatment before coming into contact with her baby, and the baby must also receive prophylactic INH.

There are no absolute contraindications to breastfeeding once the mother is noninfectious. Although antituberculosis drugs are found in breast milk, the concentrations are so low that the risk of toxicity in the infant is minimal. However, each case should be judged individually if the mother wishes to breastfeed her infant. In general, breastfeeding is not contraindicated while the mother is taking antituberculosis medications.

Immunization of the newborn with bacille Calmette-Guérin (BCG) vaccine remains controversial. If prompt use of INH as prophylaxis is unlikely or if the mother has INH-resistant disease, BCG vaccination of the infant should be considered.

Prognosis

If the pregnant patient is adequately treated with antituberculosis chemotherapy for active disease, tuberculosis generally has no deleterious effect either during the course of pregnancy or the puerperium or on the fetus. Pregnant women have the same prognosis as nonpregnant women. Tuberculosis is not a reason for recommending a therapeutic abortion.

REFERENCES

Pulmonary Disorders

Aspiration

Cohen SE et al: Does metoclopramide decrease the volume of gastric contents in patients undergoing cesarean sections? Anesthesiology 1984;61:604.

Gipson SL et al: Pharmacologic reduction of the risk of aspiration. South Med J 1986;79:11.

McCammon RL: Prophylaxis for aspiration pneumonitis. Can Anaesth Soc J 1986;33:847.

Asthma

Asthma and pregnancy—Update 2004. NAEPP working group report on managing asthma during pregnancy: Recommendations for pharmacologic treatment—Update 2004. NIH Publication No. 05-3279. 2004.

Blaiss MS: Management of rhinitis and asthma in pregnancy. Ann Allergy Asthma Immunol 2003;90(Suppl 3):16.

Carmichael SL, Shaw GM: Maternal corticosteroid use and risk of selected congenital anomalies. Am J Med Genet 1999;86:242.

Czeizel AE, Rockenbauer M: Population-based case-control study of teratogenic potential of corticosteroids. Teratology 1997;56:335.

Guidelines for the diagnosis and management of asthma. NIH Publication No. 97-4051. April 1997.

Hartert TV et al: Maternal morbidity and perinatal outcomes among pregnant women with respiratory hospitalization during influenza season. Am J Obstet Gynecol 2003;189:1705.

Kattan M et al. Cost-effectiveness of a home-based environmental intervention for inner-city children with asthma. J Allergy Clin Immunol November 2005.

Kwon HL, Belanger K, Bracken MB: Asthma prevalence among pregnant and childbearing-age women in the United States: Estimates from national health surveys. Ann Epidemiol 2002;13:317.

Li YF et al: Maternal and grandmaternal smoking patterns are associated with early childhood asthma. Chest 2005;127:1232.

Robert E et al: Malformation surveillance and maternal drug exposure: The MADRE project. Int J Risk Safe Med 1994;6:75.

Rodriguez-Pinilla E, Martinez-Frias ML: Corticosteroids during pregnancy and oral clefts: A case-control study. Teratology 1998;58:2.

Salam MT et al: Birth outcomes and prenatal exposure to ozone, carbon monoxide and particulate matter: Results from the children's health study. Environ Mental Health Perspect 2005;113:1638.

Schatz M et al: Asthma morbidity during pregnancy can be predicted by severity classification. J Allergy Clin Immunol 2003;112:283.

The use of newer asthma and allergy medications during pregnancy. The American College of Obstetricians and Gynecologists (ACOG) and The American College of Allergy, Asthma and Immunology (ACAAI). Ann Allergy Asthma Immunol 2000;84:475.

Tuberculosis

American College of Obstetricians and Gynecologists: *Pulmonary Disease in Pregnancy*. ACOG Technical Bulletin No. 224. American College of Obstetricians and Gynecologists, 1996.

Hershfield E: Tuberculosis: 9. Treatment. CMAJ 1999;161:405.

Robinson CA, Rose NC: Tuberculosis: Current implications and management in obstetrics. Obstet Gynecol Surv 1996;51:115.

Renal, Urinary Tract, Gastrointestinal, & Dermatologic Disorders in Pregnancy

Cristiane Guberman, MD, Jeffrey Greenspon, MD, & T. Murphy Goodwin, MD

■ RENAL AND URINARY TRACT DISORDERS

For a discussion of normal renal and urinary tract function in pregnancy, see Chapter 7.

URINARY TRACT INFECTION

Asymptomatic bacteriuria, acute cystitis, and acute pyelonephritis are common renal disorders in pregnancy.

Asymptomatic Bacteriuria

Asymptomatic bacteriuria is defined as the presence of actively multiplying bacteria in the urinary tract excluding the distal urethra in a patient without any obvious symptoms. The incidence is the same in nonpregnant and pregnant female and averages 2–10%. Asymptomatic bacteriuria is twice as common in pregnant women with sickle cell trait and 3 times as common in pregnant women with diabetes or with renal transplant as in normal pregnant women. Risk factors for developing asymptomatic bacteriuria include low socioeconomic status, parity, age, sexual practice, and medical conditions such as diabetes and sickle cell trait.

If asymptomatic bacteriuria is left untreated in pregnancy, up to 40% of patients will develop symptoms of urinary tract infection (UTI). Approximately 25–30% of women will develop acute pyelonephritis. With treatment, the rate is only 10%. Asymptomatic bacteriuria has been associated with preterm delivery, fetal loss, and preeclampsia. Approximately 2% percent of pregnant women with a negative urine culture will develop symptomatic cystitis and pyelonephritis. The diagnosis of asymptomatic bacteriuria is based upon isolation of microorganisms with a colony count > 10^5 organisms per milliliter of urine in a clean-catch speci-

men. The patient should be instructed to clean the vulvar area from front to back to avoid contamination of the urine sample. *Escherichia coli* is the most common offending organism for asymptomatic bacteriuria (approximately 80% of cases). The *Klebsiella-Enterobacter-Serratia* group, *Staphylococcus aureus, Enterococcus,* group B *Streptococcus,* and *Proteus* are responsible for the remainder of cases.

Acute Cystitis

Acute cystitis is uncommon in pregnancy (approximately 1%). The bacteria causing acute cystitis are similar to those in asymptomatic bacteriuria. Clinically, the patient presents with symptoms of urinary frequency, urgency, dysuria, and suprapubic discomfort. The urine often is cloudy and malodorous and should be cultured to confirm the diagnosis and to identify antibiotic sensitivities. The treatment of cystitis is the same as for asymptomatic bacteriuria.

Acute Pyelonephritis

Acute pyelonephritis occurs in 1–2% of all pregnant women (usually, although not invariably, in those with previous asymptomatic bacteriuria) and is associated with risk to the mother and fetus. It is one of the most common causes of hospitalization during pregnancy. Maternal effects include fever, bacterial endotoxemia, endotoxic shock, renal insufficiency, anemia, leukocytosis, thrombocytopenia, and elevated fibrin split product levels. Preterm labor and fetal death may be seen in severe cases. Risk factors for recurrent or severe disease are a history of pyelonephritis, urinary tract malformation, or urinary calculi.

The anemia may be due to marrow suppression, increased erythrocyte destruction, or diminished red cell production. Pulmonary dysfunction has been described in association with acute pyelonephritis. Symptoms and signs may range from minimal (mild cough and slight pulmonary infiltrate) to severe (adult respiratory distress syndrome requiring intensive therapy). Neonatal effects include prematurity and small-for-gestational-age babies.

Clinical manifestations of acute pyelonephritis include fever, shaking chills, flank pain, nausea and vomiting, headache, increased urinary frequency, and dysuria. Urine examination will reveal significant bacteriuria, with pyuria and white blood cell casts in the urinary sediment. A count of 1–2 bacteria per high-power field in unspun urine or > 20 bacteria in the sediment of a centrifuged specimen of urine collected by bladder catheterization helps in the bedside diagnosis. The diagnosis should be confirmed by urine culture. Associated hematuria may indicate urinary calculi.

Treatment

A midstream urine specimen should be collected for culture at the initial prenatal visit and repeated later in pregnancy. At each prenatal visit, dipstick testing should be performed. If proteinuria is present, urinalysis, culture, or both should be done. A pregnant woman with sickle cell trait should have urine culture and sensitivity testing every 4 weeks. The U.S. Preventive Health Task Force states that single urine culture at 12–16 weeks' gestation has 80% sensitivity. Alternatively, regular dipstick testing for leukocyte esterase and nitrites has a negative predictive value > 95% and sensitivity of 50–92%.

Pregnant women should be encouraged to maintain adequate fluid intake and to void frequently.

The initial antibiotic selection should be empiric. Based on the fact that the most common offending pathogen is *E coli*, sulfonamides, nitrofurantoin, or a cephalosporin are reasonable choices. These antibiotics should be safe for the mother and fetus, with minimal side effects. A 5- to 14-day course of one of these agents will effectively eradicate asymptomatic bacteriuria in approximately 65% of pregnant patients. A urine culture should be repeated 1–2 weeks after therapy is started and then monthly for the remainder of pregnancy. Recurrent infections occur in approximately 30% of patients treated once and in approximately 15% of patients who have been treated twice and/or have not responded to initial therapy.

Sulfa drugs must be avoided in mothers with glucose-6-phosphatase deficiency. Additionally, sulfa drugs are best avoided late in pregnancy because of the increased likelihood of neonatal hyperbilirubinemia. Tetracyclines are contraindicated during pregnancy because of dental staining in the exposed child. Trimethoprim is a folic acid antagonist; therefore, trimethoprim-sulfamethoxazole is generally avoided during organogenesis; it may be used when alternatives are limited. A pregnant woman with pyelonephritis initially should be evaluated in the hospital. Antibiotics should be given parenterally and hypovolemia corrected. Acetaminophen can be used as an antipyretic, if indicated. Vital signs, including respiratory rate, and input and output should be closely monitored. Pulse oximetry may be useful. A first-generation cephalosporin such as cefazolin 1 g parenterally every 8 hours usually is effective. However, due to increasing antibiotic resistance, the local susceptibilities should be considered when selecting the initial antibiotic. Ceftriaxone 1 g parenterally every 24 hours often is effective for most *Enterobacteriaceae* in this setting. The urine culture and sensitivities guide therapy thereafter. When the patient is afebrile for 48 hours, parenteral therapy may be changed to an effective oral antibiotic. A total course of 14 days of antibiotic is commonly administered.

If no clinical response is seen in 48–72 hours, a resistant organism can be treated by adding an aminoglycoside such as gentamicin 3–5 mg/kg per 24 hours in 3 divided doses given every 8 hours. Failure to respond may be caused by urolithiasis or a structural urinary tract abnormality. Ultrasound imaging of the kidneys and urinary tract usually is the next diagnostic test. Perinephric abscess causing persistent pain and fever can be identified by ultrasound. Perinephric abscess usually is due to obstruction complicated by infection. The perinephric abscess must be drained surgically in addition to administration of antibiotic therapy. An intravenous pyelogram is often useful if a lack of response continues. A preliminary "scout" film and a film taken 15 minutes after administration of intravenous contrast often are helpful. In selected cases of persistent infection or obstruction, cystoscopy and retrograde pyelography are needed.

Cunningham (1994) reported that following an episode of pyelonephritis, recurrent bacteriuria occurred in 28% of women, and pyelonephritis recurred in 10% during the same pregnancy. For this reason, antibiotic suppressive therapy with nitrofurantoin 100 mg orally at bedtime, or a similar regimen, is continued during the pregnancy and during the puerperium, often for 6 weeks (Table 23–1). Monthly urine cultures to identify a recurrent UTI may be similar in effectiveness to antibiotic suppression for patients who are allergic or who prefer not to take antibiotics.

Periodic culture of the urine assists in detection of recurrence. *Relapse* is defined as recurrent infection from the same species and type-specific strain of organism present before treatment; this represents a treatment failure. Most relapses occur < 2 weeks after completion of therapy. *Reinfection* is recurrent infection due to a different strain of bacteria following successful treatment of the initial infection, occurring > 3 weeks after the completion of therapy.

Table 23–1. Antibiotic regimen for pyelonephritis.

Antibiotic	Dosage	Route	Frequency
Ampicillin plus gentamicin	1–2 g	IV	q4–6h
	2 mg/kg, then 1.7 mg/kg	IV	q8h
Ampicillin/sulbactam	3 g	IV	q6h
Cefazolin	1–2 g	IV	q6–8h
Ceftriaxone	1–2 g	IV or IM	q24h
Mezlocillin	3 g	IV	q6h
Piperacillin	4 g	IV	q8h

URINARY CALCULI

The incidence of urinary calculi is not altered by pregnancy. The incidence is 0.03–0.35% of pregnancies, and the incidence increases as gestational age advances. Stones cause obstruction, infection, pain, and hematuria. Recurrent hospitalization, preterm labor and delivery, and need for operative intervention are increased. The causes of urinary calculi are the same in pregnant and nonpregnant women: chronic UTI, hyperparathyroidism or other causes of hypercalciuria, gout (uric acid), and obstructive uropathy. Congenital or familial cystinuria and oxaluria are less common causes. Most stones are composed of calcium, usually calcium oxalate.

The physiologic hydroureter of pregnancy is more prominent on the right side; however, stones occur with equal frequency on either side. The physiologic hydroureter of pregnancy increase the likelihood that a pregnant patient will spontaneously pass her stone(s).

Clinical Findings

Patients may present with a variety of symptoms, including typical renal or ureteric colic, vague abdominal or back pain that may radiate into the groin, fever, nausea, and vomiting. The patient may have a history of recurrent UTI or hematuria. Fever, bacteriuria, and flank pain may suggest coexisting pyelonephritis from obstruction. The differential diagnosis includes other acute abdominal conditions unrelated to pregnancy (eg, appendicitis, biliary colic or tract disease, adnexal torsion) and conditions related to pregnancy (eg, abruption placentae, preterm labor, chorioamnionitis). When fever attributed to pyelonephritis persists beyond 48 hours of parenteral antibiotic treatment, then obstruction due to urolithiasis must be evaluated. Hematuria, ranging for microscopic to gross, is usually present, although it is not pathognomonic for urolithiasis. The

index of suspicion should be high in the clinical situations described, in patients in whom urine culture is negative in the setting of suspected pyelonephritis, or in cases of persistent hematuria or recurrent UTI.

Clinical diagnosis is confirmed by ultrasound examination of the urinary tract. In selected cases, excretory urography includes a precontrast scout film and another image obtained 20 minutes after contrast injection. This examination exposes the fetus to 0.2 rad. The common indications for intravenous pyelography include microscopic hematuria and recurrent UTI. Sterile urine culture should be performed when pyelonephritis is suspected.

Treatment

Treatment includes hospital admission, adequate hydration, urine culture and Gram stain, appropriate antibiotic therapy, correction of electrolyte imbalances, and systemic analgesia (eg, opioids). Epidural analgesia may be considered for patients with severe pain. Most stones pass spontaneously. The patient should strain her urine so that a stone can be analyzed. Surgical intervention, such as ureteral stenting, transurethral cystoscopic stone extraction, nephrostomy drainage, or open surgery, can be performed by a urologist if indicated for unremitting pain, infection unresponsive to antibiotic therapy, or obstructive uropathy. Lithotripsy is contraindicated during pregnancy.

ACUTE RENAL FAILURE

Acute renal failure is defined as urine output < 400 mL in 24 hours. It occurs infrequently in pregnancy but carries a high mortality rate; therefore it must be prevented where possible and treated aggressively. Most cases result from acute hypovolemia associated with obstetric hemorrhage (placenta previa, placental abruption, or postpartum hemorrhage) or sepsis. Clinically, acute renal failure is a condition in which the kidneys are temporarily unable to perform their excretory and regulatory functions. Blood urea nitrogen and serum creatinine concentrations are increased. Without prompt intervention, the condition may result in abortion, low birthweight, premature labor, and stillbirth. Dialysis may be required. Although hypotension preterm contractions may occur during dialysis, numerous successful pregnancy outcomes have been reported after dialysis during pregnancy. In these cases renal failure most often is the result of intrinsic renal disease.

Based on the cause, acute renal failure can be classified as prerenal, renal, or postrenal. In the prerenal type, acute renal failure occurs due to renal hypoperfusion secondary to maternal hypovolemia (eg, hemorrhage, dehydration, abruptio placentae, septicemia), circulating nephrotoxins (eg, aminoglycosides), mismatched blood transfusion, preeclampsia–eclampsia, disseminated intravascular coagulation (DIC), and hypoxemia (eg, chronic lung disease and heart failure). In the renal type, a variety of intrinsic renal diseases such as acute glomerulonephritis, acute pyelonephritis, and amyloidosis are responsible for acute renal failure. The postrenal type is caused by urinary obstruction from ureteric stone, retroperitoneal tumor, and other diseases. Bilateral ureteral obstruction due to polyhydramnios is rare.

The state of renal hypoperfusion is reversible within 24–36 hours with volume restoration and treatment of the precipitating factors. Acute tubular necrosis may develop following reduction of the outer cortical blood flow in the absence of such treatment. The most serious condition arising secondary to acute renal failure is **acute cortical necrosis** in damaged glomerular capillaries and small kidney vessels. Acute cortical necrosis is rare but carries a poor prognosis; partial recovery can be anticipated in patients with patchy lesions.

Clinical Findings

The clinical course has been divided into an oliguric phase, a diuretic phase, and a recovery phase. In the oliguric phase, urine output drops to < 30 mL/h, with accumulation of blood urea nitrogen and potassium. The patient becomes acidotic with the increase in hydrogen ion and loss of bicarbonate. In the diuretic phase, large volumes of dilute urine are passed, with loss of electrolytes due to absence of function of the renal tubules. As tubular function returns to normal in the recovery phase, the volume and composition of urine normalize. Clinical manifestations and complications include anorexia, nausea and vomiting, lethargy, cardiac arrhythmia (secondary to electrolyte disturbance), anemia, renal or extrarenal infection, thrombocytopenia, metabolic acidosis, and electrolyte imbalance (hyperkalemia, hyponatremia, hypermagnesemia, hyperphosphatemia, hypocalcemia).

Treatment

In obstetric practice, prevention of acute renal failure should be the aim, with appropriate volume replacement to maintain adequate urine output. Proper management of high-risk obstetric conditions (eg, preeclampsia–eclampsia, abruptio placentae, chorioamnionitis), ready blood availability, and avoidance of nephrotoxic antibiotics are important.

Specific treatments include the following.

A. EMERGENCY TREATMENT

Underlying causes of acute renal failure (eg, hemorrhagic shock) may require emergency treatment.

B. SURGICAL MEASURES

Surgical measures include determination of any obstructive uropathy or sepsis due to infected products of conception. Such problems should be treated appropriately.

C. ROUTINE MEASURES

Routine measures include achieving fluid and electrolyte balance. Fluid intake can be calculated from urinary output, loss of fluid from other sources (eg, diarrhea, vomiting), and insensible loss of approximately 500 mL/d (correcting for fever may be necessary). Intake and output must be recorded carefully. The patient should be weighed daily and should maintain a constant weight or lose weight slowly (250 g/d assuming a room temperature of 22–23 °C [71–73 °F]). Hyperkalemia is a significant problem that can be controlled by giving glucose and insulin. The diet should be high in calories and carbohydrates, and low in protein and electrolytes. Parenteral feeding may be given in cases of nausea and vomiting. Prophylactic antibiotics should not be used, but infections can be treated with antibiotics without renal toxicity. Indwelling bladder catheters are to be avoided when possible.

D. DIALYSIS

Dialysis is indicated if serum potassium levels rise to 7 mEq/L or more, serum sodium levels are 130 mEq/L or less, the serum bicarbonate is 13 mEq/L or less, blood urea nitrogen levels are more than 120 mg/dL or there are daily increments of 30 mg/dL in patients with sepsis, and dialyzable poisons or toxins are present. Different criteria are applied for renal failure in the antepartum period with a continuing pregnancy. In these cases, dialysis is instituted earlier in the process in consideration of fetal well-being. Although specific criteria have not been firmly established, one commonly used figure is a blood urea nitrogen level 60 mg/dL.

GLOMERULONEPHRITIS

Acute glomerulonephritis during pregnancy is rare, with an estimated incidence of 1 in 40,000 pregnancies. The condition is associated with increased perinatal loss. The clinical course is variable during pregnancy and may be easily mistaken for preeclampsia. In some patients, the condition resolves early in pregnancy, with return to normal renal function. Microscopic hematuria with red blood cell casts is a common finding in acute glomerulonephritis. Treatment is similar to that of the nonpregnant patient and consists of controlling blood pressure, preventing congestive heart failure, administering fluids and electrolytes, and close follow-up.

The outcome of pregnancy with chronic glomerulonephritis depends on the degree of functional impairment of the kidneys, blood pressure levels prior to conception, and the exact histology of the glomerulonephritis. For patients with active glomerulonephritis, the principal risk for pregnancy is superimposed preeclampsia. Conditions associated with poor fetal outcome include preexisting hypertension, severe proteinuria during the first trimester, primary focal and segmental hyalinosis, and sclerosis. Successful pregnancy should be anticipated, although renal function is expected to decrease. The incidence of fetal intrauterine growth retardation, premature labor, abruptio placentae, and intrauterine fetal demise is increased. Routine prenatal care must include periodic renal function tests, control of blood pressure, ultrasonic evaluation of fetal growth, and biophysical monitoring of fetal well-being. Hypertension at the time of conception correlates with worsening maternal renal function during pregnancy. Early delivery is indicated after evaluation of pulmonary maturity as appropriate.

SOLITARY KIDNEY

A solitary kidney may be the result of developmental aberration or disease requiring removal of 1 kidney. A single kidney may be abnormally developed or it may be placed low, perhaps even within the true pelvis. A second small, virtually functionless kidney may not be discovered by the usual diagnostic tests. Anatomic and functional hypertrophy of the kidney usually occurs and is augmented by pregnancy. These patients should be evaluated preconceptually for the presence of infection. If renal function is normal, pregnancy is not contraindicated.

During pregnancy, infection in a solitary kidney must be treated aggressively. An increased rate of preeclampsia with a solitary kidney has been reported.

RENAL TRANSPLANTATION

Approximately 0.5% of transplanted women in the reproductive age range become pregnant. A number of large series document successful pregnancy outcomes after renal transplantation. Patients with adequate renal function prior to pregnancy will experience little if any deterioration in graft function during pregnancy. The likelihood of graft rejection during pregnancy remains the same as in nonpregnant graft recipients. For renal transplant patients considering pregnancy, a stable serum creatinine level < 1.4 mg/dL identifies a group more likely to experience an uncomplicated obstetric outcome (97% vs. 75% for patients with a higher serum creatinine level). The spontaneous abortion rate is not increased. In general, prenatal care visits should be made every 2 weeks up to 32 weeks and then weekly from 32 weeks until delivery. Laboratory examination, including complete blood count, electrolyte levels, creatinine clearance, timed protein excretion, and midstream urinalysis, should be obtained every 1–2 months. The risk of infection is considerably higher during pregnancy in renal transplant patients. Primary or reactivated herpesvirus or cytomegalovirus (CMV) infection may be seen. A higher rate of hepatitis B surface antigenemia is seen in dialysis patients as well.

Preterm delivery, both spontaneous and indicated, is common (45–60%). Intrauterine growth restriction and fetal abnormalities caused by immunosuppressive agents taken by the mother may occur. The route of delivery depends primarily on obstetric indications. A transplanted kidney in the false pelvis usually does not cause obstruction leading to dystocia. In patients with aseptic necrosis of the hip joints or other bony dystrophy secondary to long-standing disease, cesarean delivery may be required. Vaginal delivery should be the aim for patients with renal transplant.

■ SKIN DISORDERS

PHYSIOLOGIC CHANGES

Many physiologic changes that occur during pregnancy can be noted in the integumentary system and may be confused with disease processes. For example, the impressive vascular changes during pregnancy lead to *erythema* early in gestation, particularly in the midpalmar and thenar areas. Although this sign could be diagnostic of hyperthyroidism, cirrhosis of the liver, or systemic lupus erythematosus, other signs of disease are not present. Palmar erythema usually vanishes postpartum.

Venous congestion and vascular permeability during pregnancy can lead to varicosities and labial edema. Vascular proliferations such as *capillary hemangiomas* are most commonly seen around the gums, tongue, upper lip, and eyelids. Usually patients have a history of preexisting lesions, which in most cases do not recede completely after pregnancy.

Striae are normal findings during pregnancy, but they also may be observed with adrenocortical hyperactivity (eg, Cushing's syndrome, exogenous corticosteroid administration). Increased activity of the adrenal gland during pregnancy may increase their occurrence. Most physicians believe heredity is the most common predictor of the development of these pinkish or purplish lines on the abdomen, buttocks, and breasts. After pregnancy, striae usually become silvery-white and sunken, but they rarely disappear. Many remedies have been proposed (vitamin E oil, lubricants, lotions), but none are effective.

Hyperpigmentation is common in pregnancy and occurs most frequently in the localized areas of hyperpigmentation (eg, nipples, areolae, and axillas). Hyperpigmentation is related to increased levels of melanocyte-stimulating hormone, estrogen, and progesterone. Melasma gravidarum ("mask of pregnancy") has a similar cause but usually develops on the forehead and across the cheeks and nose. It tends to recur and worsen with successive pregnancies and oral contraceptive use. There is no effective treatment during pregnancy, although topical application of hydroquinone 2% after delivery may assist in lightening areas of hyperpigmentation. Pigmentation of preexisting nevi or freckles may increase during pregnancy but usually regresses afterward.

Changes in the distribution and amount of *hair* are common during pregnancy. Increased hair growth in facial areas and around the breasts is common, particularly during the second and third trimesters. Importantly, there are no signs of virilization, and hirsutism regresses slightly or remains unchanged postpartum. Postpartum loss of hair is fairly common. During pregnancy, the number of hair follicles in the resting phase (telogen) is decreased by about half and then nearly doubles in the first few weeks postpartum. This increased hair loss usually stops in 2–6 months as the hair follicles enter the growing phase (anagen). Thus, no therapy other than reassurance is required.

POLYMORPHIC ERUPTION OF PREGNANCY (PRURITIC URTICARIAL PAPULES AND PLAQUES OF PREGNANCY)

Polymorphic eruption of pregnancy may be the most common of all the pruritic skin conditions that occur during pregnancy. The lesions usually appear during the third trimester and disappear completely within 2 weeks after delivery.

Clinical Findings

The pruritic papules are generally red, unexcoriated, and found principally on the abdomen. In most lesions a marked halo surrounds the small papules and plaques. Focal lesions are uncommon and rarely appear on the face or distal extremities. The lesions may be indistinguishable from those of herpes gestationis.

Diagnosis

Immunofluorescence reveals no immunoglobulin (Ig) or complement.

Treatment

Symptomatic treatment with antihistamines, topical steroids, and antipruritic medications usually is helpful. Occasionally, oral corticosteroid therapy is necessary.

Complications & Prognosis

This disorder appears to have no ill effect on the mother or the fetus and is self-limiting. It does not tend to recur.

HERPES GESTATIONIS (PEMPHIGOID GESTATIONIS)

Herpes gestationis has an incidence of 1 in 7000 gestations and usually appears in the second and third trimesters. Despite its name, the herpes virus is not the causative agent, and the etiology is unknown. Elevated hormone levels during pregnancy are suspected to be causative because progestins can induce exacerbations.

Clinical Findings

Systemic signs of herpes gestationis may be severe and include malaise, fever, and chills. The lesion appears as erythematous plaques with vesicles that soon form bullae in the periphery of the lesion. The typical blistering eruption has a herpetiform appearance, but the vesicles are not clustered and are more peripheral than herpes. Lesions usually begin on the trunk and spread to the entire body, including the distal extremities. Lesions on mucous membranes are uncommon.

Diagnosis

Most patients with herpes gestationis have circulating IgG that will fix C3 complement. Immunofluorescence testing of bullous lesions aids in establishing the diagnosis. Pemphigus vulgaris can be differentiated by histologic examination. The pustules, fever, and hypocalcemia of impetigo herpetiformis are not present in herpes gestationis. Dermatitis herpetiformis is excluded because, although it is pruritic, the clusters of vesicles do not form bullae, and no plaques are present. In herpes gestationis a crust forms, and a hyperpigmented area but little or no scarring occurs after the lesion heals.

Treatment

Oral corticosteroids are the treatment of choice.

Complications & Prognosis

Herpes gestationis is characterized by exacerbations and remissions during pregnancy. Although significant exacerbations can occur postpartum, the condition usually abates by the sixth week postpartum. Recurrence is frequent in subsequent pregnancies, and the disorder may appear earlier in pregnancy than the other disorders discussed. Its effect on maternal and fetal morbidity is not clear because the condition is so rare, but an increase in stillbirths, premature births, and small-for-gestational-age infants has been reported. Five percent of newborns have transient blisters.

IMPETIGO HERPETIFORMIS

Impetigo herpetiformis (also called *pustular psoriasis, von Zumbusch's type*) is a pustular eruption on an erythematous base with total body distribution. It is rare and probably represents an acute form of psoriasis that occurs during pregnancy. Pregnancy may precipitate this acute manifestation, but the disease is not restricted to gestation as it has been documented in nonpregnant women and in males. Most patients with this disease also have chronic psoriasis or a family history of psoriasis.

Clinical Findings

Generalized erythematous patches covered with sterile pustules allow a presumptive diagnosis. Fever, nausea, diarrhea, and malaise often accompany this symptom complex.

Diagnosis

Spongiform pustules noted in the epidermis on biopsy distinguish this disorder from pustular dermatosis or infection. The pustules are usually sterile, but they may become secondarily infected. In addition, pruritus is not a prominent symptom. The disorder is often associated with hypocalcemia and ensuing tetany, seizures, and delirium.

Treatment

Treatment is usually limited to supportive measures, occasional corticosteroids, and appropriate antibiotics

for superimposed infection. Methotrexate, vitamin A derivatives, and tetracycline should not be used during pregnancy.

Complications & Prognosis

Data on the fetal effects of this disorder are inadequate. Increased maternal and perinatal mortality have been reported, but these cases may have been related to secondary infection and sepsis.

■ GASTROINTESTINAL DISORDERS

PEPTIC ULCER DISEASE

Pregnancy usually ameliorates extension of ulceration, and an initial attack rarely occurs during pregnancy. The salutary effect of pregnancy may be related to progesterone's ability to inhibit motility, because acid secretion remains unchanged. The incidence of peptic ulcer disease in pregnancy is rare (1 in 4000 deliveries); it seems to be more common with associated preeclampsia. If activation of previously dormant ulcer disease does occur, it usually is in the puerperium.

Clinical Findings

The classic signs of gastric or duodenal ulcer are related to a burning epigastric pain that is relieved by meals or antacids. Peptic ulcer disease must be differentiated from reflex esophagitis or simple heartburn, which commonly occurs during pregnancy. Patients with a gastric or duodenal ulcer most often report discomfort rather than pain and describe the feeling as "acid" or burning or indigestion.

Diagnosis

The symptoms of peptic ulcer disease are relieved by food but return approximately 1–2 hours later, paralleling gastric acidity. Likewise, antacids may relieve the pain and help confirm the diagnosis. Most commonly, the diagnosis is confirmed by endoscopic visualization of the ulcer crater in the stomach or duodenum. Although gastric carcinoma is rare, many physicians recommend biopsy during the endoscopic procedure. Upper gastrointestinal x-ray films with barium studies usually are avoided because of radiation exposure and because endoscopy is a more direct diagnostic method.

Helicobacter pylori is an organism associated with gastritis, ulcers, and possibly gastric adenocarcinoma and lymphoma. Diagnosis is based on biopsy histology, culture, or urease test. Noninvasive testing includes the C-urea breath test, stool antigen, or serology.

Treatment

Documented peptic ulcer disorders are treated symptomatically during pregnancy by avoiding symptom-provoking foods and using antacids and sucralfate. Supportive advice can be given regarding cessation of smoking, bed rest, and avoidance of stress. For persistent symptoms, an H_2 antagonist such as cimetidine or ranitidine can be given. As a last resort, a proton pump inhibitor such as lansoprazole can be added to the drug regimen. Eradication of *H pylori* is 90% successful with an antibiotic such as tetracycline or clarithromycin, a bismuth compound, and a proton pump inhibitor.

Complications & Prognosis

In general, the fetus is not adversely affected by peptic ulcer disease unless maternal compromise, such as perforated ulcer with bleeding, occurs. Particular vigilance in the postpartum period is necessary because ulcers become active again during this time and can become penetrating.

INFLAMMATORY BOWEL DISEASE

Inflammatory bowel disease encompasses regional enteritis (Crohn's disease), ulcerative colitis, and granulomatous colitis. In general, inflammatory bowel disease has no effect on fertility unless colonic disease has resulted in pelvic abscesses. Overall, studies show a reduced relapse rate during pregnancy compared to preconception. Relapse shows a predilection for the first trimester and postpartum. Subsequent pregnancies will not necessarily have the same course.

Clinical Findings

In these conditions, cramping, lower abdominal pain, and diarrhea are the main complaints. Weight loss and anorexia, even during pregnancy, may occur. Electrolyte imbalance with severe diarrhea also may occur.

Diagnosis

Infectious disorders that would cause diarrhea and abdominal pain must be ruled out. A personal or family history of inflammatory bowel disease is helpful in confirming the diagnosis. If the lower intestine is involved, proctoscopy or colonoscopy may be helpful. However, in some cases a small bowel series and barium enema are needed to make the diagnosis. Malignancy and infectious disease, such as tuberculosis of the small intestine, also must be considered because they have appearances similar to inflammatory bowel disease on x-ray film. Finally,

a response to trials of medication and a change in diet may be helpful in confirming the diagnosis.

Treatment

Treatment of inflammatory bowel disease usually involves dietary management and use of medications. Sulfasalazine inhibits prostaglandin synthesis, which is thought to be important in bowel disease. Although sulfasalazine and corticosteroids cross the placenta, their use during pregnancy may be preferable to acute exacerbations of disease. If sulfasalazine is used, maternal folic acid should be given daily because it inhibits brush border enzymes. Although sulfasalazine is a sulfa drug, no increased risk of neonatal jaundice has been noted. Azathioprine has not been associated with congenital malformations. There is an associated increase in fetal growth restriction and prematurity. Mercaptopurine has shown no fetal toxicity after first-trimester exposure. Methotrexate should be avoided in pregnancy. Short-term use of antibiotics such as metronidazole is allowed. Other immunosuppressant drugs have not been shown to be helpful and should not be used during pregnancy.

Complications & Prognosis

Complications during pregnancy are similar to those in the nonpregnant state: abdominal pain, cramping, and rectal bleeding. The risk of abortion and stillbirth is dependent on disease activity. Pregnancy is not contraindicated with inflammatory bowel disease, but when possible the disorder should be controlled by surgery or medication prior to conception. Pregnancy does not exert an adverse effect on inflammatory bowel disease. In most patients, pregnancy and delivery proceed smoothly. Patients with ileostomies should be followed for complications, most importantly intestinal obstruction (8%). If a patient has undergone a bowel resection, total parenteral nutrition may be required during the pregnancy. Women with active perianal disease should be delivered via cesarean section.

CHOLECYSTITIS

Cholecystitis occurs rarely during pregnancy (0.3%) because the gallbladder and biliary duct smooth muscle are relaxed by progesterone. Acute inflammation during pregnancy is treated with intravenous fluids and limitations of oral intake. If acute cholecystitis does not resolve or if pancreatitis develops, cholecystectomy should be considered. If this operation can be performed in the second trimester, the fetal loss rate probably is not increased. The laparoscopic approach in pregnancy is widely accepted. After 20 weeks' gestation, it should be performed with special care to avoid injury to the uterus. In the third trimester, surgical intervention can cause preterm delivery. Later in gestation, prolonged IV hyperalimentation can be an option to delay surgery until postpartum.

INTRAHEPATIC CHOLESTASIS OF PREGNANCY

Intrahepatic cholestasis of pregnancy is a condition characterized by accumulation of bile acids in the liver with subsequent accumulation in the plasma, causing pruritus and jaundice. It is similar to the cholestasis that occasionally occurs during combined oral contraceptive therapy. Estrogens are considered to play a role in its etiology, probably by slowing the enzymes involved in bile transport. Some cases of intrahepatic cholestasis of pregnancy result from specific mutations in bile transport genes, although common mutations or polymorphisms have not been identified in most cases. The cardinal clinical finding is total body itching involving the palms and soles. The main liver conditions that must be considered in the differential diagnosis are hepatitis and biliary tract disease, in addition to acute fatty liver of pregnancy (AFLP) and the *h*emolysis, *e*levated *l*iver enzymes, *l*ow *p*latelet count (HELLP) syndrome. Laboratory values show increased levels of alkaline phosphatase, bilirubin, and serum bile acids (chenodeoxycholic acid, deoxycholic acid, cholic acid). Aspartate transaminase (AST) and alanine transaminase (ALT) levels may be mildly elevated. Patients may be symptomatic weeks before the diagnosis laboratory abnormalities are noted.

Symptomatic treatment of pruritus with antihistamines such as diphenhydramine is useful. Ursodeoxycholic acid (10–15 mg/kg/d in 2 divided doses) has been shown to inhibit absorption of toxic bile acids and increase their biliary excretion. In doing so, the medication normalizes bile acids, improves liver function tests, and alleviates pruritus. Oral steroids also have been used to relieve symptoms. Cholestyramine is no longer routinely used because of poor compliance. Symptoms resolve postpartum.

Although controversial, it now is accepted that intrahepatic cholestasis of pregnancy is associated with fetal death, spontaneous preterm birth, and postpartum hemorrhage. The etiology is unclear, but some refer to the fetal toxicity of bile acids as a causative factor. Antenatal testing with a modified biophysical profile twice per week starting at the time of diagnosis is suggested. Because the modified biophysical profile reportedly is less effective in predicting fetal compromise in intrahepatic cholestasis of pregnancy, different strategies have been proposed: amniocentesis at 35–36 weeks, delivery at 37–38 weeks, and delivery at 37–38 weeks only if bile acid concentration is > 40 nmol/L. There is no agreement on whether to induce the pregnancy at 37–38 weeks or to await spontaneous labor.

ACUTE FATTY LIVER OF PREGNANCY

Acute fatty liver of pregnancy is a rare complication (1 in 5000 to 1 in 13,000) that occurs in the third trimester. Early recognition and termination of the pregnancy (delivery) and extensive supportive therapy have reduced the mortality rate to approximately 5–10%. Recurrence in subsequent pregnancies is rare and appears limited to women with mutations in the fatty acid transport and metabolism pathway. A number of studies have shown an association between AFLP and fetal recessive inheritance of long-chain 3-hydroxyacyl-CoA dehydrogenase (LCHAD) deficiency. In all but one reported case, the mother has been a carrier of LCHAD deficiency. AFLP shares clinical and histologic features of the broad family of disorders of fatty acid transport and mitochondrial oxidation, and several disorders of fatty acid metabolism are associated with AFLP. Nevertheless, the specific molecular basis of most cases of AFLP remains unknown.

Symptoms and signs include nausea and vomiting, malaise, epigastric pain, and jaundice. AFLP should be suspected in any patient who presents with new-onset nausea and malaise in the third trimester until the results of liver and chemistry panels are available. Laboratory values show elevated AST and ALT levels (up to 7 times normal) and may show markedly elevated bilirubin level and prolonged prothrombin time. Glucose is low in 30% of cases; levels of platelets and fibrinogen are notably decreased. Almost all women have elevated liver enzyme levels at the time of diagnosis; an elevated serum creatinine level (0.9 mg/dL in pregnancy) is universally present. Liver biopsy, which is rarely needed for diagnosis, reveals microvesicular hepatic steatosis and mitochondrial disruption on electron microscopy. Complications such as acute renal failure, DIC, encephalopathy, and sepsis can be severe. The principles of management are supportive care and prompt delivery. Glucose, blood products, broad-spectrum antibiotic coverage, and pulmonary support are critical. Importantly, the total bilirubin level may continue to rise for up to 10 days after delivery. This process is part of the natural history of recovering AFLP and should not be taken as an indication for liver transplant, which is not required in AFLP.

HELLP SYNDROME

HELLP syndrome is a disorder that in some respects mimics AFLP. This liver derangement is a variant of severe preeclampsia or eclampsia. The disorder occurs in the last trimester of pregnancy and is characterized by nausea and vomiting and right upper quadrant pain. Unlike AFLP, liver function is generally preserved as reflected by the normal prothrombin time. Stillbirth occurs frequently (10–15%) if delivery is not prompt; neonatal loss is high (20–

25%), usually because of prematurity (see Chapter 19). Corticosteroids may hasten recovery in HELLP syndrome.

HELLP syndrome occasionally persists beyond 2–3 days postpartum, in which case it takes on the characteristics of other microangiopathic hemolytic disorders, such as thrombotic thrombocytopenic purpura or hemolytic-uremic syndrome. Plasmapheresis may be required with persistent HELLP syndrome.

VIRAL HEPATITIS

Viral hepatitis complicates 0.2% of all pregnancies in the United States. Hepatitis may be caused by numerous viruses, drugs, or toxic chemicals; the clinical manifestations of all forms are similar. The development of specific serologic markers has improved the accuracy of the diagnosis. The most common viral agents causing hepatitis in pregnancy are hepatitis A virus, hepatitis B virus, hepatitis C (formerly termed non-A, non-B hepatitis virus), hepatitis E, hepatitis G, and Epstein-Barr virus. Hepatitis D (Delta) has also received increasing attention as a cause of hepatitis.

1. Hepatitis A

Hepatitis A may occur sporadically or in epidemics. A generalized viremia occurs with the infection that is predominantly hepatic. The primary mode of transmission is the fecal/oral route. Excretion of the virus in stool normally begins approximately 2 weeks prior to the onset of clinical symptoms and is complete within 3 weeks following onset of clinical symptoms. No known carrier state exists for the virus. Both blood and stool are infectious during the 2- to 6-week incubation period. Perinatal transmission does not occur.

2. Hepatitis B

Hepatitis B usually is transmitted by inoculation of infected blood or blood products, or sexual intercourse. The virus is contained in most body secretions. Infection by parenteral and sexual contact has been well documented. Groups at risk for hepatitis B infection are injection drug users; male homosexuals (or men who have sex with men [MSM]); medical, hemodialysis, blood bank, and medical laboratory personnel; spouses of hepatitis carriers; prostitutes and others with multiple sexual partners; and Southeast Asian emigrants. Approximately 5–10% of people infected with hepatitis B virus become chronic carriers of the virus. The incubation period of hepatitis B is 6 weeks to 6 months. The clinical features of hepatitis A and B are similar, although hepatitis B is more insidious. Fulminant hepatitis is very rare with hepatitis A but occurs in approximately 1% of patients infected with hepatitis B.

The hepatitis B surface antigen (HBsAg) of the largest of several pleomorphic viral structures is the marker usually measured in blood. The presence of HBsAg is the first manifestation of viral infection; it usually appears before clinical evidence of the disease and lasts throughout the infection. Persistence of HBsAg after the acute phase of hepatitis usually is associated with clinical and laboratory evidence of chronic hepatitis. The hepatitis B core antibody (HBcAb) is produced against the core of the largest viral particle. HBcAb occurs with acute hepatitis B infection at the onset of clinical illness. Hepatitis B e antigen (HBeAg) is a soluble, nonparticulate antigen that is found only when HBsAg is present. Pregnant women who are HBeAg-positive in the third trimester frequently transmit this infection to the offspring (80–90%) in the absence of immunoprophylaxis, whereas those who are negative rarely infect the their offspring.

3. Hepatitis C

Up to 85% of infected individuals become chronic carriers. The incubation period usually is 7–8 weeks but may vary from 3–21 weeks. The course of infection is similar to that of hepatitis B. Hepatitis C antibody is present in approximately 90% of patients. However, the antibody may not be detectable for weeks after infection. Polymerase chain reaction (PCR) for hepatitis C RNA then becomes useful. Vertical transmission occurs in 5–8% of infected pregnancies and is increased with concomitant HIV infection. Risk of vertical transmission is increased with higher hepatitis C viral loads. Although most studies have not demonstrated a decreased risk of vertical transmission with cesarean delivery, some studies suggest cesarean delivery may be protective.

4. Hepatitis D

Hepatitis D virus is an RNA virus that is smaller than all other known RNA viruses. The agent can cause infection only when HBsAg positivity exists. Hepatitis D is isolated in up to 50% of cases of fulminant hepatitis B infection. Hepatitis D antigen (HDAg) and hepatitis D antibody (HDAb) are serologic markers for the disease.

5. Hepatitis E

Hepatitis E is transmitted via the oral/fecal route. Hepatitis E is rare in the United states but is endemic in several developing countries. The disease is self-limited and does not result in a chronic carrier state. Pregnant patients who are acutely infected have a 15% risk of fulminant liver failure with a 5% mortality rate; the rate is higher in resource-poor settings.

6. Hepatitis G

Hepatitis G is more likely to be found in people infected with hepatitis B or C or with a history of injection drug use. There is no chronic carrier state. Vertical transmission has been noted.

Clinical Findings

The clinical picture of hepatitis is highly variable. Most patients have asymptomatic infection, but a few may present with fulminating disease and die within a few days. Frequent symptoms include general malaise, myalgia, fatigue, anorexia, nausea and vomiting, right upper quadrant pain, and low-grade fever. Mild hepatomegaly and/or splenomegaly occur in 5–10% of affected patients. The white blood cell count is depressed, and mild proteinuria and bilirubinuria occur early in the course of the disease. The levels of AST, ALT, bilirubin, and alkaline phosphatase usually are elevated. Prothrombin and partial thromboplastin times may be prolonged with severe liver involvement.

Diagnosis

The diagnosis is made using serologic markers—anti-HA IgM, HBsAg, HC PCR, anti-HBc IgM, HD PCR, anti-HE IgM, and anti-HG IgM. Liver biopsy, which should be avoided during pregnancy, shows extensive hepatocellular injury and inflammatory infiltrate. The differential diagnosis of viral hepatitis should include viruses A, B, C, and D; Epstein-Barr virus; CMV infection; cholestasis; preeclampsia; AFLP; *t*oxoplasmosis, *o*ther agents, *r*ubella, *c*ytomegalovirus, and *h*erpes simplex (TORCH) infections; secondary syphilis; autoimmune; and toxic or drug-induced hepatitis. Additionally, intrahepatic or extrahepatic bile duct obstruction should be included.

Treatment

Bed rest should be instituted during the acute phase of illness. If nausea, vomiting, or anorexia is prominent, intravenous hydration and general supportive measures are instituted. All hepatotoxic agents should be avoided. Antepartum fetal assessment should be instituted in the third trimester because of the increased risks for premature delivery and stillbirth. Immunoglobulin prophylaxis should be given to pregnant women within 2 weeks of exposure to hepatitis A. Two hepatitis A vaccines using inactivated virus are available and can be used during pregnancy. Hepatitis B Ig can be given to patients parenterally or sexually exposed to blood or secretions from hepatitis B–infected individuals. Hepatitis B vaccine also should be administered to an HBsAg-negative patient. Hepatitis B Ig 0.5 mL intramuscularly and hepatitis B vaccine with a repeat dose at 1 and 6 months should be administered to neonates born of HBsAg-positive mothers, to decrease the risk of vertical transmission. Passive and active immunization of the newborn is 85–95% effective in preventing perinatal transmission of hepatitis B virus. Breastfeeding is not contraindicated with hepatitis B as long as the infant has been immunized.

Nausea or Vomiting Interfering with Daily Routine

Vitamin B$_6$ 10–30 mg TID–QID PO

Continued symptoms after 48 hours
Add doxylamine 12.5 mg TID–QID PO

Continued symptoms after 48 hours
Substitute doxylamine with other antihistamine:

Promethazine 12.5 –25 mg q4h PO or PR

Dimenhydrinate 50–100 mg q4–6h PO or PR

Consider alternative therapies at any point in this sequence:
Acupuncture or acustimulation,
ginger tablets 250 mg QID

Persistent Symptoms, with or without Dehydration

Prochlorperazine 25 mg q12h PR
OR
Metoclopramide 5–10 mg q8h PO or IV
OR
Trimethobenzamide 200 mg q6–8h PR

Dehydration or Weight Loss

Thiamine 100 mg IV daily for 3 days
Continue thiamine in MVI daily

Ondansetron 8 mg q8–12h IV or PO
OR
Methylprednisolone up to 16 mg TID for 3 days
Taper over 2 weeks to lowest effective dose
Total duration of therapy 6 weeks

Unable to Maintain Weight

Institute total enteral or parenteral nutrition

Figure 23–1. Nausea and vomiting of pregnancy/hyperemesis gravidarum treatment sequence at the University of Southern California. PO = by mouth; PR = by rectum.

Complications & Prognosis

The acute illness usually resolves rapidly in 2–3 weeks, with complete recovery usually occurring within 8 weeks. Chronic persistent or chronic active hepatitis develops in 10% of hepatitis B and C cases. Additionally, 1–3% of patients develop acute fulminant hepatitis.

The maternal course of viral hepatitis is generally unaltered by pregnancy, except for hepatitis E in which the pregnant woman may fare worse; prematurity may be increased. In general, infertility results in patients with severe liver disease. Chronic active hepatitis does not mandate therapeutic abortion, but fetal loss is increased. All pregnant women should routinely be tested for HBsAg during an early prenatal visit in each pregnancy. Women with cirrhosis of the liver from other causes have an outcome related to the extent of maternal disease. Perinatal loss rates usually are high with a poor maternal prognosis, particularly with poor liver function or esophageal varices. Pregnancy in women with liver transplants has been reported and, in general, has an uncomplicated prenatal and delivery course. Treatment with immunosuppressants and corticosteroids is generally well tolerated in pregnancy. Interferon and ribavirin therapy improves the prognosis for chronic active hepatitis (C in particular), but both drugs are relatively contraindicated during pregnancy.

HYPEREMESIS GRAVIDARUM

Hyperemesis gravidarum is persistent, otherwise unexplained vomiting in early pregnancy associated with ketonuria weight loss. It affects 1–2% of pregnant women and is the second most common cause of antenatal hospitalization in the United States. Elevated levels of transaminases, bilirubin, amylase, lipase, and various electrolytes are seen in 15–40% of patients. Biochemical evidence of hyperthyroidism due to the effect of human chorionic gonadotropin on the thyroid-stimulating hormone receptor is seen in 60–70% of patients. The differential diagnosis includes a wide variety of conditions capable of causing persistent nausea and vomiting and must be considered carefully in each patient.

The etiology is not understood. The spectrum of maternal susceptibility to an unknown emetogenic stimulus from the placenta accounts for the variability in the condition and the difficulty in identifying a single etiologic factor. The recurrence rate is approximately 20% in prospective studies but this value probably is an underestimation because the sickest women often limit family size.

Treatment of hyperemesis gravidarum begins with supportive measures including hydration and vitamin supplementation, in particular vitamin B_1, which is needed to prevent Wernicke's encephalopathy. Nonpharmacologic measures, such as vitamin B_6, ginger, and acupressure, appear to be effective with lesser degrees of, vomiting but their role in hyperemesis gravidarum is uncertain. Antihistamines as a class have some efficacy and the best record for fetal safety. Other conventional antiemetics can be used in an algorithm that balances safety and efficacy (Fig 23–1).

Fetal status is generally not adversely affected by vomiting until persistent maternal weight loss occurs. In this setting, the rate of intrauterine growth retardation (IUGR) increases and fetal death appears to increase. Long-term effects of hyperemesis gravidarum on offspring are unknown. If weight loss persists despite therapy, nutritional supplementation by enteral tube feeding or parenteral feeding is necessary.

REFERENCES

Renal Disorders

Armenti VT et al: Report from the National Transplantation Pregnancy Registry (NTPR): Outcomes of pregnancy after transplantation. In: Cecka JM, Terasaki PI (editors): *Clinical Transplants.* UCLA Immunogenetics Center, 2002, p. 97.

Bar J et al: Prediction of pregnancy outcome in subgroups of women with renal disease. Clin Nephrol 2000;53:437.

Cohen RA, Brown RS: Microscopic hematuria. N Engl J Med 2003; 348:2330.

Cunningham FG, Lucas MJ: Urinary tract infections complicating pregnancy. Baillieres Clin Obstet Gynaecol 1994;8:353.

Hill JB et al: Acute pyelonephritis in pregnancy. Obstet Gynecol 2005; 105:18.

Lindheimer MD, Davison JM, Katz AL: The kidney and hypertension in pregnancy: twenty exciting years. Semin Nephrol 2001;21:173.

Schrier RW et al: Acute renal failure: Definitions, diagnosis, pathogenesis, and therapy. J Clin Invest 2004;114:5.

Selcuk NY et al: Outcome of pregnancies with HELLP syndrome complicated by acute renal failure (1989–1999). Ren Fail 2000;22:319.

Teichman JM: Acute renal colic from ureteral calculus. N Engl J Med 2004;350:684.

Gastrointestinal Disorders

Alsulyman OM et al: Intrahepatic cholestasis of pregnancy: Perinatal outcome associated with expectant management. Am J Obstet Gynecol 1996;175:957.

Castro MA et al: Reversible peripartum liver failure: a new perspective on the diagnosis, treatment, and cause of acute fatty liver of pregnancy, based on 28 consecutive cases. Am J Obstet Gynecol 1999;181:389.

Connell W, Miller A: Treating inflammatory bowel disease during pregnancy: Risks and safety of drug therapy. Drug Saf 1999;21:311.

European Paediatric Hepatitis C Virus Network: A significant sex—but nor elective cesarean section—effect on mother-to-child transmission of hepatitis C virus infection. J Infect Dis 2005;192:1872.

Goodwin TM: Hyperemesis gravidarum. Prog Obstet Gynecol 2006; In press.

Ibdah JA: Role of genetic screening in identifying susceptibility to acute fatty liver of pregnancy. Nat Clin Pract Gastroenterol Hepatol 2005;21:494.

Sloan D et al: Prevention of perinatal transmission of hep B to babies at high risk: An evaluation. Vaccine 2005;23:5500.

Strader D et al: Diagnosis, management, and treatment of hepatitis C. Hepatology 2004;39:1147.

Williamson C et al: Clinical outcome in a series of cases of obstetric cholestasis identified via a patient support group. BJOG 2004; 111:676.

Skin Disorders

Aronson IK et al: Pruritic urticarial papules and plaques of pregnancy: Clinical and immunopathologic observations in 57 patients. J Am Acad Dermatol 1998;39:933.

Garcia-Gonzalez E et al: Immunology of the cutaneous disorders of pregnancy. Int J Dermatol 1999;38:721.

Vaughan Jones SA, Black MM: Pregnancy dermatoses. J Am Acad Dermatol 1999;40:233.

Thyroid and Other Endocrine Disorders during Pregnancy

24

Martin N. Montoro, MD

■ THYROID DISORDERS

Thyroid diseases are among the most common endocrine disorders encountered during pregnancy. They are challenging because of the potential complications of the disease itself and of the side effects of the medications used to treat mother and fetus.

■ THYROID FUNCTION DURING NORMAL PREGNANCY

Both total thyroxine (T_4) and triiodothyronine (T_3) levels increase because the level of their carrier, thyroxine-binding globulin (TBG), becomes elevated. Estrogen causes increased TBG synthesis and decreased TBG clearance. The concentrations of free thyroxine (FT_4) and free triiodothyronine (FT_3) fluctuate but are within the normal range. The thyrotropin-stimulating hormone (TSH) level decreases and may even be low in some patients: 13% in the first trimester, 4.5% in the second trimester, and 1.2% in the third trimester. The TSH level is lowest and FT_4 level highest when the human chorionic gonadotropin (hCG) level peaks. Serum thyroglobulin level increases, more toward the end of pregnancy, because of increased thyroid mass. The larger thyroid size is rarely detectable by physical examination, but it has been documented by serial ultrasound measurements. The average increase is 18% but may be much greater in areas of iodine deficiency. Overall, the demand for T_4 increases by an estimated 1–3% above daily nonpregnant needs. The increased demand starts very early, reaching a plateau at 16–20 weeks.

The fetal hypothalamic-pituitary-thyroid axis becomes functional toward the end of the first trimester. Until then, the fetus is dependent on local monodeiodi-nation of transferred maternal T_4 to T_3. The small but effective transfer of T_4 from mother to fetus seems to be important for fetal growth, particularly early brain development. TSH does not cross the placenta. Thyrotropin-releasing hormone (TRH) crosses the placenta, but it does not have a known effect on fetal thyroid function. Iodine also crosses the placenta, and the fetal thyroid starts concentrating it by weeks 10–12. Excess iodine causes fetal goiter and hypothyroidism. At birth, dramatic changes occur; in the full-term neonate, the thyroid hormone profile reaches normal values after a few hours. Normal thyroid hormones levels in the newborn are crucial for subsequent brain maturation and intellectual development.

HYPERTHYROIDISM

The reported incidence of hyperthyroidism is 0.2–0.9%. Hyperthyroidism rarely starts during pregnancy; in the majority of patients it antedates pregnancy. In most cases (> 85%) the etiology is Graves' disease. Other causes include toxic nodular goiters, iatrogenic (excess exogenous thyroid), iodine induced, subacute thyroiditis, hyperemesis gravidarum, and hydatidiform mole or choriocarcinoma.

Potential complications of hyperthyroidism in the mother include spontaneous abortion, pregnancy-induced hypertension, preterm delivery, anemia, higher susceptibility to infections, placental abruption, and, in severe, untreated cases, cardiac arrhythmias, congestive heart failure, and thyroid storm. In the fetus, possible complications include fetal and neonatal hyperthyroidism, intrauterine growth restriction (IUGR), stillbirth, prematurity, and morbidity related to antithyroid medications. Most maternal and neonatal complications are seen in cases of uncontrolled or untreated hyperthyroidism.

Graves' disease is caused by thyroid-stimulating antibody (TSAb) belonging to the immunoglobulin (Ig)G class, which binds with high affinity to the TSH receptor. TSAb may cross the placenta, bind to fetal TSH receptors, and cause fetal or neonatal hyperthyroidism.

However, the placental acts as a partial barrier, so usually only those with high titers are likely to be affected.

The diagnosis may not be easy, particularly in mild cases, because normal pregnant women may experience symptoms resembling thyrotoxicosis, such as heat intolerance, warm and moist skin, tachycardia, and a systolic flow murmur on cardiac auscultation. More reliable findings include a goiter, a resting pulse > 100 bpm, onycholysis, eye involvement, and weight loss or failure to gain despite a good appetite. The thyroid enlargement usually is diffuse with a firm consistency. A bruit may be audible over the thyroid but disappears after effective treatment. The eyes (Grave's ophthalmopathy) may be affected in up to half of patients, but pretibial myxedema is found in only 6–10% of cases. Hand tremor, proximal muscle weakness, hyperkinesis, and a hyperdynamic cardiovascular system may be present.

Laboratory tests will confirm elevated T_4, FT_4, T_3, and FT_3 levels and a suppressed or undetectable TSH level. TSAb titers will be elevated in a significant number of patients.

Treatment during pregnancy almost always consists of antithyroid medications. Surgery is performed in exceptional situations, such as allergic reactions to all drugs available or lack of response to very large doses ("drug resistance"), which in most cases has been the result of noncompliance. The goals of treatment are to rapidly achieve and maintain euthyroidism with the minimum but effective amount of medication, provide symptomatic relief, and keep FT_4 levels in the upper third of normal. The medications available are propylthiouracil (PTU) and methimazole. Some physicians prefer PTU, but reports of large number of patients indicate that the two drugs are equally effective and have similar side effects. PTU is shorter acting, meaning more pills are required more often; therefore, methimazole may be preferable when compliance is a problem. The initial methimazole dose is 20–40 mg/d and the initial PTU dose is 200–400 mg/d. The dose is gradually reduced as improvement occurs. Most women can be effectively treated on an outpatient basis; however, hospitalization may be considered in severe, uncontrolled cases in the third trimester because of increased risk for complications. Women who have remained euthyroid while taking small amounts of PTU (≤ 100 mg/d) or methimazole (≤ 10 mg/d) for 4 weeks or longer can stop taking the medication altogether by 32–34 weeks' gestation under close surveillance. The purpose is to minimize the risk of fetal/neonatal hypothyroidism, which is otherwise uncommon with PTU doses ≤ 200 mg/d or methimazole ≤ 20 mg/d. The therapy is resumed if symptoms recur. Women with large goiters, long-standing hyperthyroidism, or significant eye involvement should remain on treatment throughout pregnancy. Other potential side effects of antithyroid medications are pruritus, skin rash, urticaria, fever, arthralgias, cholestatic jaundice, lupuslike syndrome, and migratory polyarthritis. Leukopenia may be a medication effect but is also seen in untreated Graves' disease; therefore, a white blood cell (WBC) count should be obtained before treatment is started. Agranulocytosis is the most severe complication, but fortunately it is uncommon.

β Blockers (propanolol 20–40 mg every 6–8 hours) can be used for symptomatic relief in severe cases but only for short periods (few weeks) and before 34–36 weeks' gestation.

Tests of fetal well-being are recommended for poorly controlled cases and for patients with high TSAb titers, even if they are euthyroid. Serial ultrasounds are useful for dating and fetal growth evaluation.

Breastfeeding is allowed if the total daily dose of PTU is ≤ 150 mg or methimazole ≤ 10 mg. The medication should be given immediately after each feeding and the infant monitored periodically.

Fetal and neonatal thyrotoxicosis are rare because placental transfer of IgG is limited. Usually only those with high titers are at risk. Fetal tachycardia and IUGR are the most common signs. A fetal goiter has occasionally been detected by ultrasound. High levels of fetal thyroid hormone detected by cordocentesis have been confirmed in a few cases. Treatment consists of administering to the mother antithyroid medication, which effectively crosses the placenta. If untreated, the mortality rate may reach 50%. The clinical manifestations of neonatal hyperthyroidism may appear at the time of birth or may be delayed several weeks if the mother was taking antithyroid medication until delivery. The disease will subside after several weeks or months when the maternal TSAb titer disappears, but infants require treatment in the meantime because, if untreated, the mortality rate may reach 30%.

TRANSIENT HYPERTHYROIDISM OF HYPEREMESIS GRAVIDARUM

Biochemical hyperthyroidism is seen in most women (66%) with this condition. Women in early pregnancy with weight loss, tachycardia, vomiting, and laboratory evidence of hyperthyroidism may be difficult to differentiate from early, true thyrotoxicosis. Women with transient hyperthyroidism of hyperemesis gravidarum have no previous history of thyroid disease, no palpable goiter, and, except for tachycardia, no other symptoms or signs of hyperthyroidism. Test results for thyroid antibodies are negative. TSH level may be suppressed and T_4 and T_3 levels elevated, but the T_3 level is lower than in true hyperthyroidism. The degree of thyroid function abnormalities correlates with the severity of vomiting. The time to resolution is widely variable (1–10 weeks). Treatment is symptomatic, and antithyroid medication is not recommended. The most likely etiology is thyroid stimulation by hCG (or perhaps certain hCG subfractions).

HYPOTHYROIDISM

Hypothyroidism was considered rare because of menstrual disturbances and frequent anovulatory cycles in hypothyroid women but recently has been reported to be much more common. Overt hypothyroidism (elevated TSH, low T_4) has been reported in 1 in 1000 to 1 in 1600 deliveries and subclinical hypothyroidism (elevated TSH, normal T_4) in 0.19–2.5% of pregnancies.

The most common cause of hypothyroidism is autoimmune thyroid disease, with the goitrous form more frequent than the atrophic form with nonpalpable thyroid. Most other cases are secondary to previous treatment with radioactive iodine or thyroidectomy. Less common causes are transient hypothyroidism in silent (painless) and subacute thyroiditis, drug induced, high-dose external neck radiation, congenital hypothyroidism, inherited metabolic disorders, and thyroid hormone resistance syndromes. Secondary hypothyroidism may occur in pituitary or hypothalamic disease. Drugs that may cause hypothyroidism by interfering with thyroid hormone synthesis and/or its release include antithyroid drugs (PTU, methimazole), iodine, and lithium. Increased T_4 clearance is caused by carbamazepine, phenytoin, and rifampin. Amiodarone decreases T_4 to T_3 conversion and inhibition of T_3 action. Interference with intestinal absorption is seen with aluminum hydroxide, cholestyramine, ferrous sulfate, calcium, vitamins, soy, and sucralfate. Many pregnant women take ferrous sulfate, and it is important to ensure that thyroxine is taken at least 2 hours before (even 4 hours sometimes recommended) because insoluble ferric–thyroxine complexes may form, resulting in reduced thyroxine absorption.

The clinical diagnosis is difficult and frequently unsuspected except in advanced cases. Symptoms may include fatigue, sleepiness, lethargy, mental slowing, depression, cold intolerance (very unusual in normal pregnancy), decreased perspiration, hair loss, dry skin, deeper voice or frank hoarseness, weight gain despite poor appetite, constipation, arthralgias, muscle aching, stiffness, and paresthesias. Signs include general slowing of speech and movements, dry and pale or yellowish skin, sparse thin hair, hoarseness, bradycardia (also unusual in pregnancy), myxedema, hyporeflexia, prolonged relaxation of reflexes, carpal tunnel syndrome, and a diffuse or a nodular goiter.

The best laboratory test is the TSH level; current sensitive assays allow very early diagnosis and accurate treatment monitoring. Other useful tests include FT_4 and antibody titers. Anemia occurs in 30–40%. It usually results from decreased erythropoiesis, but it may result from vitamin B_{12}, folic acid, or iron deficiency. Levels of lipids and creatine phosphokinase ([CPK] of muscle origin) may be elevated.

Implications of Hypothyroidism during Pregnancy

Some studies have reported a twofold increased rate of spontaneous abortion in women with elevated levels of thyroid antibodies, even if they are euthyroid, but this finding is not universally confirmed. These antibodies (antiperoxidase-TPO, antimicrosomal-AMA, and antithyroglobulin-ATG) may cross the placenta and cause neonatal hypothyroidism, which, if untreated, may lead to serious cognitive deficiencies. Lower IQs in infants of even very mild hypothyroid women have been reported. None of the most recent reports indicate an increased frequency of congenital anomalies. The main complication found in practically all studies is a high risk of preeclampsia, which often leads to premature delivery with its related morbidity, mortality, and high cost. Placental abruption and postpartum hemorrhage may occur. The severity of the hypertension and other perinatal complications is greater in the more severely hypothyroid woman. Early treatment and close monitoring to ensure euthyroidism will prevent or decrease perinatal complications. Hypothyroidism is frequently associated with other illnesses, particularly type 1 diabetes, chronic hypertension, and anemia; these conditions should be properly monitored and treated as well. Why hypertension occurs more frequently in hypothyroidism is unclear. Reduced cardiac output and increased peripheral resistance have been found and attributed to increased sympathetic nervous tone and α-adrenergic response.

There is no consensus on whether or not universal screening for hypothyroidism during pregnancy should be performed. We strongly recommend that certain high-risk women undergo routine screening for hypothyroidism: previous therapy for hyperthyroidism, high-dose neck irradiation, previous postpartum thyroiditis, presence of a goiter, family history of thyroid disease, treatment with amiodarone, suspected hypopituitarism, and type 1 diabetes mellitus. Because thyroxine requirements increase very early in pregnancy, hypothyroid women should be seen early and frequently during the first half of pregnancy and less often afterward in the second half.

L-Thyroxine has long been the treatment drug of choice. The hormonal content of the synthetic drugs is more reliably standardized, and they have replaced desiccated thyroid as the mainstay of therapy. Administration of T_4 alone is recommended. In the normal physiologic process, T_4 is deiodinated to T_3 in the extrathyroidal tissues. In addition, during early pregnancy the fetal brain is unable to use maternal T_3. A combination of T_4 and T_3, approximating the ratio secreted by the thyroid, was sometimes recommended but its usefulness has not been confirmed. The best time to take L-thyroxine is early in the morning, on an empty stomach. Women experiencing nausea and vomiting should be allowed to take it later in the day until they improve. Numerous reports indicate that thyroxine requirements increase during pregnancy. The initial dose should be 2 µg per kilogram of actual body weight. Further adjustments are made according to the TSH level. If the TSH level is elevated but < 10 µU/mL, add 25–50 µg/d; if the TSH level is >10 but < 20, add 50–75 µg/d; and if the TSH level is > 20, add 75–100 µg/d. Changes made at less than 4-week intervals may lead to overtreatment. Up to 85% of women receiving thyroxine replacement before pregnancy will require higher doses while they are pregnant. The levels should be checked early in pregnancy and then periodically thereafter to maintain euthyroidism. After delivery, the dosage is reduced to the prepregnancy amount, and a TSH level measured 4–8 weeks postpartum. In women with pituitary disease, the TSH level cannot be used to guide therapy. In these cases, the FT_4 level should be kept in the upper third of normal.

POSTPARTUM THYROID DYSFUNCTION

Postpartum thyroid dysfunction reportedly occurs in between 2% and 5% of all women. It occurs in autoimmune thyroid disease (usually lymphocytic thyroiditis, less frequently in Graves' disease) and often recurs in subsequent pregnancies. In general the condition resolves spontaneously immediately after delivery, but a high rate of hypothyroidism has been observed after long-term follow-up. The clinical course is characterized by mild hyperthyroid symptoms occurring 4–8 weeks postpartum and sometimes later. The TSH level is suppressed, and T_4, T_3, and antibody titers are elevated. The thyroid gland may enlarge but is painless to palpation. A needle biopsy, if performed, shows lymphocytic infiltration. A radioactive iodine uptake test, if performed, shows little or no uptake, but the test should not be performed if the patient is breastfeeding. A high uptake would be more consistent with Graves' disease. The symptoms resolve and the results of thyroid tests return to normal after a few weeks or months. However, most patients subsequently develop a hypothyroid phase with clinical symptoms, low T_4 level, elevated TSH level, and further elevation of antibody titers. Spontaneous resolution occurs in most patients after another several weeks or months. The clinical course may vary, with some patients experiencing only the hyperthyroid phase and others only the hypothy-

roid phase. Treatment in the immediate postpartum is limited to symptomatic patients only (β blockers for the hyperthyroid phase and low-dose levothyroxine or triiodothyronine for the hypothyroid phase, which is enough to alleviate symptoms and allows recovery of thyroid function when discontinued).

SOLITARY THYROID NODULE DURING PREGNANCY

Thyroid nodules are frequently first detected during pregnancy when many women see a doctor for the first time. Little information on the management of these patients is available. The recommended approach in our institution is shown in Figure 24–1. The effect of pregnancy on the natural history of thyroid cancer is not completely known, but the present consensus is that pregnancy does not affect the cancer growth rate or the long-term prognosis. The risk of malignancy for a solitary nodule varies between 5% and 43%, depending on various factors including previous radiation, rate of growth, and patient age. Surgery during pregnancy carries a higher risk if it is performed during the first and the third trimesters (miscarriage, premature delivery, and fetal death); surgery during the second trimester reportedly has a lower complication rate. Radioactive iodine should never be given during pregnancy.

■ CALCIUM DISORDERS

CALCIUM METABOLISM IN NORMAL PREGNANCY

Both, calcium (Ca) and phosphorus (P) have many metabolic functions, including maintenance of the skeletal system, neuromuscular excitability, cell membrane permeability, high-energy phosphate bonds, and blood coagulation. The daily Ca requirements are 1200 mg (400 mg more than outside of pregnancy) and the total accumulation by term is 30 g (> 25 g in the fetus). It is linearly related to fetal weight, and > 80% accumulates in late pregnancy. Of the circulating Ca, 46% is bound to albumin, 7% to other complexes (phosphate, citrate, and other anions), and 47% is free (or ionized). The protein-bound fraction decreases because of increased extracellular volume, transfer to the fetus, and, perhaps, increased renal clearance. The free fraction remains the same, although some studies have reported a slight decrease leading to increased parathyroid hormone (PTH) levels. Urinary Ca excretion increases early in gestation and decreases in late pregnancy but does not exceed the

Single Thyroid Nodule

Abnormal ← Serum TSH

Work-up for Thyroid Dysfunction

Normal

Thyroid Ultrasound

Solid Lesion > 2 cm
Cystic Lesion > 4 cm

Solid Lesion < 2 cm
Cystic Lesion < 4 cm

< 28 Weeks   > 28 Weeks

Needle Biopsy

Malignant   Not Malignant → Observation → Follow-up
                            Thyroxine Suppression?   Postpartum

Surgery
Second Trimester

Needle Biopsy if:
1) Cervical Adenopathy
2) Enlarging Nodule

Figure 24–1. Evaluation of single thyroid nodules in pregnancy.

normal range. The P level falls slightly in early pregnancy and rises to normal by 30 weeks.

The PTH level remains unchanged during the first half of pregnancy and then rises gradually until term, coinciding with the time of greatest fetal skeletal calcification. PTH promotes Ca transport from mother to fetus. The most potent factor affecting PTH secretion is the free Ca level (inverse correlation), but calcitonin, vitamin D, and magnesium (Mg) also play a role. Calcitonin is secreted by C-cells inside the thyroid, but these cells actually are of neural crest origin and migrate to the thyroid. Calcitonin is a Ca-lowering hormone whose secretion is also mainly affected by free Ca levels, but in this case the correlation is direct. Its action is antagonistic to that of PTH, and it plays a role in Ca homeostasis and bone remodeling. Vitamin D increases the efficiency of intestinal Ca absorption, plays a role in the maintenance of Ca and P levels, and has a role in the mineralization of bone matrix. In order to exert its action, vitamin D must be transformed into active metabolites $[1,25\text{-}(OH)_2D_3]$ in the kidney, and PTH is needed for the process. The requirements are 400 IU/d, the same as outside of pregnancy. Vitamin D crosses the placenta readily.

Whether Ca metabolism during pregnancy is influenced by other hormones, such as estrogen, progesterone, or hCG, is not known. The placenta plays a major role in transporting Ca against a gradient. PTH facili-

tates this transport, although neither PTH nor calcitonin crosses the placenta. The fetal Ca concentration (both total and free) increases gradually from 5.5–11.0 mg/dL from the second trimester to term. In the fetus, the PTH level is suppressed but detectable, and cord levels are 25% lower than in the mother. Calcitonin in cord is higher than in the mother, a combination favoring skeletal growth, which also causes Ca levels in the newborn to fall to normal. Given these findings, all the observed changes in normal pregnancy favor mineralization of the fetal skeleton.

DISORDERS OF CALCIUM METABOLISM

HYPERPARATHYROIDISM

Hyperthyroidism is a frequently occurring disease but has been uncommonly reported to occur during pregnancy. Just over 120 cases have been reported since 1931, with the first successful surgery performed in 1947. The etiology is an adenoma in 89–90% of cases, hyperplasia (of all the glands) in 9%, and carcinoma in 1–2%. The latter should be suspected in severe hyperparathyroidism, particularly if a palpable neck mass is present (palpable neck masses are reported in < 5% of parathyroid adenomas). Rarely it occurs in a familial pattern with or without other endocrine abnormalities (eg, multiple endocrine adenomatosis). Other causes of hypercalcemia during pregnancy are uncommon and include vitamin D toxicity, sarcoidosis, various malignancies, milk-alkali syndrome, thyrotoxicosis, adrenal insufficiency, and secondary hyperparathyroidism in those undergoing chronic hemodialysis or after renal transplantation.

Reported complications include 27.5% fetal mortality and 19% neonatal tetany. Neonatal hypocalcemia is often the initial clue to the presence of maternal hyperparathyroidism. The condition occurs because the high levels of maternal Ca inhibit the activity or the proper development of the infant's parathyroid glands. It develops between days 2 and 14 after delivery, depending on the severity of the maternal hypercalcemia, and usually resolves with appropriate therapy. One case of hypocalcemia persisting for 3 months and another case of hypocalcemia that became permanent have been reported.

Complications in the mother include 36% nephrolithiasis, 19% bone disease, 13% pancreatitis, 13% urinary tract infections and pyelonephritis, 10% hypertension (100% in all cases of carcinoma thus far reported), and 8% hypercalcemic crisis. Maternal deaths have occurred among those with complications of pancreatitis or hypercalcemic crisis. Women who developed hypercalcemic crisis had a 30% maternal death rate and 40% fetal demises. Pancreatitis is reported in only 1.5% of nonpregnant hyperparathyroid patients and in < 1% of normal pregnancies. Most pregnant women with hyperparathyroidism (76%) are symptomatic, whereas 50–80% of nonpregnant hyperparathyroid patients are asymptomatic at the time of diagnosis. Common symptoms include anorexia, nausea and vomiting, thirst, weakness, fatigue, lethargy, headaches, emotional lability, inappropriate behavior, confusion, and even delirium.

A persistently elevated serum Ca level and a normal or elevated PTH level, despite hypercalcemia, confirm the diagnosis. Hypercalciuria is commonly seen. The serum levels of P, Mg, and bicarbonate usually are low, and chloride and citrate levels often are elevated. The chloride/P ratio is sometimes used as a diagnostic clue because the ratio usually is > 30 in hyperparathyroidism but is < 30 in hypercalcemia from other causes. The levels of serum alkaline phosphatase (of bone origin) and urinary hydroxyproline will be elevated in cases with significant bone involvement.

Surgery is the treatment of choice for confirmed hyperparathyroidism. In pregnancy, the optimal time for surgery is the second trimester, when the complication risks (abortion or premature labor) are reduced. An experienced surgeon performing the neck exploration will be able to proceed appropriately in case of parathyroid hyperplasia (removal of all glands with parathyroid tissue transplantation). In addition, the complication rate should be reduced when an experienced surgeon performs the procedure. Postoperatively, hypocalcemia may occur in patients with significant osteitis fibrosa or if injury occurs to the normal parathyroid glands during surgery. When surgery is not possible, maintaining adequate hydration and administering oral phosphates may be temporary measures until surgery can be safely performed. Preventing hypercalcemic crisis is of utmost importance; if it develops, aggressive treatment is recommended.

HYPOPARATHYROIDISM

The most common cause of hypoparathyroidism is surgical removal or damage to the parathyroid glands, or their vascular supply, during thyroid surgery. Hypoparathyroidism reportedly occurs in 0.2–3.5% of cases after thyroid surgery. Idiopathic hypoparathyroidism is relatively rare and is seldom seen in pregnancy. It may be isolated or occur in association with agenesis of the thymus or as part of a familial disorder, which includes deficiencies of thyroid, adrenal and ovarian function, pernicious anemia, and mucocutaneous candidiasis. Pseudohypoparathyroidism (deficient end-organ response to PTH in bone and kidney) is a rare hereditary disorder infrequently encountered during pregnancy. The severity of symptoms depends on the degree of hypocalcemia and range from clumsiness (fingers), mental changes (mainly depression), muscle stiffness, parkinsonism, acral and perioral paresthesias, to laryngeal stridor, tetany, and convulsions. Clinical signs include dry, scaly skin, brittle nails, coarse hair, and positive Chvostek's (present in 10% of normals) and Trousseau' signs. Ectopic soft tissue calcifications and a prolonged QT interval on the electrocardiogram may be observed. Pseudohypoparathyroidism is more likely if the patient has unusual skeletal or developmental defects and if other family members affected. The diagnosis usually is evident from the history and confirmed by a "normal" or low PTH level in the presence of hypocalcemia, hyperphosphatemia, and normal renal function.

Before the availability of specific therapy, maternal morbidity and mortality rates were high, and termination of pregnancy was frequently recommended. Currently the prognosis is much improved provided the mother is kept eucalcemic. From 1–4 g/d of elemental calcium and 50,000–100,000 U/d of vitamin D usually are recommended. The synthetic vitamin D analogue $1\alpha,25\text{-}(OH)_2D_3$ at doses of 0.25–2 μg/d is considered safer by some authors. The therapeutic margin is narrow in these patients, who experience frequent episodes of hypercalcemia or hypocalcemia. Hypercalcemia, when it develops, may be long-lasting. The synthetic analogues are more active and shorter-acting, and they might be safer. In hypercalcemia, the vitamin D therapy is stopped, hydration is provided, and a course of corticosteroids is given (prednisone, or equivalent, 40–100 mg/d). If convulsions and tetany result from hypocalcemia, Ca gluconate 10–20 mg is given intravenously, followed by infusion of 15 mg of Ca gluconate per kilogram of actual body weight administered over 4–8 hours, according to the serum Ca level. Replace Mg if the serum level is low. Once the acute episode resolves, the daily oral therapy is readjusted to prevent recurrences.

These patients require frequent serum Ca determinations, and the therapy should be readjusted as often as necessary to prevent acute decompensation. If the mother is hypercalcemic, the newborn may develop hypocalcemia and tetany, the same as when the mother has hyperparathyroidism. If the mother is hypocalcemic, hyperplasia of the fetal parathyroid glands, mobilization of calcium from the skeleton and generalized demineralization, subperiosteal resorption, and even osteitis fibrosa with very high perinatal mortality will occur. With proper treatment, symptoms in surviving infants will subside by age 4–7 months.

After delivery, hypoparathyroid women may develop hypercalcemia with the same dose of calcium and vitamin D that was effective during pregnancy. Hypersensitivity to vitamin D in lactating women may result from the effect of prolactin (PRL) on 1α-hydroxylase vitamin D activity. Serum calcium levels should be monitored closely and the doses readjusted as necessary. Vitamin D travels into breast milk, even when low doses are taken, so many physicians discourage breastfeeding in these women.

ADRENAL DISORDERS

Pregnancy is rarely associated with diseases of the adrenal glands, particularly in those with excessive cortisol secretion, because of the high prevalence of infertility in these women.

CUSHING'S SYNDROME

Up to 75–80% of women with excess cortisol experience menstrual irregularities and infertility. Excess cortisol, either endogenous or exogenous, suppresses gonadotropin secretion. In addition, elevated androgen and PRL levels are contributing factors in some patients. Approximately 70 cases occurring in pregnancy have been reported, usually in the form of single cases based upon a review of the literature. Most cases (70%) of Cushing's syndrome occurring outside of pregnancy are the result of excess adrenocorticotropic hormone (ACTH) secretion, usually by

small pituitary adenomas. However, of the cases reported during pregnancy, only 40% were ACTH-dependent Cushing's syndrome; 60% were adrenal tumors (90% adenomas and 10% carcinomas). Apparently, women with ACTH-dependent Cushing's syndrome have a higher infertility rate.

The clinical diagnosis is difficult because the changes occur insidiously. During pregnancy, diagnosis is even more difficult because weight gain, skin striae (stretch marks), and fatigue are common during normal pregnancy, but all other symptoms and signs will be the same as outside of pregnancy. The laboratory diagnosis also is more difficult during pregnancy. Urinary free cortisol excretion may overlap with that seen in some cases of Cushing's syndrome, and the suppression to exogenous corticosteroids may be incomplete. However, the diurnal variations of both ACTH and cortisol are preserved; therefore, measurement of morning and evening cortisol levels remains very useful. Therefore, the diagnosis may be confirmed by the loss of diurnal variation, elevated levels of urinary free cortisol, particularly if > 250 mg per 24 hours, and lack of cortisol suppression to dexamethasone. Measurements of ACTH may be useful as well ("normal" or high in Cushing's disease and suppressed in adrenal tumors). Magnetic resonance imaging (MRI) may confirm the presence of a pituitary or adrenal tumor. A few cases of "pregnancy-induced" Cushing's syndrome with spontaneous resolution postpartum have been reported and attributed to a placental corticotropin-releasing factor. However, long-term follow-up revealed other causes of Cushing's syndrome in most of the women.

The most common complication (64%) is premature labor resulting in considerable fetal morbidity and mortality. IUGR occurs in 26–37% and fetal losses (spontaneous abortions and stillbirths) in 16%. Little information about the long-term quality of survival of those born premature but alive is available. Hypertension and diabetes mellitus complicate 70% and 32% of these pregnancies, respectively, and unfavorably influence the outcome of these pregnancies if untreated. Other potential maternal complications include congestive heart failure, thromboembolism, osteoporosis and vertebral fractures, proximal muscle weakness, electrolyte disturbances (particularly low potassium), and poor healing with wound breakdown (to be considered in case of cesarean section). Maternal mortality has occurred in 5% of cases.

An attempt at some form of treatment is advocated given the poor outcome. Surgery in the second trimester can be attempted when a pituitary or adrenal tumor is found. Few reports of these procedures performed during pregnancy are documented. Medical therapy is limited, and the potential side effects of the medications are not well known. Metyrapone, cyproheptadine, aminoglutethimide, and ketoconazole (teratogenic in animals) have been used in a few patients. All efforts should be made to control the hypertension and hyperglycemia so commonly seen with excess cortisol. Early delivery in the third trimester as soon as the fetus is mature is recommended, with postponement of definitive treatment of the mother until after delivery.

ADRENAL INSUFFICIENCY

Primary adrenocortical insufficiency (Addison's disease) more often is the result of autoimmune destruction of the adrenal glands (in the era before antibiotics, tuberculosis was the most common cause). Occasionally, it is associated with other autoimmune endocrine disorders (polyendocrine autoimmune deficiency). Other causes are exceptionally rare in fertile women of childbearing age. Secondary adrenal failure results from reduced or absent ACTH secretion caused by various pituitary disorders or inhibition from chronic exogenous steroid use. Causes of partial or complete anterior pituitary insufficiency in women of reproductive age include tumors, pituitary surgery or radiation, and postpartum infarction (Sheehan's syndrome). Less common causes are acute pituitary hemorrhage, infiltration by granulomatous diseases, thalassemia, necrosis from increased intracranial pressure, and lymphocytic hypophysitis. A few cases of pituitary necrosis in type 1 pregnant diabetic women have been reported.

Since the advent of steroid treatment, most pregnancies have been successfully managed. Even women with anterior pituitary insufficiency may conceive because of advances in infertility treatment and, with proper hormonal replacement, may carry their pregnancies to term. Infants of well-treated mothers with adrenal insufficiency appear to be normal.

The symptoms during pregnancy are similar to those in nonpregnant cases and include weakness, nausea, vomiting, abdominal pain, hyperpigmentation, hyponatremia, and hyperkalemia. The diagnosis may be delayed or missed unless there is a high index of suspicion. Acute adrenal crisis is a more dramatic presentation. If not diagnosed and treated promptly, it will become a catastrophic event resulting in maternal and/or fetal death.

The daily steroid replacement dose is 20–25 mg/m^2 by mouth (ie, 30–37.5 mg/d of hydrocortisone or equivalent steroid). Two thirds of the daily dose (20–25 mg) is given in the morning and one third (10–12.5 mg) in the late afternoon. Usually the daily dosage does not need to be changed during pregnancy. However, compensation is required for periods of stress and during labor and delivery (up to 300 mg of hydrocortisone or equivalent steroid given intravenously in divided doses the first day and gradual tapering to the maintenance dose over the next

several days). In secondary adrenal insufficiency, mineralocorticoid replacement is not necessary, but women with primary adrenal disease also should receive fludrocortisone 0.05–0.1 mg/d by mouth.

CONGENITAL ADRENAL HYPERPLASIA

Of the several inherited enzymatic deficiencies of cortisol synthesis that may cause congenital adrenal hyperplasia, the 21-hydroxylase deficiency accounts for 90–95% of cases. These enzymatic deficiencies are inherited as autosomal recessive traits (25% risk of inheriting the condition and 50% of being a carrier).

The low cortisol level stimulates excessive ACTH secretion, which in turn causes adrenal enlargement ("adrenal hyperplasia"). The excessive secretion of androgens leads to masculinization of the external genitalia (congenital sexual ambiguity) and the low cortisol level to adrenal insufficiency. Untreated, these conditions can be life-threatening. In most cases, the diagnosis is made and treatment initiated after birth when the newborn becomes ill. However, prenatal diagnosis (chorionic villous sampling and DNA testing) now is reported. If the defect is a 21-hydroxylase deficiency and the fetus is female, treatment of the mother with dexamethasone may prevent the development of adrenal hyperplasia and virilization of the external genitalia. Those born with virilization of the external genitalia will require surgical reconstruction to allow vaginal intercourse.

In affected females, the earlier the treatment is initiated, the higher the likelihood that they will be ovulatory and fertile. During pregnancy, glucocorticoid therapy should be continued and adjusted to avoid excessive androgen levels. Otherwise the steroid management is the same as described for adrenal insufficiency. If extensive surgical reconstruction of the genitalia was performed, a cesarean delivery might be necessary. Genetic counseling should be mandatory for these women, before they consider pregnancy, given the high risk of transmission and the severity of the disease.

PHEOCHROMOCYTOMA

Pheochromocytomas are rare in the general population and are the least common cause of hypertension during pregnancy. However, given the severity of the complications (48% maternal mortality and 55% fetal mortality) if untreated, the possibility of its existence must always be considered in the differential diagnosis. The symptoms are similar to those outside of pregnancy and are caused by excess catecholamines. They include sustained or paroxysmal hypertension, headaches, palpitations, diaphoresis, and anxiety. Blurred vision and convulsions are reported more commonly during pregnancy. Higher blood pressure while recumbent and lower when standing may be clues to the diagnosis during pregnancy (pressure from the gravid uterus on the tumor while lying down). Complications include spontaneous abortion, IUGR, placental abruption, and fetal and maternal death. Differentiation from preeclampsia may be difficult when proteinuria is also present. Elevated levels of free catecholamines and their metabolites metanephrine and vanillylmandelic acid (VMA) in a 24-hour urine collection confirm the diagnosis. Urinary metanephrine levels > 1.2 mg/d are considered highly suggestive of pheochromocytoma. A plasma level of total catecholamines > 2000 pg/mL, drawn after the patient has been in the supine position for > 30 minutes, also is highly suggestive. For tumor localization, MRI is the test of choice during pregnancy. Other test and scans are not considered safe during pregnancy. Most pheochromocytomas are benign and are located in the adrenal glands, but approximately 10% are located elsewhere and difficult to find. In a few patients, the pheochromocytoma may be part of a familial disorder and more likely to be bilateral.

Few of the reported cases were diagnosed during pregnancy. However, if the diagnosis is made, surgical removal during the second trimester is recommended. Blood pressure control is attempted first with adequate adrenergic blockade (usually phenoxybenzamine), followed by β-adrenergic blockade if necessary, until surgery can be performed in the second trimester or, if after 26–28 weeks, until the fetus is mature. Phenoxybenzamine is considered safe, but it does cross the placenta and has the potential to cause depression and transient hypotension in the newborn. Laparoscopic removal has been reported in a few cases, but most surgeons prefer an abdominal approach to ensure adequate adrenal visualization. Vaginal delivery is not recommended because of precipitation of hypertensive crisis by mechanical pressure on the tumor from changes in posture, contractions, and fetal movements. Cesarean delivery followed by tumor removal during the same surgery is generally advised. Adequate medical preparation for surgery is mandatory. Pheochromocytoma removal is a high-risk procedure, and an experienced surgeon and anesthesiologist are strongly recommended.

■ PITUITARY DISORDERS

PITUITARY TUMORS

Prolactinomas are the most common pituitary tumors encountered during pregnancy, particularly since the availability of effective treatments for restoring fertility. The diagnosis usually is made when the PRL level is high enough to cause galactorrhea, oligomenorrhea, or amenorrhea. MRI confirms the diagnosis. The tumors are divided into microadenomas (< 10 mm) or macroadenomas (> 10 mm). The risk of growth during pregnancy is low (1–2%) for microadenomas, in contrast to the 15–25% risk for untreated macroadenomas. Previously treated macroadenomas (bromocriptine, cabergoline, and/or surgery) have a lower risk (4%) of growth during pregnancy. In general, serial PRL measurements do not predict tumor growth and are not recommended. In actuality, pregnant women with prolactinomas tend to have lower PRL levels, a lower response to stimulation (eg, to TRH), and loss of the diurnal PRL variation.

Serial visual field examinations or MRI is not recommended for microadenomas unless symptoms appear. If severe headache occurs, MRI is recommended even if no visual field defects are detected. MRI should always be performed if visual field defects are detected. If the tumor enlarges, medical therapy (bromocriptine or cabergoline) is started and visual field examinations performed daily. If no rapid response occurs, high-dose steroid therapy is added. If still no response occurs, surgery should be strongly considered. Few reports of surgery during pregnancy are documented, but medical therapy, continued until after delivery, generally has been safe and effective. Labor and delivery are generally uncomplicated, but shortening the duration of the second stage in women experiencing tumor growth during pregnancy is recommended in an effort to prevent intracranial pressure elevation during the most active pushing.

In macroprolactinomas, monthly visual field examinations and MRI are recommended if tumor growth is suspected. In addition to headaches and visual changes, pituitary infarction and diabetes insipidus are rarely seen. Complications of tumor growth are more likely to appear during the first trimester.

Most women with prolactinomas are allowed to breastfeed. MRI usually is recommended approximately 3–4 months after delivery to reassess tumor size.

ACROMEGALY

Because menstrual disturbances are very common (up to 75%), few pregnancies during the active phase of the disease have been reported. Hyperprolactinemia, which also is commonly seen (30–40%), adds to fertility difficulties. If conception occurs, spontaneous abortion may occur due to inability to maintain implantation. Diabetes and hypertension are common complications during pregnancy, adding further serious adverse consequences.

The clinical diagnosis is infrequently made early in the disease because changes in shoe or glove size and coarsening of facial features develop slowly. Determination of growth hormone levels during pregnancy requires specific assays able to differentiate growth hormone from pituitary or placental origin. Insulinlike growth factor-I (IGF-I) levels are elevated during normal pregnancy, and their measurement is of limited usefulness in the diagnosis of acromegaly during gestation. Ideally, treatment should be accomplished before pregnancy. In general, medical therapy is stopped when pregnancy is diagnosed. However, bromocriptine administration throughout gestation without untoward effects to mother or infant has been reported. The data for octreotide are limited, so until its safety is determined, octreotide should be stopped when pregnancy is diagnosed. Elective surgery during pregnancy is safer during the second trimester. Emergency surgery is reserved for women with pregnancy-associated tumor enlargement and visual loss.

MRI should be performed in all patients before conception and after delivery. Follow-up for microadenomas during pregnancy include clinical assessments (headaches, visual changes) every trimester and no intervention unless symptoms appear. For macroadenomas, monthly assessments are recommended along with an MRI 4 months into the pregnancy. It appears that women with microadenomas can breastfeed safely.

SHEEHAN'S SYNDROME

H.L. Sheehan described the syndrome bearing his name as partial or complete pituitary insufficiency due to postpartum necrosis of the anterior pituitary gland in women with severe blood loss and hypotension during delivery. Nevertheless, up to 10% cases have no history of bleeding or hypotension. The clinical manifestations depend on the extent of pituitary destruction and hormonal deficiencies. With destruction of 90% or more, symptoms of acute adrenal insufficiency predominate (see Adrenal Insufficiency). If the condition is not treated promptly, serious complications and even death may occur. In most cases, the full-blown picture may take longer, even years, to appear. Failure to lactate, breast involution, and, if untreated, breast atrophy may occur. Loss of pubic and axillary hair (or failure of hair to regrow if it is shaved), oligomenorrhea or amenorrhea, loss of libido, and pale ("waxy") skin with premature wrinkling, especially around the eyes and mouth, are possible. Fatigue, weight loss, and postural hypotension are common complaints. Hyponatremia and anemia (usually normocytic and normochromic) are frequent laboratory abnormalities. Hormonal deficiencies point to a secondary cause, with low thyroxine, TSH, estrogen, gonadotropin, cortisol, and ACTH levels. Provocative hormonal testing may be necessary to confirm the diagnosis. Once the diagnosis of secondary hormonal deficiency is established, MRI of the pituitary and hypothalamus is necessary to exclude a tumor or other pathology.

All deficient hormones must be replaced. However, it is well known that some patients with clear panhypopituitarism may recover TSH and even gonadotropin function after cortisol replacement alone. The mechanism is unknown, but it is speculated that cortisol has a permissive effect on other hypothalamic and pituitary functions. Rare cases of spontaneous recovery have been reported.

The outcome of pregnancy in women with Sheehan's syndrome shows no increased perinatal morbidity or mortality if the mothers are treated properly. Women with persistent amenorrhea and anovulation will require fertility treatment to become pregnant.

DIABETES INSIPIDUS

Diabetes insipidus (DI) is caused by a deficiency of antidiuretic hormone (ADH), called central DI, or by renal tubule resistance to ADH action, called nephrogenic DI. A transient form of DI during pregnancy has been observed with increasing frequency and has attributed to excessive placental production of vasopressinase, perhaps decreased hepatic clearance, and, because most of the patients reported had abnormal liver function, preeclampsia, fatty liver, or hepatitis. It is possible that some of these cases represent mild preexisting DI unmasked by pregnancy. It usually resolves several weeks after delivery but may recur in subsequent pregnancies, so follow-up is recommended.

A variety of lesions may cause DI, such as pituitary surgery, radiation, trauma, tumors, granulomas, and infections. However, no etiology is found in as many as 50% of patients, and these cases are labeled as "idiopathic." Clinical symptoms include polyuria of 4–15 L/d and intense thirst, particularly for ice-cold fluids. The incidence during pregnancy has been reported as 1 in 50,000 to 1 in 80,000 deliveries. Approximately 60% of women with previously known DI worsen, 20% improve, and 20% do not change during pregnancy. Worsening is attributed to excessive placental vasopressinase production. Some women with DI who also develop placental insufficiency show DI improvement, which is attributed to decreased vasopressinase production by the damaged placenta.

The diagnosis of DI is confirmed by the standard water deprivation test. However, this test may prove hazardous during pregnancy because 3–5% of body weight may be lost during the test. This degree of dehydration, which is required to produce sufficient stimulation for ADH secretion, may lead to uteroplacental insufficiency and fetal distress. Even before fetal distress occurs, uterine contractions and even frank labor may be precipitated, forcing termination of the test before it can be properly interpreted. Uterine contractions respond rapidly to intravenous fluid administration. If the decision is made to perform a water deprivation test, continuous fetal monitoring is recommended. Because of these difficulties, a suggested alternative test is 20 µg of L-deamino-8-D-arginine vasopressin (DDAVP) given intranasal and serial urinary osmolalities determined during the next 12 hours. Any value > 700 mOsm/kg is normal. DDAVP is a synthetic analogue of ADH and is resistant to vasopressinase.

The treatment of choice is intranasal DDAVP. It also can be given subcutaneously when the intranasal route cannot be used. The usual dose is 10 to 25 µg once or twice daily (or 2–4 µg subcutaneously). The dosage is adjusted according to fluid intake, urinary output, osmolality, and plasma electrolytes. Close follow-up is necessary to prevent dehydration or the opposite, water intoxication. Many reports indicate that DDAVP is safe during pregnancy and postpartum, even while the mother is breastfeeding. Oxytocin secretion appears to be normal, and no labor difficulties have been reported. No difficulties with lactation have been reported even in women with central DI.

REFERENCES

Thyroid Disorders

Alexander EK et al: Timing and magnitude of increases in levothyroxine requirements during pregnancy in women with hypothyroidism. N Engl J Med 2004;351:241.

Mestman JH: Diagnosis and management of maternal and fetal thyroid disorders. Curr Opin Obstet Gynecol 1999;11:167.

Mestman JH, Goodwin TM, Montoro MN: Thyroid disorders of pregnancy. Endocrinol Metab Clin North Am 19945;24:41.

Montoro MN: Management of hypothyroidism during pregnancy. Clin Obstet Gynecol 1997;40:65.

Moosa M, Mazzaferri EL: Outcome of differentiated thyroid cancer diagnosed in pregnant women. J Clin Endocrinol Metab 1997;82:2862.

Calcium Disorders

Ficinski ML, Mestman JH: Primary hyperparathyroidism during pregnancy. Endocr Pract 1996;2:362.

Kovacs CS: Calcium and bone metabolism in pregnancy and lactation. J Clin Endocrinol Metab 2001;86:2344.

Montoro MN et al: Parathyroid carcinoma during pregnancy. Obstet Gynecol 2000;96(5 Suppl 2):841.

Adrenal Disorders

Buescher MA, McClamrock HD, Adashi EY: Cushing's syndrome in pregnancy. Obstet Gynecol 1992;79:130.

Garner PR: Congenital adrenal hyperplasia in pregnancy. Semin Perinatol 1998;22:46.

Grudden C, Lawrence D: Addison's disease in pregnancy. Lancet 2001;357:1197.

Hadden DR: Adrenal disorders of pregnancy. Endocrinol Metab Clin North Am 1995;24:139.

Krone N et al: Mothers with congenital adrenal hyperplasia and their children: Outcome of pregnancy, birth and childhood. Clin Endocrinol 2001;55:523.

Perlitz Y et al: Acute adrenal insufficiency during pregnancy and puerperium: Case report and literature review. Obstet Gynecol Surv 1999;54:717.

Pheochromocytoma

Keely E: Endocrine causes of hypertension in pregnancy—When to start looking for zebras. Semin Perinatol 1998;22:471.

Takahashi K, Sai Y, Nosaka S: Anesthetic management for caesarean section combined with removal of pheochromocytoma. Eur J Anesthesiol 1998;15:364.

Pituitary Diseases

Chee GH et al: Transsphenoidal pituitary surgery in Cushing's disease: Can we predict outcome? Clin Endocrinol 2001;54:617.

Durr JA et al: Diabetes insipidus in pregnancy associated with abnormally high circulating vasopressinase activity. N Engl J Med 1987;316:1070.

Iwasaki Y et al: Aggravation of subclinical diabetes Insipidus during pregnancy. N Engl J Med 1991;324:522.

Krege J, Katz VL, Bowes WA: Transient diabetes insipidus of pregnancy. Obstet Gynecol Surv 1989;44:789.

Kupersmith MJ, Rosenberg C, Kleinberg D: Visual loss in pregnant women with pituitary adenomas. Ann Intern Med 1994;121:473.

Molitch ME: Management of prolactinomas during pregnancy. J Reprod Med 1999;144:1121.

Montoro MN, Mestman JH: Pituitary diseases during pregnancy. Infertil Reprod Med Clin North Am 1994;5:729.

Randeva HS et al: Classical pituitary apoplexy: clinical features, management and outcome. Clin Endocrinol (Oxf) 1999;51:181.

Ray JG: DDAVP use during pregnancy: Analysis of its safety for mother and child. Obstet Gynecol Surv 1998;53:450.

Sheehan HL: Postpartum necrosis of the anterior pituitary. J Pathol Bacteriol 1937;45:189.

Nervous System & Autoimmune Disorders in Pregnancy

25

Laura Kalayjian, MD, & T. Murphy Goodwin, MD

■ DISORDERS OF THE NERVOUS SYSTEM

CEREBROVASCULAR DISORDERS

The causes of cerebrovascular disease include insufficiency *(arteriosclerosis, cerebral embolism, vasospasm from hypertensive disease)* and disorders associated with bleeding into the cerebral cortex *(arteriovenous malformation, ruptured aneurysm)*. The brain becomes infarcted from lack of blood flow, or intracranial bleeding results in a space-occupying lesion. The severity of such disorders can be affected by blood pressure, oxygen saturation (anemia or polycythemia), hypoglycemia, and adequacy of collateral circulation.

The overall incidence of ischemic cerebrovascular accidents in pregnancy is approximately 1 in 20,000 births, with most occurring in the last trimester or immediately postpartum. Etiologic factors for stroke include cardioembolic disorders, cerebral angiopathies, hematologic disorders, and cerebral vein thrombosis. Causes exclusive to pregnancy are eclampsia, choriocarcinoma, and amniotic fluid embolism. Although cerebral ischemic disease can occur in either the arterial or venous system, approximately 75% of occlusive cerebral disease occurs on the arterial side.

Cerebrovascular accidents involving subarachnoid hemorrhage or intraparenchymal hemorrhage similarly occur at a rate of 1 in 20,000 births. These events usually are the result of aneurysms or arteriovenous malformations. The most common aneurysm is the saccular (berry) variety, which protrudes from the major arteries in the circle of Willis, particularly at its bifurcations. Aneurysms have an increasing tendency to bleed as the pregnancy progresses, likely due to changes in hemodynamic factors. Rupture of arteriovenous malformations have been found to occur evenly throughout gestation. No consensus has been reached regarding the increased frequency of bleeding from either an aneurysm or arteriovenous malformation during pregnancy or the im-mediate postpartum period. Rupture of the malformation appears to be more frequent during pregnancy. Eclampsia can lead to cerebral hemorrhage when elevated blood pressures lead to vasospasm, loss of autoregulatory function, and rupture of the vessel wall.

Clinical Findings

Headaches, visual disturbances, syncope, and hemiparesis are among the most common presenting findings.

Diagnosis

The pattern of clinical signs and symptoms generally allows recognition of the area of the brain involved. Computed tomography (CT) scan and magnetic resonance imaging (MRI) can be used in pregnancy to increase the delineation of cerebrovascular involvement. Arteriography is considered definitive if surgical intervention is being considered because arteriography can more precisely localize the involved area. Because coagulopathies can also cause intracranial bleeding or may be secondary to the cerebrovascular lesion itself, a coagulation profile should be performed. Additionally, antinuclear antibody (ANA), lupus anticoagulant, factor V Leiden, homocysteine, anticardiolipin, proteins C and S, antithrombin 3, and plasminogen levels should be considered with thrombotic cerebral events.

Treatment

The treatment of ischemic or hemorrhagic cerebrovascular disease is best managed supportively; however, surgery is indicated for treatment of some aneurysms and arteriovenous malformations. Anticoagulation with heparin may be required depending on the etiology of the infarction; tissue plasminogen activator is relatively contraindicated in pregnancy, but it has been used successfully according to several case reports. Normalization of blood pressure, adequate respiratory support, therapy for metabolic complications, and treatment of coagulopathies or cardiac abnormalities are crucial. Dexamethasone 10 mg intravenously initially, followed by 5 mg every 6 hours for 24 hours, may decrease cerebral edema and be of some assistance prior to surgery or in recovery. Additionally, hyperventilation, mannitol infusions, phenobarbital coma, and intracerebral pressure monitoring may be helpful with severe cerebral edema. Once the patient's condition has been stabilized, physical therapy and rehabilitation should begin as soon as possible.

Appropriate surgery for aneurysms and arteriovenous malformations should be performed with the pregnancy undisturbed unless fetal maturity allows for cesarean birth just prior to the neurosurgical procedure. On the other hand, inoperable lesions during pregnancy are managed by pregnancy conservation until fetal maturity is sufficient to allow abdominal birth. Once a lesion has been surgically corrected, vaginal delivery can be attempted depending on the practitioner's comfort level. However, the second stage of labor should be modified by regional anesthesia and forceps delivery to reduce cerebral pressures associated with the Valsalva maneuver.

Complications & Prognosis

The percentage of patients with venous occlusion who recover from the initial episode without neurologic sequelae during rehabilitation equals that of patients with arterial occlusion. Thrombosis of the superior sagittal sinus is a rare complication. Its incidence is increased in pregnancy, and it has a high mortality rate of approximately 55%.

If the cerebral hemorrhagic disorder is operable, the prognosis is favorable, with few long-term neurologic deficits. In inoperable lesions or when severe maternal cerebral hemorrhage has occurred, the prognosis—although unfavorable—is better for those with aneurysms than for those with arteriovenous fistulas. If a neurosurgical procedure is performed during pregnancy, the fetus usually is not adversely affected, despite the induced hypotension that is often necessary. The prognosis for the mother and fetus is the same as that in a normal gestation once the condition has been corrected.

CEREBRAL NEOPLASMS

Cerebral neoplasms occur primarily at the extremes of life; thus primary cancer or even metastatic tumors are uncommon during the childbearing years. Although brain tumors are not specifically related to gestation, meningiomas, angiomas, and neurofibromas are thought to grow more rapidly with pregnancy. Of the primary neoplasms (half of all brain tumors), gliomas are the most common (50%), with meningiomas and pituitary adenomas accounting for 35%. Of the metastatic cerebral tumors, lung and breast tumors account for 50%. *Choriocarcinoma* commonly metastasizes to the cerebrum.

Clinical Findings

The clinical manifestations, although dependent on the type and location of the tumor, are generally characterized by a slow progression of neurologic signs with evidence of increased intracranial pressure. One of the most frequent signs is headache, which must be differentiated from that occurring in tension and in vascular or inflammatory conditions. Pain that is not relieved by analgesics or muscle relaxants (as a tension headache would be), the absence of a history of migraine headaches, and the lack of signs of infection or meningeal inflammation all point to increased intracranial pressure as a possible cause of the headache. Tumors in the pituitary gland or occipital region may be associated with visual deficits. Other presenting signs and symptoms include nausea, vomiting, double vision, vertigo, seizures, and altered mental status.

Diagnosis

CT scan and MRI are of greatest assistance in revealing space-occupying lesions. MRI is generally preferred during pregnancy, although fetal radiation exposure from CT is minimal. If the cerebrospinal fluid glucose and protein levels are normal, inflammation or infection of the central nervous system is unlikely. Similarly, an increase in the cerebrospinal fluid human chorionic gonadotropin (hCG) titer raises the suspicion of metastatic choriocarcinoma. Pleocytosis may be present with cerebral neoplasia, but usually it is lymphocytic or monocytic, without an increase in the number of polymorphonucleocytes. Finally, failure to find blood or xanthochromic fluid in the cerebrospinal fluid helps in differentiating a neoplasm from a hemorrhagic lesion, unless the tumor has undergone hemorrhagic necrosis.

Treatment

The treatment of cerebral neoplasms during pregnancy depends on the type of tumor, its location, and the stage of gestation. Anticonvulsants should be used only if seizures have occurred. Steroids can be used to decrease intracranial pressure causing focal neurologic signs or headaches. Deterioration of the patient's status in early pregnancy should prompt a discussion about the risks of continuing the pregnancy. Nevertheless, most such pregnancies can be carried through successfully. During the second trimester, treatment with surgery, chemotherapy, or directed radiation can be started and the pregnancy allowed to continue. Later in gestation, maternal treatment can be delayed until delivery. Pituitary adenomas can be treated with bromocriptine if visual problems or disabling headaches occur.

Complications & Prognosis

Brain tumors usually do not affect pregnancy or the fetus unless the neoplasm leads to early delivery or maternal death. When diagnosed in the second or third trimester, the outcome for the fetus is excellent, even though therapy may be initiated during the course of the pregnancy.

MIGRAINE HEADACHE

Chronic migraine headaches decrease during pregnancy in 50–80% of affected patients. Women with classic migraine (migraine with aura) may experience their initial onset during pregnancy.

Clinical Findings

Most often, the patient has a history of migraine headaches, which usually are described as "pounding" and may settle in the eyes, the temporal region, or occiput. The pain can be unilateral or bilateral. Frequently, migraines are associated with gastrointestinal complaints (eg, nausea, vomiting, and diarrhea) or with systemic symptoms (eg, vertigo or syncope). Light sensitivity (photophobia) and noise sensitivity (sonophobia) often accompany the pain. An aura may or may not precede the headache, but it is the most common visual phenomenon. Sleep often aborts the attack.

Diagnosis

The diagnosis of migraine headaches usually is made clinically by the characteristics of the pain, associated symptoms, event triggers (see below), and absence of neurologic signs. Tension and caffeine withdrawal headaches typically are associated with bandlike pressure pain. If vertigo is associated with migraine headaches, it is important to rule out Ménière's disease (labyrinthitis). In the latter, vertigo is accompanied by tinnitus, a fluctuating sensorineural hearing loss, and nystagmus. If vertigo is associated with ataxia of gait, it is almost always central in origin, in which case head trauma, brain tumors, seizure disorders, and multiple sclerosis must be excluded. Syncope (fainting) may occur with migraine or vascular headaches and is common during pregnancy. However, when syncope occurs with migraine headache, it usually is associated with vertigo. Rarely, ocular nerve palsy develops in association with migraine headaches; the third cranial nerve is the most commonly involved, and the palsy usually disappears with abatement of the migraine. It is important to visualize the optic disk to ensure that cerebrospinal fluid pressure is not increased. In cases where the disk borders are not sharp, *pseudotumor cerebri* or an intracranial mass lesion should be considered first.

Treatment

Treatment of migraine headaches initially includes identification of any trigger that precipitates attacks, followed by avoidance of those triggers. Common triggers for some migraine patients include missing meals, stress, aged cheeses, sausage or other nitrates, chocolate, citrus fruit, wine and other sulfites, monosodium glutamate, strong odors, lights or glare, and inadequate sleep. When this environmental manipulation fails to control migraines, drug therapy is indicated. Migraine therapy is either abortive or prophylactic depending on the frequency and severity of attacks. Preferred abortive medications during pregnancy include acetaminophen, acetaminophen and codeine or other narcotics, and magnesium. The following are more effective migraine abortive medications but are not preferred during pregnancy: butalbital, isometheptene, caffeine, aspirin, naproxen, ibuprofen, and triptan drugs (eg, sumatriptan). The nonsteroidal anti-inflammatory drugs should not be used for prolonged periods and should be avoided in the third trimester because of possible oligohydramnios or premature closure of the ductus arteriosus. Prophylactic medications should be instituted if abortive therapy is only partially effective and if disabling migraines are occurring more than once per week. Options include beta mimetic blockers, low-dose tricyclic antidepressants, calcium channel blockers, magnesium, riboflavin, and topiramate. Valproic acid or divalproate should be avoided in pregnancy.

Complications & Prognosis

Migraine headaches usually have no deleterious long-term effect on mother or fetus, and treatment of acute exacerbation usually is successful.

EPILEPSY AND SEIZURE DISORDERS

Epilepsy is defined as 2 or more unprovoked seizures and is different from eclamptic seizures sometimes seen during pregnancy. Seizures associated with epilepsy can be generalized convulsive (tonic-clonic or grand mal), complex partial (loss of awareness or staring with mild motor movements), focal motor or sensory (Jacksonian with no loss of awareness, absence or petit mal (brief eye blinking with no postictal confusion), myoclonic jerks, or auras of déjà vu, fear, or abnormal odors. The onset of epilepsy is not increased during pregnancy. More than 95% of patients who have seizures during pregnancy have a history of epilepsy or have been receiving anticonvulsant therapy. Patients whose seizures are adequately controlled are not likely to experience a deterioration of their condition during pregnancy. On the other hand, patients who have experienced frequent and uncontrolled seizures before pregnancy likely will experience the same pattern, particularly during early pregnancy.

Clinical Findings

A detailed history from the patient and observers helps to distinguish true seizures from other forms of loss of consciousness, such as syncopal episodes, hysteric attacks, or hyperventilation. These problems do not commonly involve a postictal confusional state, nor do they usually involve loss of bladder or bowel control or tongue biting. Noncentral nervous system causes, such as hypoxia, hypoglycemia, hypocalcemia, and hyponatremia, also must be excluded. Finally, seizures may result from drug withdrawal, medications, or exposure to toxic substances; thus, appropriate physical examination and screening for toxic substances are important in patients suffering an apparent first seizure during pregnancy.

Diagnosis

Detailed neurologic work-up is required in patients whose first seizure occurs during pregnancy. Electroencephalogram (EEG), CT scan with shielding or MRI, and lumbar puncture are useful for detailing the cause of the seizure and are not contraindicated during pregnancy. In established epilepsy, EEG is useful to confirm the type of epilepsy and therefore provide the appropriate drug therapy.

Treatment

Treatment of epilepsy should consist of the medication that has been most beneficial for the patient and at the lowest possible dose to maintain seizure control with some caveats. Some antiepileptic agents are more likely to cause birth defects than are others, and attempts to change medications should be made prior to conception.

During pregnancy, anticonvulsant levels change as a result of decreased protein binding, increased plasma volume, and alterations in the absorption and excretion of drugs. In addition, lamotrigine, phenytoin, phenobarbital, and carbamazepine have an increased plasma clearance that probably is related to high hepatic metabolism. These factors most often lead to low antiseizure plasma levels. Noncompliance, morning sickness, and hyperemesis gravidarum are other reasons for low drug levels. Therefore, blood level measurements of antiseizure medications are used to monitor and maintain a therapeutic range. Levels should be checked at least each trimester and prior to delivery. More frequent monitoring may be needed. Because of decreased protein binding, serum free drug levels rather than routine serum levels will be more accurate. Breakthrough seizures can result from poor sleep in the third trimester because the patient cannot obtain a comfortable sleeping position. For patients with refractory seizures while taking medication, an attempt should be made to maximize the dosage and the level of 1 medication before switching or adding another agent.

In patients with status epilepticus, control of seizures is mandatory for the safety of the patient and fetus. Lorazepam 2 mg IV push followed by 2 mg IV every minute up to 0.1 mg/kg is first-line treatment. If seizures continue, phenytoin 20 mg/kg slow IV push at a rate of 50 mg/min or fosphenytoin 20 phenytoin equivalents/kg IV at 150 phenytoin equivalents/min can be given intravenously. General anesthesia can be considered if seizures persist. In these cases, cerebral edema almost invariably is present and may be reduced with dexamethasone, mannitol, or hyperventilation. Many cases of status epilepticus in pregnancy are the result of inadequate treatment with antiepileptic drugs, abrupt withdrawal of phenobarbital or benzodiazepines, noncompliance, or failure to monitor serum levels.

Complications & Prognosis

Antiepileptic drugs and seizures can negatively affect a fetus. Seizures can cause maternal and fetal injury, spontaneous abortion, premature labor, and fetal bradycardia. All antiepileptic drugs cross the placenta, equilibrate rapidly in cord blood, and may have teratogenic effects. The risk of anomalies among infants exposed to anticonvulsants is approximately 2-fold greater than in the general population. The previous thinking that women with seizure disorders had an increased risk of fetal malformations even without exposure to anticonvulsant medication has been disproved. The most common defects fall into 2 categories: major and minor malformations. Major malformations include orofacial clefts, neural tube defects, and congenital heart disease. Minor malformations consists of craniofacial anomalies (low-set ears, widely spaced eyes, etc), short neck, and hypoplastic fingernails. The *fetal hydantoin syndrome* (associated with phenytoin) was the first described association between antiepileptic drugs and birth defects. It affects 3–5% of exposed offspring. It is characterized by mental retardation, small-for–gestational-age size, craniofacial anomalies, and limb defects. A milder phenytoin-associated syndrome may be present at a greater frequency (8–15%) but is detectable only by careful assessment during the first 3 years of life. Use of trimethadione in pregnancy has been abandoned given the high rate of anomalies (up to 30%) associated with intrauterine trimethadione exposure.

The teratogenic potential of specific antiepileptic agents has been the subject of much debate. Prospective pregnancy registries have been established around the world to clarify the risks. The older anticonvulsants—ethosuximide, carbamazepine, phenobarbital, valproic acid, primidone, and phenytoin—are all pregnancy category D because of known increased risk of birth defects in exposed fetuses. Neural tube defects are most common with carbamazepine (0.5–1%) and valproic acid (1–2%). The North American AED (antiepileptic drug) Pregnancy Registry has determined that the overall major malformation rate with exposure to valproic acid is 10.7%. Other pregnancy registries and studies have found the teratogenic potential of valproic acid increases with doses higher than 1000 mg/d or levels higher than 70 μg/mL. Besides neural tube defects, hypospadia, polydactyly, and kidney and heart malformation have been associated with valproic acid, so its use during pregnancy should be avoided if possible. Phenobarbital, previously believed to be safe during pregnancy, has a malformation rate of 6.5%, which is slightly higher than the approximately 3% rate of other antiepileptic drugs such as carbamazepine, phenytoin, and lamotrigine. Less human data on the newer antiepileptic drugs are available, with the exception of lamotrigine and oxcarbazepine. All newer antiepileptic drugs are category C, but more data are needed before they can be deemed safe.

Treatment with 2 or more antiseizure medications approximately doubles the risk for malformations.

Women with existing seizure disorders who are contemplating pregnancy should be tested to determine whether they still require anticonvulsant therapy—particularly if anticonvulsants were started during childhood or if the patient has been seizure-free for 2–5 years. If a pregnant woman requires seizure medication, she should be informed of the likelihood of fetal anomalies associated with each drug, and a discussion regarding the risks and benefits of attempting to switch to a different or safer drug, if available, should ensue. The patient should be counseled regarding folic acid supplementation (4 mg/d) starting at least 3 months preconceptionally to possibly reduce the chance of neural tube defects.

If the patient is taking an antiseizure medication metabolized by the P450 liver enzyme system, she should take vitamin K 10 mg/d from week 36 until delivery to prevent hemorrhage in her baby. This is in addition to the intramuscular vitamin K the infant will receive after delivery.

Antiepileptic drugs pass into the breast milk to varying degrees, depending on protein binding characteristics. The benefits of breast milk usually outweigh the small risk from the medication to the infant. If a breastfed infant is too sedated and not feeding well, presumably from the medication in the breast milk, breastfeeding should be suspended and supplanted with formula.

Mothers with frequent seizures must be counseled on seizure and infant safety. Sponge baths instead of tub baths and use of a strap on the changing table will decrease potential injury to an infant in case of a maternal seizure.

MULTIPLE SCLEROSIS

Multiple sclerosis is an autoimmune demyelinating process in the white matter of the central nervous system. It affects women twice as often as men and usually has its onset between the ages of 20 and 40 years. People in the Northern Hemisphere are more commonly af-

fected. The cause is not known, but possible etiologies include environmental, viral, and genetic.

Clinical Findings

The 2 patterns of disease are relapsing remitting and primary progressive. Findings include weakness in the extremities, sensory loss, difficulty with coordination, and visual problems. Increased reflexes, spasticity, and bladder control problems develop over time. Myasthenia gravis should be ruled out with an anticholinesterase (neostigmine) challenge and acetylcholine receptor antibody testing. Guillain-Barré syndrome should be ruled out if the patient has a history of recent viral infection.

Diagnosis

Laboratory tests and imaging should be performed to rule out other possible etiologies. Serum should be checked for vitamin B_{12}, Lyme and HTLV-1 (human T-cell lymphotropic virus type 1) titers, erythrocyte sedimentation rate (ESR), ANA, and rheumatoid factor. An MRI would reveal lesions (plaques) in the white matter of the brain and spinal cord. Active plaques would enhance with contrast materials. An elevated level of immunoglobulin (Ig)G in the cerebrospinal fluid is virtually diagnostic.

Treatment

Treatment options include interferon beta-1a, interferon beta-1b, and glatiramer. These medications decrease relapse rates, decrease disease activity as measured by serial MRI, and decrease disease progression. The interferon beta-1b and 1a multiple sclerosis trials showed an increased rate of spontaneous abortions of exposed fetuses. Although the increased rate did not reach statistical significance, there is good reason for caution. In patients planning to become pregnant, interferon treatment should be switched to glatiramer until conception then discontinued once pregnancy is established. Symptomatic treatment of spasticity, pain, fatigue, and bowel and bladder dysfunction will be required as well. Intravenous immunoglobulin (IVIG) has been used in the postpartum period to decrease the risk of exacerbation with some success. Short courses of corticosteroids may be helpful if the patient has optic neuritis or other disabling relapse.

Complications & Prognosis

The disease is characterized by exacerbations and remissions, with 70% of patients experiencing slow progression over a number of years. Pregnancy does not appear to exert any deleterious effect on multiple sclerosis and may improve the rate of exacerbation. The risk of exacerbations is increased in the first 3 months postpartum. Family planning should be discussed because of the progressive nature of the disease. If so desired, families should be completed or started as soon as possible.

MYASTHENIA GRAVIS

Myasthenia gravis is a chronic disorder of the neuromuscular junction of striate muscles as result of acetylcholine receptor dysfunction. Antibodies to acetylcholine receptors usually are present. It occurs more commonly in females than in males, and its peak occurrence is in the third decade of life. It is characterized by abnormal voluntary muscle function with muscle weakness after repeated effort. Although some cases of myasthenia gravis appear to be hereditary, most adult cases appear to be acquired.

Clinical Findings

The most common symptom is easily fatigued small muscles, most frequently the ocular muscles, which results in double vision. Weakness usually increases as the muscles are used repeatedly. Patients who may not have noticeable symptoms in the morning may be easily diagnosed in the afternoon. Difficulties with swallowing and speech are not uncommon, and the facial muscles are almost always affected.

Diagnosis

The diagnosis can be confirmed by administering edrophonium (Tensilon; a total of 10 mg, consisting of 2 mg followed by 8 mg 45 seconds later) to assess improvement in muscular weakness. A radioimmunoassay for the acetylcholine receptor antibody can be performed. Repetitive nerve stimulation would show a decrement greater than 15% in a person with the condition.

Treatment

Treatment with anticholinesterases (eg, neostigmine) is the same as in the nonpregnant state, although dosages must be administered more frequently during pregnancy. Other treatment options include thymectomy, steroids, plasma exchange, and IVIG. During labor, anticholinesterases should be administered parenterally rather than orally. Parenteral and regional anesthesia are not contraindicated in labor. Curarelike agents (eg, aminoglycoside antibiotics) and magnesium sulfate, as well as the older general anesthetics such as ether and chloroform, should be avoided. Women taking anticholinesterase drugs are advised not to breastfeed.

Complications & Prognosis

One-third of pregnant patients with myasthenia experience exacerbation, one-third do not change, and one-third have a remission. The disease does not affect uterine activity because the uterus consists of smooth muscle. The length of labor is not affected. However, an assisted second stage might be considered because of maternal fatigue. Exacerbations are most common during the postpartum period. Placental transfer of acetylcholine receptor antibodies can occur, so the fetus should be monitored at frequent intervals during pregnancy with fetal kick counts and ultrasound. A rare finding in neonates is arthrogryposis multiplex congenita, congenital contractures secondary to lack of movement in utero. Antibodies may affect the fetal diaphragm and lead to pulmonary hypoplasia and polyhydramnios. From 12–15% of newborns will be affected with transient myasthenia gravis. The mean duration of neonatal symptoms is 3 weeks.

SPINAL CORD DISORDERS

Spinal cord lesions that are caused by trauma, tumor, infection, or vascular disorders usually do not prevent conception. Diagnosis and therapy should be performed without regard to pregnancy. In general, pregnancy coexisting with trauma to the spinal cord from any cause, even paraplegia, proceeds unremarkably with the exception of an increased frequency of urinary tract infections and sepsis from pressure necrosis of the skin. Fetal growth usually is unimpeded even though initial maternal weight is frequently < 100 lb because of muscular wasting. Generally labor proceeds without evidence of fetopelvic disproportion. Women whose paraplegia is related to anterior horn cell damage or to cord lesions below the tenth thoracic level have appropriate perception of labor contractions and may require analgesia or anesthesia. In most patients, rapid, painless labors are the rule, with the only abnormality being a prolonged second stage because of decreased muscular effort. Paraplegic patients may develop autonomic hyperreflexia during labor due to loss of central regulation of the sympathetic nervous system below the level of the lesion. This is best managed with an epidural, continuous monitoring of the cardiac rhythm and blood pressures, and an assisted second stage.

DISORDERS OF CRANIAL NERVES

Palsies of the facial nerve due to inflammation are called *Bell's palsy*. Although patients may complain of paresthesia over the area of paralysis, this is strictly a motor disorder involving paralysis of the muscles of facial expression on 1 side that are innervated by the facial nerve. Given that approximately one-fifth of cases of Bell's palsy occur during pregnancy or shortly thereafter, it has been suggested that pregnancy increases the frequency of this disorder, although viral infections also have been causally related. Treatment with corticosteroids (prednisone 40–60 mg/d) and acyclovir is helpful if given within 1 week of onset. However, Bell's palsy usually is self-limited. Because the patient is unable to blink or close her eye on the affected side, corneal damage will occur if frequent eye drops and nighttime closure of the eye with patches and lubrication are not instituted. Rarely is surgical decompression of the nerve indicated.

GUILLAIN-BARRÉ SYNDROME

Guillain-Barré syndrome is an acute inflammatory demyelinating polyneuropathy often related to an upper respiratory or gastrointestinal infection or recent immunization. Rapid onset of weakness occurs, most frequently in an ascending pattern involving the extremities first then respiratory muscles and face. Hospitalization is required and supportive treatment aimed at preventing respiratory failure is mandatory. If the vital respiratory capacity falls to 800 mL or below, tracheostomy should be performed. Plasmapheresis or IVIG is the treatment of choice to shorten the course of illness. Most patients progress normally through pregnancy and deliver at term, so abortion is not mandated. On the other hand, if respiratory paralysis occurs near term, cesarean delivery may be indicated to improve ventilation.

PERIPHERAL NEUROPATHIES

Carpal tunnel syndrome is a neuropathic disorder related to median nerve compression by swelling of the tissue in the synovial sheaths at the wrist. Symptoms usually are limited to paresthesia over the thumb, index, and middle fingers and the medial portion of the ring finger. Most commonly, symptoms are noted at night and usually are best treated conservatively with elevation of the affected wrist and splinting. The syndrome usually abates postpartum. Surgery and corticosteroids are rarely indicated.

Compression of the femoral or obturator nerve can occur from retraction at the time of cesarean delivery or hysterectomy, but it is most commonly related to pressure of the fetus just before and during vaginal delivery. Femoral nerve palsy results in weakness of the iliopsoas and quadriceps muscles and sensory loss over the anterior thigh. Obturator nerve palsy is characterized by adduction weakness of the thigh and minimal sensory loss over the medial aspect of the affected limb. *Peroneal neuropathy* reveals footdrop and weakness on dorsiflexion of the foot, occasionally with paresthesia in the foot and second toes. This disorder usually appears 1–2 days postpartum and may be related to prolonged episiotomy repair and to pressure on the nerve from knee stirrups. Women at risk include small women with relatively large babies, those who have had midforceps rotations, and those who have had prolonged labor, especially with abnormally large infants (owing to compression of the L4–5 lumbosacral nerve trunk). The prognosis is excellent with conservative therapy, but occasionally a short leg brace is necessary.

Brachialgia or the *thoracic outlet syndrome* occurs when the brachial plexus and subclavian artery are compressed by the clavicle and first rib. Occurrence in pregnancy is increased because of the greater weight of the breasts and abdomen. The pain is referred to the lateral aspect of the hand and forearm, although motor symptoms are rare. Blanching of the fingers and exacerbation of symptoms when the hands are elevated are diagnostic. The syndrome usually is self-limited; posture instruction and strengthening of shoulder suspension muscles are helpful. Surgical removal of the rib is very occasionally necessary (as in the nonpregnant patient).

Herniation of intervertebral disks occurs more commonly in the lumbar than the cervical region. There are both motor and sensory findings along the distribution of the sciatic nerve. It is limited to 1 extremity and must be differentiated from more serious disorders such as spinal cord tumors and hemorrhage. Diagnosis usually can be made by physical examination and history. MRI of the spine is the best diagnostic modality if needed. Conservative management with bedrest and physical therapy is helpful. The process should cause no problems during pregnancy or vaginal delivery unless the patient has cervical disk disease. In that event, cesarean delivery is advised to prevent herniation and paralysis. Surgical correction should be avoided during pregnancy if possible.

■ AUTOIMMUNE DISORDERS

RHEUMATOID ARTHRITIS

Rheumatoid arthritis is a chronic autoimmune disease characterized by symmetric inflammatory synovitis. The prevalence in North America is 0.5–3.8%, and it occurs 3 times more frequently in women. Symptoms of rheumatoid arthritis are insidious, with a prodrome of fatigue, weakness, generalized joint stiffness, and myalgias preceding the appearance of joint swelling. The course is variable and unpredictable, with spontaneous remissions and exacerbations. Laboratory findings are mild leukocytosis, elevated ESR (which may not always reflect the activity of the disease), and a positive rheumatoid factor (in the majority of patients).

Treatment consists of rest, anti-inflammatory drugs, splints, physical therapy, a well-balanced diet, and adequate movement of all joints. Cyclooxygenase (COX)-1 and COX-2 inhibitors should be avoided in pregnancy. If they are used, therapy should be limited to short courses prior to 32 weeks' gestation to avoid premature closure of the ductus arteriosus. The amniotic fluid index should be followed for oligohydramnios. Low-dose oral corticosteroid therapy or hydroxychloroquine can be substituted safely for COX inhibitors. Tumor necrosis factor (TNF)-α inhibitors, penicillamine, gold, and methotrexate should be avoided. Symptoms improve during pregnancy in approximately 75% of women. However, many patients relapse within 6 months postpartum. The activity of the disease during pregnancy is best followed by assessment of duration of morning stiffness and the number of joints involved. Levels of Ro/SS$_A$ and La/SS$_B$ antibodies should be obtained to determine the fetal risk for complete heart block. In cases of severe postpartum exacerbation, early termination of breastfeeding may be necessary early in order to allow the full range of pharmacologic therapy, including TNF-α inhibitors.

SYSTEMIC LUPUS ERYTHEMATOSUS

Systemic lupus erythematosus (SLE) is an multisystem autoimmune disorder with a wide spectrum of disease manifestations. It is of interest to obstetricians because it predominantly affects women (10:1) of reproductive age. The diagnosis can be made when 4 of the following criteria are present: malar rash, discoid rash, photosensitivity, oral ulcers, serositis, renal disorders, neurologic disorders, hematologic disorders (hemolytic anemia, leukopenia, thrombocytopenia), immunologic disorders (anti-DNA, anti-SM, false-positive Venereal Disease Research Laboratory [VDRL] test), or an abnormal ANA titer. Common serologic markers of SLE are present 5 years before the diagnosis is made in up to 50% of women. Complications of pregnancy characteristic of SLE may precede the clinical diagnosis by many years as well. The differential diagnosis includes rheumatoid arthritis, drug-induced SLE syndromes, polyarteritis, chronic active hepatitis, and, late in pregnancy, preeclampsia. Common symptoms at presentation in pregnancy are malaise, fever, myalgias, and weight loss.

Management during pregnancy includes a careful history, physical examination, and laboratory evaluation. A history of prior spontaneous abortions or fetal losses should be elicited. The history should note the manifestations of SLE in the past; determination of the severity of disease activity is important in anticipating pregnancy complications. Although the fertility rate of patients with SLE is normal, patients have a higher percentage of total fetal losses. This may be associated with the presence of antiphospholipid antibodies. Physical examination should focus on signs of active disease. Laboratory evaluation should include a complete blood count, serum chemistries, and liver function tests. ANA (if the diagnosis is not previously confirmed), double-stranded DNA, urine protein, C3, C4, and CH$_{50}$ tests should be obtained. Subse-

quent changes in these values may herald a flare of lupus nephritis. The results of the SS$_A$, lupus anticoagulant, anticardiolipin antibody, and anti-β$_2$ glycoprotein I tests should be known. The presence of SS$_A$ is associated with neonatal lupus, manifested by cutaneous lesions or congenital heart block. Anticardiolipin antibody and lupus anticoagulant anti-beta 2 glycoprotein 1 tests are associated with antiphospholipid antibody syndrome (APS), which predisposes patients to thromboembolic events, fetal death, fetal growth restriction, and preeclampsia. Prophylactic treatment with daily baby aspirin and heparin is recommended when APS is diagnosed. Diagnostic criteria require a clinical event (as listed above) plus a positive lupus anticoagulant result or moderate- to high-titer anticardiolipin antibody (> 20 GPL or MPL) or a positive anti-beta 2 glycoprotein 1. These tests should be positive on two occasions 12 weeks apart. Most fetal loss in SLE appears to be due to concomitant APS, which occurs in approximately 30% of patients.

Considerable controversy exists about the effects of pregnancy on SLE and vice versa. Most patients who become pregnant while their SLE is not active for at least 6 months seem to have few problems except for a 2-to 3-fold increased risk of superimposed preeclampsia and fetal growth restriction; the risk of a lupus flare is 20%. Women with active SLE are at very high risk for superimposed preeclampsia (60–80%), fetal growth restriction, preterm birth, and lupus flare (50–80%). Women with preexisting renal disease frequently have some deterioration in renal function, but it is irreversible in only 10% of cases.

Distinguishing between superimposed preeclampsia in the third trimester and an SLE flare often is difficult. In fact, it is not possible to say with certainty that preeclampsia is not present, but careful consideration can suggest whether an SLE flare is a contributing factor. In a pregnancy remote from term, aggressive empiric therapy of presumed SLE may allow significant prolongation of pregnancy.

Serial ultrasounds for fetal growth and antenatal testing starting at 32–34 weeks should be instituted to ensure fetal well-being. Delivery is often recommended at 38–39 weeks' gestation. Uterine artery Doppler at midgestation can be used to predict early-onset preeclampsia and fetal growth restriction.

The mainstay of treatment of SLE in pregnancy consists of corticosteroids, hydroxychloroquine, and azathioprine. Corticosteroids appear to a weak teratogens resulting in 1 extra facial cleft for every 1000 first-trimester exposures. Thereafter is a risk of premature rupture of membranes (PROM) and preterm birth, but usually after 34 weeks' gestation. Little information on the use of newer agents, such as mycophenolate, is available. The chance of successful pregnancy outcome for women with SLE has improved dramatically over the years with better understanding of the natural history of the disease and medical therapy in pregnancy.

SCLERODERMA

Pregnancy in patients with scleroderma is rare, as the disorder occurs most frequently in patients beyond reproductive age. Symptoms appear to improve or remain unchanged. One study did show an increase in preterm births. Pregnancy progresses normally in otherwise stable disease. When scleroderma-related renal disease and hypertension are present, pregnancy can be complicated by malignant hypertension.

REFERENCES

Disorders of the Nervous System

Cunnington M, Tennis P, International Lamotrigine Pregnancy Registry Scientific Advisory Committee: Lamotrigine and the risk of malformations in pregnancy. Neurology 2005;64:955.

Donaldson JO: *Neurology of Pregnancy,* 2nd ed. WB Saunders, 1989.

Holmes LB, Wyszynski DF: North American Antiepileptic Drug Pregnancy Registry. *Epilepsia* 2004;45:1465.

Holms LB et al: The teratogenicity of anticonvulsant drugs. N Engl J Med 2001;344:1132.

Horton JC et al: Pregnancy and the risk of hemorrhage from cerebral arteriovenous malformations. Neurosurgery 1990;27:867.

Isla A et al: Brain tumors and pregnancy. Obstet Gynecol 1997;89:19.

Loder E: Safety of sumatriptan in pregnancy: a review of the data so far. CNS Drugs 2003;17:1.

Marcus DA, Scharff L, Turk D: Longitudinal prospective study of headache during pregnancy and postpartum. Headache 1999;39:625.

May JL, Lamy C: Stroke in pregnancy and the puerperium. J Neurol 1998;245:305.

Morrell M: Guidelines for the care of women with epilepsy. Neurology 1998;51(Suppl 5):S21.

Nei M, Daly S, Liporace J: A maternal complex partial seizure in labor can affect fetal heart rate. Neurology 1998;51:904.

Orvieto R et al: Pregnancy and multiple sclerosis: a 2-year experience. Eur J Obstet Gynecol Reprod Biol 1999;82:191.

Paonessa K, Fernand R: Spinal cord injury and pregnancy. Spine 1991;16:596.

Roelvink NC et al: Pregnancy-related primary brain and spinal tumors. Arch Neurol 1987;44:209.

Sances G et al: Course of migraine during pregnancy and postpartum: a prospective study. Cephalalgia 2003;23:197.

Sandberg-Wollheim M et al: Pregnancy outcomes during treatment with interferon beta-1a in patients with multiple sclerosis. Neurology 2005;65:802.

Wand JS: Carpal tunnel syndrome in pregnancy and lactation. J Hand Surg [Br] 1990;15:93.

Wiltin AG, Mattar F, Sibai BM: Postpartum stroke: a twenty-year experience. Am J Obstet Gynecol 2000;183:83.

Wyszynski DF et al, Antiepileptic Drug Pregnancy Registry: Increased rate of major malformations in offspring exposed to valproate during pregnancy. Neurology 2005;64:961.

Autoimmune Disorders

Arbuckle MR et al: Development of autoantibodies before the clinical onset of systemic lupus erythematosus. N Engl J of Med 2003;349:1526.

Cimaz R et al: Incidence and spectrum of neonatal lupus erythematosus: a prospective study of infants born to mothers with anti-Ro autoantibodies. J Pediatr 2003;142:678.

Clark CA et al: Decrease in pregnancy loss rates in patients with systemic lupus erythematosus over a 40-year period. J Rheumatol 2005;32:1709.

Clowse ME et al: Early risk factors for pregnancy loss in lupus. Obstet Gynecol 2006;107:293.

Clowse ME et al: The impact of increased lupus activity on obstetric outcomes. Arthritis Rheum 2005;52:514.

Doria A et al: Pregnancy, cytokines, and disease activity in systemic lupus erythematosus. Arthritis Rheum 2004;51:989.

Erkan D et al: Real world experience with antiphospholipid antibody tests: how stable are results over time? Ann Rheum Dis 2005;64:1321.

Janssen NM, Genta MS: The effects of immunosuppressive and anti-inflammatory medications on fertility, pregnancy and lactation. Arch Intern Med 2000;160:610.

Lansink M et al: The onset of rheumatoid arthritis in relation to pregnancy and childbirth. Clin Exp Rheumatol 1993;11:171.

Lassere M, Empson M: Treatment of antiphospholipid syndrome in pregnancya– systematic review of randomized therapeutic trials. Thromb Res 2004;114:419.

Miyakis S et al: International consensus statement on an update of the classification criteria for definite antiphospholipid syndrome (APS). J Thromb Haemost 2006;4:295.

Morgan GJ Jr, Chow WS: Clinical features, diagnosis, and prognosis in rheumatoid arthritis. Curr Opin Rheumatol 1993;5:184.

Ollier WE, Harrison B, Symmons D: What is the natural history of rheumatoid arthritis? Best Pract Res Clin Rheumatol 2001;15:27.

Sampaio-Barros PD et al: Gynecologic history in systemic sclerosis. Clin Rheumatol 2000;19:184.

Steen V: Pregnancy in women with systemic sclerosis. Obstet Gynecol 1999;94:15.

Venkat-Raman N et al: Uterine artery Doppler in predicting pregnancy outcome in women with antiphospholipid syndrome. Obstet Gynecol 2001;98:235.

Witter FR, Petri M: Antenatal detection of intrauterine growth restriction in patients with systemic lupus erythematosus. Int J Gynecol Obstet 2000;71:67.

Yasmeen S et al: Pregnancy outcomes in women with systemic lupus erythematosus. J Matern-Fetal Med 2001;10:91.

Hematologic Disorders in Pregnancy 26

Christina Arnett, MD, & Jeffrey S. Greenspoon, MD

ANEMIA

Anemia is a significant maternal problem during pregnancy. The Centers for Disease Control defines anemia as a hemoglobin concentration of less than 11 g/dL (hematocrit of < 33%) in the first or third trimester or a hemoglobin concentration of less than 10.5 g/dL (hematocrit < 32%) in the second trimester. A pregnant woman will lose blood during delivery and the puerperium, and an anemic woman is at increased jeopardy of blood transfusion and its related complications.

During pregnancy, the blood volume increases by approximately 50% and the red blood cell mass by approximately 33%. This relatively greater increase in plasma volume results in a lower hematocrit but does not truly represent anemia.

Anemia in pregnancy most commonly results from a nutritional deficiency in either iron or folate. Pernicious anemia due to vitamin B_{12} deficiency almost never occurs during pregnancy. Other anemias occurring during pregnancy include anemia of chronic disease; anemia due to hemoglobinopathy; immune, chronic (eg, hereditary spherocytosis or paroxysmal nocturnal hemoglobinuria), or drug-induced hemolytic anemia; and aplastic anemia.

1. Iron Deficiency Anemia

Iron deficiency is responsible for approximately 95% of the anemias during pregnancy, reflecting the increased demands for iron. The total body iron consists mostly of (1) iron in hemoglobin (approximately 70% of total iron; approximately 1700 mg in a 56-kg woman) and (2) iron stored as ferritin and hemosiderin in reticuloendothelial cells in bone marrow, the spleen, and parenchymal cells of the liver (approximately 300 mg). Small amounts of iron exist in myoglobin, plasma, and various enzymes. The absence of hemosiderin in the bone marrow indicates that iron stores are depleted. This finding is both diagnostic of anemia and an early sign of iron deficiency. Subsequent events are a decrease in serum iron, an increase in serum total iron-binding capacity, and anemia.

During the first half of pregnancy, iron requirements may not be increased significantly, and iron absorbed from food (approximately 1 mg/d) is sufficient to cover the basal loss of 1 mg/d. However, in the second half of pregnancy, iron requirements increase due to expansion of red blood cell mass and rapid growth of the fetus. Increased numbers of red blood cells and a greater hemoglobin mass require approximately 500 mg of iron. The iron needs of the fetus average 300 mg. Thus, the additional amount of iron needed due to the pregnancy is approximately 800 mg. Data published by the Food and Nutrition Board of the National Academy of Sciences show that pregnancy increases a woman's iron requirements to approximately 3.5 mg/d. This need outstrips the 1 mg/d of iron available from the normal diet and must be met by supplementation of at least 40 mg/d of elemental iron (10% of which is absorbed).

Clinical Findings

A. Symptoms and Signs

The symptoms may be vague and nonspecific, including pallor, easy fatigability, headache, palpitations, tachycardia, and dyspnea. Angular stomatitis, glossitis, and koilonychia (spoon nails) may be present in long-standing severe anemia.

B. Laboratory Findings

The hemoglobin may fall as low as 3 g/dL, but the red cell count is rarely below $2.5 \times 10^6/mm^3$. The red cells usually are hypochromic and microcytic, with mean corpuscular volumes of less than 79 fL. Serum ferritin concentrations fall to less than 15 μg/dL and transferrin saturation to less than 16%. Serum iron levels usually are less than 60 μg/dL. The total iron-binding capacity is elevated in both normal pregnancies and pregnancies affected by iron deficiency anemia and therefore is of little diagnostic value by itself. The reticulocyte count is low for the degree of anemia. Platelet counts are frequently increased, but white cell counts are normal. Bone marrow biopsy demonstrates lack of stainable iron in marrow macrophages and erythroid precursors but usually is unnecessary in uncomplicated iron deficiency anemia.

Differential Diagnosis

Anemia due to chronic disease or an inflammatory process (eg, rheumatoid arthritis) may be hypochromic and microcytic. Anemia due to thalassemia trait can be differentiated from iron deficiency anemia by normal serum iron levels, the presence of stainable iron in the marrow, and elevated levels of hemoglobin A_2. Other less common causes of microcytic, hypochromic anemia include sideroblastic anemia and anemia due to lead poisoning.

Complications

Iron deficiency anemia normally does not endanger the pregnancy unless it is severe, in which case intrauterine growth retardation and preterm labor may result.

Angina pectoris or congestive heart failure may develop as a result of marked iron deficiency anemia. **Sideropenic dysphagia (Paterson-Kelly syndrome, Plummer-Vinson syndrome)** is a rare condition characterized by dysphagia, esophageal web, and atrophic glossitis due to long-standing severe iron deficiency anemia.

Prevention

During the course of pregnancy and the puerperium, at least 60 mg/d of elemental iron should be prescribed to prevent anemia.

Treatment

In an established case of anemia, prompt adequate treatment is necessary.

A. ORAL IRON THERAPY

Ferrous sulfate 300 mg (containing 60 mg of elemental iron, of which approximately 10% is absorbed) should be given 3 times per day. If this agent is not tolerated, ferrous fumarate or gluconate should be prescribed. Therapy should be continued for approximately 3 months after hemoglobin values return to normal in order to replenish iron stores. Hemoglobin levels should increase by at least 0.3 g/dL/wk if the patient is responding to therapy.

Iron is best absorbed in the ferrous or reduced form from an empty stomach. Administering ascorbic acid at the time of iron supplementation creates a mildly acidic environment that aids the absorption of iron.

B. PARENTERAL IRON THERAPY

The indication for parenteral iron is intolerance of, or refractoriness to, oral iron. In most cases of moderate iron deficiency anemia, the total iron requirements equal the amount of iron needed to restore hemoglobin levels to normal or near normal plus 50% of that amount to replenish iron stores.

Iron dextran is the most widely available parenteral iron preparation in the United States. Each 2-mL vial provides 100 mg of elemental iron. After a 0.5-mL

test dose, iron dextran can be administered intramuscularly or intravenously at a rate not to exceed 100 mg/d of elemental iron. Intramuscular injection must always be given into the muscle mass of the upper outer quadrant of the buttock with a 2-inch, 20-gauge needle, using the Z technique (ie, pulling the skin and superficial musculature to one side before inserting the needle to prevent leakage of the solution and subsequent tattooing of the skin). Intramuscular iron raises hemoglobin concentration only slightly faster than oral iron administration due to slow and occasionally incomplete mobilization of iron from the muscle. Risks of parenteral iron administration include anaphylactic reaction, muscle necrosis, and phlebitis.

2. Folic Acid Deficiency Anemia (Megaloblastic Anemia of Pregnancy)

Megaloblastic anemia of pregnancy is almost exclusively caused by folic acid deficiency and is common where nutrition is inadequate. In the United States, access to fresh vegetables and the fortification of grains makes folate deficiency much less common than in the developing world.

In the nonpregnant woman, the minimum daily intake of folate necessary for adequate hematopoiesis and to maintain stores is 50 mg. However, this requirement increases during pregnancy. In order to meet this need and to decrease the neural tube defects associated with folate deficiency, a dietary supplement of at least 400 mg/d of folic acid is recommended.

Additional folic acid may be required in states of heightened DNA synthesis, such as multifetal gestation. Similarly, patients with a chronic hemolytic anemia such as **sickle cell anemia** require additional folate supplementation in order to meet the demand imposed by increased hematopoiesis. Other hemolytic states are also commonly complicated by folic acid deficiency, including **hereditary spherocytosis** and **malaria.**

Folic acid absorption or metabolism may be impaired by the use of oral contraceptives, pyrimethamine, trimethoprim-sulfamethoxazole, primidone, phenytoin, or barbiturates. Alcohol consumption also interferes with folate metabolism. Jejunal bypass surgery for obesity or the malabsorption syndrome (sprue) may impair folic acid absorption.

Clinical Findings

A. SYMPTOMS AND SIGNS

The symptoms are nonspecific (eg, lassitude, anorexia, nausea and vomiting, diarrhea, and depression). Pallor often is not marked. Rarely, a sore mouth or tongue is present. Occasionally, purpura may be a clinical manifestation. Megaloblastic anemia should be suspected if iron deficiency anemia fails to respond to iron therapy.

B. LABORATORY FINDINGS

Folic acid deficiency results in a hematologic picture similar to that of true pernicious anemia (due to vitamin B_{12} deficiency), which is extremely rare in women of childbearing age.

The hemoglobin may be as low as 4–6 g/dL, and the red cell count may be less than 2 million/μL in severe cases. Extreme anemia often is associated with leukocytopenia and thrombocytopenia.

The red cells are macrocytic (mean corpuscular volume usually > 100 fL) and appear as macroovalocytes on peripheral blood smear. However, in pregnancy macrocytosis may be concealed by accompanying iron deficiency or thalassemia. Up to 70% of folate-deficient patients also lack iron stores.

Serum folate levels less than 4 ng/mL are suggestive of folic acid depletion in nonpregnant patients. However, in otherwise normal pregnant patients, folate tends to fall slowly to low levels (3–6 ng/mL) with advancing gestation. The red cell folate level in megaloblastic patients is lower, but in 30% of patients the values overlap. The peripheral white blood cells are hypersegmented. Seventy-five percent of folate-deficient patients have more than 5% neutrophils with 5 or more lobes, but this also may be true for 25% of normal pregnant patients.

The urinary excretion of formiminoglutamic acid (FIGLU) has been used to diagnose folate deficiency, but levels are abnormal only in severe megaloblastic anemia. Bone marrow aspirate demonstrates megaloblastic erythropoiesis but usually is not necessary for diagnosis. Serum iron and vitamin B_{12} levels should be normal.

Treatment

Folic acid 1–5 mg/d orally is continued for several weeks after delivery or for several weeks in patients diagnosed in the puerperium. This therapy produces the maximum hematologic response, replaces body stores, and provides the minimum daily requirements. The hematocrit should rise approximately 1% each day, beginning on day 5–6 of therapy. The reticulocyte count should become elevated after 3–4 days of therapy and is the earliest morphologic sign of response. Iron supplementation should be administered as indicated.

Prognosis

Megaloblastic anemia due to folate deficiency during pregnancy carries a good prognosis if adequately treated.

The anemia usually is mild unless associated with multifetal pregnancy, systemic infection, or hemolytic disease (eg, sickle cell anemia). Low birthweight as well as fetal neural tube defects are known to be associated with maternal folic acid deficiency. The associations with placental abruption, spontaneous abortion, and preeclampsia–eclampsia are not universally accepted. Even without treatment, anemia due to folate deficiency usually resolves after delivery when folate demands normalize.

3. Aplastic Anemia

Aplastic anemia with primary bone marrow failure during pregnancy is rare. The anemia may be secondary to exposure to known marrow toxins, such as chloramphenicol, phenylbutazone, mephenytoin, alkylating chemotherapeutic agents, or insecticides. In approximately two-thirds of cases, no obvious cause is detected. Idiopathic aplastic anemia in pregnancy may have a spontaneous remission following delivery or pregnancy termination but may recur in subsequent pregnancies. The condition likely is immunologically mediated.

Clinical Findings

The rapidly developing anemia causes pallor, fatigue, tachycardia, painful ulceration of the throat, and fever. The diagnostic criteria are pancytopenia and empty bone marrow on biopsy examination.

Complications

Aplastic anemia in pregnancy may cause increased fetal wastage, prematurity, or intrauterine fetal demise. Increased maternal morbidity and death usually are due to infection and hemorrhage.

Treatment

The patient must avoid any toxic agents known to cause aplastic anemia. Blood product replacement with packed red blood cells and platelets should be utilized as needed. In some cases, delivery or termination of pregnancy may be necessary. Bone marrow transplantation is performed if remission does not occur following delivery or termination of pregnancy. Other possible treatments include antithymocyte antibody, corticosteroids, or immunosuppressive agents. Infection must be treated aggressively with appropriate antibiotics, but most authorities do not recommend giving prophylactic antibiotics.

4. Drug-Induced Hemolytic Anemia

Drug-induced hemolytic anemia usually occurs as a result of drug-mediated immunologic red cell injury. For example, a drug can act as a hapten with an erythrocyte protein to which an antidrug antibody attaches. Hemolysis occurs as a result of the subsequent immune response. Many drugs used in pregnancy can have such an effect, including cephalosporins, acetaminophen, and erythromycin.

In African-American women, drug-induced hemolytic anemia is more likely caused by drug-induced oxidative damage rather than a drug-mediated immune mechanism. The most common congenital erythrocyte enzymatic defect to cause this condition is **glucose-6-phosphate dehydrogenase (G6PD) deficiency**. This X-linked disorder causes a heterozygous state in 10–15% of African-American females, but enzyme activity is variable due to random X-chromosome inactivation.

Decreased G6PD activity in one-third of patients in the third trimester causes an increased risk of hemolytic episodes. More than 40 substances toxic to susceptible people are recognized, including sulfonamides, nitrofurans, antipyretics, some analgesics, sulfones, vitamin K analogues, uncooked fava beans, some antimalarials, naphthalene, and nalidixic acid. Specific laboratory tests to identify susceptible individuals include a glutathione stability test and cresyl blue dye reduction test.

Clinical Findings

The red blood cell count and morphology are normal until hemolysis occurs. Levels of anemia are variable depending on the degree of hemolysis.

Complications

Exposure of the G6PD-deficient fetus to maternally ingested oxidant drugs (eg, sulfonamides) may produce fetal hemolysis, hydrops fetalis, and fetal death. A black pregnant woman probably should be screened for G6PD deficiency before starting sulfonamide therapy for urinary tract infection.

Treatment

Management includes immediate discontinuation of any suspected medications, treatment of intercurrent illness, and blood transfusion where indicated.

SICKLE CELL DISEASE

Sickle cell hemoglobin (hemoglobin S) results from a genetic substitution of valine for glutamic acid at codon 6 of the β-globin chains. Decreased oxygen tension causes hemoglobin S to form insoluble polymers in curvilinear strands. These polymers deform the normal biconcave structure of the erythrocyte. The process is reversible but eventually leads to cell membrane damage and permanent sickling.

Patients homozygous for the hemoglobin S gene have **sickle cell anemia (SS disease)**, and those who are heterozygous have **sickle cell trait.** Approximately 8–

10% of African-Americans carry the sickle cell trait, whereas approximately 1 in 500 has sickle cell anemia.

Other sickling syndromes exist when the gene for hemoglobin S is inherited along with the gene for another abnormal hemoglobin, such as hemoglobin C or thalassemia. Hemoglobin C, also caused by β-globin chain mutation, is less soluble than normal hemoglobin A and has a propensity to form hexagonal crystals. Women who are heterozygous for both the S and C genes have **hemoglobin SC disease.** Maternal mortality rates are as high as 2–3%. Hemoglobin SC disease is peculiarly associated with embolization of necrotic fat and cellular bone marrow with resultant respiratory insufficiency. Neurologic symptoms from fat embolism have been reported with sickle cell disease.

In **hemoglobin S/beta thalassemia disease,** the patient is heterozygous for both hemoglobin S and beta thalassemia. The severity of complications during pregnancy is related to hemoglobin S concentrations in this particular disease.

Prenatal genetic counseling is of great importance. If both partners have the gene for S hemoglobin, their offspring have a 1 in 4 chance of having sickle cell anemia. Fetal DNA isolated from amniotic fluid cells is most useful for prenatal diagnosis of hemoglobinopathy in cases at risk.

Clinical Findings

Sickle cell disease is characterized by chronic hemolytic anemia and intermittent crises of variable frequency and severity. Although persons with sickle cell trait are not anemic and usually are asymptomatic, they have twice as many urinary tract infections as normal women and are at higher risk for preeclampsia. Additionally, their red blood cells tend to sickle when oxygen tension is significantly lowered.

A. SYMPTOMS AND SIGNS

1. Chronic anemia—Chronic anemia results from the shortened survival time of the homozygous S red blood cells due to circulation trauma and intravascular hemolysis or phagocytosis by reticuloendothelial cells in the spleen and liver.

2. Sickling of red blood cells—Intravascular sickling leads to vasoocclusion and infarction. Small blood vessels supplying various organs and tissues can be partially or completely blocked by sickled erythrocytes, resulting in ischemia, pain, necrosis, and organ damage.

3. Crises—Crises of variable frequency and severity occur. **Pain crises** involve the bones and joints. They usually are precipitated by dehydration, acidosis, or infection. An **aplastic crisis** is characterized by rapidly developing anemia. The hemoglobin may be as low as 2–3 g/dL due to cessation of red blood cell production.

An **acute splenic sequestration** crisis is associated with severe anemia and hypovolemic shock, resulting from sudden massive trapping of red blood cells within the splenic sinusoids.

4. Other manifestations—Other manifestations include increased susceptibility to bacterial infection; bacterial pneumonia and pulmonary infarction; myocardial damage and cardiomegaly; and functional and anatomic renal abnormalities in the form of sickle cell nephropathy or papillary renal necrosis, resulting in hematuria. Central nervous system manifestations include headache, convulsions, hemorrhage, or thrombosis (from vasoocclusion). Ophthalmologic abnormalities include anoxic retinal damage, retinal detachments, vitreous hemorrhages, and proliferative retinopathy. Hepatosplenomegaly or cholelithiasis may occur.

B. LABORATORY FINDINGS

Sickle cell anemia is associated with serious risks for mother and fetus. Screening for abnormal hemoglobin is imperative in the population at risk. Two screening tests are in common use. The sodium metabisulfite test uses 1 drop of fresh 2% reagent mixed on a slide with 1 drop of blood. Sickling of most red cells will occur in a few minutes with both sickle cell trait and sickle cell disease. The Sickledex test is a simple solubility test that uses 20 μL of blood mixed with 2 mL of sodium dithionite reagent. Clouding of the solution indicates the presence of hemoglobin S. If the test is positive, the homozygous and heterozygous states must be differentiated by hemoglobin electrophoresis.

C. EFFECTS ON PREGNANCY

Pregnant women with sickle cell disease face increased rates of maternal mortality and morbidity from hemolytic and folic acid deficiency anemias, frequent crises, pulmonary complications, congestive heart failure, infection, and preeclampsia–eclampsia. It is encouraging, however, that maternal mortality has decreased to 1% since 1972. There is an increased incidence of early fetal wastage, stillbirth, preterm delivery, and fetal growth restriction.

Treatment

Optimal prenatal care, including prevention or rapid treatment of complications, is necessary to increase the chance for a good outcome. Pneumococcal polyvalent vaccine has been shown to reduce the incidence of pneumococcal infection in adults with sickle disease and therefore is highly recommended. This vaccine is not contraindicated in pregnancy. Similarly, influenza vaccine should be administered annually. Folic acid 1 mg/d will prevent megaloblastic anemia, which can result from intense hematopoiesis. Serial ultrasonic evaluations are essential to assess fetal growth. Antepartum testing should begin at 32–34 weeks' gestation. Careful surveillance for asymptomatic bacteriuria and demonstration of cure is important for preventing pyelonephritis. Regional anesthesia can be safely administered to patients with sickle cell disease while they are in labor.

In the management of crises, the most common predisposing factors—infection, dehydration, and hypoxia—should be evaluated and treated. Symptomatic treatment of pain crisis consists of intravenous fluid, oxygen supplementation, and adequate analgesics (eg, morphine). Bacterial pneumonia or pyelonephritis must be treated vigorously with intravenous antibiotics. Streptococcal pneumonia is common and is a serious complication. In all cases, adequate oxygenation must be maintained by face mask as necessary.

The concentration of hemoglobin S should be less than 50% of the total hemoglobin to prevent crisis. Blood transfusion should be considered in cases of a fall in hematocrit to less than 25%, but this decision must be guided by the individual patient history and her status during pregnancy. Important considerations are repeated crisis; symptoms of tachycardia, palpitation, dyspnea, or fatigue; and evidence of inadequate or retarded intrauterine growth.

Randomized controlled trials have shown that administration of prophylactic hypertransfusion or exchange transfusion is not necessary to prevent maternal and fetal complications, except in well-defined circumstances. Transfusion carries the risks of allergic reaction, delayed hemolytic reaction, isoimmunization, and transmission of infection.

Bone marrow transplant has been limited by the complications of infection and graft-versus-host disease but shows promise as a potential long-term solution to sickle cell anemia.

Prenatal diagnosis of sickle cell disease is possible using cells obtained from amniocentesis or chorionic villus sampling. Single-blastomere DNA analysis prior to in vitro fertilization has allowed for the successful transfer of unaffected embryos. In utero stem cell therapy with normal hemoglobin stem cells is a potential future treatment for affected fetuses.

THALASSEMIA

The thalassemias are genetically determined disorders of reduced synthesis of 1 or more of the structurally normal globin chains in hemoglobin. Thalassemia is found throughout the world but is concentrated in the Mediterranean coastal areas, central Africa, and parts of Asia. The high incidence in these regions may represent a balanced polymorphism due to heterozygous advantage.

All thalassemias are inherited as an autosomal recessive trait. The two major groups are the alpha and beta thalassemias, both of which affect the synthesis of hemoglobin A, which contains two α and two β chains. The severity of the anemia varies with the type of hemoglobin abnormality.

Pathophysiology

In beta thalassemia, hemoglobin β-chain synthesis is defective, but the α chains are produced normally; in alpha thalassemia, the reverse is true. The unbalanced synthesis results in a relative excess of the normally produced chain. The normal globin chains then form tetramers that precipitate within red blood cell precursors in the bone marrow, resulting in ineffective erythropoiesis, red cell sequestration and destruction, and hypochromic anemia. The most severe forms of this disorder may cause intrauterine or childhood death. A person who is heterozygous, or a carrier, for a thalassemia trait may be asymptomatic.

A. Alpha Thalassemia

The most severe form of alpha thalassemia compatible with extrauterine life is **hemoglobin H (β_4) disease,** which results from deletion of 3 of the 4 α-globin genes. In patients with this disease, some normal hemoglobin A ($\alpha_2\beta_2$) is produced because 1 of the α-globin genes is present, but the excess of β-globin changes causes the formation of hemoglobin H (β_4) as well. Anemia of variable levels results that usually is worsened in pregnancy.

In **alpha thalassemia minor,** 2 α-globin genes are deleted, causing a mild hypochromic, microcytic anemia that must be differentiated from iron deficiency anemia. Women with this condition tolerate pregnancy well.

B. Beta Thalassemia

Beta thalassemia results from impaired β-globin chain production. **Beta thalassemia major** is the homozygous state, in which there is little or no production of β chains. At birth, the neonate usually is asymptomatic because fetal hemoglobin F ($\alpha_2\gamma_2$) contains no β-globin chain. However, this protection disappears at birth, when fetal hemoglobin production terminates. At approximately 1 year of age, a baby with defective β-globin production usually begins to show signs of thalassemia (anemia, hepatosplenomegaly) and requires frequent blood transfusions. Affected individuals often die in their late teens or early 20s because of congestive heart failure, often related to myocardial hemosiderosis and liver failure. However, improved treatment with transfusion and iron chelation have led to overall improved survival and even to successful pregnancies in women with beta thalassemia major.

Beta thalassemia minor, the heterozygous state, is frequently diagnosed only after the patient fails to respond to iron therapy or delivers a baby with homozygous disease. Such patients usually suffer from mild to moderate hypochromic microcytic anemia, with increased red blood cell count, elevated hemoglobin A$_2$ ($\alpha_2\delta_2$)concentrations, increased serum iron levels, and iron saturation greater than 20%.

Suspected adult cases of thalassemia are diagnosed by hemoglobin electrophoresis. Antenatal diagnosis of thalassemia is now possible. Molecular hybridization measures the number of intact α-globin structural genes in fetal cells obtained by amniocentesis. Preimplantation genetic diagnosis allows for the transfer of unaffected embryos after in vitro fertilization.

LYMPHOMA & LEUKEMIA

1. Hodgkin's Disease

The lymphoma of Hodgkin's disease is the most common lymphoma to affect women of childbearing age. Even so, it is uncommon during pregnancy, affecting only approximately 1 in 6000.

Clinical Features

Patients may be asymptomatic or have fever, weight loss, and pruritus. The most common finding is peripheral lymphadenopathy. Histologic evaluation of the affected nodes establishes the diagnosis.

Careful staging is essential prior to the initiation of treatment with radiotherapy or chemotherapy. Modifications of standard staging modalities, such as the use of magnetic resonance imaging (MRI), can allow for adequate staging during pregnancy. However, some procedures, such as staging laparotomy, after the first trimester impose risks to the pregnancy.

Treatment

Treatment is tailored to the individual based on the extent of disease and the gestational age. Radiotherapy is an effective treatment option if radiation scatter to the fetus can be minimized. Chemotherapy is relatively safe later in gestation but best avoided in the first trimester if the clinical situation allows. Pregnancy termination is an alternative if Hodgkin's disease is diagnosed early in gestation. Although pregnancy itself does not appear to adversely affect the lymphoma, pregnancy termination permits the aggressive radiotherapy and chemotherapy often necessary. Conversely, if the diagnosis is made later in gestation and the patient is asymptomatic, delaying therapy until fetal lung maturity is established may be reasonable.

Women with Hodgkin's disease are extremely susceptible to infection and sepsis. Sequelae of treatment include radiation pneumonitis causing restrictive lung disease, pericarditis leading to congestive heart failure, hypothyroidism, and ovarian failure. Given that 85% of relapses in Hodgkin's disease occur within 2 years, it is generally accepted that pregnancy should be deferred for 2 years following remission. The risk of second malignancies, especially leukemia, is dramatically increased.

2. Non-Hodgkin's Lymphoma

Until recently, non-Hodgkin's lymphomas were encountered infrequently in pregnancy. However, because 5–10% of individuals infected with the human immunodeficiency virus (HIV) will develop a lymphoma, the incidence of non-Hodgkin's lymphomas is rising. Similar to Hodgkin's disease, extensive staging is essential. Treatment with radiotherapy is indicated for localized disease, whereas chemotherapy is used for more extensive disease. Care of the pregnant patient with lymphoma requires a multidisciplinary approach by obstetrician gynecologists, hematologic oncologists, perinatologists, and neonatologists. With careful treatment, the fetuses of affected women appear to tolerate treatment of lymphoma quite well.

3. Leukemia

Leukemias are malignant proliferations of cells of the hematopoietic system. Acute leukemias are derived from primitive progenitor cells of either the myeloid lineage (**acute myelogenous leukemia** [AML]) or the lymphocytic lineage (**acute lymphocytic leukemia** [ALL]). Chronic leukemias are also derived from either myeloid cells (**chronic myelogenous leukemia** [CML]) or lymphocytic cells (**chronic lymphocytic leukemia** [CLL]). All leukemias are rare before age 40 years with the exception of ALL, a childhood disease with a median age at diagnosis of 10 years.

Clinical Features

Affected individuals often present with the symptoms of anemia (fatigue, weakness), thrombocytopenia (bleeding, bruising), or neutropenia (infection) caused by the replacement of normal hematopoietic cells with leukemia cells in the bone marrow. White blood cell count in the serum can be low, normal, or extremely elevated. Diagnosis is made by cytochemical, genetic, and immunochemical evaluations of the cells of a bone marrow biopsy or aspirate.

Treatment

Treatment of acute leukemia is based upon immediate initiation of chemotherapy. For example, the median survival time of untreated patients with AML is 3 months or less. Exposure to chemotherapy during orga-

nogenesis frequently results in fetal death. However, most authorities consider chemotherapy safe in the second and third trimesters. A period of pancytopenia following chemotherapy can be complicated by infection and hemorrhage. Patients often require erythrocyte and platelet transfusions, as well as antibiotic medications.

Acute leukemia during pregnancy is associated with premature delivery, fetal growth restriction, and fetal loss, but these findings are more likely due to chemotherapy and its complications rather than the leukemia itself.

HEMORRHAGIC DISORDERS

Although hemorrhagic disorders (eg, immune thrombocytopenic purpura [ITP], disseminated intravascular coagulation, circulating anticoagulants) are not common during pregnancy, these conditions could cause significant risks for both mother and fetus.

1. Gestational Thrombocytopenia

Incidental thrombocytopenia of pregnancy, also termed *gestational thrombocytopenia,* affects 5% of pregnancies. It is characterized by mild, asymptomatic thrombocytopenia with platelet levels usually greater than 70,000/μL. It usually occurs late in gestation and resolves spontaneously after delivery. Gestational thrombocytopenia has no association with fetal thrombocytopenia. Its etiology is unclear, although some authorities suspect that gestational thrombocytopenia represents a very mild form of ITP. Antiplatelet antibodies are isolated from patients in both groups and therefore do not aid in diagnosis. Routine obstetric management is appropriate.

2. Immune Thrombocytopenic Purpura

In ITP, also called **idiopathic thrombocytopenic purpura,** platelet destruction is secondary to a circulating immunoglobulin (Ig)G antiplatelet antibody that crosses the placenta and may affect fetal platelets.

Clinical Features

The maternal clinical picture varies from asymptomatic to minor bruises or petechiae, bleeding from mucosal sites, or rarely fatal intracranial bleeding. Splenomegaly may be present. In the peripheral circulation, the platelet count often is between 80,000 and 160,000/μL, but it may be lower. The bone marrow aspirate demonstrates hyperplasia of megakaryocytes, although this test is rarely indicated. The diagnosis can be made once laboratory evaluation demonstrates an isolated thrombocytopenia and other causes, such as drug-induced or HIV-related thrombocytopenia, have been excluded. Antiplatelet antibody testing is not diagnostic.

Treatment

The standard management is to initiate treatment when the platelet count falls to less than 30,000–50,000/µL, although significant bleeding does not begin until platelet levels are less than 10,000/µL. Glucocorticoids suppress the phagocytic activity in the splenic monocyte-macrophage system, increasing platelet levels in approximately two-thirds of patients. Patients refractory to steroid therapy are candidates for immunoglobulin infusion, which has been a great benefit to most patients who fail glucocorticoid therapy. Splenectomy usually is reserved for patients refractory to prednisone and intravenous immunoglobulin. Immunosuppressive agents should be used with great caution and only in extraordinary cases of ITP in pregnancy. Transfusion of platelets and whole blood may be necessary to restore losses from acute hemorrhage or to normalize low perioperative platelet counts (< 50,000/mL).

Complications

Because maternal IgG antiplatelet antibodies cross the placenta, the fetus is at risk for severe thrombocytopenia. Fortunately, only approximately 10% of infants born to women with ITP have platelet counts less than 50,000/µL at birth. Antepartum identification of severely affected fetuses has proved difficult. Maternal and fetal platelet counts do not correlate well, nor do levels of maternal antiplatelet antibody and fetal platelet levels. Given the low incidence of severe neonatal thrombocytopenia and morbidity, most authorities do not recommend direct fetal platelet determination by fetal scalp sampling or umbilical cord blood sampling.

3. Circulating Anticoagulants

Circulating anticoagulants, mainly inhibitors of factor VIII, an IgG, can cause minor to severe bleeding from various sites. Bleeding may be spontaneous or due to trauma, surgery, or sometimes delivery. Treatment may include exchange transfusion with replacement of specific factors or use of corticosteroids or immunosuppressive agents.

THROMBOEMBOLISM

Venous thromboembolism (VTE) affects approximately 1 in 1000 pregnancies. Pregnancy and the puerperium are periods of increased risk for these events because they are hypercoagulable states. Indeed, all the elements of **Virchow's triad** (circulatory stasis, vascular damage, and hypercoagulability of blood) are present. Increased venous capacity during pregnancy coupled with compression of large veins by the gravid uterus causes venous stasis. Endothelial damage occurs at delivery and is more extensive following cesarean delivery, contributing to the increased risk of VTE following cesarean section. Coagulation is favored during pregnancy due to estrogen stimulation of coagulation factors and decreased activity of the fibrinolytic.

Inherited thrombophilias such as **activated protein C resistance** (most commonly due to the **factor V Leiden** mutation), prothrombin gene mutation, **antithrombin III deficiency, protein C and protein S deficiency,** along with acquired thrombophilias such as the **antiphospholipid syndrome** (**APS**), have emerged as important risk factors for VTE. Other risk factors include prior VTE, older age, smoking, and immobilization.

1. Superficial Thrombophlebitis

Patients with thrombosis of the superficial veins of the saphenous system present with tenderness, pain, or erythema along a vein. A palpable cord is sometimes present. Because of the possibility of concurrent deep vein thrombosis (DVT), compression ultrasound is reasonable to confirm the diagnosis and exclude DVT. Treatment consists of compression stockings, ambulation, leg elevation, local heat, and analgesic medications. Of note, the superficial femoral vein belongs to the deep venous system despite its name. A thrombus in this vein requires treatment for DVT.

2. Deep Vein Thrombosis

Approximately half of DVT in pregnancy occurs antepartum and half occurs postpartum. Previous clinical practices that contributed to thrombosis, such as prolonged postpartum bed rest, likely falsely elevated the risk of DVT in the puerperium. Greater than 80% of DVT in pregnancy occurs in the left lower extremity rather than the right, a finding attributed to compression of the left iliac vein by the right iliac artery as it branches off the aorta.

Clinical Features

The presentation of DVT is variable but frequently includes lower extremity tenderness, swelling, color changes, and a palpable cord. **Homan's sign,** pain elicited by passive dorsiflexion of the foot, may be present. Occasionally, the extremity is pale and cool with decreased pulses due to reflex arterial spasm.

Diagnosis

The modality of choice for diagnosis of DVT is real-time ultrasound, used with duplex and color Doppler ultrasound. Venography remains the standard but has been largely replaced by the less invasive diagnostic tests. Magnetic resonance imaging is used when there is a strong clinical suspicion of thrombus not detected by ultrasound or if the ultrasound results are equivocal. With MRI, anatomy above the inguinal ligament can be evaluated as can pelvic blood flow.

Treatment

Anticoagulation, bed rest, and analgesia are the fundamental treatments of DVT. Ambulation with elastic stockings begins once all symptoms have abated, usually in 7–10 days. Patients are initially anticoagulated with unfractionated heparin or low-molecular-weight heparin. **Low-molecular-weight heparin** has a longer half-life and increased bioavailability, making administration easier and anticoagulant response more predictable. It is associated with fewer bleeding problems than unfractionated heparin and does not require laboratory monitoring. In the postpartum state, the patient can then transition to warfarin. Due to embryopathy and fetal hemorrhage, warfarin is contraindicated during pregnancy. Antepartum DVT is treated with anticoagulation for the rest of pregnancy and then for 6–12 weeks postpartum. Deep vein thrombosis occurring postpartum should be treated with anticoagulation for 3–6 months.

3. Pulmonary Embolism

Pulmonary embolism accounts for approximately 20% of maternal deaths in the United States. Its antepartum and postpartum prevalence are approximately equal, although postpartum pulmonary embolism is associated with higher mortality rates. Clinical evidence of DVT often precedes pulmonary embolization. However, given the prevalence of thrombosis originating in the iliac veins during pregnancy, antecedent DVT is frequently not clinically apparent.

Clinical Features

The most common presenting symptom of pulmonary embolus is dyspnea, followed by pleuritic chest pain, apprehension, cough, syncope, and hemoptysis. Associated signs include tachypnea and tachycardia.

Diagnosis

Initial evaluation of the symptoms associated with pulmonary embolism usually consists of arterial blood gas measurement, chest radiograph, and electrocardiogram. Ventilation–perfusion scintigraphy is used in most centers to evaluate for perfusion defects and ventilation mismatches that suggest pulmonary embolus. The test has negligible fetal radiation exposure. High-probability scans are indicative of pulmonary embolism in 88% of cases. Conversely, in patients with normal or near-normal scans, pulmonary embolism was detected by angiography only 4% of the time. However, the use-

fulness of this modality is limited by that fact that the majority of results are reported as intermediate- or low-probability scans, categories without much diagnostic value. Because of these limitations, spiral computed tomographic (CT) pulmonary angiography is emerging as a useful, noninvasive modality for the detection of pulmonary embolism but is limited in the detection of multiple small emboli. Pulmonary artery catheterization with angiography remains the gold standard but is used less frequently due to its invasive nature.

Treatment

Treatment of pulmonary embolism is anticoagulation. Guidelines such as those published by the American College of Chest Physicians (2004) should be followed. The factors influencing anticoagulant choice (heparin vs. warfarin [Coumadin]) are the same as those for DVT. Therapeutic anticoagulation should be continued for at least 4–6 months to prevent recurrence. Vena caval filter use may be necessary should recurrent embolization occur despite anticoagulation.

Prevention

Prophylactic anticoagulation should be considered for women at high risk for thromboembolism during pregnancy. Women with a prior VTE that was not related to a temporary risk factor (eg, prolonged immobilization after injury) should receive prophylactic anticoagulation with heparin during pregnancy and the puerperium. Women with inherited thrombophilias that confer a high risk for thrombosis during pregnancy, such as antithrombin III deficiency or protein S deficiency, also should be anticoagulated. Recommendations for women with lower risk for thrombophilias, such as activated protein C resistance and the prothrombin gene mutation (G20210A), vary based on the individual woman's past medical and obstetric history. In general, women with these disorders and prior VTE or adverse pregnancy outcome, such as fetal death or severe preeclampsia, are offered anticoagulation.

SEPTIC PELVIC THROMBOPHLEBITIS

Septic pelvic thrombophlebitis is thrombosis in the veins of the pelvis due to infection. The most important risk factor is cesarean section, especially if complicated by infection. In fact, almost 90% of cases occur after cesarean delivery. The overall incidence is low, affecting only approximately 1 in every 2000 pregnancies.

Pathophysiology

Pelvic infection leads to infection of the vein wall and intimal damage. Thrombogenesis occurs at the site of intimal damage. The clot is then invaded by microorganisms. Suppuration follows, with liquefaction, fragmentation, and, finally, septic embolization.

Both the uterine and ovarian veins may be involved, as well as the common iliac, hypogastric, and vaginal veins and the inferior vena cava. The ovarian vein is the most common site of septic thrombosis (40% of cases). The onset of symptoms may be as early as 2–3 days postpartum or as late as 6 weeks following delivery.

Clinical Findings

The condition is suspected when fever persists in the puerperium in spite of adequate antibiotic therapy for aerobic and anaerobic organisms and no other discernible cause of fever. Abdominal pain and back discomfort are common presenting symptoms. A picket-fence fever curve ("hectic" fevers) with wide swings from normal to as high as 41 °C (105.8 °F) is seen in 90% of cases. Tachycardia and tachypnea may be present. Leukocytosis usually is present. Blood cultures drawn during fever spikes yield positive results more than 35% of the time.

Diagnosis

Pelvic examination often is consistent with a normal postpartum examination and therefore not helpful in diagnosing this condition. However, in approximately 30% of cases, hard, tender, wormlike thrombosed veins may be palpable in the vaginal fornices or in one or both parametrial areas. A temperature spike may be noted following examination because of disturbance of infected pelvic veins; this may be considered a diagnostic indication of septic pelvic thrombophlebitis. Chest radiograph often reveals evidence of multiple, small septic emboli. Computed tomography or MRI may eliminate other pelvic causes, such as abscess, and assist in the diagnosis of pelvic vein thrombosis.

Differential Diagnosis

The differential diagnosis includes pyelonephritis, meningitis, systemic lupus erythematosus, tuberculosis, malaria, typhoid, sickle cell crisis, appendicitis, and torsion of the adnexa.

Complications

The serious complications associated with this condition are septic pulmonary emboli, extension of the venous clot in the pelvis, renal vein thrombosis, ureteral obstruction, and death.

Treatment

The mainstays are anticoagulation with heparin and broad-spectrum antibiotics (including coverage for anaerobes and common Enterobacteriaceae). Within 48–72 hours of initiation of heparin therapy, fever should resolve. Treatment usually is empirically continued for 7–10 days.

REFERENCES

Alfirevic Z et al: Postnatal screening for thrombophilia in women with severe pregnancy complications. Obstet Gynecol 2001;97:753.

American College of Obstetricians and Gynecologists: *Thromboembolism in Pregnancy.* ACOG Practice Bulletin No. 19. American College of Obstetricians and Gynecologists, 2000.

Aviles A, Neri N: Hematological malignancies and pregnancy: A final report of 84 children who received chemotherapy in utero. Clin Lymphoma 2001;2:173.

Bates SM, et al: Use of antithrombotic agents during pregnancy: The Seventh ACCP Conference on Antithrombotic and Thrombolytic Therapy. Chest 2004;126(3 Suppl):627S.

Bazzan M, Donvito V: Low-molecular-weight heparin during pregnancy. Thromb Res 2001;101:V175.

Burlingame J et al: Maternal and fetal outcomes in pregnancies affected by von Willebrand disease type 2. Am J Obstet Gynecol 2001;184:229.

Burns MM: Emerging concepts in the diagnosis and management of venous thromboembolism during pregnancy. J Thromb Thrombolysis 2000;10:59.

Burrows RF: Platelet disorders in pregnancy. Curr Opin Obstet Gynecol 2001;13:115.

Choi JW, Pai SH: Change in erythropoiesis with gestational age during pregnancy. Ann Hematol 2001;80:26.

Gerhardt A et al: Prothrombin and factor V mutations in women with a history of thrombosis during pregnancy and the puerperium. N Engl J Med 2000;342:374.

Greer IA: The challenge of thrombophilia in maternal-fetal medicine. N Engl J Med 2000;342:424.

Haram K, Nilsen ST, Ulvik RJ: Iron supplementation in pregnancy—Evidence and controversies. Acta Obstet Gynecol Scand 2001;80:683.

Koshy M et al: Prophylactic red-cell transfusions in pregnant patients with sickle cell disease. A randomized cooperative study. N Engl J Med 1988;319:1447.

Naylor CS et al: Cefotetan-induced hemolysis associated with antibiotic prophylaxis for cesarean delivery. Am J Obstet Gynecol 2000;182:1427.

Nizzi FA Jr, Mues G: Hemorrhagic problems in obstetrics, exclusive of disseminated intravascular coagulation. Hematol Oncol Clin North Am 2000;14:1171.

Pejovic T, Schwartz PE: Leukemias. Clin Obstet Gynecol 2002;45:866.

Rai R, Regan L: Thrombophilia and adverse pregnancy outcome. Semin Reprod Med 2000;18:369.

Rosenfeld S et al: Antithymocyte globulin and cyclosporine for severe aplastic anemia: association between hematologic response and long-term outcome. JAMA 2003;289:1130.

Serjeant GR et al: Outcome of pregnancy in homozygous sickle cell disease. Obstet Gynecol 2004;103:1278.

Sermon K, Van Steirteghem A, Liebaers I: Preimplantation genetic diagnosis. Lancet 2004;363:1633.

Sloan NL, Jordan E, Winikoff B: Effects of iron supplementation on maternal hematologic status in pregnancy. Am J Public Health 2002;92:288.

Spina V, Aleandri V, Morini F: The impact of the factor V Leiden mutation on pregnancy. Hum Reprod Update 2000;6:301.

Sun PM et al: Sickle cell disease in pregnancy: twenty years of experience at Grady Memorial Hospital, Atlanta, Georgia. Am J Obstet Gynecol 2001;184:1127.

Tichelli A et al: European Group for Blood and Marrow Transplantation Severe Aplastic Anaemia Working Party. Outcome of pregnancy and disease course among women with aplastic anemia treated with immunosuppression. Ann Intern Med 2002;137:164.

Xiong X et al: Anemia during pregnancy and birth outcome: a meta-analysis. Am J Perinatol 2000;17:137.

Surgical Diseases & Disorders in Pregnancy

27

Christine H. Holschneider, MD

Surgical interventions other than cesarean section are performed in 1.5–2.0% of all pregnancies. Altered anatomy and physiology and potential risks to the mother and fetus make diagnosis and management of surgical disorders more difficult during pregnancy. Generally, the interests of mother and fetus are best served by the obstetrician's active participation throughout the mother's course of diagnosis and management of a nonobstetric surgical disorder, although usually the responsibility is shared with other specialists. It is imperative that the obstetrician be well informed about the ways in which surgical disorders influence pregnancy and vice versa, the risks of diagnostic and therapeutic procedures to the fetus, and appropriate management of preterm labor in the immediate postoperative period.

Surgical disorders can be either incidental to or directly related to the pregnancy. Diagnostic evaluation requires gentle, sensitive elicitation of physical signs, often without resorting to sophisticated diagnostic aids that involve risk to the developing fetus. Good judgment regarding the timing, methods, and extent of treatment is important. In the absence of peritonitis, visceral perforation, or hemorrhage, surgical disorders during gestation generally have little effect on placental function and fetal development.

MATERNAL CONSIDERATIONS

Pregnancy is accompanied by physiologic and anatomic changes that alter the evaluation and management of the surgical patient. The 30–50% increase in plasma volume during pregnancy affects cardiac output and may alter drug distribution and laboratory test results. Red cell mass increases but not as much as the plasma volume, resulting in a slight physiologic anemia. Colloid osmotic pressure is decreased during pregnancy. Increased interstitial fluid is seen as mild edema, particularly in the lower extremities. Systemic vascular resistance decreases during pregnancy. Systolic and diastolic blood pressures characteristically drop during the early second trimester, with a gradual return to baseline by

term. Functional pulmonary residual capacity decreases due to limitation of diaphragmatic excursion. Minute ventilation increases due to increased tidal volume and respiratory rate. A compensated mild respiratory alkalosis exists. Increased renal blood flow is evidenced by increased glomerular filtration rate and decreased serum creatinine and blood urea nitrogen values. Gastrointestinal motility is diminished, resulting in delayed gastric emptying and constipation. The enlarging uterus may alter the anatomic relation among the different organs. When the patient is in the supine position, the enlarged uterus may compress the vena cava and result in the hypotensive vena cava compression syndrome.

FETAL CONSIDERATIONS

Optimal care of the pregnant surgical patient requires that potential hazards to the fetus be minimized. This includes risks associated with the maternal disease, diagnostic radiologic procedures, therapeutic drugs, anesthesia, and surgery. Assessment of the risks and benefits to the mother is relatively easy but less so for the fetus because of its relative inaccessibility.

A number of imaging modalities are available for diagnosis during pregnancy, including ultrasound (US), magnetic resonance imaging (MRI), computed tomography (CT), and x-ray. Although no harmful effects from the diagnostic use of US and MRI during pregnancy are reported, exposure to radiation is associated with fetal risks. Limited diagnostic CT or x-ray procedures can be undertaken with care in the pregnant patient. The fetus should be shielded whenever possible. The risk of adverse fetal effects associated with radiation exposure changes with gestational age and is related to the radiation dose to the fetus. For example, before 8 weeks the embryo is most susceptible to radiation-induced growth restriction. At 8–15 weeks the embryo is the most susceptible to mental retardation, with an approximately 4% risk upon exposure at 10 rad (radiation absorbed dose) and 60% at 150 rad. The most common fetal defects seen with direct fetal irradiation of 10 rad or more are microcephaly, mental retardation, intrauterine growth restriction, and eye abnormalities. Current evidence suggests no increased structural or developmental fetal risk with radiation doses less than 5 rad. Concern exists regarding in utero radiation exposure associated with an increase in childhood neoplasms. The risk appears dose related. Fetal exposure to 1–2 rad is estimated to translate into a relative risk of 1.5–2.0 for leukemia during childhood. Table 27–1 outlines estimates of fetal radiation exposure with various diagnostic procedures. In summary, routine preoperative x-ray procedures are not justified. However, if a significant alteration in clinical management of the patient would result from the findings of a judiciously performed radiologic procedure, the limited fetal exposure risk is generally warranted.

Fortunately, most women who require surgery during pregnancy are otherwise relatively healthy and undergo an uneventful postoperative course. Generally, the safety of nonobstetric surgery in pregnancy and general anesthesia has been well established. Nevertheless, some increased risks are associated with surgery and anesthesia during pregnancy, and purely elective surgical procedures should be postponed until after pregnancy. A population-based study from Sweden compared 5405 patients who underwent nonobstetric surgery using general anesthesia during pregnancy with 720,000 similar patients who did not receive general anesthesia. Adverse effects including low birth weight, prematurity, intrauterine growth restriction, and early neonatal death are thought to correlate with the underlying condition that necessitates the surgical procedure. Although several studies have found no increased risk of congenital anomalies with anesthesia and surgery during pregnancy, 1 study of 572 women operated at 4–5 weeks' gestation suggests a possible increase in neural tube defects. Thus, despite the general safety of anesthetic agents in pregnancy, some concern remains regarding teratogenicity in early gestation, and all but truly emergent surgery should be postponed until the second trimester. The second trimester is the preferred surgery time over the third trimester, as the risk of preterm labor is lowest at that time. Whenever possible, regional anesthesia should be performed. No known reproductive toxicity is associated with currently used local anesthetic agents at recommended dose ranges. Short-term postoperative use of narcotic analgesic agents, frequently in combination with acetaminophen or nonsteroidal anti-inflammatory drugs, generally appears to produce no adverse fetal effects.

Because intrauterine asphyxia is a major risk to the fetus consequent to maternal surgery, monitoring and maintaining maternal oxygen-carrying capacity, oxygen affinity, arterial PO_2, and placental blood flow throughout the preoperative, operative, and postoperative periods are important. Attention should be given

Table 27–1. Estimated fetal radiation exposure from common diagnostic radiologic procedures.

Procedure	Fetal Exposure	
	rad	mGY
Chest x-ray (2 views)	$2–7 \times 10^{-5}$	$2–7 \times 10^{-4}$
Mammogram (4 views)	$7–20 \times 10^{-3}$	0.02–0.07
Abdominal x-ray (1 view)	0.1	1
Hip x-ray (1 view)	$1–2 \times 10^{-3}$	0.01–0.02
Ventilation–perfusion scan	0.01–0.04	0.1–0.4
Helical CT chest	$1–10 \times 10^{-3}$	0.01–0.1
CT abdomen	1.7–3.5	17–35

Gray (Gy) is the International System unit for the radiation absorbed dose rad, which is the old but still frequently used unit (1 Gy = 100 rad). Radiographic exposure from a single diagnostic procedure to less than 5 rad (50 mGy) has not been associated with an increase in fetal abnormalities or pregnancy loss. Although concerns about exposure in the range from 5–10 rad (50–100 mGy) have been raised, serious developmental risk to the fetus is not known until the absorbed dose reaches 10 rad (100 mGy).

to providing uterine displacement to prevent venocaval compression when the patient is in the supine position. Supplemental oxygen administration and maintenance of circulating volume also assist fetal oxygenation. A reduction in maternal blood pressure can lead directly to fetal hypoxia. Greater reductions in uteroplacental perfusion by direct vascular constriction and an increase in uterine tonus are noted in association with the use of vasopressors, especially those with predominantly α-adrenergic activity. Ephedrine, with its peripheral β-adrenergic effect, produces much less vasospasm and is the vasopressor of choice in the pregnant patient, especially for treating hypotensive complications of regional anesthesia. To detect fetal hypoxia, continuous electronic fetal heart rate monitoring should be used when maternal surgery is performed in the latter half of gestation as long as the monitoring device can function outside the sterile surgical field.

The severity of the inflammatory response associated with the disease treated by the surgery appears to be more important in determining pregnancy outcome than is the use of anesthesia or the surgical procedure itself. Premature labor does not appear to be a common result of procedures such as exploratory celiotomy unless visceral perforation and peritonitis are encountered or a low pelvic procedure is performed with significant uterine manipulation. Prophylactic use of tocolytics in this setting is controversial. Often, a single dose of a β-adrenergic agent such as terbutaline is sufficient to arrest contraction. Use of indomethacin may be preferred if significant inflammation is present. If possible, uterine activity should be monitored following surgery to detect preterm labor and allow for early intervention.

DIAGNOSTIC CONSIDERATIONS

Pain

Pain is the most prominent symptom encountered with acute abdominal conditions complicating pregnancy. Generalized abdominal pain, guarding, and rebound strongly suggest peritonitis secondary to bleeding, exudation, or leakage of intestinal contents. Cramping with lower central abdominal pain suggests a uterine disorder. Lower abdominal pain on either side suggests torsion, rupture, or hemorrhage of an ovarian cyst or tumor. Right lower or midabdominal pain suggests appendicitis. Disorders of the descending and sigmoid colon with left lower quadrant pain are infrequently encountered because of the relatively young age of obstetric patients. Midabdominal pain early in gestation suggests an intestinal origin. Upper abdominal pain is often related to the liver, spleen, gallbladder, stomach, duodenum, or pancreas. Constipation is a common problem but is rarely associated with other symptoms.

Other Symptoms

Abdominal pain associated with nausea and vomiting after the first trimester usually suggests a gastrointestinal disorder. Nausea and vomiting associated with the inability to pass gas or stool points to an intestinal obstruction. Diarrhea is seldom encountered in association with acute surgical problems except as a symptom of recurrent ulcerative colitis.

Syncope associated with pain and signs of peritoneal irritation usually indicates an acute abdominal emergency with rupture of a viscus, ischemia, or hemorrhage. A temperature of over 38 °C (100 °F) suggests infection, which may be localized by other clinical findings. Vaginal bleeding usually points to an intrauterine problem. Urinary tract infection is often accompanied by urinary frequency and urgency.

History Taking & Examination

Clues to the cause of surgical disorders in pregnancy are often found in a careful review of the medical history. The stage and status of pregnancy are also relevant. The patient with an acute abdomen should undergo careful assessment of the reproductive organs, and her vital signs and general condition should be noted as well as the presence or absence of bowel sounds, abdominal rigidity or rebound tenderness, and the presence or absence of a mass. The fewest possible number of abdominal examinations should be gently performed without

haste and with adequate explanation, using the flat part of the hand and starting in an asymptomatic area.

Laboratory Studies

Several laboratory studies routinely used in the evaluation of surgical disease have altered normal values during gestation; they are discussed where appropriate for the specific disease entity. The white blood cell count is considered elevated if the value is above 16,000/μL in any trimester. An interval of several hours usually passes between onset of hemorrhage and detection of lowered hematocrit values.

GENERAL VERSUS REGIONAL ANESTHESIA

The type of anesthesia is determined primarily by the planned surgical procedure. As a general rule in pregnancy, it seems prudent to choose the anesthetic technique that requires minimal quantities of drugs and minimizes fetal exposure (eg, regional anesthesia) that is appropriate for the surgical procedure and the patient's condition. Advantages of general anesthesia include optimization of maternal and fetal oxygenation and reduction in intraoperative uterine irritability.

PRINCIPLES OF SURGICAL MANAGEMENT

Delay in diagnosis and performance of surgery is the factor primarily responsible for increased maternal morbidity rates and perinatal loss, especially with maternal abdominal trauma. With unmistakable signs of peritoneal irritation, evidence of strangulating intestinal obstruction with possible gangrene, or intra-abdominal hemorrhage, immediate surgical exploration generally is indicated. In subacute conditions, caution should be used in deciding to proceed with surgery. Surgery that is not urgent and can be delayed is best deferred until the second trimester or puerperium. Surgical techniques usually are not altered because of the pregnancy. Essentials of good preoperative care include adequate hydration, availability of blood for transfusion, and appropriate preoperative medication that will not decrease oxygenation for mother and fetus.

Gestational age, uterine size, the specific surgical disorder, and the anticipated type of surgery to be performed are important factors in the selection of the abdominal incision. At operation, the least extensive procedure necessary should be performed with as little manipulation of the uterus as possible. Unless an obstetric indication is present or the uterus interferes with performance of a procedure, it usually is best not to perform a cesarean delivery during an abdominal operation.

Postoperative care depends on the gestational age and the operation performed. For patients in the second half of gestation, electronic monitoring of fetal heart rate and uterine activity should be continued in the immediate postoperative period. Oversedation and fluid or electrolyte imbalance are to be avoided. Encouragement of early maternal activity and resumption of normal food intake are generally recommended.

LAPAROSCOPY IN PREGNANCY

Over the past decade, laparoscopy has been increasingly used during pregnancy in the management of a variety of surgical disorders, most commonly for the exploration and treatment of adnexal masses, for appendectomy, and for cholecystectomy. The major advantages are decreased postoperative morbidity, less pain, and shorter hospital stay and postoperative recovery time. Possible drawbacks are the risk of injury to the pregnant uterus, technical difficulty with exposure because of the enlarged uterus, increased carbon dioxide absorption, and decreased uterine blood flow secondary to excessive intra-abdominal pressure. Knowledge of the precise effects of laparoscopy on the human fetus is limited. During the first half of pregnancy, the risks inherent to the laparoscopic procedure do not appear to be substantially increased compared to the risks in nonpregnant patients. One population-based study of 2181 laparoscopies during pregnancy and 1522 laparotomies did not find any differential impact of laparoscopy versus laparotomy on perinatal outcome.

■ UPPER ABDOMINAL DISEASES & DISORDERS

Early accurate diagnosis of serious abdominal surgical disease during pregnancy is more difficult for the following reasons: (1) altered anatomic relationships, (2) impaired palpation and detection of nonuterine masses, (3) depressed symptoms, (4) symptoms that mimic the normal discomforts of pregnancy, and (5) difficulty in differentiating surgical and obstetric disorders. In general, elective surgery should be avoided during pregnancy, but operation should be performed promptly for definite or probable acute disorders. The approach to surgical problems in pregnant or puerperal patients should be the same as in nonpregnant patients, with prompt surgical intervention when indicated. The risk of inducing labor with diagnostic laparoscopy or laparotomy is low, provided unnecessary manipulation of the uterus and adnexa is avoided. Spontaneous abor-

tion is most likely to occur if surgery is performed before 14 weeks' gestation or when peritonitis is present.

APPENDICITIS

Acute appendicitis is the most common extrauterine complication of pregnancy for which laparotomy is performed. Suspected appendicitis accounts for nearly two-thirds of all nonobstetric exploratory celiotomies performed during pregnancy; most cases occur in the second and third trimesters.

Appendicitis occurs in 0.1–1.4 per 1000 pregnancies. Although the incidence of disease is not increased during gestation, rupture of the appendix occurs 2–3 times more often during pregnancy secondary to delays in diagnosis and operation. Maternal and perinatal morbidity and mortality rates are greatly increased when appendicitis is complicated by peritonitis.

A. SYMPTOMS AND SIGNS

The diagnosis of appendicitis in pregnancy is challenging. Signs and symptoms often are atypical and not dramatic. Right lower quadrant or middle quadrant pain almost always is present when acute appendicitis occurs in pregnancy but may be ascribed to so-called *round ligament pain* or urinary tract infection. In nonpregnant women, the appendix is located in the right lower quadrant (65%), in the pelvis (30%), or retrocecally (5%), but in pregnancy the appendix may be upwardly displaced (Fig 27–1).

The most consistent clinical symptom encountered in pregnant women with appendicitis is vague pain on the right side of the abdomen, although atypical pain

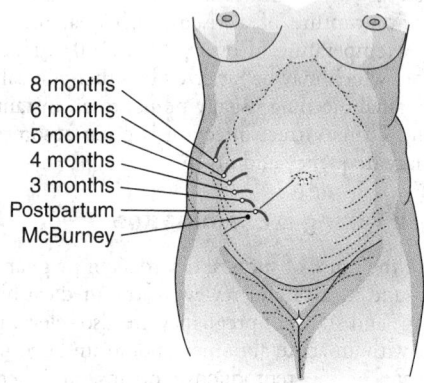

Figure 27–1. Changes in position of the appendix as pregnancy advances. After the first trimester and continuing until the 8th month of gestation, the appendix may be gradually displaced above McBurney's point and may rotate upward and toward the right subcostal area.

patterns abound. Muscle guarding and rebound tenderness are much less demonstrable as gestation progresses. Rectal and vaginal tenderness are present in 80% of patients, particularly in early pregnancy. Nausea, vomiting, and anorexia usually are present, as in the nonpregnant patient. During early appendicitis, the temperature and pulse rate are relatively normal. High fever is not characteristic of the disease, and 25% of pregnant women with appendicitis are afebrile.

B. LABORATORY FINDINGS

The relative leukocytosis of pregnancy (normal 6000–16,000/μL) clouds interpretation of infection. Although not all patients with appendicitis have white blood cell counts above 16,000/μL, at least 75% show a left shift in the differential. Urinalysis may reveal significant pyuria (20%) as well as microscopic hematuria. This is particularly true in the latter half of pregnancy, when the appendix migrates closer to the retroperitoneal ureter.

C. IMAGING

In the nonpregnant patient, CT of the abdomen with and without contrast has become an important tool aiding in the diagnosis of appendicitis. To avoid the risk of radiation to the fetus, US has a distinct role as the first-line imaging modality in pregnancy. Graded compression ultrasonography has been reported in small series to be accurate in the first and second trimesters but technically difficult in the third trimester. MRI has been found helpful in further aiding the diagnosis in patients for whom sonographic findings are nondiagnostic.

D. DIFFERENTIAL DIAGNOSIS

Pyelonephritis is the most common misdiagnosis in patients with acute appendicitis in pregnancy. The differential diagnosis of appendicitis includes ruptured corpus luteum cyst, adnexal torsion, ectopic pregnancy, abruptio placentae, early labor, round ligament syndrome, chorioamnionitis, degenerating myoma, salpingitis, cholangitis, mesenteric adenitis, neoplasm, diverticulitis, and parasitic infection of the intestine.

E. TREATMENT

The difficult clinical problem in treating appendicitis during pregnancy is making the decision to operate. Under appropriate conditions, laparoscopic appendectomy can be as safe as open appendectomy. Most large series report a negative surgical exploration rate between 13% and 35%. However, diagnostic accuracy is only approximately 50% at laparotomy or laparoscopy due to the many processes that may mimic appendicitis in pregnancy. When the appendix appears normal at laparotomy, careful exploration for other nonobstetric and obstetric conditions is important.

Treatment of nonperforated acute appendicitis complicating pregnancy is appendectomy. Prophylactic antibiotic therapy is controversial. However, broad-spectrum intravenous antibiotics are appropriate in the presence of perforation, peritonitis, or abscess formation. Induced abortion is rarely indicated. If drainage is necessary for generalized peritonitis, drains should be placed transabdominally and not transvaginally. During the first trimester, a vertical midline or paramedian incision on the right side is generally considered appropriate. Laparoscopy is an alternate surgical approach used with increasing frequency, especially in the first half of pregnancy. In the late second or third trimester, a muscle-splitting incision centered over the point of maximal tenderness usually provides optimal appendiceal exposure. As a rule, appendiceal disease is managed and the pregnancy is left alone. A Smead-Jones closure with secondary wound closure 72 hours later may be advisable when the appendix is gangrenous or perforated or in the presence of peritonitis or abscess formation.

Depending on the gestational age and expert neonatal care available, abdominal delivery occasionally is performed when peritonitis, sepsis, or a large appendiceal or cul-de-sac abscess occurs. Data are limited, so making definitive recommendations regarding the use of prophylactic tocolytics is difficult. It appears unnecessary in uncomplicated appendicitis but may be appropriate with advanced disease. Caution is indicated because of reports that tocolytics are associated with an increased risk of pulmonary edema in women with sepsis. Labor that follows shortly after surgery in the late third trimester should be allowed to progress because it is not associated with a significant risk of wound dehiscence. At times, the large uterus may help wall off an infection, which after delivery may become disrupted, leading to an acute abdomen within hours postpartum.

F. PROGNOSIS

Better fluid and nutritional support, use of antibiotics, safer anesthesia, prompt surgical intervention, and improved surgical technique have been important elements in the significant reduction of maternal mortality from appendicitis during pregnancy. Similarly, the fetal mortality rate has significantly improved over the past 50 years. Postoperative preterm labor has been reported to occur in 13–25% of second or third trimester patients. Perinatal loss may occur in association with preterm labor and delivery or with generalized peritonitis and sepsis, occurring in 0–1.5% of uncomplicated appendicitis cases. With appendiceal rupture, fetal loss rates are reportedly as high as 30%. This is of particular concern because appendiceal rupture occurs most frequently in the third trimester. Thus it is imperative to avoid surgical delay. A higher negative laparotomy or laparoscopy rate may be an acceptable trade-off for a lower fetal mortality rate.

CHOLECYSTITIS & CHOLELITHIASIS

Gallbladder disease is one of the most common medical conditions and the second most common surgical disorder during pregnancy. Acute cholecystitis occurs in 1 in 1600 to 1 in 10,000 pregnancies. It has been estimated that at least 3.5% of pregnant women harbor gallstones. Multiparas are at increased risk of gallbladder disease. Both an increase in lithogenicity of the bile and a decrease in gallbladder contractility are seen during pregnancy.

A. SYMPTOMS AND SIGNS

Signs and symptoms are similar to those seen in the nonpregnant state and include anorexia, nausea, vomiting, dyspepsia, and intolerance of certain foods, particularly those with high fat content. Biliary tract disease may cause right upper quadrant, epigastric, right scapular, and even left upper quadrant or left lower quadrant pain that tends to be episodic. Biliary colic attacks often are of acute onset, seemingly are triggered by meals, and may last from a few minutes to several hours. Fever, right upper quadrant pain, and tenderness under the liver with deep inspiration (Murphy's sign) are often present in patients with acute cholecystitis.

B. LABORATORY FINDINGS

An elevated white blood cell count with an increase in immature forms is seen with acute cholecystitis. Abnormalities of liver function tests are often encountered, such as increases in aspartate transaminase (AST) and alanine transaminase (ALT) levels. Modest increases in the alkaline phosphatase and bilirubin levels are anticipated very early in cholecystitis or common duct obstruction. However, a more characteristic pattern of relatively normal AST and ALT levels with elevated alkaline phosphatase and bilirubin levels is generally found after the first day of the attack. These changes are not diagnostic and do not signify common bile duct stone or obstruction alone, but when present they serve to support the diagnosis.

C. ULTRASOUND FINDINGS

US findings of stones in the gallbladder, a thickened gallbladder wall, fluid collection around the gallbladder, a dilated common bile duct, or even swelling in the pancreas are suggestive of cholelithiasis and cholecystitis. The diagnostic accuracy of US for detecting gallstones in pregnancy is 95%, making it the diagnostic test of choice.

D. DIFFERENTIAL DIAGNOSIS

The major diagnostic difficulty imposed by pregnancy is differentiating between cholecystitis and appendicitis. In addition to gallstones, cholecystitis can be infectious secondary to *Salmonella typhi* or parasites. A number of other lesions of the biliary tract occur rarely during gestation, including choledochal cysts, which are seen as a spherical dilatation of the common bile duct with a very narrow or obstructed distal end. Associated pancreatitis may be present. Severe preeclampsia with associated right upper quadrant abdominal pain and abnormal liver function tests, hemolysis, elevated liver enzymes, and low platelet count (HELLP) syndrome, acute fatty liver of pregnancy, and acute viral hepatitis are in the differential diagnosis. The presence of proteinuria, nondependent edema, hypertension, and sustained increases in AST and ALT levels compared with alkaline phosphatase level are clinical and laboratory features usually associated with preeclampsia.

E. COMPLICATIONS

Pancreatitis may frequently accompany cholecystitis during pregnancy. Removal of the gallbladder and gallstones may be preferred over conservative medical therapy when pancreatitis is concurrent. Other uncommon complications of cholecystitis during gestation are retained intraductal stones, cholangitis, and rupture of the cystic duct.

F. TREATMENT

The initial management of symptomatic cholelithiasis and cholecystitis in pregnancy is nonoperative with bowel rest, intravenous hydration, correction of electrolyte imbalances, intravenous antibiotics, and analgesics. This therapy results in resolution of acute symptoms in most patients. Surgical intervention is indicated if symptoms fail to improve with medical management, for recurrent episodes of biliary colic, and for complications such as recurrent cholecystitis, choledocholithiasis, and gallstone pancreatitis. Because recurrence rates for symptomatic biliary disease during pregnancy may be as high as 60%, active surgical management, especially in the second trimester, has been advocated in recent years. Recent literature has demonstrated the safety of open and laparoscopic cholecystectomy during pregnancy. Endoscopic retrograde cholangiopancreatography (ERCP) with endoscopic sphincterotomy may be an alternative for selected patients with common bile duct stones. Operative therapy for cholecystitis performed during the second and third trimesters does not appear to be associated with an appreciable increase in morbidity and mortality rates or fetal loss.

G. PROGNOSIS

The outcomes for mother and fetus following uncomplicated gallbladder surgery are excellent. Morbidity and mortality rates increase with maternal age and extent of disease.

ACUTE PANCREATITIS

The incidence of acute pancreatitis in pregnancy reportedly ranges from 1 in 1000 to 1 in 5000 deliveries. Pancreatitis occurs most frequently in the third trimester and puerperium. The mortality rate associated with acute pancreatitis may be higher during pregnancy because of delayed diagnosis. The ultimate cause of pancreatitis is the presence of activated digestive enzymes within the pancreas. Many cases of pancreatitis are idiopathic. As in the nonpregnant state, cholelithiasis is the most commonly identified cause, followed by alcoholism, lipidemia, viral- and drug-induced pancreatitis, familial pancreatitis, structural abnormalities of the pancreas or duodenum, severe abdominal trauma, vascular disease, and preeclampsia-associated pancreatitis.

A. SYMPTOMS AND SIGNS

Gravidas with pancreatitis usually present with severe, steady epigastric pain that often radiates to the back in general approximation of the retroperitoneal location of the pancreas. Often exacerbated by food intake, its onset may be gradual or acute and is frequently accompanied by nausea and vomiting. During gestation, patients may present primarily with vomiting with little or no abdominal pain. Although physical examination is rarely diagnostic, several findings of note may be present, including a low-grade fever, tachycardia, and orthostatic hypotension. The latter finding may be present with hemorrhagic pancreatitis in addition to Cullen's sign (periumbilical ecchymosis) and Turner's sign (flank ecchymosis). Epigastric tenderness and ileus also may be present.

B. LABORATORY FINDINGS

The cornerstone of diagnosis is the determination of serum amylase and lipase levels. Interpretation of serum amylase levels in pregnancy is difficult at times because of the physiologic, up to 2-fold rise in serum amylase level during pregnancy. A laboratory serum amylase level that is more than 2 times above the upper limit of normal suggests pancreatitis. However, an elevated serum amylase level is not specific for pancreatitis because cholecystitis, bowel obstruction, hepatic trauma, or a perforated duodenal ulcer can cause similar serum amylase level elevations. Serum lipase level is a pancreas-specific enzyme and is very helpful in the differential diagnosis. Serum amylase levels usually return to normal within a few days of an attack of uncomplicated acute pancreatitis. In severe pancreatitis, hypocalcemia develops as calcium is complexed by fatty acids liberated by lipase.

C. ULTRASOUND DIAGNOSIS

Sonographic examination may demonstrate an enlarged pancreas with a blunted contour, peritoneal or peripan-creatic fluid, and abscess or pseudocyst formation. Ultrasonography allows for the diagnosis of cholelithiasis, which may be etiologic for pancreatitis. The mere presence of gallstones, however, does not demonstrate etiologic relevance. US also is helpful for evaluating other differential diagnostic considerations.

D. DIFFERENTIAL DIAGNOSIS

Especially pertinent in the differential diagnosis of pancreatitis in pregnancy are hyperemesis gravidarum, preeclampsia, ruptured ectopic pregnancy (often with elevated serum amylase levels), perforated peptic ulcer, intestinal obstruction, acute cholecystitis, ruptured spleen, liver abscess, and perinephric abscess.

E. COMPLICATIONS

Although all of the usual complications of pancreatitis can occur in parturients, there is no special predisposition to complications during pregnancy. Acute complications include hemorrhagic pancreatitis with severe hypotension and hypocalcemia, acute respiratory distress syndrome, pleural effusions, pancreatic ascites, abscess formation, and liponecrosis.

F. TREATMENT

Treatment of acute pancreatitis is primarily medical and supportive, including bowel rest with or without nasogastric suction, intravenous fluid and electrolyte replacement, and parenteral analgesics. Antibiotics are reserved for cases with evidence of an acute infection. Pancreatic enzyme inhibitors have not been successful. Surgical exploration is reserved for patients with pancreatic abscess, ruptured pseudocyst, severe hemorrhagic pancreatitis, or pancreatitis secondary to a lesion that is amenable to surgery. Pregnancy does not influence the course of pancreatitis. Pancreatitis in pregnancy is managed as it is in the nonpregnant state, except that parenteral nutritional supplementation is considered at an earlier point in treatment to protect the fetus. In patients with gallstone pancreatitis, consideration is given to cholecystectomy or ERCP after the acute inflammation subsides.

G. PROGNOSIS

Maternal mortality rates as high as 37% were reported prior to the era of modern medical and surgical management. Respiratory failure, shock, need for massive fluid replacement, and severe hypocalcemia are predictive of disease severity. Perinatal losses are few, although preterm labor appears to occur in a high proportion of patients with acute pancreatitis in later gestation. Most recent single-institution series reflect a reduced maternal mortality rate of 3.4% and a fetal salvage rate of 89%.

PEPTIC ULCER DISEASE

Pregnancy appears to be somewhat protective against the development of gastrointestinal ulcers, as gastric secretion and motility are reduced and mucus secretion is increased. Close to 90% of women with known peptic ulcer disease experience significant improvement during pregnancy, but more than half will have recurrence of symptoms within 3 months postpartum. Thus, peptic ulcer disease occurring as a complication of pregnancy or diagnosed during gestation is encountered infrequently, although the exact incidence is unknown. Infection with *Helicobacter pylori* is associated with the development of peptic ulcer disease.

A. Clinical Findings

Signs and symptoms of peptic ulcer disease in pregnancy can be mistakenly dismissed as being a normal part of the gravid state. Dyspepsia is the major symptom of ulcers during gestation, although reflux symptoms and nausea are also common. Epigastric discomfort that is temporally unrelated to meals is often reported. Abdominal pain might suggest a perforated ulcer, especially in the presence of peritoneal signs and systemic shock. Endoscopy is the diagnostic method of choice for these patients if empiric clinical therapy, including lifestyle and diet modifications, antacids or sucralfate, and empiric H_2-receptor antagonist therapy, fails to lead to improvement of symptoms.

B. Differential Diagnosis

Reflux esophagitis, a common occurrence in pregnancy, and Mallory-Weiss tears may result in symptoms very similar to those of peptic ulcer disease. Gastritis and irritable bowel syndrome must be ruled out. In recent years the diagnosis of persistent hyperemesis gravidarum has been linked to *H pylori* infection.

C. Treatment

Dyspepsia during pregnancy first should be treated with dietary and lifestyle changes, supplemented with antacids or sucralfate. When symptoms persist, H_2-receptor antagonists or, in severe cases, proton pump inhibitors can be used. A 2-week course of antibiotics for *H pylori* during pregnancy is controversial. Administration of triple-drug therapy for *H pylori* often is deferred to the postpartum period because of the low risk of complications from peptic ulcer disease during pregnancy.

D. Complications

Fewer than 100 parturients with complications of peptic ulcer disease, such as perforation, bleeding, and obstruction, have been reported. Most of these cases have occurred in the third trimester of pregnancy. Gastric perforation during pregnancy has an exceedingly high mortality rate, partly because of the difficulty in establishing the proper diagnosis. Other causes of upper gastrointestinal bleeding in pregnancy are reflux esophagitis and Mallory-Weiss tears. Surgical intervention is indicated for significant bleeding ulcerations. In patients requiring surgery for complicated peptic ulcers late in the third trimester, concurrent cesarean delivery may be indicated to enhance operative exposure of the upper abdomen and to prevent potential fetal death or damage from maternal hypotension and hypoxemia.

ACUTE INTESTINAL OBSTRUCTION

Intestinal obstruction is an infrequently encountered complication of pregnancy that is estimated to occur in approximately 1–3 of every 10,000 pregnancies. However, it is the third most common nonobstetric reason for laparotomy during pregnancy (following appendicitis and biliary tract disease). It occurs most commonly in the third trimester. The most common causes of mechanical obstruction are adhesions (60%) and volvulus (25%), followed by intussusception, hernia, and neoplasm.

A. Clinical Findings

The same classic triad of abdominal pain, vomiting, and obstipation is observed in pregnant and nonpregnant women with intestinal obstruction. Pain may be diffuse, constant, or periodic, occurring every 4–5 minutes with small-bowel obstruction or every 10–15 minutes with large-bowel obstruction. Bowel sounds are of little value in making an early diagnosis of obstruction, and tenderness to palpation typically is absent with early obstruction. Vomiting occurs early with small-bowel obstruction. Guarding and rebound tenderness are observed in association with strangulation or perforation. Late in the course of disease, fever, oliguria, and shock occur as manifestations of massive fluid loss into the bowel, acidosis, and infection. The classic findings of bowel ischemia include fever, tachycardia, localized abdominal pain, and marked leukocytosis.

The diagnosis usually is confirmed by radiologic studies, which should be obtained when intestinal obstruction is suspected. A single abdominal series (upright and supine abdominal film) is nondiagnostic in up to 50% of early cases, but serial films usually reveal progressive changes that confirm the diagnosis. Volvulus should be suspected when a single, grossly dilated loop of bowel is seen. A volvulus primarily occurs at the cecum but may also be seen at the sigmoid colon. Occasionally, more extensive radiologic imaging is indicated.

B. Differential Diagnosis

The diagnosis of hyperemesis gravidarum in the second and third trimesters should be viewed with caution and made only after gastrointestinal causes of the symptoms have been excluded. Adynamic ileus of the colon (Ogilvie's syndrome) and pseudo-obstruction are included in the differential diagnosis but are rarely seen during pregnancy.

C. TREATMENT

The management of bowel obstruction in pregnancy is essentially no different from treatment of nonpregnant patients. The cornerstones of therapy are bowel decompression, intravenous hydration, correction of electrolyte imbalances, and timely surgery when indicated. The patient's condition must be rapidly stabilized. The amount of fluid loss often is underestimated and may be 1–6 L by the time obstruction is identified on a scout film. Aggressive hydration is needed to support both the mother and the fetus. A nasogastric tube should be placed. Surgery is indicated if perforation or gangrenous bowel is suspected or when the patient's symptoms do not resolve with medical management. A vertical midline incision on the abdomen provides the best operative exposure and can be extended as needed. Surgical principles for intraoperative management apply similarly to pregnant and nonpregnant patients. Cesarean delivery is performed first if the large uterus prevents adequate exposure of the bowel in term pregnancies or if indicated obstetrically. The entire bowel should be examined carefully because there may be more than one area of obstruction or limited bowel viability.

D. PROGNOSIS

Intestinal obstruction in pregnancy is associated with a maternal mortality rate of 6%, with losses occurring secondary to infection and irreversible shock. Early diagnosis and treatment are essential for an improved outcome. Perinatal mortality is approximately 20% and usually results from maternal hypotension and resultant fetal hypoxia and acidosis.

SPONTANEOUS HEPATIC & SPLENIC RUPTURE

Intra-abdominal hemorrhage during pregnancy has diverse causes, including trauma, preexisting splenic disease, and preeclampsia–eclampsia. Often, the exact cause cannot be determined preoperatively. Spontaneous hepatic rupture associated with severe preeclampsia–eclampsia may be manifested by severe abdominal pain and shock, with thrombocytopenia and low fibrinogen levels. Exploratory celiotomy should be undertaken immediately because early diagnosis, blood transfusion, and prompt operation have been associated with improved survival rates.

Bleeding from a lacerated or ruptured spleen does not cease spontaneously and requires immediate surgical attention. Evidence of a hemoperitoneum on imaging studies or a hemorrhagic peritoneal lavage in association with a falling hematocrit level and abdominal pain establish the presence of a hemoperitoneum.

RUPTURED SPLENIC ARTERY ANEURYSM

Autopsy data suggest that splenic artery aneurysm occurs in 0.1% of adults. It is estimated that 6–10% of lesions will rupture, with portal hypertension and pregnancy being the main risk factors. Twenty-five to 40% of ruptures occur during gestation, especially in the last trimester, and are a major cause of intraperitoneal hemorrhage. Pregnant women who develop ruptured splenic artery aneurysm have a 75% mortality rate, with an even higher fetal mortality rate of up to 95%. Most patients with this condition are thought preoperatively to have placental abruption or uterine rupture.

Prior to rupture, the presenting symptoms may be completely absent or vague. The most common symptom is vague epigastric, left upper quadrant, or left shoulder pain. In approximately 25% of patients a 2-stage rupture is seen, with a smaller primary hemorrhage into the lesser sac, which may allow for temporary tamponade of the bleeding until complete rupture into the peritoneal cavity occurs, causing hemorrhagic shock. A bruit may be audible. A highly diagnostic finding on flat x-ray film of the abdomen is demonstration in the upper left quadrant of an oval calcification with a central lucent area. In stable clinical situations, angiography can provide positive confirmation and is the gold standard for diagnosis. In pregnancy, however, ultrasonography and pulsed-wave Doppler studies are preferred in order to minimize fetal radiation exposure. A splenic artery aneurysm in a woman of childbearing age should be treated electively, even during pregnancy, because of the increased risk of rupture and associated mortality. The elective operative mortality rate reportedly ranges between 0.5% and 1.3%.

■ PELVIC DISEASES & DISORDERS

OVARIAN MASSES

The incidental finding of an adnexal mass in pregnancy has become more common with the routine use of ultrasonography. As many as 1–4% of pregnant women are diagnosed with an adnexal mass. The majority of the masses are functional or corpus luteum cysts and spontaneously resolve by 16 weeks' gestation. More than 90% of unilateral, noncomplex masses less than 5 cm in diameter that are noticed in the first trimester are functional and resolve spontaneously. Patients who undergo assisted reproduction present a special subgroup as their ovaries frequently have ovarian cysts in the first trimester due to ovarian hyperstimulation. More than 90% of these cysts resolve spontaneously. Pathologic ovarian neoplasms tend not to resolve. The most common pathologic ovarian neoplasms during pregnancy are benign cystic teratoma (21%), serous cystadenoma (21%), cystic corpus luteum (18%), and mucinous cystadenoma. Of the adnexal masses that persist, 1–10% will be malignant.

The three main reasons for advising surgery for an adnexal mass in pregnancy are the risks of rupture, torsion, and malignancy. The risk of malignancy can be further gauged by the ultrasonographic characteristics of the mass. Determination of the actual risk of rupture or torsion of a benign-appearing adnexal mass in pregnancy remains an unsettled issue. It is estimated that only approximately 2% of such masses will rupture during gestation, and the incidence of torsion in recent published series ranges from 0–7%. The challenge to the clinician is to weigh for each individual patient these risks against the risks of abdominal surgery during pregnancy, including miscarriage, rupture of membranes, and preterm labor. If adnexal masses diagnosed in the first trimester require surgery in pregnancy, it is generally advisable to perform the operation via laparotomy or laparoscopy in the second trimester unless signs or symptoms suggestive of torsion or highly aggressive malignancy indicate the need for more immediate intervention. Similarly, asymptomatic ovarian masses that are initially noted in the third trimester of pregnancy can be followed until the time of delivery or postpartum because the size of the uterus may present problems with access during laparotomy and because preterm labor may be inadvertently induced.

Ultrasonography usually facilitates delineation of the size and consistency of adnexal masses. If the mass is unilateral, mobile, and cystic, anaplastic elements are less likely and operation can be deferred. Ovarian masses must be differentiated from lesions of the colon, pedunculated leiomyomas, pelvic kidneys, and congenital abnormalities of the uterus. Any adnexal lesion that is present after 14 weeks' gestation, is growing in size on serial ultrasonographic evaluations, contains solid and complex components or internal papillae, is fixed, is surrounded by abdominal ascites, or is symptomatic warrants surgical exploration and pathologic diagnosis.

Torsion of the Adnexa

Torsion of the adnexa can involve the ovary, tube, and ancillary structures, either separately or together. The most common time for occurrence of adnexal torsion is between 6 and 14 weeks and in the immediate puerperium. Although torsion of a normal adnexa has been described, it commonly is associated with a cystic neoplasm. Symptoms include abdominal pain and tenderness that usually are sudden in onset and result from occlusion of the vascular supply to the twisted organ. Shock and peritonitis may ensue. Ultrasonography frequently demonstrates an adnexal mass and altered blood flow on Doppler studies. The diagnosis of torsion is ultimately made at surgery. Prompt operation is necessary to prevent tissue necrosis, preterm labor, and potential perinatal death. The right ovary is involved more frequently than is the left ovary. Benign cystic teratomas and cystadenomas are the most common histologic findings in ovaries that have undergone torsion. Traditional thinking has been that ovarian cysts that have undergone torsion must not be untwisted prior to pedicle clamping because of the concern for potential fatal thromboembolic complications. However, recent series on both nonpregnant and pregnant patients demonstrate that adnexa that had undergone torsion can safely be derotated, followed by the appropriate removal of the mass, eg, cystectomy. These adnexa are capable of recovering and being functional. Salpingo-oophorectomy can be reserved for the management of active bleeding or suspicious neoplasms.

Solid Ovarian Tumors

Solid and complex ovarian tumors with significant solid components discovered during pregnancy generally should be treated surgically because of the low but significant incidence of cancer (1–10%).

Carcinoma of Ovary

Carcinoma of the ovary occurs in less than 0.1% of all gestations and has been encountered in all trimesters. Between 1 and 10% of all ovarian tumors complicating pregnancy are malignant. Consistent with the young age of the pregnant patient population, most neoplasms are germ cell tumors (dysgerminoma, endodermal sinus tumor, malignant teratoma, embryonal carcinoma, and choriocarcinoma) and tumors of low malignant potential, but cystadenocarcinomas do occur.

The treatment of gestational ovarian cancer in the pregnant patient is no different from that for the nonpregnant patient. A generous surgical incision is important not only to remove the tumor but also to properly explore the abdomen and to reduce uterine manipulation until the definitive surgical course of management is determined. Staging is accomplished and adequate tissue obtained for histologic diagnosis. Conservative surgery is appropriate for an encapsulated tumor if no evidence of uterine or contralateral ovarian involvement is seen. In more advanced stages, the extent of surgery, including tumor debulking, will depend upon gestational age and the patient's wishes with regard to the pregnancy. In some cases, optimal surgical cytoreduction of the tumor to < 1-cm residual disease can be accomplished with the uterus and pregnancy left in situ. Neoadjuvant chemotherapy may offer an interim treatment for selected patients diagnosed at midgestation to allow for fetal maturity prior to extensive surgical cytoreduction. Elevated tumor markers, such as α-fetoprotein (AFP), lactate dehydrogenase (LDH), β-human chorionic gonadotropin (β-hCG), and cancer antigen (CA)-125, during the preoperative work-up of an adnexal mass may be misleading because pregnancy itself may cause an increase in these values.

If the tumor is benign, residual ovarian tissue is conserved if possible. The contralateral ovary must always be carefully evaluated to rule out disease. Should surgical extirpation of the corpus luteum be required in the first trimester, progestin support is recommended.

LEIOMYOMAS

Uterine leiomyomas occur in 0.1–3.9% of pregnancies. A large recent cohort study of obstetric outcomes of women diagnosed ultrasonographically with uterine leiomyomas in pregnancy found an increased risk of cesarean delivery, breech presentation, malposition, preterm delivery, placenta previa, and severe postpartum hemorrhage. Uterine leiomyomas may further complicate pregnancy by undergoing degeneration or torsion, or by causing mechanical obstruction of labor. A degenerating leiomyoma or one undergoing torsion is characterized by acute abdominal pain with point tenderness over the site of the leiomyoma. Conservative treatment with analgesia, reassurance, and supportive therapy almost always is adequate. Occasionally, surgery during pregnancy is indicated for torsion of an isolated, pedunculated leiomyoma. With the exception of a pedunculated leiomyoma on a narrow stalk, myomectomy should not be performed during pregnancy because of the risk of uncontrollable hemorrhage.

Ultrasonography is of great value to document the location, size, and consistency of leiomyomas in a pregnant uterus. Cystic changes in leiomyomas are often visualized when clinical signs of degeneration are present.

■ CANCER IN PREGNANCY

The incidence of cancer in pregnancy is approximately 1 in 1000. The most common malignancies diagnosed during pregnancy are cervical cancer (26%; see Chapter 50), breast cancer (26%), leukemias (15%), lymphomas (10%), and malignant melanomas (8%).

BREAST CANCER

Breast cancer is the most common cancer affecting women in the United States. One of every 5 cases occurs in women younger than 45 years, and 2–5% of women are pregnant when diagnosed with breast cancer. In the United States, the incidence of breast cancer in pregnancy is 3 per 10,000 live births. For this reason, careful breast examination should be performed during prenatal and postnatal care, and a family history should be obtained. Pregnancy- and lactation-related changes in the breast increase the frequency and range of breast problems and make the diagnosis of breast cancer more difficult. A painless lump is the most common presentation of gestational breast cancer. Bloody nipple discharge may be a presenting symptom and requires work-up. Any mass found by the patient or by the obstetrician should be fully evaluated without undue delay. The differential diagnoses is broad and includes lactating adenoma, galactocele, milk-filled cyst, fibroadenoma, abscess, and cancer.

Initial management of the pregnant patient with a breast mass does not differ significantly from that for nonpregnant women. When a localized lesion is present, breast ultrasonography is the preferred first imaging modality during pregnancy. It is safe and helpful in distinguishing between cystic and solid masses. Although the sensitivity of mammography is diminished by the breast changes in pregnancy, the study still may be helpful for selected patients with inconclusive clinical examinations. With low-dose mammography and appropriate shielding, fetal radiation exposure is minimal. Nonetheless, it is generally recommended that the procedure be avoided during the first trimester. Breast MRI is a promising breast imaging technique and may be indicated in selected patients, although experience with breast MRI in pregnancy is limited. Cystic lesions should be aspirated and the fluid, if bloody, examined cytologically. Malignant cells are rarely found in nonbloody fluid. Fine-needle aspiration, core biopsy, or incisional biopsy can be used in some cases, but surgical excisional biopsy may be most appropriate for clinically suspicious or cytologically equivocal lesions. The increased vascularity of the breasts is associated with a higher rate of bleeding and the lactating breast is prone to infectious complications, but neither pregnancy nor lactation appears to interfere with excisional biopsy in an outpatient setting.

Management of the pregnant woman with breast carcinoma is especially difficult because it requires careful consideration of both mother and fetus. The general approach to treatment of breast cancer in pregnancy should be similar to that in nonpregnant patients and should not be delayed because of pregnancy. Termination of pregnancy has not been shown to improve survival rates. Modified radical mastectomy is the preferred local management of pregnant patients with breast cancer, with the goal of avoiding the need for adjuvant radiation therapy. Breast-conserving surgery, which must be combined with adjuvant radiation, is limited to patients presenting in the third trimester, for whom surgery is performed during late gestation and radiation treatment can be safely postponed until after delivery. Radical mastectomy is well tolerated during pregnancy. Adjuvant chemotherapy is frequently recommended for premenopausal women with breast cancer. The recommendation of chemotherapy to a pregnant woman with breast cancer is a complex decision, but the indications for adjuvant chemotherapy for gestational breast cancer are generally the same as for the nonpregnant patient. Cyclophosphamide, doxorubicin, and 5-fluorouracil have been given successfully during the second and third trimesters, with no measurable increase in congenital malformations. However, the incidences of prematurity and intrauterine growth restriction are increased. Neoadjuvant chemotherapy may be a treatment option in select patients with locally advanced or metastatic gestational breast cancer. Use of tamoxifen in pregnancy is generally discouraged because of reports of teratogenicity and mammary tumorigenicity in rats and ambiguous genitalia in humans. There is no contraindication to breastfeeding after completion of therapy for breast cancer. Breastfeeding should be avoided during chemotherapy, hormone therapy, or radiation. The results of treatment are much the same stage for stage as they are in nonpregnant patients, but pregnancy-associated breast cancers tend to be more advanced at diagnosis (larger tumor size, more frequently involved lymph nodes), resulting in an overall worse prognosis for this group of patients as a whole. Subsequent pregnancies need not necessarily be discouraged after a suitable period of recuperation and observation, as subsequent pregnancy does not increase the risk of recurrence or death from breast cancer. For women who are breast cancer antigen (BRCA)-1 or BRCA-2 mutation carriers, there is no evidence that pregnancy decreases their breast cancer risk.

LYMPHOMAS AND LEUKEMIAS

The incidence of Hodgkin's lymphoma in pregnancy is estimated to be 1 in 1000 to 1 in 6000 pregnancies, with non-Hodgkin's lymphomas being significantly less frequent. The typical presentation is painless adenopathy, and adequate biopsy is essential for diagnosis. Prognosis and stage distribution of pregnancy-associated Hodgkin's lymphoma generally appear comparable to those in the nonpregnant patient. Approximately 70% of patients present with early-stage disease and can be treated with either single-agent chemotherapy or, in selected cases, modified supradiaphragmatic radiation. Patients in early pregnancy presenting with extensive

infradiaphragmatic disease, for which radiation therapy would be a significant component of curative therapy, should consider termination of pregnancy because of the associated significant teratogenic risks.

The incidence of leukemia in pregnancy is estimated at 1 in 100,000. The acute leukemias are more frequent. Treatment of acute leukemia should be started immediately after diagnosis. Depending on the gestational age, the management during pregnancy poses many challenges to the patient, her family, and the treating physicians.

MALIGNANT MELANOMA

Of women with melanoma, approximately 30–35% are of childbearing age, and approximately 1% of female melanoma patients are pregnant. The diagnosis is made by excision, allowing for microstaging. Tumor thickness, tumor site, and presence of metastases are the most important prognostic factors. There has been long-standing controversy regarding the prognosis of pregnancy-associated melanoma, but more recent evidence suggests that patients with early primary lesions and wide surgical excision with appropriate margins have a prognosis comparable to that of their nonpregnant counterparts. Data on higher-stage melanoma diagnosed in pregnancy are limited. Malignant melanoma is the tumor that most frequently metastasizes to the placenta or fetus, accounting for more than half of all tumors with fetal involvement.

■ CARDIAC DISEASE

Cardiac disease complicates 1–4% of all pregnancies in the United States. Rheumatic and congenital heart disease constitute the majority of cases. Patients requiring cardiac surgery should undergo the procedure prior to becoming pregnant. Nevertheless, the rare patient will require cardiac surgery during pregnancy. Most available reports on cardiac surgery during pregnancy involve closed and open mitral valvuloplasties and mitral or aortic valve replacement. Cardiac surgery can be performed with good results in pregnancy, although there is maternal and fetal risk. Operations should generally be performed early in the second trimester when organogenesis is complete and there is comparatively less hemodynamic burden and less risk of preterm labor than later in gestation. Maternal mortality rates average 4–9%, related to the specific procedure performed and the patient's preoperative cardiovascular status. Closed cardiac surgery techniques appear to be associated with better fetal outcome than open cardiac procedures. Fetal or perinatal mortality is expected in 5–10% of percutaneous balloon valvuloplasties and in 20–30% of open valvular or bypass surgery. Fetal risk is substantial because of the nonpulsatile blood flow and hypotension associated with cardiopulmonary bypass. Close fetal surveillance by electronic heart rate and uterine contraction monitoring is essential during any cardiac surgical procedure, whether or not cardiopulmonary bypass is used. During bypass, blood flow to the uterus can be assessed indirectly by changes in the fetal heart rate, and alterations in flow can be made accordingly.

NEUROLOGIC DISEASE

Intracranial hemorrhage during pregnancy is rare (1–5 per 10,000 pregnancies) but is associated with significant maternal and fetal mortality and serious neurologic morbidity in survivors. Rupture of an aneurysm or arteriovenous malformation (AVM) is the most common cause, followed by eclampsia. Other causes include coagulopathy, trauma, and intracranial tumors. During pregnancy the risk of bleeding from an AVM that had not bled previously is 3.5%, which is close to the annual bleeding rate in the nonpregnant patient. However, mortality due to a bleeding AVM in pregnancy is higher (30%) than in the nonpregnant state (10%). Intracranial hemorrhage with associated neurologic damage during pregnancy (limited capacity for decision making, persistent vegetative state, brain death) poses significant medical and ethical challenges in caring for the mother and fetus.

Most commonly, bleeding from an aneurysm occurs in the subarachnoid space, whereas bleeding from an AVM is located within the brain parenchyma. Symptoms and signs of subarachnoid hemorrhage include headache, nausea and vomiting, stiff neck, photophobia, seizures, and a decreasing level of consciousness. The headache usually is very sudden in onset, whereas the headache associated with intraparenchymal bleeding usually is somewhat less severe and is slower in onset. Focal neurologic deficits may be absent in up to 40% of patients. CT or MRI confirm the diagnosis of an intracranial bleed. Cerebral angiography may be needed to identify and characterize an aneurysm or AVM.

Early operative intervention after aneurysmal hemorrhage during pregnancy is associated with reduced maternal and fetal mortality. For patients with AVM, the decision to treat the lesion during pregnancy is less clear but should follow the same guidelines that apply to nonpregnant patients.

HEMORRHOIDS

Pregnancy is the most common cause of symptomatic hemorrhoids. Venous congestion secondary to the enlarging uterus probably is the culprit. The current management approach to hemorrhoid disease is conservative, with simple outpatient treatment preferred, particularly during pregnancy and the puerperium. Medical therapy with dietary changes, avoidance of excessive straining, stool softeners, and hemorrhoidal analgesics often is the only requirement for nonthrombosed hemorrhoids. Rubber-band ligation is a simple, minimally invasive outpatient procedure for the management of hemorrhoids. Hemorrhoidectomy is the best means of definitive therapy for hemorrhoidal disease and should be considered postpartum if the patient continues to fail to respond to conservative measures, if hemorrhoids are severely prolapsed and require manual reduction, or if associated pathology such as ulceration, severe bleeding, fissure, or fistula, is present. Thrombosis or clots in the vein lead to severe symptoms. If thrombosed external hemorrhoids remain tender and resist conservative treatment, they can be infiltrated with 1% lidocaine and a small incision made to extract the clot.

TRAUMA

Approximately 7% of pregnancies are complicated by trauma, such as motor vehicle accidents (40%), falls (30%), direct assaults to the maternal abdomen (20%), and other causes (10%). Automobile accidents are the most common nonobstetric cause of death during pregnancy. The most common cause of fetal death is death of the mother. The second most common cause of fetal death is abruptio placentae. Pregnant women with traumatic injuries may be victims of physical abuse. A pregnancy may increase family stress; therefore, the practitioner should be alert for signs of abuse.

The primary initial goal in treating a pregnant trauma victim is to stabilize the mother's condition. To optimize maternal and fetal outcome, an organized team approach to the pregnant trauma patient is essential. Maternal assessment and management are similar to those for the nonpregnant patient, keeping in mind the goal of protecting the fetus from unnecessary drug and x-ray exposure. The fetus should be evaluated early during trauma assessment, and after fetal viability is reached, continuous fetal heart rate and uterine activity monitoring should be instituted, as long as it does not interfere with maternal resuscitative efforts. Posttraumatic placental abruption usually occurs quite soon after the injury but rarely manifests as late as 5 days post trauma. The fetal heart rate and uterine contractions should be monitored for at least 4 hours after the trauma. Suspicious findings include frequent uterine contractions, vaginal bleeding, abdominouterine tenderness, postural hypotension, and fetal heart rate abnormalities. If any of these signs occur or if the trauma was severe, monitoring should be extended to 24–48 hours. A Kleihauer-Betke test may show evidence of fetomaternal hemorrhage and is recommended for Rh-negative patients. If the results of the Kleihauer-Betke cannot be obtained in a timely fashion, Rh_o (D) immunoglobulin (RhoGAM) should be given empirically to Rh-negative patients. Routine coagulation profiles are not clinically helpful.

REFERENCES

General

Naylor DF, Olson MM: Critical care obstetrics and gynecology. Crit Care Clin 2003;19:127.

Parry RA, Glaze SA, Archer BR: The AAPM/RSNA physics tutorial for residents. Radiographics 1999;19:1289.

Winer-Muram HT et al: Pulmonary embolism in pregnant patients: Fetal radiation dose with helical CT. Radiology 2002; 224:487.

Anesthesia

Goodman S: Anesthesia for nonobstetric surgery in the pregnant patient. Semin Perinatol 2002;26:136.

Kuczkowski KM: Nonobstetric surgery during pregnancy: What are the risks of anesthesia? Obstet Gynecol Surv 2003;59:52.

Rosen MA: Management of anesthesia for the pregnant surgical patient. Anesthesiology 1999;91:1159.

Laparoscopy

Fatum M, Rojansky N: Laparoscopic surgery during pregnancy. Obstet Gynecol Surv 2001;56:50.

Reynolds JD et al: A review of laparoscopy for non-obstetric-related surgery during pregnancy. Curr Surg 2003;60:164.

Rollins MD, Chan KJ, Price RR: Laparoscopy for appendicitis and cholelithiasis during pregnancy: A new standard of care. Surg Endosc 2004;18:237.

Appendicitis

Baer JL, Reis RA, Araens RA: Appendicitis in pregnancy with changes in position and axis of the normal appendix in pregnancy. JAMA 1932;98:1359.

Guttman R, Goldman RD, Koren G: Appendicitis during pregnancy. Can Fam Physician 2004;50:355.

Mourad J et al: Appendicitis in pregnancy: New information that contradicts long-held clinical beliefs. Am J Obstet Gynecol 2000;182:1027.

Oto A et al: Right-lower-quadrant pain and suspected appendicitis in pregnant women: Evaluation with MR imaging–initial experience. Radiology 2005;234:445.

Terasawa T et al: Systematic review: Computed tomography and ultrasonography to detect acute appendicitis in adults and adolescents. Ann Intern Med 2004;:537.

Tracey M, Fletcher S: Appendicitis in pregnancy. Am Surg 2000; 66:555.

Cholecystitis & Cholelithiasis

Graham G, Baxi L, Tharakan T: Laparoscopic cholecystectomy during pregnancy: A case series and review of the literature. Obstet Gynecol Surv 1998;53:566.

Kahaleh M et al: Safety and efficacy of ERCP in pregnancy. Gastrointest Endosc 2004;60:287.

Lu EJ et al: Medical versus surgical management of biliary tract disease in pregnancy. Am J Surg 2004;755.

Pancreatitis

Karsenti D et al: Serum amylase and lipase activities in normal pregnancy: A prospective case-control study. Am J Gastroenterol 2001;96:697.

Peptic Ulcer Disease

Cappell MS: Gastric and duodenal ulcers in pregnancy. Gastroenterol Clin North Am 2003;32:263.

Intestinal Obstruction

Connolly MM, Unti JA, Nora PF: Bowel obstruction in pregnancy. Surg Clin North Am 1995;75:101.

Hauspy J et al: Small bowel obstruction during pregnancy. Acta Chir Belg 2003;103:588.

Splenic/Hepatic Hemorrhage

Fender GRK et al: Management of splenic artery aneurysm during trial of labor with epidural analgesia. Am J Obstet Gynecol 1999;180:1038.

Hillemanns P et al: Rupture of splenic artery aneurysm in a pregnant patient with portal hypertension. Am J Obstet Gynecol 1996;174:1665.

Smith LG Jr et al: Spontaneous rupture of liver during pregnancy: Current therapy. Obstet Gynecol 1991;77:171.

Adnexal Disease

Bromley B, Benacerraf B: Adnexal masses during pregnancy: Accuracy of sonographic diagnosis and outcome. J Ultrasound Med 1997;16:447.

Mathevet P et al: Laparoscopic management of adnexal masses: A case series. Eur J Obstet Gynecol Reprod Biol 2003;108:217.

Schneler KM et al: Adnexal masses in pregnancy: Surgery compared with observation. Obstet Gynecol 2005;105:1098.

Zanetta G et al: A prospective study of the role of ultrasound in the management of adnexal masses in pregnancy. Br J Obstet Gynaecol 2003;110:578.

Leiomyomas

Qidwai GI et al: Obstetric outcomes in women with sonographically identified uterine leiomyomata. Obstet Gynecol 2006; 107:376.

Cancer in Pregnancy

Berry DL et al. Management of breast cancer during pregnancy using a standardized protocol. J Clin Oncol 1999;17:855.

Jernstrom H et al: Pregnancy and risk of early breast cancer in carriers of BRCA1 and BRCA2. Lancet 1999;354:1846.

Pavlidis NA: Coexistence of cancer and pregnancy. Oncologist 2002;7:279.

Psyrri A, Burtness B: Pregnancy-associated breast cancer. Cancer J 2005;11:83.

Ring AE et al: Chemotherapy for breast cancer during pregnancy: An 18-year experience from five London teaching hospitals. J Clin Oncol 2005;23:4192.

Wiesz B, Schiff E, Lishner M: Cancer in pregnancy: Maternal and fetal implications. Human Reprod Update 2001;7:384.

Malignant Melanoma

Daryanani D et al: Pregnancy and early-stage melanoma. Cancer 2003;97:2248.

Cardiac Surgery

Routray SN et al: Balloon mitral valvuloplasty during pregnancy. Int J Gynecol Obstet 2004;85:18.

Weiss BM: Managing severe mitral valve stenosis in pregnant patients—Percutaneous balloon valvuloplasty, not surgery, is the treatment of choice. J Cardiothorac Vasc Anesth 2005; 19:277.

Neurologic Disease

Finnerty JJ et al: Cerebral arteriovenous malformation in pregnancy: Presentation and neurologic, obstetric, and ethical significance. Am J Obstet Gynecol 1999;181:296.

Stoodley MA, Macdonald RL, Weir BK: Pregnancy and intracranial aneurysm. Neurosurg Clin North Am 1998; 9:549.

Tewari KS et al: Obstetric emergencies precipitated by malignant brain tumors. Am J Obstet Gynecol 2000;182:1215.

Trauma

Stone KI: Trauma in the obstetric patient. Obstet Gynecol Clin 1999;26:459.

Warner MW et al: Management of trauma during pregnancy. ANZ J Surg 2004;74:125.

Weinber L et al: The pregnant trauma patient. Anaesth Intensive Care 2005;33:167.

Complications of Labor & Delivery 28

Stacy Strehlow, MD, & Peter Uzelac, MD

■ DYSTOCIA

DEFINITION & CLASSIFICATION

Dystocia is defined as difficult labor or childbirth. It can be considered to involve the maternal pelvis *(passage)*, the fetus *(passenger)*, the expulsive forces *(powers)*, or a combination of these factors.

INCIDENCE

The overall incidence of dystocia in women in labor is difficult to determine, in part secondary to ambiguities in definition. In nulliparous patients the incidence of labor disorders is approximately 25%. The clinical diagnosis of dystocia often is retrospective. If the outcome is uneventful and spontaneous vaginal delivery occurs, dystocia may go unreported. Failure to progress and cephalopelvic disproportion are most often diagnosed after clinical identification of abnormal labor patterns.

Over the last quarter of a century, the cesarean section rate in the United States has risen to approximately 25% of deliveries per year. Approximately 50–60% of cesarean deliveries in the United States are directly or indirectly due to dystocia. Dystocia is currently the most common indication for primary cesarean section, approximately 3 times more common than either nonreassuring fetal status or malpresentation. Elective repeat cesarean section is the second most common indication, often following a primary cesarean delivery for dystocia.

ABNORMAL PATTERNS OF LABOR

Labor is a dynamic process characterized by regular uterine contractions that cause progressive dilatation and effacement of the cervix and descent of the fetus through the birth canal. The progress of labor is evaluated primarily through estimates of cervical dilatation and descent of the fetal presenting part. Normal labor patterns in primigravidas and multiparas have been described in detail by Friedman and others.

Friedman described four abnormal patterns of labor: (1) prolonged latent phase, (2) protraction disorders (protracted active-phase dilatation and protracted descent), (3) arrest disorders (arrest of dilatation, arrest of descent, and failure of descent), and (4) precipitate labor disorders.

1. Prolonged Latent Phase

The latent phase of labor begins with the onset of regular uterine contractions and extends to the beginning of the active phase of cervical dilatation. The duration of the latent phase averages 6.4 hours in nulliparas and 4.8 hours in multiparas. The latent phase is abnormally prolonged if it lasts more than 20 hours in nulliparas or 14 hours in multiparas.

Causes of prolonged latent phase include excessive sedation or sedation given before the end of the latent phase, use of conduction or general anesthesia before labor enters the active phase, labor beginning with an unfavorable cervix, uterine dysfunction characterized by weak, irregular, uncoordinated, and ineffective uterine contractions, and fetopelvic disproportion.

Treatment options in prolonged latent phase primarily consist of therapeutic rest regimens or active management of labor. After 6–12 hours of rest with sedation and hydration, 85% of patients spontaneously enter the active phase of labor, and further progression in dilatation and effacement may be expected. Ten percent of patients will have been in false labor and can be allowed to return home to await the onset of true labor if no other indications for delivery are present. In the remaining 5% of patients, uterine contractions remain ineffective in producing dilation; in the absence of any contraindication, augmentation with oxytocin infusion may be effective in progression to the active phase of labor.

Some authorities recommend oxytocin infusion as the primary treatment for all patients with prolonged latent phase. If immediate delivery is required for clinical reasons (eg, severe preeclampsia or amnionitis), oxytocin infusion is the treatment of choice.

The prognosis for vaginal delivery after therapeutic measures is excellent. After abnormalities in the latent phase have been corrected, patients are not at any greater risk of developing subsequent labor disorders than are patients who have experienced a normal latent phase.

2. Protraction Disorders

Protracted cervical dilatation in the active phase of labor and protracted descent of the fetus constitute the protraction disorders. Protracted active-phase dilatation is characterized by an abnormally slow rate of dilatation in the active phase, ie, less than 1.2 cm/h in nulliparas or less than 1.5 cm/h in multiparas. Protracted descent of the fetus is characterized by a rate of descent less than 1 cm/h in nulliparas or less than 2 cm/h in multiparas. The second stage of labor, which normally averages 20 minutes in parous women and 50 minutes in nulliparous women, is protracted when the stage exceeds 2 hours in nulliparas or 1 hour in multiparas, or 3 and 2 hours, respectively, in the presence of conduction anesthesia.

The underlying pathogenesis of protracted labor probably is multifactorial. Fetopelvic disproportion is encountered in approximately one-third of patients. Other factors include minor malpositions such as occiput posterior, improperly administered conduction anesthesia (eg, epidural anesthesia administered above dermatome T10), excessive sedation, and pelvic tumors obstructing the birth canal.

Treatment of protraction disorders depends on the presence or absence of fetopelvic disproportion, the adequacy of uterine contractions, and the fetal status. Cesarean section is indicated in the presence of confirmed fetopelvic disproportion. Patients experiencing protraction disorders generally do not respond to oxytocin infusion if adequate uterine contractions are documented by intrauterine pressure catheter monitoring. Although enhancement of uterine contractility may be possible, progression of dilatation may not improve. In the absence of fetopelvic disproportion, conservative management, consisting of support and close observation, and therapy with oxytocin augmentation both carry a good prognosis for vaginal delivery (approximately two-thirds of patients) if continued cervical dilatation and effacement occur and there is no fetal compromise. Compelling new evidence suggests a link between labor dystocia and nonreassuring fetal heart rate (FHR) patterns, so fetuses should be closely monitored in the presence of protracted labor.

3. Arrest Disorders

The two patterns of arrest in labor can be characterized as follows: (1) secondary arrest of dilatation, with no progressive cervical dilatation in the active phase of labor for 2 hours or more; and (2) arrest of descent, with descent failing to progress for 1 hour or more.

Approximately 50% of patients with arrest disorders demonstrate fetopelvic disproportion when inadequate uterine contractions have been treated. Other causative factors include various fetal malpositions (eg, occiput

posterior, occiput transverse, face, or brow), inappropriately administered anesthesia, and excessive sedation.

When an arrest disorder is diagnosed, thorough evaluation of fetopelvic relationships before initiation of treatment is crucial. Evaluation should include a careful clinical pelvic examination for pelvic adequacy and estimation of fetal weight. If fetopelvic disproportion is established in the context of an arrest disorder, cesarean section is clearly warranted because considerable trauma to both mother and baby could otherwise occur. If fetopelvic disproportion is not present and uterine activity is less than optimal, oxytocin stimulation is generally effective in producing further progress.

Arrest disorders in the presence of adequate uterine contractions carry a poor prognosis for vaginal delivery. If allowed to continue, arrest disorders are associated with increased perinatal morbidity. However, if a post-arrest rate of dilatation or descent that is equal to or greater than the prearrest rate can be established, prognosis for vaginal delivery is excellent.

4. Precipitate Labor Disorders

Precipitate labor has been defined as delivery in less than 3 hours from onset of contractions. *Precipitate dilatation* can be defined as cervical dilatation occurring at a rate of 5 cm or more per hour in a primipara or 10 cm or more per hour in a multipara. Precipitate labor may result from either extremely strong uterine contractions or low birth canal resistance. Although the initiating mechanism for extraordinarily forceful uterine contractions usually is not known, abnormal contractions may be associated with administration of oxytocin. Strong uterine contractions (both in force and increased basal tone) may accompany placental abruption. Little is known about causes of low birth canal resistance.

If oxytocin administration is the cause of abnormal contractions, it may simply be stopped. The problem typically resolves in less than 5 minutes. The patient should be placed in the lateral position to prevent compression of the inferior vena cava. If excessive uterine activity is associated with FHR abnormalities and this pattern persists despite discontinuation of oxytocin, a beta-mimetic such as 125–250 μg of terbutaline or ritodrine can be given by subcutaneous or slow intravenous injection if no contraindications are present. Physical attempts to retard delivery are absolutely contraindicated.

Maternal complications are rare if the cervix and birth canal are relaxed. However, when the birth canal is rigid and extraordinary contractions occur, uterine rupture may result. Lacerations of the birth canal are common. Furthermore, the uterus that has been hypertonic with labor tends to be hypotonic postpartum, thereby predisposing to postpartum hemorrhage.

Perinatal mortality is increased secondary to possible decreased uteroplacental blood flow, possible intracranial hemorrhage, and risks associated with unattended delivery. Persistently increased basal uterine tone can lead to decreased placental perfusion and fetal hypoxemia. Perinatal intracranial hemorrhage may result from trauma to the fetal head pushing against unyielding maternal tissue with contractions. Resuscitation equipment, infant warmers, and other supportive measures may not be readily available in cases of unattended delivery.

ABNORMALITIES OF THE PASSAGE

Abnormalities of the "passage" involve aberrations of pelvic structure and its relationship to the presenting part. Such abnormalities may be related to size or configurational alterations of the bony pelvis, soft-tissue abnormalities of the birth canal, reproductive tract masses or neoplasia, or aberrant placental location. Bony abnormalities are the most common cause of passage dystocia. The etiology and diagnosis of bony abnormalities begin with the shape, classification, and clinical assessment of the adult female pelvis.

Using roentgenographic studies, Caldwell and Moloy classified the 4 major types of adult pelvic types: gynecoid, android, anthropoid, and platypelloid. Pure forms of these pelvic types are rare; mixed elements are more often present in each type of pelvis. The **gynecoid** pelvis is considered the most typically "female" type and is the most favorable for uncomplicated vaginal delivery. Found in approximately 50% of all women, the pelvic inlet has an oval configuration with a transverse diameter slightly greater than the anteroposterior diameter. Pelvic side walls are straight, the ischial spines are not prominent, the subpubic arch is wide, and the sacrum is concave. The **android,** or "male," type of pelvis is found in approximately 33% of white women and approximately 15% of black women. The inlet is wedge-shaped with convergent side walls, the ischial spines are prominent, the subpubic arch is narrowed, and the sacrum is inclined anteriorly in its lower third. The android pelvis is associated with persistent occiput posterior position and deep transverse arrest. The **anthropoid** pelvis is present in almost half of black women and 20% of white women. The inlet is oval, with an anteroposterior diameter greater than the transverse diameter. Pelvic side walls are divergent, and the sacrum is inclined posteriorly. This pelvic type is most often associated with persistent occiput posterior position. The **platypelloid** pelvis is present in fewer than 3% of all women. This pelvis is characterized by a transverse diameter that is wide with respect to the anteroposterior diameter. Deep transverse arrest patterns of labor are commonly associated with this pelvic type.

X-ray pelvimetry has now fallen into limited use because accumulating evidence suggests that the measurements obtained do not influence the management of labor and may even increase cesarean section rates. Ultrasound, magnetic resonance imaging (MRI), and x-rays have been used to delineate pelvic size and shape, but clinical pelvimetry usually is sufficient for routine evaluation of obstetric patients. In an era of continuous fetal monitoring and safe protocols for use of dilute oxytocin to induce and augment labor, a trial of labor can be accomplished safely in most patients. The diagnosis of fetopelvic disproportion essentially has become a diagnosis of exclusion, after fetal factors and uterine dysfunction have been ruled out. However, x-ray pelvimetry may retain a role in the evaluation of a pelvis for the feasibility of vaginal breech delivery and in the assessment of gross bony distortion. If abnormal architecture is abnormal based on history and physical examination, imaging studies may be warranted. In this category, traumatic pelvic fractures are the most common abnormalities; other possibilities include rachitic pelves, chondrodystrophic dwarf pelves, kyphotic and scoliotic pelves, exostoses, and bony neoplasms.

Clinical pelvimetry is performed to estimate pelvic dimensions. To assess the pelvic inlet, the diagonal conjugate is obtained by measuring the distance from the lower edge of the symphysis pubis to the sacral promontory. The obstetric conjugate, the distance from the most prominent portion of the symphysis pubis to the sacral promontory, measures 1.5–2.0 cm less than the diagonal conjugate. The obstetric conjugate should measure greater than 10 cm. The pelvic outlet can be assessed by measuring intertuberous diameter and palpating the subpubic arch. Intertuberous diameter greater than 8 cm and a wide subpubic arch characterize an adequate pelvic outlet. The midpelvis is evaluated clinically based on convergence of side walls, prominence of ischial spines, and concavity of the sacrum. Pelvic contractions may present as a floating vertex presentation with no descent during labor, as abnormal presentation, or as a prolapsed cord or extremity. In prolonged labors complicated by pelvic contraction, considerable molding of the fetal head, caput succedaneum formation, and prolonged rupture of the membranes are possible. If allowed to continue, ultimately frank uterine rupture may occur, preceded by abnormal thinning of the lower uterine segment and development of a Bandl's retraction ring. With severely prolonged second stage, vesicovaginal or rectovaginal fistula formation may result with pressure necrosis of the surrounding tissues of the birth canal by the fetal head. Fortunately, these complications are rare in developed countries where cesarean sections are accessible. Other anatomic abnormalities of the reproductive tract may cause dystocia. So-called *soft-tissue dystocia* may be caused by uterine or vaginal congenital anomalies, scarring of the birth canal, pelvic masses, or low implantation of the placenta.

ABNORMALITIES OF THE PASSENGER

Dystocia may be caused by abnormalities of the "passenger," or fetus. Common fetal abnormalities leading to dystocia include excessive fetal size, malpositions, congenital anomalies, and multiple gestation.

Malposition and Malpresentation

Fetal malpresentations are abnormalities of fetal position, presentation, attitude, or lie. They collectively constitute the most common cause of fetal dystocia, occurring in approximately 5% of all labors. Persistent occiput posterior and occiput transverse positions, brow presentation, face presentation, transverse or oblique lies, and breech and compound presentation are included in this category.

A. Vertex Malpositions

1. Occiput posterior—The occiput posterior position may be normal in early labor, with approximately 10–20% of fetuses in occiput posterior position at onset of labor. In 87% of cases, the head rotates to the occiput anterior position when it reaches the pelvic floor. If the head does not rotate, persistent occiput anterior position may result in dystocia. Interestingly, approximately two-thirds of cases of occiput posterior presentation at delivery occur through malrotation during the active phase of labor. The mechanism of this fetopelvic disproportion is partial deflexion of the fetal head. This partial deflexion increases the diameter that must engage in the pelvis. Occiput posterior presentation may result from a contracted anthropoid or android pelvis or insufficient uterine action.

The diagnosis of occiput posterior position is generally made by manual vaginal examination of the orientation of the fetal cephalic sutures. If no gross pelvic contraction is documented on clinical pelvimetry and uterine contractions are inadequate, cautious infusion of oxytocin may be tried. A few authorities advocate midforceps rotation from the occiput posterior to the occiput anterior position. This should be attempted only when macrosomia and gross fetopelvic disproportion have been excluded, other criteria for forceps delivery have been met, and the operator is sufficiently skilled. The prognosis for the infant is excellent when these guidelines are followed; however, maternal morbidity, including extension of episiotomies, higher rates of anal sphincter injury, and other birth canal lacerations, occurs more frequently in occiput posterior deliveries.

2. Occiput transverse—Occiput transverse is frequently a transient position. In most labors, the fetal head spontaneously rotates to the occiput anterior position. Persistent occiput transverse is associated with pelvic dystocia, uterine dystocia, and platypelloid or android pelves. Diagnosis, management, and prognosis are similar to those of persistent occiput posterior presentation. When the fetal head engages but for various reasons does not rotate spontaneously in the midpelvis as in normal labor, midpelvic transverse arrest is diagnosed. Deep transverse arrest occasionally occurs at the inlet, with molding and caput succedaneum formation falsely indicating a lower descent. Cesarean section is required.

B. Brow Presentation

Brow presentations usually are transient fetal presentations with deflexion of the fetal head. During the normal course of labor, conversion to face or vertex presentation generally occurs. If no conversion takes place, dystocia is likely. Brow presentation occurs in approximately 0.06% of deliveries. In approximately 60% of cases, pelvic contraction, prematurity, and grand multiparity are associated findings. The diagnosis is made by vaginal examination. Initial management is expectant, as spontaneous conversion to vertex presentation occurs in more than one-third of all brow presentations. Oxytocin is not recommended, as arrest patterns and uterine inertia are common sequelae because pelvic contraction is often associated with this presentation, and liberal use of cesarean section should be made. Perinatal mortality rates are low when corrected for congenital anomaly, prematurity, and manipulative vaginal delivery.

C. Face Presentation

In face presentation, the fetal head is fully deflexed from the longitudinal axis. Face presentation occurs in approximately 0.2% of all deliveries and has been associated with grand multiparity, advanced maternal age, pelvic masses, pelvic contraction, multiple gestation, polyhydramnios, macrosomia, congenital anomalies including anencephaly and hydrocephaly, prematurity, cornual implantation of the placenta, placenta previa, and premature rupture of the membranes.

Diagnosis of face presentation is most often accomplished by vaginal examination. The prognosis for vaginal delivery is guarded. Complications generally arise with simultaneous pelvic contraction or persistent mentum posterior position. Mentum posterior positions in average-size fetuses are not deliverable vaginally. Arrested labor is typical when spontaneous rotation to the mentum anterior position fails to occur. With mentum anterior presentation, oxytocin augmentation can be considered for arrested labor if cephalopelvic disproportion can be ruled out. Delivery can be accomplished by spontaneous vaginal delivery or cesarean section. There is little or no place for manual flexion of the fetal head or manual rotation from the mentum posterior position to the mentum anterior position.

D. ABNORMAL FETAL LIE

In transverse or oblique lie, the long axis of the fetus is perpendicular, or at an angle, to the maternal longitudinal axis. Abnormalities in axial lie occur in approximately 0.33% of all deliveries but may occur 6 times more frequently in premature labors. Causative factors include grand multiparity, prematurity, pelvic contraction, and abnormal placental implantation.

When the diagnosis is made in the third trimester prior to labor, external cephalic version (ECV) enables a number of these patients to undergo vaginal delivery. Abnormal axial lies have a 20 times greater incidence of cord prolapse than do vertex presentations. Thus prompt cesarean delivery is mandatory with onset of labor or when the membranes rupture. Increased perinatal mortality is associated mainly with prematurity, cord prolapse, and manipulative vaginal delivery. Increased perinatal mortality rates have been consistently reported secondary to internal podalic version, other birth trauma associated with manipulation, and cord prolapse (11–20% of cases of the latter).

A prolapsed extremity alongside the presenting part constitutes **compound presentation.** Compound presentation complicates approximately 0.1% of deliveries. Prematurity and a large pelvic inlet are associated clinical findings. Compound presentations are often diagnosed during physical examination and investigation for failure to progress in labor. Most commonly, a hand is palpated beside the vertex. In most of these patients, labor ends in uncomplicated vaginal delivery, but cesarean section should be performed in the presence of dystocia or cord prolapse. Attempts to reposition the fetal extremity are discouraged, except for gentle pinching of the digits to determine whether the fetus will retract the extremity.

E. BREECH PRESENTATION

Breech presentation is a longitudinal lie with the fetal head occupying the fundus. A **frank breech** describes a breech presentation with flexed hips and extended knees. A **complete breech** describes flexion at both hips and knees. An **incomplete (footling) breech** describes extension of one or both hips. Breech presentation at term occurs in approximately 3–4% of all deliveries. The incidence increases with the degree of prematurity; the incidence at 32 weeks is 7% and at under 28 weeks is 25%. Breech presentation is associated with similar causative factors as face presentation, as well as with previous breech presentation, congenital anomalies, and any anomaly that alters the normal piriform shape of the uterus.

Management options for singleton breech presentation include vaginal breech delivery, ECV with subsequent vaginal cephalic delivery if successful, or elective cesarean section. Recently, a large international multi-

center randomized controlled trial clearly demonstrated lower rates of fetal morbidity with planned cesarean section rather than planned vaginal delivery for singleton breech fetuses, with relative risk of 0.33. In light of these findings, the American College of Obstetricians and Gynecologists (ACOG) Committee on Obstetric Practice issued a formal position that planned vaginal breech delivery may no longer be appropriate for singleton pregnancies. ACOG recommends application of ECV to reduce breech presentation or cesarean section for persistent singleton presentation.

ECV performed at 36 completed weeks of gestation or later, usually with tocolysis, may significantly reduce both the incidence of breech presentation in labor and the number of cesarean sections. Success rates range from 35–86%. Predictors of failure include nulliparity, anterior placental location, fetal weight less than 2500 g, advanced cervical dilatation, and low station. Whereas labor after successful ECV demonstrated higher rates of cesarean section for dystocia and FHR abnormalities, overall cesarean section rates for breech can be lowered.

Prospective studies have identified a subgroup of breech presentations that may be safely delivered vaginally, albeit with great caution. This group includes near-term frank breeches weighing between 2500 and 3800 g with flexed head and no concurrent congenital anomalies, maternal pelvis of adequate dimensions, and a normal labor pattern without FHR abnormalities. In addition, women with prior breech deliveries have lower risks of poor perinatal outcome with subsequent breech delivery. Complications of vaginal breech delivery, including maternal or fetal trauma, fetal head entrapment, and cord prolapse, are uncommon when limited to a properly selected group of patients. Piper forceps should be available for delivery of the aftercoming head. Continuous electronic fetal monitoring is essential, and immediate cesarean section should be available.

Fetal Macrosomia

Excessive fetal size encompasses those fetuses that are large for gestational age (LGA) and those with macrosomia. LGA implies a birth weight greater than the 90th percentile, and macrosomia implies growth beyond a certain size, usually 4000–4500 g, regardless of gestational age. It occurs in approximately 5% of deliveries. Associated risk factors include maternal diabetes, maternal obesity (> 70 kg), excessive maternal weight gain (> 20 kg), postdates pregnancy, and previous delivery of a macrosomic infant. However, fewer than 40% of macrosomic infants are born to patients with identifiable risk factors.

Diagnosis by abdominal palpation is notoriously inaccurate. A better estimated weight may be possible with real-time ultrasonography and standard measured parameters, but ultrasound lacks accuracy, particularly with increased fetal size. Whereas morbidities to infant and mother increase with increasing size between 4000 and 4500 g, perinatal mortality for fetuses weighing more than 4500 g is increased over normal weight infants, and the incidence of shoulder dystocia is at least 10% in this group.

Shoulder dystocia, or difficult delivery of the shoulders after delivery of the fetal head, is an obstetric emergency, with approximately 20% risk of fetal brachial plexus injury, hypoxia, or asphyxia. The incidence of shoulder dystocia is 0.6–1.4% of all vaginal deliveries. It may be heralded by the classic turtle sign. After the fetal head delivers, it retracts back on the maternal perineum. The first action is to call for assistance. Then if gentle inferior traction of the fetal head is not successful, the McRoberts' maneuver may be attempted, which causes rotation of the symphysis pubis. The patient's legs are sharply flexed against her abdomen in an attempt to free the anterior shoulder of the fetus. At the same time, suprapubic pressure can be applied. If shoulder dystocia persists, the shoulder can be rotated (Wood's corkscrew or Rubin's maneuver) to a transverse or oblique diameter of the pelvis, or the posterior arm can be delivered. Episiotomy usually is indicated because it may reduce soft-tissue dystocia and allow the operator to maneuver more easily. Intentional fracture of the clavicle may be required to effect delivery.

If all maneuvers fail and there is a chance for a good fetal outcome, a symphysiotomy or the Zavanelli procedure may be performed. This last maneuver consists of re-placement of the fetal head into the vagina in the flexed position, followed by urgent cesarean section.

Given the morbidity associated with shoulder dystocia and the increasing risk of dystocia with larger fetuses, estimated fetal weights greater than 4500 g in nondiabetic patients and greater than 4250 g in diabetic patients have been suggested by some as thresholds for discussing the option of elective cesarean section for macrosomia. However, because estimations of fetal size frequently are inaccurate, especially in fetuses weighting more than 4000 g, the diagnosis of dystocia secondary to macrosomia requires progression to the active phase of labor and assessment of the adequacy of uterine contractions. In addition, shoulder dystocia cannot be reliably predicted in labor, with more than half of cases occurring without identifiable risk factors. After review of the available evidence, ACOG Practice Bulletin 22 recommends considering elective cesarean section with estimated fetal weight above 5000 g in nondiabetic women or above 4500 g in diabetic women. Prolonged second stage or arrest of descent in macrosomic infants should be delivered by cesarean section rather than operative vaginal delivery, as rates of shoulder dystocia in infants greater than 4500 g delivered with midforceps have been reported to be above 50%.

Fetal Malformation

Fetal malformation may cause dystocia, primarily through fetopelvic disproportion. The most common malformation is hydrocephalus, with an incidence of 0.05%. Management is determined by the severity of the disorder and its prognosis. Other fetal anomalies that may prevent the normal progress of labor include enlargement of the fetal abdomen caused by distended bladder, ascites, or abdominal neoplasms; or other fetal masses, such as meningomyelocele or large omphalocele.

ABNORMALITIES OF THE POWERS

Abnormalities of the "powers" constitute uterine activity that is ineffective in eliciting the normal progress of labor. Ineffective uterine action characteristically falls into one of two categories: hypotonic, with a normal pattern of low-pressure contractions; or hypertonic, with a discoordinated pattern of high-pressure contractions. Studies of normal uterine activity during labor have revealed the following characteristics: (1) the relative intensity of contractions is greater in the fundus than in the midportion or lower uterine segment (**fundal dominance**); (2) the average value of the intensity of contractions is more than 24 mm Hg (in the active phase of labor, pressures often increase to 40–60 mm Hg); (3) contractions are well synchronized in different parts of the uterus; (4) the basal resting pressure of the uterus is between 12 and 15 mm Hg; (5) the frequency of contractions progresses from 1 every 3–5 minutes to 1 every 2–3 minutes during the active phase; (6) the duration of effective contraction in active labor approaches 60 seconds; and (7) the rhythm and force of contractions are regular.

Quantification of uterine activity during labor uses external tocodynamometry or intrauterine pressure catheter measurement. The external tocodynamometer is a pressure sensor placed over the fundal prominence of the uterus that gives an accurate determination of the frequency and duration of uterine contractions. This technique is not adequate for assessment of the resting tone of the uterus or the intensity of contractions. An internal uterine pressure catheter measures intra-amniotic pressure, which is transmitted through the noncompressible fluid within the catheter to a pressure sensor. This technique shows baseline uterine resting pressure, contraction intensity and duration, and frequency of uterine activity. It is the most accurate method for diagnosing uterine dysfunction and evaluating treatment. The **Montevideo unit** is the most widely used measurement of uterine activity. The Montevideo unit is defined as the product of the average intensity of uterine contractions (measured from the baseline resting pressure) multiplied by the number of contractions in a 10-minute interval. Measurements greater than 200 mm Hg should be adequate to produce normal labor progression in most patients.

Uterine dysfunction generally comprises 2 categories: hypotonic dysfunction and uncoordinated hypertonic dysfunction. Hypotonic dysfunction is characterized by contraction of the uterus with insufficient force, irregular or infrequent rhythm, or both. Seen most often in primigravidas in the active phase of labor, hypotonic dysfunction may be caused by excessive sedation, early administration of conduction anesthesia, or overdistension of the uterus (eg, twins, polyhydramnios). Hypotonic dysfunction responds well to oxytocin; however, cephalopelvic disproportion and malpresentation care must be ruled out first. Active management of labor has been shown to decrease perinatal morbidity and cesarean section rates. Less commonly than hypotonic dysfunction, hypertonic uterine contractions and uncoordinated contractions often occur together and are characterized by elevated resting tone of the uterus, dyssynchronous contractions with elevated tone in the lower uterine segment, and frequent intense uterine contractions. It is generally associated with placental abruption, overzealous use of oxytocin, cephalopelvic disproportion, fetal malpresentation, and the latent phase of labor. Treatment may require tocolysis, decrease in oxytocin infusion, or cesarean section as indicated for concomitant malpresentation, cephalopelvic disproportion, or FHR abnormalities. Oxytocin administration is generally of no value. When these patterns occur in the latent phase of labor, sedation may be effective in converting hypertonic contractions to normal labor patterns. Hypertonic labor may cause precipitate labor disorders (see Precipitate Labor Disorders).

Inadequate pushing in the second stage of labor is common and may be caused by conduction anesthesia, oversedation, exhaustion, underlying neurologic dysfunction (eg, paraplegia or hemiplegia), or psychiatric disorders. Mild sedation or a waiting period to permit analgesic or anesthetic agents to wear off may improve expulsive efforts, and outlet forceps or vacuum delivery may be effected in selected cases.

■ FETAL COMPROMISE

Fetal compromise can be defined as a complex of signs indicating a critical response of the fetus to inadequate oxygenation. It represents a continuum of metabolic derangements ranging from hypoxemia to acidosis that affect the functions of vital organs to the point of temporary or permanent injury or death.

FHR monitoring during labor can be accomplished via continuous electronic monitoring or intermittent auscultation with a DeLee stethoscope. Prompt recognition of the symptoms of fetal compromise and, when necessary, decisive, well-planned interventions are imperative for the reduction of perinatal mortality and morbidity, especially to prevent permanent damage to the central nervous system.

FHR should be regularly evaluated for baseline, presence of variability, presence of accelerations, and presence of periodic or episodic decelerations. Baseline rate is between 110 and 160 bpm. *Variability,* defined as fluctuations in the baseline FHR, is reported as absent (undetectable amplitude range), minimal (range < 5 bpm), moderate (range between 6 and 25 bpm), or marked (range greater than 25 bpm). Lack of FHR variability may be associated with a number of factors (eg, fetal immaturity, effect of drugs) that do not indicate fetal compromise. However, the absence of FHR variability may indicate decreased central nervous system control. FHR accelerations occur frequently in early labor. They usually are caused by fetal movement or fetal stimulation. In the absence of decreased variability or decelerations, accelerations are a favorable sign for fetal well-being. Early FHR decelerations result from head compression with uterine contractions and are not associated with poor outcome. Variable FHR decelerations are usually due to cord compression and are not worrisome unless they become recurrent, deeper, and longer in duration. Late decelerations are more ominous because they signify fetal hypoxemia due to uteroplacental insufficiency.

Fetal compromise is secondary to decreased oxygen perfusion, which can be classified as maternal, uterine, placental, or cord complications. Maternal hypotension, shock, heart failure, or hypoxia–hypercapnia result in decreased oxygen supply to the uterus. In cases of uterine hypertonia (tachysystole, tetanic contractions) or placental abruption, oxygen cannot cross from the maternal vessels to the placenta. Placental and cord problems include abnormal placentation such as placenta previa, lack of sufficient placental reserve to tolerate labor (postmaturity, placental infarcts), umbilical cord compression (knots, entanglement, occult or frank prolapse), and ruptured vasa previa.

Tachycardia, lack of FHR variability, and late FHR decelerations together signify fetal compromise. Recurrent variable or late decelerations despite attempted therapy and prolonged decelerations are signs of fetal compromise and may represent a fetal pH of less than 7.10, reflecting fetal acidemia. Prompt evaluation and treatment are mandatory.

MANAGEMENT OF FETAL COMPROMISE

It is important to note that although a fetal heart tracing with accelerations carries a high sensitivity and high negative predictive value for a healthy, nonacidotic fetus, the presence of decelerations and decreased variability has a low specificity for acidosis. Thus, except in cases of ominous fetal heart tracing patterns such as refractory bradycardia or a sinusoidal pattern, which mandate immediate delivery, intrauterine resuscitative measures and assessment of fetal status can be accomplished. The presence of FHR accelerations elicited by scalp stimulation or fetal acoustic stimulation strongly correlates with nonacidotic fetal status. Preliminary studies show promise for fetal pulse oximetry as an additional tool in the assessment of fetal status. In the presence of continued signs of fetal well-being, it is possible to allow labor to continue.

Intrauterine resuscitation should be tailored to the likely underlying cause of fetal compromise. In the presence of a concerning fetal tracing, vaginal examination to assess for rapid progression of labor or cord prolapse should be part of the initial assessment. A change of the mother's position may adjust fetal position and decrease compression of the umbilical cord. Variable decelerations can be improved by amnioinfusion, replacement of amniotic fluid with saline via an intrauterine pressure catheter. Maternal venous return, relative hypovolemia, and thus uterine perfusion may be improved with the patient in a lateral position. Supine hypotension, particularly after placement of epidural anesthesia, may be corrected by elevation of the maternal legs, lateral positioning, and rapid administration of fluids intravenously. These actions help to restore the gravida's arterial pressure and increase the blood flow in the intervillous space and perfusion to the fetus. Rarely, cardiotonics (eg, ephedrine) are required. Discontinuing the administration of oxytocin may improve placental perfusion, increasing the oxygenation of the fetus. Administration of high concentrations of oxygen (10 L/min by mask) will raise the maternofetal PO_2 gradient and increase maternofetal oxygen transfer, alleviating fetal hypoxia. However, evidence is insufficient to support the use of prophylactic oxygen therapy for women in the second stage of labor or to evaluate its effectiveness in alleviating fetal hypoxemia. In the rare case of maternal acidosis as the cause of fetal acidosis, administering bicarbonate to the mother may benefit both mother and infant. However, if acidosis is severe, the infant should be promptly delivered.

In summary, in cases of possible fetal compromise, vaginal examination should be performed to assess for rapid progression or cord prolapse. Intrauterine resuscitation can be accomplished by changing the position of the mother, amnioinfusion, correcting maternal hypotension by intravenous fluid administration, decreasing uterine activity by stopping oxytocin or administering tocolytics, and providing oxygen by face mask. Labor can be continued if the FHR tracing is not ominous. If fetal well-being cannot be documented, or if FHR abnormalities do not resolve with these measures, immediate delivery is indicated. Obstetric judgment must dictate how the delivery will be accomplished in accordance with the presentation, station, position, dilatation of the cervix, and presumed fetal status. Cesarean delivery, if chosen, must be accomplished rapidly.

■ VAGINAL BLEEDING IN LABOR

A small amount of bleeding associated with cervical dilatation is common in labor, but vaginal bleeding must be carefully evaluated to assess for placental abruption or placenta previa.

Placenta previa complicates approximately 0.5% of pregnancies. Diagnosis is frequently made prior to the onset of labor; the hallmark of previa is painless vaginal bleeding during the second or third trimester. Profuse painless bleeding during the course of labor may represent a previously undiagnosed placenta previa. Patients should be evaluated with abdominal ultrasound and, if indicated, vaginal ultrasound. Digital palpation of the cervix should not be done. When diagnosed remote from delivery, previa with bleeding mandates abdominal delivery.

Placental abruption should be suspected in cases of vaginal bleeding with FHR abnormalities. Patients at risk for abruption (see Chapter 20) should be surveilled closely. Abruption also may manifest as bloody fluid at the time of rupture of membranes, abdominal pain, or uterine hypertonicity. If bleeding is severe or the FHR pattern is ominous and vaginal delivery is not imminent, emergent cesarean delivery is necessary.

FETAL BLOOD LOSS IN LABOR

Blood loss occurring in labor and delivery is most commonly of maternal origin, but fetal blood loss may occur from trauma to the placenta or from vasa previa. The fetoplacental vascular volume at term is only 250–500 mL, so what appears to be minor vaginal bleeding could be rapidly fatal to the fetus. Certain FHR patterns on electronic monitoring, particularly fetal tachycardia, recurrent decelerations, prolonged bradycardia, or a sinusoidal pattern, may signify fetal compromise due to anemia. The Apt test and the Kleihauer-Betke test both can detect fetal hemoglobin. However, these tests are performed only when there is clinical suspicion of fetomaternal hemorrhage. When significant fetal bleeding is more certain, delivery must be accomplished expeditiously if the infant is to be saved.

VASA PREVIA

In approximately 1% of pregnancies, the umbilical vessels divide within the amnionic membranes before they reach the placenta. In this condition, known as a *velamentous cord insertion,* the vessels may cross the internal os in advance of the fetal presenting part (**vasa previa**). During labor, the vessels are likely to be disrupted, with rapid fetal exsanguination occurring in as many as 75% of cases. Diagnosis of vasa previa or velamentous cord insertion is rarely made before rupture of the membranes. The antenatal period is the ideal time for identification of vasa previa, but the discovery of vessels crossing the internal os is rare prior to cervical dilatation.

The diagnosis is often made after the rupture of the membranes by palpation of fetal vessels in the membranes overlying the presenting part through the partially or fully dilated cervix. The usual presentation is sudden-onset bleeding with fetal tachycardia. Fetal tachycardia alone soon after rupture of the membranes may indicate fetal bleeding. Sinusoidal FHR pattern on electronic fetal monitoring may indicate severe anemia. When vasa previa is diagnosed during labor, the infant should be delivered by emergency cesarean section. Even in the most expeditiously performed delivery, infant prognosis is poor when fetal exsanguination occurs.

REFERENCES

Dystocia

American College of Obstetricians and Gynecologists: *External Cephalic Version.* ACOG Practice Bulletin No. 13. American College of Obstetricians and Gynecologists, 2000.

American College of Obstetricians and Gynecologists: *Fetal Macrosomia.* ACOG Practice Bulletin No. 22. American College of Obstetricians and Gynecologists, 2000.

American College of Obstetricians and Gynecologists: *Mode of Term Singleton Breech Delivery.* ACOG Committee Opinion No. 265. American College of Obstetricians and Gynecologists, 2001.

American College of Obstetricians and Gynecologists: *Shoulder Dystocia.* ACOG Practice Bulletin No. 40. American College of Obstetricians and Gynecologists, 2002.

Boucher M et al: The relationship between amniotic fluid index and successful external cephalic version: a 14-year experience. Am J Obstet Gynecol 2003;189:751.

Caldwell WE, Moloy HC: Anatomical variations in the female pelvis and their effect in labor with a suggested classification. Am J Obstet Gynecol 1933;26:479.

Fitzpatrick M et al: Influence of persistent occiput posterior position on delivery outcome. Obstet Gynecol 2001;98:1027.

Friedman EA: The labor curve. Clin Perinatol 1981;8:15.

Gherman RB et al: Analysis of McRoberts' maneuver by x-ray pelvimetry. Obstet Gynecol 2000;95:43.

Gilbert WM et al: Vaginal versus cesarean delivery for breech presentation in California: A population-based study. Obstet Gynecol 2003;102:911.

Hannah ME et al: Planned caesarean section versus planned vaginal birth for breech presentation at term: A randomised multicentre trial. Lancet 2000;356:1375.

Hernandez C, Wendel GD: Shoulder dystocia. Clin Obstet Gynecol 1990;33:526.

Hofmeyr GJ: Interventions to help external cephalic version for breech presentation at term. Cochrane Database Syst Rev 2004;(2):CD000184.

Kozak LJ, Owings MF, Hall MJ: National Hospital Discharge Summary: 2001 annual summary with detailed diagnosis and procedure data. Vital Health Stat 13;156:1.

Pattinson RC: Pelvimetry for fetal cephalic presentations at term. Cochrane Database Syst Rev 2000;(2):CD000161.

Porreco RP et al: Dystocia in nulliparous patients monitored with fetal pulse oximetry. Am J Obstet Gynecol 2004;190:113.

Ramsey PS, Ramin KD, Field CS: Shoulder dystocia. Rotational maneuvers revisited. J Reprod Med 2000;45:85.

Sadler LC, Davidson T, McCowan LM: A randomised controlled trial and meta-analysis of active management of labour. Br J Obstet Gynaecol 2000;107:909.

Sizer AR, Nirmal DM: Occipitoposterior position: Associated factors and obstetric outcomes in nulliparas. Obstet Gynecol 2000;96:749.

Stubbs TM: Oxytocin for labor induction. Clin Obstet Gynecol 2000;43:489.

Fetal Compromise

American College of Obstetricians and Gynecologists: Neonatal encephalopathy and cerebral palsy: Executive summary. Obstet Gynecol 2004;103:780.

Dildy GA: Fetal pulse oximetry: A critical appraisal. Best Pract Res Clin Obstet Gynaecol 2004;18:477.

Hofmeyr GJ, Kulier R: Tocolysis for preventing fetal distress in second stage of labour. Cochrane Database Syst Rev 2000;(2):CD000037.

National Institute of Child Health and Human Development Research Planning Workshop: Electronic fetal heart rate monitoring: Research guidelines for interpretation. Am J Obstet Gynecol 1997;177:1385.

Rinehart BK et al: Randomized trial of intermittent or continuous amnioinfusion for variable decelerations. Obstet Gynecol 2000;96:571.

Sameshima H et al: Unselected low-risk pregnancies and the effect of continuous intrapartum fetal heart rate monitoring on umbilical blood gases and cerebral palsy. Am J Obstet Gynecol 2004;190:118.

Vaginal Bleeding in Labor

Kayani SI, Walkinshaw SA, Preston C: Pregnancy outcome in severe placental abruption. Br J Obstet Gynaecol 2003;110:679.

Lee W et al: Vasa previa: Prenatal diagnosis, natural evolution, and clinical outcome. Obstet Gynecol 2000;95:572.

Oyelese Y et al: Second trimester low-lying placenta and in-vitro fertilization? Exclude vasa previa. J Matern Fetal Med 2000;9:370.

Obstetric Analgesia & Anesthesia

John S. McDonald, MD, & Ralph W. Yarnell, MD, FRCPC

Analgesia is the loss or modulation of pain perception. It can be (1) local and affect only a small area of the body, (2) regional and affect a larger portion of the body, or (3) systemic. Analgesia is achieved by the use of hypnosis (suggestion), systemic medication, regional agents, or inhalational agents.

Anesthesia is the total loss of sensory perception and may include loss of consciousness. It is induced by various agents and techniques. In obstetrics, **regional anesthesia** is accomplished with local anesthetic techniques (epidural, spinal) and **general anesthesia** with systemic medication and endotracheal intubation.

The terms *analgesia* and *anesthesia* are sometimes confused in common usage. Analgesia denotes those states in which only modulation of pain perception is involved. Anesthesia denotes those states in which mental awareness and perception of other sensations are lost. Attempts have been made to divide anesthesia into various components, including analgesia, amnesia, relaxation, and loss of reflex response to pain. Analgesia can be regarded as a component of anesthesia if viewed in this way.

The use of techniques and medications to provide pain relief in obstetrics requires an expert understanding of their effects to ensure the safety of both mother and fetus.

ANATOMY OF PAIN

It may be academic to argue that pain should be defined as the parturient's response to the stimuli of labor, because agreement on a definition of pain has eluded scholars for centuries.

Nevertheless, it should be appreciated that the "pain response" is a response of the total personality and cannot be dissected systematically and scientifically. Physicians are obligated to provide a comfortable or at least a tolerable labor and delivery. Many patients are tense and apprehensive at the onset of labor, although they may have little or no discomfort. The physician must be knowledgeable of the options for pain relief and respond to the patient's needs and wishes.

The evolution of pain in the first stage of labor originally was described as involving spinal segments T11 and T12. Subsequent research has determined that segments T10–L1 are involved. Discomfort is associated with ischemia of the uterus during contraction as well as dilatation and effacement of the cervix. Sensory pathways that convey nociceptive impulses of the first stage of labor include the uterine plexus, the inferior hypogastric plexus, the middle hypogastric plexus, the superior hypogastric plexus, the lumbar and lower thoracic sympathetic chain, and the T10–L1 spinal segments.

Pain in the second stage of labor undoubtedly is produced by distention of the vagina and perineum. Sensory pathways from these areas are conveyed by branches of the pudendal nerve via the dorsal nerve of the clitoris, the labial nerves, and the inferior hemorrhoidal nerves. These are the major sensory branches to the perineum and are conveyed along nerve roots S2, S3, and S4. Nevertheless, other nerves, such as the ilioinguinal nerves, the genital branches of the genitofemoral nerves, and the perineal branches of the posterior femoral cutaneous nerves, may play a role in perineal innervation.

Although the major portion of the perineum is innervated by the 3 major branches of the pudendal nerve, innervation by the other nerves mentioned may be important in some patients. The type of pain reported may be an ache in the back or loins (referred pain, perhaps from the cervix), a cramp in the uterus (due to fundal contraction), or a "bursting" or "splitting" sensation in the lower vaginal canal or pudendum (due to dilatation of the cervix and vagina).

Dystocia, which usually is painful, may be due to fetopelvic disproportion; tetanic, prolonged, or dysrhythmic uterine contractions; intrapartum infection; or many other causes (see Chapter 28).

SAFETY OF OBSTETRIC ANESTHESIA

Substantial advances in the quality and safety of obstetric anesthesia have been made in the past 3 decades. Outdated techniques, such as "twilight sleep" and mask anesthesia, have been recognized as ineffective or unsafe and have been replaced by epidural infusion of narcotic/local anesthesia mixtures and patient-controlled analgesia during labor and postoperatively. When required, general anesthesia is provided using short-acting drugs with well-known fetal effects, and careful attention is focused on airway management.

Maternal mortality relating to anesthesia has been reduced 10-fold since the 1950s, largely because of an enhanced appreciation of special maternal risks associated with anesthesia. The overall anesthesia-related death rate in the United States now is as low as 1.3 per million live births, a 5-fold decline in the last decade. Regional anesthesia now is more commonly performed for cesarean delivery, fewer births occur in hospitals performing fewer than 500 deliveries per year, and having both in-house anesthesia and obstetric physician coverage is more common. In the face of these improvements, 2 distressing statistics have recently emerged. First, the case fatality rate for general anesthesia for cesarean delivery has risen from 20 deaths per million general anesthetics administered in the early 1980s to 32.3 deaths per million general anesthetics administered today. This increase occurred during a period when the case fatality rate for regional anesthesia in obstetrics deceased from 8.6 per million to 1.9 per million regional anesthetics administered. The case fatality rate for general anesthesia may have increased because general anesthesia now is reserved for urgent and critical situations, whereas in the past general anesthesia was more commonly used for elective obstetric delivery. Difficulty with intubation, aspiration, and hypoxemia leading to cardiopulmonary arrest are the leading causes of anesthesia-related maternal death.

The second point of concern is the increase in overall maternal mortality (not related specifically to anesthesia) in the United States since 1985. This increase in maternal mortality is most pronounced in older parturients (older than 35 years), particularly in black parturients. Cardiomyopathy, hypertension, and hemorrhage are the principal etiologies associated with these rising mortality rates and are important factors for the anesthesiologist to consider.

TECHNIQUES OF ANALGESIA WITHOUT THE USE OF DRUGS

Psychophysical Methods

Three distinct psychological techniques have been developed as a means of facilitating the birth process and making it a positive emotional experience: "natural childbirth," psychoprophylaxis, and hypnosis. So-called *natural childbirth* was developed by Grantly Dick-Read in the early 1930s and popularized in his book *Childbirth Without Fear*. Dick-Read's approach emphasized the reduction of tension to induce relaxation. The psychoprophylactic technique was developed by Velvovski, who published the results of his work from Russia in 1950. In Russia in the mid-1950s, it became evident that obstetric psychoprophylaxis was a useful substitute for poorly administered or

dangerously conducted anesthesia for labor and delivery. This method was later introduced in France by Lamaze. Hypnosis for pain relief has achieved periodic spurts of popularity since the early 1800s and depends on the power of suggestion.

Many obstetricians argue that psychoprophylaxis can largely eliminate the pain of childbirth by diminishing cortical appreciation of pain impulses rather than by depressing cortical function, as occurs with drug-induced analgesia. Relaxation, suggestion, concentration, and motivation are factors that overlap other methods of preparation for childbirth. Some of them are closely related to hypnosis.

These techniques can significantly reduce anxiety, tension, and fear. They provide the parturient with a valuable understanding of the physiologic changes that occur during labor and delivery. In addition, they provide an opportunity for closer understanding and communication between the patient and her mate, who may be an important source of comfort to her during the stressful process of childbirth. If psychophysical techniques do no more than this, they deserve the obstetrician's support.

Studies undertaken to assess the effectiveness of psychophysical techniques have reported widely divergent results, with effectiveness ranging from as low as 10–20% to as high as 70–80%. The overall benefit is best judged by the parturient herself, with validation by the observations of attendants. As is no doubt true in other aspects of medical practice in which emotional overlay and subjective reporting play a role in the evaluation of specific types of therapy, the personality and level of enthusiasm of the doctor can strongly influence the patient's reactions to a given therapy. Practitioners who are skeptical of psychophysical techniques cannot expect to accomplish very much using them.

None of these psychophysical techniques should be forced on a patient, even by a skillful practitioner. The patient must not be made to feel that she will fail if she does not choose to complete her labor and delivery without analgesic medication. It must be made clear to the patient from the outset that she is expected to ask for help if she feels she wants or needs it. All things considered, psychophysical techniques should be viewed as adjuncts to other analgesic methods rather than substitutes for them.

The effectiveness of hypnosis is partially due to the well-known, although incompletely understood, mechanisms by which emotional and other central processes can influence a person's overall responses to the pain experience. Verbal suggestion and somatosensory stimulation may help to alleviate discomfort associated with the first stage of labor. In addition, hypnotic states may provide apparent analgesia and amnesia for distressing, anxiety-provoking experiences. Finally, hypnotic techniques may substantially improve the parturient's outlook and behavior by reducing fear and apprehension. However, certain practical points with regard to hypnosis must be considered because the time needed to establish a suitable relationship between physician and patient often is more than can be made available in the course of a busy medical practice.

ANALGESIC, AMNESTIC, & ANESTHETIC AGENTS

General Comments & Precautions

1. If the patient is prepared psychologically for her experience, she will require less medication. Anticipate and dispel her fears during the antenatal period and in early labor. Never promise a painless labor.
2. Individualize the treatment of every patient, because each one reacts differently. Unfavorable reactions to any drug can occur.
3. Know the drug you intend to administer. Be familiar with its limitations, dangers, and contraindications as well as its advantages.
4. All analgesics given to the mother will cross the placenta. Systemic medications produce higher maternal and fetal blood levels than regionally administered drugs. Many drugs have central nervous system depressant effects. Although they may have the desired effect on the mother, they also may exert a mild to severe depressant effect on the fetus or newborn.

The ideal drug will have an optimal beneficial effect on the mother and a minimal depressant effect on the offspring. None of the presently available narcotic and sedative medications used in obstetrics has selective maternal effects. The regional administration of local anesthetics accomplished this goal to a large extent because the low maternal serum levels that are produced expose the fetus to insignificant quantities of drugs.

Pharmacologic Aspects

A. ROUTE OF ADMINISTRATION

Systemic techniques of analgesia and anesthesia include both oral and parenteral routes of administration. Parenteral administration includes subcutaneous, intramuscular, and intravenous injection. Sedatives, tranquilizers, and analgesics usually are given by intramuscular injection. In some cases, the intravenous route is preferred.

The advantages of intravenous administration are (1) avoidance of variable rates of uptake due to poor vascular supply in fat or muscle; (2) prompt onset of effect; (3) titration of effect, avoiding the "peak effect" of

$$R{:}NH^+ + OH^- \longrightarrow R{:}N + HOH$$

Cation   Base

$$pH = pK_a + \log \frac{Base}{Cation}$$

Figure 29–1. Local anesthetics are weak bases coexisting as undissociated free base and dissociated cation. Their proportion can be calculated by means of the Henderson-Hasselbalch equation.

an intramuscular bolus; and (4) smaller effective doses because of earlier onset of action.

The disadvantages of intravenous injection are inadvertent arterial injection and the depressant effect of overdosage, but the advantage of smaller dosage outweighs the disadvantages.

Always administer the lowest concentration and the smallest dose to obtain the desired effect.

B. PHYSICAL AND CHEMICAL FACTORS

Anesthetics penetrate body cells by passing through the lipid membrane boundary. This membrane is not permeable to charged (ionized) drugs but is permeable to unionized forms of drugs. Much of the total drug transfer is dependent on the degree of lipid solubility, so local anesthetics are characterized by aromatic rings that are lipophilic, and all are lipid-soluble. The intermediate amine radical of a local anesthetic is a weak base that in aqueous solutions exists partly as undissociated free base and partly as dissociated cation. Figure 29–1 shows the equilibrium for such an existence and the Henderson-Hasselbalch equation, with which the proportion of the anesthetic in the charged and uncharged forms can be determined. The ratio of the cation to the base form of the drug is important, because the base form is responsible for penetration and tissue diffusion of the local anesthetic, whereas the cation form is responsible for local analgesia when the drug contacts the site of action within the sodium channel on the axolemma.

The pK_a of a drug is the pH at which equal proportions of the free base and cation form occur. Most local anesthetics used in obstetric analgesia have pK_a values ranging from 7.7–9.1 (Table 29–1). Because the pH of maternal blood is equal to or greater than 7.4, the pK_a of local anesthetics is so close that significant changes in maternal and fetal acid–base balance may result in fluxes in the base versus the cation forms of the drug. For example, a rising pH shifts a given amount of local anesthetic cation to the base form; conversely, a fall in pH generates more of the cationic form.

Physical factors are important in drug transfer. Drugs with a molecular weight (MW) under 600 cross the pla-

Table 29–1. pK$_a$ values of the more commonly used local anesthetics.

Drug	Brand Name	pK$_a$
Bupivacaine	Marcaine	8.1
Chloroprocaine	Nesacaine	8.7
Etidocaine	Duranest	7.7
Lidocaine	Xylocaine	7.9
Ropivacaine	Naropin	8.0

centa without difficulty, whereas those with MW over 1000 do not. A molecule such as digoxin (MW 780.95) crosses the ovine placenta very poorly. Molecular weights of most local anesthetics are in the 200–300 range. From the physical aspect, most local anesthetics cross the maternal–fetal barrier by simple diffusion according to the principles of Fick's law (Fig 29–2), which states that the rate of diffusion of a drug depends on the concentration gradient of the drug between the maternal and fetal compartments and the relationship of the thickness and total surface available for transfer.

C. PLACENTAL TRANSFER

Factors other than the physical or chemical properties of a drug may affect its transfer across the placenta. These factors include the rate and route of drug administration and the distribution, metabolism, and excretion of the drug by the mother and fetus. Fick's law may appear to be a simple method of determining drug transfer, but other complexities exist: differential blood flow on either side of the placenta, volume of maternal and fetal blood, and various shunts in the intervillous space that are important determinants of the final amount of drug a fetus may receive. Certain maternal disorders, such as hypertensive cardiovascular disease, diabetes, and preeclampsia-eclampsia, may alter placental blood flow and in some way affect the extent of drug distribution.

As the placenta matures, the thickness of the epithelial trophoblastic layer progressively decreases. This reduction may cause the thickness of the tissue layers between the maternal and fetal compartments to decrease 10-fold (from as much as 25 μm in early gestation to 2 μm at term in some species). As gestation progresses,

$$Q/T = K\left[\frac{A(C_M - C_F)}{D}\right]$$

Figure 29–2. Fick's law. A, surface area available for drug transfer; C$_M$, maternal drug concentration; C$_F$, fetal drug concentration; D, membrane thickness; K, diffusion constant of the drug; Q/T, rate of diffusion.

the surface area of the placenta also increases. At term, these changes in physical structure tend to favor improved transfer of drugs across the placenta.

Placental transfer is affected by the pH of the blood on both sides of the placenta. The pH of the blood on the fetal side of the placenta normally is 0.1–0.2 U lower than that on the maternal side. Therefore, passage of drug to the fetal unit results in a tendency for more of the drug to exist in the ionized state. Because the maternal–fetal equilibrium is established only between the unionized fraction of the drug on either side of the barrier, this physiologic differential will expedite maternal–fetal transfer of drug. With more drug in the ionized form in the fetal unit, the new equilibrium that arises results in a greater total (ionized plus un-ionized) drug load in the fetus. Because the pK$_a$ values of commonly used local anesthetics are closer to the maternal blood pH, these agents tend to accumulate on the fetal side of the placenta. This also is true of other basic drugs such as morphine, meperidine, and propranolol. Further decreases in the fetal pH lead to additional drug entrapment in the fetus. For acidic drugs (eg, thiopental) the shift in total drug concentration is in the opposite direction, that is, toward the maternal side of the placenta.

In summary, the rate of transfer of a drug is governed mainly by (1) lipid solubility, (2) degree of drug ionization, (3) placental blood flow, (4) molecular weight, (5) placental metabolism, and (6) protein binding.

D. FETAL DISTRIBUTION

After a drug deposited in the maternal compartment passes through the maternal–fetal barrier, the drug must reach the fetus and undergo distribution (Fig 29–3). The response of the fetus and newborn depends on drug concentration in vessel-rich organs, such as the brain, heart, and liver. Drugs transferred from the maternal to the fetal compartment of the placenta are then diluted before distribution to the various fetal vital organs. Approximately 85% of the blood in the umbilical vein, which passes from the placenta to the fetus, passes through the fetal liver and then into the inferior vena cava. The remainder bypasses the liver and enters the vena cava primarily via the ductus venosus. The drug concentration is further reduced by an admixture of blood coming from the lower extremities, the abdominal viscera, the upper extremities, and the thorax. Blood from the right atrium shunts from right to left through the foramen ovale into the left atrium, resulting in a final concentration on the left side of the heart, which is only slightly lower than that in the vena cava.

The amount of drug ultimately reaching a vital organ is related to that organ's blood supply. Because the central nervous system is the most highly vascularized fetal organ, it receives the greatest amount of drug. Once the drug reaches the fetal liver, it may either be bound to protein or metabolized.

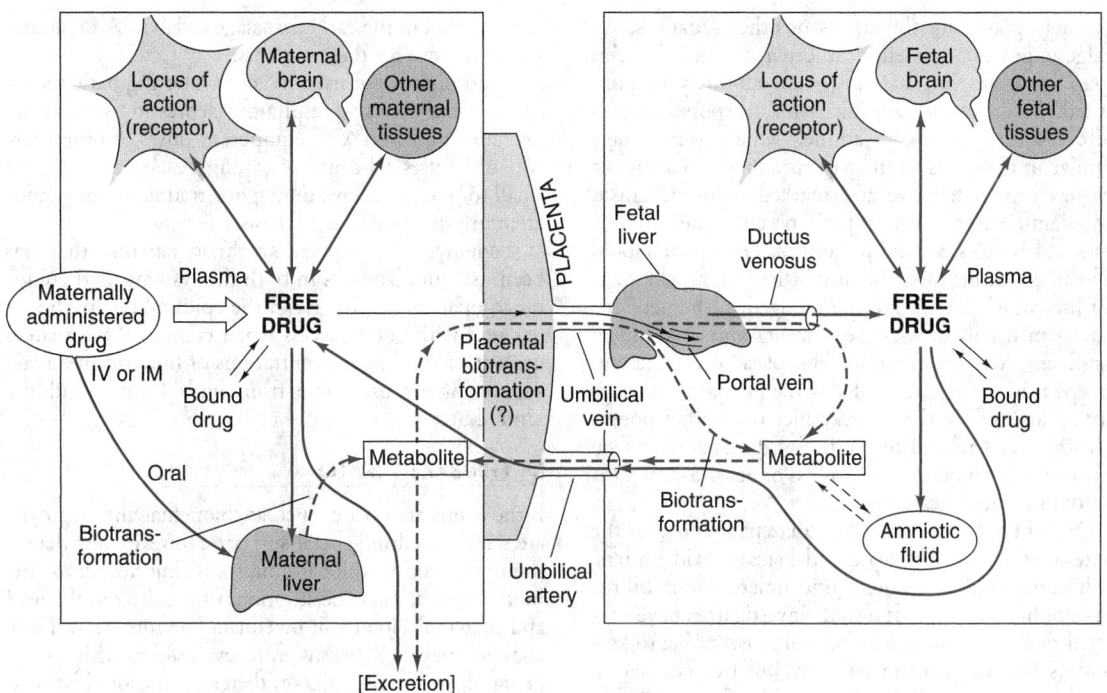

Figure 29–3. Relationship between maternal and fetal compartments and distribution of drugs between them. Drug is passed from the maternal compartment, via the placenta (a partial barrier), to the fetal compartment, where the principles of drug dynamics (ie, distribution, biotransformation, and excretion) determine the eventual specific organ tissue levels. One purely mechanical barrier exists between the maternal and fetal compartments, which attains importance in the late first and second stages of labor—the umbilical cord, which is susceptible to partial and total occlusion.

The uptake of drug by fetal tissues can be very rapid after either intravenous or epidural administration. Measurable concentrations of local anesthetics have been found in fetal tissues as early as 1–2 minutes after injection. Lipid solubility of a drug is important in developing concentrations in certain organs with high lipid content, such as the adrenal, ovary, liver, and brain.

Drug metabolism and excretion are the final features of the fetal distribution picture. The fetal liver is able to metabolize drugs and numerous substrates as early as the second trimester, an ability that improves to term. Narcotics and sedatives are metabolized much more slowly by the fetal liver, producing a prolonged effect of these drugs in the newborn who is exposed in utero. Finally, the ability of the fetus to excrete drugs is also reduced by reduced renal function.

Systemic Analgesics & Anesthetics

A. SEDATIVES (HYPNOTICS)

The principal use of sedative–hypnotic drugs is to produce drowsiness. For many years, these drugs were the only ones available to reduce anxiety and induce drowsiness. The latent phase of the first stage of labor can be managed by either psychologic support alone or utilization of sedative–hypnotic compounds. Psychologic support may be complemented by the use of sedatives. When properly used, these drugs induce tranquility and an enhanced feeling of well-being. They are poor analgesics and do not raise the pain threshold appreciably in conscious subjects. Amnesia does not occur. Labor may be slowed by large doses of sedatives, especially when given too early in the first stage.

The use of barbiturates alone for obstetric analgesia is not common practice and should be discouraged. The required dosage is dangerous to the fetus, which is extremely sensitive to central nervous system depression by these drugs. Periodic apnea and even abolition of all movements outlast the effects of the barbiturates on the mother.

B. TRANQUILIZERS AND AMNESTICS

These drugs are used principally to relieve apprehension and anxiety and to produce a calm state. Additionally, they may potentiate the effects of other sedatives. An analgesic-potentiating effect is often claimed for this group of agents but has not been definitely demonstrated. Hydroxyzine and diazepam are popular tranquilizer–amnestics. Scopolamine, which was widely popular in obstetrics in the past, produces no analgesia but has a mild sedative and marked amnestic effect. Scopolamine is no longer used because the amnesia produced is excessive and prolonged. Diazepam should be avoided during labor because it has a long chemical half-life, which is even more prolonged in the neonate. Diazepam readily crosses the placenta and is found in significant concentrations in fetal plasma. At present, diazepam is not recommended if the neonate is premature because of the threat of kernicterus. Other potential side effects related to the use of diazepam are fetal hypotonia, hypothermia, and a loss of beat-to-beat variability in the fetal heart rate.

One of the controversies over diazepam concerns the content of sodium benzoate and benzoic acid buffers. Both compounds are potent uncouplers of the bilirubin–albumin complex, and some investigators have suggested that the neonate may be more susceptible to kernicterus because of an increase level of free circulating bilirubin. However, because injectable diazepam is effective in the treatment of human newborn seizure disorders, opiate withdrawal, and tetanus and because it is regarded as a useful adjunct in obstetric analgesia, a study was undertaken in animals in which comparable quantities of sodium benzoate were injected to determine whether significant amounts of bilirubin would be made available to the circulation. Midazolam, a short-acting water-soluble benzodiazepine, appears to be devoid of the neonatal effects seen with diazepam and is more rapidly cleared. Midazolam is a relatively new agent with minimal clinical use to date in obstetrics, but in small doses it could conceivably become a useful anxiolytic for the laboring patient. Midazolam is 3–4 times more potent than diazepam, and there is a brief delay in the onset of its sedative effect after intravenous injection. Doses should be kept below 0.075 mg/kg to avoid excessive anterograde amnesia.

C. NARCOTIC ANALGESICS

Systemic analgesic drugs (including narcotics) are commonly used in the first stage of labor because they produce both a state of analgesia and mood elevation. The favored drugs are codeine 60 mg intramuscularly or meperidine 50–100 mg intramuscularly or 25–50 mg (titrated) intravenously. The combination of morphine and scopolamine was once popular for its "twilight sleep" effect but is rarely used now. Common undesirable effects of this combination of drugs are nausea and vomiting, cough suppression, intestinal stasis, and diminution in frequency, intensity, and duration of uterine

contractions in the early first stage of labor. Also, amnesia is excessive for these patients.

Morphine is not used in active laboring patients because of the excessive respiratory depression seen in the neonate compared with equipotent doses of other narcotics. Fetuses who are of young gestational age, are small for dates, or have undergone trauma or long labor are more susceptible to narcosis.

Fentanyl is a popular synthetic narcotic that has been used in obstetrics in both the systemic and epidural compartments. Its use in the epidural compartment has met with good success when combined with small quantities and low concentrations of bupivacaine. Data supporting its use come from both Europe and the United States.

D. THIOBARBITURATES

Intravenous anesthetics such as thiopental and thiamylal are widely used in general surgery. However, less than 4 minutes after a thiobarbiturate is injected into the mother's vein, the concentrations of the drug in the fetal and maternal blood will be equal. The mother will lose consciousness and airway protective reflexes with a thiopental dose of 1.5–2 mg/kg; therefore, it should be used only in association with general endotracheal anesthesia.

E. PROPOFOL

Propofol is a newer induction agent that was introduced into practice in the United States in the early 1990s. It is a hydrophobic propylphenol that is formulated as an aqueous emulsion in soybean and egg phosphatide. As an induction agent, it is similar to the barbiturates in mild cardiac depression and loss of peripheral vasomotor tone. It offers the advantages of rapid clearance, short duration of action, antiemetic properties, and reduced risk of airway reactivity. It is an ideal agent for induction of general anesthesia at a dose of 2 mg/kg in parturients. It also can be used in 10- to 20-mg increments during surgery under regional block to treat nausea and vomiting. Neonatal Apgar scores and umbilical gases are similar following induction with propofol or barbiturates.

F. KETAMINE

The phencyclidine derivative ketamine produces anesthesia by a dissociative interruption of afferent pathways from cortical perception. It has become a useful and widely used adjunctive agent in obstetrics because maternal cardiovascular status and uterine blood flow are well maintained. In low doses of 0.25–0.5 mg/kg intravenously, effective maternal analgesia results but without loss of consciousness or protective reflexes. The margin of safety is narrow, however, so it should be used only by physicians able to easily secure and protect the airway if loss of consciousness occurs. For cesarean section delivery, general anesthetic induction can be produced with 1–2 mg/kg intravenously and is followed in rapid sequence with a muscle relaxant and endotracheal intubation. Ketamine is useful in the setting of major blood loss, when rapid induction of general anesthesia is required. However, it has significant hallucinogenic effects that limit its utility in obstetrics.

Ketamine stimulates the cardiovascular system to maintain heart rate, blood pressure, and cardiac output; therefore, it is useful in complicated situations of maternal hypotension/hemorrhage.

G. Inhalation Anesthetics

Inhaled anesthetics are administered as a component of general anesthesia. In the past, inhaled anesthetics were given during labor in subanesthetic concentrations to treat contraction pain, but they are no longer used for this indication. The mask administration of these gases to the conscious laboring patient can result in airway obstruction, aspiration, and hypoxia. Also, the labor room environment would become unacceptably contaminated by the vaporized gases because effectively scavenging of exhaust gases from the room is not possible. Finally, of all the presently used volatile anesthetics, only nitrous oxide has analgesic properties at subanesthetic concentrations.

The most commonly used inhaled anesthetics in pregnancy are nitrous oxide, halothane, and isoflurane. During general anesthesia, 50% nitrous oxide in oxygen is supplemented with either 0.5% halothane or 0.7% isoflurane to provide most of the anesthetic requirements during the maintenance phase of the anesthetic. These drugs all readily cross the placenta and produce significant blood concentrations in the fetus. During the brief exposure to maternally administered anesthetic gases, the fetus is not adversely affected. Fetal cardiac output is slightly reduced by these drugs, but critical organ blood flow is unaffected, and fetal acid–base status is unchanged. Exposure to minimum alveolar concentrations of anesthetic gases for more than 15 minutes is associated with reduced Apgar scores, but other parameters of fetal and newborn well-being are unimpaired.

The term parturient is more sensitive to the anesthetic effects of all inhaled anesthetics, presumably as a result of elevated progesterone levels. This increased sensitivity of 20–30% compared to nonpregnant subjects places the patient at increased risk for obtundation and aspiration; therefore these drugs should not be administered without preparation for endotracheal intubation. Halothane and isoflurane produce uterine relaxation, and high concentrations should be avoided during delivery to prevent uterine atony and postpartum hemorrhage. At low concentrations (< 1%), they produce amnesia and their tocolytic effects are easily counteracted by standard infusions of oxytocin (Pitocin). These gases are both bronchodilators. Halothane has a more depressant effect on the myocardium, and isoflurane produces greater reduction in systemic vascular resistance (SVR).

Newer volatile anesthetics (eg, desflurane, sevoflurane) have not been used widely in the parturient. These anesthetic gases are insoluble in blood and tissue and therefore are very short acting. Whether this property is an advantage or disadvantage during cesarean surgery compared to halothane and isoflurane is not clear.

REGIONAL ANESTHESIA

Regional anesthesia is achieved by injection of a local anesthetic (Table 29–2) around the nerves that pass from spinal segments to the peripheral nerves responsible for sensory innervation of a portion of the body. More recently, narcotics have been added to local anesthetics to improve analgesia and reduce some side effects of local anesthetics. Regional nerve blocks used in obstetrics include the following: (1) lumbar epidural and caudal epidural block, (2) subarachnoid (spinal) block, and (3) pudendal block.

Infiltration of a local anesthetic drug and pudendal block analgesia carry minimal risks. The hazards increase with the amount of drug used. The safety and suitability of regional anesthesia depend on proper selection of the drug and the patient and the obstetrician–gynecologist's knowledge, experience, and expertise in the diagnosis and treatment of possible complications. Major conductive anesthesia and general anesthesia in obstetrics require specialized knowledge and expertise in conjunction with close maternal and fetal monitoring. This field of expertise has developed as a subspecialty within anesthesia, reflecting the need for specialized understanding of the obstetric patient and her response and of the fetal responses to anesthesia.

Patient Selection

Regional anesthesia is appropriate for labor analgesia, cesarean delivery, and other obstetric operative procedures (eg, postpartum tubal ligation, cervical cerclage). Most patients prefer to remain awake; however, occasionally a choice is made to provide general anesthesia.

The anesthesiologist will assess the patient to determine the relative risks of general versus regional anesthesia. For example, some forms of valvular heart disease may contraindicate regional block, and general anesthesia may be considered more appropriate. Other contraindications to regional anesthesia include infection, coagulopathy, hypovolemia, progressive neurologic disease, and patient refusal.

Table 29–2. Drugs used for local anesthesia.

	Tetracaine (Pontocaine)	Lidocaine (Xylocaine)	Bupivacaine (Marcaine)
Potency (compared to procaine)	10	2–3	9–12
Toxicity (compared to procaine)	10	1–1.5	4–6
Stability at sterilizing temperature	Stable	Stable	Stable
Total maximum dose	50–100 mg	500 mg	175 mg
Infiltration			
Concentration	0.05–0.1%	0.5–1%	0.25%
Onset of action	10–20 min	3–5 min	5–10 min
Duration	1½–3 h	30–60 min	90–120 min
Nerve block and epidural			
Concentration	0.1–0.2%	1–2%	0.5%
Onset of action	10–20 min	5–10 min	7–21 min
Duration	1½–3 h	1–1½ h	2–6 h
Subarachnoid			
Concentration	0.1–0.5%	5%	...
Dose	5–20 mg	40–100 mg	...
Onset of action	5–10 min	1–3 min	...
Duration	1½–2 h	1–1½ h	...

Modified and reproduced, with permission, from Guadagni NP, Hamilton WK: Anesthesiology. In: Dunphy JE, Way LW (editors): *Current Surgical Diagnosis & Treatment,* 4th ed: Lange, 1979.

Patient Preparation

The woman who is well informed and has a good rapport with her physician generally is a calm and cooperative candidate for regional or general anesthesia. The patient and her partner should be well informed early in her pregnancy of the options for labor anesthesia as well as for cesarean section if that circumstance arises. The anesthesiologist can be involved early in pregnancy if the patient has special concerns about anesthesia (family history of anesthetic risk, previous back surgery, coagulation problems). Some hospitals have obstetric anesthesia preassessment clinics that deal with these patient concerns.

Local Anesthetic Agents

A local anesthetic drug blocks the action potential of nerves when their axons are exposed to the medication. Local anesthetic agents act by modifying the ionic permeability of the cell membrane to stabilize its resting potential. The smaller the nerve fiber, the more sensitive it is to local anesthetics because the susceptibility of individual nerve fibers is inversely proportional to the cross-sectional diameter of the fibers. Hence, with regional anesthesia, the patient's perception of light touch, pain, and temperature and her capacity for vaso-

motor control are obtunded sooner and with a smaller concentration of the drug than is the perception of pressure or the function of motor nerves to striated muscles. The exception to this rule is the sensitivity of autonomic nerve fibers that are blocked by the lowest concentration of local anesthetic despite their being larger than some sensory nerves.

Only anesthetic drugs that are completely reversible and nonirritating and cause minimal toxicity are clinically acceptable. Other desirable properties of regional anesthetic agents include rapidity of onset, predictability of duration, and ease of sterilization. Table 29–2 summarizes the local anesthetics commonly used in obstetrics and gynecology together with their uses and doses.

All local anesthetics have certain undesirable dose-related side effects when absorbed systemically. All these drugs are capable of stimulating the central nervous system and may cause bradycardia, hypertension, or respiratory stimulation at the medullary level. Moreover, they may produce anxiety, excitement, or convulsions at the cortical or subcortical level. This response stimulates grand mal seizures because it is followed by depression, loss of vasomotor control, hypotension, respiratory depression, and coma. Such an episode of indirect cardiovascular depression often is accentuated by a direct vasodilatory and myocardial depressant effect.

The latter is comparable to the action of quinidine. This effect explains why lidocaine is useful for treatment of certain cardiac arrhythmias.

Chloroprocaine is an ester derivative that was popular in the mid-1960s but fell into disuse clinically. In the 1970s, it enjoyed a resurgence in popularity primarily because of its rapid onset and short duration of action and its low toxicity to the fetus. Its physicochemical properties are imparted by the chloro substitution of the 2-position in the benzene ring of procaine. It is metabolized by plasma cholinesterase and therefore does not demand liver enzyme degradation, as do the more complex and longer-acting amide derivatives. Chloroprocaine has a half-life of 21 seconds in adult blood and 43 seconds in neonatal blood. Direct toxic effects on the fetus are minimized because less drug is available for transfer in the maternal compartment.

The potency of chloroprocaine is comparable to that of lidocaine and mepivacaine, and the drug is 3 times more potent than procaine. Its average onset of action ranges from 6–12 minutes and persists for 30–60 minutes, depending on the amount used. Its use has been severely curtailed because of recent reports of toxicity that include arachnoiditis and associated neuropathies. The new 3% chloroprocaine is less acidic and has a reduced concentration of sodium metabisulfate (0.5 mg/mL) and is safe for epidural use.

Bupivacaine, the amide local anesthetic, is related to lidocaine and mepivacaine but has some very different physicochemical properties. It has a much higher lipid solubility, a higher degree of binding to maternal plasma protein, and a much longer duration of action. More than with other local anesthetics, the concentration of bupivacaine can be reduced to produce sensory block with minimal motor block. Because injection of bupivacaine for labor pain relief now is mostly in the form of continuous small-volume and minimal concentration administration via a pump mechanism, the complications previously of concern, such as hypotension and convulsions, are now rare.

A word of caution is needed regarding the administration of bupivacaine for cesarean section delivery. This drug has been implicated in certain cardiovascular catastrophes associated with initial drug injection, such as cardiac arrests that were refractory to full and appropriate resuscitative attempts. Although these catastrophes are rare, the practitioner is well advised to inject no more than 5 mL of the drug at any one time, to wait 4–5 minutes, then to repeat the procedure until the desired volume has been delivered. The maximum concentration of bupivacaine now allowed by the Food and Drug Administration (FDA) for obstetric epidural anesthesia is 0.5%. The toxic dose of bupivacaine now is considered 1–2 mg/kg.

Ropivacaine is a new amide local anesthetic introduced into the United States in the mid-1990s. It is less lipid soluble than bupivacaine, and initial studies suggested that it produced less motor blockade and was less cardiotoxic than its homologue bupivacaine. Later studies have been less convincing in documenting improved efficacy and safety, but ropivacaine has replaced bupivacaine in some institutions. There is ongoing study of the safety and efficacy of levobupivacaine, the levorotatory isomer of bupivacaine, which may also prove less cardiotoxic than its racemic parent molecule. Both of these newer amide local anesthetics are used in doses and concentrations similar to those of bupivacaine.

Local Infiltration Analgesia

Local tissue infiltration of dilute solutions of anesthetic drugs generally yields satisfactory results because the target is the fine nerve fibers. Nevertheless, one must keep in mind the dangers of systemic toxicity when large areas are anesthetized or when reinjection is required. It is good practice, therefore, to calculate in advance the milligrams of drug and volume of solution that may be required to keep the total dosage below the accepted toxic dose.

Infiltration in or near an area of inflammation is contraindicated. Injections into these zones may be followed by rapid systemic absorption of the drug as a result of increased vascularity of the inflamed tissues. Moreover, the injection may introduce or aggravate infection.

Regional Analgesia Techniques

A. LUMBAR EPIDURAL BLOCK

This analgesic technique has become more popular recently because it is well suited to obstetric anesthesia. Either bolus injections or continuous infusion of local anesthetics is used for labor, vaginal delivery, or cesarean surgery. Narcotics are added to supplement the quality of the block.

After the patient is evaluated, an epidural block can be placed once labor is established. Drug dosages can be adjusted as circumstances change. The catheter can be used for surgery and postoperative analgesia if necessary. The second stage of labor is prolonged by epidural anesthesia; however, the duration of the first stage is unaffected. The use of outlet forceps is increased, but fetal outcome is not adversely affected by epidural block.

The epidural block technique must be exact, and inadvertent massive (high) spinal anesthesia occasionally occurs. Other undesirable reactions include the rapid absorption syndrome (hypotension, bradycardia, hallucinations, convulsions), postpartum backache, and paresthesias. Epidural block should eradicate pain between T10 and L1 for the first stage of labor and between T10 and S5 for the second stage of labor.

The procedure is as follows. Inject 3 mL of a 1.5% aqueous solution of lidocaine or similar agent into the

Figure 29–4. Caudal catheter in place for continuous caudal anesthesia.

catheter as a test dose. If spinal anesthesia does not result after 5–10 minutes, inject an additional 5 mL. Inject 10 mL of the anesthetic solution in total to slowly accomplish an adequate degree and suitable level of anesthesia. Once the block is established, a continuous infusion of 10–12 mL/h will maintain the block for labor. Bupivacaine 0.125–0.25% is most often used for an epidural block, with fentanyl 2–5 µg/mL in the epidural mixture.

The mother is nursed in a wedged or lateral position to prevent aortocaval compression. The sympathectomy produced by the block predisposes the patient to venous pooling and reduced venous return. Maternal blood pressure must be measured frequently when the epidural is in effect.

B. CAUDAL BLOCK

Caudal anesthesia (Fig 29–4) is an epidural block approached through the caudal space. It can provide selective sacral block for the second stage of labor; however, it is rarely used now because of complications specific to the obstetric patient. The descent of the fetal head against the perineum, in addition to the sacral edema at term, obscures the landmarks of the sacral hiatus. This makes the caudal procedure technically challenging,

and reports of transfixing the rectum and fetal skull puncture with the epidural needle have led many anesthesiologists to avoid this technique. Lumbar epidural anesthesia is considered a safer alternative.

C. SPINAL ANESTHESIA

Spinal anesthesia currently is the anesthetic of choice for cesarean delivery. Spinal anesthesia can be performed more quickly than epidural anesthesia and provides ideal operating conditions, including dense sensory and motor block. The onset of sympathectomy is more abrupt than with epidural block, so care must be taken to ensure that the patient is adequately preloaded with 1.5–2 L of saline solution prior to performing the technique. Spinal anesthesia is used less commonly these days to alleviate the pain of delivery and the third stage of labor. The advantages of spinal anesthesia are that the mother remains conscious to witness delivery, no inhalation anesthetics or analgesic drugs are required, the technique is not difficult, and good relaxation of the pelvic floor and lower birth canal is achieved. Prompt anesthesia is achieved within 5–10 minutes. The dosage of spinal anesthetic is small. Complications are rare and easy to treat. However, spinal headache occurs in 1–2% of patients.

D. COMBINED SPINAL–EPIDURAL ANESTHESIA

The use of combined spinal–epidural anesthesia (CSE) became popular in the mid 1990s as an alternative to epidural anesthesia for labor. A small dose of local anesthetic and narcotic (2.5 mg bupivacaine and 25 μg fentanyl) is injected through a spinal needle, which is introduced through the epidural needle and advanced into the intrathecal space. The spinal needle is withdrawn and the epidural catheter placed for later use. The spinal medication produces immediate pain relief and minimal motor block and may allow ambulation. Later in labor, the epidural catheter is used for continuous infusion of epidural solution, similar to that described for standard epidural anesthesia in labor.

Detractors of CSE argue that the technique may increase the incidence of post–lumbar puncture headache, and that ambulation even after low-dose spinal injection is unsafe for both mother and baby. Finally, because the technique is technically cumbersome, it may be associated with higher complication rates. No data support either a benefit or a disadvantage of CSE compared with standard epidural anesthesia for labor.

The most serious consequence of spinal or epidural anesthesia is maternal mortality. Maternal deaths associated with use of 0.75% bupivacaine for cesarean section delivery and labor were reported in the late 1980s, prompting the FDA to outlaw the use of this drug in obstetrics. These deaths were attributed to venous uptake of the drug and immediate and lasting myocardial depression from the local anesthetic, which did not respond to appropriate cardiac resuscitative efforts. Today maternal mortality associated with regional anesthesia is lower, primarily because bolus dosing of high concentrations of local anesthesia is no longer performed.

Most side effects of spinal or epidural anesthesia are secondary to block of the sympathetic nerve fibers that accompany the anterior roots of the spinal thoracic and upper lumbar nerves (thoracolumbar outflow). Thus, many physiologic regulating mechanisms are disturbed. The blood lumbar pressure falls as a result of loss of arterial resistance and venous pooling—assuming no compensation is made by change of the patient's position (eg, Trendelenburg position). If high thoracic dermatomes (T1–T5) are blocked, alteration of the cardiac sympathetic innervation slows the heart rate and reduces cardiac contractility. Epinephrine secretion by the adrenal medulla is depressed. Concomitantly, the unopposed parasympathetic effect of cardiac slowing alters vagal stimulations. As a result of these and related changes, shock follows promptly, especially in hypotensive or hypovolemic patients. Moreover, a precipitous fall in the blood pressure of the arteriosclerotic hypertensive patient is inevitable.

Fluids, oxygen therapy for adequate tissue perfusion, shock position to encourage venous return, and pressor drugs given intravenously are recommended.

In the past, postdural puncture headache (PDPH) due to leakage of cerebrospinal fluid through the needle hole in the dura was an early postoperative complication in up to 15% of patients. Small-caliber needles (25F) decrease the incidence of headache to 8–10%. With the introduction of pencil-point Whitaker and Sprotte spinal needles, the incidence of PDPH has been reduced to 1–2%. Therapy for PDPH includes recumbent position, hydration, sedation, and, in severe cases, epidural injection of 10–20 mL of the patient's fresh blood to "seal" the defect.

Rarely, spinal or epidural anesthesia caused nerve injury and transient or permanent hypesthesia or paresthesia. Excessive drug concentration, sensitivity, or infection may have been responsible for some of these complications. The incidence of serious complications of spinal or epidural anesthesia is considerably lower than that of cardiac arrest during general anesthesia.

E. PARACERVICAL BLOCK

Paracervical block is no longer considered a safe technique for the obstetric patient. In the past, paracervical anesthesia was used to relieve the pain of the first stage of labor. Pudendal block was required for pain during the second stage of labor. Sensory nerve fibers from the uterus fuse bilaterally at the 4–6 o'clock and 6–8 o'clock positions around the cervix in the region of the cervical–vaginal junction. Ordinarily, when 5–10 mL of 1% lidocaine or its equivalent is injected into these areas, interruption of the sensory input from the cervix and uterus promptly follows.

Many now consider paracervical block to be contraindicated in obstetrics because of the potential adverse fetal effects. Many reports in the literature place the incidence of fetal bradycardia at 8–18%. However, recent work with accurate fetal heart rate monitoring associated with continuous uterine contraction patterns suggests that the incidence is closer to 20–25%. Some researchers have attempted to investigate the significance of the bradycardia. One explanation is that an acid–base disturbance in the fetus does not occur unless the bradycardia lasts longer than 10 minutes, and that neonatal depression is rare unless associated with delivery during the period of bradycardia. There seems to be little difference in the incidence and severity of fetal bradycardia by paracervical block between complicated and uncomplicated patients. Other disadvantages of paracervical block include maternal trauma and bleeding, fetal trauma and direct injection, inadvertent intravascular injection with convulsions, and short duration of the block.

F. PUDENDAL NERVE BLOCK

Pudendal block has been one of the most popular of all nerve block techniques in obstetrics. The infant is not depressed, and blood loss is minimal. The technique is simplified by the fact that the pudendal nerve approaches the spine of the ischium on its course to innervate the perineum. Injection of 10 mL of 1% lidocaine on each side will achieve analgesia for 30–45 minutes approximately 50% of the time.

Both the transvaginal and transcutaneous methods are useful for administering a pudendal block. The transvaginal technique has important practical advantages over the transcutaneous technique. The "Iowa trumpet" needle guide can be used, and the operator's finger should be placed at the end of the needle guide to palpate the sacrospinous ligament, which runs in the same direction and is just anterior to the pudendal nerve and artery. Appreciating the sensation of the needle puncturing the ligament usually is difficult. This facet of the technique (no definite endpoint) may make it difficult for the inexperienced clinician to perform. Aspiration of the syringe for possible inadvertent entry into the pudendal artery should be accomplished, and, if no blood is returned, 10 mL of local anesthetic solution should be injected in a fanlike fashion on the right and left sides. The successful performance of the pudendal block requires injection of the drug at least 10–12 minutes before episiotomy. Often in clinical practice, pudendal block is performed within 4–5 minutes of episiotomy, so the local anesthetic may not have adequate time to take effect.

1. Advantages and disadvantages—Advantages of pudendal nerve block are its safety, ease of administration, and rapidity of onset of effect. Disadvantages include maternal trauma, bleeding, and infection; rare maternal convulsions due to drug sensitivity; occasional complete or partial failure; and regional discomfort during administration.

The pudendal perineal block, like any other nerve block, demands some technical experience and knowledge of the innervation of the lower birth canal. Nevertheless, in spite of a well-placed bilateral block, skip areas of perineal analgesia may be noted. The possible reason is that although the pudendal nerve of S2–S4 derivation does contribute to the majority of fibers for sensory innervation to the perineum, other sensory fibers also are involved. For example, the inferior hemorrhoidal nerve may have an origin independent from that of the sacral nerve and therefore will not be a component branch of the pudendal nerve. In this case, it must be infiltrated separately. In addition, the posterior femoral cutaneous nerve (S1–S3) origin may contribute an important perineal branch to the anterior fourchette bilaterally. In instances where this nerve plays a major role in innervation, it must be blocked separately by local skin infiltration.

Two other nerves contribute to the sensory innervation of the perineum: the ilioinguinal nerve, of L1 origin, and the genital branch of the genitofemoral nerve, of L1 and L2 origin. Both of these nerves sweep superficially over the mons pubis to innervate the skin over the symphysis of the mons pubis and the labium majus. Occasionally, these nerves must also be separately infiltrated to provide optimal perineal analgesic effect. Thus it should be apparent that a simple bilateral pudendal nerve block may not be effective in many cases. For maximum analgesic effectiveness, in addition to a bilateral pudendal block, superficial infiltration of the skin from the symphysis medially to a point halfway between the ischial spines may be necessary. Thus, a true perineal block may be regarded as a regional technique.

Either lumbar epidural or caudal epidural block should eradicate pain between the T10 and S5 levels for the second stage. All of these nerves are denervated because they all are derived from L1–S5 segments.

2. Procedure (Fig 29–5)

1. Palpate the ischial spines vaginally. Slowly advance the needle guide toward each spine. After placement is achieved, the needle is advanced through the guide to penetrate approximately 0.5 cm. Aspirate and, if the needle is not in a vessel, deposit 5 mL below each spine. This blocks the right and left pudendal nerves. Refill the syringe when necessary, and proceed in a similar manner to anesthetize the other areas specified. Keep the needle moving while injecting and avoid the sensitive vaginal mucosa and periosteum.

2. Withdraw the needle and guide approximately 2 cm and redirect toward an ischial tuberosity. Inject 3 mL near the center of each tuberosity to anesthetize the inferior hemorrhoidal and lateral femoral cutaneous nerves.

3. Withdraw the needle and guide almost entirely and then slowly advance toward the symphysis pubica almost to the clitoris, keeping approximately 2 cm lateral to the labial fold and approximately 1–2 cm beneath the skin. Injection of 5 mL of lidocaine on each side beneath the symphysis will block the ilioinguinal and genitocrural nerves.

If the procedure explained is carefully and skillfully done, only slight discomfort will be felt during the injections. Prompt flaccid relaxation and good anesthesia for 30–60 minutes can be expected. A summary of anesthetic approaches in labor is shown in Figure 29–6.

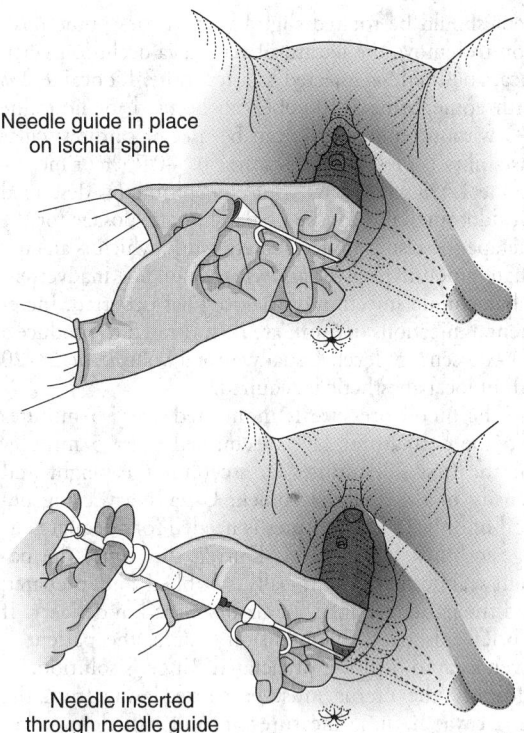

Needle guide in place
on ischial spine

Needle inserted
through needle guide

Figure 29–5. Use of needle guide ("Iowa trumpet") in pudendal anesthetic block. (Reproduced, with permission, from Benson RC: *Handbook of Obstetrics & Gynecology,* 8th ed. Lange, 1983.)

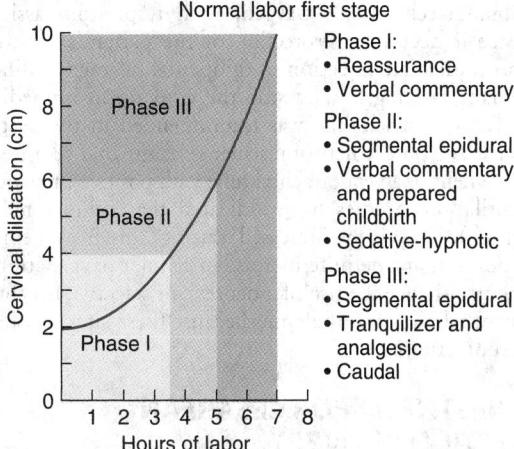

Normal labor first stage

Phase III

Phase II

Phase I

Phase I:
• Reassurance
• Verbal commentary

Phase II:
• Segmental epidural
• Verbal commentary and prepared childbirth
• Sedative-hypnotic

Phase III:
• Segmental epidural
• Tranquilizer and analgesic
• Caudal

Figure 29–6. First-stage management in a primipara can be divided into 3 phases. Phase I (early labor) should be managed by simple reassurance and verbal commentary if the patient has received adequate antepartum education. An epidural may be performed once labor is well established. Phase II can be handled by a segmental epidural block, continued reassurance, a sedative–hypnotic drug, a narcotic, or a tranquilizer. Phase III, the accentuated phase of labor, can be handled by segmental epidural block, a combination tranquilizer and analgesic, or a caudal epidural block. However, use of reassurance and verbal commentary in conjunction with prepared childbirth methods may be adequate for some patients to tolerate the discomfort of phase III labor.

Prevention & Treatment of Local Anesthetic Overdosage

The correct dose of any local anesthetic is the smallest quantity of drug in the greatest dilution that will provide adequate analgesia. The pregnant patient is more likely to have an intravascular drug injection because of venous distention in the epidural space and may be more susceptible to the toxic effects of local anesthetics (Table 29–3). Injection of the drug into a highly vascularized area will result in more rapid systemic absorption than, for example, injection into the skin. To prevent too-rapid absorption, the operator can add epinephrine to produce local vasoconstriction and prolong the anesthetic. A final concentration of 1:200,000 is desirable, especially when a toxic amount is approached. Epinephrine is contraindicated in patients with increased cardiac irritability of medical or drug origin.

Treatment of local anesthetic overdosage manifested by central nervous system toxicity (a convulsion) is generally achieved effectively and without incident. However, the clinician must be aware of certain basic principles. These include the recognition of prodromal signs of

a central nervous system toxic reaction and immediate treatment as required. A toxic central nervous system reaction to local anesthetics consists of ringing in the ears, diplopia, perioral numbness, and deep, slurred speech. An adequate airway must be maintained, and the patient

Table 29–3. Toxic doses of local anesthetics commonly used in obstetrics.

Drug	Toxic Dose
Lidocaine	5 mg/kg, plain 7 mg/kg, with epinephrine
Bupivacaine	1.5 mg/kg[1]
Chloroprocaine	10 mg/kg
Tetracaine	1 mg/kg
Ropivacaine	3 mg/kg

[1]Doses as low as 90 mg have produced cardiac arrest.

should receive 100% oxygen, with respiratory assistance if necessary. Protection of the patient's airway and immediate injection of thiopental 50 mg or midazolam 1–2 mg usually stop the convulsion immediately. Succinylcholine was recommended in the past, but it is a potent neuromuscular relaxant that requires placement of an endotracheal tube with positive-pressure ventilation. Studies have indicated that cellular metabolism is greatly increased during convulsive episodes so that a definite increase in cellular oxygenation occurs—hence the use of a depressant selective for the hypothalamus and thalamus because these sites are the foci of irritation.

ANESTHESIA FOR CESAREAN SECTION DELIVERY

With few exceptions, all cesarean section deliveries in the United States are performed with spinal, epidural, or general anesthesia. Maternal and neonatal outcomes are good when these techniques are performed effectively. In 1982, more than half of the cesarean births in the United States were performed under general anesthesia. By 1998, the rate had dropped to less than 10% of all cesarean births. Spinal anesthesia has become more common than epidural anesthesia for cesarean delivery in the past few years, primarily as a result of the introduction of newer spinal needles that prevent post–lumbar puncture headaches. Although the majority of anesthesia-related maternal mortality is associated with cesarean birth, the rate has continued to decline dramatically over the last few decades and now is less than 1.5 anesthesia-related deaths per million live births in the United States.

Regional Analgesia

A. LUMBAR EPIDURAL BLOCK

Lumbar epidural blockade can be used for cesarean section analgesia and adequate analgesia for operative delivery. As mentioned in the discussion of regional anesthesia, the major hazard of the regional analgesic technique is blockade of sympathetic fibers and a decrease in vascular resistance, along with venous pooling and hypotension. However, this can be greatly alleviated by elevating the patient's right hip to prevent compression of the vena cava by the gravid uterus when the patient is lying on the operating table. In addition, the anesthesiologist can rotate the operating table 15–20 degrees to the left to rotate the uterus away from the vena cava.

An epidural catheter can be placed immediately prior to surgery, or a catheter used to provide pain relief for labor can be reinjected for the surgery. After the catheter is suitably placed and taped in position, the pa-

tient should be rotated slightly out of the supine position to remove the hazard of vena cava occlusion when local anesthetic is injected as a test dose. Lidocaine 2% with epinephrine 1:200,000 can be used, or lidocaine 2% without epinephrine can be used if cardiovascular instability is present. Bupivacaine 0.5–0.75% or mepivacaine 1.5% with or without epinephrine (as described for lidocaine) also can be used. The total dosage for the therapeutic test is approximately 3 mL, which is an adequate amount to ascertain whether or not inadvertent subarachnoid injection of the drug has occurred. Incremental injections of 5 mL are then titrated to produce a T4–T6 sensory level. Usually a total volume of 18–20 mL of local anesthetic is required.

The blood pressure is monitored every 5 minutes and the dermatome levels examined every 5 minutes for the first 20 minutes to ascertain the height and density of the analgesic block. Usually a waiting period of only 15–20 minutes is needed for adequate analgesic block for incision. During this time, the patient's abdomen is surgically scrubbed and prepared and the patient draped for cesarean section delivery. If a brief episode of hypotension occurs, the patient is given a rapid infusion of lactated Ringer's solution. In addition, the uterus must be shifted away from the vena cava. If these measures are not sufficient to relieve a brief episode of hypotension, 5–10 mg of ephedrine intravenously can be administered for a mild vasopressor effect.

B. SUBARACHNOID BLOCK

Spinal block is now the most common anesthesia used for elective cesarean delivery in the United States. The advantages are immediate onset of analgesia, so no waiting period is needed for the block to become effective, and the absence of drug transmission from the maternal to the fetal compartment because the anesthetic is deposited in the subarachnoid space in such small quantities. In addition, subarachnoid block may be a simpler technique to perform because the endpoint is definite—the identification of fluid from the subarachnoid space. The disadvantages are a more profound and rapid onset of hypotension and more frequent nausea and vomiting due either to unopposed parasympathetic stimulation of the gastrointestinal tract or to hypotension. Subarachnoid block usually is achieved via the paramedian or midline technique, details of which are beyond the scope of this text. The agents most commonly used for subarachnoid analgesia are lidocaine 5% (50–75 mg) and bupivacaine 10–12.5%. As with the lumbar epidural technique, the patient is prehydrated with 500–1000 mL of lactated Ringer's solution.

After the technical aspects of the procedure have been completed, the patient is placed in the supine position with the uterus displaced to the left as described. If hypotension occurs, the uterus should be pushed farther to the left to improve return of blood from the lower extremities into the circulation and increase right atrial pressure and thus cardiac output, and a bolus of Ringer's lactate should be given. If these measures are not successful, the patient should receive ephedrine 5–10 mg intravenously to sustain a mild vasopressor effect. During a period of hypotension, the mother should receive oxygen by mask to increase oxygen delivery to the uteroplacental bed. Newer spinal needles are associated with a low incidence (1–2%) of spinal headache (PDPH). As a result, spinal anesthesia is becoming more popular for elective cesarean surgery.

General & Local Anesthesia

General anesthesia is indicated for cesarean section delivery when regional techniques cannot be used because of coagulopathy, infection, hypovolemia, or urgency. Some patients prefer to be "put to sleep" and refuse regional techniques.

Ideally, general anesthesia for cesarean section delivery should cause the mother to be unconscious, feel no pain, and have no unpleasant memories of the procedure; the fetus should not be jeopardized, with minimal depression and intact reflex irritability.

General anesthesia for cesarean section delivery is substantially modified from the typical nonobstetric technique. A rapid sequence technique is used with cricoid pressure to prevent aspiration, with recognition that the risks for the term obstetric patient include (1) full stomach (and aspiration), (2) difficulty with laryngoscopy and intubation, and (3) rapid desaturation if intubation is unsuccessful.

A. PATIENT PREPARATION

Preoperative medication usually is not required when the patient is brought to the cesarean section room. Alert the patient preoperatively that she may have a lucid "window" during the operative procedure when she experiences pain or hears voices. Explain that the condition results from the need to maintain a light analgesic state in order to protect the fetus from large doses of drugs. The patient should be prepared with 30 mL of nonparticulate antacid to offset gastric acidity. The patient is given 100% oxygen with a close-fitting mask for 3 minutes prior to induction.

B. PROCEDURE

When the surgeon is ready to make the incision, thiopental 2.5 mg/kg should be injected intravenously and cricoid pressure exerted by an assistant. Immediately,

succinylcholine 120–140 mg intravenously should be administered, and intubation and inflation of the cuff performed. Intubation is confirmed by auscultation and monitoring end-tidal CO_2 before the cricoid pressure is released and the incision made. After 6–8 breaths of 100% oxygen, the patient should be given nitrous oxide 50% with oxygen 50% until delivery of the fetus. Low concentrations of halothane or isoflurane (0.5%) will reduce the incidence of awareness. Intermediate-acting muscle relaxants maintain paralysis. An attempt must be made to keep the induction-to-delivery time under 10 minutes. Five minutes is required for redistribution of barbiturate back across the placenta into the maternal compartment. After delivery of the fetus, the nitrous oxide concentration can be increased to 70% if oxygen saturation is more than 98% and intravenous narcotics and benzodiazepines injected for supplemental anesthesia.

The patient should be fully awakened and on her side before extubation. Postoperative analgesia can be provided by patient-controlled administration of morphine or meperidine.

With this approach, good neonatal outcomes are anticipated if induction-to-delivery times and uterine invasion-to-delivery times are kept to a minimum.

C. SPECIAL PROBLEMS

1. Midforceps delivery—Each patient's requirements vary, and every situation must be evaluated on an individual basis. Midforceps delivery often involves both rotation and traction. Therefore, the anesthetic regimen must provide relaxation as well as analgesia for the perineum, lower vagina, and upper birth canal. In order for the obstetrician to perform the procedures necessary for delivery, optimal conditions must be provided so that maternal and fetal trauma can be minimized. Regional analgesia with a lumbar, caudal epidural, or subarachnoid block is preferred because these blocks provide analgesia and optimal relaxation.

2. The trapped head—On the rare occasion when breech delivery is complicated by a trapped head, the application of forceps or other manipulations may be required urgently. If an epidural block is in place, no further analgesia will be required; however, if one is not in place, immediate anesthesia and pelvic relaxation will be required to facilitate rapid delivery and minimize trauma. The best technique for this purpose is general anesthesia with halothane after suitable protection of the patient from the hazards of aspiration. Protection should include use of antacid 30 mL orally and adequate oxygenation, followed by thiopental 200 mg intravenously, succinylcholine 80–100 mg intravenously, and rapid intubation with cricoid pressure. Another approach described in the literature is administration of

50–100 µg intravenous nitroglycerin to relax the lower uterine segment.

Multiple Pregnancy

A. PSYCHOANALGESIA

The psychoprophylactic technique helps to prepare the patient for the intrapartum experience. When the labor progresses normally, psychoanalgesia can effectively reduce apprehension and enhance the pleasurable aspects of childbirth. It also may prepare the patient for an understanding of some of the complications of multiple pregnancy (uterine inertia in the first stage of labor, uterine atony in the third stage, and possible need for cesarean section delivery) and reduce the total amount of drugs required for analgesia.

B. PUDENDAL NERVE BLOCK

Pudendal nerve block usually is reserved for cases in which epidural block is not available. Analgesia is more limited and does not provide as effective analgesia should version or breech extractions of the second twin be required.

C. EPIDURAL BLOCK

This technique is useful as a first-stage analgesic method, but only a segmental type should be used (T10–L2) to prevent the increased hazard of hypotension secondary to a combined large-segment sympathetic block and vena cava occlusion. Ideal management entails the use of lumbar epidural block for the first stage of labor and low caudal block for the late second stage of labor. Epidural anesthesia does not affect fetal outcome with twin delivery but has the advantage of enabling the obstetrician to intervene more easily if the second twin presents abnormally. The need for a general anesthetic can be avoided if an epidural is in place and a cesarean section is required urgently for delivery of the second twin.

D. SPINAL BLOCK

The low subarachnoid block is rarely used at the end of the second stage for crowning, delivery, and episiotomy. A low spinal block does not provide a sufficiently high block for cesarean section should it be required urgently (eg, in malpresentation or cord prolapse of the second twin). Therefore, an epidural anesthetic is always preferable for the labor and delivery of multiple births.

E. INHALATION ANALGESICS

Nitrous oxide is the only inhalation anesthetic that is analgesic at low concentrations. Experience is needed to use nitrous oxide safely because the pregnant patient is sensitive to the drug's anesthetic effects and she can easily become obtunded. Loss of airway reflexes and aspiration are causes of maternal mortality.

General endotracheal anesthesia can be used for cesarean section delivery of twins. Neonatal depression is more likely if the induction-to-delivery time is long (> 8 minutes), especially if the uterine incision-to-delivery time also is prolonged (> 3 minutes).

Maternal Complications

A. PREECLAMPSIA–ECLAMPSIA

This syndrome is classically described as the triad of hypertension, generalized edema, and proteinuria. Other variants are described, the most notable being HELLP syndrome, the constellation of hemolysis, elevated liver enzymes and low platelet count. Preeclampsia–eclampsia accounts for approximately 20% of maternal deaths per year in the United States. The primary pathologic characteristic of this disease process is generalized arterial spasm. As gestation lengthens, there is a tendency toward a fluid shift from the vascular to the extravascular compartment with resultant hypovolemia—in spite of an expanded extracellular fluid space.

It is estimated that nearly 50% of eclamptic patients who die have myocardial hemorrhages or areas of focal necrosis. Major disorders of central nervous system function probably are caused by cerebral vasospasm. Optimal anesthetic management of these patients during the intrapartum period must include a careful preanesthetic evaluation of the cardiovascular and central nervous systems.

The physiologic changes of severe preeclampsia–eclampsia are exaggerated by regional block as a result of restricted intravascular volume, which may lead to considerable depression of blood pressure. A small subgroup of these patients suffer from reduced cardiac output (compared to normal pregnancy), decreased intravascular fluid space, and marked increases in SVR. Patients with severe hemodynamic changes may require direct monitoring of pulmonary artery and wedge pressures to manage labor and the effects of epidural anesthesia. Uterine blood flow is increased with epidural block because of the favorable reduction of SVR, as long as central filling pressures and mean arterial pressure are well maintained.

Regional and general anesthesia is used in the management of preeclamptic patients. Contraindications to regional anesthesia include coagulopathy and urgency for nonreassuring fetal testing. The latter may mitigate against taking excessive time for placing a spinal or epidural if the baby requires immediate delivery.

Epidural anesthesia may be preferred to spinal anesthesia in cases of severe hypertension. The more graduated onset of sympathetic block with this technique is thought to produce less hypotension than would occur with spinal block. However, recent evidence suggests that adequate volume preloading of these patients, who by definition are depleted intravascularly, results in similar hemodynamic responses to both regional techniques. More study is required to confirm these findings. However, spinal and epidural anesthesia now usually is encouraged for the management of preeclamptic patients. Obstetricians have become aware that epidural anesthesia is a valuable adjunct in the management of hypertension as a result of the pain relief as well as the vasodilation produced by epidural block. In the past, epidural anesthesia was avoided because of an exaggerated concern over hypotension; now epidural anesthesia is encouraged if the patient's volume status is well managed and if coagulopathy does not complicate the clinical picture.

B. HEMORRHAGE AND SHOCK

Intrapartum obstetric emergencies demand immediate diagnosis and therapy for a favorable outcome for the mother and fetus. Placenta previa and abruptio placentae are accompanied by serious maternal hemorrhage. Aggressive obstetric management may be indicated, but superior anesthetic management will play a major role in reducing maternal and fetal morbidity and mortality rates. The primary threat to the mother is blood loss, which reduces her effective circulating blood volume and her oxygenation potential. Similarly, the chief hazard to the fetus is diminished uteroplacental perfusion secondary to maternal hypovolemia and hypotension. The perinatal mortality rate associated with placenta previa and abruptio placentae ranges from 15–20% in some studies up to 50–100% in other studies. The overall morbidity and mortality rates for both the fetus and the mother depend on the gestational age and health of the fetus, the extent of the hemorrhage, and the therapy given.

Good anesthetic management demands early consultation. Reliable intravenous lines should be established early. In addition, recommendations for treatment and control of shock must be formulated. Prompt cesarean section delivery often is indicated. Ketamine can support blood pressure for induction. A modified nitrous oxide–oxygen relaxant method of general anesthesia will provide improved oxygenation for both the mother and the fetus and will have a minimal effect on maternal blood pressure. As surgery progresses, it may be necessary to administer large volumes of warm blood, intravenous fluids, or even vasopressors when imperative. Regional block is contraindicated in the presence of hypovolemia.

C. UMBILICAL CORD PROLAPSE

Umbilical cord prolapse is an acute obstetric emergency that is a critical threat to the fetus. Often, because of confusion, irrational behavior by the medical staff may threaten the mother's life. For example, a haphazard rapid induction of anesthesia without attention to many of the essential safety details may be attempted. Naturally, prolapse of the umbilical cord is incompatible with fetal survival unless the fetal presenting part is elevated at once and maintained in that position to avoid compression of the cord. There then should be adequate time for methodical, safe induction of anesthesia. General anesthesia is induced as soon as the abdomen is prepped and draped. In the rush of the emergency situation, the anesthesiologist must remain meticulous in his or her assessment and management of the mother's airway. A failed intubation and its consequent cardiorespiratory arrest constitute the leading cause of anesthetic maternal mortality.

D. BREECH DELIVERY

Epidural anesthesia can be used for the labor patient with a breech presentation. The need for breech extraction is not increased by the use of epidural anesthesia, and a functioning epidural may prevent the need for general anesthesia should an emergency arise at delivery.

If an epidural block is not in place at the time of delivery, the anesthesiologist must be prepared to proceed with an immediate endotracheal general anesthesia if the aftercoming fetal head becomes trapped. Drugs, monitors, and anesthetic equipment must be prepared in anticipation of such an event.

Because breech delivery is associated with a high perinatal mortality rate, excellent communication and cooperation between the obstetrician and the anesthesiologist is greatly needed to effect an atraumatic delivery.

E. ANESTHESIA FOR EMERGENCY CESAREAN SECTION

General anesthesia is the technique most suitable for the urgent cesarean section delivery. It entails placement of an endotracheal tube with an inflated cuff to protect the patient from aspiration of gastric contents into the lung after administration of adequate barbiturate and a muscle relaxant to facilitate endotracheal intubation. Several safety measures must be taken. (1) Give 30 mL of a nonparticulate antacid (sodium citrate) within 15 minutes of induction. (2) Accomplish denitrogenation with 100% oxygen by tight-fitting mask. (3) Inject thiopental 2.5 mg/kg intravenously. (4) Apply cricoid pressure. (5) Give succinylcholine 100–120 mg intravenously. (6) Intubate the trachea and inflate the cuff. (7) Give 6–8 deep breaths of 100% oxygen. (8) Continue to administer nitrous oxide 50% with oxygen 50%, 0.5% halothane or isoflurane, and maintain relaxation with vecuronium or atracurium. (9) Supplement with short-acting narcotics and midazolam after the baby is delivered.

These steps should be instituted rapidly and with effective communication between the anesthesiologist and the obstetrician, who should be scrubbed and prepared to make the incision. With this technique, anesthesia can be induced and the fetus delivered within 30 minutes from the time cesarean section is ordered. To prevent vena cava occlusion from the gravid uterus, a wedge should be placed under the patient's right hip or the operating table rotated slightly to the left.

ANESTHESIA FOR NONOBSTETRIC COMPLICATIONS

Anesthesiologists use the following classification system developed by the American Society of Anesthesiologists (ASA). It is used in both emergency and nonemergent situations to record physical status and to ascertain that proper materials are available for the anticipated procedure.

Class 1: No organic, physiologic, biochemical, or psychiatric disturbance

Class 2: Mild to moderate systemic disturbance that may or may not be related to the reason for surgery (Examples: Heart disease that only slightly limits physical activity, essential hypertension, anemia, extremes of age, obesity, chronic bronchitis)

Class 3: Severe systemic disturbance that may or may not be related to the reason for surgery (Examples: Heart disease that limits activity, poorly controlled hypertension, diabetes mellitus with vascular complications, chronic pulmonary disease that limits activity)

Class 4: Severe systemic disturbance that is life-threatening with or without surgery (Examples: Congestive heart failure, crescendo angina pectoris, advanced pulmonary, renal, and hepatic dysfunction)

Class 5: Moribund patient who has little chance of survival but is submitted to surgery as a last resort (resuscitative effort) (Examples: Uncontrolled hemorrhage as from a ruptured abdominal aneurysm, cerebral trauma, pulmonary embolus)

Emergency operation (E): Any patient in whom an emergency operation is required (Example: Otherwise healthy 30-year-old woman who requires dilatation and curettage for moderate but persistent hemorrhage [ASA class 1E])

Hypertension

Preexisting hypertensive cardiovascular disease in a pregnant woman should be differentiated from preeclampsia–eclampsia. Unlike the latter, the manifestations of hyper-

tensive disease usually are present before week 24 of pregnancy and persist after delivery. The untreated disease by itself presents a serious challenge to the obstetrician and increases maternal and fetal risk. Chronic hypertension does not specifically contraindicate any of the anesthetic options, but the anesthesiologist must assess and manage abnormalities of volume and vascular resistance to prevent hypotension. Systemic analgesia with sedatives and tranquilizers may be selected for first-stage pain relief, but a hazard still remains.

Heart Disease

Pregnancy superimposed on heart disease presents serious problems in anesthetic management. Patients with functional class I or II rheumatic or congenital heart disease usually fare well throughout pregnancy. Except for patients with fixed cardiac output (moderate to severe aortic stenosis or mitral stenosis), regional analgesia epidural block provides ideal management of first- and second-stage pain relief. This avoids undesirable intrapartum problems such as anxiety, tachycardia, increased cardiac output, and the Valsalva maneuver. The lumbar epidural catheter can be activated for first-stage analgesia with sensory levels of T10 through L2 segments. With the restricted epidural technique, wide variations in blood pressure usually will be avoided and adequate analgesia provided.

Patients with valvular heart disease must be thoroughly assessed prior to onset of labor so that the anesthesiologist can determine the risks of regional block, tolerance to volume loading, and sympathectomy and determine the need for invasive monitoring. These patients require thorough physical examination, electrocardiography, echocardiography, and Doppler assessment of valve areas and left ventricular function.

Patients with stenotic lesions may not tolerate fluid loading or sympathetic block. Epidural narcotic anesthesia does not provide complete analgesia for labor but may be an appropriate choice if the patient does not tolerate the autonomic effects of local anesthetics. Patients with regurgitant valve lesions generally do well with this afterload reduction of epidural local anesthesia. Central monitoring of preload is indicated with severe lesions.

Marfan's syndrome and ischemic heart disease require early and aggressive management of labor pain to prevent hypertension and tachycardia. Early lumbar epidural anesthesia with narcotic/local anesthetic mixtures is recommended.

Diabetes Mellitus

Diabetes presents unique problems in anesthetic management because of the hazard to the fetus. The patient with diabetes requires a detailed regimen of antepartum care that extends through the intrapartum and the neonatal period. Moreover, hypotension presents an anesthetic hazard in situations of reduced fetal reserve common to diabetes. The latent phase of labor is best managed with psychological support, mild sedatives, or tranquilizers. The latter part of the first stage can be managed with small intravenous doses of narcotics or epidural block. If labor continues without signs of fetal distress and analgesia for the second stage is desired, either local or pudendal block or epidural or saddle block is appropriate. If a patient is allowed to undergo the stress of labor but fetal decompensation is evident, operative delivery must be performed at once, with emphasis on preventing hypotension. Careful regional block can be used if time permits. If time does not permit placement of a regional block, emergency general endotracheal anesthesia is indicated. Blood glucose levels should be measured intraoperatively because the unconscious patient cannot report hypoglycemia.

Gastrointestinal Difficulties

Gastrointestinal nonstriated muscle has diminished tone and motility during pregnancy. Some medical gastrointestinal difficulties present special problems in management during the intrapartum period. Peptic ulcer often improves during pregnancy, but in some cases the disease worsens in the last trimester and causes serious problems during labor and the immediate postpartum period. Ulcer perforation and hematemesis are rare in labor. Nonetheless, good management of analgesia during delivery is necessary to decrease anxiety and apprehension.

Ulcerative colitis may worsen during pregnancy. Perinatal and maternal mortality rates are not increased because symptomatic management usually is adequate. Regional ileitis may become more severe during pregnancy.

Chronic pancreatitis may be reactivated during pregnancy. Acute pancreatitis occasionally occurs in the third trimester. The significant laboratory values are elevated serum amylase and reduced serum calcium levels, along with typical symptoms of epigastric pain and nausea and vomiting.

Sympathetic blocking techniques are not contraindicated for anesthetic management of the first and second stages of labor in these gastrointestinal disorders that may coincide with pregnancy. It is clinically desirable to alleviate anxiety and apprehension in the first stage of labor because tension may exacerbate the disease process. Therefore, a tranquilizer–narcotic combination early in the first stage of labor should be considered and then lumbar epidural block for first- and second-stage management. Subarachnoid block can be administered to manage the second stage of labor successfully, with use of a true saddle block obtunding chiefly the sacral fibers.

Psychiatric Disorders

Most patients approaching delivery look upon the experience as one of the happiest times of their lives. However, some patients undergo severe emotional stress during the third trimester and as delivery nears.

The obstetrician and the anesthesiologist should talk openly with a psychiatric patient about the problems of labor and delivery management and offer suggestions for management of discomfort so that she will have minimal emotional stress. The ideal technique is the combined use of lumbar epidural block for the first stage and lumbar or caudal epidural block for the second stage. It is best to carefully point out to the patient the reasons for choosing the technique and to review the technical points of the procedure so that she will not be alarmed when the block is attempted. These techniques are preferred because they afford early and continuous analgesia during labor and delivery.

TREATMENT OF COMPLICATIONS OF ANESTHETICS

Resuscitation of the Mother

Anesthesia is responsible for 10% of maternal mortality. The most common cause of maternal death is failure to intubate the trachea at induction of general anesthesia. Less frequently, maternal death results from inadvertent intravascular injection of local anesthetic (toxic reaction) or inadvertent intrathecal injection of anesthetic (total spinal).

When faced with maternal cardiovascular collapse, full cardiopulmonary resuscitation (CPR) is indicated:

1. Establish a patent airway.
2. Aspirate mucus, blood, and vomitus with a tracheal suction apparatus. Use a laryngoscope for direct visualization of air passages and intubate the trachea.
3. Administer oxygen by artificial respiration if respirations are absent or weak. If high spinal anesthesia has occurred, continue to ventilate the patient until paralysis of the diaphragm has dissipated.
4. Give vasopressors intravenously (ephedrine 10–20 mg). Place the patient in the wedged supine position with the feet elevated and give transfusions of plasma, plasma expanders, and blood for traumatic or hemorrhagic shock.
5. Specifically treat cardiac arrhythmias in accordance with advanced cardiac life support (ACLS) recommendations.
6. Provide external cardiac massage in the absence of adequate rhythm and blood pressure.
7. Consider immediate cesarean section delivery to salvage fetus and improve venous return if the patient does not immediately respond to efforts.

Full cardiopulmonary arrest can be averted if the prodromal symptoms are recognized and treated immediately. A total spinal block is recognized by excessive and dense sensory and motor block to a test injection of local anesthesia through the epidural catheter. Further injections are avoided, and the patient's blood pressure is supported with fluid, positioning, and vasopressors.

An intravascular injection of local anesthetic is recognized early by symptoms of drowsiness, agitation, tinnitus, perioral tingling, bradycardia, and mild hypotension. The patient should be immediately given 100% oxygen and a small dose of diazepam (5 mg), midazolam (1 mg), or pentothal (50 mg). Further treatment may not be needed. The patient must be watched closely and the epidural catheter removed.

REFERENCES

Breen TW, MacNeil T, Diernenfield L: Obstetric anesthesia practice in Canada: Occasional survey. Can J Anesth 2000;47:1230.

Chestnut DH et al: Does early administration of epidural analgesia affect obstetric outcome in nulliparous women who are in spontaneous labor? Anesthesiology 1994;80:1201.

Hood DD, Curry R: Spinal versus epidural anesthesia for cesarean section in severely preeclamptic patients: A retrospective survey. Anesthesiology 1999;90:1276.

MacKay AP, Berg CJ, Atrash HK: Pregnancy-related mortality from preeclampsia and eclampsia. Obstet Gynecol 2001;97:533.

Palmer CM et al: Postcesarean epidural morphine: A dose-response study. Anesth Analg 2000;90:887.

Practice Guidelines for Obstetrical Anesthesia: A report by the American Society of Anesthesiologists Task Force on Obstetrical Anesthesia. Anesthesiology 1999;90:600.

Operative Delivery

30

Marc H. Incerpi, MD

An *operative delivery* refers to an obstetric procedure in which active measures are taken to accomplish delivery. Operative delivery can be divided into *operative vaginal delivery* and *cesarean delivery*. The last several years have seen a trend toward a decrease in the operative vaginal delivery rate but a climb in the cesarean section rate. In addition, vacuum-assisted vaginal delivery has been increasing while vaginal delivery using forceps has started declining. The success and safety of these procedures are based upon operator skill, proper timing, and ensuring that proper indications are met while contraindications are avoided. This chapter explains how each procedure is performed, the indications and contraindications to the procedure, the potential complications, and how to minimize complications.

■ FORCEPS OPERATIONS

The obstetric forceps is an instrument designed to assist with delivery of the baby's head. It is used either to expedite delivery or to assist with certain abnormalities in the cephalopelvic relationship that interfere with advancement of the head during labor. The primary functions of the forceps are to assist with traction of the fetal head and/or to assist with rotation of the fetal head to a more desirable position.

Although forceps-assisted vaginal deliveries once were extremely popular, the most recent data demonstrate that less than half of all operative vaginal deliveries are performed using forceps. The reverse was true approximately 10 years ago. In fact, many investigators are concerned that the use of forceps is becoming a lost art. The reasons often cited as contributing to the decline in the use of forceps are (1) medicolegal implications and fear of litigation, (2) reliance on cesarean section as a remedy for abnormal labor and suspected fetal jeopardy, (3) perception that the vacuum is easier to use and less risky to the fetus and mother, and (4) decreased number of residency programs that actively train residents in the use of forceps. These factors have led to a cycle in which less teaching has led to a decrement in

technical skills, an increased fear of litigation, and a resultant further decrease in the use of forceps.

THE OBSTETRIC FORCEPS

The obstetric forceps (Fig 30–1) consists of 2 matched parts that articulate or "lock." Each part is composed of a blade, shank, lock, and handle. Each blade is designed so that it possesses 2 curves: the cephalic curve, which permits the instrument to be applied accurately to the sides of the baby's head, and the pelvic curve, which conforms to the curved axis of the maternal pelvis. The tip of each blade is called the *toe*. The front of the forceps is the concave side of the pelvic curve. The blades are referred to the left and right according to the side of the mother's pelvis on which they lie after application. During application, the handle of the left blade is held in the left hand, and the blade is applied to the left side of the mother's pelvis. Conversely, the handle of the right blade is held in the right hand and inserted so as to lie on the right side of the mother's pelvis. When the blades are inserted in this order, the right shank comes to lie atop the left so that the forceps articulate, or lock, as the handles are closed.

Physicians have been modifying 1 or more of the 4 basic parts since forceps were first invented. Although more than 600 kinds of forceps have been described, only a few are currently in use (Fig 30–2). Although it is beyond the scope of this chapter to discuss all the different varieties of forceps and their indications, a brief comment on the more common types of forceps is appropriate. Simpson or Elliot forceps are most often used for outlet vaginal deliveries, whereas Kielland or Tucker-McLane forceps are used for rotational deliveries. Piper forceps are used in the United States for delivery of the aftercoming head. The pelvic and cephalic curve, shank, blade, lock, and handle are different for each type of forceps. These features determine the type of forceps that is best suited for the appropriate indication. For example, Piper forceps, which are specifically designed for breech deliveries, have a reverse pelvic curve compared to other forceps. Simpson forceps are suited for application to the molded fetal head, whereas Tucker-McLane forceps or Kielland forceps are more appropriate for application to the fetal head with little or no molding.

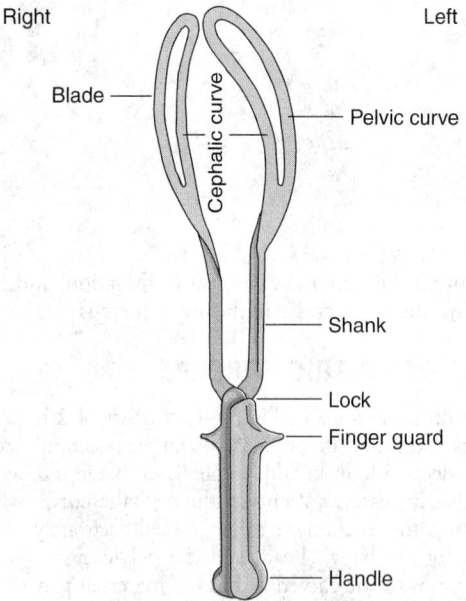

Right   Left

Blade

Cephalic curve

Pelvic curve

Shank

Lock

Finger guard

Handle

Figure 30–1. DeLee modification of Simpson forceps. (Reproduced, with permission, from Benson RC: *Handbook of Obstetrics & Gynecology*, 8th ed. Lange, 1983.)

INDICATIONS AND CONDITIONS FOR FORCEPS DELIVERY

In each of the following indications for forceps delivery, it must be emphasized that cesarean section is an alternative procedure that should be considered depending on the prevailing circumstances. Recognizing the inherent risks of both procedures, the obstetrician must decide which operation (vaginal delivery or cesarean section) will be safer for mother and baby. In modern obstetrics there is rarely, if ever, a place for the difficult forceps delivery that endangers either mother or child.

The indications for forceps delivery are as follows: (1) nonreassuring fetal heart rate pattern, (2) shortening of the second stage of labor for fetal or maternal reasons, (3) prolonged second stage of labor not due to dystocia, and (4) delivery of the aftercoming head in a breech presentation. A prolonged second stage of labor has been defined according to parity. In a nulliparous patient, a prolonged second stage is defined as more than 3 hours with a regional anesthetic or more than 2 hours without a regional anesthetic. In a multiparous patient, more than 2 hours with a regional anesthetic or more than 1 hour without a regional anesthetic constitutes a prolonged second stage of labor.

Simpson forceps

Bailey-Williamson forceps

Elliot forceps

Tucker-McLane forceps

Kielland forceps

Barton forceps and traction handle

Piper forceps

Figure 30–2. Commonly used forceps. (Reproduced, with permission, from Benson RC: *Handbook of Obstetrics & Gynecology*, 8th ed. Lange, 1983.)

In order for a patient to be considered a candidate for a forceps-assisted vaginal delivery, *all* of the following prerequisites must be met: (1) complete cervical dilatation, (2) ruptured membranes, (3) vertex presentation, (4) fetal head engaged with the fetal head position known, (5) empty bladder, (6) no evidence of cephalopelvic disproportion, (7) adequate analgesia, (8) cesarean section capability, and (9) an experienced operator.

CLASSIFICATION OF FORCEPS DELIVERIES

In 1988 the American College of Obstetricians and Gynecologists redefined the classification of forceps. As discussed later, the same classification should be applied to vacuum delivery. This classification uses the leading bony point of the fetal skull and its relationship to the maternal ischial spines in centimeters as the point of reference. Each station of the fetal head refers to the relationship of the leading bony part of the fetal skull with respect to the ischial spines. The fetal head is said to be at 0 station when the head is at the level of the spines. When the head is above this level, the station is described as −1 through −5, corresponding to the number of centimeters above the level of the ischial spines. When the head is below this level, the station is described as +1 through +5, corresponding to the number of centimeters below the level of the ischial spines.

The classification of forceps is defined as follows:

1. **Outlet forceps** is the application of forceps when (a) the fetal scalp is visible at the introitus without separating the labia, (b) the fetal skull has reached the pelvic floor, (c) the sagittal suture is in the anteroposterior diameter or in the right or left occiput anterior or posterior position, and (d) the fetal head is at or on the perineum. According to this definition, rotation of the fetal head must be equal to or less than 45 degrees.
2. **Low forceps** is the application of forceps when the leading point of the fetal skull is at station +2 or greater and not on the pelvic floor. Low forceps have two subdivisions: (a) rotation less than or equal to 45 degrees and (b) rotation greater than 45 degrees.
3. **Midforceps** is the application of forceps when the head is engaged but the leading point of the fetal skull is above station +2.

Only rarely should an attempt be made at forceps delivery above station +2. Under unusual circumstances, such as sudden onset of severe fetal or maternal compromise or transverse arrest, application of forceps above station +2 can be attempted while simultaneously initiating preparation for a cesarean delivery in case the forceps maneuver is unsuccessful. *Under no circumstances should forceps be applied to an unengaged head.*

PREPARATION OF THE PATIENT FOR FORCEPS DELIVERY

The patient must be placed in the dorsal lithotomy position. The legs should be comfortably placed in stirrups with the hips flexed and abducted. The abdomen and legs should be adequately draped, and the vagina and perineum should be prepped in usual fashion. If conduction (spinal/epidural) anesthesia is to be used, it must be administered prior to the foregoing steps in delivery. If pudendal block or local infiltration is to be used, it should be administered after the preliminary examination has been performed and all is in readiness for delivery. An appropriate and effective anesthetic is essential to the performance of any forceps delivery.

The Preliminary Examination

Before the application of forceps, a careful examination is necessary to determine the following:

1. **The position of the fetal head,** which usually is easily determined by first locating the lambdoid sutures and then determining the direction of the sagittal suture. The posterior fontanelle is readily evident after the 3 sutures running into it are identified. If the most accessible fontanelle is found to have 4 sutures running into it, it is the anterior fontanelle and the position usually is occiput posterior. In the presence of marked edema of the scalp or caput succedaneum, both sutures and fontanelles may be masked, and the position can be determined only by feeling an ear and noting the direction of the pinna. It must be emphasized that if the position of the fetal head cannot be adequately determined, then forceps should not be applied.
2. **The station of the fetal head,** which is the relationship of the presenting part to the ischial spines, must be determined. In labor that proceeds swiftly without complications, such a determination usually is simple and accurate. However, when the first or especially the second stage of labor is prolonged and is further complicated by marked molding and a heavy caput, this relationship may suggest a false level of the head in the pelvis. If the head can be felt above the symphysis pubis, forceps should not be used.
3. **The adequacy of the pelvic diameters** of the midpelvis and outlet is determined by noting the following: (a) the prominence of the ischial spines, the degree to which they shorten the transverse diameter of the midpelvis, and the amount of space between the spine and the side of the fetal head; (b) the contour of the accessible portion of the sacrum and the amount of space posterior to the head usually based on the length of the sacrospinous ligament; and (c) the width of the subpubic arch. This kind of appraisal is neither needed nor

feasible for outlet forceps but is essential for indicated low forceps or midforceps.

APPLICATION OF FORCEPS

A major concept to bear in mind is that the application of forceps should use finesse rather than force. Before the forceps are applied to the fetal head, a "phantom application" should be performed first. It is vital to inspect the forceps to ensure that they consist of a complete and matched set and that they articulate (lock) easily. Forceps should be applied in a delicate fashion in order to avoid potential injury to the vagina and perineum. The goal is for the blades to fit the fetal head as evenly and symmetrically as possible. The blades should lie evenly against the side of the head, covering the space between the orbits and ears (Fig 30–3). It is important to emphasize that correct application prevents soft tissue and nerve injury, as well as bony injuries to the fetal head. After the forceps have been applied, they should articulate easily. If the forceps cannot be easily articulated, the forceps should be removed and a second attempt made. Once the forceps articulate, the following checks should be performed for delivery of an occiput anterior position before any traction is placed on the fetal head. (1) The sagittal suture should be perpendicular to the plane of the shanks. (2) The posterior fontanelle should be 1 fingerbreadth away from the plane of the shanks, equidistant from the sides of the

Figure 30–3. Forceps correctly applied along occipitomental diameter of head in various positions of the occiput. **A:** Occiput posterior. **B:** Occiput anterior. (Reproduced, with permission, from Benson RC: *Handbook of Obstetrics & Gynecology,* 8th ed. Lange, 1983.)

blades, and directly in front of the articulated forceps. (3) If fenestrated (open) blades are used, the amount of fenestration in front of the fetal head should admit no more than the tip of 1 finger. After these checks have been performed, then traction can safely be applied to the fetal head. Traction forces should be applied in the plane of least resistance and should follow the pelvic curve. This can best be accomplished by applying downward pressure on the shanks with outward pressure exerted upon the handle of the forceps. Once the fetal head begins to emerge out of the vagina, the forceps are disarticulated, and the head is delivered via a modified Ritgen maneuver. After delivery, it is important to ensure that no vaginal or perineal lacerations go unrecognized, paying particular attention to deep lateral vaginal sidewall (sulcal) lacerations. Lacerations, if present, should be repaired in customary fashion.

A more detailed step-by-step description of a forceps-assisted vaginal delivery in the occiput anterior position is as follows (Figs 30–4 through 30–6). The left handle is held between the thumb and fingers of the left hand. Using 2 or 3 fingers of the right hand placed into the vagina, the blade is guided to its correct position on the left side of the fetal head (Fig 30–4). This maneuver is repeated with the right hand and the right blade, using the fingers of the left hand placed into the vagina to guide the blade (Fig 30–5). The handles are depressed slightly before locking, in order to place the blades properly along the optimal diameter of the fetal head (Fig 30–6).

The forceps are designed such that they lock easily as the handles are closed if the application is accurate. If the handles are askew or if any force is needed to achieve precise articulation, the application is faulty and the position must be rechecked. If simple manipulation of the blades does not permit easy articulation, the forceps should be removed, the position verified (by feeling an ear, if necessary), and the blades reapplied correctly. After these 3 checks have been adequately performed, traction can be applied.

Obstetricians hold forceps for traction in different ways. One method is to grasp the crossbar of the handle between the index and middle fingers of the left hand from underneath and to insert the middle and index fingers of the right hand in the crotch of the instrument from above. Another method is to grasp the handles with the fingers on the top of the handles or shanks and the thumbs on the bottom. Traction is made only in the axis of the pelvis along the curve of the birth canal. No more force is applied than can be exerted by the flexed forearms; the muscles of the back must not be used, and the feet must not be braced. If a greater degree of traction is needed, the cause may be cephalopelvic disproportion, asynclitism of the fetal head, or an

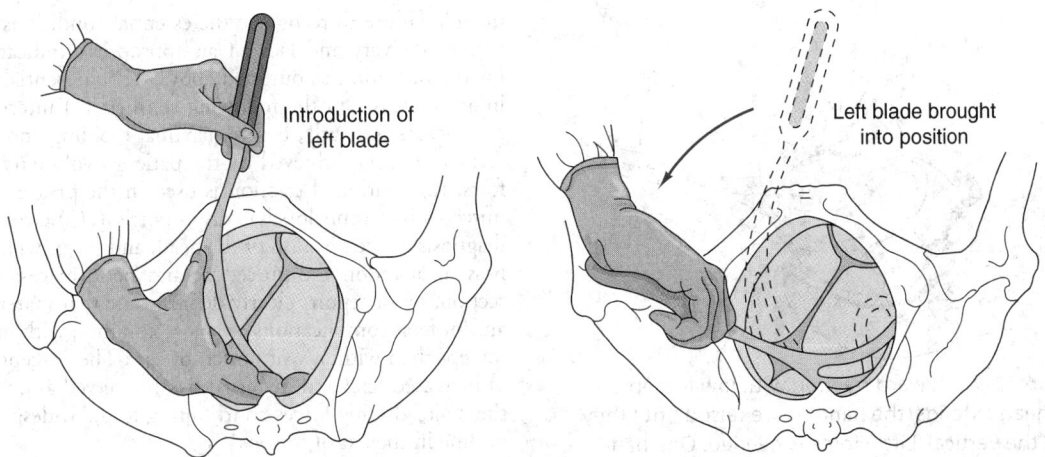

Figure 30–4. Introduction of left blade (left blade, left hand, left side of pelvis). The handle is held with the fingers and thumb, not clenched in the hand. The handle is held vertically. The blade is guided with the fingers of the right hand. Placement of blade is completed by swinging the handle down to the horizontal plane.

error in evaluation of the pelvic diameters. The obstetrician then should reassess the possibility of successful vaginal delivery.

As the head begins to distend the perineum, both the amount and direction of traction must be altered. The farther the head advances, the less the resistance offered by both the pelvis and the soft parts; hence, only minimal traction should be applied as the head is about to be delivered. The head negotiates the final position of the pelvic curve by extension, and the physician should simulate this movement by elevating the handles of the forceps more and more as the head crowns (Fig 30–7). If the forceps are allowed to remain in place throughout delivery of the fetal head, the handles will have passed the vertical plane as delivery of the head is completed. It is preferable to remove the forceps as the head crowns in the reverse order of their application by first disarticulat-

Figure 30–5. Introduction of right blade (right blade, right hand, right side of pelvis). The left blade is already in place. The handle is grasped with the fingers and thumb, not gripped in the whole hand. The handle is held vertically. (Reproduced, with permission, from Benson RC: *Handbook of Obstetrics & Gynecology*, 8th ed. Lange, 1983.)

Figure 30–6. Both blades introduced. The 2 handles are brought together and locked. If application is correct, the handles lock precisely, without the need for force. (Reproduced, with permission, from Benson RC: *Handbook of Obstetrics & Gynecology*, 8th ed. Lange, 1983.)

Figure 30–7. Upward traction with low forceps. As the head extends, the handles are raised until they pass the vertical. Little force is needed. One hand suffices; the other hand may support the perineum. (Reproduced, with permission, from Benson RC: *Handbook of Obstetrics & Gynecology*, 8th ed. Lange, 1983.)

ing the forceps and raising the right handle until the blade is delivered. The left blade is then removed in similar fashion. Early removal of the forceps reduces the size of the mass that must pass through the introitus and thus reduces the likelihood of lacerations or extension of episiotomies. After removal of the forceps, the head may recede; however, if the forceps have not been removed too soon, the head can be delivered readily by the use of the Ritgen maneuver during the next contraction. Because rotations with forceps and vaginal breech deliveries are now rarely, if ever, performed, it is beyond the scope of this chapter to discuss these techniques.

DANGER AND SAFETY OF FORCEPS

Although use of forceps has fallen into disfavor over the last few years, few studies have prospectively evaluated the safety of forceps. A number of injuries to both mother and baby can result from the use of forceps, some serious or even fatal. Maternal complications include lacerations of the vagina and cervix, episiotomy extensions involving third- and fourth-degree lacerations, pelvic hematomas, urethral and bladder injuries, and uterine rupture. In addition, blood loss and the need for blood transfusion are increased in forceps deliveries. The baby may sustain minor facial lacerations, forceps marks, facial and brachial plexus palsies, cephalhematomas, skull fractures, intracranial hemorrhage, and seizures.

Many of the serious injuries and many of the minor ones inflicted by obstetric forceps result from errors in judgment rather than lack of technical skill. Such errors

include failure to recognize the essential conditions for forceps delivery and lack of an appropriate indication for the operation as outlined above. The potential for injury increases in the following settings: (1) intervention occurs too early, before maximal molding and descent have been achieved by the patient's voluntary efforts, (2) continued traction is used in the presence of unrecognized cephalopelvic disproportion, (3) errors in diagnosis of the position of the head, and (4) unwillingness to abandon the procedure and perform cesarean section. Most reports clearly demonstrate that maternal and/or fetal complications are more common with midforceps than with low or outlet forceps. The perception of increased fetal and maternal risk has served as one of the major driving forces contributing to the widespread decline in the use of forceps.

■ THE VACUUM EXTRACTOR

The idea of using a suction device applied to the fetal scalp to help facilitate delivery of the fetal head originated in the 1700s. The first vacuum cup was not designed until 1890. As one could well imagine, the first types of vacuum devices were crude, resembling a toilet plunger. In fact, the vacuum device did not gain much popularity until Malmström introduced a metal vacuum cup in 1954. The most common type of vacuum in use today is a pliable, Silastic cup with a handheld pump and gauge that allow delivery of the proper amount of suction pressure to the fetal head to effect delivery. Two models are shown in Figures 30–8 and 30–9.

The vacuum extractor works by allowing the external traction forces applied to the fetal scalp to be transmitted to the fetal head. The traction on the vacuum apparatus increases the forces of delivery and facilitates passage of the fetus through the pelvis. In order for delivery to be accomplished, both traction on the fetal scalp and compression of the fetal head occur.

INDICATIONS AND CONTRAINDICATIONS FOR VACUUM DELIVERY

With the exception of delivery of the aftercoming head in a breech presentation, the indications for vacuum use are similar to those of forceps. In addition, as mentioned earlier, the classification of forceps deliveries is the same classification used for vacuum deliveries, and the prerequisites are similar. Contraindications for vacuum delivery include the following: face presentation,

Figure 30–8. Mityvac obstetrical vacuum delivery system includes extractor cup and pump. (Photograph reproduced with permission of Prism Enterprises, Inc, Rancho Cucamonga, Calif.)

breech presentation, true cephalopelvic disproportion, congenital anomalies of the fetal head (eg, hydrocephalus), gestational age less than 34 weeks or estimated fetal weight less than 2000 g, estimated fetal weight greater than 4000 g, and an unengaged fetal head.

VACUUM APPLICATION

Before the vacuum is applied to the fetal head, the patient is prepared and the initial patient examination is performed as discussed earlier with regard to forceps deliveries. Application of the vacuum is perceived by many to be much simpler than use of the forceps. Before application occurs, the vacuum system should be assembled to ensure that no leaks are present. The cup should then be inserted into the vagina by directing pressure toward the posterior aspect of the vagina. The objective is to place the cup directly over the sagittal suture at the median flexion point located approximately 3 cm anterior to the posterior fontanelle. This cup placement should allow for adequate maintenance of flexion of the fetal head during the entire procedure. As with forceps application, 3 checks should be undertaken prior to application of traction to the fetal head. (1) No maternal tissue should be included under the cup margin. (2) The cup should be placed in the midline over the sagittal suture and not off to the side of the head. (3) The marker or vacuum port of the suction cup should point toward the occiput.

After the cup has been appropriately placed on the fetal scalp, an initial suction is applied, and the cup edges are reexamined to ensure that no maternal tissue is trapped underneath the vacuum cup. While the cup is held firmly against the fetal head, the pressure is increased to approximately 600 mmHg at the beginning of a uterine contraction. As the mother pushes, traction is applied along the pelvic axis. If more than 1 contraction is necessary, the vacuum pressure can be decreased to low levels between contractions. While the fetal head is delivering, the cup should assume a 90-degree orientation to the horizontal as the head is extended. Once the head has completely delivered through the vagina, the suction is withdrawn and the cup removed.

EFFECTIVENESS AND SAFETY OF VACUUM

Most reports demonstrate that the vacuum is effective, with a failure rate of approximately 10%. The following

Figure 30–9. CMI Tender Touch extractor cup. (Photograph reproduced with permission of Utah Medical Products.)

factors have been implicated in determining the effectiveness of vacuum delivery: cup design, shape, size, and traction site attachment, consistency and strength of vacuum, strength of maternal expulsive efforts and coordination with traction, fetal size and extent of cephalopelvic disproportion, station and deflection of the fetal head, and angle and technique of traction.

The safety of the vacuum has been called into question. In May 1998, the United States Food and Drug Administration issued a Public Advisory Statement regarding fetal complications associated with vacuum delivery. The purpose of this statement was to advise practitioners that vacuum devices may cause serious or fatal complications when improperly used. As a result the following recommendations were made: (1) The vacuum should be used only when a specific obstetric indication is present. (2) Persons using the vacuum should be experienced and aware of the indications, contraindications, and precautions. (3) Those who use the vacuum should read and understand the instructions for the particular instrument being used. (4) The neonatal care staff should be educated about the potential complications of vacuum. (5) Individuals responsible for the care of the neonate should be alerted that vacuum has been used. (6) All adverse reactions should be reported to the Food and Drug Administration.

Use of the vacuum has been associated with a variety of neonatal injuries ranging from benign superficial scalp markings to serious and potentially life-threatening intracranial hemorrhages. The most common neonatal complication is retinal hemorrhage, which may occur in as many as 50% of deliveries. Fortunately, this complication rarely has any clinical significance. Cephalhematoma involves bleeding beneath the periosteum and complicates approximately 6% of all vacuum deliveries. Because the bleeding is located under the periosteum, significant bleeding rarely results because of the inability of the blood to cross the sutures. Subgaleal hematoma, a more serious complication, occurs in 50 of 10,000 vacuum deliveries. The condition arises when bleeding occurs in the loose subaponeurotic tissues of the scalp. Because bleeding occurs above the periosteum, it is not contained by the sutures. Consequently, there is the potential for life-threatening hemorrhage. The subgaleal space actually extends from the orbits of the eyes to the nape of the neck. This potential space can occupy over half of a newborn's blood volume. Intracranial hemorrhage occurs in approximately 0.35% of vacuum deliveries. It can be a catastrophic complication that includes subdural, subarachnoid, intraventricular, and/or intraparenchymal hemorrhage. These complications can be quite severe but fortunately are rare.

Most authorities agree that injury can be significantly decreased or eliminated if the following protocol is used. (1) Traction is applied only when the patient is actively pushing. (2) Applying torsion or twisting the cup in an attempt to rotate the head is prohibited. (3) The duration of time during which the cup is applied to the head should not exceed 20 minutes. (4) The procedure should be abandoned after the cup has dislodged from the fetal head twice. It should not be applied a third time. (5) The procedure should be abandoned if there is no fetal descent after a single pull. (6) The vacuum should not be used when the estimated fetal weight is less than 2000 g or greater than 4000 g. (7) Neonatal staff should be present at the time of the vacuum delivery. (Note: This also applies to forceps deliveries.) (8) Under no circumstances should the operator switch from vacuum to forceps or vice versa. An excellent study examining neonatal injury clearly demonstrated that the greatest incidence of neonatal injury occurred in babies in whom both vacuum and forceps were used. The practitioner must be cognizant of the risk for shoulder dystocia, which is increased with instrumental delivery. Shoulder dystocia occurs more commonly with vacuum deliveries than with forceps deliveries.

A detailed and complete delivery note should accompany each operative vaginal delivery. The medical record must document the indication for the procedure, the fetal station and head position at the time of the application(s) of forceps or vacuum, the type of device used, the total application time, the number of applications and "pop-offs" if vacuum was used, and, if unsuccessful, the subsequent mode of delivery.

Somewhat surprisingly, relatively few randomized, prospective studies have compared vacuum with forceps. In surveying the medical literature, the following conclusions can be drawn. On the whole, the vacuum extractor is less likely to achieve a successful vaginal delivery than is the forceps. The vacuum is significantly less likely to cause serious maternal injury than is the forceps. Although the vacuum is associated with a greater incidence of cephalhematoma, other facial/cranial injuries are more common with forceps. In comparing Apgar scores, the trend is toward more low 5-minute Apgar scores in the vacuum group than in the forceps group. Thus, an overall reduction in severe maternal injuries appear to be the most immediate benefit associated with use of the vacuum. However, at this time, which instrument results in fewer major adverse neonatal effects remains to be determined.

Although both forceps and vacuum have proved to be useful in assisting with vaginal delivery, the vacuum is quickly becoming the preferred instrument of choice. Both forceps and vacuum have the potential to cause fetal and neonatal injury; however, the incidence of maternal injury is less with the vacuum than with forceps. In order to minimize both maternal and fetal risks, the operator must be familiar with the indications, contra-indications, application, and use of the particular instrument. Safe and effective guidelines similar to those discussed in this chapter should exist in order to facilitate a safe and effective delivery.

CESAREAN SECTION

A *cesarean section* refers to the delivery of a fetus, placenta, and membranes through an abdominal and uterine incision. The first documented cesarean section on a living person was performed in 1610. The patient died 25 days later. Since that time, numerous advances have made cesarean section a safe procedure. In the past 35 years, the rate of cesarean section has steadily increased from 5% to approximately 25%. Over this time, the maternal mortality ratio (maternal deaths per 100,000 births) has decreased from almost 300 to less than 10. The following factors are often cited as contributing to the increasing cesarean section rate: (1) lower vaginal delivery rates, (2) lower rates of vaginal birth after cesarean section (VBAC), and (3) fewer vaginal breech deliveries. In order for the practitioner to perform this common operation safely, he or she must be aware of the indications, risks, operative technique, and potential complications of the procedure.

INDICATIONS

Cesarean section is used in cases where vaginal delivery either is not feasible or would impose undue risks to the mother or baby. Some of the indications for cesarean section are clear and straightforward, whereas others are relative. In some cases, fine judgment is necessary to determine whether cesarean section or vaginal delivery would be better. It is not practical to list all possible indications; however, hardly any obstetric complication has not been dealt with by cesarean section. The following indications are currently the most common.

Repeat Cesarean Section

A prior uterine incision from a myomectomy or previous cesarean section may weaken the uterine wall or predispose to rupture if labor is permitted. The initial dictum of "once a cesarean, always a cesarean" was held for many years. However, as multiple publications documenting the safety of VBAC began appearing in the literature, many physicians moved away from this long-held belief. In 2000, a national goal was to lower the rate of repeat cesarean sections to 3% while increasing the VBAC rate to 35%. The major incentives that led to this change in philosophy were fewer delivery risks with vaginal delivery, less need for anesthesia, less postpartum morbidity, shorter hospital stay, lower costs, and encouraging earlier and often smoother interaction and bonding between mother and infant. As more and more VBACs were performed in less than ideal settings, more complications arose. There may be no greater obstetric catastrophe than a uterine rupture resulting in maternal and/or fetal death. In fact, there appears to be a trend back toward the belief of "once a cesarean, always a cesarean." Suffice it to say, "once a cesarean, always a controversy."

In general, patients who are the most suitable candidates for trial of labor after cesarean section are those (1) with one prior low-transverse cesarean section, (2) who present in labor, (3) with nonrecurring conditions (eg, breech, fetal distress, placenta previa), and (4) with a prior vaginal delivery. Patients who are not candidates for trial of labor include women with a prior classic (vertical) uterine incision or prior myomectomy. If a trial of labor is to be conducted, the patient must be placed on continuous fetal heart rate and uterine activity monitoring, and an obstetrician and anesthesiologist must be immediately available to intervene in case uterine rupture is suspected. Prostaglandins for cervical ripening must be avoided, and oxytocin must be used in a judicious and conservative fashion, if at all. Current studies cite a maternal mortality rate of close to 1% percent in cases of uterine rupture and a perinatal mortality rate of approximately 50% in association with uterine rupture. Therefore, it is of utmost importance that equipment for both maternal and electronic fetal monitoring and appropriate obstetric and neonatal facilities be available. A large-bore intravenous catheter must be used, and blood for possible maternal transfusion must be available. Appropriate anesthesia, a fully equipped operating room, and obstetric and neonatal staff experienced in emergency care all must be immediately available.

Cephalopelvic Disproportion/Dystocia

Cases in which the fetal head is too large to traverse the pelvis should be managed by cesarean section. As discussed earlier, if the head does not engage during labor and remains at a station higher than 0 station, operative vaginal delivery should not be attempted. Rather, cesarean section must be performed. Inlet disproportion should be suspected in the primigravida if the patient begins labor with the fetal head unengaged. In a significant number of these patients, the head fails to engage and cesarean section in indicated. Midpelvic disproportion may be suspected if the anteroposterior diameter is short, the ischial spines are prominent, the sacrospinous ligament is short, and the fetus is large. Outlet disproportion usually requires a trial of forceps or vacuum before a safe vaginal delivery is determined to be impossible.

Dystocia literally means "difficult labor." This occurs when a patient's labor progresses and then either stops completely *(arrests)* or becomes prolonged *(protracted)*. When either of these situations occurs during labor, the patient warrants careful reassessment, including labor pattern, contraction pattern, evaluation of the estimated fetal weight and fetal presentation, as well as evaluation of the pelvis.

Malposition and Malpresentation

Transverse lie and breech presentations are common indications for cesarean section. The trend toward cesarean delivery for breech has been hastened by a large randomized trial comparing breech infants born vaginally versus those born by cesarean section; better outcomes were achieved after cesarean section. Although some still consider vaginal breech delivery to be an acceptable option, experience with the technique is largely disappearing from practice.

External cephalic version is a reasonable alternative for some patients and can be attempted to convert the fetus to a cephalic presentation. However, this procedure is successful in allowing vaginal birth in only 50% of cases.

Fetal Distress

Fetal monitoring before and during labor may disclose fetal problems that otherwise would not be evident. As a result of continuous fetal monitoring, the number of cesarean sections performed for the indication of fetal distress or fetal jeopardy has increased. Best estimates demonstrate that approximately 10% of cesarean sections are performed because of fetal distress.

Other Indications

In addition to the indications discussed, other conditions that can lead to cesarean section are placenta previa, preeclampsia–eclampsia if remote from term, multiple gestations, fetal abnormalities (eg, hydrocephalus), cervical cancer, and active herpes infection. One other indication that is becoming more prevalent is patient choice. The idea of primary elective cesarean section continues to increase in popularity and generate controversy.

PREOPERATIVE PREPARATION FOR CESAREAN SECTION

The following steps are generally taken before cesarean section is performed. The patient is made aware of the indications for the cesarean section, the alternatives, and the potential risks and complications. She then signs a form indicating that she has received the information and consents to the procedure ("informed consent"). An intravenous 18-gauge needle should be in place with an appropriate intravenous IV solution running before the operation begins. The patient is given a clear antacid to minimize the likelihood of aspiration during anesthesia. A Foley catheter is placed to allow for continuous bladder drainage before, during, and after surgery. Anesthesia is administered, and the abdomen is prepped and shaved. The patient is covered with sterile drapes. Tilting the patient slightly to the left moves the uterus to the left of the midline and minimizes pressure on the inferior vena cava.

OPERATIVE PROCEDURE
Abdominal Incision

Opinions differ regarding the type of abdominal incision that should be performed. Most obstetricians use the transverse (Pfannenstiel) incision with or without transection of the rectus muscles because wound dehiscence and postoperative incisional hernia are rare, and because the cosmetic result usually is better. In cases of fetal distress, especially in patients with prior abdominal surgery or marked obesity, the midline suprapubic incision is preferred because it is much quicker and the exposure for expeditious delivery and resolving uterine bleeding (by hysterectomy, if needed) usually is better. In the presence of a prior lower abdominal scar, it is important to enter the peritoneal cavity at the upper end of the incision to avoid entering the bladder, which may have been pulled upward on the abdominal wall at the time of closure of the previous incision.

Uterine Incision

Before the uterine incision is made, laparotomy pads that have been soaked in warm saline and wrung out can be placed on either side of the uterus to catch the spill of amniotic fluid. The degree of dextrorotation should also be determined by noting the position of the round ligaments so that the uterine incision will be centered. Torsion should not be corrected; instead, access to the midline should be obtained by retracting the abdominal wall to the patient's right. The different types of uterine incisions will be discussed later.

Encountering the Placenta

If the placenta is encountered beneath the uterine incision, the operator should try to avoid cutting thorough it, otherwise serious fetal bleeding may result. If the placenta cannot be avoided, an incision can be made through it. However, the baby must be delivered as quickly as possible and the cord clamped immediately to prevent significant blood loss.

Delivery

The operator delivers the baby and then the placenta delivers. Recent evidence has demonstrated that blood loss can be minimized by massaging the uterus to allow for spontaneous placental expulsion rather than by manually separating and extracting the placenta. Both methods are performed. After delivery of the placenta, the uterus should be massaged and oxytocin administered in a dilute intravenous solution at a rate sufficient to maintain a firm contraction. The uterine cavity is wiped clean with a sponge so as to remove any retained membranes. The uterus is exteriorized, and active bleeding sinuses are clamped with either Pennington clamps or ring forceps.

Closure of the Uterine Incision

The closure of the uterine incision is dependent upon the type of incision that is made. In general, the entire thickness of the myometrium should be closed. The two types of uterine incisions used most often and discussed here are the classical uterine incision and the low-transverse uterine incision.

CLASSICAL CESAREAN SECTION

This is the simplest to perform. However, it is associated with the greatest loss of blood and may result in uterine rupture with subsequent pregnancies. The currently accepted indications for classical cesarean section are placenta previa, transverse lie (especially back down), and preterm delivery in which the lower uterine segment is poorly developed. A classical cesarean section may be preferred if extremely rapid delivery is needed, because this type of incision offers the quickest means of delivering the baby. Nonetheless, the hazards of this procedure must be weighed against the additional minute or so needed to dissect the bladder away from the lower uterine segment and to make the transverse semilunar low-transverse incision.

In performing a classic procedure, a vertical incision is made in the corpus. A scalpel is used to enter the uterine cavity, and the incision is enlarged with bandage scissors. The fetus is delivered through the incision. After the placenta and membranes are removed, the uterine defect is repaired with 3 layers of running, interlocking absorbable suture. Number 0 suture is recommended for the 2 deeper layers and 2-0 suture is used for the superficial layer to reapproximate the serosal edges.

LOW-TRANSVERSE CESAREAN SECTION

Because the low-transverse uterine incision (Figs 30–10 through 30–17) is associated with less blood loss and

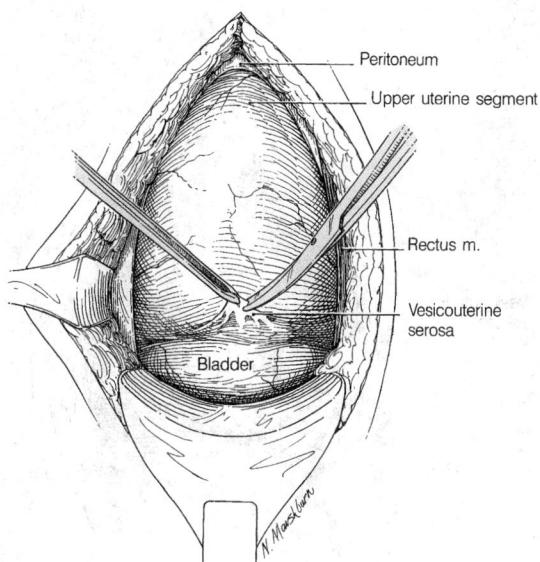

Figure 30–10. The loose vesicouterine serosa is grasped with the forceps. The hemostat tip points to the upper margin of the bladder. The retractor is firmly positioned against the symphysis. (m. = muscle.) (From Cunningham FG, Leveno KJ, Bloom SL, et al: Williams Obstetrics, 22nd ed. New York: McGraw-Hill; 2005, p 594.)

the risk of subsequent uterine rupture is less than with a classic cesarean section, this type of cesarean delivery is performed more frequently. After the peritoneal cavity is opened and the uterus identified, the bladder fold of peritoneum is picked up with tissue forceps and incised transversely. The bladder is bluntly separated from the anterior aspect of the uterus inferiorly for a distance of 3–4 cm. The bladder is held away from this area by a specially designed bladder retractor. A transverse incision is made through the anterior uterine wall with the scalpel. Using either bandage scissors or fingers, the transverse incision is extended in a semilunar fashion and extended superiorly at the lateral edges in order to avoid the uterine vessels.

If the maneuver can be easily done, the fetal presenting part is elevated with the hand, making sure not to flex the wrist, thereby increasing the possibility of extension of the incision inferiorly towards the cervix. If the head is located deep in the pelvis, the head can safely be pushed up by an assistant inserting a hand into the vagina to elevate the fetal head for ease of delivery. After the baby and placenta are delivered, the uterus is exteriorized and clamps are placed on the cut edge of the uterus in areas of significant bleeding from the uterine sinuses. The uterine incision is generally closed in 2 layers using number 0 chromic catgut or other absorb-

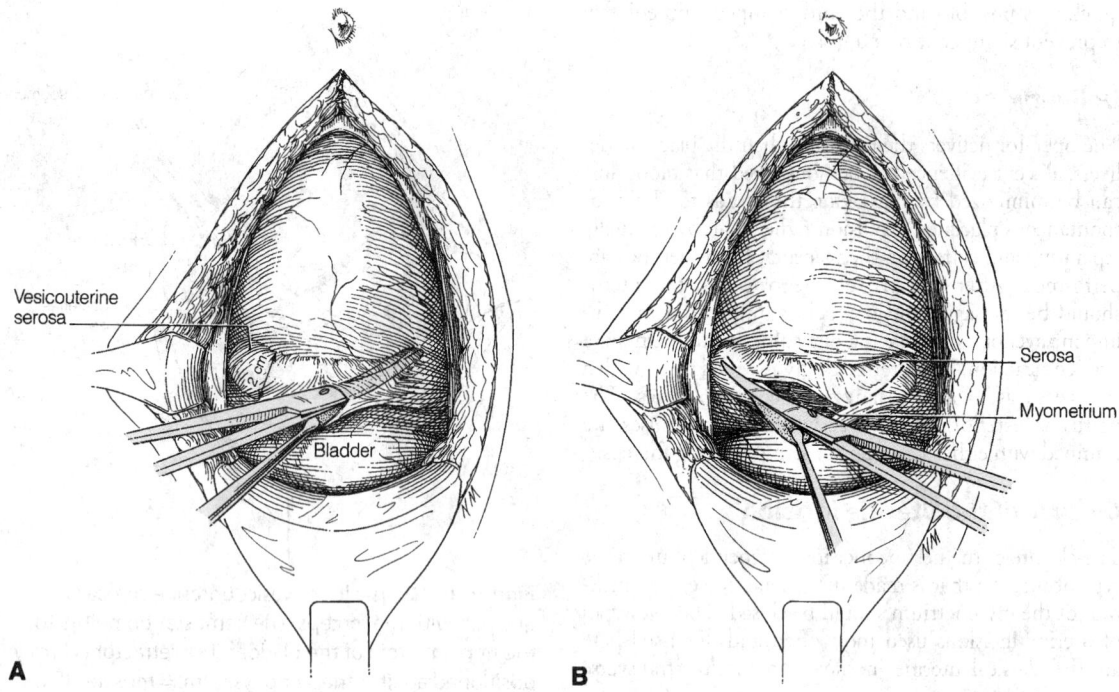

A **B**

Figure 30–11. The loose serosa above the upper margin of the bladder is elevated and incised laterally. (From Cunningham FG, Leveno KJ, Bloom SL, et al: Williams Obstetrics, 22nd ed. New York: McGraw-Hill; 2005, p 594.)

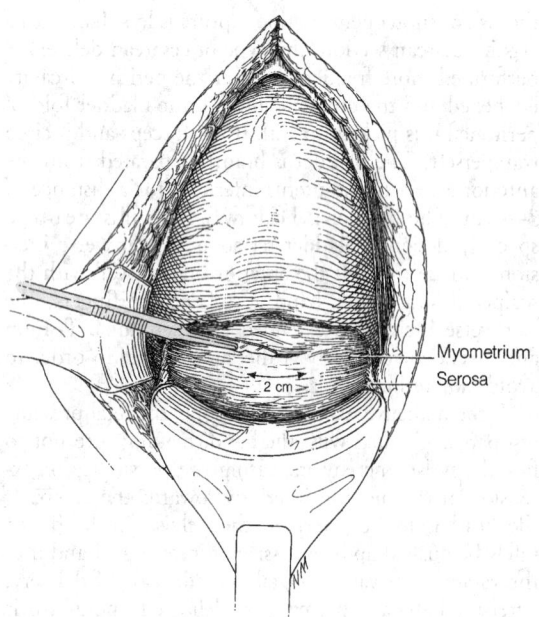

Figure 30–12. The myometrium is incised carefully to avoid cutting the fetal head. (From Cunningham FG, Leveno KJ, Bloom SL, et al: Williams Obstetrics, 22nd ed. New York: McGraw-Hill; 2005, p 595.)

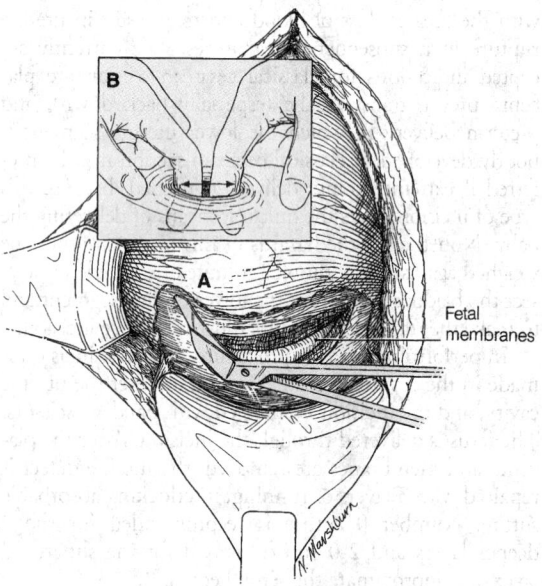

Figure 30–13. After entering the uterine cavity, the incision is extended laterally with bandage scissors (**A**) or with fingers, as shown in **B**. (From Cunningham FG, Leveno KJ, Bloom SL, et al: Williams Obstetrics, 22nd ed. New York: McGraw-Hill; 2005, p 595.)

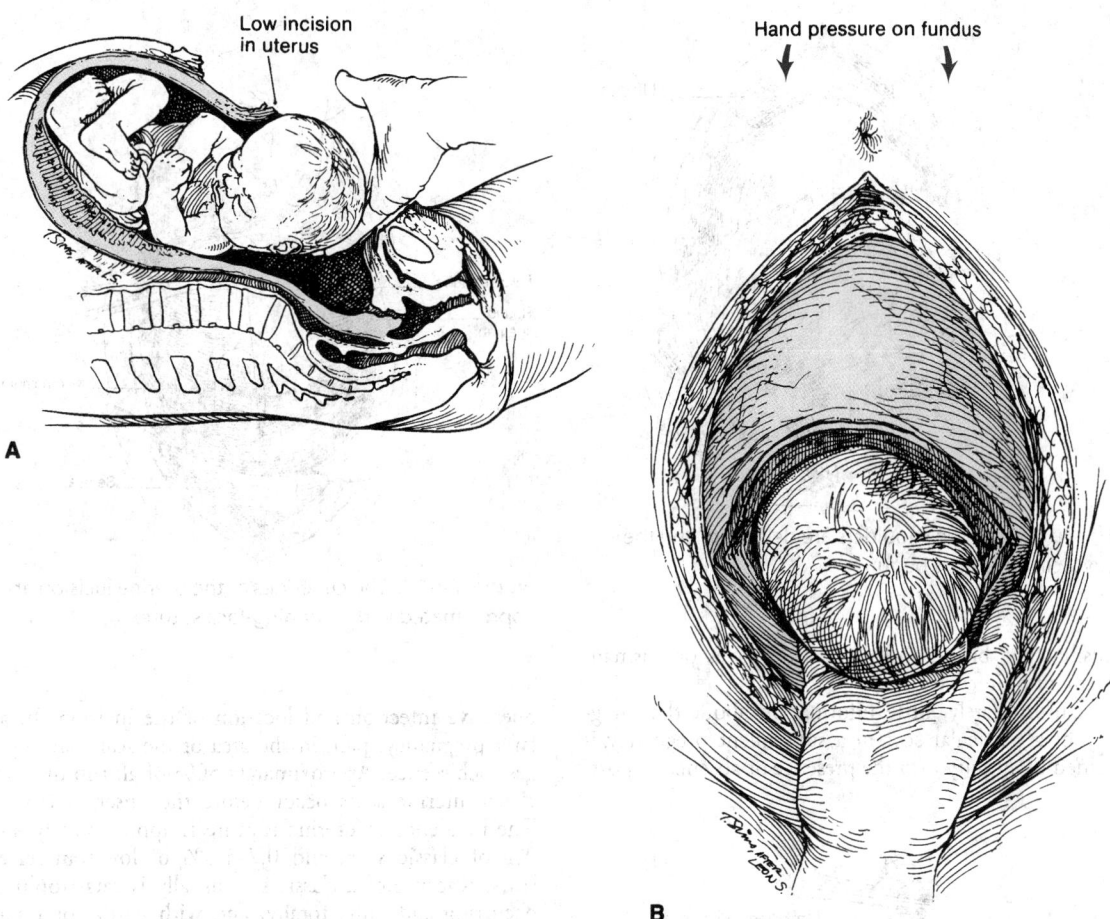

Figure 30–14. **A.** Immediately after incising the uterus and rupturing the fetal membranes, the fingers are insinuated between the symphysis pubis and the fetal head until the posterior surface is reached. The head is lifted carefully anteriorly and, as necessary, superiorly to bring it from beneath the symphysis forward through the uterine and abdominal incisions. **B.** As the fetal head is lifted through the incision, pressure usually is applied to the uterine fundus through the abdominal wall to help expel the fetus. (From Cunningham FG, Leveno KJ, Bloom SL, et al: Williams Obstetrics, 22nd ed. New York: McGraw-Hill; 2005, p 596.)

able suture. After adequate hemostasis has been achieved, the bladder peritoneum either is reapproximated with suture or left in place. Before the uterus is returned to the peritoneal cavity, the adnexa should be inspected for the presence of any pathology, such as ovarian cysts. Some practitioners prefer to close the anterior peritoneum with absorbable suture, whereas others prefer to leave it alone. The fascia, subcutaneous tissue, and skin are reapproximated in standard fashion.

COMPLICATIONS

The most common complications that result from cesarean section are postpartum hemorrhage, endometri-tis, and wound infection. Administering prophylactic antibiotics and ensuring hemostasis prior to closure of the abdomen have helped decrease the incidence of these complications. The major factors affecting healing of the uterine incision are hemostasis, accuracy of apposition, quality and amount of suture material, and avoidance of infection and tissue strangulation. It can generally be stated that the longer the operative procedure, the greater the likelihood of postoperative complications. Disasters following cesarean section are rare. Some clearly are not preventable. Others are the direct result of faulty surgical technique, especially lack of attention to hemostasis, inept or ill-chosen anesthesia, inadequate blood product replacement or transfusion of

Figure 30–15. The shoulders are delivered, and the oxytocin infusion is begun.

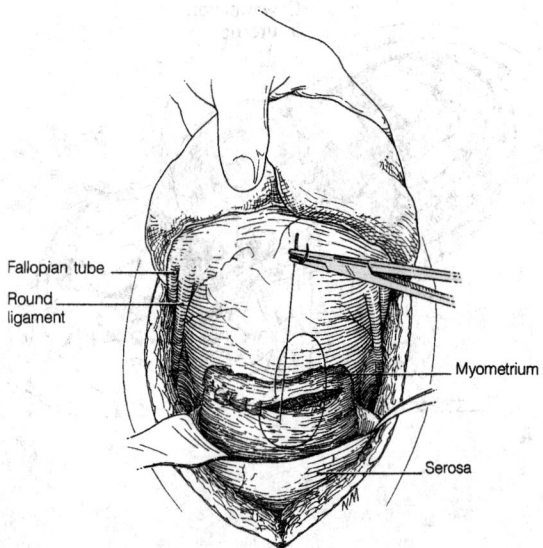

Figure 30–17. The cut edges of the uterine incision are approximated with a running-lock suture.

mismatched blood, and delayed diagnosis or mismanagement of infection.

Unfortunately, little information about the integrity of a particular scar in a subsequent pregnancy is gained by inquiry into the presence or absence of post-

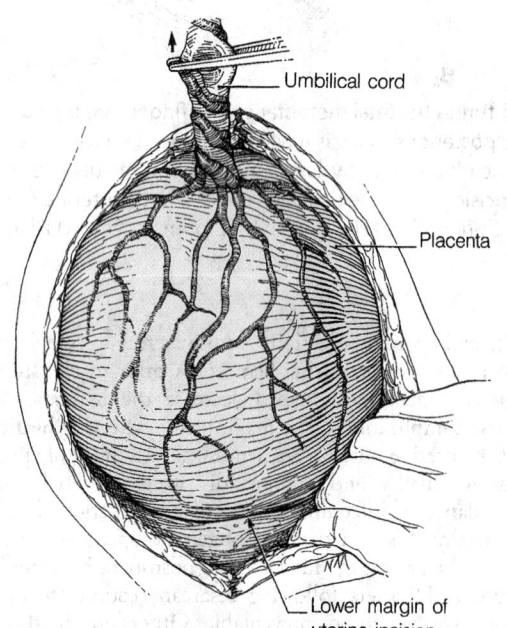

Figure 30–16. Placenta bulging through the uterine incision as the uterus contracts.

operative infection and location of the incision. In a later pregnancy, pain in the area of the scar may suggest dehiscence. Approximately 50% of all ruptures of classic uterine scars occur before the onset of labor. The incidence of uterine rupture is approximately 4–9% of classic scars and 0.7–1.5% of low-transverse scars. Rupture of a classic scar usually is catastrophic, occurring suddenly, totally, and with partial or total extrusion of the fetus into the abdominal cavity. Shock due to internal hemorrhage is a prominent sign. Rupture of the low-transverse scar usually is more subtle and almost always occurs during active labor. The most common presenting sign (present in more than 80% of cases) is a change in the fetal heart rate pattern. A newly recognized finding of variable decelerations or late decelerations should alert the obstetrician. Additional findings that might signal uterine rupture include vaginal bleeding, abdominal pain (especially over the prior incision site), and loss of fetal station. If uterine rupture is suspected, the patient must undergo surgery as soon as possible.

PERINATAL MORBIDITY AND MORTALITY

Although it may appear on the surface that cesarean delivery is the safest for the baby, this may not be entirely true. Although usually benign, transient tachypnea of the newborn is more common with cesarean section than with vaginal delivery. The risk of fetal hemorrhage and hypoxia is present when the placenta is encountered below the uterine incision and is inadvertently or purposely transected, and there is the potential risk for laceration of the baby at the time the uterine incision is made. Fetal laceration is reported to occur rather infrequently at a rate of approximately 0.2–0.4% of all cesarean sections. The usual site is on the face, in the area of the cheek, but it also may occur on the buttock, ear, head, or any other body site under the incision. Therefore it is of great importance that care be taken when incising the layers of the uterus. This is especially true in a prolonged labor, in which the uterus may be very thin. Because of the potential complications to the baby inherent with each cesarean section, each infant must be examined by a trained professional as soon as possible after delivery.

■ CESAREAN HYSTERECTOMY

A major indication for cesarean hysterectomy is the inability to stop bleeding. The most common reason for performing cesarean hysterectomy is abnormal placental implantation, such as placenta accreta, increta, and percreta. As the cesarean section rate continues to escalate, these complications are becoming more common. Other indications for cesarean hysterectomy include intractable uterine atony, inability to repair a ruptured uterus, and large uterine myomas. Cesarean hysterectomy is a potentially morbid procedure because of increased blood loss and potential for injury to the bladder or ureter.

The technical aspects of hysterectomy at the time of cesarean section are similar to those of hysterectomy in the nonpregnant patient except that all structures, cleavage planes, and pedicles are highly vascular. Therefore, there is significant risk for excessive blood loss and the need for transfusion of blood products. At least 4 units of packed red blood cells should be available. Studies have demonstrated that cesarean hysterectomy performed on a nonemergent basis is much safer than cesarean hysterectomy performed on an emergent basis. Specifically, injury to bladder and ureter and the need for blood transfusions are more common when cesarean hysterectomy is performed emergently.

REFERENCES

American College of Obstetricians and Gynecologists: *Delivery by Vacuum Extraction.* Committee Opinion No. 208. American College of Obstetricians and Gynecologists, September 1998.

American College of Obstetricians and Gynecologists: *Obstetric Forceps.* Committee Opinion No. 71. American College of Obstetricians and Gynecologists, 1989.

American College of Obstetricians and Gynecologists: *Operative Vaginal Delivery.* Technical Bulletin No. 196. American College of Obstetricians and Gynecologists, 1994.

American College of Obstetricians and Gynecologists: *Task Force on Cesarean Delivery Rates: Evaluation of Cesarean Delivery.* American College of Obstetricians and Gynecologists, 2000.

American College of Obstetricians and Gynecologists: *Vaginal Birth after Previous Cesarean Delivery.* Practice Bulletin No. 54. American College of Obstetricians and Gynecologists, 2004.

Bofill JA et al: A randomized prospective trial of the obstetric forceps versus the M-cup vacuum extractor. Am J Obstet Gynecol 1996;175:1325.

Bofill JA et al: Forceps and vacuum delivery: A survey of North American residency programs. Obstet Gynecol 1996;88:622.

Bofill JA et al: Shoulder dystocia and operative vaginal delivery. J Matern Fetal Med 1997;6:220.

Broekhuizen FF et al: Vacuum extraction versus forceps deliveries: Indications and complications. 1979–1984. Obstet Gynecol 1987;69:338.

Caughey AB, et al. Forceps compared with vacuum: rates of neonatal and maternal morbidity. Obstet Gynecol 2005; 106:908.

Chalmers JA, Chalmers I: The obstetric vacuum extractor is the instrument of first choice for operative vaginal delivery. Br J Obstet Gynaecol 1989;96:505.

Dell DL, Sighler SE, Plauche WC: Soft cup vacuum extraction: A comparison of outlet delivery. Obstet Gynecol 1985; 66:624.

Fall O et al: Forceps or vacuum extraction? A comparison of effects on the newborn infant. Acta Obstet Scand 1986;65:75.

Flamm BL: Once a cesarean, always a controversy. Obstet Gynecol 1997;90:312.

Hagadorn-Freathy AS, Yeomans ER, Hankins GDV: Validation of the 1988 ACOG forceps classification system. Obstet Gynecol 1991;77:356.

Hankins GDV, Rowe TF: Operative vaginal delivery—Year 2000. Am J Obstet Gynecol 1996;175:275.

Johnson JH, et al. Immediate maternal and neonatal effects of forceps and vacuum-assisted deliveries. Obstet Gynecol 2004; 103:513.

Lydon-Rochelle M et al: Risk of uterine rupture during labor among women with a prior cesarean delivery. N Engl J Med 2001;345:3.

Miksovsky P, Watson WJ: Obstetric vacuum extraction: State of the art in the new millennium. Obstet Gynecol Surv 2001; 56:736.

Miller DA, Diaz FG, Paul RH: Vaginal birth after cesarean: A 10-year experience. Obstet Gynecol 1994;84:255.

Nygaard I, et al. Should all women be offered elective cesarean delivery? Obstet Gynecol 2003;102:217.

Paul RH, Miller DA: Cesarean birth: How to reduce the rate. Am J Obstet Gynecol 1995;172:1903.

Plauche WC: Subgaleal hematoma—A complication of instrumental delivery. JAMA 1980;244:1597.

Seago DP et al: Planned cesarean hysterectomy: A preferred alternative to separate operations. Am J Obstet Gynecol 1999; 180:1385.

Towner D et al: Effect of mode of delivery in nulliparous women on neonatal intracranial injury. N Engl J Med 1999; 341:1709.

Vacca A et al: Portsmouth operative delivery trial: A comparison of vacuum extraction and forceps delivery. Br J Obstet Gynaecol 1983;90:1107.

Vacca A: Birth by vacuum extraction: Neonatal outcome. J Paediatr Child Heath 1996;32:204.

Williams MC: Vacuum-assisted delivery. Clin Perinatol 1995;22:933.

Postpartum Hemorrhage & the Abnormal Puerperium

Sarah B.H. Poggi, MD

POSTPARTUM HEMORRHAGE

Definition

Postpartum hemorrhage denotes excessive bleeding (> 500 mL in vaginal delivery) following delivery. Hemorrhage may occur before, during, or after delivery of the placenta. Actual measured blood loss during uncomplicated vaginal deliveries averages 700 mL, and blood loss often may be underestimated. Nevertheless, the criterion of a 500-mL loss is acceptable on historical grounds.

Blood lost during the first 24 hours after delivery is *early postpartum hemorrhage;* blood lost between 24 hours and 6 weeks after delivery is *late postpartum hemorrhage.*

Incidence

The incidence of excessive blood loss following vaginal delivery is 5–8%. Postpartum hemorrhage is the most common cause of excessive blood loss in pregnancy, and most transfusions in pregnant women are performed to replace blood lost after delivery. Hemorrhage is the third leading cause of maternal mortality in the United States and is directly responsible for approximately one-sixth of maternal deaths. In less-developed countries, hemorrhage is among the leading obstetric causes of maternal death.

Morbidity & Mortality

Although any woman may suffer excessive blood loss during delivery, women already compromised by anemia or intercurrent illness are more likely to demonstrate serious deterioration of condition, and anemia and excessive blood loss may predispose to subsequent puerperal infection. Major morbidity associated with transfusion therapy (eg, viral infection, transfusion reactions) is infrequent but is not insignificant. Moreover, other types of treatment for anemia may involve some risk.

Postpartum hypotension may lead to partial or total necrosis of the anterior pituitary gland and cause postpartum panhypopituitarism, or Sheehan's syndrome, which is characterized by failure to lactate, amenorrhea, decreased breast size, loss of pubic and axillary hair, hypothyroidism, and adrenal insufficiency. The condition is rare (< 1 in 10,000 deliveries). A woman who has been hypotensive postpartum and who is actively lactating probably does not have Sheehan's syndrome. Hypotension also can lead to acute renal failure and other organ system injury. In extreme hemorrhage, sterility will result from hysterectomy performed to control intractable postpartum hemorrhage.

Etiology

Causes of postpartum hemorrhage include uterine atony, obstetric lacerations, retained placental tissue, and coagulation defects.

A. UTERINE ATONY

Postpartum bleeding is physiologically controlled by constriction of interlacing myometrial fibers that surround the blood vessels supplying the placental implantation site. Uterine atony exists when the myometrium cannot contract.

Atony is the most common cause of postpartum hemorrhage (50% of cases). Predisposing causes include excessive manipulation of the uterus, general anesthesia (particularly with halogenated compounds), uterine overdistention (twins or polyhydramnios), prolonged labor, grand multiparity, uterine leiomyomas, operative delivery and intrauterine manipulation, oxytocin induction or augmentation of labor, previous hemorrhage in the third stage, uterine infection, extravasation of blood into the myometrium (Couvelaire uterus), and intrinsic myometrial dysfunction.

B. OBSTETRIC LACERATIONS

Excessive bleeding from an episiotomy, lacerations, or both causes approximately 20% of postpartum hemorrhages. Lacerations can involve the uterus, cervix, vagina, or vulva. They usually result from precipitous or uncontrolled delivery or operative delivery of a large infant; however, they may occur after any delivery. Laceration of blood vessels underneath the vaginal or vulvar epithelium results in hematomas. Bleeding is concealed and can be particularly dangerous because it may go unrecognized for several hours and become apparent only when shock occurs.

Episiotomies may cause excessive bleeding if they involve arteries or large varicosities, if the episiotomy is large, or if a delay occurred between episiotomy and delivery or between delivery and repair of the episiotomy.

Persistent bleeding (especially bright red) and a well-contracted, firm uterus suggests bleeding from a laceration or from the episiotomy. When cervical or vaginal lacerations are identified as the source of postpartum hemorrhage, repair is best performed with adequate anesthesia.

Spontaneous rupture of the uterus is rare. Risk factors for this complication include grand multiparity, malpresentation, previous uterine surgery, and oxytocin induction of labor. Rupture of a previous cesarean section scar after vaginal delivery may be an increasingly important cause of postpartum hemorrhage.

C. RETAINED PLACENTAL TISSUE

Retained placental tissue and membranes cause 5–10% of postpartum hemorrhages. Retention of placental tissue in the uterine cavity occurs in placenta accreta, in manual removal of the placenta, in mismanagement of the third stage of labor, and in unrecognized succenturiate placenta.

Ultrasonographic findings of an echogenic uterine mass strongly support a diagnosis of retained placental products. The technique probably is better used in cases of hemorrhage occurring a few hours after delivery or in late postpartum hemorrhage. Transvaginal duplex Doppler imaging also is effective in evaluating these patients. Some evidence indicates that sonohysterography may aid in the diagnosis of residual trophoblastic tissue. If the endometrial cavity appears empty, unnecessary dilatation and curettage may be avoided.

D. COAGULATION DEFECTS

Coagulopathies in pregnancy may be acquired coagulation defects seen in association with several obstetric disorders, including abruptio placentae, excess thromboplastin from a retained dead fetus, amniotic fluid embolism, severe preeclampsia, eclampsia, and sepsis. These coagulopathies may present as hypofibrinogenemia, thrombocytopenia, and disseminated intravascular coagulation. Transfusion of more than 8 U of blood in itself may induce a dilutional coagulopathy.

Von Willebrand's disease, autoimmune thrombocytopenia, and leukemia may occur in pregnant women.

Risk Factors

Prevention of hemorrhage is preferable to even the best treatment. All patients in labor should be evaluated for risk of postpartum hemorrhage. Risk factors include co-

agulopathy, hemorrhage, or blood transfusion during a previous pregnancy; anemia during labor; grand multiparity; multiple gestation; large infant; polyhydramnios; dysfunctional labor; oxytocin induction or augmentation of labor; rapid or tumultuous labor; severe preeclampsia or eclampsia; vaginal delivery after previous cesarean birth; general anesthesia for delivery; and forceps delivery.

Management

A. PREDELIVERY PREPARATION

All obstetric patients should have blood typed and screened on admission. Patients identified as being at risk for postpartum hemorrhage should have their blood typed and cross-matched immediately. The blood should be reserved in the blood bank for 24 hours after delivery. A large-bore intravenous catheter should be securely taped into place after insertion. Delivery room personnel should be alerted to the risk of hemorrhage. Severely anemic patients should be transfused as soon as cross-matched blood is ready.

With concerns associated with blood transfusion, autologous blood donation in obstetric patients at risk for postpartum hemorrhage has been advocated. Despite careful evaluation for risk factors, with the exception of cases of placenta previa, our ability to predict which patients will have hemorrhage and require blood transfusion remains poor; therefore, the cost of such an approach may not be justified.

B. DELIVERY

Following delivery of the infant, the uterus is massaged in a circular or back-and-forth motion until the myometrium becomes firm and well contracted. Excessive and vigorous massage of the uterus before, during, or after delivery of the placenta may interfere with normal contraction of the myometrium and instead of hastening contraction may lead to excessive postpartum blood loss.

C. THIRD STAGE OF NORMAL LABOR; PLACENTAL SEPARATION

The placenta typically separates from the uterus and is delivered within 5 minutes of delivery of the infant. Attempts to speed separation are of no benefit and may cause harm. Spontaneous placental separation is impending if the uterus becomes round and firm, a sudden gush of blood comes from the vagina, the uterus seems to rise in the abdomen, and the umbilical cord moves down out of the vagina.

The placenta then can be removed from the vagina by gentle traction on the umbilical cord. Prior to placental separation, gentle steady traction on the cord combined with upward pressure on the lower uterine segment (Brandt-Andrews maneuver) ensures that the placenta can be removed as soon as separation occurs and provides a means of monitoring the consistency of the uterus. Adherent membranes can be removed by gentle traction with ring forceps. The placenta is inspected for completeness immediately after delivery.

Manual Removal of the Placenta

Opinion is divided about the timing of manual removal of the placenta. In the presence of hemorrhage, it is unreasonable to wait for spontaneous separation, and manual removal of the placenta should be undertaken without delay. In the absence of bleeding, many advocate removal of the placenta 30 minutes after delivery of the infant.

Efforts to promote routine manual removal of the placenta were often made in the past. The rationale includes shortening the third stage of labor, decreasing blood loss, developing experience in manual removal as practice for dealing with placenta accreta, and providing a way to simultaneously explore the uterus. Evidence now indicates that manual removal of the placenta may be a risk factor for postpartum endometritis. These real or potential benefits must be weighed against the discomfort caused to the patient, the risk of infection, and the risk of causing more bleeding by interfering with normal mechanisms of placental separation.

Technique: The uterus is stabilized by grasping the fundus with a hand placed over the abdomen. The other hand traces the course of the umbilical cord through the vagina and cervix into the uterus to palpate the edge of the placenta. The membranes at the placental margin are perforated, and the hand is inserted between the placenta and the uterine wall, palmar side toward the placenta. The hand is then gently swept from side to side and up and down to peel the placenta from its attachments to the uterus. When the placenta has been completely separated from the uterus, it is grasped and pulled from the uterus.

The fetal and maternal sides of the placenta should be inspected to ensure that it has been removed in its entirety. On the fetal surface, incomplete placental removal is manifested as interruption of the vessels on the chorionic plate, usually shown by hemorrhage. On the maternal surface, it is possible to see where cotyledons have been detached. If evidence of incomplete removal is observed, the uterus must be re-explored and any small pieces of adherent placenta removed. The uterus should be massaged until a firm myometrial tone is achieved. Depending on the patient's other risk factors for postpartum endometritis, prophylactic antibiotics can be given at the time of manual removal of the placenta.

Immediate Postpartum Period

Uterotonic agents can be administered as soon as the infant's anterior shoulder is delivered. Recent studies show a significantly lowered incidence of postpartum hemorrhage in patients receiving oxytocin (either low-dose IV or IM) at the time of delivery of the anterior shoulder and controlled cord traction compared to patients receiving IV oxytocin following placental delivery. There was no greater incidence of placental retention. However, populations without ultrasound screening for twins have a potential risk for entrapment of an undiagnosed second twin, and oxytocin should only be given after placental delivery. Routine administration of oxytocics during the third stage reduces the blood loss of delivery and decreases the chances of postpartum hemorrhage by 40%. Oxytocin, 10–20 U/L of isotonic saline, or other intravenous solution by slow intravenous infusion or 10 U intramuscularly can be used. Bolus administration should not be used because large doses (> 5 U) can cause hypotension. Ergot alkaloids (eg, methylergonovine maleate 0.2 mg intramuscularly) also can be routinely used, but they are not more effective than oxytocin and pose more risk because they rarely cause marked hypertension. This occurs most commonly with intravenous administration or when regional anesthesia is used. Ergot alkaloids should not be used in hypertensive women or in women with cardiac disease.

Repair of Lacerations

If bleeding is excessive before placental separation, manual removal of the placenta is indicated. Otherwise, excessive manipulation of the uterus should be avoided.

The vagina and cervix should be carefully inspected immediately after delivery of the placenta, with adequate lighting and assistants available. The episiotomy is quickly repaired after massage has produced a firm, tightly contracted uterus. A pack placed in the vagina above the episiotomy helps to keep the field dry; attaching the free end of the pack to the adjacent drapes reminds the operator to remove it after the repair is completed.

The tendency of bleeding vessels to retract from the laceration site is the reason for 1 of the cardinal principles of repair. Begin the repair above the highest extent of the laceration. The highest suture is also used to provide gentle traction to bring the laceration site closer to the introitus. Hemostatic ligatures are then placed in the usual manner, and the entire birth canal is carefully inspected to ensure that no additional bleeding sites are present. Extensive inspection also provides time to confirm that prior hemostatic efforts have been effective.

A cervical or vaginal laceration extending into the broad ligament should not be repaired vaginally. Laparotomy with evacuation of the resultant hematoma and hemostatic repair or hysterectomy is required.

Large or expanding hematomas of the vaginal walls require operative management for proper control. The vaginal wall is first exposed by an assistant. If a laceration accompanies the hematoma, the laceration is extended so that the hematoma can be completely evacuated and explored. When the bleeding site is identified, a large hemostatic ligature can be placed well above the site. This ensures hemostasis in the vessel, which is likely to retract when lacerated. The hematoma cavity should be left open to allow drainage of blood and ensure that bleeding will not be concealed if hemostasis cannot be achieved.

If no laceration is present on the vaginal side wall when a hematoma is identified, then an incision must be made over the hematoma to allow treatment to proceed as outlined.

Following delivery, recovery room attendants should frequently massage the uterus and check for vaginal bleeding.

Evaluation of Persistent Bleeding

If vaginal bleeding persists after delivery of the placenta, aggressive treatment should be initiated. It is not sufficient to perform perfunctory uterine massage, for instance, without searching for the cause of the bleeding and initiating definitive treatment. The following steps should be undertaken without delay:

1. Manually compress the uterus.
2. Obtain assistance.
3. If not already done, obtain blood for typing and cross-matching.
4. Observe blood for clotting to rule out coagulopathy.
5. Begin fluid or blood replacement.
6. Carefully explore the uterine cavity.
7. Completely inspect the cervix and vagina.
8. Insert a second intravenous catheter for administration of blood or fluids.

A. MEASURES TO CONTROL BLEEDING

1. Manual exploration of the uterus—The uterus should be explored immediately in women with postpartum hemorrhage. Manual exploration also should be considered after delivery of the placenta in the following circumstances: (1) when vaginal delivery follows previous cesarean section; (2) when intrauterine manipulation, such as version and extraction, has been performed; (3) when malpresentation has occurred during labor and delivery; (4) when a premature infant has been delivered; (5) when an abnormal uterine contour has been noted prior to delivery; and (6) when there is a possibility of undiagnosed multiple pregnancy—to rule out twins.

Ensure that all placental parts have been delivered and that the uterus is intact. This should be done even in the case of a well-contracted uterus. Exploration performed for reasons other than evaluation of hemorrhage also should confirm that the uterine wall is intact and should attempt to identify any possible intrauterine

structural abnormalities. Manual exploration of the uterus does not increase febrile morbidity or blood loss.

Technique: Place a fresh glove over the glove on the exploring hand. Form the hand into a cone and gently introduce it by firm pressure through the cervix while stabilizing the fundus with the other hand. Sweep the backs of the first and second fingers across the entire surface of the uterus, beginning at the fundus. In the lower uterine segment, palpate the walls with the palmar surface of 1 finger. Uterine lacerations will be felt as an obvious anatomic defect. All exploration should be gentle because the postpartum uterus is easily perforated.

Uterine rupture detected by manual exploration in the presence of postpartum hemorrhage requires immediate laparotomy. A decision to repair the defect or proceed with hysterectomy is made on the basis of the extent of the rupture, the patient's desire for future childbearing, and the degree of the patient's clinical deterioration.

2. Bimanual compression and massage—The most important step in controlling atonic postpartum hemorrhage is immediate bimanual uterine compression, which may have to be continued for 20–30 minutes or more. Fluid replacement should begin as soon as a secure intravenous line is in place. Typed and cross-matched blood is given when it is available. Manual compression of the uterus will control most cases of hemorrhage due to uterine atony, retained products of conception (once the products are removed), and coagulopathies.

Technique: Place a hand on the patient's abdomen and grasp the uterine fundus; bring it down over the symphysis pubis. Insert the other hand into the vagina and place the first and second fingers on either side of the cervix and push it cephalad and anteriorly. The pulsating uterine arteries should be felt by the fingertips. Massage the uterus with both hands while maintaining compression. Prolonged compression (20–30 minutes) may be required but almost always is successful in controlling bleeding.

Insert a Foley catheter into the bladder during compression and massage because vigorous fluid and blood replacement will cause diuresis. A distended bladder will interfere with compression and massage, will contribute to the patient's discomfort, and may itself be a major contributor to uterine atony.

3. Curettage—Curettage of a large, soft postpartum uterus can be a formidable undertaking because the risk of perforation is high and the procedure commonly results in increased rather than decreased bleeding. The suction curette, even with a large cannula, covers only a small area of the postpartum uterus, and its size and shape increase the likelihood of perforation. A large blunt curette, the "banjo" curette, probably is the safest instrument for curettage of the postpartum uterus. It can be used when manual exploration fails to remove fragments of adherent placenta.

Curettage should be delayed unless bleeding cannot be controlled by compression and massage alone. Overly vigorous puerperal curettage can result in focal complete removal of the endometrium, particularly if the uterus is infected, with subsequent healing characterized by formation of adhesions and **Asherman's syndrome** (amenorrhea and secondary sterility due to intrauterine adhesions and uterine synechiae). If circumstances permit, ultrasonic evaluation of the postpartum uterus may distinguish those patients who will benefit from curettage from those who should be managed without it.

4. Uterine packing—Although once widely used for control of obstetric hemorrhage, uterine packing is no longer favored. The uterus may expand to considerable size after delivery of the placenta, thus accommodating both a large volume of packing material and a large volume of blood. The technique also demands considerable technical expertise because the uterus must be packed uniformly with 5 yards of 4-inch gauze, sometimes with the aid of special instrumentation (Torpin packer). However, this method has been used successfully, avoiding conversion to laparotomy in 9 reported cases. As a last resort, uterine packing may be particularly appropriate in centers where an interventional radiologist is not immediately available.

5. Uterotonic agents—Oxytocin 20–40 U/L of crystalloid should be infused, if not already running, at a rate of 10–15 mL/min. Methylergonovine 0.2 mg can be given intramuscularly but is contraindicated if the patient is hypertensive. Intramyometrial injection of prostaglandin $F_{2\alpha}$ ($PGF_{2\alpha}$) to control bleeding was initially described in 1976. Intravaginal or rectal prostaglandin suppositories, intrauterine irrigation with prostaglandins, and intramyometrial injection of prostaglandins also have been reported to control hemorrhage from uterine atony. Intramuscular administration of 15-methylprostaglandin analogue was successful in treating 85% of patients with postpartum hemorrhage due to atony. Failures in these series occurred in women who had uterine infections or unrecognized placenta accreta. Side effects usually are minimal but may include transient oxygen desaturation, bronchospasm, and, rarely, significant hypertension. Transient fever and diarrhea may occur. A recent randomized controlled trial showed excellent efficacy of 800 µg of rectal misoprostol, a prostaglandin E_1 analogue, in the treatment of primary postpartum hemorrhage secondary to atony.

6. Radiographic embolization of pelvic vessels—Embolization of pelvic and uterine vessels by angiographic techniques is increasingly common and has success rates from 85–95% in experienced hands. In institutions with trained interventional radiologists, the technique is worth considering in women of low parity as an alternative to hysterectomy. With the patient under local anesthesia, a catheter is placed in the aorta and fluoroscopy is used to identify the bleeding vessel. Pieces of absorbable gelatin sponge (Gelfoam) are injected into the damaged vessel or into the internal iliac vessels if no specific site of bleeding can be identified. If bleeding continues, further embolization can be performed. This technique has the advantage of being effective even when the cause of hemorrhage is extrauterine and in the presence or absence of uterine atony. Many authors recommend embolization before internal iliac ligation, because ligation obstructs the access route for angiography. Adequate recanalization can occur to maintain fertility, although fertility rates following embolization are not known.

7. Operative management—The patient's wishes regarding further childbearing should be made clear as soon as laparotomy is contemplated for the management of postpartum hemorrhage. If the patient's wishes cannot be ascertained, the operator should assume that the childbearing function is to be retained. Whenever possible, the spouse or family members should also be consulted prior to laparotomy.

a. Pressure occlusion of the aorta—Immediate temporary control of pelvic bleeding may be obtained at laparotomy by pressure occlusion of the aorta, which will provide valuable time to treat hypotension, obtain experienced assistants, identify the source of bleeding, and plan the operative procedure. In the young and otherwise healthy patient, pressure occlusion can be maintained for several minutes without permanent sequelae.

b. Uterine artery ligation—During pregnancy, 90% of the blood flow to the uterus is supplied by the uterine arteries. Direct ligation of these easily accessible vessels can successfully control hemorrhage in 75–90% of cases, particularly when the bleeding is uterine in origin. Recanalization can occur, and subsequent pregnancies have been reported.

Technique: The uterus is lifted upward and away from the side to be ligated. Absorbable suture on a large needle is placed around the ascending uterine artery and vein on 1 side of the uterus, passing through the myometrium 2–4 cm medial to the vessels and through the avascular area of the broad ligament. The suture includes the myometrium to fix the suture and to avoid tearing the vessels. The same procedure is then performed on the opposite side. If the ligation is performed during cesarean section, the sutures can be placed just below the uterine incision under the bladder flap. It is not necessary to mobilize the bladder otherwise. Bilateral uteroovarian artery ligation can also be performed in an attempt to reduce blood flow to the uterus. This technique should be performed with absorbable suture near the point of anastomoses between

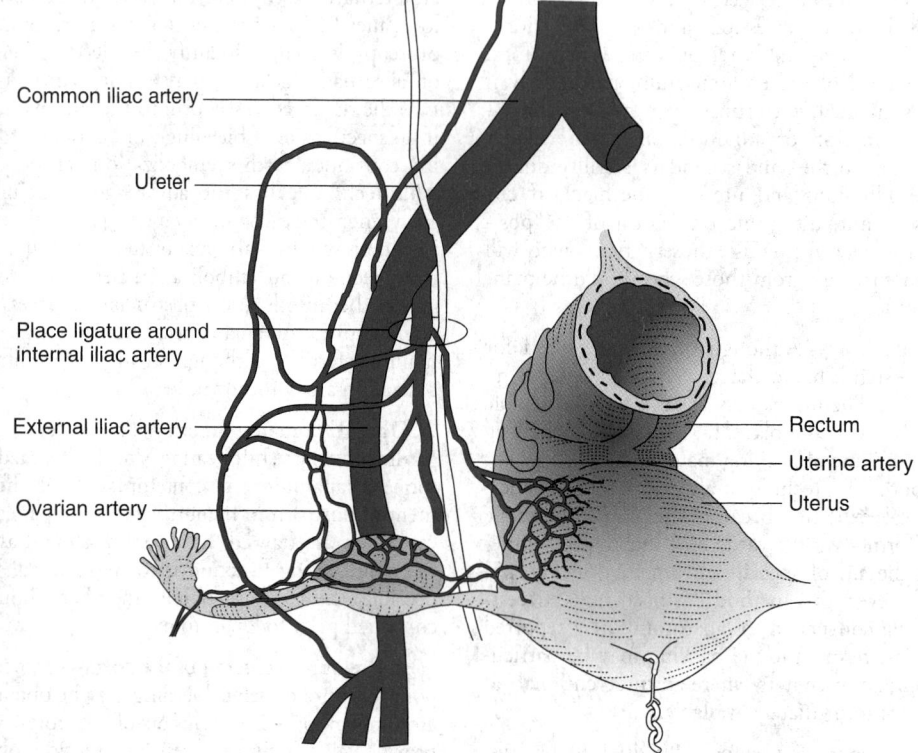

Figure 31–1. Location of ligatures for right internal iliac (hypogastric) artery ligation.

the ovarian artery and the ascending uterine artery at the uteroovarian ligament.

c. Internal iliac artery ligation—Bilateral internal iliac (hypogastric) artery ligation is the surgical method most often used to control severe postpartum bleeding (Fig 31–1). Exposure can be difficult, particularly in the presence of a large boggy uterus or hematoma. Failure rates of this technique can be as high as 57% but may be related to the skill of the operator, the cause of the hemorrhage, and the patient's condition before ligation is attempted.

Technique: The peritoneum lateral to the infundibulopelvic ligament is incised parallel with the ligament, or the round ligament is transected. In either case, the peritoneum to which the ureter will adhere is dissected medially, which removes the ureter from the operative field. The pararectal space is then enlarged by blunt dissection. The internal iliac artery on the lateral side of the space is isolated and doubly ligated (but not cut) with silk ligatures at its origin from the common iliac artery. The operator must be careful not to tear the adjacent thin veins. Blood flow distally to the uterus, cervix, and upper vagina is not occluded, but the pulse pressure is sufficiently diminished to allow hemostasis

to occur by in situ thrombosis. Fertility is preserved, and subsequent pregnancies are not compromised.

d. B-Lynch brace suture—An alternative to the vessel ligation techniques is placement of a brace suture to compress the uterus in cases of diffuse bleeding from atony or percreta (Fig 31–2). A small case series shows success and avoidance of hysterectomy using this novel approach.

Technique: Laparotomy is made in the standard way for cesarean section, and a low-transverse uterine incision is made after the bladder is taken down. The uterus is exteriorized. To test the effectiveness of the method, the uterus is compressed manually and another operator checks the vagina for decreased bleeding. Using no. 2 catgut, the uterus is punctured 3 cm from the right lower incision and 3 cm from the right lateral border. The suture is threaded to emerge 3 cm above the upper incision margin and 4 cm from the lateral border. The catgut is now visible anteriorly as it is passed over to compress the uterine fundus approximately 34 cm from the right cornual border. The suture is fed posteriorly and vertically to enter the posterior wall of the uterine cavity at the same level as the previous entry point. After manual compression, the su-

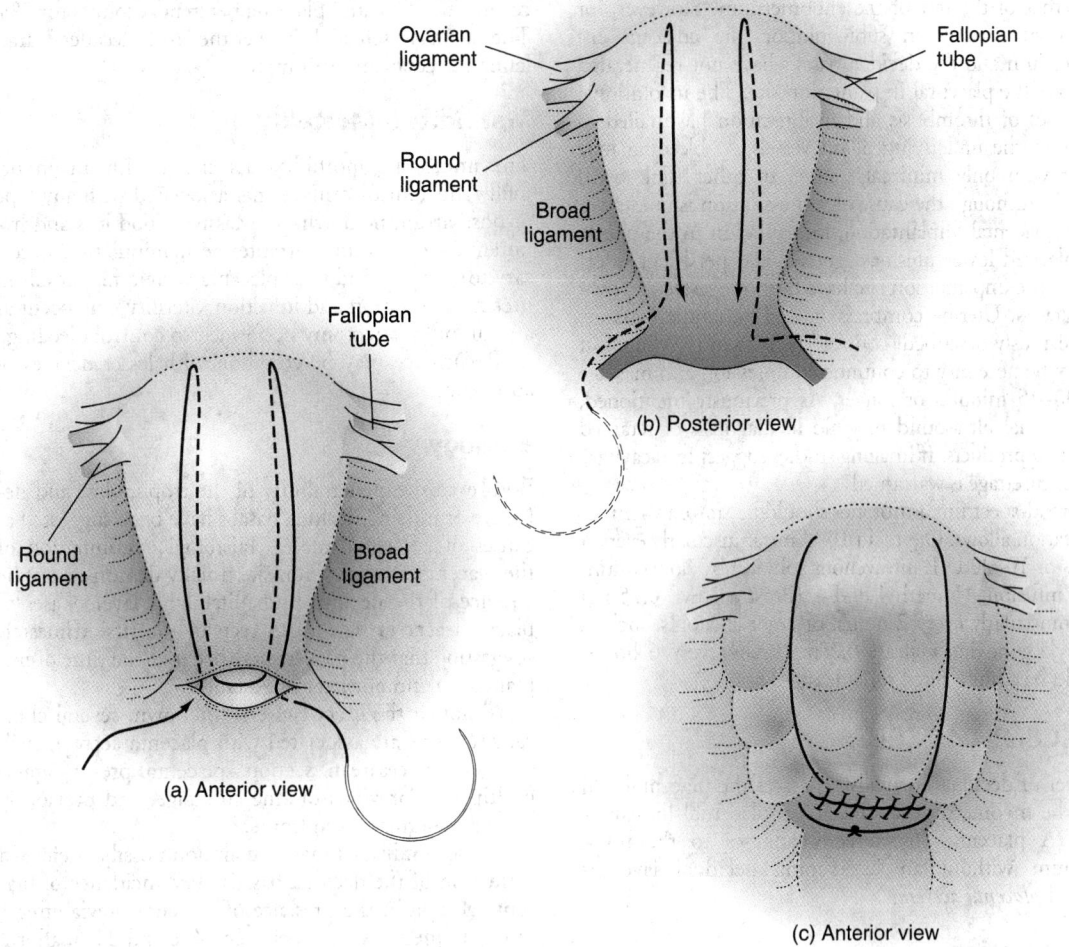

Figure 31–2. B-Lynch brace suture (see text for details).

ture is tightened and then passed posteriorly on the left side and passed around the uterine fundus again, this time on the left. The suture is brought anteriorly to puncture the uterus at the upper part of the left uterine incision and then reemerge below the lower incision in a symmetric fashion. With 1 operator providing compression, the other throws the knot. The hysterotomy is closed in the standard fashion for a cesarean section.

c. Hysterectomy—Hysterectomy is the definitive method of controlling postpartum hemorrhage. Simple hemostatic repair of a ruptured uterus with or without tubal ligation in a woman of high parity or in poor condition for more extensive surgery may be preferred unless she has intercurrent uterine disease. The procedure is undoubtedly lifesaving.

8. Blood replacement—Blood and fluid replacement are required for successful management of postpartum hemorrhage. Massive transfusions may be necessary in patients with severe hemorrhage. Component therapy is advocated, with transfusion of packed cells, platelets, fresh-frozen plasma, and cryoprecipitate when indicated. Blood products should be obtained and given without delay when needed, because postponing transfusion may only contribute to the development of disseminated intravascular coagulation.

B. MANAGEMENT OF DELAYED POSTPARTUM HEMORRHAGE

Delayed postpartum hemorrhage (bleeding ≥ 2 weeks after delivery) is almost always due to subinvolution of the placental bed or retained placental fragments. Involution of the placental site is normally delayed when compared with that of the rest of the endometrium. However, for unknown reasons, in subinvolution the adjacent endometrium and the decidua basalis have not regenerated to cover the placental implantation site. The involutional processes of thrombosis and hyalinization have failed to occur in the underlying blood vessels, so bleeding may occur with only minimal trauma or other (unknown) stimuli. Although the cause of subinvolution is unknown, faulty placental implantation, implantation in the poorly vascularized lower uterine segment, and persistent infection at the implantation site have been suggested as possible factors. Uterine compression and bimanual massage, as previously described, control this type of bleeding, but it may be necessary to continue compression and massage for 30–45 minutes or longer. As previously mentioned, transvaginal ultrasound may aid in diagnosis of retained placental products. If imaging studies suggest intracavitary tissue, curettage is warranted.

Broad-spectrum antibiotics should be started when resuscitation allows. Oxytocin 10 U intramuscularly every 4 hours or 10–20 U/L intravenous solution by slow continuous infusion, 15-methyl $PGF_{2\alpha}$ (Prostin 15M) 0.25 mg intramuscularly every 2 hours, or ergot alkaloids, such as methylergonovine maleate 0.2 mg orally every 6 hours, should be administered for at least 48 hours.

PLACENTA ACCRETA

A layer of decidua normally separates the placental villi and the myometrium at the site of placental implantation. A placenta that directly adheres to the myometrium without an intervening decidual layer is termed *placenta accreta*.

Classification

A. BY DEGREE OF ADHERENCE

1. Placenta accreta vera—Villi adhere to the superficial myometrium.

2. Placenta increta—Villi invade the myometrium.

3. Placenta percreta—Villi penetrate the full thickness of the myometrium.

B. BY AMOUNT OF PLACENTAL INVOLVEMENT

1. Focal adherence—A single cotyledon is involved.

2. Partial adherence—One or several cotyledons are involved.

3. Total adherence—The entire placenta is involved.

Incidence

Estimates of the incidence of placenta accreta (all forms) vary from 1 in 2000 to 1 in 7000 deliveries. Placenta accreta vera accounts for approximately 80% of abnormally adherent placentas, placenta increta accounts for 15%, and placenta percreta accounts for 5%. The rate has risen slightly over the last 2 decades, paralleling the cesarean section rate.

Morbidity & Mortality

The immediate morbidity associated with an abnormally adherent placenta is that associated with any type of postpartum hemorrhage. Massive blood loss and hypotension can occur. Intrauterine manipulation necessary to diagnose and treat placenta accreta may result in uterine perforation and infection. Sterility may occur as a result of hysterectomy performed to control bleeding.

Recurrence may be common with lesser degrees of adherence.

Etiology

Both excessive penetrability of the trophoblast and defective or missing decidua basalis have been suggested as causes of placenta accreta. Histologic examination of the placental implantation site usually demonstrates the absence of the decidua and Nitabuch's layer. Cases of placenta accreta have been seen in the first trimester, suggesting that the process may occur at the time of implantation and not later in gestation.

Although the exact cause is unknown, several clinical situations are associated with placenta accreta, such as previous cesarean section, placenta previa, grand multiparity, previous uterine curettage, and previously treated Asherman's syndrome.

These conditions share a common possible defect in formation of the decidua basalis. The incidence of placenta accreta in the presence of placenta previa after 1 prior uterine incision is between 14% and 24%, after 2 is 23–48%, and after 3 is 35–50%. The incidence of placenta accreta after successful treatment of Asherman's syndrome may be as high as 15%.

Diagnosis

Adverse effects from placenta accreta in pregnancy or during the course of labor and delivery are uncommon. Rarely, intra-abdominal hemorrhage or placental invasion of adjacent organs prior to labor has occurred, with the diagnosis made at laparotomy.

The diagnosis of placenta increta prior to delivery based on the lack of the sonolucent area normally seen beneath the implantation site during ultrasonographic examination is a finding confirmed in several reports. Sonographic antenatal diagnosis of the less invasive placental accreta also has been reported. Color Doppler imaging appears to be particularly helpful in diagnosis. Magnetic resonance imaging has also aided in the diagnosis of placenta accreta. The diagnosis is more often established when no plane of cleavage is found between the placenta or parts of the placenta and the myometrium in the presence of postpartum hemorrhage. Retained placental parts prevent the myometrium from contracting and thereby achieving hemostasis. Bleeding can be brisk. Inspection of the already separated placenta shows that portions are missing, and manual exploration may produce additional placental fragments.

Delayed spontaneous separation of the placenta is also an indication of an unusually adherent placenta. Focal or partial involvement may be manifested as difficulty in establishing a cleavage plane during manual removal of the placenta. Removal of a totally adherent placenta is difficult. Persistent efforts to manually remove a totally adherent placenta are futile and waste time, and they result in even more blood loss. Preparation for hysterectomy should begin as soon as the diagnosis is suspected.

Management

Fluid and blood replacement should begin as soon as excessive blood loss is diagnosed. Insertion of a second large-bore intravenous catheter may be necessary. Evaluation of puerperal hemorrhage should be performed as outlined in Evaluation of Persistent Bleeding.

Conservative treatment of placenta accreta in women of low parity has occasionally succeeded. The placenta (or portions of it) is left in situ if bleeding is minimal and will later slough off. Successful subsequent pregnancies have been reported, although the risk of recurrence of placenta accreta may be high. In up to 72% of cases of placenta accreta, particularly those associated with placenta previa, hysterectomy is required.

Successful conservative treatment of placenta percreta is rare, but the conservative approach may be a reasonable option if only focal defects are present, blood loss is not excessive, and the patient wishes to preserve fertility. In anticipated cases of severe placenta accreta, preoperative balloon occlusion and embolization of the internal iliac arteries may minimize intraoperative blood losses. Successful embolization in unpredicted cases of placenta accreta has been reported. However, additional resection of adjacent organs, such as partial cystectomy, may be necessary in placenta percreta.

UTERINE INVERSION

Definition

Uterine inversion is prolapse of the fundus to or through the cervix so that the uterus is in effect turned inside out. Almost all cases of uterine inversion occur after delivery and may be worsened by excess traction on the cord before placental separation. Nonpuerperal uterine inversion is rare and usually is associated with tumors (eg, polypoid leiomyomas).

Classification

If the uterus is inverted but does not protrude through the cervix, the inversion is *incomplete*. In *complete* inversion, the fundus has prolapsed through the cervix. Occasionally, the entire uterus may prolapse out of the vagina.

Puerperal inversion has also been classified on the basis of its duration. Acute inversion occurs immediately after delivery and before the cervix constricts. Once the cervix constricts, the inversion is termed *subacute*. Chronic inversion is noted more than 4 weeks after delivery. Today, nearly all cases of uterine inversion are of the acute variety and are recognized and treated immediately after delivery.

Incidence

In series reported within the past 30 years, the incidence of uterine inversion has varied from 1 in 4000 to 1 in 100,000 deliveries; an incidence of 1 in 20,000 is frequently cited. One worker reported no inversions in more than 10,000 personally conducted deliveries. More recent reviews indicate a greater incidence of uterine inversion, approximately 1 in 2000 to 1 in 2500 deliveries.

Morbidity & Mortality

The morbidity and mortality associated with uterine inversion correlate with the degree of hemorrhage, the rapidity of diagnosis, and the effectiveness of treatment.

The immediate morbidity is that associated with any postpartum hemorrhage; however, endomyometritis frequently follows uterine inversion. The intestines and uterine appendages may be injured if they are entrapped by the prolapsed uterine fundus. Death has occurred from uterine inversion, although with prompt recognition, definitive treatment, and vigorous resuscitation, the mortality rate in this condition should be quite low.

Etiology

The exact cause of uterine inversion is unknown, and the condition is not always preventable. The cervix must be dilated and the uterine fundus must be relaxed for inversion to occur. Rapid uterine emptying may contribute to uterine relaxation.

Conditions that may predispose women to uterine inversion include fundal implantation of the placenta, abnormal adherence of the placenta (partial placenta accreta), congenital or acquired weakness of the myometrium, uterine anomalies, protracted labor, previous uterine inversion, intrapartum therapy with magnesium sulfate, strong traction exerted on the umbilical cord, and fundal pressure.

Many cases of uterine inversion result from mismanagement of the third stage of labor in women who already are at risk for developing uterine inversion. The following maneuvers are to be avoided: excessive traction on the umbilical cord, excessive fundal pressure, excessive intra-abdominal pressure, and excessively vigorous manual removal of the placenta.

Diagnosis

The diagnosis of uterine inversion usually is obvious. Shock and hemorrhage are prominent, as is considerable pain. A dark red–blue bleeding mass is palpable and often visible at the cervix, in the vagina, or outside the vagina. A depression in the uterine fundus or even an absent fundus is noted on abdominal examination. Partial inversion in which the fundus stays within the vagina can escape immediate notice if the attendant is not aware of this complication.

Treatment

Successful management of patients with uterine inversion depends on prompt recognition and treatment. If initial measures fail to relieve the condition, it may progress to the point at which operative treatment or even hysterectomy is necessary. Shock associated with uterine inversion typically is profound. Hemorrhage can be massive, and hypovolemia should be vigorously treated with fluid and blood replacement.

A. MANUAL REPOSITIONING OF THE UTERUS

Treatment should begin as soon as the diagnosis of uterine inversion is made. Assistance is vital. An initial attempt should be made to reposition the fundus. The inverted fundus, along with the placenta if it is still attached, is slowly and steadily pushed upward in the axis of the uterus (Fig 31–3). If the placenta has not separated, do not remove it until an adequate intravenous infusion has been established.

If the initial attempt fails, induce general anesthesia, preferably with a halogenated agent (eg, halothane) to provide uterine relaxation. Alternatively, 50 μg of IV nitroglycerin can be given as a bolus to relax the uterus and avoid intubation. The dose can be repeated at least once. While awaiting anesthesiology assistance, easily available tocolytics may be used effectively. Either intravenous magnesium sulfate or terbutaline 0.25 mg given as a bolus dose intravenously has been used successfully to achieve uterine relaxation in subacute inversion, and neither has been associated with bleeding.

Technique: The operator's fist is placed on the uterine fundus, and the fundus is gradually pushed back into the pelvis through the dilated cervix. The general anesthetic or uterine relaxant is discontinued. Infusion of oxytocin or ergot alkaloids is started and fluid and blood replacement continued. Alternatively, prostaglandins can

Figure 31–3. Replacement of an inverted uterus.

be used to effect uterine contraction after repositioning. Bimanual uterine compression and massage are maintained until the uterus is well contracted and hemorrhage has ceased. The placenta can then be removed.

Antibiotics should be started as soon as is practical. Oxytocics or ergot alkaloids are continued for at least 24 hours. Frequent determinations of the hematocrit level should be made to ascertain the need for further blood replacement. Iron supplements should begin with resumption of oral intake.

B. SURGICAL REPOSITIONING OF THE UTERUS

Surgical repositioning of the uterus is rarely necessary in contemporary medical practice in the United States. However, when all other efforts have failed to reposition the everted uterus, operative intervention may be lifesaving. This is generally accomplished by a vertical incision through the lower uterine segment directly posterior. The uterus is repositioned by either pulling from above or, very rarely, pushing from below (using a sterile glove). The incision is then repaired as would be any uterine incision. Blood replacement, antibiotics, and careful monitoring are necessary for successful perioperative management.

■ ABNORMALITIES OF THE PUERPERIUM

When compared with the dramatic and climactic events of delivery, the puerperium may seem uneventful. Nevertheless, significant physiologic changes occur during this interval, and they undoubtedly influence many of the problems that often arise rapidly and without warning. Hypotension and shock demand urgent treatment and careful follow-up. Cardiac monitoring and insertion of Swan-Ganz or central venous pressure catheters may be prudent to permit rapid evaluation of hemodynamic status. Appropriate medical and surgical consultation are also recommended.

POSTPARTUM & PUERPERAL INFECTIONS

Infections are among the most prominent puerperal complications. An improved understanding of the natural history of female genital infections and the availability of powerful antibiotics may have produced a complacent attitude toward puerperal infections that is unrealistic. Postpartum infections still are costly to both patients and society, and they are associated with an admittedly small but not negligible threat of serious disability and death.

Puerperal morbidity due to infection has occurred if the patient's temperature is higher than 38 °C (100.4 °F) on 2 separate occasions at least 24 hours apart following the first 24 hours after delivery. Overt infections can and do occur in the absence of these criteria, but fever of some degree remains the hallmark of puerperal infection, and the patient with fever can be assumed to have a genital infection until proved otherwise.

Incidence

Puerperal infectious morbidity affects 2–8% of pregnant women and is more common in those of low socioeconomic status, who have undergone operative delivery, with premature rupture of the membranes, with long labors, or who have multiple pelvic examinations.

Morbidity & Mortality

Postpartum infections are responsible for much of the morbidity associated with childbirth, and they either are directly responsible for or contribute to the death of approximately 8% of all pregnant women who die each year. The costs are considerable, not only in additional days of hospitalization and medications but also in time lost from work.

Sterility may result from the sequelae of postpartum infections, such as periadnexal adhesions. Hysterectomy occasionally is required in patients with serious postpartum or postoperative infection.

Pathogenesis

The flora of the birth canal of pregnant women is essentially the same as that of nonpregnant women, although variations in culture techniques and in the study populations have produced markedly different results. The vaginal flora typically includes aerobic and anaerobic organisms that are commonly considered pathogenic (Table 31–1). Several mechanisms appear to prevent

Table 31–1. Percentage of organisms isolated from the vagina or cervix in normal pregnant and nonpregnant women.

Organism	Percentage Isolated
Aerobic bacteria	
Lactobacillus	17–97
Diphtheroids	14–83
Staphylococcus epidermidis	7–67
Staphylococcus aureus	0–12
α-Hemolytic streptococci	2–53
β-Hemolytic streptococci	0–93
Nonhemolytic streptococci	4–37
Group D streptococci	4–44
Escherichia coli	0–28
Gardnerella vaginalis	40–43
Neisseria gonorrhoeae	1–7
Mycoplasma	15–72
Ureaplasma	40–95
Anaerobic bacteria	
Lactobacillis	11–72
Bacteroides fragilis	0–20
Bacteroides species	0–50
Fusobacterium species	0–18
Peptococcus species	0–71
Peptostreptococcus species	12–40
Veillonella species	0–27
Clostridium species	0–17
Bifidobacterium species	0–32
Eubacterium species	0–36

overt infection in the genital tract, such as the acidity of the normal vagina; thick, tenacious cervical mucus; and maternal antibodies to most vaginal flora.

During labor and particularly after rupture of the membranes, some of the protective mechanisms are no longer present. Examinations and invasive monitoring apparatus probably facilitate the introduction of vaginal bacteria into the uterine cavity. Bacteria can be cultured from the amniotic fluid of most women undergoing intrauterine pressure monitoring, but overt postpartum infection is seen in fewer than 10% of these cases. Contractions during labor may spread bacteria present in the amniotic cavity to the adjacent uterine lymphatics and even into the bloodstream.

The postpartum uterus initially is devoid of mechanisms that keep it sterile, and bacteria may be recovered from the uterus in nearly all women in the postpartum period. Whether or not disease is clinically expressed depends on the presence of predisposing factors, the duration of uterine contamination, and the type and amount of microorganisms involved. The necrosis of decidua and other intrauterine contents (lochia) promotes an increase in the number of anaerobic bacteria, heretofore limited by lack of suitable nutrients and other factors necessary for growth.

Sterility of the endometrial cavity returns by the third or fourth postpartum week. Granulocytes that penetrate the endometrial cavity and the open drainage of lochia are effective in preventing infection in most patients.

Etiology

Almost all postpartum infections are caused by bacteria normally present in the genitalia of pregnant women. The lochia is an excellent culture medium for organisms ascending from the vagina. In women who have undergone cesarean section, more devitalized tissue and foreign bodies (sutures) are present, providing additional fertile ground for possible contamination and subsequent infection. Approximately 70% of puerperal soft-tissue infections are mixed infections consisting of both aerobic and anaerobic organisms; infections occurring in women undergoing cesarean section are more likely to be serious.

General Evaluation

The source of infection should be identified, the likely cause determined, and the severity assessed. Most women with fever in the postpartum period have endometritis. Urinary tract infection is the next most common infection. Neglected or virulent endomyometritis may progress to more serious infection. Generalized sepsis, septic pelvic thrombophlebitis, or pelvic abscess may be the end result of an initial infection of the endometrial cavity.

1. Endometritis

Etiology

All of the following circumstances have led to higher than normal postpartum infection rates: prolonged rupture of the membranes (> 24 hours), chorioamnionitis, an excessive number of digital vaginal examinations, prolonged labor (> 12 hours), toxemia, intrauterine pressure catheters (> 8 hours), fetal scalp electrode monitoring, preexisting vaginitis or cervicitis, operative vaginal deliveries, cesarean section, intrapartum and postpartum anemia, poor nutrition, obesity, low socioeconomic status, and coitus near term.

Cesarean section and low socioeconomic class are consistently associated with higher rates of postpartum infection, and cesarean section is easily the most common identifiable risk factor for development of puerperal infection. Some series report an infection rate of 40–80% following cesarean section delivery. Postpartum infection is more likely to be serious after cesarean section than after vaginal delivery. A history of bacterial vaginosis confers a higher risk of postcesarean endometritis.

Clinical Findings

A. SYMPTOMS AND SIGNS

Fever and a soft, tender uterus are the most prominent signs of endometritis. The lochia may or may not have a foul odor. Leukocytosis (white blood cell count > 10,000/µL) is seen. In more severe disease, high fever, malaise, abdominal tenderness, ileus, hypotension, and generalized sepsis may be seen. Movement of the uterus causes increased pain.

1. **Fever**—Although the puerperium is a period of high metabolic activity, this factor should not raise the temperature above 37.2 °C (99 °F) and then only briefly in the first 24 hours postpartum. Modest temperature elevations may occur with dehydration. Any woman with a fever over 38 °C (100.4 °F) at any time in the puerperium should be evaluated.

Endometritis results in temperatures ranging from 38 °C to over 40 °C (100.4 °F to > 104 °F), depending on the patient, the causative microorganism, and the extent of infection. The lower range of temperatures is more common. Endometritis usually develops on the second or third postpartum day. Early fever (within hours of delivery) and hypotension are almost pathognomonic for infection with β-hemolytic streptococci.

2. **Uterine tenderness**—The uterus is soft and exquisitely tender. Motion of the cervix and uterus may cause increased pain.

Abdominal tenderness is generally limited to the lower abdomen and does not lateralize. A carefully performed baseline examination should include an adnexal evaluation. Adnexal masses palpable on abdominal or pelvic examination are not seen in uncomplicated endometritis, but tubo-ovarian abscess may be a later complication of an infection originally confined to the uterus. Bowel sounds may be decreased and the abdomen distended and tympanitic.

Pelvic examination confirms the findings disclosed by abdominal examination.

B. LABORATORY FINDINGS

1. Hematologic findings—Leukocytosis is a normal finding during labor and the immediate puerperal period. White blood cell counts may be as high as 20,000/μL in the absence of infection, so higher counts can be anticipated in infection. Bacteremia is present in 5–10% of women with uncomplicated endometritis. *Mycoplasma* is frequently recovered from the blood of patients with postpartum fever. Infections with *Bacteroides* as the predominant organism are frequently associated with positive blood cultures.

2. Urinalysis—Urinalysis should be routinely performed in patients thought to have endometritis because urinary tract infections are often associated with a clinical picture similar to that of mild endometritis. If pyuria and bacteria are noted in a properly collected specimen, appropriate antibiotic therapy for urinary tract infections should be started and a portion of the specimen sent for culture.

3. Lochia cultures—Bacteria colonizing the cervical canal and ectocervix almost always can be recovered from lochia cultures, but they may not be the same organisms causing endometritis. Accurate cultures can be achieved only if specimens obtained transcervically are free from vaginal contamination. Material should be obtained using a speculum to allow direct visualization of the cervix and a gloved culture device (a swab that is covered while it is passed through a contaminated area, then uncovered to obtain a culture from the desired area). Transabdominal aspiration of uterine contents does secure an uncontaminated specimen, but routine use of this technique probably is not justified, and confirmation of placement within the uterine cavity may be difficult. Unless special means are taken to prevent cervical contamination and to ensure the recovery of anaerobic species, results of lochia cultures must be interpreted with great care.

4. Bacteriologic findings—Although the organisms responsible for puerperal infections vary considerably among hospitals, most puerperal infections are due to anaerobic streptococci, gram-negative coliforms, *Bacteroides* spp., and aerobic streptococci. *Chlamydia* and *Mycoplasma* are also implicated in many postpartum infections, but clinical isolates are rare because of the difficulty in culturing these organisms. Gonococci are recovered in vary-

Table 31–2. Percentage of organisms recovered from women with postpartum endomyometritis.

Organism	Percentage Isolated
Aerobic bacteria	
Group A streptococci	2–6
Group B streptococci	6–21
Group D streptococci	3–14
Enterococcus	12–21
Other streptococci	32
Staphylococcus epidermidis	28
Staphylococcus aureus	10
Escherichia coli	13–36
Gonococci	1–40
Gardnerella vaginalis	16
Anaerobic bacteria	
Bacteriodes fragilis	19–75
Bacteroides species	17–100
Peptococcus	4–40
Peptostreptococcus	15–54
Veillonella species	10
Clostridium species	4–32

ing degrees. The percentage of representative microorganisms recovered from women with endometritis is given in Table 31–2.

Patterns of bacterial isolates in puerperal infections in the patient's hospital are more important in guiding selection of appropriate antibiotics than are studies from the literature.

a. Aerobic bacteria—Group A streptococci are no longer a major cause of postpartum infection, but infection with these organisms still occurs occasionally. If more than an isolated instance of infection due to these streptococci occurs, immediate measures should be taken to halt a potential epidemic. Penicillin is highly effective.

In as many as 30% of women with clinically recognized endometritis, group B streptococci are partly or wholly responsible for the infection. Classic presenting signs are high fever and hypotension shortly after delivery. However, group B streptococci are commonly recovered from the vaginas of pregnant women whether or not they have endometritis. Why some women with positive cultures develop serious illness whereas others do not undoubtedly depends on the presence of predisposing factors as well as other, as yet unknown, elements. It is interesting that positive cultures in women do not correlate well with the incidence of streptococcal infection in their newborns. Penicillin is the treatment of choice for patients with endometritis.

Group D streptococci, which include *Streptococcus faecalis,* are common isolates in endometritis. Ampicillin in high doses is the treatment of choice. Aminoglycosides are also effective against this group.

Staphylococcus aureus is not commonly seen in cultures from women with postpartum infections of the uterus. *Staphylococcus epidermidis* is frequently recovered from women with postpartum infections. These organisms are typically not seen in pure culture. When established staphylococcal infections require treatment, nafcillin, cloxacillin, or cephalosporins should be used.

Among the gram-negative aerobic organisms likely to be recovered in postpartum uterine infections, *Escherichia coli* is the most common. In postpartum uterine infections, *E coli* is more likely to be isolated from seriously ill patients, whereas in urinary tract infections, it is the most commonly isolated organism but is not necessarily found in the sickest patients. Hospital-acquired *E coli* is most susceptible to aminoglycosides and cephalosporins.

The incidence of *Neisseria gonorrhoeae* is 2–8% in pregnant women antepartum. Unless repeat screening examinations and treatment of patients with positive cultures are undertaken in women near term, the incidence of asymptomatic endocervical gonorrhea at delivery probably is only slightly less, and it is reasonable to believe that some cases of puerperal endometritis are gonococcal in origin.

Gardnerella vaginalis, a cause of vaginitis, is seen in isolates from women with postpartum infections, usually in those with a polymicrobial cause, although pure isolates have been reported.

Other gram-negative bacilli that are commonly encountered on medical and surgical wards (eg, *Klebsiella pneumoniae, Enterobacter, Proteus,* and *Pseudomonas* spp.) are uncommon causes of endometritis.

b. Anaerobic bacteria—Anaerobic bacteria are involved in puerperal infections of the uterus in at least 50% and perhaps as many as 95% of cases. They are much less commonly seen in urinary tract infections. Anaerobic Peptostreptococci and Peptococci are commonly recovered in specimens from women with postpartum infection, particularly with other anaerobic species. Clindamycin, chloramphenicol, and the newer cephalosporins are active against these organisms.

Bacteroides spp., particularly *Bacteroides fragilis,* are commonly found in mixed puerperal infections. These are likely to be the more serious infections (eg, puerperal pelvic abscess, cesarean section wound infections, and septic pelvic thrombophlebitis). When infection with this organism is suspected or confirmed, clindamycin, chloramphenicol, or third-generation cephalosporins should be used.

Gram-positive anaerobic organisms are represented only by *Clostridium perfringens,* which is not infrequently isolated from an infected uterus but which is a rare cause of puerperal infection.

c. Other organisms—*Mycoplasma* and *Ureaplasma* spp. are common genital pathogens that have been isolated from the genital tract and blood of postpartum women both with and without overt infection. These pathogens are frequently found in the presence of other bacteria. The role of these organisms in puerperal infections is unknown.

Chlamydia trachomatis is now thought to be the leading cause of pelvic inflammatory disease in some populations. Because the population most at risk for pelvic inflammatory disease is the same as that most likely to become pregnant, it is not surprising that *Chlamydia* is in some way involved in puerperal infections, but it is infrequently isolated as a cause of early postpartum endometritis. *Chlamydia* is more frequently associated with mild late-onset endometritis, so cultures for this organism should be obtained from patients with endometritis diagnosed several days after delivery. *Chlamydia* is difficult to culture, and it is possible that as more effective culture techniques become available, the place of this organism in the morbidity associated with postpartum infections will be clarified.

Differential Diagnosis

In the immediate postpartum period, involuntary chills are common and are not necessarily an indication of overt infection. Lower abdominal pain is common as the uterus undergoes involution with continuing contractions.

Extragenital infections are much less common than endometritis and urinary tract infections. Most of these infections can be effectively ruled out by history and examination alone. Patients should be asked, at a minimum, about coughing, chest pain, pain at the insertion site of intravenous catheters, breast tenderness, and leg pain. Examination of the breasts, chest, intravenous catheter insertion site, and leg veins should determine whether these areas might be the source of the postpartum fever. Chest x-ray films are rarely of benefit unless signs and symptoms point to a possible pulmonary cause of the fever.

Treatment

The choice of antibiotics for treatment of endometritis depends on the suspected causative organisms and the severity of the disease. If the illness is serious enough to require antibiotics, initial therapy should consist of intravenous antibiotics in high doses. Factors reinforcing the need for this approach include the large volume of the uterus, the expanded maternal blood volume, the brisk diuresis associated with the puerperium, and the difficulty in achieving adequate tissue concentrations of the antibiotic distal to the thrombosed myometrial blood vessels. Clindamycin plus an aminoglycoside is a standard first-line regimen. Good evidence now indicates that once-a-day dosing of gentamicin is as effective as the traditional thrice-daily regimen. Single-agent therapy with second- or third-generation cephalosporins is an acceptable alternative.

The response to therapy should be carefully monitored for 24–48 hours. Deterioration or failure to respond determined both clinically and by laboratory test results requires a complete re-evaluation. Ampicillin is added when the patient has a less than adequate response to the usual regimen, particularly if *Enterococcus* spp. are suspected.

Intravenous antibiotics are continued until the patient has been afebrile for 24–48 hours. Randomized and prospective trials have shown that additional treatment with oral antibiotics after intravenous therapy is unnecessary. Patients with documented concurrent bacteremia can be treated similarly, unless they have persistently positive blood cultures or a staphylococcal species cultured. If the patient remains febrile despite the standard antibiotic regimens, further evaluation should be initiated to look for abscess formation, hematomas, wound infection, and septic pelvic thrombophlebitis.

For patients known to be infected or at extremely high risk for infection at the time of delivery, initial therapy with 2- or 3-drug regimens in which 1 of the agents is clindamycin is prudent. Single-agent intravenous infusion of broad-spectrum agents such as piperacillin or cefoxitin appears to be equally effective.

2. Urinary Tract Infection

Approximately 2–4% of women develop a urinary tract infection postpartum. Following delivery, the bladder and lower urinary tract remain somewhat hypotonic, and residual urine and reflux result. This altered physiologic state, in conjunction with catheterization, birth trauma, conduction anesthesia, frequent pelvic examinations, and nearly continuous contamination of the perineum, is sufficient to explain the high incidence of lower urinary tract infections postpartum. In many women, preexisting asymptomatic bacteria, chronic urinary tract infections, and anatomic disorders of the bladder, urethra, and kidneys contribute to urinary tract infection postpartum.

Clinical Findings

A. SYMPTOMS AND SIGNS

Urinary tract infection usually presents with dysuria, frequency, urgency, and low-grade fever; however, an elevated temperature is occasionally the only symptom. White blood cells and bacteria are seen in a centrifuged sample of catheterized urine. A urine culture should be obtained. The history should be reviewed for evidence of chronic antepartum infections. If a woman had an antepartum urinary tract infection, then her postpartum infection likely is caused by the same organism. Repeated urinary tract infections call for careful postpartum evaluation. Urethral diverticulum, kidney stones, and upper urinary tract anomalies should be ruled out.

Urinary retention postpartum in the absence of regional anesthesia or well after its effects have worn off almost always indicates urinary tract infection.

Pyelonephritis may be accompanied by fever, chills, malaise, and nausea and vomiting. Characteristic signs of kidney involvement associated with pyelonephritis include costovertebral angle tenderness, dysuria, pyuria, and, in the case of hemorrhagic cystitis, hematuria.

B. LABORATORY FINDINGS

E coli is easily the most common organism isolated from infected urine in postpartum women (approximately 75% of cases). Other gram-negative bacilli are much less likely to be recovered. *E coli* is less likely to be the causative organism in women who had repeated urinary tract infections in the recent past.

Treatment

Antibiotics with specific activity against the causative organism are the cornerstone of therapy in uncomplicated cystitis. These drugs include sulfonamides, nitrofurantoin, trimethoprim-sulfamethoxazole, oral cephalosporins (cephalexin, cephradine), and ampicillin. Some hospitals report a high incidence of microbial resistance to ampicillin. The oral combination of amoxicillin-clavulanic acid provides a better spectrum of bacterial sensitivity. Sulfa antibiotics can be used safely in women who are breastfeeding if the infants are term without hyperbilirubinemia or suspected glucose-6-phosphate dehydrogenase deficiency. High fluid intake should be encouraged.

Pyelonephritis requires initial therapy with high doses of intravenous antibiotics, such as ampicillin 8–12 g/d or first-generation cephalosporins (cefazolin 3–6 g/d, cephalothin 4–8 g/d). An aminoglycoside can be added when resistant organisms are suspected or when the patient has clinical signs of sepsis. A long-acting third-generation cephalosporin, such as ceftriaxone 1–2 g every 12 hours, also can be used. The response to therapy may be rapid, but some women respond with gradual defervescence over 48 hours or longer. Urine cultures should be obtained to guide any necessary modifications in drug therapy if the patient's response is not prompt. Even with prompt resolution of fever, antibiotic therapy should be continued intravenously or orally for a total of 10 days. Urine for culture should be obtained at a postpartum visit after therapy has been completed.

3. Pneumonia

Women with obstructive lung disease, smokers, and those undergoing general anesthesia have an increased risk for developing pneumonia postpartum.

Clinical Findings

A. SYMPTOMS AND SIGNS

Symptoms and signs are the same as those of pneumonia in nonpregnant patients: productive cough, chest pain, fever, chills, rales, and infiltrates on chest x-ray film. In some cases, careful differentiation from pulmonary embolus is required.

B. X-RAY AND LABORATORY FINDINGS

Chest x-ray film confirms the diagnosis of pneumonia. Gram-stained smears of sputum and material for culture should be obtained.

Streptococcus pneumoniae and *Mycoplasma pneumoniae* are the 2 most likely causative organisms. *S pneumoniae* can easily be identified on gram-stained smears. Infection with *M pneumoniae* can be suspected on clinical grounds.

Treatment

Appropriate antibiotics, oxygen (if the patient is hypoxic), intravenous hydration, and pulmonary toilet are the mainstays of therapy.

4. Cesarean Section Wound Infection

Incidence

Wound infection occurs in 4–12% of patients following cesarean section.

Etiology

The following risk factors predispose to subsequent wound infection in women undergoing cesarean section: obesity, diabetes, prolonged hospitalization before cesarean section, prolonged rupture of the membranes, chorioamnionitis, endomyometritis, prolonged labor, emergency rather than elective indications for cesarean section, and anemia.

Clinical Findings

A. SYMPTOMS AND SIGNS

Fever with no apparent cause that persists to the fourth or fifth postoperative day strongly suggests a wound infection. Wound erythema and tenderness may not be evident until several days after surgery. Occasionally, wound infections are manifested by spontaneous drain-age, often accompanied by resolution of fever and relief of local tenderness. Rarely, a deep-seated wound infection becomes apparent when the skin overtly separates, usually after some strenuous activity by the patient.

B. LABORATORY FINDINGS

Gram-stained smears and culture of material from the wound may be helpful in guiding selection of the initial antibiotic. Blood cultures may be positive in the patient with systemic sepsis due to wound infection. The organisms responsible for most wound infections originate on the patient's skin. *S aureus* is the organism most commonly isolated. *Streptococcus* species, *E coli,* and other gram-negative organisms that may originally have colonized the amniotic cavity are also seen. Occasionally, *Bacteroides,* which comes only from the genital tract, is isolated from material taken from serious wound infections.

Rarely, necrotizing fasciitis and the closely related synergistic bacterial gangrene can involve cesarean section incisions. They are recognized by their intense tissue destruction, lack of sensation in the involved tissues, and rapid extension. Radical debridement of necrotic and infected tissue is the cornerstone of treatment.

Treatment

A. INITIAL EVALUATION

The incision should be opened along its entire length and the deeper portion of the wound gently explored to determine whether fascial separation has occurred. If the fascia is not intact, the wound is dissected to the fascial level, debrided, and repaired. Wound dehiscence has a high mortality rate and should be treated aggressively. Dehiscence is uncommon in healthy patients and with Pfannenstiel incisions. The skin can be left open to undergo delayed closure or to heal by primary intention.

If the fascia is intact, the wound infection can be treated by local measures.

B. DEFINITIVE MEASURES

Mechanical cleansing of the wound is the mainstay of therapy for cesarean wound infection. Opening the wound encourages drainage of infected material. The wound can be packed with saline-soaked gauze 2–3 times per day, which will remove necrotic debris each time the wound is unpacked. The wound can be left open to heal, or it can be closed secondarily when granulation tissue has begun to form.

Antibiotic Prophylaxis for Cesarean Section

The high rate of infection (averaging 35–40%) following cesarean section is sufficient reason to consider prophylactic perioperative antibiotic administration in high-risk patients. If possible, a single drug should be used because of the convenience. The drug should have a wide spectrum of activity, including reasonably good activity against pathogens likely to be present at the incision site. The dosage regimen should be designed to ensure adequate tissue levels at the time the operation begins or shortly thereafter. The drug should not be one that is used to treat serious, established infections. The duration of therapy should be short. (Antibiotics administered for > 48 hours can hardly be called prophylactic.) The drug should be free of major side effects and should be relatively inexpensive.

One drug commonly used is cefazolin 1 g intravenously when the umbilical cord is clamped, followed by 2 similar doses at 6-hour intervals. A single dose has been shown to be as effective as a 3-dose regimen. Almost all studies on the use of prophylactic antibiotics in patients with cesarean section deliveries have shown significant reductions in the incidence of infection, regardless of the drugs, doses, and schedules used. However, no regimen has provided total protection against the incidence of fever and associated morbidity, nor has one completely prevented serious postoperative infections. Low-risk women, that is, those undergoing elective cesarean section who are not in active labor, do not benefit to the same degree from prophylactic antibiotics.

5. Episiotomy Infection

It is surprising that infected episiotomies do not occur more often than they do, because contamination at the time of delivery is universal. Subsequent contamination during the healing phase also should be common, yet infection and disruption of the wound are infrequent (0.5–3%). The excellent local blood supply is suggested as an explanation for this phenomenon.

Etiology

In general, the more extensive the laceration or episiotomy, the greater the chances for infection and breakdown of the wound. More tissue is devitalized in a large episiotomy, thereby providing greater opportunity for contamination. Women with infections elsewhere in the genital area probably are at greater risk for infection of the episiotomy.

Clinical Findings

A. SYMPTOMS AND SIGNS

Pain at the episiotomy site is the most common symptom. Spontaneous drainage is frequent, so a mass rarely forms. Incontinence of flatus and stool may be the presenting symptom of an episiotomy that breaks down and heals spontaneously.

Inspection of the episiotomy site shows disruption of the wound and gaping of the incision. A necrotic membrane may cover the wound and should be debrided if possible. A careful rectovaginal examination should be performed to determine whether a rectovaginal fistula has formed. The integrity of the anal sphincter should be evaluated.

B. LABORATORY FINDINGS

Infection with mixed aerobic and anaerobic organisms is common. *Staphylococcus* may be recovered from cultures of material from these infections. Culture results frequently are misleading because the area of the episiotomy typically is contaminated with a wide variety of pathogenic bacteria.

Treatment

Initial treatment should be directed toward opening and cleaning the wound and promoting the formation of granulation tissue. Warm sitz baths or Hubbard tank treatments help the debridement process. Attempts to close an infected, disrupted episiotomy are likely to fail and may make ultimate closure more difficult. Surgical closure by perineorrhaphy should be undertaken only after granulation tissue has thoroughly covered the wound site. There is an increasing trend towards early repair of episiotomy wound dehiscence, in contrast to conventional wisdom, which suggests a 3- to 4-month delay. Several large case series show excellent results once initial infection is treated.

6. Mastitis

Congestive mastitis, or breast engorgement, is more common in primigravidas than in multiparas. Infectious mastitis and breast abscesses also are more common in women pregnant for the first time and are seen almost exclusively in nursing mothers.

Etiology

Infectious mastitis and breast abscesses are uncommon complications of breastfeeding. They almost certainly occur as a result of trauma to the nipple and the subsequent introduction of organisms from the infant's nostrils to the mother's breast. *S aureus* contracted by the infant while in the hospital nursery is the usual causative agent.

Clinical Findings

A. SYMPTOMS AND SIGNS

Breast engorgement usually occurs on the second or third postpartum day. The breasts are swollen, tender, tense, and warm. The patient's temperature may be mildly elevated. Axillary adenopathy can be seen.

Mastitis presents 1 week or more after delivery. Usually only 1 breast is affected and often only 1 quadrant or lobule. It is tender, reddened, swollen, and hot. There may be purulent drainage, and aspiration may produce pus. The patient is febrile and appears ill.

B. Laboratory Findings

The organism responsible for infectious mastitis and breast abscess almost always is *S aureus*. *Streptococcus* spp. and *E coli* are occasionally isolated. Leukocytosis is evident.

Treatment

A. Congestive Mastitis

The form of treatment depends on whether or not the patient plans to breastfeed. If she does not, tight breast binding, ice packs, restriction of breast stimulation, and analgesics help to relieve pain and suppress lactation. Medical suppression of lactation probably does not hasten involution of congested breasts unless the drug is taken very early after delivery. Bromocriptine 2.5 mg twice daily orally for 10 days is an effective regimen, although concerns about its side-effect profile have curtailed its use. For the woman who is breastfeeding, manually emptying the breasts following infant feeding is all that is necessary to relieve discomfort.

B. Infectious Mastitis

Infectious mastitis is treated in the same way as congestive mastitis. Local heat and support of the breasts help to reduce pain. Cloxacillin, dicloxacillin, nafcillin, or a cephalosporin—antibiotic with activity against the commonly encountered causative organisms—should be administered. Infants tolerate the small amount of antibiotics in breast milk without difficulty. It may be prudent to check the infant for possible colonization with the same bacteria present in the mother's breast.

If an abscess is present, incision and drainage are necessary. The cavity should be packed open with gauze, which is then advanced toward the surface in stages daily. Most authorities recommend cessation of breastfeeding when an abscess develops. Antistaphylococcal antibiotics should be prescribed. Inhibition of lactation is also recommended.

DISORDERS OF LACTATION

Inhibition & Suppression of Lactation

Anatomic alteration of the breasts during pregnancy prepares them for sustained milk production shortly after delivery. The rapid decrease of serum estrogen and progesterone levels postpartum does not occur in prolactin levels, which decrease much more slowly. The breast is no longer subject to the inhibitory effects of the steroid hormones and now comes under the influence of high prolactin levels to begin sustained milk production.

Colostrum is secreted in late pregnancy and for the first 2–3 days postpartum. It is higher in protein (much of which may be antibodies) and minerals and lower in carbohydrates and fat than is later breast milk. Prior to full milk production, from the second to the fourth postpartum days, the breasts become enlarged, engorged, and tender. The breast lobules enlarge, and alveoli and blood vessels proliferate. Milk production truly begins around the third or fourth postpartum day. Fortuitously, infants may frequently take this long to feel a sensation of hunger and to develop the neuromuscular control necessary to successfully empty the breast.

In spite of the manifold benefits of breastfeeding for both infants and mothers, at least one-third of all women who give birth today do not wish to nurse, and perhaps an additional 10–20% discontinue attempts within a few weeks of delivery. For these women, inhibition of lactation for relief of breast congestion and tenderness may be necessary.

A. Physical Methods of Suppression of Lactation

Inhibition of physical stimuli that encourage milk secretion can prevent lactation. Tight breast binding, avoidance of any tactile breast stimulation, ice packs, and mild analgesics (eg, aspirin or ibuprofen) are effective in inhibiting lactation and relieving the symptoms of breast engorgement in 50% of women. Physical methods successfully inhibit lactation and prevent breast engorgement either before the onset of lactation or after it has been established for some time.

B. Hormonal Suppression of Lactation

Large doses of estrogen alone have been used to suppress lactation; they do inhibit milk production, probably by acting directly on the breast. Estrogens are somewhat more successful than physical methods alone. Side effects are tolerable in young women who have had vaginal deliveries, but increased rates of thrombophlebitis and pulmonary embolism are seen in women older than 35 years, in those who have undergone cesarean section, and in women with difficult deliveries. For these reasons, pure estrogens are no longer used for suppression of lactation as they once were. Furthermore, drug-induced suppression of lactation is not very effective after lactation has been established.

The ergot derivative bromocriptine has strong prolactin-inhibiting and thus lactation-inhibiting properties. In the dosage ranges used to suppress lactation, the drug is relatively free of serious side effects. Minor side effects include nausea and nasal congestion. More serious associations with hypertension, cerebrovascular accidents, and myocardial infarction have been reported. The risks seem to be reported frequently when bromocriptine is used in patients with pregnancy-induced hypertension. Drawbacks of bromocriptine therapy include the necessity for prolonged treatment (10–14 days) and a more rapid resumption of ovulation. A significant number of women have rebound lactation (18–40%). The Food and Drug Administration (FDA) removed painful breast engorgement as an indication for bromocriptine use in 1989. The FDA noted that although there is no clear proof of adverse effects of these medications, there is no proved health benefit, so even minor safety concerns become significant because of their potential unfavorable effects on the benefit/risk ratio. Bromocriptine may be a reasonable treatment option in women with severe congestive mastitis.

Inappropriate Lactation

Lactation is physiologic in late pregnancy and for a considerable period after delivery. In the woman who has not lactated for 1 year or more or who has never been pregnant, lactation may indicate a significant endocrinopathy.

POSTPARTUM MONITORING

Serious and acute obstetric and postanesthetic complications often occur during the first few hours immediately following delivery. Therefore the patient should be transferred to a recovery room where she can be constantly attended to and where observation of bleeding, blood pressure, pulse, and respiratory change can be made every 15 minutes for at least 1–2 hours after delivery or until the effects of general or major regional anesthesia have disappeared. On return to the patient's room or ward, the patient's blood pressure should be taken and the measurement repeated every 12 hours for the first 24 hours and daily thereafter for several days. Preeclampsia–eclampsia, infection, or other medical or surgical complications of pregnancy may require more prolonged and intensive postpartum care.

POSTPARTUM COMPLICATIONS

1. Complications of Anesthesia

The most common respiratory complications that follow general anesthesia and delivery are airway obstruction or laryngospasm and vomiting with aspiration of vomitus. Bronchoscopy, tracheostomy, and other related procedures must be performed promptly as indicated. Hypoventilation and hypotension may follow an abnormally high subarachnoid block. Because serum cholinesterase activity is lower during labor and the postpartum period, hypoventilation during the early puerperium may follow the use of large amounts of succinylcholine during anesthesia for cesarean section. Brief postpartum shivering is commonly seen after completion of the third stage of labor and is no cause for alarm. The cause of the shivering is unknown, but it may be related to loss of heat, or it may be a sympathetic response. Subcutaneous emphysema may appear postpartum after vigorous bearing-down efforts. Most cases resolve spontaneously.

If preeclampsia has been ruled out, hypertension in the immediate puerperium may be due to excessive use of vasopressor or oxytocic drugs. It must be treated promptly with a vasodilator. Hydralazine 5 mg administrated slowly intravenously usually reduces the blood pressure.

Postanesthetic complications that manifest themselves later in the puerperium include postsubarachnoid puncture headache, atelectasis, renal or hepatic dysfunction, and neurologic sequelae.

Postpuncture headache usually is located in the forehead, deep behind the eyes; occasionally, the pain radiates to both temples and to the occipital region. It usually begins on the first or second postpartum day and lasts 1–3 days. Because new mothers frequently develop various types of headache, the correct diagnosis is essential. An important characteristic of postspinal puncture headache is increased pain in the sitting or standing position and significant improvement when the patient is supine. The mild form is relieved by aspirin or other analgesics. Headache is due to leakage of cerebrospinal fluid through the site of dural puncture into the extradural space. It is advisable to supplement the daily oral intake of fluids with at least 1 L of 5% glucose in saline intravenously. Administration of 7–10 mL of the patient's own blood into the thecal space at the point of previous needle insertion will "patch" the leaking point and relieve the headache in most patients. Subdural hematoma is a rare complication of chronic leakage of cerebrospinal fluid and resultant loss of support to intracranial structures.

A small percentage of women who develop headaches during this time also show symptoms of meningeal irritation. Headache due to aseptic chemical meningitis is not relieved by lying down. Lumbar puncture reveals a slightly elevated pressure and an increase in spinal fluid protein and white blood cells but no bacteria. Symptoms usually disappear 1–3 days later, and the spinal fluid returns to normal within 4 days with no sequelae. Treatment is conservative and includes supportive measures, analgesics, and fluids.

Neurologic problems in the puerperium sometimes follow traumatic childbirth, such as injury to the femoral nerve caused by forceps when the patient was in the lithotomy position. Such complications are rarely bilateral, which aids in the differential diagnosis of a spinal cord lesion. Evidence of more serious neurologic sequelae following regional or general anesthesia for delivery requires consultation with the anesthesiologist or a neurologist.

2. Postpartum Cardiac Problems

The puerperium is relatively complicated for the patient with congenital or acquired heart disease. Following delivery, the cardiovascular system responds with sharply increased cardiac output as a result of unimpeded venous return from the lower extremities and pelvis. This produces a relative bradycardia that may persist for several days. For the initial few days after delivery, the intracellular water and sodium retained during pregnancy are mobilized and contribute to increasing cardiac output. A concomitant postpartum diuresis gradually mitigates the bradycardia and increases cardiac output (see Chapter 7).

Valvular Heart Disease

The management principles underlying treatment of valvular heart disease in the postpartum period are those instituted in the intrapartum period: antibiotic prophylaxis of bacterial endocarditis, careful fluid and electrolyte administration, accurate (often continuous invasive) monitoring, and frequent physical examinations to detect changes in cardiovascular status. Return to an ambulatory state soon after delivery reduces the possibility of thrombophlebitis. The postpartum period is also a time for the patient to carefully consider further childbearing options in light of the fetal outcome and the possible progression of heart disease during the antecedent pregnancy.

Women whose valvular heart disease required systemic anticoagulation before delivery should continue the treatment postpartum; however, oral anticoagulants can be used instead of heparin. There are no reports of problems in term breastfed infants of women taking warfarin or dicumarol. Other oral anticoagulants are contraindicated if the patient is breastfeeding.

Postpartum Cardiomyopathy

A cardiomyopathy unique to the latter half of pregnancy and the puerperium has been described by numerous investigators. The incidence is estimated to be 1 in 4000 deliveries. Congestive heart failure, cardiomegaly, and cardiac arrhythmias develop in otherwise healthy young women. This problem is addressed in Chapter 22 on cardiac disease in pregnancy.

3. Postpartum Pulmonary Problems

Return to nonpregnant pulmonary physiology occurs by 6 weeks after delivery. Except for women undergoing general anesthesia, the puerperium is not a time

of special concern. The factors placing pregnant women at risk for highly destructive chemical aspiration pneumonitis (gastric pH < 2.5 and fasting gastric contents > 25 mL) persist for at least 48 hours after delivery. Thus, women undergoing general anesthesia in the puerperium (eg, for tubal ligation) are at high risk for aspiration. A nonparticulate antacid should be used preoperatively for women undergoing general anesthesia in the puerperal period as well as other anesthetic techniques (rapid sequence induction of anesthesia, endotracheal intubation, and preanesthetic fasting) designed to prevent aspiration of gastric contents.

Pulmonary hypertension, either primary or secondary to congenital heart disease, is an overt threat to the mother's life in the intrapartum and postpartum periods. The most important management principle is to use invasive monitoring to avoid hypovolemia (see Chapter 22).

4. Postpartum Thyroiditis

Thyroid abnormalities, particularly of immunologic origin, are common in the postpartum period. Although racial differences exist, between 3% and 17% of women will develop postpartum thyroiditis, and over half of these women will have positive microsomal antibody titers. Patients with known Graves' disease are at particular risk; even if they are euthyroid at time of delivery, approximately 10% will experience postpartum hyperthyroidism. Postpartum thyroiditis usually presents with mild transient hyperthyroidism 3–8 months postpartum, followed by mild and transient hypothyroidism, although simple hypothyroidism or hyperthyroidism may be seen. Suppression of hyperthyroid symptoms or temporary thyroid hormone supplementation may be necessary, but most women recover completely and are euthyroid within 6–9 months after delivery. The recurrence risk for postpartum thyroiditis in a subsequent pregnancy is 10–25%.

5. Postpartum Thrombophlebitis & Thromboembolism

Historically, the puerperium has been known as the time for occurrence of severe thrombophlebitic conditions and pulmonary embolism, probably as a result of the once-prevalent recommendation of prolonged bed rest following parturition. Even though contemporary postpartum management encourages early ambulation, puerperal thrombophlebitis and thromboembolism remain a serious problem.

Thrombophlebitis requires careful and prolonged medical management. The risk of recurrence in a subsequent pregnancy is substantial, and a history of thrombophlebitis may prohibit the future use of oral contraceptives and replacement estrogens.

The incidence of thrombophlebitic conditions is difficult to estimate because the clinical diagnosis of these disorders is highly unreliable. One study of venographically confirmed deep venous thrombosis reported 1.3 antepartum cases per 10,000 deliveries and 6.1 postpartum cases per 10,000 deliveries. Most studies confirm that the incidence of superficial thrombophlebitis, deep vein thrombosis, and pulmonary embolism is 2–6 times higher in the postpartum period than in the antepartum period, although these data may be influenced by the effects of the prolonged postpartum bed rest once advocated. (Methods of diagnosis and treatment of thromboembolic conditions are discussed in Chapter 26.)

6. Postpartum Neuropsychiatric Complications

Peripheral Nerve Palsy

Nerve palsies involving pelvic nerves or parts of the lumbosacral plexus result from pressure by the presenting part or trauma by obstetric forceps. Typically, the palsy occurs after prolonged labor in a nullipara and presents as unilateral footdrop noted when ambulation resumes after delivery. Most cases resolve spontaneously in a matter of days or weeks. A few may have a more protracted course. Electromyography may help in predicting the course of the disorder.

Seizures

Postpartum seizures immediately raise the possibility of eclampsia, but if the interval since delivery is more than 48 hours, other etiologies should be considered. In the absence of a history of epilepsy or signs of pregnancy-induced hypertension, a thorough evaluation to determine the cause of the seizures must be performed.

Postpartum Depression

Considering the excitement, anticipation, and tension associated with imminent delivery, the marked hormonal alterations following delivery, and the substantial new burdens and responsibilities that result from childbirth, it is not surprising that some women experience depression after delivery. The incidence of postpartum depression is difficult to estimate, but the disorder is common. The disorder in its usual form is self-limited

and benign. However, hypothyroidism is emerging as a cause of some cases of postpartum depression, and screening for this disorder should be considered if suggested by clinical presentation.

In women who suffered from depression before they became pregnant and in those without effective support mechanisms, the severity of depression may be more profound and the consequences far more serious. An openly psychotic state may develop within a few days after delivery and render the woman incapable of caring for herself or her newborn. In some cases she may harm her infant and herself.

Psychiatric consultation should be obtained for the postpartum woman who shows symptoms of severe depression or overt psychosis. Nursery personnel are often the first to notice that the new mother does not devote the usual amount of attention to her newborn (see Chapter 62).

REFERENCES

B-Lynch C et al: The B-Lynch surgical technique for the control of massive postpartum hemorrhage: an alternative to hysterectomy? Five cases reported. Br J Obstet Gynaecol 1997;104:372.

Brown CS, Bertolet BD: Peripartum cardiomyopathy: A comprehensive review. Obstet Gynecol 1998;178:408.

Capella-Allouc S et al: Hysteroscopic treatment of severe Asherman's syndrome and subsequent fertility. Hum Reprod 1999;14:1230.

Dubois J et al: Placenta percreta: Balloon occlusion and embolization of the internal iliac arteries to reduce intraoperative blood losses. Am J Obstet Gynecol 1997;176:723.

Khan GQ et al: Controlled cord traction versus minimal intervention techniques in delivery of the placenta: A randomized control study. Am J Obstet Gynecol 1997;177:770.

Lokumamage AU et al: A randomized study comparing rectally administered misoprostol versus Syntometrine combined with an oxytocin infusion for the cessation of primary post partum hemorrhage. Acta Obstet Gynecol Scand 2001;80:835.

Miller DA et al: Clinical risk factors for placenta previa-placenta accreta. Am J Obstet Gynecol 1997;177:210.

Pelage J et al: Life-threatening primary postpartum hemorrhage: Treatment with emergency selective arterial embolization. Radiology 1998;208:359.

Rogers J et al: Active versus expectant management of the third stage of labour: The Hinchingbrooke randomised controlled trial. Lancet 1998;351:693.

Terry AJ, Hague WM: Postpartum thyroiditis. Semin Perinatol 1998;22:497.

The Resuscitation & Care of the Newborn at Risk

32

Elisabeth L. Raab, MD

Delivery of a high-risk fetus requires multidisciplinary prenatal decision making to ensure the best outcome for the newborn and mother. Obstetricians, neonatologists, and, in appropriate cases, pediatric medical and/or surgical subspecialists must work together to determine an appropriate plan of care for the fetus and delivery of the newborn and provide counseling for the family. Discovery of a significant complication during pregnancy often warrants referral of the mother to a perinatologist for further evaluation and possible treatment. When circumstances allow, the mother of a high-risk fetus should be transferred to a tertiary care center with experience in high-risk obstetric and neonatal care prior to delivery. Numerous studies have shown improved outcomes for low-birth-weight (LBW) infants (< 2500 g) with delivery at a center with a higher level of neonatal care.

Successful transition from fetal to ex utero life involves a complex series of hormonal and physiologic changes, many of which occur or begin before birth. Events such as cord compression, placental abruption, meconium aspiration, and premature delivery or the presence of infection or major congenital malformations may alter or prevent the essential postnatal transition. Any process that prevents or hinders the newborn from inflating the lungs with air and establishing effective ventilation, oxygenation, and/or circulation will result in a depressed newborn in need of resuscitation for survival.

RESUSCITATION OF THE HIGH-RISK INFANT

The American Academy of Pediatrics (AAP) guidelines mandate that at least 1 skilled person capable of carrying out resuscitation of a newborn be present at every delivery. When a delivery is identified as high risk, 2 or more skilled people may be required to provide adequate care. Often it is useful to assign roles to the resuscitation staff to ensure that the resuscitation flows as smoothly as possible. The equipment required for resuscitation, such as the bag and mask used for ventilation, the blender for oxygen and air delivery, the suc-

tion equipment, the radiant warmer, and the monitors, should be checked prior to the delivery. Communication between the obstetric and neonatal staff about the maternal medical and obstetric history as well as the prenatal history of the fetus is essential to ensure that the neonatal team can anticipate and interpret the problems the newborn may have in the delivery room.

Delivery Room Management

Although the expectations may be different and the need for resuscitation more common, the same principles apply to a high-risk delivery as to a routine delivery: the newborn should be kept warm and rapidly assessed to determine the need for intervention.

The initial evaluation and resuscitation may take place in the delivery room or, in centers with a high-risk delivery service, preferentially in an adjacent room specifically designed for high-risk resuscitations. Typically the newborn is brought immediately to a radiant warmer, although some institutions weigh extremely premature infants prior to transfer to the warmer bed in order to determine the birth weight if viability is in question. The infant is dried with prewarmed towels to prevent heat loss. At some centers LBW newborns are put into polyurethane bags or wrapped with polyethylene occlusive wrap after delivery; these measures have been shown to significantly improve temperature stability during stabilization and transport to the neonatal intensive care unit (NICU). In addition, a knit hat is used to prevent heat loss from the head. Preterm infants are at increased risk for thermal instability given their greater body surface area to weight ratio, thinner skin, and relative paucity of subcutaneous fat compared to term infants. Hypothermia (body temperature < 36 °C) can occur rapidly in the preterm infant and may cause complications such as hypoglycemia and acidosis.

After rapidly drying the infant and removing the wet towels, the resuscitation team should position and clear the airway. The team then assesses the newborn's respiratory effort, heart rate, color and activity to determine the need for intervention. Figure 32–1 depicts the most recent AAP algorithm for neonatal evaluation and re-

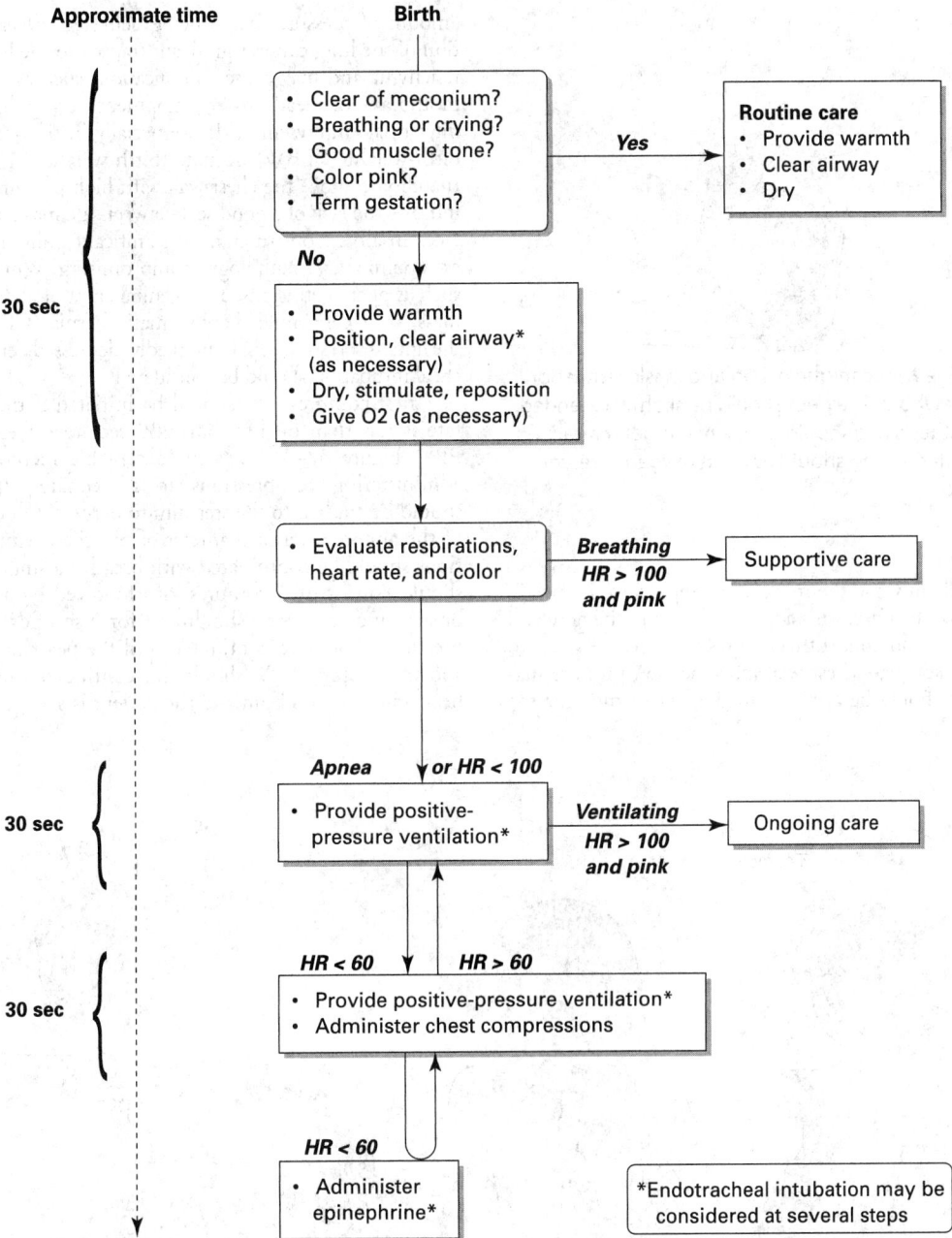

Figure 32–1. Algorithm for resuscitation of the newborn.

suscitation. Drying the patient and suctioning the airway usually provide adequate stimulation for the newborn to breathe. Rubbing the back or flicking the soles of the feet may be done to provide additional stimulus if initial respirations are irregular.

As illustrated in Figure 32–1, positive-pressure ventilation (PPV) should be started if the newborn is apneic or has a heart rate less than 100 bpm. Figure 32–2 shows the correct positioning of the neck and placement of the mask. PPV will not be effective if the airway is not ex-

Figure 32–2. Technique of bag and mask ventilation of the newborn. The neck should be slightly extended. An anesthesia bag should have a manometer attached; a self-inflating bag should have an oxygen reservoir attached.

tended slightly and the mask is not applied to the face in the correct manner, with a tight seal around the nose and mouth. In addition, sufficient pressure must be given to produce adequate chest wall movement. A pressure manometer should be attached to the bag to monitor the amount of pressure that is being delivered. Overdistention of the lung causes significant trauma to the lung parenchyma and may cause complications such as a pneumothorax or lead to development of pulmonary interstitial emphysema (PIE), especially in the very-low-birth-weight (VLBW) neonate (birth weight < 1500 g). Inability to move the chest wall with high pressures may indicate the lack of a good seal between the mask and the face, an airway obstruction, or significant pulmonary or extrapulmonary pathology compromising ventilation, such as pleural effusions, a congenital chest or abdominal mass, or a congenital diaphragmatic hernia (CDH). If the infant's respiration is markedly depressed, endotracheal intubation should be considered.

Chest compressions should be initiated if the heart rate is less than 60 bpm after 30 seconds of effective PPV. Figure 32–3 shows the acceptable methods for administering compressions to a neonate. Pressure should be applied to the sternum to depress it one-third of the anteroposterior diameter of the chest. Compressions should be coordinated with breaths: a single cycle should consist of 3 compressions followed by a single breath, and each cycle should last for 2 seconds. Compressions should be continued until the heart rate rises above 60 bpm. PPV should be continued until the heart rate is > 100 bpm and the patient is showing ade-

Thumb Placement

One Over the Other   Side by Side

A   B

Figure 32–3. **A:** Thumb technique for performing chest compressions on an infant. The two thumbs, placed either side by side or overlapping one another, are used to depress the lower third of the sternum, with the hands encircling the torso and the fingers supporting the back. **B:** Two-finger method for performing chest compressions on an infant. The tips of the middle finger and either the index finger or ring finger of one hand are used to compress the lower third of the sternum.

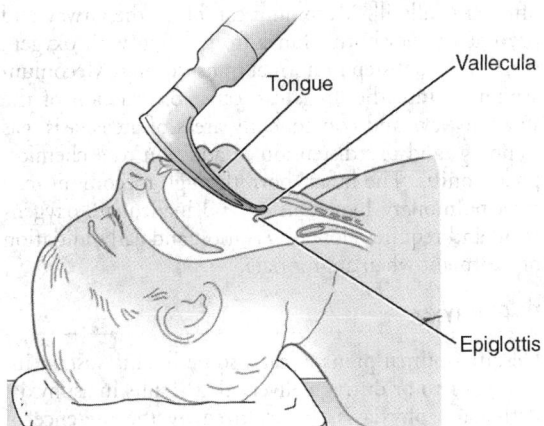

Figure 32–4. Landmarks for placement of the laryngoscope.

quate respiratory effort. If the heart rate remains < 60 bpm after 30 seconds of compressions, administration of epinephrine is indicated. Failure to respond to PPV and chest compressions is a clear indication for endotracheal intubation; intubation should be attempted at this time if it has not already been performed. Figure 32–4 shows the landmarks used to guide placement of the endotracheal tube (ETT) between the vocal cords.

Epinephrine can be given via an ETT or an umbilical venous catheter. The standard dose of epinephrine in neonates is 0.01–0.03 mg/kg. The 2006 American Academy of Pediatrics (AAP) guideline recommends using a higher dose of 0.1 mg/kg/dose of the 1:10,000 concentration solution administered rapidly if epinephrine is delivered via the ETT (Table 32–1). The dose can be repeated every 3–5 minutes until the heart rate rises above 60 bpm.

When the infant's response to resuscitation is poor, other factors that may be complicating successful resuscitation of a newborn should be considered. Naloxone should be considered if respiratory depression is thought to be secondary to maternal narcotic administration within 4 hours of delivery and there is no history of maternal narcotic abuse during pregnancy. Naloxone can cause symptoms of withdrawal, including seizures, if given to the child of a mother addicted to narcotics. Hypovolemia should be suspected if there is a perinatal history consistent with blood loss (eg, placental abruption, placenta previa) or sepsis, and the baby is hypotensive and pale, with weak pulses and cool extremities. A 10 cc/kg IV infusion of normal saline, lactated Ringer's solution, or O-negative blood, if available and anemia is suspected, can be given to treat the suspected hypovolemia. The dose can be repeated if there is minimal improvement with the initial bolus. Metabolic acidosis may be present at birth if the baby was significantly distressed in utero or may develop after birth if oxygenation and/or perfusion are compromised. Although use of bicarbonate in resuscitation is somewhat controversial, significant acidosis will cause pulmonary vasoconstriction and poor myocardial contractility and should be treated. The umbilical artery can be catheterized to provide ongoing access to blood samples for determination of the extent of acidosis and the response to treatment during resuscitation. The recommended dose of bicarbonate is 2 mEq/kg IV of a 0.5 mEq/mL (4.2%) solution. Bicarbonate should be given slowly via an intravenous line (IV) and should be used only after ventilation is established so that the CO_2 produced with bicarbonate administration can be removed. Otherwise, bicarbonate administration may result in a significant increase in intracellular acidosis. Tromethamine (Tham) may be used as an alternative to bicarbonate when there is documented or suspected hypercapnia, as occurs in neonates with conditions resulting in pulmonary hypoplasia. Tham is a buffer that increases bicarbonate while lowering $PaCO_2$ levels.

Apgar scores are assigned at 1 and 5 minutes of life and continued at 5-minute intervals for up to 20 minutes as long as the score remains below 7. However, the Apgar score does not determine the need for resuscitation. Although a depressed or distressed newborn likely will receive a low Apgar score, assessment of the need for intervention with PPV should already have been made by the time the 1-minute Apgar score was assigned, and the score may not accurately reflect the newborn's clinical status. The initial assessment of the newborn and assignment of the Apgar score are discussed in further detail in Chapter 11.

Although 100% oxygen is the current standard for neonatal resuscitation, this treatment has recently been called into question. Oxygen is known to have numerous toxic effects, and there is concern among many neonatologists that use of 100% oxygen during resuscitation may actually cause cellular injury, particularly to

Table 32–1. Neonatal resuscitation and newborn infant drug doses.

Epinephrine	(1:10,000) 0.2 mL/kg IV or ET. Give rapidly. Dilute 1:1 with saline for ET use.
Volume Expansion	(Whole blood, saline, 5% albumin, Ringer's lactate) 10 mL/kg. Give over 5–10 minutes.
$NaHCO_3$	(0.5 mEq/mL) 1–2 mEq/kg IV. Give slowly, only if ventilation adequate.
Naloxone	(0.4 mg/mL) 0.1 mg/kg = 0.25 mL/kg IV, ET, IM, SQ. Give rapidly.
Glucose	$D_{10}W$ 2 mL/kg IV. Give over 1–2 minutes.

the brain, via production of oxygen-derived radicals. In addition, a recent study of more than 50,000 children showed a slightly higher risk of a certain type of leukemia in children exposed at birth to oxygen for more than 3 minutes compared to unexposed children. A Cochrane Database meta-analysis published in 2005 analyzed the results of several clinical trials comparing neonatal resuscitation with room air (21% oxygen) versus 100% oxygen. The results showed a significant decrease in mortality in the group resuscitated with room air and no difference between the rates of moderate or severe hypoxic–ischemic encephalopathy (HIE) in the room air and 100% oxygen groups. The single study with follow-up (at 18–24 months) that was included in the meta-analysis showed no difference in neurodevelopmental outcome between the groups. However, given the small number of studies to date and the use of backup 100% oxygen in many of the infants studied, the authors concluded there currently is not enough evidence to recommend standard use of room air instead of 100% oxygen for resuscitation when oxygen is available. The debate continues, but it is clear that every effort should be made to avoid hyperoxia and to minimize any unnecessary exposure to oxygen.

Specific Considerations in the Delivery Room

A. MECONIUM

Meconium-stained fluid is present in 10–20% of deliveries. It is extremely rare if delivery takes place prior to 34 weeks' gestation. Passage of meconium in utero usually indicates fetal distress, and those personnel present at the delivery should be alerted by the presence of meconium to the possibility that the newborn may be depressed at birth.

It is no longer recommended by the AAP that all meconium-stained babies receive intrapartum suctioning. An active, crying, well-appearing infant does not require endotracheal intubation regardless of the presence of meconium staining or the thickness of the meconium. If the newborn is in distress or has depressed respiratory effort, the appropriate intervention is to intubate and suction the trachea before stimulating the baby in any way. If no meconium is suctioned from the airway, resuscitation should proceed according to the standard algorithm. If meconium is suctioned from the trachea, another attempt should be made to intubate the patient and suction the trachea again. However, if the patient has significant bradycardia it may be appropriate to defer repeated suctioning and provide PPV.

The majority (94–97%) of infants born through meconium-stained fluid will not develop meconium aspiration syndrome, but when it does occur, infants are often critically ill. Meconium can block the airway and prevent the newborn's lungs from filling with oxygen, which is a vital step in normal transitioning. Meconium aspiration into the lungs can cause obstruction of the small airways and consequently areas of atelectasis, gas trapping, and overdistention in addition to a chemical pneumonitis. The infant born through meconium may have pulmonary hypertension and inadequate oxygenation and requires close observation and early initiation of treatment when appropriate.

B. ASPHYXIA

Despite optimal prenatal care, some infants sustain injury prior to or during delivery that results in asphyxia. Perinatal asphyxia is characterized by the presence of hypoxemia, hypercapnia, and metabolic academia. It is the result of compromised oxygen delivery and blood flow to the fetus, either chronically or acutely, that stems from processes such as placental insufficiency, cord compression, trauma, and placental abruption.

If significant prepartum or peripartum hypoxic–ischemic injury has occurred, the infant likely will be depressed at birth and may not respond to initial interventions to establish respiration. The initial response in the newborn to lack of oxygen is rapid breathing, followed shortly thereafter by a period of apnea, termed *primary apnea.* Drying the infant and rubbing the back or flicking the soles of the feet is sufficient to stimulate respiration during the primary apnea phase. However, without intervention at this point, continued oxygen deprivation will lead to a series of gasps followed by a period of secondary apnea. It is important to recognize that an infant who does not respond to stimulation likely is in secondary apnea and requires further intervention. Respiration will not resume with stimulation if secondary apnea has begun and positive pressure is necessary to reverse the process. As Figure 32–5 demonstrates, heart rate changes typically begin toward the end of primary apnea, whereas blood pressure typically is maintained until the period of secondary apnea.

Effective resuscitation of an asphyxiated newborn usually requires treatment of acidosis. Perinatal asphyxia may also be complicated by hypoglycemia and hypocalcemia. Myocardial dysfunction may be present, and fluid boluses and continuous infusion of inotrope may be required for adequate blood pressure support. However, in the presence of significant myocardial dysfunction, repeated volume boluses will worsen the cardiovascular status. In these cases, early administration of an inotrope (eg, dobutamine) with or without low to moderate doses of a vasopressor (eg, dopamine) is the appropriate approach. In addition, seizures may occur in the newborn with perinatal asphyxia. Seizures usually are the result of hypoxic–ischemic injury to the cerebral cortex, but hypoglycemia and hypocalcemia also may

Figure 32–5. Heart rate and blood pressure changes during apnea.

cause seizure activity in the depressed neonate. In the newborn, phenobarbital (15–20 mg/kg IV) typically is given as the first-line treatment of seizures not caused by hypoglycemia or hypocalcemia. An additional 5–10 mg/kg bolus can be given to control status epilepticus. Asphyxiated infants are at increased risk for persistent pulmonary hypertension (discussed in detail later in the section Pathology and Care of the High Risk Term Neonate).

The severity of the insult sustained by the newborn can be difficult to assess in the neonatal period. The presence of abnormal findings on the neurologic examination and the severity and persistence of those abnormalities are the most useful measures for assessing the degree of brain injury sustained. Laboratory (umbilical cord and baby blood gases, serum creatinine level, liver function tests, blood lactate level, cardiac enzyme levels) studies, radiographic (brain magnetic resonance imaging [MRI]) studies, and electroencephalographic (EEG) findings provide additional information to help predict the likelihood and anticipated extent of an adverse neurodevelopmental outcome. Early onset of seizure activity has been shown to increase the likelihood of a poor outcome. Infants with severe HIE, which is characterized by absent reflexes, flaccid muscle tone, seizures, and a markedly altered level of consciousness, either die within several days of birth or have significant neurologic sequelae. It is a misconception that perinatal asphyxia is the cause of cerebral palsy. A minority of the cases of cerebral palsy are actually attributable to intrapartum complications. Selective hypothermia, or brain cooling, currently is under investigation as a possible intervention to improve outcome after asphyxia. Therapies aimed at inhibiting free-radical production also may have a role in preventing adverse outcomes of asphyxia in the future.

C. SHOCK

The newborn who fails to respond to initial attempts at resuscitation may be in circulatory shock. A number of different pathophysiologic processes can result in shock in the delivery room. Circulatory collapse can result from absolute (hemorrhage, capillary leak) or relative (vasodilatation) hypovolemia, cardiac dysfunction (asphyxia, congenital heart disease [CHD]), abnormal peripheral vasoregulation (prematurity, asphyxia, sepsis), or a combination of these factors. The peripartum history often helps pinpoint the etiology. The presence of risk factors for sepsis (prolonged rupture of membranes, maternal fever, chorioamnionitis), hemorrhage (placenta previa, placental abruption, trauma), or perinatal asphyxia may be informative. Pallor or peripheral hyperemia, weak pulses with tachycardia, and cool or warm extremities are present on examination. Hypotension in the newborn immediately following delivery is commonly defined as a mean arterial pressure that is equal to or less than the gestational age. It is worth noting that blood pressure is normal in the early (compensated) phase of shock; hypotension may only develop as the process progresses.

As mentioned in Delivery Room Management, a 10 cc/kg normal saline bolus typically is given to the newborn with hypotension. An additional 10–20 cc/kg is often given if the improvement in circulation is inadequate. Unmatched O-negative blood can be transfused in 10–15 cc/kg aliquots if severe anemia from blood loss is suspected. Volume should be administered slowly and judiciously to preterm infants who lack the mechanisms to autoregulate cerebral blood flow and protect the brain against reperfusion injury. Excessive volume may worsen the patient's status if cardiac dysfunction is the cause of hypotension. As discussed earlier, administration of sodium bicarbonate or Tham is frequently indicated to treat metabolic acidosis in the newborn in shock. Vasopressor/inotrope infusions should be initiated in neonates who do not respond to volume resuscitation.

D. CYANOSIS

Although acrocyanosis (cyanosis of the hands and feet) often is normal in the newborn, central cyanosis is not. Cyanosis is due to inadequate oxygen delivery to the tissue, either as a result of poor blood flow (peripheral vasoconstriction in acrocyanosis or low cardiac output in cardiogenic shock) or insufficiently oxygenated blood (pulmonary hypertension or severe parenchymal lung disease). Free-flow oxygen can be administered if a newborn has central cyanosis despite regular respirations. Free-flow oxygen can be delivered by holding a mask or oxygen tubing that is connected to a flowing source of 100% oxygen close to the baby's nose and mouth. Oxygen can be gradually withdrawn when the newborn turns pink. PPV is often indicated if the baby remains cyanotic despite free-flow oxygen. Lack of improvement of central cyanosis with administration of free-flow oxygen necessitates an evaluation of the cause of cyanosis. As discussed earlier, provision of 100% oxygen may have significant side effects if it is used for newborn resuscitation.

E. PREMATURITY

The delivery of a preterm infant requires a skilled multidisciplinary resuscitation team that has an understanding of the myriad problems associated with preterm delivery and has experience handling VLBW newborns. The presence at delivery of physicians, nurses, and a respiratory therapist trained in newborn resuscitation will optimize the early care of the newborn. Details of the delivery room care of the preterm infant are discussed in the section Delivery Room Management earlier in this chapter.

The neonatal team should meet with the family prior to delivery whenever possible. The parents should be informed about the prognosis for the fetus and need for intensive care admission if appropriate.

It is critical that the family understand the plan for resuscitation in the delivery room and the anticipated short- and long-term problems the newborn may face. Often it is helpful to families to discuss the emotional impact of the admission and the possibility of a prolonged stay of their newborn in the ICU. If the fetus is at the limits of viability, currently considered 23–24 weeks' gestation and/or weight < 500 g, it is essential that the parents understand the considerable risk of death and the serious cognitive, motor, and pulmonary complications that may occur if the newborn does survive. The neonatal team must have a clear conversation with the parents about the possible options for postnatal management. Unfortunately, it often is difficult to make definitive plans given that the margin of error for prenatal determination of birth weight and gestational age is wide enough to have a significant impact on the viability of the fetus. Although many physicians have strong feelings of their own, it is vital that the course of resuscitation of a newborn at the limits of viability incorporates the family's wishes. Nevertheless, parents should understand that the fetus' viability will be reassessed after delivery, and that the maturity of the newborn, the newborn's condition at delivery, and the response to the resuscitative efforts made, in combination with available outcomes data, ultimately will determine the management in the delivery room.

F. ABDOMINAL WALL DEFECTS

Gastroschisis is the herniation of abdominal contents through an abdominal wall defect. The defect in gastroschisis usually is small and to the right of the umbilicus, and the intestines are unprotected by the peritoneal sac. *Omphalocele* also involves the herniation of abdominal contents through the abdominal wall, but the defect is in the umbilical portion of the abdominal wall, and the herniated viscera are covered by the peritoneal sac. Both defects require emergent care in the delivery room. The extra-abdominal organs should be delicately wrapped with warm saline-soaked gauze and then covered in plastic. Care should be taken to position the bowel centrally over the area of the defect with the infant supine or lying on his or her right side to prevent compromising blood flow to the intestines by kinking mesenteric blood vessels. A nasogastric tube should be placed to prevent distention of the bowel with air. Patients will have increased heat and insensible fluid losses, and intravenous fluid should be started promptly at 1.5 times normal maintenance requirements to prevent dehydration and hypernatremia. Electrolytes and fluid status must be monitored closely. A surgical consultation should occur prenatally if the defect is diagnosed in utero. An urgent surgical evaluation should be obtained upon admission of the newborn to the NICU.

PATHOLOGY AND CARE OF THE PRETERM INFANT

In 2003, 12.3% of all births in the United States were preterm, a 16% increase since 1990. Advances in obstetric and neonatal care have markedly increased the survival of premature infants and improved outcomes. However, prematurity continues to account for a significant percent of neonatal and infant mortality in the United States. In fact, 2003 saw a slight increase in infant mortality in the United States from the previous year, a trend that has not occurred in more than 40 years and is attributable to an increased numbers of babies with birth weights < 750 g. As tinier and less mature infants survive, we face new ethical and medical challenges to continue improving the long-term and societal impact of the care provided in the NICU.

Respiratory Distress Syndrome

In 1959 Mary Ellen Avery and Jere Mead reported data showing that the severe respiratory disease seen in preterm infants, then known as hyaline membrane disease, was due in part to a deficiency of surfactant. Surfactant, a complex of phospholipids and protein secreted by type II pneumocytes, reduces surface tension in the alveoli of the lung. Its absence, or deficiency, results in diffuse microatelectasis and decreased functional residual capacity leading to the presentation of a "ground-glass" pattern and poor expansion of the lungs on chest radiograph (CXR). The lung disease of the preterm infant, now known as respiratory distress syndrome (RDS), also is a consequence of the immature architecture of the lung at the time of birth.

RDS presents as tachypnea and increased work of breathing that develops shortly after birth. Both oxygenation and ventilation are impaired, and blood gas analysis typically reveals hypoxia and a respiratory acidosis. Although most commonly seen in premature infants, RDS is associated with other conditions as well. Infants of diabetic mothers are at risk, even at term, because high levels of insulin in the fetus suppress lung maturation, including surfactant production. Without intervention, RDS typically worsens over the first few days of postnatal life. Historically, improvement was often heralded by a marked increase in urine output ("diuretic phase" of RDS).

The likelihood of RDS is inversely proportional to gestational age. It now is standard to give corticosteroids to mothers at risk of delivery before 32–34 weeks' gestation to hasten maturation of fetal organs, including the lungs, and to decrease the incidence and severity of RDS. Some larger preterm infants may require supplemental oxygen by nasal cannula or no respiratory assistance whatsoever. Babies with significant RDS typically require assisted ventilation. Ventilatory support can be given with continuous positive airway pressure (CPAP), a pressure- or volume-limited ventilator, or a high-frequency ventilator. A recent analysis concluded the data are not sufficient to recommend any mode of mechanical ventilation over the other as standard therapy for RDS. Provision of positive end-expiratory pressure (PEEP) (either as CPAP or PEEP) quickly after delivery is vital in order to prevent collapse of the lungs. If the lungs are allowed to collapse, oxygenation and ventilation will be compromised further and higher pressures will be required to reinflate the lungs, causing avoidable barotrauma and volutrauma to the lungs.

Exogenous surfactant administration has significantly reduced morbidity and mortality from RDS since its routine use began in the early 1990s. Prophylactic administration of surfactant to the preterm infant (ie, before 15 minutes of age) has been shown to reduce neonatal morbidity (pneumothorax and pulmonary interstitial edema) and mortality compared to rescue therapy (ie, waiting until after the diagnosis of RDS is made). Proposed explanations of this finding include a more homogeneous distribution of surfactant in the fluid-filled lung and the delivery of surfactant after a minimal period of PPV minimizing barotrauma and volutrauma to the lung. However, it is very important to ensure correct placement of the ETT prior to surfactant administration in the delivery room. If the ETT position cannot be determined, it may be better to delay surfactant until CXR has confirmed placement. If the degree of RDS is significant, an additional 2–4 doses of surfactant can be given every 6–12 hours depending on the surfactant preparation used. The newborn should be monitored closely after receiving surfactant because rapid changes in respiratory status usually occur, necessitating aggressive weaning of the ventilator settings. If the ventilator support is not weaned appropriately, the improving lung compliance will result in high tidal volume ventilation leading to volutrauma and hypocapnia. Complications such as obstruction of the ETT, pneumothorax, or pulmonary hemorrhagic edema may occur with surfactant. Pulmonary hemorrhagic edema likely is due to the surfactant administration-associated rapid decrease in pulmonary vascular resistance and the resulting pulmonary overcirculation through the ductus arteriosus. Blood gases should be checked frequently to prevent hypocapnia, which is associated with an increased incidence of periventricular leukomalacia (PVL) in the preterm neonate.

Despite the advances attributable to prenatal steroids, surfactant, and newer modes of ventilation, RDS continues to carry significant morbidity, including the risk of chronic lung disease, which is defined as the need for supplemental oxygen or ventilatory support at 36 weeks' postmenstrual age. New strategies have evolved over recent years to improve outcomes of newborns with RDS. Given the toxicities of oxygen, as discussed earlier, efforts are being made to limit exposure of preterm infants to hyperoxia. Many centers now aim to keep the oxygen saturation percent in the 80s or low 90s for preterm babies to prevent periods of hyperoxygenation and free-radical production. Although the data are scant and not well controlled, no current evidence suggests adverse neurologic effects of the lower saturations. However, it is recommended that saturations be kept in the high 90s once an infant's corrected gestational age reaches near-term. Future studies must be designed to investigate the potential side effects of lower saturations, including the development of pulmonary hypertension and subsequent cor pulmonale during infancy or early childhood.

Another recent change in neonatal practice has been the adoption of permissive hypercapnia. Permissive hypercapnia involves allowing CO_2 levels in the blood to rise above the normal value of 40 mm Hg in order to minimize the pressures required for ventilation and thereby reduce the lung injury caused by ventilator-induced barotrauma and volutrauma. This practice allows for infants to remain extubated who might have been reintubated in the past because of CO_2 retention. Although the procedure differs, CO_2 levels of 45–55 mm Hg are generally accepted, with some centers allowing higher CO_2 levels without a change in ventilatory management. The side effects of this approach are unknown, but hypercapnia may decrease the autoregulatory capacity of cerebral vessels, resulting in a more-or-less pressure-passive cerebral circulation. Therefore, the potential long-term neurodevelopmental effects of hypercapnia-associated pressure-passive cerebral circulation require investigation.

Encouraged by data from nonrandomized studies at Columbia University, many neonatologists are now trying to avoid intubation and/or mechanical ventilation, even in the tiniest babies. Using CPAP with nasal prongs for newborns with respiratory distress soon after birth (regardless of gestational age or birth weight) and a strategy of permissive hypercapnia, physicians at Columbia University reported a low incidence of bronchopulmonary dysplasia (BPD) compared to other tertiary care centers, without any significant increase in mortality. Because these findings require confirmation in appropriately designed randomized clinical trials, some centers have chosen an intermediate approach: VLBW infants are intubated for surfactant administration, but the ETT is removed shortly after and the period of mechanical ventilation is brief. Although approaches differ, early extubation is now a widely shared goal among neonatologists.

Dexamethasone was a key part of efforts to prevent and/or treat BPD for many years. However, a number of studies have shown a worse neurodevelopmental outcome in preterm infants who received dexamethasone treatment compared to controls with a similar degree of illness in the neonatal period. Many studies are still in progress, and data on long-term outcomes are not yet available, but the routine use of dexamethasone is no longer recommended. Dexamethasone is now reserved for those patients with the most severe lung disease al-though, in general, no data support a better pulmonary outcome with its use. The available data suggest that there may be a window for dexamethasone use at 7–14 postnatal days, categorized as "moderately early" treatment, which has not been seen to cause any adverse outcomes. However, as mentioned earlier, a significant direct benefit associated with the use of dexamethasone is not available. Steroids also are now usually given in lower doses and shorter courses than in the past. The AAP currently recommends that neonatologists counsel parents about the risks and benefits of dexamethasone prior to initiating treatment. Future studies are needed to evaluate the effect, if any, of the newer treatment regimens on neurodevelopment outcome.

Nutrition

Providing optimal nutrition is an essential and challenging part of the care of the premature baby. Preterm infants are born with minimal nutrient stores and high metabolic demands, and growth failure is a frequent complication of prematurity. Supplying adequate nutrition for growth and development is complicated by the fact that many preterm newborns are too unstable to receive enteral nutrition in the first few days of postnatal life. There may be clear contraindications to enteral feeding, such as hypotension and vasopressor requirements, or factors can arise that can raise concerns about early initiation of enteral feeds, such as cocaine exposure in utero, indomethacin administration, the presence of a patent ductus arteriosus (PDA), or respiratory instability. Parenteral hyperalimentation is used to meet the newborn's initial fluid and nutritional requirements, but the ultimate goal is to meet those needs with enteral feedings given as early as safely possible.

An IV infusion of 10% glucose typically is started soon after birth to maintain glucose homeostasis. Extremely-low-birth-weight (ELBW) babies (birth weight < 1000 g) may require lower concentrations of dextrose because of higher total fluid requirements. Calcium supplementation in the dextrose infusion is standard for VLBW babies because transfer of calcium from mother to fetus primarily occurs during the third trimester, so VLBW babies are born with inadequate stores. The infusion rate of fluids typically is begun at 80–120 cc/kg/d depending on the immaturity and severity of illness of the neonate. Excessive fluids should be avoided because they have been associated with an increased risk for RDS, PDA, intraventricular hemorrhage (IVH), and necrotizing enterocolitis (NEC). Electrolytes and fluid status must be closely monitored over the first few days of life to determine appropriate fluid management. Depending on the level of immaturity, prenatal steroid exposure, and ambient humidity, ELBW infants may have enormous insensible losses and may develop hypernatremia if fluid needs are not met.

Protein breakdown can begin within the first post-natal days in preterm infants receiving only dextrose-containing fluids as nutrition. As a result, protein supplementation should be started as soon as possible to prevent a catabolic state. Parenteral hyperalimentation containing amino acids can be safely initiated immediately after delivery without development of acidosis, hyperammonemia, or uremia. The amino acid infusion should be started at 1.5–2 g/kg/d and advanced over several days to a goal of 3–4 g/kg/d.

Preterm newborns typically require a glucose infusion rate (GIR) of 6–8 mg/kg/min. The GIR is advanced in small increments to provide additional calories. Carbohydrate should account for approximately 40% of the 90–120 kcal/kg/d provided to the neonatal patient receiving parenteral nutrition. (Caloric requirements are higher with enteral feeding, typically 120–150 kcal/kg/d.) The need for GIR in excess of 15–18 mg/kg/min for adequate caloric support is rare. Glucose levels should be monitored and the dextrose infusion adjusted to maintain normoglycemia (ie, plasma glucose concentration 60–160 mg/dL). An insulin infusion can be started in the unusual event that hyperglycemia persists despite restricting the GIR to 4–6 mg/kg/min to continue to provide adequate calories for growth.

Intralipids provide the essential fatty acids required for multiple physiologic processes. Ideally, 40–50% of the daily caloric intake for a preterm infant receiving parenteral nutrition should come from fat. Usually a continuous 20% infusion at 0.5–1 g/kg/d is started on the first or second day of life, with the ultimate goal of providing 3 g/kg/d. Triglyceride and cholesterol levels must be monitored closely; elevated levels may require lower levels of lipid supplementation. Lipid infusion of 0.5–1 g/kg/d is required to prevent essential fatty acid deficiency.

In addition to providing protein, glucose, and fats, parenteral hyperalimentation provides electrolytes, vitamins, and minerals for the preterm infant unable to tolerate enteral feeds. Electrolyte levels must be monitored periodically to ensure appropriate levels. Particular attention must be paid to providing maximal amounts of calcium and phosphorous to VLBW infants who are at risk for developing osteopenia of prematurity.

It is important to begin enteral feeds as soon as possible in preterm infants. Delayed enteral feeding has adverse effects on the gut, such as mucosal atrophy, decreased digestive enzyme activity, and altered intestinal motility. In addition, long term parenteral nutrition can cause cholestasis and presents an increased risk of infection because of the prolonged need for central venous access. Regimens for initiation of enteral feeding in VLBW infants vary but usually involve starting volumes of 10–20 cc/kg/d. Feeds are given via an orogastric or nasogastric tube for all but the most mature infants. The infant is monitored carefully for signs of feeding intolerance, such as abdominal distention, emesis, or large-volume gastric residuals while the feed volume is increased daily by 10–20 cc/kg. Some centers continue small-volume feeds for 5–10 days before advancing the volume toward the ultimate goal of 140–160 cc/kg/d.

Mothers of preterm infants should be encouraged to breastfeed. Although preterm infants almost always are unable to feed from the breast and perhaps are not able to receive any breast milk at all during the first postnatal days, preterm infants still ultimately will benefit by receiving breast milk. The advantages of breastfeeding on everything from the appropriate function of the immune system to developmental outcomes and IQ are well documented. The caloric value of human milk clearly has proved to be superior to formula, and it is the most easily digested form of infant nutrition. Many NICUs now use pasteurized human breast milk banks to provide these benefits to infants whose mothers are unable to breastfeed. Human milk fortifiers are used to increase the protein, calories, calcium, phosphorous, vitamins, and minerals of mature human milk in order to meet the needs of the growing premature infant. Breastfed infants should receive iron supplements once they reach the goal volume of enteral feeds.

Special formulas have been designed to better meet the nutritional needs of preterm infants receiving formula. Premature infant formulas contain 24 kcal/oz and provide higher amounts of protein, medium-chain triglycerides, vitamins, and minerals (eg, calcium and phosphorous) than standard formulas. If needed for adequate growth, the caloric content of preterm formula can be increased with any of a number of commercially available supplements, the majority of which provide additional calories as carbohydrate or fat. Although term infants gain an average of 30 g/d, 15–20 g/d is considered sufficient growth in the preterm infant.

Necrotizing Enterocolitis

NEC is a significant cause of morbidity and mortality in neonates. Although gastrointestinal in origin, NEC may lead to septic shock, respiratory failure, and death. Only 10% of cases occur in term newborns. The most premature and smallest infants are disproportionately affected; NEC occurs in 5–10% of all VLBW infants.

The presentation of NEC is highly variable. Signs and symptoms often are specific to the gastrointestinal tract, such as abdominal distention and/or erythema, emesis, bilious gastric residuals, and bloody stools; however, they may be nonspecific, such as apnea, temperature instability, and lethargy. Findings may be subtle initially, or the onset may be fulminant. Acidosis and thrombocytopenia are worrisome findings that may indicate necrotic bowel. Hyponatremia, due to upregulated sodium transport into the gut, and edema, due to increased capillary leak, often develop. Respiratory distress develops from abdominal competition due to inflammation and distention. The pathognomonic feature of NEC is the presence of intestinal pneumatosis on abdominal x-ray. Pneumatosis results from the production of hydrogen from bacteria in the bowel wall. Serial x-rays are obtained to follow disease progression. Air in the portal venous system or free air in the abdominal cavity indicates intestinal perforation, warranting surgical intervention for either an exploratory laparotomy to resect the necrotic bowel or placement of a right lower quadrant drain to decompress the abdomen if the patient is very small or unstable. Whether or not perforation has occurred, treatment of NEC includes at least 14 days of broad-spectrum antibiotics and discontinuation of enteral feeds, usually for 14 days. Many infants require fluid resuscitation and vasopressor/inotrope support. Seventy-five percent of infants with NEC survive, but half sustain long-term complications such as intestinal strictures and short gut syndrome.

Prematurity and enteral feeds have been clearly linked to NEC, but the pathogenesis of NEC is not well defined and is widely considered to be multifactorial. An infectious component is suggested by the association of certain organisms with outbreaks of NEC and the immature immune function of the preterm gastrointestinal tract. Mucosal injury as a result of altered intestinal and/or mucosal blood flow, either during periods of ischemia from hypotension or vascular spasm or during reperfusion and free-radical production, is believed to make the infant vulnerable. The presence of bacteria, ischemia and reperfusion, formula, and other unknown factors may all work together to trigger the inflammatory cascade responsible for the pathologic findings of NEC.

Risk factors for NEC include ELBW, polycythemia, umbilical catheters, enteral feeding, formula feeding, low Apgar scores, cyanotic heart disease, in utero cocaine exposure, and the presence of a PDA. Data on whether or not the rate of advancement of enteral feeds contributes to the development of NEC are conflicting. However, a recent study showed a decreased incidence of NEC in VLBW neonates who received small-volume feeds for 10 days before advancement compared to those who received daily 20 cc/kg advancement of feeds. The incidence of NEC has also been shown to decrease when standardized feeding regimens are instituted within a unit. The effect may be due to heightened awareness of signs and symptoms of feeding intolerance rather than to the actual specific regimen, but the effect has been reproduced and is dramatic.

NEC occurs less frequently in infants who receive breast milk. The protective effect of breast milk is speculated to result from the transfer of components of breast milk such as cytokines, immunoglobulins, growth factors, and probiotics to the infant. Recent studies have shown a decreased incidence and severity of NEC in VLBW neonates who received supplementation with probiotic bacte-ria such as lactobacillus acidophilus, *Bifidobacterium* spp., and *Streptococcus thermophilus*. However, further studies are needed to examine the safety of probiotics given recent reports of sepsis due to supplemented probiotic organisms. Antenatal steroids also have a protective effect against NEC, likely due to a demonstrated effect on gastrointestinal maturation and PDA closure.

Patent Ductus Arteriosus

During fetal life, close to 90% of the blood that leaves the right ventricle flows from the pulmonary artery to the aorta through the ductus arteriosus. After birth the pulmonary pressure falls, blood flow to the lungs increases, and the ductus arteriosus, primarily as a response to the increased oxygen tension in the blood and decreased circulating levels of prostaglandin E_2 (PGE_2), begins to close. Functional closure of the ductus arteriosus occurs within the first 1–2 days of postnatal life in the vast majority of term neonates, and definitive anatomic closure of the ductus usually is complete by the end of the first postnatal week. However, in neonates born prematurely this process takes longer and may not always occur. In preterm neonates, failure of the ductus arteriosus to close is the result of several factors, including persistent hypoxia as a result of RDS and the continued presence of PGE_2. A PDA may be asymptomatic initially, but as the pulmonary pressure continues to fall, the left-to-right shunt of blood through the ductus arteriosus increases. Increasing left-to-right shunt produces pulmonary overcirculation (often with > 50% of the left ventricular output shunting back into the lungs), worsening respiratory distress and gas exchange, an increasing oxygen requirement, and systemic hypotension. The presence of a PDA is suggested on physical examination by a hyperdynamic precordium (left ventricular overload), bounding palmar and brachial pulses, and a holosystolic precordial murmur. The pulse pressure usually is wide, and CXR typically demonstrates cardiomegaly and pulmonary congestion. Unless contraindications such as renal insufficiency, active bleeding, or thrombocytopenia are present, indomethacin, a nonselective inhibitor of the cyclooxygenase enzyme, is the first-line treatment of PDA because indomethacin effectively decreases prostaglandin synthesis. Indomethacin also has certain actions not directly related to inhibition of prostaglandin synthesis, such as a drug-induced decrease in global cerebral blood flow. This action may contribute to the indomethacin-induced decrease in severe IVH observed in ELBW neonates given indomethacin shortly after birth. However, there appears to be no significant long-term neurodevelopmental benefit of prophylactic indomethacin administration. In neonates with a PDA, fluids should be restricted to prevent worsening of pulmonary edema. Indomethacin may fail to achieve closure of the ductus, particularly in those who were born most prematurely or who received therapy later in postnatal life (beyond 10–14 days). Persistent patency of the ductus typically requires a repeat course of indomethacin followed by surgical ligation of the ductus, depending on the patient's age and clinical status.

Intraventricular Hemorrhage

IVH is one of the most feared complications of prematurity; severe IVH is a major risk for adverse long-term neurodevelopmental outcome. The incidence of IVH (approximately 20% in VLBW infants) is inversely proportional to gestational age. A number of factors combine to put the preterm neonate at risk. The blood vessels in the periventricular germinal matrix are abundant, immature, and fragile. These vessels may bleed when exposed to changes in blood flow. Sick newborns often experience periods of hypotension and hypertension, and they lack effective autoregulatory mechanisms to protect the brain during these variations in perfusion pressure. Changes in carbon dioxide levels in the blood also play an important role in regulating cerebral blood flow, and VLBW newborns may swing from hypocarbia to hypercarbia and back, particularly during the first few hours of life. In addition, bleeding may be aggravated by abnormal coagulation, particularly in the septic newborn.

Most IVH occurs during the first postnatal day; a few cases occur after 5 days of life. Recent findings suggest that, at least in the VLBW neonate, IVH during the transitional period is caused by an ischemia–reperfusion cycle. Although IVH usually occurs without any clear outward signs that the process is occurring, a large bleed may cause a sudden change in mental status, a drop in hematocrit (Hct) level, and a full fontanelle. IVH is characterized as grade I when hemorrhage is confined to the region of the germinal matrix. Grade II IVH involves both the germinal matrix and the ventricles but does not fill or distend the ventricles. IVH grades I and II usually are not associated with a poor neurologic outcome and generally resolve. Grade III IVH fills greater than 50% of the ventricles with blood and causes distention of the ventricles. Grade III IVH carries a significantly increased risk of mortality and adverse neurologic outcome because it more frequently evolves into ex vacuo or obstructive (fibrosis obstructs the ventricular system) hydrocephalus. IVH is classified as grade IV when the hemorrhage involves the brain parenchyma. This hemorrhage historically was considered to be an extension of IVH into the parenchyma but may more accurately represent a distinct process of venous infarction or severe ischemia followed by reperfusion in the periventricular white matter. Irrespective of the etiology, intraparenchymal hemorrhage results in tissue destruction and is associated with neurodevelopmental deficits in a marked majority of affected patients.

Although numerous preventative therapies have been evaluated (indomethacin, phenobarbital, vitamin E, morphine), none is currently recommended for routine prophylactic use. Every effort is made to keep blood pressure and carbon dioxide levels stable and within the normal range and to avoid unnecessary interventions, such as suctioning, which elevate intracranial pressure. Current guidelines recommend cranial ultrasound screening between postnatal days 7 and 14 days for infants less than 30 weeks' gestation and again when the infant reaches a corrected gestational age between 36 and 40 weeks. However, detection of IVH mandates repeated studies to follow the bleed for progression and the ventricles for further dilation. Performing an ultrasound study earlier in life for newborns who are particularly unstable often is useful; the presence of a significant intraparenchymal bleed may help with decisions about direction of care for those whose viability is in question. Many centers advocate brain MRI prior to discharge to evaluate for white matter injury that may go undetected on cranial ultrasound and has been shown to be predictive of significant neurologic sequelae.

Retinopathy of Prematurity

Retinopathy of prematurity (ROP) is a disorder of retinal vascular proliferation that primarily affects premature infants. It is the second most common cause of blindness in children in the United States. Under normal conditions, the retina is completely vascularized by 36–40 weeks of gestation. The earlier in gestation delivery occurs, the larger the avascular region of the retina and the greater the risk for ROP. The pathogenesis of ROP is not completely clear but seems to involve a period of vessel damage (from acidosis, hyperoxia, infection) and cessation of vessel development followed by abnormal proliferation. Hyperoxia and/or fluctuations in PaO_2 have been clearly shown to have an adverse effect on retinal development.

VLBW neonates, especially those who are critically ill and were born before 28 weeks' completed gestation, are at the highest risk for ROP. ROP tends to develop at 33 to 36 weeks' corrected gestation irrespective of the gestational age at birth. It may resolve spontaneously, as occurs on over 80–90% of cases, or it may progress to complete retinal detachment. Screening ophthalmologic examinations are recommended for infants born at less than 28 weeks' gestation or weighing less than 1500 g, or weighing 1500–2000 g but with an unstable course, to monitor the progression of retinal vascularization. The initial examination should be performed at 4–6 weeks of life or 31–33 weeks' corrected gestational age, whichever comes later. The frequency of repeat examinations is dictated by the findings, with the goal being early detection of ROP that meets criteria for surgical intervention.

PATHOLOGY AND CARE OF THE HIGH-RISK TERM NEONATE

Persistent Pulmonary Hypertension

During fetal life, oxygenated blood is delivered to the fetus from the placenta. Pulmonary vascular resistance is elevated in utero; consequently minimal blood flow goes to the lungs. Instead, as noted in PDA, close to 90% of the output from the right ventricle passes from the pulmonary artery to the aorta through the ductus arteriosus. However, successful transition from fetal to extrauterine life requires a drop in pulmonary vascular resistance. The fall in pulmonary pressures results from a series of events that begins before birth but accelerates when a baby is born, the baby cries (filling the lungs with air), and the umbilical cord is cut. A number of processes can interrupt this process, either by mechanically blocking the airways, thus preventing essential lung expansion and increase in the partial pressure of oxygen, or by preventing relaxation of the pulmonary vascular bed. Meconium aspiration syndrome, asphyxia, sepsis, pneumonia, and CDH are among the most common causes of persistently elevated pulmonary vascular resistance, termed *persistent pulmonary hypertension of the newborn* (PPHN).

PPHN results in severe hypoxia in the newborn. Blood continues to shunt away from the pulmonary circulation through the foramen ovale, ductus arteriosus, or both, bringing poorly saturated blood to the body. Treatment consists of interventions aimed at lowering the pulmonary vascular resistance. Acidosis and hypoxemia are potent pulmonary vasoconstrictors and are avoided. When possible, PaO_2 is maintained in the normal range (80–100 mm Hg). Supplemental oxygen is weaned cautiously because even relatively small changes can cause an acute decompensation. Every effort should be made to maintain left ventricular output and blood pressure (thus systemic perfusion) in the normal range and to keep the blood pH in the 7.3–7.4 range. Acidosis is to be avoided, but aggressive use of bicarbonate or Tham may not be beneficial. Although hyperventilation was used in the past to maintain an alkaline pH, concerns about ventilator-induced lung damage and the effect of hypocarbia on cerebral blood flow have altered this practice. In addition, studies have shown that it is the normalized pH, not the decreased CO_2, that improves pulmonary vasoconstriction. Most physicians adjust the ventilator support to target a $PaCO_2$ of 40–50. High-frequency ventilators are often used, allowing for higher mean airway pressures without increasing barotrauma and volutrauma to the lungs. Vasopressors, typically dopamine, are used to maintain systemic blood pressure. If there is evidence of myocardial dysfunction, an inotrope such as dobutamine typically is used, and vasopressor support is adjusted to prevent undesirable increases in systemic vascular resistance. Patients with PPHN are extremely sensitive to noise and tactile stimulation, so infusions of sedatives and analgesia are routinely used to minimize agitation. However, use of neuromuscular blockade is to be avoided because it does not appear to improve clinical outcome and is associated with significant side effects, including sensorineural hearing loss.

Nitric oxide is a selective pulmonary vasodilator. Inhaled nitric oxide (iNO) reduces the need for extracorporeal membrane oxygenation (ECMO) in term infants with PPHN. iNO is routinely started at 20 ppm, although lower doses may be as effective iNO is weaned as the patient stabilizes and the supplemental oxygen requirement falls. Despite the dramatic improvement in outcomes since the availability of iNO, a number of patients with PPHN still will require ECMO. Historically the criterion for ECMO has been a greater than 80% estimated risk of mortality with continued conventional medical management. General guidelines for the criteria for ECMO include an oxygenation index greater than 35–60 for between 0.5 and 6 hours, an alveolar–arterial oxygen difference greater than 605–620 (at sea level) for 4–12 hours, or a preductal PaO_2 less than 40 for more than 2 hours. ECMO is contraindicated in neonates less than 34 weeks' gestational age because of technical issues regarding catheter placement as well as the increased risk of intracranial bleeding in the preterm neonate. A preexisting grade II or higher IVH, signs of severe irreversible brain damage, lethal congenital anomalies, and nonreversible pulmonary disease are other contraindications to ECMO. Survival of patients with PPHN treated with ECMO varies depending on the underlying cause of PPHN. The survival rate of patients with meconium aspiration syndrome is 85–90%, but the survival rate of patients with CDH is only 50%.

Congenital Diaphragmatic Hernia

CDH is a defect that results from incomplete development and closure of the diaphragm, usually at the foramen of Bochdalek at 8–10 weeks' gestation. The defect in the diaphragm allows the contents of the abdominal cavity to migrate into the chest, resulting in compression of the lungs and, in more severe cases, the heart. The compression leads to pulmonary hypoplasia, abnormal lung development, and potentially underdevelopment of one or both ventricles. Ninety percent of CDH involves the left hemidiaphragm. CDH usually is prenatally diagnosed, but a number of cases still go undiagnosed, even with good prenatal care.

A number of features should raise suspicion about the possibility of CDH in the newborn with cyanosis and respiratory distress. Breath sounds may be absent on the left side of the chest and the heart sounds shifted to the right. The abdomen tends to be scaphoid, as some of the abdominal organs have shifted into the thorax. It may be difficult to effectively ventilate and resuscitate the patient. If a CDH is suspected, mask and bag ventilation must be avoided. The patient should be intubated and a nasogastric tube placed as soon as possible to prevent filling the stomach and bowel with air and thus compromising ventilation further. Many centers use sedation and sometimes paralysis to minimize activity, reduce the risk of pneumothorax, and prevent competition from swallowed air. CXR observation of bowel loops in the chest confirms the diagnosis

Surgical repair of the defect usually is delayed for several days to allow time for the patient's condition to stabilize and pulmonary hypertension to improve. Efforts are made to use the lowest ventilator settings tolerated to minimize ventilator-induced lung injury. Surfactant, iNO, high-frequency ventilation, and, if necessary, ECMO are often used to manage patients with CDH. However, surfactant administration has been shown to be of no benefit, and some studies suggest that it may be associated with an increased need for ECMO, so its routine use cannot be recommended. To date, the evidence also has not shown a clear benefit of iNO for patients with CDH. Additional studies are needed to evaluate the role of each of these interventions in the care of the patient with CDH.

Reported survival rates vary from approximately 35–80%, perhaps reflecting differences between centers and/or bias related to referral patterns. The prognosis depends on the severity of the pulmonary hypertension and underlying pulmonary hypoplasia as well as the presence of other anomalies or a chromosomal abnormality. Development of a pneumothorax has been shown to predict a poor outcome. Failure to achieve a preductal PaO_2 greater than 100 mm Hg or a $PaCO_2$ lower than 60 in the first 24 hours of life generally indicates a poor prognosis as well. Some physicians argue that infants in whom the $PaCO_2$ level never falls below 60 or who never achieve a preductal oxygen saturation of at least 85% for at least 1 hour have severe pulmonary hypoplasia and are not appropriate candidates for ECMO. However, the outcome of the individual patient is hard to predict, and every measure must be made to provide gentle ventilation and accept higher $PaCO_2$ and lower PaO_2 levels as long as systemic oxygen delivery is appropriate.

Transient Tachypnea of the Newborn

The differential diagnosis for the newborn with tachypnea in the first postnatal hours ranges from RDS to sepsis to CHD. One of the most common, and benign, causes of tachypnea in the newborn is transient tachypnea of the newborn (TTN). TTN results when fetal lung fluid production fails to cease with the onset of labor. The newborn presents with tachypnea, increased work of breathing, and cyanosis. Moderate supplemental oxygen may be required. CXR reveals interstitial and alveolar edema; fluid is characteristically seen in the right middle lobe fissure. Symptoms of TTN typically resolve over the first 24 hours without

intervention (fetal lung fluid production ceases in response to stress), and CXR clears by the second or third day of life. However, TTN is a diagnosis of exclusion, and other causes of tachypnea and respiratory distress must be ruled out. An evaluation for sepsis (including initiation of antibiotic therapy pending culture results) as well as other causes of tachypnea is generally warranted.

Congenital Heart Disease

CHD occurs in approximately 1 in 100 live births, and approximately 3 in 1000 have CHD that requires surgical repair or results in death within the first year of life. CHD rarely presents in the delivery room. In fact, the majority of infants with prenatally diagnosed CHD initially appear well. Nevertheless, the newborn with cyanosis that fails to respond to oxygen should be evaluated for structural heart disease. Complex CHD typically presents as cyanosis or congestive heart failure and circulatory shock and only rarely as an asymptomatic murmur in a newborn. Signs such as tachypnea, weak peripheral pulses, or cool extremities may develop quickly with closure of the ductus arteriosus if the lesion has ductal-dependent pulmonary or systemic flow. Right-sided obstructive lesions (eg, pulmonic atresia or stenosis), which are dependent on the ductus for pulmonary blood flow, tend to present with cyanosis due to diminished or absent pulmonary blood flow. Left-sided obstructive lesions (eg, coarctation of the aorta and hypoplastic left heart syndrome) typically present as shock and often are initially misdiagnosed as sepsis. However, statistically the term neonate who develops signs of shock after the first 24–48 hours of life is approximately 5 times more likely to have ductal-dependent CHD than bacterial sepsis.

The initial steps in evaluating a stable patient for suspected CHD include 4-extremity blood pressure measurements, measurement of preductal and post-ductal saturations, electrocardiogram, CXR, and hyperoxia test. If the PaO_2 level fails to increase above 100 after exposure to 100% FiO_2 for 15 minutes, cyanotic CHD is likely; if the PaO_2 level increases above 250, CHD is unlikely. CXR may reveal black lungs that signify diminished pulmonary blood flow (as occurs in right-sided obstructive lesions) or congestion (as occurs with obstructed pulmonary venous return). The diagnosis of CHD usually is established by echocardiogram, although cardiac catheterization is sometimes necessary to clarify the specifics of the abnormal anatomy in complex cases. Low-dose PGE infusion should be started when critical CHD is suspected in order to maintain or reestablish ductal patency Once the diagnosis of cyanotic heart disease has been made, supplemental oxygen should be used sparingly but as necessary to keep oxygen saturations around 75–85% until surgical repair occurs. This supplementation should provide adequate oxygen delivery to prevent the development of metabolic acidosis without decreasing pulmonary vascular resistance and causing pulmonary overcirculation.

Esophageal Atresia/ Tracheoesophageal Fistula

Esophageal atresia occurs when there is an interruption in the separation of the foregut into the trachea and esophagus during the fourth week of gestation. In its most common form, there is a proximal esophageal pouch and a fistula between the trachea and the distal segment of the esophagus. The newborn with esophageal atresia typically presents in the first few hours after birth with copious secretions and coughing or gagging with the first feed. Respiratory distress may develop if secretions or feeds are aspirated. The prenatal history often is remarkable for polyhydramnios due to the inability of the fetus to regulate amniotic fluid levels by swallowing. The diagnosis usually is apparent when a CXR reveals a nasogastric tube coiled in the proximal esophageal pouch. Absence of a gastric bubble on x-ray usually suggests that a distal fistula is not present. Emergent gastrostomy may be necessary to decompress the stomach. The feasibility of primary repair depends on the distance between the proximal and distal portions of the esophagus. If primary repair is not possible, initial surgery involves ligation of the fistula. Patients typically then undergo serial dilations of the proximal pouch and delayed anastomosis or may require colonic interposition if the gap remains too wide to close. Postoperative complications include leaking or stenosis at the anastomosis site, poor esophageal motility, and gastroesophageal reflux.

Polycythemia

Polycythemia, defined as a central venous Hct greater than 65%, results from either increased in utero erythropoiesis or from maternofetal or twin-twin transfusion. Increased in utero erythropoiesis occurs most often as a response to fetal hypoxia, usually from placental insufficiency. Erythropoiesis in the fetus is also increased with maternal diabetes, chromosomal abnormalities, and endocrine disorders such as congenital adrenal hyperplasia, thyroid disease, and Beckwith-Wiedemann syndrome. Maternofetal hemorrhage must commonly results from delayed cord clamping.

Polycythemia may cause congestive heart failure from volume overload, as in the case of the recipient twin in twin-twin transfusion syndrome. More commonly, the complications attributed to polycythemia arise from hyperviscosity rather than increased blood volume. Blood viscosity increases as the Hct level rises, placing the polycythemic infant at risk for complications from impaired blood flow and oxygen delivery. Polycythemia may present as hypoglycemia, poor feeding, respiratory distress, pulmonary hypertension, lethargy, jitteriness, or seizures. Infants are at increased risk for NEC, and thrombotic strokes may occur.

Although IV hydration may be useful, a symptomatic neonate with Hct level greater than 65% or an asymptomatic neonate with Hct level greater than 70% should undergo a partial exchange transfusion performed to decrease blood viscosity and ameliorate any symptoms. The volume of blood that should be removed and then replaced with isotonic saline (to lower the viscosity without causing hypovolemia) is determined by the following formula:

$$\text{Exchange volume} = \frac{\text{Observed Hct} - \text{Goal Hct}}{\text{Observed Hct}} \times \text{Blood volume (cc/kg)} \times \text{Weight (kg)}$$

Blood volume usually is estimated at 100 cc/kg. The goal Hct usually is 55%. The hope is that partial exchange will prevent symptoms from worsening and further complications from developing, but long-term follow-up studies have failed to show any benefit.

Hyperbilirubinemia

Hyperbilirubinemia is a common problem in the neonatal period, affecting 60–70% of all infants born in the United States to some degree. In most instances, the level of the unconjugated form of bilirubin is elevated. Although the course usually is benign and an increase in serum bilirubin level occurs in all newborns during the first postnatal days, severe unconjugated hyperbilirubinemia can cause kernicterus and long-term neurologic damage.

Bilirubin is produced when heme-containing compounds such as hemoglobin are broken down. The initial unconjugated product is fat soluble but water insoluble, a form that can cross the blood–brain barrier and cause central nervous system toxicity but cannot be excreted. The blood carries bilirubin to the liver, where it is conjugated to a water-soluble and excretable form by the enzyme glucuronyl transferase. The immature hepatic enzyme function in the newborn impairs bilirubin conjugation and thus excretion. The shorter life span of red blood cells and increased red cell mass in neonates further predispose the newborn to elevated plasma concentrations of bilirubin, as does the increased reabsorption of bilirubin that occurs in the sterile newborn intestinal tract.

Hyperbilirubinemia may be severe when other coexisting factors increase hemolysis, decrease the rate of bilirubin conjugation, or impede excretion. Hemolysis is increased by abnormal red cell enzyme function (glucose-6-phophate dehydrogenase [G6PD] deficiency, less frequently pyruvate kinase deficiency) or morphology (spherocytosis, elliptocytosis) and isoimmunization due to ABO, minor antigen, or Rh incompatibility. Sepsis can increase hemolysis. A number of inborn errors of metabolism and enzyme defects can impair conjugation. Conjugation is impaired when there is delayed maturation of the conjugating enzymes, as is thought to occur in cases of congenital hypothyroidism.

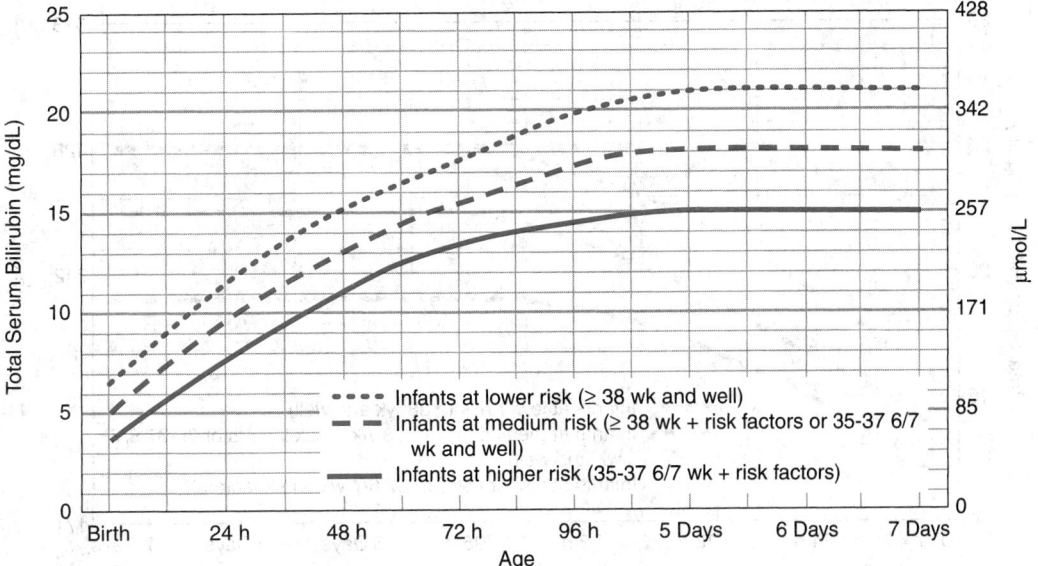

• Use total bilirubin. Do not subtract direct reacting or conjugated bilirubin.
• Risk factors = isoimmune hemolytic disease, G6PD deficiency, asphyxia, significant lethargy, temperature instability, sepsis, acidosis, or albumin < 3.0g/dL (if measured).
• For well infants 35–37 6/7 wk can adjust TSB levels for intervention around the medium risk line. It is an option to intervene at lower TSB levels for infants closer to 35 wks and at higher TSB levels for those closer to 37 6/7 wk.
• It is an option to provide conventional phototherapy in hospital or at home at TSB levels 2-3 mg/dL (35-50 mmol/L) below those shown but home phototherapy should not be used in any infant with risk factors.

Figure 32–6. Guidelines for phototherapy in hospitalized infants of 35 or more weeks' gestation.

Obstructed biliary flow, as in biliary atresia, and gastrointestinal obstruction cause decreased excretion. Many disease states are associated with hyperbilirubinemia.

Hyperbilirubinemia presents clinically as jaundice, a yellow–green discoloration of the skin and mucous membranes. A serum bilirubin level should be checked in all jaundiced newborns. It is standard policy in some nurseries to check a total serum bilirubin (TSB) level in all newborns prior to discharge. Most centers check a level within 24–48 hours of life in all VLBW infants as risk for sequelae from hyperbilirubinemia is believed to exist at lower serum bilirubin concentrations in preterm neonates. The etiology of the hyperbilirubinemia must be sought. A blood type, Coombs' test, Hct level, and reticulocyte count will provide important information, as will the parent's ethnicity, maternal blood type, and history of jaundice in siblings. It is important to determine whether it is the level of conjugated or unconjugated fraction of bilirubin that is elevated. The differential diagnosis, evaluation, and treatment are markedly different depending on whether or not the elevated portion is conjugated. A conjugated bilirubin level greater than 10% of the total value should prompt an investigation for biliary obstruction or causes of hepatocellular

damage such as TORCH (toxoplasmosis, other agents, rubella, cytomegalovirus, herpes simplex) infection, galactosemia and α_1-antitrypsin deficiency. A complete sepsis work-up is indicated in the ill-appearing patient.

The American Academy of Pediatrics (AAP) has established practice parameters to help direct the use of phototherapy and exchange transfusion for hyperbilirubinemia in infants of greater than 35 weeks' gestation. Phototherapy causes the photoisomerization of unconjugated bilirubin to a water-soluble form that can be excreted by the kidneys and gastrointestinal tract. Phototherapy is contraindicated for conjugated hyperbilirubinemia; it is not effective and can cause a bronze staining of the skin. Figure 32–6 shows the current AAP recommendations for initiation of phototherapy. A patient should receive phototherapy if the TSB level lies above the line for the appropriate risk group for the patient. A newborn is considered to have risk factors if any of the following are present: isoimmune hemolytic disease, G6PD deficiency, asphyxia, significant lethargy, temperature instability, sepsis, acidosis, or albumin level less than 3.0 g/dL.

Insensible losses increase under phototherapy, and liberal intravenous fluids should be given in anticipation of increased daily fluid needs. Infants who appear well, are

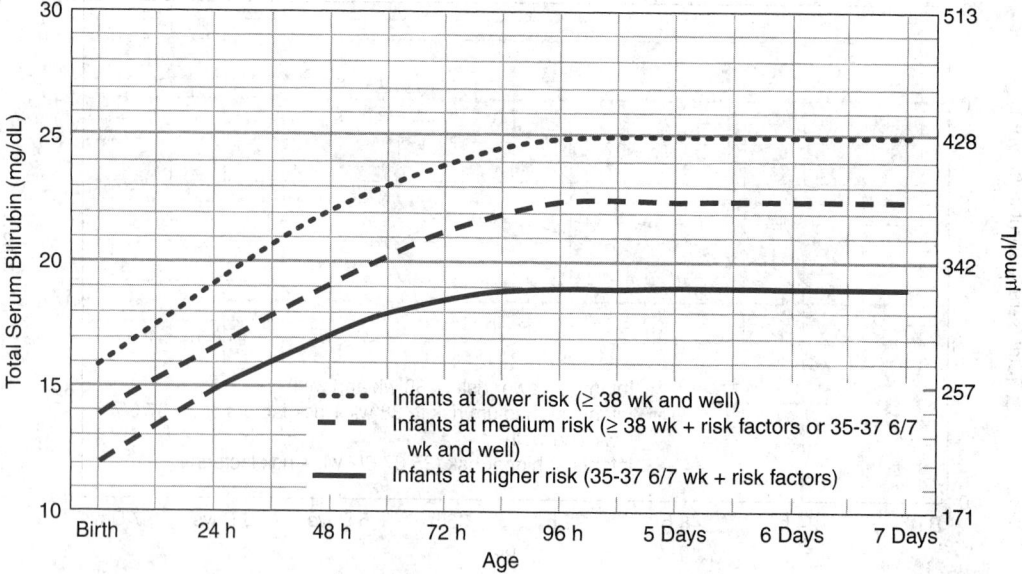

- The dashed lines for the first 24 hours indicate uncertainty due to a wide range of clinical circumstances and a range of responses to phototherapy.
- Immediate exchange transfusion is recommended if infant shows signs of acute bilirubin encephalopathy (hypertonia, arching, retrocolitis, opisthotonos, fever, high pitched cry) or if TSB is ≥5 mg/dL (85 μmol/L) above these lines.
- Risk factors—isoimmune hemolytic disease, G6PD deficiency, asphyxia, significant lethargy, temperature instability, sepsis, acidosis.
- Measure serum albumin and calculate B/A ratio.
- Use total bilirubin. Do not subtract direct reacting or conjugated bilirubin.
- If infant is well and 35-37 6/7 wk (median risk) can individualize TSB levels for exchange based on actual gestational age.

Figure 32–7. Guidelines for exchange transfusion in infants 35 or more weeks' gestation.

tolerating enteral feeds, and not likely to require an exchange transfusion should continue feeding. Enteral nutrition will increase stooling and facilitate bilirubin excretion. Intravenous fluid should be given in addition if oral intake is insufficient or if needed for adequate hydration.

Figure 32–7 shows the AAP guidelines for exchange transfusion. Exchange transfusion effectively removes bilirubin as well as anti–red cell antibodies circulating in the blood. Twice the blood volume (estimated at 85–100 cc/kg) is slowly removed from the patient in aliquots of 5–10 cc, with each aliquot followed by transfusion of an equal volume of fresh type O negative blood. The guidelines shown in Figure 32–7 are intended to apply to the newborn who has a continuous rise in TSB level despite intensive phototherapy or to a neonate readmitted to the hospital after discharge who continues to have a TSB above the exchange level for 6 hours after initiation of phototherapy. Immediate exchange is recommended if the TSB is more than 5 mg/dL greater than the exchange threshold or if the patient has abnormal findings on neurologic examination that suggest acute bilirubin encephalopathy. Complications of exchange transfusion include

hypocalcemia, hypoglycemia, hypothermia, coagulation abnormalities, apnea, and bradycardia. Many centers delay resuming oral feeds until 24–48 hours post exchange because of the increased risk of NEC after exchange.

Indications for phototherapy and exchange transfusion in preterm infants are not well established. A reasonable guideline is to begin phototherapy when the bilirubin concentration is equal to 0.5% of the birth weight (in grams) and to consider an exchange transfusion when the concentration reaches 1% of the birth weight. These numbers represent a very general guideline, however, and it is important that treatment decisions take into account the etiology of the jaundice and the patient's overall clinical status (Table 32–2). The presence of significant bruising, hemolysis, sepsis, or acidosis should lower the physician's threshold for initiating treatment.

Infection

Infection is a significant cause of morbidity and mortality in the newborn. The immature newborn immune system places the neonate at increased risk for infection. The

Table 32–2. Indirect bilirubin concentration (mg/dL).

BW (kg)	5–6	7–9	10–12	13–15	16–20	> 20
<1.0	Phototherapy		Think of exchange		Exchange transfusion	
1.0–1.5		Phototherapy		Think of exchange	Exchange transfusion	
1.5–2.0			Phototherapy		Think of exchange	Exchange transfusion
2.0–2.5				Phototherapy	Think of exchange	Exchange transfusion
> 2.5					Phototherapy	Think of exchange

Guidelines for suggested bilirubin levels for phototherapy or exchange transfusion based on birth weight (BW) and clinical course of the infant. (Reproduced, with permission, from Harvey-Wilkes K, 1993.)

preterm infant, whose immune system is markedly immature and who has diminished levels of immunoglobulin compared to the term newborn, is at particularly high risk. Typically infection is acquired when organisms ascend into the uterine cavity and come into contact with the fetus, but infection can be acquired hematogenously, from the mother's blood, or at the time of delivery when the newborn passes through the vaginal canal.

A. Sepsis

Neonatal sepsis occurs in 1 in 1000 term infants and 1 in 4 preterm infants. Risk factors for neonatal sepsis include premature delivery, multiple pregnancy, prolonged rupture of amniotic membranes (> 18 hours), maternal fever, maternal group B streptococcus (GBS) colonization, and chorioamnionitis. The most common causes of early-onset (within the first week of life) sepsis are GBS and *Escherichia coli. Listeria monocytogenes,* enterococci, and several different gram-negative rod species are other identified causes of early-onset neonatal sepsis. Late-onset infection in hospitalized infants is more often due to *Staphylococcus* spp.

Signs and symptoms of sepsis in the newborn can be very subtle and nonspecific, such as temperature instability, hypoglycemia or hyperglycemia, apnea, poor feeding, or tachypnea. In contrast, some neonates present in fulminant shock. A complete blood count and blood culture should be sent if sepsis is suspected and antibiotics should be started. A decreased or elevated white blood cell count, a predominance of immature white blood cell forms, and thrombocytopenia are suggestive of infection. Although nonspecific, an elevated C-reactive protein (CRP) level indicates the presence of an inflammatory or infectious process, and data support the value of the CRP level in the evaluation for sepsis in the neonate. In addition, CXR is indicated to evaluate for pneumonia. Often differentiating an infiltrate from atelectasis, RDS, or retained lung fluid is difficult, but serial films may be useful in differentiating the various processes. There is debate about whether a culture of cerebrospinal fluid (CSF) is necessary in the newborn evaluated for early-onset sepsis. (A CSF culture is clearly warranted in suspected late-onset sepsis because the incidence of coexisting meningitis with late-onset bacteremia is very high.) Unless signs of meningitis (eg, seizure activity or altered mental status) or a documented positive blood culture is present, meningitis is unlikely in the immediate newborn period. However, studies have reported positive CSF cultures with concurrent negative blood cultures in asymptomatic neonates. The issue has been further complicated by the current widespread use of maternal intrapartum antibiotics. Consequently, given the ramifications of failure to diagnose or only partially treatment of a case of meningitis, CSF culture is a routine part of the newborn sepsis evaluation in many institutions. Urine culture, a routine part of the sepsis evaluation for late-onset disease, is rarely useful in the first few days of life.

Antibiotics that provide broad-spectrum coverage, typically ampicillin and gentamicin in the first few days of life, should be continued for 48–72 hours pending the results of all cultures that were sent analysis. Vancomycin and gentamicin are often used for nosocomial infections. If bacteremia is documented by a positive blood culture or highly suspected based on clinical status or laboratory findings, antibiotics should be continued for 7–10 days. Intravenous antibiotics usually are continued for a minimum of 2 weeks for gram-positive meningitis and 3 weeks for gram-negative meningitis.

The Centers for Disease Control and Prevention (CDC) developed guidelines in 1996 that recommended screening for GBS colonization at 35–37 weeks' gestation. It was recommended that colonized women and those with other risk factors receive intrapartum antibiotic therapy beginning at least 4 hours prior to delivery. The incidence of early-onset GBS sepsis has been reduced by 65% in communities that have adopted the CDC GBS prevention guidelines. Currently no evidence suggests an increased incidence of non–GBS early-onset sepsis with adoption of the guidelines, as had been feared.

B. Conjunctivitis

Infection of the conjunctiva may occur within the first few weeks of life. Prophylaxis with erythromycin 0.5% ophthalmic ointment immediately after delivery is now a standard part of newborn care. Conjunctivitis usually presents with injection of the conjunctiva and discharge from the eye, usually bilaterally, in the first week of life. Erythema of the conjunctiva helps differentiate conjunctivitis from lacrimal duct obstruction, a common cause of eye discharge in the neonate.

Chlamydia trachomatis and *Neisseria gonorrhoeae* are the most notable causes of neonatal conjunctivitis. Maternal treatment of either infection during pregnancy reduces the risk of infection in the neonate. Gonococcal conjunctivitis produces a purulent discharge and may cause serious complications, including blindness. A Gram stain and culture of the discharge should be performed if there is any suspicion of infection to determine appropriate therapy. It is important to recognize that the infant with *Chlamydia* conjunctivitis may have or may develop *Chlamydia* pneumonia. *Chlamydia* pneumonia commonly presents in the first 6 weeks of life with tachypnea and cough. The infant with gonococcal conjunctivitis should receive 7 days of IV or IM treatment with a third-generation cephalosporin such as ceftriaxone. *Chlamydia* conjunctivitis is treated with oral erythromycin for 14 days.

C. VIRAL INFECTION

A number of viral infections can cause disease in the newborn. The infection may be acquired in utero or at the time of delivery. Antibody titers and cultures should be sent when congenital viral infection is suspected. A number of viruses, including cytomegalovirus (CMV), varicella, parvovirus, and toxoplasmosis, are associated with congenital infection, and the presentation varies significantly depending on the virus. Herpesvirus and enterovirus infections can present acutely with respiratory failure and/or shock. Hepatitis and coagulopathy are often seen in neonates with viral sepsis, even early in the disease process before end-organ damage is even suspected, and should raise suspicion about the possibility of a viral process. There is no maternal history of herpes simplex virus (HSV) in the majority of neonates diagnosed with HSV sepsis or encephalitis. Cultures for HSV should be sent from the asymptomatic infant born to a mother with active HSV lesions at the time of vaginal delivery. Although no clear evidence supports the practice, some experts advocate empiric therapy if the lesions are due to a primary infection. Acyclovir is used to treat herpes viruses such as HSV and varicella.

Transmission from mother to infant at birth is one of the most efficient modes of hepatitis B virus (HBV) transmission. From 80–90% of children born to mothers who are both hepatitis B surface antigen (HBsAg) and hepatitis B e antigen (HBeAg) positive will become infected, and 90% of those infants will become chronic HBV carriers. Transmission falls to less than 25% if HBeAg is negative and to 12% if anti-HBe is present. Babies born to HBsAg-positive mothers should receive hepatitis B immune globulin (HBIg) and the hepatitis B vaccine within 12 hours of delivery. If the mother's status is unknown at the time of delivery, the newborn should receive the vaccine within 12 hours of life. If the newborn weighs more than 2 kg, HBIg

can be deferred for up to 7 days to allow determination of the mother's status according to the most recent AAP *Red Book* guidelines. However, given the less reliable immune response to vaccine in the preterm host, HBIg should not be deferred in patients weighing less than 2 kg. Appropriate postexposure prophylaxis in the newborn has been shown to prevent transmission in 95% of exposures.

Perinatal infection with human immunodeficiency virus (HIV) now accounts for almost all new infections in preadolescents in the United States. The risk of perinatal transmission if a HIV-positive mother does not receive antiretroviral therapy during pregnancy is 13–39%. A trial of zidovudine during pregnancy and delivery, with continued treatment for the newborn for 6 weeks after delivery, showed a greater than 60% reduction in transmission. It is currently recommended that HIV-positive women receive zidovudine prophylaxis in addition to the standard current recommendations for antiretroviral therapy for all HIV-positive patients. Zidovudine prophylaxis/treatment of the newborn should be started and analysis for HIV DNA polymerase chain reaction sent when in utero exposure to HIV is recognized before 7 days of life.

Infant of the Diabetic Mother

From 50,000–100,000 infants are born to diabetic mothers every year in the United States. The infant of a diabetic mother (IDM) is at increased risk for congenital malformations, macrosomia, birth injury, and a number of postnatal complications, such as RDS, polycythemia, and hypoglycemia. With improved obstetric monitoring and neonatal care, perinatal mortality has decreased significantly over the past few decades. With decreased losses from stillbirths, perinatal asphyxia, and RDS, congenital malformations now represent the single most important cause of perinatal mortality and severe morbidity in IDMs.

Studies have shown that IDMs have a 2- to 8-fold higher risk of a structural malformation compared to infants born to nondiabetic mothers. The most common malformations in IDMs are neural tube defects, CHD, renal anomalies, and abnormalities of the genitourinary tract. The exact pathogenesis of the malformations is unclear, but various mechanisms, including altered levels of arachidonic acid and/or myoinositol, free-radical damage, and altered gene expression, have been proposed. The risk of structural malformations has been clearly shown to correlate with poor glycemic control in the first trimester. Consequently, tight control of glucose levels must begin prior to conception in order to decrease the risk of structural malformations.

Metabolic alterations seen in IDMs are more closely associated with glycemic control later in pregnancy. Elevated maternal glucose levels result in elevated fetal glucose levels that produce hyperinsulinism in the fetus. Insulin is a growth factor, and abnormal exposure to insulin results in fetal macrosomia. After delivery, the hyperinsulinemic state persists, but there is no longer an ongoing supply of glucose coming across the placenta and the newborn is at risk for hypoglycemia. IDMs should be closely monitored after birth to ensure that glucose requirements are met. Severe and prolonged hypoglycemia can cause significant injury to the developing brain. Poor glucose control during the second and third trimesters is associated with an increased risk for macrosomia and neonatal hypoglycemia. Other metabolic derangements frequently seen in IDMs are hypocalcemia and hypomagnesemia.

IDMs are at increased risk for RDS. Surfactant production occurs later than normal in diabetic pregnancies. Polycythemia also occurs at a higher rate. The greater red cell volume, in turn, increases the risk of hyperbilirubinemia. Hyperglycemia and the resulting hyperinsulinemia in the fetus generate a catabolic state, causing oxygen consumption. Erythropoiesis is believed to occur as a response to fetal hypoxia.

Hypertrophic cardiomyopathy is a frequent finding in IDMs. The cardiomyopathy may be asymptomatic, apparent only as cardiomegaly on CXR, or it may be clinically significant, usually as a result of left ventricular outflow tract obstruction and/or poor ventricular filling and cardiac output related to hypertrophy of the ventricular septum. The hypertrophy of the cardiac muscle resolves over time, and the only indicated treatment is supportive care.

Intrauterine Growth Restriction

Intrauterine growth restriction (IUGR) describes a pattern of aberrant and reduced fetal growth that is identified by prenatal ultrasound examinations. The growth restriction is classified as asymmetric if the head circumference, used as a marker for brain growth, is spared. IUGR refers to growth in utero, and IUGR newborns may or may not be small for gestational age (SGA). (The definition of SGA varies, but historically it has been defined as less than the 10th percentile on the growth curve.) IUGR can result from a range of processes that may originate with the fetus (chromosomal abnormalities, fetal gender, genetic inheritance, TORCH infection), the placenta (abnormal implantation or insertion of the cord, preeclampsia, placental insufficiency), or the mother (chronic disease such as diabetes, systemic lupus erythematosus, or cyanotic heart disease, smoking, abnormal uterine anatomy, low pregnancy weight gain). The etiology of IUGR in approximately 40% of patients is never determined. CMV and toxoplasmosis studies are sometimes sent for affected newborns to determine an infectious cause. However, given the number of idiopathic cases of IUGR, some have questioned the utility of sending these cultures for infants with no physical examination or imaging study findings suggestive of congenital infection. Prenatal management of the IUGR fetus is impacted by the increased risk of intrauterine demise and perinatal asphyxia with IUGR, but also requires consideration of the fact that gestational age at birth is still a major determinant

of outcome in the premature growth-restricted infant. There is currently great interest in the connection between low birth weight and the development of type 2 diabetes, hypertension, and coronary artery disease in adulthood.

The Dysmorphic Infant

It is estimated that 2% of all newborns have a serious congenital malformation. Advances in prenatal care now allow for early diagnosis of many congenital birth defects or diseases, but many are still difficult or impossible to detect in utero. Dysmorphic features and structural abnormalities may be immediately apparent, or they may be subtle and identified only upon close inspection. Every newborn should undergo a thorough examination to identify features suggestive of underlying pathology, genetic abnormalities, or specific syndromes or disorders.

Transfer of the newborn to a referral center where an evaluation by a clinical geneticist or dysmorphologist can be conducted may be warranted if abnormalities are present. The remarkable progress in our understanding of human genetics over the past decade has dramatically increased our ability to identify the genetic defects responsible for countless diseases and syndromes. In addition, each year more is understood about numerous multifactorial disorders, improving the odds that affected patients will be correctly diagnosed. A geneticist can help identify pertinent elements of the family, exposure, and prenatal history and direct a thorough but targeted radiologic and cytogenetic work-up for the newborn. It is preferable to avoid making conclusions about the diagnosis (ie, a particular syndrome or sequence) until a complete evaluation has been performed. The emotional impact of an unsuspected defect or syndrome on the new parents should not be ignored, and misinformation can only hinder the process of acceptance (Table 32–3).

Table 32–3. Elements of counseling for developmental defects.

Description of the anomalies present
Cause of the condition (if known)
Indication of the prognosis
Discussion of immediate options
Therapeutic means that may be necessary
Potential for recurrence
Mode of inheritance (if known)
Late complications to be expected
In cases of death, the autopsy findings
Thorough answering of questions
Provisions for familial emotional support

Modified and reproduced, with permission, from Pernoll ML, King CR, Prescott GH: Genetics in obstetrics and gynecology. In: Wynn RM (editor): *Obstetrics and Gynecology Annual: 1980.* Vol 9. Appleton-Century-Crofts, 1980, p. 31.

REFERENCES

Allan WC, Sobel DB: Neonatal intensive care neurology. Semin Pediatr Neurol 2004;11:119.

American Academy of Pediatrics: *AAP 2003 Red Book: Report of the Committee on Infectious Diseases,* 26th ed. American Academy of Pediatrics, 2003.

American Academy of Pediatrics, Section on Ophthalmology: Screening examination of premature infants for retinopathy of prematurity. Pediatrics 2001;108:809.

American Academy of Pediatrics, Subcommittee on Hyperbilirubinemia: Management of hyperbilirubinemia in the newborn infant 35 or more weeks of gestation. Pediatrics 2004;114:297.

American Academy of Pediatrics and American Heart Association: *Textbook of Neonatal Resuscitation,* 4th ed. American Academy of Pediatrics, 2000.

Askie LM et al: Oxygen-saturation targets and outcomes in extremely preterm infants. N Engl J Medi 2003;349:959.

Avery ME, Mead J: Surface properties in relation to atelectasis and hyaline membrane disease. Am J Dis Child 1959;97(5 Pt 1):517.

Baltimore RS et al: Early-onset neonatal sepsis in the era of group B streptococcal prevention. Pediatrics 2001;108:1094.

Berseth CL, Bisquera JA, Paje VU: Prolonging small feeding volumes early in life decreases the incidence of necrotizing enterocolitis in very low birth weight infants. Pediatrics 2003;111:529.

Bin-Nun A et al: Oral probiotics prevent necrotizing enterocolitis in very low birth weight neonates. J Pediatr 2005;147:192.

Boloker J et al: Congenital diaphragmatic hernia in 120 infants treated consecutively with permissive hypercapnia/spontaneous respiration/elective repair. J Pediatr Surg 2002;37:357.

Cifuentes J et al: Mortality in low birth weight infants according to level of neonatal care at hospital of birth. Pediatrics 2002; 109:745.

Clark RH et al: Low-dose nitric oxide therapy for persistent pulmonary hypertension of the newborn. N Engl J Med 2000;342:469.

Connor EM et al: Reduction of maternal-infant transmission of human immunodeficiency virus type 1 with zidovudine treatment. Pediatric AIDS Clinical Trials Group Protocol 076 Study Group. N Engl J Med 1994;331:1173.

Dempsey EM, Barrington KJ: Short and long term outcomes following partial exchange transfusion in the polycythemic newborn: A systematic review. Arch Dis Child Fetal Neonatal Ed 2006; 91:F2.

Halliday HL, Ehrenkranz RA, Doyle LW: Early postnatal (<96 hours) corticosteroids for preventing chronic lung disease in preterm infants. In: *The Cochrane Library. Issue 3.* John Wiley & Sons, 2004.

Halliday HL, Ehrenkranz RA, Doyle LW: Moderately early (7–14 days) postnatal corticosteroids for preventing chronic lung disease in preterm infants. In: *The Cochrane Library. Issue 3.* John Wiley & Sons, 2004.

Halliday HL, Ehrenkranz RA, Doyle LW: Delayed (>3 weeks) postnatal corticosteroids for preventing chronic lung disease in preterm infants. In: *The Cochrane Library. Issue 3.* John Wiley & Sons, 2004.

Hëller G et al: Are we regionalized enough? Early-neonatal deaths in low-risk births by the size of delivery units in Hesse, Germany 1990–1999. Int J Epidemiol 2002;31:1061.

Khan N, Khazzi S: Yield and costs of screening growth-retarded infants for TORCH infections. Am J Perinatol 2000;17:131.

Kluckow M, Evans N: Low superior vena cava flow and intraventricular hemorrhage in preterm infants. Arch Dis Child 2000;82:188.

Kunz AN, Noel JM, Fairchok MP: Two cases of Lactobacillus bacteremia during probiotic treatment of short gut syndrome. J Pediatr Gastroenterol Nutr 2004;38:457.

Lin HC et al: Oral probiotics reduce the incidence and severity of necrotizing enterocolitis in very low birth weight infants. Pediatrics 2005;115:1.

Martin JA et al: Annual summary of vital statistics—2003. Pediatrics 2005;115:619.

Ment LR, Bada HS, Barnes P: Practice parameter: Neuroimaging of the neonate: Report of the Quality Standards Subcommittee of the American Academy of Neurology and the Practice Committee of the Child Neurology Society. Neurology 2002;58:1726.

Paneth N: The evidence mounts against use of pure oxygen in newborn resuscitation. The J Pediatr 2005;147:4.

Patole S: Prevention of necrotising enterocolitis: Year 2004 and beyond. J Matern Fetal Neonatal Med 2005;17:69.

Patole S, de Klerk N: Impact of standardized feeding regimens on incidence of neonatal necrotizing enterocolitis: A systematic review and meta-analysis of observational studies. Arch Dis Child Fetal Neonatal Ed 2005;90:F147.

Polin RA, Sahni R: Newer experience with CPAP. Semin Neonatol 2002;7:379.

Saugstad OD: Oxygen for newborns: How much is too much? J Perinatol 2005;25(Suppl 2):S45.

Schmidt B et al: Trial of Indomethacin Prophylaxis in Preterms Investigators. Long-term effects of indomethacin prophylaxis in extremely-low-birth-weight infants. N Engl J Med 2001;344:1966.

Schreiber MD, Heymann MA, Soifer SJ: Increased arterial pH, not decreased $PaCO_2$, attenuates hypoxia-induced pulmonary vasoconstriction in newborn lambs. Pediatr Res 1986;20:113.

Soll RF, Morley CJ: Prophylactic versus selective use of surfactant in preventing morbidity and mortality in preterm infants. In: *The Cochrane Library. Issue 2.* John Wiley & Sons, 2005.

Spector LG et al: Childhood cancer following neonatal oxygen supplementation. J Pediatr 2005;147:27.

Tan A et al: Air versus oxygen for resuscitation of infants at birth. Cochrane Database Syst Rev 2005;(2):CD002273.

Van Meurs K: Is surfactant therapy beneficial in the treatment of the term newborn infant with congenital diaphragmatic hernia? J Pediatr 2004;145:312.

Vohra S et al: Heat loss prevention (HeLP) in the delivery room: A randomized controlled trial of polyethylene occlusive skin wrapping in very preterm infants. J Pediatr 2004;145:750.

Wunsch H, Mapstone J, Takala J: High-frequency ventilation versus conventional ventilation for the treatment of acute lung injury and acute respiratory distress syndrome: A Systematic review and Cochrane analysis. Anesth Analg 2005;100:1765.

SECTION IV
General Gynecology

Gynecologic History, Examination, & Diagnostic Procedures

33

Charles Kawada, MD

The gynecologist needs to approach each patient not just as a person requiring medical intervention for a specific presenting problem, but also as one who may have a variety of factors possibly affecting her health. The initial approach to the gynecologic patient and the general diagnostic procedures available for the investigation of gynecologic complaints are presented here. Although other aspects of the general medical examination are left to other texts, concern for the patient's total health and well-being is mandatory.

THE PERIODIC HEALTH SCREENING EXAMINATION

It is now a generally accepted part of the physician's responsibility to advise patients to have periodic medical evaluations. The frequency of visits varies according to the patient's problem.

The periodic health screening examination helps detect the following ailments of women that are especially amenable to early diagnosis and treatment: diabetes mellitus; urinary tract infection or tumor; hypertension; malnutrition or obesity; thyroid dysfunction or tumor; and breast, abdominal, or pelvic tumor. These conditions can be detected by a review of systems, with specific questions regarding recent abnormalities or any variation in function. Determination of weight, blood pressure, and urinalysis may reveal variations from the previous examination. An examination of the thyroid gland, breasts, abdomen, and pelvis, including a Papa-

nicolaou (Pap) smear, should then be performed. A rectal examination also is advisable, and a conveniently packaged test for occult blood (Hemoccult) is recommended for patients older than 40 years. Patients of an advanced age (> 50 years) may undergo blood test for lipid profile, bone density scan, pelvic ultrasound examination, and mammogram.

The physician should be concerned about conditions other than purely somatic ones. Unless a patient's problems require the services of a psychiatrist or some other specialist, the doctor should be prepared to act as a counselor and work with the patient during a mutually agreeable time when it is possible to listen to her problems without being hurried and to give support, counsel, and other kinds of help as required.

HISTORY

To adequately evaluate the gynecologic patient, it is important to establish a rapport during the history taking. The patient needs to tell her story to an interested listener who does not allow body language or facial expressions to imply disinterest or boredom. One should avoid cutting off the patient's story, because doing so may obscure important clues or other problems that may have contributed to the reasons for the visit.

The following outline varies from the routine medical history because, in evaluating the gynecologic patient, the problem often can be clarified if the history is obtained in the following order.

Identifying Information

A. AGE

Knowledge of the patient's age sets the tone for the complaint and the approach to the patient. Obviously, the problems and the approach to them vary at different stages in a woman's life (pubescence, adolescence, childbearing years, and premenopausal and postmenopausal years).

B. LAST NORMAL MENSTRUAL PERIOD

The date of onset of the last normal menstrual period (LNMP) is important to define. A missed period, irregularity of periods, erratic bleeding, or other abnormalities may all imply certain events that are more easily diagnosed when the date of onset of the LNMP is established.

C. GRAVIDITY AND PARITY

The process of taking the patient's obstetric history is detailed in Chapter 9, but the reproductive history should be recorded as part of the gynecologic evaluation. A convenient symbol for recording the reproductive history is a 4-digit code denoting the number of term pregnancies, premature deliveries, abortions, and living children (TPAL), eg, 2-1-1-3 means 2 term pregnancies, 1 premature delivery, 1 abortion, and 3 living children.

Chief Complaint

The chief complaint usually is best elicited by asking "What kind of problem are you having?" or "How can I help you?" It is important to listen carefully to the way the patient responds to this question and to allow her to fully explain her complaint. The patient should be interrupted only to clarify certain points that may be unclear.

Present Illness

Each of the problems the patient describes must be obtained in detail by questioning regarding what exactly the problem is, where exactly the problem is occurring, the date and time of onset, whether the symptoms are abating or getting worse, the duration of the symptoms when they do occur, and how these symptoms are related to or influence other events in her life. For example, the site, duration, and intensity of pain must be accurately described. Getting a sense of how the pain affects her life often is helpful in evaluating the intensity of pain: "Does the pain prevent you from standing or walking?"

It is important to maintain eye contact with the patient and to listen to every word. Do not rely on a patient's sophistication as a measure of her knowledge of anatomy and medical terminology. It is important for the physician to judiciously adjust the level of terminology according to the patient's knowledge and vocabulary. Communicating with the patient in this manner may help the physician obtain an accurate history and establish rapport.

In addition to physiologic events and the life cycle, symptoms described could be related to starting a new job, the beginning of a new relationship or difficulties in the current relationship, an exercise regimen, new medication, and any emotional changes in the patient's life.

Past History

After the physician is satisfied that all possible information concerning the present illness and the important corollaries has been obtained, the past history should be elicited.

A. CONTRACEPTION

Continuing with the history, it is important to elicit whether the patient is using or needs some form of contraception. If she is using contraception, her level of satisfaction with her chosen method should be determined. In patients taking oral contraceptives, the history should reflect the agent and dose, whether there is a great variation in the time of day she takes her pill, and any impact of the pill on other physiologic functions. Other forms of hormonal contraceptives, including vaginal rings, dermal patches, and injectable contraceptives, have become available and have their own unique issues. It is extremely important to ask questions during the remainder of the history and to key the physical examination to ascertain whether there are any contraindications to the patient's current form of contraception.

B. MEDICATIONS AND HABITS

Any medications, prescribed or otherwise, that are being taken or that were being taken when symptoms first occurred should be described. Particular attention must be directed to use of hormones, steroids, and other compounds likely to influence the reproductive tract. Herbal preparations may not be viewed by the patient as medications, so this question should be specifically asked. In addition to medications, the patient should be questioned concerning her use of street drugs. It must be ascertained whether the patient smokes and, if so, how much and for how long. It is important to ascertain the amount of alcohol ingested, if any. This questioning provides an ideal time to indicate the health risks of various habits.

C. MEDICAL

It is important to discover any history of serious medical and psychiatric illnesses and whether hospitalization was required. Particularly important are illnesses in the major organ systems. It is important to know whether there is a major endocrinopathy in the patient's history. Notable weight gain or loss prior to the onset of the patient's current symptoms should be detailed. Other important details include when she had her last physical examination, including pelvic examination and Pap smear.

D. SURGICAL

The surgical history includes all operations, the dates performed, and associated postoperative or anesthetic complications.

E. ALLERGIES

Questioning should continue relating any possible allergic reactions to drugs or specific foods. The reaction produced (eg, rash, gastrointestinal upset) must be elicited and the approximate time when it occurred ascertained. Any testing to confirm or deny the observation must be noted. Latex allergy has become more common and severe and should be considered prior to most medical procedures, such as drawing blood samples, pelvic examination, and taking blood pressures.

F. BLEEDING AND THROMBOTIC DIATHESES

Determining whether or not the patient bleeds excessively in relation to prior surgery or minor trauma is important. A history of easy bruising or of bleeding from the gums while brushing teeth may be useful in this judgment. The patient should be asked whether she or one of her close relatives experienced venous thromboembolism (VTE). A history of VTE may guide the physician as to which treatment to offer. Suspicion of a bleeding or clotting problem indicates the need for further laboratory evaluation.

G. OBSTETRICS

The obstetric history includes each of the patient's pregnancies listed in chronologic order. The date of birth; sex and weight of the offspring; duration of pregnancy; length of labor; type of delivery; type of anesthesia; and any complications should be included.

H. GYNECOLOGIC

The first item in the gynecologic past history is the menstrual history: age at menarche, interval between periods, duration of flow, amount and character of flow, degree of discomfort, and age at menopause. The menstrual history often is an important clue in the diagnosis.

A prior history of sexually transmitted disease (STD) needs to be detailed. Although in the past it was more common to note only gonorrhea and syphilis, it is important to also document exposure to human immunodeficiency virus (HIV), hepatitis, herpesvirus, chlamydia, and papillomavirus. Any treatment or admissions to the hospital for treatment of salpingitis, endometri-

tis, or tubo-ovarian abscess must be carefully documented. Attempts to assess the impact of these processes in relation to ectopic pregnancy, infertility, and type of contraception must be elicited.

Although its significance is less than that of the prior stated diseases, the occurrence of episodes of vaginitis should not be dismissed. Their frequency and the medications used to treat them should be discussed. In the case of such infections, it is important to detail whether or not the episode was pathologic or merely a misinterpreted physiologic circumstance.

I. SEXUAL

The sexual history should be an integral part of any general gynecologic history. In taking a sexual history, the physician must be nonjudgmental and not embarrassed or critical.

Questions that may be covered include the following. Is she currently sexually active? Is the relationship satisfactory to her and, if not, why not? A question regarding whether the patient is heterosexual or lesbian is important but often difficult to ask because the question may be offensive to some patients. It is important, however, not to assume that a relationship is heterosexual because a lesbian woman will lose all rapport with the physician when the physician is insensitive to such issues.

J. SOCIAL

A social history can be an extension of earlier questions pertaining to the marital and sexual history. Knowing the type of work the patient does, the type of educational background, and her community activities may assist in ascertaining the patient's relationship to her entire environment.

The patient's involvement with her own health care should be carefully elicited, including her attention and knowledge concerning diet, health screening examinations, recreation, and the degree of regular physical exercise.

Family History

The patient's family history must include the state of health of immediate relatives (parents, siblings, grandparents, and offspring). In addition to listing these relatives, it is useful in cases where genetic illnesses may be apparent to record a 3-generation pedigree.

The incidence of familial heart disease, hypertensive renal or vascular disease, diabetes mellitus (insulin dependent or non–insulin-dependent), vascular accidents, and hematologic abnormalities should be ascertained. If the patient has a problem with hirsutism or if she perceives excessive hair growth, it is important to elicit whether anyone in her family has the same distribution of hair growth. Familial history of breast, ovarian, and colon cancers is important to elicit because a close familial history may require additional testing and close follow-up. It is important to relate the time of menopause in the mother or grandmother and to ascertain a history of osteoporosis.

PHYSICAL EXAMINATION

The physical examination is most useful if it is conducted in an environment that is aesthetically pleasing to the patient. Adequate gowning and draping assist in preventing embarrassment. Often a physician's assistant conducts the patient to the dressing area and gives explicit instructions about what to take off and how to put on her gown and then may assist in draping the patient.

A physician may have a female assistant remain in the examining room to assist when necessary, but whether or not she remains solely as a chaperone depends on local custom and the preference of the patient and the physician. A chaperone is not legally required, but the physician, male or female, must use good judgement, especially during the breast and pelvic examinations. If the patient wants her partner, relative, or a friend to be present, the request should be honored unless, in the physician's judgment, such an arrangement would interfere with the examination or with obtaining an accurate history. It is highly recommended that the physician explain the steps and acts that will be taken, especially during the pelvic examination when the patient might lack a direct eye contact with the physician.

General Examination

If the gynecologist is the primary care physician for the patient, a general physical examination should be performed annually or whenever the situation warrants. A complete examination obviously provides more information, demonstrates the physician's thoroughness, and establishes rapport with the patient.

General Evaluation

A. VITAL SIGNS

As part of every examination—whether for a specific problem, routine annual examination, or a return visit for a previously diagnosed problem—the patient should be weighed and her blood pressure taken. Postmenopausal patients should have their height measured to document any loss of height from osteoporosis and vertebral fractures. Before the patient empties her bladder for the examination, determination should be made as to whether the urine will need to be sent for urinalysis, culture, or pregnancy testing.

The examination of the chest should include visual assessment for any skin lesions and symmetry of movement. Auscultation and percussion of the lungs are important for excluding primary pulmonary problems such as asthma and pneumonia. The examination of the heart includes percussion for size and auscultation for arrhythmias and significant murmurs.

Breast Examination

(See also Chapter 63.)

Breast examination should be a routine part of the physical examination. Breast cancer will occur in 1 in 8 women in the United States during her lifetime. Physicians who treat women should educate patients on the technique of self-examination, because the well-prepared patient is one of the most accurate screening methods for breast disease.

The physical examination provides an ideal time to ascertain the frequency and methodology of breast self-examination. It also is an ideal time to teach the patient how to perform breast self-examination. The patient should be advised to examine herself in the mirror, looking for skin changes or dimpling, and then carefully palpate all quadrants of the breast. Most women prefer to do this with soapy hands while showering or bathing. The examination should be repeated at the same time each month, preferably 1 week after the initiation of the menses, when the breasts are least nodular; postmenopausal women should perform self-examination on the same day each month.

The frequency of mammography or the earlier use of mammography depends on both the individual woman and her family history. Patients with a positive family history of breast cancer should have a mammogram at an earlier age, particularly those whose mother, aunt, or sister developed premenopausal breast cancer. In general, a mammogram should be obtained every 1–2 years from ages 40 to 50 years and annually thereafter. Ultrasonography now can reliably differentiate solid from cystic lesions; this technique complements but does not supplant mammography. Breast self-examination, physician examination, mammography, and ultrasonography are complementary, and all should be used for the early detection of breast cancer.

The correct technique for breast examination is shown in Figure 33–1. If abnormalities are encountered, a decision should be reached concerning the need for mammography (or other imaging methods) or direct referral to a breast surgeon unless the gynecologist is trained in performing breast biopsies. Skin lesions, particularly eczematous lesions in the area of the nipple, should be closely observed; if they are not easily cured by simple measures, they should be biopsied. An eczematous lesion on the nipple or areola may represent Paget's carcinoma.

Figure 33–1. Breast examination by the physician. **A:** Patient is sitting, arms at sides. Perform visual inspection in good light, looking for lumps or for dimpling or wrinkling of skin. **B:** Patient is sitting, hands pressing on hips so that pectoralis muscles are tensed. Repeat visual inspection. **C:** Patient is sitting, arms above head. Repeat visual inspection of breasts and perform visual inspection of axillae. **D:** Patient is sitting and leaning forward, hands on examiner's shoulders, the stirrups, or her own knees. Perform bimanual palpation, paying particular attention to the base of the glandular portion of the breast.

Abdominal Examination

The patient should be lying completely supine and relaxed; the knees may be slightly flexed and supported as an aid to relaxation of the abdominal muscles. Inspection should detect irregularity of contour or color. Auscultation should follow inspection but precede palpation because the latter may change the character of intestinal activity. Palpation of the entire abdomen—gently at first, then more firmly as indicated—should detect rigidity, voluntary guarding, masses, and tenderness. If the patient complains of abdominal pain or if unexpected tenderness is elicited, the examiner should ask her to indicate the point of maximal pain or tenderness with 1 finger. Suprapubic palpation is designed to detect uterine, ovarian, or urinary bladder en-

E

F

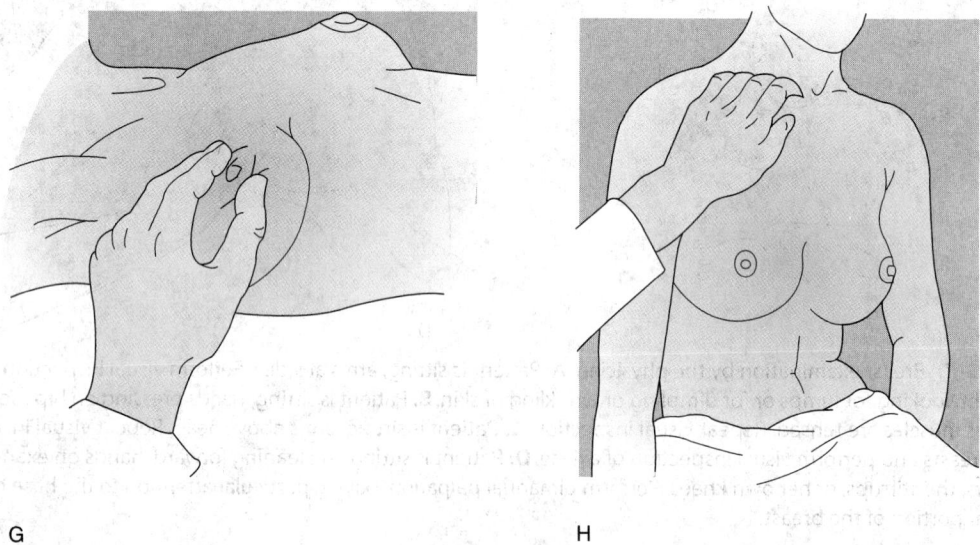

G

H

Figure 33–1 (cont'd). **E:** Patient is sitting, arms extended 60–90 degrees. Palpate axillae. **F:** Patient is supine, arms relaxed at sides. Perform bimanual palpation of each portion of breast (usually each quadrant, but smaller sections for unusually large breasts). Repeat examinations **C, E,** and **F** with patient supine, arms above head. **G:** Patient is supine, arms relaxed at sides. Palpate under the areola and nipple with the thumb and forefinger to detect a mass or test for expression of fluid from the nipple. **H:** Patient is either sitting or supine. Palpate supraclavicular areas.

largements. A painful area should be left until last for deep palpation; otherwise, the entire abdomen can be guarded voluntarily. As a final part of the abdominal examination, the physician should carefully check for any abnormality of the abdominal organs: liver, gallbladder, spleen, kidneys, and intestines. In some instances, the demonstration of an abnormality of the abdominal muscle reflexes may be diagnostically helpful. Percussion of the abdomen should be performed to identify organ enlargement, tumor, or ascites.

Pelvic Examination

The pelvic examination is a procedure feared by many women, so it must be conducted in such a way as to allay her anxieties. A patient's first pelvic examination may be especially disturbing, so it is important for the physician to attempt to allay fear and to inspire confidence and cooperation. The empathic physician usually finds that by the time the history has been obtained and a painless and nonembarrassing general examination performed, a satisfac-

tory gynecologic examination is not a problem. Relaxing surroundings; a nurse or attendant chaperone if indicated; warm instruments; and a gentle, unhurried manner with continued explanation and reassurance are helpful in securing patient relaxation and cooperation. This is especially true with the woman who has never before undergone a pelvic examination. In these patients, a 1-finger examination and a narrow speculum often are necessary. In some cases, vaginal examination is not possible; palpation of the pelvic structures by rectal examination is then the only recourse. Occasionally an ultrasound examination may be helpful in ascertaining whether the pelvic organs are normal in size and configuration in patients who cannot adequately relax the abdominal muscles. If a more definitive pelvic examination is essential, it can be performed with the patient anesthetized.

A. EXTERNAL GENITALIA (FIG 33–2)

The pubic hair should be inspected for its pattern (masculine or feminine), for the nits of pubic lice, for infected

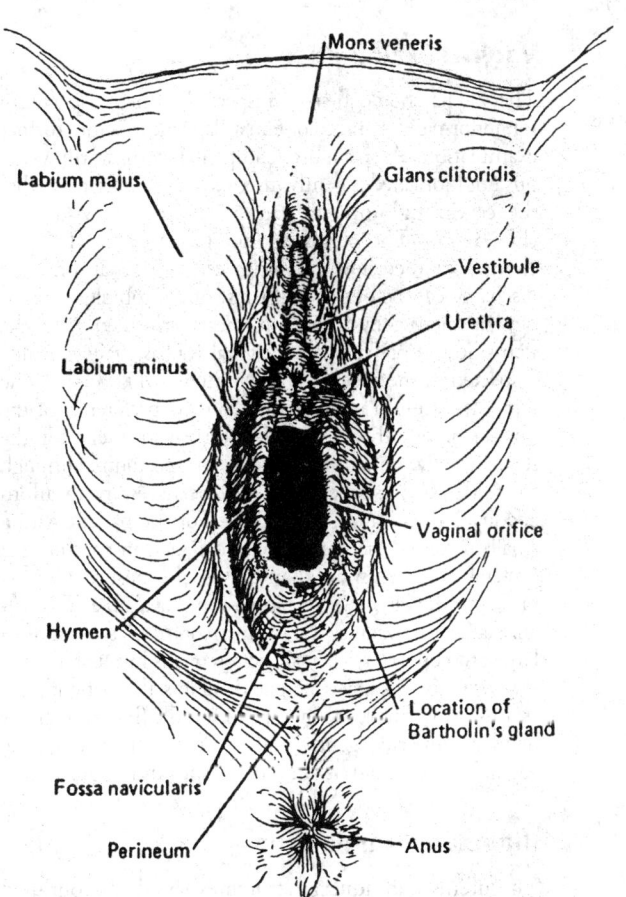

Figure 33–2. Normal external genitalia in a mature woman. (Reproduced, with permission, from Pernoll ML: *Benson & Pernoll's Handbook of Obstetrics and Gynecology,* 10th ed. McGraw-Hill, 2001.)

hair follicles, and for any other abnormalities. The skin of the vulva, mons pubis, and perineal area should be examined for evidence of dermatitis or discoloration. The glans clitoridis can be exposed by gently retracting the surrounding skin folds. The clitoris is at the ventral confluence of the 2 labia; it should be no more than 2.5 cm in length, most of which is subcutaneous. The major and minor labia usually are the same size on both sides, but a moderate difference in size is not abnormal. Small protuberances or subcutaneous nodules may be either sebaceous cysts or tumors. External condylomata are often found in this area. The urethra, just below the clitoris, should be the same color as the surrounding tissue and without protuberances. Normally, vestibular (Bartholin's) glands can be neither seen nor felt, so enlargement may indicate an abnormality of this gland system. The area of vestibular glands should be palpated by placing the index finger in the vagina and the thumb outside and gently feeling for enlargement or tenderness (Fig 33–3). The perineal skin may be reddened as a result of vulvar or vaginal infection. Scars may indicate obstetric lacerations or surgery. The anus should be inspected at this time for the presence of hemorrhoids, fissures, irritation, or perianal infections (eg, condylomata or herpesvirus lesions).

B. HYMEN

An unruptured hymen may present in many forms, but only a completely imperforate, cribriform, or septate

Figure 33–3. Palpation of vestibular glands.

hymen is pathologic. After rupture, the hymen may be seen in various forms (Fig 33–4). After the birth of several children, the hymen may disappear almost completely.

C. PERINEAL SUPPORT

To determine the presence of pelvic relaxation, the physician spreads the labia with 2 fingers and tells the patient to "bear down." This will demonstrate urethrocele, cystocele, rectocele, or uterine prolapse, although sometimes an upright position may be necessary to demonstrate significant prolapse (see Chapter 44).

D. URETHRA

Redness of the urethra may indicate infection or a urethral caruncle or carcinoma. The paraurethral glands are situated below the urethra and empty into the urethra just inside the meatus. With the labia spread adequately for better vision, the urethra may be "stripped" (ie, pressure exerted by the examining finger as it is moved from the proximal to the distal urethra) to express discharge from the urethra or paraurethral glands.

Vaginal Examination

The vagina should first be inspected with the speculum for abnormalities and to obtain a Pap smear before further examination. A speculum dampened with warm water but not lubricated is gently inserted into the vagina so that the cervix and fornices can be thoroughly visualized (Fig 33–5). The cervix should be inspected for discharge, color, erosion, and other lesions. At that time, any discharge can be obtained for test of microbiology, virology, or microscopy and a Pap smear performed. After the Pap smear is prepared, the vaginal wall is again carefully inspected as the speculum is withdrawn (Fig 33–6). The type of speculum used depends on the preference of the physician, but the most satisfactory instrument for the sexually active patient is the Pederson speculum, although the wider Graves' speculum may be necessary to afford adequate visualization (Fig 33–7). For the patient with a small introitus, the narrow-bladed Pederson speculum is preferable. When more than the usual exposure is necessary, an extra large Graves' speculum is available. To visualize a child's vagina, a Huffman or nasal speculum, a large otoscope, or a Kelly air cystoscope is invaluable.

Next, the vagina is palpated; unless the patient's introitus is too small, the index and middle fingers of either hand are inserted gently and the tissues palpated. The vaginal walls should be smooth, elastic, and nontender.

Bimanual Examination

The uterus and adnexal structures should be outlined between the 2 fingers of the hand in the vagina and the

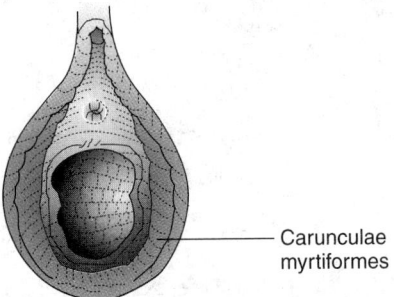

Caruncular
myrtiformes

Figure 33–4. Ruptured hymen (parous introitus).

flat of the opposite hand, which is placed upon the lower abdominal wall (Fig 33–8). Gentle palpation and manipulation of the structures will delineate position, size, shape, mobility, consistency, and tenderness of the pelvic structures—except in the obese or uncooperative patient or in a patient whose abdominal muscles are taut as a result of fear or tenderness. Tenderness can be elicited either on direct palpation or on movement or stretching of the pelvic structures.

A. CERVIX

The cervix is a firm structure traditionally described as having the consistency of the tip of the nose. Normally it is round and approximately 3–4 cm in diameter. Various appearances of the cervix are shown in Figure 33–5. The external os is round and virtually closed. Multiparous women may have an os that has been lacerated. An irregularity in shape or nodularity may be due to 1 or more nabothian cysts. If the cervix is extremely firm, it may contain a tumor, even cancer. The cervix (along with the body of the uterus) normally is moderately mobile, so it can be moved 2–4 cm in any direction without causing undue discomfort. (When examining a patient, it is helpful to warn her that she will feel the movement of her uterus but that ordinarily this maneuver is not painful.) Restricted mobility of the cervix or corpus often follows inflammation, neoplasia, or surgery.

B. CORPUS OF THE UTERUS

The corpus of the uterus is approximately half the size of the patient's fist and weighs approximately 70–90 g. It is regular in outline and not tender to pressure or moderate motion. In most women, the uterus is anteverted; in approximately one-third of women, it is retroverted (see Chapter 44). A retroverted uterus usually is not a pathologic finding. In certain cases of endometriosis or previous salpingitis, the "tipped" uterus may be the result of adhesions caused by the disease process. The uterus usually is described in terms of its size, shape, position, consistency, and mobility.

C. ADNEXA

Adnexal structures (fallopian tubes and ovaries) cannot be palpated in many overweight women because the normal tube is only approximately 7 mm in diameter and the ovary no more than 3 cm in its greatest dimension. In very slender women, however, the ovaries nearly always are palpable and, in some instances, the oviducts are as well. Usually no adnexal structures can be palpated in the postmenopausal woman. Unusual tenderness or enlargement of any adnexal structure indicates the need for further diagnostic procedures; an adnexal mass in any woman is an indication for investigation.

Rectovaginal Examination

At the completion of the bimanual pelvic examination, a rectovaginal examination should always be performed, es-

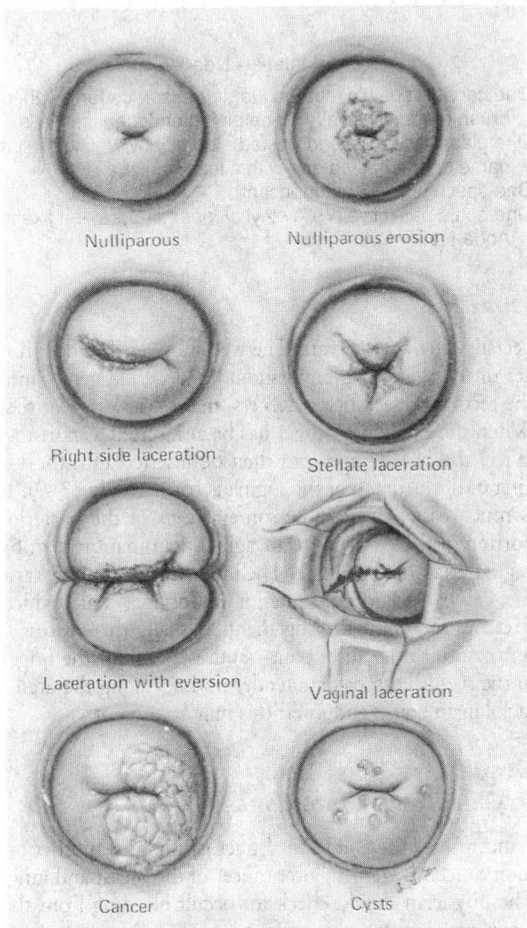

Nulliparous

Nulliparous erosion

Right side laceration

Stellate laceration

Laceration with eversion

Vaginal laceration

Cancer

Cysts

Figure 33–5. Uterine cervix: normal and pathologic appearance.

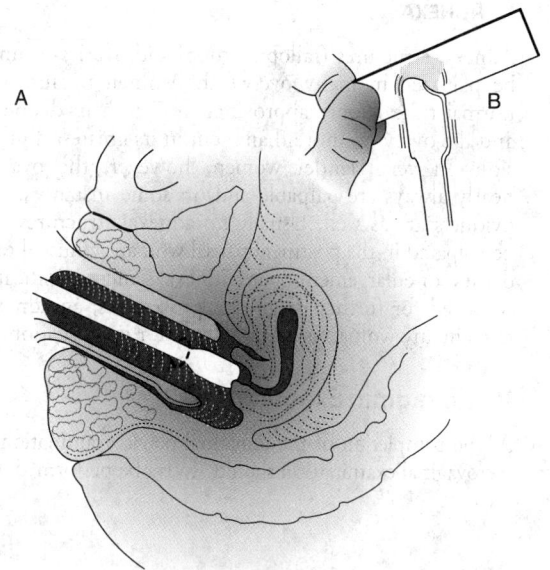

Materials Needed

One cervical spatula, cut tongue depressor, cotton swab, or small brush made especially for obtaining endocervical cells.
One glass slide (one end frosted). Identify by writing the patient's name on the frosted end with a lead pencil.
One speculum (without lubricant).
One bottle of fixative (75% ethyl alcohol) or spray-on fixative, eg, Aqua-Net or Cyto-Spray.

Figure 33–6. Preparation of a Papanicolaou (Pap) smear **A:** Obtain cervical scraping from complete squamocolumnar junction by rotating 360 degrees around the external os. **B:** Place the material 1 inch from the end of the slide and smear along the slide to obtain a thin preparation. Place a saline-soaked cotton swab or small endocervical brush into the endocervical canal and rotate 360 degrees. Place this specimen onto the same slide and quickly fix with fixative. (Reproduced, with permission, from Pernoll ML: *Benson & Pernoll's Handbook of Obstetrics and Gynecology,* 10th ed. McGraw-Hill, 2001.)

pecially after age 40 years. The well-lubricated middle finger of the examining hand should be inserted gently into the rectum to feel for tenderness, masses, or irregularities. When the examining finger has been inserted a short distance, the index finger can then be inserted into the vagina until the depth of the vagina is reached (Fig 33–9). It is much easier to examine some aspects of the posterior portion of the pelvis by rectovaginal examination than by vaginal examination alone. The index finger can now raise the cervix toward the anterior abdominal wall, which stretches the uterosacral ligaments. Usually this process is not painful; if it causes pain—and especially if the finger in the rectum can palpate tender nodules along the uterosacral ligaments—endometriosis may be present.

Occult Bleeding Due to Gastrointestinal Cancer

Cancer of the gastrointestinal tract is the third most common cancer in women, after cancer of the breast and lung. The physician should check for occult bleeding from the gastrointestinal tract by performing a guaiac test on feces adhering to the examination glove following the rectovaginal examination. Several commercial test kits are available.

An early gastrointestinal tract lesion may not bleed continuously and may be associated with a false-negative result. Therefore, testing should be done at each routine health screening visit. If the patient has recently eaten a large amount of meat, a false-positive reaction may result. Therefore, patients with a positive guaiac test should be placed on a meat-free diet for 3 days and the test repeated. Alternatively, patients can be given a test kit to take home and mail back to the physician.

DIAGNOSTIC OFFICE PROCEDURES

Certain diagnostic procedures can be performed in the office because complicated equipment and general anesthesia are not required. Other office diagnostic procedures useful in specific situations (eg, tests used in infertility evaluation) can be found in appropriate chapters elsewhere in this book.

Tests for Vaginal Infection

If abnormal vaginal discharge is present, a sample of vaginal discharge should be scrutinized. A culture is obtained by applying a sterile cotton-tipped applicator to

Graves vaginal speculum   Pederson vaginal speculum

Sims vaginal retractor   Kelly air cystoscope

Figure 33–7. Specula. (Reproduced, with permission, from Pernoll ML: *Benson & Pernoll's Handbook of Obstetrics and Gynecology,* 10th ed. McGraw-Hill, 2001.)

the suspect area and then transferring the suspect material to an appropriate culture medium. Because this procedure is inconvenient to perform in the physician's office, most laboratories supply a prepackaged kit that allows the physician to put the cotton-tipped applicator into a sterile container, which is then sent to the laboratory. The vaginal discharge can also be tested for the vaginal pH. An acidic pH of 4–5 is consistent with fungal infection, whereas an alkaline pH of 5.5–7 suggests infections such as bacterial vaginosis and *Trichomonas.* Often an endocervical infection may be perceived as a vaginal infection. Obtaining a swab for gonorrhea and chlamydia testing from the endocervix is warranted.

A. Saline (Plain Slide)

To demonstrate *Trichomonas vaginalis* organisms, the physician mixes on a slide 1 drop of vaginal discharge with 1 drop of normal saline warmed to approximately body temperature. The slide should have a coverslip. If the smear is examined while it is still warm, actively motile trichomonads usually can be seen.

The saline slide can also be used to look for the mycelia of the fungus *Candida albicans,* which appear as segmented and branching filaments. The slide can be useful in looking for bacterial vaginosis by looking for "clue cells," epithelial cells covered from edge to edge by short coccobacilli-type bacteria.

B. Potassium Hydroxide

One drop of an aqueous 10% potassium hydroxide solution is mixed with 1 drop of vaginal discharge on a clean slide and a coverslip applied. The potassium hydroxide dissolves epithelial cells and debris and facilitates visualization of the mycelia of a fungus causing vaginal infection. The slide can be brought near the nose to determine if the discharge has a "fishy" odor. This odor is strongly suggestive of bacterial vaginosis, a common vaginal infection associated with a mixed anaerobic bacterial flora. In addition, this same slide with a coverslip can be magnified with a microscope to visualize mycelia that may have been hidden by debris with just the saline smear.

C. Bacterial Infection

Bacterial infection may be present, especially if there is an ischemic lesion such as occurs after radiation therapy for cervical carcinoma, or if a patient is suspected of having bacterial vaginosis, gonorrhea, or a *Chlamydia trachomatis* infection. Material from the cervix, urethra, or vaginal lesion can be smeared, stained, and examined microscopically, or the material can be cultured.

Figure 33–8. Bimanual pelvic examination.

Figure 33–9. Rectovaginal examination.

Fern Test for Ovulation

The fern test can determine the presence or absence of ovulation or the time of ovulation. When cervical mucus is spread upon a clean, dry slide and allowed to dry in air, it may or may not assume a frondlike pattern when viewed under the microscope (sometimes it can be seen grossly). The fern frond pattern indicates an estrogenic effect on the mucus without the influence of progesterone; thus, a non-frondlike pattern can be interpreted as showing that ovulation has occurred (Fig 33–10).

Schiller Test for Neoplasia

Although colposcopy is more accurate, the Schiller test can be performed when cancer or precancerous changes of the cervix or vaginal mucosa are suspected. The suspect area is painted with Lugol's (strong iodine) solution, which interacts and marks the glycogen-rich epithelial cells of the cervix. Any portion of the epithelium that does not accept the dye is abnormal because of the presence of scar tissue, neoplasia and precursors, and columnar epithelium. Biopsy of samples taken from this area should be performed if there is any suspicion of cancer.

Biopsy

A. Vulva and Vagina

For biopsy of the vulva or vagina, a 1–2% aqueous solution of a standard local anesthetic solution can be injected around a small suspicious area and a sample obtained with a skin punch or sharp scalpel. Bleeding usually can be controlled by pressure or by Monsel's solution, but occasionally suturing is necessary.

B. Cervix

Colposcopically directed biopsy is the method of choice for the diagnosis of cervical lesions, either suspected on visualization or indicated after an abnormal Pap smear. Colposcopy should reveal the full columnar–squamous "transformation zone" (TZ) at the juncture of the exocervix and endocervix. In addition, it may be advisable to sample the endocervix by curettage. Specific instruments have been devised for cervical biopsy and endocervical curettage (Fig 33–11). The cervix is less sensitive to cutting procedures than is the vagina, so 1 or more small biopsy samples of the cervix can be taken with little discomfort to the patient. Bleeding usually is minimal and controlled with light pressure for a few minutes or by use of Monsel's solution. A "4-quadrant" biopsy sample of the squamocolumnar junction can be taken at 12, 3, 6, and 9 o'clock positions if colposcopy is not available. A Schiller test often may more quickly direct the physician to the area that should be biopsied.

C. Endometrium

Endometrial biopsy can be helpful in the diagnosis of ovarian dysfunction (eg, infertility) or irregular uterine bleeding and as a test for carcinoma of the uterine corpus. Endometrial biopsy can be performed with flexible disposable cannulas, such as the Pipelle, which have replaced most metal curettes previously used (Fig 33–12). In fact, endometrial biopsies have dramatically reduced the need for formal dilatation and curettage (D&C) because the accuracy of biopsy is nearly the same. Because the procedure causes cramping, the patient should be warned and advised to take a pain medication such as ibuprofen 1 hour prior to the procedure.

Normal cycle, 14th day

Midluteal phase, normal cycle

Anovulatory cycle with estrogen present

Figure 33–10. Patterns formed when cervical mucus is smeared on a slide, permitted to dry, and examined under a microscope. Progesterone makes the mucus thick and cellular. In the smear from a patient who failed to ovulate (**bottom**), there is no progesterone to inhibit the estrogen-induced fern pattern. (Reproduced, with permission, from Ganong WF: *Review of Medical Physiology*, 20th ed. McGraw-Hill, 2003.)

DIAGNOSTIC LABORATORY PROCEDURES

Routine procedures that are not discussed here but should be considered with periodic primary care visits include a complete blood count (including differential white cell count), glucose screening, lipid profile, and thyroid function tests. The frequency with which these tests are performed should be at the discretion of the physician, based on risk factors and presenting complaints.

Urinalysis

Urinalysis should be obtained in symptomatic patients and should include both gross and microscopic examinations. A microscopic examination may reveal crystals or bacteria, but unless the specimen is collected in a manner that will exclude vaginal discharge, the presence of bacteria is meaningless (see below).

Urine Culture

Studies have demonstrated that a significant number of women (approximately 3% of nonpregnant women and

7% of pregnant women) have asymptomatic urinary tract infections. Culture and antibiotic sensitivity testing are required for the diagnosis and as a guide to treatment of urinary tract infections.

Reliable specimens of urine for culture often can be obtained by the "clean-catch" method: the patient is instructed to cleanse the urethral meatus carefully with soap and water, to urinate for a few seconds to dispose of urethral contaminants, and then to catch a "midstream" portion of the urine. It is essential that the urine not dribble over the labia, but this may be difficult for some patients to accomplish.

A more reliable method of collecting urine for culture is by sterile catheterization performed by the physician or nurse. However, care must be exercised in catheterization to minimize the risk of introducing an infection.

Other Cultures

A. URETHRAL

Urethral cultures are indicated if an STD is suspected.

B. VAGINAL

A culture usually is unnecessary for the diagnosis of vaginal infections, as visual inspection or microscopic examination usually will enable the physician to make a diagnosis, eg, curdlike vaginal material that reveals mycelia (candidiasis). However, a culture should be obtained in questionable cases.

C. CERVICAL

As in the case of the urethra, the usual indication for a culture of cervical discharge is the suspected presence of an STD.

Specific Tests

A. HERPESVIRUS HOMINIS

Herpesvirus hominis (herpes genitalis, both types 1 and 2) is a frequently seen vulvar lesion (see Chapter 41). It can be diagnosed by the cytopathologist, who finds typical cellular changes. The most accurate method is culturing.

B. HUMAN PAPILLOMAVIRUS

Human papillomavirus (HPV) infection is associated with the development of genital warts and the occurrence of vaginal and cervical intraepithelial lesions. Some of these lesions are precancerous or cancerous in origin. Different HPV subtypes are linked to either benign or more aggressive epithelial changes. The different subtypes can be identified by the specific fingerprints obtained from the polymerase chain reaction (PCR) products.

Tischler cervical biopsy forceps

Kevorkian-Younge cervical biopsy forceps

Duncan curette

Figure 33–11. Biopsy instruments.

C. CHLAMYDIA AND GONORRHEAL INFECTIONS

These sexually transmitted infections are the two most prevalent infections, with chlamydia being the most common. They are found more often in women who have multiple sexual partners and those who do not use barrier methods of contraception. Nucleic acid amplification testing is the most commonly used method of diagnosis, with a sensitivity greater than 90%.

D. HUMAN IMMUNODEFICIENCY VIRUS

Acquired immunodeficiency syndrome (AIDS) has become one of the most difficult issues confronting all kinds of clinicians. The need to screen for HIV in the general population has become more pressing given that the largest increase in incidence is seen in young heterosexually active females with no other risk factors. An accurate blood test is available for diagnosis. Prior to drawing the blood, the physician must discuss with the patient the accuracy of the blood test for diagnosing the presence of HIV. The patient must be made aware that there are infrequent false-positive tests and a "window" during which the test may be falsely negative prior to the development of antibodies. At present, a written consent must be signed by the patient prior to drawing the blood.

Other Specific Tests

Specific diagnostic laboratory procedures may be indicated for some of the less common venereal diseases, eg, lymphogranuloma venereum and hepatitis B and C. A screening test for streptococcus B carrier is advocated at 35–37 weeks' gestation. A 1-step culture swab from the lower vagina, followed by the anus, is recommended. These tests are discussed with the specific diseases in other chapters of this book.

Pregnancy Testing

Pregnancy testing is discussed in Chapter 9.

Papanicolaou Smear of Cervix

The Pap smear is an important part of the gynecologic examination. The frequency of the need for this test has been recently revised. Epidemiologic statistics have led the US Preventive Services Task Force to recommend that for the average woman who has had 3 normal Pap smears, a Pap test every 2 or 3 years is adequate. This recommendation is based on the observation that most cervical cancers are slow growing. The American College of Obstetricians and Gynecologists recommends annual Pap smear screenings from 3 years after the start of sexual intercourse but no later than age 21 years. After age 30

Biopsy sites

Figure 33–12. Sites of endometrial biopsy. (Reproduced, with permission, from Pernoll ML: *Benson & Pernoll's Handbook of Obstetrics and Gynecology,* 10th ed. McGraw-Hill, 2001.)

years, a woman who has had 3 consecutive negative Pap smears can be screened every 2–3 years. Patients at risk, including women with multiple sexual partners, a history of STD, genital condylomata, prior abnormal Pap smears, or receiving immune suppression therapy, should undergo annual smear tests. Aside from premalignant and malignant changes, other local conditions often can be suspected by the cytologist. Viral infections, such as herpes simplex, HPV, and condylomata acuminata, can be seen as mucosal changes. Actinomycosis and *Trichomonas* infections can be detected by a Pap smear.

The Pap smear is a screening test only. Positive tests are an indication for further diagnostic procedures, such as colposcopy, endocervical curettage, cervical biopsy or conization, endometrial biopsy, or D&C. The properly collected Pap smear can accurately lead to the diagnosis of carcinoma of the cervix in approximately 95% of cases. The Pap smear also is helpful in the detection of endometrial abnormalities such as endometrial polyps, hyperplasia, and cancers, but it detects fewer than 50% of cases.

The techniques of collection of a Pap smear may vary, but the following is a common procedure.

The patient should not have douched for at least 24 hours before the examination and should not be menstruating. The speculum is placed in the vagina after it has been lubricated with water only. With the cervix exposed, a specially designed plastic or wooden spatula is applied to the cervix and rotated 360 degrees to abrade the surface slightly and to pick up cells from the squamocolumnar area of the cervical os. Next, a cotton-tipped applicator or a small brush is inserted into the endocervix and rotated 360 degrees. These 2 specimens can be mixed or placed on the slide separately according to the preference of the examiner. A preservative is applied immediately to prevent air drying, which would compromise the interpretation. The slide is sent to the laboratory with an identification sheet containing pertinent history and findings (see Fig 33–6). Another method called ThinPrep automates the preparation of the Pap smear slide so that the variability introduced by the clinician preparing the slide itself is no longer a factor. With this method, the specimen is placed in a liquid-based medium and sent to the laboratory. In addition, the ThinPrep technique decreases the rate of smears showing atypical squamous cells-undetermined significance (ASCUS), thereby decreasing the need for colposcopic evaluations. For these reasons, in many parts of the country the ThinPrep technique has replaced the conventional Pap smear.

The liquid-based medium allows for testing for high-risk HPV, the most common being subtypes 16, 18, 31, 33, and 35. Testing for high-risk HPV has been proposed by the American Society for Colposcopy and Cervical Pathology as a method of evaluating and sorting out patients with ASCUS Pap smear results. If no high-risk HPV is present in the ASCUS Pap smear, then these individuals can be followed-up with a repeat Pap smear in 1 year, similar to those who have a negative Pap smear. Patients known to have a high-risk HPV subtype would undergo colposcopic evaluation.

The laboratory reports the Pap smear using the Bethesda System, which has advocated a standardized reporting system for cytologic reports. Chapter 50 discusses the recently updated nomenclature.

Alternatives to the traditional Pap smear are being evaluated in an attempt to decrease the false-negative and false-positive Pap smear results. Evidence indicates that computerized screening of Pap smears can decrease the likelihood of missing significant pathologies. Various methods of computerized screening have been developed to aid the human eye in picking up abnormalities, although no system has yet achieved widespread acceptance.

Colposcopy

The colposcope is a binocular microscope used for direct visualization of the cervix (Fig 33–13). Magnification as high as 60× is available, but the most popular

Figure 33–13. Zeiss colposcope.

instrument in clinical use has 13.5× magnification, which effectively bridges the gap between what can be seen by the naked eye and by the microscope. Some colposcopes are equipped with a camera for single or serial photographic recording of pathologic conditions.

Colposcopy does not replace other methods of diagnosing abnormalities of the cervix; rather, it is an additional and important tool. The 2 most important groups of patients who can benefit by its use are (1) patients with an abnormal Pap smear and (2) diethylstilbestrol (DES)-exposed daughters, who may have dysplasia of the vagina or cervix (see Chapter 38).

The colposcopist is able to see areas of cellular dysplasia and vascular or tissue abnormalities not visible otherwise, which makes possible the selection of areas most propitious for biopsy. Stains and other chemical agents are also used to improve visualization. The colposcope has reduced the need to perform blind cervical biopsies for which the rate of finding abnormalities is low. In addition, the necessity for a cone biopsy, a procedure with a high morbidity rate, has been greatly reduced. Thus the experienced colposcopist is able to find focal cervical lesions, obtain directed biopsy at the most appropriate sites, and make decisions about the most appropriate therapy largely based on what is seen through the colposcope.

Hysteroscopy

Hysteroscopy is the visual examination of the uterine cavity through a fiberoptic instrument, the hysteroscope. In order to inspect the interior of the uterus with the hysteroscope, the uterine cavity is inflated with a solution such as saline, glycine, or dextran, or by carbon dioxide insufflation. Intravenous sedation and paracervical block often are adequate for hysteroscopy so long as prolonged manipulation is not required.

Hysteroscopic applications include evaluation for abnormal uterine bleeding, resection of uterine synechiae and septa, removal of polyps and intrauterine devices (IUDs), resection of submucous myomas, and endometrial ablation. Most of these therapeutic maneuvers require extensive manipulation, so regional or general anesthesia is required.

Hysteroscopy should be performed only by physicians with proper training. The tip of the instrument should be inserted just beyond the internal cervical os and then advanced slowly, with adequate distention under direct vision.

Hysteroscopy is often used in conjunction with another operative procedures, such as curettage and laparoscopy.

Failure of hysteroscopy may be the result of cervical stenosis, inadequate distention of the uterine cavity, bleeding, or excessive mucus secretion. The most common complications include perforation, bleeding, and infection. Perforation of the uterus usually occurs at the fundus. Unless a viscus is damaged or internal bleeding develops, surgical repair may not be required. Bleeding generally subsides, but fulguration following attempts to remove polyps or myomas may be required to stop bleeding in some cases. Parametritis or salpingitis, rarely noted, usually necessitates antibiotic therapy. Intravascular extravasation of fluid or gas from hysteroscopy often does not become clinically significant but has been associated with severe consequences such as hyponatremia, air embolism, cerebral edema, and even death.

Culdocentesis

The passage of a needle into the cul-de-sac—culdocentesis—in order to obtain fluid from the pouch of Douglas is a diagnostic procedure that can be performed in the office or in a hospital treatment room (Fig 33–14). The type of fluid obtained indicates the type of intraperitoneal lesion, eg, bloody with a ruptured ectopic pregnancy, pus with acute salpingitis, or ascitic fluid with malignant cells in cancer. With refinements in ul-

Figure 33–14. Culdocentesis.

trasound technology enabling more definitive evaluation of pelvic pathology, culdocentesis is performed less frequently today.

Radiographic Diagnostic Procedures

Many common radiologic procedures may be helpful in the diagnosis of pelvic conditions. The "flat film" shows calcified lesions, teeth, or a ring of a dermoid cyst and indicates other pelvic masses by shadows or displaced intestinal loops. Use of contrast media frequently is indicated to help delineate pelvic masses or to rule out metastatic lesions. Barium enema, upper gastrointestinal series, intravenous urogram, and cystogram may be helpful.

Hysterography & Sonohysterography

The uterine cavity and the lumens of the oviducts can be outlined by instillation of contrast medium through the cervix, followed by fluoroscopic observations or film. The technique was first widely used for the diagnosis of tubal disease as part of the investigation of infertile women. Its use now is being extended to the investigation of uterine disease.

To diagnose tubal patency or occlusion, the medium is instilled through a cervical cannula. Filling of the uterine cavity and spreading of the medium through the tubes are watched via a fluoroscope, with the radiologist taking spot films at intervals for subsequent, more definitive, scrutiny. If no occlusion is present, the medium will reach the fimbriated end of the tube and spill into the pelvis—evidence of tubal patency. This procedure can reveal an abnormality of the uterus, eg, congenital malformation, submucous myomas, or endometrial polyps.

Another technique that is gaining acceptance is sonohysterography, in which the uterine cavity is filled with fluid while ultrasound is used to delineate the architecture of the endometrial cavity and detect a spillage through the fallopian tubes. Thus it becomes easier to diagnose intrauterine abnormalities, such as polyps or fibroids, and tubal patency.

Angiography

Angiography is the use of radiographic contrast medium to visualize the blood vascular system. By demonstrating the vascular pattern of an area, tumors or other abnormalities can be delineated. Angiography also is used to delineate continued bleeding from pelvic vessels postoperatively, to visualize bleeding from infiltration by cancer in cancer patients, or to embolize the uterine arteries in order to decrease acute bleeding and/or reduce the size of uterine myomas. These vessels then can be embolized with synthetic fabrics to stop the bleeding or indicate therapy that can prevent the need for a major abdominal operation in a highly compromised patient.

Computed Tomography

Computed tomography (CT) scan is a diagnostic imaging technique that provides high-resolution 2-dimensional images. The CT scan takes cross-sectional images through the body at very close intervals so that multiple "slices" of the body are obtained. The beam transmission is measured and calculated through an array of sensors that are approximately 100 times more sensitive than conventional x-rays. The computer is able to translate the densities of different types of tissues into gray-scale pictures that can be read on an x-ray film or a television monitor.

Contrast media can be given orally, intravenously, or rectally. They are used to outline the gastrointestinal and urinary systems, thus helping to differentiate these organ systems from the pelvic reproductive organs. In gynecology, the CT scan is most useful in accurately diagnosing retroperitoneal lymphadenopathy associated with malignancies. It also has been used to determine the depth of myometrial invasion in endometrial carcinoma as well as extrauterine spread. It is an accurate tool for locating pelvic abscesses that cannot be located by ultrasonography. Often a needle can be placed into an abscess pocket to both drain the abscess and determine what organism may be involved. Pelvic thrombophlebitis often can be diagnosed by CT scan as an adjunct to clinical suspicion. Common abnormalities such as ovarian cysts and myomas are easily diagnosed (Fig 33–15).

Magnetic Resonance Imaging

Magnetic resonance imaging (MRI) is a diagnostic imaging technique that creates a high-resolution, cross-sectional image of the body like a CT scan. The technique is based on the body absorbing radio waves from the machine. A small amount of this energy is absorbed by the nuclei in the various tissues. These nuclei act like small bar magnets and are influenced by the magnetic field created by the machine. These nuclei then emit some of the radio waves back out of the body. The waves are picked up by sensitive and sophisticated receivers, and these signals are translated into images by computer technology.

The advantages of MRI include the fact that it uses nonionized radiation that has no adverse or harmful effects on the body. MRI is superior to CT in its ability to differentiate among various types of tissue, including inflammatory masses, cancers, and abnormal tissue me-

Figure 33–15. CT scan of the pelvis showing a large fibroid uterus with 3 calcified fibroids in the body of the uterus. (Picture courtesy of Dr. Barbara Carter, New England Medical Center, Boston.)

tabolism. Its disadvantages are mainly its high cost and its poor demonstration of calcifications. Its main use in gynecology appears to be staging and follow-up of pelvic cancers. MRI in obstetrics is limited to its use as an adjunct to prenatal diagnosis of fetal anomalies. It allows for multiple image cuts that can help decipher complex anomalies. Other potential uses of MRI include evaluation of placental blood flow and accurate performance of pelvimetry.

Ultrasonography

Ultrasonography records high-frequency sound waves as they are reflected from anatomic structures. As the sounds waves pass through tissues, they encounter variable acoustic densities. Each of the tissues returns a different echo, depending on the amount of energy reflected. This echo signal can be measured and converted into a 2-dimensional image of the area under examination, with the relative densities shown as differing shades of gray.

Ultrasonography is a simple and painless procedure that has the added advantage of freedom from any radiation hazard. It is especially helpful in patients in whom an adequate pelvic examination may be difficult, such as in children, virginal women, and uncooperative patients.

The pelvis and lower abdomen are scanned and recorded at regular intervals of distance, using a sector scanner that provides a better 2-dimensional picture than does the linear array scanner (Fig 33–16). Generally, the abdominal scan is performed with the bladder full; this condition elevates the uterus out of the pelvis, displaces air-filled loops of bowel, and provides the operator with an index of density—a sonographic "window" differentiating the pelvic organs.

Ultrasonography can be helpful in the diagnosis of almost any pelvic abnormality, as all structures, normal and abnormal, usually can be demonstrated. In most instances, a clinical picture has been developed—by history, physical examination, or both—before ultrasonograms are obtained. Thus, the scan often corroborates the clinical impression, but it also may uncover an unexpected condition of which the clinician should be aware.

There are many indications for ultrasonography. Normal early pregnancy can be diagnosed, as can pathologic pregnancies such as incomplete and missed abortions and hydatidiform moles. Ultrasonography can be extremely helpful in avoiding the placenta and fetus during midtrimester amniocentesis. The uses for ultrasound examination in obstetrics are discussed elsewhere in this book.

Ultrasonography may be used to locate a lost IUD or a foreign body in the vagina of a child. Congenital malformations such as a bicornuate uterus or vaginal agenesis are sometimes, but not always, detected. Ultrasound ex-

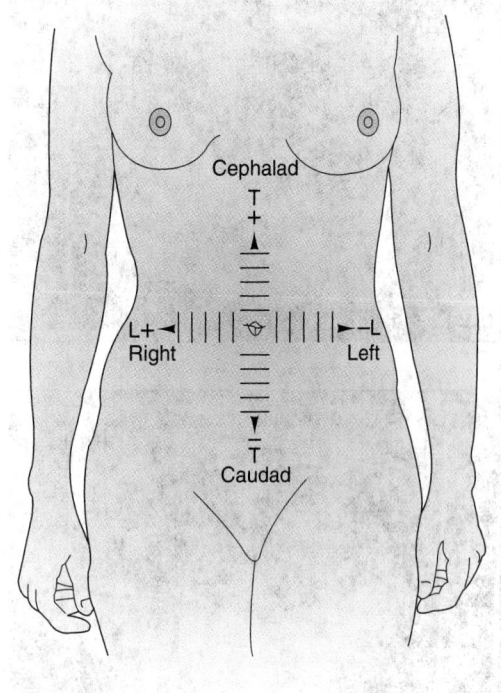

Figure 33–16. Planes of ultrasonograms.

amination is useful in the placement of uterine tandems for radiation therapy for endometrial cancer and for guidance during second-trimester abortion procedures.

One of the more common uses for ultrasonography is the diagnosis of pelvic masses. Often because of their location, attachment, and density, myomas can be diagnosed without too much difficulty (Fig 33–17A).

Adnexal masses can be found with relative ease by ultrasonography, although an accurate diagnosis is more difficult because of the various types of adnexal masses that can be found (Fig 33–17B and C).

Ovarian cysts can be described as unilocular or multilocular, totally fluid-filled, or partially solid. A common adnexal mass, the dermoid cyst, can have characteristic ultrasound findings because of fat tissue and bone densities seen in these cysts (Fig 33–17D). Pelvic abscesses can be diagnosed by ultrasonography, especially if a well-encapsulated large abscess pocket is present.

In addition to the traditional abdominal scan, the vaginal probe scan has become a useful modality. The vaginal probe is used for determining early gestations and can diagnose a pregnancy as early as 5 weeks from the LNMP. Although vaginal ultrasonography can sometimes visualize ectopic pregnancies, it is more use-

Figure 33–17. A: Longitudinal view of the uterus with anterior fibroid outlined by the x's; bladder anterior. **B:** Transverse section through an endometrioma with multiple loculations and debris. **C:** Longitudinal view of large ovarian cyst outlined by the +'s and x's with a focal multicystic area. **D:** Longitudinal view of a dermoid cyst showing areas of fat within the cyst. (Pictures courtesy of Dr. Frederick Doherty, New England Medical Center, Boston.)

ful for excluding an intrauterine gestation when there is suspicion of an ectopic pregnancy.

Ultrasonography is commonly used to diagnose ovarian cysts, especially in obese patients in whom abdominal scans are of limited use. The vaginal scan is used often to determine follicular size with in vitro fertilization and to predict the best time for ovum retrieval.

Innovations in ultrasound probes and computerizing processes of the obtained images enable the development of 3-dimensional ultrasound machines. The 3-dimensional images help to accurately evaluate normal and abnormal findings, such as uterine shape and cavity, pelvic masses, and fetal malformations.

Carbon Dioxide Laser

Controlled tissue vaporization by laser is a modality for treatment of cervical, vaginal, or perineal condylomata and dysplasia. It also can be used for conization of the cervix for diagnosis of dysplasia or carcinoma within the cervical canal.

The vaporization procedure is not difficult, but training is essential, especially in the physics of laser light and the potential risks of laser therapy not only to the patient but to the operator and others in the immediate vicinity. Antiseptic preparation of the vagina should be gentle to avoid trauma to the tissue that is to be examined histologically. Local anesthesia, with or without preliminary intravenous sedation, usually is adequate.

Advantages of the laser method of cervical conization include little or no pain; a low incidence of infection because the beam sterilizes the tissues; decreased blood loss, because the laser instrument—at a decreased energy level—is a hemostatic agent; less tissue necrosis than occurs with electrocautery (but probably the same as with excision by a sharp knife); and a decreased incidence of postoperative cervical stenosis.

Loop Electrosurgical Excision Procedure

Loop electrosurgical excision procedure (LEEP) is another modality of therapy for vulvar and cervical lesions. LEEP uses a low-voltage, high-frequency alternating current that limits thermal damage but at the same time has good hemostatic properties. It is most commonly used for excision of vulvar condylomata and cervical dysplasias and for cone biopsies of the cervix. It has displaced sharp knife and laser cone biopsies for treatment of most cervical dysplasias.

The technique requires the use of local anesthesia followed by the use of a wire loop cautery unit that cauterizes and cuts the desired tissue. Loops of various sizes are used for specimens of different size. The major advantages of LEEP are its usefulness in an office setting with lower equipment cost, minimal damage to the surrounding tissue, and low morbidity.

REFERENCES

American Cancer Society guidelines for breast cancer screening: Update 2003. CA Cancer J Clin 2003;53:141.

American College of Obstetricians and Gynecologists: Cervical cytology screening. ACOG Practice Bulletin No. 45. Obstet Gynecol 2003;102:417.

Marrazzo JM, Stine K: Reproductive health history of lesbians: implications for care. Am J Obstet Gynecol 2004;190:1298.

Nustaum MR, Hamilton CD: The proactive sexual health history. Am Fam Physicians 2002;66:1705.

Vassilakos P et al: Biopsy-based comparison of liquid-based, thin-layer preparations to conventional Pap smear. J Reprod Med 2000;45:11.

Wright T et al: Interim guidelines for the use of human papillomavirus DNA testing as an adjunct to cervical cytology screening. Obstet Gynecol 2004;103:304–309.

Pediatric & Adolescent Gynecology | 34

David Muram, MD

The field of pediatric and adolescent gynecology has expanded greatly over the past century, as increased attention has been directed to the complex roles of children and adolescents in society. Today, pediatric and adolescent gynecology has evolved from reviews of developmental physiology and case reports of aberrations to discussions that include not only these topics but also address issues related to adolescent reproductive health.

Gynecologic care begins in the delivery room, with inspection of the external genitalia during routine newborn examination. Evaluation of the external genitalia continues through routine well-child examinations, permitting early detection of infections, labial adhesions, congenital anomalies, and even genital tumors. A complete gynecologic examination is indicated when a child has symptoms or signs of a genital disorder. The American College of Obstetricians and Gynecologists recommends that adolescents should have their first visit to an obstetrician/gynecologist for health guidance, general physical screening, and the provision of preventive health care services at age 13–15 years. A pelvic examination should be performed on adolescents who are sexually active, older than 18 years, or when indicated by medical history. Specially designed equipment must be used (eg, vaginoscope, virginal vaginal speculum) to prevent undue discomfort and consequent anxiety about future examinations.

ANATOMIC & PHYSIOLOGIC CONSIDERATIONS

Newborn Infants

During the first few weeks of life, residual maternal sex hormones may produce physiologic effects on the newborn. Breast budding occurs in nearly all female infants born at term. In some cases, breast enlargement is marked, and there may be fluid discharge from the nipples. No treatment is indicated. The labia majora are bulbous, and the labia minora are thick and protruding (Fig 34–1). The clitoris is relatively large, with a normal index of 0.6 cm² or less.* The hymen initially is turgid,

---

* Clitoral index (cm²) = Length (cm) × width (cm). For example, a clitoris 1 cm long and 0.5 cm wide = 0.5 cm².

covering the external urethral orifice. Vaginal discharge is common, composed mainly of cervical mucus and exfoliated vaginal cells.

The vagina is approximately 4 cm long at birth. The uterus is enlarged (4 cm in length) and without axial flexion; the ratio between the cervix and the corpus is 3:1. Columnar epithelium protrudes through the external cervical os, creating a reddened zone of physiologic eversion. The ovaries remain abdominal organs in early childhood and should not be palpable on pelvic or rectal examination. Vaginal bleeding may occur as estrogen levels decline following birth and the stimulated endometrial lining is shed. Such bleeding usually stops within 7–10 days.

Young Children

In early childhood, the female genital organs receive little estrogen stimulation. The labia majora flatten and the labia minora and hymen become thin (Fig 34–2). The clitoris remains relatively small, although the clitoral index is unchanged. The vagina, lined with atrophic mucosa with relatively few rugae, offers very little resistance to trauma and infection. The vaginal barrel contains neutral or slightly alkaline secretions and mixed bacterial flora. Because vaginal fornices do not develop until puberty, the cervix in childhood is flush with the vaginal vault, and its opening appears as a small slit. The uterus regresses in size and does not regain the size present at birth until approximately age 6 years. As the child matures, the ovaries begin to enlarge and descend into the true pelvis. The number and size of ovarian follicles increase. They may attain significant size and then regress.

At laparotomy, the uterus may appear as merely a strip of dense tissue in the anteromedial area of the broad ligaments. Palpation may aid in delineating the uterine outline. The ovaries may appear cystic secondary to follicular development. Biopsy is not warranted.

Older Children

During late childhood (age 7–10 years), the external genitalia again show signs of estrogen stimulation: the mons pubis thickens, the labia majora fill out, and the

Figure 34–1. External genitalia of a newborn female. Note the hypertrophy and turgor of the vulvar tissues. A small catheter is inserted into the vagina to demonstrate patency. (Reproduced, with permission, from Huffman JW: *The Gynecology of Childhood and Adolescence.* WB Saunders, 1968.)

labia minora become rounded. The hymen thickens (Fig 34–3), losing its thin, transparent character. The vagina elongates to 8 cm, the mucosa becomes thicker, the corpus uteri enlarges, and the ratio of cervix to corpus becomes 1:1. The cervix remains flush with the vault. A maturation index determination at this time

Figure 34–3. External genitalia of a child 11 years of age. Early estrogen response is evidenced by the fuller labia, wrinkling of the vulvar mucosa, and thickening of the hymen.

will show not only basal cells but also a greater proportion of parabasal cells and superficial cells, in a typical ratio of 75:25:0 or 70:25:5.

By the time a girl reaches age 9–10 years, uterine growth begins, with alteration in uterine shape resulting primarily from myometrial proliferation. Rapid endometrial proliferation occurs as menarche is imminent. Prior to this time, the endometrium gradually thickens, with modest increases in the depth and complexity of the endometrial glands. As the ovaries enlarge and descend into the pelvis, the number of ovarian follicles increases. Although these follicles are in various stages of development, ovulation generally does not occur.

Young Adolescents

During early puberty (age 10–13 years), the external genitalia take on adult appearance. The major vestibular glands (Bartholin's glands) begin to produce mucus just prior to menarche. The vagina reaches adult length (10–12 cm) and becomes more distensible, the

Figure 34–2. External genitalia of a child 3 years of age.

mucosa thickens, vaginal secretions grow more acidic, and lactobacilli reappear. With the development of vaginal fornices, the cervix becomes separated from the vaginal vault, and the differential growth of the corpus and cervix becomes more pronounced. The corpus grows twice as large as the cervix. The ovaries descend into the true pelvis.

Secondary sexual characteristics develop, often rapidly, during the late premenarcheal period. Body habitus becomes more rounded, especially the shoulders and hips. Accelerated somatic growth velocity (the adolescent growth spurt) occurs. At the same time, estrogen increases adipose tissue deposition and initiates stromal and ductal growth in the breasts. Physiologic leukorrhea often is noted.

Pubic hair growth appears to be under the control of adrenal androgens. Sparse, long, slightly curly, pigmented hair over the pubic area gives way to coarse, pigmented curly hair. The pubic hair pattern assumes the characteristic triangle with the base above the mons pubis. Hair growth in the axilla appears later, also as a result of adrenocorticosteroid stimulation. The development of secondary sexual features described by Marshall and Tanner is summarized in Table 34–1 (see Fig 6–3).

GYNECOLOGIC EXAMINATION OF INFANTS, CHILDREN, & YOUNG ADOLESCENTS

Examination of the Newborn Infant

Newborns should be examined immediately upon delivery or in the nursery. When an infant is born with ambiguous genitalia, immediate actions should be to counsel the parents and to prevent dehydration, as congenital adrenal hyperplasia accounts for greater than 90% of cases of ambiguous genitalia, and salt-wasting forms may lead to rapid dehydration and fluid imbalances. In most cases, an internal examination is unnecessary, as most gynecologic abnormalities that should be recognized at this stage are limited to the external genitalia.

A. GENERAL EXAMINATION

As in adults, the first step in a genital evaluation of the newborn is a careful general examination, which may reveal abnormalities suggesting genital anomaly (eg, webbed neck, abdominal mass, edema of the hands and legs, coarctation of the aorta).

B. CLITORIS

Clitoral enlargement in the newborn almost always is associated with congenital adrenal hyperplasia. Other causes, such as hermaphroditism and neoplasms, also must be considered.

Table 34–1. Tanner classification of female adolescent development.

Stage	Breast Development	Pubic Hair Development
I	Papillae elevated (preadolescent), no breast buds	None
II	Breast buds and papillae slightly elevated	Sparse, long, slightly pigmented
III	Breasts and areolae confluent, elevated	Darker, coarser, curly
IV	Areolae and papillae project above breast	Adult–type pubis only
V	Papillae projected, mature	Lateral distribution

C. VULVA AND VAGINA

The vaginal orifice should be evident when the labia are separated or retracted. If the vaginal orifice cannot be located, the infant most likely has an imperforate hymen or vaginal agenesis. Inguinal hernias are uncommon in females, and the presence of inguinal masses suggests the possibility that the child is a genetic male.

D. RECTOABDOMINAL EXAMINATION

Usually, the uterus and adnexa in the newborn cannot be palpated on rectal examination. Occasionally, a small central mass representing the uterine cervix can be felt on examination. An ovary that is palpable denotes enlargement, and the possibility of an ovarian tumor should be investigated, even though pelvic masses in newborns likely represent a Wilms' tumor. In addition, a rectal examination can confirm patency of the anorectal canal, which is most important in newborns who have not yet passed meconium.

Examination of the Premenarcheal Child

The examination of the premenarcheal and peripubertal child should focus on the main symptoms identified in this population: pruritus, dysuria, skin color changes, and discharge.

Parents can be helpful during the examination of a young child because they provide a sense of security and they can distract the patient. Placing a child up to age 5 years on her parent's lap affords a better opportunity to perform an adequate examination (Fig 34–4). Older children can be placed on the examination table, but the use of stirrups is not generally necessary. The examiner may have adequate exposure of the genitalia when the patient is asked to flex her knees and abduct her legs. I often ask the young patient to assist in the examination, as this may distract the child as well as provide her with a sense of control. In some patients, the knee–chest position may be useful in visualizing the upper vagina and cervix.

Figure 34–4. Child is positioned on mother's lap and feels secure in mother's arms. The mother can assist by supporting the child's legs, providing an excellent view of the genital area. (Photo courtesy of Dr. T. Anglin.)

Studies indicate that young patients and adolescents tend to prefer physicians who wear white coats. As a uniform, the white coat identifies the physician in his or her role, which may involve inspection and occasional palpation of private areas. This is even more important today when many children have been instructed in personal safety programs.

In older girls, explaining procedures, demonstrating the various instruments, and providing health information during the examination may decrease apprehension and help establish a good patient–physician relationship.

A. PHYSICAL EXAMINATION

1. General inspection—The examination begins with an evaluation of the patient's general appearance, nutritional status, body habitus, and any gross congenital anomalies.

2. Breasts—Breast budding usually begins at approximately age 8–9 years. Prominence of the nipple and breast development at an earlier age may be early signs of sexual precocity. Appropriate monitoring may include assessment of bone age, as well following height and breast development at 3-month intervals.

3. Abdomen—Inspection and palpation of the abdomen should precede examination of the genitalia. If the child is ticklish, having her place one hand on or under the examiner's hand usually will overcome the problem.

The ovary of a premenarcheal child is situated high in the pelvis. This location and the small size of the pelvic cavity tend to force ovarian tumors above the true pelvic brim. Thus, large neoplasms of the ovary are likely to be mistaken for other abdominal masses (eg, polycystic kidney). Although inguinal hernias are less common in females than in males (approximately 1: 10), they may occur, usually without discomfort. An excellent method of demonstrating an inguinal hernia is to have the child stand up and increase the intra-abdominal pressure by blowing up a balloon.

4. Genitalia—The vulva and vestibule can be exposed by light lateral and downward pressure on each side of the perineum, a technique referred to as *labial separation.* When exposure of the vaginal walls is necessary, the labia can be grasped between the examiner's thumb and forefinger and pulled forward, downward, and sideways, a technique called *labial traction.* Particular attention should be paid to the adequacy of perineal hygiene, because poor hygiene may predispose a child to local inflammation. The examiner should look for skin lesions, perineal excoriations, ulcers, and tumors. Signs of hormonal stimulation in early childhood and absence of such signs later in childhood are important signs of endocrine disorders associated with precocious or delayed puberty. Enlargement of the clitoris is of diagnostic significance, especially during early pubertal development, because it alerts the clinician to the presence of an endocrinopathy.

Special attention should be paid to vulvar inflammation and vulvar and vaginal discharge. In some patients the vestibule or the vaginal orifice may not be visible because of labial adhesions or congenital anomalies. The former condition is frequently mistaken for vaginal agenesis or imperforate hymen.

It is extremely difficult to perform a digital vaginal examination in a child whose vagina is of normal size for her age. The hymeneal orifice is small, and the tissue is thin, friable, and extremely sensitive. Gentle rectal digital examination can be accomplished, but the small size of the uterus and ovaries and the resistance most children offer to the examination render accurate intrapelvic evaluation difficult. If the uterus and ovaries are not palpable, the child likely does not have a genital tumor. If the presence of a pelvic tumor is suspected and the neoplasm cannot be palpated on rectal examination, other diagnostic procedures (eg, sonography, laparoscopy) should be performed.

B. VAGINOSCOPY

Instrumentation is required when it is necessary to carefully visualize the upper third of the vagina for a source of abnormal vaginal bleeding, to confirm patency of the genital tract, to detect and remove foreign bodies, or to exclude penetrating injuries. In the latter case, the examination is often performed under general anesthesia. Figure 34–5 shows the office vaginoscope in use. I prefer to use a water cystoscope, which distends the vagina and permits visualization of the vaginal mucosa, while washing away secretions, blood, and debris (Fig 34–6). Alternatively, a urethroscope or laparoscope can be used.

Figure 34–5. Huffman vaginoscope used for examination of a premenarcheal child.

Figure 34–6. Performing vaginoscopy under anesthesia using a water cystoscope.

In infancy and childhood, the hymenal orifice normally will admit a 0.5-cm vaginoscope. An instrument 0.8 cm in diameter can be used to examine older premenarcheal girls. Topical lidocaine gel can be used to anesthetize the vulva and provide lubrication. If the aperture is too small to allow instrument passage without patient discomfort, vaginoscopy should not be further attempted without general anesthesia.

Examination of the Adolescent

The adolescent's first trip to the gynecologist is often laden with fear and apprehension. Time spent putting the patient at ease and winning her confidence will save time and frustration in the examining room. The physician should make it clear that the adolescent is the patient. She, the patient, rather than an accompanying adult if present, is asked for information that will go on the medical record. Questions about high-risk behaviors, including sexual behavior and sexually transmitted diseases (STDs), should be asked privately.

After the history is taken, the patient should be given a brief description of what the examination entails. She should be assured that the examination will not be painful. The examination is performed in the presence of a female chaperone.

A breast examination is an integral part of the physical examination of every female patient. Controversy exists over whether self-examination techniques should be taught to adolescents at this time, as the risks of a mass being cancerous in this age group are extremely low and evaluation at the time of routine examination most likely is sufficient.

The examination is also used to provide the patient with health maintenance instructions and explanations about her body and its various functions. Many adolescents are not familiar with the appearance of their own genitalia. Some physicians use mirrors during the examination to show normal anatomic details, to demonstrate abnormalities, to explain treatment plans, and to provide explanations regarding health maintenance. Others use a colposcope attached to a video monitor for the genital examination of young children. This provides an enlarged image seen simultaneously by the examiner and the patient and permits direct communication, particularly in difficult cases.

Following inspection of the genitalia, a speculum is inserted into the vagina. The introitus of most virginal adolescents is approximately 1 cm in diameter and will admit a narrow speculum. The Huffman-Graves and Pedersen specula both are designed to allow for easy inspection of the cervix in adolescents, in whom the vagina is 10–12 cm long (Fig 34–7). The larger Graves speculum, although useful in parous women, is generally not appropriate for most younger patients. In a patient with a large hymenal opening, bimanual examination is performed by inserting a finger into the vagina. If the hymenal orifice is too small for digital examination, rectal examination can be performed.

Following the examination, the patient is given an opportunity to speak alone with the examiner. Confidentiality is essential to the physician–patient relationship, and problems can be discussed with the patient's guardians only with the patient's consent. Physical or sexual abuse, however, is a legal issue, which may require breach of confidentiality.

The gynecologic visit serves as an excellent opportunity to review basic health care maintenance. For example, current recommendations advise universal vaccination for hepatitis B for all adolescents at ages 11–12 years, with immunization for older adolescents based on risk status. Tetanus and measles-mumps-rubella (MMR) vaccinations also should be updated. In addition, screening for eating disorders, depression, and behavioral risks including sexual activity and tobacco, alcohol, and substance abuse should be done routinely. To assist providers of adolescent health care, the American Medical Association has issued recommendations based on annual health guidance, screening, and immunization schedules.

Examination of the Young Victim of Sexual Abuse

Studies show that approximately 38% of girls are sexually victimized before age 18 years. Among adolescent girls in grades 9–12, 26% report experiencing physical or sexual abuse. Therefore, all adolescents should be asked about history of abuse. Many children who are possible victims of sexual abuse are brought to a hospital emergency room or to their physician's office for a comprehensive medical evaluation. Statutes vary from state to state as to the need for legal consent from a parent or guardian to perform a genital examination and collect evidence in cases of suspected abuse.

Figure 34–7. The Huffman-Graves speculum (**middle**) is as long as the adult Graves speculum (**right**) and as narrow as the short pediatric Graves speculum (**left**).

A. HISTORY

In some facilities, a designated individual conducts an investigative interview, to minimize repetitive questioning of the child. When asking young children about abuse, line drawings, dolls, or other aids are generally used only by professionals trained in interviewing young children. However, this does not preclude the physician from asking relevant questions to obtain a detailed history, a review of systems, and basic information about the assault. An account of the incident is extremely valuable, as it can later be used in court as evidence, or it may reveal an unusual area of injury and thus uncommon sites for collection of evidence. It is important to know how and from whom the patient sustained the injury and whether the child is in a safe environment.

It is imperative that the clinician use questions that are not leading, avoid showing strong emotions such as shock or disbelief, and maintain a "tell me more" or "and then what happened" approach. The courts have allowed physicians to testify regarding specific details of the child's statements obtained in the course of taking a medical history to provide a diagnosis and treatment. The American Academy of Child and Adolescent Psychiatry and the American Professional Society on the Abuse of Children have published guidelines for interviewing sexually abused children.

The examiner should note the patient's composure, behavior, and mental state, as well as how she interacts with her parents and other persons. Victims of physical or sexual abuse must be removed immediately from an unsafe environment.

The information should be recorded carefully, using the patient's own words. Written notes in the medical record or audiotape or videotape should be used to document the questions asked and the child's responses. Although a detailed history is desirable, the victim should not be made to repeatedly recount the incident. When obtaining a history from a very young child is not possible, the physician should obtain accounts of the incident from other sources.

B. Physical Examination

The physical examination has 2 purposes: to detect and treat injuries and to collect samples that later can be used as evidence.

1. Detection of injuries—Nonspecific findings are relatively common in young children. Vulvar irritation is often seen in small children as a result of poor local hygiene, maceration of the skin because of wetness from diapers, or excoriations caused by local infection. Such nonspecific findings should not be regarded as diagnostic of sexual abuse. It is important to remember that the examination is often normal in most children who were sexually abused. In one study of 2384 children who were seen in a tertiary referral center, less than 5% had genital findings suggesting abuse. The examination was deemed normal in 96.3% of children referred for the evaluation. Even so, interviews of the children indicated that 68% of the girls reported penetration of vagina or anus.

The physician should be able to recognize hymenal trauma. A lacerated hymen usually is discontinuous from 3 to 9 o'clock. In postpubertal girls, penetration and stretch trauma can result in hymeneal remnants.

2. Collection of evidence—During the general inspection, all foreign material (eg, sand and grass) should be removed and placed in clearly labeled envelopes. Scrapings from underneath the fingernails and loose hairs on the skin are collected. Semen can be detected on the skin many hours after the assault. A Wood's lamp can be used to detect the presence of seminal fluid on the patient's body, as the ultraviolet light causes semen to fluoresce. The stain can be lifted off the skin with moistened cotton swabs for further analysis.

If vaginal penetration is suspected, vaginal fluid is collected and sent for sexual disease evaluation, wet-mount preparation, cytology, acid phosphatase determination, and enzyme p30. To avoid additional psychological trauma in a prepubescent child, these specimens can be collected without the insertion of a pediatric speculum, via vaginal aspiration using a feeding tube or Angiocath. An immediate wet-mount preparation done by the examining physician may detect motile sperm.

Culture swabs are obtained from the rectum, vagina, urethra, and pharynx. Current data indicate that a prepubertal child with gonorrhea or trichomonas most likely had genital–genital contact. The mode of transmission of other STDs is controversial. Testing for

STDs, including human immunodeficiency virus (HIV), should be offered.

All specimens must be clearly labeled and the containers and envelopes sealed and signed by the examiner. All persons handling the materials must sign for them. Such a system is necessary to maintain the chain of evidence; otherwise, these specimens may not be admissible in court. Some hospitals provide preassembled "rape kits" that guide the examiner in documenting and collecting specimens in a manner suitable for legal uses.

If an STD or other signs of abuse are found, all states require that the findings be reported to child protective service agencies for investigation of sexual abuse. Furthermore, it is important to keep in mind that a normal physical examination does not exclude the possibility of sexual abuse.

■ CONGENITAL ANOMALIES OF THE FEMALE GENITAL TRACT

Congenital anomalies of the genitalia can be divided into those that suggest sexual ambiguity (intersex problems) and those that do not. Intersex individuals have significant ambiguity of the external genitalia such that the true gender cannot be immediately determined. Detailed discussion on intersex conditions is beyond the scope of this chapter.

ANOMALIES OF THE VULVA & LABIA

Minor differences in the contour or size of vulvar structures are not unusual. Often there is considerable variation in the distance between the posterior fourchette and the anus or between the urethra and the clitoris. Rare anomalies of the vulva include bifid clitoris, which occurs in conjunction with bladder exstrophy; a caudal appendage resembling a tail; congenital prolapse of the vagina; and variations in the insertion of the bulbocavernosus muscle, which may alter the appearance of the labia majora and at times obliterate the fossa navicularis. Duplication of the vulva is an extremely rare anomaly, which may be associated with duplication of the urinary or intestinal tracts.

There is considerable variation in the size and shape of the labia minora. One of the labia may be considerably larger than the other, or both labia may be unusually large. These variations usually require no treatment (Fig 34–8). If asymmetry is significant or if large labia are pulled into the vagina during intercourse, the hypertrophied labia can be trimmed surgically to provide a more symmetric appearance or to relieve dyspareunia. Surgical reduction can be accomplished by amputating the protu-

Figure 34–8. Labial asymmetry resulting from enlargement of the left labium minor.

berant segment, excising a wedge of protuberant labial tissue, or simply removing the central portion.

ANOMALIES OF THE CLITORIS

Clitoral enlargement almost invariably suggests exposure to elevated levels of androgens. Such enlargement is often associated with fusion of the labioscrotal folds. Recklinghausen's neurofibromatosis, lymphangiomas, and fibromas may also involve the clitoris and cause enlargement. When an isolated neoplasm causes enlargement of the clitoris, therapy consists of excision of the neoplasm with reduction of the clitoris to normal size.

Clitoral splitting is caused by a midline fusion defect. Bifid clitoris usually occurs in conjunction with bladder exstrophy, epispadias, and absence or cleavage of the symphysis pubis. The labia majora are widely separated, and the labia minora are separated anteriorly but can be traced posteriorly around the vaginal orifice. The uterus often shows a fusion deformity, and the vaginal orifice is narrow. The vagina is shortened and rotated anteriorly. The pelvic floor is incomplete, and uterine prolapse is often observed in these patients. Other congenital anomalies may be present. Clitoral agenesis is extremely rare.

Finally, children with clitoral enlargement must be fully evaluated to exclude the presence of an intersex condition. Clitoral reduction is often performed as part of therapy once the diagnosis is made and a female gender is assigned. Many techniques have been described. Although the surgery is often performed in early childhood, the long-term effects on sexual function are unknown. A recent study of 39 adults who had intersex conditions with ambiguous genitalia and who were living as females showed that those who had undergone clitoral surgery had higher rates of nonsensuality and of inability to achieve orgasm. The authors concluded that sexual function of adult females could be compromised by clitoral surgery.

ANOMALIES OF THE HYMEN

Hymenal anomalies result from incomplete degeneration of the central portion of the hymen. Variations include imperforate, microperforate, septate, and cribriform hymens. Although most of these variants are not clinically significant, hymenal anomalies require surgical correction if they block vaginal secretions or menstrual fluid, interfere with intercourse, or prevent treatment of a vaginal disorder.

Imperforate Hymen

Imperforate hymen represents a persistent portion of the urogenital membrane. It occurs when the mesoderm of the primitive streak abnormally invades the urogenital portion of the cloacal membrane. It is one of the most common obstructive lesions of the female genital tract. When mucocolpos develops from accumulation of vaginal secretions behind the hymen, the membrane is seen as a shiny, thin bulge (Fig 34–9). The distended vagina forms a large mass that may interfere with urination and at times may be mistaken for an abdominal tumor. The diagnosis is quite easy, and the condition can treated in the nursery. Topical anesthetic is used to prevent discomfort to the newborn, and the central portion of the obstructing membrane is excised. When imperforate hymen is corrected in infants, the central portion of the membrane is excised; sutures usually are not necessary (Fig 34–10).

If missed during the newborn period, imperforate hymen often is not diagnosed until an adolescent presents with complaints of primary amenorrhea and cyclic pelvic pain. It may present as back pain or difficulty with defecation or urination secondary to mass effect from vaginal distention. Inspection of the vulva may reveal a purplish-red hymenal membrane bulging outward as a result of accumulation of blood above it (hematocolpos). Blood may fill the uterus (hematometra)

Figure 34–9. Mucocolpos in a newborn infant.

Figure 34–10. Newborn infant following excision of an imperforate hymen. Forward traction on the labia majora provides an unimpaired view of the hymenal ring. Note the large opening created. No bleeding was noted, and no sutures were required.

and spill through the fallopian tubes into the peritoneal cavity. Endometriosis and vaginal adenosis are known but not inevitable complications.

Repair of imperforate hymen is facilitated if the tissue has undergone estrogen stimulation and the membrane is distended. When the procedure is performed in an adolescent, a large central portion of the membrane should be removed because the edges of a small incision may coalesce, allowing the obstructing membrane to reform.

ANOMALIES OF THE VAGINA

1. Transverse Vaginal Septum

Transverse vaginal septa result from faulty fusion or canalization of the urogenital sinus and müllerian ducts. The incidence is approximately 1 in 30,000 to 1 in 80,000 women. Approximately 46% occur in the upper vagina, 40% in the midportion, and 14% in the lower vagina. When the septum is located in the upper vagina, it is likely to be patent, whereas those located in the lower part of the vagina are more often complete.

A complete septum results in signs and symptoms similar to those of an imperforate hymen. An undiscovered imperforate transverse septum may lead to the formation of a large mucocolpos in infancy. Diagnosis is often delayed until after menarche, when menstrual blood is trapped behind an obstructing membrane. An incomplete septum usually is asymptomatic, as the central aperture allows for vaginal secretions and menstrual flow to egress from the vagina. Excision is indicated in the sexually active patient with dyspareunia.

Treatment

If the diagnosis of a complete septum is established prior to menarche, it should be incised, creating an aperture to allow drainage. Incision of a complete septum is most easily accomplished when the upper vagina is distended and the membrane is bulging, reducing the risk of injury to adjacent structures. Because of the technical difficulties in performing intravaginal surgery on immature structures, it is best to limit the procedure only to allow the establishment of vaginal drainage.

Surgical correction of vaginal narrowing should be performed only when the patient is contemplating initiation of sexual activity. The membrane should be excised with its surrounding ring of subepithelial connective tissue at the level of partition. End-to-end reanastomosis of the upper and lower vaginal mucosa, which may be accomplished with the aid of a Lucite bridge, is then undertaken.

2. Longitudinal Vaginal Septum

Duplication of the vagina is an extremely rare condition, often associated with duplication of the vulva, bladder, and uterus. More commonly, a longitudinal vaginal septum forms when the distal ends of the müllerian ducts fail to fuse properly. Both parts of the vagina are encircled by one muscular layer, and a fibrous septum lined with epithelium divides the vagina. The uterus may be bicornuate, with 1 or 2 cervices (Fig 34–11).

Asymptomatic longitudinal septa require no treatment. Division of the septum is indicated when dyspareunia is present, when obstruction of drainage from half of the vagina is noted, or when it appears that the septum will interfere with vaginal delivery.

Figure 34–11. Longitudinal septum dividing the vagina.

3. Vaginal Agenesis

The incidence of vaginal agenesis is approximately 1 in 5000. The external genitalia of patients with vaginal agenesis (**Mayer-Rokitansky-Kuster-Hauser [MRKH] syndrome**) are normal, with a ruffled ridge of tissue representing the hymen (Fig 34–12). Variable levels of uterine development are present, with most cases accompanied by cervical and uterine agenesis. Other developmental defects are often present, affecting the urinary tract (45–50%), the spine (10%), and, less frequently, the middle ear and other mesodermal structures. Evaluation of the urinary tract and spine, as well as a hearing test, should be performed after diagnosis.

Persons with vaginal agenesis typically have normal female karyotypes with normal ovaries and ovarian function; thus, they develop normal secondary sexual attributes. Patients often present with primary amenorrhea or, in women with functioning uteri, with cyclic pelvic pain. Serum testosterone level and karyotyping may identify the rare instances in which müllerian agenesis represents the effects of testicular activity, indicating male pseudohermaphroditism.

Treatment

Creation of a satisfactory vagina is the objective of treatment of vaginal agenesis. Treatment should be deferred until the patient is contemplating sexual activity. Nonoperative creation of a vagina using serial vaginal dilators, in a method described by Frank and later modified by Ingram, is relatively risk-free but requires patient motivation and cooperation. The procedure takes a few months to complete. Repetitive coitus can also be used to create a functioning vagina.

The McIndoe procedure involves the creation of a cavity by surgical dissection between the urethra and bladder anteriorly and the perineal body and rectum posteriorly. The cavity is lined by a split-thickness skin graft overlying a plastic or soft silicone mold. The labia minora are secured around the mold for 7 days prior to removal. Postoperatively the patient must continue to use dilators for several months to maintain vaginal patency. Patient satisfaction rates greater than 80% have been reported. Complications include graft failure, hematoma, fistula formation, and rectal perforation.

The Williams vulvovaginoplasty utilizes the labia majora to construct a coital pouch. Placing the labia under tension, a U-shaped incision is carried from the level of the urethra along the margins of the labia majora to the midpoint between the posterior fourchette and the anus. The vulvar skin is dissected from the subcutaneous fat to allow approximation without tension. The vagina is closed in 3 layers. This procedure is not performed as often as the McIndoe procedure because

Figure 34–12. Vaginal agenesis in a girl 16 years of age.

the vaginal pouch created is only 4–5 cm in length and positioned at an unusual angle for intercourse.

Alternative procedures, such as sigmoid vaginoplasty and laparoscopic approaches using the Vecchietti procedure and the Davydov procedure, have been described. Limited data on success and complications rates are available.

Few studies address the long-term success of both vaginal dilatation and surgical correction in patients with vaginal agenesis. Unfortunately, each medical center has only limited experience with such patients. Morgan and Quint identified 14 patients with vaginal agenesis, but only 7 could be contacted. In this small series, the authors noted that sexual functioning was variable and patients had unique psychosocial and psychosexual concerns. In another series, Crouch et al. sent questionnaire to 43 women who underwent vaginal dilatation. The authors reported that 23% of the patients never used the dilators they were given, compliance was poor, and only 50% of users were satisfied with their dilators. Sexual difficulties were common irrespective of dilator use or vaginal length.

4. Partial Vaginal Agenesis

Partial vaginal agenesis occurs when a large portion of the vaginal plate, usually the distal part, fails to canalize.

The affected vaginal segment of the vagina is replaced by a soft mass of tissue. The cause of this uncommon anomaly is unknown. Absence of the distal vagina may be identified when the infant is examined at birth, and sonographic visualization of the upper vagina, cervix, and uterus serves to distinguish the condition from Rokitansky syndrome.

If the uterus has developed normally, the upper part of the vagina fills with blood when menstruation begins. The symptoms are similar to those associated with imperforate hymen after the menarche. Vulvar inspection reveals findings identical with those of vaginal agenesis, but rectoabdominal palpation reveals a large, boggy pelvic mass. Diagnostic imaging using sonography, computed tomography, or magnetic resonance imaging will confirm the diagnosis.

Treatment

Surgery is indicated because obstruction to menstrual flow may occur. In some patients, drainage of the uterus can be achieved through a reconstructed vagina. In others, particularly when the uterus is rudimentary, consideration may be given to performing a hysterectomy.

ANOMALIES OF THE UTERUS

Uterine anomalies result from agenesis of the müllerian duct or a defect in fusion or canalization. These anomalies include bicornuate uterus (37%), arcuate uterus (15%), incomplete septum (13%), uterine didelphys (11%), complete septum (9%), and unicornuate uterus (4%).

Most uterine anomalies are asymptomatic and therefore are not detected during childhood or early adolescence. Symptoms during adolescence are primarily caused by retention of menstrual flow. Asymptomatic abnormalities often escape detection until they interfere with reproduction.

1. Unicornuate Uterus and Rudimentary Uterine Horn

A unicornuate uterus is a single-horned uterus with its corresponding fallopian tube and round ligament. It results from agenesis of one müllerian duct, with absence of structures on that side. When the other hemiuterus is present, it often creates a small rudimentary uterine horn. If this rudimentary horn does not communicate with the other uterine cavity or the vagina, menstrual blood cannot escape, resulting in severe dysmenorrhea, hematometra, or pyometra. A pregnancy that occurs in a rudimentary horn may result in rupture, a complication that is potentially fatal for both mother and fetus (Fig 34–13). Women with unicornuate uteri are at higher risk for preterm labor, infertility, endometriosis, and malpresentation.

Figure 34–13. Pregnancy in a noncommunicating rudimentary uterine horn that has resulted in rupture.

Ideally, a rudimentary horn should be resected before conception. The tube and ovary on the affected side can be preserved, provided that the blood supply is not impaired. If the endometrial cavity of the remaining horn is entered during the operation, cesarean section is a reasonable mode of delivery for any subsequent pregnancies.

A unicornuate uterus occasionally is accompanied by an anomaly of the opposite paramesonephric duct, creating a lateral vaginal wall cyst with an endometrial lining. As a result, the cyst fills with blood following menarche and produces a vaginal mass (Fig 34–14). Excision of a small segment of the wall between the cyst and the vagina often provides adequate drainage. Attempts to remove the cyst may involve extensive dissection, with potential damage to the urethra, bladder, or ureter.

2. Uterine Didelphys

Failure of fusion of the müllerian duct may result in 2 separate uterine bodies. The fusion defect usually is limited to the uterine body and cervix. Duplication of the bladder, urethra, vagina, anus, and vulva may also occur.

Women with uterine didelphys generally have good reproductive outcomes. Vaginal septae may require resection if they cause difficulty with sexual intercourse or vaginal delivery or if pain results from obstructed menstrual flow.

3. Bicornuate Uterus and Septate Uterus

Bicornuate uterus results from partial fusion of the müllerian ducts, leading to varying degrees of separation of the uterine horns. Uterine septa result from failures of canalization or resorption of the midline septum between the 2 müllerian ducts. Although reproductive function is good overall in bicornuate uterus, the risk for miscarriage is higher with increasing length of septa. Hysteroscopic resection of septa or metroplasty may be considered for infertility.

Figure 34–14. Unicornuate uterus with paramesonephric vaginal cyst. The endometrium lining the upper part of the cyst bleeds at menarche, and the blood filling the lower part of the cyst forms a mass that protrudes into the vagina.

ANOMALIES OF THE OVARIES

At approximately week 5 of gestation, the midportion of the urogenital ridge, close to the mesonephric duct, thickens to form the gonadal ridge. Located along the urogenital ridge, an additional ovary is infrequently found, separated from the normal ovaries (supernumerary ovary). Similarly, excess ovarian tissue may be observed near a normally placed ovary and connected to it (accessory ovary).

During development, the testes are drawn into the scrotum by the gubernaculum testis. Similarly, an ovary may be drawn by the round ligament into the inguinal canal or the labium major. A firm inguinal mass should alert the examiner to the possible presence of an aberrant gonad, possibly containing testicular elements, even in the presence of female external genitalia. A karyotype should be obtained. At the time of hernia repair, the gonad should be biopsied. If it proves to be an ovary, it should be returned to the peritoneal cavity and the hernia repaired. If a testis is identified, the gonad should be removed.

Patients with gonadal dysgenesis may demonstrate typical physical manifestations. These include cutis laxa and edema of the dorsal surfaces of the hands and feet in infants, height and weight below the third percentile, broad chest and small nipples, webbed neck, coarctation of the aorta, prominent epicanthal folds, nevi, and other somatic anomalies (eg, short fourth metacarpal). In most adults with gonadal dysgenesis, the normal gonad is replaced by a white fibrous streak, 2–3 cm long and approximately 0.5 cm wide, located in the gonadal ridge. Histologically, the streak gonad is characterized by interlacing waves of dense fibrous stroma, indistinguishable from normal ovarian stroma.

Although oocytes are present in children, they usually are absent in 45,X adults. Increased atresia and failure of germ cell formation deplete oocyte supply, but when atresia is incomplete, pubertal changes, spontaneous menstruation, and even pregnancies have been reported.

ANOMALIES OF THE URETHRA & ANUS

Failure of a newborn infant to pass meconium or urine demands investigation. Passage of feces or urine through the vagina suggests a fistulous communication, and usually either the urethra or the anus is imperforate.

Anal and rectal anomalies are classified according to Ladd and Gross (Table 34–2). In general, anomalies are divided into 2 major groups: those that form

Table 34–2. Malformations of the anus and rectum.

	Female	Male
Anal stenosis		
Imperforate anal membrane		
Anal agenesis	With fistula Anoperineal (ectopic perineal anus, anovulvar)	With fistula Anoperineal (ectopic perineal anus, anocutaneous [covered anus]), or anourethral (bulbar or membranous)
	Without fistula	Without fistula
Rectal agenesis	With fistula Rectovestibular, rectovaginal, rectocloacal (urogenital sinus)	With fistula Rectourethral, rectovesical
	Without fistula	Without fistula
Rectal atresia		

Reproduced, with permission, from Ladd WE, Gross RE: Congenital malformations of the anus and rectum: Report of 162 cases. Am J Surg 1934;23:167.

complete obstruction of the intestinal tract and those that are associated with some type of abnormal opening or fistula.

Because findings are so diverse, only broad generalizations on the management of urogenital anomalies of this type can be offered. The following principles may serve as guidelines. (1) Obstruction of the intestinal tract must be corrected. (2) Obstruction of the urinary tract must be relieved (this may require an initial ureterostomy or cystostomy). (3) If the urogenital sinus cannot be used later as a urethra, a permanent diversion (eg, ileal conduit) must be created. (4) Fecal contamination of the urinary tract, if present, must be corrected, usually with a temporary colostomy.

Epispadias & Bladder Exstrophy

Epispadias denotes the failure of normal fusion of the anterior wall of the urogenital sinus, resulting in a urethra that opens cephalad to a bifid clitoris under the symphysis pubis (Fig 34–15). Occasionally, the defect is more extensive, involving the bladder and the anterior abdominal wall, causing exstrophy of the bladder. Both conditions may be associated with defects involving the anterior pelvic girdle, resulting in diminished pelvic support. Uterine and vaginal vault prolapse as well as anterior displacement of the vagina are common gynecologic complications. Rarely, vaginal and uterine prolapse occur in the absence of other malformations. Major urologic reconstruction is required promptly, although gynecologic defects can be repaired later, usually during adolescence.

■ GYNECOLOGIC DISORDERS IN PREMENARCHEAL CHILDREN

VULVOVAGINITIS

Pruritus vulvae and vulvovaginitis are common gynecologic disorders in children. Pruritus vulvae refers to itching of the external female genitalia. Vulvovaginitis, although inconsistently delineated in the literature, generally involves prominent vaginal discharge. The child is susceptible to both these conditions for several reasons: the prepubertal vulva is thin without labial fat pads and pubic hair, as well as anatomically in close proximity to the anus and its contaminants; the unestrogenized vagina is atrophic with pH ranges excellent for bacterial growth; and perineal hygiene often is suboptimal as supervision declines with age. Table 34–3 lists classification of vulvovaginitis according to cause.

Figure 34–15. Adolescent girl following repair of bladder exstrophy. Note the bifid clitoris and anterior displacement of the vagina.

Clinical Findings

Acute vulvovaginitis may denude the thin vulvar or vaginal mucosa; however, bleeding usually is minimal. Mucopurulent or purulent discharge usually is present. Vaginal discharge may vary from minimal to copious, and at times it is bloodstained. Symptoms vary from minor discomfort to relatively intense perineal pruritus. The child often complains of a burning sensation accompanied by a foul-smelling discharge. The irritating discharge inflames the vulva and often causes the child to scratch the area to the point of bleeding. Inspection of the vagina reveals an area of redness and soreness that may be minimal or may extend laterally to the thighs and backward to the anus. Many patients experience a burning sensation when urine flows over the inflamed tissues, and vulvovaginitis should be excluded in children prior to treatment for urinary tract infection.

Table 34–3. Classification of vulvovaginitis according to cause.

Nonspecific vulvovaginitis
Polymicrobial infection associated with disturbed homeostasis: secondary to poor perineal hygiene or a foreign body

Vulvovaginitis due to secondary inoculation
Infection resulting from inoculation of the vagina with pathogens affecting other areas of the body by contact or bloodborne transmission: secondary to upper respiratory tract infection or urinary tract infection

Specific vulvovaginitis
Specific primary infection, most commonly sexually transmitted: *Neisseria gonorrhoeae*, *Gardnerella vaginalis*, herpesvirus, *Treponema pallidum*, others

---

Diagnosis is suspected by the typical appearance of the inflamed tissue. A wet-mount preparation reveals numerous leukocytes and occasional red blood cells. Culture of vaginal secretions sometimes identifies the offending organism.

Evaluation of the vaginal secretions may include smears for Gram's stain, bacterial cultures, cultures for mycotic organisms, wet prep, *Trichomonas,* and parasitic ova.

Improvement of perineal hygiene is important to relieve the symptoms and to prevent recurrences. Most cases of nonspecific pruritus vulvae resolve with improvements in hygiene and avoidance of irritants, including soaps.

Amoxicillin (20–40 mg/kg/d in 3 divided doses) is effective against a variety of potentially pathogenic organisms in nonspecific vulvovaginitis. When the infection is severe and extensive mucosal damage is seen, a short course of topical estrogen cream is given to promote healing of vulval and vaginal tissues. When irritation is intense, hydrocortisone cream may be necessary to alleviate the itch. In recurrent infections refractory to treatment or associated with a foul-smelling, bloody discharge, vaginoscopy is necessary to exclude a foreign body or tumor.

FOREIGN BODIES

Vaginal foreign bodies induce an intense inflammatory reaction and result in blood-stained, foul-smelling discharge. Usually, the child does not recall inserting the foreign object or will not admit to it. Radiographs are not reliable for revealing a foreign body because many objects are not radiopaque. Foreign bodies in the lower third of the vagina can be flushed out with warm saline irrigation. If the vagina cannot be adequately inspected in the office even after removal of the foreign body, vaginoscopy is indicated to confirm that no other foreign bodies are present in the upper vagina.

URETHRAL PROLAPSE

Occasionally, vulvar bleeding is the result of urethral prolapse. The urethral mucosa protrudes through the meatus and forms a hemorrhagic, sensitive vulvar mass. Urethral prolapse can be definitively diagnosed without laboratory or radiographic evaluation by demonstrating that the edematous tissue surrounds the meatus circumferentially and is separated from the vagina. When the lesion is small and urination is unimpaired, treatment consists of parental reassurance, observation, warm soaks, and a short course of therapy using estrogen cream. When urinary retention is present, if the lesion is large and necrotic, if medical therapy fails, or if the child is being examined under anesthesia, resection of the prolapsed tissue should be performed and an indwelling catheter inserted for 24 hours.

LICHEN SCLEROSUS

Lichen sclerosus of the vulva is a hypotrophic dystrophy. More common in postmenopausal women, it is occasionally seen in children. Histologically, the findings in both age groups are similar, with flattening of the rete pegs, hyalinization of the subdermal tissues, and keratinization. In children, the lesion has no known malignant potential if only hypoplastic dystrophy is present.

The clinical presentation includes flat papules that may coalesce into plaques or, in extreme cases, involve the entire vulva (Fig 34–16). Usually, the lesion does not extend beyond the middle of the labia majora laterally or into the vagina medially. The clitoris, posterior fourchette, and anorectal areas are frequently involved. Occasionally, lesions affect extragenital areas. Although most lesions are predominantly white, some have pronounced vascular markings. They tend to bruise easily, forming bloody blisters, and they are susceptible to secondary infections. Symptoms consist of vulvar irritation, dysuria, and pruritus. Scratching is common and occasionally provokes bleeding or leads to secondary infection.

Histologic confirmation is necessary in postmenopausal women but is not always mandatory in children. Treatment usually consists of improved local hygiene, reduction of trauma, and short-term use of hydrocortisone cream to alleviate the pruritus. Topical testosterone or newer androgen-containing skin patches

Figure 34–16. Lichen sclerosus of the vulva in a 6-year-old child.

have also been used, but longer-term exposure may induce androgen-dependent secondary sex characteristics. Over half of children improve significantly or recover during puberty.

LABIAL ADHESION

Labial adhesion is common in prepubertal children. The cause is not known but probably is related to low estrogen levels. The skin covering the labia is extremely thin, and local irritation may induce scratching, which may denude the labia. The labia then adhere in the midline, and reepithelialization occurs on both sides (Fig 34–17). It is important to differentiate this condition from congenital absence of the vagina.

Most children with small areas of labial adhesions are asymptomatic. When symptoms occur, they usually relate to interference with urination or accumulation of urine behind the adhesion. Dysuria and recurrent vulvar and vaginal infections are cardinal symptoms. Rarely, urinary retention may occur.

Figure 34–17. Labial adhesion in a young girl. Note the translucent vertical line in the center where the labia are fused together.

Figure 34–18. Management of labial adhesions.

Asymptomatic minimal to moderate labial fusion does not require treatment. Symptomatic fusion may be treated with a short course of estrogen cream applied twice daily for 7–10 days; this may separate the labia. Some girls may require manual separation once they have been treated with topical estrogen. When medical treatment fails or if severe urinary symptoms exist, surgical separation of the labia is indicated. This can be performed in the operating room under anesthesia, or as an office procedure using 1–2% topical lidocaine (Xylocaine) gel. A schematic approach to the management of labial adhesions is shown in Fig 34–18.

Because of low estrogen levels, recurrences of labial adhesion are common until puberty. Following puberty, the condition resolves spontaneously. Improved perineal hygiene and removal of vulvar irritants may help prevent recurrences.

GENITAL INJURIES

Most injuries to the genitalia during childhood are accidental. Many are of minor significance, but a few are life-threatening and require surgical intervention. The physician must determine how the child sustained the injury, bearing in mind that the child requires protection if she is the victim of physical or sexual abuse.

1. Vulvar Injuries

Contusion of the vulva usually does not require treatment. A hematoma manifests as a round, tense, ecchymotic, tender mass (Fig 34–19). A small vulvar hematoma usually can be controlled by pressure with an ice pack. The vulva should be kept clean and dry. A hematoma that is large or continues to increase in size may require incision, with removal of clotted blood and ligation of bleeding points. If the source of bleeding cannot be found, the cavity should be packed with gauze and a firm pressure dressing applied. The pack is removed in 24 hours. Prophylactic broad-spectrum antibiotics may be advisable.

When a large hematoma obstructs the urethra, insertion of a catheter is necessary, usually by a suprapubic approach. Radiography of the pelvis may be necessary to rule out pelvic fracture.

2. Vaginal Injuries

Usually, only a small amount of bleeding results from a hymenal injury. However, when the hymen is lacerated or other evidence indicates an object has entered the vagina or penetrated the perineum, a detailed examination is necessary to exclude injuries to the upper vagina or intrapelvic viscera (Fig 34–20).

Most vaginal injuries involve the lateral walls. Generally, there is relatively little blood loss, and the child does not have much pain if only the mucosa is damaged. If the laceration extends beyond the vaginal vault, exploration of the pelvic cavity is necessary to rule out extension into the broad ligament or peritoneal cavity. Bladder and bowel integrity must be confirmed by catheterization and rectal palpation. Because of the small caliber of the organs involved, special instruments, as well as proper exposure and assistance, may be required for repair of vaginal injuries in young girls. Many vaginal lacerations are limited to the mucosal and submucosal tissues and are repaired with fine suture material after complete hemostasis is secured.

A vaginal wall hematoma from a small vessel may stop bleeding spontaneously. Larger vessels may form large, tense hematomas that distend the vagina and require evacuation and ligation of the bleeding vessel. When a vessel is torn above the pelvic floor, a retroperitoneal hematoma may develop. If the hematoma is enlarging, laparotomy must be performed, the clot removed, and the bleeding vessel ligated. Alternatively, the bleeding may be controlled by angiographic embolization of the bleeding vessel.

Figure 34–20. Transvaginal perforation of cul-de-sac and penetration of peritoneal cavity by a fall on a mop handle. Scanty bleeding from a hymenal tear was the only symptom on admission.

3. Anogenital Injuries Caused by Abuse

Many children who are victims of sexual abuse do not sustain physical injuries, and an examination is not expected to detect signs of abuse. Even when injured, many of these children may not be seen for weeks, months, or even years after the incident. The delay allows for semen and debris to wash away and for most, if not all, injuries to heal.

Injuries to the vulva may be caused by manipulation of the vulva or introitus, without vaginal penetration, or by friction of the penis against the child's vulva ("dry intercourse"). Erythema, swelling, skin bruising, and excoriations are found on the labia and vestibule. These injuries are superficial and often limited to the vulvar skin; they should resolve within a few days and require no special treatment.

Meticulous perineal hygiene is important in the prevention of secondary infections. Sitz baths should be used to remove secretions and contaminants. In some patients with extensive skin abrasions, broad-spectrum antibiotics should be given as prophylaxis. Large vulvar tears require suturing, which is best performed under general anesthesia, using fine absorbable sutures. Bite wounds on the genitalia should be irrigated copiously and necrotic tissue cautiously debrided. A noninfected fresh wound often can be closed primarily, but most bite wounds should be left open. Closure is completed when granulation tissue is formed. After 3–5 days, secondary debridement may be required to remove necrotic tissues. Antitetanus immunization should be given if the child is not already immunized. Broad-spectrum antibiotics should be used for therapy rather than prophylaxis.

Most vaginal injuries occur when an object penetrates the vagina through the hymenal opening. Such

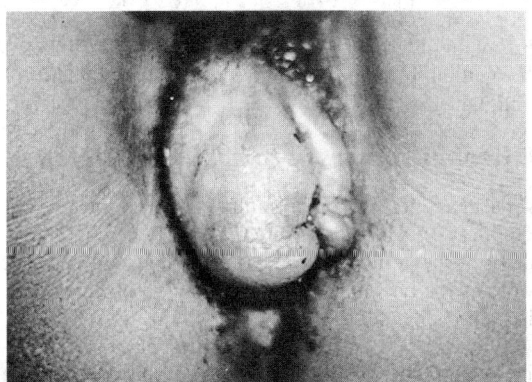

Figure 34–19. Large vulvar hematoma secondary to bicycle injury.

penetration may result in a laceration or a tear of the hymenal ring as well as associated vaginal injuries. A detailed examination is necessary to exclude injuries to the upper vagina.

Examination of the anus and rectum is easier than is examination of the vagina, and most children tolerate it well. Because the anal sphincter and anal canal allow for some dilatation, a tear of the anal mucosa or sphincter rarely occurs following a digital assault. However, penetration by a larger object almost always results in some degree of injury, which varies from swelling of the anal verge to gross tearing of the sphincter. In the period immediately following penetration, the main findings are sphincter laxity and swelling and small tears of the anal verge. If the sphincter is not severed, it may be in spasm and will not permit a digital examination. Within days, the swelling subsides and the mucosal tears heal, occasionally forming skin tags. If not severed, the anal sphincter regains function. Repeated anal penetration over a prolonged period may cause the anal sphincter to become loose, forming an enlarged opening. The anal mucosa thickens and loses its normal folds. Although some investigators suggest that many of the children who experienced anal assault exhibit perianal scars and tags, longitudinal studies showed that anal injuries heal completely in most children.

Occasionally, child victims of abuse contracts an STD. The risk of a prepubertal child contracting an STD after sexual assault is relatively low, estimated to range from 2–5%. Treatment of gonorrhea, chlamydia, and syphilis may be deferred until the results of tests become available. If vulvovaginitis is clinically suspected on the initial visit, appropriate antibiotic therapy is given. If the infection is severe, a short course of topical estrogen cream is given to promote healing of vulval and vaginal tissues. When irritation is intense, hydrocortisone cream may be necessary to alleviate itching. A repeat VDRL (Venereal Disease Research Laboratory) test to detect seroconversion is required 6 weeks later. Prophylaxis for hepatitis B with hepatitis B vaccination is recommended following sexual assault. For nonimmune victims with a high-risk exposure, practitioners may also consider adding hepatitis B immune globulin to the regimen.

The Sexually Transmitted Diseases Treatment Guidelines from 2002 do not recommend the routine screening for HIV for all child victims of sexual abuse. In view of recent data, the CDC issued a revised policy (2005) which recommends that people exposed to AIDS virus from rapes, accidents, occasional drug use, or unsafe sex receive drug cocktails that can keep them from becoming infected. Clinicians should try to identify children who are at high risk for HIV exposure and consider offering them counseling and prophylactic therapy.

Protective Services & Counseling

It is imperative to ensure that the child will be discharged to a safe environment. Sometimes it is advisable to admit the child to the hospital or to utilize temporary placement. All patients who are suspected of being victims of child sexual abuse must be referred to child protective services for further evaluation.

In the period immediately following sexual assault or disclosure of sexual abuse, the child and her family often require intensive day-to-day emotional support, counseling, and guidance. Child victims often show signs of depression and have feelings of guilt, fear, and low self-esteem. Appropriate referral for counseling is imperative. The major emphasis of emotional support involves strengthening the child's ego, improving her self-image, and helping her to learn to trust others and feel secure again. To begin the strengthening process, the child needs to realize that she was a victim. She must be encouraged to express her feelings of anger and hurt so that these feelings can be later expressed without experiencing further guilt. Often, the child has both positive and negative feelings toward the perpetrator and may need help in sorting out these feelings. Sometimes the child blames her parents for not protecting her. The child's relationships with her parents and other family members are critical and may need restructuring. Following this crisis intervention phase, a treatment program using individual and peer-group therapy is initiated. The patient and her family should be offered treatment.

GENITAL NEOPLASMS

Genital tumors are uncommon but must be considered when a girl is found to have a chronic genital ulcer, nontraumatic swelling of the external genitalia, tissue protruding from the vagina, a fetid or bloody discharge, abdominal pain or enlargement, or premature sexual maturation. Virtually every type of genital neoplasm reported in adults has also been found in girls younger than 14 years. Approximately 50% of the genital tumors in children are premalignant or malignant.

1. Benign Tumors of the Vulva & Vagina

Teratomas, hemangiomas, simple cysts of the hymen, retention cysts of the paraurethral ducts, benign granulomas of the perineum, and condylomata acuminata are some of the benign vulvar neoplasms observed in children and adolescents.

Obstruction of a paraurethral duct may form a relatively large cyst that distorts the urethral orifice. The recommended treatment is incision and drainage, marsupialization, or excision.

Teratomas usually present as cystic masses arising from the midline of the perineum. Although a teratoma in this area may be benign, local recurrence is likely. To prevent recurrences, a generous margin of healthy tissue is excised about the periphery of the mass.

Capillary hemangiomas usually disappear as the child grows older and thus require no therapy except reassurance. Cavernous hemangiomas, in contrast, are composed of vessels of considerable size, and injury to them may cause serious hemorrhage. They are best treated surgically.

Most benign tumors of the vagina in children are unilocular cystic remnants of the mesonephric duct (Fig 34–21). Small cysts of the mesonephric duct (Gartner's duct) do not require surgery when they are asymptomatic. Large cysts (eg, those that block the vagina) must be treated surgically. The technical difficulties associated with excision of a large mesonephric cyst from the wall of the vagina in an infant may be considerable. Removal of a large portion of the cyst wall and marsupialization of the edges, which prevents reaccumulation of fluid, usually are sufficient.

2. Malignant Tumors of the Vagina & Cervix

Embryonal Carcinoma of the Vagina (Botryoid Sarcoma)

Embryonal vaginal carcinomas are most commonly seen in very young girls (< 3 years old). The tumor usually involves the vagina, but the cervix may be affected as well, particularly in an older child. The tumors arise

Figure 34–22. Botryoid sarcoma presenting as a hemorrhagic growth extruding from the vagina.

in the submucosal tissues and spread rapidly beneath an intact vaginal epithelium. The vaginal mucosa then bulges into a series of polypoid growths (thus the term botryoid sarcoma; Fig 34–22). The diagnosis is made on the basis of histologic evaluation of a biopsy specimen, but routine microscopic evaluation may lead to an erroneous diagnosis of these lesions as benign. Striated muscle fibers are not always seen, and most of the tumor demonstrates myxomatous changes. Electron microscopy may be required to confirm the diagnosis of embryonal rhabdomyosarcoma.

Combination chemotherapy regimens—often, vincristine, dactinomycin (actinomycin D), and cyclophosphamide—have been used with success. Following a course of chemotherapy lasting for at least 6 months, the tumor is reexamined and rebiopsied. If following chemotherapy no residual tumor is found, surgical extirpation may not be required. If a tumor is present and is amenable to surgical removal, radical hysterectomy and vaginectomy may be performed. The ovaries are preserved, and exenteration is not recommended. If the tumor is unresectable, radiation therapy is used to further shrink and control tumor growth. Following surgery, chemotherapy should be continued for another 6–12 months.

Other Malignant Tumors of the Vagina

Three types of vaginal carcinoma may appear during childhood and the early teens. Endodermal carcinoma occurs most often in young children. Carcinoma arising in a remnant of a mesonephric duct (mesonephric carcinoma) occurs more often in girls 3 years of age or older. Clear cell adenocarcinoma of müllerian origin, often associated with a history of antenatal exposure to diethylstilbestrol (DES), is encountered most frequently in postmenarcheal teenage girls. The clinical

Figure 34–21. Simple vulvar or hymeneal cyst arising posterior to the urethra of a newborn infant.

features and treatment of malignant lesions of the vagina and cervix are similar to those in adult women.

3. Ovarian Tumors

With the increasing use of antenatal imaging modalities, greater numbers of fetal ovarian cysts are being diagnosed. Although many of these cysts are small, some may pose a risk of acute and long-term complications, such as torsion or rupture. Because many of the cysts regress after birth, many clinicians prefer to observe such cysts and intervene only infrequently. The decision to intervene is based on cyst size, ultrasound characteristics, and clinical symptoms. Treatment options include antenatal or neonatal cyst aspiration, laparoscopic cystectomy, and laparotomy.

Even though ovarian tumors are the most common genital neoplasm encountered in children and adolescents, they represent only 1% of all neoplasms in premenarcheal children. Ovarian tumors of all varieties (except Brenner's tumors) have been reported in premenarcheal children, with benign cystic teratomas accounting for at least 30%. Seventy percent of ovarian cancers in youth are of germ cell origin. The most common symptoms of ovarian tumors are abdominal pain and an abdominal mass. The small pelvic cavity of a child causes most ovarian tumors to rise above the pelvic inlet and present abdominally. Acute symptoms of severe pain, peritoneal irritation, or intra-abdominal hemorrhage resulting from a tumor accident (torsion, rupture, or perforation) may lead to an erroneous diagnosis of appendicitis, intussusception, or volvulus. At least 25% of all childhood ovarian tumors elude diagnosis until exploratory laparotomy is performed. Tumors of the ovary should be considered in the differential diagnosis of most disorders causing abdominal pain or mass in a child. Pelvic (rectal) examination may be helpful if the tumor is in the pelvis but will not detect most abdominal tumors. Imaging is a critical step in the evaluation of the adolescent or child with an adnexal mass. The use of serum markers, such as inhibin or α-fetoprotein, may be helpful in children with ovarian enlargement.

The management of ovarian neoplasms in premenarcheal children varies from that in older patients because continued ovarian function is necessary to complete sexual and somatic maturation in children. Although laparoscopy is an acceptable option if an adnexal mass is thought to be benign, suspicion of malignancy should prompt laparotomy. Conservative surgery (unilateral salpingo-oophorectomy) is justified for most premenarcheal patients with stage I cancer of the ovary, provided the tumor can be shown to be limited to the ovary. If a tumor has extended beyond the ovary, more radical surgery (bilateral salpingo-oophorectomy with hysterectomy) is indicated, regardless of age. Germ cell tumors are highly responsive to chemotherapy, with the exception of dysgerminomas, which respond well to radiation.

■ DISORDERS OF SEXUAL MATURATION

ACCELERATED SEXUAL MATURATION

Puberty is the process by which sexually immature persons become capable of reproduction. These changes occur largely as the result of maturation of the hypothalamic-pituitary-gonadal axis. As a rule, breast development, cornification of the vaginal mucosa, and growth of genital hair precede uterine bleeding by approximately 2 years. The normal sequence of events in sexual development is outlined in Fig 34–23. Accelerated growth and early estrogen effects of the genitalia occur first, but the most obvious sign of early puberty usually is breast enlargement, which initially may be unilateral. Pubic and axillary hair may appear before, at about the same time, or well after the appearance of breast tissue. The vaginal mucosa, which in prepubertal girls is a deep red color, takes on a moist pastel-pink appearance as estrogen exposure increases. Menses are a late event, usually not occurring until 2–3 years after onset of breast enlargement.

In young Northern American girls, breast budding occurs between ages 7 and 11 years and is followed by pubarche and a marked increase in growth rate, often referred to as the *adolescent growth spurt.* Secondary sexual features often occur earlier in African-American girls. The first menstrual period occurs at an average age of 12.8 years in girls in the United States. Regular ovulatory cycles, 20 months later, mark the end of the pubertal changes.

Sexual precocity is the onset of sexual maturation at any age that is 2.5 SD earlier than the normal age for that population. It may be classified as gonadotropin-releasing hormone (GnRH)-dependent precocious puberty (true precocious puberty) or GnRH-independent precocious puberty (pseudoprecocious puberty).

GnRH-Dependent Precocious Puberty

GnRH-dependent precocious puberty is normal pubertal development that occurs at an early age. Premature activation of the hypothalamic-pituitary axis is followed by gonadotropin secretion, which in turn stimulates the gonads to produce steroid hormones and, subsequently, pubertal changes. GnRH-dependent precocious puberty is seen more frequently in girls than in boys. The cause of such early development often remains unclear and has been labeled central precocious puberty (CPP) . Most girls suspected of having CPP are otherwise healthy children whose pubertal maturation begins at the early end of the normal distribution curve. In general, the older the child,

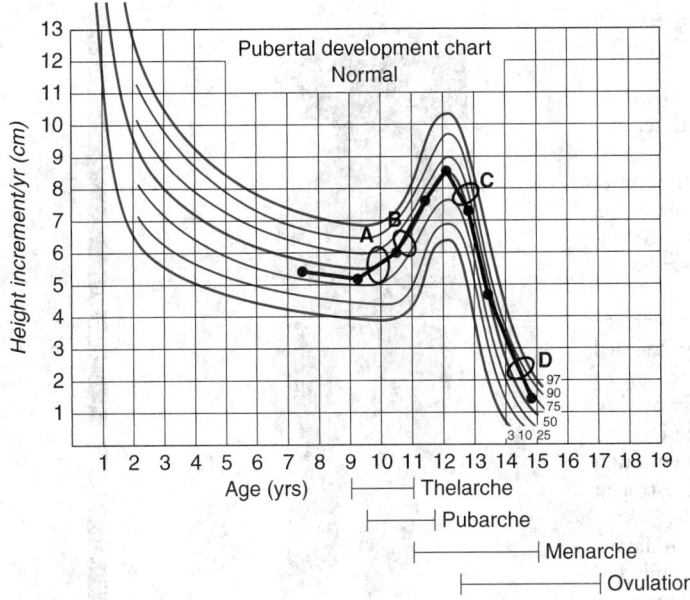

Figure 34–23. Pubertal development chart for a normally developing female adolescent. Growth data are converted to growth velocity and plotted. The growth velocity curve shows initial acceleration in growth, followed by the growth spurt and subsequent deceleration. Superimposed on this curve are the following pubertal events: **A,** thelarche; **B,** pubarche; **C,** menarche; **D,** onset of ovulation. (Reproduced, with permission, from Reindollar RH, McDonough PG: Delayed sexual development: Common causes and basic clinical approach. Pediatr Ann 1981;10:178.)

the less the chance of finding an organic etiology for CPP. Central nervous system (CNS) imaging studies of these otherwise healthy 6- to 8-year-old girls usually reveal no structural abnormalities.

Occasionally, precocious puberty is associated with CNS abnormalities, including hypothalamic hamartomas, optic gliomas, and neurofibromas, as well as other CNS neoplasms. Cranial irradiation and CNS injuries may also be associated with precocious puberty. Prolonged excessive therapy with exogenous sex steroids may accelerate hypothalamic-pituitary axis maturation, resulting in precocious puberty.

The diagnosis is made with the help of a careful history and physical examination in conjunction with radiologic and laboratory evaluations.

GnRH-Independent Precocious Puberty

GnRH-independent precocious puberty is the appearance of pubertal development, but the presence of sex steroids is independent of pituitary gonadotropin release. Causes of precocious pseudopuberty include congenital adrenal hyperplasia, tumors that secrete human chorionic gonadotropin, tumors of the adrenal gland or gonads, McCune-Albright syndrome (MAS), and exposure to exogenous sex steroid hormones.

A. Endogenous Estrogens

The ovary in the newborn female contains 1–2 million primordial follicles, most of which undergo atresia during childhood without producing significant quantities of estrogen. However, large follicular cysts capable of estrogen production occur occasionally and may cause early feminization. Benign tumors of the ovary (eg, teratoma, cystadenoma) may produce estrogen or may induce surrounding ovarian tissue to produce steroids. Circulating sex steroids cause secondary sexual development. The sex steroids (estrogen or testosterone) come from either the adrenal gland or the gonad, independent of the hypothalamic-pituitary portion of the pubertal axis. Sex steroids also may be ingested or absorbed from exogenous sources.

Granulosa cell tumors capable of estrogen production are a rare cause of prepubertal feminization. Other rare tumors of extragonadal origin, including adrenal adenomas and hepatomas, may produce estrogens as well. In rare instances, the neoplasm secretes GnRH, which in turn stimulates the gonad to produce sex hormones.

B. Exogenous Estrogens

Ingestion of estrogens or prolonged use of creams containing estrogens is a possible, but uncommon, cause of early feminization. Prompt discontinuation is indicated.

C. McCune-Albright Syndrome

McCune-Albright syndrome (MAS) in its classic form consists of at least 2 features of the triad of polyostotic fibrous dysplasia, café-au-lait skin pigmentation, and autonomous endocrine hyperfunction, the most common form of which is GnRH secretion and subsequent precocious puberty. Although changes in ovary, bone, and skin tissue are most common, other endocrine and nonendocrine tissues also may be affected, including the adrenal, thyroid, pituitary, liver, and heart.

The fibrous dysplasia seen in children, MAS most commonly affects the long bones, ribs, and skull. The lesions range in size from small asymptomatic areas to markedly disfiguring lesions that can result in pathologic fractures.

The café-au-lait spots in children with MAS are large melanotic macules with irregular outline, described as "coast of Maine" (Fig 34–24).

MAS is caused by a postzygotic somatic mutation in the gene coding for the a subunit of the stimulatory G protein, which is involved in transmitting hormone signals. In patients with MAS, the signaling cascades are activated in the absence of hormone stimulation.

Affected children usually present at a younger age than those with idiopathic precocious puberty. Vaginal bleeding occurs early and in most is the first sign of puberty. The diagnosis is made on the basis of skin pigmentation and demonstration of bone lesions or pathologic fractures. The exact cause is unknown, but a primary ovarian abnormality with premature estrogen production has been suggested.

The prognosis for children with MAS is unfavorable. Adult height is significantly reduced, not only because of early epiphyseal closure but also because of pathologic bone fractures. Multiple endocrinopathies often exist as well. As in adults, most patients have menstrual abnormalities and many are infertile.

D. INCOMPLETE FORMS OF PUBERTAL DEVELOPMENT

Occasionally, for reasons that remain unclear, only 1 sign of pubertal development is present (breast development, pubic hair, or menstruation). Premature thelarche and premature pubarche, which are more common conditions than true precocious puberty, are 2 benign normal variant conditions that can look like precocious puberty but are nonprogressive or very slowly progressive. It possibly results from transient elevations of the levels of circulating steroid hormones or from extreme sensitivity of the end organ (eg, breast tissue) to the low, prepubertal levels of sex hormones. Such isolated development, however, may represent the initial sign of precocious puberty, and these patients should be reevaluated at regular intervals.

E. PREMATURE THELARCHE

Premature thelarche is the isolated development of breast tissue prior to age 8 years, most commonly occurring between 1 and 3 years of age. It may affect 1 or both breasts (Fig 34–25). A thorough history, physical examination, and growth curve review can help distinguish this normal variant from true sexual precocity. On examination, the somatic growth pattern is not accelerated, bone age is not advanced, and smear of vaginal secretions fails to show estrogen effect. The diagnosis is made by exclusion of other disorders. Surgical biopsy of the breast is not indicated,

Figure 34–24. Four-year-old child with idiopathic precocious puberty.

as extensive excision of tissue may cause permanent damage to the breast. Occasionally, premature thelarche occurs when the child is exposed to exogenous estrogens. In Puerto Rico, an epidemic of premature thelarche in the 1970s was suspected to have been caused by exposure to estrogens in the food chain.

F. PREMATURE PUBARCHE

Premature pubarche previously was defined as the appearance of pubic or axillary hair prior to age 8 years, without other signs of precocious puberty (Fig 34–26). However, new guidelines suggest that this presentation should not be considered precocious unless noted before age 7 years in white girls and before age 6 years in black girls. Such hair growth may be idiopathic and of no clinical significance.

Premature pubarche probably results from an earlier-than-usual increase in the secretion of androgens by the adrenal glands. Regulation of adrenal androgen secretion is distinct from that of gonadal steroids; therefore, early appearance of pubic hair may not correlate with true precocious puberty and generally is not a cause for concern. Thorough evaluation of adrenal and gonadal function

Figure 34–25. Premature thelarche in a child 5 years of age.

and assessment of androgen production are necessary to exclude such abnormalities. The diagnosis of idiopathic premature pubarche is made only after such an evaluation fails to detect an abnormality.

Signs of severe androgen excess (eg, clitoral enlargement, growth acceleration, acne) should prompt further investigation for a rare virilizing tumor (Leydig cell tumor), or a variant form of congenital adrenal hyperplasia.

G. PREMATURE MENARCHE

Premature menarche denotes the appearance of cyclic vaginal bleeding in children in the absence of other signs of secondary sexual development. The cause is unknown but may be related to increased end-organ sensitivity of the endometrium to low prepubertal levels of estrogens. Alternatively, bleeding may be related to transient elevation of estrogens due to premature follicular development. These patients have estradiol levels in the prepubertal range, and cytologic smears of vaginal secretions indicate lack of estrogenic stimulation. When patients are given GnRH, the response of the pituitary gland is similar to that seen in prepubertal children.

The diagnosis of premature menarche is formulated by exclusion following investigation of other causes of vaginal bleeding and is confirmed when the cyclic nature of the bleeding becomes apparent. The prognosis is excellent. Adult height is uncompromised, the menstrual pattern is normal, and fertility potential remains unimpaired.

Evaluation of the Patient with Precocious Puberty

When evaluating the patient with sexual precocity, the age at onset, duration, and progression of signs and symptoms constitute important historical information. Family history and review of systems may add important facts.

A. GENERAL CHANGES

Enhancement of general growth is coincident with the onset of estrogen-stimulated change. The child often exhibits accelerated growth velocity, tall stature for age, and advanced skeletal maturation.

B. SKIN

Additional androgen-dependent findings include acne and adult-type body odor.

C. BREAST DEVELOPMENT

Breast development is at least at Tanner stage II, with the areolae having a broadened, darkened appearance.

D. GENITALIA

Genital changes reflect estrogen-induced thickening of the genital tissues. Increased vaginal secretions may result in leukorrhea. Dark, coarse pubic hair may be present.

Diagnosis

The diagnosis of GnRH-dependent precocity requires demonstration of pubertal gonadotropin secretion. The diagnostic evaluation required to document early pubertal development and differentiate central from peripheral causes includes the determination of serum luteinizing hormone (LH), follicle-stimulating hormone (FSH), and estradiol levels, and a GnRH stimulation test. In patients with GnRH-dependent precocious puberty, the results of these tests will be in the normal pubertal range. In addition, these patients will require diagnostic imaging to document skeletal age and the absence of gonadal or CNS lesions.

Figure 34–26. Premature pubarche in a child 4 years of age.

With the improvement in imaging technology, clinicians often order such studies to help establish the diagnosis. Sonography may aid in the evaluation of the ovaries and adrenal glands. Uterine size is estrogen dependent and is a good bioassay to determine the length of time and magnitude of estrogen exposure. Ovarian cysts and tumors are also visible. Sonography of the adrenal glands is less sensitive than abdominal computed tomography (CT) and magnetic resonance imaging (MRI). A skeletal survey and bone scan may identify areas of fibrous dysplasia in patients with MAS. Brain MRI is indicated in patients with sexual precocity or with neurologic signs.

Treatment of GnRH-Dependent Precocious Puberty

The treatment of choice for GnRH-dependent precocious puberty is GnRH analogues. Analogues of GnRH are modifications of the native hormone, which have greater resistance to degradation and increased affinity for the pituitary GnRH receptors. They induce downregulation of receptor function, resulting in temporary, reversible inhibition of the hypothalamic-pituitary-ovarian axis, as reflected by minimal or no response to GnRH stimulation and regression of the manifestations of puberty.

Treatment with GnRH analogues decreases gonadotropins and sex steroids to prepubertal levels, which is followed by regression of secondary sexual features. Treatment also causes a deceleration in the skeletal maturation rate, preserving or even improving predicted height, unless bone age is so advanced that further growth is precluded. All published evidence indicates a gain of adult height over height predicted before treatment or over untreated historical controls. However, ascertaining the exact height increment is difficult because of the inaccuracy of height prediction methods. Use of GnRH agonists in girls who begin pubertal development only 1 or 2 years earlier than normal is of limited or no benefit. Treatment is continued until puberty is appropriate based on age, emotional maturity, height, and height potential. Resumption of puberty occurs promptly after discontinuation of GnRH analogue therapy.

DELAYED SEXUAL MATURATION

Delayed sexual development has been defined as the absence of normal pubertal events at an age 2.5 SD later than the mean. The absence of thelarche by age 13 years or the absence of menarche by age 15 years is an indication for investigation. Some degree of sexual maturation occurs in more than 30% of patients with gonadal dysgenesis; therefore, a patient who presents following thelarche with a delay in the orderly progression of pubertal development should undergo investigation. Delayed sexual development can be classified according to gonadal function (Table 34–4).

Table 34–4. Classification of patients with delayed sexual maturation.

Delayed Menarche with Adequate Secondary Sexual Development
Anatomic genital abnormalities
Inappropriate positive feedback
Androgen insensitivity syndromes (complete forms)
Delayed Puberty with Inadequate or Absent Secondary Sexual Development
Hypothalamic-pituitary dysfunction (low FSH)
  Reversible: Constitutional delay, weight loss due to extreme dieting, protein deficiency, fat loss without muscle loss, drug abuse
  Irreversible: Kallmann's syndrome, pituitary destruction
Gonadal failure (high FSH)
  Abnormal chromosomal complement (eg, Turner's syndrome)
  Normal chromosomal complement: chemotherapy, irradiation, infection, infiltrative or autoimmune disease, resistant ovary syndrome
Delayed Puberty with Heterosexual Secondary Sexual Development (Virilization)
Enzyme deficiency (eg, 21α-hydroxylase deficiency), neoplasm, male pseudohermaphroditism

FSH, follicle-stimulating hormone.

1. Delayed Menarche with Adequate Secondary Sexual Development

Patients with functioning gonads and delayed sexual maturation usually consult a physician while they are in their mid-teens because of amenorrhea. Most have well-formed female configuration with adequately developed breasts. Many of these patients suffer from an inappropriate hypothalamic-pituitary-ovarian feedback mechanism leading to anovulation and androgen excess. Primary amenorrhea may persist until a progestin challenge is given. Patients should be monitored for continued menstrual shedding. Persistent amenorrhea is treated with progestins administered every other month to prevent endometrial hyperplasia. A sexually active girl should be given oral contraceptives rather than cyclic progestins. Further evaluation is required in patients with persistent menstrual abnormalities, because similar clinical manifestations are encountered in adolescents with adult-onset congenital adrenal hyperplasia and those with polycystic ovarian disease.

The possibility of pregnancy in an adolescent who has not begun to menstruate is highly unlikely but must be borne in mind when considering causes of delayed menarche in patients with normal pubertal development.

Most patients with congenital anomalies of the paramesonephric (müllerian) structures complain of primary amenorrhea. The most common defect is congenital absence of the uterus and vagina. Other causes are obstructive abnormalities, such as imperforate hymen, transverse vaginal septa, and agenesis of the cervix. Gynecologic examination supplemented by pelvic sonogram or MRI establishes the diagnosis of these congenital anomalies.

The complete forms of androgen insensitivity (Fig 34–27) are also associated with amenorrhea and normal breast development. Affected persons have normal testicular function but are not responsive to male concentrations of testosterone, and the development of breasts is secondary to the small amounts of unopposed estrogens produced by the testis. Pubic and axillary hair is scant or often absent. A short blind vaginal pouch is present. Once pubertal development has been completed, surgical extirpation of the gonads and reconstruction of the vagina are necessary. Recent data suggest that regardless of the technique used, sexual function may be impaired in some of these young women. A study of 66 women with complete forms of androgen insensitivity showed that 90% had sexual difficulties, most commonly sexual infrequency and vaginal penetration difficulty. Furthermore, most women perceived the newly created vagina to be too small, even though the vagina was of adequate size in many of the women.

2. Delayed Puberty with Inadequate or Absent Secondary Sexual Development

Hypothalamic-Pituitary Dysfunction

Both reversible and irreversible causes of delayed puberty secondary to lack of maturation or function of the hypothalamus and pituitary have been described.

The onset of puberty depends on an ill-defined stage of maturity that is reflected in skeletal age. Maturation is partly genetically determined but also depends on multiple environmental factors; thus the chronologic age of puberty varies considerably. Statistical limits of normal variation in a defined population group indicate that, by definition, 2.5% of all normal adolescents will develop later than the age defined as "normal." This group has been labeled "late bloomers" or as having a constitutional growth delay (CGD). These girls often have retarded linear growth within the first 3 years of life, and then their growth resumes at a normal rate. As a result, these girls grow either along the lower growth percentiles or beneath the curve but parallel to it for the remainder of the prepubertal years.

At the expected time of puberty, the height of children with CGD begins to drift further from the growth curve because of delayed onset of the pubertal growth spurt. Catch-up growth, onset of puberty, and pubertal growth spurt occur later than average, resulting in normal adult stature and sexual development. Although CGD is a variant of normal growth rather than a disor-

Figure 34–27. XY sisters with androgen insensitivity syndrome. (Courtesy of C.J. Dewhurst.)

der, absence of signs of puberty (including the growth spurt) often concerns the patient when her adolescent friends have developed secondary sexual features and gained the characteristic increase in height.

The diagnosis of hypothalamic-pituitary dysfunction is made by exclusion of other causes of delayed sexual maturation. Growth charts, bone age, and the GnRH challenge test differentiate constitutional delay from similar conditions associated with GnRH deficiency. Reassurance is the only treatment necessary, but the patient must be kept under observation until regular menstrual cycles are established. Occasionally, an adolescent requires hormonal replacement therapy because of emotional distress over her condition.

Kallmann's syndrome is a genetic condition characterized by hypogonadotrophic hypogonadism and anosmia. It affects approximately 1 in 40,000 females, with most presentations of the "sporadic" type. Various forms of Kallmann's syndrome are inherited, and the gene responsible for the X-linked form has been identified.

The clinical features include deficiency of GnRH associated with anosmia. Because GnRH neurones originate extracranially within the olfactory system, both can be simultaneously affected, and the defects are believed to be secondary to abnormalities of neuronal migration during development. Patients with Kallmann's syndrome fail to develop secondary sexual features, and blood levels of gonadotropins are very low.

Patients with Kallmann's syndrome have a diminished gonadotropin response to the GnRH stimulation test. Pulsatile administration of GnRH for 1 week usually restores subsequent pituitary responsiveness to GnRH. All postpubertal-age patients with Kallmann's syndrome are candidates for gonadal steroid replacement therapy in the absence of specific contraindications. Estrogen replacement therapy is used to initiate and sustain sexual development. Induction of ovulation with human menopausal gonadotropins or GnRH is necessary when pregnancy is desired.

A pituitary or parasellar tumor, particularly craniopharyngioma or pituitary adenoma, must be considered in the evaluation of a patient with delayed sexual maturation. Craniopharyngiomas are rapidly growing tumors that often develop in late childhood. Pituitary adenomas are slow growing, may become symptomatic during puberty, and may interfere with sexual maturation. An occult pituitary prolactinoma in adolescents with unexplained delayed sexual maturation must be ruled out. Serum prolactin levels should be measured yearly in patients with unexplained delayed sexual maturation.

Weight loss due to extreme dieting, marked protein deficiency, and fat loss without notable loss of muscle (often seen in athletes) may delay or suppress hypothalamic-pituitary maturation. Heroin addiction may cause amenorrhea, but its effects on sexual maturation have not been documented.

Gonadal Failure

Most patients with gonadal dysgenesis present during adolescence with delayed puberty and primary amenorrhea. For young women with gonadal failure the most common cause is Turner's syndrome, which occurs with an incidence of 1 in 2500 to 1 in 10,000 live births. If untreated, estrogen and androgen levels are decreased and FSH and LH levels are increased. Estrogen-dependent organs show the predictable effects of hormonal deficiency. Breasts contain little parenchymal tissue, and the areolar tissue is only slightly darker than the surrounding

skin. The well-differentiated external genitalia, vagina, and müllerian derivatives remain small. Pubic and axillary hair fail to develop in normal quantity.

However, normal pubertal development, menstruation, and even pregnancies have been reported in adults with gonadal dysgenesis. It is possible that a few of these persons maintain some germ cells into adulthood. Spontaneous development is more commonly observed in patients with mosaicism with a 46,XX line. The rare offspring of these women probably do not have an increased risk for chromosomal abnormalities.

Some patients may have ovarian failure even though they have a normal chromosome complement and two intact sex chromosomes (46,XX). An autosomal recessive form of ovarian failure has been demonstrated in some families. Other causes of follicular depletion include chemotherapy, irradiation, infections (eg, mumps), infiltrative disease processes of the ovary (eg, tuberculosis), autoimmune diseases, and unknown environmental agents.

A karyotype is necessary to rule out the presence of Y chromosome material. DNA probes and assays for the minor histocompatibility antigen H-Y have also been used to identify Y chromosome material. A high incidence of neoplastic changes in the gonadal ridge has been reported in the presence of a Y chromosome (Fig 34–28), so prophylactic gonadectomy is recommended. Replacement hormonal therapy is then given in a cyclic manner.

Some patients have similar features, yet follicles are present but unresponsive, a condition called the *resistant ovary syndrome*. It is characterized by delayed menarche or primary amenorrhea, a 46,XX chromosome complement, high FSH levels, and ovaries with apparently normal follicular apparatus that do not respond to endogenous gonadotropins. Absence of follicular receptors for gonadotropins is assumed to be responsible for ovarian dysfunction in these patients. These individuals may have normally developed secondary sexual characteristics.

Figure 34–28. Gonadoblastoma developing in a gonadal ridge in a patient with gonadal dysgenesis and 45,XO/46,XY karyotype.

Estrogen replacement therapy is required to prevent long-term complications of estrogen deficiency (eg, vaginal dryness, osteoporosis). Pregnancies have been reported in some patients treated with menotropins or following discontinuation of estrogen therapy.

3. Delayed Puberty with Heterosexual Secondary Sexual Development

Virilization refers to the concomitant presentation of hirsutism with various signs of androgen excess, including acne, frontotemporal balding, deepening of the voice, decrease in breast size, clitoral hypertrophy, increase in muscle mass, and amenorrhea. Virilization at puberty is the result of elevated levels of androgens from adrenal or gonadal sources. These may be the result of an enzyme deficiency (eg, late-onset congenital adrenal hyperplasia) or a neoplasm (eg, Leydig cell tumor).

A small group of patients are male pseudohermaphrodites. These adolescents are being reared as girls and have female external genitalia, intra-abdominal or ectopic malfunctioning testes, and a normal 46,XY chromosomal complement. The diagnosis and treatment of intersex disorders are discussed in Chapter 5.

Evaluation of the Patient with Delayed Sexual Development

Determination of gonadal function can be accomplished by obtaining a medical history and performing a detailed physical examination, supplemented by selected laboratory studies. Historical information should center around previous growth and pubertal development. Linear and velocity growth charts as well as a pubertal development chart clarify previous growth patterns and are useful in subsequent follow-up. Knowledge of previous medical disorders may immediately identify the cause of aberrant puberty.

Physical examination must include height and weight assessments and a careful search for somatic anomalies. Staging of pubertal development by Tanner criteria is most important in the determination of gonadal function. Presence of breast development signifies prior gonadal function. A vaginal smear for cytohormonal evaluation can determine whether the gonad is continuing to produce estrogen. Pelvic and rectal examination will identify patients with an obstructed outflow tract, as well as patients with congenital absence of the vagina and uterus. Further confirmation of patients with Rokitansky sequence is dependent on a karyotype to identify normal 46,XX complement and a pelvic sonogram to confirm uterine absence and ovarian presence.

Absence of pubic hair is suggestive of the androgen insensitivity syndrome. Karyotype will identify the 46,XY cell line in patients with testicular feminization syndrome (Fig. 34–27). Patients with complete pubertal development, evidence of continued estrogen production, and normal müllerian systems probably have inappropriate positive feedback and thus chronic anovulation. Progesterone challenge in such patients is helpful. A withdrawal bleed signifies a normal müllerian system and continued estrogen production.

When breast development is minimal, the usual diagnosis is lack of gonadal function. Serum gonadotropin assays are performed for further elucidation. Elevated FSH levels suggest gonadal failure. Other endocrine profiles should be obtained if hypothyroidism, congenital adrenal hyperplasia, or Cushing's syndrome is suspected. Karyotype is necessary in all patients with gonadal failure and will identify both normal and abnormal chromosome complements. The presence of a Y chromosome in either group dictates gonadal removal.

Low FSH levels suggest interference with hypothalamic-pituitary maturation and gonadotropin release. Skull films and prolactin assays must be obtained for all patients to rule out the presence of pituitary or hypothalamic tumors. Appropriate endocrine evaluation identifies the occasional patient with hypothyroidism or congenital adrenal hyperplasia and the rare patient with Cushing's syndrome. Diagnosis of Kallmann's syndrome is suspected in hypogonadotrophic patients who have an associated anosmia, and the diagnosis is confirmed by GnRH challenge tests. The presumed diagnosis of constitutional delay is made by exclusion of all other causes and by the typical GnRH release patterns after GnRH challenge.

Evaluation of the Patient with Vaginal Bleeding

A. VAGINAL BLEEDING IN CHILDREN

When vaginal bleeding occurs in children, 2 sources generally should be suspected: (1) the endometrium (bleeding usually is a manifestation of precocious puberty) and (2) a local vulvar or vaginal lesion (eg, vulvovaginitis, foreign bodies, urethral prolapse, trauma, botryoid sarcoma, adenocarcinoma of the cervix or vagina, and vulvar skin disorders).

Vaginal bleeding during childhood should always alert the physician to the possibility of a genital tumor. Vaginoscopy and examination under anesthesia are the mainstays of evaluation to exclude the presence of tumors, foreign bodies, and other local lesions. Benign tumors of the vulva and vagina are rare in childhood, and those that do occur seldom cause bleeding. Malignant neoplasms usually bleed from necrotic or ulcerative areas that appear early in their development. Suspicious lesions require biopsy for diagnosis.

B. BLEEDING DISORDERS IN ADOLESCENTS

One of the most common gynecologic complaints of adolescents is a problem with the menstrual period. In most cases, there is no true medical disorder, especially in the first 2 years after menarche, when 50–80% of periods are anovulatory. Evaluation of abnormal bleeding is indicated if the menstrual interval is less than 22 days or more than 44 days, lasts longer than 1 week, menses is so heavy that anemia develops, or if the cycle interval is still unstable 2 years after menarche. Dysfunctional uterine bleeding accounts for 95% of abnormal vaginal bleeding in teenagers. Screening for inherited coagulation disorders, such as von Willebrand's disease, may be indicated, as 18% of adolescents hospitalized for menorrhagia have an underlying bleeding disorder. When menstrual irregularity is accompanied by symptoms such as acne, hirsutism, and obesity, polycystic ovarian syndrome should be suspected, and treatment may need to address some of these symptoms as well.

Pregnancy should always be considered in a young woman with abnormal bleeding or amenorrhea until proven otherwise. Nonmenstrual causes of bleeding, such as hypothyroidism, cervicitis, condylomas, polyps, cervical cancer, estrogen-producing ovarian tumors, and vaginitis, also should be considered.

Management of anovulatory bleeding is directed toward controlling symptoms and preventing anemia. Oral contraceptive pill tapers, cyclic oral contraceptives, and medroxyprogesterone acetate have been used to control bleeding. In severe cases, hospitalization and intravenous conjugated equine estrogen in doses of 25 mg every 4–6 hours until bleeding stops for 24 hours have been used successfully. If oral contraceptives are given for secondary amenorrhea, they should be continued for at least 9–12 months before attempting to stop. If menses do not resume within 8 weeks, oral contraceptive pills should be resumed for another 9–12 months.

■ SEXUALITY AND PREGNANCY IN CHILDREN AND ADOLESCENTS

PRECOCIOUS (JUVENILE) PREGNANCY

Precocious, or juvenile, pregnancy is rare. The youngest known patient was a Peruvian girl aged 5 years 8 months, who in 1939 delivered at term by cesarean section a healthy male infant weighing 2950 g (6 lb 8 oz). Both mother and infant survived. In every reported instance, the underage mothers were sexually precocious, and most had menstruated for several years before becoming pregnant. Juvenile pregnancy per se does not increase the chance of congenital anomalies in the offspring. However, in many cases the mother is a victim of sexual abuse, and if the pregnancy is the result of incest, there is a greater likelihood of genetic malformations carried by recessive genes.

Most precocious mothers and their babies have not done well, with increased incidences of spontaneous abortion, pregnancy-induced hypertension, and premature labor and delivery. In patients younger than 9 years, less than 50% have normal labor, with a 35% likelihood of neonatal loss.

The underage mother and her family may need psychiatric counseling, both during pregnancy and following delivery. Lessening the emotional, social, and medical trauma associated with such a gestation is an important task for all who assist in the care of the pregnant child.

SEXUALLY TRANSMITTED DISEASES

STDs are the most common infectious diseases in adolescents today. Approximately 25% of all sexually active adolescents aged 13–19 years become infected each year. By age 15 years, 1 in 4 girls in the United States has sexual relations. The younger the age of first intercourse, the higher the risk for STDs. Chlamydia is the most prevalent of the bacterial STDs, with almost 30% of inner-city female adolescents aged 12–19 showing positive cultures in a longitudinal 2-year study of family planning, school-based, and STD clinics. Sequelae of chlamydial infections include pelvic inflammatory disease (PID), ectopic pregnancy, and infertility. This age group accounts for 8% of cases of HIV in females, with the majority of these women asymptomatic at the time of positive testing. In the United States, 15- to 24-year-olds accounted for approximately 60% of gonorrhea cases, 25% of syphilis cases, and 17% of hepatitis B cases in 1996. By the time they reach college age, 43% of women are infected with human papillomavirus (HPV).

Nearly 70% of patients with PID are younger than 25 years. The estimated incidence of PID in sexually active females is approximately 1 in 8 for 15-year-olds and 1 in 10 for 16-year-olds. PID in adolescents should be treated with hospitalization and intravenous antibiotics. Tubo-ovarian abscess has been found in 2–4% of adolescents with adnexal masses. Treatment includes broad-spectrum antibiotics and possible surgical drainage. Patients who have had PID or tubo-ovarian abscess are at high risk for pelvic pain, pelvic adhesive disease, infertility, and ectopic pregnancy.

CERVICAL CANCER SCREENING IN ADOLESCENTS

Because infection with certain strains of HPV is the most important risk factor for the development of cervical cancer and HPV infection in women usually is acquired via heterosexual transmission, cervical cancer screening with a Papanicolaou (Pap) test should be initiated soon after the onset of sexual activity. Pap smear screening is underutilized in sexually active adolescents. Although measures that include teen clinics have increased the rate of surveillance, efforts at both prevention by encouraging condom use and increased availability of services are still needed.

If a Pap smear is abnormal, colposcopic evaluation may be indicated. STD screening should be incorporated as part of the evaluation. Low-grade lesions usually can be followed with serial Pap smears. Ablative or excisional procedures are indicated for moderate- to high-grade lesions, regardless of age. Cryotherapy offers a 92–95% cure rate for cervical intraepithelial neoplasia (CIN) 2–3 in young women. Loop electrosurgical excisional procedure (LEEP) offers similar cure rates and does not appear to impact cervical competence in future pregnancies with depths of excision of 1.5 cm or less. Teens with abnormal Pap smears should be advised regarding smoking cessation and follow-up.

CONTRACEPTION IN ADOLESCENTS

More than 95% of adolescent pregnancies are unintended. By age 18 years, 1 in 4 experiences a pregnancy. Half of adolescent pregnancies occur in the first 6 months after initiation of sexual activity. Despite a decline in teenage pregnancy rates during the 1990s, teenage pregnancy rates remain higher in the United States than in other Western countries. In addition, teenagers in the United States use contraceptives less frequently and use less effective methods of contraception than do their European counterparts. Although great inroads in adolescent access to health care have been made over the last decade, problems of cost and fears of lack of confidentiality still appear to inhibit young women from obtaining contraceptives, ultimately resulting in high teenage pregnancy rates.

Contraception is the voluntary prevention of impregnation. As such, postponing sexual activity is an appropriate option to suggest. If this is not realistic, counseling regarding various methods of contraception requires consideration not only of the side effects and efficacy of the various methods but also of the personal requirements of each teenager. For example, a teenager who has difficulty remembering to take pills or who must hide pill packs may be better served by medroxyprogesterone acetate injections. Health benefits of adolescents taking oral contraceptive pills include decreased menstrual pain; increased menstrual regularity; decreased risk of PID, anemia, and fibrocystic breast disease; improved long-term fertility; and treatment of acne and hirsutism. The importance of both contraception and STD prevention should be reviewed, and the use of barrier methods should be encouraged. Adolescents with chronic medical illnesses represent an especially high-risk group, as issues of both fertility and contraceptive risks and efficacy may be affected by these illnesses.

Emergency contraception regimens with progestin-only regimens or combined estrogens and progestins are highly effective means of preventing pregnancy after intercourse if taken at the appropriate interval. Improving access through education or prescribing pills in advance or over the telephone may give a young woman a second chance at preventing unintended pregnancy.

PREGNANCY TERMINATION

The rate of teenage abortion remains higher in the United States than in other Western countries for which data are available. The U.S. Supreme Court initially ruled in favor of a minor's right to have an abortion in 1976. Although this ruling has been amended to allow states to require parental notification before abortion, a system of judicial bypass for minors who do not want parental involvement is required in these states.

ADOLESCENT PREGNANCY

For years it has been accepted that adolescent pregnancy is a high-risk pregnancy. Many pregnant adolescents come from low socioeconomic backgrounds and have poor education and perhaps poor general health due to inadequate nutrition, cigarette smoking, drug abuse, or STDs. Nutrition is an important problem. Bone mineral content, iron stores, and caloric intake often are reduced among adolescent girls, and iron deficiency anemia is frequently found. Proper education and dietary counseling may improve nutritional status and prevent anemia.

Optimal care should be given to teenage mothers, not only to improve the pregnancy outcome but also to enhance their social, educational, and emotional adjustment. Complications of labor and delivery are highly dependent on the quality of prenatal care. Preeclampsia–eclampsia, which is more common in a first pregnancy, occurs more frequently among adolescents than among adult women. Prematurity and small-for-dates infants are a major problem in adolescent pregnancies. Predisposing factors are high-risk factors such as low prepregnancy weight, poor weight gain, adverse socioeconomic conditions, cigarette smoking, anemia, first pregnancy, and deficient prenatal care, all of which occur more commonly in adolescents. To minimize prenatal complications and to improve maternal and fetal outcome, the young patient should be enrolled in an aggressive prenatal care program that addresses the unique problems of the adolescent patient.

REFERENCES

Acquavella AP, Braverman P: Adolescent gynecology in the office setting. Pediatr Clin North Am 1999;46:489.

American Academy of Child and Adolescent Psychiatry. Practice parameters for the forensic evaluation of children and adolescents who may have been physically or sexually abused. J Am Acad Child Adolesc Psychiatry 1997;36:423.

American Professional Society on the Abuse of Children. *Guidelines for Psychosocial Evaluation of Suspected Sexual Abuse in Young Children.* American Professional Society on the Abuse of Children, 1990.

Antiretroviral postexposure prophylaxis after sexual, injection-drug use, or other nonoccupational exposure to HIV in the United States. MMWR 2005;54(RR02):1.

Apter D, Hermanson E: Update on female pubertal development. Curr Opin Obstet Gynecol 2002;14:475.

Arbel-DeRowe Y et al: The contribution of pelvic ultrasonography to the diagnostic process in pediatric and adolescent gynecology. J Pediatr Adolesc Gynecol 1997;10:3.

Bamberger J et al: HIV postexposure prophylaxis following sexual assault. Am J Med 1999;106:323.

Bays J, Chadwick D: Medical diagnosis of the sexually abused child. Child Abuse Negl 1993;17:91.

Bechtel K, Podrazik M: Evaluation of the adolescent rape victim. Pediatr Clin North Am 1999;46:809.

Bravender T, Emans SJ: Menstrual disorders. Pediatr Clin North Am 1999;46:545.

Bruni M. Anal findings in sexual abuse of children (a descriptive study). J Forensic Sci 2003;48:1343.

Bryant AE, Laufer MR: Fetal ovarian cysts: Incidence, diagnosis and management. J Reprod Med 2004;49:329.

Carel JC et al: Precocious puberty and statural growth. Hum Reprod Update 2004;10:135.

Chan LF et al: Pseudo-precocious puberty caused by a juvenile granulosa cell tumour secreting androstenedione, inhibin and insulin-like growth factor-I. J Pediatr Endocrinol Metab 2004;17:679.

Choi HY, Kim KT: A new method for aesthetic reduction of labia minora (the deepithelialized reduction of labioplasty). Plast Reconstr Surg 2000;105:419.

Cothran MM, White JP: Adolescent behavior and sexually transmitted diseases: The dilemma of human papillomavirus. Health Care Women Int 2002;3:306.

Craighill MC: Pediatric and adolescent gynecology for the primary care physician. Pediatr Clin North Am 1998;45:1659.

Crouch N, Minto C, Creighton S: Vaginal dilation therapy for vaginal hypoplasia: Success, satisfaction, compliance and sexual function outcomes. J Pediatr Adolesc Gynecol 2003;16:175.

Cutler GB Jr, Laue L: Congenital adrenal hyperplasia due to 21-hydroxylase deficiency. N Engl J Med 1990;323:1806.

Edmonds DK: Congenital malformations in the genital tract. Obstet Gynecol Clin North Am 2000;27:49.

Edmonds DK, Muram D: Sexual developmental anomalies and their reconstruction: Upper and lower tracts. In: Sanfilippo J et al (editors): *Pediatric and Adolescent Gynecology,* 2nd ed. WB Saunders, 2001:553.

Elster AB, Kuznets NJ: AMA Guidelines for Adolescent Preventative Services (GAPS): recommendations and rationale, 1994:93.

English A: Reproductive health services for adolescents. Obstet Gynecol Clin North Am 2000;27:195.

Fallat ME, Donahoe PK: Intersex genetic anomalies with malignant potential. Curr Opin Pediatr 2006;18:305.

Frank R: Formation of artificial vagina without operation. Am J Obstet Gynecol 1938;35:1053.

Gellert GA et al: Situational and sociodemographic characteristics of children infected with human immunodeficiency virus from pediatric sexual abuse. Pediatrics 1993;91:39.

Gevelber MA, Biro FM: Adolescents and sexually transmitted diseases. Pediatr Clin North Am 1999;46:747.

Giardino AP, Finkel MA. Evaluating child sexual abuse. Pediatr Ann 2005;34:382.

Gold MA: Prescribing and managing oral contraceptive pills and emergency contraception for adolescents. Pediatr Clin North Am 1999;46:695.

Gordon CM: Menstrual disorders in adolescents. Pediatr Clin North Am 1999;46:519.

Griffin JE et al: Congenital absence of the vagina: The Mayer-Rokitansky-Kuster-Hauser syndrome. Ann Intern Med 1976;85:224.

Hampton HL: Examination of the adolescent patient. Obstet Gynecol Clin North Am 2000;27:1.

Harel Z, Cromer B: The use of long-acting contraceptives in adolescents. Pediatr Clin North Am 1999;46:719.

Heger A et al: Children referred for possible sexual abuse: Medical findings in 2384 children Child Abuse Negl 2002;26:645.

Heger A et al (editors): *Evaluation of the Sexually Abused Child,* 2nd ed. Oxford University Press, 2000.

Heller ME, Dewhurst J, Grant DB: Premature menarche without other evidence of precocious puberty. Arch Dis Child 1979;54:472.

Heppenstall-Heger A et al: Healing patterns in anogenital injuries: A longitudinal study of injuries associated with sexual abuse, accidental injuries, or genital surgery in the preadolescent child. Pediatrics 2003;112:829.

Hewitt G, Cromer B: Update on adolescent contraception. Obstet Gynecol Clin North Am 2000;27:143.

Hu Y et al: Kallmann's syndrome: Molecular pathogenesis. Int J Biochem Cell Biol 2003;35:1157.

Imperato-McGinley J et al: The diagnosis of 5 alpha-reductase deficiency in infancy. J Clin Endocrinol Metab 1986;63:1313.

Ingram JM: The bicycle seat stool in the treatment of vaginal agenesis and stenosis: A preliminary report. Am J Obstet Gynecol 1981;140:867.

Joishy M, Ashtekar CS, Jain A, Gonsalves R: Do we need to treat vulvovaginitis in prepubertal girls? BMJ 2005;330:186.

Kahn JA et al: Intention to return for Papanicolaou smears in adolescent girls and young women. Pediatrics 2001;108:333.

Kahyaoglu S, Turgay I, Ertas E, Batioglu S: Swyer syndrome with SRT +Y chromosome and rudimentary internal genitalia demonstrating temporary action of antimüllerian hormone in utero: a case report. J Reprod Med 2006;51:510.

Kapoor R, Sharma DK, Singh KJ, et al: Sigmoid vaginoplasty: long-term results. Urology 2006;67:1212.

Lang ME, Darwish A, Long AM: Vaginal bleeding in the prepubertal child. CMAJ 2005;172:1289.

Lavery JP et al: Pregnancy outcome in a comprehensive teenage parent program. Adolesc Pediatr Gynecol 1988;1:34.

Lawson MA, Blythe MJ: Pelvic inflammatory disease in adolescents. Pediatr Clin North Am 1999;46:767.

Marshall WA, Tanner JM: Variation in the pattern of pubertal changes in girls. Arch Dis Child 1969;44:291.

McCann J, Voris J: Perianal injuries resulting from sexual abuse: A longitudinal study. Pediatrics 1993;91:390.

McCann J, Voris J, Simon M: Genital injuries resulting from sexual abuse: A longitudinal study. Pediatrics 1992;89:307.

McCann J et al: Comparison of genital examination techniques in prepubertal girls. Pediatrics 1990;85:182.

McCann J et al: Perianal findings in prepubertal children selected for nonabuse: A descriptive study. Child Abuse Negl 1989;13:179.

McCann J et al: Genital findings in prepubertal girls selected for nonabuse: A descriptive study. Pediatrics 1990;86:428.

McDonough PG, Tho PT: The spectrum of 45,X/46,XY gonadal dysgenesis and its implications (a study of 19 patients). Pediatr Adolesc Gynecol 1983;1:1.

Meneses MF, Ostrowski ML: Female splenic-gonadal fusion of the discontinuous type. Hum Pathol 1989;20:486.

Minjarez DA, Bradshaw KD: Abnormal uterine bleeding in adolescents. Obstet Gynecol Clin 2000;27:63.

Minto CL et al: The effect of clitoral surgery on sexual outcome in individuals who have intersex conditions with ambiguous genitalia: A cross-sectional study. Lancet 2003;361:1252.

Minto CL et al: Sexual function in women with complete androgen insensitivity syndrome. Fertil Steril 2003;80:157.

Morgan E, Quint E: Psychosocial and psychosexual concerns at diagnosis and treatment for women with vaginal agenesis J Pediatr Adolesc Gynecol 2004;17:232.

Moscicki A: Human papillomavirus infection in adolescents. Pediatr Clin North Am 1999;46:783.

Muram D: Genital tract trauma in pre-pubertal children. Pediatr Ann 1986;15:616.

Muram D: Child sexual abuse: Correlation between genital findings and sexual acts. Child Abuse Negl 1989;13:211.

Muram D: Treatment of labial adhesions in prepubertal girls. Adolesc Pediatr Gynecol 1999;12: 67.

Muram D, Dewhurst J: The inheritance of intersexuality. CMAJ 1984;130:121.

Muram D, Elias S: The treatment of labial adhesions in prepubertal girls. Surg Forum 1988;34:464.

Muram D, Rau F: Anatomic variations of the bulbocavernosus muscle. Adolesc Pediatr Gynecol 1991;4:85.

Muram D, Grant DB, Dewhurst J: Precocious puberty: A follow-up study. Arch Dis Child 1984;59:77.

Muram D, Speck PM, Dockter M: Child sexual abuse examination: Is there a need for routine screening for N. gonorrhoeae? J Pediatr Adolesc Gynecol 1996;9:79.

Muram D et al: Ovarian cancer in children and adolescents. Adolesc Pediatr Gynecol 1992;5:21.

Muram D et al: Genital injuries. J Pediatr Adoles Gynecol 2003;16:149.

Muram D et al: The medical evaluation of sexually abused children: Roundtable discussion. J Pediatr Adolesc Gynecol 2003;16:5.

Neinstein LS: Breast disease in adolescents and young women. Pediatr Clin North Am 1999;46:607.

Nyirjesy P: Vaginitis in the adolescent patient. Pediatr Clin North Am 1999;46:733.

Owens K, Honebrink A: Gynecological care of the medically complicated adolescents. Pediatr Clin North Am 1999;46:631.

Paek SC, Merritt DF, Mallory SB: Pruritus vulvae in prepubertal children. J Am Acad Dermatol 2001;44:795.

Papadimitriou A, Beri D, Tsialla A, et al: Early growth acceleration in girls with idiopathic precocious puberty. J Pediatr 2006;149:43.

Persaud D et al: Delayed recognition of human immunodeficiency virus infection in preadolescent children. Pediatrics 1992; 90:688.

Pfeifer SM, Gosman GG: Evaluation of adnexal masses in adolescents. Pediatr Clin North Am 1999;46;573.

Pinsky L, Kaufman M: Genetics of steroid receptors and their disorders. Adv Hum Genet 1987;16:299.

Pinsky L, Kaufman M, Levitsky LL: Partial androgen resistance due to a distinctive qualitative defect of the androgen receptor. Am J Med Genet 1987;27:459.

Pinto SM, Garden AS: Prepubertal menarche: a defined clinical entity. Am J Obstet Gynecol 2006;195:327.

Pletcher JR, Slap GB: Menstrual disorders. Pediatr Clin North Am 1999;46:505.

Plouffe L: Disorders of excessive hair growth in the adolescent. Obstet Gynecol Clin 2000;27:79.

Pokorny S: Anatomic detail of the prepubertal hymen. Am J Obstet Gynecol 1987;157:950.

Quint EH, Smith YR: Vulvar disorders in adolescent patients. Pediatr Clin North Am 1999;46:593.

Reider J, Coupey SM: The use of nonhormonal methods of contraception in adolescents. Pediatr Clin North Am 1999;46:671.

Reindollar RH, Tho SPT, McFonough PG: Abnormalities of sexual differentiation. Clin Obstet Gynecol 1987;30:697.

Rock JA, Azziz R: Genital anomalies in childhood. Clin Obstet Gynecol 1987;30:682.

Russo JF: Pediatric and adolescent gynecology. Curr Opin Obstet Gynecol 2001;13:449.

Schroeder B: Vulvar disorders in adolescents. Obstet Gynecol Clin North Am 2000;27:35.

Shulman L et al: Marker chromosomes in gonadal dysgenesis: Avoiding unnecessary surgery. Adolesc Pediatr Gynecol 1992;5:39.

Shurtleff BT, Barone JG. Urethral prolapse: four quadrant excisional technique. J Pediatr Adolesc Gynecol 2002;15:209.

Siegel SF et al: Assessment of clinical hyperandrogenism in adolescent girls. Adolesc Pediatr Gynecol 1992;5:13.

Siegel SF et al: Premature pubarche: Etiological heterogeneity. J Clin Endocrinol Metab 1992;74:239.

Slyper AH. The pubertal timing controversy in the USA, and a review of possible causative factors for the advance in timing of onset of puberty. Clin Endocrinol (Oxf) 2006;65:1.

Smith YR, Berman DR, Quint EH: Premenarchal vaginal discharge: Findings of procedures to rule out foreign bodies. J Pediatr Adolesc Gynecol 2002;15:227.

Smith YR, Haefner HK: Vulvar lichen sclerosus: Pathophysiology and treatment. Am J Clin Dermatol. 2004;5:105.

Spiegel AM: Inborn errors of signal transduction: Mutations in G proteins and G protein-coupled receptors as a cause of disease. J Inherit Metab Dis 1997;20:113.

Templeman C, Hertweck SP: Breast disorders in the pediatric and adolescent patient. Obstet Gynecol Clin North Am 2000;27:19.

Ulloa-Aguirre A et al: Incomplete regression of müllerian ducts in androgen insensitivity syndrome. Fertil Steril 1990;53:1024.

Verp MS, Simpson JL: Abnormal sexual differentiation and neoplasia. Cancer Genet Cytogenet 1987;25:191.

Vermillion ST, Holmes MM, Soper DE: Adolescents and sexually transmitted diseases. Obstet Gynecol Clin 2000;27:163.

White ST et al: Sexually transmitted diseases in sexually abused children. Pediatrics 1983; 72:16.

Winer-Muram HT et al: The sonographic features of the peripubertal ovaries. Adolesc Pediatr Gynecol 1989;2:158.

Complications of Menstruation; Abnormal Uterine Bleeding

35

Caroline M. Colin, MD, & Asher Shushan, MD

■ COMPLICATIONS OF MENSTRUATION

PREMENSTRUAL SYNDROME

 ESSENTIALS OF DIAGNOSIS

- Symptoms include mood symptoms (irritability, mood swings, depression, anxiety), physical symptoms (bloating, breast tenderness, insomnia, fatigue, hot flushes, appetite changes), and cognitive changes (confusion and poor concentration).
- Symptoms must occur in the second half of the menstrual cycle (luteal phase).
- There must be a symptom-free period of at least 7 days in the first half of the cycle.
- Symptoms must occur in at least two consecutive cycles.
- Symptoms must be severe enough to require medical advice or treatment.

General Considerations

Premenstrual syndrome (PMS) is a psychoneuroendocrine disorder with biologic, psychologic, and social parameters. It is both difficult to define adequately and quite controversial. One major difficulty in detailing whether PMS is a disease or a description of physiologic changes is its extraordinary prevalence. Up to 75% of women experience some recurrent PMS symptoms; 20–40% are mentally or physically incapacitated to some degree, and 5% experience severe distress. The highest incidence occurs in women in their late 20s to early 30s. PMS is rarely encountered in adolescents and resolves after menopause. Evidence suggests that women who have suffered with

PMS and premenstrual dysphoric disorder are more likely to suffer from perimenopausal symptoms.

The symptoms of PMS may include headache, breast tenderness, pelvic pain, bloating, and premenstrual tension. More severe symptoms include irritability, dysphoria, and mood lability. When these symptoms disrupt daily functioning, they are clustered under the name *premenstrual dysphoric disorder* (PMDD).

Other symptoms commonly included in PMS are abdominal discomfort, clumsiness, lack of energy, sleep changes, and mood swings. Behavioral changes include social withdrawal, altered daily activities, marked change in appetite, increased crying, and changes in sexual desire. In all, more than 150 symptoms have been related to PMS. Thus the symptom complex of PMS has not been clearly defined.

Pathogenesis

The etiology of the symptom complex of PMS is not known, although several theories have been proposed, including estrogen–progesterone imbalance, excess aldosterone, hypoglycemia, hyperprolactinemia, and psychogenic factors. A hormonal imbalance previously was thought to be related to the clinical manifestations of PMS/PMDD, but in the most recent consensus, physiologic ovarian function is believed to be the trigger. This is supported by the efficacy of ovarian cyclicity suppression, either medically or surgically, in eliminating premenstrual complaints.

Further research has shown that serotonin (5-hydroxytryptamine [5-HT]), a neurotransmitter, is important in the pathogenesis of PMS/PMDD. Both estrogen and progesterone have been shown to influence the activity of serotonin centrally. Many of the symptoms of other mood disorders resembling the features of PMS/PMDD have been associated with serotonergic dysfunction.

Diagnosis

No objective screening or diagnostic tests for PMS and PMDD are available; thus special attention must be paid to the patient's medical history. Certain medical conditions (eg, thyroid disease and anemia) with symptoms that can mimic those of PMS/PMDD must be ruled out.

The patient is instructed to chart her symptoms for at least 2 symptomatic cycles. The classic criteria for PMS require that the patient have symptoms in the luteal phase and a symptom-free period of at least 7 days in the first half of the cycle for a minimum of 2 consecutive symptomatic cycles. To meet the criteria for PMDD, in addition to the criteria for PMS, she must have a chief complaint of at least 1 of the following: irritability, tension, dysphoria, or mood lability; and 5 of 11 of the following: depressed mood, anxiety, affective lability, irritability, decreased interest in daily activities, concentration difficulties, lack of energy, change in appetite or food cravings, sleep disturbances, feeling overwhelmed, or physical symptoms (eg, breast tenderness, bloating).

Clinical Findings

A careful history and physical examination are most important to exclude organic causes of PMS localized to the reproductive, urinary, or gastrointestinal tracts. Most patients readily describe their symptoms, but careful questioning may be needed with some patients who may be reluctant to do so. Although it is important not to lead a patient to exaggerate her concerns, it is equally important not to minimize them.

Symptoms of PMS may be specific, well localized, and recurrent. They may be exacerbated by emotional stress. Migrainelike headaches may occur, often preceded by visual scotomas and vomiting. Symptomatology varies among patients but often is consistent in the same patient.

A psychiatric history should be obtained, with special attention paid to a personal history of psychiatric problems or a family history of affective disorders. A mental status evaluation of affect, thinking, and behavior should be performed and recorded. A prospective diary correlating symptoms, daily activities, and menstrual flow can be useful to document changes and to encourage patient participation in her care.

If underlying psychiatric illness is suspected, a psychiatric evaluation is indicated. The most common associated psychiatric illness is depression, which generally responds to antidepressant drugs and psychotherapy. Recall that psychiatric illnesses have premenstrual exacerbations, so medications should be altered accordingly.

Treatment

Treatment of PMS/PMDD depends on the severity of the symptoms. For some women, changes in eating habits—limiting caffeine, alcohol, tobacco, and chocolate intake, and eating small, frequent meals high in complex carbohydrates—may be sufficient. Decreasing sodium intake may alleviate edema. Stress management, cognitive behavioral therapy, and aerobic exercise have all been shown to improve symptoms.

Low-risk pharmacologic interventions that may be effective include calcium carbonate (1000–1200 mg/d) for bloating, food cravings, and pain; magnesium (200–360 mg/day) for water retention; vitamin B_6 (note that prolonged use of 200 mg/d may cause peripheral neurotoxicity) and vitamin E; nonsteroidal anti-inflammatory drugs (NSAIDs); spironolactone for cyclic edema; and bromocriptine for mastalgia. Herbal preparations have been proposed. St. John's wort has potential given its selective serotonin reuptake inhibitor (SSRI)-like effects but should be used with caution given its enzyme-inducing property on cytochrome P450. Chaste berry fruit *(Vitex agnus-castus)* 20 mg/day has been shown to be more effective than placebo and has minimal side effects but is not as effective as fluoxetine.

For symptoms of severe PMS and PMDD, further pharmacologic intervention may be necessary. Psychotropic medications that are effective include SSRIs, desipramine, and L-tryptophan. SSRIs have minimal side effects and provide symptom improvement in more than 60% of patients studied. Treatment should be given 14 days prior to the onset of menstruation and continued through the end of the cycle. Anxiolytics such as alprazolam and buspirone also have been shown to be efficacious, but their side effects and potential for dependence must be seriously considered.

Hormonal interventions have been shown to be effective. Use of gonadotropin-releasing hormone (GnRH) agonists leads to a temporary "medical menopause" and an improvement in symptoms. Their limitations lie in a hypoestrogenic state and a risk for osteoporosis, although "add-back" therapy with estrogen and progesterone may obviate these problems. Danazol may improve mastalgia. Finally, bilateral oophorectomy is a definitive surgical treatment option; again, estrogen replacement would be recommended.

Use of oral contraceptives has been suggested because they suppress ovulation. However, studies have found little difference between women taking a low-dose birth control pill and women who do not take pills, and oral contraceptives currently are not recommended for treatment of PMS/PMDD.

MASTODYNIA

Pain, and usually swelling, of the breasts caused by edema and engorgement of the vascular and ductal systems is termed *mastodynia,* or mastalgia. A positive correlation between degree of ductal dilatation and degree of breast pain has been documented. Mastodynia specifically refers to a cyclical occurrence of severe breast pain, usually in the luteal phase of the menstrual cycle. It is common in women with PMS/PMDD, and it may be the primary symptom of this syndrome in some. It has been shown to be related to high gonadotropin levels. Estrogen stimulates the ductal elements, whereas progesterone stimulates the stroma. An augmented response to prolactin has also been suggested. Examination is always necessary to rule out neoplasm, although most malignant tumors are painless. In postpartum patients, mastitis must be considered.

The presence of solitary or multiple cystic areas suggests fibrocystic change. The diagnosis usually can be confirmed by aspiration, but excisional biopsy occasionally is necessary. Serial mammograms or ultrasound examinations can be used to help monitor these patients (see Chapter 64).

Treatment

Management of painful breasts due to fibrocystic changes consists of support of the breasts, avoidance of methylxanthines (coffee, tea, chocolate, cola drinks), avoidance of nicotine, and occasional use of a mild diuretic. Patients with mastodynia have improved with topical NSAIDs, tamoxifen, danazol, bromocriptine, oral contraceptives, and vitamins, but with limited success. Recent data suggest goserelin (Zoladex) is an effective short-term treatment; however, the side-effect profile indicates continued treatment with alternative therapies.

DYSMENORRHEA

Dysmenorrhea, or painful menstruation, is one of the most common complaints of gynecologic patients. Many women experience mild discomfort during menstruation, but the term *dysmenorrhea* is reserved for women whose pain prevents normal activity and requires medication, whether an over-the-counter or a prescription drug.

There are 3 types of dysmenorrhea: (1) primary (no organic cause), (2) secondary (pathologic cause), and (3) membranous (cast of endometrial cavity shed as a single entity). This discussion focuses mainly on primary dysmenorrhea. Secondary dysmenorrhea is discussed elsewhere in this book in association with specific diseases and disorders (eg, endometriosis, adenomyosis, pelvic inflammatory disease, cervical stenosis, fibroids, and endometrial polyps). Membranous dysmenorrhea is rare; it causes intense cramping pain due to passage of a cast of the endometrium through an undilated cervix. Another cause of dysmenorrhea that should be considered is cramping due to the presence of an intrauterine device (IUD).

Pathogenesis

Pain during menstruation has long been known to be associated with ovulatory cycles. The mechanism of pain has been attributed to prostaglandin activity. Prostaglandins are present in much higher concentrations in women with dysmenorrhea than in those with mild or no pain.

Other studies have confirmed increased leukotriene levels as a contributing factor. Vasopressin was thought to be an aggravating agent, but atosiban, a vasopressin antagonist, has shown no effect on menstrual pain.

Psychologic factors may be involved, including attitudes passed from mother to daughter. Girls should receive accurate information about menstruation before menarche; this can be provided by parents, teachers, physicians, or counselors. Emotional anxiety due to academic or social demands may be a cofactor.

Clinical Findings

Reactions to pain are subjective, and questioning by the physician should not lead the patient to exaggerate or minimize her discomfort. History taking is most important and should include the following questions: When does the pain occur? What does the patient do about the pain? Are there other symptoms? Do oral contraceptives relieve or intensify the pain? Does the pain become more severe over time?

Because dysmenorrhea almost always is associated with ovulatory cycles, it does not usually occur at menarche but rather later in adolescence. As many as 14–26% of adolescents miss school or work as a result of pain. Typically, pain occurs on the first day of the menses, usually about the time the flow begins, but it may not be present until the second day. Nausea and vomiting, diarrhea, and headache may occur. The specific symptoms associated with endometriosis are not present.

The physical examination does not reveal any significant pelvic disease. When the patient is symptomatic, she has generalized pelvic tenderness, perhaps more so in the area of the uterus than in the adnexa. Occasionally, ultrasonography or laparoscopy is necessary to rule out pelvic abnormalities such as endometriosis, pelvic inflammatory disease, or an accident in an ovarian cyst.

Differential Diagnosis

The most common misdiagnosis of primary dysmenorrhea is secondary dysmenorrhea due to endometriosis. With endometriosis, the pain usually begins 1–2 weeks before the menses, reaches a peak 1–2 days before, and is relieved at the onset of flow or shortly thereafter. Severe pain during sexual intercourse or findings of adnexal tenderness or mass or cul-de-sac nodularity, particularly in the premenstrual interval, help to confirm the diagnosis (see Chapter 43). A similar pain pattern occurs with adenomyosis, although in an older age group and in the absence of extrauterine clinical findings.

Treatment

NSAIDs or acetaminophen may relieve mild discomfort. Addition of continuous heat to the abdomen in addition to NSAIDs decreases pain significantly. For severe pain, codeine or other stronger analgesics may be needed, and bed rest may be desirable. Occasionally, emergency treatment with parenteral medication is necessary. Analgesics may cause drowsiness at the dosages required.

A. ANTIPROSTAGLANDINS

Antiprostaglandins are now used for treatment of dysmenorrhea. The newer, stronger, faster-acting drugs appear to be more useful than aspirin. Ibuprofen, an NSAID that is available over the counter and in prescription strength, has been extremely effective in reducing menstrual prostaglandin and relieving dysmenorrhea. Less frequently dosed naproxen (550 mg/day) also is effective. Cyclooxygenase-2 (COX-2) inhibitors such as valdecoxib (20–40 mg/day) is equally effective and has fewer gastrointestinal side effects, but it is more costly. The drug must be used at the earliest onset of symptoms, usually at the onset of, and sometimes 1–2 days prior to, bleeding or cramping.

Antiprostaglandins work by blocking prostaglandin synthesis and metabolism. Once the pain has been established, antiprostaglandins are not nearly as effective as with early use.

B. ORAL CONTRACEPTIVES

Cyclic administration of oral contraceptives, usually in the lowest dosage but occasionally with increased estrogen, prevents pain in most patients who do not obtain relief from antiprostaglandins or cannot tolerate them. The mechanism of pain relief may be related to absence of ovulation or to altered endometrium resulting in decreased prostaglandin production. In women who do not require contraception, oral contraceptives are given for 6–12 months. Many women continue to be free of pain after treatment has been discontinued. NSAIDs act synergistically with oral contraceptive pills to improve dysmenorrhea.

C. SURGICAL TREATMENT

In a few women, no medication controls dysmenorrhea. Cervical dilatation is of little use. Laparoscopic uterosacral ligament division and presacral neurectomy are infrequently performed, although some physicians consider these procedures to be important adjuncts to conservative operation for endometriosis.

Adenomyosis, endometriosis, or residual pelvic infection unresponsive to medical therapy or conservative surgical therapy eventually may require hysterectomy with or without ovarian removal in extreme cases. Rarely a patient with no organic source of pain eventually requires hysterectomy to relieve symptoms.

D. ADJUVANT TREATMENTS

Continuous low-level topical heat therapy has been shown to be as effective as ibuprofen in treating dysmenorrhea, although its practicality in daily life may be questionable. Many studies have indicated that exercise decreases the prevalence and/or improves the symptomatology of dysmenorrhea, although solid evidence is lacking.

Diets low in fat and meat products have been shown to decrease serum sex-binding globulin and decrease the duration and intensity of dysmenorrhea.

ABNORMAL UTERINE BLEEDING

Abnormal uterine bleeding includes abnormal menstrual bleeding and bleeding due to other causes such as pregnancy, systemic disease, or cancer. The diagnosis and management of abnormal uterine bleeding present some of the most difficult problems in gynecology. Patients may not be able to localize the source of the bleeding from the vagina, urethra, or rectum. In childbearing women, a complication of pregnancy must always be considered, and one must always remember that more than 1 entity may be present, such as uterine myomas and cervical cancer.

Patterns of Abnormal Uterine Bleeding

The standard classification for patterns of abnormal bleeding recognizes 7 different patterns.

(1) **Menorrhagia** (**hypermenorrhea**) is heavy or prolonged menstrual flow. The presence of clots may not be abnormal but may signify excessive bleeding. "Gushing" or "open-faucet" bleeding is always abnormal. Submucous myomas, complications of pregnancy, adenomyosis, IUDs, endometrial hyperplasias, malignant tumors, and dysfunctional bleeding are causes of menorrhagia.

(2) **Hypomenorrhea** (**cryptomenorrhea**) is unusually light menstrual flow, sometimes only spotting. An obstruction such as hymenal or cervical stenosis may be the cause. Uterine synechiae (Asherman's syndrome) can be causative and are diagnosed by a hysterogram or hysteroscopy. Patients receiving oral contraceptives occasionally complain of light flow and can be reassured that this is not significant.

(3) **Metrorrhagia** (**intermenstrual bleeding**) is bleeding that occurs at any time between menstrual periods. Ovulatory bleeding occurs midcycle as spotting

and can be documented with basal body temperatures. Endometrial polyps and endometrial and cervical carcinomas are pathologic causes. In recent years, exogenous estrogen administration has become a common cause of this type of bleeding.

(4) **Polymenorrhea** describes periods that occur too frequently. This usually is associated with anovulation and rarely with a shortened luteal phase in the menstrual cycle.

(5) **Menometrorrhagia** is bleeding that occurs at irregular intervals. The amount and duration of bleeding also vary. Any condition that causes intermenstrual bleeding can eventually lead to menometrorrhagia. Sudden onset of irregular bleeding episodes may be an indication of malignant tumors or complications of pregnancy.

(6) **Oligomenorrhea** describes menstrual periods that occur more than 35 days apart. Amenorrhea is diagnosed if no menstrual period occurs for more than 6 months. Bleeding usually is decreased in amount and associated with anovulation, either from endocrine causes (eg, pregnancy, pituitary-hypothalamic causes, menopause) or systemic causes (eg, excessive weight loss). Estrogen-secreting tumors produce oligomenorrhea prior to other patterns of abnormal bleeding.

(7) **Contact bleeding** (**postcoital bleeding**) is self-explanatory but must be considered a sign of cervical cancer until proved otherwise. Other causes of contact bleeding are much more common, including cervical eversion, cervical polyps, cervical or vaginal infection (eg, *Trichomonas*), or atrophic vaginitis. A negative cytologic smear does not rule out invasive cervical cancer, and colposcopy, biopsy, or both may be necessary.

EVALUATION OF ABNORMAL UTERINE BLEEDING

Detailed history, physical examination, cytologic examination, pelvic ultrasound, and blood tests are the first steps in the evaluation of abnormal uterine bleeding. The main aim of the blood tests is to exclude a systemic disease, pregnancy, or a trophoblastic disease. The blood tests usually include complete blood count, assay of the β subunit of human chorionic gonadotropin (hCG), and thyroid stimulating hormone (TSH).

A. HISTORY

Many causes of bleeding are strongly suggested by the history alone. Note the amount of menstrual flow, the length of the menstrual cycle and menstrual period, the length and amount of episodes of intermenstrual bleeding, and any episodes of contact bleeding. Note also the last menstrual period, the last normal menstrual period, age at menarche and menopause, and any changes in general health. The patient must keep a record of bleeding patterns to determine whether bleed-

ing is abnormal or only a variation of normal. However, most women have an occasional menstrual cycle that is not in their usual pattern. Depending on the patient's age and the pattern of the bleeding, observation may be all that is necessary.

B. PHYSICAL EXAMINATION

Abdominal masses and an enlarged, irregular uterus suggest myoma. A symmetrically enlarged uterus is more typical of adenomyosis or endometrial carcinoma. Atrophic and inflammatory vulvar and vaginal lesions can be visualized, and cervical polyps and invasive lesions of cervical carcinoma can be seen. Rectovaginal examination is especially important to identify lateral and posterior spread or the presence of a barrel-shaped cervix. In pregnancy, a decidual reaction of the cervix may be the source of bleeding. The appearance is a velvety, friable erythematous lesion on the ectocervix.

C. CYTOLOGIC EXAMINATION

Although most useful in diagnosing asymptomatic intraepithelial lesions of the cervix, cytologic smears can help screen for invasive cervical (particularly endocervical) lesions. Although cytology is not reliable for the diagnosis of endometrial abnormalities, the presence of endometrial cells in a postmenopausal woman is abnormal unless she is receiving exogenous estrogens. Likewise, women in the secretory phase of the menstrual cycle should not shed endometrial cells. Of course, a cytologic examination that is positive or suspicious for endometrial cancer demands further evaluation.

Tubal or ovarian cancer can be suspected based on a cervical smear. The technique of obtaining a smear is important, because a tumor may be present only in the endocervical canal and may not shed cells to the ectocervix or vagina. Laboratories should report the presence or absence of endocervical cells. The current use of a spatula and endocervical brush has significantly increased the adequacy of cytologic smears from the cervix. Any abnormal smear requires further evaluation (see Chapter 50).

D. PELVIC ULTRASOUND SCAN

Pelvic ultrasonography has become an integral part of the gynecological pelvic examination. The scan can be performed either transvaginally or transabdominally. The transvaginal examination is performed with an empty bladder and enables a closer look with greater details at the pelvic organs. The transabdominal examination is performed with a full bladder and enables a wider, but less discriminative, examination of the pelvis. The ultrasound scan can add many details to the physical examination, such as a description of the uterine lining and its width and regularity (Fig 35–1), and the presence of intramural or submucous fibroids

Figure 35–1. Typical ultrasound scan of a uterine fibroid (**left**) and normal endometrial lining (**right**).

(Fig 35–1), intrauterine polyps, and adnexal masses. Persistent thick and irregular endometrium is one of the preoperative predictors of endometrial pathology and demands further evaluation and tissue biopsy.

Sonohysterography is a modification of the pelvic ultrasound scan. The ultrasound is performed following injection of saline by a thin catheter into the uterus. This technique increases significantly the sensitivity of transvaginal ultrasonography and has been used to evaluate the endometrial cavity for polyps, fibroids, and other abnormalities.

F. Endometrial Biopsy

Methods of endometrial biopsy include use of the Novak suction curette, the Duncan curette, the Kevorkian curette, or the Pipelle. Cervical dilatation is not necessary with these instruments. Small areas of the endometrial lining are sampled.

If bleeding persists and no cause of bleeding can be found or if the tissue obtained is inadequate for diagnosis, hysteroscopy and, in some cases, formal dilatation and curettage (D&C) must be performed.

E. Hysteroscopy

Placing an endoscopic camera through the cervix into the endometrial cavity allows direct visualization of the cavity. Because of its higher diagnostic accuracy and suitability for outpatient investigation, hysteroscopy is increasingly replacing D&C for the evaluation of abnormal uterine bleeding. Hysteroscopy currently is regarded as the gold standard evaluation of pathology in the uterine cavity. Resection attachments allow immediate capability to remove or biopsy lesions.

G. Dilatation and Curettage

For many years D&C has been regarded as the gold standard for the diagnosis of abnormal uterine bleeding. It can be performed with the patient under local or general anesthesia, almost always in an outpatient or ambulatory setting. With general anesthesia, relaxation of the abdominal musculature is greater, allowing for a more thorough pelvic examination, more precise evaluation of pelvic masses, and more complete curettage. Nevertheless, D&C is a blind procedure, and its accuracy, particularly when the cause of the abnormal uterine bleeding is a focal lesion such as a polyp, is debateable.

General Principles of Management (Fig 35–2)

In making the diagnosis, it is important not to assume the obvious. A careful history and pelvic examination are vital. The possibility of pregnancy must be considered, as well as use of oral contraceptives, IUDs, and hormones. Adequate sampling of the endometrium is essential for a definitive diagnosis.

Improved diagnostic techniques and treatment have resulted in decreased use of hysterectomy to treat abnormal bleeding patterns. If pathologic causes (eg, submucous myomas, adenomyosis) can be excluded, if there is no significant risk for cancer development (as from atypical endometrial hyperplasia), and if there is no acute life-threatening hemorrhage, most patients can be treated with hormone preparations. Myomectomy can be suggested for treatment of myoma if the patient wishes to retain her childbearing potential. Endometrial ablation and endometrial resection may offer successful outpatient and in-office alternatives.

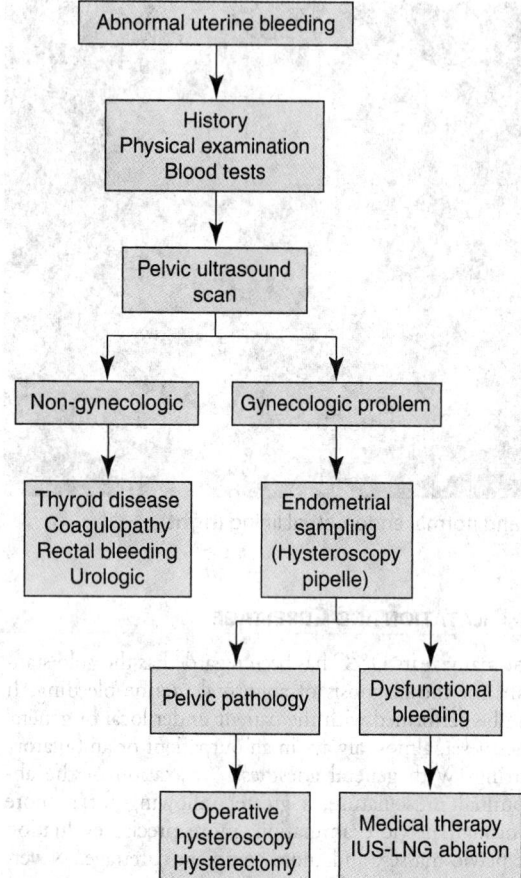

Figure 35–2. General principles of management of abnormal uterine bleeding. IUS-LNG = intrauterine system-levonorgestrel releasing.

For menorrhagia, prostaglandin synthetase inhibitors have been shown to significantly decrease blood loss during menses, as has antifibrinolytic therapy. Long-acting intramuscular progestin administration (Depo-Provera) can be given but may result in erratic bleeding or even amenorrhea. Finally, levonorgestrel-releasing IUDs are as effective as endometrial resection in decreasing blood loss.

ABNORMAL UTERINE BLEEDING DURING PREGNANCY

See Chapter 20.

ABNORMAL BLEEDING DUE TO NONGYNECOLOGIC DISEASES & DISORDERS

In the differential diagnosis of abnormal bleeding, nongynecologic causes of bleeding (eg, rectal or urologic disorders) must be ruled out, because patients may have difficulty differentiating the source of bleeding. Gynecologic and nongynecologic causes of bleeding may coexist. Systemic disease may cause abnormal uterine bleeding. For example, myxedema usually causes amenorrhea, but less severe hypothyroidism is associated with increased uterine bleeding. Liver disease interferes with estrogen metabolism and may cause variable degrees of bleeding. Both of these conditions are usually clinically apparent before gynecologic symptoms appear. Blood dyscrasias and coagulation abnormalities can also produce gynecologic bleeding. Patients receiving anticoagulants or adrenal steroids may expect abnormalities. Extreme weight loss due to eating disorders, exercise, or dieting may be associated with anovulation and amenorrhea.

DYSFUNCTIONAL UTERINE BLEEDING

Exclusion of pathologic causes of abnormal bleeding establishes the diagnosis of dysfunctional uterine bleeding. Although a persistent corpus luteum cyst or short luteal phase can produce abnormal bleeding associated with ovulation, most patients are anovulatory. The exact cause of anovulation is not truly understood but probably represents dysfunction of the hypothalamic-pituitary-ovarian axis, resulting in continued estrogenic stimulation of the endometrium. The endometrium outgrows its blood supply, partially breaks down, and is sloughed in an irregular manner. Conversion from proliferative to secretory endometrium corrects most acute and chronic bleeding problems. Organic causes of anovulation must be excluded (eg, thyroid or adrenal abnormalities).

Dysfunctional bleeding occurs most commonly at the extremes of reproductive age (20% of cases occur in adolescents and 40% in patients over age 40 years). Management depends on the age of the patient (adolescent, young woman, or premenopausal woman). The diagnosis is made by history, absence of ovulatory temperature changes, low serum progesterone level, and results of endometrial sampling in the older woman.

Treatment

A. ADOLESCENTS

Because the first menstrual cycles frequently are anovulatory, the menses not unusually are irregular, and explanation of the reason is all the treatment that is necessary. Heavy bleeding—even hemorrhage—may occur. Invasive diagnostic procedures usually are not necessary in young patients, but physical (pelvic if possible) examination and ultrasonography must be performed to exclude pregnancy or pathologic conditions. Estrogens given orally should be adequate for all patients except those requiring curettage to control hemorrhage. Numerous regimens are available, including estrogens followed by progesterone, progesterone alone, or combination oral contraceptives. For acute hemorrhage, high-dose estrogen given intravenously (25 mg conjugated estrogen every 4 hours) gives rapid response. In hemodynamically stable patients, the oral dose of conjugated estrogens is 2.5 mg every 4–6 hours for 14–21 days. Once bleeding has stopped, medroxyprogesterone acetate 5 mg once or twice per day should be given for 7–10 days.

Oral contraceptives, 3–4 times the usual dose, are just as effective and may be simpler to use than sequential hormones. Again, the dose is lowered after a few days and the lower dose is continued for the next few cycles, particularly to raise the hemoglobin levels in an anemic patient. Medroxyprogesterone acetate 10 mg/d for 10 days can be given to patients who have proliferative endometrium on biopsy. In patients receiving cyclic therapy, 3–6 monthly courses are usually administered, after which treatment is discontinued and further evaluation performed if necessary. In adolescents in whom the bleeding is not severe, oral contraceptives can be used as normally prescribed.

B. YOUNG WOMEN

In patients 20–30 years old, pathologic causes are similarly not very common and the appropriate diagnostic procedures should be considered following the initial evaluation by history, physical and cytologic examination, and pelvic ultrasound. Hormonal management is the same as for adolescents.

C. PREMENOPAUSAL WOMEN

In the later reproductive years, even more care must be given to excluding pathologic causes because of the possibility of endometrial cancer. The initial evaluation should be complemented by hysteroscopy and endometrial biopsy and should clearly establish anovulatory or dyssynchronous cycles as the cause before hormonal therapy is started. Recurrences of abnormal bleeding demand further evaluation.

D. SURGICAL MEASURES

For patients whose bleeding cannot be controlled with hormones, who are symptomatically anemic, and whose lifestyle is compromised by persistence of irregular bleeding, D&C may temporarily stop bleeding. If bleeding persists, levonorgestrel-releasing IUDs or a minimal invasive procedure such as endometrial ablation may be offered. Studies have shown that approximately 80% of patients scheduled for hysterectomy changed their minds following endometrial ablation. However, if these minimally invasive procedures fail or if the patient prefers a definitive solution, hysterectomy may be necessary. Definitive surgery may also be needed for coexistent endometriosis, myoma, and disorders of pelvic relaxation.

POSTMENOPAUSAL BLEEDING

Postmenopausal bleeding may be defined as bleeding that occurs after 12 months of amenorrhea in a middle-aged woman. When amenorrhea occurs in a younger person for 1 year and premature ovarian failure or menopause has been diagnosed, episodes of bleeding may be classified as postmenopausal, although resumption of ovulatory cycles can occur. Follicle-stimulating hormone (FSH) levels are particularly helpful in the differential diagnosis of menopausal versus hypothalamic amenorrhea. An FSH level greater than 30 mIU/mL is highly suggestive of menopause.

Postmenopausal bleeding is more likely to be caused by pathologic disease than is bleeding in younger women and must always be investigated. Nongynecologic causes must be excluded; these causes are more likely to result from pathologic disease in older women, and patients may be unable to determine the site of bleeding. The source of bleeding should not be assumed to be nongynecologic unless there is good evidence or proper evaluation has excluded gynecologic causes.

Neither normal ("functional") bleeding nor dysfunctional bleeding should occur after menopause. Although pathologic disorders are more likely, other causes may also occur. Atrophic or proliferative endometrium is not unusual. Secretory patterns should not occur unless the patient has resumed ovulation or has received progesterone therapy.

After nongynecologic causes of bleeding are excluded, gynecologic causes must be considered.

Exogenous Hormones

The most common cause of postmenopausal uterine bleeding is the use of exogenous hormones. In the past, face creams and cosmetics contained homeopathic amounts of estrogens, but today this cause is highly unlikely. Careful history taking becomes vital, because patients may not follow specific instructions on the use of estrogen and progesterone therapy.

In light of the new caution placed on postmenopausal hormone replacement therapy (HRT) because of cardiovascular risks, long-term estrogen/progesterone administration for prevention of osteoporosis is no longer recommended. Women continue HRT for menopausal symptoms to improve their quality of life. Regular menstrual bleeding may resume if they take HRT agents cyclically. Not uncommonly, these patients present with vaginal bleeding as many as 6–12 months after initiation of HRT. If bleeding is still occurring by that time, further investigation is warranted to determine its etiology. If endometrial hyperplasia is found, specific attention must be paid to the presence of atypia and treatment started by increasing the progesterone component or by hysterectomy.

Vaginal Atrophy and Vaginal and Vulvar Lesions

Bleeding from the lower reproductive tract almost always is related to vaginal atrophy, with or without trauma. Examination reveals thin tissue with ecchymosis. Rarely, a tear at the introitus or deep in the vagina requires suturing. With vulvar dystrophies, a white area and cracking of the skin of the vulva may be present. Cytologic study of material obtained from the cervix and vagina will reveal immature epithelial cells with or without inflammation. After coexisting upper tract lesions are excluded, treatment can include local or systemic estrogen therapy for vaginal lesions. Vulvar lesions require further diagnostic evaluation to determine the proper treatment.

Tumors of the Reproductive Tract

The differential diagnosis of organic causes of postmenopausal uterine bleeding includes endometrial hyperplasias (simple, complex, and atypical), endometrial polyps, endometrial carcinoma or other more rare tumors such as cervical or endocervical carcinoma, uterine sarcomas (including mixed mesodermal and myosarcomas), and, even more rarely, uterine tube and ovarian cancer. Estrogen-secreting ovarian tumors also should be considered.

Uterine sampling must be done and tissue obtained. Endocervical curettage should be performed, along with any endometrial sampling technique. If a diagnosis cannot be established or is questionable with office procedures, D&C is necessary. Hysteroscopy performed in the office or operating room may prove helpful in locating endometrial polyps or fibroids that could be missed even by fractional curettage. Pelvic ultrasonography may be extremely helpful in the diagnosis of ovarian tumors and in evaluation of the thickness of the endometrium, as well as in discerning between uterine myomas and adnexal tumors. Recurring episodes of postmenopausal bleeding may rarely require hysterectomy, even when a diagnosis cannot be established by endometrial sampling.

REFERENCES

Abu JI et al: Leukotrienes in gynaecology: The hypothetical value of anti-leukotriene therapy in dysmenorrhea and endometriosis. Hum Reprod Update 2000;6:200.

Akin MD et al: Continuous low-level topical heat in the treatment of dysmenorrhea. Obstet Gynecol 2001;97:343.

Barnard ND et al: Diet and sex-hormone binding globulin, dysmenorrhea, and premenstrual symptoms. Obstet Gynecol 2000;95:245.

Chan WY et al: Prostaglandins in primary dysmenorrhea. Comparison of prophylactic and nonprophylactic treatment with ibuprofen and use of oral contraceptives. Am J Med 1981;70:535.

Daniels SE et al: Valdecoxib, a cyclooxygenase-2-specific inhibitor, is effective in treating primary dysmenorrhea. Obstet Gynecol 2002;100:350.

Davis AR et al: Oral contraceptives for dysmenorrhea in adolescent girls: A randomized trial. Obstet Gynecol 2005;106:97.

Di Carlo C et al: Use of leuprolide acetate plus tibolone in the treatment of severe premenstrual syndrome. Fertil Steril 2001;75:380.

Ecochard R et al: Gonadotropin level abnormalities in women with cyclic mastalgia. Eur J Obstet Gynecol Reprod Biol 2001;94:92.

Golumb LM et al: Primary dysmenorrhea and physical activity. Med Sci Exerc 1998;30:906.

Jensen JT et al: Health benefits of oral contraceptives. Obstet Gynecol Clin North Am 2000;27:705.

Johnson S: Premenstrual syndrome, premenstrual dysphoric disorder, and beyond: A clinical primer for practitioners. Obstet Gynecol 2004;104:845.

Kaleli S et al: Symptomatic treatment of premenstrual mastalgia in premenopausal women with lisuride maleate: A double-blind placebo-controlled randomized study. Fertil Steril 2001;75:718.

Mansel RE et al: European randomized, multicenter study of goserelin (Zoladex) in the management of mastalgia. Am J Obstet Gynecol 2004;191:1942.

Peters F et al: Severity of mastalgia in relation to milk duct dilatation. Obstet Gynecol 2003;101:54.

Rauramo I, Elo I, Istre O: Long-term treatment of menorrhagia with levonorgestrel intrauterine system versus endometrial resection. Obstet Gynecol 2004;104:1314.

Revel A, Shushan A: Investigation of the infertile couple. Hysteroscopy with endometrial biopsy is the gold standard investigation for abnormal uterine bleeding. Hum Reprod 2002;17:1947.

Schwayder JM: Pathophysiology of abnormal uterine bleeding. Obstet Gynecol Clin North Am 2000;27:219.

Steiner M, Born L: Diagnosis and treatment of premenstrual dysphoric disorder: An update. Int Clin Psychopharmacol 2000;15(Suppl 3):S5.

Valentin L et al: Effects of a vasopressin antagonist in women with dysmenorrhea. Gynecol Obstet Invest 2000;50:170.

Yuk VJ et al: Frequency and severity of premenstrual symptoms in women taking birth control pills. Gynecol Obstet Invest 1991;31:42.

Contraception & Family Planning

Ronald T. Burkman, MD

■ CONTRACEPTION

Decision-making concerning fertility control is, for many people, a deeply personal and sensitive issue, often involving religious or philosophical convictions. Thus, it is important for the clinician to approach the subject with particular sensitivity, empathy, maturity, and nonjudgmental behavior.

Despite the introduction of modern contraceptives, unintended or unplanned pregnancies continue to be a major problem in the United States. According to the 1995 National Survey of Family Growth, there were a total of 6.3 million pregnancies in the United States, of which 49.2% were unintended. Among the unintended pregnancies, nearly half result in a pregnancy termination and over 10% in spontaneous abortion, a substantial degree of pregnancy wastage. Unintended and unplanned pregnancies have social and economic ramifications; they also have a significant impact on public health. Approximately 40% of unintended pregnancies occur among women who do not desire pregnancy yet do not use a method of contraception. Approximately 60% of unintended pregnancies occur among women using some form of birth control. Such data suggest that many women and couples are inadequately motivated to use contraception, that side effects may be problematic for some, that access may be an issue for others, or that some methods may be difficult for women to use correctly.

Individual Indications for Birth Control

Contraception is practiced by most couples for personal reasons. Many couples use contraception to space their children or to limit their family size. Others desire to avoid childbearing because of the effects of preexisting illness on the pregnancy, such as severe diabetes or heart disease. For all of these types of decisions, clinicians must provide accurate information about the benefits and risks of both pregnancy and contraception. However, medical conditions that may substantially increase the risk of using some form of contraception usually increase the risks associated with pregnancy to an even greater extent. As a matter of public policy, some countries, especially those that are less developed, promote contraception in an effort to curb undesired population growth.

Legal Aspects of Contraception

Contraceptives are prescribed, demonstrated, and sold throughout most of the United States without restriction. Despite high rates of unprotected intercourse and unintended pregnancy, the pros and cons of providing contraceptive information and materials to teenagers have been vigorously debated. Most states either have legislation that permits access to contraception for persons under 18 years or have not addressed the issue legislatively. There is a general consensus among physicians that teenagers should be given contraceptive advice and prescriptions within the limits of the law. Physicians must be careful to avoid imposing their own religious or moral views on their patients.

Health care providers are obliged to provide all persons requesting contraception with detailed information about use of the method(s) and its benefits, risks, and side effects so that the patient can make an informed choice relative to a particular method. Not only is the provision of this information of ethical and legal importance, but such counseling is likely to increase the likelihood the method will be used appropriately with overall improved compliance. Documentation of the discussion with the patient and her understanding of what has been said is important both clinically and legally. In particular, when using methods that require instrumentation or surgery and that also may require intervention by a health care professional for discontinuation (eg, intrauterine contraceptive device [IUD], injectable progestin, or sterilization), signed consent forms that outline the information discussed and the patient's understanding of it may reduce potential legal issues should a problem occur. If needed, the signed consent form serves as evidence that the patient was given counseling about use of a particular birth control method, that she appeared competent to understand what was said to her, and that she consented to receive contraceptive management in the manner specified.

■ METHODS OF CONTRACEPTION

The available methods of contraception can be classified in many ways. For this discussion, traditional or folk methods are coitus interruptus, postcoital douche, lactational amenorrhea, and periodic abstinence (rhythm or natural family planning). Barrier methods include condoms (male and female), diaphragm, cervical cap, vaginal sponge, and spermicides. Hormonal methods encompass oral contraceptives and injectable or implantable long-acting progestins. In addition, the IUD and sterilization (tubal ligation or vasectomy) are part of the contraceptive armamentarium. Sterilization is discussed in Chapter 48.

COITUS INTERRUPTUS

One of the oldest contraceptive methods is withdrawal of the penis before ejaculation. This process results in deposition of the semen outside the female genital tract. It has the disadvantage of demanding sufficient self-control by the man so that withdrawal precedes ejaculation. Although the failure rate probably is higher than that of most methods, reliable statistics are not available. Failure may result from escape of semen before orgasm or the deposition of semen on the external female genitalia near the vagina.

POSTCOITAL DOUCHE

Plain water, vinegar, and a number of "feminine hygiene" products are widely used as postcoital douches. Theoretically, the douche flushes the semen out of the vagina, and the additives to the water may possess some spermicidal properties. Nevertheless, sperm have been found within the cervical mucus within 90 seconds after ejaculation. Hence, the method is ineffective and unreliable.

LACTATIONAL AMENORRHEA

The lactational amenorrhea method can be a highly efficient method for breastfeeding women to utilize physiology to space births. Suckling results in a reduction in the release of gonadotropin-releasing hormone, luteinizing hormone (LH), and follicle-stimulating hormone (FSH). β-Endorphins induced by suckling also induce a decline in the secretion of dopamine, which normally suppresses the release of prolactin. This results in a condition of amenorrhea and anovulation. During the first 6 months, if breastfeeding is exclusive, menses are mostly anovulatory and fertility remains low. A recent World Health Organization (WHO) study on lactational amenorrhea revealed that during the first 6 months of nursing, cumulative pregnancy rates ranged from 0.9–1.2%. However, at 12 months, pregnancy rates rose as high as 7.4%. When using lactation as a method of birth control, the mother must provide breastfeeding as the only form of infant nutrition. Supplemental feedings may alter both the pattern of lactation and the intensity of infant suckling, which secondarily may affect suppression of ovulation. Second, amenorrhea must be maintained. Finally, the method should be practiced as the only form of birth control for a maximum of 6 months after birth. If another pregnancy is undesired, most practitioners advise lactating women to use a reliable contraceptive method starting 3 months after delivery.

MALE CONDOM

The condom, or contraceptive sheath, serves as a cover for the penis during coitus and prevents the deposition of semen in the vagina. The most common material used for male condom manufacture is latex, although available condoms are also made from polyurethane material and lamb ceca. The advantages of the condom are that it provides highly effective and inexpensive contraception as well as protection against sexually transmitted infections (STIs). Some condoms now contain a spermicide, which may offer further protection against failure, particularly if the condom breaks. Given the concern about STIs, including human immunodeficiency virus (HIV), condom use should be recommended for all couples except those in a mutually monogamous relationship.

The condom probably is the most widely used mechanical contraceptive in the world today. Condoms made of latex or polyurethane are impervious to both sperm and most bacterial and viral organisms that cause sexually transmitted diseases (STDs) or HIV infection. However, the less commonly used lamb's cecum condom is not impermeable to such organisms. The failure of all condoms results from imperfections of manufacture (approximately 3 in 1000); errors of technique, such as applying the condom after some semen has escaped into the vagina; and escape of semen from the condom as a result of failure to withdraw before detumescence. In typical use, failure rates with condoms range from 10–30% in the first year of use.

When greater contraceptive effectiveness is desired, a second method such as contraceptive vaginal jelly or foam should be used in conjunction with the condom. This combination significantly reduces the chances for condom failure due to mechanical or technical deficiencies. No association has been established between the use of vaginal contraceptives (spermicides) and the occurrence of congenital malformations if a pregnancy occurs.

FEMALE CONDOM

The female condom is made of thin polyurethane material with 2 flexible rings at each end. One ring fits into the depth of the vagina, and the other ring sits outside the vagina near the introitus. Female condoms have the advantage of being under the control of the female partner and of offering some protection against STDs. Significant disadvantages may be their cost and overall bulkiness. Comparisons of the female condom with other female barrier methods such as the diaphragm and cervical cap indicate that typical use failure rates are comparable. The 6-month probability of failure during perfect use of the condom is 2.6%, which is much lower than the initial prediction of 15%. Perfect use of the female condom may reduce the annual risk of acquiring HIV by more than 90%.

VAGINAL DIAPHRAGM

The diaphragm is a mechanical barrier between the vagina and the cervical canal. Diaphragms are circular rings ranging from 50–105 mm in diameter. They are designed to fit in the vaginal cul-de-sac and cover the cervix. Although the designs vary, the arcing spring version probably is the easiest for most women to use. A contraceptive jelly or cream should be placed on the cervical side of the diaphragm before insertion because the device is ineffective without it. This medication also serves as a lubricant for insertion of the device. Additional jelly should be introduced into the vagina on and around the diaphragm after it is securely in place. The diaphragm can be inserted up to 6 hours prior to intercourse and should be left in place for at least 6–24 hours after intercourse. When the diaphragm is of proper size (as determined by pelvic examination and trial with fitting rings) and is used according to directions, its failure rate is as low as 6 pregnancies per 100 women per year of exposure. With typical use, however, the pregnancy rate is 15–20 pregnancies per 100 woman-years. The diaphragm has the disadvantages of requiring fitting by a physician or a trained paramedical person and the necessity for anticipating the need for contraception. Weight alterations and deliveries might change the vaginal diameter. Therefore, the fit of the diaphragm to the user must be assessed yearly during the routine pelvic examination. Failures may result from improper fitting or placement and dislodgment of the diaphragm during intercourse. It cannot be used effectively by women with significant pelvic relaxation, a sharply retroverted or anteverted uterus, or a shortened vagina. As with condoms, diaphragms offer some protection against STDs. The only side effects are vaginal wall irritation, usually with initial use or if the device fits too tightly, and an increased risk of urinary tract infections due to pressure of the rim against the urethra and alterations in the composition of the vaginal flora.

CERVICAL CAP

Cervical caps are small cuplike diaphragms placed over the cervix that are held in place by suction. To provide a successful barrier against sperm, they must fit tightly over the cervix. Because of variability in cervical size, individualization is essential. Tailoring the cap to fit each cervix is difficult, greatly limiting the practical usefulness of the method. In addition, many women are unable to feel their own cervix and thus have great difficulty in placing the cap correctly over the cervix. Because of these problems, the cervical cap has few advantages over the traditional vaginal diaphragm. Although some advocates of the cervical cap recommend that it remain in place for 1 or 2 days at a time, a foul discharge often develops after approximately 1 day of use. With proper use, the efficacy of the cervical cap is similar to that of the diaphragm, with dislodgment being the most frequently cited cause of failure in most reports. The cap should be left in place for 8–48 hours after intercourse, and its proper placement over the cervix should be confirmed by digital self-examination after each sexual act.

SPERMICIDAL PREPARATIONS

Spermicidal vaginal jellies, creams, gels, suppositories, vaginal sponge, and foams, in addition to their toxic effect on sperm, act as a mechanical barrier to entry of sperm into the cervical canal. The only spermicide available in the United States contains nonoxynol 9, which is a long-chain surfactant that is toxic to spermatozoa. Spermicides can be used alone or in conjunction with a diaphragm or condom. Some foam tablets and suppositories require a few minutes for adequate dispersion throughout the vagina, and failures may result if dispersion is not allowed to occur. In general, when used alone, spermicides have a failure rate of approximately 15% per year with perfect use but double that rate with typical use. These chemical agents may irritate the vaginal mucosa and external genitalia. Recent evidence indicates that spermicides containing nonoxynol 9 are not effective in preventing cervical gonorrhea, chlamydia, or HIV infection. In addition, frequent use of spermicides containing nonoxynol 9 without a barrier has been associated with genital lesions that may be linked to increased risk of HIV transmission.

PERIODIC ABSTINENCE

It has long been known that women are fertile for only a few days of the menstrual cycle. The periodic abstinence (rhythm or natural family planning) method of contraception requires that coitus be avoided during the time of the cycle when a fertilizable ovum and motile sperm could meet in the oviduct. Fertilization takes place within the tube, and the ovum remains in the tube for approximately 1–3 days after ovulation; hence the fertile period is from the time of ovulation to 2–3 days thereafter.

Accurate prediction or indication of ovulation is essential to the success of the periodic abstinence method. Data from surveys in developed and developing countries performed during the past decade indicate the use of natural family planning methods varies from 0–11%. Pregnancy rates vary, but most reliable studies report 1-year life table pregnancy rates between 10 and 25 per 100 woman-years.

(1) The **calendar method** predicts the day of ovulation by means of a formula based on the menstrual pattern recorded over a period of several months. Ovulation ordinarily occurs 14 days before the first day of the next menstrual period. The fertile interval should be assumed to extend from at least 2 days before ovulation to no less than 2 days after ovulation. An overlap of 1–2 days of abstinence either way increases the likelihood of success. Successful use of this approach is based on the knowledge that the luteal phase of a menstrual cycle is relatively constant at 14 days for normal women. Furthermore, for this approach to be successful as the only form of contraception requires regular menstrual cycles so that the various timing schedules retain validity. Although this is the most commonly used method of periodic abstinence, it is also the least reliable, with failure rates as high as 35% in 1 year's use.

(2) A somewhat more efficacious approach to periodic abstinence is the **temperature method,** as more reliable evidence of ovulation can be obtained by recording the basal body temperature (BBT). The vaginal or rectal temperature must be recorded upon awakening in the morning before any physical activity is undertaken. Although it is often missed, a slight drop in temperature occurs 24–36 hours after ovulation. The temperature then rises abruptly approximately 0.3–0.4 °C (0.5–0.7 °F) and remains at this plateau for the remainder of the cycle. The third day after the onset of elevated temperature is considered the end of the fertile period. For reliability, care must be taken by the woman to ensure that true basal temperatures are recorded, ie, that temperature elevations due to other causes such as fever do not provide misleading information. A distinct limitation of this technique is that prediction of timing of ovulation in any given cycle is retrospective, making it difficult to predict the onset of the fertile period.

(3) The **combined temperature and calendar method** uses features of the 2 methods to more accurately predict the time of ovulation. Failure rates of only 5 pregnancies per 100 couples per year have been reported in studies of well-motivated couples.

(4) The **cervical mucus (Billings) method** uses changes in cervical mucus secretions as affected by menstrual cycle hormonal alterations to predict ovulation. Starting several days before and until just after ovulation, the mucus becomes thin and watery, whereas at other times the mucus is thick and opaque. Women using this approach are trained to evaluate their mucus on a daily basis. Success rates are similar to those described for the combined temperature and calendar method. Advantages of this approach include relative simplicity and lack of a requirement for charting. Disadvantages include difficulty in evaluating mucus in the presence of vaginal infection and the reluctance of some women to evaluate such secretions.

(5) The **symptothermal method,** if used properly, probably is the most effective of all the periodic abstinence approaches. It combines features of both the cervical mucus and the temperature methods. In addition, symptoms that may occur just prior to ovulation, such as bloating and vulvar swelling, are used as adjuncts to predict the likely occurrence of ovulation.

The most accurate method of determining ovulation time is to demonstrate the LH peak in serum specimens. Because of the cost and the time required for serial measurements of LH level that are essential to indicate the abrupt rise, this method is impractical as a method of birth control. It is valuable in the treatment of infertility, however, when the optimal time for coitus or artificial insemination is of great importance.

Figure 36–1 shows the relationships among ovulation, BBT, serum levels of LH and FSH, and menses. At least 20% of fertile women have enough variation in their cycles that reliable prediction of the fertile period is impossible.

Epidemiologic studies of women using periodic abstinence have suggested an increased incidence of congenital anomalies, such as anencephaly and Down syndrome, among children resulting from unplanned pregnancies. Animal experiments have shown delayed fertilization results in an increased incidence of aneuploidy and polyploidy in offspring, thus suggesting a possible explanation for similar human fetal anomalies. However, despite a theoretical explanation for the occurrence of such birth defects, it is important to recognize that much of the data are subject to bias, and concluding that such associations have been conclusively proved would be inappropriate.

ORAL HORMONAL CONTRACEPTIVES

Oral contraceptives when placed in general use in 1960 heralded the modern era of contraception. Oral contraceptives provide an estrogen, ethinyl estradiol, and a progestin. The most commonly used progestins in the United States are the estranes: norethindrone and norethindrone acetate; the gonanes: levonorgestrel, desogestrel, and norgestimate; and the spironolactone analogue drospirenone. When first developed, the 2 principal regimens of oral contraception were combined and sequential. The sequential method has been abandoned in the United States because several studies

Figure 36–1. Relationships among ovulation, basal body temperature, and luteinizing hormone (LH) and follicle-stimulating hormone (FSH) surges in the normal menstrual cycle.

showed a higher than normal incidence of endometrial cancer in women using this method of contraception. In the most commonly used combined method, pills containing both estrogen and progestin are taken each day for 21 days, followed by 7 days of placebo pills during which time most women experience withdrawal bleeding. Over the past several decades the estrogen content has been reduced by a factor of 3-fold to 4-fold, such that the current dose of ethinyl estradiol ranges between 20 and 35 μg. Similarly, the progestin content has been substantially reduced. In general use, the combined regimen is started either with the onset of the menstrual cycle or on the Sunday closest to the start of menses. Because most oral contraceptive preparations are packaged in 28-day regimens, the Sunday start approach may be easier to follow for some women. However, a good practice is to recommend use of an additional form of contraception during the first week of the cycle to maximize efficacy. Recently, some practitioners have initiated an approach in which birth control pills are started on the day of the office visit if pregnancy is unlikely. It appears this approach may reduce unwanted pregnancies. However, backup contraception is required for at least 7 days after initiation of the method. The newest approach with combined oral contraceptives is to administer active pills for 84 days followed by 7 days (extended-use regimen) to allow for withdrawal bleeding to occur. Although this approach is designed to reduce the number of withdrawal bleeding episodes to 4 per year, a significant number of

women experience irregular bleeding, especially during the first few cycles of use. With standard oral contraceptive preparations, withdrawal bleeding can be expected within 3–5 days after completion of the 21-day regimen of active pills.

The serum levels of FSH and LH throughout the normal menstrual cycle are shown in Figure 36–2A. During a typical cycle under the combined oral contraceptive regimen (Fig 36–2B), there is no rise during the first half of the cycle; thus the growth of the dominant follicle and ovulation do not occur, and there are no midcycle alterations of FSH and LH levels. Oral contraceptives change the consistency of cervical mucus, resulting in less sperm penetration; make the endometrial lining less receptive to implantation; and alter tubal transport of both sperm and oocytes. During the sequential oral contraceptive regimen (Fig 36–2C), the estrogen stimulates LH secretion in an irregular manner. There is no concomitant early rise in FSH level when progestin is added, and another LH surge usually is produced. When a progestin-only regimen (Fig 36–2D) is followed (see Progestin Only Pill), there are multiple LH surges but no significant changes in FSH levels.

Advantages

Benefits that are reasonably established include reduction in risk of ovarian and endometrial cancer, ectopic pregnancy, pelvic inflammatory disease (PID),

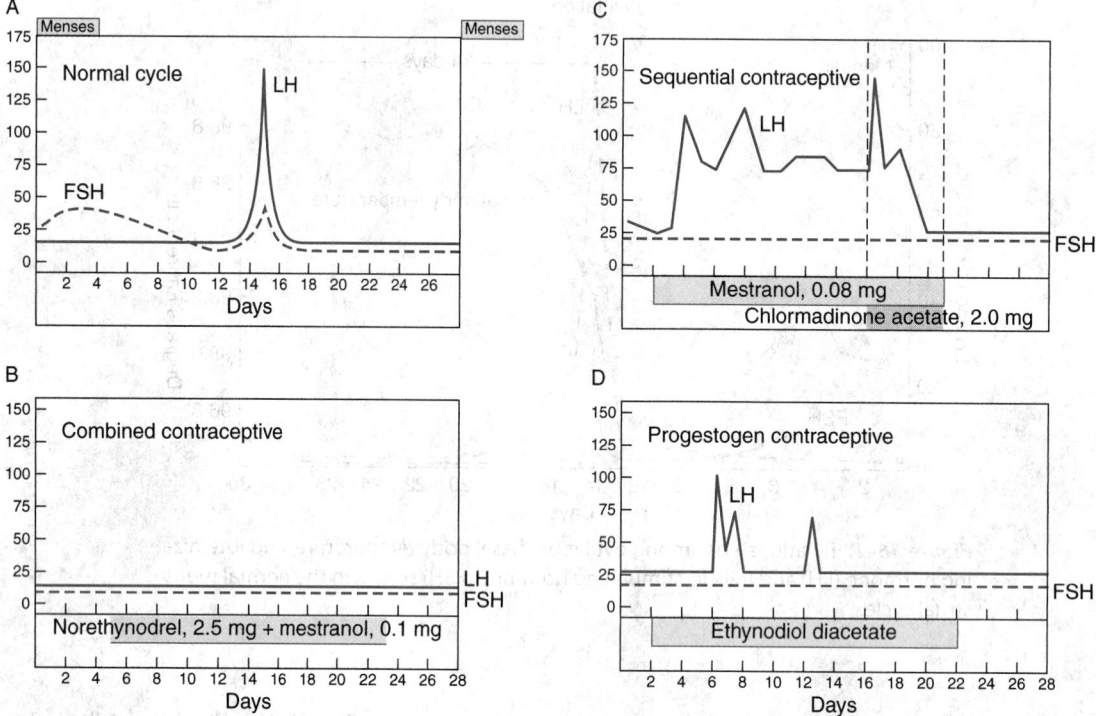

Figure 36–2. Serum levels (in mIU/mL) of follicle-stimulating hormone (FSH) and luteinizing hormone (LH) during the menstrual cycle, with and without oral contraception. **A:** During a normal cycle without medication. **B:** During a typical cycle with combined medication (see text). **C:** During a typical cycle with sequential medication (see text). **D:** During progestin-only medication. (Reproduced, with permission, from Odell WD, Moyer DL: *Physiology of Reproduction.* Mosby, 1971.)

menstrual disorders, benign breast disease, and acne. Emerging benefits include protection against bone mineral density loss, development of colorectal cancer, and progression of rheumatoid arthritis. Multiple observational studies have documented that combination oral contraceptives decrease the risk of ovarian cancer by 40–80% and endometrial cancer by approximately 50%. These effects take place after 1 year of use, and protection persists for a significant period after oral contraceptive use is discontinued. Oral contraceptives also reduce the risk of ectopic pregnancy by approximately 90% and the risk of acute salpingitis by as much as 50–80% in some studies, although other studies suggest the protection occurs to a lesser extent. However, birth control pills do not offer protection against lower tract infections such as gonorrhea or chlamydia. Oral contraceptives reduce menstrual blood loss as well as dysmenorrhea. There is a 30–50% overall decrease in benign fibrocystic conditions of the breast. Randomized placebo controlled trials have demonstrated a reduction in acne lesions with some oral contraceptive preparations. Evidence

from several studies indicates that oral contraceptives maintain bone mineral density. Other recent studies suggest that oral contraceptive use offers protection against colorectal cancer and that they also prevent the progression of rheumatoid arthritis to more severe varieties.

Disadvantages & Side Effects

Much attention has been paid to a possible relationship between the use of oral contraceptives and the incidence of thromboembolic disease, including pulmonary embolism. Use of most current combination oral contraceptives roughly triples a user's risk of venous thromboembolism (VTE) from approximately 3 to 9 events per 100,000 users annually, although some studies of formulations containing desogestrel suggest that the risk could climb as high as 7-fold. However, it is important to recognize that even with the worst case scenarios, the attributable risk annually is approximately 18 additional events per 100,000 users compared with nonusers of combination oral contraceptives. VTE risk is enhanced by risk factors such as recent leg trauma, pelvic surgery, stasis (but not varicose veins), and the presence of the mutation known as factor V Leiden. Although the presence of this latter clotting abnormality markedly elevates a user's risk of VTE, the absolute risk is still low such that routine screening for the disorder among all potential oral contraceptive users would not be cost effective.

Myocardial infarction (MI) is a rare condition that occurs among combination oral contraceptive users only in the presence of risk factors such as hypertension, diabetes, severe dyslipidemia, and, in particular, cigarette smoking. Age above 35 years and smoking also act synergistically to increase risk; thus, prescribing combination oral contraceptives to women over 35 years who smoke is not recommended. However, even with a 20- to 30-fold relative risk of MI among smoking combination oral contraceptive users, this risk equates to only a maximum of 500–600 events per million woman-years. However, unlike VTE in which the case fatality rate in the reproductive age group is less than 1%, the case fatality rate for MI is approximately 50%.

Stroke is a rare condition among women in the reproductive age group, with hemorrhagic stroke somewhat more common than ischemic stroke. Among nonsmoking women, the rates range from 6–46 events per million woman-years; combination oral contraceptive use increases that risk only if risk factors such as age, cigarette smoking, migraine headaches (for ischemic but not hemorrhagic stroke), and especially hypertension are present. Overall, the relative risk of stroke varies between 2-fold and 10-fold, depending on the number of risk factors present.

Although cancer of the cervix among users of oral contraceptives has been a matter of concern, a major problem with many studies attempting to examine this relationship is confounding factors such as multiple sexual partners, age at first intercourse, and frequency of sexual activity and the concomitant use of barrier contraceptive methods. A recent meta-analysis determined that the risk of cervical cancer among oral contraceptive users compared to nonusers increased with duration of use, reaching a relative risk of approximately 4 after 10 years. For several decades, concern has been expressed regarding the possible association between oral contraceptive use and breast cancer. In 1996, a collaborative project representing a reanalysis of 54 studies demonstrated that for current users of oral contraceptives, the relative risk of breast cancer for users compared with women who had never used oral contraceptives was 1.24. This small increase in risk persisted for approximately 10 years after discontinuation of oral contraceptive use, with the risk essentially disappearing after that time. In addition, there was no overall effect of oral contraceptive use by dosage, specific formulation, duration of use, age at first use, age at time of cancer diagnosis, or family history of breast

cancer. The pattern of disappearance of risk after 10 years coupled with a tendency toward localized disease suggests that the overall effect may represent detection bias or perhaps a promotional effect. Another recent, large population-based case-control study showed that neither current nor past use of any type of oral contraceptive increased the risk of breast cancer compared to population-based controls. Further, the results did not vary according to potential risk factors such as estrogen dose, duration of use, family history of breast cancer, or age at initiation of use. Other infrequent problems occasionally noted with oral contraceptive use include hypertension, cholelithiasis, and benign liver tumors. However, none of these problems occurs frequently enough to be of significant concern to most users.

Because the current formulations are associated with significant reductions in risk of serious sequelae, side-effect control will be of greater importance to most users in the future. Furthermore, studies have shown that compliance is affected by occurrence of side effects and that such "minor" problems, particularly spotting and breakthrough bleeding, account for approximately 40% of the discontinuations. Approximately 10–20% of women experience intermenstrual bleeding, including breakthrough bleeding and spotting, in the first few months of use. With today's formulations, such problems stabilize after approximately 6 months and are seen in only approximately 5% of users. Missed menstrual periods or amenorrhea are relatively infrequent and of little clinical significance, except that these problems can raise concern as regarding contraceptive failure. Nausea may be seen in up to 10% of users; as with intermenstrual bleeding, this is a duration effect that declines rapidly after several months of use. Significant headaches and weight gain are far less frequent than reported with higher-dose preparations.

Contraindications for use of oral contraceptives include pregnancy; undiagnosed vaginal bleeding; prior history of VTE, MI, or stroke; women at increased risk for cardiovascular sequelae, such as active systemic lupus erythematosus, uncontrolled diabetes, or hypertension, and cigarette smokers over age 35 years; current or prior breast cancer; and active liver disease.

Because compliance and a clear understanding of how to take oral contraceptives are important to their successful use, health care providers should take the time at the initial visit to explain the packaging of the brand being prescribed, discuss the side effects, review how to start the first cycle, and discuss what to do when pills are missed. It should be emphasized that the patient package insert provides useful information on these topics. In addition, users should be encouraged to contact their provider or someone in the office or clinic who is familiar with oral contraceptive health care if problems occur. Finally, users should be advised to use alternate forms of contraception if oral contraceptive

Table 36–1. Oral contraceptive agents in use. The estrogen-containing compounds are arranged in order of increasing content of estrogen (ethinyl estradiol and mestranol have similar potencies).

	Estrogen (mg)	Progestin (mg)	
Combination tablets			
Loestrin 1/20	Ethinyl estradiol 0.02	Norethindrone acetate	1
Loestrin 1.5/30	Ethinyl estradiol 0.03	Norethindrone acetate	1.5
Ovcon-35	Ethinyl estradiol 0.035	Norethindrone	0.4
Brevicon	Ethinyl estradiol 0.035	Norethindrone	0.5
Modicon			
Nordette	Ethinyl estradiol 0.03	L-Norgestrel	0.15
Ortho-Cept, Desogen	Ethinyl estradiol 0.30	Desogestrel	0.15
Ortho-Cyclen	Ethinyl estradiol 0.35	Norgestimate	0.25
Lo/Ovral	Ethinyl estradiol 0.03	DL-Norgestrel	0.3
Ovral	Ethinyl estradiol 0.05	DL-Norgestrel	0.5
Demulen 1/50	Ethinyl estradiol 0.05	Ethynodiol diacetate	1
Demulen 1/35	Ethinyl estradiol 0.35	Ethynodiol diacetate	1
Ovcon 50	Ethinyl estradiol 0.05	Norethindrone	1
Ovcon 35	Ethinyl estradiol 0.35	Norethindrone	0.4
Norinyl 1/50	Mestranol 0.05	Norethindrone	1
Norinyl 1/35	Ethinyl estradiol 0.35	Norethindrone	1
Ortho-Novum 1/50			
Ortho-Novum 1/35	Ethinyl estradiol 0.35	Norethindrone	0.4
Alesse	Ethinyl estradiol 0.20	Levonorgestrel	0.1
Levlite	Ethinyl estradiol 0.20	Levonorgestrel	0.1
Levlen	Ethinyl estradiol 0.30	Levonorgestrel	0.15
Nordette	Ethinyl estradiol 0.30	Levonorgestrel	0.15
Yasmin	Ethinyl estradiol 0.30	Drosperinone	3
Yaz	Ethinyl estradiol 0.20	Drosperinone	3*
Combination tablets—multidose			
Biphasic			
Ortho-Novum 10/11			
Day 1–10	Ethinyl estradiol 0.035	Norethindrone	0.5
Day 11–21	Ethinyl estradiol 0.035	Norethindrone	1
Jenest-28			
Day 1–7	Ethinyl estradiol 0.35	Norethindrone	0.5
Day 8–21	Ethinyl estradiol 0.35	Norethindrone	1
Mircette			
Day 1–21	Ethinyl estradiol 0.20	Desogestrel	0.15
Day 22–26	Ethinyl estradiol 0.10	None	
Triphasic			
Tri-Norinyl			
Day 1–7	Ethinyl estradiol 0.035	Norethindrone	0.5
Day 8–16	Ethinyl estradiol 0.035	Norethindrone	1
Day 17–21	Ethinyl estradiol 0.035	Norethindrone	0.5
Day 22–28		Placebo	
Triphasil, Trilevlen			
Day 1–6	Ethinyl estradiol 0.030	Levonorgestrel	0.05
Day 7–11	Ethinyl estradiol 0.040	Levonorgestrel	0.075

(continued)

Table 36–1. Oral contraceptive agents in use. The estrogen-containing compounds are arranged in order of increasing content of estrogen (ethinyl estradiol and mestranol have similar potencies). (continued)

	Estrogen (mg)	Progestin (mg)	
Triphasic (cont'd)			
Day 12–21	Ethinyl estradiol 0.030	Levonorgestrel	0.125
Day 22–28		Placebo	
Ortho-Novum 7/7/7			
Day 1–7	Ethinyl estradiol 0.035	Norethindrone	0.5
Day 8–14	Ethinyl estradiol 0.035	Norethindrone	0.75
Day 15–21	Ethinyl estradiol 0.035	Norethindrone	1
Day 22–28		Placebo	
Ortho-Tri-Cyclen			
Day 1–7	Ethinyl estradiol 0.35	Norgestimate	0.180
Day 8–14	Ethinyl estradiol 0.35	Norgestimate	0.215
Day 15–21	Ethinyl estradiol 0.35	Norgestimate	0.250
Combination Estrophasic			
Estrostep Fe			
Day 1–5	Ethinyl estradiol 0.20	Norethindrone	1
Day 6–12	Ethinyl estradiol 0.30	Norethindrone	1
Day 13–21	Ethinyl estradiol 0.35	Norethindrone	1
Daily progestin tablets			
Micronor	...	Norethindrone	0.35
Nor-QD	...	Norethindrone	0.35
Ovrette	...	DL-Norgestrel	0.075
Daily combination tablet (84 days)			
Seasonale	Ethinyl estradiol 0.03	Norgestrel	0.15

Some of the above oral contraceptives are available as generic formulations. *Active pills take 24 out of 28 days.

use is interrupted because of forgotten pills or the occurrence of side effects.

Table 36–1 lists the currently available oral contraceptives and their contents.

Progestin-Only Pill (Minipill)

Several studies have demonstrated that a small daily quantity of a progestin alone, usually norethindrone or levonorgestrel, provides reasonably good protection against pregnancy without suppressing ovulation. The method has several advantages: the side effects attributable to the estrogen component of conventional oral contraceptives are eliminated because no estrogen is given, and no special sequence of pill-taking is necessary because the minipill is taken every day. Although the mechanism of action of progestin-only pills is not known, it has been postulated that the cervical mucus becomes less permeable to sperm and that endometrial activity goes out of phase so that nidation is thwarted even if fertilization does occur. In clinical trials, progestin-only oral contraceptives result in a pregnancy rate of approximately 2–7 pregnancies per 100 woman-years. Unlike combined oral contraceptives, which permit a certain margin of patient error and forgetfulness, minipill progestin agents must be taken each day promptly. Even a delay of 2–3 hours diminishes the contraceptive effectiveness for the for coming 48 hours. Progestins given alone are associated with side effects, particularly irregular bleeding. Progestin-only contraceptives are ideal for women for whom estrogen is contraindicated. Ideal candidates include older women who smoke; women with sickle cell anemia, mental retardation, migraine headache, hypertension, or systemic lupus erythematosus; or women who are breastfeeding.

Emergency Contraception

Postcoital or emergency contraception is a therapy used to prevent unwanted pregnancy after unprotected intercourse or after a failure to use a contraceptive method appropriately. The major methods used for emergency contraception include combination oral contraceptives containing the progestin levonorgestrel (also known as the Yuzpe method), levonorgestrel tablets given alone, or the copper T 380A intrauterine contraceptive device. The hormonal methods prevent pregnancy by delaying or inhibiting ovulation or by disrupting the function of the corpus luteum. The usual combination hormonal formulation consists of 100 μg ethinyl estradiol and 500–600 μg levonorgestrel in several tablets administered twice, 12 hours apart. Under current recommendations, the first dose is administered within 72 hours of intercourse. The levonorgestrel-alone formulation requires administration of 750 μg of the progestin twice, also 12 hours apart. Many authorities currently recommend initial dosing within 72 hours, although data suggest this approach may be effective as long as 5 days after intercourse. Furthermore, data suggest that a single dose of 1500 μg levonorgestrel may be as effective as the 2-dose regimen. The intrauterine device may inhibit implantation or possibly interfere with sperm function. The T 380A is inserted within 7 days from the time of unprotected intercourse.

Nausea occurs in approximately 50% and vomiting in 20% of the combination hormonal emergency contraception users. Administration of an antiemetic (eg, meclizine) 1 hour before may reduce this effect. The levonorgestrel-only approach is associated with rates of nausea and vomiting that are 50% and 70% lower than the rates experienced by combination emergency contraception users, respectively.

HORMONAL CONTRACEPTION BY INJECTION

Depot medroxyprogesterone acetate (DMPA), an aqueous suspension of 17-acetoxy-6-methyl progesterone, has been used as a contraceptive in the United States for at least 4 decades. The usual dose is 150 mg administered intramuscularly into the gluteus maximus or deltoid every 3 months. The mechanisms of action include suppression of ovulation by suppressing the surge of gonadotropins, thickening cervical mucus to impede ascent of sperm, and thinning of the endometrium such that implantation of a blastocyst is less likely. Although labeled as effective for up to 13 weeks, the contraceptive activity actually persists for approximately 4 months after an injection, allowing some leeway for providers to schedule follow-up injections. During 1 year of use, the perfect use failure rate is 0.3 pregnancies per 100 woman-years, whereas the failure rate with typical use is 3 pregnancies per 100 woman-years.

Use of DMPA is associated with several health benefits. The risk of ectopic pregnancy is significantly lower among users compared to women who do not use contraception. The risk of endometrial cancer is reduced by as much as 80%, an effect that is long term and increases with duration of use. Studies have shown as much as a 70% reduction in the frequency of sickle cell crises; the mechanism for this effect is not known. Some women with endometriosis have improvement of symptoms with use of DMPA.

Use of DMPA does not increase the risk for arterial or venous disease. The most significant potential risk associated with DMPA use is a reduction in bone mineral density. Overall, prospective studies of at least 1 year's duration have shown a maximum reduction of 1.5–2.3% in bone mineral density. No studies have shown any increase in fracture risk. Finally, retrospective studies have shown improvement in bone mineral density when DMPA was discontinued. Until further data become available, adequate calcium intake should be encouraged for DMPA users, particularly young patients and longer-term users. Irregular bleeding and prolonged menstrual flow are not uncommon during the first 6 months of use. However, with continued use, many women become amenorrheic, and up to 70% of users experience no menses after 1 year. Mood change and depression have been reported in association with DMPA use. However, most studies are uncontrolled. Although earlier studies suggested DMPA users gained an average of 5 lb after 1 year of use, a recent randomized clinical trial demonstrated that DMPA was not associated with significant weight gain or changes in variables that might lead to weight gain. Finally, when DMPA users stop injections in an effort to achieve pregnancy, the return to baseline fertility may take an average of 10 months.

Implants

Although no implantable contraceptives currently are available in the United States, clinical trials of a single rod implant 4 cm long and 2 mm in diameter have been completed. This system releases etonogestrel, the major metabolite of desogestrel, and maintains its efficacy for up to 3 years. The rod usually is inserted in the upper arm, using a trocar. Removal is easier than with other implants because it is a single rod system. The likely mechanism of action is similar to that of DMPA. Overall efficacy is extremely high, with no reported pregnancies in more than 70,000 cycles of use. No major complications have been reported to date. Side effects include menstrual abnormalities and weight gain.

Vaginal Ring

The vaginal ring is approximately 5 cm in diameter and 4 mm thick. The ring is flexible. It releases ethinyl estradiol and etonogestrel at fairly constant rates. The ring is worn for 3 weeks per month, although the ring's reservoir contains enough contraceptive steroid for approximately 14 more days. The ring maintains its efficacy even if it is removed for up to 3 hours, although it is designed to be left in place even during intercourse. Users are instructed to insert the ring high into the vagina; fitting by a health professional is not required. The overall pregnancy rate over 1 year of use is 0.65 pregnancies per 100 woman-years.

No published data indicate the rates of major side effects or potential noncontraceptive benefits. However, because the vaginal ring contains steroids that are used in combination oral contraceptives, rates of serious side effects may be similar, and some of the noncontraceptive benefits may accrue to users of this method. Minor side effects are similar to those seen in users of combination oral contraceptives, although the frequency of breakthrough bleeding and spotting appears lower. Approximately 10–15% of users report vaginal-related symptoms, such as slight discomfort, a sensation of a foreign body, leukorrhea, vaginitis, or coital problems.

Transdermal Patch

The transdermal contraceptive patch is 20 cm², roughly the size of a small adhesive-back (Post-It) pad consisting of 3 layers. The transdermal contraceptive patch is designed to deliver norelgestromin, the active metabolite of norgestimate, and ethinyl estradiol daily for a 7-day period. After 7 days, the patch is removed and a new patch is applied to another skin site. Three consecutive 7-day patches are applied in a typical cycle, followed by a 7-day patch-free period to allow withdrawal bleeding. Application sites include the buttocks, lower abdomen, upper outer arm, and upper torso except for the breasts. Because this is a combination steroid preparation, the same contraindications noted for combination oral contraceptives use apply.

The transdermal contraceptive patch has a method use rate of 0.70 and a typical use rate of 0.88 pregnancies per 100 woman-years. These rates are comparable to pregnancy rates achieved with current oral contraceptives. However, a failure rate approaching the typical use failure rate seen with combination oral contraceptive users was noted for women weighing over 198 pounds who used the patch.

Although few reports have documented the rates of serious adverse events, one should assume that the events and risks will be similar to those noted for combination oral contraceptives. To date, one published study has indicated that the risk of venous thromboembolism is similar to that of an oral contraceptive. Similarly, no data on noncontraceptive benefits are available. The frequency of side effects such as headache and nausea are similar to that seen among users of combination oral contraceptives, although contraceptive patch users have application site reactions, more breast symptoms (only during the first 2 cycles), and more dysmenorrhea than combination oral contraceptive users. The pattern of breakthrough bleeding and spotting with the transdermal contraceptive patch is similar to that seen with oral contraceptive users. No evidence indicates that use of the patch influences body weight. Among users, 1.8% of women required replacement for complete detachment and 2.9% became partially detached. Detachment rates were similar for women living in warm, humid climates and for women who were subjected to vigorous exercise, swimming, and sauna use compared to other users. When patches do become detached, users should attempt to reattach them if possible, without using ancillary adhesives or tape. If detachment has occurred for 24 hours or less, the cycle continues as usual, with the patch changed on the previously determined change day. If detachment has occurred for more than 24 hours, a new patch should be applied, backup contraception should be used for 1 week, and the day that the new patch is applied now becomes the patch change day.

INTRAUTERINE CONTRACEPTIVE DEVICES

Two types of IUDs are available in the United States: the copper T 380A device and a levonorgestrel-releasing device (Fig 36–3). The T 380A is a T-shaped device approximately 36 mm in length and 32 mm in diameter that contains 380 mm² of copper on its vertical and side arms. Two monofilament strings are attached to the vertical arm to ascertain placement in the uterus over the course of use. This IUD has a useful lifespan of at least 10 years. The exact mechanism of action is unknown, although current theories include spermicidal activity, interference with either normal development of ova or the fertilization of ova, and activity on the endometrium that may promote phagocytosis of sperm and which may impede sperm migration or capacitance.

Figure 36–3. Intrauterine contraceptive devices currently available in the United States. **Left**: The copper T 380A device; **Right**: the levonorgestrel device.

Figure 36–4. Insertion of the ParaGard T 380A intrauterine copper contraceptive device.

No data support this or other IUDs as abortifacients. The perfect use failure rate with the T 380A is 0.6 pregnancies per 100 woman-years and approximately 0.8 for typical use. In the past, IUDs were associated with an increased risk for PID around the time of insertion. However, by restricting use to mutually monogamous couples and couples currently at low risk of STIs, the absolute risk of PID in association with IUD use is almost negligible. PID appears to be associated primarily with the insertion of the device (Fig 36–4) and not with its duration of use. Currently, with appropriately selected users, the rate of PID is approximately 1 case per 1000 insertions. Women at risk for HIV infection or who are already infected are not believed to be candidates for use of this device. Other ideal candidates are women in whom combination hormonal contraception is contraindicated. The other major risks reported in association with use of this IUD include ectopic pregnancy, spontaneous abortion, uterine perforation, and expulsion. Although 5–8% of pregnancies that occur with use of this IUD are ectopic, overall, because of the high effectiveness of this device, the absolute risk of ectopic pregnancy in users is substantially less than that experienced by nonusers of contraception. In addition, if a user becomes pregnant with the device in place, the risk of a spontaneous abortion is approximately 50%. Removing the device when the strings can be readily identified will reduce this risk by approximately 50%. If the pregnancy continues with the IUD in place, users should be apprised of an increased risk for premature rupture of the membranes and preterm delivery. Uterine perforation, which occurs at the time of insertion, has been reported at a rate of 1–2 events per 1000 insertions. This risk is minimized by performing a preinsertion pelvic examination to determine the position of the uterus and by using a tenaculum to straighten the uterine axis during insertion. Expulsions of the device are more common in the first few weeks of use, with rates of approximately 5%. Minor side effects include abnormal bleeding and cramping. Use of nonsteroidal anti-inflammatory drugs often will reduce the overall amount of flow as well as reduce cramping.

The levonorgestrel-releasing intrauterine device (LNG-20 IUD) has a T-shaped frame with a reservoir on the vertical arm that releases the progestin levonorgestrel daily. Two monofilament strings are attached to the vertical arm. Blood levels of levonorgestrel among users are approximately 25% the levels seen among users of oral contraceptives containing this progestin. In contrast to the copper T 380A device, the LNG-20 IUD has a life span of 5 years in clinical trials. The primary mechanisms of action of the LNG-20 IUD are thickening the cervical mucus to impede ascent of sperm and altering the uterotubal fluid to also interfere with sperm migration. This IUD causes anovulation in approximately 10–15% of cycles and changes the characteristics of the endometrium to reduce the likelihood of implantation. Candidates for use of this IUD fit the same profile as those who would consider use of the T 380A. The perfect and typical use pregnancy rates are 0.1 pregnancies per 100 woman-years after 1 year of use, and the cumulative pregnancy rate over 5 years is 0.7 pregnancies per 100 woman-years. Approximately 50% of the pregnancies that occur are ectopic. However, as with the T 380A device, the absolute risk of ectopic pregnancy still is substantially lower than that experienced by nonusers of contraception. Because the LNG-20 IUD releases a potent progestin at the endometrial level, the bleeding pattern is substantially different from that seen with the T 380A. During the initial 3–4 months of use, some women experience irregular bleeding that may be heavy at times. However, after a few months of use, most women experience a significant decrease in menstrual flow by as much as 70%. In some studies, 20–25% of users become amenorrheic in the second year of use. In addition, dysmenorrhea tends to improve with use of this device. Because of the effectiveness of the LNG-20 IUD in reducing menstrual blood flow, it has been used for treatment of menorrhagia, a significant noncontraceptive benefit. Major risks with this IUD are similar to those noted for the copper T 380A, except that PID has not been associated with use of this device. The minor side effects of bleeding and cramping are less frequent with this device, except for irregular bleeding patterns during the first few months of use. Some women have reported headache, acne, or mastalgia, which could be related to the systemic effects of the progestin.

A not infrequent issue with IUD use is the management of missing strings. First, the patient should be encouraged to use a backup contraceptive method until she is evaluated. If the IUD strings cannot be seen even with gentle probing of the endocervical canal, one should perform a pregnancy test if indicated and consider ordering a transvaginal ultrasound to determine if the IUD is intrauterine, intraperitoneal, or likely has undergone expulsion. If the patient is pregnant, an ectopic pregnancy must be excluded. If the IUD is determined to be intra-peritoneal in location, removal usually is indicated because of likely peritoneal irritation by the device.

◼ INDUCED ABORTION

Induced abortion is the deliberate termination of pregnancy in a manner that ensures that the embryo or fetus will not survive. Societal attitudes toward elective abortion have changed markedly in the past few decades. In some situations the need for abortion is accepted by most people, but political and medical attitudes regarding induced abortion have continued to lag behind changing attitudes. Certain religious objections continue to prevail, resulting in personal, medical, and political conflicts.

Approximately one-third of the world's population lives in nations with nonrestrictive laws governing abortion. Another third live in countries with moderately restrictive abortion laws, ie, in countries where unwanted pregnancies may not be terminated as a matter of right or personal decision but only on broadly interpreted medical, psychologic, and sociologic indications. The remainder live in countries where abortion is illegal without qualification or is allowed only when the woman's life or health would be severely threatened if the pregnancy were allowed to continue.

An estimated 1 of every 4 pregnancies in the world is terminated by induced abortion, making it perhaps the most common method of reproduction limitation. In the United States, estimates of the number of criminal abortions performed prior to legalization of the procedure ranged from 0.25–1.25 million per year. The number of legal abortions now being performed in the United States approximates 1 abortion per 4 live births. In 1997, there were 1.33 million induced abortions compared to 3.88 million live births.

The procedures being used in the United States for legally induced abortions during the first trimester are relatively safe. Table 36–2 shows that first-trimester legal abortions are consistently safer for the woman than if she used no birth control method and gave birth. Table 36–2 also shows that although the number of maternal deaths related to births steadily increased from 5.6 to 22.6 per 100,000 women as age increased, the age-related increase in number of deaths per 100,000 women per year from legal abortions was insignificant.

In general, the risk of death from legal abortion is lowest when it is performed at 8 menstrual weeks or sooner. Table 36–3 shows the relationship between death from legal abortion and the gestational age at the time of the procedure.

Paracervical anesthesia has replaced general anesthesia in many health settings, resulting in fewer complica-

Table 36–2. Pregnancy-related deaths per 100,000 women per year in developed countries compared with deaths resulting from legal abortion as a means of contraception.

Type of Birth Control	Age Groups (Years)					
	15–19	20–24	25–29	30–34	35–39	40–44
No birth control; birth related	5.6	6.1	7.4	13.9	20.8	22.6
First-trimester abortion only; method related	1.2	1.6	1.8	1.7	1.9	1.2

Adapted from Tietze C: Induced abortion: 1977 supplement, Table 11. Rep Popul Fam Plann 1977; 14[2nd ed. Suppl]:16.

tions related to anesthesia. Midtrimester abortion techniques still are problematic and are associated with a higher mortality rate. Hysterectomy carries a far greater risk than does induction of labor by amnioinfusion or dilatation and evacuation.

Legal Aspects of Induced Abortion in the United States

The United States Supreme Court ruled in 1973 that the restrictive abortion laws in the United States were invalid, largely because these laws invaded the individual's right to privacy, and that an abortion could not be denied to a woman in the first 3 months of pregnancy. The Court indicated that after 3 months a state may "regulate the abortion procedure in ways that are reasonably related to maternal health" and that after the fetus reaches the stage of viability (approximately 24 weeks) the states may refuse the right to terminate the pregnancy except when necessary for the preservation of the life or health of the mother. Still, much opposition

Table 36–3. Death-to-case for legal abortions by weeks of gestation (in the United States, 1972–1975).

Weeks of Gestation	Deaths per 100,000 Procedures
8 or less	0.7
9–10	1.9
11–12	4.1
13–15	7.5
16–20	19.6
21 or more	22.9

Adapted from Tyler CW Jr: In: *Abortion Surveillance, 1975.* Center for Disease Control, United States Department of Health, Education, and Welfare Annual Summary 1975, April 1977, p. 36.

is raised by various "right-to-life" groups and religious groups. In spite of this opposition, more than 1 million procedures are still performed annually in the United States, with approximately one-third performed on teenaged women. This dramatically emphasizes the inadequacy of sex education and the need for greater availability of adequate contraceptive methods in order to avoid such pregnancy wastage.

The patient must be informed regarding the nature of the procedure and its risks, including possible infertility or even continuation of pregnancy. The rights of the spouse, parents, or guardian also must be considered and permission obtained when indicated (until the individual woman's rights are clearly established). State laws must be obeyed with special reference to residence, duration of pregnancy, indications for abortion, consent, and consultations required.

Evaluation of Patients Requesting Induced Abortion

Patients give varied reasons for requesting abortion. Because in some cases the request is made at the urging of the woman's parents, in-laws, husband, or peers, every effort should be made to ascertain that the patient herself desires abortion for her own reasons. In addition, one should be certain that the patient knows she is free to choose from among other methods of solving the problem of unplanned pregnancy, such as adoption or single-parent rearing.

Although the majority of abortions are performed as elective procedures, ie, because of social or economic reasons as opposed to medical reasons, some women still request such services for medical or surgical indications. For example, continuation of pregnancy may pose a threat to the life of women with certain medical conditions, such as Eisenmenger's syndrome and cystic fibrosis. Other indications are pregnancy resulting from a rape or pregnancy with a fetus affected with a major disorder, such as trisomy 13. In any event, the ultimate decision rests with the pregnant woman. Help from social agencies should be made available as necessary. A complete social history, medical history, and physical examination are required. Particular attention must be given to uterine size and position; the importance of accurate calculation of the duration of pregnancy (within 2 weeks but preferably within 1 week) cannot be overstated. With uncertainty, pelvic sonography should be used liberally. Routine laboratory tests should include pregnancy tests, urinalysis, hematocrit level, Rh typing, serologic tests for syphilis, culture for gonorrhea, and Pap smear.

Methods of Induced Abortion

Numerous methods are used to induce an abortion: suction or surgical curettage; induction of labor by means of intraovular or extraovular injection of a hypertonic solution or other oxytocic agent; dilatation and evacuation; extraovular placement of devices such as catheters, bougies, or bags; hysterotomy—abdominal or vaginal; hysterectomy—abdominal or vaginal; and menstrual regulation.

The method of abortion used is determined primarily by the duration of pregnancy, with consideration for the patient's health, the experience of the physician, and the available physical facilities.

Suction curettage on an outpatient basis performed under local or light general anesthesia can be accomplished with a high degree of safety. The safety of outpatient abortion and the shortage of hospital beds have led to the development of single-function, "freestanding" abortion clinics. In addition to providing more efficient counseling and social services, these clinics have effectively reduced the cost of abortion. Many hospitals have "short-stay units," which match the efficiency of outpatient clinics but also offer the backup facilities of the general hospital.

A. Suction Curettage

Suction curettage is the safest and most effective method for terminating pregnancies of 12 weeks' duration or less. This technique has gained rapid worldwide acceptance, and over 90% of induced abortions in the United States are now performed by this method. The procedure involves dilatation of the cervix by instruments or by hydrophilic *Laminaria* tent (see Induction of Labor by Intra-amniotic Instillation), followed by insertion of a suction cannula of the appropriate diameter into the uterine cavity (Fig 36–5). Most procedures are performed using a paracervical block with local anesthesia with or without additional medication for sedation. Standard negative pressures used range from 30–50 mm Hg. Many physicians follow aspiration with light instrumental curettage of the uterine cavity.

The advantages of suction over surgical curettage are that suction curettage empties the uterus more rapidly, minimizes blood loss, and reduces the likelihood of perforation of the uterus. However, failure to recognize perforation of the uterus with a cannula may result in serious damage to other organs. Knowledge of the size and position of the uterus and the volume of the contents is mandatory for safe suction curettage. Moreover, extreme care and slow minimal dilatation of the cervix, with special consideration for the integrity of the internal os, should prevent injury to the cervix or uterus. Attention to the decrease in uterine size that occurs with rapid evacuation helps to avoid uterine injury.

When performed in early pregnancy by properly trained physicians, suction curettage should be associated with a very low failure rate. The complication rate should be less than 1% for infection, approximately 2% for excessive bleeding, and less than 1% for uterine perforation. The risk of major complications, such as persistent fever, hemorrhage requiring transfusion, and unintended major surgery, ranges between 0.2% and 0.6% and is proportional to pregnancy duration. The incidence of mortality for suction curettage is approximately 1 in 100,000 patients.

B. Surgical Curettage

Surgical ("sharp") curettage has been used for first-trimester abortion in the absence of suction curettage equipment. This procedure is performed as a standard dilatation and curettage, such as for the diagnosis of abnormal uterine bleeding or for the removal of endometrial polyps. The blood loss, duration of surgery, and likelihood of damage to the cervix or uterus are greatly increased when surgical curettage is used. In addition, the risk of uterine synechiae or Asherman's syndrome is increased with this approach. Accordingly, suction curettage is generally preferred over sharp curettage for first-trimester termination procedures.

C. Medical Abortion with Methotrexate and Misoprostol

Women with first-trimester pregnancies less than 49 days from their first day of the last menstrual period may be eligible for medical abortion. An alternative method of medical abortion consists of the administration of an oral antiprogestin (RU-486 [mifepristone]) followed by oral misoprostol 48 hours later. The reported success rate of this method is greater than 90%, provided the protocol is started prior to 7 weeks from the last menstrual period. Complications include cramping, bleeding due to incomplete abortion, and failure to evacuate the uterus necessitating completion by suction curettage. With one of the more common protocols, 50 mg methotrexate is administered orally, followed by 800 mg misoprostol per vagina (by the patient at home) 3–7 days later using the same tablets as those used for oral dosing. The patient is seen at least 24 hours after the misoprostol administration; a vaginal ultrasound is performed to determine if there has been passage of the

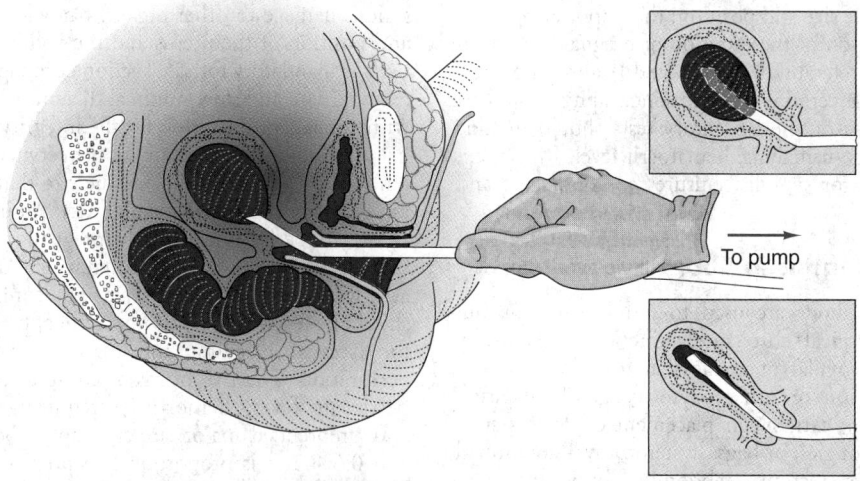

To pump

Figure 36–5. Suction method for induced abortion.

gestational sac. If abortion has not occurred, the misoprostol dose is repeated. The patient is then followed-up in 4 weeks; if abortion has not occurred by this time, a suction curettage is typically performed. If fetal cardiac activity is noted on ultrasound, office follow-up is more frequent. Efficacy with this method is up to 98% for pregnancies up to 49 days' gestation; complete abortion rates are inversely proportional to duration of gestation. Nausea is the most frequently reported side effect. Contraindications include active liver disease, active renal disease, severe anemia, acute inflammatory bowel disease and coagulopathy, or anticoagulant therapy.

D. INDUCTION OF LABOR BY INTRA-AMNIOTIC INSTILLATION

The Japanese developed this technique for induced abortion after the first trimester. Currently, the technique is used almost exclusively for initiating midtrimester abortion. The original procedure consisted of amniocentesis, aspiration of as much fluid as possible, and instillation into the amniotic sac of 200 mL hypertonic (20%) sodium chloride solution. In most (80–90%) cases, spontaneous labor and expulsion of the fetus and placenta occur within 48 hours. This technique has been modified, primarily to reduce the injection–abortion interval, and as a result of the development of other agents that initiate labor when instilled intra-amniotically.

Because of the problems associated with hypertonic sodium chloride, many clinicians have used intra-amniotic hyperosmolar (59.7%) urea, usually with oxytocin or prostaglandin or intra-amniotic prostaglandin alone. These approaches result in injection–abortion intervals of 16–17 hours for urea and 19–22 hours for prostaglandin. The

urea is instilled in a fashion similar to that described for hypertonic sodium chloride. The prostaglandin, most frequently prostaglandin F_{2a} (PGF_{2a}), usually is instilled as a single dose of 40–50 mg or as 2 doses of 25 mg instilled 6 hours apart. When oxytocin is used to augment these agents, doses as high as 332 mU/min are required to produce uterine contractions because of the relative insensitivity of the myometrium to oxytocin at this stage of pregnancy. To avoid water intoxication, the oxytocin is made up in highly concentrated solutions and given at slow rates.

It is advantageous to soften the unripe cervix with *Laminaria* tents placed in the cervix a few hours before amniocentesis is performed. Such an approach markedly reduces the risk of cervical injury.

Midtrimester abortion induced by this method must be accomplished with scrupulous aseptic surgical technique, and the patient must be monitored until the fetus and placenta are delivered and postabortion bleeding is under control. The complication rate is high—up to 20% in some institutions—and the mortality rate is comparable to that of term parturition. Fortunately, because first-trimester abortion is now more readily available, more women are consulting their physicians early and thus availing themselves of the much safer suction curettage.

Several types of complications are associated with the use of instillation agents. Retained placenta is the most common problem; rates ranging from 13–46% have been reported. The placenta usually can be removed without difficulty using ring forceps and large curettes with the patient under local anesthesia. Hemorrhage may be caused by retained products or atony; coagulopathy is seen in up to 1% of patients in whom hypertonic sodium chloride is used. Infection can occur but is reduced significantly by use of prophylactic antibiotics in high-risk situations, eg, in patients with early ruptured membranes and during injection–abortion intervals greater than 24 hours. Cervical laceration can occur but is reduced by the use of *Laminaria* tents. Hypernatremia can occur with the use of hypertonic sodium chloride if the drug is absorbed rapidly by the placental bed or if it is given intravascularly by mistake.

Failure of labor to expel the products of conception necessitates either a repetition of the procedure if the membranes are still intact or oxytocin stimulation, usually by intravenous injection or use of the dilatation and evacuation technique.

Emotional stress is an important factor for many women because they are awake at the time of the expulsion of the fetus and the fetus is well formed. (The emotional stress is also a factor for hospital personnel—a problem impossible to avoid.)

E. INDUCTION OF LABOR WITH VAGINAL PROSTAGLANDINS

Prostaglandin E_2 given intravaginally can be used to induce midtrimester abortion. Vaginal suppositories containing 20 mg are used every 3–4 hours until abortion occurs; the presence or absence of labor determines whether the prostaglandin E_2 should be stopped. Misoprostol, a synthetic prostaglandin E_1 analogue, is also used. Treatment–abortion intervals, rates of incomplete abortion, and complications are similar to those described for instillation agents. The major disadvantages are significant gastrointestinal side effects, a higher incidence of live abortion, and a more frequent occurrence of fever.

F. DILATATION AND EVACUATION

This technique for inducing midtrimester abortion is essentially a modification of suction curettage. Because fetal parts are larger at this stage of pregnancy, most operators use serial placement of *Laminaria* tents to effect cervical dilatation with less likelihood of injury. Larger suction cannulas and specially designed forceps are used to extract tissue. In most instances, the operation can be performed in the outpatient setting using paracervical block anesthesia and intravenous sedation on patients with pregnancies up to 18 weeks' gestation. Complications include hemorrhage (usually due to atony or laceration), perforation, and rarely infection. Retained tissue is uncommon, especially when tissue is carefully inspected for completion at the end of each procedure. Compared with instillation techniques or vaginal prostaglandin, the overall incidence of complications (in pregnancies up to 18 weeks' gestation) is less with dilatation and evacuation. In addition, most patients prefer the technique because it is an outpatient procedure and the woman does not undergo labor.

G. HYSTEROTOMY AND HYSTERECTOMY

The use of hysterotomy and hysterectomy is currently reserved for special circumstances such as the failure to complete a midtrimester abortion due to cervical stenosis or the management of other complications. Both approaches, compared with other techniques discussed, have unacceptably high rates of morbidity and mortality, and neither should be used as a primary method.

H. MENSTRUAL REGULATION

Menstrual regulation consists of aspiration of the endometrium within 14 days after a missed menstrual cycle or within 42 days after the beginning of the last menstrual period by means of a small cannula attached to a source of low-pressure suction, such as a syringe or other suction machine. This is a simple and safe procedure that can be readily performed in the office or outpatient clinic, usually without any anesthetic, although paracervical block can be used if necessary. Menstrual regulation was used extensively in the 1970s and 1980s before reliable, inexpensive, and sensitive urine pregnancy tests became available. It offered a safe early approach to pregnancy termination; however, approximately 40% of women were not pregnant at the time of the procedure. With the advent of urine pregnancy tests that have the ability to document pregnancy even before a missed menstrual period, standard first-trimester suction curettage probably is more widely used. Complications are similar to those described for suction curettage except that persistent pregnancy is more common, particularly when very early menstrual regulation procedures are performed.

I. RU-486

RU-486 (mifepristone) is a synthetic drug, developed by French pharmacologists, that acts at least partially as an antiprogestational agent. When given orally in conjunction with a prostaglandin such as misoprostol, it effects first-trimester abortion. Complications include failure to terminate a pregnancy, incomplete abortion, and significant uterine cramping.

Follow-Up of Patients after Induced Abortion

Follow-up care after all procedures must be ensured. After abortion by all methods, human Rho (D) immune globulin (RhoGAM) should be administered promptly if the patient is Rh-negative, unless the male partner is known to be Rh-negative. The patient should take her temperature several times daily and report fever or unusual bleeding at once. She should avoid intercourse or the use of tampons or douches for at least 2 weeks. The physician should discuss with the patient the possibility that emotional depression, similar to that following term pregnancy and delivery, may occur after induced abortion. Follow-up care should include pelvic examination to rule out endometritis and parametritis, salpingitis, failure of involution, or continued uterine growth. Finally, effective contraception should be made available according to the patient's needs and desires.

Long-Term Sequelae of Induced Abortion

Many studies during the past 2 decades have examined the possible long-term sequelae of elective induced abortion. Most of the attention has focused on subsequent reproductive function; unfortunately, many of the studies had inherent biases and serious methodologic flaws. Despite these problems, enough information is available to provide relative estimates of potential risks. Data from some studies suggest that midtrimester pregnancy loss is more common in women who have undergone 2 or more induced or spontaneous abortions. However, women who have undergone 1 procedure have essentially the same risk as women who have experienced a single term pregnancy. Regarding low birthweight, only women who have undergone a first-trimester procedure by sharp curettage under general anesthesia appear to have increased risks. The reason for this association might be related to the method of dilatation used. Finally, studies that have examined both ectopic pregnancy and infertility have failed to show any consistent association between these adverse events and prior induced abortion.

REFERENCES

General

Burkman RT: Clinical pearls: Factors affecting reported contraceptive efficacy rates in clinical studies. Int J Fertil Womens Med 2002;47:153.

Chandra A, Martinez GM, Mosher WD, Abma JC, Jones J. Fertility, family planning, and reproductive health of US women: data from the 2002 National Survey of Family Growth. National Center for Health Statistics. Vital Health Stat 2005;23.

Fulfilling the Promise. The Alan Guttmacher Institute, 2002.

Henshaw SK: Unintended pregnancy in the United States. Fam Plann Perspect 1998;30:24.

Kubba A et al: Contraception. Lancet 2000;356:1913.

Lethbridge DJ: Coitus interruptus. Considerations as a method of birth control. J Obstet Gynecol Neonatal Nurs 1991;20:80.

Mishell DR: Contraception. N Engl J Med 1989;320:777.

Piccinino LJ, Mosher WD: Trends in contraceptive use in the United States: 1982–1995. Fam Plann Perspect 1998;30:4.

Trussell J, Vaughan B: Contraceptive failure, method-related discontinuation and resumption of use: Results from the 1995 National Survey of Family Growth. Fam Plann Perspect 1999;31:64.

Contraception in the Adolescent

Kahn JG, Brindis CD, Glei DA: Pregnancies averted among U.S. teenagers by the use of contraceptives. Fam Plann Perspect 1999;31:29.

Lactational Amenorrhea

Van der Wijden C, Kleijnen J, Van den Berk T: Lactational amenorrhea for family planning. Cochrane Database Syst Rev 2003;(4):CD001329.

Vekeman M: Postpartum contraception: the lactational amenorrhea method. Eur J Contracept Reprod Health Care 1997;2:105.

World Health Organization Task Force on Methods for the Natural Regulation of Fertility: World Health Organization Multinational Study of Breast-feeding and Lactational Amenorrhea. III. Pregnancy during breastfeeding. Fertil Steril 1999;72:431.

Condom

Bounds W: Female condoms. Eur J Contracept Reprod Health Care 1997;2:113.

Gilliam ML, Derman RJ: Barrier methods of contraception. Obstet Gynecol Clin North Am 2000;27:841.

Kulig J: Condoms: The basics and beyond. Adolesc Med 2003;14:633.

Diaphragms

Allen RE: Diaphragm fitting. Am Fam Physician 2004;69:97.

Hooten TM et al: A prospective study of risk factors for symptomatic urinary tract infection in young women. N Engl J Med 1996;335:468.

Spermicidal Preparations

Jick H et al: Vaginal spermicides and congenital disorders. JAMA 1981;245:1329.

Raymond EG, Chen PL, Luoto J: Contraceptive effectiveness and safety of five nonoxynol-9 spermicides: A randomized trial. Obstet Gynecol 2004;103:430.

Richardson BA: Nonoxynol-9 as a vaginal microbicide for prevention of sexually transmitted infections. JAMA 2002;287:1171.

Periodic Abstinence

Gray RH, Kambic RT: Epidemiologic studies of natural family planning. Hum Reprod 1988;3:693.

Klaus H: Natural family planning: A review. Obstet Gynecol Surv 1982;37:128.

Hormonal Contraceptives

Anderson FD, Hait H: A multicenter, randomized study of an extended cycle oral contraceptive. Contraception 2003;68:89.

Audet M et al: Evaluation of contraceptive efficacy and cycle control of a transdermal contraceptive patch vs an oral contraceptive. JAMA 2001;285:2347.

Breast cancer and hormonal contraceptives: Collaborative reanalysis of individual data on 53 297 women with breast cancer and 100 239 women without breast cancer from 54 epidemiological studies. Collaborative Group on Hormonal Factors in Breast Cancer. Lancet 1996;347:1713.

Breast cancer and hormonal contraceptives: Further results. Collaborative Group on Hormonal Factors in Breast Cancer. Contraception 1996;54:1S.

Burkman RT: Cardiovascular issues with oral contraceptives: Evidenced-based medicine. Int J Fertil Womens Med 2000;45:166.

Burkman RT: The transdermal contraceptive system. Am J Obstet Gynecol 2004;190:S49.

Burkman R, Schlesselman JJ, Zieman M: Safety concerns and health benefits associated with oral contraception. Am J Obstet Gynecol 2004;190:S5.

Chang CL, Donaghy M, Poulter N: Migraine and stroke in young women: Case-control study. The World Health Organization Collaborative Study of Cardiovascular Disease and Steroid Hormone Contraception. BMJ 1999;318:13.

Croxatto HB. Clinical profile of Implanon: a single-rod etonogestrel contraceptive implant. Eur J Contracept Reprod Health Care 2000;5(Suppl 2):21.

Croxatto HB et al, and the Implanon Study Group: A multicentre efficacy and safety study of the single contraceptive implant Implanon. Hum Reprod 1999;14:976.

Darney PD: Implantable contraception. Eur J Contracept Reprod Health Care 2000;5(Suppl 2):2.

DeCherney A: Bone-sparing properties of oral contraceptives. Am J Obstet Gynecol 1996;174:15.

Dunn S et al: Emergency contraception. J Obstet Gynaecol Can 2003;25:673.

Fernandez E et al. Oral contraceptive use and risk of colorectal cancer. Epidemiology 1998;9:295.

Harrison-Woolrych M, Hill R: Unintended pregnancies with etonogestrel implant (Implanon): a case series from postmarketing experience in Australia. Contraception 2006;73:223.

Kaunitz AM: Current concepts regarding use of DMPA. J Reprod Med 2002;47:785.

Jick SS, Kay JA, Russmann S, Jick H: Risk of nonfatal venous thromboembolism in women using a contraceptive transdermal patch and oral contraceptives containing norgestimate and 35 microg of ethinyl estradiol. Contraception 2006;73:223.

Kuohung W, Borgatta L, Stubblefield P: Low-dose oral contraceptives and bone mineral density: An evidence-based analysis. Contraception 2000;61:77.

Lara-Torre E: "Quick Start," an innovative approach to the combination oral contraceptive pill in adolescents. Is it time to make the switch? J Pediatr Adolesc Gynecol 2004;17:65.

Le J, Tsourounis C: Implanon: A critical review. Ann Pharmacother 2001;35:329.

Marchbanks PA et al: Oral contraceptives and the risk of breast cancer. N Engl J Med 2002;346:2025.

Meckstroth KR, Darney PD: Implant contraception. Semin Reprod Med 2001;19:339.

Moreno V et al: Effect of oral contraceptives on risk of cervical cancer in women with human papillomavirus infection: The IARC multicentric case-control study. Lancet 2002;359:1085.

Mulders TMT, Dieben TO: Use of the novel combined contraceptive vaginal ring NuvaRing for ovulation inhibition. Fertil Steril 2001;75:865.

Parsey KS, Pong A. An open-label, multicenter study to evaluate Yasmin, a low-dose combination of oral contraceptive containing drospirenone, a new progestogen. Contraception 2000;6:105.

Rosenberg MJ et al: Compliance and oral contraceptives: A review. Contraception 1995;52:137.

Roumen FJ, Apter D, Mulders TM, Dieben TO: Efficacy, tolerability and acceptability of a novel contraceptive vaginal ring releasing etonogestrel and ethinyl oestradiol. Human Reproduction 2001;16:469.

Sanchez-Guerrero J, Uribe AG, Jimenez-Santana L, et al. A trial of contraceptive methods in women with systemic lupus erythematosus. NEJM 2005;353:2539.

Shoupe D et al: The significance of bleeding patterns in Norplant implant users. Obstet Gynecol 1991;77:256.

Webb AM: Emergency contraception. BMJ 2003;326:775.

Westhoff C: Clinical practice. Emergency contraception. N Engl J Med 2003;349:1830.

Yuzpe AA, Lancee WI: Ethinyl estradiol and dl-norgestrel as a postcoital contraceptive. Fertil Steril 1977;28:932.

Intrauterine Contraceptive Devices

Backman T et al: Pregnancy during the use of levonorgestrel intrauterine system. Am J Obstet Gynecol 2004;190:50.

Barbosa I et al: Ovarian function after seven years' use of a levonorgestrel IUD. Adv Contracept 1995;11:85.

Dardano KL, Burkman RT: The intrauterine contraceptive device: An often-forgotten and maligned method of contraception. Am J Obstet Gynecol 1999;181:1.

Lee NC, Rubin GL, Borucki R: The intrauterine device and pelvic inflammatory disease revisited: New results from the Women's Health Study. Obstet Gynecol 1988;72:1.

Sivin I, Schmidt F: Effectiveness of IUDs: A review. Contraception 1987;36:55.

Sivin I, Tatum HJ: Four years' experience with the TCU 380A intrauterine contraceptive device. Fertil Steril 1981;36:159.

Induced Abortion

Burkman RT et al: Hyperosmolar urea for elective midtrimester abortion: Experience in 1913 cases. Am J Obstet Gynecol 1978;131:10.

Centers for Disease Control: Mortality vital statistics. Volume 37, No. 6, Supplement. U.S. Department of Health and Human Services, 1988.

Creinin MD: Randomized comparison of efficacy, acceptability and cost of medical versus surgical abortion. Contraception 2000;62:117.

Creinin MD: Current medical abortion care. Curr Womens Health Rep 2003;3:461.

Grimes DA, Cates W Jr: Complications from legally-induced abortion: A review. Obstet Gynecol Surv 1979;34:177.

Grimes DA, Cates W Jr: The comparative efficacy and safety of intraamniotic prostaglandin F_{2a} and hypertonic saline for second-trimester abortion: A review and critique. J Reprod Med 1979;22:248.

Grimes DA, Creinin MD: Induced abortion: An overview for internists. Ann Intern Med 2004;140:620.

Grimes DA et al: Midtrimester abortion by dilatation and evacuation: A safe and practical alternative. N Engl J Med 1977;296:1141.

Grimes DA et al: Local versus general anesthesia: Which is safer for performing suction curettage abortions? Am J Obstet Gynecol 1979;135:1030.

Hogue CJW, Cates W, Tietze C: The effects of induced abortion on subsequent reproduction. Epidemiol Rev 1982;4:66.

Hubacher D, Grimes DA: Noncontraceptive health benefits of intrauterine devices: a systematic review. Obstet Gynecol Survey 2002;57:120.

Segal SJ: Mifepristone (RU 486). N Engl J Med 1990;322:691.

Benign Disorders of the Vulva & Vagina

37

Fariborz Mazdisnian, MD

Benign vulvar and vaginal disorders are common gynecologic conditions. These disorders may present with significant clinical symptoms or may be asymptomatic and noted only during routine examination. A thorough understanding of vulvar and vaginal pathophysiology is of clinical importance in diagnosing and treating these disorders. This chapter reviews the predisposing factors that contribute to the development of these disorders as well as the evaluation, diagnosis, and treatment of the different benign vulvovaginal disorders. The premalignant and invasive vulvar and vaginal disorders are discussed in Chapter 49.

ANATOMY & PHYSIOLOGY

The anatomy of the vagina and vulva is described in Chapter 2. The development of vulvar and vaginal disorders is influenced in part by the presence or absence of endogenous and exogenous estrogen. Estrogen thickens the vaginal epithelium and results in the presence of large quantities of glycogen in the epithelial cells. The collection of intraepithelial glycogen results in the production of lactic acid. This acid environment (pH 3.5–4.0) promotes the growth of normal vaginal flora, chiefly lactobacilli and acidogenic corynebacteria. *Candida* organisms may be present, but only in small quantities, because of the preponderance of the bacteria. The absence of endogenous estrogen in prepubertal girls results in a thin vaginal epithelium, which predisposes this age group most commonly to bacterial infections. In postmenopausal women, endogenous estrogen production declines, the cells of the vaginal epithelium and vulvar skin lose glycogen, and the vaginal acidity declines. The resulting atrophic vaginal and vulvar tissue is prone to trauma and infection, and the lactobacilli are replaced by a mixed flora consisting chiefly of pathogenic cocci. Vulvar irritation also occurs with urinary and fecal soiling, which can be an underlying factor in this age group.

EVALUATION

Evaluation of a patient with vulvar and/or vaginal symptoms requires a detailed history and physical examination, including inspection of other mucosal and skin surfaces. Specific questions regarding symptoms of vulvar or vaginal pain, itching, discharge, and previous infections should be elicited. Sexual activity, the use of feminine hygiene products (douching, soaps, perfumes), and medications (oral contraceptive pills, antibiotics) can alter the normal vaginal flora. Any underlying medical conditions, such as diabetes, can impact the development of certain vulvovaginal disorders. Overlying garments made of synthetic fabrics that retain heat and moisture can exacerbate vulvovaginal symptoms.

The first symptom of vaginal irritation is often vulvar pruritus, which often results from contact with vaginal discharge. Any variance from the normal, physiologic milky vaginal discharge should be noted. Before menarche, a scant vaginal discharge occurs that normally does not cause irritation and is not considered abnormal. Inspection in the adolescent girl may reveal a small amount of white mucoid material in the vaginal vault that is the result of normal desquamation and accumulation of vaginal epithelial cells. The most common cause of leukorrhea (vaginal discharge) is a vaginal infection. The presence or absence of odor, pruritus, and the color can help determine the etiology.

A vaginal discharge is considered abnormal by the patient if there is an increase in the volume (especially if there is soiling of the clothing), an objectionable odor, or a change in consistency or color. Specific characteristics depend on the cause (Table 37–1). Secondary irritation of the vulvar skin may be minimal or extensive, causing pruritus or dyspareunia. Ideally, evaluation should occur after the onset of symptoms if the patient is not menstruating. She should be instructed not to douche. After the clinical history is obtained, the vulva, vagina, and cervix should be thoroughly inspected (Table 37–2). The pH of the vaginal secretions in the speculum blade should be determined, and a small amount of secretion should be placed on each of 2 glass slides. One slide should be treated with 10% room-temperature potassium hydroxide (KOH) and the other diluted with room-temperature normal saline. A transient "fishy odor" after KOH application is characteristic of bacterial vaginosis, the "sniff test" or

Table 37–1. Diagnosis of major causes of vaginitis.

	Symptom	pH	Discharge	Wet Smear
Candida	Pruritus	4.0–5.0	Thick, curdy	Hyphae
Tricho-monas	Discharge	5.0–7.0	Thin, copious	Motile pro-tozoa
Bacterial vaginosis	Odor	4.0–6.0	Scant, nonir-ritating	Clue cells

"whiff test." White blood cells and epithelial cells are digested by the KOH; therefore, the candidal pseudo-hyphae and spores are easier to detect (Figs 37–1 and 37–2). Motile trichomonads may be detected under low power on the saline-diluted slide (Fig 37–3). Bacterial vaginosis is diagnosed by the presence of "clue cells," which are epithelial cells that have bacteria attached to their cell membranes (Fig 37–4). The relative number of white blood cells and the maturity of the epithelial cells should be determined. Patients with vaginitis or cervicitis show many white blood cells, and the presence of intermediate or basal cells indicates inflammation of the vaginal epithelium. Selective cultures may be performed for trichomoniasis, bacterial infection, and candidiasis.

VAGINAL DISORDERS

Candidiasis

It is estimated that approximately 75% of women will experience an episode of vulvovaginal candidiasis. *Candida albicans* is the most common *Candida* species causing symptomatic candidiasis in approximately 90% of cases (Table 37–3). *C albicans* frequently inhabits the mouth, throat, large intestine, and vagina normally. Clinical infection may be associated with a systemic disorder (diabetes mellitus, human immunodeficiency virus [HIV], obesity), pregnancy, medication (antibiotics, corticosteroids, oral contraceptives), and chronic debilitation.

Vulvovaginal candidiasis presents with intense vulvar pruritus; a white curdlike, cheesy vaginal discharge; and vulvar erythema. A burning sensation may follow urination, particularly if there is excoriation of the skin from

Table 37–2. Diagnosis of vaginitis.

Obtain history, symptoms.
Examine vulva, vaginal walls, and cervix.
Check pH of discharge.
Prepare wet smear with saline.
Prepare potassium hydroxide smear ("sniff test").

Figure 37–1. Saline wet mount demonstrating *Candida albicans*.

scratching. Widespread involvement of the skin adjacent to the labia may suggest an underlying systemic illness such as diabetes. The labia minora may be erythematous, excoriated, and edematous. The ubiquitous nature of the organism allows for repeated infections that may be interpreted as a recurrent vulvovaginal candidiasis. Diagnosis is based on demonstration of candidal mycelia and a normal vaginal pH ≤ 4.5. Identification of *C albicans* requires finding filamentous forms (pseudohyphae) of the organism (Fig 37–2) when vaginal secretions are mixed with 10% KOH solution. The gold standard for its diagnosis is a vaginal culture.

Treatment is reserved for symptomatic patients (Table 37–4). Underlying metabolic illnesses (diabetes) should be well controlled, and complicating medications (antibiotics) should be discontinued if possible. Nonabsorbent undergarments should be avoided, as should douching. Treatment of yeast infections consists of 3 echelons. (1) **Chemicals and dyes**—1% Gentian violet is an aniline dye that when painted over vaginal sur-

Figure 37–2. Potassium hydroxide preparation showing branched and budding *Candida albicans*.

Figure 37–3. Saline wet mount with mobile trichomonads in the center.

faces once per week is effective against *C albicans* and *Candida glabrata*. Boric acid compounded in a suppository form is also effective therapy for all candida infections. (2) **Polyenes**—Nystatin is not absorbed from the gastrointestinal tract and may be used orally to reduce the intestinal colonization. As topical agents, they have been largely replaced by imidazoles. (3) **Imidazoles**—Include clotrimazole and oral agents such as ketoconazole. They are mostly used as topical agents and are effective against *C albicans*. However resistant strains of *C glabrata* and *Candida tropicalis* are found with increasing frequency. Inclusion of a topical steroid (Mycolog [triamcinolone acetonide, nystatin], Lotrisone [betamethasone dipropionate, clotrimazole]) also may be beneficial in the patient who remains symptomatic to help decrease inflammation and relieve itching externally. A single 150-mg oral dose of fluconazole has been shown to be

Figure 37–4. Bacterial vaginosis. Saline wet mount of clue cells. Note the absence of inflammatory cells.

Table 37–3. Causes of vaginitis.

Infectious
  Vulvovaginal candidiasis
  Bacterial vaginosis
  Bacterial infections
  Trichomoniasis
  Viral infections
  Desquamative inflammatory vaginitis (clindamycin
    responsive)
  Secondary bacterial infection associated with foreign body
    or atrophic vaginitis
  Parasitic
Noninfectious
  Atrophic vaginitis
  Allergic vaginitis
  Foreign body
  Desquamative inflammatory vaginitis (steroid responsive)
  Collagen vascular disease, Behçet's syndrome, pemphigus
    syndromes

effective in treating symptomatic candidiasis in nonpregnant patients. With severe cases of vaginal candidiasis, a 2-dose sequential regimen has been proposed.

During pregnancy, vulvovaginal candidiasis may be more difficult to eradicate. The azoles have not been well studied for use during the first trimester; therefore, treatment should be avoided until the second trimester, or 1 tablet of nystatin 100,000 units may be administered vaginally at night for 2 weeks during the first trimester.

Table 37–4. Medications used in the treatment of vulvovaginal candidiasis.

Butoconazole 2% cream, 1 applicator vaginally, for 3–5 days
Clotrimazole 1% cream, 1 applicator (5 g) vaginally, for 7
  days (14 days if chronic)
Clotrimazole 100-mg tablet, vaginally, for 7 days
Clotrimazole 100-mg tablets, 2 tablets vaginally, for 3 days
Clotrimazole 500-mg tablet, vaginally, for 1 dose
Miconazole 2% cream, 1 applicator vaginally, for 7 days
Miconazole 100-mg suppository, vaginally, for 7 days
Miconazole 200-mg suppository, vaginally, for 3 days
Tioconazole 2% cream, 1 applicator vaginally, for 3 days
Tioconazole 6.5% cream, 1 applicator vaginally, for 1 dose
Terconazole 0.4% cream, 1 applicator vaginally, for 7 days
Terconazole 0.8% cream, 1 applicator vaginally, for 3 days
Terconazole 80-mg suppository, vaginally, for 3 days
Boric acid 600-mg gelatin capsule, vaginally at night, for 2
  weeks or nightly for 1 week then 2 times per week
  for 3 weeks
Ketoconazole 200 mg, orally 2 times per day for 5 days
Itraconazole 200 mg, orally 2 times per day for 1 day
Fluconazole 150-mg tablet, orally, for 1 day

Chronic or recurrent infections ($\geq$ 4 infections per year) may occur in 5% of the population. Recurrent disease may result from insufficient duration of therapy, recontamination, and/or resistant strains. In evaluating the patient with recurrent vulvovaginal candidiasis, underlying predisposing disease processes should be ruled out. Additionally, cultures of the vagina should be obtained to identify possible resistant strains. High-dose estrogen or oral contraceptive use may precipitate infections and therefore should be discontinued. Treatment includes prolonging antifungal therapy for at least 2 weeks but preferably for 3 weeks to cover the life cycle of yeast, self-medication for 3–5 days at the first evidence of symptoms, and prophylactic treatment for several days prior to menstruation or during antibiotic therapy. Ketoconazole 100 mg orally each day for 6 months, fluconazole 150 mg weekly for 6 months, or itraconazole 100 mg orally daily for 6 months may reduce the frequency of recurrence to 10% during maintenance therapy. Unfortunately, within 6 months of discontinuation of prophylaxis, close to 57% of patients develop recurrences. Liver function tests should be monitored during prolonged oral therapy. Treatment of the partner may be considered in cases of symptomatic balanitis. Chronic or recurrent infections are secondary to *C tropicalis* or *C glabrata* may be resistant to topical imidazoles. In this case, ketoconazole or fluconazole should be given. Acidification of the vagina may also help.

Bacterial Infections

In the premenarcheal and postmenopausal hypoestrogenic vagina, a mixed bacterial flora may be expected, particularly in the presence of trauma or a foreign body. Specific diagnosis can be made through stained smears and cultures, although culture reports can be misleading in the presence of mixed flora. Bacterial vaginosis, previously referred to as *Gardnerella* vaginitis or nonspecific vaginitis, is the most common cause of symptomatic bacterial infection in reproductive-age women. In bacterial vaginosis the normal vaginal flora is altered. The concentration of the hydrogen peroxide–producing lactobacilli is decreased, and there is overgrowth of *Gardnerella vaginalis*, *Mobiluncus* spp., anaerobic gram-negative rods (*Prevotella* spp., *Porphyromonas* spp., *Bacteroides* spp.), and *Peptostreptococcus* spp. Other significant causes of bacterial infections are *Neisseria gonorrhoeae*, *Chlamydia*, *Mycoplasma hominis*, and *Ureaplasma urealyticum*.

In the hypoestrogenic vagina, bacterial infection may present as discharge and spotting. Inspection of the vagina will rule out a foreign body. Microscopic examination of the vaginal secretions is necessary to detect the more common causes of vaginitis and will demonstrate intermediate and parabasal epithelial cells.

A. BACTERIAL VAGINOSIS

Bacterial vaginosis presents as a "fishy" vaginal discharge, which is more noticeable following unprotected intercourse. The patient complains of a malodorous, nonirritating discharge, and examination reveals homogeneous, gray-white secretions with a pH of 5.0–5.5. A transient "fishy" odor can be released on application of 10% KOH to the vaginal secretions on a glass slide. A wet mount of the vaginal secretions using normal saline under microscopy demonstrates the characteristic clue cells, decreased lactobacilli, and few white blood cells. Clue cells are identified as numerous stippled or granulated epithelial cells (Fig 37–4). This appearance is caused by the adherence of *G vaginalis* organisms to the edges of the vaginal epithelial cells. Gram stain reveals a large number of small gram-negative bacilli and a relative absence of lactobacilli. Gram stain provides a more sensitive (93%) and specific (70%) diagnosis than does wet mount. Whether bacterial vaginosis is a true sexually transmitted disease is controversial, although women who are not sexually active are rarely affected.

Treatment in symptomatic patients should be implemented and should be considered in asymptomatic patients. Treatment regimens in nonpregnant women include metronidazole 500 mg orally twice daily for 7 days, metronidazole gel 0.75% (1 full applicator, 5 g) intravaginally once or twice daily for 5 days, or clindamycin cream 2% (1 full applicator, 5 g) intravaginally at bedtime for 7 days. (Clindamycin is oil based, so patients should be told that condoms or diaphragms might be weakened during treatment.) Alternative regimens include metronidazole 2 g orally in a single dose, clindamycin 300 mg orally twice daily for 7 days, or clindamycin ovules 100 g intravaginally once at bedtime for 3 days. In pregnant women, the recommended treatment is metronidazole 250 mg orally 3 times daily for 7 days. Alternatively, clindamycin 300 mg orally twice daily for 7 days can be given. Existing data do not support the use of topical agents during pregnancy. Possible management strategies for recurrent vaginosis includes use of condoms, longer treatment periods, prophylactic maintenance therapy, oral or vaginal application of yogurt containing lactobacillus acidophilus, intravaginal planting of other exogenous lactobacilli, and hydrogen peroxide douches. Treatment of the male does not help in preventing recurrence in the female.

Bacterial vaginosis has been reported to increase the risk of preterm delivery, although not all studies have confirmed that metronidazole treatment of asymptomatic pregnant women reduces the occurrence of preterm delivery or adverse pregnancy outcomes. In nonpregnant women, bacterial vaginosis has been related to posthysterectomy vaginal cuff cellulitis, postabortion infection, and pelvic inflammatory disease.

B. *NEISSERIA GONORRHOEAE*

Symptoms of infection by *N gonorrhoeae* may be quite severe, but up to 85% of women are asymptomatic. The incidence of the disease is rising and depends on the patient population. Family planning clinics report a 10% prevalence; private practitioners report 2–3%. The glandular structures of the cervix, urethra, vulva, perineum, and anus are most commonly infected. In acute disease, patients present with a copious mucopurulent discharge, and Gram's stain reveals gram-negative diplococci within leukocytes. However, diagnosis should be confirmed with a culture or with nucleic acid amplification. The specimen is collected from the endocervix. Cultures may also be taken from the urethra, rectum, and mouth. An estimated 15–20% of women with lower tract disease will develop upper tract disease presenting with salpingitis, tubo-ovarian abscess, and peritonitis. Ectopic pregnancy and infertility may result. If active infection is present during delivery, the newborn may develop conjunctivitis by contamination during vaginal delivery. Treatment of uncomplicated gonococcal infections of the cervix consists of ceftriaxone 125 mg IM in a single dose. Cefixime 400 mg orally in a single dose, ciprofloxacin 500 mg orally in a single dose, ofloxacin 400 mg orally in a single dose, or levofloxacin 250 mg orally in a single dose are other recommended regimens. Because of quinolone-resistant strains of *N gonorrhoeae* in parts of Asia and the Pacific, quinolones are no longer recommended for patients residing in, or who may have acquired infection while in, Asia and the Pacific (including Hawaii). The prevalence of quinolone resistance in California is increasing; therefore, the use of fluoroquinolones in California probably is inadvisable. Spectinomycin 2 g IM in a single dose can be given to patients sensitive to cephalosporins and quinolones. Treatment of *Chlamydia trachomatis* infection should be considered.

C. *CHLAMYDIA TRACHOMATIS*

C trachomatis infections can be asymptomatic, or they can present with a mucopurulent cervicitis, dysuria, and/or postcoital bleeding. Sexually active young women should be screened. *C trachomatis* can be identified by culture (50–90% sensitivity), a direct fluorescent antibody (50–80% sensitivity) and enzyme immunoassay (40–60% sensitivity), or most recently using nucleic acid amplification tests (polymerase chain reaction or ligase chain reaction, 60–100% sensitivity). All tests have a specificity > 99%. *Chlamydia* can also cause an ascending infection, salpingitis, in 20–40% of untreated patients. More than 50% of upper tract infections may be caused by *C trachomatis,* leading to tubal occlusion, ectopic pregnancy, or infertility. *C trachomatis* also can cause neonatal conjunctivitis if untreated

and atypical cytologic findings on Papanicolaou smear. *C trachomatis* may present as lymphogranuloma venereum (LGV), which most commonly affects the vulvar tissues. Retroperitoneal lymphadenopathy may be present. The initial lesion in LGV presents as a transient, painless vesicular lesion or shallow ulcer at the inoculation site. More advanced disease is characterized by anal or genital fistulas, stricture, or rectal stenosis. The disease is uncommon in the United States but is endemic in Southeast Asia and Africa.

If *C trachomatis* is suspected or diagnosed, both the patient and partner should be treated. In addition, a concurrent gonococcal infection should be considered. Recommended therapy includes azithromycin 1 g orally in a single dose or doxycycline 100 mg orally twice daily for 7 days. Erythromycin base 500 mg orally 4 times daily for 7 days, ofloxacin 300 mg orally twice daily, or levofloxacin 50 mg once daily for 7 days are alternative regimens. Doxycycline, levofloxacin, and ofloxacin should be avoided in pregnancy and during lactation. Patients should abstain from intercourse for 7 days. Test of cure is required in cases of possible reinfection or persistent symptoms and in pregnancy. Repeat testing can be considered 3 weeks after treatment with erythromycin. Women should be rescreened 3–4 months after treatment. For LGV, the recommended regimen is doxycycline 100 mg twice daily for 21 days.

D. OTHER

M hominis and *U urealyticum* also cause genital disease. Identification using polymerase chain reaction can increase the sensitivity over culture. Mycoplasma infections may cause infertility, spontaneous abortion, postpartum fever, nongonococcal urethritis in men, and possibly salpingitis and pelvic abscess. The most effective treatment is doxycycline 100 mg orally twice daily for 10 days.

Trichomonas Vaginitis

Trichomonas vaginalis is a unicellular flagellate protozoan (Fig 37–5). *T vaginalis* organisms are larger than polymorphonuclear leukocytes but smaller than mature epithelial cells. *T vaginalis* infects the lower urinary tract in both women and men. It is the most prevalent nonviral sexually transmitted disease in the United States. Nonsexual transmission is infrequent because large numbers of organisms are required to produce symptoms.

A persistent vaginal discharge is the principal symptom with or without secondary vulvar pruritus. The discharge is profuse, extremely frothy, greenish, and at times foul-smelling. The pH of the vagina usually exceeds 5.0. Involvement of the vulva may be limited to the vestibule and labia minora. The labia minora may become edematous and tender. Urinary symptoms may occur; however, burning with urination is most often associated with severe vulvitis. Examination of the vagi-

A   B   C

Figure 37–5. *Trichomonas vaginalis* as found in vaginal and prostatic secretions. **A:** Normal trophozoite. **B:** Round form after division. **C:** Common form seen in stained preparation. Cysts not found. (Reproduced, with permission, from Brooks GF, Butel JS, Ornston LN: *Jawetz, Melinick, & Adelberg's Medical Microbiology,* 19th ed. Appleton & Lange, 1991.)

nal epithelium and cervix shows generalized vaginal erythema with multiple small petechiae, the so-called strawberry spots, which may be confused with epithelial punctation. Wet mount with normal saline reveals an increase in polymorphonuclear cells and characteristic motile flagellates in 50–70% of culture-confirmed cases (Fig 37–3). Papanicolaou smears have a sensitivity of approximately 60% and may yield false-positive results. Culture is the gold standard, providing 95% sensitivity and 100% specificity. DNA probes and monoclonal antibodies may assist with accurate diagnosis.

Systemic therapy with metronidazole is the treatment of choice as trichomonads can be present in the urinary tract system. Partners should be treated simultaneously, with intercourse avoided or a condom used until treatment is completed. Metronidazole is the only Food and Drug Administration (FDA)-approved treatment in the United States, with cure rates of approximately 90–95%. A single-dose regimen of 2 g may assure compliance. Other regimens include a 500-mg tablet orally twice daily for 7 days. In resistant cases, which most likely are related to reinfection, oral metronidazole can be repeated after 4–6 weeks if the presence of trichomonads has been confirmed and the white blood cell count and differential are normal. Side effects of metronidazole include nausea or emesis with alcohol consumption. Contraindications include certain blood dyscrasias (neutropenia) and central nervous system diseases. An oncogenic effect has been demonstrated in animals but not in humans. Resistance to metronidazole therapy is rare but is rising and can be confirmed in vitro. A maximal dose of metronidazole 2–4 g daily should be given for 10 to 14 days if the patient tolerates

it. If treatment fails, consultation with the Centers for Disease Control is recommended. Nonoxynol 9 and other spermicidal agents have been demonstrated to decrease the transmission of *Trichomonas.*

Trichomoniasis is associated with many perinatal complications and an increased incidence in the transmission of HIV. Women with trichomoniasis should be evaluated for other sexually transmitted diseases, including *N gonorrhoeae, C trachomatis,* syphilis, and HIV.

Viral Infections

The viruses that affect the vulva and vagina are the herpesvirus (herpes simplex, varicella-zoster, and cytomegalovirus), poxvirus (molluscum contagiosum), and papovavirus types.

A. HERPESVIRUS

The herpesvirus (HSV) may cause superficial ulcerations or an exophytic necrotic mass involving the cervix, which may cause a profuse vaginal discharge. The cervix may be tender to manipulation and bleed easily. The primary lesion lasts 2–6 weeks and heals without scarring. Recurrent infections may cause cervical lesions. The virus may be cultured from ulcers or ruptured vesicles. Cervical cytologic examination may reveal multinucleated giant cells with intranuclear inclusions. The herpesvirus hominis has 2 immunologic variants, type I and type II. In general, most genital lesions are secondary to the type II virus. The type I virus is responsible for only 10–15% of genital herpes infections. Approximately 83% of patients will develop antibodies to herpesvirus type II in a minimum of 21 days following a primary infection. HSV is responsible for recurrent and disabling symptomatic disease, venereal transmission, and infection to the neonate (ie, herpes encephalitis). Further discussion of HSV is reviewed later in the chapter.

B. Human Papillomavirus

Human papillomavirus (HPV) is responsible for condyloma acuminata of the vagina, cervix, vulva, perineum, and perianal areas as well as for dysplasia and cancer. The rate of HPV infection is high and is rising. Approximately 30–60% of people may have been infected with HPV at some point in their lives, but the gross clinical prevalence of HPV is less than 1%. The virus is small and contains all its genetic material on a single double-stranded molecule of DNA. More than 20 types of HPV have been identified using viral DNA probes that can infect the genital tract. Types 16, 18, 31, 33, and 35 appear to have the most oncogenic potential. Types 6 and 11 are associated with genital condyloma. Most types cause an asymptomatic infection. The viruses are sexually transmitted and infect both partners.

The typical lesion is an exophytic or papillomatous condyloma. Colposcopic examination permits identification of flat, spiked, and inverted condyloma (Fig 37–6). The florid, papillomatous condyloma shows a raised white lesion with fingerlike projections often containing capillaries. Although large lesions may be seen with the naked eye, the colposcope is necessary to identify smaller lesions. The flat condyloma appears as a white lesion with a somewhat granular surface. A mosaic pattern and punctation also may be present, suggesting vaginal intraepithelial neoplasia (VAIN), which must be excluded by biopsy. Spiked lesions present as a hyperkeratotic lesion, with surface projections and prominent capillary tips. An inverted condyloma grows into the glands of the cervix but has not been identified on the vaginal epithelium. Condylomatous vaginitis causes a rough vaginal surface, demonstrating white projections from the pink vaginal mucosa. Vaginal discharge and pruritus are the most common symptom with florid condylomas. Postcoital bleeding may occur. No specific symptoms are related to the other types of condylomas. The entire lower tract usually is involved with subclinical or florid lesions when vulvar lesions are present. States of immunosuppression (pregnancy, HIV infection, diabetes, renal transplant) are associated with massive proliferation of condyloma and often are difficult to treat. Laryngeal papilloma and vulvar condylomas in infants delivered through an infected vaginal canal have been reported; however, unlike herpetic lesions, the presence of HPV lesions is not a contraindication to a vaginal delivery.

HPV infection is associated with dysplasia. The presence of koilocytes is pathognomonic for HPV infection. Koilocytes are superficial or intermediate cells on biopsy

Figure 37–6. Vaginal condylomata acuminata as seen with a colposcope ($\times$ 13).

characterized by a large perinuclear halo. Colposcopic-directed biopsies must be taken to exclude intraepithelial neoplasia. The chief histologic difference between dysplasia and condyloma is the progression of cellular atypia. In dysplasia, the dysplastic cells move toward the surface, whereas in condyloma the changes progress from the surface inward toward the basal membrane.

Prior to treatment, a colposcope can be used to inspect the lower genital tract. Lesions may extend to the anal canal or urethral meatus. The virus is present in normal cells as well as those with condylomatous changes; therefore, recurrence is common. Cure of clinically identifiable disease depends on the responsiveness of the patient's immune system. On gross examination, condylomas cannot always be distinguished from dysplastic warts. Therefore, biopsy should be considered, especially if the cervix is involved, if the condyloma has not responded to standard treatment, or if the lesion is pigmented, indurated, fixed, and/or ulcerated. Normal micropapillae of the inner labia minora (vestibular micropapillomatosis) may be confused with papillary HPV. True HPV disease is patchy and has koilocytes and more intense acetowhite changes.

Multiple therapies are available for treatment (Table 37–5); however, whether treatment actually affects the natural progression or eradicates HPV infection is unclear. Coexistent vulvovaginitis should be treated. Treatment should be based on patient preference and convenience. If treatment fails with an initial regimen, a different agent can be used. Patients should be informed that complications with treatment are rare but can result in scarring and pigmentation changes.

Prevention of recurrence is difficult in patients who are immunosuppressed or receiving lifelong corticosteroid therapy. Examination of sex partners is not necessary as most partners are likely to have subclinical infection. The use of condoms may help in reducing transmission to partners who are not already infected.

Condylomas may complicate pregnancy. In most cases if the lesions are small, therapy is not necessary. Treatment with trichloroacetic acid (TCA) may be applied in the last 4 weeks of pregnancy to avoid cesarean section with larger lesions. Electrocoagulation, cryotherapy, or laser therapy should be used prior to 32 weeks to avoid posttreatment necrosis, which may last as long as 4–6 weeks. Podophyllin, podofilox, and imiquimod should not be used during pregnancy.

Atrophic Vaginitis

Prepubertal, lactating, and postmenopausal women lack the vaginal effects of estrogen production. The pH of the vagina is abnormally high, and the normally acidogenic flora of the vagina may be replaced by mixed flora. The vaginal epithelium is thinned and more susceptible to infection and trauma. Although most patients are asymptomatic, many postmenopausal women

Table 37–5. Treatment of condyloma acuminata.

Applied by Provider
Bichloroacetic acid (BCA) or trichloroacetic acid (TCA), 50–80% solution
A lower percentage solution is generally applied to the cervix and vagina, a higher percentage to the vulva. One should be careful to avoid excessive amounts, which may burn normal skin. Xylocaine 1% gel can be applied around the wart to prevent damage to adjacent skin. Repeat treatments are given weekly as necessary.
Podophyllin 10–25% in tincture of benzoin
Cryosurgery, electrosurgery, simple surgical excision, laser vaporization
Applied by Patient
Podofilox 0.5% solution or gel
Imiquimod 5% cream (topically active immune enhancer that stimulates production of interferon and other cytokines)

report vaginal dryness, spotting, presence of a serosanguineous or watery discharge, and/or dyspareunia. Some of the symptoms of irritation are caused by a secondary infection. On examination, the vaginal mucosa is thin, with few or absent vaginal folds. The pH is 5.0–7.0. The wet mount shows small, rounded parabasal epithelial cells and an increased number of polymorphonuclear cells.

Treatment includes intravaginal application of estrogen cream. Approximately one-third of the vaginal estrogen is systemically absorbed; therefore, this treatment may be contraindicated in women with a history of breast or endometrial cancer. The estradiol vaginal ring, which is changed every 90 days, may provide a more preferable route of administration for some women, or estradiol hemihydrate (Vagifem) 1 tablet intravaginally daily for 2 weeks and then 2 times per week for at least 3–6 months may be less messy. Systemic estrogen therapy should be considered if there are no contraindications.

Foreign Bodies

Foreign bodies commonly cause vaginal discharge and infection in preadolescent girls. Paper, cotton, or other materials may be placed in the vagina and cause secondary infection. Children may require vaginal examination under anesthesia to identify or rule out a foreign body or tumor high in the vaginal vault. The vaginal canal can be flushed in the office using a small catheter in an attempt to remove a foreign body. In adults, a forgotten menstrual tampon or contraceptive device may cause a malodorous discharge. The diagnosis usually can be made by pelvic examination.

Clinical symptoms associated with foreign bodies include abnormal vaginal discharge and intermenstrual spotting. Symptoms are generally secondary to drying of the vaginal epithelium and micro-ulcerations, which can be detected by colposcopy. Ulcerative lesions, particularly associated with tampon use, are typically located in the vaginal fornices and have rolled, irregular edges with a red granulation tissue base (Fig 37–7). Regenerating epithelium at the ulcer edge may shed cells that may be interpreted as atypical, suggesting dysplasia. The lesions heal spontaneously once tampon use is discontinued. A foreign body retained in the vagina for a prolonged period may erode into the bladder or rectum.

Treatment involves removal of the foreign body. Rarely, antibiotics are required for ulcerations or cellulitis of the vulva or vagina. Dryness or ulceration of the vagina secondary to use of menstrual tampons is transient and heals spontaneously.

Toxic shock syndrome (see Chapter 41) is the most serious complication of improper use of vaginal

Figure 37–7. Colposcopic view of ulcer anterior to cervix caused by prolonged use of a vaginal tampon.

tampons. The syndrome has been linked to staphylococcal vaginal infection in healthy young women who use high-absorbency tampons continuously throughout the menstrual period. Some of the clinical manifestations are secondary to the release of staphylococcal exotoxins. Symptoms consist of a high fever ($\geq$ 38.9 °C [102 °F]) possibly accompanied by severe headache, sore throat, myalgia, vomiting, and diarrhea. The disease may resemble meningitis or viremia. Palmar erythema and a diffuse sunburn-like rash have been described. The skin rash usually disappears within 24–48 hours, but occasionally a patient has a recurrent maculopapular, morbilliform eruption between days 6 and 10. Superficial desquamation of the palms and soles often follows within 2–3 weeks. Progressive hypotension may occur and proceed to shock levels within 48 hours. Multisystem organ failure may occur, including renal and cardiac dysfunction. The incidence of toxic shock syndrome was 1 in 100,000 among females 15 to 44 years old in 1986. Any menstruating woman who presents with sudden onset of a febrile illness should be evaluated and treated for toxic shock syndrome. The tampon should be removed, cultures sent, and the vagina cleansed to decrease the organism inoculum. Appropriate supportive measures should be provided and β-lactamase–resistant penicillin or vancomycin (if the patient is allergic to penicillin) administered. Women who have been treated for toxic shock syndrome are at considerable risk for recurrence. Therefore, these women should avoid tampon use until *Staphylococcus aureus* has been eradicated from the vagina.

Desquamative Inflammatory Vaginitis

This disorder demonstrates clinical and microscopic features of postmenopausal atrophic vaginitis; however, it presents in premenopausal women with normal estrogen levels. The cause is unknown. Patients complain of a profuse purulent vaginal discharge, vaginal burning or irritation, dyspareunia, and occasional spotting. The process is patchy and usually localized to the upper half of the vagina. The purulent discharge contains many immature epithelial and pus cells without any identifiable cause. Vaginal erythema is present and synechiae may develop in the upper vagina, causing partial occlusion. The diagnosis is one of exclusion. Vaginal pH may be elevated, with wet mount and Gram's stain demonstrating an increased number of parabasal cells, an absence of gram-positive bacilli, and presence of gram-positive cocci, usually streptococci. Treatment often is unsatisfactory but has included local application of estrogen, antibiotics (particularly clindamycin cream 2% 5 g intravaginally daily for 7 days), and corticosteroids.

Noninfectious Vaginitis

Chemical vaginitis secondary to multiple irritating offenders, including topical irritants (sanitary supplies, spermicides, feminine hygiene supplies, soaps, perfumes), allergens (latex, antimycotic creams), and possibly excessive sexual activity can cause pruritus, irritation, burning, and vaginal discharge. The etiology may be confused with vulvovaginal candidiasis. The offending agent should be removed for treatment. A short course of corticosteroid treatment may be used along with sodium bicarbonate sitz baths and topical vegetable oils.

Cervical Mucorrhea or Vaginal Epithelial Discharge

Cervicitis due to cervical polyps or cervical or vaginal cancer can cause a mucopurulent discharge and bleeding. Excessive cervical ectropion may cause excessive discharge of cervical mucus from normal endocervical cells. Vaginal adenosis may cause the same type of clear, mucoid-type discharge with no associated symptoms. Excessive desquamation of the vaginal epithelium may produce a diffuse gray-white pasty vaginal discharge, which may be confused with candidiasis. Vaginal pH is normal. Microscopic evaluation shows normal bacterial flora, mature vaginal squamae, and no increase in the number of leukocytes. Excessive but normal vaginal discharge should be treated with reassurance and, if required at times, with cryosurgery or carbon dioxide treatment of the cervix. Continuous use of a tampon should be avoided.

Parasitic Infection

Less common causes of vaginitis are parasitic infections with pinworms (*Enterobius vermicularis*) and with *Entamoeba histolytica*. Pinworm infection usually is seen in children. Fecal contamination at the introitus is the source of infection. The perineal area is extremely pruritic. The parasite is generally detected by pressing a strip of adhesive cellulose tape to the perineum. The tape is then adhered to a slide, allowing the double-walled ova to be identified under the microscope. *E histolytica* infection of the vagina and cervix is rare in the United States but is quite common in developing countries. Severe infection may resemble cervical cancer, but symptoms generally are due to vulvar involvement. Trophozoites of *E histolytica* may be demonstrated on wet-mount preparations or occasionally on a Papanicolaou smear.

PRINCIPLES OF DIAGNOSIS OF VULVAR DISEASES

A complete history of potential causes of vulvar irritation, such as creams, powders, soaps, type of underwear, and cleansing techniques, should be reviewed. Physical examination should include careful inspection, palpation, and liberal use of colposcope at low magnification, followed by biopsy of any suspicious areas, lesions, or discolorations if indicated.

Pruritus

Pruritus is the most common symptom of vulvar disease. The term **pruritus vulvae** denotes intense itching of the vulvar epithelium and mucous membranes from any cause. Specific diagnosis depends on a thorough history, a physical examination that includes inspection of all body surfaces, and, in some cases, a biopsy.

Ulceration, Tumor, Dystrophy

Ulcerative lesions suggest a granulomatous sexually transmitted disease or cancer. Therefore, appropriate tests for sexually transmitted disease should be conducted along with biopsy to rule out primary or coexisting cancer. Well-circumscribed solid tumors should be excised widely and submitted for microscopic evaluation. Diffuse, dystrophic white lesions may demonstrate great histologic variability. A colposcope at low magnification or a simple magnifying glass should be used to select the most suitable biopsy site(s). A satisfactory full-thickness biopsy of the skin and tumor can be obtained with a dermatologic punch biopsy of the skin under local anesthesia.

Abnormalities of Pigmentation

A. WHITE

The color of vulvar epithelium or lesions depends principally on the vascularity of the dermis, the thickness of the overlying epidermis, and the amount of intervening pigment, either melanin or blood pigments. A dystrophic lesion of the vulva may have a white appearance primarily due to a decrease in the vascularity (lichen sclerosus) or an increase in the keratin layer (squamous hyperplasia) that has undergone maceration from the increased moisture in the vulvar area. During the acute phase of lichen sclerosus, the vulvar epithelium is moderately erythematous. As the lesion matures, it becomes hyperkeratotic and develops a typical white appearance resembling cigarette paper. The epidermal thickening of neoplasia obscures the underlying vasculature and, in conjunction with the macerating effects of the moist environment, usually produces a hyperplastic white lesion. A diffuse white lesion of the vulva is also produced by the loss or absence of melanin pigmentation as with vitiligo, a hereditary disorder. Leukoderma is a localized white lesion resulting from transient loss of pigment in a residual scar after healing of an ulcer.

B. RED

A red lesion results from thinning or ulceration of the epidermis, the vasodilation of inflammation or an immune response, or the neovascularization of a neoplasia. With ulceration of the epithelium, epidermal areas are lost, and the vascular dermis is apparent. Acute candidal vulvovaginitis, as seen with diabetes, is a typical example of vulvar erythema secondary to inflammation and the local immune response. Paget's disease (adenocarcinoma in situ of the vulva) is characterized by the velvety red lesion that spreads over the vulvar skin. Psoriasis involving the vulva is another lesion that can take on a red appearance.

C. BLUE/BLACK

Dark lesions are the result of an increased amount or concentration of melanin or blood pigments, which may occur following trauma. A persistent dark lesion on the vulva skin likely represents a nevus or a melanoma. **Melanosis,** or **lentigo,** is a benign, darkly pigmented flat lesion that may be mistaken for a melanoma. With carcinoma in situ of the vulva, the atypical squamous cells are unable to contain the melanin pigment. Instead it is concentrated in the local macrophages, causing dark coloration of the tumor. Vulvar epithelium may darken following use of estrogen cream or oral contraceptive pills.

VULVAR DISORDERS (TABLE 37–6)

Vascular & Lymphatic Diseases

The vulva and vagina have a rich vascular and lymphatic blood supply. These channels may undergo obstruction, dilatation, rupture, or infection, or they may develop into tumorous lesions, which usually are malformations rather than true neoplasms.

A. VARICOSITIES

Varicosities of the vulva involve 1 or more veins. Severe varicosities of the legs and vulva may be aggravated during pregnancy. Symptomatic vulvar varices in a patient who is not pregnant are uncommon and may signify an underlying vascular disease in the pelvis, either primary or secondary to a tumor in the pelvis. Regardless of the cause, varicosities can cause considerable discomfort, consisting of pain, pruritus, and a sense of heaviness. On examination a large mass of veins may be apparent, which is best diagnosed with the patient standing to distend the veins. Rupture of a vulvar varicosity during pregnancy may cause profuse hemorrhage. Pain and tenderness may be caused by acute phlebitis or thrombosis.

Treatment of vulvar and vaginal varicosities is seldom necessary, although symptoms might be quite severe during pregnancy. Support clothing such as panty hose or leotards usually provides adequate relief of symptoms. Operative intervention is usually required only in cases of rupture and hemorrhage, which are rare. Management of the pregnancy should be guided

Table 37–6. Vulvar disorders.

Vascular and lymphatic diseases
   Varicosities, hematoma, edema, granuloma pyogenicum, hemangioma, lymphangioma
Vulvar manifestation of systemic diseases
   Leukemia, dermatologic disorders (disseminated lupus erythematosus, pemphigus vulgaris, contact dermatitis, psoriasis), obesity, diabetes mellitus, Behçet's syndrome
Viral infections
   Herpes genitalis, herpes zoster, molluscum contagiosum, condyloma acuminatum
Infestations of the vulva
   Pediculosis pubis, scabies, enterobiasis
Mycotic infections of the vulva
   Candidiasis, fungal dermatitis
Other infections of the vulva
   Impetigo, furunculosis, erysipelas, hidradenitis, tuberculosis
Vulvar nonneoplastic epithelial disorders
   Lichen sclerosus, squamous cell hyperplasia, other dermatoses (lichen planus, lichen simplex chronicus)
Benign cystic tumors
   Epidermal cysts, sebaceous cysts, apocrine sweat gland cysts, Skene duct cyst, urethral diverticulum, inguinal hernia, Gartner's duct cyst, Bartholin's duct cyst and abscess
Benign solid tumors
   Acrochordon, pigmented nevi, leiomyoma, fibroma, lipoma, neurofibromas, granular cell myoblastoma

by standard obstetric care, with vaginal delivery advised. Persistent postpartum cases may be alleviated by injection of a sclerosing agent.

B. HEMATOMA

The vulva has a rich blood supply arising predominately from the pudendal vessels. If a vessel is ruptured, especially in a pregnant patient, significant bleeding and hematoma formation can occur because of the distensible nature of the vulvar tissue. Following trauma, an ice pack should be applied. If the hematoma continues to expand, the area should be incised and any bleeders (which may be multiple) ligated. The wound can be packed and left open or closed with a drain in place, if appropriate. Antibiotics should be administered on an individual basis, depending on the initiating event and contamination in the area.

C. EDEMA

The loose integument of the vulva predisposes to the development of edema. Vascular or lymphatic obstruction may be the result of an underlying neoplasm or infection such as LGV, which can cause extensive lymphatic obstruction and gross deformity of the vulvar tissues. If edema persists following appropriate antibiotic treatment, vulvectomy may be indicated.

Accidental trauma from a bicycle accident (saddle injury) in a young girl or a kick to the pudendum may cause painful swelling. An ice pack applied to the perineum after an acute trauma tends to retard the development of significant edema. Warm packs or warm sitz baths may then be applied after 1–2 days to help resolve the associated inflammation and/or hematoma.

Severe generalized vulvar edema may represent an underlying systemic illness such as congestive heart failure, nephrotic syndrome, preeclampsia, or eclampsia. Acute development of edema may result from a systemic or local allergic reaction. Dependent edema is occasionally seen with prolonged bed rest.

D. GRANULOMA PYOGENICUM

Pyogenic granuloma is considered to be a variant of a capillary hemangioma. It usually is single, raised, and dull red. Its size seldom exceeds 3 cm (Fig 37–8). Pyogenic granuloma is important because it tends to bleed easily if traumatized. Wide excisional biopsy is indicated to alleviate symptoms and to rule out a malignant melanoma.

Figure 37–8. Pyogenic granuloma.

E. HEMANGIOMA

1. Senile—Senile (cherry) hemangiomas usually are multiple, small, dark blue, asymptomatic papules discovered incidentally during examination of the older patient. Excision biopsy is needed only if the hemangiomas bleed repeatedly. A cryosurgical probe or carbon dioxide laser can also be used.

2. Childhood—Childhood hemangiomas usually are diagnosed in the first few months of life. They may vary in size from small strawberry hemangiomas to large cavernous ones. They tend to be elevated and bright red or dark, depending on their size and the thickness of the overlying skin. Those that tend to increase in size during the first few months of life often will become static or regress without therapy after approximately age 18 months. Although most of these hemangiomas can be observed without therapy, larger ones may require treatment with cryosurgery, argon laser therapy, or sclerosing solutions.

F. LYMPHANGIOMA

Lymphangiomas are tumors of the lymphatic vessels. They may be difficult to differentiate from hemangiomas microscopically unless blood cells are present within the blood vessels. Lymphangioma cavernosum may cause a diffuse enlargement of 1 side of the vulva and extend down over the remainder of the vulva and perineum. A tumor that is sufficiently enlarged should be surgically excised. Lymphangioma simplex tumors (circumscription tumors) usually are small, soft, white or purple nodules or small wartlike lesions most commonly seen on the labia majora. They usually are asymptomatic and do not require excision unless intense pruritus and excoriation are present and are not alleviated with topical measures.

Vulvar Manifestation of Systemic Diseases

A. LEUKEMIA

Rarely, nodular infiltration and ulceration of the vulva and rectovaginal septum occur with acute leukemia.

B. DERMATOLOGIC DISORDERS

Recurrent ulcerations of the mucous membranes of the mouth and vagina may be a manifestation of **disseminated lupus erythematosus.** Bullous eruptions of apparently normal skin and mucous membrane surfaces of the vulva may be one of the first signs of **pemphigus vulgaris** (a rare, chronic autoimmune disease).

Contact dermatitis is an inflammatory response of the vulvar tissue to agents that may either be locally irritating or induce sensitivity on contact. The local reaction to a systemically administered drug is called **dermatitis medicamentosa.**

Psoriasis is a chronic relapsing dermatosis that may also affect the scalp, the extensor surfaces of the extremities, the trunk, and the vulva. The vulvar skin may be the only body surface affected, and the primary lesions are raised and appear typically erythematous, resembling a candidal infection. Most lesions are sharply demarcated. The silver scaly crusts that are present on other parts of the body usually are absent (Fig 37–9). Treatment includes topical corticosteroids.

C. Obesity

Acanthosis nigricans is a benign hyperpigmented lesion characterized by papillomatous hypertrophy. It may be associated with an underlying adenocarcinoma. **Pseudoacanthosis nigricans** is a benign process that may appear on the skin of the vulva and inner thighs in obese and darkly pigmented women. Glucose intolerance, insulin resistance, chronic anovulation, and androgen disorders may be associated. **Intertrigo** is an inflammatory reaction involving the genitocrural folds or the skin under the abdominal panniculus. It is common in obese patients and results from persistent moistness of the skin surfaces. An associated superficial fungal or bacterial infection may be present. The area may be either erythematous or white from maceration. Measures to promote dryness, such as wearing absorbent cotton undergarments and dusting with cornstarch powder, may be helpful.

D. Diabetes Mellitus

Diabetes mellitus is the systemic disease most commonly associated with chronic pruritus vulvae. The chronic vulvitis that develops may be termed **diabetic vulvitis.** It is caused by a chronic vulvovaginal candidiasis. A diagnosis of diabetes should be considered in any patient who responds poorly to antifungal treatment or who has recurrent fungal infections. Such patients should undergo glucose tolerance testing. In uncontrolled diabetes, the vulvar epithelium often undergoes lichenification and secondary bacterial infection. Occasionally, a vulvar abscess, chronic subcutaneous abscesses, and draining sinuses develop from a bacterial infection. Treatment should include controlling the underlying diabetes and specific therapy for the bacterial or fungal infection. Suppressive antifungal therapy using fluconazole should be initiated in diabetic patients with recurrent vulvovaginal candidiasis.

Necrotizing fasciitis is seen most commonly in diabetics. It is an uncommon, acute, rapidly spreading, frequently fatal polymicrobial infection of the superficial fascia and subcutaneous fascia. It may be seen following a surgical procedure such as an episiotomy or after minor trauma. It presents as an extremely painful, tender, and indurated region with central necrosis and peripheral purplish erythema. Treatment requires

Figure 37–9. Typical lesions of psoriasis with a sharp outline and bright red surface.

E. Behçet's Syndrome

Behçet's syndrome is a rare inflammatory disorder of unknown cause characterized by recurrent oral and genital ulcerations and uveitis. The painful genital ulcers are preceded by small vesicles or papules and last for variable periods. The borders are irregular, with deep ulcers that, following healing, may result in scarring. Ocular lesions begin as superficial inflammation and may proceed to iridocyclitis and even blindness. Monoarticular arthritis and central nervous system symptoms are manifestations of severe disease. Susceptibility to Behçet's disease is strongly associated with the presence of the *HLA-B51* allele and is primarily seen in Eastern Europe and the Mediterranean. The exact etiology is unknown, but it likely represents an underlying autoimmune process. No specific viral infection has been implicated.

Behçet's syndrome, together with disseminated lupus erythematosus and pemphigus, should be included in the differential diagnosis of recurrent aphthous ulcers of the oral and vaginal mucosa. There is no specific therapy—only palliative care. Topical and systemic corticosteroids provide the most consistent relief. Patients with Behçet's syndrome require consultation and long-term management by a dermatologist.

Viral Infections

Systemic infections in children, such as varicella and rubeola, may involve the skin and mucosa of the vulva. The principal viruses that affect the vulva are DNA viruses, primarily of the herpesvirus, poxvirus, and papovavirus types. In adults, the principal viral infections of the lower genital tract are herpes genitalis, herpes zoster, molluscum contagiosum, and condyloma acuminatum.

A. HERPES GENITALIS

Herpesvirus hominis infection of the lower genital tract (herpes genitalis) is the most common cause of genital ulcer disease in the United States. In private practice 10% of women demonstrate serologic prior exposure to the virus. Approximately 85% of primary infections are secondary to herpesvirus hominis type II, with the remainder by type I.

Infection occurs through direct contact with secretions or mucosal surfaces contaminated with the virus. The virus enters the skin through cracks or other lesions but can enter through an intact mucosa. The virus initially replicates in the dermis and epidermis. Incubation time is 2–7 days. Prodromal symptoms of tingling, burning, or itching may occur shortly before vesicular eruptions appear. The vesicles erode rapidly, resulting in painful ulcers distributed in small patches, or they may involve most of the vulvar surfaces (Fig 37–10). Bilateral inguinal adenopathy may be present. Dysuria or other urinary symptoms may develop, including urinary retention. Approximately one-third of patients demonstrate systemic manifestations such as fever, malaise, headaches, and myalgia. In other cases the primary infection is asymptomatic. Lesions may persist for 2–6 weeks with no subsequent scarring.

Diagnosis is based on clinical presentation and laboratory results. The virus can be cultured from vesicle fluid during the acute phase. However, organisms usually cannot be cultured after the primary vesicles heal, which occurs by 2 weeks. A scraping taken from the ulcer and stained Giemsa or Papanicolaou stain (Tzanck test) can also demonstrate the characteristic giant cells indicative of viral infection. This test is less sensitive than the culture.

Approximately 85% of patients develop immunoglobulin (Ig)M antibodies to type II virus within 21 days of exposure. Serologic tests are best used to determine whether the patient has been infected in the past. A 4-fold or higher increase in neutralizing complement fixation antibody titers between acute and convalescent scra may be useful to document a primary infection. Only 5% of patients with recurrent infection demonstrate a 4-fold or higher rise in antibody titer. New type-specific serologic tests for herpes simplex virus are available. The serologic type-specific glycoprotein G–based assays should be specifically requested when se-

Figure 37–10. Ulcerating vesicles of herpes genitalis.

rology is performed to distinguish between herpes simplex types I and II.

Despite the presence of adequate humoral and cell-mediated immunity, reactivation of the virus occurs. Following replication in the skin, the viral particles are transported along the peripheral sensory nerves to the dorsal root ganglion, where latent infection is established. Exogenous factors known to contribute to activation of herpesvirus include fever, emotional stress, and menstruation. Immunocompromised patients are prone to develop extensive local disease and systemic dissemination. Whether frequent coitus promotes recurrent disease is unknown. Type II virus is more likely to recur than is type I virus, with men more likely to have recurrent symptoms than women. Approximately 50% of patients will have a recurrence within 6 months of the primary infection. The ulcers tend to be smaller, fewer in number, and confined to 1 area in the vulva, cervix, or vagina. Healing is generally complete in 1–3 weeks. Virus is not recoverable within 7 days after healing of recurrent lesions. Inguinal adenopathy and systemic symptoms generally do not occur. Primary infection usually can be distinguished from secondary infection based on clinical findings. Extragenital sites, such as the fingers, buttocks, and trunk (eczema herpeticum), have been described.

1. Pregnancy—The incidence of neonatal simplex virus infection ranges from 1 in 5000 to 1 in 20,000 live births. Infection in the newborn is associated with a 60% mortality rate, and at least half of the survivors have significant neurologic and/or ocular sequelae. The risk of infection to an infant born vaginally in a mother with active primary genital infection is 40–50%; for recurrent infection the risk is 5%. However, most infants who develop herpetic infection are born to women who have no history or clinical evidence of infection during pregnancy. Therefore, identifying women whose infants may be in jeopardy is difficult. All pregnant women should be asked whether they or their partners have had genital herpetic lesions. Women with a history of herpes can deliver vaginally if no clinical signs or symptoms of infection are present. Obtaining routine vaginal cultures to detect herpes is not standard. However, suppressive antiviral therapy may be initiated at 36 weeks to decrease the need for cesarean section (Table 37–7).

2. Treatment—The lesions of herpesvirus infection are self-limiting, and they heal spontaneously unless they become infected secondarily. Symptomatic treatment includes good genital hygiene, loose-fitting undergarments, cool compresses or sitz baths, and oral analgesics. Indications for hospitalization for a severe primary infection include urinary retention, severe headache or other systemic symptoms, and temperature greater than 38.3 °C (101 °F). Immunosuppressed patients are more prone to systemic dissemination and should be carefully managed. Treatment includes intravenous acyclovir for hospitalized patients and oral and/or topical antivirals for outpatient treatment. Recurrent herpes should be treated at the onset of prodromal symptoms or vesicle formation. Studies have indicated a decrease in the frequency and severity of recurrences with antiviral treatment. Once-daily dosing may be considered for frequent recurrent outbreaks, with 40–70% of patients free of recurrence at 1 year (Table 37–7).

Table 37–7. Oral treatment of herpes genitalis.

First episode of genital herpes	
Acyclovir	400 mg orally 3 times daily for 7–10 days
Famciclovir	250 mg orally 3 times daily for 7–10 days
Valacyclovir	1000 mg orally twice daily for 10 days
Recurrent genital herpes	
Acyclovir	400 mg orally 3 times daily for 5 days
Famciclovir	125 mg orally twice daily for 5 days
Valacyclovir	500 mg orally twice daily for 5 days
Genital herpes prophylaxis	
Acyclovir	400 mg orally twice daily
Famciclovir	250 mg orally twice daily
Valacyclovir	500–1000 mg orally daily

Avoidance of direct contact with active lesions prevents spread of the disease. However, contact with an individual with subclinical disease can result in primary infections. The general rules for prevention of dissemination are as follows:

1. Precautions are unnecessary in the absence of active lesions.
2. Small lesions situated away from the oral or vaginal orifices can be covered with adhesive or paper tape during coitus.
3. In the presence of active lesions, whether or not the partner contracts the disease depends on previous exposure to herpes. A nonimmune partner usually will be infected. If a regular partner has had genital herpes or has not been infected after prolonged exposure, no precautions are necessary. If a casual partner has had a history of genital herpes, a contraceptive cream or foam should be used, followed by genital cleansing with soap and water. If a partner has no past history of genital herpes, a condom can be used but may be of limited value.

B. HERPES ZOSTER (SHINGLES)

Herpes zoster is an inflammatory disorder in which a painful eruption of groups of vesicles is distributed over an area of skin corresponding to the course of 1 or more peripheral sensory nerves. The causative agent is varicella-zoster virus. The lesion is commonly unilateral and not infrequently attacks 1 buttock, 1 thigh, or 1 side of the vulva. The vesicles may rupture and crust over, although they usually dry, forming a scab that ultimately separates. The primary purposes of treatment (antivirals) are alleviation of pain, resolution of vesicles, and prevention of secondary infection and ulceration.

C. MOLLUSCUM CONTAGIOSUM

These benign epithelial poxvirus-induced tumors are dome-shaped, often umbilicated, and vary in size up to 1 cm. The lesions often are multiple and are mildly contagious. The microscopic appearance is characterized by numerous inclusion bodies (molluscum bodies) in the cytoplasm of the cells. Each lesion can be treated by desiccation, freezing, or curettage and chemical cauterization of the base. Topical imiquimod can be used as alternative therapy.

D. CONDYLOMA ACUMINATUM

Condylomata acuminata (genital warts) are caused by the papovavirus group. Papillary growths, small at first, tend to coalesce and form large cauliflower-like masses that may proliferate profusely during pregnancy.

Before treatment is undertaken, the entire lower genital tract should be examined with the colposcope and a cytologic smear taken from the cervix. Considering the frequent coexistence of other sexually transmitted diseases, appropriate studies are indicated. There is considerable variation in the oncogenic potential of human papovaviruses; therefore, a biopsy may be indicated. The incubation period for appearance of clinical disease after exposure is 3 months or longer. Apparent clinical disease may represent only a small area of the infected surface. Prompt recurrences after treatment may represent reinfection or clinical manifestation of latent disease. During treatment, the patient should keep the area as clean as possible and abstain from sexual intercourse or have her partner use a condom. If clinical disease recurs, then the sexual partner should be examined and treated as necessary. Penile, urethral, and perianal warts in the male may be overlooked.

Standard treatment is to cover the wart with bichloroacetic or trichloroacetic acid every week until the wart is gone. Alternative forms of treatment include cryosurgery, electrosurgical destruction, excision, and laser vaporization. Some authors recommend laser ablation of all visible lesions plus a margin of normal adjacent skin under colposcopic guidance. Intralesional interferon has been shown to be effective in refractory cases. Self-administered medication includes podofilox 0.5% solution or gel or imiquimod 5% cream (Table 37–5). Chemotherapeutic agents such as 5-fluorouracil ointment or bleomycin in the form of intralesional injections can be used as second-line therapies. Vaccine against certain high-risk HPV types has been recently developed. Preliminary studies have proved the vaccine to be safe and effective in the prevention of persistent HPV infection as well as cervical intraepithelial neoplasia (CIN).

Condyloma lata, a variation of secondary syphilis, should be considered in the differential diagnosis of condyloma acuminata.

Condylomatous warts may grow rapidly during pregnancy. Warts at the vaginal introitus may bleed during delivery and predispose the newborn to genital warts or laryngeal papillomatosis. Condylomata recognized early in pregnancy should be treated early enough to allow healing prior to delivery. If treatment is not successful, delivery by cesarean section should be considered.

Infestations of the Vulva

A. PEDICULOSIS PUBIS

The crab louse (*Phthirus pubis*) is transmitted through sexual contact or from shared infected bedding or clothing. The louse eggs are laid at the base of a hair shaft near the skin. The eggs hatch in 7–9 days, and the louse must attach to the skin of the host to survive. The result is intense pubic and anogenital itching.

Minute pale-brown insects and their ova may be seen attached to terminal hair shafts. Treatment consists of permethrin 1% cream, lindane 1% shampoo, or pyrethrins with piperonyl butoxide. Lindane is not recommended for pregnant or lactating women or for children younger than 2 years. Treat all contacts and sterilize clothing that has been in contact with the infested area.

B. SCABIES

Sarcoptes scabiei causes intractable itching and excoriation of the skin surfaces in the vicinity of minute skin burrows where parasites have deposited ova. The itch mite is transmitted, often directly, from infected persons. The patient should take a hot soapy bath, scrubbing the burrows and encrusted areas thoroughly. Treatment consists of permethrin cream (5%), which should be applied to the entire body from the neck down, with particular attention to the hands, wrists, axillae, breasts, and anogenital region. It should be washed off after 8–14 hours. Alternatively, lindane (1%) in the lotion or cream form can be applied in a thin layer to all areas of the body and washed off after 8 hours. All potentially infected clothing or bedding should be washed or dry-cleaned. All contacts or persons in the family must be treated in the same way to prevent reinfection. Therapy should be repeated in 10–14 days if new lesions develop.

C. ENTEROBIASIS (PINWORM, SEATWORM)

E vermicularis infection is common in children. Nocturnal perineal itching is described by the patient, and perianal excoriation may be observed. Apply adhesive cellulose tape to the anal region, stick the tape to a glass slide, and examine under the microscope for ova. Patients should wash their hands and scrub their nails following each defecation. Underclothes must be boiled. Apply ammoniated mercury ointment to the perianal region twice daily for relief of itching. Pinworms succumb to systemic treatment with pyrantel pamoate, mebendazole, or pyrvinium pamoate.

Mycotic Infections of the Vulva

A. FUNGAL DERMATITIS (DERMATOPHYTOSES)

Tinea cruris is a superficial fungal infection of the genitocrural area that is more common in men than in women. The most common organisms are *Trichophyton mentagrophytes* and *Trichophyton rubrum*. The initial lesions usually are located on the upper inner thighs and are well circumscribed, erythematous, dry, scaly areas that coalesce. Scratching causes lichenification and a gross appearance similar to neurodermatitis. The diagnosis depends on microscopic examination (as for *Can-*

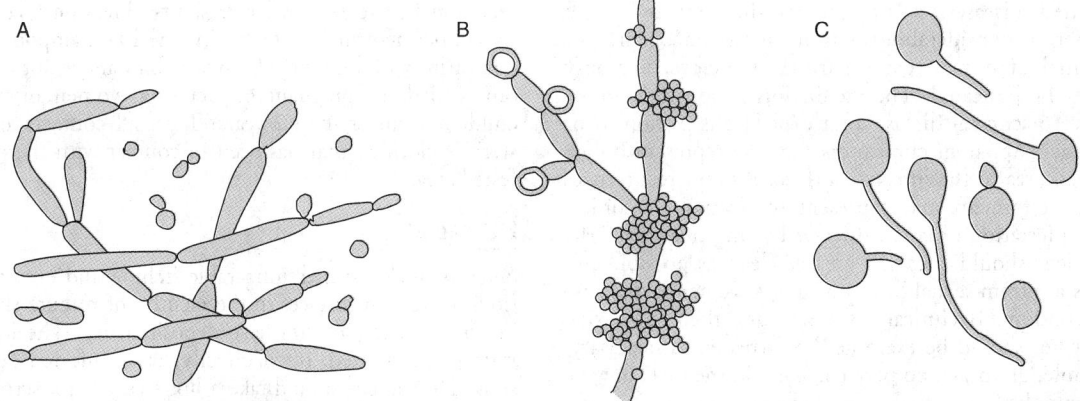

Figure 37–11. *Candida albicans.* **A:** Blastospores and pseudohyphae in exudate. **B:** Blastospores, pseudohyphae, and conidia in culture at 20 °C. **C:** Young culture forms germ tubes when placed in serum for 3 hours at 37 °C. (Reproduced, with permission, from Brooks GF, Butel JS, Ornston LN: *Jawetz, Melinick, & Adelberg's Medical Microbiology,* 19th ed. Appleton & Lange, 1991.)

dida) (Fig 37–11). Culture on Sabouraud's medium confirms the diagnosis. Treatment with 1% haloprogin, tolnaftate, or a similar agent is effective. Topical imidazole preparation at twice-daily application for 2–3 weeks also is highly effective.

Tinea versicolor usually involves the skin of the trunk, although occasionally the vulvar skin is involved. The lesions usually are multiple and may have a red, brown, or yellowish appearance. Diagnosis is the same as for other fungal infections. Treatment with selenium sulfide suspension daily for 5–7 days usually is curative. Topical imidazole preparations are most effective when used for 4 weeks. Ketoconazole has been used in recalcitrant cases.

B. DEEP CELLULITIS CAUSED BY FUNGI

Blastomycosis and actinomycosis are examples of deep mycoses that usually affect internal organs but also may involve the skin. Involvement of the vulvar epithelium in these diseases is rare in the United States. The diagnosis usually is made by laboratory exclusion of the granulomatous sexually transmitted diseases, tuberculosis, and other causes of chronic infection.

Treatment of blastomycosis with amphotericin B or hydroxystilbamidine is not very satisfactory. Actinomycosis usually can be treated successfully with penicillin.

Other Infections of the Vulva

A. IMPETIGO

Impetigo is caused by the hemolytic *S aureus* or streptococci. The disease is autoinoculable and spreads quickly to other parts of the body, including the vulva. Thin-walled

vesicles and bullae develop that display reddened edges and crusted surfaces after rupture. The disease is common in children, particularly on the face, hands, and vulva.

The patient must be isolated and the blebs incised or crusts removed aseptically. Neomycin or bacitracin should be applied twice daily for 1 week. Bathing with an antibacterial soap is recommended.

B. FURUNCULOSIS

Vulvar folliculitis is caused by a staphylococcal infection of hair follicles. Furunculosis occurs if the infection spreads into the perifollicular tissues, producing a localized cellulitis. Some follicular lesions are palpable as tender subcutaneous nodules that resolve without suppuration. A furuncle begins as a hard, tender subcutaneous nodule that ruptures through the skin, discharging blood and purulent material. After expulsion of a core of necrotic tissue, the lesion heals. New furuncles may appear sporadically over years.

Minor infections can be treated by applications of topical antibiotic lotions. Deeper infections can be brought to a head with hot soaks, after which the pustules should be incised and drained. Appropriate systemic antibiotics are warranted when extensive furunculosis is present.

C. ERYSIPELAS

Erysipelas is a rapidly spreading erythematous lesion of the skin caused by invasion of the superficial lymphatics by β-hemolytic streptococci. Erysipelas of the vulva is exceedingly rare and is most commonly seen after trauma to the vulva or a surgical procedure. Systemic symptoms of chills, fever, and malaise associated with an erythematous vulvitis suggest the diagnosis. Vesicles and bullae may appear, and erythematous streaks leading to the regional lymph nodes are typical.

The patient should be given systemic (preferably parenteral) penicillin or tetracycline orally in large doses.

D. HIDRADENITIS

Hidradenitis suppurativa is a refractory process of the apocrine sweat glands, usually associated with staphylococci or streptococci. The apocrine sweat glands of the vulva become active following puberty. Inspissation of secretory material and secondary infection may be related to occlusion of the ducts. Initially, multiple pruritic subcutaneous nodules appear that eventually develop into abscesses and rupture. The process tends to involve the skin of the entire vulva, resulting in multiple abscesses and subsequent chronic draining sinuses and scars. Treatment early in the disease consists of drainage and administration of antibiotics based on organism sensitivity testing. Long-term therapy with isotretinoin may be considered. Antiandrogen therapy with cyproterone acetate or ethinyl estradiol may be an alternate but highly effective treatment. Severe chronic infections may not respond to medical therapy, and the involved skin and subcutaneous tissues must be removed down to the deep fascia. This may necessitate a filet and curettage or a complete vulvectomy. The area generally will not heal after a primary closure; therefore, the wound must be left open and allowed to heal by secondary intention, or a split-thickness graft may be placed. Squamous cell carcinoma is rarely associated with hidradenitis suppurativa.

E. TUBERCULOSIS (VULVOVAGINAL LUPUS VULGARIS)

Pudendal tuberculosis is manifested by chronic, minimally painful, exudative "sores" that are tender, reddish, raised, moderately firm, and nodular, with central "apple jelly"-like contents. Ulcerative, necrotic discharging lesions develop later. There is some tendency toward healing with heavy scarring. Induration and sinus formation are common in the scrofulous type of infection. Cancer and sexually transmitted disease must be ruled out, and evaluation for tuberculosis at other sites must be performed.

Wet compresses of aluminum acetate solution (Burow's solution) are helpful. Systemic antituberculosis therapy should be given.

Vulvar Nonneoplastic Epithelial Disorders

The term **vulvar dystrophies** was previously used to define the nonneoplastic epithelial disorders of the vulva. As characterized by the International Society for the Study of Vulvovaginal Disease (ISSVD), these lesions include (1) lichen sclerosus (previously lichen sclerosus et atrophicus), (2) squamous cell hyperplasia (previously hyperplastic dystrophy), and (3) other dermatoses (lichen simplex chronicus, lichen planus). These lesions present classically with intense pruritus with or without pain and vulvar epithelial changes. Differentiating from among these disorders and ruling out an underlying malignant process require histopathologic diagnosis. The risk of an underlying malignancy is less than 5%. Patients must be reexamined periodically, and one should not hesitate to take additional biopsy specimens. Table 37–8 lists a classification of these lesions.

A. LICHEN SCLEROSUS

Lichen sclerosus is a benign, chronic, inflammatory process and the most common vulvar dermatologic disorder. Although its etiology is unknown, a multifactorial process is most likely involved in its development. Köbner's phenomenon occurs in lichen sclerosus; therefore, scarring or trauma may elicit its development. The skin of the vulva is most commonly involved, although other sites may be affected. Lichen sclerosus can affect both sexes and individuals of any age. However, the disease is clinically more prevalent in older patients. During the acute phase, the lesion may appear red or purple and classically involves the non–hair-bearing areas of the vulva, perineum, and perianal area in an hourglass pattern (Fig 37–12). With acute disease, erythema and edema of vulvar skin occur. The patient experiences intense pruritus leading to scratch cycle, ulcerations, and ultimately scar formation. With chronic disease, the skin is thin, wrinkled, and white and has a cigarette-paper appearance. The vulvar structures contract with agglutination of the labia minora and prepuce and introital stenosis. Symptoms of pain, including dyspareunia, may occur, mostly from decreased skin elasticity with loss of elastin from the upper dermis. Although skin atrophy ultimately may develop, the underlying disease is inflammatory in nature, and consequently areas of dysplasia may develop. Therefore, suspicious areas must be biopsied (Fig 37–13). Repeat biopsies should be taken as indicated because this is a chronic condition. Patients should be monitored for possible malignant changes because of an estimated 4–6% risk of developing squamous cell carcinoma.

Definitive diagnosis depends on histologic examination of the biopsy. The differential diagnosis includes pemphigoid, pemphigus, advanced scleroderma, lupus erythematosus, advanced lichen planus, and radiation fibrosis. In the well-developed lesion, lichen sclerosus is characterized by hyperkeratosis, epithelial atrophy, and flattening of the rete pegs. The upper dermis is edematous, pale staining with fibrin deposition. The deeper dermis has an inflammatory infiltrate, mainly monocytic. Beneath the epidermis is a zone of homog-

Table 37–8. Nonneoplastic epithelial disorders of the vulva.

Dermatosis	Physical Exam	Histology	Treatment
Lichen sclerosus	Thin, white, wrinkled tissue, with a cigarette-paper appearance Agglutination of the labia minora and prepuce Introital stenosis	*Epidermis*—Hyperkeratosis, epithelial atrophy, and flattening of the rete pegs; cytoplasmic vacuolization of the basal layer of cells *Upper dermis*—Edematous, pale-staining, acellular, homogenous collagen tissue *Deeper dermis*—Inflammatory infiltrate, mainly lymphocytic	Clobetasol propionate 0.05% twice daily for 1 month, then once daily for 2 months Not proven—2% testosterone cream, 1.25% topical progesterone
Squamous cell hyperplasia	Circumscribed, single or multifocal Raised white lesion on vulva or adjacent tissue (generally of labia majora and clitoris)	*Epidermis*—Hyperkeratosis and acanthosis, producing thickening of the epithelium and elongation of the rete pegs *Dermis*—No inflammatory infiltrate present	Medium-potency topical steroids twice daily
Lichen simplex chronicus	Thickened white epithelium on vulva Generally unilateral and localized	*Epidermis*—Hyperkeratosis and acanthosis, producing thickening of the epithelium and elongation of the rete pegs *Superficial dermis*—Chronic inflammatory cells, fibrosis, and collagenization Presence of cellular atypia signifies vulvar intraepithelial neoplasia (VIN I–III)	Medium-potency topical steroids twice a daily
Lichen planus	Erosive lesions at vestibule ± vaginal synechiae resulting in stenosis May have associated oral mucocutaneous lesions and desquamative vaginitis	Mild, localized, lichenoid, chronic inflammatory process at the epidermal-dermis junction to ulcerative process with fibrosis Immunofluorescent staining should be considered to exclude pemphigus and pemphigoid	Vaginal hydrocortisone suppository 25 mg Betamethasone cream 0.1% vaginally at bedtime for 2 weeks Vaginal estrogen cream in cases of atrophic epithelium Vaginal dilators in cases of stenosis
Psoriasis	Red moist lesions ± scales	*Epidermis*—Parakeratosis with clubbing of the rete pegs *Dermis*—Microabscesses of Munro	Topical corticosteroids

enized collagenous tissue that is acellular and pink in appearance (Fig 37–14).

Treatment involves initially stopping the itch-scratch cycle and minimizing the dermal inflammation. An oral antihistamine agent can be given at bedtime. Several studies have found treatment with ultra-potent steroid cream or ointment to be very effective in treating lichen sclerosus. Clobetasol propionate 0.05%, twice daily for 1 month and then daily for 3 months, has been shown to be most effective for treatment of lichen sclerosus, with ap-

proximately 75% success. A subsequent taper to lower-potency topical steroids is necessary for maintenance of therapy. Atrophic degeneration of the skin secondary to the steroid paradoxically does not occur. Although 2% testosterone or progesterone cream have been used to treat lichen sclerosus, they are minimally effective and should not be used as first-line therapy. In addition, patients should avoid tight undergarments, they should cleanse daily with mild soap, and they should use a hair dryer to keep the vulvar skin dry. In refractory cases, intralesional

Figure 37–12. Early lesion of lichen sclerosus—typical hourglass configuration.

injection of steroids may be attempted. Other alternative therapies for refractory lichen sclerosus include tacrolimus cream, retinoids, cryotherapy, antimalarial agents, and photodynamic therapy. Surgical therapy should be limited to treatment of introital narrowing, pseudocysts, and associated squamous cell carcinoma.

B. SQUAMOUS CELL HYPERPLASIA

Vulvar squamous cell hyperplasia is known by various names—hyperplastic dystrophy, atopic dermatitis, atopic eczema, and neurodermatitis. The benign epithelial thickening and hyperkeratosis may be the result of chronic vulvovaginal infections or other causes of chronic irritation. During the acute phase, as in diabetic vulvitis, the lesions may be red and moist and demonstrate evidence of secondary infection. The condition is exacerbated by the accompanying pruritus, which leads to rubbing and scratching. This becomes involuntary over time. As epithelial thickening develops, the environment of the vulva causes maceration, and a raised white lesion may be circumscribed or diffuse and may involve any portion of the vulva, adjacent thighs, perineum, or perianal skin. Biopsy must be performed to eliminate intraepithelial neoplasm or invasive tumor. With squamous cell hyperplasia, histologic examination demonstrates hyperkeratosis and acanthosis,

producing thickening of the epithelium and elongation of the rete pegs. No dermal inflammatory infiltrate is present as with lichen sclerosus. Atypical hyperplasia or cancer is characterized by nuclear pleomorphism and loss of cellular polarity in the epithelium.

Treatment of squamous cell hyperplasia seeks to achieve symptomatic relief. Sitz baths and lubricants can help restore moisture to cells and reconstruct the epithelial barrier. Oral antihistamines or antidepressants (ie, selective serotonin reuptake inhibitors) may help relieve pruritus. Local application of medium-potency topical steroids twice per day can decrease the inflammation and pruritus. Vulvar epithelium takes at least 6 weeks to heal. In intractable cases, subcutaneous intralesional injection of steroids can be considered. Differential diagnosis includes lichen simplex chronicus, lichen planus, condyloma acuminatum, psoriasis, and vulvar intraepithelial neoplasia.

C. OTHER DERMATOSES

Lichen planus of the vulva is a relatively common mucocutaneous dermatosis characterized by the presence of

Figure 37–13. Advanced lesion of lichen sclerosus. The labia minora and prepuce of the clitoris have blended into the labial skin. Focal dysplasia was present in the posterior third of the right labium majus.

Figure 37–14. Microscopic appearance of lichen sclerosus, characterized by hyperkeratosis, flattened epidermis, and hyalinization of the dermis.

sharply margined violaceous, flat-topped papules on the skin and less sharply marginated white plaques on oral and genital mucous membranes. The pathogenesis is unknown. In the vulva two clinical aspects can be observed: classic leukoplastic lesions and erosive lesions. Vulvar erosive lichen planus seems to be more frequent but often ignored. The clinical appearance of vaginal erosive lichen planus is similar to that of desquamative inflammatory vaginitis. It is a chronic, recalcitrant disease with associated vulvar burning and pruritus that is only partially ameliorated by therapy. Although mild forms are sometimes controlled with topical corticosteroids, the course of usual erosive lichen planus is one of exacerbations with slow healing. Treatment of lichen planus is mainly topical, using fluorinated corticosteroids or ultra-potent corticosteroids for the vulva and hydrocortisone foam for the vagina (Colofoam). Careful and frequent examination of the vagina for early adhesions is important. In cases of severe pruritus and intensive mucocutaneous involvement, systemic steroids should be used. Recently, topical treatment with tacrolimus 0.1% has been tried with success. Introital stenosis and vaginal adhesions sometimes benefit from home use of vaginal dilators in graduated sizes or from surgical release of scars.

Lichen simplex chronicus is another chronic inflammatory process of the vulva that presents as a white lesion associated with vulvar pruritus. Biopsy is generally necessary for the diagnosis. Histologically, the features are similar to those of squamous cell hyperplasia. Again, treatment is with medium-strength topical corticosteroid cream.

Benign Cystic Tumors

The diagnosis of small cystic structures on the vulva is ordinarily made by clinical examination or by excision biopsy, which also serves as treatment.

A. EPIDERMAL CYSTS

Cysts of epidermal origin are lined with squamous epithelium and filled with oily material and desquamated epithelial cells. Epidermal inclusion cysts may result from traumatic suturing of skin fragments during closure of the vulvar mucosa and skin after trauma or episiotomy. However, most epidermal cysts arise from occlusion of pilosebaceous ducts. These cysts usually are small, solitary, and asymptomatic.

B. SEBACEOUS CYSTS

A sebaceous cyst develops when the sebaceous gland's duct becomes occluded and accumulation of the sebaceous material occurs. These cysts are frequently multiple and almost always involve the labia majora. They are generally asymptomatic; however, acutely infected cysts may require incision and drainage.

C. APOCRINE SWEAT GLAND CYSTS

Apocrine sweat glands are numerous in the skin of the labia majora and the mons pubis. They become functional after puberty. Occlusion of the ducts with keratin results in an extremely pruritic, microcystic disease called **Fox-Fordyce disease.** Chronic infection in the apocrine glands, usually with staphylococci or streptococci, results in multiple painful subcutaneous abscesses and draining sinuses. This condition is called **hidradenitis suppurativa,** which is generally treated with a broad-spectrum antibiotic. Hidradenoma and syringoma are included in a diverse group of benign cystic or solid tumors of apocrine sweat gland origin present as small subcutaneous and asymptomatic tumors.

D. BARTHOLIN'S DUCT CYST AND ABSCESS

Obstruction of the main duct of Bartholin's gland results in retention of secretions and cystic dilatation. Infection is an important cause of obstruction; however, other causes include inspissated mucus and congenital narrowing of the duct. Secondary infection may result in recurrent abscess formation.

The gland and duct are located deep in the posterior third of each labium majus. Enlargement in the postmenopausal patient may represent a malignant process (although the incidence is < 1%), and biopsy should be considered.

Acute symptoms ordinarily result from infection, which leads to pain, tenderness, and dyspareunia. The surrounding tissues become edematous and inflamed. A fluctuant, tender mass is usually palpable. Unless an extensive inflammatory process is present, systemic symptoms or signs of infection are less likely.

Primary treatment consists of drainage of the infected cyst or abscess, preferably with insertion of a Word catheter (an inflatable bulb-tipped catheter) or by marsupialization (Fig 37–15). Simple incision and drainage may provide temporary relief. However, the end may become obstructed and recurrent cystic dilatation may recur. Appropriate antibiotics should be given if considerable surrounding inflammation develops. Excision of the cyst may be required in recurrent cases or in the postmenopausal patient.

Recurrent infection resulting in cystic dilatation of the duct is the rule unless a permanent opening for drainage is established.

E. Other

A variety of other infrequent cystic vulvar tumors must be considered in the differential diagnosis. Anteriorly, a **Skene duct cyst** or **urethral diverticulum** may be visible, suggesting a vulvar tumor. An **inguinal hernia** may extend into the labium majus, causing a large cystic dilatation. Occlusion of a persistent processus vaginalis (canal of Nuck) may cause a cystic tumor or hydrocele. Dilatation of the mesonephric duct vestiges produces lateral vaginal wall cysts, **Gartner's duct cyst.** Supernumerary mammary tissue that persists in the labia majora may form a cystic or solid tumor or even an adenocarcinoma; engorgement of such tissue in the pregnant patient can be symptomatic.

Benign Solid Tumors

A benign solid tumor may be an incidental finding at the time of pelvic examination, or it may be of sufficient size to cause symptoms of irritation and/or bleeding. The diagnosis should be established by excision or biopsy to rule out an underlying malignancy.

A. Acrochordon

An acrochordon is a flesh-colored, soft polypoid tumor of the vulvar skin that has been called a *fibroepithelial polyp* or simply a *skin tag.* The tumor does not become malignant and is of no clinical importance, unless it becomes traumatized, causing bleeding. Simple excision biopsy in the office is ordinarily adequate therapy.

B. Pigmented Nevus

Pigmented lesions, suggestive of nevi, should be removed by wide local excision or biopsied to diagnose or exclude a melanoma. A nevus on the vulvar skin may be flat, slightly elevated, papillomatous, dome-shaped, or pedunculated. Melanomas of the vulva are uncommon neoplasms constituting only 1–3% of vulvar cancers. They are extremely aggressive malignant lesions and may arise from pigmented nevi of the vulva. Melanosis of the vaginal or vulvar epithelium is a benign, flat, darkly pigmented lesion that usually can be differentiated from a nevus without histologic examination.

Figure 37–15. Marsupialization of a vestibular duct (Bartholin's) cyst.

C. Leiomyoma, Fibroma, and Lipoma

Tumors of mesodermal origin occur infrequently on the vulva, but they can become extremely large. **Leiomyomas** arise from muscle in the round ligament and appear as firm, symmetric, freely mobile tumors deep in the substance of the labium majus. **Fibromas** arise from proliferation of fibroblasts and vary in size from small subcutaneous nodules found incidentally to large polypoid tumors. Large tumors often undergo myxomatous degeneration and are very soft and cystic to palpation. **Lipomas** consist of a combination of mature fat cells and connective tissue. They cannot be differentiated from degenerated fibromas except by histopathologic examination.

Small tumors can be removed under local anesthesia in the office. Large tumors require general anesthesia and operating room facilities. The diagnosis of sarcoma depends on histologic examination.

D. Neurofibroma

Neurofibromas are fleshy polypoid lesions and may be solitary, solid tumors of the vulva or associated with generalized neurofibromatosis (Recklinghausen's disease). They arise from the neural sheath and usually are small lesions of no consequence. Multiple disfiguring tumors of the vulva may interfere with sexual function and require excision or vulvectomy.

E. Granular Cell Myoblastoma (Schwannoma)

Granular cell myoblastoma is usually a solitary, painless, slow-growing, infiltrating but benign tumor of neural sheath origin, most commonly found in the tongue or integument, although approximately 7% involve the vulva. The usual picture consists of small subcutaneous nodules 1–4 cm in diameter. With increasing size, they erode through the surface and result in ulcerations that may be confused with cancer. The margins of the tumor are indistinct, and wide local excision is necessary to completely excise the cells extending into contiguous tissues. The area of resection must be periodically re-examined and secondary excision performed promptly if recurrence is suspected.

VULVAR PAIN SYNDROME

Vulvar pain in the absence of relevant, visible physical findings is termed *vulvodynia*. The patient suffering from vulvodynia describes her symptoms as burning, rawness, irritation, dryness, and hyperpathia (pain provoked by very light touch). Approximately 16% of the female population has experienced vulvodynia and approximately 1.5% currently suffer from the disorder. The ISSVD has classified vulvodynia into **generalized vulvodynia** (**provoked or unprovoked**) and **localized vulvodynia** (**provoked and unprovoked**). When interviewing a patient suffering from vulvodynia, a detailed history and examination are important to help determine the etiology (Table 37–9) and to direct the diagnosis and treatment.

The time of onset, the type of pain (burning, stinging, irritation), timing (constant or cyclic), associated activities (eg, intercourse), inciting agents (eg, perfumes, lotions, detergents, clothing), and relieving factors (eg, antifungal medications) should be elicited. In addition, past or current infections (HPV, herpes, *Candida*), medications (eg, trichloroacetic acid, 5-fluorouracil), local and systemic dermatologic disorders, neurologic disorders (eg, herniated disks, herpes zoster, pudendal or genitofemoral neuralgia), urologic disorders (eg, interstitial cystitis, urethral syndrome), and physical trauma (eg, vaginal delivery, episiotomy, vaginal surgery) should be ascertained. In many cases the vulva appears normal on physical examination. The patient should be tested for allodynia and hyperalgesia in the vulvar area. Mapping of tender surfaces should be performed using a cotton-tipped swab. Vaginal pH and microscopic examination of vaginal secretions with KOH and normal saline can help evaluate for vaginitis. Acetowhite changes with application of 5% acetic acid should be biopsied as well as any distinct lesions to evaluate for an underlying dermatosis, infectious, or neoplastic process.

Localized Provoked Vulvodynia

The condition was formerly known as vulvar vestibulitis and clitorodynia. The vestibule is the nonpigmented, nonkeratinized squamous epithelium of the vulva between the labia minora and the hymen. Localized provoked vulvodynia is characterized by 3 criteria: (1) introital pain on vestibular or vaginal entry (entry dyspareunia), (2) vestibular erythema or inflammation of the vestibule, commonly involving the posterior fourchette, and (3) vestibular tenderness—pressure from a cotton-tipped applicator at the vestibule reproduces the pain.

Table 37–9. Etiologies of vulvodynia.

Infections
  Bartholin's gland abscess, vulvovaginal candidiasis, herpes, herpes zoster, human papillomavirus, molluscum contagiosum, trichomoniasis
Trauma
  Sexual assault, prior vaginal deliveries, hymenectomy
Systemic Illness
  Behçet's disease, Crohn's disease, Sjögren's syndrome, systemic lupus erythematosus
Neoplasia
  Vulvar intraepithelial neolplasia and invasive squamous cell carcinoma
Allergens/toxic medications
  Soaps, sprays, douches, antiseptics, suppositories, creams, laser treatment, podophyllin, trichloroacetic acid, 5-fluorouracil
Dermatologic conditions
  Allergic and contact dermatitis, eczema, hidradenitis suppurativa, lichen planus, lichen sclerosus, pemphigoid, pemphigus, psoriasis, squamous cell hyperplasia
Urinary tract syndromes
  Interstitial cystitis and urethral syndrome
Neurologic
  Referred pain from urethra, vagina, and bladder; dysesthesias secondary to herpes zoster, spinal disk problems; specific neuralgias (pudendal, genitofemoral)
Psychological
  Sexual/physical abuse history

This syndrome generally affects women in their 20s and 30s who complain of introital dyspareunia (severe pain on vaginal penetration by their partner). It may present as persistent vaginal discharge and burning. On biopsy, the subepithelial tissue demonstrates a nonspecific, chronic inflammatory infiltrate, consisting predominately of lymphocytes without direct glandular inflammation. The etiology remains undetermined.

Although numerous medical options are available for treatment, the success of many of these modalities are not substantiated by properly conducted studies (Table 37–10). Patients should be instructed on proper vulvar hygiene (cotton underwear, keeping area dry, avoidance of constrictive garments and irritating agents). The initial conservative approach to therapy includes topical estradiol with twice-daily application, 5% lidocaine ointment daily, calcium citrate 400 mg 3 times daily to decrease the urinary oxalate crystal concentration, oral antifungal therapy using fluconazole 150 mg weekly, and pelvic floor therapy with biofeedback. The injectable forms of therapy include intralesional interferon injection to treat possible HPV, trigger point injections with long-acting injectable anesthetics, and injection of botulism toxin to treat vaginismus as the source of vulvodynia. The

Table 37–10. Treatment of vulvodynia.

Supportive measures—warm sitz baths, Burrow's solution, topical anesthetic agents (2% topical xylocaine gel or 5% ointment) and other lubricants with intercourse

Vulvar hygiene—cotton underwear, avoidance of constrictive garments

Treat underlying cause:

    Human papillomavirus (HPV)[1]—trichloroacetic acid, topical 5-fluorouracil, interferon 1 million IU per injection site with total of 12 injection sites over 4 weeks, laser, and cream

    Candida—fluconazole 150 mg once per week for 6 weeks then once per month for 6 months (for cyclic vulvodynia)

    Allergens—avoidance of agent (also of local creams and suppositories containing propylene glycol), hydroxyzine or other antihistamine, hydrocortisone 1% cream twice daily, 5% aspirin cream

    Atrophy—topical estrogen vaginal cream, oral hormone replacement therapy

Diet modification—low-oxalate diet with calcium citrate 400 mg orally twice daily

Tricyclic antidepressants—amitriptyline 10–25 mg three times daily (use lowest dose possible)

Psychological and behavioral pain management

Biofeedback

Surgery—vestibuloplasty, partial vestibulectomy with vaginal advancement, total vestibulectomy with vaginal advancement

---

[1]Current studies do not substantiate HPV as a causative factor in vulvodynia; however, its treatment, particularly with interferon, is still supported in the literature.

surgical treatment of localized provoked vulvodynia in the form of vulvar vestibulectomy with vaginal advancement is most effective (70% success rate) in patients who have been refractory to more conservative therapies.

CO_2 laser vaporization is no longer recommended for this condition.

Up to two-thirds of patients may be cured following a variety of treatments. Recalcitrant cases even subsequent to surgery may occur, resulting in continued dyspareunia. In these cases, acupuncture and referral to a pain treatment center may be an option.

Generalized Unprovoked Vulvodynia

This condition was formerly known as pudendal neuralgia. Its etiology is unknown. The pain involves a larger surface area than that of localized vulvodynia. The average patient is in her 40s. The typical patient complains of intermittent or constant burning sensation with periods of unexplained relief and/or flares. The diagnosis is made by exclusion. Infections and dermatosis should be ruled out.

A test for allodynia and hyperalgesia using a cotton-tipped swab should be performed. It is believed to be a neuropathic pain, but other organic causes, including pudendal nerve entrapment, pudendal nerve injury due to child birth, referred pain from ruptured disk, neuropathic viruses such as herpes simplex or varicella-zoster, and neurologic disease such as multiple sclerosis, are possible.

Treatment of generalized unprovoked vulvodynia is mostly unsuccessful. The patient should be counseled on elimination of irritants and on self-care. Topical local anesthetics, tricyclic antidepressants, or anticonvulsants such as gabapentin can be tried. If the patient is refractory to such treatment, acupuncture or referral to a pain center may be attempted.

REFERENCES

General

Centers for Disease Control and Prevention: Sexually transmitted diseases treatment guidelines. MMWR Recomm Rep 2002; 51(RR-6):1.

Gilson RJ, Mindel A: Recent advances: Sexually transmitted infections. BMJ 2001;322:1160.

Sobel JD: Vaginitis. N Engl J Med 1997;337:1896.

Wilkinson EJ: Vulvar nonneoplastic epithelial disorders. ACOG Educational Bulletin 1997;241:1.

Specific

ACOG practice bulletin. Management of herpes in pregnancy. Clinical management guidelines for obstetrician-gynecologists. Int J Gynaecol Obstet 2000;68:165.

ACOG practice bulletin. Gynecologic herpes simplex virus-clinical management guidelines for obstetrician-gynecologists. Obstet Gynecol 2004;104(5 Pt 1):1111.

Baker DA, Blythe JG, Miller JM: Once-daily valacyclovir hydrochloride for suppression of recurrent genital herpes. Obstet Gynecol 1999;94:103.

Boer J, van Gemert MJ: Long-term results of isotretinoin in the treatment of 68 patients with hidradenitis suppurativa. J Am Acad Dermatol 1999;40:73.

Bohm M et al: Successful treatment of anogenital lichen sclerosus with topical Tacrolimus. Arch Dermatol 2003;139:922.

Braig S et al: Acyclovir prophylaxis in late pregnancy prevents recurrent genital herpes and viral shedding. Eur J Obstet Gynecol Reprod Biol 2001;96:55.

Brocklehurst P, Hannah M, McDonald H: Interventions for treating bacterial vaginosis in pregnancy (Cochrane Review). In: *The Cochrane Library.* Update Software, 2001, p. 3.

Carey JC et al: Metronidazole to prevent preterm delivery in pregnant women with asymptomatic bacterial vaginosis. N Engl J Med 2000;342:534.

Edwards L et al: Self-administered topical 5% imiquimod cream for external anogenital warts. Human Papillomavirus Study Group. Arch Dermatol 1998;134:25.

Forna F, Gülmezoglu AM: Interventions for treating trichomoniasis in women (Cochrane Review). In: *The Cochrane Library.* Update Software, 2001, p. 3.

Franco EL et al: Vaccination against human papillomavirus infection: a new paradigm in cervical cancer control. Vaccine 2005;32:S72.

Funaro D: Lichen sclerosus: A review and practical approach. Dermatol Ther 2004;17:28.

Ghazizadeh S et al: Botulinum toxin in the treatment of refractory vaginismus. Obstet Gynecol 2004;104(5 Pt 1):922.

Goodman A: Role of routine human papillomavirus subtyping in cervical screening. Curr Opin Obstet Gynecol 2000;12:11.

Gülmezoglu AM: Interventions for trichomoniasis in pregnancy (Cochrane Review). In: *The Cochrane Library.* Update Software, 2001, p. 3.

Hajjeh RA et al: Toxic shock syndrome in the United States: Surveillance update, 1979–1996. Emerg Infect Dis 1999;5:807.

Haley JC, Mirowski GW, Hood AF: Benign vulvar tumors. Semin Cutan Med Surg 1998;17:196.

Handa VL, Stice CW: Fungal culture findings in cyclic vulvitis. Obstet Gynecol 2000;96:301.

Hanson JM et al: Metronidazole for bacterial vaginosis. A comparison of vaginal gel vs. oral therapy. J Reprod Med 2000;45:889.

Harlow BL et al: A population-based assessment of chronic unexplained vulvar pain: Have we underestimated the prevalence of vulvodynia? J Am Med Womens Assoc. 2003;5882.

Harper DM et al: Efficacy of a bivalent L1 virus like particle vaccine in prevention of infection with human papillomavirus type 16 and 18 in young women: A randomized trial. Obstet Gynecol Surv 2005;60:171.

Kamarashev JA, Vassileya SG: Dermatologic diseases of the vulva. Clin Dermatol 1997;15:53.

Lotery HE et al: Erosive lichen planus of the vulva and vagina. Obstet Gynecol 2003;101:1121.

Lotery HE et al: Vulvodynia. Lancet 2004;363:1058.

Lynch PJ: Lichen simplex chronicus (atopic neurodermatitis)of the anogenital region. Dermatol Ther 2004;17:8.

Marrazzo JM, Stamm WE: New approaches to the diagnosis, treatment, and prevention of chlamydial infection. Curr Clin Top Infect Dis 1998;18:45.

Mazdisnian F et al: Intralesional injection of triamcinolone in the treatment of lichen sclerosus. J Reprod Med 1999;44:332.

McGregor JA, French JI: Bacterial vaginosis in pregnancy. Obstet Gynecol Surv 2000;55(5 Suppl 1):S1.

Morris MC, Rogers PA, Kinghorn GR: Is bacterial vaginosis a sexually transmitted infection? Sex Transm Infect 2001; 77:63.

Ninia JG: Treatment of vulvar varicosities by injection—Compression sclerotherapy. Dermatol Surg 1997;23:573.

Pandit L, Ouslander JG: Postmenopausal vaginal atrophy and atrophic vaginitis. Am J Med Sci 1997;314:228.

Petrin D et al: Clinical and microbiological aspects of *Trichomonas vaginalis.* Clin Microbiol Rev 1998;11:300.

Rioux JE et al: 17-beta-estradiol vaginal tablet versus conjugated equine estrogen vaginal cream to relieve menopausal atrophic vaginitis. Menopause 2000;7:156.

Sakane T et al: Behçet's disease. N Engl J Med 1999;341:1284.

Sobel JD et al: Treatment of complicated candida vaginitis, comparison of single and sequential dose of fluconazole. Am J Obstet Gynecol 2001;185:363.

Sobel JD et al: Maintenance fluconazole therapy for recurrent vulvovaginal candidiasis. N Engl J Med 2004;351:876.

Theos AU et al: Effectiveness of imiquimod cream 5% for treating childhood molluscum contagiosum in a double-blind randomized pilot trial. Cutis 2004;74:134.

Wiseman MC: Hidradenitis suppurativa: A review. Dermatol Ther 2004;17:50.

Young GL, Jewell D: Topical treatment for vaginal candidiasis in pregnancy (Cochrane Review). In: *The Cochrane Library.* Update Software, 2001, p. 3.

Benign Disorders of the Uterine Cervix

Anna Kogan, MD, Avi Ben-Shushan, MD, & Martin L. Pernoll, MD

CONGENITAL ANOMALIES OF THE CERVIX

The cervix develops from the paramesonephric ducts in the sixth week of embryologic development. After fusion of the 2 müllerian ducts in the midline, there is resorption of the septum (Fig 38–1). In the absence of the development of paramesonephric ducts, there is agenesis of the cervix and uterus. Other anomalies may result from incomplete fusion of these ducts or failure of resorption of the midline septum.

Cervical Agenesis

Cases of an absent uterine cervix with a normal uterine corpus and normal vagina have been reported. These cases presumably result from either failure of müllerian duct canalization or abnormal epithelial proliferation after canalization. More common is the absence of a cervix along with the absence of a uterine corpus and upper vagina. Because most of the vagina is derived from müllerian ducts, the vagina may be shortened in müllerian aplasia. Women with müllerian aplasia have normal ovaries and are able to contribute oocytes for in vitro fertilization with their partner's sperm. This allows for a transfer to a uterus of a surrogate woman who may carry the pregnancy to term. Female offspring of women with müllerian aplasia have been studied to identify a possible genetic contribution to this disorder. Because no offspring with müllerian aplasia have been reported, this disorder is assumed to be result from a polygenic multifactorial inheritance pattern.

Cervical agenesis with a normal functioning uterine corpus must be differentiated from müllerian aplasia (Figs 38–2 and 38–3). In the former, menstrual blood may accumulate, leading to retrograde flow and development of endometriosis. Ultrasonography, magnetic resonance imaging (MRI), and laparoscopy can help with the diagnosis by defining the anatomy. Many of these patients also have urinary tract abnormalities and require an intravenous pyelogram.

Nonsurgical treatment involves the use of vaginal dilators. Using a bicycle stool designed by Ingram, special dilators are placed that are under constant perineal pressure. The most common surgical approach is the McIndoe technique for creation of a neovagina. The Vecchietti operation combines a surgical and nonsurgical approach to creating a neovagina and has been recently performed by laparoscopy.

Incomplete Müllerian Fusion

If the müllerian ducts fail to completely fuse and canalize, a variety of anomalies may occur. Complete failure of fusion of the ducts results in uterine didelphys; there are 2 separate uterine horns, each with a distinct cervix and vagina. The 2 vaginas are separated by a midline septum. If incomplete fusion results in a uterine horn ending blindly, a hematocolpos can develop (Fig 38–4).

Bicornuate uterus and arcuate uterus are due to partial incomplete fusion of the müllerian ducts. In the bicornuate uterus, 2 discrete uterine cavities lead to the same cervix (Fig 38–5). The arcuate uterus may demonstrate minimal depression of the uterine fundus and is often clinically insignificant. Renal abnormalities are found in 20–30% of women with müllerian defects.

Failure of Resorption

After fusion of the müllerian ducts, resorption of the intervening septum proceeds both caudal and cephalic. A septate uterus results from failure of resorption of the intervening septum (Fig 38–6). The septum may project from the uterine fundus through the cervical canal, completely dividing the uterine cavity in 2, or it may be segmental.

The septum consists of fibromuscular tissue. Failure or incomplete resorption of this septum is associated with reproductive and obstetric complications. First- and second-trimester spontaneous miscarriages are common and usually occur between 8 and 16 weeks' gestation. It is hypothesized that the septum interferes with placental implantation. Obstetric complications can include premature labor, malpresenta-

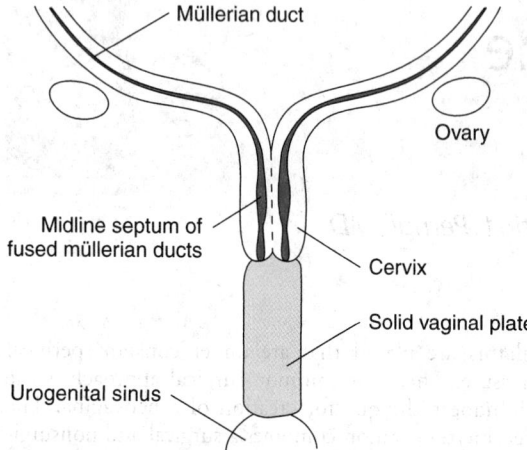

Figure 38–1. Fusion of müllerian ducts to form cervix and corpus uteri.

tion, and intrauterine growth restriction. Approximately 15–25% of spontaneous miscarriages are due to müllerian abnormalities, and the majority are associated with the septate uterus (70–88%).

If a septate uterus is identified in association with reproductive or obstetric complications, surgical therapy is recommended. Imaging studies including ultrasound, MRI, sonohysterography, and hysterosalpingogram provide information to differentiate the septate uterus from other uterine abnormalities. Combined laparoscopy and hysteroscopy remains the most reliable method for accurately differentiating the septate uterus from a bicornuate uterus. Hysteroscopic resection of the uterine septum has been demonstrated to improve reproductive outcome in women with recurrent spontaneous miscarriages. Whether a hysteroscopic metroplasty improves fertility in those infertile women is controversial.

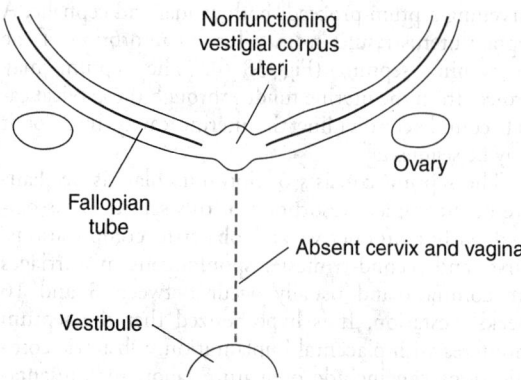

Figure 38–2. Congenital absence of vagina.

Figure 38–3. Cervical aplasia with hematometra and retrograde menstruation.

CERVICAL ABNORMALITIES DUE TO DIETHYLSTILBESTROL EXPOSURE IN UTERO

Diethylstilbestrol (DES) is a synthetic nonsteroidal estrogen that was first synthesized in 1938. Although the number of pregnant women treated with DES is unknown, estimates range from 2–10 million. DES has been shown to cause uterine and cervical abnormalities. Common structural changes of the cervix include collars, hoods, cockscombs, and pseudopolyps (Fig 38–7). Multiple anomalies of the uterus and vagina are also reported in association with DES exposure in utero.

Women who are exposed to DES in utero and have cervical abnormalities are at increased risk for infertility. These women are also at increased risk for adverse out-

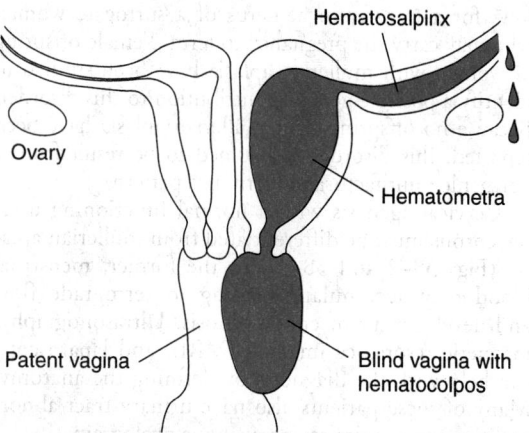

Figure 38–4. Uterus didelphys with blind vagina hematocolpos, hematometra, hematosalpinx, and retrograde menstruation.

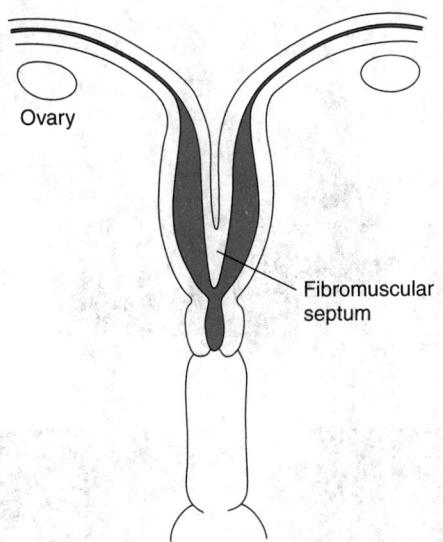

Figure 38–5. Complete bicornuate uterus with fibromuscular septum at the level of internal cervical os.

comes in pregnancy, including miscarriage, ectopic pregnancy, and premature delivery. The use of prophylactic cervical cerclage for cervical incompetence related to DES exposure in utero is not recommended.

CERVICAL INJURIES

Lacerations

Cervical lacerations most frequently occur after a normal or abnormal vaginal delivery, but they can occur in the nonobstetric patient as well. With delivery, the most common tears occur at the 3 and 6 o'clock posi-

Figure 38–6. Complete septate uterus.

tions. Lacerations are more commonly found after an operative vaginal delivery requiring forceps or vacuum. It is important to carefully inspect the entire cervix after delivery to identify any lacerations. Most lacerations can be easily repaired with suture technique. Often a laceration is asymptomatic and does not require repair. More severe lacerations that may extend into the broad ligament have been reported and may require more extensive surgical repair.

Performance of dilatation and curettage (D&C), particularly on the postmenopausal patient, can result in cervical laceration. The use of cervical laminaria preoperatively may decrease the risk of trauma and laceration of the cervix. Preoperative use of misoprostol to reduce the force required to dilate the cervix, potentially reducing the incidence of cervical lacerations, has been reported.

Cervical lacerations are reported with use of the resecting loop in hysteroscopic surgery. Use of the rollerball and other instruments for ablating the endometrium for treatment of menorrhagia has been found to increase the incidence of cervical lacerations. Excessive traction on the anterior lip of the cervix with a single-tooth tenaculum may lead to a laceration.

Perforations

Perforation of the cervix may occur during self-induced abortion with sharp objects (eg, wires or darning or knitting needles), or inadvertently during sounding of the uterus, cervical dilatation, insertion of radioactive sources, or conization of the cervix. The urinary bladder and the rectum are at risk for injury because of their close proximity to the cervix.

Ulcerations

Ulceration of the cervix may result from pressure necrosis due to a vaginal pessary or a cervical stem pessary. Cervical ulceration may also develop with uterine prolapse when the cervix protrudes through the vaginal introitus.

Cervical Stenosis

Cervical stenosis usually occurs at the level of the internal os and may lead to significant symptoms. In the premenopausal woman, cervical stenosis may be responsible for obstruction of menstrual flow, leading to amenorrhea and pelvic pain. Additionally, infertility may result from cervical stenosis. A postmenopausal woman with cervical stenosis may have pyometra, requiring evacuation of uterine contents and biopsy to rule out endometrial carcinoma.

Cervical surgery such as cone biopsy, loop excision, or ablative techniques for treatment of dysplasia may lead to cervical stenosis. Excision by loop diathermy tends to re-

Figure 38–7. Cervical changes in women exposed to diethylstilbestrol in utero. **A:** Circular sulcus. **B:** Central depression and ectopy. **C:** Portio vaginalis covered by columnar epithelium (ectopy). **D:** Anterior cervical protuberance (rough). **E:** Anterior cervical protuberance (smooth).

move less cervical stroma and therefore is less likely to cause cervical stenosis than a cold knife cone biopsy. Radiation therapy, neoplasia, and atrophic changes are more common causes in the postmenopausal woman.

The diagnosis of cervical stenosis is made by the inability to pass a small cervical dilator. Ultrasonography may indicate the presence of uterine contents that are obstructed. Treatment is usually with dilators under ultrasound guidance. Use of various techniques such as laser treatment, loop diathermy, and the hysteroscope with resecting loop to remove areas of cervical stenosis has been reported. After successful dilatation, placement of a pediatric Foley catheter in the cervix for a few weeks may be beneficial in order to maintain patency.

Annular Detachment

Annular detachment of the cervix is a rare complication resulting from compression necrosis of the cervix during labor. It occurs when the external os fails to dilate and the blood supply is compromised by pressure of the fetal head. The diagnosis is made when the detached ring or portion of cervix is expelled prior to delivery of the presenting part of the fetus.

Complications of Cervical Injuries

Hemorrhage is the most immediate and serious complication of cervical laceration. Although external bleeding usually is present, intraperitoneal or extraperitoneal hemorrhage may occur when the cervical tear extends into the uterus. The clinical picture is that of hypovolemic shock out of proportion to visible blood loss.

Cervical incompetence results from unrecognized or improperly repaired lacerations at the level of the internal os. Repeated or habitual abortion, often occurring during the second trimester of pregnancy, may be due to cervical incompetence.

CERVICAL INFECTIONS

General Considerations

Advances in colposcopy and sensitive testing for infectious diseases has allowed better assessment of the causes of acute and chronic cervicitis. Hypervascularity, erythema, and ectopy are more consistent with squamous metaplasia than is an inflammatory change requiring therapy. Histologic diagnosis of cervicitis is common enough to be considered a normal finding. The cervix is in direct contact with the vagina and therefore is exposed to viral, bacterial, fungal, and parasitic agents. Cervical infections of these types may be found in the absence of vaginal disease. The cervix is a reservoir for infections with *Neisseria gonorrhoeae, Chlamydia trachomatis,* herpes simplex virus (HSV), human papillomavirus (HPV), and *Mycoplasma* spp. Because many of these women are asymptomatic, screening of women at risk is important.

Etiology and Pathogenesis

C trachomatis is sexually transmitted and invades the columnar epithelium of the cervix; thus, the condition is best categorized as endocervicitis. With the cervix as a reservoir, the organism may infect the fetus during its passage through the birth canal, or it may ascend via the endometrial cavity to the fallopian tubes to cause salpingitis as well as pelvic and perihepatic peritonitis. It has been implicated as the agent responsible

for the Fitz-Hugh and Curtis syndrome (violin-string adhesions between the liver and the parietal peritoneum). *C trachomatis* and *N gonorrhoeae* often are coinfecting agents in the etiology of acute and chronic cervicitis and salpingitis. *C trachomatis* may be transmitted to the eyes, where it causes trachoma and inclusion conjunctivitis.

N gonorrhoeae is a common cause of cervicitis also infecting the columnar epithelium of the endocervix. The mature squamous epithelium of the adult cervix and vagina is resistant to the invading organism. As in the case of *Chlamydia* infections, the cervix acts as a nidus for ascending infection of the endometrium and the fallopian tubes, with upward invasion often occurring after a menstrual period and loss of the protective mucus plug.

HSV infection produces cervical lesions similar to those found on the vulva. The lesion is vesicular at first and then becomes ulcerative. Primary infections may be extensive and severe, producing constitutional symptoms of low-grade fever, myalgia, and malaise lasting approximately 2 weeks. The ulcers eventually heal, but recurrences of lesser severity and duration are common. Herpes simplex virus type 2 (HSV-2) is the etiologic agent in more than 90% of genital herpes infections; the remainder are due to herpes simplex virus type 1 (HSV-1), the cause of the common cold sore or fever blister. Orogenital contact is thought to be responsible. After the initial infection has healed, the virus continues to reside in the epithelial cells of the cervix, and viral shedding occurs in asymptomatic patients. Infection of infants during their passage through the birth canal has led to the practice of cesarean section in women who have evidence of active infection at term. Women with antibodies to HSV-2 have a higher incidence of intraepithelial neoplasia as well as invasive malignancy, although a direct etiologic link has not been established.

The cervical lesions of HPV are sexually transmitted. They are flatter and moister than the typical genital warts (condylomata acuminata) seen on the vulva and perianal skin. In fact, they often are invisible to the naked eye, becoming visible only after application of a dilute solution of acetic acid (acetowhite epithelium) or by colposcopic examination (white epithelium, mosaicism, and coarse punctation). More than 65 types of HPV have been identified. Benign lesions of the cervix are associated with types 6, 11, 42, 43, 44, 53, 54, and 55, whereas types 16, 18, 31, 33, 35, 39, 45, and 56 are more often found in association with cervical intraepithelial neoplasia and invasive cancers.

Approximately one-third of women with HPV infection have coexistent cervicitis caused by other organisms. The presence of cervicitis does not significantly affect the clinical course of HPV lesions.

Cytopathology

The Papanicolaou (Pap) smear often reflects the pathologic changes of cervical infections. A few inflammatory cells normally are seen on the smear, particularly immediately before, during, and immediately after the menses. However, the presence of large numbers of polymorphonuclear leukocytes and histiocytes indicate an acute cervicitis. At times the inflammatory exudate may be so dense that it obscures the epithelial cells, in which case the smear should repeated after the inflammatory process has been treated and cleared. Epithelial cell changes are commonly associated with cervical inflammation and must be distinguished from those related to neoplastic disease. Nuclear enlargement, clumping of chromatin, hyperchromatism, and nucleoli, as well as cytoplasmic eosinophilia and poorly defined cell membranes, are often seen. These are the findings of "cytologic atypia" and are nonspecific. Frequently, however, a specific diagnosis can be made either by directly identifying the offending organism(s) or by noting typical changes in the epithelial cells characteristic of a specific type of infection. For example, the organism of trichomoniasis and moniliasis can be identified directly on the Pap smear. HPV cannot be seen, but the infection is characterized by squamous epithelial cell enlargement, multinucleation, and the perinuclear "halo" effect of koilocytosis. The so-called "balloon cell" is almost pathognomonic of this condition. Cellular changes of mild dysplasia (low-grade squamous intraepithelial lesion [SIL]), moderate or severe dysplasia (carcinoma in situ [CIS], high-grade SIL), and even invasive cancer may be associated findings.

Greatly enlarged, multinucleated cells with ground-glass cytoplasm and nuclei containing characteristic inclusion bodies are indicative of HSV infection.

Histopathology of Cervical Infections

Histopathologic findings of cervical infection are both nonspecific and specific. Characteristically, both *N gonorrhoeae* and *C trachomatis* infections produce a nonspecific acute inflammatory reaction. Because of edema and increased vascularity, the cervix becomes swollen and reddened. Stromal edema and infiltration by polymorphonuclear leukocytes are seen microscopically, and there may be focal loss of overlying mucous membrane.

As the acute process subsides, the swelling and redness disappear, and the polymorphonuclear leukocytes are replaced by lymphocytes, plasma cells, and macrophages—the histologic picture of chronic cervicitis. Irritation due to infection causes the glandular epithelium to hyperfunction, and mucus mixed with inflammatory cells produces a copious purulent or mucopurulent exudate, which may be clinically apparent only by introducing a cotton swab into the cervical canal. Because the infected clefts and crypts drain poorly, they become dilated and often obstructed,

leading to microabscess formation. With longstanding inflammation, proliferation of fibrous connective tissue in the cervical stroma occurs. This results in hypertrophy and elongation of the cervix. If this process is extreme, the portio vaginalis may actually protrude beyond the vaginal introitus, giving the impression of a prolapse of the uterus.

On numerous occasions a histopathologic diagnosis of chronic cervicitis is made based on the finding of small collections of lymphocytes in the cervical stroma. This finding is characteristic of the cervix of almost all parous women and probably is not significant unless some clinical manifestation of cervicitis is present.

The gross appearance of acute cervicitis must be distinguished clinically and at times histologically from the red, granular inflamed-appearing cervix of cervical ectopy, in which variable portions of the cervical portio vaginalis are covered by endocervical, mucus-secreting epithelium or by a thin layer of immature metaplastic epithelium. Particularly in younger women, the squamocolumnar junction, instead of being located at or near the external os, is found on the surface of the portio. Being covered only by a single layer of columnar cells, the underlying vascular stroma is clearly visible, producing a red, granular appearance. In the past this has been called a cervical "erosion." "Erosion" is not a proper term for cervical redness except as an acute, limited denudation of mucous membrane as might be seen with an especially virulent acute cervicitis or following punch biopsy, cauterization, cryotherapy, laser treatment, loop excision, cone biopsy, or radiation therapy.

The location of squamocolumnar tissue of the cervix is not static throughout life; instead it undergoes continuous change. Through the process of squamous metaplasia, columnar epithelium on the portio vaginalis is gradually converted to stratified squamous epithelium. Initially the stratified metaplastic epithelium is thin and immature, but with time it becomes thicker and more mature, eventually taking on the appearance of original squamous epithelium. Microscopically, the squamocolumnar junction rarely demonstrates an abrupt transition from squamous to columnar epithelium, but instead is marked by a zone of immature squamous metaplasia (Figs 38–8 and 38–9). This change from a mucous membrane covered by a single layer of columnar epithelium to one of the stratified squamous epithelium is not only a continuously ongoing process but is accelerated during 3 periods of a woman's life: fetal existence, adolescence, and during the first pregnancy.

By the time a woman reaches her fifth decade, the squamocolumnar junction has receded into the endocervical canal, and the portio vaginalis is completely covered by squamous epithelium. In the process, however, the deeper crypts and clefts of columnar epithelium are bridged over and occluded by metaplastic epithelium, obstructing the egress of mucus, producing the common, typical nabothian cysts of the cervix. To the naked eye,

Figure 38–8. Abrupt transition, squamocolumnar junction.

the presence of nabothian cysts indicates that this area at one time was occupied by columnar epithelium that has undergone transformation. Therefore, the nabothian cyst is the hallmark of the "transformation zone," the area in which epithelial neoplasia first appears.

Certain pathologic findings are specific in that they implicate specific organisms. For example, microscopic examination of a cervical biopsy obtained from a vesicular lesion may demonstrate intraepithelial, multinucleated giant cells containing nuclear inclusions surrounded by a clear halo typical of HSV infection. Colposcopically directed biopsy of an area of white epithelium, coarse punctation, or mosaicism may show a flat, thickened, squamous epithelium whose superficial layers are occupied by cells demonstrating large cytoplasmic vacuoles that are devoid of glycogen, surrounding shrunken, hyperchromatic nuclei, and cell membranes that are thickened and eosinophilic. These are the typical histologic findings of HPV infection (Fig 38–10). They may be associated with the findings of intraepithelial neoplasia (see Chapter 50).

Clinical Findings

A. SYMPTOMS AND SIGNS

1. Acute cervicitis—The primary symptom of acute cervicitis is a purulent vaginal discharge. The appearance of the discharge is variable—often thick and creamy as in gonorrheal infection; foamy and greenish-white as in trichomonal infection; white and curdlike as in candidiasis; and thin and gray as in bacterial vaginosis. Chlamydia infections often produce a purulent discharge from an angry, reddened, congested cervix. The discharge is often indistinguishable from that due to gonorrheal cervicitis and has been characterized as mucopurulent. Other pathogens that have recently been identified as possible causes of cervicitis are *Mycoplasma genitalium*, HSV-1 and HSV-2, cytomegalovirus, and bacterial vaginosis. Mucopurulent cervicitis, however, may be present in 40–60% of women in whom no infection is identified.

Inspection of the cervix initially infected by *N gonorrhoeae* generally reveals an acutely inflamed, edematous cervix with a purulent discharge escaping from the external os. In trichomonal infection, the classic strawberry-like appearance may be visible on the squamous epithelial surface of the portio vaginalis as well as the adjacent vaginal mucosa. In candidiasis, there is likely to be a white cheesy exudate that is difficult to wipe away and, if scraped off, usually leaves punctate hemorrhagic areas. Colposcopic findings of acute cervicitis are those primarily of an altered microangioarchitecture with marked increase in the surface capillaries, which when viewed end-on may show a pattern of diffuse "punctation." Trichomoniasis is typified by characteristic double-hairpin capillaries. The capillary pattern of inflammation should not be confused with that of neoplasia. In an inflammatory process, the colposcopic picture is diffuse with ill-defined margins in contrast with the localized and sharply demarcated vascular changes associated with

Figure 38–9. Metaplastic epithelium at the squamocolumnar junction.

Figure 38–10. Squamous epithelium showing histologic changes of human papillomavirus infection.

intraepithelial neoplasia. It should be emphasized that invasive cancers often are secondarily infected, so in addition to the colposcopic changes associated with frank malignancy, those related to inflammation are also present. Colposcopy also readily identifies the fine villiform pattern of cervical ectopy (Fig 38–11).

Infertility may be a consequence of cervicitis. A thick, glutinous, acidic, pus-laden cervical mucus is noxious to sperm and prevents fertilization.

Vulvar burning and itching may be prominent symptoms. Gonorrheal cervicitis may be accompanied by urethritis with frequency, urgency, and dysuria. If associated with acute salpingitis, the symptoms and signs will be those of pelvic peritonitis. Hyperemia of the infected cervix may be associated with freely bleeding areas. Cervical ooze may account for intermenstrual (often postcoital) spotting. Bleeding commonly occurs due to cervical friability when endocervical smears are obtained.

2. Chronic cervicitis—In chronic cervicitis, leukorrhea may be the chief symptom. Although it may not be as profuse as in acute cervicitis, the discharge may cause vulvar irritation. The discharge may be frankly purulent and variable in color, or it may present simply as thick, tenacious, turbid mucus. Intermenstrual bleeding may occur.

Associated eversion may present as a velvety to granular redness or as patchy erythema due to scattered squamous metaplasia (epithelialization or epidermization). Nabothian cysts in the area of the so-called transformation zone often occur. The Schiller test may show poorly staining or nonstaining areas. Often some tenderness and thickening in the region of the uterosacral ligaments are noted on pelvic examination, and motion of the cervix may be painful.

Lower abdominal pain, lumbosacral backache, dysmenorrhea, or dyspareunia may occur occasionally related to an associated parametritis. Infertility may be due to inflammatory changes that result in a tacky cervical mucus that is acidic and otherwise hostile (toxic) to sperm. Urinary frequency, urgency, and dysuria may be seen in association with chronic cervicitis. These symptoms are related to an associated subvesical lymphangitis, not to cystitis.

Inspection of the chronically infected cervix often reveals only abnormal discharge. Fibrosis and stenosis of the cervix may follow chronic cervical infection. Patulousness of the deeply lacerated external os often exposes the endocervical canal, which may bleed when wiped with a cotton applicator. The portio and the upper vagina usually appear normal in cervicitis.

B. LABORATORY FINDINGS

1. Stains and smears—Mucopurulent cervicitis is defined as gross evidence of purulent material at an inflamed cervix along with a microscopic presence of 10

Figure 38–11. Colposcopic view of villiform pattern of cervical ectopy.

or more polymorphonuclear leukocytes per microscopic field on Gram's stain of material obtained from the endocervical canal. In the absence of mucopurulent discharge, routine use of Gram's stain is not recommended because of its low sensitivity in detecting infection. Cervicovaginal infections with *Trichomonas vaginalis* can often be identified on wet smear preparations by identification of the motile flagellated organisms. Bacterial vaginosis can be seen on wet mount by the hallmark trait of a speckled periphery to the epithelial "clue cells." Candidal infections can be seen on potassium hydroxide preparations, with the distinctive presence of hyphae.

In acute cervicitis with *N gonorrhoeae*, the sensitivity of Gram's stain for detection is only 50%.

2. Detection of *N gonorrhoeae* and *C trachomatis*—Previously, culture of *C trachomatis* was the preferred method for detection of infection and was considered the gold standard for diagnosis. Although it has excellent specificity, the sensitivity is no higher than 70% in females. Variables are involved in the testing, such as the manner of specimen collection, transport condition, culture procedures, and identification of a positive culture.

More recently, new techniques for detection of *C trachomatis* include nucleic acid amplification methods such as polymerase chain reaction (PCR), transcription-mediated amplification (TMA), and strand displacement amplification (SDA). The benefit of using nucleic acid amplification is its high sensitivity (82–100%) and specificity. The specimen can be noninvasively obtained from either a vulvar swab or urine. These tests also allow for simultaneous detection of *N gonorrhoeae* from the same specimen, although sensitivity with urine samples is not as high as with cervical swab. Enzyme immunoassay (EIA) and direct fluorescent antibody (DFA) rely on antigen detection and have a sensitivity ranging from 70–80%, but the specimen still requires invasive testing using a swab from the cervix or urethra.

N gonorrhoeae may also be diagnosed by direct culture of the endocervical mucus. The culture is performed on Thayer-Martin or blood agar medium. Proper transport medium and timing are essential for accurate diagnosis. Most laboratories are moving toward nonculture assays such as PCR, which offer high sensitivity and specificity.

3. Blood studies—In uncomplicated cervicitis not accompanied by salpingitis, the white count may be normal, or the leukocytosis sedimentation rate may be slightly elevated.

Patients with gonorrhea or chlamydia are at risk for infection with other sexually transmitted diseases (STDs). Counseling and testing should be offered for syphilis, hepatitis B, and human immunodeficiency virus (HIV).

Differential Diagnosis

Noninfectious cervicitis is most commonly due to the effects of endogenous or exogenous hormones on the maintenance of integrity of cervicovaginal mucosa. Bimanual examination should be performed to distinguish the signs and symptoms of pelvic tenderness, induration, and mass formation about the cervix when discharge is noted from the cervix.

Cervicitis must be distinguished from early neoplastic processes. This may not be easy because inflammatory conditions may alter the epithelial cells to produce atypia on cytologic examination. Colposcopy is useful (see Chapter 50). Cervical cytology and histologic examination by endocervical curettage and biopsy should be performed to help distinguish chronic cervicitis from developing cancer of the cervix.

Lesions of syphilis and chancroid as well as the chronic granulomatous ulcerations of tuberculosis and granuloma inguinale also should be considered.

Complications

Leukorrhea, cervical stenosis, and infertility are sequelae of chronic cervicitis. Patients with acute or chronic cervicitis may complain of vaginal discharge and vaginal bleeding, most frequently after sexual intercourse. With *N gonorrhoeae* or *C trachomatis* cervicitis, salpingitis is a common complication, with long-term consequences including infertility and chronic pelvic pain. Gonorrheal and chlamydial cervicitis causing increased shedding of HIV 1 in HIV infected women has been reported. A history of genital infections is more common among women with carcinoma of the cervix; however, no current evidence suggests that these agents increase the risk of developing cancer in women with cervicitis.

Prevention

Gonorrheal, herpetic, and chlamydial cervicitis can be prevented by educating those at risk about ways to reduce their risk. Avoidance of sexual contact with infected persons and the use of condoms for protection during coitus are the most important recommendations for changing the sexual behaviors of women at risk for infection. Clinicians should be aware of the importance of detection in the asymptomatic patient, followed by effective treatment and counseling of the patient and her sexual partners. The avoidance of surgical or obstetric trauma and the prompt recognition and proper repair of cervical lacerations help to prevent the subsequent development of a chronically infected cervix.

When surgical removal of the corpus of the uterus is indicated, the cervix should also be removed if this is feasible. Recommendations to retain the cervix at the time of hysterectomy in order to maintain sexual function or vaginal support are controversial.

Treatment

Selection of the most appropriate treatment depends on the age of the patient and her desire for pregnancy; whether she is presently pregnant or is breastfeeding; the severity of the cervical infection; the presence of complicating factors (eg, salpingitis); and previous treatment. Instrumentation and vigorous topical therapy should be avoided during the acute phase of cervicitis and before the menses, when ascending infection may occur.

A. ACUTE CERVICITIS

When acute cervicitis is associated with vaginitis due to a specific organism, treatment must be directed accordingly. Metronidazole is specific for treatment of *T vaginalis* infection. Metronidazole can be administered as 2 g orally in a single dose or alternatively as 500 mg twice daily for 7 days. This has resulted in cure rates of approximately 90–95%. Ensuring treatment of sex partners might increase the cure rate. Topical forms of metronidazole appears to be less efficacious than the oral preparations. Candidiasis is most effectively treated with topically applied azole drugs. This will result in relief of symptoms and negative cultures in 80–90% of patients. Treatment may continue for 1, 3, or 7 days, depending on the severity of infection. Oral fluconazole in a 150-mg oral tablet has been shown to be effective treatment.

Bacterial vaginosis can be treated with oral metronidazole 500 mg twice daily for 7 days, or with topical clindamycin cream or metronidazole gel. Treatment of bacterial vaginosis in pregnancy is particularly important because of its association with adverse outcomes such as preterm labor and premature rupture of the membranes. Pregnant women without risk of premature delivery should be treated if they have symptomatic bacterial vaginosis. High-risk women should be tested and treated regardless of the presence of symptoms. Treatment in pregnancy is metronidazole 250 mg orally 3 times daily for 7 days. Metronidazole has not been shown to be teratogenic in humans.

C trachomatis can be treated with azithromycin 1 g orally in a single dose or alternatively with doxycycline 100 mg twice daily for 7 days. Alternative treatments with erythromycin or ofloxacin are suggested. In pregnancy, azithromycin may be given. Amoxicillin for 7 days has also been shown to be effective and well tolerated. Cervicitis due to *N gonorrhoeae* can be treated with single oral doses of ofloxacin 400 mg or ciprofloxacin 500 mg. An intramuscular injection of ceftriaxone 125 mg may also be used. In pregnancy, fluoroquinolones should be avoided. Fluoroquinolones also should not be used in patients residing in, or who may have acquired infections in, Asia, the Pacific (including Hawaii), or California. This is due to increasing quinolone-resistant *N gonorrhoeae* (QRNG) in these areas (see Chapters 41 and 42 and the 2002 Centers for Disease Control guidelines for treatment of STDs for full recommendations). Because of the high rate of coinfection with *C trachomatis* (up to 42%), it is recommended that patients also receive treatment for *C trachomatis* when *N gonorrhoeae* infection is found.

B. CHRONIC CERVICITIS

Several studies using more sensitive testing for *N gonorrhoeae* and *C trachomatis* have demonstrated that microscopic findings of 10 or more polymorphonuclear leukocytes per high-power field do not correlate with infection. Therefore it is not necessary to treat an asymptomatic patient with chronic cervicitis who does not test positive for an STD.

Surgical procedures may be useful for treatment of symptomatic chronic cervicitis or in the absence of an infectious pathogen or evidence of dysplasia. Techniques including cryosurgery, electrocauterization, and laser therapy may be of use, although significant disadvantages include the high risk for recurrence and risk for cervical injury.

Treatment of Complications

A. CERVICAL HEMORRHAGE

This may follow electrocauterization, loop excision, cryosurgery, or laser vaporization and may require suture and ligation of the bleeding vessels. Usually, point coagulation of bleeding areas with Monsel's solution or silver nitrate applied topically is successful. Repeat electrocauterization may also be beneficial.

B. SALPINGITIS

Inflammation of the uterine tubes usually necessitates the administration of a broad-spectrum antibiotic.

C. LEUKORRHEA

Significant cervical discharge may be due to persistent infection with a pathogen. Appropriate testing should be performed and selective antibiotic treatment administered.

D. CERVICAL STENOSIS

The gentle passage of graduated sounds through the cervical canal at weekly intervals during the intermenstrual phase for 2–3 months following treatment will prevent or correct stenosis.

E. INFERTILITY

The absence of cervical mucus necessary for sperm migration often causes infertility and may be due to extensive destruction (cauterization, freezing, or vaporization) or removal (conization or loop excision) of the endocervical glandular cells. Treatment includes low-dose estrogen for 1 week prior to ovulation or intrauterine insemination with washed and incubated sperm.

Prognosis

With conservative, systemic, and persistent therapy, cervicitis can almost always be cured. With neglect or overtreatment, the prognosis is poor.

GRANULOMATOUS INFECTIONS OF THE CERVIX

Tuberculosis, tertiary syphilis, and granuloma inguinale may on rare occasions be manifested by chronic cervical lesions. These lesions usually take the form of nodules, ulcerations, or granulation tissue. They produce a chronic inflammatory exudate characterized histologically by lymphocytes, giant cells, and histiocytes. They may simulate carcinoma of the cervix and must be distinguished from this and other neoplastic diseases.

Tuberculosis

Since 1986, the steadily decreasing incidence of tuberculosis in the United States over the previous several decades has reversed, and the risk has increased, particularly for blacks, Hispanics, and Asians. Some of this increase has been attributed to the epidemic spread of HIV.

Genitourinary tuberculosis is almost always secondary to infection elsewhere in the body, usually pulmonary, but active pulmonary disease can be documented in only one-third of patients. Vascular dissemination is responsible for infection of the fallopian tubes in almost all patients with genital tuberculosis, and involvement of the endometrium follows in 90%. Cervical disease can occur by direct extension or lymphatic spread but is rare, occurring in only 1% of cases. In the past, genital tuberculosis has accounted for only 1% of patients with pelvic inflammatory disease; however, in European and Asian countries, the occurrence ranges from 5–13%. With increasing numbers of immigrants to the United States and with the rise in incidence of AIDS in American women, an increase in the incidence of pelvic tuberculosis can be expected.

The chief clinical manifestations of pelvic and cervical involvement are abdominal pain, irregular bleeding, and constitutional symptoms. The cervix may be hypertrophied and nodular, without any visible lesion on the portio vaginalis. Speculum examination may demonstrate either an ulcerative or a papillary lesion, thus resembling neoplastic disease.

The diagnosis of tuberculosis of the cervix must be made by biopsy. Histologically, the disease is characterized by tubercles undergoing central caseation. Because such lesions may be caused by other entities such as amoebiasis, schistosomiasis, brucellosis, tularemia, sarcoidosis, and foreign body reaction, the tubercle bacillus must be demonstrated by acid-fast stains or culture.

The reader is referred to other texts for the details of medical therapy of genital tuberculosis. Most patients are cured by medical management alone. Patients who respond poorly or who have other problems (eg, tumors, fistulas) may require total hysterectomy and bilateral salpingo-oophorectomy after a trial of chemotherapy.

RARE INFECTIOUS DISEASES OF THE CERVIX

Lymphogranuloma venereum, a chlamydial infection, and chancroid, caused by *Haemophilus ducreyi*, may attack the cervix along with other areas of the reproductive tract.

Cervical actinomycosis may occur as a result of contamination by instruments and by intrauterine devices. The cervical lesion may be a nodular tumor, ulcer, or fistula. Prolonged penicillin or sulfonamide therapy is recommended.

Schistosomiasis of the cervix usually is secondary to involvement of the pelvic and uterine veins by the blood fluke *Schistosoma haematobium*. Cervical schistosomiasis may produce a large papillary growth that ulcerates and bleeds on contact, simulating cervical cancer. In other instances, it may be found in endocervical polyps, causing intermenstrual and postcoital bleeding. An ovum occasionally can be identified in a biopsy specimen taken from the granulomatous cervical lesion. However, the diagnosis usually is made

by recovering the parasite from the urine or feces. Chemical, serologic, and intradermal tests for schistosomiasis are available.

Echinococcal cysts may involve the cervix. Treatment consists of surgical excision.

CYSTIC ABNORMALITIES OF THE CERVIX

Nabothian Cysts

Nabothian cysts develop when a tunnel or cleft of tall columnar endocervical epithelium becomes covered by squamous metaplasia. They appear grossly as translucent or yellow and may vary in diameter from a few millimeters to 3 cm.

Mesonephric Cysts

Microscopic remnants of the mesonephric (wolffian) duct are often seen deep in the stroma externally in the normal cervix. Occasionally they become cystic, forming structures up to 2.5 mm in diameter, lined by ragged cuboid epithelium. They may be confused with deeply situated nabothian cysts, but their location and the wolffian-type cells lining the cysts serve as useful distinguishing features.

CERVICAL STENOSIS

Cervical stenosis of congenital, inflammatory, neoplastic, or surgical origin may be partially or even completely occlusive. Most cases of cervical stenosis follow extensive surgical manipulation of the cervix (eg, electrocoagulation, cryotherapy, laser vaporization, conization, or cervical amputation) or radiation therapy. Cervical stenosis is not uncommon, however, in postmenopausal women with prolonged estrogen deficiency. Marked to complete obstruction of menstrual drainage will result in hematometra, typified by cryptomenorrhea or amenorrhea; abdominal discomfort; and a soft, slightly tender midpelvic mass. Pyometra may develop in the postmenopausal woman with cervical stenosis and always raises the suspicion of an associated endometrial carcinoma. Both hematometra and pyometra are readily confirmed by pelvic ultrasonography.

Cautious dilatation of the cervix is recommended, with drainage of the entrapped fluid. Cultures and sensitivity tests should be performed and, with appropriate antibiotic coverage, cervical endometrial tissue or both should be obtained to rule out cancer. The endocervical canal should receive minimal caustic therapy or electrotherapy for chronic cervicitis to prevent cervical stenosis. Removal of the cicatrix by laser vaporization and loop excision has been effective in cases of postconization stenosis.

BENIGN NEOPLASMS OF THE CERVIX

1. Microglandular Hyperplasia of the Endocervical Mucosa

Microglandular hyperplasia (MGH) usually occurs in women of reproductive age, but 6% of known cases are detected in postmenopausal women. MGH has been linked to hormonal stimulus of oral contraceptive use and pregnancy, although reports have questioned this association. MGH also may result from inflammation. Grossly, adenomatous hyperplasia appears as exuberant granular tissue within the cervical canal, often extruding beyond the cervical os. The disorder may be mistaken for cancer, but biopsy should be performed to make the distinction. Microscopically, it presents as a collection of closely packed cystic spaces lined by nonneoplastic columnar epithelium and filled with mucus.

2. Cervical Polyps

ESSENTIALS OF DIAGNOSIS

- *Intermenstrual or postcoital bleeding.*
- *A soft, red pedunculated protrusion from the cervical canal at the external os.*
- *Microscopic examination confirms the diagnosis of benign polyp.*

General Considerations

Cervical polyps are small, pedunculated, often sessile neoplasms of the cervix. Most originate from the endocervix; a few arise from the portio (Fig 38–12). They are composed of a vascular connective tissue stroma and are covered by columnar, squamocolumnar, or squamous epithelium. Polyps are relatively common, especially in multigravidas over 20 years of age. They are rare before menarche, but an occasional polyp may develop after menopause. Asymptomatic polyps often are discovered on routine pelvic examination. Most are benign, but all should be removed and submitted for pathologic examination because malignant change may occur. Moreover, some cervical cancers present as a polypoid mass.

Polyps arise as a result of focal hyperplasia of the endocervix. Whether this is due to chronic inflammation, an abnormal local responsiveness to hormonal stimulation, or a localized vascular congestion of cervical blood vessels is not known. They are often

Figure 38–12. Cervical polyp.

found in association with endometrial hyperplasia, suggesting that hyperestrogenism plays a significant etiologic role.

Endocervical polyps usually are red, flame-shaped, fragile growths. The polyps vary from a few millimeters in length and diameter to larger tumors 2–3 cm in diameter and several centimeters long. These polyps usually are attached to the endocervical mucosa near the external os by a narrow pedicle, but occasionally the base is broad. On microscopic examination, the stroma of a polyp is composed of fibrous connective tissue containing numerous small vessels in the center. There is often extravasation of blood and marked infiltration of the stroma by inflammatory cells (polymorphonuclear neutrophils, lymphocytes, and plasma cells). The surface epithelium resembles that of the endocervix, varying from typical picket-fence columnar cells to areas that show squamous metaplasia and mature stratified squamous epithelium. The surface often is thrown into folds, as is much of the normal endocervical mucosa.

Ectocervical polyps are pale, flesh-colored, smooth, and rounded or elongated, often with a broad pedicle. They arise from the portio and are less likely to bleed than are endocervical polyps. Microscopically, they are more fibrous than endocervical polyps, with few or no mucus glands. They are covered by stratified squamous epithelium.

Metaplastic alteration is common. Inflammation, often with necrosis at the tip (or more extensively), is typical of both polyp types.

The incidence of malignant change in a cervical polyp is estimated to be less than 1%. Squamous cell carcinoma is the most common type, although adenocarcinomas have been reported. Endometrial cancer may involve the polyp secondarily. Sarcoma rarely develops within a polyp.

Botryoid sarcoma, an embryonal rhabdomyosarcoma tumor of the cervix (or vaginal wall) resembling small pink or yellow grapes, contains striated muscle and other mesenchymal elements. It is extremely malignant. Most polypoid structures are vascular, often are infected, and are subject to displacement or torsion. Discharge commonly results, and bleeding, often metrorrhagia of the postcoital type, follows.

Chronic irritation and bleeding are annoying and cause cervicitis, endometritis, and parametritis. Salpingitis may develop if conditions these are not treated successfully.

Because polyps are a potential focus of cancer, they must be examined routinely for malignant characteristics upon removal.

Clinical Findings

A. Symptoms and Signs

Intermenstrual or postcoital bleeding is the most common symptom of cervical polyps. Leukorrhea and hypermenorrhea have also been associated with cervical polyps.

Abnormal vaginal bleeding is often reported. Postmenopausal bleeding is frequently described by older women. Infertility may be traceable to cervical polyps and cervicitis.

Cervical polyps appear as smooth, red, fingerlike projections from the cervical canal. They usually are approximately 1–2 cm in length and 0.5–1 cm in diameter. Generally they are too soft to be felt by the examiner's finger.

B. X-Ray Findings

Polyps high in the endocervical canal may be demonstrated by hysterosalpingogram or saline infusion sonohysterography. They often are significant findings in hitherto unexplained infertility.

C. Laboratory Findings

Vaginal cytology will reveal signs of infection and often mildly atypical cells. Blood and urine studies are not helpful.

D. Special Examination

A polyp high in the endocervical canal may be seen with the aid of a special endocervical speculum or by hysteroscopy. Some polyps are found only at the time of diagnostic D&C in the investigation of abnormal bleeding.

Differential Diagnosis

Masses projecting from the cervix may be polypoid but not polyps. Adenocarcinoma of the endometrium or endometrial sarcoma may present at the external os or even beyond. Discharge and bleeding usually occur.

Typical polyps are not difficult to diagnose by gross inspection, but ulcerated and atypical growths must be distinguished from small submucous pedunculated myomas or endometrial polyps arising low in the uterus. These often result in dilatation of the cervix, presenting just within the os and resembling cervical polyps. The products of conception, usually decidua, may push through the cervix and resemble a polypoid tissue mass, but other signs and symptoms of recent pregnancy generally are absent. Condylomata, submucous myomas, and polypoid carcinomas are diagnosed by microscopic examination.

Complications

Cervical polyps may be infected, some by virulent staphylococci, streptococci, or other pathogens. Serious infections occasionally follow instrumentation for the identification or removal of polyps. A broad-spectrum antibiotic should be administered at the first sign or symptom of spreading infection.

Acute salpingitis may be initiated or exacerbated by polypectomy.

It is unwise to remove a large polyp and then perform a hysterectomy several days thereafter. Pelvic peritonitis may complicate the latter procedure. A delay of several weeks or 1 month between polypectomy and hysterectomy is recommended.

Treatment

A. Medical Measures

Appropriate testing for cervical discharge should be performed as indicated and treatment administered if infection is identified.

B. Specific Measures

Most polyps can be removed in the physician's office. This is done with little bleeding by grasping the pedicle with a hemostat or long grasping instrument and twisting it until the growth is avulsed. Large polyps and those with sessile attachments may require excision in an operating room. This will allow for administration of anesthesia for further visualization, treatment using the hysteroscope, and control of any hemorrhage.

If the cervix is soft, patulous, or definitely dilated and the polyp is large, hysteroscopy should be performed, especially if the pedicle is not readily visible. Exploration of the cervical and uterine cavities with the hysteroscope allows for further identification of other polyps. All tissue must be sent to a pathologist to be examined for possible underlying malignant or premalignant conditions.

Prognosis

Simple removal of cervical polyps is usually curative.

3. Papillomas of the Cervix

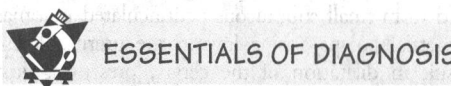

ESSENTIALS OF DIAGNOSIS

- Asymptomatic.
- Papillary projection from the exocervix.
- The presence of koilocytes with or without cyto-logic atypia.
- Colposcopic identification.

General Considerations

Cervical papillomas are benign neoplasms found on the portio vaginalis of the cervix. The neoplasms consist of 2 types. (1) The typical solitary papillary projection from the exocervix, composed of a central core of fibrous connective tissue covered by stratified squamous epithelium. This is a true benign neoplasm, and the cause is unknown. (2) Condylomata of the cervix, which may be present in various forms ranging from a slightly raised area on the exocervix that appears white after acetic acid application (on colposcopy) to the typical condyloma acuminatum. These usually are multiple and are caused by HPV infection, an STD. Similar lesions of the vagina and vulva are often, but not always, present. Evidence of HPV infection can be found in 1–2% of cytologically screened women. The incidence is much higher in women attending STD clinics.

Clinical Findings

A. Symptoms and Signs

There are no characteristic symptoms of cervical papillomas; they are often discovered on routine pelvic examination or colposcopic examination for dysplasia revealed by Pap smear.

B. Laboratory Findings

Cytologic findings of koilocytes—squamous cells with perinuclear clear halos—are strongly suggestive of HPV infection. Dysplastic squamous cells are frequently found in association with koilocytes. Biopsy of involved epithelium reveals papillomatosis and acanthosis. Mitoses may be frequent, but in the absence of neoplastic change, the cells are orderly with regular nuclear features. Koilocytes predominate in the superficial cells.

Complications

Intraepithelial neoplasia is associated with certain types of HPV infection (see Cervical Intraepithelial Neoplasia, Chapter 50). The presence of condylomata of the portio vaginalis substantially increases the risk for squamous cell carcinoma of the cervix.

Prevention

Contraception with condoms and other barrier methods may prevent primary infection and reinfection.

Treatment

Solitary papillomas should be surgically excised and submitted for pathologic examination. Likewise, biopsies of flat condylomata should be submitted for histopathologic examination. Flat condylomata may be completely removed with a biopsy instrument if they are small. More extensive lesions may require cryotherapy, loop excision, or laser vaporization. Dysplasia associated with HPV infection should be managed according to the severity and extent of the dysplastic process (see Cervical Intraepithelial Neoplasia, Chapter 50).

Prognosis

Because the entire lower genital tract is a target area for HPV infection, long-term follow-up with attention to the cervix, vagina, and vulva is necessary. Excision of solitary, non–PV-related papillomas is curative.

4. Leiomyomas of the Cervix

The paucity of smooth muscle elements in the cervical stroma makes leiomyomas that arise in the cervix uncommon. The corpus leiomyoma/cervical leiomyoma ratio is in the range of 12:1.

Although myomas usually are multiple in the corpus, cervical myomas are most often solitary and may be large enough to fill the entire pelvic cavity, compressing the bladder, rectum, and ureters (Fig 38–13). Grossly and microscopically they are identical to leiomyomas that arise elsewhere in the uterus.

Clinical Findings

A. Symptoms and Signs

Cervical leiomyomas are often silent, producing no symptoms unless they become very large. Symptoms result from pressure on surrounding organs such as the bladder, rectum, or soft tissues of the parametrium, or obstruction of the cervical canal. Frequency and ur-

Figure 38–13. Large cervical leiomyoma filling true pelvis.

gency of urination are the result of bladder compression. Urinary retention occasionally occurs as a result of pressure against the urethra. Hematometra may develop with obstruction of the cervix.

If the direction of growth is lateral, there may be ureteral obstruction with hydronephrosis. Rectal encroachment causes constipation. Dyspareunia may occur if the tumor occupies the vagina. In pregnancy, because of their location, large cervical leiomyomas, unlike those involving the corpus, are apt to cause soft-tissue dystocia, preventing descent of the presenting part in the pelvis. Cervical leiomyomas of significant size can be readily palpated on bimanual examination.

B. IMAGING

A plain film may demonstrate the typical mottled calcific pattern associated with cervical leiomyomas. Hysterography may define distortion of the endocervical canal. Intravenous urography may demonstrate ureteral displacement or obstruction. MRI is diagnostic.

Treatment

Small, asymptomatic cervical leiomyomas do not require treatment. If the leiomyomas become symptomatic, removal may be possible via hysteroscopic resection. If additional multiple leiomyomas are present that cannot be resected with the hysteroscope, uterine artery embolization, abdominal myomectomy, or hysterectomy may be indicated, depending on the patient's desire for preservation of fertility.

Because of the proximity of the pelvic ureter to the cervix, this structure may be in jeopardy in any operation involving a cervical leiomyoma, and precautions should be taken to prevent its injury.

Prognosis

Recurrence of cervical myomas after surgical removal is rare.

REFERENCES

Anomalies of the Cervix

ACOG Practice Bulletin. Cervical insufficiency. Obstet Gynecol 2003;102:1091

Deffarges JV et al: Utero-vaginal anastomosis in women with uterine cervix atresia: Long-term follow-up and reproductive performance. A study of 18 cases. Hum Reprod 2001;16:1722.

Folch M, Pigem I, Konje JC: Müllerian agenesis: Etiology, diagnosis and management. Obstet Gynecol Surv 2000;55:644.

Fujimoto VY et al: Congenital cervical atresia: Report of seven cases and review of the literature. Am J Obstet Gynecol 1997;177:1419.

Gell JS: Mullerian anomalies. Semin Reprod Med 2003;21:375.

Goldberg JM, Falcone T: Effect of diethylstilbestrol on reproductive function. Fertil Steril 1999;72:1.

Homer HA, Li TC, Cooke ID: The septate uterus: A review of management and reproductive outcome. Fertil Steril 2000;73:1.

Kaufman RH et al: Continued follow up of pregnancy outcomes in diethylstilbestrol-exposed offspring. Obstet Gynecol 2000;96:483.

Keser A et al: Treatment of vaginal agenesis with modified Abbe-McIndoe technique: Long-term follow-up in 22 patients. Eur J Obstet Gynecol Reprod Biol 2005;121:110.

Preutthipan S, Herabutya Y: Vaginal misoprostol for cervical priming before operative hysteroscopy: A randomized controlled trial. Obstet Gynecol 2000;96:890.

Propst AM, Hill JA: Anatomic factors associated with recurrent pregnancy loss. Semin Reprod Med 2000;18:341.

Simpson JL: Genetics of the female reproductive ducts. Am J Med Genet 1999;89:224.

Troiano RN, McCarthy SM: Mullerian duct anomalies: Imaging and clinical issues. Radiology 2004;233:19.

Cervical Infections

Adair CD et al: Chlamydia in pregnancy: A randomized trial of azithromycin and erythromycin. Obstet Gynecol 1998;91:165.

Anttila T et al: Serotypes of *Chlamydia trachomatis* and risk for development of cervical squamous cell carcinoma. JAMA 2001; 285:47.

Black CM: Current methods of laboratory diagnosis of *Chlamydia trachomatis* infections. Clin Microbiol Rev 1997;10:160.

Black CM et al: Head-to-head multicenter comparison of DNA probe and nucleic acid amplification tests for Chlamydia trachomatis infection in women performed with an improved reference standard. J Clin Microbiol 2002;40:3757.

Bohmer JT et al: Cervical wet mount as a negative predictor for gonococci- and *Chlamydia trachomatis*-induced cervicitis in a gravid population. Am J Obstet Gynecol 1999;181:283.

Cates W Jr: Estimates of the incidence and prevalence of sexually transmitted diseases in the United States. American Social Health Association Panel. Sex Transm Dis 1999;26(4 Suppl):S2.

Centers for Disease Control and Prevention: Sexually transmitted disease treatment guidelines. MMWR Recomm Rep 2002; 51(RR-6):1.

Chow TW, Lim BK, Vallipuram S: The masquerades of female pelvic tuberculosis: Case reports and review of literature on clinical presentations and diagnosis. J Obstet Gynaecol Res 2002;28:203.

Cook RL et al: Systematic review: Noninvasive testing for Chlamydia trachomatis and Neisseria gonorrhoeae. Ann Intern Med 2005;142:914.

Dalgic H, Kuscu NK: Laser therapy in chronic cervicitis. Arch Gynecol Obstet 2001;265:64.

Gaydos CA et al: *Chlamydia trachomatis* infections in female military recruits. N Engl J Med 1998;339:739.

Hook EW III et al: Diagnosis of genitourinary *Chlamydia trachomatis* infections by using the ligase chain reaction on patient-obtained vaginal swabs. J Clin Microbiol 1997;35:2133.

Kaufman RH et al: Human papillomavirus testing as triage for atypical squamous cells of undetermined significance and low-grade squamous intraepithelial lesions: Sensitivity, specificity, and cost-effectiveness. Am J Obstet Gynecol 1997;177:930.

Kerry L et al: Embryonal rhabdomyosarcoma (sarcoma botryoides) of the cervix presenting as a cervical polyp treated with fertility-sparing surgery and adjuvant chemotherapy. Gynecol Oncol 2004;95:243.

Lamba H et al: Tuberculosis of the cervix: Case presentation and a review of the literature. Sex Transm Infect 2002;78:62.

Lanham S et al: Detection of cervical infections in colposcopy clinic patients. J Clin Microbiol 2001;39:2946.

Marrazzo JM: Mucopurulent cervicitis: No longer ignored, but still misunderstood. Infect Dis Clin North Am 2005;19:333.

Marrazzo JM et al: Predicting chlamydial and gonococcal cervical infection: Implications for management of cervicitis. Obstet Gynecol 2002;100:579.

McClelland RS et al: Treatment of cervicitis is associated with decreased cervical shedding of HIV-1. AIDS 2001;15:105.

Mehta SD et al: Unsuspected gonorrhea and chlamydia in patients of an urban adult emergency department: A critical population for STD control intervention. Sex Transm Dis 2001; 28:33.

Modarress KJ et al: Detection of *Chlamydia trachomatis* and *Neisseria gonorrhoeae* in swab specimens by the Hybrid Capture II and PACE 2 nucleic acid probe tests. Sex Transm Dis 1999; 26:303.

Moore SG et al: Clinical utility of measuring white blood cells on vaginal wet mount and endocervical gram stain for the prediction of chlamydial and gonococcal infections. Sex Transm Dis 2000;27:530.

Myziuk L, Romanowski B, Brown M: Endocervical Gram stain smears and their usefulness in the diagnosis of *Chlamydia trachomatis*. Sex Transm Infect 2001;77:103.

Nucci MR: Symposium part III: Tumor-like glandular lesions of the uterine cervix. Int J Gynecol Pathol 2002;21:347.

Paavonen J et al: Cost-benefit analysis of first-void urine *Chlamydia trachomatis* screening program. Obstet Gynecol 1998;92:292.

Sellors J et al: Chlamydial cervicitis: Testing the practice guidelines for presumptive diagnosis. CMAJ 1998;158:41.

Stary A: Chlamydia screening: Which sample for which technique? Genitourin Med 1997;73:99.

Tyndall MW et al: Predicting *Neisseria gonorrhoeae* and *Chlamydia trachomatis* infection using risk scores, physical examination, microscopy, and leukocyte esterase urine dipsticks among asymptomatic women attending a family planning clinic in Kenya. Sex Transm Dis 1999;26:476.

US Preventive Services Task Force: Screening for Chlamydial infection: Recommendations and rationale. Am J Prev Med 2001; 20(3 Suppl):90.

Woodman CB et al: Natural history of cervical human papillomavirus infection in young women: A longitudinal cohort study. Lancet 2001;357:1831.

Wright TC Jr et al: Human immunodeficiency virus 1 expression in the female genital tract in association with cervical inflammation and ulceration. Am J Obstet Gynecol 2001;184:279.

Cervical Polyps and Leiomyomas

Ozsaran AA, Itil IM, Sagol S: Endometrial hyperplasia co-existing with cervical polyps. Int J Gynaecol Obstet 1999;66:185.

Tiltman AJ: Leiomyomas of the uterine cervix: A study of frequency. Int J Gynecol Pathol 1998;17:231.

Varasteh NN et al: Pregnancy rates after hysteroscopic polypectomy and myomectomy in infertile women. Obstet Gynecol 1999;94:168.

Varras M et al: Clinical considerations and sonographic findings of a large nonpedunculated primary cervical leiomyoma complicated by heavy vaginal haemorrhage: A case report and review of the literature. Clin Exp Obstet Gynecol 2003;30:144.

Benign Disorders of the Uterine Corpus

39

Jamie S. Drinville, MD, & Sandaz Memarzadeh, MD

LEIOMYOMA OF THE UTERUS (FIBROMYOMA, FIBROID, MYOMA)

 ESSENTIALS OF DIAGNOSIS

- *Mass: irregular enlargement of the uterus.*
- *Bleeding: menorrhagia, metrorrhagia, dysmenorrhea.*
- *Pain: torsion or degeneration.*
- *Pressure: symptoms from neighboring organs.*

General Considerations

Uterine leiomyomas are benign clonal neoplasms arising from smooth muscle cells in the uterine wall. They contain an increased amount of extracellular collagen and elastin. A thin pseudocapsule composed of areolar tissue and compressed muscle fibers surrounds the tumor. Leiomyomas may enlarge to cause significant distortion of the uterine surface or cavity. These tumors are present in 20–25% of reproductive-age women. However, for unknown reasons, leiomyomas occur 2–3 times more frequently in black than in white women. By their fifth decade, as many as 50% of black women will have leiomyomata.

Leiomyomas are not detectable before puberty and, being hormonally responsive, normally grow only during the reproductive years. Although they can occur as isolated growths, they are more commonly multiple. They usually are less than 15 cm in size but in rare cases may reach enormous proportions, weighing more than 45 kg (100 lb)

Although usually asymptomatic, leiomyomata can produce a wide spectrum of problems, including metrorrhagia and menorrhagia, pain, and infertility. Excessive uterine bleeding from leiomyomas is one of the most common indications for hysterectomy in the United States.

Asymptomatic leiomyomas may mask other concomitant and potentially lethal pelvic tumors, so the physician should not be deceived into following "asymptomatic myomas" without verifying that an underlying uterine tube, ovarian, or bowel carcinoma does not coexist. Occasionally it is necessary to differentiate leiomyomata from leiomyosarcoma. The latter occurs infrequently (<1% of cases) and is malignant.

Pathogenesis

The cause of uterine leiomyomata is not known. Glucose-6-phosphate dehydrogenase studies suggest that each individual leiomyoma is unicellular in origin (monoclonal). Although no evidence suggests that estrogens cause leiomyomas, estrogens certainly are implicated in growth of myomas. Leiomyomas contain estrogen receptors in higher concentrations than the surrounding myometrium but in lower concentrations than the endometrium. Progesterone increases the mitotic activity of myomas in young women. Progesterone may allow for tumor enlargement by downregulating apoptosis in the tumor. Estrogens may contribute to tumor enlargement by increasing the production of extracellular matrix. Leiomyomas may increase in size with estrogen therapy and during pregnancy but do not always do so. There is speculation that leiomyoma growth in pregnancy is related to synergistic activity of estradiol and human placental lactogen (hPL). They usually decrease in size after menopause.

Pathology

Leiomyomas are usually multiple, discrete, and either spherical or irregularly lobulated. Their pseudocapsule usually clearly demarcates them from the surrounding myometrium. They can be often easily and cleanly enucleated from the surrounding myometrial tissue. On gross examination in transverse section, they are buff-colored, rounded, smooth, and usually firm. Generally, they are lighter in color than the myometrium (Fig 39–1). When a fresh specimen is sectioned, the tumor surface

Figure 39–1. Multiple leiomyomas. Cervix is opened at the bottom.

projects above the surface of the surrounding musculature, revealing the pseudocapsule.

A. CLASSIFICATION

Uterine leiomyomas originate in the myometrium and are classified by anatomic location (Fig 39–2). Submucous leiomyomas lie just beneath the endometrium and tend to compress it as they grow toward the uterine lumen. Their impact on the endometrium and its blood supply most often leads to irregular uterine bleeding. Leiomyomata may develop pedicles and protrude fully into the uterine cavity. Occasionally they pass through the cervical canal while still attached within the corpus by a long stalk. When this occurs, leiomyomata are subject to torsion or infection, conditions that must be taken into onsideration before treatment.

Intramural or interstitial leiomyomas lie within the uterine wall, giving it a variable consistency. Subserous or subperitoneal leiomyomata may lie just at the serosal surface of the uterus or may bulge outward from the myometrium. The subserous leiomyomata may become pedunculated. If such a tumor acquires an extrauterine blood supply from omental vessels, its pedicle may atrophy and resorb; the tumor is then said to be *parasitic*. Subserous tumors arising laterally may extend between the 2 peritoneal layers of the broad ligament to become intraligamentary leiomyomas. This may lead to compromise of the ureter and/or pelvic blood supply.

B. MICROSCOPIC STRUCTURE

Nonstriated muscle fibers are arranged in interlacing bundles of varying size running in different directions (whorled appearance). Individual cells are spindle-shaped, have elongated nuclei, and are uniform in size. Varying amounts of connective tissue are intermixed with the smooth muscle bundles. Leiomyomata are sharply demarcated from surrounding normal musculature by a pseudocapsule of areolar tissue and compressed myometrium. The arterial density of a leiomyoma is less than that of the surrounding myometrium, and the small arteries that supply the tumor are less tortuous than are the adjacent radial arteries. The arteries penetrate the myoma randomly on its surface and are oriented in the direction of the muscle bundles; thus, they present no regular pattern. One or 2 major vessels may be found in the base or pedicle. The venous pattern appears to be even more sparse, but this may be in part artifactual because of the difficulty encountered in filling the venous circulation under artificial conditions.

C. SECONDARY CHANGES

There may be areas of hyalinization, liquefaction (cystic degeneration), calcification, hemorrhage, fat, or inflammation within leiomyomata. Although these secondary alterations are histologically interesting, they usually have little clinical significance. Whether leiomyosarco-

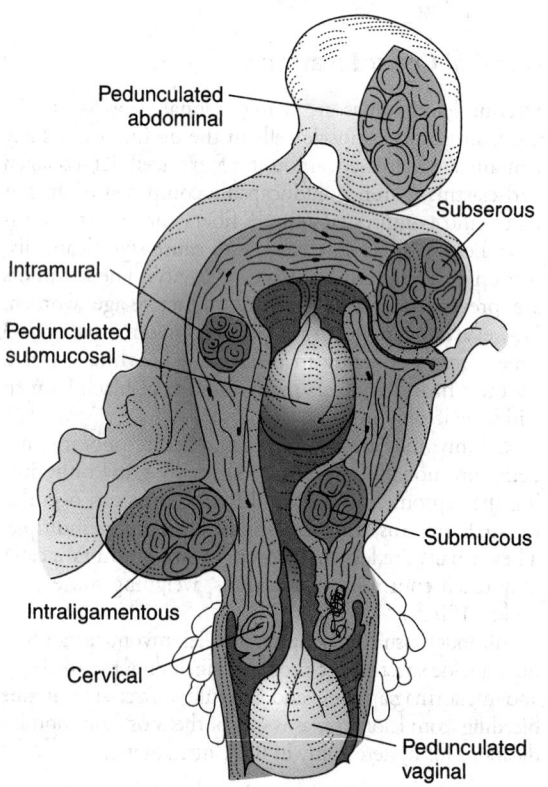

Figure 39–2. Myomas of the uterus.

mas are a malignant alteration within a mature leiomyoma, as is commonly stated, or arise de novo remains an unsettled issue. Extraordinarily cellular myomas have often been misinterpreted as sarcomas because the criteria used to differentiate leiomyoma from sarcoma are imprecise and often subjective. Ultrastructural studies suggest that leiomyoma and leiomyosarcoma are distinct entities and that the cellular leiomyoma is merely a variety of the common leiomyoma.

1. Benign degeneration—Benign degeneration consists of the following types:

a. Atrophic—Signs and symptoms regress or disappear as tumor size decreases at menopause or after pregnancy.

b. Hyaline—Mature or "old" leiomyomas are white but contain yellow, soft, and often gelatinous areas of hyaline change. These tumors are usually asymptomatic.

c. Cystic—Liquefaction follows extreme hyalinization, and physical stress may cause sudden evacuation of fluid contents into the uterus, the peritoneal cavity, or the retroperitoneal space.

d. Calcific (calcareous)—Subserous leiomyomata are most commonly affected by circulatory deprivation, which causes precipitation of calcium carbonate and phosphate within the tumor.

e. Septic—Circulatory inadequacy may cause necrosis of the central portion of the tumor followed by infection. Acute pain, tenderness, and fever result.

f. Carneous (red)—Venous thrombosis and congestion with interstitial hemorrhage are responsible for the color of a leiomyoma undergoing red degeneration (Fig 39–3). During pregnancy, when carneous degeneration is most common, edema and hypertrophy of the myometrium occur. The physiologic changes in the leiomyoma are not the same as in the myometrium; the resultant anatomic discrepancy impedes the blood supply, resulting in aseptic degeneration and infarction. The process is usually accompanied by pain but is self-limited. Potential complications of degeneration in pregnancy include preterm labor and, rarely, initiation of disseminated intravascular coagulation.

g. Myxomatous (fatty)—This uncommon and asymptomatic degeneration follows hyaline and cystic degeneration.

2. Metastasizing leiomyomata—Rarely, myomas spread beyond the uterus to distant locations such as the peritoneum, distant vasculature, and lung. Histologically these leiomyomas appear benign and have a low mitotic rate, and they are often asymptomatic. Most women with these tumors have undergone a prior dilatation and curettage (D&C), myomectomy, or hysterectomy, suggesting the possibility of surgically induced vascular spread of leiomyoma cells. Another theory suggests a multifocal origin from smooth muscle in blood vessels anywhere in the body.

Figure 39–3. Carneous (red) degeneration. Note the congested, dark appearance compared with Figure 39–1.

Clinical Findings

A. SYMPTOMS

Symptoms are present in only 35–50% of patients with leiomyomas. Thus, most leiomyomata do not produce symptoms, and even very large ones may remain undetected, particularly in obese patients. Symptoms from leiomyomas depend on their location, size, state of preservation, and whether the patient is pregnant.

1. Abnormal uterine bleeding—Abnormal uterine bleeding is the most common and most important clinical manifestation of leiomyomas, being present in up to 30% of patients. The abnormal bleeding commonly produces iron deficiency anemia, which may not be uncontrollable even with iron therapy if the bleeding is heavy and protracted.

Bleeding from a submucous leiomyoma may occur from interruption of the blood supply to the endometrium, distortion and congestion of the surrounding vessels, particularly the veins, or ulceration of the overlying endometrium. Most commonly, the patient has prolonged, heavy menses (menorrhagia), premenstrual spotting, or prolonged light staining following menses; however, any type of abnormal bleeding is possible.

Minor degrees of metrorrhagia (intermenstrual bleeding) may be associated with a tumor that has areas of endometrial venous thrombosis and necrosis on its surface, particularly if it is pedunculated and partially extruded through the cervical canal.

2. Pain—Leiomyomata may cause pain when vascular compromise occurs. Thus, pain may result from degeneration associated with vascular occlusion, infection, torsion of a pedunculated tumor, or myometrial contractions to expel a subserous myoma from the uterine cavity. The pain associated with infarction from torsion or red degeneration can be excruciating and produce a clinical picture consistent with acute abdomen.

Large tumors may produce a sensation of heaviness or fullness in the pelvic area, a feeling of a mass in the pelvis, or a feeling of a mass palpable through the abdominal wall. Tumors that become impacted within the bony pelvis may press on nerves and create pain radiating to the back or lower extremities; however, backache is such a common general complaint that it is usually difficult to ascribe it specifically to myomas.

Pain with intercourse may result, depending on the position of the tumors and the pressure they exert on the vaginal walls.

3. Pressure effects—Pressure effects are unusual and difficult to directly relate to leiomyomata, unless the tumors are very large. Intramural or intraligamentous leiomyomata may distort or obstruct other organs. Parasitic tumors may cause intestinal obstruction if they are large or involve omentum or bowel. Cervical tumors may cause serosanguineous vaginal discharge, vaginal bleeding, dyspareunia, and infertility. Large tumors may fill the true pelvis and displace or compress the ureters, bladder, or rectum.

Compression of surrounding structures may result in urinary symptoms or hydroureter. Large tumors may cause pelvic venous congestion and lower extremity edema or constipation. Rarely, a posterior fundal leiomyoma carries the uterus into extreme retroflexion, distorting the bladder base and causing urinary retention. This may present as intermittent overflow incontinence produced by elongation of the urethra with loss of sphincter control—a situation identical to sacculation of the uterus during early pregnancy. The condition is relieved by dislodging the uterus from the true pelvis with the patient in the knee–chest position.

4. Infertility—The relationship between fibroids and infertility remains uncertain. Between 27% and 40% of women with multiple leiomyomas are reported to be infertile, but other causes of infertility are present in a majority of cases. When fibroids are entirely or mostly endocavitary, a strong rationale supports the use of surgery to improve fertility.

5. Spontaneous abortion—The incidence of spontaneous abortion secondary to leiomyoma is unknown but is possibly 2 times the incidence in normal pregnant women. For example, the incidence of spontaneous abortion prior to myomectomy is approximately 40% and following myomectomy is approximately 20%.

B. Examination

Most myomas are discovered by routine bimanual examination of the uterus or sometimes by palpation of the lower abdomen. Uterine retroflexion and retroversion may obscure the physical examination diagnosis of even moderately large leiomyomata. When the cervix is pulled up behind the symphysis, large fibroids are usually implicated. The diagnosis is obvious when the normal uterine contour is distorted by 1 or more smooth, spherical, firm masses, but often it is difficult to be absolutely certain that such masses are part of the uterus. A pelvic ultrasound generally assists in establishing the diagnosis, as does excluding pregnancy as a cause of uterine enlargement. Magnetic resonance imaging (MRI) may better delineate the size and position of myomas but is not always clinically necessary.

C. Laboratory Findings

Anemia is a common consequence of leiomyomata due to excessive uterine bleeding and depletion of iron reserves. However, occasional patients display erythrocytosis. Hematocrit levels return to normal following removal of the uterus, and elevated erythropoietin levels have been reported in such cases. Moreover, the recognized association of polycythemia and renal disease has led to speculation that leiomyomas compress the ureters, causing ureteral back pressure and thus inducing renal erythropoietin production.

Leukocytosis, fever, and an elevated sedimentation rate may be present with acute degeneration or infection.

D. Imaging

Pelvic ultrasound examinations are useful in confirming the diagnosis of leiomyomata. Although ultrasound should never be a substitute for a thorough pelvic examination, it can be extremely helpful in identifying leiomyomata, detailing the cause of other pelvic masses, and identifying pregnancy. Moreover, ultrasonography is particularly useful in obese individuals. Saline sonohysterography can identify submucosal myomas that may be missed on ultrasound.

Large leiomyomata typically appear as soft tissue masses on x-ray films of the lower abdomen and pelvis; however, attention is sometimes drawn to the tumors by calcifications. Hysterosalpingography may be useful in detailing an intrauterine leiomyoma in the infertile patient.

Intravenous urography may be useful in the workup of any pelvic mass because it frequently reveals ureteral deviation or compression and identifies urinary anomalies. MRI can also be used to evaluate the urinary tract and is highly accurate in depicting the number, size, and location of leiomyomata.

E. Special Examinations

Hysteroscopy may assist in identification, and may also be used for removal, of submucous leiomyomata. Laparoscopy is often definitive in establishing the precise origin of leiomyomata and is increasingly being used for myomectomy (see later).

Differential Diagnosis

The diagnosis of uterine myoma usually is not difficult, although any pelvic mass, including pregnancy, may be mistaken for a leiomyoma. Indeed, leiomyoma is a common preoperative diagnosis for ovarian carcinoma, endolymphatic stromal meiosis, tubo-ovarian abscess, and endometriosis. Modern imaging techniques may clarify the diagnosis, particularly in obese women or in patients in whom palpation is difficult for other reasons, eg, when the abdominal muscles are tense.

Ovarian cysts or neoplasia must be considered in the differential diagnosis of uterine leiomyomata. Other adnexal considerations include tubo-ovarian inflammatory or neoplastic masses. Uterine enlargement simulating leiomyomata may be due to pregnancy (including subinvolution), endometrial cancer, adenomyosis, myometrial hypertrophy, or congenital anomalies. Adnexa, omentum, or bowel adherent to the uterus may be erroneously diagnosed as leiomyomata. Because a fetus may exist within an obviously myomatous uterus, a pregnancy test should be obtained in all women of childbearing age with a suspected pelvic mass.

The most common symptom of leiomyomata, recurrent abnormal bleeding, may be caused by any of the numerous conditions that affect the uterus. Adenocarcinoma of the endometrium or uterine tube, uterine sarcomas, and ovarian carcinomas are the most lethal and therefore the most important to be excluded. Hyperplasia, polyps, irregular shedding, dysfunctional (nonorganic) bleeding, ovarian neoplasms, endometriosis, adenomyosis, and exogenous estrogens or steroid hormones may all cause abnormal bleeding.

The definitive diagnosis in cases of uterine bleeding usually can be established by endometrial biopsy or fractional D&C. Some form of endometrial evaluation should be considered essential in the work-up of any patient with abnormal bleeding or a pelvic mass, particularly those over age 35 years, in whom endometrial cancer may be a serious concern. Even in the presence of uterine leiomyomas, other conditions can coexist and must be ruled out before definitive therapy is undertaken.

Complications

A. MYOMAS AND PREGNANCY

Slightly less than two-thirds of women with uterine leiomyomas and otherwise unexplained infertility conceive after myomectomy, and approximately half of these women go on to deliver term infants. However, comparisons with expectant management are needed before drawing conclusions on the effectiveness of the procedure.

During the second and third trimesters of pregnancy, myomas may rapidly increase in size and undergo vascular deprivation and subsequent degenerative changes. Clinically this most commonly leads to pain and localized tenderness (see Benign Degeneration—Carneous) but also may initiate preterm labor. Expectant management with bed rest and narcotics almost always is successful in alleviating the pain, but tocolytics may be necessary to control the uterine contractions. Once the acute episode is over, most patients can carry to term without further complications.

During labor, leiomyomas may produce uterine inertia, fetal malpresentation, or obstruction of the birth canal. In general, leiomyomas tend to rise out of the pelvis as pregnancy progresses, and vaginal delivery may be accomplished. Nevertheless, a large cervical or isthmic myoma may be immobile and may necessitate cesarean delivery. Leiomyomas may interfere with effective uterine contraction immediately after delivery; therefore, the possibility of postpartum hemorrhage should be anticipated.

B. COMPLICATIONS IN NONPREGNANT WOMEN

Heavy bleeding with anemia is the most common complication of myomas. Urinary or bowel obstruction from large or parasitic myomas is much less common, and malignant transformation is rare. Ureteral injury or ligation is a well-recognized complication of surgery for leiomyomas, particularly cervical.

Precautions

Exogenous hormones must be used with caution in postmenopausal patients with leiomyomas. The dose should be the lowest necessary to control symptoms, and the size of the tumors should be closely followed with pelvic examinations (every 6 months) and imaging studies as necessary. No evidence links oral contraceptive use with an increase in myoma size. However, close clinical follow-up of these patients is reasonable given the potential for exogenous hormones to affect growth of myomas.

Treatment

Asymptomatic leiomyomas are usually managed expectantly. Choice of treatment depends on the patient's symptoms, age, parity, pregnancy status, reproductive plans, and general health, as well as the size and location of the leiomyomas. Other causes of pelvic masses must be ruled out.

A. EMERGENCY MEASURES

Blood transfusions may be necessary to correct anemia. Transfusion of packed red blood cells is preferred over whole blood. Surgery is usually indicated for these patients when they become hemodynamically stable. Emergency surgery is indicated for infected leiomyomata, acute torsion, or intestinal obstruction caused by a pedunculated or parasitic myoma.

B. SPECIFIC MEASURES

1. Medical therapy—The goal of medical treatment is to relieve or reduce symptoms. Although no definitive medical therapy is currently available for leiomyomata, the gonadotropin-releasing hormone (GnRH) agonists have proven very useful for limiting growth or temporarily decreasing tumor size. GnRH agonists induce hypogonadism through pituitary desensitization, downregulation of receptors, and inhibition of gonadotropins. GnRH treatment of uterine fibroids for 3 months usually will achieve maximal shrinkage of the myomatous uterus to approximately 35–60% of its volume and amenorrhea with resulting improvement in hematologic parameters. GnRH treatment is limited by hypoestrogenic side effects and bone loss, especially with treatment for more than 6 months. There is a rapid resumption of uterine volume and menses upon discontinuation of therapy. GnRH agonists may be useful for controlling bleeding from leiomyomata (acutely or preoperatively); improving the preoperative hematocrit level, act as a temporizing measure until surgery can be scheduled or menopause is anticipated; or shrinking myomas sufficiently to allow vaginal hysterectomy. Oral contraceptive pills are commonly prescribed to control abnormal uterine bleeding, but they do not appear to be effective in the treatment of fibroids. They may assist in treating coexisting conditions such as pelvic pain or anovulatory bleeding, which may otherwise be contributed to leiomyomas.

Small observational studies have shown good results with use of the levonorgestrel-releasing intrauterine device for treatment of menorrhagia related to multiple smaller leiomyomata.

C. SURGICAL MEASURES

Surgery is the mainstay of treatment of leiomyomas. Imaging most often must be accompanied by endometrial evaluation to rule out other pelvic neoplastic processes. All patients should undergo cervical Papanicolaou smear test and evaluation of the endometrium if bleeding is irregular. Before definitive surgery, necessary blood volume should be replenished, and other measures such as administration of prophylactic antibiotics or heparin should be considered. Mechanical and antibiotic bowel preparation can be used when difficult pelvic surgery is anticipated.

1. Myomectomy—Myomectomy is an option for the symptomatic patient who wishes to preserve fertility or conserve the uterus. The disadvantage is the significant risk for future leiomyomas. Five years postmyomectomy, 50–60% of patients will have new myomas detected on ultrasound, and up to 25% will require a second major surgery. Couples should undergo a thorough infertility evaluation before the woman undergoes myomectomy to improve fertility.

Most women are counseled to delay pregnancy for 3–6 months after abdominal myomectomy and to plan for cesarean deliveries after removal of a transmural fibroid. The risk of uterine rupture prior to labor after abdominal myomectomy is reported to be 0.0002%. Myomectomy is increasingly being performed through the hysteroscope in cases of submucous leiomyomata and through the laparoscope for small numbers of subserous or intramural leiomyomata. These less invasive procedures are liberalizing the surgical indications for myomectomy. The strength of the uterine closure in laparoscopic myomectomies is controversial, and uterine rupture has been reported starting at 33 weeks' gestation. Patients desiring fertility should be counseled carefully regarding these risks.

A pedunculated submucous myoma protruding into the vagina can sometimes be removed vaginally with a looped wire snare or by hysteroscopy. This is most useful if other tumors do not obviously require removal. If the pedunculated myoma cannot be removed vaginally, careful biopsy should be performed to rule out leiomyosarcoma or a mixed mesodermal sarcoma. Both of these tumors are known to protrude through the cervix in older women and may be clinically indistinguishable from an infarcted prolapsed myoma (Fig 39–4).

Surgical intervention for properly diagnosed uterine fibroids should normally be avoided in pregnancy. The only indication for myomectomy in pregnancy is torsion of a pedunculated fibroid in which transection and hemostasis of the stalk can be achieved with relative safety. Similarly, myomectomy has traditionally been discouraged during cesarean section, except perhaps to facilitate access to the lower uterine segment. A few small studies have recently challenged the theoretical increased risk for hemorrhage and transfusion.

2. Hysterectomy—Leiomyomas are the most common indication for hysterectomy, with a cumulative risk of 7% for all women between 25 and 45 years old. More than 50% of hysterectomies in black women are performed for fibroids, with a cumulative risk of 20% until age 45 years. Hysterectomy eliminates the symptoms and recurrence.

Uteri with small myomas may be removed by total vaginal hysterectomy, particularly if vaginal relaxation demands repair of cystocele, rectocele, or enterocele.

Figure 39–4. Prolapsed and partially infarcted myoma.

When numerous large tumors (especially intraligamentary myomas) are found, total abdominal hysterectomy is indicated. Ovaries generally are preserved in premenopausal women. There is no consensus about the virtue of conserving or removing ovaries in postmenopausal women.

3. Uterine fibroid embolization—Embolic occlusion of the uterine arteries is an alternative to major surgery in premenopausal women not desiring fertility but who wish to retain their uterus or avoid the side effects of medical therapy. In this procedure, an arteriogram is performed to identify the blood supply to the fibroid. A catheter is then advanced into the distal uterine artery under fluoroscopic guidance, usually through the right femoral artery. The artery is infused with an embolizing agent (polyvinyl alcohol particles or tris-acryl gelatin microspheres) until flow ceases. The average procedure lasts 1 hour. Long-term follow-up is currently available for 5 years, with reports indicating that 95% of patients have significant improvement in symptoms and quality of life. Seven percent experience amenorrhea. Observational studies suggest the treatment is as effective as hysterectomy and myomectomy, with more frequent minor complications, fewer major complications, and shorter hospital stays. Frequency of leiomyoma recurrence is lower with embolization (10–15%) compared to myomectomy (20–50%).

4. Endometrial ablation—For women not desiring fertility, ablation of the endometrium may control the symptoms of bleeding. The procedure is more effective when combined with myolysis.

5. Myolysis—This technique of laparoscopic thermal coagulation of leiomyomas does not require suturing and is easy to perform. Localized tissue destruction may contribute to increase postoperative adhesions or chance of rupture during pregnancy.

6. Laparoscopic uterine artery occlusion—This method of cauterizing the uterine arteries at laparoscopy (with or without concurrent myomectomy) has been recently reported. Experience is limited.

7. Magnetic resonance-guided focused ultrasound surgery—This method was approved by the Food and Drug Administration (FDA) in October 2004 for the treatment of leiomyoma in premenopausal women who have completed childbearing. The outpatient procedure uses MRI for real-time thermal monitoring of the thermoablative technique, which converges multiple waves of ultrasound energy on a small volume of tissue to be destroyed. Studies of long-term outcomes of this procedure are ongoing.

Prognosis

Hysterectomy with removal of all leiomyomas is curative. Following myomectomy, the uterus and its cavity gradually return to normal contour. One major concern is the risk of recurrence after myomectomy. Recent studies suggest a rate of 2–3% per year of symptomatic myomas after myomectomy.

ADENOMYOSIS

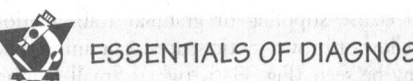

ESSENTIALS OF DIAGNOSIS

- *Premenstrual and comenstrual dysmenorrhea.*
- *Uniform and symmetric uterine enlargement.*
- *Menorrhagia.*

General Considerations

Adenomyosis is defined by the presence of endometrial glands and stroma within the myometrium of the uterus, ie, beneath the basement membrane. It may exist as either diffuse disease detected at hysterectomy only by microscopy or as distinct nodules known as *adenomyomas*. Adenomyosis is generally thought to affect 20% of women, although meticulous sectioning of hysterectomy specimens has yielded an incidence as high as 65%.

In adenomyosis, the uterus becomes diffusely enlarged and globular due to induced hypertrophy and hyperplasia of the smooth muscle elements adjacent to the ectopic glands.

The pathogenesis of adenomyosis is unknown. It is more common in women with a history of childbirth, although increasing parity does not seem to correlate with a higher risk for the disease. It is thought that postpartum endometritis might cause the initial break in the normal boundary, allowing endomyometrial invasion of the endometrium . A separate theory of metaplastic origin speculates an arrest of müllerian cells in the myometrium and later de novo development of endometrial glands in this site. Animal models suggest prolactin and follicle-stimulating hormone stimulate growth of adenomyosis and play a role in its pathogenesis.

Adenomyosis causes symptoms in approximately 70% of proved cases; approximately 30% of cases are asymptomatic and are discovered incidentally. Symptoms typically develop in patients between 40 and 50 years of age and later regress after menopause.

Pathology

On gross inspection, the uterus is uniformly enlarged and boggy. The myometrial thickening produced by adenomyosis is of uniform consistency rather than irregularly nodular, as seen with leiomyomas. The fundus generally is the site of adenomyosis. It may involve either or both walls of the uterus, creating a globular enlargement (usually 10–12 cm in diameter; Fig 39–5, left). The uterus has enhanced vascularity. The cut surface appears convex (bulging) and exudes serum. The cut surface may have a whorl-like or granular trabecular pattern, and coarse stippling or granular trabeculation with small yellow or brown cystic spaces containing fluid or blood may be seen (Fig 39–5, right). Small hemorrhagic areas represent endometrial islands in which menstrual bleeding has occurred. The endometrial–myometrial juncture often is indiscernible, making excision of adenomyosis difficult. Leiomyomas and adenomyosis coexist in the same specimen in up to 50% of cases.

The microscopic pattern is one of endometrial islands scattered throughout the myometrium, at a distance of least 1 low-power field from the basement membrane of the endometrium (some experts demand a distance of 2 low-power fields). Depth of penetration can be graded. Endometrial ablation distorts the normal endometrium–myometrium junction and makes the diagnosis of adenomyosis more difficult.

Myometrial hypertrophy and hyperplasia are almost invariably apparent around the endometrial is-

lets, and phagocytosed hemosiderin occasionally is seen in the muscularis. The ectopic endometrium usually has an immature proliferative pattern, but if the degree of involvement is marked, the embedded endometrium may show cyclic changes identical to those of normal endometrium. The ectopic glands appear to respond fairly well to estrogen and to progesterone to a lesser degree. The ectopic endometrium may participate in the decidual changes characteristic of pregnancy.

Although both adenomyosis and endometriosis are disorders of ectopic endometrium, the 2 diseases are unrelated. They frequently coexist.

Clinical Findings

A. Symptoms and Signs

Significant degrees of adenomyosis are associated with menorrhagia in 60% of patients, and approximately 25% have an acquired, increasingly severe form of dysmenorrhea. One-third of patients are asymptomatic. The classic patient with adenomyosis is a parous, middle-aged woman with menorrhagia and dysmenorrhea who has a symmetrically enlarged uterus.

Despite widespread knowledge of the major symptoms of adenomyosis, the correct preoperative diagnosis is made in less than one-third of all instances. Failure to make the diagnosis preoperatively usually results from attributing symptoms to coexisting lesions. Leiomyomas, endometrial polyps, endometrial hyperplasia, endometrial carcinoma, and endometriosis may all disguise the symptomatology.

1. Menorrhagia—It is claimed that even minimal myometrial invasion by endometrial glands subbasalis may produce hypermenorrhea in a high proportion of cases. There is direct correlation between the degree of involvement of adenomyosis (as opposed to depth of penetration), vascularity of the uterus, and the occurrence of menorrhagia. The increased surface area of the endometrium in the enlarged uterus likely contributes to the menorrhagia.

2. Dysmenorrhea—Dysmenorrhea is directly related to the depth of penetration and degree of involvement. It probably results from myometrial contractions invoked by premenstrual swelling and menstrual bleeding in endometrial islands. The uterus is usually tender and slightly softened under bimanual examination performed premenstrually (Halban's sign).

B. Imaging

Transvaginal ultrasonography may suggest the diagnosis but is not highly accurate (sensitivity 83% and specificity 67%). MRI is the most accurate noninva-

Figure 39–5. Adenomyosis. **Left:** Gross view showing globular mass. **Right:** Close-up view showing stippled trabeculation with small cystic spaces containing fluid or blood.

sive diagnostic test for detecting adenomyosis, but the cost of the procedure must be weighed against the information gathered. It is best reserved for the symptomatic patient with a negative or equivocal sonogram or for the patient with leiomyomas.

Differential Diagnosis

Pregnancy can be ruled out with a pregnancy test.

Submucous leiomyomas may be present in 50–60% of cases of adenomyosis. Leiomyomas may cause excessive and progressive menorrhagia and pain. The uterus is usually firm and nontender, even during menstruation, unless degenerating myomas are a confounder. Diagnosis is confirmed by hysteroscopy and/or curettage. Endometrial cancer is diagnosed by endometrial biopsy or curettage.

Pelvic congestion syndrome (Taylor's syndrome) is characterized by chronic complaints of continuous pelvic pain and menometrorrhagia. In some instances, the uterus is enlarged, symmetric, and minimally softened; the cervix may be cyanotic and patulous. At operation, the pelvic vessels may appear enlarged or tortuous.

Pelvic endometriosis is marked by premenstrual and intramenstrual dysmenorrhea, adherent adnexal masses, and "shotty" cul-de-sac or uterosacral ligament nodulations. The disorder is often associated with adenomyosis.

Complications

Chronic severe anemia may result from persistent menorrhagia.

Primary adenocarcinoma has rarely been observed in islands of aberrant endometrium within myometrium, provided the surface endometrium is normal. On the other hand, endometrial adenocarcinoma is often associated with islands of malignant glands in the muscularis, but it may be impossible to determine whether myometrial metastasis from the primary surface tumor or development of carcinoma within a focus of adenomyosis has occurred. However, if the urface tumor is markedly anaplastic and the myometrial islets exhibit well-differentiated glands, it seems reasonable to conclude that the latter are not metastases.

When the stromal component of endometrium, without glands, invades the myometrium, the resulting "tumor" is referred to as *endolymphatic stromal myosis,* or stromatosis. This entity is not dependent on ovarian hormonal production and therefore is not truly comparable to adenomyosis.

Prevention

Adenomyosis cannot be prevented.

Treatment

A. Hysterectomy

Although focal adenomyomas occasionally can be successfully removed, hysterectomy is the only other definitive treatment of adenomyosis. Hysterectomy is also the only method for establishing the diagnosis with certainty. Whether the ovaries should be removed depends, as in many other situations, on the patient's age and the presence of obvious ovarian lesions or generalized pelvic endometriosis. Small series on uterine artery embolization suggest hysterectomy is not an effective treatment.

B. HORMONAL THERAPY

Medical treatment with hormones has not been successful in the treatment of adenomyosis. Some foci of adenomyosis have shown pseudodecidual reaction to progestins with no symptomatic relief. GnRH agonists can provide temporary relief of symptoms if the focus of adenomyosis is estrogen- and progesterone-receptor positive. However, symptoms recur after the medication is discontinued. Oral contraceptives may exacerbate the symptoms.

Prognosis

Hysterectomy is curative.

ENDOMETRIAL POLYPS

ESSENTIALS OF DIAGNOSIS

- *Menometrorrhagia or postmenopausal bleeding.*
- *Visualization by imaging and/or biopsy.*

General Considerations

"Polyp" is a general descriptive term for any mass of tissue that projects outward or away from the surface of surrounding tissues. An endometrial polyp is a hyperplastic overgrowth of endometrial glands visible as a spheroidal or cylindric structure that may be either pedunculated (attached by a slender stalk) or sessile (relatively broad-based) (Fig 39–6).

Benign endometrial polyps are rare among women younger than 20 years. Their incidence increases directly with age, peaks in the fifth decade, and slowly declines after menopause. Risk factors include hypertension and obesity. A higher incidence of endometrial polyps is noted in patients undergoing tamoxifen therapy for breast cancer. Endometrial polyps must be differentiated from submucous myomas, malignant neoplasms (especially mixed sarcomas), and even retained fragments of placental tissue (which may grossly assume a polypoid architecture).

Polyps may be single or multiple and may range in diameter from a few millimeters to masses that fill or even distend the uterine cavity. Most polyps arise

Figure 39–6. Endometrial polyps.

in the fundal region and extend downward. Occasionally, an endometrial polyp projects through the external cervical os and even extends to the vaginal introitus (Fig 39–7). Postmortem examinations have shown that approximately 10–24% of uteri contain presumably asymptomatic polyps.

Polyps rarely undergo malignant change, and isolated endometrial carcinomas and sarcomas have been identified in solitary polyps. When this occurs, the prognosis is more favorable than for uterine carcinoma or sarcoma in general, providing there is no evidence of spread beyond the polyp on analysis of the hysterectomy specimen. In one large series of 509 women undergoing hysteroscopic resection of polyps, 70% were benign, 26% had hyperplasia without atypia, 3% had hyperplasia with atypia, and 0.8% harbored a malignancy.

The histogenesis of endometrial polyps is not clear. Unresponsive areas of endometrium often remain in situ, along with the basalis, during menstrual shedding, and such an area may serve as the nidus of a polyp. However, not even the smallest polyps studied by histologic sectioning have given a wholly acceptable clue as to the precise mechanism of their formation. Polyps are considered to be estrogen-sensitive; their response to estrogen is similar to that of the surrounding endometrium, and their association with other proliferative endometrial lesions (eg, hyperplasia and endometrial carcinoma) is well recognized.

Figure 39–7. Large, partially infarcted endometrial polyp prolapsed through the cervical os.

Pathology

Grossly, an endometrial polyp is a smooth, red or brown, ovoid body with a velvety texture, ranging from a few millimeters to many centimeters in widest diameter. A large polyp usually tapers to an obvious pedicle. A small polyp, when cut longitudinally, often presents a cylindrical silhouette, with rounding at the distal end. Uterine polyps are the same color as the surrounding endometrium unless they are infarcted, in which case they are dark red. A sectioned polyp may have a spongy appearance if it contains many dilated glandular spaces.

The microscopic pattern of an endometrial polyp is a mixture of (1) generally dense fibrous tissue—the stroma, (2) impressively large and thick-walled vascular channels, and (3) glandlike spaces, of variable size and shape, lined with endometrial epithelium. The relative amounts of these 3 components vary considerably. The surface of an intact polyp in a functioning uterus usually is covered by a layer of endometrium resembling that of the remainder of the endometrial surface, but beneath this exterior are glandular components that are seemingly much older but apparently do not participate in menstrual shedding.

Squamous metaplasia of the surface epithelium is not uncommon. The subsurface epithelial spaces are often compared with basal endometrial glands unresponsive to progesterone, but they tend to form bizarre shapes and become dilated. Hence, a fragment of polyp may be mistaken for the cystic variety of endometrial hyperplasia ("Swiss cheese" endometrium). The distal or dependent portion of a polyp may show marked engorgement of blood vessels, hemorrhage into the stroma, inflammatory cells, and ulceration at the surface.

Adenocarcinoma may develop within an otherwise benign polyp, usually at some distance from its base or pedicle. On the other hand, a benign polyp may exist in an area of endometrial carcinoma. Thus, recovery of a harmless-appearing polyp from the bleeding uterus of a postmenopausal woman does not guarantee that a more serious lesion does not exist elsewhere in the cavity.

Polyps that contain interlacing bands of smooth muscle are called *pedunculated adenomyomas*. Generally, these polyps have broad bases and are associated with adenomyosis of the uterus. In the same uterine cavity, endometrial polyps may coexist with pedunculated leiomyomas. In cases of hyperplasia of the endometrium, the abundant overgrowth of tissue may produce a gross pattern called *multiple polyposis*. Curettage of such lesions may suggest the presence of adenocarcinoma because of the unexpected volume of tissue obtained.

Clinical Findings

A. SYMPTOMS AND SIGNS

Metrorrhagia (irregular bleeding) is the most common presentation of symptomatic polyps, occurring in half of patients. Menorrhagia, postmenopausal bleeding, or a prolapsed mass may also be the presenting complaint. Presumably, a large polyp, with its central vascular component, contributes to menstrual bleeding and adds greatly to the total blood loss. Polyps may be the source of minor premenstrual and postmenstrual bleeding, allegedly because the dependent tip of the polyp is the first endometrial area to degenerate and the last to obtain a new epithelial covering and cease bleeding after the menstrual slough.

In the postmenopausal woman, bleeding from polyps is usually light and is often described as "staining" or "spotting." A polyp should be suspected when bleeding continues following a D&C that has produced only benign normal tissue.

B. IMAGING

Sonohysterography is the most useful imaging modality used to evaluate for the presence of polyps in women with abnormal uterine bleeding. It has a higher sensitivity (93% vs 65%) and specificity (94% vs 76%) than transvaginal ultrasound. Polyps appear as a homogeneous hyperechoic intracavitary mass on both transvaginal ultrasound and sonohysterogram. Polyps may be evident on hysterosalpingogram as irregularities in the outline of the uterine cavity or as filling defects. However, this technique has largely been replaced by office hysteroscopy and saline sonohysterography. No imaging modality can reliably distinguish between benign and malignant polyps.

Treatment

A. SURGICAL EXCISION

Hysteroscopic resection of polyps followed by curettage is the gold standard for diagnosis and treatment of symptomatic polyps, as small polyps can be missed on blind curettage. Direct visualization of polyps by hysteroscopy has greatly aided in their identification and removal. The stalk may be identified, and hysteroscopic instruments used under direct visualization to remove the polyp. With larger polyps, sectioning the tumor into portions that can be removed through the cervix may be necessary. Many authorities recommend curettage of the point of insertion of the stalk into the endometrium–myometrium. Direct visualization of the endometrium and selected biopsies can rule out endometrial atypias or dysplasias.

If hysteroscopy is not available and a blind curettage is planned, the endometrial cavity must be explored separately using a grasping forceps (such as an Overstreet polyp forceps [Fig 39–8] or a Randall stone clamp), preferably at the beginning of the curettage procedure.

Despite this precaution, polyps are frequently missed and remain in the uterus after curettage, only to be discovered later when menorrhagia persists and a hysterectomy is performed. At other times, only a portion of a polyp is removed by curettage, and brisk bleeding continues postoperatively from the residual basal portion of the lesion. A very large polyp may have to be severed at its base using a wire snare or scissors. In all cases, a fractional curettage should follow any nonvisualizing attempt at polyp removal, whether or not it was successful, in order to rule out endometrial carcinoma.

Figure 39–8. Overstreet polyp forceps.

A polyp should be labeled as such, preserved separately in fixative solution, and sent to the pathology laboratory as a separate specimen because it may prove to be the most significant portion of the total tissue sample. If it is intermingled with other curettings or biopsies, there is no assurance that the polyp specimen will be part of the material chosen for histologic sectioning.

Hysteroscopic resection of polyps prior to intrauterine insemination in infertility patients has been associated with a significantly higher pregnancy rate (63% vs 28% in controls), even when the polyp is asymptomatic. Therefore, infertility patients should be offered excision of polyps before initiating assisted reproductive technologies.

B. MEDICAL THERAPY

GnRH agonists may be useful for short-term treatment of polyps, but symptoms tend to recur after cessation of treatment. Progestin therapy may also cause some regression. Prospective studies have shown that some polyps less than 1 cm regress spontaneously.

C. HYSTERECTOMY

Simple excision is adequate for a benign polyp, but if areas of carcinoma or sarcoma are discovered, hysterectomy should be performed. In a premenopausal patient, persistence of abnormal uterine bleeding after removal of an apparently benign polyp (or some portion of it) may require further diagnostic steps and/or more invasive treatment (Fig 39–9). Uteri removed for this reason occasionally contain additional polyps, submucous leiomyomata, or rarely a small area of carcinoma in a relatively inaccessible location.

Prognosis

Removal is curative for that polyp, but recurrence is frequent. Hysterectomy is definitive but usually unnecessary if cancer has been ruled out.

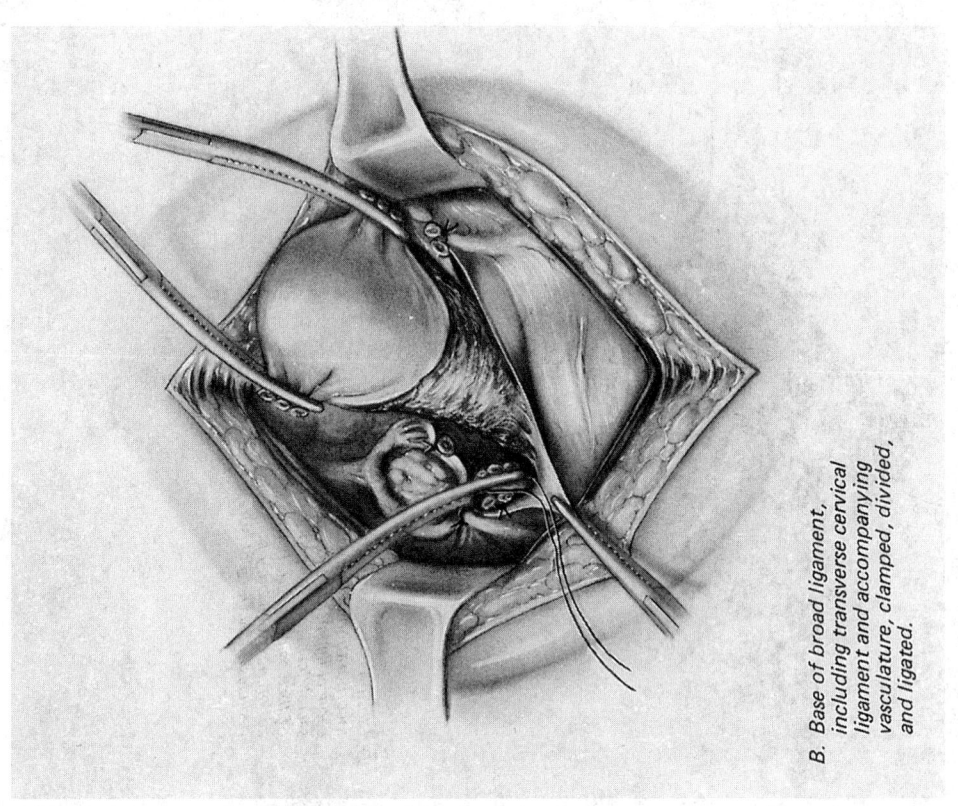

B. Base of broad ligament,
including transverse cervical
ligament and accompanying
vasculature, clamped, divided,
and ligated.

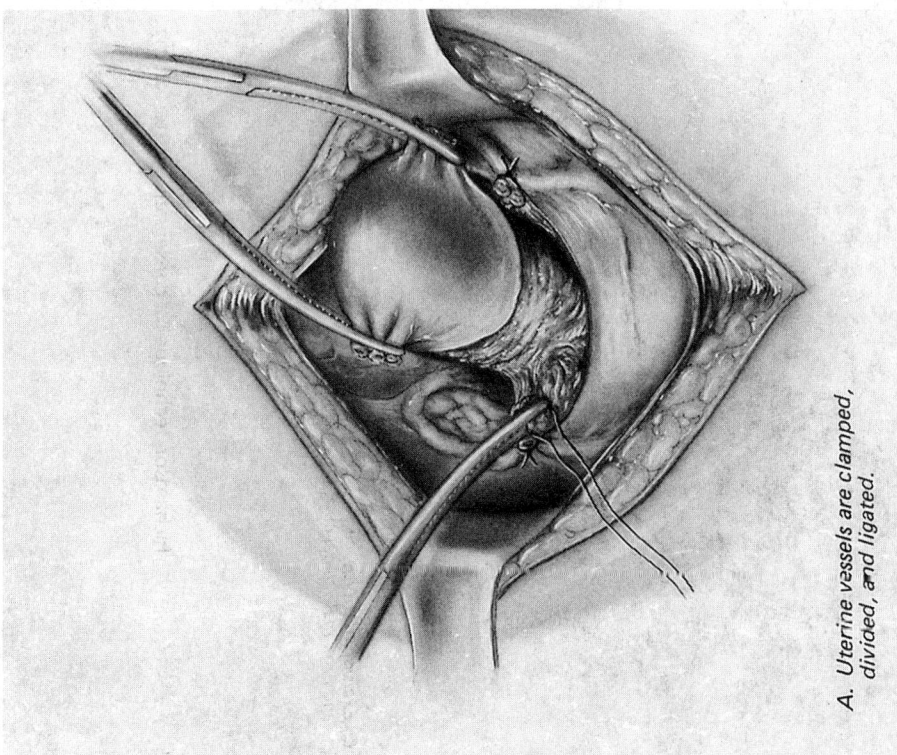

A. Uterine vessels are clamped,
divided, and ligated.

Figure 39-9. Richardson technique for conservative hysterectomy.

D. Closure of vaginal vault and incorporation of transverse cervical ligaments and uterosacral ligaments for support of the vaginal vault. Peritonization next will bury adnexal pedicles and vaginal closure.

C. Excision of uterus, cervix, and proximal vaginal cuff.

Figure 39–9 (cont'd). Richardson technique for conservative hysterectomy.

REFERENCES

Uterine Leiomyomas

Agency for Healthcare Research: Management of uterine fibroids. Summary, evidence report/technology assessment: No. 34. AHRQ Publication No. 01-E051, 2001.

Ang WC et al: Effect of hormone replacement therapies and selective estrogen receptor modulators in postmenopausal women with uterine leiomyomas: A literature review. Climacteric 2001;4:284.

Bachman G: Expanding treatment options for women with symptomatic uterine leiomyomas: Timely medical breakthroughs. Fertil Steril 2006;85:46.

DeWaay DJ et al: Natural history of uterine polyps and leiomyomata. Obstet Gynecol 2002;100:3.

Ryan GL et al: Role, epidemiology, and natural history of benign uterine mass lesions. Clin Obstet Gynecol 2005;48:312.

Schwartz SM: Epidemiology of uterine leiomyomata. Clin Obstet Gynecol 2001;44:316.

Stewart E: Epidemiology, pathogenesis, diagnosis, and natural history of uterine leiomyomas. UpToDate Online Version 14.1. Available at: www.utdol.com.

Adenomyosis

Ascher SM et al: Benign myometrial conditions: Leiomyomas and adenomyosis. Top Magn Reson Imaging 2003;14:281.

Devlieger R et al: Uterine adenomyosis in the infertility clinic. Hum Reprod Update 2003;9:139.

Matalliotakis IM et al: Adenomyosis: What is the impact on fertility? Curr Opin Obstet Gynecol 2005;17:261.

Pelage JP et al: Midterm results of uterine artery embolization for symptomatic adenomyosis: Initial experience. Radiology 2005;234:948.

Stewart E: Adenomyosis and endometrial polyps. UpToDate Online Version 14.1. Available at: www.utdol.com.

Endometrial Polyps

Perez T et al: Endometrial polyps and their implication in the pregnancy rates of patients undergoing intrauterine insemination: A prospective randomized study. Hum Reprod 2005;20:1632.

Savelli L et al: Histopathologic features and risk factors for benignity, hyperplasia and cancer in endometrial polyps. Am J Obstet Gynecol 2003;188:927.

Stewart E: Adenomyosis and endometrial polyps. UpToDate Online Version 14.1. Available at: www.utdol.com.

Benign Disorders of the Ovaries & Oviducts

40

Mor Tzadik, MD, Karen Purcell, MD, PhD, & James E. Wheeler, MD

Benign adnexal masses are common in women in the reproductive age group and are caused by physiologic cysts or benign neoplasms. The management of these benign masses is dictated by their presentation. Operative intervention is indicated when a patient is symptomatic because of hemorrhage of a ruptured cyst or ovarian torsion. Most adnexal masses, however, are discovered incidentally, and the risk of malignancy must always be assessed and excluded (see Chapter 52 for proper evaluation). For instance, sonographic indices such as septations, solid components, and Doppler flow within a neoplasm are suspicious for malignancy. When malignancy is not suspected, expectant management is indicated, as many of these cysts are physiologic in nature and thus are expected to regress over time. Patients should be re-evaluated 6 weeks after initial presentation, and persistent masses should be considered potentially benign or malignant neoplasms that warrant operative evaluation. Pathologic diagnosis by frozen section during surgery can aid in making a final diagnosis and determining what type of surgery is indicated. For most benign ovarian cysts, laparoscopy is the preferred method because of its shorter recovery time, as well as less pain, blood loss, and overall cost compared to laparotomy. Even extremely large ovarian cysts (reaching the umbilicus and higher) currently are being managed laparoscopically. Laparoscopic approach is recommended if the cyst appears benign by preoperative evaluation. For most patients, ovarian cystectomy is favored over oophorectomy in order to retain fertility.

■ PHYSIOLOGIC ENLARGEMENT

FUNCTIONAL CYSTS

Follicular Cysts

Follicular cysts (Fig 40–1) are common and vary in diameter from 3 to 8 cm. Histologically, they are seen to be lined by an inner layer of granulosa cells and an outer layer of theca interna cells that may or may not be luteinized. These cysts result from a failure in ovulation, most likely secondary to disturbances in the release of the pituitary gonadotropins. The fluid of the incompletely developed follicle is not reabsorbed, producing an enlarged follicular cyst. Typically they are asymptomatic, although bleeding and torsion can occur. Large cysts may cause aching pelvic pain, dyspareunia, and occasionally abnormal uterine bleeding associated with a disturbance of the ovulatory pattern. Most follicular cysts disappear spontaneously within 60 days without treatment. Use of oral contraceptive pills (OCPs) has often been recommended to help establish a normal rhythm; however, recent data show that this practice may not produce more rapid resolution than expectant management.

Corpus Luteum (Granulosa Lutein) Cysts

These are thin-walled unilocular cysts ranging from 3–11 cm in size. Following normal ovulation, the granulosa cells lining the follicle become luteinized. In the stage of vascularization, blood accumulates in the central cavity, producing the corpus hemorrhagicum. Resorption of the blood then results in a corpus luteum, which is defined as a cyst when it grows larger than 3 cm. A persistent corpus luteum cyst may cause local pain or tenderness. It can also be associated with either amenorrhea or delayed menstruation, thus simulating the clinical picture of an ectopic pregnancy. A corpus luteum cyst may be associated with torsion of the ovary, causing severe pain; or it may rupture and bleed, in which case laparoscopy or laparotomy is usually required to control hemorrhage into the peritoneal cavity. Unless acute complications develop, symptomatic therapy is indicated. As with follicular cysts, corpus luteum cysts usually regress after 1 or 2 months in menstruating patients, and OCPs have been recommended but may be of questionable benefit.

Theca Lutein Cysts

Elevated levels of chorionic gonadotropin can produce theca lutein cysts and thus are seen in patients with hydatidiform mole or choriocarcinoma and in

Figure 40–1. Wall of a follicular cyst showing the proliferating granulosa cells with tiny cystic Call-Exner bodies in the upper portion of the figure. They have artifactually pulled away from the underlying theca cells.

patients undergoing chorionic gonadotropin or clomiphene therapy. Rarely, they are seen in normal pregnancy. The cysts are lined by theca cells that may or may not be luteinized, and they may or may not have granulosa cells. They are usually bilateral and are filled with clear, straw-colored fluid. Abdominal symptoms are minimal, although a sense of pelvic heaviness or aching may be described. Rupture of the cyst may result in intraperitoneal bleeding. Continued signs and symptoms of pregnancy, especially hyperemesis and breast paresthesias, are reported. The cysts disappear spontaneously following termination of the molar pregnancy, treatment of the choriocarcinoma, or discontinuation of fertility therapy; however, such resolution may take months to occur. Surgery is reserved for complications such as torsion and hemorrhage.

Endometriomas

In women with endometriosis, ovarian endometrial cysts can develop and grow up to 6–8 cm. These endometriomas are also referred to as "chocolate cysts" because they contain thick, brown blood debris inside.

HYPERTHECOSIS

Hyperthecosis, or thecomatosis, commonly produces no gross enlargement of the ovary (Fig 40–2). Thus, the lesions are demonstrable only by histologic examination of the excised gonad. They are characterized by nests of stromal cells demonstrating increased cytoplasm, simulating the changes seen in

the normal theca after stimulation by pituitary gonadotropin. In the premenopausal woman, hyperthecosis is associated with virilization and clinical findings similar to those seen in polycystic ovarian disease (see following text). These alterations may also be associated with postmenopausal bleeding and endometrial hyperplasia.

POLYCYSTIC OVARIAN SYNDROME (STEIN-LEVENTHAL SYNDROME)

Polycystic ovarian syndrome (PCOS) is characterized by persistent anovulation that can lead to clinical manifestations, including enlarged polycystic ovaries, secondary amenorrhea or oligomenorrhea, and infertility. The syndrome has a prevalence of 5–10%, with variance among races and ethnicities. Approximately 50% of patients are hirsute, and 30–75% are obese. A presumptive diagnosis of PCOS often can be made based on the history and initial examination. According to an international consensus group, the syndrome can be diagnosed if at least 2 of the following conditions are present: oligomenorrhea or amenorrhea, hyperandrogenism, and polycystic ovaries on ultrasound. Polycystic ovaries have been called "oyster ovaries" because they are enlarged and "sclerocystic" with smooth, pearl-white surfaces without indentations. Many small, fluid-filled follicle cysts lie beneath the thickened fibrous surface cortex (Fig 40–3). Luteinization of the theca interna is usually observed,

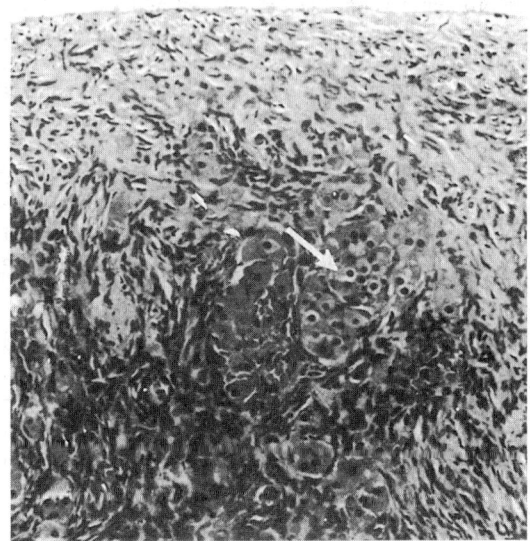

Figure 40–2. In hyperthecosis, nests of rounded eosinophilic luteinized stroma cells are found in the ovarian cortex.

Figure 40–3. Polycystic ovary with a thickened capsule and prominent subcapsular cysts. Note lack of corpora lutea or corpora albicantia due to anovulation.

and occasionally focal stromal luteinization is seen. Laboratory testing often reveals imildly elevated serum androgen levels, an increased ratio of luteinizing hormone to follicle-stimulating hormone (LH/FSH), lipid abnormalities, and insulin resistance. Anovulation is identified in women with persistently high concentrations of LH and low concentrations of FSH, a low day-21 progesterone level, or on sonographic follicular monitoring. PCOS is presumably related to hypothalamic pituitary dysfunction and insulin resistance. A primary ovarian contribution to the problem has not been clearly defined.

Most patients with PCOS seek treatment for either hirsutism or infertility. The hirsutism can be treated with any agent that lowers androgen levels, and OCPs are typically the first choice in patients not desiring pregnancy. Infertility in PCOS patients is often responsive to clomiphene citrate. In the recalcitrant case, the experienced clinician can add human menopausal gonadotropin to produce the desired ovulation. Recent studies indicate that therapy with metformin improves fertility rates both when given alone and, even more so, when given in conjunction with clomiphene. Studies show that a small reduction in body weight, as little as 2–7%, is associated with improved ovulatory function in women with PCOS. As patients with PCOS are chronically anovulatory, the endometrium is stimulated by estrogen alone. Thus endometrial hyperplasia, both typical and atypical, and endometrial carcinoma are more frequent in patients with PCOS and long-term anovulation. Many of these markedly atypical endometrial features can be reversed by large doses of progestational agents, such as megestrol acetate 40–60 mg/d for 3–4 months. Follow-up endometrial biopsy is mandatory to determine endometrial response and subsequent recurrence.

LUTEOMA OF PREGNANCY

Tumorlike nodules of lutein cells may form in the ovaries during pregnancy and are often both multifocal and bilateral. The nodules range up to 20 cm in diameter, but most often they range from 5–10 cm. On section they reveal well-delineated, soft, brown masses with focal hemorrhage. Microscopically, they are formed of sheets of large luteinized cells with abundant cytoplasm and relatively uniform nuclei with occasional mitoses. Clinically, they appear ominous to the obstetrician, who becomes aware of them only when the abdomen is open at the time of cesarean delivery. Unilateral salpingo-oophorectomy can be performed for frozen section in the belief that the large masses are malignant. A confirmatory biopsy is adequate, and follow-up will reveal total regression a few months later.

■ OVARIAN NEOPLASMS

TREATMENT OF OVARIAN TUMORS

The preferred treatment of all ovarian tumors is surgical excision with careful exploration of the abdominal contents. If the risk of malignant neoplasia is confidently low, laparoscopy is preferred. In patients requesting future fertility, cystectomy is performed if possible; otherwise a unilateral oophorectomy is performed. Frozen section is helpful in identifying the type and neoplastic potential of the tumor. However, because adequate sampling of a large ovarian neoplasm often is impossible, final opinion and prognosis *must* be based on analysis of permanent, rather than frozen, sections. Therefore, in a patient desirous of retaining fertility, the surgeon must err on the side of retention of the uterus and contralateral ovary if the pathologist has the slightest doubt as to tumor malignancy.

EPITHELIAL TUMORS

Epithelial tumors account for approximately 60–80% of all true ovarian neoplasms and include the common serous, mucinous, endometrioid, clear cell, and transitional cell (Brenner) tumors, and the stromal tumors with an epithelial element. The epithelium of these tumors arises from a common anlage, ie, the mesothelium lining the coelomic cavity and ovarian surfaces (Fig 40–4). This basic thesis explains the similarity of the epithelia of the upper genital canal—endocervix, endometrium, and endosalpinx—to those found in the ovarian tumors. Most tumors presumably arise from invaginated surface epithelium (Fig 40–4) and proliferation or malignant degeneration in the epithelial lining of the resulting sur-

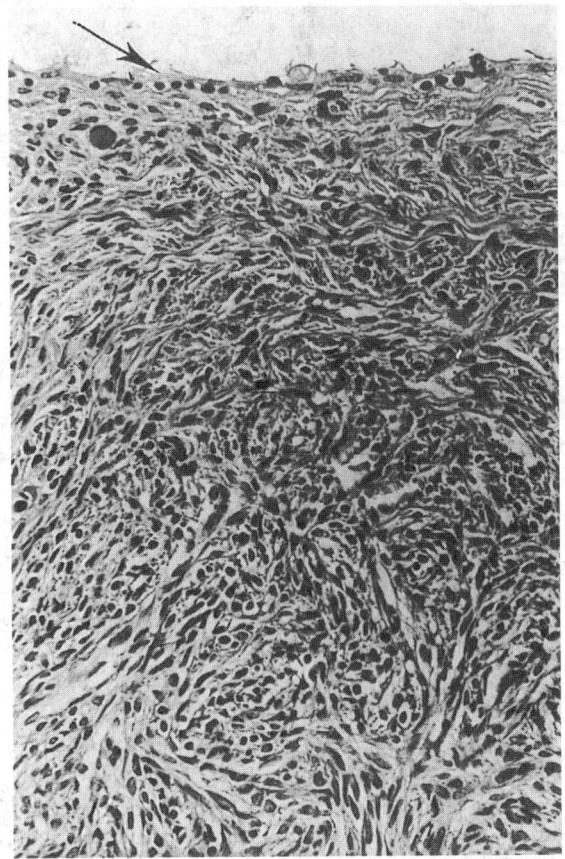

Figure 40–4. Surface epithelium (mesothelium; indicated by the arrow) of the ovary forms an inconspicuous, usually flat, layer of cells over the underlying ovarian cortex.

Figure 40–5. Most surface (germinal) inclusion cysts, such as the one shown here, undergo a serous (tubal) metaplasia. By definition, cysts larger than 1 cm in diameter are termed cystadenomas.

face inclusion cyst (Fig 40–5). The epithelial tumors are classified on the basis of their histologic appearance.

Serous Tumors

Serous tumors have been reported in all age groups and are responsible for approximately 30% of all epithelial ovarian neoplasms. Low-grade neoplasms generally are found in patients in their 20s and 30s, whereas their anaplastic counterparts occur more commonly in perimenopausal and postmenopausal women. Serous cystadenomas are benign lesions, commonly unilocular, with a smooth surface, and containing thin, clear yellow fluid. The cells lining the cyst are a mixed population of ciliated and secretory cells similar to those of the endosalpinx. They may grow large enough to fill the abdominal cavity, but usually they are smaller than their mucinous counterparts. Approximately 10–15% are bilateral. Focal proliferation of the underlying stroma may produce firm papillary projections into the cyst, forming a serous cysta-

denofibroma (Fig 40–6). It is important to study these papillary projections thoroughly to rule out atypical proliferation. Some serous tumors consist of benign stromal proliferation interspersed with tiny serous cysts; these are known as *serous adenofibromas*.

Mucinous Tumors

Mucinous tumors account for approximately 10–20% of all epithelial ovarian neoplasms, of which approximately 75%–85% are benign. The benign tumors are typically found in women in their 30s through 50s. Bilateral tumor development occurs in 8–10% of all cases, whether the tumors are benign or malignant. They are the largest tumors found in the human body; 15 re-

Figure 40–6. Serous cystadenofibromas usually form unilocular cysts with firm white papillations protruding into the cyst, seen here microscopically.

ported tumors have weighed more than 70 kg (154 lb). Consequently, the more massive the tumor, the greater the possibility that it is mucinous. They generally are asymptomatic, and patients present with either an abdominal mass or nonspecific abdominal discomfort. In postmenopausal patients, luteinization of the stroma rarely may result in hormone production (usually estrogen) leading to associated endometrial hyperplasia with vaginal bleeding. During pregnancy, hormonal stimulation may result in virilization.

Histologically, they are usually smooth-walled; true papillae are rare (compared with the serous variety). The tumors generally are multilocular, and the mucus-containing locules appear blue through the tense capsule (Fig 40–7). The internal surface is lined by tall columnar cells with dark, basally situated nuclei and mucinous cytoplasm (Fig 40–8).

The epithelium of mucinous cysts resembles that of the endocervix in approximately 50% of cases; in the other 50%, mucin-containing goblet cells resembling intestinal epithelial cells are present. Careful study of mucinous neoplasms has shown that the histologic appearance may vary greatly from area to area; some areas appear benign whereas others are of low malignant potential or are frankly malignant. Hence, sampling must be more extensive than in the typical serous tumor. Me-

Figure 40–8. Mucinous cystadenoma. The lining cells are tall and columnar with basally situated nuclei. Generous sampling of these tumors is necessary to rule out a higher-grade lesion.

tastases from appendiceal and other primary tumors may simulate closely a mucinous cystadenoma.

Endometrioid Lesions

Endometrioid tumors are characterized by proliferation of benign nonspecific stroma in which bland endometrial-type glands may be found. The only clearly recognizable benign endometrioid tumors are the uncommon endometrioid adenofibroma and the proliferative endometrioid adenofibroma. If the epithelial growth is exuberant but cytologically benign, it is termed a *proliferative* rather than a low malignant potential tumor as the prognosis appears to be invariably excellent (Fig 40–9).

Endometriosis of the ovary (see Chapter 43) represents a benign "tumorlike" condition rather than a true neoplasm.

Clear Cell (Mesonephroid) Tumors

Like the endometrioid tumors, clear cell tumors in their benign form are rare and are virtually limited to clear cell adenofibromas in which a solid proliferation of nonspecific stroma contains small cytologically bland glands formed by columnar cells with clear cytoplasm. Clinically they appear like any other benign ovarian mass and are diagnosed only on histologic examination. The prognosis is excellent.

Transitional Cell (Brenner) Tumors

Transitional cell tumors are adenofibromas in which the proliferating epithelial element has a transitional cell appearance, which represents metaplasia. Brenner tumors account for 1–2% of primary ovarian tumors; more than 98% are benign, and nearly 95% of cases are unilateral.

Figure 40–7. Multilocular mucinous cystadenoma of the ovary.

Figure 40–9. Endometrioid cystadenomas contain a proliferation of bland endometrial-like glands without the stroma of endometriosis.

They frequently are so small that they are incidental operative findings. However, the tumor may reach 5–8 cm in diameter and present as an adnexal mass on pelvic examination. On section they are firm and pale yellow or white (Fig 40–10). The epithelium is composed of nests of cells with ovoid nuclei having a prominent longitudinal groove ("coffee-bean nuclei"; Fig 40–11). Occasionally there is a mucinous metaplasia of the cells in the center of one or more of these nests, which may account for the 10% incidence of mucinous cystadenomas found associated with Brenner tumors.

SEX CORD-STROMAL TUMORS

Thecoma

This type of tumor can occur at any age, although they are most commonly found in postmenopausal women. They account for only 2% of all ovarian tumors and may not be a true neoplasm but instead a condition of hyperplasia of the cortical stroma. Histologically, the mass is filled with lipid-containing cells that are similar to theca cells, and the tumor is known to produce estrogen. As such, these tumors often present with dysfunctional uterine bleeding or postmenopausal bleeding. Occasionally they have presented with adenocarcinoma of the endometrium given the unopposed estrogen production by the tumor. The tumors range from nonpalpable to more than 20 cm in size. They are rarely bilateral and rarely malignant.

Fibroma

Unlike thecomas, fibromas produce no hormones. They can occur at any age but most often in the years prior to menopause. They range in size from incidental findings to greater than 20 cm. They are multinodular and whorled, and they are formed from bundles of collagen-producing spindle cells. They can be found as part of Meigs' syndrome, in which a patient is found to have a pelvic mass in concert with ascites and hydrothorax. Fibromas are also part of a hereditary basal cell nevus syndrome in which basal cell carcinoma is found with mesenteric cysts, calcification of the dura, and keratocysts of the jaw.

Hilus Cell Tumor

These tumors are a subset of Leydig cell tumors, which originate from the ovarian hilum or less frequently from the ovarian stroma. The typical presentation includes hirsutism, virilization, and menstrual irregularities. Hilus cell tumors rarely attain a palpable size. Histologically, groups of steroid cells containing eosinophilic cytoplasm and lipochrome pigment are found. For the tumor to be defined as a Leydig cell neoplasm, elongated eosinophilic crystalloids of Reinke must be found.

GERM CELL TUMORS

Mature Teratomas

Mature cystic teratomas, commonly referred to as *dermoid cysts,* compose some 40–50% of all benign ovarian neoplasms. They contain well-differentiated tissue derived from any of the 3 germ cell layers, including hair and teeth as ectodermal derivatives. They account for the majority of benign ovarian neoplasms in reproductive-age women and usually are asymptomatic unless complications such as torsion or

Figure 40–10. Cut surface of a Brenner tumor is firm, solid, and yellowish-white, and resembles a fibrothecoma.

Figure 40–11. In a transitional cell (Brenner) tumor, islands of bland transitional cells (arrows) proliferate, accompanied by prominent proliferation of benign spindly fibroblast-like cells.

rupture occur. Transvaginal ultrasound is known to be very accurate in the diagnosis of dermoid cysts, with the hair and sebum, rather than calcium, creating highly reflective irregular solid components within fluid-containing masses.

Studies have detailed several advantages to the laparoscopic approach to removal of dermoids, including less postoperative pain and blood loss, shorter hospital stay, and lower overall cost. Recent studies have shown that dermoid cysts can usually be removed laparoscopically without intraperitoneal spillage. If intraoperative spillage does occur, the potential for chemical peritonitis or excess adhesion formation has led to the recommendation of copious saline irrigation until the lavage is clear. The risk of peritonitis, however, is quite low (< 0.2%) with laparoscopic removal of dermoid cysts.

Although most mature teratomas contain cells from all germ cell layers, a subset of monodermal teratomas exists. Those tumors composed mostly or entirely of thyroid tissue are called *struma ovarii*. These tumors account for only 3% of all teratomas, and only 5% of these will produce symptoms of thyrotoxicosis.

■ BENIGN TUMORS OF THE OVIDUCT

Benign lesions of the uterine tube are routinely asymptomatic and rarely large enough to be palpable—with the exception of the paratubal or parovarian cyst—so the diagnosis is made incidentally at the operating table or in the pathology laboratory.

CYSTIC TUMORS

Hydatid cysts of Morgagni are cystic tumors of the uterine tube located at or near the fimbriated end. They are lined by tubal-type epithelium, filled with clear fluid, and are usually approximately 1 cm in diameter. They are most often found inadvertently during a pelvic operative procedure. On rare occasions, torsion produces an acute surgical emergency.

Occasionally, larger paratubal or parovarian cysts develop, especially in the broad ligament (Fig 40–12). These cysts are almost always serous tumors of low malignant potential with a benign clinical outcome.

A third type of cyst associated with the fallopian tubes is the *Walthard rest*. This type is found as a 1-mm cyst beneath the serosa of the fallopian tube. It appears to represent an inclusion cyst in which the mesothelium has undergone metaplasia similar to transitional cell (Brenner) tumors.

EPITHELIAL TUMORS

Benign epithelial tumors of the uterine tube are extremely rare. The polyps that occur in the cornual portion appear to be of endometrial rather than tubal origin.

ADENOMATOID TUMORS

The adenomatoid tumor probably is the most common benign tumor found in the uterine tube. It actually represents a benign mesothelioma, but the compact nature of the adenomatous pattern may be mistaken for malignancy (Fig 40–13). Adenomatoid lesions rarely measure more than 1–1.5 cm. They are always incidental findings when the adnexa are removed for other purposes. Similar lesions, usually cystic, may involve the myometrium or ovary.

OTHER BENIGN TUBAL AND PARATUBAL TUMORS

Other benign tubal tumors, such as leiomyomas and teratomas, are rare, as are benign adnexal tumors of

Figure 40–12. Parovarian cyst. Note the orientation of the cyst to the fimbriated end of the oviduct.

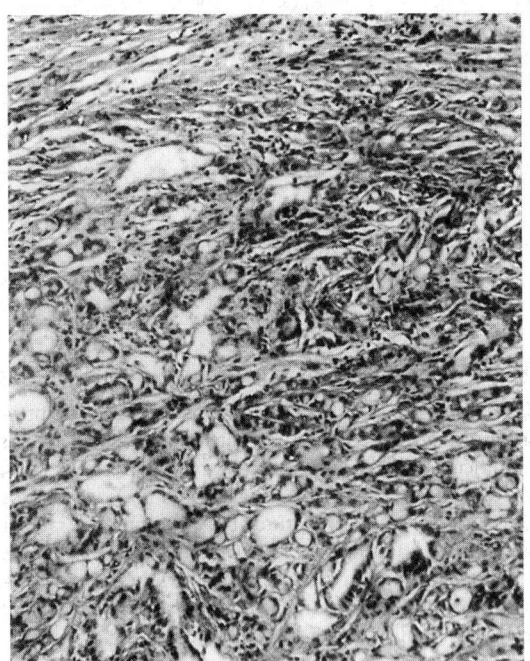

Figure 40–13. Adenomatoid tumor (benign mesothelioma) with tiny slitlike spaces and glands invading the muscular wall of the tube.

probable wolffian origin. Adrenal cortical nests, however, are common incidental embryologic rests found in the broad ligament, seen as yellowish ovoid nodules 3–4 mm in diameter.

SUMMARY

Ovarian neoplasms may arise from any histologic element of the ovary and are most often benign, especially in premenopausal women. The characteristics of the mass and the age of the patient are important factors guiding diagnosis and treatment. The overall risk of malignancy of an ovarian cyst is 13% in a premenopausal woman versus 45% in a postmenopausal woman. Therefore, vigilant work-up of these masses with the aid of ultrasound and close follow-up is essential. Use of cancer antigen-125 (CA-125) for diagnostic purposes is controversial. With the increased use of imaging studies has come discovery of incidental, asymptomatic, small ovarian cysts. These cysts should be evaluated by ultrasound. If they do not contain septa or solid components, they can be closely followed. However, any mass that enlarges or changes in character, especially in postmenopausal women, should be explored surgically.

REFERENCES

Allias F et al: Value of ultrasound-guided fine-needle aspiration in the management of ovarian and paraovarian cysts. Diag Cytopathol 2000;22:70.

Canis M et al: Management of adnexal masses: Role and risk of laparoscopy. Semin Surg Oncol 2000;19:28.

Canis M et al: Laparoscopic management of adnexal masses: a gold standard? Curr Opin Obstet Gynecol 2002;14:423.

Ehrmann D: Medical progress: Polycystic ovary syndrome. N Engl J Med 2005;352:1223.

Ginsburg KA, McGinnis KT: Ovarian cystectomy: Perioperative considerations and operative technique. Oper Tech Gynecol Surg 2000;5:224.

Jermy K, Luise C, Bourned T: The characterization of common ovarian cysts in premenopausal women. Ultrasound Obstet Gynecol 2001;17:140.

Lewis V: Polycystic ovary syndrome. A diagnostic challenge. Obstet Gynecol Clin North Am 2001;28:1.

Sagiv R et al: Laparoscopic management of extremely large ovarian cysts. Obstet Gynecol 2005;105:1319.

Scully RE et al: *Tumors of the Ovary, Maldeveloped Gonads, Fallopian Tube, and Broad Ligament. AFIP Atlas of Tumor Pathology, 3rd Series.* Armed Forces Institute of Pathology, 1998.

Templeman CL et al: Managing mature cystic teratomas of the ovary. Obstet Gynecol Surv 2000;55:738.

Sexually Transmitted Diseases & Pelvic Infections

41

Steven W. Ainbinder, MD, Susan M. Ramin, MD, & Alan H. DeCherney, MD

■ SEXUALLY TRANSMITTED DISEASES

The term "sexually transmitted diseases" is used to denote disorders spread principally by intimate contact. Although this usually means sexual intercourse, it also includes close body contact, kissing, cunnilingus, anilingus, fellatio, mouth–breast contact, and anal intercourse. Many sexually transmitted diseases (STDs) can be acquired by transplacental spread, by passage through the birth canal, and via lactation during the neonatal period. The organisms involved are peculiarly adapted to growth in the genital tract and are present in body secretions or blood.

Physicians have a critical role in preventing as well as treating STDs. The clinician's role is 4-fold. First, to understand the microbiology of STDs in order to appropriately diagnose and treat patients. Second, to alleviate the symptoms and prevent future sequelae. Third, to prevent the transmission to others including health care professionals. Finally, to do all of the above combined with patient education and counseling. As the future continues to bring advancements in therapy, the physician must be able to adapt to these changes. Today, preexposure vaccinations appear to be the trend in future therapy. For now, however, prevention through lifestyle and behavioral modification is the primary weapon against the spread of STDs. Multiple cohort studies have demonstrated the protective effects of both male and female condoms.

The list of organisms traditionally thought of as causing STDs has been extended to include cytomegalovirus, herpes simplex virus type 1 (HSV-1) and type 2 (HSV-2), *Chlamydia*, group B *Streptococcus*, molluscum contagiosum virus, *Sarcoptes scabiei*, hepatitis viruses, and human immunodeficiency virus (HIV). Some diseases spread by body contact but not necessarily by coitus—eg, pediculosis pubis and molluscum contagiosum—are discussed with the dermatitides rather than here; herpes genitalis is discussed in Chapter 37.

VULVAR LESIONS & GENITAL ULCERS

Genital herpes, syphilis, and chancroid are the most prevalent ulcerative lesions in the United States. The diagnosis is difficult to make by physical examination alone. Thus, the work-up for all genital ulcers should include serologic screening for syphilis, culture/antigen testing for HSV-1 and HSV-2, and culture for *Haemophilus ducreyi*. More than one infectious etiology may be present in a single lesion. In today's environment it is important to recognize HIV as a risk factor for genital ulcers.

1. Herpes Simplex

Vulvovaginal infections with HSV have assumed a primary role in STDs. HSV (types 1 and 2) is a highly prevalent (5 million cases in the United States), incurable, recurrent viral disease. Patient education and clinical skills are mandatory in obstetrics in order to prevent vertical transmission to the fetus or newborn. Systemic antiviral agents are commonly used during the first clinical episode to reduce symptoms, shorten duration of the lesion, and decrease the number of cesarean deliveries among infected mothers. These infections are discussed in Chapter 37.

2. Condylomata Acuminata (Venereal Warts)

See Chapter 37.

3. Chancroid (Soft Chancre)

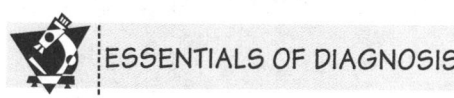

ESSENTIALS OF DIAGNOSIS

- *Painful, tender genital ulcer.*
- *Culture positive for H ducreyi.*
- *Inguinal adenitis with erythema or fluctuance.*

General Considerations

Chancroid is an STD characterized by a painful genital ulcer. However, studies have shown asymptomatic carriers among commercial sex workers. Although this condition can be difficult to diagnosis clinically, suppurative inguinal adenopathy with painful ulcers is pathognomonic and may assist with a preculture diagnosis. It is endemic in many areas of the United States, although it occurs more frequently in Africa, the West Indies, and Southeast Asia. The causative organism is the gram-negative rod *H ducreyi*. Exposure is usually through coitus, but accidentally acquired lesions of the hands have occurred. The incubation period is short: the lesion usually appears in 3–5 days or sooner. An increased rate of HIV infection has been reported among patients with this genital ulcer disease; chancroid is a cofactor for HIV transmission. Moreover, 10% of patients with genital chancroid may have coinfection with herpes or syphilis.

Clinical Findings

A. SYMPTOMS AND SIGNS

The early chancroid lesion is a vesicopustule on the pudendum, vagina, or cervix. Later, it degenerates into a saucer-shaped ragged ulcer circumscribed by an inflammatory wheal. Typically, the lesion is very tender and produces a heavy, foul discharge that is contagious. A cluster of ulcers may develop. Lesions typically occur on the vulva, cervix, and perianal area in women.

Painful inguinal adenitis is noted in over 50% of cases. The buboes may become necrotic and drain spontaneously.

B. LABORATORY FINDINGS

Syphilis must first be ruled out. Clinical diagnosis is more reliable than smears or cultures because of the difficulty of isolating this organism. Isolation of *H ducreyi* is diagnostic, but isolation occurs in less than one-third of cases. Aspirated pus from a bubo is the best material for culture. Serum adsorption enzyme immunoassays have been evaluated and currently have a limited sensitivity. However, polymerase chain reaction (PCR) testing of genital samples is becoming widely available. Multiplex PCR is a technique that can simultaneously screen for HSV, *Treponema pallidum,* and *H ducreyi* using a single swab but is not yet commercially available.

Differential Diagnosis

Syphilis, granuloma inguinale, lymphogranuloma venereum, and herpes simplex may coexist with chancroid and must be ruled out.

Prevention

Chancroid is a reportable disease. Routine antibiotic prophylaxis is not warranted. Condoms can give protection. Liberal use of soap and water is relatively effective. Education is essential.

Treatment

A. LOCAL TREATMENT

Good personal hygiene is important. The early lesions should be cleansed with mild soap solution. Sitz baths are beneficial.

B. ANTIBIOTIC TREATMENT

The susceptibility of *H ducreyi* to antimicrobial agents varies by locality. Consultation with the nearest STD clinic may reveal information about current susceptibilities and effective treatment regimens. Guidelines issued by the Centers for Disease Control and Prevention (CDC) for genital chancroid are as follows. *Recommended regimen*—(a) azithromycin 1 g orally once; (b) ceftriaxone 250 mg intramuscularly (IM) as a single dose; (c) erythromycin base 500 mg orally 3 times daily for 7 days; and (d) ciprofloxacin 500 mg orally twice daily for 3 days in nonpregnant patients over age 17 years who are not lactating. The course may have to be repeated. Fluctuant lymph nodes may need to be aspirated through normal adjacent skin. Incision and drainage of the nodes is not recommended because it will delay healing.

Prognosis

Untreated or poorly managed cases of chancroid may persist, and secondary infection may develop. Frequently, the ulcers heal spontaneously. They should improve within 7–10 days. If no improvement is noted, coinfection, HIV, resistant strains, and noncompliance must be considered. If not treated, they may cause deep scarring with sequelae in men.

4. Granuloma Inguinale (Donovanosis)

 ESSENTIALS OF DIAGNOSIS

- Ulcerative vulvitis, chronic or recurrent.
- Donovan bodies revealed by Wright's or Giemsa's stain.

General Considerations

Granuloma inguinale is a chronic ulcerative granulomatous disease that usually develops in the vulva, perineum, and inguinal regions (Fig 41–1). The disease is almost

Figure 41–1. Granuloma inguinale.

nonexistent in the United States. It is most common in India, Brazil, the West Indies, some South Pacific islands, and parts of Australia, China, and Africa. The causative organism is *Calymmatobacterium granulomatis* (Donovan body). Donovan bodies are bacteria encapsulated in mononuclear leukocytes. Transmission is via coitus, and the incubation period is 8–12 weeks.

Clinical Findings

A. Symptoms and Signs

Although granuloma inguinale most often involves the skin and subcutaneous tissues of the vulva and inguinal regions, cervical, uterine, orolabial, and ovarian sites have been reported. A malodorous discharge is characteristic. The disorder often begins as a papule, which then ulcerates, with the development of a beefy-red granular zone with clean, sharp edges. The ulcer shows little tendency to heal, and the patient usually has no local or systemic symptoms. Healing is very slow, and satellite ulcers may unite to form a large lesion. Lymphatic permeation is rare, but lymphadenitis may result when the cutaneous lesion becomes superimposed on lymphatic channels. Inguinal swelling is common, with late formation of abscesses (buboes). Rarely, granuloma inguinale is manifested by chronic cervical lesions.

These lesions usually take the form of redness or ulceration, or they form granulation tissue. They produce a chronic inflammatory exudate characterized histologically by lymphocytes, giant cells, and histiocytes. They may mimic carcinoma of the cervix and must be distinguished from this as well as other neoplastic diseases.

The chronic ulcerative process may involve the urethra and the anal area, causing marked discomfort. Introital contraction may make coitus difficult or impossible; walking or sitting may become painful. The possibility of the coexistence of another venereal disease must be considered. Spread to other areas occurs in approximately 7% of patients.

B. Laboratory Findings

Direct smear from beneath the surface of an ulcer may reveal gram-negative bipolar rods within mononuclear leukocytes. These are seen best in Wright-stained smears. When smears are negative, a biopsy specimen should be taken. Biopsy of the lesion generally shows granulation tissue infiltrated by plasma cells and scattered large macrophages with rod-shaped cytoplasmic inclusion bodies (Mikulicz cells). Pseudoepitheliomatous hyperplasia often is seen at the margin of the ulcer.

The diagnosis of granuloma inguinale is made by demonstrating, in biopsy or smear material stained with Wright's, Giemsa's, or silver stain, large mononuclear cells having one or more cystic inclusions containing the so-called Donovan bodies—small round or rod-shaped particles that stain purple in traditional hematoxylin and eosin preparations.

Prevention

Personal hygiene is the best method of prevention. Therapy immediately after exposure may abort the infection.

Treatment

Trimethoprim-sulfamethoxazole, 1 double-strength tablet orally twice daily for at least 3 weeks or doxycycline 100 mg twice daily for 3 weeks are the CDC-recommended agents. Ciprofloxacin 750 mg twice daily for 3 weeks, erythromycin base, 500 mg 4 times daily for 2–3 weeks, or azithromycin 1 g orally once per week for 3 weeks are alternate regimens. Penicillin is not effective.

Sex partners must be considered for treatment. Partners who had sexual contact during the 60 days preceding the onset of symptoms or are clinically symptomatic should be treated by 1 of the regimens. Special consideration for HIV and gravid women should be made. Recommendations to add intravenous gentamicin to the oral protocol have been made.

5. Lymphogranuloma Venereum

ESSENTIALS OF DIAGNOSIS

- Rectal ulceration, inguinal lymphadenopathy, or rectal stricture.
- Positive complement fixation test.

General Considerations

The causative agent of lymphogranuloma venereum is 1 of the aggressive L serotypes (L1, L2, or L3) of *Chlamydia trachomatis*. It is encountered more frequently in the tropical and subtropical nations of Africa and Asia but is also seen in the southeastern United States. Transmission is via sexual contact; men are affected more frequently than are women (6:1). The incubation period is 7–21 days.

Clinical Findings

A. SYMPTOMS AND SIGNS (FIG 41–2)

Early in the course of the disease, a vesicopustular eruption may go undetected. With inguinal (and vulvar) ulceration, lymphedema, and secondary bilateral invasion, excruciating conditions arise. Sitting or walking may cause pain. During the inguinal bubo phase, the groin is exquisitely tender. A hard cutaneous induration (red to purplish-blue) is a notable feature. This usually occurs within 10–30 days after exposure and may be bilateral. Anorectal lymphedema occurs early; defecation is painful, and the stool may be blood-streaked.

Later, as the lymphedema and ulceration undergo cicatrization, rectal stricture makes defecation difficult or impossible. Vaginal narrowing and distortion may end in severe dyspareunia. In the late phase, systemic symptoms—fever, headache, arthralgia, chills, and abdominal cramps—may develop.

B. LABORATORY FINDINGS

The diagnosis can be proved only by isolating *C trachomatis* from appropriate specimens and confirming the immunotype. These procedures are seldom available, so less specific tests are used.

A complement fixation test using a heat-stable antigen that is group-specific for all *Chlamydia* species is available. This test is positive at a titer ≥ 1:16 in more than 80% of cases of lymphogranuloma venereum. If acute or convalescent sera are available, a rise in titer is

Figure 41–2. Lymphogranuloma venereum. Note involvement of perineum and spread over buttocks.

particularly helpful in making the diagnosis. Application of the microimmunofluorescent test may also be useful.

Differential Diagnosis

As with any disseminated disease, the systemic symptoms of lymphogranuloma venereum may resemble meningitis, arthritis, pleurisy, or peritonitis. The cutaneous lesions must be differentiated from those of granuloma inguinale, tuberculosis, early syphilis, and chancroid. In the case of colonic lesions, proctoscopic examination and mucosal biopsy are needed to rule out carcinoma, schistosomiasis, and granuloma inguinale.

Complications

Perianal scarring and rectal strictures—late complications—can involve the entire sigmoid, but the urogenital diaphragm is rarely involved. Vulvar elephantiasis (esthiomene) produces marked distortion of the external genitalia.

Prevention

Lymphogranuloma venereum is reportable. Avoiding infectious contact with a carrier is achieved by use of a condom or by refraining from coitus. Definite exposure can be treated with sulfonamides or tetracyclines.

Treatment

A. CHEMOTHERAPY

Doxycycline 100 mg twice daily orally should be given for 21 days according to tolerance. If disease persists, the course should be repeated. An alternative regimen is erythromycin 500 mg orally 4 times daily for 21 days.

B. Local and Surgical Treatment

Anal strictures should be dilated manually at weekly intervals. Severe stricture may require diversionary colostomy. If the disease is arrested, complete vulvectomy may be done for cosmetic reasons. Abscesses should be aspirated, not excised.

6. Syphilis

ESSENTIALS OF DIAGNOSIS

Primary Syphilis

- *Painless genital sore (chancre) on labia, vulva, vagina, cervix, anus, lips, or nipples.*
- *Painless, rubbery, regional lymphadenopathy followed by generalized lymphadenopathy in the third to sixth weeks.*
- *Dark-field microscopic findings.*
- *Positive serologic test in 70% of cases.*

Secondary Syphilis

- *Bilaterally symmetric extragenital papulosquamous eruption.*
- *Condyloma latum, mucous patches.*
- *Dark-field findings positive in moist lesions.*
- *Positive serologic test for syphilis.*
- *Lymphadenopathy.*

Tertiary Syphilis

- *Cardiac, neurologic, ophthalmic, and auditory lesions.*
- *Gummas.*

Congenital Syphilis

- *History of maternal syphilis.*
- *Positive serologic test for syphilis.*
- *Stigmata of congenital syphilis (eg, x-ray changes of bone, hepatosplenomegaly, jaundice, anemia).*
- *Normal examination or signs of intrauterine infection.*
- *Often stillborn or premature.*
- *Enlarged, waxy placenta.*

Latent Syphilis

- *History or serologic evidence of previous infection.*
- *Absence of lesions.*
- *Serologic test usually reactive; titer may be low.*

General Considerations

According to CDC data, the rate of primary and secondary syphilis in the United States declined by 90% during 1990–2000, but the rate increased from 2000–2004. Overall increases in rates during 2000–2004 were observed only among men. In 2004, for the first time in more than 10 years, the rate of primary and secondary syphilis among women did not decrease; it remained the same between 2003 and 2004 at 0.8 cases per 100,000 population. Syphilis is caused by *T pallidum*, which is transmitted by direct contact with an infectious moist lesion. Treponemes pass through intact mucous membranes or abraded skin. Ten to 90 days after the treponemes enter, a primary lesion (chancre) develops. The chancre persists for 1–5 weeks and then heals spontaneously, but it may persist with signs of secondary disease. Serologic tests for syphilis are usually nonreactive when the chancre first appears but become reactive 1–4 weeks later. Two weeks to 6 months (average, 6 weeks) after the primary lesion appears, the generalized cutaneous eruption of secondary syphilis may appear. The skin lesions heal spontaneously in 2–6 weeks. Serologic tests are almost always positive during the secondary phase. Latent syphilis may follow the secondary stage and may last a lifetime, or tertiary syphilis may develop. The latter usually becomes manifest 4–20 or more years after disappearance of the primary lesion.

In one-third of untreated cases, the destructive lesions of late (tertiary) syphilis develop. These involve skin or bone (gummas), the cardiovascular system (aortic aneurysm or insufficiency), and the nervous system (meningitis, tabes dorsalis, paresis). The complications of tertiary syphilis are fatal in almost one-fourth of cases, but one-fourth never show any ill effects.

Clinical Findings

A. Symptoms and Signs

1. Primary syphilis—The chancre (Fig 41–3) is an indurated, firm, painless papule or ulcer with raised borders. Groin lymph nodes may be enlarged, firm, and painless. Genital lesions are not usually seen in women unless they occur on the external genitalia; however, careful examination may reveal a typical cervical or vaginal lesion. Primary lesions may occur on any mucous membrane or skin area of the body (nose, breast, perineum), and dark-field examination is required for all suspect lesions. Serologic tests should be done every week for 6 weeks or until positive.

2. Secondary syphilis—Signs of diffuse systemic infection become evident as the spirochetes spread hematogenously. A "viral syndrome" presentation, often with diffuse lymphadenopathy, is not uncommon.

Figure 41–3. Chancre of primary syphilis (arrow).

The characteristic dermatitis appears as diffuse, bilateral, symmetric, papulosquamous lesions that often involve the palms and soles. Lesions may also cover the trunk and be macular, maculopapular, papular, or pustular. Other systemic manifestations include patchy alopecia, hepatitis, and nephritis. Moist papules can be seen in the perineal area (condyloma lata). Mucous patches may also be seen; like condyloma lata, they are dark-field–positive, infectious lesions. Serologic tests for syphilis are invariably reactive in this stage.

3. Latent syphilis—With resolution of the lesions of primary and secondary infection or the finding of a reactive serologic test without a history of therapy, a patient passes into latency. Persons are infectious in the first 1–2 years of latency, with clinical relapses resembling the secondary stage occurring in approximately 25% of cases in the first year. The U.S. Public Health Service defines early latent syphilis as disease of less than 1 year's duration and includes it in the category of "early or infectious syphilis, with primary and secondary lues." Late latent syphilis is an infection of indeterminate or greater than 1 year's duration; consideration must be given to possible asymptomatic neurosyphilis in this setting, and cerebrospinal fluid (CSF) examination is recommended.

4. Neurosyphilis—Although the central nervous system is always vulnerable to *T pallidum*, it is most commonly infected during latent syphilis. Neurologic involvement of ophthalmic and auditory systems can be detected. Cranial nerve palsy and meningeal signs should be evaluated on physical examination. All patients require CSF sampling with laboratory testing for cell count, protein, Venereal Disease Research Laboratory (VDRL), and fluorescent treponemal antibody absorption (FTA-ABS). FTA-ABS is less specific but very sensitive when diagnosing neurosyphilis.

5. Syphilis during pregnancy—The course of syphilis is unaltered by pregnancy, but misdiagnoses are common. The chancre is often unnoticed or internal and not brought to medical attention. Chancres, mucous patches, and condyloma lata are often thought to be herpes genitalis. The dermatoses can resolve prior to diagnosis, or they may be misdiagnosed.

The effect of syphilis on pregnancy outcome can be profound. The risk of fetal infection depends on the degree of maternal spirochetemia (greater in the secondary stage than in the primary or latent stages) and the gestational age of the fetus. Treponemes may cross the placenta at all stages of pregnancy, but fetal involvement is rare before 18 weeks because of fetal immunoincompetence. After 18 weeks, the fetus is able to mount an immunologic response, and tissue damage may result. The earlier in pregnancy the fetus is exposed, the more severe the fetal infection and the greater the risk of premature delivery or stillbirth. Antepartum infection in late pregnancy does not necessarily result in congenital infection, as only 40–50% of such infants will have definite congenital infection. Placental infection can occur with resultant endarteritis, stromal hyperplasia, and immature villi. Grossly, the placenta looks hydropic (pale yellow, waxy, and enlarged). Because hydramnios is frequently associated with symptomatic congenital infection, fetuses are ultrasonographically followed throughout pregnancy.

6. Congenital syphilis—Between 2003 and 2004, the overall rate of congenital syphilis decreased 17.8% in the United States, from 10.7 to 8.8 cases per 100,000 live births, which reflects the overall decrease in primary and secondary syphilis in women over the past decade. Most infants with congenital syphilis are born to women of low socioeconomic status with inadequate or no prenatal care. Either these neonates may be affected at birth from intrauterine infection (hepatosplenomegaly, osteochondritis, jaundice, anemia, skin lesions, rhinitis, lymphadenopathy, nervous system involvement), or symptoms may develop weeks or months later. The clinical spectrum of congenital infection is analogous to adult secondary disease, as the disease is systemic from onset due to transplacental hematogenous inoculation.

Because the antibodies from the maternal compartment are of the immunoglobulin (Ig)G class, they freely cross the placenta, giving most neonates a reactive serologic test if the mother's test was reactive. With symptomatic neonatal infection, often the cord blood serologic test will be higher in titer than the maternal test. No clinically reliable neonatal IgM serologic test is available. Other diagnostic aids include long-bone survey and lumbar puncture, which may help diagnose asymptomatic systemic infection requiring more intense therapy.

The newborn may have lymphadenitis and an enlarged liver and spleen. The bones usually reveal signs of osteochondritis and an irregular epiphyseal juncture on x-ray. The eyes, central nervous system structures, and other organs may reveal abnormalities at birth, or defects may develop later in untreated cases.

Any infant with the stigmata of syphilis should be placed in isolation until a definite diagnosis can be made and treatment administered.

Newborns with congenital syphilis may appear healthy at birth but often develop symptoms weeks or months later. Examine the body for stigmata of syphilis at intervals of 3 weeks to 4 months. If the mother's serologic test is positive at delivery, the baby's test will also be positive. Obtain serial quantitative serologic tests of the infant's blood for 4 months. A rising titer indicates congenital syphilis, and treatment is indicated.

B. LABORATORY FINDINGS

1. Identification of the organism—*T pallidum* can usually be identified by dark-field examination of specimens from cutaneous lesions, but the recovery period of the treponeme is brief; in most cases, diagnosis depends on the history and serologic tests. An immunofluorescent technique is now available for dried smears. Silver staining for *T pallidum* of biopsy specimens, placental sections, or autopsy material may confirm the diagnosis in difficult cases. Motile spirochetes can be identified in amniotic fluid obtained transabdominally in women with syphilis and fetal death. PCR is extremely specific for detection of *T pallidum* in amniotic fluid and neonatal serum and spinal fluid. Newer techniques involving molecular methods are now being used to diagnosis early syphilis. Multiplex PCR is such an assay that can simultaneously detect *T pallidum*, *H ducreyi*, and herpes simplex but is not yet commercially available.

2. Serologic tests—Diagnostic tests after the primary or secondary moist lesion has disappeared are confined largely to serologic testing. Serologic tests become positive several weeks after the primary lesion appears.

a. Nontreponemal tests—These measure reaginic antibody detected by highly purified cardiolipin-lecithin antigen. They can be performed rapidly, relatively easily, and inexpensively. Nontreponemal tests are used principally for syphilis screening, but they are relatively specific, so they are not absolute for syphilis, and false-positive reactions may occur. Nontreponemal tests currently in use are flocculation procedures that include the VDRL slide test, rapid reagin test, and automated reagin test for screening procedures in the field. The latter tests are more sensitive but less specific than the VDRL. If they are positive, the activity should be verified, and the degree of reactivity should be checked by the VDRL test. Complement

fixation tests (eg, Kolmer) are no longer used in the United States.

The VDRL test (the nontreponemal test in widest use) generally becomes positive 3–6 weeks after infection, or 2–3 weeks after the appearance of the primary lesion; it is almost invariably positive in the secondary stage. The VDRL titer is usually high in secondary syphilis and tends to be lower or even nil in late forms of syphilis, although this is highly variable. A 4-fold falling titer in treated early syphilis or a falling or stable titer in latent or late syphilis indicates satisfactory therapeutic progress. False-positive serologic reactions are frequently encountered in a wide variety of situations, including collagen diseases, infectious mononucleosis, malaria, many febrile diseases, leprosy, vaccination, drug addiction, old age, and possibly pregnancy. False-positive reactions are usually of low titer and transient and may be distinguished from true-positive results by specific treponemal antibody tests.

b. Treponemal antibody tests—The FTA-ABS test and microhemagglutination assay for *Treponema pallidum* (MHA-TP) detect antibody against *Treponema* spirochetes. Both tests are more sensitive and specific than nontreponemal tests (except the MHA-TP test with primary disease; Table 41–1). These tests remain positive despite therapy, so they are not given in titers or used to follow serologic response to treatment.

Differential Diagnosis

Primary syphilis must be differentiated from chancroid, granuloma inguinale, lymphogranuloma venereum, herpes genitalis, carcinoma, scabies, trauma, lichen planus, psoriasis, drug eruption, aphthosis, mycotic infections, Reiter's syndrome, and Bowen's disease.

Secondary syphilis must be differentiated from pityriasis rosea, psoriasis, lichen planus, tinea versicolor, drug eruption, "id" eruptions, perlèche, parasitic infections, iritis, neuroretinitis, condyloma acuminatum, acute exanthems, infectious mononucleosis, alopecia, and sarcoidosis.

Table 41–1. Percent sensitivity of serologic tests in untreated syphilis.

Type of Test	Stage of Disease			
	Primary	Secondary	Latent	Late
VDRL	59–87	100	73–91	37–94
FTA–ABS	86–100	99–100	96–99	96–100
MHA–TP	64–87	96–100	96–100	94–100

Reproduced, with permission, from Holmes KK et al (editors): *Sexually Transmitted Diseases.* McGraw-Hill, 1984.

Prevention

If the patient is known to have been exposed to syphilis, do not wait for the disease to develop to the clinical or reactive serologic stage before giving preventive treatment. Even so, every effort should be made to reach a diagnosis, including a complete physical examination, before administering preventive treatment. It is recommended that any patient who is exposed and becomes symptomatic within 90 days of sexual contact and is seronegative should still be treated. Also, if the exposure occurred more than 90 days earlier and seroconversion takes place, the exposed person should be treated. Finally, if the duration since exposure is unknown and the nontreponemal antibody titer is greater than 1:32, treatment is indicated.

Prenatal care is often underutilized or unavailable in geographic areas where congenital syphilis occurs. Education on the preventive value of prenatal care in these high-risk, generally low socioeconomic groups is essential. All pregnant women should undergo a routine serologic test for syphilis at the first visit. The test should be repeated between 28 and 32 weeks' gestation in high-risk regions. If the test result is positive, attention must be given to the patient's prior serologic test and therapy (if any) for syphilis. If doubt exists as to whether the patient has active syphilis, repeat therapy is far better than the risk of congenital syphilis.

Syphilis is still a serious public health problem. Teaching young people about the disease and its consequences is still the best method of control. Use of a condom, together with soap and water decontamination after coitus, would prevent most cases. If a lesion develops, a physician should be notified at once. All exposed persons must be sought and treated and the case reported to the communicable disease service in the city or state. The United States Preventive Services Task Force (USPSTF) updated syphilis screening guidelines in 2004. Further evidence was found to support the strategy of screening all pregnant women and people at higher risk for acquiring syphilis (men who have sex with men who engage in high-risk behaviors, commercial sex workers, persons who exchange sex for drugs, and those in adult correctional facilities). Several new screening tests are currently being studied, including the immunochromatographic strip (ICS), line immunoassay (LIA), enzyme-linked immunosorbent assay (ELISA), rapid plasma reagent (RPR) card, and rapid syphilis test (RST). New screening tests currently being studied for use in pregnant women and infants include IgM immunoblotting and PCR assay of serum and CSF for central nervous system infection in infants, placenta histopathology, and umbilical cord blood testing.

Treatment

A. EARLY SYPHILIS AND CONTACTS

Primary, secondary, and early latent syphilis (<1 year's duration):

1. Benzathine penicillin G 2.4 million units IM once.
2. Tetracycline hydrochloride 500 mg orally 4 times daily or 100 mg doxycycline twice daily for 14 days, for nonpregnant penicillin-allergic patients.

Erythromycin estolate should not be administered to pregnant women because of potential drug-related hepatotoxicity.

Ceftriaxone 1 g daily IM or IV for 8–10 days may be effective, but data on this regimen are limited.

B. LATE SYPHILIS

Includes latent syphilis of indeterminate duration or more than 1 year's duration, except neurosyphilis.

1. Benzathine penicillin G 2.4 million units IM weekly for 3 successive weeks (7.2 million units total).
2. Tetracycline hydrochloride 500 mg orally 4 times daily or 100 mg doxycycline twice daily for 14 days, for penicillin-allergic patients.

C. SYPHILIS IN PREGNANCY

Treat as indicated above, except that tetracycline or erythromycin is not recommended. If serologic tests are equivocal (eg, possible biologic false-positive result), it is better to err on the side of early treatment. Because of the increased risk for treatment failure, a second dose of 2.4 million units of penicillin IM is often recommended. Penicillin-allergic patients can be given oral desensitization therapy using gradually larger doses of phenoxymethyl penicillin suspension to achieve a temporary tolerant state that allows parenteral penicillin therapy. This is particularly useful in circumventing compliance problems due to hyperemesis or drug-induced gastric upset.

D. CONGENITAL SYPHILIS

Adequate maternal treatment before 16–18 weeks' gestation prevents congenital syphilis. Treatment thereafter may arrest fetal syphilitic infection, but some stigmata may remain.

1. Benzathine penicillin G 50,000 U/kg IM as a single injection, for asymptomatic infants without neurosyphilis.
2. Aqueous crystalline penicillin G 50,000 U/kg IV every 8–12 hours, or procaine penicillin G 50,000 U/kg IM once daily for 10–14 days, for symptomatic infants or those with neurosyphilis.

E. JARISCH-HERXHEIMER REACTION

A febrile reaction may occur in 50–75% of patients with early syphilis treated with penicillin. This occurs 4–12 hours after injection and is completed by 24 hours. Its cause is uncertain but may involve a release of treponemal toxic products upon organism lysis. The reaction is generally benign but may trigger labor or fetal distress. Prophylaxis with antipyretics or corticosteroids is of unknown value.

F. COEXISTING INFECTION WITH HIV

No specific changes in treatment are currently necessary, but close follow-up is necessary to ensure adequate treatment. Recommendations include serology tests every 3 months for 1 year and twice during the second year.

VAGINITIS

Vaginitis is a clinical syndrome characterized by vaginal discharge, vulvar irritation, or malodorous discharge. This is often broken down into 2 entities: infectious vaginitis and atrophic vaginitis. This chapter focuses on infectious vaginitis. Infectious vaginitis is most frequently caused by 1 of 3 diseases: trichomoniasis, bacterial vaginosis, or candidiasis.

1. Bacterial Vaginosis (Corynebacterium vaginale *Vaginitis*; Gardnerella vaginalis *Vaginitis*)

Although bacterial vaginosis is the most prevalent vaginal infection, almost 50% of affected women are asymptomatic. The term *bacterial vaginosis* refers to the intricate changes of vaginal bacterial flora with a loss of lactobacilli, an increase in vaginal pH (pH > 4.5), and an increase in multiple anaerobic and aerobic bacteria. Clinical criteria for diagnoses include (1) homogeneous white, noninflammatory discharge; (2) microscopic presence of > 20% clue cells; (3) vaginal discharge with pH > 4.5; and (4) fishy odor with or without addition of 10% potassium hydroxide (KOH). *Gardnerella vaginalis* (formerly designated *Corynebacterium vaginale* and *Haemophilus vaginalis*) is a small, nonmotile, nonencapsulated, pleomorphic rod that stains variably with Gram's stain. It may be spread by sexual contact and, although of low virulence, causes vaginitis. The disorder may be atypical and even more troublesome when *G vaginalis* coexists with more virulent organisms. *G vaginalis* is not the only cause of bacterial vaginosis. The characteristic fishy odor of bacterial vaginosis is due to anaerobic bacteria, such as *Bacteroides, Prevotella, Peptostreptococcus,* and *Mobiluncus* spp., and genital mycoplasmas.

G vaginalis infection is often overlooked. It may be suspected on the basis of the microscopic appearance of unstained exfoliated vaginal cells in a wet preparation

that appears to be dusted with many small dark particles, actually *G vaginalis* organisms. These "clue cells" are presumptive evidence of the presence of this organism. In case of mixed infection (eg, with *Candida albicans*), it may not be possible to make the diagnosis except by culture. Gram's stain is another method useful for making the diagnosis of bacterial vaginosis. Observational studies have consistently shown an association between bacterial vaginosis and adverse pregnancy outcomes, including preterm delivery, preterm premature rupture of membranes, spontaneous abortion, and preterm labor. However, 2 large randomized, placebo-controlled trials demonstrated that treatment of bacterial vaginosis in asymptomatic, pregnant women with metronidazole does not prevent preterm deliveries. The CDC recommends that pregnant women with a history of preterm delivery and asymptomatic bacterial vaginosis be evaluated for treatment.

Treatment

Specific therapy for vaginal infection caused by *G vaginalis* and *C vaginale* has been neglected, in part because of the rather innocuous symptoms reported. Therapy should always be initiated for symptomatic relief. Pregnant women who are at high risk for preterm labor may benefit from treatment. Treatment is recommended for low-risk groups during pregnancy if patients are infected and symptomatic. A third cohort of patients who are thought to benefit from therapy are asymptomatic carriers before pelvic/abdominal surgery. Guidelines issued by the CDC for therapy are as follows. (1) *Recommended regimen*—(a) oral metronidazole 500 mg twice daily for 7 days; (b) clindamycin cream 2%, 1 applicatorful (5 g) intravaginally at night for 7 days; and (c) metronidazole gel 0.75%, 1 applicatorful (5 g) intravaginally once daily for 5 days. (2) *Alternative regimens*—(a) oral metronidazole 2 g in a single dose; (b) oral clindamycin 300 mg twice daily for 7 days; (c) clindamycin ovules 100 g intravaginally once at bedtime for 3 days. Four randomized controlled trials have demonstrated overall cure rates of 95% for the 7-day metronidazole regimen and 84% for the single 2-g regimen. During pregnancy, oral treatment is preferred to local agents to ensure adequate tissue levels of the bactericidal drug. The recommended regimen is metronidazole 250 mg orally 3 times daily for 7 days or clindamycin 300 mg orally twice daily for 7 days.

2. Trichomonas vaginalis

See Chapter 37.

3. Candidiasis

See Chapter 37.

URETHRITIS AND CERVICITIS

Urethral mucopurulent or purulent discharge is commonly caused by *Neisseria gonorrhoeae, C trachomatis,* or genital herpes. Although asymptomatic infections are common, some patients experience slow-onset dysuria with vaginal discharge and/or irregular bleeding. Urethritis and cervicitis are often coinfections. Both are reportable STDs, and clinicians must mandate that partners of patients obtain diagnostic and therapeutic interventions.

Cervicitis is an inflammation of either the ectocervical cells or the glandular cells composing the cervical epithelium. The ectocervical squamous cells are contiguous with the vaginal epithelium and can be infected by the same organisms that cause inflammatory vaginitis. The glandular cells of the endocervix are more commonly inflamed by *N gonorrhoeae* and *C trachomatis*.

1. Gonorrhea

ESSENTIALS OF DIAGNOSIS

- *Most affected women are asymptomatic carriers.*
- *Purulent vaginal discharge.*
- *Urinary frequency and dysuria.*
- *Recovery of organism in selective media.*
- *May progress to pelvic infection or disseminated infection.*

General Considerations

N gonorrhoeae is a gram-negative diplococcus that forms oxidase-positive colonies and ferments glucose. The organism may be recovered from the urethra, cervix, anal canal, or pharynx. Optimal recovery of the organism is with use of Thayer-Martin or Martin-Lester (Transgrow) medium. *N gonorrhoeae* is rapidly killed by drying, sunlight, heat, and most disinfectants.

The columnar and transitional epithelium of the genitourinary tract is the principal site of invasion. The organism may enter the upper reproductive tract (Fig 41–1), causing salpingitis with its attendant complications. Approximately 600,000 new infections occur each year in both men and women. It has been estimated that after exposure to an infected partner, 20–50% of men and 60–90% of women become infected. Without therapy, 10–17% of women with gonorrhea develop pelvic infection. Depending on the geographic location and population involved, *N gonorrhoeae* is often present with other STDs. Traditionally, women with gonorrhea are considered to be at risk for incubating syphilis. It has been shown that 20–40% also have *Chlamydia* infection.

Clinical Findings

A. SYMPTOMS AND SIGNS

1. Early symptoms—Most women with gonorrhea are asymptomatic. When symptoms occur, they are localized to the lower genitourinary tract and include vaginal discharge, urinary frequency or dysuria, and rectal discomfort. The incubation period is only 3–5 days.

2. Discharge—The vulva, vagina, cervix, and urethra may be inflamed and may itch or burn. Specimens of discharge from the cervix, urethra, and anus should be taken for culture from the symptomatic patient. A stain of purulent urethral exudate may demonstrate gram-negative diplococci in leukocytes. Similar findings in a purulent cervical discharge are less conclusively diagnostic of *N gonorrhoeae*.

3. Bartholinitis—Unilateral swelling in the inferior lateral portion of the introitus suggests involvement of Bartholin's duct and gland. In early gonococcal infections, the organism may be recovered by gently squeezing the gland and expressing pus from the duct. Enlargement, tenderness, and fluctuation may develop, signifying abscess formation. *N gonorrhoeae* is then less frequently recovered; however, the prevalence of infection with other bacteria merits a search for these pathogens. Spontaneous evacuation of pus often occurs if the incision is not drained. The infection may result in asymptomatic cyst formation.

4. Anorectal inflammation—Anal itching, pain, discharge, or bleeding occurs rarely. Most women are asymptomatic and acquire infection by perineal spread of vaginal secretions rather than by anal intercourse.

5. Pharyngitis—Acute pharyngitis and tonsillitis rarely occur; most infections are asymptomatic.

6. Disseminated infection—For unknown reasons, asymptomatic carriers can develop systemic infection. Commonly, a triad of polyarthralgia, tenosynovitis, and dermatitis is seen, or purulent arthritis without dermatitis. Septicemia is more common in the former clinical setting and *N gonorrhoeae* cultured from joint aspirates in the latter. Endocarditis and meningitis have been described.

7. Conjunctivitis—In adults, ophthalmic infection is usually due to autoinoculation. Ophthalmia neonatorum may result from delivery through an infected birth canal.

8. Vulvovaginitis in children—Gonococcal invasion of nonkeratinized membranes in prepubertal girls produces severe vulvovaginitis. The typical sign is a purulent vaginal discharge with dysuria. The genital mucous membranes are red and swollen. Infection is commonly introduced by adults, and in such cases the physician must consider the possibility of child abuse.

B. LABORATORY FINDINGS

A presumptive diagnosis of gonorrhea can be made based on examination of the stained smear; however, confirmation requires positive identification on selective media. Secretions are examined under oil immersion for presumptive identification. Gram-negative diplococci that are oxidase-positive and obtained from selective media (Thayer-Martin or Transgrow) usually signify *N gonorrhoeae*. Carbohydrate fermentation tests may be performed, but in addition to being time-consuming and expensive, they occasionally yield other species of *Neisseria*. Therefore, cultures are reported as "presumptive for *N gonorrhoeae*." Chlamydial cultures or direct smear testing (ELISA or immunofluorescent staining) of the cervix and a serologic test for syphilis should also be obtained. In addition, other techniques for detecting gonorrhea include enzyme immunoassay from cervical swab or urine specimens, DNA probes from endocervical swabs, and nucleic acid amplification tests (NAATs) from endocervical swabs, liquid Papanicolaou (Pap) specimens, vaginal swabs, and urine specimens.

Complications

The major complication in the female is salpingitis and the complications that may arise from salpingitis (see Acute Salpingitis-Peritonitis). *N gonorrhoeae* can be recovered from the cervix in approximately 50% of women with salpingitis. It is important to note that asymptomatic carriers can also develop tubal scarring, infertility, and increased risk for ectopic gestations. Resistant strains of *N gonorrhoeae* have emerged in some geographic areas because of their capacity to produce penicillinase or because of chromosome-mediated resistance. Some strains are resistant to spectinomycin and tetracycline. Follow-up cultures are essential in these settings, at least by 7 days to 3 weeks after completion of therapy.

Differential Diagnosis

See Chapter 37.

Prevention

Gonorrhea is a reportable disease that can be controlled only by detecting the asymptomatic carrier and treating her and her sexual partners. It is crucial to instruct patients to abstain from sexual relations for the 7 days after therapy is initiated. All high-risk populations should be screened by routine cultures. Re-examination 3 weeks after treatment is mandatory to rule out reinfection or failure of therapy. Use of condoms will protect against gonorrhea.

Treatment

Any patient with gonorrhea must be suspected of having other STDs (eg, syphilis, HIV, and chlamydial infection) and managed accordingly. Treatment should cover *N gonorrhoeae*, *C trachomatis*, and incubating syphilis. Dual therapy has contributed greatly to the declining prevalence of chlamydial infections. Therefore, if chlamydial infection is not ruled out, the following regimens should be given with doxycycline (for nonpregnant patients) or azithromycin.

Quinolone-resistant *N gonorrhoeae* is common in parts of Asia and the Pacific. It is becoming increasingly common in areas on the west coast of the United States, particularly California. Because of this, quinolones are no longer recommended for treatment of gonorrhea acquired in Asia and the Pacific (including Hawaii). Quinolones may not be advisable for treatment of gonorrhea acquired in California.

A. UNCOMPLICATED INFECTIONS

Guidelines issued by the CDC for therapy of uncomplicated infection in adults are as follows. (1) *Recommended regimens*—(a) ceftriaxone 125 mg IM once, plus doxycycline 100 mg orally twice daily for 7 days (for nonpregnant patients), or azithromycin 1 g orally in a single dose if chlamydial infection is not ruled out; (b) cefixime 0.4 g orally once, plus doxycycline or azithromycin as above; and (c) ofloxacin 0.4 g, levofloxacin 0.25 g, or ciprofloxacin 0.5 g orally once in nonpregnant, nonlactating patients over 17 years old, plus doxycycline or azithromycin as above. Quinolones should not be given to patients residing in, or who may have acquired infection in, Asia and the Pacific (including Hawaii). Use of fluoroquinolones in California probably is inadvisable. According to one study, the advantage of oral cefixime over ceftriaxone is the reduced potential for needlesticks (HIV, hepatitis C) and increased patient comfort. (2) *Alternative regimens*—(a) spectinomycin 2 g IM once, followed by doxycycline or azithromycin as above, for patients who cannot take cephalosporins or quinolones (not reliable for pharyngeal infection); (b) ceftizoxime 0.5 g, cefotaxime 0.5 g, or cefoxitin 2 g IM once with probenecid 1 g orally, plus doxycycline or azithromycin as above; and (c) gatifloxacin 0.4 g, norfloxacin 0.8 g, or lomefloxacin 400 mg orally once in nonpregnant, nonlactating patients over 17 years old, plus doxycycline or azithromycin as above. Azithromycin 2 g orally is equally effective for *N gonorrhoeae* but may be limited because of its higher cost and potential for gastrointestinal distress.

Pregnant women should not be treated with quinolones or tetracyclines. They should be treated with a recommended or alternate cephalosporin. If cephalosporins are not tolerated, spectinomycin 2 g IM should be given along with treatment for diagnosed or presumptive *C trachomatis*.

The incidence of penicillinase-producing strains of *N gonorrhoeae* (PPNGs) is increasing and is spreading from coastal areas to the center of the United States. They are unresponsive to previously recommended conventional therapy such as penicillin, ampicillin, or amoxicillin. Currently recommended cephalosporins and quinolones and regimens with β-lactamase inhibitors are effective therapy against PPNG strains.

B. ACUTE SALPINGITIS

See Acute Salpingitis-Peritonitis.

C. DISSEMINATED INFECTIONS

Disseminated gonococcal infection should be treated in the hospital initially. Evidence for endocarditis or meningitis should be sought. Recommended regimens include ceftriaxone 1 g IM or IV every 24 hours, or cefotaxime or ceftizoxime 1 g IV every 8 hours. For patients with β-lactamase allergy, spectinomycin 2 g IM every 12 hours can be used. Testing for chlamydia should be performed or therapy given. Therapy should be given for a total of 1 week; oral medications include cefixime 0.4 g every 12 hours, ciprofloxacin 0.5 g every 12 hours, ofloxacin 0.4 g every 12 hours, or levofloxacin 0.5 g once daily in women who are not pregnant or lactating.

D. NEONATES AND CHILDREN

Infants born to women with untreated gonorrhea should be treated with ceftriaxone 25–50 mg/kg IV or IM, not to exceed 125 mg. It should be given cautiously to premature or hyperbilirubinemic infants.

Prognosis

The prognosis is excellent for patients with gonorrhea who receive prompt treatment. Infertility may result from even a single episode. Fewer cases have been reported to the CDC in recent years than previously reported.

2. Chlamydial Infections

ESSENTIALS OF DIAGNOSIS

- Mucopurulent cervicitis.
- Salpingitis.
- Urethral syndrome.
- Nongonococcal urethritis in males.
- Neonatal infections.
- Lymphogranuloma venereum.

General Considerations

The spectrum of genital infections caused by serotypes of *C trachomatis* has only recently become appreciated. *C trachomatis* infections are the most commonly reported notifiable disease in the United States. In 2004, 929,462 chlamydia infections were reported to the CDC, which is 2.5 times greater than the number of cases of gonorrhea. Genital infection with this organism is the most common sexually transmitted bacterial disease in women. Chlamydiae are obligate intracellular microorganisms that have a cell wall similar to that of gram-negative bacteria. They are classified as bacteria and contain both DNA and RNA. They divide by binary fission, but like viruses they grow intracellularly. They can be grown only by tissue culture. With the exception of the L serotypes, chlamydiae attach only to columnar epithelial cells without deep tissue invasion. As a result of this characteristic, clinical infection may not be apparent. For example, infections of the eye, respiratory tract, or genital tract are accompanied by discharge, swelling, erythema, and pain localized to these areas only. *C trachomatis* infections are associated with many adverse sequelae due to chronic inflammatory changes as well as fibrosis (eg, tubal infertility and ectopic pregnancy). The proposed mechanism for the pathogenesis of chlamydial disease is an immune-mediated response. This mechanism has been supported *C trachomatis* vaccine studies in humans and monkeys as well as other animal model studies. Evidence indicates that a 57-kDa chlamydial protein, which is a member of 60-kDa heat shock proteins, plays a role in the immunopathogenesis of chlamydial disease.

Certain factors may be predictive of women with a greater likelihood of acquiring *C trachomatis*. Sexually active women younger than 20 years have chlamydial infection rates 2–3 times higher than the rates of older women. The number of sexual partners and, in some studies, lower socioeconomic status are associated with higher chlamydial infection rates. Persons who use barrier contraception are less frequently infected by *C trachomatis* than are those who use no contraception, and women who use oral contraceptives may have a higher incidence of cervical infection than women not using oral contraceptives. Cervical infection in pregnant women varies from 2–24% and is most prevalent in young, unmarried women of lower socioeconomic status in inner-city environments. The CDC recommends screening sexually active adolescent girls at their routine yearly gynecologic examination, as well as women 20–24 years old, especially those who have new or multiple partners, and those who inconsistently use barrier contraceptives.

Clinical Findings

A. SYMPTOMS AND SIGNS

Women with chlamydial infection not uncommonly are asymptomatic. Women with cervical infection generally have a mucopurulent discharge with hypertrophic cervical inflammation. Salpingitis may be unassociated with symptoms.

B. LABORATORY FINDINGS

The diagnosis of chlamydial infection is based solely on laboratory tests. Diagnosis of *C trachomatis* using cell culture isolation has a sensitivity of 70–90%; however, this specialized modality is not widely available. Cell culture is the detection method of greatest specificity (almost 100%), but the cost can be prohibitive, and a 3- to 7-day delay in diagnosis is required. Despite its disadvantages, cell culture is presently the standard for quality assurance of nonculture chlamydia tests. The CDC recommends cell culture for specimens from the urethra, rectum, and vagina of prepubertal girls and from the nasopharynx of infants. In infants with inclusion conjunctivitis, Giemsa stain of purulent discharge from the eye is used to identify chlamydial inclusions, but similarly stained slides of exudates in adults with genital infections are only approximately 40% accurate in the diagnosis of these infections. Serologic methods, either the complement fixation or microimmunofluorescence test, are not totally accurate, as 20–40% of sexually active women have positive antibody titers. In fact, most women with microimmunofluorescent antibody do not have a current infection.

Moss and colleagues examined antibody responses to chlamydia species in patients who attended a genitourinary clinic and found that up to 50% of all chlamydia IgG-positive cases were due to nongenital chlamydiae (*C pneumoniae* and *C psittaci*). The low specificity of the chlamydia serology tests is attributed to these antibodies as well as to the presence of group-specific antibodies. Therefore, it is of utmost importance to use serologic tests capable of distinguishing antibodies to *C trachomatis* from antibodies to *C pneumoniae* and *C psittaci* (nongenital chlamydial pathogens). Direct smear fluorescent antibody testing requires a fluorescence microscope, and processing time is only 30–40 minutes. Sensitivity is 90% or higher, with a specificity of 98% or higher if an experienced microscopist and a satisfactory specimen are available. This test appears to be the most promising, and when tissue samples (endometrial or uterine tube) are being evaluated, it has been reported to be more accurate. PCR, ligase chain reaction, and current DNA probes used for detection of *C trachomatis* may be more rapid and less expensive. Nucleic acid hybridization methods (DNA probe) require only 2–3 hours of processing time. The DNA probe assay is specific for *C trachomatis;* cross-reactivity with *C pneumoniae* and *C psittaci* has not been reported. To ensure high specificity, a competitive probe assay has been produced and is currently being evaluated in clinical trials. Recent reports indicate PCR positivity with negative culture.

PCR may be the most sensitive and specific test method for chlamydia.

Differential Diagnosis

Mucopurulent cervicitis is frequently caused by *N gonorrhoeae,* and selective cultures for this organism should be performed. As discussed above, *C trachomatis* alone may be associated with as many as 20–35% of cases of acute salpingitis in the United States. In both cervicitis and salpingitis, cultures frequently may be positive for both organisms.

Complications

Adverse sequelae of salpingitis, specifically infertility due to tubal obstruction and ectopic pregnancy, are the most dire complications of these infections. Pregnant women with cervical chlamydial infection can transmit infections to their newborns; evidence indicates that up to 50% of infants born to such mothers will have inclusion conjunctivitis. In perhaps 10% of infants, an indolent chlamydial pneumonitis develops at 2–3 months of age. This pathogen may cause otitis media in the neonate. Whether maternal cervical infection with *Chlamydia* causes significantly increased fetal and perinatal wastage by abortion, premature delivery, or stillbirth is uncertain.

Increasing evidence indicates that chlamydial infection in pregnancy is a risk marker for premature delivery and postpartum infections. Women at greatest risk are those with recent chlamydial infection detected by antichlamydial IgM. Those with chronic or recurrent infection do not have increased risk for preterm delivery. It is hypothesized that asymptomatic cervicitis predisposes to mild amnionitis. This event activates phospholipase A_2 to release prostaglandins, which cause uterine contractions that may lead to premature labor. Chlamydial infection is associated with higher rates of early postpartum endometritis as well as delayed infection from *Chlamydia* that often presents several weeks postpartum.

Treatment

In most cases, *Chlamydia* can be eradicated from the cervix by doxycycline 100 mg orally twice daily for 7 days (for nonpregnant patients), or azithromycin 1 g orally as a single dose. Compliance with treatment may play a major role in controlling chlamydial infections. One group of researchers evaluated the compliance with antichlamydial and antigonorrheal therapy and found that 63% of patients treated with the standard 7-day regimen of tetracycline or erythromycin were compliant. An alternate regimen is erythromycin base 500 mg or erythromycin ethylsuccinate 800 mg orally 4 times daily given for a minimum of 7 days. Patients who cannot tolerate erythromycin should consider ofloxacin 300 mg twice daily or levofloxacin 500 mg orally once daily for 7 days. Administration of high doses of ampicillin has resulted in elimination of *C trachomatis* from the cervices of women with acute salpingitis. Addition of the irreversible β-lactamase enzyme inhibitor sulbactam increases in vitro antichlamydial activity.

Pregnant women are advised to take erythromycin base 500 mg 4 times daily for 7 days, or amoxicillin 500 mg 3 times daily for 7 days. Alternate regimens include erythromycin base 250 mg orally 4 times daily for 14 days, erythromycin ethylsuccinate 800 mg orally 4 times daily for 7 days, erythromycin ethylsuccinate 400 mg orally 4 times daily for 14 days, or azithromycin 1 g orally as a single dose.

Current studies indicate that 3–5% of pregnant women and as many as 15% of sexually active nonpregnant women have an asymptomatic chlamydial cervical colonization. Whether attempts to eradicate asymptomatic colonization will prevent chlamydial cervicitis, salpingitis, or neonatal infections is not known. Posttreatment cultures are not usually advised if doxycycline, azithromycin, or ofloxacin is taken as described above and symptoms are not present; cure rates should be higher than 95%. Retesting may be considered 3 weeks after completing treatment with erythromycin. A positive posttreatment culture is more likely to represent noncompliance by the patient or sexual partner or reinfection rather than antibiotic resistance. It is important to ensure that the sexual partner is treated, as most posttreatment reinfections occur because the sexual partner was not treated. Clinicians should advise all women with chlamydial infection to be re-screened 3–4 months after treatment.

PELVIC INFECTIONS

Because of their common occurrence and often serious consequences, infections are among the most important problems encountered in the practice of gynecology. A wide variety of pelvic infections, ranging from uncomplicated gonococcal salpingo-oophoritis to septicemic shock following rupture of a pelvic abscess, confront the general physician as well as the gynecologist.

The following is a general classification of pelvic infections by frequency of occurrence:

1. Pelvic inflammatory disease
   a. Acute salpingitis
      i. Gonococcal
      ii. Nongonococcal
   b. Intrauterine device (IUD)-related pelvic cellulitis
   c. Tubo-ovarian abscess (TOA)
   d. Pelvic abscess

2. Puerperal infections
   a. Cesarean section (common)
   b. Vaginal delivery (uncommon)
3. Postoperative gynecologic surgery
   a. Cuff cellulitis and parametritis
   b. Vaginal cuff abscess
   c. TOA
4. Abortion-associated infections
   a. Postabortal cellulitis
   b. Incomplete septic abortion
5. Secondary to other infections
   a. Appendicitis
   b. Diverticulitis
   c. Tuberculosis

Pelvic inflammatory disease (PID) is a general term for acute, subacute, recurrent, or chronic infection of the oviducts and ovaries, often with involvement of adjacent tissues. Most infections seen in clinical practice are bacterial, but viral, fungal, and parasitic infections occur. The term PID is vague at best and should be discarded in favor of more specific terminology, which should include identification of the affected organs, the stage of the infection, and, if possible, the causative agent. This specificity is especially important in light of the rising incidence of venereal disease and its complications.

The three proposed pathways of dissemination of microorganisms in pelvic infections are depicted in Figs 41–4, 41–5, and 41–6. Lymphatic dissemination (Fig 41–5), typified by postpartum, postabortal, and some IUD-related infections, results in extraperitoneal parametrial cellulitis. In Fig 41–4, the endometrial-endosalpingeal-peritoneal spread of microorganisms is depicted. This represents more common forms of nonpuerperal PID, in which pathogenic bacteria gain access to the lining of the uterine tubes, with resultant purulent inflammation and egress of pus through tubal ostia into the peritoneal cavity. These infections are represented by endometritis, adnexal infection, and peritonitis. In rare instances, certain diseases (eg, tuberculosis) may gain access to pelvic structures by hematogenous routes (Fig 41–6).

Early recognition and treatment of the various entities that constitute PID are mandatory so that specific therapy can be instituted to prevent damage to the reproductive system. Laparoscopic studies have confirmed a 65–90% positive predictive value for tubal disease among patients with the diagnosis of presumed PID. Repeated sexual contacts with multiple partners predispose to subsequent reinfection or superinfection, spreading the disease throughout the reproductive system and resulting in sterility and an increased risk for tubal pregnancy.

The initial gonococcal infection (more common in young single women of low parity) may be relatively

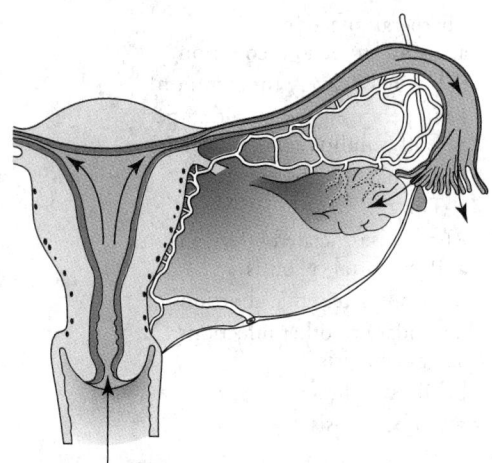

Figure 41-4. Intra-abdominal spread of gonorrhea and other pathogenic bacteria.

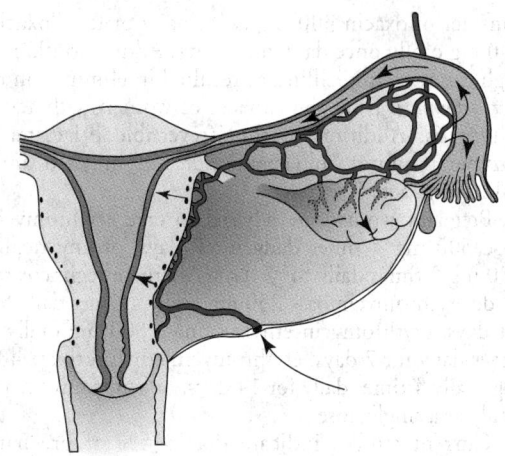

Figure 41-6. Hematogenous spread of bacterial infection (eg, tuberculosis).

asymptomatic, and the patient may not be seen until recurrent infection with irreversible pathologic changes has occurred. Gonorrhea involving only the lower genital tract and urethra is often asymptomatic; severe symptomatic gonorrhea implies tubal and peritoneal involvement. If the initial infection is limited to the lower tract, proper therapy may prevent further sequelae. The presence of endosalpingitis or ovarian infection carries a graver prognosis with regard to future fertility.

Originally, gonococcus was thought to be the only organism responsible for nonpuerperal acute pelvic inflammation. More recent data indicate that *N gonorrhoeae* is isolated in only 40–60% of women with acute salpingitis. In Sweden, *C trachomatis* was estimated to cause 60% of cases of salpingitis. Although direct evidence of such infection, eg, recovery from

tubal culture, is lacking in most studies performed in the United States, authorities believe that this pathogen may be responsible for 20–35% of such pelvic infections. How frequently salpingitis is caused by chlamydiae alone or by chlamydia in association with other invasive microorganisms is unclear. Regardless of the initiating factors, nongonococcal pathogens that compose the normal vaginal flora may be involved in many cases of acute salpingitis-peritonitis.

N gonorrhoeae was present alone or with other pathogens in 65% of the specimens. One group of researchers reported positive cul-de-sac fluid cultures in 18 (90%) of 20 patients with acute salpingitis compared with 8 normal patients with negative results.

If the infectious process continues, pelvic adhesions become more pronounced, and tissue planes are lost. Identification of the tubes and ovaries in the inflammatory mass, which may include omental and intestinal attachments, becomes difficult. Further progression causes tissue necrosis with abscess formation. Containment of the purulent exudate under pressure becomes impossible at certain sites, and pus is released into the peritoneal cavity. This usually is at the site of an adhesion to a nearby organ, and the point of rupture often can be identified at operation. Abscess formation may be localized in either or both of the tubes and ovaries without leakage or rupture. Another possibility is accumulation of purulent material walled off in the cul-de-sac.

Recent observations have shown these pelvic infections are polymicrobial with mixed anaerobic and aerobic bacteria. Anaerobes predominate and frequently coexist with aerobes. In some cases, aerobes alone are isolated. With further advanced disease, such as abscess formation, anaerobic organisms seem to predominate. All these bacteria are members of the normal vaginal and endocervical

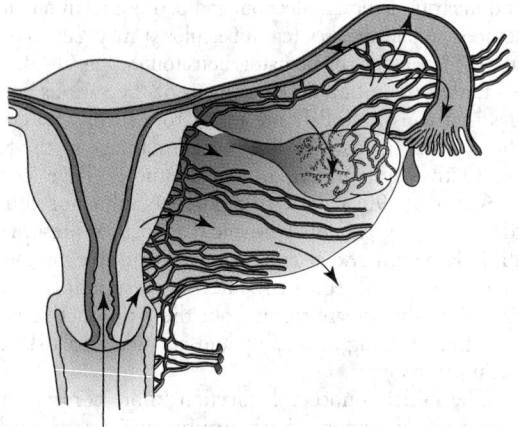

Figure 41-5. Lymphatic spread of bacterial infection.

flora and include *Bacteroides, Escherichia coli,* aerobic streptococci, and anaerobic cocci (*Peptostreptococcus* and *Peptococcus*). Virtually any organism indigenous to the normal vaginal or gastrointestinal flora may be isolated if specific techniques are used. Direct immunofluorescent antibody testing of cervical smears of 500 asymptomatic women showed *C trachomatis* in 10%. Moreover, among women recently treated as outpatients for acute salpingitis, 16% had *C trachomatis* in endocervical specimens and 8% had the organism in the endometrial cavity (obtained with a double-lumen catheter-protected brush). These numbers should not be taken lightly when considering the cost of chlamydia-related PID. Also, many retrospective studies point to recurrent infections and delays in treatment as the major behavioral risk factors contributing to PID. From the same sites, *N gonorrhoeae* was identified in 68% and 65% of specimens, respectively. Great numbers of both aerobes and anaerobes were recovered from endometrial cultures; 10% had group B *Streptococcus,* 10% had *Bacteroides fragilis,* 55% had *Streptococcus faecalis,* 65% had *Staphylococcus epidermidis,* 75% had anaerobic *Streptococcus* spp., and 65% had *Prevotella bivius* in that location. Whether this is a result of infection or is flora from the lower tract and endometrium is under evaluation.

Many factors may account for adverse sequelae of these pelvic infections, eg, infertility and pain. Delay in initiation of treatment is associated with later symptomatology. Likewise, inadequate therapy because of improper antimicrobial selection, insufficient dosage, or inadequate duration of therapy may be responsible for subsequent problems. An inflammatory process that is allowed to continue—for whatever reason—results in anatomic derangements with adhesive attachments to nearby organs. An ovulation site in an ovary may serve as a portal of entry for extension of the infection into the ovarian stroma, and this sets the stage for formation of TOAs.

The most important factor in the diagnosis of women with pelvic infections is clinical awareness by the physician. For patients with high-risk factors (eg, postoperative pelvic surgery, postpartum, or postabortal), fever is usually the first clue. For women without these factors, a high index of suspicion is important. If gonorrhea is suspected, a Gram-stained smear of endocervical purulent material or fluid obtained by culdocentesis may be helpful. The Gram-stained smear may be lifesaving, especially in the woman seen with a rare serious infection due to *Clostridium perfringens.* Except for isolation of *N gonorrhoeae* with specialized media, cultures taken from women with pelvic infections currently are not useful for clinical management. Because these infections are usually polymicrobial, sophisticated techniques are necessary for microbiologic identification. These techniques are time-consuming, and by the time the results become available to the clinician, the woman has usually been cured with empiric antimicrobial drug therapy.

PELVIC INFLAMMATORY DISEASE

1. Acute Salpingitis-Peritonitis

 ESSENTIALS OF DIAGNOSIS

- Onset of lower abdominal and pelvic pain, usually following onset or cessation of menses and associated with vaginal discharge, abdominal, uterine, adnexal, and cervical motion tenderness, plus one or more of the following:

  a. Temperature above 38.3 °C (101 °F).

  b. Leukocyte count greater than 10,000/μL or elevated C-reactive protein.

  c. Inflammatory mass (examination or sonography).

  d. Gram-negative intracellular diplococci in cervical secretions.

  e. Purulent material (white blood cells) from peritoneal cavity (culdocentesis or laparoscopy).

  f. Elevated erythrocyte sedimentation rate.

General Considerations

There is generally an acute onset of pelvic infection, often associated with invasion by *N gonorrhoeae* and involving the uterus, tubes, and ovaries, with varying degrees of pelvic peritonitis. In the acute stage, there is redness and edema of the tubes and ovaries with a purulent discharge oozing from the ostium of the tube.

Clinical Findings/Diagnosis

A. SYMPTOMS AND SIGNS

The insidious or acute onset of lower abdominal and pelvic pain usually is bilateral and only occasionally is unilateral. There may be a sensation of pelvic pressure, with back pain radiating down 1 or both legs. In most cases, symptoms appear shortly after the onset or cessation of menses. There is often an associated purulent vaginal discharge.

Nausea may occur, with or without vomiting, but these symptoms may be indicative of a more serious problem (eg, acute appendicitis). Headache and general lassitude are common complaints.

Fever is not necessary for the diagnosis of acute salpingitis, although its absence may indicate other disorders, specifically ectopic pregnancy. In 1 study, only 30% of women with laparoscopically confirmed acute salpingitis had fever. Although standardization of criteria for diagnosis of acute salpingitis to include fever greater than 38.3 °C (101 °F) may greatly aid clinical research, such a distinction may result in many women with acute pelvic infection being erroneously diagnosed and inadequately treated.

Abdominal tenderness is often encountered, usually in both lower quadrants. The abdomen may be somewhat distended, and bowel sounds may be hypoactive or absent. Pelvic examination may demonstrate inflammation of the periurethral (Skene) or Bartholin's glands as well as a purulent cervical discharge. Bimanual examination typically elicits extreme tenderness on movement of the cervix and uterus and palpation of the parametria.

B. LABORATORY FINDINGS

Leukocytosis with a shift to the left is usually present; however, the white blood cell count may be normal. A smear of purulent cervical material may demonstrate gram-negative kidney-shaped diplococci in polymorphonuclear leukocytes. These organisms may be gonococci, but definitive cultures on selective media are advised. Penicillinase production should be confirmed.

Culdocentesis generally is productive of "reaction fluid" (cloudy peritoneal fluid) that, when stained, reveals leukocytes with or without gonococci or other organisms. Culture and sensitivity testing of organisms from culdocentesis samples may be done.

C. RADIOLOGIC FINDINGS

X-ray examination of the abdomen may show signs of ileus, but this finding is nonspecific. Air may be seen under the diaphragm with a ruptured tubo-ovarian or pelvic abscess and demands immediate laparotomy in addition to combination antimicrobial therapy.

D. ULTRASOUND

With the introduction of transvaginal sonography, the female reproductive tract now can be visualized at bedside. Markers for acute and chronic PID can be differentiated. Incomplete septation of the tubal wall ("cogwheel sign") is a marker for acute disease, and a thin wall ("beaded string") indicates chronic disease. Thickening is noted in the pelvic areas during the inflammatory process. Ultrasound diagnosis is approximately 90% accurate compared with laparoscopic diagnosis. Ultrasonography is most valuable in following the progression or regression of an abscess after it has been diagnosed. The borders of an abscess conform to the surrounding pelvic structures and as such do not give a well-defined border as noted in an ovarian cyst.

E. CULDOCENTESIS

Culdocentesis (cul-de-sac tap) may be helpful in the diagnosis of suspected pelvic infection. Other conditions that may simulate infection can be ruled out using this simple procedure. The rectouterine pouch (of Douglas) is punctured with a long spinal needle to obtain a sample of the contents of the peritoneal cavity after vaginal membrane preparation with povidone-iodine or similar agents. Culdocentesis is easy to perform and can be performed with or without local anesthesia in the hospital or in the office. One milliliter of sterile saline anesthetizes the vaginal membrane and peritoneum. Culdocentesis is indicated whenever peritoneal material is needed for diagnosis. Cultures for aerobic and anaerobic organisms may also be obtained. Contraindications include a cul-de-sac mass or a fixed retroflexed uterus. The differential evaluation of fluid obtained by culdocentesis is given in Table 41–2.

Differential Diagnosis

Acute salpingitis must be differentiated from acute appendicitis, ectopic pregnancy, ruptured corpus luteum cyst with hemorrhage, diverticulitis, infected septic abortion, torsion of an adnexal mass, degeneration of a leiomyoma, endometriosis, acute urinary tract infection, regional enteritis, and ulcerative colitis.

Complications

Complications of acute salpingitis include pelvic peritonitis or generalized peritonitis, prolonged adynamic ileus, severe pelvic cellulitis with thrombophlebitis, abscess formation (pyosalpinx, TOA, cul-de-sac abscess) with adnexal destruction and subsequent infertility, and intestinal adhesions and obstruction. Rarely, dermatitis, gonococcal arthritis, or bacteremia with septic shock occurs.

Table 41–2. Differential evaluation of fluid contained by culdocentesis.

Finding	Implications for Diagnosis
Blood	Ruptured ectopic pregnancy. Hemorrhage from corpus luteum cyst. Retrograde menstruation. Rupture of spleen or liver. Gastrointestinal bleeding. Acute salpingitis.
Pus	Ruptured tubo-ovarian abscess. Ruptured appendix or viscus. Rupture of diverticular abscess. Uterine abscess with myoma.
Cloudy	Pelvic peritonitis (such as is seen with acute gonococcal salpingitis). Twisted adnexal cyst. Other causes of peritonitis: appendicitis, pancreatitis, cholecystitis, perforated ulcer, carcinomatosis, echinococcosis.

Prevention

Approximately 15% of women with asymptomatic gonococcal cervical infection develop acute salpingitis. Detection and treatment of these women and their sexual partners should therefore prevent a substantial number of cases of gonococcal pelvic infection. Early diagnosis and eradication of minimally symptomatic disease (cervicitis, urethritis) also usually prevent salpingitis.

Treatment

As with most female pelvic infections, the microbial etiologic agents are not readily apparent when clinical infection is diagnosed, and because of the myriad of pathogens described, empiric therapy is given as soon as a presumptive diagnosis is made. It is important to note that negative cultures do not preclude upper reproductive tract disease. The majority of women who present with acute salpingitis-peritonitis have clinical disease of mild to moderate severity that usually responds well to outpatient antibiotic therapy. Hospitalization usually is warranted for women who are more severely ill as well as for women in whom the exact diagnosis is uncertain. Prepubertal children and pregnant women with this diagnosis should be hospitalized for therapy, as should women with a suspected abscess, women unable to tolerate outpatient oral therapy, and women who have not responded to outpatient therapy. Although it has not been clinically proved that inpatient therapy is associated with improved future fertility, women who desire future fertility may benefit from inpatient therapy if only by reason of compliance. Some authors believe that all women with this infection should receive inpatient therapy.

A. OUTPATIENT THERAPY

Outpatient therapy for women with acute salpingitis may be undertaken if the temperature is less than 39 °C (102.2 °F), lower abdominal findings are minimal, and the patient is not "toxic" and can take oral medication. These women can be treated with antibiotics, IUD removal, analgesics, and bed rest. Regimens recommended by the CDC include (1) ofloxacin 400 mg orally twice daily or levofloxacin 500 mg orally once daily for 14 days, plus clindamycin 450 mg orally 4 times daily or metronidazole 500 mg orally twice daily for 14 days; (2) ceftriaxone 250 mg IM or equivalent cephalosporin (eg, ceftizoxime or cefotaxime) IM, with probenecid 1 g orally, followed by 14 days of doxycycline 100 mg orally twice daily, with or without metronidazole 500 mg twice daily; or (3) cefoxitin 2 g IM, plus probenecid 1 g orally, followed by 14 days of doxycycline 100 mg orally twice daily, with or without metronidazole 500 mg twice daily. If a response to therapy is not observed after 72 hours, the patient should be admitted for inpatient therapy. Refer the patient to the city or county health department or STD clinic for contact surveillance. All male sexual partners of women treated for this acute infection should be examined for STDs and promptly treated with a regimen effective against uncomplicated gonococcal and chlamydial infections.

B. INPATIENT THERAPY

Inpatient therapy is prudent for patients with a temperature over 39 °C (102.2 °F), for those with guarding and rebound tenderness in lower quadrants, or for patients who look "toxic." Hospitalization of these patients is necessary to administer therapy and to observe for signs of complications or deterioration. Patients who do not respond to outpatient therapy should be evaluated for a suspected TOA. The following measures should be taken:

(1) Maintain bed rest.

(2) Restrict oral feeding.

(3) Administer intravenous fluids to correct dehydration and acidosis.

(4) Use nasogastric suction in the presence of abdominal distention or ileus.

(5) No standardization of inpatient antimicrobial therapy for women with acute salpingitis has been established. Symptomatic response and adverse sequelae are related to the severity of tubal inflammatory disease and the development of adnexal abscesses. The CDC recommends one of the following regimens: (1) doxycycline 100 mg IV or orally twice daily, plus cefoxitin 2 g IV 4 times daily, or cefotetan 2 g IV twice daily, for at least 24 hours after the patient shows clinical improvement, followed by doxycycline 100 mg orally twice daily to complete 14 days of therapy; (2) clindamycin 900 mg IV 3 times daily, plus gentamicin 2 mg/kg IV and then 1.5 mg/kg IV every 8 hours (single daily dosing of gentamicin may be substituted), given as above in women with normal renal function, followed by doxycycline 100 mg twice daily or clindamycin 450 mg orally 4 times daily for 14 days. The incidence of infertility after the first episode of salpingitis is approximately 12%. Because infertility increases with the degree of inflammatory response, intensive broad-spectrum therapy should reduce complications. If suspicion for TOA is elevated, a regimen consisting of metronidazole or clindamycin should be used both for inpatient therapy and for continued outpatient therapy for increased anaerobic coverage.

(6) Exploratory laparotomy should be performed if there is clinical suspicion of abscess rupture. More gynecologists are successfully performing just a linear salpingostomy, as might be done for ectopic pregnancy, when pyosalpinx is identified. Percutaneous drainage may avoid operation.

(7) Continual evaluation by the same experienced clinician is of paramount importance to maintain accuracy and continuity of clinical observation.

Prognosis

A favorable outcome is directly related to the promptness with which adequate therapy is begun. For example, the incidence of infertility is directly related to the severity of tubal inflammation judged by laparoscopic examination. A single episode of salpingitis has been shown to cause infertility in 12–18% of women. Tubal occlusion was demonstrated in only approximately 10% of these patients regardless of the presence of a gonococcal or nongonococcal infection. Nongonococcal infection predisposed more commonly to ectopic pregnancy and thus carried a worse prognosis for subsequent viable pregnancy. The ability and willingness of patients to cooperate with their physicians are important to the outcome of patients with milder cases who are adequately treated on an outpatient basis. Follow-up care and education are necessary to prevent reinfection and complications.

2. Recurrent or Chronic Pelvic Infection

ESSENTIALS OF DIAGNOSIS

- History of acute salpingitis, pelvic infection, or postpartum or postabortal infection.
- Recurrent episodes of acute reinfection or recurrence of symptoms and physical findings less than 6 weeks after treatment for acute salpingitis.
- Chronic infection may be relatively asymptomatic or may provoke complaints of chronic pelvic pain and dyspareunia.
- Generalized pelvic tenderness on examination; usually less severe than with acute infection.
- Thickening of adnexal tissues, with or without hydrosalpinx (often).
- Infertility (commonly).

General Considerations

Recurrent PID begins as does primary disease, but pre-existing tubal tissue damage may result in more severe infection. Chronic pelvic infection implies the presence of tissue changes in the parametria, tubes, and ovaries. Adhesions of the peritoneal surfaces to the adnexa as well as fibrotic changes in the tubal lumen are usually present. Hydrosalpinx or tubo-ovarian "complexes" may be present. Chronic inflammatory lesions usually are secondary to changes induced by previous acute salpingitis but may represent an acute reinfection.

The diagnosis of chronic pelvic infection generally is difficult to make clinically. It has been erroneously applied to almost any cause of chronic pelvic pain. However, it may be the cause of pain in less than 50% of such women.

Clinical Findings

A. SYMPTOMS AND SIGNS

Recurrent infection usually has the same manifestations as acute salpingitis, and a history of pelvic infection can usually be obtained. Pain may be unilateral or bilateral, and dyspareunia and infertility are often reported. The patient may be febrile, with tachycardia; however, unless an acute reinfection is present, the fever is minimal. Tenderness is noted upon movement of the cervix, uterus, or adnexa. Adnexal masses may be present, as well as thickening of the parametria.

B. LABORATORY FINDINGS

Cultures from the cervix usually do not show gonococci unless reinfection is present. Leukocytosis may be demonstrated if active infection is superimposed on chronic changes.

Differential Diagnosis

Any patient with suspected chronic pelvic infection who presents with pelvic tenderness but without fever must be suspected of having an ectopic pregnancy. Other conditions to be considered include endometriosis, symptomatic uterine relaxation, appendicitis, diverticulitis, regional enteritis, ulcerative colitis, ovarian cyst or neoplasm, and acute or chronic cystourethritis.

Complications

The complications of chronic or recurrent pelvic infection include hydrosalpinx, pyosalpinx, and TOA; infertility or ectopic pregnancy; and chronic pelvic pain of varying degrees.

Prevention

Prompt and adequate treatment of acute pelvic infections is the essential preventive measure. Education about avoidance of STDs is also important.

Treatment

A. RECURRENT CASES

Treat as for acute salpingitis. If an IUD is in place, it should be removed and treatment started.

B. Chronic Cases

Long-term antimicrobial administration is of questionable benefit but is worthy of trial in young women of low parity. Therapy with a tetracycline, ampicillin, or a cephalosporin occasionally is beneficial, but changes responsible for symptoms are usually not due to active infection. Symptomatic relief can be achieved with analgesics such as ibuprofen or acetaminophen with or without codeine. Careful follow-up, preferably by the same physician, may detect serious sequelae, eg, TOA.

If the patient remains symptomatic after 3 weeks of antibiotic therapy, other causes must be considered. Consider laparoscopy or exploratory laparotomy to rule out other causes, eg, endometriosis.

If infertility is a problem, verify tubal patency by hysterosalpingography or laparoscopy and retrograde injection of methylene blue solution. It is important to prescribe antibiotics prior to and following either procedure because acute retrograde reinfection is common.

Total abdominal hysterectomy with bilateral adnexectomy may be indicated if the disease is far advanced and the woman is symptomatic or if an adnexal mass is demonstrated. Consideration can be given to resection or drainage of the abscess if preservation of fertility is desired. In many instances, computed tomography (CT)- or ultrasound-directed percutaneous drainage may avoid laparotomy.

Prognosis

With each succeeding episode of recurrent pelvic infection, the prognosis for fertility dramatically decreases. Likewise, the chances of an ectopic gestation increase with ensuing episodes of acute infection. These sequelae are undoubtedly due to chronic infection, which is the postinflammatory end result of 1 or multiple infections. Superimposition of acute infection on chronic disease is also associated with a higher incidence of tubo-ovarian and other pelvic abscesses.

3. Pelvic (Cul-De-Sac) Abscess

Pelvic abscess is an uncommon complication of chronic or recurrent pelvic inflammation. It may occur as a sequela to acute pelvic or postabortal infection. Abscess formation is frequently associated with organisms other than gonococcus, commonly anaerobic species, especially *Bacteroides*. Occasionally, resistant gram-negative bacteria such as *Bacteroides bivius* and *Bacteroides fragilis* are found.

Any of the symptoms of acute or chronic pelvic inflammation may be present together with a fluctuant mass filling the cul-de-sac and dissecting into the rectovaginal septum. These patients usually have more severe symptoms. They may complain of painful defe-

cation and severe back pain, rectal pain, or both. The severity of symptoms is often directly proportionate to the size of the abscess, but occasionally even a large pelvic abscess may be totally asymptomatic. One woman who was admitted to the obstetric service with "fetal heart tones" ultimately was drained of 3000 mL of pus through a colpotomy incision.

Differential Diagnosis

The following conditions must be considered in the differential diagnosis: TOA, periappendiceal abscess, ectopic pregnancy, adnexal torsion, ovarian neoplasm, uterine leiomyoma (especially those undergoing torsion or degeneration), retroflexed and incarcerated uterus, endometriosis, carcinomatosis, and diverticulitis with perforation.

Treatment

In addition to the measures already outlined, the following are required:

(1) Antibiotics to include anaerobic as well as aerobic microorganisms: (a) penicillin G 20–30 million units or ampicillin 2 g IV 4 times daily; clindamycin 900 mg IV 3 times daily; and gentamicin, 5 mg/kg IV per 24 hours. Metronidazole can be substituted for clindamycin at a dose of 15 mg/kg loading dose, then 7.5 mg/kg 4 times daily; (b) cefoxitin, 8–12 g IV per 24 hours (2 g every 4–6 hours), and gentamicin or tobramycin 5 mg/kg IV per 24 hours; (c) cefotaxime, 6–8 g IV per 24 hours in divided doses. With almost any effective therapeutic regimen, antibiotic-associated enterocolitis (diarrhea) is a complication that demands immediate evaluation, including testing for the presence of *Clostridium difficile* toxin. Pseudomembranous colitis is rare.

(2) Re-evaluate abdominal findings frequently to detect peritoneal involvement.

(3) If the abscess is dissecting the rectovaginal septum and is fixed to the vaginal membrane, colpotomy drainage with dissection of sacculations is indicated. This space should be actively drained with a large catheter, such as a Cook catheter, and preferably irrigated with sterile saline solution every 4 hours until the space is obliterated.

(4) If fever persists in the face of altered antimicrobial therapy but no evidence of abscess rupture or dissection of the rectovaginal septum is seen, percutaneous drainage and irrigation may obviate laparotomy (Figs 41–7, 41–8, and 41–9).

(5) If the patient's condition deteriorates despite aggressive management, perform exploratory laparotomy. In patients with recurrent infections and loss of reproductive function, total abdominal hysterectomy with bilateral salpingo-oophorectomy and lysis of adhesions offers the only cure. The patient's age and parity

Figure 41–7. Pelvic CT scan, with bladder and contrast medium on top, uterus and thickened broad ligaments centrally, and the posterior pelvis filled with abscess.

and the degree of involvement of the tubes and ovaries determine the extent of surgery when there is some likelihood of preservation of reproductive function. Clinical judgment is difficult and tends to favor surgery. Conservative surgery for women desiring future fertility is appropriate in many cases.

Prognosis

With early treatment, the prognosis for the woman with a well-localized abscess is good. Antibiotic treatment is essential; drainage may be necessary. Rupture into the peritoneum is a serious complication and demands im-

Figure 41–8. Pelvic CT scan with percutaneous drainage in process.

Figure 41–9. Cook catheter in abscess cavity. Note mild bilateral hydroureter caused by abscess compression at the pelvic brim.

mediate abdominal exploration. The prognosis for fertility is very poor following this type of abscess.

4. Tubo-Ovarian Abscess

 ESSENTIALS OF DIAGNOSIS

- *History of pelvic infection. TOA may present as a complication of acute salpingitis, including the initial episode.*
- *Lower abdominal and pelvic pain of varying degrees.*
- *Nausea and vomiting.*
- *Adnexal mass, usually extremely tender.*
- *Fever and tachycardia.*
- *Rebound tenderness in lower quadrants.*
- *Adynamic ileus.*
- *Culdocentesis productive of gross pus in case of rupture. (Contraindicated in cases of posterior pelvic abscess.)*

General Considerations

TOA formation may occur following an initial episode of acute salpingitis, but it is usually seen with recurrent infection superimposed on chronically damaged adnexal tissue. It is strongly believed that fallopian tube necrosis and epithelial damage by bacterial pathogens create the environment necessary for anaerobic invasion and growth. Initially there is salpingitis with or without ovarian involvement. The inflammatory process may subside spontaneously or in response to therapy; however, the result may be anatomic derangement, with fibrinous attachments to nearby organs (Figs 41–10 and 41–11). Involvement of the adjacent ovary, usually at an ovulation site, may serve as the portal of entry for extension of infection and abscess formation. Pressure of the purulent exudate may cause rupture of the abscess with resultant fulminating peritonitis, necessitating emergency laparotomy.

Slow leakage of the abscess may cause formation of a cul-de-sac abscess (see previous text). Culdocentesis into an abscess of this type will yield exudate like that of a ruptured TOA. Clinical appraisal usually will differentiate the 2 conditions, but if any doubt exists, treatment should be as specified for ruptured TOA.

These abscesses may occur in association with IUD use or in the presence of granulomatous infection (eg, tuberculosis, actinomycosis). Disease can be bilateral, although unilateral disease is more common than previously observed and may account for up to 60% of such abscesses even in the absence of IUD usage. Abscesses are usually polymicrobial.

Actinomyces israelii, a normal anaerobic commensal of the gastrointestinal tract, has been identified in 8–20% of women who have an IUD. Most patients

Figure 41–11. Uterus with myoma, unruptured right tubo-ovarian abscess, and chronic inflammatory left tubo-ovarian cyst.

are asymptomatic, but up to 25% reportedly develop symptoms of pelvic infection. Controversy exists as to whether an IUD should be removed from an asymptomatic woman with evidence of *Actinomyces* on Pap smear or culture. If the IUD is removed, a new IUD should not be inserted until the organism is no longer present; this rarely takes longer than 1 menstrual cycle. Antimicrobial therapy with penicillin should be reserved for symptomatic patients. Surgical drainage is usually required for actinomycotic abscesses, which are almost always the result of intestinal infections such as appendicitis but may be associated with IUD use.

Clinical Findings

A. SYMPTOMS AND SIGNS

The clinical spectrum varies greatly and may range from total absence of symptoms in a woman who, on routine pelvic examination, is found to have an adnexal mass to a moribund patient presenting with acute abdomen and septicemic shock.

The typical patient with TOA is usually young and of low parity, with a history of previous pelvic infection. However, no age group is exempt. The duration of symptoms for these women is usually approximately 1 week, and the onset is usually approximately 2 weeks or more after a menstrual period. This in contrast to what occurs in uncomplicated acute salpingitis, in which symptoms usually appear shortly after the onset or cessation of menses. The typical symptoms are pelvic and abdominal pain, fever, nausea and vomiting, and tachycardia. Four-quadrant abdominal tenderness and guarding may be present. Adequate pelvic examination is often impossible because of tenderness, but an adnexal mass may be palpated. Culdocentesis may lacerate (rupture) a pelvic abscess, so this procedure must be performed with extreme caution, if at all.

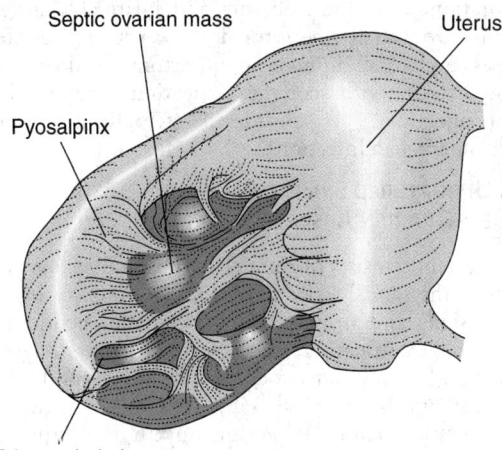

Figure 41–10. Tubo-ovarian abscess. (Reproduced, with permission, from Benson RC: *Handbook of Obstetrics & Gynecology,* 8th ed. Lange, 1983.)

Septic ovarian mass

Uterus

Pyosalpinx

Tube occluded

Signs and symptoms of ruptured TOA may resemble those of any acute surgical abdomen. A careful history and an alert clinician are essential to ensure an accurate diagnosis. Signs of actual or impending septic shock frequently accompany a ruptured abscess and include fever (occasionally hypothermia), chills, tachycardia, disorientation, hypotension, tachypnea, and oliguria.

B. LABORATORY FINDINGS

Laboratory findings are generally of little value. The white count may vary from leukopenia to marked leukocytosis. Urinalysis may demonstrate pyuria without bacteriuria. Mean erythrocyte sedimentation rate of at least 64 mm/h and mean acute C-reactive protein level of at least 20 mg/L can assist in making the diagnosis of TOA. Monitoring these levels has proven useful in following disease course.

C. X-RAY FINDINGS

Plain films of the abdomen (kidneys, ureter, bladder [KUB]) usually demonstrate findings of a dynamic ileus and may arouse suspicion of adnexal mass. Free air may be seen under the diaphragm with ruptured TOA.

D. ULTRASONOGRAPHY

Ultrasonography is the radiologic modality of choice and can be used with fewer complications to the patient. It can be of great help in following the patient and detecting changes that may occur, such as progression, regression, formation of pus pockets, and rupture.

E. SPECIAL EXAMINATIONS

Culdocentesis fluid obtained in a woman with an unruptured TOA may demonstrate the same cloudy "reaction fluid" seen in acute salpingitis. With a leaking or ruptured TOA, however, grossly purulent material may be obtained.

Differential Diagnosis

An unruptured TOA must be differentiated from an ovarian cyst or tumor with or without torsion, unruptured ectopic pregnancy, periappendiceal abscess, uterine leiomyoma, hydrosalpinx, perforation of the appendix, perforation of a diverticulum or diverticular abscess, perforation of peptic ulcer, and any systemic disease that causes acute abdominal distress (eg, diabetic ketoacidosis, porphyria). If an abscess does not respond to medical therapy and colpotomy is not possible, CT or magnetic resonance imaging (MRI) scanning may disclose the cause (Fig 41–12).

Complications

Unruptured TOA may be complicated by rupture with sepsis, reinfection at a later date, bowel obstruction, infertility, and ectopic pregnancy.

Figure 41–12. CT scan showing thickened appendix with intraluminal purulence. The source of this woman's pelvic abscess was a ruptured appendix.

Ruptured TOA is a surgical emergency and is frequently complicated by septic shock, intra-abdominal abscess (eg, subphrenic abscess), and septic emboli with renal, lung, or brain abscess.

Treatment

A. UNRUPTURED ASYMPTOMATIC TUBO-OVARIAN ABSCESS

Treatment is similar to that of chronic salpingitis: long-term antibacterial therapy and close follow-up. If the mass does not begin to subside within 15–21 days or becomes larger, drainage is indicated. At exploration, total hysterectomy and bilateral adnexectomy are usually performed; however, in selected cases, unilateral salpingo-oophorectomy or linear salpingostomy with copious irrigation and suction drainage may be considered (see Recurrent or Chronic Pelvic Infection).

B. UNRUPTURED SYMPTOMATIC TUBO-OVARIAN ABSCESS

Treatment consists of immediate hospitalization, bed rest in the semi-Fowler position, close monitoring of vital signs and urinary output, frequent gentle abdominal examination, nasogastric suction if necessary, and intravenous sodium-containing fluids. Intensive antimicrobial therapy should be instituted and should include either clindamycin or metronidazole because of their specific activity against anaerobes. The following combinations, given in appropriate intravenous doses, are recommended for these severely ill patients: penicillin G or ampicillin, and gentamicin plus metronidazole or clindamycin. One group of researchers suggests a regimen of 48–72 hours of triple antibiotics. If the patient demonstrates clinical rupture (peritonitis), an increase in the size of the abscess, or persistent fever, she should be taken to the operating room.

Laparoscopy or laparotomy is mandatory in all cases of suspected leakage or rupture as well as in all cases that do not respond to medical management and percutaneous drainage.

If initial therapy is successful, the patient is maintained on antibiotics (eg, oral tetracycline 500 mg 4 times daily, or doxycycline 100 mg twice daily) for a minimum of 10–14 days and must have frequent follow-up examinations. If the abscess persists—and many do—laparotomy may be necessary. The reported incidence of surgery for clinically diagnosed, unruptured TOA varies from 30–100%. On one service, approximately 57% of cases undergo surgery, and the remaining 43% seemingly respond to aggressive medical management. A recent prospective study found that aggressive antimicrobial treatment with cefotaxime was successful in 95% of 40 women, with abscesses ranging in size from 4 × 4 cm to 13 × 15 cm. Only 12% of these patients underwent hysterectomy and bilateral adnexectomy 1–33 months following initial therapy because of a persistent adnexal mass. These patients did not wish to retain reproductive function. Of the remainder, 7 conceived and delivered a mean of 26 months after study entry; 6 of the 7 had bilateral abscesses at sonography. These data support the theory that conservative therapy can be successful.

C. Ruptured Tubo-Ovarian Abscess

This is an acute life-threatening catastrophe requiring immediate medical therapy associated with operation. The following steps may be necessary:

(1) Monitoring of hourly urinary output with an indwelling catheter in place.

(2) Monitoring of central venous pressure.

(3) Administration of oxygen by mask.

(4) Rapid replacement of fluid and perhaps blood to maintain blood pressure and ensure urine output of 30 mL/h.

(5) Rapid evaluation and preparation for immediate operation. The patient's systemic deficiencies should first be corrected by intravenous fluids and blood if needed.

(6) Surgical measures: The anesthesiologist must be well informed of the patient's condition. A low midline incision is made to allow for cephalad extension. When the abdomen is opened, pus is obtained for aerobic and anaerobic cultures. The bowel is inspected and all loculated abscesses identified and drained. The subphrenic and subhepatic spaces are explored and loculations lysed to allow drainage of

pus. Careful irrigation and suction are performed to minimize spread of infection. Total hysterectomy and bilateral salpingo-oophorectomy were standard treatment; however, occasional supracervical hysterectomy may significantly shorten the operating time. The abscess wall is dissected from the adjacent structures. This is usually thick, indurated, and densely adherent to bowel, in which case it is best to dissect within the abscess wall, leaving a small portion of outer rim, rather than risk perforation of bowel wall. Careful surgical technique is necessary to avoid perforation of the bowel or ligation and transection of the ureters. The vaginal cuff is left open after a hemostatic interlocking continuous suture has been applied around the edge of the cuff.

Active drainage of the pelvis is performed routinely. Active suction through the abdominal wall provides the best result with the least contamination. The drains are left in place as long as purulent material is recovered. The fascia is closed with wide monofilament synthetic or wire sutures. Retention sutures may be used. The subcutaneous space is left open. In some cases, only drainage may be possible.

Prognosis

A. Unruptured Abscess

Generally the patient with an unruptured abscess has an excellent prognosis. Medical therapy, followed by judicious surgical treatment, yields good results in most cases. Unruptured localized abscesses that do not respond to aggressive medical management by improvement in signs and symptoms and decreasing size are best drained or removed surgically if inaccessible to percutaneous or transvaginal drainage. Many clinically diagnosed unruptured TOAs may represent only acute salpingitis with omental and intestinal adhesions, which respond promptly to adequate antibiotic therapy. Serial ultrasonography may help to identify true unruptured TOAs. The outlook for fertility, however, is greatly reduced, ranging from 5–15% from retrospective analysis. There is also an increased risk for ectopic pregnancy. The risk of reinfection must be considered if definitive surgical treatment has not been performed, but the incidence of reinfection in our prospectively studied patient population is less than 10%.

B. Ruptured Abscess

Before effective means of treating overwhelming septicemia became available and the need for immediate surgical intervention was recognized, the mortality rate from ruptured TOA was 80–90%. With modern therapeutic resources, both medical and surgical, the mortality rate should be less than 2%.

5. Postoperative Pelvic Infections

 ESSENTIALS OF DIAGNOSIS

- *Recent pelvic surgery.*
- *Pelvic or low abdominal pain or pressure.*
- *Fever and tachycardia.*
- *Purulent, foul discharge.*
- *Constitutional symptoms: malaise and chills.*
- *Vaginal cuff tenderness with cellulitis or abscess.*

General Considerations

Patients who have undergone gynecologic surgery, especially hysterectomy, may develop postoperative infections of the remaining pelvic structures. These infections include simple cuff induration (cellulitis), infected cuff hematoma (cuff abscess), salpingitis, pelvic cellulitis, suppurative pelvic thrombophlebitis, and TOA with or without rupture. The incidence of such infections has been significantly reduced, from 32% after abdominal hysterectomy and 57% after vaginal hysterectomy in women given placebo to approximately 5% in women given a single dose of antimicrobial prophylaxis. It is important to note that severe pelvic abscess formation may occur following the relatively benign procedure of oocyte pickup used with in vitro fertilization.

The pathogenesis of posthysterectomy infection is simple and straightforward. The apex of the vaginal vault consists of crushed, devitalized tissue, and the loose areolar tissue in the parametrial areas usually oozes postoperatively. These conditions provide an ideal medium for the myriad of pathogens that normally inhabit the vagina and are inoculated into the operative site during surgery.

The term "pelvic cellulitis" implies that the soft tissue of the vaginal apex and adjacent parametrial tissues have been invaded by bacteria. In addition, the serum and blood at the cuff apex may become infected, resulting in an infected hematoma, which in essence is a cuff abscess. The infection is treated at this point by establishing adequate drainage combined with antibiotic therapy. Infection may extend via lymphatic channels to the adnexa, resulting in salpingitis. Pelvic veins may become involved in the infectious process, particularly if *Bacteroides* or anaerobic streptococci are predominant pathogens. Rarely, septic emboli to the lungs, brain, spleen, and elsewhere occur.

Clinical Findings

The diagnosis of postoperative pelvic infection is made clinically. Laboratory studies may be useful in establish-

ing the specific etiologic diagnosis and determining the sensitivity of the recovered bacteria to various antibiotics.

A. SYMPTOMS AND SIGNS

Any postoperative gynecologic patient who develops fever may have atelectasis, phlebitis, upper urinary tract infection, or pelvic infection. These conditions may or may not require antimicrobial therapy. Although some investigators have stated that fever due to postoperative pelvic infection usually does not occur before the third or fourth postoperative day, up to 50% of patients develop temperatures of 38.3–39.4° C (101–103 °F) by the 24th–36th postoperative hour. Recurrent temperature elevation without symptoms occurs a mean of 50 hours after hysterectomy in our patient population and disappears without therapy. Temperature elevations associated with symptoms and physical findings of infection occur later. The mean time of this diagnosis in our patients is approximately 80 hours. Patients who ultimately require parenteral antimicrobial therapy do not experience early asymptomatic temperature elevation.

Within 2 days following hysterectomy, the surgical margin of the vagina (vaginal cuff) appears hyperemic and edematous, and there is almost always a purulent or seropurulent exudate, regardless of the clinical condition of the patient and the presence of fever. When palpated, this site is usually indurated and tender—findings common to most healing wounds and not indicative of the need for antimicrobial therapy. When natural defense mechanisms of the host are inadequate for the inoculum, lymphatic extension of the infection to adjacent tissues results in pelvic cellulitis, demonstrable on pelvic examination as tender induration in the parametrial areas. The infection may involve the tubes and ovaries, with resultant abscess formation in unresponsive patients. At this point, the patient begins to complain of lower abdominal, pelvic, or back pressure or pain. Abdominal distention due to ileus may develop, as may urinary symptoms due to perivesical irritation.

The diagnosis of suppurative pelvic thrombophlebitis is rare and usually is not apparent until after the sixth postoperative day, at which time the patient continues to have hectic spiking fever of 39–40.5 °C (102.2–105 °F) with a diurnal variation. The pelvic findings are usually unrevealing except for mild pelvic tenderness. Surprisingly, the woman's general health often is good unless septic embolization has occurred. CT scan is the diagnostic tool of choice for these diagnoses.

An infected pelvic hematoma is impossible to palpate early, but it can be diagnosed by sonography. Recurring temperature elevation is the principal indicator of this type of infection. Rarely do these patients have symptoms, and their examination is usually unremarkable. This problem can be suspected when the hematocrit level is lower than anticipated. Onset frequently is the same time as when other pelvic infections begin.

B. LABORATORY FINDINGS

Unfortunately, the polymicrobial nature of these infections prohibits accurate identification of the offending microorganisms in a reasonable time. For this reason, broad-spectrum empirical antimicrobial administration is necessary.

Serial complete blood counts (CBCs) usually demonstrate leukocytosis but occasionally enable the physician to detect concealed hemorrhage, which may harbor a large pelvic abscess. Urinalysis is rarely helpful.

C. X-RAY FINDINGS

Chest films are unrevealing in most cases but can be useful if pulmonary complications are suspected.

D. ULTRASONOGRAPHY

Pelvic sonograms may prove helpful in detecting hematomas or either retroperitoneal or TOAs that develop as a complication of cuff infection.

Differential Diagnosis

Pulmonary atelectasis may become manifest within 12–36 hours after operation. This can usually be detected by auscultation and confirmed by chest x-ray film. Aspiration pneumonitis must always be considered if pulmonary problems develop.

Deep vein thrombophlebitis of the lower extremities is rarely detected clinically and, when present, is seldom accompanied by significant fever. Superficial phlebitis of the upper extremity due to an indwelling venous catheter may cause significant pyrexia. Long-term (48–72 hours) infusion of intravenous antimicrobials increases the likelihood of phlebitis. Routine changing of the intravenous site every 48 hours may prevent this complication, but if it develops it will respond to warm soaks and anti-inflammatory drugs, such as aspirin.

Upper urinary tract infection may account for the fever. Because of the liberal use of indwelling catheters in gynecologic surgery, significant bacteriuria commonly develops; however, this rarely causes fever unless pyelonephritis develops.

Fever from abdominal wound infection usually becomes manifest on or after the fourth postoperative day. Examination of the abdominal wound is mandatory in all febrile patients. Careful probing of the abdominal incision may be necessary, regardless of the incision's appearance, especially if the pelvic examination is unrevealing.

Complications

Complications of postoperative pelvic infection include extensive pelvic or intra-abdominal abscesses, TOA with or without rupture, intestinal adhesions and obstruction, septic pelvic thrombophlebitis with metastatic abscesses, and septicemia.

Prevention

Many attempts have been made to decrease infectious morbidity following gynecologic surgical procedures. None has been uniformly successful, but the following measures may be helpful:

(1) Preoperative insertion of antibacterial vaginal creams or suppositories, especially if cervicitis, bacterial vaginosis, or vulvovaginitis is present.

(2) Preparation of the vagina with hexachlorophene or povidone-iodine solution just prior to surgery.

(3) Meticulous attention to hemostasis at operation and gentle handling of tissues. Use of large, strangulating hemostatic sutures should be avoided; nonreactive suture material should be used.

(4) If hemostasis is less than desirable but is maximal under given circumstances, suction drainage of that area should be accomplished. This can be done with the vaginal surgical margin left open or closed at hysterectomy.

(5) Antimicrobial prophylaxis beginning preoperatively has been shown by many to significantly reduce pelvic infectious morbidity following vaginal and abdominal hysterectomy. However, some controversy regarding this treatment still exists. Before prophylaxis is used, consider these guidelines. (a) Morbidity on a specific service should be significant enough to warrant attempts to decrease it. (b) Antimicrobials of relatively insignificant toxicity but proved value should be used. (c) The first dose should be given preoperatively to ensure adequate tissue concentrations at the time of surgery. Increasingly, studies show that a single preoperative dose is as effective as multiple doses in preventing major infection. Use of many different antimicrobials has been associated with dramatic lowering of pelvic infection morbidity rates. Recent comparative studies indicate that the newer, more expensive semisynthetic cephalosporins and penicillins are more effective than the older agents. In otherwise uncomplicated cases, pelvic infections developing despite prophylaxis generally are mild in nature, although severe infections and resultant complications are not always prevented.

(6) Severe, more advanced infections may be prevented by early diagnosis, drainage (including an open vaginal cuff), and prompt treatment of mild infections.

Treatment

If a cuff hematoma or abscess is found, adequate drainage can be established by separating the apposed vaginal edges with ring forceps or some other suitable instrument. Care must be taken not to disrupt the intact peritoneum. The usual supportive measures are instituted, and antibiotic therapy is begun. Many of the newer semisynthetic cephalosporins and expanded spectrum penicillins have proved valuable as single-agent therapy for these infections. Rarely, the addition of metronidazole to these regimens is necessary to effect a cure.

In most cases, the patient with postoperative pelvic infection becomes afebrile within 48–72 hours. If a large, infected pelvic hematoma has developed, more prolonged treatment will be necessary. Large hematomas can be drained and irrigated from below by means of a Foley catheter or Penrose drain introduced into the abscess cavity. Suction drains should be used whenever possible.

A postoperative TOA is treated expectantly as outlined for unruptured TOA. If intra-abdominal rupture of a pelvic abscess or TOA is suspected, immediate laparotomy is indicated.

Persistent fever and clinical signs of unresponsiveness to therapy may indicate septic pelvic thrombophlebitis, which is generally a diagnosis of exclusion after a 7- to 10-day course of antibiotics. Intermittent intravenous heparin therapy, 5000 U every 4 hours, should be given. Persistence of fever in spite of heparin therapy suggests abscess formation. Abscesses—as well as septic thrombophlebitis—are usually associated with anaerobic bacteria, and antimicrobial therapy should include clindamycin or metronidazole in addition to other agents effective against aerobic microorganisms.

6. Pelvic Tuberculosis

ESSENTIALS OF DIAGNOSIS

- *Infertility.*
- *Active or healed pulmonary tuberculosis.*
- *Findings by hysterosalpingography or laparoscopy.*
- *Recovery of* Mycobacterium tuberculosis *from either menstrual fluid or biopsy specimen.*

General Considerations

In the United States, pelvic tuberculosis is becoming a rare entity. When it does occur, it usually represents secondary invasion from a primary lung infection via the lymphohematogenous route (Fig 41–6). The overall incidence of pelvic tuberculosis in patients with pulmonary tuberculosis is approximately 5%. Prepubertal tuberculosis rarely results in genital tract infection.

Figure 41–13. Miliary tuberculosis involving the uterus and peritoneum.

After the pelvic organs become affected (Fig 41–13), direct extension to adjacent organs may occur. Older studies in the United States indicated that the oviducts were most frequently involved (90%) and the endometrium next most frequently (70%). More recent studies in Scotland, where the disease is still prevalent, showed endometrial involvement in more than 90% of cases and tubal involvement in only 5%.

Clinical Findings

A. SYMPTOMS AND SIGNS

The only complaint may be infertility, although dysmenorrhea, pelvic pain, and evidence of tuberculous peritonitis may also be present. Endometrial involvement may result in amenorrhea or some other disturbance of the cycle. Abdominal or pelvic pain from this infection is commonly associated with low-grade fever, asthenia, and weight loss. The diagnosis can usually be established on the basis of a complete history and physical examination, chest x-ray and lung scan, and appropriate tests such as a tuberculin (Mantoux) test, sputum smears, and sputum cultures. Tuberculosis of the female genital tract is usually secondary to hematogenous spread involving the endometrium, tubes, and ovaries. The manifestations are usually those of chronic pelvic disease and sterility. Gross ascites with fluid containing more than 3 g of protein per 100 mL of peritoneal fluid is characteristic of tuberculous peritonitis.

Pelvic tuberculosis is usually encountered in the course of a gynecologic operation performed for other reasons. Although pelvic tuberculosis may be mistaken for chronic pelvic inflammation, some distinguishing features usually can be found: extremely dense adhesions without planes of cleavage, segmental dilatation of the tubes, and lack of occlusion of the tubes at the ostia. If the internal genitalia are involved, with disseminated granulomatous disease of the serosal surfaces, ascites usually is present. Clinical diagnosis is difficult.

B. LABORATORY FINDINGS

The best direct method of diagnosis in suspected genital tuberculosis is detection of acid-fast bacteria by Ziehl-Neelsen stain followed by culture on Lowenstein-Jensen medium. The specimen may be from menstrual discharge, from curettage or biopsy, or from peritoneal biopsy in cases where ascites is present. A rapid sedimentation rate, peripheral blood eosinophilia, and a strongly positive Mantoux test are additional evidence of tuberculous infection.

C. X-RAY FINDINGS

1. Chest x-ray film—A chest x-ray film should be taken in any patient with proved or suspected tuberculosis of other organs or tissues.

2. Hysterosalpingography—The tubal lining may be irregular, and areas of dilatation may be present. Saccular diverticula extending from the ampulla and giving the impression of a cluster of currants are characteristic of granulomatous salpingitis. Other findings that should arouse suspicion are calcifications of the periaortic or iliac lymph nodes.

D. SPECIAL EXAMINATIONS

Visual inspection (laparoscopy) as well as aspiration of fluid for culture and biopsy of affected areas is possible and often diagnostic.

Differential Diagnosis

Pelvic tuberculosis should be differentiated from schistosomiasis, enterobiasis, lipoid salpingitis, carcinoma, chronic pelvic inflammation, and mycotic infections.

Complications

Sterility and tuberculous peritonitis are possible sequelae of pelvic tuberculosis.

Treatment

A. MEDICAL MEASURES

To prevent the emergence of drug-resistant strains, the initial therapy of tuberculous infection should include 4 drugs. The drug regimen for the first 2 months of treatment should include isoniazid, rifampin, pyrazinamide, and streptomycin or ethambutol. Once drug sus-

ceptibility results are available, the drug regimen can be appropriately changed. Treatment should be continued for 24–36 months because extrapulmonary tuberculosis is more difficult to eradicate.

B. SURGICAL MEASURES

The primary mode of treatment for pelvic tuberculosis is medical therapy; however, surgical intervention may be necessary. Medical therapy should be attempted for 12–18 months prior to evaluation for surgery. The ultimate indications for surgery include (1) masses not resolving with medical therapy, (2) resistant or reactivated disease, (3) persistent menstrual irregularities, and (4) fistula formation.

Prognosis

The prognosis for life and health is excellent if chemotherapy is instituted promptly, although the prognosis for fertility is poor.

7. Toxic Shock Syndrome

 ESSENTIALS OF DIAGNOSIS

- *Fever of 38.9 °C (102 °F) or higher.*
- *Diffuse macular rash.*
- *Desquamation (1–2 weeks after onset of illness; particularly affects palms and soles).*
- *Hypotension (systolic < 90 mm Hg for adults or orthostatic syncope).*
- *Involvement of 3 or more of the following organ systems: gastrointestinal, muscular, mucous membrane, renal, hepatic, hematologic, central nervous system.*

General Considerations

Toxic shock syndrome was first described in children in 1978 but was quickly identified as an illness occurring primarily in menstruating women 12–24 years of age. An association with use of superabsorbent tampons was made by the CDC. The majority of cases have occurred in California, Minnesota, Wisconsin, Utah, and Iowa. Peak incidence was reported in August 1980. Whether the abrupt decline in incidence has been the result of changes in tampon use, improvements in manufacture, or reduction in disease severity due to early recognition is not known. Of the approximately 30 million menstruating women in the United States, it is estimated that 70%

use tampons and more than 50% of those women use superabsorbent types. Almost 1 million women are at theoretic risk. The incidence in menstruating women is now 6–7:100,000 annually. Toxic shock syndrome has also been reported in women after delivery and in those using a diaphragm, in men and women following surgical procedures, or in patients with soft-tissue abscesses or osteomyelitis. The incidence of nonmenstrual disease has increased only slightly in the past 10 years.

The cause of toxic shock syndrome is preformed toxins produced by *Staphylococcus aureus* so that colonization or infection by this microorganism must occur. A pyrogenic toxin induces high fever and may enhance susceptibility to endotoxins that cause shock as well as liver, kidney, and myocardial damage. Other unrecognized toxins may play a role. How toxins gain access to the circulatory system is unknown. Tampon use has been associated with this syndrome, but evidence for the mechanism of toxin entry remains obscure. Insertion could cause mucosal damage. Vaginal ulcerations due to pressure changes usually are not observed, although vaginal erythema commonly is present. Superabsorbent tampons may obstruct the vagina, resulting in retrograde menstruation and peritoneal absorption of bacteria or toxin. Tampons may be associated with increased numbers of aerobic bacteria due to oxygen trapped in interfibrous spaces. The longer a tampon is left in place, the greater the risk for development of this syndrome.

Clinical Findings

A. SYMPTOMS AND SIGNS

Onset is usually sudden, with high fever, watery diarrhea, and vomiting—the triad often seen with viral gastroenteritis. Myalgia, headache, and sometimes sore throat may be present as well as erythroderma and conjunctivitis, as frequently seen with viral infections. Unlike most viral infections, however, this disorder may progress to hypotensive shock within several hours (usually < 48 hours). Timely diagnosis is critical, and the key is the fact that the woman is menstruating or using tampons. The patient will appear acutely ill, with a fever of 39 °C (102.2 °F) or higher. An erythematous, sunburnlike rash is seen over the face, proximal extremities, and trunk. Dehydration is evident, and the patient will have tachycardia and perhaps hypotension. The conjunctiva will be erythematous as will the pharynx, and usually muscle and abdominal tenderness is noted. A vaginal examination must be performed; if a tampon is present, it must be removed. Mucosal lesions should be sought, and a culture for *S aureus* performed. If nuchal rigidity, headache, or disorientation unexplained by hypotension or fever is present, a lumbar puncture must be performed to rule out meningitis. During convalescence, desquamation can be striking.

B. LABORATORY FINDINGS

Tests should include a CBC with differential, electrolyte measurements, urinalysis, urea nitrogen measurement, creatinine measurement, and hepatic function tests. Other tests are performed as indicated by clinical symptoms and signs. Cultures should be made of blood, throat secretions, and probably CSF. A vaginal culture will yield penicillinase-producing *S aureus*.

Differential Diagnosis

Other systemic diseases characterized by rash, fever, and systemic complications should be considered. Most patients will not have an obvious source of infection such as a recent incision, soft-tissue abscess, or osteomyelitis, but these should be sought. Kawasaki's disease of young children is similar but not as severe, as hypotension, renal failure, and thrombocytopenia do not occur and the incidence of myalgia, diarrhea, and hepatic damage is greatly decreased. Scarlet fever must be excluded. Rocky Mountain spotted fever, leptospirosis, and measles can be excluded by appropriate serologic tests. Gram-negative sepsis must be excluded by both blood and CSF cultures.

Complications

Approximately 30% of women who develop toxic shock syndrome have recurrences. The greatest risk for recurrence is during the first 3 menstrual periods following treatment, and the recurrent episode may be less or more severe than the initial one. The incidence is reduced to less than 5% if antistaphylococcal antibiotic therapy is given during therapy of the initial occurrence. Half of the women who developed this disease in Wisconsin during the infancy of its recognition have experienced 3 recurrences. Cervicovaginal and nasal cultures for *S aureus* should be negative twice, 4 weeks apart, prior to resumption of tampon use. Women can almost entirely eliminate the risk of this illness by not using tampons and may substantially reduce the risk by using tampons only intermittently during menstruation.

Treatment

Aggressive supportive therapy is imperative for a successful outcome. Appropriate initial management begins with fluid and electrolyte resuscitation—up to 12 L/d. Packed red blood cells and coagulation factors may be necessary. Central venous or pulmonary wedge pressures and urine output must be monitored to guide therapy. Laboratory studies and appropriate cultures must be obtained early. Dopamine infusion at 2–5 μg/kg/min may be necessary if fluid volume alone does not correct hypotension. Mechanical ventilation may be necessary if acute respiratory syndrome develops, and hemodialysis may be necessary if renal failure develops. Corticosteroid therapy (methylprednisolone 30 mg/kg or dexamethasone 3 mg/kg as a bolus and repeated every 4 hours as necessary), if instituted early, may reduce the severity of illness and duration of fever. Naloxone has resulted in reversal of hypotension in seriously compromised patients by antiendorphin activity. Although *S aureus* is not present in the blood, treatment with a β-lactamase–resistant antibiotic such as nafcillin or oxacillin (2 g IV every 4 hours) should be given. If penicillin allergy is present, vancomycin should be given. Dose reduction is necessary with renal impairment. Until gram-negative sepsis has been excluded, an aminoglycoside should be included with caution because of altered renal function. The mortality rate associated with toxic shock syndrome is 3–6%. The 3 major causes of death are acute respiratory distress syndrome, intractable hypotension, and hemorrhage secondary to disseminated intravascular coagulopathy.

8. Human Immunodeficiency Virus Infection

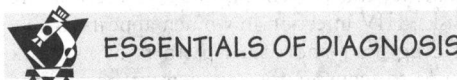

ESSENTIALS OF DIAGNOSIS

Asymptomatic Infection

- *HIV antibody, antigen, or ribonucleic acid or culture.*
- *High-risk group member.*
- *Mononucleosis-like syndrome with weight loss, fever, night sweats.*
- *Neurologic involvement.*
- *Lymphadenopathy.*
- *Pharyngitis.*
- *Erythematous maculopapular rash.*
- *Extragenital lymphadenopathy.*

Acquired Immunodeficiency Syndrome (AIDS)

- *HIV antibody, antigen, ribonucleic acid, or culture.*
- *Any of the above signs or symptoms of asymptomatic infection.*
- *Opportunistic infections.*
- *Cognitive difficulties or depression.*
- *Kaposi's sarcoma.*
- *CD4$^+$ counts below 200 CD4 lymphocytes/mm^3.*
- *Cervical neoplasia.*

General Considerations

The World Health Organization (WHO) and The Joint United Nations Program on HIV/AIDS (UN-AIDS) estimate that the total number of people living with HIV worldwide in 2005 is just over 40 million. Worldwide, women represent half of the people infected with HIV. Globally, fewer than 1 in 5 people at risk for becoming infected with HIV has access to basic prevention services. Only 1 in 10 people living with HIV has been tested and knows his or her HIV status. According to 2003 data, the CDC estimates that up to 1,185,000 persons in the United States were living with HIV/AIDS. In 2004, 25% of all AIDS diagnoses in the United States were made in women. The best estimates of the incidence of HIV infection in the United States are likely to come from ongoing serologic surveillance studies in sentinel areas and hospitals. In the general population, HIV infection is most prevalent in gay or bisexual men, intravenous drug abusers, and hemophiliacs. The high-risk groups of women are intravenous drug abusers, those with heterosexual contacts with men in high-risk groups, recipients of unscreened transfusions, and prostitutes.

Over 80% of the female AIDS cases occur in women of reproductive age, making heterosexual and perinatal transmission important concerns. Minorities are disproportionately represented in the reported AIDS cases. Most HIV infections in the United States are due to HIV-1. The prevalence of HIV-2 in this country is very low. HIV-2 is endemic in parts of West Africa and has been reported increasingly in Angola, Mozambique, Portugal, and France.

Modes of Transmission

Although there has been much speculation about the modes of HIV transmission, HIV infection can be acquired in only 3 ways.

First, HIV infection can be acquired by sexual contact. Transmission has been reported from male to male, male to female, female to male, and, recently, female to female. The risk appears to be greatest for the female sexual partners of men with AIDS, followed in decreasing order by intravenous drug abusers, bisexual men, transfusion recipients, and hemophiliacs. Other factors that increase the risk for heterosexual acquisition of HIV infection are the number of exposures to high-risk sexual partners; anal-receptive intercourse; and infection with other STDs such as syphilis, genital herpes, chancroid, and condylomata acuminata.

The second means by which HIV transmission can occur is by parenteral exposure to blood or bodily fluids, such as with intravenous drug use or occupational exposure.

The third means by which HIV infection can occur is by transmission from an infected woman to her fetus or infant.

Course of Infection

The chance of acquiring HIV infection through sexual contact is unknown. In women in the United States, approximately 40% of the reported cases appear to be acquired through heterosexual contact; some of the cases without risk factors may be heterosexually acquired. The percentage of cases arising from heterosexual contact is significantly larger in women than in men, probably because transmission can occur more easily from male to female. This is due to 2 reasons: (1) the concentration of HIV in semen is high, and (2) coitus causes more breaks in the introital mucosa than in the penile skin. It is hypothesized that these breaks in the mucosa, similar to those that occur with anal-receptive intercourse, increase the chances for acquiring HIV through sexual contact. The presence of a genital ulcerative disease also increases the risk of infection in a similar fashion.

The natural course of HIV infection is becoming better understood. HIV is a single-stranded RNA-enveloped retrovirus that attaches to the CD4 receptor of the target cell and integrates into the host genome. Most patients who become infected develop anti-HIV antibody within 12 weeks and 95% within 6 months after exposure. As many as 45–90% of patients develop an acute HIV-induced retroviral infection in the first few months after infection. This is similar to mononucleosis, with symptoms of weight loss, fever, night sweats, pharyngitis, lymphadenopathy, erythematous maculopapular rash, and extragenital lymphadenopathy. Critical awareness of this acute syndrome is important because of improved prognoses associated with early antiretroviral treatment. This syndrome usually resolves within several weeks, and the patient becomes asymptomatic. HIV-infected individuals ultimately show evidence of progressive immune dysfunction, and the condition progresses to AIDS as immunosuppression continues and systemic involvement becomes more severe and diffuse. AIDS develops in the majority of untreated HIV-infected individuals within 17 years after contracting the virus. All women diagnosed with HIV require counseling, an extensive STD work-up, Pap smear, CBC, chemistry panel, toxoplasma antibody, hepatitis panel, purified protein derivative, and chest radiograph. All patients should be offered vaccinations for hepatitis B, influenza, and pneumococcus. The CDC case definition of AIDS is an HIV-infected person with a specific opportunistic infection (eg, *Pneumocystis carinii* pneumonia, central nervous system toxoplasmosis), neoplasia (eg, Kaposi's sarcoma), dementia, encephalopathy, wasting syndrome, rapid progression of cervical dysplasia to cancer, or CD4 lymphocyte count less than 200/mm^3. A patient without laboratory evidence of infection may also be diagnosed with AIDS if one of the indicator diseases is present and there is no explanation for the immune dysfunction.

Unfortunately, the mortality rate for patients with established AIDS is high and at present does not appear to be altered by antiviral agents such as zidovudine. Further research in the development of antivirals and vaccines is in progress.

Prevention

"Safer sex" guidelines have been established to decrease the risk of acquiring HIV infection through sexual contact. These guidelines include a reduction in the number of sexual partners, especially those who are in high-risk groups, and use of condoms for all coital activity. Latex condoms are the most effective. Condoms lubricated with spermicides such as nonoxynol 9 are no more effective than other lubricated condoms in protecting against transmission of HIV. In addition, recent data indicate that nonoxynol 9 may increase the risk for HIV transmission during vaginal intercourse, possibly via development of genital lesions that have been associated with nonoxynol 9 use.

Education and counseling for detection of HIV-infected patients and prevention of HIV infection are difficult tasks. HIV infection in women appears to be a disease of drug users and sexual partners of high-risk men. Groups to whom information must be targeted are intravenous drug users and ethnic minorities, particularly blacks and Hispanics. Counseling must not only stress behavior modification but also reinforce those behavioral changes through culturally significant and sensitive messages. In general, reduction of high-risk behavior and use of safer sex guidelines have been the two main areas of education and counseling.

The general preventive guidelines for seropositive women include the following:

(1) Refraining from donating blood, plasma, organs, or tissue.

(2) Being in a mutually monogamous sexual relationship.

(3) Using condoms with spermicide.

(4) Avoiding pregnancy.

HIV Infection During Pregnancy

Maternal transmission of HIV can occur transplacentally before birth, peripartum by exposure to blood and bodily fluids at delivery, or postpartum through breast-feeding. Hence, all pregnant women should be offered HIV testing. In the absence of any intervention, an estimated 15–30% of mothers with HIV infection will transmit the infection during pregnancy and delivery, and 10–20% will transmit the infection through breast milk. Vertical transmission of HIV-1 occurs mostly during the intrapartum period (50–70%) but also can occur in the antepartum period (15–30%), especially in untreated women who seroconvert during pregnancy. The risk appears to be higher in subsequent pregnancies if a patient has delivered 1 infected infant; in this setting the risk may be 37–65%. The mode of delivery may play a role in increasing or decreasing the risks of developing pediatric AIDS. It is recommended that membranes not be ruptured longer than 4 hours. Fetal scalp electrodes and scalp sampling are contraindicated.

Many of the concerns about the effect of pregnancy on HIV infection are unanswered. Does the altered immune status of pregnancy accelerate the progression of HIV infection? Clinically, progression from asymptomatic infection to AIDS is uncommon in pregnancy. However, 45–75% of women will develop symptomatic HIV infection within 2–3 years postpartum if their child was infected. Whether this represents an accelerated progression of HIV infection or demonstrates more effective perinatal transmission in women with longstanding infection is unknown. Diagnosis of acute HIV infection may be delayed because some of the symptoms of early HIV infection may mimic those of the first trimester of pregnancy.

Prenatal care must be individualized, with referral to support systems ideally occurring during the pregnancy rather than postpartum. Screening for other STDs (eg, syphilis, gonorrhea, and HSV infection) is important. Other specific HIV-related infections must be sought, including *P carinii* pneumonia, *Mycobacterium* tuberculosis, cytomegaloviral infection, toxoplasmosis, and candidiasis. At a minimum, HIV-infected patients should undergo shielded chest radiography, a tuberculin skin test with controls, and cytomegalovirus and toxoplasmosis baseline serologic tests. Susceptible patients should receive hepatitis B virus, pneumococcal, and influenza vaccines. CD4+ lymphocyte cell counts should be monitored each trimester. A CD4+ count less than 200/mm^3 is an indication for prophylaxis against *P carinii* pneumonia. Plasma viral load (HIV-1 RNA) is also monitored throughout pregnancy. HIV-1 RNA levels should be monitored every 3–4 months or every trimester. In addition, the levels should be evaluated at 34–36 weeks to determine mode of delivery.

Zidovudine (ZDV) administered during the second and third trimesters, during labor, and for 6 weeks to the newborn has been shown to decrease vertical transmission from 25–30% to 5–8%. Newer protocols that use a combination of drugs are now being used and compose what is referred to as highly active anti-retroviral therapy (HAART). HAART in patients has been shown to reduce the overall transmission to 1.2–1.3%. The 3 main classes of drugs used in HAART are nucleoside analogue reverse transcriptase inhibitors, non-nucleoside reverse transcriptase inhibitors (NNRTIs), and protease inhibitors. Perinatal transmission rates appear to have declined even further with use of HAART. Pregnant women should be treated according to standard guidelines for antiretroviral therapy in adults, with the goal being reduction of plasma viral load (plasma HIV-1 RNA). However, specific recommendations for antiretroviral treatment in pregnant patients continue to evolve, so all pregnant patients with HIV infection should be under the supervision of experts in the management of HIV in pregnancy. Although individual treatment regimens may vary, ZDV plus lamivudine (3TC) are the recommended dual nucleoside reverse transcriptase inhibitor (NRTI) backbone for pregnant women. Nevirapine is an NNRTI that should be initiated in pregnant women with CD4+ counts greater than 250 cells/mm^3.

Data suggest that cesarean section prior to onset of labor and rupture of membranes further decreases the risk of vertical transmission. However, the bulk of these data were obtained prior to the routine use of viral load testing and combination antiretroviral therapy. More recent data suggest that the risk of vertical transmission is proportional to the viral load. In 2 separate analyses, when the viral load was less than 1000 copies per milliliter, the perinatal transmission rate was zero (upper limits of 95% confidence interval were 2.8% and 5.1%). Therefore, it is reasonable to offer scheduled cesarean section prior to onset of labor and rupture of membranes to HIV-infected women with viral loads greater than 1000 copies per milliliter. The American College of Obstetricians and Gynecologists (ACOG) recommends that a scheduled cesarean section be performed at 38 weeks' gestation in order to prevent HIV transmission. For patients receiving ZDV, adequate levels of the drug in the blood should be achieved if the infusion is begun 3 hours preoperatively. The increased maternal morbidity associated with cesarean section must be taken into account, however, when making decisions regarding mode of delivery. Whether cesarean section is beneficial when the mother has received HAART and/or has low to undetectable viral loads is unclear. Also unclear is whether cesarean section after rupture of membranes or onset of labor confers a decrease in HIV transmission.

Peripartum care should include universal application of infection control guidelines to prevent exposure to blood and bodily fluids. These measures include water-repellant gowns, double gloves, handwashing between patient contacts, goggles for significant splash exposures, and wall or bulb suction. Needles should not be recapped. A 1:10 sodium hypochlorite solution should be used to clean instruments. Fetal scalp sampling and scalp electrodes should be avoided because they could become portals of entry for infection.

Postpartum care should entail a continuance of blood and bodily fluids precautions with proscription of breastfeeding. Family planning and safer sex counseling can be continued in the postpartum period with consideration given to tubal ligation. Medical and support system referrals should be initiated prior to discharge from the hospital, if possible.

Pediatric HIV Infection

As of 2004, approximately 93% of pediatric AIDS cases in the United States were perinatally acquired, occurring in infants born to women in high-risk groups (intravenous drug users, partners of high-risk men, and women with AIDS). The progression to infection appears to be faster than in adults, and pediatric AIDS carries a mortality rate similar to that in adults.

Identification of infected neonates is difficult because maternal anti-HIV IgG crosses the placenta. Thus, most infants are born with HIV seropositivity, which may persist up to 15 months by the enzyme immunoassay technique. Nucleic acid or antigen HIV studies are necessary to help identify fetal infection. An HIV embryopathy similar to the fetal alcohol syndrome has been described. Because many the high-risk mothers have multifactorial perinatal problems, assigning the cause of the syndrome to HIV is uncertain.

Infant care involves many of the same guidelines as for maternal peripartum care. Blood and bodily fluid precautions, as well as immunosuppression care guidelines, should be exercised. Consultation with a pediatric immunologist to plan neonatal and follow-up care should begin prior to discharge from the hospital. Circumcision should be discouraged. Prior to discharge, detailed home-care instruction regarding avoidance of bodily secretions should be given.

Guidelines for HIV Testing

HIV serologic testing should include pretest and posttest counseling about interpretation of test results. After obtaining informed consent from the patient, confidentiality must be maintained concerning the test results. Situations in which HIV testing should be offered include the following:

(1) Women who have used intravenous drugs.

(2) Women who have engaged in prostitution.

(3) Women with sex partners who are HIV-infected or are at risk for HIV infection.

(4) Women who have STDs.

(5) Women who have lived in communities or were born in countries where the prevalence of HIV infection (especially heterosexually acquired HIV infection) among women is high.

(6) Women who received blood transfusions between 1978 and 1985.

(7) Women undergoing medical evaluation or treatment for clinical signs and symptoms of HIV infection.

(8) Women who have been inmates in correctional systems.

(9) Women who consider themselves at risk.

(10)Pregnancy: In 2003, the CDC revised its guidelines to recommend the opt-out approach whereby pregnant women have the option of declining universal HIV testing as part of routine prenatal blood tests.

HIV Antibody Testing

The diagnosis of HIV infection is usually by HIV-1 antibody tests. Routine testing for HIV-2, other than at blood banks, is currently not recommended unless a patient is at risk for HIV-2 infection or has clinical findings of HIV disease and has had a negative HIV-1 antibody test. Refer to recent reviews cited in the references for details of the criteria for HIV antibody detection. In general, the ELISA functions as a screening test for exposure to HIV. Most patients exposed to HIV develop detectable levels of antibody against the virus by 12 weeks after exposure. The presence of antibody indicates current infection, although the patient may be asymptomatic for years. The sensitivity and specificity of the ELISA test is 99% when it is repeatedly reactive. Thus, the test for HIV antibody is considered negative if the ELISA is nonreactive, and it indicates a lack of HIV infection unless the period is too early for detection of antibody production.

The probability of a false-negative test in an uninfected woman is remote unless she is in the "window" before antibody is produced. A positive test result occurs when an ELISA is repeatedly reactive followed by a positive Western blot assay. The Western blot assay is reactive when a critical pattern of specific antibodies is detected against the 3 main gene products of HIV. The probability that an abnormal testing sequence will falsely identify a patient as HIV-infected is less than 1 in 100,000 to 5 in 100,000 persons. Individuals in high-risk groups should be retested in 3 months; they are likely to become positive. The status of those without associated risk factors is likely to remain indeterminate, but persistent indeterminate status is not diagnostic of HIV infection.

Rapid HIV testing can be used to identify HIV infection in women who arrive at labor and delivery with undocumented HIV status and to provide an opportunity to begin prophylaxis of previously undiagnosed infection before delivery. Test results are available within a few hours. Most rapid assays have a sensitivity and specificity comparable to ELISA.

REFERENCES

General

Centers for Disease Control and Prevention: 2002 Sexually transmitted diseases, treatment guidelines. MMWR Recomm Rep 2002;51:RR-6;1.

Fontanet AL et al: Protection against sexually transmitted diseases by granting sex workers in Thailand the choice of using the male or female condom: results from a randomized controlled trial. AIDS 1998;12:1851.

Levinson ME, Bush LM: Peritonitis and other intra-abdominal infections. In: Mandell GL, Douglas RG, Bennett JE (editors): *Principles and Practice of Infectious Diseases,* 3rd ed. Churchill Livingstone, 1990, p. 643.

McGregor JA et al: Assessment of office-based care of sexually transmitted diseases and vaginitis and antibiotic decision making by obstetrician-gynecologists. Infect Dis Obstet Gynecol 1988;6:247.

Miller HG et al: Correlates of sexually transmitted bacterial infections among U.S. women in 1995. Fam Plann Perspect 1999;31:4.

Gonorrhea

Friedland LR et al: Cost-effectiveness decision analysis of intramuscular ceftriaxone versus oral cefixime in adolescents with gonococcal cervicitis. Ann Emerg Med 1996;27:299.

Chlamydial Infections

Centers for Disease Control and Prevention: Chlamydia trachomatis genital infections—United States, 1995. MMWR Morb Mortal Wkly Rep 1997;46:193.

Faaunders A et al: The risk of inadvertent intrauterine device insertion in women carriers of endocervical *Chlamydia trachomatis.* Contraception 1998;58:105.

Lea AP, Lamb HM: Azithromycin: A pharmacoeconomic review of its use as a single-dose regimen in the treatment of uncomplicated urogenital *Chlamydia trachomatis* infections in women. Pharmacoeconomics 1997;12:596.

Chancroid

Chen CY et al: Comparison of enzyme immunoassays for antibodies to *Haemophilus ducreyi* in a community outbreak of chancroid in the United States. J Infect Dis 1997;175:1390.

Hawkes S et al: Asymptomatic carriage of *Haemophilus ducreyi* confirmed by the polymerase chain reaction. Genitourin Med 1995;71:224.

Mertz KJ et al: An investigation of genital ulcers in Jackson, Mississippi, with the use of a multiplex polymerase chain reaction assay: high prevalence of chancroid and human immunodeficiency virus infection. J Infect Dis 1998;178:1060.

Genital Ulcers

Dillon SM et al: Prospective analysis of genital ulcer disease in Brooklyn, New York. Clin Infect Dis 1997;24:945.

Mertz KJ et al: Etiology of genital ulcers and prevalence of human immunodeficiency virus coinfection in 10 U.S. cities. The Genital Ulcer Disease Surveillance Group. J Infect Dis 1998;178:1795.

Human Immunodeficiency Virus

American College of Obstetricians and Gynecologists: Scheduled cesarean delivery and the prevention of vertical transmission of HIV infection. ACOG Committee Opinion No. 234, 2000.

Anderson JR (editor): *A Guide to the Clinical Care of Women with HIV.* U.S. Department of Health and Human Services, HIV/AIDS Bureau, 2001, pp. 1, 77.

Blattner W et al: Effectiveness of potent antiretroviral therapies on reducing perinatal transmission of HIV-1. XIII International AIDS Conference, Durban, South Africa (Abstr. LbOr4), July 9–14, 2000.

The European Mode of Delivery Collaboration: Elective caesarean section versus vaginal delivery in prevention of vertical HIV-1 transmission: A randomized clinical trial. Lancet 1999;353:1035.

Garcia PM et al: Maternal levels of plasma human immunodeficiency virus type 1 RNA and the risk of perinatal transmission. Women and Infants Transmission Study Group. N Engl J Med 1999;341:394.

Mofenson LM et al: Risk factors for perinatal transmission of human immunodeficiency virus type 1 in women treated with zidovudine. Pediatric AIDS Clinical Trial Group Study 185 Team. N Engl J Med 1999;341:385.

Staszewski S et al: Safety and efficacy of lamivudine-zidovudine combination therapy in zidovudine-experienced patients: A randomized controlled comparison with zidovudine monotherapy. JAMA 1996;276:111.

U.S. Department of Health and Human Services—Centers for Disease Control and Prevention: Estimated incidence of AIDS and deaths of persons with AIDS, adjusted for delays in reporting, by quarter-year of diagnosis/death, United States, January 1985 through June 1997. HIV AIDS Surveil Rep 1997;9:1.

U.S. Department of Health and Human Services—Centers for Disease Control and Prevention: Guidelines for the use of antiretroviral agents in pediatric HIV infection. MMWR Recomm Rep 1998;47:RR-4:1.

Pelvic Inflammatory Disease

Aral SO, Wasserheit JN: Social and behavioral correlates of pelvic inflammatory disease. Sex Transm Dis 1998;25:378.

Arredondo JL et al: Oral clindamycin and ciprofloxacin versus intramuscular ceftriaxone and oral doxycycline in the treatment of mild-to-moderate pelvic inflammatory disease in outpatients. Clin Infect Dis 1997;24:170.

McNeeley SG, Hendrix SL, Mazzoni MM: Medically sound, cost effective treatment for pelvic inflammatory disease and tuboovarian abscesses. Am J Obstet Gynecol 1998;178:1272.

Reljic M, Gorisek B: C-reactive protein and the treatment of pelvic inflammatory disease. Int J Gynecol Obstet 1998;60:143.

Teisala K, Heinonen PK: C-reactive protein in assessing antimicrobial treatment of acute pelvic inflammatory disease. J Reprod Med 1990;35:955.

Timor-Tritsch IE et al: Transvaginal sonographic markers of tubal inflammatory disease. Ultrasound Obstet Gynecol 1998;12:56.

Tubo-Ovarian Abscess

Golde SH, Israel R, Ledger WJ: Unilateral tubo-ovarian abscess: A distinct entity. Am J Obstet Gynecol 1977;127:807.

Henry-Suchet J, Soler A, Loffredo V: Laparoscopic treatment of tuboovarian abscesses. J Reprod Med 1984;29:579.

Landers VD, Sweet LR: Current trends in the diagnosis and treatment of tuboovarian abscess. Am J Obstet Gynecol 1985;151:1098.

Lavy G, Hilsenrath RE: Management of tubo-ovarian abscess. Infertil Reprod Med Clin North Am 1992;3:821.

Reed SD, Landers DV, Sweet RL: Antibiotic treatment of tuboovarian abscess: comparison of broad-spectrum lactam agents versus clindamycin containing regimens. Am J Obstet Gynecol 1991;164:1556.

Wilson JR, Black RJ: Ovarian abscess. Am J Obstet Gynecol 1964;90:34.

Younis JS et al: Late manifestation of pelvic abscess following oocyte retrieval for in vitro fertilization, in patients with severe endometriosis and ovarian endometriomata. J Assist Reprod Genet 1997;14:343.

Antimicrobial Chemotherapy

42

Ronald S. Gibbs, MD

ANTIMICROBIAL CHEMOTHERAPY

Although microbial infection has always been a threat to obstetric and gynecologic patients, gratifying developments in antimicrobial therapy have led to decreases in puerperal and postoperative morbidity and perinatal mortality.

PRINCIPLES OF SELECTION OF ANTIMICROBIAL DRUGS

Several special conditions are pertinent to most infections encountered in obstetric and gynecologic practice. First, patients (except for some elderly and some oncology patients) are generally healthy and free of debilitating illness. Second, most infections, such as postpartum or postoperative infection and pelvic inflammatory disease, are polymicrobial in origin, involving an array of aerobes, anaerobes, genital mycoplasmas, and, in some conditions, *Chlamydia trachomatis*. Third, when a clinical diagnosis of infection is made, empiric antibiotic therapy is usually indicated before culture results are available. Fourth, because of limitations in laboratory technique, culture results may not be available in a timely fashion, or tests may not even be performed at all.

To serve as a guide to antibiotic selection, 4 tables are provided. Table 42–1 provides the classification of β-lactam and related antibiotics. Table 42–2 provides a classification of antibiotics commonly used in obstetric and gynecologic practice and their main adverse effects, both in the adult and in the fetus. Table 42–3 shows recommended drugs and alternatives for suspected or proved etiologic microorganisms. Table 42–4 shows appropriate selections by clinical diagnosis.

The following steps merit consideration in each patient.

A. ETIOLOGIC DIAGNOSIS

The physician must attempt to decide on clinical grounds (1) whether the patient has a microbial infection that might be influenced by antimicrobial drugs and (2) the most probable infectious agent causing the disorder ("best guess") (Table 42–4).

B. "BEST GUESS"

Based on a best guess about the probable cause of the patient's infection, the physician should choose a drug (or drug combination) that is likely to be effective against the suspected microorganism.

C. LABORATORY CONTROL

Before beginning antimicrobial drug treatment, obtain meaningful specimens, if available, for laboratory examination to determine the causative infectious organism and, if appropriate, its susceptibility to antimicrobial drugs.

D. CLINICAL RESPONSE

Based on the clinical response of the patient, evaluate the laboratory reports and consider the desirability of changing the antimicrobial drug regimen. Laboratory results should not automatically overrule clinical judgment.

E. DRUG SUSCEPTIBILITY TESTS

Some microorganisms are uniformly susceptible to certain drugs; if such organisms are isolated from the patient, they need not be tested for drug susceptibility. For example, group A and B streptococci and clostridia are uniformly susceptible to penicillin. On the other hand, enteric gram-negative rods are sufficiently variable in their response to warrant drug susceptibility testing when they are isolated from a significant specimen, and group B streptococci have variable susceptibility to erythromycin and clindamycin.

Antimicrobial drug susceptibility tests can be performed on solid media as "disk tests," in broth tubes, or in wells of microdilution plates. The latter method yields results usually expressed as minimal inhibitory concentration (MIC). In some infections, the MIC provides a better estimate of the amount of drug required for therapeutic effect in vivo. Disk tests usually indicate whether an isolate is susceptible or resistant to drug concentrations achieved in vivo with conventional dosage regimens, thus providing valuable guidance in selecting therapy.

When marked discrepancies are noted between in vitro test results and in vivo response, the following possibilities must be considered:

Table 42–4. Drugs used to treat suspected or proved infections.

Suspected or Proved Infection	Recommended Drug(s)	Alternative Drug(s)
Sexually Transmitted Infections		
Syphilis	Benzathine penicillin	A tetracycline
Genital herpes	Acyclovir, famciclovir, valacyclovir	
Gonorrhea	See Table 42–3	
C trachomatis	Azithromycin, tetracycline	Erythromycin, ofloxacin; amoxicillin or clindamycin in pregnancy
Pelvic inflammatory disease	Cefoxitin (or alternate) plus doxycycline OR clindamycin plus gentamicin for parenteral treatment; ofloxacin plus metronidazole OR ceftriaxone (or alternate) plus doxycycline for oral treatment.	See CDC Guidelines for multiple alternatives.[1]
Vaginitis		
Trichomonas vaginalis	Metronidazole	
Candidiasis	Topical imidazoles; fluconazole	
Bacterial vaginosis	Metronidazole, clindamycin	
Obstetric Infection		
Puerperal endometritis	Clindamycin plus gentamicin	Several including cefoxitin or cefotetan; ampicillin plus sulbactam
Clinical chorioamnionitis	Ampicillin plus gentamcin, plus clindamycin if cesarean delivery	As for endometritis
Sepsis	Clindamycin plus gentamicin, plus ampicillin	Metronidazole plus gentamicin, plus ampicillin
Pyelonephritis, first episode	Ceftriaxone, TMP-SMX,[2] ofloxacin or ciprofloxacin	Third-generation cephalosporin
Urinary Tract Infection		
Recurrent	Ampicillin plus gentamicin	Same
Gynecologic Infection		
Posthysterectomy cuff infection	As for endometritis	As for endometritis
Abdominal wound infection	Drainage with or without antibiotics as for endometritis	

[1]Reproduced, with permission, from Centers for Disease Control and Prevention: 1998 guidelines for treatment of sexually transmitted diseases. MMWR Recomm Rep 1998;47:(RR–1).
[2]TMP-SMX is a mixture of 1 part trimethoprim and 5 parts sulfamethoxazole.

F. ADEQUATE DOSAGE

To determine whether the proper drug is being used in adequate dosage, a serum assay can be performed. However, in obstetric-gynecologic practice, testing antibiotic levels usually is unnecessary. However, with dosing of an aminoglycoside every 24 hours, determination of serum levels is standard. Determination of drug levels may also be useful in obese women, in women with renal insufficiency, in patients with longer courses (> 7 days), and in patients not responding to therapy.

G. ROUTE OF ADMINISTRATION

The absorption of oral penicillins, tetracyclines, and erythromycin is impaired by food. Therefore, these oral drugs should be given between meals.

H. DURATION OF ANTIMICROBIAL THERAPY

In general, effective antimicrobial treatment results in marked clinical improvement within a few days. However, continued treatment for varying periods may be necessary to effect cure. For most postoperative and postpartum infections, intravenous antibiotics can be discontinued after the patient has been afebrile for 24–48 hours. Furthermore, in most patients who respond promptly to intravenous treatment, oral antibiotic therapy is unnecessary.

I. ADVERSE REACTIONS

The administration of antimicrobial drugs is occasionally associated with untoward reactions (Table 42–2). These reactions can be divided into several groups.

1. Hypersensitivity—The most common reactions are fever and skin rashes. Hematologic or hepatic disorders and anaphylaxis are rare.

2. Direct toxicity—Most common are nausea, vomiting, and diarrhea. More serious toxic reactions are impairment of renal, hepatic, or hematopoietic function or damage to the eighth nerve.

3. Suppression—Suppression of normal microbial flora and "superinfection" by drug-resistant microorganisms, or continued infection with the initial pathogen through the emergence of drug-resistant variants.

Oliguria, Impaired Renal Function, & Uremia

Oliguria, impaired renal function, and uremia have an important influence on antimicrobial drug dosage, because most of these drugs are excreted by the kidneys. Only minor adjustment in dosage or frequency of administration is necessary with renally excreted drugs when relatively nontoxic drugs (eg, penicillins) are used. On the other hand, the dosage or frequency of administration of aminoglycosides (gentamicin, tobramycin, and amikacin), tetracyclines, and vancomycin must be reduced if toxicity is to be avoided in the presence of nitrogen retention. Administration of such drugs during renal failure should be guided by assay of drug concentrations in serum.

Antimicrobial Drugs

PENICILLINS

The penicillins are a large group of antimicrobial substances, all of which share a common chemical nucleus (6-aminopenicillanic acid) that contains a β-lactam ring essential to their biologic activity (Table 42–1). All β-lactam antibiotics inhibit formation of microbial cell walls. In particular, they block the final transpeptidation reaction in the synthesis of cell wall mucopeptide (peptidoglycan), and they activate autolytic enzymes in the cell wall. These reactions result in bacterial cell death.

One million units of penicillin G equals 0.6 g. Other penicillins are prescribed in grams or milligrams. A blood level of 0.01–1 μg/mL of penicillin G or ampicillin is lethal for most susceptible gram-positive microorganisms. Most β-lactamase–resistant penicillins are 5–50 times less active against penicillin G–susceptible organisms.

Absorption, Distribution, & Excretion

After parenteral administration, absorption of most penicillins is complete and rapid. After oral administra-tion, only a portion of the dose is absorbed (from 1/20 to 1/3, depending on acid stability, binding to foods, and presence of buffers). To minimize binding to foods, oral penicillins should not be preceded or followed by food for at least 1 hour.

After absorption, penicillins are widely distributed in body fluids and tissues. With parenteral doses of 3–6 g (5–10 million units) per 24 hours of any penicillin injected by continuous infusion or divided intramuscular injections, average serum levels of the drug reach 1–10 units (0.6–6 μg) per milliliter.

In many tissues, penicillin concentrations are equal to those in serum. Lower levels are found in the central nervous system. However, with active inflammation of the meninges, as in bacterial meningitis, penicillin levels in the cerebrospinal fluid exceed 0.2 μg/mL with a daily parenteral dose of 12 g.

Most of the absorbed penicillin is rapidly excreted by the kidneys into the urine—90% by tubular secretion. Tubular secretion can be partially blocked by probenecid 0.5 g every 6 hours by mouth, to achieve higher systemic levels.

Renal excretion of penicillin results in very high levels in the urine.

Indications, Dosages, & Routes of Administration

The penicillins have been among the most effective and the most widely used antimicrobial drugs.

A. PENICILLIN G

In obstetric-gynecologic practice, penicillin is the drug of choice for treatment of infections caused by group A and B streptococci, *Treponema pallidum,* aerobic gram-positive rods, clostridia, and *Actinomyces.*

Penicillin G has not been recommended to treat gonococci for more than 25 years because of widespread resistance. Enterococci are not susceptible to penicillin G alone, but they are susceptible to a synergistic combination of penicillin G and an aminoglycoside or, in milder infections (particularly in the urinary tract), to ampicillin alone.

1. Intramuscular or intravenous—Although most of the infections respond to aqueous penicillin G in daily doses of 0.6–5 million units administered by intermittent intramuscular injection, larger amounts (6–50 g daily) given by intermittent intravenous infusion are usually used. Sites for intravenous administration are subject to thrombophlebitis and must be rotated every 2–3 days. In enterococcal infections, an aminoglycoside is given simultaneously with large doses of a penicillin.

2. Oral—Penicillin V is indicated in minor infections (eg, of the respiratory tract or its associated structures) in daily doses of 1–4 g (1.6–6.4 million units).

B. BENZATHINE PENICILLIN G

This penicillin is a salt with low water solubility. It is injected intramuscularly to establish a depot that yields low but prolonged drug levels. An injection of 2.4 million units intramuscularly once per week for 1 or 3 weeks is the recommended treatment for early and late syphilis, respectively.

C. AMPICILLIN, AMOXICILLIN, CARBENICILLIN, TICARCILLIN, PIPERACILLIN, MEZLOCILLIN, AZLOCILLIN

These drugs have greater activity against gram-negative aerobes than does penicillin G but are destroyed by penicillinases (β-lactamases).

Ampicillin can be given orally in divided doses, 2–3 g daily, to treat urinary tract infections with susceptible coliform bacteria, enterococci, or *Proteus mirabilis*. It is ineffective against *Enterobacter* and *Pseudomonas*. Amoxicillin, 500 mg every 8 hours, is similar to ampicillin but is better absorbed. Thus, it can be given at less frequent intervals. Because of widespread gram-negative bacterial resistance to ampicillin, susceptibility testing should be performed.

Carbenicillin is more active against *Pseudomonas* and *Proteus,* but resistance emerges rapidly. Ticarcillin resembles carbenicillin but gives higher tissue levels. Because carbenicillin and ticarcillin also possess moderate activity against the wide array of bacteria involved in pelvic infections, they have been used with fairly good success as single-agent therapy. Carbenicillin indanyl sodium can be given orally for some urinary tract infections. Piperacillin resembles ticarcillin but is somewhat more active against some gram-negative aerobes, especially *Pseudomonas.* Combinations of clavulanic acid with amoxicillin or ticarcillin are somewhat protected against destruction by β-lactamases and have been used for treatment of some lactamase producers, eg, *Haemophilus influenzae.*

D. β-LACTAMASE–RESISTANT PENICILLINS

Cloxacillin, nafcillin, and others are relatively resistant to destruction by β-lactamase. The main indication for use of these drugs is infection by β-lactamase–producing staphylococci.

1. Oral—Oxacillin, cloxacillin, dicloxacillin, or nafcillin can be given in doses of 0.25–0.5 g every 4–6 hours in mild or localized staphylococcal infections. Food markedly interferes with absorption.

2. Intravenous—For serious systemic staphylococcal infections, nafcillin 6–12 g is given intravenously, by adding 1–2 g every 2 hours to a continuous infusion of 5% dextrose in water.

E. COMBINATIONS OF PENICILLINS PLUS β-LACTAMASE INHIBITORS

Because of their wide spectrum of activity against bacteria involved in pelvic infections, these combinations have been successful in many circumstances, particularly pelvic infections. For example, ampicillin plus sulbactam (Unasyn), 3 g every 6 hours, carbenicillin plus clavulanic acid (Timentin), 3.1 g every 6 hours, or piperacillin plus tazobactam (Zosyn), 4 g piperacillin plus 0.5 g tazobactam IV every 8 hours may be the regimen given in such polymicrobial infections (Table 42–1).

Adverse Effects

Most of the serious side effects of the penicillins are due to hypersensitivity.

A. ALLERGY

All penicillins are cross-sensitizing and cross-reacting. In general, sensitization occurs in direct proportion to the duration and total dose of penicillin received in the past. Skin tests with penicilloylpolylysine, with alkaline hydrolysis products (minor antigen determinants), and with undegraded penicillin can identify many hypersensitive individuals. Among positive reactors to skin tests, the incidence of subsequent immediate (immunoglobulin [Ig]E-mediated) penicillin reactions is high. Although many persons develop IgG antibodies to antigenic determinants of penicillin, the presence of such antibodies is not correlated with allergic reactivity (except rare hemolytic anemia). A history of a penicillin reaction in the past is not reliable; however, in such cases the drug should be administered with caution. Allergic reactions may occur as anaphylactic shock, serum sickness-type reactions (urticaria, fever, joint swelling, angioneurotic edema, intense pruritus, and respiratory embarrassment occurring 7–12 days after exposure), skin rashes, oral lesions, fever, nephritis, eosinophilia, hemolytic anemia and other hematologic disturbances, and vasculitis. The incidence of hypersensitivity to penicillin is estimated to be 3–5% among adults. Acute anaphylactic life-threatening reactions are rare (0.05%). Ampicillin produces skin rashes (mononucleosis-like) 3–5 times more frequently than do other penicillins, but some ampicillin rashes are not allergic. Methicillin and other penicillins can induce interstitial nephritis; nafcillin is less nephrotoxic than methicillin. In circumstances where penicillin is the clear drug of choice and where alternatives are likely to be less effective, an oral desensitization protocol may be used safely. One such indication is the treatment of a patient with syphilis. One widely used protocol is administration of penicillin V suspensions orally starting at 100 units and giving incremental doses over 4 hours.

B. Toxicity

Because the action of penicillin is directed against a unique bacterial structure, the cell wall, penicillin has virtually no effect on animal cells. The toxic effects of penicillin G are due to the direct irritation caused by intramuscular or intravenous injection of exceedingly high concentrations (eg, 1 g/mL). A patient receiving more than 50 g of penicillin G daily parenterally may exhibit signs of cerebrocortical irritation as a result of the passage of large amounts of penicillin into the central nervous system. With doses of this magnitude, direct cation toxicity (Na^+, K^+) can also occur. Potassium penicillin G contains 1.7 mEq of K^+ per million units (2.7 mEq/g), and potassium may accumulate in the presence of renal failure. Carbenicillin contains 4.7 mEq of Na^+ per gram—a risk in heart failure.

Large doses of penicillins given orally may lead to gastrointestinal upset, particularly nausea and diarrhea. These symptoms are most marked with oral ampicillin or amoxicillin. Oral therapy may be accompanied by luxuriant overgrowth of staphylococci, *Pseudomonas, Proteus,* or yeasts, which may cause enteritis. Penicillins have caused pseudomembranous colitis. Superinfections in other organ systems may occur. Carbenicillin and ticarcillin may damage platelet function, cause bleeding, or result in hypokalemic alkalosis.

CEPHALOSPORINS

The cephalosporins are structurally related to the penicillins. They consist of a β-lactam ring attached to a dihydrothiazoline ring. Substitutions of chemical groups at various positions on the basic structure have resulted in a proliferation of drugs with varying pharmacologic properties and antimicrobial activities.

The mechanism of action of cephalosporins is analogous to that of the penicillins: (1) binding to specific penicillin-binding proteins that serve as drug receptors on bacteria, (2) inhibition of cell wall synthesis, and (3) activation of autolytic enzymes in the cell wall that result in bacterial death.

Cephalosporins have been divided into 3 major groups or "generations," based mainly on their antibacterial activity (Table 42–1). First-generation cephalosporins have good activity against aerobic gram-positive organisms and many community-acquired gram-negative organisms. Second-generation drugs have a slightly extended spectrum against gram-negative bacteria, and some are active against anaerobes. Third-generation cephalosporins have less activity against gram-positives but are extremely active against most gram-negative bacteria. Not all cephalosporins fit neatly into this grouping, and there are exceptions to the general characterization of the drugs in the individual generations. However, the generational classification of cephalosporins is useful for discussion purposes.

1. First-Generation Cephalosporins

Antimicrobial Activity

These drugs are very active against gram-positive cocci, including pneumococci, viridans streptococci, group A and B streptococci, and *Staphylococcus aureus*. Like all cephalosporins, they are inactive against enterococci and methicillin-resistant staphylococci. Among gram-negative bacteria, *Escherichia coli, Klebsiella pneumoniae,* and *Proteus mirabilis* are usually sensitive except for some hospital-acquired strains. There is no activity against such gram-negatives as *Pseudomonas aeruginosa,* indole-positive *Proteus* spp., *Enterobacter* spp., *Serratia marcescens, Citrobacter* spp., and *Acinetobacter* spp. Anaerobic cocci are usually sensitive, but most *Bacteroides* species are not.

Pharmacokinetics & Administration

A. Oral

Cephalexin, cephradine, and cefadroxil are absorbed from the gut to a variable extent. After a 500-mg oral dose, serum levels range from 15 to 20 μg/mL. Urine concentrations are usually very high, but in other tissues the levels are variable and usually lower than in the serum. Cephalexin and cephradine are given orally in doses of 0.25–0.5 g 4 times daily (15–30 mg/kg/d). Cefadroxil can be given in doses of 0.5–1 g twice daily.

Dosage should be reduced in marked renal insufficiency: for creatine clearance (Cl_{cr}) 20–50 mL/min, give half the normal dose; for Cl_{cr} less than 20 mL/min, give one-fourth the normal dose.

B. Intravenous

Cefazolin has a longer half-life than cephalothin or cephapirin. After an intravenous infusion of 1 g, the peak serum level of cefazolin is 90–120 μg/mL, whereas cephalothin and cephapirin levels reach 40–60 μg/mL. The usual dose of cefazolin for adults is 1–2 g intravenously every 8 hours (50–100 mg/kg/d) and for cephalothin and cephapirin is 1–2 g every 4–6 hours (50–200 mg/kg/d). In patients with impaired renal function, dosage adjustment as for oral dosage is needed.

C. Intramuscular

Both cephapirin and cefazolin can be given intramuscularly, and pain on injection is less than with cefazolin.

Clinical Uses

Although the first-generation cephalosporins have a broad spectrum of activity and are relatively nontoxic, they are rarely the drugs of choice. Oral drugs are indicated for treatment of urinary infections in patients who are allergic to trimethoprim-sulfamethoxazole (TMP-

SMX) or penicillins, and they can be used for minor staphylococcal infections in penicillin-allergic patients. Oral cephalosporins may be preferred for minor polymicrobial infections (eg, cellulitis, soft-tissue abscess).

Cefazolin or an alternative cephalosporin is the drug of choice for group B streptococcal infection or for prophylaxis in patients who cannot take penicillin, but who are at low risk for anaphylaxis.

Intravenous first-generation cephalosporins penetrate most tissues well and are among the drugs of choice for gynecologic and cesarean section prophylaxis. More expensive second- and third-generation cephalosporins offer no advantage over the first-generation drugs for surgical prophylaxis and should not be used for that purpose.

Other major uses of intravenous first-generation cephalosporins include infections for which they are the least toxic drugs (eg, *Klebsiella* infections) and infections in persons with a history of mild penicillin allergy (not anaphylaxis).

2. Second-Generation Cephalosporins

Second-generation cephalosporins are a heterogeneous group with marked individual differences in activity, pharmacokinetics, and toxicity. In general, all of them are active against organisms also covered by first-generation drugs, but they have an extended gram-negative coverage. Indole-positive *Proteus* and *Klebsiella* spp. (including cephalothin-resistant strains) are usually sensitive. In addition, cefoxitin and cefotetan are active against *Bacteroides fragilis,* other gram-negative anaerobes, and some strains of *Serratia,* but they have poor activity against *Enterobacter* and *H influenzae.* Against gram-positive organisms, these drugs are less active than the first-generation cephalosporins. Like the latter, second-generation drugs have no activity against *P aeruginosa* or enterococci.

Pharmacokinetics & Administration

After an intravenous infusion of 1 g, serum levels range from 75–125 μg/mL. Because of differences in drug half-life and protein binding, intervals between doses vary greatly. For cefoxitin (short half-life), the interval is 4–6 hours; cefoxitin, 50–200 mg/kg/d

Drugs with longer half-lives can be injected less frequently: cefotetan, 1–2 mg every 8–12 hours; and cefonicid or cefonide, 1–2 g (15–30 mg/kg/d) once or twice daily. In renal failure, dosage adjustments are required.

Clinical Uses

Because of their activity against anaerobes, cefoxitin and cefotetan are widely used to treat polymicrobial ob-

stetric and gynecologic infections. They are not more effective than first-generation cephalosporins for perioperative prophylaxis, and they are more expensive.

3. Third-Generation Cephalosporins

Antimicrobial Activity

These drugs are active against staphylococci (not methicillin-resistant strains) but less so than first-generation cephalosporins. They have no activity against enterococci but inhibit nonenterococcal streptococci. Most of these drugs are active against *N gonorrhoeae.* A major advantage of the new cephalosporins is their expanded gram-negative coverage. In addition to organisms inhibited by other cephalosporins, they are consistently active against *Enterobacter* spp., *Citrobacter freundii, S marcescens, Providencia* spp., *Haemophilus* spp., and *Neisseria* spp., including β-lactamase–producing strains. Two drugs—ceftazidime and cefoperazone—have good activity against *P aeruginosa,* whereas the others inhibit only 40–60% of strains. *Listeria* spp., *Acinetobacter* spp., and non-*aeruginosa* strains of *Pseudomonas* are variably sensitive to third-generation cephalosporins. Only ceftizoxime and moxalactam have good activity against *B fragilis.* Several of these drugs have relatively long half-lives.

Pharmacokinetics & Administration

After an intravenous infusion of 1 g, serum levels of these drugs range from 60–140 μg/mL. They penetrate well into body fluids and tissues. The half-life of these drugs is variable: ceftriaxone, 7–8 hours; cefoperazone, 2 hours; the others, 1–1.7 hours. Consequently, ceftriaxone can be injected every 12–24 hours in a dose of 15–30 mg/kg/d (or 30–50 mg/kg every 12 hours in adult meningitis and 50 mg/kg every 12 hours in infants). Cefoperazone can be given every 8–12 hours in a dose of 25–100 mg/kg/d, and the other drugs of the group every 6–8 hours in doses ranging from 2–12 g/d depending on the severity of infection. Cefoperazone and ceftriaxone are eliminated primarily by biliary excretion, and no dosage adjustment is required in renal insufficiency. The other drugs in this generation are eliminated by the kidney and thus require dosage adjustments in renal insufficiency.

Clinical Uses

Ceftriaxone 250 mg intramuscularly and cefixime 400 mg orally are two recommended regimens for treating uncomplicated gonorrhea. They are combined with doxycycline or azithromycin for cotreatment of chlamydia.

In obstetric-gynecologic practice, these agents have been used to treat urinary infection.

ADVERSE EFFECTS OF CEPHALOSPORINS

Allergy

Cephalosporins are sensitizing, and a variety of hypersensitivity reactions occur, including anaphylaxis, fever, skin rashes, nephritis, granulocytopenia, and hemolytic anemia. The incidence of cross-allergy between cephalosporins and penicillins is estimated to be approximately 6–10%. Persons with a history of anaphylaxis to penicillins should not receive cephalosporins.

Toxicity

Local pain can occur after intramuscular injection, or thrombophlebitis can occur after intravenous injection. Hypoprothrombinemia is a potential adverse effect of cephalosporins that have a methylthiotetrazole group (eg, cefamandole, moxalactam, cefoperazone), but these are infrequently used in obstetric-gynecologic practice.

Superinfection

Many newer cephalosporins have little activity against gram-positive organisms, particularly staphylococci and enterococci. Superinfection with these organisms—as well as with fungi—may occur. Pseudomembranous colitis has occurred with use of these antibiotics.

NEW β-LACTAM DRUGS

Monobactams

Monobactams are drugs with a monocyclic β-lactam ring, which are resistant to β-lactamases and are active against gram-negative organisms (including *Pseudomonas*) but not against gram-positive organisms or anaerobes. Aztreonam resembles aminoglycosides in activity. The usual dose is 1–2 g intravenously every 6–8 hours. Clinical uses of aztreonam alone are limited because of the availability of third-generation cephalosporins with a broader spectrum of activity and minimal toxicity. However, in combination with a drug such as clindamycin, aztreonam provides a regimen with broad activity and appears equivalent to clindamycin–gentamicin in efficacy. Although aztreonam has potentially less toxicity than gentamicin, gentamicin is much less expensive, and the majority of obstetric-gynecologic patients are at low risk for gentamicin toxicity. The place of aztreonam in obstetric-gynecologic practice remains limited.

Carbapenems

This class of drugs is structurally related to β-lactam antibiotics. Imipenem, the first drug of this type, has a wide spectrum with good activity against many gram-negative rods, gram-positive organisms, and anaerobes. It is resistant to β-lactamases but is inactivated by dipeptidases in renal tubules. Consequently, it must be combined with cilastatin, a dipeptidase inhibitor, for clinical use.

The half-life of imipenem is 1 hour. Penetration into body tissues and fluids, including the cerebrospinal fluid, is good. The usual dose is 0.5–1 g intravenously every 6 hours. Dosage adjustment is required in renal insufficiency. Because imipenem has an unusual spectrum, it should be reserved for special cases such as treatment of highly resistant organisms. It should not be used as a first-line treatment for pelvic infections.

The most common adverse effects of imipenem are nausea, vomiting, diarrhea, reactions at the infusion site, and skin rashes. Seizures can occur in patients with renal failure. Patients allergic to penicillins may be allergic to imipenem as well.

MACROLIDES (ERYTHROMYCIN, AZITHROMYCIN, CLARITHROMYCIN)

The erythromycins inhibit protein synthesis and are bacteriostatic or bactericidal against gram-positive organisms in concentrations of 0.02–2 μg/mL. *Chlamydia, Ureaplasma urealyticum, Legionella,* and *Campylobacter* are also susceptible. Activity is enhanced at alkaline pH.

Erythromycins are the drugs of choice in pneumonia caused by mycoplasmas or *Legionella.* They are useful as substitutes for penicillin in persons who are allergic to penicillin and for tetracyclines in pregnancy for treatment of *Chlamydia* and *Ureaplasma.* Erythromycin preparations can be used parenterally for prophylaxis of group B streptococcal perinatal infection in patients with penicillin allergy. However, because the likelihood of erythromycin resistance to group B streptococci is up to 15%, erythromycin should not be used unless susceptibility has been established.

Dosages

A. ORAL

Erythromycin base, stearate, or estolate, 0.25–0.5 g every 6 hours (for children, 40 mg/kg/d), or erythromycin ethylsuccinate, 0.4–0.6 g every 6 hours. The estolate derivative should not be used during pregnancy because it elevates hepatic enzyme levels.

B. INTRAVENOUS

Erythromycin lactobionate, 0.5 g every 6 hours.

Adverse Effects

Nausea, vomiting, and diarrhea may occur after oral intake. Erythromycin estolate probably more than the other salts can produce acute cholestatic hepatitis (fever, jaundice, impaired liver function) because of hypersensitivity. Most patients recover completely.

AZITHROMYCIN

Azithromycin is the first of the azalide antibiotics that are chemically similar to the macrolides such as erythromycin. With excellent in vitro activity against *C trachomatis* and with favorable kinetics including sustained high concentration in tissue (even though serum concentrations are low), azithromycin (1 g orally once) has been as effective as doxycycline (100 mg twice daily for 7 days), 97% versus 95%, respectively, in treating chlamydia urethritis and cervicitis. Side effects were similar, mainly gastrointestinal, and were mild to moderate. Accordingly, azithromycin has become one of the recommended regimens for treatment of chlamydial infection as a 1-g dose given orally. In pregnancy, the 1-g dose of azithromycin is an alternative regimen to the recommended regimens in pregnancy of erythromycin base or amoxicillin. Because this 1-g dose of azithromycin is not adequate for treating gonorrhea, cotreatment with single-dose ceftriaxone (250 mg intramuscularly) is necessary.

CLINDAMYCIN

Clindamycin resembles erythromycin and is active against gram-positive organisms (except enterococci). Clindamycin 0.15–0.3 g orally every 6 hours yields serum concentrations of 2–5 μg/mL. The drug is widely distributed in tissues. Excretion is through the bile and urine. Group B streptococcal resistance to clindamycin has become common. Thus, as with erythromycin, clindamycin should not be used for group B streptococcus prophylaxis unless susceptibility has been established. It is also effective against most strains of *Bacteroides* and is an excellent drug in polymicrobial aerobic-anaerobic infections, when used in combination with an aminoglycoside. Seriously ill patients are given clindamycin intravenously during a 1-hour period, 900 mg every 8 hours. Vaginal clindamycin cream (2%) when used nightly (5–7 mL) for 5–7 days is highly effective in treating bacterial vaginosis. A clindamycin ovule is indicated for treatment of bacterial vaginosis for 3 days.

Common side effects of systemic clindamycin are diarrhea, nausea, and skin rashes. Impaired liver function and neutropenia have been noted. If 3–4 g is given rapidly intravenously, cardiorespiratory arrest may occur. Pseudomembranous colitis has been associated with clindamycin administration. This is due to necrotizing toxin produced by *Clostridium difficile*, which is clindamycin-resistant and increases in the gut with the selection pressure exerted by administration of this drug. *C difficile* is sensitive to vancomycin and

metronidazole, and the colitis rapidly regresses during oral treatment with metronidazole, which is preferred to vancomycin because of its lower cost.

TETRACYCLINE GROUP

The tetracyclines have common basic chemical structures, antimicrobial activity, and pharmacologic properties. Microorganisms resistant to one tetracycline show cross-resistance to all tetracyclines.

Antimicrobial Activity

Tetracyclines are inhibitors of protein synthesis and are bacteriostatic for many gram-positive and gram-negative bacteria. They are strongly inhibitory for the growth of mycoplasmas, rickettsiae, chlamydiae, and some protozoa (eg, amoebas). Equal concentrations of all tetracyclines in blood or tissue have approximately equal antimicrobial activity. However, there are great differences in the susceptibility of different strains of a given species of microorganism, so laboratory tests are important. Because of the emergence of resistant strains, tetracyclines have lost some of their former usefulness against gram-negative and gram-positive bacteria, but they have ongoing usefulness in treating sexually transmitted organisms. Tetracyclines alone are no longer considered adequate therapy for gonorrhea, but they are recommended for chlamydia.

Absorption, Distribution, & Excretion

Tetracyclines are absorbed somewhat irregularly from the gut. Absorption is limited by the low solubility of the drugs and by chelation with divalent cations, eg, Ca^{2+} or Fe^{2+}. A large proportion (80%) of orally administered tetracycline remains in the gut lumen, modifies intestinal flora, and is excreted in feces. With full systemic doses (2 g/d), levels of active drug in serum reach 2–10 μg/mL. Tetracyclines are specifically deposited in growing bones and teeth, bound to calcium.

Absorbed tetracyclines are excreted mainly in bile and urine. Up to 20% of oral doses may appear in the urine after glomerular filtration. With renal failure, doses of tetracyclines must be reduced or intervals between doses increased.

Minocycline and doxycycline are well absorbed from the gut but are excreted more slowly than others, leading to accumulation and prolonged blood levels. Doxycycline does not accumulate greatly in renal failure.

Indications, Dosages, & Routes of Administration

Tetracyclines are the drugs of choice in chlamydial and genital mycoplasmal infections in nonpregnant women.

A. ORAL

Tetracycline hydrochloride is dispensed in 250-mg capsules. Give 0.25–0.5 g orally every 6 hours. Doxycycline 100 mg twice daily is as effective as tetracycline hydrochloride 2 g/d.

B. INTRAVENOUS

Several tetracyclines are formulated for parenteral administration in individuals unable to take oral medication. The dose is generally similar to the oral dose (see manufacturer's instructions).

Adverse Effects

A. ALLERGY

Hypersensitivity reactions with fever or skin rashes are uncommon.

B. GASTROINTESTINAL SIDE EFFECTS

Gastrointestinal side effects are common. They can be diminished by reducing the dose or by administering tetracyclines with food. After a few days of oral use, the gut flora is modified so that drug-resistant bacteria and yeasts become prominent. This may cause functional gut disturbances, anal pruritus, and even enterocolitis.

C. BONES AND TEETH

Tetracyclines are bound to calcium deposited in growing bones and teeth, causing fluorescence, discoloration, enamel dysplasia, deformity, or growth inhibition. Tetracyclines are contraindicated in pregnant women.

D. LIVER DAMAGE

Tetracyclines can impair hepatic function or even cause liver necrosis, particularly during pregnancy, in the presence of preexisting liver damage, or with doses of more than 3 g intravenously.

E. KIDNEY DAMAGE

Outdated tetracycline preparations have been implicated in renal tubular acidosis and other renal damage. Tetracyclines may increase blood urea nitrogen when diuretics are administered.

F. OTHER

Tetracyclines may induce photosensitization, especially in fair-complected individuals. Intravenous injection may cause thrombophlebitis, and intramuscular injection may induce local inflammation with pain. Minocycline causes vestibular reactions (dizziness, vertigo, nausea) in 30–60% of cases after doses of 200 mg daily.

AMINOGLYCOSIDES

This group includes widely used drugs such as gentamicin and tobramycin. These agents inhibit protein synthesis in bacteria by attaching to and inhibiting the function of the 30S subunit of the bacterial ribosome. Anaerobic bacteria are resistant to aminoglycosides because transport across the cell membrane is an oxygen-dependent, energy-requiring process.

All aminoglycosides are potentially ototoxic and nephrotoxic, although to different degrees. All can accumulate in renal failure; therefore, dosage adjustments must be made in uremia.

Aminoglycosides are used widely against presumed or established gram-negative enteric bacteria. In the treatment of bacteremia or endocarditis caused by fecal streptococci or by some gram-negative bacteria, the aminoglycoside is given together with penicillin to enhance permeability and facilitate the entry of the aminoglycoside.

General Properties of Aminoglycosides

A. PHYSICAL PROPERTIES

Aminoglycosides are water soluble and stable in solution. If they are mixed in solution with β-lactam antibiotics, they may form complexes and lose some activity. Aminoglycosides may be mixed with clindamycin in IV solutions.

B. ABSORPTION, DISTRIBUTION, METABOLISM, AND EXCRETION

Aminoglycosides are well absorbed after intramuscular or intravenous injection but are not absorbed from the gut. They are distributed widely in tissues and penetrate pleural, peritoneal, or joint fluid in the presence of inflammation. They accumulate in amniotic fluid, but not for 6 hours after maternal injection. They enter the central nervous system to only a slight extent after parenteral administration. There is no significant metabolic breakdown of aminoglycosides. The serum half-life is 2–3 hours; excretion is mainly by glomerular filtration. Urine levels are 10–50 times higher than serum levels.

C. DOSE AND EFFECT IN CASES OF IMPAIRED RENAL FUNCTION

In the past, the dose of gentamicin for a person with normal renal function was 3–7 mg/kg/d divided in 3 equal injections every 8 hours. In the past several years, dosing every 24 hours has become the usually recommended regimen. The usual initial dose of gentamicin is 4.0–5.0 mg/kg intravenously once daily, in an infusion given over a 30-minute period. Reasons for the once-daily administration of gentamicin are the potentially less toxicity, less cost, and equivalent clinical efficacy. In persons with impaired renal function, excretion is diminished and the dosing interval may be prolonged beyond 24 hours.

Because of the increased glomerular filtration rate in pregnancy and the subsequent rapid excretion of aminoglycosides in pregnancy, doses greater than 5 mg/kg every 24 hours may be necessary. When 24-hour dosing is used, gentamicin levels are usually determined and plotted on a nomogram to ascertain appropriateness of the dose. Studies of gentamicin in postpartum individuals have been performed, but there have been few studies of 24-hour dosing of gentamicin during pregnancy. Accordingly, some clinicians prefer to continue to use dosing at 8-hour intervals for gentamicin in the pregnant patient.

D. ADVERSE EFFECTS

All aminoglycosides can cause varying degrees of ototoxicity and nephrotoxicity. Ototoxicity can present either as hearing loss (cochlear damage) that is noted first as a deficiency in hearing high frequencies or as vestibular damage, as evidenced by vertigo, ataxia, and loss of balance.

In very high doses, aminoglycosides can be neurotoxic, producing a curarelike effect with neuromuscular blockage that results in respiratory paralysis. This has been most common in gynecologic surgery when solutions containing aminoglycosides have been used for peritoneal irrigation. Calcium gluconate or neostigmine can serve as antidote. Rarely, aminoglycosides cause hypersensitivity and local reactions.

1. Gentamicin

Gentamicin is the most widely used aminoglycoside antibiotic on obstetric-gynecologic services. In concentrations of 0.5–5 µg/mL, gentamicin is bactericidal not only for staphylococci and coliform organisms but also for many strains of *Pseudomonas, Proteus,* and *Serratia.* Enterococci are resistant to gentamicin alone, but they are susceptible to gentamicin plus penicillin. With doses of 3–7 mg/kg/d, serum levels reach 3–8 µg/mL. Gentamicin may be synergistic with ticarcillin against *Pseudomonas.* However, the 2 drugs should not be mixed in vitro.

Indications, Dosages, & Routes of Administration

Gentamicin is used for severe infections caused by gram-negative bacteria, including *Klebsiella-Enterobacter, Proteus, Pseudomonas,* and *Serratia.* The dosage is usually 4–5 mg/kg every 24 hours in a single IV infusion. It is necessary to monitor renal function by checking serum creatinine levels every few days and to reduce the dosage or lengthen the interval between

doses if renal function declines. Approximately 2–3% of patients develop vestibular dysfunction and loss of hearing when peak serum levels exceed 10 µg/mL. Serum concentrations should be monitored in selected circumstances.

2. Tobramycin

Tobramycin is an aminoglycoside that closely resembles gentamicin in antibacterial activity and pharmacologic properties and exhibits partial cross-resistance. Tobramycin may be effective against some gentamicin-resistant gram-negative bacteria, especially *Pseudomonas.* Tobramycin may be less nephrotoxic than gentamicin; their ototoxicity is similar.

SPECTINOMYCIN

Spectinomycin is an aminocyclitol antibiotic, related to the aminoglycosides. Its sole indication is for treatment of β-lactamase–producing gonococci or gonorrhea in a penicillin-hypersensitive person. One injection of 2 g (40 mg/kg) is given. Pain at the injection site is usual, and nausea and fever may occur.

SULFONAMIDES-TRIMETHOPRIM

The combination of sulfonamides, particularly sulfamethoxazole with trimethoprim, offers a combination of 2 folic acid antagonists that is useful in a number of circumstances. The indications are as follows:

(1) Urinary tract infection: Many coliform organisms that are the most common causes of urinary tract infections are susceptible to the combination of TMP-SMX. For lower urinary tract infection, TMP-SMX 160/800 mg is often given every 12 hours for a 3-day regimen. For uncomplicated pyelonephritis in women who do not have evidence of sepsis, TMP-SMX 160/800 mg can be given orally every 12 hours for 10–14 days. Women who have pyelonephritis requiring hospitalization can be treated with TMP-SMX 160/800 mg intravenously every 12 hours until the patient is able to tolerate oral nourishment and oral therapy, which should be continued to complete a 10- to 14-day course.

(2) Parasitic diseases: The combination of trimethoprim with sulfamethoxazole is often effective for prophylaxis or treatment of *Pneumocystis carinii* pneumonia. The combination of pyrimethamine with sulfadiazine is used for treatment of toxoplasmosis. It should be given in combination with folinic acid in pregnant women.

(3) Sexually transmitted diseases: Sulfonamides are no longer considered for treatment of infection by *C trachomatis.*

Because trimethoprim and sulfonamides both are folate antagonists, there is a hypothetical possibility of teratogenesis. Accordingly, this combination should be avoided in the first trimester of pregnancy. Sulfonamides may lead to hemolysis in persons with glucose-6-phosphate (G6PD) enzyme deficiency. Sulfonamides also compete with bilirubin for binding sites. Accordingly, long-acting sulfonamides should not be given at term in order to avoid the unusual complication of low-level kernicterus in the newborn infant. These infants do not develop hyperbilirubinemia, but they do develop kernicterus at low bilirubin levels because of displacement of bilirubin from its binding sites to free bilirubin.

Adverse Effects

Sulfonamides produce a wide variety of side effects—due partly to hypersensitivity and partly to direct toxicity—which must be considered whenever unexplained symptoms or signs occur in a patient who may have received these drugs. Except in the mildest reactions, fluids should be forced and, if symptoms and signs progressively increase, the drugs should be discontinued.

A. SYSTEMIC SIDE EFFECTS

Side effects may include fever, skin rashes, urticaria; nausea and vomiting or diarrhea; stomatitis, conjunctivitis, arthritis, exfoliative dermatitis; hematopoietic disturbances, including thrombocytopenia, hemolytic (in G6PD deficiency) or aplastic anemia, granulocytopenia, leukemoid reactions; hepatitis, polyarteritis nodosa, vasculitis, Stevens-Johnson syndrome; and psychosis.

B. URINARY TRACT DISTURBANCES

Sulfonamides may precipitate in urine, especially at neutral or acid pH, producing hematuria, crystalluria, or even obstruction. They have been implicated in various types of nephritis and nephrosis. Sulfonamides and methenamine salts should not be given together.

Precautions in the Use of Sulfonamides

(1) There is cross-allergenicity among all sulfonamides. Obtain a history of past administration or reaction. Observe for possible allergic responses.

(2) Keep the urine volume above 1500 mL/d by encouraging fluid intake. Check urine pH—it should be 7.5 or higher. Give alkali by mouth (sodium bicarbonate or equivalent, 5–15 g/d). Examine fresh urine for crystals and red cells every 5–7 days.

(3) Check hemoglobin, white blood cell count, and differential count once weekly to detect possible disturbances early in high-risk patients.

METRONIDAZOLE

Metronidazole is an antiprotozoal drug that also is active against most anaerobes, including *Bacteroides* species. Metronidazole is well absorbed after oral administration and is widely distributed. The drug is metabolized in the liver, and dosage reduction is required in the presence of hepatic insufficiency. Metronidazole can also be given intravenously or by rectal suppository, with serum levels equivalent for both routes. It is used to treat amebiasis and the following:

(1) *Trichomonas* vaginitis: The recommended dose is 2 g orally (single dose). The alternative is 500 mg twice daily for 7 days. Both sexual partners should be treated.

(2) Bacterial vaginosis: Recommended regimens for nonpregnant women are 500 mg orally 2 times daily for 7 days or vaginal gel 0.75%, 5 g vaginally twice daily for 5 days. In pregnant women, the CDC-recommended regimen is 250 mg orally 3 times daily. Topical treatment of BV is not recommended in pregnancy. Single-dose treatment is less effective, and treatment of sexual partners is not recommended because it does not decrease recurrences in the female.

(3) In anaerobic or mixed infections, metronidazole can be given intravenously, 500 mg 3 times daily.

(4) For pseudomembranous colitis, give 500 mg 3 times daily orally.

Adverse effects of metronidazole include stomatitis, nausea, diarrhea, and disulfiram-like reactions. With prolonged use, peripheral neuropathy may develop.

VANCOMYCIN

Vancomycin is bactericidal for most gram-positive organisms, particularly staphylococci. Resistant mutants had been rare, but development of vancomycin-resistant enterococci has become a major cause for concern since the late 1980s. In many institutions, policies for control of vancomycin use have been developed. Vancomycin is an alternative to metronidazole in the treatment of pseudomembranous colitis. For this indication, it is given 2 g/d orally, but metronidazole is preferred because it is less expensive and because of the concern that oral vancomycin may lead to increased selection pressure for vancomycin-resistant enterococci in the gut. For systemic effect, the drug must be administered intravenously. After intravenous infusion of 0.5 g over 20 minutes, blood levels of 10 μg/mL are maintained for 1–2 hours. Vancomycin is excreted mainly through the kidneys, but it may accumulate in the kidneys in patients with liver failure. In renal insufficiency, the half-life may be up to 8 days. Thus, only 1 dose of 0.5–1 g can be given every 4–8 days to a uremic individual undergoing hemodialysis.

The chief indications for parenteral vancomycin are serious staphylococcal infection and enterococcal endocarditis (in combination with an aminoglycoside). Vancomycin is the recommended drug for group B streptococcus prophylaxis in patients who are at high risk for a serious penicillin allergic reaction and when the group B streptococcus isolate is resistant to clindamycin or erythromycin or when the susceptibility is unknown. Vancomycin 0.5 g is infused intravenously over 20 minutes every 6–8 hours (for children, 20–40 mg/kg/d).

Vancomycin is irritating to tissues; chills, fever, and thrombophlebitis sometimes follow intravenous injection. Rapid infusion may result in diffuse hyperemia (red man syndrome); this can be avoided by giving infusions over 1 hour. Vancomycin is sometimes ototoxic and (perhaps) nephrotoxic.

LINEZOLID

Linezolid (Zyvox) is an antibiotic of the new class providing clinical use in the treatment of aerobic gram-positive infections, especially those resistant to more common antibiotics. The potential use of linezolid is for treatment of resistant enterococcal, staphylococcal, and other streptococcal infections. Linezolid is available in preparations for both intravenous and oral administration. Its use in obstetric and gynecologic practice currently is limited.

QUINOLONES

Quinolones are synthetic analogues of nalidixic acid and are active against many gram-positive and gram-negative bacteria. All quinolones inhibit bacterial DNA synthesis by blocking the enzyme DNA gyrase. The earlier quinolones (nalidixic acid, oxolinic acid, cinoxacin) did not achieve systemic antibacterial levels and thus were useful only as urinary antiseptics. The newer fluoroquinolones (eg, norfloxacin, ciprofloxacin, enoxacin, oxofloxacin, pefloxacin, levofloxacin, and trovafloxacin) have greater antibacterial activity, achieve clinically useful levels in blood and tissues, and have low toxicity. They are active against a wide variety of aerobic bacteria, and some members of this group are active against clinically important anaerobes. After oral administration, these newer fluoroquinolones are well absorbed and widely distributed, with a serum half-life of 3–8 hours. They are excreted mainly by tubular renal secretion or glomerular filtration. Up to 20% of the dose is metabolized by the liver.

Indications for fluoroquinolones have been developed over the last few years and are as follows:

(1) Urinary tract infection: Use of quinolones should be reserved for infection due to organisms resistant to first-line treatment with nitrofurantoin, trimethoprim, and TMP-SMX. Quinolones should be used when resistant organisms are suspected (eg, for treatment of documented resistant strains), treatment failures, recurrent infection, or infection in patients with allergy to preferred drugs of choice. For complicated pyelonephritis, an oral quinolone can be used. For women with evidence of sepsis requiring hospitalization, a regimen including a fluoroquinolone can be used. For example, ofloxacin or ciprofloxacin in a dose of 200–400 mg IV every 12 hours can be used until the patient's course improves. Thereafter, when the patient can take oral nourishment, oral therapy should be started and continued to complete a 10- to 14-day course.

(2) Fluoroquinolones are widely used for treatment of sexually transmitted diseases. For example, for treatment of pelvic inflammatory disease, quinolones fit among the alternative parenteral regimens such as ofloxacin 400 mg IV every 12 hours with or without other antibiotics such as IV metronidazole, plus doxycycline. Another alternative regimen is levofloxacin 500 mg IV every 24 hours with or without the other combinations. Fluoroquinolones are also recommended in combination with other agents for treatment of pelvic inflammatory disease on an ambulatory basis. One recommended regimen is ofloxacin 400 mg orally twice daily or levofloxacin 500 mg once daily for 14 days plus metronidazole 500 mg orally twice daily for 14 days.

For treatment of chlamydial infections in adolescents and adults, ofloxacin 300 mg twice daily for 7 days is an alternative regimen.

Several fluoroquinolones are listed as recommended regimens for treatment of uncomplicated gonococcal infection of the cervix, urethra, and rectum. For example, 1 regimen is ciprofloxacin 500 mg orally in a single dose or ofloxacin 400 mg orally in a single dose. Either of these regimens should be combined with either azithromycin or doxycycline if chlamydial infection is not ruled out. Because they inhibit DNA gyrase, quinolones should be avoided in pregnancy.

The most pronounced adverse effects are nausea, vomiting, diarrhea, headache, dizziness, insomnia, occasional skin rashes, impairment of liver function, seizures, and anaphylaxis.

NITROFURANTOIN

Nitrofurantoin is bacteriostatic and bactericidal for both gram-positive and gram-negative bacteria in urine. The drug has no systemic antimicrobial activity. Its activity in urine is enhanced at pH 5.5 or below. Microbial resistance does not emerge rapidly.

The usual daily dose for treatment of urinary tract infections is 100 mg orally twice daily for 3 days, taken with food. Nitrofurantoin is also useful for continuous or postcoital suppression of urinary infection.

Oral nitrofurantoin may cause nausea and vomiting. Hemolytic anemia occurs in G6PD deficiency. Hypersensitivity may produce skin rashes and pulmonary infiltration. In uremia, there is virtually no excretion of nitrofurantoin into the urine and no therapeutic effect.

ANTIFUNGAL DRUGS

Most antibacterial drugs have no effect on yeasts and fungi. Others (eg, amphotericin B) are relatively effective in some systemic mycotic infections but are difficult to administer because of toxicity. New imidazoles are fairly effective and relatively nontoxic. Many topical preparations, such as 2% miconazole, 1% clotrimazole, 2% butoconazole, and 0.4% terconazole, all have been used effectively for treatment of vaginal candidiasis. Ketoconazole can be given orally, 200–600 mg once daily, preferably with food. It is well absorbed, reaches serum levels of 2–4 μg/mL, and is degraded in tissues, thus requiring no renal or biliary excretion. It has a dramatic therapeutic effect on chronic vaginal candidiasis. Ketoconazole blocks the synthesis of adrenal steroids and can cause gynecomastia. Adverse effects are mild, with nausea, headache, skin rashes, and occasional elevations in transaminase levels. If evidence of liver dysfunction persists, the drug should be discontinued.

Fluconazole (Diflucan) is an effective single-dose treatment of uncomplicated yeast infection. The dose is 150–200 mg orally as a single dose. The drug is also effective for treatment of recurrent or refractory vulvovaginal candidiasis and is less hepatotoxic than ketoconazole. One regimen for recurrent or refractory yeast infection is fluconazole 150 or 200 mg taken on days 1, 4, and 8. Because of its unusually long half-life, it does not need to be given more frequently. One prophylactic regimen for patients with frequent recurrent yeast infections (ie, > 4–6 per year) is fluconazole 150 mg taken once weekly for up to 6 months.

ANTIMICROBIAL CHEMOPROPHYLAXIS IN SURGERY

A major portion of all antimicrobial drugs used in hospitals are used on surgical services with the stated intent of "prophylaxis." Several general features of "surgical prophylaxis" are applicable.

(1) Prophylactic administration of antibiotics should generally be considered only if the expected rate of infectious complications is high or where a possible infection would have a catastrophic effect.

(2) If prophylactic antimicrobials are to be effective, a sufficient concentration of drug must be present at the operative site to inhibit or kill bacteria that might settle there. Thus, it is essential that drug administration begin immediately before (or in cesarean section just after) operation begins.

(3) Prolonged administration of antimicrobial drugs tends to alter the normal flora of organ systems, suppressing the susceptible microorganisms and favoring the implantation of drug-resistant ones. Thus, antimicrobial prophylaxis should last only 1–3 doses.

(4) Systemic antimicrobial levels usually do not prevent wound infection, pneumonia, or urinary tract infection if physiologic abnormalities or foreign bodies are present.

In hysterectomy and nonelective cesarean section, administration of a broad-spectrum bactericidal drug from just before until 1 day after the procedure has been found effective. Thus, for example, cefazolin 1 g intravenously given before pelvic operations and again for 1–2 doses after the end of the operation results in a demonstrable lowering of the risk of deep infections at the operative site.

Other forms of surgical prophylaxis are used to reduce normal flora or existing bacterial contamination at the site. Thus, the colon is routinely prepared not only by mechanical cleansing through cathartics and enemas but also by oral administration of poorly absorbed drugs (eg, neomycin 1 g, plus erythromycin base 0.5 g, every 6 hours) for 1–2 days before operation.

In all situations in which antimicrobials are administered with the hope that they may have a prophylactic effect, the risk from these same drugs (eg, allergy, toxicity, selection of superinfecting microorganisms) must be evaluated daily, and the course of prophylaxis must be kept as brief as possible.

ANTIVIRAL CHEMOPROPHYLAXIS & THERAPY

Several compounds can suppress development of viral diseases. Of these, acyclovir is important in gynecologic practice.

Acyclovir (acycloguanosine [Zovirax]) inhibits replication of herpesviruses in infected cells. When given intravenously (15 mg/kg/d), acyclovir is effective in controlling disseminating herpesvirus infections in immunocompromised patients. It can also markedly reduce pain and the extent of lesions in primary genital herpes infections of women. In herpetic encephalitis and neonatal herpetic dissemination, acyclovir is more effective than vidarabine. Acyclovir has no effect on cytomegalovirus or Epstein-Barr virus infections, but acyclovir can arrest the progression of varicella and herpes zoster, especially in immunocompromised patients.

Oral acyclovir, 200 mg 5 times daily for adults, has therapeutic effects similar to those of intravenous acyclovir, particularly in primary genital herpes simplex infections. When taken prophylactically in patients with frequent (> 6 per year) episodes, it can reduce the frequency of recurrent lesions for up to 3 years. However, no regimen of acyclovir can block the establishment of latency or permanently eliminate recurrences.

Two additional antiviral drugs have become available: famciclovir and valacyclovir. The advantage of these preparations is that they have longer half-lives, and they can be given at less frequent dosing intervals than acyclovir. However, they appear to be no more effective. Valacyclovir, famciclovir, and acyclovir are all recommended for first-episode genital herpes, for recurrent episodes of genital herpes, and for daily suppressive therapy of frequent recurrences. Their use in pregnancy has not been extensive, but available data are reassuring for no side effects peculiar to the pregnant woman or the fetus. Valacyclovir has also been established as a means of preventing herpes simplex virus HSV-2 transmission from 1 sexual partner to the other when the HSV-2–infected partner has taken daily valacyclovir (500 mg) for 8 months.

REFERENCES

American College of Obstetricians and Gynecologists: *Antibiotic Prophylaxis for Gynecologic Procedures.* ACOG Practice Bulletin No. 23. American College of Obstetricians and Gynecologists, 2001.

American College of Obstetricians and Gynecologists: *Prophylactic Antibiotics in Labor And Delivery.* ACOG Practice Bulletin No. 47. American College of Obstetricians and Gynecologists, 2003.

Centers for Disease Control and Prevention: 2002 Guidelines for treatment of sexually transmitted diseases. MMWR Recomm Rep 2002;51(RR-6):1.

Corey L et al: Once-daily valacyclovir to reduce the risk of transmission of genital herpes. N Engl J Med 2004;350:11.

Kucers A et al: *The Use of Antibiotics: A Clinical Review of Antibacterial, Antifungal and Antiviral Drugs,* 5th ed. Butterworth-Heinemann, 1997.

Sweet RL, Gibbs RS: *Infectious Diseases of the Female Genital Tract,* 4th ed. Lippincott Williams & Wilkins, 2001.

Wendel GD et al: Penicillin allergy and desensitization in serious infections during pregnancy. N Engl J Med 1985;312:1230.

Endometriosis

Susan Sarajari, MD, PhD, Kenneth N. Muse, MD, & Alan H. DeCherney, MD

Endometriosis is a disorder in which abnormal growths of tissue, histologically resembling the endometrium, are present in locations other than the uterine lining. Although endometriosis can occur very rarely in post-menopausal women, it is found almost exclusively in women of reproductive age. All other manifestations of endometriosis exhibit a wide spectrum of expression. The lesions are usually found on the peritoneal surfaces of the reproductive organs and adjacent structures of the pelvis, but they can occur anywhere in the body (Fig 43–1). The size of the individual lesions varies from microscopic to large invasive masses that erode into underlying organs and cause extensive adhesion formation. Similarly, women with endometriosis can be completely asymptomatic, or may be crippled by pelvic pain and infertility.

Epidemiology

Endometriosis is a common and important health problem of women. Its exact prevalence is unknown because surgery is required for its diagnosis, but it is estimated to be present in 3–10% of women in the reproductive age group and 25–35% of infertile women. It is seen in 1–2% of women undergoing sterilization or sterilization reversal, in 10% of hysterectomy surgeries, in 16–31% of laparoscopies, and in 53% of adolescents with pelvic pain severe enough to warrant surgical evaluation. Endometriosis is the most common single gynecologic diagnosis responsible for hospitalization of females 15–44 years old, being found in over 6% of patients.

Pathogenesis

The cause of endometriosis is unknown. The leading theories include retrograde menstruation with transport of endometrial cells, metaplasia of coelomic epithelium, hematogenous or lymphatic spread, and direct transplantation of endometrial cells. A combination of these theories likely is responsible.

A theory of retrograde menstruation was proposed during the 1920s. It was postulated that endometriosis occurred because viable fragments of endometrium were shed at the time of menstruation and passed through the uterine tubes. Once in the pelvic cavity, the tissue became implanted on peritoneal surfaces and grew into endometriotic lesions. Subsequent observations have confirmed that some degree of retrograde menstruation normally occurs in women with patent tubes, that outflow tract obstructions (cervical stenosis, transverse vaginal septa) increase the incidence of endometriosis, and that intentional deposition of endometrium onto peritoneum can initiate endometriosis. Also, the risk of developing the disease is higher in women with prolonged menstrual flow and in those with short menstrual cycle lengths (more menses per year). This theory is simple, attractive, and easily explains why endometriosis is most commonly found on the peritoneal surfaces of the ovaries, cul-de-sac, and bladder and why lesions may develop in episiotomies and other incisions. However, it does not explain why all women do not develop endometriosis, nor does it explain the rare cases of endometriosis in the lung, brain, or other soft tissues or in nonmenstruating subjects (women with Turner's syndrome or with absent uteri).

Evidence indicates that altered humoral and cell-mediated immunity plays a role in the pathogenesis of endometriosis. The activity of natural killer cells may be reduced, and deficient cellular immunity may cause an inability to recognize endometrial tissue in abnormal locations. Endometriosis may occur when the deficiency in cellular immunity allows menstrual tissue to implant and grow on the peritoneum. Some evidence also indicates increased concentration of leukocytes and macrophages in the ectopic endometrium and the peritoneal cavity, which secrete growth factors and cytokines into the peritoneal fluid. These cytokines and growth factors are postulated to lead to proliferation of the endometriotic implants and the inflammatory reaction, of which oxidative stress may be another component. Patients with endometriosis have been described as having a higher rate of autoimmune inflammatory disorders compared to the general population. Genetic influences in the development of endometriosis also have been described. Studies have found that 7–9% of first-degree female relatives of patients with endometriosis are diagnosed with the disease; this rate is significantly greater than the control rate of 1–2%. Further

Figure 43–1. Common sites of endometrial implants (endometriosis). (Reproduced, with permission, from Way LW [editor]: *Current Surgical Diagnosis & Treatment*, 7th ed. Lange, 1985.)

investigation has revealed a possible role for the HLA-B7 allele. Expression of HLA-B7 has been shown to inhibit the cytotoxic activity of natural killer-like T lymphocytes, suggesting that growth of ectopic endometrial cells might be under genetic control.

Pathology

The gross appearance of endometriosis at operation is usually quite characteristic and, to an experienced surgeon, is sufficient for diagnosis. The smallest (and presumably earliest) implants are red, petechial lesions on the peritoneal surface. With further growth, menstrual-like detritus accumulates within the lesion, giving it a cystic, dark brown, dark blue, or black appearance. The surrounding peritoneal surface becomes thickened and scarred. These "powder burn" implants typically attain a diameter of 5–10 mm. With progression of disease, the number and size of lesions increase, and extensive adhesions may develop. When present on the ovary, cysts may enlarge to several centimeters in size and are called "endometriomas" or "chocolate cysts." Severe disease can erode into underlying tissues and distort the remaining organs with extensive adhesions. In addition to these traditional presentations, endometriosis lesions can have a variety of nonclassical appearances: clear vesicles, white or yellow spots or nodules, circular folds of peritoneum ("pockets"), and visually normal perito-

neum (lesions so small they can only be detected microscopically).

The distribution of lesions also exhibits a characteristic pattern. Solitary lesions are possible, but multiple implantations are the rule. The most common site of disease is the ovary (approximately half of all cases), followed by the uterine cul-de-sac, posterior broad ligament, uterosacral ligaments, uterus, fallopian tubes, sigmoid colon, appendix and round ligaments. Implants may occur over the bowel, bladder, and ureters; rarely, they erode into underlying tissue and cause blood in the stool or urine, or their associated adhesions result in stricture and obstruction of these organs. Implants can occur deep in tissue, especially on the cervix, posterior vaginal fornix, or within wounds contaminated by endometrial tissue (see Fig 43–1). Very rarely, endometriosis is found distant from the pelvis, in such sites as the lung, brain, and kidney. Pleural implantations are associated with recurrent right pneumothoraces at the time of menses, termed "catamenial pneumothorax." Similarly, lesions in the central nervous system can cause catamenial seizures.

The microscopic finding that these lesions are composed of tissue histologically resembling endometrial glands and stroma gives endometriosis its name (Fig 43–2). The normal endometrial appearance is best seen in small, early lesions. With advanced disease, cyst formation, and fibrosis, the wall of the implant is lined by a monolayer of cells, if at all. Blood is present inside the cyst, and hemosiderin-laden macrophages are found in the cyst wall.

Pathologic Physiology

It is generally agreed that pelvic pain occurs premenstrually in endometriosis patients. Because of this, pain from endometriosis is thought to be due to stimulation from estrogen and progesterone during the menstrual cycle; the tissue of the implant is stimulated to grow in much the same way as is the endometrium. The implants enlarge and may undergo secretory change and bleeding; however, the fibrotic tissues surrounding the implants prevent the expansion and escape of hemorrhagic fluid that occurs in the uterus. With subsequent cycles, this process repeats itself. Pain is produced by pressure and inflammation within and around the lesion, by traction on adhesions associated with the lesions, by the number of implants and their proximity to nerves and other sensitive structures, and by the mass effect of large lesions. Although this sequence of events explains why premenstrual pelvic pain can occur in endometriosis, it is incomplete, because many patients with extensive endometriosis have no pain. It is a common observation that the occurrence and severity of pain from endometriosis bear little relationship to the amount and distribution of the disease. Severe pain in

Figure 43–2. Histologic appearance of endometriosis. **Left:** Endometriosis of ovary. **Right:** Endometriosis of cervix. (Courtesy of Eugene H. Ruffolo, MD.)

patients with endometriosis is associated with deeply infiltrating lesions, and it is thought that the degree of pain is perhaps determined by the depth of invasion.

The relationship between endometriosis and infertility has been more extensively investigated. Moderate and severe endometriosis is associated with pelvic adhesions that distort pelvic anatomy, prevent normal tubo-ovarian apposition, and encase the ovary. Implants can destroy ovarian and tubal tissue, although occlusion of uterine tubes is rare.

It is not difficult to understand how advanced disease can result in infertility, but minimal or mild endometriosis, in which pelvic anatomy is entirely normal except for a few peritoneal surface lesions, can also cause infertility. The mechanism by which this occurs is unknown. Various theories explaining this phenomenon have been proposed.

Several investigators have examined peritoneal fluid abnormalities. The peritoneal fluid is an ultrafiltrate of plasma, with less than 5 mL normally present in the pelvis. After ovulation, a transient rise to approximately 20 mL occurs. The volume of peritoneal fluid and the concentrations of various hormones and other substances in it affect the processes of ovulation, ovum pickup, tubal function, and so on. The normal role of

the peritoneal fluid and its constituents in these processes, and how it is altered by endometriosis, are largely unknown. Peritoneal fluid volume has been reported to be altered in endometriosis patients, but studies have led to inconsistent results.

Similarly, reports are contradictory as to whether endometriosis patients have elevations in peritoneal fluid prostaglandins F_2 and E_2. Prostaglandins are normally secreted by the endometrium and by endometriosis lesions; an increase in peritoneal fluid prostaglandin levels could theoretically decrease fertility by altering ovulation, tubal motility, nidation, and luteal phase adequacy. The conflicting reports may result from fluctuations that normally occur across the cycle in prostanoid production, as well as variations in the lesions' synthesis of prostaglandins; small red petechial implants have been found to secrete more prostaglandins than larger, powder burnlike ones.

Several disorders of menstrual cyclicity and ovulation have been suggested as a basis for the infertility caused by mild endometriosis. The rate of ovulation among endometriosis patients is 11–27%. Nearly half of patients become pregnant when this problem is also treated. More subtle problems in folliculogenesis in endometriosis patients have been reported, including lower serum estradiol levels, smaller follicle size during follicular growth, and lower oocyte fertilization rates and pregnancy rates in assisted reproduction. Problems with ovum pickup by the fallopian tube and embryo implantation in the endometrium have also been suggested.

Clinical Findings

Endometriosis is common among women of reproductive age, and its prevalence increases to 30–40% among infertile women. Clinical findings vary greatly depending on the number, size, and extent of the lesions and on the patient population being examined.

The diagnosis of endometriosis is often strongly suspected from a patient's initial history. Infertility, dysmenorrhea, and dyspareunia are the main presenting complaints. Most patients complain of constant pelvic pain or a low sacral backache that occurs premenstrually and subsides after menses begins. Dyspareunia is often present, particularly with deep penetration. Lesions involving the urinary tract or bowel may result in bloody urine or stool in the perimenstrual interval. Implantations on or near the external surfaces of the cervix, vagina, vulva, rectum, or urethra may cause pain or bleeding with defecation, urination, or intercourse at any time in the menstrual cycle. Adhesions from endometriosis may cause discomfort at any time during the cycle, and a sensation of pelvic pressure may result if large masses are present. Premenstrual spotting may occur and is more likely to be associated with endometriosis than with luteal phase inadequacy. It must be emphasized, however, that many patients either have no symptoms or have infertility as their only symptom and that the extent of disease often has little correlation with the severity of symptoms.

The physical examination may be helpful in discerning whether endometriosis is present. Classically, pelvic examination reveals tender nodules in the posterior vaginal fornix and pain upon uterine motion. The uterus may be fixed and retroverted due to cul-de-sac adhesions, and tender adnexal masses may be felt because of the presence of endometriomas. Careful inspection may reveal implants in healed wounds, especially episiotomy and cesarean section incisions, in the vaginal fornix, or on the cervix. Biopsy may be required to prove that the lesions are due to endometriosis. However, many patients have no abnormal findings on physical examination.

For the vast majority of patients, endometriosis is included in the differential diagnosis of infertility or pelvic pain. Endometriosis should be suspected in any patient of reproductive age complaining of pain or infertility. Medical treatment can be given for pelvic pain thought to be due to endometriosis, but the specific diagnosis of endometriosis should not be made unless documented by direct visualization. The final diagnosis of endometriosis can only be made at laparoscopy or laparotomy, by direct observation of the implants. Occasionally, an isolated endometrioma is removed, and the diagnosis must be made histologically by the demonstration of "endometrial" glands and stroma or of hemosiderin-laden macrophages in the cyst wall.

Except for special circumstances, such as urography or sigmoidoscopy for suspected bowel or urinary involvement, ancillary diagnostic studies (ultrasound, x-ray films, computed tomographic scans) are of little help in diagnosis. Cancer antigen-125 (CA-125) is often elevated in women with endometriosis. However, it has been shown that this marker is elevated in many other pelvic diseases and therefore has little specificity in the diagnosis of endometriosis. Elevated CA-125 levels that return to normal after medical or surgical treatment can be helpful in the evaluation for recurrences.

Complications

True complications of endometriosis are few. Implants over the bowel or ureters may cause obstruction and silent impairment of renal function. The erosive nature of the lesions in advanced aggressive disease can cause a myriad of symptoms, depending on the tissue damaged. Endometriomas can cause ovarian torsion, or they can rupture and spill their irritating contents into the peritoneal cavity, resulting in a chemical peritonitis. Excision of endometriosis causing catamenial seizures or pneumothorax may be necessary.

Differential Diagnosis

The varied presentations of endometriosis mandate that its consideration in the differential diagnosis of virtually all pelvic disease. In particular, the pain, infertility, and adhesions associated with endometriosis must be distinguished from similar symptoms accompanying pelvic inflammatory disease and pelvic tumors. Usually this requires operative evaluation. A patient with a persistent adnexal mass larger than 5 cm should never be presumed to have an endometrioma even if endometriosis has been diagnosed previously. Such masses require surgical diagnosis.

Prevention

Prevention of endometriosis is not currently possible. Traditionally, women with relatives affected by endometriosis—or in whom the diagnosis has recently been made—are advised not to postpone childbearing. The merits of this advice have not been proved. A more thorough understanding of the pathophysiology of endometriosis is required before preventive strategies can be devised.

Classification

Several classification schemes to assist in describing the anatomic location and severity of endometriosis at operation have been created. Although none is entirely satisfactory, the scoring systems are useful for reporting operative findings and for comparing the results of various treatment protocols. The revised American Society for Reproductive Medicine classification is given in Table 43–1 and Fig 43–3. Note that this system does not correlate with the severity of pain but is mainly designed to predict the chance of pregnancy.

Treatment

Treatment options are dictated by the patient's desire for future fertility, her symptoms, the stage of her disease, and to some extent her age. It must be emphasized that therapy for endometriosis requires operative inspection of the lesions for correct diagnosis and staging and to ensure that the patient's symptoms are attributable to endometriosis only.

A. EXPECTANT MANAGEMENT

In asymptomatic patients, those with mild discomfort, or infertile women with minimal or mild endometriosis, expectant management may be appropriate. Although endometriosis is generally believed to be a progressive disease, no evidence indicates that treating an asymptomatic patient will prevent or ameliorate the onset of symptoms later. Many reports have found expectant management of infertile women with minimal or mild endometriosis to be as successful as medical or surgical therapies.

B. ANALGESIC THERAPY

Analgesic treatments include nonsteroidal anti-inflammatory drugs. These drugs are appropriate sole therapy for endometriosis when the patient has mild premenstrual pain from minimal endometriosis, no abnormalities on pelvic examination, and no desire for immediate fertility.

C. HORMONAL THERAPY

The goal of treatment with hormonal therapy is to interrupt the cycles of stimulation and bleeding of endometriotic tissue. This can be achieved with various agents.

1. Oral contraceptive pills—Oral contraceptive pills (OCPs) are a good choice for patients with minimal or mild symptoms. In general, monophasic products are prescribed either cyclically or continuously for 6–12 months. The continuous exposure to combination OCPs results in decidual changes in the endometrial glands. Continuous use of OCPs has been shown to be effective in decreasing dysmenorrhea and may retard progression of endometriosis.

Table 43–1. American Society for Reproductive Medicine revised classification of endometriosis.

	Endometriosis	< 1 cm	1–3 cm	> 3 cm
Peritoneum	Superficial	1	2	4
	Deep	2	4	6
Ovary	R Superficial	1	2	4
	Deep	4	16	20
	L Superficial	1	2	4
	Deep	4	16	20

	Posterior Cul-de-sac Obliteration	Partial	Complete
		4	40

	Adhesions	< 1/3 Enclosure	1/3–2/3 Enclosure	> 2/3 Enclosure
Ovary	R Filmy	1	2	4
	Dense	4	8	16
	L Filmy	1	2	4
	Dense	4	8	16
Tube	R Filmy	1	2	4
	Dense	4[1]	8[1]	16
	L Filmy	1	2	4
	Dense	4[1]	8[1]	16

[1]If the fimbriated end of the fallopian tube is completely enclosed, change the point assignment to 16. Staging: Stage I (minimal): 1–5; stage II (mild): 6–15; stage III (moderate): 16–40; stage IV (severe): > 40. (Reproduced, with permission, from Revised American Society for Reproductive Medicine classification of endometriosis: 1996. Fertil Steri 1997; 67:819.)

2. Progestins—These agents work via a mechanism similar to that of the OCPs, causing decidualization in the endometriotic tissue. Oral medroxyprogesterone acetate can be prescribed as a 10- to 30-mg daily dose. An alternative regimen is norethindrone acetate 5 mg daily or megestrol acetate prescribed as a 40-mg daily dose. Depot medroxyprogesterone acetate 150 mg IM can also be given as a single injection every 3 months.

In a few small studies, the levonorgestrel-releasing intrauterine device has been shown to relieve dysmenorrheal and pelvic pain. Eighty percent of women treated with progestins have a partial or complete relief of pain.

3. Danazol—Danazol is a 19-nortestosterone derivative with progestinlike effects. Danazol acts via several mechanisms to treat endometriosis. It acts at the hypo-

STAGE I (MINIMAL)	STAGE II (MILD)	STAGE III (MODERATE)

STAGE I (MINIMAL)

PERITONEUM
  Superficial Endo   –   1-3cm   -2
R. OVARY
  Superficial Endo   –   < 1cm   -1
  Filmy Adhesions   –   < 1/3   -1
        TOTAL POINTS   4

STAGE II (MILD)

PERITONEUM
  Deep Endo   –   > 3cm   -6
R. OVARY
  Superficial Endo   –   < 1cm   -1
  Filmy Adhesions   –   < 1/3   -1
L. OVARY
  Superficial Endo   –   < 1cm   -1
        TOTAL POINTS   9

STAGE III (MODERATE)

PERITONEUM
  Deep Endo   –   > 3cm   -6
CULDESAC
  Partial Obliteration   -4
L. OVARY
  Deep Endo   –   1-3cm   -16
        TOTAL POINTS   26

STAGE III (MODERATE)

PERITONEUM
  Superficial Endo   –   > 3cm   -4
R. TUBE
  Filmy Adhesions   –   < 1/3   -1
R. OVARY
  Filmy Adhesions   –   < 1/3   -1
L. Tube
  Dense Adhesions   –   < 1/3   -16*
L. OVARY
  Deep Endo   –   < 1cm   -4
  Dense Adhesions   –   < 1/3   -4
        TOTAL POINTS   30

STAGE IV (SEVERE)

PERITONEUM
  Superficial Endo   –   > 3cm   -4
L. OVARY
  Deep Endo   –   1-3cm   -32**
  Dense Adhesions   –   < 1/3   -8**
L. Tube
  Dense Adhesions   –   < 1/3   -8**
        TOTAL POINTS   52

*Point assignment changed to 16
**Point assignment doubled

STAGE IV (SEVERE)

PERITONEUM
  Deep Endo   –   > 3cm   -6
CULDESAC
  Complete Obliteration   -40
R. OVARY
  Deep Endo   1-3cm   -16
  Dense Adhesions   –   < 1/3   -4
L. Tube
  Dense Adhesions   –   > 2/3   -16
L. OVARY
  Deep Endo   –   1-3cm   -16
  Dense Adhesions   –   > 2/3   -16
        TOTAL POINTS   114

Figure 43–3. Staging of endometriosis. Determination of stage or degree of endometrial involvement is based on a weighted point system (see Table 43–1 for point values). Distribution of points has been arbitrarily determined and may require further revision or refinement as knowledge of the disease increases. To ensure complete evaluation, inspection of the pelvis in a clockwise or counterclockwise fashion is encouraged. Number, size, and location of endometrial implants, plaques, endometriomas, and/or adhesions are noted. For example, 5 separate 0.5-cm superficial implants on the peritoneum (2.5 cm total) would be assigned 2 points. (The surface of the uterus should be considered peritoneum.) The severity of the endometriosis or adhesions should be assigned the highest score only for peritoneum, ovary, tube, or cul-de-sac. For example, a 4-cm superficial and a 2-cm deep implant of the peritoneum should be given a score of 6 (not 8). A 4-cm deep endometrioma of the ovary associated with more than 3 cm of superficial disease should be scored 20 (not 24). In patients with only 1 set of adnexa, points applied to disease of the remaining tube and ovary should be multiplied by 2. Points assigned may be circled and totaled. Aggregation of points indicates stage of disease (minimal, mild, moderate, or severe). The presence of endometriosis of the bowel, urinary tract, fallopian tube, vagina, cervix, and skin should be documented under "additional endometriosis." Other pathology, such as tubal occlusion, leiomyomata, and uterine anomaly, should be documented under "additional pathology." All pathology should be depicted as specifically as possible on the sketch of pelvic organs, and the means of observation (laparoscopy or laparotomy) should be noted. (Copyright 1996, American Society for Reproductive Medicine. From: Revised American Society for Reproductive Medicine classification of endometriosis: 1996. Fertil Steril 1997;67:820.)

thalamic level to inhibit gonadotropin release, inhibiting the midcycle surge of luteinizing hormone and follicle-stimulating hormone. Danazol also inhibits steroidogenic enzymes in the ovary responsible for estrogen production. As a result, a hypoestrogenic environment is created. This, in addition to the androgenic effects of danazol, prevents the growth of endometriotic tissue.

The dosage of danazol is 400 to 800 mg/d in divided doses for 6 months.

Side effects of danazol include acne, oily skin, deepening of the voice, weight gain, edema, and adverse plasma lipoprotein changes. Most changes are reversible upon cessation of therapy, but some (such as deepening of the voice) may not be.

Pain relief is achieved in up to 90% of patients taking danazol.

4. GnRH agonists— Gonadotropin-releasing hormone (GnRH) agonists are analogues of the 10-amino-acid peptide hormone GnRH. With continuous administration of GnRH analogues, suppression of gonadotropin secretion occurs, resulting in elimination of ovarian steroidogenesis and suppression of endometrial implants. Pain related to endometriosis is relieved in most cases by the second or third month of therapy. GnRH agonists can be administered intramuscularly as leuprolide acetate 3.75 mg once per month, intranasally as nafarelin 400 to 800 mg daily, or subcutaneously as goserelin 3.6 mg once per month.

Use of these agents is generally limited to 6 months because of the adverse effects associated with a hypoestrogenic state, particularly loss of bone mineral density. Other side effects include vasomotor symptoms, vaginal dryness, and mood changes.

Many side effects can be minimized by providing add-back therapy in addition to the GnRH agonists in the treatment of endometriosis. The addition of 2.5 mg of norethindrone or 0.625 mg of conjugated estrogens with 5 mg/d of medroxyprogesterone acetate seems to relieve vasomotor symptoms and decrease bone mineral density loss in a 6-month treatment period. The addition of 5 mg daily of norethindrone acetate alone or in conjunction with low-dose conjugated equine estrogen seems to eliminate the loss of bone mineral density effectively as well.

5. Aromatase inhibitors— Anastrozole 1 mg daily or letrozole 2.5 mg daily are the most commonly used aromatase inhibitors. They act by inhibiting the enzyme aromatase, which converts androgens to estrogens. Endometriosis lesions may contain aromatase and be deficient in the enzymes that degrade estrogen, which promotes their own growth by creating an estrogen-rich microenvironment within the lesions. This may explain why some patients continue to have symptoms on therapies that lower systemic estrogen levels. Aromatase inhibitors have not been studied extensively in endometriosis;

they can be used singly or as an adjunct to other therapies. Adverse effects on bone mass limit their use.

6. Surgical treatment— In women with complaints of infertility who have severe disease or adhesions or who are older, conservative surgical therapy is the treatment of choice. This surgery attempts to excise or destroy all endometriotic tissue, remove all adhesions, and restore pelvic anatomy to the best possible condition. Conservative surgery has traditionally been performed at laparotomy, but a laparoscopic approach is associated with a shorter hospital stay and less morbidity, and it may be more cost effective. This is particularly true in contemporary practice, where this therapy is usually performed at the time of the initial diagnostic laparoscopy. Reported pregnancy rates following conservative surgery are inversely proportional to the severity of disease and vary greatly. In counseling patients, approximate pregnancy rates of 75% for mild disease, 50–60% for moderate disease, and 30–40% for severe disease should be quoted; however, individualization of therapy is stressed.

Presacral neurectomy to relieve pain should be performed only in selected cases, such as women with recurrent endometriosis, severe incapacitating dysmenorrhea, or disease that did not respond to initial treatment, because the efficacy of this treatment is controversial.

If the patient does not desire future childbearing and has severe disease or symptoms, definitive surgery is appropriate and often curative. This entails total abdominal hysterectomy, bilateral salpingo-oophorectomy, and excision of remaining adhesions or implants. If endometriosis remains after excision, postoperative medical therapy may be indicated. After this or after complete excision, hormone replacement therapy is indicated. Estrogen–progestin therapy can be used without reactivating the endometriosis, but individualization of therapy is required.

7. Assisted reproduction— Infertile women with endometriosis who are older, or who have not responded to other therapies for infertility, can undergo assisted reproduction, such as ovulation induction with intrauterine insemination or in vitro fertilization (IVF). However, women with endometriosis undergoing IVF were found to have significantly lower pregnancy rates, fertilization rates, implantation rates, mean number of oocytes retrieved, and peak estradiol concentrations compared to women with tubal factor infertility. The need to treat women surgically or medically prior to starting an IVF cycle remains unclear.

Prognosis

Proper counseling of patients with endometriosis requires attention to several aspects of the disorder. Of primary importance is the initial operative staging of the disease to obtain adequate information on which to base future decisions about therapy. The patient's symptoms and desire for childbearing dictate appropriate therapy. Most patients can be told that they will be able to obtain significant relief from pelvic pain and that treatment will assist them in achieving pregnancy.

Long-term concerns must be more guarded because all current therapies offer relief but not cure. Even after definitive surgery, endometriosis may recur, but the risk is very low (approximately 3%). Estrogen replacement therapy does not significantly increase the risk of recurrence. After conservative surgery, reported recurrence rates vary greatly but usually exceed 10% in 3 years and 35% in 5 years. Pregnancy delays but does not preclude recurrence. Recurrence rates after medical treatment vary and are similar to or higher than those reported following surgical treatment.

Although many patients are concerned that endometriosis will progress inexorably, experience has been that conservative surgery prevents the necessity for hysterectomy in the great majority of cases. The course of endometriosis in any individual cannot be predicted at present, and future treatment options should greatly improve upon what is offered now.

REFERENCES

Introduction & Epidemiology

Giudice LC, Kao LC: Endometriosis. Lancet 2004;364:1789.

Kuohung W et al: Characteristics of patients with endometriosis in the United States and the United Kingdom. Fertil Steril 2002;78:767.

Prentice A: Endometriosis. BMJ 2001;323:93.

Pathogenesis

McLaren J, Prentice A: New aspects of pathogenesis of endometriosis. Curr Obstet Gynecol 1996;6:85.

Osteen KG, Bruner-Tran KL, Eisenberg E: Endometrial biology and the etiology of endometriosis. Fertil Steril 2005;88:33.

Stefansson H et al: Genetic factors contribute to the risk of developing endometriosis. Hum Reprod 2002;17:555.

Witz CA: Current concepts in the pathogenesis of endometriosis. Clin Obstet Gynecol 1999;42:566.

Pathology

Bergqvist A, Ferno M: Estrogen and progesterone receptors in endometriotic tissue and endometrium: Comparison according to localization and recurrence. Fertil Steril 1993; 60:63.

Murphy AA et al: Unsuspected endometriosis documented by scanning electron microscopy in visually normal peritoneum. Fertil Steril 1986;46:52.

Pathologic Physiology

D'Hooghe TM, Debrock S, Hill JA: Endometriosis and subfertility: Is the relationship resolved? Semin Reprod Med 2003;21:243.

Schindler AE: Pathophysiology, diagnosis, and treatment of endometriosis. Minerva Ginecol 2004;56:419.

Sharpe-Timms KL: Haptoglobin expression by shed endometrial tissue fragments found in peritoneal fluid. Fertil Steril 2005;84:22.

Vercellini P et al: Endometriosis and pelvic pain: relation to disease stage and localization. Fertil Steril 1996;65:299.

Clinical Findings

Porpora MG et al: Correlation between endometriosis and pelvic pain. J Am Assoc Gynecol Laparosc 1999;6:429.

Vlahos N, Fortner KB: Emerging issues in endometriosis. Postgrad Obstet Gynecol 2005;25:4.

Complications

Schorlemmer GR, Battaglini JW: Pneumothorax in menstruating females. Contemp Surg 1982;20:53.

Zwas FR, Lyon DT: Endometriosis: An important condition in clinical gastroenterology. Dig Dis Sci 1991;36:353.

Classification

American Society for Reproductive Medicine: Revised American Society for Reproductive Medicine classification of endometriosis: 1996. Fertil Steril 1997;67:817.

Treatment

Abbott JA et al: The effects and effectiveness of laparoscopic excision of endometriosis: A prospective study with 2-5 year follow-up. Human Reprod 2003;18:1922.

ACOG Committee on Adolescent Health Care: Endometriosis in adolescents. Obstet Gynecol 2005;105:921.

Adamsom D: Surgical management of endometriosis. Semin Reprod Med 2003;21:223.

Barbieri RL: Hormonal treatment of endometriosis: The estrogen threshold hypothesis. Am J Obstet Gynecol 1992;166:740.

Brosens I: Endometriosis and the outcome of in vitro fertilization. Fertil Steril 2004;81:1198.

Lessey BA: Medical management of endometriosis and infertility. Fertil Steril 2000;73:1089.

Marcoux S et al: Laparoscopic surgery in infertile women with minimal or mild endometriosis. N Engl J Med 1997;337:217.

Practice Committee of the American Society for Reproductive Medicine: Endometriosis and infertility. Fertil Steril 2004;81:1441.

Surrey ES, Hornstein MD: Prolonged GnRH agonist and add-back therapy for symptomatic endometriosis: Long-term follow-up. Obstet Gynecol 2002;99:709.

Yates M, Vlahos N: Endometriosis and in vitro fertilization. Postgrad Obstet Gynecol 2003;23:22.

Zupi E et al: Add-back therapy in the treatment of endometriosis-associated pain. Fertil Steril 2004;82:1303.

Pelvic Organ Prolapse

Christopher M. Tarnay, MD

Pelvic organ prolapse (POP) is a common group of clinical conditions affecting women. The prevalence rates increase with age and POP currently affects millions of women. In the United States, POP is responsible for more than 200,000 surgeries per year. The lifetime risk that a woman will undergo surgery for prolapse or urinary incontinence is 11%, with a third of surgeries representing repeat procedures. The risk of requiring a repeat procedure for POP may be as high as 29%. As our population ages, quality-of-life-altering conditions such as POP will demand more attention from our health care services. The ability to screen, diagnose and treat these entities will become increasingly important for clinicians.

Defects in the pelvic supporting structures result in a variety of clinically evident pelvic relaxation abnormalities. Pelvic support defects can be classified by their anatomic location.

Anterior Vaginal Wall Defects

- *Anterior vaginal prolapse* describes an anterior vaginal wall defect where the bladder is associated with the prolapse. It is also known as a cystocele (Fig 44–1).
- *Urethrocele* describes a distal anterior vaginal wall defect where the urethra is associated with the prolapse. It is essentially a very distal anterior wall defect.
- *Paravaginal/midline/transverse prolapse* indicate the location of anterior vaginal wall defect (Fig 44–2)

Apical Prolapse

- *Uterine prolapse* (Fig 44–3)
- *Vaginal vault prolapse* (posthysterectomy)
- *Enterocele* describes an apical vaginal wall defect in which bowel is contained within the prolapsed segment (Fig 44–4). Generally occurs in posthysterectomy women, but can occur with the uterus in situ.

Posterior Vaginal Wall Prolapse

- *Posterior vaginal wall prolapse* describes a posterior vaginal wall defect. It is also known as a rectocele (Figs 44–5 and 44–6).

Description and Staging of Pelvic Organ Prolapse

Two general classifications are used to describe and document the severity of pelvic organ prolapse.

The most current system employs objective measurements from fixed anatomic points. The Pelvic Organ Prolapse Quantification (POP-Q) system standardizes terminology of female pelvic organ prolapse. This is accepted as the most objective method for quantifying prolapse as it provides a more precise description of the anatomy. This descriptive system contains series of site-specific measurements of vaginal and perineal anatomy. Prolapse in each segment is evaluated and measured relative to the hymen, which is a fixed anatomic landmark that can be consistently identified. The anatomic position of the six defined points for measurement should be in centimeters above the hymen (negative number) or centimeters beyond the hymen (positive number). The plane at the level of the hymen is defined as zero (Fig 44–7 and Table 44–1). Stages are assigned according to the most severe portion of the prolapse when the full extent of the protrusion has been demonstrated. An ordinal system is utilized for measurements of different points along the vaginal canal that facilitates communication among clinicians and enables objective tracking of surgical results. The POP-Q system has generally replaced the "1/2 way" system designed by Baden and Walker.

A better understanding of the pathophysiology of the pelvic supportive defects, their causes, and clinical presentations allows the individualization of the therapy most likely to successfully affect long-term therapy for each patient. As POP is a disease impacting the quality of life, obtaining a detailed symptom history is an essential starting point.

PELVIC ORGAN PROLAPSE

General Considerations

The cause of POP is most assuredly caused by multiple factors. This is the clearest model to explain the vast discrepancies in the incidence of POP and variety of anatomic findings despite shared risk factors. Proven risk factors include age, increasing parity, obesity, and

Figure 44–1. Anterior vaginal prolapse, known as a cystocele.

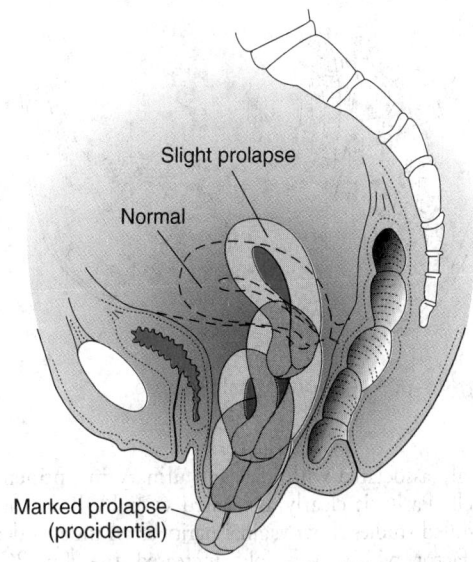

Figure 44–3. Prolapse of the uterus.

history of pelvic surgery, specifically hysterectomy. Additionally, certain lifestyle or disease conditions can promote the development of POP. Chronic coughing from lung disease and straining from chronic constipation for example, may increase the pressures on the pelvic floor. Acting as a constant piston, driving forces exerted onto the pelvic support tissues can cause herniation of the vaginal walls. In a similar manner, occupational activity requiring repetitive heavy lifting (e.g. environmental service workers or care providers of the elderly) may promote the development of POP with this daily insult of frequent pelvic pressure.

Furthermore, menopausal status, physical debilitation and even neurologic decline can contribute to the development of POP. Yet even with a multitude of risk

factors, certain women are predisposed to developing POP. As prolapse has been demonstrated in women with no identifiable risk factors, the inherent quality of a woman's connective tissue plays a large role in the susceptibility to the development of prolapse and related conditions. Investigating the consistency and composition of the endopelvic "fascial" tissues and the interplay of enzymatic remodeling is an area of intense interest and current research.

Parity has long been recognized as a prime risk factor for the development of POP. Not surprisingly, it is also

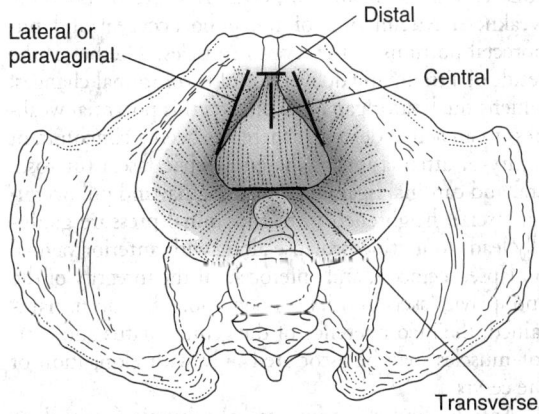

Figure 44–2. Four areas in which pubocervical fascia can break or separate—four defects.

Figure 44–4. Enterocele and prolapsed uterus.

Figure 44–5. Posterior vaginal prolapse.

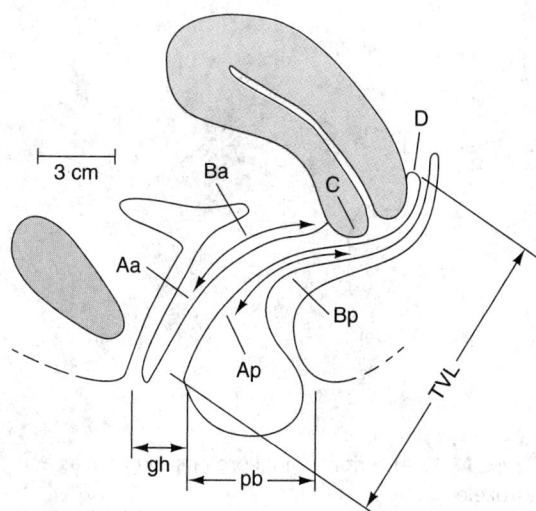

Figure 44–7. Six sites (points *Aa, Ba, C, D, Bp,* and *Ap*), genital hiatus *(gh)*, perineal body *(pb)*, and total vaginal length *(TVL)* used for pelvic organ quantitation. (Reproduced with permission from Bump RC et al: The standardization of terminology of female pelvic organ prolapse and pelvic floor dysfunction. Am J Obstet Gynecol 1996;175:10.)

strongly associated with anal and urinary incontinence as well. Parity is clearly associated with POP, as case-controlled studies show vaginal parity as an independent risk factor with a threefold increased risk for POP amongst parous women compared to nullipara controls. This risk increases up to 4.5-fold with more than two vaginal deliveries. The question as to whether it is the pregnancy, the size of the baby, or the mode of delivery that plays the largest role in the development of POP is still not clear. During labor, as the vertex descends through the vagina, the physical forces on the pelvic tissues can be severe. The muscles, viscera, connective tissue, and nerves are all potentially susceptible to injury. Forces of compression and stretching combine to injure pelvic-floor nerves, leading to ischemia and neurapraxia. Myofascial fibers can be disrupted or torn because of distention of the fetal head and body. When tissues are injured, the body will repair them. Factors impairing adequate tissue repair and wound healing may also play an as yet undetermined role in the development of POP.

The principal components of the basin-like pelvic floor are the pelvic bones (including the coccyx), the endopelvic fascia, and the levator and perineal muscles. These structures normally support and maintain the position of the pelvic viscera despite great increments in intra-abdominal pressure that occur with straining, coughing, and heavy lifting when the patient is in the erect position. The urogenital hiatus ("anterior levator muscle gap"), which permits the urethra, vagina, and anus to emerge from the pelvis, is a site of potential weakness. Attenuation of the pubococcygeal and puborectal portions of the levator muscles, whether as the result of a traumatic delivery or of involutional changes, widens the levator gap and converts this potential weakness to an actual defect. If there has been a concomitant injury or attenuation of the endopelvic fascia (uterosacral and cardinal ligaments, rectovaginal and pubocervical fascia), heightened intra-abdominal pressure gradually leads to uterine prolapse along with anterior vaginal prolapse, rectocele, and enterocele. If the integrity of the endopelvic fascia and its condensations has been maintained, the incompetency of the genital hiatus and levator muscles may be associated only with elongation of the cervix.

Anterior and posterior vaginal relaxation, as well as incompetence of the perineum, often accompanies prolapse of the uterus. Large anterior vaginal prolapse is

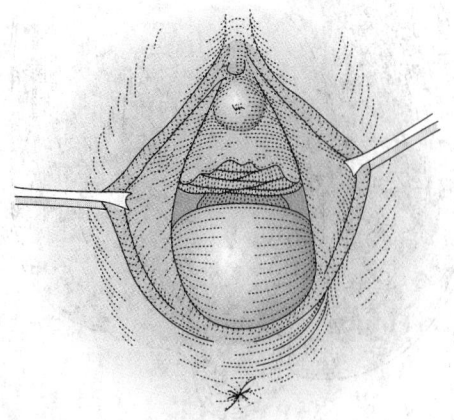

Figure 44–6. Posterior vaginal prolapse.

Table 44–1. Staging of pelvic organ prolapse.

Stage 0	No prolapse is demonstrated. Points Aa, Ap, Ba, and Bp are all at –3 cm and either point C or D is between –TVL (total vaginal length) cm and –(TVL–2) cm (ie, the quantitation value for point C or D is ≤–[TVL–2] cm).
Stage I	The criteria for stage 0 are not met, but the most distal portion of the prolapse is > 1 cm above the level of the hymen (ie, its quantitation value is < –1 cm).
Stage II	The most distal portion of the prolapse is ≤ 1 cm proximal to or distal to the plane of the hymen (ie, its quantitation value is ≥–1 cm but ≤+1 cm).
Stage III	The most distal portion of the prolapse is > 1 cm below the plane of the hymen but protrudes no further than 2 cm less than the total vaginal length in centimeters (ie, its quantitation value is > +1 cm but < +[TVL–2] cm).
Stage IV	Essentially, complete eversion of the total length of the lower genital tract is demonstrated. The distal portion of the prolapse protrudes to at least (TVL–2) cm (ie, its quantitation value is ≥+[TVL–2] cm). In most instances, the leading edge of stage IV prolapse is the cervix or vaginal cuff scar.

Reproduced, with permission, from Bump RC et al: The standardization of terminology of female pelvic organ prolapse and pelvic floor dysfunction, Am J Obstet Gynecol 1996;175:10.

more common than posterior vaginal prolapse because the bladder is more easily carried downward than is the rectum. Prior to the menopause, the prolapsed uterus hypertrophies and is engorged and flaccid. After the menopause, the uterus atrophies. In procidentia, the vaginal mucosa thickens and cornifies, coming to resemble skin.

 ESSENTIALS OF DIAGNOSIS

Symptoms

The symptoms of POP are in general not unique to any particular vaginal defect. Often the symptoms are a reflection of only the most prominent point of prolapse. Most women become symptomatic only when the prolapse nears the vaginal opening. A critical concept is that the functional complaints may not always relate to the anatomic findings.

Symptoms of POP include:

- *Sensation of vaginal fullness, pressure, "something falling out," or "heaviness."*
- *Sensation of "sitting on a ball."*
- *Discomfort in the vaginal area.*
- *Presence of a soft, reducible mass bulging into the vagina and distending through vaginal introitus.*
- *With straining or coughing, increased bulging and descent of the vaginal wall.*
- *Back pain and pelvic pain are often also associated with POP. It is important in women with these complaints to investigate other causes, as a direct link in mild to moderate prolapse is unproven.*
- *Urinary symptoms are also common.*
  - *Feeling of incomplete emptying of the bladder*
  - *Stress incontinence*
  - *Urinary frequency*
  - *Urinary hesitancy*
  - *Perhaps a need to push the bladder up in order to void (splinting)*
  - *Patients with advanced prolapse may have "potential" stress urinary incontinence. A condition in which underlying urinary incontinence is masked by kinking of the urethra and causing functional continence.*

Defecatory symptoms may also occur, more commonly in posterior vaginal prolapse. The sense of incomplete emptying, need to strain or manually splint in the vagina or on the perineal body (space between vagina and anus) in order to defecate. The history may include prolonged, excessive use of laxatives, or frequent enemas. Other nonspecific symptoms such as low back pain, dyspareunia, or even fecal and gas incontinence may be reported.

Symptoms of sexual function may also be elicited. Coital laxity or a sense of feeling "loose" may be reported. Avoiding intercourse as a consequence of embarrassment may occur. Attention to this aspect of a woman's symptoms is especially critical if any surgical intervention is considered.

Clinical Findings

A. PHYSICAL EXAMINATION

Examination for pelvic organ prolapse should begin in the dorsal lithotomy position. Inspection of the vulva and perineum should focus on evaluation of vulvar architecture, the presence of pressure ulceration or erosions or of other skin lesions. Epithelial skin lesions, particularly in the elderly should be biopsied.

At first with the patient at rest the labia should be separated and any prolapse noted (Figs 44–1 and 44–6). Examination of the patient with vaginal prolapse reveals a relaxed and open genital hiatus with a thin-walled, rather smooth, bulging mass. Vaginal rugae are normally present. A loss of rugation denotes disruption of the connective tissue attachment below the epithelium.

During evaluation for urinary incontinence, a stress test is performed at this initial portion of the examination. The patient should be asked to cough forcefully and any loss of urine noted.

For prolapse assessment, when using the POP-Q system, the genital hiatus, perineal body, and vaginal length can be recorded. (Use of a wooden PAP spatula and tape measure can be helpful.) Vaginal support can then be assessed with strain (cough or Valsalva) and the point of maximal protrusion should be noted in centimeters relative to the hymen and recorded. A speculum can also be used to "usher" the prolapse out during straining. This is also the most effective way to evaluate uterocervical support. In posthysterectomy patients, the cuff can often be visualized by the presence of "dimples" in the vaginal epithelium at the apex. Discriminate examination of the vaginal walls using the posterior blade of a Graves speculum or similar retractor should then be used to evaluate the anterior and posterior walls separately, again noting the point of maximal prolapse during strain. For evaluation of the anterior wall compress the posterior wall and have the patient strain. For evaluation of the posterior wall, elevate the anterior wall and have the patient strain. Complete examination should also include a rectovaginal palpation. In this way, one can evaluate for the presence of concurrent enterocele in addition to a rectocele. The septal defect may involve only the lower third of the posterior vaginal wall, but it often happens that the entire length of the rectovaginal septum is thinned out. The finger in the rectum confirms sacculation into the vagina. A deep pocket into the perineal body may be noted, so that on apposition of the finger in the rectum and the thumb on the outside, the perineal body seems to consist of nothing but skin and rectal wall.

Assessment of anal sphincter tone should also be performed both at rest and with squeeze contraction. The presence of perianal lesions or hemorrhoids should be noted.

If during examination the prolapse is not able to be reproduced based on symptoms, examination with the woman in the standing position should be performed. With the patient facing the seated examiner, knees slightly bent, and with strain, prolapse not demonstrable in the supine position because of poor Valsalva, can often be confirmed in the upright position.

Assessment of the pelvic floor strength is accomplished by vaginal or rectovaginal palpation of the levator ani musculature. Within 2 to 3 cm from the hymen, the bulk of the pubococcygeus component of the levator ani muscle can be palpated. The patient should be asked to contract the muscle and the tone, symmetry, and duration should be recorded. This portion of the examination is often a valuable time to provide feedback to the patient about the volitional ability to contract the pelvic floor muscles. If the patient's ability to identify and contract the muscles is inadequate, the examiner may facilitate isolation of the proper muscles using verbal cues and manual feedback.

Evaluation of urinary function is also important in patients with POP. This is most germane in patients with large anterior vaginal defects. With prolapse of the anterior vagina, the bladder and urethra may herniate into the vagina. The urethra can bend and kink as it is fixed distally at the level of the pubourethral ligament. This "kinking" can alter normal voiding function in two fundamental ways. One, it will increase outflow resistance and impair normal emptying. After voiding, simple catheterization should be performed and the residual volume measured. The specimen should then be sent for routine urinalysis and culture. Although not standardized, postvoid residual volumes over 100 mL are considered elevated and may indicate abnormal voiding, and require referral for more sophisticated testing.

The second way urethral kinking can impact voiding, is by masking underlying stress urinary incontinence. With increased outflow resistance functional continence is created. Reduction of the prolapse during examination can be performed (elevation of anterior segment with a pessary, ring forceps, or speculum). The patient strains/coughs and the presence of urinary loss confirms the condition of stress urinary incontinence. This is commonly referred to as "potential" stress urinary incontinence and should be addressed with an anti-incontinence procedure at the same time if surgery is offered for POP.

B. IMAGING STUDIES

In general, a complete discriminative gynecologic examination is all that is necessary to accurately assess pelvic organ prolapse. In certain cases, further diagnostic studies can be employed.

Recent advances in radiologic medicine have allowed assessment of the pelvic floor with sonography, computed tomography (CT), and magnetic resonance imaging (MRI).

Despite newer techniques, intravenous pyelogram (IVP) still holds great value, as it is a simple and safe method to visualize the urinary tract. It can be used to evaluate the bladder and ureters. The course of the ureters can be identified preoperatively if obstruction caused by pelvic mass or scarring is suspected. IVP can be used to evaluate for fistulae, congenital anomalies, or suspected damage as a result of operative injury. However, it lacks sensitivity in imaging the pelvic floor and its associated defects, and does not yield much information regarding vaginal support, pelvic floor musculature and lacks dynamic capabilities.

Ultrasound techniques can be an important tool to the urogynecologist. Compared to other radiologic techniques, ultrasound is noninvasive and inexpensive, and does not require contrast media. Its main disadvantage is that the quality of the study depends heavily on the skill of the operator. When performed transabdominally, transvaginally, or transperineally and combined with Doppler or endoluminal transducers, the bladder, urethra, and surrounding structures can be visualized.

1. Videocystourethrography (VCUG)—VCUG combines a fluoroscopic voiding cystourethrogram with simultaneous recording of intravesical, intraurethral, and intra-abdominal pressure and urine flow rate. The contrast in the bladder allows dynamic evaluation of the bladder and bladder support.

2. Computed tomography (CT)—CT can be used in the evaluation of ureteral obstruction, urolithiasis, and the kidneys. It has poor resolution of soft tissues and has limited value in imaging the pelvic floor and associated defects.

3. Magnetic resonance imaging (MRI)—MRI has evolved into an important tool for the evaluation of the pelvic floor. It is an ideal modality because its resolution of soft tissues is superior to that of other radiologic techniques. The capability to image in multiple planes is also an advantage, particularly when visualizing the complex three-dimensional relationships of the pelvic floor. As this modality becomes less costly and techniques evolve to allow evaluation of patients in the upright position, the information provided by MRI will be invaluable in increasing our knowledge and understanding of functional pelvic support.

Differential Diagnosis

Prolapse of the vagina is generally a straightforward diagnosis. However, less common disease entities may present as bulges in the vagina. Tumors of the urethra and bladder are much more indurated and fixed than is anterior vaginal prolapse.

A large urethral diverticulum may look and feel like an anterior vaginal prolapse but usually is more focal, and may be painful. With urethral diverticulum, compression may express some purulent material from the urethral meatus. Anterolateral defects can represent embryologic remnants such as a Gartner's duct cyst.

Skene's and Bartholin's glands can become obstructed and enlarge to form cysts or abscesses. Rarely, hemangiomas will present as vaginal bulging, although they will often have characteristic purple discoloration on the overlying epithelium.

Soft tumors (lipoma, leiomyoma, sarcoma) of the vagina are more fixed and are nonreducible.

Cervical tumors—as well as endometrial tumors (pedunculated myoma or endometrial polyps)—if prolapsed through a dilated cervix and presenting in the lower third of the vagina, may be confused with mild or moderate uterine prolapse. Myomas or polyps may coexist with prolapse of the uterus and cause unusual symptoms.

Despite the variety of possibilities, the history and physical findings in uterine prolapse are so characteristic that diagnosis is usually not a problem.

Prevention

Prevention of genital prolapse is the focus of much debate. Antepartum and intrapartum and postpartum exercises, especially those designed to strengthen the levator and perineal muscle groups (Kegel), often help improve or maintain pelvic support. Obesity, chronic cough, straining, and traumatic deliveries must be corrected or avoided. Estrogen therapy following the menopause may help to maintain the tone and vitality of pelvic musculofascial tissues and thereby prevent or postpone the appearance of anterior vaginal prolapse and other forms of relaxation.

Treatment

Pelvic organ prolapse, except in rare situations, is a condition that impacts only the quality of life. Consequently, the extent and type of treatment should reflect and be commensurate with the degree of negative impact on the quality of life the patient experiences. Patient perception is also a critical component, and self-image and conceptual discomfort are relevant to any discussion of therapy. Common reasons to intervene are when function is impaired because of the prolapse. Anterior prolapse can contribute to urinary incontinence or, when severe, urinary obstruction. Bulging vaginal epithelium can come into contact with undergarments and clothing and over time develop pressure sores and erosion, leading to cellulitis. A posterior vaginal defect can become so large that fecal evacuation is difficult, or the patient finds it necessary to manually reduce the posterior vaginal wall into the vagina to expedite expulsion of feces. Mobility can be impaired by a large prolapse. All of the above complaints are reasons to discuss surgical repair.

Chronic decubitus ulceration of the vaginal epithelium may develop in procidentia. Urinary tract infection may occur with prolapse because of anterior vaginal prolapse; and partial ureteral obstruction with hydronephrosis may occur in procidentia. Hemorrhoids result from straining to overcome constipation. Small-bowel obstruction from a deep enterocele is rare.

A. CONSERVATIVE MEASURES

The patient with a small or moderate-sized POP requires reassurance that the pressure symptoms are not the result of a serious condition and that, in the absence of urinary retention or severe skin pressure ulceration, no serious illness will result. The natural history of POP is such that it either will stay the same or progress. There is some evidence that a small subset of patients may experience regression of the prolapse after the menopause or postpartum if the prolapse is noted shortly after delivery. Reassurance and observation of prolapse should be encouraged in the absence of symptoms.

If prolapse presents in the reproductive years, surgical correction of POP is rarely indicated in women who may still wish to have children. If the young woman does present with significant symptoms related to POP or with a disturbing degree of urinary incontinence—temporary medical measures may provide adequate relief until she has completed childbearing, whereupon a definitive operative procedure can be accomplished.

1. Pessary—Pessary use in selected patients may provide adequate relief of symptoms. There are a variety of available pessary types and sizes that allow for individualization of therapy (Fig 44–8). For the most common type of POP of the anterior or apical segment, a ring pessary is usually a sensible starting point for treatment. For the patient with complicating medical factors who is a poor operative risk, the temporary use of a vaginal pessary may provide relief of symptoms until her general condition has improved.

Prolonged use of pessaries, if improperly managed, may lead to pressure necrosis and vaginal ulceration.

The vaginal pessary is a prosthesis of ancient lineage, now made of rubber, plastics, and silicone-based material, often with a metal band or spring frame. Many types have been devised, but fewer than a dozen are basically unique and specifically helpful.

Pessaries are principally used to support the uterus and vaginal walls. They are effective because they reduce vaginal prolapse and increase the tautness of the pelvic floor structures. Little or no leverage is involved. Either by placement behind the pubic bone and perineal body or by filling the vaginal vault, pessaries remain in place to hold up the prolapsing vaginal walls or uterus. In most cases, adequate support anteriorly and a reasonably good perineal body are required; otherwise, the pessary may slip from behind the symphysis and extrude from the vagina.

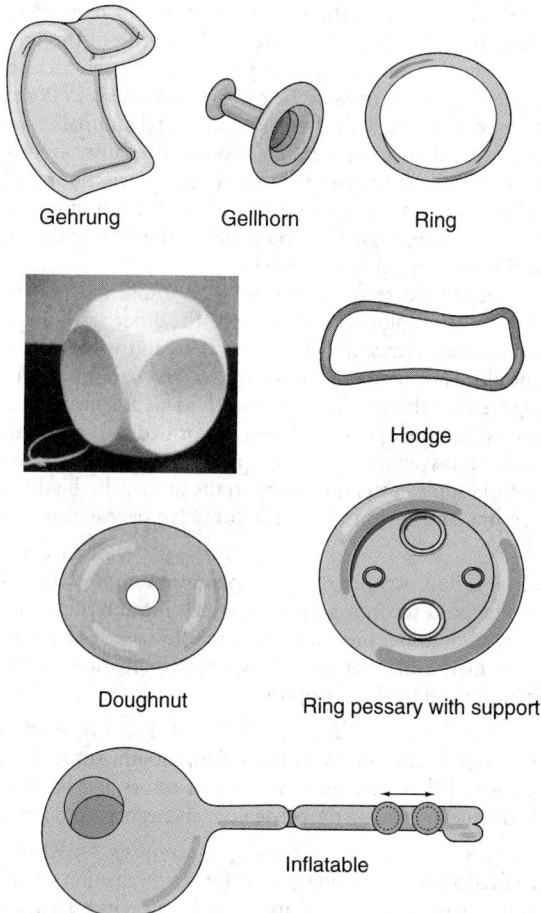

Figure 44–8. Types of pessaries.

Pessaries are contraindicated in acute genital tract infections and in adherent retroposition of the uterus.

Several pessary types are available:

- **Ring Pessary** A ring pessary with or without support provides relief of uterine prolapse or anterior vaginal prolapse.

- **Gellhorn Pessaries** These types are uniquely shaped like a collar button and provide a ringlike platform for the cervix or apex. The pessary is stabilized by a stem that rests on the perineum. These pessaries are used to correct marked prolapse when the perineal body is reasonably adequate.

- **Doughnut** The doughnut is made of soft rubber or silicone, and this type of pessary provides support for severe uterine prolapse or vault prolapse.

- **Gehrung Pessary** The Gehrung pessary resembles two firm letter Us attached by crossbars. It rests in the vagina with the cervix cradled between the long arms; this arches the anterior or posterior vaginal wall and helps reduce the vaginal prolapse.

- **Hodge Pessary (Smith-Hodge, or Smith and Other Variations)** This is an elongated, curved ovoid. One end is placed behind the symphysis and the other in the posterior vaginal fornix. The anterior bow is curved to avoid the urethra; the cervix rests within the larger, posterior bow. This type of pessary is used to hold the uterus in place after it has been repositioned.

- **Inflatable Pessary** The inflatable pessary functions much like a doughnut pessary. The ball valve is moved up and down; when the ball is in the down position, air inflates the pessary; when in the up position, the air is sealed in and inflation is maintained.

- **Cube** This is a flexible rubber cube, with suction cups on each of its six sides that adhere to the vaginal walls. This is useful in women with severe prolapse. However, vaginal erosions are common and can be severe. Frequent monitoring initially to identify pressure ulcers is critical.

a. Fitting of pessaries—Medicine is known as both an art and a science. Pessary fitting (Fig. 44–9) falls into the art category. Pessaries that are too large cause irritation and ulceration; those that are too small may not stay in place and may protrude.

In general, fitting a pessary is very much a trial-and-error endeavor. Once a type is selected based on the defects in the vaginal anatomy and on symptoms, sizing is best done with an office sizing set. This task is somewhat complicated as each pessary has its own measurement system, but familiarity with each pessary over time simplifies this task. The pessary should be lubricated and inserted with its widest dimension in the oblique diameter of the vagina to avoid painful distention at the introitus. With a finger of the opposite hand, depress the perineum to widen the introitus. Each pessary type has an optimal method for insertion.

Once a pessary is in place, the forefinger should pass easily between the sides of the frame and the vaginal wall at any point; if it cannot, the pessary is too large. After the pessary has been fitted, the patient should be asked to stand, walk, and squat to determine whether

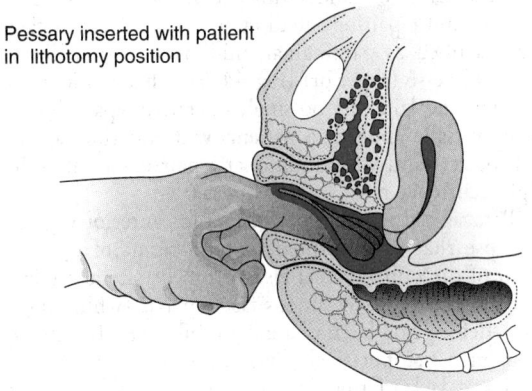
Pessary inserted with patient in lithotomy position

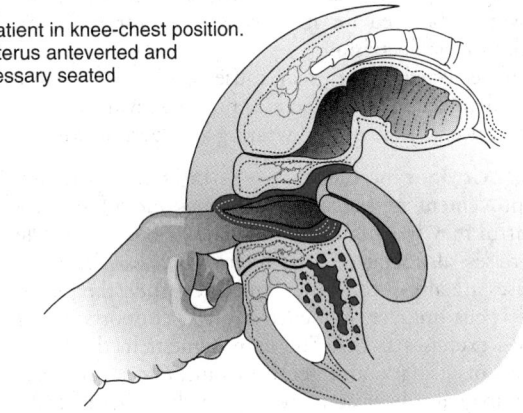
Patient in knee-chest position. Uterus anteverted and pessary seated

Final seating of pessary and support of uterus

Figure 44–9. Insertion of Hodge-type pessary.

pain occurs or whether the pessary becomes displaced. The patient should be shown how to withdraw the pessary if it becomes displaced or is uncomfortable, and cautioned that a contraceptive vaginal diaphragm cannot be used while a vaginal pessary is in place.

During the initial period of pessary wear, any discomfort, bleeding, or disturbance in defecation or urinary function should be reported immediately. The patient should be examined 1–2 weeks after insertion to inspect for the presence of pressure and inflammatory or allergic reactions. A repeat exam in 4 weeks can be done, then visits should be done at 3- to 6-month intervals to assess for continued proper fit and to evaluate for vaginal erosion and inflammation as a result of pessary use. For women who are unable to remove and clean the pessary themselves, the pessary should be changed about every 2–3 months.

The pessary should be maintained with an acidic pH gel such as Trimo-San (Milex Products, Inc., Chicago, Illinois). In postmenopausal patients, topical estrogen can vitalize the vaginal mucosa and reduce ulceration. An estrogen-containing ring can also be used in conjunction by "piggybacking" the ring with the pessary and then changing it every 3 months.

Vaginal pessaries are not curative of prolapse, but they may be used for months or years for palliation with proper supervision.

A neglected pessary may cause fistulas or promote genital infections, but there is no clear evidence that cancer occurs as a result of wearing a modern pessary.

2. Pelvic floor muscle exercises—In some patients, improvement of pressure symptoms and of urinary control may be obtained by using pelvic floor muscle exercises, also referred to as Kegel exercises. These exercises are aimed to tighten and strengthen the pubococcygeus muscles. Evidence strongly supports use of Kegel exercises as first-line management in the treatment of urinary and fecal incontinence; however, they may also have some benefit in the relief of POP symptoms. Kegel exercises work best after specific instruction on how to perform them as most women do not perform them either correctly or in optimal fashion without supervised instruction and feedback.

3. Estrogens—In postmenopausal women, local estrogen therapy for a number of months may improve the tone, quality, and vascularity of the musculofascial supports. It is available in cream, parvule, and ring insert forms. With counseling, local estrogen can be offered to all postmenopausal women to reduce urogenital atrophy. For postmenopausal patients with exposed prolapse, who are awaiting surgery, or using a pessary, local therapy should be recommended to promote healthy epithelium.

B. SURGICAL MEASURES

1. Anterior vaginal prolapse—

a. Anterior vaginal colporrhaphy—Anterior vaginal colporrhaphy is the most common surgical treatment for anterior vaginal prolapse (Fig 44–10). Traditional anterior colporrhaphy (anterior repair) is a vaginal approach that involves dissecting the vaginal epithelium from the underlying fibromuscular connective tissue and bladder, then plicating the vaginal muscularis across the midline. Excess vaginal epithelium is excised and the wound closed. Recurrence of anterior prolapse as high as 52% has been reported and has always been a limitation of all reparative procedures. Modifications involving permanent suture material and most recently graft materials have been introduced in the hope of increasing durability.

b. Paravaginal repair—The etiology of the anterior vaginal prolapse has been much debated, beginning with White in 1912. The repair of defects in the anterior vaginal segment has traditionally been done by midline plication. An alternative method based on the anatomic observations by Richardson and colleagues advocates identification of the specific defect in the pubocervical fascia underlying the anterior vaginal epithelium and repairing the discrete breaks. These breaks are described as paravaginal, midline (central), distal, and transverse (superior) (Fig 44–2). This relationship may help explain why no single operative repair should be universally applied to patients with anterior vaginal wall defects and why traditional repair has resulted in high recurrence rates.

Paravaginal repair is performed for anterior vaginal prolapse that is confirmed to be a result of detachment of the pubocervical fascia from its lateral attachment at the arcus tendineus fascia pelvis (white line). This defect can be unilateral or bilateral. It can be confirmed preoperatively by noting loss of the lateral sulci and lack of rugation over the epithelium along the base of the bladder and elongation to the anterior vaginal wall. Clinically, vaginal examination using a speculum reveals a preponderance of the prolapse lateralized to one side as the speculum is withdrawn. In addition, a ring forceps can be used by gently exerting anterior traction along the vaginal sulci. If the defect is reduced, then the defect is consistent with a paravaginal defect and can be approached with a paravaginal repair technique.

The surgery can be performed either abdominally or vaginally. Both require identification of the white line and placement of serial sutures from the medial portion of the pubocervical fascia to the lateral sidewall at the level of the white line as it runs from the ischial spine over the obturator internus muscle to the

Figure 44–10. Repair of anterior vaginal prolapse.

posterior and inferior aspect of the pubic bone on the ipsilateral side. Reapproximation of the detached pubocervical fascia should reduce the anterior vaginal prolapse. This procedure can be done with other reconstructive procedures in the vagina as well as surgery to alleviate incontinence. Short-term surgical studies have shown good results but no long-term or comparative data exist for this repair.

Transabdominal approach to the paravaginal repair may be elected to correct the anterior vaginal prolapse when an abdominal approach is necessary for other pelvic conditions such as abdominal hysterectomy, adnexal surgery, or, most commonly, with sacral colpopexy for apical prolapse repair.

2. Posterior vaginal prolapse—There are two main surgical methods of a posterior vaginal defect (rectocele) repair. The traditional repair (Fig. 44–11) for colpoperineorrhaphy is the one described in most texts and involves posterior midline incision, often high, to the level of the posterior fornix. The vaginal epithelium is separated off the underlying fibromuscular layer and endopelvic fascia. Repair often includes plication of the levator ani muscles and bulk lateral plication of tissue oversewing the rectovaginal fascia. No attempt at identifying specific fascial defects is made.

An alternate method of posterior vaginal defect (rectocele) repair relies on the identification of discrete defects in the rectovaginal fascia (Fig 44–12). This anatomic description was first introduced by gynecologists advocating that rectoceles were caused by a variety of breaks in the rectovaginal fascia and that repairing these defects primarily was critical to anatomic restoration and lasting cure. This surgical technique included separating the vaginal epithelium off the underlying rectovaginal fascia as in a traditional colpoperineorrhaphy. Efforts are made to leave as much fascia on the rectum as possible. The surgeon inserts a finger of the nondominant hand into the rectum to inspect the rectovaginal fascia for defects. The rectal wall is brought forward to distinguish the uncovered muscularis (fascial defect) from the muscularis that was covered by the smooth semitransparent rectal vaginal septum. The defects are then repaired with interrupted sutures to plicate over the rectal wall. In this manner, the isolated defects are repaired and the functional anatomy is optimally restored. Notably absent is any effort to plicate the levator ani musculature as this often results in a bandlike stricture over the posterior wall—a likely cause of dyspareunia.

Perineorrhaphy is generally combined with posterior vaginal repairs. This procedure is principally aimed at restoring the perineal body, and reducing the vaginal outlet (genital hiatus) to more normal caliber. Reapproximation of the superficial transverse perinei muscle and the bulbocavernosus muscle rebuilds the perineum, and lengthens the distance between vaginal opening and anal verge.

Postoperative factors—The prognosis after vaginal repair is excellent in the absence of a subsequent pregnancy or comparable factors (eg, constipation, obesity, large pelvic tumors, bronchitis, bronchiectasis, heavy manual labor) that increase intra-abdominal

A

Incision in
mucocutaneous
border

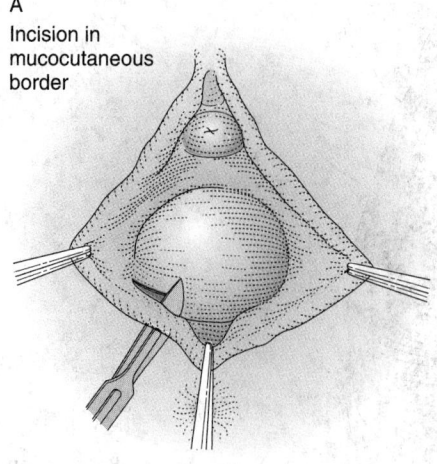

B

Flap reflected
and rectocele
exposed

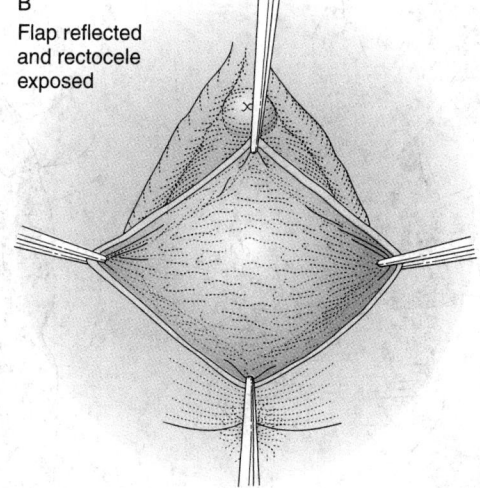

C

Manual
depression
of rectocele

Pubococcygeal
area of
levator ani

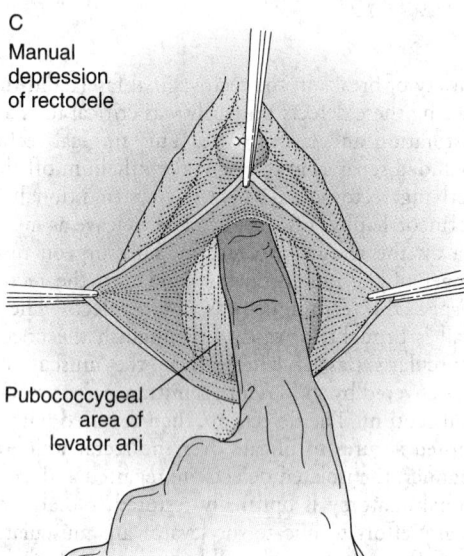

D

Fascial edges
closed and
interrupted
mattress
sutures laid
in levator ani

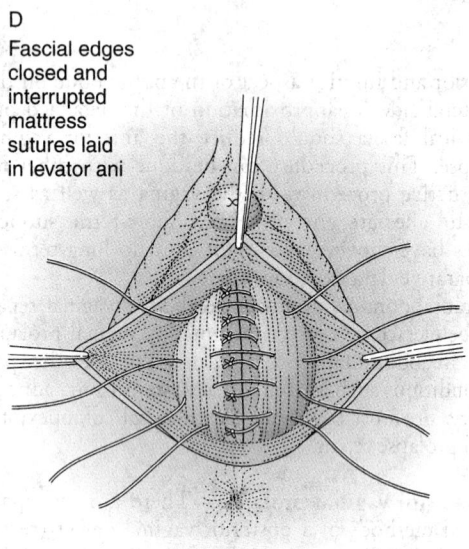

Figure 44–11. Repair of rectocele.

pressure. The recurrence of the POP is probable when a specific defect of pelvic supports has been overlooked or ignored; in such cases, subsequent progression of the overlooked site may itself lead to new symptoms, or even to disruption of the previously repaired segment.

Postoperative avoidance of straining, coughing, and strenuous activity is advisable. Careful instruction about diet to avoid constipation, about intake of fluids, and about the use of stool-softening laxatives and lubricating suppositories is necessary to ensure durable integrity of the rectocele repair.

3. Apical vaginal repair—Prolapse of the vaginal apex includes:

Uterine prolapse
Posthysterectomy vaginal cuff prolapse
Enterocele

All of the clinical conditions above indicate a failure of apical support. The procedures used to address surgical repair requires a knowledge of the specific support structures available to reestablish normal anatomy.

Apical prolapse may be congenital or acquired; the latter is much more common. The congenital form rarely

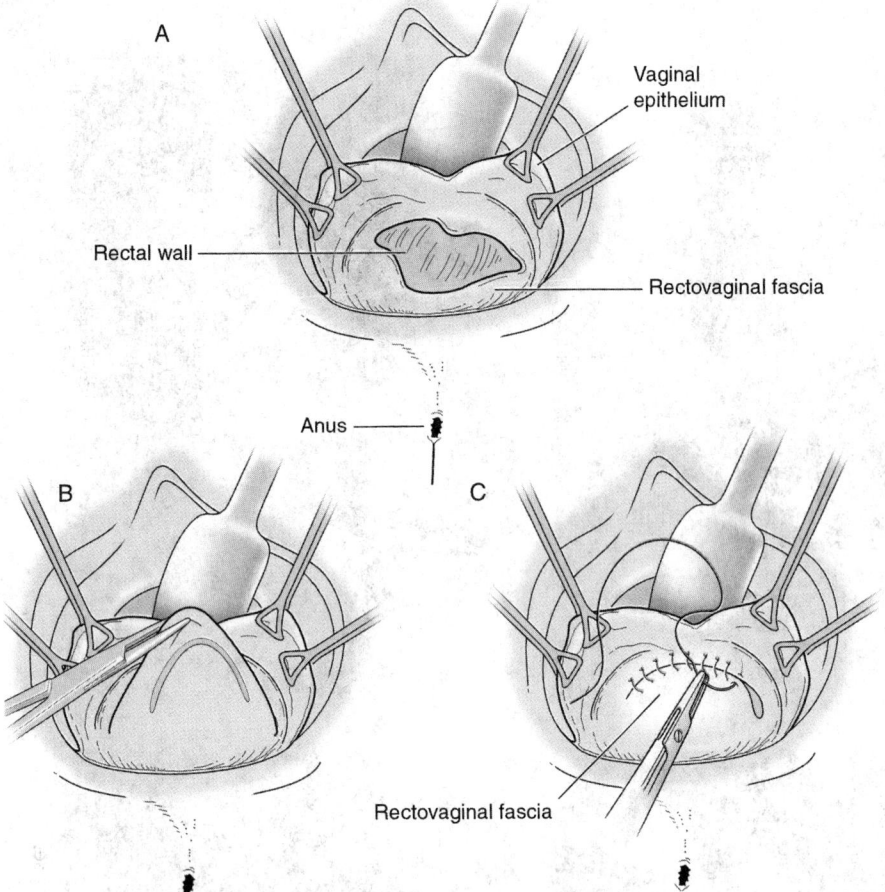

Figure 44–12. Site-specific repair of posterior vaginal prolapse. **A:** Dissection below vaginal epithelium exposes defect in rectovaginal (RV) fascia. **B:** Reflection of detached RV fascia. **C:** Restoration of the continuity of RV fascia by reapproximation with delayed absorbable suture.

causes symptoms. The acquired form of enterocele occurs in multiparous premenopausal or postmenopausal women and almost invariably is associated with other manifestations of pelvic organ prolapse. The trauma of many pregnancies and vaginal deliveries (particularly operative deliveries), large pelvic tumors, marked obesity, ascites, chronic bronchitis, and other factors that increase intra-abdominal pressure are of etiologic importance.

Uterine prolapse is almost always accompanied by some degree of enterocele, and, as the degree of uterine descent progresses, the size of the hernial sac increases. Similarly, posthysterectomy prolapse of the vaginal vault usually is the result of an enterocele that was overlooked (not repaired) at the time of hysterectomy or develops as a result of poor repair and identification of cuff support structures. Consequently, it is critical to always address apical cuff support at the time of surgery if

a hysterectomy is being performed because of prolapse. Rarely, after hysterectomy, the enterocele is located anterior to the vaginal vault, where it may be easily confused with ordinary anterior vaginal prolapse.

Apical vaginal repair may be accomplished transabdominally or transvaginally. A review of vaginal operations includes, among others, sacrospinous ligament suspension, iliococcygeal fixation, and high uterosacral ligament suspension (high McCall culdoplasty; Fig 44–13).

Because the normal vaginal axis is directed some distance posteriorly (almost horizontally when the patient is in an erect position) over the levator plate, operative correction by any means, whether by the vaginal or the abdominal route, should restore a normal vaginal axis. This is accomplished by suspension of the vaginal apex far back on the uterosacral ligaments, the presacral fascia, or the sacrospinous ligaments.

Figure 44-13. Vaginal hysterectomy for uterine prolapse.

732

a. Sacrospinous ligament fixation—A popular method of vaginal vault suspension is that of unilateral fixation to the sacrospinous ligament. In this technique, the vaginal mucosa is separated from the rectovaginal tissues, and the associated enterocele is identified and repaired (as previously described). Perforation through the right or left rectal pillar is usually easily accomplished by directing blunt dissection toward the ischial spine through the loose areolar tissue. After an appropriate location on the sacrospinous ligament is identified (usually 2–3 cm medial to the ischial spine), one of several techniques may be used to safely pass 2 or more permanent (or delayed absorbable) ligatures through the ligament to the submucosal apex of the vagina. Tying the sutures brings the vaginal apex to that sacrospinous ligament, and a posterior colporrhaphy is then performed (as noted previously). Closing the dead space by intermittently suturing the vaginal mucosa to the underlying reconstituted rectovaginal septum may be useful. Patients who have concomitant stress urinary incontinence should have a corrective procedure at this time.

Bilateral vaginal connection to both sacrospinous ligaments has been described, but may result in excessive lateral stretching of the vaginal apex or posterior impingement on the distal sigmoid colon. Vaginal vault suspension to one or both sacrospinous ligaments has the potential of injury to the pudendal nerve or pudendal vessels and is often technically difficult. Because gluteal and posterior leg pain is a potential complication of this procedure, it requires a skilled surgeon and should be undertaken only by those familiar with the technique.

b. Iliococcygeal vaginal suspension—First described in 1962, this procedure uses the fascia overlying the iliococcygeal muscle. Although not as commonly used as other procedures, this point of attachment allows reliable apical fixation without the need to gain peritoneal access. It is generally a safe procedure requiring a posterior vaginal incision in the midline with wide dissection of the overlying epithelium. Bilateral placement of permanent or delayed absorbable suture can be used.

c. Bilateral uterosacral ligament suspension—The use of the uterosacral ligaments to attach the vaginal cuff has become a reappreciated technique in apical repairs. Several modifications of the procedure have been described since its introduction in 1938. This technique, as with the other vaginal procedures, can be done at the time of vaginal hysterectomy or to correct posthysterectomy apical cuff prolapse. After entrance into the peritoneum is complete, traction on the ipsilateral posterior vaginal wall with rectal digital examination will facilitate transperitoneal identification of the uterosacral ligament. Placement of a pair of permanent sutures in a lateral-to-medial fashion, one at the level of the ischial spine and another placed more cephalad, can

be performed bilaterally. These sutures are then brought to the ipsilateral vaginal apices. Fixation of the cuff at this level reproduces cuff placement to the normal position of the cervicovaginal junction. Anterior vaginal repair should be peformed prior to tying down the vaginal cuff.

A risk of this procedure is medial displacement and kinking of the ureters, which has been reported to occur in up to 11% of patients undergoing this procedure. Cystoscopic assessment of ureteral function without and with tension on the fixation sutures, prior to tying down the vaginal apices, is critical. If ureteral flow compromise is identified, removal of the sutures on the affected side will often restore normal function.

d. Abdominal sacrocolpopexy—Vaginal vault suspension can also be performed abdominally by attaching the vaginal cuff to the sacral promontory. Abdominal sacrocolpopexy is an excellent primary procedure for apical vaginal prolapse and enterocele, and is the procedure of choice for those who are already having an abdominal approach for hysterectomy or for another indication. In this procedure, a laparotomy is performed, and the cul-de-sac and peritoneum overlying the sacrum is visualized. A window in the peritoneum over the sacral promontory is created and two permanent sutures are placed through the anterior longitudinal ligament, approximately at the level of S1. The vaginal cuff is then exposed by dissecting off the overlying peritoneum. Fixation of a graft over the anterior and posterior vagina is then performed fashioning a Y-shape. This Y graft is then brought posteriorly along the hollow of the sacrum and affixed to the anterior longitudinal ligament sutures overriding the sacral promontory. Avoidance of undue tension is critical.

Many different graft types have been described, as well as different methods of attaching these grafts to the vagina. Synthetic grafts have higher erosion complication rates than biologic grafts. Biologic grafts, however, have high failure rates when placed at the apex. As graft technologies evolve, identification of the optimal graft material that maximizes durability and compatibility may materialize. Numerous studies demonstrate this technique to be curative (Table 44–2).

In addition to concerns about graft complications, operative hemorrhage is a significant risk. Specifically, during placement of the sacral sutures, the nearby fragile sacral veins may be lacerated. Bleeding from these veins is difficult to control if the veins retract into the bone. Use of sterile thumbtacks to occlude these veins has been an operative technique used to stem potentially life-threatening hemorrhage.

e. Obliterative vaginal operations (colpocleisis and Le Fort's operation)—These are used primarily for severe uterovaginal prolapse in elderly patients

Table 44–2. Follow-up and cure rate after abdominal sacral colpopexy.

Author (Year)	Duration of Follow-Up	No. Patients	No. Cured (%)
Cowan and Morgan (1980)	≤ 60 mo	39	38 (97)
Addision et al (1985)	6–126 mo	56	54 (96)
Baker et al (1990)	1–45 mo	51	51 (100)
Snyder and Krantz (1991)	≥ 6 mo	116	108 (93)
Timmons et al (1992)	9–216 mo	162	161 (99)
Iosif (1993)	12–120 mo	40	39 (96)
Grunberger et al (1994)	3–91 mo	48	45 (94)
Valatis and Stanton (1994)	3–91 mo	41	38 (96)

Adapted from Walters MD, Karram MM: *Urogynecology and Reconstructive Pelvic Surgery,* 2nd ed. Mosby, 1999.

and chronically ill patients who no longer desire coital function. It has the advantage of being done with either regional or local anesthesia. These procedures are highly effective and generally well tolerated. Traction produced by the obliterating scar tissue under the bladder neck and the urethra that may actually cause or aggravate stress incontinence is associated with these operations. Closing the genital hiatus may reduce the chance of recurrence and can be achieved by performing an "extended" perineorrhaphy concomitantly.

REFERENCES

Bump RC et al: The standardization of terminology of female pelvic organ prolapse and pelvic floor dysfunction. Am J Obstet Gynecol 1996;175(1):10.

Burrows LJ et al: Pelvic symptoms in women with pelvic organ prolapse. Obstet Gynecol 2004;104(5 Pt 1):982.

Cundiff GW et al: An anatomic and functional assessment of discrete defect rectocele repair. Am J Obstet Gynecol 1998;179:1451.

Ellerkmann RM et al: Correlation of symptoms with location and severity of pelvic organ prolapse. Am J Obstet Gynecol 2001;185(6):1332; discussion 1337.

Fitzgerald MP et al: Colpocleisis: A review. Int Urogynecol J Pelvic Floor Dysfunct 2006;17(3):261.

Handa VL et al: Progression and remission of pelvic organ prolapse: A longitudinal study of menopausal women. Am J Obstet Gynecol 2004;190(1):27.

Luber KM, Boero S, Choe JY: The demographics of pelvic floor disorders: Current observations and future projections. Am J Obstet Gynecol 2001;184(7):1496; discussion 1501.

Lukacz ES, et al: Parity, mode of delivery, and pelvic floor disorders. Obstet Gynecol 2006;107:1253.

Maher C et al: Surgical management of pelvic organ prolapse in women. Cochrane Database Syst Rev. 2004;(4):CD004014.

Nygaard IE et al: Abdominal sacrocolpopexy: A comprehensive review. Obstet Gynecol 2004;104(4):805.

Shull BL: Pelvic organ prolapse: Anterior, superior, and posterior vaginal segment defects. Am J Obstet Gynecol 1999;181:6.

Sze EH, Karram MM: Transvaginal repair of vault prolapse: A review. Obstet Gynecol 1997;89:466.

Webb MJ et al: Posthysterectomy vaginal vault prolapse: Primary repair in 693 patients. Obstet Gynecol 1998;92:281.

Weber AM, Richter HE: Pelvic organ prolapse. Obstet Gynecol 2005;106:615.

Weber AM, Walters MD: Anterior vaginal prolapse: Review of anatomy and techniques of surgical repair. Obstet Gynecol 1997;89:311.

Wheeless CR Jr: Total vaginal hysterectomy. In: *Atlas of Pelvic Surgery.* Lea & Febiger, 1981.

Urinary Incontinence

45

Christopher M. Tarnay, MD, & Narender N. Bhatia, MD

Urinary incontinence affects well over 13 million adult women in the United States. It is estimated to affect 30–40% of American women during their lifetime. Despite its prevalence and estimated costs in excess of $19.5 billion annually, up to 70% of women do not seek help for incontinence, primarily because of social embarrassment or because they are unaware that help is available. Because of increasing awareness by both patients and physicians, the societal concept that incontinence is part of the "normal" aging process is no longer acceptable. Advances in modern medicine during the last 80 years have increased the life expectancy of women well into the eighth and ninth decades. We are caring for patients longer and better than ever, effectively managing chronic medical problems such as hypertension, cardiovascular disease, and diabetes, enabling women to enjoy longer and more productive lives. This results in a large population of women living up to one-third of their life after menopause, thereby introducing a whole host of medical issues and health concerns. A prime example of this is the problem of urinary incontinence, which has become more prevalent as the population of aging women grows. In this chapter we focus on the evaluation and treatment of women with urinary incontinence.

ANATOMY

The urinary and reproductive tracts are intimately associated during embryologic development. The lower urinary tract can be divided into 3 parts: the bladder, the vesical neck, and the urethra (Fig 45–1). The bladder is a hollow muscular organ lined with transitional epithelium designed for urine storage. The bladder musculature consists of 3 layers of smooth muscle, which are densely intertwined and constitute the detrusor muscle. The bladder stays relaxed to facilitate urine storage and contracts periodically to completely evacuate its contents when appropriate and acceptable. At the bladder base is the trigone, which is embryologically distinct from the bladder.

The 2 ureteral orifices and the internal urethral meatus form the boundaries of the trigone. The trigone has 2 distinct muscular layers: superficial and deep. The deep layer shares a similar cholinergic autonomic innervation as the detrusor muscle, whereas the superficial layer is densely innervated by noradrenergic nerves. This distinct difference in receptor distribution is important, as it provides opportunities to target more specific sites for pharmacotherapeutic intervention. The superficial detrusor layer extends muscular fibers that contribute to the distal urethra and posterior to the proximal urethra. The urethral "sphincter" itself is not a well-delineated structure; rather, it is a complex and intricate meshwork of intertwining smooth and striated muscle fibers that functionally responds neurophysiologically to variable degrees of vesicle pressures and facilitates urine storage and voiding.

The female urethra is approximately 3–4 cm long. The composition and support of the urethra and bladder neck play key roles in the function and maintenance of urinary continence. Together the striated urethral and periurethral muscles compose the extrinsic urethral sphincter mechanism. The urethral sphincter, along with the levator ani, function in the reflex contraction. The urethra is surrounded by dense vasculature that contributes to the urethral mucosal seal and urethral closure pressure. An abundance of submucosal glands are found along the dorsal surface. Most of the urethral diverticula arise from this area. The uroepithelium is stratified squamous (Fig 45–2).

Neuroanatomy

Neuronal innervation of the lower urinary tract is considered part of the autonomic and somatic nervous systems. The autonomic system (ie, the parasympathetic and sympathetic components) receives visceral sensation and regulates smooth muscle actively during conscious and involuntary lower urinary tract functions. The autonomic nervous system constitutes the bulk of neural control of the lower urinary tract. Sympathetic contributions from T1–L2 and parasympathetic contributions from S2–4 compose the neuronal control system (Fig 45–3). Voluntary control of micturition is controlled by the central nervous system. Cortical control of the detrusor muscle rests in the supramedial portion of the frontal lobes and in the genu of the corpus callosum. Receiv-

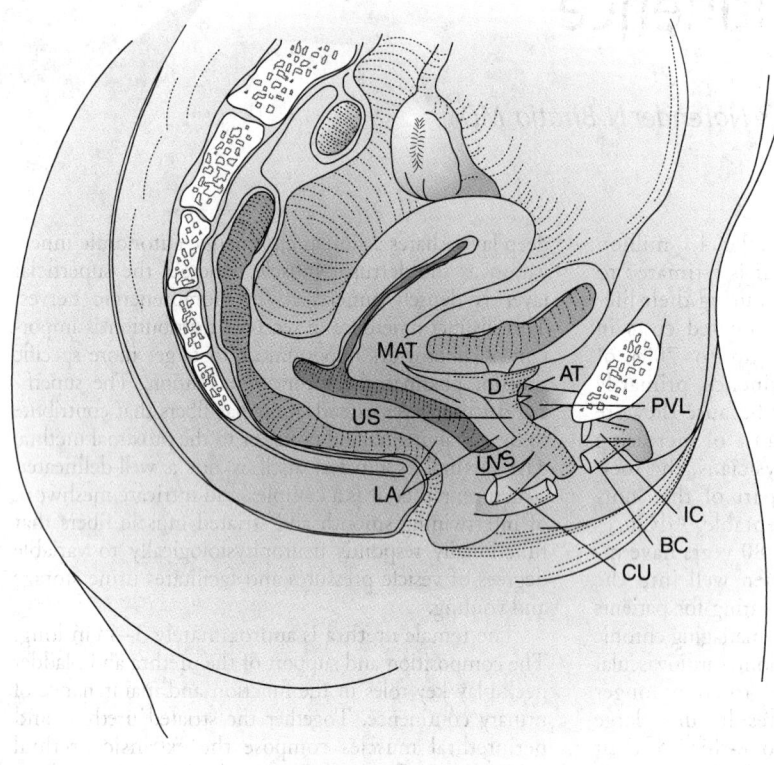

Figure 45–1. Interrelationships and approximate location of paraurethral structures. Levator ani muscles are shown as light lines running deep to the pelvic viscera. AT, arcus tendineus fasciae pelvis; BC, bulbocavernosus muscle; CU, compressor urethrae; D, detrusor loop; IC, ischiocavernosus muscle; LA, levator ani muscles; MAT, muscular attachment of the urethral supports; PVL, pubovesical ligament (muscle); US, urethral sphincter; UVS, urethrovaginal sphincter.

ing both sensory afferent and modulating motor efferent nerves, the net effect is that the brain provides tonic inhibition of detrusor contraction. Lesions in the frontal lobe chiefly cause loss of voluntary control of micturition and thus loss of suppression of the detrusor reflex, resulting in uncontrolled voiding or urge urinary incontinence. The pons and mesencephalic reticular formation in the brainstem constitute the micturition center. A reflex activation in the central brainstem and peripheral spinal cord mediate a coordinated series of events, consisting of relaxation of the striated urethral musculature and detrusor contraction that result in opening of the bladder neck and urethra. Lesions that interrupt these pathways

Smooth muscle

Striated muscle

Smooth   Striated

Figure 45–2. Urethral anatomy. The submucosal vascular plexus matures after puberty but undergoes great changes after menopause. The amount of smooth and especially striated muscles decreases with age, and the striated components become almost rudimentary. (Reproduced, with permission, from Rud T, Asmussen M: Neurophysiology of the lower urinary tract as measured by simultaneous urethral cystometry. In: Ostergard DR, Bent AE [editors]: *Urogynecology and Urodynamics: Theory and Practice*, 4th ed. Williams & Wilkins, 1996, p. 55.)

TH$_{11}$ – L$_2$

S$_2$ – S$_4$

Hypogastric
nerve
(sympathetic)

Micturition center

Smooth muscle
relaxants

Anticholinergics

Calcium
channel
blockers

β

α

Pudendal
nerve
(somatic)

Pelvic nerve
(parasympathetic)

Alpha-adrenergic
agonists

Figure 45–3. Schematic neuroanatomy of the lower urinary tract, with major sites of drug action. (Reproduced, with permission, from Sourander LB: Treatment of urinary incontinence. Gerontology 1990;36[Suppl 2]:19. Copyright Karger S, with permission.)

have various effects depending on the level of interruption, essentially resulting in dyscoordination or dyssynergia of detrusor function.

URINARY INCONTINENCE—OVERVIEW

Definition

Urinary incontinence as defined by the International Continence Society (ICS) is the complaint of any involuntary leakage of urine. Incontinence can be a sign, a symptom (patient complaint), or a condition diagnosed by an examiner. There are many types and causes of urinary incontinence (Table 45–1). The reported incidence of urinary incontinence varies widely, ranging from 8–41% in women over 65 years. Incontinence becomes more common as women age, particularly after menopause. In light of projections that the percentage of postmenopausal women in the population will increase from 23% in 1995 to 33% in 2050, it is apparent that the problem of urinary incontinence will be a major health and quality-of-life issue well into the future.

Etiology

Numerous factors play a role in maintaining urinary continence; therefore, the development of incontinence is frequently not attributable to any single cause. Gender, age, hormonal status, birthing trauma, and genetic differences in connective tissue all contribute to the development of incontinence. Urinary incontinence is 2–3 times more common in women than in men because of women's shorter urethral length and the risk of connective tissue, muscle, and nerve injury associated with childbirth. Observational studies have consistently noted a high incidence of incontinence in the elderly population, with 1 study finding a 30% higher prevalence for each 5-year increase in age. The association of childbirth with urinary incontinence has long been suspected and has generated new interest in identifying the causes. In 1 study of over 15,000 women, the risk of developing urinary incontinence was 2.3 times higher in women who had a vaginal delivery compared to nulliparous women. Damage to the pelvic floor neuromusculature during vaginal delivery may lead to loss of pelvic muscle strength and nerve function, resulting in both stress urinary incontinence (SUI) and pelvic floor support defects. Although muscle strength may be regained over time or with the help of pelvic floor muscle exercises, dysfunction may be permanent.

Table 45–1. Classification and causes of urinary incontinence.

Genuine stress incontinence
  Bladder neck displacement
  Intrinsic sphincter dysfunction (ISD)
Detrusor instability/urge incontinence
  Idiopathic
  Neurologic detrusor hyperreflexia
Mixed incontinence (genuine stress and detrusor instability combined)
Overflow incontinence with urinary retention
  Obstruction
  Bladder hyporeflexia
Bypass incontinence
  Genitourinary fistulas
Urethral diverticulum
Congenital urethral abnormalities (eg, epispadias, bladder exstrophy, ectopic ureter)
Functional and transient incontinence
  Infection
  Pharmacologic
  Restricted mobility
  Dementia/delirium
  Excessive urine production (diabetes mellitus, diabetes insipidus, resorption of extravascular fluid as with lower extremity edema)
  Stool impaction

Table 45–2. Lower urinary tract symptoms (LUTS).

Urinary incontinence: the complaint of any involuntary leakage
Stress urinary incontinence: the complaint of involuntary leakage on effort or exertion, or on sneezing or coughing
Urge urinary incontinence: the complaint of involuntary leakage accompanied by or immediately preceded by urgency
Mixed urinary incontinence: the complaint of involuntary leakage associated with urgency and also with exertion, effort, sneezing or coughing
Increased daytime frequency: the complaint by the patient who considers she voids too often by day
Nocturia: the complaint that the individual has to wake one or more times to void
Urgency: the complaint of a sudden compelling desire to pass urine.
Nocturnal enuresis: complaint of loss of urine occurring during sleep

Aging and incontinence are closely associated. The prevalence of incontinence increases as women age, but the specific cause is unclear. Global decrease in the storage capacity, reduced receptor response, general loss in muscle tone, or latent manifestation from denervation during parturition may all be important factors. The state of hypoestrogenism as a woman transitions to the menopause may also contribute to urinary incontinence. Although estrogen reduces urinary urgency, results from studies specifically examining menopausal status have been equivocal, with some studies showing a positive association and others showing no association.

Abnormalities in the muscular components and innervation of the pelvic floor and the connective tissue to this region likely contribute to the multifactorial etiology of incontinence. Initial observations that the prevalence of abdominal hernias, lower leg varices, and uterine prolapse was higher in women with SUI suggested that connective tissue weakness may identify women at risk for developing incontinence. Subsequent studies have supported a connection between relative collagen deficiencies in the connective tissues of incontinent patients versus continent controls.

Incontinence affects a woman's quality of life, and it is an uncomfortable and embarrassing problem. The psychosocial impact on the patient as well as her family is enormous. Women with urinary incontinence are reported to be more depressed, to have lower self-esteem, and to be ashamed about their appearance and the odor. Urinary incontinence impacts sexual desire and reduces sexual activity. This can curb social interactions to the point where individuals become isolated and even entirely homebound.

History

The first step in evaluating an incontinent patient is a thorough history. The nature and extent of the patient's lower urinary tract symptoms (LUTS) should be elucidated. Knowledge of the duration, frequency, and severity of the urinary incontinence is essential to understanding the social implications and its impact on the patient's life and aids the clinician in determining the direction and extent of diagnostic and therapeutic measures (Table 45–2). A multitude of diagnostic and imaging studies are available, but taking a thorough but focused urogynecologic history can isolate many of the easily reversible causes of incontinence (Table 45–3). Knowledge of the use of protective items, such as sanitary napkins, panty liners, absorbent pads, or adult diapers, is useful in quantitating urinary loss. Including questions about menopausal status and use of hormone treatment, history of urinary tract infections, previous surgery to remedy incontinence, and the patient's mental and functional status are essential.

Patient Questionnaires

Survey instruments can be valuable in helping to identify and determine the severity of patient symptoms. Although initially designed for clinical research, short forms of longer questionnaires exist and can be used for clinical care. Surveys such as the Urinary Distress Inventory (UDI-6) and Incontinence Impact Questionnaire (IIQ-7) can be easily filled out

Table 45–3. Helpful questions when taking history of incontinence.

• Do you leak urine when you cough, sneeze, or laugh?
• Do you ever have such an uncomfortably strong need to urinate that if you don't reach the toilet you leak?
• How many times during the day do you urinate?
• How many times do you get up to void during the night after going to bed?
• Have you ever wet the bed?
• Do you leak during sexual intercourse?
• Do you wear a pad to protect your clothing?
• If yes, how often do you change the pad: when it has only a few drops, when it is damp, or when it is totally wet?
• After you urinate do you have dribbling or still feel the presence of urine in your bladder?
• Does it hurt when you urinate?
• Do you lose urine without the urge to go?

by a patient to facilitate diagnosis and to follow treatment interventions.

Voiding Diary

A voiding diary, or urolog, that quantitates frequency and volume is a helpful tool. For a 24- to 48-hour period the patient records all fluid intake, and measures and records all urine output, including frequency and episodes of leakage (Fig 45–4). Numerous studies have validated the voiding diary as a reliable tool in the diagnosis and management of urinary urgency or urge incontinence. These data are beneficial to the physician because they clarify home voiding patterns, particularly in the elderly. They are often useful to patients as well because

they provide a focus on the problem and can serve as a baseline for treatment interventions such as behavioral training, bladder drills, and pharmacologic management.

Urinalysis

Examination of the urine is an essential part of the workup of urinary incontinence for any patient with LUTS. Infection is a common cause of urinary complaints, including frequency, urgency, and incontinence. A clean-catch voided specimen is suitable for routine urinalysis; however, a sterile "in and out" catheterized specimen is appropriate for patients unable to correctly perform collection or if urine culture has been previously equivocal because of skin flora contamination.

Urolog

Date	Time	Fluids (type and how much) ounces	Urine (how much) ounces or mL	Accidents/ Leaks
example 9/1/00	8:00	Water 8 oz		
9/1/00	8:30		150 mL	

Figure 45–4. Urinary diary (urolog).

Urinary protein, glucose, ketones, hemoglobin, casts, and nitrates can indicate primary renal disease or injury. Microscopic evaluation of the urinary sediment may indicate renal tubular damage with the presence of casts or indicate infection by the presence of leukocytes and red blood cells. More than 6–8 white blood cells per high-power field along with the presence of bacteria are very suggestive of urinary tract infection.

Physical Examination

A general gynecologic and neurologic examination should be performed on all patients, with a focus on the vaginal walls and pelvic floor. The patient should come to the clinic with a comfortably full bladder for spontaneous uroflowmetry and postvoid residual assessment. An examination should be performed with the patient in the lithotomy position. The examination should begin with an assessment of the vulvar area. In postmenopausal patients, atrophy and change in labial architecture may be due to estrogen deficiency. Vulvar dermatoses may be coexistent with vulvar complaints ascribed to incontinence. The presence of inflammation or irritation from chronic moisture or pad usage should be noted. The presence of discharge should be noted because this may mimic urinary incontinence. Examination of the urethra with palpation of the anterior vaginal wall under the urethra for fluctuance, masses, or discharge may reveal signs of urethral diverticulum, infection of the urethra, or rarely carcinoma. Tenderness may point to urethral pain syndrome, a condition marked by episodic urethral pain usually with voiding, and by daytime frequency and nocturia.

Vaginal wall integrity must be assessed. Vaginal rugae, or the folds in the epithelium, are normal and tend to be absent if the underlying supportive endopelvic fascia is detached. The presence of anterior wall defects (cystoceles), posterior vaginal wall defects (rectoceles), and apical defects (enteroceles) can be quantified. The uterocervical position, or, if the woman has had a hysterectomy, the cuff position and its descent should be recorded. The position of the vaginal walls should be noted in the lithotomy position at rest and with Valsalva/straining maneuver. A Sims' speculum or the lower blade of a Graves' speculum allows easy visualization of either the anterior or posterior vaginal wall. The severity of vaginal laxity, which may be masked in the supine position, can often best be elicited by repeating the examination in the standing position while the patient places 1 foot on the step of the examination table or on a small portable step.

Cotton Swab Test

Mobility at the level of the bladder neck can be quantified with the use of a sterile cotton-tipped swab (Q-tip) test. The Q-tip test is 1 of the most commonly used tests to evaluate women with urinary problems because it effectively quantifies the degree of anatomic rotation of the support of the urethra and bladder neck. With the patient in the dorsolithotomy position, the labia are separated and urethral meatus swabbed with antiseptic. A sterile Q-tip lubricated with 1–2% lidocaine (Xylocaine) jelly is inserted transurethrally into the bladder and then withdrawn slowly until definite resistance is felt. This places the tip of the Q-tip at the level of the bladder neck just distal to the internal urethral meatus. Using a standard protractor, resting angle is measured. The patient is then asked to perform a Valsalva maneuver or to cough, and the maximum straining angle is noted. Net deflection is equal to the change from resting to maximum straining position (Fig 45–5). An angle greater than 30 degrees is considered abnormal. Urethral hypermobility must be interpreted with caution because it may be present in women without incontinence. The utility of this simple test is that an angle greater than 30 degrees is certainly present in the majority of women with genuine stress incontinence. In the absence of hypermobility, the physician must question the diagnosis of anatomic stress incontinence and entertain the possibility of a fixed and damaged urethral sphincter (also called *intrinsic sphincteric deficiency*) to explain stress-related urinary loss.

Urinary Cough Stress Test

Having the patient perform a Valsalva maneuver or to cough forcefully multiple times to reproduce urine loss at the beginning of the examination may reveal the presence of incontinence. Observation of urine lost immediately with the cough or Valsalva maneuver may obviate the need for more complex urodynamic testing if the complaint is minor. If no urine loss is exhibited, the patient is asked to stand with legs shoulder width apart and asked to cough. Immediate loss of urine suggests a diagnosis of SUI.

Bimanual examination to evaluate the uterine size, position, and descent within the vaginal canal and palpation of the ovaries should be performed. A rectovaginal examination permits adequate assessment of the posterior vaginal wall. Anal sphincter tone can be assessed at rest and with anal tightening. The presence of fecal impaction must be ruled out because this condition has been shown to be a contributing factor to urinary incontinence, particularly in the elderly population.

The description of pelvic organ prolapse is critical. (For details see Chapter 44 and Table 44–1.)

Neurologic Examination

The control of micturition is complex and multitiered, with both autonomic and voluntary control. In addition to a complete history and screening for neurologic

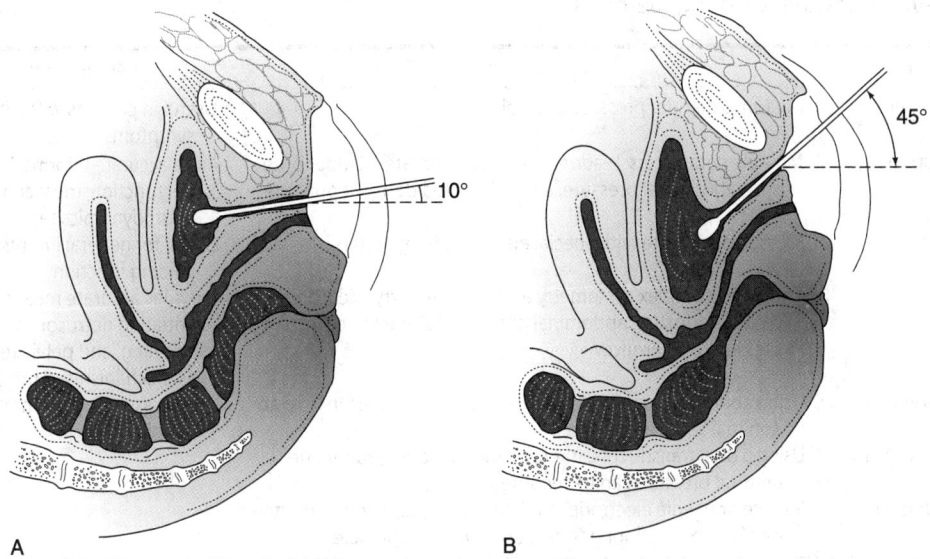

Figure 45–5. The cotton-tipped swab (Q-tip) test for assessment of urethral and bladder support. **A:** Angle of the Q-tip at rest. **B:** Angle of the Q-tip with Valsalva maneuver or cough (straining). The urethrovesical junction descends, causing upward deflection of the Q-tip.

symptoms, a thorough physical examination is important because many neurologic diseases may present with voiding dysfunction in the absence of overt neurologic findings.

Mental status, cranial nerves, motor strength, sensory function, deep tendon reflexes, and sacral spinal cord integrity should all be assessed. Testing the patient's orientation to place and time and assessing speech and comprehension skills will help to ascertain her mental status. Motor control may be diminished in focal brain or cord lesions, most commonly Parkinson's disease, multiple sclerosis, and cerebrovascular accident. Motor strength is tested in the lower extremities by assessing hip, knee, and ankle flexion, as well as ankle eversion and inversion. Deep tendon reflexes are tested at the patella, ankle, and foot planus. Sensation can be tested at the dermatomes using light touch and pinprick over the perineum and thigh area. Deficits should be noted, but it should be kept in mind that there is considerable overlap in sensory innervation in the sensory nerve roots. The sacral spinal cord nerve roots 2–4 contain vital neurons controlling micturition. The anal wink reflex and the bulbocavernosus reflex can confirm integrity of neurovisceral and urethral reflex functions. These reflexes can be evoked by stroking the perianal area and looking for an external anal sphincter contraction, and by tapping or gently squeezing the clitoris and watching for contraction of the bulbocavernosus muscle, respectively. These reflexes are often easier to elicit at the beginning of the examination, but their absence is not always indicative of neurologic deficit. Clinically observed neurologic deficits should lead to a neurologic consultation.

Urodynamics

A urodynamic study is any test that provides objective dynamic information about lower urinary tract function. Many methods and tests are available (Table 45–4). Some methods are simple, such as diaries that track frequency and volume of urination, and some methods are more complex, requiring special equipment and training. A cystometrogram is necessary to rule out unstable bladder, overflow incontinence, reduced bladder capacity, or abnormalities of bladder sensation. A cystometrogram can be performed using water manometry or more advanced methods. Complex urodynamic testing increases the diagnostic accuracy and may often identify the reason for failure of previous therapy. Uroflowmetry can be performed to measure detrusor pressure and flow rate to evaluate for voiding dysfunction. If a poorly functioning urethra, such as intrinsic sphincter deficiency (ISD), is suspected, urethral pressure profile (UPP) or abdominal leak point pressure (ALPP) can be measured to evaluate urethral closure pressures. Such testing is particularly helpful in difficult or complex cases.

The indications for more complex testing in the form of multichannel urodynamics are not standardized, and each patient must be assessed individually (Table 45–5). However, some basic criteria, if met, in-

Table 45–4. Urodynamic testing methods.

Test	Purpose	Indications
Simple cystometry	Measures bladder pressure and volume	Useful in patients with clear-cut symptoms
Complex cystometry	Multiple parameters: bladder volume, filling rate, bladder pressure, abdominal pressure, and subtracted detrusor pressure	More accurate information on bladder function; most common type of urodynamics test
Uroflowmetry	Measures flow rate with special electronic flow-meters	Useful for general impression of voiding function
Pressure-flow	Combines complex cystometry and uroflowmetry. Measures bladder pressure, abdominal pressure, subtracted detrusor pressure, and uroflow	Provides accurate means of differentiating detrusor contraction, straining, and pelvic relaxation as mechanisms of urination
Leak point pressure	Using abdominal or bladder pressures, urethral resistance to abdominal strain is measured	Used in assessing urethral sphincter function
Urethral pressure profilometry	Using a dual transducer catheter, simultaneous bladder and urethral pressure can be recorded	
Electromyography	Surface or needle electrodes to determine striated muscle activity of the pelvic floor or the anal or urethral sphincters	

dicate a need for urodynamic evaluation, which can aid in more accurate diagnosis and thus appropriate medical or surgical management.

Cystourethroscopy

Endoscopic evaluation is an invaluable adjunct for the diagnosis and management of the urogynecologic patient. It is a simple office procedure that can yield important data when performed by experienced operators. Cystourethroscopy is indicated for hematuria, irritative voiding symptoms, obstructive voiding, suspicion of diverticula or fistula, persistent incontinence, and as a preoperative evaluation prior to reconstructive pelvic surgery.

Imaging Tests

Radiologic studies can be an integral component of the evaluation of lower urinary tract dysfunction and abnormalities. However, these modalities are of limited use in the evaluation of all but the most complex of incontinent patients. Magnetic resonance imaging (MRI) has become more extensively used in patients with pelvic floor dysfunctions and prolapse. As the technique becomes less costly, applications for the uses of MRI to aid in the urogynecological work-up will expand.

STRESS URINARY INCONTINENCE

The International Continence Society (ICS) defines SUI as the complaint of involuntary leakage on effort or exertion, or on coughing or sneezing.

Normally, at rest the intraurethral pressure is greater than the intravesical pressure. The pressure difference between the bladder and the urethra is known as the *urethral closure pressure*. If intra-abdominal pressure increases as it does with a cough, sneeze, or strain, and if this pressure is not equally transmitted to the urethra, then continence is not maintained and leakage of urine occurs. What is thought to cause this inequity of pressure transmission is not universally accepted, and the discussion of the proposed mechanisms are beyond the scope of this chapter.

Treatment of Stress Urinary Incontinence

A. NONSURGICAL MEASURES

For most patients with SUI, consideration of the simplest, least invasive, and least costly interventions is appropriate (Table 45–6). Dietary measures can be instituted, with identification of items that can be modified.

Table 45–5. Indications for multichannel urodynamic testing.

- Complicated symptoms and history
- Use when considering surgery for correction of incontinence or pelvic organ prolapse
- Underlying neurologic disease
- Urge incontinence refractive to initial conservative therapies
- Continuous leakage
- Previous anti-incontinence surgery
- Clinical findings do not correlate with symptoms
- Elderly patients > 65 years old

Table 45–6. Nonsurgical management of urinary incontinence.

Behavioral therapy
Fluid management
Bladder training
Pelvic floor muscle training
• Biofeedback
• Vaginal cones
Functional electrical stimulation
Anti-incontinence pessary
Pharmacotherapy

Reduction in consumption of caffeinated beverages and alcoholic drinks should be encouraged. Fluid restriction in patients without chronic medical problems, such as cardiovascular, renal, or endocrinologic disease, can be attempted. Timed voiding to prevent filling the bladder to a capacity that causes urine loss should be undertaken with the use of a urine diary. The diary can also facilitate discussion between patient and clinician as therapy progresses.

Pelvic floor muscle exercises or Kegel exercises have been found to be extremely helpful in patients with mild to moderate forms of incontinence. Focused repetitive voluntary contractions of the levator ani muscles (pubococcygeus, coccygeus, and iliococcygeus) created by having the patient contract or "squeeze" the muscle as if to prevent the passage of rectal gas is an effective therapy. The contractions exert a closing force on the urethra and increase muscle support to the pelvic organs. The patient should be provided written and verbal instructions on performing the exercises. Repetitions, with each contraction held for 3–5 seconds alternated with periods of relaxation, should be begun at 45–100 repetitions daily. In settings in which the patient is motivated and has individual instruction and thorough follow-up and support, results for cure or improvement of bladder control (reduction in urine loss) can be up to 75%.

1. Biofeedback—Biofeedback is an adjunct to pelvic floor exercises that is used to facilitate the patient's comprehension of the proper muscles to contract. By using a pressure catheter and myographic monitoring, a visual or auditory signal of the physiologic response can be provided to the patient to help refine exercise skills. Using surface electromyography on the perineum to measure levator contraction and a pressure monitor in the vagina or rectum to indicate abdominal pressure, the patient can be instructed to preferentially contract the pelvic floor without concomitant abdominal contraction. Studies using a variety of techniques demonstrate a 54–95% cure rate or improvement in

SUI. The efficacy of this modality is highly dependent on patient motivation and compliance. Pelvic floor muscle exercises with or without biofeedback require continued implementation and practice or effectiveness will wane.

2. Electrical stimulation—As an alternative to active patient contraction of the levator muscles, electrical stimulation of the muscles via small electrical currents can be used to help both SUI and mixed incontinence. Using intravaginal or transrectal electrodes with stimulators, the pelvic muscles automatically contract and are thereby artificially "trained." When used long term, weakened muscles are strengthened and innervation re-established during activation. Experiences with the devices are variable, but they generally show a positive impact on incontinence and acceptable patient tolerance.

3. Pessaries—Intravaginal devices or pessaries to correct the anatomic deficits associated with stress incontinence have long been used to address this vexing problem. Many devices have been proffered, but long-term solutions to incontinence have yet to be proven in the general population. Pessaries, traditionally used for treatment of genital prolapse, have also been shown to have a potential role in supporting the bladder neck and urethra and preventing stress incontinence. Many pessary devices designed to fit within the vagina and elevate the bladder neck are available. Continence can often be achieved because many devices adequately obstruct the bladder neck and urethra. As with all intravaginal devices, maintenance is essential to avoid urinary obstruction and vaginal erosion if the pessary is too compressive.

Occlusive devices are commercially available. External devices, such as urethral plugs that are placed over the external urethral meatus or internal occlusive devices placed transurethrally with an internal balloon, are available and have been shown to be partially helpful in reducing wetting episodes.

B. Surgical Management

Surgical treatment should be offered for moderate to severe incontinence. Urinary incontinence is not a life-threatening condition, and the decision to operate must be based on the patient's symptoms and the impact on daily life. Many patients are able to tolerate slight urine loss, and what often provokes a desire for treatment is an increase in loss above a tolerable threshold. If medical management to improve bladder control is possible and symptoms are reduced to below this threshold, then medical management is most desirable. If not, surgery should be considered.

At least 130 operative procedures have been described for treatment of female urinary stress incontinence. It is therefore not surprising that many of these procedures have not resulted in long-term success. For patients who desire surgical correction, the options can be categorized by method of surgical approach (Table 45–7). Common to most surgical procedures is restoration of bladder neck support by elevation of the urethrovesical junction. Some procedures reconstruct bladder neck supports and provide a stable suburethral layer.

Assessment of the cure rate of any surgical treatment for genuine stress incontinence must take into account the selection of patients, accuracy of the preoperative diagnosis, length of postoperative follow-up, and criteria for cure. Reported cure rates for abdominal procedures range from 60–100%, with 75–90% being the generally accepted rate. Most failures appear to result from incorrect preoperative diagnosis, poor surgical technique, and healing failures.

1. Anterior repair—Anterior colporrhaphy with Kelly plication is one of the oldest methods of surgical correction, introduced in 1914. Used for anterior vaginal defects (cystocele), the technique involves vaginal dissection of the epithelium below the bladder and bladder neck, identifying the perivesical fascia and pubocervical fascia, and plicating each side over the midline. The Kelly plication involves specific support at the bladder. Numerous studies have evaluated this approach, and long-term analysis does not support this method as an effective cure for stress incontinence, with greater than 60% failure rates over 5 years.

2. Needle urethropexy—Since the introduction of this procedure in 1957 by Armand Pereyra and its modifications with contributions by Thomas Lebherz, needle urethropexy has become a fixture in anti-incontinence surgery. Numerous authors have published alterations of this technique (eg, Raz, Stamey, Gittes, and Musznai). All rely on vaginal incision, dissection and mobilization of periurethral tissues, entry into the space of Retzius (retropubic space), and passage of a needle ligature carrier from a small abdominal incision into the vaginal incision. The periurethral tissues and fascia are identified, secured with delayed absorbable suture, and brought through retropubically and secured above the abdominal rectus fascia. In this manner the bladder neck is elevated and continence restored. The heterogeneity of procedure and technique make generalized statements about this procedure difficult, but prospective long-term studies for individual procedures are available. The procedures appear to be effective initially, with cure rates of approximately 80–85% with variable follow-up. When examining some studies (including 1 large prospective study) with at

Table 45–7. Surgical treatment of SUI.

Retropubic urethropexy
   Burch
   Marshall-Marchetti-Krantz (MMK)
Needle urethropexy
Suburethral sling
Midurethral sling
   Retropubic (TVT, Uretex, SPARC, Advantage)
   Transobturator
Urethral bulking agents

least 2 years of follow-up, the cure rates drop dramatically to less than 65%.

3. Abdominal retropubic colpopexy—The Marshall-Marchetti-Krantz (MMK) and Burch colposuspension are the two classic retropubic surgeries for incontinence. They share the same mechanism of correction. First, both suspend the periurethral and paravaginal tissue at the level of the urethrovesical junction, and second, both use a firm point of attachment for fixation of these suspension sutures. In the MMK procedure, the sutures are fixed to the periosteum of the pubic bone, and in the Burch procedure, the iliopectineal ligament (Cooper's ligament) (Fig 45–6). The Burch colposuspension has become the first choice for treatment of patients with hypermobility of the bladder neck and genuine SUI. In both longitudinal studies and randomized comparative trials against other procedures, the Burch procedure maintains the highest objective and subjective cure rates of 80% after 5 years and 68% after 10 years of follow-up.

A laparoscopic approach to Burch colposuspension offers the benefit of minimally invasive surgery with the same level of efficacy. With the laparoscopic approach, hospital stay and postoperative recovery are minimized. Using the transperitoneal or preperitoneal approach, this method has demonstrated cure rates comparable to the open procedure. Success rates with variable follow-up range between 87% and 97%, with 85% at 5 years of follow-up reported by 1 prospective study. The procedure requires advanced laparoscopic skills, and the results are highly dependent on the skill of the operator. Accordingly, some reports report lower cure rates and higher complications compared with the open procedure.

4. Suburethral slings—The suburethral sling was one of the original surgical procedures developed for correction of SUI. The SUI concept of restoring continence by encircling the urethra with supportive tissue, either from the patient or foreign material, was introduced at the beginning of the 20th century. Contemporary techniques have used a patient's own fascia har-

Figure 45–6. Abdominal surgical procedure to correct stress incontinence. **A:** Anterior vaginal wall has been mobilized. Two sutures have been placed on either side and far lateral from the midline. Distal sutures are opposite the midurethra. Proximal sutures are at the end of the vesicourethral junction. Sutures are attached to Cooper's ligament. **B:** Cross-section shows urethra free in the retropubic space, with anterior vaginal wall lifting and supporting it. **C** and **D:** Urethra is compressed and strangulated against pubic bone when vaginal sutures are applied close to the urethra and then fixed to the pubic symphysis. (Reproduced, with permission, from Tanagho EA: Colpocystoure-thropexy. J Urol 1876;116:751. Copyright 1976 by The Williams and Wilkins Co.)

vested from the leg or rectus fascia, or donor fascia in the form of cadaveric fascia lata. Cure rates of suburethral sling procedures for genuine stress incontinence vary from 70–95%. Reported rates vary because of the heterogeneity of patients, and many are previous surgical failures. Variations in sling material and technique have made cure rates among sling techniques difficult to interpret. Furthermore, most studies vary in the definition of cure and may not distinguish between cure and improvement.

In a large review study summarizing cure rates of surgical treatments for SUI, 16 studies comparing sling procedures to colposuspension were reviewed. Of the 4 that were randomized controlled trials comprising 150 patients, none reported a difference in cure. The remaining 12 were retrospective studies, with only 1 demonstrating a difference in outcome between procedures, 79% versus 95% cure for sling and colposuspension, respectively.

5. Midurethral slings—The latest modification of the sling is the use of tension-free vaginal mesh made of polypropylene placed at the level of the midurethra. This pioneering technique, developed in Sweden, was introduced to the United States in the late 1990s. Use of tension-free vaginal tape (TVT) (Fig 45–7) was de-

Figure 45–7. **A:** Placement of midurethral sling in the sagittal view. **B:** Retropubic passage of midurethral sling. **C:** Transobturator passage of midurethral sling.

veloped as a minimally invasive technique for surgical correction of genuine SUI. The initial study had an 84% cure rate in 75 women with 2-year follow-up. Considerable data now support a high subjective cure of 85–93% and objective cure rate of 75–85% with up to 7-year follow-up.

Because of the success of TVT, numerous other devices using the same principles and technique have been introduced. All use a polypropylene mesh but have different designs of delivery needle/trocar, mesh construction, and sheath type. Comparative data between devices are scanty.

The newest variation of the midurethral sling is the transobturator approach. Rather than retropubic passage, the sling is passed through the obturator foramen laterally. This creates a more lateral point of fixation. The purported advantage is reduction in bladder, bowel, or major vascular injury because this method avoids the space of Retzius and does not traverse the peritoneal space. Early data suggest similar short-term cure rates to

retropubic passage (94%). Long-term comparative studies will determine the role of the transobturator approach as a viable alternative to retropubic midurethral slings (Fig 45–7).

C. PERIURETHRAL AND TRANSURETHRAL INJECTION

Periurethral or transurethral injection of a bulking agent into the submucosal space of the bladder neck causes narrowing or coaptation of the proximal urethra and bladder neck opening. This increases urethral resistance to involuntary urine loss without changing resting urethral closure pressure. Currently glutaraldehyde cross-linked bovine collagen is the most commonly used material. This procedure is generally reserved for genuine SUI caused by intrinsic sphincteric deficiency. The injections can be performed with the patient under sedation with local anesthetic in an outpatient or office setting. The bovine collagen degrades over 9–19 months, and repeat "booster" injections are often required. Improvement and cure rates are very high in the short term, and complications are minimal. Pyrolytic carbon beads (Durasphere) is a permanent and hypoallergenic bulking agent that may obviate the need for repeat injections, but long-term cure rates are equally disappointing. Newer formulations are being introduced. Inert gel formulations that become firm after injection are being studied in clinical trials.

D. ARTIFICIAL SPHINCTERS

The artificial urethral sphincter is an effective option for patients with incontinence not amenable to standard surgical treatment because of urethral scarring or atony. The artificial urinary sphincter is best used in patients with incontinence due to poor urethral sphincter function. The sphincter obstructs the urethra by compressing the bladder neck via a pressure-regulated balloon and releases the compression when the patient desires to void. Reported success rates are up to 91%, but complication rates are high, with 21% of patients requiring surgical replacement of parts or the entire sphincter.

URGE URINARY INCONTINENCE

Definition

Urge urinary incontinence is the complaint of involuntary leakage accompanied by or immediately preceded by urgency. Urge urinary incontinence is usually associated with involuntary contractions of the bladder or detrusor contractions. Strictly speaking, detrusor instability (DI) is an urodynamic definition and term. Recent questions about the relevance and reproducibility of the role of involuntary contractions in the clinical presentation of incontinence have been raised. The literature is at times confusing concerning the methodology (catheter type, bladder filling rate, provocative maneuvers, etc) for data acquisition. The literature is filled with many different terms describing DI, such as overactive bladder (OAB), bladder dyssynergia, uninhibited detrusor, and unstable bladder. In addition, when the cause of involuntary detrusor contractions is due to an underlying neurologic lesion, DI is called detrusor hyperreflexia. OAB is a term that lends itself to encompassing all conditions related to bladder urgency, frequency with and without incontinence. Overactive bladder has become a preferred term because it comprises symptoms of urgency, urge urinary incontinence, frequency, and nocturia.

Etiology

The incidence of OAB varies depending on the population studied and the definition applied. Consequently, the reported prevalence varies widely from 8–50% in the general population, and in women over 65 years it is esti-

mated to be at least 38%. An important concept is that involuntary detrusor contractions for bladder emptying are normally overridden by cortical inhibition of reflex bladder activity. In the majority of cases the cause of OAB symptoms is unknown. Patients with underlying neurologic disease may manifest with urinary incontinence. Although neurologic disease is not a common cause of OAB, multiple sclerosis, cerebrovascular disease, Parkinson's disease, and Alzheimer's disease are most often associated with involuntary bladder contractions.

Diagnosis

Diagnosis of OAB is suggested by urinary frequency often associated with a strong urge or a sense of impending urine loss. Incontinence often occurs prior to reaching the toilet. Loss of urine may occur seconds after stress, such as a cough or strain. Physical or environmental stimuli, such as running water, cold weather, or hand washing, may elicit an urge. Patients often describe "key in lock" syndrome. This is typically characterized by an uncontrollable urge to void when unlocking the door after returning from a trip out of the house. The first thing done upon return is to immediately rush to the toilet or risk losing urine.

Treatment

Adequate therapy depends greatly on accuracy of diagnosis of OAB. History is most often suggestive, and the diagnosis can be confirmed with office cystometry or more precisely with multichannel urodynamics.

Patients with OAB first should be offered simple treatments. Behavioral modifications and medical treatment are the standard first-line therapy for urge urinary incontinence.

A. BEHAVIORAL THERAPY

Behavioral therapy includes bladder training, timed voiding, and pelvic floor muscle exercises. Bladder training is an educational program that combines written and verbal instruction to educate patients about the mechanisms of normal bladder control with the teaching of relaxation and distraction skills to resist premature signals to urinate. Creating a voiding schedule for which the patient urinates at preset intervals while attempting to ignore the urge to urinate may progressively lead to re-establishment of cortical voluntary control over the micturition reflex.

Timed voiding is a form of bladder retraining that again mandates regularly scheduled voiding and attempts to match the person's natural voiding schedule. No effort is made to motivate the patient to delay voiding by resisting the urge. This method is geared more toward elderly patients with more challenging problems who have skilled help available.

Pelvic floor exercises may aid in the treatment of OAB. Evidence supports the utility of this modality in all types of incontinence. Particularly when augmented with biofeedback, pelvic floor exercises can greatly reduce symptoms of urinary frequency and urge incontinence, by up to 54–85%.

B. PHARMACOLOGIC THERAPY

One of the most effective and popular treatments for urge urinary incontinence and OAB is drug therapy. Numerous agents for the treatment of these patients have been tried over the years, but only a few have demonstrated substantial impact on reduction of symptoms in controlled trials. One of the main difficulties in treating OAB is that the cause of OAB is still under investigation. The drugs available can be divided into classes by mechanism of action (Table 45–8).

Antimuscarinics, or anticholinergics, have become the mainstay of drug treatment of OAB. Acetylcholine is the primary neurotransmitter involved with bladder contraction. The detrusor muscle of the bladder is heavily populated with cholinergic receptors. Anticholinergic activity, therefore, is a property of most drugs used to treat OAB. The prototype medicine is propantheline. Used for many years, it has excellent results in uncontrolled case series but only modest efficacy in controlled trials, providing benefit in up to 53% of patients.

The mainstays of drug therapy for OAB include oxybutynin chloride and tolterodine. Oxybutynin chloride has been shown in randomized placebo-controlled trials to be effective in increasing bladder capacity, decreasing the frequency of detrusor contractions, and improving symptoms of urinary urgency in approximately 70% of patients. It is effective for both idiopathic and neuropathic etiologies of DI.

Tolterodine is a medication designed specifically for OAB. It also has anticholinergic activity with specificity for the bladder, and it acts through muscarinic receptors as well as smooth muscle relaxation. In a multicenter randomized controlled trial, the medication compared favorably with oxybutynin in terms of reducing the number of micturitions in 24 hours and the number of incontinent episodes. Because of its bladder specificity, tolterodine has a more favorable side effect profile than oxybutynin. It is also dosed less frequently and improves patient compliance. Both are available in immediate-release and long-acting formulations. Oxybutynin is also available for delivery in a transdermal patch. Recently, a third antimuscarinic, trospium, has become available in the United States for treatment of OAB.

A large randomized comparative trial evaluating the performance of the long-acting formulations of oxybutynin and tolterodine demonstrated similar efficacy. Both reduced weekly urge incontinence episodes, but patients randomized to oxybutynin had a

Table 45–8. Pharmacologic treatment of urge incontinence.

Drug Name	Trade Name	Drug Type	Dosage	Potential Side Effects
Oxybutynin chloride	Ditropan	Anticholinergic (antimuscarinic)/smooth muscle relaxant; tertiary amine	15–30 mg daily	Dry mouth, blurry vision, constipation, tachycardia, drowsiness, dizziness
Oxybutynin chloride (OROS)	Ditropan XL	See above	5–30 mg daily	See above, less CNS side effects
Transdermal oxybutynin	Oxytrol	See above	3.9 mg/day patch	See above
Tolterodine	Detrol	Antimuscarinic/smooth muscle relaxant	1–2 mg BID	See above
Tolterodine (long acting)	Detrol LA	See above	2–4 mg Q day	See above
Trospium chloride	Sanctura	Antimuscarinic; quaternary amine	20 mg BID	Dry mouth, constipation, headache
Darifenacin	Enablex	Antimuscarinic selective; tertiary amine	7.5–15 mg Q day	Dry mouth, constipation, blurred vision No CNS effects
Imipramine hydrochloride	Tofranil	Tricyclic antidepressant: anticholinergic, alpha-adrenergic, antihistamine	25–100 mg daily	Drowsiness, orthostatic hypotension, hepatic dysfunction, xerostomia

significant reduction in micturition frequency compared with patients receiving tolterodine, and significantly more patients taking oxybutynin became totally dry (23% vs 16%). Adverse events were similar, but the occurrence of dry mouth was higher in the oxybutynin group.

Two new antimuscarinics are solifenacin and darifenacin. Both significantly improve OAB symptoms compared to placebo. Evidence suggests that their side effects will be similar or lower than those of currently available antimuscarinics.

Imipramine hydrochloride is a tricyclic antidepressant that acts through its anticholinergic properties to increase bladder storage. The drug improves bladder compliance rather than counteracting uninhibited detrusor contractions. It is given in doses greatly reduced from those recommended for use as an antidepressant. It also has pharmacologic activity in the blockade of postsynaptic noradrenaline uptake and thereby increases bladder outlet resistance. With its dual action, imipramine may be effective in patients with both stress incontinence and DI (mixed incontinence). It has a low rate of discontinuation because of the main side effects of tremor and fatigue, but it should be dosed in the evening because it may have a sedative effect, and it should be used with caution in elderly patients because of potential orthostatic hypotension.

Surgical measures are methods of last resort for severe intractable DI. Recently, the InterStim surgically implantable device has been found to be effective in patients with intractable urinary urgency and voiding dysfunction.

MIXED INCONTINENCE

Mixed incontinence occurs when both stress incontinence and DI occur simultaneously. Patients may present with symptoms of both types of incontinence. These patients present both a diagnostic and therapeutic dilemma. The prevalence of mixed incontinence is more common than most practitioners realize. A detailed history will reveal symptoms of SUI with urine loss associated with cough, sneeze, or other increase in Valsalva pressure, as well as urinary urgency, frequency, and concomitant incontinence. The coexistence of these 2 conditions may be brought about by many causes. Patients with stress incontinence often preemptively urinate to avoid a full bladder and subsequent urine loss, thereby conditioning the bladder to habituate to a low functional capacity. This may promote premature signaling of bladder fullness and result in frequent urge symptoms. Patients may have DI that is precipitated by coughing or laughing. Patients may have indolent involuntary bladder contractions that

only manifest with the additional pressure of a cough, sneeze, or laugh. The cause is often difficult to ascertain, but the diagnosis should be confirmed with urodynamic studies that can assist in identifying the cause of urine loss.

Treatment

For mixed incontinence, treatment should be based on the patient's worst symptoms. Often patients can prioritize their symptoms, stating that one component impacts their life more than the other. By having the patient separate the symptoms, a practical management plan with realistic expectations can be devised. A great disservice can be done by operating on a patient to restore bladder neck support and remove stress symptoms, when the patient's main concern is daily urge incontinence while she is at work. Conservative measures should be tried first, and if symptoms do not improve surgical measures can be entertained to target alleviation of the stress component. However, there is a 50–60% chance that urge symptoms may resolve after a midurethral sling is performed. Occasionally the involuntary contractions are alleviated by restoration of bladder support and vaginal anatomy.

OVERFLOW INCONTINENCE
Definition

Overflow incontinence is defined as the involuntary loss of urine associated with bladder overdistention in the absence of detrusor contraction. This condition classically occurs in men who have outlet obstruction secondary to prostatic enlargement that progresses to urinary retention. In women this is a relatively uncommon cause of urinary incontinence. When it does occur, it can be from increased outlet resistance from advanced vaginal prolapse causing a "kink" in the urethra or after an anti-incontinence procedure which has overcorrected the problem. Additionally, it can result from bladder hyporeflexia from a variety of neurologic causes (Table 45–9).

Etiology

Overflow incontinence most often occurs due to postoperative obstruction if the bladder neck is overcorrected, or with a hyporeflexic bladder due to neurologic disease or spinal cord injury. The normal act of voiding is controlled centrally by sacral and pontine micturition centers. Impaired emptying can be the result of disruption of either central or peripheral neurons mediating detrusor function. Failure to iden-

Table 45–9. Causes of overflow incontinence.

Neurologic	Anatomic	Iatrogenic
Spinal cord trauma	Extrinsic compression	Surgery
Cerebral cortical lesions	Urethral mass	Obstetric
Diabetes mellitus		Anesthetic
Multiple sclerosis		
Infectious	**Pharmacologic**	
Cystitis	Anticholinergics	
Urethritis	α-Adrenergics	

tify the cause early may lead to permanent dysfunction and may lead to injury to the detrusor muscle or compromise in the parasympathetic ganglia in the bladder wall.

Diagnosis

Usually symptoms are loss of urine without awareness or intermittent dribbling and constant wetness. Suprapubic pressure or pain may be associated. Patients will often note a sensation of a full bladder and the need to strain in order to empty or apply suprapubic pressure to void. Patients are at risk for urinary tract infection secondary to persistent residual urine in the bladder, which acts as a medium for bacterial growth. It is commonly seen after a bladder neck suspension. Complaints of poor urinary stream and sense of incomplete emptying combined with having to strain or apply hand pressure to void are likely.

Evaluation should always include a postvoid residual and, if the diagnosis is questionable, voiding pressure flow studies. An imaging study of the upper urinary tract to evaluate the ureters and kidney should follow, because persistent high-volume retention can lead to reflux and hydroureter or hydronephrosis and renal injury if left unchecked.

Treatment

Bladder drainage to relieve retention is the first priority. Self-intermittent or prolonged catheterization may be necessary, depending on resolution of the inciting cause. In cases of postoperative urinary retention, bladder function can be evaluated by serial postvoid residual urine determinations. Although no normal volume for residual urine is universally accepted, it less than 100 mL is generally considered to be within normal limits and greater than 150 mL is considered abnormal. More than one value is needed because per-

sistently high residual volumes will require prolonged catheterization.

When urinary retention occurs in the setting of neurologic disease, diabetes, or stroke, correction of the underlying cause is often impossible; therefore, the goal is to prevent injury or damage to the upper urinary tract. Intermittent self-catheterization is preferable to an indwelling catheter, which may predispose to infection, bladder spasms, or erosion.

Medical therapy may assist in the care of these patients. Acetylcholine agonists can stimulate detrusor contractions in patients that have vesical areflexia. α-Adrenergic blockers can facilitate bladder emptying by relaxing tone at the bladder neck.

Behavior modification in the form of timed voiding on a preset schedule to empty regardless of urge will prevent accumulation of excess urine. Usually a voiding pattern of every 2–3 hours is preferable. In bladder areflexia, manual pressure or abdominal splinting may facilitate emptying.

BYPASS INCONTINENCE

Urinary loss due to abnormal anatomic variations is uncommon but extremely important to consider in the evaluation of the incontinent woman. Bypass incontinence may often mimic other forms of urinary incontinence but usually presents as constant dribbling or dampness. Patients may complain of positional loss of urine without urge or forewarning. Diagnosing this type of incontinence requires a high level of suspicion and an understanding of the underlying anatomic deviation in the lower urinary tract. Genitourinary fistulas (vesicovaginal or ureterovaginal) can be a debilitating cause of incontinence and are formed because of poor wound healing after a traumatic insult (eg, obstetric laceration, pelvic surgery, perineal trauma, or radiation exposure). Leakage due to fistulas is generally continuous, although it may be elicited by position change or stress-inducing activities. Evaluation should include a careful examination of the vaginal walls for fistulas. This can be facilitated by filling the bladder with milk or dilute indigo carmine dye and looking for pooling in the vaginal canal. Pad testing can be performed by having the patient ingest 200 mg of oral phenazopyridine hydrochloride (Pyridium) several hours before a subsequent examination. By placing a tampon in the vagina and on the perineum, the diagnosis may be confirmed by inspection of the pads after a period of time. Further imaging (intravenous urography) and cystoscopy can identify the exact location of the aberrant communication. If diagnosis is made early, the fistulous tract may heal with prolonged catheterization. However, if this procedure is unsuccessful or if diagnosis is made late, surgical correction is generally the only hope for cure.

DIVERTICULUM

Another important but uncommon cause of involuntary urine loss is urethral diverticula. Diverticula are essentially weaknesses or "hernias" in the supportive fascial layer of the bladder or urethra. Urethral diverticulum is most likely to cause symptoms of urinary loss. It has an incidence of 0.3–3% in women and is thought to be largely an acquired condition resulting from obstruction and expansion of the paraurethral Skene's glands. The symptoms of constant small amounts of leakage or urethral discharge are often described. A suburethral mass is visible and palpable on physical examination. Urine or discharge may often be "milked" by palpation of the suburethral mass. Treatment is usually surgical excision of the diverticulum.

FUNCTIONAL AND TRANSIENT INCONTINENCE

Incontinence may be caused by factors outside the lower urinary tract and is particularly significant in the geriatric population, because often a multitude of special circumstances affect the health of the elderly. Physical impairment, cognitive function, medication, systemic illness, and bowel function are all factors that may contribute to incontinence. Many immobile patients are incontinent because of the inability to toilet. Cognitive disturbances limit a patient's ability to respond normally to the sensation to void. Numerous medications have effects on the bladder that may reduce capacity, inhibit bladder function, increase diuresis and bladder load, or relax the urinary sphincter. Additionally, stool impaction and constipation both have been associated with increased prevalence of urinary incontinence. Treatments should first identify the etiologic factors of the incontinence and then reduce or remove the cause.

REFERENCES

Abrams P et al: The standardisation of terminology in lower urinary tract function: Report from the standardisation sub-committee of the International Continence Society. Urology 2003;61:37.

Diokno A et al: Prevention of urinary incontinence by behavioral modification program: A randomized, controlled trial among older women in the community. J Urol 2004;171:1165.

Diokno AC et al, OPERA Study Group: Prospective, randomized, double-blind study of the efficacy and tolerability of the extended-release formulations of oxybutynin and tolterodine for overactive bladder: Results of the OPERA trial. Mayo Clin Proc 2003;78:687.

Goode PS et al: Effect of behavioral training with or without pelvic floor electrical stimulation on stress incontinence in women: A randomized controlled trial. JAMA 2003;290:345.

Hofmeyr GJ, Hannah ME: Planned caesarean section for term breech delivery. Cochrane Database Syst Rev 2003;(3):CD000166.

Holmgren C et al: Long-term results with tension-free vaginal tape on mixed and stress urinary incontinence. Obstet Gynecol 2005;106:38.

Holroyd-Leduc JM, Straus SE: Management of urinary incontinence in women: Scientific review. JAMA 2004;291:986.

Hunskaar S et al: Epidemiology and natural history of urinary incontinence. Int Urogynecol J Pelvic Floor Dysfunct 2000; 11:301.

Rortveit G et al: Urinary incontinence after vaginal delivery or cesarean section. N Engl J Med 2003;348:900.

Ulmsten U: An introduction to tension-free vaginal tape (TVT)— A new surgical procedure for treatment of female urinary incontinence. Int Urogynecol J Pelvic Floor Dysfunct 2001; 12(Suppl 2):S3.

Ward K, Hilton P, United Kingdom and Ireland Tension Free Vaginal Tape Trial Group: Prospective multicentre randomised trial of tension-free vaginal tape and colposuspension as primary treatment for stress incontinence. BMJ 2002;325:67.

Weidner AC et al: Which women with stress incontinence require urodynamic evaluation? Am J Obstet Gynecol 2001; 184:20.

WEBSITE RESOURCES

National Association for Continence: www.nafc.org
The Simon Foundation: www.simonfoundation.org
American Urogyneoclogic Society: www.augs.org

Perioperative Considerations in Gynecologic Surgery

Mikio Nihira, MD, MPH, Muriel Boreham, MD, & Peter Drewes, MD

The gynecologic surgeon focuses on the normal and pathologic anatomy and function of the female reproductive system. However, because no organ system functions independently, the gynecologist must also be familiar with many pathologic conditions not directly related to the reproductive system. At no time is this more crucial than during the perioperative period, i.e., just before, during, and immediately after gynecologic surgery.

The differential diagnosis of abdominopelvic pain and dysfunction not directly related to the reproductive system must be fully understood by the gynecologist because many of these entities can present with symptoms suggestive of uterine or adnexal origin. Conversely, the first evidence of nongynecologic disease may be an alteration in the function of the female reproductive system.

This chapter covers the perioperative period: the decision to operate (emergently or electively), and the pre- and immediate postoperative management of these patients. Selected medical and surgical disorders of importance to the gynecologist are reviewed as they relate to management of the surgical patient.

■ ACUTE ABDOMEN

ESSENTIALS OF DIAGNOSIS

Essential Elements:
- *Acute onset of severe abdominal pain.*
- *Signs of peritoneal irritation with guarding and rebound tenderness.*

Frequently Seen:
- *Anemia or hypovolemic shock if intraperitoneal hemorrhage exists.*
- *Varying degrees of gastrointestinal irritation, nausea, and vomiting.*

- *Elevated white blood cell count (if cause is inflammatory or infectious).*
- *Fever (occasionally).*
- *Possible complication of pregnancy.*

General Considerations

The diagnosis of acute abdomen has traditionally been based on signs and symptoms of peritonitis, which can be caused by a diverse array of disease processes. Although the acute abdomen always requires an immediate surgical or medical decision, some patients suffer from a major intra-abdominal pathologic process not associated with peritonitis and should not be considered to have an acute abdomen. An example is the patient with acute gastrointestinal bleeding who requires emergency care but does not have an acute abdomen in the strictest sense. Although the acute abdomen is not precisely defined, a number of signs and symptoms generally accompany this diagnosis (Table 46–1).

It is important to note that although many physicians perceive the acute abdomen as a problem always requiring surgical intervention, in many instances medical management is more appropriate. The presence of an acute abdomen does not dictate the type of management, only the need to come to a rapid decision and implement appropriate therapy as expeditiously as possible.

Finally, it should be stated that an abdomen with generalized peritonitis in all four quadrants is commonly termed a "surgical abdomen." If the patient has a rigid abdomen with guarding and rebound tenderness in all four quadrants, a clear diagnosis usually cannot be achieved except in the operating room. Ultrasonography, computed tomography (CT), culdocentesis, and other routine tests can often establish whether the process is hemorrhagic or inflammatory, but the specific diagnosis can typically be determined only during laparotomy or laparoscopy.

Table 46–1. Differential diagnosis of acute gynecologic intra-abdominal disease.

	Clinical and Laboratory Findings						
Disease	CBC	Urinalysis	Pregnancy Test	Ultrasound	Culdocentesis	Fever	Nausea and Vomiting
Ruptured ectopic pregnancy	Hematocrit low after treatment of hypovolemia.	Red blood cells rare.	Positive. β-hCG low for gestational age.	Possible adnexal mass. Possible sac-like decidual reaction in uterus. Possible increased free fluid in cul-de-sac.	High hematocrit. Defibrinated, non-clotting sample with no platelets. Crenated red blood cells.	No.	Unusual.
Salpingitis	Rising white blood cell count.	White blood cells occasionally present.	Generally negative.	Negative unless pyosalpinx or tubo-ovarian abscess present.	Yellow, turbid fluid with many white blood cells and some bacteria.	Progressively worsening. Spiking.	Gradual onset with ileus.
Ruptured ovarian cyst (hemorrhagic)	Hematocrit may be low after treatment of hypovolemia.	Normal.	Usually negative.	No masses. Increase free fluid in cul-de-sac.	Hematocrit generally less than 10%.	No.	Rare.
Ruptured ovarian cyst (non-hemorrhagic)	Normal.	Normal.	Generally negative	No masses. Increased free fluid in cul-de-sac.	Increased clear fluid.	No.	Rare.
Torsion of adnexa	Normal or elevated white blood cell count with necrosis.	Normal.	Generally negative.	Adnexal mass common. Decreased flow on Doppler study.	Minimal clear fluid if obtained early.	Possibly with necrosis.	Possibly.
Degenerating leiomyoma	Normal or elevated white blood cell count.	Normal.	Generally negative.	Pedunculated or uterine mass often with central fluid areas.	Normal clear fluid.	Possibly.	Rare.

The patient with a surgical abdomen should never be delayed. The operating room should be notified, large-bore intravenous access obtained, and blood work, including a complete blood count (CBC) and blood for cross-matching, should be sent as the patient is being moved to the operating room. This is the exceptional case that demands the gynecologic surgeon's total attention and skills. For most patients with localized peritoni-tis, however, a diagnosis can be made outside the operating room, allowing more time for consideration of therapeutic options.

Etiology and Pathogenesis

The acute abdomen can be caused by a wide variety of problems. Their similar clinical presentation reflects the stimulation of pain receptors in the peritoneum by leakage of purulent matter into the peritoneal cavity, intraperitoneal bleeding, necrosis of an intra-abdominal structure, or inflammation because of infection. Stomach acid, bile, and pancreatic secretions cause intense peritoneal irritation when released into the peritoneal cavity, but urine and ascitic fluid generally do not.

Clinical Findings

A. SYMPTOMS AND SIGNS

The most common symptom of a patient with acute abdomen is pain. It can be generalized or have a maximum intensity in a specific area. The presence of guarding, rebound tenderness, or referred tenderness on abdominal examination can be helpful in localizing the area of greatest peritoneal irritation. On pelvic examination, the patient may exhibit uterine motion tenderness. Although commonly associated with pelvic inflammatory disease, this sign is nonspecific and is likely to be present with a number of irritative pelvic processes.

The irritated peritoneum is most sensitive to stretching and movement, so patients often minimize motion to reduce these stimuli. The patient's position may provide a useful clue to the site of greatest irritation. Patients with pelvic peritonitis are frequently most comfortable with one or both hips flexed, depending on the site and extent of the peritonitis.

The quality of the patient's pain is important. Patients with intermittent torsion of the adnexa or ruptured ovarian cyst may have had such pain before. The temporal relationship of the onset of pain to the patient's last menstrual period may give valuable clues, especially regarding possible complications of early pregnancy.

Gastrointestinal symptoms that often accompany the acute abdomen are anorexia, nausea, vomiting, and/or diarrhea. The extent of bowel involvement depends on the severity of the peritonitis. Patients with mild bowel irritation note decreased appetite. Nausea and vomiting may develop as the bowel becomes more directly involved in the inflammatory process. Further progression leads to inhibition of peristalsis with associated abdominal distention secondary to gas- and fluid-filled loops of bowel. As peristalsis decreases, bowel sounds may be decreased, and eventually may be absent. High-pitched bowel sounds and rushes may be heard if obstruction is present.

If the peritoneum covering the bladder or rectosigmoid is irritated first, the patient's initial complaint may be of painful bladder or bowel function. It can be a mistake to assume that a patient complaining of painful bladder filling and emptying merely has cystitis. For example, it is not unusual for a patient to note an episode of urinary or bowel urgency at the time of initial rupture of an ectopic pregnancy or an ovarian cyst.

When taking the history, keep in mind the progression and timing of the appearance of the patient's symptoms. When performing the physical examination, it is necessary to realize that the patient has an evolving process occurring, and a single examination only assesses one stage of that process. Several serial examinations may be necessary to guide clinical decision making.

B. LABORATORY FINDINGS

Routine laboratory studies for all women with pelvic peritonitis should include CBC, urinalysis, and rapid pregnancy test. The CBC may demonstrate either acute blood loss or, if the white blood cell count is elevated, an infectious process.

A rapid, reliable pregnancy test should always be performed immediately in the female patient with pelvic pain. A patient whose history suggests salpingitis may actually have a ruptured ectopic pregnancy. In addition, a pregnancy may coexist with an independent pathologic process, in which case the pregnancy may influence management. For example, elective surgery for a degenerating leiomyoma in a pregnant patient should be deferred until the second trimester if possible.

Urinalysis may demonstrate urinary tract infection, but pyuria may also result from an abscess adjacent to the ureter, as occurs in ruptured retrocecal appendicitis. Gross or microscopic hematuria can reflect the passage of a stone, or perhaps exacerbation of an underlying pathologic process such as interstitial cystitis.

Patients with diabetic ketoacidosis may present with severe acute abdominal pain, making testing the blood and urine for glucose and ketones essential. It is also possible for the stress of an acute abdomen from other causes to initiate or aggravate ketoacidosis in a normally well-controlled diabetic patient. Prior to operating on such patients every effort must be made to fully correct their fluid, glucose, electrolyte, and acidotic status.

Cervical cultures for *Neisseria gonorrhoeae* and *Chlamydia trachomatis* should also be obtained. Although not useful for immediate management decisions, they may aid in guiding antibiotic therapy if the patient is determined to have a pelvic infection. The erythrocyte sedimentation rate is a nonspecific test for the presence of inflammation and is not very useful in the initial evaluation of the acute abdomen.

C. SPECIAL EXAMINATIONS

1. Culdocentesis—Culdocentesis is an easily performed and important diagnostic procedure that is often overlooked in the modern era of high-resolution imaging studies, but it may be useful when those studies are not available. The contents of the peritoneal cavity can be evaluated by means of culdocentesis in any patient with pelvic peritonitis or pain during uterine and adnexal movement.

Clear, straw-colored peritoneal fluid represents a negative culdocentesis, indicating no intraperitoneal bleeding. An unruptured ectopic gestation could still be present. Large amounts of fluid of this type can indicate a ruptured, nonhemorrhagic ovarian cyst or ascites. Turbid peritoneal fluid containing white blood cells on Gram-stained smear suggests an intrapelvic inflammatory process.

A bloody, nonclotting peritoneal fluid sample with a hematocrit in the range of 15–40% reflects recent hemorrhage into the peritoneal cavity, possibly from ruptured ectopic pregnancy or a bleeding ovarian cyst. In this case, prior clotting of blood in the peritoneal cavity results in crenated red blood cells, defibrination, absence of platelets, and lack of clotting factors in the hemorrhagic fluid aspirated from the cul-de-sac. A bloody aspirate that forms a clot may represent blood inadvertently drawn from vaginal or uterine vessels. An attempted culdocentesis that returns no fluid at all is termed "nondiagnostic."

Given the increasing availability of transvaginal ultrasonography, the role of culdocentesis for the detection of hemoperitoneum is currently being reassessed. A review of 252 consecutive cases, in which patients underwent culdocentesis and subsequent surgery for presumed ectopic pregnancy revealed that 86% of the patients with a positive culdocentesis had a hemoperitoneum. However, 25 of the 42 patients with a negative result from culdocentesis were found to have a hemoperitoneum, a false-negative rate of 54%.

More recently, another study compared the sensitivity and specificity of culdocentesis and transvaginal ultrasound to identify hemoperitoneum. Among 46 patients who underwent surgery for the treatment of suspected ectopic pregnancy, the presence of "echogenic fluid" on transvaginal ultrasound had a sensitivity of 95% and a specificity of 100% for the detection of hemoperitoneum. A positive culdocentesis was found to have a sensitivity of 62% and a specificity of 89% for the detection of hemoperitoneum. Because culdocentesis is an invasive procedure whose sensitivity may be lower than previously thought, it should be primarily used when transvaginal ultrasound is not available.

2. Radiographic studies—Transvaginal and transabdominal ultrasound studies have become extremely useful over the past decade for diagnosis of the acute abdomen. In the pelvis, ultrasonography is useful for characterizing the location and gestational age of early pregnancies, identifying adnexal or uterine masses, and determining the presence or absence of pelvic abscesses or excessive free fluid in the cul-de-sac. Outside the pelvis, ultrasonography is often the initial diagnostic modality used to investigate possible cholecystitis, choledocholithiasis, and appendicitis. In patients too uncomfortable to allow adequate abdominal or biman-

ual pelvic examination, ultrasound examination plays an even more important role. A number of CT techniques have also proved useful in the evaluation of the acute abdomen.

Plain radiograph films of the abdomen are less helpful in diagnosing gynecologic causes of acute abdomen, but may be helpful in detecting bowel obstruction or paralytic ileus if dilated loops of bowel with air-fluid levels are seen. Free air under the diaphragm on an upright film indicates perforation of a viscus organ and requires immediate intervention. An upright film that does not show the diaphragms should be considered inadequate in the work-up of the acute abdomen. Occasionally, loss of the psoas shadow on the right side is seen, supporting a diagnosis of appendicitis. In addition, renal calculi may be seen on plain films.

3. Microbiologic studies—In the acute patient, Gram stains and cultures assume a role of lesser importance. Cervical cultures for *N. gonorrhoeae* should be done; however, because this organism can be found on the cervix of asymptomatic as well as symptomatic patients, Gram-stained smears of cervical secretions to detect gram-negative diplococci may be unreliable. Finding *N. gonorrhoeae* on the cervix does not prove that peritonitis is caused by salpingitis. Conversely, many patients with laparoscopically proven pelvic infections have negative cervical cultures. In the patient who proves to have salpingitis, cervical cultures or cultures of washings done at laparoscopy may help to sharpen the focus of subsequent antibiotic therapy. Cervical material should be submitted for culture in all patients suspected of having gonococcal salpingitis, if only to determine the need for treatment of the sexual partner. Chlamydial culture or enzymatic assay is frequently done as well.

GYNECOLOGIC CAUSES OF ACUTE ABDOMEN

Ruptured ectopic pregnancy, salpingitis, and hemorrhagic ovarian cyst are the three most commonly diagnosed gynecologic conditions presenting as acute abdomen in the emergency room. Degenerating leiomyomas occur less frequently. Table 46–1 lists typical clinical and laboratory findings for these conditions. These gynecologic entities are discussed fully in their respective chapters.

Torsion, or twisting, of the ovary or both the ovary and tube is an unusual cause of acute abdomen. The most common etiology is ovarian enlargement by a benign mass. Patients present with acute, severe abdominal, pelvic pain which may be accompanied by nausea and vomiting. With progressive torsion venous and lymphatic obstruction occurs. Interruption of the arterial supply may follow, resulting in hypoxia, necrosis, fever and leukocytosis. Diagnosis is aided by ultrasound, where an adnexal mass is usually seen. Management is surgical. In a patient of reproductive age with a benign mass, it is acceptable to untwist the ovary and if the ovary is viable, remove the mass and stabilize the remaining ovary with sutures.

The challenge of the acute abdomen is expeditious arrival at an accurate diagnosis and the rapid implementation of a treatment plan. The gynecologist may be the only physician to evaluate the patient and must be capable of entertaining all possible diagnoses in the differential—both gynecologic and nongynecologic. The next section and Table 46–2 review the most common nongynecologic entities that need to be considered by the gynecologist evaluating the patient with an acute abdomen.

NONGYNECOLOGIC CAUSES OF ACUTE ABDOMEN

1. Appendicitis

More than 10% of the general population will develop appendicitis at some time in their lives. Appendicitis is widely recognized as a disease of childhood and is the most common reason for laparotomy in infants and children. In the older patient, however, appendicitis can manifest later and in a more subtle fashion. This can be of great clinical significance in these patients, who often have other significant underlying diseases. It is wise to consider the possibility of appendicitis in every patient—regardless of age—who presents in the emergency room with an acute abdomen.

In pregnancy the need to consider appendicitis is of paramount importance. One researcher found in a 10-year experience at a large teaching hospital a perinatal mortality rate of less than 3% for uncomplicated appendicitis as well as for negative laparotomy. When perforation occurred before surgery, the perinatal mortality rate rose to 20%. As the researcher put it, "the maxim regarding acute appendicitis—if in doubt, take it out—is never more true than in pregnancy."

Clinical Findings

A. SYMPTOMS AND SIGNS

It is prudent for the gynecologist to remember that the patient may not present with the "classic" symptoms of appendicitis, but may present with many variations that closely mimic other diagnostic entities.

The patient's first symptom may be nausea and loss of appetite. Pain typically begins in the periumbilical area and then gradually shifts to the right lower quadrant. Fever is usually not significant unless the appendix has ruptured. Bowel sounds are reduced, and often no bowel movement will have occurred since the onset of pain. After the patient's pain migrates to the right lower quadrant, tenderness to palpation is most severe at McBurney's point, approximately 5 cm medial to the right anterior superior iliac spine on a line between the anterior superior iliac spine and the umbilicus. As inflammation increases, guarding and rebound tenderness appear at this location. Palpation in the left lower quadrant may produce referred pain in the right lower quadrant.

Some patients note marked discomfort upon uterine motion, as well as right adnexal tenderness on pelvic examination. These symptoms develop because the inflamed appendix irritates the peritoneum adjacent to the uterus and oviduct, and they may be improperly interpreted as signs of salpingitis. The patient is generally most comfortable in the supine position with the right hip flexed to minimize tension on the peritoneum adjacent to the appendix.

B. LABORATORY FINDINGS

The CBC may be normal, but an elevated white blood cell count may develop, especially after rupture of the appendix. Urinalysis results are usually normal unless the inflamed appendix rests adjacent to the ureter, or unless an abscess has formed near the ureter, producing pyuria. If the pregnancy test is positive, the presentation of appendicitis may be significantly altered.

C. RADIOLOGIC FINDINGS

High-resolution ultrasonography with graded compression has proven useful in the diagnosis of acute appendicitis. In one study, researchers claimed a diagnostic sensitivity varying from 80–95%, a specificity of 95–100%, and an accuracy rate of 91–95%. Ultrasonography also allows some differentiation between the acute appendix and the gangrenous and perforated appendix.

X-ray films of the abdomen may demonstrate an oval calcified fecalith up to 1–2 cm in diameter in the right lower quadrant. A dilated, gas-filled "sentinel loop" of the bowel may also be seen as a result of localized inflammation near the cecum on plain films.

D. SPECIAL EXAMINATIONS

Culdocentesis may demonstrate straw-colored, turbid peritoneal fluid containing numerous white blood cells. This finding is not diagnostic for appendicitis but merely reflects the existence of an intraperitoneal inflammatory process; similar findings may be seen in salpingitis and acute regional enteritis.

Laparoscopy may be appropriate in young, nulligravid patients in whom a missed diagnosis may have an adverse effect on future fertility. Considerable technical skill may

Table 46–2. Differential diagnosis of acute nongynecologic intra-abdominal disease.

Disease	CBC	Urinalysis	Pregnancy Test	Culdocentesis	Fever	Nausea and Vomiting
			Clinical and Laboratory Findings			
Appendicitis	Normal early; high white blood cell count later.	Normal.	If patient is pregnant, presentation of disease is atypical.	Yellow, turbid fluid with many white blood cells and no bacteria.	Not early in course.	Yes.
Retrocecal appendicitis	Normal early; high white blood cell count later.	Many white blood cells if abscess forms.	Not helpful.	May be normal.	Yes in advanced diseases.	Variable.
Regional enteritis (Crohn's disease)	High white blood cell count.	Normal.	Not helpful.	Yellow, turbid fluid with many white blood cells.	Yes if severe.	Yes if severe. Recent history of diarrhea.
Colonic diverticulitis	High white blood cell count.	Normal.	Not helpful.	Yellow, turbid fluid with many white blood cells and no bacteria.	Yes if severe.	Variable.
Bowel obstruction	High if ischemic bowel damage is present.	Normal.	Not helpful.	Increased amount of fluid with many white blood cells if bowel is ischemic.	Only if bowel is ischemic.	Yes.

be required to establish or rule out a diagnosis of appendicitis, depending on the location of the appendix and other intra-abdominal conditions. Removal of the appendix through the laparoscope may then also be possible as well.

Differential Diagnosis

On the basis of physical examination alone, it may be difficult to distinguish acute salpingitis from appendicitis. The irritation associated with pelvic inflammatory disease usually extends to both lower quadrants unless unilateral salpingitis (possibly associated with an intrauterine device) is suspected. In contrast to the patient with appendicitis, the patient with salpingitis is more likely to have a fever with an elevated white blood cell count at an earlier stage of her disease. The woman with salpingitis usually develops gastrointestinal symptoms later, as pelvic inflammation spreads from the oviducts to secondarily involve the bowel in the pelvic cavity.

A history of early gastrointestinal symptoms, decreased appetite, and nausea and vomiting are often the most reliable factors in establishing a diagnosis of appendicitis rather than early pelvic inflammatory disease.

The possibility of a ruptured right ovarian cyst must be entertained as well.

In the emergency setting, it is occasionally impossible to differentiate appendicitis from acute regional enteritis (Crohn's disease) with involvement of the terminal ileum. At laparotomy for suspected appendicitis in the patient with regional enteritis, the appendix is normal but the terminal ileum is inflamed. In contrast to the patient with appendicitis, a patient with regional enteritis usually has a history of recent diarrhea (Table 46–2).

Ruptured retrocecal appendicitis may be misdiagnosed as pyelonephritis. The fever, nausea, right-sided back pain, and pyuria from a retrocecal abscess may be mistakenly assumed to be of renal origin.

In the pregnant patient, the enlarging uterus displaces the appendix upward, thereby changing the site of the pain of appendicitis. Pregnant patients with appendicitis also demonstrate less dramatic gastrointestinal symptoms and may even continue to have an appetite. For these reasons, the diagnosis of appendicitis in the pregnant patient is much more likely to be made after appendiceal rupture and abscess formation have occurred than in the nonpregnant patient. This most often leads to premature labor. The risk of early surgical intervention in the gravid patient must be weighed against the considerable risk of premature delivery if appendicitis is indeed present and rupture occurs.

Treatment

The diagnosis of acute appendicitis requires immediate surgical removal of the appendix either by laparotomy or laparoscopy.

Complications

Early diagnosis and surgery are essential to prevent rupture of the appendix and the possible complications of recurrent pelvic abscess, wound infection, pelvic adhesions, and occasionally, infertility.

2. Acute Bowel Obstruction

Bowel obstruction may result from an intrinsic or extrinsic expanding neoplasm, compression of a segment of bowel by a hernia, constriction of the lumen by extrinsic bowel adhesions, or volvulus or intussusception of a segment of bowel. Because of the wide range of causes, all age groups or populations should be considered at risk for development of bowel obstruction. The cause is often not clear until laparotomy is performed. Obstruction caused by adhesions is always a possibility if the patient has undergone previous abdominal surgery, especially if the previous surgery was complicated by peritonitis.

Clinical Findings

A. Symptoms and Signs

Nausea and vomiting associated with abdominal distention and severe abdominal pain are the hallmarks of bowel obstruction. Bowel sounds may be absent if obstruction is total, or high-pitched if it is partial. The patient may complain of constipation and usually ceases to have bowel movements. A hernia or abdominal mass may be evident on physical examination. Abdominal palpation produces guarding and rebound tenderness.

B. Laboratory Findings

Loss of hydrochloric acid through protracted vomiting results in alkalosis with respiratory compensation. Serum bicarbonate levels may be high. Serum potassium levels may be low, indicating general depletion of electrolytes.

C. X-Ray Findings

A supine x-ray view of the abdomen demonstrates one or more loops of gas-filled bowel. Air-fluid levels are evident in these loops in upright films (Fig 46–1).

Nasogastric tube

R

Air-fluid levels

Figure 46–1. Upright abdominal film demonstrating air-fluid levels in a patient subsequently found to have small-bowel obstruction.

Differential Diagnosis

Peritonitis with secondary inhibition of peristalsis, generally termed paralytic ileus, must be distinguished from bowel obstruction. The patient with paralytic ileus usually experiences constant abdominal pain rather than the cramping abdominal pain associated with bowel obstruction. Treatment of the condition causing peritonitis also results in gradual resolution of paralytic ileus.

Complications

Marked distention of a segment of bowel may result in vascular compromise, strangulation, and, eventually, bowel perforation with spillage of toxic bowel contents into the abdominal cavity. Dehydration and loss of electrolytes are associated with accumulation of fluid within the bowel lumen. Hypokalemia may produce electrocardiographic abnormalities if the serum potassium level is lower than 3 mEq/L.

Treatment

Nasogastric suction may be effective in decompressing the distended bowel and may relieve the persistent vomiting and cramping pain associated with bowel obstruction. Surgical correction of the structural abnormality responsible for obstruction is the only definitive treatment. Partial bowel obstruction caused by adhesions occasionally subsides while the patient is undergoing nasogastric or long-tube suction. Fluid or electrolyte imbalance must also be corrected, and losses must be compensated for during prolonged suction drainage. Evidence of a perforated viscus organ requires immediate surgical intervention.

3. Inflammatory Bowel Disease (Ulcerative Colitis & Regional Enteritis [Crohn's Disease])

Ulcerative colitis and regional enteritis represent two distinct forms of inflammatory bowel disease. Inflammation restricted to the colon is termed ulcerative colitis. Regional enteritis (Crohn's disease, terminal ileitis) is characterized by multiple sites of small bowel or colonic inflammation, especially in the terminal ileum. Women are twice as likely to develop regional enteritis but carry the same risk as men for ulcerative colitis. Inflammatory bowel disease is most likely to develop during the reproductive years.

Clinical Findings

A. SYMPTOMS AND SIGNS

Patients suffering from inflammatory bowel disease generally complain of episodic bloody diarrhea and abdominal pain. Abdominal guarding and rebound tenderness are noted on palpation of the localized area of peritonitis associated with the inflamed segment of bowel. The severity of recurrent episodes of abdominal pain and diarrhea varies widely. Acute regional enteritis with terminal ileitis may mimic appendicitis, although the patient with acute regional enteritis is far more likely to give a history of recent diarrhea.

B. LABORATORY FINDINGS

The CBC generally shows an elevated white blood cell count with an increased number of polymorphonuclear leukocytes. Culdocentesis should be avoided if inflammatory bowel disease is suspected. If done, however, it would yield turbid fluid containing numerous white cells—largely a result of inflammatory transudate from the inflamed bowel.

C. X-RAY FINDINGS

Barium enema and an upper gastrointestinal study with small-bowel follow-through may demonstrate either mucosal changes of the bowel consistent with acute inflammation, or induration and narrowing of bowel segments, suggesting chronic disease. Involvement of only one segment of colon suggests a diagnosis of ulcerative colitis; multiple sites of involvement, often including the terminal ileum, suggest regional enteritis. X-ray studies may be normal in patients with early or inactive inflammatory bowel disease.

D. SPECIAL EXAMINATIONS

Endoscopic evaluation with biopsy of areas of inflamed bowel mucosa is the most direct method of diagnosis.

Differential Diagnosis

Appendicitis, diverticulitis, torsion of the adnexa, and salpingitis may produce physical findings similar to those of acute terminal ileitis. Because of the great difference in appropriate therapy for each of these conditions and because of the serious results of inappropriate treatment, each disease must be ruled out whenever the diagnosis of acute inflammatory bowel disease is suspected.

Complications

Perforation of the colon and small bowel fistulas are serious inflammatory complications. Appendectomy in a patient with terminal ileitis carries an additional risk of poor healing, abscess formation, and fistula development, especially if the cecum and base of the appendix are involved in the inflammatory process.

Treatment

Acute inflammatory bowel disease generally responds to administration of corticosteroids. Intravenous metronidazole has been effective in some patients with acute illness. Recurrence may be prevented by long-term administration of sulfasalazine. Therapy is complex, however, and should be directed by a gastroenterologist. Surgical excision of segments of inflamed bowel may be appropriate in cases of stricture with obstruction, perforation, or massive hemorrhage, or in severe cases unresponsive to corticosteroids. Reanastomosis of bowel after resection for inflammatory bowel disease is often unsuccessful, and resection fails to prevent recurrence, which often occurs just proximal to the anastomotic site. Supportive care, including intravenous fluids, electrolytes, transfusion, antibiotics if sepsis is present, and nutritional replacement for patients with malabsorption, are essential general measures.

4. Colonic Diverticulitis

Diverticula of the distal colon are uncommon in women during the reproductive years, but as many as one-third of postmenopausal women have colonic diverticula demonstrable by barium enema or colonoscopy. Colonic diverticula appear to result from herniation of the bowel mucosa at a site of weakness of the colonic muscularis. The mucosa may be disrupted as the diverticulum enlarges, with resulting bleeding or localized infection. Bleeding may require partial colonic resection. Superficial infection may be self-limiting and associated with mild left lower quadrant pain, which spontaneously subsides as the bowel mucosa heals over a period of 2 or 3 days. Broad-spectrum antibiotics may be necessary if the patient with diverticulitis develops severe left lower quadrant pain, guarding, rebound tenderness, fever, and leukocytosis. Patients not responding to antibiotics or patients with associated pelvic abscess formation require surgical management, including drainage of the pelvic abscess, temporary colostomy, and possible resection of the segment of inflamed or obstructed colon. The surgeon must also rule out carcinoma of the colon, especially in the case of bowel obstruction.

5. Meckel's Diverticulitis

Meckel's diverticulum, a remnant of the vitelline duct, is found in 2–3% of the general population but is three times more common in men than in women. The diverticulum is generally found on the antimesenteric surface of the small bowel, about 8 cm from the ileocecal valve, although the exact distance from the cecum varies greatly. Ectopic secretory gastric mucosa may be found in 20% of patients with Meckel's diverticulum.

If secretory gastric mucosa is present in the diverticulum, ulceration of adjacent bowel mucosa may result in bleeding. Bleeding is an indication for laparotomy in 50% of patients subjected to surgery for complications arising from Meckel's diverticulum. Intestinal obstruction from intussusception of Meckel's diverticulum or obstruction due to volvulus around a vestigial band from the diverticulum to the umbilicus is the reason for an additional 25% of surgical procedures, and Meckel's diverticulitis is the reason for the remaining 25% of surgical cases.

Meckel's diverticulitis is associated with symptoms similar to those of appendicitis, except that abdominal pain is located more medially. Inflamed Meckel's diverticulum may rupture earlier than an inflamed appendix. If the cause of inflammatory peritonitis is unclear at the time of laparotomy, it is important to inspect the entire length of the small bowel for a possible inflamed Meckel's diverticulum. An inflamed Meckel's diverticulum should be resected. The base of the diverticulum may be broader than the base of the appendix, so simple ligation may not be possible.

6. Nephrolithiasis

Various metabolic factors, in combination with dehydration, may frequently produce supersaturated solutions of relatively insoluble substances that subsequently crystallize in the urine. Men are two to three times more likely than women to develop calcium renal stone disease. The

less-frequently detected struvite (magnesium-ammonium-phosphate), uric acid, and cystine stones are associated with chronic *Proteus* infection of the urinary tract, gout, and cystinuria, respectively.

Clinical Findings

A. Symptoms and Signs

Renal stones may be discovered in any portion of the urinary tract but are most likely to be symptomatic in the ureter. A renal stone passing from the ureteropelvic junction to the bladder usually causes severe ureteral spasm. Ureteral colic generally radiates from the flank on the affected side to the labia or bladder and may occur episodically over several hours or days until the stone passes into the bladder. Although the pain is usually prostrating, the patient experiences no peritonitis and may sometimes be able to remain mobile during the attack. A renal stone may remain lodged at the ureterovesical junction for a long time. In a patient with partial ureteral obstruction, symptoms caused by a renal stone at the ureterovesical junction may mimic the urinary frequency, urgency, bladder discomfort, and hematuria of hemorrhagic cystitis.

Abdominal and pelvic examinations remain normal during an acute attack of ureteral colic, but gentle flank percussion worsens ureteral pain.

B. Laboratory Findings

The most helpful initial laboratory test is evaluation for hematuria; blood is found in the urine sample of every patient with a renal stone unless total ureteral obstruction exists. Abdominal x-rays are helpful in locating calcium- and magnesium-containing stones. An intravenous pyelogram is useful in assessing ureteral obstruction and secondary renal structural damage. Intravenous pyelogram may also be necessary to locate stones not containing calcium or magnesium (< 10% of all stones), as these are not visible on x-rays. Renal ultrasonography will reveal hydronephrosis or hydroureter if distal obstruction is present.

C. Special Examinations

After acute pain has subsided, efforts should be directed toward establishing the cause of renal stone disease. All urine should be filtered to collect stones for analysis of their mineral content. Appropriate metabolic studies to detect hyperuricosuria, hypercalciuria, hyperoxaluria, etc, are dictated by the composition of the stones.

Treatment

Treatment to prevent recurrent stone formation includes correction of any metabolic abnormalities in the minority of patients who demonstrate such disorders.

The most helpful therapy for most patients appears to be conscientious efforts to maintain adequate hydration; consumption of more than 2 L of water daily is advised. Efforts to maintain hydration are especially important after meals and during the night. The pain caused by passage of a stone can be excruciating; adequate pain control is very important.

Obstructing stones lodged in the ureter must occasionally be removed surgically, either by laparotomy or through a cystoscope with the aid of a wire snare attached to a ureteral catheter. Large stones in the renal pelvis or proximal ureter may be pulverized by high-energy shockwave therapy (extracorporeal shockwave lithotripsy) to facilitate passage through the ureter.

7. Other Nongynecologic Causes

Other causes of acute onset of abdominopelvic pain in the female must also be entertained. Perforation of a peptic ulcer will allow entry of gastric secretions into the peritoneal cavity with resultant severe peritonitis. Acute cholecystitis is most often associated with right upper quadrant pain subsequent to a fatty ingestion. Always keep in mind the remote possibility of a nongynecologic intra-abdominal hemorrhage—either spontaneous or secondary to trauma. Trauma to the left upper quadrant can lead to intraperitoneal splenic hemorrhage that is delayed significantly from the event secondary to capsular containment. Sickle cell crisis can present with severe abdominal pain, as interstitial cystitis does occasionally.

THE DECISION TO OPERATE: SCHEDULED GYNECOLOGIC SURGERY

Emergent operations represent a small fraction of all the gynecologic surgical procedures performed. Most operations are planned in an elective fashion with varying degrees of urgency. The patient with a gynecologic malignancy does not have to be rushed to the operating room in the middle of the night, but will need to have her procedure planned within a reasonable period of time. On the other hand, the patient who is having a uterovaginal prolapse repaired has much more leeway to fit her operation into her life rather than having to fit her life around her operation.

Scheduled surgery allows a patient time to get mentally prepared for the procedure. Patients should be encouraged to assemble support and assistance to help with their recovery, to help cover their responsibilities at work, and to help with child care during the postoperative period. The date for an elective gynecologic procedure should always be selected by the patient for the time that is most convenient in her life.

Patients should be encouraged to optimize their physical and emotional conditions prior to scheduled surgery. There is time to attempt to stop smoking, to donate autologous blood for surgery, to lose weight, to take preoperative estrogen or iron, and to take care of any concurrent medical problems before their surgery. In addition, the option exists to postpone a patient's surgery if a respiratory infection or other medical problem develops as the date for surgery approaches.

The indications, work-ups, and operations for benign and malignant gynecologic conditions are well documented elsewhere in this text. Hysterectomy, laparoscopy, hysteroscopy, and dilatation and curettage; surgery for pelvic floor relaxation (Chapter 44); infertility surgery (Chapter 55); and surgery for urinary incontinence (Chapter 45) make up a large portion of procedures done for benign disease or dysfunction. Surgeries for gynecologic malignancies are well covered in Chapters 49 through 52.

■ PREOPERATIVE CARE

GENERAL CONSIDERATIONS IN PREOPERATIVE EVALUATION

Preoperative evaluation should include a general medical and surgical history, a complete physical examination, and appropriate laboratory tests. An anesthesiologist routinely sees patients preoperatively; however, a patient's medical status may warrant earlier consultation with an anesthesiologist and possibly with physicians in other specialties as well. The medical evaluation must be carried out in such a way as to identify all disorders that might complicate the operative procedure or convalescence. Although "diagnostic overkill" should be avoided, the responsibility of the operating gynecologist is to adequately assess—and take steps to minimize—a given patient's operative risk.

Records of prior hospitalizations should be obtained. Past records may be essential to the interpretation of present findings and may significantly influence the management plan. Patients' ability to recall illnesses and the details of previous surgeries is notoriously inaccurate.

Laboratory Studies

Although the efficacy of various preoperative testing regimens has not been established in a prospective, randomized fashion, most gynecologists would agree that preoperative laboratory studies should include, at a minimum, a CBC, a blood typing and antibody screen, and a urinalysis and culture. Further laboratory tests should be performed only when indicated by the patient's medical condition or by the type of surgery to be performed. A Papanicolaou smear should also be obtained.

A routine chest x-ray and electrocardiogram for all preoperative patients should be discouraged. One set of researchers found an overall positive yield for routine chest x-ray of 6%: 17% in patients older than 60 years of age, and 2% in patients younger than 60 years of age. Routine electrocardiograms showed an overall positive yield of 7%: 7.4% in those older than 40 years of age and 4.5% in those younger than 40 years of age. Finally, they found that investigations prompted by history or physical findings yielded a high positive rate (34% for chest x-ray and 31% for electrocardiograms) and included most of the younger patients who would be missed by an age-only criterion for preoperative testing. It seems reasonable to obtain a preoperative chest x-ray and electrocardiogram on all patients older than 45 years of age, as well as on all patients whose medical history or physical findings are matters of concern, regardless of their age.

Blood should be drawn for typing and cross-matching if a need for transfusion is anticipated, especially in patients with abnormal antibodies that would make intraoperative cross-matching time-consuming. If the patient's preoperative hematocrit and physical status permit, and if there is an appropriate interval before the anticipated surgery, the possibility of autologous blood donation should be discussed. Directed donor programs can be discussed as well.

Patients scheduled for surgery for menorrhagia with low hematocrit can often be allowed the time to build up their own blood supply through the use of a gonadotropin-releasing hormone (GnRH) agonist and iron supplementation. This can significantly lower the patient's risk for requiring transfusion by starting with a larger red blood cell mass. A GnRH agonist-induced reduction in the size of fibroids, if present, may also help reduce intraoperative blood loss or enable the patient to have a vaginal hysterectomy.

More extensive testing tailored to the individual patient's needs can improve the safety of surgical procedures. Fasting and 2-hour postprandial plasma glucose determinations are helpful to exclude diabetes. Platelet count, bleeding time, prothrombin time, and partial thromboplastin time evaluate the adequacy of the clotting system. Liver, renal, and endocrine function testing should be obtained as indicated. A patient with poor pulmonary function might benefit from a baseline arterial blood gas determination. If prolonged parenteral dependency is anticipated, a preoperative laboratory assessment of the patient's nutritional status would be useful. Liver function tests and tumor markers are often obtained in the gynecologic cancer patient (see Chapters 49–52). Finally, testing for human immunodeficiency virus (HIV) antibodies and hepatitis B surface antigen, and a serologic test for syphilis, although controversial, may also be appropriate.

Further imaging studies should be obtained only as indicated. Ultrasonography is particularly useful for characterization of pelvic masses. Important morphologic characteristics most often associated with cancer include thick septation, solid tumors and papillary projections. Ascites has been found to have a positive predictive value (95%) for ovarian cancer. Hysterosonography can be used to differentiate between endometrial polyps, focal hyperplasia, and submucosal leiomyomata, and to determine if leiomyomata can be approached hysteroscopically. CT is more commonly used to estimate the extent of ovarian cancer, and can also provide information regarding the course of the ureters and an assessment of retroperitoneal adenopathy. Intravenous pyelogram demonstrates renal function and architecture and provides information on the course of the ureters and presence of urinary tract abnormalities. Magnetic resonance imaging, with its superb soft-tissue differentiation, can give much information regarding uterine, adnexal, and retroperitoneal architecture. Its use is mainly reserved for situations with nondiagnostic ultrasound studies. It is also helpful for evaluation of colorectal endometriosis and anterior vaginal wall cysts. Double-contrast barium enema can be useful in identifying bowel lesions or colonic involvement with pelvic masses.

Imaging studies as well as functional studies (eg, pulmonary function tests, stress electrocardiograms, multichannel urodynamics, and anal manometry) are informative but costly. They should be obtained on an individualized basis when the information they yield would decrease the patient's perioperative risk, influence the choice of the surgical procedure to be performed, or increase the chances for a successful surgical outcome for the patient. See the following section on Assessment and Minimization of Surgical Risk for further discussion of the extended preoperative evaluation.

Consultations

Patients should be seen well in advance of their surgical date by a member of the anesthesia team. This allows for the optimal selection of the type of anesthesia by considering the patient's physical status, prior anesthesia history, proposed surgery, and personal preferences. Consultation also gives the anesthesia team an opportunity to allay the patient's anxieties.

Consultations with other physicians should be requested if the surgeon desires advice or assistance with a particularly high-risk surgical candidate or if the proposed procedure involves high risk. Medical preoperative consultation is of particular importance for the older surgery patient as well as the younger patient with known cardiovascular, pulmonary, renal, hematologic, or endocrinologic problems.

Preoperative urogynecologic consultation, individualized as noted in Chapter 45, can be considered in many cases requiring surgery for urinary incontinence. Consultation with a gynecologic oncologist should be considered preoperatively when the index of suspicion for malignancy is high.

Patient–Physician Communication

A. INFORMED CONSENT

It is imperative for every patient to have a complete understanding of exactly what her procedure will involve, why it is proposed, what alternatives are available, what the chances are for success, and what all the possible complications of the proposed procedure might mean to her in terms of further surgery, disability, or even death. It is important that this dialogue be carried out in lay terms in the patient's native language and that the patient have ample opportunity to ask any questions that she may have.

To document that this important interaction took place to the satisfaction of the patient, she or her legal guardian should sign a consent form or note. All major points covered in the preoperative discussion should be written on the consent form or within the consent note before it is signed by the patient and the physician. If an interpreter was used, the interpreter should sign this document as well. Permission should be considered as being granted only for the procedures discussed in the preoperative conversation and designated in the consent form or note. This includes optional procedures such as appendectomy.

B. PATIENT EDUCATION

In view of the increasing complexity of operative procedures and the associated short- and long-term risks, audiovisual aids may be helpful in the patient counseling process. These aids can supplement, but should never replace, the actual communication between the gynecologic surgeon and the patient as outlined above.

A well-prepared videotape with simple diagrams can provide a consistent, in-depth presentation. Patient education pamphlets can serve a similar function. The patient should have an opportunity to ask questions about the videotape or pamphlet, and any modifications pertinent to her particular case should be explained. As documentation that this patient education was accomplished, it is appropriate to have the patient sign a form indicating that she has viewed the videotape, discussed it with the physician, and understands its content. If necessary, the videotape and signed form may serve as evidence that adequate preoperative counseling has been provided.

C. DOCUMENTATION

All details of the history, physical examination, and diagnostic and therapeutic formulations and conclusions of all preoperative consultations must be entered in the patient's chart. This history and physical, or preoperative note, must include a problem-oriented assessment and a clearly delineated plan to address each problem. A note, or consent form as just described, documenting the scope of preoperative counseling must also be entered in the admission record. A carefully completed record is important for health care team communication and continuity of the patient's care, as well as for hospital quality assurance.

ASSESSMENT AND MINIMIZATION OF SURGICAL RISK

1. Cardiovascular System

Cardiac Disease

The perioperative period is associated with significant cardiovascular stress. Annually, it has been estimated that 1 million patients undergoing noncardiac surgery have a perioperative cardiac complication, and 50,000 of these have a myocardial infarction. Therefore, any patient with heart disease should be considered a high-risk surgical candidate and must be fully evaluated preoperatively. The goal of the preoperative cardiac evaluation is to evaluate the patient's current medical status and identify the most appropriate testing and treatment strategies to optimize care of the patient, identify short- and long-term cardiac risk, minimize cardiac risk from surgery, and yet avoid unnecessary testing and intervention in this era of cost containment. In patients with known cardiac disease, this evaluation should take place in consultation with the patient's internist or a cardiologist.

Goldman's 1977 landmark study identified patients most at risk for a perioperative cardiac ischemic event. Since then, other models have been developed to stratify perioperative cardiac risk. In 2002, the American College of Cardiology and the American Heart Association (ACC/AHA) issued a practice guideline update regarding perioperative cardiovascular evaluation in the noncardiac surgical patient. The guideline offers an algorithm for deciding which patients are candidates for preoperative cardiac testing. The algorithm takes into account clinical markers, functional capacity, and surgery-specific risk. Patients most at risk are those with a recent unstable coronary syndrome such as acute myocardial infarction (MI) less than 7 days previously, a recent MI less than 1 month previously, unstable or severe angina, evidence of a large ischemic burden, decompensated heart failure (HF), significant arrhythmias (eg, high-grade atrioventricular block, supraventricular tachycardia with uncontrolled rate), and severe valvular disease. Intermediate predictors of increased risk are mild angina, MI more than 1 month previously, compensated HF, preoperative serum creatinine ≥ 2 mg/dL, and diabetes mellitus (DM). Minor predictors of risk are advanced age, abnormal electrocardiogram (ECG), nonsinus rhythm, low functional capacity, history of stroke, and uncontrolled systemic hypertension.

Functional capacity is expressed in metabolic equivalent (MET) levels. Perioperative cardiac risk is increased in patients unable to meet a 4-MET demand. The Duke Activity Status Index is a useful scale to help determine a patient's functional status. For instance, asking a patient if she can climb a flight of stairs demonstrates at least 4-MET tolerance.

Surgery-specific cardiac risk is related to the type of surgery itself and the associated hemodynamic stress it produces intraoperatively and in the immediate postoperative period. Most benign gynecologic surgeries are considered intermediate or low-risk procedures from a cardiac standpoint, with a cardiac risk of less than 5%. Many factors may adversely affect cardiovascular function during and after surgery; for example, fluid shifts, hypotension, electrolyte imbalance, infection, severe pain, apprehension, and tachycardia. Perioperative monitoring, anesthesia induction, maintenance techniques, and postoperative care can be tailored to the specific cardiovascular disease, thus improving the patient's chances for a good surgical outcome. *If a recent stress test does not indicate residual myocardium at risk, the likelihood of reinfarction after noncardiac surgery is low. Although there are no adequate clinical trials on which to base firm recommendations, it appears reasonable to wait at least 4–6 weeks after MI to perform elective surgery.*

Special Studies

A. ELECTROCARDIOGRAPHY

The need for a preoperative ECG in an asymptomatic patient without a history of cardiac disease is controversial, as the literature to support this practice is lacking. In 2002, the American Society of Anesthesiologists Task Force on Preanesthesia Evaluation did not reach consensus on a specific minimum age in those patients without specific risk factors, and recognized that age alone may not be an indication for an electrocardiogram. The aforementioned ACC/AHA practice guideline also concluded that evidence supporting routine preoperative ECG on asymptomatic patients is not well established. Nonetheless, a common practice is to obtain a preoperative ECG on all patients older than 50 years of age. It should also be obtained on younger patients with a history of symptoms of cardiovascular disease or diabetes mellitus. The ECG is of value in identifying the patient with coronary artery disease, ventricular hypertrophy, electrolyte disturbance, arrhythmia, and digitalis or other drug effect. Comparison with older ECGs is important when significant

changes do exist. The preoperative ECG should serve as a baseline for subsequent studies if postoperative complications develop. In patients with important abnormalities on their resting ECG (eg, left bundle-branch block, left ventricular hypertrophy with strain), other techniques such as exercise ECG or exercise myocardial perfusion imaging should be considered.

B. ECHOCARDIOGRAPHY

Echocardiography demonstrates any valvular or ventricular wall motion abnormalities resulting from coronary artery insufficiencies or cardiomyopathy. Left ventricular ejection fraction can also be estimated from an echocardiogram. Resting left ventricular function has not been a consistent predictor of perioperative ischemic events. Echocardiography may be of value in patients with current or poorly controlled heart failure, or dyspnea of unknown etiology.

C. DIPYRIDAMOLE/THALLIUM STRESS TEST

Patients with a significant cardiac history or an abnormal ECG should have a preoperative stress ECG under the direction of the patient's cardiologist. Dipyridamole or thallium stress-tolerance scanning demonstrates older, fibrosed, fixed lesions, or areas subject to ischemia and potential infarct. This test identifies ischemia under stress before the patient is subjected to the stress of surgery. The result will guide the gynecologist and anesthesiologist in their invasive monitoring and surgical anesthesia maintenance decisions.

D. INTRAOPERATIVE CENTRAL MONITORING

Invasive catheter measurements of intracardiac pressures can often provide useful information regarding cardiovascular dynamics. In most cases, the need for this intraoperative information can be evaluated simply by careful attention to aspects of the physical examination such as blood pressure, pulse, pulse pressure, heart rate, status of neck veins when supine, auscultation and percussion of the chest, presence or absence of edema, and size of the liver. If the preoperative evaluation raises a significant question, direct central venous pressure monitoring should be considered. A Swan-Ganz pulmonary artery catheter is particularly useful when surgery is likely to be prolonged, and the history, physical examination, and cardiology testing indicate depressed myocardial function or pulmonary artery hypertension. In patients at high risk for heart failure, the information provided by a pulmonary artery catheter can help optimize stroke volume without excessive hydration. However, use of a pulmonary artery catheter is not without risk. Moreover, the 2002 ACC/AHA Guidelines Update confirms that there is no general agreement that the pulmonary artery catheter monitoring is effective and useful for noncardiac surgery. The decision to use a pulmonary artery catheter should be made in consultation with the anesthesiologist and a critical care specialist, taking into account the patient's underlying disease, the planned surgery, and expected fluid shifts.

Prophylaxis for Venous Thromboembolism

Venous thromboembolism (VTE) is a relatively common postoperative complication. Because of the clinically silent nature of the disease in the majority of patients, the morbidity, and potential mortality associated with unprevented thrombi, perioperative prophylaxis against the development of this condition is always an important consideration. The major risk factors that have been identified for the development of VTE include increasing age; prolonged immobility, stroke, or paralysis; previous VTE; cancer and its treatment; major surgery (particularly operations involving the abdomen, pelvis, and lower extremities); trauma (especially fractures of the pelvis, hip, or leg); obesity; varicose veins; cardiac dysfunction; indwelling central venous catheters; inflammatory bowel disease; nephrotic syndrome; and pregnancy or estrogen use. Without prophylaxis, the patients considered to be at highest risk after major surgery, eg, patients older than the age of 40 years with VTE, cancer, or hypercoagulable state, are estimated to have a risk of calf deep venous thrombosis (DVT) between 40% and 80% and a risk of fatal DVT between 0.2% and 5%. Among patients younger than age 40 years without other risk factors, the risk of calf DVT is estimated to be as high as 10–20%, with a risk of fatal DVT estimated to be between 0.1% and 0.4%. One researcher reviewed 2 meta-analyses of more than 70 published trials of deep venous thrombosis prophylaxis in general surgical patients. Both studies concluded that prophylaxis significantly reduced the rates of deep venous thrombosis and fatal pulmonary embolism and resulted in improved overall survival. Physical methods such as compression stockings and intermittent pneumatic compression were shown to be as effective as pharmacologic prophylaxis with heparin. Surgeons in the United States tend to avoid pharmacologic prophylaxis because of concerns of bleeding complications. The disadvantages to their routine administration of heparinoids include prolonged lymph leak, lymphocele, and hematoma formation, and epidural hematoma when epidural analgesia is employed.

Prophylactic administration of unfractionated heparin, 5000 units subcutaneously initiated just before surgery and every 8–12 hours thereafter until full ambulatory status is achieved, may be used to prevent thromboembolization in high-risk cases. With this standardized approach, it is unnecessary to check the partial thromboplastin or activated partial thromboplastin times. Low-molecular weight heparin is an alternative to unfractionated heparin. The benefit of these agents is that they are dosed less often than unfractionated heparin, typically once a day rather than every 8 or 12 hours. Also, there is some data that indicates that low-molecular-weight heparin is less likely to cause heparin-induced thrombocytopenia. In a large multicenter, double-blind trial, 936 patients undergoing resection of part or all of the colon or rectum were randomized to receive, by subcutaneous injection, 5000 units of unfractionated heparin or 4000 units of low-molecular-weight heparin once daily (plus two additional saline injections so that the dosing regimens would be equal). Treatment was initiated 2 hours prior to surgery. Deep vein thrombosis was assessed by routine bilateral contrast venography performed between postoperative days 5 and 9, or earlier if clinically suspected. The venous thromboembolism rates were the same in both groups. There were no deaths from pulmonary embolism or bleeding complications. Although the proportion of all bleeding events in the low-molecular-weight heparin group was significantly greater than in the unfractionated heparin group, the rates of major bleeding and reoperation for bleeding were not significantly different. Because unfractionated heparin is considerably less expensive than low-molecular-weight heparin, many authors deem unfractionated heparin to be the agent of choice.

Given the variety of thromboprophylaxis regimens available, how should the gynecologic surgeon choose which approach to employ. In their exhaustive review article on the subject, Geerts et al. conclude that the decision as to which option(s) to choose should be tailored to the risk of VTE for each individual patient. For example, for patients younger than 40 years of age who are undergoing procedures that are shorter than 1 hour in duration, early ambulation may be all that is required. In contrast, an elderly patient with a gynecologic malignancy may warrant dual therapy in which a heparinoid and a mechanical antithrombotic device is employed.

Varicose Veins and History of Deep Vein Thrombosis

Patients with large, extensive varicosities or a history of thrombophlebitis or thromboembolic events are at risk for developing lower-extremity thrombophlebitis or thromboembolic phenomena. This risk may be minimized by prevention of dehydration, early ambulation, and prompt and adequate treatment of cardiac disorders. Discontinuation of oral contraceptives 3 to 4 weeks preoperatively should be considered.

Before the operation, the patient should wear support stockings from toe to thigh. After surgery, these stockings should be worn continuously and discarded only after full ambulation is restored. Pressure on the calf or thigh should be avoided during a long operative procedure. Postoperative leg exercises should be initiated as soon as possible to prevent phlebitis. These may be begun even before ambulation by having the patient press against a footboard whenever supine. When discharged the patient should be advised to avoid prolonged sitting (eg, auto, train, or air travel) during the first month after surgery. Similarly, the use of sequential compression boots intraoperatively and postoperatively or the use of subcutaneous heparinoids until the patient is fully ambulatory may help to prevent thrombosis in high-risk patients.

Valvular Heart Disease

Patients with a history of valvular heart disease or a heart murmur should have echocardiography performed to determine the severity of the valvular lesion. Antibiotic prophylaxis should be administered according to the American Heart Association (AHA) guidelines. The most recent AHA guidelines (1997) regarding endocarditis prophylaxis stratify valvular lesions by risk and recommend a treatment regimen based on the type of proposed surgery. Most gynecologic surgeries, in contrast to dental, respiratory, or urinary tract procedures, do not represent a high risk for development of endocarditis.

2. Pulmonary System

Elective surgery should be postponed if acute upper or lower respiratory tract infection is present. Even mild upper airway infection is associated with an irritable airway, which predisposes to laryngospasm or severe coughing on induction or emergence from anesthesia. Pulmonary infection causes poor ciliary motility, which predisposes to postoperative bronchitis and pneumonia. If emergency surgery is necessary in the presence of a respiratory tract infection, regional anesthesia should be used if possible and aggressive measures should be taken to avoid postoperative atelectasis or pneumonia. If the infection is severe, appropriate antibiotic therapy should be initiated promptly and modified as necessary when the results of cultures become available. The patient should be free from respiratory infection for at least 1–2 weeks, and preferably for 1 month, before elective surgery.

Chronic obstructive pulmonary disease, including chronic bronchitis, and emphysema, puts the patient at increased risk in the perioperative period. Optimizing the patient's pulmonary status with chest physical therapy, breathing exercises such as incentive spirometry, and appropriate antibiotic prophylaxis decreases the potential for prolonged postoperative ventilation and su-

ture line strain from coughing. Bronchiectasis, relatively uncommon at present, requires the patient to have rigorous chest physiotherapy and antibiotics before surgery. Preoperative pulmonary function tests should be performed to assess the severity and type of disease and to have as a baseline for reference in the postoperative period.

Those who smoke are at particular risk of developing pulmonary complications during or after surgery. These complications include increased airway reactivity that can result in coughing, bronchospasm, increased sputum production, atelectasis, and an increased risk of postoperative pulmonary infection. Furthermore, up to 15% of smokers' hemoglobin is combined with carbon monoxide to form carboxyhemoglobin, thus diminishing oxygen-carrying capacity. Patients who smoke and for whom general anesthesia by endotracheal intubation is planned should be encouraged to stop smoking for as long as possible before their surgery. Prolonged operations involving general anesthesia increases the risk of postoperative hypoventilation. Careful evaluation, including chest x-rays and pulmonary function tests, enable the surgeon and the surgeon's consultant to decide when the operation may be safely undertaken, and may influence the mode of anesthesia selected.

Asthmatics typically have intermittent symptoms of expiratory airflow obstruction. The preoperative medical history should include frequency of attacks, any hospitalizations or intubations, steroid use, and regular medication use. In patients with a significant asthma history, preoperative pulmonary function tests help gauge the severity of the disease, and assess the benefit of bronchodilators. A forced vital capacity in 1 second (FEV_1) of less than 50% normal indicates moderate to severe disease. After recent exacerbation, patients should be given adequate time to return to baseline before proceeding with elective surgery.

3. Renal System

Renal function should be appraised if there is a history of kidney disease, diabetes mellitus, or hypertension; if the patient is older than 60 years of age; or if routine urinalysis reveals proteinuria, casts, or red cells. Functional examination of renal function include measurement of creatinine clearance, blood urea nitrogen, and plasma electrolytes. Radiographic examinations, such as intravenous pyelogram or CT scan, may sometimes be indicated for functional or anatomic evaluation, especially in patients with a history of prior reconstructive urologic surgery.

Most patients with chronic renal failure are anemic, and many have hypertension. Hypertension should be controlled, and any electrolyte imbalances corrected prior to surgery. In dialysis patients, the optimum time for elective surgery is 24 hours after dialysis. Care should be taken not use the arm with the arteriovenous fistula for intravenous access.

4. Hematologic System

Anemia

Anemia diagnosed in the preoperative obstetric or gynecologic patient usually is of the iron-deficiency type caused by inadequate diet, chronic blood loss, or chronic disease. Care must be taken to differentiate iron-deficiency anemia from other anemias such as sickle cell anemia. Iron-deficiency anemia is the only type of anemia in which stained iron deposits cannot be identified in the bone marrow. Megaloblastic, hemolytic, and aplastic anemias usually are easily differentiated from iron-deficiency anemia on the basis of the history and simple laboratory examinations. The diagnosis of obscure anemias may require the help of a hematologic consultation.

Anemia mainly impacts surgery and anesthesia by decreasing oxygen-carrying capacity. Chronically anemic patients can partially compensate by expanding plasma volume, however this mechanism fails when hemoglobin falls below 10 g/dL. Although, traditionally, a hemoglobin of at least 10 mg/dL was a prerequisite for elective surgery, some authorities now accept a hemoglobin as low as 7–8 g/dL in young, healthy patients. Patients with iron-deficiency anemia respond to oral or parenteral iron therapy. Before elective surgery for menorrhagia, the patient's blood loss might be stopped with a GnRH agonist long enough to allow reversal of the anemia. In emergencies or urgent cases, preoperative blood transfusions, preferably with packed red cells, may be given.

von Willebrand's Disease

von Willebrand's disease is a family of congenital bleeding disorders characterized by altered factor VIII activity and deficient platelet function. Inheritance is generally autosomal dominant, although more rare autosomal recessive forms have been identified. Clinical manifestations include epistaxis, easy bruising, hypermenorrhea, and postpartum hemorrhage. von Willebrand's disease is reported to be the most common congenital cause of hypermenorrhea. Menstrual abnormalities are generally persistent and severe but may be intermittent or moderate, so that milder cases are less likely to be diagnosed. Hypermenorrhea may develop in affected persons at menarche and persist until the menopause or may not develop until after the second or third decade of life. von Willebrand's disease is diagnosed in 10 persons per 100,000, but the true prevalence may be as high as 1–2% of the general population. It is possible that the true cause of menstrual abnormalities is undetected in some women with undi-

agnosed von Willebrand's disease who undergo hysterectomy for hypermenorrhea.

The diagnosis of von Willebrand's disease is confirmed by a prolonged bleeding time, decreased factor VIII activity, and abnormal platelet function. The platelet count is normal. All patients should avoid aspirin and nonsteroidal anti-inflammatory medications preoperatively, but this is especially true of the patient with von Willebrand's disease. For patients with the most common types of von Willebrand's disease, types 1 and 2a, treatment with desmopressin, or desmopressin acetate (DDAVP), 0.3 μg/kg intravenously immediately before surgery may help to improve platelet function. This should only be done in patients known to respond to DDAVP. DDAVP is a synthetic analogue of antidiuretic hormone, and must be used judiciously, as fluid overload and hyponatremia may result. Patients with more severe forms of this disease, or who have not responded to DDAVP, should be given factor VIII concentrates or cryoprecipitate intraoperatively, if needed. Preoperative consultation with a hematologist is helpful.

Thrombocytopenia

The normal platelet count ranges from 150,000–350,000/mm^3. In the patient with thrombocytopenia but normal capillary function, platelet deficiency begins to manifest itself clinically as the count falls below 100,000/mm^3. Typical manifestations include petechiae on easily traumatized areas of the body, epistaxis, and menorrhagia. Epistaxis and hypermenorrhea may be severe enough to require transfusion. Bleeding into deep muscle and hemarthroses usually does not result spontaneously from thrombocytopenia, but intracranial hemorrhage is a serious risk if the platelet count is very low. The thrombocytopenic patient may require transfusion of platelets before surgery if the platelet count falls too low.

If thrombocytopenia is severe, the deficiency of platelet-produced factors involved in the coagulation cascade may result in some prolongation of clotting time. Transfusion of fresh-frozen plasma or cryoprecipitate may be useful in the acute patient with a prothrombin time and partial thromboplastin time greater than 1.5 times normal. The most sensitive early clinical measure of platelet deficiency was thought to be the bleeding time. More recent literature suggests that bleeding time may not be a reliable indicator of platelet function and no study has established that bleeding time will predict the risk of hemorrhage in individual patients. Spontaneous hemostasis is not expected if the platelet count falls to 10,000/mm^3 or less, and the patient may begin to bleed from all old puncture wounds as the platelet count approaches this threshold.

Bone marrow suppression, autoimmune disease, and platelet consumption are the chief causes of thrombocytopenia. Treatment revolves around treating the underlying cause and support with platelet transfusion and clotting factors as necessary.

Patients Receiving Oral Anticoagulation

Dunn and Turpie performed a systematic review of the 31 English-language reports regarding the perioperative management and outcomes of patients receiving long-term oral anticoagulant therapy. The available literature supports the continuation of oral anticoagulants without increasing the risk of major bleeding for single and multiple dental extractions, joint and soft-tissue injections, cataract surgery, and upper endoscopy or colonoscopy with or without biopsy. However, if oral anticoagulants are continued for one of these procedures, the international normalized ratio should not be beyond the therapeutic range at the time of the procedure.

For invasive surgical procedures, oral anticoagulation should be withheld. The surgeon faces the decision as to how to manage perioperative anticoagulation. There are three options: (a) Hold the oral anticoagulant until after the patient is determined to be a low risk for postoperative hemorrhage. (b) Pursue an aggressive strategy of therapeutic anticoagulation with perioperative intravenous heparin or subcutaneous low-molecular-weight heparin and re-initiate anticoagulation as soon as possible after surgery. (c) Employ subcutaneous unfractionated or low-molecular-weight heparin to achieve partial, but not therapeutic, anticoagulation. The decision as to which management strategy to employ should be individualized and should result as a compromise between the risk of arterial and venous thrombosis as a result of the condition that warrants anticoagulation and the potential consequences of postoperative hemorrhage.

5. Endocrine System

Diabetes Mellitus

Diabetes is the most common disease of disordered metabolism, arising largely from altered pancreatic islet cell function. The incidence increases with age, and occurs in up to 4% of the general population. The American Diabetes Association adopted new criteria for diagnosis in 1997. Diabetes is diagnosed by a fasting plasma glucose of greater than or equal to 126 mg/dL, or a random plasma glucose above 200 mg/dL. The oral glucose tolerance test (OGTT) is no longer required for diagnosis, but it may still be of some value in identifying at-risk patients with nondiabetic fasting plasma glucose values. Fifty percent of diabetics are treated by diet alone, with the remaining 50% evenly divided between oral hypoglycemic use and insulin use.

Diabetes can lead to the long-term complications of both large and small vessels. Conditions such as atherosclerosis, neuropathy, and nephropathy, may negatively impact the diabetic patient during the perioperative period. Control of diabetes is made especially difficult by the stress of operation, acute infection, anesthesia, and electrolyte imbalance. The operative diabetic patient must be carefully observed and promptly treated before fluid and electrolyte abnormalities, ketosis, hyperglycemia, and infection develop. Diabetics whose disease is out of control are especially susceptible to postoperative sepsis. Preoperative consultation with an internist may be considered to ensure control of insulin-requiring diabetics before, during, and after surgery.

Type I diabetes accounts for approximately 90% of cases and is seen in the older, usually more obese, patient population. Insulin production is close to or at normal values, but not appropriate for the blood sugar level. There is also peripheral insulin resistance. These patients develop neither ketoacidoses nor hyperosmolar states. The blood sugar is controlled by diet or oral medication. The oral medications most commonly used are the sulfonylurea derivatives, glyburide or glipizide. Their duration of action can be greater than 24 hours, and chlorpropamide may be effective for up to 50 hours. Consequently, it is important to avoid hypoglycemia by closely monitoring blood sugar on the day of surgery, and possibly by not using the longer-acting agents for up to 2 days preoperatively.

Type I diabetics tend to be younger, are less likely to be obese, and have little or no insulin production. They require insulin to avoid development of ketoacidoses, nonketotic hyperosmolar states, and hyperglycemia. Insulin-dependent diabetics with good control should be given half of their total morning insulin dose as regular insulin on the morning of surgery. This is preceded or immediately followed by the initiation of a 5% dextrose solution intravenously to prevent hypoglycemia in a fasting patient. Regular insulin should then be given by continuous infusion at a rate dictated by plasma glucose or fingerstick determinations.

If the diabetes is severe, it may be necessary to admit the patient to the hospital before the operation for glycemic control. Regular insulin may be substituted for long-acting insulin to achieve tighter control. Serum electrolyte determinations should be recorded as points of reference for postoperative management. Fasting plasma glucose should be determined prior to surgery. The insulin/dextrose infusion is continued postoperatively until the patient is eating.

Some controversy exists regarding how tightly the blood sugar should be controlled perioperatively. It is generally accepted that keeping the blood sugar in the 100–250 mg/dL range in the perioperative period is adequate for most types of surgery. Impaired neutrophil phagocytic activity has been reported when blood glucose is above 200–250 mg/dL. Cardiopulmonary bypass surgery, procedures in pregnancy or after a cerebral ischemic episode, and neurosurgical operations in which maintenance of cerebral autoregulation is important, have better results if the blood sugar is more tightly controlled at about 80–130 mg/dL. Tight control is achieved by using an intravenous insulin infusion based on frequent blood sugar estimations.

Occasionally, surgery is required emergently in a patient who presents in a hyperglycemic ketoacidotic state. It is important to first correct the fluid and electrolyte status, particularly the potassium levels, but it is not necessary to hold off surgery until complete resolution has occurred. The surgical condition may be the precipitating factor, and final correction may not be possible until surgery is completed. The hyperglycemic ketoacidotic state is treated by giving 10 U of regular insulin intravenously followed by an infusion of insulin based on the formula of the blood sugar level divided by 150 U/h. Normal saline solution is given to correct dehydration. Potassium must be supplemented because the insulin drives it into the cells. Total-body potassium, despite its initial elevated serum level, may be significantly depleted. Because there are a fixed number of insulin receptors, there is nothing to gain by using higher doses of insulin. Blood glucose levels usually fall at a maximum rate of 100 mg/dL/h, except during the initial rehydration period, when the fall is more precipitous.

Chronic medical conditions associated with diabetes may also complicate the perioperative period, eg, hypertension and coronary artery disease. Myocardial ischemia may often be silent in the diabetic with autonomic neuropathy. Autonomic neuropathy is also associated with gastric paresis and increased risk of aspiration. These patients should have an extended cardiac work-up and receive metoclopramide as well as a nonparticulate antacid before surgery. Intubation in some patients may be difficult because the atlantooccipital joint may be involved with the diabetic process.

Thyroid Disease

Elective surgery should be postponed when thyroid function is suspected of being either excessive or inadequate. Hyperthyroidism is suspected clinically when the patient has a history of weight loss, muscle weakness, a persistently rapid pulse, agitation, tremor, heat intolerance, nervousness, or warm skin. The gland either may be diffusely enlarged, as in Graves' disease, or may have only an unobtrusive adenoma. Exophthalmos may be evident. Cardiac signs may be the only clue in the elderly patient (apathetic hyperthyroidism) and may include an unexplained atrial fibrillation or other tachyarrhythmia or dysrhythmia. A varying level of ventricular dysfunction is present in all patients with hyperthyroidism.

The patient should be rendered euthyroid before surgery if possible. This may take up to 2 months if antithyroid medications are used in combination with potassium iodide (Lugol's solution). The combination of a blocker, usually propranolol, and potassium iodide allows surgery in about 14 days. Propranolol blocks the peripheral effects of hyperthyroidism (ie, nervousness, sweating, tachycardia) and may slow the response to atrial fibrillation. It also impairs the conversion of thyroxine (T_4) to triiodothyronine (T_3) peripherally. Care must be exercised in the use of propranolol in patients with asthma or congestive heart failure. If surgery is immediately required, propranolol is titrated slowly intravenously in 0.5-mg aliquots until the peripheral signs of thyrotoxicosis are brought under control. Regional or local anesthesia is preferable. If general anesthesia is required, the airway should be adequately assessed clinically and by x-ray or CT scan for severe tracheal compression or any deviation that might interfere with placement of an intratracheal airway.

Severe stress, such as that provided by surgery and anesthesia, can precipitate a thyroid storm in a person with hyperthyroidism. Thyroid storm is a life-threatening event that manifests itself as hyperpyrexia, tachycardia, and cardiovascular instability, and it may be mistaken for malignant hyperthermia.

Hypothyroidism is relatively common in the elderly. It is usually of insidious onset; 95% of cases are caused by primary failure of the thyroid to produce adequate T_4 and T_3. Goiter may be present, and a history of surgery or radioactive iodine treatment may be elicited. There is a slowing down of the metabolism that affects both mental and physical abilities, including a slowing of the heart rate and diminished ventricular contractility in response to catecholamines. Patients are very sensitive to respiratory-depressant medications. There is blunting of the stress response, and corticosteroid supplementation may be needed.

In mild to moderate hypothyroidism, surgery and anesthesia need not be delayed before treatment is started. If the disease is severe, treatment should be started before surgery, if possible. In all cases, treatment must be started with a very low dose of thyroid-replacement therapy to avoid sudden large demands on the myocardium, which may not yet be able to respond appropriately. The usual tests of thyroid function include total T_4 and T_3 levels, free T_4, T_3 resin uptake, and thyroid-stimulating hormone (TSH) levels. Preoperative consultation regarding the management of patients with thyroid dysfunction should be sought before major surgery.

Recent or Current Corticosteroid Use

It has been a long-held medical tenet that patients taking corticosteroids require supraphysiologic stress-dose steroids perioperatively. The origin of this belief stems from a case report in 1952 in which a steroid-dependent patient died postoperatively of intractable hypotension. Autopsy revealed bilateral adrenal cortical atrophy. Other case reports and biochemical studies confirming suppression of the hypothalamic–pituitary–adrenal (HPA) axis in steroid-dependent patients have reinforced the practice of administering perioperative stress-dose steroids. However, high-dose steroids, even if given for only a relatively short period of time, can potentially cause harm and are not without risk. Risks of high-dose steroid regimens can include immunosuppression, poor wound healing, and acute psychiatric disturbances. Brown and Buie reviewed the available literature and concluded that there is little evidence to support the practice of administering high-dose perioperative steroids to patients that have been on long-term steroids preoperatively. Hypotensive crisis can occur, but the literature supports a rate of only 1–2%, and these patients generally do well with a rescue dose of steroid when needed. The authors concluded that the current literature supports continuing patients on their normal daily dose of steroids through the perioperative period, instead of traditional high-dose regimens. An exception is critically ill patients who require pressors preoperatively—they should be given supraphysiologic dosing. As with other serious medical conditions preoperative consultation with the anesthesia team regarding perioperative medical management is always prudent.

6. Other Conditions Affecting Operative Risk

Pregnancy

The diagnosis of early pregnancy must be considered in the decision to do elective major surgery in the female. Elective surgery generally should be postponed until after delivery. Scheduled surgery that cannot be delayed, such as exploration for an adnexal mass, is best performed in the second trimester whenever possible.

Diagnostic or evaluative procedures necessary in the proper work-up for urgently needed surgery override theoretical fetal hazards in the pregnant patient. Appropriate protective measures should be taken to minimize these dangers, such as shielding the uterus from radiation during x-ray studies, using tocolytic agents to prevent premature labor, and considering possible fetal effects when pharmacologic and anesthetic agents are to be used. Hypotension and hypoxia must be meticulously avoided during anesthetic administration or surgical manipulation. Surgery should be performed in the left lateral decubitus position to optimize uterine perfusion. If the surgery is being performed after fetal viability, intraoperative fetal heart rate monitoring should be performed.

The new and more sensitive radioreceptor assay and radioimmunoassay for pregnancy are positive within 10 days of conception, ie, before the anticipated menstrual period. This capability may be important in scheduling elective surgery, especially in gynecologic procedures such as tubal ligation and hysterectomy.

Age

The 65-year-old and older segment of the population is currently undergoing the most rapid expansion of any demographic group in the United States. This expansion is projected to continue and accelerate. The majority of individuals in this age group are women. It has been estimated that more than 50% of this older population will at some point undergo some surgical intervention. In the future, the gynecologic surgeon will be caring increasingly for older patients requiring or desiring surgical procedures.

Care of the older patient can present a significant challenge. These women often have multiple medical problems against a background of a general decline of their physiologic reserve. However, if care is taken during preoperative evaluation and perioperative management, these patients can do quite well. Age itself is not an independent predictor of surgical risk. Neither the healthy elderly patient nor the carefully evaluated and managed elderly patient with medical problems should not be discouraged from pursuing a beneficial elective procedure.

A careful history and review of systems must be taken and may require the assistance of family members or caretakers. A review of past medical records is crucial. A thorough physical examination must be performed. Appropriate preoperative consultation and extended preoperative evaluation as previously described should be obtained. The results should be reviewed with, and the patient seen by, the anesthesiologist well before the operative date so that an intraoperative management plan can be developed. Care should be taken when positioning older women to reduce the risk of postoperative complications. Finally, meticulous and expeditious technique must be used during surgery to limit blood loss, hypothermia, operative time, and fluid shifts.

The principles and general considerations of good surgical practice become critically important when operating on the older patient. Serum electrolytes must be determined preoperatively and any imbalances corrected by appropriate parenteral solutions. Care should be taken not to overload the elderly patient's circulation when administering intravenous fluids, as cardiac, pulmonary, and renal reserves are often diminished. Nutritional deficiencies should be corrected before elective surgery is undertaken if possible. In older patients who are found to be significantly nutritionally deprived, total parenteral nutrition (TPN) may be required before and after surgery.

Fluid intake and urinary output should be monitored carefully and the patient's weight recorded daily. Early ambulation of the patient is very important. Care must be taken that items the patient uses at home, such as glasses, hearing aids, walkers, or canes, are brought to or available in the hospital. The older patient, or one who has been bedridden, requires frequent change of position to prevent the development of decubitus ulcers. Early ambulation and aggressive active and passive physical therapy may prevent many vascular and pulmonary complications.

The elderly patient often requires smaller dosages of medications such as narcotics and anesthetic agents; however, optimum pain relief must be ensured. Use of nonsteroidal anti-inflammatories can help reduce narcotic requirements. Barbiturates should especially be prescribed with caution, as even small doses can cause mental confusion.

In addition, the woman and her family should be prepared for postoperative recovery. It is often helpful to have a family member stay with the patient in the hospital to assist with orientation. This might involve arranging for postdischarge care in the patient's home or a skilled nursing facility. All arrangements should be made prior to surgery.

Obesity

Obesity puts the patient and every member of the hospital team at a disadvantage. Obese surgical patients are at increased risk of mortality and morbidity. Every system in the body is affected by this disease. Obese patients have an increased potential for cardiovascular disease, diabetes, and deep venous thrombosis.

Risk factors that may affect the perioperative course must be ascertained during the preoperative assessment. Recommendations for preoperative testing in the obese patient include a complete blood cell count, chemistry panel, liver function test, coagulation studies, and urinalysis; a chest radiograph and electrocardiograph are required. Additionally, prior to surgery the weight capacity of the operating table should be determined.

When treating the obese patient, the anesthesiologist is often challenged by difficult intravenous access. Occasionally, preoperative central access must be obtained by interventional radiologists. These patients have markedly decreased functional residual capacity, making hypoxia a major concern, particularly in a supine or Trendelenburg position. Increased volume and acidity of gastric secretions, along with poor gastroesophageal sphincter tone, increases the risk of pulmonary aspiration. Poor neck extension makes intubation more difficult.

The gynecologic surgeon should arrange for extra assistants and long instruments. To reduce the risk of trauma to adjacent organs, the surgeon must ensure adequate exposure through appropriate incisions. Care must be taken to avoid incisions below the pannus. In selected women, a panniculectomy may be performed in conjunction with the planned surgery. A mass closure technique with a delayed absorbable or permanent suture should be considered. Wound healing is inhibited, and there is an increased risk of postoperative wound seroma and infection.

Postoperatively, nursing personnel are also at a serious disadvantage. Attempts to achieve ambulation and to prevent respiratory and thromboembolic complications are much more difficult. Again, planning beforehand and extra personnel may be the key to a successful postoperative course.

Drug Allergies & Sensitivities

The obstetric or gynecologic patient who is being evaluated and prepared for a major operation may receive a variety of medications. Drug allergies, sensitivities, incompatibilities, and other adverse effects must be anticipated and prevented if possible. A history of serious reaction or sickness after injection, oral administration, or other use of any of the following substances should be noted and the medication avoided: antibiotic medications; narcotics; anesthetics; analgesics; sedatives; antitoxins or antisera; and antiseptics. Untoward reactions to other medications, foods (eg, milk, chocolate), adhesive tape, and antiseptic solutions, especially iodine, should also be noted.

Latex allergy is increasingly prevalent. The two main categories of latex sensitivity are type I and type IV. Type I reactions involve immediate urticaria, airway obstruction, systemic symptoms, or anaphylaxis; type IV reactions are generally limited to the skin that has come into contact with the latex and are delayed in onset. Patients with a history of atopy and/or allergies to avocado, kiwi, banana, or chestnuts have a higher incidence of latex allergy. Preoperative evaluation by an allergist is advisable in women with a history of latex sensitivity. Latex allergy is confirmed by a positive test of sensitization in a symptomatic individual. Sensitization can be identified by an in vitro assay for serum-specific immunoglobulin (Ig) E; positive skin-prick test reaction to latex antigen; or a provocative test, such as glove use or inhalation tests. Premedication with steroids and antihistamines has not proven effective. Consequently, surgery in latex-allergic individuals should take place in a latex-free environment. Most hospitals have latex-free packs or carts available for patients with latex allergy. These patients should also be scheduled as the first case of the day in the operating room.

Immunologic Compromise

A patient may be considered an immunologically compromised or altered host if her capacity to respond normally to infection or trauma has been significantly impaired by disease or therapy. Obviously, preoperative recognition and special evaluation of these patients are important.

A. Increased Susceptibility to Infection

Certain drugs may reduce a patient's resistance to infection by interfering with host defense mechanisms. Corticosteroids, immunosuppressive agents, cytotoxic drugs, and prolonged antibiotic therapy are associated with an increased incidence of superinfection by fungi or other resistant organisms. It is possible that the synergistic combination of radiation, corticosteroids, and serious underlying disease may set the stage for clinical fungal infection.

A high rate of wound, pulmonary, and other infections is seen in renal failure, presumably as a result of decreased host resistance. Granulocytopenia and diseases associated with immunologic deficiency (eg, lymphomas, leukemias, and hypogammaglobulinemia) are frequently complicated by sepsis. The uncontrolled diabetic is also observed clinically to be more susceptible to infection. The acquired immunodeficiency syndrome (AIDS) is associated with increased susceptibility to infection.

B. Delayed Wound Healing

This problem can be anticipated in certain categories of patients whose tissue repair process may be compromised. Many systemic factors have been alleged to influence wound healing; however, only the following are of clinical significance: protein depletion, ascorbic acid deficiency, marked dehydration or edema, and severe anemia. It has been shown experimentally that hypovolemia, vasoconstriction, increased blood viscosity, and increased intravascular aggregation and erythrostasis caused by remote trauma interfere with wound healing, probably by reducing oxygen tension and diffusion within the wound.

Large doses of corticosteroids depress wound healing. This effect apparently is increased by starvation and protein depletion. Wounds of patients who have received large doses of corticosteroids preoperatively should be closed with special care to prevent disruption that might delay healing.

Patients who have received anticancer chemotherapeutic agents are just as apt to require surgery as any other population group. Cytotoxic drugs may interfere with cell proliferation and may decrease the tensile strength of the surgical wound. It is wise to assume that healing may be delayed in patients receiving antitumor drugs.

Poor control of blood sugar in diabetic patients is associated with slow healing, poor scar formation, and an increased rate of wound infection. Slow healing sometimes is observed in debilitated patients, ie, those with advanced cancer, renal failure, gastrointestinal fistulas, or chronic infection. Protein and other nutritional deficiencies may be major causes of poor wound repair. Decreased vascularity and other local changes occur after a few weeks or months in tissues that have been heavily irradiated. These are potential deterrents to wound healing as well.

OTHER PREOPERATIVE CONSIDERATIONS

Autologous Blood Donation & Ovarian Preservation

Women undergoing hysterectomy must choose whether or not to undergo prophylactic oophorectomy. Specific groups of women whom will benefit from prophylactic oophorectomy have been identified. Women with the *BRCA1* or *BRCA2* mutation are at increased risk of ovarian cancer and prophylactic oophorectomy allows early ovarian cancer diagnosis and reduces the risk of ovarian and breast cancer. Women with endometriosis who are undergoing a hysterectomy without oophorectomy are at increased risk of requiring further surgery and recurrence of pain compared with women with an oophorectomy at the time of hysterectomy.

For most women however, this is a complex decision that must be fully discussed with the gynecologic surgeon. The advantage of oophorectomy is reduction of ovarian cancer risk (1 in 70 women); the disadvantage is loss of estrogen. This dilemma is compounded by the Women's Health Initiative findings. Risk factors for ovarian cancer, the potential for further surgery without performing a prophylactic oophorectomy, and a patient's age, must be considered when assisting the patient in decision making.

Supracervical Hysterectomy

The popularity and patient demand for supracervical hysterectomy has fluctuated over time. Recent randomized, controlled studies have compared supracervical with total hysterectomy. These studies found no significant differences in complication rate, symptom improvement, sexual function, bowel function, or urinary incontinence.

Preoperative Orders

Most patients are admitted to the hospital on the day of their surgery, or they have their surgery as outpatients. Much of the preoperative preparation of the patient that was formerly done in the hospital is now done at home by the patient and her family, as only a small percentage of gynecologic surgical patients are admitted before their surgical date. The following discussion reviews several areas of surgical concern that were formerly addressed in a patient's inpatient, night-before-surgery, preoperative orders.

A. SKIN PREPARATION

Many gynecologic surgeons choose to have patients wash the skin over the operative site with povidone-iodine or hexachlorophene the night before the procedure is to be performed, and follow with a povidone-iodine preparation just before surgery. In addition, a povidone-iodine vaginal preparation is performed in the operating suite. Twenty milliliters of povidone-iodine gel placed at the vaginal apex after vaginal preparation reduces the risk of pelvic abscess formation after abdominal hysterectomy.

Wound infection incidence is decreased by shaving the operative site in surgery rather than the night before the procedure. The wound infection rate is lower still with the use of clippers in the operating room or with no hair removal at all.

B. DIET

The patient should receive nothing by mouth for at least 8 hours before the operation so the stomach will be empty at the time of anesthesia.

C. PREPARATION OF THE GASTROINTESTINAL TRACT

Although there is relatively little data to support its routine use prior to gynecologic surgery, bowel preparation is currently an established practice before abdominal surgery. In the literature there is scant evidence to support the use of mechanical bowel preparation before elective colorectal surgery. In fact, there is evidence based on randomized trials and a meta-analysis report, that a significantly higher incidence of wound infection in patients receiving mechanical bowel preparation versus no bowel preparation. As to gynecologic surgery, data are minimal. There is a single, randomized trial that demonstrated a lack of efficacy of mechanical bowel preparation when compared to no bowel preparation at the time of laparoscopy. Based on this evidence, the routine use of mechanical bowel preparation should be reconsidered both in general and gynecologic surgery. However, gynecologic surgeons need to be aware of the local customs of their colleagues who practice general surgery. Currently, the majority of colorectal surgeons currently employ mechanical bowel preparations before elective anastomotic surgery. If the gynecologic surgeon is performing a procedure in which there is a strong possibility of intraoperative consultation, the surgeon should consider the preferences of the available general surgical consultants. On the other hand, many gynecologic surgeons recommend

that a patient use a cleansing enema the night before surgery to make certain that the examination under anesthesia will be accurate and to reduce the need for straining with a bowel movement during the early postoperative period.

If mechanical bowel preparation is deemed necessary, sodium phosphate preparation is better tolerated than polyethylene glycol. In 1997, Oliveira et al. compared sodium phosphate and polyethylene glycol in a prospective, randomized study involving 200 patients who underwent elective colorectal surgery. Sodium phosphate was better tolerated and judged equally effective by the operative surgeon. Wound complication rates were equal. Cohen et al. studied the safety, efficacy and tolerability of sodium phosphate compared to polyethylene glycol for precolonoscopy bowel preparation. Four hundred fifty patients were prospectively randomized to receive either 4 L of a polyethylene glycol solution or a 90-mL oral sodium phosphate preparation. The mean age of the participants was 71 years. Ninety-one percent of patients who had previously used polyethylene glycol preferred the sodium phosphate preparation. Mild hyperphosphatemia occurred in the sodium phosphate group but it was without clinical sequelae. Electrolyte imbalance, however, may be valid concern in the frail elderly.

D. SEDATION

A sedative-hypnotic can be prescribed to ensure restful sleep the night before the operation.

E. PREANESTHETIC MEDICATION

Preanesthesia medication is not administered until after an intravenous line has been started on the day of surgery. It generally consists of a sedative such as midazolam, titrated to effect.

F. OTHER MEDICATIONS

At least 25% of surgical patients take regularly scheduled medications, and this figure undoubtedly is much higher in the older patient populations. The most common medications are cardiovascular drugs, central nervous system (CNS) agents, and gastrointestinal medications. The patient is generally advised to take all of her regular medications on the morning of surgery with sips of water sufficient to swallow them unless there are specific contraindications.

Most cardiovascular medications can and should be continued through the morning of surgery. In particular, β blockers are protective in the perioperative period. An exception is the angiotensin-converting enzyme (ACE) inhibitor/angiotensin-receptor blocker (ARB) class. Conflicting data indicate that this class of antihypertensive has the potential to intensify the hypotensive effect of anesthesia. It is therefore recommended that ACE inhibitors and ARBs be discontinued 24 hours prior to surgery, or for at least one scheduled dose. Diuretics are also typically withheld the morning of surgery.

Oral anticoagulants should be stopped 3–5 days prior to major gynecologic surgery. If necessary, such patients can be "bridged" before and after surgery with low molecular weight or unfractionated heparin. Surgery is generally considered safe when the preoperative international normalized ratio (INR) is below 1.5. The warfarin is then restarted on postoperative days 3–5, with the heparin bridge, if used, continued until the patient's INR is again within the therapeutic range. A general rule is to discontinue the heparin bridge 12 hours prior to surgery, and restart it 12 hours after surgery. It should be noted that regional block in patients receiving preoperative anticoagulation is generally contraindicated. Discontinuing warfarin is probably not needed for minor gynecologic surgery; the ophthalmology and dermatology literature shows that continuing warfarin preoperatively is not detrimental.

Antiplatelet medications with irreversible binding, such as aspirin and ticlopidine, should be discontinued 7–10 days prior to surgery. Other nonsteroidal anti-inflammatory drugs (NSAIDs), which bind platelets reversibly, can be continued until within 24–72 hours of surgery. Although the newer cyclooxygenase-2 (COX-2) inhibitor NSAIDs, such as celecoxib, theoretically have no adverse effect on platelet function, they, too, should be discontinued 72 hours prior to surgery because of concerns about renal function perioperatively.

The biggest concern regarding CNS agents is the development of withdrawal symptoms when the medication is withheld. This is especially true of benzodiazepines. Tricyclic antidepressants (TCAs) and serotonin reuptake inhibitors (SSRIs) are generally safe to take up to the day of surgery, although there are reports linking TCAs with intraoperative hypotension.

Asthma, antiseizure, endocrine, and gastrointestinal medications are typically continued through the morning of surgery, and restarted as soon as practical postoperatively. Oral hypoglycemic agents are routinely withheld the morning of surgery. Metformin is withheld for up to 48 hours preoperatively because of the small but significant risk of lactic acidosis. Insulin, as noted above, is dosed differently on the morning of surgery.

The clinician should specifically ask the patient preoperatively about intake of herbal medicines. Some of these, such as ephedra (ma huang), ginseng, gingko, kava kava, St. John's wort, and even garlic and ginger, are reported to have cardiovascular, coagulation or sedative effects in the perioperative period. To be safe, patients should discontinue all herbal medications at least 2 weeks prior to surgery.

G. Antibiotics

Preoperative or prophylactic antibiotics are of value, especially in cases of expected bowel surgery, abdominal hysterectomy, all major vaginal surgery, and certain cesarean section deliveries. In contrast to mechanical bowel preparation, the positive effects of prophylactic antibiotics in case of bowel surgery is undisputed. The first- and second-generation cephalosporins have been particularly effective in decreasing postoperative febrile morbidity. Recent experience indicates that single-dose prophylaxis may be as effective as multiple doses.

H. Blood Transfusions

In circumstances in which transfusions are not usually required, a type and screen is satisfactory and cost-effective. If major blood loss is anticipated, a full cross-match should be performed. Keep in mind that more blood can be prepared as you are transfusing the units you already ordered.

Because of concerns about the risk of transmitting AIDS via transfusion, elective gynecologic surgery patients should be offered the option of autologous blood donation preoperatively. In addition, acute intraoperative autotransfusion should be considered if excessive intraperitoneal blood loss occurs either preoperatively, as in the case of ruptured ectopic pregnancy, or intraoperatively, as in the case of certain radical surgical procedures. Use of a cell-saver device, which processes blood aspirated from the surgical field and allows return of the patient's own red blood cells after washing in normal saline, is useful in these large-blood-loss situations and significantly cuts down on blood bank demand. The device is contraindicated in certain patients, such as those with infection near the operative site or those undergoing cesarean section or cesarean hysterectomy, because thromboplastins from decidual or amniotic fluid may become mixed with the blood.

I. Bladder Preparations

For minor procedures, the patient voids prior to being moved to the operating room. If major pelvic surgery is planned, an indwelling Foley catheter should be placed when the vaginal preparation is done in the operating room. For prolonged bladder drainage, a suprapubic catheter provides a lower urinary tract infection rate along with the ability to allow voiding trials without multiple urethral catheterizations. Intermittent, clean self-catheterization is another bladder drainage modality that can be taught preoperatively and offers a low postoperative infection rate.

DAY OF SURGERY

Positioning the Patient

Care must be taken to ensure adequate access to the surgical sites during positioning. Many gynecologic procedures are performed in lithotomy position for vaginal access. The risk of neurologic injury can be reduced through proper positioning. The coccyx should be well supported on the operative table (and not hanging off) to avoid hyperextension of the back. The lateral calf should not come into contact with the candy cane stirrup post to reduce the risk of compression injury of the common peroneal nerve. To reduce sciatic nerve stretch, exaggerated hip flexion, knee extension, and hip abduction should be avoided. The femoral nerve can become compressed under the inguinal ligament with excessive thigh flexion. When using universal boot stirrups, the surgeon must ensure that the weight of the leg rests upon the heel, with no pressure on the lateral or posterior calf. A prospective study found patients in dorsal lithotomy position for longer than 2 hours were at increased risk of neurologic injury; consequently, steps should be taken to minimize operative time when feasible.

■ POSTOPERATIVE CARE

IMMEDIATE POSTOPERATIVE CARE

During the immediate postoperative period, maintenance of normal pulmonary and circulatory function should be emphasized. Vital signs and fluid balance should be monitored frequently to facilitate the early diagnosis of shock or pulmonary problems. Bleeding from the surgical site and persisting pulmonary or cardiovascular effects from anesthesia are risks that mandate careful surveillance of all patients in the immediate postoperative period.

Postoperative Orders

The postsurgical patient is taken to the recovery room, accompanied by the anesthesiologist and the surgeon or other qualified attendant, as soon as she responds. Patients with medical problems may require postoperative admission to an intensive care unit for prolonged ventilation or central monitoring. The nurse receiving the patient should be given a verbal report of her condition, as well as an operative summary and postoperative orders. The postoperative orders should include the following elements.

A. VITAL SIGNS

Record the blood pressure, pulse, and respiratory rate every 15–30 minutes until the patient is stable and hourly thereafter for at least 4–6 hours. Any significant change must be reported immediately. These measurements, including the oral temperature, should then be

recorded 4 times a day for the remainder of the postoperative course.

B. WOUND CARE

Watch for excessive bleeding (inspect abdominal dressing or perineal pads). Determine the hematocrit the day after major surgery and, if there is a question of continued bleeding, repeat as indicated. An abdominal wound should be inspected daily. Skin sutures or clips generally are removed 3–5 days postoperatively and replaced with Steri-Strips.

C. MEDICATIONS

Following major surgery, give narcotic analgesics as needed (eg, meperidine, 75–100 mg intramuscularly every 4 hours, or morphine, 10 mg intramuscularly every 4 hours) to control pain. Injectable nonsteroidal anti-inflammatory drugs are available for postoperative pain control as well. Antiemetics such as promethazine or hydroxyzine may be helpful to suppress nausea, as well as to potentiate analgesics.

Patient-controlled analgesia (PCA) is widely available. With PCA, patients are able to give themselves intravenous pain medication as they need it within the parameters set by the physician. Many patients prefer PCA because it allows them to avoid the "peak and valley" effect of scheduled or on-demand pain injections.

Many centers are now using intrathecal or epidural opiate injection for relief of postoperative pain. This technique is particularly appropriate for patients who have been given regional anesthesia. A minimal dosage of less than 5 mg of morphine may allow several hours of complete pain relief without compromise of motor activity (ambulation, coughing). Respiratory depression is a hazard, however, and close monitoring of the patient is necessary. Patient-controlled epidural analgesia is becoming available in many centers as an alternative to single-dose spinal analgesics. Following minor surgery, give mild analgesics as needed. Other medications required by the patient that were taken prior to surgery (insulin, digitalis, cortisone, or others) should be resumed as required.

D. POSITION IN BED

The patient is usually placed on her side to reduce the risk of inhalation of vomitus or mucus. Other positions desired by the surgeon should be clearly stated, eg, flat with foot of bed elevated.

E. DRAINAGE TUBES

Connect the bladder catheter to the gravity drainage system. Written orders for other postoperative drainage and suction catheters should be specific and clear, setting forth the degree of negative pressure desired and the intervals for measurement of drainage volume.

F. INTAKE AND OUTPUT

The total fluid intake and output as well as daily weights are important clinical measures postoperatively.

G. FLUID REPLACEMENT

Administer fluids orally or intravenously as needed. When deciding how to replace a particular patient's fluid needs, always take into account factors such as intraoperative blood loss and urine output, operating time, intraoperative fluid replacement, and the amount of fluid received in the recovery area. Although each patient and operation are different, an average healthy young patient who has been appropriately replaced intraoperatively will do well with 2400 mL to 3 L of a balanced crystalloid and glucose solution, such as 5% dextrose in half-normal saline over the first 24 hours. The rate of intravenous hydration must always be individualized, as many patients require less volume and may become fluid overloaded at a faster rate. In the patient with normal renal function, adequate fluid replacement should result in a urine output of at least 30 mL/h.

H. DIET

Following minor surgery, offer food as desired and tolerated, when the patient is fully awake. Disagreement exists on how fast to advance a patient's diet after major surgery. This again must be individualized to the patient and depends on many factors.

One possible regimen is to allow the patient only sips of tap water on the day of surgery. Do not give ice water, because it may decrease bowel motility significantly. Give clear liquids on the first postoperative day if good bowel sounds are noted and until intestinal gas is passed. Change the diet thereafter to full regular. The time needed to progress to a full diet depends on the extent of the procedure, the duration of anesthesia, and individual variation among patients. Two randomized, controlled trials support the safety and efficacy of early oral feeding on postoperative day 1 following intra-abdominal gynecologic surgery in selected patients.

I. RESPIRATORY CARE

Encourage deep breathing every hour for the first 12 hours and every 2–3 hours for the next 12 hours. Incentive spirometry and the assistance of a respiratory therapist may be of great value, particularly in elderly, obese, or otherwise compromised or immobilized patients.

J. AMBULATION

Encourage early ambulation and bathroom privileges. If possible, require ambulation on the day of the operation after major surgery.

RECOVERY FROM MAJOR SURGERY

Even with the trend toward shorter hospital stays, the patient generally remains hospitalized until recovery of all bodily functions. Normal pulmonary function usually returns after resolution of inhalation anesthesia but may be influenced to some extent by surgical pain during the early postoperative period. Two or 3 days may pass before return of normal bowel function after laparotomy. The patient with febrile complications generally will not be discharged until she has remained asymptomatic and afebrile for 24 hours.

OUTPATIENT SURGERY

With the increasing number of outpatient procedures, the observation period following minor surgery becomes more critical. Following outpatient surgery, patients generally remain hospitalized until mental status and pulmonary and bladder functions return to normal. Occasionally, admission to the hospital becomes necessary for overnight observation or for further therapy. Although "ambulatory surgery" is designed for the healthy patient who is scheduled for less-extensive surgery, to become casual in preparation is to court disaster.

Because these patients play a more active role in the preparation and management of their surgery, the following additional elements must be considered: (a) Preoperative counseling should encompass the same information given the inpatient, but another responsible adult who will provide transportation and postoperative care for the patient should also be present at the session. (b) Emphasis should be placed on the importance of the "nothing by mouth" requirement and on the avoidance of any medications that the surgeon has not prescribed or approved. (c) A hospital must be available for backup if the facility is not hospital-based, and the patient must know where to report if problems arise; this entails establishing 24-hour telephone service for access to medical advice and care. (d) A follow-up call from the physician within 24 hours is often beneficial for picking up early postoperative problems as well as for emotional support for the patient. (e) All postoperative instructions should be reviewed with the patient before her surgery.

POSTOPERATIVE COUNSELING & RELEASE FROM THE HOSPITAL

Following operation, the patient should receive a careful explanation (both oral and written) of the surgical procedure performed, the findings at surgery, and any postoperative procedures or findings. The postoperative course may be negatively influenced by the patient's anxiety regarding lack of information or unanswered questions. It may be helpful for the physician to refer to preoperative audiovisual aids during the postoperative counseling session.

Every postoperative patient should have a complete physical examination (including a pelvic assessment) before release from the hospital. Findings can be used as a baseline for subsequent follow-up examinations.

The patient should receive oral and written instructions regarding postoperative care at home, including which physical activities she may perform. Appointments should be made for outpatient or office follow-up examinations.

REFERENCES

Acute Abdomen

Ahmad TA et al: Experience of laparoscopic management in 100 patients with acute abdomen. Hepatogastroenterology 2001; 48:733.

Mindelzun RE, Jeffrey RB: The acute abdomen: current CT imaging techniques. Semin Ultrasound CT MR 1999;20:63.

Tarraza HM, Moore RD: Gynecologic causes of the acute abdomen and the acute abdomen in pregnancy. Surg Clin North Am 1997;77:1371.

Appendicitis

Salky BA, Edye MB: The role of laparoscopy in the diagnosis and treatment of abdominal pain syndromes. Surg Endosc 1998; 12:911.

Urbach DR, Cohen MM: Is perforation of the appendix a risk factor for tubal infertility and ectopic pregnancy? An appraisal of the evidence. Can J Surg 1999;42:101.

Viktrup L, Hee P: The diagnosis of appendicitis during pregnancy and maternal and fetal outcome after appendectomy. Int J Gynaecol Obstet 1999;65:129.

Diverticulitis and Inflammatory Bowel Disease

Farrell RJ, Farrell JJ, Morrin MM: Diverticular disease in the elderly. Gastroenterol Clin North Am 2001;30:475.

Iki K et al: Preoperative diagnosis of acute appendiceal diverticulitis by ultrasonography. Surgery 2001;130:87.

Lindner AE: Inflammatory bowel disease in the elderly. Clin Geriatr Med 1999;15:487.

Schoetz DJ Jr: Diverticular disease of the colon: a century-old problem. Dis Colon Rectum 1999;42:703.

Perioperative Evaluation and Care

Abir F, Bell R: Assessment and management of the obese patient. Crit Care Med 2004;32:S87.

American College of Obstetricians and Gynecologists. *Prophylactic oophorectomy*. ACOG Practice Bulletin Number 7. American College of Obstetricians and Gynecologists, 1999.

Chan LY: Influence of the Women's Health Initiative trial on the practice of prophylactic oophorectomy and the prescription of estrogen therapy. Fertil Steril 2004;81:1699.

Chen PC et al: Sonographic detection of echogenic fluid and correlation with culdocentesis in the evaluation of ectopic pregnancy. Am J Roentgenol 1998;170:1299.

Crapo RO: Pulmonary function testing. N Engl J Med 1994;331:25.

Dunn AS, Turpie AGG: Perioperative management of patients receiving oral anticoagulants. Arch Intern Med 2003;163:901.

Eagle KA et al. ACC/AHA guideline update for perioperative cardiovascular evaluation for noncardiac surgery—Executive summary a report of the American College of Cardiology/American Heart Association Task Force on Practice Guidelines (Committee to Update the 1996 Guidelines on Perioperative Cardiovascular Evaluation for Noncardiac Surgery). Circulation 2002;105:1257.

Elliott BA: Latex allergy: the perspective from the surgical suite. J Allergy Clin Immunol 2002;110:S117.

Graham GW, Unger BP, Coursin DB: Perioperative management of selected endocrine disorders. Int Anesthesiol Clin 2000;38:31.

Halaszynski TM, Juda R, Silverman DG: Optimizing postoperative outcomes with efficient preoperative assessment and management. Crit Care Med 2004;32(4 Suppl):S76.

Irvin W et al: Minimizing the risk of neurologic injury in gynecologic surgery. Obstet Gynecol 2004;103:374.

Jacober SJ, Sowers JR: An update on perioperative management of diabetes. Arch Intern Med 1999;159:2405.

Jeong YY, Outwater EK, Kang HK: From the FSNA refresher courses: Imaging evaluation of ovarian masses. Radiographics 2000;20:1445.

Learman LA et al: A randomized comparison of total or supracervical hysterectomy: surgical complications and clinical outcomes. Obstet Gynecol 2003;102:453.

Leone FP, Lanzani C, Ferrazzi E: Use of strict sonohysterographic methods for preoperative assessment of submucous myomas. Fertil Steril 2003;79:998.

Martin JT: Geriatric anesthesia: Positioning aged patients. Anesthesiol Clin North America 2000;18:105.

Muravchick S: Preoperative assessment of the elderly patient. Anesthesiol Clin North Am 2000;18:71.

Namnoum AB et al: Incidence of symptom recurrence after hysterectomy for endometriosis. Fertil Steril 1995;64:898.

Olopade OI, Fackenthal JD: Breast cancer genetics: Implications for clinical practice. Hematol Oncol Clin North Am 2000;14:705.

Powell JL, Kasparek DK, Connor GP: Panniculectomy to facilitate gynecologic surgery in morbidly obese women. Obstet Gynecol 1999;94:528.

Shen-Gunther J, Mannel RS: Ascites as a predictor of ovarian malignancy. Gynecol Oncol 2002;87:77.

Smetana GW: Preoperative pulmonary evaluation. N Engl J Med 1999;340:937.

Southorn PA: Preoperative management of the medically at-risk patient. Clin Obstet Gynecol 2002;45:449.

Thakar R et al: Outcomes after total versus subtotal abdominal hysterectomy. N Engl J Med 2002;347:1318.

Thomassin I et al: Symptoms before and after surgical removal of colorectal endometriosis that are assessed by magnetic resonance imaging and rectal endoscopic sonography. Am J Obstet Gynecol 2004;190:1264.

Warner MA et al: Lower extremity neuropathies associated with lithotomy positions. Anesthesiol 2000;93:938.

Antibiotic Prophylaxis

American College of Obstetricians and Gynecologists: *Antibiotics and Gynecologic Infections*. ACOG Educational Bulletin No. 237. American College of Obstetricians and Gynecologists, June 1997.

Eason E et al: Antisepsis for abdominal hysterectomy: a randomized controlled trial of povidone-iodine gel. Br J Obstet Gynaecol 2004;111:695.

Faro S: Can postoperative infection be prevented? Infect Dis Obstet Gynecol 1999;7:215.

Kamat AA, Brancazio L, Gibson M: Wound infection in gynecologic surgery. Infect Dis Obstet Gynecol 2000;8:230.

Smaill F, Hofmeyr GJ: Antibiotic prophylaxis for cesarean section. Cochrane Database Syst Rev 2000:CD000933.

Bowel Preparation

Cohen SM et al: Prospective, randomized, endoscopic-blinded trial comparing precolonoscopy bowel cleansing methods. Dis Col Rectum 1994;37:689.

Muzii L et al: Bowel preparation for gynecological surgery. Crit Rev Onc Heme 2003;48:311.

Oliveira L et al: Mechanical bowel preparation for elective colorectal surgery. A prospective, randomized, surgeon-blinded trial comparing sodium phosphate and polyethylene glycol-based oral lavage solutions. Dis Col Rectum 1997;40:585.

Thromboprophylaxis

Decousus H et al: Superficial vein thrombosis: Risk factors, diagnosis, and treatment. Curr Opin Pulm Med 2003;9:393.

Galvin DJ, Mulvin D, Quinlan DM: Thromboprophylaxis for radical prostatectomy: A comparative analysis of present practice between the USA, the UK, and Ireland. Prostate 2004;60:338.

Geerts WH et al: Prevention of venous thromboembolism. Chest 2001;119:1.

McLeod RS et al: Subcutaneous heparin versus low-molecular-weight heparin as thromboprophylaxis in patients undergoing colorectal surgery: Results of the Canadian colorectal DVT prophylaxis trial: A randomized, double-blind trial. Ann Surg 2001;233:438.

Nicolaides AN et al: Prevention of VTE: International consensus statement (guidelines according to scientific evidence). Int Angiol 1997;16:3.

Corticosteroid Use

Brown CJ, Buie WD: Perioperative stress dose steroids: Do they make a difference? J Am Coll Surg 2001;193:678.

Nicholson G, Burrin JM, Hall GM: Peri-operative steroid supplementation. Anaesthesia 1998;53:1091.

Schiff RL, Welsh GA: Perioperative evaluation and management of the patient with endocrine dysfunction. Med Clin North Am 2003;87:175.

Medications

Pass SE, Simpson RW: Discontinuation and reinstitution of medications during the perioperative period. Am J Health-Syst Pharm 2004;61:899.

Postoperative Care

Schilder JM et al: A prospective controlled trial of early postoperative oral intake following major abdominal gynecologic surgery. Gynecol Oncol 1997;67:235.

Intraoperative & Postoperative Complications of Gynecologic Surgery

47

Michael P. Aronson, MD, David Chelmow, MD, & Uchechi Wosu, MD

■ INTRAOPERATIVE COMPLICATIONS

The intimate anatomic relationship of the genital tract with urologic, gastrointestinal, vascular, and neurologic structures makes occasional injury during gynecologic surgery almost inevitable. The surgeon must do everything possible to prevent such complications and, if they do occur, recognize and treat them in an organized and timely fashion. The keys to avoiding surgical misadventure, and to recognizing it when it has occurred, are understanding pelvic anatomy, using methodical meticulous surgical technique, handling tissues gently, and maintaining constant vigilance. A detailed description of the management of every possible complication of gynecologic surgery is beyond the scope of this text. For this, the reader is referred to the many excellent references at the end of this chapter.

URINARY TRACT INJURY

Ureteral Damage

Ureteral injury occurs in association with most major gynecologic surgical procedures including hysterectomy for benign indications, pelvic cancer surgery, oophorectomy, and suspension of both the vaginal apex and of the bladder neck. The incidence of ureteral injury is reported to be 0.5% for simple hysterectomies for benign disease, up to 1.6% for laparoscopically assisted hysterectomies, and as high as 30% in some older series of Wertheim radical hysterectomies. Isolated statistics such as these have little clinical significance; rather, the knowledge, skill, and diligence of the surgeon, as well as the difficulty of the surgical procedure, determine the risk for any given patient.

The ureter may be accidentally ligated, kinked, transected, crushed, burned, or devascularized. In gynecologic surgery, injury to the ureter most often occurs at the level of the infundibulopelvic ligament, the uterine artery, the uterosacral ligament, or the anterolateral fornix of the vagina as the ureter crosses it to enter the trigone of the bladder. Early recognition of ureteral injury is crucial for preservation of function of the associated kidney. Repair is also more likely to be successful if performed at the time of injury.

The best defense against injury to the ureter is knowledge of its anatomic relations and use of the avascular spaces of the pelvis to identify it intraoperatively (see Chapter 2). This requires good exposure, proper lighting and definitive visualization or palpation.

Despite this careful attention, the need to confirm ureteral integrity may still arise. This can be done at the end of the procedure with a cystoscope or other endoscope. While the patient is being given 5 mL of indigo carmine intravenously, the bladder should be filled with 300 mL of normal saline. If vaginal surgery is being performed, a 70-degree endoscope can be introduced transurethrally. If an abdominal procedure is being performed, patency can be demonstrated by introducing an endoscope through a purposeful cystotomy. To do this, the extraperitoneal dome of the bladder is dissected away from the symphysis pubis and a pursestring suture is placed and small purposeful cystotomy made within it. A 0-degree or 30-degree endoscope is placed in the bladder and the pursestring suture cinched tightly. The ureteral orifices are visualized and a blue effluent can be seen emanating from the orifices if the ureters are patent. The rest of the bladder should also be examined for gross abnormality or evidence of operative trauma. If cystotomy was performed, the pursestring suture is tied and imbricated after the endoscope is removed. Postoperative catheter management is unchanged.

If cystoscopy is not diagnostic, or if injury is strongly suspected, the dome of the bladder can be opened and a stent placed retrograde through each ureteral orifice. If ureteral patency cannot be demonstrated by any of these techniques, further steps, such as retrograde pyelography and transurethral stenting, can be initiated while the patient is still under anesthesia and the injury is fresh.

Patients who develop flank pain in the postoperative period should be strongly suspected of having a ureteral injury. However, a patient with an obstructed ureter may not experience any flank pain at all. Urinary tract injury can be detected postoperatively by intravenous pyelogram (IVP) or retrograde x-ray studies. Renal ultrasonography may reveal hydronephrosis or hydroureter. A continuous postoperative watery vaginal discharge is suggestive of vesicovaginal or ureterovaginal fistula. A urinary fistula should also be suspected if fluid draining from a surgical wound or drain demonstrates much higher creatinine concentration than the patient's blood.

A. URETERAL LIGATION

Ureters may be directly ligated during surgery. They can also be kinked by suture placement and functionally obstructed without actually being ligated. As soon as pressure within the renal pelvis builds to > 40 cm H_2O, renal function will begin to be lost. If renal function is to recover, ureteral ligation or obstruction must be discovered within a few weeks at the latest. Postoperative signs of ureteral obstruction can include flank or pelvic pain, pyelonephritis and sepsis, abdominal swelling secondary to collection of urine (urinoma), or development of a ureterocutaneous fistula. Again, ureteral obstruction and subsequent kidney failure can occur without associated warning signs.

B. TRANSECTION

Transection of the ureter may be detected intraoperatively if urine is noted to be leaking into the operative field. Hematuria may occur after transection but cannot be considered a reliable sign. If not repaired, ureteral transection can result in either a pelvic urinoma or ureterocutaneous fistula. Postoperatively such patients may present with ileus and distention. A ureteroneocystostomy should be performed if the transection occurs within 5 cm of the bladder. Otherwise, the transected ureter above the pelvic brim may be repaired with an end-to-end anastomosis over a ureteral stent.

C. CRUSH INJURY

There is a significant risk of segmental ureteral necrosis following a surgical clamp crush injury to the ureter. The smaller the amount of other tissue involved in the clamp along with the ureter, the greater the chance that the ureter has been seriously compromised. Resection of the crushed ureteral segment and reanastomosis, or performance of ureteroneocystostomy, depending on the site of injury, should be considered unless (a) the ureter was clamped for only a brief time as part of a larger pedicle, (b) there is no visible damage, and (c) peristalsis persists at the site of injury. In such a case, a double-J

ureteral stent can be placed and removed after 4–6 weeks with outpatient cystoscopy. An intravenous pyelogram should be obtained after removal to rule out extravasation and evaluate ureteral patency.

D. DEVASCULARIZATION

Extensive retroperitoneal dissection of the ureter may injure its adventitial vascular supply with subsequent necrosis of the devitalized segment. This risk is greatest in cancer surgery. In the 1950s, Viennese physician Dr. A. H. Palmrich anatomically defined the complex of vessels and nerves that supply the ureter. Later series of radical hysterectomies that preserved this complex by avoiding skeletonization of the ureter resulted in a dramatic decline in ureteral complications.

Bladder Injury

Laceration of the bladder can be confirmed by filling the bladder with sterile milk or methylene blue through a urethral catheter and observing leakage of fluid. Milk has the advantage of not staining the operative field if an injury is present. All edges of the cystotomy must be visualized and mobilized as necessary. The bladder defect can then be repaired with two layers of absorbable suture after which the bladder is again filled to test for leakage. Uncomplicated recovery is generally the rule. Five to 10 days of catheter drainage, depending on the site and extent of injury, helps to promote healing by preventing bladder distention.

Very small bladder injuries caused by Veress needle insertion or small trocar insertion during laparoscopy or bladder neck suspension procedures can sometimes be managed conservatively with dependent drainage with a transurethral catheter. Although small extraperitoneal defects may respond to drainage, intraperitoneal injuries require closure as described above.

GASTROINTESTINAL TRACT INJURY

Bowel is highly susceptible to injury during laparotomy, laparoscopy, and vaginal surgery. The moment of entry into the peritoneal cavity is a crucial step and should be approached cautiously. Patients with adhesions caused by previous surgery, endometriosis, or salpingitis are at high risk for bowel injury as adherent bowel is dissected away from the operative site. The risk of bowel laceration is even greater during the acute phase of pelvic infection because of the increased friability of the secondarily inflamed bowel. These factors should be taken into account when deciding on the operative approach: transvaginal versus laparotomy versus open or closed laparoscopy.

Tight abdominal packing, exposure of the bowel serosa with subsequent dehydration, indiscriminate use of unipolar electrocautery and superficial abrasions from manipulation may be associated with apparently minimal trauma, yet ultimately result in postoperative bowel adhesions. Bowel exposure and manipulation should be minimized during laparotomy.

Complications associated with accidental penetration of bowel arise from bacterial and chemical peritonitis from spillage of bowel contents into the peritoneal cavity. Postoperative fever, abdominal distention, paralytic ileus, and diffuse peritonitis can develop within 24 hours after unrecognized bowel injury. Fecal contamination from colonic injury can prevent successful primary repair. Copious irrigation of the abdomen followed by placement of a closed drainage system at the repair site decreases the risk of generalized postoperative peritonitis. If unprepared colon is entered, or if the injury is extensive, a temporary diverting colostomy proximal to the site of injury may be necessary to allow healing. Abdominal abscess formation, wound infection, enterocutaneous fistula, and extensive bowel adhesions may follow fecal contamination of the abdominal cavity. The risk of bacterial peritonitis is clearly greater if the colon is the site of injury.

Small-bowel injury may produce chemical peritonitis from leakage of secretions from the stomach, gallbladder, and pancreas. Injury to the small bowel or stomach can be successfully repaired with two layers of interrupted suture. It may be necessary to convert a longitudinal small bowel laceration into a transverse repair to avoid constriction of the bowel lumen. Larger injuries and thermal injuries may require segmental resection using suture techniques or stapling devices.

Unrecognized covert injury, such as thermal-bowel injury from electrocoagulation, is particularly dangerous. A patient with such an injury may appear well in the immediate postoperative period. The delayed onset of symptoms of perforation may be misinterpreted or even overlooked. Such unrecognized injuries can prove lethal. Whether operating transvaginally, by laparotomy, or laparoscopically, keep in mind the possibility of unrecognized overt or covert intraoperative bowel injury as the patient moves through the postoperative period.

NEUROLOGIC INJURY

Damage from Patient Positioning

Unnatural positioning of the patient while under anesthesia can cause significant sensory and motor defects in the extremities. Hyperextension or hyperabduction of an extremity may stretch the corresponding major nerve trunk as it exits the thorax or pelvis. The upper roots of the brachial plexus are especially vulnerable to injury, and transient shoulder pain may occur postoperatively if the shoulder has remained hyperextended during surgery. Femoral neuropathy occasionally follows procedures carried out in the lithotomy position when

the hip has been hyperflexed and hyperabducted, stretching and compromising the nerve as it travels under the inguinal ligament.

Nerves in the extremities are also vulnerable to injury where they cross over a skeletal prominence. External pressure on these sites during surgery may produce prolonged sensory and motor defects. A common nerve injury results from compression of the common peroneal nerve at the head of the fibula when the lateral aspect of the leg below the knee rests against a hard leg brace with the patient in lithotomy position. The result is loss of sensation in the dorsum of the ankle often associated with footdrop as a result of loss of motor function of the peroneus longus and brevis muscles. Proper positioning and the use of sequential compression boots may help to avoid this complication.

Prolonged pressure transmitted through the gluteal muscles may injure the sciatic nerves. Compression of the ulnar nerve against the medial epicondyle of the humerus occurs if the elbow is extended with the wrist pronated and results in nerve injury if the patient's arm remains in this position for prolonged periods.

Damage during Surgery

The tips of the blades of an improperly placed self-retaining retractor may rest on the psoas muscles. Prolonged pressure may be transmitted to the femoral, ilioinguinal, iliohypogastric, or genitofemoral nerve with resulting painful neuropathy, sensory loss, and muscle weakness. The risk is especially great in the thin patient. To prevent this, the external part of the retractor can be bolstered with folded sterile towels to relieve this pressure. Alternatively, shorter lateral blades could be used if possible.

The sciatic or obturator nerves may be at significant risk during radical pelvic cancer surgery, and the long thoracic nerve can be easily damaged during surgery for breast cancer. Careful dissection and a strong anatomic background are the best defenses against these injuries.

VASCULAR INJURY

Major Vessel Injury

Incidental injury of major pelvic blood vessels is a rare but potentially catastrophic complication of pelvic surgery. The arteries, with their thick, muscular walls are less often damaged than the thin-walled veins. The inferior vena cava and iliac veins are delicate and are easily injured during lymphadenectomy and other procedures for invasive disease, whereas injury during procedures for benign disease is much less common.

Bleeding from even small injuries to these major vessels can be extremely heavy. If injury occurs, direct pressure should be applied to the injured vessel or the blood supply should be temporarily cut off by applying pressure proximal to the site of injury. This allows the surgeon time to obtain adequate exposure for repair, to carefully assess the nature and extent of the injury, to consult if necessary, and to have blood products delivered to the operating room while limiting the patient's blood loss. Keeping up with replacement of blood volume with packed red blood cells and blood products is essential.

If the injury occurs during laparoscopy with penetration of a vessel by a Veress needle or trocar, the instrument should not be removed while the laparoscopy is being converted to a laparotomy. This allows the instrument to provide some tamponade while aiding subsequent identification of the site of penetration. A midline incision, which can be easily extended as necessary, should be made to provide adequate exposure.

Small injuries often can be repaired with carefully placed, very fine sutures after adequate exposure is obtained and the patient is stabilized. Larger injuries might require emergent consultation with a vascular surgeon about the need for vessel grafts. In the pregnant patient, many vessels are engorged, making them behave like major vessels. The uterine vessels carry 500 mL/min of blood at term. Laceration of these vessels during cesarean delivery or cesarean hysterectomy can cause massive bleeding.

Hemorrhage

Even if major vessels are not injured, unexpected and hard-to-control bleeding from other sources can occur during any gynecologic surgery. The gynecologic surgeon should be comfortable with the technique of hypogastric artery ligation, which will frequently control such bleeding (see Fig 31–1). This technique involves dissection of the hypogastric artery distal to the bifurcation of the common iliac artery. Two silk ties are then passed under the internal iliac artery from lateral to medial and tied approximately 1 cm apart. The artery itself should not be cut. Great care must be taken not to damage the delicate internal iliac vein located immediately posterior and lateral to the hypogastric artery. This ligation acts by decreasing the pulse pressure at the distal bleeding site sufficiently to allow clot formation. Rich collateral circulation exists distal to the ligation, especially from the lumbar and middle sacral circulations. Enough perfusion to the pelvis remains so that not only will the pelvic organs remain viable, but also the potential for future pregnancy is preserved.

Another technique often employed to control massive hemorrhage after a cesarean section is uterine artery ligation. It involves taking large purchases with a stitch through the uterine wall at the level of the cervical isthmus to ligate the uterine artery. One must remain ever mindful of the course of the ureter during this procedure.

Angiographically guided arterial embolization is another technique that may be useful for lesser degrees of bleeding. This technique can be used either intraoperatively or postoperatively in an attempt to avoid a subsequent return to the operating room. Arterial catheters are placed using fluoroscopic guidance, the bleeding sites identified, and embolization done by a variety of techniques. If hypogastric ligation has already been performed, angiographic catheters may not be able to reach the bleeding site and angiographic embolization may not be possible.

Massive hemorrhage, defined as bleeding requiring transfusion of more than 10 units of blood, may occur in extensive pelvic and abdominal surgery such as tumor debulking, lymph node dissections, and pelvic exenteration. This heavy bleeding can occur any time the deep pelvic venous plexus are encountered. When other measures are unsuccessful, packing of the pelvis at the site of hemorrhage with long packs or with gauze rolls inside a bowel bag has been described. The abdomen is closed after it has been packed, and the patient brought back to the operating room 48–72 hours later for removal of the packing.

ANESTHETIC COMPLICATIONS

Malignant Hyperthermia

One surgical patient in 14,000 has a congenital defect of calcium metabolism that presents as life-threatening hyperthermia during general anesthesia. In these patients, the administration of succinylcholine or the volatile anesthetic agents can prevent the reuptake of calcium by the sarcoplasmic reticulum in skeletal muscle cells. Massive calcium levels stimulate a dramatic increase in cell metabolism, causing the characteristic symptoms of elevated body temperature, generalized skeletal muscle rigidity, and metabolic acidosis. Fatal cardiac arrhythmias may occur as hyperkalemia develops in association with acidosis.

If malignant hyperthermia develops, all anesthetic agents should be immediately discontinued and intravenous dantrolene given promptly. Dantrolene exerts its effects by interfering with the release of calcium from the sarcoplasmic reticulum. The dose should be repeated until symptoms subside or until a maximum of 10 mg/kg has been given. Dantrolene should be continued postoperatively. Treatment should also be directed toward stabilization of the patient through correction of cardiac arrhythmias, metabolic acidosis, hyperkalemia, and hyperthermia.

Bronchospasm

Bronchospasm is caused by increased airway reactivity and is detected by wheezing and increased difficulty in ventilating the patient. Patients with known asthma and cardiopulmonary disease are at increased risk for bronchospasm with general anesthesia. However, bronchospasm can also occur in patients without a known history of pulmonary disease. In patients with known disease, consideration is often given to performing procedures under regional anesthesia whenever possible. When bronchospasm does occur intraoperatively, pharmacologic measures such as inhaled beta-mimetics and intravenous corticosteroids should be instituted immediately.

Hypothermia

Prolonged exposure of the lightly covered, anesthetized patient with an open abdomen to the relatively cool operating room environment can result in a drop of several degrees in core body temperature. Severe hypothermia is unusual, but even minor hypothermia has important implications. The return to normal body temperature, which often involves shivering, can cause a large increase in oxygen requirements, which, in turn, can cause cardiovascular stress, particularly for patients with underlying cardiac or pulmonary disease. These problems can be reduced with careful attention to patient temperature, including covering the patient and using warmed intravenous fluids and warmed, humidified ventilation.

Regional Anesthesia

Regional anesthetic techniques are being used with increasing frequency for primary anesthesia, as well as for relief of postoperative pain. Both epidural and spinal anesthetics are being used with increasing frequency in gynecologic surgery. The most common and worrisome problem is respiratory depression. This occurs when the anesthetic level reaches to C3-C5, the level of innervation of the diaphragm. Whenever regional anesthesia is planned, equipment for intubation and mechanical ventilation must be readily available in the event of respiratory depression. These patients must be closely observed both during the procedure and afterward, until the anesthetic agents have been completely metabolized and the anesthetic block resolved, because delayed respiratory depression can occur.

The most common and aggravating postoperative problem with regional anesthesia is spinal headache, caused by persistent leakage of cerebrospinal fluid through the hole made by the spinal or epidural needle. In most instances, headache can be avoided by the use of very-small-caliber needles and adequate hydration before, during, and after the procedure. Use of an epidural blood patch often gives immediate relief.

Other Complications

Teeth can be broken or chipped during intubation. Careful technique with the laryngoscope is always required. Some patients, particularly obese patients and patients with short necks, can be very difficult to intubate, resulting in laryngeal damage, laryngospasm, or abandonment of the procedure because of an inability to intubate the patient. Esophageal intubation can be catastrophic if unrecognized, but can be avoided by careful attention to laryngeal visualization, CO_2 monitoring of exhalation, and careful auscultation. Pneumothorax and aspiration pneumonia, two other common complications, are discussed at length in the section on pulmonary complications. It is thought that death caused by anesthetic complication occurs in approximately 1 in 1500–2000 surgical procedures.

COMPLICATIONS OF ENDOSCOPIC PROCEDURES

Laparoscopy and hysteroscopy are among the most frequently performed gynecologic procedures. These procedures are perceived as less invasive, with faster recovery times, and are frequently performed in an outpatient setting. It is clear, however, that despite being termed minimally invasive, major complications do occur with endoscopic surgery. Recognized complications include bowel, bladder, and ureteral injuries; hernias at the trocar sites; catastrophic major vessel injury at the time of trocar insertion; and CO_2 embolism. In addition to complications specific to endoscopy, any of the complications associated with traditional gynecologic surgery can occur.

Great care is necessary to minimize complications from endoscopic procedures. When inserting the Veress needle, careful attention should be paid to keeping the tip in the midline. The needle should be directed downward at approximately 45 degrees to avoid the bifurcations of the aorta and inferior vena cava, usually located 1–3 cm below the umbilicus. The umbilicus provides the shortest distance between skin and peritoneum because anatomic layers fuse there. Veress needle insertion at this site helps avoid the complication of extraperitoneal insufflation which can, in some cases, lead to respiratory acidosis, pneumothorax, and pneumomediastinum.

Many of the most serious complications occur at the time of trocar insertion. In patients with a high risk of bowel adhesions to the anterior abdominal wall, some surgeons advocate using an open trocar placement technique, although no published evidence exists to support this. All subsequent trocars should be placed under direct visualization, with careful attention paid to avoiding the inferior epigastric vessels. When performing laparoscopic procedures the same attention must be paid to identification of the ureters and other anatomy as in open procedures. Bowel, bladder, and ureter, as well as major vessels, can be injured just as easily during endoscopic procedures as during laparotomy.

Hysteroscopy has some unique complications in addition to the risks of uterine perforation, visceral damage, and hemorrhage. The uterine distention medium may cause life-threatening electrolyte imbalances as well as introduce air emboli into the uterine venous sinuses. Air emboli arise from bubbles in the distention media, room air introduced into the uterine cavity when the hysteroscope is placed, or from bubbles generated from vaporization or coagulation procedures within the distention media. Air emboli can cause pulmonary hypertension and hypoxic vasoconstriction, and result in pulmonary edema and respiratory distress. During the procedure, a drop in both oxygen saturation and end-tidal CO_2 should be recognized as a hallmark of air embolization.

Hyponatremia, hypokalemia, hypoosmolality, and fluid overload develop when electrolyte-free distention media such as glycine and sorbitol enter into the venous circulation. The patient can present with headache, nausea, vomiting, arrhythmias, and altered mental status secondary to hyponatremic encephalopathy. The most effective means to avoid these complications is to closely record hysteroscopic fluid inputs and outputs. When a deficit of 1000–2000 mL of fluid is noted, the procedure should be abandoned. Serum sodium will decrease by 10 mmol/L per 1000 mL of hypotonic solution retained. Complications from fluid overload occur at a rate of 1–4% of all hysteroscopies.

■ POSTOPERATIVE COMPLICATIONS

CARDIOVASCULAR COMPLICATIONS

1. Myocardial Infarction

Myocardial infarction is an infrequent but severe perioperative complication with significant risk of mortality. It usually occurs within the first 4 days after surgery. Its diagnosis should be considered whenever a postoperative patient demonstrates:

Chest pain
Hypotension refractory to fluid administration
Acute pulmonary edema
New-onset cardiac dysrhythmia

It is important to note that many postoperative myocardial infarctions are pain free.

The primary approach is risk stratification and prevention. The American College of Cardiology and American Heart Association have guidelines for the perioperative cardiology assessment. Patients at risk should have preoperative evaluation by their primary care provider, and high-risk patients may need consultation with a cardiologist. In at-risk patients, perioperative β blocker administration at a dose that keeps the patient's heart rate at 50–60 bpm decreases risk.

Patients suspected of having myocardial infarction need immediate evaluation with electrocardiogram and cardiac enzymes, including the myocardial band (MB) fraction of creatinine phosphokinase (CPK) and troponin. The American College of Cardiology has revised the definition of myocardial infarction and outlines use of the electrocardiogram (ECG) and enzymes for making the diagnosis. Early diagnosis and treatment are important for decreasing the amount of infarcted myocardium, thereby decreasing the risk of sequelae and mortality. Immediate treatment usually includes oxygen, nitroglycerin, and morphine. Other treatments include angiographic revascularization procedures such as balloon angioplasty and stent placement. The use of thrombolytic therapy is limited in immediate postoperative patients by the risk of surgical site bleeding.

THROMBOEMBOLIC COMPLICATIONS

1. Superficial Thrombophlebitis

Postoperative superficial thrombophlebitis is the most common complication of peripheral intravenous catheters and can also occur in the lower extremities of women with varicosities. The affected vein becomes inflamed, with erythema, localized heat, swelling, and tenderness. This disorder is generally limited to the superficial veins, and concomitant deep vein involvement or pulmonary embolism is very unusual. When superficial thrombophlebitis is diagnosed, treatment includes moving the intravenous access site, application of warm, moist packs, elevation of the extremity, and analgesics. Anticoagulants are rarely indicated when only the superficial vessels are involved. Tagalakis reviews the epidemiology of peripheral vein infusion thrombophlebitis and summarizes the Centers for Disease Control and Prevention (CDC) recommendations for prevention.

2. Deep Vein Thrombosis

Thrombosis of the deep veins occurs most often in the calf but may also occur in the thigh or pelvis. It may be primary or an extension of more peripheral disease. Age older than 40 years, obesity, cancer, pregnancy, estrogen use, diabetes, prior thromboembolism, prolonged surgery, prolonged immobilization, and thrombophilias (eg, antithrombin III deficiency, protein C and S deficiencies, factor V Leiden and prothrombin mutations, and the lupus anticoagulant) are predisposing factors, but the disease frequently occurs in otherwise healthy patients. The major complication of deep thrombophlebitis is pulmonary embolism. Chronic venous insufficiency of the affected extremity may also develop as a long-term consequence. As noted in Chapter 46, there are a number of proven prophylactic strategies that should be routinely used perioperatively to minimize the risk of deep vein thrombosis (DVT) and pulmonary embolism (PE).

A. CLINICAL FINDINGS

Symptoms may be localized to the involved extremity, or the thrombus may be asymptomatic. Pulmonary embolism may be the first sign. The patient may complain of a dull ache or more significant pain in the leg or calf. There may be tenderness or spasm in the calf muscle. Examination may reveal swelling of the calf, which may require measurement of the circumference of both calves at the same level to detect. Dorsiflexion of the foot may elicit pain in the calf (Homans' sign). Although a positive Homans' sign is specific, the test is not very sensitive (approximately 25%). Slight elevation of temperature and pulse is frequently noted. If the clot is in the femoral vein or in the pelvis, swelling of the extremity may be more severe. It is a difficult diagnosis to make clinically, with most episodes of suspected DVT unconfirmed, and a large fraction of DVTs asymptomatic.

B. DIAGNOSIS

Compression ultrasonography or impedance plethysmography usually provide a definite diagnosis. Both are noninvasive and are sensitive and specific. D-dimers have also been studied as a diagnostic test because the test is noninvasive. A normal D-dimer level is strongly predictive of the absence of thromboembolism. Unfortunately it is nonspecific, and can be elevated by recent surgery. If these tests are not diagnostic, contrast venography is the gold standard and should be performed. Chunilal and Ginsberg extensively review these tests and their use in combination in general, and Davis specifically reviews their use in gynecologic surgical patients.

C. TREATMENT

1. Medical treatment—Once the diagnosis of a deep vein thrombosis extending into the veins proximal to the calf has been made, anticoagulant therapy should be started immediately. Bates and Ginsberg extensively review therapeutic options. Traditionally, intravenous unfractionated heparin has been the first-line therapy. Recently, subcutaneous low-molecular-weight heparin has gained acceptance. Coagulation studies, including international normalized ratio (INR) and partial thromboplastin time (PTT), should be measured before anticoagulant therapy is started; these tests provide a basis for interpreting the degree of anticoagulation achieved. When using unfractionated heparin, the PTT should be kept to 1.5–2.5 times the control value. The more predictable bioavailability, clearance, and activity of low-molecular-weight heparins obviates the need for laboratory monitoring except in unusual circumstances. Unfortunately, they are quite expensive despite costs savings from decreased need for laboratory monitoring. Heparin should be continued until effective long-term therapy is established.

Oral anticoagulants, particularly warfarin, are often started at the same time as heparin. The therapeutic effect of these agents is measured by the INR. Whereas heparin prolongs the clotting time almost immediately, the oral anticoagulants do not exert their full effect for 48–72 hours. Heparin is usually started for its immediate short-term effect, then replaced with oral anticoagulants for long-term treatment. Low-molecular-weight heparin can be used long-term in patients for whom bleeding is a particular risk or laboratory monitoring is problematic. If using warfarin, the INR should be determined daily until equilibrium levels of 2.0–3.0 are attained. Anticoagulation is usually continued empirically for 3–6 months.

Anticoagulation presents significant risks, and anticoagulated patients must be thoroughly counseled to recognize possible complications of therapy, including hematuria, hemoptysis, hematemesis, melena, and easy bruisability. These patients should be provided with a means of identification indicating that they are receiving anticoagulant therapy, in case of an accident in which they become unconscious. Patients should also be given a list of over-the-counter medications to avoid, including nonsteroidal anti-inflammatory drugs, aspirin, and antibiotics, which may affect their anticoagulation.

Management of calf vein thromboses is somewhat controversial. They are often viewed as not being a problem unless they extend into the proximal veins. When suspected or confirmed, serial compression ultrasound can be performed with reservation of anticoagulation for the approximately 10% of patients whose clots eventually extend into the proximal circulation.

2. Local measures—Local measures include elevation of the legs to provide good venous drainage and the application of full-leg gradient-pressure elastic hose. Full activities may be permitted when inflammation has subsided, usually within 1–2 weeks of starting therapy. The patient should be encouraged to continue to elevate her legs whenever she can. Prolonged sitting and the use of constrictive garments, especially knee-high support stockings or hosiery, should be avoided.

3. Surgical treatment—Thrombectomy occasionally may be considered for persistent severe swelling of the extremity. An inferior vena cava filter or vena cava ligation may be considered for repeated episodes of pulmonary embolism that occur in spite of adequate anticoagulation or when anticoagulation is absolutely contraindicated.

3. Septic Pelvic Thrombophlebitis

Septic pelvic thrombophlebitis is a complication that is almost unique to pelvic surgery. It occurs most frequently related to cesarean delivery and is discussed in detail in Chapter 23.

4. Pulmonary Embolism

Pulmonary embolism is a critical complication of pelvic surgery. This diagnosis should be suspected if cardiac or pulmonary symptoms occur abruptly. Risk factors are the same as noted above for DVT. It is a complication of pelvic or proximal lower-extremity deep vein thromboembolism; nonetheless, pulmonary embolism may precede the diagnosis of peripheral disease. Pulmonary embolism may occur at any time. With the reduction in length of hospital stay, it is being noted more frequently after discharge. The differential diagnosis includes atelectasis, pneumonia, myocardial infarction, and pneumothorax.

Clinical Findings

A. SYMPTOMS AND SIGNS

The diagnosis of pulmonary embolism is suggested by pleuritic chest pain, dyspnea, tachypnea, and tachycardia. Unfortunately, these symptoms are neither specific nor consistent. Patients with large emboli can have chest pain, severe dyspnea, cyanosis, tachycardia, hypotension or shock, restlessness, and anxiety. If the embolus is massive, sudden death may result from acute cor pulmonale. The combination of risk factors and symptoms will prompt an evaluation. Fedullo and Tapson extensively review the diagnostic approach.

B. DIAGNOSIS

In the patient suspected of having a pulmonary embolus, an arterial blood gas, 12-lead ECG, and chest radiograph should be obtained. Chest film and ECG can show signs of pulmonary embolism, but are predominantly performed to eliminate other diagnostic possibilities, particularly myocardial infarction and pneumonia. Spiral chest computerized tomography (CT) is now the diagnostic procedure of choice. Lower-extremity studies, as discussed above, can also be performed. In a symptomatic patient, the diagnosis is also confirmed by the confirmation of thrombus in a proximal lower-extremity vein.

C. LABORATORY FINDINGS

A low arterial PO_2 should raise suspicion of pulmonary embolus. D-Dimer assays have high negative predictive value for ruling out deep venous thrombosis and pulmonary embolism; their role in the postoperative setting needs further clarification as recent surgery can also elevate the D-dimer level, and false positives are likely.

D. RADIOGRAPH FINDINGS

Chest radiography frequently shows no abnormality, and changes may be delayed 24–48 hours. Its primary role is to rule out pneumonia. In approximately 15% of patients, a pulmonary density is present, which is in the periphery of the lung and roughly in the shape of a triangle with its base at the lung surface. Other possible findings are enlargement of the main pulmonary artery, small pleural effusion, and elevated diaphragm.

E. ELECTROCARDIOGRAPHY

The ECG may show characteristic changes of pulmonary embolism in one-third of cases. These changes include $S_1Q_3T_3$ patterns, right bundle-branch block, and T-wave inversion in leads V_1 through V_4. The ECG is principally of use in ruling out myocardial infarction.

F. LUNG SCAN

The ventilation-perfusion (V/Q) scan was, until recently, the study of choice. Its use has largely been supplanted by spiral chest CT. The V/Q scan's main limitation is that it is frequently equivocal, although it still is useful in patients with allergy or a contraindication to contrast agents.

G. SPIRAL CHEST CT

Thin-section CT imaging of the chest with third-generation scanners has become the modality of choice for diagnosing pulmonary embolism. It frequently can visualize the emboli, as well as eliminate other diagnostic possibilities like pneumonia. High sensitivities and specificities have been reported.

H. ANGIOGRAPHY

Pulmonary angiography should be done in the rare instances when lower-extremity studies and spiral CT are nondiagnostic in a patient with high clinical suspicion. It is considered the "gold standard." It is invasive, with risks of catheter and contrast complications, and its use should be reserved for when noninvasive studies have been inadequate.

Treatment

Cardiopulmonary resuscitation measures should be instituted as necessary. Close monitoring is essential, as is treatment of acid–base abnormalities and shock. Because of the high mortality, patients with strong clinical suspicion of pulmonary embolism should be started immediately on heparin, and the heparin continued until the appropriate studies rule out the diagnosis. Management of anticoagulation follows the same procedure as for deep vein thrombosis. Goldhaber reviews current treatment in detail, as well as developing new alternatives.

Prevention

As discussed in Chapter 46, effective prophylactic measures exist, and should be routinely used. International consensus recommendations exist for prevention of venous thromboembolism and include specific recommendations for gynecologic surgery. Patients undergoing minor gynecologic surgery without risk factors may or may not receive prophylaxis. Patients at moderate and high risk (major surgery, age older than 40 years, use of oral contraceptives) should receive prophylaxis with intermittent pneumatic compression stockings or heparin.

PULMONARY COMPLICATIONS

1. Pulmonary Edema

Pulmonary edema is a serious complication that if improperly managed can be fatal. In general, it can be categorized as noncardiogenic and cardiogenic in origin. Noncardiogenic causes include diffuse pulmonary infection, aspiration, and shock, and can lead to the adult respiratory distress syndrome (ARDS). These etiologies are discussed elsewhere throughout this chapter and in other chapters.

Most postoperative pulmonary edema is cardiogenic in origin, resulting from congestive heart failure. This can be caused by fluid overload, as well as cardiac dysfunction from myocardial infarction or valvular disease such as mitral regurgitation. In many instances, it is likely a preventable complication resulting from less than full attention to fluid administration.

Pulmonary edema usually initially presents as mild tachypnea. An arterial blood gas will usually show decreased PO_2 and PCO_2 and increased alveolar–arterial gradient. These changes occur before physical or radiologic findings can be detected. If untreated, and the fluid content of the lungs further increases, symptoms worsen, blood gas parameters worsen, and the patient will develop physical findings of rales and chest radiograph findings of Kerley-B lines, development of a butterfly pattern, and opacities. At its worst, patients may have pink froth emerge from their mouth.

Strict monitoring of fluid balance may help prevent pulmonary edema. Patients suspected of having pulmonary edema should be diuresed, usually with furosemide. Patients being treated with furosemide also need careful monitoring of their potassium, and frequently need potassium supplementation. Patients with definitive signs of rales and radiographic findings should receive diuresis. Consideration should be given to diuretics in patients

where there is a strong suspicion of pulmonary edema even in the absence of these findings, as patients can have early pulmonary edema prior to the development of these findings. Patients who have gone into pulmonary edema in the absence of volume overload, or who respond poorly to diuretics should be ruled out for myocardial infarction, and consideration given to echocardiography to check for valvular dysfunction.

2. Atelectasis

Atelectasis is largely an intraoperative problem, but can also occur during the postoperative period. It consists of areas of airway collapse and occurs because of diminished functional residual capacity in the supine position and splinting caused by pain from abdominal surgery. The blood that traverses the areas with atelectasis is not oxygenated, resulting in shunting and hypoxia. Massive atelectasis may occur when a mucus plug or aspirated vomitus occludes a large bronchus. Predisposing factors include chronic obstructive pulmonary disease, obesity, smoking, and general anesthesia. In the postoperative period, atelectasis can result in hypoxemia, and more importantly, prevention may decrease the incidence of other postoperative pulmonary complications, particularly pneumonia.

Clinical Findings

The clinical findings vary with the extent of atelectasis. Mild atelectasis is the most common cause of fever in the immediate postoperative period. As the patient begins ambulating and her secretions decrease, it usually resolves. On auscultation, the patient can have diminished breath sounds, particularly at the lung bases. They may also have areas of dullness to percussion, together with bronchial breathing and inspiratory rales. Chest radiograph findings include patchy opacities. Atelectasis and bronchopneumonia have a similar clinical picture, and may occur together.

Prevention

The prevention of postoperative atelectasis begins in the preoperative period. Patients should be encouraged to stop smoking preoperatively. Patients with chronic lung disease should be given antibiotics and chest physical therapy if an acute or chronic infection is suspected. Bronchospasm should be treated with bronchodilators. Elective surgery should be postponed if upper respiratory infection is present.

Intraoperatively, the patient should be ventilated with adequate tidal volumes with the addition of positive end-expiratory pressure if signs of atelectasis such as decreasing oxygen saturation become apparent. Intraoperative atelectasis or small airway collapse is more commonly seen in patients with chronic lung disease or obesity and can be aggravated by the Trendelenburg position. Intraoperative humidification and suctioning of secretions are helpful.

Postoperatively, atelectasis is best avoided by minimizing pain, placing patients in the sitting position, and encouraging deep breathing and early ambulation. Incentive spirometry devices help patients to perform deep inspiration exercises. Patient-controlled analgesia or use of an epidural catheter for postoperative pain management can help by reducing respiratory depression.

Treatment

Treatment consists of intensive chest physical therapy and supplemental oxygen. Pain should be controlled because it is an obstacle to deep breathing. Patients should be monitored for pneumonia, for which they are at increased risk. In the rare instance of massive atelectasis, bronchoscopy can be used to manage mucous plugging. Very rarely, if there is inadequate tissue oxygenation, intubation and mechanical ventilation may be necessary.

3. Pneumonia

Postoperative pneumonia may follow atelectasis and is usually caused by aspiration of bacteria colonizing the oropharynx or upper gastrointestinal tract. Abundant tracheobronchial secretions from preexisting bronchitis also predispose to this complication. Other risk factors relevant to gynecologic surgery include obesity, age older than 70 years, chronic obstructive pulmonary disease, abdominal surgery, and smoking. Mortality rates as high as 10% have been suggested, particularly if sepsis ensues.

Fever in the first few postoperative days is usually from atelectasis. If it persists or is followed by higher temperatures, systemic toxicity, or respiratory difficulty, the patient may have pneumonia. Patients with pneumonia may have progressively worsening respiratory secretions and productive cough, although these symptoms can be masked if the patient's ability to cough is suppressed by medications or pain. Physical examination may reveal evidence of pulmonary consolidation, and numerous coarse rales are often present. Although the chest radiograph may show diffuse patchy infiltrates or lobar consolidation, this appearance may lag behind the clinical picture by as much as 24 hours.

The treatment of pneumonia includes deep breathing and coughing to mobilize secretions. The patient should be encouraged to change position frequently. Nasotracheal suction may be used to stimulate the cough reflex. Specific broad-spectrum antibiotic therapy should be instituted based on Gram stain and knowledge of pathogens specific to the institution, and revised as indicated by subsequent sputum culture and sensitivity tests. Induced sputum is more reliable as oral contamination of expectorated specimens occurs frequently. Positive-pressure ventilation may improve the depth of respiration and reduce the work of breathing in extremely ill patients.

A number of measures are supported by evidence and are suggested to decrease postoperative pneumonia, including the following:

Preoperative instruction, especially in patients with risk factors for postoperative pneumonia, in taking deep breaths and early ambulation.

Encouraging all postoperative patients to take deep breaths, move about the bed, and ambulate as soon as medically safe.

Incentive spirometry for patients with risk factors for postoperative pneumonia.

4. Aspiration Pneumonitis

Aspiration pneumonitis is the acute lung injury that occurs after sterile gastric contents are inhaled into the lung. Essentially, gastric acid creates a chemical "burn" to the lung tissue. It occurs approximately once every 3000 surgeries where general anesthesia is used. It is responsible for 10–30% of anesthetic related deaths. It can also occur in patients whose gag reflex or ability to cough may be depressed, as in the immediate postoperative period. Risk factors include difficult intubations, passive regurgitation in the patient with an incompletely empty stomach, poor gastroesophageal sphincter tone in patients with hiatal hernia, inflation of the stomach with air, and pregnancy. Other risk factors include vomiting in patients with neurologic disease, sedation, and other causes of decreased gag reflex.

The chance of pulmonary aspiration at time of surgery can be minimized by:

1. Performing awake fiberoptic intubation on patients with predictably difficult airways.
2. Speeding the process of gastric emptying by intravenously administering metoclopramide 10 mg.
3. Increasing the pH of gastric contents by means of a nonparticulate antacid and use of H_2 blockers (this helps minimize pulmonary damage if aspiration does occur).
4. Using a rapid sequence induction with pentothal and cricoid pressure. Cricoid pressure closes off the esophagus to prevent passively regurgitated material from reaching the larynx. This pressure is maintained until the proper positioning of the tube in the trachea is verified.

Generally, a small amount of aspiration may be associated with mild atelectasis and cause temporary hypoxia. Some patients will have only arterial desaturation and radiologic findings without other symptoms. Other symptoms may include shortness of breath, wheezing, coughing, and pulmonary edema. More severe aspiration may lead to serious hypoxia requiring mechanical ventilation. Some patients will progress to ARDS (Chapter 60).

If known aspiration of gastric contents occurs during intubation, the upper airway should be suctioned. Prophylactic antibiotic use is not recommended, as gastric contents are usually sterile owing to the inhibition of bacterial growth by the elevated gastric pH. Broad-spectrum antibiotics should be considered in patients whose symptoms do not resolve after 48 hours. Routine corticosteroid administration is no longer recommended. Supportive measures, sometimes including mechanical ventilation, may be necessary.

5. Tension Pneumothorax

Tension pneumothorax is an uncommon complication and is most likely to occur during the first 24–48 hours after surgery. Pneumothorax can occur during positive-pressure ventilation and may not be apparent until the ventilation is stopped. Pneumothorax presents as acute respiratory distress with distant breath sounds on the affected side and frequently a marked mediastinal shift away from the affected side. The diagnosis is made by chest radiography. Immediate placement of a chest tube is essential; temporary improvement can be obtained by inserting one or more large-bore angiocatheters under local anesthesia through the intercostal space at approximately T6-T8 to allow escape of air until a chest tube can be inserted. Chest tube drainage is usually continued for several days, until the air leak has sealed.

6. Acute Respiratory Distress Syndrome

ARDS, a frequently catastrophic postoperative complication, is considered in Chapter 60.

GASTROINTESTINAL TRACT COMPLICATIONS

Gastrointestinal complications are most likely to occur after transabdominal operations, but they may also complicate vaginal procedures. Any serious illness or surgical procedure may cause malfunction of the gastrointestinal tract.

1. Ileus

Ileus is defined as transient impairment of bowel motility. Some degree of postoperative ileus occurs whenever the peritoneal cavity is entered. There does not appear to be any physiologic benefit to ileus as part of postoperative healing.

Clinical Findings

Ileus is characterized by decreased or absent bowel sounds, and can progress to include abdominal cramps and distention. Flatus and bowel movement are usually reassuring signs that ileus is resolving, but can occur with an ileus, reflecting incomplete return of bowel function. Some patients may have nausea and vomiting. On plain abdominal radiograph (kidneys, ureters, bladder), there is generalized dilatation and gaseous distention of both small and large bowels, although the small-bowel component may be more prominent.

Prevention

Holte and Kehlet present a number of strategies effective in decreasing postoperative ileus. In particular, opioid anesthetics clearly decrease bowel motility and may prolong an ileus. Strategies of minimizing opiates by using nonsteroidal anti-inflammatory drugs, or using postoperative epidural for pain relief have been shown effective in shortening the time to return of bowel function. Routine use of nasogastric intubation does not prevent ileus, and may lengthen hospitalization. Early ambulation is beneficial for many other reasons, but does not shorten the time to return of bowel function. They reviewed a number of studies on patients undergoing gynecologic surgery suggesting that rapid advancement of diet does not worsen ileus, and likely hastens return of bowel function. Early feeding may decrease ileus by stimulating overall gastrointestinal motility through initiation of propulsive reflexes and the secretion of intestinal hormones.

Treatment

If nausea, vomiting, or abdominal distention becomes severe, a nasogastric tube should be inserted into the stomach. Postoperative small bowel obstruction can present the same way, and should be ruled out by kidneys, ureters, bladderfilms. Electrolytes should be monitored and corrected in patients undergoing prolonged nasogastric suctioning. Enemas and suppositories are frequently used, but can obscure the diagnosis of a small-bowel obstruction by placing air and fluid in the rectum, and have not been proven effective. If the ileus is persistent, especially if accompanied by a febrile course, a retained foreign body should be considered, and can usually be ruled out by the same radiologic study. Urologic trauma with resultant extravasation of urine may be an unusual cause of persistent ileus, and can be diagnosed with an intravenous urogram.

2. Postoperative Intestinal Obstruction

Small-bowel obstruction may occur as a complication of any intraperitoneal operation. It most frequently occurs as a consequence of adhesion formation. Obstruction results when these adhesions trap or kink a segment of intestine. The resultant partial or complete bowel obstruction is usually noted between the fifth and sixth postoperative days; however, obstruction can occur sooner. Other causes include herniation through a laparoscopic trocar site, internal herniation, and inflammation, for instance from an intra-abdominal abscess. Most concerning is the risk that the involved bowel can strangulate. Delayed small-bowel obstruction can also happen years after hysterectomy. Dense, fibrous adhesions develop after 8–12 weeks and can entrap bowel and cause delayed obstruction with a high incidence of bowel ischemia.

Clinical Findings

Obstruction is frequently characterized by abdominal pain, vomiting, distention, and obstipation. On examination, the bowel is distended. High-pitched bowel sounds heard on auscultation are noted to be synchronous with cramping pain. It is frequently difficult to differentiate from postoperative ileus. Obstruction should be suspected if the symptoms develop in a patient previously doing well, particularly if they were previously passing stool or flatus and are no longer doing so.

Diagnosis

Sajja and Schein review diagnostic modalities in their general review of early postoperative small-bowel obstruction. A plain abdominal radiograph usually reveals distention of a portion of the small bowel with air–fluid levels. In general, the colon is free of air. Upper gastrointestinal contrast studies can be used. If no contrast is visualized in the large bowel, obstruction is present. However, as contrast can pass through a partial obstruction, visualization of contrast in the large bowel does not eliminate the possibility. Gastrografin, a hyperosmolar agent, increases motility, and may help resolution of ileus or small-bowel obstruction. CT scan with oral contrast can differentiate ileus from small-bowel obstruction with a high degree of sensitivity and specificity, and can also detect other causes of obstruction including tumor, abscess, or hematoma.

Treatment

Small-bowel obstruction, with its risk of resultant bowel ischemia and infarction, is a serious complication requiring immediate intervention. It is frequently possible to treat postoperative bowel obstruction conservatively by bowel decompression with a nasogastric or long intestinal tube. Long intestinal tubes do not offer any advantage over nasogastric tubes unless they are properly placed, which generally requires fluoroscopic guidance. Tube decompression can result in realignment of the bowel and relief of the obstruction, or adhesions may relax or be released sufficiently to allow spontaneous decompression. If the obstruction does not respond to conservative management, or signs of bowel infarction occur, the patient will need to return to the operating room. Obstruction is associated with large fluid shifts into the bowel lumen, requiring vigorous hydration and careful electrolyte replacement. A special case is obstruction after laparoscopy. If herniation of bowel through a trocar site is suspected, early return to the operating room is warranted.

3. Constipation and Fecal Impaction

A reduction in the number of bowel movements is to be expected in the early postoperative period because of low food intake and ileus. In a postoperative patient with obstipation, where ileus and small-bowel obstruction are not suspected, a mild laxative (milk of magnesia, 30 mL orally) may be prescribed. A clear water enema or rectal bisacodyl suppository can also be used.

Fecal impaction can also cause diarrhea in the postoperative patient. If suspected, a digital rectal examination should be performed. If hard stool is encountered in the ampulla, the diagnosis of fecal impaction is verified. The condition is caused by limitation of oral fluids and is especially common in elderly patients and others confined to bed. It may be aggravated by previous gastrointestinal series or barium enema with accumulation of barium in the colon. The treatment of fecal impaction is digital disimpaction of the firm fecal masses after an oil-retention enema.

4. Diarrhea

Most postoperative diarrhea is likely related to antibiotic administration. Oral contrast agents can also cause diarrhea. Most antibiotic-related diarrhea is mild. Antibiotic administration alters the bacterial flora of the gastrointestinal tract. If overgrowth with *Clostridium difficile* occurs, a range of diseases may present, from asymptomatic colonization to mild diarrhea to pseudomembranous enterocolitis. This more significant complication may occur as a complication of any antibiotic administration, with penicillins and cephalosporins the most frequently implicated agents. This disease may be particularly devastating for the geriatric or debilitated patient.

Diagnosis

The diagnosis is made by detection of the *C. difficile* toxin in stool specimens. Enzyme immunoassays used in most labs are quite specific, but have false-negative rates of 10–20%. Pseudomembranous changes may be seen on colonoscopy.

Treatment

For any suspected antibiotic-related diarrhea, the patient should receive adequate rehydration with monitoring and repletion of electrolytes as necessary. When possible, the antibiotic should be discontinued, or changed to an antibiotic less likely to cause diarrhea. If *C. difficile* is detected or strongly suspected, oral metronidazole, 250 mg 4 times a day for 10 days, is the first-line therapy. Oral vancomycin, 125 mg every 6 hours for 10 days, is equally effective, but considerably more expensive. If the patient is unable to tolerate anything by mouth, only IV metronidazole is effective. Significant concentrations of vancomycin are not built up in the gastrointestinal tract if given intravenously. The infection is easily spread throughout hospitals, with up to 20% of hospitalized patients colonized after 1 week in the hospital. Once diagnosed, patients must be isolated and infection precautions initiated.

5. Fistulas

A full discussion of genital fistulas is beyond the scope of this chapter. Risk factors for fistulas after gynecologic surgery include malignancy, prior radiation therapy, intraoperative bowel, bladder, or ureteral injury, and obstetric trauma (eg, fourth-degree lacerations, breakdown of episiotomy repairs). Vesicovaginal, rectovaginal, and enterocutaneous fistulas are rare, but are the most commonly seen.

Vesicovaginal fistula should be suspected if the patient presents with a continuous watery discharge from the vagina. It can be diagnosed by direct observation or instillation of methylene blue into the bladder and placement of cotton balls or a tampon in the vagina. Discoloration of the cotton or tampon indicates a communication between bladder and vagina. Approximately 20% of fresh postoperative vesicovaginal fistulas will close spontaneously with prolonged catheter drainage. The remainder are usually repaired with a transvaginal surgical approach, which has a good success rate.

Rectovaginal fistulas occur after obstetric trauma or vaginal surgery. Primary transvaginal repair has an approximately 90% success of closure. Larger, recurrent, or irradiated defects may require diverting colostomy while the repair heals.

Enterocutaneous fistulas may present initially with wound erythema, followed by feculent drainage from the incision site. Treatment of enterocutaneous fistulas consists of keeping the patient from oral intake over a period of 2–4 weeks, supplementation with total parenteral nutrition, and nasogastric decompression. If spontaneous closure does not occur, surgical repair will be necessary.

URINARY TRACT COMPLICATIONS

1. Urinary Retention

Postoperative pain or surgery at the bladder neck can result in bladder dysfunction impairing bladder emptying. Urinary retention should be considered if the patient is unable to void postoperatively or after urinary catheter removal. Most patients should be able to void by 4–6 hours after completion of minor surgery, or removal of the urinary catheter after a major case. The patient should be encouraged to get out of bed to void. If the normal capacity of the bladder is exceeded (500 mL) and the bladder overdistended, serious bladder dysfunction may result. Overdistention of the bladder can also occur in the patient with a kinked or clotted suprapubic tube or transurethral catheter.

Inability of the patient to void or difficulty in voiding often is a result of pain caused by using the voluntary muscles to start the urinary stream. With transvaginal procedures or bladder neck suspension procedures, sutures near the urethra or urethral edema may make voiding difficult or impossible. Occasionally retention after urinary incontinence procedures are caused by obstruction secondary to overcorrection of the bladder neck.

Treatment

The treatment for urinary retention is immediate bladder drainage with sterile catheterization. If more than 500 mL of urine is drained, the bladder muscle has likely lost tone, and 24–48 hours of continued drainage should be considered before another voiding trial. Decompression of the distended bladder can be complicated by hematuria, transient hypotension, and postobstructive diuresis. Patients with recurrent difficulties may have underlying urinary tract infections.

Prevention

After a major procedure in which postoperative bleeding or operative damage to the urinary tract is a possibility, bladder drainage by means of a urethral catheter or suprapubic cystotomy tube should be instituted despite the small risk of bladder infection. The catheter usually can be removed within 24–48 hours.

If prolonged drainage is required, intermittent self-catheterization or suprapubic drainage is preferable to transurethral catheter drainage because of increased patient comfort, ease of care, and a reduced incidence of infection. These modalities also may be useful in facilitating postoperative voiding trials after urogynecologic procedures. If a patient is facing a prolonged return to normal voiding function and has adequate visual acuity and manual dexterity, intermittent clean self-catheterization is the most attractive alternative.

Anxiety is thought to play a role in patients with difficulty voiding after surgery. Some providers believe benzodiazepines may be helpful in management due to both their anxiolytic and skeletal muscle-relaxant effects, although a recent randomized trial failed to show an effect.

2. Oliguria and Anuria

Oliguria is typically defined as urinary output of less than 30 mL/h. It usually results from intravascular volume depletion. Disturbances of electrolyte balance (eg, "water intoxication syndrome") or diminished renal blood flow (cardiac failure, shock) also can cause oliguria, as can volume overload causing congestive heart failure and pulmonary edema. After these possible causes of oliguria have been eliminated, an underlying serious disorder of the urinary tract should be considered.

Rarely, anuria may be caused by bilateral ureteral obstruction, a complication that must be considered when there is no urinary output on the operating table or during the immediate postoperative period. If an intravenous pyelogram (IVP) fails to reveal the cause of this serious postoperative complication, underlying kidney disease (eg, acute tubular necrosis) should be suspected.

Diagnosis

Patients with low or absent urine output should be evaluated immediately. Volume status since surgery should be assessed by tallying and comparing fluids administered with total fluids lost (blood loss, urine output, and estimated insensible losses). Patients suspected of having fluid overload should be managed as in the pulmonary edema section above. Clinical signs suggestive of intravascular depletion can include tachycardia and hypotension, as well as dry mucous membranes and poor skin turgor. In patients who are suspected of being intravascularly depleted but whose calculated fluid intake and output appears balanced, there should be concern for continued blood loss. Patients can be diagnosed with an empiric trial of intravenous fluid challenge with 500–1000 mL of isotonic fluid. If there is concern regarding bleeding, hemoglobin and hematocrit should be checked immediately. They should also be checked if the patient fails to respond appropriately to the fluid challenge. Patients suspected of having bilateral ureteral injury should have an intravenous pyelogram.

Treatment

Major surgery predisposes to intravascular depletion, although most anesthesiologists will replace accordingly during the surgery. Prohibition of fluids before surgery, large insensible water losses during the operation, and inability to tolerate food or fluids postoperatively require major adjustments. Preoperative bowel preparations also cause large fluid losses.

In general, patients should initially have fluid administration that replaces their recognized and estimated insensible losses. This replacement must be individualized to the patient and her underlying medical issues. The healthy 28-year-old myomectomy patient will tolerate aggressive fluid replacement that could prove fatal to a frail 68-year-old patient with cardiopulmonary disease undergoing reconstructive vaginal surgery. Postoperative fluid replacement must be individualized, but in general, should maintain a urine output greater than 30 mL/h.

The composition of these fluids should address both electrolyte and glucose needs. Subsequent fluid requirements should be based on replacement of an average of 1000 mL of daily insensible water loss (higher in febrile patients) plus urinary output. A clinical estimate of the state of hydration can be made by noting the vital signs, urinary output, moistness of the mucous membranes, and skin turgor. If the patient is unable to take fluids orally in adequate amounts after 48 hours, potassium may need to be added to the intravenous fluids based on measurement of the serum electrolytes. If a complicated major procedure with substantial blood loss has been performed, blood product replacement will be necessary.

Patients who have abnormally low urine output despite being euvolemic may have underlying renal disease. In these patients, assessment of a urinalysis for casts to rule out acute tubular necrosis, as well as serial measurements of blood urea nitrogen (BUN) and creatinine are helpful. Consultation with a renal specialist can also be helpful.

3. Urinary Tract Infection

Urinary tract infection (UTI) may develop in the immediate postoperative period in any patient. Patients are at risk because of the urinary retention that follows surgery, anesthesia, or immobilization. The bladder usually is sterile before surgery and remains so unless bacteria are introduced by instrumentation or catheterization. Catheter-associated urinary tract infection is the most common nosocomial infection.

Although cystitis can cause frequency and dysuria, it should not cause fever. Pyelonephritis, however, can cause extremely high fever. UTI should be considered in the evaluation of any patient with postoperative fever. Clinical signs such as high fever and flank tenderness may be present. Patients with urosepsis may very rapidly become quite toxic. White blood cells and bacteria are seen on urinalysis. Postvoid residual urine, which is sometimes seen, tends to perpetuate the infection and predisposes to ascending infection and pyelonephritis.

Hydration should be increased and activity encouraged to facilitate complete emptying of the bladder. After urine specimens are obtained for culture, appropriate antibiotic therapy should be instituted. Antibiotic coverage may have to be adjusted based on culture and sensitivity results. Gram-negative organisms from the lower urogenital tract predominate. Reinstitution of catheter drainage may be necessary in patients with a postvoid residual urine of 100 mL or more, although, in general, discontinuing the catheter at the earliest possible time is useful for preventing and treating infection.

OTHER INFECTIOUS COMPLICATIONS

1. Hematoma and Pelvic Abscess

Small hematomas or seromas are frequent and usually resolve spontaneously, but some become infected. Insidious accumulations may occur either in the pelvis or under the fascia of the rectus abdominis muscles. They may first be suspected because of a falling hematocrit in association with a low-grade fever. Abscess should be considered in the postoperative patient with fever and no other source, particularly if they have not responded to initial antibiotic treatment for presumed cuff infection or endometritis. Hematoma may be suspected if there has been an unexpectedly large drop in hemoglobin levels postoperatively, or where there is significant unexplained postoperative pain.

Patients in whom hematoma or abscess is suspected should have an imaging procedure. Ultrasound is excellent for pelvic collections, but as patients can also have collections located in their abdomen, CT with contrast is usually the preferred method.

A collection under the rectus muscles, seen most frequently after a Pfannenstiel or Maylard incision or in conjunction with a retropubic urethropexy, may be difficult to outline clinically but can be clearly delineated by ultrasound.

Pelvic hematomas are not usually drained unless they fail to resolve on their own, or become infected. Some abscesses may respond to broad-spectrum antibiotic coverage, but many, especially large ones, will not resolve without drainage. If a posthysterectomy pelvic hematoma is easily accessible via the vaginal vault, it can often be managed by reopening the cuff. If an abscess is present this sometimes can be accomplished easily with finger or clamp, but may require a return to the operating room. Percutaneous drainage of intrapelvic and intra-abdominal collections are often possible via insertion of a large-caliber "pigtail" catheter under ultrasound or CT guidance. If percutaneous or transvaginal drainage is not possible and the abscess does not respond to antibiotics alone, the patient will usually need laparotomy with opening of the abscess, irrigation, and drain placement. In procedures at high risk for abscess or hematoma formation, many providers will place closed-suction drainage systems at the time of initial surgery.

2. Wound Infection

Risk factors for wound infection include the patient's age, health, nutritional status, and personal hygiene habits, as well as the presence of malignancy, history of smoking or diabetes, the use of corticosteroid medications, history of radiation therapy, and surgical technique. Active infection at the operative site (eg, pelvic abscess, ruptured appendix) or at a distant site will increase the risk of wound infection by direct contamination or hematogenous spread.

Appropriate preparation of the surgical site and prophylactic antibiotics are important preventative measures. Preoperative shaving of the operative site may cause microabscesses, resulting in increased risk of wound infection. Using clippers or omitting shaving entirely yields a lower wound infection rate. Extensive guidelines have been drafted by the CDC for prevention of surgical site infection. The use of antibiotic prophylaxis decreases infection risk with both abdominal and vaginal hysterectomy. Some providers use subcutaneous drains to decrease postoperative wound disruption.

The diagnosis of wound infection is usually made during investigation of postoperative fever, often on about the fourth or fifth day. This diagnosis is based on the physical findings of redness, induration at the operative site, or purulent drainage. Facultative and anaerobic gram-negative rods, β-hemolytic streptococci, and staphylococci are the pathogens most commonly cultured from infected wounds. If an infected hematoma or seroma is present, the wound should be opened enough to allow easy packing. Antibiotics should be started if cellulitis is present. If the vaginal cuff has been opened or urogenital flora are suspected, then broad spectrum coverage is necessary. If cellulitis is not present, wound opening and local care are adequate therapy. Damp to dry dressings should be changed two to three times a day and the wound debrided daily until definite improvement is noted. Hydrogen peroxide, iodine compounds, antibiotics, or other chemicals in the wound-irrigating solution may be toxic or impede healing and should not be used. A drain or gauze packing may be required to keep the skin from prematurely sealing the wound. This should be continued until healing by secondary intention is complete. To decrease time to healing, secondary closure of wounds after all infection is resolved and healing has begun may be considered. Delayed primary closure can be considered for cases with obvious contamination or infection.

3. Wound Dehiscence and Evisceration

Rupture of transverse lower abdominal incision is quite rare, but can occur. Vertical incisions may carry a greater risk of breakdown. Risk factors for wound dehiscence and breakdown are similar to those for wound infections: age, nutritional status, diabetes, smoking, malignancy, steroid use, and presence of a prior scar at the incision site.

Evisceration is disruption of all layers of the abdominal wall with protrusion of the intestines through the incision; it is a life-threatening postoperative emergency. The hallmark of this complication is a profuse serosanguineous discharge exuding from the abdominal incision. Proper exploration and treatment of this problem should take place in the operating room and not on the ward or in the examining room. When the diagnosis of fascial dehiscence or evisceration is made, secondary closure must be performed immediately under general anesthesia. Interrupted nonabsorbable sutures through all layers of the abdominal wall are usually used. Broad-spectrum antibiotics should be initiated. When risk factors are present, consideration should be given to a mass closure technique at the time of initial surgery.

4. Necrotic Phenomena

Necrotizing fasciitis, a synergistic mixed facultative and anaerobic infection that involves the fascia and subcutaneous tissue, has been described in both abdominal and perineal sites and is extremely destructive and rapidly progressive. Despite early recognition, mortality is high. Group A streptococcus and anaerobes are important causes.

The skin near the incision site and surrounding area is usually cool, gray, and boggy. The patient usually appears floridly septic with fever and high white count. If necrotizing fasciitis is suspected, the patient should be brought to the operating room and fascial biopsy performed. If confirmed, radical debridement in the operating room is essential, followed by treatment with broad-spectrum antibiotics. Healing is usually by secondary intention with skin grafts often being necessary. This is a potentially lethal complication that requires timely intervention, and it should always be considered in the differential diagnosis when wound problems occur.

A second necrotic complication can result from a poorly planned incision. When a new incision is made near and parallel to an existing scar, sloughing of tissue secondary to ischemia can result. New incisions should either be made through the old incision, or at least several centimeters away to allow adequate blood supply for proper healing.

REFERENCES

ACC/AHA guideline update for perioperative cardiovascular evaluation for noncardiac surgery—Executive summary. A report of the American College of Cardiology/American Heart Association Task Force on Practice Guidelines (Committee to Update the 1996 Guidelines on Perioperative Cardiovascular Evaluation for Noncardiac Surgery). Circulation 2002;105:1257. Full document available at www.acc.org.

Aronson MP, Bose TM: Urinary tract injury in pelvic surgery. Clin Obstet Gynecol 2002;45(2):428.

Barbour LA, Hassell KL: Prevention of deep vein thrombosis and pulmonary embolism. American College of Obstetrics and Gynecology Practice Bulletin #21, 2000.

Bartlett JG: Antibiotic-associated diarrhea. N Engl J Med 2002; 346:334.

Bates SM, Ginsberg JS: Treatment of deep vein thrombosis. N Engl J Med 2004;351:268.

Chan JK, Manetta A: Prevention of femoral nerve injuries in gynecologic surgery. Am J Obstet Gynecol 2002;186:1.

Chunilal SC, Ginsberg JS: Strategies for the diagnosis of deep vein thrombosis and pulmonary embolism. Thromb Res 2000; 97:V33.

Davis JD: Prevention, diagnosis, and treatment of venous thromboembolic complications of gynecologic surgery. Am J Obstet Gynecol 2001;184:759.

Eagle KA, Brundage BH, Chaitman BR, et al: Guidelines for perioperative cardiovascular evaluation for noncardiac surgery. Report of the American College of Cardiology/American Heart Association Task Force on Practice Guidelines. Committee on Perioperative Cardiovascular Evaluation for Noncardiac Surgery. Circulation 1996;93:1278.

Fedullo PF, Tapson VF: The evaluation of suspected pulmonary embolism. N Engl J Med 2003;349:1247.

Fleisher LA, Beckman JA, Brown KA, et al: ACC/AHA 2006 guideline update on perioperative cardiovascular evaluation for noncardiac surgery: focused update on perioperative beta-blocker therapy: a report of the American College of Cardiology/American Heart Association Task Force on Practice Guidelines (Writing Committee to Update the 2002 Guidelines on Perioperative Cardiovascular Evaluation for Noncardiac Surgery): developed in collaboration with the American Society of Echocardiography, American Society of Nuclear Cardiology, Heart Rhythm Society, Society of Cardiovascular Anesthesiologists, Society for Cardiovascular Angiography and Interventions, and Society for Vascular Medicine and Biology. Circulation 2006;113:2662.

Gallup DG et al: Necrotizing fasciitis in gynecologic and obstetric patients: A surgical emergency. Am J Obstet Gynecol 2002; 187:305.

Geerts WH et al: Prevention of venous thromboembolism. Sixth ACCP consensus conference on antithrombotic therapy. Chest 2001;119:132S.

Goldhaber SZ, Elliot CG: Acute pulmonary embolism: Part I—Epidemiology, pathophysiology, and diagnosis. Circulation. 2003;108:2726.

Goldhaber SZ, Elliot CG: Acute pulmonary embolism: Part II—Risk stratification, treatment, and prevention. Circulation 2003;108:2734.

Hershberger JM, Milad MP: Randomized clinical trial of lorazepam for the reduction of postoperative urinary retention. Obstet Gynecol 2003;102:311.

Holte K, Kehlet H: Postoperative ileus: A preventable event. Br J Surg 2000;87(11):1480.

Hurley BW, Nguyen CC: The spectrum of pseudomembranous enterocolitis and antibiotic-associated diarrhea. Arch Intern Med 2002;162:2177.

Joshi GP: Complications of laparoscopy. Anesth Clin N Am 2001; 19(1):89.

Magnusson L, Spahn DR: New concepts of atelectasis during general anaesthesia. Br J Anaesth 2003;91:61.

Mangram AJ et al: Guidelines for prevention of surgical site infection, 1999. Infect Control Hosp Epidemiol 1999;4:247.

Marik PE: Aspiration pneumonitis and aspiration pneumonia. N Engl J Med 2001;344:665.

Sajja SBS, Schein M: Early postoperative small bowel obstruction. Br J Surg 2004;91:683.

Seal DV: Necrotizing fasciitis. Curr Opin Dis 2001;14:127.

Smith A: Postoperative pulmonary infections. Clin Evid 2005; 14:1712.

Soper D: Antibiotic prophylaxis for gynecologic procedures. American College of Obstetrics and Gynecology Practice Bulletin #23, 2001.

Tablan OC, Anderson LJ, Besser R, et al: Guidelines for preventing health-care–associated pneumonia, 2003: recommendations of CDC and the Healthcare Infection Control Practices Advisory Committee. MMWR Recomm Rep 2004;53(RR-3):1.

Tagalakis V et al: The epidemiology of peripheral vein infusion thrombophlebitis: A critical review. Am J Med 2002;113:146.

The Joint European Society of Cardiology/American College of Cardiology Committee. Myocardial infarction redefined—A consensus document of the Joint European Society of Cardiology/American College of Cardiology Committee for the redefinition of myocardial infarction. J Am Coll Cardiol 2000; 36:959.

Tomacruz RS, Bristow RE, Montz FJ: Management of pelvic hemorrhage. Surg Clin North Am 2001;81:925.

Therapeutic Gynecologic Procedures

48

Cecilia K. Wieslander, MD, Dipika Dandade, MD, & James M. Wheeler, MD, MPH

Four of the 10 most commonly performed operations in the United States are dilatation and curettage (D&C), tubal sterilization, abdominal hysterectomy, and vaginal hysterectomy. This chapter reviews these procedures, as well as other therapeutic operations. Indications, contraindications, technique, and complications are discussed for each procedure.

DILATATION AND CURETTAGE

Indications

The procedure of cervical dilatation and uterine curettage is usually performed for one of the following indications: diagnosis and treatment of abnormal uterine bleeding, management of abortion (incomplete, missed, or induced), stenosis, or cancer of the uterus. The diagnosis of abnormal bleeding is discussed in Chapters 35 and 39; D&C as a method of induced abortion is discussed in Chapter 36. This section discusses the remaining therapeutic uses of D&C.

Technique

A. CERVICAL DILATATION

Dilatation of the cervix may be conducted under paracervical, epidural, spinal, or general anesthesia, depending largely on the indication for the procedure. Cervical dilatation usually precedes uterine curettage but may be performed as a therapeutic maneuver for acquired or congenital cervical stenosis, dysmenorrhea, or insertion of an intrauterine contraceptive device (IUD) or radium device for treatment of cancer. Dilatation may also precede hysterography or hysteroscopy.

The patient is placed in the dorsal lithotomy position, with the back and shoulders supported and the extremities padded. The inner thighs, perineum, and vagina are prepared as for any vaginal operation; the surgeon and assistant should adhere to surgical principles of asepsis. A thorough pelvic examination under anesthesia is mandatory prior to performing cervical dilatation, so as to determine the size and position of the cervix, uterus, and adnexa and the presence of any abnormalities. The patient voids normally before the operation if possible; urinary catheterization is used only if significant residual urine is suspected.

A right-angle retractor is placed anteriorly to gently retract the bladder. A weighted speculum is placed posteriorly to reveal the cervix. Under direct vision, the anterior lip of the cervix is grasped with a tenaculum, avoiding the vascular supply at the 3 and 9 o'clock positions. The cervix is grasped firmly but with care taken not to compromise, or especially perforate, the endocervical canal. With gentle traction, the cervix can be brought down toward the introitus. Before proceeding further, a complete visual examination should be made of the cervix and the four vaginal fornices, because the latter areas (especially posteriorly) are otherwise difficult to examine. Areas that appear abnormal (even benign inclusion cysts) should be noted and followed as appropriate. Areas that are clearly abnormal should be biopsied. After the cervix and vagina are evaluated, the uterine cavity is examined. A uterine sound is gently inserted into the endocervix and then advanced into the uterine cavity in the plane of least resistance and most compatible with the position of the uterus as revealed by pelvic examination. The depth of the uterine cavity is recorded as well as any abnormalities such as leiomyomas or septa.

Perforation of the uterus during D&C is most likely to occur at the time of uterine sounding or cervical dilatation. According to two large classical studies, recognized uterine perforations during D&C occur at a rate of 0.63–1.0%. The majority of perforations are thought to be caused by misdirected or excessive force. Perforation is more likely to occur if the woman is postmenopausal (1 in 38), has cancer (1 in 48), or is postpregnancy (1 in 122). Other risk factors include having a retroverted or anteverted uterus or having cervical stenosis. Unless there is evidence of hemorrhage, injury to the bowel, or evulsion of the omentum, conservative treatment of uterine perforation is best. If severe cervical stenosis is suspected from the preoperative office examination, cervical softening agents such as misoprostol or *Laminaria* tents may be used. Both oral and vaginal misoprostol and laminaria tents have demonstrated a benefit over placebo in the ease of cervical dilatation in pregnant and premenopausal women. Preoperative vaginal and oral misoprostol do not reduce the need for cervical dilatation prior to diagnostic hysteroscopy or D&C in postmenopausal women. However, oral misoprostol does increase the ease of cervical dilatation prior to operative hysteroscopy in both postmenopausal women and in those who have been pretreated with gonadotropin-releasing hormone analogue. The most common dilators used are the Hegar, Pratt, and Hanks dilators. Hegar dilators are relatively blunt, gently curved, and numbered sequentially according to width (ie, a No. 7 dilator is 7 mm wide). For most purposes, particularly preceding curettage, dilatation to a No. 9 dilator suffices; if dilatation is being performed for dysmenorrhea, infertility, or stenosis, dilatation should proceed to a No. 11 dilator.

Pratt and Hanks dilators differ from Hegar dilators in being more gradually tapered ("sharper"); they may have a solid core (Pratt) or a hollow center (Hanks), allowing egress of trapped blood and air. Pratt or Hanks dilators are measured in French sizes (a No. 20F Hanks dilator is approximately the same diameter as a No. 9 Hegar dilator). The choice of dilator is largely based on surgical training; many prefer not to use the more pointed Hanks dilators in a small postmenopausal uterus.

B. ENDOCERVICAL CURETTAGE

Fractional curettage should be used for abnormal uterine bleeding or if genital tract neoplasia is suspected. The cervical canal should be curetted prior to dilatation of the cervix and curettage of the endometrial cavity, so as to preserve the histologic characteristics of the endocervix and prevent contamination of the endometrial sample with endocervical cells. If cervical conization is planned for diagnosis or treatment of cervical intraepithelial neoplasia, uterine sounding precedes conization, but cervical dilatation and fractional curettage follow in order to minimize denuding of the endocervical epithelium. The Gusberg curet is a small, slightly curved instrument that is particularly well suited for endocervical curettage. The curet is placed in the endocervical canal to the level of the internal os; with a firm touch, each of the four walls is curetted with a single stroke, with the specimen delivered onto a coated cellulose sponge with a twirling motion of the curet. (The coated cellulose sponge is preferred over ordinary surgical sponges because tissue is less likely to adhere to it.) The cervix is then dilated as described earlier and curettage of the endometrium performed. The endocervical and endometrial specimens are immersed in fixative in separate containers and submitted to the pathologist.

Complications from endocervical curettage are rare in nongravid patients. Because of obvious risks to the fetus and membranes, endocervical curettage is contraindicated in pregnant women. Healing of the curetted endocervix may take 3 weeks or more; the cervical epithelium commonly takes 2 weeks to heal following a routine Papanicolaou smear. Tissue should be allowed to heal before follow-up Papanicolaou smears are taken, because regenerating cells are often mistaken for dysplastic cells.

C. ENDOMETRIAL POLYPECTOMY

The uterine cavity is explored with polyp forceps prior to diagnostic or therapeutic endometrial curettage. It is easier to remove polyps prior to curettage, preserving the histologic integrity necessary to differentiate benign uterine polyps from neoplasia. In a large series advocating routine exploration of the endometrial cavity preceding curettage, 64% of 130 diagnosed endometrial polyps were removed by ureteral stone forceps. Twenty-five percent of the polyps were removed before curettage and 39% were removed after curettage, illustrating how difficult it is to remove polyps via curettage alone. Pedunculated or submucous leiomyomas, intrauterine and intracervical synechia, and uterine anomalies may be first suspected at passage of the polyp forceps.

The technique of polypectomy includes gentle insertion of the forceps in the plane most compatible with the position of the uterus (as for uterine sounding). The forceps are opened slightly, rotated 90 degrees, and removed. Many clinicians repeat this procedure through 360 degrees, completely exploring the uterine cavity.

Skillful use of hysteroscopy for diagnosis and treatment of synechia, septa, leiomyomas, and polyps is preferred to blind polypectomy and curettage. With the new, narrow hysteroscope, the procedure is easily done as an office procedure similar to colposcopy for biopsy or laser conization.

D. ENDOMETRIAL CURETTAGE

Endometrial curettage is often both diagnostic and therapeutic. It is indicated for treatment of complications of pregnancy, including incomplete or missed abortion, postpartum retention of products of conception, and placental polyps. The procedure is also useful to stop the acute bleeding in women with menorrhagia who are hypovolemic. D&C should not be used to treat dysfunctional uterine bleeding in women without hypovolemia, because it has no effect on mean blood loss in subsequent periods (with the exception of the first period following the D&C) and is inferior to medical management. D&C is inferior to hysteroscopy in diagnosing and treating abnormal uterine bleeding caused by uterine fibroids or endometrial polyps. It is contraindicated in infection, such as acute endometritis, salpingitis, and pyometra. If infected placental tissue must be removed, the D&C should follow a period of parenteral antibiotics. The technique of endometrial curettage is tailored to the individual patient. In determining the hormone responsiveness of the endometrium, a small but representative sample may be obtained from the anterior and posterior walls. When curettage is being performed therapeutically, a systematic, thorough approach is indicated. The largest sharp curet that can comfortably fit through the dilated cervix is chosen. A serrated curet may cause injury to the underlying basalis layer of the endometrium and myometrium. The anterior, lateral, and posterior walls are scraped with firm pressure in a clockwise or counterclockwise fashion from the top of the uterine fundus down to the internal os. The top of the cavity is curetted with a side-to-side motion. The curettings are retrieved onto the waiting gauze and immersed in fixative as soon as possible. If endometrial curettage is being used for diagnosis of infection (eg, tuberculous endometritis), a portion of the curettings should be placed in containers appropriate for culture (without fixative).

A single curettage will not remove the entire endometrium. Thorough curettage by an experienced gynecologist often removes 50–60% of the endometrium, as determined by immediate postcurettage hysterectomy. If risk factors for endometrial cancer are present and clinical suspicion for neoplasia persists despite a histologic diagnosis of benign endometrium, further evaluation with hysteroscopically guided biopsy or hysterectomy is indicated.

Perforation of the uterus occurred in 0.63% of a large series of D&Cs. Perforation is suspected when the sound or curet meets no resistance at the point expected by uterine size, consistency, and position determined by preoperative bimanual examination. Curettage may be continued if the area of suspected perforation is avoided. Should suction curettage be associated with perforation, laparoscopy must be used to continue the procedure to avoid aspiration of bowel into the uterine cavity. In the case of suspected perforation, the patient should be observed for at least 24 hours in the hospital for possible infection or hemorrhage. In a series of 70 uterine perforations, 55 were treated expectantly, and only 1 patient developed complications (pelvic abscess drained via colpotomy). In 7 patients, hysterectomy was elected but not indicated by operative findings. Today, laparoscopy is the method of choice for evaluating perforations in the hemodynamically stable patient.

E. ENDOMETRIAL BIOPSY

Outpatient curettage, or endometrial biopsy, should always be a diagnostic and not a therapeutic technique. The many techniques available, all compared to D&C under adequate anesthesia, are discussed in Chapter 33.

HYSTEROSCOPY

This section discusses the therapeutic uses of hysteroscopy.

Indications & Contraindications

See Table 48–1.

Technique

The hysteroscope is a rigid endoscope similar in design to an operating laparoscope or a urologic resectoscope. Typically 6–10 mm in external diameter, the outer sleeve encloses a fiberoptic light source, a channel used to introduce a medium to distend the uterus, and a channel through which probes, forceps, and electrocautery or laser instruments may be visually directed in the uterine cavity. Viewing angles vary from 10 to 45 degrees.

The uterine cavity, which is normally collapsed, must be distended by a medium: dextran-70, CO_2, sodium chloride, lactated Ringer's solution, glycine, mannitol, or sorbitol. Two disadvantages to the use of electrolyte solutions such as sodium chloride and lactated Ringer's solution are mixing of blood, which limits visualization, and the inability to use electrosurgery because these solutions are electroconductors. Consequently, they should only be used for diagnostic, not operative, hysteroscopy. Pressure no greater than 100 mm Hg is required to achieve adequate uterine distention. Instillation of high-viscosity dextran can be done via a 50-mL syringe attached to the hysteroscope. The advantage of using dextran is that it is immiscible with blood, which allows for clear visualization in the presence of bleeding. However, dextran can cause rare but serious complications, including anaphylactic reactions, fluid overload, pulmonary edema, and coagulopathy. The manufacturer recommends that the patient be followed closely for pulmonary edema if the procedure lasts longer than 45 minutes, more than 250 mL of dextran-70 is absorbed, large areas of endometrium were resected, or intravenous fluids were administered at more than maintenance rate. If pulmonary edema develops, the patient may need plasmapheresis, because dextran-70 contains mainly high-molecular-weight molecules that are excreted slowly—or not at all—from the kidneys. CO_2 gas insufflation is favored by some gynecologic surgeons for both office and outpatient hysteroscopy. The addition of a cervical suction cup to prevent leakage has lost favor. The average flow rate needed to distend the uterus is 60 mL/min, and to avoid uterine injury or gas embolism, the maximum flow rate should not exceed 100 mL/min; thus laparoscopic insufflators must never be connected to a hysteroscope. The advantages of CO_2 gas over dextran are easier cleaning of

Table 48–1. Indications and contraindications for hysteroscopy.

Indications	Contraindications
Evaulation and treatment of abnormal uterine bleeding	**Absolute contraindications**
Premenopausal/postmenopausal bleeding with negative D&C.	Pelvic inflammatory disease, especially tubo–ovarian complex.
Directed biopsy in patient with atypical adenomatous hyperplasia but at high risk for hysterectomy.	Uterine perforation.
Evaulation of endocervix versus endometrium as origin of biopsy–proved adenocarcinoma.	Sensitivity to anesthetic or distention medium.
Suspicion (on history or hysterography) of uterine polyp or submucous leiomyoma amenable to hysteroscopic resection.	Lack of proper equipment, specifically, low–pressure insufflator for CO_2 distention.
Evaluation and treatment of infertility	Operator inexperience.
Habitual abortion.	**Relative contraindications**
Known uterine septum on previous hysterography or curettage.	Heavy bleeding limiting visual field.
Suspected foreign body (eg, broken or imbedded IUD).	Known gynecologic cancer, especially endometrial, cervical, tubal, and ovarian, because of theoretic risk of flushing cancer cells into the peritoneal cavity.
Suspected submucous leiomyoma on history, pelvic examination, or laparoscopy.	
Suspected cornual occlusion on hysterography.	
Suspected intracervical, intrauterine, or intracornual adhesions.	
Suspected congenital anomaly (eg, with known urologic anomaly).	
Possible intrauterine infection (eg, tuberculosis).	
Intrauterine insemination or embryo transfer in selected patients with known uterine fusion anomaly.	
Suspected endometrial polyp.	

instruments and improved comfort for the surgeon. A disadvantage is more difficult visualization because of mixing with blood or debris.

An increasing number of instruments are available for use in hysteroscopic procedures, including blunt probes, microscissors, alligator clamps with electrocautery attachment, rollerball electrode, and a wire loop for excision and coagulation (resectoscope). The argon laser is useful for lysing septa, and the neodymium:YAG (yttrium, aluminum, garnet) laser is available for polyp and myoma removal and endometrial ablation (Table 48–2).

Local or general anesthetics are chosen on the basis of expected hysteroscopic findings or procedures, concomitant operations planned, and the desires and cooperation of the patient. Most hysteroscopic examinations and virtually all therapeutic procedures are performed under general anesthesia. Following administration of anesthesia, the urinary bladder is drained, and the anterior lip of the cervix is grasped with a tenaculum. The cervix should then be gradually dilated to the same diameter as the external sleeve of the hysteroscope so as to provide a snug fit. Concomitant laparoscopy is an option in any patient in whom a hysteroscopic therapeutic procedure is

planned. Uterine perforation may be observed through the laparoscope, and excess distention media may be aspirated from the posterior cul-de-sac after a prolonged procedure.

An assistant must be constantly present during hysteroscopy to monitor uterine insufflation so that the pressure never exceeds 100 mm Hg, and the flow rate of the distending medium never exceeds 100 mL/min. The

Table 48–2. Comparison of lasers used in treatment of endometriosis.

	CO_2	Argon	Nd:YAG
Laser wavelength	10.6 μm	0.5 μm	1.06 μm
Depth of tissue destruction	0.1 mm	0.5 mm	4 mm
Beam scattering	None	Slight	Significant
Effect dependent on tissue color	None	Yes	Yes
Delivery by fiberoptic systems	Experimental	Yes	Yes

chance of fluid overload is markedly increased when the mean infusion pressure exceeds the mean arterial pressure. The lowest infusion pressure needed to obtain good visualization, should be used. The surgeon must be sitting comfortably, with all instruments available to perform the hysteroscopic procedure safely and expeditiously. Following the procedure, intrauterine instruments should be inspected for their integrity. The microscissors, in particular, are delicate and could break within the uterus. If dextran is used, it must be immediately flushed from the hysteroscope before it is allowed to dry.

Complications

Hysteroscopic surgery is generally safe in experienced hands. With laparoscopic observation, the serious complication of uterine perforation can almost always be prevented. If overt bleeding occurs during resection of a septum, polyp, or leiomyoma, the laparoscopic probe can be held against the uterine vessels to slow the blood flow. A Foley catheter may be inserted into the uterine cavity and inflated to provide a tamponade for heavy endometrial bleeding. Infection is an unusual complication following hysteroscopy, and prophylactic antibiotics are not recommended. Complications of distending media include hyponatremia and pulmonary edema if an excessive amount results in vascular intravasation. The procedure should be expedited and electrolytes should be checked if the fluid deficit exceeds 1 L. When the fluid deficit reaches 1500 mL or the serum sodium is less than 125 mmol/L, the procedure must be terminated. These risks can be prevented with close monitoring of fluid use intraoperatively.

Prognosis

With proper selection of patients, hysteroscopic surgery has high success rates. Small pedunculated leiomyomas and polyps are usually retrieved by an experienced, patient surgeon. Submucous leiomyomas may be destroyed if they are not too vascular. In the treatment of intrauterine adhesions, the chance for success and restoration of a normal endometrial cavity depends on the density and extent of the adhesions and the area of normal endometrium remaining after dissection.

Following hysteroscopic surgery for infertility in which the endometrium is denuded, many physicians prescribe postoperative estrogen therapy to promote rapid endometrial growth.

LAPAROSCOPY

Laparoscopy is a transperitoneal endoscopic technique that provides excellent visualization of the pelvic structures and often permits the diagnosis and management of gynecologic disorders without laparotomy.

Most basic laparoscopes are 4–12 mm in diameter and have a 180-degree viewing angle. The instrument has an effective length of over 25 cm and can be utilized with a fiberoptic light box. In order to facilitate visualization, CO_2 must be instilled into the peritoneal cavity to distend the abdominal wall.

Use of a pneumatic insufflator permits continuous monitoring of the rate, pressure, and volume of the gas used for inflation. In addition to the equipment used for observation, a variety of other instruments for resection, biopsy, coagulation, aspiration, and manipulation can be passed through separate cannulas or inserted through the same cannula as the laparoscope. A laser (CO_2 or Nd:YAG) may be used with the laparoscope.

Although the laparoscope is an invaluable tool in both diagnostic and operative gynecologic procedures, its use requires considerable expertise, and it should always be used by a surgeon familiar with the management of complications. Laparoscopic procedures are *major* intra-abdominal operations performed through small incisions. This technique is rapidly performed and has a low morbidity rate and a short convalescence period. In many cases, laparoscopy may replace conventional laparotomy for diagnosis and treatment of gynecologic problems. It is a cost-effective outpatient procedure.

Indications

The indications will increase with the clinician's experience and as technical innovations permit even more complicated procedures.

A. DIAGNOSIS

1. Differentiation between ovarian, tubal, and uterine masses, eg, ectopic pregnancy, ovarian cyst, salpingitis, myomas, endometriosis, and tuberculosis.
2. Pelvic pain, eg, possible adhesions, endometriosis, ectopic pregnancy, twisted or bleeding ovarian cyst, salpingitis, appendicitis, and nongynecologic pelvic pain.
3. Genital anomalies, eg, ovarian dysgenesis, uterine maldevelopment.
4. Ascites, eg, ovarian diseases versus cirrhosis.
5. Secondary amenorrhea of possible ovarian origin, eg, polycystic ovarian syndrome, arrhenoblastoma.
6. Pelvic injuries after penetrating or nonpenetrating abdominal trauma.
7. Staging of Hodgkin's disease and lymphomas.
8. Diagnosis of occult cancer.

B. EVALUATION

1. Infertility, eg, tubal patency, ovarian biopsy.
2. "Second look" after tubal surgery or treatment of endometriosis.

3. Assessment of pelvic and abdominal trauma.
4. Appraisal of bowel for viability after surgery, for mesenteric thrombosis.
5. Study of pelvic nodes after lymphography.
6. Peritoneal washings for cytology study.
7. Peritoneal culture.
8. Evaluation of uterine perforation.
9. Evaluation of pelvic viscera to determine the feasibility of vaginal hysterectomy.

C. THERAPY

1. Tubal sterilization:
   a. Electrical: unipolar or bipolar technique.
   b. Mechanical: Silastic bands, Silastic rings, or metal clips.
2. Lysis of adhesions, with or without laser.
3. Fulguration of endometriosis by laser or thermal cautery.
4. Aspiration of small unilocular ovarian cyst or of fluid for culture.
5. Removal of extruded intrauterine device.
6. Uterosacral ligament division (denervation).
7. Treatment of ectopic pregnancy.
8. Myomectomy.
9. Salpingostomy for phimotic fimbriae.
10. Removal of tuboplastic hoods or splints.
11. Ova collection for in vitro fertilization.
12. GIFT (gamete intrafallopian transfer for fertilization).
13. Mini-wedge resection of ovary.
14. Biopsy of tumor, liver, ovary, spleen, omentum, etc.
15. Placement of intraperitoneal clips as markers for radiotherapy.
16. Oophorectomy.
17. Ovarian cystectomy.
18. Laparoscopic-assisted vaginal hysterectomy, laparoscopic subtotal hysterectomy, and laparoscopic hysterectomy.
19. Reconstructive surgery for pelvic organ prolapse and urinary incontinence.

Contraindications

A. ABSOLUTE

Intestinal obstruction, generalized peritonitis, massive hemorrhage.

B. RELATIVE

Severe cardiac or pulmonary disease, previous periumbilical surgery, shock, cancer involving anterior abdominal wall.

Additional factors weighing against performing laparoscopic surgery include extremes of weight, intrauterine pregnancy after the first or early second trimester,

presence of a large mass, inflammatory bowel disease, and known severe intraperitoneal adhesions.

Preparation for Laparoscopy

Careful explanation of the contemplated procedure must be given to each patient prior to surgery. Unless the individual is a poor operative risk, laparoscopy is usually an outpatient operation. Preparation includes no solid food for at least 8 hours prior to surgery, no liquids for more than 6 hours preoperatively, a history and physical examination, and routine blood studies. Abdominal or perineal shaving is usually unnecessary, but skin preparation with an antiseptic is routine.

Anesthesia

Local anesthesia, local anesthesia with systemic analgesia, spinal or epidural block techniques, or general anesthesia with or without endotracheal intubation may be used. Special hazards of anesthesia exist, eg, reduced diaphragmatic excursion because of the pneumoperitoneum and because the patient may be operated on in the Trendelenburg position. Because of these factors, most procedures in the United States are performed with the patient under general anesthesia with endotracheal intubation. With adequate understanding of the physiology involved, effective anesthesia and laparoscopy can be accomplished safely.

An alternative to general anesthesia is local anesthesia with intravenous sedation. The patient may experience transient discomfort during manipulation of the uterine tubes, but in selected patients this discomfort is easily tolerated.

Surgical Technique

The patient should be placed with her arms at her sides in the dorsal lithotomy position and draped after induction of anesthesia and preparation of the abdomen and pelvic area. The video monitor should be placed in a position that allows for easy viewing by the surgeon, usually at the patient's feet or side. The bladder must be emptied by catheterization to decrease the risk of injury during subsequent introduction and use of other instruments. After careful bimanual examination, a tenaculum is attached to the cervix, and a uterine manipulator (eg, olive-tipped, Hasson, Harris-Kronner uterine manipulator-injector [HUMI], Hulka) is placed into the cervical canal to elevate the uterus, which places tissue on tension. A 1-cm incision is made within or immediately below the umbilicus The peritoneal cavity can be entered blindly with a Veress needle or a trocar-cannula system, or under direct visualization via a mini-laparotomy called "open laparoscopy." Direct insertion of a cannula-trocar system can be accomplished safely if there have been no previous peritonitis or abdominopelvic surgeries. Open laparoscopy minimizes the risk of vascular injuries, but does not eliminate intestinal injuries. Carbon dioxide should then be introduced and monitored by the pneumatic insufflator. The amount of gas insufflated will vary with the patient's size, the laxity of the abdominal wall, and the planned procedure. In most patients, 2–3 L of gas will be needed to obtain adequate visualization. The maximum insufflation pressure should not exceed 15 mm Hg. If a Veress needle is used, it is withdrawn and the laparoscopic trocar and cannula inserted. After proper abdominal entry, the trocar may be withdrawn and replaced with the fiberoptic laparoscope. The examiner manipulates the intrauterine cannula so that the pelvic organs can be observed. To test for tubal patency, methylene blue or indigo carmine solution can be injected through the intrauterine cannula. Direct observation of dye leakage attests to tubal patency. A second trocar with a cannula may be inserted under direct laparoscopic vision through a 5-mm transverse midline incision at the pubic hairline. Additional punctures are used as necessary for the placement of other instruments. A number of instruments are available, including irrigators, the harmonic scalpel, forceps, scissors, and staple applicators. Surgical knots may be tied and sutures placed using specially made equipment.

The operation is terminated by evacuating the insufflated gas through the cannula, followed by removal of all instruments and closure of the incisions. The skin can be closed with 3-0 subcuticular suture, skin glue or Steri-Strips. Incisions greater than 10 mm require fascial closure to avoid incisional hernias. A small dressing is applied to the wound. In uncomplicated cases involving diagnosis only, operating time is about 10 minutes.

A. STERILIZATION

Electrical cautery, Silastic rings or bands, and metal spring clips achieve sterilization by occluding the uterine tubes. The advantages or disadvantages of the different techniques are of less significance than the skill with which a physician can perform a particular technique; therefore, choice of method should depend on which technique is most comfortable for the physician. The failure rate of most sterilization methods is greater in women younger than 28 years old.

1. Cautery—Laparoscopic sterilization with electrical cautery is one of the most common laparoscopic sterilization methods. Although unipolar coagulation has a significantly lower pregnancy rate than bipolar coagulation (7.5 per 1000 vs 24.8 per 1000 over 10 years), bipolar coagulation is less likely to cause injury to adjacent structures (eg, bowel). Excessive tubal destruction is associated with an unacceptably high incidence of ectopic pregnancy, as it may create a tiny fistula from the uterus into the peritoneal cavity through which sperm may travel.

Thus when using either form (unipolar or bipolar) of electrical coagulation, one should destroy only a short section of the midportion of the uterine tube, avoiding the uterine cornu if possible. Generally, the tube is burned at two to three different locations, and division of the tube by cutting is not necessary.

2. Silastic bands—Tubal occlusion with Silastic bands or rings results in a slightly higher pregnancy rate (17.7 per 1000 over 10 years) but fewer ectopic pregnancies. Mechanical problems in placement of the bands and bleeding from the tubes during the procedure are more common.

3. Clips—Tubal occlusion with clips (Hulka or Filshie clips) have a wide range of failure. Failure rates are higher for the Hulka clip (36.5 per 1000 over 10 years) than for the Filshie clip (0–4 per 1000 over 6–10 years). The advantages of using clips are that only a small portion of the tube is damaged (thus increasing the chance of successful sterilization reversal if the patient has regret) and that inadvertent burn injury to the bowel is avoided.

4. Interval partial salpingectomy—Compared to postpartum tubal ligation, interval partial salpingectomy has a higher failure rate of 20.1 per 1000 over 10 years.

B. INFERTILITY

In procedures of sterilization reversal, laparoscopic visualization may be needed prior to reanastomosis, particularly if the ligation procedure involved electrocautery. Peritubal adhesions may be lysed with electric scissors, and salpingostomy may be accomplished. The minimal trauma of these procedures using laparoscopy and the saving of a major operative procedure are obvious benefits. Laparoscopy should be considered for women with complaints of abnormal bleeding and unexplained pelvic pain. More liberal use of the laparoscope has led to the diagnosis of many unsuspected cases of endometriosis.

Electrical fulguration of areas of endometriosis or laser destruction of these diseased areas by laparoscopy is a safe, effective, and rapid treatment. The use of laser obviously allows implants on structures such as bowel, bladder, and the fallopian tubes to be treated with a fairly wide margin of safety. Relief may be immediate and striking, whether the woman has complained of dysmenorrhea, dyspareunia, or generalized pelvic pain. Among infertile patients with lesser stages of endometriosis, pregnancy rates are similar to those in other published studies of treatment with danazol.

In infertility, the laparoscope has been important for ova collection for in vitro fertilization, GIFT, and other procedures. However, it is used less frequently now, as most egg retrievals for in vitro fertilization are performed under ultrasound guidance.

C. Ectopic Pregnancy

In hemodynamically stable patients, laparoscopic linear salpingostomy is the preferred method for conservative management of tubal pregnancies. According to a recent Cochrane Database Systematic Review, the laparoscopic approach is less successful than the open approach in the elimination of tubal pregnancy as a cause of the higher rate of persistent trophoblast tissue. However, it is feasible in virtually all patients, is safe, and is less costly compared to the open approach. Long-term follow-up shows a comparable intrauterine pregnancy rate and a lower repeat ectopic pregnancy rate. Persistent trophoblast tissue after laparoscopic salpingostomy can be significantly reduced after a prophylactic single dose of systemic methotrexate. An alternative conservative approach for those who meet the criteria is methotrexate administration.

D. Laparoscopic Hysterectomy

Laparoscopy can be used for total laparoscopic hysterectomy (LH), laparoscopic-assisted vaginal hysterectomy (LAVH), and laparoscopic subtotal hysterectomy (LSH; see section on hysterectomy). Other procedures that can be done via the laparoscope include vault suspension and pelvic reconstruction such as retropubic Burch colposuspension and abdominal sacral colpopexy.

E. Abdominal and Pelvic Pain

Laparoscopy has proved invaluable in differentiating various causes of acute and chronic pain. The technique may save the patient the necessity of a major exploratory operation. Fluid aspiration and tissue biopsy are possible through laparoscopy. Also, pelvic and intestinal disease can be differentiated. The appendix may be visualized and acute appendicitis may be diagnosed. Numerous cases of pain caused by intra-abdominal adhesions also have been diagnosed by laparoscopy, and relief has been obtained following laparoscopic adhesion resection.

F. Trauma

In cases of intra-abdominal trauma, laparoscopy can be used to exclude the need for a major abdominal operation.

G. Miscellaneous

"Missing" IUDs have been removed from the intra-abdominal cavity, Mulligan plastic hoods from tuboplasty procedures, "lost" drains, and other foreign material have been removed from the abdomen by operative laparoscopy.

Postsurgical Care

Patients may be sent home following full recovery from anesthesia, usually in 1–2 hours. Recovery from more extensive procedures such as LH may require a longer hospital stay of 1–2 days. Postoperative pain is usually minimal, and patients are discharged with a prescription for a simple oral analgesic. The most common complaint is shoulder pain secondary to subdiaphragmatic accumulation of gas. Patients are encouraged to resume full activity, except for sexual relations, the day following surgery. Sexual relations may be resumed several days postoperatively after a simple procedure, eg, tubal ligation. Following extensive operative laparoscopy or other gynecologic procedures, coitus should be delayed for an appropriate interval, ie, until it is unlikely to cause discomfort or damage to the operative site. Patients should routinely be seen in the office 1–2 weeks postoperatively.

Complications

A review of the world experience of laparoscopic gynecologic operations, including 1,549,360 patients, showed an overall complication rate ranging from 0.2–10.3%. Higher complications rates were noted with prospective studies. The frequency of complications was less for nonoperative or minor procedures (0.06–7.0%) than for major operations (0.6–18%). Complications requiring conversion to laparotomy has been estimated to be 2.1% and is most commonly due to major vascular and intestinal injuries. The readmission rate to the hospital has been quoted to be 0.4–0.5%. The mortality rate for laparoscopy including 1,374,827 patients is 4.4 per 100,000 laparoscopies. The major causes of death are due to intestinal and vascular complications, and due to anesthesia.

A. Vascular Injuries

Major vascular injuries are infrequent (0.04–0.1%), and are almost five times more frequent during blind entry than during the laparoscopic operation itself. Catastrophic bleeding can occur if the aorta, the inferior vena cava, the common, internal and external iliac arteries and veins are injured. The mortality rate as a consequence of major vascular injuries is between 9% and 17%, and immediate conversion to laparotomy is almost always needed. Massive bleeding is often concealed in large retroperitoneal hematomas, and often only small amounts of intraperitoneal bleeding is seen. Open laparoscopic technique minimizes the risk of major vascular injury, but aortic injury has been reported in thin patients caused by the scalpel during the incision. The incidence of abdominal wall bleeding is 0.5%, and most injuries involve the inferior epigastric vessels (deep and superficial) and muscular vessels. Major bleeding requiring transfusion has been observed. The inferior epigastric vessels run in the lateral umbilical ligaments, and contrary to common belief, the inferior epigastric vessels cannot be seen via transillumination by the laparoscope. They are best avoided by placing the trocars lateral to the insertion of the round ligament into the anterior abdominal wall or 1–2 cm lateral to McBurney's point (one-third the way between the anterior superior iliac spine and the umbilicus).

B. INTESTINAL INJURY

Bowel injuries are uncommon (0.06–0.5%), but have a mortality rate of 2.5–5%. The colon and small bowel are injured at about the same rate, and they can be injured sharply or via thermal burns. About one third are related to entry and the rest are caused by operative procedures. Unfortunately, most bowel injuries are not recognized intraoperatively (mean 4.4 postoperative days), likely as a result of most patients with laparoscopic intestinal injury not presenting with the typical clinical signs of bowel perforation. Most patients present with low-grade fever, leukopenia, or normal leukocyte count. In a review of 266 cases of intestinal injury, pain at the trocar site near the injury, abdominal distention, and diarrhea with normal bowel sounds were commonly seen, but peritoneal signs, severe pain, nausea, vomiting and ileus were uncommon. Open laparoscopy has a similar rate of bowel injuries, but they are recognized more commonly intraoperatively.

C. URINARY INJURIES

Urinary injuries during laparoscopy have a similar rate to open procedures (0.02–1.7%). Bladder injuries are more common than ureteral injuries and are recognized more frequently intraoperatively. About two-thirds of urinary injuries occur during laparoscopic-assisted vaginal hysterectomy.

D. HERNIA AT SITE OF ABDOMINAL WALL TROCHAR

Ventral hernia formation is about 10 times lower with laparoscopy than with laparotomy (0.06–1% vs 11–13%). Trocar wounds of 5 mm or less do not require closure, whereas larger trocar wounds do. Most surgeons close incisions greater than 10 mm because of the high rate of hernias. Richter's hernias, where only a portion of the intestinal wall is entrapped in a defect of the peritoneum or posterior fascia, can be difficult to diagnose, because an externally visible bulge is often absent. The condition needs a high index of suspicion and can be diagnosed with an ultrasound of computed tomography scan.

E. SUBCUTANEOUS EMPHYSEMA AND GAS EMBOLISMS

Localized or generalized subcutaneous emphysema occurs in 0.3–2% of cases and generally has no clinical consequence. However, subcutaneous emphysema of the neck, face, and chest may be a manifestation of a pneumothorax or pneumomediastinum.

F. POSTOPERATIVE SHOULDER PAIN

Pain from diaphragmatic irritation can be referred to the shoulder causing discomfort. Irritation of the diaphragm by the formation of carbonic acid (because of use of CO_2), stretching of the phrenic nerve by pneumoperitoneum or pressure from the abdominal organs during Trendelenburg position are possible etiologies. It can be treated with mild analgesics and reassurance.

■ OPERATIONS FOR STERILIZATION OF WOMEN & MEN

Sterilization is a permanent method of contraception, and is the most commonly used contraceptive method used in the United States. Approximately 700,000 tubal sterilizations and 500,000 vasectomies are performed in the United States annually.

TUBAL STERILIZATION

Tubal sterilization was first performed in 1823 to prevent pregnancy in women who would need repeated cesarean sections. Since the first tubal sterilization was performed, more than 200 different techniques have been described. Table 48–3 lists the most common methods of tubal sterilization and their failure rates.

Preoperative Counseling

Clear, comprehensive counseling is essential for women who are considering tubal sterilization. Possible medical and psychologic complications must be carefully out-

Table 48–3. Overall failure rates with tubal sterilization (over 10 years per 1000 procedures).

Postpartum partial salpingectomy	7.5
Unipolar coagulation	7.5
Bipolar coagulation	24.8
Spring clip	36.5
Silicone rubber band	17.7
Interval partial salpingectomy	20.1
All methods	18.5

Reproduced with permission from Peterson HB et al: The risk of pregnancy after tubal sterilization: findings from the U.S. Collaborative Review of Sterilization. Am J Obstet Gynecol 1996;174:1161.

lined (see Complications, later); women are more likely to regret having had the operation if they do not know what to expect.

The physician should be alert to signs that the patient is undecided about having the operation or is being pressured by her husband or others. Regret or dissatisfaction is more common if the procedure is done postpartum than at another time, and these women are more than twice as likely to feel that preoperative counseling was inadequate. Temporary stress associated with the pregnancy may have influenced a premature decision for sterilization in these women.

Patients should be told that tubal sterilization is usually irreversible. Some methods are sometimes reversible. Most studies estimate that approximately 1–2% of women who undergo tubal sterilization request reversal. The major risk factor for subsequent regret of sterilization is young maternal age (younger than age 30 years) at the time of sterilization. Collaborative Review of Sterilization (CREST) study data showed that women who were younger than 30 years at the time of sterilization were twice as likely to seek information about reversal as women between the ages of 30 and 34 years. Another major risk factor for regret is marital disharmony at the time of sterilization. In addition, women who have postpartum sterilization are more prone to regret than are women who have interval sterilization. Parity has not been found to be a significant risk factor for regret when controlling for maternal age. Pregnancy rates after tubal ligation reversals range from 55–90% by laparotomy and 31–78% via laparoscopy. Success of tubal ligation reversal depends on the woman's age at the time of reversal (younger than 35 years old) and length of remaining fallopian tube segment (> 4 cm). Some studies have found improved pregnancy results when the initial sterilization procedure was performed using mechanical techniques rather than electrocautery.

Complications

Pain and menstrual disturbances (postbilateral tubal ligation syndrome) have been reported following tubal sterilization. The theory holds that destruction of the mesosalpinx might alter the blood supply and subsequent gonadotropin delivery to the ovary. Ovarian function and hormone production may then be altered. However, prospective controlled studies show that these problems are no more common than in women who have not undergone sterilization. Menstrual changes seem to be related to use of contraceptives—before sterilization. Oral contraceptives are associated with decreased menstrual flow and relief of dysmenorrhea; once they are discontinued, heavier flow and pain may recur. Complaints of menstrual changes are much less frequent in the second half of the first postoperative year. Patients should be told that pelvic pain or menstrual disturbances may develop after tubal sterilization but are no more common than in other women of similar age and parity.

Patients who have undergone tubal sterilization require hysterectomy more often than patients who have not undergone this procedure. This is probably because most women who have tubal sterilizations have had children and thus are more likely to have disorders typically treated with hysterectomy (eg, symptomatic pelvic relaxation, adenomyosis). Patients may have been sterilized secondary to medical reasons and gynecologic disorders that might eventually require further surgery. Some studies suggest that women are more likely to accept a surgical treatment if they have been sterilized.

Failure of sterilization is most often secondary to poor technique such as improper application of a clip or ring. Fistula formation may occur. A complication of failure is ectopic pregnancy (7.3 per 1000).

Several studies show an association between decreased risk of ovarian cancer and tubal sterilization.

Technique (See Figs 48–1 through 48–4.)

Postpartum tubal ligation uses a small infraumbilical incision to access the tubes. Minilaparotomy involves a 2–3 cm incision made above the symphysis pubis. The incision is closed in two layers.

OTHER METHODS OF FEMALE STERILIZATION

Because of relatively high morbidity and mortality rates in comparison with tubal occlusion procedures, hysterectomy is justified for sterilization only if there is another unequivocal indication for hysterectomy. Transvaginal tubal ligation via culdotomy or culdoscopy is technically more difficult than transabdominal sterilization and has a higher infection rate. However, there may be less discomfort postoperatively. A hysteroscopic tubal sterilization technique (Essure) was recently approved by the Food and Drug Administration (FDA) (Fig 48–5). It is an expanding spring device made of titanium, stainless steel, and nickel that contain Dacron fibers that induce an inflammatory response and final fibrosis of the intramural tubal lumen. It can be successfully placed in 95% of patients and its effectiveness at 1 year is 99.5%.

VASECTOMY

Vasectomy, or vas occlusion, accounts for 8% of sterilizations worldwide. Partial vasectomy is usually done under local anesthesia via a small incision in the upper outer as-

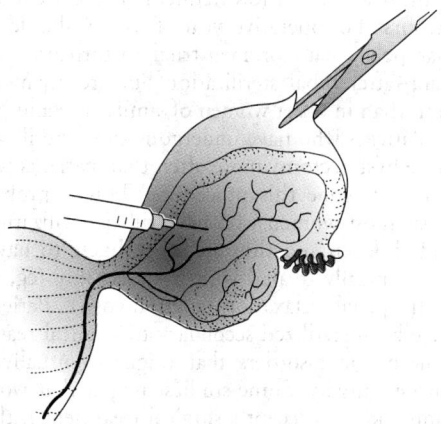

Saline with epinephrine injected below serosa, which becomes inflated locally. Muscular tube, and even blood vessels, can be separated from serosa, which is then cut open.

Muscular tube emerges through opening or is pulled out to form a U shape.

Fimbriated end is untouched, while the end leading to the uterus is stripped of serosa. This can usually be done without damaging blood vessels.

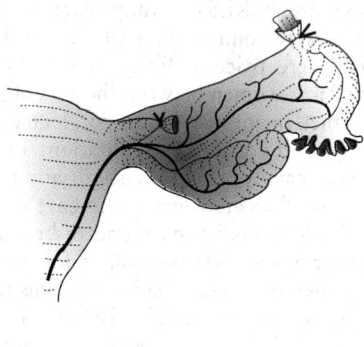

About 5 cm of muscular tube is cut away; the end is buried automatically in serosa. Fimbriated end and serosa opening are closed and tied together.

Blood supply continues normally between ovary and uterus. Hydrosalpinx or adhesion has not been noticed.

Figure 48–1. Uchida method of sterilization. (Reproduced with permission from Benson RC: *Handbook of Obstetrics & Gynecology,* 8th ed. Lange, 1983.)

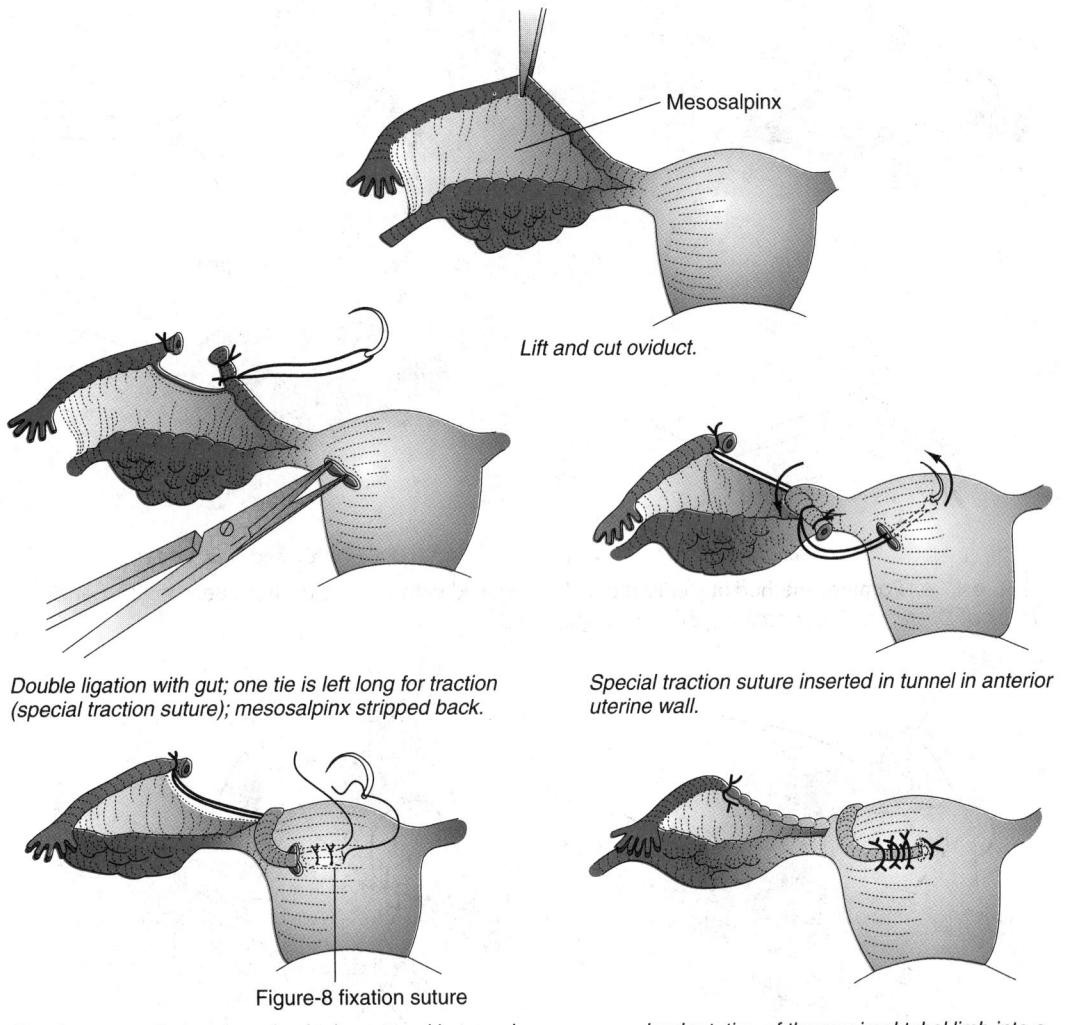

Mesosalpinx

Lift and cut oviduct.

Double ligation with gut; one tie is left long for traction (special traction suture); mesosalpinx stripped back.

Special traction suture inserted in tunnel in anterior uterine wall.

Figure-8 fixation suture

Traction suture tied and proximal tube sutured in tunnel.

Implantation of the proximal tubal limb into a tunnel in the anterior uterine wall.

Figure 48–2. Irving method of sterilization. (Reproduced with permission from Benson RC: *Handbook of Obstetrics & Gynecology,* 8th ed. Lange, 1983.)

pect of the scrotum (Fig 48–6). Sutures or clips are placed tightly around the vas, demarcating a 1–1.5-cm segment, which is then excised. The ligated and fulgurated ends are tucked back into the scrotal sac, and the incision is closed. The same procedure is performed on the opposite side. The no-scalpel technique requires no incision because a sharpened dissection forceps is used to pierce the skin and dissect the vas. Studies are being done on the efficacy of intravasal plugs to confer sterility. Microscopic examination confirms excision of vasal tissue.

The failure rate after vasectomy is 9.4 per 1000 at 1 year and 11.3 per 1000 at years 2, 3, and 5. Half of the vasectomy failures in the CREST study occurred

within 3 months of the procedure. Thus, sterility is assumed only after ejaculates are completely free of sperm after 3 months and after periodic microscopic analysis.

Complications are infrequent, usually involving slight bleeding, hematoma formation, skin infection, and reactions to sutures or local anesthetics.

When vasal anastomosis is attempted (vasovasostomy), patency is achieved in 86–97% of patients, depending on the interval between vasectomy and vasovasostomy. Pregnancy rates are lower (18–60%). Skillful microsurgery performed by an experienced urologist optimizes the chances of pregnancy.

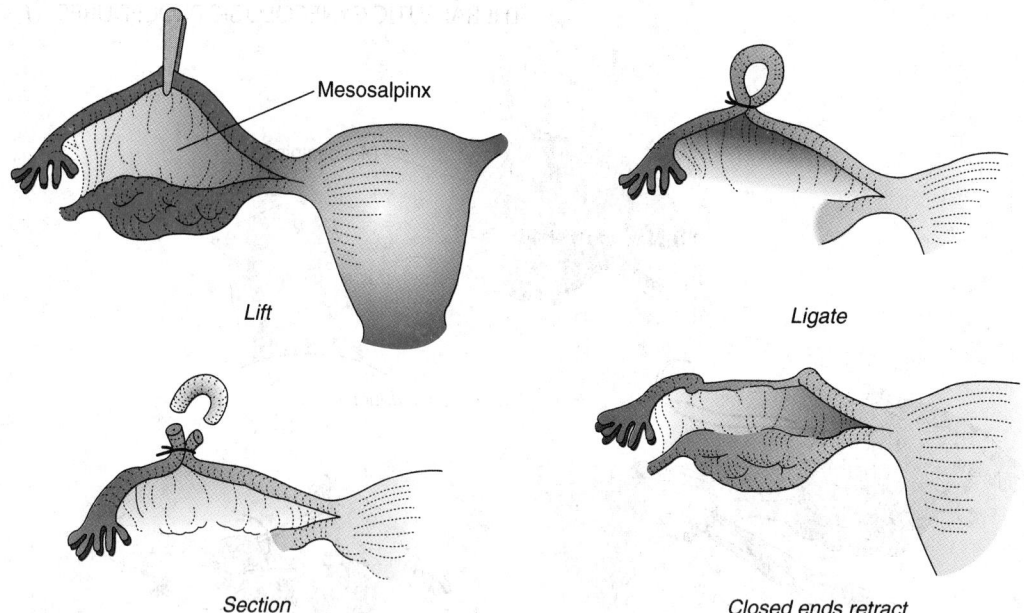

Lift

Ligate

Mesosalpinx

Section

Closed ends retract

Figure 48–3. Pomeroy method of sterilization. (Reproduced with permission from Benson RC: *Handbook of Obstetrics & Gynecology,* 8th ed. Lange, 1983.)

Figure 48–4. Sterilization by fimbriectomy.

Indications

The indications for hysterectomy can be practically divided into those for the treatment of gynecologic cancer, benign gynecologic conditions, and obstetric complications. Hysterectomy for cancer of the uterus, ovary, and cervix is discussed in Chapters 53–54B. Hysterectomy for obstetric complications, including excessive bleeding and molar pregnancy, is becoming less common (see Chapter 31).

Table 48–4 lists the most common benign diseases and disorders that warrant hysterectomy.

Preoperative Evaluation

A. DIAGNOSTIC TESTS TO DETECT OCCULT CANCER

All patients anticipating hysterectomy should have a baseline evaluation to detect occult cancer. A Papanicolaou smear should be performed within 3 months before the operation, and abnormalities should be followed with colposcopic examination and biopsy before surgery. Cervical conization is indicated prior to hysterectomy if (a) colposcopy fails to demonstrate the entire squamocolumnar junction, where cervical cancers typically arise; (b) colposcopically guided biopsies reveal dysplasia that differs by two or more grades than that shown on the Papanicolaou smear (eg, carcinoma in situ on smear but mild dysplasia on biopsy); (c) endocervical curettage demonstrates dysplastic endocervical cells; and (d) biopsy reveals microinvasive squamous cell carcinoma or squamous adenocarcinoma in situ.

Cervical conization for the previous indications is performed to ensure that occult invasive cancer is not present within the endocervical canal. Frozen-section analysis of cervical conization tissue correlates well enough with "permanent" (hematoxylin and eosin) slide analysis so that if intraepithelial neoplasia with clear margins is found, the surgeon may, with reasonable certainty, perform a hysterectomy that will totally include the tumor.

Biopsy for endometrial neoplasia must also be considered. Generally any woman older than age 35 years who presents with abnormal uterine bleeding should have endometrial evaluation (D&C, directed biopsies) before hysterectomy. However, certain clinical situations that produce an unopposed estrogen effect on the endometrium warrant preoperative endometrial evaluation at any age: chronic anovulation and secondary oligomenorrhea, unopposed estrogen therapy for menopause, and known ovarian disorders associated with endometrial neoplasia (eg, polycystic ovarian syndrome, granulosa cell tumors). Unfortunately, frozen-section analysis of endometrial curettings is neither practical nor accurate, so hysterectomy usually must wait for permanent section.

Figure 48–5. Hysteroscopic tubal sterilization technique. (Reproduced with permission from Essure, Conceptus Incorporated.)

■ HYSTERECTOMY

Hysterectomy is complete removal of the uterus. With more than 598,929 procedures done each year, hysterectomy is the second most common major operation performed in the United States. With advancements in medical and conservative surgical therapy of gynecologic conditions, the need for hysterectomy has declined. More women now wish to avoid major surgery if equally efficacious alternatives exist. Regulatory boards of gynecologists now support the use of hysterectomy as treatment for conditions refractory to more conservative management.

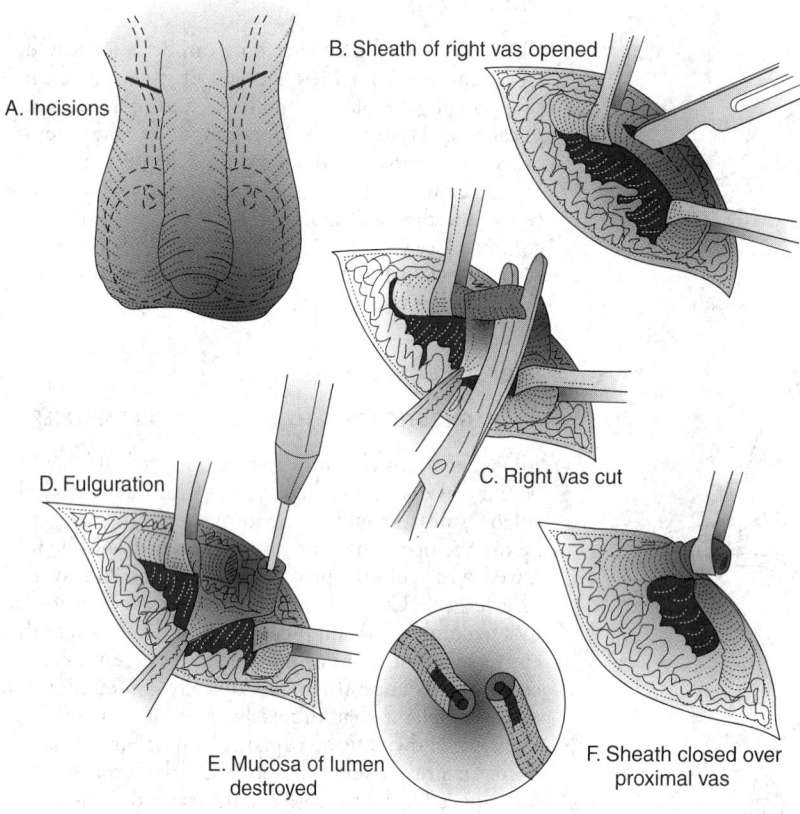

A. Incisions

B. Sheath of right vas opened

D. Fulguration

C. Right vas cut

E. Mucosa of lumen destroyed

F. Sheath closed over proximal vas

Figure 48–6. Steps in vasectomy. (Modified from a drawing by S. Taft. Reproduced with permission from Schmidt S: Vasectomy should not fail. Contemp Surg 1974;4:13.)

Occult cancer may also be present outside the genital tract. All patients should have their stool checked for occult blood preoperatively. In women 40 years of age or older, mammography is standard.

B. PREOPERATIVE EVALUATION OF THE PELVIS

In the woman with a small, mobile uterus with mobile adnexa, little diagnostic evaluation beyond bimanual examination is indicated. However, pelvic disease may have caused disturbance of normal tissue planes that endanger the urologic and gastrointestinal tracts. The following conditions may indicate the need for more extensive evaluation of the pelvis prior to hysterectomy: (a) pelvic inflammatory disease, especially if repeated, chronic, or associated with a tuboovarian complex; (b) endometriosis; (c) pelvic adhesions from other causes of pelvic inflammation (eg, appendicitis, cholecystitis, previous pelvic surgery); (d) chronic pelvic pain; (e) questionable origin of a palpable pelvic mass; and (f) clinical suspicion of cancer (eg, palpable adnexa in a postmenopausal woman).

The most commonly used preoperative adjunctive diagnostic evaluation is pelvic ultrasound, which has advantages over computed tomography (CT) scan. Ul-

trasound is helpful in detecting masses in the difficult-to-examine patient (eg, obese) and in confirming a pelvic mass detected on bimanual examination.

Intravenous pyelography (IVP) is helpful in delineating the course of the ureters through the pelvis. A preoperative intravenous pyelogram is especially useful for inflammatory conditions that could distort or obstruct the ureters. Also, patients with genital developmental anomalies should have a preoperative IVP to look for concomitant urologic anomalies.

Prehysterectomy evaluation of the colon (beyond screening for occult blood in the stool) is indicated in any patient with symptoms for rectal disease. In most cases, proctoscopy or flexible proctosigmoidoscopy is sufficient. In cases of severe pelvic inflammation, chronic pelvic pain, or suspected cancer, complete colonoscopy or barium enema is indicated. Preoperative diagnosis of bowel disease will aid in the selection of the incision. If necessary, a consultant gastrointestinal surgeon can be present during the operation.

C. PREOPERATIVE BOWEL PREPARATION

See Chapter 46.

Table 48–4. Benign diseases and disorders for which hysterectomy may be performed.

Uterine leiomyomas
    Symptomatic (abnormal bleeding or pelvic pressure)
    Asymptomatic (presenting as a large uterus obscuring palpation of the adnexa and ultrasound unavailable)
    Rapid growth of the uterus
    Failed conservative management of bleeding (eg, cyclic progestin, D&C) or uterine pain (eg, nonsteroidal anti-inflammatory medications)
Symptomatic adenomyosis
Symptomatic endometriosis refractory to conservative surgical or medical therapy
Symptomatic pelvic relaxation syndromes
Chronic incapacitating central pelvic disorder refractory to conservative treatment (eg, hormonal suppression and nonsteroidal anti-inflammatory drugs) in a woman with a normal urologic and gastrointestinal evaluation
Definitive treatment of severe pelvic inflammatory disease or any pelvic abscess involving the genitalia if conservative therapy is not possible or desired by the patient

D. PROPHYLACTIC ANTIBIOTICS

The incidence of febrile morbidity occurs in approximately 18% of patients undergoing abdominal hysterectomy versus 8% with vaginal hysterectomy. Certain risk factors are associated with a higher likelihood of operative site infection. These factors include an abdominal surgical approach, blood loss greater than 750 mL, and no preoperative antibiotics. The American College of Obstetricians and Gynecologists (ACOG) also recommends giving additional doses of Intraoperative antibiotics during lengthy operations, given at intervals of 1 or 2 half-lives of the drug. A second dose of the prophylactic antibiotic may also be given in surgical cases with an increased blood loss > 1500 mL. Patients diagnosed with a vaginal infection during preoperative evaluation should be treated prior to surgery.

A broad-spectrum antibiotic should be chosen that will be effective against common (but not necessarily *all*) pathogens causing pelvic infection. The agent should have a low incidence of toxicity and side effects and should be easily administered and cost-effective. The proper dosage should be administered 30 minutes prior to surgery. Therapeutic levels must be achieved in tissue at the surgical site. It should *not* be an antibiotic reserved for serious infection. ACOG recommends intravenous cefazolin, cefoxitin, cefotetan, or metronidazole prior to vaginal or abdominal hysterectomy.

E. THROMBOEMBOLISM PROPHYLAXIS

The risk of calf vein thrombosis, proximal vein thrombosis, and pulmonary embolism can be minimized with the use of graduated compression stockings perioperatively and early ambulation postoperatively. Sequential compression devices will help prevent stasis as well. For patients at high risk for thromboembolic disease, a dose of 5000 U subcutaneous heparin is given preoperatively and then every 8–12 hours postoperatively. Risk factors include malignancy, obesity, previous radiation therapy, immobilization, estrogen use, prolonged anesthesia, radical surgery, history of thromboembolism, and personal or family history of hypercoagulability. Other less-often-used prophylactic modalities include low-dose dihydroergotamine-heparin, dextran-70, and low-molecular-weight heparin.

F. BLOOD PRODUCTS

It may not be necessary to preoperatively cross-match all patients undergoing hysterectomy. Women who are not at particular risk of needing a transfusion during hysterectomy should at least have blood typing and antibody screening prior to surgery. Patients undergoing peripartum hysterectomy or hysterectomy for gynecologic cancer are more likely to need blood transfusion. Patients undergoing elective hysterectomy are more likely to need a transfusion if the hematocrit is low (30%), if they have pelvic inflammatory disease or pelvic abscess or adhesions, or if colporrhaphy is performed at the time of vaginal hysterectomy.

G. INFORMED CONSENT

Many women desire, and most insurance companies require, a second opinion prior to scheduling an elective hysterectomy. The patient must understand the diagnosis and be aware of alternative therapies and the risks and benefits of the operation. Common risks of surgery such as cuff cellulitis and blood loss are usually explained during preoperative counseling. The current medicolegal climate mandates the discussion of unusual complications, including the possibility of completing a vaginal operation via an abdominal route and the risks of viral illness following transfusion, severe postoperative infection (including adnexal abscess), ectopic pregnancy, and vaginal vault prolapse (see also Chapter 64).

TECHNIQUE

Vaginal versus Abdominal Hysterectomy

The route of hysterectomy is chosen according to the following guidelines.

A. PELVIC ANATOMY

The ideal candidate for vaginal hysterectomy has a gynecoid pelvis with a wide pubic arch, and a vaginal apex > 2 fingerbreadths at the apex. Some descent of the uterus is helpful but not mandatory; procidentia makes for a more complicated vaginal hysterectomy because of the greater vulnerability of the prolapsed ureters.

B. UTERINE SIZE

Most gynecologists will perform vaginal hysterectomy on a uterus equivalent in size to a uterus at 12 weeks' gestation or smaller, or a uterine weight of less than 280 g. More experienced surgeons have successfully removed uteri of up to 700 g vaginally using bivalve and morcellation techniques.

C. ADNEXA

In patients with symptoms or pelvic findings suggesting adnexal disease that may indicate adnexectomy, the abdominal route for hysterectomy is preferred. Such patients may be candidates for LAVH.

D. GASTROINTESTINAL TRACT

Especially in older patients or those with significant history of gastrointestinal complaints, the abdominal approach offers an opportunity for complete examination of the bowel.

E. UROLOGIC DISORDERS

If a retropubic urethropexy is planned, a laparoscopic or abdominal approach can be used. If anterior vaginal colporrhaphy only is planned, vaginal hysterectomy is preferred. Advanced degrees of cystocele, with marked prolapse of the urethrovesical angle, may be best treated with a combined vaginal and abdominal approach (see Chapters 44 and 45).

F. PELVIC RELAXATION

In the case of isolated rectocele, a vaginal approach is preferred. Culdoplasty for enterocele may be performed by either route.

G. PLASTIC PROCEDURES

As more women choose to undergo procedures such as abdominoplasty or suction-assisted lipectomy, an abdominal approach is indicated. Perineorrhaphy and vaginal repairs usually accompany vaginal hysterectomies but can also be done after abdominal hysterectomy.

H. MEDICAL DISORDERS

In patients with significant heart or lung disease, the vaginal approach is preferable when possible because of a lower incidence of postoperative pulmonary complications and earlier ambulation.

I. PREVIOUS SURGERY

Most surgeons are willing to perform a vaginal hysterectomy in patients with previous tubal ligation or cesar-

ean section. The surgery would be more problematic in patients with a history of multiple cesarean births or complications (eg, postpartum endomyoparametritis) or with probable abdominal adhesions from previous laparotomy. LAVH may be used in these situations.

The preceding guidelines may certainly be adjusted to the individual patient based on the surgeon's experience and abilities. An examination performed under anesthesia when the physician first sees the patient may help to decide on the approach. Uterine size can be assessed with transvaginal ultrasound. Laparoscopic evaluation of the adnexa further aids in the decision-making process. All patients anticipating vaginal hysterectomy, LH, or LAVH should be told that the operation may have to be completed abdominally if difficulties arise.

Abdominal Hysterectomy

The technique of abdominal hysterectomy varies according to the indication for the operation, the size and placement of vital structures, including the ureters (which may be distorted), and the pelvic anatomy. A standard, well-organized approach to abdominal hysterectomy is essential to avoid incidental injury. Modifications are made as necessary, always within an organized plan of operation.

The anesthetic of choice typically includes general endotracheal intubation, an inhalation agent, and an analgesic. Hysterectomies are of such duration and risk that using a mask alone is unwise. In patients with pulmonary compromise, spinal or epidural anesthesia may be used.

A sterile scrub of the abdomen and vagina is done, and a urinary catheter is placed so that the anesthesiologist can monitor urine output intraoperatively. The choice of incision is based on the suspected disease or disorder; most hysterectomies for benign disease can be accomplished through a transverse incision. However, a midline incision extending from 2 fingerbreadths above the pubic symphysis to the umbilicus offers the greatest exposure. Two modifications of the low transverse incision that improve exposure are the Maylard muscle-splitting procedure and the Cherney detachment of the rectus muscles from their insertion on the pubic symphysis.

The surgeon and assistants should rinse excessive talcum powder from their gloves before making the incision to prevent granulomatous tissue reaction in the wound. Once the incision is complete, peritoneal fluid may be aspirated if the possibility of gynecologic cancer exists. The pelvic organs are then inspected and the upper abdomen palpated in a systematic fashion: right gutter, right hemidiaphragm, liver, gallbladder, pancreas, stomach (assessing the position of the indwelling gastric decompression tube if present), and spleen and right hemidiaphragm (gently, because of the risk of trauma to the spleen), left gutter, paraaortic lymph nodes, and omentum. Excessive bowel manipulation should be avoided to decrease the severity of postoperative adynamic ileus; at the least, the appendix and cecum should be inspected, as well as the terminal meter of ileum. Older patients and those with gastrointestinal complaints would benefit from careful palpation and inspection of the bowel from rectum to ligament of Treitz. If desired, the wound may be protected with moist towels, a self-retaining retractor placed, and the bowel packed into the upper abdomen.

The classic extrafascial hysterectomy performed by Richardson remains the mainstay of surgical technique in abdominal hysterectomy. Choice of suture and needle is made according to surgeon experience and preference; 2-0, 0, or 1 absorbable sutures on half-curved taper needles are standard choices. The uterus is grasped either by the fundus with a Massachusetts double-toothed clamp or at the cornu with Ochsner or Kocher clamps. The round ligament is clamped proximal to the uterus; at its midportion, it is ligated by suture, and the suture is tagged with a small hemostat. The round ligament is divided about 0.5-cm proximal to the suture, thus opening the broad ligament at its apex. The anterior uterine peritoneum may be incised at the vesicouterine junction in preparation for advancement of the bladder. Only the peritoneum should be incised; the potentially vascular areolar tissue should be avoided. When this procedure is repeated on the contralateral side, the anterior leaves of the broad ligament are opened, the uterine vessels first become apparent, and attention is then directed to the posterior leaf of the broad ligament.

The posterior leaf of the broad ligament is incised beginning at the ligated round ligament. The extent of the incision is determined by the decision to preserve or remove the adnexa. If the adnexa are to be removed, the peritoneum is incised parallel to the infundibulopelvic ligament to the pelvic sidewall; the loose areolar tissue is dissected medial to the internal iliac (hypogastric) artery, which is typically 0.5-cm thick with a visually appreciable (and certainly palpable) pulse. The dissection will reveal a clear area of peritoneum under the infundibulopelvic ligament; below this area at a variable distance lays the ureter on this medial flap of peritoneum.

The intimate proximity of the ureters to the uterus makes ureteral dissection important. Whereas the ureter is usually 4–6 cm deep to the infundibulopelvic ligament at the lateral margin of the uterus, it is only 0.5–2 cm below this vascular bundle at the level of the pelvic brim. Observing the ureter through the peritoneum or palpating the characteristic "snap" of the ureter should serve only to guide dissection and should not be a substitute for identification of the entire ureter through its pelvic course. The ureter tolerates careful dissection well as long as its blood-carrying adventitia is not stripped away. The ureter can always be found and dissection begun at the pelvic brim, where the ureter passes over the bifurcation of the iliac artery. The most

serious ureteral injury is the unrecognized insult. The most common ureteral injuries during hysterectomy occur during ligation of the uterine artery, ligation of the infundibulopelvic ligament, and placement of the vaginal angle sutures.

Once the course of the ureters is well established, the adnexal component of the operation is completed. If the adnexa are to be removed, a ligating suture may be passed beneath the infundibulopelvic ligament and above the ureter; this step is repeated for a double ligature as a precaution. Traditionally, the infundibulopelvic ligament is clamped, divided, and ligated; the direct suture technique may avoid undue crushing of tissue. The ligament is ligated again adjacent to the uterus to avoid back bleeding; the infundibulopelvic ligament is divided and the peritoneum incised to the back of the uterine fundus, always cognizant of the proximity of the ureter. If the adnexa are to be preserved, a hole is made in the avascular portion of the posterior leaf of the broad ligament superior to the ureter. The uteroovarian ligament and fallopian tube are doubly clamped, divided, and ligated, with care taken to avoid incorporation of ovarian tissue into the ligature.

The final step is extending the peritoneal incision posteriorly around the uterus between the medial portions of the uterosacral ligaments. If the incision of the posterior leaf of the broad ligament is extended over the uterosacral ligaments, there is typically significant bleeding just lateral to the insertion of the ligament at the uterus. The advantages of making an incision between the uterosacrals include clear identification of the rectum and its separation from the uterus, ease of suturing the vaginal cuff, and improved mobility of the peritoneum to allow reperitonealization under less tension.

The bladder is advanced down off of the lower uterine segment prior to clamping the uterine vessels. Surgeons-in-training have more difficulty with advancement of the bladder than with other aspects of abdominal hysterectomy. The principal difficulty in mobilization of the bladder is failure to identify the proper cleavage plane between the bladder and the uterus. At the attachment of the bladder to the lower uterine segment, a median raphe is variably present; it is typically a 1-cm longitudinal band of thick connective tissue. The raphe is attenuated in pregnant or postmenopausal patients. The raphe is divided at midportion, and loose avascular fibroareolar tissue is seen immediately between the cervix and bladder. The uterus is retracted posteriorly and superiorly, roughly at an angle of 30 degrees to the long axis of the vagina. The midpoint of the peritoneal incision of the bladder flap is gently lifted with forceps; the avascular plane of the vesicovaginal and vesicocervical areolar spaces is continuous once the median raphe is divided. Metzenbaum scissors are pointed to the uterus, and sharp dissection reveals the shiny white pubocervical fascia overlying the cervix. Properly done, the dissection is bloodless, and the plane is recognized by the ease with which the bladder falls away from the cervix. The vesicouterine space is developed 2 cm beyond the anterior vaginal fornix. Care must be exercised in any dissection laterally, because the vesicouterine ligaments ("bladder pillars") may bleed because of the paracervical and paravaginal veins present laterally.

The uterine vessels may be skeletonized by separating the loose avascular areolar connective tissue from the vessels. The intraligamentous course of the ureter is again checked; it is typically 2–3 cm inferolateral to the insertion of the uterine vessels into the uterus. The uterine vessels are clamped with a curved crushing clamp (eg, Heaney, Phaneuf, or curved Ballantine clamp). Double-clamping is used for larger vessels. It is not necessary to place another clamp on the uterine side of the pedicle to prevent back bleeding if the uterine arteries on both sides of the uterus are clamped before either pedicle is incised. The clamp is applied at the level of the internal os, with the tip of the clamp at a right angle to the long axis of the cervix; the temptation to clamp the entire cervix and "slide off" dragging paracervical tissue into the pedicle should be avoided in order to minimize the risk of the pedicle slipping out of the clamp. The uterine vessels are then ligated by suture at the tip of the clamp. Occasionally, a second application of the curved clamp is necessary to complete ligation of the uterine vessels.

Next, the cardinal ligament is assessed. Ordinarily, a single application of a straight clamp (Ochsner, Kocher, or Ballantine clamp) will include the cardinal ligament to the level of its attachment at the lateral edge of the cervix and upper vagina. A deep knife is often useful in dividing the cardinal ligament adjacent to the uterus, leaving a larger pedicle, which is less likely to slip out of the suture than one remaining after cutting with scissors flush to the clamp. The suture ligature of the cardinal ligament is often tagged to aid in manipulation of the vaginal cuff.

The uterosacral ligaments are clamped at their insertion into the lower cervix, divided at their insertion, and ligated. Alternatively, they may be transected with large Mayo scissors while the vagina is entered posterolaterally. If division and suture ligation of either pedicle of the cardinal–uterosacral ligament complex fails to enter the vagina, the safest approach is to enter the vagina with the knife in the midline, either anteriorly or posteriorly, at the confluence of the vagina with the cervix. Once entered, the cervix is circumferentially incised, with long Ochsner clamps used to control point bleeders and elevate the vaginal cuff. The cervix is inspected to ensure complete excision.

Sutures are placed at each lateral vaginal angle to ligate small paravaginal vessels coursing upward through the paravaginal tissues and to provide vaginal vault sup-

port. The suture is begun inside the vagina 1 cm from the upper border, incorporates the cardinal and uterosacral ligaments, and, finally, transverses the vagina again to end up within the vagina. This suture is tagged, and the procedure is repeated on the contralateral side.

Surgical management of the cuff is individualized. In the case of marked pelvic inflammation and persistent oozing, the cuff may be left open to afford retroperitoneal drainage or allow egress of a closed drain system. In most cases, closing the cuff may reduce granulation tissue and possibly minimize ascension of bacteria from the vagina. The cuff may be closed with either interrupted figure-of-eight sutures or a double running suture; the key points with either closure are inversion of the cut edges into the vagina and hemostasis.

The pelvis is irrigated and hemostasis checked in a systematic fashion from one lateral pedicle to the ipsilateral round ligament pedicle to the cuff and on to the other side. Small bleeding vessels must be ligated to minimize the risk of retroperitoneal hematoma formation, which may expand or become infected. For diffuse oozing, hemostatic agents such as thrombin powder or thrombostatic absorbable sponges may be useful. There is no advantage to closing the parietal peritoneum.

Retained ovaries may be suspended to minimize the risk of torsion and adherence to the vaginal cuff. The uteroovarian ligament can be conveniently attached to the round ligament stump to suspend the ovaries above the pelvis without placing the infundibulopelvic ligament under tension.

The abnormal appendix should be removed. In cases of hysterectomy for endometriosis, appendectomy will reveal microscopic endometriotic foci in some 3% of cases.

Supracervical Hysterectomy

Prior to the 1940s, 95% of hysterectomies were either supracervical/subtotal hysterectomy or removal of the uterine corpus without the cervix. Despite Papanicolaou's introduction of his cervical smear, concern over neoplastic changes occurring in the retained cervix made total abdominal hysterectomy (TAH) the leading approach to surgery from the 1950s and on. Debate has been renewed about which approach leads to decreased morbidity. Proponents of supracervical hysterectomy believe that there is less damage to sympathetic and parasympathetic innervation than might occur with paracervical dissection. Thus, bladder function and orgasm are less likely to be affected with supracervical hysterectomy. Also, by leaving the cervix, vault prolapse and vaginal shortening might be avoided. Those in favor of TAH suggest that it decreases the risk of cervical cancer, especially in women who might not follow up for routine Papanicolaou

(Pap) smears. It also eliminates the small risk of cyclical bleeding (6.8%) that can occur after supracervical hysterectomy, if residual endometrium is left behind. A randomized, double-blind controlled trial showed no statistically significant difference in bladder, bowel, and sexual function between women who had undergone total versus supracervical hysterectomy. Current indications for supracervical hysterectomy include difficulty dissecting the cervix, distorted anatomy secondary to pelvic inflammatory disease or endometriosis, and compromised medical condition.

Following ligation of the uterine vessels, the uterine fundus may be amputated from the cervix; the level of amputation should be below the internal cervical os to avoid postoperative uterine bleeding from endometrial remnants. The cervical stump is closed with figure-of-eight sutures.

Vaginal Hysterectomy

Most vaginal hysterectomies are performed under general anesthesia. In the patient with medical complications, particularly pulmonary problems, spinal anesthesia may be elected. Following administration of the anesthetic, a bimanual examination is mandatory before beginning surgery. The perineum is shaved or trimmed as necessary and a sterile wash performed. The patient is placed in a modified dorsal lithotomy position and draped; the surgeon should participate in proper positioning of the patient, because excessive flexion of the hips can stretch the obturator and sciatic nerves and compress the femoral nerve; and excessive extension of the knee can jeopardize the peroneal nerves. All bony prominences and soft tissues in contact with the leg stirrups should be carefully padded.

The urinary bladder may be drained by catheter, but this step is optional. The cervix is grasped with a tenaculum. Passage of a uterine sound will aid in determining the size and position of the uterus; some surgeons advocate performing a D&C at this point to rule out pyometra or endometrial neoplasia.

As the surgeon exerts gentle traction downward on the cervix, two assistants maintain exposure with lateral vaginal retractors and protect the bladder with an anterior Heaney retractor. If desired, the junction of the vagina and cervix can be injected with a 1% 1:1000 epinephrine solution to minimize blood loss during incision of the cervix. Beginning posteriorly to minimize obscuring the field with blood, the surgeon circumferentially incises the cervix down to the level of the pubovesicocervical fascia. Gentle traction with the bladder retractor and downward traction of the cervix will allow exposure of the fibers of fascia between bladder and cervix, which are incised. When the bladder has been advanced up off of the cervix, attention is given to the posterior attachment of the cervix. While the assistant pulls the uterus upward, the posterior vaginal mucosa is tented away from the cervix. With the patient in the Trendelenburg position to allow as much emptying of the posterior cul-de-sac as possible, the posterior cul-de-sac is incised with a single stroke of the scissors. A retractor is placed within the opening, exposing the uterosacral ligaments. The uterosacral ligaments are grasped with Heaney clamps, making certain that the peritoneum posterior to the ligament is within the clamp. The ligament is cut and ligated with 2-0 or 0 absorbable suture and tagged with a hemostat for later manipulation of the cuff.

The cardinal ligament may be clamped next if the bladder is safely advanced; likewise, the uterine vessels are included in the next application of the Heaney clamps. The anterior cul-de-sac is entered by blunt and sharp dissection to the anterior vesicouterine fold of peritoneum. The anterior retractor is placed within this opening and the bladder is gently lifted upward. The surgeon now clamps, incises, and ligates in pedicles the remaining portions of the broad ligaments bilaterally, incorporating the tissue between the anterior and posterior leaves of the broad ligament. The round ligament, uteroovarian ligament, and fallopian tube are excised from the uterus and incorporated into these pedicles, and the uterus is removed from the field. A larger uterus may require special manipulation for delivery through the vaginal introitus (eg, bivalving the uterus in the midline, morcellation of the uterus into multiple extractable segments, or myomectomy).

The final suture on the uteroovarian ligament is tagged to allow careful inspection of the tubes and ovaries. If ovarian disease is suspected or if prophylactic oophorectomy is planned, a clamp is placed above the ovary and uterine tube on the infundibulopelvic ligament for suture ligature, while traction is placed on the last stay suture. The entire ovary must be removed, because an ovarian remnant may become cystic and produce pain many years after the hysterectomy.

Once all pedicles are inspected and found to be hemostatic, some surgeons advocate closing the peritoneum with a running 2-0 absorbable suture, incorporating the cardinal and uterosacral ligament pedicles for support of the vaginal vault. Lateral vaginal angle sutures are placed from the vaginal mucosa at the 2 o'clock position, inside the cuff and including the uterosacral pedicle, then out through the cuff to the 4 o'clock position. If anterior or posterior colporrhaphy is planned, that operation is completed prior to complete closure of the cuff. The cuff may be closed by an interrupted absorbable 0 suture, a running simple suture, or a running vertical mattress technique. The goals of closure are obliteration of the cuff's dead space back to the peritoneum and approximation of the cut edges of the vagina to afford healing and minimize postoperative granulation tissue. Modifications of the just-described technique are made by virtually every gynecologic surgeon based on operative findings and experience. Many surgeons will close the posterior cul-de-sac to prevent development of an enterocele or will shorten the uterosacral ligaments to suspend the vaginal vault. As in abdominal hysterectomy, the cuff can be left open to promote drainage with a running locked absorbable 0 suture. Another technique to drain the closure is insertion of a T-tube above the cuff, which is associated with a demonstrable reduction in postoperative febrile morbidity.

After the operation is completed, the vagina and perineum are gently cleansed. An indwelling bladder catheter is inserted and a vaginal pack may be placed. The patient is returned slowly to the dorsal supine position.

Laparoscopic Hysterectomy

The laparoscope can be used to aid vaginal hysterectomy by freeing abdominal adhesions (LAVH) or to free the uterus in its entirety with removal via the vagina (total LH). Supracervical hysterectomy can also be done laparoscopically with morcellation and removal by culdotomy or through extended trocar sites. Advantages to LH include decreased length of hospital stay, decreased postoperative analgesia, and decreased convalescence period. There may be a lower complication rate compared to TAH but there is no difference versus vaginal hysterectomy. However, the laparoscopic approach requires significantly more operating time and a well-trained, experienced surgeon. Because of the costs for the endoscopic equipment, LH has been found to be more expensive despite the shorter hospital stay. Complications with LH include hemorrhage and bowel or urinary tract damage. Conversion to abdominal hysterectomy may occur, especially in cases with large leiomyomas obstructing access to upper pedicles.

Postoperative Care of the Hysterectomy Patient

The details of postoperative care are dictated by the indications for surgery and the individual patient's overall medical condition. General guidelines include the following:

1. A Foley catheter is left indwelling for 24 hours.
2. Prophylactic antibiotics are given only within the first 24 hours postoperatively.
3. Hydration, 2–3 L/d of balanced electrolyte solution, is given intravenously, depending on blood loss and intraoperative replacement.
4. Sips of water may be given the first night, followed by clear liquids or regular diet on the next postoperative day depending on the patient's appetite. The diet is advanced based on return of bowel sounds and appetite, toleration of the diet, and the passage of flatus.
5. Prophylactic heparin therapy, sequential compression device, or antiembolic stockings are used in patients according to risk for thromboembolic complications.
6. Ambulation is begun on the first postoperative day.
7. Adequate analgesia is given parenterally. Once the patient can tolerate a regular diet, she can be switched to oral analgesics.

Complications

Perioperative deaths may be a result of cardiac arrest, coronary occlusion, or respiratory paralysis. Postoperative deaths are usually the result of hemorrhage, infection, pulmonary embolus, or intercurrent disease. A recent study of factors contributing to the risk of death found that abdominal hysterectomies performed for complications of pregnancy or cancer (8% of all hysterectomies) account for 61% of deaths caused by hysterectomy. Overall mortality rates for abdominal or vaginal hysterectomy are 0.1–0.2%. Mortality rates increase with age and medical complications for both vaginal and abdominal hysterectomies.

The bladder may be injured in 1–2% of all hysterectomies. Consequences are slight if the injury is to the dome of the bladder—which is usually the case—away from the trigone. Ureteral injury occurs in 0.7–1.7% of abdominal hysterectomies and 0–0.1% of vaginal hysterectomies. The essential point is to recognize urologic injuries and correct them intraoperatively, avoiding the serious postoperative complications that occur from urinary extravasation.

Damage to the bowel is quite uncommon, particularly with vaginal hysterectomy. In preparation for abdominal hysterectomy for suspected extensive or inflammatory pathologic process (eg, ovarian cancer, endometriosis, pelvic inflammatory disease), preoperative bowel preparation will allow incidental colon surgery without the necessity of colostomy. Small-bowel injuries, assuming no obstruction, are closed in layers perpendicular to the long axis of the bowel; a running layer of 3-0 sutures in the mucosa is supported by interrupted 2-0 silk sutures in the serosa. If a transmural large-bowel injury occurs and no preoperative bowel preparation was given, a temporary diverting colostomy may be indicated to protect the suture line and lower the risk of peritonitis and sepsis.

The most serious postoperative complication is hemorrhage (0.2–2% of patients). Bleeding usually originates at the lateral vaginal angles and is amenable to vaginal resuturing in most cases. Blood products are replaced as needed.

Infection remains the most common complication following hysterectomy. Even with immaculate technique and careful patient selection, the gynecologic surgeon can still expect a 10% rate of postoperative febrile morbidity. A postoperative temperature of 38 °C (100.4 °F) or higher on two consecutive determinations 6 hours apart must be investigated by (a) careful interview of the patient for localizing symptoms (eg, productive cough, intravenous line pain), (b) thorough physical examination (including pelvic examination for inspection and palpation of the cuff), and (c) appropriate laboratory studies (eg, urinalysis, Gram-stained smear of sputum, or complete blood count).

Antibiotics are begun only if a focus of infection is identified or highly suspected. Broad-spectrum antibiotics covering anticipated pathogens are prescribed; single-agent semisynthetic penicillins (eg, piperacillin) and cephalosporins (eg, cefoxitin) offer sufficient coverage. In the presence of sepsis, multiagent comprehensive coverage (eg, a penicillin, an aminoglycoside, and an anaerobic agent such as clindamycin or metronidazole) must be prescribed.

Granulation of the vaginal vault is part of the normal healing process and is evident on speculum examination in over half of cases. The granulation is rarely troublesome; light cauterization with silver nitrate sticks or electrocautery eliminates the granulation tissue promptly in most cases. Many suggestions have been made on ways to minimize granulation, including management of the cuff (open vs closed), choice of suture (plain gut vs chromic vs newer synthetics), and drainage techniques. The most important common denominator is close apposition of the cut vaginal edges, which can be accomplished with any of the techniques.

REFERENCES

American College of Obstetricians and Gynecologists: Antibiotic prophylaxis for gynecologic procedures. ACOG Practice Bulletin No. 23, 2001.

American College of Obstetricians and Gynecologists: Benefits and risks of sterilization. ACOG Practice Bulletin No. 46, 2003.

Aronsson A et al: Sublingual compared with oral Misoprostol for cervical dilation prior to vacuum aspiration: A randomized comparison. Contraception 2004;69:165.

Bronz L: Hysteroscopy in the assessment of postmenopausal bleeding. Contrib Gynecol Obstet 2000;20:519.

Bunnasathiansri S et al: Vaginal Misoprostol for cervical priming before dilation and curettage in postmenopausal women: A randomized controlled trial. J Obstet Gynaecol Res 2004;30(3):221.

Cheong YC, Bajekal N, Li TC. Peritoneal closure—To close or not to close. Hum Reprod 2001;16:154852.

Christman GM, Uechi H: Female sterilization. Female Patient 2000;25:4856.

Cooper JM et al: Intraoperative and early postoperative complications of operative hysteroscopy. Obstet Gynecol Clin 2000;27(2):347.

Cosson M et al: Vaginal, laparoscopic, or abdominal hysterectomies for benign disorders: immediate and early postoperative complications. Eur J Obstet Gynecol Reprod Biol 2001;98:2316.

Darai A et al: Vaginal hysterectomy for enlarged uteri, with or without laparoscopic assistance: randomized study. Obstet Gynecol 2001;997:712.

Darwish AM et al: Cervical priming prior to operative hysteroscopy: A randomized comparison of laminaria versus misoprostol. Hum Reprod 2004;19(10):2391.

Ewies AA, Olah KS: Subtotal abdominal hysterectomy: A surgical advance or a backward step. Br J Obstet Gynaecol 2000; 107:13169.

Farquhar CM, Steiner CA: Hysterectomy rates in the United States 1990–1997. Obstet Gynecol 2002;99:229.

Fung TM et al: A randomized placebo-controlled trial of vaginal misoprostol for cervical priming before hysteroscopy in postmenopausal women. Br J Obstet Gynaecol 2002;109:561.

Hajenius PJ et al: Interventions for tubal ectopic pregnancy [review]. Cochrane Database Syst Rev 2000;(2):CD0000324.

Hillis SD et al: Poststerilization regret: Findings from the United States Collaborative Review of Sterilization. Obstet Gynecol 1999;93:889.

Jamieson DJ et al: The risk of pregnancy after vasectomy. Obstet Gynecol 2004;103:848.

Josey WE: Routine intrauterine forceps exploration at curettage. Obstet Gynecol 1958;11(1):108.

Kovac SR: Hysterectomy outcomes in patients with similar indications. Obstet Gynecol 2000;95:787.

Kovac SR: Transvaginal hysterectomy: Rationale and surgical approach. Obstet Gynecol 2004;103:1321.

Loffer FD: Hysteroscopy with selective endometrial sampling compared with D&C for abnormal uterine bleeding: the value of a negative hysteroscopic view. Obstet Gynecol 1989;73(16):16.

Magrina JF: Complications of laparoscopic surgery. Clin Obstet Gynecol 2002;45(2):469.

Makinen J et al: Morbidity of 10,110 hysterectomies by type of approach. Hum Reprod 2001;16:14738.

Marana R et al: Current practical application of office endoscopy. Curr Opin Obstet Gynecol 2001;13:3837.

Marlow JL: Media and delivery systems. Obstet Gynecol Clin North Am 1995;22:409.

McElin TW et al: Diagnostic dilation and curettage. A 20-year study. Obstet Gynecol 1969;33(6):807.

Meeks GR: Advanced laparoscopic gynecologic surgery. Surg Clin North Am 2000;80(5):1443.

Mintz PD, Sullivan MF: Preoperative crossmatch ordering and blood use in elective hysterectomy. Obstet Gynecol 1985;65:389.

Munro MG: Laparoscopic access: Complications, technologies, and techniques. Curr Opin Obstet Gynecol 2002;14:365.

Ngai SW et al: Oral misoprostol for cervical priming in non-pregnant women. Hum Reprod 1997;12(11):2373.

Ngai SW et al: The use of misoprostol for pre-operative cervical dilation prior to vacuum aspiration: A randomized trial. Hum Reprod 1999;14(8):2139.

Ngai SW et al: The use of misoprostol prior to hysteroscopy in postmenopausal women. Hum Reprod 2001;16(7):1486.

Nilsson L, Rybo G: Treatment of menorrhagia. Am J Obstet Gynecol 1971:110(5):713.

Palmer RH et al: Cost and quality in the use of blood bank services for normal deliveries, cesarean sections, and hysterectomies. JAMA 1986;256:219.

Peipert JF et al: Risk factors for febrile morbidity after hysterectomy. Obstet Gynecol 2004;103:86.

Penfield AJ: The Filshie clip for female sterilization: A review of world experience. Am J Obstet Gynecol 2000;182:485.

Peterson HB et al: The risk of pregnancy after tubal sterilization: Findings from the U.S. Collaborative Review of Sterilization. Am J Obstet Gynecol 1996;174:1161.

Peterson HB et al: The risk of ectopic pregnancy after tubal sterilization. N Engl J Med 1997;336:762.

Propst AM et al: Complications of hysteroscopic surgery: Predicting patients at risk. Obstet Gynecol 2000:96(4):517.

Rhodes JC et al: Hysterectomy and sexual functioning. JAMA 1999;282:20.

Rioux JE et al: Female sterilization: An update. Curr Opin Obstet Gynecol 2001;13:377.

Rowlands S: Counseling and consent in vasectomy. J R Soc Med 2002;95:567.

Sakellariou P et al: Management of ureteric injuries during gynecological operations: 10 years experience. Eur J Obstet Gynecol Reprod Biol 2002;101:17984.

Stock RJ, Kanbour A: Prehysterectomy curettage. Obstet Gynecol 1975;45(5):537.

Summit RL et al: A multicenter randomized comparison of laparoscopically assisted vaginal hysterectomy and abdominal hysterectomy in abdominal hysterectomy candidates. Obstet Gynecol 1998;92:321.

Tadir Y et al: Actual effective CO_2 laser power on tissue in endoscopic surgery. Fertil Steril 1986;45:492.

Thakar R et al: Outcomes after total versus abdominal hysterectomy. N Engl J Med 2002;347:1318.

Thomas JA et al: The use of oral misoprostol as a cervical ripening agent in operative hysteroscopy: A double-blind, placebo-controlled trial. Am J Obstet Gynecol 2002; 186:876.

Tittel A et al: New adhesion formation after laparoscopic and conventional adhesiolysis: A comparative study in the rabbit. Surg Endosc 2001;15:446.

Ubeda A et al: Essure: A new device for hysteroscopic tubal sterilization in an outpatient setting. Fertil Steril 2004; 82(1):196.

Van Voorhis BJ: Comparison of tubal reversal procedures. Clin Obstet Gynecol 2000;43(3):641.

Wadstrow J, Gerdin B: Closure of the abdominal wall: How and why? Acta Clin Scand 1990;156:75.

Westhoff C et al: Tubal sterilization: Focus on the U.S. experience. Fertil Steril 2000;73:913.

Wingo PA et al: The mortality risk associated with hysterectomy. Am J Obstet Gynecol 1985;152:803.

Word B et al: The fallacy of simple uterine curettage. Obstet Gynecol 1958;12(6):642.

SECTION V
Gynecologic Oncology

Premalignant & Malignant Disorders of the Vulva & Vagina

49

Melanie Landay, MD, Wendy A. Satmary, MD, Sanaz Memarzadeh, MD, Donna M. Smith, MD, & David L. Barclay, MD

PREINVASIVE DISEASE OF THE VULVA

General Considerations

The vulvar skin is one component of the anogenital epithelium, extending from the distal vagina to the perineum and perianal skin. The lower genital tract epithelium is of common cloacogenic origin. Neoplasia of the vulvar skin is often associated with multiple foci of dysplasia in the lower genital tract. A strong association exists between sexually transmitted diseases and vulvar intraepithelial neoplasia (VIN), primarily human papillomavirus (HPV), but also gonorrhea, syphilis, *Gardnerella vaginalis*, trichomonas, and human immunodeficiency virus (HIV). Approximately 80% of VIN lesions are positive for high-risk HPV types, primarily HPV-16. Other risk factors include smoking and other genital precancers or cancers. VIN can also be classified into viral and nonviral etiologies. Younger women are more commonly affected by viral VIN than older women and are also more likely to exhibit multifocal disease. Although the incidence of VIN and HPV has increased over the past decade, the incidence of vulvar carcinoma has remained relatively constant. The long-term risk of malignant transformation of treated VIN III has been estimated at 3.4–7% and the risk for progression of untreated VIN is thought to be higher.

Premalignant lesions of the vulva occur in both premenopausal and postmenopausal women, with the median age being approximately 40 years. The average age is shifting toward younger women, with 75% of lesions occurring during the premenopausal period. There is no racial predisposition to VIN and the disease process is often asymptomatic. The most common presenting symptom is pruritus, which is seen in more than 60% of patients with VIN. The diagnosis is made by careful inspection of the vulvar area followed by biopsy of suspicious lesions.

Pathology

In 1989, the International Congress of the International Society for the Study of Vulvar Disease (ISSVD) adopted a standard of reporting vulvar dysplastic lesions as VIN I, II, or III, depending on the degree of epithelial cellular maturation. The degree of loss of epithelial cellular maturation in a given lesion defines the grade of VIN. In VIN I, immature cells occur in the lower one-third of the epithelium. Complete loss of cellular maturation in the full thickness of epithelium is defined as VIN III, which is synonymous with carcinoma in situ of the vulva, or Bowen's disease. VIN II is intermediate between VIN I and VIN III.

In contrast to intraepithelial carcinoma of the cervix, which seems to arise from a single point of origin, dysplasia of the vulva is often multicentric. These lesions may be discrete or diffuse, single or multiple, flat or raised. They even form papules and vary in color from the white appearance of hyperkeratotic tumors to a velvety red or black.

Figure 49–1. Carcinoma in situ demonstrating hyperkeratosis, acanthosis, and parakeratosis. The rete ridges are elongated and thickened, and individual cells are atypical.

The microscopic appearance of dysplastic vulvar lesions is characterized by cellular disorganization and loss of stratification that involves essentially the full thickness of the epithelium. Cellular density is increased, and individual cells vary greatly in size, with giant and multinucleated cells, numerous mitotic figures, and hyperchromatism (Fig 49–1). HPV cytopathic changes, such as perinuclear halos with displacement of nuclei, are also common.

Diagnosis

Possibly 1–2% of young women with cervical dysplasia have multifocal disease that tends to involve the upper third of the vagina and the vulva, perineum, and perianal areas—these surfaces arising from a common cloacogenic origin. A spectrum of disease may be found ranging from mild dysplasia to carcinoma in situ. Involvement may not be appreciated without careful inspection with and without the green colposcopy filter. Clinically, the appearance of VIN can be quite variable. Lesions are typically white and hyperkeratotic, but may also appear gray, pink, or brown. Colposcopy and biopsy of any suspicious lesion should be performed and is considered the gold standard for diagnosis. In premenopausal women, lesions tend to be more multifocal, whereas in postmenopausal women, they are more often unifocal. An abnormal vascular pattern is most frequently associated with a severe degree of dysplasia, carcinoma in situ, or early invasive disease.

Treatment

Treatment options for VIN are individualized based on biopsy results and include wide local excision, laser ablation, topical application of 5-fluorouracil (5-FU) or imi-

quimod, or superficial vulvectomy with or without split-thickness skin grafting. Untreated VIN has the potential for progression to invasive carcinoma. This risk may be high for women older than age 40 years. In younger patients, spontaneous regression may occur.

Treatment modality depends on the extent of involvement of the vulva, perineum, and perianal skin, which is defined by colposcopy. Wide local excision of small foci of VIN is preferred. For unifocal lesions, a 1-cm margin of uninvolved skin is usually curative. Carbon dioxide laser may be used for multifocal disease. Disadvantages of the laser include painful recovery and lack of pathology specimens. The incidence of foci of microinvasion in VIN III has been reported to range from 10–22% in different series. Extensive disease may be best treated by superficial vulvectomy. The surgical goal is to preserve as much of the normal anatomy as possible. In the superficial "skinning" vulvectomy procedure, the excised vulvar skin can be closed with fine suture or may need to be replaced with a split-thickness skin graft (Figs 49–2 and 49–3) if the defect is too large.

Figure 49–2. Diffuse, hypertrophic carcinoma in situ of the vulva and perianal skin. A skinning vulvectomy was performed.

Figure 49–3. Appearance after skinning vulvectomy and split-thickness skin grafting of the lesion shown in Figure 49–2.

Topical application of 5-FU, cryotherapy, and photodynamic therapy have each historically been proven useful in the treatment of some lesions, but surgery remains the hallmark treatment modality for VIN. Promising future directions for treatment of VIN involve the development of a vaccine for HPV, which is currently in the experimental phase, and use of immunomodulating agents, such as topical imiquimod.

Follow-Up

Intraepithelial carcinoma of the vulva is often one manifestation of multifocal disease. For this reason, affected patients must be examined periodically for a number of years. Recommended follow-up includes thorough pelvic examinations with colposcopy every 3–4 months until the patient is disease-free for 2 years. If the patient is disease-free for a 2-year period, examinations can be done every 6 months.

EXTRAMAMMARY PAGET'S DISEASE

General Considerations

Paget's disease of the skin is an intraepithelial neoplasia, or adenocarcinoma in situ, and accounts for less than 1% of all vulvar malignancies. Reports of long-term survivals suggest that the in situ stage of the disease persists for a long time or that invasive disease is a different clinico-

pathologic entity. It appears that there are two separate lesions: (a) intraepithelial extramammary Paget's disease and (b) pagetoid changes in the skin associated with an underlying adenocarcinoma. Experts believe that an adenocarcinoma associated with Paget's disease arises as a primary adenocarcinoma of an underlying apocrine gland, Bartholin's gland, or anorectum, and represents two separate disease entities, not a spectrum. Unlike mammary Paget's disease, less than 20% of vulvar Paget's disease is associated with an underlying adenocarcinoma. Paget's disease with an underlying adenocarcinoma metastasizes frequently to regional lymph nodes and distally. Paget's disease without an underlying adenocarcinoma behaves like an intraepithelial neoplasia and can be treated as such. However, patients with Paget's disease should be carefully examined for the presence of synchronous primaries elsewhere; 20–30% of these patients will be found to have carcinomas at other sites, including the breast, rectum, bladder, cervix, ovary, and urethra.

Pathology

The initial lesion may be confused with a number of benign forms of chronic vulvar pruritus. It is a pruritic, slowly spreading, velvety-red discoloration of the skin that eventually becomes eczematoid in appearance with secondary maceration and development of white plaques; it may spread to involve the skin of the perineum, the perianal area, and the adjacent skin of the thigh. Grossly, the lesion gives the impression of "cake icing." Because of the serpiginous growth pattern of Paget cells in the basal layer of the epidermis, the true extent of disease is difficult to assess.

Paget's disease of the vulvar skin is an intraepithelial disease. The typical Paget cell, pathognomonic of the disease process, apparently arises from abnormal differentiation of the cells of the basal layer of the epithelium (Fig 49–4). The appearance of malignant cells varies from that of the clear cell of the apocrine gland epithelium to a totally undifferentiated basal cell. It has been suggested that there may be both an intraepithelial and an invasive variety of the disease. The intraepithelial stage of the disease persists for years without evidence of an underlying adenocarcinoma.

Diagnosis

Paget's disease primarily affects postmenopausal white women in the seventh decade of life, but can be seen in younger patients. Pruritus and vulvar soreness are the most frequent symptoms. These symptoms may persist for years before the patient seeks medical attention. The lesion may be localized to one labium or involve the entire vulvar area. The lesion usually has an eczematoid appearance macroscopically and usually begins on the hair-bearing portions of the vulva. It is not unusual for

Figure 49–4. Paget's disease with typical cells in the basal layer of the epidermis.

the disease process to extend beyond the vulva to involve the perirectal area, buttocks, thighs, inguinal area, and mons. Intraepithelial extramammary Paget's disease presents as a lesion with hyperemic areas associated with a superficial white coating to give the impression of "cake icing." Although these lesions can be very extensive, most are confined to the epithelial layer. The diagnosis is made by vulvar biopsy. It is important to palpate the lesion in its entirety. A generous biopsy should be taken of any area that appears to be thickened to rule out an underlying adenocarcinoma.

Treatment

Because extramammary Paget's disease is an intraepithelial neoplasia it can be treated as such. Wide local excision is the primary treatment modality for this disease process. The lesion needs to be excised in its entirety; however, wide margins need to be removed around the primary lesion as disease often extends beyond the clinically visible erythematous area. The underlying dermis should be removed for adequate histologic evaluation. Often such a resection involves a complete vulvectomy. Careful histologic examination of the entire operative specimen is necessary to delineate the true extent of disease, ensure free surgical margins, and detect the remote possibility of underlying adenocarcinoma. For this reason, laser therapy is unsatisfactory. Patients who have Paget's disease with underlying adenocarcinoma should be treated with radical local excision of the vulva and bilateral inguinal lymph node dissection as they would for any other invasive tumor involving the vulvar area.

Prognosis

Paget's disease of the vulva has a great propensity for local recurrence, which may represent persistence of the disease or development of new disease in the remaining vulvar skin. Extramammary Paget's disease characteristically requires repeated local excisions of recurrent disease after treatment of the primary disease by total vulvectomy. Invasive disease without evidence of lymph node metastases has a favorable prognosis; however, with nodal metastases, the disease is almost invariably fatal.

CANCER OF THE VULVA

 ESSENTIALS OF DIAGNOSIS

- *Typically occurs in postmenopausal women.*
- *Long history of vulvar irritation with pruritus, local discomfort, and bloody discharge.*
- *Appearance of early lesions like that of chronic vulvar dermatitis.*
- *Appearance of late lesions like that of a large cauliflower, or a hard ulcerated area in the vulva.*
- *Biopsy necessary for diagnosis.*

General Considerations

Cancer of the vulva may arise from the skin, subcutaneous tissues, glandular elements of the vulva, or the epithelium of the lower third of the vagina. Approximately 90% of these tumors are squamous cell carcinomas. Less common tumors are extramammary Paget's disease with underlying adenocarcinoma, carcinoma of Bartholin's gland, basal cell carcinoma, melanoma, sarcoma, and metastatic cancers from other sites.

Cancer of the vulva is uncommon, accounting for approximately 5% of gynecologic cancers. Vulvar cancer is more common in the poor and elderly in most parts of the world, and no race or culture is spared. Vulvar cancer is primarily a disease of postmenopausal women, with a peak incidence in women ages 60–70 years. The average age at the time of diagnosis is 65 years, and 75% of patients are older than the age of 50 years. In general, the mean age of patients with carcinoma in situ is approximately 10 years less than that for patients with invasive cancer. Intraepithelial cancer of the vulva in women ages 20–40 years has increased remarkably in recent years, coincidentally with an increase in the incidence of diagnosis of dysplasia and carcinoma in situ of the cervix. HPV is strongly associated in younger women, though not in older women with vulvar cancer. Also, older women are more likely to have squamous hyperplasia in the tissue adjacent to the tumor.

Considering that cancer of the vulva is a disease of a body surface readily accessible to diagnostic procedures, early diagnosis should be the rule. This is not the case, however, and a 6- to 12-month delay in reporting symptoms of discovery of a tumor is common. Despite the advanced age of many of these patients and the frequent finding of a moderately large tumor, the disease is usually amenable to surgical therapy. In stages I and II disease, the corrected 5-year survival rate is greater than 90%. A 75% corrected 5-year survival rate for all stages of vulvar cancer is reported by most institutions.

Associated disorders found most frequently with carcinoma of the vulva are obesity, hypertension, and chronic vulvar irritation secondary to diabetes mellitus, granulomatous venereal disease, or vulvar dystrophy.

Pathology

The gross appearance of vulvar cancer depends on the origin and histologic type. These tumors spread by local extension and, with few exceptions, by lymphatic embolization. The primary route of lymphatic spread is by way of the superficial inguinal, deep femoral, and external iliac lymph nodes (Fig 49–5). Contralateral spread may occur as a result of the rich intercommunicating lymphatic system of the vulvar skin. Direct extension to the deep pelvic lymph nodes, primarily the obturator nodes, occurs in approximately 3% of patients and seems to be related to midline involvement around the clitoris, urethra, or rectum, or to cancer of a vestibular (Bartholin's)

gland. Extension of the tumor to the lower and middle thirds of the vagina may also allow access of tumor cells to lymph channels leading to the deep pelvic lymph nodes.

The following sections describe the gross and histologic appearance of the various types of vulvar cancers.

A. SQUAMOUS CELL CARCINOMA

Squamous cell carcinoma is by far the most common type of tumor and most frequently involves the anterior half of the vulva. In approximately 65% of patients, the tumor arises in the labia majora and minora, and in 25% the clitoris or perineum is involved. More than one-third of tumors involve the vulva bilaterally or are midline tumors. These tumors are most frequently associated with nodal spread, particularly bilateral nodal metastases. Midline tumors that involve the perineum do not worsen the outlook unless they extend into the vagina or to the anus and rectum.

Squamous cell carcinoma of the vulva varies in appearance from a large, exophytic, cauliflowerlike lesion to a small ulcer crater superimposed on a dystrophic lesion of the vulvar skin (Figs 49–6 and 49–7). Ulcerative lesions may begin as a raised, flat, white area of hypertrophic skin that subsequently undergoes ulceration. Exophytic lesions may become extremely large, undergo necrosis, and become secondarily infected and malodorous. A third variety arises as a slightly elevated, red, velvety tumor that gradually spreads over the vulvar skin. There does not appear to be a positive correlation between the gross appearance of the tumor and either histologic grade or frequency of nodal metastases. The primary determinant of nodal metastases is tumor size.

Squamous cell cancers may be graded histologically from I to III. Grade I tumors are well differentiated, often forming keratin pearls; grade II tumors are moderately well differentiated; grade III tumors are composed of poorly differentiated cells. The extent of underlying inflammatory cell infiltration into the stroma surrounding the invasive tumor is variable. The histologic grade of the tumor may be of some significance in tumors less than 2 cm in diameter. However, the lymph node status is the most significant prognostic factor.

A variant of squamous cell carcinoma, **verrucous carcinoma,** is a locally invasive tumor that seldom metastasizes to regional lymph nodes. Grossly, the tumor looks like a mature condylomatous growth. It is distinguished from squamous cell cancer by histopathology of the tumor base, which reveals papillary fronds without a central core. Local recurrence is common if a wide vulvectomy is not performed; lymphadenectomy is usually not recommended.

An attempt has been made to define a group of early vulvar cancers that might be described as microinvasive cancer and that exhibit little tendency for local recur-

Figure 49–5. Lymphatic spread of cancer of the vulva.

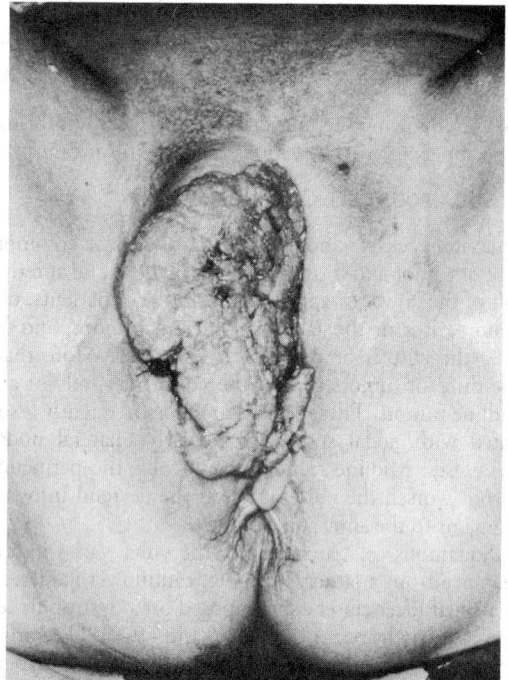

Figure 49–6. Large, exophytic, squamous cell carcinoma of the vulva, which was treated by radical vulvectomy and regional lymphadenectomy.

rence or nodal metastases. Depth of stromal penetration has proved to be the key factor in determining invasive potential of the tumor. Early authors accepted 5 mm or less of dermal invasion as the definition of microinvasion, but this has not been universally accepted. A task force of the International Society for the Study of Vulvar Diseases suggested that the term "microinvasive cancer of the vulva" be discarded. The ISSVD defined stage IA carcinoma of the vulva as a single lesion measuring 2 cm or less in diameter and exhibiting one focus of invasion to a depth of 1 mm or less. The depth of invasion was measured from the epidermal–stromal junction of the most superficial dermal papilla to the deepest point of tumor invasion.

B. Carcinoma of Bartholin's Gland

Carcinoma of Bartholin's gland accounts for approximately 1% of vulvar cancers, and although rare, is the most common site for vulvar adenocarcinoma. Approximately 50% of Bartholin's gland tumors are squamous cell carcinomas. Other types of tumors arising in the Bartholin's glands are adenocarcinoma, adenoid cystic (an adenocarcinoma with specific histologic and clinical characteristics), adenosquamous, and transitional cell.

Because it may be difficult to differentiate by clinical examination a tumor of Bartholin's gland or duct from a benign Bartholin's cyst, any woman older than age 40 years should undergo biopsy to rule out cancer, as inflammatory disease is not common in this age group. Because of its location deep in the substance of the labium, a tumor may impinge on the rectum and directly spread into the ischiorectal fossa. Consequently, these tumors have access to lymphatic channels draining directly to the deep pelvic lymph nodes as well as to the superficial channels draining to the inguinal lymph nodes.

C. Basal Cell Carcinoma

Basal cell carcinomas account for 1–2% of vulvar cancers. Most tumors are small elevated lesions with an ulcerated center and rolled edges. Some are described as pigmented tumors, moles, or simply pruritic maculopapular eruptions. These tumors arise almost exclusively in the skin of the labia majora, although occasionally a tumor can be found elsewhere in the vulva. The tumor is derived from primordial basal cells in the epidermis or hair follicles and is characterized by slow growth, local infiltration, and a tendency to recur if not totally excised. Most basal cell carcinomas of the vulva are of the

Figure 49–7. Ulcerative squamous cell carcinoma of the vulva.

primordial histologic type. Other histologic varieties that may be found are the pilar, morphealike, superficially spreading, adenoid, and pigmented cell tumors.

On microscopic examination the typical tumor consists of nodular masses and lobules of closely packed, uniform-appearing basaloid cells with scant cytoplasm and spherical or oval dark nuclei. Peripheral margination by columnar cells is usually prominent. In larger tumor nodules, there may be areas of central degeneration and necrosis.

If a sufficiently wide local excision is not performed, there is a tendency for local recurrence, estimated to be approximately 20%. If a basal-squamous cell-type tumor is diagnosed, appropriate therapy for invasive epidermoid cancer of the vulva should be undertaken.

D. Malignant Melanoma

Approximately 5% of vulvar cancers are malignant melanomas, the second most common vulvar cancer. Because only 0.1% of all nevi in women are on vulvar skin, the disproportionate frequency of occurrence of melanoma in this area may be a result of the fact that nearly all vulvar nevi are of the junctional variety. Malignant melanoma most commonly arises in the region of the labia minora and clitoris, and there is a tendency for superficial spread toward the urethra and vagina. A nonpigmented melanoma may closely resemble squamous cell carcinoma on clinical examination. A darkly pigmented, raised lesion at the mucocutaneous junction is a characteristic finding; however, the degree of melanin pigmentation is variable, and amelanotic lesions do occur. The lesion spreads primarily through lymphatic channels and tends to metastasize early in the course of the disease; local or remote cutaneous satellite lesions may be found. In contrast to squamous cell cancers, melanoma is staged according to depth of invasion. All small pigmented lesions of the vulva are suspect and should be removed by excision biopsy with a 0.5- to 1-cm margin of normal skin. In the case of large tumors, the diagnosis should be confirmed by a generous biopsy.

E. Unusual Vulvar Malignancies

Sarcomas of the vulva constitute a variety of malignant neoplasms that account for 1–2% of vulvar cancers. The most common is leiomyosarcoma, followed in frequency of occurrence by the fibrous histiocytoma group and an array of other sarcomas. Clinically, sarcoma may present as a subcutaneous nodule or may be exophytic and fleshy. Prognosis is usually poor and depends on histologic type, extent of local invasion, and treatment. In general, radical vulvectomy and regional lymphadenectomy are indicated, with the exception of tumors such as dermatofibrosarcoma protuberans, which is a locally aggressive tumor that tends to recur locally but does not metastasize.

Adenocarcinoma of the vulva is exceptionally rare unless it arises from the Bartholin's gland or the urethra. Primary cancer of the breast from ectopic breast tissue has been reported. Rarely, a malignant tumor will arise from a vulvar sweat gland.

Metastatic cancers of the vulva constitute 8% of all vulvar tumors. They usually originate from a genital tract tumor, and 18% arise from the kidney or urethra. Advanced cervical cancer is the most common primary tumor. Other primary tumors have been reported, including malignant melanoma, choriocarcinoma, and adenocarcinoma of the rectum or breast. Cloacogenic carcinoma is primarily an anorectal neoplasm, occurring twice as often in women than in men; it may arise in anal ducts and present as a submucosal mass.

Metastatic epidermoid cancer tends to form nests of cells within the dermis. Adenocarcinoma, regardless of the primary site, invades the surface squamous epithelium. Because these tumors are a manifestation of advanced disease, the prognosis is uniformly grave.

Clinical Findings

The patient with vulvar cancer characteristically has had infrequent medical examinations. Approximately 10% are diabetic, and 30–50% are obese or hypertensive or demonstrate other evidence of cardiovascular disease. The incidence of complicating medical illness exceeds that expected in the age group under consideration.

Invasive squamous cell cancer is a disease mainly of the seventh and eighth decades of life, although approximately 15% of patients are age 40 years or younger. Approximately 20% of patients have a second primary cancer that was diagnosed prior to, at the time of, or subsequent to the diagnosis of vulvar cancer; 75% of these second primary cancers are in the cervix.

A. Symptoms and Signs

Pruritus vulvae or a vulvar mass is the presenting complaint in more than 50% of patients with vulvar cancer. Other patients complain of bleeding or vulvar pain, whereas approximately 20% of patients have no complaints, and the tumor is found incidentally during routine pelvic examination. A significant number of patients, approximately 25%, have seen a physician and received various medical treatments without benefit of a biopsy of the tumor or have undergone incomplete therapy consisting of a simple excision biopsy of an invasive tumor. The importance of performing a biopsy of any vulvar lesion cannot be overemphasized.

B. Differential Diagnosis

Differential diagnosis of vulvar disease and exclusion of cancer depend on an adequate biopsy. The tumor may be a diffuse white lesion, a discrete tumor, an ulcer, or diffuse papules, which may not be appreciated without thorough colposcopic examination of the skin of the vulva, perineum, and perianal area.

Benign ulcerative lesions may be the result of a sexually transmitted disease (syphilis, herpes, or granuloma inguinale), pyogenic infections, or a benign tumor, such as a granular cell myoblastoma.

Treatment

Staging and treatment for vulvar cancer is surgical (Table 49–1). The primary treatment for invasive vulvar cancer is complete surgical removal of all tumor whenever possible. The recent trend is toward a more conservative surgical approach, departing from traditional en bloc resections.

The number of preoperative studies ordered prior to surgery depends on the extent of disease and the general condition of the patient. A complete history and a thorough physical examination that includes cytologic study of the cervix and vulvoscopy should be performed. A large tumor may interfere with adequate pelvic examination. Bleeding may be caused by a lesion higher in the genital tract rather than the obvious vulvar tumor. In that case, the pelvic examination may be performed under anesthesia, and endometrial biopsy or dilatation and curettage (D&C) considered.

Chest radiography, complete blood count, and urinalysis are performed on all patients. Older patients require an electrocardiogram (ECG) and a biochemical profile. Other studies such as proctoscopy, pyelography, barium enema, and computed tomography (CT) scans are ordered on an individual basis. Enlarged lymph nodes do not require biopsy; they will be excised by lymphadenectomy or thoroughly sampled at the time of operation. Mechanical bowel cleansing is recommended for most patients, particularly if the perineal skin is involved. An antibiotic bowel preparation is prescribed if extensive perianal dissection, skin grafting, or intestinal surgery (such as abdominoperineal resection) is anticipated. At least 2 units of packed red cells should be available for transfusion. Less than 50% of patients require a transfusion during or after the operation.

Historically, the basic operation was radical vulvectomy and regional lymphadenectomy. The trend, however, is shifting away from standard en bloc radical vulvectomy and bilateral lymph node dissection toward wide radical local excision of the primary tumor with inguinal lymph node dissection. For a unifocal stage I lesion with less than 1 mm stromal invasion, wide radical local excision with surgical margins of at least 1–2 cm should be performed. Patients with unilateral lesions with a depth of invasion greater than or equal to 1 mm should undergo ipsilateral groin dissection in addition to the above to determine nodal status. For patients with bilateral lesions or lesions impinging on or crossing the

Table 49–1. International Federation of Gynecology and Obstetrics (FIGO) staging of vulvar cancer.

Stage 0			
Cis			Carcinoma in situ, intraepithelial carcinoma
Stage I			
T1	N0	M0	Tumor confined to the vulva and/or perineum—2 cm or less in greatest dimension (no nodal metastasis)
Stage II			
T2	N0	M0	Tumor confined to the vulva and/or perineum—more than 2 cm in greatest dimension (no nodal metastasis)
Stage III			
T3	N0	M0	Tumor of any size with
T3	N1	M0	(1) Adjacent spread to the lower urethra and/or the vagina, or the anus, and/or
T1	N1	M0	(2) Unilateral regional lymph
T2	N1	M0	node metastasis
Stage IVA			
T1	N2	M0	Tumor invades any of the following: Upper urethra, bladder mucosa, rectal mucosa, pelvic bone, and/or bilateralregional node metastasis
T2	N2	M0	
T3	N2	M0	
T4	Any N	M0	
Stage IVb			
Any T	Any N	M1	Any distant metastasis including pelvic lymph nodes

midline, bilateral inguinal femoral lymphadenectomy can be performed. When disease has spread to lymph nodes, adjuvant radiation therapy is generally recommended. The role of sentinel node mapping is also being evaluated for patients with squamous vulvar carcinoma and melanomas. In general, lymphatic spread occurs in a sequential manner from the superficial to the deep inguinal lymph nodes. Consequently, if the superficial nodes harbor no metastatic disease, there is reasonable assurance that the deeper nodes are not involved.

When the disease involves the anus, rectum, rectovaginal septum, proximal urethra, or bladder, an adequate surgical resection is only possible with pelvic exenteration combined with radical vulvectomy. Operative mortality is high for these procedures and the postoperative psychologic impact is significant. In addition, with advanced stage disease where ulcerated or fixed lymph nodes are palpated, attempts at lymphadenectomy have yielded very poor results. Based on data from the Gynecologic Oncology Group, this group of patients may benefit from preoperative chemoradiation resulting in higher rates of successful resection and reduced need for more radical surgery. Chemotherapeutic agents such as cisplatin and 5-FU have been combined with radiation therapy. These chemotherapeutic agents are used as radiation sensitizers in large necrotic tumor beds, enhancing the radiation effects.

There is controversy concerning the extent of surgery required for treatment of malignant melanoma of the vulva. For some years, standard treatment consisted of vulvectomy with superficial and deep inguinal and pelvic lymphadenectomy. It is also generally treated with a more conservative surgical approach. If depth of the vulvar lesion is less than 1 mm, vulvar melanoma may be adequately treated with local incision using a 1-cm margin. However, if the depth of invasion is between 1 and 4 mm, excision requires a 2-cm margin in addition to a bilateral groin node dissection. Advanced or recurrent melanoma may be best treated with chemotherapy, radiation, or immunotherapy.

Locally invasive but nonmetastasizing sarcomas such as dermatofibrosarcoma protuberans can be removed by wide local resection. Most other sarcomas are treated by radical vulvectomy and regional lymphadenectomy. The primary determinant of cure appears to be adequate wide removal of the primary lesion.

Operative Morbidity & Mortality

The most frequently encountered complication is wound breakdown, which occurs in well over 50% of patients undergoing radical vulvectomy and bilateral inguinal dissection. This complication is related to the amount of skin removed during the procedure, particularly at the groin areas. Separate groin incisions and careful handling of skin flaps have reduced the incidence of wound breakdown. Vigorous wound care with debridement almost always results in adequate healing.

Lymphedema occurs in approximately 65% of patients who have had radical vulvectomy. Hemorrhage, lymphocyst formation, thromboembolic disease, urinary tract infections, and sexual dysfunction are other commonly associated morbidities.

Follow-Up

After the immediate postoperative period, patients should be examined every 3 months for 2 years and every 6 months thereafter to detect recurrent disease or a second primary cancer. Nearly 80% of recurrent vulvar cancer occurs in the first 2 years. Treatment modalities depend on the location of recurrence. Malignant melanomas and sarcomas may recur locally or metastasize to the liver or lungs.

Prognosis

The principal prognostic factors in cancer of the vulva are the presence or absence of regional lymph node metastases, size and location of the lesion, and the histologic type.

A 5-year survival rate of 75% and a 10-year survival rate of approximately 58% should be expected after complete surgical treatment of primary invasive squamous vulvar cancer. Lymph node status is the most important prognostic variable. Overall, the survival rate for patients with vulvar cancer and negative inguinal-femoral nodes is 90%, whereas rates drop to almost 40% with nodal metastasis. Several authors have reported no deaths from cancer among patients who were found to have negative lymph nodes. With tumors less than 2 cm in diameter, the incidence of nodal metastases is 10–15%. In general, approximately 30% of patients undergoing surgery will have positive lymph nodes. With nodal metastases, the approximate 5-year cure rates are as follows: 1 node, 94%; 2 nodes, 80%; and 3 nodes or more, less than 15%. Patients who have 3 or more positive lymph nodes in the groin usually demonstrate palpably suspicious nodes preoperatively. These patients have a high incidence of metastases to the pelvic lymph nodes; however, pelvic lymphadenectomy apparently does not improve survival rates. Involvement of contiguous organs such as the bladder or rectum increases the incidence of nodal metastases and worsens the prognosis accordingly.

The cure rate for adequately treated cancer of Bartholin's gland has not been established. There is a propensity for unresectable local recurrences under the pubic ramus despite a thorough primary operation.

Wide local excision of basal cell carcinoma should be curative. Some authors have reported an approximately 20% recurrence rate after local excision that may represent cases of incomplete excision.

Results of treatment of malignant melanoma are related to the level of penetration of the tumor into the dermis of the vulvar skin or the lamina propria of the vaginal mucosa and to the presence or absence of nodal metastases. The 5-year survival rate ranges from 14–50%, but patients who have metastases to groin lymph nodes have a survival rate below 14%. Amelanotic cutaneous melanomas are particularly virulent tumors. The survival rate for patients with superficial spreading melanomas is much better than for those with the nodular variety, which tend to have a smaller diameter and exhibit aggressive vertical invasion, increased incidence of nodal metastases, treatment failures, and distant recurrences. The most common site of recurrence is at the site of resection or the groin lymph nodes (if not previously resected).

Sarcomas of the vulva tend to recur locally, particularly if the initial resection is not extensive, and metastasize to the liver and lungs.

PREINVASIVE DISEASE OF THE VAGINA

General Considerations

Vaginal intraepithelial neoplasia (VAIN) can occur as an isolated lesion, but multifocal disease is more common. Although little is known regarding the natural history of VAIN, it is thought to be similar to that of cervical intraepithelial neoplasia (CIN). Many patients may have similar intraepithelial neoplastic lesions involving the cervix or vulva. At least one-half to two-thirds of patients with VAIN have been treated for similar disease in either the cervix or the vulva. In addition, VAIN can reappear several years later, necessitating long-term follow-up in these patients. Several investigators have recognized a "field response" involving the squamous epithelium of the lower genital tract including the cervix, vagina, and vulva to be affected simultaneously by the same carcinogenic agent. The vagina lacks a transformation zone, whereas in the cervix immature epithelial cells are infected with HPV. Some theorize that the HPV entry mechanisms involve abrasions from coitus or tampon use. HPV may begin its growth in a healing abrasion in a similar fashion as in the transformation zone.

The upper third of the vagina is vulnerable to the development of dysplasia and carcinoma in situ whether or not hysterectomy has been performed previously for intraepithelial neoplasia. Each of these entities has a potential for progression to invasive cancer. For this reason, women who have had a hysterectomy with a history of HPV or intraepithelial neoplasia should continue to have periodic cytologic screening of the vaginal apex. A similar lesion may develop after prior irradiation for a pelvic malignancy; some authors report a 20% incidence of cervical or vaginal dysplasia. These tumors are usually asymptomatic and detected by routine vaginal cytologic studies. New invasive tumors in an irradiated field usually develop 15–30 years after therapeutic irradiation.

Condylomatous lesions of the lower genital tract often demonstrate associated dysplasias. For this reason a biopsy should be made of condylomatous growth of the vagina prior to treatment.

Pathology

As with other intraepithelial neoplasias occurring in the lower genital tract, VAIN is characterized by a loss of epithelial cell maturation. This is associated with nuclear hyperchromatosis and pleomorphism with cellular crowding. The thickness of the epithelial abnormality designates the various lesions as VAIN I, II, or III. VAIN III is synonymous with carcinoma in situ of the vagina.

Diagnosis

Almost all lesions of VAIN are asymptomatic. Lesions often accompany HPV infection, so patients may complain of vulvar warts. An abnormal Papanicolaou (Pap) smear is usually the first sign of disease. The diagnosis is made by colposcopic examination of the vagina with a directed biopsy. Colposcopic examination of the vagina can be difficult to perform, particularly if a hysterectomy has already been done. Techniques similar to those used for colposcopic examination of the cervix are used for examination of the vagina. After application of 3–5% acetic acid to the vagina, a lesion under the colposcope may appear as white epithelium, and may have mosaicism or punctation. Lugol's iodine may also help to identify the borders of a lesion. Lesions are often located along the vaginal ridges; they may appear to be raised or have spicules. Because the disease process tends to be multifocal, a thorough examination of the vagina from the introitus to the apex must be conducted.

Treatment

The primary treatment modality for VAIN is surgical excision or carbon dioxide laser ablation. VAIN I lesions usually do not require treatment, as lesions typically regress, are multifocal, and often recur. VAIN II and III can be treated by laser ablation or excision. VAIN III lesions are more often associated with an early invasive lesion; therefore, adequate sampling should be performed before any ablative procedure is employed. If the lesion is focal, it is best removed in its entirety with local excision. When carcinoma in situ of the cervix extends to the upper vagina, the upper third of the vagina can be removed at the time of hysterectomy. If multifocal disease is present, a total vaginectomy may be performed with a split-thickness skin graft vaginal reconstruction. Topical 5-FU may also be used in treating multifocal VAIN. Approximately 80% of patients can expect to have evidence of regression of disease after one to two courses of treatment.

Follow-Up

Intraepithelial neoplasia of the vagina tends to be multifocal, with involvement of the cervix and vulva in many cases. These lesions can be difficult to eradicate with only one treatment modality or treatment session. This group of patients must be monitored closely every

3–4 months with colposcopic examinations of not only the vagina but also the entire lower genital tract.

CANCER OF THE VAGINA

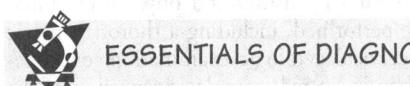

ESSENTIALS OF DIAGNOSIS

- *Asymptomatic: abnormal vaginal cytology.*
- *Early: painless bleeding from ulcerated tumor.*
- *Late: bleeding, pain, weight loss, swelling.*

General Considerations

Primary cancers of the vagina are rare, representing approximately 3% of gynecologic cancers. Approximately 85% are squamous cell cancers, and the remainder, in decreasing order of frequency, are adenocarcinomas, sarcomas, and melanomas. A tumor should not be considered a primary vaginal cancer unless the cervix is uninvolved or only minimally involved by a tumor obviously arising in the vagina. By convention, any malignancy involving both cervix and vagina that is histologically compatible with an origin in either organ is classified as cervical cancer. Secondary carcinoma of the vagina is seen more frequently than primary vaginal cancers. Secondary, or metastatic, tumors may arise from cervical, endometrial, or ovarian cancer, breast cancer, gestational trophoblastic disease, colorectal cancer, or urogenital or vulvar cancer. Extension of cervical cancer to the vagina is probably the most common malignancy involving the vagina. HPV, early hysterectomy, and prior radiation are possible risk factors for vaginal cancer, but no specific etiologic agent has been identified.

Pathology

Squamous cell carcinoma may be ulcerative or exophytic. It usually involves the posterior wall of the upper third of the vagina, but may be multicentric. Direct invasion of the bladder or rectum may occur. The incidence of lymph node metastases is directly related to the size of the tumor. The route of nodal metastases depends on the location of the tumor in the vagina. Tumors in the lower third metastasize like cancer of the vulva, primarily to the inguinal lymph nodes (Fig 49–8). Cancers of the upper vagina, which is the most common site, metastasize in a manner similar to cancer of the cervix. The lymphatic drainage of the vagina consists of a fine capillary meshwork in the mucosa and submucosa with multiple anastomoses. As a conse-

Figure 49–8. An ulcerated epidermoid cancer of the lower third of the vagina.

quence, lesions in the middle third of the vagina may metastasize to the inguinal lymph nodes or directly to the deep pelvic lymph nodes.

Melanomas and sarcomas of the vagina metastasize like squamous cell cancer, although liver and pulmonary metastases are more common. Nevi rarely occur in the vagina; therefore, any pigmented lesion of the vagina should be excised or biopsied. The anterior surface and lower half of the vagina are the most common sites. Grossly, the tumors are usually exophytic and described as polypoid or pedunculated with secondary necrosis.

Sarcomas of the vagina occur in children younger than 5 years of age and in women in the fifth to sixth decades. Embryonal rhabdomyosarcomas or sarcoma botryoides, replace the vaginal mucosa of young girls and consist of polypoid, edematous, "grapelike" masses that may protrude from the vaginal introitus. Leiomyosarcomas, reticulum cell sarcomas, and unclassified sarcomas occur in older women. The upper anterior vaginal wall is the most common site of origin. The appearance of these tumors depends on the size and the extent of disease at the time of diagnosis.

Figure 49–9. A clear cell adenocarcinoma of the vagina in a 19-year-old patient. The lesion is on the posterior wall of the upper third of the vagina.

Clear cell adenocarcinomas arise in conjunction with vaginal adenosis, which, in recent years, has been detected most frequently in young women with a history of exposure to diethylstilbestrol (DES) in utero (Fig 49–9). The Registry of Clear Cell Adenocarcinoma of the Genital Tract in Young Females was established in 1971 to study the clinicopathologic and epidemiologic aspects of these tumors in girls born in 1940 or later, the years during which DES was used during pregnancy. The risk of developing clear cell adenocarcinoma by age 24 years has been calculated to be 0.14–1.4 per 1000 exposed female fetuses. Adenosis vaginae and adenocarcinoma do occur in sexually mature and postmenopausal women.

Metastatic adenocarcinoma to the vagina may arise from the urethra, Bartholin's gland, the rectum or bladder, the endometrial cavity, the endocervix, or an ovary, or it may be metastatic from a distant site. Hypernephroma of the kidney characteristically metastasizes to the anterior wall of the vagina in the lower third. These tumors are not primary vaginal cancers.

Clinical Findings

Vaginal cancer is often asymptomatic, discovered by routine vaginal cytologic examination, and confirmed by biopsy after delineation of the location and extent of the tumor by colposcopy.

Postmenopausal vaginal bleeding and/or bloody discharge are the most common presenting symptoms. Approximately 50% of patients with invasive vaginal cancer report for examination within 6 months after symptoms are noted. Less commonly, advanced tumors may impinge upon the rectum or bladder or extend to the pelvic wall, causing pain or leg edema.

A diagnosis of primary cancer of the vagina cannot be established unless metastasis from another source is eliminated. A complete history and physical examination should be performed, including a thorough pelvic examination, cervical cytologic examination, endometrial biopsy when indicated, complete inspection of the vagina, including colposcopy, and biopsy of the vaginal tumor. Careful bimanual examination with palpation of the entire length of the vagina can detect small submucosal nodules not visualized during the examination.

The staging system for cancer of the vagina is clinical and not surgical (Table 49–2).

Differential Diagnosis

Benign tumors of the vagina are uncommon, are usually cystic, arise from the mesonephric (wolffian) or paramesonephric ducts, and are usually an incidental finding on examination of the anterolateral wall of the vagina (Gartner's duct cyst).

An ulcerative lesion may occur at the site of direct trauma, following an inflammatory reaction caused by prolonged retention of a pessary or other foreign body, or, occasionally, following a chemical burn. Granulomatous venereal diseases seldom affect the vagina but may be diagnosed with appropriate laboratory studies and a biopsy.

Endometriosis that penetrates the cul-de-sac of Douglas into the upper vagina cannot be differentiated from cancer except by biopsy.

Table 49–2. FIGO staging of carcinoma of the vagina.

Preinvasive carcinoma	
Stage 0	Carcinoma in situ, intraepithelial carcinoma.
Invasive carcinoma	
Stage I	The carcinoma is limited to the vaginal mucosa.
Stage II	The carcinoma has involved the subvaginal tissue but has not extended to the pelvic wall.
Stage III	The carcinoma has extended to the pelvic wall.
Stage IV	The carcinoma has extended beyond the true pelvis or has involved the mucosa of the bladder or rectum. A bullous edema as such does not permit allotment of a case to stage IV.
Stage IVA	Spread of the growth to adjacent organs.
Stage IVB	Spread to distant organs.

FIGO, Federation of Gynecology and Obstetrics.

Cancer of the urethra, bladder, rectum, or Bartholin's gland may penetrate or extend into the vagina. Cloacogenic carcinoma is a rare tumor of the anorectal region originating from a persistent remnant of the cloacal membrane of the embryo. The tumor accounts for 2–3% of anorectal carcinomas and occurs more than twice as often in women. Although these metastatic tumors often penetrate into the vagina as fungating or ulcerating lesions, they may present as a submucosal mass.

Biopsy should be performed to establish a histologic diagnosis.

Treatment

Following biopsy confirmation of disease, all patients should undergo a thorough physical examination and evaluation of the extent of local and metastatic disease. Pretreatment evaluation may include the following studies: chest radiography, intravenous pyelogram, cystoscopy, proctosigmoidoscopy, and CT scan of the abdomen and pelvis. The treatment of patients with invasive vaginal cancer primarily consists of combined external-beam and internal radiation therapy. In patients in whom coitus is an important factor, surgery should be considered. Also in patients with stages I and IIA lesions, radical hysterectomy with an upper vaginectomy may be performed. Therapy is complicated by the anatomic proximity of the vagina to the rectum, bladder, and urethra. Most primary invasive epidermoid cancers of the vagina are treated by irradiation. Irradiation consists of whole-pelvis external therapy supplemented by internal radiation treatment. Interstitial therapy is commonly used unless there exists a small vault lesion, which may be adequately managed by a tandem and ovoid implant.

A select group of patients with stage III or IV disease may benefit from preoperative whole-pelvic radiation followed by radical surgery. However, most affected patients are treated by irradiation, which consists of whole-pelvis external irradiation followed by intracavitary or interstitial implants, or additional external therapy through a treatment field that has been reduced in size and localized to the affected parametrium. In some cases, carcinoma at the introitus may be treated like cancer of the vulva, using radical vulvectomy and bilateral superficial and deep inguinal lymphadenectomy. A very small and early lesion may be treated by total vaginectomy. However, the close proximity of the bladder and the rectum often precludes conservative surgery. Irradiation is essentially the same as that used for cancers of the upper vagina. When the lower third of the vagina is involved, the inguinal nodes must be treated with either irradiation or inguinal lymphadenectomy.

The principles of treatment of primary adenocarcinoma of the vagina are the same as those for squamous cell cancer. However, preferred therapy for clear cell carcinoma of the vagina and cervix in young women has not been established. Approximately 60% of tumors occur in the upper half of the vagina, and the remainder occur in the cervix. The incidence of nodal metastases is approximately 18% in stage I and 30% or more in stage II disease. If the disease is found sufficiently early and is confined to the upper vagina and cervix, radical abdominal hysterectomy, upper vaginectomy, and pelvic lymphadenectomy with ovarian preservation can be performed. More advanced lesions are treated with irradiation.

Sarcoma botryoides, a variety of rhabdomyosarcoma, is usually seen in patients who are younger than 5 years of age. Radiation therapy or local excision has yielded poor results; thus, historically, pelvic exenteration was the standard of therapy. Primary chemotherapy with vincristine, actinomycin D, and cyclophosphamide plus radiation leads to excellent results in treating patients with this disease. Melanoma of the vagina may be treated with radiation, conservative excision, and/or radical surgery.

Epidermoid cancers that recur after primary radiation therapy are usually treated by pelvic exenteration. Chemotherapy for recurrent disease has been relatively ineffective, but multidrug regimens incorporating cisplatin may prove to be more useful.

Prognosis

The size and stage of the disease at the time of diagnosis are the most important prognostic indicators in squamous cell cancers. The 5-year survival rate is approximately 77% in patients with stage I disease, 45% in patients with stage II disease, 31% in patients with stage III disease, and 18% in patients with stage IV disease.

Melanomas—even small ones—are very malignant, and few respond to therapy. The tumor recurs locally and metastasizes to the liver and lungs. Chemotherapy and immunotherapy have been used as adjunctive treatment.

Too few sarcomas of the vagina have been reported to generate survival data. These tumors have a propensity for local recurrence and distant metastases, and the prognosis is usually poor.

REFERENCES

General

Berek JS: *Novak's Gynecology.* Philadelphia: Williams & Wilkins, 2002.

Preinvasive Disease of the Vulva & Vagina

Davis G, Wentworth J, Richard J: Self-administered topical imiquimod treatment of vulvar intraepithelial neoplasia. J Reprod Med 2000;45:619.

Hart WR: Vulvar intraepithelial neoplasia: Historical aspects and current status. Int J Gynecol Pathol 2001;20:116.

Hillemanns P et al: Integration of HPV-16 and HPV-18 DNA in vulvar intraepithelial neoplasia. Gynecol Oncol [2005; Epub ahead of print]. 2006;100:276.

Jones RW, Rowan DM: Spontaneous regression of vulvar intraepithelial neoplasia 2–3. Obstet Gynecol 2000;96:470.

Joura EA et al: Increasing incidence of vulvar intraepithelial neoplasia and squamous cell carcinoma of the vulva in young women. J Reprod Med 2000;45:613.

McNally OM et al: VIN 3: A clinicopathologic review. Int J Gynecol Cancer 2002;12:490.

Muderspach L et al: A phase I trial of a HPV peptide vaccine for women with high grade cervical and vulvar intraepithelial neoplasia who are HPV 16 positive. Clin Cancer Res 2000;6:3406.

Murta EF et al: Vaginal intraepithelial neoplasia: Clinical-therapeutic analysis of 33 cases. Arch Gynecol Obstet 2005;272:261.

Rome RM et al: Management of vaginal intraepithelial neoplasia: A series of 132 cases with long-term follow-up. Int J Gynecol Cancer 2000;10:382.

Extramammary Paget's Disease

Parker LP et al. Paget's disease of the vulva: Pathology, pattern of involvement and prognosis. Gynecol Oncol 2000;77:183.

Cancer of the Vulva

Ansink A, van der Velden J: Surgical interventions for early squamous cell carcinoma of the vulva. Cochrane Database Syst Rev 2000:CD002036.

Balat O, Edwards C, Delclos L: Complications following combined surgery (radical vulvectomy versus wide local excision) and radiotherapy for the treatment of carcinoma of the vulva: Report of 73 patients. Eur J Gynaecol Oncol 2000;21:501.

Benedet JL et al: FIGO staging classifications and clinical practice guidelines in the management of gynecologic cancers. FIGO Committee on Gynecologic Oncology. Int J Gynaecol Obstet 2000;70:209.

Fisher M, Marsch WC: Vulvodynia: An indicator or even an early symptom of vulvar cancer. Cutis 2001;67:235.

Groff DB: Pelvic neoplasms in children. J Surg Oncol 2001;77:65.

Lea JS, Miller DS: Optimum screening interventions for gynecologic malignancies. Tex Med 2001;97:49.

Leminen A, Forss M, Paavonen J: Wound complications in patients with carcinoma of the vulva. Comparison between radical and modified vulvectomies. Eur J Obstet Gynecol Reprod Biol 2000;93:193.

Mirhashemi R, Nieves-Neira W, Averette HE: Gynecologic malignancies in older women. Oncology 2001;15:580, discussion 592, 597.

Montana GS et al: Preoperative chemo-radiation for carcinoma of the vulva with N2/N3 nodes: A Gynecologic Oncology Group Study. Int J Radiat Oncol Biol Phys 2000;48:1007.

Moscarini M et al: Surgical treatment of invasive carcinoma of the vulva. Our experience. Eur J Gynaecol Oncol 2000;1:393.

Nucci MR, Fletcher CDM: Vulvovaginal soft tissue tumors: Update and review. Histopathology 2000;36:97.

Rodolakis A et al: Squamous vulvar cancer: A clinically based individualization of treatment. Gynecol Oncol 2000;78(3 Pt 1):346.

Rouzier R et al: Prognostic significance of epithelial disorders adjacent to invasive vulvar carcinomas. Gynecol Oncol 2001;81:414.

Selman TJ et al. A systematic review of the accuracy of diagnostic tests for inguinal lymph node status in vulvar cancer. Gynecol Oncol 2005;99:206.

Senkus E et al: Second lower genital tract squamous cell carcinoma following cervical cancer. A clinical study of 46 patients. Acta Obstet Gynecol Scand 2000;79:765.

Cancer of the Vagina

Miner TJ et al: Primary vaginal melanoma: A critical analysis of therapy. Ann Surg Oncol 2004;11:34.

Samant R et al: Radiotherapy for the treatment of primary vaginal cancer. Radiother Oncol 2005;77:133.

Tjalama WA et al: The role of surgery in invasive squamous carcinoma of the vagina. Gynecol Oncol 2001;81:360.

Premalignant & Malignant Disorders of the Uterine Cervix

Christine H. Holschneider, MD

CERVICAL INTRAEPITHELIAL NEOPLASIA

ESSENTIALS OF DIAGNOSIS

- *The cervix often appears grossly normal.*
- *Infection with the human papillomavirus is present.*
- *Dysplastic or carcinoma in situ cells are noted in a cytologic smear preparation (traditional Pap smear or liquid-based cytology).*
- *Colposcopic examination reveals an atypical transformation zone with thickened acetowhite epithelium and coarse punctate or mosaic patterns of surface capillaries.*
- *Iodine-nonstaining (Schiller-positive) area of squamous epithelium is typical.*
- *Biopsy diagnosis of cervical intraepithelial neoplasia (dysplasia or carcinoma in situ).*

General Considerations

Lower genital tract squamous intraepithelial neoplasia is often multicentric (ie, affecting multiple anatomic sites which embryologically are derived from the same anogenital epithelium): cervical intraepithelial neoplasia (CIN), vaginal intraepithelial neoplasia (VAIN, see Chapter 49), vulvar intraepithelial neoplasia (VIN, see Chapter 49), and perianal intraepithelial neoplasia (PAIN). Approximately 10% of women with CIN have concomitant preinvasive neoplasia of the vulva, vagina, or anus. Conversely, 40 60% of patients with VIN or VAIN have synchronous or metachronous CIN.

Cervical intraepithelial neoplasia (CIN), formerly called dysplasia, means disordered growth and development of the epithelial lining of the cervix. There are various degrees of CIN. Mild dysplasia, or CIN I, is defined as disordered growth of the lower third of the epithelial lining. Abnormal maturation of the lower two-thirds of the lining is called moderate dysplasia, or CIN II. Severe dysplasia, CIN III, encompasses more than two-thirds of the epithelial thickness with carcinoma in situ (CIS) representing full-thickness dysmaturity (Fig 50–1). While histologically evaluated lesions are characterized using the CIN nomenclature, cytologic smears are classified according to the Bethesda system, which was most recently revised in 2001 (Table 50–1). Briefly, atypical squamous cells are divided into those of undetermined significance (ASC-US) and those in which a high grade lesion cannot be excluded (ASC-H). Low-grade squamous intraepithelial lesion (LSIL) encompasses cytologic changes consistent with koilocytic atypia or CIN I. High-grade squamous intraepithelial lesion (HSIL) denotes the cytologic findings corresponding to CIN II and CIN III. CIN may be suspected because of an abnormal cytologic smear, but the diagnosis is established by cervical biopsy. Spontaneous regression, especially of CIN I, occurs in a significant number of patients, allowing for expectant management with serial cytologic smears in the reliable patient. A certain percentage of all dysplasias, especially high-grade lesions, will progress to an invasive cancer if left untreated. Because it is not presently possible to predict which lesions will progress, it is recommended that all patients with CIN II and CIN III be treated when diagnosed. The only exception to this recommendation concerns adolescents, in whom CIN II may be followed, as spontaneous regression is substantial and the risk of cancer almost nil.

Epidemiology & Etiology

Prevalence figures for CIN vary according to the socioeconomic characteristics and geographic area of the population studied, from as low as 1.05% in some family planning clinics to as high as 13.7% in women attending sexually transmitted disease (STD) clinics. CIN is most commonly detected in women in their 20s, the peak incidence of carcinoma in situ is in women ages 25–35 years, whereas the incidence of cervical cancer rises most significantly after the age of 40 years.

LSIL	HSIL	
CIN I lower 1/3 of epithelial lining	lower 2/3 of lining **CIN II**	>2/3 lining **CIN III**
Mild Dysplasia	**Moderate Dysplasia**	**Severe Dysplasia**

Figure 50–1. Changes in the terminology for cervical intraepithelial neoplasia. (Courtesy of UpToDate in Oncology.)

The epidemiologic risk factors for CIN are similar to those for cervical cancer and include multiple sexual partners, early onset of sexual activity, a high-risk sexual partner (history of multiple sexual partners, human papillomavirus (HPV) infection, lower genital tract neoplasia, or prior sexual exposure to someone with cervical neoplasia), a history of STDs, as well as cigarette smoking, human immunodeficiency virus (HIV) infection, acquired immune deficiency syndrome (AIDS), other forms of immunosuppression, multiparity, and long-term oral contraceptive pill use.

HPVs are a prime etiologic factor in the development of CIN and cervical cancer. In fact, most of the above behavioral and sexual risk factors for cervical neoplasia become statistically insignificant as independent variables after adjusting for HPV infection. Analyses of cervical neoplasia lesions show the presence of HPV in more than 80% of all CIN lesions and in 99.7% of all invasive cervical cancers.

Infection with HPV is extremely common and varies with the patient's age. In the United States, the prevalence of detectable HPV infection rises from 1% in newborns, to 20% in teenagers, to 40% in women 20–29 years of age, with a slow decline thereafter to a plateau of 5% in women age 50 years and older. Condoms are not as protective against HPV as they are against other sexually transmitted diseases as transmission can occur from labial-scrotal contact.

More than 90% of immunocompetent women will have a spontaneous resolution of their HPV infection over a 2-year period and only approximately 5% will have cytologically detectable CIN. Women who have persistent HPV infections, especially with high viral loads, have a higher likelihood of developing CIN and cervical cancer.

The vast majority of women infected with HPV do not develop CIN or cervical cancer. This suggests that infection with HPV alone is insufficient for the development of CIN or cervical cancer and underscores the importance of other cofactors, such as cigarette smoking or immunosuppression.

There are more than 100 HPV types, half of which infect the anogenital epithelium. Based on their malignant potential, HPV subtypes are categorized into low-risk and high-risk types. Low-risk HPV types (eg, types 6, 11, 42, 43, and 44) are associated with condylomata

Table 50–1. The Bethesda System 2001.

Specimen Type
Indicate conventional smear (Pap smear) vs. liquid-based vs. other
Specimen Adequacy
    Satisfactory for evaluation (*describe presence or absence of endocervical transformation zone component and any other quality indicators, eg, partially obscuring blood, inflammation, etc*)
    Unsatisfactory for evaluation… (*specify reason*)
        Specimen rejected/not processed (*specify reason*)
        Specimen processed and examined, but unsatisfactory for evaluation of epithelial abnormality because of (*specify reason*)
General Categorization (optional)
Negative for intraepithelial lesion or malignancy
Epithelial cell abnormality: See Interpretation/Result (*specify squamous or glandular as appropriate*)
Other: See Interpretation/Result (*eg, endometrial cells in a woman ≥40 years of age*)
Automated Review
If case examined by automated device, specify device and result
Ancillary Testing
Provide a brief description of the test methods and report the result so that it is easily understood by the clinician
Interpretation/Result
    NEGATIVE FOR INTRAEPITHELIAL LESION OR MALIGNANCY
    (*when there is no cellular evidence of neoplasia, state this in the General Categorization above and/or in the Interpretation/Result section of the report, whether or not there are organisms or other non-neoplastic findings*)
        ORGANISMS:
          Trichomonas vaginalis
          Fungal organisms morphologically consistent with *Candida* spp.
          Shift in flora suggestive of bacterial vaginosis
          Bacteria morphologically consistent with *Actinomyces* spp.
          Cellular changes consistent with herpes simplex virus
        OTHER NON-NEOPLASTIC FINDINGS (*Optional to report; list not inclusive*):
        Reactive cellular changes associated with inflammation (includes typical repair)

        Radiation
        Intrauterine contraceptive device (IUD)
        Glandular cells status posthysterectomy
        Atrophy
    OTHER
        Endometrial cells (in a woman ≥ 40 years of age)
        (*Specify if negative for squamous intraepithelial lesion*)
    EPITHELIAL CELL ABNORMALITIES
        SQUAMOUS CELL
          Atypical squamous cells of undetermined significance (ASC-US) cannot exclude HSIL (ASC-H)
          Low-grade squamous intraepithelial lesion (LSIL) encompassing: HPV/mild dysplasia/CIN
          High-grade squamous intraepithelial lesion (HSIL) encompassing: moderate and severe dysplasia, CIN 2 and CIN 3/CIS
          Squamous cell carcinoma
        GLANDULAR CELL
          Atypical (AGC)
            endocervical cells
            endometrial cells
            glandular cells not otherwise specified (NOS)
          Ayptical, favor neoplastic
            endocervical cells
            glandular cells NOS
          Endocervical adenocarcinoma in situ (AIS)
          Adenocarcinoma
            endocervical
            endometrial
            extrauterine
            not otherwise specified (NOS)
        OTHER MALIGNANT NEOPLASMS: (*specify*)
    Educational Notes and Suggestions (*optional*)
    Suggestions should be concise and consistent with clinical follow-up guidelines published by professional organizations (references to relevant publications may be included)

and low-grade lesions (CIN I), whereas high-risk HPV (such as types 16, 18, 31, 33, 35, 39, 45, 51, 52, 56, 58, 59, 68, 73, and 82) is, in addition to high-grade lesions (CIN II and CIN III), found in invasive cancer.

    Cigarette smoking and HPV infection have synergistic effects on the development of CIN, and cigarette smoking is associated with a 2- to 4-fold increase in the relative risk for developing cervical cancer. Cigarette smoke carcinogens have been found to accumulate locally in the cervical mucus, and the cumulative exposure as measured by pack-years smoked is related to the

risk of developing CIN or carcinoma in situ. However, the mechanisms by which cigarette smoking contributes to cervical carcinogenesis are poorly understood.

    The incidence of cervical neoplasia is increased in HIV-infected women, who, in some studies, have a 20–30% incidence of colposcopically confirmed CIN. With increasing immunosuppression there is an increased risk of de novo HPV infection, persistent HPV infection, and progressive cervical neoplasia. Since 1993, invasive cervical cancer has been included as an AIDS-defining illness.

Pathology

On cytologic examination, the dysplastic cell is characterized by anaplasia, an increased nuclear-to-cytoplasmic ratio (ie, the nucleus is larger), hyperchromatism with changes in the nuclear chromatin, multinucleation, and abnormalities in differentiation.

Histologically, involvement of varying degrees of thickness of the stratified squamous epithelium is typical of dysplasia. The cells are anaplastic and hyperchromatic, and show a loss of polarity in the deeper layers as well as abnormal mitotic figures in increased numbers. Benign epithelial alterations, particularly those of an inflammatory nature, the cytopathic effects of HPV, and technical artifacts may be mistaken for CIN I and CIN II.

The columnar epithelium of the mucus-secreting endocervical glands can also undergo neoplastic transformation. Adenocarcinoma in situ (ACIS) is defined as the presence of endocervical glands lined by atypical columnar epithelium that cytologically resembles the cells of endocervical adenocarcinoma, but that occur in the absence of stromal invasion. The diagnosis of ACIS can be made only by cone biopsy.

Clinical Findings

A. Symptoms and Signs

There are usually no symptoms or signs of CIN, and the diagnosis is most often based on biopsy findings following an abnormal routine cervical cytology smear. Because high-grade dysplasia probably is a transitional phase in the pathogenesis of many cervical cancers, early detection is extremely important. Based on the American Cancer Society guidelines, which were last revised in 2002, all women who have reached age 21 years, or who are 3 years past coitarche, should have a pelvic examination and collection of a cytologic smear. The cervical cytology smear should be performed annually in case of conventional Papanicolaou (Pap) smears, and biannually if using liquid-based cytology. Once a patient is age 30 years or older and has had 3 consecutive negative smears, the time interval between cervical cytology smears can be extended to every 3 years. Cervical cytology screening may be discontinued at age 70 years if the patient had 3 or more consecutive normal smears in the preceding 10 years. Screening cytology smears may also be discontinued if the patient has undergone a total hysterectomy, unless it was done for the treatment of cervical dysplasia or cancer.

B. Special Examinations

All abnormal Pap smears require further evaluation, such as visual inspection of the cervix, repeat cytology, HPV testing, staining with Lugol's solution (Schiller test) or toluidine blue, colposcopy, directed biopsy, endocervical curettage, or diagnostic conization (see treatment section) (Fig 50–2). The objective is to exclude the presence of invasive carcinoma and to determine the degree and extent of any CIN.

1. Repeat cervical cytology—There are three acceptable initial evaluation steps for patients with minimally abnormal cervical cytology smears (eg, ASC-US): accelerated serial cytology smears, triage to colposcopy based on a positive HPV testing result, or immediate referral to colposcopy. All patients with ASC-H, LSILs, HSILs, atypical glandular cells (AGCs), or smears suspicious for cancer should be referred for immediate colposcopy.

Prior to performing a repeat smear for a patient with ASC-US, she should be evaluated and treated for potential underlying conditions that might contribute to an atypical smear, such as antimicrobials for infections or hormones for atrophic vaginitis. The cervical cytology smear should be repeated every 6 months until there are two consecutive normal smears. The use of serial cytologic smears is important, as the false-negative rate of a single repeat smear following an ASC-US diagnosis is as high as 33% for biopsy-proven high-grade squamous intraepithelial lesions (CIN II/III). A second abnormal smear (atypical squamous cell [ASC] or worse) should be evaluated by colposcopy.

2. HPV testing—Testing for low-risk HPV types has no role in cervical cancer prevention. Testing for high-risk HPV types has been investigated as an intermediary test for patients with minimally abnormal cervical cytology smears (ASC-US, LSIL). For patients with ASC-US, reflex HPV testing is the preferred approach, with triage of women who test positive for high-risk HPV to colposcopy. Reflex HPV testing refers to the concurrent collection of a specimen for cervical cytology and HPV testing, with the HPV testing being performed only in case of an abnormal cytologic screen. For ASC-US, this approach is the most cost-effective and has an equal or higher sensitivity for CIN II/III at the lowest referral rate to colposcopy compared to the two alternate approaches (accelerated serial cytology or immediate colposcopy). Women with an ASC-US smear and a negative HPV test are followed with a cervical cytology smear at 1 year. The value of HPV testing for the triage of patients with LSIL is limited because nearly 85% of the lesions are HPV positive. HPV testing combined with a cervical cytology smear has been approved as a primary screening approach in the patient age 30 years and older, who still has her uterus and has no immunosuppression. If both results are negative, combined screening should not be repeated for 3 years. If cytology and HPV testing are positive, triaging to colposcopy is as outlined above. If cytology is normal, but HPV test is positive, repeat cytology and HPV test in 6–12 months is recommended, with colposcopy at that point if either test is abnormal.

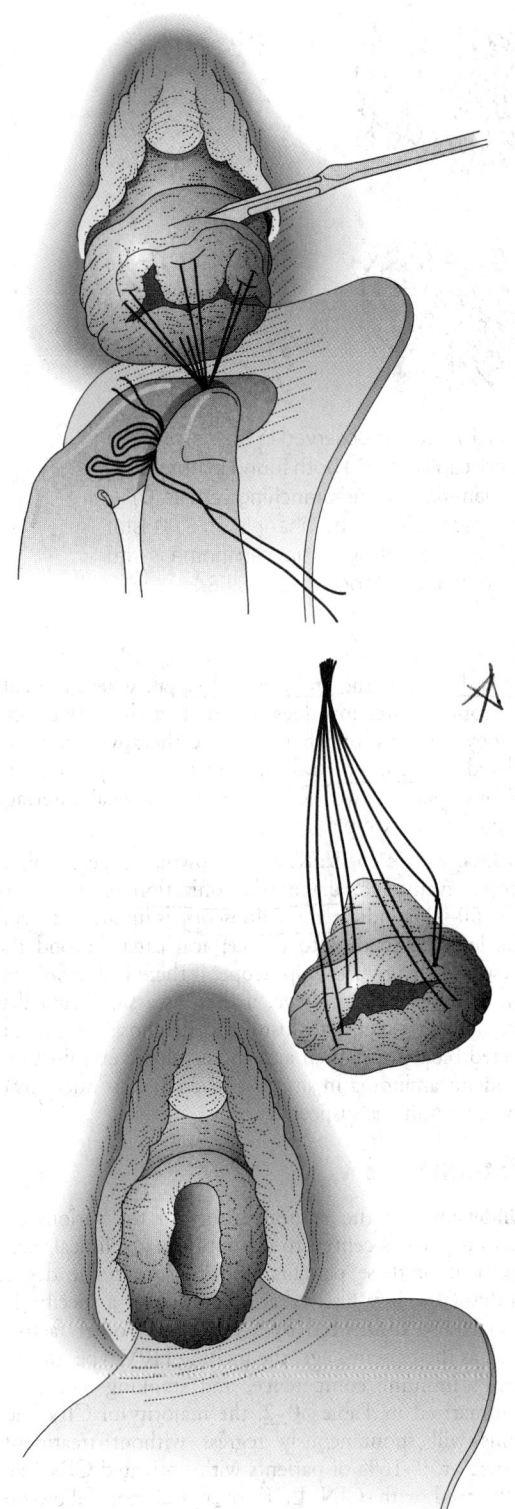

Figure 50–2. Conization of the cervix.

3. Schiller test—The Schiller test is based on the principle that normal mature squamous epithelium of the cervix contains glycogen, which combines with iodine to produce a deep mahogany-brown color. Nonstaining, therefore, indicates abnormal squamous (or columnar) epithelium, scarring, cyst formation, or immature metaplastic epithelium, and constitutes a positive Schiller test. Lugol's solution is an aqueous iodine preparation and is commonly used for the Schiller test.

4. Colposcopic examination—Colposcopy is the primary technique for the evaluation of an abnormal cervical cytology smear. The colposcope is an instrument that uses illuminated low-power magnification (5–15×) to inspect the cervix, vagina, vulva, or anal epithelium. Abnormalities in the appearance of the epithelium and its capillary blood supply often are invisible to the naked eye but can be identified by colposcopy, particularly after the application of 3–5% aqueous acetic acid solution. CIN produces recognizable abnormalities of the cervical epithelium in the majority of patients.

Indications for colposcopy are:

1. Abnormal cervical cytology smear or HPV testing;
2. Clinically abnormal or suspicious-looking cervix;
3. Unexplained intermenstrual or postcoital bleeding;
4. Vulvar or vaginal neoplasia; or
5. History of in utero diethylstilbestrol (DES) exposure.

Details of the colposcopy technique are described in Chapter 38.

Normal colposcopic findings are those of:

a) The original squamous epithelium, which extends from the mucocutaneous vulvovaginal junction to the original squamocolumnar junction.

b) The transformation zone, which is the metaplastic squamous epithelium between the original squamocolumnar junction and the active squamocolumnar junction. The original squamocolumnar junction is the junction between the stratified squamous epithelium of the vagina and ectocervix, and the columnar epithelium of the endocervical canal. In two-thirds of female infants, this original squamocolumnar junction is located on the ectocervix, in close to a third in the endocervical canal, and in a very small subset out in the vaginal fornices. During a woman's life cycle the squamocolumnar junction "migrates" as a consequence of various hormonal and environmental influences that alter the cervical volume and cause squamous metaplasia of everted endocervical columnar cells. Following menarche, the squamocolumnar junction is generally found on the ectocervix, with further eversion during pregnancy. In the postmenopausal patient, the squamocolumnar junction is frequently within the endocervical canal. This squamous metaplasia is a dynamic process and cervical neoplasia almost invariably originates within the transformation zone. If the new squamoco-

Figure 50–3. Schematic of different types of terminal vessels as observed in the normal squamous epithelium: hairpin capillaries (**A**), network capillaries (**B**) both found in normal states, double capillaries (**C**) seen in *Trichomonas* inflammation, and branching vessels (**D**) seen in the transformation zone. (Reproduced with permission from Johannisson E, Kolstat P, Soderberg G: Cytologic, vascular, and histologic patterns of dysplasia, carcinoma in situ and early invasive carcinoma of the cervix. Acta Radiol Suppl [Stockh] 1966;258.)

lumnar junction is visualized in its entirety, the colposcopic examination is called satisfactory; if it cannot be fully visualized, the examination is called unsatisfactory.

c) The columnar epithelium of the endocervical canal.

Abnormal findings indicative of dysplasia and carcinoma in situ (CIS) are those of:

1. Leukoplakia or hyperkeratosis, which is an area of white, thickened epithelium that is appreciated prior to the application of acetic acid and may indicate underlying neoplasia.

2. Acetowhite epithelium, which is epithelium that stains white after the application of acetic acid.

3. Mosaicism or punctation reflecting abnormal vascular patterns of the surface capillaries. As a general rule, capillary thickness and intercapillary distances correlate with the severity of the lesion and thus tend to be larger and coarser in higher-grade lesions.

4. Atypical vessels with bizarre capillaries with so-called corkscrew, comma-shaped, or spaghetti-like configurations suggest early stromal invasion (Figs 50–3 through 50–5).

A colposcopically directed punch biopsy of the most severely abnormal areas should be done. The transformation zone extends into the endocervical canal beyond the field of vision in 12–15% of premenopausal women and in a significantly higher percentage of postmenopausal women. Evaluation of the nonvisualized portion of the endocervical canal by endocervical curettage (ECC) should be performed using a brush or curette, at a minimum, in every case in which colposcopy is unsatisfactory, where the lesion is extending into the endocervical canal, where the colposcopic impression does not explain the cervical cytology findings, or where ablative therapy is contemplated. ECC is not indicated in pregnancy. In up to 20% of patients with CIN, the endocervical curettage is positive for dysplasia.

5. Diagnostic conization—Following expert colposcopic evaluation, diagnostic conization of the cervix (Fig 50–2) is indicated if colposcopy is unsatisfactory, if the lesion extends into the cervical canal beyond the view afforded by the colposcope, if there is dysplasia on the endocervical curettage, if there is a significant discrepancy between the histologic diagnosis of the directed biopsy specimen and the cytologic examination, if adenocarcinoma in situ is suspected, or if microinvasive carcinoma is suspected.

Natural History

Understanding the natural history of the various degrees of CIN is central to the appropriate clinical management of these patients. In addition to the degree of dysplasia, it is likely that the course of a specific lesion is also influenced by a number of other factors, such as the patient's age, the inciting HPV type, the patient's immune competence, and smoking habits. As summarized in Table 50–2, the majority of CIN I lesions will spontaneously regress without treatment. However, 9–16% of patients with untreated CIN I are diagnosed with CIN II/III over a 2-year follow-up. Spontaneous regression rates of CIN I overall are 60%; in young women, the rates are as high as 91%. There-

Figure 50–4. Schematic of punctation terminal vessels (**A**) and mosaic terminal vessels (**B**). (Reproduced with permission from Johannisson E, Kolstat P, Soderberg G: Cytologic, vascular, and histologic patterns of dysplasia, carcinoma in situ and early invasive carcinoma of the cervix. Acta Radiol Suppl [Stockh] 1966;258.)

fore, it is generally reasonable to expectantly follow the compliant patient with CIN I using surveillance with serial cervical cytology smears at 6-month intervals or an HPV test at 12 months. In the adolescent patient, observation is the preferred management approach. Because we currently lack the means to identify individuals at risk for progressive disease, immediate treatment might be appropriate for high-risk patients likely to be lost to follow-up, because up to 40% of these women may have persistent or progressive disease that will eventually require therapy. The majority of high-grade lesions will persist or progress (Table 50–2), so immediate treatment is generally warranted.

Treatment

Patient management is based on the correlation of the results of the cervical cytology smear, findings at colposcopy and biopsy, and ECC results, as well as individual patient characteristics, such as pregnancy, HIV infection, and the likelihood of compliance with management recommendations.

Figure 50–5. Schematic of atypical vessels: hairpinlike (**A**); networklike (**B**); and branching type (**C**). (Reproduced with permission from Johannisson E, Kolstat P, Soderberg G: Cytologic, vascular, and histologic patterns of dysplasia, carcinoma in situ and early invasive carcinoma of the cervix. Acta Radiol Suppl [Stockh] 1966;258.)

Table 50–2. Approximate rates of spontaneous regression, persistence, and progression of CIN.

	CIN I	CIN II	CIN III
Regression to normal	60%	40%	30%
Persistence	30%	35%	48%
Progression to CIN III	10%	20%	—
Progression to cancer	< 1%	5%	22%

Treatment options fall into one of two main categories: procedures that ablate the abnormal tissue and do not produce a tissue specimen for additional histologic evaluation and procedures that excise the area of abnormality, allowing for further histologic study. Prior to any therapeutic intervention an assessment has to be made as to whether a patient qualifies for ablative therapy (eg, satisfactory diagnostic evaluation has excluded invasive disease) or if she requires an excisional procedure (conization) for further diagnostic work-up. In most cases, conization is also the appropriate therapeutic intervention. If the intraepithelial lesion is confined to the ectocervix, treatment with cryotherapy, laser ablation, or a superficial excision by the loop electrosurgical excision procedure (LEEP) is appropriate. If the lesion extends into the endocervical canal, the endocervical curettage contains dysplastic epithelium, or the colposcopic examination is otherwise unsatisfactory, the endocervical canal must be included in the treatment by a deeper LEEP or cone biopsy (Fig 50–6). A conization procedure is also indicated in cases of a significant discrepancy between cervical cytology and colposcopy/biopsy results, in cases of suspected microinvasive carcinoma or adenocarcinoma in situ.

The five most common techniques for the treatment of CIN include two ablative techniques—cryotherapy and laser ablation—and three excisional procedures—cold knife conization, laser cone excision, and LEEP. Evidence from controlled trials show that these techniques are of equal efficacy, averaging 80–90% success rates in the treatment of CIN. Cure depends on the size of the lesion, endocervical gland involvement, margin status of any excisional specimen, and ECC results.

A. Cryotherapy

In cryotherapy, an office procedure not requiring anesthesia, nitrous oxide or carbon dioxide is used as the refrigerant for a supercooled probe. The cryoprobe is positioned on the ectocervix where it must cover the entire lesion, which at times is not easily achieved. It is then activated until blanching of the cervix extends at least 7 mm beyond the probe in all directions in order

to assure that freezing extends beyond the depth of the crypts of the glands into which the dysplasia might be extending. Introduction of a two-cycle freeze–thaw–freeze technique has improved efficacy. The advantages of cryotherapy include ease of use, low cost, widespread availability, and a low complication rate. Side effects include mild uterine cramping and a copious watery vaginal discharge for several weeks. Infection and cervical stenosis are rare. Follow-up colposcopic examinations can be unsatisfactory because of the inability to visualize the squamocolumnar junction.

B. Carbon Dioxide Laser

Carbon dioxide (CO_2) laser can be used either to ablate the transformation zone or as a tool for cone biopsies. The laser destroys tissue with a very narrow zone of injury around the treated tissue, and is therefore both precise and flexible. The tissue is vaporized to a depth of at least 7 mm to assure that the bases of the deepest glands are destroyed. Posttreatment vaginal discharge may last 1–2 weeks, and bleeding that requires reexamination can occur in a small percentage of patients. The technique is expensive and requires significant training and attention to safety, as well as local or general anesthesia.

C. Loop Electrosurgical Excision Procedure

LEEP is the procedure of choice for treating CIN II and CIN III because of its ease of use, low cost, and provision of tissue for histologic evaluation. LEEP uses a small, fine, wire loop attached to an electrosurgical generator to excise the tissue of interest. Various sizes of wire loop are available. Following LEEP excision of the transformation zone, frequently an additional narrow endocervical specimen is removed to allow for histologic evaluation while avoiding excessive damage to the cervical stroma. Fulguration with a roller ball electrode is then used to achieve complete hemostasis in the excision bed. LEEP can be performed as an office procedure under local anesthesia. An insulated speculum to prevent conduction of electricity, a grounding pad, and a vacuum to remove the smoke are necessary. Complications are less frequent than with cold knife conization and include bleeding, infection, and cervical stenosis.

D. Cold Knife Conization

Cold knife conization of the cervix refers to the excision of a cone-shaped portion of the cervix using a scalpel. This technique can be individualized to accommodate the cervical anatomy and the size and shape of the lesion. For example, a wide, shallow cone specimen can be obtained from a young patient whose squamocolumnar junction is on the ectocervix. In an older patient, in whom the squamocolumnar junction tends to move more cephalad into

Figure 50–6. Plan for management of the abnormal cytologic smear with visible or no visible cervical lesion. SCCA = squamous cell carcinoma.

the endocervical canal, a narrower, deeper cone is preferable. An endocervical curettage is performed after the conization to assess the remaining endocervical canal. Cervical cone biopsy is generally done in the operating room under local or general anesthesia. Complications include bleeding, infection, cervical stenosis, and cervical incompetence. The need to perform the procedure in the operating room and a higher complication rate are distinct disadvantages of cold knife conization. However, it results in a specimen devoid of any thermal artifact that may complicate the histologic diagnosis and margin assessment seen with LEEP and laser conization. This becomes particularly im-

portant with suspected microinvasive carcinoma and adenocarcinoma in situ.

Follow-Up

Most treatment failures are diagnosed within the first 1–2 years after therapy. Patients with positive margins or positive ECC after an excisional procedure are at higher risk for persistent/recurrent disease than are women with negative margins, necessitating close follow-up, including repeat endocervical sampling but not re-excision. Therefore, careful examination should be performed, with Pap smears every 6 months for 18 to 24 months and endocervical curettage if the endocervix was involved. Alternatively, HPV testing may be performed along with the first cytology smear 6 months after therapy. If both are negative, annual follow-up can be established. Management of recurrent dysplasia follows the same guidelines outlined in Fig 50–6. If a woman has completed childbearing, recurrent dysplasia can be treated by a simple hysterectomy after invasion has been ruled out. Women with a history of cervical dysplasia have a higher incidence of vaginal dysplasia. These women continue to need Pap smears after hysterectomy.

SPECIAL SITUATIONS

A. PREGNANCY

Pregnant women routinely undergo cervical cytology screening at their first prenatal visit. As a result, it is not uncommon that an abnormal cervical cytology smear is first discovered during pregnancy. Colposcopy is performed for the same indications as in the nonpregnant patient. However, biopsies are limited unless there are colposcopic signs suggestive of carcinoma in situ or invasive disease. Endocervical curettage is not performed in pregnancy because of the potential risk of abortion and infection. The physiologic changes of pregnancy render the transformation zone easily accessible for satisfactory colposcopy by 20 weeks' gestation in almost all women. Colposcopy during pregnancy can be challenging because pregnancy may produce changes in the cervical epithelium that mimic those of cervical dysplasia. Although the gravid cervix is more vascular, directed ectocervical biopsies can be performed safely with minimal increase in the risk of significant bleeding. After the diagnosis of dysplasia has been established, the patient can be carefully followed with colposcopic examinations and cervical cytology smears each trimester. Repeat biopsies are only performed for progressive lesions. Treatment is deferred into the postpartum period. Even high-grade lesions discovered during pregnancy have a high rate of regression in the postpartum period. Conization during pregnancy is indicated only if early invasive disease is suspected. Complications of a cone biopsy in pregnancy include abortion, hemorrhage, infection, and incompetent cervix.

B. ATYPICAL GLANDULAR CELLS ON CERVICAL CYTOLOGY SMEAR

Patients with atypical glandular cells on a cervical cytology smear have a up to 50% risk of having high-grade cervical neoplasia. The underlying lesion is most commonly CIN II or III, which is diagnosed in up to 34% of cases. Cervical adenocarcinoma in situ, invasive cervical adenocarcinoma, and endometrial disease, including hyperplasia and cancer, comprise the remaining 16%.

The 2001 Bethesda System divides glandular cell abnormalities into AGCs, AGC-favor neoplasia, endocervical adenocarcinoma in situ (AIS), and adenocarcinoma. Given the high risk for significant pathology, any patient with glandular cell abnormalities on a cervical cytology smear requires immediate evaluation, which includes, at a minimum, colposcopy with careful evaluation of the endocervical canal. Assessment of the endometrium is recommended in all patients older than age 35 years, in patients at any age with abnormal bleeding, in women with AGC (endometrial cells), and in women with AGC (nonspecified cell type) (see Table 50–1). Diagnostic conization is indicated in all cases of AGC-favor neoplasia, AIS, or suspected adenocarcinoma as well as persistent atypical glandular cell–not otherwise specified (AGC-NOS), unless a definitive diagnosis has been made on the colposcopy directed biopsy or endometrial sampling.

C. ADENOCARCINOMA IN SITU

The reported incidence of glandular neoplasia of the cervix is increasing, especially in young women, with up to 30% of cases occurring in women younger than 35 years of age. Adenocarcinoma of the cervix represents approximately 25% of all cervical cancers and there is convincing evidence that ACIS is a precursor lesion. Half of the women with ACIS have concomitant squamous CIN. Management is difficult. The lesion may be located high in the endocervical canal, involve the deeper portions of the endocervical clefts, or be multifocal with skip lesions. Conization is required to make the diagnosis. Follow-up surveillance after conization is difficult, as cervical cytology, endocervical curettage, or endocervical cytobrush sampling each have a sensitivity of only approximately 50%. This is of particular concern because the incidence of residual ACIS or invasive adenocarcinoma following conization for ACIS is as high as 58% with positive conization margins, and 19% with negative conization margins. Therefore, conservative management should be undertaken only in the young patient with a negative conization margin who is fully counseled and desires to maintain her fertility. In all other patients, hysterectomy should be performed as a definitive therapeutic intervention because even with negative margins, as many as 8–16% may have invasive disease on the hysterectomy specimen. For the same reason, consideration should be given to the performance of a modified radical hysterectomy, especially if extensive disease and positive margins were found on the preceding conization specimen.

D. HIV INFECTION

Management of CIN in the HIV-infected patient presents a great challenge. Following treatment, the risk of recurrent CIN is high, especially in the immunocompromised patient with low CD4 counts and high viral loads. Recurrence rates may reach 80% within 3 years in markedly immunocompromised women. Use of highly active antiretroviral therapy (HAART) appears to reduce the risk of recurrent or progressive cervical neoplasia.

CANCER OF THE CERVIX

ESSENTIALS OF DIAGNOSIS

- *Early disease is frequently asymptomatic, underscoring the importance of cervical cytology screening.*
- *Abnormal uterine bleeding and vaginal discharge are the most common symptoms.*
- *A cervical lesion may be visible on inspection as a tumor or ulceration; cancer within the cervical canal may be occult.*
- *Diagnosis must be confirmed by biopsy.*

General Considerations

Cancer of the cervix is the sixth most common solid cancer in American women. In the United States, an estimated 10,370 new cases of invasive cervical cancer are diagnosed annually, and there are 3710 deaths from the disease. In contrast, with more than 370,000 new cases diagnosed annually and a 50% mortality rate, cervical cancer is the second most common cause of cancer-related morbidity and mortality among women in developing countries. This dichotomy is largely the result of a 75% decrease in the incidence of cervical cancer in developed countries following the implementation of population-based screening programs and treatment of preinvasive disease. The average age at diagnosis of patients with cervical cancer is 51 years. However, the disease can occur in the second decade of life and during pregnancy. More than 95% of patients with early cancer of the cervix can be cured.

Etiology & Epidemiology

The major epidemiologic risk factors for cervical cancer are the same as those for CIN and were discussed above. HPV is central to the development of cervical neoplasia. HPV DNA is found in 99.7% of all cervical carcinomas. HPV 16 is the most prevalent HPV type in squamous cell carcinoma, and HPV 18 the most prevalent in adenocarcinoma. Other associated risk factors are immunosuppression, infection with HIV or a his-

tory of other sexually transmitted diseases, tobacco use, high parity, and oral contraceptive use.

Pathogenesis & Natural History

HPV is epitheliotropic. Once the epithelium is acutely infected with HPV, one of three clinical scenarios ensues:
 a) Asymptomatic latent infection;
 b) Active infection in which HPV undergoes vegetative replication but not integration into the genome (eg, leading to condyloma or CIN I); or
 c) Neoplastic transformation following integration of oncogenic HPV DNA into the human genome.

Integration of HPV into the human genome is associated with cell immortalization allowing for malignant transformation. This involves an upregulation of the viral oncogenes E6 and E7. These oncoproteins interfere with cell-cycle control in the human host cell. E6 and E7 have the ability to complex with the tumor suppressor genes p53 and Rb, respectively. The disabling of these two major tumor suppressor genes is thought to be central to host cell immortalization and transformation induced by HPV.

Incipient cancer of the cervix is generally a slowly developing process. Most cervical cancers probably begin as a high-grade dysplastic change (see previous section) or carcinoma in situ with gradual progression over a period of several years. At least 90% of squamous cell carcinomas of the cervix develop from the intraepithelial layers, almost always within 1 cm of the squamo-columnar junction of the cervix either on the portio vaginalis of the cervix or slightly higher in the endocervical canal.

Early stromal invasion (stage IA1) up to a depth of 3 mm below the basement membrane is a localized process, provided there is no pathologic evidence of lymphovascular space involvement. Penetration of the stroma beyond this point carries an increased risk of lymphatic metastasis (Table 50–3). When the lymphatics are involved, tumor cells are carried to the regional pelvic lymph nodes

Table 50–3. Risk of any lymph node metastasis for patients with microscopic squamous cell carcinoma of the cervix.

Depth of Tumor Invasion	Risk of Lymph Node Metastasis
FIGO stage IA1	
Early stromal invasion (< 1 mm)	3/1543 (0.2%)
Microinvasion (1–3 mm)	5/809 (0.6%)
FIGO stage IA2	
Microscopic 3–5 mm invasion	14/214 (6.5%)

Figure 50–7. Lymphatic spread of carcinoma of the cervix.

(parametrial, hypogastric, obturator, external iliac, and sacral) (Fig 50–7). The more pleomorphic or extensive the local disease, the greater the likelihood of lymph node involvement. As the tumor grows, it also spreads by direct extension to the parametria.

Squamous cell carcinoma clinically confined to the cervix involves the regional pelvic lymph nodes in 15–20% of cases. When the cancer involves the parametrium (stage IIB), tumor cells can be found in the pelvic lymph nodes in 30–40% and in the paraaortic nodes in approximately 15–30% of cases. The more advanced the local disease, the greater the likelihood of distant metastases. The paraaortic nodes are involved in approximately 45% of patients with stage IVA disease.

Ovarian involvement is rare, occurring in approximately 0.5% of squamous cell carcinomas and 1.7% of adenocarcinomas. The liver and lungs are the most common sites of blood-borne metastasis, but the tumor may involve the brain, bones, bowels, adrenal glands, spleen, or pancreas.

When cancer of the cervix is untreated or fails to respond to treatment, death occurs in 95% of patients within 2 years after the onset of symptoms. Death can occur from uremia, pulmonary embolism, or hemorrhage from direct extension of tumor into blood vessels. Life-threatening sepsis from complications of pyelonephritis or vesicovaginal and rectovaginal fistulas is possible. Large-bowel obstruction from direct extension of tumor into the rectosigmoid can be the terminal event. Pain from perineural extension is a significant management problem of advanced disease.

Pathology

Approximately 70–75% of cervical carcinomas are squamous cell; the remainder are composed of various types of adenocarcinomas (20–25%), adenosquamous carcinomas (3–5%), and undifferentiated carcinomas.

A. SQUAMOUS CELL CARCINOMAS

Cervical squamous cell carcinomas have been classified according to the predominant cell type: large cell nonkeratinizing, large cell keratinizing, and small cell carcinomas. The large cell nonkeratinizing variety accounts for the majority of tumors.

B. VERRUCOUS CARCINOMA

Verrucous carcinoma, which has been associated with HPV 6, is a rare subtype of well-differentiated squamous carcinoma. It is a slow-growing, locally invasive neoplasm. Histologically, this tumor is composed of well-differentiated squamous cells with frondlike papillae and little apparent stromal invasion, but it is potentially lethal. Radical resection is the mainstay of therapy.

C. ADENOCARCINOMA

Adenocarcinoma of the cervix is derived from the glandular elements of the cervix. The incidence of adenocarcinomas, including the mucinous, endometrioid, clear cell, and serous types, has been rising over the last several decades, especially in women younger than 35 years of age. Part of this increase may be a result of an increasing prevalence of HPV infection and part may be a result of improvements in screening and prevention of squamous preinvasive disease, thus leading to a histologic shift toward adenocarcinoma. When the initial growth of adenocarcinoma of the cervix is within the endocervical canal and the ectocervix appears normal, this lesion might not be diagnosed until it is advanced and ulcerative. The so-called clear cell variety may be related to in utero exposure to DES. It has a prognosis comparable to that of other adenocarcinomas of the cervix. The villoglandular-papillary variety of adenocarcinoma of the cervix tends to occur in younger women and have a more favorable prognosis.

D. ADENOMA MALIGNUM

Adenoma malignum or minimal deviation adenocarcinoma is an extremely well-differentiated adenocarcinoma that may be difficult to recognize as a malignant process. It represents approximately 1% of adenocarcinomas of the cervix and has been associated with Peutz-Jeghers syndrome. It occurs mainly in the fifth and sixth decades of life. Diagnosis is often delayed because of frequently normal cervical cytology smears. Punch biopsies are often nondiagnostic, requiring conization for further evaluation.

E. Adenoid Cystic Carcinoma

Another uncommon variant of adenocarcinoma is adenoid cystic carcinoma. This lesion is considered more aggressive than most cervical adenocarcinomas and occurs more commonly in black women of high parity in their sixth and seventh decades of life. It should not be confused with adenoid basal carcinomas, which have an indolent growth pattern.

F. Adenosquamous Carcinoma

Adenosquamous carcinomas contain an admixture of malignant squamous and glandular cells. Glassy cell carcinoma is a poorly differentiated form of adenosquamous carcinoma and is considered to have an extremely aggressive course. It accounts for approximately 1–2% of cervical cancers. Synchronous adenocarcinomas and squamous cell carcinomas that invade each other are called collision tumors.

G. Neuroendocrine Carcinomas

Approximately one-third of small cell carcinomas of the cervix stain positive for neuroendocrine markers. These tumors need to be distinguished from small cell type of squamous tumors. They have a high frequency of lymphovascular space invasion, lymph node metastases, recurrence, and poor survival. Carcinoid tumors, arising from the argyrophil cells of the endocervical epithelium, are malignant but have rarely been associated with the carcinoid syndrome. Because of their propensity for early systemic spread, systemic chemotherapy is an integral part of the treatment of neuroendocrine tumors of the cervix.

H. Other Malignant Tumors

Direct extension of metastatic tumors to the cervix include those originating from the endometrium, rectum, and bladder. Lymphatic or vascular metastases occur less often but are associated with endometrial, ovarian, gastric, breast, colon, kidney, and pancreas carcinomas. Sarcomas, lymphomas, choriocarcinomas, and melanomas are encountered rarely in the cervix.

Clinical Findings

A. Symptoms and Signs

Abnormal vaginal bleeding is the most common symptom of invasive cancer and may take the form of a blood-stained leukorrheal discharge, scant spotting, or frank bleeding. Leukorrhea, usually sanguineous or purulent, odorous, and nonpruritic, is frequently present. A history of postcoital bleeding may be elicited on specific questioning.

Pelvic pain, often unilateral and radiating to the hip or thigh, is a manifestation of advanced disease, as is the involuntary loss of urine or feces through the vagina, a sign of fistula formation. Weakness, weight loss, and anemia are characteristic of the late stages of the disease, although acute blood loss and anemia may occur in an ulcerating stage I lesion.

Physical examination findings include a grossly normal-appearing cervix with preclinical disease. As the local disease progresses, physical signs appear. Infiltrative cancer produces enlargement, irregularity, and a firm consistency of the cervix and eventually of the adjacent parametria. The growth pattern can be endophytic, leading to a barrel-shaped enlargement of the cervix, or exophytic, where the lesion generally appears as a friable, bleeding, cauliflowerlike lesion of the portio vaginalis. Ulceration may be the primary manifestation of invasive carcinoma; in the early stages the change often is superficial, so that it may resemble an ectropion or chronic cervicitis. With further progression of the disease, the ulcer becomes deeper and necrotic, with indurated edges and a friable, bleeding surface. The adjacent vaginal fornices may become involved next. Eventually, extensive parametrial involvement by the infiltrative process may produce a nodular thickening of the uterosacral and cardinal ligaments with resultant loss of mobility and fixation of the cervix.

B. Biopsy

Because of the failure of malignant cells to desquamate and the obscuring effect of inflammatory cells, it is not uncommon for an invasive carcinoma of the cervix to exist despite a negative cytologic smear. Any suspicious lesion of the cervix should be sampled by adequate biopsy, regardless of cytologic examination result. Biopsy of any Schiller-positive areas or of any ulcerative, granular, nodular, or papillary lesion provides the diagnosis in most cases. Colposcopically directed biopsies with endocervical curettage or conization of the cervix may be required when reports of suspicious or probable exfoliated carcinoma cells are made by the pathologist and a visible or palpable lesion of the cervix is not evident. Colposcopic warning signs of early invasive cancer in a field of CIN include capillaries that are markedly irregular, appearing as commas, corkscrews, and spaghetti-shaped vessels with great variation in caliber and abrupt changes in direction, often causing acute angles. Ulcerations or a markedly irregular appearance of the cervix with a waxy, yellowish surface and numerous bizarre, atypical blood vessels are common. Bleeding may occur also after slight irritation.

C. Conization

In the setting of a biopsy revealing carcinoma in situ, where invasion cannot be ruled out, or in the setting of a negative colposcopy in the face of a significantly abnormal cervical cytology smear, conization of the cervix should be performed to determine the presence or absence of invasion. If a cervical biopsy shows microinvasive cancer (< 3 mm of invasion), a cone biopsy is necessary to rule out deeper invasion. The conization specimen should be properly marked for the pathologist (eg, with a pin or small suture), so that the area of involvement can be specifically localized in relation to the circumference and margins of the cervix. Conization for a lesion grossly suggestive of invasive cancer is not indicated, as it only delays the initiation of appropriate therapy and predisposes the patient to serious pelvic infections and bleeding. The diagnosis of such a lesion can almost always be confirmed by simple cervical biopsy.

D. RADIOLOGIC FINDINGS

Chest radiographs are indicated in all patients with cervical cancer and an intravenous pyelogram (IVP) or computed tomography (CT) urogram should be performed to determine if there is any ureteral obstruction producing hydroureter and hydronephrosis. Magnetic resonance imaging (MRI), CT scan, lymphangiography, or positron emission tomography (PET) scanning may demonstrate involvement of the pelvic or periaortic lymph nodes or other sites of metastases. The sensitivities of CT, MRI, and PET for lymph node metastases in cervical cancer are approximately 45%, 60%, and 80%, respectively. Although the latter imaging studies are not used to assign disease stage in the International Federation of Gynecology and Obstetrics (FIGO) classification, they may be of value for planning treatment, particularly the extent of the radiation therapy field or scope of surgery.

Clinical Staging

It is important to estimate the extent of the disease not only for prognostic purposes but also for treatment planning. Clinical staging also affords a means of comparing methods of therapy for various stages of the disease worldwide. The classification adopted by FIGO is the most widely used staging system (Table 50–4). Cer-

Table 50–4. FIGO staging of cervical cancer (adopted from FIGO Annual Report on the Results of Treatment in Gynecologic Cancer 1998).

FIGO Stage	Definition
Stage 0	Carcinoma in situ
Stage I	Cervical carcinoma confined to the cervix (extension to the corpus would be disregarded)
Stage IA[1]	Invasive cervical cancer diagnosed by microscopy only
Stage IA1	Stromal invasion no deeper than 3 mm, no wider than 7 mm in horizontal spread
Stage IA2	Stromal invasion greater than 3, but less than 5 mm and no wider than 7 mm in horizontal spread
Stage IB	Clinically visible lesion confined to the cervix or microscopic disease greater than stage IA
Stage IB1	Lesion not greater than 4 cm
Stage IB2	Lesion greater than 4 cm
Stage II	Tumor extends beyond uterus but not to pelvic sidewall or lower third of vagina
Stage IIA	Vaginal involvement without parametrial involvement
Stage IIB	Parametrial involvement
Stage III	Tumor extends to pelvic sidewall and/or causes hydronephrosis and/or extends to lower third of vagina
Stage IIIA	Involvement of lower third of vagina with no extension to sidewall
Stage IIIB	Extension to pelvic sidewall and/or hydronephrosis
Stage IV	Extension beyond the true pelvis or into mucosa of rectum or bladder
Stage IVA[2]	Extension into adjacent organs
Stage IVB	Distant metastases

[1]The depth of invasion should be no more than 5 mm from the epithelial basement membrane of the adjacent most superficial epithelial papilla to the deepest point of invasion where the cancer originates. Vascular space invasion, venous or lymphatic, does not affect staging, but should be noted as it may affect future therapy. All macroscopically visible lesions (even with superficial invasion only) are allotted to stage IB.
[2]The presence of bullous edema is not sufficient to classify a tumor as stage IVA. The finding of malignant cells in cytologic bladder washings requires further histologic confirmation in order to be considered stage IVA.

vical cancer is staged by clinical examination, and evaluation of the bladder, ureters, and rectum. If the lesion is clearly confined to the cervix by office examination, only chest radiography and evaluation of the ureters by IVP or CT scan with intravenous contrast is necessary to assign the stage. If it is not possible to evaluate the extent of local disease in the office, examination under anesthesia with cystoscopy and proctoscopy may be necessary. Although CT scan, MRI, lymphangiography, and PET scan may offer information helpful for treatment planning, these findings do not change the FIGO stage of disease. The FIGO stage of disease is also not changed by surgicopathologic findings of metastatic disease at the time of radical hysterectomy or lymphadenectomy.

Differential Diagnosis

A variety of lesions of the cervix can be confused with cancer. Entities that must sometimes be ruled out include cervical ectropion, acute or chronic cervicitis, condyloma acuminata, cervical tuberculosis, ulceration secondary to sexually transmitted disease (syphilis, granuloma inguinale, lymphogranuloma venereum, chancroid), abortion of a cervical pregnancy, metastatic choriocarcinoma or other cancers, and rare lesions such as those of actinomycosis or schistosomiasis. Histopathologic examination is usually definitive.

Complications

The complications of cervical cancer, for the most part, are those related to tumor size or invasion, necrosis of the tumor, infection, and metastatic disease. The natural history of the disease was outlined above. There are also problems pertaining to treatment of the disease (eg, radical surgery or radiation therapy; see Treatment, below).

Prevention

Until now, prevention of morbidity and death from cervical cancer largely involved recognition and treatment of preinvasive and early invasive disease. Currently, approximately 60% of women who develop cervical cancer in developed countries either never had been screened or had not been screened in the preceding 5 years. Risk factors must be recognized, and screening, treatment intervention, and patient education must be modified respectively.

Universal cytologic screening of all postpubertal women must be continued on a regular basis until better, more sensitive and specific means of screening are found, and outreach into underserved areas is improved. Women with preinvasive cervical neoplasia should be treated and followed up closely (Fig 50–6). It is important to remember that cervical cytology smears are of limited value in detecting frankly invasive disease, with some studies finding false-negative rates up to 50%. Sexual abstinence is an effective but impractical prophylactic measure. Education of young women and men about risk factors and the necessity for regular screening, as well as information about the association of HIV infection and smoking with the development of cervical cancers, is crucial.

Several HPV vaccines are currently in advanced stages of development. Gardasil a quadrivalent vaccine against HPV 16/18/6/11 received FDA approval in the United States in June 2006 for use in girls and women 9–26 years old. To date, large trials have demonstrated that the vaccines are generally safe, well tolerated and highly immunogenic with excellent efficacy in the prevention of persistent HPV infection and against the development of cytologic abnormalities.

Treatment

Invasive carcinoma of the cervix spreads primarily by direct extension and lymphatic dissemination. The therapy of patients with cervical cancer needs to address not only the primary tumor site, but also the adjacent tissues and lymph nodes. This is generally accomplished by either radical hysterectomy and pelvic lymphadenectomy, radiation with concomitant chemotherapy, or a combination thereof.

A. TREATMENT OF EARLY STAGE DISEASE (STAGE IA2 TO IIA)

Patients with early stage cervical cancer may be treated with either radical hysterectomy and pelvic lymphadenectomy or with primary radiation with concomitant chemotherapy. The overall 5-year cure rates for surgery and for radiation therapy in operable patients are approximately equal. The advantage of surgery is that the ovaries may be left intact and be transposed out of the radiation field if adjuvant postoperative therapy appears necessary, that the extent of disease can be determined surgicopathologically, and that grossly metastatic lymph nodes can be resected. Furthermore, surgery may be more appropriate in sexually active women with early stage disease as radiation causes vaginal stenosis and atrophy. Adjuvant radiation with concomitant chemotherapy is administered to selected patients at increased risk for recurrence following radical hysterectomy.

1. Radical hysterectomy and therapeutic lymphadenectomy—Radical hysterectomy (techniques initially described by Wertheim, Meigs, and Okabayashi) with pelvic lymphadenectomy is the surgical procedure for invasive cancer limited to the cervix (stages I and II). The operation is technically difficult and should be performed only by those experienced in radical pelvic surgery. Surgery involves dissection of the ureters from the paracervical structures so that the ligaments supporting the uterus and upper vagina can be removed. When the operation is done vaginally, a deep Schuchardt (paravaginal) incision is required for exposure. Five different types of hysterectomy have been described based upon the extent of parametrial dissection and vaginal tissue removed (Table 50–5). Typically, a type I hysterectomy is indicated for patients with stage IA1 disease. An alternative treatment is cervical conization in the young patient wishing to preserve fertility. Stage IA2 to II A are treated with a type II (modified radical) or type III (radical) hysterectomy. It is rarely necessary to remove as much vaginal tissue as was initially recommended. As long as complete tumor clearance can be provided, a modified radical hysterectomy appears to provide therapeutic outcomes comparable to a radical hysterectomy for stage IB and IIA disease, but with shorter operating time and lower urologic morbidity. Full pelvic lymphadenectomy is indicated at the time of radical hysterectomy, followed by paraaortic lymphadenectomy for tumors larger than 2 cm or those with suspicious pelvic lymph nodes. Resection of all grossly involved lymph nodes provides a distinct survival advantage. Microscopic evaluation of the lymph nodes allows for tailoring of the postoperative radiation field, if indicated.

2. Adjuvant postoperative radiation— Postoperative adjuvant radiation therapy with concomitant chemotherapy is indicated in women with localized cervical cancer at high risk for recurrent disease, such as positive lymph nodes, positive or close resection margins, or microscopic parametrial involvement. In this setting, adjuvant radiation with platinum-based chemotherapy is superior to adjuvant radiation alone, with an improvement in the 4-year progression-free interval from 63% to 80%. Women with intermediate-risk factors for recurrent disease, such as large tumor size, deep cervical stromal invasion, and lymphovascular space invasion, also benefit from postoperative adjuvant radiation. These patients have an improved 2-year recurrence-free survival of 88% with adjuvant radiation versus 79% without adjuvant therapy.

3. Primary radiation with concomitant chemotherapy—For the treatment of early cervical cancer (stages IA to IIA), primary therapy with definitive radiation or radical surgery followed by tailored radiation if indicated by the surgical findings produce comparable outcomes. The choice of treatment depends on the tumor size, the general condition of the patient, and preferences of the oncologists at the treating institution. Surgery is often preferred for young patients in the hope of preserving ovarian function. If it is likely that the patient will need postoperative radiation therapy, transposition of the ovaries to a location outside the radiation field can be performed. For primary radiation of cervical cancer, external beam radiation is used in combination with intracavitary irradiation (see Chapter 54). At least five controlled trials have demonstrated the superi-

Table 50–5. Types of hysterectomy based on radicality.

Type of Hysterectomy	Principles of Procedure
Type I	Extrafascial hysterectomy with removal of all cervical tissue without dissecting into the cervix itself.
Type II	The uterine artery is ligated where it crosses over the ureter. The uterosacral and cardinal ligaments are divided midway towards their attachment to sacrum and pelvic sidewall. The upper third of the vagina is resected.
Type III	The uterine artery is ligated at its origin from the superior vesical or internal iliac artery. Uterosacral and cardinal ligaments are resected at their attachments to the sacrum and pelvic sidwall. The upper half of the vagina is resected.
Type IV	The ureter is completely dissected from the vesicouterine ligament, the superior vesical artery is sacrificed, and three fourths of the vagina is resected.
Type V	Involves the additional resection of a portion of the bladder or the distal ureter with ureteral reimplantation into the bladder

ority of radiation with concomitant platinum-based chemotherapy over radiation alone. This has led to the adoption of radiation plus concomitant chemotherapy as the standard of care whenever radiation therapy is given for the treatment of cervical cancer over a broad spectrum of disease stages.

Special Situations

A. Stage IA1 Disease

The definitive diagnosis of microinvasive squamous cell carcinoma of the cervix can only be made by conization. These patients may be treated by simple abdominal or vaginal hysterectomy. For a young woman desiring to maintain fertility, only conization is an acceptable treatment modality for microinvasive squamous cell carcinoma with a depth of invasion of 3 mm or less, if the conization margins are negative, and if there is no evidence of lymphovascular space invasion. If margin and endocervical curettage are positive, the risk of residual disease is as high as 33%. In this case, repeat conization should be performed if uterine preservation is the goal. FIGO staging is not influenced by the presence of lymphovascular space invasion, which occurs in close to 10% of patients with stage IA1 disease. These patients have a small but significant risk for lymph node metastases to parametrial and pelvic lymph nodes. This subgroup of patients should therefore be treated like patients with stage IA2 disease. There is considerable controversy regarding the existence of microinvasive adenocarcinoma and its pathologic diagnostic criteria, which is beyond the scope of this chapter.

B. RADICAL TRACHELECTOMY

During the last decade, radical trachelectomy has evolved as an alternative to radical hysterectomy in carefully selected young women with early stage (IA2 or small IB1) cervical cancer who wish to preserve fertility. A therapeutic lymphadenectomy is performed and following radical resection of the cervix a cerclage is placed. Experience with this technique is growing, and the oncologic outcome appears comparable to radical hysterectomy in carefully selected patients. A review of pregnancy outcomes in women who underwent radical trachelectomy revealed 16% first trimester miscarriages, 10% second trimester losses, 19% preterm deliveries, and a 49% term delivery rate.

C. BULKY CERVICAL CANCER

The management of patients with stage IB2 and bulky IIA disease is a matter of considerable debate. Proposed management strategies include the following.

1. Primary radiation therapy with concomitant chemotherapy and the option of a subsequent adjuvant extrafascial hysterectomy—Radiation therapy is usually recommended for patients with bulky cervical cancers, recently with the addition of concomitant chemotherapy. Many of these tumors, however, contain hypoxic central areas that do not respond well to radiation, as is reflected in a 15–35% pelvic failure rate. This provides the rationale for the performance of an adjuvant hysterectomy following radiation, which is associated with a significant reduction in pelvic recurrences to 2–5%. However, the impact of adjuvant hysterectomy on extrapelvic recurrences and survival is less-well established.

2. Primary radical hysterectomy and therapeutic lymphadenectomy, followed by tailored radiation with concomitant chemotherapy when indicated by pathologic findings—The potential benefits of this approach include the removal of the large primary tumor, complete surgical staging with the opportunity to resect any grossly involved lymph nodes, and the preservation of ovarian function as ovarian transposition can be performed if adjuvant radiation therapy is likely. If postoperative radiation becomes necessary, the radiation field can be tailored to the surgicopathologic findings. The resection of macroscopically involved lymph nodes has a therapeutic benefit because it improves survival to that of patients with microscopic

lymph node metastases only. A primary surgical approach should be taken in patients with acute or chronic pelvic inflammatory disease, an undiagnosed coexistent adnexal mass, or anatomic alterations that make radiation therapy difficult.

3. Neoadjuvant chemotherapy followed by radical hysterectomy and lymphadenectomy and subsequent chemoradiation when indicated by pathologic findings—Neoadjuvant chemotherapy, frequently three cycles of platinum-based combination therapy followed by radical hysterectomy and lymphadenectomy, was recently proposed as a novel treatment strategy for these patients. Neoadjuvant chemotherapy is reported to improve the resectability of bulky lesions, pelvic disease control, and possibly long-term survival. Although this is a provocative treatment strategy, in most studies, patients ultimately received multimodality treatment with chemotherapy, radical surgery, and radiation. Further randomized studies are needed to determine the precise role of neoadjuvant chemotherapy in the treatment of these patients.

B. TREATMENT OF LOCALLY ADVANCED DISEASE (STAGE IIB TO IVA)

Patients with locally advanced cervical cancer are best treated with primary radiation (external beam plus brachytherapy; see Chapter 54A) with concomitant chemotherapy. Extended field radiation should be considered in the presence of paraaortic lymph node metastases documented at surgical staging or by imaging, especially when biopsy confirmed and in the absence of other systemic metastases. The benefit of cisplatin-based combined modality therapy over radiation alone for advanced disease has been demonstrated in at least three randomized controlled trials, which found a 30–50% reduction in the risk of death from cervical cancer for patients treated with chemoradiation compared to those treated with radiation alone. This difference is most significant for patients with stage II disease (and bulky IB disease) in whom, in one study, chemoradiation, compared to radiation alone, improved 5-year survival rates from 58% to 77%. For patients with more advanced disease, the benefits associated with chemoradiation versus radiation alone appear less pronounced, with the same study showing a small, statistically insignificant improvement in 5-year survival from 57% to 63%. The optimal drug regimen is not known, but combination therapy did not show superior results over weekly single-agent cisplatin, and the latter was associated with substantially less toxicity.

C. TREATMENT OF DISSEMINATED PRIMARY (STAGE IVB) AND PERSISTENT OR RECURRENT DISEASE

The use of chemotherapeutic agents in the treatment of cervical carcinoma has been discouraging. This is partly because most patients who may be candidates for this type of treatment either present with disseminated disease or have cancer that has already failed to respond to radical surgery or radiation therapy. Modest activity in recurrent or disseminated cervical cancer has been observed with single-agent cisplatin, ifosfamide, paclitaxel, and vinorelbine. There is a small therapeutic survival advantage to multiagent chemotherapy with cisplatin and topotecan. Combination therapy using paclitaxel and platinum offers very similar outcomes, with response rates of 36% compared to 27% for cisplatin and topotecan, and a median survival of 9.7 months compared to 9.6 months with cisplatin and topotecan. Palliative pelvic radiation therapy may be indicated, especially for the control of hemorrhage. If a patient develops a palpable mass in the left supraclavicular region, it can be palliated with radiation therapy with concomitant chemotherapy, with or without resection.

D. TOTAL PELVIC EXENTERATION FOR ISOLATED CENTRAL PELVIC RECURRENCE OF DISEASE

Patients who develop a central recurrence of cervical cancer after primary therapy with radiation or after surgery followed by radiation may be candidates for this extensive, potentially curative surgical procedure if a complete evaluation fails to reveal evidence of metastatic disease. In a small proportion of patients with cancer of the cervix treated initially with radiation, a small recurrence of the cancer may be noted centrally within the cervix. A radical hysterectomy may be an alternative to total pelvic exenteration in this selected subgroup of patients. Surgery is the only potentially curative method of treating cancers that persist or recur centrally following adequate radiation therapy. In such instances, pelvic exenteration is often necessary to make certain that all of the cancer has been removed.

Pelvic exenteration is one of the most formidable of all gynecologic operations and requires removal of the bladder, rectum, and vagina, along with the uterus if hysterectomy has not yet been performed. This is followed by the reconstructive phase of the procedure. Urinary diversion needs to be provided, necessitating the creation of either a continent ileocolonic pouch or a noncontinent ileal conduit. In either case, a stoma is created in the anterior abdominal wall. If extensive rectal resection was required, a sigmoid colostomy serves for the passage of feces. If a low rectal anastomosis could be accomplished, a temporary diverting colostomy should be performed in all patients who had received prior radiation. The vagina can be reconstructed using various myocutaneous flaps, such as transverse rectus abdominis or gracilis myocutaneous flaps. Depending on the location of the lesion, an anterior (preservation of the rectosigmoid) or posterior (preservation of the bladder) exenteration is at times an alternative.

Because of the high surgical morbidity and mortality rates, stringent criteria are necessary to justify these procedures. Pelvic exenteration should be reserved primarily for problems that cannot be effectively managed in any other manner. In essence, this means (a) a biopsy-proven persistence or recurrence of cervical cancer following an adequate course of radiation therapy or radical surgery in which the recurrent or persistent tumor occupies the central portion of the pelvis (without metastases) and is completely removable; and (b) a patient who is able to cope with the urinary and fecal stomas in the abdomen created by the operation. Both psychological and physical preparation of the patient for this operation and its aftermath are of vital importance. Because of the extreme difficulties encountered in making an accurate assessment preoperatively, only about half of the patients explored for a total pelvic exenteration will intraoperatively be confirmed to have resectable, nonmetastatic disease. The 5-year survival rate following pelvic exenteration for recurrent cervical cancer averages 30–40%.

E. PALLIATIVE CARE

Comprehensive care of a patient with cancer involves in addition to antitumor therapy, good symptom relief, as well as personal and family support. The palliative care for patients with progressive cervical cancer poses many challenges. The emphasis should be to facilitate comfort, dignity, autonomy, and personal rehabilitation and development, especially in the face of an incurable disease.

Most patients with progressive cervical cancer eventually develop symptoms related principally to the site and extent of the malignant disease. Ulceration of the cervix and adjacent vagina produces a foul-smelling discharge. Tissue necrosis and slough may initiate life-threatening hemorrhage. If the bladder or rectum is involved in the tissue breakdown, fistulas result in incontinence of urine and feces. Pain caused by involvement of the lumbosacral plexus, soft tissues of the pelvis, or bone is frequently encountered in advanced disease. Ureteral compression leading to hydronephrosis and, if bilateral, to renal failure and uremia is a common terminal event. The comfort and well-being of the patient can be considerably enhanced even though cure cannot be effected. A foul, purulent discharge may be ameliorated by astringent douches and antimicrobial vaginal creams or suppositories. Hemorrhage from the vagina often can be controlled by packing the area with gauze impregnated with a hemostatic agent; occasionally emergent radiation or hypogastric artery embolization is indicated.

Current management of severe pain combines the use of a long-acting narcotic such as morphine or a transdermal fentanyl patch with short-acting narcotics for breakthrough pain and nonsteroidal anti-inflammatory agents. Anxiolytics and antidepressants may be of considerable value. For patients with significant pain who are no longer responding to oral medications, a subcutaneous or intravenous morphine drip can be started. In patients with lower back or extremity pain, a peridural catheter can be placed and connected to a subcutaneous pump with a reservoir for continuous morphine instillation. This method gives pain relief without the sedating effects of oral and parenteral narcotics.

Radiation therapy may be very helpful in the relief of pain caused by bony metastases and in the treatment of lesions that recur following primary surgical treatment of cervical cancer. In general, if initial therapy was accomplished by adequate radiation therapy, retreatment is contraindicated because it does little good and carries the potential of massive radiation necrosis.

Special Situations

A. CARCINOMA OF THE CERVIX DURING PREGNANCY

Invasive carcinoma of the cervix in pregnancy is found more frequently in areas where routine prenatal cytologic examination is done. Abnormal cervical cytology in pregnancy calls for immediate colposcopic evaluation and any other diagnostic modalities necessary to exclude invasive cancer (see section on preinvasive disease).

Invasive cervical cancer complicates approximately 0.05% of pregnancies. As is the case with nonpregnant patients, the principal symptom is bleeding, but the diagnosis is frequently missed because the bleeding is assumed to be related to the pregnancy rather than to cancer. The possibility of cancer must be kept in mind. The diagnosis and management of invasive cervical cancer during pregnancy presents the patient and the physician with many challenges. Pregnancy does not appear to affect the prognosis for women with cervical cancer and the fetus is not affected by the maternal disease, but may suffer morbidity from its treatment (eg, preterm delivery).

If the pregnancy is early and the disease is stage I to IIA, radical hysterectomy and therapeutic lymphadenectomy can be performed with the fetus left in situ, unless the patient is unwilling to terminate the pregnancy. Women at a gestational age closer to fetal viability or who are unwilling to lose the baby may decide to continue the pregnancy after careful discussion regarding the maternal risks. Delivery in patients with cervical dysplasia and carcinoma in situ may be via the vaginal route. Patients with invasive cervical cancer should be delivered by cesarean section to avoid potential cervical hemorrhage and dissemination of tumor cells during vaginal delivery. A cesarean radical hysterectomy with therapeutic lymphadenectomy is the procedure of choice for patients with stages IA2–IIA disease as soon as adequate fetal maturity is established.

As in the nonpregnant patient, radiation with concomitant chemotherapy is used for the treatment of more advanced disease. In the first trimester, irradiation may be carried out with the expectation of spontaneous abortion. In the second trimester, interruption of the pregnancy by hysterotomy prior to radiation therapy is preferred, although some physicians advocate proceeding with immediate radiation treatment, again awaiting spontaneous evacuation of the uterus. In selected cases with locally advanced disease in which the patient declines pregnancy termination, consideration may be given to neoadjuvant chemotherapy in an effort to prevent disease progression during the time needed to achieve fetal maturity. Delivery should be by cesarean section. A lymphadenectomy can be performed at the same time. Postpartum the patient should receive chemoradiation following guidelines established for the nonpregnant patient.

B. CARCINOMA OF THE CERVICAL STUMP

Early stage cervical cancer noted on a cervical stump (left in situ following supracervical hysterectomy for an unrelated indication) should be treated with radical trachelectomy and therapeutic lymphadenectomy in the medically fit patient. Surgery is preferred over chemoradiation in this setting as the delivery of an adequate radiation dose may be difficult in a patient with a short cervical stump. However, radiation with concomitant chemotherapy is the preferred treatment modality for patients with more advanced disease.

C. CERVICAL CANCER INCIDENTALLY DIAGNOSED AFTER SIMPLE HYSTERECTOMY

Women who are found to have microinvasive disease after a simple hysterectomy do not require any additional therapy. Patients with invasive disease who do not have gross parametrial disease are candidates for a radical parametrectomy, upper vaginectomy, and lymphadenectomy. This approach may be particularly desirable for young women in whom ovarian function can be preserved or for any surgically fit women with enlarged lymph nodes that should be resected prior to chemoradiation. Indications for chemoradiation follow the same guidelines as outlined above.

Complications of Therapy

A. RADICAL SURGERY

The operative mortality rate in radical hysterectomy with lymphadenectomy has been reduced to less than 1%. The most common complication is prolonged bladder dysfunction. Approximately 75% of patients have adequate recovery of bladder function within 1–2 weeks after radical hysterectomy, and most patients will have satisfactory voiding function by 3 weeks. Serious complications include fistula formation; ureterovaginal

Table 50–6. Survival of patients with cervical cancer based on FIGO stage.

Stage	Number of Patients (%)	Survival		
		1 year	2 years	5 years
IA1	860	99.8%	99.5%	98.7%
IA2	227	98.2%	97.7%	95.9%
IB	3480	98.1%	94.0%	86.5%
IIA	881	94.1%	85.6%	68.8%
IIB	2375	93.3%	80.7%	64.7%
IIIA	160	82.8%	58.8%	40.4%
IIIB	1949	81.5%	62.2%	43.3%
IVA	245	56.1%	35.6%	19.5%
IVB	189	45.8%	23.9%	15.0%

fistula is the most common type (1–2%), followed by vesicovaginal and rectovaginal fistulas. Modified radical hysterectomy as compared to radical hysterectomy is associated with a shorter operating time, a more rapid return of bladder function, and fewer fistulas. Other complications are urinary tract infections, lymphocysts and lymphedema, wound sepsis, dehiscence, thromboembolic disease, ileus, postoperative hemorrhage, and intestinal obstruction.

The surgical mortality rate from pelvic exenteration has been reduced from approximately 25% to less than 5%, but as many as 50% of patients experience major morbidity. Complications include intraoperative and postoperative hemorrhage, infectious morbidity, urinary fistulas or obstruction, urinary pouch dysfunction, pyelonephritis, bowel obstruction or intestinal leaks and fistulas, stomal retraction, electrolyte disturbances, and other less common occurrences.

B. RADIATION THERAPY WITH CONCOMITANT CHEMOTHERAPY

See Chapters 54A and B.

Posttreatment Follow-Up

Approximately 35% of patients with invasive cervical cancer will have recurrent or persistent disease following therapy. Approximately 50% of deaths from cervical cancer occur in the first year after treatment, another 25% in the second year, and 15% in the third year. This explains the generally accepted schedule of posttreatment surveillance in asymptomatic patients of every 3 months in the first year, every 4 months in the second year, and every 6 months in years 3–5. Symptomatic patients should be evaluated with appropriate examinations immediately when symptoms occur. The most common signs and symptoms of recurrent malignant disease are positive cytologic examination, palpable tumor in the pelvis or abdomen, ulceration of the cervix or vagina, pain in the pelvis, back, groin, and lower extremity, unilateral lower extremity edema, vaginal bleeding or discharge, supraclavicular lymphadenopathy, ascites, unexplained weight loss, progressive ureteral obstruction, and cough (especially with hemoptysis or chest pain).

Prognosis

The major prognostic factors affecting survival are stage, lymph node status, tumor volume, depth of cervical stromal invasion, lymphovascular space invasion and, to a lesser extent, histologic type and grade. After stage of disease, lymph node status is the most important prognostic factor. For example, following radical surgery, patients with stage IB or IIA disease have a 5-year survival of 88–96% with negative lymph nodes, compared to 64–73% in the presence of lymph node metastases.

Table 50–6 summarizes survival rates by stage of disease. These are based on the FIGO Annual Report on the Results of Treatment in Gynecological Cancer, in which results of treatment for each stage of cervical cancer are reported by more than 100 participating institutions worldwide. The results are equated in terms of 5-year cure rates, or those patients who are living and show no evidence of cervical cancer 5 years after beginning therapy.

Recurrences following radiation therapy are not often centrally located and thus amenable to exenteration procedures. Only approximately 25% of recurrences are localized to the central portion of the pelvis. The most common site of recurrence is the pelvic side wall.

REFERENCES

Cervical Intraepithelial Neoplasia

Ahdieh L et al: Cervical neoplasia and repeated positivity of human papillomavirus infection in human immunodeficiency virus-seropositive and -seronegative women. Am J Epidemiol 2000; 151:1148.

American College of Obstetricians and Gynecologists. Management of abnormal cervical cytology and histology. Practice Bulletin Number 66. Obstet Gynecol 2005;106:645.

Arbyn M et al: Virologic versus cytologic triage of women with equivocal Pap smears: A meta-analysis of the accuracy to detect high-grade intraepithelial neoplasia. J Natl Cancer Inst 2004;96:280.

Arends MJ, Buckley CH, Wells M: Etiology, pathogenesis, and pathology of cervical neoplasia. J Clin Pathol 1998;51:96.

The Atypical Squamous Cell of Undetermined Significance/Low-Grade Squamous Intraepithelial Lesions Triage Study (ALTS) Group: Human papillomavirus testing for triage of women with cytologic evidence of low-grade squamous intraepithelial lesions: baseline data from a randomized trial. J Natl Cancer Inst 2000;92:397.

The Atypical Squamous Cell of Undetermined Significance/Low-Grade Squamous Intraepithelial Lesions Triage Study (ALTS) Group: Results of a randomized trial on the management of cytology interpretations of atypical squamous cells of undetermined significance. Am J Obstet Gynecol 2003;188:1383.

Denehy TR, Gregori CA, Breen JL: Endocervical curettage, cone margins, and residual adenocarcinoma in situ of the cervix. Obstet Gynecol 1997;90:1.

Gage JC et al: Number of cervical biopsies and sensitivity of colposcopy. Obstet Gynecol 2006;108:264.

Guido R et al: Postcolposcopy management strategies for women referred with low-grade squamous intraepithelial lesions or human papillomavirus DNA-positive atypical squamous cells of undetermined significance: A two-year prospective study. Am J Obstet Gynecol 2003;188:1401.

Harper DM et al: Efficacy of a bivalent L1 virus-like particle vaccine in prevention of infection with human papillomavirus types 16 and 18 in young women: A randomised controlled trial. Lancet 2004;364(9447):1757.

Ho GY et al: Natural history of cervicovaginal papillomavirus infection in young women. N Engl J Med 1998;338:423.

Holowaty P et al: Natural history of dysplasia of the uterine cervix. J Natl Cancer Inst 1999;91:252.

Im DD, Duska LR, Rosenshein NB: Adequacy of conization margins in adenocarcinoma in situ of the cervix as a predictor of residual disease. Gynecol Oncol 1995;59:179.

Koutsky LA et al: A controlled trial of a human papillomavirus type 16 vaccine. N Engl J Med 2002;347(21):1645.

Maiman M et al: Cervical cancer as an AIDS-defining illness. Obstet Gynecol 1997;89:76.

Martin-Hirsch PL, Paraskevaidis E, Kitchener H: Surgery for cervical intraepithelial neoplasia. Cochrane Database Syst Rev 2000;CD001318.

McIndoe WA et al: The invasive potential of carcinoma in situ of the cervix. Obstet Gynecol 1984;64:451.

Melnikow J et al: Natural history of cervical squamous intraepithelial lesions: A meta-analysis. Obstet Gynecol 1998;92:727.

Moscicki AB et al: Regression of low-grade squamous intraepithelial lesions in young women. Lancet 2004;364:1678.

Munoz N et al: Epidemiologic classification of human papillomavirus types associated with cervical cancer. N Engl J Med 2003; 348:518.

Olsen AO et al: Combined effect of smoking and human papillomavirus type 16 infection in cervical carcinogenesis. Epidemiology 1998;9:346.

Poynor EA, Barakat RR, Hoskins WJ: Management and follow-up of patients with adenocarcinoma in situ of the uterine cervix. Gynecol Oncol 1995;57:158.

Prokopczyk B et al: Identification of tobacco-specific carcinogen in the cervical mucus of smokers and nonsmokers. J Natl Cancer Inst 1997;89:868.

Saslow D et al: American Cancer Society guideline for the early detection of cervical neoplasia and cancer. CA Cancer J Clin 2002;52(6):342.

Solomon D et al: The 2001 Bethesda system terminology for reporting results of cervical cytology. JAMA 2002;287:2114.

Solomon D, Schiffman M, Tarone R: Comparison of three management strategies for patients with atypical squamous cells of undetermined significance: Baseline results from a randomized trial. J Natl Cancer Inst 2001;93:293.

Soutter WP et al: Invasive cervical cancer after conservative therapy for cervical intraepithelial neoplasia. Lancet 1997;349: 978.

Wallin KL et al: Type-specific persistence of human papillomavirus DNA before the development of invasive cervical cancer. N Engl J Med 1999;341:1633.

Wolf JK et al: Adenocarcinoma in situ of the cervix: Significance of cone biopsy margins. Obstet Gynecol 1996;88:82.

Wright TC Jr et al: 2001 Consensus guidelines for the management of women with cervical intraepithelial neoplasia. Am J Obstet Gynecol 2003;189:295.

Wright TC Jr et al: 2001 Consensus guidelines for the management of women with cervical cytological abnormalities. JAMA 2002;287:2120.

Ylitalo N et al: Consistent high viral load of human papillomavirus 16 and risk of cervical carcinoma in situ: A nested case-control study. Lancet 2000;355:2194.

Yost NP et al: Postpartum regression rates of antepartum cervical intraepithelial neoplasia II and III lesions. Obstet Gynecol 1999;93:359.

Cancer of the Cervix

Anderson B et al: Ovarian transposition in cervical cancer. Gynecol Oncol 1993;49:206.

Ault KA: Vaccines for the prevention of human papillomavirus and associated gynecologic diseases: a review. Obstet Gynecol Surv 2006;61(6 Suppl 1):S26.

Averette HE et al: Radical hysterectomy for invasive cervical cancer: A 25-year prospective experience with the Miami technique. Cancer 1993;71:1422.

Benedet JL et al: FIGO annual report: Carcinoma of the cervix uteri. Int J Gynaecol Obstet 2003;83(Suppl 1):41.

Benedet JL et al: FIGO staging classifications and clinical practice guidelines in the management of gynecologic cancers. FIGO Committee on Gynecologic Oncology. Int J Gynaecol Obstet 2000;70:209.

Cosin JA et al: Pretreatment surgical staging of patients with cervical carcinoma: the case for lymph node debulking. Cancer 1998;82: 2241.

Dargent D et al: Laparoscopic vaginal radical trachelectomy: a treatment to preserve the fertility of cervical carcinoma patients. Cancer 2000;88:1877.

Eifel PJ et al: The relationship between brachytherapy dose and outcome in patients with bulky endocervical tumors treated with radiation alone. Int J Radiat Oncol Biol Phys 1994;28:113.

Feeney DD et al: The fate of the ovaries after radical hysterectomy and ovarian transposition. Gynecol Oncol 1995;56:3.

Gallion HH et al: Combined radiation therapy and extrafascial hysterectomy in the treatment of stage IB barrel-shaped cervical cancer. Cancer 1985;56:262.

Hacker NF, Wain GV, Nicklin JL: Resection of bulky positive lymph nodes in patients with cervical carcinoma. Int J Gynaecol Cancer 1995;5:250.

Hopkins MP, Lavin JP: Cervical cancer in pregnancy. Gynecol Oncol 1996;63:293.

Hricak H et al: Role of imaging in pretreatment evaluation of early invasive cervical cancer: results of the intergroup study American College of Radiology Imaging Network 6651-Gynecologic Oncology Group 183. J Clin Oncol 2005;23:9329.

Jemal A et al: Cancer statistics 2005. CA Cancer J Clin 2005;55(1):10.

Keys HM et al: Cisplatin, radiation, and adjuvant hysterectomy compared with radiation and adjuvant hysterectomy for bulky stage IB cervical carcinoma. N Engl J Med 1999; 340:1154.

Landoni F et al: Class II versus class III radical hysterectomy in stage IB–IIA cervical cancer: A prospective randomized study. Gynecol Oncol 2001;80:3.

Landoni F et al: Randomised study of radical surgery versus radiotherapy for stage IB–IIA cervical cancer. Lancet 1997;350:535.

Lazo PA: The molecular genetics of cervical carcinoma. Br J Cancer 1999;80:2008.

Lee YN et al: Radical hysterectomy with pelvic lymph node dissection for treatment of cervical cancer: A clinical review of 954 cases. Gynecol Oncol 1989;32:135.

Long HJ 3rd et al: Randomized phase III trial of cisplatin with or without topotecan in carcinoma of the uterine cervix: A Gynecologic Oncology Group Study. J Clin Oncol 2005;23(21):4626.

Metcalf KS et al: Site specific lymph node metastasis in carcinoma of the cervix: Is there a sentinel node? Int J Gynecol Cancer 2000;10:411.

Moore DH et al: Phase III study of cisplatin with or without paclitaxel in stage IVB, recurrent, or persistent squamous cell carcinoma of the cervix: A gynecologic oncology group study. J Clin Oncol 2004;22(15):3113.

Morris M et al: Pelvic radiation with concurrent chemotherapy compared with pelvic and para-aortic radiation for high-risk cervical cancer. N Engl J Med 1999;340:1137.

Omura GA: Chemotherapy for stage IVB or recurrent cancer of the uterine cervix. J Natl Cancer Inst Monogr 1996;21:123.

Omura GA et al: Randomized trial of cisplatin versus cisplatin plus mitolactol versus cisplatin plus ifosfamide in advanced squamous carcinoma of the cervix: A Gynecologic Oncology Group study. J Clin Oncol 1997;15:165.

Parkin DM, Pisani P, Ferlay J: Global cancer statistics. CA Cancer J Clin 1999;49:33.

Perez CA et al: Irradiation alone or combined with surgery in stage IB, IIA, and IIB carcinoma of uterine cervix: Update of a nonrandomized comparison. Int J Radiat Oncol Biol Phys 1995;31:703.

Peters WA III et al: Concurrent chemotherapy and pelvic radiation therapy compared with pelvic radiation therapy alone as adjuvant therapy after radical surgery in high-risk early-stage cancer of the cervix. J Clin Oncol 2000;18:1606.

Piver MS, Rutledge F, Smith JP: Five classes of extended hysterectomy for women with cervical cancer. Obstet Gynecol 1974;44:265.

Plante M et al: Vaginal radical trachelectomy: An oncologically safe fertility-preserving surgery. An updated series of 72 cases and review of the literature. Gynecol Oncol 2004;94(3):614.

Plante M et al: Vaginal radical trachelectomy: A valuable fertility-preserving option in the management of early-stage cervical cancer. A series of 50 pregnancies and review of the literature. Gynecol Oncol 2005;98(1):3.

Roman LD et al: Risk of residual invasive disease in women with microinvasive squamous cancer in a conization specimen. Obstet Gynecol 1997;90:759.

Rose PG et al: Concurrent cisplatin-based radiotherapy and chemotherapy for locally advanced cervical cancer. N Engl J Med 1999;340:1144.

Rotman M et al: A phase III randomized trial of postoperative pelvic irradiation in stage IB cervical carcinoma with poor prognostic features: follow-up of a gynecologic oncology group study. Int J Radiat Oncol Biol Phys 2006;65:169.

Sardi JE et al: Long-term follow-up of the first randomized trial using neoadjuvant chemotherapy in stage IB squamous carcinoma of the cervix: The final results. Gynecol Oncol 1997;67:61.

Sasieni PD, Cuzick J, Lynch-Farmery E: Estimating the efficacy of screening by auditing smear histories of women with and without cervical cancer. The National Co-ordinating Network for Cervical Screening Working Group. Br J Cancer 1996;73:1001.

Sedlis A et al: A randomized trial of pelvic radiation therapy versus no further therapy in selected patients with stage IB carcinoma of the cervix after radical hysterectomy and pelvic lymphadenectomy: A Gynecologic Oncology Group Study. Gynecol Oncol 1999;73:177.

Sood AK et al: Cervical cancer diagnosed shortly after pregnancy: Prognostic variables and delivery routes. Obstet Gynecol 2000;95:832.

Sutton GP et al: Ovarian metastases in stage IB carcinoma of the cervix: A Gynecologic Oncology Group study. Am J Obstet Gynecol 1992;166:50.

Tewari K et al: Neoadjuvant chemotherapy in the treatment of locally advanced cervical carcinoma in pregnancy: A report of two cases and review of issues specific to the management of cervical carcinoma in pregnancy including planned delay of therapy. Cancer 1998;82:1529.

Vizcaino AP et al: International trends in the incidence of cervical cancer: I. Adenocarcinoma and adenosquamous cell carcinomas. Int J Cancer 1998;75:536.

Walboomers JM et al: Human papillomavirus is a necessary cause of invasive cervical cancer worldwide. J Pathol 1999;189:12.

Whitney CW et al: Randomized comparison of fluorouracil plus cisplatin versus hydroxyurea as an adjunct to radiation therapy in stage IIB–IVA carcinoma of the cervix with negative para-aortic lymph nodes: A Gynecologic Oncology Group and Southwest Oncology Group study. J Clin Oncol 1999;17:1339.

Premalignant & Malignant Disorders of the Uterine Corpus

51

Oliver Dorigo, MD, PhD, & Annekathryn Goodman, MD

■ ENDOMETRIAL HYPERPLASIA & CARCINOMA

ESSENTIALS OF DIAGNOSIS

- *Abnormal uterine bleeding: menorrhagia, metrorrhagia, or postmenopausal bleeding.*
- *Risk factors: hyperestrogenism—long-term exposure to unopposed estrogens (polycystic ovarian syndrome, chronic anovulation, obesity, late menopause, and exogenous estrogens); metabolic syndrome including diabetes, hypertension; nulliparity; increasing age; history of breast cancer; genetic predisposition (hereditary nonpolyposis colon cancer syndrome).*
- *Diagnosis: endometrial sampling, ultrasonography.*

General Considerations

In the United States, white women have a lifetime risk of endometrial carcinoma of 2.4% compared with 1.3% for black women. The peak incidence of onset is in the seventh decade, but 25% of cancers occur in premenopausal women and the disease has been reported in women ages 20–30 years. Endometrial carcinoma is the most common pelvic genital cancer in women. A doubling of the incidence of endometrial cancer in the 1970s correlated with unopposed estrogen use in hormone replacement and sequential oral contraceptives over the previous 10 years. The declining incidence in the 1980s paralleled progesterone use in hormone replacement regimens and low-dose estrogen combination birth control pills. The estimated incidence for the year 2005 is 40,300 new cases with 7000 deaths occurring from the disease. The onset of endometrial bleed-

ing facilitates detection in the earlier stages of disease. Consequently, the overall prognosis is considerably better than for the other major gynecologic cancers.

Estrogens are implicated as a causative factor in endometrial carcinoma because there is a high incidence of this disease in patients with presumed alterations in estrogen metabolism and in those who take exogenous estrogens. Furthermore, patients with anovulatory cycles are at higher risk of developing endometrial cancer because of prolonged periods of estrogenic stimulation of the endometrium without the opposing effects of progesterone. Progesterone has an antiproliferative effect on the endometrium and can induce apoptosis of endometrial cells. Classically, endometrial carcinoma affects the obese, nulliparous, infertile, hypertensive, and diabetic white woman, but it can occur in the absence of all these factors. Unlike cervical cancer, it is not related to sexual history. The most common presenting symptom is abnormal vaginal bleeding, particularly postmenopausal bleeding. Less frequently, severe cramps from hematometra or pyometra caused by an obliterated endocervical canal in elderly patients may be the presenting symptom. In the asymptomatic patient, a diagnosis may be made incidentally from an abnormal Papanicolaou (Pap) smear, but cytologic discovery of endometrial cancer is not consistent and should not be relied on for early diagnosis. Screening for endometrial cancer in the general population is not recommended, but should be performed for patients with a hereditary nonpolyposis colon cancer (HNPCC) syndrome. The mainstay of treatment is surgery, including a total hysterectomy with bilateral salpingo-oophorectomy and staging with pelvic and periaortic lymphadenectomy. Further postoperative therapy depends on the particular histologic characteristics and the extent of the tumor.

Etiology

Most endometrial carcinomas arise on the background of endometrial hyperplasia and are well differentiated tumors. There are two major types of endometrial cancer. Type I is associated with either endogenous or exogenous unopposed estrogen exposure, and usually consists of a low-grade or well-differentiated tumor with a favorable prognosis. Type II tumors grow independent of estrogen and are associated with endometrial atrophy. The histology of this type is either poorly differentiated endometrioid or nonendometrioid and confers a high risk of relapse with poor prognosis.

Estrogens and progesterone are the two main hormones that influence the metabolic and proliferative state of the endometrium. In general, estrogens stimulate the endometrium, unlike progesterone, which has an antiproliferative effect. Long-term exposure to estrogens can lead to endometrial hyperplasia and, subsequently, to hormone-driven atypical endometrial hyperplasia and endometrial cancer. Clinical circumstances with chronically high levels of estrogenic stimulation include the metabolic syndrome, polycystic ovary syndrome, exogenous, unopposed estrogen replacement therapy, and chronic anovulation in the premenopausal women. Granulosa cell tumors of the ovary can produce high levels of estrogens but are a rare cause of hyperestrogenism. The antiestrogen tamoxifen has a weak estrogenic effect and increases the incidence of endometrial cancer by about 2- to 3-fold.

More than a dozen case-control studies indicate an association between estrogen administration and endometrial carcinoma. These studies report a 2- to 10-fold increase in the incidence of endometrial carcinoma in women receiving exogenous unopposed estrogens. The risk of cancer is related to both the dose and the duration of exposure and diminishes with cessation of estrogen use. The risk seems to be neutralized by the addition of cyclic progestin for 10 days at least every 1–3 months. In women without a hysterectomy, progestin should be added to the treatment to oppose the effect of estrogens on the endometrium. Endometrial biopsies to rule out endometrial hyperplasia or pelvic ultrasonography to evaluate the thickness of the endometrial stripe should be obtained if abnormal bleeding occurs.

Evidence is accumulating that there is a genetic factor in the development of endometrial cancer. Those women with a personal history of ovarian, colon, or breast cancer as well as those with a family history of endometrial cancer may be at higher risk. In HNPCC, there is an autosomal dominant pattern of inheritance for colon and endometrial cancers. Most cases of HNPCC are a result of alterations in mismatch repair genes MSH2 and MLH1. Certain oncogenes, such as Ha-, K-, and N-*ras, c-myc,* and Her-2/neu, have been found in endometrial cancers. Furthermore, alterations in the p53 and even more frequently in the PTEN tumor suppressor gene were recently identified. Certain vascular growth promoting factors like VEGF (vascular endothelial growth factor) have been found to be overexpressed in endometrial cancer.

Table 51–1. FIGO surgical staging of carcinoma of the corpus uteri (1988).

Stage I
  Stage Ia G123 Tumor limited to endometrium
  Stage Ib G123 Invasion to less than one-half the myometrium
  Stage Ic G123 Invasion to more than one-half the myometrium
Stage II
  Stage IIa G123 Endocervical glandular involvement only
  Stage IIb G123 Cervical stromal invasion
Stage III
  Stage IIIa G123 Tumor invades serosa and/or adnexa, and/or positive peritoneal cytology
  Stage IIIb G123 Vaginal metastases
  Stage IIIc G123 Metastases to pelvic and/or paraaortic lymph nodes
Stage IV
  Stage IVa G123 Tumor invades bladder and/or bowel mucosa
  Stage IVb Distant metastases including intra-abdominal and/or inguinal lymph nodes

From Internatinal Federation of Gynecology and Obstetrics: Annual Report on the results of treatment in gynecologic cancer. Int J Gynecol Obstet 1991;36(Suppl):132.

Surgical Staging (Table 51–1)

In 1988, the Cancer Committee of FIGO (International Federation of Gynecology and Obstetrics) introduced a surgical staging system for endometrial carcinoma based on abdominal exploration, pelvic washings, total hysterectomy with salpingo-oophorectomy, and selective pelvic and periaortic lymph node biopsies. Grade of the tumor is included in the staging description. The grade of the tumors refers to the architecture and nuclear atypia. The architecture of the tumor is judged by the percentage of differentiated (glandular) versus nondifferentiated (solid) elements within the tumor specimen. Grade 1 tumors consist of at least 95% glandular tissue and have less than 5% of a nonsquamous solid growth pattern. Areas of squamous differentiation are not considered to be solid tumor growth. Grade 2 tumors contain 6–50% of a nonsquamous solid growth pattern. Tumors with more than 50% of a solid pattern are classified as grade 3. The nuclear grade depends on the appearance of the nucleus, eg, size of nucleus, chromatin pattern, and is more subjective. An architectural grade of 1 or 2 is raised by 1 point in the presence of significant nuclear atypia (nuclear grade 3).

Surgical stage I tumors account for 75% of all endometrial carcinomas, which explains the relatively good overall prognosis. Eleven percent of cancers are surgical stage II, and the remaining 11% and 3% are surgical stages III and IV, respectively.

Classification

A. ENDOMETRIAL HYPERPLASIA

The glandular hyperplasias of the endometrium are benign conditions that can be classified as simple or complex and either with or without atypia. Because of their association with hyperestrogenic states, the atypical hyperplasias are considered premalignant lesions. Because endometrial hyperplasia and endometrial carcinoma present clinically as abnormal bleeding, thorough endometrial sampling or fractional curettage is always necessary when hyperplasia is present to rule out coexisting carcinoma.

1. Hyperplasia without atypia—Microscopically, this type of hyperplasia shows crowding of glands in the stroma without nuclear atypia. This type of hyperplasia is frequently asymptomatic and found incidentally in hysterectomy specimens. When followed without treatment over a 15-year period, approximately 1% progressed to endometrial cancer whereas 80% spontaneously regressed.

Complex hyperplasia without atypia (previously designated "adenomatous hyperplasia") describes a complex, crowded appearance to the glands with very little intervening stroma. Complex hyperplasia regresses under progestin therapy in approximately 85% of cases, but progresses to cancer in 3–5% if untreated.

2. Hyperplasia with atypia—The histology of hyperplasia with atypia is characterized by endometrial glands that are lined with enlarged cells. An increased nuclear-to-cytoplasmic ratio is a sign of increased nuclear activity, eg, transcription. The nuclei may be irregular with coarse chromatin clumping and prominent nucleoli. These hyperplasias are generally considered premalignant. Progression to carcinoma occurs in 10% of simple atypical and in 30–40% of complex atypical hyperplasias. The majority of lesions regress with progestin therapy but have a higher rate of relapse when therapy is stopped compared to lesions without atypia. In peri- and postmenopausal patients with atypical hyperplasias who relapse after progestin therapy, or who cannot tolerate the associated side effects, vaginal or abdominal hysterectomy is recommended.

A recent study demonstrated that in patients with untreated atypical endometrial hyperplasia on preoperative biopsy, 62.5% had a concurrent endometrial carcinoma at hysterectomy. Of women with endometrial hyperplasia without atypia who underwent hysterectomy, 5% had cancer. This new data will significantly alter how we counsel women with atypical endometrial hyperplasia.

The term *atypical endometrial hyperplasia* should be applied to endometrial neoplasia without invasion.

Severe atypical endometrial hyperplasia or adenocarcinoma in situ describe preinvasive histologies that are frequently difficult to distinguish from early invasive endometrial cancer. It is still a matter of debate whether the term *adenocarcinoma in situ* should be used for endometrial pathology. In contrast, the precursor lesion for serous carcinomas in endometrial intraepithelial carcinoma shows pleiomorphic tumor cells in the epithelium of the endometrial surface and the underlying glands without stromal invasion.

B. ENDOMETRIAL CARCINOMA

Endometrial cancer is characterized by obvious hyperplasia and anaplasia of the glandular elements, with invasion of underlying stroma, myometrium, and vascular spaces. Although atypical complex hyperplasia is thought to be a precursor lesion, only approximately 25% of patients with endometrial carcinoma have a history of hyperplasia.

Important prognostic factors include stage, histologic grade and cell type, depth of myometrial invasion, presence of lymph vascular space involvement, lymph node status, involvement of the lower uterine segment, and size of tumor. Other prognosticators relate to tumor ploidy and the proportion of cells in S phase as determined by DNA flow cytometry.

Endometrial cancers of endometrioid histology of any grade are almost never associated with lymph node metastases if there has been no myometrial invasion. The depth of myometrial invasion and histologic grade are correlated with the incidence of pelvic and aortic lymph node metastases. Patients with poorly differentiated deeply invasive cancers have about a 35% incidence of involved pelvic nodes and a 10–20% incidence of aortic node metastases. Because patients with lymph node metastases are at very high risk for recurrence, these pathologic features have serious implications for treatment planning.

Endometrial cancer can spread by four possible routes: direct extension, lymphatic metastases, peritoneal implants after transtubal spread, and hematogenous spread. Undifferentiated lesions (grade 3) may spread to the pelvic and aortic nodes while still confined to the superficial myometrium. In serous and clear cell subtypes the spread pattern is similar to that of ovarian cancer, and upper abdominal metastasis are common. Hematogenous metastases to the lungs are uncommon with primary tumors limited to the uterus but do occur with recurrent or disseminated disease. In contrast to the former belief that endometrial carcinoma spreads primarily to the aortic lymph nodes through infundibulopelvic and broad ligament lymphatics, recent studies indicate a dual pathway of spread to the pelvic and aortic lymph nodes (Fig 51–1). The aortic nodes are rarely involved when the pelvic nodes are free of metastases, but the pelvic nodes are sometimes involved when the aortic nodes are not. The

Figure 51–1. Dual lymphatic spread pattern of endometrial carcinoma.

lymph nodes most commonly involved in endometrial cancer are found in the obturator space.

Vaginal metastases occur by submucosal lymphatic or vascular metastases in approximately 3–8% of patients with clinical stage I disease. The concept that these metastases occur by spillage of tumor through the cervix at the time of surgery lacks convincing support. However, vaginal metastases are more common with higher histologic grade and with lower uterine segment or cervical involvement.

Malignant cells identified in the peritoneal washings obtained at the time of hysterectomy are usually associated with the finding of other risk factors, such as deep myometrial invasion or lymph node metastases. Pathologists recognize various histologic types of endometrial carcinoma. Approximately 80% of all endometrial cancers are of the endometrioid type with several variants: villoglandular, secretory, with squamous differentiation, and with ciliated cells. These types have similar presenting symptoms and signs, patterns of spread, and general clinical behavior. For this reason, they can be consid-

ered collectively for purposes of clinical work-up, differential diagnosis, and treatment. Endometrial adenocarcinomas of the nonendometrioid phenotype show mucinous, serous, clear cell, squamous, small cell, mixed, or transitional cell differentiation.

1. Adenocarcinoma—The most common type of endometrial carcinoma is adenocarcinoma, composed of malignant glands that range from very-well-differentiated (grade 1), barely distinguishable from atypical complex hyperplasia to anaplastic carcinoma (grade 3). To determine stage and prognosis, the tumor is usually graded by the most undifferentiated area visible under the microscope (Fig 51–2). In the United States, adenocarcinoma comprises 80% of endometrial carcinomas.

2. Adenocarcinoma with squamous differentiation—Approximately 25% of endometrioid carcinomas contain focal to extensive squamous elements, ranging from bland squamous cells to foci that could be viewed as squamous carcinoma. The behavior of the tumors with squamous differentiation is dependent on the grade of the glandular component.

3. Serous carcinoma—Histologically, this cancer is identical to the complex papillary architecture seen in serous carcinomas of the ovary. The frequency of this subtype varies from 1–10%. Women with serous carcinoma are more likely to be older and less likely to have hyperestrogenic states. These tumors account for 50% of all relapses in stage I tumors. Serous tumors spread early and involve peritoneal surfaces of the pelvis and abdomen. The tumors also have a propensity for myometrial and lymphatic invasion. The prognosis is unfavorable, and patients with serous tumors should be treated in a manner similar to that of patients with ovarian tumors.

4. Clear cell carcinoma—This subtype is not associated with clear cell carcinomas of the cervix and vagina that are seen in young women with diethylstilbestrol exposure. Clear cell carcinomas encompass approxi-

Figure 51–2. Adenocarcinoma of the endometrium. Note the sharp demarcation of the tumor at the isthmus.

mately 1% of all endometrial carcinomas. Its microscopic appearance is significant for clear cells or hobnail cells. Solid, papillary, tubular, and cystic patterns are possible. Clear cell carcinoma is commonly high grade and aggressive with deep invasion and is seen at an advanced stage. It occurs in older women (average age: 67 years), and like the serous subtype is not associated with a hyperestrogenic state.

5. Miscellaneous subtypes—Mucinous carcinomas make up 9% of endometrial adenocarcinomas; they contain periodic acid-Schiff (PAS)-positive, diastase-resistant, intracytoplasmic mucin. Secretory carcinoma, present in 1–2% of cases, exhibits subnuclear or supranuclear vacuoles resembling early secretory endometrium. These rare cancers behave in a manner similar to that of typical endometrial carcinomas. Pure squamous cell carcinomas are extremely rare and are associated with cervical stenosis, pyometra, and chronic inflammation.

Clinical Findings

A. SYMPTOMS AND SIGNS

Abnormal bleeding occurs in approximately 80% of patients and is the most important and early symptom of endometrial carcinoma. An abnormal vaginal discharge, especially after menopause or intermittent spotting, is reported by some patients. During the premenopausal years, the bleeding is usually described as excessive flow at the time of menstruation. However, bleeding may occur as intermenstrual spotting or premenstrual and postmenstrual bleeding. Approximately 5–10% of patients with postmenopausal bleeding have underlying cancer, but the probability increases with age and depends on underlying risk factors. Approximately 10% of patients complain of lower abdominal cramps and pain secondary to uterine contractions caused by detritus and blood trapped behind a stenotic cervical os (hematometra). If the uterine contents become infected, an abscess develops and sepsis may supervene.

Physical examination is usually unremarkable but may reveal medical problems associated with advanced age. Speculum examination may confirm the presence of bleeding, but because it may be minimal and intermittent, blood might not be present. Atrophic vaginitis is frequently identified in these elderly women, but postmenopausal bleeding should never be ascribed to atrophy without a histologic sampling of the endometrium to rule out endometrial carcinoma. Bimanual and rectovaginal examination of the uterus in the early stages of the disease will be normal unless hematometra or pyometra is present. If the cancer is extensive at the time of presentation, the uterus may be enlarged, and may be misdiagnosed as a benign condition such as leiomyomata. In advanced cases, the uterus may be fixed and immobile from parametrial extension.

Vaginal, vulvar, or inguinal–femoral lymph node metastases are rarely identified in early disease, but are not uncommon in advanced cases or with recurrence following treatment. Ovarian metastases may cause marked enlargement of these organs.

B. LABORATORY FINDINGS

Routine laboratory findings are normal in most patients with endometrial carcinoma. If bleeding has been prolonged or profuse, anemia may be present. Cytologic study of specimens taken from the endocervix and posterior vaginal fornix can reveal adenocarcinoma in symptomatic patients. More important, endometrial carcinoma will be missed in 40% of symptomatic patients by routine cytologic examination. Accuracy has been greatly increased by aspiration cytologic study or biopsy (discussed under Special Examinations). Nevertheless, the Pap smear is an integral part of the examination of all patients, because it identifies a small but definite percentage of patients with asymptomatic disease. Furthermore, the presence of benign endometrial cells in the cervical or vaginal smear of a menopausal or postmenopausal woman is associated with occult endometrial carcinoma in 2–6% of cases and in up to 25% with postmenopausal bleeding. Thus, any postmenopausal woman who shows endometrial cells on a routine cervical Pap smear requires evaluation for endometrial cancer, including endometrial sampling.

Routine blood counts, urinalysis, endocervical and vaginal pool cytology, chest radiography, stool guaiac, and sigmoidoscopy are useful ancillary diagnostic tests in patients with endometrial carcinoma. Liver function tests, blood urea nitrogen, serum creatinine, and a blood glucose test (because of the known relationship to diabetes) are considered routine. Serum CA-125 (cancer antigen-125), a well-established tumor marker for epithelial ovarian cancer, might be useful for endometrial cancer. Approximately 20% of patients with clinical stage I (preoperatively, the tumor appears to be confined to the uterus) have an elevated CA-125. In cases with extensive intraperitoneal spread or enlarged uterus, the tumor marker CA-125 may be markedly elevated. However, in contrast to patients with ovarian cancer, the value of CA-125 in the management of patients with endometrial cancer is limited.

C. IMAGING STUDIES

Chest radiography might reveal metastases in patients with advanced disease but is rarely positive in the early stages. Colonoscopy is usually unnecessary in a patient with a negative stool guaiac test and normal sigmoidoscopic examination, but should always be performed in the patient with gross or occult gastrointestinal bleeding or symptoms. In patients from families with HNPCC, a colonoscopy should be performed preoperatively, particularly if the patient screens positive for the HNPCC-associated DNA mismatch repair gene mutations.

Hysteroscopy can increase the diagnostic accuracy over office endometrial biopsy or dilatation and curettage. Hysteroscopy promotes the transtubal spread of tumor cells into the peritoneal cavity. However, the presence of a positive peritoneal cytology after hysteroscopy does not seem to alter the prognosis. Computer tomography is useful in assessing pelvic anatomy, visualizing enlarged lymph nodes in the pelvis and periaortic areas, and diagnosing distant metastasis in the liver and lungs. Magnetic resonance imaging (MRI) is particularly helpful in identifying myometrial invasion and lower uterine segment or cervical involvement.

D. Special Examinations

1. Fractional curettage—Dilatation and fractional curettage (D&C) is the definitive procedure for diagnosis of endometrial carcinoma. It should be performed with the patient under anesthesia to provide an opportunity for a thorough and more accurate pelvic examination. It is carried out by careful and complete curettage of the endocervical canal followed by dilatation of the canal and circumferential curettage of the endometrial cavity. When obvious cancer is present with the first passes of the curette, the procedure should be terminated as long as sufficient tissue for analysis has been obtained from the endocervix and endometrium. Perforation of the uterus followed by intraperitoneal contamination with malignant cells, blood, and bacteria is a common complication in patients with endometrial carcinoma and can usually be avoided by gentle surgical technique and limitation of the procedure to the extent necessary for accurate diagnosis and staging. D&C is never considered curative in these circumstances and should not be performed with the same vigor as therapeutic curettage.

2. Endometrial biopsy—This procedure is attractive because it can be performed in an outpatient setting, resulting in a substantial savings in cost. It can usually be done without anesthesia, although paracervical block is

Figure 51–3. Technique of endometrial biopsy with Novak curet.

effective when necessary. There is a false-negative rate of approximately 10% and all symptomatic patients with a negative endometrial biopsy need to undergo a formal D&C. There are many types of office biopsy techniques including a Pipelle, Novak Curet (Fig 51–3), and Vabra aspirator (Fig 51–4). All types of endometrial biopsy are notoriously inaccurate for diagnosing polyps and will miss a significant number of cases of endometrial hyperplasia as well.

3. Pelvic ultrasonography—Ultrasonography can be helpful in the surveillance of asymptomatic, high-risk patients, eg, breast cancer patients on tamoxifen and

Figure 51–4. Vabra aspirator.

women with strong family histories of endometrial cancer. Pelvic and transvaginal ultrasonography yield information about the size and shape of the uterus, as well as the thickness and surface contour of the endometrium. In postmenopausal women, an endometrial thickness of more than 5 mm is considered to be suspicious for hyperplasia or malignancy and should be further evaluated with an endometrial biopsy. Transvaginal ultrasound, however, can yield a high false-positive rate in women who have been on tamoxifen for more than 2 years. The subendometrial edema that develops from tamoxifen use is indistinguishable from a thickened endometrial stripe. A sonohysterogram, which involves instilling sterile saline into the endometrial cavity prior to transvaginal ultrasound, can reduce false-positive results and better delineate the endometrial cavity.

4. Estrogen and progesterone receptor assays—Estrogen and progesterone receptor assays should be obtained from the neoplastic tissue. This information helps in planning adjuvant or subsequent hormone therapy. Estrogen and progesterone receptor content are inversely proportional to histologic grade. In general, patients with tumors positive for one or two receptors have longer survival than patients with receptor-negative tumors. Furthermore, patients with receptor positive tumors might be candidates for hormone based therapy of recurrent tumor disease.

Differential Diagnosis

Clinically, the differential diagnosis of endometrial carcinoma includes all the various causes of abnormal uterine bleeding. In the premenopausal patient, complications of early pregnancy, such as threatened or incomplete abortion, must be considered initially. Other causes of bleeding in premenopausal patients are leiomyomata, endometrial hyperplasia and polyps, cervical polyps, an intrauterine device, and various genital or metastatic cancers. Cervical, endometrial, tubal, and ovarian neoplasms all can cause abnormal uterine bleeding. Although rare, metastatic cancers from the bowel, bladder, and breast have also been reported to cause abnormal uterine bleeding. After exclusion of anatomical causes for vaginal bleeding, a work-up for hemophilias should be performed. In the postmenopausal age group, the differential diagnosis includes atrophic vaginitis, exogenous estrogens, endometrial hyperplasia and polyps, and various genital neoplasms. The likelihood of cancer increases with age. In the patient with a normal pelvic examination and recurrent postmenopausal bleeding following a recent negative D&C, tubal and ovarian cancer must be strongly considered. Patients with recurrent unexplained episodes of postmenopausal uterine bleeding should be considered for total hysterectomy and bilateral salpingo-oophorectomy.

Complications

Patients with advanced disease and deep myometrial invasion may present with severe anemia secondary to chronic blood loss or acute hemorrhage. If bleeding is significant and continuous, a short-term boost of radiation therapy is usually effective in slowing the hemorrhage.

The presence of a hematometra can be confirmed by sounding the uterus under anesthesia, followed by dilatation of the cervix to allow adequate drainage. When a pyometra is present, the patient may present with peritonitis or generalized sepsis, with all the consequent complications.

Perforation of the uterus at the time of dilatation and fractional curettage or endometrial biopsy is not an uncommon problem. If the perforating instrument is large, loops of small bowel may be inadvertently retrieved through the cervical canal. A large perforation warrants laparoscopy or laparotomy to evaluate and repair the damage. If significant contamination of the peritoneal cavity with blood or necrotic tumor has occurred, the patient should be treated with broad-spectrum antibiotics to prevent peritonitis. Perforation in the patient with endometrial cancer should be viewed as a serious complication, as spillage of tumor into the peritoneal cavity may alter her prognosis.

Prevention

Several modifiable risk factors for endometrial carcinoma have been described; in particular, obesity, diabetes, hypertension, and nulliparity. Prevention of endometrial cancer is primarily based on weight control, physical exercise, adequate control of diabetes and hypertension, and increased surveillance of women at high risk. In addition, a careful family history of each patient will help identify patients with a genetic predisposition for endometrial cancer, for example, as part of the HNPCC syndrome. If appropriate, these patients should undergo genetic counseling and genetic testing. A hysterectomy after the completion of childbearing is appropriate for patients with HNPCC syndrome given the lifetime risk for endometrial cancer of 60%. Hormone therapy in postmenopausal patients without hysterectomy should always include a progestational agent to oppose the action of estrogens on the endometrium. Estrogens should be administered either continuously or cyclically using the lowest dose that controls symptoms. Progesterone (10 mg of medroxyprogesterone acetate or 200 mg of micronized progesterone) should be added for the last 10–14 days of the cycle to neutralize the risk of endometrial carcinoma. Alternatively, if estrogen and progesterone are administered continuously, 2.5 mg of medroxyprogesterone acetate is given daily.

Treatment

The majority of endometrial cancer cases is diagnosed at an early stage and can be treated with high cure rates. The most important treatment modality is surgery with total simple or radical hysterectomy, bilateral salpingo-oophorectomy, and staging, including pelvic and periaortic lymphadenectomy. Primary radiation therapy is used only in patients with medical contraindications for surgery or advanced pelvic disease. It has been repeatedly demonstrated that radiation therapy can cure endometrial carcinoma in some patients. However, radiation therapy averages about a 20% lower cure rate compared to surgery in stage I disease. Primary chemotherapy is used infrequently and mostly in patients with metastatic disease.

Adjuvant treatment is dependent on the results of surgical staging and histology. For example, radiation therapy is frequently used in endometrioid type endometrial cancers to prevent pelvic recurrences. Advanced pelvic disease may be treated with radiation followed by chemotherapy. Serous cancers of the endometrium behave biologically similar to ovarian cancer and are treated with adjuvant platinum-based chemotherapy possibly in conjunction with radiation.

Radiation therapy alone can cure endometrial carcinoma in some patients, and when used preoperatively it completely eradicates the primary tumor in more than 50% of stage I cases. Furthermore, adjuvant radiation therapy has reduced the incidence of vaginal vault recurrence following surgery for stage I patients from an average of 3–8% to 1–3%. Intracavitary vaginal irradiation can be performed by using a vaginal cylinder to deliver a surface dose of 5500–6000 cGy. Also, regional radiation therapy has eliminated microscopic nodal metastases in other tumor systems, and some patients with surgically proved nodal metastases from endometrial carcinoma are now alive more than 5 years following adjuvant radiation therapy to pelvic and aortic nodes. Accordingly, in the presence of extrauterine extension, lower uterine segment or cervical involvement, poor histologic differentiation, papillary serous or clear cell histology, or myometrial penetration greater than one-third of the full thickness, adjuvant radiation therapy is recommended. In the absence of these findings, it is difficult to justify the risk and morbidity of any additional treatment beyond simple total abdominal hysterectomy and bilateral salpingo-oophorectomy.

A. Emergency Measures

Patients with endometrial adenocarcinoma may present with severe anemia after prolonged periods of vaginal bleeding. Acute and massive blood loss may lead to hypovolemic shock. The management of these patients includes stabilization of vital signs with volume substitution and blood transfusion. A tamponade of the uterus using vaginal packing might be useful, particularly in the presence of a bleeding cervical or vaginal tumor. Monsel's solution or silver nitrate can further aid in obtaining hemostasis. An emergency dilatation and fractional curettage might help to control the bleeding, but has to be performed with great caution to avoid perforation. If bleeding does not subside, a high-dosage radiation boost to the whole pelvis is usually the treatment of choice to acutely control uterine bleeding in this situation. Rarely, in the face of very advanced lesions, embolization of the hypogastric arteries via percutaneous selective angiography may be required to control hemorrhage before treatment can be initiated. Hysterectomy should always be considered if it can be accomplished safely without jeopardizing curative therapy.

Elderly patients may present with severe lower abdominal pain and cramping secondary to hematometra or pyometra; these complications result from endometrial carcinoma in more than 50% of cases. When adequate blood levels of broad-spectrum antibiotics are established, the cervix should be dilated and the endometrial cavity adequately drained. In this setting, vigorous D&C is contraindicated because of the high risk of uterine perforation. If the cervix is well dilated, an indwelling drain is usually unnecessary, but if sepsis is not controlled within 24–48 hours, the patient should be re-examined to ascertain cervical patency. Once the infection has completely subsided and the patient has been afebrile for 7–10 days, gentle fractional curettage should be performed if the diagnosis was not confirmed at the initial procedure.

B. Radiation Therapy

Radiation therapy is used as primary therapy in patients considered too medically unstable for laparotomy. Adjuvant preoperative radiation is no longer used unless the patient presents with gross cervical involvement. In this situation, after preoperative whole-pelvic radiation and an intracavitary implant, an extrafascial hysterectomy is performed. Relative contraindications to preoperative radiation therapy include the presence of a pelvic mass, a pelvic kidney, pyometra, history of a pelvic abscess, prior pelvic radiation, and previous multiple laparotomies (see Chapter 54).

C. Surgical Treatment

Because bleeding is usually an early sign of endometrial carcinoma, most patients present with early disease and can be adequately and completely treated by simple hysterectomy. Staging includes a bilateral salpingo-oophorectomy, peritoneal washings for cytology, and removal of pelvic and periaortic lymph nodes. Recently, laparoscopic-assisted vaginal hysterectomy with lymphadenectomy has been performed in patients with endometrial cancer. Initial studies show no difference in overall long-term survival when laparoscopy was compared to laparotomy. Patients undergoing laparoscopy tend to have a significantly shorter hospital stay and less blood loss.

Pelvic and paraaortic lymphadenectomy play an important role in the surgical staging of endometrial cancer. A gross pathologic assessment of the uterus should be performed during surgery to determine the need for surgical staging in patients with endometrioid adenocarcinomas grade 1 or 2. Patients who require surgical staging are patients with stage 1 disease with grade 3 lesions, tumors greater than 2 cm in maximum dimension, tumors with greater than 50% myometrial invasion, cervical extension, and evidence of extrauterine spread. Furthermore, staging should be performed in clear cell and papillary serous carcinomas in all cases because of a high incidence of lymphatic spread. However, the criteria for lymphadenectomy are not universally accepted and are under constant investigation. The therapeutic role of lymphadenectomy is still under investigation. Several studies have suggested that external-beam therapy may be omitted or the radiation field be reduced to the central pelvis if the lymph nodes are negative. Brachytherapy via a cylinder to the vaginal cuff is performed to prevent vaginal vault recurrence but has not been shown to alter long-term survival. Bulky, positive nodes, which are unlikely to respond to external-beam radiation, should be removed during surgery.

Radical hysterectomy for stage II tumors is an accepted procedure that has the potential to omit adjuvant radiation therapy. A radical hysterectomy can also be an effective treatment for patients with recurrence following treatment with radiation therapy alone or for those who have previously received therapeutic doses of pelvic radiation therapy for other pelvic cancers. The high risk of bowel or urinary tract injury in this setting must be understood and accepted by both patient and physician.

Patients who present with significant cervical involvement or vaginal and parametrial involvement should receive initial pelvic radiation. Exploratory laparotomy should then be considered in patients whose disease seems resectable. Hormonal therapy or chemotherapy is most appropriate for patients with clinical evidence of extrapelvic metastases. Palliative radiation to bone or brain metastases is beneficial for symptomatic relief. Pelvic radiation can be helpful for local tumor control and alleviation of bleeding.

D. HORMONE THERAPY

Progesterone has shown some efficacy in the treatment of recurrent endometrial carcinoma not amenable to irradiation or surgery. This type of therapy can be administered orally or parenterally. Oral megestrol, parenteral medroxyprogesterone acetate suspension, and parenteral hydroxyprogesterone caproate appear to have similar effectiveness. Overall, approximately 13% of patients with recurrent disease appear to achieve long-term remission with progesterone therapy. The average duration of response is 20 months and up to 30% of responders survive for 5 years. In general, the clinical response is better in patients with localized recurrence, well-differentiated tumors, and late recurrences. Because some patients do not achieve remission until after 10–12 weeks of therapy, the minimum duration of treatment should be longer than 3 months. Although progesterones have a somewhat encouraging record in the treatment of recurrent endometrial adenocarcinoma, they are disappointing as prophylactic agents. They have not improved survival or decreased recurrence when used following definitive treatment of early stage disease.

Tamoxifen either alone or in combination with progesterones has been used in advanced or recurrent endometrial cancer. Patients with well-differentiated, estrogen receptor-positive tumors and long disease-free intervals tend to have a better response to tamoxifen. Tamoxifen is administered orally at 10–20 mg twice daily. For single-agent tamoxifen, the overall response rate is approximately 15–20%. Studies using combination tamoxifen-progestin therapy suggest a possibly better clinical response.

E. CHEMOTHERAPY

Doxorubicin and cisplatin are the two most active agents in the treatment of advanced or recurrent endometrial cancer. Doxorubicin used as a single agent has an overall response rate of 38%, with 26% of the patients achieving a complete response. The combination of cisplatin and doxorubicin shows slightly longer survival than either agent alone. The addition of Taxol to cisplatin and doxorubicin shows an overall response rate of 57% with improved long-term survival compared to the same regimen without Taxol. Other agents with antitumor activity against endometrial cancer include carboplatin, cyclophosphamide, hexamethylmelamine, and 5-fluorouracil.

Prognosis

The most important prognosticators for endometrial cancer are stage, histologic type, grade, myometrial invasion, and the presence of lymphvascular space invasion. Identification of these risk factors is crucial for treatment decisions, surveillance, and counseling of the patient. The prognosis is worse with increasing age, higher pathologic grade, advanced stage disease, increasing depth of myometrial invasion, and presence of lymphvascular space invasion. Because the prognosis for each patient is dependent on a variety of factors, overall

5-year survival stratified by stage is indicated as a range of percentages. The overall 5-year survival rates are 81–95% for surgical stage I, 67–77% for stage II, 31–60% for stage III, and 5–20% for stage IV.

These figures underline the increasing risk for treatment failure and recurrence with increasing bulk and extension of tumor. In the absence of risk factors, a simple total abdominal hysterectomy and bilateral salpingo-oophorectomy should result in survival greater than 95% at 5 years. However, in the presence of risk factors, a more aggressive surgical approach, and using adjuvant radiation and chemotherapy may be warranted.

■ SARCOMA OF THE UTERUS (LEIOMYOSARCOMA, ENDOMETRIAL SARCOMAS)

ESSENTIALS OF DIAGNOSIS

- *Bleeding: metrorrhagia, menorrhagia, postmenopausal or preadolescent bleeding.*
- *Mass: rapid enlargement of the uterus or a leiomyoma.*
- *Pain: pelvic discomfort as a result of mass effect from the enlarged uterus.*
- *Malignant tissue: histology confirmed by dilatation and curettage or in hysterectomy specimen.*

General Considerations

The uterine sarcomas are mesodermally derived highly malignant tumors and account for approximately 3–4% of all uterine malignancies. No common etiology has been identified in uterine sarcomas, but prior pelvic radiation therapy is associated with the mixed forms of uterine sarcoma.

Sarcomas can occur at any age but are most prevalent after age 40. They are well known as a source of hematogenous metastases, but with the exception of leiomyosarcomas, lymphatic permeation and contiguous spread are probably the most common methods of extension. Endometrial sarcomas can usually be diagnosed by endometrial biopsy or dilatation and fractional curettage, but the sarcomas derived from the myometrium (leiomyosarcoma) frequently require hysterectomy to obtain adequate tissue for analysis.

In general, uterine sarcomas follow a very aggressive growth pattern with early metastasis to the abdomen, liver and lung. There is no universal agreement on the histologic features that determine outcome, but most authorities agree that the number of mitotic figures per high-power field, vascular and lymphatic invasion, serosal extension, and degree of anaplasia are all helpful. Surgery is the most common primary treatment approach, followed by radiation and chemotherapy. Chemotherapeutic agents reported to be active against sarcomas include doxorubicin, cisplatin, ifosfamide, gemcitabine, and the taxanes. Clinical response rates for combination chemotherapy in recurrent and advanced disease are reported to be as high as 54%. However, most responses are partial and only temporary.

Histogenesis, Classification, & Staging

Although several classification systems exist for uterine sarcomas, they can be separated into four major categories: leiomyosarcomas (LMSs), endometrial stromal sarcomas (ESSs), malignant mixed mesodermal tumors (MMMTs), and adenosarcomas. LMSs are thought to arise from the myometrial smooth muscle cell or a similar cell lining blood vessels within the myometrium. The ESS and MMMT arise from undifferentiated endometrial stromal cells, which retain the potential to differentiate into malignant cell lines that histologically appear native (homologous) or foreign (heterologous) to the human uterus. Because the undifferentiated stromal cells of the endometrium arise from specialized mesenchymal cells of the müllerian apparatus in the genital ridge, and ultimately from the mesoderm during embryogenesis, endometrial sarcomas have been variously termed "mesodermal," "müllerian," or "mesenchymal" sarcomas. The prognoses of patients with homologous and heterologous tumors is similar stage for stage, and this terminology has limited clinical usefulness. ESSs have been categorized in the older literature as "pure" and homologous endometrial sarcomas because they are composed of a single cell line. MMMTs, previously designated as "mixed" because of containing two or more cell lines, arise from an undifferentiated malignant stem cell. MMMTs contain both a carcinomatous or epithelium derived element and a sarcomatous or mesenchymal element and have also been called "carcinosarcomas." The carcinomatous element is usually an undifferentiated adenocarcinoma. The concept of this terminology is better understood by study of Fig 51–5, which graphically represents the histogenesis of uterine sarcomas. Table 51–2 combines the prevailing histogenetic terminology for endometrial sarcomas and depicts the various possibilities in each category.

Pure heterologous sarcomas, such as rhabdomyosarcoma, chondrosarcoma, osteosarcoma, and liposarcoma, are extremely rare. Other uterine sarcomas, like

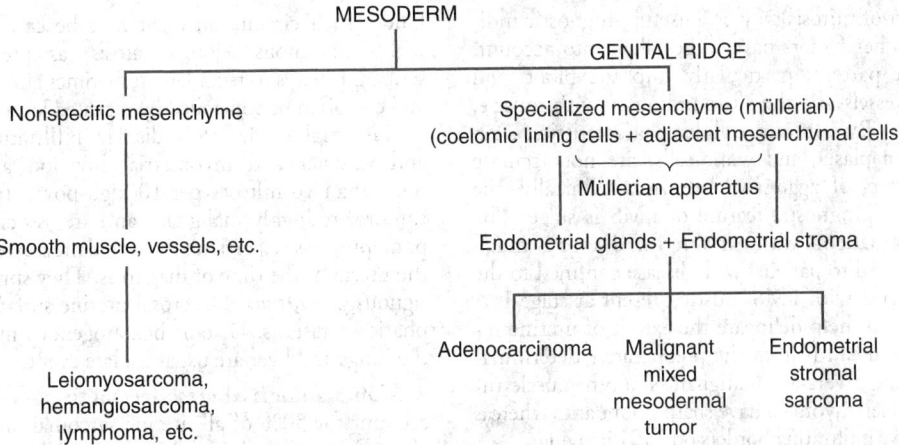

Figure 51–5. Histogenesis of uterine sarcomas.

hemangiosarcomas, fibrosarcomas, reticulum cell sarcomas, and lymphosarcomas, are indistinguishable from identical sarcomas elsewhere in the body and are therefore not considered specialized tumors of the uterus.

The commonly used staging system for uterine sarcomas follows the FIGO staging system for endometrial carcinoma (Table 51–1).

Major Types of Sarcomas of the Uterus

A. Leiomyosarcomas

LMSs make up 35–40% of all uterine sarcomas and 1–2% of all uterine cancers. LMS usually occurs between ages 25 and 75 years, with a mean incidence at about age 50 years. Younger patients with this disease seem to have a more favorable outcome than postmenopausal women. Like the benign leiomyomas, LMSs are 1.5 times more common in African American patients than in the white population. Leiomyomas are commonly

Table 51–2. Classification of uterine sarcomas.

Leiomyosarcoma (tumors of the uterine smooth muscle)
Endometrial stromal sarcoma (pure homologous endometrial sarcoma)
  High grade
  Low grade (endolymphatic stromal myosis)
Malignant mixed mesodermal tumor (mixed epithelial/stromal tumors)
  Homologous carcinosarcoma
  Heterologous carcinosarcoma
Adenosarcoma (mixed epithelial/stromal tumors)
  Homologous
  Heterologous

identified in uteri containing leiomyosarcomas, but the incidence of malignant transformation of a leiomyoma is only 0.1–0.5%. Only approximately 5–10% of LMSs are reported to originate in a leiomyoma.

Abnormal uterine bleeding is the most common symptom of LMS, occurring in approximately 60% of patients; pelvic or abdominal pain and discomfort is reported by approximately 50% of all patients. Only approximately 10% of patients are aware of an abdominal mass. The diagnosis is by made by biopsy. Occasionally, a pedunculated tumor prolapses through the cervix and is easily accessible for biopsy. The deeply situated intramural position of most tumors impedes diagnosis by D&C, which is accurate in only 25% of cases. Abnormal cells might be identified on Pap smear. The diagnosis is more commonly made after pathologic analysis of a hysterectomy specimen.

LMSs spread by contiguous growth, invading the myometrium, cervix, and surrounding supporting tissues. Lymphatic dissemination is common in the late stages. Pelvic recurrence and peritoneal dissemination following resection are also common. In the more malignant types, hematogenous metastasis to the lungs, liver, kidney, brain, and bones probably occurs early but is clinically evident only in the lungs until the advanced stages.

The clinical behavior of the tumor is generally aggressive with some correlation with the number of mitotic figures identified on microscopic examination. Low-grade LMSs are those with less than 5 mitoses per 10 high-power fields, with pushing rather than infiltrating margins. LMSs with 5–10 mitoses per 10 high-power fields are considered to be of intermediate grade, and tumors with mitotic counts greater than 10 per 10 high-power fields are highly malignant and usually lethal; less than 20% of these patients are alive at 5 years.

The number of mitosis may be a useful prognostic indicator, but other factors have to be taken into account. An invasive pattern, particularly into the blood and lymphatic vessels and the surrounding smooth muscle, is important. By contrast, cellular characteristics, such as atypia, anaplasia, and giant cells, are not accurate prognosticators of aggressive behavior. Clinically, the most reliable prognostic feature of LMS is stage. The prognosis of patients with extrauterine disease is much worse compared to patients with disease confined to the uterus. Patients with LMS mostly present at stage I. A pelvic MRI can help delineate the extent of uterine involvement and can help in the preoperative determination of a benign versus a malignant smooth muscle tumor. Benign leiomyomata have sharp boundaries whereas sarcomas have infiltrating borders on MRI imaging.

Other unusual smooth muscle tumors of the uterus such as benign metastasizing leiomyoma and intravenous leiomyomatosis should be considered low-grade LMS. Although they are histologically benign, they are notorious for local recurrence and can cause death by compression of contiguous or distant vital structures. Intravenous leiomyomatosis has been known to grow up the vena cava into the right atrium, impeding venous return and precipitating congestive heart failure. Because of their slow growth, they can frequently be controlled by repeated local excision. The metastatic lung lesions of benign metastasizing leiomyoma have disappeared following resection of the primary lesion in some cases, perhaps indicating hormone dependency.

B. ENDOMETRIAL SARCOMAS

1. Endometrial stromal sarcomas—ESSs make up 8% of all sarcomas. They occur predominantly in postmenopausal women. Patients with these tumors most commonly present with bleeding or lower abdominal discomfort and pain. The diagnosis can be made accurately by D&C in approximately 75% of cases. Although no etiologic relationship to hormones has been established, a small number of metastatic lesions has responded to progesterone therapy.

ESSs can be divided into two distinct subtypes: low grade and high grade. The indolent low-grade ESSs—also called endolymphatic stromal myosis—have fewer than 10 mitoses per 10 high-power fields, with infiltrating margins and myometrial invasion. A benign form, the stromal nodule, contains pushing rather than infiltrating margins and fewer than 3 mitoses per 10 high-power fields, with no vascular or myometrial invasion.

The mean age at *onset* for endolymphatic stromal myosis is 5–10 years earlier than for high-grade sarcomas. This tumor infiltrates surrounding structures and is characterized by indolent growth and a propensity to vascular invasion. Patients frequently present with yellowish wormlike extensions into the periuterine vascular spaces.

Under such circumstances, it may be confused grossly with intravenous leiomyomatosis, as previously described. It tends to recur late, sometimes after 5–10 years, and can often be controlled by repeated local excisions.

The high-grade ESSs display infiltrating margins and vascular and myometrial invasion and contain more than 10 mitoses per 10 high-power fields. These tumors are highly malignant and are associated with a poor prognosis, particularly when they extend beyond the uterus at the time of diagnosis. They spread by contiguous growth via the serosal uterine surface and lymphatic metastasis. Distant hematogenous metastases to the lungs and liver are usually a late event.

2. Malignant mixed mesodermal tumors—MMMTs account for 50% of all uterine sarcomas and 3–6% of all uterine tumors. They characteristically occur in postmenopausal women, with the exception of embryonal rhabdomyosarcoma of the cervix or vagina (sarcoma botryoides), which occurs also in infants and children. The incidence is about 3 times greater in black than in white women. Radiation therapy may be a predisposing cause, but the etiology of MMMTs is unknown. Many published series are available containing a significant number of patients with a history of pelvic radiation for benign or malignant conditions (Fig 51–6).

As with the other types, the presenting symptom of MMMT is usually bleeding. Abdominal discomfort and pain or a neoplastic mass prolapsed into the vagina also occur. Because the tumors are endometrial in origin, approximately 75% can be diagnosed accurately by D&C. Histologically, MMMTs are usually highly anaplastic, with many bizarre nuclei and mitotic figures. They contain an epithelial and a sarcomatous component, hence the term malignant mixed mesodermal, or müllerian tumor, or carcinosarcoma. If the sarcomatous component is derived from the smooth muscle tissue of the uterus, they are called homologous MMMTs. If the sarcomatous component contains bone, striated muscle, cartilage, or fat, the term heterologous MMMT is ap-

Figure 51–6. Mixed sarcoma of the uterine fundus. Prior full-pelvic radiation therapy had little effect on the tumor.

plied. Clinically, this distinction does not influence treatment or prognosis. MMMTs spread by contiguous infiltration of the surrounding tissues and by early hematogenous and lymphatic dissemination. The metastatic deposits are usually composed of the epithelial malignant glands, but sarcomatous elements have been identified in some cases. The prognosis depends mainly on the extent of the tumor at the time of primary surgery; there are virtually no long-term survivors among those whose tumor has extended beyond the confines of the uterus at the time of diagnosis. Treatment includes total abdominal hysterectomy with bilateral salpingo-oophorectomy, lymphadenectomy, and tumor debulking if necessary and technically feasible. Active chemotherapeutic agents include cisplatin, ifosfamide, Adriamycin, epirubicin, carboplatin, Taxol, and gemcitabine.

C. Adenosarcomas

Adenosarcoma is a distinctive mixed müllerian tumor that accounts for 1–2% of uterine sarcomas. It arises from the endometrium and is composed of a combination of benign-appearing glands and a stromal sarcoma or fibrosarcoma. Adenosarcomas usually occur in the postmenopausal age group but have been reported in adolescents and women of reproductive age. Bleeding is the most common symptom. Recurrence occurs in 25% of patients and is usually late. The primary treatment is removal of uterus, tubes, and ovaries. Postoperative radiation therapy is recommended for those tumors with deep myometrial invasion.

D. Other Uterine Sarcomas

Embryonal rhabdomyosarcoma of the cervix (sarcoma botryoides), which occurs in infants and children, was previously lethal. However, combination therapy using surgery, radiation, and chemotherapy has considerably improved the outlook for these patients.

Fibrosarcoma, hemangiosarcoma, reticulum cell sarcoma, hemangiopericytoma, and other esoteric and bizarre uterine sarcomas are rare. In general, these sarcomas behave like the other intermediate-grade uterine sarcomas, but treatment must be individualized according to age, histologic type, and the patient's state of health.

Clinical Findings

A. Symptoms and Signs

Abnormal uterine bleeding is the most common manifestation of uterine sarcoma. Other recurring complaints include pelvic discomfort or pain, constipation, urinary frequency and urgency, and the presence of a mass low in the abdomen. Uterine sarcoma should be suspected in any nonpregnant woman with a rapidly enlarging uterus. Severe uterine cramps may exist if the tumor has prolapsed into the endometrial cavity or through the cervix. Pelvic examination may reveal the characteristic grapelike structures of sarcoma botryoides protruding from the cervix or the presence of velvety fronds of ESS in the cervical canal. A necrotic fungating mass at the vaginal apex should suggest an infarcted myoma, LMS, or MMMT. The uterus is usually enlarged and often soft and globular. If the cancer has involved the cervix, cul-de-sac, or cardinal ligaments, fixation or asymmetry of the parametria may be found. In advanced cases, inguinal or supraclavicular node metastases may be evident. Patients with advanced uterine sarcomas may present with a large omental mass or ascites secondary to abdominal carcinomatosis.

B. Laboratory Findings

Standard laboratory evaluation of patients with uterine sarcoma should include a complete blood count and urinalysis, liver function studies (especially serum alkaline phosphatase, prothrombin time, and serum lactic dehydrogenase), blood urea nitrogen, and serum creatinine. CA-125 may be elevated. Estrogen and progesterone receptor analysis may indicate which patients are likely to respond to hormone therapy. Office endometrial biopsy or punch biopsy of a prolapsed vaginal mass is helpful only if positive.

C. Radiograph Findings

The chest radiography may contain metastatic coin lesions characteristic of uterine sarcomas. Because uterine sarcomas commonly metastasize to the lung, a chest computed tomography (CT) scan should be considered when the routine films are negative, particularly before any radical extirpative surgery in the pelvis is performed. CT scan of the abdomen and pelvis is helpful in assessing the extent of abdominal disease, evaluating the kidneys for hydronephrosis, identifying enlarged retroperitoneal nodes, and identifying liver metastases. MRI scans are not routinely performed but may provide an accurate preoperative assessment of uterine size and degree of involvement.

D. Special Examinations

Pelvic ultrasonography may confirm the presence of a pelvic mass or help to differentiate an adnexal from a uterine mass in the obese patient. Sigmoidoscopy should always be performed in older women, and in young women if gastrointestinal bleeding or masses suspected of being malignant are present. Cystoscopy is indicated in locally advanced disease or in the presence of gross or microscopic hematuria.

Differential Diagnosis

The clinical diagnosis of uterine sarcoma is frequently overlooked. Diagnostic accuracy can be increased if the physician keeps these tumors in mind while investigating any pelvic mass. The tumor frequently does not present the classic picture of abnormal bleeding accompanied by a symmetrically enlarged soft globular uterus. It can masquerade as any condition causing uterine enlargement or a pelvic mass; of these, pregnancy, leiomyoma, adenomyosis, and adherent ovarian neoplasms or pelvic inflammatory disease are most likely to cause misinterpretation. When cytologic studies, endometrial biopsy, or dilatation and fractional curettage fail to provide the diagnosis—a situation not uncommon with LMS—laparotomy is necessary. At laparotomy, thorough evaluation is critical to the future management of the patient with uterine sarcoma and must include inspection (where possible) and palpation of all abdominal viscera, peritoneal and mesenteric surfaces, liver, both diaphragms, and retroperitoneal structures, especially the pelvic and aortic lymph nodes. Cytologic examination of peritoneal exudate is indispensable for treatment planning; if no free fluid is present, samples may be obtained by instilling 50–100 mL of normal saline into the abdominal cavity (pelvic washings). If a sarcoma is identified on frozen section of the hysterectomy specimen, suspicious lymph nodes should be removed. This information, gathered at the time of the initial exploration and carefully documented in the operative records, is critical for identification and staging of the neoplasm and for predicting outcome.

The pathologic diagnosis of uterine sarcoma is often extremely difficult and may require consultation with a gynecologic pathologist familiar with these tumors. As each cancer becomes more anaplastic, the parent cell or tissue becomes more difficult to identify histologically. Because proper treatment is predicated on accurate histologic diagnosis, every effort should be expended to identify the cell of origin.

Complications

Severe anemia from chronic blood loss or acute hemorrhage may be present. The severity and extent of other complications caused by uterine sarcomas are directly related to the size and virulence of the primary tumor. A pedunculated mass may protrude into the uterine cavity or prolapse through the cervix, causing bleeding or uterine cramps as the uterus attempts to expel the tumor. Infarction with subsequent infection and sepsis may ensue. Rupture of the uterus as a consequence of rapidly growing uterine sarcomas has been reported. Obstructed labor and postpartum uterine inversion secondary to endometrial sarcomas have also been noted. Extensive pulmonary metastases can produce hemoptysis and respiratory failure. Ascites is common in advanced disease with peritoneal metastases.

A wide variety of complications has been reported secondary to pressure or compression of a neighboring viscus or resulting from extension or metastases to other vital structures. Urethral elongation caused by stretching of the bladder over a rapidly growing mass can simultaneously produce obstruction and loss of sphincter control, with subsequent overflow incontinence. Colon compression may result in ribbon stools and, eventually, complete bowel obstruction. Ureteral obstruction is common, especially with recurrent pelvic sarcomas. Urinary diversion or colostomy may be required prior to treatment if life-threatening viscus obstruction is present in an untreated patient, but urinary diversion should not be performed unless there is some hope for cure or meaningful palliation, because it precludes a painless death from uremia.

Prevention

Indiscriminate use of radiation therapy for benign conditions in the pelvis should be avoided, as several clinical studies have suggested an etiologic role of pelvic radiation in the development of MMMT.

Treatment

A. EMERGENCY MEASURES

Hemorrhage from uterine sarcomas can be severe and requires prompt attention. In acute hemorrhage, blood volume should be replaced rapidly, using packed red blood cells, crystalloid solutions, volume expanders, and fresh-frozen plasma.

Emergency D&C should be used only to obtain tissue for analysis. Vigorous curettage is likely to aggravate or provoke bleeding. High-dose bolus radiation is a more reliable and safe method of controlling bleeding. A dose of 400–500 cGy administered daily to the whole pelvis over 2–3 days usually controls acute hemorrhage; this does not appreciably interfere with future management. If these measures are not successful, emergency embolization or ligation of the hypogastric arteries sometimes controls hemorrhage when hysterectomy is not indicated or technically feasible.

B. SURGICAL MEASURES

Extirpative surgery provides the best chance for long-term palliation or cure for patients with uterine sarcomas. Surgery is the cornerstone of the treatment plan and should be the central focus of attack against these cancers.

Because low-grade uterine sarcomas (some LMSs, endolymphatic stromal myosis, intravenous leiomyomatosis) have a propensity for isolated local spread and central pelvic recurrence, such patients should be considered for radical hysterectomy and bilateral salpingo-oophorectomy. The benefits of this type of therapy have not been conclusively shown, but, theoretically, the problem of local recurrence should be improved by more radical excision of the primary tumor. Lymph node metastases in these low-grade tumors are negligible; consequently, pelvic lymphadenectomy can be reserved for patients with enlarged or suspicious nodes. Pelvic recurrences of low-grade uterine sarcomas have been successfully treated by repeated excisions of all resectable tumor. Patients have been known to survive for many years following this type of conservative treatment. Partial or complete pelvic exenteration may occasionally be useful for recurrence of indolent tumors.

The high-grade uterine sarcomas (some LMSs, ESSs, all MMMTs) display early lymphatic, local, and hematogenous metastases, even when apparently confined to the uterus. For this reason, radical surgery has been abandoned in favor of simple total abdominal hysterectomy and bilateral salpingo-oophorectomy preceded or followed by adjunctive radiation therapy. At the time of surgical exploration, a thorough examination and evaluation of the abdominal contents must be performed and documented. Cytologic specimens and omental tissue should be obtained, and suspicious papillations, excrescences, and adhesions should be excised for pathologic analysis. A thorough staging procedure is important for prognosis and a postoperative treatment plan.

When uterine sarcomas recur in the lung and the metastatic survey is negative, unilateral isolated metastases can be excised after a chest CT scan has ruled out other lesions not apparent on the routine chest radiograph. Considering all sources, resection of isolated sarcoma metastases to the lung carries about a 25% 5-year cure rate.

C. CHEMOTHERAPY

Adjuvant doxorubicin reduces the distant recurrence rate for LMS. Although the data are not statistically significant, some authorities recommend the use of doxorubicin-based chemotherapy in high-grade LMS.

Because of the high hormone receptor content in ESS, adjuvant progestin or tamoxifen therapy is recommended. For receptor-negative tumors, doxorubicin-based chemotherapy is used.

Doxorubicin, cisplatin, carboplatin, paclitaxel, gemcitabine, and ifosfamide display significant activity against MMMTs. Cyclophosphamide and vincristine also show activity. Some data suggest that combination chemotherapy is more effective than single-agent therapy. In advanced or metastatic disease, adjuvant combination chemotherapy is recommended. ET-743, a new agent, has been actively evaluated in sarcomas and appears to show some modest promise. Treatment with tyrosine kinase inhibitors like imatinib has been attempted.

D. RADIATION THERAPY

When used as the only modality of treatment for uterine sarcomas, radiation has produced dismal results—very few survivors are reported in the literature following treatment with radiation therapy alone for any of the uterine sarcomas. Radiation therapy does provide local tumor control and reduces local recurrences when used in combination with surgery for the treatment of some endometrial sarcomas. However, it is unclear whether a combined surgical and radiation approach changes overall survival. Collected data indicate that adjuvant radiation therapy improves the 2-year survival rate in patients with ESS by approximately 20% and may also improve survival for those with MMMTs, although less convincingly. Although an occasional 5-year survivor with LMS has been reported following radiation therapy alone, analysis of large numbers of patients from different institutions does not support its use for these tumors. Nevertheless, in advanced forms of LMS, radiation may prove useful for palliation and control of pelvic symptoms such as massive bleeding or pain.

Prognosis

In determining the prognosis for patients with uterine sarcomas, a constellation of factors must be examined simultaneously. Such considerations as the patient's age, state of health, and ability to withstand major surgery or radiation therapy (or both) must be evaluated. The most important clinical characteristic—and probably the overriding prognostic feature affecting the prognosis of these patients—is the stage of the disease at the time of diagnosis. In the high-grade sarcomas (LMS and mixed endometrial sarcoma), the presence of tumor outside the uterus at the time of diagnosis is a clear prognostic omen: fewer than 10% of patients survive 2 years. Even when the disease is apparently limited to the uterus, the prognosis is poor: 10–50% survive 5 years. In intermediate-grade LMS and high-grade ESS, the outcome is improved, with up to 80–90% of patients surviving 5 years if the disease is clinically limited to the uterus at the time of surgery. Low-grade ESS and low-grade LMS have a generally favorable outcome: 80–100% of patients survive 5 years following complete excision of the uterus. Low-grade stromal tumors have been known to recur locally after 10–20 years; this confuses the survival statistics. Undoubtedly, these patients must be followed closely for life.

REFERENCES

Endometrial Hyperplasia & Carcinoma

Amant F et al: Endometrial cancer. Lancet 2005;366(9484):491.

Duska LR et al: Pilot trial of TAC (paclitaxel, doxorubicin, and carboplatin) chemotherapy with filgrastim (r-metHuG-CSF) support followed by radiotherapy in patients with "high-risk" endometrial cancer. Gynecol Oncol 2005;96(1):198.

Fung MFK et al: Prospective longitudinal study of ultrasound screening for endometrial abnormalities in women with breast cancer receiving tamoxifen. Gynecol Oncol 2003;91:154.

Jemal A et al: Cancer statistics 2004. CA Cancer J Clin 2004;54:8.

Karamursel BS et al: Which surgical procedure for patients with atypical endometrial hyperplasia? Int J Gynecol Cancer 2005;15:127.

Koh WJ et al: Radiation therapy in endometrial cancer. Baillieres Best Pract Res Clin Obstet Gynaecol 2001;15:417.

Kurman RJ, Kaminski PF, Norris HJ: The behavior of endometrial hyperplasia: A long-term study of "untreated" hyperplasia in 170 patients. Cancer 1985;56:403.

Lalloo F, Evans G: Molecular genetics and endometrial cancer. Baillieres Best Pract Res Clin Obstet Gynaecol 2001;15:355.

Mariani A, Webb MJ, Keeney GL, Podratz KC. Routes of lymphatic spread: a study of 112 consecutive patients with endometrial cancer. Gynecol Oncol 2001;81:100–104.

Montz FJ: Significance of "normal" endometrial cells in cervical cytology from asymptomatic postmenopausal women receiving hormone replacement therapy. Gynecol Oncol 2001;81:33.

Pothuri B et al: Development of endometrial cancer after radiation treatment for cervical carcinoma. Obstet Gynecol 2003;101:941.

Sakuragi N et al: Prognostic significance of serous and clear cell adenocarcinoma in surgically staged endometrial carcinoma. Acta Obstet Gynecol Scand 2000;79:311.

Takeshima N et al: Positive peritoneal cytology in endometrial cancer: Enhancement of other prognostic indicators. Gynecol Oncol 2001;82:470.

Thigpen JT et al: Phase III trial of doxorubicin with or without cisplatin in advanced endometrial carcinoma: A gynecologic oncology group study. J Clin Oncol 2004;22(19):3902.

Sarcoma of the Uterus

Brooks SE et al: Surveillance, epidemiology, and end results analysis of 2677 cases of uterine sarcoma 1989–1999.Gynecol Oncol 2004;93(1):204.

Demetri GD: ET-743: The US experience in sarcomas of the soft tissues. Anticancer Drugs 2002;13:S7.

Dinh TA et al: The treatment of uterine leiomyosarcoma. Results from a 10-year experience (1990–1999) at Massachusetts General Hospital. Gynecol Oncol 2004;92:648.

Giuntoli RL et al: Retrospective review of 208 patients with leiomyosarcoma of the uterus: Prognostic indicators, surgical management, and adjuvant therapy. Gynecol Oncol 2003;89:460.

Hensley ML et al: Gemcitabine and docetaxel in patients with unresectable leiomyosarcoma: Results of a phase II trial. J Clin Oncol 2002;20(12):2824.

Kushner D et al: Safety and efficacy of adjuvant single-agent ifosfamide in uterine sarcoma. Gynecol Oncol 2000;78:221.

Look KY et al: Phase II trial of gemcitabine as second line chemotherapy of uterine leiomyosarcoma: An Gynecologic Oncology Group (GOG) study. Gynecol Oncol 2004;92:644.

Manolitsas TP et al: Multimodality therapy for patients with clinical stage I and II malignant mixed müllerian tumors of the uterus. Cancer 2001;15:1437.

O'Meara AT: Uterine sarcomas: Have we made any progress? Curr Opin Obstet Gynecol 2004;16(1):1.

Premalignant & Malignant Disorders of the Ovaries & Oviducts

52

Kathleen M. Brennan, MD, Vicki V. Baker, MD, & Oliver Dorigo, MD

Ovarian cancer accounts for 3–4% of cancer in women, and is the fourth most frequent cause of cancer-related death in females in the United States. In the year 2005, an estimated 22,220 new ovarian cancer cases were diagnosed in the United States and 16,210 patients succumbed to the disease. Ovarian cancer is the second most common gynecologic malignancy, endometrial cancer being the most common, but is the most common cause of death among women who develop a gynecologic malignancy. From 1985–2001, the incidence of ovarian cancer declined at a rate of 0.8% per year, the greatest decline seen among women age 65 years and older. In general, ovarian cancer is a disease of the postmenopausal woman, with the highest incidence among patients ages 65–74 years. The lifetime risk of developing ovarian cancer is approximately 1.4%, and the lifetime risk of dying from ovarian cancer is almost 1%.

ETIOLOGY OF OVARIAN CANCER

Incessant ovulation is thought to play an important role in the underlying mechanism in the development of ovarian cancer. The repeated disruption and repair of the germinal epithelium may provide ample opportunity for somatic gene deletions and mutations to occur, which, in turn, can contribute to tumor initiation and progression. Supporting this theory are the observations that multiparity, use of oral contraceptive pills, and a history of breastfeeding are protective. Pregnancy is associated with a risk reduction of 13–19% per pregnancy, and in women who use oral contraceptives for 5 years or longer, the risk of epithelial ovarian cancer decreases by 50%. Considerable controversy surrounds the idea of whether infertility treatment is associated with an increased risk of ovarian cancer. A large pooled analysis of 5207 women with cancer and 7705 controls showed no associated increased risk with fertility drug exposure. Rather, infertility itself confers a higher risk of ovarian cancer as nulliparity compared to multiparity (> 4) and infertility for longer than 5 years (compared

to < 1 year) carried relative risks of 2.42 and 2.7, respectively. Hormone replacement therapy was found to have a nonsignificant increase in risk for ovarian cancer.

A number of different studies suggest an association between dietary factors and ovarian cancer. Diets high in saturated animal fats seem to confer an increased risk by unknown mechanisms. Interestingly, Japanese women who move to the United States have an increased ovarian cancer risk. A recent Norwegian study of more than 1 million women showed a positive association between body mass index, height, and risk of ovarian cancer, particularly the endometrioid type in women younger than age 60 years. Other factors, like alcohol and milk product consumption, have been hypothesized as risk factors but never confirmed. Exposure to talc has also been proposed as a risk factor in women who place talcum powder on the external genitalia. The presence of talc granulomas in the ovaries of patients who have never been previously operated on is well documented and can be explained by the continuity of the introitus and peritoneal cavity via the endocervical canal, the endometrial cavity, and the fallopian tubes (Fig 52–1). The ability of foreign materials, including talc and asbestos, to act as carcinogenic substances is established in several models, but their role in ovarian carcinogenesis remains speculative. Bilateral tubal ligation reduces the incidence of ovarian cancer, possibly by preventing carcinogenic substances from ascending into the müllerian ductal system.

Approximately 90% of ovarian cancer develops sporadically. However, an estimated 10–12% of epithelial ovarian cancer patients have a genetic predisposition. Chromosomal abnormalities are commonly associated with ovarian malignancies. Patients with Turner's syndrome (45,XO) are at increased risk of dysgerminoma and gonadoblastoma. Hereditary ovarian cancer occurs in two forms, either as breast and ovarian cancer (BOC) syndrome, or the less common Lynch II syndrome, also known as hereditary nonpolyposis colorectal cancer (HNPCC) syndrome. BOC is most often associated

Figure 52–1. Papillary lesion with incorporated talc granules.

with germ line mutations in the *BRCA1* gene located on chromosome 17 and less commonly with *BRCA2* mutations on chromosome 13. The overall frequency of *BRCA1* mutation carriers in the United States is approximately 1 in 800 women. Greater mutation frequencies have been found in Ashkenazi Jews and Icelandic women. Because these mutations are inherited in an autosomal dominant fashion, they require a careful pedigree analysis. Women with *BRCA1* mutations from high-risk families have a lifetime risk of ovarian cancer as high as 44%. The risk in women with *BRCA2* mutations have a lifetime risk of up to 27%.

The HNPCC syndrome involves a combination of familial colon cancer (Lynch I syndrome) and a high rate of ovarian, endometrial, gastrointestinal, and genitourinary malignancies. Genes involved in this syndrome include mainly DNA mismatch repair genes like *MLH1, MSH2, MSH3, MSH6, PMS1,* and *PMS2*. A woman who is a member of a family affected by this syndrome appear to have a lifetime risk for developing ovarian cancer of approximately 12%. Hereditary ovarian cancers generally occur in women about 10 years younger than those with nonhereditary tumors.

A number of molecular mechanisms related to ovarian cancer pathogenesis have been described. Allelic loss and mutations of the p53 tumor suppressor gene are found in approximately 55% of all ovarian cancers, with the highest frequency noted in serous and endometrioid ovarian cancers, particularly in advanced stage disease. The c-*erb*-B2 (HER2/*neu*) proto-oncogene is activated in a fraction of ovarian cancers, providing the potential for increased proliferation and metastasis. The anti-HER2/*neu* antibody therapy Herceptin, which is active against breast cancer, is currently being investigated as a therapeutic agent in ovarian cancer. Other molecular pathways include decreased expression of CDK (cyclin-dependent kinase) inhibitors, k-*ras* mutations, *p16* deletions, and activation of the *PI3kinase/Akt* pathway. These molecular pathways may provide targets for novel therapeutic approaches to ovarian cancer.

HISTOPATHOLOGY OF OVARIAN CANCER

Ovarian cancer can be divided into three major categories based on the cell type of origin (Table 52–1). The ovary may also be the site of metastatic disease by primary cancer from another organ site. Unlike carcinomas of the cervix and endometrium, precursor lesions of ovarian carcinoma have not been defined.

1. Epithelial Neoplasms

Epithelial neoplasms are derived from the ovarian surface mesothelial cells and include several cell types: **serous, mucinous, endometrioid, clear cell, transitional cell, and undifferentiated.** Epithelial tumors account for more than 60% of all ovarian neoplasms and for more than 90% of malignant ovarian tumors.

Ovarian **serous cystadenocarcinoma** is the most common malignant tumor of the ovary, accounting for 75–80% of all epithelial cancers. Grossly, these neoplasms are bilateral in 40–60% of cases, and 85% are associated with extraovarian spread at the time of diagnosis. More than 50% of serous tumors exceed 15 cm in diameter, and cut section reveals solid areas, areas of hemorrhage, necrosis, cyst wall invasion, and adhesions to adjacent structures. Unilocular or multilocular cysts often contain coarse papillae that project into the cystic lumen (Fig 52–2).

Histologically, serous carcinomas of the ovary resemble the endosalpinx and exhibit mild to moderate

Table 52–1. Major histopathologic categories of ovarian cancer.

Epithelial
Serous, mucinous, endometrioid, clear cell, transitional cell (Brenner), undifferentiated
Germ Cell
Dysgerminoma, endodermal sinus tumor, teratoma (immature, mature, specialized), embryonal carcinoma, choriocarcinoma, gonadoblastoma, mixed germ cell, polyembryona
Sex Cord and Stromal
Granulosa cell tumor, bibroma, thecoma Sertoli-Leydig cell, gynandroblastoma
Neoplasms Metastatic to the Ovary
Breast, colon, stomach, endometrium, lymphoma

Figure 52–2. Internal papillae characteristic of the papillary serous cystadenocarcinoma.

nuclear atypia and occasional mitotic figures of the stratified squamous epithelium, which often forms budding tufts. Psammoma bodies, irregular lamellar calcifications, are frequently found in serous tumors. The grade of differentiation of these neoplasms is based on the degree of preservation of the papillary architecture. Most serous carcinomas are poorly differentiated with trabecular and solid growth patterns.

Serous ovarian neoplasms of low malignancy potential exhibit histologic features suggestive of both carcinoma and benignity. Although marked cellular pleomorphism and mitotic figures are often present, there is no stromal invasion. Psammoma bodies are often present. These tumors may be associated with metastatic implants, invasive or noninvasive, although most remain confined to the ovary. Seen predominantly in premenopausal women, these tumors are associated with a good prognosis.

Mucinous neoplasms of the ovary account for 10% of all epithelial ovarian tumors. In contrast to serous tumors, mucinous tumors are bilateral in less than 10% of cases.

Mucinous tumors are notable for the large size that they may attain; neoplasms weighing more than 150 pounds have been reported. However, the median size of these lesions is 18–20 cm. Cut sections of these tumors typically reveal multilocular cysts filled with viscous mucin (Fig 52–3). The lining of these tumors is composed of atypical cells with numerous mitotic figures.

Histologically, mucinous adenocarcinoma of the ovary resembles endocervical epithelium. The cells have large hyperchromatic nuclei and prominent nucleoli. Invasive mucinous ovarian carcinoma exhibits marked histologic variability from area to area within the tumor, and extensive sampling is required. It is recom-

mended that at least one section per centimeter of tumor be examined to find the most malignant focus. The differentiation of mucinous cystadenocarcinoma is related to the preservation of glandlike architecture of the tumor. These tumors must be distinguished from

Figure 52–3. Mucinous cystadenocarcinoma. Note the obvious mucinous component and the solid, more malignant areas.

Figure 52–4. Endometrioid carcinoma as seen with high-power field. Note the tall epithelium—not a tubal type or the mucoid variety.

metastatic mucinous tumors originating in the colon and rectum, appendix, endocervix, and pancreas because of similar cell architecture.

Both invasive carcinomas and tumors of low malignancy potential of the mucinous variety are recognized. Mucinous tumors of low malignancy potential are characterized histologically by several cell types, including endocervical-like columnar cells, intestinal-like columnar cells with eosinophilic cytoplasm, goblet cells, and basal endocrine cells. Although cellular atypia may be present with a moderate number of mitotic figures, cellular stratification does not exceed 2–3 layers and stromal invasion is absent.

Pseudomyxoma peritonei is an unusual condition that may occur in association with mucinous neoplasms of the ovary resulting from the progressive accumulation of mucin in the abdominal cavity following its slow leakage from a neoplasm. It most commonly occurs in association with lesions of low malignancy potential; however, it is also reported to occur in association with cystadenocarcinoma of the ovary and appendix as well as mucocele of the appendix. Although rare and histologically benign in appearance, pseudomyxoma peritonei has a protracted and potentially morbid course frequently secondary to bowel obstruction, with a mortality rate that approaches 50%.

Endometrioid neoplasms of the ovary, accounting for 10% of epithelial tumors, exhibit an adenomatoid pattern that resembles endometrial adenocarcinoma (Fig 52–4). It is bilateral in 30–50% of cases. Rarely, this neoplasm arises in foci of endometriosis (less than 10% of cases). The degree of differentiation is based on the extent to which the glandular architecture is retained. As many as 30% of patients with endometrioid carcinoma of the ovary also have a synchronous endometrial carcinoma of the uterus that is a second primary rather than a metastatic focus of disease. A recent study showed that 25% of women 45 years or younger with type I endometrial cancer had coexisting ovarian malignancies. Of these tumors, 88% were classified as synchronous primaries and 92% showed endometrioid histology.

Clear cell carcinoma of the ovary, also referred to as **mesonephroid carcinoma** of the ovary because their histologic features include "clear cells," as seen in renal cell carcinomas, accounts for less than 1% of epithelial ovarian cancers. These tumors rarely attain the size of serous and mucinous neoplasms of the ovary. Clear cell carcinomas of the ovary are biologically aggressive and can be associated with hypercalcemia and hyperpyrexia. On cut section, both cystic and solid areas are present. The external surface is smooth but has a bosselated contour. Histologically, two cell types may be present: the clear cell and the "hobnail cell" (Fig 52–5). Occasionally, clear cell carcinomas are difficult to differentiate from mucinous neoplasms. The periodic acid-Schiff reaction can be used to differentiate the two as it is only weakly positive in clear cell neoplasms but strikingly positive in mucinous tumors.

Transitional cell (Brenner) carcinoma of the ovary, accounting for < 1% of epithelial cancers, is composed of cells that resemble low-grade transitional

Figure 52–5. Adenomatous pattern with papillary infolding and "hobnail epithelium." In many areas, clear cells can be seen with transitions to the hobnail type.

cell carcinoma of the urinary bladder. Patients typically present with advanced stage disease and exhibit a poorer prognosis when compared with that of other histologic types of epithelial ovarian cancer.

Undifferentiated carcinoma of the ovary accounts for less than 10% of epithelial neoplasms. This neoplasm is characterized by the absence of any distinguishing microscopic features that permit its placement in one of the other histologic categories.

2. Germ Cell Neoplasms

Germ cell neoplasms arise from the germ cell elements of the ovary and include dysgerminoma, endodermal sinus tumor, embryonal cell carcinoma, choriocarcinoma, teratoma, polyembryoma, and mixed germ cell tumors. Unlike the epithelial neoplasms, which tend to occur during the sixth decade of life, this group of tumors tends to occur during the second and third decades and as a group is associated with a better prognosis. Many of these neoplasms produce biologic markers that can be monitored to assess response to therapy (Table 52–2).

Dysgerminoma of the ovary is the female counterpart of the seminoma in the male. It occurs primarily in young females and accounts for approximately 30–40% of germ cell tumors. Grossly, the tumor is rather rubbery in consistency, smooth, rounded, and thinly encapsulated, with a brown or grayish-brown color. This neoplasm is unilateral in 85–90% of cases. It is a solid neoplasm which may contain areas of softening as a result of degeneration.

Histologically, dysgerminoma mimics the pattern seen in the primitive gonad, with nests of germ cells that appear as large, rounded cells with central nuclei that contain one or two prominent nucleoli surrounded by undifferentiated stroma (Fig 52–6). Lymphocytes may invade the stroma and occasionally giant cells are identified. A lymphocytic infiltrate is considered a favorable prognostic indicator.

Figure 52–6. Classic histologic picture of dysgerminoma. Note nests of germ cells of various sizes separated by fibrous trabeculae.

Table 52–2. Tumor markers that may be elevated in the presence of germ cell neoplasms.

Neoplasm	AFP	hCG
Dysgerminoma	*	+/–
Endodermal sinus tumor	+	–
Immature teratoma	+/–	
Mixed germ cell tumor	+/–	+/–
Choriocarcinoma	–	+
Embryonal carcinoma	+/–	+

AFP, α-fetoprotein; hCG, human chorionic gonadotropin.
– = negative (not elevated);
+ = positive (elevated above normal level).
* = borderline (<16 ng/mL) elevations in case reports

Endodermal sinus tumor of the ovary, previously called a **yolk sac tumor,** is the third most common germ cell neoplasm. It is bilateral in nearly 100% of cases. It holds the distinction of being the most rapidly growing neoplasm that occurs at any site. These lesions are friable, focally necrotic, and hemorrhagic. Patients commonly present with an acute abdomen.

Microscopically, endodermal sinus tumor is composed of primitive epithelial cells that form architectural patterns that recapitulate the primitive gut and the primitive liver. The pathognomonic finding is the Schiller-Duval body, which is a single papilla lined by tumor cells with a central blood vessel. This neoplasm commonly contains cells that produce α-fetoprotein (AFP), which as a serum marker is useful in following the response to therapy.

Immature teratomas of the ovary are the malignant counterpart of the mature cystic teratoma, or dermoid, and are the second most common germ cell malignancy. Malignant teratomas are found most commonly in patients younger than 20 years old. This malignancy is bilateral in less than 5% of cases, although the contralateral ovary commonly contains a dermoid cyst. The serum AFP is usually elevated in patients with an immature teratoma.

Microscopic examination reveals a disordered collection of tissues derived from the three germ layers, with at least some of the components having an immature, embryonic appearance. The immature elements are commonly neuroectodermal and consist of small, round, malignant cells that may be associated with glia formation. Hyaline bodies stain positive for AFP. Immature teratomas can be graded from 1 to 3 based on the amount of immature neural tissue they contain. Tumor grade is correlated with prognosis and also guides recommendations regarding the need for chemotherapy. Metastatic implants may be composed entirely of mature neuroectodermal tissue. In this circumstance, the stage of the tumor is not increased and the prognosis is not diminished.

Mature teratomas or dermoids are common ovarian neoplasms, occurring primarily in women ages 20–30 years. They represent the most common neoplasm diagnosed during pregnancy. Less than 1% of all teratomas are malignant.

Embryonal carcinoma of the ovary is a very rare germ cell tumor with a mean age of diagnosis at 15 years. The neoplasm has a highly aggressive growth pattern with early extensive spread. Histologically, this neoplasm consists of solid sheets of large polygonal cells with pale, eosinophilic cytoplasms that appear to merge together as a syncytium because the cell membranes are poorly defined. Serum human chorionic gonadotropin (hCG) and serum AFP levels are usually elevated. In addition, estrogens can be produced by these tumors and may serve as a serum marker.

Choriocarcinoma of the ovary is another rare germ cell tumor that is unrelated to pregnancy. Unlike gestational choriocarcinoma, primary ovarian choriocarcinoma is associated with somewhat lower elevations of hCG. The endocrine activity of this neoplasm may cause precocious puberty, uterine bleeding, or amenorrhea. Microscopically, this neoplasm is composed of cytotrophoblasts, intermediate trophoblasts, and syncytiotrophoblasts.

Gonadoblastoma of the ovary is a rare neoplasm composed of nests of germ cells and sex cord derivatives that are surrounded by connective tissue stroma (Fig 52–7). These tumors are more common in the right ovary than in the left, and usually occur during the second decade of life. Gonadoblastomas are found in patients with abnormal gonadal development in the presence of a Y chromosome.

Mixed germ cell tumors of the ovary account for approximately 10% of germ cell neoplasms. As implied by the name, these neoplasms contain two or more germ cell elements. A dysgerminoma and endodermal sinus tumor occur together most frequently. These neoplasms must be meticulously evaluated by the pathologist to identify all elements correctly, as different components may require treatment with different chemotherapeutic regimens.

Figure 52–7. Gonadoblastoma with folliculoid pattern, focal calcifications, and concretions.

Polyembryoma of the ovary is an extremely rare tumor most commonly seen in premenarchal girls with signs of pseudopuberty. The tumor secretes AFP and hCG, is composed of "embryoid bodies," and mimics the structures of the three somatic layers of early embryonic differentiation.

SEX CORD-STROMAL TUMORS OF THE OVARY

Sex cord-stromal tumors of the ovary account for 5–8% of all ovarian malignancies. Granulosa cell tumors are the most common malignant tumors of the sex cord-stromal tumor category, accounting for 70% of these tumors. They are associated with hyperestrogenism and may cause precocious puberty in young girls and adenomatous hyperplasia and vaginal bleeding in postmenopausal women. Microscopically, the granulosa cells, which exhibit characteristic grooved or coffee bean nuclei, can exhibit microfollicular, macrofollicular, trabecular, insular, or solid growth patterns. Call-Exner bodies are associated with the microfollicular growth pattern and represent multiple small cavities that contain eosinophilic fluid. Theca cells are present in varying amounts.

Like granulosa cell tumors, ovarian thecomas are associated with hyperestrogenism. This mostly benign ovarian tumor consists of lipid-laden stromal cells, which confer a yellow appearance on cut section. An ovarian fibroma is another benign tumor that is noteworthy because of its association with Meigs' syndrome. Meigs' syndrome refers to the occurrence of an ovarian fibroma, ascites, and pleural effusion, which collectively mimic the presentation of ovarian cancer.

Sertoli-stromal cell tumors are rare and consist of testicular structures at different stages of development. They are usually virilizing and occur most commonly during the third and fourth decades of life, with average age at diagnosis being 25 years. They are rarely bilateral. Microscopically, both Sertoli and Leydig cells are present. A variety of architectural patterns have been described.

NEOPLASMS METASTATIC TO THE OVARY

Cancer metastatic to the ovary accounts for 5–6% of all ovarian malignancies, most commonly from the female genital tract, the breast, or the gastrointestinal tract. Microscopically, the origin of an ovarian metastasis might be difficult to determine. In metastatic breast carcinoma, for example, the histologic appearance of the ovary may be different when compared to the primary breast tumor. Gastrointestinal carcinoma metastatic to the ovary often simulates a primary mucin-secreting adenocarcinoma of the ovary with the presence of characteristic signet ring cells (Fig 52–8). Large locules lined by tall columnar mucin-secreting epithelial cells are separated by fibrous trabeculae. The epithelium shows various degrees of differentiation.

By definition, Krukenberg tumors represent carcinomas of the stomach metastatic to the ovary. However, the eponym is commonly used to denote any gas-

Figure 52–8. Metastatic ovarian cancer. Note the "signet cells," characteristic of the mucocellular nature of the tumor.

trointestinal carcinoma metastatic to the ovary. Immunohistochemistry is commonly used to facilitate the characterization of ovarian tumors. The cytokeratin expression pattern can help to distinguish between a primary mucinous ovarian and a metastatic colon cancer. The ovarian tumor is expected to stain positive for cytokeratin 7 (CK7) and negative for CK20. In contrast, a metastatic lesion from a primary mucinous adenocarcinoma of the colon is likely to show the reverse pattern (CK7 negative, CK20 positive).

■ DIAGNOSIS OF OVARIAN CANCER

Ovarian cancer typically develops as an insidious disease, with few warning signs or symptoms. Most neoplastic ovarian tumors produce few symptoms until the disease is widely disseminated throughout the abdominal cavity. A history of nonspecific gastrointestinal complaints, including nausea, dyspepsia, and altered bowel habits, is particularly common. Early satiety and abdominal distention as a result of ascites are generally signs of advanced disease. A change in bowel habits, such as constipation and decreased stool caliber, is occasionally noted. Large tumors may cause a sensation of pelvic weight or pressure. Rarely, an ovarian tumor may become incarcerated in the cul-de-sac and cause severe pain, urinary retention, rectal discomfort, and bowel obstruction.

Menstrual abnormalities may be noted in as many as 15% of reproductive-age patients with an ovarian neoplasm. Abnormal vaginal bleeding may occur in patients with ovarian cancer in the presence of a synchronous endometrial carcinoma or as a consequence of metastatic disease to the lower genital tract. Rarely, excess androgens or estrogens are present in women with ovarian neoplasms, presumably because of stimulation of normal theca, granulosa, or hilar cells that surround the neoplasm. Ovarian stromal hyperplasia or hyperthecosis also may be associated with excess androgen production, which alters the normal menstrual cycle. Granulosa theca cell tumors are classically estrogen-producing tumors that present with abnormal vaginal bleeding.

The prognosis of ovarian cancer is significantly improved when the disease is detected while still confined to the ovary. However, despite the availability of various clinical test as outlined below, general screening for the early detection of ovarian cancer so far is not an efficient strategy. Ultrasonographic evaluation can detect the majority of ovarian neoplasms but has poor specificity. The best-characterized tumor marker in epithelial ovarian cancer is cancer antigen-125 (CA-125). CA-

125 is a secreted glycoprotein present in fetal amniotic and coelomic epithelium and its level can be detected in serum using immunoassay. The accepted upper limit of normal is 35 IU/mL, but this is a rather arbitrary cut-off. Routine screening using CA-125 of low-risk, asymptomatic women cannot be recommended at this time. However, CA-125 might play a role in screening of high-risk patients with genetic predisposition. Ovarian cancer screening to detect early stage disease will remain difficult until more specific and sensitive markers are defined. Unfortunately, routine pelvic examination is a notoriously poor screening method with limited sensitivity and specificity. Ten percent of masses less than 10 cm in size are missed on routine examination, and the size of a mass is correctly predicted within 2 cm in only 68% of patients. Current strategies for screening focus on the detection of tumor-associated antigens, such as CA-125, and ultrasound examinations of the adnexa. However, the limited prevalence of ovarian cancer and the lack of sensitivity and specificity of currently available tests have so far prevented the implementation of routine ovarian cancer screening in the general population.

EVALUATION OF THE PATIENT WITH A SUSPECTED OVARIAN NEOPLASM

A patient found to have a pelvic mass must be evaluated in a timely and cost-effective manner that is tailored to a realistic list of possible diagnoses. The differential diagnosis of a pelvic mass is influenced by the age of the patient, the characteristics of the mass on pelvic examination, and the radiographic appearance of the mass. In general, the prepubescent child and the postmenopausal woman are at greatest risk for a malignant ovarian neoplasm. The reproductive age woman is more likely to have a functional ovarian cyst or endometrioma.

Physical Examination

Although the focus of the physical examination in a patient with a suspected adnexal neoplasm is the pelvis, it is important to perform a comprehensive examination. Particular attention should be paid to the lymph-node-bearing areas, particularly the supraclavicular and inguinal areas. Metastatic disease to the skin rarely occurs in the presence of ovarian cancer. Sister Mary Joseph's nodule refers to a metastatic implant in the umbilicus.

Examination of the abdomen often provides important information. Abdominal distention is one of the more common findings. The presence of flank fullness and shifting dullness implies the presence of ascites or a large pelvic-abdominal mass. Together with these signs, tympanitic percussion noted over the lateral abdomen is consistent with a large mass that displaces the bowel to the periphery. In contrast, a central tympanitic percus-

Table 52–3. Characteristics of a pelvic mass that should be noted on physical examination.

Benign	Malignant
Mobility	Fixed
Consistency	Solid or form
Cul-de-sac	Bilateral
Mobile	Nodular
Cystic	
Smooth	
Unilateral	

sion note is suggestive of ascites. Recent eversion of the umbilicus in a patient with abdominal distention may result from an increase in intra-abdominal pressure secondary to ascites.

A careful and thorough pelvic examination provides many helpful clues regarding the etiology of a pelvic mass. Table 52–3 lists the characteristics of the mass that should be noted on pelvic examination.

Unilateral, cystic masses in reproductive-age women are benign in up to 95% of cases. These masses, particularly when less than 6–8 cm in size, are observed through a menstrual cycle as many represent functional cysts and spontaneously resolve. An enlarging mass or one that is associated with pain merits prompt intervention. A cystic, somewhat immobile adnexal mass may represent a hydrosalpinx or tuboovarian abscess. Fixed, bilateral masses and firm masses with nodularity are suggestive of, but not diagnostic of, an ovarian malignancy. Because no features seen on physical examination consistently distinguish malignant from benign neoplasms, further characterization must be accomplished with select radiographic examinations.

Radiographic Evaluation

Ultrasonography is the most common radiographic test to evaluate adnexal masses. Transabdominal examinations require a full bladder as an acoustic window for optimal visualization of the adnexa. In contradistinction, a transvaginal examination does not have this requirement but may not be as useful for the assessment of large adnexal masses. Table 52–4 provides examples of ultrasonographic characteristics of benign compared to malignant ovarian masses. A number of different scoring systems are used, that include characteristics like ovarian volume, number and thickness of septations, presence of papillary projections, and solid components. Persistence of ultrasonic findings on a repeat scan after 4–6 weeks may help reduce the false-positive rate. However, there is no standardized system for evaluation of ovarian

Table 52–4. Radiographic characteristics that help to differentiate benign and malignant adnexal masses.

Benign	Malignant
Simple cyst, < 10 cm in size	Solid or cystic and solid
Septations < 3 mm in thickness	Multiple septations > 2–3
Unilateral	mm in size
Calcification, especially teeth	Bilateral
Gravity-dependent layering of cyst contents	Ascites

masses. The correlation between the ultrasonic appearance of an adnexal mass and the pathologic findings is imprecise. Color-flow Doppler studies that evaluate the vascular patterns of adnexal masses show promise as a means to improve the sensitivity and specificity of the radiographic diagnosis of benign and malignant lesions. Angiogenesis accompanying malignancy results in vascular abnormalities and increased blood flow compared with the vascular architecture and patterns of blood flow in nonmalignant lesions.

Characterization of adnexal masses by computed tomography (CT) or magnetic resonance imaging (MRI) may provide clinically useful information in select instances. CT scanning provides information about the retroperitoneal structures in addition to the pelvic organs. MRI scans can add more information regarding the nature of the ovarian neoplasm. Because of the high cost and questionable benefit, this diagnostic procedure is infrequently used for ovarian tumors. However, it may be of particular benefit in the evaluation of pregnant patients because it avoids radiation exposure of the fetus.

A patient with suspected ovarian malignancy should undergo a radiograph of the chest to exclude metastatic parenchymal disease and to detect a pleural effusion.

If the patient notes a change in bowel habits or if guaiac-positive stools are detected, a barium enema should be obtained. Patients who appear to have advanced ovarian cancer, evidenced by a nodular pelvic mass with or without ascites may actually have colon cancer. Because of the genetic links among ovarian cancer, colon cancer, and breast cancer, a patient with a suspected ovarian malignancy should also undergo a screening mammogram study.

Laboratory Evaluation

If an ovarian malignancy is suspected, laboratory tests including complete blood count (CBC) and serum electrolyte test should be obtained in all patients. The serum hCG level should be measured in any female in whom pregnancy is a possibility. In addition, a serum

AFP and lactate dehydrogenase (LDH) should be measured in young girls and adolescents who present with adnexal masses because of the greater likelihood of a malignant germ cell tumor. The serum CA-125 level should also be determined whenever an ovarian malignancy is included in the differential diagnosis. An elevated CA-125 in the postmenopausal patient is particularly suggestive of the presence of an ovarian malignancy, although it is not specific for the diagnosis. Cancers of the colon, breast, pancreas, stomach, uterus, and fallopian tube are also associated with an elevated CA-125 value. Benign conditions commonly diagnosed in younger women, including pregnancy, endometriosis, leiomyomata, and adenomyosis, limit the usefulness of this test in premenopausal women. A normal CA-125 level does *not* exclude the diagnosis of cancer and does not represent a reason to delay surgery.

Paracentesis is not advocated as a routine procedure for the patient with ascites and a pelvic mass and in whom renal, cardiac, and hepatic failure has been excluded. False-negative results may occur in as many as 40% of patients with widespread intra-abdominal disease. In contrast to the role of paracentesis, diagnostic thoracentesis for cytology is recommended for staging purposes. In the presence of malignant pleural effusions, the patient has stage IV disease.

■ SURGICAL TREATMENT OF EPITHELIAL OVARIAN CANCER

Surgery is the cornerstone of therapy for ovarian cancer, regardless of cell type or stage of disease. Whenever ovarian cancer is considered a likely diagnosis, a gynecologic oncologist should be consulted and actively involved in the evaluation and subsequent management of the patient. A gynecologic oncologist is trained to address both the surgical and the medical needs of these patients.

Intraoperatively, several features have been described that assist in the differentiation of malignant from benign adnexal masses (Table 52–5). However, gross examination of a mass is never a substitute for histologic examination. Whenever the pathology of a pelvic or adnexal mass is in question, a frozen-section pathologic study should be requested. In the hands of experienced pathologists, false-positive and false-negative diagnoses occur in less than 5% of cases. Patients diagnosed with ovarian cancer have to undergo surgical staging to reduce the amount of disease and evaluate the extent of spread. Removal of the primary tumor, as well as the associated metastatic disease, is referred to as tumor debulking or cytoreductive surgery. In early stages and when fertility is desired, removal of the involved adnexa alone may be considered.

Table 52–5. Intraoperative differentiation of benign and malignant masses.

Benign	Malignant
Simple cyst	Adhesions
Unilateral	Rupture
No adhesions	Ascites
Smooth surfaces	Solid areas
Intact capsule	Areas of hemorrhage or necrosis
	Papillary excrescences
	Multiloculated mass
	Bilateral

The full extent of disease must be carefully documented. At the time of diagnosis, more than 70% of patients with epithelial ovarian cancer have metastases beyond the pelvis. The most common locations of metastases secondary to advanced stage ovarian cancer are the peritoneum (85%), omentum (70%), liver (35%), pleura (33%), lung (25%), and bone (15%). Lymphatic metastasis occurs frequently, with up to 80% involving pelvic lymph nodes and 67% involving paraaortic lymph nodes, depending on the stage of disease.

The information gained from accurate surgical staging guides discussion of prognosis and also influences treatment decisions. Surgical staging requires documentation of the primary neoplasm and determination of the extent of disease by inspection, biopsy of peritoneal and intra-abdominal lesions, and biopsy of the retroperitoneal lymph nodes. Table 52–6 lists the procedures included in surgical staging of ovarian cancer. Any fluid in the peritoneal cavity should be aspirated. If no free fluid is present, "peritoneal washings" should be obtained by instilling 50–100 mL of saline into the right

Table 52–6. Procedures in the surgical staging of ovarian cancer.

Sample of ascites or peritoneal washings from the paracolic gutters and pelvic and subdiaphragmatic surface for cytology
Complete abdominal exploration
Intact removal of tumor
Hysterectomy
Infracolic omentectomy
Biopsies of abdominal peritoneal implants; if none present, random biopsies from the paracolic gutter peritoneum, pelvic peritoneum, and right subdiaphragmatic peritoneal surface
Pelvic and paraaortic lymph node biopsies
Cytoreductive surgery to remove all visible disease

paracolic gutter, the left paracolic gutter, the pelvic cul-de-sac, and beneath each hemidiaphragm. The fluid is subsequently collected and submitted to the laboratory for cytologic examination. Complete surgical staging of ovarian cancer requires biopsy of pelvic and paraaortic lymph nodes. It is emphasized that palpation of the retroperitoneal node-bearing areas is inaccurate and is not a substitute for biopsy and histologic examination. Table 52–7 lists the current staging of ovarian cancer approved by the International Federation of Gynecology and Obstetrics (FIGO).

In general, the contralateral adnexa should be removed even when they are grossly normal. They are often the site of occult metastatic disease, and there is a significant risk of subsequent cancer. Exceptions to this generalization are made for young women with an apparent stage I epithelial ovarian neoplasm. If future fertility is desired and the patient is informed about a higher risk of recurrent disease, a more conservative surgical approach may be chosen. The histology and grade of the neoplasm, as well as the findings at the time of surgery, guide these decisions. Well-differentiated stage I lesions are associated with a much better 5-year survival rate than are moderately and poorly differentiated

Table 52–7. International Federation of Gynecology and Obstetrics (FIGO) staging of ovarian neoplasms.

Stage I. Growth limited to the ovaries
 Ia—one ovary involved
 Ib—both ovaries involved
 Ic—Ia or Ib and ovarian surface tumor, ruptured capsule, malignant ascites, or peritoneal cytology positive for malignant cells
Stage II. Extension of the neoplasm from the ovary to the pelvis
 IIa—extension to the uterus or fallopian tube
 IIb—extension to other pelvic tissues
 IIc—IIa or b and ovarian surface tumor, ruptured capsule, malignant ascites, or peritoneal cytology positive for malignant cells
Stage III. Disease extension to the abdominal cavity
 IIIa—abdominal peritoneal surfaces with microscopic metastases
 IIIb—tumor metastases < 2 cm in size
 IIIc—tumor metastases > 2 cm in size or metastatic disease in the pelvic, paraaortic, or inguinal lymph nodes
Stage IV. Distant metastatic disease
 Malignant pleural effusion
 Pulmonary parenchymal metastases
 Liver or splenic parenchymal metastases (not surface implants)
 Metastases to the supraclavicular lymph nodes or skin

lesions. Mucinous and endometrioid neoplasms are associated with a better prognosis than serous and clear cell carcinomas of the ovary. If the frozen section during surgery does not reveal a reliable diagnosis of malignancy, the surgical procedure should be limited until the pathology results are finalized.

A hysterectomy is generally performed because the uterus is a common site for metastatic disease. There is also a risk of synchronous endometrial cancer in patients with endometrioid carcinoma of the ovary. In addition, removal of the uterus facilitates subsequent follow-up examinations and obviates potential problems secondary to uterine bleeding.

An infracolic omentectomy is recommended, even in the absence of gross tumor involvement, because it is a common site of microscopic metastatic disease. Removal of the omentum facilitates the distribution of intraperitoneal agents, may decrease the rate of accumulation of ascites postoperatively, and provides palliation to those patients with omental metastases.

Cytoreductive surgery should always be attempted if possible. The rationale for aggressive reduction of tumor burden is based on three main considerations. First, the removal of tumor mass often relieves gastrointestinal symptoms and improves the overall nutritional status. Reduction of tumor cell mass also leads to a therapeutically favorable change in tumor cell kinetics because large bulky tumors are often poorly vascularized and oxygenated and thus are more resistant to chemo- and radiation therapy. Furthermore, large tumor masses consist of a higher proportion of cells in the resting phase of the cell cycle. Finally, a number of tumors including ovarian cancer are known to produce immunosuppressive factors that block antitumor immune responses by inhibiting the generation of cytotoxic T lymphocytes.

Peritoneal implants should always be sampled to confirm the clinical impression of metastatic disease. The differential diagnosis of peritoneal implants include endometriosis, tuberculous peritonitis, and talc or suture granulomas. Nodular, roughened, or otherwise suspicious areas should be biopsied.

After completion of initial therapy with surgery followed by chemotherapy, patients without clinical evidence of disease may undergo a second-look operation to determine the therapeutic response and assess the persistence of tumor disease. This is usually done in the setting of an investigational protocol. A laparotomy is performed to obtain multiple specimens from peritoneal surfaces and suspicious areas. Approximately 30% of patients without evidence of macroscopic disease are found to have microscopic metastasis. Patients with negative second-look laparotomy have significantly longer survival than those with residual disease. The likelihood of negative findings at second-look laparotomy is higher in patients that were initially diagnosed with early stage disease, low-grade tumors, residual tumor disease < 5 mm, and chemotherapy containing paclitaxel. However, even patients with negative biopsies have a recurrence rate of 30–50% after 5 years.

The indications for and realistic benefits of surgery in the patient with recurrent or persistent ovarian cancer require individualization and considerable surgical judgment. Removal of tumor disease after primary surgery is called secondary cytoreductive surgery. These procedures are performed in selected patients for whom resection may prolong life expectancy by reducing tumor burden to less than 5 mm, or for whom resection of tumor will relieve symptoms like gastrointestinal obstruction. Patients in whom complete resection of residual tumor burden is possible have a significantly longer survival compared to patients without complete resection.

■ SURGICAL TREATMENT OF GERM CELL NEOPLASMS

In contrast to epithelial ovarian neoplasms, most germ cell neoplasms are early stage at the time of diagnosis. This observation, in conjunction with the low incidence of bilaterality and the young age of most patients, for whom future fertility is desired, influences the surgical management of this group of neoplasms. For young women with a germ cell neoplasm of the ovary, removal of the involved adnexa with preservation of the normal-appearing contralateral adnexa and uterus is generally advocated. In view of the low incidence of bilaterality, biopsy or bivalving the contralateral ovary is not recommended because of the risk of peritubal and periovarian adhesions. Complete surgical staging of germ cell neoplasms is the same as for epithelial ovarian neoplasms and should be performed in all cases.

Certain characteristics unique to germ cell neoplasms make an impact on their surgical management. Dysgerminoma of the ovary has a propensity to metastasize to the pelvic and paraaortic lymph nodes in the absence of other evidence of metastatic disease. Biopsies of these structures is particularly important. Endodermal sinus tumor of the ovary is the most rapidly growing neoplasm known to occur at any site. This diagnosis must be considered in a young woman with a rapidly enlarging pelvic or abdominal mass. Immature teratoma of the ovary may present with numerous peritoneal implants consistent with metastatic disease. It is important to adequately sample these lesions to determine whether or not they contain malignant elements.

CHEMOTHERAPY OF EPITHELIAL OVARIAN CANCER

In patients with stage Ia disease and grade 1 tumors, chemotherapy following initial surgical treatment has no influence on survival. Therefore, this group of patients, if selected carefully, does not require chemotherapeutic treatment. However, all other patients should undergo systemic chemotherapy. Agents shown to be active against epithelial ovarian cancer include cisplatin, carboplatin, cyclophosphamide, and paclitaxel. Combination therapies have been demonstrated to be superior to single-agent treatment.

Currently the most effective regimen uses a combination of paclitaxel and carboplatin. This combination has replaced the former treatment with cyclophosphamide and cisplatin because it was shown to more efficacious in a number of clinical trials. A typical regimen includes systemic administration of carboplatin and paclitaxel for 6 cycles at 3-week intervals. Potential toxicities of this treatment include nausea, vomiting, diarrhea, alopecia, nephrotoxicity, and myelosuppression.

Carboplatin is a second-generation platinum analogue that shows clinical efficacies and survival rates similar to cisplatin when used in combination with paclitaxel. However, the frequency of gastrointestinal side effects and neurotoxicity associated with carboplatin were found to be lower compared to cisplatin.

Assessment of response to combination chemotherapy is based on physical examination, changes in size of palpable or radiographically measurable lesions, and changes in the CA-125 level. Although the preoperative CA-125 level does not correlate with tumor burden, changes in response to chemotherapy appear to be of some prognostic benefit. An elevated CA-125 (> 35 IU/mL) predicts persistent disease at second look in more than 97% of patients. However, a normal CA-125 level does not completely exclude the possibility of residual, subclinical disease.

Most patients develop resistance to platin-based regimens during the course of treatment. Salvage therapy for ovarian cancer is rarely curative, although significant prolongation of survival may be achieved in some instances. The response to re-treatment with platinum-based chemotherapy is influenced by the time interval between completion of the initial regimen and subsequent disease recurrence: the greater the interval, the greater the likelihood of a beneficial response.

Patients with platinum- or paclitaxel-sensitive tumors as evidenced by the clinical response to initial chemotherapy will likely benefit from re-treatment with a platinum- or paclitaxel-based regimen.

Chemotherapy of Germ Cell Neoplasms

Significant advances have been made in the treatment of germ cell neoplasms of the ovary. Once associated with 5-year survival rates of less than 20–30%, these neoplasms are now considered curable in a majority of cases following the introduction and refinement of combination chemotherapy.

Dysgerminoma is the most radiation-sensitive neoplasm identified. Historically, it has been treated with whole abdominal radiation therapy with excellent results. More recently, chemotherapy with cisplatin-containing regimens has been administered with excellent results. A significant advantage of chemotherapy is the potential to preserve future reproductive potential compared with radiation therapy.

The other germ cell neoplasms are rare, and the optimal chemotherapy and duration of therapy have not been established. Regimens including vinblastine-bleomycin-cisplatin, vincristine-actinomycin D-cyclophosphamide, and bleomycin-etoposide-cisplatin have been used with encouraging results. Response to chemotherapy is based on physical examination and the decrease in serum tumor markers, if initially elevated.

Complications of Chemotherapy

Combination chemotherapy invariably makes an impact on the patient's day-to-day activities and can be associated with a variety of potentially life-threatening side effects. Table 52–8 lists the most common toxicities of some of the more commonly used drugs in the treatment of ovarian cancer.

Nausea, vomiting, and alopecia are side effects anticipated and feared by many patients. The development of new, more effective antiemetics permits improved control of nausea and a reduction in the number of emesis episodes. Unfortunately, suggested strategies to prevent alopecia, such as scalp tourniquets and local hypothermia, are generally ineffective. Patients should be

Table 52–8. Chemotherapy-associated toxicities.

Agent	Toxicity
Cisplatin	Nephrotoxicity, neurotoxicity, ototoxicity
Carboplatin	Thrombocytopenia, neutropenia
Cyclophosphamide	Hemorrhagic cystitis, pulmonary fibrosis
Paclitaxel	Myelosuppression
Altretamine	Peripheral neuropathy
Etoposide	Myelosuppression
Bleomycin	Pulmonary fibrosis
Doxorubicin	Cardiac toxicity
Vincristine	Neuropathy
Ifosfamide	Hemorrhagic cystitis, central neurotoxicity

counseled that all chemotherapy regimens do not invariably result in hair loss.

Myelosuppression is another common side effect of chemotherapy. Complete blood counts with differential and platelet counts are typically monitored between cycles of therapy. Most regimens cause granulocytopenia and thrombocytopenia between days 10 and 18. Synthetic erythropoietin and colony-stimulating factor can be administered to lessen the severity and duration of anemia and granulocytopenia.

RADIATION THERAPY

Currently, radiation therapy plays a limited role in the treatment of patients with epithelial ovarian cancer mainly because of radiation damage to the small bowel, liver, and kidneys. Radioisotopes such as intraperitoneal ^{32}P may be of benefit in patients with stage Ic disease and those with microscopically positive second-look operations.

With respect to germ cell neoplasms, radiation therapy has been used successfully in the treatment of patients with dysgerminoma.

ALTERNATIVE THERAPIES

A number of alternative therapies have been applied for the treatment of epithelial ovarian cancer. Cytokines like interleukin-2 and interferon-γ either alone or in combination with chemotherapy have shown some promising effects. Monoclonal antibodies directed against ovarian cancer-associated antigens, including CA-125, HMFG (human milk-fat globulin), and HER-2/*neu* have been used with variable clinical responses. Recently, antibodies against vascular epithelial growth factor (VEGF) have shown efficacy in patients with ovarian cancer. Anti-VEGF antibodies are currently being tested in combination with carboplatin and paclitaxel in first-line chemotherapy for ovarian cancer patients. Gene therapy trials have used different antitumor approaches, including the delivery of tumor suppressor gene p53 via recombinant adenovirus into the peritoneal cavities. The early trials have not shown significant clinical response, mainly as a result of the inefficiency of intraperitoneal and intratumoral gene transfer.

PROGNOSIS

The prognosis for patients with ovarian cancer is primarily related to the stage of disease. The 5-year survival rate for patients with stage I epithelial ovarian cancer is, depending on tumor grade, between 76% and 93%. The 5-year survival rate for those with stage II disease is 60–74%. Stage III ovarian cancer is associated with a 5-year survival rate of approximately 23–41%.

The survival rate for a patient with stage IV disease is approximately 5–11%. Within each stage of disease, other factors are related to response to chemotherapy, disease-free survival, and overall survival. In general, patients with well-differentiated, diploid neoplasms with an S-phase fraction of less than 8–10% do better than patients who have poorly differentiated, aneuploid, rapidly proliferating (eg, high S-phase fraction) neoplasms.

In general, germ cell tumors are associated with better 5-year survival rates than epithelial ovarian neoplasms. Patients with dysgerminoma have a 5-year survival rate of 95%. Immature teratomas are associated with 5-year survival rates of 70–80%. An endodermal sinus tumor is associated with a 5-year survival rate of 60–70%. Embryonal carcinoma, choriocarcinoma, and polyembryoma are very rare lesions, and it is difficult to assess 5-year survival estimates. Epithelial ovarian neoplasms of low malignancy potential are characterized by 5-year survival rates of 95%, reflecting their protracted and indolent biologic behavior.

DIAGNOSIS AND MANAGEMENT OF CANCER METASTATIC TO THE OVARY

Typically, patients with cancer metastatic to the ovary present as if they have primary ovarian cancer. Several clinical scenarios may be encountered. Primary colon cancer or gastric carcinoma may present as a pelvic mass, ascites, and a change in bowel habits or early satiety. Recurrent metastatic breast cancer may present as an asymptomatic pelvic mass.

The role of surgery in patients with cancer metastatic to the ovary must be individualized. When the diagnosis is unclear, exploratory laparotomy to establish the diagnosis is appropriate in most cases. However, the role of tumor-reductive surgery in patients with known metastatic disease is less clear. No long-term survivors of gastric cancer metastatic to the ovary are known, regardless of treatment. Survival following surgery and combination chemotherapy for breast and colon cancer metastatic to the ovary is poor, ranging from 4–12 months.

■ MALIGNANT NEOPLASMS OF THE FALLOPIAN TUBE

Etiology

Primary carcinoma of the fallopian tube is the least-common cancer arising in the female genital tract, accounting for approximately 0.3% of all such cancers. Fallopian tube cancers are similar to epithelial ovarian cancer in regards clinical presentation and biologic behavior.

Clinical Presentation

The patient with carcinoma of the fallopian tube is usually in the fifth or sixth decade of life. The signs and symptoms are often similar to those noted in patients with ovarian cancer. In fact, it is difficult to differentiate tubal from ovarian carcinomas preoperatively.

Fewer than 15% of patients are noted to have the classic triad of symptoms and signs associated with fallopian tube cancer including **hydrops tubae profluens** (a watery vaginal discharge), pelvic pain, and a palpable adnexal mass.

Positive vaginal cytology in the absence of endometrial or cervical neoplasia suggests the possibility of a tubal cancer, but this is rarely diagnostic.

Histopathology

At least 95% of all primary carcinomas of the fallopian tube are papillary carcinomas. Bilaterality is found in 40–50% of cases, and this is believed to represent synchronous neoplasms rather than metastatic disease from one tube to the other. Grossly, the affected tube is fusiform or sausage-shaped. On initial inspection, these neoplasms resemble pyosalpinx or tuboovarian inflammatory disease. However, there is usually little associated serosal reaction with adhesion formation, as is noted with an inflammatory process.

Classically, the neoplastic fallopian tube contains solid or necrotic cancer tissue and a dark-brown or serosanguineous fluid. The fimbriated end of the fallopian tube is patent in as many as 50% of cases, and often tumor extrudes from the ostium to adhere to adjacent structures. Histologically, papillary carcinomas may exhibit papillary, papillary–alveolar, and alveolar growth patterns. There is no prognostic significance attached to these differences. Of note, women with *BRCA1* and *BRCA2* mutations are at substantially higher risk of fallopian tube cancer; consequently, women who have prophylactic oophorectomies should also have complete resection of the oviducts.

Treatment

The surgical therapy of fallopian tube carcinoma is the same as that recommended for epithelial ovarian cancer. In addition, the same type of surgical staging should be performed if for no other reason than it is often not clear at the time of surgery whether the primary cancer is of ovarian or fallopian tube origin. The staging system for ovarian cancer is often applied to neoplasms of the fallopian tube, although this is by custom rather than FIGO recommendations.

Chemotherapy for fallopian tube cancer has evolved along the same lines as that for epithelial ovarian cancer. The currently used chemotherapeutic regimen is similar to that of epithelial ovarian cancer and includes platinum combination chemotherapy. Radiation may also be used in select cases with no residual disease after surgery. Because there is little data on well-staged tubal lesions, it is unclear if patients with early stage disease benefit from adjuvant therapy.

Prognosis

The prognosis for patients with fallopian tube carcinoma is based on the stage of disease. The overall 5-year survival rate is approximately 56%. The prognosis for early stage disease is much better than for advanced disease, as 5-year survival with stage I disease is 84%, with stage II, 52%, and with stage III, 36%.

REFERENCES

Berek JS, Schultes BC, Nicodemus CF: Biologic and immunologic therapies for ovarian cancer. J Clin Oncol 2003;21:168.

Bookman MA et al: Evaluation of monoclonal humanized anti-HER2 antibody, trastuzumab, in patients with recurrent or refractory ovarian or primary peritoneal carcinoma with overexpression of HER2: A phase II trial of the Gynecologic Oncology Group. J Clin Oncol 2003;21:283.

Christian J, Thomas H: Ovarian cancer chemotherapy. Cancer Treat Rev 2001;27:99.

Engeland A, Tretli S, Bjorge T: Height, body mass index, and ovarian cancer: A follow-up of 1.1 million Norwegian women. J Natl Cancer Inst 2003;95:1244.

Jemal A et al: Cancer statistics 2005. CA Cancer J Clin 2005; 55(1):10.

Ness RB et al: Infertility, fertility drugs, and ovarian cancer: A pooled analysis of case-control studies. Am J Epidemiol 2002; 155:217.

Runnebaum IB, Stickeler E: Epidemiological and molecular aspects of ovarian cancer risk. J Cancer Res Clin Oncol 2001;127:73.

Walsh C et al: Coexisting ovarian malignancy in young women with endometrial cancer. Obstet Gynecol 2005;106(4):693.

Windbichler G et al: Interferon-gamma in the first-line therapy of ovarian cancer: A randomized phase III trial. Br J Cancer 2000;82:1138.

Gestational Trophoblastic Diseases

Paola Aghajanian, MD

ESSENTIALS OF DIAGNOSIS

- *Uterine bleeding in first trimester.*
- *Absence of fetal heart tones and fetal structures.*
- *Rapid enlargement of the uterus or uterine size greater than anticipated by dates.*
- *β-human chorionic gonadotropin (β-hCG) titers greater than expected for gestational age.*
- *Vaginal expulsion of vesicles.*
- *Hyperemesis gravidarum.*
- *Theca lutein cysts.*
- *Onset of preeclampsia in the first trimester.*

General Considerations

Gestational trophoblastic neoplasms include the tumor spectrum of hydatidiform mole (complete and partial), invasive mole (chorioadenoma destruens), choriocarcinoma, and placental-site trophoblastic tumor (PSTT). These tumors are unique in that they develop from an aberrant fertilization event and hence arise from fetal tissue within the maternal host. They are composed of both syncytiotrophoblastic and cytotrophoblastic cells, with the exception of PSTT, which is derived from intermediate trophoblastic cells. In addition to being the first and only disseminated solid tumors that have proved to be highly curable by chemotherapy, they elaborate a unique and characteristic tumor marker, human chorionic gonadotropin (hCG).

Hydatidiform mole is the most common form of gestational trophoblastic disease and is benign in nature. Its incidence varies worldwide from 1 in 125 deliveries in Mexico and Taiwan to 1 in 1500 deliveries in the United States. The incidence is higher in women younger than 20 and older than 40 years of age, in nulliparous women, in patients of low economic status, and in women whose diets are deficient in protein, folic acid, and carotene. The most remarkable findings are that blood group A women impregnated by group O men have an almost 10-fold greater risk of developing choriocarcinoma than group A women impregnated by group A partners. Furthermore, women with blood group AB tend to have a relatively worse prognosis.

Hydatidiform mole should be suspected in any woman with bleeding in the first half of pregnancy, passage of vesicles, hyperemesis gravidarum, or onset of preeclampsia prior to 24 weeks. Absent fetal heart tones and a uterus too large for the estimated gestational age on physical examination further support the diagnosis. Ultrasonography and serial β-hCG determinations are necessary to establish a firm diagnosis of hydatidiform mole.

Invasive mole is reported in 10–15% of patients who have had primary molar pregnancy. Although considered a benign neoplasm, invasive mole is locally invasive and may produce distant metastases.

Choriocarcinoma and PSTT comprise the spectrum of gestational trophoblastic neoplasia. Choriocarcinoma is rare, being reported in 2–5% of all cases of gestational trophoblastic neoplasia. The incidence in the United States is 1 in 40,000 pregnancies, but it is higher in Asia. In about half of all cases of choriocarcinoma, the antecedent gestational event is hydatidiform mole. One-fourth of cases follow a term pregnancy, and the remaining one-fourth follow an abortion.

PSTT is a rare variant of gestational trophoblastic tumor. It may arise either from a hydatidiform mole or, less commonly, from a normal-term pregnancy. The tumor is generally confined to the uterus and metastasizes late in its course. Syncytiotrophoblastic cells are generally absent from this tumor, resulting in minimal secretion of β-hCG in relation to tumor burden. However, human placental lactogen (hPL) is secreted and its levels can be monitored to follow response.

A generalization worth repeating is that any woman with a recent history of molar pregnancy, abortion, or normal pregnancy who presents with vaginal bleeding or a tumor in any organ should have at least one β-hCG assay to ensure that metastatic gestational trophoblastic neoplasia is not the cause. This is important given that the cure rate of properly treated metastatic gestational trophoblastic neoplasia approaches 90%.

Etiology & Pathogenesis

Gestational trophoblastic tumors arise in fetal rather than maternal tissue. Cytogenetic studies demonstrate that complete moles are usually (perhaps always) euploid, paternal in origin, and sex chromatin-positive—46 XX or 46 XY. A complete mole arises when an empty ovum (with an absent or inactivated nucleus) is fertilized by a haploid sperm that duplicates its chromosomes or by two haploid sperm. A partial mole, on the other hand, is triploid—69 XXY (70%), 69 XXX (27%), or 69 XYY (3%). It arises when an ovum with an active nucleus is fertilized by a duplicated sperm or two haploid sperm. This cytogenic information provides important insight into the pathogenesis of gestational trophoblastic neoplasms, because this process results in a homozygous conceptus with a propensity for altered growth.

Hydatidiform mole is thought to arise from extraembryonic trophoblasts. Histologic similarities between molar vesicles and chorionic villi support the view that one is derived from the other. However, a detailed morphologic study of a hysterectomy specimen containing an intact molar pregnancy presents a new concept regarding the genesis of hydatidiform mole as a transformation of the embryonic inner cell mass at a stage just prior to the laying down of endoderm. At this stage in embryogenesis, the inner cell mass has the potential to develop into trophoblasts, ectoderm, or endoderm. If normal development is interrupted, such that the inner cell mass loses its capacity to differentiate into embryonic ectoderm and endoderm, a divergent development pathway is created. This pathway may then result in formation of trophoblasts (from the inner cell mass) that develop into cytotrophoblasts and syncytiotrophoblasts. Sufficient differentiation can lead to the production of extraembryonic mesoderm and molar vesicles with loose primitive mesoderm in their villous core.

Pathology

As stated earlier, four distinct forms of gestational trophoblastic neoplasia are recognized: hydatidiform mole, invasive mole (chorioadenoma destruens), choriocarcinoma, and PSTT.

A. HYDATIDIFORM MOLE

Hydatidiform mole is an abnormal pregnancy characterized grossly by multiple grapelike vesicles filling and distending the uterus, usually in the absence of an intact fetus (Fig 53–1). Most hydatidiform moles are recognizable on gross examination, but some are small and may seem to be ordinary abortuses.

Microscopically, moles may be identified by three classic findings: edema of the villous stroma, avascular villi, and nests of proliferating syncytiotrophoblastic or cytotrophoblastic elements surrounding villi (Fig 53–2). Today with earlier clinical diagnosis, the classic pathologic presentation of molar pregnancies is less common. Therefore, it can be more difficult to differentiate histo-

Figure 53–1. Hysterectomy specimen with anterior wall incised, displaying typical miliary, clear, "grapelike" vesicles filling the uterine cavity. Hysterectomy was performed for primary treatment for molar gestation.

logically between a molar pregnancy and a nonmolar hydropic abortion. The likelihood of malignant sequelae is higher in patients whose trophoblastic cells show increased proliferation and anaplasia. Although histologic study of the trophoblast provides some basis for predicting a benign or malignant course for the mole, the correlation is not absolute, and it is essential to ob-

Figure 53–2. Photomicrograph of hydatidiform mole characterized by well-developed but avascular villi with stromal edema and minimal trophoblastic proliferation.

Table 53–1. Comparison of complete and partial hydatidiform moles.

	Complete	Partial
Karyotype	Diploid (46,XX or 46,XY)	Triploid (69,XXX or 69,XXY)
Embryo	Absent	Present
Villi	Hydropic	Few hydropic
Trophoblasts	Diffuse hyperplasia	Mild focal hyperplasia
Implantation-site trophoblast	Diffuse atypia	Focal atypia
Fetal RBCs	Absent	Present
β-hCG	High (> 50,000)	Slight elevation (< 50,000)
Frequency of classic clinical symptoms[1]	Common	Rare
Risk for persistent GTT	20–30%	< 5%

[1]Hyperemesis, hyperthyroidism, excessive uterine enlargement, anemia, and preeclampsia. The frequency of these symptoms has decreased as a consequence of earlier diagnosis of molar pregnancies through evaluating β-hCG levels and ultrasonography.
GTT = gestational trophoblastic tumor.

tain accurate, sensitive gonadotropin assays in all patients who have had hydatidiform moles.

Two forms of hydatidiform moles exist: complete (true) and partial moles. Table 53–1 outlines the clinical, pathologic, and genetic characteristics of both.

B. INVASIVE MOLE (CHORIOADENOMA DESTRUENS)

An invasive mole occurs in 20% of patients who have undergone evacuation of a molar pregnancy. It is essentially a hydatidiform mole that invades the myometrium or adjacent structures. It has the potential to completely penetrate the myometrium and cause subsequent uterine rupture and hemoperitoneum (Fig 53–3). However, it also has the ability to spontaneously regress. The microscopic findings are similar to that of a hydatidiform mole (Fig 53–4). Because adequate myometrium is rarely obtained at curettage and fewer hysterectomies are being performed in patients with trophoblastic disease, the diagnosis is less often made by histologic analysis.

C. CHORIOCARCINOMA

Choriocarcinoma is a pure epithelial tumor composed of syncytiotrophoblastic and cytotrophoblastic cells. It may accompany or follow any type of pregnancy. It usually presents as late vaginal bleeding in the postpartum period. An enlarged uterus, enlarged ovaries, and vaginal lesions may be noted during the physical exam.

Figure 53–3. Hysterectomy specimen showing invasive mole penetrating the myometrium and serosal surface of the uterus that resulted in life-threatening intraperitoneal hemorrhage.

Histologic examination of the tumor discloses sheets or foci of trophoblasts on a background of hemorrhage and necrosis but no villi.

Assessment of trophoblastic tissue following or accompanying pregnancy may prove difficult because of the histologic similarities of the trophoblastic patterns in very early pregnancy and choriocarcinoma. Consequently, the curettage specimen must be processed in its entirety as the specimens may contain only small, isolated areas of choriocarcinoma.

A histopathologic diagnosis of choriocarcinoma in any site is an indication for prompt treatment after confirmation by gonadotropin excretion measurements. In perplexing situations, β-hCG testing may clarify the diagnosis as well as the need for therapy.

Figure 53–4. Photomicrograph of invasive mole. The pattern of hydatidiform mole is maintained with avascular villi and stromal edema, but they are deep within the uterine wall, interspersed among smooth-muscle bundles.

D. PLACENTAL-SITE TROPHOBLASTIC TUMOR

PSTT is derived from the intermediate trophoblasts of the placental bed, with minimal or absent syncytiotrophoblastic tissue. Histologically, local invasion occurs into the myometrium and lymphatics and less commonly into the vasculature. PSTT may occur with any type of pregnancy or present months to years thereafter.

Clinical Findings

A. SYMPTOMS AND SIGNS

Abnormal uterine bleeding, usually during the first trimester, is the most common presenting symptom, occurring in more than 90% of patients with molar pregnancies. Three-fourths of these patients present prior to the end of the first trimester.

Nausea and vomiting have been reported in 14–32% of patients with hydatidiform mole and may be confused with nausea and vomiting of pregnancy. Ten percent of these patients may have nausea and vomiting severe enough to require hospitalization.

About half of patients will have a uterine size that is greater than that appropriate for their gestational age. However, in one-third of patients, the uterus may be smaller than expected.

Multiple theca lutein cysts causing enlargement of one or both ovaries are seen in 15–30% of women with molar pregnancies. In about half these cases, both ovaries are enlarged and may be a source of pain. Involution of the cysts proceeds over several weeks and usually parallels the decline of β-hCG values. Surgical treatment of these cysts is indicated only if rupture, torsion, or hemorrhage occur, or if the enlarged ovaries become infected. In studies, patients with theca lutein cysts appear to have a greater likelihood of developing malignant sequelae of gestational trophoblastic neoplasia.

Preeclampsia in the first trimester or early second trimester—an unusual finding in normal pregnancy—has been said to be pathognomonic for a hydatidiform mole. It is seen in 10–12% of patients.

Hyperthyroidism from stimulation of thyrotropin receptors by hCG occurs in up to 10% of patients with hydatidiform mole. The disease is usually subclinical and most patients remain asymptomatic. Treatment involves evacuation of the mole. An occasional patient may require brief antithyroid therapy.

Because of the earlier diagnosis of molar pregnancies, the classic presenting symptoms and signs of gestational trophoblastic disease are now less prevalent. For instance, at the New England Trophoblastic Disease Center, the incidence of excessive uterine enlargement, hyperemesis, and preeclampsia was 28%, 8%, and 1%, respectively. The incidence of hyperthyroidism and respiratory insufficiency was negligible. Although the number of cases presenting with these classic signs and symptoms has decreased, the incidence of persistent postmolar gestational trophoblastic disease has remained static. This highlights the importance of vigilant postmolar β-hCG surveillance.

B. LABORATORY FINDINGS

The principal characteristic of gestational trophoblastic neoplasms is their capacity to produce β-hCG. This hormone may be detected in the serum or urine of virtually all patients with hydatidiform mole or malignant trophoblastic disease and its levels correlate closely with the number of viable tumor cells present. Consequently, monitoring of β-hCG levels is a necessary tool for the diagnosis, treatment, and follow-up of the disease process.

The usefulness of a serum gonadotropin assay depends on the level of the patient's β-hCG titer and the sensitivity of the test. Today, sensitive and specific immunoassays are available to differentiate β-hCG from luteinizing hormone (LH) by measuring the beta chain of hCG. Serial β-hCG levels are best monitored in the same laboratory using the same immunoassay technique.

The rate of the decline in β-hCG titers is also important. Using the serum β-hCG radioimmunoassay, a normal postmolar pregnancy hCG regression curve highlighting the weekly hCG levels in patients undergoing spontaneous remission has been constructed (Fig 53–5).

Figure 53–5. Normal postmolar pregnancy regression curve of serum β-hCG measured by radioimmunoassay. Vertical bars indicate 95% confidence limits. (Reproduced with permission of the American College of Obstetricians and Gynecologists from Schlaerth JB et al: Prognostic characteristics of serum human chorionic gonadotropin titer regression following molar pregnancy. Obstet Gynecol 1981;58:478.)

This provides a reference for the comparison of random or serial values. In most instances, the β-hCG values exhibit a progressive decline to nondetectable levels within 14 weeks following evacuation of a molar pregnancy. If the hCG titer rises or plateaus, it must be concluded that viable tumor continues to persist. If the levels of hCG are very low and not responsive to treatment, a false-positive hCG result caused by cross-reaction of heterophilic antibodies with the hCG test should be considered.

C. Ultrasonograph Findings

The simplicity, safety, and reliability of ultrasonography define it as the diagnostic method of choice for patients with suspected molar pregnancy. In a complete molar pregnancy, the characteristic ultrasound pattern consists of multiple hypoechoic areas corresponding to hydropic villi, at times described as a "snowstorm" pattern. A normal gestational sac or fetus is not present. Theca lutein cysts may also be seen. In a partial mole, focal areas of trophoblastic changes and fetal tissue may be noted. An ultrasonogram of a choriocarcinoma reveals an enlarged uterus with a necrotic and hemorrhagic pattern, whereas that of PSTT can show an intrauterine mass.

An ultrasonograph should be obtained in any patient who presents with bleeding in the first half of pregnancy and has a uterus greater than 12 weeks gestational size. Even when the uterus is appropriate for gestational age, ultrasonography can be key in differentiating between a normal pregnancy and a hydatidiform mole.

Differential Diagnosis

Gestational trophoblastic disease must be distinguished from a normal or ectopic pregnancy. Ultrasonography is useful, and quantitative β-hCG levels improve the accuracy of the diagnosis.

Analysis of tissue obtained from a dilatation and curettage for histology and DNA content will prove invaluable.

Treatment

A. Hydatidiform Mole

1. Evacuation—When the diagnosis has been confirmed and a complete blood count, liver and renal function tests, and preevacuation chest radiograph have been obtained, the molar pregnancy should be terminated. Suction curettage is the method of choice. It is safe, rapid, and effective in nearly all cases. Intravenous oxytocin should be started after a moderate amount of tissue has been removed and may be continued for 24 hours postevacuation if necessary. Suction curettage with the largest curette possible should be followed by gentle sharp curettage, and tissue from the decidua

basalis should be submitted separately for pathologic study. Suction curettage can be safely accomplished even when the uterus is the size of a 28-week gestation. Blood loss usually is moderate, but precautions should be taken for the possibility of a transfusion. When a large hydatidiform mole (> 12 weeks in size) is evacuated by suction curettage, a laparotomy setup should be readily available, as hysterotomy, hysterectomy, or bilateral hypogastric artery ligation may be necessary if perforation or hemorrhage occurs.

Before the use of suction curettage, hysterectomy was frequently used for patients with uteri beyond 12–14 weeks in size. Hysterectomy remains an option for good surgical candidates not desirous of future pregnancy and for older women (who are more likely to develop malignant sequelae). If theca lutein cysts are encountered at hysterectomy, the ovaries should remain intact, because regression to normal size will occur as the hCG titer diminishes. Hysterectomy does not eliminate the need for careful follow-up with β-hCG testing, although the likelihood of metastatic disease following hysterectomy for gestational trophoblastic disease decreases from 20% to 3.5%.

Hysterotomy is no longer a method of choice in typical cases. Current recommendations restrict hysterotomy to cases complicated by hemorrhage.

Medical induction of labor with prostaglandin, oxytocin, intra-amniotic instillation of prostaglandin or hypertonic solutions (eg, saline, glucose, urea) are no longer acceptable methods for evacuation of a molar pregnancy.

After the completion of the evacuation, all Rh-negative patients should receive Anti-D immune globulin.

2. Complications—The maternal–fetal barrier contains leaks large enough to permit passage of cellular and tissue elements. As a result, deportations of trophoblastic tissue to the lungs are frequent. Spontaneous regression of these ectopic trophoblastic tissues will occur. However, less commonly, a syndrome of acute pulmonary insufficiency may result. A patient can present with dyspnea and cyanosis within 4–6 hours after evacuation of the molar pregnancy as a result of massive deportation of trophoblasts to the pulmonary vasculature and subsequent formation of pulmonary emboli. Pulmonary edema leading to high-output congestive heart failure can also result from excessive fluid administration, preeclampsia, anemia or hyperthyroidism.

3. Prophylactic chemotherapy—It is controversial whether prophylactic chemotherapy (with methotrexate or dactinomycin) following a complete hydatidiform molar pregnancy should be offered to patients considered at high risk for persistent gestational trophoblastic disease (age > 35 years, history of prior molar pregnancy, trophoblastic hyperplasia) or in whom poor follow-up is anticipated. Several studies indicate that the incidence of postmolar gestational trophoblastic disease may be decreased with prophylactic chemotherapy. However, further studies are required to determine if the potential side effects warrant such treatment.

4. Surveillance following molar pregnancy—Regardless of the method of termination, close monitoring with serial β-hCG titers is essential for every patient because of the 20–30% incidence of malignant disease. Following evacuation of a hydatidiform mole, the patient should have serial β-hCG determinations, beginning within 48 hours after evacuation and then at weekly intervals until serum β-hCG declines to nondetectable levels on three successive assays. If titer remission occurs spontaneously within 14 weeks and without a titer plateau, the β-hCG titer should then be repeated monthly for at least 1 year before the patient is released from close medical supervision (in cases of partial moles, β-hCG may be followed for 6–12 months). Thereafter, the patient may enter into a regular gynecologic care program.

Despite earlier diagnosis of molar pregnancies, the incidence of persistent gestational trophoblastic disease has not decreased. Three-fourths of patients with malignant nonmetastatic trophoblastic disease and half of patients with malignant metastatic disease develop these tumors as sequelae to a hydatidiform mole. In the remainder, disease arises following term pregnancy, abortion, or ectopic pregnancy.

Several clinical features of hydatidiform mole are recognized as having a high association with malignant trophoblastic neoplasia. In general, at diagnosis, the larger the uterus and the higher the β-hCG titer, the greater the risk for malignant gestational trophoblastic disease. The combination of theca lutein cysts and uterine size excessive for gestational age is associated with an extremely high risk (57%) of malignant sequelae. Pathologic specimens with marked nuclear atypia, presence of necrosis or hemorrhage, and trophoblastic proliferation may also increase the risk of persistent disease.

Effective contraceptive measures should be implemented and maintained throughout the period of surveillance in these patients. Oral contraceptives are the most widely used method.

A gynecologic examination should be done 1 week after evacuation, at which time blood may be taken for the β-hCG titer. Estimates of uterine size and presence of adnexal masses (theca lutein cysts) and a careful search of the vulva, vagina, urethra, and cervix should be made for evidence of genital tract metastases. Unless symptoms develop, the examination should be repeated at 4-week intervals throughout the observation period.

If preevacuation chest radiography reveals pulmonary metastases, chest radiographs should be repeated at 4-week intervals until spontaneous remission is confirmed, then at 3-month intervals during the remainder of the surveillance period.

A patient who has entered into spontaneous remission with negative titers, examinations, and chest radiographs for 1 year and who is desirous of becoming pregnant may terminate contraceptive practices. Successful pregnancy is usual, and complications are similar to those of the general population.

Therapy for progressive gestational trophoblastic neoplasia after evacuation of a hydatidiform mole is usually instituted because of an abnormal β-hCG regression curve. The most critical period of observation is the first 4–6 weeks postevacuation. Although the β-hCG titer usually returns to normal by 1–2 weeks after evacuation of a hydatidiform mole, it should normalize by the 8th week. Approximately 70% of patients achieve a normal β-hCG level within 8 weeks postevacuation. Few patients whose β-hCG titers are normal during this interval will require treatment.

In the past, therapy was recommended if the β-hCG titer remained elevated at or beyond 8 weeks after termination of the molar pregnancy. However, current data suggest that an additional 15% of patients demonstrate a continuous decline in titers and ultimately achieve normal titers without treatment. Approximately 15% of patients who have elevated titers at 8 weeks postevacuation demonstrate a rising or plateauing titer. Nearly half of these patients will have histologic evidence of an invasive mole, and the other half will have choriocarcinoma.

Delayed postevacuation bleeding is uncommon after molar pregnancy and signifies the presence of an invasive mole or choriocarcinoma. It is invariably attended by an enlarging uterus and abnormal β-hCG regression pattern. On pelvic examination, the enlarged uterus may have the characteristics of an intrauterine pregnancy. Curettage is effective in stopping the bleeding, although little intracavitary tissue will be present in most of these cases.

The indications for initiating chemotherapy during the postmolar surveillance period are (a) β-hCG levels rising for 2 successive weeks or constant for 3 successive weeks; (b) β-hCG levels elevated at 15 weeks postevacuation; (c) rising β-hCG titer after reaching normal levels; and (d) postevacuation hemorrhage. Treatment should also be instituted whenever there is a tissue diagnosis of choriocarcinoma. However, histologic confirmation is unnecessary, because the development of metastases is a sufficient justification for chemotherapy.

B. MALIGNANT GESTATIONAL TROPHOBLASTIC NEOPLASIA

Malignant gestational trophoblastic neoplasia may be diagnosed in the setting of invasive mole, choriocarcinomas, placental-site trophoblastic tumors, and plateauing or rising postmolar β-hCG values (a plateau of 4 values ± 10% over a period of 3 weeks, a rise in β-hCG of > 10% of 3 values over a period of 2 weeks, or persistence of detectable β-hCG > 6 months after evacuation).

Once the diagnosis of malignant trophoblastic disease is established, an accurate history and physical examination are crucial. Most patients will have an enlarged uterus as well as ovarian enlargement caused by theca lutein cysts. Sites of metastasis must be sought, especially in the lower genital tract. A chest radiograph can diagnose lung metastases, whereas liver metastases may be diagnosed with ultrasonography or computerized tomography (CT) scan. Brain metastases are best evaluated with a CT scan or magnetic resonance imaging (MRI). The ratio of serum β-hCG values to the concentration of β-hCG in cerebrospinal fluid (normal > 60:1) may prove helpful. Baseline hematologic counts, coagulation studies, and hepatic and renal function tests are critical in assessing the risk for drug toxicity.

After all sites of metastases have been identified and the patient's desires for preservation of reproductive function are determined, specific therapy should be initiated.

1. Nonmetastatic gestational trophoblastic disease—Trophoblastic disease confined to the uterus is the most common malignant lesion seen in gestational trophoblastic neoplasia. The diagnosis is usually made during the follow-up period after evacuation of a molar pregnancy. Therapy for patients with nonmetastatic malignant trophoblastic disease includes (a) single-agent chemotherapy and (b) combined chemotherapy and hysterectomy, with surgery done on the third day of drug therapy if the patient does not wish to preserve reproductive function and her disease is known to be confined to the uterus.

Table 53–2 summarizes the recommended chemotherapy regimens available for nonmetastatic gestational trophoblastic disease (and low-risk gestational trophoblastic disease). Single-agent chemotherapy using methotrexate or dactinomycin has demonstrated clear-cut superiority over other protocols. The therapeutic efficacy of the two drugs is apparently equivalent; however, no randomized controlled studies have compared the response rate and side-effect profiles of single-agent chemotherapy with methotrexate to that of dactinomycin. Thus the regimen of choice has not been established. However, weekly intramuscular methotrexate injections provide a convenient and cost-effective alternative to the more intense 5-day regimens with methotrexate or dactinomycin, and with minimal side effects. Treatment failure (indicated by rising β-hCG or presence of new metastases) or intolerable side effects should result in administration of the alternative agent. Overall, the complete response rate ranges from 60–98% with salvage rates approaching 100%. Metho-

Table 53–2. Chemotherapy regimens for nonmetastatic or low-risk gestational trophoblastic disease.

Drug/dosage:

Methotrexate 30–60 mg/m^2 IM once a week.[1]

Methotrexate 0.4 mg/kg/d IV or IM for 5 days, repeat every 14 days

Methotrexate 1 mg/kg IM on days 1, 3, 5, and 7 and folinic acid 0.1 mg/kg IM on days 2, 4, 6, and 8, repeat every 15–18 days

Dactinomycin 1.25 mg/m^2 IV every 14 days

Dactinomycin 10–12 µg/kg/d IV for 5 days, repeat every 14 days

Follow-up:

Follow β-hCG titer weekly. Switch to alternative drug if β-hCG titer rises 10-fold or more, titer plateaus at an elevated level, or new metastasis appears.

Obtain labs daily during treatment cycle or weekly as indicated. Hold chemotherapy for WBC count < 3000 (absolute neutrophil count < 1500); platelets < 100,000; significantly elevated BUN, Cr, AST, ALT, or bilirubin; or for significant side effects (severe stomatitis, gastrointestinal ulceration, or febrile course).

Oral contraceptive agents or other form of birth control should be taken concurrently, and continued for at least 1 year following remission.

Chemotherapy continued for one course after negative β-hCG titer.

Follow-up program: β-hCG titer weekly until 3 consecutive normal titers; monthly β-hCG titer for 12 months thereafter; β-hCG titer every 2 months for 1 additional year or every titer for 6 months indefinitely.

Physical examination including pelvic examination and chest radiography monthly until remission is induced; at 3-month intervals for 1 year thereafter; then at 6-month intervals indefinitely.

[1]For nonmetastatic disease only.

trexate is contraindicated in the presence of hepatocellular disease or when renal function is impaired. Each treatment cycle should be repeated as soon as normal tissues (bone marrow and gastrointestinal mucosa) have recovered, with a minimum 7-day window between the last day of one course and the first day of the next course.

During treatment, weekly quantitative β-hCG titers and complete blood counts should be obtained. Before each course of therapy, liver and renal function assessments should be done. At least one additional course of drug therapy should be given after the first normal β-hCG value is obtained. The number of treatment cycles necessary to induce remission is proportionate to the magnitude of the β-hCG concentration at the start of therapy. An average of 3 or 4 courses of single-agent therapy is required. After remission has been induced and treatment is completed, β-hCG assays should be obtained monthly for 1 year.

2. Metastatic gestational trophoblastic disease— Treatment in metastatic disease uses either single-agent chemotherapy (Table 53–2) or multiple-agent chemotherapy. Multiple-agent chemotherapy is used in cases where resistance to a single agent is anticipated. Several systems have been developed to help determine which patients will, at onset, require more aggressive therapy.

3. Clinical classification of malignant gestational trophoblastic disease—

National Cancer Institute—This system is used in the United States to determine if the patient will have a good or poor prognosis in response to single-agent chemotherapy (Table 53–3).

World Health Organization (WHO)—This scoring system is based on an individual's risk factors, including age, type of antecedent pregnancy, interval from antecedent pregnancy to initiation of chemotherapy, pretreatment β-hCG level, size of largest tumor, site of metastases, number of metastases, and prior chemotherapy. Patients are categorized into low- or high-risk categories based on their total score. A total score of 0–6 is considered low-risk and a total score ≥ 7 is categorized as high-risk (Table 53–4).

Revised FIGO (International Federation on Gynecology and Obstetrics)—The revised 2000 FIGO staging system combines the use of both anatomic and nonanatomic factors. A patient is assigned a stage based on the anatomic location of disease and given a risk factor score based on the WHO prognostic scoring system.

Table 53–3. Categorization of gestational trophoblastic neoplasia.

A. Nonmetastatic disease: No evidence of disease outside uterus.

B. Metastatic diease: Any disease outside uterus.

  1. Good-prognosis metastatic disease—
    a. Short duration (< 4 months).
    b. Serum β-hCG < 40,000 mIU/mL.
    c. No metastasis to brain or liver.
    d. No significant prior chemotherapy.

  2. Poor-prognosis metastatic disease
    a. Long duration (> 4 months).
    b. Serum β-hCG > 40,000 mIU/mL.
    c. Metastasis to brain or liver.
    d. Unsuccessful prior chemotherapy.
    e. Gestational trophoblastic neoplasia following term pregnancy.

The goal of the revised FIGO staging is to improve the assessment and clinical management of patients. It also aims to unify staging to allow for comparisons in treatment success internationally (Table 53–5).

a. Good-prognosis patients—Based on the clinical classification of malignant disease, patients can be expected to respond satisfactorily to single-agent chemotherapy if (a) metastases are confined to the lungs or pelvis, (b) serum β-hCG levels are below 40,000 mIU/mL at the onset of treatment, and (c) therapy is started within 4 months of apparent onset of disease.

The most common site of metastases is the lung. When a patient develops pulmonary metastases and elevation of the β-hCG titer, choriocarcinoma is a more likely cause than metastatic mole. Invasive mole may also metastasize to the lungs, and hydatidiform mole has occasionally been reported to metastasize to the chest. Probably any form of metastases (even benign deportation) should suggest metastatic trophoblastic disease.

In these patients, single-agent chemotherapy (Table 53–2) is generally successful. Methotrexate is considered the drug of choice. Ideally, the 5-day treatment cycle is given every other week, because tumor regrowth becomes significant after treatment gaps of 2 weeks or longer. Once negative titers have been achieved, an additional course is administered. If resistance to methotrexate occurs, manifested either by rising or plateauing titers or by the development of new metastases, or if negative titers are not achieved by the fifth course of methotrexate, the patient should be given dactinomycin. Dactinomycin also should be initiated for patients who experience severe side effects with methotrexate.

The advantage of single-agent chemotherapy is that it is less toxic and its toxicity is less apt to be irreversible than is the case with multiple-agent chemotherapy.

There is a tendency not to be aggressive in treating these patients, probably because of the "good-prognosis" (low-risk) designation. But failure of drug therapy does occur in approximately 10% of cases, and meticulous care by physicians familiar with these problems is necessary for good results.

b. Poor-prognosis patients—Poor-prognosis patients, based on the Clinical Classification of Malignant Disease, are those with any of the following risk factors: (a) serum β-hCG titers greater than 40,000 mIU/mL at the onset of treatment; (b) diagnosis of disease more than 4 months after molar pregnancy; (c) brain or liver metastases; (d) prior unsuccessful chemotherapy; or (e) onset following term gestation. These patients respond poorly (< 40% response rate) to single-agent therapy. A poor response is also seen in patients with advanced revised FIGO stages and WHO scores ≥ 7. These patients present a serious challenge. Many have been previously treated with chemotherapy and have developed resis-

Table 53–4. Modified WHO prognostic scoring system as adapted by FIGO.

Scores	0	1	2	4
Age	< 40	≥ 40	—	—
Antecedent pregnancy	Mole	Abortion	Term	—
Interval months from index pregnancy	< 4	4–< 7	7–< 13	≥ 13
Pretreatment serum hCG (IU/mL)	$< 10^3$	10^3–$< 10^4$	10^4–$< 10^5$	$≥ 10^5$
Largest tumor size (including uterus)	—	3–< 5 cm	≥ 5 cm	—
Site of metastases	Lung	Spleen, kidney	Gastrointestinal	Liver, brain
Number of metastases	—	1–4	5–8	>8
Previous failed chemotherapy	—	—	Single drug	2 or more drugs

Reproduced with permission from FIGO Committee Report: FIGO staging for gestational trophoblastic neoplasia 2000. Int J Gynecol Obstet 2002;77:286.

tance to that treatment while accumulating considerable toxicity and depleting bone marrow reserves. Prior unsuccessful chemotherapy is one of the worst prognostic factors.

Generally, these patients require prolonged hospitalization and multiple courses of chemotherapy. They often need specialized care and other life-support measures, including hyperalimentation, antibiotics, and transfusions, to correct the effects of marrow depression.

Central nervous system involvement, particularly brain metastases with focal neurologic signs suggestive of intracranial hemorrhage, is common in choriocarcinoma. Because patients with brain or liver metastases are at great risk of sudden death from hemorrhage from these lesions, it is standard practice when treating them to include immediate institution of whole-brain or whole-liver irradiation concomitantly with combination chemotherapy. It is uncertain whether radiation therapy exerts its beneficial effect by destroying tumor in combination with drug therapy or by preventing fatal hemorrhage and thus keeping the patient alive until remission with chemotherapy can be achieved. For acute bleeding episodes, surgical intervention or angiographic embolization can be considered.

Table 53–5. FIGO anatomic staging.

Stage I	Disease confined to the uterus
Stage II	GTN extends outside of the uterus, but is limited to the genital structures (adnexa, vagina, broad ligament)
Stage III	GTN extends to the lungs, with or without known genital tract involvement
Stage IV	All other metastatic sites

Reproduced with permission from FIGO Committee Report: FIGO staging for gestational trophoblastic neoplasia 2000. Int J Gynecol Obstet 2002;77:286.

Cerebral metastases should be treated over a 2-week period with radiation given in a dosage of 3 Gy daily, 5 days a week, to a total organ dose of 30 Gy. Whole-liver irradiation is usually accomplished over 10 days to attain a 20-Gy whole-organ dose given at a rate of 2 Gy daily, 5 days a week. Other treatment options include selective hepatic artery chemotherapy infusion.

Prior treatments for poor prognosis/high-risk gestational trophoblastic disease have included MAC (methotrexate, dactinomycin, and chlorambucil or cyclophosphamide) and the modified Bagshawe protocol (CHAMOCA: cyclophosphamide, hydroxyurea, methotrexate, vincristine, cyclophosphamide, and dactinomycin). Currently, EMACO (etoposide, methotrexate, actinomycin D, cyclophosphamide, and vincristine) chemotherapy (Table 53–6) provides the best response rate (approximately 80%) with the lowest side-effect profile. The cycle is repeated every 2 weeks. The same tests must be employed to detect toxicity as are used when single-agent chemotherapy is given, but monitoring must be even more vigilant because of the possibility of combined toxicity.

Treatment of malignant trophoblastic disease must be continued with repeated courses of combination chemotherapy until β-hCG titers return to nondetectable levels. Complete remission is documented only after three consecutive weekly normal β-hCG titers have been achieved. It is recommended that all high-risk patients receive at least three courses of triple-agent chemotherapy after β-hCG titers have returned to normal. After remission is achieved, follow-up is the same as for hydatidiform mole and nonmetastatic or good-prognosis disease.

Salvage therapy for disease not responsive to EMACO substitutes cisplatin and etoposide (EP-EMA) for cyclophosphamide and vincristine (CO) (Table 53–6). Close monitoring of renal function is required because of nephrotoxicity secondary to cisplatin and as methotrexate is renally excreted. Other treatment op-

Table 53–6. Current treatment regimens for high-risk gestational trophoblastic disease.

EMA/CO[1]
Day

1	Etoposide	100 mg/m^2 IV (infused over 30 min)
	Actinomycin D	0.5 mg IV bolus
	Methotrexate[2]	100 mg/m^2 IV bolus
		200 mg/m^2 IV (infused over 12 h)
2	Etoposide	100 mg/m^2 IV (infused over 30 min)
	Actinomycin D	0.5 mg IV bolus
	Folinic acid	15 mg IM infusion or orally every 12 hours for 4 doses beginning 24 hours after start of methotrexate
8	Cyclophosphamide	600 mg/m^2 IV infusion
	Vincristine	1 mg/m^2 IV bolus

Other options:

Salvage therapy: Substituting etoposide (100 mg/m^2 IV) and cisplatin (80 mg/m^2 IV) (EMA-EP) for cyclophosphamide and vincristine. Adjuvant surgery (hysterectomy and thoracotomy) for chemotherapy-resistant disease.

With failure of EMA-EP, treatment with: BEP (cisplatin 20 mg/m^2 IV, etoposide 100 mg/m^2 IV on days 1–4 every 21 days, with bleomycin 30 units IV on day 1 then every week), G-CSF (granulocyte colony-stimulating factor) 300 µg SC on days 6–14.

VIP (etoposide 75 mg/m^2 IV, ifosfamide 1.2 g/m^2 IV, cisplatin 20 mg/m^2 IV each day for 4 days every 21 days). Mesna 120 mg/m^2 IV bolus prior to first ifosfamide dose, followed by 1.2 mg/m^2 12-hour IV infusion daily after each ifosfamide dose, G-CSF 300 µg SC on days 6–14.

High-dose chemotherapy with autologous bone marrow transplantation.

Taxanes (paclitaxel and docetaxel) and camptothecins (topotecan and irinotecan).

---

[1]Mild toxicity with 5-year survival 80%. Repeat cycles on days 15, 16, and 22 (every 2 weeks).

[2]Increase to 1 g/m^2 as 24-h infusion with CNS metastases, with folinic acid increased to 15 mg every 8 h for nine doses beginning 12 h following completion of methotrexate infusion. Also may receive methotrexate 12.5 mg by intrathecal injection on day 8. Another option is whole-brain irradiation 3000 cGY in 200-cGY fractions given over 10–14 days during chemotherapy.

Chemotherapy should be continued for at least 3 cycles after negative β-hCG.

As with nonmetastatic and low-risk disease, oral contraceptive pills or other form of birth control should be utilized if not contraindicated.

---

tions include such agents as paclitaxel, topotecan, and high-dose chemotherapy with autologous bone marrow transplantation.

In resistant cases, adjunctive measures along with chemotherapy may include hysterectomy, resection of metastatic tumors, or irradiation of unresectable lesions.

4. Placental-site trophoblastic tumor—Because treatment of PSTT generally is resistant to chemotherapy, hysterectomy is the recommended route of treatment. Partial uterine resection involving the tumor is possible if the patient desires to retain fertility. Chemotherapy is indicated in cases of metastatic disease. EP-EMA is the preferred regimen over EMACO, with paclitaxel and topotecan used when resistance develops. The greatest adverse outcomes are associated with an interval > 2 years from antecedent pregnancy to diagnosis.

Prognosis

The prognosis for hydatidiform mole following evacuation is uniformly excellent, although surveillance is needed as outlined in the text. The prognosis for malignant nonmetastatic disease with appropriate therapy is also quite good, as almost all patients are cured. More than 90% of patients can preserve reproductive func-

tion, but first-line therapy fails in 6.5% of patients with nonmetastatic disease. In one large reported series, no death from toxicity occurred, and only one patient died of the disease.

In poor-prognosis metastatic disease, the best results are with EMACO chemotherapy and concurrent radiation as indicated. Seventy-five percent to 85% of patients achieve remission with a 69% salvage rate. This is a similar response to agents used previously (MAC) but with fewer side effects. Brain and liver metastases have the worst prognosis with reports of survival ranging from 0–60% for hepatic involvement and 50–80% for central nervous system (CNS) involvement at diagnosis. Survival decreases to < 20% when prior chemotherapy agents have been used or if CNS metastases develop while undergoing treatment. Deaths from toxicity have decreased considerably. Recurrence, when it happens, is usually in the first several months after termination of therapy but may be as late as 3 years.

Secondary Tumors

Multiple-agent chemotherapy (specifically using etoposide) but not single-agent chemotherapy is associated with a 50% increased risk for secondary tumors. One retrospective study found that the relative risk for developing myeloid leukemia and colon cancer was 16.6 and 4.6, respectively. When survival exceeded 25 years, the relative risk for developing breast cancer was 5.8.

Subsequent Pregnancy Outcome

Subsequent pregnancies are not at increased risk for complications such as preterm labor, anomalies, or stillbirth. These pregnancies should, however, be monitored early with ultrasonography and β-hCG levels because there is a 1–2% risk of recurrent gestational trophoblastic disease following one molar pregnancy and a 25% risk of recurrence following two molar pregnancies. Following delivery, the placenta should be sent to pathology and a β-hCG level should be checked at the 6-week postpartum visit.

In cases where pregnancy occurs prior to the completion of standard postmolar surveillance (<1 year), the pregnancy may be continued with close observation, and the risks discussed with the patient. Most pregnancies end with a good outcome, but there is a small risk for delayed diagnosis of recurrence.

REFERENCES

ACOG Committee on Practice Bulletins. Practice Bulletin #53. Diagnosis and treatment of gestational trophoblastic disease. Obstet Gynecol 2004;104:1422.

Altieri A et al: Epidemiology and aetiology of gestational trophoblastic diseases. Lancet Oncol 2003;4:670.

Baergen RN et al: Placental site trophoblastic tumor: A study of 55 cases and review of the literature emphasizing factors of prognostic significance. Gynecol Oncol 2006; 100(3):511.

Berek J: Staging and treatment of gestational trophoblastic disease. www.uptodate.com. Version 13.3; August 2005.

Cohn DE, Herzog TJ: Gestational trophoblastic diseases. New standards for therapy. Curr Opin Oncol 2000;12:492.

Dorigo O, Berek J: Pathology of gestational trophoblastic disease. www.uptodate.com. Version 13.3; August 2005.

FIGO Committee Report: FIGO staging for gestational trophoblastic neoplasia 2000. Int J Gynaecol Obstet 2002; 77:285.

Ghaemmaghami F et al: Management of patient with metastatic gestational trophoblastic tumor. Gynecol Oncol 2004; 94:187.

Homesley HD: Single-agent therapy for nonmetastatic and low-risk gestational trophoblastic disease. J Reprod Med 1998;43:69.

Shapter AP, McLellan R: Gestational trophoblastic disease. Obstet Gynecol Clin North Am 2001;28(4):805.

Smith HO et al: Choriocarcinoma and gestational trophoblastic disease. Obstet Gynecol Clin North Am 2005;32:661.

Wang J, Berek J. Epidemiology, clinical manifestations and diagnosis of gestational trophoblastic disease. www.uptodate.com. Version 13.3; August 2005.

Wolfberg AJ et al: Low risk of relapse after achieving undetectable hCG levels in women with complete molar pregnancy. Obstet Gynecol 2004;104:551.

Radiation Therapy for Gynecologic Cancers

Sujatha Pathi, MD, & Oliver Dorigo, MD

Two European discoveries in the late 1800s led to future radiation treatment of human malignancies. While studying the penetrating power of cathode ray emission in Germany, Wilhelm Roentgen discovered x-rays on November 8, 1895. In France, the Curies isolated radium from uranium ore in 1898. Soon thereafter, Robert Abbe of New York City introduced radium for medical therapy, and Howard Kelly of Baltimore pioneered radium treatment of cervical cancer. Since then radiation therapy has evolved to become a major modality in the treatment of many cancers, particularly those of the female reproductive tract.

Types of Radiation

Radiation oncology may be defined as the therapeutic manipulation of radiation delivered to a target for cure or for palliation. Such radiation may be electromagnetic or particulate, both of which transfer energy to the electrons or nuclei of the target atoms.

Electromagnetic radiation is energy that is transmitted at the speed of light through oscillating electric and magnetic fields. The energy contained in these fields can be described as discrete units known as photons. The energy of each photon is proportional to the frequency of the wave associated with that photon. Because radiation with a shorter wavelength has greater frequency, it carries greater energy per photon, allowing deeper tissue penetration. The most clinically relevant forms of electromagnetic radiation are x-rays and gamma rays. For therapeutic applications, x-rays are mechanically produced by linear accelerators that accelerate electrons to very high energies. These electrons then strike a target within the accelerator, usually tungsten, to produce a beam of x-rays which is targeted at the patient. Gamma rays are produced by the decay of radioactive substances. Currently, the most commonly used radioisotopes for gynecologic cancer treatments are cesium-137 and iridium-192.

Particulate radiation uses subatomic particles (electrons, neutrons, protons), instead of photons, to deliver the dose of radiation. Compared with electromagnetic radiation, particle-beam therapy enables more precise dose localization and better depth dose distribution.

Interaction of Photons with Matter

The first step in the absorption of an incident photon with matter is the conversion of the energy of that photon into the kinetic energy of an electron, or electron–positron pair. Depending on the energy of the photon, this conversion takes place either through the photoelectric effect, the Compton effect, or pair production. In the **photoelectric effect,** an incident photon interacts with a tightly bound inner shell electron of the target tissue. The energy of the photon is completely absorbed and the electron is ejected from the atomic orbit with kinetic energy equal to the photon energy. With the photoelectric effect, absorption is influenced by atomic number; the tissues bearing elements of higher atomic number (eg, calcium in bone) absorb proportionately greater and possibly detrimental levels of radiation. In the **Compton effect,** an incident photon transfers energy to an outer-shell electron in the target tissue, causing ejection of this electron. The photon is incompletely absorbed; instead, it is scattered at an angle to its original path. This secondary photon interacts with tissue multiple times in the same manner, ionizing with each interaction (Fig 54A–1). The atomic number of the tissue elements does not determine the amount of absorbed radiation. The Compton effect accounts for the biologic effects on tissues seen in radiation therapy. **Pair production** refers to the complex interaction of an incident photon with the nucleus of a target atom, resulting in an electron–positron pair. Because the pair production interaction typically predominates at energy levels above the range that is usually used in therapy, it plays a small role in most clinical settings.

In the lower range of energy transfer, the photoelectric effect predominates, while in the transfer of higher levels of energy, the Compton effect and pair production are more prevalent.

Interaction of Photons with Tissue

As a radiation beam travels through a patient, it deposits energy in the tissue through interactions such as the

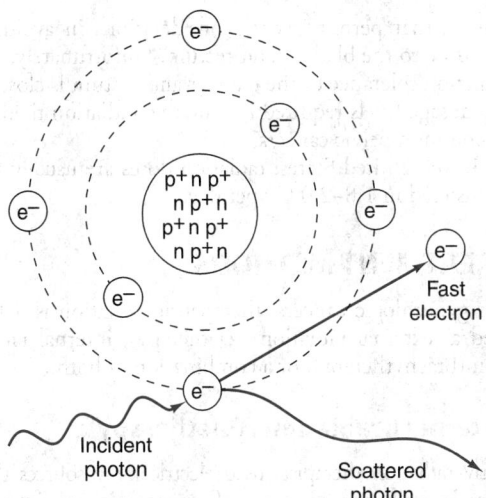

Figure 54A–1. Absorption of an x-ray photon by the Compton process. The photon interacts with a loosely bound planetary electron of an atom of the absorbing material. Part of the photon energy is given to the electron as kinetic energy. The photon, deflected from its original direction, proceeds with reduced energy. e⁻ = electron; p⁺ = proton; n = neutron. (Reproduced with permission from Hall EJ: *Radiobiology for the Radiologist*, 4th ed. JB Lippincott, 1994, p. 7.)

Compton effect. These interactions set secondary electrons in motion which result in further ionizations. These ionizations lead to the breakage of chemical bonds and subsequent damage to molecules and structures within the cell. The most significant result of cell damage is cell death.

The most critical target for damage within the cell is DNA. Direct damage occurs when a photon becomes absorbed by the an atom in the DNA and the DNA becomes ionized and damaged. More commonly, however, DNA damage is indirect. The water surrounding the DNA is ionized by the radiation, creating oxygen radicals, hydroxyl radicals, peroxide, and hydrated electrons. These highly reactive species then interact with the DNA to cause damage.

Dosage Theory

Normal tissue as well as malignant cells are susceptible to toxicity induced by radiation therapy, the extent of which depends on total dose, fractionization, and tumor volume.

After exposure to radiation, tissue survival follows a predictable curve that essentially constitutes the number of viable clone cells (Fig 54A–2). The shoulder represents the cell's enzymatic ability to reverse radiation-

induced damage. As radiation increases, cells become incapable of self-repair and a logarithmic pattern of cell destruction occurs. Importantly, for every increase in dosage that occurs beyond the shoulder, a constant fraction of cells is eliminated (**log-kill hypothesis**).

The implications of these observations provide some of the rationale for dividing (fractionating) the total dose of radiation therapy administered in the clinical setting. It is helpful to consider the so-called 4 Rs of radiobiology to understand the effects of fractionated doses at the cellular level.

Figure 54A–2. Typical radiation survival curve for mammalian cells. These cells have been irradiated and then plated out in culture, and the number of survivors has been determined by measuring the colonies (clones) of cells that survive. The curve is characterized by an initial shoulder followed by a log-linear region. Cells irradiated in air are considerably more sensitive than those irradiated in nitrogen (hypoxic), and the difference between the levels of killing is frequently about 3-fold. It is believed that most clinically demonstrable tumors have areas of hypoxia that lead to radioresistance. (Reproduced with permission from Morrow CP, Curtin JP, Townsend DE [editors]: *Synopsis of Gynecologic Oncology*, 4th ed. Churchill Livingstone, 1993, p. 449.)

A. REPAIR OF SUBLETHAL INJURY

When a specified radiation dose is divided into two doses given at separate times, the number of cells surviving is higher than that seen when the same total dose is given at one time. Fractionation allows the administration of amounts of radiation that would not be tolerated if the specified dose were given in only one treatment.

B. REPOPULATION

The reactivation of stem cells that occurs when radiation is stopped is necessary for further tissue growth; thus those tissues with increased numbers of progenitor cells have a greater ability to regenerate.

C. REOXYGENATION (OXYGEN EFFECT)

Hypoxic cells are known to be relatively resistant to radiation. Experimental and clinical evidence has confirmed that molecular oxygen must be present before radiation damage can occur. Cells located farther than 100 mm from capillary flow are at risk for hypoxia and may not be killed by radiation therapy. If these hypoxic cells are malignant, they may not be killed by radiation therapy. For this reason, it is important to correct anemia in patients undergoing radiation treatment so that tissue oxygen perfusion will be enhanced and tissues will become more radiosensitive. As tumor regresses with radiation treatment, previously anoxic areas may be brought into contact with capillary flow and increased oxygenation.

D. RADIATION-INDUCED SYNCHRONY

Malignant cells are most sensitive to radiation while in the mitotic phase of the cell cycle. If a segment of the malignant cell population can be destroyed in this phase of the cell cycle, the remaining malignant cells may be synchronized for selective destruction at a later time.

Clinical experience shows that prolonged interruption of radiation therapy has a deleterious effect on cure, as malignant cells have a greater chance to regenerate.

Dosimetry

Dosimetry is the measurement of the amount of radiation absorbed by target tissue. The unit of absorbed dose is the Gray (Gy), which is defined as the joules of energy absorbed in a kilogram of tissue (J/kg). One Gy is equal to 100 rads. External pelvic irradiation is expressed in those terms, whereas internal irradiation is also described in milligram hours. This latter unit is obtained by multiplying the number of milligrams of radioactive substance used in the internal applicators by the number of hours the applicators have been in place.

The exact conversion factor between milligram hours and Gray is difficult to determine, but computer-directed dosimetry permits the calculation of isodose curves, points of equal dose surrounding a radioactive source, that permit critical considerations in avoiding overdose to the bladder and rectum. Unfortunately, the radiation tolerance of the bladder and rectum is close to the dosage levels required for curative radiation therapy of common pelvic cancers.

In the United States, radiation doses are usually administered in 1.8–2.0 Gy per day.

TREATMENT METHODS

For gynecologic cancers, therapeutic radiation is delivered as external radiation (teletherapy), internal radiation (brachytherapy), or a combination of both.

External Irradiation (Teletherapy)

Early radiation therapists used electric x-ray sources that were basically modifications of Roentgen's experimental apparatus. Electrons were accelerated across a vacuum tube to strike a tungsten target with the subsequent liberation of photons. These orthovoltage (140–400 keV) units were limited in their power to penetrate tissue effectively because of their relatively low energy output. Consequently, pronounced fibrotic skin changes and high absorbed bone radiation levels limited their usefulness in some patients.

As units generating higher levels of energy were developed, the penetrating power of the x-rays produced was enhanced, and less scattering of radiation was seen at the margins of the treatment area. The surface skin dose was also diminished, of particular importance in the treatment of obese patients, and less-toxic bone radiation was achieved (Fig 54A–3).

The goal of external radiation treatment is to ensure that radiation is delivered to the target tissue without affecting uninvolved tissues and that the amount of radiation received is as uniform as possible. Traditionally, the planning of radiation treatment has been done in two dimensions (height and width). Today, this is achieved by optimized three-dimensional conformal planning to more precisely target a tumor with radiation beams (height, width, and depth). Patients undergo computed tomography (CT) scanning in the treatment position and the volume of abnormal tissue, that is, the gross tumor volume (GTV), is delineated. Given the possibility of microscopic extension along tissue planes, a margin of tissue is added to the GTV. This larger volume, the clinical tumor volume (CTV), is the volume of tissue to be irradiated. Using information from these images, special computer programs design radiation beams that "conform" to the shape of the tumor.

Internal Irradiation (Brachytherapy)

Brachytherapy is radiation therapy in which the source of therapeutic ionizing radiation is placed close to the treatment area.

Figure 54A–3. Typical isodose curves for orthovoltage (250 keV), cobalt 60, and a 6-MeV linear accelerator (LINAC). The most important difference between the megavoltage (cobalt 60 and LINAC) beams in comparison with the 250-keV beam is the movement of the 100% isodose line several millimeters beneath the surface. This results in elimination of the severe skin reactions characteristic of earlier radiation sources. In addition, the higher energy leads to deeper penetration as the energy of the beam increases.

The chief advantage of local irradiation is that a relatively high dose of radiation can be applied to a limited anatomic region. The **inverse square law** has critical implications in clinical applications. The principle of the inverse square law states that the intensity of radiation is inversely proportional to the square of the distance from the source. An important implication is that the rapid falloff of radiant energy supplied by a central source precludes the achievement of cancerocidal doses at the margins of the pelvis. Consequently, external therapy must be used to provide adequate radiation to eliminate tumor at the periphery of large lesions and at the pelvic side walls, where metastatic disease may be present.

Brachytherapy can be delivered using an intracavitary approach with a variety of applicators, or via an interstitial approach using needles or catheters. Most applicators for intracavitary brachytherapy consist of an intrauterine tandem and paired colpostats or ovoids which are placed in the lateral vaginal fornices. Interstitial applicators consist of multiple needles that are inserted into the tissue at or near the target site. Radioactive isotopes are then loaded into the applicators at the beginning of the treatment.

Several isotopes are available for brachytherapy. The most commonly used in the United States is a low-dose rate (LDR) approach employing cesium-137. However, acceptance of a high-dose rate (HDR) therapy, usually with iridium-192, is quickly gaining acceptance. HDR brachytherapy offers some significant advantages over LDR as it can be employed on an outpatient basis, eliminates radiation exposure to medical personnel, and has shorter treatment times.

TREATMENT OF GYNECOLOGIC CANCER

Cervical Cancer

Treatment of cervical cancer is considered a prime example of the successful application of radiation therapy. The relative accessibility of the central lesion, a metastatic pattern of cervical squamous cell carcinoma that can be predicted with reasonable accuracy, and the radiation tolerance of the cervix and surrounding tissues often permit curative radiation therapy.

Radiation therapy with curative intent uses both external-beam and intracavitary radiation. Palliative radiation for advanced cervical cancer may use either modality for control of bleeding, management of disease in the pelvis, and relief of pain.

The goal of external irradiation in cervical cancer is to sterilize metastatic disease to pelvic lymph nodes and the parametria and/or to decrease the size of the cervix to allow optimal placement of intracavitary radioactive sources.

The size of the radiation field used to treat a patient with carcinoma of the cervix must be carefully designed to encompass those structures at risk for regional spread of the cancer.

Definitive radiation therapy is an acceptable alternative to radical surgery for women with early stage disease (stages IA, IB1, and nonbulky IIA). However, concurrent cisplatin-based chemotherapy should be employed whenever radiation therapy is administered for the treatment of cervical cancer. Numerous studies show that concomitant radiation therapy and chemotherapy (chemoradiation) improves overall and progression-free survival in patients with cervical cancer. Advantages of combined treatment theoretically include no delay time in starting definitive irradiation; decreased treatment time overall; and possible interaction of chemotherapy with radiotherapy by mechanisms such as repair of sublethal and lethal damage, cell phase distribution changes, effect on vascularity of tumor, effects on repopulation, effects on hypoxic cells, alteration of cell survival curve, and modification of apoptosis.

The treatment volume for women undergoing adjuvant external radiation therapy usually involves the whole pelvis, with larger fields for patients with higher stage disease.

Patients with known or suspected metastatic disease to periaortic lymph nodes may be considered for extended field irradiation.

Endometrial Cancer

The decision to use radiation treatment for endometrial cancer is often made after adequate surgical staging has been performed and is dependent on the estimated risk of recurrent disease.

Patients who have adnexal or pelvic metastases, involvement of lymphovascular space, grade 2 disease with invasion > 50% into the myometrium, or grade 3 disease with any amount of myometrial invasion, are deemed to be at high risk of recurrence. These patients may benefit from adjuvant radiation therapy. For high-risk disease confined to the uterus, whole-pelvic therapy or vaginal brachytherapy may be used. For high-risk disease outside of the uterus but confined to the pelvis, whole-pelvis radiation with or without vaginal brachytherapy should be employed. Women with more extensive disease undergo extended-field radiation or whole-abdomen radiation.

Women who have a grade 1 or 2 tumor at either stage IC or stage II, no lymphovascular involvement, and no evidence of metastases are at intermediate risk of recurrence. The use of adjuvant radiation therapy is very controversial in this group. Studies show that use of adjuvant radiation therapy may improve local control, but overall survival is not significantly improved. Adjuvant therapy is not routinely used for women at low risk of recurrence.

Primary radiation therapy may be employed in women who are considered to be at high surgical risk, such as the elderly and those with significant comorbidities. Patients with well-differentiated adenocarcinoma may be managed with tandem and ovoids or intrauterine Simon capsules. Patients with moderately or poorly differentiated cancers or those with involvement of the cervix are at risk for parametrial and pelvic lymph node spread and should receive whole-pelvic irradiation prior to brachytherapy.

Ovarian Cancer

Since the introduction of combination chemotherapy, the role of radiation therapy in the management of ovarian cancer has become controversial. There are no well-structured trials that demonstrate the benefit of external radiation in the treatment of ovarian cancer.

Several studies have compared the use of intraperitoneal chromic phosphate (^{32}P) with platinum-based chemotherapy in early stage ovarian cancer. None of these trials showed a difference in 5-year survival rates, but they did show late bowel complications in the ^{32}P group.

Vaginal Cancer

Radiotherapy remains the primary treatment for vaginal cancer, which is one of the rarest human malignancies, and historically one of the gravest. A 1954 review of a published series of 992 patients reported an overall 5-year survival rate of 18%. More recent studies, however, have show overall 5-year cure rates of 40–50%. Such improvement in survival rates is attributed to megavoltage external therapy along with physical and technical advances in local irradiation. Despite radiation therapy being the primary treatment modality for vaginal cancers, there are no standardized treatment protocols. With squamous cell carcinoma comprising the most common form of vaginal cancer, most of these patients undergo whole-pelvic radiation therapy followed by intracavitary or interstitial brachytherapy. Patients with lesions involving the lower third of the vagina should have the inguinal and femoral lymph nodes included in the external-beam treatment field. Extended field radiation to include periaortic lymph nodes may be needed if imaging studies reveal bulky pelvic or periaortic disease.

Vulvar Cancer

Slightly more common than vaginal cancer (5% vs 2% of female malignancies), vulvar cancer also is usually squamous cell in origin. However, the mainstay of treatment of stages I and II vulvar cancer is surgical, often consisting of radical vulvectomy plus inguinal and pelvic lymphadenectomy. Adjuvant radiation therapy benefits patients with close or positive surgical margins, as well as patients with positive inguinal lymph nodes.

In patients with more advanced vulvar squamous cancer (stage III or IV) chemoradiation may reduce the need for more radical surgery, including primary pelvic exenteration.

Complications of Radiation Therapy

Radiation therapy regimens are formulated to maximize the chances for cure while incurring the smallest amount of damage to normal tissues. The effects of radiation on normal tissue is what limits the doses of therapeutic radiation that can be administered. In gynecologic cancers, the most serious complications are those involving the gastrointestinal or genitourinary systems.

Complications of radiation therapy are classified as early or delayed. Acute effects result from direct damage of parenchymal cells in organs that are sensitive to radiation. These include enteritis, proctosigmoiditis, cystitis, vulvitis, and, occasionally, depression of bone marrow elements. Bowel side effects usually comprise cramping and diarrhea that require dietary adjustments and the judicious use of antidiarrheal agents. Such problems usually respond to appropriate medication, but occasionally radiation therapy must be interrupted or curtailed because of fulminant acute reactions.

Late radiation effects are believed to be caused by slow vascular damage along with direct damage of parenchymal cells. Such injury may be manifested by chronic proctosigmoiditis, hemorrhagic cystitis, small- and large-bowel strictures, and the formation of rectovaginal and vesicovaginal fistulas. Pelvic fibrosis and loss of ovarian function may affect sexual activity in younger patients.

New Directions in Radiation Therapy

In addition to radiation sensitizers, neutron beam therapy and altered fractionation schemes are being evaluated for effectiveness against the tumor-protective effects of hypoxia, which is a common problem with gynecologic cancers. Intensity-modulated radiotherapy has emerged as a new teletherapy technique that can use radiation beams of varying intensities to deliver different doses of radiation to small areas of tissue at the same time. This allows for the delivery of higher doses of radiation within a tumor while sparing adjacent normal tissue. As newer computer technologies are wedded to imaging techniques, further advances in anatomic contouring for planning and treatment are expected to translate into better local control rates, as well as improved survival with a wider margin of safety.

REFERENCES

Ahamad A, Jhingran A: New radiation techniques in gynecological cancer [review]. Int J Gynecol Cancer 2004;14(4):569.

Cardenes H, Randall ME: Integrating radiation therapy in the curative management of ovarian cancer: Current issues and future directions. Semin Radiat Oncol 2000;10:61.

Cmelak AJ, Kapp DS: Long-term survival with whole abdominopelvic irradiation in platinum-refractory persistent or recurrent ovarian cancer. Gynecol Oncol 1997;65:453.

Creutzberg CL et al: Surgery and postoperative radiotherapy versus surgery alone for patients with stage-1 endometrial carcinoma: Multicentre randomised trial. PORTEC Study Group. Post Operative Radiation Therapy in Endometrial Carcinoma. Lancet 2000;355(9213):1404.

Eifel PJ et al: Pelvic irradiation with concurrent chemotherapy versus pelvic and para-aortic irradiation for high-risk cervical cancer: an update of radiation therapy oncology group trial (RTOG) 90-01. J Clin Oncol 2004;22(5):872.

Frank SJ et al: Definitive radiation therapy for squamous cell carcinoma of the vagina. Int J Radiat Oncol Biol Phys 2005;62(1):138.

Frumovitz M et al: Quality of life and sexual functioning in cervical cancer survivors. J Clin Oncol 2005;23(30):7428.

Green JA et al: Survival and recurrence after concomitant chemotherapy and radiotherapy for cancer of the uterine cervix: A systematic review and meta-analysis. Lancet 2001;358(9284):781.

Greven KM, Corn BW: Endometrial cancer. Curr Prob Cancer 1997;21:94.

Hareyama M et al: High-dose-rate versus low-dose-rate intracavitary therapy for carcinoma of the uterine cervix: A randomized trial. Cancer 2002;94(1):117.

Keys H et al: Cisplatin, radiation, and adjuvant hysterectomy compared with radiation and adjuvant hysterectomy for bulky stage IB cervical carcinoma. N Engl J Med 1999;340:1154.

Landoni F et al: Randomised study of radical surgery versus radiotherapy for stage Ib-IIa cervical cancer. Lancet 1997;350(9077):535.

Lertsanguansinchai P et al: Phase III randomized trial comparing LDR and HDR brachytherapy in treatment of cervical carcinoma. Int J Radiat Oncol Biol Phys 2004;59(5):1424.

Moore DH et al: Preoperative chemoradiation for advanced vulvar cancer: A phase II study of the Gynecologic Oncology Group. Int J Radiat Oncol Biol Phys 1998;42:79.

Morris M et al: Pelvic radiation with concurrent chemotherapy compared with pelvic and para-aortic radiation for high-risk cervical cancer. N Engl J Med 1999;340:1137.

Nag S et al: The American Brachytherapy Society recommendations for low-dose-rate brachytherapy for carcinoma of the cervix. Int J Radiat Oncol Biol Phys 2002;52(1):33. [Erratum: Int J Radiat Oncol Biol Phys 2002;52(4):1157.]

Nag S et al: The American Brachytherapy Society recommendations for high-dose-rate brachytherapy for carcinoma of the cervix. Int J Radiat Oncol Biol Phys 2000;48(1):201.

National Institutes of Health Consensus Development Conference Statement on Cervical Cancer. Gynecol Oncol 1997;66:351.

Okada M et al: Indication and efficacy of radiation therapy following radical surgery in patients with stage IB to IIB cervical cancer. Gynecol Oncol 1998;70:61.

Peters WA 3rd et al: Concurrent chemotherapy and pelvic radiation therapy compared with pelvic radiation therapy alone as adjuvant therapy after radical surgery in high-risk early-stage cancer of the cervix. J Clin Oncol 2000;18(8):1606.

Pickel H et al: Consolidation radiotherapy after carboplatin-based chemotherapy in radically operated advanced ovarian cancer. Gynecol Oncol 1999;72:215.

Pinilla J: Cost minimization analysis of high-dose-rate versus low-dose-rate brachytherapy in endometrial cancer. Int J Radiat Oncol Biol Phys 1998;42:87.

Rose P et al: Concurrent cisplatin-based radiotherapy and chemotherapy for locally advanced cervical cancer. N Engl J Med 1999;340:1144.

Thomas G et al: A randomized trial of standard versus partially hyperfractionated radiation with or without concurrent 5-fluorouracil in locally advanced cervical cancer. Gynecol Oncol 1998;69:137.

U.S. Department of Health and Human Services: Concurrent chemoradiation for cervical cancer. National Cancer Institute Clinical Announcement, Feb 1999.

Young RC et al: Adjuvant treatment for early ovarian cancer: A randomized phase III trial of intraperitoneal ^{32}P or intravenous cyclophosphamide and cisplatin—A Gynecologic Oncology Group study. J Clin Oncol 2003;21(23):4350.

Chemotherapy for Gynecologic Cancers

Sujatha Pathi, MD, & Oliver Dorigo, MD

Effective chemotherapy for gynecologic cancers exploits characteristic differences between tumor cells and normal cells to selectively kill malignant cells without producing serious, irreversible harm to vital organs and tissues. Knowledge of the scientific basis of cancer chemotherapy is derived from research in molecular biology and cell kinetics and is indispensable to the development of better drugs, establishment of a more rational basis for the design of protocols, and the optimal use of presently available antineoplastic drugs.

Long-lasting remissions and occasional cures for several types of cancer have been achieved with antitumor drugs. For example, up to 90% of patients with metastatic choriocarcinoma achieve a normal life expectancy, and almost 100% of patients without metastases are cured now that the effect of drugs can be monitored by the level of β-hCG (β-human chorionic gonadotropin), which provides a reliable index of tumor growth. For most tumors, however, no such specific and sensitive assay or tumor marker exists. Now that multiple-drug regimens are being used for primary chemotherapy of carcinoma of the ovary, objective response rates of 60–80% are achieved. The objective response rate of 20–40% achieved by chemotherapy in patients with primary carcinoma of the breast and endometrium warrants the use of chemotherapy as an integral part of an initial treatment program.

In spite of extensive experience, the use of cytotoxic agents for carcinomas of the vagina and vulva is still on a clinical trial basis, as these tumors usually grow more slowly, and cytotoxic drug treatment has been palliative but not curative; these types of cancer are better controlled by surgery and radiation therapy, and chemotherapy should be considered only when these standard methods have proved ineffective.

Among the uncommon gynecologic cancers that may require chemotherapy are germ cell tumors of the ovary and primary ovarian, uterine, vaginal, or vulvar sarcomas. Because these tumors are rare, little is known about their sensitivity to antitumor drugs.

The Normal Cell Cycle

Figure 54B–1 represents the cell cycle in a clockwise progression. The phases and their durations are depicted, and the phases during which some specific chemotherapeutic agents exert their effects are included for reference.

Cell Kinetics

Knowledge of tumor cells has been derived from clinical and laboratory methods of tumor growth measurement, including direct measurement of cell-cycle parameters, clinical measurement of doubling times, and use of biologic markers, such as hormone production or polyamines and other abnormal proteins. A knowledge of the terminology of cell kinetics is helpful in understanding the dynamics of tumor cells, in which some cells divide more slowly than others, some cells enter or leave a nondividing state, and some are lost from the tumor population entirely.

The **mitotic index (MI)** is the fraction of cells in mitosis in a steady-state condition. The MI may be calculated by giving a drug such as a *Vinca* alkaloid that halts further cellular progression through mitosis and then counting the number of cells in mitosis. Another method uses tritiated thymidine, which is incorporated only into the DNA of cells in the S phase; the tritiated thymidine emits rays that can then expose the silver in a photographic emulsion during cell mitosis to produce **percent-labeled mitosis (PLM)** curves. Radioactive tagging of DNA during synthesis provides the **labeling index (LI)**, which is the percentage of cells in the S phase at a particular time.

Growth fraction (GF) is the overall proportion of proliferating tumor cells in a given tumor. The growth fraction is important because most antitumor drugs inhibit only proliferating cells. Thus a major difference between tumor and normal cell populations may be the relative percentage of each in the growth fraction. The selective effect of antitumor drugs on tumor cells may be explained by the characteristic higher growth fraction of tumor cells. Toxicity results from the effects of antitumor

1. *Vinca* alkaloids
   (vincristine,
   vinblastine)
2. Podophyllotoxins
   (teniposide [VM-26],
   etoposide [VP-16])
3. Taxanes
   Paclitaxel
   Docetaxel

Bleomycin

Cellular
differentiation
of clones

Nitrosoureas
(carmustine [BCNU],
lomustine [CCNU],
semustine [MeCCnu])

G_0
Resting
stem cell

(Recruitment)

1 hr

3 hrs

G_2 Stem
         cell G_1

18 hrs

S

20 hours

1. Steroids?
2. Asparaginase
3. Diglycoaldehyde

Cell cycle (phase)-nonspecific agents
1. Alkylating agents
   (mechlorethamine, melphalan, busulfan,
   chlorambucil, cyclophosphamide)
2. Anthracycline antibiotics
   (doxorubicin, daunomycin, rubidazone,
   dactinomycin)
3. Miscellaneous
   (DTIC, cisplatin, carboplatin)
4. Nitrosoureas (also G_0)

Antimetabolites
1. Antifolates (methotrexate)
2. Antipyrimidines (cytarabine, fluorouracil, azacitidine)
3. Antipurines (mercaptopurine, thioguanine)
4. Miscellaneous (hydroxyurea, procarbazine, cisplatin,
   carboplatin)

G_1–Enzymes produced necessary
      for DNA production
S –DNA synthesis
G_2–Specialized protein and RNA
      synthesis
M –Mitosis
G_0–Resting phase (cell not com-
      mitted to division)

Figure 54B–1. Model of the cell cycle with progression proceeding clockwise. Phases and their durations are depicted, along with points in the cell cycle at which some chemotherapeutic agents exert their effects.

drugs on normal cells in the mitotic cycle or growth fraction; consequently, the toxicity of most antitumor drugs occurs in those normal cell populations with rapid turnover, eg, the hematopoietic and gastrointestinal systems. Consequently, alopecia, bone marrow suppression and diarrhea are common side effects.

Cell-cycle time denotes the amount of time needed by a proliferating cell to progress through the cell cycle and produce a new daughter cell. Cell cycle times vary widely according to histologic type (18–217 hours in solid tumors), but are relatively constant for a specific tumor type.

Doubling time is the time required for the tumor cell population to double. Human tumors often have doubling times greater than those of comparable normal tissues and, in advanced stages of disease, may exhibit a range of doubling times, but 30–60 days is typical. In the model ascites system, cell doubling time remains constant at near 100% throughout almost the entire life cycle of the tumor, whereas in solid tumor systems, a gradual slowing of the tumor doubling time and reduction of the proliferation rate of cells occur with tumor enlargement as a result of decreased accessibility to nutrients.

Cell loss may be a major determinant of the tumor growth rate. Cells are lost from a tumor mass in various ways, including death, migration, and metastases. Cell loss is frequently high in advanced tumors.

Stem Cell Theory

The stem cell theory states that only certain relatively undifferentiated cells, or stem cells, of a particular tissue type are able to divide and reproduce the entire tissue. Examples include rapidly proliferating tissues such as bone marrow, the lining of the gastrointestinal tract, and the basal cell layer of the skin. In other words, most cells making up a particular tissue have matured or have become highly differentiated after clonal division from the reproducing cell or a specific stem cell.

Not all cells of a particular stem cell population are committed to division at a given time. A significant proportion of stem cells are in the G_0, or resting phase, as is the case in normal bone marrow, in which at any one time from 15–50% of stem cells are in G_0. Numerous stimuli may recruit this reserve (resting) population of stem cells into the cell cycle. The equilibrium between the number of cells in division and those at rest, and the requirement for controls on such growth, are important. Some of the controls are understood, whereas others are unknown.

The stem cell theory also describes neoplastic growth. The clonality of many tumors such as epithelial ovarian cancer suggests that tumors originate from single stem cells. Therefore, tumors may consist of a small percentage of stem cells that, as a result of failed growth control mechanisms, continuously provide malignant cells. Based on this assumption, any therapeutic intervention should target this stem cell population to avoid recurrences.

Cell-Kill Hypothesis

The fundamental kinetic consideration in cancer chemotherapy is the cell-kill hypothesis, which states that the effects of cancer chemotherapy on tumor cell populations demonstrate first-order kinetics; ie, the proportion of tumor cells killed is a constant percentage of the total number of cells present. In other words, chemotherapy kills a constant proportion of cells, not a constant number of cells. The number of cells killed by a particular agent or combination of drugs is proportional to one variable: the dose used. The relative sensitivity of cells is not considered, and the growth rate is assumed to be constant.

Because chemotherapy follows an exponential (log-kill) model, treatment may be said to have a specific exponential, or log-kill, potential. For example, a log kill of 2 reduces a theoretical human tumor burden of 10^9 cells to 10^7 cells. Although this represents a reduction of 99%, at least 10 million (10^7) viable cells remain. A log kill of 3 achieves a reduction of 99.9%, but 1 million (10^6) cells remain. Theoretically, therefore, such fractional reductions by antineoplastic agents can never reduce a tumor cell population to zero. This traditional cell-kill model is based mainly on exponentially growing tumors in laboratory models, eg, L-1210 murine leukemia.

Although the cell-kill hypothesis probably explains some aspects of drug selectivity, other mechanisms are involved. The more responsive tumors are those with large growth fractions. Normal tissue can withstand greater cell loss caused by chemotherapy than can tumors, although the proportion killed in both systems may be identical.

Another theory states that clinical tumor regression as a result of chemotherapy is best explained by the relative growth fraction in the tumor at the time of treatment. Thus very small and very large tumors are less responsive than those of intermediate size, which have the biggest growth fraction. Consequently, log kills occur only at times of maximal tumor growth fraction. Although this hypothesis has not been directly confirmed clinically, it

explains some clinical observations of responses to chemotherapy in large and small human tumors.

Gompertzian Model of Tumor Growth

Gompertz, a German insurance actuary, depicted the relationship of an individual's age to the expected time of death by means of an asymmetric sigmoid curve. This mathematical model approximates tumor proliferation in experimental systems wherein tumors initially grow rapidly. As the tumor increases in size, a plateau effect develops, and the apparent doubling time is much longer than at the beginning.

Figure 54B–2 demonstrates several current chemotherapeutic principles plotted against a gompertzian tumor growth curve and the large tumor cell burden required to produce clinical expression of symptoms. The minimum palpable subcutaneous lesion is about 60 mg and contains 6×10^7 cells. In superficial tumors, 1 cm^3 or 1 g of tumor is not an uncommon size at the time of diagnosis and contains about 10^9 cells, whereas most patients with visceral tumors of 10–100 g are estimated to have 10^{10}–10^{11} tumor cells at the time of diagnosis. Because death occurs with a tumor burden of 10^{12} cells, which is only 1–2 orders of magnitude less than the total number of cells in the human adult, a significant proportion of the life cycle of a clinically recognizable tumor has already transpired when it is finally detected. The importance of early diagnosis of malignant disease is, therefore, even more essential.

Figure 54B–2 illustrates the outcome of the two chemotherapeutic treatment regimens, A and B, the influence of the fractional kill achieved by drug therapy, and the effect of volume of tumor at the onset of therapy. Chemotherapy treatment A in a patient with a visceral solid tumor composed of 10^{11} cells achieves a good response when the tumor cell population is reduced by the characteristic percentage of first-order kill, regardless of the actual number of tumor cells present. Thus, an agent with a 1-log cell kill reduces the cell concentration by 90% from a palpable 10-g mass to a nonpalpable 1-g mass and induces an apparently tumor-free state, yet a residual tumor burden remains that may contain more than 1 billion cells. After a brief delay, the remaining 10% of tumor cells resume their former rate of proliferation. After tumor cell repopulation has occurred, treatment again results in reduction of tumor volume, but resistance develops that results in death of the host at a predictable time.

Although normal tissues do not develop resistance to antitumor drugs, the larger the initial tumor volume and the smaller the fractional kill, the more likely is the development of resistance in tumor cells. The effect of successive drug doses in sensitive tumors depends on the number of existing cells when treatment is begun, the fractional kill, the number of cells surviving the pre-

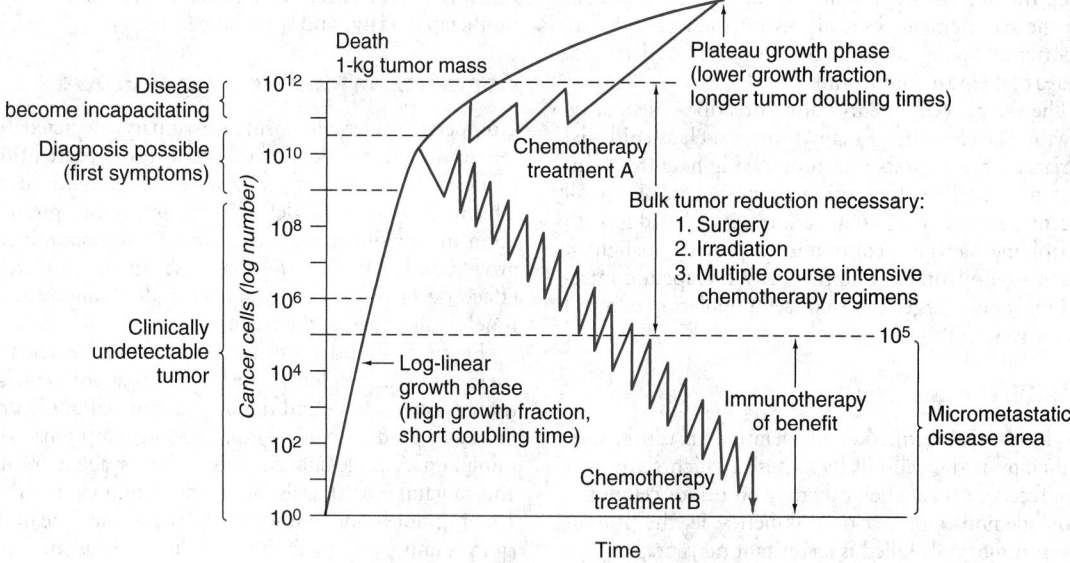

Figure 54B–2. Gompertzian tumor growth curve. The model depicts the relationship between tumor growth and diagnosis, appearance of symptoms, and various treatment regimens.

ceding treatment, and the tumor cell production between treatment cycles. Obviously, cell destruction must exceed cell production for chemotherapy to be successful.

Nonlethal damage to cells can occur as a consequence of chemotherapy and is well known after radiation therapy. Consequently, a key principle of theory is to schedule chemotherapy, radiation therapy, or both at appropriate intervals to allow normal cells to recover from nonlethal damage but to preclude the recovery of tumor cells, which is slower. It is important that the interval between treatments be reduced to the bare minimum required for restoration and recovery of normal tissues.

In chemotherapy treatment B, repeated doses of a chemotherapeutic agent are used to destroy a large tumor cell population. Such consecutive log-kill reductions cannot be consistently achieved because the cell-kill potential of a drug is limited in comparison with the size of the tumor cell population in most clinical situations; however, in Fig 54B–2, a reduction of a 10^{10} (10 billion)-cell population by 90% as a result of a single course of drug therapy produces complete clinical remission. Repeated treatment at shorter intervals may result in enhanced destruction of tumor cells as long as toxic effects remain tolerable and resistant cell lines are not selected out by the drug. A drug becomes curative once the tumor cell kill exceeds the order of magnitude of repopulation and (statistically) less than one tumor cell remains. Additional courses of drug therapy are re-

quired to eradicate the last surviving cell of the so-called exponential iceberg if each course kills the same fraction of cells and not the same number.

On the other hand, fewer cycles of chemotherapy may produce a tumor-free host if subclinical tumor containing only 10^4 cells is present at diagnosis. Unfortunately, the usual inability to detect tumors so early in clinical situations makes this model less realistic.

Alternatively, the tumor population may be reduced by surgery or radiation so that subsequent adjuvant chemotherapy has a rational basis. Initial therapy for many solid tumors involves surgery or irradiation to reduce tumor bulk. Adjuvant chemotherapy, immunotherapy, or both are added as appropriate to eradicate micrometastatic or subclinical tumor masses. The same general principle guides therapy of hematologic cancer, in which intensive induction chemotherapy is used to achieve reduction of tumor bulk and induce remission; less-intensive consolidation and remission maintenance doses of chemotherapy are then used to control subclinical tumor burdens.

Effects of Chemotherapy on the Cell Cycle

Knowledge of the site of action of antitumor drugs within the mitotic cell cycle may help to explain the mechanism of their effectiveness and may suggest ways to enhance their carcinostatic properties. Chemotherapy and radiation therapy are thought to alter the proliferation kinetics of both tumor and normal cells. Initially, individual sensitive cells are killed or incapacitated, thereby leaving a more resistant residual population. This large reduction in tumor cell mass stimulates recruitment of quiescent cells from G_0 into G_1. This shift favors an increased growth fraction in the tumor, so that the LI and the MI are increased and tumor doubling times are decreased (ie, the tumor mass doubles in less time than before). The effect is a shift to the left along the gompertzian curve.

Some drugs may not kill cells but can halt or slow the progression of a cell through a particular phase of the cell cycle. Because cells accumulate in a particular phase, this process has been termed **cell-cycle synchronization.** Generally, these effects occur at lower doses than those necessary for cell killing. Blockage may be either temporary or permanent and does not occur predictably in all cell populations treated.

The effects of various classes of anticancer agents on tumors depend on the basic events occurring in the four main phases of the cell cycle and the pharmacologic mechanisms of drug action, and these cytotoxic effects influence the design of rational drug regimens. Two basic classes of antineoplastic drugs are recognized: cell cycle (phase)-specific agents and cell cycle (phase)-nonspecific agents.

A. CELL CYCLE (PHASE)-SPECIFIC DRUGS

Cell cycle (phase)-specific drugs are much more effective in tumors in which a large proportion of cells are actively dividing, as occurs when the cell mass is low. The major cytotoxic activities of anticancer drugs in this class are manifested during a particular phase of the cell cycle, and these drugs are technically **phase-specific** rather than **cycle-specific** agents. These drugs have been termed **schedule-dependent** agents because they produce a greater cell kill if the drug is given in multiple, repeated fractions rather than as a large single dose.

In pharmacologic terms, these cell cycle (phase)-specific agents are most often described as antimetabolites, because each drug causes some type of unique biochemical blockade of a particular reaction that occurs in a single phase of the cell cycle.

Most cell cycle (phase)-specific agents, such as methotrexate and fluorouracil, exert their most significant effects in the S phase. Corticosteroids and asparaginase appear to be most active in G_1, bleomycin appears to be most active in G_2, and the *Vinca* and podophyllin alkaloids have marked activity in the M and G_2 phases.

B. CELL CYCLE (PHASE)-NONSPECIFIC AGENTS

In contrast, the cell cycle (phase)-nonspecific agents are effective in large tumors in which the growth fraction, LI, and MI are low. Drugs in this group are dose-dependent, as a single bolus injection generally kills the same number of cells as do repeated doses totaling the same amount; ie, the degree of cell kill is directly proportional to the absolute dose given. In pharmacologic terms, the alkylating agents are the prototypes of this class, which also includes the nitrosoureas, the anthracyclines, and others.

The cell cycle (phase)-nonspecific drugs do not require a large growth fraction to exert maximal effects. The effectiveness of their cytotoxic activities generally depends on cellular attempts either to divide or to repair drug-induced damage. The attempt to perform these activities triggers expression of the damage already sustained, and the cell dies. This mechanism of cell death is important, because cancer cells in G_0 (resting phase) are not generally susceptible to cytotoxic agents, with the possible exception of the cell cycle (phase)-nonspecific mustard-type alkylators and the nitrosoureas.

Selectivity of Anticancer Drugs

There is a common belief that cancer chemotherapy is generally nonselective and kills both normal and cancerous tissues. However, most anticancer drugs are more active against tumor than normal tissues. The cell-kill hypothesis probably explains some drug selectivity, but other mechanisms also are involved. The selectivity of cytotoxic agents appears to correlate inversely with cell-cycle specificity, as cell cycle (phase)-nonspecific agents, such as the nitrosoureas and mechlorethamine (an alkylator), tend to be more toxic in normal bone marrow than in tumor cells. The selectivity of most antitumor drugs must still be based largely on differences in the cell kinetics of normal and neoplastic cell lines. Normal systems can withstand greater cellular losses caused by chemotherapy than can tumors, even though the proportion of cells killed in both might be identical. Recovery from damage produced by a tumor-inhibiting drug may be more protracted in tumor cells than in normal host cells. Increased antitumor selectivity can be provided by the judicious use of a second dose of drug following return of normal tissue function but before recovery of tumor cell function. This approach to selective recovery from chemotherapeutic damage may provide enormous benefit by enhancing the antitumor activity of presently available drugs.

Most agents are equally effective at key enzymatic sites in either normal or neoplastic cells, but some anticancer drugs kill cancer cells by taking advantage of unique biochemical differences in the cancer cells; eg, the enzyme asparaginase takes advantage of a relative deficiency of aspartic acid synthetase in some leukemic cells to cause cell death. Cancer cells demonstrate a selective uptake of high concentrations of methotrexate, and this selectivity can be experimentally enhanced by vincristine or asparaginase and inhibited by aminoglycosides and cephalosporins.

Sensitivity to drugs based on the type of tissue is recognized in some anticancer agents; eg, the antimetabolite fluorouracil is more active in neoplasms arising from endodermal tissues such as the gastrointestinal tract and the breast. Dacarbazine has some selective action for melanoma cells, and bleomycin is active against epithelial tumors such as squamous cell cancers of the lung and cervix. When a tumor is derived from an organ characterized by a distinct biochemical feature (eg, the thyroid gland's ability to accumulate iodine, the sensitivity of the adrenal cortex to mitotane, or the selective destruction of the pancreatic islet cells by streptozocin), chemotherapy can be devised that attacks that tumor preferentially.

Although individual differences between the cells of a particular tumor and normal cells have been discovered, no single biochemical feature has been detected that pertains exclusively to one or the other. Studies suggest numerous possibilities for exploiting small quantitative differences between tumor and normal tissue. These include selective uptake of drugs into tumors, enhanced anabolism in tumors of "prodrugs" requiring activation, diminished catabolism of drugs by tumors, diminished repair of tumor cell damage, and reduced availability of a protecting metabolite in tumor tissue.

Chemotherapy Resistance of Cancer Cells

A major problem in the treatment of cancers with chemotherapeutic agents is the development of drug resistance. According to the Goldie-Coldman hypothesis, most mammalian cells start with intrinsic sensitivity to antineoplastic agents but subsequently develop resistance at variable rates. This model has important clinical implications; tumors are only curable if no resistant cell lines are present or develop during the course of chemotherapy. To minimize the development of drug resistance, multiple-drug regimens are preferred to single-drug therapies.

Development of resistance is mainly based on the occurrence of spontaneous mutations, which occur at a frequency of 1 in 10,000 to 1 in 1,000,000 cells. Mechanisms of drug resistance involve decreased cellular uptake or increased efflux of the chemotherapeutic agents via cellular pumps, decrease in drug activation, increase in drug degradation, inactivation of active metabolites by binding to sulfhydryl compounds, increase in DNA repair mechanisms, or increase in level of target enzyme (dihydrofolate reductase). Several genes have been implicated in drug resistance, eg, the multiple-drug resistance (MDR) gene. Gene therapy approaches are currently being studied to reverse drug resistance in tumor cells. Alternatively, the transfer of drug resistance genes into normal cells like bone marrow cells might confer increased protection to chemotherapeutic agents and possibly allow a dose increase.

Poor Host Defenses

The normal individual's immunologic defenses against an invading tumor cell population are unreliable and still poorly understood. They operate only if the tumor mass is relatively small, and they become less effective as the person ages. As tumor growth progresses, the body's diminishing immunocompetence compounds the difficulties of therapy. A complicating factor is the immunosuppressant properties of most antitumor drugs. Treatment schedules to minimize immunosuppression while permitting adequate therapeutic effectiveness should be more intensive but actually must be practiced sparingly because of the lack of antitumor selectivity.

Protected Tumor Sanctuaries

Antitumor drugs frequently fail to reach all sites of tumor cells, and so-called sanctuaries may exist that permit the establishment and unimpeded proliferation of a tumor once it has been successfully eradicated from the remainder of the body. Sanctuaries may develop because of the metastatic spread of tumors to distant sites, and the problem may be accentuated by a lack of knowledge regarding the mechanism of drug access to such secondary neoplasms and their susceptibility to various drugs.

The central nervous system is impermeable to many drugs and often represents such a protected site. Attempts to reach sequestered cells have included intrathecal administration of drugs or use of more highly lipid-soluble drugs capable of rapidly penetrating the blood–brain barrier. The success of peripheral chemotherapy in the leukemias is partly a result of the ease with which high levels of drug can be achieved in tumor cells; on the other hand, leukemic cells that have penetrated the central nervous system are no longer affected by most drugs and the disease progresses.

A more common problem, however, is the diminished blood supply in many solid tumors that blocks delivery of antitumor drugs to the tumor core, which, although necrotic, may still contain active cells sensitive to antitumor drugs. It should be remembered that high doses of radiation (as used in the primary treatment of many gynecologic cancers) produce vascular damage leading to the formation of ischemic sanctuaries for cells that might otherwise be sensitive to drug treatment.

Secondary Malignancies

Antineoplastic agents have the potential to induce secondary malignancies. The alkylating agent melphalan is associated with a cumulative 7-year risk of acute non-lymphocytic leukemia in 9.6% of patients treated for more than 1 year. The development of acute leukemia is also associated with combined chemotherapy and radiation. Secondary malignancies usually occur between 4 and 7 years after successful therapy.

Route of Administration

Chemotherapeutic drugs can be administered orally, intravenously, intramuscularly, intraperitoneally, or intra-arterially. Pleural and intraperitoneal clearance of the agent is usually slower than plasma clearance, leading to prolonged and increased concentrations of the drug. Clinical trials in ovarian cancer have used intraperitoneal cisplatin and paclitaxel with significantly improved survival compared to systemic chemotherapy. The treatment is usually well tolerated. Frequent local side effects include peritoneal irritation with abdominal discomfort and complications related to the intraperitoneal administration, such as infection at the catheter site. Systemic side effects were unexpectedly reported to be worse with intraperitoneal treatment.

Principles of Clinical Chemotherapy

The chief aim of therapy is to achieve maximum cell kill with minimum toxicity. To this end, the dose and schedule of drugs critically influence the therapeutic index. The steep dose–response curve for most drugs indicates that the highest tolerable dose producing an acceptable degree of reversible toxicity should be used in the treatment of sensitive tumors, in which a 2-fold increase in dose may produce a 10-fold increase in the fractional kill.

Therapy must also take into account the length of time a therapeutic concentration of drug is maintained. The maximal effectiveness of some oncolytic drugs depends mainly on peak tissue concentration, whereas that of others depends on the duration of exposure.

In principle, a therapeutic concentration of the cell cycle (phase)-specific drugs is best maintained by 5-day courses of treatment (about 2 average cell-generation times). Such prolonged exposure permits a higher fraction of proliferating cells to pass through vulnerable phases of the cell cycle, as proliferating cells do not progress through the cell cycle in a synchronized fashion. In contrast, the cell cycle (phase)-nonspecific drugs are best administered as an intravenous bolus of the highest tolerable dose, and the dose repeated when normal target tissues have recovered.

High-dose, intermittent therapy has been the most successful schedule against tumors with a large growth fraction. Slow-growing tumors have a large component of permanently nondividing cells and a small growth fraction. Theoretically, drugs active against cells in G_0 and given on a continuous basis should produce the best results in these tumors.

Chronic therapy is feasible only if toxicity is negligible. Some myelosuppression is acceptable, as recovery occurs between treatment cycles. Immunosuppression is a side effect of most cytotoxic drugs and is more pronounced when drugs are given continuously.

Antitumor drugs have been combined concurrently or sequentially in an effort to increase their effectiveness. It is logical to assume that drugs with different dose-limiting toxicities and different modes of action may increase the fractional cell kill without a parallel rise in damage to normal tissues and immunocompetent cells. Because tumors are composed of numerous cell clones that vary in their sensitivity to drugs, the use of multiple agents should lessen the chance of development of resistance and repopulation of the tumor by a resistant cell clone. Sequential, concomitant, or complementary blockade of metabolic pathways should avoid the problem of drug resistance secondary either to the use of alternative pathways or the emergence of a protective random mutation.

As a rule, drugs selected for multidrug therapy must be effective as single agents if improved results are to be expected. Unfortunately, the toxicities of most antitumor drugs are similar, and selecting drugs that have no overlapping side effects is usually not possible. Nevertheless, combination chemotherapy has proved superior to single-agent therapy in leukemia, lymphoma, and some rapidly proliferating solid tumors, including ovarian cancer.

In summary, successful drug therapy requires the administration of an effective agent using the best possible dose and schedule. The tumor must have a high growth fraction and must be accessible to drugs so that they can exert their antitumor effects (ie, cells must not be in tumor sanctuaries). The tumor volume must be small or the fractional cell kill large to avoid the emergence of a resistant cell clone or the development of tolerance in previously sensitive cell clones. Normal tissue must recover from drug injury faster than tumor can regenerate to pretreatment levels.

CANCER CHEMOTHERAPEUTIC AGENTS

Cancer chemotherapeutic agents are commonly classified into six general categories on the basis of their mechanism of action: alkylating agents, antimetabolites, plant alkaloids, miscellaneous agents, hormonal agents, and immunotherapeutic agents. This section presents a broad overview of the mechanism of action and general toxicities of the four major groups of cytotoxic cancer chemotherapy drugs.

Alkylating Agents

A. Classic Alkylating Agents

The alkylating agents evolved from products developed for chemical warfare. The parent chemical, dichlorethyl sulfide (sulfur mustard), was first synthesized during the mid-19th century and used during World War I because of its blistering properties on skin and mucous membranes. These agents also produced atrophy of lymphoid and myeloid tissues, a finding that led workers to explore their use in treating lymphomas and leukemias.

The 3 chemical subgroups of classic alkylating agents in use today are (a) the bis(chloroethyl)amines, which include chlorambucil, cyclophosphamide, ifosfamide, mechlorethamine, melphalan, and uracil mustard; (b) the ethyleneimines, which include triethylenethiophosphoramide (thiotepa); and (c) the alkylsulfonates, which include busulfan and improsulfan hydrochloride.

Alkylating agents induce cytotoxic effects on cells by binding to DNA, particularly at the N-7 position of guanine. This binding interferes with correct base pairing and produces single- and double-stranded DNA breaks. Consequently, DNA replication in S phase is inhibited. In addition to these cytotoxic and mutagenic effects, alkylating agents also inhibit cellular glycolysis, respiration, and synthesis of various enzymes, protein, and nucleic acids.

Most alkylating agents are cell cycle (phase)-nonspecific drugs that are active against both resting and dividing cells; thus they are effective in tumors with a small growth fraction. Cyclophosphamide is unique in that it appears to inhibit DNA synthesis in certain tumors and may therefore have some cell cycle (phase) specificity in the S phase not possessed by the other alkylating agents.

The major toxicities associated with the classic alkylating agents are related to their cytotoxic effects, although each drug has its own unique side effects. Normal tissues most affected are those with a rapid growth rate, eg, the hematopoietic system, the gastrointestinal tract, and gonadal tissue. Nausea and vomiting occur with use of most of these agents, particularly with the intravenous route, and may result from a direct effect on the chemoreceptor trigger zone in the medulla. If extravasation of mechlorethamine occurs during administration or if skin or mucous membranes are exposed to this agent, tissue necrosis develops, and sloughing will occur later, producing a slow-healing ulcer. The myelosuppression associated with classic alkylating agents is mainly a leukopenia, with the lowest cell counts occurring in 10–14 days and recovery occurring in 21–28 days. Busulfan and chlorambucil have slightly more prolonged myelosuppressive effects. Bone marrow depression causes the most serious complications of therapy associated with the alkylating agents; patients are at increased risk for bleeding episodes caused by thrombocytopenia and infection caused by leukopenia. Anemia from depressed levels of erythrocyte production occurs less frequently.

B. Nitrosoureas

The nitrosoureas include carmustine (BCNU), lomustine (CCNU), semustine (methyl CCNU), estramustine, streptozocin, and chlorozotocin. Although nitrosoureas probably act mainly as alkylating agents, they may also cause the inhibition of several key enzymatic steps necessary for the formation of DNA. The cytotoxic activity of these drugs is thought to be mediated through the action of metabolites that can alkylate DNA. Like other alkylating agents, the nitrosoureas are cell cycle (phase)-nonspecific. The nitrosoureas are lipid-soluble and cross the blood–brain barrier. These agents may undergo some enterohepatic circulation, but they are rapidly metabolized. The largest fraction of these drugs is excreted in the urine as metabolites, with only a small fraction excreted in the active form. Streptozocin is a naturally occurring nitrosourea that is particularly useful in the treatment of insulinomas because of its marked specificity for pancreatic β and exocrine cells.

The major adverse reaction associated with the nitrosoureas is a notable delayed and dose-dependent depression of the hematopoietic system occurring with commonly used dosage levels. In contrast to the classic alkylating agents, maximal depression of the white cell count occurs in 3–5 weeks with use of the nitrosoureas; it may persist for several weeks or longer. Severe nausea and vomiting may limit the dosage that can be given. Pain at the injection site is associated with the use of carmustine.

C. Antitumor Antibiotics

The antitumor antibiotics are products of microbial fermentation and include the anthracyclines and the chromomycins. Although most antitumor antibiotics exert some antimicrobial properties, the cytotoxic effects of these agents generally preclude their use as such.

1. Anthracyclines—The anthracyclines include daunorubicin, doxorubicin, and rubidazone. These drugs effectively interfere with nucleic acid synthesis and block DNA-directed RNA and DNA transcription. The anthracyclines are probably effective in all phases of the cell cycle and are therefore cell cycle (phase)-nonspecific.

Disposition kinetics of the anthracyclines are complex. Their half-life is relatively long, ranging from 15 hours to several days for doxorubicin. These drugs are extensively metabolized in the liver, and some of the metabolites retain antitumor activity. Biliary excretion appears to be the major means of elimination, but a small portion of drug is excreted in the urine.

Many of the adverse effects of the anthracyclines are similar to those of the alkylating agents. Acute toxicity is manifested as bone marrow depression that may be severe enough to require limiting of dosage; the nadir usually occurs in 10–14 days, with recovery by 21 days in most patients. The anthracyclines also produce tissue necrosis and sloughing if extravasation occurs during intravenous injection. A unique cardiomyopathy has been observed when high cumulative doses of the anthracyclines have been administered.

2. Chromomycins—Another group of antitumor antibiotics is the chromomycins, which include chromomycin A_3, mithramycin (plicamycin), and dactinomycin. All act similarly to block DNA-directed RNA synthesis by intercalating and anchoring in DNA, as do the anthracyclines. Bone marrow depression because of use of chromomycins is a significant, but usually not dose-limiting, toxicity characterized by thrombocytopenia with some leukopenia.

Chromomycin A_3 (totomycin) is rapidly cleared from plasma, is excreted via the urinary and biliary tracts, and causes nausea and vomiting, renal toxicity, and severe local reactions at the injection site.

Mithramycin crosses the blood–brain barrier and is well distributed in the cerebrospinal fluid. It is excreted mainly in the urine. Gastrointestinal effects include nausea and vomiting, anorexia, and diarrhea. Liver and kidney toxicity is common. A toxicity unique to this agent is a hemorrhagic syndrome heralded by facial flushing. Mithramycin has been used to lower serum calcium levels in patients with hypercalcemia.

Dactinomycin is rapidly cleared from serum and is excreted mainly in the bile with minimal biotransformation. Gastrointestinal effects include mucositis characterized by oral ulceration. Nausea and vomiting may be severe enough to limit the dosage. Other toxicities include bone marrow depression and alopecia.

3. Other antitumor antibiotics—Other antitumor antibiotics include mitomycin, piperazinedione, and bleomycin. Mitomycin probably functions as an alkylating agent by causing cross-linking of DNA. Mitomycin is rapidly cleared from the vascular compartment and is found in most body tissues except the brain; it is excreted via the kidneys and in bile. Delayed bone marrow depression may occur, with the nadir occurring 3–5 weeks after administration. Myelosuppression may be more severe with repeated doses and is the major dose-limiting toxicity. Renal toxicity may be observed, whereas gastrointestinal effects and alopecia occur less frequently.

Piperazinedione appears to function as an alkylating agent by inhibiting the incorporation of several DNA nucleotides into DNA synthesis. Although cell progression through G_2 is delayed, piperazinedione is probably not cell cycle (phase)-specific. Myelosuppression is the major dose-limiting toxic effect and is manifested as granulocytopenia followed by thrombocytopenia, with the nadir and recovery from myelosuppression varying by patient. The level of activity against neoplasms resistant to alternative alkylating agents and antimetabolites has not been high enough to warrant expanded clinical trials.

Bleomycins are antineoplastic antibiotics produced by fermentation of *Streptomyces verticillus.* More than a dozen fractions have been isolated, but the major constituent of commercially available preparations is bleomycin A_2. Inasmuch as the exact composition of the drug may vary, the drug is rated in units of activity. Bleomycin contains DNA- and ion-binding moieties. The mechanism of action most likely involves the production of single- and double-stranded breaks leading to inhibition of DNA synthesis, and to a lesser extent, inhibition of RNA and protein synthesis. Bleomycin is cell cycle (phase)-specific for mitosis and G_2. This cycle specificity has been useful experimentally to achieve cell-cycle synchronization in combination chemotherapy. Bleomycin appears to exert much less myelosuppressive activity than most other antineoplastic drugs and is therefore useful in patients who already have depressed bone marrow counts. Cutaneous reactions are dose-related and include hyperpigmentation, edema, erythema, and thickening of the nail beds. They are the most common side effects because the drug is concentrated in the skin. The most serious toxicity is pneumonitis related to the total dose received; the disease is characterized by dyspnea, rales, and infiltrates that progress to fibrosis. A high incidence of hypersensitivity reactions ranging from fever and chills to anaphylaxis is also associated with bleomycin.

Antimetabolites

The antimetabolites exert their major activity during the S phase and therefore are most effective against tumors that have a high growth fraction. The antimetabolites are structural analogues of naturally occurring metabolites and interfere with normal synthesis of nucleic acids by substituting different compounds for the normal purines or pyrimidines in metabolic pathways. The antimetabolites are subdivided into the folate antagonists, the purine antagonists, and the pyrimidine antagonists.

A. FOLATE ANTAGONISTS

Methotrexate is a 4-amino-4-deoxy-N-methyl analogue of folic acid and is the classic antimetabolite prototype. Methotrexate is a cell cycle (phase)-specific agent that exerts its cytotoxic effect in the S phase by binding to dihydrofolate reductase, thereby blocking the reduction of folic acid. Thymidine and purine synthesis are halted, thus arresting DNA, RNA, and protein synthesis. For maximal effect, intracellular levels of methotrexate must be sufficiently high to bind almost all of the dihydrofolate reductase, of which only small quantities are required to maintain adequate levels of the reduced folate pool. Resistance is thought to develop as a consequence either of increased levels of dihydrofolate reductase or of decreased cell uptake.

Methotrexate enters the cell through an active carrier-mediated cell membrane transport system that it shares with leucovorin calcium (folinic acid, citrovorum factor) and its metabolite, 5-methyltetrahydrofolate. When this transport system is functional in tumor cells, adequate intracellular levels of methotrexate are easily achieved. Because some tumors lack or have reduced transport capabilities, high levels of methotrexate are required to facilitate transport by a passive method instead. To limit toxicity, treatment requiring high doses of methotrexate is followed by "rescue" of normal cells with leucovorin calcium.

Another antifolate is ethane sulfonic acid compound, or Baker's antifol (triazinate). It is actively transported into the cell by a different transport carrier than is methotrexate, but the target enzyme is the same. Thus, these two antifolates may have different tumor specificity, even though their general mechanism of action is the same.

Both compounds produce bone marrow depression, with the lowest cell counts occurring in 7–14 days. Stomatitis and gastrointestinal distress are frequent. Skin rashes are common side effects of ethane sulfonic acid compound, but occur in fewer patients treated with methotrexate. Central nervous system abnormalities may also occur with either agent.

B. Purine Antagonists

Mercaptopurine and thioguanine are analogues of the natural purines hypoxanthine and guanine. The purine antagonists have specific antitumor effects on the S phase.

Mercaptopurine acts as a false metabolite because of its close chemical similarity to hypoxanthine. It competes for the enzymes responsible for the conversion of inosinic acid to adenine and xanthine ribotides, and thus interferes with normal DNA and RNA synthesis. Simultaneous administration of allopurinol may block the metabolism of mercaptopurine and azathioprine by xanthine oxidase and require reduction of the dose to one-fourth or one-third the normal amount. This drug interaction does not occur with thioguanine, because its detoxification occurs by methylation.

Thioguanine also acts as a false metabolite; its substitution for the corresponding guanine nucleotide blocks purine synthesis.

The indications for use and efficacy of thioguanine and mercaptopurine are the same. Their toxicities are identical, and the two drugs are mutually cross-resistant.

Azathioprine is an imidazolyl derivative. It is used as an immunosuppressant but has cytotoxic properties similar to those of mercaptopurine and thioguanine because it is extensively metabolized to mercaptopurine.

The major dose-limiting toxicity of the purine antagonists is myelosuppression consisting mainly of leukopenia, with lesser effects on platelets and red blood cells. Gastrointestinal distress is common, and hepatotoxicity may occur with use of any of the purine antagonists.

C. Pyrimidine Antagonists

Fluorouracil (5-fluorouracil, 5-FU) is the classic antimetabolite. It is cell cycle (phase)-specific and inhibits the enzyme thymidylate synthetase to block DNA synthesis. It is catabolized in the liver by dihydrouracil dehydrogenase.

Ftorafur is hydrolyzed to 5-FU in the liver and stomach and therefore may act as a depot form of 5-FU.

Fluorouracil and ftorafur cause myelosuppression that reaches a nadir in 1–14 days, but ftorafur appears to cause less myelosuppression, which may be a result of its slower release of 5-FU. Both agents commonly produce gastrointestinal toxicities, including occasional glossitis and stomatitis. Neurotoxicities may also occur because these drugs cross the blood–brain barrier.

The cytidine and deoxycytidine analogues include gemcitabine, cytarabine, cyclocytidine (ancitabine), and azacitidine. The active form of these nucleoside analogues stops DNA synthesis by competitively inhibiting DNA polymerase and production of deoxycytidine. Cytarabine is metabolized by cytidine deaminase in the liver, granulocytes, and gastrointestinal tract. Small amounts of cytarabine cross the blood–brain barrier. Because cyclocytidine is not inactivated by cytidine deaminase, it slowly releases the more active cytarabine, which prolongs plasma levels; cyclocytidine can therefore be regarded as a depot form of cytarabine that has a biphasic half-life occurring at 3–15 minutes and at 2 hours.

Cytarabine and cyclocytidine are active only in the S phase. Although azacitidine is most active during the S phase, it appears to exert activity in all phases of the cell cycle by inhibiting DNA, RNA, and protein synthesis. Although it has some cross-resistance with the other cytidine analogues, this is not complete. These facts suggest that azacitidine has an additional mechanism of action not found in cytarabine and cyclocytidine.

The toxicities of gemcitabine, cytarabine, cyclocytidine, and azacitidine are similar to those of other pyrimidine antagonists and include myelosuppression and gastrointestinal abnormalities, which may be severe. Cytarabine produces a flulike syndrome, and cyclocytidine commonly produces unusual jaw pain and hypotension.

Plant Alkaloids

A. *VINCA* ALKALOIDS

Although the periwinkle plant has a long history in folklore medicine, clinical research to evaluate its possible therapeutic effects was not begun until 1945; by 1958, several active alkaloids had been isolated, but to date, only vinblastine and vincristine have had extensive clinical use. Although they are quite similar chemically and structurally, vincristine and vinblastine have markedly different clinical activities and toxicities. The precise mechanism of action of these compounds is not clearly understood, but they appear to cause arrest of metaphase by crystallization of the microtubular spindle proteins. *Vinca* alkaloids may also inhibit nucleic acid and protein synthesis, but these effects become apparent only after high concentrations are reached. There appears to be no cross-resistance between the *Vinca* alkaloids and radiation therapy, alkylating agents, or each other. The differences in their therapeutic spectrum, toxicity, and potency may be related to each drug's ability to enter different types of cells.

The dose-limiting toxicity of vinblastine and vindesine is bone marrow depression, manifested chiefly by leukopenia 4–10 days after administration, with recovery occurring within 10–21 days. Vincristine does not usually cause leukopenia and can be given with relative safety to leukopenic patients.

Neurotoxicity is a major dose-limiting effect of vincristine and vindesine, but occurs infrequently with vinblastine. Vincristine neurotoxicity consists of peripheral neuropathy with loss of deep tendon reflexes, numbness, and, eventually, severe weakness. Cranial nerve palsies, vocal cord paralysis, and autonomic nervous system dysfunction, manifested as urinary retention, tachycardia, or gastrointestinal symptoms of constipation or paralytic ileus may occur. All of the *Vinca* alkaloids cause severe local necrosis if extravasation occurs, and vindesine may produce pain and phlebitis even without evidence of infiltration.

B. PODOPHYLLOTOXINS

The two podophyllotoxins presently used are semisynthetic compounds derived from the root of the mayapple plant. The mechanism of action of etoposide (VP-16) and teniposide (VM-26) is similar to that of *Vinca* alkaloids in that they cause a mitotic spindle toxicity resulting in arrest of metaphase. Podophyllotoxins prevent cells from entering mitosis, thereby causing an increase in the MI; at high concentrations, the drugs cause lysis of cells entering mitosis. They also suppress DNA synthesis and, to a lesser degree, RNA and protein synthesis. Thus both the *Vinca* alkaloids and podophyllotoxins are cell cycle (phase)-specific and exert their major activity in the M phase; they also demonstrate some activity in the G_2 and S phases.

Etoposide and teniposide are extensively protein-bound and are mainly eliminated by biliary excretion, with some enterohepatic recirculation. Both drugs may cause severe hypotension if infused too rapidly. Other adverse effects include nausea and vomiting, diarrhea, alopecia, and phlebitis at the injection site. The podophyllotoxins produce mild bone marrow depression and leukopenia, with the nadir occurring from 3–14 days following therapy.

C. TAXANES

The taxanes, paclitaxel and docetaxel, are relatively novel antimitotic agents. Taxanes arrest cells at the G_2/M phase of the cell cycle by preventing depolymerization of the microtubuli structure. The cells therefore are unable to divide and will eventually undergo apoptosis. Both taxanes have demonstrated significant activity against many solid tumors as single agents and in combination with other chemotherapeutic agents. In addition, taxanes have been used in combination with chemotherapy in a variety of cancers including non-small cell lung cancer (NSCLC), cancers of the head and neck, and cancers of the gastrointestinal tract.

Paclitaxel has been used extensively in patients with gynecologic malignancies, particularly ovarian and endometrial cancer. Major side effects include bone marrow toxicity, hypersensitivity reactions, arthralgias, peripheral neuropathy, and alopecia.

Miscellaneous Agents

Cisplatin was the first inorganic compound to be used to treat human cancers. Crosslinking of DNA may be somewhat different from that of other alkylators, in that the interatomic distance is much smaller than with the traditional alkylating agents; this characteristic may account for some of the toxicity associated with cisplatin. Cisplatin is cell cycle (phase)-nonspecific and is excreted mainly unchanged in the urine. Adverse reactions include anaphylaxis, nausea and vomiting, nephrotoxicity, ototoxicity, and myelosuppression that is usually mild.

Carboplatin is a derivative of cisplatin with equal clinical efficacy. Compared to cisplatin, it causes more hematopoietic toxicity but less ototoxicity, neuropathy, and nephrotoxicity.

Dacarbazine was originally thought to be an antimetabolite but is now recognized as an alkylating agent that is activated in the liver and excreted in the urine. It has somewhat less bone marrow toxicity than standard alkylating agents but typically causes severe nausea and vomiting similar to that caused by cisplatin.

Hexamethylmelamine does not act as an alkylating agent in vitro, even though it is structurally similar to triethylenemelamine, which is an alkylator. Although the precise mechanism is unknown, it is possible that hexamethylmelamine is activated to an alkylating agent in vivo. Hexamethylmelamine is rapidly metabolized in the liver and excreted in the urine. Gastrointestinal, neurologic, and hematologic toxicities occur.

Hydroxyurea is cell cycle (phase)-specific for the S phase. In addition to holding cells in G_1, the drug exerts a lethal effect on cells in the S phase by inhibiting ribonucleotide reductase and DNA synthesis without interfering with RNA or protein synthesis. Hydroxyurea may also act as an antimetabolite in that incorporation of thymidine into DNA appears to be inhibited. The major adverse reactions are bone marrow depression, gastrointestinal disturbances, and rarely, dermatologic reactions and renal impairment.

Procarbazine appears to be cell cycle (phase)-specific for the S phase; it apparently interferes with DNA synthesis, but its exact mechanism of action is unclear. Oxidative breakdown products, hydrogen peroxide, formaldehyde, azoprocarbazine, and free hydroxyl radicals may be responsible for the characteristic chromosomal breakage observed after use of procarbazine. Procarbazine may demonstrate dangerous interactions with a number of other drugs. Adverse reactions include myelosuppression, a flulike syndrome, and dermatologic and various central nervous system reactions.

Topotecan is a semisynthetic inhibitor of topoisomerase I. It is cycle (phase)-specific for the S phase and is excreted in urine. Myelosuppression is a dose-limiting reaction. Nausea and vomiting are common, but mild.

Most normal cells possess the ability to synthesize the amino acid asparagine. Some tumor cells, such as those in acute lymphoblastic leukemia, do not possess this ability and require exogenous asparagine. Asparaginase converts asparagine to nonfunctional aspartic acid, thereby depriving the tumor cell of this crucial amino acid to block protein synthesis. Side effects include protein depletion and pancreatic and hepatic damage. Allergic reactions are frequent, as asparaginase is a biologic product obtained from bacteria.

Chemotherapy in Gynecologic Cancers

A. Ovarian Cancer

Chemotherapy is standard in most ovarian cancers after initial surgery. Of all gynecologic malignancies, ovarian cancer responds best to chemotherapeutic regimens. A wide variety of antineoplastic drug regimens have been studied during the past two decades to determine the optimal choice of drugs, route, and timing of administration.

Currently, systemic chemotherapy with a platinum-based drug (cisplatin or its derivative, carboplatin) and paclitaxel is the most commonly used drug regimen in epithelial ovarian cancer. In patients with hypersensitivity to paclitaxel, an alternative drug like cyclophosphamide or topotecan is substituted.

Another modality being used in the first-line treatment of epithelial ovarian cancer is intraperitoneal chemotherapy. The rationale for intraperitoneal therapy is for the peritoneum, the primary site of ovarian cancer, to receive sustained exposure to the chemotherapeutic agent while sparing normal tissues such as the bone marrow. In optimally debulked stage III ovarian cancer patients, intraperitoneal and intravenous administration of paclitaxel/cisplatin has shown a statistically significant increase in survival when compared to administration of intravenous chemotherapy alone.

Treatment of malignant germ cells of the ovary are currently platinum-based chemotherapy combinations such as bleomycin, etoposide, and cisplatin (BEP). The treatment of refractory or recurrent ovarian cancer is not standardized. Patients that are resistant to platinum-based regimens are likely to be resistant to other drugs. Agents that have shown effects in these clinical situations include the topoisomerase I inhibitor topotecan, etoposide, the semisynthetic taxane docetaxel, liposome-encapsulated doxorubicin, and gemcitabine. In general, these drugs show a 13–26% clinical response rate in cisplatin-refractory and recurrent ovarian cancer.

B. Endometrial Cancer

Chemotherapy in endometrial cancer is mainly confined to patients with advanced or recurrent metastatic disease. The most active single agents are doxorubicin, platinum-based regimens, and paclitaxel.

C. Cervical Cancer

Chemotherapy combined with concurrent radiation therapy (chemoradiation) is an important modality in the treatment of cervical cancer. The chemotherapeutic agents shown to be most effective are cisplatin or a combination of cisplatin and 5-FU. In a series of clinical trials, the combination of platinum-based chemotherapy with radiation showed increased survival rates in cervical cancer in early stage disease. Patients with bulky stage IB cervical cancer showed significantly prolonged survival and disease-free intervals when preoperative radiation was combined with cisplatin chemotherapy. Patients with locally advanced cervical cancer showed a 30% reduction in the risk of death for women receiving platinum-based chemoradiation compared with radiation therapy alone.

REFERENCES

Armstrong DK et al: Intraperitoneal cisplatin and paclitaxel in ovarian cancer. N Engl J Med 2006;354(1):34.

Christian J, Thomas H: Ovarian cancer chemotherapy. Cancer Treat Rev 2001;27:99.

Eifel PJ et al: Pelvic irradiation with concurrent chemotherapy versus pelvic and para-aortic irradiation for high-risk cervical cancer: an update of radiation therapy oncology group trial (RTOG) 90–01. J Clin Oncol 2004;22(5):872.

Green JA et al: Survival and recurrence after concomitant chemotherapy and radiotherapy for cancer of the uterine cervix: A systematic review and meta-analysis. Lancet 2001;358(9284):781.

Keys HM et al: Cisplatin, radiation, and adjuvant hysterectomy compared with radiation and adjuvant hysterectomy for bulky stage IB cervical carcinoma. N Engl J Med 1999;15:1154.

Lehne G: P-glycoprotein as a drug target in the treatment of multidrug resistant cancer. Curr Drug Targets 2000;1:85.

Lanciano R et al: Randomized comparison of weekly cisplatin or protracted venous infusion of fluorouracil in combination with pelvic radiation in advanced cervix cancer: A Gynecologic Oncology Group study. J Clin Oncol 2005;23(33):8289.

Peters WA 3rd et al: Concurrent chemotherapy and pelvic radiation therapy compared with pelvic radiation therapy alone as adjuvant therapy after radical surgery in high-risk early-stage cancer of the cervix. J Clin Oncol 2000;18(8):1606.

Rose PG et al: Concurrent cisplatin-based radiotherapy and chemotherapy for locally advanced cervical cancer. N Engl J Med 1999;340(15):1144. Erratum in N Engl J Med 1999;341(9):708.

SECTION VI
Reproductive Endocrinology & Infertility

Infertility

55

Ashim Kumar, MD, Shahin Ghadir, MD, Niloofar Eskandari, MD, & Alan H. DeCherney, MD

The number of infertility visits has increased over the past decades. In some cases, couples have voluntarily delayed childbearing in favor of establishing careers and may experience an age-related decline in fertility. There have been significant advances in assisted reproductive technologies, from improved embryo culture media to intracytoplasmic sperm injection (ICSI) and preimplantation genetic diagnosis (PGD), which have resulted in remarkable increases in in vitro fertilization-embryo transfer (IVF-ET) pregnancy rates. This coupled with increasing public awareness and acceptance of assisted reproductive technology (ART) have spurred women or couples with infertility to seek medical care.

Definition

Infertility is defined as the inability of a couple to conceive within 1 year. **Sterility** implies an intrinsic inability to achieve pregnancy, whereas infertility implies a decrease in the ability to conceive and is synonymous with **subfertility**. **Primary infertility** applies to those who have never conceived, whereas **secondary infertility** designates those who have conceived at some time in the past.

Fecundity is the probability of achieving a live birth in 1 menstrual cycle. **Fecundability** is expressed as the likelihood of conception per month of exposure. Fertility, as well as infertility, of a woman or couple is best perceived as fecundability, as few infertile patients are sterile. It also allows for a direct comparison of treatment options over a more functional time frame.

Epidemiology

The prevalence of women diagnosed with infertility is approximately 13%, with a range from 7–28%, depending on the age of the woman. It has remained stable over the past 40 years; ethnicity or race appears to have little effect on prevalence. However, the incidence of primary infertility has increased, with a concurrent decrease in secondary infertility, most likely as a result of social changes such as delayed childbearing.

In normal fertile couples having frequent intercourse, the fecundability is estimated to be approximately 20–25%. Approximately 90% of couples with unprotected intercourse will conceive within 1 year. Sterility affects 1–2% of couples.

Etiology

Infertility can be due to either partner, or both. Overall, an etiology for infertility can be found in 80% of cases with an even distribution of male and female factors, including couples with multiple factors. A primary diagnosis of male factor is made in approximately 25% of cases. Ovulatory dysfunction and tubal/peritoneal factors comprise the majority of female factor infertility. In 15–20% of infertile couples, the etiology cannot be found and a diagnosis of unexplained infertility is made.

The success rates of treatment for infertility depends on a variety of factors, including cause of infertility, woman's age, duration of infertility, and treatment modality. Health insurance plans vary a great deal in the amount and type of infertility treatments that are covered. For those couples without infertility coverage, treatment choices are dictated by medical and financial considerations. Not uncommonly, infertility treatment does not actually make the difference between conceiving and not conceiving, but allows for conception in the more immediate future rather than at a delayed point of time (increasing fecundability).

PSYCHOLOGIC ASPECTS

A diagnosis of infertility can be an assault on self-image, sexuality, and relationships. The emotional roller coaster ride begins with high hopes at the initiation of a cycle and culminates positively, but often negatively, on the day of the pregnancy test result. The couple may progress through stages as described by Kubler-Ross, including denial, anger, grief, and resolution. Recognition of these stages may assist the practitioner in providing appropriate support and counseling or referral for the additional therapy.

DIAGNOSIS

The armamentarium of diagnostic tests available for the evaluation of an infertile couple is large. Therefore, a clinician should be judicious in his/her use of tests. The history and physical exam shape the endocrinologic and radiologic testing algorithm specific to each patient. Other factors to consider include patient age, risks associated with the test, invasiveness, expense, and probabilities of significant findings (Table 55–1). The patient(s) should be included in the decision-making process.

New Patient Assessment

The initial aspect of the interview includes discussion of the factors (ie, ovulation, sperm concentration, ovarian reserve, etc.) that affect fertility so that the patient(s) is aware of the potential etiologies. In this light, the physician can present an algorithm for the diagnostic evaluation that the patient will understand. This will help the patient grasp the peculiarities of the specific tests, such as timing the hysterosalpingogram to the day of the menstrual cycle, provide an opportunity for the patient(s) to ask fertility-related questions, and to address any information learned from friends, family, or the Internet.

The initial clinical assessment should begin with a thorough history of both partners. Factors to consider while obtaining the medical history are outlined in Table 55–2 for the female and in Table 55–3 for the male. The history should guide the physical examination beyond the general evaluation; for example, a rectovaginal exam to detect uterosacral ligament nodularity associated with endometriosis is indicated if a

woman presents with a history of severe dysmenorrhea. However, a thorough physical exam may divulge key information such as acanthosis nigricans and its association with insulin resistance.

The laboratory and radiologic tests assess four key aspects for fertility in a couple: the sperm (male factor), the oocyte (ovulatory factor and ovarian reserve), transport and implantation of ova (pelvic factor including fallopian tubes and uterus). In many cases, the couple will be attempting to absorb significant amounts of information, some of which may be highly technical, at a time of heightened emotion. It is therefore helpful to offer literature or a written summary of the discussion. Frequently, the initial history will indicate a probable diagnosis or a contributing cause of infertility, but it is important to complete a basic evaluation of all of the major factors so a secondary diagnosis is not ignored.

Evaluation of Male Factors

Male factor is diagnosed in 25–40% of infertile couples. The majority of the diagnoses involve testicular pathology such as varicocele. Although validation is incomplete, there is a trend toward increasing use of molecular techniques to quantify the fertility potential of semen as our knowledge of fundamental molecular genetics expands. Experience and investigation have relegated several tests previously used to assess fertilization to historical interest. Beyond the history and physical exam, the initial evaluation of male factor is through semen analysis. If abnormal, the semen analysis should be repeated in 2–3 months to confirm findings.

A. SEMEN ANALYSIS

The male partner should abstain from coitus for 2–5 days before collecting the sample and the specimen should be received in the lab within 1 hour of collection. Table 55–4 lists normal sperm values. If fundamental parameters of count and motility are normal, the assessment of the morphology of the sperm becomes more critical. Specialized expertise in determining sperm morphology and strict application of criteria should be used before declaring the semen normal. The percent of sperm with normal morphology is the semen analysis parameter, which best correlates with pregnancy.

The semen parameters in normal fertile males may vary significantly over time, and the first response to any abnormal result should be to wait an interval of several weeks to months and repeat the test. A normal semen analysis will usually exclude significant male factor. Although low counts, decreased motility, and increased numbers of abnormal forms are most frequently associated with infertility, unfavorable semen parameters may still be found in 20% of males undergoing vasectomy after having completed their families.

Table 55–1. Causes of infertility.

Male Factor	**Peripheral defects**
Endocrine disorders	Gonadal dysgenesis
Hypothalamic dysfunction (Kallmann's syndrome)	Premature ovarian failure
Pituitary failure (tumor, radiation, surgery)	Ovarian tumor
Hyperprolactinemia (drug, tumor)	Ovarian resistance
Exogenous androgens	Metabolic disease
Thyroid disorders	Thyroid disease
Adrenal hyperplasia	Liver disease
Anatomic disorders	Renal disease
Congenital absence of vas deferens	Obesity
Obstruction of vas deferens	Androgen excess, adrenal or neoplastic
Congenital abnormalities of ejaculatory system	**Pelvic Factor**
Abnormal spermatogenesis	Infection
Chromosomal abnormalities	Appendicitis
Mumps orchitis	Pelvic inflammatory disease
Cryptorchidism	Uterine adhesions (Asherman's syndrome)
Chemical or radiation exposure	Endometriosis
Abnormal motility	Structural abnormalities
Absent cilia (Kartagener's syndrome)	Diethylstilbestrol (DES) exposure
Varicocele	Failure of normal fusion of the reproductive tract
Antibody formation	Myoma
Sexual dysfunction	**Cervical Factor**
Retrograde ejaculation	Congenital
Impotence	DES exposure
Decreased libido	Müllerian duct abnormality
Ovulatory Factor	Acquired
Central defects	Surgical treatment
Chronic hyperandrogenemic anovulation	Infection
Hyperprolactinemia (drug, tumor, empty selia)	
Hypothalamic insufficiency	
Pituitary insufficiency (trauma, tumor, congenital)	

If the semen analysis reveals abnormal or borderline parameters, the history should be reviewed for any proximate cause of an abnormality, keeping in mind that the cycle of spermatogenesis takes about 74 days. A male with less than 5 million sperm per milliliter warrants an endocrinologic evaluation including follicle-stimulating hormone (FSH), leuteinizing hormone (LH), and testosterone, or a karyotype in selected cases. The patient should be referred to an urologist with a special interest and expertise in infertility as indicated.

B. DNA ASSAYS

Several tests, including sperm chromatin structure assay (SCSA), comet, and terminal dUTP nick-end labeling (TUNEL), have been developed to quantify the damage to DNA or chromatin (packaged DNA). There is some evidence associating increased DNA damage as determined by these tests to poor fertility outcome. The SCSA determines the percent of chromatin that is fragmented by exposing sperm DNA to acid denaturation (fragmented DNA is more vulnerable). Clinical experience has not matched initial expectations although the test may be useful for couples with unexplained infertility with repeated in vitro fertilization (IVF) failures. The comet assay consists of placing the sperm DNA on gel electrophoresis; DNA with increased strand breaks will be smaller and therefore travel further on the slide. The TUNEL assay identifies DNA strand breaks by their incorporation of labeled deoxyuridine triphosphate (dUTP). The comet and TUNEL assay are not in wide clinical use.

C. OTHER TESTS

More detailed assessment of sperm function may include postcoital test, antibody studies, a sperm penetration assay (hamster egg penetration assay). Such assessments are designed to investigate more subtle problems or abnormalities of function not revealed by the assessment of sperm number and motility. Although helpful in some cases, the sensitivity of these assays in detecting fertility is still uncertain and varies with the particular

Table 55–2. Medical history for female factor infertility.

In utero diethylstilbestrol (DES) exposure
History of pubertal development
Present menstrual cycle characteristics (length, duration, molimina)
Contraceptive history
Prior pregnancies, outcomes
Previous surgeries, especially pelvic
Prior infection
History of abnormal Papanicolau (Pap) smear, treatment
Drugs and medications
General health (diet, weight stability, exercise patterns, review of systems)

laboratory where the test is performed. Because no universal methodology has yet been accepted, the interpretation of these tests requires close communication with the laboratory selected.

Cervical mucus is a heterogeneous secretion containing more than 90% water. It has intrinsic properties including consistency, spinnbarkeit (stretchability), and ferning. When mucus is obtained from the cervical canal in the preovulatory phase, it normally exhibits a response to the high estrogen environment. The mucus is thin, watery, and acellular; it dries in a crystalline pattern (ferning), and acts as a facilitative reservoir for the sperm.

The functional sperm must interact normally with the egg and surrounding cells in the uterine tube. The normal migration of sperm is affected by attrition and filtering, and it is estimated that less than 1000 sperm will be found in the environment of the oocyte. The initial interaction of sperm and female genital tract can be determined by postcoital examination of the cervical mucus (Sims-Huhner test).

The purpose of the postcoital test is to determine the number of active spermatozoa in the cervical mucus

Table 55–3. Medical history for male factor infertility.

Congenital abnormalities
Undescended testes
Prior paternity
Frequency of intercourse
Exposure to toxins
Previous surgery
Previous infections, treatment
Drugs and medications
General health (diet, exercise, review of systems)
Decreased frequency of shaving

Table 55–4. Normal semen parameters.

Liquification	30 minutes
Count	20 million/mL or more
Motility	> 50%
Volume	2 mL or more
Morphology	≥ 30% normal
Strict criteria	> 14% normal
pH	7.2–7.8
White blood cell count	< 1 million/mL

and the length of sperm survival (in hours) after coitus. The test should be performed as close to ovulation as possible. The test involves aspirating cervical mucus with a syringe 6–8 hours after coitus and checking under a microscope for the number and the motility of the sperm; less than 10 motile sperm per high-power field is considered abnormal. The postcoital test is controversial and has limited use in the infertility work-up. Its value in assessing cervical hostility to sperm has never been proven.

Tests developed to predict the fertilizing ability of sperm include the zona-free hamster egg penetration test (the sperm penetration assay) and the hemizona test. These assays compare the ability of sperm to penetrate the zona-free hamster egg (a hamster egg in which the zona pellucida has been enzymatically digested) or to bind to human zona with sperm from a known fertile donor. The value of these tests remains controversial, and they are not in general clinical use.

Sperm possess antigens and semen may contain antibodies including sperm-agglutinating, sperm-immobilizing, or cytotoxic antibodies. The antibodies can be measured in semen or in serum. The immunobead test is the antibody assay used in most labs, and is considered positive when only 20% or more of motile spermatozoa have immunobead binding. However, the test is considered to be clinically significant when 50% of sperm are coated with immunobeads.

Evaluation of Female Factors

A. OVULATORY FACTOR

An ovulatory dysfunction is responsible for approximately 20–25% of infertility cases (~40% of female factor infertility). The problem should be investigated first by review of historical factors, including the onset of menarche; present cycle length (intermenstrual interval); and presence or absence of premenstrual symptoms (molimina), such as breast tenderness, bloating, or dysmenorrhea. Signs and symptoms of systemic disease, particularly of hyperthyroidism or hypothyroidism, and physical signs of endocrine disease (ie, hirsutism, galactorrhea, and obesity) should be noted. The degree and intensity of exercise, a history of weight loss, and complaints of hot flushes all are clinical clues to possible endocrine or ovulatory dysfunction.

1. Follicular pool—Early in gestation, the germ cells undergo mitosis to produce oogonia. The oogonia undergo meiosis in their transformation to oocytes but arrest at prophase of meiosis I until the time of ovulation. A layer of granulosa cells encircles the oocytes creating the follicle. A female will have the highest number of germ cells, approximately 6 million, in her ovaries at 20 weeks gestational age. Henceforth, atresia depletes the follicular pool at a brisk pace with only 1–2 million oocytes remaining at the time of birth. The ovaries contain approximately 500,000 oocytes at the time of first ovulation. Menopause signals the complete depletion of germ cells, with a woman having ovulated about 500 oocytes during her reproductive years.

2. Ovarian reserve—An inverse relationship exists between fecundity and the age of the woman. The decline in fecundity is a result of progressive follicular atresia through apoptosis, which accelerates in the early thirties and progresses rapidly in the late thirties and early forties. Concomitantly, there is a decrease in follicular quality as a result of an increase in oocytes with chromosomal anomalies and progressive deletions in mitochondrial DNA. The concept of ovarian reserve represents the remaining follicular pool of the ovaries. As ovarian reserve decreases, the ovaries' responsiveness to gonadotropins decreases necessitating higher amounts of FSH to achieve follicular growth and maturation.

Ovarian reserve should be evaluated in women older than 35 years of age who are seeking fertility. Evaluation of the level of FSH and estradiol in the early follicular phase (cycle days 2–4)may provide helpful guidance in terms of the likelihood of achieving success, as mild elevations in either FSH or estradiol may precede overt ovulatory dysfunction but still indicate a poor prognosis for successful pregnancy. Use of the clomiphene challenge test has gone out of favor, while newer tests such as inhibin-B remain to be validated in large studies. The specific cause of oligo-ovulation or anovulation is determined by the history, the physical examination, and appropriate laboratory studies.

3. Confirmation of ovulation—If the patient reports a history of mittelschmerz and/or regular menses with molimina (headaches, bloating, cramping, and emotional lability) and mild dysmenorrhea occur at intervals of 28–32 days, the likelihood of the patient having regular ovulatory cycles is very high. Otherwise, ovulation can be confirmed with a serum progesterone assay performed in the mid-luteal phase, or the third week of the cycle. Progesterone levels of 3 ng/mL or greater are consistent with ovulation.

Pelvic **ultrasonography** can provide evidence for ovulation. In the follicular phase, the developing follicle can be monitored to maturation and subsequent rupture. The disappearance of, or change in, the follicle and free fluid in the cul-de-sac can document ovulation.

To detect the LH surge, the patient can use commercially available urinary LH kits or serum LH assay. Ovulation occurs 24–36 hours after the onset of the LH surge and 10–12 hours after the peak of the LH surge. The kits can be used to time intercourse or intrauterine insemination.

The **basal body temperature** (BBT) is the temperature obtained in the resting state, and should be taken shortly after awakening in the morning after at least 6 hours of sleep and prior to ambulating. Progesterone has a central thermogenic effect; it elevates the BBT by an average of 0.8 °F during the luteal phase. The luteal phase is thus characterized by a temperature elevation lasting about 10 days. When a biphasic monthly temperature pattern is recorded, it is confirmatory evidence of luteinization, but the absence of a biphasic pattern may be seen in ovulatory cycles.

The finding of secretory endometrium confirms ovulation. The use of an **endometrial biopsy** (EMB) near the end of the luteal phase can provide reassurance of an adequate maturational effect on the endometrial lining. Generally, the EMB is performed 2–3 days before the expected onset of menses. It should be within 1–2 days of the pathologically diagnosed cycle day determined by morphology of glands and stroma.

Within 48 hours of ovulation, the **cervical mucus** changes under the influence of progesterone to become thick, tacky, and cellular, with loss of the crystalline fernlike pattern on drying.

The only absolute documentation of release of an oocyte is pregnancy. In the case of oligomenorrhea, amenorrhea, short or very irregular menstrual cycles, or when ovulation is not confirmed, evaluation of the hypothalamic-pituitary-ovarian axis is warranted. A usual initial assessment includes the serum concentrations of FSH, estradiol, prolactin, and thyroid-stimulating hormone.

4. Luteal phase defect—The subject of the inadequate luteal phase remains an area of controversy. There is disagreement on how to make the diagnosis, when the diagnosis is significant, and how best to treat the problem if diagnosed. Luteal phase defect is a histologic diagnosis made when the endometrium lags 3 days or more behind the expected pattern at the time of EMB.

B. THE PELVIC FACTOR

The pelvic factor includes abnormalities of the uterus, fallopian tubes, ovaries, and adjacent pelvic structures. Factors in the **history** that are suggestive of a pelvic factor include any history of pelvic infection, such as pelvic inflammatory disease (PID) or appendicitis, use of intrauterine devices, endometritis, and septic abortion. Endometriosis is included as a pelvic factor in infertility and may be suggested by worsening dysmenorrhea, dyspareunia, or previous surgical reports. Any history of ectopic pregnancy, adnexal surgery, leiomyomas, or exposure to diethylstilbestrol (DES) in utero should be noted as possibly contributory to the diagnosis of a pelvic factor. A **pelvic examination** can be informative, yielding information such as a fixed uterus suggestive of adhesions, leiomyomas, or adnexal masses.

A transvaginal **ultrasound** examination can be an efficient means of supplementing information gained from the standard bimanual examination. Hydrosalpinges, leiomyoma, and ovarian cysts, including endometriomas, can often be observed, and the appropriate focused evaluations initiated.

A **hysterosalpingogram** (HSG) is a fluoroscopic study performed by instilling radiopaque dye into the uterine cavity through a catheter to determine the contour of the endometrial cavity and patency of the fallopian tubes. Sensitivity and specificity of an HSG are approximately 65% and 85%, respectively. Abnormal findings include congenital malformations of the uterus, submucous leiomyomas, intrauterine synechiae (Asherman's syndrome), intrauterine polyps, salpingitis isthmica nodosa, and proximal or distal tubal occlusion. The hysterosalpingogram can be obtained in an outpatient setting, with minimal analgesia consisting of premedication with an nonsteroidal anti-inflammatory drug (NSAID). The test is usually scheduled for the interval after menstrual bleeding and prior to ovulation. Either water- or oil-based dye may be selected; Table 55–5 summarizes the advantages and disadvantages of each. There is evidence for a fertility-enhancing effect of HSG using the oil-based dye.

Peritonitis is a risk of the procedure observed in up to 1–3% of patients; many clinicians use a short-course doxycycline during the immediate period before and after the procedure to minimize risk. A HSG is contraindicated in the presence of an adnexal mass or an allergy to iodine or radiocontrast dye.

A sonohysterogram, a transvaginal ultrasound of the uterus with instillation of saline into the uterine cavity, is a sensitive and specific test for the detection of intrauterine lesions, specifically space-occupying lesions. Hysterosalpingo contrast sonography, transcervical injection of sonopaque material during ultrasonography, is used to determine tubal patency as well as detect intrauterine defects; more commonly used in Europe, the procedure's sensitivity is comparable to HSG.

Laparoscopy with chromotubation (dye instillation) is the gold standard for the evaluation of tubal factor, and when performed in conjunction with hysteroscopy, information on uterine contour can be obtained simultaneously. Tubal abnormalities such as aggluti-

Table 55–5. Comparison of oil-based versus water-based dye used in the hysterosalpingogram.

Fertility enhancement	Oil: higher pregnancy rates
Patient discomfort	Water: less cramping
Image quality	Water: rugae seen Oil: better image
Embolization	Minimal risk with either dye
Granuloma	Greater risk for retained oil

nated fimbria or adhesions (which restrict motion of the tubes) or peritubal cysts may suggest tubal disease that would not necessarily be detected on hysterosalpingogram. The diagnosis of endometriosis is usually based on laparoscopic findings.

The necessity of laparoscopy in an infertility workup is controversial. There is significant evidence that pelvic pathology may exist in almost one-third of patients with normal HSG and ultrasound; consequently, some believe that with laparoscopy one can treat the pathology (such as adhesions) found at the time of procedure, or can spare a patient needless cycles of ovulation induction that are unlikely to succeed by providing knowledge of severe pelvic disease. Others believe that although pelvic disease may be present, a stepwise empiric approach is more cost-effective.

C. THE CERVICAL FACTOR

A cervical factor may be indicated by a history of abnormal Papanicolaou (Pap) smears, postcoital bleeding, cryotherapy, conization, or DES exposure in utero. The major evaluation of the cervical factor is by physical examination and properly timed postcoital test. In some cases of apparently normal cervical mucous that repeatedly fails to yield reassuring numbers of sperm, a crosscheck of donor sperm and donor mucous can be performed to determine the possible contribution of the cervical mucous as opposed to that of the sperm. The value of routine cervical cultures is controversial, and the role of infectious agents, such as *Chlamydia* and *Ureaplasma,* is not universally accepted, particularly when the organisms are identified in cervical or vaginal cultures.

Combined Factors & Unexplained Infertility

After the completion of the diagnostic workup, the findings should be reviewed with the patients and a treatment plan finalized based on guidance from the physician and input from the patient(s). In approximately 20% of couples, a combination of factors found may be suboptimal, and multiple therapies may need to be instigated, either sequentially or simultaneously. For the couple with unexplained infertility, an empiric step-wise approach is an excellent option. However, depending upon the history, workup, and individual situation, additional test(s) including surgery should be discussed.

THERAPY FOR INFERTILITY

Male Factor Infertility

Treatment options progress from least to most invasive or use of donor sperm. Mild to moderate disease can be treated with **intrauterine insemination** (IUI). Prior to the insemination, the semen is prepared to select for highly motile sperm, concentrate sperm, and remove seminal fluid (with prostaglandins). The prepared sperm is transcervically injected into the uterus.

ICSI is used in conjunction with IVF for treatment of severe disease (< 2 million motile sperm). In this procedure, a sperm is individually injected into each oocyte. The sperm can be retrieved from the testes by microsurgical epididymal sperm aspiration (MESA) or testicular sperm aspiration (TESA); a minimum number of sperm are necessary.

Indications for ICSI include poor semen analysis parameters (low number of motile sperm, poor morphology), fertilization failure with standard IVF, and spermatozoal defects leading to poor fertilization. A decade of experience with the procedure has proven its overall safety. However, offspring conceived using ICSI may be at increased risk of imprinting disorders (eg, Angelman's syndrome), and male children are at risk for inheriting the genetic disorder (eg, Y chromosome microdeletions) that rendered their father infertile.

The initial evaluation of FSH, LH, testosterone, and prolactin helps to differentiate between obstructive defects, primary hypogonadism (testicular defect), and secondary hypogonadism (hypothalamic or pituitary). **Obstructive defects** may be addressed through surgical reanastomosis or through retrieval of sperm via MESA or TESA for use with ICSI. **Retrograde ejaculation** can be treated with alpha sympathomimetics or urine can be centrifuged to collect sperm for IUI. Patients with **primary hypogonadism** should have a karyotype, as Klinefelter's syndrome (47,XXY) is the most common etiology.

Secondary hypogonadism, or hypogonadotropic hypogonadism, may be a result of a pituitary lesion such as prolactinoma or a hypothalamic etiology such as Kallman's syndrome. Most prolactinomas respond to medical management. Pulsatile gonadotropin-releasing hormone (GnRH) administration with a pump or FSH replacement restores testosterone and sperm production in disorders leading to hypogonadotropic hypogonadism.

A **varicocele** is a dilatation of scrotal veins in the pampiniform plexus and is postulated to impair fertility through elevation of scrotal temperature. A clinical varicocele is one that is detected by examination and is present in 15% of men. Subclinical varicoceles can be detected by ultrasound or venography. There is contradicting evidence if ligation of clinical varicoceles leads to improved pregnancy rates; infertility is a questionable indication for the correction of subclinical varicoceles.

When male infertility is not amenable to therapy, **donor sperm** for insemination or IVF offers an opportunity for pregnancy. The use donor sperm is common in clinical practice and experience has lessened some of the medical, emotional, ethical, and legal issues. The American Society for Reproductive Medicine (ASRM) advocates use of frozen semen to reduce risk of transmission of infectious disease.

Female Factor Infertility

A. THE OVULATORY FACTOR

The treatment and success of specific ovulatory disorders is determined by the age of the patient and the etiology of the anovulation. A stepwise approach, from least to most invasive (and expensive), usually starts with clomiphene citrate and progresses to ovulation induction with gonadotropins and, ultimately, IVF. The risk to the patient, cost of therapy, and fecundability increase with each step closer to IVF. If premature ovarian failure or early menopause is the etiology, the options include oocyte or embryo donation.

Induction of ovulation can be accomplished in 90–95% of patients with chronic anovulation, normal ovarian reserve, and absence of other endocrine abnormalities (eg, hyperprolactinemia or hypothyroidism). Clomiphene citrate is the agent of choice for women younger than 36 years of age with oligomenorrhea or amenorrhea and normal FSH, including women with polycystic ovary syndrome (PCOS). Clomiphene citrate blocks the feedback inhibition of estradiol on the hypothalamus and pituitary leading to an increase in endogenous FSH. It is administered orally for 5 days starting on day 3 to 5 of the cycle; approximately half of the patients will ovulate at 50 mg/d and another 25% at 100 mg/d. Ultrasonographic and hormonal monitoring of follicular development is an option, which provides more information and allows greater control of the cycle. After a regimen has achieved ovulation, 3–4 cycles with timed intercourse should be attempted. Side effects with clomiphene are common, including hot flushes, emotional lability or depression, bloating, and visual changes; most are mild and all disappear with discontinuation of the drug. The incidence of twin gestation is 8% and triplets or higher-order multiple pregnancy (HOMP) is less than 1%.

A patient in whom there is no response to clomiphene, response to clomiphene but no pregnancy, pituitary insufficiency, or hypothalamic insufficiency should undergo ovulation induction with gonadotropins, often used in conjunction with IUI. Human menopausal gonadotropin (hMG) consists of FSH and LH isolated from the urine of postmenopausal women to various levels of purification (and LH content); recombinant FSH (rFSH) contains purely FSH. Gonadotropins are administered by subcutaneous (rFSH) or intramuscular injection (hMG) and the overall evidence indicates that the two preparations have similar efficacy.

Because of an increased risk of side effects such as multiple gestation and ovarian hyperstimulation syndrome, the use of gonadotropins requires close monitoring with ultrasonography and estradiol levels. Consequently, it is more time-consuming and expensive than clomiphene. The monitoring reveals both the number of developing follicles and their level of maturity. Mimicking the effects of the LH surge, human chorionic gonadotropins (hCG) is used to trigger ovulation. With perseverance, cumulative pregnancy rates of 45–90% can be achieved over 3–4 cycles with gonadotropin treatment; but even with careful monitoring there is a 25% risk of a multiple gestation. Ovarian hyperstimulation syndrome is a rare complication that occurs in less than 2% of cycles.

If pregnancy is not achieved with ovulation induction, IVF-ET is the next modality in the treatment algorithm. Development of the follicular cohort is induced with higher doses of FSH (hMG or rFSH). Follicular growth is monitored by ultrasonography and estradiol levels. When the leading follicles are mature, ovulation is triggered with hCG. The oocytes are retrieved from the follicles prior to ovulation by ultrasound-guided transvaginal aspiration of the follicular fluid. The oocytes are incubated with sperm for fertilization. Alternatively, ICSI is performed if male factor is also a concern. On average, several (from 1 to >3) embryos are transferred into the uterine cavity on day 3–5 after retrieval of the oocytes. Ovarian hyperstimulation syndrome (OHSS) is minimized by withholding hCG if there is a high number of follicles or elevated estradiol levels. Another option to limit the extent of OHSS is to cryopreserve the embryos for transfer at a later time, as pregnancy can prolong the course of OHSS.

When modification of lifestyle or body habitus does not successfully restore ovulation in the patient diagnosed with hypothalamic insufficiency, pulsatile GnRH is another viable option with high likelihood of restoring normal ovulation. Normal fertility is then restored during cycles of treatment, and most pregnancies occur within 3–6 cycles.

Hypothyroidism and hyperprolactinemia can lead to ovulatory dysfunction. Primary hypothyroidism leads to elevated thyroid-stimulating hormone (TSH) levels, which is a secretogogue of prolactin. Elevated prolactin levels inhibit GnRH secretion, causing oligomenorrhea or amenorrhea. If elevated prolactin levels are detected in a woman with normal thyroid function, a full work-up including thorough history (to rule out drugs like psychotropics), physical exam (galactorrhea), and imaging (magnetic resonance imaging [MRI] to rule out a prolactinoma or other central nervous system [CNS] tumors) is likely to reveal the etiology. The elevated prolactin can be medically managed with dopamine agonist, leading to normalization of the cycle.

There is concern about a possible association between ovulation induction agents, specifically greater than 12 cycles of clomiphene citrate, and **ovarian cancer.** The possibility that ovulation induction increases the risk of ovarian cancer remains unproven. Primary infertility and endometriosis are independent risk factors for ovarian cancer. Although additional investigation is necessary, the low incidence of ovarian cancer makes it difficult to design an adequate study to detect an association of infertility drugs with ovarian cancer.

B. THE PELVIC FACTOR

Adhesions resulting from **endometriosis** or **tubal occlusion** after salpingitis are two of the most common problems confronting infertile couples. With increasing pregnancy rates, IVF represents improved fecundability and lower risk over surgical repair except in unique circumstances. The role of surgical treatment is mostly limited to what can be accomplished at the time of diagnostic laparoscopy. There is some evidence to suggest that resection of mild endometriosis results in improved pregnancy rates. Laparoscopic resection or ablation of moderate or advanced endometriosis enhances fecundity in infertile women for the period immediately following surgery. Reversal of tubal sterilization is indicated in young women with adequate residual tubal length. Tubal interruption or resection increases IVF pregnancy rates in women with hydrosalpinx.

The role of **fibroids** in infertility is unclear, and most surgeons reserve myomectomy for treatment of recurrent abortion, repeated implantation failure, or with distortion of the endometrial cavity by a submucosal leiomyoma. The fibroids which distort the endometrial cavity are considered to be significant. These may be diagnosed by hysterosalpingogram, sonohysterogram, hysteroscopy, or magnetic resonance imaging.

C. THE CERVICAL FACTOR

The absence of nurturing mucus at midcycle can be treated by bypassing the mucus with intrauterine insemination. When the cervical mucus appears to be affected by cervicitis and inflammatory changes, some physicians advocate empiric treatment of patient and partner with doxycycline. When the cervix is altered by congenital malformation or past surgical treatment that has rendered endocervical glands absent or nonfunctional, intrauterine insemination with washed sperm can be anticipated to result in pregnancy in 20–30% of patients per cycle in each of the first 3 cycles of treatment. Cervical factor patients who do not respond to these therapies can be offered IVF, gamete intrafallopian transfer (GIFT), or zygote intrafallopian transfer (ZIFT), although GIFT and ZIFT are now rarely used.

Unexplained Infertility

A diagnosis of unexplained infertility is assigned to couples with normal results of a standard infertility work-up. The main treatment options include expectant observation with timed intercourse, ovarian stimulation with or without IUI, and IVF. Studies support the use of clomiphene with intrauterine insemination for up to 4 cycles. The next step is usually hMG with intrauterine insemination for 3 cycles; if unsuccessful, IVF should be considered. The rationale for treatment with superovulation in women with documented ovulation is that by increasing the number of oocytes available, the likelihood of pregnancy is increased. In instances in which unexplained infertility may be the result of a fundamental defect in fertilization or in embryo transfer to the uterus, IVF may play a role in treatment. Donor oocytes or donor sperm may be considered in couples with continued difficulties in achieving pregnancy. For many, the hardest course to contemplate is no therapy at all.

REFERENCES

Chen D et al: Ovarian hyperstimulation syndrome: Strategies for prevention. Reprod Biomed Online 2003;7(1):43.

Chow GE, Criniti AR, Soules MR: Antral follicle count and serum follicle-stimulating hormone levels to assess functional ovarian age. Obstet Gynecol 2004;104(4):801.

Coutifaris C et al: NICHD National Cooperative Reproductive Medicine Network. Histological dating of timed endometrial biopsy tissue is not related to fertility status. Fertil Steril 2004;82(5):1264.

Devroey P et al: Reproductive biology and IVF: Ovarian stimulation and endometrial receptivity. Trends Endocrinol Metab 2004;15(2):84.

Devroey P, Van Steirteghem A: A review of ten years experience of ICSI. Hum Reprod Update. 2004;10(1):19.

Erenpreiss J et al: An evidence-based evaluation of endometriosis-associated infertility. Endocrinol Metab Clin North Am 2003;32(3):653.

Evers JL, Collins JA: Surgery or embolisation for varicocele in subfertile men. Cochrane Database Syst Rev 2004;(3):CD000479.

Homburg R, Insler V: Ovulation induction in perspective. Hum Reprod Update 2002;8(5):449.

Marcoux S et al: Laparoscopic surgery in infertile women with minimal or mild endometriosis. N Engl J Med 1997;337:217.

Oliveira FG et al: Impact of subserosal and intramural uterine fibroids that do not distort the endometrial cavity on the outcome of in vitro fertilization-intracytoplasmic sperm injection. Fertil Steril 2004;81(3):582.

Rossing MA et al: A case-control study of ovarian cancer in relation to infertility and the use of ovulation-inducing drugs. Am J Epidemiol 2004;160(11):1070.

Toner JP: Ovarian reserve, female age and the chance for successful pregnancy. Minerva Ginecol 2003;55(5):399.

Amenorrhea

Wendy Y. Chang, MD, & Alan H. DeCherney, MD

Menstruation has long been an important societal marker of female sexual development, as well as one of the most tangible signs of female endocrine and reproductive tract maturation. Regular and spontaneous menstruation requires (a) an intact hypothalamic–pituitary–ovarian endocrine axis; (b) an endometrium competent to respond to steroid hormone stimulation; and (c) an intact outflow tract from internal to external genitalia.

The human menstrual cycle is susceptible to environmental influences and stressors. Thus, missing a single or occasional menstruation rarely reflects a significant pathology. However, prolonged or persistent absence of menses may be one of the earliest signs of neuroendocrine or anatomic abnormality.

DEFINITION & INCIDENCE

Amenorrhea is literally defined as the absence of menses. **Primary amenorrhea,** seen in approximately 2.5% of the population, is clinically defined as the absence of menses by age 13 years in the absence of normal growth or secondary sexual development; or the absence of menses by age 15 years in the setting of normal growth and secondary sexual development. Traditionally, evaluation was usually initiated by age 16 years if normal growth and secondary sexual characteristics were present, and at age 13 years if absent. However, because of secular trends toward earlier menarche over the past half century, the evaluation should begin at age 15 years, the age when more than 97% of girls should have experienced menarche. Certainly, the decision to evaluate should be made with a full understanding of the patient's clinical presentation. For example, evaluation should not be delayed in the setting of neurologic symptoms (suggestive of hypothalamic–pituitary lesion) or pelvic pain (suggestive of outflow obstruction). **Secondary amenorrhea** is clinically defined as the absence of menses for more than 3 cycle intervals, or 6 consecutive months, in a previously menstruating woman. The incidence of secondary amenorrhea can be quite variable, from 3% in the general population to 100% under conditions of extreme physical or emotional stress. Table 56–1 lists the most common causes of secondary amenorrhea.

Diagnosing and treating amenorrhea is important because of the implications for future fertility; risks of un-

opposed estrogen, including endometrial hyperplasia and neoplasia; risks of hypoestrogenism, including osteoporosis and urogenital atrophy; and impact on psychosocial development. Because of their significant overlap in etiology and treatment, primary and secondary amenorrhea are discussed collectively in this chapter.

ETIOLOGY & PATHOGENESIS

Pregnancy is the most common cause of amenorrhea and must be considered in every patient presenting for evaluation of amenorrhea. Amenorrhea caused by aberrations of the normal menstrual cycle is discussed in Chapter 6. Chapters 34 and 57 discuss developmental anomalies of the reproductive organs and masculinization, respectively. This chapter discusses amenorrhea associated with 46,XX and 46,XY karyotypes, anatomic defects, and defects in the hypothalamic–pituitary–ovarian axis, as well as systemic disorders that affect menstruation.

Hypothalamic Defects

Gonadotropin-releasing hormone (GnRH) secreting neurons of the hypothalamus originate in the olfactory bulb and migrate along the olfactory tract into the mediobasal hypothalamus and the arcuate nucleus. Under normal physiologic circumstances, the arcuate nucleus releases pulses of GnRH into the hypophyseal portal system approximately every hour. Discharge of GnRH releases luteinizing hormone (LH) and follicle-stimulating hormone (FSH) from the pituitary; LH and FSH, in turn, stimulate ovarian follicular growth and ovulation. **The ovarian hormones estradiol and progesterone stimulate the development and shedding of the endometrium, culminating in the withdrawal bleeding of menses.** Anovulation and amenorrhea occur as a result of interference with GnRH transport, GnRH pulse discharge, or congenital absence of GnRH (Kallmann's syndrome). Any of these situations leads to hypogonadotropic hypogonadism.

A. DEFECTS OF GnRH TRANSPORT

Interference with the transport of GnRH from the hypothalamus to the pituitary may occur with pituitary

Table 56–1. Causes of secondary amenorrhea.

Common
  Pregnancy
  Hypothalamic amenorrhea
  Androgen disorders: polycystic ovarian syndrome, congenital adrenal hyperplasia
  Galactorrhea-amenorrhea syndrome
Less Common
  Premature ovarian failure
  Asherman's syndrome
  Sheehan's syndrome
Rare
  Diabetes
  Hyperthyroidism or hypothyroidism
  Cushing's syndrome or Addison's disease
  Cirrhosis
  Tuberculosis
  Malnutrition
  Irradiation or chemotherapy
  Surgery

stalk compression or destruction of the arcuate nucleus. Pituitary stalk transsection from trauma, compression, radiation, tumors (craniopharyngioma, germinoma, glioma, teratomas), and infiltrative disorders (sarcoidosis, tuberculosis) may either destroy areas of the hypothalamus or prevent transport of hypothalamic hormones to the pituitary.

B. DEFECTS OF GnRH PULSE PRODUCTION

The metabolic consequence of any significant reduction in the normal GnRH pulse frequency or amplitude is that little or no LH or FSH can be released, with the result that no ovarian follicles develop, virtually no estradiol is secreted, and the patient is amenorrheic. This is the biochemical status in normal prepubertal girls and those with constitutional delayed puberty, such as in anorexia nervosa, severe stress, extreme weight loss, or prolonged vigorous athletic exertion, and in hyperprolactinemia. Amenorrhea on this basis may also be an idiopathic phenomenon.

Less-severe reductions in GnRH pulse amplitude and frequency result in diminished LH and FSH secretion with some follicular stimulation. The stimulation is insufficient to result in full follicular development and ovulation, but estradiol is secreted. This may occur with stress, hyperprolactinemia, as a result of vigorous athletic activity, or in the early stages of eating disorders. It may also be idiopathic.

Functional or hypothalamic amenorrhea results from abnormal hypothalamic GnRH secretion in the absence of pathologic processes. As a result, patients demonstrate decreased gonadotropin pulsations, absent follicular development and ovulation, and low estradiol secretion. Serum FSH levels are usually in the normal range; the setting of high FSH:LH ratio is consistent with prepubertal patterns. A number of environmental stressors are associated, including eating disorders and physical or psychological stress. Weight loss, especially to a level of at least 10% below ideal body weight, and excessive exercise are also associated with hypothalamic amenorrhea. The female athlete triad syndrome is defined by amenorrhea, eating disorder, and osteopenia or osteoporosis.

Congenital GnRH deficiency is called idiopathic hypogonadotropic hypogonadism when it occurs as an isolated phenomenon, and **Kallmann's syndrome** when it is associated with anosmia. These patients lack GnRH secretion, and express low, prepubertal levels of serum gonadotropins. Follicular recruitment and ovulation do not occur. Although more than 60% of cases are sporadic, congenital GnRH deficiency can also be inherited in an autosomal or X-linked pattern.

More common in boys with delayed puberty, **constitutional delay** of puberty is an uncommon etiology of primary amenorrhea in girls. Patients demonstrate delayed adrenarche and gonadarche, but ultimately go on to have normal, albeit delayed, pubertal development.

Pituitary Defects

Pituitary causes of amenorrhea are rare; most are secondary to hypothalamic dysfunction. However, acquired pituitary dysfunction can ensue from previous local radiation or surgery. Excess iron deposition due to hemochromatosis or hemosiderosis may destroy gonadotropes.

A. CONGENITAL PITUITARY DYSFUNCTION

Congenital absence of the pituitary is a rare and lethal condition. Isolated defects of LH or FSH production do occur (rarely), resulting in anovulation and amenorrhea.

B. ACQUIRED PITUITARY DYSFUNCTION

Sheehan's syndrome, characterized by postpartum amenorrhea, results from postpartum pituitary necrosis secondary to severe hemorrhage and hypotension and is a rare cause of amenorrhea. Surgical ablation and irradiation of the pituitary as management of pituitary tumors also can cause amenorrhea.

Iron deposition in the pituitary may result in destruction of the cells that produce LH and FSH. This occurs only in patients with markedly elevated serum iron levels (ie, hemosiderosis), usually resulting from extensive red cell destruction. Thalassemia major is an example of a disease that causes hemosiderosis.

Pituitary microadenomas and macroadenomas also lead to amenorrhea because of elevated prolactin levels, but the mechanism(s) underlying this cause of amenorrhea are unclear. Isolated hyperprolactinemia in the absence of adenoma is an uncommon cause of primary amenorrhea. However, the diagnosis is strongly suggested by a history of galactorrhea. Diagnosis is readily made by evaluating a serum prolactin level. Hypothyroidism may also lead to elevated prolactin levels and thereby lead to amenorrhea.

Ovarian and Ovulatory Dysfunction

A variety of gonadal disorders can result in amenorrhea. The most common cause of primary amenorrhea is gonadal dysgenesis. This group of disorders is usually associated with sex chromosomal abnormalities, resulting in streak gonad development, premature depletion of ovarian follicles and oocytes, and absence of estradiol secretion. Patients usually present with hypergonadotropic amenorrhea regardless of degree of pubertal development. Primary ovarian failure is characterized by elevated gonadotropins and low estradiol (**hypergonadotropic hypogonadism**). Secondary ovarian failure is almost always caused by hypothalamic dysfunction and is characterized by normal or low gonadotropins and low estradiol (**hypogonadotropic hypogonadism**).

Table 56–2 lists the causes of primary ovarian failure.

A. OVARIAN DYSGENESIS

If the primitive oogonia do not migrate to the genital ridge, the ovaries fail to develop. Streak gonads, which do not secrete hormones, develop instead, and the result is primary amenorrhea. Cytogenetic abnormalities of the X chromosome account for the majority of abnormal ovarian development and function, and studies show that two intact X chromosomes are required to maintain normal oocytes. Fetuses with 45,X karyotype demonstrate normal oocyte number at 20–24 weeks' gestation, but there is rapid atresia resulting in absence of oocytes at birth. Similarly, women with deletions in either the long or short arm of one X chromosome also develop either primary or secondary amenorrhea.

Gonadal dysgenesis with no Y chromatin—Turner's syndrome (45,XO or 45,XO,XX mosaics) and 46,XX gonadal dysgenesis are the most common karyotypes. Patients with Turner's syndrome usually present with primary amenorrhea. However, some patients with mosaic abnormalities may menstruate briefly and a few have conceived.

Gonadal dysgenesis with Y chromatin—Normal female sexual differentiation depends on testicular secretion of antimüllerian hormone (AMH) by Sertoli cells and testosterone by Leydig cells. AMH causes regression of müllerian structures, whereas testosterone and its metabolite dihydrotestosterone (DHT) promote differentiation of male internal and external genitalia, re-

Table 56–2. Causes of primary ovarian failure (hypergonadotrophic hypogonadism).

Idiopathic premature ovarian failure
Steroidogenic enzyme defects (primary amenorrhea)
   Cholesterol side-chain cleavage
   3β-ol-dehydrogenase
   17-hydroxylase
   17-desmolase
   17-ketoreductase
Testicular regression syndrome
True hermaphroditism
Gonadal dysgenesis
   Pure gonadal dysgenesis (Swyer's syndrome) (46,XX and
     46,XY)
   Turner's syndrome (45,XO)
   Turner variants
Mixed gonadal dysgenesis
Ovarian resistance syndrome (Savage's syndrome)
Autoimmune oophoritis
Postinfection (eg, mumps)
Postoophorectomy (also wedge resections and bivalving)
Postirradiation
Postchemotherapy

spectively. A variety of disorders can result in the presentation of amenorrhea in phenotypic females possessing Y chromatin material.

The vanishing testes syndrome occurs in 46,XY males with failed gonadal development. Although anorchia commonly occurs around 7 weeks' gestational age, the patient's presentation depends on the timing of gonadal regression. Failure occurring later in development might result in male genitalia at birth, but absence of puberty as a consequence of gonadal failure. On the other hand, typical early gonadal failure prior to testicular development would result absent secretion of testis-determining factor (TDF) and AMH. These patients would demonstrate feminization of internal and external genitalia, and primary amenorrhea.

Ullrich-Turner syndrome, which presents as a form of early onset vanishing testes syndrome, results from a deletion mutation in the TDF region of Y chromosome. These patients possess the 46,XY genotype but do not secrete testosterone or AMH, resulting in feminization of internal and external genitalia. Patients present with primary amenorrhea and gonadal failure. The syndrome is diagnosed by DNA hybridization studies showing abnormality in the short arm of the Y chromosome.

B. PREMATURE OVARIAN FAILURE

Menopause occurs when the ovaries fail secondary to depletion of ova. If this occurs before age 40 years, it is

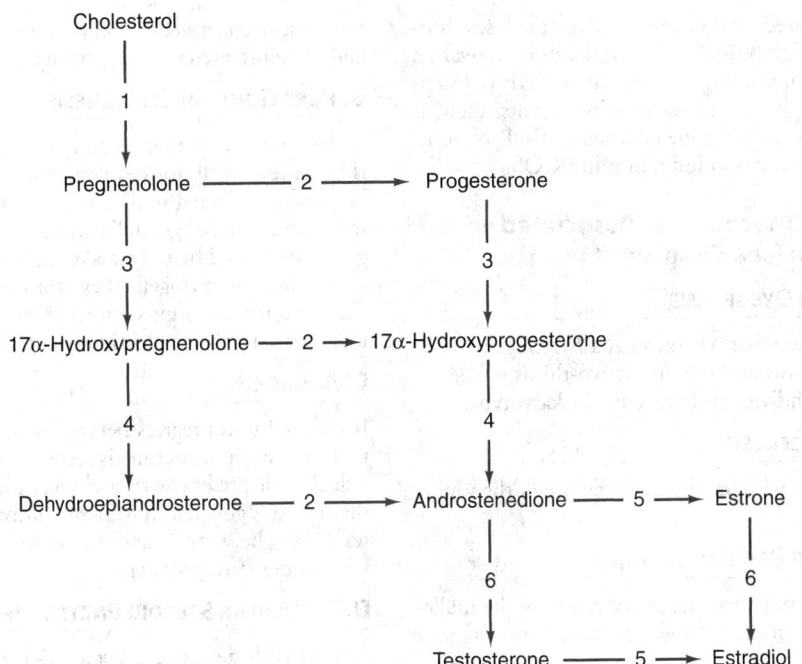

Key to enzymes
1 = Cholesterol 20- and 22-desmolase and 20-hydroxylase
2 = 3β-Hydroxysteroid dehydrogenase
3 = 17α-Hydroxylase
4 = 17- and 20-Desmolase
5 = Aromatase
6 = 17-Hydroxysteroid dehydrogenase

Figure 56–1. Steroidogenesis in the ovary.

considered premature. It is marked by amenorrhea, increased gonadotropin levels, and estrogen deficiency.

C. STEROID ENZYME DEFECTS

Figure 56–1 depicts normal steroidogenesis in the ovary. Genetic females with defects in enzymes 1–4 have normal internal female genitalia and 46,XX karyotype. However, they cannot produce estradiol and thus they fail to menstruate or have breast development.

Congenital lipoid adrenal hyperplasia describes one of fifteen known defects in the steroidogenic acute regulatory (STAR) protein, which facilitates cholesterol transport from the outer to the inner mitochondrial membrane. This enzyme catalyzes an early, rate-limiting step in tropic hormone-stimulated steroidogenesis. Patients thus present with hyponatremia, hyperkalemia, and acidosis in infancy. Both XX and XY individuals are phenotypically female. These patients can survive into adulthood given appropriate glucocorticoid and mineralocorticoid supplementation. XX patients may exhibit some secondary sexual characteristics at puberty, but present with amenorrhea and premature

ovarian failure due to intraovarian accumulation of cholesterol.

D. OVARIAN RESISTANCE (SAVAGE'S SYNDROME)

Patients with this syndrome have elevated LH and FSH levels, and the ovaries contain primordial germ cells. A defect in the cell receptor mechanism is the presumed cause.

E. POLYCYSTIC OVARY SYNDROME

One of the most common causes of secondary amenorrhea is **polycystic ovary syndrome** (**PCOS**). PCOS is the most common cause of ovulatory dysfunction in reproductive-age women. Diagnosis is based on the presence of at least two of the following characteristics. (a) oligo- or anovulation; (b) clinical and/or biochemical signs of hyperandrogenism; (c) polycystic ovaries; and (d) exclusion of other etiologies (congenital adrenal hyperplasia, androgen-secreting tumors, Cushing's syndrome). Although the exact mechanism is unknown, it appears that insulin resistance and hyperinsulinemia play a permissive role. Abnormally elevated baseline insulin leads to increased androgens via decreased sex hormone-binding globulin, and stimulation of ovarian insulin and insulinlike growth factor-I (IGF-I) receptors. Increasingly, insulin-sensitizing agents such as metformin and rosiglitazone are used as a sole or adjuvant agent for ovulation induction in PCOS.

Anatomic Abnormalities Associated with Amenorrhea (see Chapter 34)

A. MÜLLERIAN DYSGENESIS

Müllerian dysgenesis is characterized by congenital absence of the uterus and the upper two-thirds of the vagina. Affected individuals have a 46,XX karyotype.

B. VAGINAL AGENESIS

Vaginal agenesis is characterized by failure of the vagina to develop.

C. TRANSVERSE VAGINAL SEPTUM

This anomaly results from failure of fusion of the müllerian and urogenital sinus-derived portions of the vagina.

D. IMPERFORATE HYMEN

If the hymen is complete, menstrual efflux cannot occur.

E. ASHERMAN'S SYNDROME

In Asherman's syndrome, amenorrhea is caused by intrauterine synechiae. The usual cause is a complicated dilatation and curettage (D&C) (eg, infected products of conception, vigorous elimination of the endometrium), but the syndrome can occur after myomectomy, cesarean section, and tuberculous endometritis.

Amenorrhea in Women with 46,XY Karyotype

The details of embryonic sexual differentiation are discussed in Chapter 4. Briefly, the sexually undifferentiated male fetal testis secretes müllerian-inhibiting factor (MIF) and testosterone. MIF promotes regression of all müllerian structures: the uterine tubes, the uterus, and the upper two-thirds of the vagina. Testosterone and its active metabolite DHT are responsible for embryonic differentiation of the male internal and external genitalia.

A. TESTICULAR FEMINIZATION

In testicular feminization, all müllerian-derived structures are absent. The external genital anlagen and mesonephric ducts cannot respond to androgens, because androgen receptors are either absent or defective. Affected individuals are therefore phenotypic females lacking a uterus and a complete vagina. They produce some estrogen, develop breasts, and are reared as girls, and therefore present with primary amenorrhea.

B. PURE GONADAL DYSGENESIS

If the primitive germ cells do not migrate to the genital ridge, a testis will not develop, and a streak gonad will be present. Affected individuals have normal female internal and external genitalia, as neither MIF nor androgens are secreted by the streaks. Because these individuals produce no estrogen, they will not develop breasts. They are reared as girls and present clinically with either delayed puberty or primary amenorrhea.

C. ANORCHIA

If the fetal testes regress before 7 weeks' gestation, neither MIF nor testosterone is secreted, and affected individuals will present with a clinical picture identical to that of pure gonadal dysgenesis. Individuals whose testes regress between 7 and 13 weeks' gestation present with ambiguous genitalia.

D. TESTICULAR STEROID ENZYME DEFECTS

A testis with defective enzymes 1–4 will produce MIF but not testosterone (Fig 56–1). Affected individuals have female external genitalia and no müllerian structures. They will be reared as girls and present clinically with either delayed puberty or primary amenorrhea.

A defect in enzyme 6 (17-hydroxysteroid dehydrogenase) results in ambiguous genitalia and virilization at puberty.

DIAGNOSIS

Figures 56–2 to 56–4 summarize the diagnostic workup for amenorrhea. It is important at the outset to determine which organ is dysfunctional and then to identify the exact cause. Once this has been done, specific therapy can be planned.

Any patient with amenorrhea who has a uterus should be tested for pregnancy and for serum levels of thyroid-stimulating hormone (TSH) and prolactin. Galactorrhea should be identified or ruled out by physical examination.

Diagnosis of Primary Amenorrhea

Figure 56–2 outlines the diagnostic scheme for primary amenorrhea. Pelvic examination should be done to establish the presence of a vagina and uterus and no vaginal septum or imperforate hymen that might account for the failure of appearance of menses. Because pelvic examination of an adolescent girl may be difficult, pelvic ultrasound or examination under anesthesia may be required to establish the presence of a uterus.

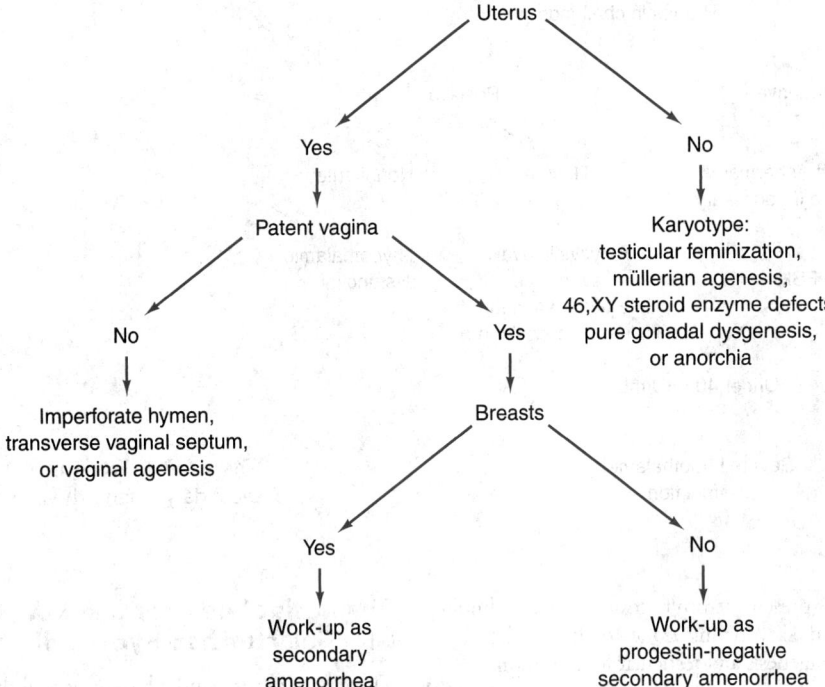

Figure 56–2. Work-up for patients with primary amenorrhea.

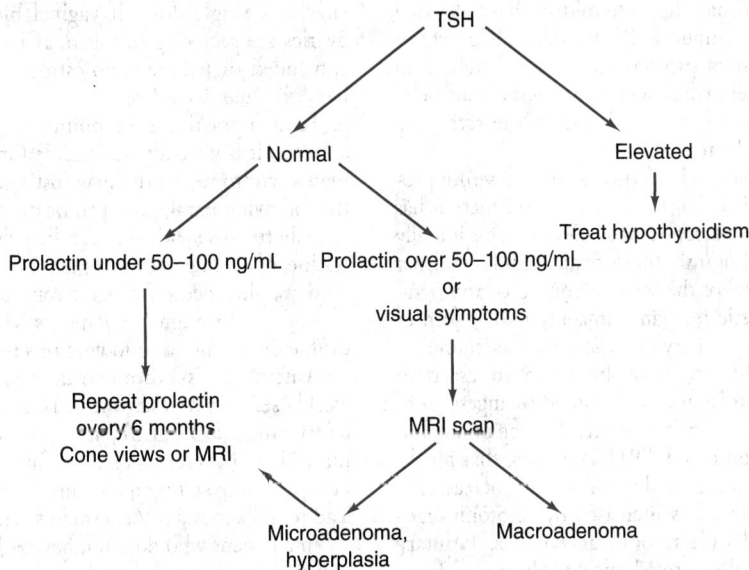

Figure 56–3. Work-up for patients with amenorrhea–galactorrhea–hyperpro-lactinemia.

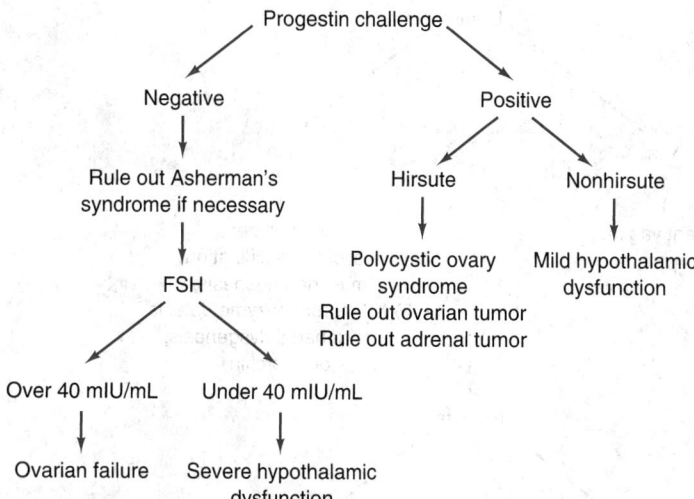

Figure 56–4. Work-up for patients with secondary amenorrhea.

If no uterus is present, serum testosterone levels should be measured and karyotyping done to differentiate between müllerian agenesis and testicular feminization.

Diagnosis of Amenorrhea Associated with Galactorrhea-Hyperprolactinemia

Figure 56–3 outlines the diagnostic work-up of patients with galactorrhea or hyperprolactinemia. Table 56–3 summarizes the differential diagnosis of galactorrhea-amenorrhea.

Patients with primary hypothyroidism have elevated thyroid-releasing hormone (TRH) levels. TRH acts to stimulate the release of prolactin and may thereby lead to galactorrhea-amenorrhea syndrome. TSH is also elevated and easier to measure and thus is the screening test for hypothyroidism.

Once hypothyroidism is adequately treated serum prolactin must be measured again after thyroid function has become normal. If prolactin remains elevated or is initially higher than 50–200 ng/mL, the patient should be further studied via cone view of the sella, or computed tomography (CT) or magnetic resonance imaging (MRI) scan of the sella, to rule out pituitary micro- or macroadenoma.

A meticulous history must be taken to ascertain whether the hyperprolactinemia is caused by ingestion of drugs. Prolactin secretion is inhibited by dopamine and stimulated by serotonin and TRH. Any drug that blocks the synthesis or binding of dopamine will increase the prolactin level. Prolactin is increased by serotonin agonists and decreased by serotonin antagonists. Pituitary macroadenoma should be ruled out if prolactin levels are higher than 50–100 ng/mL, even if the patient is taking drugs that lead to raised prolactin levels.

Diagnosis of Amenorrhea Not Associated with Galactorrhea-Hyperprolactinemia

These patients are studied according to the scheme outlined in Figure 56–4.

The first step is the progestin challenge, which indirectly determines whether the ovary is producing estrogen. If the endometrium has been primed with estrogen, exogenous progestin will produce menses. Give either medroxyprogesterone acetate, 10 mg orally daily for 5 days, or progesterone, 100–200 mg intramuscularly as a single dose. If vaginal bleeding follows, the ovaries are secreting estrogen. If it does not, it can be concluded that there is no estrogen or that the patient has Asherman's syndrome.

From a practical standpoint, if a patient has not had a D&C, it is virtually impossible for her to have Asherman's syndrome, so the diagnostic steps summarized in the following paragraphs can be disregarded.

Asherman's syndrome can be ruled out by administration of conjugated estrogen, 2.5 mg orally daily for 25 days, plus medroxyprogesterone acetate, 10 mg orally on days 16 through 25. Patients with Asherman's syndrome do not bleed following this regimen.

Asherman's syndrome can also be diagnosed by weekly serum progesterone tests. Any value in the ovulatory range (> 3 ng/mL) not associated with menses is indicative of Asherman's syndrome. Hysterosalpingography, sonohysterography, and hysteroscopy can also lead to a diagnosis of Asherman's syndrome.

In a patient who does not have Asherman's syndrome and who does not respond to the progestin challenge, ovarian dysfunction may be of hypothalamic or ovarian origin. The distinction is based on the FSH level. Pri-

Table 56–3. Differential diagnosis of galactorrhea-hyperprolactinemia.

Pituitary tumors secreting prolactin
   Macroadenomas (> 10 mm)
   Microadenomas (< 10 mm)
Hypothyroidism
Idiopathic hyperprolactinemia
Drug-induced hyperprolactinemia
   Dopamine antagonists
      Phenothiazines
      Thioxanthenes
      Butyrophenone
      Diphenylbutylpiperidine
      Dibenzoxazepine
      Dihydroindolone
      Procainamide derivatives
   Catecholamine-depleting agents
   False transmitters (α-methyldopa)
Interruption of normal hypothalamic–pituitary relationship
   Pituitary stalk section
Peripheral neural stimulation
   Chest wall stimulation
      Thoracotomy
      Mastectomy
      Thoracoplasty
      Burns
      Herpes zoster
      Bronchogenic tumors
      Bronchiectasis
      Chronic bronchitis
   Nipple stimulation
      Stimulation of nipples
      Chronic nipple irritation
   Spinal cord lesion
      Tabes dorsalis
      Syringomyelia
   Central nervous system disease
      Encephalitis
      Craniopharyngioma
      Pineal tumors
      Hypothalamic tumors
      Pseudotumor cerebri

mary ovarian dysfunction resulting in low estradiol secretion is associated with high serum FSH. Values vary in different laboratories, but in general an FSH level higher than 40 mIU/mL indicates primary ovarian failure.

Diagnosis of Amenorrhea Caused by Primary Ovarian Failure

Table 56–2 lists the causes of primary ovarian failure.

Karyotyping is indicated for all women who present with premature menopause, particularly if their amenorrhea is primary. Patients with primary amenorrhea may have a steroid enzyme defect. Autoimmune oophoritis is a reversible cause of ovarian failure that must be investigated.

Diagnosis of Amenorrhea Associated with Hypothalamic–Pituitary Dysfunction

Table 56–4 summarizes the differential diagnosis of hypoestrogenic amenorrhea. The category includes amenorrhea associated with athletic activity, weight loss, or stress. Differentiation of hypothalamic from pituitary dysfunction can be achieved by giving GnRH, but is generally not a worthwhile effort, as pituitary causes are rare and can often be diagnosed on the basis of the history. Moreover, in Kallmann's syndrome, a single bolus dose of GnRH may not elicit a normal response. Up to 40 doses of GnRH have been required to prime the pituitary so that it will respond normally. A GnRH pump also has been used.

If there is a significant history consistent with Sheehan's syndrome, pituitary function testing is indicated in order to determine the functional capacity of the gland—particularly the integrity of the pituitary–adrenal axis.

In girls with primary amenorrhea, observing the pattern of LH and FSH release after administration of GnRH will help to determine whether the patient is undergoing late pubertal changes.

Patients who bleed in response to the progestin challenge (ie, whose ovaries are secreting estrogen) fit into one of 4 categories: (a) virilized, with or without ambiguous genitalia; (b) hirsute, with polycystic ovaries, hyperthecosis, or mild maturity-onset adrenal hyperplasia; (c) nonhirsute, with hypothalamic dysfunction; or (d) amenorrheic secondary to systemic disease.

Table 56–4. Differential diagnosis of hypoestrogenic amenorrhea (hypogonadotropic hypogonadism).

Hypothalamic dysfunction
   Kallmann's syndrome
   Tumors of hypothalamus (craniopharyngioma)
   Constitutional delay of puberty
   Severe hypothalamic dysfunction
   Anorexia nervosa
   Severe weight loss
   Severe stress
   Exercise
Pituitary disorder
   Sheehan's syndrome
   Panhypopituitarism
   Isolated gonadotropin deficiency
   Hemosiderosis (primarily from thalassemia major)

Table 56–5. Differential diagnosis of eugonadotropic eugonadism (progestin-challenge positive).

Mild hypothalamic dysfunction
　Emotional stress
　Psychological disorder
　Weight loss
　Obesity
　Exercise induced
　Idiopathic
Hirsutism-virilism
　Polycystic ovary syndrome (Stein-Leventhal syndrome)
　Ovarian tumor
　Adrenal tumor
　Cushing's syndrome
　Congenital and maturity-onset adrenal hyperplasia
Systemic disease
　Hypothyroidism
　Hyperthyroidism
　Addison's disease
　Cushing's syndrome
　Chronic renal failure
　Many others

Table 56–5 sets forth the differential diagnosis. Clinical examination and transvaginal ultrasound may be helpful in making the diagnosis of PCOS. However, 25% of normal patients have polycystic ovaries; consequently, ultrasound cannot be the sole criterion for diagnosis.

TREATMENT

1. Management of Patients Desiring Pregnancy—Ovulation Induction

Ovulation Induction in Patients with Amenorrhea-Galactorrhea with Pituitary Macroadenoma

Dopamine agonist drugs such as cabergoline and bromocriptine remain the first-line treatment of hyperprolactinemia of any cause, including macroadenomas. These drugs can decrease prolactin secretion and tumor size. Surgical therapy, transsphenoidal or frontal removal of the pituitary adenoma or the entire gland, may be required if tumor size or secretion are resistant to dopamine agonists; the lesion is rapidly enlarging or causing symptoms such as visual changes or headaches; or in women with giant adenomas (> 3 cm) who wish to discontinue agonist treatment for conception and the duration of pregnancy. About half of surgically treated patients will menstruate normally after this procedure.

Ovulation Induction in Patients with Amenorrhea-Galactorrhea without Macroadenoma (Including Patients with Microadenomas)

These patients ovulate readily in response to dopamine agonist treatment, with dose titrated until serum prolactin is normal. Patients are maintained on the lowest dose necessary to maintain normal prolactin levels. Once pregnancy has been achieved, the agent can be discontinued. Patients with macroadenomas may need to continue therapy throughout pregnancy to avoid further growth of the lesion.

Patients taking drugs that raise the prolactin level should discontinue them if possible, but continued use of such drugs is not a contraindication to therapy.

Ovulation Induction in Patients with Hypothyroidism

Amenorrheic patients with hypothyroidism frequently respond to thyroid replacement therapy.

Ovulation Induction in Patients with Primary Ovarian Failure

According to Rebar and associates, patients with primary ovarian failure can be made to ovulate only under very rare circumstances. Patients with reversible ovarian failure include those with autoimmune oophoritis, who can be successfully treated with corticosteroids. Otherwise, almost all patients with primary ovarian failure fall into the category of idiopathic premature ovarian failure and cannot be made to ovulate. In vitro fertilization (IVF) with donor oocytes is the only way they can have children.

Any patient with a Y chromosome should undergo oophorectomy to prevent tumor development.

Ovulation Induction in Patients with Hypoestrogenic Hypothalamic Amenorrhea (Progestin-Challenge Negative)

In these patients with low estrogen levels, the pituitary does not release high quantities of LH and FSH (as would be expected with an intact, normally functioning, negative feedback mechanism). Therefore, even though clomiphene citrate (an antiestrogen) is unlikely to stimulate gonadotropin release, many reproductive endocrinologists treat such patients successfully with a single course of clomiphene citrate, 150 or 250 mg daily for 5 days, on the chance that ovulation will occur.

Injections of exogenous gonadotropins (human recombinant follicle-stimulating hormone [hrFSH] or human menopausal gonadotropin [hMG]) is usually first-line therapy. Patients showing some ovarian stimulation by clomiphene can be treated with a combination of clomiphene and hMG—the advantage being a reduction in the amount of hMG required and thus a substantial cost savings. Ovulation induction with gonadotropins must be carefully monitored with serial ultrasound and estradiol determinations to avoid hyperstimulation. Hyperstimulation is the stimulation of too many follicles, with associated ovarian enlargement and ascites, as well as other systemic abnormalities.

If a specific and potentially reversible cause of amenorrhea can be identified (eg, marked weight loss), it should be corrected.

Ovulation Induction in Patients Who Bleed in Response to Progestin Challenge

Virtually all of these patients respond to clomiphene citrate. The starting dose is 50 mg orally daily for 5 days. This can be increased to a maximum of 250 mg orally daily in 50-mg increments until ovulation is induced. Efficacy of clomiphene, however, plateaus at 100 mg/d. This medication is FDA-approved for use up to 150 mg/d. Ovulation occurs 5–10 days after the last dose. Patients with elevated androgens who do not respond to clomiphene citrate may respond to combined treatment with an oral hypoglycemic agent and clomiphene. If clomiphene therapy with or without oral hypoglycemic agents is ineffective, gonadotropin therapy may be attempted. Care must be taken in using FSH in these patients, as they are likely to become hyperstimulated.

Laparoscopic ovarian drilling (LOD) is a surgical method of ovulation induction in PCOS patients. LOD involves electrocautery or laser drilling of the ovarian cortex, with the goal of creating foci of laser or thermal damage in the cortex and ovarian stroma. In general, at least 6 puncture sites 2–4 mm in depth are made in the ovary away from the hilum. The mechanism of action is unknown, but may involve destruction of androgen-producing stromal cells, a sudden drop in ovarian androgen levels, improved follicular microenvironment, or increased gonadotropin secretion. This procedure may cause postoperative pelvic adhesions, resulting in tubal compromise.

2. Management of Patients Not Desiring Pregnancy

Patients who are hypoestrogenic must be treated with a combination of estrogen and progesterone to maintain bone density and prevent genital atrophy. The dose of estrogen varies with the age of the patient. Oral contraceptives are good replacement therapy for most women. Combinations of 0.625–1.25 mg of conjugated estrogens orally daily on days 1 through 25 of the cycle with 5–10 mg of medroxyprogesterone acetate on days 16 through 25 are a suitable alternative. Calcium intake should be adjusted to 1–1.5 g of elemental calcium daily.

Patients who respond to the progestin challenge require occasional progestin administration to prevent the development of endometrial hyperplasia and carcinoma. Oral contraceptive pills may be used to regulate the menstrual cycle. Oral contraceptives also help with management of hirsutism. Alternatively, medroxyprogesterone acetate, 10 mg orally daily for 10–13 days every month or every other month, is sufficient to induce withdrawal bleeding and to prevent the development of endometrial hyperplasia. Patients with hyperprolactinemia need periodic prolactin measurements and radiographic cone views of the sella turcica to rule out the development of macroadenoma.

COMPLICATIONS

The complications of amenorrhea can be numerous, including infertility and psychosocial developmental delays with lack of normal physical sexual development. Hypoestrogenic patients can develop severe osteoporosis and fractures, the most hazardous to life being femoral neck fracture (see Chapter 59). The complications associated with amenorrhea in patients who respond to progestin challenge are endometrial hyperplasia and carcinoma (see Chapter 50) resulting from unopposed estrogen stimulation.

PROGNOSIS

The prognosis for amenorrhea is good. It is not usually a life-threatening clinical event, as with proper evaluation, tumors can be recognized and treated. Many patients with hypothalamic amenorrhea will spontaneously recover normal menstrual cycles.

Virtually all amenorrheic women who do not have premature ovarian failure can be made to ovulate with a dopamine agonist, clomiphene citrate, insulin-sensitizing agents, and gonadotropins.

REFERENCES

Abrahamson MJ, Snyder PJ: Treatment of hyperprolactinemia due to lactotroph adenoma and other causes. UpToDate Online 2005;13.1. Available at www.uptodate.com.

Bose SH et al: The pathophysiology and genetics of congenital lipoid adrenal hyperplasia. N Engl J Med 1996;335:1870.

Crowley WF, Jameson JL: Clinical counterpoint: Gonadotropin-releasing hormone deficiency: Perspectives from clinical investigation. Endocr Rev 1992;13:635.

The Practice Committee of the American Society for Reproductive Medicine: Current evaluation of amenorrhea. Fertil Steril 2004;82(Suppl 1):33.

Reindollar RH, Byrd JR, McDonough PG: Delayed sexual development: A study of 252 patients. Am J Obstet Gynecol 1981;140:371.

The Rotterdam ESHRE/ASRM-Sponsored PCOS Consensus Workshop Group: Revised 2003 consensus on diagnostic criteria and long-term health risks related to polycystic ovary syndrome. Fertil Steril 2004;81:19.

Simpson JL: Phenotypic-karyotypic correlations of gonadal determinants: Current status and relationship to molecular studies. In Vogel F, Sperling K (editors): *Proceedings of the International Congress of Human Genetics.* Springer-Verlag, 1987.

Singh RP, Carr DH: The anatomy and histology of XO human embryos and fetuses. Anat Rec 1966;155:369.

Warren MP et al: Osteopenia in exercise-associated amenorrhea using ballet dancers as a model: A longitudinal study. J Clin Endocrinol Metab 2002;87:3162.

Hirsutism

57

*Marsha K. Guess, MD, D. Ellene Andrew, MD, Carol L. Gagliardi, MD,
& Adelina M. Emmi, MD*

■ HIRSUTISM

Definition

Hirsutism is defined as excessive growth of androgen-dependent sexual hair. This is most often manifested as increased "midline hair" on the upper lip, chin, ears, cheeks, lower abdomen, back, chest, and proximal limbs. The interpretation of what constitutes excessive growth is subjective and may range from an occasional hair on the upper lip to a full male-pattern beard. The psychological implications of hirsutism must not be underestimated. In Western society, excessive facial or body hair in women is unacceptable. Women who do not conform to a prevailing feminine ideal of physical appearance because of hirsutism may feel unattractive and suffer from low self-esteem, and such women may find social interactions difficult. Hirsutism is more than a cosmetic problem, however, because it usually represents a hormonal imbalance, resulting from a subtle excess of androgens that may be of ovarian origin, adrenal origin, or both.

Etiology

Excessive growth of sexual hair may be due to excessive production of androgens, increased sensitivity of the hair follicle to androgens, or increased conversion of weak androgens to potent androgens. Potential sources of increased androgens include the ovaries, the adrenal glands, exogenous hormones and other medications (Table 57–1).

A. OVARIAN DISORDERS CAUSING HIRSUTISM

1. Nonneoplastic disorders—The most common cause of hirsutism is **polycystic ovary syndrome.** Polycystic ovary syndrome is typically associated with menstrual irregularities, infertility, obesity, and hirsutism. The histologic changes seen in polycystic ovary disease include a thickened ovarian capsule and numerous follicular cysts surrounded by a hyperplastic, luteinized theca interna. The pathophysiology of this disease is not fully

understood; proposed causes include ovarian dysregulation, a disturbance of the hypothalamic-pituitary axis, adrenal androgen excess, and increased insulin resistance. Regardless of the underlying defect, the degree of hyperandrogenism and the individual's sensitivity to androgens may result in the complaint of hirsutism in 80% of these patients.

Other nonneoplastic ovarian disorders associated with hirsutism include stromal hyperplasia and stromal hyperthecosis. **Stromal hyperplasia** results in the hypersecretion of androgens from hypertrophic ovaries. It has a peak incidence between 60 and 70 years of age and is usually associated with uniform enlargement of both ovaries. **Stromal hyperthecosis** is a proliferation of stroma with foci of luteinized thecal cells, and also results in bilateral ovarian involvement. It frequently results in the clinical manifestations of virilism, obesity, hypertension, and disturbances of glucose metabolism, with most patients showing histologic evidence of concurrent stromal hyperplasia. A syndrome known as *Hyper*Androgenism, *I*nsulin *R*esistance, *A*canthosis *N*igricans (HAIR-AN) has also been described; however, this is thought to most likely represent a variation of one of the nonneoplastic disorders, rather than denoting a separate disease entity.

2. Neoplastic disorders—Androgen-secreting ovarian neoplasms usually present with rapidly developing hirsutism, amenorrhea, and virilization, and are rare causes of hirsutism. The most common androgen secreted by these tumors is testosterone, with serum testosterone levels usually in excess of 200 ng/dL. Most hormone-secreting neoplasms are palpable on pelvic examination and are unilateral.

Sertoli-Leydig cell tumors and **hilar (Leydig) cell tumors** are ovarian neoplasms typically associated with hirsutism and virilization. Sertoli-Leydig cell tumors constitute less than 0.5% of all ovarian tumors and occur mainly in young, menstruating females. Hilar cell tumors are rare neoplasms and are usually encountered in older women. Their presentation is often more indolent and less dramatic than that of Sertoli-Leydig cell tumors. Other ovarian neoplasms that may be associated with hirsutism are the gynandroblastomas, germ cell tumors, granulosa cell tumors, and gonadoblasto-

937

Table 57–1. Differential diagnosis of hirsutism.

Ovarian nonneoplastic causes
  Polycystic ovary syndrome
  Stromal hyperplasia
  Stromal hyperthecosis
  Hyperandrogenism, insulin resistance, acanthosis nigricans (HAIR-AN)
Ovarian neoplastic causes
  Sertoli-Leydig cell tumors
  Hilar cell tumors
  Germ cell tumors
  Gynandroblastomas
  Granulosa cell tumors
  Gonadoblastomas
  Ovarian tumors with functional stroma
Pregnancy-related causes
  Theca lutein cysts
  Luteoma of pregnancy
Adrenal causes
  Congenital adrenal hyperplasia (CAH)
  Adrenal tumors
  Cushing's syndrome
  Hyperprolactenemia
Iatrogenic causes
  Methyltestosterone
  Danazol
  Anabolic steroids
  19-Nortestosterones
Idiopathic hirsutism

mas. The latter occur mainly in male patients, with gonadal dysgenesis and resultant female phenotypes.

Ovarian tumors with functional stroma are categorized as germ cell tumors containing syncytiotrophoblast cells and idiopathic and pregnancy-related tumors (see below). In these tumors, the neoplastic cells do not secrete steroid hormones directly, but stimulate secretion by the ovarian stroma either within or immediately adjacent to the tumor. These tumors have been described in essentially all tumors that occur in the ovary, whether benign or malignant, metastatic or primary.

3. Pregnancy-related disorders—During pregnancy, elevated androgen levels that lead to severe hirsutism and virilization may be due to any of the above-mentioned conditions; however, pregnancy-specific disorders also exist. **Theca lutein cysts** (hyperreactio luteinalis) are benign neoplasms that can cause bilateral ovarian enlargement, hirsutism, and infrequently, virilization. These cysts occur almost exclusively in pregnancy and have an increased incidence in pregnancies complicated by gestational trophoblastic disease. Ovarian biopsy reveals cysts lined mostly with luteinized theca cells, but luteinized granulosa cells may also be present. Typically, resolution of the cysts occurs after pregnancy.

Luteoma of pregnancy is a benign human chorionic gonadotropin (hCG)–dependent ovarian tumor that may develop during pregnancy. High levels of testosterone and androstenedione are present, and virilization may occur in up to 25% of affected mothers and 65% of female fetuses. In most patients, spontaneous regression of the neoplasm and return of androgen levels to normal occur in the postpartum period.

B. ADRENAL DISORDERS CAUSING HIRSUTISM

1. Enzyme deficiencies—Enzyme deficiencies affecting adrenal and ovarian steroidogenesis represent the second most common cause of hyperandrogenism in postmenarchal females and **congenital adrenal hyperplasia** (**CAH**) represents the most common disorder in this group. CAH is inherited as an autosomal recessive trait, and is present in 1–5% of women who complain of hirsutism. It results from mutations in enzymes required for adrenal steroidogenesis. The most common form of CAH is characterized by a deficiency of 21-hydroxylase with case reports of similar occurrences in patients with 3β-hydroxysteroid dehydrogenase and 11β-hydroxylase deficiencies. These defects prohibit cortisol synthesis from its precursor 17β-hydroxyprogesterone. The expectant decrease in serum cortisol stimulates pituitary secretion of adrenocorticotropic hormone (ACTH) in an effort to normalize cortisol levels. Higher levels of ACTH stimulate adrenal production of intermediates in the biosynthetic pathway of cortisol. Consequently, these intermediates cannot be used for cortisol production because of enzyme defects, and are instead shunted into the biosynthetic pathways for androgens, with resultant increases in testosterone and androstenedione.

Classical CAH is usually diagnosed in females during the neonatal period because of androgen-induced ambiguous genitalia (pseudohermaphroditism); however, a minor enzyme deficiency may go unrecognized until puberty or later when hirsutism, amenorrhea, and virilization may occur. Such disease is termed acquired, late-onset, or adult-onset CAH.

2. Neoplastic disorders—Adrenal tumors are a rare cause of hirsutism, although when present, symptoms may be acute and quite severe. The main androgen produced by adrenal neoplasms is dehydroepiandrosterone sulfate adrenocorticotropic hormone (DHEAS), with serum levels usually greater than 700–800 μg/dL. Rarely, adrenal neoplasms may secrete testosterone; when this occurs, testosterone values are usually higher than 200 ng/dL.

3. Cushing's syndrome—Cushing's syndrome and the associated overproduction of cortisol may increase androgen levels and cause hirsutism. The syndrome has three known etiologies: (1) adrenal tumor, (2) ectopic production of ACTH by a nonpituitary tumor, or (3) excess production of ACTH by the pituitary (**Cushing's disease**). Since androgens are formed from intermediates in the synthesis of cortisol, increased serum and tissue levels of cortisol and its intermediates may result in hyperandrogenism and clinically present as hirsutism, regardless of the underlying cause of this syndrome.

4. Other causes—Hyperprolactinemia has been shown to produce mild hirsutism. Several investigators have reported increased DHEAS levels with hyperprolactinemia. This likely results from adrenal stimulation after prolactin binds to its numerous receptors on the adrenal gland. Despite increased androgen secretion, clinical manifestations are mild or absent, due to the inhibitory effects of prolactin on the conversion of testosterone to dihydrotestosterone (DHT) and its metabolites.

The adrenal gland may be the source of excess androgen production in the absence of an identifiable cause. The cause of this adrenal hyperactivity is not clear, but mild enzyme deficiencies, stress and hyperfunctioning of the entire adrenal gland, have been postulated as probable causes.

C. IATROGENIC MECHANISMS CAUSING HIRSUTISM

Exogenous sources of androgens should also be considered as possible causes of hirsutism. Methyltestosterone, danazol, and anabolic steroids such as oxandrolone may lead to excessive hair growth. The 19-nortestosterones in low-dose oral contraceptives rarely cause hirsutism or acne.

D. IDIOPATHIC HIRSUTISM

Hirsutism that occurs without adrenal or ovarian dysfunction, in patients with normal menstrual cycles and in the absence of any exogenous source of steroid hormones is termed **idiopathic hirsutism.** The term idiopathic hirsutism is thought to be a misnomer, since a likely cause has been elucidated. When normal levels of testosterone, unbound testosterone, DHEAS, dihydrotestosterone, and androstenedione are present, increased 5α-reductase enzyme activity appears to be the major mechanism of action. This enzyme converts testosterone to the more potent dihydrotestosterone in the hair follicle. Many patients with idiopathic hirsutism have an elevated level of plasma 3α-androstanediol glucuronide, a metabolite of dihydrotestosterone, thought to reflect the increased peripheral androgen metabolism, which is responsible for the clinical manifestation of hirsutism.

In summary, hirsutism may result from an ovarian disorder, an adrenal disease, an iatrogenic cause, or an increase in peripheral androgen metabolism. Rarely, other endocrinologic disturbances such as hypothyroidism or acromegaly may be associated with excessive hair growth. An important clinical correlation is that hirsutism may be accompanied by infertility as a result of the underlying abnormality. Since infertility may be the inciting factor triggering a patient to seek medical care, questions regarding a history of hirsutism should be a part of any infertility work-up.

Physiology of Androgens

Androgens are steroids that stimulate the development of male secondary sex characteristics and consequently promote the growth of sexual hair. The major androgens are testosterone, dihydrotestosterone, androstenedione, dehydroepiandrosterone (DHEA), and DHEAS. In order to comprehend the role played by elevated levels of androgens in the development of hirsutism, one must understand the sources of androgens, their metabolic pathways and sites of action, and their interrelationship with other steroid hormones such as estrogens and corticosteroids.

A. PRODUCTION

All steroid hormone production begins with the two-stage rate-limiting step of cholesterol conversion to pregnenolone, which is regulated by trophic hormones. In the nonpregnant woman, androgens are produced by both the ovaries and the adrenals, as well as by peripheral conversion. The rate-limiting step in androgen formation is the regulation of P450c17 gene expression, which is dependent on the concentrations of luteinizing hormone (LH) in the ovary and ACTH in the adrenal cortex.

1. Ovarian production of androgens—Androgens are produced by the normal ovary as precursors in the synthesis of estrogens. When gonadotropin-releasing hormone (GnRH) is secreted in a pulsatile fashion, thecal cells are stimulated to secrete and bind LH. In response to ligand binding, the theca cells of the preantral follicle produce androstenedione, DHEA, and testosterone. In the normal female, follicle-stimulating hormone (FSH) secreted from granulosa cells stimulates the granulosa cells to aromatize these androgens to the estrogens, estrone and estradiol. This relationship produces a system of androgen anabolism and catabolism balanced and coordinated to meet the needs of the follicular cycle.

2. Adrenal production of androgens—Stimulation of the adrenal gland by ACTH results in androgen production in the zona reticularis and zona fasciculata of the adrenal cortex. The main androgen manufactured is DHEAS, with smaller amounts of DHEA and androstenedione. A phenomena called adrenarche occurs and is usually chronologically timed before menarche in females. During this period, the adrenal cortex has a significant increase in adrenal hormone production, as a result of increased responsiveness of androgens and their precursors to the circulating levels of ACTH. This results in adrenocortical secretion of DHEAS at a level similar to that of cortisol secretion. Controversy remains regarding the causative factors.

B. CIRCULATION

1. Testosterone—Testosterone, by virtue of its plasma concentration and its potency, is one of the major androgens. It is the second most potent androgen after dihydrotestosterone, and circulating levels are 20–80 ng/dL in adult women. The ovary and the adrenals contribute equally to testosterone production, with each supplying about 25% of the total circulating level. The other 50% of circulating testosterone is derived from peripheral conversion of androstenedione, although the ovarian contribution to testosterone levels may increase during the periovulatory portion of the menstrual cycle. Peripheral levels of testosterone display a slight diurnal variation that parallels that of cortisol. In normal women, 99% of testosterone is protein-bound, of which 80% is bound to sex hormone-binding globulin (SHBG) and 19% is loosely bound to albumin. The remaining 1% is free and unbound. The free and albumin-bound testosterone are the biologically active forms of circulating testosterone.

2. Dihydrotestosterone—Circulating levels of dihydrotestosterone, the most potent androgen, are 2–8 ng/dL or one-tenth those of testosterone. Although both the ovary and the adrenal gland secrete it, most dihydrotestosterone is produced by peripheral conversion of testosterone by 5α-reductase.

3. Androstenedione—Androstenedione, one of the 17-ketosteroids, is not very potent, with only 20% of the effectiveness of testosterone. Synthesis and secretion occur mostly in the ovaries and adrenals in equal amounts, with the remaining 10% being produced peripherally. Androstenedione levels display a diurnal variation paralleling that of cortisol and may simultaneously increase by as much as 50% when cortisol levels rise. Moreover, periovulatory increases in androstenedione levels can also be observed. In contrast to testosterone, androstenedione is bound mainly to albumin and secondarily to SHBG.

4. DHEA and DHEAS—DHEA and DHEAS, both weak androgens, have approximately 3% of the effectiveness of testosterone, and are the other major precursors of 17-ketosteroids. DHEA is primarily produced by the adrenals (60–70%), with ovarian production and hydrolysis of DHEAS accounting for the remainder. DHEA has a large diurnal variation similar to that of cortisol. Conversely, DHEAS is derived almost entirely from the adrenal, has only slight diurnal variation, and circulates in high concentrations. The DHEAS level may provide a good clinical assessment of adrenal function.

C. ACTION

The skin and hair follicles are androgen-responsive and thus have the capacity to metabolize androgens. DHEA, androstenedione, and testosterone enter the target cell and are reduced to dihydrotestosterone by 5α-reductase. Dihydrotestosterone is then bound to a cytoplasmic receptor protein that transports the androgen into the cell nucleus, where it is bound to chromatin and initiates transcription of stored genetic information. In the hair follicle, this promotes hair growth, leading to increased hair growth and initiating the conversion of vellus to terminal hair.

In females a certain amount of androgenic stimulation is expected, with the greatest levels noted at puberty, when these increased levels result in the clinical appearance of pubic hair and axillary hair. Similarly, androgens stimulate the facial pilosebaceous glands resulting in the pubertal development of acne.

Metabolic conversion of androgens to dihydrotestosterone may be accelerated. This results in irreversible conversion of vellus hair to terminal hair in areas of androgen-sensitive skin. Thus, in excess androgens are pathologic, and the clinical signs and symptoms of hirsutism and virilization result.

Physiology of Hair Growth

The hair follicle and its sebaceous gland together make up the pilosebaceous unit. The hair follicle begins to develop within the first 2 months of gestation, and by birth, a child possesses all of the hair follicles he or she will ever have. Hair first appears as vellus hair, which is fine, short, and lightly pigmented. During puberty, adrenal and ovarian androgen levels rise, converting vellus hair to terminal hair, which is coarse, long, and more heavily pigmented.

Hair growth is cyclic. The three phases of the cycle are (1) anagen (growth), (2) catagen (rapid involution), and (3) telogen (inactivity). The length of each hair is determined by the relative duration of anagen and telogen and varies with different locations on the body, although each hair follicle has its own growth cycle independent of adjacent hair follicles. Scalp hair has a long anagen, from 2 to 6 years, with a short telogen.

The growth and development of the hair follicle may be influenced by several factors. First, the pilosebaceous unit is sensitive to the effects of sex hormones, especially androgens. During puberty, adrenal and ovarian androgen levels rise, converting testosterone to dihydrotestosterone, which can initiate growth and increase both the diameter and pigmentation of hair. Although conversion of vellus hair to terminal hair is essentially irreversible, removal of the androgenic stimulus will slow hair growth and stop the conversion of vellus to terminal hair. Conversely, estrogens can retard the growth rate and result in finer hair with less pigmentation.

Genetic factors may also influence the pilosebaceous unit. Although males and females are born with equal numbers of hair follicles, racial and ethnic differences are noted in the concentration of hair follicles; Caucasians have a greater number of hair follicles than African-Americans, who in turn have a greater number than Asians. Different ethnic groups within each race may also exhibit differences in hair follicle concentrations (eg, Caucasians of Mediterranean ancestry have a greater concentration of hair follicles than those of Nordic ancestry).

Understanding the role of exogenous factors on the pilosebaceous unit allows one to better understand how pathologic hirsutism develops, and what factors may affect the severity of the disease process.

Diagnosis & Clinical Findings

Appropriate questioning allows one to rule out any history of drug ingestion that might cause excessive hair growth, to determine the speed of onset of symptoms, and to correlate the timing of symptoms with age and puberty. Specific inquiry into the patient's menstrual history allows the classification of patients who are amenorrheic or oligomenorrheic, and to distinguish those whose pathology began with puberty from those with a later onset of hirsutism. Knowledge of a family history of hirsutism or of abnormal menstrual cycles may also be informative.

Finally, a physical examination should be performed to differentiate hypertrichosis from hirsutism and to evaluate for acanthosis nigricans or additional signs of virilization such as clitorimegaly, male pattern balding, deepening voice, or decreased breast contour. Particular attention should be paid to body habitus, hair distribution, and the pelvic examination. Employing the Ferriman-Gallwey grading system provides a subjective determination of the severity of hirsutism and may also be followed to determine treatment effectiveness.

A. SIGNS AND SYMPTOMS

Many of the disorders involving hirsutism have characteristic presentations that may aid in diagnosis. For example, in classical congenital adrenal hyperplasia, the stigmata are identified at birth and include clitorimegaly, labial fusion, and an abnormal urethral course. Hirsutism presenting in childhood may be due to androgen-producing tumors and usually presents with other pronounced signs of virilization and the presence of a pelvic mass. However, an androgen-producing tumor should also be suspected when a woman with a normal menstrual history presents with sudden onset of irregular menses followed by amenorrhea, hirsutism, and virilization. Genetic anomalies such as mosaic cells containing Y chromosomes or incomplete androgen insensitivity syndrome may produce signs of androgen stimulation associated with primary amenorrhea at puberty. Moreover, if a patient presents with a long history of irregular menses with slow onset of hirsutism beginning at puberty or in the early 20s, polycystic ovary syndrome or

late-onset congenital adrenal hyperplasia are suggested. A higher index of suspicion for CAH should be considered in individuals with a genetic predisposition (Ashkenazi Jews and Eskimos), short stature, or a strong family history of hirsutism. Similarly, menstrual irregularities, in the presence of galactorrhea or visual changes, should cause suspicion of hyperprolactinemia. Hirsutism or virilization during pregnancy raises the suspicion of a luteoma of pregnancy or bilateral thecalutein cysts. The physical signs of Cushing's syndrome, including centripetal obesity, wasting of the extremities, fat deposition in supraclavicular areas and in the neck and face, facial plethora, and wide cutaneous striae are usually apparent if this syndrome exists. When acromegaly is present, overgrowth of the viscera and soft body tissues, as well as enlargement of the bones of the hands, feet, and face can be seen. Finally, if hypothyroidism is present, thickening of the skin of the lips, fingers, lower legs, or lower eyelids may be present, along with complaints of lethargy, cold intolerance, constipation, and voice changes.

While the medical history, the menstrual history, and the physical examination are directive and informative, significant overlap exists and laboratory studies and sometimes imaging studies are needed before a diagnosis can be confirmed.

B. LABORATORY FINDINGS

Investigators disagree about which androgens should be measured in the evaluation of hirsutism. Laboratory evaluation should seek to identify life-threatening conditions associated with hyperandrogenism, such as Cushing's syndrome, congenital adrenal hyperplasia, and ovarian or adrenal tumors. Serum testosterone, DHEAS, and 17β-hydroxyprogesterone levels can be obtained for screening purposes.

1. Screening tests

a. Testosterone—A serum testosterone level of less than 200 ng/dL will rule out almost all of the testosterone-secreting neoplasms. A total testosterone level higher than 200 ng/dL should be considered evidence of an ovarian tumor until proven otherwise; few adrenal tumors produce testosterone.

The presence of hirsutism in a patient with a normal testosterone level indicates increased androgen effects. In hirsute women, increased androgen levels may decrease production of SHBG by the liver, and the free, biologically active fraction of testosterone may increase 2–3%. Therefore, normal total serum levels of testosterone in a hirsute woman can reflect a decreased level of SHBG, with an increase in the free testosterone fraction. However, the determination of the serum free testosterone level is expensive and does not add any useful clinical information.

b. DHEAS—A normal or slightly elevated DHEAS level excludes significant adrenal pathology. Adrenal tumors usually produce DHEAS with plasma levels markedly elevated to greater than 700–800 µg/dL. The plasma DHEAS level is reliable and convenient and has replaced 24-hour urine collection for measurement of 17-ketosteroids in most laboratories.

c. 17α-hydroxyprogesterone—17α-Hydroxyprogesterone is the single most accurate diagnostic test for congenital adrenal hyperplasia due to 21-hydroxylase deficiency. It is a cost-effective screen for women whose history suggests CAH. 17α-Hydroxyprogesterone should be measured immediately upon awakening, in the morning, and only during the follicular phase of the menstrual cycle. Normal levels are less than 200 ng/dL. Levels ranging between 200 and 400 ng/dL warrant further evaluation. Levels greater than 400 ng/dL are virtually diagnostic of 21-hydroxylase deficiency.

2. Directed tests—Further testing should be ordered based on history and physical examination. If a woman is oligo-ovulatory or anovulatory, determination of FSH, LH, thyroid-stimulating hormone (TSH), and prolactin levels is helpful. In patients with a mild enzyme deficiency or a partial block at the 21-hydroxylation step in the biosynthesis of cortisol, 17α-hydroxyprogesterone levels may not be elevated and ACTH stimulation may be required for diagnosis. If the DHEAS level is elevated or if Cushing's syndrome is suspected, then either an overnight dexamethasone suppression test or a 24-hour urinary free cortisol level should be obtained. If the above laboratory tests are normal in a hirsute female, the diagnosis of idiopathic hirsutism must be considered and an androstanediol glucuronide level may be evaluated.

a. FSH and LH—An elevated level of LH, particularly when the LH:FSH ratio is 3 or higher, suggests polycystic ovary syndrome; however, this value is neither sensitive nor specific and is not required for the diagnosis. Newer diagnostic tests being employed include the evaluation of the glusose:insulin ratio and SHBG. Low levels of these values indicate insulin resistance, which is often a contributing factor in the development of polycystic ovarian syndrome.

b. Prolactin—A mildly elevated prolactin level may be seen in patients with polycystic ovarian syndrome or those with increased adrenal stimulation. However, prolactin elevation above 200 µg/dL usually suggests a prolactinoma.

c. TSH—An increased TSH level is strongly suggestive of hypothyroidism. A free T_4 and T_4 index should be obtained to confirm the diagnosis in these individuals.

d. ACTH stimulation test—The ACTH-induced increase in 17α-hydroxyprogesterone is a sensitive diagnostic test for congenital adrenal hyperplasia. Generally, this test is reserved for individuals in high-risk populations, given the low prevalence of disease among hirsute women. For diagnosis, 17α-hydroxyprogesterone is measured 30 minutes after an intravenous injection of 250 µg of synthetic ACTH. Values rarely exceed 400 ng/dL in normal women and values above 1000 ng/dL are indicative of disease. Once the diagnosis is made, the nomogram by Marie New can be used to differentiate nonclassical and classical disease.

e. Tests used to diagnose Cushing's syndrome

(1) Overnight dexamethasone suppression test—An overnight dexamethasone suppression test may be used as a simple outpatient screening test. A baseline morning plasma cortisol level is drawn, then dexamethasone, 1 mg orally, is given at 11:00 PM. A second plasma cortisol level is obtained at 8:00 AM the next morning. In normal patients, cortisol levels are suppressed to 5 µg/dL, whereas in patients with Cushing's syndrome, cortisol levels fall but do not go below 5 µg/dL. This test is easily performed on an outpatient basis, but may result in false-negative results, particularly in patients with mild disease. The false-positive rate is much higher in obese patients, chronically ill or depressed patients, and patients taking carbamazepine.

(2) 24-hour urinary free cortisol—The most accurate screening test for documentation of hypercortisolism is measurement of urinary free cortisol over a 24-hour period. Values greater than 100 ng/24 h are considered abnormal and further evaluation is warranted. Values greater than 250 ng/24 h are virtually diagnostic of Cushing's syndrome. The 24-hour urinary free cortisol determination is an excellent screening test because it has a low incidence of false-negative results; however, false-positive values may occur in the presence of depression, polycystic ovarian syndrome, carbamazepine therapy, or increased fluid intake.

(3) Low-dose dexamethasone suppression test—If the above screening tests yield equivocal results, the low-dose dexamethasone suppression test may be employed. Low-dose suppression of urinary free cortisol to less than 25 mg/24 h or 17-hydroxycorticosteroids to less than 3 mg/24 h after the administration of 0.5 mg of dexamethasone every 6 hours for 2 consecutive days rules out Cushing's syndrome. Unfortunately, this test also has remarkably low sensitivity and specificity, and some investigators questions its benefit in patient evaluation.

(4) Additional tests—Alternatively, newer tests may be employed. These include (1) evaluation of late night plasma or salivary cortisol levels; (2) assessment of plasma cortisol after dexamethasone and corticotropin-

releasing hormone are given; and (3) evaluation of ACTH after administration of intravenous and oral hydrocortisone. While all of the above tests may assist when verification of disease is required, the ideal test for evaluation has yet to be identified.

f. Tests used to differentiate Cushing's disease from Cushing's syndrome

(1) High-dose dexamethasone test—Once the diagnosis of Cushing's syndrome has been made, the etiology should be further elucidated. The high-dose dexamethasone test is usually used for this purpose, although it is currently being reevaluated. It requires 6 days of urine collection and the sensitivity and specificity are poor. Despite efforts by many investigators to improve this test, limitations continue to exist. When this test is used diagnostically, Cushing's disease is diagnosed when urinary free cortisol and 17-hydroxycorticosteroid are suppressed by 90%.

(2) Corticotropin-releasing hormone (CRH) stimulation test—Measuring plasma ACTH levels before and after the administration of CRH yields better results than the high-dose dexamethasone test; however, the diagnostic accuracy is no better than 85–90%. Therefore, the addition of imaging studies or inferior petrosal sinus sampling may be justified (see below).

g. Androstanediol glucuronide levels—The measurement of serum androstanediol glucuronide has been proposed as a good marker of peripheral androgen production and activity in hirsutism. Serum androstanediol glucuronide may be elevated in idiopathic hirsutism as a result of altered metabolism or increased utilization of androgen in the skin and hair follicles. Although this test is useful for research, its clinical applicability remains limited. Because of high cost and limited usefulness, the test for androstanediol glucuronide levels is not currently recommended in the routine evaluation of hirsutism.

C. IMAGING STUDIES

Ultrasonography is usually reserved for patients suspected of having a pelvic mass contributing to their disease process. In general, pelvic examination reveals a palpable ovarian mass; however, if the examination is limited by the individual's body habitus, pelvic ultrasonography may help delineate an abnormal structure. Although patients with polycystic ovarian syndrome have characteristic small, peripheral ovarian follicles, the specificity of ultrasonography is extremely limited, since many individuals without this syndrome have been found to have polycystic ovaries. Hence, routine ultrasonography in the diagnosis of this syndrome is not a universal practice.

If the testosterone level is higher than 200 ng/dL and no ovarian mass is identified, computed tomography (CT) or magnetic resonance imaging (MRI) of the adrenal glands should be performed before laparotomy to rule out the rare testosterone-producing adrenal tumor. CT scan and MRI of the adrenal glands have proven to be sensitive diagnostic techniques that have generally replaced selective venous sampling and selective angiography. Selective bilateral venous catheterization of adrenal and ovarian veins has limited clinical usefulness, since it is technically difficult and hazardous to perform, and its diagnostic sensitivity is poor.

Primary adrenal disease is most often confirmed with adrenal CT scan. CT scan or MRI of the lung is indicated with ectopic ACTH secretion, since this is the most common site of ectopic ACTH production. Similarly, a CT scan or MRI of the sella turcica may be used to localize an ACTH-secreting tumor. Currently, MRI is the preferred study due to its increased sensitivity when enhancement and dynamic imaging are judiciously used. Still, detection of the more centrally located ACTH-secreting microadenomas is only about 45–71%, and only 40–50% of these lesions are visualized before surgical correction of the problem. Due to limitations in biochemical testing and conservative imaging studies for Cushing's disease, simultaneous bilateral inferior petrosal sinus sampling is usually necessary to confirm the disease and to localize the lesion. A petrosal sinus:peripheral venous ACTH ratio greater than 2 in the absence of CRH, or greater than 3 when CRH is administered, is diagnostic of Cushing's disease.

Differential Diagnosis

Hirsutism should be differentiated from both virilization and hypertrichosis, since the cause and treatment of these disorders may be different. **Virilization** is characterized by more extensive androgen-induced changes than hirsutism alone. These changes include acne, increased oiliness of the skin, temporal balding, clitorimegaly, deepening of the voice, development of male muscular pattern and body habitus (in extreme cases), and atrophy of the breasts.

Hypertrichosis is also characterized by excessive growth of hair, but the term denotes increased growth of nonsexual hair (eg, hair on the forehead, lower leg, or forearm). The hair is usually fine-textured and is not caused by androgen excess or abnormal androgen metabolism. Heredity, certain drugs, physical irritation (trauma to the skin), or even starvation may be responsible. However, drug ingestion is the most common cause. Phenytoin, diazoxide, and minoxidil are known to cause a generalized increase in hair growth. Penicillamine and streptomycin have been associated with increased hair growth in infants and children. In addition, inadvertent ingestion of the fungicide hexachlorobenzene has also caused hypertrichosis. Disorders such as porphyria, hypothyroidism, dermatomyositis, acromegaly, Hurler's syndrome, trisomy E, and Cornelia de Lange's syndrome may be associated with hypertrichosis.

Treatment

The selection of therapy for hirsutism depends on the physical and laboratory findings, as well as on the patient's desire for childbearing. After evaluation has ruled out neoplasm or a serious disease process, a mildly hirsute woman with normal menstrual cycles may require only reassurance. A moderately or severely hirsute woman with menstrual irregularities requires treatment. For women not desiring childbearing in the near future, medical therapy consisting of adrenal or ovarian suppression or the blocking of peripheral androgen effects is advised. If infertility is a major concern, ovulation induction with the appropriate drug (eg, clomiphene, bromocriptine, human menopausal gonadotropin [hMG], or gonadotropin-releasing hormone [GnRH]) is started after appropriate evaluation. In many patients, simultaneous use of mechanical depilators and rarely surgery may be necessary.

D. MEDICAL MANAGEMENT

The medical treatment of hirsutism is not completely successful. The response rate has been reported to be between 23% and 95%, depending on the drug and dosage used. The drugs most commonly used to treat hirsutism include oral contraceptives, GnRH analogs, androgen receptor antagonists, and corticosteroids.

All drug therapy should seek to alter at least one of the 5 major aspects of androgen metabolism: (1) decrease production; (2) increase the metabolic clearance rate; (3) inhibit androgen receptors; (4) inhibit the enzymes involved in the peripheral production of testosterone or dihydrotestosterone; or (5) increase SHBG.

1. Combination oral contraceptives—Oral contraceptives have been extensively used to treat hirsutism. Their effect is exerted through a wide range of actions. The combination pill contains both estrogen and progestins and prevents ovulation by inhibiting gonadotropin secretion. Inhibition of LH secretion is mainly accomplished by the addition of the progestational component. When adequate suppression of LH is achieved, ovarian steroidogenesis is suppressed, leading to decreased testosterone production by the ovary. A decline in plasma testosterone can be seen as early as 1 week after treatment has been started; levels may decrease to normal by 3 months. Hair growth is reportedly decreased 50–60% in patients taking combination birth control pills. This effect is seen with the administration of all combination oral contraceptives, regardless of the individual steroid concentrations. Use of a low-dose pill (less than or equal to 35 ng of estrogen) allows for suppression of testosterone production while minimizing estrogen-related side effects.

The estrogen component decreases the androgenic effects of plasma testosterone by increasing hepatic SHBG synthesis. Since only the unbound form of testosterone is available to initiate a biologic response, increasing the bound fraction of testosterone by increasing SHBG levels leads to a decrease in testosterone-mediated effects. However, this increase has not been shown to have a direct effect on hirsutism.

Several studies suggest that combination birth control pills may exert a significant suppressive effect on adrenal androgen synthesis. Although the mechanism of action is presently unclear, this effect is probably due (at least in part) to suppression of ACTH release. The ability of combination birth control pills to lower the serum levels of DHEAS has several therapeutic implications. First, although DHEAS is low in biologic potency, it can serve as a precursor for peripheral conversion to more biologically potent androgens, and elevated levels of DHEAS can therefore be clinically manifested as hirsutism. Second, the ability of combination birth control pills to suppress both adrenal and ovarian androgen production, resulting in a significant reduction of androstenedione, DHEAS, and testosterone, may make these pills an even more attractive therapeutic option.

Older combination pills contain progestins, which are derivatives of testosterone. These 19-nortestosterones have some androgenic properties, which may result in hirsutism, acne, or oily skin. However, newer generation oral contraceptives contain desogestrel, gestodene, norgestimate or drospirenone. These drugs have fewer androgenic side effects, but have not consistently been shown to be more beneficial in the treatment of hirsutism.

2. Gonadotropin-releasing hormone (GnRH) agonists—GnRH analogs inhibit the secretion of gonadotropins from the pituitary gland, thereby inhibiting the secretion of androgens and estrogens from the ovary. Although GnRH agonists acutely stimulate ovarian production of androgens and estrogens, continued therapy causes a sustained decrease in ovarian steroid production compared with pretreatment levels. This suppression continues for the duration of GnRH agonist therapy. Significant decreases in serum levels of estradiol, testosterone, and androstenedione occur during treatment, although adrenal androgens are usually unaffected.

As a result of the hypoestrogenism associated with ongoing GnRH therapy, a potential risk of osteoporosis and menopausal symptoms exists with long-term therapy. However, concomitant use of estrogen and progesterone replacement therapy may counteract the adverse effects. Newer studies suggest that spironolactone may also simulate this effect.

Most studies have shown greater improvement of hirsutism with the use of GnRH agonists alone or in combination with oral contraceptives as compared with combination oral contraceptives alone; however, some studies show comparable efficacy.

3. Androgen receptor antagonists—There are four androgen receptor antagonists currently being used for the treatment of hirsutism. Despite proven efficacy in numerous clinical trials, none of these drugs has been approved by the U.S. Food and Drug Administration for this indication. Additionally, similar reported efficacy has been reported with all of these medications. Hence the agent of choice should be dictated by the individual's response, reported side effects, and known contraindications.

a. Cyproterone acetate—This potent agent was the first androgen receptor antagonist used to treat hirsutism and is widely prescribed in Europe to treat hirsutism. Antiandrogenic effects result from competitive displacement of dihydrotestosterone from its receptor and reduction of 5α-reductase activity in the skin. Progestational activity results in gonadotropin suppression with subsequent suppression of ovarian testosterone secretion. Cyclical administration of 50–100 mg on days 1–10 of the menstrual cycle combined with oral estrogen on days 1–21 produces therapeutic levels. Additionally, this method counters hypoestrogenism and irregular bleeding and prevents pregnancy and the potential teratogenic complications that may result. Although effective in 50–75% of hirsute women, significant side effects include decreased libido, mental depression, and hepatotoxicity, which is rarely seen when cyclic administration is performed. Clinical studies have shown efficacy equivalent to that of spironolactone, with the latter showing fewer side effects (see below). Currently, cyproterone acetate is not available in the U.S.

b. Spironolactone—Spironolactone, an aldosterone antagonist traditionally used as a diuretic in the treatment of hypertension, is also used to treat hirsutism. It possesses antiandrogenic properties and exerts its peripheral antiandrogenic effects in the hair follicle by competing for androgenic receptors and displacing dihydrotestosterone at both nuclear and cytosol receptors. It also lowers testosterone levels by inhibiting the cytochrome P450 monooxygenases that are required for biosynthesis of androgens in gonadal and adrenal steroid-producing cells. Serum levels of SHBG, DHEAS, and DHEA are unaltered by treatment with spironolactone. The dosage used for treatment of hirsutism has varied between 50 and 200 mg/d. Serum androgen levels will drop within a few days of the start of treatment, and a clinical response can usually be seen within 2–5 months. Side effects are mild—transient diuresis

and polydipsia have been noted in the first few days of treatment, and disturbances in the menstrual cycle, breast tenderness, and fatigue have also been reported, but no long-term problems have been encountered. Because spironolactone is a potent antiandrogen, all women using it should use effective contraception.

c. Flutamide—Flutamide is a potent, highly specific, nonsteroidal antiandrogen with no intrinsic hormonal or antigonadotropin activity. Although the exact mechanism of action is unknown, it competitively inhibits target tissue androgen receptor sites. Recent studies suggest that 250 mg 1–3 times daily is a highly effective treatment for moderate to severe hirsutism. Side effects include decreased appetite, amenorrhea, decreased libido, or dry skin. A rare but serious reported side effect is hepatotoxicity. Consequently, flutamide is usually reserved for resistant cases of hirsutism, and liver enzymes should be checked regularly in patients on the drug. Additionally, because of possible teratogenic effects, contraception must be used with this therapy.

d. Finasteride—Finasteride is the newest antiandrogenic agent used for hirsutism. It is a selective type 2 5α-reductase inhibitor that blocks the conversion of testosterone to dihydrotestosterone. It has proven efficacy in up to 86% of patients with a subjective improvement rate of 21–45% when 5 mg is administered orally over 3 months to 1 year. Side effects at this dosage are usually mild or absent and include headaches, transient gastrointestinal upset, and an unexplained increase in total testosterone.

4. Glucocorticoids—Dexamethasone is used mainly to treat hirsutism in patients with hyperandrogenism of adrenal origin. Chronic low-dose dexamethasone, 0.5–1 mg orally taken at bedtime, will provide adequate adrenal androgen suppression. Diminution of hair growth is reported in 16–70% of patients. Glucocorticoid therapy has fallen out of favor due to frequent side effects, potential for adrenal suppression, and evidence that these agents are less effective than antiandrogens, even when there is a clear adrenal cause of hyperandrogenism. However, their use may be justified in some patients, since recent data suggest that concomitant use of glucocorticoids with GnRH agonists may prolong the disease-free interval when therapy is discontinued. Moreover, glucocorticoids are the treatment of choice to decrease ACTH levels and thereby decrease formation of androgenic precursors of cortisol for patients with congenital adrenal hyperplasia.

5. Other

a. Dopamine—Dopamine is a centrally acting inhibitor of prolactin secretion and is frequently used in the treatment of hyperprolactinemia. Recently, hirsutism scores were shown to decrease significantly during dopamine treatment of hyperandrogenic women with hyperprolactinemia.

b. Troglitazone—Troglitazone is an insulin-sensitizing agent of the thiazolidinedione class, which results in a dose-related decrease in androgen level in patients with polycystic ovarian syndrome. Additionally, it has been shown that the administration of 600 mg/d results in significant improvement of hirsutism in this population.

c. Cimetidine—Cimetidine, an H_2-receptor antagonist, has weak antiandrogenic properties. Recent studies show minimal or no beneficial effect in hirsutism.

d. Ketoconazole—Ketoconazole is a synthetic imidazole derivative that blocks adrenal and gonadal steroidogenesis; it has been advocated by some as a treatment for hirsutism. However, serious side effects result in poor compliance and preclude long-term use. Its use should be avoided since safer therapeutic regimens exist.

E. Mechanical Therapy

The goal of mechanical therapy is to limit new hair growth without affecting existing hair. For this reason, mechanical depilators such as lasers, electrolysis devices, creams, and waxes are often used as supplemental therapy. Recent technology has made this procedure faster, easier, less painful, and generally free of any serious adverse effects.

F. Surgical Treatment

In the minority of hirsute patients in whom a specific cause can be identified, therapy should be directed toward the underlying disorder. For example, ovarian and adrenal tumors should be surgically excised. Additionally, women with Cushing's disease are treated with transsphenoidal pituitary microsurgery. Alternatively, when Cushing's syndrome is caused by an adrenal tumor, simple adrenalectomy is sufficient. Finally, acromegaly can be treated by transsphenoidal hypophysectomy. For persistent disease, bilateral adrenalectomy or pituitary irradiation is appropriate.

Similarly, a minority of older women may fail to respond to medical management for hyperthecosis despite good compliance. For these women, bilateral oophorectomy may be justified as definitive therapy.

Although wedge resection of the ovary has been successfully used to induce ovulation, it is not recommended for the treatment of hirsutism. This surgical procedure exposes patients to the risks of both anesthesia and possible formation of adhesions. More importantly, this procedure results in only a transient decrease in androgen levels and has successfully reduced the rate of hair growth in only 16% of patients. Wedge resection should not be used as a treatment for hirsutism.

Complications & Prognosis

The treatment for hirsutism can be frustrating for both patient and physician because of the physiologic properties of hair itself. The growth cycle of hair is long, varying between 6 and 24 months, and the conversion of vellus hair to terminal hair is essentially irreversible. Also, once hair growth has been stimulated by excessive androgen levels, maintenance of that same growth rate requires much less androgen. Patients must be advised that a response to therapy may not be seen for 6–12 months and that although it is possible to prevent further conversion of vellus hair to terminal hair, little change will be seen in the total number of terminal hairs. Some patients may note lightening of hair color and a decrease in the diameter of the hair shaft with therapy. Cosmetic treatment of excess hair consists of shaving, plucking, bleaching, waxing, or use of depilatories; however, shaving and plucking may cause infection and scarring and are not recommended. Permanent hair removal may be accomplished only by electrolysis (electrocoagulation of the hair root, or papilla), which is costly and uncomfortable, or by depilation. Unless there is excessive hirsutism, electrolysis should be delayed until after 6–12 months of medical therapy have been completed.

Patients who exhibit progressive hirsutism while receiving hormonal therapy or patients whose circulating androgen levels fail to decrease as expected should undergo further evaluation. If androgen levels are not suppressed with appropriate therapy, the possibility of a slow-growing neoplasm should be considered. Levels of testosterone and DHEAS should be monitored and the adrenal glands and ovaries reevaluated.

When adequate suppression of DHEAS and testosterone has been maintained for 6–12 months but a satisfactory reduction in new hair growth has not occurred, several options are available. The dose of the current medication can be increased, a new medication can be substituted, or a new medication can be added. It is frequently impossible to increase the dose of the initial medication, since the incidence of side effects may increase as the drug dosage increases. Likewise, it is not always easy to switch medications, since choice of the initial drug may have been guided by specific therapeutic considerations (eg, hirsute women who desire contraception may be treated with combination contraceptive pills, whereas hirsutism associated with hypertension may be treated with spironolactone). Some authors have recommended adding a second medication to the treatment regimen for hirsutism unresponsive to therapy. Newer evidence suggests that combination drug treatment for hirsutism with concomitant use of drugs that act at different sites may produce the best results (eg, combination birth control pills that act chiefly through decreased production of ovarian steroids may be combined with spironolactone, which acts mainly at the peripheral androgen receptors).

Treatment for hirsutism must be individualized and based on the results of a thorough history, physical examination, and laboratory studies. After therapy has begun, the patient's progress can be monitored on the basis of both clinical appearance and laboratory values. The patient should be educated about her disorder in order to prevent unrealistic expectations of therapy and to make her aware of any side effects that might manifest during therapy. Adjunctive therapy is almost always necessary with any medical treatment for hirsutism. Depilatories and electrolysis are frequently needed to remove the terminal hair already present; these methods, when combined with medical therapy, offer the best cosmetic result.

REFERENCES

Azziz R et al: Troglitazone improves ovulation and hirsutism in the polycystic ovary syndrome: a multicenter double blind, placebo-controlled trial. J Clin Endocrinol Metab 2001; 86:1626. [PMID: 11297595]

Barnes R: Diagnosis and therapy of hyperandrogenism. Balliere's Clin Obstet Gynaecol 1997;11:369.

Bencini PL et al: Long-term epilation with long-pulsed neodymium:YAG laser. Dermatol Surg 1999;25:175. [PMID: 10193962]

Carmina E, Lobo R: The addition of dexamethasone to antiandrogen therapy for hirsutism prolongs the duration of remission. Fertil Steril 1998;69:1075. [PMID: 9627295]

Castelo-Branco C et al: Gonadotropin-releasing hormone analog plus an oral contraceptive containing desogestrel in women with severe hirsutism: effects on hair, bone, and hormone profile after 1-year use. Metabolism 1997;46:437. [PMID: 9109850]

DeLeo V et al: Hormonal and clinical effects of GnRH agonist alone, or in combination with a combined oral contraceptive or flutamide in women with severe hirsutism. Gynecol Endocrinol 2000;14:411. [PMID: 11228061]

Deplewski D et al: Role of hormones in pilosebaceous unit development. Endocr Rev 2000;21:363. [PMID: 10950157]

Escobar-Morreale HF et al: Treatment of hirsutism with ethinyl estradiol-desogestrel contraceptive pills has beneficial effects on the lipid profile and improves insulin sensitivity. Fertil Steril 2000;74:816. [PMID: 11020530]

Falsetti L et al: Comparison of finasteride versus flutamide in the treatment of hirsutism. Eur J Endocrinol 1999;141:361. [PMID: 10526249]

Findling JW, Raff J: Newer diagnostic techniques and problems in Cushing's disease. Endocrinol Metab Clin North Am 1999;28:191. [PMID: 10207691]

Fox R: Transvaginal ultrasound appearances of the ovary in normal women and hirsute women with oligomenorrhoea. Aust N Z J Obstet Gynaecol 1999;39:63. [PMID: 10099753]

Fruzzetti F et al: Treatment of hirsutism: comparisons between different antiandrogens with central and peripheral effects. Fertil Steril 1999;71:445. [PMID: 10065780]

Gregoriou O et al: The effect of combined oral contraception with or without spironolactone on bone mineral density of hyperandrogenic women. Gynecol Endocrinol 2000;14:369. [PMID: 11109976]

Hagag P et al: Androgen suppression and clinical improvement with dopamine agonists in hyperandrogenic-hyperprolactinemic women. J Reprod Med 2001;46:678. [PMID: 11499189]

Hock DL et al: New treatments of hyperandrogenism and hirsutism. Obstet Gynecol Clin North Am 2000;27:567. [PMID: 10958004]

Judd HL et al: The effects of ovarian wedge resection on circulating gonadotropin and ovarian steroid levels in patients with polycystic ovary syndrome. J Clin Endocrinol Metab 1976; 43:347. [PMID: 950366]

Lunde O et al: Polycystic ovarian syndrome: a follow-up study on fertility and menstrual pattern in 149 patients 15–25 years after ovarian wedge resection. Hum Reprod 2001;16:1479. [PMID: 11425833]

Moghetti P et al: Comparison of spironolactone, flutamide, and finasteride efficacy in the treatment of hirsutism: a randomized, double blind, placebo-controlled trial. J Clin Endocrinol Metab 2000;85:89. [PMID: 10634370]

Moran C et al: 21-Hydroxylase-deficient nonclassic adrenal hyperplasia is a progressive disorder: a multicenter study. Am J Obstet Gynecol 2000;183:1468. [PMID: 11120512]

Naidich MJ, Russell EJ: Current approaches to imaging of the sellar region and pituitary. Endocrinol Metab Clin North Am 1999;28:45. [PMID: 10207685]

Pazos F et al: Prospective randomized study comparing the long-acting gonadotropin-releasing hormone agonist triptorelin, flutamide, and cyproterone acetate, used in combination with an oral contraceptive in the treatment of hirsutism. Fertil Steril 1999;71:122. [PMID: 9935128]

Shin Y et al: Comparison of Diane 35 and Diane 35 plus finasteride in the treatment of hirsutism. Fertil Steril 2001; 75:496. [PMID: 11239530]

Simberg N et al: High bone density in hyperandrogenic women: effect of gonadotropin-releasing hormone agonist alone or in conjunction with estrogen-progestin replacement. J Clin Endocrinol Metab 1996;81:646. [PMID: 8636283]

Sonino N, Boscaro M: Medical therapy for Cushing's disease. Endocrinol Metab Clin North Am 1999;28:211. [PMID: 10207692]

Spritzer PM et al: Spironolactone as a single agent for long-term therapy of hirsute patients. Clin Endocrinol (Oxf) 2000; 52:587. [PMID: 10792338]

Tulandi T, Took SA: Surgical management of ovarian syndrome. Baillière's Clin Obstet Gynaecol 1998;12:541.

Venturoli S et al: A prospective randomized trial comparing low dose flutamide, finasteride, ketoconazole, and cyproterone acetate-estrogen regimens in the treatment of hirsutism. J Clin Endocrinol Metab 1999;84:1304. [PMID: 10199771]

Assisted Reproductive Technologies: In Vitro Fertilization & Related Techniques

58

Catherine M. DeUgarte, MD, Alan H. DeCherney, MD, & Alan S. Penzias, MD

Assisted reproductive technologies (ART) include many techniques that allow gamete manipulation outside the body, and have evolved greatly over the past two decades.

IN VITRO FERTILIZATION

In vitro fertilization (IVF) involves the removal of eggs from the ovary, fertilizing them in the laboratory, and replacing them in the patient's uterus. The first live birth resulting from this technique occurred in June 1978. Since then, thousands of children have been born throughout the world.

Assisted reproductive techniques have come a long way with more programs reporting, an increasing number of cycles treated, an increasing pregnancy rate, and an increase in live births per cycle (from 6.6% in 1985 to 28% in 2003) for IVF. In 2003 there were 122,872 ART cycles (99.4% were IVF cycles and the rest were gamete intrafallopian transfer for fertilization (GIFT) and zygote intrafallopian transfer (ZIFT) cycles. Approximately half of the IVF cycles were IVF/ICSI. From all these cycles, 33,141 deliveries resulted in 45,751 babies. Among the ART cycles using fresh non-donor eggs or embryos, from 91,032 cycles that were started, there were 79,602 retrievals, 74,296 transfers, and 31,348 pregnancies, which resulted in 25,775 live births. The most important prognostic indicator for pregnancy rates is the age of the female partner. After age 43 years, the live birth rate with IVF is 2.4%.

Approximately 39% of patients who undergo egg retrieval will become pregnant with sonographic documentation of an intrauterine pregnancy (clinical pregnancy); 82% of these patients will carry to term. Many "biochemical pregnancies" occur, but these should not be included in pregnancy statistics. (A biochemical pregnancy is one in which serum levels of human chorionic gonadotropin [hCG] rise and then fall before sonographic detection of pregnancy is possible.) Eggs are almost always obtained by aspiration, and under ordinary circumstances, approximately 75% of

eggs will fertilize and cleave. The clinical pregnancy rate of approximately 34% per embryo transfer per IVF cycle is greater than the 20–25% pregnancy rate per cycle observed in spontaneous conceptions in the general population.

The success rate in IVF has been improved by replacing more than 1 embryo, but doing so increases the likelihood of multiple gestations. Among the 31,348 pregnancies that resulted from fresh nondonor cycles in 2002, 54.1% were singletons, 28.1% were twins, and the rest were triplets or more. Although multiple gestations are often welcomed by the infertility couples, they are riskier pregnancies that often result in preterm births.

Indications

In vitro fertilization-embryo transfer (IVF-ET) bypasses the mechanical transport functions of the female reproductive tract. It was first developed for patients with severe tubal disease, and it clearly offers the only hope of conception to patients who have had a bilateral salpingectomy or whose tubes are so badly damaged that they cannot function. Subsequently, in vitro fertilization has been applied to a variety of other infertility problems. Indications for IVF include (a) male factor infertility, (b) tubal disease, (c) decreased ovarian reserve, (d) endometriosis, (e) genetic diseases with need for genetic testing of the embryos, (f) need for third-party reproduction-donor eggs or gestational surrogate, and (g) unexplained infertility. When the probability of conception by IVF exceeds that of conception by conventional therapy, IVF appears to be the procedure of choice. Because of an increased incidence of infertility in our modern society in which women work earlier and conceive later and there is an increased awareness and availability of ART, the demand for these technologies has grown.

Although IVF is successful in treating many infertility problems, its success hinges on entry of sperm into the egg. It was initially hoped that routine IVF could be used to compensate for severe oligospermia (< 5 million sperm/mL). However, early results were highly variable. Advances in this area are now being applied in clinical practice. Modern microsurgical techniques permit placement of sperm directly into the cytoplasm of the oocyte. This is discussed in detail below. In addition to male factor issues, another barrier to success with IVF is hydrosalpinx (fluid collection in the fallopian tube). This condition may interfere with implantation and additional surgery may be needed so that implantation and pregnancy rates improve.

Technique

A. Superovulation

All ART programs use superovulation to stimulate production of several eggs and to improve timing of egg aspiration. The type of ovulation-induction therapy varies from group to group and is constantly changing. The following methods are used alone or in combination:

1. Clomiphene citrate;
2. Human menopausal gonadotropins—urinary or recombinant;
3. Follicle-stimulating hormone (FSH) products—urinary or recombinant; and
4. Leuteinizing (LH) agonists (mostly used in Europe).

Superovulation is carefully monitored with ultrasound scans to monitor the number and growth of follicles, as well as the uterine lining, and serum estradiol is drawn to assess the function of the follicles. At least 2 or 3 follicles should be developing before proceeding with egg aspiration; otherwise, the cycle is usually abandoned and an alternative stimulation regimen is selected for a subsequent cycle. Serum estradiol levels are complementary to ultrasonography in evaluating the maturation and growth of the developing follicles (200 pg/mL per mature follicle is expected). There is evidence that the pattern of serum estradiol may predict the cycles most likely to result in pregnancy. A declining estradiol level prior to hCG administration is associated with a lower pregnancy rate. hCG (either urinary or recombinant) is usually administered when the mature follicles have reached at least 17 mm in diameter to induce ovulation. Ovulation usually occurs 36 hours after hCG injection.

The introduction of gonadotropin-releasing hormone (GnRH) agonists or antagonists to superovulation regimens has drastically reduced the likelihood of a premature LH surge; consequently, they are used in the majority of IVF patients in the United States. The GnRH agonists are usually administered on day 21 or the previous cycle (long protocol) or at the beginning of menses, along with the addition of gonadotropins

(short protocol), and they are continued until the day of hCG. When GnRH antagonists are used, treatment with antagonists begins after 5–6 days of gonadotropins or when the lead follicle is 13 mm. The antagonists have the advantage of requiring fewer injections; however, there may not be a difference in pregnancy rates when using the agonists versus the antagonists.

B. Oocyte Retrieval

Aspiration of the preovulatory follicles is performed approximately 34–36 hours after the hCG injection.

Egg aspiration is performed using either of two methods. Laparoscopy was the first method to be used and is rarely used today. The second method uses ultrasonography to direct transvaginal aspiration. In transvaginal aspiration, a needle is passed through the posterior vaginal fornix using a vaginal ultrasound probe and directed into the ovary. The advantage of ultrasound aspiration is that it can be performed on an outpatient basis, it is simpler, less invasive, and less expensive.

C. Fertilization with Capacitated Sperm and Intracytoplasmic Sperm Injection (ICSI)

Freshly ejaculated sperm cannot fertilize an egg; the sperm must be capacitated. Fortunately, capacitation is a very simple process in humans and involves only a short incubation period in a culture medium.

Because of the nature of the superovulatory process, eggs will be in different stages of maturation. Once the eggs have been identified, the embryologist classifies them as either mature (preovulatory) or immature. Mature eggs have an expanded cumulus oophorus, whereas immature eggs have a very compact cumulus. Mature eggs have undergone the first meiotic division and the first polar body is visible; immature eggs have not. Mature eggs are usually fertilized 5 hours after aspiration. Immature eggs can be incubated in the laboratory for up to 36 hours prior to fertilization. If sperm and eggs are mixed too early, fertilization and cleavage will not take place. Between 50,000 and 150,000 motile sperm are placed with each egg.

For male factor infertility (< 5 million total normal motile sperm/mL), intracytoplasmic sperm injection has emerged as an effective solution, resulting in higher fertilization rates and expanded possibilities for cryopreservation. In this procedure, 1 normal motile sperm is selected per oocyte and injected directly into the cytoplasm away from the polar body. Other indications for ICSI include surgically retrieved sperm (for men with azoospermia who need testicular or epididymal biopsy), cryopreserved oocytes, or cases in which preimplantation genetic diagnosis (PGD) is performed for single gene disorders.

D. Embryo Culture

Embryos are incubated in an atmosphere of ≤ 5% carbon dioxide. Various culture media are used and are often supplemented with either the patient's serum or synthetic albumin as well as essential and nonessential amino acids and sugars. At various intervals after the attempted fertilization, the embryos are examined in order to identify pronuclei, which confirm fertilization, as well as the stage of cleavage.

E. Embryo Transfer

After 3–5 days of laboratory culture, the embryos are replaced into the patient's uterus, a procedure named *embryo transfer*. Prior to transfer, the embryos are graded from A to D depending on their appearance and on the degree of fragmentation. If day 5 or 6 transfers are performed, the embryos are at the blastocyst stage. The decision to transfer on day 3 or 5 depends on the success rates of the lab and the physicians. The decision of how many embryos to transfer is done by the patient in conjunction with the physician and the embryologist in conjunction with the American Society for Reproductive Medicine (ASRM) recommendations based on the patient's age (Table 58–1).

Most embryo transfers are performed under direct visualization with 2-dimensional (2-D) or 3-dimensional (3-D) ultrasounds. Before the embryo transfer is performed, the patient is usually asked to drink water so as to fill the bladder. A full bladder helps straighten the uterus as well as to improve visualization by ultrasound during the transfer. The embryologist prepares the best embryos by aspirating them into a small catheter with some media, and after the physician cleans the cervix with culture media and aspirates the extra cervical mucous, the catheter is passed transcervically into the uterus, and the embryos are injected into the uterine cavity under direct visualization. The probability of pregnancy after embryo transfer can be affected by the patient's age, the cause of infertility, the endometrial thickness, and the average embryo grade.

In some patients, assisted hatching or an opening in the zona is performed in order to improve implantation. This is thought to be beneficial in older patients (age 38 years and older) who have harder zonae; however, it is not routinely performed in all IVF centers.

F. Luteal Phase Support

After embryo transfer is performed, progesterone supplementation is usually recommended by most physicians until approximately 7 weeks' gestation. Progesterone is usually administered by an intramuscular injection or by a vaginal suppository or gel.

Table 58–1. Recommended number of embryos to transfer

Age (years)	Number
< 35	2 (consider 1 if previous successful IVF cycle, great embryos, 1st IVF cycle)
35–37	2–3
38–40	3–4
> 40	5
Age independent	In some cases, such as previous failed IVF cycles or unfavorable prognosis, OK to transfer more

Complications

Few risks are associated with ART. Some of the complications and drawbacks of ART are as follows:

1. Multiple gestations—Transferring more embryos does not necessarily lead to a greater IVF success rate. If embryos are left over, they can be either frozen for later use or be donated to another couple. A frozen embryo is thought to have one-half the potential for successful implantation of a fresh embryo. Recently, the methods for oocyte freezing have been improved as well, with some labs reporting comparable pregnancy rates in fresh or frozen cycles.

2. Ectopic and heterotopic pregnancies—Patients who undergo ART procedure are at twice the risk for having an ectopic pregnancy as the general population. Heterotypic pregnancies, which are rare but seen more commonly with ART, involve cases in which there is an intrauterine pregnancy and an ectopic pregnancy in the same patient.

3. Cost—Currently only a few states allow health insurance to cover infertility treatment, which leaves many couples with tremendous expenses (the estimated cost per delivery is $66,667).

4. Preterm birth and low-birth-weight infants—These are higher in patients undergoing IVF.

5. Ovarian hyperstimulation syndrome—This syndrome is characterized by ovarian enlargement, ascites, and hemoconcentration. Risk factors include polycystic ovary syndrome, multiple follicles, and high estradiol levels. The prognosis is usually worse in patients who get pregnant and have this syndrome. Patients with this syndrome may be at risk for blood clots.

6. Congenital abnormalities—The risk of congenital abnormalities may be slightly higher in patients who use ART; however, this concept is still controversial. In patients who have ICSI performed,

the risk of imprinting disorders may be increased (such as Angelman's syndrome and Beckwith-Wiedemann syndrome).

OTHER TECHNIQUES RELATED TO IVF-ET

Ovum Donation

Embryos have been donated from one woman to another with many resultant live births. Women who receive donated embryos include those with ovarian failure or absence (eg, gonadal dysgenesis), diminished ovarian reserve, or genetically transmitted disorders.

Ovum donation can occur under either of two circumstances. One circumstance is the infertile patient who produces a large number of oocytes during her own IVF or GIFT cycle and elects to donate some of them to another woman who is otherwise incapable of producing eggs. The other, more common circumstance involves the recruitment of a woman who undergoes superovulation and oocyte retrieval purely for the purpose of donating her oocytes. The donor may be known to the patient (a family member or friend), or more commonly may be anonymous. Although the genetics of the resulting pregnancy are derived from the husband and the donor, the infertile woman incapable of producing her own eggs goes through the pregnancy. In these cases, the endometrium of the recipient must be primed with estrogen and progesterone prior to transfer of the donated embryos, and progesterone and estrogen supplementation must be maintained for at least 10 weeks. The number of embryos transferred is decided based on the age of the donor, not the age of the recipient.

Gestational Surrogacy

Sometimes a woman may be able to make eggs but may not be able to carry the gestation. These are women with certain medical conditions that are medically unfit to carry pregnancy or women who have no uterus, or have a uterus that is unsuitable for pregnancy. In these cases, a gestational surrogate may be used and transfer of the embryo is done into a uterus of a woman who has agreed to carry the pregnancy.

Gamete Intrafallopian Tube Transfer (GIFT)

GIFT is similar to IVF. It was first used in 1984 and the number of cycles in North America increased 75-fold from 75 in 1985 to 5767 in 1992, and the pregnancy rate rose from 4% to 29.5%. However with the improved pregnancy rates in IVF, GIFT procedures are rarely done now. Usual indications for GIFT nowadays include patients who have moral or religious objections to IVF and want to have fertilization in vivo rather than in vitro. As with IVF, superovulation is induced and the follicles are aspirated vaginally under ultrasound guidance. The eggs are then identified in the laboratory. Thereafter, sperm is collected and capacitated, and laparoscopy is performed. Sperm are then mixed with the eggs and drawn up into a catheter. The sperm and eggs can also be separated by an air bubble in the catheter, after which they are transferred into one of the fallopian tubes, permitting in vivo fertilization and cleavage. A 20–30% pregnancy rate per cycle has been reported for this technique.

Obviously, GIFT is useful only in patients who have normal tube function and are not of advanced age. It has been argued that the requirement of normal tubal function renders the direct comparison of IVF-ET and GIFT results impossible. Among proponents of each technique, there is vigorous ongoing debate as to the advantages of GIFT over IVF-ET.

In unexplained infertility, IVF-ET will differentiate the etiology of fertilization problems between egg and sperm; GIFT will not. Additionally, GIFT exposes patients to the risks of general anesthesia and laparoscopy. GIFT is now rarely used.

Zygote Intrafallopian Transfer

ZIFT is a procedure that combines IVF and GIFT. Ovulation is induced and the oocytes are removed and fertilized in vitro. Soon thereafter the zygotes are placed into the fallopian tubes by laparoscopy similar to GIFT and the embryo travels to the uterine cavity. ZIFT also is now rarely used.

Preimplantation Genetic Diagnosis

PGD is a technology that has been around since early 1990. It allows many genetically heritable diseases to be identified using a variety of molecular biologic techniques. These techniques include but are not limited to polymerase chain reaction (PCR) and fluorescent in situ hybridization (FISH). Recent advances in embryo manipulation have made possible the removal of 1 or 2 cells, or blastomeres, from a developing 8-cell human embryo without harm to the embryo. Biopsy of the first and/or second polar bodies can also be done for several single-gene defects. In patients at risk of passing along a heritable genetic disease, PGD has made possible the identification of normal embryos (those with no risk of passing the heritable disease). These normal embryos are then transferred back to the patient. More than 1000 live births have been reported following application of these techniques. The number of centers performing these techniques are few but growing. PGD is also performed for patients with recurrent miscarriages, previous failed IVF cycles, aneuploidy diagnosis for patients with advanced maternal age, and for sex selection, but these indications are still controversial.

Cryopreservation

Cryopreservation is the process by which embryos or eggs are frozen to be used at a later time after thawing (unfreezing). Cryopreservation of embryos is very successful and has greatly improved since the first case in 1983. Survival rates of frozen embryos have been reported to be between 50% and 90%. Before thawing embryos, the patient's cycle is usually synchronized so that embryo transfer occurs during the implantation window of the uterus. Consequently, pretreatment with estrogen and progesterone is recommended. In 2003, the live birth rate per transfer of frozen embryos was 27%.

Cryopreservation of oocytes has been gaining attention and has improved over the past few years; however, it remains investigational. The same is true for ovarian cryopreservation and autologous transplantation (when the ovary is removed and transferred to a different location such as the forearm or abdomen).

REFERENCES

In Vitro Fertilization and ART

Abusheikha N, Salha O, Brinsden P: Extra-uterine pregnancy following assisted conception treatment. Hum Reprod Update 2000;6:80.

Agrawal R, Holmes J, Jacobs HS: Follicle-stimulating hormone or human menopausal gonadotropin for ovarian stimulation in in vitro fertilization cycles: a meta-analysis. Fertil Steril 2003; 80:1086.

Akande VA et al: Biologic versus chronological aging of oocytes, distinguishable by raised FSH levels in relation to the success of IVF treatment. Hum Reprod 2002;17:2003.

Albuquerque LE et al: Depot versus daily administration of GnRH agonist protocols for pituitary desensitization in assisted reproduction cycles: a Cochrane review. Hum Reprod 2003; 18:2008.

American Society for Reproductive Medicine: *Guidelines on Number of Embryos Transferred*. Birmingham, AL, 2004.

Balasch J, Barri PN: Reflections on the cost-effectiveness of recombinant FSH in assisted reproduction. The clinician's perspective. J Assist Reprod Genet 2001;18:45.

Baird DT: Is there a place for different isoforms of FSH in clinical medicine? IV. The clinician's point of view. Hum Reprod 2001;16:1316.

Barnhart K, Dunsmoor-Su R, Coutifaris C: Effect of endometriosis on in vitro fertilization. Fertil Steril 2002;77:1148.

Camus E et al: Pregnancy rates after in-vitro fertilization in cases of tubal infertility with and without hydrosalpinx: a meta-analysis of published comparative studies. Hum Reprod 1999;14:1243.

CDC Report 2005. National Summary and Fertility Clinic Report. http://www.cdc.gov/ART/ART/ART2005.

Chen D et al: Ovarian hyperstimulation syndrome: strategies for prevention. Reprod Biomed Online 2003;7:43.

Coroleu B et al: Embryo transfer under ultrasound guidance improves pregnancy rates after in-vitro fertilization. Hum Reprod 2000;15:616.

Cox GF et al: Intracytoplasmic sperm injection may increase the risk of imprinting defects. Am J Hum Genet 2002;71:162.

Desai NN et al: Morphological evaluation of human embryos and derivation of an embryo quality scoring system specific for day 3 embryos: a preliminary study. Hum Reprod 2000;15: 2190.

Edi-Osagie E, Hooper L, Seif MW: The impact of assisted hatching on live birth rates and outcomes of assisted conception: a systematic review. Hum Reprod 2003;18:1828.

Engel JB et al: Use of cetrorelix in combination with clomiphene citrate and gonadotropins: a suitable approach to "friendly IVF." Hum Reprod 2002;17:2022.

Engmann L et al: Trends in the incidence of births and multiple births and the factors that determine the probability of multiple birth after IVF treatment. Hum Reprod 2001;16:2598.

Ericson A, Kallen B: Congenital malformations in infants born after IVF: a population-based study. Hum Reprod 2001;16:504.

Filicori M et al: Comparison of controlled ovarian stimulation with human menopausal gonadotropin or recombinant follicle stimulating hormone. Fertil Steril 2003;80:1100.

Friedler S et al: Factors influencing the outcome of ICSI in patients with obstructive and non-obstructive azoospermia: a comparative study. Hum Reprod 2002;17:3114.

Garcia-Velasco JA, Isaza V, Requena A: High doses of gonadotrophins combined with stop versus non-stop protocol of GnRH analogue administration in low responder IVF patients: a prospective, randomized, controlled trial. Hum Reprod 2000;15:2292.

Gleicher N et al: Reducing the risk of high-order multiple pregnancy after ovarian stimulation with gonadotropins. N Engl J Med 2000;343:2.

Hansen M et al: The risk of major birth defects after intracytoplasmic sperm injection and in vitro fertilization. N Engl J Med 2002;346:725.

Hugues JN, Bry-Gauillard H, Bstandig B: Comparison of recombinant and urinary follicle-stimulating hormone preparations in short-term gonadotropin releasing hormone agonist protocol for in vitro fertilization-embryo transfer. J Assist Reprod Genet 2001;18:191.

Ingerslev HJ et al: A randomized study comparing IVF in the unstimulated cycle with IVF following clomiphene citrate. Hum Reprod 2001;16:696.

Langley MT et al: Extended embryo culture in human assisted reproduction treatments. Hum Reprod 2001;16:902.

Ludwig M, Doody KJ, Doody KM. Use of recombinant human chorionic gonadotropin in ovulation induction. Fertil Steril 2003;79:1051.

Ludwig M, Rietmuller-Winzen H, Felberbaum RE: Health of 227 children born after controlled ovarian stimulation for in vitro fertilization using the luteinizing hormone-releasing hormone antagonist cetrorelix. Fertil Steril 2001;75:18.

Milki AA et al: Accuracy of day 3 criteria for selecting the best embryos. Fertil Steril 2002;77:1191.

Muasher SJ, Abdallah RT, Hubayter ZR: Optimal stimulation protocols for in vitro fertilization. Fertil Steril 2006;86(2)267.

Nargund G, Waterstone J, Bland J: Cumulative conception and live birth rates in natural (unstimulated) IVF cycles. Hum Reprod 2001;16:259.

Nikolettos N et al: Gonadotropin-releasing hormone antagonist protocol: A novel method of ovarian stimulation in poor responders. Eur J Obstet Gynecol Reprod Biol 2001;97:202.

Olivennes F et al: The use of GnRH antagonists in ovarian stimulation. Hum Reprod Update 2002;8:279.

Plachot M et al: Outcome of conventional IVF and ICSI on sibling oocytes in mild male factor infertility. Hum Reprod 2002;17:362.

Pritts E, Atwood AK: Luteal phase support in infertility treatment: a meta-analysis of the randomized trials. Hum Reprod 2002; 17:2287.

Propst AM et al: A randomized trial comparing Crinone 8% and intramuscular progesterone supplementation in in vitro fertilization-embryo transfer cycles. Fertil Steril 2001;76:1144.

Schieve LA et al: Low and very low birth weight in infants conceived with use of assisted reproductive technology. N Engl J Med 2002;346:731.

Schoolcraft WB, Surrey ES, Gardner DK: Embryo transfer: techniques and variables affecting success. Fertil Steril 2001;76:863.

Sharlip ID et al: Best practice policies for male infertility. Fertil Steril 2002;77:873.

Shoham Z: The clinical therapeutic window for luteinizing hormone in controlled ovarian stimulation. Fertil Steril 2002;77:1170.

Speroff L, Fritz MA: *Clinical Gynecologic Endocrinology and Infertility*, 7th ed. Lippincott Williams & Wilkins, 2005.

Stelling JR et al: Subcutaneous versus intramuscular administration of human chorionic gonadotropin during an in vitro fertilization cycle. Fertil Steril 2003;79:881.

Steptoe PC, Edwards RG: Birth after the reimplantation of a human embryo. Lancet 1978;2:366.

Strehler E, Abt M, El-Danasouri I: Impact of recombinant follicle-stimulating hormone and human menopausal gonadotropins on in vitro fertilization outcome. Fertil Steril 2001;75:332.

Surrey ES, Schoolcraft WB. Laparoscopic management of hydrosalpinges before in vitro fertilization-embryo transfer: salpingectomy vs. proximal tubal occlusion Fertil Steril 2001;75:612.

Tarlatzis BC, Bili H: Intracytoplasmic sperm injection. Survey of world results. Ann N Y Acad Sci 2000;900:336.

Taylor RC, Berkowitz J, McComb PF: Role of laparoscopic salpingectomy in the treatment of hydrosalpinx. Fertil Steril 2001;75:594.

Terriou P et al: Embryo scoring is a better predictor of pregnancy than the number of transferred embryos or female age. Fertil Steril 2001;75:525.

The ESHRE Capri Workshop Group: Multiple gestation pregnancy. Hum Reprod 2000;15:1856.

Vahratian A et al: Live-birth rates and multiple-birth risk of assisted reproductive technology pregnancies conceived using thawed embryos, USA 1999–2000. Hum Reprod 2003;18:1442.

Van Voorhis BJ, Barnett M, Sparks AE: Effect of the total motile sperm count on the efficacy and cost-effectiveness of intrauterine insemination and in vitro fertilization. Fertil Steril 2001;75:661.

Wigert M et al: Comparison of stimulation with clomiphene citrate in combination with recombinant follicle-stimulating hormone and recombinant luteinizing hormone to stimulation with a gonadotropin-releasing hormone agonist protocol: a prospective, randomized study. Fertil Steril 2002;78:34.

Wilson M et al: Integration of blastocyst transfer for all patients. Fertil Steril 2002;77:693.

Yim SF, Lok IH, Cheung LP: Dose-finding study for the use of long-acting gonadotrophin-releasing hormone analogues prior to ovarian stimulation for IVF. Hum Reprod 2001;16:492.

Zayed F, Ghazawi I, Francis L: Predictive value of human chorionic gonadotrophin in early pregnancy after assisted conception. Arch Gynecol Obstet 2001;265:7.

Zuppa AA, Maragliano G, Scapillati ME: Neonatal outcome of spontaneous and assisted twin pregnancies. Eur J Obstet Gynecol Reprod Biol 2001;95:68.

Other Techniques Related to IVF

Aubard Y et al: Ovarian tissue cryopreservation and gynecologic oncology: A review. Eur J Obstet Gynecol Reprod Biol 2001;97:5.

Farhi J, Weissman A, Nahum H: Zygote intrafallopian transfer in patients with tubal factor infertility after repeated failure of implantation with in vitro fertilization-embryo transfer. Fertil Steril 2000;74:390.

Licciardi F et al: A two versus three embryo transfer: the oocyte donation model. Fertil Steril 2001;75:510.

Oktay K, Kan MT, Rosenwaks Z: Recent progress in oocyte and ovarian tissue cryopreservation and transplantation. Curr Opin Obstet Gynecol 2001;13:263.

Oktay K, Karlikaya G: Ovarian function after the transplantation of frozen, banked autologous ovarian tissue. N Engl J Med 2000;342:1919.

Pantos K et al: Cryopreservation of embryos, blastocysts, and pregnancy rates of blastocysts derived from frozen-thawed embryos and frozen-thawed blastocysts. J Assist Reprod Genet 2001;18:579.

Schoolcraft WB, Gardner DK: Blastocyst culture and transfer increases the efficiency of oocyte donation. Fertil Steril 2000;74:482.

Senn A: Prospective randomized study of two cryopreservation policies avoiding embryo selection: the pronuclear stage leads to a higher cumulative delivery rate than the early cleavage stage. Fertil Steril 2000;74:946.

Shenfield F, Pennings G, Sureau C: The cryopreservation of human embryos. Hum Reprod 2001;16:1049.

Silva PD, Olson KL, Meisch JK: Gamete intrafallopian transfer. A cost-effective alternative to donor oocyte in vitro fertilization in women aged 40–42 years. J Reprod Med 1998;43:1019.

Soderstrom-Antilla V: Oocyte donation in infertility treatment—a review. Acta Obstet Gynecol Scand 2001;80:191.

Soderstrom-Antilla V: Pregnancy and child outcome after oocyte donation. Hum Reprod Update 2001;7:28.

Speroff L, Fritz MA: *Clinical Gynecologic Endocrinology and Infertility*, 7th ed. Lippincott Williams & Wilkins, 2005.

Tarlatzis BC, Pados G: Oocyte donation: clinical and practical aspects. Mol Cell Endocrinol 2000;161:99.

Thornhill AR et al: Best practice guidelines for clinical preimplantation diagnosis (PGD) and preimplantation genetic screening (PGS) Hum Reprod 2005;20:35

Verlinsky Y et al: Over a decade of experience with preimplantation genetic diagnosis: a multicenter report. Fertil Steril 2004;82:292.

Menopause & Postmenopause

Lauren Nathan, MD, & Howard L. Judd, MD

According to the 2002 U.S. census, of the 144 million women in this country, 33 million were 55 years of age or older. Most of these women had or shortly would have their last menstrual period, thus becoming post-menopausal. As a woman at age 55 years can expect to live another 28 years, a large portion of the female population is without ovarian function and lives about one-third of their lives after this function ceases. Consequently, physicians caring for women must understand the hormonal and metabolic changes associated with the menopause, or "change of life," and the potential benefits and risks of hormone therapy (HT).

According to the Comite des Nomenclatures de la Federation Internationale de Gynecologie et d'Obstetrique, the **climacteric** is the phase of the aging process during which a woman passes from the reproductive to the nonreproductive stage. The signals that this period of life has been reached are referred to as "climacteric symptoms" or, if more serious, as "climacteric complaints." **Perimenopause,** or **menopausal transition,** refers to the part of the climacteric before the menopause occurs when the menstrual cycle is likely to be irregular and when other climacteric symptoms or complaints may be experienced. The **menopause** is the final menstruation, which occurs during the climacteric. **Postmenopause** refers to the phase of life that comes after the menopause.

To develop a more functional staging system of reproductive aging, the Stages of Reproductive Aging Workshop (STRAW) was held in 2001. The specific goals of the workshop were to (a) develop a useful staging system, (b) revise nomenclature, and (c) identify knowledge gaps that should be addressed by the research community. According to STRAW, reproductive aging is divided into 7 stages (−5 to +2), with −5 beginning with menarche and +2 being defined as the late menopause. This staging system is not applicable to women who smoke, who are at the extremes of weight, who engage in heavy aerobic exercise, who have chronic menstrual irregularity, who have undergone hysterectomy, or who have abnormal uterine or ovarian anatomy.

The **menopausal transition,** or **perimenopause,** is divided into two stages—early (−2) and late (−1) and encompasses a wide age range. Both stages vary in length and both are characterized by an elevation in early follicular phase follicle-stimulating hormone (FSH). In stage −2, the menstrual cycles remain regular, but the cycle length changes by 7 days or more (ie, cycle length becomes 24 days instead of 31). Stage −1 (late menopausal transition) is characterized by two or more skipped menstrual cycles and at least one intermenstrual interval of 60 days or more. Many women begin to experience symptoms during this time which may include vasomotor symptoms, and sleep disturbance. The early postmenopausal period (stage +1) includes the first 5 years following the final menstrual period and the late postmenopausal period (stage +2) begins 5 years after the final menstrual period and continues until death.

Etiology & Pathogenesis

A. PREMENOPAUSAL STATE

The decades of mature reproductive life are characterized by generally regular menses and a slow, steady decrease in cycle length. Mean cycle length at age 15 years is 35 days, at age 25 years it is 30 days, and at age 35 years it is 28 days. This decrease is a result of shortening of the follicular phase of the cycle, with the luteal phase length remaining constant. After age 45 years, altered function of the aging ovary is detectable in regularly menstruating women (Fig 59–1). The mean cycle length is significantly shorter than in younger women and is attributable to a shortened follicular phase. The luteal phase is of similar length, and progesterone levels are no different from those observed in younger women. Estradiol levels are lower during portions of the cycle, including active follicular maturation, the midcycle peak, and the luteal phase. Concentrations of FSH are strikingly elevated during the early follicular phase and fall as estradiol increases during follicular maturation. FSH levels at the midcycle peak and late in the luteal phase are also consistently higher than those found in younger women and decrease during the midluteal phase. Luteinizing hormone (LH) concentrations are indistinguishable from those observed in younger women. The mechanism responsible for this early rise of FSH is probably related to inhibin. **Inhibin** is a polypeptide hormone that is synthesized and secreted by granulosa cells. It causes negative feedback on FSH re-

Figure 59–1. Mean and range of LH, FSH, estradiol (E₂), and progesterone levels in women over age 45 with regular menstrual cycles. Shaded area represents the mean (±2 SEM) in cycles found in young women. (Reproduced with permission from Sherman BM, Korenman SG: Hormonal characteristics of the human menstrual cycle throughout reproductive life. J Clin Invest 1975;55:699.)

lease by the pituitary. As the oocyte number decreases, inhibin levels fall, resulting in a rise in FSH levels.

The transition from regular cycle intervals to the permanent amenorrhea of menopause is characterized by a phase of marked menstrual irregularity. The duration of this transition varies greatly among women. Those experiencing the menopause at an early age have a relatively short duration of cycle variability before amenorrhea ensues. Those experiencing it at a later age usually have a phase of menstrual irregularity characterized by unusually long and short intermenstrual intervals and an overall increase of mean cycle length and variance.

The hormonal characteristics of this transitional phase are of special interest and importance. The irregular episodes of vaginal bleeding in premenopausal women represent the irregular maturation of ovarian follicles with or without hormonal evidence of ovulation. The potential for hormone secretion by these remaining follicles is diminished and variable. Menses are sometimes preceded by maturation of a follicle with limited secretion of both estradiol and progesterone.

Vaginal bleeding also happens after a rise and fall of estradiol without a measurable increase in progesterone, such as is seen during anovulatory menses.

From these findings, it is clear that the transitional phase of menstrual irregularity is not one of marked estrogen deficiency. During the menopausal transition, high levels of FSH appear to stimulate residual follicles to secrete bursts of estradiol. Occasionally, estradiol levels will rise to concentrations 2 or 3 times higher than is normally seen, probably reflecting the recruitment of more than 1 follicle for ovulation. This may be followed by corpus luteum formation, often with limited secretion of progesterone. Because the episodes of follicular maturation and vaginal bleeding are widely spaced, premenopausal women may be exposed to persistent estrogen stimulation of the endometrium in the absence of regular cyclic progesterone secretion.

B. MENOPAUSE

The two types of menopause are classified according to cause.

1. Physiologic menopause—In the human embryo, oogenesis begins in the ovary around the third week of gestation. Primordial germ cells appear in the yolk sac, migrate to the germinal ridge, and undergo cellular divisions. It is estimated that the fetal ovaries contain approximately 7 million oogonia at 20 weeks' gestation. After 7 months' gestation, no new oocytes are formed. At birth, there are approximately 1–2 million oocytes, and by puberty this number is reduced to 300,000–500,000. Continued reduction of oocyte numbers occurs during the reproductive years through ovulation and atresia. Nearly all oocytes vanish by atresia, with only 400–500 actually being ovulated. Very little is known about oocyte atresia. Animal studies show that estrogens prevent the atretic process while androgens enhance it.

Menopause apparently occurs in the human female because of two processes. First, oocytes responsive to gonadotropins disappear from the ovary, and second, the few remaining oocytes do not respond to gonadotropins. Isolated oocytes can be found in postmenopausal ovaries on very careful histologic inspection. Some of them show a limited degree of development, but most reveal no sign of development in the presence of excess endogenous gonadotropins.

The average age at menopause in the United States is 50–51 years. There does not appear to be any consistent relationship between age at menarche and age at menopause. Marriage, childbearing, height, weight, and prolonged use of oral contraceptives do not appear to influence the age of menopause. Smoking, however, is associated with early menopause.

Spontaneous cessation of menses before age 40 years is called **premature menopause,** or **premature ovarian**

failure. It appears that approximately 0.9% of women in the United States may experience this early cessation of function. Cessation of menstruation and the development of climacteric symptoms and complaints can occur as early as a few years after menarche. The reasons for premature ovarian failure are unknown.

Disease processes, especially severe infections or tumors of the reproductive tract, can occasionally damage the ovarian follicular structures so severely as to precipitate the menopause. The menopause can also be hastened by excessive exposure to ionizing radiation, chemotherapeutic drugs, particularly alkylating agents, and surgical procedures that impair ovarian blood supply. The possibility of associated endocrine or chromosomal abnormalities should also be considered.

2. Artificial menopause—The permanent cessation of ovarian function brought about by surgical removal of the ovaries or by radiation therapy is called an artificial menopause. Irradiation to ablate ovarian function is rarely used today. Artificial menopause is employed as a treatment for endometriosis and rarely may be used to treat estrogen-sensitive neoplasms of the breast and endometrium. More frequently, artificial menopause is a side effect of treatment of intra-abdominal disease; eg, ovaries are removed in premenopausal women because the gonads have been damaged by infection or neoplasia. When laparotomy is being performed for intra-abdominal or pelvic disease (ie, hysterectomy for leiomyomata), elective bilateral oophorectomy is sometimes employed to prevent ovarian cancer. In some women who are genetically predisposed to ovarian cancer, elective laparoscopic oophorectomy is also performed.

C. CHANGES IN HORMONE METABOLISM ASSOCIATED WITH THE MENOPAUSE

Following the menopause, there are major changes in androgen, estrogen, progesterone, and gonadotropin secretion, much of which occurs because of cessation of ovarian follicular activity (Fig 59–2).

1. Androgens—During reproductive life, the primary ovarian androgen is androstenedione, the major secretory product of developing follicles. In postmenopausal women, there is a reduction of circulating androstenedione to approximately 50% of the concentration found in young women, reflecting the absence of follicular activity. In the year following the last menstrual period, the levels of this hormone are steady. In older women, there is a circadian variation of androstenedione, with peak concentration between 8:00 AM and 12 noon, and the nadir occurring between 3:00 PM and 4:00 AM. This rhythm reflects adrenal activity. The clearance rate of androstenedione is similar in pre- and postmenopausal women; therefore, the change in levels of circulating hormone reflects changes in production. Thus, the average production rate of androstenedione is

Figure 59–2. Serum androgen and estrogen levels in 16 postmenopausal women with endometrial cancer before and after oophorectomy. (Reproduced with permission from Judd HL: Hormonal dynamics associated with the menopause. Clin Obstet Gynecol 1976; 1:775.)

approximately 1.5 mg/24 h in older women, a rate that is 50% of the rate found in premenopausal women. The source of most of this circulating androstenedione appears to be the adrenal glands, but continued secretion by the postmenopausal ovary accounts for approximately 20%.

For testosterone, the level found in postmenopausal women is only minimally lower than that found in premenopausal women before oophorectomy and is distinctly higher than the level observed in ovariectomized young women. There is also a prominent circadian variation of this androgen, with the highest levels occurring at 8:00 AM and the nadir at 4:00 PM. There is no difference in the clearance rate of testosterone before and after the menopause. Thus, the production rate in older women is approximately 150 μg/24 h, a rate that is only one-third lower than the rate seen in young women.

The source of circulating testosterone is more complex than that of androstenedione. Oophorectomy following menopause is associated with a nearly 60% decrease in testosterone. There is no change in the metabolic clearance rate of the androgen with oophorectomy; therefore, the fall in the circulating level reflects alterations of its production rate. Approximately 15% of circulating androstenedione is converted to testosterone. The small simultaneous fall of androstenedione after oophorectomy can only account for a small portion of the total decrease of testosterone. The remainder of the loss presumably represents loss from direct ovarian secretion of testosterone. Direct ovarian secretion in the postmenopausal ovary is larger than the amount secreted directly by the premenopausal ovary. Large increments in testosterone have been found in the ovarian compared with the peripheral veins of postmenopausal women. These increments are greater than those observed in premenopausal women, supporting the hypothesis that the postmenopausal ovary secretes more testosterone directly than the premenopausal ovary. Hilar cells and luteinized stromal cells (hyperthecosis) are present in most postmenopausal ovaries and have been shown to produce testosterone in premenopausal women. Presumably, these cells could do the same in postmenopausal subjects.

A proposed mechanism for increased ovarian testosterone production by postmenopausal ovaries is the stimulation of gonadal cells still capable of androgen production by excess endogenous gonadotropins, which, in turn, are increased because of reduced estrogen production by the ovaries. This increased ovarian testosterone secretion, coupled with a reduction of estrogen production, and decrease in sex hormone-binding globulin (SHBG) may partly explain the development of symptoms of defeminization, hirsutism, and even virilism occasionally seen in older women.

Levels of the adrenal androgens dehydroepiandrosterone (DHEA) and dehydroepiandrosterone sulfate (DHEAS) are reduced by 60% and 80%, respectively, with age. Whether these reductions are related to the menopause or to aging has not been determined. Again, a marked circadian variation of DHEA has been observed. Whether a similar rhythm is present for DHEAS is unknown. As with younger subjects, the primary source of these two androgens is thought to be the adrenal glands, with the ovary contributing less than 15%. Thus, the marked decreases of DHEA and DHEAS reflect altered adrenal androgen secretion, and this phenomenon has been called the *adrenopause*. The mechanism responsible for it is unknown.

In premenopausal women, plasma androstenedione is approximately 1.5 ng/mL. Plasma testosterone is about 0.3 ng/mL. Mean DHEA and DHEAS levels are approximately 4 ng/mL and 1600 ng/mL, respectively, in samples drawn at 8:00 AM.

In postmenopausal women, the mean plasma androstenedione concentration is reduced by at least 50%, to approximately 0.6 ng/mL. Plasma testosterone levels are only slightly reduced (to about 0.25 ng/mL). Plasma DHEA and DHEAS levels are decreased to mean levels of 1.8 ng/mL and 300 ng/mL in women in their sixties and seventies.

2. Estrogens—After a woman has passed the menopause, there is good clinical evidence of reduced endogenous estrogen production in most subjects. When circulating levels have been assessed, the greatest decrease is in estradiol. Its concentration is distinctly lower than that found in young women during any phase of their menstrual cycle and is similar to the level seen in premenopausal women following oophorectomy. A decrease of this estrogen occurs up to 1 year following the last menstrual period. There does not appear to be a circadian variation of the circulating concentration of estradiol following the menopause. The metabolic clearance rate of estradiol is reduced by 30%. The average production rate is 12 μg/24 h.

The source of the small amount of estradiol found in older women has been established. Direct ovarian secretion contributes minimally, but the adrenal glands are the major source. Investigators who have examined the concentrations of estradiol in adrenal veins have reported minimal increments, arguing against direct adrenal secretion being a major contributor. Although both estrone and testosterone are converted in peripheral tissues to estradiol, it is conversion from estrone that accounts for most estradiol in older women.

After the menopause, the circulating level of estrone decreases—not as much as that of estradiol—and overlaps with values seen in premenopausal women during the early follicular phase in menstrual cycles. There is a circadian variation of circulating estrone, with the peak in the morning and the nadir in late afternoon or early evening. This variation is not as prominent as that observed for the androgens. In postmenopausal women, there is a 20% reduction of estrone clearance, and the average production rate is approximately 55 μg/24 h.

The adrenal gland is the major source of estrone. Direct adrenal or ovarian secretion is minimal. Most estrone results from the peripheral aromatization of androstenedione. The average percent conversion is double that found in ovulatory women and can account for the total daily production of this estrogen. Aromatization of androstenedione occurs in fat, muscle, liver, bone marrow, brain, fibroblasts, and hair roots. Other tissues may also contribute but have not been evaluated. To what extent each cell type contributes to total conversion has not been determined, but fat cells and muscle may be responsible for only 30–40%. This conversion correlates with body size, with heavy women having higher conversion rates and circulating estrogen levels than slender women.

During normal menstrual life, the mean plasma estradiol fluctuates from 50–350 pg/mL and estrone from 30–110 pg/mL. In postmenopausal women, the mean estradiol level is approximately 12 pg/mL, with a range of 5–25 pg/mL. The mean estrone level is approximately 30 pg/mL, with a range of 20–70 pg/mL. Estradiol levels in normal young women do not overlap with those observed in postmenopausal subjects. The finding

of estradiol levels below 20 pg/mL can be helpful in establishing the diagnosis of menopause, as the fall of this
estrogen is the last hormonal change associated with
loss of ovarian function. There is substantial overlap of
estrone levels in younger and older women. Measurement of this estrogen is not helpful in determining the
ovarian status of a patient.

3. Progesterone—In young women, the major source
of progesterone is the ovarian corpus luteum following
ovulation. During the follicular phase of the cycle,
progesterone levels are low. With ovulation the levels
rise greatly, reflecting the secretory activity of the corpus luteum. In postmenopausal women, the levels of
progesterone are only 30% of the concentrations seen
in young women during the follicular phase. Because
postmenopausal ovaries do not contain functional follicles, ovulation does not occur and progesterone levels
remain low. The source of the small amount of progesterone present in older women is felt to be caused by
adrenal secretion, as dexamethasone suppresses its level,
adrenocorticotropic hormone (ACTH) increases its
level, and human chorionic gonadotropin (hCG) administration has no effect.

In young menstruating women, the mean progesterone level is approximately 0.4 ng/mL during the follicular phase of the cycle, with a range of 0.2–0.7 ng/mL.
During the luteal phase, progesterone levels rise and
fall, reflecting corpus luteum function; the mean level is
approximately 11 ng/mL with a range of 3–21 ng/mL.
In postmenopausal women, the mean progesterone
level is 0.17 ng/mL. To date, no clinical use has been
established for the measurement of progesterone in
postmenopausal women.

4. Gonadotropins—With the menopause, both LH
and FSH levels rise substantially, with FSH usually
higher than LH. This is thought to reflect the slower
clearance of FSH from the circulation. The reason for the
marked increase in circulating gonadotropins is the absence of the negative feedback of ovarian steroids and inhibin on gonadotropin release. As in young women, the
levels of both gonadotropins are not steady, but instead
show random oscillations. These oscillations are thought
to represent pulsatile secretion by the pituitary. In older
women, these pulsatile bursts occur every 1–2 hours, a frequency similar to that seen during the follicular phase of
premenopausal subjects. Although the frequency is similar,
the amplitude is much greater. This increased amplitude is
secondary to increased release by the hypothalamic hormone gonadotropin-releasing hormone (GnRH) and enhanced responsiveness of the pituitary to GnRH because
of low estrogen levels. Studies with rhesus monkeys suggest that the site governing pulsatile GnRH release is in
the arcuate nucleus of the hypothalamus. The large
pulses of gonadotropin in the peripheral circulation are
believed to maintain the high levels of the hormones
found in postmenopausal women.

During reproductive life, the levels of both FSH and
LH range from 4–30 mU/mL except during the preovulatory surge, when they may exceed 50 mU/mL and
100 mU/mL, respectively. After the menopause, both
rise to levels above 100 mU/mL, with FSH rising earlier
and to higher levels than LH.

When contradictory or uncertain clinical findings
make the diagnosis of the postmenopausal state questionable, measurement of plasma FSH, LH, and estradiol levels may be helpful. This situation occurs frequently in women following hysterectomy without
oophorectomy. The findings of plasma estradiol below
20 pg/mL and elevated FSH and LH levels are consistent with cessation of ovarian function. In practical
terms, it is not necessary to measure LH.

D. PHYSICAL CHANGES ASSOCIATED WITH THE MENOPAUSE

1. Reproductive tract—Because estrogen functions as
the major growth factor of the female reproductive
tract, there are substantial changes in the appearance of
all the reproductive organs. Most postmenopausal
women experience varying degrees of atrophic changes
of the vaginal epithelium. The vaginal rugae progressively flatten and the epithelium thins. This may lead to
symptomatic atrophic vaginitis (see Atrophic Vaginitis).

There are also atrophic changes of the cervix. It usually decreases in size, and there is a reduction of secretion of cervical mucous. This may contribute to excessive vaginal dryness, which may cause dyspareunia.

Atrophy of the uterus is also seen, with shrinkage of
both the endometrium and myometrium. This shrinkage
can be beneficial to women who enter the climacteric
with uterine myomas. Reduction in size and elimination
of symptoms frequently prevent the necessity for surgical
treatment. The same applies to adenomyosis and endometriosis, both of which usually become asymptomatic following the menopause. Palpable and symptomatic areas of endometriosis generally become
progressively smaller and less troublesome. With cessation of follicular activity, hormonal stimulation of the
endometrium usually ceases. Endometrial biopsy may reveal anything from a very scanty, atrophic endometrium
to one that is moderately proliferative. Spontaneous postmenopausal bleeding may occur in the presence of any of
these patterns. Endometrial tissue revealing glandular hyperplasia (with or without uterine bleeding) is an indication of enhanced estrogenic stimulation from either endogenous estrogen production (eg, increased conversion
of androgen), or from exogenous intake of estrogen.

The oviducts and ovaries also decrease in size postmenopausally. Although this produces no symptoms, the
small size of the ovaries makes them difficult to palpate

during pelvic examination. A palpable ovary in a post-menopausal woman must be viewed with suspicion, and the presence of an ovarian neoplasm must be considered.

The supporting structures of the reproductive organs suffer loss of tone as estrogen levels decline. Postmenopausal estrogen deficiency may lead to symptomatic progressive pelvic relaxation.

2. Urinary tract—Estrogen plays an important role in maintaining the epithelium of the bladder and urethra. Marked estrogen deficiency may produce atrophic changes in these organs similar to those that occur in the vaginal epithelium. This may give rise to atrophic cystitis, characterized by urinary urgency, frequency, incontinence, and dysuria. Recurrent urinary tract infection may also develop in the setting of estrogen deficiency. Loss of urethral tone, with pouting of the meatus and thinning of the epithelium, favors the formation of a urethral caruncle with resultant dysuria, meatal tenderness, and occasionally hematuria. Treatment of symptomatic women involves topical vaginal estrogen (see Estrogen Therapy).

3. Mammary glands—Regression of breast size during and after menopause is psychologically distressing to some women. For those who have been bothered by cyclic symptoms of breast pain and cyst formation, the disappearance of these symptoms postmenopausally is a great relief.

Clinical Conditions Associated with Menopause

A. Atrophic Vaginitis

1. Pathogenesis—As the epithelium thins following menopause, the capillary bed shines through as a diffuse or patchy reddening. Rupture of surface capillaries produces irregularly scattered petechiae, and a brownish discharge may be noted. Further atrophy of the vaginal epithelium renders its capillary bed increasingly sparse, so that the hyperemic appearance gives way to a smooth, shiny, pale epithelial surface. The epithelium lacks glycogen which leads to a reduction in lactic acid production and an increase in the vaginal pH to 5.0–7.0. This is associated with disappearance of lactobacilli. Early in the process, local bacterial invasion may initiate vaginal pruritus and leukorrhea. Vaginal burning, soreness, dyspareunia, and a thin watery or serosanguineous discharge may also occur. Minimal trauma with examinations or coitus may result in slight vaginal bleeding. Urinary complaints, including urinary frequency, urgency, dysuria, and urge incontinence, have also been described in association with atrophic vaginitis.

2. Diagnosis—There is no specific test that reliably quantifies the degree of atrophy. Clinical decision making is therefore generally based on patient symptomatology and findings on physical examination. However, vaginal cytology has been used to assist in the diagnosis of atrophic vaginitis. The degree of maturation of exfoliated vaginal epithelial cells, as revealed by stained vaginal smears, is an index of estrogenic activity. Among the various methods of assessing the smears, the following are most commonly used: the **maturation index** consists of a differential count of three types of squamous cells—parabasal cells, intermediate cells, and superficial cells, in that order—expressed as percentages (eg, 10/85/5); a greater percentage of parabasal cells reflects a greater degree of atrophy. The **cornification count** is the percentage of precornified and cornified cells among total squamous cells counted. This is actually a simplified maturation index, because this percentage is essentially the same as that of the superficial cells.

The assessment of exfoliated vaginal epithelial cells is influenced not only by the level of estrogenic activity, but also by other hormones (particularly progesterone and testosterone), local vaginal inflammation, local medication, vaginal bleeding, the presence of genital cancer, the location of the vaginal area sampled, and variations in end-organ (epithelial) responses to estrogenic influence. Thus, women with identical levels of circulating estrogens may have quite different cytograms.

The great variation in cytologic findings leads to the following conclusions regarding the use of smears in the clinical management of postmenopausal women: (a) The smear is only a rough measure of estrogenic status, and it may sometimes be grossly misleading. (b) The vaginal cytogram cannot predict whether or not an individual woman is experiencing menopausal signs and symptoms. (c) The smear cannot be used as the sole guide to steroid supplementation therapy; clinical signs and symptoms are more dependable for this purpose.

3. Treatment—Symptomatic atrophic vaginitis may be managed with water-soluble lubricants and/or topical vaginal estrogens, which are available in the form of creams, tablets, or estradiol-releasing rings (see Estrogen Therapy). Systemic estrogens may also be utilized in the treatment of atrophic vaginitis, but vaginal preparations are preferred when estrogen therapy is being utilized solely for the treatment of vulvovaginal atrophy.

B. Hot Flushes

1. General considerations—The most common and characteristic symptom of the climacteric is an episodic disturbance consisting of sudden flushing and perspiration, referred to as a **hot flash** or **flush.** It is observed in approximately 75% of women who go through the physiologic menopause or have a bilateral ovariectomy. Of those having flushes, 82% experience the disturbance for more than 1 year and 25–50% complain of the symptom for more than 5 years. Most women indicate that hot flushes begin with a sensation of pressure in the head, much like a headache. This increases in intensity until the physiologic flush occurs. Palpitations may also be experienced. The actual flush is characterized as a feeling of heat or burning in the face, neck, and chest, followed immediately by an outbreak of sweating that affects the entire body but is particularly prominent over the head, neck, upper chest, and back. Less-common symptoms include weakness, fatigue, faintness, and vertigo. The duration of the whole episode varies from momentary to as long as 10 minutes; the average length is 4 minutes. The frequency varies from 1–2 per hour to 1–2 per week. In women with severe flushes, the mean frequency is 54 minutes.

Investigators have characterized the physiologic changes associated with hot flushes and have shown that the symptoms result from true alterations in cutaneous vasodilation, perspiration, reductions of core temperature, and elevations of pulse rate. Fluctuations in electrocardiographic data probably reflect changes in skin conductance. Changes in heart rhythm and blood pressure have not been observed.

The patient's awareness of symptoms does not correspond exactly with physiologic changes. Women become conscious of symptoms approximately 1 minute after the onset of measurable cutaneous vasodilation, and discomfort persists for an average of 4 minutes, whereas physical changes persist for several minutes longer.

2. Pathogenesis—The exact mechanism responsible for hot flushes is unknown, but physiologic and behavioral data indicate that symptoms result from a defect in central thermoregulatory function. Several observations support this conclusion: (a) The two major physiologic changes associated with hot flushes—perspiration and cutaneous vasodilation—are the result of different peripheral sympathetic functions. Excitation of sweat glands results from sympathetic cholinergic fibers, and cutaneous vasodilation is under the control of tonic α-adrenergic fibers. It seems unlikely that any peripheral event could cause both cholinergic excitation of sweat glands and α-adrenergic blockade of cutaneous vessels, and it is well recognized that these are the two basic functions triggered by central thermoregulatory mechanisms that lower the central temperature. (b) During a hot flush, the central temperature decreases because of cutaneous vasodilation and perspiration. If hot flushes were the result of some peripheral event, the body's regulatory mechanisms would be expected to prevent such a decrease. (c) There is also a change in behavior associated with hot flushes. Women feel warm and have a conscious desire to cool themselves by throwing off the bedcovers, standing by open windows or doors, fanning themselves, or by other means. This behavior is observed even in the presence of a steady or decreasing central temperature.

Most investigators believe the core temperature of the body is maintained near a central set point that is

controlled by central thermoregulatory centers, particularly those in the rostral hypothalamus. This central set point temperature is analogous to a thermostat setting. Hot flushes appear to be triggered by a sudden lowering of the central hypothalamic "thermostat." As a consequence, heat loss mechanisms, both physiologic and behavioral, are activated so that the core temperature will be brought in line with the new set point; this results in a fall of central temperature.

Because hot flushes occur after the spontaneous cessation of ovarian function or following oophorectomy, it is presumed that the underlying mechanism is endocrinologic, related either to reduction of ovarian estrogen secretion or to enhancement of pituitary gonadotropin secretion. Low estrogen levels alone do not appear to trigger hot flushes; prepubertal children and patients with gonadal dysgenesis have low estrogen levels but not flushing. Patients with gonadal dysgenesis do experience symptoms if they are given estrogens that are later withdrawn. Thus, it appears that estrogen must be present and then withdrawn for hot flushes to be experienced.

Hot flushes appear to be related to gonadotropins. A close temporal association between the occurrence of flushes and the pulsatile release of LH has been demonstrated. The observation that flushes occur after hypophysectomy suggests that they are not directly caused by LH release (Fig 59–3). The appearance of hot flushes in women with defects in GnRH release or synthesis (Kallmann's syndrome) also suggests GnRH itself

Figure 59–3. Skin temperature and LH and FSH levels in a woman with hot flushes. Note the close temporal relationship between the rises in skin temperature and the occurrence of pulsatile LH release. (Reproduced with permission from Tataryn IV et al: LH, FSH, and skin temperature during the menopausal hot flash. J Clin Endocrinol Metab 1979;49:152.)

is not involved in the flushing mechanism. The absence of hot flushes in women with hypothalamic amenorrhea and hypoestrogenemia is intriguing. These women have defects in neurotransmitter or neurochemical input to their GnRH neurons. In particular, excessive endogenous opioid and dopamine input to GnRH neurons may account for chronic suppression of GnRH release, leading to hypothalamic amenorrhea. The absence of hot flushes in these women suggests that altered afferent input of neurotransmitters or neurochemicals to the GnRH neuron that is secondary to hypogonadism leads to hot flushes. Two likely candidates are norepinephrine and endogenous opioids.

Hot flushes are a greater annoyance than most physicians recognize. Patients frequently complain of night sweats and insomnia. There is a close temporal relationship between the occurrence of hot flushes and nighttime awakening. Women with frequent flushes may experience flushes and awakening episodes hourly, which may cause a profound sleep disturbance that may, in turn, cause cognitive (memory) and affective (anxiety) disorders in some women.

3. Treatment—Estrogens are the principal medications used to relieve hot flushes. Estrogens block both the perceived symptoms and the physiologic changes. Their use also relieves some aspects of the sleeping disorder. Estrogen administration has been shown to enhance hypothalamic opioid activity in postmenopausal women. This increase of hypothalamic opiates may be involved in the relief of hot flushes with estrogen administration.

Progestins also block hot flushes and represent a reasonable form of substitutional therapy in women who can't take estrogens. **Clonidine,** a centrally acting alpha agonist, is more effective than a placebo but is associated with side effects. More recently, certain **selective serotonin reuptake inhibitors (SSRIs)** have been shown to be effective in the treatment of hot flashes. Their side effects may limit their overall benefit, but they are one of the first alternative choices in women who are not taking estrogen. **Black cohosh** may have modest effects in decreasing hot flashes, but concerns remain regarding its potential to stimulate breast and uterine tissue. **Gabapentin** also decreases hot flashes. **Tibolone** is a synthetic steroid with estrogenic, progestogenic, and androgenic properties that alleviates menopausal symptoms and has been used in other countries for this purpose, as well as to preserve bone mineral density. However, its long-term safety profile with regard to breast and endometrial cancer remains controversial. Its mechanism of action would suggest that it is unlikely to increase the risk of breast cancer. This idea has been supported by results from studies showing that tibolone does not increase mammographic density. Furthermore, no increased risk of breast cancer has been observed in phase III/IV trials of ti-

bolone. However, the Million Women Study reported an increased risk of breast cancer among participants using tibolone as compared to controls. Tibolone's action on the endometrium also suggests that it is unlikely to cause endometrial proliferation. This is supported by findings from studies demonstrating a low incidence of vaginal bleeding and an absence of endometrial hyperplasia on histology. However, rates of endometrial cancer were also increased in the Million Women's Study. Further study is required to ascertain whether tibolone can be used long-term without increased risks for breast and endometrial cancer. Tibolone's potential to modify risk for cardiovascular disease is also unknown. However, a recent study evaluating the effect of tibolone on myocardial blood flow demonstrated that tibolone improved myocardial blood flow in women with ischemic heart disease. Vitamins E and K, mineral supplements, and phytoestrogens have all been tried to alleviate menopausal symptoms, but have not been proven beneficial.

C. Osteoporosis

1. General considerations—As defined by the Consensus Development Center in 1993, osteoporosis is a systemic skeletal disorder characterized by low bone mass and microarchitectural deterioration of bone tissue, with a consequent increase in fragility of bone and susceptibility to risk of fracture. This loss occurs primarily in trabecular bone and is therefore most noticeable in the vertebra and distal radius. Although gradual bone loss occurs in all humans with aging, this loss is accelerated in women after cessation of ovarian function. Following attainment of peak bone mass by age 25–30 years, bone loss begins, accelerates in women at menopause, and then slows again but continues into advanced years at a rate of 1–2% per year (Fig 59–4). Women can lose up to 20% of their bone mass in the 5–7 years following menopause.

Osteoporosis affects an estimated 10 million Americans 50 years of age or older, 80% of whom are women. Of Americans 50 years of age or older, 34 million are estimated to have low bone mass, placing them at increased risk for osteoporosis. Osteoporosis is most severe in women who have had early oophorectomy or premature ovarian failure, and in those with gonadal dysgenesis. Osteoporosis occurs most often in whites, followed by Asians, Hispanics and African Americans. Estrogen loss, smoking, family history, eating disorders, abnormal or absent menstrual periods, hyperthyroidism, excessive alcohol consumption, low lifetime calcium intake, vitamin D deficiency, use of certain medications (ie, corticosteroids, chemotherapy), slender body size, advanced age, and other chronic medical conditions are also risk factors.

Bone loss produces minimal symptoms, but leads to reduced skeletal strength. Thus, osteoporotic bones are

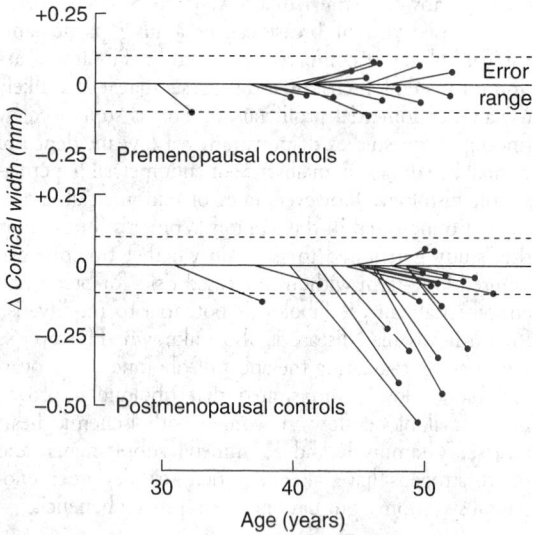

Figure 59–4. Changes in metacarpal cortical width, as determined by sequential measurements in pre- and postmenopausal women, age range 30–50 years. Note bone loss in postmenopausal women. (Reproduced with permission from Nordin BEC et al: Postmenopausal osteopenia and osteoporosis. Front Horm Res 1975; 3:131.)

more susceptible to fractures. The most common site of fracture is in the vertebral body; however, fractures also occur in the hip, upper femur, distal forearm, humerus and ribs (Fig 59–5). Recent figures from the National Osteoporosis Foundation show that osteoporosis is responsible for more than 1.5 million fractures per year, including 300,000 hip fractures, 700,000 vertebral fractures, 250,000 wrist fractures, and more than 300,000 fractures at other sites. Approximately 1 in 2 women older than the age of 50 years will have an osteoporosis-related fracture in her remaining lifetime. The incidence of hip fractures in women is 2–3 times that in men. The mortality rate associated with hip fractures is between 5% and 20% within 12 months following the injury. Of survivors, 15–25% are permanently disabled. The estimated cost for osteoporosis-related fractures in the United States totals more than $17 billion per year.

2. Pathogenesis—Bone loss occurs because bone resorption is excessive, bone formation is decreased, peak bone mass is low or because of a combination of all three factors. Bone remodeling is regulated by many factors, including systemic hormones, local cytokines, prostaglandins, and local growth factors. Of the systemic hormones, sex steroids, parathyroid hormones, glucocorticoids, thyroid hormones, and growth hormone/insulinlike growth factors likely play a role.

Ovarian estrogen and estrogen administered postmenopausally are protective against osteoporosis. The exact mechanisms by which estrogen regulates bone remodeling are incompletely understood. Estrogens likely modulate osteoclast and osteoblast function possibly via effects on cytokines and growth factors such as transforming growth factor-β (TGFβ) and tumor necrosis factor-α (TNFα).

Interleukin-1 (IL-1) and TNFα derived from bone marrow macrophages stimulate bone resorption and may inhibit bone formation. There is evidence to suggest they may be regulated by estrogen as IL-1 activity in bone increases immediately after the menopause or oophorectomy. The levels remain increased in osteoporotic women, whereas they return to the premenopausal range after 2–3 years in those who do not develop the disease. Furthermore, it has been shown in animal models that inhibition of IL-1 and TNFα following ovariectomy attenuates bone loss. IL-6 and prostaglandins, especially prostaglandin E₂ (PGE₂), are also involved in bone remodeling and are regulated by sex steroids. Other factors, such as insulinlike growth factor and fibroblast growth factor, also likely play a role in the pathogenesis of osteoporosis and may be regulated by sex steroids.

Androgens play a role in bone remodeling as androgen deficiency is associated with increased bone loss. The precise mechanism by which androgens alter bone remodeling is unknown.

Progestins may affect bone remodeling in a similar way to estrogens and androgens, but the mechanisms underlying these effects are not well understood.

Parathyroid hormone (PTH) also plays a role in bone remodeling. PTH stimulates bone resorption and

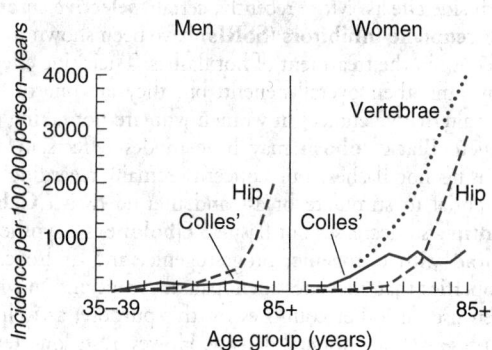

Figure 59–5. Incidences of the 3 common osteoporotic fractures (Colles', hip, and vertebral) in men and women, plotted as a function of age at time of fracture in the community population of Rochester, Minnesota. (Reproduced, with permission, from Riggs BL, Melton LJ III: Involutional osteoporosis. N Engl J Med 1986; 314:1677.)

absence of this hormone inhibits development of osteoporosis in animal and human studies. Thus far, it does not appear that PTH is elevated in most women with osteoporosis or that the sensitivity of bone to PTH is enhanced. It is interesting that the amino-terminus of PTH (1-34) inhibits bone resorption.

Growth hormone stimulates bone remodeling; however, studies evaluating the effect of exogenous growth hormone administration on established osteoporosis are inconclusive. Recently, new factors were discovered that are involved with the regulation of bone remodeling: osteoprotegerin, a naturally occurring protein, and RANKL (receptor activator of nuclear factor kappa beta ligand), both regulate osteoclastogenesis and bone resorption.

Genetic factors may also affect risk for osteoporosis. Variants in the estrogen receptors α and β expressed in bone are associated with altered risk for osteoporosis and fracture. Variants in the vitamin D receptor gene and bone morphogenetic protein 2 (BMP2) may also play a role in the pathogenesis of osteoporosis.

3. Diagnosis—Although much has been done to study urinary and serum factors as predictors of osteoporosis, the most predictive test remains bone densitometry. Several different types of densitometry are available. Single-photon absorptiometry can be used to measure appendicular bone mineral density (BMD). However, to measure axial bone, dual-energy x-ray absorptiometry is required for an accurate assessment. The variability of soft-tissue density around the spine and pelvis decreases the accuracy of single-photon testing. Results are given in grams or g/cm². In 1994, the World Health Organization created a clinically useful definition of osteoporosis. Bone mineral density results are reported using T and Z scores. The T score is the number of standard deviations (SD) above or below the mean bone mineral density for gender-matched young controls. The Z score compares the patient with a population adjusted for age, and gender. Normal bone density is defined as a T score greater than –1.0 SD. Osteopenic patients have T scores between –1.0 and –2.5, whereas osteoporotic patients have T scores below –2.5. In most studies, a decrease by 1 SD in mass increases the risk of fracture 2–3-fold.

Assessment of risk factors has not been nearly as predictive of fracture risk as density measurement. Assessment of serum osteocalcin and bone-specific alkaline phosphatase, markers of bone formation, or of urinary deoxypyridinoline (DPD) cross-links and serum/urinary cross-linked N-telopeptides (NTX) of type I collagen, markers of bone resorption, have not been shown to be useful for diagnosing osteoporosis but may give some indication of future risk for bone loss and/or be useful for monitoring response to antiresorptive therapy.

In 1998 the National Osteoporosis Foundation created a set of guidelines for the use and interpretation of measurement of bone mineral density. Measurements of bone mineral density are recommended for the following groups: (a) all postmenopausal patients younger than age 65 years who have one or more additional risk factors for osteoporosis (other than being white, postmenopausal, and female); (b) all women age 65 years and older regardless of additional risk factors; (c) postmenopausal women who present with fractures; (d) women considering therapy for osteoporosis if testing would facilitate the decision; and (e) women who have been on hormone replacement therapy for prolonged periods.

4. Prevention and treatment—All individuals at risk for or who have been diagnosed with osteoporosis should be advised to consume adequate **calcium** (minimum of 1200 mg elemental calcium per day) and **vitamin D** (400–800 IU/d). Smoking cessation, avoidance of excessive alcohol intake, and participation in regular weight-bearing exercise should be encouraged. Pharmacologic therapy should be strongly considered in women with BMD scores below –2.0 with no risk factors, and in women with BMD T-scores below –1.5 with 1 or more risk factors. Current pharmacologic therapy for osteopenia/osteoporosis, listed in alphabetical order, includes (a) **bisphosphonates,** (b) **calcitonin,** (c) **estrogens** (with or without progestogens), (d) **parathyroid hormone,** and (e) **raloxifene.**

Bisphosphonates are excellent choices for prevention and treatment of osteoporosis. They are potent antiresorptive agents that bind to hydroxyapatite crystals on the surface of bones, enter osteoclasts, and decrease resorptive actions by reducing the production of hydrogen ions and lysosomal enzymes. In addition, they have indirect effects, causing osteoblasts to produce substances that inhibit osteoclasts. They increase bone mineral density at the spine, wrist, and hip in a dose-dependent manner and decrease the risk of vertebral fractures by 30–50%. In addition, they reduce the risk of subsequent nonvertebral fractures in women with osteoporosis. There are three bisphosphonates currently available for oral administration. Alendronate is approved by the Food and Drug Administration for the prevention of osteoporosis (5 mg daily and 35 mg weekly) and for the treatment of established osteoporosis (10 mg daily or 70 mg weekly). Risedronate is approved by the FDA for prevention and treatment of postmenopausal osteoporosis. The recommended daily dose is 5 mg daily or 35 mg weekly. Ibandronate was recently approved for both prevention and treatment of postmenopausal osteoporosis. It has the advantage of being available in both a daily and monthly dosing regimen. The daily dose is 2.5 mg and the monthly dose is 150 mg. Intestinal absorption of bisphosphonates is poor and therefore these medications should be taken in the morning with 8 ounces of water, prior to consumption of any food or beverage. Nothing else should be taken by mouth for at least 30–60 minutes after oral dosing. The patient should also remain upright for 30 minutes after administration. The most common side effects of bisphosphonates are gastrointestinal. Pain in the joints, bone, and muscle may also occur. Risks include gastric and esophageal ulceration and, rarely, osteonecrosis of the jaw. Most cases of osteonecrosis of the jaw have been described in cancer patients being treated with intravenous bisphosphonates, but some cases have occurred in patients being managed for postmenopausal osteoporosis.

Calcitonin is a peptide hormone that inhibits osteoclast activity and therefore inhibits bone resorption. It demonstrates positive effects on bone mineral density at the lumbar spine, although less effectively than estrogen or bisphosphonates. Salmon calcitonin is the most potent form and is available for intranasal administration or as a subcutaneous injection. Calcitonin 100 IU is given subcutaneously daily or every other day; the intranasal calcitonin dose is 200 IU daily. The most frequent side effect with the intranasal route is rhinitis. Other antiresorptive therapies, such as bisphosphonates, are preferred over calcitonin, as they produce greater increases in bone mineral density. However, because of calcitonin's analgesic properties, calcitonin is the preferred therapy in patients with pain from vertebral fracture.

Until recently **estrogen** was the mainstay of therapy for prevention and treatment of postmenopausal osteoporosis. However, with the findings from the Women's Health Initiative (WHI) trial demonstrating overall greater health risks than benefits from hormone therapy, it is no longer first-line therapy for prevention of osteoporosis. Osteoporosis prevention does remain an FDA-approved indication for estrogen therapy, however. It is best used in women who would otherwise use estrogen/hormone therapy for management of menopausal symptoms, or in women who cannot tolerate alternate antiresorptive therapies.

In observational studies, estrogen decreases the risk of hip fractures by 25–50%, of vertebral fractures by approximately 50%, and reduces the risk of other fractures. Daily dosages of 0.3–0.625 mg of conjugated estrogens, 0.5–1 mg micronized estradiol, 1.25 mg piperazine estrone sulfate, 0.025–0.05 mg of transdermal estradiol, and a new low dose (0.014 mg) of transdermal estradiol all are appropriate for the prevention of osteoporosis. The lower doses (ie, 0.3 mg conjugated equine estrogens) are not as effective as higher doses but do prevent bone loss. For best results, therapy should begin soon after the menopause.

Parathyroid hormone, teriparatide (PTH [1-34]) has been approved by the FDA for use in women and men who are at high risk for fracture, including those with previous fracture, multiple risk factors for fracture, and previous failed treatment. Despite its potential del-

eterious effect on bone, intermittent administration of recombinant PTH stimulates bone formation and clinical trials support its use in the treatment of osteoporosis. It should only be used in high-risk patients because of its high cost, the need for daily injection, and a possible risk for osteosarcoma.

Selective estrogen receptor modulators (SERMs) are nonhormonal agents that bind to estrogen receptors and may exhibit either estrogen agonist or antagonist activity. Currently, there are three SERMs approved for use in humans (tamoxifen, toremifene, and raloxifene); however, raloxifene is the only SERM approved for the prevention and treatment of osteoporosis. It exhibits estrogen agonist properties in the bone (inhibits osteoclast function) and the liver (decreases low-density lipoprotein cholesterol), and acts as an antagonist in the breast and uterus. Raloxifene 60 mg daily for 24 months is associated with a 1–2% increase in lumbar spine and hip bone density.

Other therapies have been proposed for osteoporosis treatment and prevention, some without proven benefit. **Progestins** decrease biochemical markers of bone resorption and preserve bone density. When used as monotherapy for osteoporosis, they may be more effective at preserving bone in the wrist than in the spine.

Fluoride has been used in Europe and the United States and is associated with a marked increase in trabecular bone, but did not improve fracture rates, and in some studies fracture rates were increased. This may be a result of a lack of increase in cortical bone. Sodium fluoride is generally not recommended for the treatment of osteoporosis.

Phytoestrogens are plant-derived compounds that have weak estrogenlike effects. Although some animal studies are promising, no effects on the incidence of fractures in humans have been shown.

Tibolone (see Hot Flushes) also increases lumbar spine and femoral neck bone density. Its effects on bone are comparable to those of estrogens. As discussed previously, however, issues regarding long-term safety are currently being evaluated.

D. SEXUAL DYSFUNCTION

The determinants of sexual behavior are complex and interrelated. Sexual function is believed to be regulated by three general components: the individual's motivation (also called desire or libido), endocrine competence, and social-cultural beliefs. Decreased libido is reported with increasing age. However, the relative contributions of the primary decrease in desire, anatomic limitations to sexual function, or beliefs that sexual behavior is inappropriate in older women to this decreased libido are unknown.

The hypoestrogenemic state leads to atrophy of the internal genitalia. Although dyspareunia is the most obvious symptom of vaginal atrophy, suboptimal sexual functioning can occur without frank dyspareunia. Diminished genital sensation (and therefore decreased sensory output in the arousal phase), lessened glandular secretions, less vasocongestion, and decreased vaginal expansion may not be perceived as discrete symptoms by the postmenopausal female, but may influence her perception that she is less responsive.

Genital atrophy, one cause of postmenopausal sexual dysfunction, responds to estrogen therapy. The specific impact of estrogen on libido has been difficult to determine. Improved anatomy may also have a positive psychologic impact and may indirectly encourage sexual motivation. The role of androgen therapy in female sexual dysfunction is an active area of investigation.

Common Clinical Conditions of the Aged, Postmenopausal Woman: Controversial Role of Estrogens

A. Coronary Heart Disease (CHD)

Heart disease affects approximately 6 million women in the United States. Deaths caused by CHD in women number more than 230,000 per year. The incidence of death from CHD increases with age in all populations and both sexes. Substantially more heart disease is seen in younger men, with the onset of cardiovascular problems occurring an average of 10 years later in women. Before the age of menopause, very few women die of a heart attack. After the menopause, a woman's risk increases progressively such that CHD rates in women after menopause are 2–3 times those of women of the same age before menopause. Statistics such as these, indicating a role for both gender and menopause on the development of CHD, have led to the suggestion that estrogen deficiency that occurs following menopause is at least partially responsible for the increased risk of CHD in postmenopausal women.

Until recently, two types of studies have attempted to ascertain whether cessation of ovarian function is associated with an increased incidence of heart disease. The first examined the relationship between the menopause and carefully defined cardiovascular disease in an entire population. For example, the Framingham study, in which nearly 3000 women were examined biennially, revealed that following the menopause, there is indeed an increased incidence of heart disease that is not just age-related. In this study, the impact of the menopause was abrupt, and further (age-related) increases in incidence occurred only slowly, if at all. In the Nurses' Health Study cohort of 121,700 women, after controlling for age and cigarette smoking, women who had a natural menopause had no appreciable increase in risk compared to that of premenopausal women. However, women who underwent a bilateral oophorectomy and no estrogen replacement had an increased risk (relative risk [RR] 2.2) compared with that seen in premenopausal women.

In the second type of investigation, case-control studies were performed comparing the degree of coronary heart disease or the incidence of myocardial infarction in women who had undergone early oophorectomy with age-matched premenopausal controls. Most of these studies revealed an increased risk of cardiovascular disease after ovarian excision. All these reports have been criticized because of patient selection bias, particularly of the controls.

Numerous case-control and large-cohort studies have been published, with most showing a beneficial impact of estrogens. A meta-analysis found that estrogen use provided a 50% decrease in risk of mortality from heart disease. Although the magnitude of change and the consistency of results appear compelling, it must be recognized that all these studies are observational, and that the choice of controls has been questioned. In particular, women who take estrogens are more health conscious and must see a doctor regularly to receive their medication, whereas women who don't take estrogens may or may not receive regular medical checkups. Thus, some or all of the apparent benefits of estrogens on heart disease may have been a consequence of these other considerations.

Based on these observational/case-controlled studies suggesting a beneficial effect of estrogens, numerous experimental studies were performed attempting to elucidate the mechanism(s) by which estrogens could prevent coronary heart disease. Evidence for both an indirect effect on circulating lipids and a direct action on the vascular system was found. For years, the greatest emphasis of research had been to study the impact of estrogens on lipoproteins. Orally administered estrogens influence hepatic lipid metabolism and raise high-density lipoprotein (HDL) cholesterol and triglycerides and lower low-density lipoprotein (LDL) cholesterol. The impact of nonorally administered estrogens is of lesser magnitude and takes longer to become apparent. The Lipid Research Clinic study suggested that approximately 50% of the benefit of estrogen on heart disease was elicited through the action of estrogens on lipoproteins, whereas the remainder was through other mechanisms.

The PEPI (Postmenopausal Estrogen Progestin Intervention) Trial showed that there is a significant lowering of LDL cholesterol with oral conjugated equine estrogens (CEEs), even with the addition of medroxyprogesterone acetate (MPA) or micronized natural progesterone. Of the four regimens studied, continuous CEE 0.625 mg without the addition of progestin had the most favorable effect on lipid profiles. All active HT regimens lowered LDL cholesterol and fibrinogen levels.

Numerous studies show that estrogen and progesterone receptors are present in the heart and aorta. Thus, the subcellular components necessary for hormonal action exist in these tissues. Studies in castrated cynomolgus monkeys given atherogenic diets have shown estradiol administered by subcutaneous pellets prevents coronary atherogenesis in the absence of any measurable change in circulating lipoproteins. Endothelial cells of the arteries produce factors in response to estrogen. One of the most potent of these is believed to be nitric oxide (NO). NO exerts several effects on the arterial wall. It increases intracellular cyclic guanosine monophosphate in the arterial smooth muscle, which results in vasodilation. It also inhibits platelet adhesion and aggregation, as well as monocyte adherence to the arterial endothelium. Estrogen appears to increase NO production. Basal release of NO is greater in intact female rabbits than in either male rabbits or castrated females. Acetylcholine is known to stimulate vasodilation of the coronary arteries of humans and monkeys. This effect is dependent on an intact vascular endothelium and mediated via NO. It has been theorized that estrogens may increase muscarinic receptors on endothelial cells, leading to acetylcholine-induced, endothelial-dependent, NO-mediated vasodilation, which may be important in preventing vasospasm. Estrogen has also been shown in an animal model to prevent two of the earliest steps in the atherogenic process—adhesion and migration of monocytes. Estrogens also likely have adverse effects on the vessel wall. Estrogens lead to a hypercoagulable state which may increase the risk of coronary events. Although these mechanisms are only partially understood, they emphasize the importance of studying the direct effects of estrogen on the vascular system.

Interestingly, use of estrogen had been widespread for many years, yet it was not until recently that large-scale, prospective, randomized, placebo-controlled studies evaluating the effect of hormone therapy on relevant clinical endpoints in humans were performed. One of the first of these studies was the Heart and Estrogen/Progestin Replacement Study (HERS) which studied the use of estrogen and progestin in the secondary prevention of coronary events in women with known coronary heart disease. HERS showed that treatment with oral conjugated equine estrogen (CEE) plus medroxyprogesterone acetate (MPA) did not reduce the overall rate of coronary heart disease events in postmenopausal women with established heart disease. In addition, there was an early increased risk of CHD events within the first year of starting HT. In addition, the ERA (Estrogen Replacement and Atherosclerosis) Trial, which was the first randomized angiographic end point trial to test the effect of HT on the progression of atherosclerosis in postmenopausal women with documented coronary stenosis, showed no benefit of CEE either alone, or in combination with MPA, on angiographic progression of disease. Consequently, it is sug-

gested that physicians not prescribe estrogen therapy (ET)/HT for the sole purpose of *secondary* prevention of coronary events.

The primary prevention of CHD by HT also had not been evaluated in a prospective, randomized fashion until recently. The WHI, a large, multicenter, prospective, randomized, placebo-controlled trial of primarily healthy postmenopausal women, was initiated to assess the effects of a specific regimen of CEE alone or in combination with MPA on several health-related outcomes, including CHD. The combined estrogen/progestin portion of the study was stopped after 5.2 years as overall health risks exceeded benefits. The increased risks included a greater number of cardiovascular events. Although the absolute risk of harm was small, the authors concluded that this regimen of HT should not be initiated or continued for the primary prevention of CHD. The estrogen-only arm of the study was continued for approximately 7 years. This arm of the study was stopped early because of an increased risk of stroke. Overall, there was no reduction in the risk of coronary events. Interestingly, there appeared to be a trend toward a decreased risk of coronary events in the younger subset of postmenopausal women. This finding was confirmed in a subanalysis of the data for the 50–59-year-old age group where the investigators reported a lower relative risk for the combined end points of myocardial infarction, coronary death, coronary revascularization, and confirmed angina among women ages 50–59 years using estrogen alone.

There were several limitations of the WHI study. It did not assess different dosages, types of estrogens and progestogens, nor different routes of administration (ie, transdermal vs. oral). Finally, many of the subjects had become menopausal several years before entry into the study. Consequently, it was not possible to precisely ascertain whether starting HT with the onset of menopause, when initiation or more rapid acceleration of atherosclerosis may take place, is beneficial. Because estrogen has been shown in experimental models to prevent the very earliest steps in atherogenesis, but to raise cardiovascular risk in the setting of established atherosclerosis (possibly via increases in clotting factors), it is possible that the adverse cardiovascular effects seen in this study may have been a result of the possibility that many women started HT following the onset of menopause when subclinical atherosclerotic changes and irreversible endothelial damage may have already set in. In support of this concept, a recent analysis from the ongoing Nurses Health Study, a long-term prospective observational study, demonstrated that women who used HT had a decrease in the risk of CHD relative to women who did not use HT. The majority of these women started HT/ET close to menopause. This is in contrast to the WHI where the majority of women started HT/ET remote from menopause. This emphasizes the importance of continuing to study the effects of estrogen, particularly in younger, recently postmenopausal women. Additional studies are currently underway to assess whether estrogen administration to younger, healthy, recently postmenopausal women is safe from a cardiovascular standpoint.

The decision to use HT should be based primarily on the proven benefits of ET/HT on other systems, the potential risks of therapy, and patient preference. Short-term use of HT for relief of postmenopausal symptoms is still an option for women without contraindications.

B. Mood Disorders

Studies assessing the effects of estrogen on depression and other mood disorders are conflicting. Although some studies suggest beneficial effects of estrogen, others, including the recent WHI, do not. Early cross-sectional surveys of community or large, general, medical practice–based populations attempted to measure the temporal association of depression and irritability to the cessation of menses. Some reports indicated an increased incidence of minor symptoms such as irritability, dysphoria, and nervousness early in the menopausal transition.

Reports from community-based cohort studies have refined knowledge in the area of mood, mentation, and menopause. The initial longitudinal report of the U.S. cohort found an increase in overall nonspecific symptom reporting at the menopause. Depression for more than two interviews was noted in 26% of the cohort. Perceived health, rather than menopause or coincident life stresses, was most related to depression in this study. These findings are consistent with the concept of variability in a woman's response to the menopause; individual characteristics and self-perceptions appear to be important determinants of each woman's experience of the climacteric.

Hypotheses as to the etiology of the affective complaints at the menopause also include a primary biologic cause (eg, an alteration in brain amines). Studies using the opioid antagonist naloxone have demonstrated that estrogen deficiency is associated with low levels of endogenous opioid activity and that estrogen supplementation increases opioid activity. These findings suggest that central neurotransmitters may contribute to the etiology of affective and cognitive complaints. Sociologic factors postulated to cause psychologic symptoms, such as negative cultural values attached to aging, may also promote a negative climacteric experience.

Double-blind studies have found improvements in self-reported irritability, mild anxiety, and dysphoria in women treated with estrogen alone or when combined with progestin. Improvement of the Beck depression score in women without hot flushes indicates that estrogens likely have direct effects on brain function.

Depression and other quality of life outcomes were studied in the Women's Health Initiative trial. Overall, conjugated equine estrogen alone, or in combination with medroxyprogesterone acetate, did not improve depressive symptoms amongst postmenopausal women ages 50–79 years after 1 and 3 years. In a subgroup analysis of 50–54-year-old women experiencing hot flashes, estrogen plus progestin improved hot flashes and sleep disturbance, but no other quality-of-life outcomes. In the estrogen-alone group, there was a slight improvement in sleep disturbance and social functioning, but no other quality-of-life outcomes measured. Therefore, a role for HT/ET in improving depressive symptoms following the menopause remains unproven.

C. Cognitive Decline

As life expectancy in women has risen, there has been more research regarding the effects of estrogen on cognitive functioning in postmenopausal women. Research indicates that estrogen influences areas of the brain known to be important for memory. However, recent data from the WHI suggests that estrogen alone or in combination with progestin does not decrease, and in fact may increase, the risk of cognitive decline in women older than 65 years of age.

D. Skin and Hair Changes

With aging, noticeable changes occur in the skin. There is generalized thinning and an accompanying loss of elasticity, resulting in wrinkling. These changes are particularly prominent in the areas exposed to light (ie, the face, neck, and hands). "Purse-string" wrinkling around the mouth and "crow's feet" around the eyes are characteristic. Skin changes on the dorsum of the hands are particularly noticeable. In this area, the skin may be so thin as to become almost transparent, with details of the underlying veins easily visible.

Histologically, the epidermis is thinned, and the basal layers become inactive with age. Dehydration is typical. Reduction in the number of blood vessels to the skin is also seen. Degeneration of elastic and collagenous fibers in the dermis also appears to be part of the aging process.

These skin changes are of cosmetic importance and are of great concern to many women. It is unclear if these changes are primarily caused by the menopause, aging, or a combination of both factors. It is commonly stated that women undergoing estrogen replacement look younger, and the cosmetic industry has been putting estrogens in skin creams for years for precisely this reason.

The possibility that estrogens may have effects on skin was suggested by the demonstration of estrogen receptors in skin. The number of receptors is highest in facial skin, followed by skin of the breasts and thighs.

This gives credence to the hypothesis that estrogens affect the skin.

Skin circulation is decreased in women after oophorectomy. Radiolabeled thymidine incorporation (an index of new DNA metabolism) is reported to decrease during the several months following oophorectomy. In some animal studies, estrogens increase the mitotic rate (a reflection of growth) of skin. Estrogens may alter the vascularization of skin. They also change the collagen content of the dermis, as reflected by mucopolysaccharide incorporation, hydroxyproline turnover, and alterations of the ground substance. In addition, dermal synthesis of hyaluronic acid and dermal water content are enhanced.

Skin collagen content and thickness have been studied in postmenopausal women. Decreases of both have been observed at a rate of 1–2% per year. The losses correlated with the number of years since the menopause, but not with chronologic age. Estrogen replacement prevents these losses or restores both parameters to premenopausal values. The greatest recovery is observed in women who began with low values. These data were interpreted to indicate that estrogen can prevent loss in women with high skin collagen levels, whereas it can restore content as well as prevent further loss in women with low collagen levels. Although these results are promising, it remains unclear whether they are clinically relevant. Estrogen should not be prescribed to improve the appearance of skin.

After the menopause, most women note some change in patterns of body hair. Usually there is a variable loss of pubic and axillary hair. Often there is loss of lanugo hair on the upper lip, chin, and cheeks, together with increased growth of coarse terminal hairs; a slight moustache may become noticeable. Hair on the body and extremities may either increase or decrease. Slight balding is seen occasionally. All of these changes may be partly a result of reduced levels of estrogen in the face of fairly well-maintained levels of testosterone.

E. Miscellaneous Symptoms

Many other symptoms are attributed to the endocrine changes of the postmenopausal state, but a direct cause-and-effect relationship has not been established for them. Some of these so-called climacteric symptoms are so common that they deserve brief mention.

Symptoms possibly related to specific autonomic nervous system instability—but equally attributable to anxiety or other emotional disturbances—are paresthesia (pricking, itching, formication), dizziness, tinnitus, fainting, scotomas, and dyspnea. Symptoms clearly not of endocrine origin are weakness, fatigue, nausea, vomiting, flatulence, anorexia, constipation, diarrhea, arthralgia, and myalgia.

Many women erroneously believe that the endocrine changes accompanying menopause will produce a steady weight gain. Women and men do tend to gain weight at this time of life, but the cause is usually a combination of decreased exercise and possibly increased caloric intake. There may be some redistribution of body weight occasioned by the deposition of fat over the hips and abdomen. Perhaps this is partly an endocrine effect, but more likely it is the result of decreased physical activity, reduced muscle tone, and other effects of aging.

Many of the previously mentioned symptoms occasionally respond promptly to administration of estrogen. This should not mislead physicians into assuming a specific endocrine action for what is actually a placebo effect.

Differential Diagnosis of Common Signs and Symptoms during Menopause

Signs and symptoms similar to those of the climacteric can be caused by a variety of other diseases. In general, seeing the entire clinical picture is helpful in establishing the proper diagnosis. The absence of evidence of other disease points to cessation of ovarian function, whereas the presence of prominent features of other conditions, in the absence of other climacteric symptoms, suggests a nonclimacteric origin.

A. Amenorrhea

By definition, the primary symptom of the menopause is the absence of menstruation. Amenorrhea can occur for many reasons, of which physiologic menopause is only one. Cessation of ovarian function is by far the most common reason for amenorrhea to occur in women in their forties or early fifties. Persistent amenorrhea in younger women may be a result of premature cessation of ovarian function, but must be differentiated from other causes. Obvious features of specific disease often suggest the proper diagnosis (eg, extreme weight loss in anorexia nervosa, galactorrhea in hyperprolactinemia, hirsutism and obesity in polycystic ovarian disease).

B. Hot Flashes

Several diseases can produce sensations of flushing that may be misinterpreted as hot flushes. Notable are hyperthyroidism, pheochromocytoma, carcinoid syndrome, diabetes mellitus, tuberculosis, and other chronic infections. None of these disorders produces the specific symptoms associated with the climacteric (ie, short duration and specific body distribution). Moreover, the absence of other signs or symptoms of the climacteric suggest some other cause of the flushes should be sought.

C. Abnormal Vaginal Bleeding

Prior to the menopause, irregular vaginal bleeding is expected and does not necessitate a diagnostic work-up in many cases. However, organic disease can occur at this time, and some patients require evaluation. If a woman is in her forties or fifties and experiences an increase in cycle length and a decrease in the quantity of bleeding, menopausal involution can be presumed and endometrial sampling is usually not necessary. However, if menses become more frequent and heavier, spotting between menses occurs, or any pattern of irregular bleeding persists, assessment of the endometrium should be performed. The usual procedure is an endometrial biopsy or dilatation and curettage (D&C) to rule out endometrial hyperplasia or cancer. The disadvantage of the former is that entry into the endometrial cavity may not be accomplished in the setting of a stenotic os, and the drawbacks of the latter are greater expense, risk and need for anesthesia.

It is most unusual for a woman to experience vaginal bleeding because of ovarian activity by 6 months after the menopause. Thus, postmenopausal bleeding is much more ominous and necessitates evaluation each time it occurs. The only exception to this rule is the uterine bleeding associated with estrogen replacement therapy. Other guidelines are recommended for this type of bleeding (see Estrogen Therapy).

Organic disease is commonly associated with postmenopausal bleeding. Endometrial polyps may be found, which can be resected via the hysteroscope. Endometrial hyperplasia may be discovered, frequently in obese women. This can be treated by the periodic administration of progestin or by hysterectomy. If hyperplasia develops in a woman taking estrogens, the addition of progestins should be considered. If hyperplasia develops unrelated to hormone replacement, surgery should be considered if the patient is a good surgical risk or is not reliable in taking progestins. The finding of endometrial cancer necessitates appropriate therapy depending on the stage and grade of the tumor.

D. VULVOVAGINITIS

Many specific vulvar and vaginal diseases (eg, trichomoniasis and candidiasis) may mimic the atrophic vulvovaginitis of estrogen deficiency. Their special clinical characteristics usually suggest more specific diagnostic testing. When pruritus and thinning of the vaginal epithelium or the vulvar skin are the only manifestations, therapeutic testing with local applications of estrogen may help to establish the diagnosis of vulvovaginitis. When any whitening, thickening, or cracking of vulvar tissues is present, biopsy to rule out carcinoma is mandatory. Raised or erosive lesions should also be sampled. Biopsy to rule out carcinoma is also necessary for suspicious looking vaginal or cervical lesions.

E. BACK PAIN

Occasionally, the pain of vertebral compression from osteoporosis may mimic that of gastric ulcer, renal colic,

pyelonephritis, pancreatitis, spondylolisthesis, acute back strain, or herniated intervertebral disk.

Prevention of Menopause

Nothing can prevent the physiologic menopause (ie, ovarian function cannot be prolonged indefinitely), and nothing can be done to postpone its onset or slow its progress. However, artificial menopause can often be prevented. When ionizing radiation is used for the treatment of intra-abdominal disease, incidental ablation of ovarian function often cannot be avoided. In such cases, if an operation will serve equally well to treat intra-abdominal disease, it should be used in preference to radiation therapy in order to preserve the ovaries.

Elective removal of the ovaries to prevent ovarian cancer is frequently performed at laparotomy or laparoscopy in premenopausal women, with deliberate acceptance of artificial menopause. This form of therapy, however, remains controversial.

Estrogen Therapy

Every woman with menopausal symptoms deserves an adequate explanation of the physiologic event she is experiencing, so as to dispel her fears and address symptoms such as hot flashes and sleep disturbance. Reassurance should be emphasized. Specific reassurance about continued sexual activity is important.

As long as ovarian function is sufficient to maintain some uterine bleeding, no treatment is usually required. Occasionally, women complain of hot flushes while menstrual function is still present. Treatment with low-dose oral contraceptive pills, if no contraindications exist, will relieve these symptoms and help to regulate menstrual cycles during the menopausal transition.

A. INDICATIONS

Estrogen therapy has been used for many years for a variety of symptoms and conditions seen in the aged female population. However, despite suggestions from observational and experimental studies that estrogens prevent many common conditions of aging, such as Alzheimer's disease and CHD, estrogen therapy has only been proven to be effective in the prevention of osteoporosis, treatment of vasomotor symptoms, and treatment of vulvovaginal atrophy. Results from the WHI further call into question the degree to which estrogen can act as a "cure-all" for the common conditions of aging, particularly those affecting the brain and heart. Benefits beyond those already established are still possible, but await proof in large-scale studies in humans. Therefore, use of estrogens should be limited to the currently approved Food and Drug Administration (FDA) indications: prevention of osteoporosis, treatment of vasomotor symptoms, and treatment of vulvovaginal atrophy (see D. Management Guidelines for Estrogen Therapy).

B. COMPLICATIONS

Before discussing the management of estrogen replacement, it is necessary to review the complications of and contraindications to this type of therapy. These play an important role in the ultimate decision regarding treatment for all patients.

1. Endometrial cancer—The role of estrogen therapy in the development of endometrial cancer is one of the most highly charged issues related to the menopause. Current concerns are based on several lines of investigation. The scope of investigative efforts lead to the conclusion that estrogen stimulation of the endometrium, unopposed by progesterone, causes endometrial proliferation, hyperplasia, and, finally, neoplasia. Consequently, it is recommended that a progestin be added to ET to reduce the risk of endometrial hyperplasia or carcinoma.

The reports of estrogen replacement and endometrial carcinoma have received the greatest attention. In most studies, a strong association has been found, with 2- to 8-fold overall risk ratios. High dosage and prolonged treatment increase the risk. Disease is local in most cases, although more widespread invasive tumors have been reported. Concerns have been raised about these studies, particularly regarding the selection of controls. In most studies, controls had not undergone sampling of the endometrium to rule out asymptomatic endometrial cancer. Thus, debates persist, and prudent physicians should discuss the risks with their patients and employ preventive measures.

2. Breast cancer—Early age at menarche and older age at menopause are known risk factors for breast cancer, and early oophorectomy is known to give protection against this disease. Ovarian activity is an important determinant of risk, thus estrogen may play a role in the development of breast cancer. Studies in rodents support that view. More than 30 epidemiologic studies have been published since 1974 to determine the possible link between postmenopausal estrogen use and breast cancer. In general, the later studies have had better design, quality, and analytic strategies. The number of subjects in more recent studies has also been larger. At least 6 meta-analyses of this topic also have been conducted. These results have not always agreed. The recent prospective, randomized Women's Health Initiative trial also addressed this issue. In this study there was an increased risk of invasive breast cancer in the estrogen/progestin arm. However, in the estrogen-alone arm, the risk of breast cancer was not increased compared to controls.

Despite this inconsistency in studies, some trends have been observed: (a) The overall risk of breast cancer with estrogen use has not uniformly been shown to be increased. (b) Long-term use (ie, 4–10 years) has been associated with mild increased risk (RR 1.2–1.5) in some of the meta-analyses and the Women's Health Initiative. (c) The addition of a progestin does not appear to decrease risk and may increase risk. (d) Finally, risk does not vary in strata of family history of breast cancer or with benign breast disease.

It must be remembered that all women are at risk for breast cancer. Thus, instructions for breast self-examination, a careful breast assessment, and routine screening mammography should be a part of the medical care of all older women.

3. Thromboembolic disease—Use of oral contraceptives increases the risk of overt venous thromboembolic disease and subclinical disease extensive enough to be detected by laboratory procedures such as ^{125}I fibrinogen uptake and plasma fibrinogen chromatography. The risk of venous thromboembolic disease was also increased among users of ET/HT in the WHI, as well as among users of HT in the HERS trial.

The effects of estrogen on the clotting mechanism may contribute to or be responsible for a generalized hypercoagulable state. Oral estrogens affect synthesis of coagulation factors through a first-pass effect in the liver, an effect associated with an increased risk of thromboembolic disease. The risk for thromboembolic events with use of ET/HT is also likely further increased amongst patients with inherited thrombophilias.

Use of transdermal estrogens is probably associated with a lowered risk for thromboembolic events as compared to use of oral estrogens. However, randomized trials are needed to better characterize the effects of transdermal estrogens on risk for clinical thromboembolic events.

4. Stroke—Several recent studies suggest that hormone therapy is associated with an increased risk of stroke. In the combined HT arm of the WHI, there was an increased risk of ischemic stroke amongst those using combined HT when compared to the placebo. In the estrogen alone arm of the WHI, there was also a statistically significant increased risk of stroke after approximately 7 years of follow-up, and this outcome led to the trial being terminated.

5. Uterine bleeding—If patients are given sequential estrogen and progestins, the majority will experience some uterine bleeding, particularly soon after initiation of therapy. This bleeding can occur during the treatment-free interval (scheduled bleeding) or while the medications are being administered (unscheduled bleeding). Hyperplastic endometrium can develop with this type of therapy. If the bleeding is heavy or prolonged, a biopsy should be performed. In women using a combined continuous regimen of estrogen and progestin, bleeding is common in the first several months of therapy and usually doesn't indicate endometrial pathology. However, if bleeding persists in these patients, or is prolonged or heavy at any time, endometrial sampling should be performed. If endometrial hyperplasia is present, the medications can be discontinued, progestin dose can be increased or a progestin can be given each day of estrogen administration. Whichever approach is adopted, a repeat biopsy should be performed to make certain that the hyperplastic endometrium has resolved. The cost-effectiveness ratio for periodic biopsy in women who do not bleed or bleed only during the medication-free interval is poor and indicates that such biopsy is probably unnecessary.

In women taking estrogen only, the incidence of endometrial hyperplasia can be as high as 25% after only 12 months of therapy. Hyperplasia occurs in women who do not experience vaginal bleeding, bleed only during the medication-free interval, or bleed during drug administration. Thus, a pretreatment biopsy and yearly endometrial biopsies are necessary in all women receiving estrogens alone to assess for the presence of hyperplasia. Again, estrogen withdrawal or combined estrogen-progesterone therapy may be employed to treat the hyperplasia. The incidence of endometrial cancer will likely be reduced if the programs discussed above are instituted.

6. Gallbladder disease—An increased incidence of gallbladder disease has been reported following estrogen replacement therapy. Estrogens cause increased amounts of cholesterol to collect in bile. Two primary bile salts, cholate and chenodeoxycholate, are produced by liver cells. In women taking estrogen, decreased levels of chenodeoxycholate and increased levels of cholate are found in bile. Chenodeoxycholate inhibits activity of the enzyme β-hydroxy-β-methylglutaryl-CoA reductase, which regulates cholesterol synthesis, and a decrease in chenodeoxycholate may therefore cause increased activity of β-hydroxy-β-methylglutaryl-CoA reductase, leading to increased synthesis of cholesterol. Bile normally has a 75–90% saturation in cholesterol, and even small increases of this substance can initiate cholesterol precipitation and stone formation. Three-fourths of gallstones are composed predominantly of cholesterol.

7. Lipid metabolism—Estrogen replacement also has an impact on circulating lipids. As discussed above, many of these effects are favorable. However, others may pose increased risk. Most lipids are bound to proteins in the blood, and the concentrations of the various types of lipoproteins are associated with varying risks of heart disease. Lower levels of HDL cholesterol and higher concentrations of total cholesterol, LDL cholesterol, very-low-density lipoprotein (VLDL) cholesterol, and triglycerides are associated with increased risk of atherosclerosis and coronary artery disease. Estrogen replacement decreases LDL cholesterol and increases HDL cholesterol and triglycerides. Use of conjugated estrogens, 0.625 mg/d or less, causes approximately a 10% increase in HDL cholesterol. Much attention has been focused on the impact of estrogens on lipoproteins to explain what appeared to be a beneficial effect of HT on heart disease in earlier observational studies of younger postmenopausal women. The impact of estrogen-induced increases in triglycerides on cardiovascular risk is unclear. In patients with familial defects of lipoprotein metabolism, estrogen replacement therapy is associated with massive elevations of plasma triglycerides, leading to pancreatitis and other complications. However, this is a very unusual complication of estrogen replacement. Transdermal estrogens are probably less likely to raise triglyceride levels and thus are preferred in women with an elevation in triglyceride levels.

8. Miscellaneous—Other side effects of estrogen therapy include uterine bleeding, generalized edema, mastodynia and breast enlargement, abdominal bloating, signs and symptoms resembling those of premenstrual tension, headaches (particularly of a "menstrual migraine" type), and excessive cervical mucous. These side effects may be dose related or idiosyncratic, and are managed by lowering the dosage, by use of another agent, or by discontinuation of the medication.

C. CONTRAINDICATIONS TO ESTROGEN REPLACEMENT THERAPY

Contraindications to estrogen therapy are as follows: (a) Undiagnosed abnormal vaginal bleeding; (b) known, suspected or history of cancer of the breast; (c) known or suspected estrogen-dependent neoplasia; (d) active deep vein thrombosis, pulmonary embolism, or a history of these conditions; (e) arterial thromboembolic disease (myocardial infarction, stroke); and (f) liver dysfunction or disease. In general, estrogen therapy should be avoided in patients with a diagnosis of endometrial cancer. Estrogen therapy may stimulate growth of malignant cells remaining after treatment of breast or endometrial carcinoma and may thus hasten the recurrence of cancer. Therefore, it is prudent to avoid systemic estrogen therapy in breast cancer patients and most endometrial cancer patients. Recently, it was suggested that women with early (stage 1) and well-differentiated (grade 1) endometrial cancer can be administered estrogens following primary treatment of the cancer. Care must be exercised in following this recommendation until it has been properly studied. Any decision to use ET/HT following a diagnosis of endometrial cancer should be made in consultation with the patient's oncologist. Patients who have had estrogen receptor-positive malignant tumors of the breast probably should not receive systemic estrogen supplements. Topical vaginal estrogens to treat symptoms of urogenital atrophy in breast/endometrial cancer patients might be acceptable, but should first be discussed with the patient's oncologist. A history of treated carcinoma of the cervix or ovary is not a contraindication to estrogen therapy. Estrogens may have undesirable effects on some patients with preexisting seizures, hypertension, fibrocystic disease of the breast, uterine leiomyoma, collagen disease, familial hyperlipidemia, diabetes mellitus, migraine headaches, chronic thrombophlebitis, and gallbladder disease. At the low dosages recommended for replacement therapy, increased growth of uterine myomas, endometriosis, or chronic cystic mastitis is rarely a concern.

D. MANAGEMENT GUIDELINES FOR ESTROGEN THERAPY

1. General—Only general guidelines can be offered, because risks and benefits must be evaluated for each patient. Numerous formulations of estrogen and estrogen plus progestin are available (Table 59–1). Current indications for estrogen therapy are relief of menopausal symptoms (including hot flushes and vaginal atrophy) and prevention of osteoporosis. Caution should be exercised in providing therapy for other conditions until more definitive studies have been performed. If symptoms of hot flushes and vaginal atrophy are moderate to severe, therapy may be used for the shortest duration possible; minimal or no symptoms may not require hormones.

In women who require pharmacologic intervention for prevention of **osteoporosis,** estrogen may be used. However, estrogen therapy for osteoporosis prevention is generally reserved for those women who are otherwise using estrogen for menopausal symptoms and/or who cannot tolerate other antiresorptive therapies. Lower dosages of estrogen are being increasingly used for prevention of osteoporosis so as to minimize the risks of estrogen therapy. There are several options available for use of estrogen or estrogen plus progestin for prevention of osteoporosis (Table 59–1). In the past, standard doses included 0.625 mg of conjugated equine estrogens, 0.05 mg of transdermal estradiol, and 1 mg of micronized estradiol. However, 0.3 mg of conjugated equine estrogens, 0.5 mg of micronized estradiol, and 0.025-mg transdermal patches also prevent bone loss, although not as well as higher doses. A new **lowdose** (0.014 mg/d) transdermal formulation of estradiol was recently FDA approved for prevention of osteoporosis. Early commencement of prophylaxis following cessation of ovarian function will maintain the highest bone density. Initiation of HT well after the menopause will stop bone loss, but will not return bone density to that which was present at the time of the menopause.

For women with **hot flashes,** a standard dosage of estrogen, such as 0.3–0.625 mg of conjugated equine estrogens, 0.025 mg transdermal estradiol, or 0.5 mg oral estradiol should be given daily (Table 59–1). Higher doses may be necessary to relieve hot flashes. Progressive reduction of dosage should be attempted as soon as feasible. Additional formulations containing estradiol, synthetic estrogens and estrogens plus progestins are also available (Table 59–1).

In women who are suffering from **atrophic vaginitis,** vaginal preparations can be used and are preferred over systemic estrogens. These preparations are available in the form of creams (ie, conjugated equine estrogens or estradiol 0.25–2 g given nightly for 2 weeks, followed by twice weekly), tablets (25 μg estradiol given nightly for 2 weeks, followed by twice weekly), and rings (estradiol releasing rings which remain in place for 3 months at a time) (Table 59–1). With the tablets, rings, and lowest-dose creams, endometrial proliferation is rare. However, higher doses, presence of vaginal bleeding, or other risk factors may necessitate periodic endometrial biopsy or ultrasound to assess the endometrial thickness. Progestins may be necessary to prevent endometrial proliferation in some cases.

2. Progestogen-estrogen therapy—One of the most serious concerns about estrogen replacement is the occurrence of endometrial hyperplasia or cancer. Progestins oppose the action of estrogen on the endometrium. Progestins reduce the number of estrogen receptors in glandular and stromal cells of the endometrium. These agents also block estrogen-induced synthesis of DNA, and they induce the intracellular enzymes estradiol dehydrogenase and estrogen sulfotransferase. The former reduces estradiol to the much less potent estrone, whereas the latter converts estrogen to estrogen sulfates for rapid elimination from endometrial cells. In addition, full secretory transformation occurs if the progestin is given at a large enough dosage for a sufficient length of time.

Progestins reduce the occurrence of endometrial cancer. Epidemiologic studies show significant reduction of the occurrence of endometrial cancer with estrogen plus progestin compared with estrogen alone. One study indicated use of the progestin for more than 10 days a month reduced the occurrence more than use for a shorter interval. In treating women with hormones, a more practical concern is the prevention of endometrial hyperplasia. Initially, British investigators showed that high-dose estrogens (1.25 mg or greater of conjugated equine estrogens) resulted in 32% hyperplasia, whereas low doses (0.625 mg or less) stimulated 16% hyperplasias in women followed for 15 months. In women given estrogen plus progestins, the occurrence of hyperplasia was 6% and 3%, respectively. In comparing length of therapy, 7 days of progestin reduced the occurrence of hyperplasia to 4%, 10 days reduced it to 2%, and 12 days eliminated hyperplasia. Direct comparisons in drug trials have also shown reductions of hyperplasia in women given estrogens and progestins compared with those given estrogen alone. It should be pointed out that the majority of endometrial lesions observed in women in these trials were either cystic or simple hyperplasias, which could be reversed by giving a progestin or discontinuing the estrogen.

One option is to administer a progestin such as medroxyprogesterone acetate at a dosage of 5–10 mg/d for 12–14 days each month (see Table 59–1). If this is

Table 59–1. Preparations of estrogens and progestins available in the United States for hormone therapy.

Agent	How Supplied	Special Features
Oral estrogens		
Conjugated equine estrogens	0.3 mg, 0.45 mg, 0.625 mg, 0.9 mg, 1.25 mg tablets	Well studied, well tolerated; approved for prevention of osteoporosis, 0.625 mg dose used in WHI study
Estradiol	0.5 mg, 1 mg, 2 mg tablets	Well tolerated; approved for prevention of osteoporosis
Piperazine estrone (estropipate)	0.75 mg, 1.5 mg tablets	
Synthetic conjugated estrogens	0.3 mg, 0.45 mg, 0.625 mg, 0.9 mg, 1.25 mg tablets	Not approved for prevention of osteoporosis
Transdermal estrogens		
Estradiol patch (mg/day)	0.014 mg, 0.025 mg, 0.0375 mg, 0.05 mg, 0.06 mg, 0.075 mg, 0.1 mg patches	Well tolerated, 10% skin rash, available in weekly and biweekly formulations; approved for prevention of osteoporosis; new low dose (0.014 mg) also approved for prevention of osteoporosis
Estradiol gel	0.06% gel	Not approved for prevention of osteoporosis
Vaginal estrogens		
Creams		
Conjugated equine estrogens	0.625 mg/g cream	Not approved for prevention of osteoporosis
Estradiol	0.1 mg/g cream	Not approved for prevention of osteoporosis
Tablets		
Estradiol	0.025 mg tablet	Not approved for prevention of osteoporosis
Rings		
Estradiol	0.05 mg/day, 0.1 mg/day	Remains in place for 3 months; not approved for prevention of osteoporosis
Oral Progestogens		
Medroxyprogesterone acetate	2.5 mg, 5 mg, 10 mg tablets	Well tolerated, well studied
Micronized progesterone	100 mg, 200 mg capsules	Well tolerated, possible somnolence
Megestrol acetate	20 mg, 40 mg scored tablets	Not used routinely for postmenopausal hormone therapy
Norethindrone	0.35 mg tablets	Available as contraceptive "minipill"
Norethindrone acetate	5 mg scored tablets	Dosage probably too large for routine hormone therapy
Intrauterine Progestin		
Levonorgestrel releasing IUD	20 µg/day	Not routinely used for postmenopausal hormone therapy, approved for use as contraceptive; remains in place for 5 years; may prevent endometrial hyperplasia with fewer side effects but not approved for this use.

(continued)

Table 59–1. Preparations of estrogens and progestins available in the United States for hormone therapy. (continued)

Agent	How Supplied	Special Features
Estrogen/Progestogen Combination Formulas		
Oral		
Conjugated equine estrogens (CEE)/medroxyprogesterone acetate (MPA)	0.3 mg CEE/1.5 mg MPA; 0.45 mg CEE/1.5 mg MPA; 0.625 mg CEE/2.5 mg MPA; 0.625 mg CEE/5 mg MPA; 0.625 mg CEE days 1–14, then 0.625 mg CEE/5 mg MPA days 15–28	Well tolerated, well studied, approved for prevention of osteoporosis, 0.625 mg/2.5 mg preparation used in WHI study
Estradiol/norethindrone acetate	1 mg estradiol/0.5 mg norethindrone	Approved for prevention of osteoporosis
Estradiol/norgestimate	1 mg estradiol × 3 days, alternating with 1 mg estradiol/0.09 mg norgestimate × 3 days	Intermittent progestin; approved for prevention of osteoporosis
Ethinyl estradiol/norethindrone acetate	2.5 μg ethinyl estradiol/ 0.5 mg norethindrone; 5 μg ethinyl estradiol/1 mg norethindrone	Approved for prevention of osteoporosis
Esterified estrogens/methyl testosterone	0.625 mg esterified estrogens/1.25 mg methyl testosterone; 1.25 mg esterified estrogens/2.5 mg methyl testosterone	Not approved for prevention of osteoporosis
Transdermal patches		
Estradiol/norethindrone acetate	0.05 mg estradiol/0.14 mg norethindrone per day; 0.05 mg estradiol/ 0.025 mg norethindrone per day	Not approved for prevention of osteoporosis
Estradiol/levonorgestrel	0.045 mg estradiol/0.015 mg levonorgestrel per day	Not approved for prevention of osteoporosis

accomplished, 80–90% of women will experience some vaginal bleeding monthly toward the end of or after the progestin is administered. An alternative is to prescribe a lower dosage, 2.5 mg, continuously. Many newer formulations of hormone therapy contain both estrogen and progestin (Table 59–1). The combined, continuous administration of estrogen plus progestin is the most common mode of administration today. This regimen promotes endometrial atrophy and results in amenorrhea in 70–90% of women who use continuous therapy for more than 1 year. The remainder will bleed occasionally, with the bleeding usually being less frequent, shorter, and lighter than with sequential therapy.

Administration of progestins can be associated with other uncomfortable side effects including fatigue, depression, breast tenderness, bloating, menstrual cramps, and headaches. It is also important to keep in mind that it was a progestin-containing regimen that was used in the WHI trial that was discontinued largely because of a trend toward an increased risk of breast cancer. In the estrogen-only arm, breast cancer rates were not increased over control levels. This raises concerns about the potential role of progestogens in increasing breast cancer risk. This concern combined with potential progestogen side effects may lead to elimination of or nonstandard progestogen administration. If lower dosages or shorter duration of progestogens are used, endometrial sampling

to diagnose the development of hyperplasia or cancer should be performed. Use of locally administered progestins through the use of the levonorgestrel intrauterine device is also being considered as an alternative strategy to minimize systemic side effects and risks while maintaining endometrial protection.

Prognosis

The prognosis for the postmenopausal woman who does not develop clinically manifest estrogen deficiency includes only the ordinary hazards of disease and aging. For the woman who does develop signs of estrogen deficiency, hormone therapy can correct physical symptoms and signs, and prevent the development of osteoporosis. Correction of minor distressing symptoms and signs can improve the general well-being of the postmenopausal woman and help her to pursue a vigorous life. However, hormone therapy for the postmenopausal woman who does not need it serves no purpose and can cause unpleasant side effects and impose unnecessary risks to her health.

REFERENCES

Abraham GE, Maroulis GB: Effect of exogenous estrogen on serum pregnenolone, cortisol, and androgens in postmenopausal women. Obstet Gynecol 1975;45:271.

Adams MR et al: Inhibition of coronary artery atherosclerosis by 17-beta estradiol in ovariectomized monkeys: lack of an effect of added progesterone. Arteriosclerosis 1990;10:1051.

American Heart Association. *Heart Disease and Stroke Statistics, 2000 Update.* American Heart Association, 2006.

Antunes CM et al: Endometrial cancer and estrogen use. N Engl J Med 1979;300:9.

Arias E: United States Life Tables, 2002, National Vital Statistics Reports. Centers for Disease Control and Prevention. 53(6), 2004.

Avioli LV: The role of calcitonin in the prevention of osteoporosis. Endocrinol Metab Clin North Am 1998;27:411.

Barrett-Connor E, Bush TL: Estrogen replacement and coronary heart disease. Cardiovasc Clin 1989;19:159.

Barrett-Connor E, Miller V: Estrogens, lipids, and heart disease. Clin Geriatr Med 1993;9:57.

Beral V, Million Women Study Collaborators: Breast cancer and hormone-replacement therapy in the Million Women Study. Lancet 2003;362:419.

Dimitrakakis C et al: Clinical effects of tibolone in postmenopausal women after five years of tamoxifen therapy for breast cancer. Climacteric 2005;8:342.

Bergkvist L et al: The risk of breast cancer after estrogen and estrogen-progestin replacement. N Engl J Med 1989;321:293.

Bolognia J: Aging skin, epidermal and dermal changes. Prog Clin Biol Res 1989;320:121.

Bone HG et al: Alendronate and estrogen effects in postmenopausal women with low bone mineral density. Alendronate/Estrogen Study Group. J Clin Endocrinol Metab 2000;85:720.

Brincat M et al: Long-term effects of the menopause and sex hormones on skin thickness. Br J Obstet Gynecol 1985;92:256.

Brincat M et al: A study of the decrease of skin collagen content, skin thickness, and bone mass in the postmenopausal woman. Obstet Gyneol 1987;70:840.

Brunner RL et al: Effects of conjugated equine estrogen on health-related quality of life in postmenopausal women with hysterectomy: Results from the Women's Health Initiative Randomized Clinical Trial. Arch Intern Med 2005; 165:1976.

Campisi R et al: Tibolone improves myocardial perfusion in postmenopausal women with ischemic heart disease: an open-label exploratory pilot study. J Am Coll Cardiol 2006;47:559.

Cauley JA et al: Estrogen replacement therapy and mortality among older women: the study of osteoporotic fractures. Arch Intern Med 1997;157:2181.

Chetkowski RJ et al: Biologic effects of transdermal estradiol. N Engl J Med 1986;314:1615.

Collaborative group on hormonal factors in breast cancer: Breast cancer and hormone replacement therapy. Lancet 1997;350:1047.

Creasman WT: Estrogen replacement therapy: Is previously treated cancer a contraindication? Obstet Gynecol 1991;77:308.

Delmas PD: Biochemical markers of bone turnover: methodology and clinical use in osteoporosis. Am J Med 1991;91:59S.

Delmas PD et al: Effects of raloxifene on bone mineral density, serum cholesterol concentrations, and uterine endometrium in postmenopausal women. N Engl J Med 1997; 337:1641.

Erickson GE: Normal ovarian function. Clin Obstet Gynecol 1978;21:31.

Espeland MA et al: Conjugated equine estrogens and global cognitive function in postmenopausal women: the Women's Health Initiative Memory Study. JAMA 2004;291:2959.

Ettinger B et al: Low-dosage micronized 17β-estradiol prevents bone loss in postmenopausal women. Am J Obstet Gynecol 1992;166:479.

Ettinger B et al: Reduction of vertebral fracture risk in postmenopausal women with osteoporosis treated with raloxifene: results from a 3-year randomized clinical trial. Multiple Outcomes of Raloxifene Evaluation (MORE) Investigators. JAMA 1999;282:637.

Falkeborn M et al: The risk of acute myocardial infarction after estrogen and estrogen-progesterone replacement. Br J Obstet Gynaecol 1992;99:821.

Feyen JH: Prostaglandin production by calvariae from sham operated and oophorectomized rats: effect of 17 beta-estradiol in vivo. Endocrinology, 1987; 121:819.

Field CS et al: Preventive effects of transdermal 17-estradiol on osteoporotic changes after surgical menopause: a two-year placebo-controlled trial. Am J Obstet Gynecol 1993;168:114.

Fogelman I et al: Risedronate reverses bone loss in postmenopausal women with low bone mass: results from a multinational, double-blind, placebo-controlled trial. BMD-MN Study Group. J Clin Endocrinol Metab 2000;85:1895.

Furchgott RF, Vanhoutte PM: Endothelium-derived relaxing and contracting factors. FASEB J 1989;3:2007.

Gambone J et al: Further delineation of hypothalamic dysfunction responsible for menopausal hot flashes. J Clin Endocrinol Metab 1985;59:1097.

Grodstein F et al: Postmenopausal hormone therapy and mortality. N Engl J Med 1997;336:1769.

Grodstein F et al: Hormone therapy and coronary heart disease: The role of time since menopause and age at hormone initiation. J Women's Health 2006;15:35.

Guttuso T et al: Gabapentin's effects on hot flashes in postmenopausal women: a randomized controlled trial. Obstet Gynecol 2003;101:337

Harris ST et al: Effect of combined risedronate and hormone replacement therapies on bone mineral density in postmenopausal women. J Clin Endocrinol Metab 2001;86:1890.

Harris ST: Effects of risedronate treatment on vertebral and non-vertebral fractures in women with postmenopausal osteoporosis: a randomized controlled trial. Vertebral Efficacy with Risedronate (VERT) Study Group. JAMA 1999;282:1344.

Hayashi T et al: Basal release of nitric oxide from aortic rings is greater in female rabbits than in male rabbits: implications for atherosclerosis. Proc Natl Acad Sci U S A 1992;89:11259.

Hays J et al: Effect of estrogen plus progestin on health-related quality of life. N Engl J Med 2003;348:1839.

Hemminki E et al: Impact of postmenopausal hormone therapy on cardiovascular events and cancer: pooled data from clinical trials. BMJ 1997;315:149.

Herrington DM et al: The effects of estrogen replacement on the progression of coronary-artery atherosclerosis. N Engl J Med 2000;343;522.

Holloway L: Skeletal effects of cyclic recombinant human growth hormone and salmon calcitonin in osteopenic postmenopausal women. J Clin Endocrinol Metab 1997;82:1111.

Horwitz RI et al: Necropsy diagnosis of endometrial cancer and detection-bias in case-control studies. Lancet 1981;2:66.

Hulley S et al: Randomized trial of estrogen plus progestin for secondary prevention of coronary heart disease in postmenopausal women. Heart and Estrogen/Progestin Replacement Study research group. JAMA 1998;280:605.

Ioannidis JP et al: Association of polymorphisms of the estrogen receptor alpha gene with bone mineral density and fracture risk in women: a meta-analysis. J Bone Miner Res 2002;17:2048.

Ioannidis JP et al: Differential genetic effects of ESR1 gene polymorphism on osteoporosis outcome. JAMA 2004;292:2105.

Jensen J et al: Long-term effects of percutaneous estrogens and oral progesterone on serum lipoproteins in postmenopausal women. Am J Obstet Gynecol 1987;156:66.

Johnston CC Jr, Slemenda CW, Melton LJ III: Clinical use of bone densitometry. N Engl J Med 1991;324:1105.

Judd HL: Hormonal dynamics associated with the menopause. Clin Obstet Gynecol 1976;19:775.

Judd HL et al: Endocrine function of the postmenopausal ovary: concentrations of androgens and estrogens in ovarian and peripheral vein blood. J Clin Endocrinol Metab 1974;39:1020.

Judd HL et al: Origin of serum estradiol in postmenopausal women. Obstet Gynecol 1982;59:680.

Judd HL et al: Serum androgens and estrogens in postmenopausal women with and without endometrial cancer. Am J Obstet Gynecol 1980;136:859.

Kado DM et al: Vertebral fractures and mortality in older women: a prospective study. Study of Osteoporotic Fractures Research Group. Arch Intern Med 1999;159:1215.

Kenemans P, Speroff L: Tibolone: clinical recommendations and practical guidelines. A report of the International Tibolone Consensus Group. Maturitas 2004;51:21.

Kimble RB: Simultaneous block of interleukin-1 and tumor necrosis factor is required to completely prevent bone loss in the early postovariectomy period. Endocrinology 1995;136:3054.

Laufer LR et al: Effect of clonidine on hot flashes in postmenopausal women. Obstet Gynecol 1982;60:583.

Lindsay R et al: Bone response to termination of estrogen treatment. Lancet 1978;1:1325.

Lindsay R et al: Sustained vertebral fracture risk reduction after withdrawal of teriparatide in postmenopausal women with osteoporosis. Arch Intern Med 2004;164:2024.

Loprinzi CL et al: Venlafaxine in management of hot flashes in survivors of breast cancer: a randomized controlled trial. Lancet 2000;356:2059.

Loprinzi CL et al: Phase III evaluation of fluoxetine for treatment of hot flashes. J Clin Oncol 2002;20:1578.

Manson JE et al: Estrogen plus progestin and the risk of coronary heart disease. N Engl J Med 2003;349:523.

Meldrum DR et al: Elevations in skin temperature of the finger as an objective index of postmenopausal hot flashes: standardization of the technique. Am J Obstet Gynecol 1979;135:713.

Mendelsohn ME et al: The protective effects of estrogen on the cardiovascular system. N Engl J Med 1999;340:1801.

Meunier PJ: Fluoride salts are no better at preventing new vertebral fractures than calcium-vitamin D in postmenopausal osteoporosis: the FAVO study. Osteoporos Int 1998;8:4.

Miller et al: Estrogen therapy and thrombotic risk. Pharmacol Ther 2006;111:792.

Million Women Study Collaborators. Endometrial cancer and hormone-replacement therapy in the Million Women Study. Lancet 2005;365:1543.

Nabulsi AA et al: Association of hormone-replacement therapy with various cardiovascular risk factors in postmenopausal women. N Engl J Med 1993;328:1069.

National Osteoporosis Foundation: *Physician's Guide To Prevention and Treatment of Osteoporosis.* National Osteoporosis Foundation, 2005.

Nathan L et al: Estradiol inhibits leukocyte adhesion and transendothelial migration in vivo: possible mechanisms for gender differences in atherosclerosis. Circ Res 1999; 85:377–385.

Neer RM et al: Effect of parathyroid hormone (1-34) on fractures and bone mineral density in postmenopausal women with osteoporosis. N Engl J Med 2001;344:1434.

Osteoporosis Prevention, Diagnosis, and Therapy. National Institutes of Health Consensus Development Conference Statement 2001;17:1.

Pandya KJ et al: Gabapentin for hot flashes in 420 women with breast cancer: a randomized double-blind placebo-controlled trial. Lancet 2005;366:818.

Phillips SM, Sherwin BB: Effects of estrogen on memory function in surgically menopausal women. Psychoneuroendocrinology 1992;17:485.

Rapp SR et al: Effect of estrogen plus progestin on global cognitive function in postmenopausal women: the Women's Health Initiative Study: a randomized trial. JAMA 2003; 289:2663.

Rickard DJ, Gowen M, MacDonald BR: Proliferative responses to estradiol IL-1 alpha and TGF beta by cells expressing alkaline phosphatase in human osteoblast-like cell cultures. Calcif Tissue Int 1993;52:227.

Roberts WC, Giraldo AA: Bilateral oophorectomy in menstruating women and accelerated coronary atherosclerosis: An unproved connection. Am J Med 1979;67:363.

Rosen CJ: Emerging anabolic treatments for osteoporosis. Rheum Dis Clin North Am 2001;27:215.

Ross RK, Paganini-Hill A, Wan PC et al: Effect of hormone replacement therapy on breast cancer risk: Estrogen versus estrogen plus progestin. J Natl Cancer Inst 2000;92:328.

Roux S: Bone loss. Factors that regulate osteoclast differentiation: An update. Arthritis Res 2000;2:6.

Scarabin PY et al: Differential association of oral and transdermal oestrogen-replacement therapy with venous thromboembolism risk. Lancet 2003;362:428.

Shahrad P, Marks R: A pharmacologic effect of estrogen on human epidermis. Br J Dermatol 1977;97:383.

Sherman BM, Korenman SG: Hormonal characteristics of the human menstrual cycle throughout reproductive life. J Clin Invest 1975;55:669.

Shearman AM et al: Estrogen receptor beta polymorphisms are associated with bone mass in women and men: the Framingham Study. J Bone Miner Res 2004;19:773.

Shermin BB: Estrogen effects on cognition in menopausal women. Neurology 1997;48(5 Suppl 7):S21.

Soules MR et al: Executive summary: Stages of Reproductive Aging Workshop (STRAW). Fertil Steril 2001;76:874.

Stearns V et al: Paroxetine controlled release in the treatment of menopausal hot flashes: a randomized controlled trial. JAMA 2003;289:2827.

Stock JL et al: Calcitonin-salmon nasal spray reduces the incidence of new vertebral fractures in postmenopausal women: three year interim results of the "PROOF" study group. J Bone Miner Res 1997;12(Suppl 1):S187.

Storm T et al: Effect of intermittent cyclical etidronate therapy on bone mass and fracture rate in women with postmenopausal osteoporosis. N Engl J Med 1990;322:1265.

Sunyer T: Estrogen's bone-protective effects may involve differential IL-1 receptor regulation in human osteoclast-like cells. J Clin Invest 1999;103:1409.

Tataryn IV et al: LH, FSH, and skin temperature during the menopausal hot flash. J Clin Endocrinol Metab 1979;49:152.

Tsai KS, Ebeling PR, Riggs BL: Bone responsiveness to parathyroid hormone in normal and osteoporotic postmenopausal women. J Clin Endocrinol Metab 1989;69:1024.

U.S. Census Bureau, Current Population Survey, Special Populations Branch, Population Division, March, 2002.

Vermeulen A: The hormonal activity of the postmenopausal ovary. J Clin Endocrinol Metab 1976;42:247.

Weiss NS et al: Decreased risk of fractures of the hip and lower forearm with postmenopausal use of estrogen. N Engl J Med 1980;302:551.

Williams JK, Adams MR, Klopfenstein HS: Estrogen modulates responses of atherosclerotic coronary arteries. Circulation 1990; 81:1680.

Williams JK et al: Short-term administration of estrogen and vascular responses of atherosclerotic coronary arteries. J Am Coll Cardiol 1992;20:452.

Woitge HW et al: Biochemical markers to survey bone turnover. Rheum Dis Clin North Am 2001;27:49.

The Women's Health Initiative Steering Committee: Effects of conjugated equine estrogen in postmenopausal women with hysterectomy. JAMA 2004;291:1701.

The Women's Health Initiative Study Group: Design of the Women's Health Initiative clinical trial and observational study. Control Clin Trials 1998;19:61.

Woo SB et al: Osteonecrosis of the jaw and bisphosphonates. N Engl J Med 2005; 353:99.

World Health Organization: Assessment of fracture risk and its application to screening for postmenopausal osteoporosis. Report of a WHO Study Group. World Health Organ Tech Rep Ser 1994;843:1.

Writing Group for the Women's Health Initiative: Risks and benefits of estrogen plus progestin in healthy postmenopausal women: Principal results from the Women's Health Initiative randomized controlled trial. JAMA 2002;288:321.

SECTION VII
Contemporary Issues

Critical Care Obstetrics

60

Johanna Weiss Goldberg, MD, & Ramada S. Smith, MD

CRITICAL CARE OBSTETRICS: INTRODUCTION

Critical care medicine has increasingly become an area of interest to the obstetrician-gynecologist. Pregnancy complications such as shock, thromboembolism, acute respiratory distress syndrome (ARDS), and coagulation disorders can lead to significant morbidity. Furthermore, the approach to these patients can be influenced by a variety of physiologic changes that are unique to pregnancy. This chapter provides a basic approach to some of the common clinical problems that often require complex multidisciplinary care and a knowledge of invasive hemodynamic monitoring.

PULMONARY ARTERY CATHETERIZATION

The flow-directed pulmonary artery catheter has been a major addition to the clinician's armamentarium because of its applicability to a wide range of cardiorespiratory disorders. The catheter allows simultaneous measurement of central venous pressure (CVP), pulmonary artery pressure (PAP), pulmonary capillary wedge pressure (PCWP), cardiac output, and mixed venous oxygen saturation. The pulmonary artery catheter is a 7F triple lumen polyvinyl chloride catheter with a balloon and thermodilution cardiac output sensor at the tip. The distal port is used to measure PAP when the balloon is deflated and PCWP when inflated. A proximal lumen is present 30 cm from the balloon tip; this can be used to monitor the CVP and to administer fluids and drugs. Both ports can be used to withdraw blood.

Oximetric catheters also have 2 optical fibers that permit continuous measurement of mixed venous oxygen saturation by reflection spectrophotometry.

Insertion Technique

A 16-gauge catheter is used to gain access to the internal jugular or subclavian vein (Fig 60–1). Pertinent anatomic landmarks for the internal jugular vein approach are shown in Figure 60–2. A guidewire is then introduced into the vein through the catheter, and the 16-gauge catheter sheath is removed. A pulmonary artery catheter is inserted over the guidewire, and the guidewire is removed. The central venous and pulmonary artery ports are connected to a pressure transducer, so that the characteristic waveforms of the various heart chambers can be identified as the catheter is advanced (Fig 60–3). When the catheter is in the superior vena cava, the balloon is inflated with 1–1.5 mL of air, and the catheter is advanced forward into the main pulmonary artery. Table 60–1 shows the average distance in centimeters the catheter must be advanced from various insertion sites. From the main pulmonary artery, the flow of blood moves the catheter into a branch of the pulmonary artery, where it wedges and records the PCWP.

Criteria for verification of the true PCWP include (1) x-ray confirmation of catheter placement, (2) characteristic left atrial waveform configuration, (3) mean PCWP lower than mean PAP, (4) respiratory variation demonstrated by fluctuation of the PCWP waveform baseline with inspiration and expiration, and (5) blood samples showing higher oxygen tension and lower CO_2 tension than in arterial blood.

Figure 60–1. Comparison of right internal jugular vein and subclavian vein vascular access sites for right heart catheterization.

Internal jugular vein

Subclavian vein

Sternal head

Clavicle

Common carotid artery

Internal jugular vein

Clavicular head

Figure 60–2. Important anatomic landmarks associated with the internal jugular vein approach for right heart catheterization.

Figure 60–3. Changes in waveforms observed during placement of a pulmonary artery catheter. RA, right atrium; RV, right ventricle; PA pulmonary artery; PAW, pulmonary artery wedge. (Reproduced, with permission, from Rosenthal MH: Intrapartum intensive care management of the cardiac patient. Clin Obstet Gynecol 1981;24:796.)

After deflation of the balloon, the pulmonary artery waveform should again be visualized. Fiberoptic catheters allow verification of PCWP by showing a sudden increase in mixed venous saturation to 95% or greater.

Indications for Invasive Monitoring

According to the American College of Obstetricians and Gynecologists, invasive hemodynamic monitoring may provide useful information for critical conditions during pregnancy such as:

- Shock (septic, hemorrhagic, cardiogenic, unexplained).
- Pulmonary edema (eg, severe pregnancy-induced hypertension [PIH], congestive heart failure [CHF], unexplained or refractory).
- Severe PIH with persistent oliguria unresponsive to fluid challenge.
- ARDS.
- Severe cardiac disease.

Hemodynamic Parameters Available with Pulmonary Artery Catheterization

During the diastolic period of the cardiac cycle, the left ventricle, left atrium, and pulmonary vascular bed essentially become a common chamber (Fig 60–4). In a normal cardiovascular system, the left ventricular end-diastolic pressure (LVEDP), left atrial pressure, and PCWP are essentially interchangeable. A disparity may develop between PCWP and LVEDP when LVEDP is greater than 15 mm Hg; however, for clinical purposes, the

PCWP provides a fairly accurate index of LVEDP, especially if the "a" wave (caused by retrograde transmission of the left atrial contraction) can be identified in the wedge tracing. The relationships described earlier can be substantially altered by mitral or aortic valvular disease.

A. CARDIAC OUTPUT

The thermal sensing device in the tip of a pulmonary artery catheter allows for rapid determination of cardiac output by the thermodilution method. Five milliliters of 5% dextrose in water is injected through the central venous port at a constant distance from the thermistor tip. The use of this solution at room temperature can minimize sources of potential error associated with inaccurate temperature measurements and catheter warming. The change in pulmonary artery temperature is detected by the thermistor. The cardiac output is inversely proportional to the fall in temperature and is computed by planimetric or computerized methods. The average of 3 values within 10% of each other is typically utilized to calculate cardiac output.

B. SYSTEMIC VASCULAR RESISTANCE

Systemic vascular resistance (SVR) represents the total resistance to forward flow of blood through the body's vascular tree. SVR is calculated as follows:

$$SVR = \frac{[(MAP - CVP)] \times 80}{CO}$$

During pregnancy, this parameter is usually in the range of 800–1200 dynes $\cdot$ s $\cdot$ cm^{-5}. Depending on the clinical condition, a reduction or increase in SVR may be desirable in the presence of normal blood pressure (eg, septic shock), in which a very low SVR may be seen despite normal or low blood pressure. In order to maintain vital organ perfusion, vasopressor therapy may be indicated to increase SVR.

C. PULMONARY CAPILLARY WEDGE PRESSURE

The PCWP provides important information on 2 basic parameters of cardiopulmonary function: (1) pulmonary venous pressure, which is a major determinant of pulmonary congestion; and (2) the left atrial and left ventricular filling pressures, from which ventricular function curves can be constructed.

Pulmonary capillary wedge pressure can be reliably assessed by CVP monitoring only in the absence of significant myocardial dysfunction. The measurement of PCWP has certain advantages over measurement of CVP alone. A disparity between right and left ventricular function may be seen in conditions such as myocardial infarction, valvular disease, sepsis, and severe PIH. Under these circumstances, the management of

Table 60–1. Distance to right atrium from various sites of insertion in pulmonary artery catheterizaton.

Vein	Distance to Right Atrium[1] (cm)
Internal jugular	15
Subclavian	15
Right antecubital	40
Left antecubital	50
Femoral	30

[1]Distance from right atrium to pulmonary artery is 8–15 cm.

fluid therapy based on CVP alone could have adverse results. Additionally, cardiac output and mixed venous oxygen tension cannot be determined with a simple CVP catheter.

D. VENTRICULAR FUNCTION CURVES

Myocardial performance is best interpreted in terms of left ventricular function curves (ie, the Frank-Starling relationship). The cardiac output and PCWP are used to construct the ventricular function curve by plotting the ventricular stroke work index against the mean atrial pressure or ventricular end-diastolic pressure (usu-ally the PCWP). The left ventricular stroke work index is calculated by the following formula:

$$LVSWI = SVI \times (MAP - PCWP) \times 0.0136$$

(LVSWI = left ventricular stroke work index [g-m/m^2]; SVI = stroke volume index [mL/beat/m^2]; MAP = mean arterial pressure [mm Hg]; PCWP = pulmonary capillary wedge pressure [mm Hg]).

Ventricular function curves provide a useful index of cardiovascular status to guide inotropic and vasoactive drug therapy. Evaluation of myocardial contractility by ventricular function curves allows one to obtain optimal filling pressures and stroke volume index in critically ill patients. The effects of therapy (eg, diuretics, antihypertensive agents, or volume expanders) can be evaluated on the basis of performance. Under normal conditions, a small rise in filling pressure is accompanied by a rapid rise in stroke work. Unfavorable conditions such as hypoxia or myocardial depression produce a shift in the curve to the right and downward such that lower stroke work indices are seen at higher filling pressures.

E. MIXED VENOUS OXYGEN SATURATION

The mixed venous oxygen saturation (SvO$_2$) reflects the body's capacity to provide adequate tissue oxygenation.

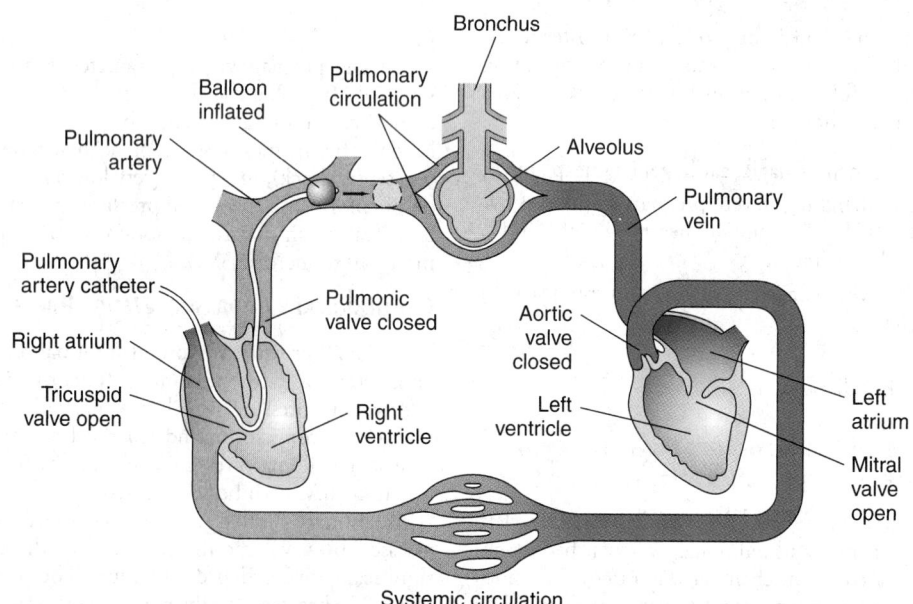

Figure 60–4. Pulmonary capillary wedge pressure in diastole. (ventricles relaxed). (Reproduced, with permission, from *Understanding Hemodynamic Measurements Made With the Swan-Ganz Catheter.* American Edward Laboratories, 1982.)

This parameter is affected by cardiac output, hemoglobin concentration, arterial oxygen saturation, and tissue oxygen consumption. An SvO_2 of 60–80% usually indicates normal oxygen delivery and demand with adequate tissue perfusion. An SvO_2 greater than 80% reflects increased oxygen delivery and decreased oxygen utilization. This situation may be seen in patients with hypothermia or sepsis who are receiving supplemental oxygen. A high SvO_2 may also provide confirmatory evidence that the pulmonary artery catheter is in the wedge position. Finally, a low SvO_2 (< 60%) indicates increased oxygen demands with decreased oxygen delivery due to anemia, low cardiac output, or decreased arterial oxygen saturation.

Measurement of SvO_2 allows for continuous monitoring of cardiorespiratory reserve by providing an index of tissue oxygen delivery and utilization. Changes in SvO_2 will be apparent with infusion of vasoactive drugs, volume loading, or afterload reduction. While many intensive care units rely on direct measurement of cardiac output alone, this parameter does not always accurately reflect tissue oxygenation. For instance, normal cardiac output might not be adequate to meet increased oxygen requirements in malignant hyperthermia or thyroid storm.

F. MATERNAL OXYGEN CONSUMPTION

Mixed venous oxygen saturation results can be used with arterial blood gas analysis to provide useful information about the metabolic status of the critically ill obstetric patient. Resting maternal oxygen consumption progressively increases during pregnancy. Occasionally, one needs to pay particular attention to the metabolic status of critically ill women or those with ARDS. Factors such as tachycardia or fever that are associated with increased oxygen consumption should be minimized under these circumstances.

The Fick relationship:

$$CO = \frac{Vo_2}{Avo_2 \text{ diff.}} \times 100$$

provides a method for calculating oxygen consumption (Vo_2), if the cardiac output (CO) and systemic arteriovenous oxygen (Avo_2) concentration difference is known. The Avo_2 difference can be calculated by subtracting the oxygen content of desaturated mixed venous blood from that of arterial blood that passes through the pulmonary artery catheter. For example, a patient with a cardiac output minus Avo_2 difference of 5 mL would have an oxygen consumption (Vo_2) of 300 mL.

$$6000 \text{ mL min}^{-1} \times 5 \text{ mL per 100 mL blood}$$

$$Vo_2\ 100 = 300 \text{ mL min}^{-1}$$

Table 60–2. Serum colloid oncotic pressure during pregnancy.

	Normotensive (mm Hg)	Hypertensive (mm Hg)
Antepartum (term)	22.4 ± 0.5	17.9 ± 0.7
Postpartum (first 24 hours)	15.4 ± 2.1	13.7 ± 0.5

An understanding of these relationships will allow the clinician to better understand how to use physiologic variables for interpreting the hemodynamic and pulmonary condition of critically ill patients.

G. COLLOID OSMOTIC PRESSURE

The plasma colloid oncotic pressure (COP) is another measurement that can be useful in critical care (Table 60–2). Plasma COP is the pressure exerted by certain plasma proteins that hold fluid in the intravascular space. Albumin accounts for 75% of the oncotic pressure of plasma, with the rest coming from globulin and fibrinogen. It has been demonstrated in dogs that iatrogenic reduction in plasma proteins resulted in pulmonary edema with only minimal increases in left atrial pressure. Subsequent studies in humans identified cases of pulmonary edema in which normal or slightly elevated PCWP was present. From these studies, the important concept of a COP-PCWP gradient evolved. It appears that when the COP-PCWP gradient is less than 4 mm Hg, the likelihood of pulmonary edema is increased, although not all patients with a decreased gradient will develop pulmonary edema. The determination of COP and its relationship to the PCWP can play a crucial role in the detection of patients likely to develop pulmonary edema in the face of normal left-sided filling pressures.

Studies of pregnant women have demonstrated that patients with certain conditions in which the risk of pulmonary edema is markedly increased tend to have lowered COP (eg, hypovolemic shock, severe PIH, prolonged tocolytic therapy, and frank pulmonary edema).

Complications

The most common complication associated with pulmonary artery catheter placement is dysrhythmia. More serious complications also include pulmonary infarction, thromboembolism, balloon rupture with air embolism, pulmonary artery or valve rupture, catheter knotting, infection, arterial puncture, thromboembolism, pneumothorax, and pulmonary hemorrhage. Table 60–3 summarizes the complication rates for pulmonary artery catheterization.

Table 60–3. Complications of pulmonary artery catheterization.[1]

Complication	Incidence (%)
Premature ventricular contractions	15–27
Arterial puncture	8
Superficial cellulitis	3
Thromboembolism	?
Pneumothorax	1–2
Balloon rupture	< 1
Pulmonary infarction/ischemia	1–7
Pulmonary artery rupture	< 1
Catheter knotting	< 1
Catheter-related sepsis	1

[1]Reproduced, with permission, from Hankins GDV, Cunningham FG: Severe preeclampsia and eclampsia: Controversies in management. Williams Obstetrics 1991;18(suppl):11. Appleton & Lange.

A. DYSRHYTHMIA

Premature ventricular contractions may transiently occur as the catheter tip enters the right ventricle. However, they usually resolve following advancement of the catheter into the pulmonary artery. If the dysrhythmia is refractory to lidocaine, 50–100 mg given intravenously, the catheter should be withdrawn from the cardiac chambers.

B. PULMONARY INFARCTION

Pulmonary infarction may occur when the catheter migrates distally and wedges spontaneously for a prolonged period. This complication, as well as thromboembolism, may be avoided by monitoring the PCWP at regular intervals and by using a continuous heparinized flow system.

C. BALLOON RUPTURE

Balloon rupture can be avoided by limiting the number of balloon inflations and by inflating only to the smallest necessary volume. Inflation of the balloon beyond 2 mL of air is unnecessary and may be harmful. To avoid rupture of a pulmonary artery branch, inflation of the balloon should be stopped immediately when the wedge tracing is seen.

D. CATHETER KNOTTING

Catheter knotting is usually the result of advancing the catheter 10–15 cm farther than is necessary to reach the right ventricle or pulmonary artery. Withdrawing the catheter while the balloon is still inflated may cause tricuspid rupture or chordae tendineae tears.

E. INFECTION AND PHLEBITIS

Infection and phlebitis can be minimized by using aseptic technique. The risk of associated sepsis is related to excessive catheter manipulation and the duration of catheterization.

NONINVASIVE MONITORING FOR CRITICALLY ILL PATIENTS

Pulse oximetry is a simple tool that can be used with invasive monitoring for patients with cardiovascular or respiratory compromise. The correlation between pulse oximetry and direct blood oxygen saturation is excellent when oxygen saturation is greater than 60%. Factors adversely affecting the accuracy of pulse oximetry include movement, peripheral vasoconstriction, hypotension, anemia, hypothermia, intravascular dye, and possibly nail polish.

OBSTETRIC SHOCK

Shock may be defined as an imbalance between oxygen supply and demand. The basic underlying defect is a significant reduction in the supply of oxygenated blood to various tissues due to inadequate perfusion. In obstetrics, this reduction often results from hemorrhage, sepsis, or pump failure. The physiologic compensation common to all shock states involves tachycardia and peripheral vasoconstriction to maximize cerebral and cardiac perfusion by way of the sympathetic nervous system. Failure of these compensatory mechanisms will lead to a predominance of anaerobic metabolism and lactic acidosis, which can be potentially devastating to the patient and fetus. Cardiogenic shock may be seen in pregnant women with cardiac dysrhythmias, congenital heart disease, peripartum cardiomyopathy, and congestive heart failure. The following discussion will focus on 2 of the more common shock syndromes complicating pregnancy—those related to hemorrhage and sepsis.

Hypovolemic Shock

 ESSENTIALS OF DIAGNOSIS

- *Recent history of acute blood loss or excessive diuresis.*
- *Hypotension, tachycardia, tachypnea, and oliguria with progression to altered mental status.*
- *Precipitous drop in hematocrit.*

General Considerations

Hypovolemic shock is a leading cause of maternal mortality in the U.S. and is most commonly associated with obstetric hemorrhage. Bleeding severe enough to cause hemorrhagic shock may result from a wide variety of conditions, including ruptured ectopic pregnancy; abruptio placentae; placenta previa; placenta accreta; rupture, atony, or inversion of the uterus; surgical procedures; obstetric lacerations; or retained products of conception.

Pathophysiology

During normal pregnancy, the blood volume expands by approximately 1500 mL. This hypervolemia results from hormonal alterations and may be considered protective against peripartum bleeding. During acute hemorrhage, the body responds to volume loss by hemodynamic, volume-altering, and hormonal mechanisms.

Hemodynamic adjustments result from activation of the sympathetic nervous system. These changes include vasoconstriction of arteriolar resistance vessels, constriction of venous capacitance vessels, and redistribution of blood flow away from peripheral organs to preserve adequate cerebral and cardiac blood flow.

Volume adjustments occur from extravascular fluid shifts into the intravascular compartment. The rate of plasma refill depends on the magnitude of volume depletion.

If these mechanisms are insufficient to restore circulatory function, other compensatory effects, such as secretion of antidiuretic hormone (ADH), cortisol, aldosterone, and catecholamines will occur. Epinephrine, in addition to causing peripheral vasoconstriction, will have inotropic and chronotropic effects on the heart. ADH, cortisol, and aldosterone will help conserve water and salt, which may then result in reduced blood flow to the kidneys and decreased urine output.

These homeostatic mechanisms serve to maintain adequate tissue perfusion until approximately 25–30% of the circulating blood volume is lost. Inadequate tissue perfusion and oxygenation will then lead to anaerobic metabolism and lactic acidosis. Over a prolonged period of vasoconstriction, there may be decompensation of the peripheral vasculature leading to damaged or leaky capillaries. Observations of blood flow regulation during pregnancy suggest that uterine arteries have limited capacity to autoregulate fetoplacental perfusion. Thus uteroplacental blood flow is critically dependent upon systemic maternal cardiac output.

Clinical Findings

The clinical manifestations of hemorrhagic shock depend on the quantity and rate of volume depletion. Orthostatic signs and symptoms may be masked by the hypervolemia of pregnancy, especially if a source of bleeding is not evident. Obvious hypotension and tachycardia in the presence of external bleeding should alert the clinician to the possibility of shock. A careful physical examination will identify decreased tissue per-

fusion in several different organ systems, including the heart, brain, kidneys, lungs, and skin. Altered mental status, dizziness, diaphoresis, and cold, clammy extremities, as well as a fast, "thready" pulse are common findings in significant hemorrhagic shock. Oliguria (< 30 mL/h), CVP of less than 5 cm H_2O, and PCWP of less than 5 mm Hg are all consistent with significant volume depletion. The identification of intra-abdominal bleeding may require culdocentesis or peritoneal lavage. Fetal heart monitoring may reveal bradycardia or late decelerations.

Differential Diagnosis

Hypovolemic shock should be differentiated from other shock syndromes resulting from sepsis or heart failure. Usually, there is a history of profound bleeding. Since shock may affect several organ systems, it is essential that its underlying cause be identified. Patients with septic shock will tend to be febrile, with associated abnormal white blood cell counts and clinical evidence of infection. Cardiogenic shock may be associated with clinical and radiographic evidence of pulmonary congestion or a previous history of heart disease.

Complications

Electrolyte imbalance, acidosis, acute tubular necrosis, stress-induced gastric ulceration, pulmonary edema, and ARDS are common complications associated with hemorrhagic shock. Myocardial infarction is a rare complication in the obstetric population.

Treatment

The treatment of hemorrhagic shock should be directed toward replacing blood volume and optimizing cardiac performance. The source of bleeding should be controlled. Uterine atony that is unresponsive to massage and oxytocin may benefit from methylergonovine (0.2 mg intramuscularly), or 15-methyl prostaglandin $F_{2\alpha}$ (0.25 mg intramuscularly). Persistent bleeding may require uterine artery ligation, hypogastric artery ligation, or even cesarean hysterectomy (see Fig 28–1). Decisions regarding blood and fluid replacement should be guided by central pressures and urine output, although pulmonary artery catheterization is rarely necessary. Military antishock trousers (MAST) suit will mobilize blood pooled in the lower body and return it to the central circulation, improving systemic cardiac output and organ perfusion. Supplemental oxygen will minimize tissue hypoxia and fetal acidosis.

Initial rapid volume replacement with crystalloid solution given through a large-bore intravenous site is a temporizing measure until blood replacement is possible. Typically, 1–2 L of lactated Ringer's solution can be administered as rapidly as possible. Compared with normal saline, the electrolyte composition of lactated Ringer's solution more closely approximates plasma, and the metabolism of lactate to bicarbonate provides some buffering capacity for acidosis.

Guidelines for perioperative transfusion of red blood cells have been defined by the National Institutes of Health. Initial treatment of hemorrhagic shock should involve volume replacement by crystalloid or colloid solutions that do not carry risks for disease transmission or transfusion reaction. The use of perioperative red blood cell transfusion should not rely solely upon the dogma of "transfusing to a hematocrit above 30%" as the sole criterion since there is poor evidence supporting its usefulness. The decision whether or not to transfuse red cells should also take into account other factors such as patient age, hemodynamic status, anticipated bleeding, and medical or obstetrical complications. If it is necessary to transfuse large amounts of blood, it is important to note and correct the presence of electrolyte imbalances, acid-base abnormalities, hypothermia, and the dilution of platelets and coagulation factors, which may require the transfusion of other blood products.

The risk of posttransfusion hepatitis has been dramatically decreased by testing blood products with a commercially available hepatitis C assay. The test is a qualitative, enzyme-linked imunosorbent assay (ELISA) for the detection of antibody to hepatitis C virus (anti-HCV) in human serum or plasma. The ELISA test has a specificity of 99.84% in a low prevalence population. A supplemental assay, the recombinant immunoblot assay (RIBA), can be performed on blood that has a repeat reactive anti-HCV.

Fluid balance from intravenous infusions or urine output should be meticulously recorded with daily weights. Oliguria refractory to volume loading may be improved by the addition of intravenous dopamine in low doses (2–5 µg/kg/min) to improve renal perfusion. A diuretic such as bumetanide 0.5–1 mg IV, not to exceed 10 mg/day, should be considered for patients with prolonged oliguria despite normal elevated pulmonary capillary wedge pressures.

Blood tests should include complete blood count, serum electrolytes, creatinine, arterial blood gas analysis, and coagulation profile. Urinalysis is also important. A baseline chest radiograph and electrocardiogram are desirable. Typed and cross-matched transfusion products should be available from the blood bank. One to two ampules of sodium bicarbonate (50–100 mEq) can be administered intravenously to correct acidosis (pH < 7.20). Frequent serial hematocrits may provide an index of acute blood loss. A baseline hematologic profile (PT, partial thromboplastin time [PTT], fibrinogen, platelets) is necessary to evaluate the possibility of coagulopathy.

Prognosis

Maternal and fetal survival rates are directly related to the magnitude of volume depletion and length of time the patient remains in shock. If the hemorrhage is controlled and intravascular volume is restored within a reasonable interval, the prognosis is generally good in the absence of associated complications. However, the return of fetal blood flow may lag behind correction of maternal flow.

Septic Shock

 ESSENTIALS OF DIAGNOSIS

- History of recent hospitalization or surgery.
- Pelvic or abdominal infection with positive confirmatory cultures.
- Temperature instability, confusion, hypotension, oliguria, cardiopulmonary failure.

General Considerations

Septic shock is a life-threatening disorder secondary to bacteremia. The American College of Obstetricians and Gynecologists defines septic shock as sepsis with hypotension despite adequate fluid resuscitation, with the presence of perfusion abnormalities including (but not limited to) lactic acidosis and oliguria. The incidence of bacteremia in obstetric patients has been estimated to be between 0.7% and 10%. Although gram-negative bacteria are usually responsible for most of these infections, septic shock may also result from infection with other bacteria, fungi, protozoa, or viruses. The most common cause of obstetric septic shock is postoperative endometritis (85%). Other commonly associated conditions include antepartum pyelonephritis, septic abortion, and chorioamnionitis.

Pathophysiology

Sepsis may lead to a systemic inflammatory response that can be triggered not only by infections but also by noninfectious disorders, such as trauma and pancreatitis. However, there is strong evidence to support the concept that endotoxin is responsible for the pathogenesis of gram-negative septic shock. *Escherichia coli* has been implicated in 25–50% of cases of septic hypotension, but a variety of other organisms may be causative, including *Klebsiella, Enterobacter, Serratia, Proteus, Pseudomonas, Streptococcus, Peptostreptococcus, Staphylococcus, Fusobacterium, Clostridium,* and *Bacteroides*. The gram-negative endotoxin theory does not explain gram-positive shock, although an understanding of the proposed mechanisms will serve to exemplify the multisystemic effects of this disorder.

Endotoxin is a complex lipopolysaccharide present in the cell walls of gram-negative bacteria. The active component of endotoxin, lipid A, is responsible for initiating activation of the coagulation, fibrinolysis, complement, prostaglandin, and kinin systems. Activation of the coagulation and fibrinolysis systems may lead to consumptive coagulopathy. Complement activation leads to the release by leukocytes of mediators that are responsible for damage to vascular endothelium, platelet aggregation, intensification of the coagulation cascade, and degranulation of mast cells with histamine release. Histamine will cause increased capillary permeability, decreased plasma volume, vasodilatation, and hypotension. Release of bradykinin and β-endorphins also contributes to systemic hypotension. Early stages of septic shock involve low SVR and high cardiac output with a relative decrease in intravascular volume. Late or cold shock subsequently involves an endogenous myocardial depressant factor that has not been isolated. This factor is associated with decreased cardiac output and continued low SVR in the absence of pressor agents. Recent studies suggest that tumor necrosis factor (TNF) may lead to depressed myocardial function during septic shock. Monocytes and macrophages incubated with endotoxin produce this 17-kDa polypeptide within 40 minutes. Direct injection of TNF into animals leads to many of the changes seen in endotoxic shock. Other possible factors include IL-1, IL-6, IL-8, interferon gamma, and granulocyte stimulating factor.

Clinical Findings

A. SYMPTOMS AND SIGNS

Septic shock can be divided into 3 stages: preshock, early shock (warm shock), and late (or cold) shock. In preshock, patients present with tachypnea and respiratory alkalosis. Their condition is best described as a moderate hyperdynamic state, with elevated cardiac output, decreasing SVR, and normal blood pressures. Response to therapy will be greatest at this stage. Early shock is a more hyperdynamic state. Blood pressure drops (SBP < 60 mm Hg), and SVR decreases dramatically (< 400 dynes · s · cm⁻⁵). Altered mental status, temperature instability, and sinusoidal fluctuations in arterial blood pressure may be seen at this stage. As this condition progresses into late shock, activation of the sympathetic nervous system with release of catecholamines will lead to intense vasoconstriction, which serves to shunt blood from the peripheral tissues to the heart and brain (cold shock). The compensatory vasoconstriction results in increased cardiac work. Lactic acidosis, poor coronary perfusion, and the influence of myocardial depressant factor may also contribute to

poor cardiac performance (Fig 60–5). The fetus is more resistant to the effects of endotoxin than the mother; however, alterations in uteroplacental flow can lead to hypoxia, acidosis, placental abruption, intracranial hemorrhage, and fetal demise.

The clinical manifestations of septic shock depend on the target organs affected (Table 60–4). The most common cause of death in patients with this condition is respiratory insufficiency secondary to ARDS.

B. LABORATORY FINDINGS

Complete blood cell count, serum electrolytes, urinalysis, baseline arterial blood gases, chest radiograph, and a coagulation profile are laboratory studies important in the management of these patients. Hematologic findings may include significant anemia, thrombocytopenia, and leukocytosis. Serum electrolytes are often abnormal because of acidosis, fluid shifts, or decreased renal perfusion. Urinalysis permits evaluation of renal involvement. In addition to urine cultures, aerobic and anaerobic blood cultures may be helpful to confirm the diagnosis and guide antibiotic therapy.

Arterial blood gas measurements and a chest radiograph will facilitate clinical assessment of the ventilatory and oxygenation status. Early stages of septic shock will be associated with respiratory alkalosis, which later progresses to metabolic acidosis.

A baseline electrocardiogram (ECG) should be performed to rule out myocardial infarction or cardiac dysrhythmia. Abdominal radiographic studies may be useful to rule out other intrapelvic or intra-abdominal sources of obstetric sepsis (eg, bowel perforation, uterine perforation, tubo-ovarian abscess). Significant disseminated intravascular coagulation (DIC) will be identified by abnormal PT, PTT, or fibrinogen levels.

Differential Diagnosis

The differential diagnosis should include other hypovolemic and cardiogenic shock syndromes. Additional causes of acute cardiopulmonary compromise include amniotic fluid embolism, pulmonary thromboembolism, cardiac tamponade, aortic dissection, and diabetic ketoacidosis. The history, physical examination, and laboratory studies will usually be sufficient to distinguish between these diagnoses.

Complications

Numerous complications may occur with septic shock, depending on the target organs involved. Aside from ARDS, some of the more serious complications include congestive heart failure and cardiac dysrhythmias. Systemic hypotension and ischemic end-organ damage can lead to hepatic failure or renal insufficiency. Fetal or maternal demise are the most dire outcomes.

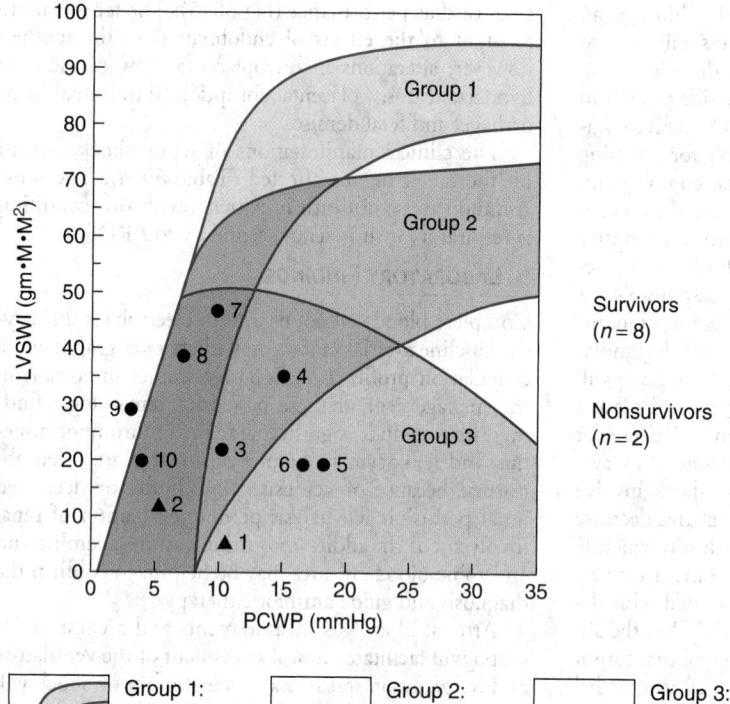

Survivors ●
(n = 8)

Nonsurvivors ▲
(n = 2)

Group 1:
Normal
ventricular
function

Group 2:
Mildly
depressed
ventricular
function

Group 3:
Markedly
depressed
ventricular
function

Figure 60–5. Presenting left ventricular function of 10 pregnant women with septic hypotension. LVSWI, left ventricular stroke work index; PCWP, pulmonary capillary wedge pressure. (Reproduced, with permission, from Lee W et al: Septic shock during pregnancy. Am J Obstet Gynecol 1988;159:410.)

Table 60–4. Effects on target organs in septic shock.[1]

Organ System	Clinical and Laboratory Findings
Brain	Confusion, obtundation
Hypothalamus	Hypothermia, hyperthermia
Cardiovascular	Myocardial depression, arrhythmias, tachycardia, hypotension
Pulmonary	Tachypnea, arteriovenous shunting, hypoxemia
Gastrointestinal	Vomiting, diarrhea
Hepatic	Increased AST (SGOT) and bilirubin
Kidneys	Oliguria, renal failure
Hematologic	Hemoconcentration, thrombocytopenia, leukocytosis, coagulopathy

[1]Adapted and reproduced, with permission, from American College of Obstetricians and Gynecologists: Septic shock. ACOG Technical Bulletin No. 75, March 1984.

Treatment

Successful management of obstetric septic shock depends on early identification and aggressive treatment focused on stabilization of the patient, removal of underlying causes of sepsis, broad-spectrum antibiotic coverage, and treatment of associated complications. Febrile patients with mild hypotension who respond rapidly to volume infusion alone do not require invasive monitoring. In other cases, the pulmonary artery catheter should be used to guide specific therapeutic maneuvers for optimizing myocardial performance and maintaining systemic cardiac output and blood pressure. A hemodynamic approach for stabilizing pregnant women with septic shock should include (1) volume repletion and hemostasis; (2) inotropic therapy with dopamine on the basis of left ventricular function curves; and (3) addition of peripheral vasoconstrictors (phenylephrine first, then norepinephrine) to maintain afterload (Fig 60–6).

A. GENERAL MEASURES

Septic shock during pregnancy should be treated with a broad-spectrum antibiotic regimen such as ampicillin, gentamicin, and clindamycin. Aminoglycoside mainte-

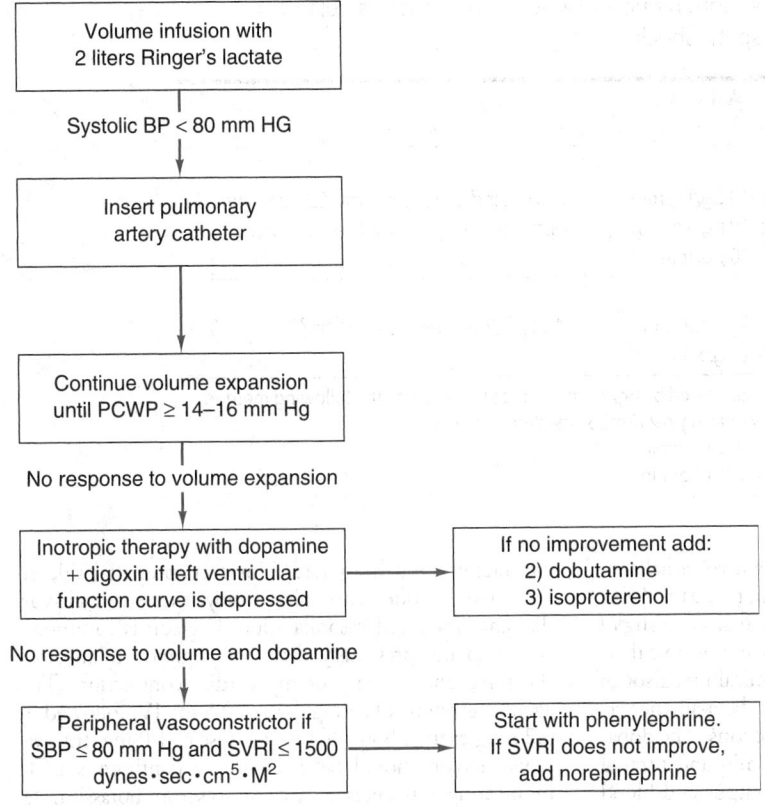

Figure 60–6. Hemodynamic algorithm for treatment of obstetric septic shock. SVRI = systemic vascular resistance index. PCWP = pulmonary capillary wedge pressure; SBP = systolic blood pressure. (Reproduced, with permission, from Lee W et al: Septic shock during pregnancy. Am J Obstet Gynecol 1988;159:410.)

nance doses should be titrated in relation to serum peak and trough levels or a 24-hour dosing regimen may be used. Newer antibiotics such as imipenem, cilastatin, vancomycin, and the extended spectrum penicillins (eg, ticarcillin) are also proving to be effective therapies. There must be a careful search for infected or necrotic foci that can result in persistent bacteremia, and surgical intervention may be necessary. In one study, 40% of septic obstetric patients required surgical removal of infected products of conception, and all survived. If chorioamnionitis is present in the septic obstetric patient, prompt delivery is necessary. However, if the pregnancy is not the cause of infection, immediate delivery is usually not required. Supportive care should also include control of fever with antipyretics, hypothermic cooling blankets, or both. Correction of maternal acidosis, hypoxemia, and systemic hypotension will usually improve any abnormalities in the fetal heart tracing.

B. CARDIOVASCULAR SUPPORT

Aggressive treatment of obstetric septic shock must rapidly and effectively reverse organ hypoperfusion, improve oxygen delivery, and correct acidosis. Priority should be given to cardiopulmonary support with the

additional understanding that other major organ systems can also be severely affected.

A sequential hemodynamic approach for stabilizing obstetric septic shock with volume repletion, inotropic therapy, and peripheral vasoconstrictors is recommended. Volume therapy initially begins with 1–2 L of lactated Ringer's solution infused over approximately 15 minutes. However, it is important that volume infusion not be withheld in a hypotensive patient pending placement of a pulmonary artery catheter. The total amount of crystalloid administered should be guided by the presence or absence of maternal hypoxemia secondary to pulmonary edema and left ventricular filling pressures, as estimated by PCWP.

In general, myocardial performance will be optimized according to the Starling mechanism at a PCWP of 14–16 mm Hg. Such preload optimization is mandatory prior to the initiation of inotropic therapy. Blood component therapy can also be an important adjunctive measure if the patient has experienced significant hemorrhage and has developed an associated coagulopathy.

If the shock state persists despite volume replacement and adequate hemostasis, efforts should be directed toward improving myocardial performance and vascular tone. Inotropic agents such as dopamine, dobutamine, or isopro-

Table 60–5. Sympathomimetic and vasopressor drugs useful for therapy of obstetric spetic shock.

Agent	Maintenance Dose Range[1]	Therapeutic Goals
Inotropic		
Dopamine	2–10 µg/kg/min	Cardiac index ≥ 3 L/min/m² SBP ≥ 80 mm Hg
Dobutamine	2–10 µg/kg/min	Optimize left ventricular function curves
Isoproterenol	1–20 µg/min	
Vasopressors		
Phenylephrine	1–5 µg/kg/min	SVRI ≥ 1500 dynes · 5 · cm⁻⁵· m²
Norepinephrine	1–4 µg/min	

[1]Drug dosages that are administered by µg/kg/min can be prepared by the following method:
1.5 mg × body weight (kg) = total mg in 250 mL 5% dextrose in water
10 mL/h = 1 µg/kg/min
20 mL/h = 2 µg/kg/min

terenol are excellent choices for improving myocardial contractility in an obstetric patient with a failing heart (Table 60–5). We recommend dopamine as the first-line drug of choice for treating septic hypotension when inotropic therapy is indicated. This substance is a chemical precursor of norepinephrine that has alpha-adrenergic, beta-adrenergic, and dopaminergic receptor stimulating actions. The dopamine infusion is initiated at 2–5 µg/kg/min and titrated against its effect on improving cardiac output and blood pressure in patients with obstetric septic shock. At low doses (0.5–5.0 µg/kg/min), this sympathomimetic amine acts primarily on the dopaminergic receptors, leading to vasodilation and improved perfusion of the renal and mesenteric vascular beds. Higher dopamine doses (5.0–15.0 µg/kg/min) are associated with predominant effects on the β receptors of the heart. The beta-adrenergic effects are responsible for improved myocardial contractility, stroke volume, and cardiac output. Much higher dopamine dosages (15–20 µg/kg/min) will elicit an alpha-adrenergic effect, similar to a norepinephrine infusion, and result in generalized vasoconstriction. Vasoconstrictive action associated with high doses of infused dopamine can actually be detrimental to organ perfusion and will rarely be useful under these clinical circumstances. Although myocardial performance after dopamine therapy is best evaluated by ventricular function curves, it is reasonable to maintain a systemic cardiac index above 3 L/min/m².

If satisfactory ventricular function is not achieved with dopamine, a second inotropic agent such as dobutamine (2–20 µg/kg) should be added to the dopamine regimen. Dobutamine is a direct myocardial $β_1$ stimulant that increases cardiac output with only minimal tachycardia. Isoproterenol should be considered a third-line agent, which can be titrated at 1–20 µg/min. This drug acts primarily on beta-adrenergic receptors to increase contractility and heart rate. However, potential side effects may include ventricular ectopy, excessive tachycardia, and undesired vasodilatation. Digoxin is commonly added to the previously described regimen to improve the force and velocity of myocardial contraction. This agent is given in a loading dose of 0.5 mg IV, followed by 0.25 mg every 4 hours for a total dose of 1.0 mg. Intravenous digoxin should be given under continuous ECG monitoring with special attention to serum potassium levels. The usual maintenance dosage during pregnancy is 0.25–0.37 mg/dL depending on plasma drug levels.

A peripheral vasoconstrictor may be initiated if there is a reduced systemic vascular resistance index (SVRI; less than 1500 dynes · s · cm⁻⁵) accompanied by a systolic blood pressure of less than 80 mm Hg despite inotropic therapy. It should be emphasized that maintenance of afterload appears to be a major hemodynamic determinant associated with maternal survival. Because of its pure alpha-adrenergic activity (which increases SVR), phenylephrine (1–5 µg/kg/min) is the initial drug of choice. Norepinephrine is only indicated for septic shock patients with decreased afterload who do not respond to volume loading, inotropic therapy, and phenylephrine. This drug is a mixed adrenergic agonist with a primary effect on the alpha receptors, which leads to generalized vasoconstriction and increased SVR. Although the therapy of septic shock should focus primarily on stabilization of maternal factors, vasopressor agents should be administered cautiously during pregnancy since they have been reported to decrease uterine blood flow in animals with experimentally-induced spinal hypotension.

Some investigators have advocated large doses of corticosteroids for the acute management of septic shock, but human clinical trials have failed to demonstrate any conclusive benefit.

Newer investigational agents include corticosteroids and antiendotoxin therapy. Multicenter trials of endotoxin antibodies have suggested a possible improvement in mortality rate and organ failure in some subgroups of nonpregnant septic patients.

Prognosis

Despite all medical and surgical therapeutic options, the overall maternal mortality rate in septic shock is approximately 50%. The prognosis is worsened by the presence of ARDS or preexisting medical problems.

AMNIOTIC FLUID EMBOLISM

 ESSENTIALS OF DIAGNOSIS

- *Sudden, unexplained peripartum respiratory distress, cardiovascular collapse, and coagulopathy.*
- *Bleeding secondary to coagulopathy or uterine atony (common).*
- *Amniotic fluid debris in right side of the heart on autopsy.*

General Considerations

Amniotic fluid embolism is a rare but potentially devastating complication of pregnancy that often results in poor obstetric outcome. Most of the information about amniotic fluid embolism has been derived from clinical reports, because the rarity of the disorder does not allow for clinical trials, and no suitable animal model exists. The first major review of the literature regarding this condition was by Morgan in 1979. This evaluated 272 cases. Since that time, a national registry was initiated by Clark. The incidence of amniotic fluid embolism is difficult to estimate, and may be anywhere from 1:8000 to 1:30,000.

Pathophysiology

The basic mechanism of disease is related to the effects of amniotic fluid on the respiratory, cardiovascular, and coagulation systems. One of the classic theories hypothesized that the following 3 primary acute events occur: (1) pulmonary vascular obstruction, leading to sudden decreases in left ventricular filling pressures and cardiac output; (2) pulmonary hypertension with acute cor pulmonale; and (3) ventilation-perfusion inequality of lung tissue, leading to arterial hypoxemia and its metabolic consequences.

Only a small volume of amniotic fluid (1–2 mL) is transferred to the maternal circulation during normal labor. Thus, enhanced communication between the amniotic fluid sac and the maternal venous system is necessary for amniotic fluid embolism to occur. Sites of entry may include endocervical veins lacerated during normal labor, a disrupted placental implantation site, and traumatized uterine veins. Squamous cells and trophoblastic tissue are often found in the maternal pulmonary vasculature of patients who underwent pulmonary artery catheterization. However, one must see more specific material like mucin, fetal debris, vernix, lanugo, and squamous cells coated with white blood cells and granular debris to confirm the diagnosis. If meconium is present, a more dramatic response is seen. Fetal demise has also been shown to worsen this condition. Once amniotic debris enters the venous system, it travels rapidly to the cardiopulmonary circulation, leading to shock and arterial hypoxemia. Myocardial dysfunction may result from ischemic injury or right ventricular dilatation. Some experimental evidence suggests that amniotic fluid may have a direct myocardial depressant effect. Endothelin, a vasoconstrictive peptide found in vascular endothelial cells, has been implicated. Other factors that may play a role include proteolytic enzymes, histamine, prostaglandins, complement, and biogenic amines (eg, serotonin). These mediators are seen in other shock states like sepsis and anaphylaxis, leading Clark to suggest that amniotic fluid embolism be termed "anaphylactoid syndrome of pregnancy." The effects of systemic hypotension and hypoxemia may lead to cardiopulmonary collapse, renal insufficiency, hepatic failure, seizures, and coma.

Amniotic fluid embolism is almost always associated with some form of DIC. The etiology of coagulopathy associated with amniotic fluid embolism is incompletely understood, but it is known that amniotic fluid has potent total thromboplastin and antifibrinolytic activity, both of which increase with advancing gestational age. Once clotting is triggered in the pulmonary vasculature, local thrombin generation can cause vasoconstriction and microvascular thrombosis.

Limited hemodynamic observations with pulmonary artery catheterization suggest that in humans with amniotic fluid embolism, left ventricular dysfunction is the only significant hemodynamic alteration that is consistently documented. The response to amniotic fluid embolus in humans may be biphasic, initially resulting in intense vasospasm, severe pulmonary hypertension, and hypoxia. The transient period of right heart failure with hypoxia is later followed by a secondary phase of left heart failure, as reflected by elevated pulmonary artery pressure with subsequent return of right heart function. This biphasic theory may account for the extremely high maternal mortality rate within the first hour (25–34%) and explains why pulmonary hypertension can be difficult to document in patients with this disorder.

Clinical Findings

A. SYMPTOMS AND SIGNS

In his classic review of 272 patients with amniotic fluid embolus, Morgan characterized the main presenting clinical features: 51% presented with respiratory distress and cyanosis, 27% with hypotension, and only 10% with seizures. The Clark national registry noted 30% of patients presented with seizures or seizure-like activity, 27% with dyspnea, 17% with fetal bradycardia, and 13% with hypotension. Between 37% and 54% of patients exhibited an associated bleeding diathesis. Risk factors identified in the Morgan study included multiparity, tumultuous labor, or tetanic uterine contractions. Other studies have noted risk factors including advanced maternal age, use of uterine stimulants, cesarean section, uterine rupture, high cervical lacerations, premature separation of the placenta, and intrauterine fetal demise. Clark, however, was unable to identify any notable risk factors. Other presenting signs that have been described include tachypnea, peripheral cyanosis, bronchospasm, and chest pain.

B. LABORATORY FINDINGS

Arterial blood oxygen tension typically indicates severe maternal hypoxemia. This hypoxemia may result from ventilation-perfusion inequality with atelectasis and associated pulmonary edema. The diagnosis of significant coagulopathy is manifested by the presence of microangiopathic hemolysis, hypofibrinogenemia, prolonged clotting times, prolonged bleeding time, and elevated fibrin split products. The chest radiograph is nonspecific, although pulmonary edema is often noted. The ECG typically reveals unexplained tachycardia, nonspecific ST- and T-wave changes, and a right ventricular strain pattern. Lung scans occasionally identify perfusion defects resulting from amniotic fluid embolism even though chest radiographic findings are normal.

Differential Diagnosis

Many conditions may mimic the effects of amniotic fluid embolism on the respiratory, cardiovascular, and coagulation systems. Pulmonary thromboembolism can result in severe hypoxemia with pulmonary edema. In contrast to amniotic fluid embolism, chest pain is a relatively common finding. Congestive heart failure due to fluid overload or preexisting heart disease may mimic the cardiorespiratory compromise observed during amniotic fluid embolism. Hypotension may result from several disorders, including septic chorioamnionitis or postpartum hemorrhage. Pulmonary aspiration (Mendelson's syndrome) is associated with tachycardia, shock, respiratory distress, and production of a frothy pink sputum, but is usually also associated with bronchospasm and wheezing. Other conditions in the differential diagnosis include air embolism, myocardial infarc-

tion, anaphylaxis, placental abruption, eclampsia, uterine rupture, transfusion reaction, and local anesthesia toxicity.

Treatment

Amniotic fluid embolism remains one of the most devastating and unpreventable conditions complicating pregnancy. Therapeutic measures are supportive and should be directed toward minimizing hypoxemia with supplemental oxygen, maintaining blood pressure, and managing associated coagulopathies. Patients with poor oxygenation often require intubation and positive end-expiratory pressure. Adequate oxygenation will minimize related cerebral and myocardial ischemia and acidosis-induced pulmonary artery vasospasm. Pulmonary artery catheterization should be considered in the absence of coagulopathy to guide inotropic therapy with dopamine. If invasive hemodynamic monitoring is not available, rapid digitalization should be considered. Finally, the development of consumptive coagulopathy may require replacement of depleted hemostatic components in cases with significant uncontrollable bleeding or abnormal clotting parameters.

Prognosis

Maternal mortality rates range from 60–80%; however, a recent study quoted a 26.4% mortality rate. Of those patients who do not survive, 25% die within the first hour, and 80% within the first 9 hours. Correspondingly high perinatal morbidity and mortality rates would be expected.

PULMONARY THROMBOEMBOLISM

 ESSENTIALS OF DIAGNOSIS

- *Unexplained chest pain and dyspnea (most frequent presenting symptoms).*
- *History of pulmonary embolism, deep venous thrombosis, prolonged immobilization, or recent surgery.*
- *Physical examination: usually nonspecific, depending on extent of cardiopulmonary involvement, but may include tachycardia, wheezing, pleural friction rub, and pulmonary rales.*
- *Laboratory evaluation: decreased arterial blood oxygen tension to less than 90 mm Hg in the sitting position.*
- *Diagnostic studies: pulmonary radionuclide ventilation-perfusion scanning, spiral CT, and angiography.*

General Considerations

Pulmonary thromboembolism is a rare complication of pregnancy (0.09%) but is a significant cause of maternal morbidity and mortality. Mortality has been documented as 12.8% if untreated, and 0.7% if therapy is instituted. The diagnosis of deep venous thrombosis (DVT) occurs in the antepartum period approximately half the time, and is evenly distributed throughout each trimester. Pulmonary embolism has a higher incidence in the postpartum period. Predisposing factors commonly include advanced maternal age, obesity, traumatic delivery, abdominal delivery, thrombophlebitis, and endometritis. Patients with underlying thrombophilias or previous thrombotic events are at greater risk for this condition.

Pathophysiology

More than 100 years ago, Virchow postulated that the basic mechanism of thrombus formation is related to a combination of vessel injury, vascular stasis, and alterations in blood coagulability. Venous thrombi consist of fibrin deposits and red blood cells with varying amounts of platelet and white blood cell components. In most cases, lower extremity and pelvic thrombi are responsible for the pathologic sequelae.

Ordinarily, the vascular endothelium does not react with either platelets or the blood coagulation system unless it is disrupted by vessel injury. Such injury exposes subendothelial cells to blood elements responsible for activation of the extrinsic coagulation cascade. Disruption of the vascular endothelium may occur during traumatic vaginal delivery or cesarean section.

Pregnancy is also associated with venous stasis, especially in the lower extremities, because the enlarging uterus reduces blood return to the inferior vena cava by direct mechanical effects. Hormonal factors may contribute to venodilatation and stasis during pregnancy. Stasis prevents the hepatic clearance of activated coagulation factors and minimizes mixing of these factors with their serum inhibitors. In this manner, venous stasis becomes another predisposing factor for the formation of thrombi. Stasis secondary to prolonged bedrest for medical or obstetric complications will predispose a pregnant woman to increased venous stasis and formation of vascular thrombi. The period of greatest risk for thrombosis and embolism appears to be the immediate postpartum, especially after cesarean delivery.

The maternal circulation becomes hypercoagulable from alterations in the coagulation and fibrinolytic systems. Serum concentrations of most coagulation proteins, such as fibrinogen and factors II, VII, VIII, IX, and X, increase during pregnancy. These changes are also associated with decreased fibrinolytic activity, which is responsible for the conversion of plasminogen to the active proteolytic enzyme plasmin.

Women with congenital or acquired thrombophilias are at increased risk for thrombosis; in fact, up to half of women who have these events in pregnancy may have an underlying disorder. The most commonly recognized thrombophilia in the Caucasian population is factor V Leiden mutation (5%). Other less common but significant disorders include: prothrombin gene mutation G20210A (2–4%), antithrombin III deficiency (0.02–0.2%), protein C deficiency (0.2–0.5%), protein S deficiency (0.08%), and hyperhomocysteinemia (1%). The antiphospholipid antibody syndrome also significantly increases maternal risk.

Once a venous thrombus is formed, it may dislodge from its peripheral vascular origin and enter the central maternal circulation. Propagation of the original venous clot or recurrent pulmonary emboli are possible. DVTs limited to the calf rarely embolize, but approximately 20% extend to the proximal lower extremity.

Clinical Findings

A. Symptoms and Signs

The subsequent cardiopulmonary effects of pulmonary embolus will depend on the location and size of thrombi in the lung. A patient with a large embolus affecting the central pulmonary circulation may present with acute syncope, respiratory embarrassment, and shock. Smaller emboli may not have significant clinical sequelae.

No single symptom or combination of symptoms is specific for the diagnosis of pulmonary embolus. Classic triads (hemoptysis, chest pain, and dyspnea; or dyspnea, chest pain, and apprehension) are rarely seen (Table 60–6). Chest pain and dyspnea were the most common symptoms in patients with angiographically documented pulmonary emboli (over 80%). Physical findings include tachycardia, tachypnea (rate > 16/min), pulmonary rales, wheezing, and pleural friction rub.

B. Laboratory Findings

There are no specific routine laboratory findings associated with the diagnosis of pulmonary embolus, although arterial blood gas measurements will often reveal significant hypoxemia. In the upright position, almost all healthy young pregnant women will have an arterial blood oxygen tension greater than 90 mm Hg. An alveolar-atrial (A-a) gradient of greater than 20 is suspicious for pulmonary embolus. The ECG may reveal unexplained tachycardia associated with cor pulmonale (right axis deviation, S wave in lead I, Q wave plus T wave inversion in lead III). A chest roentgenogram may be normal or may show infiltrates, atelectasis, or effusions. Thirty percent of patients with a pulmonary embolus will have a normal chest x-ray.

It is generally accepted that a normal radionuclide perfusion study can effectively rule out pulmonary

Table 60–6. Symptoms and signs in 327 patients with pulmonary embolus confirmed by angiography.[1]

Symptom or Sign	Frequency (%)
Chest pain	88
Pleuritic	74
Nonpleuritic	14
Dyspnea	84
Apprehension	59
Cough	53
Hemoptysis	30
Sweating	27
Syncope	13
Respiration more than 16/min	92
Pulmonary rales	58
Pulse more than 100/min	44
Fever (> 37.8 °C [99.7 °F])	43
Phlebitis	32
Heart gallop	34
Diaphoresis	36
Edema	24
Heart murmur	23
Cyanosis	19

[1]Adapted and reproduced, with permission, from Bell WR, Simon TL, DeMets DL: The clinical features of submassive and massive pulmonary emboli. *Am J Med* 1977;62:355.

embolus. Perfusion studies are occasionally equivocal, and ventilation scanning may be required to clarify the diagnosis. Ventilation scanning will improve the specificity of the perfusion study, since this will rule out airway disorders that may be responsible for reduced pulmonary perfusion. The radiation exposure is minimal (< 0.1 rad). Unfortunately, a V/Q scan can only confirm a diagnosis if it is normal or indicates high probability of embolus. Therefore, 40–60% of patients will require further testing.

Spiral computed tomography is a newer form of imaging that has a sensitivity and specificity of 94% in the nonpregnant patient. Spiral CT may also be helpful in detecting other abnormalities causing pulmonary symptoms (eg, pleural effusions, consolidation, emphysema, pulmonary masses). However, this study may miss emboli below the segmental level. Magnetic resonance imaging has limited value in pregnancy because it has not been well studied.

If the above studies are equivocal, pulmonary angiography should be considered. Subsequent exposure of the fetus to the relatively low levels of ionizing radiation from angiography can be minimized with appropriate

pelvic shielding and selective angiography on the basis of prior radionuclide scanning.

Noninvasive Doppler should be considered as an initial diagnostic test for suspected DVT involving the lower extremities. Compression ultrasound uses firm compression with the transducer probe to detect intraluminal filling defects. Imaging is most useful for the distal iliac, femoral, and popliteal veins. Doppler is also useful for the proximal iliac veins. Sensitivity is 95%, with a 96% specificity. Impedance plethysmography measures impedance flow with pneumatic cuff inflation. Sensitivity and specificity are 83% and 92%, respectively. Compression of the inferior vena cava by the gravid second- or third-trimester uterus may cause false-positive results.

If the above noninvasive tests are inconclusive, it may be helpful to confirm the extent of the original thrombotic event by venography with pelvic shielding. The soleal calf sinuses and the valves involving the popliteal and femoral veins are the sources of most deep venous thrombi. Venography is associated with induced phlebitis in approximately 3–5% of procedures performed. Radiofibrinogen methods to detect thrombus formation will result in placental transfer of radioactive iodine and are contraindicated in pregnant or nursing women.

Differential Diagnosis

Any condition potentially related to cardiopulmonary compromise during pregnancy should be included in the differential diagnosis. This includes amniotic fluid and air emboli, spontaneous pneumothorax, septic shock, and preexisting heart disease.

Treatment

A. Preventive Treatment

Once predisposing risk factors to pulmonary embolus are identified, it is important to minimize the possibility of further complications. In patients at higher risk for DVT, prophylactic measures should be directed toward preventing venous stasis that leads to clot formation. Mechanical maneuvers such as raising the lower extremities 15 degrees above the horizontal, keeping the legs straight rather than bent at the knees when sitting, or performing calf flexion exercises may be useful, as may external pneumatic compression. One method used to prevent perioperative thrombophlebitis includes minidose heparin prophylaxis, 5000 U subcutaneously 2 hours before surgery and every 12 hours until routine ambulation is achieved. Minidose heparin prophylaxis significantly decreases not only the incidence of DVT but also the incidence of fatal pulmonary emboli. Subcutaneous minidose heparin may be reinstituted approximately 6 hours after delivery. Postpartum or postoperative ambulation is important in minimizing thromboembolic complications during this high-risk period. Some women may require therapeutic anticoagulation during pregnancy to prevent a thromboembolic event. Included in this category are women with artificial heart valves, antithrombin III deficiency, antiphospholipid antibody syndrome, history of rheumatic heart disease and atrial fibrillation, homozygosity for factor V Leiden or prothrombin gene mutation, and recurrent thromboembolic disease. Therapeutic anticoagulation can be achieved by using subcutaneous heparin 2–3 times a day, adjusting for a PTT of 2.0–3.0 times normal. Low molecular weight heparin (LMWH) can also be used. LMWH does not cross the placenta, and it has been shown to be relatively safe in pregnancy. In addition, complications of heparin therapy (osteoporosis, thrombocytopenia) are not seen with this medication, and dosing in pregnancy usually does not require many adjustments. The PTT does not need to be followed; instead, peak antifactor Xa levels can be checked every 4–6 weeks. It is controversial whether other disorders, like protein C or S deficiency, or a family history of thrombophilias, require anticoagulation therapy. These patients may benefit from minidose heparin prophylaxis.

B. TREATMENT OF DOCUMENTED PULMONARY EMBOLISM

Once pulmonary embolism is documented, therapeutic intervention should be directed to correction of arterial hypoxemia and any associated hypotension. Other measures should prevent clot propagation or recurrent emboli. Supplemental oxygen should be given to achieve an arterial oxygen tension of at least 70 mm Hg. A loading dose of 5000–10,000 U of heparin should be given intravenously by continuous infusion, followed by a maintenance dose of approximately 1000 U/h. The PTT should be maintained at 1.5–2.5 times control values. Other investigators recommend the use of heparin levels for monitoring anticoagulation therapy. Heparin levels may be measured on the third or fourth day and should be about 0.2 µg/mL, not to exceed 0.4 µg/mL. Leg elevation, bedrest, and local heat will be beneficial to patients who have associated DVT. Intravenous morphine may be helpful in alleviating anxiety and ameliorating chest pain.

Intrapartum care of pulmonary embolus is complicated, and individual treatment approaches may vary. Selected patients with recent pulmonary thromboembolism, ileofemoral DVT, or heart valve prosthesis should probably continue full anticoagulation with high-dose heparin during labor or surgical procedures. Under these circumstances, the risk for potential bleeding complications from anticoagulant needs to be balanced against the risk of thromboembolism. Although there is a higher incidence of wound hematomas associated with peripartum anticoagulation, there is no clear evidence that this regimen is associated with excessive postpartum hemorrhage after normal vaginal delivery.

Postpartum patients receiving heparin may be switched over to warfarin once oral intake is tolerated. Heparin should be continued for the first 5–7 days of warfarin therapy. By the time heparin is discontinued, the international normalized ratio (INR) should be 2.0–3.0 times the normal value. Alternatively, it may be desirable to continue moderate doses of subcutaneous heparin (10,000 U twice daily), especially in nursing mothers. Postpartum anticoagulation should be continued for at least 3 months if the patient developed pulmonary embolus in the third trimester.

C. COMPLICATIONS OF TREATMENT

The major complication of anticoagulant therapy is maternal or fetal hemorrhage. Heparin does not cross the placenta due to its large molecular weight, but it has been associated with maternal thrombocytopenia and osteoporosis. These effects can be avoided with low molecular weight heparin. Warfarin is known to cross the placental barrier, and its use in the first trimester has been associated with embryopathy (nasal hypoplasia and stippled epiphyses). Fetal nervous system abnormalities (eg, hydrocephalus) have also been noted with the use of warfarin during pregnancy.

A small percentage of patients will experience recurrent pulmonary emboli despite full anticoagulation. These patients may be candidates for vena caval ligation by a transabdominal approach under general or regional anesthesia. If the pelvis is suspected as the source of embolus, the right ovarian vein should also be ligated. It has been estimated that approximately 95% of patients with pulmonary embolism massive enough to cause hypotension eventually die. In this context, pulmonary artery embolectomy may be life-saving.

Placement of a vena caval umbrella via the internal jugular vein is an option for unstable patients with recurrent emboli who would not be prime surgical candidates. Although abdominal radiography is required for this procedure, placement of the umbrella filter does not require general anesthesia. This strategy will prevent larger emboli from reaching the pulmonary circulation.

Prognosis

Pulmonary embolus, with a mortality rate of 12–15% if left untreated, will develop in approximately one-fourth of untreated patients with antenatal DVT. In a review of pregnancies complicated by DVT treated with anticoagulant therapy, the incidence of pulmonary embolus was 4.5% of patients, with a maternal mortality rate of less than 1%.

DISSEMINATED INTRAVASCULAR COAGULATION (DIC)

ESSENTIALS OF DIAGNOSIS

- *History of recent bleeding diathesis, especially concurrent with placental abruption, amniotic fluid embolism, fetal demise, sepsis, preeclampsia-eclampsia, or saline abortion.*
- *Clinical evidence of multiple bleeding points associated with purpura and petechiae on physical examination.*
- *Laboratory findings classically include thrombocytopenia, hypofibrinogenemia, and elevated PT, elevated D-dimer, and fibrin split products.*

General Considerations

DIC is a pathologic condition associated with inappropriate activation of coagulation and fibrinolytic systems. It should be considered a secondary phenomenon resulting from an underlying disease state. The most common obstetric conditions associated with DIC are intrauterine fetal death, amniotic fluid embolism, preeclampsia-eclampsia, HELLP (hemolysis, elevated liver enzymes, and low platelet count syndrome), placenta previa, and placental abruption. Saline-induced abortion is also a cause.

Pathophysiology

The most widely accepted theory of blood coagulation entails a "cascade theory" (Fig 60–7). Basically, the coagulation system is divided into intrinsic and extrinsic systems. The intrinsic system contains all the intravascular components required to activate thrombin by sequential activation of factors XII, XI, IX, X, V, and II (prothrombin). The extrinsic system is initially activated by tissue thromboplastin, leading to sequential activation of factors VII, X, V, and prothrombin. Both the intrinsic and extrinsic pathways converge to activate factor X, which subsequently reacts with activated factor V in the presence of calcium and phospholipid to convert prothrombin to thrombin.

Thrombin is a proteolytic enzyme responsible for splitting fibrinogen chains into fibrinopeptides, leading to the formation of fibrin monomer. This central enzyme is capable of activating factor XIII to stabilize the newly formed fibrin clot and will enhance the activity of factors V and VIII.

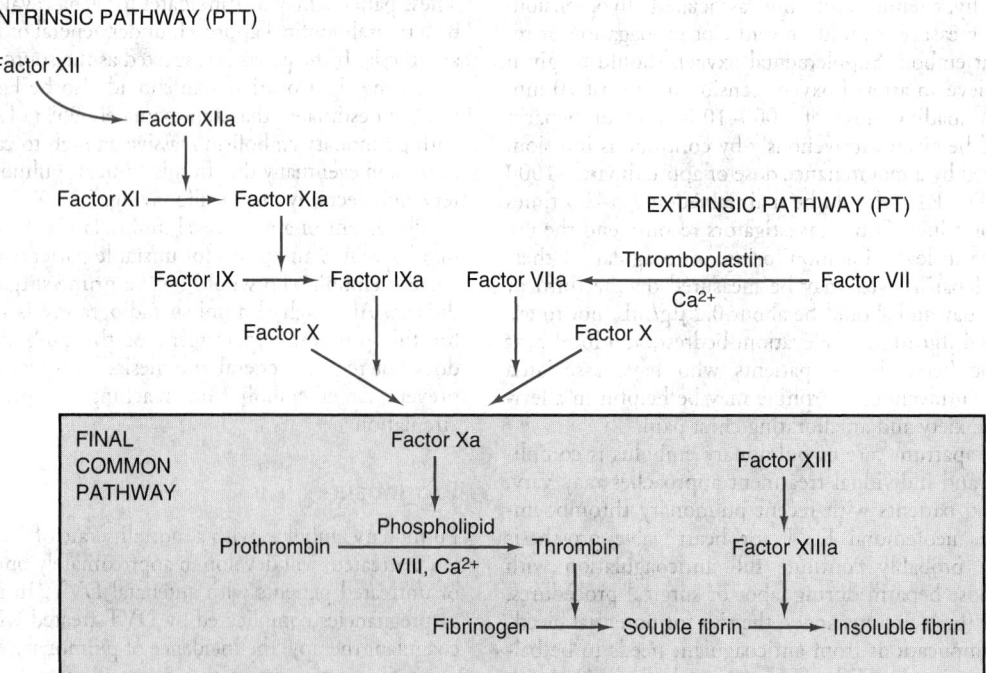

Figure 60–7. Coagulation cascade mechanism.

Activation of the coagulation system also stimulates the conversion of plasminogen to plasmin as a protective mechanism against intravascular thrombosis. Plasmin is an enzyme that inactivates factors V and VIII and is capable of lysing fibrin and fibrinogen to form degradation products. Thus, the normal physiologic hemostatic mechanism represents a delicate and complex balance between the coagulation and fibrinolytic systems.

Pregnancy is considered to represent a hypercoagulable state. With the exception of factors XI and XIII, there is an overall increase in the activity of coagulation factors. Fibrinogen rises as early as 12 weeks' gestation and reaches a peak level of 400–650 mg/dL in late pregnancy. The fibrinolytic system is depressed during pregnancy and labor but returns to normal levels within 1 hour of placental delivery. The early puerperium is accompanied by a secondary rise in fibrinogen, factors VIII, IX, X, and antithrombin III; a return to nonpregnant levels occurs by 3–4 weeks postpartum.

The complex pathophysiology of DIC is characterized by (1) procoagulant system activation; (2) fibrinolytic system activation; (3) inhibitor consumption; (4) cytokine release; (5) cellular activation; and (6) resultant end-organ damage. DIC occurs as a secondary event in a wide variety of illnesses associated with excess production of circulating thrombin. The pathophysiologic factors responsible for inappropriate activation of the clotting mechanism include endothelial cell injury, liberation of thromboplastin from injured tissue, and release of phospholipid from red cell or platelet injury. All these mechanisms may contribute to development of a bleeding diathesis resulting from increased thrombin activity. Additionally, widespread DIC will cause increased platelet aggregation, consumption of coagulation factors, secondary activation of the fibrinolytic system, and deposition of fibrin into multiple organ sites, which can result in ischemic tissue damage. The associated thrombocytopenia and presence of fibrin split products will impair hemostasis.

Specific obstetric conditions associated with DIC include the following.

A. PLACENTAL ABRUPTION

DIC may occur in placental abruption involving liberation of tissue thromboplastin or possible intrauterine consumption of fibrinogen and coagulation factors during the formation of retroplacental clot. This leads to activation of the extrinsic coagulation mechanism. Placental abruption is one of the most common obstetric causes of DIC.

B. RETAINED DEAD FETUS SYNDROME

Another cause of DIC is retained dead fetus syndrome involving liberation of tissue thromboplastin from nonviable tissue. This cause is less common in recent years due to advanced ultrasound technology and the earlier detection of this condition.

C. AMNIOTIC FLUID EMBOLISM

This involves not only the release of tissue thromboplastin but also the intrinsic procoagulant properties of amniotic fluid itself. It is likely that the associated hypotension, hypoxemia, and tissue acidosis will encourage the activation of coagulation factors.

D. PREECLAMPSIA-ECLAMPSIA

This condition is associated with chronic coagulation abnormalities that may lead to thrombocytopenia and elevation of fibrin degradation products. It is uncertain whether endothelial damage activates procoagulant proteins and platelets or the reverse, although the former is more likely. Eclampsia is associated with DIC 11% of the time; with HELLP syndrome this increases to 15%. Preeclampsia together with placental abruption also significantly increases this association.

E. SALINE OR SEPTIC ABORTION

Saline-induced abortion has been associated with subclinical DIC. Severe cases of DIC have occurred in 1:400–1:1000 cases. Disease may be related to the release of tissue thromboplastin from the placenta. Septic abortion may also cause release of tissue thromboplastin or release of bacterial endotoxin (phospholipids).

F. OTHER

Other triggers of DIC include septicemia, viremias (eg, HIV, varicella, CMV, hepatitis), drugs, and acidosis.

Clinical Findings

A. SYMPTOMS AND SIGNS

Acute clinical manifestations of DIC are variable and include generalized bleeding, localized hemorrhage, purpura, petechiae, and thromboembolic phenomena. Also, fever, hypotension, proteinuria, hypoxia, hemorrhagic bullae, acral cyanosis, and frank gangrene have been described. Widespread fibrin deposits may affect any organ system, including the lungs, kidneys, brain, and liver. Chronic DIC (eg, fetal demise) is associated with slower production of thrombin and may be associated with minimal or absent clinical signs and symptoms.

B. LABORATORY FINDINGS

Although histologic diagnosis of fibrin deposits is the only definitive manner by which DIC may be confirmed, there are a host of indirect tests suitable for the clinical evaluation of coagulopathy.

1. Platelets—Platelets are decreased (< 100,000/μL) in more than 90% of cases. In the absence of other causes, spontaneous purpura usually does not occur when platelet counts are greater than 30,000/μL.

2. Prothrombin time (PT)—PT measures the time required for clotting by the extrinsic pathway and is dependent on the ultimate conversion of fibrinogen to fibrin. It is prolonged in only 50–75% of patients with DIC. The explanations for the normal PTs are, first, the presence of circulating activated clotting factors like thrombin or factor Xa, that accelerate the formation of fibrin; and second, the presence of early degradation products, which are rapidly clottable by thrombin; these may cause the test to register a normal or fast PT.

3. Partial thromboplastin time (PTT)—PTT is frequently normal in DIC (40–50% of the time) and is not as helpful for establishing the diagnosis. This test measures the function of the intrinsic and final common pathways of the coagulation cascade.

4. Thrombin time (TT)—TT is elevated in 80% of patients with DIC. It is affected only by the amount of circulating fibrinogen or the presence of thrombin inhibitors such as fibrin degradation products and heparin. This test specifically measures the time necessary for conversion of fibrinogen to fibrin.

5. Fibrinogen—Fibrinogen is often decreased, with approximately 70% of patients with DIC having a serum level less than 150 mg/dL. The normal physiologic increase of serum fibrinogen levels during pregnancy may mask a pathologic decrease in this parameter.

6. Fibrin split products—Values greater than 40 μg/mL are suggestive of DIC. These are elevated in 85–100% of patients with DIC. These degradation products are diagnostic of the plasmin biodegradation of fibrinogen or fibrin, so indicate only the presence of plasmin.

7. Clotting time and clot retraction—Observation of clotting time and ability of the clot to retract can be performed by using 2 mL of blood in a 5-mL glass test tube. These are relatively simple bedside tests that can provide qualitative evidence of hypofibrinogenemia. When the clot forms, it is usually soft but not reduced in volume (adding celite will hasten this reaction). Over the next half hour, the clot should retract, with the volume of serum exceeding that of the formed clot. If this phenomenon does not occur, low serum fibrinogen levels can be suspected.

8. Peripheral blood smear—A peripheral blood smear reveals schistocytes in approximately 40% of patients with DIC.

9. Bleeding time—The time required for hemostasis after skin puncture will become progressively prolonged as the platelet count falls below 100,000/μL. Spontaneous continuous bleeding from puncture sites may develop if the platelet count falls below 30,000/μL.

10. Newer tests—Several of these laboratory findings are more reliable than the classic studies.

    a. D-Dimer—This is a neoantigen formed as a result of plasmin digestion of cross-linked fibrin when thrombin initiates the transition of fibrinogen to fibrin, and activates factor XIII to cross-link the fibrin formed. The test is specific for fibrin (not fibrinogen) degradation products, and is abnormal in 90% of cases.

    b. Antithrombin III Level—This is abnormal in 89% of cases.

    c. Fibrinopeptide A—This is abnormal 75% of the time.

Differential Diagnosis

Most acute episodes of generalized bleeding in obstetric patients will be related to pregnancy, but other rare causes of congenital or acquired coagulopathies need to be considered. These include idiopathic thrombocytopenic purpura, hemophilia, and von Willebrand's disease. Placental abruption is often associated with uterine tenderness, fetal bradycardia, and uterine bleeding. DIC associated with fetal demise usually does not become apparent until at least 5 weeks after the absence of heart tones has been documented. Amniotic fluid embolus is typically associated with acute onset of respiratory distress and shock. Preeclampsia is characterized by hypertension and proteinuria, which may lead to eclamptic seizures.

Complications

In addition to the potential complications of uncontrolled hemorrhage previously discussed, widespread fibrin deposition may affect any major organ system. This may include the liver (hepatic failure), kidneys (tubular necrosis), and lungs (hypoxemia).

Treatment

Although individual measures will be dictated by the specific obstetric condition, the primary, most important treatment of pregnancy-related DIC is correction of the underlying cause. In most cases, prompt termination of the pregnancy is required. Moderate or low-grade DIC may not be associated with clinical evidence of excessive bleeding and often will require close observation but no further therapy.

    Supportive therapy should be directed to the correction of shock, acidosis, and tissue ischemia. Cardiopulmonary support, including inotropic therapy, blood replacement, and assisted ventilation, should be implemented with the patient in close proximity to a delivery suite. Fetal monitoring, careful recording of maternal fluid balance, and serial evaluation of coagulation parameters are extremely important. If sepsis is suspected, antibiotics should be employed. Central monitoring with a pulmonary artery catheter is relatively contraindicated due to potential bleeding complications. Vaginal delivery, without episiotomy if possible, is preferable to cesarean section. Failure of improvement in the coagulopathy within several hours after delivery suggests sepsis, liver disease, retained products of conception, or a congenital coagulation defect.

Blood component therapy should be initiated on the basis of transfusion guidelines reported by the National Institutes of Health. Criteria for red cell transfusions were discussed earlier (see Hypovolemic Shock). Fresh-frozen plasma has only limited and specific indications, which include massive hemorrhage, isolated factor deficiencies, reversal of warfarin, antithrombin II deficiency, immunodeficiencies, and thrombocytopenic purpura. Although most cases of severe obstetric hemorrhage will lead to laboratory evidence of coagulation abnormalities, transfusion of fresh-frozen plasma may not always benefit these patients; the amount transfused is usually insufficient for replacing coagulation factors lost by dilution or clot formation. Even with massive obstetric hemorrhage, most procoagulant levels are above 30% of normal values, which is sufficient for maintaining clinical hemostasis in most patients. Specific replacement of fibrinogen should be accomplished by cryoprecipitate. Each unit of cryoprecipitate carries approximately 250 mg of fibrinogen. Platelets should only be administered in the face of active bleeding with a platelet count < 50,000/μL or prophylactically with platelet count 20–30,000/μL or less or following massive transfusion (> 2 times blood volume). Platelets should be transfused on the basis of 1 U/10 kg body weight to raise the cell count above 50,000/μL. However, it should be noted that clotting factors containing fibrinogen may be associated with enhanced hemorrhage and also with thrombosis when given to patients with DIC. For this reason, they should be administered with extreme caution. Obstetricians should remember that Rh immune globulin should be given to Rh-negative recipients of platelets from Rh-positive donors.

Subcutaneous low-dose heparin or low molecular weight heparin may be effective in treating the intravascular clotting process of DIC. Heparin acts as an anticoagulant by activating antithrombin III but has little effect on activated coagulation factors. Anticoagulation is contraindicated in patients with fulminant DIC and central nervous system insults, fulminant liver failure, or obstetric accidents. The one instance, however, in which heparin has been demonstrated to benefit pregnancy-related DIC is in the case of the retained dead fetus with an intact vascular system, where heparin may be administered to interrupt the coagulation process and thrombocytopenia for several days until safe delivery may be implemented.

Prognosis

Most cases of obstetric DIC will improve with delivery of the fetus or evacuation of the uterus. The maternal and fetal prognosis will be more closely related to the associated obstetric condition than to the coagulopathy.

ACUTE RESPIRATORY DISTRESS SYNDROME (ARDS)

 ESSENTIALS OF DIAGNOSIS

- *History of gastric aspiration, infection/sepsis, preeclampsia-eclampsia, seizures, hemorrhage, coagulopathy, or amniotic fluid embolism.*
- *Progressive respiratory distress with decreased lung compliance.*
- *Severe hypoxemia refractory to oxygen therapy.*
- *Diffuse infiltrates on chest roentgenogram.*
- *Normal PCWP, with absence of radiographic evidence of congestive heart failure.*

General Considerations

ARDS is a severe form of lung disease with acute onset, characterized by bilateral infiltrates on chest X-ray, no evidence of intravascular volume overload (PCWP no greater than 18 mm Hg), and severely impaired oxygenation, demonstrated by a ratio of arterial oxygen tension (PaO_2) to the fraction of inspired oxygen (FIO_2) of less than 200 mm Hg. ARDS appears to occur more commonly in obstetric patients than in the general population. Its incidence in the nonpregnant population is 1.5 per 100,000, but it has been estimated to occur in between 1:3000 and 1:10,000 pregnant patients. ARDS has many causes, including gastric aspiration, amniotic fluid embolism, sepsis, coagulopathy, massive blood transfusion, and shock. It can be easily confused with cardiogenic pulmonary edema secondary to alterations in preload, myocardial contractility, or afterload. A basic understanding of the differences between cardiogenic and noncardiogenic pulmonary edema is essential before rational therapeutic intervention may be implemented.

Pathophysiology

The basic underlying pathologic change responsible for ARDS is lung injury that results in damage to the pulmonary epithelium and endothelial tissue. This, in turn, leads to enhanced vascular permeability. Factors determining the net flux of lung fluid between the capillary lumen and interstitial space are quantitatively related by the Starling equation:

Net fluid flux = k[(Pcap – Pis) – (πcap – πis)]

(k = filtration coefficient, Pcap = pulmonary capillary hydrostatic pressure, Pis = interstitial space hydrostatic pressure, πcap = pulmonary capillary serum colloid osmotic pressure, πis = interstitial space fluid colloid osmotic pressure)

Normally, fluid flows from the capillary system to the interstitial space and is returned to the systemic circulation by the pulmonary lymphatic system. An increase in left atrial pressure is observed when the left ventricle is unable to pump all the returning blood into the left atrium. Accordingly, the pulmonary capillary hydrostatic pressure increases, facilitating net movement of lung fluid into the interstitial space. When capillary fluid efflux into the interstitial space exceeds lymphatic resorption, the clinical presentation of pulmonary edema will occur. Although colloid osmotic pressure in the interstitial space and serum also plays a role in pulmonary edema, the most common factor is increased capillary hydrostatic pressure secondary to increased preload (fluid overload), afterload (severe hypertension), and decreased myocardial contractility (postpartum cardiomyopathy).

Capillary membrane permeability plays a much larger role in the genesis of noncardiogenic pulmonary edema (ARDS). Such injury due to hypoxic ischemia, vasoactive substances, chemical irritation, or microthrombi facilitates further efflux of capillary fluid and plasma proteins into the interstitium. This increase in permeability acutely produces atelectasis and diminished compliance of the lung, and damage is usually non-uniform. As the functional capability of atelectatic bronchioles diminishes, shunting and hypoxemia develop.

Maternal physiologic changes can contribute to the severity of ARDS. It has been suggested that decreased extrathoracic compliance, decreased functional residual capacity, higher oxygen deficit, limited cardiac output increases, and anemia may adversely affect the clinical presentation and course of ARDS during pregnancy.

Clinical Findings

A. SYMPTOMS AND SIGNS

Classic signs of respiratory distress are tachypnea, intercostal retractions, and even cyanosis, depending on the degree of hypoxemia. Fetal tachycardia or late decelerations may reflect maternal hypoxemia and uteroplacental insufficiency. Pulmonary rales in noncardiogenic pulmonary edema will be indistinguishable from those of cardiogenic pulmonary edema, but physical findings consistent with the cardiogenic disorder (ventricular gallop, jugular venous distention, and peripheral edema) are not typical features of ARDS. Unfortunately, the physiologic changes of pregnancy may mask the significance of these physical findings during the more subtle stages of respiratory distress.

B. LABORATORY FINDINGS

Arterial blood gas determinations will reveal a progressive moderate to severe hypoxemia despite oxygen therapy. Depending on the obstetric cause of ARDS, other laboratory findings will be variable or nonspecific. The initial chest roentgenogram will often be normal, even in the presence of clinically significant respiratory distress. Within the next 24–48 hours, patchy or diffuse infiltrates will progress to prominent alveolar infiltrates (Fig 60–8). Unlike in cardiogenic pulmonary edema, the heart will most likely be of normal size in a patient with ARDS. PCWP measured by right heart catheterization is the procedure most helpful in differentiating ARDS and pulmonary edema. The PCWP is elevated (> 20 mm Hg) in cardiogenic pulmonary edema but is often normal in ARDS.

Measurement of endobronchial fluid COP has also been utilized to differentiate capillary permeability-induced pulmonary edema from hydrostatic or cardiogenic pulmonary edema. In pulmonary edema secondary to capillary permeability, the COP of endobronchial fluid obtained from endotracheal tube suctioning is usually greater than 75% of the simultaneously obtained plasma COP. In cardiogenic pulmonary edema, the COP of the endobronchial fluid is usually less than 60% that of plasma.

Histopathologically, idiopathic pulmonary fibrosis and ARDS are remarkably similar. Both show evidence of acute alveolar injury, which is characterized by interstitial inflammation, hemorrhage, and edema. This is followed by a hypercellular phase, loss of alveolar structure, and pulmonary fibrosis.

Differential Diagnosis

ARDS should be differentiated from infectious pneumonitis and cardiogenic causes of pulmonary edema. Cardiogenic pulmonary edema will usually respond more rapidly to diuretic therapy than will ARDS, in which abnormalities in capillary membrane permeability are not quickly resolved by such intervention.

Treatment

Therapy should be directed toward the prevention of hypoxemia, correcting acid-base abnormalities, removal of inciting factors, and hemodynamic support appropriate for the specific cause (eg, amniotic fluid embolus, DIC). Cardiogenic pulmonary edema is usually treated with a combination of diuretics, inotropic therapy, and afterload reduction. If a hemodynamic profile is not immediately available by pulmonary artery catheter, the clinician may elect to begin oxygen and furosemide (20 mg IV) for the presumptive diagnosis of cardiogenic pulmonary edema. By contrast, it should be apparent that the basic therapy for ARDS is

Figure 60–8. Sequence of chest radiographs from a 21-year-old woman during her first pregnancy with antepartum pyelonephritis and ARDS. **A:** Normal chest film. **B:** Bilateral patchy pulmonary densities have developed consistent with the diagnosis of ARDS. Much of the apparent increase in heart size is related to shallow inspiration and supine technique. **C:** ARDS has improved dramatically with only minimal residual pulmonary densities.

supportive. Endotracheal intubation with mechanical ventilation is almost always required. The pulmonary artery catheter will be helpful in guiding fluid management and optimizing cardiac performance. Additionally, mixed venous oxygen saturation from the distal port of the pulmonary artery catheter will provide an index of oxygen utilization.

In obstetric patients, reasonable therapeutic goals for cardiorespiratory support include a mechanical ventilator tidal volume of less than 10 mL/kg, PCWP 8–12 mm Hg, arterial blood oxygen tension greater than 60 mm Hg, and mixed venous oxygen tension greater than 30 mm Hg. If unable to maintain PaO_2 of at least 60 mm Hg on 50% or less inspired oxygen, positive end-expiratory pressure (PEEP) in amounts of up to 15 cm H_2O may be helpful. However, it is important to avoid barotrauma to the remaining functional alveolar units, so high tidal volumes and pressures should be avoided. If the mixed venous tension is low, transfusion of red blood cells or inotropic therapy may improve oxygen transport and delivery.

Since the presence of capillary membrane abnormalities in ARDS is associated with rapid equilibration of proteinaceous material between the capillaries and interstitial spaces, intravenous colloid replacement should be discouraged in lieu of crystalloid resuscitation. A policy of relative fluid restriction should be followed, but only if the following criteria are met: stable fetus, no evidence of metabolic acidosis, normal renal function, and no need for vasopressor therapy or PEEP. Sedation and pain relief should be used liberally, and may help to decrease oxygen consumption. Nutritional support for patients on prolonged mechanical ventilation must be considered; enteral feeding is preferred as it may reduce the translocation of gut bacteria into the body. Prospective controlled studies have not demonstrated the benefit of steroid therapy for ARDS. Once therapy for cardiopulmonary support has been implemented, a thorough search for predisposing factors to ARDS must be identified for specific intervention.

Potential future therapies for ARDS include high frequency ventilation, extracorporeal membrane oxygenation (ECMO), intravenous oxygen, inhaled nitric oxide, surfactant replacement, oxygen-free radical scavengers, arachidonic acid metabolite inhibitors, antiprotease agents, antiendotoxin antibodies, anti-tumor necrosis factor antibodies, and other immunologic therapies for sepsis.

The timing of delivery in these patients is unclear from the literature. Based on the high rates of fetal death, preterm labor, fetal heart rate abnormalities, and perinatal asphyxia, most authorities recommend delivery after a gestational age of 28 weeks. In one review, only 10 of 39 patients with antepartum ARDS were discharged undelivered, and all had pyelonephritis or

Varicella. Cesarean section should be reserved for standard obstetrical indications.

Prognosis

Older series suggested a mortality rate as high as 50–60% for patients with ARDS. More recent reviews show rates of 39–44%. One study of 41 patients demonstrated a 24.4% mortality rate; this has been attributed to possible differences in patient population as well as improvements in critical care. Many affected patients developed pulmonary complications that included barotrauma and pneumothorax. Fortunately, survivors of ARDS usually do not demonstrate permanent long-term pulmonary dysfunction.

CARDIOPULMONARY RESUSCITATION DURING PREGNANCY

Many of the critical conditions discussed in this chapter can lead to cardiopulmonary arrest. Cardiopulmonary resuscitation should follow standard protocols, with some modifications for the pregnancy. It may be difficult to perform cardiac compressions due to a large uterus and engorged breasts. Compressions should not be performed in the supine position, as the gravid uterus may cause aortocaval compression, diminished venous return, and subsequent decreased cardiac output. Patients should be positioned with a left lateral tilt before compressions are applied. This can be accomplished using a moving table, a wedge, or with manual displacement of the uterus. Defibrillation and cardioversion been successfully used during pregnancy without disturbance of the fetal cardiac conduction system. It is important, however, to remove fetal monitors to prevent arcing. Finally, the decision to perform a perimortem cesarean section should be made rapidly, within 4–5 minutes of cardiac arrest. This extreme measure can maximize maternal survival by relieving aortocaval compression and increasing blood flow return back to the heart.

REFERENCES

Hypovolemic Shock

American College of Obstetricians and Gynecologists: Hemorrhagic shock. ACOG Educational Bulletin No. 235. ACOG, April 1997.

Amniotic Fluid Embolism

Clark LD et al: Amniotic fluid embolism: analysis of the national registry. Am J Obstet Gynecol 1995;172;1158. [PMID: 7726251]

Davies SD: Amniotic fluid embolus: a review of the literature. Canadian J Anesth 2001;48:88.

Locksmith GJ: Amniotic fluid embolism. Obstet Gynecol Clin North Am 1999;26:435. [PMID: 10472063]

Morgan M: Amniotic fluid embolism. Anaesthesia 1979;34:20. [PMID: 371460]

Pulmonary Thromboembolism

American College of Obstetricians and Gynecologists: Thromboembolism in pregnancy. ACOG Practice Bulletin No. 19. ACOG, August 2000.

Disseminated Intravascular Coagulation

Bick RL: Syndromes of disseminated intravascular coagulation in obstetrics, pregnancy, and gynecology. Hematol Oncol Clin North Am 2000;13:5.

Ginsberg JS, Greer I, Hirsh J: Use of antithrombotic agents during pregnancy. Chest 2001;119:122S. [PMID: 11157646]

Ray JG, Chan WS: Deep vein thrombosis during pregnancy and the puerperium: a meta-analysis of the period of risk and the leg of presentation. Obstet Gynecol Surv 1999;54:265. [PMID: 10198931]

Acute Respiratory Distress Syndrome

Catanzarite V et al: Acute respiratory distress syndrome in pregnancy and the puerperium: causes, courses, and outcome. Obstet Gynecol 2001;97:760. [PMID: 11339930]

Perry KG: Maternal mortality associated with adult respiratory distress syndrome. South Med J 1998;91:441. [PMID: 9598851]

Van Hook JW: Acute respiratory distress syndrome in pregnancy. Semin Perinatol 1997;21:320. [PMID: 9298721]

Psychological Aspects of Obstetrics & Gynecology

61

Alexandra Haessler, MD, & Miriam B. Rosenthal, MD

■ PSYCHOLOGICAL ASPECTS OF GYNECOLOGY

Human sexual behavior and reproduction have long been influenced by culture, taboos, religion, and civil forces. For this reason, the psychological aspects of obstetrics and gynecology deserve special consideration. Recent changes in gynecologic practice and the growing number of female practitioners have greatly influenced women's care. This chapter addresses normal and pathologic psychological issues that are seen in the scope of obstetric and gynecologic practice.

Gynecologists care for women throughout their life cycle—from menarche through adolescence, young adulthood, pregnancy, menopause, and old age. Thus it is critical that they understand the psychosexual and physical development of women. The obstetrician and gynecologist will often fill the role of a general physician, surgeon, sexual counselor, educator, and confidant. Gynecologists must be sensitive to their own attitudes, values, prejudices, and personality style, as these tendencies will influence their practice and their patients' willingness to work collaboratively with them.

THE DOCTOR–PATIENT RELATIONSHIP IN GYNECOLOGY

Traditionally, doctors and patients related to each other in accordance with a model in which a compliant patient viewed the doctor as omnipotent. Today, many women reject this model and demand a more active role in making health care decisions. Health and disease-related information are widely available. Thus, patients are often better informed than they have been in the past. However, there are many sources of misinformation. The lay media can confuse patients by oversimplifying the data or jumping to conclusions. Pharmaceutical advertisements are often biased. A patient may arrive at a first visit with a physician having preconceived ideas about what her diagnosis is and how it should be treated. However, there are still many women who do not want to participate in decisions about health care and who view their physicians as an all-knowing protector. Although these beliefs may be flattering to the physician, unrealistic expectations often lead to anger and disappointment on the part of the patient.

The doctor–patient relationship is an essential part of the therapeutic process and can lead to healthy compliance with medical and surgical regimens. To achieve this relationship, it is essential to have some understanding of the personality style of each patient and her approach to thinking about her body and medical interventions. The collaborative model of doctor–patient interaction is usually most effective for both doctor and patient. The patient interview is the place to begin this collaboration and to evaluate the woman's personality.

The Patient Interview

The first task of any physician is to take the patient's history. The more comfortable the patient feels, the more personal and detailed information she will give. The clinician must use both direct and indirect methods in history taking. It is important to actively listen, noting not only the words, but also the affect and the nonverbal cues. Facial expressions, body posture, gestures, voice quality, and tears are examples. The physician also needs to learn why the patient is seeking help with her problem at this time. Did the patient recently undergo a hardship, did the condition worsen, or did she lose her ability to cope with a preexisting problem?

It is most useful to start with open-ended questions, followed by more specific ones. For example, in interviewing a woman with pelvic pain, it is better to ask the open-ended question, "What is the pain like and what is it associated with?" than the close-ended question, "Does the pain hurt badly, and does it happen in the morning or at night?" Psychological symptoms, such as problems with sleep or eating, fatigue, libido, and anxiety, may relate to physical disorders. If open-ended questions are asked, the interviewer gleans a better understanding of all the factors that play a role in the patient's complaint.

1003

Understanding a patient's social context can also shed light on the medical issues at hand. It may be difficult for the patient to bring up these topics. In these circumstances, it is often best to ask personal questions in a direct way that demonstrates that the interviewer is comfortable discussing the topic. For example, instead of assuming a patient is in a monogamous relationship, ask her if she has intimate sexual relations with men, women, or both. You will likely get to the core of the issue by using this technique when discussing personal topics.

Personality Style

The following personality styles are commonly seen across the scope of medical practice. These descriptions are rather extreme, but are useful outlines. The insightful physician will consider how each patient copes with illness and relate to her in a way that benefits that patient.

A. The Dependent Personality

These patients have a lack of self-confidence and require significant reassurance. This patient becomes increasingly dependent on the physician, calls frequently and often creates frustration. The physician needs to set limits, but with some concessions such as telling the patient she can call at specific times. Interviews can be limited in frequency and duration. The dependent patient can make the physician angry by venting hostility in an indirect way. Illness is seen as a threat of abandonment. Assuring her of continued care that has definite limits is helpful.

B. The Obsessive or Anxious Personality

These patients have an unusual need for control. They tend to employ the defense mechanisms of isolation and intellectualization. This patient seeks copious medical information and is particularly active in medical decision making. Illness is seen as a punishment for letting things get out of control. Her participation in the management of her illness will likely help.

C. The Histrionic or Dramatic Personality

These patients are dramatic and attention seeking. They are often flirtatious and can be quite emotional. A caring physician with a firm professional manner is ideal for this patient. She needs support, but not overly detailed explanations.

D. Borderline Personality Disorder

This patient poses one of the most difficult personality types for physicians. Borderline patients suffer from an unstable self-image. As a result they have unstable moods and often alternate between kindness and volatility. They tend to identify some medical staff as "good" and others as "bad." They come across as un-

predictable and manipulative. These patients possess deep loneliness and impulsivity. Not uncommonly, they self-mutilate or attempt suicide. Physicians often need to manage these patients in conjunction with a psychiatrist.

E. The Paranoid Personality

This patient is suspicious, blaming, hypersensitive and is threatened by intimacy. A respectful distance is necessary to help this individual. Illness is viewed as an annihilating assault coming from outside the self. Helpful techniques include honest, simple explanations and assuring her that the medical team is there to help her.

F. The Schizoid Personality

This patient is remote, unsociable, and uninvolved. She may be very eccentric or have an unusual style of dress. These patients are often in denial of their illness and present late. Illness is viewed as a force that threatens to invade her privacy. It is important to screen for a more serious psychiatric illness, such as schizophrenia. A respect for privacy and distance is helpful.

PSYCHOLOGICAL ASPECTS OF SPECIFIC GYNECOLOGIC PROBLEMS

Acute Gynecologic Emergency

When urgent medical or surgical care is needed, the relationship with the patient changes to one that requires submission of the patient to the physician. In these cases the patient has likely never met the physician. This role may be one the physician is comfortable with, but that terrifies the patient. Once the emergency has passed, it is essential to help the patient gradually resume a role in her care. Prolongation of the dominant role by the physician may easily lead to continued dependency after its justification has ceased. The patient recovering from surgery or a serious illness must not be suddenly abandoned to her own devices as long as she needs her doctor's help and support. Every effort should be made to hasten her return to full health without dependency on her doctor.

Emergent care for the sexual-assault survivor deserves special mention. In this circumstance, the care provider needs not only to be concerned with patient care, but also with obtaining important legal evidence. Many states require that at least the physician, a police representative, and a patient advocate be present during the interview and examination. It is essential to be familiar with your local government's guidelines and to take appropriate steps to ensure proper data collection. Obviously, sedatives and narcotic medications should only be used once the patient has given a full, recorded statement. Counseling services should be arranged.

Chronic Pelvic Pain

Chronic pelvic pain (CPP) is generally defined as pelvic pain that persists for at least 6 months. The pain cannot be limited to the dysmenorrhea, although an exacerbation of baseline pain during this time is consistent with the diagnosis. This is a diagnosis of exclusion and is made once another etiology cannot be identified. Between 3.8% and 14.7% of women suffer from this syndrome. In primary care practices, 39% of women complain of CPP. The differential diagnosis for CPP is broad. The most likely gynecologic causes of CPP are endometriosis, masses, and infection. Neoplasia and less-common diagnoses should be ruled out with imaging and biopsy when indicated. Other common causes of CPP are irritable bowel syndrome (up to 79%), urinary tract complaints, and musculoskeletal pain. CPP can be extremely frustrating for the patient and her physician, as a clear etiology cannot be identified. It is important to remember that there are at least three reasons why women complain of pain in the apparent absence of organic pelvic disease: (a) Disease processes are present but have not been detected; (b) pain may be associated with disorders that are not accompanied by objective evidence (migraine variant, neurologic problem, limited medical technology, chronic/episodic syndrome); and (c) complaints may be psychogenic or a manifestation of a somatization disorder.

The gynecologic work-up includes a careful history that allows the patient to explain the course of her symptoms. The timing of symptom onset and exacerbation should be noted. The severity of pain is best assessed by pain scales. Visual analogue scales, or a 0–10 scale, is useful in tracking pain fluctuation. Pretreatment assessments (like the one provided by the International Pelvic Pain Society) are often used in research to quantify pain and identify response to treatment. The nature and quality of the pain may give a clue to the source of the pain. Somatic pain (musculoskeletal, cutaneous) is sharp and usually localized. Visceral pain (intraperitoneal, upper reproductive tract) is vague, aching, and difficult to isolate and describe. Obstetrical, surgical, menstrual, and sexual histories often give important clues to the etiology. The perception of pain can be influenced by several psychosocial variables. Examples include the anxiety that accompanies pain, childhood experiences with pain and punishment, the ability of an individual to control pain by cognitive and behavioral means, experiences with physical and sexual abuse, previous painful illnesses, the patient's current psychic state, and the patient's cultural expression of pain. These patients often have histories of childhood and adult sexual abuse. Patients with chronic pelvic pain are more often found to be depressed and suffer from substance abuse, sexual dysfunction and somatization disorders.

Women without a clear cause of their pain are often labeled as having psychiatric problems. In such cases, pain is seen as a result of emotional conflicts or a depression. Despite our limited understanding of the mechanism of pelvic pain, the syndrome has been included as a psychiatric diagnosis in the *Diagnostic and Statistical Manual of Mental Disorders, 4th edition* (DSM-IV). This is a very controversial classification. The fact that CPP pain patients are more likely to suffer from psychiatric conditions leads many to suspect the conditions are part of one syndrome. This finding neither clarifies that they are part of one syndrome nor whether there is a causal relationship between the conditions. Sadly, patients with pain syndromes and depression are less likely to have their depression identified and treated. One should determine which organic and psychiatric disorders are present and treat distinct symptoms. Research suggests that depression and pain share neurotransmitters and biologic pathways that may shed light on how these conditions interact.

The management of chronic pain and somatization requires a complete evaluation of possible etiologies, psychological assessment (and treatment), and a multidisciplinary approach that incorporates specialists. Unnecessary surgery should be avoided, and psychological treatments along with suitable medications are helpful. Narcotics should be used as appropriate, usually in conjunction with the care of a pain specialist. Biofeedback, relaxation training, hypnosis, and psychotherapy can be helpful. Antidepressants have been used with good results. Advances in this field will come from research that integrates the biologic, psychological, and cultural approaches. A multidisciplinary approach appears to be the most effective in managing intractable pelvic pain syndromes.

Eating Disorders

Eating disorders are 10 times more likely to occur in women than men. The incidence of eating disorders is believed to have increased in recent years, although changing diagnostic criteria makes these conditions difficult to track. Anorexia, bulimia, and obesity are heterogeneous conditions with biologic, psychological, and social dimensions. For each patient being evaluated particular attention should be paid to history of the eating problem, weight history, physical examination, and family dynamics, including affective mental disturbances in the family, personality style, substance abuse, physical abuse, and cultural background. Life changes (ie, pregnancy, relationship trouble) can trigger recurrence of an eating disorder. Although these patients present to the OB/GYN, psychiatric consultation should be obtained.

A. ANOREXIA NERVOSA

Ninety-five percent of patients are female, and occurrence is rare in heterosexual males. Its prevalence is 0.13–

1% in females 12–18 years old. Usually these patients are in their teens with the overwhelming majority being younger than age 30 years. Anorexia nervosa is a disorder characterized by refusal to maintain a body weight within 85% of ideal body weight for age and height. Firm control over one's diet distinguishes this disorder form the others. Generally, anorexia is seen in the cultural context of a society where food is abundant and thinness is desirable. The fact that minority women are more likely to develop an eating disorder the more assimilated they are into American society supports this assertion.

Anorexia is characterized by markedly decreased food intake, a preoccupation with a fear of becoming obese, a distorted body image, and often by amenorrhea for at least 3 consecutive menstrual cycles. The subtypes include restricting (food avoidance) and binge eating/purging. Although the weight loss is generally dramatic, the patient does not consider it concerning. Because these patients are secretive and in denial of their problem, experts suspect the incidence of anorexia is higher than reported. These patients often come to the attention of the gynecologist for evaluation of amenorrhea, infertility, or other endocrine disorders. Associated physiologic signs may include hypothermia, bradycardia, hypotension, edema, lanugo, and other metabolic changes. Not uncommonly, these patients develop osteopenia during the important years of bone deposition. Anorexics are 2.9 times more likely to suffer a fracture than controls.

Typically, anorexia nervosa presents in early adolescence or the early twenties. The course may be episodic or chronic: Approximately 40% of patients recover, 30% significantly improve, 20% remain ill, and death occurs in more than 5%. Family patterns demonstrate that these disorders are more prevalent in sisters and mothers of affected individuals. Other family members may have a history of major depression or bipolar affective disorder. The onset may or may not coincide with a stressful life event. The associated family model has included parental pressure for the child to be perfect (perceived), poor communication within the family, and a devalued mother role. Research does not clearly demonstrate that this is the case.

Management consists of referral to specialists trained in the treatment of this disorder, usually as a team with behavioral medicine specialists and nutritionists. Hospital treatment is indicated for severe cases. Inpatients should be managed by specialists, as they can develop complicated medical problems. The primary physician should remain involved throughout each phase of treatment to provide continuity of care. Better prognosis is associated with earlier age of onset and poor prognosis with premorbid obesity, bulimia, vomiting, and laxative abuse.

B. BULIMIA

The estimated incidence of bulimia nervosa is 1–1.5%. Bulimia is characterized by recurrent bouts of rapid consumption of large amounts of food in a short time. This behavior alternates with self-induced vomiting, use of laxatives and diuretics, dieting, fasting, and/or vigorous exercise. These behaviors are all intended to keep weight down. The subtypes include purging (eg, laxative, vomiting) and nonpurging type (fasting, excessive exercise). They are generally accompanied by depression, anxiety, lack of control over the eating, low self-esteem, and/or social isolation. Preoccupation with food, weight, and body shape are common. The diagnosis is made when there are at least 2 large binge-eating episodes per week for at least 3 months. The food eaten is usually high in calories and eaten secretly. The binge may be followed by abdominal pain, distention, and vomiting. The individual may be obese, thin, or of normal weight. Stress or eating itself may precipitate binges.

Many bulimics are depressed or are afflicted with other affective disorders. Alcohol or drug abuse is often associated with bulimia and often involves sedatives, amphetamines, and cocaine. A variety of personality types, including those with borderline personality disorders, develop this condition. Subjective complaints may include lethargy, impaired concentration, and abdominal pain. Dehydration and electrolyte disturbances (ie, hypokalemia, metabolic alkalosis, hypochloremia, and, rarely, metabolic acidosis) may result from fasting, diuretic use, and acute diarrhea. Arrhythmias may result from significant electrolyte disturbances. Other complications are gastric rupture, salivary gland swelling (usually the parotid), and dental problems including decalcification of teeth that result from frequent vomiting. The neuroendocrine abnormalities include blunted thyroid-stimulating hormone response to thyroid-releasing hormone (TRH) administration, increase in growth hormone following TRH or glucose administration, and elevated basal serum prolactin. Menstrual dysfunction may be due to disturbed gonadotropin production.

An exact etiology is unknown, but associated factors include a history of traumatic events, especially separation or loss and a history of being overweight. The mild form of bulimia is fairly common among women in college (one study of college freshmen reported 4.5% of women and 0.4% of men). The course is chronic and intermittent over many years. The differential diagnosis must include schizophrenia, certain neurologic diseases such as central nervous system tumors, and epileptic equivalent seizures. A history of sexual assault is common. A recent survey of girls demonstrated that sexual assault survivors were three times more likely to binge and purge than girls who did not report a history of sexual abuse.

1. Eating disorder (not otherwise specified)—Between 3% and 5% of women between 15 and 30 have an unspecified eating disorder. They can have any of the complications that anorexics and bulimics have. They also need a complete evaluation to determine any precipitating causes or stressors along with a psychiatric consultation.

2. Binge eating disorder—Binge eating disorder (BED) is a new diagnosis that is characterized by rapid binge eating to the point of discomfort and self-disgust. It is identified in 3% of people in a community population, but up to 30% in obese patients in the weight-loss clinic population. Men are much more likely to have this condition than any other eating disorder.

For each of these conditions management and treatment begin with a very careful history of eating patterns, stressors, and screening for mental disorders, substance abuse and physical/sexual abuse. Behaviors to inquire about include binge eating and use of diuretics, laxatives, diet pills, and enemas. The next step is careful physical examination including a neurologic work-up, noting the state of hydration, teeth, salivary glands, and cardiac function. Minimal laboratory work should include plasma glucose, complete blood count, liver function tests, thyroid function, brain imaging (if needed), and an amenorrhea work-up if indicated. Hospitalization may be necessary for cardiac complications (heart failure, arrhythmia), severe electrolyte disturbances, seizures, gastrointestinal bleeding, and initiating feeding in severe anorexia. Psychological approaches are usually cognitive-behavioral therapy, group therapy, family counseling, and nutrition education. This requires continuity of care and a multidisciplinary approach. Drug treatment consists of antidepressants/antianxiety medications, anticonvulsants, and appetite suppressants.

Sleep Disorders

A national survey indicates that one-third of the U.S. population has some degree of sleep disturbance. Over the course of a woman's life she goes through different hormonal and physiologic phases that may affect sleep (ie, puberty, pregnancy, postpartum, menopause). Sleep disturbance is not only uncomfortable, but also associated with affective disorders. Complaints are frequently presented to gynecologists and may represent a minor problem or exist as part of a more serious physical or psychiatric disorder. Considerable diagnostic and treatment options are available.

Recent advances in the study of sleep have related sleep physiology and the stages of the sleep cycle. Stage 0 is wakefulness with closed eyes, high muscle tone, and some eye movement. Stages 1–4 are non-REM (rapid eye movement) sleep in humans and are characterized by specific encephalographic changes. REM, or "desynchronized," sleep is characterized by extreme hypotonia, rapid eye movements, blood pressure and heart rate variability, muscle twitches, and nocturnal penile tumescence. There is high dream recall if one awakens during REM sleep. Sleep cycles vary with age, sex, and numerous other influences. In an ordinary 8-hour period of sleep, a 25-year-old adult will go through 4–6 cycles, with the average cycle taking 90 minutes with REM 15-minute periods.

Sleep and arousal problems have been classified into 4 groups. (a) The insomnias are disorders of initiating and maintaining sleep. They are a heterogeneous group associated with organic and psychiatric conditions. A history of the sleep–wakefulness pattern helps with diagnosis. A disturbance in falling asleep may be caused by anxiety or worry. Staying asleep or early morning awakening is often seen in depressive illness. Myoclonus or central apnea can disturb sleep. (b) Disorders of excessive somnolence can be caused by narcolepsy, obstructive airway syndrome, depression, substance abuse, and other conditions. (c) Disorders of the sleep–wake schedule are those in which there is a misalignment between the individual's usual sleep–wake cycle and the internal circadian rhythms (eg, jet lag). (d) Parasomnias are a group of clinical conditions that happen during sleep, sleep stages, and partial arousals. Examples include somnambulism (sleep walking) and asthma (which may get worse during sleep). They are manifestations of atypical central nervous system activation during sleep with discharge into skeletal muscle or into channels of autonomic activity.

Women have fluctuations in the quality and quantity of sleep that associate with their life phases. For example, sleep disturbance is reported in 16–42% of premenopausal, 39–47% of perimenopausal, and 35–60% of postmenopausal women. Of women in the third trimester of pregnancy, 66–97% suffer from insomnia. Very little is known about how the changing hormone environment affects sleep. For example mood changes, fetal movement, raised body temperature (luteal phase), caring for a newborn at night, hot flashes, and the stress that can accompany life changes are some of the main causes of the sleep disorders. Subjective and objective measures of sleep correlate poorly, making it difficult to study sleep.

Treatment of sleep problems requires an accurate diagnosis. After ruling out medical problems that contribute to sleep disturbances behavior modification (sleep hygiene) should be the nest step in treatment. Sleep hygiene generally includes curtailing excess sleep; maintaining regular awake and bed times; regular exercise; maintaining a quiet sleep environment; avoiding hunger, caffeine, smoke, and alcohol. Relaxation techniques are also useful. Hypnotic drugs are among the most widely used drugs in the United States. The three most commonly used groups are the barbiturates, the benzodiazepines, and nonbarbiturate nonbenzodiazepines (eg, chloral hydrate, methaqualone). It is essential to be familiar with their pharmacology, action, potential for addiction or use for suicide, and teratogenicity before prescribing these drugs. Hormonal therapies have not been clearly shown to alleviate sleep disturbances. Insomnias that do not respond to treatment with relaxation techniques, sleep hygiene methods, and a short course of medication should be referred to a sleep specialist for diagnosis and treatment.

Premenstrual Syndrome and Premenstrual Dysphoric Disorder

Premenstrual syndrome and premenstrual dysphoric disorder are psychoneuroendocrine disorders that accompany the menstrual cycle. A complete discussion is found in Chapter 35.

PSYCHOLOGICAL ASPECTS OF GYNECOLOGIC SURGERY

Most people are afraid of the prospect of surgery. There are several sources of fear: the unknown, separation from family, forced dependency, and injury or death. It is not abnormal to have a recurrence of childhood fears. Patients often experience these as punishment or abandonment and may exhibit aggressive and controlling behaviors. Patients who have a clear understanding of why they are having surgery, the risks of surgery, appropriate expectations about outcome, motivation to be healthy, and a lack of psychiatric conditions cope best with the stress of the perioperative period.

Preoperative Preparation

Patients who are well prepared for surgery show less postoperative pain, use fewer pain medications, and have shorter hospital stays. Preparation means more than reassurance. It includes a careful description of the indications for surgery and an explanation of the preferred surgical approach. A clear preoperative discussion about patient preferences and concerns may prevent a great deal of anxiety, miscommunication, and dissatisfaction after the procedure.

It is ideal to review these topics while obtaining informed consent. Informed consent occurs when the patient agrees to certain procedures after a complete discussion with the physician delineating the risks, benefits, and alternatives to the procedures. The process of obtaining consent allows the patient to make an informed decision about whether she understands and accepts the medical implications of the surgery. When the physician and patient sign the document, it serves as a legal statement of the patient's permission to proceed. Answering all of the patient's questions is a necessary component of informed consent. Patients often have strong feelings about their preferred surgical approach; for example, where the incision should be made. Such issues should be

discussed and documented before the patient has received any sedating or antianxiety medications.

Because patients who are anxious do not assimilate information well, it is necessary to communicate effectively with the patient. Consideration of a patient's social context and personality type may help the physician navigate this communication successfully. It can be helpful to have a family member or friend assist the patient in asking questions and assimilating information. A representative of the professional staff or translation services (24-hour availability via telephone services) should be used for translation whenever possible. The physician cannot be sure that his or her words are being properly communicated by the patient's family or friends.

Postoperative Preparation

Patients need a clear explanation of their procedure and potential postoperative outcomes. They also need to know what to expect in the hospital and how to transition once home. Anticipatory guidance includes a brief orientation to hospital procedures, rehabilitation, medication instructions, follow-up arrangements, expectations about pain management and activity limitations. They should also understand how their body will change. For example, the possibility of hormone replacement after oophorectomy should be discussed preoperatively.

Hysterectomy: A Special Case

It is important to remember that hysterectomy has not been shown to cause psychopathology. New evidence actually suggests it improves quality of life in patients with appropriate indications for hysterectomy.

This being said, many women are afraid that removing their reproductive organs will divest them of their womanhood. For some this may be because they consider menstruation an important confirmation of their feminine identity. For others, the reproductive years represent sexuality and vitality. Of course cultural influences affect how one interprets the significance of hysterectomy. The prospect of having a hysterectomy may bring sadness to an infertile patient who held onto hope or to someone who places religious importance on childbearing. A woman who views the world from a more analytical or medical perspective may feel liberated after hysterectomy, knowing her symptoms will not return or that her risk of cancer has been lowered. A woman's adaptation to hysterectomy is related to her age, stage of development, personality, style of coping, ideas regarding fertility, sexuality, experiences with surgery, and the rapport she establishes with medical personnel.

Preoperatively, it is helpful to inquire about attitudes toward femininity, prior losses, attitudes and expectations about surgery, baseline sexual functioning, and past history of anxiety or depression. Patients at high risk for psychological difficulties after hysterectomy are those who seek surgery without a clear indication, suffer from chronic pelvic pain, have a psychiatric history, have conflicts over sexuality/childbearing, have inappropriate levels of preoperative anxiety, and who do not want surgery. Of course, surgery should be avoided unless a clear indication exists and the patient desires surgery. In the operating room, patients may perceive comments made despite being under anesthesia. Care should be taken when conversing in the operating room, even when the patient is thought to be unconscious.

Postoperatively the surgeon may note that a previously high-functioning patient has developed delirium. This is a transient form of encephalopathy that is characterized by an alteration in consciousness, disorientation, perceptual abnormalities, and agitation or withdrawal. An excess of pain medications and electrolyte imbalances can also create an altered mental state. Other postoperative syndromes include tremors, postoperative depression or psychosis, and excessive pain.

Sexual function is a common concern for patients undergoing gynecologic surgery. It is important to address concerns directly and to reassure patients that sexual function is minimally altered by hysterectomy. The best predictor of sexual functioning postoperatively is a patient's level of sexual functioning preoperatively. Patients who had bothersome pelvic symptoms before hysterectomy often have improved sexual functioning. Patients complaining of a worse sexual functioning after hysterectomy should be encouraged to consider other contributing factors, such as changes in relationship, body image, age, medications, libido, and stress.

Gynecologic Oncology

The improved prognosis for many cancers makes quality of life an increasingly important issue in the management of malignancy. The physician who cares for patients with gynecologic cancer needs to be familiar with the most current technical data, and must be able to respond to the patient with empathy and understanding at all stages of the illness. A multidisciplinary team of physicians, social workers, nurses, research coordinators, and counselors may be required at times along the course of disease. Sometimes the patient's family members also need counseling. Suffering should be minimized and a lower threshold for prescribing medications and work-release may be appropriate.

With the diagnosis there is often a grief response characterized by shock, disbelief, anger, and fears of death, pain, losing a body part, and abandonment. This can occur even when the malignancy is treatable. A discussion of the treatment plan should cover expected functional losses, side effects of treatment, and effects on sexual functioning. Psychiatric disorders that may occur in the course of malignant disease (eg, organic brain syndromes, depressive syndromes, and anxiety syndromes) need recognition and treatment. When the physician suspects a patient is not going to survive her cancer, she should be informed and allowed to make the necessary adjustments in her and her family's life.

SEXUALITY IN GYNECOLOGIC PRACTICE

The most available resource for the woman with sexual difficulties is her gynecologist or family physician. Thus, a sexual history is part of every gynecologic history. The gynecologist should be familiar with the sexual response cycle, taking a sexual history, the ability to make diagnoses of the most common sexual disorders, the effects of organic problems and drugs on sexuality, and the kind of sexual therapies that are available. Most sexual problems are managed by education, corrections of organic problems, and reassurance. More serious psychological problems should be managed by gynecologists with added training in sexual therapy. Certain common dimensions of sexual identity warrant discussion for those providing primary sexual counseling. Sexuality and reproduction are central to one's identity as a male or female, whether or not one wants children. The sexual identity can be described along three major dimensions: gender identity, sexual orientation, and sexual intention.

Gender identity is the earliest aspect of sexual identity to form. Core gender identity is the sense one has of being male or female. It develops in the second year of life and is the result of (a) biologic factors originating in fetal life and with the organization of the fetal brain; (b) sex assignment at birth by parents and medical staff; (c) parental attitudes; (d) conditioning and imprinting; and (e) development of body ego and body image, which comes in part from sensations from the genitals and other body parts. Masculinity and femininity are those behaviors that a person, parents, society, or the culture define as male or female. These may change from time to time. While many children show some evidence of gender confusion, 90% develop a core gender identity consistent with their biologic sex. **Gender role** is the sum of what one does that indicates to others the degree of maleness or femaleness. Gender identity continues to be influenced by identification with important adults as the child grows to adulthood.

Sexual orientation refers to the sex of the person in fantasy or reality that causes sexual arousal. Heterosexual individuals are sexually aroused by persons of the opposite sex, homosexual individuals by persons of the same sex, and bisexual individuals by persons of both sexes. There is increasing evidence of biologic contributions to sexual orientation, but further research is needed in this area.

Sexual intention refers to what a person wants to do with his or her sexual partner, eg, kissing, caressing, or intercourse. There are two dimensions: fantasy and real-life behavior. The usual intention is giving and receiving pleasure. Some examples of abnormal sexual intention related to aggression are sadism, exhibitionism, rape, and pedophilia.

The ability to function sexually in adulthood is formed at birth with the earliest parent–infant bonds. The loving care a person receives in infancy and childhood prepares him or her for intimate relationships in adult life.

Phases of the Sexual Response Cycle*

Stages in the sexual response cycle are described below. A more detailed description can be found in the classic work of Masters and Johnson, *Human Sexual Response.*

A. EXCITEMENT PHASE

In the woman, arousal in the excitement phase is associated with vaginal lubrication. This lubrication, previously thought to be of uterine or cervical origin, has been demonstrated by Masters and Johnson to be a "sweating reaction" of the vagina; it is probably a true transudation that continues throughout sexual excitement. Coalescence of droplets provides a lubricating film. Later in the response cycle, Bartholin's glands make a small contribution. The glans clitoridis swells, often to almost double its size, as a result of engorgement. The degree of enlargement is apparently unrelated either to the woman's capacity for sexual response or to her ability to achieve orgasm. The shaft of the clitoris also increases in diameter. Engorgement of the glans clitoridis and shaft occur most rapidly with direct manual stimulation of the glans clitoridis and the mons veneris.

Breast changes in the sexually aroused woman consist of nipple erection and, later in the excitement phase, an increase in total size of the breasts. The labia majora, which in a resting state meet in the midline of the vagina, gape slightly and may be displaced toward the clitoris. In nulliparous women, the outer labia may also thin out and flatten against the surrounding tissue. In multiparous women, they may extend and be engorged to an exaggerated degree. The labia minora also swell. The vagina, which is in a collapsed state normally, now begins to expand in the inner two-thirds of the vaginal canal, alternating with a tendency to relax. As excitement increases, progressive distention of the vagina occurs. The vaginal walls also "tent" in response to upward and backward posterior movement of the cervix and uterus, so that the inner portion of the vagina swells dramatically. Engorgement changes the color of the vaginal wall to dark purple and causes the vaginal rugae to become smooth.

In both men and women, erotic tension causes increased muscle tone accompanied by tachycardia and blood pressure elevation. A "sex flush" begins over the upper abdomen and later spreads over the breasts as a morbilliform rash; this occurs in approximately 75% of women and 25% of men before orgasm.

Early sexual arousal in the male, whether initiated by tactile, visual, or psychic stimuli, results in engorgement and erection of the penis and an increase in penile size and in the angle of protrusion from the body. In the late phase, the man experiences shortening of the spermatic cords and retraction of the testes. The scrotum thickens and is flattened against the body.

B. THE PLATEAU PHASE

The delineation between the excitement and the plateau phases is imprecise. Ordinarily, the penis is completely erect in the first phase. In the plateau phase, there is usually a slight increase in the diameter of the coronal ridge and, in some men, a deepening of color of the glans to reddish-purple. Progressive excitement may increase testicular size by approximately 50%; at this point, the man is very close to orgasm and approaches an inevitable stage. In the late plateau phase, respiratory rate, muscle tone, pulse rate, and blood pressure changes intensify, and muscle tension increases in the buttocks and anal sphincter. A few drops of fluid may appear in the male urethra from the bulbourethral (Cowper's) gland. Although this is not semen, it can contain large numbers of active sperm, which means that impregnation is possible before ejaculation.

In the woman, the "orgasmic platform" is formed by increased engorgement and swelling of the tissues of the outer third of the vagina, which reduces its interior diameter by 30–50%, tightening the grip on the penis and indicating that she is rapidly approaching orgasm. Elevation and ballooning of the inner two-thirds of the vagina increase, as does the size of the uterus (especially in multiparous women). The clitoris, now erect, rises from its position over the pubic bone, and retracts into its hood, shortening by approximately 50%. In this position, the clitoris continues to respond to either manual stimulation or penile thrusts. Engorgement of the labia continues until they take on a deep wine color, indicating that climax is imminent.

C. ORGASMIC PHASE

Orgasm consists of rhythmic contractions (1 per second) of pelvic musculature, uterine and vaginal contractions, and increased lubrication, all accompanied by pleasurable feelings. Because of the connection between brain and spinal cord centers for orgasm, learned inhibition can occur as with other reflexes. Orgasm is under voluntary control so there may be neural connections between the orgasm center and the voluntary motor perception areas of the brain. Occasionally, rhythmic contractions in the

---

*This section contributed by Ralph Benson.

anal sphincter occur. The reflex centers are close to those for bowel and bladder control, so that injuries to the lower cord may affect all three functions.

In the man, the rhythmic contractions stimulate a discharge in the perineal floor, particularly in the bulbocavernosus muscle. Just before orgasm, increasing tension in the seminal vesicles causes the semen to empty into the bulbous urethra. Simultaneously, the prostate begins to contract, expelling fluid and distending the bulbous portion of the urethra as semen and prostatic fluid mingle. A series of rhythmic contractions at the bulb now eject the semen. A series of minor contractions persists in the urethra for several seconds, continuing even after complete expulsion of the semen.

Changes in pulse rate, blood pressure, and respiratory rate reach a peak and quickly dissipate, but for both the man and the woman the height of orgasm is marked by generalized muscle tension. The facial muscles tighten, and the muscles of the neck, extremities, abdomen, and buttocks are strongly contracted. There may be grasping movements by both partners, followed by clutching and even carpopedal spasm. A fleeting period occurs in which each individual withdraws psychologically, concentrating almost solely on genital sensation.

D. RESOLUTION PHASE

Muscle tension is released and engorgement subsides in the genitals and skin. The "sexual flush" slowly fades and perspiration may occur. In some women, perspiration appears uniformly over the entire body, whereas men frequently perspire on the soles and palms. In either case, the amount of perspiration is unrelated to the degree of muscular effort expended before or during orgasm.

In the woman, the clitoris promptly returns to its unstimulated state but will not reach normal size for 5–10 minutes. Relaxation of the orgasmic platform then occurs, and the diameter of the outer third of the vagina increases. Vaginal ballooning diminishes, the uterus shrinks, and the cervix descends into its normal position. The slight enlargement of the cervical canal is maintained. Total resolution time varies; as much as 30 minutes may elapse before the woman is in a truly unstimulated state.

In men, loss of erection occurs in two stages: In the first, most of the erectile volume is lost; the second is a refractory stage during which he is unable to be aroused again, and the remainder of the shrinkage occurs. In young men, the refractory period may be very short, but it lengthens with age. In most men it will last for several minutes, in others it may last for hours, or even days. Women are generally capable of multiple orgasms.

Sexual History Taking

A sexual history should be part of every gynecologic examination. This history provides information that may relate to a patient's medical problem, identifies high-risk sexual practices, provides a opportunity to discuss contraception, gives insight into a patient's domestic situation, and provides a forum for the patient to bring up her personal concerns. Sexual dysfunction is very common, and patients usually appreciate suitable inquiry.

A physician's own anxiety may get in the way of adequate questioning. The sexual history belongs in the review of systems. Language should begin with biologic terms and then move to simpler terms. General questions precede more specific ones. The physician should maintain a positive, empathetic, and professional manner with a patient and ask questions in a logical sequence. The sexual history can cover (a) areas of the sexual response cycle: sexual desire, sexual arousal (erection in males, lubrication in females), orgasm, and satisfaction; (b) concerns about gender identity and sexual orientation; (c) classification of problems: onset, course, best and worst functioning, frequency of sexual behaviors, and relationship of sexual behaviors to other life circumstances (ie, relationships, losses, financial problems, illness, medication, surgery, family difficulties, infertility, and contraception).

Sexual history taking should include the following information:

1. Identifying data
   a. Patient: age, sex, number of pregnancies and marriages
   b. Parents and family
   c. Partner
   d. Children
2. Childhood sexuality
   a. Family and religious attitudes toward sex
   b. Sexual learning
   c. Childhood sexual activity
   d. Childhood sexual abuse or incest
3. Adolescence
   a. Preparation for menses
   b. Menarche
   c. Masturbation
   d. Consent to sexual activity
   e. Intercourse
   f. Gender issues
4. Adolescence and adulthood
   a. Sexual fantasies
   b. Sexual orientation (heterosexual, homosexual)
   c. Partner choice
   d. Sexual activity
   e. Sexual deviations
   f. Sexual orientation
   g. Sexual function and dysfunction
   h. Contraception
5. Recent life changes
   a. Losses
   b. Moves
   c. Pregnancy
   d. Other

Validated questionnaires and scales are available for screening and determining a patient's baseline and post-treatment level of functioning (eg, pain or sexual function).

Sexual Dysfunction

In the past, women had been so inhibited by their culture that some had lived through courtship, marriage, childbearing, and menopause without ever experiencing or feeling comfortable with sexual arousal, orgasm, or a sense of sexual freedom. Although more women are comfortable exploring their sexual side, sexual dysfunction does persist. Considerable advances in the knowledge of female sexuality have occurred in the past decade. The major contributions of researchers William Masters and Virginia Johnson to the physiology and psychology of sexuality are well recognized. Sexual dysfunction includes psychogenic and organic causes of decreased sexual desire, arousal, orgasm, and pain causing personal distress. Table 61–1 lists the most common types of female sexual dysfunction. When evaluating these patients, it is important to determine if the problem is lifelong or acquired; generalized or situational; and organic, psychogenic, mixed, or unknown. It is important to remember that many drugs contribute to sexual dysfunction, such as antihypertensives, gastrointestinal agents, chemotherapy, anticonvulsants, antipsychotic drugs, antidepressants, sedatives, anxiolytics, cannabis, alcohol, and heroin.

A. Inhibited Sexual Desire

This condition may be lifelong (primary) or occur after a period of normal functioning (secondary). Its presence

Table 61–1. Classification of female sexual dysfunctions.

Component	Symptom	Term
Desire	Decreased interest in sex	Inhibited sexual desire (ISD)
Excitement or arousal	Decreased lubrication	Excitement-phase dysfunction
Orgasm	No orgasm	Orgasmic dysfunction
Satisfaction	Decreased satisfaction	—
Other	Pain with intercourse	Dyspareunia
	Spasm of circum-vaginal musculature	Vaginismus
	Fear of sex; fear of penetration	Sexual phobias Sexual panic

All: Primary or seondary, situational or absolute.

does not necessarily imply a lack of ability to respond physiologically. Many women with primary inhibited sexual desire come from very sexually repressive backgrounds, have been sexually traumatized in childhood or adolescence, or have a poor partner relationship. They may avoid relationships in order to avoid sex. Treatment consists of behavioral and psychological methods. Secondary inhibited sexual desire often develops after problems with a partner, physical or emotional traumas, physical illnesses, drug or alcohol abuse, surgery, or psychological depression. A careful history will usually reveal recent life changes, losses, and medical or drug problems. Other contributions to difficulties in sexual desire come from concern about pregnancy, partners with very different sexual appetites, and changes in body image. A dramatic change in libido should be evaluated by a physician.

Sexual phobias occur in many women who then develop patterns of avoidance and are thought to have low desire. The thought of sex arouses panic and anxiety. There may be avoidance of any mention of sex and social isolation. Treatment consists of education, support, psychotherapy, medications, and behavioral desensitization.

B. Arousal Disorders

Arousal disorder represents an inability to achieve or maintain satisfactory sexual excitement. They are often caused by vasomotor phenomena or inadequate lubrication. Nitric oxide contributes to the engorgement of the genitals and many medical and herbal therapies aim to increase local production of nitric oxide. Any process that contributes to small vessel disease or neuropathy also impedes the arousal response.

C. Orgasmic Disorder

Orgasmic problems are very common. Approximately 8–10% of adult women in the United States have never been orgasmic; another 10% may achieve orgasm with fantasy alone. Most women fall somewhere in between these two extremes, demonstrating a variety of responses. Women with primary orgasmic problems have never experienced orgasm in any situation, even after prolonged and effective sexual stimulation. Those with secondary orgasmic problems have had periods of normal functioning. In both primary and secondary cases, the women may lubricate easily, enjoy lovemaking, and feel satisfaction. Somehow, they get "stuck" in the plateau phase of the sexual-response cycle. Some women are not sure if they have reached orgasm; others regularly "fake" orgasm in order to please their partner or live out their own fantasies. A number of women are orgasmic with clitoral stimulation but not during intercourse; this is a normal variant. For others, the presence of the penis or other erotic stimulus is necessary for orgasm.

There are innumerable orgasmic variations. Theories that labeled vaginal orgasms mature and clitoral orgasms immature have been laid to rest. The goal of any treatment is to help the individual achieve her first orgasm, often without a partner present. Although most women are physiologically capable of having an orgasm, the focus that our culture places on the achievement of orgasm may actually inhibit a woman's ability to reach orgasm. Pressure may also come from partners who insist that a woman's lack of orgasm is because of her partner's failure.

Treatment is aimed at enhancing sensory stimulation and extinguishing the woman's involuntary inhibitions. The therapist's first task is to make certain that the woman understands that sufficient clitoral stimulation is required and is able to communicate her needs to her partner. She needs to know that it is normal to be sexual. Sometimes these educational techniques alone are enough to overcome the problem. Barbach's book *For Yourself* has been very helpful to many women.

A woman with primary orgasmic dysfunction needs to learn what it feels like to have an orgasm. She may have to disregard her obsessive thoughts and distractions and focus on the erotic thoughts and premonitory feelings that directly precede orgasm. The use of fantasy can be very helpful. Women with very religious backgrounds may find the idea of erotic fantasy (ie, thinking of other partners and being overcome by a loving partner) more guilt-provoking than sex itself. Self-stimulation is often recommended as a means of learning what feels good and helps the woman become sexually aroused. The long-standing prohibition against masturbation in her value system may be difficult to overcome. She may prefer to masturbate in private, rather than with a partner. Some women have marked success with a vibrator, at first alone and then possibly with the partner. In addition to mastering the physical aspects of achieving orgasm, women need to address their fears. Many patients find it helpful to join a women's discussion group. Besides discussing educational issues, members are assigned specific sexual tasks to do at home alone. Tasks are performed in privacy and responses are later shared with the group members. They may also be able to share fantasies and give one another support.

Transferring orgasmic achievement to a partner situation is the final step in most treatment situations. Heterosexual women are encouraged to heighten arousal before penetration. They learn the clitoris may be stimulated by indirect friction of the hood being pulled back and forth over this organ, eg, during penile thrusting. Each woman needs to learn the most effective means of increasing her own pleasure, eg, active thrusting and use of pelvic and thigh musculature, avoidance of distracting thoughts, and free use of erotic and exciting fantasies. When there is a beloved, trusted partner, the prognosis is good.

D. DYSPAREUNIA

Pain during sexual intercourse can be especially distressing. After the pain has subsided the memory of pain

Table 61–2. Some physical reasons for dyspareunia.

Vaginal opening
    Hymen—rare
    Tender episiotomy scar
    Aging—with decreased elasticity
    Labia—Bartholin's gland abscess
    Other lesions
Clitoris
    Irritation
    Infections
Vagina
    Infections
    Sensitivity reactions
    Atrophic reactions
    Decreased lubrication
Uterus, uterine tubes, ovaries
    Endometriosis
    Pelvic inflammatory disease
    Ectopic pregnancy
Numerous others

may persist and interfere with pleasure. Some women with no background of trauma or major inhibitions may assume that sex will be painful because they associate menstruation and childbirth with pain. Inadequate lubrication (45% of women) is one of the main sources of dyspareunia. Low estrogen states, such as the postpartum and menopausal stages, is often to blame. Luckily, estrogen replacement (transdermal, oral, vaginal) is usually very helpful. A careful history and physical examination are essential. Table 61–2 lists the physical reasons for dyspareunia. Management consists of treating the specific problem.

E. VAGINISMUS

Vaginismus is the painful, involuntary reflex spasm of the pubococcygeal muscles that occurs in anticipation of vaginal penetration. It occurs most often in young women. Some patients may have been subjected to rape or incest as children or adults. Severe pain secondary to trauma, surgical procedures, or medical disorders in the vaginal area may sometimes cause the problem. Insufficient lubrication from lack of arousal or sexual phobias may also cause pain with intercourse and vaginismus.

Vaginismus must be diagnosed by history and physical examination. Gynecologists often institute a program of gradual vaginal dilatation using dilators or the patient or her partner's finger. Not all women will respond to this prescription. Some may have more serious problems that require psychotherapy. It is not unusual for a woman who has overcome her difficulty to find that her partner has developed erectile problems. This

Table 61–3. Classification of male sexual dysfunctions.

Component	Symptom	Term
Desire	Decreased interest in sex	Inhibited sexual desire (ISD)
Arousal of excitement	Difficulty with erection	"Impotence," erectile difficulty
Orgasm	No ejaculation No emission	Premature ejaculation, inhibited orgasm, retrograde ejaculation
Satisfaction	Decreased satisfaction	—

All: primary or secondary, situational or absolute.

finding supports the belief that sexual problems are rarely limited to one partner.

Male Sexual Dysfunction

The term **impotence** used to refer to most male performance problems. Today, the word has an imprecise meaning as there has been a great increase in knowledge about sexual dysfunction and classification based on the physiology of the sexual response cycle (Table 61–3). The term impotence usually refers to erectile problems or the inability to sustain an erection for the time necessary for a desired sexual act. Erectile problems are common and increase with age.

Male sexual dysfunctions have been classified on the basis of an understanding of the sexual response cycle. The classification includes (a) problems of desire—diminished or excessive; (b) problems with arousal, ie, erectile difficulties; and (c) problems with orgasm—premature ejaculation, inhibited orgasm, or retrograde ejaculation. These conditions may be caused by psychogenic, organic, or mixed psychogenic and organic factors. Performance anxiety leads to "spectatoring" in which a person becomes preoccupied in watching his or her own sexual responses. They may be primary (present all of one's life) or secondary (having developed after a period of normal functioning). The history should focus on the stage of life of the man, the quality of his sexual desire, the role of his partner, and significance of early and past life experiences. Organic contributions are more common than was previously thought and are related to illness, surgery, medication, drugs, alcohol, vascular disorders, and neuropathies.

Psychological causes include performance anxiety, fear of women and intimacy, relationship problems, and depression or other mental illnesses. The purely psychogenic dysfunctions show more variability in erectile responses and are associated with normal nocturnal tumescence studies. An evaluation by a urologist knowledgeable about sexual function is often indicated.

Treatment is based on etiology. Organic causes need treatment if possible. The psychogenic forms of dysfunction are best managed by behavioral treatment approaches. Partners are seen together and their relationship helped with improved communication as well as special techniques for specific problems.

Sexual Activity with Aging

Generally, the sexual response diminishes with age. Older women may have less sexual desire, with fewer sexual fantasies and a slower and lessened lubrication response to arousal. The vaginal walls are thinner and less pliable. Orgasm may be less intense, with weaker muscle contractions, and may be uncomfortable. Atrophic skin changes and altered peripheral nerve endings may diminish sensory perceptions. The gynecologist can help the aging couple by educating them about normal changes and alternative techniques. Estrogen and progesterone replacement (when indicated) may diminish vaginal discomfort. Estrogen and testosterone therapy may increase a woman's libido.

Men show decreased sexual activity with aging. By age 60 years men have about 1 erection a week. Sexual desire may diminish and erections take longer, require more stimulation, and are less firm. Ejaculation takes longer, with the feeling of ejaculatory inevitability less pronounced. There is less ejaculate, and the refractory period is longer.

Despite these normal changes with aging, the capacity for sexual activity and enjoyment persists. Many couples, freed from the worries of pregnancy, feel more able than ever to have the pleasure of an active sex life. Noncoital sexual activity may be a very satisfying form of intimacy and pleasure for some couples. However, 30–78% of 60-year-olds are sexually active. Never make an assumption regarding a patient's sexual activity.

■ PSYCHOLOGICAL ASPECTS OF OBSTETRICS

A woman's psychology cannot be understood without considering the stage she is in the course of her reproductive life. Pregnancy affects nearly all aspects of her life. Her body, family, relationships, job, financial status, and life plans are all impacted by pregnancy. Changes in our modern social structure also influence psychological aspects of pregnancy. Many women now work outside the home, are single or divorced, or are having first babies in the teenage years or after age 35 years. Women have more knowledge about their bodies, and most want to participate in important decisions regarding fertility, pregnancy, delivery, and infant care. Many men want a greater part in sharing their partner's pregnancy. Finally, the legal climate has greatly affected medical practice. These alterations significantly influence the practice of obstetrics and gynecology. Indeed, the clinician is faced with new challenges and stresses in caring for women from diverse ethnic, economic, and social backgrounds.

Good obstetric and gynecologic care requires the consideration of each woman as an individual. To establish an effective working alliance with women who seek treatment, the clinician must not only be knowledgeable in medicine but also be a good observer and an able communicator. With a biopsychosocial approach, the clinician sees a person and not a disease. Objectivity, compassion, and a nonbiased approach are essential principles that foster appropriate care. Often a multidisciplinary approach is useful in evaluating and managing patients when psychological issues are intertwined with their medical problems. This involves employing physicians along with nurses, social workers, and psychiatrists or psychologists in the process of evaluation and treatment.

This section presents an overview of the important normal and abnormal psychological aspects of pregnancy and the puerperium, and describes some of the syndromes and clinical situations that tend to affect female patients. It is important to remember that many women only see physicians during their pregnancies. They may lack insurance, time, or interest, and may not seek medical care outside of pregnancy. Every effort should be made to screen for medical, social, and psychiatric problems that need attention after pregnancy.

MOTIVATIONS FOR PREGNANCY

Pregnancy may be a welcomed and fulfilling experience for many women, but not for all. Motivations for pregnancy are varied and complex, and only some of them are conscious. The desire for a pregnancy is not always the same as the wish for a child. For example, a pregnancy may be wanted to confirm one's sexual identity or to give proof of one's reproductive integrity and capability. Desire for a pregnancy may also be a response to loss or feelings of loneliness. A woman may have a child so that she will always have someone to love who will love her in return. She may wish to preserve a relationship with a partner or she may be responding to family or cultural pressures to have a baby. In adolescents, peer pressure, rebellion against family, and feelings of depression are frequent motivations for pregnancy. Toward the end of their reproductive years, women may feel pressured to

conceive before their personal and professional lives are ready to incorporate a child. Many of these feelings also exist in men. In some cultures, children represent immortality for parents, and it is natural as they grow older for many people to hope that some part of them will live on in future generations. Regardless of the multifactorial forces that play a role in women's reproductive choices, many women face similar stresses as the stages of pregnancy unfold.

Pregnancy as a Developmental Transition

Pregnancy is a major developmental step in the lives of women, often providing fulfillment of deep and powerful wishes that allow creativity, self-realization, and an opportunity for new growth. Although pregnancy may bring a sense of joy and well-being, it is also a stressful experience. Conflicts may arise. How a woman responds to pregnancy is related to her early childhood experiences, coping mechanisms, personality style, life situation, emotional supports, and physical problems.

The father-to-be is also presented with challenges and conflicts. Men may have unusual symptoms during their partner's pregnancy and visit physicians more often with complaints reflecting their own anxieties and concerns about their new role. Infidelity often manifests when the female partner is pregnant. Men may envy their partner's new condition, have conflicts with sexuality and pregnancy, or may feel threatened by the baby's potential to replace them as the mother's focus of attention.

Although prenatal classes, friendships, and office visits are useful ways for patients to learn about the process of pregnancy and alleviate fears, professional consultation may be necessary. With a full understanding of the psychological aspects of pregnancy, an insightful physician will be able to identify these issues and help a patient navigate though this developmental stage.

Normal Psychological Processes during Pregnancy and the Puerperium

The basic developmental and psychological tasks of pregnancy vary with the stage of pregnancy. During the first trimester, a woman tends to incorporate the fetus as an integral part of her body and self. Ultrasonography has led to earlier maternal and paternal bonding. In the second trimester, with recognition of fetal movement, it is necessary to perceive the fetus as a separate entity and to begin to visualize the fetus as a baby with needs of its own. In the third trimester and postpartum, the patient comes to see herself as a mother and begins to establish a nurturing relationship with the infant. She may have to resolve some lingering conflicts with her own parents. Her relationship with her partner may also change for better or worse.

A. FIRST TRIMESTER

The diagnosis of a wanted pregnancy is usually accompanied by a sense of excitement and anxiety. Even the most wanted pregnancy may cause ambivalence on the part of both parents because of the recognized major life transition. An unplanned pregnancy is not necessarily unwanted and may be readily accepted. However, the woman and her partner need time to process their feelings and thoughts. If a termination is being considered, counseling should begin as soon as possible and without ambivalence on the part of the professional staff. Such counseling should allow the woman, and her partner if possible, to understand the implications of each of their possible choices and to weigh the risks, benefits, and alternatives before making a decision. If a physician is unable to provide an unbiased approach to counseling, the patient should be referred for appropriate counseling.

The first trimester, with its attendant fatigue, breast tenderness, nausea, and urinary frequency, is often accompanied by an increased preoccupation with self and with the growth of the fetus. There may be a sense of fulfillment and well-being, but emotions may be labile. Sexual interest may decline, while a desire for affection may increase. Concern about weight gain may manifest. Apprehension concerning miscarriage, the baby's health, and changing roles is common. Interestingly, even the most educated individuals may harbor superstitious beliefs that serve to help patients understand or feel control over the process of pregnancy.

B. SECOND TRIMESTER

During the second trimester, there is an increased sense of well-being and the resumption of outside interests. Fetal movement, commencing at approximately 16–18 weeks, often results in a greater sense of reality about the pregnancy. The fetus is perceived as a separate entity, and the parents fantasize about how the baby will look. The mother may experience increased feelings of dependency; sexual desire varies greatly, and changes in body image may be distressing.

C. THIRD TRIMESTER

During the latter part of pregnancy, fear or anxiety about labor and delivery may increase. Concerns arise about pain, injury, and the baby's health; about being a responsive mother; and about how relationships may be changed. Sleep is often disturbed, and somatic preoccupations may increase.

Childbirth education is invaluable. Ideally, the woman will be in a setting where she and her partner feel free to ask questions, regardless of how inconsequential she may think they are. Questions to the mother-to-be should be open-ended, not "yes" or "no"

questions. For example, "What worries or concerns are you having?" is far more likely to evoke a meaningful response than "Is everything going well?" In high-risk pregnancies, a patient should have realistic expectations about her options and their implications before entering the labor and delivery floor.

There is an increasingly high parental expectation that modern obstetric technology will prevent anything untoward from disrupting their expectation of a positive birth experience. Because patients think of childbirth as a natural process, patients often have a limited understanding of the inherent dangers involved. For these reasons it is essential to obtain informed consent before performing procedures. Obtaining informed consent not only offers an opportunity for physicians to explain all of the risks, benefits, and alternatives to procedures, but it also allows patients to discuss their concerns and make their preferences clear. It is important to respect a patient's wishes and incorporate her desired approach whenever possible. Good communication is essential for an informed exchange. Patience in listening is an invaluable aid to lessening patient anxiety and fear and improving the chance of successful communication.

D. LABOR AND DELIVERY

Each woman has a different experience on labor and delivery. The professional support team's goals are to enhance the health and safety of mother and infant while fostering a fulfilling experience. The emphasis today is on active family involvement in the birth experience. Women differ in their interest in obtaining medical information and even in making decisions about labor or pain management. Fear and unfamiliarity can increase tension and pain. Generally, fear can be minimized by educating patients about what to expect. Childbirth education classes, relaxation techniques, knowledge of both usual and unusual obstetric procedures, and familiarity with hospital facilities and delivery rooms can alleviate some fear. Some difficulties arise when a woman does not fulfill her own expectations concerning birth options and delivery methods. For example, she may feel like a failure if she requires anesthesia or surgical intervention during labor and delivery. Prospective discussion of these issues may prevent the patient from placing value judgments on treatment options. It is essential to remind patients that the ultimate goal is having a healthy baby and a healthy mother.

The presence during the labor of the partner, a close friend, or a family member offers invaluable support to the mother. Even having a doula (professional labor coach) improves a woman's birth experience and is associated with decreased epidural use. It is important to remember that each person has a different pain tolerance level. The perception of pain can be influenced by fear, past experiences, personality, style of expression, and cultural factors. The reassuring presence of a labor companion and childbirth preparation classes can help the mother handle the pain of labor and delivery.

The patient's attitude during pregnancy may *not* be a good predictor of her emotional state in labor. Some women report that the loss of unity (the "oneness" with the child) is a stressor that saddens them. Fears exist about death, bodily injury, loss of adequacy or control, and, especially, about exposing bodily functions. Other women feel the pressure of the importance of their labor for their family. Often family members insist on being present at the delivery and are convinced that the patient is comforted by their presence. This may not be the case. Care givers should ask the patient if she prefers privacy in labor. It is appropriate for the medical professional to request that guests vacate the labor room, as the patient is often uncomfortable doing so.

Although the safety of mother and infant must be the first concern, hospitals should strive to provide a more homelike and less institutional atmosphere for the birthing experience. The number of home births in the United States remains low. The major concern is that there may be complications that require hospital-level care. One-third of infants requiring immediate intensive care after home deliveries have been products of normal pregnancies. Electronic fetal monitoring during labor is now commonly employed. Some patients find this practice intrusive, whereas others find it reassuring. Women who have experienced prior fetal loss are more accepting of its presence and find it reduces their anxiety. However, highly technical equipment does not eliminate the possibility of complications, nor is it a replacement for human skill. Patients may need to be reminded that though birth is a beautiful process, it can be a dangerous process.

E. Puerperium

Attachment between mother and infant begins long before birth. The term **bonding** refers to a sensitive period after birth, during which interactions between mother and infant facilitate a powerful connection. The attachment direction is from mother to infant, making her a more effective parent. Early visual and physical contact between mother and baby facilitates the attachment. Attachment behaviors include fondling, kissing, cuddling, breastfeeding, and gazing—practices that maintain contact between mother and infant. Factors that can interfere with early bonding include lack of instinctual response, psychological problems, inadequate preparation, unrealistic scheduling, physical illness in mother or baby, and hospital practices that separate mother and infant. To facilitate early bonding, sedation and separation should be minimal. Separation may have physical, biologic, and emotional consequences. However, a mother should not believe she will be a failure because something has interfered with her earliest contact with her infant. There is evidence that later bonding is also successful.

Bonding is especially important for women and infants who may have attachment problems. Some of these high-risk individuals are mothers who are very young, ill, or ambivalent about pregnancy, or who have suffered child abuse, have relational difficulties with their partner, or have a psychiatric disorder. Intervention includes recognition of the problem and referral to an appropriately trained mental health professional or support services.

The father's presence in the labor and delivery room contributes to earlier father–infant bonding, but fathers must be prepared for attending the delivery and should have a role in it (eg, coaching the mother's efforts). Whether the father will be present when complications occur or when operative delivery is required should be discussed in advance.

F. Transition to Motherhood

Mothering has instinctual roots, but it is largely a learned behavior. A mother's early experiences with a loving caregiver in her own infancy strengthen her capacity for mothering. Mothers of young infants in our culture are often isolated from family and friends, which makes the early days even more difficult. During this stressful time, the new mother needs supportive individuals in her environment. It is helpful if the professional staff knows about unusual home circumstances. Indeed, an evaluation of this environment should be part of discharge planning. Will this new mother be alone or with numerous relatives? Are there religious or cultural practices that will interfere with sexuality, reproduction, nursing, or motherhood? Will this woman be returning to work? If so, when? Finally, have her personality and coping ability undergone abrupt changes?

Breastfeeding has many advantages, but once a woman decides to bottle-feed her decision should be supported.

It is helpful for a woman to review her labor and delivery experience with her physician. She just completed one of life's greatest challenges and may need a forum to process her feelings. Such communication may be encouraged by asking the woman, "How do you feel about your labor and delivery?" Often patients have expectations for the perfect labor and may not realize that some procedures are normal. Clarification can put a patient at ease.

Sources of Stress in Pregnancy and the Puerperium

Endocrinal, psychological, and body changes contribute to making pregnancy and the puerperium times of stress. The confirmation of pregnancy may be thrilling for some but devastating for others. Indeed, some degree of ambivalence is probably the usual response. Anticipatory guidance can assist the new mother in navigating the coming challenges.

Women with preexisting health problems may be concerned about withstanding the physical demands. Most healthy women have some physical distress from the discomforts of abdominal enlargement, nausea, heartburn, musculoskeletal pain, and urinary frequency. Most women also experience psychological distress from worries about body image, genetic problems, and role changes, as well as the effect of the pregnancy on her partner, career, education plans, finances, or her ability to be a mother. A worry often not voiced, especially by a primigravida, is "Can I do this?"

Interpersonal relationships with the patient's partner, mother, coworkers, and friends change during and after the pregnancy. Her partner's sexual satisfaction may decline during pregnancy. Women who are sexually responsive are more likely to enjoy sex during pregnancy. Pregnancy is a public statement of a woman's sexual activity, which may be a source of pride or embarrassment.

Although anxiety, emotional lability, and worries are normal during this time, the ability to cope depends on each woman's life experiences, personality style, social supports, and the care and technical expertise of the obstetric staff.

A. Denial of Pregnancy

Good prenatal care improves pregnancy outcome. Early recognition of pregnancy by a woman and her family leads her to seek prenatal health care, take extra care of herself, eat well, and get sufficient rest. Denial of pregnancy may interfere with the patient obtaining proper care. The woman most prone to denial of pregnancy may be psychotic, have borderline personality, or be from an extremely rigid background. The denial is usually an unconscious process in which the individual keeps the unpleasant reality of an unwanted pregnancy out of her awareness. She is often joined in this negativity by family and, on rare occasions, by physicians. She may go through an entire pregnancy forgetting missed periods, and unaware of breast changes, abdominal enlargement, or fetal movements. She may present in the emergency room in labor or deliver the infant at home. With the birth, a psychotic reaction may occur. These neonates are at higher risk for injury or death. Obviously, these women need extra support in the postnatal period and, if identified during the course of pregnancy, may benefit from psychological assistance.

B. Sexuality

There are many variations in sexual functioning during pregnancy and the puerperium. In general, women note a decrease of sexual interest during the first trimester,

which is related to fatigue, nausea, and a feeling of turning inward. Women without a history of miscarriage, genital bleeding, or dyspareunia need not fear that intercourse will harm the fetus. In the second trimester there is often an increased interest and desire for sexual activity. Many women have an increased wish to be held or to masturbate. Some become orgasmic for the first time, possibly because of increased pelvic vasocongestion.

In the third trimester, sexual interest and performance are even more variable. The woman may feel awkward and have increased fears of harming the fetus. If there are no obstetric complications or physical discomfort, intercourse is not contraindicated; there is no evidence that intercourse precipitates premature labor, although orgasm does cause uterine contractions. Some men lose their sexual interest during their partner's pregnancy, or they fear harming the fetus. Noncoital techniques can be satisfying to the couple. Couples should be told that oral–genital sex must not include air blown into the vagina as this practice may cause an air embolism, which is potentially fatal to mother and fetus.

Sexual desire postpartum may not return for many weeks or months. This may be a consequence of new interest in the baby, fatigue, depression, hormonal status, pain, or concerns about body image. Breastfeeding may alter sexual feelings in the new mother or her partner. Fathers may feel excluded. The obstetrician can be helpful to a couple by discussing changes in sexuality with them.

C. Vomiting in Pregnancy

Vomiting in pregnancy can have several causes: the same as those seen in the nonpregnant state (eg, viral, dietary, drug reactions); hormonal changes in the first trimester (which affect approximately 80% of pregnant women); preeclampsia, liver disease, or other obstetric complication; or hyperemesis gravidarum (pernicious vomiting of pregnancy).

Hyperemesis gravidarum is a severe form of nausea that may occur at any time during pregnancy. The woman may become severely dehydrated, lose weight, and have metabolic disturbances and electrolyte imbalances. The incidence in the United States is 1 in 1000 pregnancies. Biologic, psychological, and social etiologies have been suggested for hyperemesis gravidarum. Disturbances in the endocrine, metabolic, or immune system likely play a role. There is some support for an association with multiple birth and past pregnancy loss. Treatment may require rehydration, hospitalization, and correction of electrolyte imbalance. Antiemetics are the most effective treatment. In fact, hyperemesis gravidarum is one of the only approved indications for droperidol. Ginger, steroids, antihistamines, vitamin B_6 (pyridoxine), and acupuncture may be helpful. It is important to review the teratogen risk before prescribing medications in pregnancy.

At times this condition may represent a somatization disorder in which dysphoric feelings or psychic conflicts are expressed via physical symptoms. There is often a history of early life experience colored by abdominal pain and nausea. The condition is not related to any one psychiatric diagnosis, although more severe psychiatric illness may be present. Social stress may contribute to its severity. Many practitioners believe that the most effective aspect of hospitalization is actually isolating the patient from the stressors of her life at home. A good response has been noted with hypnosis and relaxation techniques. Identification of stress in the individual's life and help with stress reduction are often useful.

D. SLEEP IN PREGNANCY AND THE PUERPERIUM

Sleep disturbances during pregnancy and the puerperium are common. There is often increased sleepiness in the early prepartum period associated with high levels of estrogen and progesterone. In the postpartum period, a demanding infant together with decreased ovarian hormone levels may lead to sleep deficiency. During pregnancy and the puerperium, sleep latency, the frequency of awakening, and stage 0 sleep are increased; REM sleep is decreased. Hormonal fluctuations are related to sleep pattern changes. Medication should be used cautiously. Developing a routine for baby and mom is useful. Often the patient's partner needs education as well. Family meetings may be necessary for both parents to fully understand the impact of the patient's inadequate sleep on the family and to develop a schedule.

ADOLESCENT PREGNANCY: PSYCHOLOGICAL ISSUES

Approximately 1 million adolescents 15–19 years old (10% of all women in this age range in the United States) become pregnant each year. Half of them will give birth. This high teenage pregnancy rate is a result of many factors, including a subculture in which there is glorification of sexual activity without education of young people regarding its consequences. Other motivations for pregnancy in adolescence may be related to peer pressure, rebellion, keeping a relationship, and desiring more emotional intimacy. Unfortunately, teen pregnancy is associated with many bad outcomes. These include premature birth, infant homicide, domestic violence, substance abuse, low maternal educational achievement, low socioeconomic status, and maternal depression. Interestingly, the teen pregnancy rate has declined over the last 50 years (89.1/1000 vs. 45.9/1000 in 1960 vs. 2001). This trend is seen across age groups and races. As a result, the abortion rate has also dropped. Access to birth control appears to be the most important factor.

Half of all teen pregnancies are conceived within 6 months of first intercourse. Because the average delay between intercourse and initiation of contraception is 6–18 months, contraception counseling is essential whenever caring for a teen. Psychological traits associated with contraceptive use in adolescents are high self-esteem, an orientation toward the future, feelings of control over life, and acceptance of the sexual self.

Three psychological subsets of adolescent mothers have been described. "Problem-prone" adolescents are those who use alcohol or drugs, are truant from school, and get poor grades. They act on impulse and are often part of a peer counterculture that rejects conventional values. The adequate copers are those who are competent and open to alternative lifestyles but characteristically go through life transitions at an earlier age than their peers. The depressed or lonely adolescents are those who idealize pregnancy as a way of dealing with their feelings of loss, sadness, and emptiness. It is useful to distinguish among these three groups and to offer assistance in response to their various needs.

Adolescents often strain the patience of health care personnel because they may be difficult to talk with, have values very different from those of the staff, arrive late for prenatal care, or be noncompliant. If the physician understands adolescent development and sexuality well, adolescent care can be extremely gratifying. The importance of taking a responsible approach to prenatal care should be stressed. Counseling adolescents requires an ability to educate and communicate with them while offering privacy and confidentiality. Many states consider a pregnant adolescent to be an emancipated minor. It is important for practitioners to be familiar with the laws in their state.

PSYCHIATRIC DISORDERS OF PREGNANCY AND THE PUERPERIUM

Pregnancy and the puerperium are emotionally stressful periods for many women. Mood swings are commonly manifested by emotional lability, weepiness, irritability, and feeling blue or high. Prenatal assessment for psychological difficulties should include the following:

(1) Prior personal or family history of psychiatric illness.
(2) Psychiatric disorder.
(3) Psychological problems that accompanied maturational periods, eg, puberty.
(4) History of early maternal deprivation or mother's death.
(5) Difficulty separating from parents.
(6) Conflicts about mothering.
(7) Marital or family difficulties, including separation.

(8) Past difficulty with pregnancy, delivery, or post-partum depression.

(9) Recent death of family member or close friend.

(10) Familial or congenital disorders.

(11) History of infertility.

(12) History of repeat abortion.

(13) History of pseudocyesis or hyperemesis.

(14) Prior fetal death, miscarriage, or congenital abnormality.

(15) History of sexual, physical, or emotional abuse, current or past.

(16) History of premenstrual syndrome.

Psychiatric disorders during pregnancy and in the puerperium have been described throughout history, although there is disagreement as to whether these disorders are the same or different from those occurring at other times. Because untreated maternal mental illness is associated with deleterious effects on maternal–infant attachment and synchrony in child development, it is essential to diagnose and appropriately treat psychological disorders. Although some psychotropic medications appear to be safe when used in breastfeeding mothers, few randomized controlled trials have been performed. For this reason, it is important to involve a pediatrician in the infant's care when treating a breastfeeding mother with psychotropic medications.

Depressive Disorders

Depressive symptoms are part of human experience and relate to sadness, frustration, discouragement, and feeling "down." Many women experience such moods in the weeks following delivery. The **symptom** can be related to another illness such as alcoholism, pain, or a worsening medical condition. A **syndrome,** such as major depression, is characterized by a specific set of mood symptoms that persists and is severe enough to interfere with activities of daily living. A wide range of mood changes occur during the postpartum period. The severity can vary considerably from a transient period of feeling blue to major clinical depression with thoughts of infanticide.

A. POSTPARTUM BLUES

This condition (also called 3-day blues or baby blues) is a transitory mood disturbance following delivery (within 2 weeks) and usually occurs at the height of hormonal changes. It is frequent, occurring in approximately 50–85% of women. It is characterized by irritability, feeling trapped, sensitivity to criticism, despondence, anxiety, sadness, anger, guilt, or elation. It is unrelated to the health of mother or baby, obstetric complications, hospitalization, social class, or breast-feeding. However, any of these factors can affect the patient's mood. It occurs cross-culturally, but is less noticeable in cultures where emotions are expressed freely and when relatives and friends surround the new mother, offering care and support. It may last a few days to 2–3 weeks. Although it is generally self-limited, 20% of women who suffer from this disorder will go on to develop depression in the first postpartum year. Treatment consists of support from family, health care providers, and other mothers.

B. MAJOR DEPRESSION

Major depression is a depressive syndrome (without psychosis) that can occur during pregnancy or the postpartum period. It is estimated that this syndrome develops at the following rates during each phase of pregnancy: 7.4% first trimester, 12.8% second trimester, 12.0% third trimester, 10–20% postpartum. Its symptoms include change in mood, sleep patterns, eating, mental concentration, and libido, and may involve somatic preoccupations, phobias, and fear of harming self or infant. Diagnosis is best made through standardized self-report or physician screens. The syndrome is profoundly under diagnosed (< 15%) and often left untreated. Postpartum depression is likely to go undiagnosed because the syndrome develops weeks to months after delivery when the patient is not under the routine medical care.

Clear risk factors for pregnancy-associated depression include a history of depression, a family history of depression, prior pregnancy-associated depression. Precipitating factors such as ambivalence about pregnancy, marital problems, financial problems, and limited social support may contribute. Postpartum depression has a high rate of recurrence in subsequent pregnancies. Treatment may include psychotherapy, antidepressant medication, support groups, and the involvement services that take some of the child care burden off of the patient. Suicidal or homicidal patients should be immediately referred to a mental health professional. Of course they should not be left alone. Hospitalization may be necessary.

Initiating a conversation regarding a patient's depressive symptoms may be difficult. It may be useful to start by acknowledging that the transition to motherhood is difficult for most parents. Next the physician should ask more specific questions, aimed at screening for depression. To elicit suicidal or homicidal ideas, the physician might ask "Have you felt so overwhelmed or that you might hurt yourself or your baby?" Patients tend to view parenting as a process that should come naturally. They often underestimate the challenges and pressure that accompanies a new baby. They should be reminded that they are under more stress than they realize and that it is acceptable to ask for help. The mother of today generally has more responsibility than raising children. Many balance careers and/or single parent. Often simply redistributing child care responsibilities or adjusting the patients work responsibilities can relieve tremendous pressure.

Postpartum Psychoses

A woman is more likely to suffer from new-onset psychosis during the postpartum period than during any other time of her life. Interestingly, the antenatal period is not associated with increased risk of psychosis. Psychosis is a severe mental illness characterized by a false reality and can be associated with fear and impulsivity. Patients usually require admission to mental hospitals for delusions and the concern that the woman may harm herself or the infant. Psychosis is most frequently associated with depressive illness (70–80%) but must be differentiated from bipolar disorder, schizophrenia, drugs and organic brain disease. Contributing factors include a family history of mental illness, past psychiatric disorders, marital and family problems, recent stressful life situations, and a lack of social supports, although none of these risk factors may be present. These individuals appear to be biologically vulnerable to mental disease. Risk of recurrence in subsequent pregnancies may be as high as 20–30%.

Symptoms develop most commonly from a few days to 4–6 weeks postpartum, although a careful history may reveal that the illness began in the third trimester of pregnancy. The woman may become restless, unable to sleep, irritable, have pressured speech, unusual behavior, obsessional or delusional thinking, or become very withdrawn. Drug-dependency, endocrinopathies, such as thyroid diseases, and other neurologic disorders must be ruled out. Infant injury or infanticide by the mother is rare but does occur. Treatment of affective disorders is with antidepressant drugs or lithium and care in a psychiatric care facility.

Schizophrenia is a psychiatric disorder of at least 6 months' duration, characterized in its acute phase by delusions, hallucinations, incoherent speech, catatonia, or flat affect. Generally, the level of the individual's function declines, with withdrawal and social isolation. The onset is usually during adolescence or young adulthood. Genetic as well as environmental and psychological factors are involved. Schizophrenic women may have exacerbations during pregnancy and the puerperium and should be carefully monitored. Delusions in pregnancy often relate to bodily changes and fetal movements. The disease is considered to have an organic basis with biochemical abnormalities, and drug treatment is usually with neuroleptic antipsychotics such as phenothiazines, butyrophenones, and thioxanthenes. A psychiatric referral is indicated. Suicidal risk should be assessed.

Organic brain disease (delirium, organic brain syndrome) is often confused with acute psychosis. Toxic states, drugs, metabolic disorders, infection, and hemorrhage can cause neurodysfunction. There may be impairment of orientation, memory, intellectual function, and judgment, as well as emotional lability. The individual is usually conscious and symptoms fluctuate. A neuropsychiatric consultation is indicated. It is best to avoid sedative drugs until an evaluation and diagnosis are made and treatment of the underlying disorder is begun.

In-hospital management includes keeping the surroundings familiar, the room well lit, and the woman oriented by using her name. The clinician must be alert to changes in mood, behavior, and thinking.

Psychoses require specialized psychiatric care. If a patient becomes acutely disturbed or confused, she requires emergency management until the psychiatric consultation can be performed. Such patients can be divided into five categories according to the following features:

(1) Acute psychoses with disordered thought, hallucinations, and fear, possibly caused by psychotic illness or drug reaction.
(2) Delirium caused by an underlying medical problem with fluctuating disorientation to time, place, and person.
(3) Severe anxiety with somatic symptoms.
(4) Anger and belligerence with or without alcohol or drug abuse.
(5) Depression with suicidal ideas.

A medical and drug history should be obtained from relatives or friends. Accuracy in diagnosis is essential (eg, insulin shock in a diabetic may be confused with psychogenic seizures). If possible, a blood sample should be drawn for drug and toxicity screening. The patient is calmed, and a relative or friend may remain with her unless she becomes violent. In such instances, security personnel should be alerted and the patient transferred to a psychiatric care facility as quickly as possible. Haloperidol may be given orally or parenterally to facilitate immediate management.

Anxiety Disorders in Pregnancy

Anxiety during pregnancy and the puerperium is normal; its total absence is as pathologic as is its excess. When anxiety increases enough to be considered a disorder, there are two major classifications: phobic disorders and anxiety state disorders. Phobic disorders include persistent and irrational fear of a specific object, activity, or situation that may lead to avoidance. In pregnancy, irrational fears are often related to the fetus (eg, unsubstantiated worries about food that might harm the fetus). Treatment ranges from simple reassurance to behavior modification to medication.

Anxiety states are divided into three categories. Panic disorders include recurrent attacks of anxiety with sudden onset of intense fear and apprehension. There may be physical symptoms such as dyspnea, chest pains, palpitations, choking, and dizziness. Attacks may last minutes to hours with anxiety between attacks. They are thought to have a biochemical basis, but there is often a precipitating event. Panic disorders may be part of the syndrome of depression. Generalized anxiety disorders last a month or more with signs of motor tension, vigilance, scanning, autonomic hyperactivity, and apprehension. Other conditions causing anxiety must be ruled out. Obsessive-compulsive disorder is characterized by repetitive behaviors that result from anxiety or preoccupation with particular irrational fears.

These disorders may interfere with function and compliance. Treatment of anxiety disorder is initiated with a psychiatric evaluation, reassurance, and behavioral modification. Cognitive behavioral therapy is an effective treatment for these syndromes, but requires patient commitment and compliance. Selective serotonin reuptake inhibitor (SSRI) antidepressants are the first-line medical therapies. Benzodiazepines are useful for an acute anxiety crisis, but should be avoided during pregnancy. They are highly addictive and there is some evidence that they are associated with fetal malformations.

Posttraumatic Stress Disorder

After an emotionally traumatic experience, some patients develop a constellation of symptoms typical of posttraumatic stress disorder (PTSD). These symptoms include a sense of recurrently experiencing the event (flashbacks, dreams), avoiding stimuli associated with the trauma (activities, people, places), and heightened arousal (anxiety, irritability, trouble concentrating). Treatments include cognitive behavioral therapy and medical therapy with SSRIs. The traumatic event may have been a traumatic medical experience, fetal loss, infertility, sexual assault, or the death of a close relative or friend that the patient associates with pregnancy or labor.

When counseling a woman with any of the above disorders, the clinician needs to address several questions: Is there a medical condition causing the disorder? Is there a basic psychiatric disorder, such as depression or schizophrenia, present? Does substance abuse complicate the clinical presentation? Is this patient abusing alcohol or other drugs? Consultation with a mental health professional is recommended. Some sexual assault survivors may strongly prefer a cesarean section to a vaginal delivery.

Psychotropic Medications during Pregnancy and Lactation

No psychotropic medication has been approved by the Food and Drug Administration for use in pregnancy.

Because of the unknown risk of medications to the fetus, medications have not traditionally been studied in pregnancy. As no definitive treatment regimen for the treatment of psychiatric disorders exists, each patient's treatment must be custom tailored. Consideration must be given to each patient with regard to her psychiatric history, past pregnancy history, the severity of her symptoms, her response to medication in the past, the likelihood that nonpharmacologic treatments will be effective, and her compliance. The risk of treatment must be less than the risk that psychiatric illness places on the patient and the baby. Given the mounting evidence that untreated psychiatric illness hinders pregnancy outcome and infant development, physicians have lowered the treatment threshold.

Ideally, these discussions regarding the use of psychiatric medications in pregnancy start before the patient is pregnant. Patients with psychiatric illness may benefit from a planned pregnancy, during a time when stressors are minimal and support is adequate. In general, medications should be avoided during the first trimester, given that the fetus is undergoing organogenesis. Certain medications, such as lithium, should be avoided. Anticonvulsants (teratogens) should be used only after careful consideration of the risks and benefits and in conjunction with folic acid supplementation.

Antidepressants are the most commonly used psychotropic medications in pregnancy and the postpartum period. Although they cross the placenta, they are not teratogens. In the few studies that have been performed, no clear morbidity outcomes were associated with the use of SSRIs (mainly fluoxetine) and tricyclic antidepressants (TCAs). Both SSRI and TCA use in the third trimester is associated with a perinatal syndrome in neonates. Symptoms include irritability, gastrointestinal problems, urinary retention, sweating, jerky movements, tachycardia and tachypnea. Antidepressants may be tapered in the third trimester to minimize these symptoms (when appropriate). SSRIs are the first-line medical treatment for depression, as they are less often associated with the perinatal syndrome and side effects than the TCAs. A pregnant patient may require higher doses than a nonpregnant women, given her increased metabolism and liver function.

With regard to lactation, one may not assume that drug concentrations are lower in breast milk than in maternal circulation. Drugs are excreted in breast milk at differing rates, depending on the specific drug's pharmacokinetics and the patient. Infant serum drug concentrations do not correlate well with maternal drug concentration. For this reason, there are no clear guidelines regarding psychotropic medication use in lactating women. However, when using lithium to treat bipolar disorder, breastfeeding should be discontinued.

As a general rule, a patient and her physician should carefully discuss the risks and benefits on a case-by-case basis before prescribing psychotropic drugs during pregnancy or lactation. Psychiatric and pediatric consultation may be an important component of your evaluation, assessment, and planning. It is important to remember that psychiatric illness has deleterious effects on pregnancy and infant outcomes and that proper treatment is warranted.

Substance and Alcohol Abuse

Substance abuse can cause major problems in pregnancy and the puerperium. These problems may be mild or may be severe enough to lead to fetal abnormalities, morbidity, and death of infant and mother. Therefore, inquiry concerning drug use should be made during prenatal visits and documented in the record.

GRIEF & GRIEVING: PERINATAL LOSS

Grief in pregnancy can accompany an elective or therapeutic abortion, still birth, neonatal loss, or neonatal illness. Relinquishment of a baby for adoption may have the same psychological effect as loss as a result of death. Death of a fetus or baby is often felt to be a loss of part of the mother's self. Grief is the process of adapting to such a loss by detaching little by little through anger, pain, and sadness. The mother and father may feel an emptiness. Thoughtless comments such as "you can always have another," "you didn't know the baby anyway," or "plan another pregnancy right away" may only serve to increase the couple's emotional pain.

Parents grieve for the lost fetus or infant in their own way and in their own time. One difficulty in grieving for a lost pregnancy is the lack of identification that is useful in detaching from a known person. Parents should be encouraged to make their own decisions concerning seeing or holding the baby, disposition of the remains (burial or cremation), religious observances, and naming the baby. They should not be discouraged from seeing a malformed infant; they often recall the positive aspects. Photos should be obtained if desired. Autopsies often give parents more information about the normal as well as the abnormal features. Mothers, perhaps more than fathers, suffer from guilt and helplessness. Participation in decision making can help them achieve more control in dealing with their loss.

Physicians may also feel helpless and sad. They must talk with patients, give them as much information as possible, and assure them (if possible) that nothing the mother did caused the fetal or infant demise. Often, the anger that is part of the grieving process is displaced to hospital staff, especially physicians. It is important to deal with each set of parents individually, to meet with them, and encourage them to grieve in their own way. If severe grief persists beyond several months, psychiatric consultation should be obtained.

PSEUDOCYESIS

Pseudocyesis is a syndrome in which a nonpregnant woman believes she is pregnant and develops signs and symptoms suggestive of pregnancy. Pseudocyesis is a conversion reaction in which a psychic conflict is expressed in physical terms. It is an example of how a false belief may affect physiologic processes. It has been known since ancient times, and many cases have been described in women ages 7–79 years. The most common symptoms include menstrual abnormalities (oligomenorrhea, amenorrhea), abdominal enlargement, and breast changes. There may be nausea and vomiting. On examination, the uterus is not enlarged; the abdomen is firm to palpation and often tympanic to percussion. "Fetal movement" has been reported; it is usually intestinal activity or contractions of abdominal muscles. A supposed fetal heart rate may be maternal tachycardia. Galactorrhea may be present because of increased prolactin levels from other causes (eg, pituitary adenomas), long-term breast stimulation, or use of drugs such as phenothiazines. There are usually neuroendocrine abnormalities (eg, hypothalamic amenorrhea). Duration varies from 9 months to several years. Diagnosis of true pregnancy can be obtained with pregnancy tests and ultrasonography. However, negative test results may not convince a woman with this syndrome that she is not pregnant.

The clinical variants of pseudocyesis include "true" pseudocyesis, which should be distinguished from psychosis in women in whom the false belief in pregnancy is a delusion; factitious illness in which the woman knows she is not pregnant but simulates pregnancy for some secondary gain (eg, to keep a straying partner); organic diseases such as a pelvic tumor; and iatrogenic pseudopregnancy caused by administration of human chorionic gonadotropin to produce positive pregnancy tests in infertile women.

Management consists of a careful history, physical examination, and laboratory tests to rule out pregnancy and organic disease. Psychological assessment and treatment are also indicated.

THE REFERRAL PROCESS

Referral to mental health professionals may be indicated for any psychological process the gynecologist believes to be beyond his or her ability, training, or willingness to treat. The gynecologist may prefer to work closely with a psychiatrist, psychologist, social worker, or psychiatric nurse. The attitude taken should be comfort in the belief that counseling would be helpful, not that the patient is bothersome and therefore should be labeled or stigmatized by such referrals. Consultation–liaison psychiatrists have expertise in the psychological aspects of medical and surgical problems, as well as in the use of psychopharmacologic drugs. Most hospital staffs include social workers and psychiatric nurses who specialize in psychosocial issues. Marriage counselors offer much to those with relationship problems. As with obstetrics, the biopsychosocial approach is extremely useful.

REFERENCES

Psychological Aspects of Gynecology

American Psychiatric Association, *Diagnostic and Statistical Manual of Mental Health Disorders*, 4th ed. American Psychological Association, 1994.

Bair MJ et al: Depression and pain comorbidity. Arch Intern Med 2003;103:2433.

Gunter J: Chronic pelvic pain: An integrated approach to diagnosis and treatment. Obstet Gynecol Surv 2003;58(5):615.

Masters W, Johnson V: *Human Sexual Response*. Little, Brown, 1966.

Moline ML, Broch L, Zak R: Sleep in women across the life cycle from adulthood through menopause. Med Clin North Am 2004;88:706.

Morely J, Kaiser F: Female sexuality. Med Clin North Am 2003; 87:1077.

NIH State-of-the Science Conference Statement: Management of the menopause-related symptoms. Ann Intern Med 2005; 142(12):1003.

Nusbaum MR: The proactive sexual health history. Am Fam Physician 2002;66(9):1705.

Rannestad T: Hysterectomy: Effects on quality of life and psychological aspect. Best Pract Res Clin Obstet Gynaecol 2005; 19(3):419.

Psychological Aspects of Obstetrics

Bennett HA et al: Prevalence of depression during pregnancy: Systematic review. Obstet Gynecol 2004;103:698.

Cott AD, Wisner KL: Psychiatric disorders during pregnancy. Int Rev Psychiatry 2003;15:217.

Elfenbein D, Felice M: Adolescent pregnancy. Pediatr Clin North Am 2003;50:781.

Gordon N et al: Effects of providing hospital-based doulas in HMOs. Obstet Gynecol 1999;93:422.

Howard LM et al: Antidepressant prevention of postnatal depression. Cochrane Database Syst Rev 2005;2:CD004363.

Jewell D, Young G: Interventions for nausea and vomiting in early pregnancy. Cochrane Database Syst Rev 2003;1: CD000145.

Domestic Violence & Sexual Assault 62

Michael C. Lu, MD, MPH, Jessica S. Lu, MPH, & Vivian P. Halfin, MD

For many victims of domestic violence and sexual assault, the first contact with the health care system is with the obstetrician-gynecologist or primary care doctor. Consequently, it is critical that these physicians be knowledgeable in the identification, evaluation, and treatment of such patients.

DOMESTIC VIOLENCE

While the home is often thought of as a safe haven, it is the site of the most common manifestations of violence in our society today. Domestic or intimate partner violence typically refers to violence perpetrated against adolescent and adult females within the context of family or intimate relationships. Although victims of domestic violence may be male or female, 90–95% of the victims are women. It is a behavior pattern that is manifested in physical and sexual attacks, as well as psychological and economic coercion. The abuser uses the behavior in order to establish and maintain domination and control over the victim. Because abuse is usually accompanied by shame and guilt, the victim often does not report the abuse.

As a result of significant underreporting, it is difficult to compile exact data on the incidence of domestic violence. Every year, approximately 4–5 million women are believed to be battered by their intimate partners. Violence by an intimate partner accounts for approximately 21% of all the violent crime experienced by women. More than 40% of all female murder victims are murdered by their husbands, boyfriends, or ex-partners. It is estimated that at least one-fifth of all American women will be physically assaulted by a partner or ex-partner during their lifetime.

Violent acts may include threats, throwing objects, pushing, kicking, hitting, beating, sexual assault, and threatening with or using a weapon. Domestic violence frequently includes verbal abuse, intimidation, progressive social isolation, and deprivation of things such as food, money, transportation, or access to health care. The violence typically occurs in a predictable, progressive cycle. The tension-building phase is characterized by arguing and blaming as anger intensifies. This leads to the battering phase that may involve verbal threats, sexual abuse, physical battering, and use of weapons. The battering phase is followed by a honeymoon phase

during which the abuser may deny the violence, make excuses for battering, apologize, buy gifts, and promise never to do it again, until the next cycle begins. Although unemployment, poverty, and alcohol and substance abuse increase the likelihood of abuse, domestic violence cuts across all racial, ethnic, religious, educational, and socioeconomic lines. Domestic violence often occurs within a framework of family violence that can include child abuse, elder abuse, or abuse of adults who are disabled. It is estimated that child abuse occurs in 33–77% of families where adults are abused.

Clinical Presentation

Survivors of domestic violence or sexual abuse may present to health care professionals in a variety of clinical settings. The prevalence of domestic violence among patients in ambulatory care settings is estimated to be between 20% and 30%.

Such patients commonly report chronic pelvic pain to their gynecologists. A history of sexual abuse is found in significantly more women with chronic pelvic pain as compared with other gynecologic conditions. Others may complain of sexual dysfunctions such as decreased interest or arousal, dyspareunia, or anorgasmia. Incest victims have a very high rate of sexual dysfunction and may avoid sex or seek it out compulsively. Still others may present with chronic or recurrent vaginitis. Some women may present for a routine gynecologic appointment but become anxious and tearful before or during the pelvic examination.

Some women present to their primary care physicians with persistent multiple bodily complaints, such as chronic headaches, palpitations, abdominal complaints, or sleep and appetite disturbances. Eating disorders may be more common among abuse victims. Others may have a somatoform disorder. This condition is characterized by physical symptoms suggesting a physical condition for which there are no demonstrable organic findings or physiologic mechanisms. In the face of a negative work-up, there may be evidence of or a presumption that the symptoms are linked to psychological factors or conflicts. Women who meet the criteria for somatoform disorder often have a history of abuse.

In a mental health setting, victims of domestic violence or sexual assault may note feeling depressed or suicidal. They may have anxiety or sleep disorders that they may self-medicate with alcohol or other substances. Most commonly, these women may have post-traumatic stress disorder (PTSD), which occurs in individuals who have experienced a psychologically distressing event that is outside the range of usual human experience. Symptoms of PTSD include re-experiencing the traumatic event through intrusive memories, dreams, flashbacks, or exposure to events symbolic of the trauma. Patients with PTSD also exhibit a "psychic numbing," ie, they are detached from other people and have difficulty feeling emotions, especially those associated with intimacy or sexuality. Other clinical syndromes include personality disorders characterized by maladaptive character traits. In very extreme cases, patients may have multiple personality disorder (MPD), characterized by having two or more distinct personalities existing within them. This disorder is marked by a disturbance in the normally integrated functions of identity, memory, and consciousness as the result of dissociation from traumatic experiences.

The problem of domestic violence in pregnancy merits special mention because it is a threat to both the mother and her developing fetus. Estimates of prevalence of domestic violence in pregnancy are in the range of 1–20%, with most studies identifying rates between 4% and 8%. These estimates suggest that violence is a more common problem for pregnant women than preeclampsia, gestational diabetes, and placenta previa, conditions for which pregnant women are routinely screened and evaluated. Some evidence suggests that violence may escalate during pregnancy, especially in the postpartum period. Abuse is associated with increased physical and psychological stress, inadequate prenatal care utilization, poor nutrition and weight gain, and increased maternal behavioral risks (cigarette, alcohol, and substance abuse). These may lead to problems with fetal growth and development. Physical trauma can cause abruptio placentae, preterm labor, preterm premature rupture of membranes, and maternal and fetal injuries and demise.

Diagnosis & Treatment

Although battered women seek medical care frequently, as few as 1 in 20 are correctly identified by the practitioner to whom they turn for help. Barriers to diagnosis include the practitioner's lack of knowledge or training, lack of recognition of the widespread prevalence of the problem, time constraints, fear of offending the patient, and a feeling of powerlessness in the area of treatment. Research suggests that the use of abuse assessment questions on standard medical records may increase screening and documentation. In addition, because many women will not voluntarily disclose abuse, asking each patient directly about prior or ongoing victimization increases the likelihood of disclosure.

The screening assessment should be prefaced with a statement to establish that screening is universal, such as, "I would like to ask you a few questions about physical, sexual, and emotional trauma because we know that these are common and affect women's health." Direct questioning using behaviorally specific phrasing should follow:

- Has anyone close to you ever threatened to hurt you?
- Has anyone ever hit, kicked, choked, or hurt you physically?
- Has anyone, including your partner, ever forced you to have sex?
- Are you ever afraid of your partner?

Disclosure rates will be higher when the questions are asked face to face by the health care provider rather than through a questionnaire, and when behaviorally specific descriptions rather than the terms "abuse," "domestic violence," or "rape" are used. Abuse victims are often accompanied to health care appointments by the perpetrator, who may appear overprotective or overbearing, and may answer questions directed toward the woman. It is important to ask the patient questions in private, apart from the male partner. It is also important to ask the patient questions apart from children, family, or friends, and to avoid using them as interpreters when asking questions about violence.

In the office setting, the most effective and efficient strategy for providing assistance to a woman who has disclosed abuse involves acknowledging and documenting the trauma, assessing immediate safety and establishing a safety plan, and providing patient education and referrals to community support services. An essential first step is to acknowledge the trauma. It is important to reinforce to the victim that she is not to blame as many victims have trouble believing that they are not responsible for the abuse.

Documenting domestic violence is no different from documenting other patient interactions, but such documentation may provide important supportive evidence in the courtroom to put an end to the violence. Direct quotations of the patient's explanation of her injuries should be recorded. Photographs may be taken after consent is granted. Every effort should be made to maintain confidentiality to avoid retaliation by the perpetrators when they suspect disclosure of abuse. The physician or health care professional may be required by state law to report actual or suspected domestic violence.

Once domestic violence is acknowledged and documented, the next step is to assess immediate safety and to establish a safety plan. Lethality of the violence should be assessed by asking questions such as:

- Has your partner ever threatened to kill you or your children?
- Are there weapons in the house?

- Does your partner abuse alcohol or use drugs?
- Is it safe for you to go home?
- Are the children (or other dependents) safe?

If the violence has escalated to the point where she is afraid for her safety or that of her children, she should be offered shelter.

An important step in addressing ongoing violence is to help the victim establish a safety plan. The American College of Obstetricians and Gynecologists (www.acog.org) distributes pocket cards with suggested steps for making an exit plan. These cards can be handed to the patient or left in patient restrooms where a woman can pick it up without concern of being seen by an accompanying partner.

Providing educational materials about domestic violence and its consequences can sometimes help victims take action toward ending the violence. These materials demonstrate to women that their physicians' offices are both a resource and a safe place should they decide to take action. A list of referral resources should be readily available in medical offices. The list should include telephone numbers for police departments, emergency departments, shelters for battered women, rape crisis centers, counseling services, self-help programs, and advocacy agencies that can provide legal, financial, and emotional support.

Given the high rate of psychiatric symptomatology in this population, referral for psychiatric screening and counseling can be useful. Patients who are experiencing posttraumatic stress disorder can benefit from psychotherapy and possibly medication as well. Those with depression, substance abuse, or anxiety, personality, or dissociative disorders will also require ongoing treatment. Psychiatrists or other mental health professionals can serve to coordinate a variety of treatment modalities for the victims: individual, couples, and family therapy, detoxification and substance abuse treatment, and advocacy groups.

Despite the best efforts of physicians and other health care professionals, some women may initially be unable to extirpate themselves from victimization. For such women, an encounter with a health care system that they experience as nonblaming, accessible, and supportive will help to maximize the chances of their making a positive life change at some future point.

SEXUAL ASSAULT

Sexual assault is any sexual act performed by one person on another without the person's consent. Sexual assault includes genital, oral, or anal penetration by a part of the accused's body or by an object. It may result from force, the threat of force either on the victim or another person, or the victim's inability to give appropriate consent. Many states have now adopted the gender-neutral legal term *sexual assault* in favor of *rape,* which traditionally referred to forced vaginal penetration of a woman by a male assailant.

An estimated 700,000 to 1,000,000 American women are sexually assaulted every year. These estimates are higher than official crime reports because the majority of cases go unreported. According to one estimate, only 30% of rapes are reported to the police, and 50% of rape victims tell no one. At least 20% of adult women, 15% of college-age women, and 12% of adolescent girls have experienced sexual abuse and assault during their lifetime. Sexual assault occurs in all age, racial-ethnic, and socioeconomic groups, but its incidence may be higher for African American women and for adolescent females. In several studies, about one-fourth to one-half of the victims of sexual assault were younger than the age of 18 years. The very young, the elderly, and the physically or developmentally disabled may be particularly vulnerable to sexual assault.

Several variants of sexual assault deserve special mention. **Marital rape** is defined as forced coitus or related sexual acts within a marital relationship without the consent of a partner. **Acquaintance rape** refers to those sexual assaults committed by someone known to the victim. More than 75% of adolescent rapes are committed by an acquaintance of the victim. When the acquaintance is a family member, including step-relatives and parental figures living in the home, the sexual assault is referred to as **incest.** When the forced or unwanted sexual activity occurs in the context of a dating relationship, it is referred to as **date rape.** In this situation, the woman may voluntarily participate in sexual play but coitus occurs, often forcibly, without her consent. Alcohol use is frequently associated with date rape. "Date rape drugs" such as flunitrazepam (Rohypnol) and gamma-hydroxybutyrate (GHB) have also been used to diminish a woman's ability to consent or to remember the assault.

Statutory rape refers to sexual intercourse with a female under an age specified by state law (ranging from 14–18 years of age); the consent of an adolescent younger than this age is legally irrelevant because she is defined as being incapable of consenting. **Child sexual abuse** is defined as contact or interaction between a child and an adult when the child is being used for the sexual stimulation of that adult or another person. All 50 states and the District of Columbia mandate reporting of child abuse, including child sexual abuse. Nearly half of the states also require physicians to report statutory rape. Physicians should be familiar with the laws in their states; failure to report sexual assault against children may subject the physicians to fines and incarceration for up to 1 year.

Our society has many misperceptions about sexual assault. The victims are often blamed for having encouraged the assault by their behavior or dress, for not sufficiently resisting the assault, for being promiscuous, or for having ulterior motives for pressing charges. This misplaced culpability is often internalized by the victims, which (in addition to fear of retribution) may explain their reluctance to report the violent crime to the authorities. Another common misperception is that rape is an impulsive or aggressive extension of normal sex drive on the part of the rapist. The motivation for most sexual assault, however, seems not to be sexual gratification but rather degradation, terrorization, and humiliation of the victim. The assault is often a demonstration of power (power rape), anger (anger rape), or sadism manifested in ritualized torture or mutilation of the victim (sadistic rape) on the part of the rapist.

Clinical Presentation

The majority of rape victims who come to emergency rooms do not openly admit to having been sexually assaulted. Instead, they may complain of having been mugged or may voice concerns about acquired immune deficiency syndrome (AIDS) or other sexually transmitted diseases. Others may present with psychiatric symptoms including depression, anxiety, or a suicide attempt. Unless the primary care physician, obstetrician-gynecologist, or psychiatrist obtains a sexual history, assault victims will remain unidentified as such, and will be inadequately treated.

A "rape-trauma" syndrome often occurs after a sexual assault. The initial response (acute phase) may last for hours or days and is characterized by a distortion or paralysis of the individual's coping mechanisms. The initial outward responses vary from complete loss of emotional control (crying, uncontrolled anger) to an unnatural calm and detachment (although some physical signs such as shaking or lowered skin temperature are usually present). The latter behavior represents the victim's need to reestablish control over herself and her environment while simultaneously abandoning the defense mechanism of denial and allowing the renewed invasion of privacy represented by the questioning and examination. The initial reactions of shock, numbness, withdrawal and denial typically abate after the first 2 weeks. However, studies suggest there is a period, occurring from 2 weeks to several months postassault, in which symptomatology returns and may intensify. It is at this time that the victim may begin to seek help for her symptoms, often without telling the health care provider of the sexual assault that precipitated these symptoms.

The next phase (delayed phase) may occur months or years after the sexual assault and is characterized by chronic anxiety, feelings of vulnerability, loss of control, and self-blame. Long-term reactions include anxiety, nightmares, flashbacks, catastrophic fantasies, feelings of alienation and isolation, sexual dysfunction, psychological distress, mistrust of others, phobias, depression, hostility, and somatic symptoms. More than half of rape victims experience substantial difficulty in reestablishing sexual and emotional relationships with spouses or boyfriends. Thirty-three percent to 50% of victims report suicidal ideation; suicide attempts have been reported in nearly 1 in 5 rape victims who do not seek treatment.

PTSD is a common long-term sequela of sexual assault, characterized by psychic numbing, intrusive re-experiencing of the trauma, avoidance of stimuli associated with the trauma, and intense psychological distress. Women with prior victimization histories often have more severe sequela. Women assaulted sexually by family members or dates experience as severe levels of distress as women assaulted by acquaintances or strangers.

Up to 40% of victims who are sexually assaulted sustain injuries. Although most injuries are minor, approximately 1% of the injuries require hospitalization and major operative repair, and 0.1% are fatal. Somatic symptoms are common during the acute phase and include disturbed sleeping and eating patterns, gastrointestinal irritability (with nausea predominating), musculoskeletal soreness, fatigue, tension headaches, and intense startle reactions. Symptoms of vaginal irritation occur in more than 50% of victims, and rectal pain and bleeding are frequent in patients subjected to anal penetration. Ongoing health concerns include gynecologic trauma, risk of pregnancy, and the potential for contracting infections or sexually transmitted diseases, including human immunodeficiency virus (HIV). Victims may also seek to escape the pain of rape's effects through the use of alcohol and drugs.

Rape victims appear to be frequent users of medical services in the months and years following the assault. In one study, visits to physicians increased 18% in the year of the assault, 56% in the following year, and 31% in the year after, compared to previctimization levels. Reintegration of the self following sexual assault is a slow process that may take months to years as the victim works through the trauma and the loss of the event and replaces it with other life experiences. The prognosis for complete recovery is improved if health care professionals responsible for the victim's care have a supportive, nonjudgmental approach and a well-developed understanding and competent treatment of the emotional, as well as physical, consequences of sexual assault.

Diagnosis & Treatment

The physician evaluating the victim has both medical and legal responsibilities, and should be aware of state statutory requirements. Such requirements may involve the use of sexual assault assessment kits, which list the steps necessary and the items to be obtained for forensic purposes. If personnel trained in collecting samples and information are available, it is appropriate to request their assistance.

Informed consent must be obtained prior to examining a sexual assault victim. A careful history and physical examination should be performed in the presence of a chaperon or victim advocate. The patient should be asked to state in her own words what happened, and to identify or describe her attacker, if possible. The history should include inquiry about last menstrual period, contraceptive use, preexisting pregnancy and infection, and last consensual intercourse before the assault. The patient's activities in the interval between the assault and the examination—whether the patient has eaten, drunk, bathed, douched, voided, or defecated—might affect findings on physical examination; such activities must be recorded.

A careful physical examination of the entire body should be performed. The physician should search for bruises, abrasions, or lacerations about the neck, back, buttocks, and extremities. Bite marks should be noted, particularly about the genitalia and breasts. Injuries to the mouth and pharynx may result from oral penetration. Injuries should be documented with photographs or drawings in the medical record. *Rape* and *physical assault* are legal terms that should not be used in medical records. Instead, the physician should report findings as "consistent with the use of force."

A pelvic examination should be performed. Injuries to the vulva, hymen, vagina, urethra, and rectum should be noted. Occasionally, foreign objects may be found in the orifices. The speculum must be moistened only with saline. Two milliliters of normal saline are injected into the vaginal vault. Nonabsorbent cotton swabs should be used to sample fluid from this vaginal pool and should then be placed in sterile glass tubes and refrigerated. Air-dried, nonfixed smears of this same fluid should be placed on glass slides. A Papanicolaou (Pap) test may also be obtained. Evidence of coitus will be present in the vagina for as long as 48 hours after the attack. Motile sperms may be noted in the vagina for up to 8 hours after intercourse, but may be present in the cervical mucous for as long as 2–3 days. Nonmotile sperm may be noted in the vagina for up to 24 hours and in the cervix for up to 17 days. Acid phosphatase is an enzyme found in high concentrations in the seminal fluid. Evidence of acid phosphatase should be sought by swabbing the vaginal secretions, even in the absence of sperm because the attacker may have had a vasectomy. DNA evaluation may also be performed from the vaginal swab. Nonmotile sperm may be found in the rectum for up to 24 hours after the assault, and acid phosphatase can also be detected in the rectum.

A wet mount or vaginal swab should be obtained to detect *Trichomonas vaginalis*. Testing for *Neisseria gonorrhoeae* and *Chlamydia trachomatis* should be performed from specimens from any sites of penetration or attempted penetration. A serum sample should be collected for subsequent serologic analysis if test results are positive. The risk of acquiring gonorrhea from sexual assault is estimated to be between 6% and 12%. Baseline serologic tests for hepatitis B virus, HIV, and syphilis should also be offered. The risk of acquiring syphilis from sexual assault is estimated to be 3%; the risk of acquiring HIV is undetermined.

An important part of the physician's legal responsibilities is to collect samples for forensic purposes. Pubic hair combings should be collected to look for pubic hair from the assailant. Fingernail scrapings should be obtained to look for skin or blood of the attacker. Skin washings and clothing should be investigated for the presence of blood or semen. A Wood light may be helpful because dried semen will fluoresce under its light. Saliva should be collected from the victim. Because seminal fluid is rapidly destroyed by salivary enzymes, identification of seminal fluid in the mouth after a few hours is difficult. Consequently, victims should be encouraged to come to a medical facility immediately following an assault, where they can be evaluated before they bathe, urinate, defecate, wash out their mouths, or clean their fingernails.

Proper processing and labeling of collected specimens is crucial. All collected specimens are placed in a larger sealed container and processed in a "chain of evidence" fashion. The person who collects the specimens verifies their completeness by signature on the sealed master container. The individual to whom they are transferred must verify by signature that all specimens were received in an untampered state. Thus, each individual who has "custody" of the specimens during processing must verify that they were transmitted without alteration until they are turned over to the responsible law enforcement agency. The name of the law enforcement agent who receives the specimens should be noted in the medical record.

Treatment of physical injuries sustained at the time of assault should be initiated immediately; prophylactic medical treatment may be indicated for prevention of sexually transmitted infections and pregnancy. For prophylaxis against sexually transmitted infections, empiric recommended antimicrobial therapy for chlamydial, gonococcal, and trichomonal infections may be given. One such regimen consists of

- Ceftriaxone 125 mg intramuscularly in a single dose, plus
- Metronidazole 2 g orally in a single dose, plus
- Doxycycline 100 mg orally 2 times a day for 7 days.

Alternative treatment may be given as recommended by the Centers for Disease Control and Prevention. In addition, it is recommended that hepatitis B immunoglobulin be administered intramuscularly as soon as possible, but certainly within 14 days of exposure. It should be followed by the standard three-dose active immunization series with hepatitis B vaccine at 0, 1, and 6 months, beginning at the time of passive immunization. Prophylaxis against HIV is controversial.

Emergency contraception can be offered as prophylaxis against pregnancy. The risk of pregnancy after sexual assault has been estimated to be 2–4% in victims who were not using some form of contraception at the time of the assault. A serum pregnancy test should be obtained prior to administration of emergency contraception to evaluate for preexisting pregnancy. Emergency contraception should be given within 72 hours of the assault, although it can still be effective up to 120 hours later. There are several different methods of emergency contraception. For many years, the most common method (Yuzpe method) involved the use of high-dose combined oral contraceptives within 72 hours of unprotected coitus, repeated 12 hours following the first dose. More recently, use of a progestin-only method has become popular. This method involves the use of levonorgestrel 0.75 mg, in 2 doses 12 hours apart, within 72 hours of unprotected coitus. A randomized study showed that this is more effective and better tolerated than the Yuzpe method. Levonorgestrel prevented 85% of pregnancies that would have occurred without treatment.

As most patients suffer significant psychological trauma as a consequence of sexual assault, the physician must be prepared to provide access to counseling. It is preferable that follow-up psychological counseling be provided by individuals who have extensive experience in the management of crisis-response to rape. Even if the victim appears to be in control emotionally, she will probably experience aspects of rape-trauma syndrome at some time in the future. She should be made aware of the symptoms that she may experience, and advised to seek help if and when these symptoms occur. No patient should be released from the facility until specific follow-up plans are made and agreed upon by the patient, physician, and counselor.

A follow-up visit should be scheduled approximately 2 weeks after the assault for repeat physical examination and collection of additional specimens. Testing for *N. gonorrhoeae, C. trachomatis,* and *T. vaginalis* should be repeated unless prophylactic antimicrobials have been provided. Follow-up counseling should be discussed again at the second visit. Additional visits may be scheduled according to the victim's needs; an additional follow-up visit approximately 12 weeks following the sexual assault is advisable to collect sera for detection of antibodies against *T. pallidum,* hepatitis B virus (unless vaccine was given), and HIV (repeat test at 6 months). During each of these visits, assessment of the patient's psychological symptoms should be performed, and referrals for further counseling are made as indicated.

Much of this chapter addresses the role and responsibilities of the health care professional in caring for victims of domestic violence and sexual assault after they have occurred. One of the greatest challenges for health care and public health professionals working to improve women's health continues to be the epidemic of violence against women in our society and around the world. A great deal remains to be learned and done about the primary prevention of violence.

REFERENCES

American College of Obstetricians and Gynecologists: Emergency oral contraception. ACOG Practice Bulletin No. 25, 2001.

American College of Obstetricians and Gynecologists: Domestic violence. ACOG Educational Bulletin No. 257, 1999.

American College of Obstetricians and Gynecologists: Sexual assault. ACOG Educational Bulletin No. 242, 1997.

Burgess AW, Holmstrom LL: Rape trauma syndrome. Am J Psychiatry 1974;131:981.

Campbell JC: Health consequences of intimate partner violence. Lancet 2002;359:1331.

Centers for Disease Control and Prevention: 2002 Sexually transmitted disease treatment guidelines. MMWR 2002;51(RR06):1.

Jones RF 3rd, Horan DL: The American College of Obstetricians and Gynecologists: Responding to violence against women. Int J Gynaecol Obstet 2002;78:S75.

Kaplan DW et al: Care of the adolescent sexual assault victim. Pediatrics 2001;107:1476.

Patel M, Minshell L: Management of sexual assault. Emerg Med Clin North Am 2001;19:817.

Riggs N et al: Analysis of 1076 cases of sexual assault. Ann Emerg Med 2000;35:358.

Rhodes KV, Levinson W: Interventions for intimate partner violence against women: Clinical applications. JAMA 2003;289:601.

United States Preventive Services Task Force: Screening for family and intimate partner violence: Recommendation statement. Ann Fam Med 2004;2:156.

Wathen CN, MacMillan HL: Interventions for violence against women: Scientific review. JAMA 2003;289:589.

The Breast

Matthew M. Poggi, MD, & Kathleen Harney, MD

ANATOMY OF THE FEMALE BREAST

The breasts are secondary reproductive glands of ectodermal origin. They are frequently referred to as modified sweat glands. Each breast lies on the superior aspect of the chest wall. In women the breasts are the organs of lactation, whereas in men the breasts are normally functionless and undeveloped.

HISTOLOGY

The adult female breast contains glandular and ductal elements, stroma consisting of fibrous tissue that binds the individual lobes together and adipose tissue within and between the lobes.

Each breast consists of 12–20 conical lobes. The base of each lobe is in close proximity to the ribs. The apex, which contains the major excretory duct of the lobe, is deep to the areola and nipple. In turn, each lobe consists of a group of lobules. The lobules have several lactiferous ducts, which unite to form a major duct that drains the lobes as they course toward the nipple–areolar complex. Each of the major ducts widens to form an ampulla as they travel toward the areola and then narrow at its individual opening in the nipple. The lobules are held in place by a meshwork of loose, fatty areolar tissue. The fatty tissue increases toward the periphery of the lobule and gives the breast its bulk and hemispheric shape.

Approximately 80–85% of the normal breast is adipose tissue. The breast tissues are joined to the overlying skin and subcutaneous tissue by fibrous strands.

In the nonpregnant, nonlactating breast, the alveoli are small and tightly packed. During pregnancy, the alveoli hypertrophy and their lining cells proliferate in number. During lactation, the alveolar cells secrete proteins and lipids, which comprise breast milk.

The deep surface of the breast lies on the fascia that covers the chest muscles. The fascial stroma, derived from the superficial fascia of the chest wall, is condensed into multiple bands that run from the breast into the subcutaneous tissues and the corium of the skin overlying the breast. These fascial bands—Cooper's ligaments—support the breast in its upright position on the chest wall. These bands may be distorted by a tumor, resulting in pathologic skin dimpling.

HISTOLOGIC CHANGES IN THE FEMALE BREAST DURING THE LIFE SPAN

In response to multiglandular stimulation during puberty, the female breast starts to enlarge and eventually assumes its conical or spherical shape. Growth is the result of an increase in acinar tissue, ductal size and branching, and deposits of adipose, the main factor in breast enlargement. Also during puberty, the nipple and areola enlarge. Smooth muscle fibers surround the base of the nipple, and the nipple becomes more sensitive to touch.

Once menses is established, the breast undergoes a periodic **premenstrual phase** during which the acinar cells increase in number and size, the ductal lumens widen, and breast size and turgor increase slightly. Many women have breast tenderness during this phase of the menstrual cycle. Menstrual bleeding is followed by a **postmenstrual phase,** characterized by a decrease in size and turgor, reduction in the number and size of the breast acini, and a decrease in diameter of the lactiferous ducts. Cyclic hormonal influences to the breast are quite variable. This is true for changes in breast size and turgor, as well as the degree of hypertrophic and regressive histologic changes that may occur.

In response to progesterone during pregnancy, breast size and turgidity increase considerably. These changes are accompanied by deepening pigmentation of the nipple–areolar complex, nipple enlargement, areolar widening, and an increase in the number and size of the lubricating glands in the areola. The breast ductal system branches markedly, and the individual ducts widen. The acini increase in number and size. In late pregnancy, the fatty tissues of the breasts are almost completely replaced by cellular breast parenchyma. After delivery, the breasts, now fully mature, start to secrete milk. With cessation of nursing or administration of estrogens, which inhibit lactation, the breast rapidly returns to its prepregnancy state, with marked diminution of cellular elements and an increase in adipose deposits.

When menses ceases between the fifth and sixth decades of life, the breast undergoes a gradual process of

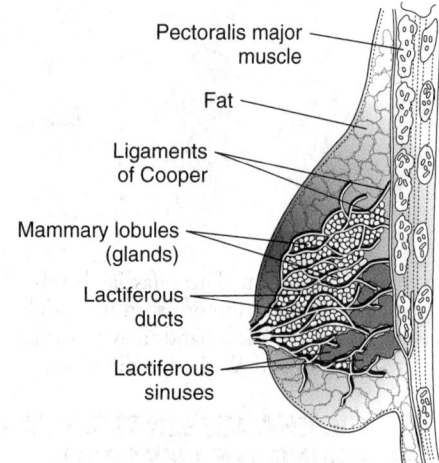

Pectoralis major
muscle

Fat

Ligaments
of Cooper

Mammary lobules
(glands)

Lactiferous
ducts

Lactiferous
sinuses

Figure 63–1. Sagittal section of mammary gland.

atrophy and involution. There is a decrease in the number and size of acinar and ductal elements, so that the breast tissue regresses to an almost infantile state. Adipose tissue may or may not atrophy, with disappearance of the parenchymal elements.

GROSS ANATOMY (FIG 63–1)

The adult female breast mound characteristically forms a near hemispheric contour on each side of the chest wall, usually extending from just below the level of the second rib inferiorly to the sixth or seventh rib. The breast mound is usually situated between the lateral sternal border and the anterior axillary fold. The breast tissue extends over a larger anatomic area than the more obvious breast mound. The superior portion of the breast tissue emerges gradually from the chest wall inferior to the clavicle, whereas the lateral and inferior borders are better defined. The major portion of the breast tissue is located superficial to the pectoralis major muscle and projects laterally and ventrally toward the tail of Spence. Smaller portions of breast tissue extend laterally and inferiorly to lie superficial to the serratus anterior and external oblique muscles and as far caudad as the rectus abdominis. The tail of Spence is a triangular tongue-shaped portion of breast tissue that extends superiorly and laterally toward the axilla, perforating the deep axillary fascia, and enters the axilla, where it terminates in close proximity to the axillary lymph nodes and vessels as well as the axillary blood vessels and nerves.

The Nipple & Areola

The areola is a circular pigmented zone 2–6 cm in diameter at the tip of the breast. Its color varies from pale pink to deep brown depending on age, parity and skin

pigmentation. The skin of the areola contains multiple small, elevated nodules beneath which are located the sebaceous glands of Montgomery. The glands are responsible for lubrication of the nipple and help prevent cracks and fissures in the nipple–areolar complex that occur during breastfeeding. During the third trimester of pregnancy, the sebaceous glands of Montgomery markedly hypertrophy.

A circular smooth muscle band surrounds the base of the nipple. Longitudinal smooth muscle fibers branch out from this ring of circular smooth muscle to encircle the lactiferous ducts as they converge toward the nipple. The many small punctate openings at the superior aspect of the nipple represent the terminals of the major lactiferous ducts. As discussed earlier, the ampullae of the lactiferous ducts are deep to the nipple and the areola.

Blood Vessels, Lymphatics, & Nerves

A. ARTERIES (FIG 63–2)

The breast has a rich blood supply with multiple arteries and veins. Branches from the internal thoracic artery that penetrate the second, third and fourth intercostal interspaces supply blood to the medial half of the breast. These arteries perforate the intercostal muscles and the anterior intercostal membrane to supply both the breast and the pectoralis major and minor muscles. During pregnancy, and not infrequently in advanced breast disease, the intercostal perforators may enlarge from engorgement. Small branches from the anterior intercostal arteries also supply the medial aspect of the breast. Laterally, the pectoral branch of the thoracoacromial branch of the axillary artery and the external mammary branch of the lateral thoracic artery, which also is a branch of the second segment of the axillary artery, supply the breast. The external mammary artery passes along the lateral free edge of the pectoralis major muscle to reach the lateral half of the breast. The artery usually is located medial to the long thoracic nerve.

The medial and lateral arteries, as they reach the breast, tend to arborize mainly in the supra-areolar area; consequently, the arterial supply to the upper half of the breast is almost twice that of the lower half.

B. VEINS

Venous return from the breast closely follows the routes of the arterial system. Blood returns to the superior vena cava via the axillary and internal thoracic veins. It also returns via the vertebral venous plexuses, which are fed by the intercostal and azygos veins. Through the azygos veins, there is also some minor flow into the portal system. A rich anastomotic plexus of superficial breast veins is located in the subareolar region. In thin-skinned, fair individuals, these veins are normally visible, and they are

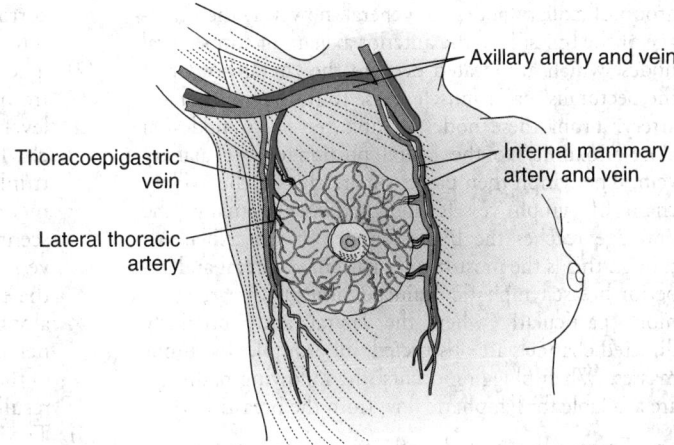

Figure 63–2. Arteries and veins of the breast.

almost always visible during pregnancy. Their presence makes for marked vascularity of sub- and para-areolar incisions. Venous return flow is greater in the superior quadrants than in the inferior quadrants of the breast.

C. LYMPHATICS (FIG 63–3)

A thorough knowledge of the lymphatic drainage of the breast is of critical importance to the clinician. This is true because the lymphatic drainage has significant implications in several disease etiologies, including breast cancer. To a large extent, modern, less-invasive surgical management techniques such as sentinel lymph node biopsy are based on a solid understanding of the pattern of lymphatic drainage in the breast.

Lymphatic drainage in the breast may be divided into 2 main categories: superficial (including cutaneous) drainage and deep parenchymatous drainage.

1. Superficial drainage—A large lymphatic plexus exists in the subcutaneous tissues of the breast deep to the nipple–areolar complex. This plexus drains the areola and nipple regions, including the cutaneous and subcutaneous tissues adjacent to the nipple–areolar complex. In addition, the superficial plexus drains the deep central parenchymatous region of the breast.

2. Deep parenchymatous drainage—The deep parenchymatous lymph vessels drain the remainder of the breast as well as some portion of the skin and subcutaneous tissues of the nipple–areolar complex not served by the superficial plexus. Small periductal and periacinal lymph vessels collect parenchymal lymph and deliver it to the larger interlobar lymphatics. Lymph from the cutaneous and nipple–areolar regions may drain either directly into the subareolar plexus or deeply into the parenchymatous lymph system. Once in the deep parenchymatous drainage, the lymph is delivered to the subareolar plexus for efferent transport.

The majority of lymphatic drainage from both the retroareolar and the deep interlobar lymphatics of the breast travel to the ipsilateral axillary lymph nodes. The route of drainage to the highest axillary node or nodes is not reproducible from patient to patient. For example, lymph flowing in either the superior or inferior mammary trunk may bypass the inferior or central group of axillary nodes and flow directly to the highest

Figure 63–3. Lymphatics of the breast and axilla.

group of axillary nodes. In general, however, the drainage of the breast is to the anterior axillary or subpectoral nodes, which are located deep to the lateral border of the pectoralis major muscle, close to the lateral thoracic artery. From these nodes, lymph travels to nodes in close proximity to the lateral portion of the axillary vein. The lymph then passes superiorly, via the axillary chain of lymph vessels and nodes. Eventually, the drainage reaches the highest nodes of the axilla. Although this is the most regular pattern of lateral and superior breast lymphatic drainage, other paths are common, particularly when the lateral and superiorly directed channels are obstructed, for example, by tumor masses. When plugging occurs, the following pathways are available for lymphatic flow from the breast:

a. From the breast directly to the highest axillary node, completely bypassing all other axillary nodal tissue. This may occur with superior quadrant breast tumors.

b. From the breast directly to the subscapular group of axillary nodes, subsequently progressing ventrally and superiorly through channels lying close to the axillary vein.

c. From the breast directly to the most inferior group of supraclavicular cervical nodes. Supraclavicular nodes, however, are more commonly involved via direct extension from the apical axillary nodes.

d. From the breast across the sternal midline to the lymphatics of the contralateral breast.

e. From the breast directly to the contralateral axilla.

f. From the breast to the internal mammary group of nodes when the primary breast tumor is in a medial quadrant.

g. Rarely, from the breast to lymphatics that drain to lymphatics closely related to the sheaths of the superior segments of the rectus abdominis and external oblique muscles and in turn drain inferiorly toward the upper abdominal wall, the diaphragm, and the intra-abdominal viscera (especially the liver).

D. NERVES ENCOUNTERED DURING AXILLARY DISSECTION

The lateral and anterior cutaneous branches of T4–6 supply the cutaneous tissues covering the breasts. Two major nerves and two smaller groups of nerves are in close proximity to the breast area and thus assume importance in breast surgery:

(1) The **thoracodorsal nerve,** a branch of the posterior cord of the brachial plexus (C5–7), runs inferiorly along with the subscapular artery lying close to the posterior axillary wall and the ventral surface of the subscapular muscle. The nerve innervates the superior half of the latissimus dorsi muscle and is usually surrounded by a large venous plexus that drains into the subscapular veins.

(2) The **long thoracic nerve** (nerve of Bell) arises from the anterior primary divisions of C5–7 at the level of the lower half of the anterior scalene muscle. In the neck, the nerve descends dorsal to the trunks of the brachial plexus on the inferior segment of the middle scalene muscle. Further descent places it dorsal to the clavicle and the axillary vessels. On the lateral thoracic wall, it descends on the external surface of the serratus anterior muscle along the anterior axillary line. The long thoracic nerve supplies filaments to each of the digitations of the serratus anterior muscle. Injury to this nerve results in a "winged" scapula.

(3) The **intercostal brachial nerves** are three relatively minor cutaneous nerves that supply the skin of the medial surface of the upper arm. They transverse the lateral chest wall to the upper inner surface of the arm, passing across the base of the axilla.

(4) The **medial and lateral pectoral nerves** supply the two pectoral muscles and pass from the axilla to the lateral chest wall. At the lateral chest wall, they pierce the costocoracoid membrane. The medial pectoral nerve arises from the medial cord of the brachial plexus; the lateral pectoral nerve arises from the lateral cord of the plexus.

■ DISEASES OF THE BREAST

FIBROCYSTIC CHANGE

ESSENTIALS OF DIAGNOSIS

- *Painful, often multiple, usually bilateral mobile masses in the breast.*
- *Rapid fluctuation in the size of the masses is common.*
- *Frequently, pain occurs or increases as does size during the premenstrual phase of the cycle.*
- *Most common age is 30–50 years; occurrence is rare in postmenopausal women.*

General Considerations

Fibrocystic disease, or chronic cystic mastitis, formerly known as mammary dysplasia, is the most frequent benign condition of the breast. It is most common in

Figure 63–4. Algorithm for the use of fine-needle aspiration (FNA) and fine-needle aspiration cytology (FNAC) for office triage of breast lumps. (Reproduced with permission from Hindle WH: *Breast Disease for Gynecologists.* Appleton & Lange, 1990.)

women 30–50 years of age, but rare in postmenopausal women; this suggests that it is related to ovarian activity. The term **mammary dysplasia,** or **fibrocystic disease,** is imprecise and encompasses a wide spectrum of pathologic entities. The lesions are always associated with benign changes in the breast epithelium, some of which are found so frequently in normal breasts that they are probably variants of normal breast histology, but have, unfortunately, been termed a "disease."

The microscopic findings of fibrocystic change include cysts (gross and microscopic), papillomatosis, adenosis, fibrosis, and ductal epithelial hyperplasia.

Clinical Findings

Fibrocystic change may produce an asymptomatic lump or lumps in the breast that are discovered by palpation, but pain or tenderness is often the presenting symptom and calls attention to the mass. There may be discharge from the nipple. In many cases, discomfort occurs or is increased during the premenstrual phase of the cycle, at which time the cysts tend to enlarge. Some women seem to have more severe pain that is constant and not related to the menstrual cycle (**mastodynia**). Fluctuation in size and rapid appearance or disappearance of a breast mass are common in cystic changes. Multiple or bilateral masses are also common, and many patients give a history of a transient lump in the breast or cyclic breast pain. In many women, caffeine seems to potentiate these symptoms. However, the role of caffeine as a direct cause of these symptoms has never been proven. Pain, fluctuation in size, and multiplicity of lesions are the features most helpful in differentiation from carcinoma. However, if a dominant mass is present, it should be evaluated by biopsy.

Differential Diagnosis

Pain, fluctuation in size, and multiplicity of lesions help to differentiate these lesions from carcinoma and the benign entity of fibroadenoma. Final diagnosis often rests on biopsy and pathologic determination. Mammography may be helpful, but the breast tissue in these young women may be too radiodense to allow a meaningful evaluation. Aspiration and/or sonography may be useful in differentiating a cystic from a solid mass.

Treatment

Because the condition of fibrocystic change is frequently indistinguishable from carcinoma on the basis of clinical findings, it is often advisable to proceed with biopsy and histologic examination of suspicious lesions, which is usually done under local anesthesia. Surgery should be conservative, as the primary objective is to exclude a malignant process. Simple mastectomy or extensive removal of breast tissue is rarely, if ever, indicated for fibrocystic change.

When the diagnosis of fibrocystic change has been established by previous biopsy or is practically certain, because the history is classic, aspiration of a discrete mass suggestive of a cyst is another option. The patient is reexamined at intervals thereafter. If no fluid is obtained or if the fluid is bloody, if a mass persists after aspiration, or if anytime during follow-up a persistent lump is noted, biopsy should be performed (Fig 63–4).

Breast pain associated with generalized fibrocystic change is best treated by avoiding trauma and by wearing a bra with adequate support.

The role of caffeine consumption in the development and treatment of fibrocystic change is controversial. Many patients report relief of symptoms after abstinence from coffee, tea, and chocolate.

Prognosis

Exacerbations of pain, tenderness, and cyst formation may occur at any time until menopause, when symptoms subside. The patient should be advised to examine her own breasts each month just after menstruation, conventionally 5 days after the last day of bleeding, and to inform her physician if a mass appears. Because the risk of breast cancer in women with fibrocystic change showing proliferative or atypical changes in the epithelium is higher than that of women in general, follow-up examinations at regular intervals should be arranged.

FIBROADENOMA OF THE BREAST

This common, benign neoplasm occurs most frequently in young women, usually within 20 years after puberty. It is somewhat more frequent and tends to occur at an earlier age in black women than in white women. Multiple tumors in one or both breasts are found in 10–15% of patients.

The typical fibroadenoma is a round, firm, discrete, relatively movable, nontender mass 1–5 cm in diameter. The tumor is usually discovered accidentally. Clinical diagnosis in young patients is generally not difficult. In women older than age 30 years, cystic disease of the breast and carcinoma of the breast must be considered in the differential. Cysts can be identified by ultrasound examination and aspiration. Fibroadenoma does not normally occur after menopause, but postmenopausal women may occasionally develop fibroadenoma after administration of estrogenic hormone.

Treatment is either excision under local anesthesia or close, careful, clinical observation.

Cystosarcoma phyllodes is a type of fibroadenoma with cellular stroma that tends to grow rapidly. This tumor may reach a large size and if inadequately excised will recur locally. The lesion can be, but rarely is, malignant. Treatment is by local excision of the mass with a margin of surrounding normal breast tissue. The treatment of malignant cystosarcoma phyllodes is more controversial. In general, complete removal of the tumor and a rim of normal tissue should prevent recurrence. Because these tumors tend to be large, simple mastectomy is often necessary to achieve complete local control.

NIPPLE DISCHARGE

General Considerations

The most common causes of nipple discharge in the nonlactating breast are carcinoma, intraductal papilloma, and fibrocystic change with ectasia of the ducts. The important characteristics of the discharge and some other factors to be evaluated by history and physical examination are as follows:

(1) Nature of discharge (serous, bloody, or other)
(2) Association with or without a mass
(3) Unilateral or bilateral
(4) Single duct or multiple duct discharge
(5) Discharge that is spontaneous, persistent or intermittent, or must be expressed
(6) Discharge produced by pressure at a single site or by general pressure on the breast
(7) Relation to menses
(8) Premenopausal or postmenopausal
(9) History of oral contraceptive use or estrogen replacement for postmenopausal symptoms

Differential Diagnosis

Unilateral, spontaneous serous or serosanguineous discharge from a single duct is usually caused by an intraductal papilloma or, more infrequently, by an intraductal malignancy. In either case, a palpable mass may not be present. The involved duct may be identified by pressure at different sites around the nipple at the margin of the areola. Bloody discharge is more suggestive of cancer but is usually caused by a benign papilloma in the duct. Cytologic examination of the discharge should be accomplished and may identify malignant cells, but negative findings do not rule out cancer, which is more likely in women older than age 50 years. In either situation, the involved duct, and a mass if present, should be excised.

In premenopausal women, spontaneous multiple duct discharge, unilateral or bilateral, most markedly just prior to menstruation, is often caused by fibrocystic change. Discharge may be green or brownish. Papillomatosis and ductal ectasia are also diagnostic possibilities. Biopsy may be necessary to establish the diagnosis of a diffuse nonmalignant process. If a mass is present, it should be surgically removed.

Milky discharge, galactorrhea, from multiple ducts in the nonlactating breast may occur in certain syndromes (Chiari-Frommel syndrome, Argonz-Del Castillo [Forbes-Albright] syndrome), usually as a result of increased secretion of pituitary prolactin. An endocrine work-up is generally indicated. Drugs of the chlorpromazine family and contraceptive pills may also cause milky discharge that ceases on discontinuance of the medication. Other medical illnesses may less frequently cause galactorrhea (Table 63–1).

Oral contraceptive agents may cause clear, serous, or milky discharge from a single duct, but multiple duct discharge is more common. The discharge is most prevalent prior to menstruation and ceases with discontinuation of the medication. If it does not and the discharge is from a single duct, surgical exploration should be considered.

Purulent discharge can originate in a subareolar abscess and may require excision of the abscess and related lactiferous sinus.

When localization is not possible and no mass is palpable, the patient should be re-examined every week for 1 month. When unilateral discharge persists, even without definite localization or palpable mass, exploration must be considered. The alternative is careful follow-up at intervals of 1–3 months with accompanying mammography. Cytologic examination of nipple discharge for exfoliated cancer cells may be helpful in yielding a diagnosis.

Table 63–1. Causes of galactorrhea.

Idiopathic

Drug induced
    Phenothiazines, butyrophenones, reserpine, methyldopa, imipramine, amphetamine, metoclopramide, sulpride, pimozide, oral contraceptive agents

Central nervous system (CNS) lesions
    Pituitary adenoma, empty sella, hypothalamic tumor, head trauma

Medical conditions
    Chronic renal failure, sarcoidosis, Schuller-Christian disease Cushing's disease, hepatic cirrhosis, hypothyroidism

Chest wall lesions
    Thoracotomy, herpes zoster

Reproduced, with permission, from Hindle WH: *Breast Disease for Gynecologists.* Appleton & Lange, 1990.

Chronic unilateral nipple discharge, especially if bloody, is an indication for resection of the involved ducts.

FAT NECROSIS

Fat necrosis is a rare condition of the breast but is of clinical importance because it produces a mass, often accompanied by skin or nipple retraction, that is clinically indistinguishable from carcinoma. Trauma is the presumed etiology, although only about half of patients recall a history of injury to the breast. Ecchymosis is occasionally observed in conjunction with the mass. Tenderness may or may not be present. If untreated, the mass associated with fat necrosis gradually disappears. Should the mass not resolve after several weeks, a biopsy should be considered. The entire mass should be excised, primarily to rule out malignant processes.

BREAST ABSCESS

During lactation and nursing, an area of redness, tenderness, and induration may develop in the breast. In its early stages, the infection can often be resolved while continuing nursing with the affected breast and administering an antibiotic. If the lesion progresses to form a palpable mass with local and systemic signs of infection, an abscess has developed and needs to be drained. At this point, nursing should be discontinued.

Less frequently, a subareolar abscess may develop in young or middle-age women who are not lactating. These infections tend to recur after simple incision and drainage unless the area is explored in a quiescent interval with excision of the involved lactiferous duct or ducts at the base of the nipple. Except for the subareolar type of abscess, infection in the breast is very rare unless the patient is lactating. Therefore, findings suggestive of abscess in the nonlactating breast require surgical evaluation with biopsy of indurated tissue.

MALFORMATION OF THE BREAST

Many women consult their physicians for abnormalities in either the size or the symmetry of their breasts. Difference in size between the two breasts is common. If extreme, however, these differences may be corrected by cosmetic surgery, although the breast tissue in these individuals is otherwise normal.

Similarly, woman may complain of overly large breasts (macromastia). Studies fail to show any endocrinologic or pathologic abnormalities, and these patients may also be considered candidates for cosmetic surgery such as breast-reduction mammoplasty.

Less-common malformations of the breast include amastia, complete absence of one or both breasts, or the presence of accessory nipples and breast tissue along the embryologic milk line, which occurs in 1–2% of whites.

PUERPERAL MASTITIS

See Chapter 31.

■ CARCINOMA OF THE FEMALE BREAST

 ESSENTIALS OF DIAGNOSIS

- *Early findings: Single, nontender, firm to hard mass with ill-defined margins; mammographic abnormalities and no palpable mass.*
- *Later findings: Skin or nipple retraction; axillary lymphadenopathy; breast enlargement, redness, edema, brawny induration, peau d'orange, pain, fixation of mass to skin or chest wall.*
- *Late findings: Ulceration; supraclavicular lymphadenopathy; edema of arm; bone, lung, liver, brain, or other distant metastases*

General Considerations

Cancer of the breast is the most common cancer in women, excluding nonmelanoma skin cancers. After lung cancer, it is the second most common cause of cancer death for women. The American Cancer Society estimates 212,930 new cases of cancer of the breast and 40,870 deaths in 2005. These figures include male breast cancer, which accounts for less than 1% of annual breast cancer incidence. Despite a slight increase in yearly incidence, the cancer death rate for malignancies of the breast decreased an average of 2.3% per year from 1990 to 2001. The probability of developing the disease increases throughout life. The mean and the median age of women with breast cancer is 60–61 years.

At the present rate of incidence, a woman's risk of developing invasive breast cancer in her lifetime from *birth* to *death* is 1 in 8. This figure is from the Surveillance, Epidemiology, and End Results Program (SEER) of the National Cancer Institute (NCI) and is often cited but needs clarification. The data include all age groups in 5-year intervals with an open-ended interval at 85 years and above. When calculating risk, each age interval is weighted to account for the increasing risk of breast cancer with increasing age. A woman's risk of being diagnosed with breast cancer by age is as follows:

- By age 30: 1 in 2000
- By age 40: 1 in 233
- By age 50: 1 in 53
- By age 60: 1 in 22
- By age 70: 1 in 13
- By age 80: 1 in 9
- In a lifetime: 1 in 8

Although a woman's lifetime risk of developing breast cancer is 1 in 8, it must be emphasized that she still has a 7 in 8 chance of never developing breast cancer. Women whose mothers or sisters had breast cancer are more likely to develop the disease than controls. The presence of an inherited genetic mutation in the *BRCA1* and *BRCA2* genes, which accounts for approximately 5% of all breast cancers, also places women at increased risk of being diagnosed with breast cancer. Risk is increased when breast cancer has occurred before menopause, was bilateral, or was present in two or more first-degree relatives such as a mother and sister. However, there is no history of breast cancer among female relatives in more than 90% of patients with newly diagnosed breast cancer. Nulliparous women and women whose first full-term pregnancy was after age 30 years have a slightly higher incidence of breast cancer than multiparous women. Late menarche and artificial menopause are associated with a lower incidence of breast cancer, whereas early menarche (before age 12 years) and late natural menopause (after age 50 years) are associated with a slight increase in risk of developing breast cancer. Fibrocystic change of the breast, when accompanied by proliferative changes, papillomatosis, or atypical epithelial hyperplasia, is associated with an increased incidence of cancer. A personal history of breast cancer is the greatest risk factor for subse-

quent breast cancer events. A woman who has had cancer in one breast is at increased risk of recurrence and second primary in that ipsilateral breast, as well as developing cancer in the contralateral breast. Women with cancer of the uterine corpus have a breast cancer risk significantly higher than that of the general population, and women with breast cancer have a comparably increased risk of endometrial cancer. In the United States, breast cancer is more common in whites than in nonwhites. The incidence of the disease among nonwhites, mostly African Americans, however, is increasing, especially in younger women. In general, rates reported from developing countries are low, whereas rates are high in developed countries, with the notable exception of Japan. Some of the variability may be a result of underreporting in the developing countries, but a real difference probably exists. Lifestyle factors such as diet, exercise, and increasing extent of antibiotic use are implicated as possible causes for this observed difference.

Women who are at greater-than-normal risk of developing breast cancer should be identified by their physicians and followed carefully. Screening programs involving periodic physical examination and mammography of asymptomatic high-risk women increase the detection rate of breast cancer and may improve the survival rate, although this has not yet been demonstrated. Unfortunately, more than 50% of women who develop breast cancer do not have significant identifiable risk factors.

Growth potential of tumor and resistance of host vary over a wide range from patient to patient and may be altered during the course of the disease. The doubling time of breast cancer cells ranges from several weeks in a rapidly growing lesion to nearly a year in a slowly growing one. If one assumes that the rate of doubling is constant and that the neoplasm originates in one cell, a carcinoma with a doubling time of 100 days may not reach clinically detectable size (1 cm) for about 8 years. On the other hand, rapidly growing cancers have a much shorter preclinical course and a greater tendency to metastasize to regional nodes or more distant sites before a breast mass is discovered.

The relatively long preclinical growth phase and the tendency of breast cancers to metastasize have led many clinicians to believe that breast cancer is a systemic disease at the time of diagnosis. Although it may be true that breast cancer cells are released from the tumor prior to diagnosis, variations in the host–tumor relationship may prohibit the growth of disseminated disease in many patients. For this reason, a pessimistic attitude concerning the management of localized breast cancer is not warranted, and many patients can be cured with proper treatment.

Staging

The physical examination of the breast and additional preoperative studies are used to determine the clinical stage of a breast cancer. Clinical staging is based on the TNM (tumor, node, metastasis) system of the Interna-

Table 63–2. Clinical staging of breast carcinoma.

Tis carcinoma in situ		**Stage 0**			
		Tis	N0	M0	
T1					
T1mic microinvasion ≤ 0.1 cm		**Stage I**			
T1a > 0.1 but ≤ 0.5 cm		T1	N0	M0	
T1b > 0.5 but ≤ 1.0 cm					
T1c > 1.0 but ≤ 2.0 cm		**Stage IIa**			
		T0	N1	M0	
T2 > 2 but ≤ 5 cm		T1	N1	M0	
		T2	N0	M0	
T3 > 5 cm					
		Stage IIb			
T4		T2	N1	M0	
T4a extension to chest wall		T3	N0	M0	
T4b edema or ulceration of skin					
T4c both T4a & T4b		**Stage IIIa**			
T4d inflammatory carcinoma		T0	N2	M0	
		T1	N2	M0	
N1 movable ipsilateral axillary lymph nodes; fixed ipsilateral axillary lymph nodes or clinically apparent[a] ipsilateral internal mammary nodes in the absence of clinically evident axillary lymph node metastasis		T3	N1	M0	
		T3	N2	M0	
		Stage IIIb			
		T4	N0	M0	
N2a fixed ipsilateral axillary lymph nodes		T4	N1	M0	
N2b clinically apparent ipsilateral internal mammary nodes and in the absence of clinically evident axillary lymph node metastasis		T4	N2	M0	
N3 ipsilateral infraclavicular lymph node(s) with or without axillary lymph node involvement, or in clinically apparent[a] ipsilateral internal mammary lymph node(s) and in the presence of clinically evident axillary lymph node metastasis; or metastasis in ipsilateral supraclavicular lymph node(s) with or without axillary or internal mammary lymph node involvement		**Stage IIIc**			
		Any T	N3	M0	
		Stage IV			
		Any T	any N	M1	
N3a ipsilateral infraclavicular lymph node(s)					
N3b ipsilateral internal mammary lymph node(s) and axillary lymph node(s)					
N3c ipsilateral supraclavicular lymph node(s)					

M1 distant metastasis

[a]Clinically apparent as shown by MRI.
Reproduced with permission from Fleming ID et al (editors): *AJCC Cancer Staging Manual*, 6th ed. Springer, 2002, p. 174.

tional Union Against Cancer. This classification considers tumor size, clinical assessment of axillary nodes, and the presence or absence of distant metastases. The assessment of the clinical stage is important in planning therapy. Histologic (or pathologic) staging is determined following surgery and along with clinical staging helps determine prognosis (Table 63–2).

Clinical Findings

The patient with breast cancer usually presents with a lump in the breast or an abnormal screening mammogram. Clinical evaluation should include assessment of the local lesion, including a bilateral mammogram, if not previously performed, and a search for evidence of metastases in regional nodes or distant sites. After the diagnosis of breast cancer has been confirmed by tissue biopsy, additional studies are often needed to complete the evaluation for distant metastases or an occult primary lesion in the other breast. Then, before any decision is made about treatment, all the available clinical data are used to determine the extent or "stage" of the patient's disease.

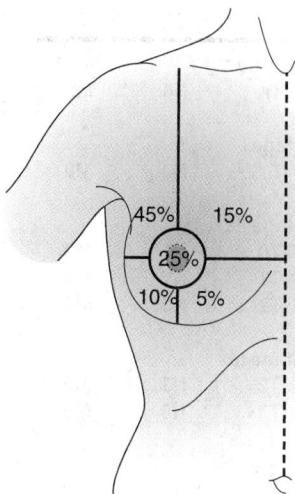

Figure 63-5. Frequency of breast carcinoma at various anatomic sites.

Figure 63-6. Palpation of axillary region for enlarged lymph nodes.

A. SYMPTOMS

When the history is taken, special note should be made of the onset and duration of menarche, pregnancies, parity, artificial or natural menopause, date of last menstrual period, previous breast lesions and/or biopsies, hormonal supplementation, radiation exposure, and a family history of breast cancer. Back or other bone pain may be the result of osseous metastases. Systemic complaints or weight loss should raise the question of metastases, which may involve any organ but most frequently the bones, liver, and lungs. The more advanced the cancer in terms of aggressive histologic features, size of primary lesion, local invasion, and extent of regional node involvement, the higher is the incidence of metastatic spread to distant sites. Lymph node involvement is the single most significant prognostic feature and increases with increasing tumor size and aggressive histologic features such as pathological grade.

The presenting complaint in approximately 70% of patients with breast cancer is a lump (usually painless) in the breast. Approximately 90% of breast masses are discovered by the patient herself. Less-frequent symptoms are breast pain; nipple discharge; erosion, retraction, enlargement, or itching of the nipple; and redness, generalized hardness, enlargement, or shrinking of the breast. Rarely, an axillary mass, swelling of the arm, or bone pain (from metastases) may be the first symptoms. Approximately 35–50% of women involved in organized screening programs have cancers detected by mammography only.

B. SIGNS

Figure 63–5 shows the relative frequency of carcinoma in various anatomic sites in the breast.

Inspection of the breast is the first step in physical examination and should be carried out with the patient sitting, arms at sides and then overhead. Abnormal variations in breast size and contour, minimal nipple retraction, and slight edema, redness, or retraction of the skin can be identified. Asymmetry of the breasts and retraction or dimpling of the skin can often be accentuated by having the patient raise her arms overhead or press her hands on her hips in order to contract the pectoralis muscles. Axillary and supraclavicular areas should be thoroughly palpated for enlarged nodes with the patient sitting (Fig 63–6). Palpation of the breast for masses or other changes should be performed with the patient both seated and supine with the arm abducted (Fig 63–7).

Breast cancer usually consists of a nontender, firm or hard lump with poorly delineated margins generally

Figure 63-7. Palpation of breasts. Palpation is performed with the patient supine and the arm abducted.

caused by local infiltration. Slight skin or nipple retraction is an important sign as it may affect staging. Minimal asymmetry of the breast may be noted. Very small (1–2-mm) erosions of the nipple epithelium may be the only manifestation of Paget's carcinoma. Watery, serous, or bloody discharge from the nipple is an occasional early sign but is more often associated with benign disease as discussed earlier.

A lesion smaller than 1 cm in diameter may be difficult or impossible for a clinical examiner to feel and yet may be discovered by the patient's self-examination. She should always be asked to demonstrate the location of the mass; if the physician fails to confirm the patient's suspicions, radiographic evaluation should be attempted and the examination should be repeated in 1 month. During the premenstrual phase of the cycle, increased innocuous nodularity may suggest neoplasm or may obscure an underlying lesion. If there is any question regarding the nature of an abnormality under these circumstances, the patient should be asked to return after her period.

The following are characteristic of advanced carcinoma: edema, redness, nodularity, or ulceration of the skin; the presence of a large primary tumor (> 5 cm); fixation to the chest wall; enlargement, shrinkage, or retraction of the breast; marked axillary lymphadenopathy; edema of the ipsilateral arm; supraclavicular lymphadenopathy; and distant metastases.

Spread of disease is often, though not always, systematic. Most frequently, metastases initially tend to involve regional lymph nodes first, which may be clinically palpable, before spreading to distant sites. With regard to the axilla, 1 or 2 movable, nontender, not particularly firm lymph nodes 5 mm or less in diameter are frequently present and are generally of no clinical significance. Any firm or hard nodes larger than 5 mm in diameter are highly suspicious for nodal metastases. Axillary nodes that are matted or fixed to skin or deep structures indicate locally advanced disease (at least stage III). Histologic studies show that microscopic metastases are present in approximately 40% of patients with clinically negative nodes. Conversely, if the examiner believes that the axillary nodes are involved, this is confirmed in approximately 85% of cases on pathologic examination. The incidence of positive axillary nodes increases with the size of the primary tumor, the degree of local invasiveness of the neoplasm and certain aggressive histologic features such as tumor grade.

Usually no nodes are palpable in the supraclavicular fossa. Firm or hard nodes of any size in this location or just beneath the clavicle (infraclavicular nodes) are indicative of locally advanced disease and suggest the strong possibility of distant metastatic sites of cancer. Biopsy or fine-needle aspiration to confirm nodal involvement in these areas is paramount. Ipsilateral supraclavicular nodes containing cancer indicate that the patient is in an advanced stage of the disease (stage IIIC). Edema of the ip-silateral arm, commonly caused by metastatic infiltration of regional lymphatics, is also a sign of advanced cancer.

C. SPECIAL CLINICAL FORMS OF BREAST CARCINOMA

1. Paget's disease—This refers to eczematous changes about the nipple and is associated with cancer in 99% of cases. An underlying mass is palpable in 60% of patients with Paget's disease. Of these masses, 95% are found to be an invasive cancer, mostly infiltrating ductal. For patients with Paget's disease and no palpable mass, 75% of breast biopsies are found to harbor ductal carcinoma in situ, a noninvasive breast malignancy. The nipple epithelium is infiltrated, but gross nipple changes are often minimal, and a tumor mass may not be palpable. The first symptom is often itching or burning of the nipple, with a superficial erosion or ulceration. The diagnosis is established by biopsy of the erosion.

Paget's disease is not common (approximately 1% of all breast cancers), but it is important because it appears innocuous. It is frequently diagnosed and treated as dermatitis or bacterial infection, leading to an unfortunate delay in detection. If detected early, Paget's disease rarely involves the axillary lymph nodes. Treatment can be modified radical mastectomy or breast-conservation therapy, which includes postlumpectomy radiation, with an expected 8-year disease-free survival of 90% or greater.

2. Inflammatory carcinoma—This is a clinical, pathologic entity defined as diffuse, brawny edema of the skin of the breast with an erysipeloid border, usually without an underlying palpable mass. Generally this is a clinical diagnosis with pathologic confirmation of tumor embolization in the dermal lymphatics by biopsy of the overlying skin. Inflammatory breast cancer is the most aggressive form of breast cancer. Luckily, it represents less than 5% of cases. At presentation, nearly 35% of patients with inflammatory breast cancer have evidence of metastases. The inflammatory component, often mistaken for an infectious process, is caused by the blockage of dermal lymphatics by tumor emboli, which results in edema and hyperemia. If a suspected skin infection does not rapidly respond (1–2 weeks) to a course of antibiotics, biopsy must be performed. Treatment usually consists of several cycles of neoadjuvant polychemotherapy followed by surgery or radiation depending on tumor response. Because of its severity and relatively small incidence, patients should be encouraged to enter into protocol therapy.

3. Occurrence during pregnancy or lactation—Cancer of the breast diagnosed in pregnancy has a ratio of occurrence from 1:3000 to 1:10,000. The association of pregnancy and breast cancer presents a therapeutic dilemma for the patient and the physician. Numerous studies differ regarding the prognosis; some show poorer outcome, while others demonstrate no difference. Termination of the pregnancy, formerly performed routinely in the first two trimesters, has not been demonstrated to improve outcome. In addition, the use of radiotherapy is contraindicated because of the potential for fetal damage. The use of most chemotherapy, for similar reasons, is debatable but generally accepted as safe based on retrospective reviews and experience.

In most instances, modified radical mastectomy in pregnancy is the minimal treatment of choice, with the possible exception of the latter part of the third trimester, wherein lumpectomy and radiotherapy in the puerperium may be considered.

4. Bilateral breast cancer—Clinically evident simultaneous bilateral breast cancer occurs in less than 1% of cases, but there is a 5–8% incidence of later occurrence of cancer in the second breast. Bilaterality occurs more often in women younger than age 50 years and is more frequent when the tumor in the primary breast is lobular. The incidence of second breast cancers increases directly with the length of time the patient is alive after her first cancer and is approximately 1.0% per year.

In patients with breast cancer, mammography should be performed before primary treatment and at regular intervals thereafter to search for occult cancer in the opposite breast. Routine biopsy of the opposite breast is usually not warranted.

D. MAMMOGRAPHY

Mammography is the most reliable means of detecting breast cancer before a mass can be palpated in the breast. Some breast cancers can be identified by mammography as early as 2 years before reaching a size detectable by palpation.

Although false-positive and false-negative results are occasionally obtained with mammography, the experienced radiologist can interpret mammograms correctly in approximately 90% of cases. For women with a history of mammographically occult lesions or otherwise at high risk for harboring cancer that is not detectable by mammogram, magnetic imaging resonance (MRI) and ultrasound may be warranted but they are not recommended for screening the general population.

Other than for screening, indications for mammography are as follows: (a) to evaluate each breast when a diagnosis of potentially curable breast cancer has been made, and at yearly intervals thereafter; (b) to evaluate a questionable or ill-defined breast mass or other suspicious change in the breast; (c) to search for an occult breast cancer in a woman with metastatic disease in axillary nodes or elsewhere from an unknown primary; (d) to screen at regular intervals a selected group of women who are at high risk for developing breast cancer (see below); (e) to screen women prior to cosmetic operations or prior to biopsy; and (f) to follow women who have been treated with breast-conserving surgery and radiation.

Patients with a dominant or suspicious mass must undergo biopsy regardless of mammographic findings. The mammogram should be obtained prior to biopsy so that other suspicious areas can be noted and the contralateral breast can be checked. Mammography is never a substitute for biopsy because it may not reveal clinical cancer in a very dense breast, as may be seen in young women with fibrocystic change, and it often does not reveal medullary-type histology breast cancer.

E. CYTOLOGY

Cytologic examination of nipple discharge or cyst fluid may be helpful on rare occasions. As a rule, mammography and breast biopsy are required when nipple discharge or cyst fluid is bloody or cytologically equivocal.

F. BIOPSY

The diagnosis of breast cancer depends ultimately on examination of tissue removed by biopsy. Treatment should never be undertaken without an unequivocal histologic diagnosis of cancer. The safest course is biopsy examination of all suspicious masses found on physical examination and, in the absence of a mass, of suspicious lesions demonstrated by mammography. Approximately 30% of lesions thought to be definitely cancer prove on biopsy to be benign, and approximately 15% of lesions believed to be benign are found to be malignant. These findings demonstrate the fallibility of clinical judgment and the necessity for biopsy.

The simplest method is needle biopsy, either by fine-needle aspiration (FNA) of tumor cells or by obtaining a small core of tissue with a stereotactic core-needle biopsy. A negative FNA should be followed by open biopsy because false-negative needle biopsies may occur in 10% of cancers.

The definitive diagnostic method is open biopsy under local anesthesia as a separate procedure prior to deciding on treatment. Palpable masses are readily evaluated by a general surgeon. With the aid of diagnostic radiology, a nonpalpable, radiographically detected mass may be biopsied with the use of needle localization. The patient need not be admitted to the hospital. Decisions on additional work-up for metastatic disease and on definitive therapy can be made and discussed with the patient after the histologic diagnosis of cancer is established. This approach has the advantage of avoiding unnecessary hospitalization and diagnostic procedures in many patients as cancer is found in the minority of patients who require biopsy for diagnosis of a breast lump.

In general, outpatient biopsy followed by definitive surgery at a later date gives patients time to adjust to the diagnosis of cancer, meet with members of the multidisciplinary team involved with managing breast cancer, and consider a second opinion, as well as alternative forms of treatment. Studies show no adverse effects from the short (1–2 weeks) delay of the two-step procedure, and this is the current recommendation of the NCI.

At the time of the initial biopsy of breast cancer, it is important for the physician to preserve a portion of the specimen for immunohistochemical staining for hormone and growth factor (eg, HER-2-Neu) receptors. Tumor analysis using reverse transcriptase polymerase chain reaction (RT-PCR) technology from pathologic specimens to assess the tumor recurrence risk is now available. Such tests can aid the patient and physician in the decision for further adjuvant therapy or not. At the time of pathologic confirmation of a breast cancer diagnosis, patients on hormone replacement therapy (HRT) should be instructed to stop hormone use until counseled by an oncologist.

G. Laboratory Findings

A complete blood cell count (CBC), chemistry panel including liver function tests (LFTs), and a β-human chorionic gonadotropin (β-hCG) in premenopausal patients to diagnose pregnancy should be obtained as part of the initial evaluation. An elevation in alkaline phosphatase or liver function may be an indication of distant metastatic disease and warrants further investigation. Hypercalcemia may be seen in advanced cases of metastatic cancer.

H. Radiographic Findings

A baseline posteroanterior and lateral chest radiograph may reveal pulmonary disease involvement, which could include parenchymal metastases, plural thickening or studding, and effusions. A chest x-ray also provides for a radiographic evaluation of the cardiac silhouette prior to interventions, which could tax the cardiovascular system such as anthracycline chemotherapy, trastuzumab (Herceptin) and radiation therapy. Computed tomography (CT) scans of the brain and liver should be obtained sparingly and are generally reserved for locally advanced cases (stage IIA or IIB or greater), as well as early stage cases in which there is a strong clinical suspicion of metastatic disease. Magnetic resonance imaging (MRI) scans of the previously surgically altered breast in which there is a question of malignancy, or in the T0 N1 patient, may be helpful in better characterizing the soft tissue of the breast, but are otherwise not routinely used.

I. Radionuclide Scanning

Bone scans using technetium 99m–labeled phosphonates are an important tool for the evaluation of metastatic breast cancer. There is no role for this imaging in screening or in the routine work-up of a patient. The incidence of a positive bone scan increases with advancing disease stage. Stages I and II patients have a 7% and 8% possibility, respectively, of having a positive bone scan, whereas a stage III patient has roughly a 25% risk. Therefore bone scans are reserved for the locally advanced patient (stage IIB [T3 N1 M0] or greater) with

elevated alkaline phosphatase, or for the patient in whom there is clinical suspicion for metastatic disease.

Positron emission tomography (PET) is a promising tool in the staging and metastatic evaluation of breast cancer. Most often it is used for defining the extent of recurrent or metastatic disease and monitoring treatment response. PET is a diagnostic modality that is complementary to conventional studies such as bone scintigraphy and CT. Its role has not yet been firmly established or defined in the setting of breast cancer. Consequently, clinicians should resist the inclination to consider PET a substitute for the conventional staging studies and metastatic evaluation of patients with breast cancer.

Early Detection

A. Screening Programs

Mammography remains the single best screening procedure for the early detection of breast cancer. Both physical examination and mammography are necessary for maximum yield in detecting early breast cancer, as approximately 40% of early malignancies can be discovered only by mammography and another 40% can be detected by palpation. In general, depending on a woman's age and the density of her breasts, the sensitivity of mammography is 70–90% and its specificity is greater than 90%. Yearly mammogram screening among women continues to increase so that in 1997, roughly 85% of women had had a mammogram at least once previously. This was an increase of 15% from 1990 and of 47% from 1987. Women of color, however, have more advanced stages of disease at the time of diagnosis and are less likely to engage in screening practices than white women. It is postulated that socioeconomic status, education, and medical access may account for these differences.

Despite a consensus on the importance of mammographic screening, mammography has still not been demonstrated unequivocally to decrease breast cancer mortality across all age groups. In women between 50 and 69 years of age, there is reasonable evidence, based largely on 8 randomized controlled trials, that screening mammography is beneficial. In elderly patients, however, the optimal frequency of screening is still unknown. For younger women, the evidence is also not entirely clear. In the age group 40–49 years, there appears to be a small benefit, but this benefit emerges only after meta-analyses with varying levels of statistical significance and confidence intervals. Nevertheless, in the Health Insurance Plan of Greater New York screening study from the United States, which with 18 years has the longest follow-up of any randomized mammography screening study, there was a 30% reduction in mortality in women older than 50 years of age. Despite academic debate and challenges and controversy in the news media, the consensus that screening mammography saves lives has been upheld.

Current screening recommendations from the American College of Radiology, the American Cancer Society, and the American Medical Women's Association call for annual mammograms starting at age 40 years. The American College of Obstetricians and Gynecologists calls for screening mammography every 1–2 years for women age 40–49 and annually thereafter. There is no recommendation for a "baseline" examination prior to age 40 years, nor is there any evidence to support this practice in women younger than this age. Women with a first-degree relative who had breast cancer typically are requested to obtain a first mammogram 5 years prior to the age at which the relative was diagnosed with breast cancer. Mammographic patterns are an unreliable predictor of the risk of developing breast cancer.

Breast ultrasonography is very useful in distinguishing cystic from solid lesions but should be used only as a supplement to physical examination and mammography in screening for breast cancer.

B. SELF-EXAMINATION

Once women have reached puberty and start to develop breasts, breast self-examination should be encouraged. Initially, this allows the woman to become acquainted with her body and foster good self-examination habits for the future. All women older than age 20 years should be advised to examine their breasts monthly. Premenopausal women should perform the examination 5–7 days after the completion of the menstrual cycle when breast tissue is less dense. High-risk patients may wish to perform another self-examination in mid-cycle. Postmenopausal women should pick a particular date each month, perhaps the anniversary of a special occasion, to perform breast self-examination.

Breast self-examination consists of two parts: inspection and palpation. Using a mirror, the breasts should be inspected while standing with arms at sides, with arms overhead and palms pressed together, and with hands on hips pressing firmly to contract the pectoralis muscles. Gross asymmetry of the breasts, masses, and skin dimpling and/or retraction may be more apparent through the use of these maneuvers. In the supine position, each breast should be palpated with the fingertips of the opposite hand. Numerous techniques are advocated but methodical palpation is the goal.

The American Cancer Society publishes instructive guides, which can be viewed online at www.cancer.org. Their recommendations, along with breast self-examination starting at age 20 years, are for a clinical breast examination to be performed by a health professional at least once every 3 years between the ages of 20 and 39 years. After age 40 years, a clinical breast examination should be performed annually. Physicians should instruct women in the technique of self-examination and advise them to report at once for medical evaluation if a mass or other abnormality is discovered. Many women report easier detection of breast abnormalities when the skin is moist while bathing or showering.

C. GENETIC TESTING

A positive family history of breast cancer is recognized as a risk factor for the subsequent development of breast cancer. With the discovery of two major breast cancer predisposition genes, *BRCA1* (17q21) and *BRCA2* (13q12-13), there has been increasing interest in genetic testing. Mutations in these two genes are associated with an elevated risk for breast cancer, as well as ovarian, colon, prostate, and pancreatic cancers. Of all women with breast cancer, approximately 5–10% may have mutations in *BRCA1* or *BRCA2*. The estimated risk of a patient developing cancer with a *BRCA1* or *BRCA2* mutation is believed to be between 40% and 85%. Particular mutations may be more common in specific ethnic groups like the Ashkenazi Jewish population. Genetic testing is available and may be considered for members of high-risk families. Currently, there are no established guidelines or recommendations for genetic testing. In general, women diagnosed with breast cancer before age 40 years, women with a first-degree relative diagnosed with breast cancer before age 50 years, and women with a family history that includes male breast or multiple, significant neoplasms such as ovarian, colon, and pancreatic cancer, are potential candidates for testing. Because of the complexities of genetic testing, genetic counseling before and after testing is necessary.

Differential Diagnosis

The lesions most often to be considered in the differential diagnosis of breast cancer include, in order of frequency, fibrocystic change, fibroadenoma, intraductal papilloma, and fat necrosis. The differential diagnosis of a breast lump should be established without delay by biopsy, either open or with localization guidance, or aspiration. Observation—even for a short, defined period—should be entertained with considerable caution.

Pathologic Types

Numerous pathologic subtypes of breast cancer can be identified histologically (Table 63–3). These pathologic types are distinguished by the histologic appearance and growth pattern of the tumor. In general, breast cancer arises either from the epithelial lining of the large or intermediate-sized ducts (ductal) or from the epithelium of the terminal ducts of the lobules (lobular). The cancer may be invasive or in situ. Most breast cancers arise from the intermediate ducts and are invasive (invasive ductal or infiltrating ductal), and most histologic types are merely subtypes of invasive ductal cancer with unusual growth patterns (colloid, medullary, scirrhous, etc). Ductal carcinoma that has not invaded the extraductal tissue is in-

Table 63–3. Histologic types of breast cancer.

Type	Percent Occurrence
Invasive ductal (not otherwise specified)	80–85
Medullary	3–6
Colloid (mucinous)	3–6
Tubular	3–6
Papillary	3–6
Invasive lobular	4–10
Noninvasive	15–20
Intraductal	80
Lobular in situ	20

traductal or ductal in situ. Lobular carcinoma may be either invasive or in situ.

The histologic subtypes have only slight bearing on prognosis when outcomes are compared after accurate staging. Colloid (mucinous), medullary, papillary, adenoid cystic, and tubular histologies are generally believed to have a more favorable prognosis. Other histologic criteria have been studied in an attempt to substratify patients based on features such as tumor differentiation, lymph vascular space invasion, and tumor necrosis. Although these characteristics are important, stage is predominant and paramount in predicting outcome.

The noninvasive cancers by definition lack the ability to spread. However, in patients whose biopsies show noninvasive intraductal cancer, associated invasive ductal cancers are present in 1–3% of cases. Lobular carcinoma in situ is considered by some to be a premalignant lesion that by itself is not a true cancer. It lacks the ability to spread but is associated with the subsequent development of invasive ductal cancer in 25–30% of cases within 15 years.

Hormone Receptor Sites

The presence or absence of estrogen receptors in the cytoplasm of tumor cells is of critical importance in managing patients with initial, recurrent and metastatic disease. To further emphasis this point, up to 60% of patients with metastatic breast cancer will respond to hormonal manipulation if their tumors contain estrogen receptors. However, fewer than 10% of patients with metastatic, estrogen receptor–negative tumors can be successfully treated with hormonal manipulation.

Progesterone receptors may be an even more sensitive indicator than estrogen receptors of patients who may respond to hormonal manipulation. Up to 80% of patients with metastatic progesterone receptor-positive tumors seem to respond to hormonal manipulation. Receptors probably have no relationship to response to chemotherapy.

Estrogen receptors may be of prognostic significance, especially in the node-negative patient, but current evidence is still unclear. If there is a survival benefit, it is of a small magnitude, less than 10%. The defined role of establishing a tumor's hormone status is to help guide hormonal and systemic therapies. Two randomized trials (National Surgical Adjuvant Breast Project [NSABP] B-14 and B-20) have shown a disease-free survival and an overall survival advantage for women with node-negative, estrogen-positive tumors who received tamoxifen.

It is advisable to obtain an estrogen-receptor assay for every breast cancer at the time of initial diagnosis. Receptor status may change after hormonal therapy, radiotherapy or chemotherapy. The specimen requires special handling, and the laboratory should be prepared to process the specimen correctly.

Curative Treatment

All oncologic treatment may be classified as curative or palliative. Curative treatment intent is advised for early stage and locally advanced disease (clinical stages I to IIIC disease; see Table 63–2). Treatment intent is palliative for patients in stage IV disease and for previously treated patients who develop distant metastases or unresectable local recurrence.

A. THERAPEUTIC OPTIONS

1. Radical mastectomy—Historically, Halsted is credited with performing the first modern **radical mastectomy** in 1882 in the United States. This surgical procedure was the en bloc removal of the breast, pectoral muscles, and axillary lymph nodes. It was the standard surgical procedure performed for breast cancer in the United States from the turn of the 20th century until the 1950s. During the 1950s, emerging information about lymph node drainage patterns prompted surgeons to undertake the **extended radical mastectomy,** which is a radical mastectomy and the removal of the internal mammary lymph nodes. It was postulated that a more extensive dissection of the draining lymphatics would improve control rates and translate into improved survival. A randomized trial, however, proved no benefit to the extended radical mastectomy versus the radical mastectomy, and the former was abandoned. Moreover, the failure of the extended radical mastectomy underscored the complications and morbidity of breast cancer surgery. This morbidity coupled with inadequate disease control led surgeons to explore less invasive and disfiguring techniques. Currently, radical mastectomy is rarely indicated or performed. Even in settings where radical resection may be entertained, such as invasion of the pectoralis muscles or large tumors, less-invasive surgery coupled with adjuvant or neoadjuvant treatments like radiation and chemotherapy are preferred.

2. Modified radical mastectomy—Replacing radical mastectomy, the **modified radical mastectomy** (MRM) is the removal of the breast, underlying pectoralis major fascia but not the muscle, and evaluation of selected axillary lymph nodes. Variations of this procedure include sacrificing the pectoralis minor muscle or not, and retracting, splitting, or transecting the pectoralis major to access the apex of the axilla for dissection. Because it is less invasive and less disfiguring, MRM provides a better cosmetic and functional result than radical mastectomy. Two prospective randomized trials, single-institution data, and several retrospective studies all demonstrate no difference in disease-free or overall survival rates between radical mastectomy and MRM for early stage breast cancer. Until the early 1980s and the emergence of breast-conservation therapy (BCT), MRM was the standard treatment available to women for early stage cancer. For locally advanced breast cancer and when the patient is not a candidate for BCT, or if the patient is not motivated for breast conservation, MRM remains a valid treatment option. A **total mastectomy** (simple mastectomy) is the removal of the whole breast, like a MRM, without the axillary dissection. Because an axillary evaluation is critical for staging purposes, total mastectomy is not performed for invasive cancers and is generally reserved for in situ lesions with their low metastatic potential.

3. Breast conservation therapy—BCT involves a surgical procedure such as a **lumpectomy**—an excision of the tumor mass with a negative surgical margin—an axillary evaluation, and postoperative irradiation. Several other operations, more limited in the scope of surgical dissection than MRM, such as **segmental mastectomy, partial mastectomy,** and **quadrantectomy,** are also used in conjunction with radiation and are part of the surgical component of BCT. As a result of six prospective randomized trials that showed no significant difference in local relapse, distant metastases, or overall survival between conservative surgery with radiation and mastectomy, BCT has gained increasing acceptance as a treatment option for stages I and II breast cancers.

B. CHOICE OF LOCAL THERAPY

Breast cancer is a multidisciplinary disease in which surgeons, medical and radiation oncologists, radiologists, pathologists, nurses, and psychosocial support staff all play fundamental roles. Working with the patient, this team recommends the most appropriate treatment strategy. Clinical and pathologic stage (see Table 63–2), as well as biologic aggressiveness, are the principal determinants guiding local therapy, treatment strategy, and, ultimately, outcome. For early stage breast cancer, including node-positive cases, much of the decision for initial local therapy rests with the patient. MRM is always a valid choice for addressing the local treatment of breast cancer. A patient's decision to undergo MRM

does not necessarily obviate the role of radiation in the further management of breast cancer, and postmastectomy irradiation may still be recommended in approximately 20–25% of cases. To be a candidate for BCT, the patient must not be pregnant and cannot have multicentric breast cancer (evidence of cancer in more than 1 quadrant of the breast), locally advanced disease, diffuse microcalcifications on mammogram, or a prior history of ipsilateral breast irradiation. Relative contraindications are collagen-vascular disorders that could lead to a poor cosmetic outcome with irradiation and breast implants or psychiatric issues that would make close follow-up and surveillance difficult. These restrictions are only a portion of the decision-making process that must be completed before embarking on BCT.

Perhaps most importantly, the patient must be motivated and desire to maintain her breast in the face of a cancer diagnosis. This may entail some degree of physical, emotional, and psychological distress. For example, a patient may have to endure multiple re-excisions to obtain a negative surgical margin on the lumpectomy specimen. A patient may also experience resistance to BCT in areas where it is not commonly offered and where a multidisciplinary approach to breast cancer is not practiced. It has been shown that the surgical management of breast cancer differs considerably based on geographic location in the United States, independent of patient and tumor characteristics. Nevertheless, both physicians and patients pursue BCT because it allows the patient to preserve her breast without any decrement to survival, and the vast majority of women are pleased with the cosmetic result.

Because the treatment options for locally advanced and inflammatory breast cancers are in some ways less flexible than those for early stage breast cancer, it is even more critical to engage the patient in the decision-making process for the choice of initial therapy. Many different strategies, which include mastectomy and less-invasive surgeries, with or without neoadjuvant chemotherapy and adjuvant chemotherapy, radiation, and further maintenance interventions, are commonly used. In many settings, protocol therapy may be the most desirable treatment option.

Mastectomy

For about three-quarters of a century, radical mastectomy was considered standard therapy for breast cancer. The procedure was designed to remove the primary lesion, the breast in which it arose, the underlying muscle, and, by dissection in continuity, the axillary lymph nodes that are most often are the first site of regional spread beyond the breast. When radical mastectomy was introduced by Halsted, the average patient presented for treatment with locally advanced disease, and a relatively extensive procedure was often necessary just to remove all gross cancer. This is no longer the case. Patients now present with much smaller, less locally advanced lesions. Most of the patients in Halsted's original series would now be considered incurable by surgery alone, because they had extensive involvement of the chest wall, skin, and supraclavicular regions.

Although radical mastectomy is rarely performed today, MRM is a common initial local treatment for breast cancer. Radical mastectomy is seldom, if ever, indicated given advances in surgical technique and other more modern treatment modalities. Radical mastectomy has the disadvantage of being one of the most deforming of any of the available treatments for the management of primary breast cancer. Since the 1960s, MRM has supplanted the radical mastectomy because of its comparable disease control and a substantial decrease in morbidity and disfiguration.

In many cases, adjuvant therapy following MRM, eg, radiation, can even further reduce the incidence of local recurrence in certain patients with unfavorable tumor characteristics. In addition, three recent randomized trials of postmastectomy radiation, which confirmed a local-control advantage, demonstrated an overall survival benefit in certain subsets of both pre- and postmenopausal women. For patients with ≥ 4 positive lymph nodes or an advanced primary tumor, postmastectomy radiation is strongly recommended. The role of postmastectomy radiation in patients with 1–3 positive nodes is more nebulous. However, with increasing duration of follow-up of the three aforementioned randomized studies, the weight of evidence in favor of postmastectomy radiation for 1–3 nodes seems to be gathering strength. In addition, a prospective randomized intergroup trial enrolling patients with 1–3 nodes recently closed to accrual. Although it will take years to mature, definitive data surrounding the extent of benefit of postmastectomy chest wall radiation is forthcoming. When deciding on initial local therapy, therefore, a patient must keep in mind that choosing MRM does not necessarily exclude a recommendation for adjuvant radiation.

Breast-Conservation Therapy

As studies comparing radical mastectomy and MRM demonstrated no decrement in local control or survival, radical mastectomy has given way to MRM. With less-invasive surgery, there are fewer side effects, less morbidity, and, ultimately, an improvement in quality of life. Simple mastectomy performed alone, however, has an unacceptably high failure rate. (In part, this is because the lymph nodes are not removed. As many as 40% of patients with clinically negative nodes will have evidence of metastatic spread within these nodes at dissection, and roughly half of these patients subsequently develop regional recurrences.)

In the 1980s, six prospective randomized trials were conducted worldwide that showed no significant difference in local–regional relapse or overall survival between breast-conserving surgery and radiation versus MRM for early stage invasive breast cancer. Two of these studies included patients with node-positive breast cancer. With the addition of radiation to breast-conserving surgery techniques such as lumpectomy with an axillary evaluation, local failure is reduced to rates comparable to MRM with no compromise to overall survival.

The next step has been to perform breast-conserving surgery without the addition of adjuvant radiation. Two recent randomized trials confirmed the existence of a continuum of local control benefit to subsets of postmenopausal women treated with adjuvant tamoxifen and radiation versus tamoxifen without radiation. Similarly, in the setting of in situ breast cancer, radiation confers a local control benefit although the magnitude may vary from patient to patient. Several trials including a seminal study by the NSABP established the efficacy of BCT for noninvasive breast cancer. For in situ disease, a group from Van Nuys, California, has proposed a prognostic index to determine which patients might not benefit from or need radiation after excision. With the exception of a small number of highly selected cases, the work of this group has not yet produced reproducible results sufficient to justify omitting radiation as standard practice.

Axillary Evaluation

It is important to recognize that axillary evaluation is valuable both in planning therapy and in staging of the cancer. Surgery is extremely effective in preventing axillary recurrences. Although the removal of even occult cancer in axillary lymph nodes generally does not translate into an improvement in overall survival rates, regional failures will be lower. In addition, lymph nodes removed during the procedure can be pathologically assessed. This assessment is essential for the planning of adjuvant therapy, which is often recommended for patients with gross or occult involvement of axillary nodes.

A standard alternative to formal axillary dissection for the pathologic assessment of the clinically negative axilla is sentinel lymph node biopsy (SLNB). This procedure uses a tracer material that is injected into the tumor bed to map the tumor drainage to the primary or "sentinel" axillary lymph node(s). The sentinel lymph node is excised and pathologically examined. If the sentinel lymph node is found to harbor metastatic disease, a subsequent formal dissection is done. Conversely, if the sentinel lymph node is negative, no further surgical evaluation need be performed. Although this procedure relies heavily on the surgeon's expertise with a new technique and has some inherent limitations, SLNB is another step toward less-invasive breast-cancer management. Potential side effects and complications are minimized, and recovery is quick without sacrificing diagnostic or therapeutic results. A practical example of the benefits of SLNB is that, when used in conjunction with BCT, reported rates of lymphedema are lower than with axillary dissection.

Current Recommendations

I believe that BCT, which includes radiation, with an axillary evaluation or MRM is the best initial local treatment for most patients with potentially curable carcinoma of the breast. It cannot be overemphasized, however, that a diagnosis of breast cancer should be managed with a multidisciplinary approach and treatment should be individualized. Treatment of the axillary nodes is not indicated, although evaluation may be given size and grade of the primary lesion, for noninvasive cancers, because by definition in situ lesions do not have metastatic potential. Nevertheless, axillary nodal metastases are detected in a small minority of cases, most of which are subsequently found to harbor microinvasive disease.

Preoperatively, full discussion with the patient regarding the rationale for BCT and mastectomy, as well as the manner of coping with the cosmetic and psychological effects of the operation, is essential. Patients often have numerous questions about BCT and MRM and wish detailed explanations of the risks and benefits of the various procedures. If a patient decides on MRM, breast reconstruction should be discussed. Time spent preoperatively in educating the patient and her family is time well spent.

Adjuvant Systemic Therapy

A. CHEMOTHERAPY

Cytotoxic chemotherapy is commonly offered to women as adjuvant treatment for early stage, as well as locally advanced, breast cancer. The goal of adjuvant chemotherapy is to eliminate occult microscopic metastases that are often responsible for late recurrences. It is systemic treatment and should not be confused with efforts to address known local disease. In the past, only premenopausal women with lymph node-positive cancers were routinely candidates for cytotoxic chemotherapy. For a host of reasons, recent guidelines recommend the use of chemotherapy on a more individualized basis and thus broaden the scope of who may be a candidate for therapy. Node-negative patients are now stratified into risk categories to help guide the decisions for adjuvant systemic therapy (Table 63–4).

The National Institutes of Health (NIH) Consensus Statement on Adjuvant Therapy for Breast Cancer recommends that chemotherapy be offered to most women with localized breast cancer > 1 cm regardless of nodal, menopausal or hormone receptor status. Polychemotherapy (≥ 2 agents) is superior to single-agent

Table 63–4. NIH consensus conference on adjuvant treatment for women with breast cancer risk categories for node-negative patients.

	Low Risk (All listed factors)	Intermediate Risk	High Risk (≥ 1 factor)
Tumor size	< 1.0 cm	1–2 cm	> 2 cm
ER or PR	+	+	–
Tumor grade	Grade I	Grade I–II	Grade II–III

Abbreviations: ER, estrogen receptor; NIH, National Institutes of Health; PR, progesterone receptor.

chemotherapy. Duration for 3–6 months or 4–6 cycles appears to offer optimal benefit without subjecting the patient to undue toxicity associated with more prolonged treatment, which adds little benefit in terms of overall outcome. Cytotoxic chemotherapy with an anthracycline-based (doxorubicin [A] or epirubicin [E]) regimen is favored, as a small but statistically significant improvement in survival has been demonstrated compared with nonanthracycline-containing regimens. The cardiac toxicity caused by anthracyclines is not considered detrimental in women without significant cardiac disease but does occur in 1% of cases or less. Nevertheless, traditional regimens using 6 cycles of cyclophosphamide, methotrexate, and 5-fluorouracil (CMF), which do not cause alopecia, are not necessarily inferior to regimens now commonly used, such as 4 cycles of doxorubicin and cyclophosphamide (AC). Alterations in dose schedule (eg, "dose-dense" regimens) also offer advantages over other combinations and administrations of chemotherapy for well-defined patient populations. The choice of adjuvant chemotherapy is complex. The medical oncologist must consider multiple tumor and patient features and individualize treatment for breast cancer patients.

Several areas concerning chemotherapy have generated considerable interest but lack conclusive evidence. For instance, the current data support the administration of taxanes (paclitaxel or docetaxel) in node-positive patients with estrogen receptor-negative tumors. By extrapolation and some inference, however, most node-positive patients are offered a taxane in addition to other standard chemotherapy agents. For node-negative patients, there is no direct evidence to justify their routine use but consideration is often given to individual cases. High-dose chemotherapy with bone marrow or stem cell rescue is also not recommended. There is no evidence that high-dose regimens are superior to standard-dose polychemotherapy. Stem cell support or bone marrow transplant should be offered only on protocol.

Table 63–5. Summary of NIH conference on adjuvant treatment for women with axillary node–negative breast cancer.

Patient Group	Low Risk	Intermediate Risk	High Risk
Premenopausal ER/PR–	None or TAM	TAM + CT TAM Ablation GnRH	CT + TAM CT + Ablation/GnRH CT + TAM + Ablation/GNRH
Premenopausal ET/PR–	N/A	N/A	CT
Postmenopausal ER/PR +	None or TAM	TAM + CT TAM	TAM + CT TAM
Postmenopausal ER/PR–	N/A	N/A	CT
> 70 years	None or TAM	TAM TAM ± CT	TAM ± CT if receptor–

Abbreviations: Ablation, ovarian ablation; CT, chemotherapy; ER, estrogen receptor; GnRH, gonadotropin-releasing hormone analogue; PR, progesterone receptor; TAM, tamoxifen.

Further investigations need to be performed to clarify the role of high-dose regimens and new chemotherapy as well as biologic agents and dosing schedules. Trials need to enroll more patients older than age 70 years to assess the benefits and toxicities of adjuvant chemotherapy in this population. Finally, studies designed to measure quality of life need to be done to place the benefits versus toxicity question of adjuvant therapies into context.

B. HORMONAL THERAPY

Adjuvant hormonal therapy or manipulation is recommended for all women whose breast cancer expresses hormone receptors. Even if the tumor does not express estrogen hormone receptor protein but only progesterone, hormonal therapy may be beneficial. This recommendation is made regardless of age, menopausal status, involvement or number of positive lymph nodes, or tumor size. The benefit of adjuvant hormonal therapy is seen across all subgroups of breast cancer patients, with both invasive and in situ lesions. Although the absolute decrease in recurrence, second primary breast cancer, and death may vary from group to group, there is a firmly established role for adjuvant hormonal intervention. Two possible exceptions, according to the NIH Consensus Conference, are the premenopausal patient with a tumor < 1 cm who wants to avoid estrogen loss and the elderly patient with a similar-size tumor and a history of thromboembolic events. Because of the overwhelming benefit of hormonal therapy, however, this determination should be made by an experienced medical oncologist (Tables 63–5 and 63–6).

Five years of tamoxifen is currently the most common regimen of hormonal therapy, although other forms of manipulation, such as ovarian ablation, exist. Randomized trials support the 5-year duration, which is superior to shorter courses and does not expose the patient to the increased risk of adverse effects associated with longer use. Furthermore, use longer than 5 years doesn't appear to enhance the long-term benefit seen with just 5 years of use. Although tamoxifen carries a slight increased risk of endometrial cancer and venous thromboembolism (5–6 events per 1000 patient-years of treatment), the benefits outweigh the risks for the vast number of patients. Surveillance screening procedures such as transvaginal ultrasound and endometrial biopsy are not necessary in asymptomatic patients on tamoxifen.

More recently, aromatase inhibitors (AI) such as anastrozole have been shown to be superior to tamoxifen in postmenopausal women with early stage, invasive breast cancer. In fact, anastrozole is superior to tamoxifen and was found to be superior to the combination of

Table 63–6. Summary of NIH consensus conference on adjuvant treatment for women with axillary node–positive breast cancer.

Patient Group	Treatment
Premenopausal ER/PR +	CT + TAM CT + Ablation/GnRH CT + TAM + Ablation/GnRH
Premenopausal	CT
Postmenopausal ER/PR +	TAM + CT
Postmenopausal ER/PR–	CT
> 70 years	TAM + CT if ER/PR–

Abbreviations: See Table 63–5.

anastrozole and tamoxifen, in terms of disease-free survival, time to recurrence, and the incidence of contralateral breast cancer. The toxicity profile of AIs is also favorable. Compared to tamoxifen, the use of AIs confers a smaller risk of endometrial cancer, venous thromboembolic events, and hot flashes for patients. However, AIs have a higher risk of musculoskeletal disorders and fractures when compared to tamoxifen. Ongoing studies seek to answer questions about the role of AIs in noninvasive, in situ cancers and in premenopausal patients.

Follow-Up Care

After primary treatment, breast cancer patients should be followed for life because of the long, insidious natural history of breast cancer. The goals of close breast cancer follow-up are to detect recurrences and second primaries after treatment in the ipsilateral breast and to detect new cancers in the contralateral breast. The risk of a second primary in the contralateral breast of a patient with a history of breast cancer is believed to be roughly 0.5–1% per year. Although there are no universally accepted guidelines, several consensus conferences have met to establish recommendations. After the completion of treatment, it is recommended that the patient undergo a physical examination every 4 months for the first 2 years, then every 6 months until year 5, and annually thereafter. A mammogram should be obtained annually for all patients. For patients who received irradiation, a chest radiograph is also obtained yearly. Routine laboratory tests including CBC, chemistry profile, and liver function tests can be ordered yearly, especially if the patient received chemotherapy, or else as needed. There is no role for routine bone scans or additional imaging unless the patient is symptomatic or there is clinical suspicion of an abnormality. Patients taking tamoxifen should have annual pelvic examinations and be counseled to report any irregular vaginal bleeding. Patients on AIs need periodic, usually annual, bone density studies to monitor their risk of developing osteopenia.

A. LOCAL RECURRENCE

The development of local recurrence correlates with stage and thus tumor size as well as the presence and number of positive axillary lymph nodes, margin status, nuclear grade, and histologic type. The median time to recurrence is roughly 4 years, with a 1–2% risk per year for the first 5 years and a 1% risk per year thereafter. Late failures occurring 15–20 years or more after treatment, however, do occur. The risk of local recurrence following BCT or MRM is generally < 15% 20 years after treatment. Positive axillary lymph nodes are prognostic for local failure at the chest wall following MRM, but they are not prognostic for a local failure following BCT.

The treatment of local recurrences depends on the initial local therapy. In the breast, failures after BCT can be treated with salvage mastectomy with salvage rates of approximately 50%. In general, there is no difference in overall survival for an isolated breast recurrence successfully treated with salvage mastectomy. Node failures are more ominous. Axillary failures have roughly a 50% 3–5-year disease-free survival and supraclavicular failures 0–20% 3-year disease-free survival. All chest wall abnormalities should be biopsied to rule out recurrence and resected with a wide local excision if possible. Adjuvant salvage therapies such as radiation, cytotoxic chemotherapy, and hormonal therapy may also be instituted.

Local recurrence may signal the presence of widespread disease and is an indication for bone and liver scans, posteroanterior and lateral chest x-rays, and other examinations as needed to search for evidence of distant metastases. When there is no evidence of metastases beyond the chest wall and regional nodes, radical irradiation for cure and complete local excision should be attempted. Most patients with locally recurrent tumors will develop distant metastases within 2 years. For this reason, many physicians use systemic therapy for treatment of patients with local recurrence. Although this seems reasonable, it should be pointed out that patients with local recurrence may be cured with local resection and/or radiation. Systemic chemotherapy or hormonal treatment should be used for patients who develop disseminated disease or for patients in whom local recurrence occurs following adequate local therapy.

B. EDEMA OF THE ARM

Lymphedema of the arm is a significant and often dreaded complication of breast cancer treatment. Lymphedema occurs as a result of lymphatic disruption and insult caused primarily by local treatment modalities like surgery and radiation. Although each of these modalities carries its own a risk with respect to arm edema, a combined modality approach further increases this risk. With a typical level I/II axillary lymph node dissection and radiation, the risk of lymph edema is roughly < 10%. This risk approached 30% when a more aggressive level III dissection was more commonly performed in the past. The rates of clinically significant lymphedema—that is edema, that affects function and is not merely detectable with sophisticated measurement tools—are generally considered to be much lower. With the advent of SLNB, lymphedema rates are expected to continue to improve.

Late or secondary edema of the arm may develop years after MRM, as a result of axillary recurrence or of infection in the hand or arm, with obliteration of lymphatic channels. Interestingly, there is usually no obvious initiating event causing late arm swelling in a patient with a history of breast cancer treatment.

C. Breast Reconstruction

Breast reconstruction, with the implantation of a prosthesis or transverse rectus abdominis myocutaneous flap (TRAM), is usually feasible after MRM. Reconstruction should be discussed with patients prior to mastectomy because it offers an important psychological focal point for recovery. Reconstruction is not an obstacle to the diagnosis of recurrent cancer.

Prognosis

The stage of breast cancer is the single most reliable indicator of prognosis. Patients with disease localized to the breast and no evidence of regional spread after microscopic examination of the lymph nodes have by far the most favorable prognosis. Estrogen and progesterone receptors appear to be an important prognostic variable because patients with hormone receptor-negative tumors and no evidence of metastases to the axillary lymph nodes have a much higher recurrence rate than do patients with hormone receptor-positive tumors and no regional metastases. The histologic subtype of breast cancer (eg, medullary, lobular, comedo) seems to have little significance in prognosis once these tumors are truly invasive.

As mentioned above, several different treatment regimens achieve approximately the same results when given to the appropriately selected patient. Localized disease can be controlled with local therapy—either MRM or BCT, which includes radiation. However, the criteria for selection of patients to be treated with conservative resection and radiation therapy require further clarification.

Many patients who develop breast cancer will ultimately die of breast cancer. The mortality rate of breast cancer patients exceeds that of age-matched normal controls for nearly 20 years. Thereafter, the mortality rates are equal, although deaths that occur among the breast cancer patients are often directly the result of tumor. Five-year statistics do not accurately reflect the final outcome of therapy.

When cancer is localized to the breast, with no evidence of regional spread after pathologic examination, the clinical cure rate with most accepted methods of therapy is 75–80%. Exceptions to this may be related to the hormonal receptor content of the tumor, tumor size, host resistance, or associated illness. Patients with small estrogen and progesterone receptor-positive tumors and no evidence of axillary spread probably have a 5-year survival rate of nearly 90%. When the axillary lymph nodes are involved with the tumor, the survival rate drops to 50–60% at 5 years, and probably to less than 25% at 10 years. In general, breast cancer appears to be somewhat more aggressive in younger than in older women, which may be related to the fact that relatively fewer younger women have estrogen receptor-positive tumors.

PALLIATIVE TREATMENT OF RECURRENT AND METASTATIC BREAST CANCER

This section discusses palliative therapy of disseminated disease incurable by surgery (stage IV).

Radiotherapy

Palliative radiotherapy may be advised for locally advanced cancers with distant metastases in order to control ulceration, pain and other manifestations in the breast and regional nodes. As part of multimodality treatment, radical irradiation of the chest wall and the axillary, internal mammary, and supraclavicular nodes should be undertaken in an attempt to cure locally advanced and inoperable lesions when there is no evidence of distant metastases. A small number of patients in this group are cured in spite of extensive breast and regional node involvement. Adjuvant chemotherapy also plays a valuable role in the treatment of such patients.

Palliative irradiation is also of value in the treatment of certain bone or soft tissue metastases to control pain or avoid pathological fracture. Radiotherapy is especially useful in the treatment of the isolated bony metastasis and chest wall recurrences.

Hormonal Therapy

Disseminated disease may respond to prolonged endocrine therapy such as ovarian ablation or administration of drugs that block hormone receptor sites or that block hormone synthesis or production. Hormonal manipulation is usually more successful in postmenopausal women. If treatment is based on the presence of estrogen receptor protein in the primary tumor or metastases, however, the rate of response is nearly equal in premenopausal and postmenopausal women. A favorable response to hormonal manipulation occurs in about one-third of patients with metastatic breast cancer. Of those whose tumors contain estrogen receptors, the response is approximately 60%, and perhaps as high as 80%, for patients whose tumors contain progesterone receptors as well. Tumors negative for both estrogen and progesterone receptors have response rates to hormonal therapy that are 10% or less.

Because the quality of life during a remission induced by endocrine manipulation is usually superior to a remission following cytotoxic chemotherapy, it may be best to try endocrine manipulation as a first-line systemic treatment for tumor recurrence or palliation.

As a general rule, only one type of systemic therapy should be given at a time. The systemic modality may be given in combination with a local or regional treatment if symptomatic lesions develop. For instance, it may be necessary to irradiate a destructive lesion of weight-bearing bone while the patient is taking a hormonal agent or chemotherapy. The palliative systemic regimen should be changed only if the disease is clearly progressing but not if disease appears stable. This is especially important for patients with destructive bone metastases, because minor changes in the status of these lesions are difficult to determine radiographically. A plan of therapy that would simultaneously minimize toxicity and maximize benefits is often best achieved by hormonal manipulation.

The choice of endocrine therapy depends on the menopausal status of the patient. Women within 1 year of their last menstrual period are considered to be premenopausal, whereas women whose menstruation ceased more than 1 year ago are usually classified as postmenopausal. The initial choice of therapy is referred to as primary hormonal manipulation; subsequent endocrine treatment is called secondary or tertiary hormonal manipulation.

A. PRIMARY HORMONAL THERAPY

In the past, ovarian ablation usually by bilateral surgical oophorectomy, chemical means or radiation was the standard method of hormone manipulation employed in premenopausal women with advanced breast cancer. However, it has subsequently become clear that tamoxifen is equally effective and has none of the attendant risks of surgical ablation of the ovaries. Tamoxifen is recommended as the treatment of choice for hormonal therapy in the premenopausal woman with advanced breast cancer. For postmenopausal patients, AIs and tamoxifen are the initial therapy of choice for metastatic breast cancer amenable to endocrine manipulation.

B. SECONDARY OR TERTIARY HORMONAL THERAPY

A favorable response to initial hormonal therapy with tamoxifen is predictive of future responses to hormonal maneuvers.

Other hormonal agents have been found effective in premenopausal patients. Gonadotropin-releasing hormone (GnRH) agonists that act on the pituitary to eventually suppress follicle-stimulating hormone (FSH) and leutenizing hormone (LH) and the pituitary–ovarian axis, thereby decreasing estrogen production, have been used since the 1980s. They are an alternative to oophorectomy if used alone or can be combined with tamoxifen to provide a slight improvement in progression-free survival and overall survival.

The use of AIs, which work by blocking the conversion of testosterone to estradiol and androstenedione to estrogen both in the adrenal cortex and in peripheral tissue, including breast cancers themselves, are effective in postmenopausal patients.

Progestins, megestrol acetate, and medroxyprogesterone acetate are alternative agents reserved mainly for cases resistant to tamoxifen.

Chemotherapy

Cytotoxic drugs should be considered for the treatment of metastatic breast cancer in the following instances: (a) if visceral metastases are present (especially brain or lymphangitic pulmonary spread), (b) if hormonal treatment is unsuccessful or the disease has progressed after an initial response to hormonal manipulation, or (c) if the tumor is estrogen and progesterone receptor-negative. With response rates of 35–55% in many series, the taxanes are quickly eclipsing the anthracyclines in the single-agent treatment of hormone-refractory metastatic breast cancer. Where once doxorubicin could achieve response rates of 40–50%, in some trials the taxanes seem to offer a small overall survival advantage. In addition, they are generally well tolerated with an acceptable side-effect profile. Questions about dosing, schedule of administration, and use with other agents, however, still have to be thoroughly answered.

Combination chemotherapy using multiple agents is appealing because, theoretically, the risk of drug resistance and cumulative toxicity is decreased. When compared to single-agent doxorubicin therapy, combination chemotherapy provides higher response rates and longer intervals until first progression. Nevertheless, the use of combination chemotherapy has never been shown to decrease drug resistance or toxicity in breast cancer. When combination chemotherapy has been compared to single-agent taxane therapy, although response rates were slightly lower, quality-of-life measurements were higher for the single agent. Thus, either a single-agent taxane or an anthracycline-containing combination regimen is frequently used as a first-line treatment. The use of cytotoxic chemotherapy or any other treatment modality should always be highly individualized, especially in the palliative setting.

Bisphosphonate Therapy

Subsequent to a definitive treatment of primary breast cancer, bone is the most common site of disseminated breast cancer recurrence. It is also the most common site of metastatic disease at initial presentation. Bone metastases are often detected with a bone scan obtained in the staging of locally advanced cases or obtained because of clinical suspicion in the previously treated patient. Confirmation with plain radiographs, MRI, and/or CT is frequently needed as nearly 10% of lytic lesions may not be detected with a nuclear medicine scan. These other radiographic studies also help to delineate the extent of the metastatic disease. After bone metastases are confirmed, bisphosphonate therapy should be started.

Although no survival advantage has been demonstrated, bisphosphonates have been shown to reduce bony as well as visceral metastases. Bisphosphonate therapy should be administered with other palliative systemic treatments such as hormonal manipulation or chemotherapy. It is typically given intravenously every 3–4 weeks for 2 years or for the duration of other systemic treatment.

REFERENCES

American Cancer Society. *Cancer Facts and Figures 2005.* American Cancer Society; 2005.

American College of Obstetricians and Gynecologists (ACOG) Breast Cancer Screening. ACOG Practice Bulletin, 42. Washington, DC: ACOG, 2003.

Andersson M et al: Tamoxifen in high-risk premenopausal women with primary breast cancer receiving adjuvant chemotherapy. Report from the Danish Breast Cancer Co-operative Group DBCG 82B Trial. Eur J Cancer 1999;35:1659.

Bishop JF et al: Initial paclitaxel improves outcome compared with CMFP combination chemotherapy as front-line therapy in untreated metastatic breast cancer. J Clin Oncol 1999;17:2355.

Baum M et al: Anastrozole alone or in combination with tamoxifen versus tamoxifen alone for adjuvant treatment of postmenopausal women with early-stage breast cancer: results of the ATAC (Arimidex, Tamoxifen Alone or in Combination) trial efficacy and safety update analyses. Cancer 2003;98:1802.

Citron ML et al: Randomized trial of dose-dense versus conventionally scheduled and sequential versus concurrent combination chemotherapy as postoperative adjuvant treatment of node-positive primary breast cancer: first report of Intergroup Trial C9741/Cancer and Leukemia Group B Trial 9741. J Clin Oncol 2003;21:2226.

Diel IJ et al: Reduction in new metastases in breast cancer with adjuvant clodronate treatment. N Engl J Med 1998;339:357.

Elmore JG et al: Screening for breast cancer. JAMA 2005;293:1245.

Erickson VS et al: Arm edema in breast cancer patients. J Natl Cancer Inst 2001;93:96.

Eubank WB, Manoff DA: Evolving role of positron emission tomography in breast cancer imaging. Semin Nucl Med 2005;35:84.

Fisher B et al: Twenty-year follow-up of a randomized trial comparing total mastectomy, lumpectomy, and lumpectomy plus irradiation for the treatment of invasive breast cancer. N Engl J Med 2003;347:1233.

Fisher B et al: Five versus more than five years of tamoxifen for lymph node-negative breast cancer: Updated findings from the National Surgical Adjuvant Breast and Bowel Project B-14 randomized trial. J Natl Cancer Inst 2001;93:684.

Fisher B et al: Tamoxifen and chemotherapy for lymph node-negative, estrogen receptor-positive breast cancer. J Natl Cancer Inst 1997;89:1673.

Fisher B et al: Tamoxifen in treatment of intraductal breast cancer: National Surgical Adjuvant Breast and Bowel Project B-24 randomized controlled trial. Lancet 1999;353:1993.

Fisher ER et al: Fifteen-year prognostic discriminates for invasive breast carcinoma. Cancer 2001;91:1679.

Fisher ER et al: Pathologic findings from the National Surgical Adjuvant Breast Project (NSABP) eight-year update of Protocol B-17: Intraductal carcinoma. Cancer 1999;86:429.

Freedman DA, Petitti DB, Robins JM: On the efficacy of screening for breast cancer. Int J Epidemiol 2004;33:43.

Freedman GM, Fowble BL: Local recurrence after mastectomy or breast-conserving surgery and radiation. Oncology (Huntingt) 2000;14:1561.

Fyles AW et al: Tamoxifen with or without breast irradiation in women 50 years of age or older with early breast cancer. N Engl J Med 2004;351:963.

Greene FL et al (editors): *AJCC Cancer Staging Manual*, 6th ed. Springer, 2002, p. 221.

Haagensen CD: *Diseases of the Breast*, 2nd ed. Saunders, 1971.

Harris JR et al: Consensus statement on postmastectomy radiation therapy. Int J Radiat Oncol Biol Phys 1999;44:989.

Hayes DF: Evaluation of patients after primary therapy. In: Harris JR et al (editors): *Diseases of the Breast*, 3rd ed. Lippincott, 2004.

Hughes KS et al: Lumpectomy plus tamoxifen with or without irradiation in women 70 years of age or older with early breast cancer. N Engl J Med 2004;351:971.

Kerlikowske K: Efficacy of screening mammography among women aged 40 to 49 years and 50 to 69 years: Comparison of relative and absolute benefit. J Natl Cancer Inst Monogr 1997;22:79.

Klauber-DeMore N et al: Sentinel lymph node biopsy: Is it indicated in patients with high-risk ductal carcinoma-in-situ and ductal carcinoma-in-situ with microinvasion? Ann Surg Oncol 2000;7:636.

Krag D et al: The sentinel node in breast cancer. N Engl J Med 1998;339:941.

McCarthy EP et al: Local management of invasive breast cancer. In: Harris JR et al (editors): *Diseases of the Breast*, 3rd ed. Lippincott, 2004.

Miner TJ et al: Sentinel lymph node biopsy for breast cancer: the role of previous biopsy on patient eligibility. Am Surg 1999;65:493.

Moskowitz MA: Mammography use helps to explain differences in breast cancer stage at diagnosis between older black and white women. Ann Intern Med 1998;128:729.

Myers RE et al: Baseline staging tests in primary breast cancer: a practice guideline. CMAJ 2001;164:1439.

National Institutes of Health Consensus Development Conference: *Adjuvant Therapy for Breast Cancer*, November 1–3, 2000.

Overgaard M et al: Postoperative radiotherapy in high-risk postmenopausal breast-cancer patients given adjuvant tamoxifen: Danish Breast Cancer Cooperative Group DBCG 82c randomised trial. Lancet 1999;353:1641.

Paik S et al: A multigene assay to predict recurrence of tamoxifen-treated, node-negative breast cancer. N Engl J Med 2004;351:2865.

Pendas S et al: Sentinel node biopsy in ductal carcinoma in situ patients. Ann Surg Oncol 2000;7:15.

Petrek JA, Pressman PI, Smith RA: Lymphedema: Current issues in research and management. CA Cancer J Clin 2000;50:292.

Ragaz J et al: Locoregional radiation therapy in patients with high-risk breast cancer receiving adjuvant chemotherapy: 20-year results of the British Columbia randomized trial. J Natl Cancer Inst 2005;97:116.

Recht A et al: Locoregional failure 10 years after mastectomy and adjuvant chemotherapy with or without tamoxifen without irradiation: experience of the Eastern Cooperative Oncology Group. J Clin Oncol 1999;17:1689.

Ries LAG et al (editors): SEER Cancer Statistics Review, 1973–1998, National Cancer Institute. Available at http://seer.cancer.gov/Publications/CSR1973_1998/. Last accessed October 2001.

Roetzheim RG et al: Effects of health insurance and race on early detection of cancer. J Natl Cancer Inst 1999;9:1409.

Sakorafas GH, Tsiotou AG: Selection criteria for breast conservation in breast cancer. Eur J Surg 2000;166:835.

Schrenk P et al: Morbidity following sentinel lymph node biopsy versus axillary lymph node dissection for patients with breast carcinoma. Cancer 2000;88:608.

Self-reported use of mammography and insurance status among women aged > or = 40 years—United States, 1991–1992 and 1996–1997. MMWR 1998;47:825.

Shapiro S: Periodic screening for breast cancer: The HIP randomized controlled trial. J Natl Cancer Inst Monogr 1997;22:27.

Silverstein MJ et al: A prognostic index for ductal carcinoma in situ of the breast. Cancer 1999;77:2267.

Swenson KK et al: Prognostic factors after conservative surgery and radiation therapy for early stage breast cancer. Am J Clin Oncol 1998;21:111.

Theriault RL: Medical treatment of bone metastases. In: Harris JR et al (editors): *Diseases of the Breast,* 3rd ed. Lippincott, 2004.

Velicer CM et al. Antibiotic use in relation to the risk of breast cancer. JAMA 2004;291:827.

The Borderland Between Law & Medicine

64

John P. O'Grady, MD, Dennis R. Anti, JD, Heather Beattie, RN, JD, & James E. Fanale, MD

"The time has come," the Walrus said,
"To talk of many things:
Of shoes—and ships—and sealing wax—
Of cabbages—and kings—
And why the sea is boiling hot—
And whether pigs have wings."

The Walrus and the Carpenter,
Alice's Adventures in Wonderland (1865)

Lewis Carroll (Charles Lutwidge Dodgson)
(1832–1898)

The practice of medicine and the governing standards for medical care have changed rapidly in recent years as a result of many influences. Advances in medical science are continuous. Useful techniques have been rapidly disseminated and promptly applied. New government regulations and protocols and practice guidelines by specialty societies affecting medical practice have been introduced. Finally, society expects a continuation of the medical advances of recent years.

Advances in the technical and scientific aspects of medicine and improvements in the actual provision of care have been accompanied by other, less desirable trends. In parallel with advances in medicine, novel legal theories have also evolved. This process has fostered innovative theories of causation and put new areas at risk for potential legal action.

Even the past had to endure medicolegal problems for practitioners of obstetrics. Legal cases claiming medical malpractice were uncommon in the United States before the early 1800s. Cases filed in the late 18th and early 19th centuries often involved specific medical complications: poor outcomes after vaccination, malunion and deformities following fractures, and serious obstetric outcomes. Early obstetric cases focused on injury and/or death to the mother, usually associated with instrumental delivery. It is interesting in regards to the capabilities of medicine and the expectations of the public that these cases were brought for maternal injuries as opposed to fetal injury or death. While parturition was recognized as a risky life event, both the public

and the courts considered the assisted delivery of an infant to be a routine mechanical skill, a belief that increased the expectation of a competent and error-free performance. The judge in *Sumner v. Utley* (7 Conn. 256 at 260 [1828]), noted that a "...physician may mistake the symptoms of a patient or may misjudge as to the nature or disease; and even as to the powers of a medicine; and yet his error may be of that pardonable kind that will do him no essential justice." However, the judge also noted that although a physician was part of a profession often "...beset by great difficulties...yet..., the employment of a man mid-wife and surgeon for the most part, is merely mechanical, and therefore held to a higher standard of performance."

As the science of obstetric care evolved, and the capabilities of medicine improved, the public's call for the specialty changed. The anticipation has become that all mothers and infants will not only survive childbirth but also remain unharmed. Unfortunately, not all of the techniques introduced into obstetric medicine have fulfilled the expectations of their inventors or of society. Medical-legal issues in modern obstetrics focus heavily on birth injury, especially permanent neuralgic injury to infants. Despite evidence exonerating the events of labor and delivery in the etiology of most neonatal injuries, bad-baby cases are most feared by practitioners. These cases can result in multimillion-dollar verdicts. Unfortunately, the false impression persists that the events of labor and delivery are a merely mechanical process, meaning practitioners are held to a higher standard of performance than is true for other medical specialties.

This chapter discusses the interdependent and contentious relationship between law and medicine. The presentation is not intended as an exhaustive compendium of legal wisdom or as a primer for clinicians seeking to avoid legal entanglements. It is, however, a review of selected legal issues important for practitioners combined with a critique of several contemporary medicolegal problems likely to involve practitioners in legal proceedings. Also briefly discussed is the impact of recent governmental regulations, some newly identified potential risks of previously accepted standard treatments, and the current efforts toward the assurance of patient safety and the proper stewardship of medical records.

IMPORTANT LEGAL CONCEPTS

Most malpractice claims proceed under rules of **common law,** the body of legal judicial opinion derived from precedent cases rather than statutory or legislative rules. As standards of care change and new legal arguments develop; common law continually redefines the potential grounds for litigation. There are a number of important legal concepts in tort law that clinicians should be familiar with. A selected number of these issues are briefly reviewed below.

Burden of Proof

In negligence torts, medical liability is established by proving the elements of **duty, breach of duty, causation,** and **damages.** To prevail, the plaintiff must demonstrate that all four of these basic elements of a negligence tort are present by a preponderance of the evidence. This demand for proof is the simple requirement that one side is stronger than the other. The testimony of expert medical witnesses concerning breach of one or more standards of care and how these deviations relate to causation is central to establishing liability.

Causation

Causation is the link or **proximal cause** between an alleged breach of duty and an injury. Unless there is proof of causation, no liability exists, not even when improper care is provided. Proving causation in obstetric cases is usually contentious because the cause of many birth injuries is not established, the range of acceptable practice is wide, and experts willing to promote unusual theories of causation are easily recruited.

Damages

The damages suffered as a result of alleged malpractice must constitute a demonstrable injury. Damages can either be purely economic (medical expenses, lost wages, and the like) or noneconomic (emotional distress, loss of consortium, pain and suffering, and the like). Compensation awarded for noneconomic injuries is subjective. These amounts depend largely on the response of the judge and jury to the plaintiff's presentation, and in some jurisdictions, may also be subject to statutory limits.

Statute of Limitations

The statute of limitations is a state-specific legislative act requiring that a legal action must be brought within a specified period of time. This period of time is usually calculated from either the date of the alleged incident or from the date when the alleged negligence was, or should have been, discovered. Most states also incorporate an extension into their statute of provisions for what is termed "incapacity." This could be the incapacity of a minor because of age, or the incapacity of an adult because of medical confinement. Once a lawsuit has been filed against one defendant, courts often allow other defendants to be added at a later date as the claims against these new defendants relate back to the original claim and date of filing.

Vicarious Liability

Vicarious liability claims are founded on the theory of *respondeat superior.* This doctrine professes that, in certain cases, a master is liable for the wrongful acts of the master's employee, servant, or agent. Under the theory of vicarious liability, an individual, an institution, or the employer of a practitioner can be held liable for the negligent acts of those over whom direction or control is exerted. The doctrine is usually inapplicable if the employee or agent is acting outside his or her scope of authority when the injury occurs. In a health care situation, a physician commonly directs nurse practitioners, residents, and other health care providers. Because physicians arguably retain direction and control over the actions of the other health care workers, they are potentially subject to vicarious liability for maloccurrences. Hospitals or physician group-practice corporations are also at risk of liability, either based on their employing a physician or midlevel practitioner or, in a nonemployment situation, by merely exerting direction or control over the practitioner's care. Allegations of negligent supervision, hiring, and training are usually separate claims from those of vicarious liability and are also an added potential liability to supervising physicians.

Standard of Care

The term *standard of care* defines a plan of management for a specified medical condition that is employed by the average qualified physician. Obstetric and gynecologic clinicians are held to national standards, not simply a standard specific to their state or local area. In the face of rapid innovation, determining the standard of care is not always easy. Even when clinicians identify the broad outlines of acceptable or standard practice, there is often professional disagreement concerning details.

Information contained in legislative statutes and regulations, textbook chapters, peer review articles, institution protocols and practice guidelines, and publications by groups such as The American College of Obstetricians and Gynecologists (ACOG) are used in medical malpractice cases as evidence of the current standards of practice.

Standards affect clinical practice as they are major influences on the content of institutional protocols and practice guidelines. Such guidelines and protocols are an effort by institutions to improve patient care, reduce costs, encourage compliance with scientifically sound medicine, and regularize practice. Another potential source for evidence of the standard of care is the institution's or individual practitioner's web site. Web sites are innocently created to increase the public's awareness of health issues and available health care but frequently contain information that arguably reflects the provider's own declaration of the standard of care.

NEW LEGAL THEORIES

In response to advances in science, the continuous expectations of society, new governmental regulations and statutes, and improvements in treatment, legal theories of liability continually evolve. A brief discussion of the nature and complexity of a selected number of these claims exemplifies the type of novel legal problems now possible in obstetric and gynecologic practice.

Wrongful Birth

A wrongful birth is an alleged claim against a clinician for the fact of the birth as opposed to a specific birth injury. These claims are usually brought by the patients following the birth of an infant with serious disabilities. The allegation is usually that the genetic or hereditary basis for the serious condition that afflicts the child was not recognized by the clinician and thus proper counseling did not occur. Alternatively, it might be claimed that appropriate screening or definitive testing was not offered early enough to the family to permit either pregnancy prevention or termination. To prevail, the parents must prove that if they had been informed of the potential for fetal defects or abnormality, they would have sought to either avoid pregnancy or to seek a termination. Because of these claims, the personal convictions of the parents concerning both prenatal testing and pregnancy termination become legitimate areas of examination by the defense.

If a wrongful birth claim is successful, potential damages depend upon both the condition of the infant as well as precedents in the jurisdiction where the action is brought. Wrongful birth claims are uncommon proceedings and are not permitted in all jurisdictions.

The potential for allegations of wrongful birth emphasize the importance of obtaining a complete family and genetic history and timely counseling for at-risk pregnant women concerning the available methods of genetic testing. When antepartum screening is performed, the physician should also be mindful of the limitations of any given test and counsel patients accordingly. The physician must also carefully document that a discussion took place and truthfully note the information given during all informed consent discussions. Routine referral to genetics counselors is not considered the standard of care. However, in the event of a legal claim, genetic counseling

by practitioners will likely be against the current measured standard of a trained geneticist as opposed to that of an obstetric generalist. Given the complexity and sophistication of genetic evaluations, the trend toward referral to perinatal geneticists for all but routine genetic testing and counseling can accelerate.

New protocols performed at less than 12 weeks' gestation combine ultrasound examinations (for the measurement of nuchal lucency), limited study of fetal anatomy, and maternal blood tests. The purpose of these examinations is to identify if a fetus is a member of a high-risk population. If it is, the mother and fetus will undergo additional, definitive testing. First trimester procedures have several advantages. A larger percentage of the abnormal fetuses found in the pool of normal fetuses are more accurately identified by these new tests than was possible using traditional methods. Because of technical improvements, fewer invasive tests, such as chorionic villus biopsy or amniocentesis, are required. This reduces the number of normal pregnancies lost as a result of test complications. These tests are performed early enough to permit less-risky pregnancy terminations if the parents' choice is not to continue.

There are, as usual, several pitfalls. The specific ultrasound techniques for performing nuchal lucency measurements are critical. Proper measurements are not easy to obtain and retraining, independent of their prior experience, is required for those conducting these ultrasound examinations.

As first trimester pregnancy evaluation becomes a standard of care, the implications must be thoroughly understood by clinicians. Although there is great promise in these novel methods, the potential for error is also substantial. Proper patient counseling, the assurance that the testing performed is offered in a timely fashion to at-risk women, and the requirement that the ultrasound studies are properly conducted are critical to accurate predictions. Yet, these new methods will never entirely supersede current midtrimester maternal blood testing and ultrasonic fetal surveys. Irregular menstrual cycles are common. The time of conception cannot be accurately estimated except in assisted-reproduction cases. Consequently, pregnancies do not often present for clinical evaluation until well beyond the appropriate period. It will require years to retrain clinicians in the appropriate ultrasound techniques. Also, as first trimester genetic and anatomic analysis becomes popular, it is possible that the demand for diagnostic procedures such as chorionic villus biopsy could overpower existing capacity. In sum, neither institutions nor practitioners should offer these tests without thoughtful preparation and retraining.

Wrongful Life

Wrongful life is an action claiming that negligent prenatal testing on the part of the health care provider resulted in the birth of a damaged child. Wrongful life differs from wrongful birth in that the claim is brought in the name of the physically or mentally disabled child, and not in the name of the parents. These cases commonly involve infants with serious inherited disorders or those born with major injuries as a result of undiagnosed maternal disease or drug exposure that adversely effects the infant. The underlying legal theory is that the duty of the clinician owed to the unborn child is similar to that owed to the parents.

The Netherlands Supreme Court recently recognized the validity of a wrongful life claim for a child born with mental and physical disabilities. The court held that the midwife attending the mother was liable for failing to recommend genetic testing. The court held that not only was the mother entitled to compensation under a theory of wrongful birth, but the child was also entitled to compensation for emotional damage under the theory of wrongful life. The arguments and reasoning behind this decision may eventually make their way into more courts in the United States.

Wrongful Conception

Wrongful conception claims are brought by the parents of a healthy, normal infant. In this instance, the alleged negligence is in the performance of a failed sterilization operation or the improper provision of contraceptive techniques leading to the birth of an otherwise normal but unwanted child. A common problem is a woman who becomes pregnant following a postpartum tubal ligation. Another possible scenario involves a woman who undergoes tubal ligation only to discover that an early, undiagnosed pregnancy was already present at the time the surgery was performed. In a wrongful conception suit, potentially all costs relating to prenatal treatment and labor and delivery are recoverable as damages, including the expenses related to the failed sterilization. Courts remain divided on whether parents may recover damages for the economic expenses of rearing a normal infant. The unique facts of each case, the jurisdiction in which the case is brought, and the amount of credit the court assigns as a benefit for the delivery of a normal child, versus the deduction for this unwanted pregnancy, determines the final judgment.

CURRENT ISSUES

This section discusses a number of important topics concerning the provision of medical care, the public perception of medicine, and the effects of recent legislation. Familiarity with these developing trends is important, as change in obstetric and gynecologic management is inevitable.

Changing Roles

Nonphysician health workers such as Certified Nurse Midwives (CNMs) and nurse practitioners are performing greater numbers of increasingly complex tasks. These personnel have been introduced into outpatient clinics and intrapartum and intraoperative levels, and it is likely that their numbers and responsibilities will accelerate in coming years. Such ancillary personnel function under an umbrella of state statutes and hospital rules written to delineate practice and limit prescribing privileges.

An important example of changing responsibilities in the field of obstetrics is the expansion of the nurse's role. With the arrival of advanced-degree nurses, the establishment of nursing diagnoses, and the expectation that nurses have a duty to perform as patient advocates, both the public and the courts are holding nurses to a higher standard of performance than in the past. In obstetric malpractice cases, nurses caring for patients during labor and delivery commonly become codefendants. In the absence of blatantly negligent action, nurses are often sued for failure to access the chain of command when there are signs of problems, particularly acute fetal jeopardy. The plaintiff will allege that the nurse has sufficient knowledge to determine when fetal problems exist and has a responsibility to advocate for both mother and child. Once persistent heart rate abnormalities or nonreassuring tracing are noted, for example, the nurse is responsible for addressing these findings with the attending physician. If the attending physician does not respond appropriately, the nurse must refer the issue up the chain of command to the nursing supervisor or the senior obstetric consultant or departmental chair. In theory, this all must be accomplished within minutes in order to prevent permanent injury to the child. Notwithstanding the obvious absurdity of this formulation, practitioners need to recognize the possibility of such claims. Effective communication among team members optimizes patient care, improves risk prevention, and helps offset this type of claim.

When a midlevel practitioner is sued for malpractice, the supervising or assigned physician and practice entity may also be sued under vicarious liability statutes or for negligent supervision, hiring, or training. The individual physician additionally may be sued for medical negligence because, in the collaborative relationship with the nurse practitioner, or midwife, the practitioner retains an independent duty to the patient. The specific practice protocol that delineates the relationship between the physician and the midlevel practitioner, together with individual state statutes, influences the success of such claims. Given these complexities, great care should be taken when drafting institutional and practice rules for nonphysician clinicians. Both legislative requirements and risk of liability need to be considered.

Practice Guidelines, Standards, and Protocols

Nonphysician practitioners, especially nurses and nurse practitioners, are accustomed to working under specific guidelines and protocol restraints. However, the experience is relatively new for physicians. The most common experience for clinicians are pharmacy and procedure lists prepared by insurance companies or other third-party payers.

Operating under the constraints of protocols and guidelines, practitioners are being forced to forgo unique or idiosyncratic drug-use management plans. This is probably all to the good. However, some doctors have not fared well in changing their methods of practice or with the introduction of new techniques. Part of the problem is the content of new practice guidelines and protocols. Poorly written documents may do more harm than good. Despite good intentions, documents from institutions and groups can increase the clinician's legal risk if the protocols or guidelines are overly rigid, inappropriate, or not reflective of best practice. These restrict the options available for covered drugs and procedures.

PATIENT SAFETY

The issue of medical errors attracted a great deal of attention following the 1999 Institute of Medicine (IOM) publication, *To Err is Human: Building a Safe Health System.* The report electrified the public and dismayed physicians with the claim that up to 98,000 deaths occurred annually in U.S. hospitals as a result of avoidable medical error. These assertions concerning the death rate state that hospital-based fatal errors are the eighth leading cause of death in the United States, ahead of breast cancer, acquired immune deficiency syndrome (AIDS), and motor vehicle accidents.

In March 2001, the IOM issued a subsequent medical safety report that outlined quality issues germane to health care and suggested specific improvement strategies. Although the issues that were highlighted in both the 1999 and 2001 reports had been mulled over for years, the timing, the call for reform, and the professional standing of the IOM found a ready public and governmental audience. Progress in the initiation of the slow, painful process of change by practitioners and institutions has begun.

The scope of the problem and the challenge of modifying established institutional practices are immense. There are almost 5000 community hospitals in the United States, including nongovernmental nonprofits,

for-profit institutions, and hospitals owned by state and local governments. The number of urban and rural community hospitals is similar. There are wide variations in bed number, financial resources, complexity, and staffing levels among these institutions. Because of these factors, institutions have experienced difficulty as they abandon traditional practices, institute new ones, and retrain their staff.

Issues of safety have not escaped federal attention. In 1999, Congress mandated the Agency for Healthcare Research and Quality (AHRQ) of the Department of Health and Human Services to prepare annual reports on the quality of health care.

The IOM report of 2001 suggested important redesigns for medical care. Several levels for attention are specified: the patient experience in the institution, the systems that provide care, support organizations, and the matrix of laws, rules, and training that shape or direct organizational action.

The goals of the IOM report of 2001, since revised, require that several steps are implemented. The principal suggestions focus on the redesign of the care process, the use of new information technologies, development of an effective team approach, better coordination of care, and the effective use of performance and outcomes measurements. There are also calls for specific programs to assure patient safety, foster the development of a blame-free culture for error review, promote a learning environment, and initiate specific planning for health care quality.

Part of the safety problem is appropriately attributed to institutional culture and the survival of outdated standard operating procedures and part to limitations in available personnel, especially nurses.

The impact of the nurse-staffing crisis on maintaining patient safety and the incidence of medical errors is not to be underestimated. The 2002 Joint Commission on Accreditation of Healthcare Organizations (JCAHO) Analysis of Patient Safety highlights the issue of nursing shortages in acute care. This report listed recommendations to reduce the shortage and highlighted the threats of too few personnel. Currently, 90% of long-term care organizations lack sufficient numbers of nurses, and more than 125,000 nursing positions remain unfilled, impacting patient safety and the quality of health care; nursing shortages cause emergency departments to divert patients, and hospitals to reduce beds or discontinue programs and services, and cancel elective surgeries. However, in the face of current political and financial constraints and the natural shortage of nurses, the staffing recommendations cited by JCAHO are unlikely to be rapidly implemented.

In terms of patient safety, the IOM suggests that combined and complex factors are usually involved when serious errors are made. Human error remains a common thread in many maloccurrences, but this is certainly not the only factor. Additional barriers to reducing medical errors include misunderstandings or incorrect data concerning causation; the traditional blame culture of many quality assurance systems; faults in error reporting systems; a general fear of litigation; and the failure of important members of the healthcare team to agree on goals and even the need for concerted action. A large part of the problem is directly attributable to hospital organization.

Most American hospitals are professional bureaucracies where considerable power resides with the clinical staff and not the institution's officers. Thus, programs for fundamental change must be accepted by more than one constituency and cannot simply be imposed. In such a system interpersonal contacts, working relationships between important individuals who represent different interests, and a motivated hospital administration are critical to success when major changes are implemented. New quality improvement programs cannot succeed unless they are clearly aligned with the core objectives of the organization, made a priority by its administrative leaders, and supported by influential members of the medical staff.

Experience with institutional bureaucracies indicates that a basic requirement in avoiding errors is to develop effective systems for identifying problems and seeking the cause both for errors and "near misses." When properly functioning, surveillance systems permit learning from errors and the subsequent modification of behaviors or policies to avoid recurrences. Once collected, data on errors, nears misses, and maloccurences can serve as the basis for a following critical analysis of how quality and safety are to be improved.

Physicians are not infallible and flaws in the process of patient care are prominent in patient injury. The heralded case of a young heart transplant patient at Duke University Medical Center who succumbed because of an incorrectly typed blood transfusion is an obvious example. Mismatching blood types is a significant, serious medical error. A process improvement and/or the use of currently available information technology for patient identification would most certainly have prevented this outcome.

The Institute for Healthcare Improvement (IHI) recently started a national program for hospitals to "save 100,000 lives." IHI's plan revolves around standard, scientifically sound policies and treatments that are intended to reduce medical errors and improve patient safety. For example, to reduce ventilator-associated pneumonias (VAPs), hospitals are asked to adopt a set of care principles applicable to all ventilated patients. Adoption of these standards is anticipated to reduce the incidence of VAP. A large number of hospitals have signed up to participate in either this or another of the six current IHI initiatives.

National accrediting organizations have also been active in patient safety. The JCAHO has tremendous influence as their approval of an institution is required for Medicaid reimbursement. Drawing on the IOM reports, the JCAHO has established patient safety goals. These goals focus on avoidance of both error and reduction in patient injury. No one practicing in an institution can avoid the impact of the changes. The JCAHO goals include (a) the improvement of patient identification (two patient identifiers required for procedures and lab work approval); (b) improvement in care giver communication (read-back of telephone reports, standardized abbreviations, periodic assessment of report timeliness); (c) improvement in medication safety (standardization and limitation of available drug concentrations, avoidance of look or sound-alike drugs, and prohibition against adding concentrated salt solutions to intravenous solutions on care units); (d) the introduction of improved infusion pump technology; (e) the reduction in the risks of infection for institutionalized patients; (f) the documentation and reliable communication of data concerning patient medications between caregivers; and (g) programs to reduce patient risk from accidental falls.

The type of medical error that particularly caught public attention was "wrong-site" surgery. JCAHO defines "wrong-site surgery" as operative procedures that are performed on the wrong side or site of the body, the performance of an incorrect procedure, and surgeries erroneously performed on the wrong patient On review, many of the "wrong-site" cases arose from errors either in the transfer of patient information or in imperfect communication between caregivers concerning orders or procedures.

The JCAHO now demands specific protocols for patient identification prior to administering medications, blood products, or obtaining blood samples and other specimens. The most immediate impact for surgeons is the introduction of special methods for correct patient identification in the operating room. These patient identification protocols have not met universal approval from surgeons. A common complaint is that the techniques are burdensome and waste time. Such opinions cannot prevail against the case reports of surgery incorrectly performed either on the wrong individual or the incorrect body part.

At first glance, the issue of correct patient identification seems to be of less importance in obstetric practice. Procedures such as cesarean delivery are usually conducted only after the parturient has been hospitalized for some time and nursing personnel have been in immediate attendance. This should make misidentification a very remote risk. Obviously, in obstetric practice, marking the lower abdomen over the gravid uterus to verify the appropriate site for a cesarean delivery is nonsensical. However, there are other considerations. In busy clinical services, especially when patients may not speak or understand English, when surgery often occurs as an emergency, or when procedures are performed on individuals incapable of identifying themselves, such as newborns or unresponsive adults, patient identity verification techniques are as necessary in obstetric practice as in general surgery. The meticulous identification of any individual undergoing surgery and the verification of the surgical site is a reasonable and necessary requirement for all surgeons for all procedures, despite the redundancies of the methods currently employed. The rare egregious errors of the past necessitate the use of these procedures.

Perhaps the most commonly observed change in hospital practices is the manner in which medications are ordered, stocked, and administered. Institutions have now abandoned the onward addition of electrolytes and drugs to intravenous solutions, moving these procedures back to the pharmacy. In some instances premixed solutions are directly ordered from manufacturers. Again, this is in an effort to reduce errors, avoiding inadvertent wrong drug or wrong dose administration.

As part of the process of improving care and assuming patient safety, various types of electronic and computer-based programs have been introduced to hold clinical data, regularize and limit pharmacy ordering, or provide assistance in decision making. Information technologies are underused in modern health care and we still largely rely on handwritten records and methods of data archiving, recording, and retrieval that are prone to include missing or outdated items, or old or forgotten protocols. The arrival of electronic health records holds great promise.

There are potential problems with electronic records. Although computerized physician order entry systems have been enthusiastically promoted and rapidly introduced into many institutions, in some instances, the architecture of some programs, paradoxically, has facilitated making errors rather than reducing them. Difficulties ensue when programs do not reflect the realities of patient care, are hard to access, are not up to date, or have no established system for timely revision. Many programs, even newly written, are often poor at identifying problems inherent in their own structure and the supporting technicians are invariably reluctant to revise the original programs.

With time, clinicians find ways to work around to the various computer system limitations. Although these applications of human ingenuity facilitate day to-day care, they also help conceal major system shortcomings to the computer mavens. Problems are particularly common when the computerized physician order entry programs are not written with close attention to how practitioners actually perform, what orders are most fre-

quently entered, and the usual and customary sequence in which care is provided. Thus, an absolute requirement for success for any health information system is the inclusion of flexibility and continuous surveillance of its own function.

Despite potential problems, data solutions based on modern information technologies have the potential to address several issues including information availability, transfer of data, accurate administration of medications, and adherence to clinical guidelines. The allure of technology must not blind us to the requirement that electronic systems exist to facilitate care and should not make the provision of care more difficult.

The process of safety improvement has not been without its own difficulties and missteps. Reviews of institutional actions provides ample examples of foolish protocols and administrative overreaching. There are other problems as well. Both institutions and physician groups have failed to discipline egregious behavior by clinicians who willingly violate new procedures and protocols. There are also important unintended consequences of changing practices that have interfered with the acceptance of new systems and limited both their flexibility and success. Despite these and other difficulties, there are data documenting that adherence to guidelines for obstetric care does reduce the risk of litigation. In one study, in cases in which deviations from guidelines occurred, the likelihood of litigation was 6-fold greater. At present, several states, including Kentucky, Florida, and Maine, have enacted legislation that establishes adherence to guidelines as a defense to claims of malpractice.

The JCAHO incorporated into its accreditation process patient safety goals and has studied the extent to which the medical liability system either supports or undermines these recommendations. It comes as no surprise that the effects of legal oversight on safety are both ineffective and counterproductive.

The JCAHO proposes that litigation can only be controlled by combining programs for injury reduction with the creation of new mechanisms for early settlement of claims outside of litigation; the resolution of disputes through a special no-fault administrative health court system; and the shifting of liability away from individuals to organizations.

Similar to the current workers' compensation system, negligence would be excluded as the basis for compensation. Case resolution would be by a no-trial, administrative process. Compensation for unavoidable complications would rely on expert guidelines. Damages would be awarded based on an established fee schedule for avoidable events. In problem cases, special health courts may hear legal arguments concerning specific cases as well as consider the opinions of independent, court-appointed experts. Finally, all decisions or settlements would be a public record.

It is unclear how to develop a no-blame system for medical errors. At present, the fear of litigation colors the willingness of practitioners to both report and investigate maloccurences. The same may be said for institutions. When errors are identified in institutional protocols or procedures, we need new methods to hold institutions accountable for bad practices without destroying them in the light of adverse publicity. It also remains uncertain as to how institutions should manage physicians, nurses, and other providers who behave poorly. Whatever system evolves must distinguish clinicians who have simply made errors and who would profit from retraining from the small number of those whose behavior requires discipline, practice restriction, or dismissal. Anyone who has sat on a hospital review panel realizes that the distinction between simple human error and poor practice can be surprisingly difficult to establish.

The existing tort system has proven to be a very poor method to control or remove from practice incompetent practitioners. Unfortunately, removing fault as the driving force behind recovery for injuries such as suggested in the JCAHO report does not address this problem. Other nationally accredited bodies are taking the first tentative steps. The American Board of Medical Specialties is implementing new requirements for the maintenance of board certifications. These include time-limited certifications and the requirement for the periodic reassessment of the competence of practicing specialists. Much more needs to be done in this regard.

Hospitals need to develop a systems approach to safety issues. Maloccurences should undergo analysis to identify process problems. A partial system is already in place as the JCAHO requires that institutions recognize sentinel events and institute preventative policies to avoid recurrences. Sentinel events include medication errors, treatment delays, and operative and wrong-site surgical complications, among others. Recent case analysis links a host of chronic institutional problems to these adverse sentinel events, including limited staffing, unavailability of patient data, inadequate staff training and orientation, and various communication lapses. In response to the issue of problem identification, several states, including Pennsylvania and New York, have instituted mandatory reporting systems for hospital errors. Other hospital specific systems for reporting of maloccurences exist at a number of other sites across the United States.

An unresolved and inadequately studied problem is the response of clinicians to these various management strategies and protocol changes. Skeptical physicians accustomed to idiosyncratic practices also must become convinced—and in some instances required—to accept new protocols, techniques, and methods. And all this must be done without generating serious resistance.

There has been a great deal of recent interest in crew resource management. This is a model for managing complex events developed in the aviation industry in response to accident analysis. As applied to medical care, this team approach involves the organization of new multidisciplinary professional teams (MedTeams) with special group training. This reorganization is claimed to ease communication, encourage unrestrained questioning up the hierarchy, and various redundancies to better assure quality and safety. This technique deserves additional study in medical settings where extreme complexity and rapidly changing events are commonplace such as emergency rooms, intensive care units and obstetric services.

HEALTH INSURANCE PORTABILITY AND ACCOUNTABILITY ACT OF 1996

The Health Insurance Portability and Accountability Act of 1996 (HIPAA) directly affects all providers of medical care. The requirements of HIPAA on institutional stewardship of confidential patient information were gradually introduced, with the last major implementation in mid 2003. Unfortunately, securing the privacy of personal medical information was not an established priority in the past. Various egregious examples of commercial and otherwise improper use of personal medical information resulted in the political pressure leading to the HIPAA statute. Similar efforts to make medical records more secure yet accessible to patients are underway in a number of countries, including Ireland, Australia, Canada, the United Kingdom, and South Africa.

The HIPAA mandates are federally established rules concerning the privacy of medical information. Both practitioners and institutions become a covered entity when they conduct any medical business either via paper or by electronic means. Thus, no one involved in health care escapes the HIPAA umbrella.

The act defines protected health care information and specifies the manner in which these data can be accessed by caregivers and others. HIPAA also requires the development of procedures or administrative protocols restricting access to health care records. The intention of the legislation is also to give patients greater control over access to information within their medical records.

The enforcement muscle for HIPAA includes both fines and the threat of imprisonment for willful violations of patient privacy rules. There are severe criminal penalties written into the law. Fines of $50–$250,000 and 1–10 years of imprisonment are possible for the willful or malicious release of medical records for commercial or other reasons.

Basically, the law requires that only minimally necessary individually identifiable health information can be released or requested for a specific purpose. This requirement excludes information disclosures authorized by the individual, the transmission of information between health care providers, and various other disclosures as required by law.

HIPAA has limits. The law does not supersede family law statutes. These state laws include regulations concerning matters such as parent–child relationships and the rights of children, among other important matters. State regulations still apply in the laws governing informed consent. In general, if local rules and regulations are more protective or restrictive than HIPAA, the more limiting laws and not the HIPAA regulations apply.

HIPAA also requires that patients be informed of their privacy rights and be provided with a written privacy policy notice. This document reveals who has access to an individual's records and under what circumstances a specific signed release for record use will be required. Patients are also informed of their right to inspect, copy, or amend their own records, or to obtain an accounting of prior record disclosures. Stewards of medical information must specifically identify a privacy officer. Finally, and coming as a surprise to many when the document is read closely, patients are notified that their health information may be released without their specific authorization for various health care operations, including institutional performance evaluations, quality control assessments, and various other management procedures such as billing. The vagueness of this permitted operations section permits wide interpretation.

HIPAA applies to all medical research activities in the United States, regardless of the funding source, but local institutional review boards retain substantial discretion in providing consent waivers. These waivers allow researchers access to patient records without a specific prior authorization. What is usually required for researchers is a set of specified measures to protect the identity of the individuals whose charts have been included in the approved study. This is usually easily accomplished by assigning each case a number and keeping the name and number code in a restricted site. This waiver loophole was added because of the recognition that without chart access many studies, including those necessary for quality assurance, became essentially impossible to conduct.

HIPAA represents a series of political compromises, and the statute has its fair share of inconsistencies and fuzzy definitions. These ambiguities, along with the threat of fines and even imprisonment, have frightened both institutions and practitioners, leading to the prompt appearance of a cadre of compliance consultants.

In theory, a more patient-accessible medical record has the potential to improve health care, principally by enhancing doctor–patient communication. Other benefits have been suggested, including reducing chart errors and improving care quality. Published research papers evaluating the success of these new regulations is limited, but suggest a modest benefit from enhanced patient chart access. So far, the associated risks have been limited or inconsequential. However, the full impact of these HIPAA regulations on health care quality, the associated benefits to individuals, if any, and the unintended consequences of these rules will not be known for years.

The federal HIPAA statute and its accompanying regulations influence the day-to-day actions of healthcare providers. Physicians, nurses, and hospital employees must recognize that their world is now profoundly different. They must discipline both themselves and others on a daily basis. A casual elevator conversation between a nurse and physician regarding a patient's laboratory results is a potential HIPAA violation. The resident's notes from morning rounds, jotted on a scrap of paper, and inadvertently taken home in a lab coat pocket might threaten the privacy of patient information. A hospital clerk accessing a friend's laboratory results from the computer is violating HIPAA rules and will be terminated as an employee because hospital toleration of such behavior is also a HIPAA violation. These are just a few examples of the potential misuse of patient information that HIPAA rules now cover.

The behavioral changes required for compliance with this new law are vexing for caregivers and will doubtlessly prove burdensome. Nonetheless, because of the wide scope of HIPAA, neither institutions nor individual practitioners can avoid its requirements or evade its punishments. Whether these regulations will actually improve health care on balance, proving worthy of this large investment, remains for future reviewers to determine.

LIABILITY

There is consternation at both the national and local levels of medicine concerning professional liability. Skyrocketing insurance rates and the continued pressure of medicolegal risk influence medical practice and practitioners. The issue of securing insurance coverage and the potential for increased legal exposure in high-risk settings has restricted practices and increased patient referrals. Clinicians are justifiably reluctant to perform certain procedures and to manage certain types of cases when it is perceived that there is substantial legal risk to themselves and to their institutions. Insurance and legal concerns have also trimmed the ranks of older practitioners of obstetrics and gynecology and steered otherwise interested students into less-risky specialties.

No subject better illustrates the thorny problems that occur when medical decision making becomes entangled with litigation fears than the issue of trials of labor after cesarean delivery, popularly known as VBAC trials (vaginal birth after cesarean).

Dozens of articles have been published in recent years concerning the maternal and fetal risk associated with VBAC trials. The general consensus is that VBAC trials involve a greater relative risk of serious or fatal fetal injury than does elective, repeat cesarean delivery. Yet the magnitude of these risks remains low. Studies vary in assigning an enhanced risk of maternal morbidity to VBAC trials. However, failed VBAC trials going to cesarean delivery clearly increase both maternal febrile and infectious morbidity, as well as other surgical complications. Prolonged labor, multiple examinations, tissue injury, enhanced blood loss, and the need for anesthesia are important associated factors.

Drawing data from a number of sources, the risk for uterine rupture for an intended VBAC trial in a pregnancy at term with a prior low, transverse scar is approximately 0.35–0.75%. In cases where the uterus ruptures, the likelihood for significant perinatal injury or death is 10% or less. In general terms:

Risk of rupture/VBAC trial = 1/150–1/200
Risk of serious or fatal fetal injury/VBAC trial
    = 1/1500–2600

These trial-associated risks are well documented in the literature. However, it was the practice guideline published by the American College of Obstetricians and Gynecologists in 1999 that initiated rapid change in the behavior of practitioners and institutions. This document stipulated that institutions offering trials were required to have both anesthesia and obstetric personnel *immediately available* during the trial. Many obstetric services, both with and without house staff, could not meet this requirement. Once the potential implications of failing to comply with the guidelines were understood there was a precipitous decline in the number of VBAC trials. Many doctors and institutions decided that the risk was too high to permit these trials to be conducted and simply barred them. The exceptions have been training institutions with house staff when close fetal monitoring and rapid surgical intervention in emergencies is possible.

Whether VBAC-associated risks are considered small or not depends on how the risk is interpreted. The question for clinicians and potential parturients concerning potentially hazardous medical procedures where the complication rate is low is not the relative risk of a specific procedure versus a specified alternative,

but the magnitude of the actual risk. Put into perspective, the risk of a complication could be doubled or even tripled for specific procedures. However, if the net magnitude of that change was to leave the individual's actual risk as still uncommon or even rare (ie, 1/5000–1/1000 or less), the increase in the relative risk might or might not be perceived as significant.

So, when does a risk become so high that it is unacceptable? Or fall low enough to be acceptable? Might properly counseled individuals decide that a 1/1500 to 1/2600 risk of a serious complication with a VBAC trial is of such a low magnitude as to be acceptable?

Adverse outcomes with VBAC trials will invariably come under legal scrutiny, regardless of the artfully written consent forms, documentation concerning the consent process in the medical record, or evidence of assiduous attention to clinical detail by the birth attendants. The central problem is that when large numbers of VBAC trials are permitted, inevitably but very infrequently, a few otherwise normal infants and mothers will be seriously injured, although rarely fatally.

The reluctance of providers and institutions to accept cases for VBAC trial means that women seeking VBACs will have a progressively more difficult time locating practitioners willing to attend their labors and, more importantly, institutions willing to permit the labor to take place. This is best seen in the State of Florida. The passed referendum specifying loss of licensure for physicians with a fixed number of lost malpractice cases, in conjunction with the demands for immediate hospital and clinic coverage, have essentially closed the door on VBAC trials in that state. As a consequence of the sum total of these problems, VBAC trials are simply no longer considered to be worth the legal risk for many institutions and practitioners.

PREMATURE LABOR AND DELIVERY

Complications associated with either the prevention of preterm labor and delivery or diagnosis and treatment constitute fertile ground for lawsuits. The onset of human labor is a complicated and extensively studied process that is slowly becoming better understood. Based on recent data, it is theorized that infection plays a role in initiating at least 25% of preterm labors. Histologic evidence for inflammation in the amniotic membrane is common in cases of early labor. Also, bacterial vaginosis (BV), a polymicrobial overgrowth of anaerobic bacteria in the birth canal, is a recognized risk factor. However, it remains unclear if treatment of BV can successfully reduce the incidence of premature delivery. Current studies remain inconclusive. BV may function as a marker for preterm labor risk and not be the direct cause for premature uterine activity. Infection also plays an important role in birth injury. Epidemiologic data supports a causal relationship between chorioamnionitis and permanent neurologic injury in term and perhaps also in premature pregnancies. A number of inflammatory substances, including interferon, cytokines, interleukin-6, and tumor necrosis factor, are implicated in this process.

The various treatments to control or avert early labor have led to legal entanglements. The introduction, 20 years ago, of tocolytic drugs was initially hailed as a great advance in preterm delivery prevention. The complications and failures of tocolysis are now better recognized and hard-won experience indicates that the role for tocolysis in preterm labor is quite limited. Following disillusionment with tocolysis, it was believed that the answer to premature delivery could be found in the medical and social protocols championed by Papernik et al. These French investigators reported success in early delivery prevention by screening women for risk based largely on history, social, and environmental factors. In theory, this allowed a high-risk group to be identified, closely observed, and treated early. This initially promising approach is now considered suspect due to the evidence of its limited efficacy in several U.S. studies.

Recently, specific types of maternal infection and clinical markers, such as cervical length and fetal fibronectin (FFN), have been promoted for the identification of the at-risk population for early labor. Despite these innovations, success in the prematurity prevention remains a difficult goal. However, some recent developments have proven encouraging and The March of Dimes has now introduced a new national campaign for prematurity prevention.

New tests such as FFN assays have proven useful in preterm labor prediction. Fetal fibronectin is a glycoprotein located in the extracellular matrix at the choriodecidual interface. Normally, FFN is not detected in cervical/vaginal secretions between 24 and 34 weeks' gestation as its presence indicates activation of the labor cascade. When the test is performed, and is negative, the probability of delivery within 7–10 days is very low (ie, the negative predictive value is very good). However, the positive predictive value is fair to poor (20–50%). New data indicates that a short cervix diagnosed by ultrasound scanning and a positive FFN are independent risk factors for premature labor/delivery. Thus, combining test results is a good idea and probably enhances the identification of a high-risk population.

While these and other promising new tests may better identify an at risk population, there is no consensus concerning how best to employ these tests, the order in which they should be used, what clinical decisions should follow a positive or negative result, and what is to be done if the tests disagree.

Bed rest, the traditional management for untimely labor, is now recognized to be of uncertain efficacy. Treatment of bacterial vaginosis early in pregnancy may be effective in some cases, but recent data are not encouraging. Administration of steroids to the mother to enhance fetal pulmonic maturity is usually prudent. Some preterm labors may be avoided by progesterone therapy.

Recent reports using various progesterone compounds, administered either by vaginal suppositories of natural progesterone or by muscular injection of a synthetic form (17α-hydroxyprogesterone caproate), claim efficacy as a prophylaxis against preterm labor. Much remains uncertain. The ideal type of progesterone and how to administer it is not established. Which at-risk women might benefit from treatment and at what gestational age treatment should begin remains to be determined. Despite the attractiveness of the concept, progesterone therapy is no panacea. Considering the bitter experience with other treatments for preterm labor that were enthusiastically promoted in past years, caution is needed before embracing yet another drug regimen before its safety and efficacy is firmly established.

Other issues relate to potential risks from tocolytics. Terbutaline, an inexpensive and commonly administered beta-mimetic tocolytic drug has recently come under scrutiny. This drug was extensively used in past years in both infusion pump and oral medication protocols that have now largely been abandoned. Problems now arise as new questions are raised concerning unintended adverse effects of such chronic beta-mimetic treatment. This is because many preterm labor cases are associated with cytokine release. These vasoactive substances have the potential for direct cellular injury, believed to be exacerbated by hypoxia and ischemia. It is theorized that in glutamate predominate sites in the fetal brain (putamen, caudate, thalami, etc.) beta-agonist mediated increases in blood flow could promote additional brain damage. Magnesium sulfate might be protective, at least for this effect.

In experimental models, rats on high terbutaline doses do develop suspicious central nervous system (CNS) changes. How this experimental model relates to humans is unclear as complex and poorly understood events in both the maternal and fetal environment affect the risk for CNS injury. The causes of human preterm labor are so varied and primate central nervous system blood flow is so different from common laboratory animals as to make a link between the rat model and clinical observations tenuous. Much more data are required to properly investigate this alleged beta-mimetic CNS injury link. Despite the distinct data limitations, enterprising attorneys are now advertising for women who previously delivered an injured premature neonate and who were treated in their pregnancy for preterm labor by one of the now largely abandoned protocols using either terbutaline or other beta-mimetics.

Where does this leave clinicians? The standard of care for years was to employ various tocolytics to at least temporarily arrest labor and clinicians faced liability claims if they failed to administer these drugs. As it is now recognized, tocolytic drug treatment to inhibit early or established preterm labor is largely ineffective. In fact, long-term treatment was never feasible except in a small part of the preterm labor population as clinical circumstances rendered most cases inappropriate for treatment. Currently, labor arrest is attempted for specific and limited reasons and for brief periods. These include allowing time for steroid administration, facilitating obstetric procedures, or permitting patient transfer. Tocolytics can also briefly arrest uterine activity in instances of spontaneous or induced uterine tachysystole or presumed fetal distress. In the latter case, treatment is for the purpose of temporary in utero resuscitation.

The tocolytic experience provides further proof of the cost of initiating new therapies before the benefits and risks of treatment versus nontreatment are well established. This is an egregious error that obstetric medicine seems destined to repeat. Re-emphasizing time-worn admonishments for limited goals, careful patient counseling, and concern for the unknown risks remains the best practice.

Appropriate management for preterm labor remains illusive. As obstetric medicine struggles to implement new management protocols, the high incidence of complications from prematurity, the uncertainties and inconsistencies in current management and the problems arising from the use of well-intentioned, yet incompletely tested, therapies will assure a continuous supply of legal claims.

ECTOPIC PREGNANCY

Ectopic pregnancy is a common complication, with approximately 110,000 cases diagnosed each year. More than 95% of ectopic pregnancies occur in the fallopian tube, with 80% in the ampullary region. The frequency of ectopic gestation has increased 6-fold in the last 20 years. Ectopic pregnancies now occur in 2% of all gestations and result in nearly 60,000 hospital admissions per year.

Risk factors for ectopic pregnancy include a history of pelvic inflammatory disease, previous tubal surgery, prior ectopic gestation, use of fertility drugs or other assisted-reproductive technologies, presence of an intrauterine device, increasing maternal age, smoking, and a number of other factors.

Serious complications following the rupture of an ectopic pregnancy include internal hemorrhage, cardiovascular collapse, and, in rare instances, maternal death. The maternal fatality rate is approximately 2.6 per 10,000 cases. The small numbers of nontubal ectopic pregnancies occurring at an interstitial site are especially problematic. Once an ectopic pregnancy is diagnosed,

either medical management (methotrexate or other drug administration) or surgery (laparoscopy or laparotomy with salpingostomy or salpingectomy) must be promptly undertaken. Unfortunately, the correct diagnosis is often difficult to establish.

Because of recent biochemical advances and improvements in ultrasound scanning techniques, the presence of a normal early pregnancy is usually easy to establish. Problems in separating ectopic symptoms from other causes of abdominal pain ensue when the patient's menstrual dating is inexact or when other common complications of early pregnancy exist such as threatened abortion. Unfortunately for clinicians, irregular ovulation and unreliable menstrual dating are common.

Most problems arise when the menstrual dating is uncertain and vaginal spotting or cramping are present but the gestational sac is not visualized when an ultrasound examination is performed. Under these circumstances, other conditions such as a ruptured corpus luteum, appendicitis, ovarian torsion, and pelvic inflammatory disease should be considered.

Establishing the correct diagnosis may prove difficult. A review of the history, serial physical examinations, special laboratory tests, updated ultrasound studies, or exploratory surgery (laparoscopy) may be required. In the absence of reliable menstrual dating, specialized laboratory testing for levels of human chorionic gonadotropin (hCG) or progesterone are often combined with serial abdominal or vaginal ultrasound examinations with or without color-flow Doppler to establish the correct diagnosis.

All these studies include the potential for error. Although there is no single hCG level value that is diagnostic for ectopic pregnancy, when the value is greater than 1500 mIU/mL (1st, 2nd IRP [International Reference Preparation]), an intrauterine sac and fetal pole should be seen by transvaginal ultrasonography. In uncertain cases, serial blood tests to detect a doubling of the hCG concentration, done approximately every 48 hours, are occasionally helpful. However, serial study can simply delay establishing the correct diagnosis and such tests should not be used in isolation. Use of serial hCG levels is also problematic as only about a third of ectopic pregnancies have declining hormone levels at the time of presentation.

Serum progesterone concentrations are currently a popular test. However, there is no consensus of opinion concerning the discriminatory level for progesterone. As a consequence of biologic variability, the serum progesterone levels for ectopics and either normal or failing intrauterine pregnancies show considerable overlap, limiting the diagnostic utility of these tests.

As a result of the associated morbidity and the rising incidence of ectopic gestations, there are substantial legal risks for erroneous or delayed diagnoses. Delay risks morbidity and additional surgery, which the plaintiff will charge was unnecessary. Despite the complexities in establishing the true status of a pregnancy, it is most often the failure of a clinician to suspect an ectopic pregnancy that leads to trouble, not a lack of familiarity with the methods for diagnosis and treatment.

ONCE A PREGNANCY, ALWAYS A CESAREAN?

To avoid the maternal and fetal risks of labor, to protect pelvic structures or function, and to permit scheduling, there is pressure for elective cesarean delivery on demand. Although purely elective cesarean deliveries are an uncommon practice in the United States, in other countries, especially countries in South America, elective operative delivery is a practice norm, resulting in operative delivery rates often exceeding 50% in private clinics.

Cesarean delivery rates in the United States now hover at approximately 22–25%. Large increases in the number of elective procedures would have major effects on obstetric services, especially in terms of the availability of nursing and anesthesia personnel.

The resistance to major increases in elective operative deliveries is likely to prove less than was originally anticipated. The ability of practitioners, parturients, and other birth attendants to have a fixed, elective schedule has appeal. A large number of elective operations would also free beds normally used for labor. Anesthesia services might applaud the change to cesarean on demand because of easier case scheduling, increased clinical activity, and increased billing. If cesarean on demand became popular, deliveries would increasingly become scheduled events more akin to other surgical procedures. The demand for surgery could also prompt the hiring of more house doctors and an expansion of surgical facilities. How institutions would implement new protocols for a large number of purely elective surgical deliveries while retaining the ability to respond to emergencies remains to be seen. There are potential legal implications to such a major change in routine obstetric management. If labor and vaginal delivery are identified as major risk factors in long-term bladder or perineal dysfunction or rectal incontinence, then scheduled operative deliveries delayed by human error or other mischance until the onset of labor or an unplanned vaginal delivery might come under legal review. Alternatively, early elective deliveries resulting in infant morbidity because of iatrogenic prematurity could easily prompt legal claims. It is safe to predict that the number of purely elective cesarean deliveries will increase and that legal complications will follow.

CONCLUSIONS

The recent improvements in reproductive technologies, prenatal genetics and other scientific advances in obstetric surgery and management, and the promotion of these capabilities by clinicians and the media have led to increased public expectations of medicine and a general down playing of risk. However, our scientific knowledge remains incomplete and the inherent limitations in the reproductive process remain unchanged. Biologic variations in presentation, the occurrence of human error, uncertainties inherent in establishing firm diagnoses, complications in surgery, and the imperfections of medical treatment have not disappeared. Thus it is safe to predict that the complex, interdependent, and contentious confrontation between the law and obstetric and gynecologic medicine will continue.

REFERENCES

2004 Compendium of Selected Publications. American College of Obstetrical and Gynecology, 2004.

Allen VM et al: Maternal morbidity associated with cesarean delivery without labor compared with spontaneous arrest of labor at term. Obstet Gynecol 2003;102:477.

Asinas GJ: HIPAA regulations—a new era of medical record privacy? N Engl J Med 2003;348:1486.

Banta DH, Thacker SB: Historical controversy in health technology assessment: the case of electronic fetal monitoring. Obstet Gynecol Surv 2001;56:707.

Benham BN et al: Risk factors for preterm delivery in patients demonstrating sonographic evidence of premature dilation of the internal os, prolapse of the membranes in the endocervical canal and shortening of the distal cervical segment by second trimester ultrasound. Aust N Z J Obstet Gynaecol 2002;42:46.

Bloche MG, Studdert DM: A quiet revolution: law as an agent of health system change. Health Aff (Millwood) 2004;23:29.

da Fonseca EB et al: Prophylactic administration of progesterone by vaginal suppository to reduce the incidence of spontaneous preterm birth in women at increased risk: a randomized placebo-controlled study. Am J Obstet Gynecol 2003;188:419.

Devers K, Pham HH, Liu G: What is driving hospitals' patient-safety efforts? Health Aff (Millwood) 2004;23:103.

DeVille KA: *Medical Malpractice in Nineteenth Century America.* New York University Press, 1990.

Dugoff L et al: First-trimester maternal serum PAPP-A and free-beta subunit human chorionic gonadotropin concentrations and nuchal translucency are associated with obstetric complications: a population-based screening study (the FASTER Trial). Am J Obstet Gynecol 2004;191(4):1446.

Garland SM et al: Mechanisms, organisms and markers of infection in pregnancy. J Reprod Immunol 2002;57:169.

Ghetti C, Chan BK, Guise JM: Physician's responses to patient-requested cesarean delivery. Birth 2004;31:280.

Goffinet F et al: Bacterial vaginosis: prevalence and predictive value for premature delivery and neonatal infection in women with preterm labour and intact membranes. Eur J Obstet Gynecol Reprod Biol 2003;108:146.

Gomez R et al: Cervicovaginal fibronectin improves the prediction of preterm delivery based on sonographic cervical length in patients with preterm uterine contractions and intact membranes. Am J Obstet Gynecol 2005;192:350.

Hankins GD: The long journey: defining the true pathogenesis and pathophysiology of neonatal encephalopathy and cerebral palsy. Obstet Gynecol Surv 2003;58:435.

Haram K, Mortensen JH, Wollen AL: Preterm delivery: an overview. Acta Obstet Gynecol Scand 2003;82:687.

Health Insurance Portability and Accountability Act of 1996. Pub Law No. 104-191, 110 Stat 1936 (1996).

Iams JD et al: The Preterm Prediction Study: recurrence risk of spontaneous preterm birth. Am J Obstet Gynecol 1998;178:1035.

Illingworth RS: Why blame the obstetrician? A review. Br Med J 1979;24:797.

Joint Commission on Accreditation of Healthcare Organizations: *Healthcare at the crossroads: strategies for addressing the nursing crisis.* 2002 August. Available at www.JCAHO.org.

Joint Commission on Accreditation of Healthcare Organizations: *Healthcare at the crossroads: strategies for improving the medical liability system and preventing patient injury.* 2005. Available at www.JCAHO.org.

Kiss H, Petricevic L, Husslein P: Prospective randomized controlled trial of an infection screening program to reduce the rate of preterm delivery. BMJ 2004;329: 371.

Kohn L, Corrigan J, Donaldson M (editors): *To Err is Human: Building a Safer Health System.* National Academies Press, 2001.

Koppel R et al: Role of computerized physician order entry systems in facilitating medication errors. JAMA 2005;293:1197.

Mello MM, Kelly CN: Effects of a malpractice crisis on residents' practice decisions. Am J Obstet Gynecol 2005;105:1287.

Morey JC et al: Error reduction and performance improvement in the emergency department through formal teamwork training: results of the Med Teams project. Health Serv Res 2002; 37:1553.

Nicolaides KH: Nuchal translucency and other first-trimester sonographic markers of chromosomal abnormalities. Am J Obstet Gynecol 2004;19:45.

Office of Civil Rights, Department of Health and Human Services: *Standards for privacy of individually identifiable health information: final rules.* Fed Reg 2002;67:53182.

Petrinc JR et al: Estimated effect of 17 alpha-hydroxyprogesterone caproate on preterm birth in the United States. Obstet Gynecol 2005;105:267.

Ransom SR et al: Reduced medicolegal risk by compliance with obstetric clinical pathways: a case-controlled study. Obstet Gynecol 2003;104:751.

Redline RW: Severe fetal placental vascular lesions in term infants with neurologic impairment. Am J Obstet Gynecol 2005;192:452.

Ross SE, Lin Chen T: The effects of promoting patient access to medical records: a review. J Am Med Inform Assoc 2003;10: 129.

Sepilian V, Wood E: Ectopic pregnancy. 2004 Nov 24. Available at www.imedicine.com.

Sosa C et al: Bed rest in singleton pregnancies for preventing preterm birth. Cochrane Database Syst Rev 2004;(1)CD003581.

Studdert DM, Mello MM, Brennan TA: Medical malpractice. N Engl J Med 2004;350:283.

To MS et al: Cervical cerclage for prevention of preterm delivery in women with short cervix: Randomized controlled trial. Lancet 2004;363:1849.

Tsoi E et al: Ultrasound assessment of cervical length in threatened preterm labor. Ultrasound Obstet Gynecol 2003;21:552.

Tucker JM et al: Etiologies of preterm birth in an indigent population: Is prevention a logical expectation? Obstet Gynecol 1991;77:343.

Wachter RM, Shojania KG: *Internal Bleeding.* Rugged Land, LLC, 2004.

Index

Note: Page numbers in **boldface** indicate a major discussion; page numbers followed by *f* indicate figures; page numbers followed by *t* indicate tables.

Anal orifice, 89
Anal sphincter, external, 22f, 92f
Anal stenosis, 551t
Analgesia, 441
  obstetric. *See* Obstetric analgesia
  patient controlled, postoperative, 775
Analgesics
  administration route for, 443
  fetal distribution of, 444–445, 445f
  narcotic, postoperative, 775
  physical and chemical factors and, 443f,
      443–444, 444f, 444t
  placental transfer of, 444
  precautions for, 443
  systemic, 445–447
    narcotic, 446
    sedatives, 445
Anaphase, in mitosis, 99, 100f
Anaphase I, in meiosis, 100, 101f
Anaphase II, in meiosis, 100–101, 101f
Ancitabine, 912–913
Androgen(s), 73, 939–940
  action of, 940
  bone remodeling and, 962
  circulation of, 940
  estrogen and, 138
  exogenous sources of, hirsutism and, 939
  metabolism of, changes associated with
      menopause, 956f, 956–957
  production of, 939
  puberty and, 126, 127f
Androgen insensitivity (syndrome), 122,
      123f, 563, 563f
Androgen receptor agonists, for hirsutism,
      945
Android pelvis, 30, 30f, 434
Androstanediol glucuronide, serum level of, to
      differentiate Cushing's syndrome
      from Cushing's disease, 943
Androstenedione, circulation of, 940
Anemia
  assessment and minimization of surgical
      risk and, 767
  physiologic, of the newborn, 171
  in pregnancy, **406–409**
    aplastic, 408
    folic acid deficiency, 407–408
    hemolytic, drug-induced, 408–409
    iron deficiency, 406–407
    multiple, hypochromic normocytic,
      308–309
    sickle cell, 407, 409–410
Anesthesia, 441
  agents for. *See* Anesthetics
  complications associated with, 782–783
    bronchospasm, 782–783
    hypothermia, 783
    malignant hyperthermia, 782
    with regional anesthesia, 783
  general, 441
  for laparoscopy, 801
  obstetric. *See* Obstetric anesthesia
  in pregnancy, general versus regional, 419

Anesthetics, **443–447**
  administration route for, 443
  fetal distribution of, 444–445, 445f
  physical and chemical factors and, 443f,
      443–444, 444f, 444t
  placental transfer of, 444
  precautions for, 443
  regional. *See* Regional anesthesia
  systemic, 445–447
    inhalation, 447
    ketamine, 446–447
    propofol, 446
    sedatives, 445
    thiobarbiturates, 446
    tranquilizers and amnestics, 445–446
Aneuploidy
  screening for, 254
  spontaneous abortion and, 259
Aneurysms, ruptured, in pregnancy, 397–
      398, 429
Angelman's syndrome, with assisted repro-
      duction, 951
Angiography
  in gynecologic evaluation, 535
  with pulmonary embolism, 786
Angiotensin II, during pregnancy, 154
Angiotensin-converting enzyme inhibitors,
      for chronic hypertension, during
      pregnancy, 321
Angiotensinogen, estrogens and, 136
Annular detachment, cervical, 627
Anococcygeal ligament, 22f
Anogenital injuries, caused by abuse, in pre-
      menarcheal children, 555–556
Anorchia, amenorrhea and, 930
Anorectal agenesis, 89
Anorectal canal, 72f, 76
Anorectal inflammation, in gonorrhea, 671
Anorexia nervosa, 1005–1006
Anovulation, dysfunctional uterine bleeding
      with, 576–577
Anovulatory cycles, 132
Anoxia, with breech delivery, 349–350
Anthracyclines, 910–911
Anthropoid pelvis, 30, 30f, 434
Antibiotics. *See also* Antimicrobial chemo-
      therapy
  antitumor, 910–911
  for premature rupture of membranes, 281,
      281t
  for preterm labor, 278
  prophylactic
    for cesarean section, 492–493
    following rape, 1029
    for hysterectomy, 811
    preoperative, 492–493, 774, 811
Antibody studies, in infertility, 919–920
Anticancer drugs. *See* Chemotherapy
Anticoagulants
  circulating, in pregnancy, 413
  oral
    assessment and minimization of surgi-
      cal risk and, 768

for deep vein thrombosis, 785
  discontinuing before surgery, 774
Antidiuretic hormone, deficiency of, in preg-
      nancy, 395–396
Antiepileptic drugs, teratogenic potential of,
      400–401
Antifungal drugs, **170.** *See also specific drugs*
Antihypertensive therapy
  in chronic hypertension, during preg-
      nancy, 320–321
  for preeclampsia, 325
Antimetabolites, 911–913
  folate antagonists, 911–912
  purine antagonists, 912
  pyrimidine antagonists, 912–913
Antimicrobial chemotherapy, **696–711.** *See
      also* Antibiotics; *specific drugs*
  aminoglycosides for, **706–707**
  antifungal drugs for, **710**
  antiviral drugs for, **710–711**
  cephalosporins for, **702–704**
  clindamycin for, **705**
  drug selection principles for, 696–697,
      697t–699t, 699–700
    administration route and, 699
    adverse reactions and, 699–700
    "best guess" and, 696
    clinical response and, 696
    dosage adequacy and, 699
    drug susceptibility tests and, 696–
      697
    duration of therapy and, 699
    etiologic diagnosis and, 696
    laboratory control and, 696
    oliguria and, 700
    renal function impairment and, 700
    uremia and, 700
  linezolid for, **709**
  metronidazole for, **708**
  monobactams for, **704**
    carbapenems for, 704
    macrolides for, 704–705
  nitrofurantoin for, **709–710**
  penicillins for, **700–702**
  quinolones for, **709**
  spectinomycin for, **707**
  sulfonamides-trimethoprim for, **707–
      708**
  for surgical chemoprophylaxis, 710
  tetracyclines for, **705–706**
  vancomycin for, **708–709**
Antimüllerian hormone, 73, 74
Antiphospholipid syndrome, 413
Antiplatelet drugs, discontinuing before sur-
      gery, 774
Antiprostaglandins, for dysmenorrhea, 573
Antithrombin III
  deficiency of, 413
  in disseminated intravascular coagulation,
      998
Antitumor antibiotics, 910–911
Antiviral drugs, **710–711**
Anuria, postoperative, 792

MW00753793

a LANGE medical book

CURRENT
Diagnosis & Treatment
in Orthopedics

Fourth Edition

Edited by

Harry B. Skinner, MD, PhD
Professor and Chairman
Department of Orthopaedic Surgery
University of California, Irvine
Irvine, California

Lange Medical Books/McGraw-Hill
Medical Publishing Division

New York   Chicago   San Francisco   Lisbon   London   Madrid   Mexico City
Milan   New Delhi   San Juan   Seoul   Singapore   Sydney   Toronto

Current Diagnosis & Treatment in Orthopedics, Fourth Edition

Previous editions copyright © 2003, 2000 by The McGraw-Hill Companies; © 1995 by Appleton & Lange.

ISBN: 0-07-143833-5 (Domestic)
ISSN: 1081-0056

3 4 5 6 7 8 9 0 DOC/DOC 0 9 8 7

Notice

This book was set in Garamond by Silverchair Science + Communications, Inc.
The editors were Hilarie Surrena, Christie Naglieri, and Regina Y. Brown.
The production supervisor was Catherine Saggese.
The index was prepared by Ann Blum.
The cover designer was Mary McKeon.
RR Donnelley was printer and binder.

This book is printed on acid-free paper.

INTERNATIONAL EDITION ISBN 0-07-110451-8

Contents

Authors

Juan F. Agudelo, MD
Resident, Department of Orthopedic Surgery,
   University of Colorado School of Medicine,
   Oakland, California
Musculoskeletal Trauma Surgery

Michael S. Bednar, MD
Associate Professor, Department of Orthopaedic
   Surgery and Rehabilitation, Loyola University
   Medical Center, Maywood, Illinois
Mbednar@lumc.edu
Hand Surgery

Nitin N. Bhatia, MD
Assistant Clinical Professor; Chief, Spine Service;
   Director, The UC Irvine Spine Center, Department
   of Orthopaedic Surgery, University of California,
   Irvine, Medical Center, Orange, California
bhatian@uci.edu
Disorders, Diseases, and Injuries of the Spine

Vincent J. Caiozzo, PhD
Professor, Department of Orthopaedic Surgery,
   School of Medicine, University of California, Irvine
vjcaiozz@uci.edu
Basic Science in Orthopedic Surgery

Loretta B. Chou, MD
Assistant Professor, Division of Orthopaedic
   Surgery, Stanford University School of Medicine,
   Stanford, California
lchou@stanford.edu
Foot & Ankle Surgery

Ranjan Gupta, MD
Associate Professor, Department of Orthopaedic
   Surgery, Center for Biomedical Engineering,
   University of California, Irvine
ranjang@uci.edu
*Basic Science in Orthopedic Surgery; Adult
Reconstructive Surgery*

Bang H. Hoang, MD
Assistant Professor, Department of Orthopaedic
   Surgery, School of Medicine, University of
   California, Irvine
Musculoskeletal Oncology

Serena S. Hu, MD
Professor of Clinical Orthopaedics, Department of
   Orthopaedic Surgery, University of California,
   San Francisco
Hus@orthosurg.ucsf.edu
Disorder, Diseases, & Injuries of the Spine

Lee D. Kaplan, MD
Sports Medicine

Mary Ann E. Keenan, MD
Chief, Neuro-Orthopaedics Surgery,
   Department of Orthopaedic Surgery,
   University of Pennsylvania School of
   Medicine, Philadelphia
maryann.keenan@uphs.upenn.edu
Rehabilitation

Terry R. Light, MD
Dr. William M. Scholl Professor and Chairman,
   Department of Orthopaedic Surgery and
   Rehabilitation, Loyola University Medical
   Center, Maywood, Illinois
tlight@lumc.edu
Hand Surgery

Jeffrey Mann, MD
Alta-Bates Summit Medical Center, Oakland,
   California
Jeffmann@msn.com
Foot & Ankle Surgery

Patrick J. McMahon, MD
Assistant Professor, Divisions of Sports
   Medicine, and Shoulder and Elbow Surgery,
   Department of Orthopedic Surgery, University
   of Pittsburgh School of Medicine, Pittsburgh,
   Pennsylvania
mcmahonp@msx.upmc.edu
Sports Medicine

Samir Mehta, MD
Administrative Chief Resident; Instructor,
   Department of Orthopaedic Surgery, University
   of Pennsylvania, Philadelphia
Samir.mehta@uphs.upenn.edu
Rehabilitation

Robert S. Namba, MD
Associate Clinical Professor of Orthopaedic
    Surgery, University of California, Irvine, School
    of Medicine; Attending Surgeon, Southern
    California Permanente Medical Group,
    Anaheim, California
Robert.s.namba@kp.org
Adult Reconstructive Surgery

Anand Parekh, MRCS
Research Fellow, Department of Orthopedic
    Surgery, University of Colorado School of
    Medicine, Denver Colorado, Denver Health
    Medical Center, Denver, Colorado
Anand.parekh@dhha.org
Musculoskeletal Trauma Surgery

George T. Rab , MD
Ben Ali Shriners Professor of Pediatric
    Orthopedics, Chair, Department of
    Orthopedic Surgery, Chief, Division of
    Pediatric Orthopedics, University of
    California, Davis, School of Medicine;
    Consulting Physician, Shriners Hospitals for
    Children, Northern California
George.rab@ucdmc.ucdavis.edu
Pediatric Orthopedic Surgery

R. Lor Randall, MD, FACS
Associate Professor, Director, Sarcoma Services
Chief, SARC Lab, Huntsman Cancer Institute and
Primary Children's Medical Center, University of
Utah, Salt Lake City, Utah
Musculoskeletal Oncology

Steven D. K. Ross, MD
Clinical Professor, Department of Orthopaedic
    Surgery, University of California, Irvine, College
    of Medicine, Orange, California
Sdross@uci.edu
Foot & Ankle Surgery

John R. Shank, MD
Private Practice, Colorado Springs, Colorado
johnrshank@yahoo.com
Musculoskeletal Trauma Surgery

Harry B. Skinner, MD, PhD
Professor and Chairman, Department of Orthopaedic
    Surgery, University of California, Irvine
hskinner@uci.edu
*Basic Science in Orthopedic Surgery; General
Considerations in Orthopedic Surgery; Sports
Medicine; Adult Reconstructive Surgery;
Orthopedic Infections*

Douglas G. Smith, MD
Harborview Medical Center, Department of
    Orthopedics and Sports Medicine, Seattle,
    Washington
dgsmith@u.washington.edu
Amputations

Wade R. Smith, MD
Associate Professor of Orthopedic Surgery,
    University of Colorado School of Medicine,
    Denver, Colorado; Director of Orthopedic
    Surgery, Denver Health Medical Center,
    Denver, Colorado
Wsmith@dhha.org
Musculoskeletal Trauma Surgery

Robert K-B Tay, MD
Assistant Professor in Residence, Department of
    Orthopaedic Surgery, University of California,
    San Francisco
tayb@orthosurg.ucsf.edu
Disorder, Diseases, & Injuries of the Spine

Clifford B. Tribus, MD
Associate Professor, Division of Orthopedics,
    University of Wisconsin School of Medicine,
    Madison, Wisconsin
tribus@surgery.wisc.edu
Disorder, Diseases, & Injuries of the Spine

Scott C. Wilson, MD
Assistant Professor of Orthopedic Surgery, Tulane
    University School of Medicine, New Orleans,
    Louisiana
mshinn@Tulane.edu
Orthopedic Infections

Preface

This *Current Diagnosis and Treatment in Orthopedics* is the Fourth Edition of the orthopedic surgery contribution to the Lange Current Series of books. It is surprising to realize that it has been 10 years since the first edition of this book. The goal of this book has not changed. It is intended to fill a need for a ready source of up-to-date information on disorders and diseases treated by orthopedic surgeons and related physicians. The format in this edition is unchanged from previous: there is emphasis on the major diagnostic features of disease states, the natural history of the disease where appropriate, the work-up required for definitive diagnosis, and, finally, definitive treatment. The book focuses on orthopedic conditions, de-emphasizing the treatment of the patient from a general medical viewpoint, except when it pertains to the orthopedic problem under consideration. Importantly, pathophysiology, epidemiology, and pathology are included when they assist in arriving at a definitive diagnosis or an understanding of the treatment of the diseases or condition. In many conditions, such as infection or neoplasm, it is extremely important to understand the pathophysiology because the disease may be encountered at various time points in the progression of the disease.

This edition of the *Current Diagnosis and Treatment in Orthopedics* is truly current.

The entire book has been updated in its references to include only those references since 2000, except in cases where classic articles are necessary to refer back to major advances in understanding or treatment, or in situations where there has been little change in the sub-specialization in orthopedics, such as rehabilitation. These selected references to the older literature represent landmarks in the advancement of the understanding of orthopedic diseases and conditions, and serve as useful sources of the fundamental basis for understanding these diseases and conditions.

INTENDED AUDIENCE

The unique format of the Lange series textbooks allows readers of many levels of understanding to derive benefit from the information.

Students will find that the book encompasses virtually all aspects of orthopedics that they will encounter in classes and as sub-interns in major teaching institutions. Residents and house officers can use the book as a ready reference covering the majority of disorders and conditions in emergency and elective orthopedic surgery. Despite its small size, it is truly comprehensive. Because of the organization of the book on a sub-specialty basis, review of individual chapters will provide house officers rotating on sub-specialty orthopedic services with an excellent basis for further in-depth study.

For emergency room physicians, especially those with medical backgrounds, the text provides an excellent resource in managing orthopedic problems seen on an emergent basis. Similarly, family practice, pediatricians, general practitioners, and internists will find the book particularly helpful in the referral decision process, and as a resource to explain disorders to patients. Finally, practicing orthopedic surgeons, particularly those in sub-specialties of orthopedics, will find the book a helpful resource in reassuring them that their treatment in areas outside their sub-specialty interest is current and up-to-date.

ORGANIZATION

The book is structured similarly to the structure of orthopedic surgery. Natural sub-specialization has occurred in orthopedic surgery over the years, which has resulted in some overlap in anatomic areas. This has resulted in the book having some overlap and some artificial division of subjects. Because of the primarily sub-specialization structure, the reader is encouraged to read entire chapters, or for more discrete topics, go directly to the index for information. For example, the house officer rotating on the pediatric orthopedic service would find reading the pediatric chapter to be a prudent method of developing a baseline knowledge in pediatric orthopedic surgery. Knee problems however, might be best approached by looking in the sports medicine chapter, or in the adult reconstruction chapter, since these areas overlap, mostly in age of patient.

The first chapter serves as a basis for the rest of the book because it summarizes current basic information that is fundamental in the understanding of orthopedic surgery. Chapter Two introduces aspects of interest in the perioperative care of the orthopedic patient, including social aspects of the patient/physician relationship. Management of orthopedic problems arising from trauma is covered in Chapter Three, while Chapter Four deals with sports medicine with an emphasis on the knee and shoulder. Chapter Five covers all aspects of spine surgery, including degenerative spinal problems, spinal deformity, and spinal trauma.

Chapter Six provides comprehensive coverage of tumors in orthopedic surgery, including benign and malignant soft tissue and hard tissue tumors. Adult joint reconstruction, including the disorders that lead to joint reconstruction are covered in Chapter Seven. In Chapter Eight, infections, with their special implications for orthopedic surgery are covered. Chapter Nine discusses foot and ankle surgery, and Chapter Ten, hand surgery. Chapter Eleven covers diseases in orthopedics unique to children. The final two chapters deal with amputation and all aspects of rehabilitation fundamental to orthopedic surgeons in returning patients to full function.

OUTSTANDING FEATURES

- Illustrations have been carefully selected to maximize their benefits in pointing out orthopedic principles and concepts. The effect of changes in imaging technology on optimal diagnostic studies is emphasized, including cost-effectiveness.
- Bone and soft tissue tumor differential diagnoses are simplified by comprehensive tables that categorize tumors by age, location, and imaging characteristics. The molecular basis of the current understanding of tumor etiology is expanded.
- Concise, current, and comprehensive treatment of the basic sciences underlying the understanding of orthopedic surgery is provided.

NEW TO THIS EDITION

- Information on shoulder evaluation has been widely expanded, including tables to elucidate the diagnosis of shoulder problems.
- Advances in treatment of back pain, including disk replacement, are included.
- The latest on molecular biology of neoplasm has been expanded in the musculoskeletal tumor section.
- Surgical management of osteoporosis, including techniques such as kyphoplasty and vertebroplasty, and information on shoulder replacement have been widely expanded.
- Guidelines for predicting function, such as ambulatory capability after spinal cord injury, are updated.
- New materials in orthopedics that are making changes in the way replacement arthroplasty is performed are included.
- The latest information on important growth factors in orthopedics is elucidated with current usage.

I am pleased to be able to say, with the concurrence of my co-authors, that these new features added to the information in the previous edition, make this edition a significant improvement over the last.

Harry B. Skinner, MD, PhD

Basic Science in Orthopedic Surgery

Ranjan Gupta, MD, Vincent J. Caiozzo, PhD, & Harry B. Skinner, MD, PhD

BIOMECHANICS & BIOMATERIALS

*Ranjan Gupta, MD, Vincent Caiozzo, PhD,
Stephen D. Cook, PhD, Robert L. Barrack, MD, &
Harry B. Skinner, MD, PhD*

Orthopedic surgery is the branch of medicine concerned with restoring and preserving the normal function of the musculoskeletal system. As such, it focuses on bones, joints, tendons, ligaments, muscles, and specialized tissues such as the intervertebral disk. Over the last half century, surgeons and investigators in the field of orthopedics have increasingly recognized the importance that engineering principles play both in understanding the normal behavior of musculoskeletal tissues and in designing implant systems to model the function of these tissues. The goals of the first portion of this chapter are to describe the biologic organization of the musculoskeletal tissues, examine the mechanical properties of the tissues in light of their biologic composition, and explore the material and design concepts required to fabricate implant systems with mechanical and biologic properties that will provide adequate function and longevity. The subject of the second portion of the chapter is gait analysis.

BASIC CONCEPTS & DEFINITIONS

Most biologic tissues are either **porous materials** or **composite materials.** A material such as bone has mechanical properties that are influenced markedly by the degree of porosity, defined as the degree of the material's volume that consists of void. For instance, the compressive strength of osteoporotic bone, which has increased porosity, is markedly decreased in comparison with the compressive strength of normal bone. Like composite materials, **alloys** consist of two or more different metallic elements that are in solution. Although composite materials can be physically or mechanically separated, alloyed materials cannot.

Generally, composites are made up of a matrix material, which absorbs energy and protects fibers from brittle failure, and a fiber, which strengthens and stiffens the matrix. The performance of the two materials together is superior to that of either material alone in terms of mechanical properties (eg, strength and elastic modulus) and other properties (eg, corrosion resistance). The mechanical properties of various types of composite materials differ, based on the percentage of each substance in the material and on the principal orientation of the fiber. The substances in combination, however, are always stronger for their weight than is either substance alone. Microscopically, bone is a composite material consisting of hydroxyapatite crystals and an organic matrix that contains collagen (the fibers).

The mechanical characteristics of a material are commonly described in terms of stress and strain. **Stress** is the force that a material is subjected to per unit of original area, and **strain** is the amount of deformation the material experiences per unit of original length in response to stress. These characteristics can be adequately described by a **stress–strain curve** (Figure 1–1), which plots the effect of a uniaxial stress on a simple test specimen made from a given material. Changes in the geometric dimensions of the material (eg, changes in the material's area or length) have no effect on the stress–strain curve for that material.

Mechanical characteristics can also be illustrated by a **load-elongation curve,** in which the slope of the initial linear portion depicts the **stiffness** of a given material. Although similar in appearance to the stress–strain curve, the load-elongation curve for a given material can be altered by changes in the material's diameter (cross-sectional area) or length. For instance, doubling the cross-sectional area of a test specimen while maintaining the original length will double the stiffness because the increased diameter doubles the **load to failure** (ie, it doubles the force that a material can withstand in a single application) without changing the total elongation. Conversely, doubling the length of the test specimen while maintaining the original diameter will decrease the stiffness by half because doubling the length in turn doubles the elongation without changing the load to failure.

Because of this difference between the stress–strain curve and load-elongation curve, any comparison of the characteristics of specimens requires that the same type of curve be used in the evaluation. If the load-elongation curve is used, the geometric dimensions of the specimens must also be the same. In this chapter, subsequent

Figure 1–1. A generalized stress–strain diagram illustrating the mechanical properties of a material subjected to stress. The proportional limit (σ_p) of a material is the stress at which permanent or plastic deformation begins. Because the proportional limit is difficult to measure accurately for some materials, a 0.2% strain offset line parallel to the linear region of the curve is constructed. The stress corresponding to this line is defined as the yield stress (σ_y). If stress is removed after the initiation of plastic deformation (point A), only the elastic deformation denoted by the linear portion of the stress–strain curve is recovered. The ultimate tensile strength (σ_u) is the maximal stress that a material can withstand in a single application before it fails.

measure accurately for some materials. Therefore, a 0.2% strain offset line parallel to the linear region of the curve is constructed, as shown in Figure 1–1. The stress corresponding to this line is defined as the **yield stress,** or σ_y. If stress is removed after the initiation of plastic deformation (point A in Figure 1–1), only the elastic deformation denoted by the linear portion of the stress–strain curve is recovered. The **ultimate tensile strength** (failure load), or σ_u, is the maximal stress that a material can withstand in a single application before it fails.

When subjected to repeated loading in a physiologic environment, a material may fail at stresses well below the ultimate tensile strength. The **fatigue curve,** or **S-N curve,** demonstrates the behavior of a metal during cyclic loading and is shown in Figure 1–2. Generally, as the number of cycles (**N**) increases, the amount of applied stress (**S**) that the metal can withstand before failure decreases. The **endurance limit** of a material is the maximal stress below which fatigue failure will never occur regardless of the number of cycles. Fatigue failure will occur if the combination of local peak stresses and number of loading cycles at that stress are excessive. Although most materials exhibit a lower stress at failure with cyclic loading, some do not, such as pyrolytic carbon, making it appropriate for high-cycle applications such as heart valves. Environmental conditions strongly influence fatigue behavior. The physiologic environment, which is corrosive, can significantly reduce the number of cycles to failure and the endurance limit of a material.

Materials can be evaluated in terms of ductility, toughness, viscoelasticity, friction, lubrication, and wear.

discussions pertain to the stress–strain curve, although differing terminology in the load-elongation curve is noted parenthetically.

The initial linear or elastic portion of the stress–strain curve (see Figure 1–1) depicts the amount of stress a material can withstand before permanently deforming. The slope of this line is termed the **modulus of elasticity** (stiffness) of the material. A high modulus of elasticity indicates that the material is difficult to deform, whereas a low modulus indicates that the material is more pliable. The modulus of elasticity is an excellent basis on which different materials can be compared. When materials such as those used in implants are compared, however, it is important to remember that the modulus of elasticity is a property only of the material itself and not of the structure. Implant stiffness in bending—or, more correctly, flexural rigidity—is a function both of material elastic modulus and of design geometry.

The **proportional limit,** or σ_p, of a material is the stress at which permanent or plastic deformation begins. The proportional limit, however, is difficult to

Figure 1–2. A generalized diagram comparing two fatigue curves, or S-N curves, for the same material. Curve A illustrates the material's endurance limit in a noncorrosive environment, and curve B illustrates its endurance limit in a corrosive environment. The body is an example of a corrosive environment for implant materials.

These properties are introduced here, and many of them are explored in detail in subsequent sections.

Ductility is defined as the amount of deformation that a material undergoes before failure and is characterized in terms of total strain. A brittle material will fail with minimal strain caused by propagation of a crack because the yield stress is higher than the tensile stress. A ductile material, however, will fail only after markedly increased strain and decreased cross-sectional area. Polymethylmethacrylate (PMMA, a polymer) and ceramics are brittle materials, whereas metals exhibit relatively more ductility. Environmental conditions, especially changes in temperature, can alter the ductility of materials.

Toughness is defined as the energy imparted to a material to cause it to fracture and is measured by the total area under the stress–strain curve.

Because all biologic tissues are viscoelastic in nature, a thorough understanding of **viscoelasticity** is essential. A viscoelastic material is one that exhibits different properties when loaded at different strain rates. Thus, its mechanical properties are time-dependent. Bone, for example, absorbs more energy at fast loading rates, such as in high-speed motor vehicle accidents, than at slow loading rates, such as in recreational snow skiing.

Viscoelastic materials have three important properties: hysteresis, creep, and stress relaxation. When a viscoelastic material is subjected to cyclic loading, the stress–strain relationship during the loading process differs from that during the unloading process (Figure 1–3). This difference in stress–strain response is termed **hysteresis.** The deviation between loading and unloading processes depends on the degree of viscous behavior. The area between the two curves is a measure of the energy lost by internal friction during the loading process. **Creep,** which is also called **cold flow** and observed in polyethylene components, is defined as a deformation that occurs in a material under constant stress. Some deformation is permanent, persisting even when the stress is released. The decrease in stress associated with a constant strain over time is a result of **stress relaxation,** a phenomenon evident, for example, in the loosening of fracture fixation plates. The time necessary to attain creep, or stress relaxation equilibrium, is an inherent property of the material.

Friction refers to the resistance between two bodies when one slides over the other. Friction is greatest at slow rates and decreases with faster rates. This is because the surface asperities (peaks) tend to adhere to one another more strongly at slower rates. Mechanisms of **lubrication** reduce the friction between two surfaces. Several lubrication mechanisms are present in articular cartilage to overcome friction processes in normal joint motion. Similarly, mechanisms are present in polyethylene-metal articulations to overcome friction in joint replacements.

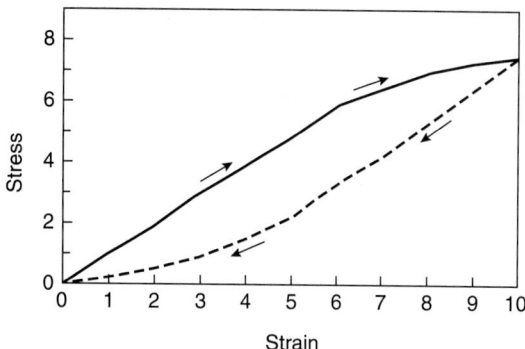

Figure 1–3. When a viscoelastic material is subjected to cyclic loading, the stress–strain curve during the loading process (solid lines) differs from that during the unloading process (dotted lines). This difference in stress–strain response is called **hysteresis.** The area between the two curves is a measure of the energy lost by internal friction during the loading process.

Wear can occur from friction and is defined as the removal of surface material by mechanical motion. Wear is always observed between two moving surfaces, but lubrication mechanisms act to reduce the detrimental effects of excessive wear. Three types of wear mechanisms are apparent in normal and prosthetic joint motion: abrasive, adhesive, and three-body wear. **Abrasive wear** is the generation of material particles from a softer surface when it moves against a rougher, harder surface. An example of the product of abrasive wear is sawdust, which results from the movement of sandpaper against a wood surface. The amount of wear depends on factors such as contact stress, hardness, and finish of the bearing surfaces.

Adhesive wear results when a thin film of material is transferred from one bearing surface to the other. In prosthetic joints, the transfer film can be either polyethylene or the passivated (corrosion-resistant) layer of metal. Regardless of the material, wear occurs in the surface that loses the transfer film. If the particles from the transfer film are shed from the other surface as well, they behave as a third body and also result in wear.

Three-body wear occurs when another particle is located between two bearing surfaces. Cement particles act as third bodies in prosthetic joints. Implant designers continue to search for compatible substances that reduce friction at articulating surfaces and thereby reduce the amount of wear debris generated. Wear of polyethylene is the dominant problem in total joint replacement today because the wear debris generated is biologically active and leads to osteolysis.

BIOMECHANICS IN ORTHOPEDICS

An analysis of the factors that influence normal and prosthetic joint function requires an understanding of free-body diagrams as well as the concepts of force, moment, and equilibrium.

Force, Moment, & Equilibrium

Forces and moments are vector quantities—that is, they are described by point of application, magnitude, and direction. A force represents the action of one body on another. The action may be applied directly (eg, via a push or a pull) or from a distance (eg, via gravity). A normal tensile or compressive force is applied perpendicular to a surface, whereas a shear force is applied parallel to a surface. A force that is applied eccentrically produces a moment.

The force generated by gravity on an object acts at the center of gravity. An object that is symmetric has its center of gravity in the geometrically centered position, whereas an object that is asymmetric has its center of gravity closer to its "heavier" end. The center of gravity for the human body is the resultant of the individual centers of gravity from each segment of the body. Therefore, as the body segments move, the center of gravity changes accordingly and may even lie outside the body in extreme positions, such as encountered in gymnastics. A moment is defined as the product of the quantity of force and the perpendicular distance between the line of action of the force and the center of rotation. A moment usually results in a rotation of the object about a fixed axis.

Newton's first law states that a body (or object) is in equilibrium if the sum of the forces and moments acting on the body are balanced; therefore, the sum of forces and moments for each direction must equal zero. The concept of equilibrium is important in understanding and determining force–body interactions, such as the increased joint reaction force occurring in an extended arm because of an external weight and such as the increased joint reaction force occurring in the hip at a specific moment during walking.

Free-Body Diagrams

A free-body diagram can be used schematically to represent all the forces and moments acting on a joint. The concepts of equilibrium can be extended to determine joint reaction or muscle forces for different conditions, as demonstrated in the following two examples.

Example 1: Determine the force on the abductor muscle of a person's hip joint (the abductor force, or F_{AB}) and the joint reaction force (the F_J) when the person is standing on one leg. The weight of the trunk,

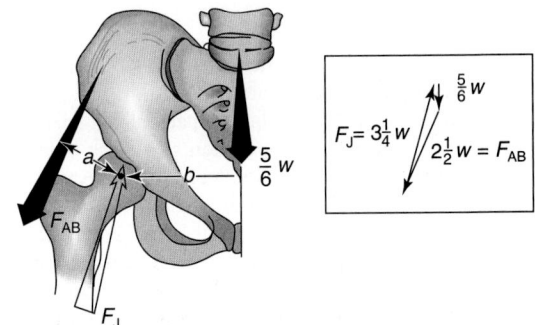

Figure 1–4. A free body diagram and force triangle illustrating the method for determining the force of the abductor muscle of a person's hip joint (F_{AB}) and the joint reaction force (F_J) when the person is standing on one leg and the total weight (w) of the person is known. See the discussion of example 1 in the text.

both arms, and one leg is $5/6$ of the total weight (w) of the person. As illustrated in Figure 1–4, this weight will tend to rotate the body about the femoral head and is counteracted by the pull of the abductor muscles on the pelvis. The necessary equation to solve for F_{AB} is as follows:

$$F_{AB} \times a = \frac{B}{nw} \times b$$

In solving the equation, assume that a = 5 cm and that b = 15 cm.

After this equation is solved, two of the three forces are known. The remaining force (the F_J) can be determined from a force triangle (see Figure 1–4) because, according to Newton's first law, the sum of forces must equal zero.

Example 2: Determine the force on a person's deltoid muscle (the deltoid force, or F_D) and the force of the joint acting about the shoulder (F_J) when the person holds a metal weight (w) at arm's length (Figure 1–5). The weight of the arm is ignored because only the increase in forces about the shoulder caused by the metal weight is to be determined. F_D is determined by summing the moments about the joint center. The necessary equation is as follows:

$$F_D \times a = w \times b$$

In solving the equation, assume that a = 5 cm and that b = 60 cm.

After this equation is solved, an F_J of 1150 N is determined using a force triangle (see Figure 1–5).

Figure 1–5. A free body diagram and force triangle illustrating the method for determining the force of a person's deltoid muscle (F_D) and the force of the joint acting about the shoulder (F_J) when the person holds a metal weight (w) at arm's length. See the discussion of example 2 in the text.

Moments of Inertia

The orientation of the bone's or implant's cross-sectional area with respect to the applied principal load also greatly influences the biomechanical performance. Bending and torsion occur in long bones and are important considerations in the design of implants. In general, the farther that material mass is distributed from the axis of bending or torsion while still retaining structural integrity, the more resistant the structure will be to bending or torsion. The **area moment of inertia** is a mathematical expression for resistance to bending, and the **polar moment of inertia** is a mathematical expression for resistance to torsion. Both types of moment of inertia relate the cross-sectional geometry and orientation of the object with respect to the applied axial load. The larger the area moment of inertia or the polar moment of inertia, the less likely the material will fail. Figure 1–6 summarizes the area moments of inertia for representative shapes important to orthopedic surgery. Creating an open slot in an object will significantly decrease the polar moment of inertia of the object.

Knowledge of moments of inertia is important for understanding mechanical behavior in relation to object geometry. For instance, the length of the long bones predisposes them to high bending moments. Their tubular shape helps them resist bending in all directions, however. This resistance to bending is attributable to the large area moment of inertia because the majority of bone tissue is distributed away from the neutral axis. The concept of moment of inertia is crucial in the design of implants that are exposed to excessive bending and torsional stresses.

Hills BA: Boundary lubrication in vivo. Proc Inst Mech Eng [H] 2000;214:83. [PMID: 10718053]

BIOLOGIC TISSUES IN ORTHOPEDICS

The functions of the musculoskeletal system are to provide support for the body, to protect the vital organs, and to facilitate easy movement of joints. The bone, articular cartilage, tendon, ligament, nerve, and muscle all interact to fulfill these functions. The musculoskeletal tissues are integrally specialized to perform their duties and have excellent regenerative and reparative processes. They also adapt and undergo compositional changes in response to increased or decreased stress states. Specialized components of the musculoskeletal system, such as the intervertebral disk, are particularly suited for supporting large stress loads while resisting movement.

Bones

Bones are dynamic tissues that serve a variety of functions and have the ability to remodel to changes in internal and external stimuli. Bones provide support for the trunk and extremities, provide attachment to ligaments and tendons, protect vital organs, and act as a mineral and iron reservoir for the maintenance of homeostasis.

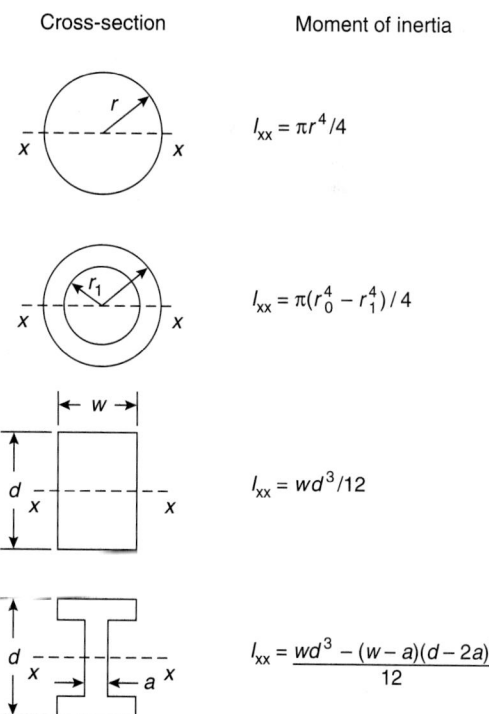

Figure 1–6. Summary of the area moments of inertia for representative shapes important to orthopedic surgery.

A. Structural Composition

Bone is a composite consisting of two types of material. The first material is an organic extracellular matrix that contains collagen, accounts for approximately 30–35% of the dry weight of bone, and is responsible for providing flexibility and resilience to the bone. The second material consists primarily of calcium and phosphorous salts, especially hydroxyapatite $[Ca_{10}(PO_4)_6(OH)_2]$, accounts for approximately 65–70% of the dry weight of bone, and contributes to the hardness and rigidity of the bone. Microscopically, bone can be classified as either woven or lamellar.

Woven bone, which is also called **primary bone,** is characterized by a random arrangement of cells and collagen. Because of its relatively disoriented composition, woven bone demonstrates isotropic mechanical characteristics, with similar properties observed regardless of the direction of applied stress. Woven bone is associated with periods of rapid formation, such as the initial stages of fracture repair or biologic implant fixation. Woven bone, which has a low mineral content, remodels to lamellar bone.

Lamellar bone is a slower forming, mature bone that is characterized by an orderly cellular distribution and regular orientation of collagen fibers (Figure 1–7). The lamellae can be parallel to one another or concentrically organized around a vascular canal called a **Haversian system** or **osteon.** At the periphery of each osteon is a cement line, a narrow area containing ground substance primarily composed of glycosaminoglycans. Neither the canaliculi nor the collagen fibers cross the cement line. Biomechanically, the cement line is the weakest link in the microstructure of bone. The organized structure of lamellar bone makes it anisotropic, as seen in the fact that it is stronger during axial loading than it is during transverse, or shear, loading.

Bone can be classified macroscopically as cortical tissue and cancellous (trabecular) tissue. Both types are morphologically lamellar bone. Cortical tissue relies on osteons for cell communication. Because trabecular width is small, however, the canaliculi can communicate directly with blood vessels in the medullary canal. The basic differences between cortical tissue and cancellous tissue relate to porosity and apparent density. The porosity of cortical tissue typically ranges from 5% to 30%, and that of cancellous tissue ranges from 30% to 90%. The apparent density of cortical tissue is approximately 1.8 g/cm, and that of cancellous tissue typically ranges from 0.1 to 1.0 g/cm. The distinction between cortical tissue and cancellous tissue is arbitrary, however, and in biomechanical terms, the two tissues are often considered as one material with a specific range in porosity and density.

The organization of cortical and cancellous tissue in bone allows for adaptation to function. Cortical tissue

Figure 1–7. The structure of bone. **A:** A section of the diaphysis of a long bone, depicted without inner marrow. Each osteon is bounded by a cement line. **B:** Each osteon consists of lamellae, concentric rings composed of mineral matrix surrounding the Haversian canal. **C:** Along the boundaries of the lamellae are small cavities known as lacunae, each of which contains a single osteocyte. Radiating from the lacunae are tiny canals, or canaliculi, into which the cytoplasmic processes of the osteocytes extend. (Reproduced, with permission, from Nordin M, Frankel VH: Biomechanics of bone. In: Nordin M, Frankel VH, eds: *Basic Biomechanics of the Musculoskeletal System.* Lea & Febiger, 1989.)

always surrounds cancellous tissue, but the relative quantity of each type of tissue varies with the functional requirements of the bone. In long bones, the cortical tissue of the diaphysis is arranged as a hollow cylinder to best resist bending. The metaphyseal region of the long bones flares to increase the bone volume and surface area in a manner that minimizes the stress of joint contact. The cancellous tissue in this region provides an intricate network that distributes weight-bearing forces and joint reaction forces into the bulk of the bone tissue.

B. Biomechanical Behavior

The mechanical properties of cortical bone differ from those of cancellous bone. Cortical bone is stiffer than cancellous bone. Cortical bone fractures in vivo when the strain exceeds 2%, but cancellous bone does not until the strain exceeds 75%. The larger capacity for energy storage (area under the stress–strain curve) of cancellous bone is a function of porosity. Despite different stiffness values for cortical and cancellous bone, the following axiom is valid for all bone tissue: Because the compressive strength of the tissue is proportional to the square of the apparent density, and the elastic modulus or material stiffness of the tissue is proportional to the cube of the apparent density, any increase in porosity, as occurs with aging, will decrease the apparent density of bone, which, in turn, will decrease the compressive strength and elastic modulus of bone.

Variations in the strength and stiffness of bone also result from specimen orientation (longitudinal versus transverse) and loading configuration (tensile, compressive, or shear). Generally, the strength and stiffness of bone are greatest in the direction of the common load application (longitudinally for long bones). With regard to orientation, cortical bone (Figure 1–8) is strongest in the longitudinal direction. With regard to loading configuration, cortical bone is strongest in compression and weakest in shear.

Tensile loading is the application of equal and opposite forces (loads) outward from the surface. Maxi-

mal stresses are in a plane perpendicular to the load application and result in elongation of the material. Microscopic studies show that the tensile failure in bones with Haversian systems is caused by debonding of the cement lines and pullout of the osteons. Bones with a large percentage of cancellous tissue demonstrate trabecular fracture with tensile loading.

The converse of tensile loading is **compressive loading,** which is defined as the application of equal and opposite forces toward the surface. Under compression, a material shortens and widens. Microscopic studies show that compressive failure occurs by oblique cracking of the osteons in cortical bone and of the trabeculae in cancellous bone. Vertebral fractures, especially associated with osteoporosis, are associated with compressive loading.

The application of either a tensile load or a compressive load produces a shear stress in the material. **Shear loading** is the application of a load parallel to a surface, and the deformation is angular. Clinical studies show that shear fractures are most common to regions with a large percentage of cancellous bone, such as the tibial plateau.

Figure 1–8. The effects of specimen orientation and loading configuration on the strength and elastic modulus of cortical bone from the diaphyseal region of a long bone.

Bone is a viscoelastic material, and its mechanical behavior is therefore influenced by strain rate. Bones are approximately 50% stiffer at high strain rates than at low strain rates, and the load to failure nearly doubles at high strain rates. The result is a doubling of the stored energy at high strain rates. Clinical studies show that the loading rate influences the fracture pattern and the associated soft-tissue damage. Low strain rates, characterized by little stored energy, result in undisplaced fractures and no associated soft-tissue damage. High strain rates, however, are associated with massive damage to the bone and soft tissue owing to the marked increase in stored energy.

Bone fractures can be produced either from a single load that exceeds the ultimate tensile strength of the bone or from repeated loading that leads to fatigue failure. Because bone is self-repairing, fatigue fracture occurs only when the rate of microdamage resulting from repeated loading exceeds the intrinsic repair rate of the bone. Fatigue fractures are most common during strenuous activity when the muscles have become fatigued and are therefore unable to store energy adequately and absorb the stress imposed on the bone. When the muscles are fatigued, the bone is required to carry the increased stress.

C. Remodeling Mechanisms

Bone has the ability to alter its size, shape, and structure in response to mechanical demands. According to Wolff's law regarding bone remodeling in response to stress, bone resorption occurs with decreased stress, bone hypertrophy occurs with increased stress, and the planes of increased stress follow the principal trabecular orientation. Thus, bone remodeling occurs under a variety of circumstances that alter the normal stress patterns. Clinically, altered stress patterns resulting from fixation devices or joint prostheses have caused concern about effects on the long-term bone architecture.

Bone mass and body weight are positively correlated, especially for weight-bearing bones. Therefore, immobilization or weightlessness (as experienced by astronauts) decreases the strength and stiffness of bone. The subsequent loss in bone mass results from the alteration or absence of normal stress patterns. Bone mass, however, is regained with the return of normal stress patterns. The loss of bone mass in response to immobilization or weightlessness is a direct consequence of Wolff's law. Associated bone resorption in response to orthopedic implants can be deleterious to bone healing, however. Although bone plates provide support for fractured bone, the altered stress patterns associated with stiff metal plates cause resorption of bone adjacent to the fracture or underneath the plate. Therefore, removal of the plate may precipitate another fracture. Resorption of bone is also reported in total hip and knee replacements. This is particularly common with larger diameter noncemented femoral stems, which have an increased moment of inertia and thus have less flexibility than do smaller diameter cemented stems.

The resorption of bone in response to a stiff implant, which alters the stress pattern the bone carries, is termed **stress shielding.** The degree of stress shielding does not depend on the absolute flexibility of the prosthesis but, rather, on the amount of reduced flexibility in the implant in relation to the flexibility of the bone. Clinically, stress shielding could also be detrimental to the longevity of implant fixation. In an effort to reduce stress shielding, designers of implants are using materials with a degree of flexural rigidity that approximates the flexibility of bone.

D. Healing Mechanisms

The fracture healing process involves five stages: impact, inflammation, soft callus formation, hard callus formation, and remodeling. Impact begins with the initiation of the fracture and continues until energy has completely dissipated. The inflammation stage is characterized by hematoma formation at the fracture site, bone necrosis at the ends of the fragments, and an inflammatory infiltrate. Granulation tissue gradually replaces the hematoma, fibroblasts produce collagen, and osteoclasts begin to remove necrotic bone. The subsidence of pain and swelling marks the initiation of the third, or soft callus, stage. This stage is characterized by increased vascularity and abundant new cartilage formation. The end of the soft callus stage is associated with fibrous or cartilaginous tissue uniting the fragments. During the fourth, or hard callus, stage, the callus converts to woven bone and appears clinically healed. The final stage of the healing process involves slow remodeling from woven to lamellar bone and reconstruction of the medullary canal.

Three types of fracture healing are described. The first type, endochondral fracture healing, is characterized by an initial phase of cartilage formation, followed by the formation of new bone on the calcified cartilage template. The second type, membranous fracture healing, is characterized by bone formation from direct mesenchymal tissue without an intervening cartilaginous stage. Combinations of endochondral healing and membranous healing are typical of normal fracture healing. The former process is observed between fracture gaps, whereas the latter is observed subperiosteally. The third type of fracture healing, primary bone healing, is observed with rigid internal fixation and characterized by the absence of visible callus formation. The fracture site is bridged by direct Haversian remodeling, and there are no discernible histologic stages of inflammation or soft and hard callus formation.

Articular Cartilage

Articular cartilage is primarily avascular and has an abnormally small cellular density. The chief functions of articular cartilage are to distribute joint loads over a large area and to allow relative movement of the joint surfaces with minimal friction and wear.

A. Structural Composition

Articular cartilage is composed of chondrocytes and an organic matrix. The chondrocytes account for less than 10% of the tissue volume, and they manufacture, secrete, and maintain the organic component of the cellular matrix. The organic matrix is a dense network of type II collagen in a concentrated proteoglycan solution. Collagen accounts for 10–30% of the organic matrix; proteoglycan accounts for 3–10%; and water, inorganic salts, and matrix proteins account for the remaining 60–87%.

The basic collagen unit consists of tropocollagen molecules, which form covalent cross-links between collagen molecules to increase the tensile strength of the fibrils. The most important mechanical properties of the collagen fiber are tensile strength and stiffness. Fiber resistance to compression is relatively ineffective because the large ratio of length to diameter (slenderness ratio) predisposes the fibers to buckling. The anisotropic nature of cartilage is thought to be related to several factors, including variations in fiber arrangements within the planes parallel to the articular surface, the collagen fiber cross-link density, and the collagen–proteoglycan interactions.

The mechanical properties of the cartilage are attributed to the inhomogeneous distribution of collagen fibrils (Figure 1–9). The superficial tangential zone contains sheets of fine, densely packed collagen fibers that are ran-domly woven in planes parallel to the articular surface. The middle zone contains randomly oriented and homogeneously dispersed fibers that are widely spaced to account for increased matrix content. Finally, the deep zone contains larger, radially oriented collagen fiber bundles that eventually cross the tidemark, enter the calcified cartilage, and anchor the tissue to the underlying bone.

Proteoglycans are monomers that consist of a protein core with glycosaminoglycan units (either keratan sulfate or chondroitin sulfate units) covalently bound to the core. Proteoglycan aggregation promotes immobilization of the proteoglycans within the collagen network and adds structural rigidity to the matrix. There are numerous age-related changes in the structure and composition of the proteoglycan matrix, including the following: a decrease in proteoglycan content from approximately 7% at birth to half that by adulthood, an increase in protein content with maturity, a dramatic drop in the ratio of chondroitin sulfate to keratan sulfate with aging, and a decrease in water content as proteoglycan subunits become smaller with aging. The overall effect is that the cartilage stiffens. The development of osteoarthritis is associated with dramatic changes in cartilage metabolism. Initially, there is increased proteoglycan synthesis, and the water content of osteoarthritic cartilage is actually increased.

The water content of normal cartilage permits the diffusion of gases, nutrients, and waste products between the chondrocytes and the nutrient-rich synovial fluid. The water is primarily concentrated (80%) near the articular surface and decreases in a linear fashion with increasing depth, such that the deep zone is 65% water. The location and movement of water are important in controlling mechanical function and lubrication properties of the cartilage.

Figure 1–9. Orientation of the collagen fiber network in the three zones of the articular cartilage. (Modified and reproduced, with permission, from Mow VC et al: Biomechanics of articular cartilage. In: Nordin M, Frankel VH, eds: *Basic Biomechanics of the Musculoskeletal System.* Lea & Febiger, 1989.)

Important structural interactions occur between proteoglycans and collagen fibers in cartilage. A small percentage of the proteoglycans may serve as a bonding agent between the collagen fibrils that span distances too great for the maintenance or formation of cross-links. These structural interactions are thought to provide strong mechanical interactions. In essence, the proteoglycans and collagen fibers interact to form a porous, composite, fiber-reinforced matrix, possessing all the essential mechanical characteristics of a solid that is swollen with water and able to resist the stresses and strains of joint lubrication.

B. BIOMECHANICAL BEHAVIOR

The biomechanical behavior of articular cartilage is best understood when the cartilage is considered as a viscoelastic and composite material consisting of a fluid phase and a solid phase. The compressive behavior of cartilage is primarily caused by the flow of interstitial fluid, whereas the shear behavior of cartilage is primarily caused by the motion of collagen fibers and proteoglycans. The creep behavior of cartilage is characterized by the exudation of interstitial fluid, which occurs with compressive loading. The applied surface load is balanced by the compressive stress developed within the collagen–proteoglycan matrix and the frictional drag generated by the flow of the interstitial fluid during exudation. Typically, human cartilage takes 4–16 hours to reach creep equilibrium, and the amount of creep is inversely proportional to the square of the tissue thickness.

Similar to creep, stress relaxation is the response of the tissue to compressive forces on the articular surface. An initial compressive phase, characterized by increased stress, is associated with fluid exudation. In the subsequent relaxation phase, stress decay is associated with fluid redistribution within the porous collagen–proteoglycan matrix. The rate of stress relaxation is used to determine the permeability coefficient of the tissue, and the equilibrium stress is used to measure the intrinsic compressive modulus of the solid matrix. Microstructural changes in osteoarthritic cartilage reduce the compressive stiffness of cartilage.

Under uniaxial tension, articular cartilage demonstrates anisotropic and inhomogeneous properties. The tissue is stronger and stiffer parallel to the split lines and in superficial regions. Variations in the material characteristics are a result of the structural organization of the collagen–proteoglycan matrix in layering arrangements throughout the tissue. For example, the superficial tangential zone appears to provide a tough, wear-resistant, protective zone for the tissue. To examine the tissue's intrinsic response to tension, the biphasic viscoelastic effects of the tissue must be negated. This can be achieved by testing the tissue at low strain rates or by performing incremental testing and allowing for stress

relaxation equilibrium to be achieved before continuing. The tissue tends to stiffen with increasing strain. Typically, specimens are pulled to the failure point at a displacement rate of 0.5 cm/min.

The shape of the stress–strain curve (Figure 1–10) can be described in morphologic changes of the collagen fibers: (1) the toe region designates collagen fiber pullout, (2) the linear region designates stretching of the aligned collagen fibers, and (3) failure is the point at which all of the collagen fibers have ruptured. The tensile properties of the tissue are thus changed by an alteration of the molecular structure of collagen, an alteration in the organization of the fibers within the collagenous network, or a change in collagen fiber cross-linking. For this reason, disruption of the collagen network may be a key factor in the initial development of osteoarthritis.

When the cartilage is tested in pure shear under infinitesimal strain conditions, no pressure gradients or volume changes are observed within the tissue as they are during tension or compression conditions. Thus, the viscoelastic shear properties of cartilage can be determined in a steady-state dynamic shear experiment. Cartilage shear stiffness is a function of collagen content or collagen–proteoglycan interaction. Increased collagen content reduces frictional dissipation of the load, and this in turn results in increased shear loading.

C. LUBRICATION MECHANISMS

Sophisticated lubrication processes are responsible for the minimal wear of normal cartilage under large and

Figure 1–10. A stress–strain diagram for articular cartilage during tensile loading. The schematic representations on the right illustrate the orientation of the collagen fibrils in response to loading. (Reproduced, with permission, from Mow VC et al: Biomechanics of articular cartilage. In Nordin M, Frankel VH, eds: *Basic Biomechanics of the Musculoskeletal System.* Lea & Febiger, 1989.)

varied joint stresses. Four types of lubrication mechanisms are related to articular cartilage: boundary, fluid film, mixed, and self-lubrication. These mechanisms are inherent properties of the composition of the tissue with respect to water content and collagen–proteoglycan matrix orientation. Normal joints display all of the lubrication mechanisms just mentioned, whereas artificial joints are thought primarily to display elastohydrodynamic and boundary lubrication mechanisms.

The boundary mechanism protects the joint from surface-to-surface wear by means of an adsorbed lubricant. This mechanism, which depends chiefly on the chemical properties of the lubricant, is most important under severe loading conditions when contact surfaces must sustain high loads.

The fluid film mechanism relies on a thin layer of lubricant that causes greater surface separation. The load on the joint surface is supported by the pressure on the film. Fluid film lubrication occurs with rigid (squeeze-film or hydrodynamic) bodies as well as with deformable (elastohydrodynamic) bodies. When two rigid surfaces are nonparallel and move tangentially with respect to each other, the pressure generated by the lubricant in the gap between the two surfaces is sufficient to raise one surface above the other. Moreover, when two rigid surfaces are parallel and move perpendicular to each other, the pressure generated by the lubricant is sufficient to keep the surfaces separated. This squeeze-film or hydrodynamic lubrication mechanism is able to carry high loads for short durations. When the squeeze-film mechanism generates a pressure great enough to deform the surface and thereby increase the amount of bearing surface area, elastohydrodynamic lubrication mechanisms begin to make the necessary adjustments. Increased bearing surface area allows less lubricant to escape from between the surfaces, decreasing the stress and increasing the duration associated with motion.

The mixed lubrication mechanism is a combination of the boundary and fluid film mechanisms. Boundary lubrication is essential in areas of asperity contact, and fluid film lubrication is present in areas of no contact. Therefore, most of the friction is generated in the boundary lubricated areas, whereas most of the load is carried by the fluid film.

Self-lubrication, or weeping, relies on the exudation of fluid in front of and beneath the surface of the rotating joint. Once the area of peak stress passes a given point, the cartilage reabsorbs the fluid and returns to its original dimensions. This lubrication mechanism results from the inhomogeneous character of the collagen and water distribution throughout the cartilage. When the pressure rises and strains are low, the tissue is most permeable and a large amount of water is exuded in front of the leading contact edge of the joint. As the joint advances, the load increases in the region of expelled fluid and the increased pressure and strains decrease the tissue permeability to fluid. This prevents the fluid on the articular surface from returning to the cartilage. As the contact surface moves past the point of contact, the pressure and strains are again low and the tissue permeability is increased, resulting in the return of fluid to the cartilage in preparation for the cycle to start again.

Synovial fluid is a key component in the lubrication process in joints. It is non-Newtonian, indicating that the resistance to flow increases more slowly than the flow of the fluid. Joint fluid in normal joints, abnormal joints, and artificial joints is different. Hence, different mechanisms of lubrication come into play in each situation with implications for joint surface damage and artificial joint wear.

D. WEAR MECHANISMS

Wear is the removal of material from a surface and is caused by the mechanical action of two surfaces in contact. The principal types of wear experienced in articular cartilage are interface wear and fatigue wear.

Interface wear occurs when bearing surfaces come into direct contact with no lubricating film separating them. This type of wear may be found in an impaired or degenerated synovial joint. When ultrastructural surface defects in articular cartilage result in softer tissue with increased permeability, the fluid from the lubricant film may easily leak through the cartilage surface, thereby increasing the probability of direct contact between asperities. There are two forms of interface wear: adhesive wear, which occurs when surface fragments adhere to one another and are torn from the surface during sliding, and abrasive wear, which occurs when a soft material is scraped by a harder one.

Fatigue wear results from the accumulation of microscopic damage within the bearing material under repetitive stress. In the cartilage, three mechanisms are primarily responsible for fatigue wear. First, repetitive stress on the collagen–proteoglycan matrix can disrupt the collagen fibers, the proteoglycan molecules, or the interface between the two. In this case, cartilage fatigue is caused by the tensile failure of the collagen network, and proteoglycan changes could be considered part of the accumulated tissue damage. Second, repetitive and massive exudation and inhibition of interstitial fluid may cause a proteoglycan washout from the cartilage matrix near the articular surface. This results in decreased stiffness and increased tissue permeability. Third, during synovial joint impact loading, insufficient time for internal fluid redistribution to relieve high stress in the compacted region may result in tissue damage.

Numerous structural defects of the articular cartilage are caused or exacerbated by wear and damage. For example, fibrillations (splitting of the articular surface) are associated with wear and will eventually extend the full thickness of the cartilage. Destructive smooth-surface thinning is apparent when layers erode rather than split. In these and other types of surface damage of the cartilage, more than a single wear mechanism is likely to be responsible.

Several biomechanical hypotheses cover cartilage degradation. Factors associated with progressive failure of the tissue include the magnitude of imposed stress, the total number of sustained stress peaks, changes in the intrinsic molecular and microscopic structure of the collagen–proteoglycan matrix, and changes in the intrinsic mechanical property of the tissue. Failure-initiating mechanisms include a loosening of the collagen network, which allows for abnormal expansion of the proteoglycan matrix and swelling of the tissue, and a decrease in cartilage stiffness, which is accompanied by an increase in tissue permeability.

Biomechanically, conditions that cause excessive stress concentrations may result in increased tissue damage or wear. Joint surface incongruity, such as the incongruity of the hip joint in patients who had Perthes disease during childhood, can result in abnormally small contact areas, which are associated with increased stress and increased tissue damage. Moreover, the presence of high contact pressures between the articular surfaces, such as that seen in patients with a shallow acetabulum (acetabular dysplasia), can reduce the probability of fluid film lubrication, allow for continued tissue damage, and also increase the risk of early degenerative arthritis.

Tendons & Ligaments

Tendons and ligaments are similar both structurally and biomechanically and differ only in function. Tendons attach muscle to bone; transmit loads from the muscle to the bone, which results in joint motion; and allow the muscle belly to remain an optimal distance from the joint on which it acts. Ligaments attach bone to bone, augment mechanical stability of the joint, guide joint motion, and prevent excessive joint displacement.

A. STRUCTURAL COMPOSITION

Both the tendons and the ligaments are parallel-fibered collagenous tissues that are sparsely vascularized. They contain relatively few fibroblasts (constituting approximately 20% of their volume) and an abundant extracellular matrix. The matrix consists of approximately 70% water and 30% collagen, ground substance, and elastin.

The fibroblasts secrete a precursor of collagen, procollagen, which is cleaved extracellularly to form type I collagen. Cross-links between collagen molecules provide strength to the tissue. The arrangement of the collagen fibers determines tissue function. In tendons, a parallel arrangement of the collagen fibers provides the tissues with the ability to sustain high uniaxial tensile loads. In ligaments, the nearly parallel fibers, which are intimately interlaced with one another, provide the ability to sustain loads in one predominant direction but allow for carrying small tensile loads in other directions.

Tendons and ligaments are surrounded by loose areolar connective tissue. The paratenon forms a protective sheath around the tissue and enhances gliding. At places where the tendons are subjected to large friction forces, a parietal synovial membrane is found just beneath the paratenon and additionally facilitates gliding. Each individual fiber bundle is bound by the endotenon. At the musculotendinous junction, the endotenon continues into the perimysium. At the tendoosseous junction, the collagen fibers of the endotenon continue into the bone as perforating fibers (Sharpey fibers) and become continuous with the periosteum.

Tendons and connective tissues of the musculotendinous junction help determine the mechanical characteristics of whole muscle during contraction and passive extension. The muscle cells are extensively involuted and folded at the junction to provide maximal surface area for attachment, thereby allowing for greater fixation and transmission of forces. The sarcomeres directly adjacent to the junction of fast contracting muscles are shortened in length. This may represent an adaptation to decrease the force intensity within the junction. A complex intracellular and extracellular transmitting membrane consisting of a glycoprotein links the contractile intracellular proteins to the extracellular protein connective tissue.

The tendon insertions and ligament insertions to the bone are structurally similar. The collagen fibers from the tissue intermesh with fibrocartilage. The fibrocartilage gradually becomes mineralized, and this mineralized cartilage merges with cortical bone. These transition zones produce a gradual alteration in the mechanical properties of the tissue, resulting in a decreased stress concentration effect at the insertion of the tendon or ligament to the bone.

B. MECHANICAL BEHAVIOR

Tendons and ligaments are viscoelastic structures that have specific mechanical properties related to their function and composition. Tendons are strong enough to sustain high tensile forces resulting from muscle contraction during joint motion, but they are also sufficiently flexible to angulate around bone surfaces, to change the final direction of muscle pull. Ligaments are pliant and flexible enough to allow natural movements of the bones they connect; however, they are strong, are

Figure 1–11. The load-elongation curve for progressive failure of the anterior cruciate ligament. (Reproduced, with permission, from Carlstedt CA, Nordin M: Biomechanics of tendons and ligaments. In: Nordin M, Frankel VH, eds: *Basic Biomechanics of the Musculoskeletal System*. Lea & Febiger, 1989.)

not extensible, and offer suitable resistance to applied forces and large joint movements. Because tendons and ligaments are viscoelastic structures, the injury they sustain is affected by the rate of loading as well as the amount of the stress load. The stress–strain and load-elongation curves for ligaments and tendons, like those for articular cartilage, have several regions that characterize the tissue behavior.

Figure 1–11 shows the load-elongation curve for progressive failure of the anterior cruciate ligament. Like the curve in Figure 1–10, the curve in Figure 1–11 has a toe region (correlating with the region labeled clinical test, when the anterior drawer test was administered) and a linear region preceding the failure region. In Figure 1–11, the curve in the toe region represents large elongations with small changes in load. This pattern is thought to reflect the straightening of the wavy, relaxed collagen fibers with increased loads. Within the linear region, the collagen fibers continue to become more parallel in orientation as physiologic loading proceeds. At the end of the linear region, small force reductions can be observed in the load-deformation curve. These dips are caused by the early sequential failure of a few maximally stretched fiber bundles. The final region represents major failure of fiber bundles in an unpredictable manner. Complete failure occurs rapidly, and the load-supporting ability of the tissue is substantially reduced.

The mechanical behavior characteristics of the anterior cruciate ligament differ somewhat from those of soft tissues that contain a high proportion of elastin fibers. These tissues can elongate up to 50% before stiffness markedly increases. After 50% elongation, however, the stiffness increases greatly with increased loading, and failure is abrupt with minimal further elongation. Load-elongation curves for several soft tissues are shown in Figure 1–12.

The viscoelastic behavior of ligaments is best exemplified in the bone-ligament-bone complex. Anterior

Figure 1–12. Load-elongation curves for several soft tissues. The range in mechanical properties of the tissues is attributable to collagen fiber orientation and interaction with the extracellular matrix.

cruciate ligaments in primate knee specimens were tested in tension to failure at both slow and fast loading rates to determine the viscoelastic nature of the bone-ligament-bone complex. At slow loading rates the bony insertion of the ligament was the weakest link, and an avulsion resulted. At fast loading rates, the ligament was the weakest link, and a midsubstance rupture generally was found. At slow rates, the load to failure was decreased by 20% and the stored energy was decreased by 30% in comparison with results with fast rates. The stiffness of the bone-ligament-bone complex was relatively unaffected by strain rate, however. Increased strain rates demonstrated a greater increase in strength for bone as compared with ligaments.

The mechanical properties of ligaments are closely related to the number and quality of the cross-links within the collagen fibers. Therefore, any process that affects collagen formation or maturation directly influences the properties of the ligaments. As aging continues, the number and the quality of cross-links increase, thereby increasing the tensile strength of the tissue. Moreover, the diameter of the collagen fibril increases with age. As aging progresses, however, collagen reaches a mechanical plateau, after which point tensile strength and stiffness decrease. There is also a decrease in the tissue collagen content, and this contributes to the continued decline in the mechanical properties of the tissue.

Tendons and ligaments remodel in response to mechanical demand. Physical training increases the tensile strength of the tendons and the ligament-bone interface, whereas immobilization decreases tensile strength. Even if the tissue maintains a relatively constant cross-sectional area during immobilization, the increased tissue metabolism results in proportionately more immature collagen and a decrease in the amount and quality of cross-links between molecules. Investigators who studied ligaments that were immobilized for 8 weeks and control ligaments found that the previously immobilized ligaments required 12 months of reconditioning before they demonstrated strength and stiffness values comparable to those of the control ligaments.

Studies of nonsteroidal antiinflammatory drugs (NSAIDs) such as indomethacin demonstrated that treatment results in increases in the proportion of insoluble collagen and the total collagen content in tissue. It also leads to increased tensile strength, which is probably attributable to increased collagen molecule cross-links. Therefore, short-term NSAID therapy may increase the rate of biomechanical restoration of the tendons and ligaments.

C. INJURY MECHANISMS

Tendons and ligaments are subjected to less than a third of their ultimate stress during normal physiologic loading. The maximal physiologic strain ranges from 2% to 5%. Several factors lead to tissue injury, however. When tendons and ligaments are subjected to stresses that exceed the physiologic range, microfailure of collagen bundles occurs before the yield point of the tissue is reached. When the yield point is reached, the tissue undergoes gross failure and the joint simultaneously becomes displaced. The amount of force produced by the maximal contraction of the muscle results in a maximal tensile stress in the tendon. The extent of tendon injury is influenced by the amount of tendon cross-sectional area compared with that for muscle. The larger the muscle cross-sectional area, the higher the magnitude of the force produced by the contraction and thus the greater the tensile load transmitted through the tendon.

Clinically, ligament injuries are characterized according to degree of severity. First-degree sprains are typified by minimal pain and demonstrate no detectable joint instability despite microfailure of collagen fibers. Second-degree sprains cause severe pain and demonstrate minimal joint instability. This instability is most likely masked by muscle activity, however. Therefore, testing must be performed with the patient under anesthesia for proper evaluation. Second-degree sprains are characterized by partial ligament rupture and progressive failure of the collagen fibers, with the result that ligament strength and stiffness decrease by 50%. Third-degree sprains cause severe pain during the course of the injury and minimal pain afterward. The joint is completely unstable. Most collagen fibers have ruptured, but a few may remain intact, giving the ligament the appearance of continuity even though it is incapable of supporting loads. Abnormally high stress on the articular cartilage results if pressure is exerted on a joint that is unstable owing to ligament or joint capsule rupture.

D. HEALING MECHANISMS

During tendon and ligament healing and repair, fibroblastic infiltration from the adjacent tissues is essential. The healing events are initiated by an inflammatory response, which is characterized by polymorphonuclear cell infiltration, capillary budding, and fluid exudation and continues during the first 3 days following the injury. After 4 days, fibroplasia occurs and is accompanied by the significant accumulation of fibroblasts. Within 3 weeks, a mass of granulation tissue surrounds the damaged tissue. During the next week, collagen fibers become longitudinally oriented. During the next 3 months, the individual collagen fibers form bundles identical to the original bundles.

Sutured tendons heal with a progressive penetration of connective tissue from the outside. The deposited collagen fibers become progressively oriented until eventually they form tendon fibers like the original ones. This orientation of collagen fibers is essential because the tensile strength of repaired tendon depends on collagen content and orientation. If tendon is sutured during the first 7–10 days of healing, the strength of the suture maintains the fixation until adequate callus forms.

Tendon mobilization during healing is important to avoid adhesion of the tendon to adjacent tissue, particularly in cases involving the flexor tendons of the hand. Motion can be passive to prevent adhesion and at the same time to prevent putting excessive tensile stress on the suture line. The gliding properties of flexor tendons that were mobilized are consistently superior to those of flexor tendons that were immobilized during the healing process.

Direct apposition of the surfaces of a divided ligament provides the most favorable conditions for healing because it minimizes scar formation, accelerates repair, hastens collagenization, and comes closer to restoring normal ligamentous tissue. Care must be taken during the repair of ligaments to avoid subsequent common problems with healing, however. For instance, divided and immobilized ligaments heal with a fibrous tissue gap between the two ends, whereas sutured ligaments unite without a fibrous tissue gap. If excessive tension is placed on a suture, necrosis and failure to heal are observed. Unsutured ligaments can retract, shorten, and become atrophic, however, making repair difficult 2 weeks following the injury. In spite of this, many ligaments are not routinely repaired in orthopedic surgery.

The anterior cruciate ligament is often severely damaged in cases of midsubstance rupture and generally does not fare well following repair. The ligament is intraarticular, with synovial fluid tending to disrupt the repair. Instability of the knee also tends to place excessive stress on the repair unless the knee is immobilized, which leads to joint stiffness and muscle atrophy.

Bellucci G, Seedhom BB: Tensile fatigue behaviour of articular cartilage. Biorheology 2002;39:193. [PMID: 12082282]

Ding M: Age variations in the properties of human tibial trabecular bone and cartilage. Acta Orthop Scand 2000;292:1. [PMID: 10951715]

Ding M et al: Mutual associations among microstructural, physical and mechanical properties of human cancellous bone. J Bone Joint Surg Br 2002;84:900. [PMID: 12211688]

Fung YCB: *Biomechanics: Mechanical Properties of Living Tissues.* Springer-Verlag, 1981.

Jay GD et al: Lubricating ability of aspirated synovial fluid from emergency department patients with knee joint synovitis. J Rheumatol 2004;31:557. [PMID: 14994405]

Kjaer M: Role of extracellular matrix in adaptation of tendon and skeletal muscle to mechanical loading. Physiol Rev 2004;84:649. [PMID: 15044685]

Kopperdahl DL et al: Quantitative computed tomography estimates of the mechanical properties of human vertebral trabecular bone. J Orthop Res 2002;20:801.

Mazzuco D, Spector M: The role of joint fluid in the tribology of total joint arthroplasty. Clin Orthop 2004;429:17. [PMID: 15577461]

Mountney J et al: Tensile strength of the medial patellofemoral ligament before and after repair or reconstruction. J Bone Joint Surg Br 2005;87:36. [PMID: 15686235]

Mow VC, Guo XE: Mechano-electrochemical properties of articular cartilage: Their inhomogeneities and anisotropies. Annu Rev Biomed Eng 2002;4:175. [PMID:12117756]

Musgrave DS et al: Gene therapy and tissue engineering in orthopedic surgery. J Am Acad Orthop Surg 2002;10:6. [PMID: 11809046]

Shinar H et al: Mapping the fiber orientation in articular cartilage at rest and under pressure studied by 2H double quantum filtered MRI. Magn Reson Med 2002;48:322. [PMID: 12210941]

Silva MJ et al: Recent progress in flexor tendon healing. J Orthop Sci 2002;7:508. [PMID: 12181670]

Silver FH, Bradica G, Tria A: Viscoelastic behavior of osteoarthritic cartilage. Connect Tissue Res 2001;42:223. [PMID: 11913493]

Vanwanseele B et al: Knee cartilage of spinal cord-injured patients displays progressive thinning in the absence of normal joint loading and movement. Arthritis Rheum 2002; 46:2073. [PMID: 12209511]

Wu JZ, Herzog W: Elastic anisotropy of articular cartilage is associated with the microstructures of collagen fibers and chondrocytes. J Biomech 2002;35:931. [PMID: 12052395]

Skeletal Muscle

Skeletal muscles perform a wide variety of mechanical and biologic functions. From a mechanical perspective, it is obvious that skeletal muscles generate force and length changes. The generation of force and length change gives rise to the production of mechanical work and power. Less obvious is the fact that skeletal muscles are often subjected to so-called lengthening or eccentric contractions. During these types of contractions, muscles may act as so-called dynamic joint stabilizers and may store energy. From a biologic perspective, skeletal muscles are believed to secrete various growth factors such as insulin-like growth factor 1 (IGF-1), which is thought to play an important autocrine/paracrine role in regulating muscle fiber size. Additionally, it has been proposed that skeletal muscles play a key role in maintaining the health of motor neurons.

A. SKELETAL MUSCLE STRUCTURE

1. Macroscopic anatomy—Figure 1–13 provides both a macroscopic and microscopic perspective of the structure of skeletal muscle. From a macroscopic perspective, skeletal muscles are composed of tens of thousands of individual muscle fibers (muscle cells). Muscles that are involved in fine motor control usually contain a small number of muscle fibers compared with those muscles involved in activities requiring the generation of large forces and power outputs. Muscle fibers are usually found in so-called bundles that are also referred to as **fascicles.** Each fascicle typically contains approximately 10–30 muscle fibers that are encased in a connective tissue sheath known as the **endomysium.**

Figure 1–13. Overview of macroscopic and microscopic structure of skeletal muscle. (Reprinted, with permission, from McMahon TA: *Muscles, Reflexes, and Locomotion.* Princeton University Press, 1984.)

From an architectural perspective, muscles are often classified on the basis of the orientations of the muscle fibers' longitudinal axes relative to that of the entire muscle. For instance, **longitudinal** muscles are composed of muscle fibers whose longitudinal axis runs parallel to that of the whole muscle. Good examples of this type of architecture are the rectus abdominis and the sartorius muscles. In **fusiform** muscles, the fibers run parallel to the longitudinal axis throughout most of the muscle, but they taper at the ends of the muscle. The soleus and brachioradialis muscles are typical of this architecture. Muscles can also exhibit a so-called **pennate** (unipennate, bipennate) architecture whereby the longitudinal axis of the individual muscle fibers runs diagonal to that of the whole muscle. A good example of a bipennate muscle is the gastrocnemius muscle. The muscle fibers of **angular** or **fan-shaped** muscles radiate from a narrow attachment at one end and fan out, resulting in a broad attachment at the other end as is seen in muscles like the pectoralis major.

Consistent with the theme of structure–function relationships, muscle architecture can be an important determinant of the mechanical properties of skeletal muscle. For instance, fusiform muscles typically have longer muscle fibers than bipennate muscles. Functionally, this means that a fusiform muscle should be able to generate greater shortening velocities and muscle length excursions at the whole muscle level. In contrast, muscles with a pennate or bipennate architecture have shorter fibers, but the fibers are packed in such a manner that a larger number of muscle fibers are in parallel to one another, resulting in a larger physiologic cross-sectional area. Hence, the pennate muscle has a greater capacity for generating force.

2. Molecular anatomy of the myofibril—The structure of skeletal muscle at the molecular level is quite complex (see Figure 1–13). Each muscle fiber is made up of thousands of so-called **myofibrils** that are arranged in parallel to one another. Each myofibril has a cross-sectional area of approximately 1 μm^2. Hence, a muscle fiber with a cross-sectional area of approximately 1000 μm^2 would contain approximately 1000 myofibrils. Typically, the cross-sectional area of a muscle fiber can range from approximately 1000 to 7000 μm^2. Each myofibril consists of a repeating series of striations that are caused by the arrangement of so-called **sarcomeres** in series. Each sarcomere is approximately 2–3 μm in length. Sarcomeres are often referred to as the contractile units of skeletal muscle.

In a general sense, sarcomeres consist of Z-lines, thin filaments, and thick filaments. The interdigitation of thick and thin filaments along with the presence of Z-lines is primarily responsible for the striation pattern of skeletal muscle. As shown in Figure 1–14, the Z-lines are dense thin structures that are found in the middle of the so-called I-band. In reality, each Z-line represents

an anchor point to which thin filaments are attached. By definition, the collection of proteins between each Z-line is known as a sarcomere. Hence, the I-band represents a region where no overlap occurs of the thin filaments (by thick filaments), yielding a relatively light band. The A-band is composed of the thick filament and is strongly birefringent, producing a dark band on microscopic inspection. By definition, the length of the A-band is equivalent to the length of the thick filament. Normally, the thick and thin filaments partially overlap, and as a result a lighter region occurs in the middle of the A-band known as the H-zone.

Changes in sarcomere length and, as a result, muscle fiber length are caused by the sliding of the thick and thin filaments relative to one another. In its most simplistic sense, this model states that contraction takes place not because of changes in the individual lengths of thick and thin filaments, but rather by the sliding of thin filaments past thick filaments. This model of contraction is known as the **sliding-filament hypothesis.** The changes in striation patterns during shortening contractions played a central role in developing the sliding-filament hypothesis. In this context, Table 1–1 summarizes the changes in the striation pattern that occur during isometric, shortening (isotonic), and lengthening (eccentric) contractions.

3. Molecular anatomy of the sarcomere—As shown in Figure 1–14 and in Table 1–2, the overall structure of the sarcomere became quite complex as more sophisticated techniques for studying skeletal muscle evolved. On a basic level, the sarcomeric proteins and those associated with the sarcomere can be placed into four different categories: (1) contractile; (2) regulatory contractile; (3) structural; and (4) costameric.

As shown in Table 1–2, the primary contractile proteins are simply **actin** and **myosin.** These are referred to as contractile proteins, given their central role in the contractile process. Individual monomers of actin bind to one another to form so-called actin filaments. In contrast, the thick filament is composed primarily of myosin heavy-chain molecules packed in an antiparallel arrangement. A more detailed description of myosin is provided later. Regulatory contractile proteins are defined as those that turn the contractile apparatus on or off and those that can modulate the activity of the myosin heavy chain. In skeletal muscle, the regulatory contractile proteins involved in turning the contractile apparatus on or off are associated exclusively with the actin filament, and these proteins include **tropomyosin, troponin-T, troponin-I,** and **troponin-C.** Collectively, the thin filament is composed of the actin filament and these (ie, tropomyosin, troponin-T, troponin-I, and troponin-C) regulatory contractile proteins. Other regulatory contractile proteins are associated with the myosin heavy chain, and these are referred to collectively as **myosin light**

Figure 1–14. Striation pattern and various proteins associated with sarcomere. Electron micrograph of sarcomeres is shown in (**A**). A schematic illustration of the various structures and proteins of the sarcomere is shown in (**B**). p94 = muscle-specific calpain. MURF-1 = muscle ring finger-1, which is believed to be part of the ubiquitin-proteosome complex involved in protein degradation. MyBP-C = myosin-binding protein-C, otherwise known as C-protein. CARP = cardiac adriamycin-responsive protein. (A reproduced, with permission, from Aidley DJ: *The Physiology of Excitable Cells.* Cambridge University Press, 1998. B reproduced, with permission, from Clark KA et al: Striated muscle cytoarchitecture: An intricate web of form and function. Ann Rev Cell Dev Biol 2002;18:637.) Also, see Table 1–2.

Table 1–1. Effect of different types of contractions on the various bands, zones, lines, and length.

Type of Contraction	Z-line	I-band	A-band	H-zone	M-line	Sarcomere Length
Isometric	↔	↔	↔	↔	↔	↔
Shortening (isotonic)	↔	↓	↔	↓	↔	↓
Lengthening (eccentric)	↔	↑	↔	↑	↔	↑

↔ = no change in length; ↑ = increase in length; ↓ = decrease in length.

Table 1–2. Overview of proteins involved with the sarcomere and cytoskeletal-extracellular matrix interactions.

Classes and Types of Sarcomeric Proteins	Molecular Wt (kDa)	Location	Function
Contractile proteins			
Myosin heavy chain	~200	Thick filament	Molecular motor; binds to actin; generates force and length change
Actin	~42	Thin filament	Binds myosin and translates force and/or length changes
Regulatory contractile proteins			
Tropomyosin	~37	Thin filament	Regulates interaction between actin and myosin; stabilizes thin filament
Troponin-T	~30	Thin filament	Couples troponin complex to actin?
Troponin-I	~22	Thin filament	Influences position of tropomyosin
Troponin-C	~18	Thin filament	Binds Ca^{+2}, influences position of tropomyosin
Myosin light chain-1	~22	Thick filament	Influences V_{max}?
Myosin light chain-2	~20	Thick filament	Influences tension–pCa^{+2} relationship
Myosin light chain-3	~18	Thick filament	Influences V_{max}
Structural proteins			
Associated with thin filament			
CapZ-α, CapZ-β	~36, ~32	Z-line	Caps free end of actin, regulates actin filament length; binds to α-actinin
Tropomodulin	~40	Thin filament	Caps pointed end of actin filament
Nebulin	~600–900	I-band	Anchors actin to Z-line; molecular ruler of actin filament length?
Associated with thick filament			
Myosin binding protein-C	~140	Thick filament	Binds to lever arm and rod region of MHC; titin binding site
Myomesin	~185	M-line	Binds to myosin and titin; may play role in linking myosin and titin
MurF-1	~40	M-line	May play key role in degradation
Calpain-3; p94		M-line	Binds to titin
Titin	~3000–4000	Spans A–I bands	Molecular spring? Sarcomere template?
Associated with Z-line			
α-Actinin	~97	Z-line	Major protein of Z-line
LIM	~23	Z-line	Binds α-actinin, zyxin, β-spectrin
FATZ	~32	Z-line	Binds calcineurin to Z-line
Intermediate filaments			
Desmin	~53	Z-line	Longitudinal and lateral alignment of sarcomeres
Skelemin	~200	M-band	M-line integrity
Vimentin	~53	Z-line	Periodicity of Z-lines
Costameric proteins			
Ankyrin	17–440	Costamere	Localization
α-Dystrobrevin	~87	Costamere	Membrane stabilization; transmembrane signaling involved with NOS
α/β-Dystroglycan	~156, 43	Costamere	Prevents injury to sarcolemma
Dystrophin	427	Costamere	Stabilizes cytoskeleton and sarcolemma
α-Fodrin	85	Costamere	Attachment of cytoskeleton to ECM; signaling
Integrins	~90 and 150	Costamere	Stabilization of cytoskeleton
α-Sarcoglycan	~240	Costamere	Binds dystrophin and α-dystrobrevin; associated with NOS
α/β-Spectrin	~250	Costamere	Stabilization of sarcomere
Syntrophins	~57–60	Costamere	NOS?
Talin	~235	Costamere/MTJ	Role in stabilizing link between muscle fiber and tendon fibrils?
Vinculin	116 ~130	Costamere/MTJ	Role in stabilizing link between muscle fiber and tendon fibrils?

MHC = myosin heavy drain; LIM = cysteine-rich double zinc finger motifs that mediate protein binding; FATC = filamin, α-actinin and telethonin-associated Z-line protein; NOS = nitric oxide synthase; ECM = extracellular matrix.

chains (MLCs) because of their relatively low molecular weight. These MLCs may possibly be involved in regulating the kinetics of crossbridge cycling.

Structural and costameric proteins play several essential roles. First, electron micrographs (see Figure 1–14) demonstrate that sarcomeres are organized in a very orderly fashion such that the Z-lines of adjoining sarcomeres appear to be in register with one another. As noted in Table 1–2, key intermediate filaments like **desmin** and **vimentin** are believed to play key roles in aligning the Z-line of one sarcomere with that of another. Other proteins like **synemin** are also thought to be involved in the alignment of sarcomeres. Structural proteins also play a key role in developing a mechanical linkage between sarcomeres and the extracellular matrix. These sites of connectivity between the sarcomere, cell membrane, and extracellular matrix are referred to as **costameres** (see section 5. Molecular anatomy of the connection between the cytoskeleton and the extracellular matrix).

4. Molecular anatomy of myosin molecule—Although the term *myosin molecule* is often used, in reality the myosin molecule is a hexameric structure composed of two myosin heavy chains, two so-called essential light chains (MLC$_1$ or MLC$_3$), and two regulatory light chains (MLC$_2$). The term *heavy* or *light* is used in reference to the molecular weights of each of these proteins. Each myosin heavy chain is composed of a rod region, lever arm (also known as S$_2$), and a globular head (also known as S$_1$). The rod region plays an important role in the packing of individual myosin heavy chains into thick filaments. The globular head contains the key functional domains of this molecular motor. Within the globular head (Figure 1–15) are domains that contain (1) the actin-binding site, (2) the nucleotide (adenosine triphosphate [ATP])-binding site, and (3) the enzymatic (adenosine triphosphatase [ATPase]) properties responsible for converting chemical energy in the form of ATP into mechanical work and heat. The essential and regulatory light chains are bound to the so-called lever arm or S$_2$ region (see Figure 1–15). Each globular head has bound to it one essential and one regulatory light chain. Mutations of some of these domains (eg, the actin-binding site) are thought to play roles in diseases such as familial hypertrophic cardiomyopathy. As noted earlier, the light chains are thought to play modulatory roles in regulating the kinetics of the crossbridge cycle.

The complexity of the myosin molecule is further complicated by the presence of isoforms for both the myosin heavy and light chains. Although it has long been recognized that muscles could be classified as **slow** or **fast twitch** (based on twitch properties), the importance of myosin heavy-chain isoforms has only been intensely studied during the past 20 years. In many smaller adult mammals (eg, mice, rats, rabbits), four myosin heavy-chains isoforms are identified and classified as **slow Type I, fast Type IIA, fast Type IIX,** and **fast Type IIB** (in order of increasing ATPase activities and associated maximal shortening velocities). In adult humans, the slow Type I, fast Type IIA, and fast Type IIX myosin heavy-chain isoforms are expressed. This scheme of classifying myosin heavy-chain isoforms forms the basis for the nomenclature typically used to identify different muscle fiber types. Hence, a slow Type I muscle fiber would exclusively express the slow Type I myosin heavy-chain isoform.

Note that there are isoforms for myosin heavy chains, myosin light chains, tropomyosin, troponin-T, troponin-I, and troponin-C. Hence, by mixing and matching these contractile and regulatory contractile proteins, the complexity that can arise in the design of sarcomeres becomes readily apparent.

The sequence of the crossbridge cycle is shown in Figure 1–15. First, myosin is detached from actin. Second, the head of the myosin heavy chain is attached to actin and releases Pi, leading to the power stroke (change in position of head between Figure 1–15B and 1–15C). Following completion of the power stroke, adenosine diphosphate (ADP) is released, and subsequently ATP binds to the nucleotide-binding site (Figure 1–15D, E). The hydrolysis of ATP ultimately leads to the globular head of the myosin heavy chain returning to its original position. The magnitude of crossbridge cycling that occurs during a single contraction is enormous and can approach rates equivalent to 10^{17}–10^{18} crossbridge cycles per gram of muscle per second.

In thinking about the plasticity of the sarcomere and its constituent proteins, note that mechanical unloading and denervation lead to a decrease in the number of sarcomeres in parallel. From a functional perspective, this leads to a decrease in the capacity to produce force. In contrast, resistance training leads to an increase in the number of sarcomeres in parallel, and, as a consequence, increased capacity to produce force.

Factors such as mechanical unloading (eg, as accompanies cast immobilization) and altered thyroid hormone status produce shifts in the contractile and regulatory contractile protein isoform profiles such that they become faster. For instance, cast immobilization may lead to a transition from the slow type I to the fast type IIX myosin heavy-chain isoform. From a functional perspective, this will lead to an increase in maximal shortening velocity. Although it is commonly thought that strength training is an effective tool for increasing sprint speed, note that this will produce fast-to-slow transitions in myosin heavy-chain isoform expression.

5. Molecular anatomy of the connection between the cytoskeleton and the extracellular matrix—Costameres are important structures that link the cytoskeleton of skeletal muscle with the extracellular matrix

Figure 1–15. Molecular anatomy of myosin molecule (**A**) and stop-motion movie of the crossbridge cycle (**B–E**). The orientation in the stop-frame movie is inverted from that shown in (**A**). (The ribbon structure of the S2 [lever arm] and S1 [globular head/motor domain] regions of the myosin heavy chain are reproduced, with permission, from Tyska MJ, Warshaw DM: The myosin power stroke. Cell Motil Cytoskeleton 2002;51:1. The stop-frame movie is reproduced, with permission, from Vale RD, Milligan RA: The way things move: Looking under the hood of molecular motor proteins. Science 2000;288:88.)

(Figure 1–16). Currently, it is believed that the costameres serve at least three different functions: (1) aligning the sarcolemma with the cytoskeleton; (2) maintaining membrane integrity during different types of contractions, preventing injury to the sarcolemma; and (3) possibly playing a role in the lateral transmission of force. From a structural perspective, costameres are found aligned with the Z- and M-lines. This linkage occurs as a result of so-called intermediate filaments. Note that mutations in the costameric structure are

Figure 1-16. Molecular anatomy of a costamere, a structure believed to play a key role in maintaining the mechanical integrity of the membrane during various types of contractions. They are localized at points of contact between the Z-line, M-line, and membrane (sarcolemma). They are also found at myotendinous junctions. The major proteins found localized at the costamere include ankyrin, cytokeratin, desmin, α-dystroglycan, β-dystroglycan, dystrophin, α-fodrin, β-spectrin, α and β subunits of the Na⁺/K⁺ ATPase pump, sarcoglycan, sarcospan. The costamere forms a mechanical link between the sarcomeres within the muscle fiber and laminin located in the extracellular matrix. (Reproduced, with permission, from Clark KA et al: Striated muscle cytoarchitecture: An intricate web of form and function. Ann Rev Cell Dev Biol 2002;18:637.)

22

thought to be involved in some of the muscular dystrophies. Additionally, these structures may play an important role in protecting muscle fibers from eccentrically induced muscle damage.

6. The on-and-off switch of the molecular motor: Excitation-contraction coupling—From a mechanical perspective, all of the sarcomeres must become activated in a synchronous fashion. An asynchronous activation of sarcomeres would lead to large heterogeneities in sarcomere length along the length of a muscle fiber with some sarcomeres actively shortening, whereas the nonactivated sarcomeres would be lengthened. The net result might be a contraction, whereby there is little overall shortening of the muscle fiber. The synchronous activation of all sarcomeres requires an elaborate reticulum that functionally couples the depolarization of the sarcolemma (cell membrane) with activation of the sarcomere. The coupling between excitation and contraction involves extensive invaginations of the sarcolemma known as **transverse tubules** (T-tubules), which are associated with the **sarcoplasmic reticulum.** The sarcoplasmic reticulum is a network of membranes wrapped around the myofibrils, containing a large store of Ca^{2+}. When a skeletal muscle fiber is excited, the depolarization of the sarcolemma is propagated into the T-tubules. Excitation of the T-tubules then leads to the release of Ca^{2+} from the ends of the sarcoplasmic reticulum via so-called **Ca^{2+} release channels** (also known as ryanodine receptors). The Ca^{2+} quickly diffuses into the space occupied by the sarcomere, binding to troponin-C. This then causes tropomyosin to rotate about the longitudinal axis of the actin filament, uncovering the myosin binding sites of each actin molecule. The globular head of the myosin heavy chain attaches to this binding site and goes through its power stroke, leading to the production of force or length change. Simply stated it is the binding of Ca^{2+} to troponin-C that turns on the contractile apparatus.

The contractile activity of the sarcomere is turned off by resequestering Ca^{2+} back into the sarcoplasmic reticulum via **Ca^{2+} ATPase pumps** located along the length of the sarcoplasmic reticulum. The dissociation of Ca^{2+} from troponin-C causes tropomyosin to rotate back into its original position, once again covering up or blocking the myosin-binding sites of each actin molecule. In this manner, the globular head of the myosin heavy chain is prevented from binding to actin, leading to decay in force production and causing the muscle to relax.

As mentioned earlier, there are a number of isoforms for the contractile and regulatory contractile proteins. Isoforms are also identified for the Ca^{2+} release channels and Ca^{2+} ATPase pumps of the sarcoplasmic reticulum. These different isoforms play a key role in determining the rate of activation (ie, the release of Ca^{2+}) and relax-

ation (resequestration of Ca^{2+}). Mechanical unloading of skeletal muscle typically leads to an increased expression of the fast isoforms of the Ca^{2+} release channels, whereas reloading or strength training produces the opposite effect.

B. SKELETAL MUSCLE FUNCTION

In a general sense, the mechanical activity of skeletal muscle depends on two factors: the pattern of stimulation and the extent of loading. The most basic unit of contractile response is known as a twitch. Simply stated, a twitch is the mechanical response of skeletal muscle to a single brief stimulus (Figure 1–17). This single stimulus leads to a single pulse of Ca^{2+} released from the sarcoplasmic reticulum. This single pulse of Ca^{2+} is nonsaturating, meaning that it binds to only some of the troponin-C molecules. In turn, this causes only some of the tropomyosin molecules to rotate about the longitudinal axis of the actin filament, uncovering only some of the myosin-binding sites. From a mechanical perspective, this leads to a submaximal force transient called a **twitch** (see Figure 1–17A). The Ca^{2+} is quickly resequestered by the sarcoplasmic reticulum, and force returns to resting levels.

The amount of Ca^{2+} released by the sarcoplasmic reticulum can be modulated by the pattern of stimulation. If a muscle is repetitively stimulated but with long durations between each stimulus, then the mechanical response will appear as a series of individual twitches, and the force produced will be submaximal. If the muscle is stimulated using a moderate frequency, however, then the mechanical response caused by one stimulus will fuse with that of the second stimulus, leading to a mechanical response known as **tetanus,** and the amplitude depends on the balance between Ca^{2+} release and resequestration. A greater frequency of stimulation leads to a greater release of Ca^{2+} and production of force (Figure 1–17B). Tetanus has two types: one in which partial relaxation occurs between each stimulus (unfused) and another in which no discernible relaxation happens between stimuli (fused) (Figure 1–17B). During fused tetanus, all of the Ca^{2+}-binding sites of troponin-C are saturated, causing all of the myosin-binding sites to be exposed. This results in the greatest production of force.

As noted earlier, the loading of skeletal muscle also plays a key role in determining the mechanical response. For instance, if a muscle contracts against an immovable object, the muscle does not shorten, and hence muscle length remains constant. This type of contraction is referred to as **an isometric contraction** (iso = same; metros = length), and it is under these loading conditions that the muscle produces maximal force. If a muscle contracts against a load that is submaximal (ie, less than the maximal force the muscle can generate), then the muscle shortens. This type of contraction is often

Figure 1–17. Various mechanical measurements that are typically made. The kinetics of a twitch are shown in (**A**). P_t = maximal twitch tension; TPT = time-to-peak tension; $1/2$ RT = one-half relaxation time. The importance of stimulation frequency in regulating the release of Ca^{2+} from the sarcoplasmic reticulum and ultimately force production is shown in (**B**). Methods used to determine the force–velocity relationship are shown in (**C**). V_{max} = maximal shortening velocity; P_o = maximal isometric tension. The mechanical response of a fully activated muscle to a strain of approximately 6% is shown in (**D**). σ = yield stress; ε = yield strain.

referred to as either a **shortening** or an **isotonic contraction.** Muscles not only work under these types of loading conditions, but they work almost as often under conditions in which the muscle is activated and forcibly lengthened. These types of contractions are known as **lengthening** or **eccentric contractions.**

1. Conceptual framework of factors that determine muscle function—From an orthopedics perspective, it would be beneficial to have a framework that would include the key factors that determine the mechanical function of skeletal muscle. Such a framework is laid out in Figure 1–18 and revolves around the context of net mechanical work. In a general context, the net mechanical work produced by skeletal muscle during cyclic length changes (eg, cyclic sinusoidal length changes) is determined by those factors that determine the positive amount of work produced during the shortening phase and those factors that determine the amount of mechanical work done on relengthening the muscle (ie, negative work).

The four determinants of the amount of positive work that can be produced during the shortening phase are (1) the length–tension relationship, (2) the rate of

activation, (3) the force–velocity relationship in the shortening domain, and (4) the rate of relaxation. Two factors determine the amount of work done on the muscle during lengthening: (1) the force–velocity relationship in the lengthening domain and (2) the passive stiffness of the muscle. From an engineering perspective, each of these factors can be thought of as representing design constraints, one of which is static (the length–tension relationship) and others are dynamic. The term *static* in reference to the length–tension relationship implies that the basic dimensions of the sarcomere (and hence length–tension relationship) do not appear to be malleable. In contrast, the other factors can all be altered by factors influencing the mechanical loading of skeletal muscle (eg, immobilization), innervation (partial/complete denervation), and hormonal milieu (eg, thyroid, steroids).

2. Length–tension relationship—The amount of force a muscle can generate depends on muscle length; this length–tension relationship is shown in Figure 1–19. Typically, three regions of the length–tension relationship are described. The ascending limb extends from a sarcomere length of approximately 1.3–2.0 μm. In this region,

Figure 1–18. Various factors that limit the production of mechanical work and power. S.R. = sarcoplasmic reticulum. dP/dx = stiffness of series elastic component. MHC = myosin heavy chain. MLC = myosin light chain. (Modified, with permission, from Caiozzo VJ: Phenotypic plasticity of skeletal muscle: Mechanical consequences. Muscle Nerve 2002;26:740.)

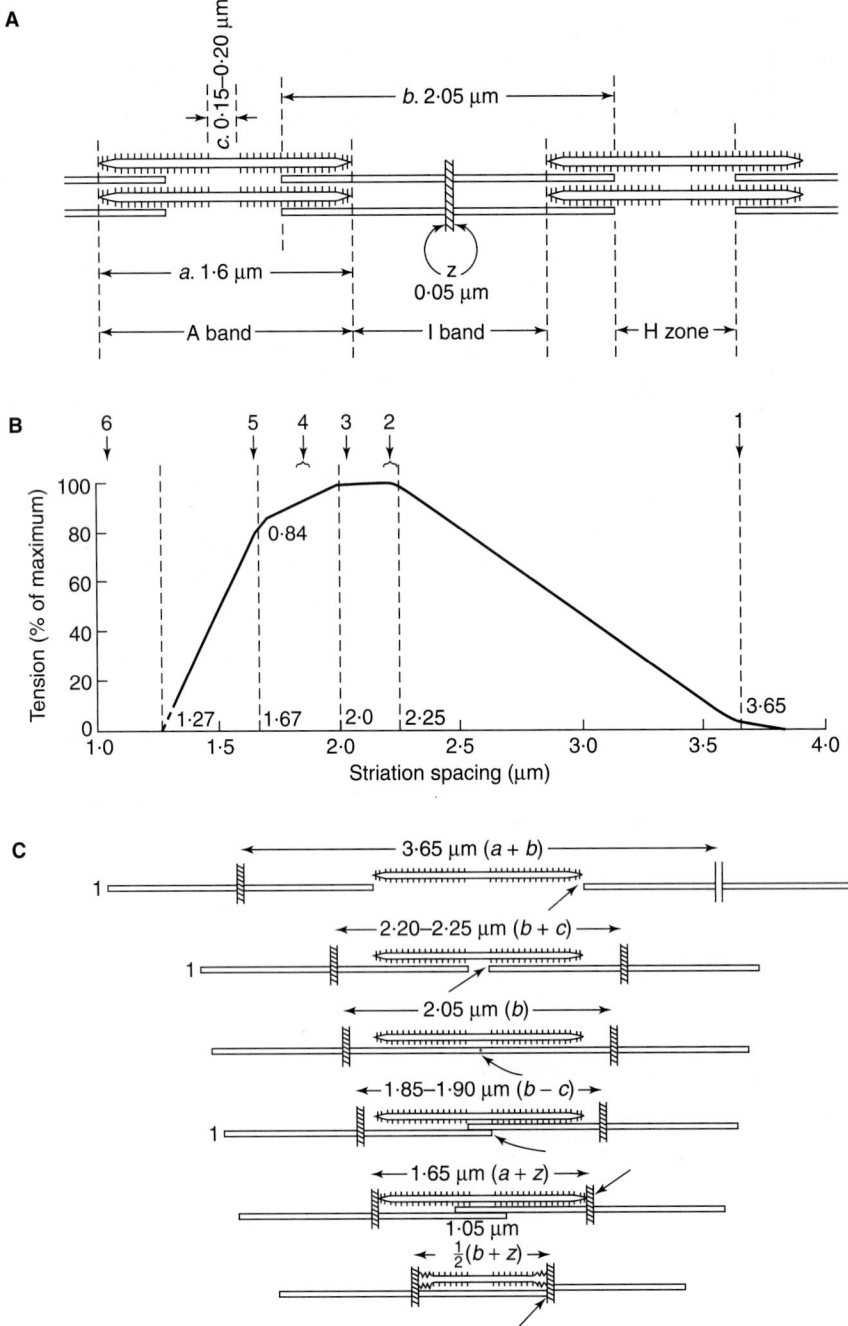

Figure 1–19. Length–tension relationship. (Reproduced, with permission, from Gordon AM et al: The variation in isometric tension with sarcomere length in vertebrate muscle fibres. J Physiol 1966;184:170.)

the amount of isometric tension increases in direct proportion to the increase in sarcomere length. The plateau region extends from approximately 2.0 to 2.5 μm in mammalian fibers, and in this range there is an optimal overlap between the thick and thin filaments. Beyond a sarcomere length of 2.5 μm, the isometric force that can be produced decreases as a linear function of increases in sarcomere length, reflecting a progressive decrease in overlap between the thick and thin filaments.

The length–tension relationship of the sarcomere is thought to represent a static design criteria, implying that it does not change with various types of interventions such as mechanical unloading. However, it is well known that muscles immobilized in a lengthened position increase the number of sarcomeres in series, leading to the longitudinal growth of the fiber. In contrast, immobilization in a shortened position reduces the number of sarcomeres in series and results in a shorter muscle fiber. Hence, such manipulations have the potential for influencing the overall length–tension relationships of muscle fibers and whole muscles. Clearly, contractures may have a large effect on the number of sarcomeres in series and result in various clinical complications such as equinus contractures.

3. Force–velocity relationship in the shortening domain—When a muscle contracts against a light load, it is able to shorten at a relatively high velocity. However, when a muscle contracts against a heavy load, it shortens at a relatively slow velocity. The relationship between the force and shortening velocity is shown in Figure 1–17C and reveals that the force–velocity relationship in the shortening domain can be described by a rectangular hyperbola. Importantly, the shape and dimensions of this relationship depend on the types of contractile protein isoforms and how they are packaged. As noted earlier, **maximal shortening velocity** is primarily determined by the types of myosin heavy-chain isoforms present in the muscle fiber. For instance, a muscle fiber that expresses only the slow type I myosin heavy chain has a much slower V_{max} than one that expresses only the fast type IIX or IIB myosin heavy-chain isoforms. V_{max} does not depend on the cross-sectional area of the muscle fiber. The **maximal isometric tension** that a muscle can produce, often referred to as P_o, is largely independent of myosin heavy-chain isoforms but is heavily dependent on the number of sarcomeres in parallel (ie, cross-sectional area). Hence, in an individual who has marked atrophy, P_o would be expected to be significantly reduced but V_{max} would be unchanged. In this context, the force–velocity relationship can be referred to as a dynamic design criterion, meaning that changes in either cross-sectional area or myosin heavy-chain isoform expression can alter the shape and dimensions of this relationship. Importantly, this relationship represents a design crite-

rion because the muscle can only operate on or below the force–velocity relationship.

The product of force × velocity is mechanical power. Hence, the force–velocity relationship also defines the maximal amount of mechanical power that can be produced under any given loading condition. This has important implications for a wide variety of movements.

4. Force–velocity relationship in the lengthening domain—When a muscle is maximally activated and then forcibly lengthened, the tension that can be generated is much greater than that observed under isometric conditions. However, at velocities beyond a relatively low lengthening velocity, tension does not rise any further. This is shown in Figure 1–20. Although muscles commonly perform lengthening contractions, our understanding of the factors that determine the shape of the force–velocity relationship in the lengthening domain is relatively poor. The shape and dimensions of the force–velocity relationship in the lengthening domain are much more complicated than these same dimensions in the shortening domain. In the shortening domain, the force–velocity relationship can be described by a planar curve with the axes of force and velocity. In the lengthening domain, the relationship is three-dimensional, dependent on force, velocity, and time.

An example of the response of skeletal muscle to a lengthening contraction is shown in Figure 1–17D. Note that the muscle is stimulated, and force is allowed to move onto its isometric plateau. A constant-velocity

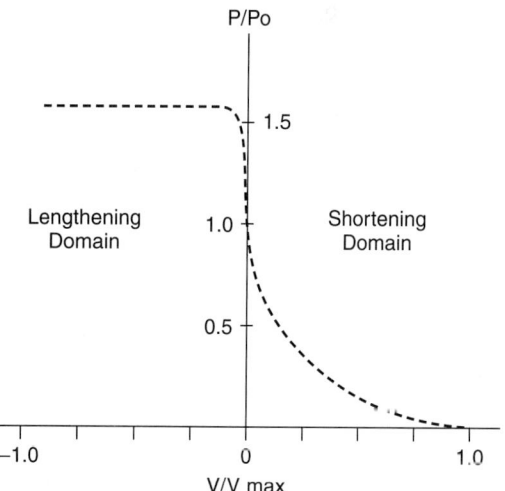

Figure 1–20. Force–velocity relationship in both the shortening and lengthening domains. (Reproduced, with permission, from Caiozzo VJ: Phenotypic plasticity of skeletal muscle: Mechanical consequences. Muscle Nerve 2002;26:740.)

stretch is then imposed on the muscle, and tension rises rapidly. However, at a strain of approximately 1–2%, a sudden change occurs in the rise in tension such that the slope decreases dramatically. The initial force response is often referred to as short-range stiffness. Note that both before and after the yield, force is constantly changing but the velocity of lengthening remains constant. This demonstrates the complexity of understanding the force–velocity relationship in the lengthening domain.

From a functional perspective, the force–velocity relationship in the lengthening domain is important because it determines the amount of work done on relengthening a muscle that is either fully or partially activated. Additionally, muscles are thought to act as dynamic joint stabilizers, so it might be hypothesized that stiffer muscles might better protect joints and ligaments (ie, anterior cruciate ligament) that are susceptible to injury. Newer studies show that mechanical unloading dramatically reduces both the stiffness and elastic modulus of skeletal muscle. The loss of elastic modulus occurs either because of a decrease in crossbridge density or to changes in the unitary stiffness of crossbridges.

5. Passive stiffness of skeletal muscle—The passive stiffness of skeletal muscle is influenced by both sarcomeric and extracellular matrix proteins. **Titin** is the largest known protein identified to date, and it attaches the thick filaments to the Z-line. Within the titin molecule is a unique region, the PEVK region, that functions like a molecular spring. The term *PEVK* refers to the abundance of proline (P), glutamate (E), valine (V), and leucine (K) found in this region. The passive tension of skeletal muscle fibers during stretch may, in part, be caused by the properties of titin. Newer evidence suggests that titin also acts as a molecular blueprint for the organization and structure of the sarcomere, and that titin may play a key role in regulating mechanosensitivity and mechanotransduction in skeletal muscle. For instance, titin contains a kinase domain near the M-line, and this appears to play a prime role in regulating the response of skeletal muscle to increased/decreased mechanical loading by providing a signaling bridge between the sarcomere and nucleus. Newer data suggest that mechanical unloading of skeletal muscle (especially slow type I fibers) results in a loss of titin relative to other myofibrillar proteins such as myosin, but it does not produce shifts in the types of titin isoforms. This, in turn, is believed to impact the passive stiffness of skeletal muscle, but it should be emphasized that the loss in stiffness associated with mechanical unloading is relatively small.

Although the extracellular matrix (ECM) is composed of a number of proteins, the major constituents are collagen and laminin. Fifteen different collagens are

identified to date, and the most prevalent types found in skeletal muscle are types I and III. Type I collagen is more common in slow skeletal muscle, whereas type III is more abundant in fast skeletal muscles. Type I and III collagens are each composed of three individual chains that are arranged in a triple helical fashion. Type I collagen is composed of two α1 chains and one α2 chain. In contrast, type III is composed of three α1 chains. Each of the different types of chains (eg, Iα1) is a product of its own specific gene. From a mechanical perspective, type I collagen is known to have a high tensile strength, whereas type III is more compliant.

Skeletal muscle fibers can be exposed to a variety of forces (eg, normal and shear stress) and strains (normal and shear strain). In a simplistic sense, isometric contractions are associated with high stresses and no strain. Alternatively, passive stresses can be imposed on a skeletal muscle fiber that result in stretch, producing a given amount of strain (relative change in length). To date, the scientific community only has a basic understanding of the effects of different loading conditions on the collagen content of skeletal muscle and associated regulatory pathways. Several studies show that mechanical unloading via hindlimb suspension results in a downregulation of the expression of type I and III collagens. In contrast, the responses of collagen genes/proteins to chronic stretch have not been studied in any detail, yet knowledge in this area may have important clinical ramifications. For instance, orthopedic surgeons commonly use distraction osteogenesis (Ilizarov procedure) as a method to correct limb length deformities. Unfortunately, such procedures (ie, distraction osteogenesis) often result in complications like equinus contractures, which are hypothesized to occur in skeletal muscle because of a proliferation of collagen content.

Anderson JB et al: Physiology: Postprandial cardiac hypertrophy in pythons. Nature 2005;434(7029):37.

Caiozzo VJ: Phenotypic plasticity of skeletal muscle: Mechanical consequences. Muscle Nerve 2002;26:740. [PMID: 12451599]

Clark KA et al: Striated muscle cytoarchitecture: An intricate web of form and function. Ann Rev Cell Dev Biol 2002;18:637. [PMID: 12142273]

Gordon AM et al: The variation in isometric tension with sarcomere length in vertebrate muscle fibres. J Physiol 1966;184:170. [PMID: 5921536]

Tyska MJ, Warshaw DM. The myosin power stroke. Cell Motil Cytoskeleton 2002;51:1. [PMID: 11810692]

Vale RD, Milligan RA. The way things move: Looking under the hood of molecular motor proteins. Science 2000;288:88. [PMID: 10753125]

Intervertebral Disks

The intervertebral disks sustain and distribute loads and also prevent excessive motion of the spine. An individual's intervertebral disks account for 20–33% of his or her spinal column height. The disks are subjected to high stresses during normal daily activity, and stress may double during increased activity, lifting, or trauma. Whether intervertebral disk failure occurs depends on loading rate and stress distribution.

A. STRUCTURAL COMPOSITION

Each intervertebral disk has a nucleus pulposus surrounded by a thick capsule called the annulus fibrosus (Figure 1–21). End-plates composed of hyaline cartilage separate the intervertebral disk from the vertebral body. The unique interplay of the nucleus pulposus, annulus fibrosus, and end-plates accounts for the ability of the disk to withstand compressive, rotational, and shear forces. It is likely that hedgehog genes and the bone morphogenetic protein (BMP) inhibitors, including Pax-1, sonic hedgehog, Indian hedgehog, and Noggin genes, are key factors involved with intervertebral disc formation.

The nucleus pulposus lies in the center of the intervertebral disk, except in the lumbar spine, where it lies slightly posterior, at the junction of the middle and posterior thirds of the sagittal diameter. The nucleus pulposus is composed of a loose network of fine fibrous strands in a gelatinous matrix that contains water-binding glycosaminoglycans. The number of glycosaminoglycans decreases with age, thereby decreasing the hydration of the nucleus pulposus.

The annulus fibrosus is the ringlike outer portion of the disk and consists of fibrocartilage and fibrous tissue. The fibrocartilage is in a series of concentric laminated bands. In the first band, the collagen fibers are principally oriented at a 30-degree angle in one direction; in the second band, they are oriented at a 30-degree angle in the opposite direction; and the pattern continues (Figure 1–21A), with the result that the annular fibers form an intricate crisscross arrangement (Figure 1–21B). Centrally, the collagen fibers of the annulus fibrosus are attached to the cartilaginous end plates. Peripherally, the fibers are attached to the bone of the vertebral body by Sharpey fibers.

B. BIOMECHANICAL BEHAVIOR

The interaction between the nucleus pulposus and the annulus fibrosus accounts for the mechanical behavior of the intervertebral disk. The mechanical properties of the disk are viscoelastic and therefore depend on the loading rate and duration.

During compressive loading, the stress is transferred from the vertebral end plates to the intervertebral disk. With compression, pressure increases in the nucleus pulposus, and the fluid exerts hydrostatic pressure on the annulus fibrosus. As a result, the central portion of the vertebral end plates are pushed away from one

A

B

Figure 1–21. The intervertebral disk consists of a nucleus pulposus surrounded by the annulus fibrosus. In the first band of the annulus fibrosus, the collagen fibers are principally oriented at a 30-degree angle in one direction; in the second band, they are oriented at a 30-degree angle in the opposite direction; and the pattern continues (**A**), with the result that the annular fibers form an intricate crisscross arrangement (**B**). (Reproduced, with permission, from White AA, Panjabi MM: *Clinical Biomechanics of the Spine.* Lippincott, 1978.)

another, and the annular bands are pushed radially outward. The bulging annular bands develop tensile stress in all directions, the optimal orientation for maximal mechanical strength for the collagen fibers.

When the nucleus pulposus ages, its hydration decreases and its hydrostatic properties change. The load-transferring mechanism of the disk is greatly altered if sufficient hydrostatic pressure does not develop. In this situation, the annulus fibrosus transfers the stress to the periphery of the intervertebral disk; however, the fibers are subjected to compressive stress, which is not the optimal loading orientation for collagen fibers. This situation could lead to inadequate stress transfer from successive vertebral bodies, and this in turn could result in compression fractures of the vertebral bodies.

The nucleus pulposus has no effect during tensile loading of the intervertebral disk. Tensile loads are supported by tensile and shear stresses in the annulus fibrosus. The orientation of the collagen fibers of the annulus fibrosus provides no ability to resist shear stresses. Therefore, disk failure is greater with tensile loading than with compressive loading. Excessive shear stresses in the intervertebral disk may cause failure in pure rotational loading when the nucleus pulposus has insufficient load to apply its hydrostatic effects to the annulus fibrosus.

C. DISC REPLACEMENT

Pain located in the low back or neck, without radiation to the extremities, is frequently attributed to the structures in the area, namely the intervertebral disk and/or the facet joints. The relief of pain achieved by joint replacement in other areas of the body has provided an impetus to replace the joints in the spine. Tight regulation of these interventions has resulted in a delay in getting these types of prostheses to the U.S. market. Other countries are actively marketing prostheses for the cervical disc and the lumbar disc. Several designs for each area are now in clinical studies in the United States. In addition to pain relief, these prostheses offer the maintenance of at least some motion in the disc space, compared to fusion. Some of these replacements are metal on metal; others are designed like a traditional joint replacement with a polyethylene bearing component. The efficacy of these devices remains to be seen, especially when compared to the potential complications that might ensue.

Bass EC et al: Biaxial testing of human annulus fibrosus and its implications for a constitutive formulation. Ann Biomed Eng 2004;32:1231. [PMID: 15493511]

Carl A et al: New developments in nucleus pulposus replacement technology. Spine J 2004;4(Suppl 6):325S. [PMID:15541685]

Dipaola CP et al: Molecular signaling in intervertebral disk development. J Orthop Res 2005;23:1112. [PMID: 15936916]

Kumaresan S et al: Contribution of disc degeneration to osteophyte formation in the cervical spine: A biomechanical investigation. J Orthop Res 2001;19:977. [PMID: 11562150]

Kurtz SM et al: Analysis of a retrieved polyethylene total disc replacement component. Spine J 2005;5:344. [PMID: 15863092]

Lee SH et al: In vitro measurement of pressure in intervertebral discs and annulus fibrosus with and without annular tears during discography. Spine J 2004;4:614. [PMID: 15541691]

Simunic DI, Broom ND, Robertson PA: Biomechanical factors influencing nuclear disruption of the intervertebral disc. Spine 2001;26:1223. [PMID: 11389387]

Zigler JE: Lumbar spine arthroplasty using the ProDisc II. Spine J 2004;4(Suppl 6):260S. [PMID: 15541675]

Peripheral Nerves

Peripheral nerves are heterogeneous composite structures comprised of multiple cell types including neurons, Schwann cells, macrophages, and fibroblasts. The primary function of peripheral nerves is the propagation of action potentials. To improve the speed of action potential propagation (ie, nerve conduction velocity) without increasing the diameter of the axon, the Schwann cell, the primary glial cell of the peripheral nervous system, forms a myelin sheath around the axon to insulate the axon and reduce dissipation of the action potential.

A. STRUCTURAL COMPOSITION

The peripheral nerve is composed of motor, sensory, and sympathetic nerve fibers. Such fibers can be either myelinated or unmyelinated. The average diameter of myelinated fibers is 2–22 μm, and unmyelinated axons are 0.4–1.25 μm. Surrounding the individual myelinated nerve fibers or the group of unmyelinated nerve fibers is the endoneurium, a collection of thin collagen strands that provides adequate nourishment and protects the individual axons. Multiple nerve fibers collect to form a group of fibers called a *fascicle*. Such fascicles are bound and encircled by the perineurium, a collection of a connective tissue sheath composed of perineurial cells. The perineurium is the major contributor to the nerve's tensile integrity and strength and is also the blood–nerve barrier. Several fascicles may be arranged into a group fascicle surrounded by connective tissue, termed the internal or interfascicular epineurium. The connective tissue that surrounds the periphery of the entire nerve is called the external or extrafascicular epineurium. The primary function of this connective tissue structure is to nourish and protect the fascicles. Fascicular patterns are divided into the following three types: monofascicular, oligofascicular, and polyfascicular. Monofascicular patterns consist of one large fascicle, whereas oligofascicular patterns consist of a few fascicles; polyfascicular patterns consist of many fascicles of varying sizes that can be arranged with or without groupings of fascicles. Nerves found in the upper arm are routinely polyfascicular. In its course from the upper arm to the fingertips, a peripheral nerve undergoes changes from polyfascicular pattern in the upper arm, oligofascicular in the elbow region, and monofascicular in the hand and fingers. For example, the ulnar nerve is polyfascicular as it exits the brachial plexus until just before the elbow, at which point it becomes oligofascicular. After the division into the motor branch at the wrist, the pattern is monofascicular. These patterns may help determine which type of nerve repair is appropriate for a particular nerve injury. In surgical nerve repair, proper identification of fascicular arrangement is crucial to achieving a successful outcome. Peripheral nerves are extensively vascularized with separate yet interconnected microvascular systems in the epineurium, perineurium, and endoneurium. The vascular pattern of the peripheral nerve is characterized by longitudinally oriented groups of vessels, with a great number of communicating anastomoses. The vasculature is composed of an intrinsic vascular system consisting of vascular plexa in the epineurium, perineurium, and endoneurium and an extrinsic system derived from closely associated vessels running with the nerve. From a surgical perspective, the role of the intraneural microvascular system is vital in regard to the effects of chronic irritation, compression, mobilization, stretching, and transection. If considering a group fascicular or fascicular repair technique, the effects of intraneural vascular damage secondary to surgical manipulation need to be considered.

B. ROLE OF MYELIN SHEATH

One of the primary functions of a myelin sheath is to provide faster, more efficient transmission of the nerve impulse. Myelin itself acts as an insulator around the axon, reducing the dissipation of the action potential into the surrounding medium as it propagates through the axon. There are discontinuities in the myelin sheath along the nerve fiber that are known as nodes of Ranvier and contain high concentrations of voltage-gated sodium channels. The arrival of an action potential at a node depolarizes the membrane, opening the sodium channels to induce a massive influx of sodium ions into the axon. This generates an electrical pulse that is propagated down the axon to the next node of Ranvier, a process termed *saltatory conduction.* Saltatory conduction allows not only for an increased speed of nerve impulse transmission, but also reduces the energy requirement as well. Myelin is not just a conduit for conduction, however. Several myelinopathies, including type I Charcot-Marie-Tooth disease and multiple sclerosis, feature axonal pathology secondary to myelin dysfunction. Although the reciprocal relationship between neurons and glial cells is maintained, many of the clinical manifestations of these diseases are directly related to secondary axonal loss rather than to primary myelin dysfunction. Furthermore, mice with mutations in genes that encode the myelin-specific proteins myelin-associated glycoprotein (MAG), proteolipid protein (PLP), and ciliary neurotrophic factor (CNTF) exhibit evidence of axonal degeneration. MAG localizes to the periaxonal membrane and has a similar structure to members of the immunoglobulin family that participate in cell adhesion. MAG-deficient mice seem to develop apparently normal myelin sheaths and appear phenotypically normal. However, the caliber of myelinated axons decreases, and by 8 months functional contact between the axon and myelin is disrupted and the axons undergo a degenerative process similar to many human peripheral neuropathies. PLP is the major protein constituent of central nervous system myelin. PLP-deficient mice initially appear phenotypically normal and exhibit only minor myelin abnormalities, but they eventually develop behavioral motor abnormalities resulting from ongoing swelling and degeneration of small-diameter myelinated axons. CNTF is a neurotrophic factor that plays an important role in the neural response to injury. Adult CNTF-null mutant mice exhibit a progressive atrophy and degeneration of large-diameter motor neurons, in addition to disruption of the axon–Schwann cell communication network in the paranodal region, resulting in a small reduction in muscle strength. This evidence suggests a functional role for myelin in regulating the maturation, maintenance, and viability of myelinated axons.

Myelin is formed from the extension of the plasma membrane of Schwann cells. Myelin is unique in its high lipid-to-protein ratio, including high contents of galactosphingolipids and saturated long-chain fatty acids. For myelin to achieve its insulating properties, nonconducting structures as well as aqueous cytosolic molecules must be removed. Myelin excludes much of its conductive extracellular and cytoplasmic material by fusing large surfaces of the cytoplasmic leaflets of its plasma membrane, forming a morphological structure called the major dense line. The apposing exoplasmic surfaces of the plasma membrane also fuse to form intraperiod lines. Schmidt-Lanterman incisures are cytoplasmic channels that extend from the internal limit to the external limit of the major dense line. These channels facilitate communication between the axon and Schwann cell body and assure adequate nutritional supply within the regions of compacted myelin.

Gupta R et al: Schwann cells up-regulate vascular endothelial growth factor secondary to chronic nerve compression injury. Muscle Nerve 2005;31(4):452. [PMID: 15685607]

Rowshan K et al: Current surgical techniques in nerve repair. Operative Techniques in Orthopaedics 2004;14(3):163.

Rummler LS et al: The anatomy and biochemistry of myelin and myelination. Operative Techniques in Orthopaedics 2004;14(3):146.

IMPLANT MATERIALS IN ORTHOPEDICS

The body is a harsh chemical environment for foreign materials. An implanted material can have its mechanical and biologic properties significantly altered by body fluids. Degradation mechanisms, such as corrosion or leaching, can be accelerated by ion concentrations and pH changes in body fluids. The body's response to an implant can range from a benign to a chronic inflammatory reaction, with the degree of biologic response largely dependent on the implanted material. For optimal performance in physiologic environments, implant materials should have suitable mechanical strength, biocompatibility, and structural biostability. As the field of biomaterials science developed, various classification schemes for implantable materials were proposed, including schemes based on chemical composition and biologic response.

Implant materials can be classified as biotolerant, bioinert, and bioactive. **Biotolerant materials,** such as stainless steel and PMMA, are usually characterized by a thin fibrous tissue layer along the bone-implant interface. The fibrous tissue layer develops in part as a result of leaching processes that produce chemicals that irritate the surrounding tissues. **Bioinert materials,** such as cobalt-based alloys, titanium, and aluminum oxide, are characterized by direct bone contact, or osseointegration, at the interface under favorable mechanical conditions. Osseointegration is achieved because the material surface is chemically nonreactive to the surrounding tissues and body fluids. **Bioactive materials,** such as calcium phosphate ceramics, particularly hydroxyapatite, have a bone-implant interface characterized by direct chemical bonding of the implant with surrounding bone. This chemical bond is believed to be caused by the presence of free calcium and phosphate ion groups at the implant surface. The calcium phosphate materials can be used as implants or coatings. Other bioactive materials are the growth factors, which are finding application in stimulating desired responses from connective tissues.

Minimizing the local and systemic response to an implanted material through improved biocompatibility is only one engineering concern for reconstructive implant surgery. A prosthetic implant must appropriately transfer stress at the bone-implant surface to ensure long-term implant stability. Nonphysiologic stress transfer may cause pressure necrosis or resorption at the bone-implant interface. Necrotic and resorbed bone may lead to implant loosening and migration, thus compromising implant longevity. Polyethylene wear particles are linked to osteolysis, also compromising implant longevity. Moreover, it is essential that materials have properties capable of sustaining the cyclic forces to which the implant will be subjected. For example, if the material properties are not adequate for load sharing, the implant may fail because of fracture. If the geometry and material properties of the implant make it too rigid in comparison with the bone, then stress shielding of the bone is likely to occur, making bone resorption and implant loosening inevitable.

In addition to acceptable biocompatibility characteristics, biomaterials must demonstrate material properties suitable for their desired use. Materials used to manufacture total joint replacement systems must demonstrate a yield stress that is greater than the stress expected from joint forces but must also have a flexural rigidity that will not result in unacceptable amounts of stress shielding of the bone. General stress–strain curves for the classes of materials allow for the comparison of material properties (Figure 1–22). For instance, ceramics are characterized by a high elastic modulus but are extremely brittle. In contrast with ceramics, metals have a lower elastic modulus but demonstrate increased ductility.

The most commonly used biomaterial combinations for orthopedic joint replacement are metals and metal

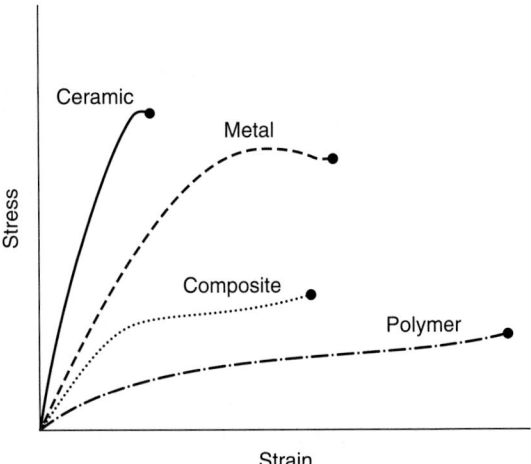

Figure 1–22. Representative stress–strain curves for the classes of materials used in orthopedic implants.

alloys articulating with ultrahigh-molecular-weight polyethylene (UHMWPE). Stainless steel, an iron-based alloy, was used in Charnley's original hip prosthesis and is the material most commonly used for internal fixation plates, rods, and screws. Advances in materials science have produced stronger cobalt-based and titanium-based alloys. The wear resistance of cobalt-based alloys makes them desirable for applications involving articulating surfaces. Titanium-based alloys, which have a modulus of elasticity closer to that of bone than the other metal alloys do, are currently being manufactured as femoral hip stems to reduce the effects of stress shielding.

Polymers and ceramics are also important classes of materials for orthopedic implant applications. UHMWPE has a low coefficient of friction, making it ideal for an articulating surface. PMMA is used as a grouting agent in total joint arthroplasty to provide immediate fixation of total joint components to the skeleton. Porous-coated components require ingrowth of tissue to the porous coating over a period of weeks or months to obtain stability. Aluminum oxide and zirconium oxide have gained popularity as materials for ceramic femoral heads because of their high wear resistance and low coefficient of friction. Finally, calcium phosphate ceramics, particularly hydroxyapatite, are used in monolithic form as an augmentation material for metaphyseal bone defects and as a coating on metal devices for total joint arthroplasty.

Metals

The suitability of a metal component for maintaining longevity of a total joint replacement depends on the design of the implant and the biocompatibility, strength, wear, and corrosion characteristics of the metal. Materials scientists can improve on one or several of the characteristics of a metal alloy by varying the composition or by using different manufacturing processes.

An understanding of the terminology used to describe the strength and stiffness characteristics of a metal is essential in making informed decisions about the different metal alloys. The most important characteristics are elastic modulus, yield stress, ultimate tensile stress, and fatigue stress. As discussed at the beginning of this chapter, these properties can be determined from stress–strain curves and fatigue curves. The composition specifications and mechanical characteristics of all metals and their alloys used for orthopedic implants were standardized by the American Society for Testing and Materials (ASTM).

The grain size, inclusion content, and surface porosity influence the strength characteristics of a metal. In general, the larger the grain size, the lower the tensile and fatigue strength at fracture. Excessive inclusions or a high surface porosity weakens the metal by acting as stress risers and by providing areas for crevice corrosion. Manufacturing processes can be used to control these factors. For example, heating metal to a temperature near its melting point increases the grain size, whereas forging processes decreases the grain size.

Corrosion is a chemical reaction process that weakens the metal. Three types of corrosion are prevalent in implant materials: fatigue, galvanic, and crevice corrosion. Although all metals corrode in the physiologic environment, the severity of corrosion is determined by the chemical composition of the metal. Stainless steel corrodes more readily than either cobalt-based or titanium-based alloys. The chromium and molybdenum content of both stainless steel and cobalt-based alloys produces a corrosion-resistant surface layer. Titanium-based alloys have an adherent oxide passive film layer that provides their corrosion resistance.

The surfaces of all metallic implants are passivated (made passive to corrosion) with nitric acid to form an oxide surface layer that increases corrosion resistance. **Fatigue corrosion** may occur, however, if this passive film layer on the implant surface was scratched or cracked and does not self-passivate in vivo. The ability to self-passivate may be hindered by wear processes or micromovement between modular components, a process called *fretting*. Once corrosion begins, the implant weakens and will fail at a stress level below the endurance limit of the metal.

Galvanic corrosion occurs when an electric current is established between two metals that have different chemical or metallurgic compositions. Some differences arise from manufacturing processes and may be subtle, as in the difference between annealed bone plates and

cold-worked screws made of stainless steel. Other differences that lead to galvanic corrosion arise from the close contact of two different metals in an implant, such as a titanium alloy femoral stem in contact with a cobalt alloy head. An evaluation of retrieved mixed metal femoral hip components consisting of a cobalt-chromium modular head on a titanium alloy stem demonstrated some degree of corrosion in the majority of the components. Further evaluation determined that corrosion occurred in all components that were implanted for longer than 40 months. The long-term clinical significance of the presence of corrosion caused by femoral component modularity is unknown. To avoid catastrophic galvanic corrosion, however, stainless steels should never be used with either cobalt-based or titanium-based alloys.

Crevice corrosion generally occurs when the fluid in contact with a metal becomes stagnant, resulting in a local oxygen depletion and a subsequent decrease in pH in relation to the rest of the implant. This form of corrosion is most prevalent underneath bone plates at the screw-plate junction. The mechanism of crevice corrosion, however, is apparent in point or structural defects in a metal. Corrosion of a defect results in progressive deepening of the defect, leading to the development of large stress concentrations and catastrophic failure of the implant.

A. IRON-BASED ALLOYS

There are four major groups of iron-based alloys or stainless steels, classified according to their microstructure. The group III (austenitic) stainless steels, which are labeled 316 and 316L, are used for orthopedic implants. The difference between 316 and 316L is that the latter contains a smaller percentage of carbon. Lowering the carbon content increases the corrosion resistance. Among the various elements contained in 316 and 316L stainless steels is molybdenum, which hardens the passive layer and increases pitting corrosion resistance.

Iron-based alloys have a wide range of mechanical properties (Table 1–3) that make them desirable for implant applications. Despite composition modifications, stainless steels are susceptible to corrosion inside the body, however. Therefore, they are most appropriate for temporary devices such as bone plates, bone screws, hip nails, and intramedullary nails.

Corrosion of stainless steels occurs for one of several reasons. The most common reason is incorrect metal composition, which increases the chance that galvanic corrosion processes will occur. Molybdenum is added to these metals to increase corrosion resistance; however, too much molybdenum can embrittle the alloy. Chromium carbide may form between the grain boundaries and result in grain boundary corrosion. This phenomenon is referred to as **sensitization.**

Table 1–3. Minimum mechanical requirements for metal implant materials, as standardized by the American Society for Testing and Materials (ASTM).

Material Type	ASTM Number	Ultimate Elastic Modulus (GPa)	0.2% Offset Tensile Strength (MPa)	Yield Strength (MPa)	Elongation (%)	Reduction of Area (%)
Iron-based alloys						
Annealed stainless steel 316	F55-82	200	515	205	40	—
Annealed stainless steel 316L	F55-82	200	480	170	40	—
Cold-worked stainless steel 316 and 316L	F55-82	200	860	690	12	—
Cobalt-based alloys						
Cast Co-Cr-Mo alloy	F75-87	250	655	450	8	8
Wrought Co-Ni-Cr-Mo alloy	F562-84	240	793–1000	241–448	50	65
Titanium and titanium-based alloys						
Unalloyed titanium	F67-89	105	240–550	170–483	15–24	25–30
Cast Ti-6Al-4V alloy	F1108-88	110	860	858	8	14
Wrought Ti-6Al-4V ELI alloy	F136-84	110	860–896	795–827	10	25

Another reason for corrosion is mismatch of implant components, especially when bone plates and screws are used, because even implants manufactured by the same company in different lots can be susceptible to corrosion processes caused by compositional differences. Crevice corrosion can occur at the junction of the screw with the bone plate and develops from local changes in pH and oxygen concentration that may result from slightly different manufacturing processes of the components.

Leaving plates and screws used to fix fractures in younger patients increases the risk of slow progressive corrosion over the years. Failure of the plate resulting from corrosion processes may also lead to bone fracture because stress shielding invariably occurs under the plate. Titanium alloy plates and rods are gaining popularity because of their corrosion resistance and lower elastic modulus, properties that lower the degree of stress shielding.

B. COBALT-BASED ALLOYS

The mechanical properties that make cobalt-based alloys suitable for load-bearing implant applications are summarized in Table 1–3. Among the elements contained in these alloys is molybdenum, which is added to produce finer grains and thereby results in higher strength. The cobalt-based alloys are characterized by high fatigue resistance and high ultimate tensile strength levels, properties that make them appropriate for applications requiring a long service life and ability to resist fracture. The high

wear resistance of these alloys also makes them desirable for load-bearing and articulating surface applications. Cobalt-chromium alloys are primarily used for components in total joint implants.

Despite the advantages of cobalt-based alloys, some reported cases show that surface porosities act as stress risers and lead to premature fatigue failure. Hot isostatic pressing (HIP)—a process that involves simultaneously applying both heat and pressure to consolidate powder into a solid form—was adapted to significantly reduce surface porosity in cast metals. After this process is performed, the material must be heat treated to attain maximal benefit. When performed properly, HIP increases the fatigue resistance, static strength characteristics, and corrosion resistance of cobalt-based alloys. Unfortunately, the heat treatment necessary to apply porous coatings, such as beads, obviates much of the benefit of HIPing.

C. TITANIUM AND ZIRCONIUM ALLOYS

Commercially pure titanium and titanium-based alloys are metals of low density (4.5 g/cm^3) and have chemical properties suitable for implant applications. Zirconium is in the same group in the periodic table. Both metals form an adherent, highly stable oxide surface layer that makes them extremely resistant to corrosion and chemically nonreactive to the surrounding tissues.

The mechanical properties of titanium and titanium-based alloys are summarized in Table 1–3. The elastic modulus value for titanium-based alloys is approximately 110 GPa, which is approximately half the value for iron-based or cobalt-based alloys but is still at least five times greater than the value for bone. Zirconium, when alloyed with niobium (2.5%) and oxygen (0.11%), has a modulus of 97.9 GPa. The higher the impurity content of the metal, the higher the strength and brittleness. Titanium and zirconium can be alloyed together and in combination with a variety of other metals, including niobium, tantalum, molybdenum, and iron. Because of their low density, these alloys have superior specific strength (strength per density) over all other metals. Titanium has poor shear strength and wear resistance, however, making it unsuitable for applications involving articulating surfaces. It also exhibits notch sensitivity, which means that a small flaw or crack on the surface, such as might occur with mechanical damage, can cause a tremendous reduction in strength and increase the susceptibility to fracture.

New manufacturing techniques are attempting to improve titanium-based alloys as bearing surfaces. Nitrogen ion implantation techniques were evaluated for their ability to increase the wear resistance and surface hardness of the alloys. The ion implantation process embeds elemental nitrogen ions in the surface, which causes distortions or strains within the crystal lattice of the metal and results in increased surface microhardness. The results are not adequate to allow titanium or its alloys to be used as bearing surfaces. However, an oxidized zirconium alloy (ASTM F2384) has produced a bearing surface that is showing promise in clinical trials for the last several years. In vitro studies show that the increased surface hardness from the oxide layer significantly improves the wear resistance of the treated implant. The surface oxide layer is very thin (approximately 0.004 mm) but extremely adherent.

Polymers

Polymers have a wide range of properties attributable to variations in their chemical composition, structure, and manufacturing process, which make them suitable for several different implant applications. The choice of polymer for application is dictated by the effect of the physiologic environment on the stability of the material. Some polymers, such as PMMA, leach toxic substances into the surrounding tissues. Conversely, other polymers, such as silicone, absorb fluids from the body, and this absorption alters the mechanical properties. Despite the possible consequences of polymer implantation, the use of polymers as implant materials has been successful.

All polymers are composed of long chains of repeating units. These units may form linear, cross-linked, or branched chains. The individual chains may be organized in an orderly crystalline form having parallel or folded chains, or they may have an amorphous structure or a mixed structure. The molecular weight, chemical composition, degree of crystallinity, size and polarity of side groups, and degree of cross-linking determine the mechanical properties of the polymer. In general, as the molecular weight and crystallinity increase, the tensile strength and the resistance to cracking increase. The crystallinity is decreased by copolymerization, branching of chains, and large side groups.

A. Ultrahigh-Molecular-Weight Polyethylene

UHMWPE possesses an array of properties, including high abrasion resistance, low friction, high impact strength, excellent toughness, low density, ease of fabrication, biocompatibility, and biostability, that makes it an attractive material for use in fabricating bearing surfaces for total joint replacements. UHMWPE is the material of choice for the liner of acetabular cups in total hip arthroplasties, the tibial insert, patellar components in total knee arthroplasties, and other load-bearing interfaces. The clinical performance of these components for nearly three decades has been excellent; however, there are concerns about the long-term wear of these devices. The concern is not only that the materials will wear out, but also that the wear debris generated will evoke an undesirable biologic reaction. It is known that particles in the submicron size undergo phagocytosis, resulting in a variety of biologic reactions. The reactions can include granulomatous lesions, osteolysis, and bone resorption. The phenomenon of wear of UHMWPE in total joint replacement is widely regarded as one of the most challenging problems in contemporary orthopedics.

A variety of factors influence the wear of polyethylene. These include the nature or quality of the starting material; the degree of cross-linking, strength, and toughness of the material; the manufacturing technique; the thickness of the polyethylene; the component sterilization conditions; and the storage environment and age of the component. The composition and physical properties of the starting materials used in the fabrication of UHMWPE components—in particular, molecular weight—have a profound effect on the material's performance. It is widely agreed that low-molecular-weight impurities and a high crystallinity are detrimental to the clinical performance. Increased crystallinity causes less resistance to crack initiation, crack propagation, and oxidation-enhanced wear.

UHMWPE is either machined from ram-extruded bar stock or compression molded directly from the starting powder. Ram extrusion is a two-step process in which the starting powder is first heated and pressurized in a polymerizing chamber followed by extrusion of bar stock. The second step, usually performed by the implant manufacturer, is the machining of the component with a precision cutting tool. By contrast, direct compression molding is a one-step process. A preshaped component and premeasured volume of starting powder are placed into a heated mold, and the component is then formed under pressure. Each manufacturing process has its own unique characteristics and problems. Some engineers believe that compression-molded components, although more expensive to produce, result in products with enhanced in vivo wear performance.

In general, as the thickness of the UHMWPE components decreases, the stresses increases, and therefore, the wear also increases. This is because with an increase in thickness, the structural stiffness of the component increases, even when the value of the modulus of elasticity of the material remains unchanged. This effect has resulted in a recommendation for the minimal thickness of acetabular liners of approximately 5–6 mm and tibial inserts of 7–8 mm.

Several manufacturers choose gamma irradiation for sterilizing UHMWPE components at doses between 25,000 and 40,000 Gy. Gamma radiation causes both cross-linking and chain fission and is the major contributor to subsequent surface and subsurface oxidative degradation of the components. Other manufacturers choose surface sterilization techniques, such as ethylene oxide, or one of the several plasma techniques, which have no effect on the bulk properties of the polyethylene. There is considerable literature on the effect of a number of variables associated with sterilization, packaging, and aging of polyethylene on the in vivo and in vitro physical and mechanical properties. These include the method of sterilization, sterilization dosage, packaging atmosphere, and aging conditions. For example, irradiation and storage in an inert atmosphere reduces the oxidative degradation before implantation. Because of this volume of work, no consensus has yet emerged on these effects. As noted, gamma sterilization, particularly in air, causes significant reduction of the various mechanical characteristics that are related to the subsequent wear and performance of the material. These parameters include crystallinity, melting temperature, oxidation strength, tensile properties, and density.

Irradiation of polyethylene at much higher doses (50,000–150,000 Gy) followed by an annealing process results in a cross-linked polyethylene with different properties. Early hip simulator wear studies indicate that this cross-linked polyethylene has very low wear rates and superior wear properties compared with conventional polyethylene. Early clinical trials seem to confirm a reduction in wear rates but not to the magnitude predicted by the wear simulator studies.

B. POLYMETHYLMETHACRYLATE

Self-curing PMMA, commonly used as a grouting agent, is often called the weak link in total joint arthro-plasty. Compared with cortical bone, bone cement has a lower elastic modulus and significantly inferior mechanical strength properties. The tensile strength of PMMA is similar to that of cancellous bone. The low modulus of elasticity allows for gradual transfer of stress from implant to bone. Mechanically, PMMA is weakest in shear loading and strongest in compression loading configurations.

Implant design and cementing technique must compensate for weakness in tension, to avoid catastrophic failure of the cement. The poor fatigue strength of PMMA can be attributed primarily to porosity. Studies show that PMMA porosity is increased and fatigue strength is further decreased by mixing the cement with chilled monomer, rather than with monomer at room temperature. Therefore, if chilled monomer must be used, it is crucial to use porosity reduction techniques, such as centrifugation or vacuum mixing, concurrently. The fatigue strength of PMMA is also decreased by the presence of inclusions, such as bone chips and blood.

Aside from the inherent mechanical weakness of PMMA, the polymerization process causes local and systemic biologic effects. Locally, adjacent tissues can become necrotic because of the extreme heat of polymerization, which can generate temperatures approaching 100° C. Systemically, the leaching of monomer during the curing process may cause hypotension.

The fatigue properties of PMMA manufactured by different companies vary because of intrinsic compositional differences, such as the size of the polymer beads, the addition of copolymers, and the presence of additives and radiopacifiers. In a study of the fatigue life of five commonly used bone cements (CMW, LVC, Palacos R, Simplex P, and Zimmer Regular), investigators prepared each cement in the manner suggested by its manufacturer. They found that Palacos R and Simplex P had equivalent fatigue strengths and that these two products had significantly greater fatigue strengths than the other three products. For each product, investigators compared the fatigue life of a regular sample with that of a sample that had undergone a process to reduce its porosity. In the case of each product, a reduction in the cement's porosity increased its fatigue life. Moreover, when investigators centrifuged two packages of Simplex P mixed with chilled monomer for 60 s, they found a fivefold increase in the fatigue properties of this cement.

Antibiotics were added to bone cement at the time of surgery for years to reduce the risk of infection or to treat infection. Heat-stable antibiotics that are eluted from the bone cement inhibit antibiotic growth for variable periods from days to weeks. To obtain more uniform formulations, manufacturers have now obtained permission from the Food and Drug Administration

(FDA) to make the bone cement with premixed antibiotics. Studies show that the fatigue strength of the cement is not reduced with these additions.

Ceramics

Ceramics are wear resistant and strong in compression, but they are extremely brittle and susceptible to cracking. Ceramic materials must be carefully chosen for specific implant applications because chemical composition affects the mechanical properties and biologic responses of each ceramic. For instance, in calcium phosphate ceramics, an alteration in the ratio of calcium to phosphorous can significantly alter the in vivo dissolution rate of the ceramic.

The mechanical properties of ceramics depend on grain size, porosity, density, and crystallinity. Strength is normally improved with increased density, increased crystallinity, and decreased porosity. The hardness and wettability of ceramics and the fact that ceramics can be polished to smooth surfaces make them ideal candidates for bearing surfaces. Nevertheless, for a ceramic implant to be reliable, its design must avoid sharp corners and notches, to overcome the predictable mechanical flaws of the material.

A. ALUMINUM OXIDE

The catastrophic effects of implant loosening associated with polyethylene wear debris led to interest in using other materials at the articulating surface. The use of aluminum oxide (Al_2O_3) was explored because it is a highly biocompatible material with high frictional resistance. In fact, the coefficient of friction for alumina-on-alumina articulations is approximately 2.3 times less than the coefficient for metal-on-polyethylene articulations. Studies show that alumina-on-alumina articulations demonstrate approximately 5000 times less wear than metal-on-polyethylene articulations do under experimental loading conditions.

In clinical practice, all-alumina acetabular components have not performed well, probably because of loosening caused by the modulus mismatch between aluminum oxide and bone. Designs to circumvent this problem have fixed an alumina bearing component inside a metal ingrowth cup, so the bone can grow into a porous metal surface. Ceramic-on-polyethylene articulations show clinical promise, however. Aluminum oxide has excellent wear characteristics, and any ceramic wear debris that does accumulate at the interface may be less bioreactive than polyethylene or PMMA wear debris. Alumina-on-alumina articulations demonstrate very low wear rates when clinically applied with a metal shell for attachment to acetabular bone. Although the alumina wear rates are low, problems have occurred because of placement of the components, allowing

impingement and abrasion of the neck of the femoral component.

Despite the excellent wear and friction characteristics of aluminum oxide, its fracture toughness and tensile strength are relatively low. The fracture rate of alumina is low but significant. In one series, the authors reported 13 failures out of 5500 implantations over 25 years (0.23%), and disturbingly, they were unable to attribute some of the fractures to any rational explanation. Fracture can be a result of microstructural flaws, which are statistical in nature. The elastic modulus of aluminum oxide is approximately 20 times greater than that of cortical bone. Increased grain size decreases strength and a large grain size is linked to reported cases of catastrophic wear. Careful regulation of manufacturing processes is necessary to obtain reliable aluminum oxide implants with small grain size, high density, high purity, adequate strength, and adequate component size. With these caveats, these alumina-on-alumina implants may have a role in hip replacement in younger patients because of their reduced rate of particulate wear production. The high strength and hardness of alumina also recommend it for use with polyethylene bearings.

B. ZIRCONIUM OXIDE

Zirconium oxide (Zirconia) temporarily became an attractive material for highly loaded joint replacement applications. Pure zirconium oxide can be maintained in a metastable, tetragonal crystal structure with fine grain structure, with the addition of a stabilizing oxide, such as yttrium oxide (Y_2O_3).

In comparison with aluminum oxide, zirconium oxide exhibits increased fracture toughness, increased bending strength, and decreased elastic modulus. Moreover, Zirconia-to-polyethylene articulations demonstrate favorable wear characteristics compared with alumina-to-polyethylene articulations in vitro. Because the mechanical and wear properties of zirconium oxide are superior to those of aluminum oxide, it is possible to manufacture smaller femoral heads for low-friction total hip arthroplasty. However, several studies show an increase in the monoclinic phase of Zirconia over time in vivo, calling into question the long-term biostability of the material. Further, the phase change was associated with an increase in surface roughness and wear rates of polyethylene bearing surfaces. Other problems have plagued proponents of Zirconia as a bearing material. Catastrophic failure was seen in a high proportion of Zirconia heads produced in a tunnel kiln in Europe, which were shown on retrieval to have high (21–68%) monoclinic phase present. Zirconia femoral heads may need significant research to demonstrate safety and regain consumer confidence. Although still available in some markets, Zirconia femoral heads may have a very limited place in the orthopedic market.

C. HYDROXYAPATITE

Calcium phosphate ceramics, classified as polycrystalline ceramics, have a material structure derived from individual crystals that become fused at the grain boundaries during high-temperature sintering processes.

Tribasic calcium phosphate [$Ca_{10}(PO_4)_6(OH)_2$], which is commonly called **hydroxyapatite,** is a geologic mineral that closely resembles the natural mineral in vertebrate bone tissue. Tribasic calcium phosphate should not be confused with other calcium phosphate ceramics, especially tricalcium phosphate [$Ca_3(PO_4)_2$], which is chemically similar to hydroxyapatite but is not a natural bone mineral.

Bulk hydroxyapatite (HA) is manufactured from a starting powder, and the manufacturing process consists of compression molding and subsequent sintering. Macroporous ceramics can be obtained by combining the starting mixture with hydrogen peroxide. Otherwise, a dense structure with a small percentage of micropores results. Dense HA ceramics have a compressive strength greater than that of cortical bone; however, their tensile strength is approximately 2.5 times less than their compressive strength. Small reductions in density can significantly reduce tensile characteristics of the ceramic. Bulk HA can also be formed with a very uniform pore structure by the chemical conversion of calcium carbonate coral structures. This material can be used to augment bone graft in cancellous bone areas.

Although the static mechanical properties of bulk HA are good, the resistance to fatigue failure is low in physiologic conditions, as is common with sintered ceramics and particularly bioactive ceramics. Therefore, bulk HA is not suitable for applications requiring mechanical loading. Bulk HA is used successfully in clinical practice as a bone graft substitute to fill defects associated with fractures or as a bone graft extender for fractures or fusions. A composite prosthesis made by plasma spraying thin (approximately 50 μm) coatings of HA or other calcium phosphate compounds onto a metal substrate was developed and is able to withstand the physiologic stresses imposed on it while providing an osteoconductive surface to achieve optimal bone apposition and ingrowth. These coatings can be applied by other means including chemical deposition from solution. Generally, HA coatings do not provide adequate fixation of bone when applied to smooth metal surfaces, and they require a roughened or porous surface for long-term fixation. Experimental results indicate that HA stimulates more extensive and uniform growth of bone into a porous-surfaced femoral stem or acetabular cup and probably aids bone growth across gaps between implants and surrounding bone. The durability of the fixation of the prosthesis to bone may be related to the quality and durability of the coating. HA coatings on ingrowth/ongrowth surfaces is probably not needed in the primary procedure but is considered by many surgeons to be helpful in the revision procedure, to obtain more reliable bone ingrowth.

Several formulations of an injectable hydroxyapatite are now available for minimally invasive surgery. These materials are similar to PMMA in that the setting process is a chemical reaction that yields the final product, in this case hydroxyapatite, or a similar calcium phosphate compound.

D. PYROLYTIC CARBON

Carbon occurs naturally in many forms, each having different structures, material properties, and uses. Coal is an example of carbon in its amorphous form with no crystalline structure. Graphite has an organized crystalline structure, in which carbon atoms are arranged in two-dimensional hexagonal sheets tightly joined by strong covalent bonds. Diamond is a third form of carbon having a three-dimensional cubic crystal structure with increased atomic bonds.

Pyrolytic carbon is a manufactured material formed by the pyrolysis, or heating, of gaseous hydrocarbons, causing them to decompose to a stable gas and carbon. The resulting pyrolytic carbon is usually deposited on a graphite substrate in a turbostatic, two-dimensional crystalline structure with a high concentration of three-dimensional diamond cross-link bonding. In general, the physical properties of pyrolytic carbon fall between those of graphite and diamond. The form of pyrolytic carbon used as a surgical implant material has a very fine grain structure (approximately 50 Å), and isotropic physical and mechanical properties. Pyrolytic carbon is chemically inert and resistant to wear and mechanical fatigue with a fatigue strength at 10^9 cycles close to its failure strength. It also has a high fracture strength, and low elasticity modulus (21–26 GPa), which falls within the range of moduli reported for cortical bone. Its biocompatibility is well documented and has been confirmed clinically in extensive use in cardiovascular implants for more than 30 years. Pyrolytic carbon has also proved to be extremely biocompatible in both osseous and soft tissues.

Pyrolytic carbon was evaluated in cardiovascular, dental, soft-tissue, and orthopedic implants. It is the material of choice for the construction of mechanical artificial heart valves. The human heart beats on an average of 100,000 times per day, or 35 million times per year. The carbon-on-carbon pivot systems in heart valves must resist stress and wear each time the heart beats. The history of successful function in heart valve components demonstrates the outstanding wear resistance of the carbon-on-carbon articulation, biocompatibility, high fatigue strength, and structural durability of the pyrolytic carbon material. Pyrolytic carbons were evaluated clinically in orthopedics for replacement of the small bones and joints of the hands and feet. Non-constrained pyrolytic carbon metacarpophalangeal joint replacements were evaluated in human clinical trials with results at long-term follow-up demonstrating excellent performance of the implants with a 15-year survival rate of more than 70%. The long-term clinical results of the metacarpophalangeal joint arthroplasties verify the biologic and biomechanical compatibility of pyrolytic carbons in a demanding orthopedic application. With FDA approval, these joints are now being marketed for general use.

Baleani M et al: Fatigue strength of PMMA bone cement mixed with gentamicin and barium sulphate vs pure PMMA. Proc Inst Mech Eng (H) 2003;217:9. [PMID: 12578214]

Catledge SA et al: Surface crystalline phases and nanoindentation hardness of explanted femoral heads. J Mater Sci Mater Med 2003;14:863. [PMID: 15348523]

Cook SD et al: Long-term follow-up of pyrolytic carbon metacarpophalangeal implants. J Bone Joint Surg Am 1999;81:635. [PMID: 10360692]

Endo MM et al: Comparative wear and wear debris under three different counterface conditions of crosslinked and non-crosslinked ultra high molecular weight polyethylene. Biomed Mater Eng 2001;11:23. [PMID: 11281576]

Ezzet KA et al: Oxidized zirconium femoral components reduce polyethylene wear in a knee simulator. Clin Orthop 2004;428.120. [PMID: 15534531]

Food and Drug Administration, HHS: Medical devices; reclassification of polymethylmethacrylate (PMMA) bone cement. Final rule. Fed Regist 2002;67:46852. [PMID: 12125716]

Friedman RJ et al: Current concepts in orthopaedic biomaterials and implant fixation. J Bone Joint Surg Am 1993;75:1086. [PMID: 11132264]

Gott VL, Alejo DE, Cameron DE: Mechanical heart valves: 50 years of evolution. Ann Thorac Surg 2003;76:S2230. [PMID: 14667692]

Hannouche D et al: Fractures of ceramic bearings: History and present status. Clin Orthop 2003;417:19. [PMID: 14646699]

Haraguchi K et al: Phase transformation of a Zirconia ceramic head after total hip arthroplasty. J Bone Joint Surg Br 2001;83:996. [PMID: 11603539]

Hernigou P, Bahrami T: Zirconia and alumina ceramics in comparison with stainless-steel heads. Polyethylene wear after a minimum ten-year follow-up. J Bone Joint Surg Br 2003;85:504. [PMID: 12793553]

Jeffers JR, Browne M, Taylor M: Damage accumulation, fatigue and creep behaviour of vacuum mixed bone cement. Biomaterials 2005;26:5532. [PMID: 15860209]

Kurtz SM et al: In vivo degradation of polyethylene liners after gamma sterilization in air. J Bone Joint Surg Am 2005;87:815. [PMID: 15805212]

Laskin RS: An oxidized Zr ceramic surfaced femoral component for total knee arthroplasty. Clin Orthop 2003;416:191. [PMID: 14646761]

Lewis G, Carroll M: Rheological properties of acrylic bone cement during curing and the role of the size of the powder particles. J Biomed Mater Res 2002;63(2):191. [PMID: 11870653]

Lim TH et al: Biomechanical evaluation of an injectable calcium phosphate cement for vertebroplasty. Spine 2002;27:1297. [PMID: 12065977]

Ma L, Sines G: Fatigue behavior of a pyrolytic carbon. J Biomed Mater Res 2000;51(1):61. [PMID: 10813746]

Mashoof AA et al: Supplementation of autogenous bone graft with coralline hydroxyapatite in posterior spine fusion for idiopathic adolescent scoliosis. Orthopedics 2002;25:1073. [PMID: 12401014]

Masonis JL et al: Zirconia femoral head fractures: A clinical and retrieval analysis. J Arthroplasty 2004;19:898. [PMID: 15483807]

McKellop H et al: Development of an extremely wear-resistant ultra high molecular weight polyethylene for total hip replacements. J Orthop Res 1999;17(2):157. [PMID: 10221831]

Morscher EW, Wirz D: Current state of cement fixation in THR. Acta Orthop Belg 2002;68:1. [PMID: 11915452]

Murphy BP, Prendergast PJ. The relationship between stress, porosity, and nonlinear damage accumulation in acrylic bone cement. J Biomed Mater Res 2002;59:646. [PMID: 11774326]

Oonishi H, Kadoya Y: Wear of high-dose gamma-irradiated polyethylene in total hip replacements. J Orthop Sci 2000;5(3):223. [PMID: 10982661]

Porter AE et al: Bone bonding to hydroxyapatite and titanium surfaces on femoral stems retrieved from human subjects at autopsy. Biomaterials 2004;25:5199. [PMID: 15109844]

Ries MD et al: Polyethylene wear performance of oxidized zirconium and cobalt-chromium knee components under abrasive conditions. J Bone Joint Surg Am 2002;84(Suppl 2):129. [PMID: 11712832]

Ries MD et al: Relationship between gravimetric wear and particle generation in hip simulators: Conventional compared with cross-linked polyethylene. J Bone Joint Surg Am 2001;83 (Suppl 2, Pt 2):116. [PMID: 11712832]

Sakoda H et al: A comparison of the wear and physical properties of silane cross-linked polyethylene and ultra-high molecular weight polyethylene. J Arthroplasty 2001;16:1018. [PMID: 11740757]

Schulz M et al: Early results of proximal interphalangeal joint replacement with pyrolytic carbon prosthesis (Ascension) idiopathic and post-traumatic arthritis. Handchir Mikrochir Plast Chir 2005;37:26. [PMID: 15744654]

Sharkey PF et al: The bearing surface in total hip arthroplasty: Evolution or revolution. Instr Course Lect 2000;49:41. [PMID: 10829160]

Smith SL, Unsworth A: An in vitro wear study of alumina-alumina total hip prostheses. Proc Inst Mech Eng [H] 2001;215:443. [PMID: 11726044]

Spector BM et al: Wear performance of ultra-high molecular weight polyethylene on oxidized zirconium total knee femoral components. J Bone Joint Surg Am 2001;83(Suppl 2, Pt 2):80. [PMID: 11712839]

Sun L et al: Material fundamentals and clinical performance of plasma-sprayed hydroxyapatite coatings: A review. J Biomed Mater Res 2001;58:570. [PMID: 11505433]

Urban JA et al: Ceramic-on-polyethylene bearing surfaces in total hip arthroplasty. Seventeen to twenty-one-year results. J Bone Joint Surg Am 2001;83:1688. [PMID: 11701792]

Vallo CI: Flexural strength distribution of a PMMA-based bone cement. J Biomed Mater Res 2002;63:226. [PMID: 11870658]

Weisman DL et al: In vitro evaluation of antibiotic elution from polymethylmethacrylate (PMMA) and mechanical assessment of antibiotic-PMMA composites. Vet Surg 2000;29:245. [PMID:10871226]

Yamamoto T et al: Wear analysis of retrieved ceramic-on-ceramic articulations in total hip arthroplasty: Femoral head makes contact with the rim of the socket outside of the bearing surface. J Biomed Mater Res B Appl Biomater 2005;73:301. [PMID: 15742373]

GROWTH FACTORS

Biology

Growth factors hold great promise for the treatment of a variety of musculoskeletal conditions. The response of bone to structural damage is nearly unique in biology. The vast majority of tissues, when traumatized, heal with a fibrous scar, the cells and structure of which are not normal and are unable to assume fully the function of the tissue. In contrast, bone, the cornea, and the liver are capable of true cellular, morphologic, and functional regeneration. The initial phase of bone healing is characterized by an inflammatory response in consolidation of the hematoma within the fracture site. This is followed by the proliferation of periosteal, endosteal, and marrow stromal cells adjacent to the site, and recruitment of undifferentiated mesenchymal cells from nearby soft tissues. These cells and their progeny differentiate to become chondroblasts, chondrocytes, osteoblasts, and osteocytes. The cartilage formed is eventually replaced by bone, and the early woven bone is remodeled to a more mature lamellar structure.

Growth factors are polypeptides that serve as signaling agents for cells. These local proteins bind to specific receptors, occasionally with the assistance of extracellular binding proteins, to stimulate or inhibit functions inside the cell during development and throughout an organism's life. For example, growth/differentiation factor-5 (GDF-5) is essential for normal appendicular skeletal and joint development in humans. GDF-5 acts at two stages of skeletal development and by two distinct mechanisms: (1) promoting the initial stages of chondrogenesis by promoting cell adhesion and (2) increasing the size of the skeletal elements by increasing proliferation within the epiphyseal cartilage adjacent to its expression within the joint interzone. The discovery of these substances revolutionized the field of cell biology by revealing the mechanisms of regulation of cell activities. Growth factors are present in plasma or tissues, in concentrations measured in billionths of a gram; yet, they are the principal effectors of critical cellular functions, such as cell proliferation, matrix synthesis, and tissue differentiation. Cytokines are similar to growth factors because they are receptor-activating locally act-

ing polypeptides. Although cytokines were originally characterized from cells of the hematopoietic and immune cell systems, the distinction is rather artificial because most authors currently consider growth factors to be a subset of cytokines.

Although the same growth factor is often found throughout the body, they are named based on their function and tissue of origin. Several growth-promoting substances are identified in bone matrix and at the site of fracture healing. These growth factors are believed to play a role in the healing process. Among these are the transforming growth factor beta (TGF-β), BMP, fibroblast growth factors (FGF), IGFs, and platelet-derived growth factor (PDGF). These growth factors are produced by osteoblasts and incorporated into the extracellular matrix during bone formation. Small amounts of growth factors can also be trapped systemically from serum and incorporated into the matrix. The present hypothesis is that growth factors are located within the matrix until remodeling or trauma causes solubilization and release of the proteins.

A. TRANSFORMING GROWTH FACTOR BETA

TGF-βs are a family of dimeric polypeptide growth factors and coded by closely related genes. The family includes at least five molecules known as TGF-β 1–4, and, by itself, it is a member of a superfamily that includes BMPs, activins, and GDFs, among others, that regulate morphogenesis in early development. The broad range of cellular activities regulated by TGF-βs include the proliferation and expression of differentiated phenotypes of many of the cell populations that make up the skeleton. Among these are the mesenchymal precursor cells for chondrocytes, osteoblasts, and osteoclasts. The presence of TGF-βs in normal fracture healing suggests they play a role in the repair process. TGF-βs are secreted in an inactive form requiring acid pH or heat for activation. These dimeric, disulfide bonded molecules mediate their function through receptors that act as serine/threonine kinases. The receptors autophosphorylate, after forming a complex with TGF-β, activate Smad intracellular pathways that translocate to the nucleus and regulate gene transcription. Thus far, eight mammalian Smad proteins are identified. After oligomerization, these proteins enter the nucleus to regulate transcription following assembly with transcriptional cofactors and comodulators. Because articular cartilage has limited potential for repair, TGF-β 1 is used in animal studies for its stimulatory effect on chondrogenesis in periosteal explants.

B. BONE MORPHOGENETIC PROTEIN

Related to the TGF-βs, the bone morphogenic proteins constitute a family of at least 15 growth factors originally identified for their ability to stimulate de novo bone formation. The BMPs are also referred to as osteogenic proteins (OPs); hence, there is some name confusion because BMP-7 is also called OP-1. BMPs are the only growth factors that can stimulate differentiation of mesenchymal stem cells into a chondroblastic (BMP-2) and osteoblastic (BMP-5, -6, and -7) direction. These BMP molecules are also quite effective osteoinductive agents. Noggin and chordin are extracellular binding proteins that alter binding of BMP molecules with their receptors. When implanted, most BMPs can stimulate a cascade of cellular events that closely mimics the process of endochondral ossification in normal fracture healing. Precursor cells are recruited and differentiated into chondrocytes that manufacture cartilage matrix. The cartilage is then gradually replaced by bone as osteoblasts populate the site. Eventually, bone marrow elements fill the newly formed intertrabecular spaces, and the bone remodels. Overexpression of BMP-4 in inflammatory cells is responsible for fibrodysplasia ossificans progressiva.

C. FIBROBLAST GROWTH FACTORS

Fibroblast growth factors are currently a group of eleven polypeptides that were originally discovered on the basis of their mitogenic effect on fibroblasts and have four known receptors. Acid fibroblast growth factor and basic fibroblast growth factor, also termed FGF-1 and FGF-2, respectively, are both implicated in cartilage and bone regulation. Basic FGF is generally more potent than acid FGF. FGFs have a significant proliferative effect on osteoblasts but less effect on protein synthesis. FGFs probably enhance bone formation by increasing the number of cells capable of synthesizing bone collagen. FGFs are also angiogenic factors, which are important for neovascularization during bone healing. A defect in the FGF receptor 3 is implicated as the cause for achondroplasia.

D. INSULIN-LIKE GROWTH FACTOR

The pivotal role of IGF in regulating endochondral ossification in skeletal growth suggests that this factor may also participate in endochondral ossification of bone healing. IGF regulates both bone matrix formation and cell replication. Of all the growth factors present in bone matrix, IGF-2 has the highest concentration; however, IGF-1 is four to seven times more potent than IGF-2. IGF-1, also known as somatomedin C, is produced in the liver and by skeletal tissue in response to stimulation with growth hormone. The cells that secrete IGFs also secrete any one of the six IGF-binding proteins that actually regulate the effectiveness of this growth factor.

Both IGF-1 and IGF-2 stimulate preosteoblastic cell replication by increasing the number of cells capable of synthesizing bone matrix. However, their mitogenic

effect is less pronounced than those of other growth factors. IGFs also have independent effects on the differentiation of osteoblasts, increasing bone collagen production and inhibiting collagen degradation. Recent studies evaluating the endogenous tissue levels of different growth factors within healing tendon lesions show that there are low endogenous levels of IGF-I. As such, the exogenous administration of IG-1 during the first 2 weeks following injury may provide a therapeutic advantage by bolstering low endogenous tissue levels and thereby enhancing the metabolic response of individual tendon fibroblasts.

E. PLATELET-DERIVED GROWTH FACTOR

PDGF was discovered in serum as having a major mitogenic activity responsible for growth of cultured mesenchymal cells. It is a dimeric molecule that exists in two isoforms (A and B). When it is overproduced with some tumors, the protooncogene name is c-*sis*. PDGF is a potent regulator of bone cells and chondrocytes and plays a role in tendon healing.

F. VASCULAR ENDOTHELIAL GROWTH FACTOR

Vascular endothelial growth factor (VEGF), a potent angiogenic agent, is found in endothelial cells and responsible for the formation of new vasculature. It is involved with the angiogenesis of calcified cartilage and distraction angiogenesis. Although not significantly involved in the formation of normal bone, VEGF is involved with angiogenesis of malignancy. Clinical trials are being performed to evaluate the effectiveness of VEGF therapy into ischemic areas and the role of anti-VEGF therapy for treating malignancy. Studies show that administering autologous platelet-rich clots through the action of VEGF may be beneficial to the treatment of tendon injuries by inducing cell proliferation and promoting the synthesis of angiogenic factors during the healing process.

Applications

Extensive efforts are being made to find methods by which growth factors can be used to stimulate local bone healing and bone formation in a variety of clinical models. The growth factors TGF-β, BMP, IGF-1, and basic FGF are currently the only growth factors that are demonstrated to possess substantial capacity for in vivo bone stimulation. Growth factors are probably best able to exert a stimulatory effect when used in conditions associated with impaired healing. Research has begun to show increasing evidence that growth factors can be used in vivo to stimulate bone healing and bone formation. The growth factors BMP-2 and BMP-7, also known as **osteogenic protein-1 (OP-1),** are in the final stages of pivotal human trials. Issues of the best delivery system are currently being debated from the use of collagen gel/sponge carrier to ex vivo adenoviral-mediated delivery systems.

There are many challenges to the clinical application of growth factors. It is unlikely that cell-signaling molecules act independently of one another or are present in isolation from one another at their sites of action. Although therapeutic measures that employ single agents may be efficacious in some circumstances, it is likely that most clinical applications will require the development of combination or serial treatment regimens. In addition, because the specific actions of growth factors are context dependent, it is critical to distinguish appropriate from inappropriate indications. Considerable effort is directed at altering the method of treating anterior cruciate ligament (ACL) ruptures. Certain growth factors such as TGF-β 1, PDGF-AB, and FGF-2 can alter the biologic functions of human ACL cells in a collagen-glycosaminoglycan (CG) scaffold implanted as a bridge at the site of an ACL rupture. The addition of these selected growth factors to an implantable CG scaffold may actually facilitate ligament healing in the gap between the ruptured ends of the human ACL.

The therapeutic application of growth factors must also accommodate the fact that most factors have a widespread and variable distribution of target cells. A growth factor administered to elicit a desired response from one cell type may also influence other cell types, possibly in unintended or undesirable ways. Finally, in addition to demonstrating acceptable safety profiles and providing a physician-friendly delivery system in the current era of cost consciousness in health care, a growth factor treatment must demonstrate cost effectiveness along with clinical efficacy. Growth factors have many potential orthopedic applications. As challenges are met, it is plausible, if not probable, that growth factors will provide a means of treating patients with a variety of musculoskeletal disorders.

Anitua E et al: Autologous preparations rich in growth factors promote proliferation and induce VEGF and HGF production by human tendon cells in culture J Orthop Res 2005;23(2): 281. [PMID: 15779147]

Buxton B et al: Growth/differentiation factor-5 (GDF-5) and skeletal development. J Bone Joint Surg 2001;83A:S23. [PMID: 11263662]

Dahlgren LA et al: Temporal expression of growth factors and matrix molecules in healing tendon lesions. J Orthop Res 2005; 23(1):84. [PMID: 15607879]

Meaney Murray M et al: The effect of selected growth factors on human anterior cruciate ligament cell interactions with a three-dimensional collagen-GAG scaffold. J Orthop Res 2003;21:238. [PMID: 12568954]

Miura Y et al: Brief exposure to high-dose transforming growth factor-beta 1 enhances periosteal chondrogenesis in vitro: A preliminary report. J Bone Joint Surg Am 2002;84:793. [PMID: 12004023]

Musgrave DS et al: Gene therapy and tissue engineering in orthopaedic surgery. J Am Acad Orthop Surg 2002;10:6. [PMID: 11809046]

Yoon ST, Boden SD: Osteoinductive molecules in orthopaedics: Basic science and preclinical studies. Clin Orthop 2002;395: 33. [PMID: 11937864]

IMPLANT DESIGN & BIOLOGIC ATTACHMENT PROPERTIES

Total joint arthroplasty requires the type of implant materials and design that can support large functional loads. The implant must remain stable and rigid with respect to the bone while sustaining these loads. Adequate interface fixation requires interface micromotion of less than 100 μm or gap spaces less than a fraction of a millimeter. Precise and uniform contact between the device and surrounding bone depends on the skill of the surgeon and the design of the instrumentation with which the site is prepared. The surface area of actual contact is probably small relative to the surface area of the implant. The contact points tend to induce areas of stress concentration rather than distribute the stress evenly. Bone maintains its structural integrity by responding to stress. In areas of stress concentration, bone resorption often occurs. Additionally, fibrous encapsulations of varying thicknesses are commonly found, and these further alter the ability of the implant to distribute stress uniformly. Implant loosening and migration may eventually occur and cause discomfort to the patient, in which case the implant may need to be removed.

Implant Fixation Mechanisms

Several types of implant fixation methods and surface texture designs were investigated to obtain better surgical fit and stress distribution at the implant-bone interface. The methods include the use of a grouting agent, direct bone apposition to the implant surface, bone growth into porous-surfaced implants, and chemical bonding between bone and surface-active ceramic implant coatings.

A. GROUTING AGENTS

PMMA bone cement provides a mechanical interlock between the metal prosthesis and adjacent bone. Bone cement is not an adhesive; therefore, mechanical interlocking depends on the amount of interdigitation of the cement with trabecular bone and the quality of the fixation between the cement and the metal. The most favorable effect of cement fixation is immediate stability of the implant. Bone cement allows for load distribution over a larger area of bone, which reduces stress concentrations that may result in pressure necrosis and remodeling. Despite the early clinical advantages of cement fixation, the long-term results (15–25 years) are not as encouraging. The poor fatigue properties of cement lead to fractures of the cement. These fractures result in altered stress patterns in the bone, eventually leading to bone remodeling and implant loosening. Particulate debris that results from cement fracture is associated with osteolysis and aseptic loosening.

Improvements in the mechanical properties of cement and cementing techniques over the past two to three decades are leading to more promising results regarding the longevity of cemented prostheses. Femoral stems that were implanted with modern cement techniques maintain stability and function beyond 10 years in 95–98% of the cases.

B. DIRECT BONE APPOSITION

Optimal osseointegration at the bone-implant interface is affected by the material properties and design of the implant. Implant design encompasses both the surface texture and geometry of the implant. The mechanical properties of the implant-bone interface were investigated with various surface preparations, including smooth finishes, roughened or grit-blasted finishes, and grooved surfaces. Histologically, implants with smooth finishes have interfaces characterized by fibrous encapsulation, whereas implants with grit-blasted finishes have interfaces characterized by areas of direct bone apposition. Numerous studies demonstrated that surface texture is a significant factor in obtaining adequate implant fixation with direct bone apposition methods.

Evaluation of implant materials, including PMMA, commercially pure titanium, aluminum oxide, and low-temperature isotropic pyrolytic carbon with various surface finishes, demonstrated that the implant elastic modulus or surface composition did not significantly affect the interface attachment strength or histologic response. Surface texture significantly affected the interface mechanical properties, however. Implants with grit-blasted surfaces exhibited significantly higher interface attachment strengths than implants with polished surfaces did. Histologically, all implants with grit-blasted surfaces demonstrated areas of direct bone apposition, whereas all implants with polished surfaces demonstrated fibrous encapsulation (Figure 1–23), indicating that bone apposition required textured interface surface for attachment.

C. POROUS INGROWTH ATTACHMENT

The long-term problems associated with implant fixation with PMMA led to the development the porous coating as a method for permanent biologic fixation of prostheses. It is generally accepted that an implant can achieve stabilization by tissue growth into the surface porous structure if (1) the material is bioinert, (2) there is direct apposition of the bone at the implant interface,

Figure 1–23. Histologic appearance of mechanically tested grit-blasted titanium alloy implants 10 weeks after implantation. Areas of direct bone apposition (N) and minimal fibrous tissue (F) were observed at the implant interface. The undecalcified histologic section was photographed using simultaneous transmitted and reflected illumination (basic fuchsin and toluidine blue stain; original magnification × 160).

(3) there is minimal or no movement at the implant site, and (4) the porous structure has appropriate pore size and morphology.

Porous coatings are effective as a means of biologic fixation because their interface attachment strength of fixation is at least an order of magnitude higher than that of nonporous implants relying on direct bone apposition for fixation.

To maintain optimal bone growth into a porous structure, the pores must be large enough to accommodate the development of bone tissue. Several groups of investigators concluded that a pore size of 100 μm allowed bone ingrowth but that a pore size greater than 150 μm was necessary for osteon formation. Another group investigated the optimal pore size range for cobalt-based alloys by observing the rate of bone ingrowth and time necessary to attain maximal attachment strength. The results indicated that although a pore size range of 50–400 μm obtained the maximal attachment strength in the shortest time, osteon formation was not demonstrated histologically at this range. In addition to a minimal pore size, an effective porous coating must also have appropriate pore morphology. The available porous layer for bone growth must be large enough to accommodate a sufficient quantity of bone to maintain adequate fixation, and a volume fraction porosity of 35–40% is accepted as optimal for effective biologic fixation of an implant with a strongly bonded porous layer. The volume fraction porosity is related to the interconnection pore size, particle interconnectivity, and particle size of the porous coating. Particle interconnectivity is important for ensuring adequate strength within the coating and between the coating and substrate. Too much particle interconnectivity can decrease the interconnection pore size and restrict the amount and type of ingrown tissue, however. A two-layer porous surface creates an interconnected and open porosity that is effective in creating a three-dimensional mechanical interlock of the ingrown bone.

Several different types of porous coatings were evaluated, including the fiber mesh, beaded porous, and irregular plasma-sprayed types. The fiber mesh type of porous coating is composed of wires that are cut and kinked to form the specific shape of the coating. The wires are then bonded to a solid metal substrate of the same metallic alloy through a sintering process in an inert gas environment or vacuum. The porosity obtained with this technique ranges from 40% to 50% with a mean pore size of 270 μm. A void type of porous coating was obtained using a cobalt-based or titanium-based alloy. Magnesium microspheres are mixed with the base alloy by means of an investment casting technique. Under high temperatures, the magnesium evaporates, leaving pores on the surface of the alloy. This technique produces pores with different depths and connectivities. The most frequently studied porous coating is the beaded type. Cobalt-based alloy or titanium metal powder or macrobeads are either gravity compacted or applied with an organic binder onto a substrate. The beads are then sintered to the substrate at a submelting temperature for the base metal. The porosity ranges from 30% to 45% with pore diameters ranging from 100 to 400 μm. Production of another type of porous coating involves plasma-spraying titanium to either a titanium-based or cobalt-based alloy substrate. The plasma-spray technique is further discussed with regard to ceramic coatings (see following section).

The extent to which implants are covered with porous coating varies. On femoral stems, it ranges anywhere from complete coverage to coverage of the proximal third. The extent of porous coating to achieve optimal stability is not determined. Circumferential coverage is preferable, however, to prevent wear debris migration toward the distal portion of the prosthetic stem.

Clinically, the short-term results for porous-coated prostheses are comparable to those for cemented prostheses. Histologically, retrieved human prostheses demonstrated variable amounts of bone ingrowth, ranging from limited to extensive, with large amounts of fibrous tissue (Figure 1–24). Some retrieved prostheses exhibited complete fibrous tissue infiltration into the porous surface. Components with limited bone ingrowth showed fibrous tissue that was oriented in a fashion capable of load transmission. The bone ingrowth and extensive fibrous ingrowth are most likely effective mechanisms for early implant stabilization. A histologic analysis performed on six retrieved, noncemented, porous-coated femoral hip components demonstrated a significant increase in bone ingrowth from 19 to 53 months after implantation. The data showed that human bone remodels slowly and advances appositionally with limited endochondral ossification. Therefore, to achieve reproducible bone ingrowth, the porous coating must be adjacent to cortical bone.

D. SURFACE TOPOGRAPHY AND COATINGS

Calcium phosphate coatings on metal surfaces were developed to overcome the mechanical problems of the ceramic as well as the biologic shortcomings of the metal. Many composite implants are manufactured to have the mechanical properties of the metal and the biologic properties of the bioactive ceramics. However, evidence is mounting from animal studies suggesting that quantity of ingrowth is approximately 80% dependent on the microscopic surface morphology and only modestly (approximately 20%) dependent on the hydroxyapatite (HA) chemistry. The bone formation is apparently encouraged by a microscopically rough surface, which is routinely produced with a crystalline HA surface coating. Titanium ingrowth was enhanced by acid etching the surface of implants, which changes its microscopic topography. Biological coatings of HA (calcium phosphates) may still enhance the chemistry of the surface, and they are the standard method of inducing ingrowth.

The bond between a metal substrate and a HA coating is critical to the success of a coated prosthesis. The processes and techniques of coating a prosthesis vary, and for this reason not all HA coatings perform equivalently.

A coating thickness of 50 μm is generally accepted as adequate for coverage of nonporous surfaces; thinner coatings are necessary for porous coatings to keep from blocking the pores. Coating thickness >50 μm tend to separate from the substrate and can cause debris that compromises the bearing surfaces. A coating thickness of 25–45 μm does not occlude the pores or alter the mechanical bone ingrowth properties of the porous surface.

Chemical dissolution of an HA surface within the first few months of implantation occurs when coating thicknesses of 15 μm or less are used. Calcium phosphate coatings are applied to substrates by a variety of methods, including dip coating, vacuum deposition, and plasma spraying. In dip coating, the substrate can either be dipped into a suspension of ceramic powder in a carrier or be dipped into a liquid form of glass ceramic. In vacuum deposition, ceramic material is removed from a source and deposited onto the target substrate.

Plasma-spraying methods are used by most manufacturers to apply calcium phosphate coatings to metal surfaces, particularly for load-bearing applications. A plasma or ionized gas is created by passing a gas or mix-

A

B

C

Figure 1–24. Four years after implantation, an uncemented porous-coated femoral stem was removed for revision because the patient suffered persistent thigh pain and limp. **A:** The radiograph taken prior to stem removal showed a relatively poor fit, without subsidence but with the presence of nonanatomic remodeling, as evidenced by the so-called pedestal sign. **B:** Gross specimen (posterior aspect) analysis suggested that the component was well fixed, as demonstrated by large amounts of bone. **C:** Histologic examination demonstrated extensive bone ingrowth (basic fuchsin and toluidine blue stain; original magnification× 24).

ture of gases (usually argon or a mixture of nitrogen and hydrogen) through a high-energy, direct current (DC) electric arc struck between two electrodes. Then the coating powder suspended in a carrier gas is introduced into this plasma stream, melted, and propelled onto the substrate target, usually at high velocities. The coating is applied in several layers, each approximately 5–10 μm thick.

Because of the high temperatures necessary for plasma spraying, the ceramic coating material may be chemically or structurally altered from the original ceramic. For this reason, all HA coatings are not identical and may vary among manufacturers in their composition, crystallinity, density, purity, and structure. These differences may affect the surface topography, bioactivity, and bioresorbability of coatings and make it nearly impossible to predict their long-term in vivo behavior. To ensure the correct composition of HA coatings, manufacturers perform a variety of tests, including radiograph diffraction, infrared spectroscopy, scanning electron microscopy, and atomic absorption spectroscopy. Several studies showed that HA-coated implants are superior to uncoated implants in terms of interface attachment strength and bone apposition. In newer research, HA coating improved bone purchase and bone-screw interface strength in healthy and osteopenic animals. Also, the properties of HA-coated implants with larger surface areas (macrotextured or porous surfaces) are superior to the properties of HA-coated implants with smaller surface areas (smooth surfaces). IGF-1, basic fibroblast growth factor (bFGF) and TGF-β 1, alone and in combination, were tested to augment osseointegration and were absorbed onto a carrier of β-tricalcium phosphate (β-TCP). These composites were implanted into a defect around a hydroxyapatite-coated, stainless steel implant in the proximal tibia of rat in a model of revision arthroplasty. Although no growth factor combination significantly enhanced new bone formation or the mechanical strength of the implant, of the growth factors tested, only bFGF had any beneficial effect on the host response to the implant, perhaps by delaying osteoblast differentiation and thereby prolonging osteoclast access to the ceramic.

Clinical experience with HA-coated orthopedic prostheses is limited. Therefore, only short-term studies based on clinical follow-ups and radiographic evaluations exist. In a prospective bilateral total hip replacement study, a titanium prosthesis with and without HA coating was evaluated. At a mean of 6.6 years after implantation, there was no difference in clinical or radiographic results. Similar short-term results were reported for HA-coated, porous, cobalt-chromium primary and revision femoral hip stems. Other findings in early clinical studies of HA-coated porous implants included decreased pain, decreased radiolucent lines

around the implant (Figure 1-25), and improved bone remodeling.

Not all studies in patients with HA-coated implants have reported positive findings. In fact, some newer studies reported cell-mediated osteolysis, implant loosening, and other negative effects linked with the degradation or delamination of the HA coating, the generation and migration of HA particles, and the subsequent three-body wear of the implant that is caused by these particles. These findings suggest that changing the surface topology might be an effective way of achieving the same or nearly the same goal with less potential problems.

A

B

Figure 1–25. Histologic appearance of an HA-coated implant with a defect shown at two points in time: at 10 weeks after implantation (**A**) and at 32 weeks after implantation (**B**). Bone is observed in direct apposition to the HA coating and extending continuously from the edge of the HA material into the defect and along the metal substrate. The undecalcified histologic sections were photographed using simultaneous transmitted and reflected illumination (basic fuchsin and toluidine blue stain; original magnification × 160).

Factors That Affect Biologic Attachment

Attachment at the bone-implant interface is affected by the material properties and design of the implant, surgical technique, initial implant stability, and direct contact with the surrounding bone. Initial implant stability and apposition with bone are not always achievable but are vital for implant longevity. Persistent micromotion at the bone-implant interface causes bone resorption and necrosis, which can in turn result in fibrous tissue infiltration at the interface and in implant loosening. Moreover, any initial gap between the implant and surrounding bone may adversely alter the amount of osseointegration and the rate at which it occurs.

A. Motion at the Bone-Implant Interface

Motion of an implant within the surgical site has a primary influence on biologic fixation and implant longevity. Initial implant stability is essential for the early tissue infiltrate within the porous structure to differentiate into bone by either direct bone formation or appositional bone growth. When excessive early movement occurs at the bone-implant interface, bone formation within the pores is inhibited. The majority of research concerning motion at the interface involves porous implants; however, the findings are applicable for press-fit implant systems.

Studies of implants suggest that relative motion of greater than 150 μm at the bone-implant interface prevents bone formation, although a well-ordered fibrous tissue interface was maintained and provided adequate implant attachment. When interface motion was 40 μm, bone ingrowth occurred, but the calcified ingrown bone was not continuous with the surrounding bone. These findings support the concept that in optimal bone growth into porous surfaces or bone apposition onto press-fit surfaces requires little or no initial micromotion at the interface.

In a study of HA coating in a continuous loaded implant model, investigators found that when interface motion led to the formation of a fibrous membrane, the HA coating was able to convert the membrane to bone. Furthermore, pulsed electromagnetic fields accelerated HA osteointegration in trabecular bone.

B. Surgical Fit

The technical difficulties in cutting bone precisely to provide an exact fit around the implant often result in a poor surgical fit. Implant and instrumentation design may also make it difficult to achieve initial implant-bone interface apposition. When a femoral stem is press-fit into the femoral canal, only 10–20% of the prosthesis comes into direct contact with bone.

The effects of interface gaps and poor surgical fit of implants were investigated by numerous groups. In stud-

ies of HA-coated prostheses, researchers found that the HA coating does not compensate for improper implant placement or poor surgical technique. The cell populations necessary for bone formation are identical across large interface gaps and in press-fit situations. In large gaps, the rate of gap filling and subsequent ingrowth is delayed, and the quality of bone at the interface may also be reduced. Such studies indicate the potential benefits of robot-controlled surgery, where much better initial apposition can be obtained.

Aldini NN et al: Pedicular fixation in the osteoporotic spine: A pilot in vivo study on long-term ovariectomized sheep. J Orthop Res 2002;20:1217. [PMID: 12472232]

Bach CM et al: No functional impairment after Robodoc total hip arthroplasty: Gait analysis in 25 patients. Acta Orthop Scand 2002;73:386. [PMID: 12358109]

Bobyn JD et al: The optimum pore size for the fixation of porous-surfaced metal implants by the ingrowth of bone. Clin Orthop 1980;150:263. [PMID: 7428231]

Clarke SA et al: The effect of osteogenic growth factors on bone growth into a ceramic filled defect around an implant. J Orthop Res 2004;22:1016. [PMID: 15304274]

DeGroot K et al: Plasma sprayed coatings of hydroxylapatite. J Biomed Mater Res 1987;21:1375.

Fernandez-Pradas JM et al: Characterization of calcium phosphate coatings deposited by Nd-YAG laser ablation at 355 nm: Influence of thickness. Biomaterials 2002;23:1989. [PMID: 11996040]

Freels DB et al: Animal model for evaluation of soft tissue ingrowth into various types of porous coating. Clin Orthop 2002;397:315. [PMID: 11953623]

Geesink RG: Osteoconductive coatings for total joint arthroplasty. Clin Orthop 2002;395:53. [PMID: 11937866]

Hacking SA et al: Acid-etched microtexture for enhancement of bone growth into porous-coated implants. J Bone Joint Surg Br 2003;85:1182. [PMID: 14653605]

Hacking SA et al: Relative contributions of chemistry and topography to the osseointegration of hydroxyapatite coatings. Clin Orthop 2002;405:24. [PMID: 12461353]

Jinno T et al: Comparison of hydroxyapatite and hydroxyapatite tricalcium-phosphate coatings. J Arthroplasty 2002;17:902. [PMID: 12375251]

Karabatsos B et al: Osseointegration of hydroxyapatite porous-coated femoral implants in a canine model. Clin Orthop 2001;392:442. [PMID: 11716420]

Kim YH et al: Comparison of porous-coated titanium femoral stems with and without hydroxyapatite coating. J Bone Joint Surg Am 2003;85:1682. [PMID: 12954825]

LeGeros RZ: Properties of osteoconductive biomaterials: Calcium phosphates. Clin Orthop 2002;395:81. [PMID: 11937868]

Manso M et al: Biological evaluation of aerosol-gel-derived hydroxyapatite coatings with human mesenchymal stem cells. Biomaterials 2002;23:3985. [PMID: 12162331]

Nevelos JE et al: Wear of HIPed and non-HIPed alumina-alumina hip joints under standard and severe simulator testing conditions. Biomaterials 2001;22:2191. [PMID: 11456058]

Noble PC et al: The anatomic basis of femoral component design. Clin Orthop 1988;235:148. [PMID:3416522]

Paprosky WG, Burnett RS. Extensively porous-coated femoral stems in revision hip arthroplasty: Rationale and results. Am J Orthop 2002;31:471. [PMID: 12216970]

Pilliar RM et al: Observations on the effect of movement on bone ingrowth into porous-surfaced implants. Clin Orthop 1986; 208:108. [PMID: 3720113]

Soballe K et al: Hydroxyapatite coating converts fibrous tissue to bone around loaded implants. J Bone Joint Surg Br 1993; 75:270. [PMID: 8444949]

Thomas KA et al: The effect of surface macrotexture and hydroxy-lapatite coating on the mechanical strengths and histologic profiles of titanium implant materials. J Biomed Mater Res 1987;21:1395. [PMID: 3429474]

Thomsen MN et al: Robotically-milled bone cavities: A compari-son with hand-broaching in different types of cementless hip stems. Acta Orthop Scand 2002;73:379. [PMID: 12358108]

TISSUE RESPONSE TO IMPLANT MATERIALS

The effect of an implanted material on adjacent tissues depends on the amount and type of substance released into the tissues, the histologic response to the material, and the wear and corrosion properties of the material. The type of response to the implant determines the bio-logic classification of the material.

Biocompatibility

Biotolerant materials, such as stainless steel, PMMA, and UHMWPE, elicit the worst tissue response. When these materials are used, a fibrous tissue layer may form between the bone and the implant. This fibrous layer is generally observable as a radiolucent line on radio-graphs. Examination with light microscopy shows the presence of numerous macrophages near resorbing adja-cent bone and the resulting fibrous tissue that contains macrophages and foreign body giant cells.

PMMA elicits adverse local and systemic effects from the moment of its introduction into the body. At the time of implantation, PMMA causes local tissue necro-sis because of the extreme heat of polymerization. Dur-ing the polymerization process, monomer may leach into the surrounding tissues and cause hypotension. Finally, PMMA fragmentation particles elicit a chronic macrophage response at the implant-bone interface, which can result in progressive osteoclasis and eventual aseptic loosening of the implant. Macrophages are stim-ulated by cell necrosis, bacteria, and foreign particulate matter. Particulate matter is the primary cause of aseptic loosening in cemented joint arthroplasties. In spite of this, bulk PMMA is well tolerated by the body, whereas particulate PMMA is not.

Bioinert materials, such as titanium and cobalt-chromium alloys, usually cause minimal tissue irritation. With stable implants of either titanium or cobalt-chromium alloys, appositional bone growth or osseo-integration occurs. If titanium implants are used in articulating surface applications, however, they have poor wear resistance, and the excessive wear particles behave as biotolerant materials. These particles elicit a chronic macrophage response, which can lead to implant loosening. However, newer animal studies showed that coating titanium implants with autologous osteoblasts accelerates and enhances the osseointegra-tion of these implants and could be a successful bio-technology for future clinical applications.

Bioactive materials, such as calcium phosphate ceramics, offer the best biologic advantage of implant materials. The biocompatibility of the calcium phos-phate ceramics is well documented. In response to these implanted ceramics, the body typically responds (1) with-out local or systemic toxicity, (2) without inflammatory or foreign body reaction, (3) without alteration of natu-ral mineralization processes, (4) with functional integra-tion of bone, and (5) with chemical bonding to bone via natural bone cementing mechanisms. Implant sur-faces coated with HA are characterized as being capable of forming direct, intimate bonds with the surrounding bone. The bonding area (approximately 50–200 µm) contains biologic apatite crystals that are highly ori-ented at the interface with a 10-µm periodicity similar to that of calcified tissue, as determined by electron dif-fraction studies. The bone apatite crystals are arranged against the implant surface in a palisade fashion, resem-bling the natural bonding between two bone fragments. The bonding area contains a ground substance that is heavily mineralized, although devoid of collagen fibrils, and is likened to the natural bone cementing substance, which is amorphous in structure, heavily mineralized, and rich in mucopolysaccharides.

One study used animal models to characterize tissue-specific reactions to particles of bone-substitute mate-rials for osteocompatibility. Tested particles included demineralized bone powder (DBP), nonresorbable cal-cium phosphate (nrCP), PMMA, polyethylene (PE), and resorbable calcium phosphates (rCPs). Although both DBP and nrCP were incorporated into the reactive medullary and cortical bone, DBP also induced enchon-dral osteogenesis, and nrCP evoked a fibrous reaction. Although PMMA particles were surrounded with a fibrous layer, they did not impair bone healing. PE shards and rCPs were inflammatory and inhibited osse-ous repair. rCPs, PMMA, and PE shards all generated inflammatory reactions with each particle being sur-rounded by fibrous tissue and large multinucleated giant cells. DBP showed both osteoinductive as well as osteo-compatible properties. Although nrCP was shown to be osteocompatible, rCPs stimulated various degrees of inflammatory responses. PMMA was osteocompatible and did not interfere with the bone healing process. PE was not osteocompatible and generated foreign body reactions in both sites. It is important to distinguish among the osteoinductive, osteocompatible, and inflammatory properties of particles that may be used as bone-substitute materials.

Problems Associated with Maintaining Implant Longevity

Implant loosening, which can result from bone loss that is caused either by stress shielding or by osteolysis, has been a problem associated with total joint arthroplasty since its inception. Periprosthetic osteolysis presents radiographically as diffuse femoral cortical thinning or as a focal cystic lesion.

Although the exact cause of osteolysis is unknown, it is thought to be a result of movement of the implant, primarily at the bearing surface, with generation of wear particles that migrate to the implant-bone interface, where they cause a tissue reaction. Movement at taper joints, or between the implant and bone cement, can cause particulate material. Particulate debris in the 0.1–1.0 μm range are most active in stimulating bone resorption and eventually causing implant loosening. Macrophages play a key role in the osteoclastic process by elaborating cytokines in host defense and in forming precursors for osteoclasts. TNF-α is a key cytokine in the osteolysis process. The prevalence of osteolysis in stable cemented femoral components ranges from 3% to 8%. It appears, however, that osteolysis is observed earlier in patients with stable uncemented components and that the prevalence increases with time in vivo. The prevalence in uncemented systems ranges from 10% to 20% after 2–9 years in vivo. Newer studies suggest that hydrostatic pressure may play a far greater role in the induction of osteolysis than previously thought.

In addition to osteolysis, another problem with total joint implants is the increase in metal ions released into the body. This problem is especially associated with uncemented porous-coated implants. Systemic and long-term effects caused by wear and corrosion are just being discovered. An understanding of the wear and corrosion mechanisms associated with decreasing implant longevity is vital for the development of improved implant designs and material manufacturing methods.

A. SURFACE DAMAGE OF POLYETHYLENE IMPLANTS

Osteolysis, loosening, and other complications that reduce implant longevity are attributed to polyethylene wear particles. Careful examination of retrieved polyethylene components demonstrated a variety of modes by which surface damage occurs. These include scratching, burnishing, embedding of debris, pitting (the presence of shallow, irregular surface voids in the surface), surface deformation (permanent deformation on the articulating surface), abrasion (characterized by a tufted

or shredded appearance of the polyethylene), and delamination (separation of large, thin surface sheets of polyethylene from implant components).

Fatigue is suggested as the primary mechanism of polyethylene surface damage because the damage was correlated with the length of time since implantation (number of cycles in the fatigue curve shown in Figure 1–2) and with patient weight (applied load or stress in Figure 1–2). Surface damage is noticeably less in acetabular components than in tibial components. The increased polyethylene damage in total knee arthroplasties can be attributed to reduced surface conformity and to compression-tension loading patterns. Nonconformity of articulating components in total knee arthroplasties results in contact stresses that approximate or exceed the yield strength of the polyethylene. Cruciate-retaining designs vary the location of contact over the entire articulating surface, thereby subjecting the implant components to alternating compression-tension contact stresses throughout the loading cycle. This cyclic process could contribute to the beginning and spread of cracks, which may lead to pitting, delamination, and other fatigue failure modes.

The elastic modulus and thickness of the polyethylene are significant predictors of contact stresses large enough to cause surface damage. An increased elastic modulus, as is found with enhanced (Hylamer) polyethylene, raises contact stresses and can be expected to result in increased wear. This is important in component design because the elastic modulus of polyethylene near the surface may increase up to 100% over 10 years in vivo. A reduced level of polyethylene thickness, as is found in metal-backed acetabular and tibial components, can result in increased wear and creep, eventually leading to cracking and separation of the polyethylene from the metal. To avoid the high stresses that cause cracking, acetabular polyethylene thickness should be greater than 6 mm, and tibial polyethylene thickness should be greater than 8 mm. Another concern regarding metal-backed components is that loosening of the metal backing may cause the screws to break and migrate into the polyethylene insert, and this in turn can result in the generation of large amounts of metal and polyethylene wear debris.

The current practice is to try to minimize polyethylene wear debris through the use of highly cross-linked polyethylene for total hip applications, with some trials for total knee applications. The higher contact stresses on knee components is concerning from a materials viewpoint because the cross-linked material has a lower ductility and fatigue strength, although even in this application, early reports are encouraging. Other strategies to reduce particulate wear include alternative bearings, such as ceramic on ceramic, metal on metal, and ceramic on polyethylene, either as bulk ceramic (alumina) or as a surface treatment(oxidized zirconium).

B. FATIGUE OF POROUS-COATED IMPLANTS

The primary failure mode of load-bearing orthopedic implants is fatigue. The majority of hip and knee systems have sintered porous coatings to maximize biologic fixation or cement impregnation. The fatigue properties of these porous-coated implants are influenced not only by the sintering treatment but also by a notch effect from the coating.

Sintering affects the fatigue properties of coated implants by altering the microstructure of their metal substrate. With titanium-based alloys, sintering requires that the material be heat treated above the beta phase transition temperature, which reduces the fatigue properties of the material by approximately 40%. When postsintering heat treatments are performed, the fatigue strength of the previously sintered titanium-based alloy increases by 25%. With cobalt-based alloys, sintering does not necessarily result in a reduction of fatigue strength. A dissolution of carbides and an increase in porosity occur, however, when cobalt-based alloys with less than 0.3% carbon are exposed to sintering temperatures. Additionally, with improper cooling, the sintered cobalt-based alloys can develop continuous grain boundary precipitates.

Investigators performed studies to determine the effects of sintering, postsintering heat treatments, and HIP techniques on the fatigue properties of nonporous and porous-coated cobalt-based alloys. They reported that sintered materials exhibited severe porosity and continuous grain boundary precipitates, which resulted in reduced fatigue and tensile strength. HIP eliminated the porosity and grain boundary precipitation resulting from sintering, however. Moreover, HIP of the sintered materials increased the tensile and fatigue properties in implants with or without a porous coating.

Aside from manufacturing processes, which may alter the fatigue properties of the substrate, porous coatings demonstrate a notch effect at the contact regions. These regions are susceptible to the initiation of cracks, which may continue to propagate along surface grain boundaries. This effect is most significant for the titanium-based alloys.

The fatigue properties that are caused by sintering and the notch effect of coating in load-bearing implants can be reduced by the following measures: (1) avoiding the use of porous coating in regions of maximal tensile stress, (2) using an additional heat treatment process on previously sintered titanium-based alloys, and (3) using HIP on previously sintered cobalt-based alloys.

The fatigue properties have to be considered in relation to newer animal studies that evaluated the roles of sex and estrogen therapy on the amount of bone ingrowth into porous cobalt-chromium implants. Histological examination showed significantly more bone ingrowth in areas with cortical bone contact than in areas with cancellous bone contact, with no difference between male and female animals. However, ovariectomized animals showed less overall bone ingrowth than male and female controls, and bone ingrowth in areas with cortical bone contact did not decrease significantly, whereas bone ingrowth in areas with cancellous bone contact was significantly impaired. In another study evaluating osseointegration, osteoblasts from patients older than 60 years were less able to form bone on Ti-6Al-4V implants. Taken together, these data suggest that extensively coated or full-coated porous prostheses are recommended to achieve enough cortical bone contact and ingrowth for postmenopausal patients.

C. METAL IMPLANTS: ION RELEASE, METAL-ON-METAL BEARINGS, AND IMMUNOLOGY

Any metal exposed to the physiologic environment will corrode. Corrosion is most evident in fracture fixation devices. Retrieval studies of stainless steel components revealed evidence of pitting and crevice corrosion in approximately 75% of the components.

Apart from potential implant mechanical failure, the clinical significance of corrosion is determined by the type and quantity of metal ion that is released and by the local and systemic effects of ion release. The widespread use of porous coatings on metallic implants and the popularity of metal-on-metal bearing surfaces has raised additional concerns regarding metal ion release. Porous coatings increase the amount of surface area that is exposed to body fluids by a factor of 1.2 to 7.2. Depending on the type and morphology of the porous coating, the increased surface area could increase the corrosion and ion release rates by a factor of 1.2 to 5.2. Unlike the metallic surface of cemented implants, the metallic surface of porous implants is in direct contact with the endosteal bone surface and vasculature, creating an environment in which a cellular response to metallic ions is possible. Another significant source of metal ions in the systemic circulation is the loose prosthesis. Local synovial fluid levels were increased in most prostheses at revision, but examination of blood showed that metal ion concentrations were elevated only in cases involving loose components. The metal-on-metal (MOM) bearing does not directly increase the corrosion area but does produce metal particulate debris that has a very large surface area to volume ratio. This debris then is available to dissolve and put ions into the systemic circulation. Significantly increased levels of implant elements are documented in serum and urine after implantation of these devices. Reference values for two of these elements in blood are cobalt, <0.15 µg/L, and chromium, <0.26 µg/L. Blood cobalt levels are reported to be 5–20 times higher and chromium levels 5–10 times higher than reference levels for MOM bearing total hips.

Released metal ions (Al, Co, Cr, Fe, Mn, Ni, Ti, and V ions) have one of four types of possible effects on the body: metabolic, bacteriologic, immunogenic, or oncogenic. With the possible exception of titanium, the metallic elements used to fabricate implants are either essential or toxic to processes of metabolism. Although it is known that excessive concentrations of essential elements can produce toxic effects, the ultimate fate of the released ions locally, systemically, or in remote organ systems remains to be determined. There is a reported increase in chromosome translocations and aneuploidy in peripheral lymphocytes after MOM hip arthroplasties, but the risk of cancer does not seem to be increased in the few underpowered studies available.

Metal sensitivity induced by metal ion release is not a common problem causing prosthesis loosening. The prevalence of dermal sensitivity in patients with joint replacements is greater than in the general population, and dermal patch testing is not accepted for identifying patients at risk for hypersensitivity to the implant materials. Nickel, chromium, and cobalt (present in cobalt-chromium [Co-Cr] alloy) are the ions most frequently responsible for metal sensitivity reactions. When investigators studied porous-coated hip and knee devices retrieved from patients, they reported the finding of a cellular response in interfacial and interstitial tissues. Although none of the components were removed because of infection and none had shown clinical or radiographic evidence of loosening, the investigators identified an inflammatory infiltrate with accompanying vascular proliferation in 22% of the components. The predominant cell types within the porous coatings were lymphocytes and histiocytes, although giant cells were also present. Several groups reported that delayed hypersensitivity can produce an immunologic reaction in which T cells recognize a metal ion-protein complex, release a variety of lymphokines, and stimulate a mononuclear infiltration. Further research is necessary, however, to determine if an allergic or hypersensitivity response to metal ions is responsible for inflammatory infiltrates. Various tests were proposed to determine if a particular patient is likely to have a sensitivity reaction. However, sensitivity is rare, so routine testing would be expensive and unrewarding, and in the case of a positive history, the surgeon would still be likely to use a component that does not contain the potentially offending elements, such as titanium alloy or zirconium alloy, with ceramic as a femoral head.

MOM bearing surfaces, on the one hand, have the potential to reduce the wear debris problem, but, on the other hand, they are certain to raise levels of circulating ions and raise issues of long-term safety from an organ viewpoint. Hypersensitivity issues may also be increased.

Anissian L et al: Cobalt ions influence proliferation and function of human osteoblast-like cells. Acta Orthop Scand 2002;73:369. [PMID: 12143988]

Berzins A et al: Surface damage in machined ram-extruded and net-shape molded retrieved polyethylene tibial inserts of total knee replacements. J Bone Joint Surg Am 2002;84:1534. [PMID: 12208909]

Brown SR et al: Long-term survival of McKee-Farrar total hip prostheses. Clin Orthop 2002;402:157. [PMID: 12218479]

Cook SD et al: Inflammatory response in retrieved noncemented porous coated implants. Clin Orthop 1991;264:209. [PMID: 1997238]

Cook SD et al: The effect of post-sintering heat treatments on the fatigue properties of porous coated Ti-6Al-4V alloy. J Biomed Mater Res 1988;22:287. [PMID: 3372550]

Dorr LD et al: Histologic, biochemical, and ion analysis of tissue and fluids during total hip arthroplasty. Clin Orthop 1990;261:82. [PMID: 2173987]

Edwards SA et al: Analysis of polyethylene thickness of tibial components in total knee replacement. J Bone Joint Surg Am 2002;84:369. [PMID: 11886905]

Eid K et al: Tissue reactions to particles of bone-substitute materials in intraosseous and heterotopic sites in rats: Discrimination of osteoinduction, osteocompatibility, and inflammation. J Orthop Res 2001;19:962-9. [PMID: 11562148]

Friberg L et al: Handbook on the Toxicology of Metals. Elsevier, 1986.

Frosch KH et al: Autologous osteoblasts enhance osseointegration of porous titanium implants. J Orthop Res 2003;21:213. [PMID: 12568951]

Georgette FS, Davidson JA: The effect of hot isostatic pressing on the fatigue and tensile strength of a cast, porous coated Co-Cr-Mo alloy. J Biomed Mater Res 1986;20:1229. [PMID: 3782180]

Goldberg JR et al: A multicenter retrieval study of the taper interfaces of modular hip prostheses. Clin Orthop 2002;401:149. [PMID: 12151892]

Hallab NJ, Mikecz K, Jacobs JJ: A triple assay technique for the evaluation of metal-induced, delayed-type hypersensitivity responses in patients with or receiving total joint arthroplasty. J Biomed Mater Res 2000;53:480. [PMID: 10984695]

Hallab NJ et al: Immune responses correlate with serum-metal in metal-on-metal hip arthroplasty. J Arthroplasty 2004;19 (Suppl):88. [PMID: 15578560]

Hallab NJ et al: Metal sensitivity in patients with orthopaedic implants. J Bone Joint Surg Am 2001;83:428. [PMID: 11263649]

Huang CH et al: Particle size and morphology of UHMWPE wear debris in failed total knee arthroplasties—A comparison between mobile bearing and fixed bearing knees. J Orthop Res 2002;20:1038. [PMID: 12382971]

Ingrahm F, Fisher J: The role of macrophages in osteolysis of total joint replacement. Biomaterials 2005;26:1271. [PMID: 15475057]

Ladon D et al: Changes in metal levels and chromosome aberrations in the peripheral blood of patients after metal-on-metal hip arthroplasty. J Arthroplasty 2004;19(Suppl):78. [PMID: 15578558]

MacDonald SJ: Can a safe level for metal ions in patients with metal-on-metal total hip arthroplasties be determined? J Arthroplasty 2004;19(Suppl):71. [PMID: 15578557]

Merritt K, Rodrigo JJ: Immune response to synthetic materials. Sensitization of patients receiving orthopaedic implants. Clin Orthop 1996;326:71. [PMID: 8620661]

Muratoglu OK et al: Optical analysis of surface changes on early retrievals of highly cross-linked and conventional polyethylene tibial inserts. J Arthroplasty 2003;18(Suppl 1):42. [PMID: 14560410]

Murray DW, Rushton N: Macrophages stimulate bone resorption when they phagocytose particles. J Bone Joint Surg Br 1990; 72:988.

Rao AR et al: Tibial interface wear in retrieved total knee components and correlations with modular insert motion. J Bone Joint Surg Am 2002;84:1849. [PMID: 12377918]

Santavirta S et al: Alternative materials to improve total hip replacement tribology. Acta Orthop Scand 2003;74:380. [PMID: 14521286]

Shih LY et al: The effects of sex and estrogen therapy on bone ingrowth into porous coated implant. J Orthop Res 2003;21:1033. [PMID: 14554216]

Shrivastava R et al: Effects of chromium on the immune system. FEMS Immunol Med Microbiol 2002;34:1. [PMID: 12208600]

Skoglund B et al: PMMA particles and pressure—A study of the osteolytic properties of two agents proposed to cause prosthetic loosening. J Orthop Res 21(2):196. [PMID: 12568949]

Wright TM, Bartel DL: The problem of surface damage in polyethylene total knee components. Clin Orthop 1986;205;67. [PMID: 3698394]

Wroblewski BM, Siney PD, Fleming PA: Wear of enhanced ultrahigh molecular-weight polyethylene (Hylamer) in combination with a 22.225 mm diameter zirconia femoral head. J Bone Joint Surg Br 2003;85:376. [PMID: 12729113]

Zhang H et al: The effects of patient age on human osteoblasts' response to Ti-6Al-4V implants in vitro. J Orthop Res 2004; 22:30. [PMID: 14656656]

■ GAIT ANALYSIS

Harry B. Skinner, MD, PhD

The science of studying human walking is called gait analysis. This science evolved as a means of quantitating the individual components of gait. As measurement techniques were refined to permit the determination of forces, moments, and movements of the human body, these techniques were applied to functions other than walking. Thus, it has been possible to measure the functional demands of wheelchair motion and running, as well as activities as diverse as pitching a baseball. The study of gait analysis was assisted by the development of devices that are able to measure gait in terms of (1) movement in space, (2) metabolic energy consumed during movement, (3) functional patterns of muscles during movement, and (4) forces applied to the ground during movement. Direct measurements of these factors permit the secon-

dary determination of quantities concerning mechanical work, joint moments, and center of pressure, which in turn are helpful in quantifying the function of prostheses and the effects of ataxia. The techniques of gait analysis are applied to other facets of human function. Motion analysis, for example, is applied to elucidate the kinesthetic changes in the spine occurring with fatigue in a study of repetitive lifting.

GAIT CYCLES, PHASES, & EVENTS

For uniformity in the reporting of gait measurements, investigators adopted several definitions concerning gait cycle. One **gait cycle** is defined as the time from initial ground contact of one foot to subsequent ground contact of the same foot. This is then normalized to 100%, with the intervening phases, periods, and events (Figure 1–26) defined on this basis. Ground contact is chosen as the beginning of the cycle because it is easily defined. The duration of the gait cycle varies, depending on the height, weight, and age of the individual whose gait is being analyzed as well as on any pathologic process affecting the individual's movement. Normalization of the gait cycle into percentages facilitates comparison among individuals.

Two **gait phases** are recognized: the stance phase and the swing phase. The normal **stance phase,** when the extremity is on the ground, accounts for approximately 62% of the cycle, and the normal **swing phase** of that extremity accounts for the remainder. The proportions vary with speed. Each phase is divided into periods. The stance phase starts with double-limb support, is followed by single-limb support, and ends with a second period of double-limb support. Each period of double-limb support accounts for an estimated 10% of the gait cycle. The swing phase is divided into early, mid, and late periods, with each period accounting for approximately 13% of the gait cycle. Swing phase for one limb corresponds to stance phase for the opposite limb.

The swing and stance phases are also divided into **gait events** (see Figure 1–26). Terms such as **heel strike** and **toe-off,** which are used to describe the events in the gait cycle, were initially derived from the observation of normal gait. The nomenclature of gait analysis, however, is evolving to take into account the fact that these terms are inadequate in describing the gait of individuals who have joint contractures, joint instability, pain, spasticity, or other conditions that alter the gait so the heel may never strike the floor or the heel and toe may strike simultaneously or depart simultaneously. In gait analysis, the various events are recognized by observation and can be correlated with measurements of the ground reaction force and motion variables. Observation is greatly enhanced through the use of slow-motion photography or video equipment.

Figure 1–26. The typical normal gait cycle, with the phases, periods, and events of gait shown. (From DH Sutherland.)

Phases ———————— Stance phase ———————— | ———————— Swing phase ————————

Periods — Initial double support — | — Single limb stance — | — Second double support — | — Swing —

Events Foot strike | Opposite toe off | [Reversal of fore-aft shear] | Opposite foot strike | Toe off | | Foot strike

Periods |— Mid-stance —|— Terminal stance —|— Pre-swing —|— Initial-swing —|— Mid-swing —|— Terminal swing —|

53

GAIT MEASUREMENTS

The quantities measured in a complete analysis of gait include three-dimensional translation, velocity, acceleration for all motion segments, forces exerted on the ground, electromyographic response of muscles during the gait cycle, and metabolic energy consumption. Obviously, a complete gait analysis is an expensive and time-consuming procedure and perhaps is not even possible within the endurance limits of some patients studied. A typical gait analysis is problem oriented and focuses on information relevant to the disorder being addressed by the clinician.

Movement during Gait

A. STRIDE CHARACTERISTICS

The fundamental data needed for almost any gait analysis are basic measurements termed *stride characteristics*. These are necessary because they form a baseline for interpreting all of the other aspects of gait. The stride characteristic variables are velocity (speed), gait cycle, cadence, stride length, step length, single- and double-limb support time, and swing and stance time.

Velocity of gait is the measure of forward progression of an individual's center of gravity, which is generally located midline and anterior to the sacrum. Velocity is expressed as an average number of meters per minute, although it is obvious that the instantaneous velocity can vary somewhat.

Gait cycle is measured as the number of seconds from the initial ground contact of one foot until the subsequent ground contact of the same foot. **Cadence** is the number of steps per minute (the number of times both feet strike the ground per minute) and is different from the number of strides per minute (the number of times the same foot strikes the ground per minute).

Step length is measured as the distance (number of meters) covered from the time one foot strikes the ground until the opposite foot strikes. It differs from stride length, which is the distance (number of meters) covered from the time one foot strikes the ground to the next time the same foot strikes the ground. In normal individuals, the length of each step is half of the stride length. But in people with pathologic processes that affect gait, the lengths of the two steps are different.

Single-limb and double-limb support times are periods of the gait cycle that can be measured in terms of seconds or in terms of percentage of the gait cycle (Table 1–4 and Figure 1–26). These periods in patients with a painful condition such as an ankle sprain generally differ from periods in normal individuals. Less obvious is the fact that the two double-limb support times (one following left foot strike and the other following right foot strike), which are usually of the same length in normal individuals, may be of two different

Table 1–4. Gait characteristics of normal men and women at free walking speed.

Component (Unit of Measure)	Men (Mean ± 1SD)	Women (Mean ± 1SD)
Velocity (m/min)	91 ± 12	74 ± 9
Gait cycle (s)	1.06 ± 0.09	1.03 ± 0.08
Cadence (steps/min)	113 ± 9	117 ± 9
Step length (cm)[a]	78 ± 6	62 ± 5
Stride length (cm)	160	137
Single-limb support[a]		
Time (s)	0.44	0.39
As proportion of gait cycle (%)	40	38
Swing (s)[a]	0.41 ± 0.04	0.39 ± 0.03
Stance (s)[a]	0.65 ± 0.07	0.64 ± 0.06
Lateral motion of the head (cm)	5.9 ± 1.7	4.0 ± 1.1
Vertical motion of the head (cm)		
During right stance	4.8 ± 1.1	4.1 ± 0.9
During left stance	4.9 ± 1.1	4.1 ± 0.9
Hip flexion-extension used (degree)	48 ± 5	40 ± 4
Anteroposterior pelvic tilting (degree)	7.1 ± 2.4	5.5 ± 1.3
Transverse pelvic rotation (degree)	12 ± 4	10 ± 3

[a]Right equals left in normal individuals.

Data adapted, with permission, from Murray MP, Gore DR: Gait patients with hip pain or loss of hip joint motion. In: Black J, Dumbleton JH, eds: *Clinical Biomechanics: A Case History Approach*, Churchill Livingstone, 1981; and from Rancho Los Amigos Hospital data on normal values.

lengths in patients with pathologic processes that affect gait. **Swing and stance times** can also be measured in terms of seconds or in terms of percentage of gait cycle.

Gait characteristics of normal men and women at free walking speed are shown in Table 1–4, and a sampling of these data for normal children at selected ages is presented in Table 1–5. Gait measurements are generally made at the **free walking speed** for each person because that speed is selected by the person to minimize energy consumption and is therefore considered the optimal gait velocity. Velocities that are slower or faster can be continuously maintained by individuals as long as the metabolic energy consumption remains in the aerobic range. These velocities are more costly in terms of energy expenditure, however.

Stride characteristics are sensitive indicators of diseases and disorders that affect gait. Many variables have a bearing on the stride measurements. Age, height, weight, and shoe wear are physiologic variables that help define the

Table 1–5. Gait characteristics of normal children at free walking speeds for selected ages.

Component (Unit of Measure)	1 Year	2 Years	3 Years	4 Years	5 Years
Velocity (m/min)	38.2	43.1	51.3	64.8	68.6
Gait cycle (s)	0.68	0.78	0.77	0.77	0.83
Cadence (steps/min)	175.7	155.8	153.5	153.4	143.5
Step length (cm)[a]	21.6	27.5	32.9	42.3	47.9
Stride length (cm)	43.0	54.9	66.8	84.3	96.5
Single-limb support as proportion of gait cycle (%)[a]	32.1	33.5	34.8	36.5	37.6

[a]Right equals left in normal individuals.

Data adapted, with permission, from Sutherland DH et al: The development of mature gait. J Bone Joint Surg Am 1980;62:336; and from Sutherland DH et al: The development of mature walking. Clin Dev Med 1988;104:1.

basic parameters of velocity, cadence, and gait cycle. Abnormalities resulting from an anatomic change, such as joint replacement, degenerative disease of the lower extremities, or knee fusion, can be demonstrated as non-specific and asymmetric variations in the stride characteristics. External variables such as those affecting the walking surface (eg, sand, concrete, and ice) can markedly alter stride measurements and must be considered in comparing data from different treatment groups or locations. Data are also sensitive to measurement technique. "Free" walking behavior in a laboratory may be different from that which takes place unobserved on a street and is definitely different from walking on a treadmill. Thus, to eliminate extraneous variables, care must be exercised not only in measuring stride characteristics but also in interpreting them.

B. Motion Analysis

Motion analysis is necessary for the complete characterization of gait. Aside from simply recording motions, quantification of the dynamic range of motion of a joint or body segment is called *kinematics*. Rather than measuring all limb segments, investigators generally focus on motion in certain limb segments and the trunk. Although major displacements of the lower extremities and upper extremities are occurring during gait, the center of mass of the body is only moving approximately 2–4 cm in a mediolateral direction and 2 cm in a superoinferior direction. Simultaneously, pelvic and trunk motion is occurring around the center of mass in a sinusoidal fashion. To conserve angular momentum, the upper extremity moves forward with the contralateral lower extremity.

Motion analysis has benefits and limitations. On the one hand, it provides more information to the clinician than does simple analysis of stride characteristics. For example, although stride analysis may show that the single-limb support time is reduced, motion analysis can clarify whether this is caused by decreased hip or knee motion, weakness of knee or ankle musculature, or some other condition, and it can also permit documentation of

the benefit of intervention. On the other hand, motion analysis equipment is expensive, although this is improving, as is the need for human input to the data analysis. It also presents difficulties in defining motion segments accurately and sometimes in measuring relatively small movements. There are problems, for example, in placing the markers to determine mediolateral pelvic rotation or anteroposterior pelvic rotation and in measuring these movements, whereas measuring knee flexion and extension is much easier. Highly sophisticated motion analysis systems were developed to maximize the accuracy and efficiency of these measurements, with a significant improvement. One study was able to discern abnormal tibial motion during gait in ACL-deficient knees.

Motion analysis has taken on new functions with the interest in upper extremity motion, especially in sports. Training problems and injuries in baseball pitching, golf, and racquet sports, among others, can be defined in terms of motions (rotations, displacements, and angular velocities) of the upper extremity joints. For example, world-class tennis players achieve ball velocities of 40–50 meters per second (m/s), with elbow extension and shoulder internal rotation angular velocity peaks of 1510 degrees per second (deg/s) and 2400 deg/s, respectively. Motion analysis can lead to methods of prevention and treatment, as well as improvement in technique.

Energy Consumption during Gait

Energy expenditure results from muscle function and is possible as a direct result of the body's use of food. Steady-state aerobic metabolism is the optimal means of using oxygen to metabolize food, although less efficient anaerobic mechanisms are available. Measurements of oxygen consumption per unit of time can be converted to measurements of energy expenditure or power. An oxygen consumption measurement of 1 L/min is approximately equivalent to an energy consumption measurement of 5 kcal/min.

Figure 1–27. Rate of oxygen uptake as a function of velocity.

Energy expenditure per unit of body mass can be expressed per step, per unit of distance, or per unit of time. Most commonly, energy expenditure is measured in terms of **rate of oxygen uptake,** expressed as milliliters of oxygen per kilogram per minute (mL O_2/kg/min), and **net oxygen cost,** expressed as milliliters of oxygen per kilogram per meter (mL O_2/kg/m). Both the rate of oxygen uptake and the net oxygen cost depend on the velocity (v) of walking, expressed in terms of m/min. The approximate relations are as follows:

$$\text{Rate of oxygen uptake} = 0.001\,v^2 + 6.0$$

$$\text{Net oxygen cost} = \frac{6.0}{v} + 0.0011\,v$$

The rate of oxygen uptake for normal adults is 11.9 ± 2.3 mL O_2/kg/min, and the net oxygen cost is 0.15 mL O_2/kg/m.

The rate of oxygen uptake increases with the square of the velocity (Figure 1–27). Body mass is obviously important in determining energetics, but location of the mass is even more important. An increase in weight around the center of mass (ie, the waist) is not nearly as energy costly as an increase around the ankles. This is because the center of mass moves at a near constant velocity with relatively small motions. Conversely, the ankles must be accelerated and decelerated constantly during gait, with each acceleration and deceleration requiring energy. When net oxygen cost for normal individuals is expressed as a function of velocity, there is a minimum in the energy consumption curve at approximately 80 m/min (1.3 m/s) at approximately 0.16 mL O_2/kg/m (approximately 1.1 J/kg/m), indicating that this is the most efficient velocity of ambulation (Figure 1–28). Similarly, the most efficient running speed is

between 3 and 4 m/s at an energy consumption rate of approximately 3.1 J/kg/m.

Energy expenditure in gait assumes importance when gait efficiency decreases or when the most efficient attainable gait velocity is markedly below normal. Attempts to increase velocity can increase energy costs to the point that sustained ambulation cannot be maintained. This can be seen, for example, in the case of traumatic transfemoral amputation. Although the amputee may ambulate with a net oxygen cost of approximately 0.28 mL O_2/kg/m, which is nearly 100% above normal (0.15 ± 0.02 mL O_2/kg/m), attempts to increase the speed could push the amputee into the anaerobic consumption range and thereby limit the ambulation distance. A similar problem can be seen in the case of a paraplegic who has adequate muscle function to ambulate before gaining weight but finds that the net oxygen cost of increased weight makes wheelchair mobility more energy efficient.

Muscle Function during Gait

Measurement of the function of muscles during gait is helpful in understanding and treating problems associated with cerebral palsy, stroke, poliomyelitis, and other diseases that alter the normal pattern of muscle function. The activity of muscles during gait is determined by **dynamic electromyography** through the use of either surface electrodes or fine-wire electrodes inserted into muscles. Electrical activity generated from these muscles is monitored and recorded in an on-off fashion as a function of the gait cycle. Activity does not necessarily indicate agonistic (contracting) or antagonistic (lengthening) function, but this determination can be made with simultaneous motion analysis. At present, it is not possible to quantify the relationship between electromyographic activity and force.

Normal functioning of the muscles can be presented as a function of the gait cycle and is shown in Figure 1–29.

Figure 1–28. Net oxygen cost as a function of velocity.

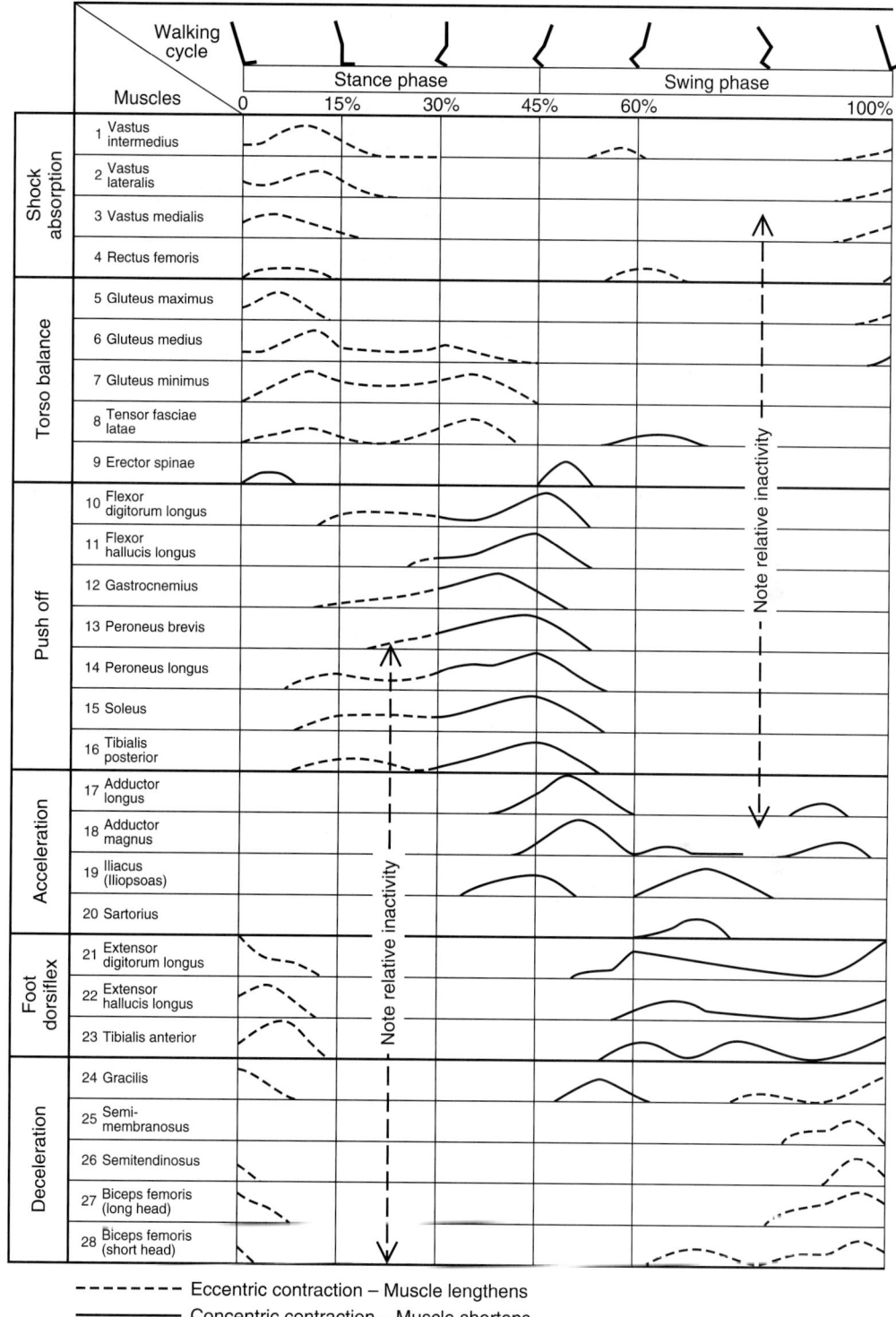

Figure 1–29. Tabulation of the on-off activity of the major muscles in the lower extremity during gait. Dashed lines show eccentric contraction (muscle lengthens); solid lines show concentric contraction (muscle shortens). (Reproduced, with permission, from Charles O Bechtel, Los Angeles, CA. American Academy of Orthopaedic Surgeons: *Atlas of Orthotics: Biomechanical Principles and Application.* Mosby, 1975.)

Most muscle activity is generated at the beginning and end of the stance and swing phases of gait because it is necessary at these times to accelerate and decelerate the extremities.

Dynamic electromyography is particularly useful in disorders associated with spasticity, such as cerebral palsy and cerebral vascular accident. In these disorders, the results of functional muscle testing of the patient in the supine position can be markedly different from the results of testing in the upright ambulating position. For example, the tibialis anterior may function normally when the patient is supine, but dynamic electromyography may reveal a varus-deforming force of the hindfoot during ambulation.

Forces during Gait: Kinetics

Forces acting during ambulation arise from gravity, inertia, and ground reaction. At ambulation speeds, viscous drag can be ignored. The **gravitational force** (mass × gravity) must be considered because it causes moments around centers of rotation for limb segments and body segments. The **inertial force** is proportional to the acceleration of the body segment and acts in the opposite direction because it resists acceleration. The **ground reaction force** is a measurement of the load applied to a device such as a force platform and has three components: vertical ground reaction force, fore-aft shear, and mediolateral shear.

Typical curves for the three components of the ground reaction force are shown in Figure 1–30. The dip in the vertical force curve (Figure 1–30A) during the single-limb stance phase of gait occurs because the inertial forces reduce the ground reaction force below body weight. The fore-aft shear (Figure 1–30B) is negative after the heel strike because the foot is pushing the plate anterior. On toe-off, the converse is occurring so the shear force is in the opposite direction. Again, correlation of ground reaction forces to stride characteristics can be beneficial in interpreting gait data. Force platform data show variations with walking speed, shoe wear, and compensatory mechanisms of gait, such as the avoidance of weight bearing on a painful extremity. The components of the ground reaction force in gait can be an indication of dynamic aspects of gait. The vertical ground reaction force tends to increase in magnitude and higher frequency content with increasing velocity and flatten with lower velocity and/or lower extremity pain. Examination of the frequency content especially in the medial-lateral shear component is an indicator of balance control, as in scoliosis. Static measurements provide center of pressure variations, also as a measure of balance control.

More sophisticated force measurement devices were developed to permit measurement of pressure (force per

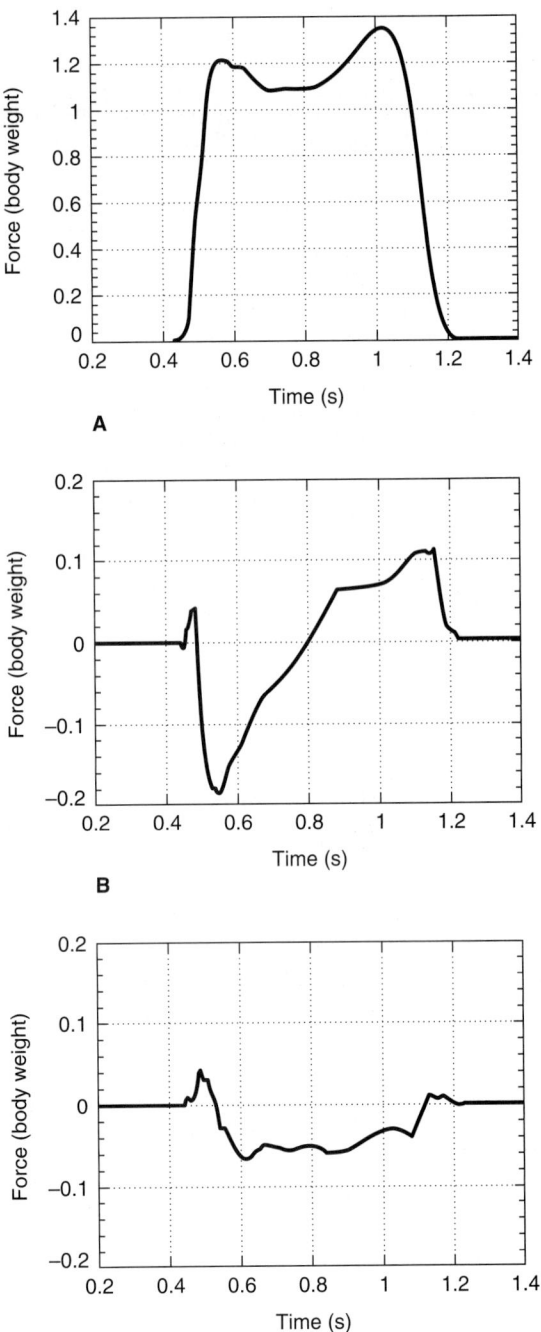

A

B

C

Figure 1–30. The typical ground reaction force for the left foot, shown with its three components. **A:** Vertical force. **B:** Fore-aft shear, which in this plot is negative for heel strike and positive for toe-off. **C:** Mediolateral shear, which in this plot is negative in the lateral direction. (Courtesy of S. Rossi.)

unit area). These devices can yield both in-shoe pressures and pressures applied to the external surface of the shoe by a force platform. Thus discrimination of measures at the 1-cm^2 level is possible, allowing studies of feet of diabetic patients to discern differences shoe wear can have on the risk of skin breakdown.

Andriacchi TP, Alexander EJ: Studies of human locomotion: past, present, future. J Biomech 2000;33:1217. [PMID: 10899330]

Anglin C, Wyss UP: Review of arm motion analysis. Proc Inst Mech Eng (H) 2000;214:541. [PMID: 11109862]

Burdett RG et al: Comparison of mechanical work and metabolic energy consumption during normal gait. J Orthop Res 1983; 1:63. [PMID: 6679577]

Chambers HG, Sutherland DH: A practical guide to gait analysis. J Am Acad Orthop Surg 2002;10:222. [PMID: 12041944]

Fleisig G et al: Kinematics used by world class tennis players to produce high-velocity serves. Sports Biomech 2003;2:51. [PMID: 14658245]

Marshall RN, Elliott BC: Long-axis rotation: The missing link in proximal-to-distal segmental sequencing. J Sports Sci 2000; 18:247. [PMID: 10824641]

Park SS et al: The shoulder in baseball pitching: Biomechanics and related injuries-part 1. Bull Hosp Jt Dis 2002-3;61:68. [PMID:12828383]

Park SS et al: The shoulder in baseball pitching: Biomechanics and related injuries-part 2. Bull Hosp Jt Dis 2002-3;61:80. [PMID: 12828384]

Perry J et al: Functional evaluation of the pes anserinus transfer by electromyography and gait analysis. J Bone Joint Surg Am 1980;62:973. [PMID: 7430186]

Saibene F, Minetti AE: Biomechanical and physiological aspects of legged gait in humans. Eur J Appl Physiol 2003;88:297. [PMID: 12527959]

Sutherland DH et al: The development of mature gait. J Bone Joint Surg Am 1980;62:336. [PMID: 7364807]

ROLE OF GAIT ANALYSIS IN THE MANAGEMENT OF GAIT DISORDERS

Gait analysis was traditionally been a research tool and continues to find its primary use in the research arena. However, the impetus to document the benefit of medical intervention has resulted in a reliance on gait analysis to quantify gains made by surgery or other treatments. There continue to be proponents of gait analysis as a clinical diagnostic tool. New areas in which gait analysis is under investigation include Parkinson's disease, cervical myelopathy, high-heeled gait, and even depression. The publication of normative data permits the definition of pathologic gait and thereby defines a goal in the rehabilitation of a patient with a gait disorder. Analysis in gait laboratories can measure the initial deviation from normal as well as the improvements occurring through the rehabilitation process. Even as gait laboratories assume a more prominent role in evaluation of patients, however, the data generated from

research laboratories have already affected clinical practice in a variety of ways.

New techniques of analysis were developed as computer sophistication and availability evolved. Gait is a process with inherent variability, which must be understood and accounted for to maximize its utility. Fractal analysis is one approach and may result in a better description of gait rhythm variations during maturation from childhood to adulthood. Understanding and predicting muscle activation patterns can be accomplished using artificial neural network models. These are particularly exciting because their use may lead to active control of prostheses. Part of the variability of gait arises from differences in body size. Scaling the gait data to body size can reduce intersubject variability and provide a tighter evaluation of abnormality. Identification of "abnormal" gait can be subtle in some cases in view of the variable and voluminous data generated. The common method of evaluation is principal component analysis, which quantifies the deviation of variables from normal. A newer report evaluates variability based on an index that used the squared distance from the mean obtained from joint angle measurements of many subjects. These techniques promise to improve the usefulness of gait analysis in the evaluation and treatment of orthopedic patients.

Gait studies of patients with transfemoral and transtibial amputations resulted in an objective evaluation of ambulatory potential after prosthetic replacement. Early studies demonstrated that amputations at more proximal levels resulted in greater loss of symmetry and increased energy expenditure (Table 1–6). These findings stimulated renewed attempts to maintain amputations at the most distal level. Other studies showed that strengthening the muscles of the residual limb in patients with transtibial amputations resulted in velocities that were improved although still lower than normal. Recent electromyographic studies of gait in transfemoral amputees demonstrated the importance of reattaching biarticular muscles that are transected at the amputation site to bone to maintain their function.

Techniques for gait analysis of amputees also provide the objective means of comparing various prosthetic components, such as the solid ankle cushion heel (SACH) foot, and the multiaxial and uniaxial feet.

Gait analysis is now a common tool in the treatment and evaluation of patients who have cerebral palsy or have suffered from a cerebrovascular accident or head injury. For disorders such as these, gait improvement can be expected for 6 months or more. Studies suggest that the natural history of gait in child and adolescent cerebral palsy is one of deterioration with aging, an important finding when evaluating long-term effects of intervention to improve gait. The use of electromyographic gait data can improve the results of muscle transfers in this group

Table 1–6. Results of free walking gait analysis in patients with transfemoral (TF) and transtibial (TT) amputations.

Cause and Level of Amputation	Velocity (m/min)	Cadence (steps/min)	Stride Length (m)	Gait Cycle (s)	Rate of Oxygen Uptake (mL/kg/min)	Net Oxygen Cost (mL/kg/m)
Traumatic TF amputation	55	86	1.26	1.42	12.7	0.28
Dysvascular TF amputation	36	72	1.00	1.66	12.6	0.35
Traumatic TT amputation	68	98	1.38	1.22	12.4	0.22
Dysvascular TT amputation	45	87	1.02	1.36	11.7	0.26

Data adapted, with permission, from Bagley AM, Skinner HB: Progress in gait analysis in amputees: A special review. Crit Rev Phys Rehabil Med 1991;3:101.

of patients. Knowledge of the activity period of a muscle (swing phase/stance phase) can allow prediction of the effect of transfer of that muscle. Thus, gait analysis is applied to spastic equinovarus feet to determine the efficacy of transfers of tibialis anterior and tibialis posterior. Similarly, gait analysis can be used to evaluate different surgical interventions, such as selective dorsal rhizotomies and orthopedic surgical interventions in spastic diplegic patients, showing improvement in energy cost and gait kinematics with both interventions.

Clinicians can use gait analysis to provide objective clinical data whenever orthotics are prescribed. Gait analysis before and after the application of an orthosis can quantify the effects in an objective manner. In evaluating the results, clinicians should remember that an orthosis that eliminates motion of a joint may improve function by putting the joint in a better position without bringing the patient back to a normal state. With orthotic fitting, lack of motion at a joint such as the ankle results in an increase in energy consumption and an alteration of gait symmetry, compared to normal. But without orthotic fitting, a poor joint position such as ankle equinus may make the gait even more inefficient and asymmetric. Similarly, ankle-foot orthoses (AFOs) thought to work through changes in spastic reflexes are shown with gait studies to be less effective than hinged AFOs in children with cerebral palsy. Other studies also showed that design of orthoses can be evaluated. In hemiplegic stroke patients, the use of a cane or the combination of a cane and an AFO were found to decrease energy consumption significantly.

Gait analysis is also improving surgical decision making. One study allowed experienced clinicians to review videotape and clinical examination data before recommending a treatment plan. After reviewing complete gait data, the same clinicians changed recommendations in 52% of patients. A second study showed 39% of planned surgical procedures on children were deemed unnecessary after gait analysis. Evaluation of a patient's

gait before and after a procedure can demonstrate the efficacy of the procedure and assist in postoperative care. A newer study demonstrated that the Van Nes rotational osteotomy allowed ambulation in children with proximal femoral focal deficiency at a more energy efficient rate than children with a Syme amputation. Gait analysis can allow objective comparisons of various procedures. This is primarily applicable, however, to those procedures in which the end point is an improvement of function. For example, walking efficiency as determined by velocity statistically is the same for transfemoral amputation and for proximal tibial replacement for tumor, but below normal for both treatments for age. Such a comparison of therapy choices can aid in the surgical decision process or the informed consent process. Procedures such as joint replacement have pain as the primary indication for surgery, although improvement of function is also a desirable by-product.

The results of surgical procedures such as total knee arthroplasty and total hip arthroplasty depend on a whole host of variables, including the surgeons' experience and the patients' age, preexisting disease, cooperation, and motivation. Clinical evaluation of the results of these procedures is at best crude from a functional viewpoint. For example, evaluation criteria include walking distance and the ability to climb stairs sequentially. Although the application of sophisticated gait analysis techniques to total joint replacement is relatively new, normative data on total knee and total hip replacement surgery have appeared in the literature for some time. These data are shown in Tables 1–7, 1–8, and 1–9. To date, gait analysis is unable to settle controversies that concern prosthesis design and are related to the efficacy of one type of cemented hip prosthesis versus another, the efficacy of cemented versus uncemented hip prostheses. Another controversy is the issue of the efficacy of prostheses that sacrifice the posterior cruciate ligament of the knee versus those that preserve this ligament and whether mobile bearing knee designs

Table 1–7. Results of free walking gait analysis in patients with total knee arthroplasty.

Study[a]	Patient Diagnosis	Time Since Surgery (yr)	Velocity (m/min)	Cadence (steps/min)	Stride Length (m)	Prosthesis Design
(1) Collopy et al (1977)	OA	1	57	100	1.2	Geometric
	RA	1	46	98	0.9	Geometric
(2) Simon et al (1983)	OA	3.3	63	100.6	1.2	Duopatellar
(3) Skinner et al (1983)	OA or RA	Preop	38.9	87.6	0.864	—
	OA or RA	5	46.5	91.5	1.01	Multiple
(4) Skinner et al (1983)	OA or RA	5.5	50.7	91	1.30	Polycentric
(5) Olsson and Barck (1986)	OA	9	62.4	107	1.14	Gunston-Hult
(6) Berman et al (1987)	OA, with normal contralateral knee	1.5	49.6	—	1.07	Total condylar
	OA, with asymptomatic diseased contralateral knee	2.0	35.2	—	0.958	—
	OA in both knees	1.3	54.5	—	1.07	—
(7) Waters et al (1987)	RA	0.9	63	103	1.31	—
(8) Kroll et al (1989)	OA	1.1	64.1	109.7	1.18	—
(9) Steiner, Simon, and Pisciotta (1989)	OA or RA	1.0	69	114	1.18	Total condylar or unicompartmental

[a]References are as follows: (1) Collopy MC et al: Kinesiologic measurements of functional performance before and after geometric total knee replacement. Clin Orthop 1977;126:196. (2) Simon SR et al: Quantitative gait analysis after knee arthroplasty for monoarticular degenerative arthritis. J Bone Joint Surg Am 1983;65:605. (3) Skinner HB et al: Ambulatory function in total knee arthroplasty. South Med J 1983;76:1237. (4) Skinner HB et al: Correlation of gait analysis and clinical evaluation of polycentric total knee arthroplasty. Orthopedics 1983;6:576. (5) Olsson E, Barck A: Correlation between clinical examination and quantitative gait analysis in patients operated upon with the Gunston-Hult knee prosthesis. Scand J Rehab Med 1986;18:101. (6) Berman AT et al: Quantitative gait analysis after unilateral or bilateral total knee replacement. J Bone Joint Surg Am 1987;69:1340. (7) Waters RL et al: The energy cost of walking with arthritis of the hip and knee. Clin Orthop 1987;214:278. (8) Kroll MA et al: The relationship of stride characteristics to pain before and after total knee arthroplasty. Clin Orthop 1989;239:191. (9) Steiner ME, Simon SR, Pisciotta JC: Early changes in gait and maximum knee torque following knee arthroplasty. Clin Orthop 1989;238:174.
OA = osteoarthrosis; RA = rheumatoid arthritis.
Reproduced, with permission, from Skinner HB: Pathokinesiology and total joint arthroplasty. Clin Orthop 1993;288:78.

demonstrate a benefit over nonmobile bearing knee designs. Thus far, variability in the data has prevented demonstration of a clear difference in designs. As advances in prosthesis design and gait analysis continue, improvements in the management of patients with gait disorders will also continue.

Andriacchi TP et al: The influence of total knee replacement design on walking and stair climbing. J Bone Joint Surg Am 1982; 64:1328. [PMID: 7142241]

Bagley AM, Skinner HB: Progress in gait analysis in amputees: A special review. Crit Rev Phys Rehabil Med 1991;3:101.

Chambers HG, Sutherland DH: A practical guide to gait analysis. J Am Acad Orthop Surg 2002;10:222. [PMID: 12041944]

Chau T: A review of analytical techniques for gait data. Part I: Fuzzy, statistical and fractal methods. Gait Posture 2001; 13:49. [PMID: 11166554]

DeLuca PA et al: Alterations in surgical decision making in patients with cerebral palsy based on three-dimensional gait analysis. J Pediatr Orthop 1997;17:608.

Dennis DA et al: Multicenter determination of in vivo kinematics after total knee arthroplasty. Clin Orthop 2003;416:37. [PMID: 14646738]

De Visser E et al: Gait and electromyographic analysis of patients recovering after limb-saving surgery. Clin Biomech 2000;15: 592. [PMID: 10936431]

Gefen A et al: Analysis of muscular fatigue and foot stability during high-heeled gait. Gait Posture 2002;15:56. [PMID: 11809581]

Hesse S et al: Non-velocity-related effects of a rigid double-stopped ankle-foot orthosis on gait and lower limb muscle activity of hemiparetic subjects with an equinovarus deformity. Stroke 1999;30:1855. [PMID: 10471436]

Huang G-F et al: Gait analysis and energy consumption of below-knee amputees wearing three different prosthetic feet. Gait Posture 2000;12:162. [PMID: 10998614]

Table 1–8. Results of free walking gait analysis in patients with total hip arthroplasty.

Study[a]	Patient Diagnosis	Time Since Surgery (yr)	Velocity (m/min)	Cadence (steps/min)	Stride Length (m)	Prosthesis Design
(1) Murray, Brewer, and Zuege (1972)	NA	—	50.0	—	0.98	McKee-Farrar
(2) Stauffer, Smidt, and Wadsworth (1974)	NA	0.5	37.1	80.4	—	Charnley
(3) Murray et al (1975)	OA or RA	2	65	106	1.23	McKee-Farrar
(4) Murray et al (1976)	OA or RA	0.5	62	102	—	Charnley
	OA or RA	0.5	57	102	—	Müller
	OA or RA	0.5	55	100	—	McKee-Farrar
(5) Murray et al (1979)	OA or RA	2	68	110	—	Charnley or Müller
(6) Brown et al (1980)	OA	1	55	101	1.12	—
(7) Olsson, Goldie, and Wykman (1986)	OA or RA	1	53.4*	97.2	1.08	Charnley
	NA	—	48.0*	93	1.00	H.P. Garches
(8) Mattsson, Brostrom, and Linnarsson (1990)	OA	1	80*	—	—	Charnley or H.P. Garches

[a]References are as follows: (1) Murray MP, Brewer BJ, Zuege RC: Kinesiologic measurements of functional performance before and after McKee-Farrar total hip replacement. J Bone Joint Surg Am 1972;54:237. (2) Stauffer RN, Smidt GL, Wadsworth JB: Clinical and biomechanical analysis of gait following Charnley total hip replacement. Clin Orthop 1974;99:70. (3) Murray MP et al: Kinesiology after McKee-Farrar total hip replacement: A two-year follow-up of one hundred cases. J Bone Joint Surg Am 1975;57:337. (4) Murray MP et al: Comparison of functional performance after McKee-Farrar, Charnley, and Müller total hip replacement: A six-month follow-up of one hundred sixty-five cases. Clin Orthop 1976;21:33. (5) Murray MP et al: Comparison of the functional performance of patients with Charnley and Müller total hip replacement. Acta Orthop Scand 1979;50:563. (6) Brown M et al: Walking efficiency before and after total hip replacement. Phys Ther 1980;60:1259. (7) Olsson E, Goldie I, Wykman A: Total hip replacement: A comparison between cemented (Charnley) and noncemented (H.P. Garches) fixation by clinical assessment and objective gait analysis. Scand J Rehab Med 1986;18:107. (8) Mattsson E, Brostrom LA, Linnarsson D: Walking efficiency after cemented and noncemented total hip arthroplasty. Clin Orthop 1990;254:170.
*Asterisk indicates velocity at fast walking speed; otherwise, velocity is at free walking speed.
NA = diagnostic data not available; OA = osteoarthritis; RA = rheumatoid arthritis.
Reproduced, with permission, from Skinner HB: Pathokinesiology and total joint arthroplasty. Clin Orthop 1993;288:78.

Table 1–9. Results of energy consumption analysis during gait in patients with total hip arthroplasty.

Study[a]	Patient Diagnosis	Time Since Surgery (yr)	Velocity (m/min)	Rate of Oxygen Uptake (mL/kg/min)	Net Oxygen Cost (mL/kg/m)
(1) Pugh (1973)	OA	—	—	10.0	0.15
(2) Brown et al (1980)	OA	1	55	11.86	0.22
(3) McBeath, Bahrke, and Balke (1980)	NA	2	64.5	12.13	0.186
(4) Mattsson, Brostrom, and Linnarsson (1990)	OA	1	80*	—	0.221

[a]References are as follows: (1) Pugh LG: The oxygen intake and energy cost of walking before and after unilateral hip replacement with some observations on the use of crutches. J Bone Joint Surg Br 1973;55:742. (2) Brown M et al: Walking efficiency before and after total hip replacement. Phys Ther 1980;60:1259. (3) McBeath AA, Bahrke MS, Balke B: Walking efficiency before and after total hip replacement as determined by oxygen consumption. J Bone Joint Surg Am 1980;62:807. (4) Mattsson E, Brostrom LA, Linnarsson D: Walking efficiency after cemented and noncemented total hip arthroplasty. Clin Orthop 1990;254:170.
*Asterisk indicates velocity at fast walking speed; otherwise, velocity is at free walking speed.
OA = osteoarthritis; NA = diagnostic data not available.
Reproduced, with permission, from Skinner HB: Pathokinesiology and total joint arthroplasty. Clin Orthop 1993;288:78.

Johnson DC et al: The evolution of gait in childhood and adolescent cerebral palsy. J Pediatr Orthop 1997;17:392. [PMID: 9150031]

Kay RM et al: Impact of postoperative gait analysis on orthopedic care. Clin Orthop 2000;372:259. [PMID: 10818985]

Kay RM et al: The effect of preoperative gait analysis on orthopedic decision making. Clin Orthop 2000;372:217. [PMID: 10738430]

Nowak MD et al: Design enhancement of a solid ankle-foot orthosis: Real-time contact pressures evaluation. J Rehabil Res Dev 2000;37:273. [PMID: 10917259]

Pierrynowski MR, Galea V: Enhancing the ability of gait analyses to differentiate between groups: Scaling gait data to body size. Gait Posture 2001;13:193. [PMID: 11323225]

Prentice SD et al: Artificial neural network model for the generation of muscle activation patterns for human locomotion. J Electromyogr Kinesiol 2001;11:19. [PMID: 11166605]

Reitman JS, Postema K, Geertzen JH: Gait analysis in prosthetics: opinions, ideas and conclusions. Prosthet Orthot Int 2002; 26:50. [PMID: 12043926]

Romkes J, Brunner R: Comparison of a dynamic and a hinged ankle-foot orthosis by gait analysis in patients with hemiplegic cerebral palsy. Gait Posture 2002;15:18. [PMID: 11809577]

Sanders JE et al: Effects of changes in cadence, prosthetic componentry, and time on the interface pressures and shear stresses of three trans-tibial amputees. Clin Biomech 2000;15:684. [PMID: 10946102]

Schmalz T et al: Energy expenditure and biomechanical characteristics of lower limb amputee gait: The influence of prosthetic alignment and different prosthetic components. Gait Posture 2002;16:255. [PMID: 12443950]

Simon SR: Quantification of human motion: gait analysis-benefits and limitations to its application to clinical problems. J Biomech 2004;37:1869.

Thomas SS et al: A 2-year follow-up of outcomes following orthopedic surgery or selective dorsal rhizotomy in children with spastic diplegia. J Pediatr Orthop B 2004;13:358. [PMID: 15599225]

Tingley M et al: An index to quantify normality of gait in young children. Gait Posture 2002;16:149. [PMID: 12297256]

REFERENCES

Cristal P et al, eds: *Biological and Biomechanical Performance of Biomaterials.* Elsevier, 1986.

Friberg L et al: *Handbook on the Toxicology of Metals.* Elsevier, 1986.

Fung YCB: *Biomechanics: Mechanical Properties of Living Tissues.* Springer-Verlag, 1981.

Gage JR et al: Instructional course lecture, The American Academy of Orthopaedic Surgeons. Gait Analysis: Principles and applications emphasis on its use in cerebral palsy. J Bone Joint Surg Am 1995;77:1607.

Perry J: *Gait Analysis: Normal and Pathological Function.* Slack, 1992.

Rose J, Gamble JG, eds: *Human Walking,* 2nd ed. Williams & Wilkins, 1994.

General Considerations in Orthopedic Surgery

Harry B. Skinner, MD, PhD

Orthopedic surgery encompasses the entire process of caring for the surgical patient, from diagnostic evaluation to the preoperative evaluation and through the postoperative and rehabilitative period. Although the surgical procedure itself is the key step toward helping the patient, the preliminary and follow-up care can determine whether the surgery is successful.

DIAGNOSTIC WORK-UP

History and Physical Exam

Although it may seem obvious, the history and physical exam are still important in the evaluation of the patient. Every office visit is a history and physical exam, whether a new or a return visit. The completeness of the history and physical has assumed new importance in view of the complexities required for compliance with federal regulations. Regulations require that a chief complaint be specified, and this must be clearly defined because it determines the direction for the rest of the history and physical. The history must address the key features of the problem, both to elucidate the medical problem and to cover the subsidiary requirements for billing purposes. The social history and past medical history are similarly important because they change billing codes without necessarily affecting outcome or success of care. The physical again must cover the essentials necessary for diagnosis, and frequently the confirmation of the diagnosis is based on physical exam, but such considerations as skin condition and blood supply must be documented, despite the fact that this process is also part of the surgical evaluation. The next step is imaging and laboratory exams. The most important point here is to use the most cost-effective examination possible while keeping patient safety, satisfaction, and convenience in mind.

Imaging Studies

A. ROENTGENOGRAPHY

Roentgenography is still the most cost-effective and most important initial diagnostic test in the orthope-

dist's armamentarium. Almost every patient should have a radiograph prior to going to a more sophisticated imaging study. Certain situations are obvious; for example, a 68-year-old man with knee pain should have standing, flexed-knee posteroanterior (PA), lateral, and merchant plain film views taken. If those views show normal joint spaces, consideration of intraarticular pathology, such as a degenerative meniscus tear, can be worked up with magnetic resonance imaging (MRI). The normal views usually ordered are as follows:

1. **Neck pain**—No history of trauma, more than 4 weeks' duration.

    Younger than 35 years: anteroposterior (AP) lateral, odontoid

    Older than 35 years: obliques

    History of trauma: flexion/extension laterals (obtain on first visit)

2. **Thoracic spine pain and tenderness**—

    Younger than 40 years, no reason to suspect malignancy: AP and lateral (if history of trauma, or possibility of osteoporosis on first visit, otherwise at 4 weeks).

    Consider cervical (C)-spine as a source of referred pain to thoracic (T)-spine if no tenderness in T-spine.

3. **Lumbar (L)-sacral (S)-spine**—

    Younger than 40 years, no reason to suspect malignancy after 4 weeks duration of the pain. With significant trauma, at first visit, or possible malignancy (ie, weight loss, malaise, fatigue): AP, lateral.

    Add obliques for chronic low back pain (ie, spondylolisthesis).

4. **Hips**—

    AP pelvis, lateral of affected hip.

    Consider lumbar-sacral (L-S) series if pain is in the buttock rather than in the groin.

5. **Knees—**

Older than 40 years or history of meniscectomy: Rosenberg, lateral, and sunrise films. Merchant views are similar to sunrise. The Rosenberg view is a 10-degree down shot of the PA of the knees while standing at 45 degrees of flexion.

For other knees: AP, lateral, and sunrise.

In the child, up to age 16, consider a pelvis film with the complaint of knee pain and negative physical exam referable to the knee.

6. **Femur, tibia, humerus, forearm—**AP and lateral are indicated for trauma, palpable lesions, or suspected tumors.

7. **Ankle—**AP lateral and mortise.

8. **Foot—**AP, lateral, and oblique for routine evaluation.

9. **Shoulder—**AP, axillary, scapular Y, and outlet views.

10. **Elbow—**AP and lateral (true lateral).

11. **Hand/wrist—**

Hand: PA and lateral.

Wrist: PA, lateral, and oblique

For suspected instability: clenched fist PA in radial and ulnar deviation.

Follow-up radiographs are obtained when a change in the radiographic findings is expected. Remember that bone changes occur slowly, so radiographic changes take a comparable length of time. Radiographs are obtained in view of the clinical picture. For example, closed treatment of a distal radius fracture would not be expected to show changes because of healing for a minimum of 2 weeks. However, displacement of the fracture could occur sooner. Hence, radiographs to show displacement might be obtained at 1 week and 2 weeks. If no displacement is observed, the fracture position could be considered stable, and the next films might be obtained at 6 weeks—the earliest time healing might be observed. Similarly, closed treatment of an adult tibia fracture might be followed with radiographs at 2-week intervals, checking for displacement and healing, whereas a tibia fracture treated with an intramedullary rod might be followed at monthly intervals to check for healing.

B. MAGNETIC RESONANCE IMAGING

This imaging modality is very useful, but like electron beam computed tomography (CT), MRI is sometimes too revealing. This method should be reserved for clarifying a particular problem. Frequently in orthopedics, a bony lesion can be localized with a radiograph or bone scan, which then provides a focus for the MRI. MRI is useful for some bony lesions, such as osteonecrosis, tumors, fatigue fractures, and osteomyelitis. It is also

helpful in some soft-tissue problems, such as knee meniscus tears and shoulder rotator cuff tears. MRI should not be used when the diagnosis can be made with a less expensive test. For example, the use of the MRI in knee studies in patients older than 45 years should always be preceded by plain films of the knee, as noted earlier. An MRI of an arthritic knee adds little additional information because the meniscus and anterior cruciate ligament are likely to be damaged from the arthritic process already. However, the MRI can be very helpful in determining soft-tissue extension of tumors or infection.

The advent of new portable MRI units that perform limited studies with more resolution adds a new dimension to their use. These can provide data on the progression of disorders such as rheumatoid arthritis or osteomyelitis in a timely and cost-effective way. The possibility of osteomyelitis in the bones adjacent to ulcers on the foot is easily determined with this test because it shows the changes, typically edema, in the bone with osteomyelitis. A bone scan usually does not have the resolution to distinguish the inflammatory response in the soft tissue from the bony involvement. Osteomyelitis should be treated much differently from a soft-tissue ulcer, which does not affect the bone.

C. COMPUTED TOMOGRAPHY

The CT scan is an extremely important imaging modality for examining bony lesions such as fractures. Frequently, plain films provide some information about the fracture of interest, but the CT scan provides the three-dimensional information that can only otherwise be determined from the integration of the plain films in the surgeon's mind. The CT scan adds significantly to the management of such fractures as tibial plateaus, scapular fractures, ankle fractures, and cervical and lumbar spine fractures, as well as many others. Again, if little information can be gained that cannot be already discerned from the plain films, the CT scan only adds expense and patient inconvenience. The spiral CT makes imaging with this modality less expensive and much more rapid. The CT scan is also now the method of choice for determining whether a pulmonary embolus (PE) has occurred. Again, a CT for this indication is easier on the patient, more accurate, and less invasive than angiography.

D. TECHNETIUM-99M BONE SCAN

The bone scan finds many uses in orthopedic surgery. Keep in mind that the bone scan labels the osteoblast activity with the radioactive tracer, technetium-99; thus, bone formation activity is recorded and little or no bone resorption activity is noted. Any disorder that results in increased bone formation, therefore, results in a "hot" bone scan. This means that a disorder such as multiple myeloma may not show up on a bone scan because only osteoclastic activity is involved in the majority of lesions. This test is helpful in discerning loose total hip and total knee prostheses, however, even though the findings are nonspecific. It is very helpful in examining probable benign bone lesions because a cold bone scan largely rules out an aggressive process such as a malignancy. The bone scan is also helpful in diagnosing any disorder of unknown origin when there is pain localized to a particular region. A cold bone scan implies that the problem is a soft-tissue one, whereas a hot bone scan points to a region that may benefit from MRI.

Laboratory Exams

The two most important laboratory exams are for C-reactive protein and the erythrocyte sedimentation rate. These two tests indicate whether an inflammatory process, malignancy, or rheumatologic disorder are diagnostic considerations. If these tests are negative, systemic causes of a complaint can frequently be ruled out. In that situation, a more localized disorder should be identified. The next most important test is the complete blood count, which provides the general indication of the patient's health, revealing information about anemia, infectious processes, and so on. The next most useful laboratory test for the orthopedic surgeon is the synovial fluid analysis. This test typically should include a culture and sensitivity. If there is any concern about infection, a cell count, differential, protein, and glucose measurement should be performed. Crystals should be looked for because they indicate chondrocalcinosis or gout. Elevated protein and reduced glucose levels suggest infection. The final factor that should be considered with any major surgery is the patient's nutritional status, which is evaluated with several tests, including lymphocyte count and levels of prealbumin, albumin, and serum iron transferrin.

Educating & Informing Patients & Their Families

Surgical procedures in orthopedics have varying degrees of difficulty and importance, ranging from a relatively simple clawtoe correction to the performance of a multilevel complex spinal fusion. After the decision to employ surgery as a therapeutic modality is made, it is important to help the patient completely understand what to expect before, during, and after surgery. This process, which the legal profession calls **informed consent,** has the more important purpose of ensuring the patient's cooperation and satisfaction.

To comply with the requirements of the legal profession and accrediting organizations, such as the Joint Commission on Accreditation of Healthcare Organiza-tions (JCAHO), the surgeon must provide an explanation of the risks, prognosis, alternatives, and complications that might be encountered. The risks should be reviewed in some detail for the general risks encountered in typical orthopedic surgical procedures. The risks and the complications that occur in surgery are intimately associated and thus must be dealt with together. The alternatives are sometimes straightforward. For example, a patient with an open fracture has a high risk of infection if not adequately treated with irrigation, debridement, and antibiotics. Thus, in such a situation, any reasonable and prudent person would consent to the procedure. The choice between alternatives can become significantly more subtle, however. For example, it is possible that a choice must be made between two different procedures or between a particular procedure and no procedure. In this situation, the surgeon must consider the psychosocial and physical attributes of the patient so as to assist him or her in making this decision. For example, consider men, both 75 years of age, with severe degenerative disease in the right knee noted on radiograph. One individual is now at the point where he cannot play golf, a situation that is reducing his physical exercise and a number of his social outlets. The other individual leads a relatively sedentary lifestyle, seldom walks more than a block, and obtains cardiorespiratory exercise by swimming, an activity in which his knee does not bother him. The surgeon should recommend knee replacement to one individual but not the other. At the same time, both men must be offered the alternatives, which include continued nonsteroidal antiinflammatory medicine, bracing, sleeping medication, and analgesics.

Patients with an active lifestyle are becoming much more concerned about what will happen to them in the postoperative period, including how soon they can safely travel, when they can work, and when they will be fully able to take care of themselves. They are also concerned about what social services are available to help them if they cannot care for themselves fully. The surgeon must be prepared to address these questions and also advise patients with lower extremity or spinal problems about when they will be able to walk. In the same manner, after procedures on the hand or upper extremity, patients must be advised about when they will be able to use the hand. Advising the patient of these situations before surgery can prevent unexpected surprises in the postoperative period.

The patient should also be informed about the range of expectations for ambulation or use of the upper extremity because individuals vary in their response to surgery. For example, patients should be advised that after surgery on the hip or knee, they will need a walker for a few days, move to crutches, and typically be done with the crutches in the range of 2–4 weeks. They will use a cane before 6 weeks and be done with the cane before 3 months. Patients should be cautioned about travel after surgery, particularly with lower extremity injuries, because of the risk of deep venous thrombosis (DVT). In such cases, discourage (for the first 6 weeks) plane trips longer than an hour and extended car trips made without stopping perhaps every 45 minutes. Antiinflammatory medication (to reduce platelet adhesion) or anticoagulants should be recommended if such travel is unavoidable.

A. EXPLAINING THE PROCEDURES

An essential part of the patient's presurgical preparation and postsurgical cooperation is knowing what to expect at every step in the process. Nuances become important in the process of explaining the surgical procedures and their implications. For example, scheduling a bunion procedure 2 weeks prior to a patient's participation in her daughter's wedding could upset the patient if she fails to realize that she will be unable to wear the shoes she purchased for the event. Similarly, lifestyle considerations can affect the decision-making process in cases of medial gonarthrosis, in which the choice between a unicompartmental knee replacement and a high tibial osteotomy could be influenced by whether the patient plays tennis and holds a physically strenuous job or, alternatively, whether the patient is sedentary and works behind a desk most of the day.

B. REVIEWING THE RISKS AND POSSIBLE COMPLICATIONS

Reviewing the perioperative risks is important for all patients and optimally should be done well in advance and then repeated closer to the time of surgery. Some patients require more detailed explanations, particularly if their relatives have undergone surgery in the past and had a problem with anesthesia or a complication such as a PE or infection. Based on the patient's responses to explanations, the health care team members needs to alter their approach to reach a balance between inadequately informing the patient and inducing unnecessary alarm that could make the patient refuse to undergo a procedure judged to be both beneficial and necessary.

Risk is a poorly understood concept in our culture. Some situations are considered to be higher in risk than they actually are. Some risks are understood better than others. It can help the patient to understand if these risks are put in perspective. The risks can be surprisingly high or low but still disturbing to the patient. For example, many people have moved away from California to avoid an earthquake or refuse to fly commercial aircraft because of the risk, not realizing that the risk of death is 10–100 times higher while driving a car (Table 2–1). This lack of understanding of the risk can contribute to significant differences in the perception of lia-

Table 2–1. Rates of death and complications associated with common activities.

Death or Complication	Percentage
Death (from MI after previous MI)	1
Major bleed (7 days, warfarin, INR 2.65)	0.02
GI ulcer/bleed perforation (naproxen 6 months)	1
Paralysis (from epidural)	0.02
Death (frequent flying professor/year)	0.001
Death (automobile/year)	0.016
Earthquake in California/per year	0.00018

GI = gastrointestinal; INR = international normalized ratio; MI = myocardial infarction.

bility associated with these activities. For example, the death benefit from a commercial airline accident might reach several million dollars per passenger, whereas death in an automobile accident might have no death benefit at all. Thus, the *perception* of risk is very important and must be clarified in the patient's mind. Similarly, patients can understand and accept having a myocardial infarction after a major surgery because they can clearly see the strain on the heart from the surgery. However, they are not nearly as understanding of a lower extremity paralysis that can result from the epidural anesthetic for that surgery. The explanation of risks must be individualized for each patient. The patient with a previous myocardial infarction is clearly different from the healthy 20-year-old (see Table 2–1). Across-the-board rates of problems do not translate into direct risks for the individual patient.

Although all procedures carry some risks, the incidence and type of risks and complications vary with the surgical procedure as well as with the patient's age and general health. Potential problems are listed and discussed here in alphabetical order.

1. Amputation—The potential problem of amputation is seldom of acute concern except in cases of significant trauma. The topic of amputation can frequently be discussed with the risk of infection because ischemia and infection can increase the risk of amputation.

2. Anesthesia—One of the major risks in orthopedic surgery is associated with anesthesia, not because complications of anesthesia are frequent but because they can be devastating. Death occurs at a rate of approximately 1 in 200,000 patients undergoing elective anesthesia. Other complications include but are not limited to the following: nerve damage and paraplegia from nerve blocks; headaches from dural leaks following use of spinal anesthetics; aspiration of stomach contents;

and cardiac problems, including ischemia and arrhythmias. The surgeon should discuss these problems with the patient only in general terms, allowing the anesthesiologist to provide the most detailed explanations.

3. Arthritis—Virtually any procedure that enters a joint, other than to replace it, has the potential to cause damage to that joint. In some instances, as in an intraarticular fracture, the surgery will likely lessen the risk of arthritis. Even in these instances, the patient should be told that the risk of damage is still real because the joint surface healing will not result in a normal cartilage surface.

4. Blood loss—Patients should be given a reasonably accurate estimate of blood loss as well as the opportunity to donate autologous blood prior to surgery. Designated donor blood is probably not safer but gives the patient who receives it a sense of security. The use of erythropoietin can elevate preoperative hemoglobin (Hgb) levels (usually for patients with Hgb <13) and thereby reduce postoperative homologous blood transfusion needs. Other alternatives include the use of intraoperative blood salvage for reinfusion (OrthoPAT, Antovac). The use of erythropoietin is generally accepted by Jehovah's Witness patients, whereas the autologous reinfusion acceptance is variable. To help minimize blood loss during surgery, the patient's use of nonsteroidal antiinflammatory drugs (NSAIDs) should be discontinued approximately 2 weeks before surgery. Discontinuation of NSAIDs can significantly compromise comfort and incite rheumatoid flares in many patients who rely on these drugs. To minimize the risk, newer COX-II inhibitor NSAIDs may be used as a substitute during this period; no platelet disorders or bleeding time derangement occurs with these drugs because they do not affect platelet function or inhibit thromboxane A_2.

5. Blood vessel damage—Arterial and venous damage take on greater significance as the size of the vessel increases and the arterial supply becomes more calcified with age and vascular disease. Patients generally understand this, but it must be emphasized where appropriate. Hip and knee replacement put unusual strains on the femoral and popliteal vessels, from positioning, and may damage calcified arteries.

6. Deep venous thrombosis/pulmonary embolism—Virtually all lower extremity and spine procedures in orthopedics involve some risk of DVT, which should be explained to the patient. As many as 25% of patients who undergo a relatively high-risk procedure such as total hip arthroplasty have venographically diagnosed DVT. The risk of PE is much less, however, and is in the range of 0.3% for fatal emboli. This rate of fatal PE is approximately a 10-fold increase over the rate of fatal PE in the U.S. population in men older than 65 years. The risks associated with other procedures may be lower. In any case, the patient should be reassured that prevention procedures commensurate with risk will be undertaken.

7. Fracture—Many procedures in orthopedic surgery carry the risk of a bone fracture. Some procedures, such as uncemented hip replacement, present a higher risk for this complication, but virtually any orthopedic procedure could result in fracture of a bone. The patient must be informed of the risk in relation to the probability of the occurrence of such a problem.

8. Infection—The risk of infection in orthopedic surgery ranges from near zero in procedures such as arthroscopy to several percent in open fracture surgery. The problem of infection should be emphasized in proportion to risk. For example, if a diabetic patient is to undergo knee replacement, he or she should not only be assured that all steps will be taken to prevent infection (eg, administration of prophylactic antibiotics, use of ultrafiltration of air, or ultraviolet lights in the operating room) but should also be told of the various techniques that would be considered if infection occurred. These options include debridement, prosthesis removal, gastrocnemius flap, reinsertion, arthrodesis, and amputation. The common use of external fixation devices for fracture care is accompanied by the frequent problems associated with pin care. The patient and family should be informed about the problems caused by percutaneous devices to prevent the presumption that something has gone wrong. Skin problems are frequently associated with infection but may arise from other causes, such as adjacent scars compromising the blood supply to a surgical flap. Older patients and individuals who are smokers, have diabetes, or have wounds on the distal lower extremity are at increased risk. In such cases, the patient may be warned that delayed healing or necrosis of the skin edges may occur.

9. Loss of reduction—Although fracture care continues to improve, displacement of hardware or fracture fragments may necessitate a second procedure. The explanation of this risk should be individualized, based on the type of fracture. Loss of reduction may contribute to delayed union or nonunion of fractures. These problems may occur despite optimal care by the orthopedic surgeon. Poor vascular supply or smoking can be a factor leading to nonunion. The rate of nonunion is site dependent but is only a few percent.

10. Nerve damage—Certain procedures are associated with nerve damage, although the damage is usually minor. For example, medial parapatellar incisions on the knee cause some numbness from cutting the infrapatellar branch of the saphenous nerve. The patient should be informed in advance if some degree of minor nerve damage is anticipated in association with the particular surgical procedure being pursued and should also be informed of the risks of unexpected nerve damage that accompany all surgical procedures.

C. PROGNOSIS

The prognosis of the procedure is intimately related to the procedure. However, certain guidelines may be given. The expected time off work or time away from activities is important to the patient and depend on the patient's occupation, age, and available sick leave. The bank president with more control over her agenda will be able to return to work activities sooner than the day laborer. Driving is an important activity for many people, and limitations placed by a procedure can determine how much postoperative assistance a patient will need.

The patient should be given reasonable expectations about range of motion, strength, possible disability, and when these should return to normal, if at all. Furthermore, walking or writing ability, ability to use a computer keyboard, and the time to expect to be able to do such activities may be appropriate for some patients. Again, these have to be individualized for each patient and determined for each home situation.

D. KEEPING THE PATIENT AND FAMILY INFORMED

Immediately before elective surgery, the surgeon can help comfort the patient and family by meeting them in the preoperative area and appearing relaxed, well rested, and positive about the outcome of the surgery. Giving the family a good estimate of the surgery time is important, but they should also be reassured that delays do not necessarily indicate the occurrence of complications that are detrimental to the patient. If the family members wish to be notified about delays, they should be encouraged to leave instructions about where they can be contacted. When surgery is completed and the patient is no longer at risk of untoward accidents such as aspiration during extubation, a member of the surgical team should apprise the family of the outcome. At this time, it is appropriate to emphasize particular concerns to the family, such as the need to continue vigilance for infection in a diabetic patient who has undergone foot surgery.

Johnson BF et al: Relationship between changes in the deep venous system and the development of the postthrombotic syndrome after an acute episode of lower limb deep vein thrombosis. A one- to six-year follow-up. J Vasc Surg 1995;21:307. [PMID: 7853603]

Lilienfeld DE: Decreasing mortality from pulmonary embolism in the United States, 1979–1996. Int J Epidemiol 2000;29:465. [PMID: 10869318]

Lilienfeld DE, Godbold JH: Geographic distribution of pulmonary embolism mortality rates in the United States, 1980 to 1984. Am Heart J 1992;124:1068. [PMID: 1529881]

McKee MD et al: The effect of smoking on clinical outcome and complication rates following Ilizarov reconstruction. J Orthop Trauma 2003;17:663. [PMID: 14600564]

Nosanchuk JS: Quantitative microbiologic study of blood salvaged by intraoperative membrane filtration. Arch Pathol Lab Med 2001;125(9):1204. [PMID: 11520273]

Salvati E et al: Recent advances in venous thromboembolic prophylaxis during and after total hip replacement. J Bone Joint Surg Am 2000;82:252. [PMID: 10682733]

Tamir L et al: Recombinant human erythropoietin reduces allogeneic blood transfusion requirements in patients undergoing major orthopedic surgery. Haematologia (Budap) 2000;30(3):93. [PMID: 11128112]

Warner C: The use of the orthopaedic perioperative autotransfusion (OrthoPAT) system in total joint replacement surgery. Orthop Nurs 2001;20(6):29. [PMID: 12025800]

SURGICAL MANAGEMENT

Preoperative Care

A. THE TEAM APPROACH

Inclusion of nurses, residents, anesthesiologists, and other members of the surgical team in the planning process can improve the efficiency and therefore affect the outcome of a surgical procedure. Good estimates of the length of the operative procedure and of the patient's anticipated blood loss and muscle relaxation requirements minimizes the risks from anesthesia and surgery. Reviewing the site of the operation and assessing the need for any special supplies and equipment, such as prostheses, lasers, or fracture tables, also contributes to efficiency and optimal results. Special care must be exercised by all members of the operative team to prevent "wrong side" surgery. It is now a JCAHO standard to have the surgical team "mark" the surgical site.

B. PREPARING AND POSITIONING THE PATIENT

Once the patient is in the operating room, every effort should be made to make him or her comfortable. A calm, efficient, and professional demeanor by everyone involved is necessary both before and after anesthesia is induced. If the anesthesiologist indicates that placement of the antithromboembolic hose, intermittent pneumatic compression stockings, or tourniquets will improve efficiency, these can be put in place prior to induction. Placement of arterial lines, central lines, and Foley catheters should be done after the patient is anesthetized, if possible. Location of the operating table must be adjusted to ensure good lighting, optimize the efficiency of the surgeon and staff, and allow for maintenance of surgical sterile technique.

Positioning of the patient is the responsibility of both the surgeon and the anesthesiologist to facilitate the operation and to ensure the patient's safety. A perfectly executed operation can be marred by a nerve palsy that results from the failure to pad a remote area appropriately. If the patient is placed in the lateral decubitus position, the peroneal nerve at the knee and the brachial plexus of the downside shoulder girdle must be protected. During shoulder surgery, the surgeon must take care to avoid stretching the patient's brachial plexus or cervical nerve roots while attempting to maximize the operative field. Similarly, the patient's shoulder should not be abducted past 90 degrees, and joints with contractures should not be forced into unusual positions. These precautions are particularly necessary in treating rheumatoid patients or older osteoporotic patients. Injury to the extremities and loss of lines can be avoided by careful planning and synchronization when positioning patients into the lateral decubitus position or prone position.

C. USE OF ANTIBIOTICS

Except in cases in which concern about infection requires unambiguous cultures to be obtained, prophylactic antibiotics should be started prior to skin incision. A first- or second-generation cephalosporin antibiotic is considered appropriate for orthopedic procedures.

D. USE OF A TOURNIQUET

A tourniquet can be extremely helpful in some procedures and is practically mandatory for others. The tourniquet stops the flow of blood to and from an extremity. To achieve this, the pneumatic tourniquet is inflated to a pressure that must be significantly higher than the arterial pressure because the pressure is dissipated in the soft tissue underneath the tourniquet.

1. Tourniquet size and placement—The tourniquet should be wide enough for the extremity while still permitting adequate exposure of the extremity. Particularly in cases involving surgery on muscles that cross the elbow or knee, the tourniquet should be placed as proximal as possible to ensure the muscles have adequate stretch to permit full joint motion. When a tourniquet is used on a large extremity with a great deal of adipose tissue, care must be taken to ensure that the tourniquet does not slip distally, which could result in wrinkles in the tourniquet and localized pressure on the skin. Slippage can be prevented by applying 5-cm (2-inch) adhesive tape to the skin in a longitudinal direction below the cast padding placed under the tourniquet.

2. Tourniquet time and pressure—The effects of tourniquets on tissues are a combination of time and pressure on individual structures. Neural and muscle tissue are most sensitive, with deleterious effects arising from direct pressure to structures and from distal ischemia.

Several considerations are involved in the selection of the level of tourniquet pressure. First, the level must be low enough to avoid pressure damage to sensitive neural structures but high enough so the pressure around the arterial supply to the extremity is greater than systolic pressure (Figure 2–1). Second, if the patient's blood pressure is labile, a margin of safety is usually necessary. In a patient with a stable blood pressure, tourniquet pressures of 75 mm Hg above preinduction systolic pressure are typically adequate, although some surgeons use pressures as high as twice systolic. If the tourniquet is on an extremity with a great deal of adipose tissue, higher pressures are necessary to achieve adequate pressure at the artery to stop blood flow. Tourniquets should be calibrated and can be tested with an independent pressure measurement device or alternatively by palpation of the pulse and gradual elevation of pressure until the pulse disappears.

Complications will arise if tourniquets are used at high pressure for too long. The effects can sometimes

Figure 2–1. Distribution of tissue fluid pressure at four depths beneath pneumatic tourniquet with cuff pressure of 300 mm Hg applied on arms (**top**) and thighs (**bottom**). Values represent means for six limbs on each graph. (Reproduced, with permission, from Hargens AR et al: Local compression patterns beneath pneumatic tourniquets applied to arms and thighs of human cadavers. J Orthop Res 1987;5:247.)

be mitigated by using wider cuffs and curved cuffs, which allow for higher and more uniform pressure below the tourniquet. A rule of thumb is that tourniquet pressures should not be elevated for longer than 2 hours, and less time is preferable. In a canine study of the muscle tissue distal to the tourniquet, investigators found that 90-minute tourniquet times with 5 minutes between reinflation minimized the ischemic damage. This finding points to the need for efficiency in performing surgical procedures under tourniquet. After tourniquet release, reflex hyperemia and edema are frequently encountered, making closure more difficult. Exsanguination with an Esmarch bandage prior to tourniquet inflation facilitates emptying of large veins of the thigh and arm, although it is not recommended to use an Esmarch in trauma cases. Careful exsanguination may help prevent DVT, especially when reinflation of the tourniquet is planned.

Barwell J et al: The effects of early tourniquet release during total knee arthroplasty: A prospective randomized double-blind study. J Bone Joint Surg Br 1997;79:265. [PMID: 9119854]

Classen DC et al: The timing of prophylactic administration of antibiotics and the risk of surgical wound infection. N Engl J Med 1992;326:281. [PMID: 1728731]

Darmanis S, Papanikolaou A, Pavlakis D: Fatal intra-operative pulmonary embolism following application of an Esmarch bandage. Injury. 2002 ;33:761. [PMID: 12379384]

Fernandez AH, Monge V, Garcinuno MA: Surgical antibiotic prophylaxis: effect in postoperative infections. Eur J Epidemiol 2001;17:369. [PMID: 11767963]

Hargens AR et al: Local compression patterns beneath pneumatic tourniquets applied to arms and thighs of human cadavers. J Orthop Res 1987;5:247. [PMID: 3572594]

Idusuyi OB, Morrey BF: Peroneal nerve palsy after total knee arthroplasty. Assessment of predisposing and prognostic factors. J Bone Joint Surg Am 1996;78:177. [PMID: 8609107]

Ostman B et al: Tourniquet-induced ischemia and reperfusion in human skeletal muscle. Clin Orthop 2004;418:260. [PMID: 15043128]

Pedowitz RA et al: The use of lower tourniquet inflation pressures in extremity surgery facilitated by curved and wide tourniquets and an integrated cuff inflation system. Clin Orthop 1993;287:237. [PMID: 8448950]

Sapega AA et al: Optimizing tourniquet application and release times in extremity surgery. J Bone Joint Surg Am 1985;67:303. [PMID: 3968122]

Wakai A et al: Pneumatic tourniquets in extremity surgery. J Am Acad Orthop Surg 2001;9:345. [PMID: 11575914]

Operative Care

The surgical team should make every effort to work efficiently during the period between the administration of anesthesia and the conclusion of the final steps of preoperative preparation, which may take from 10 to 30 minutes or longer. It is in the best interests of the patient to minimize the time between onset of anesthesia and the beginning of surgery.

A. INCISION SITES AND APPROACHES

Although the surgical wound "heals side-to-side, not end-to-end," the incorrect placement or the excessive length of a surgical incision for a given procedure only serves to increase surgical trauma to the patient, slow the healing process, and lengthen the rehabilitation period. If there is any doubt about the surgical incision site, roentgenographic examination should be considered. Use of an image intensifier should be considered in obese patients or in patients with previous surgery and retained hardware.

The incision should be made perpendicular to the skin, generally longitudinally, and with a sharp knife. In tumor biopsies, longitudinal incisions are always made. The approach by the surgeon through the subcutaneous fatty layer is variable and depends on the location on the body. In most areas, sharp dissection with a knife through the subcutaneous tissue to the fascial layer is indicated. In the upper extremity and in areas where cutaneous nerves can be troublesome if injured, blunt dissection is used because cutaneous nerves travel in the fatty tissue. Many surgeons prefer blunt dissection with scissors used to spread tissue perpendicular to the wound. Hemostasis is obtained layer by layer. Subcutaneous fat usually is not dissected from the skin, because this might devascularize it.

Surgeons must be extremely careful with the skin, making sure to avoid crushing it when forceps are used. The skin should never be clamped, nor should it be excessively stretched. A larger incision is much better for the skin than extreme tension. Care of the soft tissues includes keeping them moist, avoiding excessive retraction, and being especially careful of neurovascular bundles. Nerves suffer damage from both traction and compression. Nerve palsies and paresthesias can spoil an otherwise well-performed operation in the eyes of both the surgeon and the patient. Care of the cartilage includes keeping it moist because drying has a deleterious effect.

Surgical approaches that go through internerve planes, such as between the deltoid and the pectoralis major, should be used to avoid denervation of muscles. The splitting of muscles in the surgical approach should also be avoided because splitting is generally more traumatic and more likely to denervate the muscle. This rule does not always apply in tumor surgery because it is important to keep tumor cells in a single compartment.

B. ORTHOPEDIC INSTRUMENTS AND DRAINS

It is mandatory that tools be sharp at all times because the sharpness enables the surgeon to avoid the excessive pressure that creates problems by plunging into the depths of the wound. When an osteotome or elevator is needed, the concurrent use of a hammer is preferred because achieving exact control is possible by the strength and number of hammer taps, whereas control is difficult to achieve by pushing on an osteotome. With drill points and power saws, the sharpness of the instruments should be maintained to reduce necrosis secondary to heating and to facilitate the operation. Unless using a drill guide, the surgeon should start drilling bone in a perpendicular direction even though the final direction may be at some angle to the direction of the bone. This prevents slipping off the desired bone entry point. Holes in long bones are stress concentration sites. Care should be taken to minimize the likelihood and degree of stress concentration by rounding holes and using drill holes to terminate saw cuts (Figure 2–2). When holes were made in bone, especially in the lower extremity, the patient should be advised against torsional loading.

Obtaining hemostasis in bone can be troublesome, and the use of microcrystalline collagen is preferred to bone wax because of the foreign body response. Postoperative bleeding is common from bony surfaces. Despite the traditional use of drains by surgeons, evidence is accumulating that at least for some operations, such as total hip or total knee replacement, wound drainage may not be necessary and may lead to increased blood loss. If drains are used, they should be secured to prevent accidental removal and should be large enough to prevent clogging by clot formation. Drains are generally removed within 48 hours of surgery unless they are used to eliminate dead space.

C. CLOSURE AND DRESSING

Wound closure should be done quickly and efficiently to minimize total operative and anesthesia time. It should also be accomplished carefully to avoid damage to the skin. When a previous scar is entered, it is sometimes worthwhile to remove scar tissue from the edge of the skin, as well as from the subcutaneous tissue, to provide a more vascular area for healing. Meticulous subcutaneous wound closure is necessary to avoid tension on the skin in many areas on the extremities. Four-throw square knots are important for knot security, especially when plans call for use of continuous passive motion machines or early motion, which may apply repetitive stress to the wound before it heals. Tissue adhesives are an advent in wound closure. One study found no difference between adhesives and sutures for closure of incisions, although the adhesives generally resulted in a more cosmetic wound.

Dressings should be padded with cotton or gauze to discourage the formation of hematomas. Closed wound suction drainage does not change outcome and is associated with a higher infection rate in total knee arthro-

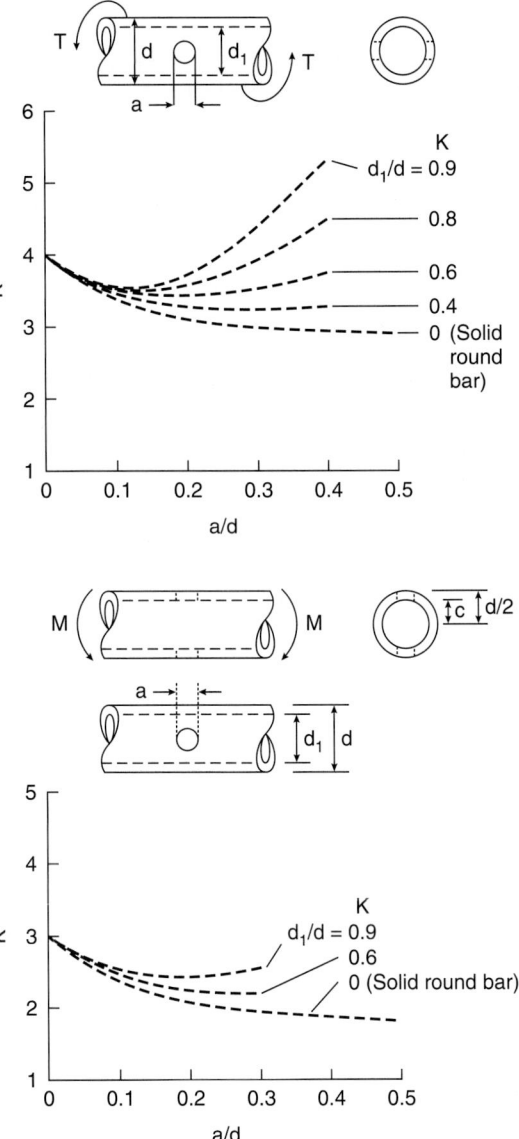

Figure 2–2. Stress concentration factors for torsion (**top**) or bending (**bottom**) of a round bar or tube with a transverse hole, where a = the size of the hole; d = the outside diameter of the tube; d_1 = the inside diameter of the tube; K = the stress concentration factor, defined as the factor by which stress is increased by the hole; M = the bending moment; and T = the torsional load. (Modified and reproduced, with permission, from Peterson RE: *Stress Concentration Factors: Charts and Relations Useful in Making Strength Calculations for Machine Parts and Structural Elements.* Wiley, 1974.)

plasty. Tape should be avoided when possible because it sometimes causes allergic reactions, and also the combination of wound swelling and shear from the tape can lead to blistering and other problems.

Batra EK et al: Influence of surgeon's tying technique on knot security. J Appl Biomater 1993;4:241. [PMID: 10146307]

Brown MD, Brookfield KF: A randomized study of closed wound suction drainage for extensive lumbar spine surgery. Spine 2004;29(10):1066. [PMID: 15131430]

Coulthard P et al: Tissue adhesives for closure of surgical incisions. Cochrane Database Syst Rev 2004;(2):CD004287. [PMID: 15106245]

Kolt JD: Use of adhesive surgical tape with the absorbable continuous subcuticular suture. ANZ J Surg 2003;73(8):626. [PMID: 12887534]

Minnema B et al: Risk factors for surgical site infections following primary total knee arthroplasty. Infect Control Hosp Epidemiol 2004;25:477. [PMID:15242195]

Ong CC, Jacobsen AS, Joseph VT: Comparing wound closure using tissue glue versus subcuticular suture for pediatric surgical incisions: A prospective randomized trial. Pediatr Surg Int 2002; 18:553. Epub accessed June 14, 2002. [PMID: 12415411]

POSTOPERATIVE CARE

Inpatient Care

Postoperative care begins in the postanesthesia room and is the same for both inpatients and outpatients. It is imperative that the orthopedic surgeon takes an active and early role in the treatment of the postoperative patient, including pain management, blood management, and DVT prophylaxis. As soon as practicable, neurologic and vascular evaluation of the operated area should be made. Sensory and motor exam of the pertinent upper or lower extremity nerves should be documented as soon as practical. Early vascular surgery consultation is indicated if pulses are absent or diminished. The wound site should be checked for excessive drainage, and, when appropriate, compartment syndrome should be considered. The general medical condition of the patient, although primarily the concern of the anesthesiologist, should be evaluated to be sure the anesthesiologist is aware of special concerns regarding the individual patient.

During the subsequent postoperative period, orthopedic aspects of care are relatively routine for most procedures. The main responsibility of the orthopedic surgeon is the evaluation of the vascular and neural status of the extremities affected by the surgery, as well as pain control and vigilance for disorders such as DVT or PE. The frequency of postsurgical examinations depends on the clinical setting. Hourly examinations may be necessary in the face of a potential compartment syndrome, although daily examinations are usually adequate. Epidural morphine analgesia may significantly mute or alter the pain picture in a compartment syndrome, making clinical evaluation difficult if not impossible in the immediate postoperative period.

A. PAIN MANAGEMENT

Pain management is a major issue in the United States. There is a growing concern that patients are undermedicated for pain control and suffering unnecessarily. The public has embraced this concept, resulting in litigation and disciplinary action by state medical boards for undermedication. Physicians traditionally were seen as being reluctant to prescribe narcotic medication as a result of concerns that they would be disciplined by state medical boards. This concept has lead to a major initiative by the JCAHO to address pain control as a patient "right." JCAHO mandates that pain control be a factor in the total evaluation of the patient and pain evaluation be performed as the fifth vital sign. The scale used is the numeric scale from 0 to 10, similar to the visual analogue scale, with 0 being no pain and 10 being unbearable pain. Acceptable pain levels are defined as 4 and below.

Pain is a very subjective sensation that is an emotional response to the process of nociception: the sum of four separate components beginning with tissue damage, which results in the first component, transduction to a nerve impulse. The next component is transmission to the spinal cord, where the third component occurs: modulation. This modulated signal is then perceived in the cerebral cortex (perception). Pain perception depends on culture, ethnicity, and gender. It is nonlinear, in that a stimulus two times higher does not necessarily result in twice the pain. Pain perception is also based on patient expectations. Studies show that preoperative patient education can reduce patients' pain after major (eg, total knee arthroplasty [TKA]) orthopedic surgery.

Traditional postoperative pain management included the administration of intravenous (IV) or intramuscular narcotic analgesics until oral narcotics were able to control the pain. The patient-controlled analgesia (PCA) is now a mainstay. In this system, morphine is used as the analgesic and typically administered IV at a rate of 1 mg/hour with a patient-controlled dose of 1 mg, which can be administered as often as every 10 minutes. Doses can be increased or decreased to tailor the dose to the patient. Dosing at this level can result in depressed respiration in some patients. However, more cautious dosing can result in insufficient pain relief that can stress the heart, leading to myocardial ischemia in some patients. Other problems can result from traditional pain management with narcotics. Patient rehabilitation can be delayed; nausea, vomiting, constipation, hallucinations, and disorientation can result in lengthened hospital stay and patient dissatisfaction.

Alternative postoperative analgesic methods are proposed. These include epidural and intrathecal administration of local anesthetics and analgesics on a continuous and one-shot basis. These methods have the potential of providing significant pain relief but must be balanced against the alternatives available and the drawbacks that each presents. The one-shot method of adding morphine to the spinal or epidural anesthetic provides pain relief for a limited time, usually on the order of 12 hours, although longer acting forms of morphine (DepoDur) are coming on the market for epidural use, providing pain relief for up to 48 hours. It has the additional problem of limiting additional narcotic analgesia by other routes because overdosing may be possible. Long-term use of continuous epidural or intrathecal analgesia poses the problem of inhibiting rehabilitation. Nurses and physical therapists tend not to mobilize patients with catheters into the spinal canal, and in some hospitals these patients are mandated to go to the intensive care unit. Nerve blocks and injections into joint cavities are limited by the length of action of the local anesthetic agent. Nerve blocks must address all nerves to an area to control postoperative pain. Hence, studies show best results with a longer term effect achieved by the use of pumps that provide a continuous anesthetic flow into the joint or body cavity, with some designs allowing an intermittent bolus for more pain relief. These pumps typically use a long-acting agent such as bupivacaine (0.25% or 0.5%) and infuse at the rate of 2–4 mL/hour. Ropivacaine is reported to have vasoconstrictive properties and less cardiotoxicity than bupivacaine, although at a higher cost.

In the past, non-narcotic pharmacologic treatment of acute postoperative pain was largely restricted to ketorolac, which can be administered by the IV or intramuscular (IM) route in the patient who is restricted in oral intake. Although ketorolac is an effective analgesic through the reduction in the need for morphine, it also increases the perioperative blood loss. After oral intake is permitted, other NSAIDs can be used for analgesics. Neither ketorolac nor other NSAIDs play a routine role in the acute pain management for most orthopedic surgical patients because of the effect these drugs have on the platelets and subsequent blood loss. The availability of COX-2 selective NSAIDs has opened up the possibility of using these drugs as major analgesics for postoperative pain control, without fear of bleeding problems. These drugs act to reduce the need for narcotics with improved pain relief and decreased narcotic side effects. On the horizon are new COX-2 drugs that can be administered parenterally, and these drugs may be of major assistance in the management of early postoperative pain. Such a drug is parecoxib, which is undergoing trials for approval by the Food and Drug Administration (FDA). The use of highly specific COX-2 inhibi-

tors or analgesics came into question with the withdrawal of rofecoxib and valdecoxib from the market because of concern over increased cardiovascular events with long-term use. At this time, other less specific NSAIDs may be considered as alternatives (celecoxib, diclofenac, meloxicam, etodolac) because their effect on platelet function is minimal.

Other analgesics and techniques do not get sufficient recognition for their role in pain control. Acetaminophen is thought to be a central prostaglandin synthase inhibitor and thereby achieves significant relief of pain. It can be tolerated in doses up to 4 g/day, and because it does not act in the same pathway as narcotics, its effect is additive to that of morphine or other narcotics and can reduce the requirement for narcotics. Another analgesic that should be used more often for analgesia is tramadol. This analgesic has very low abuse potential but provides significant analgesia, acting through inhibition of norepinephrine reuptake as well as a weak μ-agonist (similar to morphine) action. Again this mechanism of action is additive to that of traditional opioids and acetaminophen in its analgesic effect. Glucocorticoids are naturally increased in periods of stress such as surgery and are provided exogenously for those patients with suppressed adrenal function. One study showed an increase in cortisol production of 17-fold after TKA, but no such increase after knee arthroscopy. Divided doses of approximately 200 mg of hydrocortisone (8 days normal production) are typically prescribed for such patients. High doses (20 mg) of dexamethasone (equivalent to 400 mg of hydrocortisone) reduce the early postoperative pain in tonsillectomy patients. Although such doses may reduce postoperative nausea, swelling, and pain, as well as create a feeling of well-being, an increased susceptibility to infection may result from longer term dosing. Short courses of relatively high doses of glucocorticoids may be beneficial in reducing postoperative pain. Other methods of pain control may be indirect, such as controlling swelling and pain through hemostasis and cold therapy. Hemostasis may be achieved through the use of bone wax on cancellous bone or through the use of fibrin glue. Vasoconstriction from cold therapy can reduce swelling and also have a direct effect on nociceptive transduction.

A comprehensive approach to pain management can lead to beneficial effects. Multimodal analgesic regimens are suggested using several analgesics that address different points in the nociception process. Combinations of medications can include narcotics, acetaminophen, tramadol, COX-2 inhibitors, and local anesthetics administered through the use of pain pumps. Consideration should be given to administering these medications in the preanesthesia room to preempt the pain of surgery. This can also assist in diminishing peripheral sensitization that occurs with tissue damage. In addition to pharmacological interventions, patient education can reduce preoperative anxiety, reducing pain and increasing satisfaction.

Bianconi M et al: Pharmacokinetics and efficacy of ropivacaine continuous wound instillation after joint replacement surgery. Br J Anaesth 2003;91:830. [PMID: 14633754]

Cook P, Stevens J, Gaudron C: Comparing the effects of femoral nerve block versus femoral and sciatic nerve block on pain and opiate consumption after total knee arthroplasty. J Arthroplasty 2003;18:583. [PMID: 12934209]

Leopold SS et al: Endogenous cortisol production in response to knee arthroscopy and total knee arthroplasty. J Bone Joint Surg Am 2003;85:2163. [PMID: 14630847]

Mallory TH et al: Pain management for joint arthroplasty: Preemptive analgesia. J Arthroplasty 2002;17:129. [PMID: 12068423]

Rasmussen S et al: Increased flexion and reduced hospital stay with continuous intraarticular morphine and ropivacaine after primary total knee replacement: Open intervention study of efficacy and safety in 154 patients. Acta Orthop Scand 2004; 75:606-9. [PMID: 15513495]

Reuben SS et al: Evaluation of the safety and efficacy of the perioperative administration of rofecoxib for total knee arthroplasty. J Arthroplasty 2002;17:26. [PMID: 11805921]

Reuben SS, Sklar J: Pain management in patients who undergo outpatient arthroscopic surgery of the knee. J Bone Joint Surg Am 2000;82:1754. [PMID:11130650]

Sinatra RS, Torres J, Bustos AM: Pain management after major orthopedic surgery: Current strategies and new concepts. J Am Acad Ortho Surg 2002;10:117. [PMID: 11929206]

Sjoling M et al: The impact of preoperative information on state anxiety, postoperative pain and satisfaction with pain management. Patient Educ Couns 2003;51:169. [PMID: 14572947]

B. Deep Venous Thrombosis/Pulmonary Embolus

DVT, a potentially life-threatening disorder, frequently accompanies orthopedic surgery. It is much more of a problem for total joint replacements, spine surgery, and lower extremities immobilized after surgery. This is one of the expected risks after surgery. Venous thromboembolic phenomenon can result in three problems: postphlebitic syndrome, nonfatal PE, and fatal PE. It is necessary to put the risks of PE into appropriate perspective because, contrary to prevailing assumptions in the public and among orthopedic surgeons, PE can occur without surgery (Table 2–2). The risk of having a PE depends on a number of risk factors, including age, weight, the presence of varicose veins, immobility, smoking, previous DVT joint replacement, the season of the year, estrogen therapy, and the location. There is an uncertain relationship between DVT and the probability of having a PE. Obviously one cannot have a PE without having a clot, but which clots are likely to break off and become emboli, and which ones will cause problems are still unresolved issues. It is thought that thigh

Table 2–2. Rates of complications associated with total hip replacement at the Mayo Clinic.

Complication	Percentage
Death (overall)	0.5
Myocardial infarction	0.5
Pulmonary embolism	0.4
Deep venous thrombosis	1.1

Reproduced, with permission, from Mantilla et al: Poster presented at the Am Acad of Orthopedic Surgeons Annual Mtg; 2001.

clots are more important than calf clots because of their size and the potential damage they can do. It is generally conceded, however, that DVT is a marker for PE, and that is the surrogate variable used to determine the effectiveness of treatment of PE. A nonfatal PE can cause cor pulmonale, but this is thought to be an unlikely circumstance, and it is speculated that nonfatal PE would result in a residual effect in the range of 0.1–0.01% of cases. Deep venous thrombosis itself is thought to be a significant problem that results in incompetence of the valves in the deep veins of the calf and thigh. This results in persistent edema, which can progress to brawny edema and ulceration over time. However, many things are thought to cause these changes in addition to DVT. There is a uneven geographic distribution of fatal PE without surgery in the United States, with the West Coast census region having the lowest fatal PE rate. The rate of fatal PE increases with age, although age may simply be a marker for health and activity level. The rate of fatal PE in the general population older than 65 years is in the range of 0.03%, whereas approximate total joint PE rates are typically approximately 0.3%. Thus, there is a 10-fold increase in risk of having a fatal PE with a total hip or knee replacement.

Three classes of drugs can be used for chemoprophylaxis of DVT: warfarin (the vitamin K inhibitor), the low-molecular-weight heparins (dalteparin, enoxaparin, and similar drug fondaparinux), and the platelet aggregation inhibitors (aspirin, naproxen, other NSAIDs). Each approach has its advantages and disadvantages. Sodium warfarin has a slow onset of action, sometimes taking several days to reach therapeutic levels, but its oral route of administration is convenient. However, monitoring of the prothrombin time is necessary to ensure appropriate therapeutic levels. The low-molecular-weight heparins do not affect the prothrombin time or the partial thromboplastin time but do affect factor IIa and Xa levels. These do not have to be monitored because the medications are given in standard doses. These medications are provided parenterally. Both warfarin and the low-molecular-weight heparins are associated with bleeding problems. Aspirin and naproxen and other NSAIDs, although causing problems with bleeding at the time of surgery, are really not effective in prevention of DVT. Mechanical means of preventing DVT include compression hose and intermittent pneumatic compression. These are efficacious as adjunctive therapies.

The American College of Chest Physicians regularly performs and publishes metaanalyses of the data available on DVT with updated recommendations. Generally for orthopedic indications after high-risk surgery, either warfarin with an international normalized ratio (INR) of 2–3, a low-molecular-weight heparin starting 12–24 h after surgery, and elastic stockings and intermittent pneumatic compression are useful as supplemental protection against DVT. The recommended period is a minimum of 7 days. Occasionally, use of heparin or vena cava filters is recommended in high-risk situations. Table 2–3 lists the current recommendations.

The community standard in orthopedic surgery probably differs somewhat from that recommended by the American College of Chest Physicians. Newer orthopedic literature seems to suggest that warfarin is the drug of choice but with lower INR values. However, the choice of prophylactic agent is made by the doctor and the

Table 2–3. Recommendations for management of DVT prophylaxis for high-risk orthopedic patients

Procedure	Grade	Recommendation
THA/TKA	1A	LMWH started 12–24 h after surgery
		Or
	1A	Fondaparinux 2.5 mg started 6–8 h after surgery
		Or
	1A	Warfarin started immediately after surgery (Target INR 2.5, range 2.0–3.0)
Hip Fractures	1A	Fondaparinux
	1B	LDUH
	1C+	LMWH (As above when safe to use)
	2B	Warfarin (As above)
Trauma	1A	LMWH (As above when safe to use)
	1B	Elastic stockings (ES) and intermittent pneumatic compression (IPC) until LMWH is safe
Acute SCI	1B	LMWH
	1C	ES and IPC

THA = total hip arthroplasty; TKA = total knee arthroplasty; LMWH = low-molecular-weight heparin; LDUH = low dose unfractionated heparin; SCI = spinal cord injury; 1A Grade = clear risk/benefit ratio based on randomized trials without important limitations; 1B Grade = same as 1A but with inconsistent results or methodologic flaws; 1C Grade = clear risk/benefit ratio based on observation studies; 1C+ Grade = same as 1C but based on indirect evidence.
Derived from Geerts WH et al: Prevention of Venous Thromboembolism Seventh ACCP Consensus Conference. Chest (Suppl) 2004;126:338S.

patient and is influenced by their interpretation of the risk of thromboembolism and bleeding problems.

Both warfarin and heparin, either low-molecular-weight or regular, have problems that can cause catastrophic side effects in rare cases. Warfarin can cause skin necrosis and venous limb gangrene syndromes unrelated to the operative site. Heparin can induce thrombocytopenia. This is apparently an IgG antibody formation that occurs 5–10 days after starting the drug and can result in a hypercoagulable state that can result in serious problems of coagulation in unintended areas. Some new agents are becoming available, some of which are on the market at the time of this writing but are not indicated for DVT prophylaxis. These drugs are related to the antithrombin drug produced by leeches. Two of these are desirudin and bivalirudin, and they are indicated for anticoagulation in the presence of heparin-induced thrombocytopenia.

In addition, ximelagatran is an antithrombin drug that may soon be available for DVT prophylaxis as an oral prescription. A pentasaccharide (fondaparinux) is approved for DVT prophylaxis and acts in a manner similar to heparin.

1. Diagnosis—DVT is diagnosed with ultrasound in the postsurgical patient with calf swelling or with Homan's sign in the appropriate clinical setting. Several risk factors can be elicited from the history to increase the suspicion of DVT. These include immobilization, lower extremity or pelvic surgery (in the previous 4 weeks), previous history of DVT, and history of cancer. Ultrasound is a reliable screen for DVT of the thigh veins but less reliable for calf veins. The gold standard for DVT is the venogram, but this method should be used sparingly because it can be quite uncomfortable for patients. Testing for PE has evolved. In nonsurgical patients, d-dimer can be helpful in the diagnosis of PE, but the risk of PE continues for weeks after surgery so there may be a role for it in the late postoperative period. Previously, ventilation/perfusion scans were the standard method, followed by pulmonary angiography, if the probability was intermediate. Now spiral CT is quite reliable but is still only reported to be 70% sensitive and 91% specific. In outpatients with a normal ultrasound and a normal lung scan, spiral CT has only a 7% false-positive rate and 5% false-negative rate. Furthermore, evidence from a preliminary study suggests that fibrin monomer discriminates between total hip arthroplasty patients with PE and those without PE. The d-dimer was also higher in PE patients but not significantly until 7 days postoperatively.

Ananthasubramaniam K, Shuafra M, Prasad A: Heparin-induced thrombocytopenia and thrombosis. Prog Cardiovasc Dis 2000;42:247. [PMID: 10661778]

Ballard JO: Anticoagulant-induced thrombosis. JAMA 1999;282: 310. [PMID: 10432014]

Brookenthal KR et al: A meta-analysis of thromboembolic prophylaxis in total knee arthroplasty. J Arthroplasty 2001;16:293. [PMID: 11307125]

Freedman KB et al: A meta-analysis of thromboembolic prophylaxis following elective total hip arthroplasty. J Bone Joint Surg Am 2000;82:929. [PMID: 10901307]

Geerts WH et al: Prevention of venous thromboembolism: The Seventh ACCP Conference on Antithrombotic and Thrombolytic Therapy. Chest 2004;126;338S. [PMID: 15383478]

Johnson BF et al: Relationship between changes in the deep venous system and the development of post thrombotic syndrome after an acute episode of lower limb deep vein thrombosis: A one- to six-year follow-up. J Vasc Surg 1995;21:307. [PMID: 7853603]

Kane RE: Neurodeficits following epidural or spinal anesthesia. Anesth Analg 1981;60:150. [PMID: 7011100]

Kubo T et al: Fibrin monomer could be a useful predictor of pulmonary embolism after total hip arthroplasty: Preliminary report. J Orthop Sci 2001;6:119. [PMID: 11484095]

Lilienfeld DE: Decreasing mortality from pulmonary embolism in the United States, 1979–1996. Int J Epidemiol 2000;29:465. [PMID: 10869318]

Lilienfeld DE, Godbold JH: Geographic distribution of pulmonary embolism with mortality rates in the United States, 1980–1984. Am Heart J 1992;124:1068. [PMID: 1529881]

Perrier A et al: Performance of helical computed tomography in unselected outpatients with suspected pulmonary embolism. Ann Intern Med 2001;135:88. [PMID: 11453707]

Salvati E et al: Recent advances in venous thromboembolic prophylaxis during and after total hip replacement. J Bone Joint Surg Am 2000;82:252. [PMID: 10682733]

Turpie AG et al: A synthetic pentasaccharide for the prevention of deep-vein thrombosis after total hip replacement. N Engl J Med 2001;344:(9)619. [PMID: 11228275]

Weitz JI, Hirsh J: New anticoagulant drugs. Chest 2001;119;95S. [PMID: 11157644]

Wells PS et al: Excluding pulmonary embolism at the bedside without diagnostic imaging: Management of patients with suspected pulmonary embolism presenting to the emergency department by using a simple clinical model and D-dimer. Ann Intern Med 2001;135:98. [PMID: 11453709]

Outpatient Care

Economic realities today mandate earlier discharge from the hospital after some procedures and after outpatient surgery in procedures previously done on an inpatient basis. This trend suggests that patients must take more responsibility for their care, and surgeons must provide outpatient access for patients previously treated as inpatients. The indications for discharge have broadened just as the reasons for admission have narrowed. The reasons for keeping a postoperative patient in the acute-care setting are few. The main indications for hospitalization are pain control requiring parenteral narcotics, presence of hemodynamic instability, a need for traction, or a need for frequent physician observation (drains, infection, etc.). Even extended administration of IV antibiotic therapy is not an adequate reason for an acute-care stay. Thus timing of follow-up visits is important, to ensure that the patient is not only unnecessarily inconvenienced but also does not suffer delayed

recognition of a complication. In most cases, the first visit should be for suture removal (10–14 days). Again, economic realities mandate a 90-day follow-up as part of the global surgical fee. Follow-up for a total hip replacement patient might be at 2 weeks, 6 weeks, and 12 weeks after surgery. Longer or shorter intervals may be necessary, depending on how the patient is progressing and how much external support the patient is receiving (physical therapy, home nurse visits, home caregivers, and home environment). Joint-replacement patients should be followed up at least yearly on a permanent basis. The American Academy of Orthopedic Surgeons recommends prophylactic antibiotics for joint-replacement patients for procedures such as dental cleaning in which bacteremia may occur, for 2 years after joint replacement, although some surgeons recommend prophylaxis for life, especially when immune compromise is likely (eg, diabetes or renal transplant).

Long-term follow-up for patients with plates, screws, pins, rods, or other fracture devices is not typically necessary after healing of the fracture and rehabilitation of the affected muscles and joints. Antibiotic prophylaxis is not necessary for these patients. In cases of painful hardware, removal may be indicated after healing. Removal of hardware in older (more than 75 years) patients is generally not indicated. In younger (less than 50 years), active patients, hardware removal may be justified to reduce the stress concentration or stress shielding effects of the metal devices to prevent fracture prophylactically. An adequate period (12 weeks or more, depending on activity) of stress protection, especially in torsion, is indicated to reduce the risk of fracture through defects induced in the bone during removal of hardware. For a detailed discussion of rehabilitation, see Chapter 13.

Harrington P et al: Acute compartment syndrome masked by intravenous morphine from a patient-controlled analgesia pump. Injury 2000;31:387. [PMID: 10775698]

Pacheco RJ et al: Gluteal compartment syndrome after total knee arthroplasty with epidural postoperative analgesia. J Bone Joint Surg Br 2001;83:739. [PMID: 11476317]

Richards H et al: Does patient controlled analgesia delay the diagnosis of compartment syndrome following intramedullary nailing of the tibia? Injury 2004;35:296. [PMID: 15124799]

Blood Loss & Replacement

Because blood replacement is now a complicated issue, it is fortunate that not all orthopedic procedures require blood replacement. In California, the surgeon is obligated to give the patient a brochure from the state that describes the blood management options available to the surgeon and the patient when blood transfusion is likely after surgery. Many California hospitals instituted a form for the patient to sign, verifying receipt of this information. Patient involvement in the decision on how to manage blood loss is certainly a good idea. The data on when to transfuse are conflicting, however, and generally the decision is based on the physician's clinical assessment to determine the need for transfusion. Blood volume is approximately 7–8% of body weight, or approximately 5 L in a 70-kg individual. Normal individuals can be resuscitated from acute blood losses of up to 25% with crystalloid/colloid. Greater blood losses can be tolerated if the euvolemic state is maintained, but transfusion should be considered. The status of the clotting system must be monitored in the acute blood loss phase to prevent accelerated blood loss. Blood loss in the postoperative subacute phase can be managed with volume replacement and evaluation of symptomatology to determine the need for transfusion of red cell mass. Patients at risk of stroke, myocardial infarction, or those with decreased cardiac output may need transfusion at higher hemoglobin levels. Younger (less than 50 years), healthier patients may tolerate lower hemoglobin levels unless they have postural hypotension, tachycardia, dizziness, or fainting.

A. CRITERIA FOR BLOOD TRANSFUSION

The decision to transfuse in the immediate postoperative period is predicated on numerous factors, including age, medical condition and cardiac status, estimated blood loss, projected blood loss, availability of blood (autologous, designated donor, or bank), and the patient's perception of risk. Consideration of all factors argues against transfusion in the younger (less than 50 years) or healthier patient until the patient has a hematocrit level of 20–22% or has symptoms that include tachycardia, early and postural hypotension, and dizziness or fainting. Older (more than 60 years) patients at risk of stroke or myocardial infarction would be candidates for transfusion at higher hematocrit levels or with a lower threshold of symptoms.

B. STRATEGIES FOR MINIMIZING THE RISKS ASSOCIATED WITH BLOOD TRANSFUSION

Blood loss is an inevitable part of surgery. With the realization that the banked blood supply is at low risk, but still at risk, of containing infectious agents, strategies to minimize the risk of transmission were developed.

An obvious method of accomplishing this goal is to reduce blood loss. Anesthetic techniques to reduce mean arterial blood pressure can reduce blood loss by reducing the time of surgery as well as the actual blood loss. The patient has to be counseled to avoid antiplatelet drugs in the period prior to surgery. These medications include baby aspirin but also all of the ubiquitous NSAIDs that are in over-the-counter analgesics, cough and cold remedies, and arthritis medications. In the operative period, topical agents such as bone wax, Gelfoam and similar collagen products, thrombin, tranex-

amic acid and aminocaproic acid (antifibrinolytic), and fibrin glue should be considered. Tranexamic acid can be administered IV or locally to help control bleeding. Surgical technique should be efficient and meticulous to reduce time and therefore blood loss. The patient should be positioned to minimize venous pressure and blood loss, such as positioning a postoperative total knee in flexion to reduce blood loss.

Presurgical banking of autologous blood by the patient (with or without hematopoietic growth factors), immediate preoperative autodonation by hemodilution, and salvage of the patient's intraoperative and postoperatively lost blood with infusion of either washed or unwashed red cells can reduce the patient's exposure to the risks of designated donor blood or homologous banked blood. The problems with autologous blood begin with the cost, but there are other issues. Older (more than 70 years) patients sometimes do not tolerate the anemia from donation. Perhaps the greatest risks are bacterial contamination and clerical error, in which someone gets a potentially fatal ABO-incompatible unit instead of his or her own. Autologous blood that is not used is discarded and not put into the general blood bank pool.

Preoperative hemodilution has the cost associated with the operating room time to draw off the blood and that of the anesthesiologist in supervising the process. Preoperative hematocrit can be boosted through parenteral erythropoietin, which can minimize the effect of surgical blood loss. Erythropoietin is estimated to cost $900 per unit of blood saved, which is more than the cost of autologous blood at $300–400/unit. Furthermore, there may be risks with abnormally high hematocrits. Thus it is only considered when there is little other choice, such as for surgery on Jehovah's Witnesses who refuse transfusions.

Despite initial resistance and continued questions about cost effectiveness by blood bank officials, autologous blood donation has achieved considerable acceptability from patients, physicians, and blood bank administrators. There are disadvantages of autologous donation that counterbalance the obvious advantages of eliminating transfusion-related disease and incompatibility. These are possible bacterial contamination of the blood, perioperative anemia with increased risk of transfusion, administrative error resulting in blood incompatibility from receiving the wrong blood, cost, and wastage of autologous blood that is not used. Blood can be stored for 35 days or can be frozen as a red cell mass for up to 1 year, but loss in viability of the red cells occurs with both storage methods. Use of autologous blood can eliminate the need for banked blood for many but not all orthopedic patients. Some patients, for example, have marginal laboratory test results (eg, Hgb level of 10 g/dL and hematocrit level of 30%) that preclude their predonation of blood. The ability of patients to predonate blood and the amount of blood donated can sometimes be increased through the use of recombinant human erythropoietin therapy. Injections can be given twice weekly and may result in a higher red cell mass collected and a higher hematocrit level at the time of hospital admission. Although expensive, this therapy can be of benefit to patients, especially those who have blood types that are difficult to match or have religious beliefs that conflict with the practice of receiving blood from others.

Red blood cells can be salvaged by suction in the operating room or collected via surgical drains in the recovery room. Adequate loss of blood must be present to make these procedures cost effective. The salvaged blood is generally washed to remove cell debris, fat, and bone fragments. Newer filtration techniques permit the transfusion of blood collected from drains without the washing process.

Bezwada HP et al: Preoperative use of recombinant human erythropoietin before total joint arthroplasty. J Bone Joint Surg Am 2003;85:1795. [PMID: 12954840]

Goodnough LT: Autologous blood donation. Crit Care 2004;8 (Suppl 2):S49. [PMID: 15196325]

Keating EM, Ritter MA: Transfusion options in total joint arthroplasty. J Arthroplasty 2002;17:125. [PMID: 12068422]

Sparling EA et al: The use of erythropoietin in the management of Jehovah's witnesses who have revision total hip arthroplasty. J Bone Joint Surg Am 1996;78:1548. [PMID: 8876583]

Strumper D et al: Clinical efficacy of postoperative autologous transfusion of filtered shed blood in hip and knee arthroplasty. Transfusion 2004;44:1567. [PMID: 15504161]

Zohar E et al: The postoperative blood-sparing efficacy of oral versus intravenous tranexamic acid after total knee replacement. Anesth Analg 2004;99:1679. [PMID: 15562053]

Ethics in Orthopedic Surgery

Ethics in medicine started with Hippocrates and was codified by Thomas Percival in 1803, with the publication of his Code of Medical Ethics. This was extended by the American Medical Association in 1847 and has undergone several revisions over time. Ethics basically define the standards of conduct of honorable or moral behavior by the physician. Many areas of medical ethics, such as abortion or artificial insemination, have little to do with orthopedics. Although many areas of ethics are more restrictive than the law, litigation and legislation have in some cases become the standard by which orthopedists have to abide, with tighter constraints than ethics alone would place. Although ethics as a field is too broad a subject for a text such as this, certain areas that impinge on orthopedics are addressed here.

Clinical Trials

A particularly difficult ethical area is the clinical research study. Although many of these are now more than ade-quately controlled by institutional review boards (IRBs), the federal government's Office for Human Research Protections, and sponsors of research, the single practitioner in a small orthopedic group is still at risk of performing human, or even animal, research without appropriate ethical controls. The three main areas for concern are the use of ionizing radiation for exams that are not clinically indicated, the use of patient or third-party-payer funds for exams that are not clinically indicated, and the use of patient data in a manner that does not maintain confidentiality. Certainly, ionizing radiation can be used, even for control subjects, if adequate IRB review and patient/subject consent is obtained. This must be done in a formal manner. However, the use of third-party-payer funds for research or revealing patient confidentiality is never ethical. Performing unindicated studies (laboratory, radiographs) at patient expense is certainly unethical. Also, patient confidentiality is fundamental to the doctor–patient relationship. The Health Insurance Portability and Accountability Act changed the way physicians have to look at confidentiality. Verbal, written, and electronic privacy must be maintained in the office and hospital setting. Patient data have to be closely controlled with care taken regarding personal data assistants, scraps of paper with patient identifiers and data, and roentgenographic images. Photos or slides of football injuries in the public domain may be acceptable for presentation, although in some situations this may not be true. Certainly, photos or slides of radiographs with patient identifiers for professional presentations or publications cannot be used without written patient permission. The electronic medical record will produce many potential areas that might violate Health Insurance Portability and Accountability Act (HIPAA) regulations, especially with local area networks that permit laptop access in an entire office or building.

The typical orthopedic clinical research study is a retrospective review of a surgeon's cases. This model of research is considered to be of modest value by researchers doing multicenter, randomized, controlled, double-blind studies, but until the funding is found to do this type of study on something as common as knee replacement, retrospective reviews will have to serve as the database for decision making. This is especially be true for low-volume procedures. These types of studies raise several issues. The main issues are paying for the study (not through patient or third-party funds), maintaining patient confidentiality, and conflict of interest. The first two issues can be resolved by IRB oversight, and private practitioners are advised to obtain that help from their hospital. Conflict of interest has at least two aspects. Physicians may be consultants or designers of the prosthesis or drug and have a financial interest in the success of the product, and they have ego invested in their surgery, that is, they do not want to look like "bad" surgeons and hence may be hesitant to report poor results. Furthermore, they may be professors and need to demonstrate clinical research publications as part of promotion requirements or simply want to "advertise" their abilities through publication. The latter aspects are implied conflicts of interest but are probably as important as a financial conflict. The potential financial conflict should be disclosed to the patient and to other parties such as the hospital and to the journal of publication. Surgeons have an ethical obligation to share medical advances, and presenting surgeons' results with a procedure certainly meets that standard.

Gifts from Industry

The concept that gifts from industry may affect the choice of medication, prosthesis, and so on, is of concern. Generally, the guidelines recommended by the American Medical Association allow gifts, other remuneration, subsidies for meetings, and so on, if the primary purpose is education or of benefit to the patient. Gifts should be of minimal value and related to the physician's work. The pharmaceutical and orthopedic manufacturers are now self-regulated by industry organizations regarding the type of meetings that they can sponsor. Meetings directly sponsored by the company are only allowed to discuss "label" applications of the

drug or device, whereas continuing medical education credit courses, which can only be done through an educational institution, can discuss "off-label" uses of products. Payment for travel costs, lodging, and honoraria to attend such meetings is considered inappropriate unless the physician is performing a service, such as faculty duties or consulting. Although it seems unlikely that a physician would change his or her prescribing practice based on a free meal, the appearance of impropriety is important and should be kept in mind.

Cartwright JC et al: Navigating federalwide assurance requirements when conducting research in community-based care settings. J Am Geriatr Soc 2004;52:1567. [PMID: 15341563]

Council on Ethical and Judicial Affairs: *Code of Medical Ethics: Current Opinions with Annotations* (2000–2001 edition). American Medical Association, 2000.

Epps CH: Ethical guidelines for orthopedists and industry. Clin Orthop 2003;412:14. [PMID: 12838046]

Laskin RS, Davis JP: The use of a personal digital assistant in orthopaedic surgical practice. Clin Orthop 2004;421:91. [PMID: 15123932]

Oyama L, Tannas HS, Moulton S: Desktop and mobile software development for surgical practice. J Pediatr Surg 2002;37:477. [PMID:11877671]

Pancoast PE, Patrick TB, Mitchell JA: Physician PDA and the HIPAA privacy rule. J Am Med Inform Assoc 2003;10:611. [PMID: 14631929]

Musculoskeletal Trauma Surgery 3

Wade R. Smith, MD, Juan F. Agudelo, MD, Anand Parekh, MRCS (Eng), & John R. Shank, MD

The High Cost of Musculoskeletal Trauma

Trauma is the "neglected disease." It is the leading cause of death for people age 1 to 34 years of all races and socioeconomic levels and the third leading cause of death for all age groups. Injuries create a substantial burden on society in terms of medical resources used for treating and rehabilitating injured persons, productivity losses caused by morbidity and premature mortality, and pain and suffering of injured persons and their caregivers. Each year in the United States, one in six residents requires medical treatment for an injury, and one in 10 residents visits a hospital emergency department (ED) for treatment of a nonfatal injury. Data on injury prevalence and costs from the 2000 Medical Expenditure Panel Survey (MEPS) and the National Health Accounts (NHA) reported that injury-attributable medical expenditures cost as much as $117 billion in 2000, approximately 10% of total U.S. medical expenditures. In 2001, there were 157,078 trauma-related deaths, 64% of which were due to unintentional trauma, half of which were caused by motor vehicle crashes. An estimated 29.7 million persons sustained nonfatal injuries during the same period. In 2001, the death rates for motor vehicle-related injuries were 15.3 per 100,000 people, totalling 43,987. Crash injuries result in about 500,000 hospitalizations and four million emergency department visits annually. The economic burden of motor vehicle-related deaths and injuries is also enormous, costing the United States more than $150 billion each year. In 2001, approximately 140,000 Americans sustained gunshot injuries. Twenty-nine thousand of these (21%) died as a result. In the pediatric population, 10,000 deaths associated with trauma are recorded annually in the United States. Trauma accounts for 30% of pediatric emergency room visits and is the most common cause of mortality in the noninfant child.

Musculoskeletal disorders generated 3.5 million admissions to acute-care hospitals in the United States in 1988, more than 40% of which were trauma-related. Musculoskeletal injuries have a tremendous effect on the patient, the family, and the society in general because of the

1. physical and psychologic effects of pain, limitation of daily activities, loss of independence, and reduced quality of life;
2. direct expenditures for diagnosis and treatment; and
3. indirect economic costs associated with lost labor and diminished productivity.

Musculoskeletal injuries occur frequently, result in significant disability, and consume a major portion of health care resources. For example, the cost of hip fracture is estimated at $8.7 billion, or 43% of the total cost of all fractures. Direct costs are about 80% of the total, of which inpatient hospital care amounts to $3.1 billion and nursing home care $1.6 billion. More recent estimates show an increasing effect on the U.S. economy, including over $150 billion per year in direct and indirect cost from lost labor productivity due to trauma.

Mass casualty situations as a result of terrorism are the challenge of the new millennium, requiring a highly organized and effective trauma system. The capability to respond in an organized manner has gained importance after terrorist attacks within United States. In a mass casualty situation, limited resources must be allocated for a great number of victims. The terrorist attacks in Oklahoma City (1995) and at the World Trade Center (1993, 2001) showed the inefficiencies of the civilian disaster response system. The Orthopaedic Trauma Association has developed strategies to educate and optimize the response to mass casualties.

Surveillance for fatal and nonfatal injuries-United States, 2001. Vyrostek SB, Annest JL, Ryan GW. MMWR September 3, 2004/Vol. 53/No. SS-7. CDC.

Medical expenditures attributable to injuries-United States, 2000. MMWR January 16,2004. CDC.

Engelhardt S et al: The 15-year evolution of an urban trauma center: What does the future hold for the trauma surgeon? J Trauma 2001;51:633. [PMID: 11586151]

Praemer A, Furner S, Rice DP: Musculoskeletal conditions in the United States. Am Acad Orthop Surg, Park Ridge IL, 1992.

Soderstrom CA, Cole FJ, Porter JM: Injury in America: The role of alcohol and other drugs—an EAST position paper prepared by the injury control and violence prevention committee. J Trauma 2001;50:1. [PMID: 11253757]

Wynn A et al: Accuracy of administrative and trauma registry database. J Trauma 2001;51:464. [PMID: 11535892]

THE HEALING PROCESS

Bone Healing

Bone is a unique tissue because it heals by the formation of normal bone, as opposed to scar tissue. In fact, it is considered a nonunion when a bone heals by a fibroblastic response instead of by bone formation. Whatever part of the skeleton it comes from, bone has a fine fibroid structure. This is true for cortical and cancellous bone from the diaphysis, epiphysis, or metaphysis. Bone will, therefore, heal by the same mechanism wherever it breaks.

Fracture healing can be divided into primary and secondary healing. In primary healing, the cortex attempts to reestablish itself without the formation of callus (osteonal or haversian healing). This occurs when the fracture is anatomically reduced, the blood supply is preserved, and the fracture is rigidly stabilized by internal fixation. Secondary fracture healing results in the formation of callus and involves the participation of the periosteum and external soft tissues. This fracture healing response is enhanced by motion and is inhibited by rigid fixation.

Fracture healing can be conveniently divided, based on the biologic events taking place, into the following four stages

1. Hematoma formation (inflammation) and angiogenesis.
2. Cartilage formation with subsequent calcification
3. Cartilage removal and bone formation
4. Bone remodeling

A. HEMATOMA FORMATION AND ANGIOGENESIS

Initially, there is an inflammatory phase characterized by an accumulation of mesenchymal cells around the fracture site. The formed hematoma is a source of growth factors. Transforming growth factor beta (TGF-β) and platelet derived-growth factor (PDGF) are released from platelets at the fracture site. TGF-β induces mesenchymal cells and osteoblasts to produce type II collagen and proteoglycans. PDGF recruits inflammatory cells at the fracture site. Bone morphogenetic proteins (BMPs) are osteoinductive mediators inducing metaplasia of mesenchymal cells into osteoblasts. IL-1 (interleukin-1) and IL-6 recruit inflammatory cells to the fracture site. In fractures where the periosteum is intact, these cells probably come from the cambium. In higher energy fractures where the periosteum has been compromised, the appearance of spindle-shaped cells that are able to differentiate into osteogenic cells has been found to coincide with the appearance of capillary buds. These cells are possibly derived from the pericytes found around capillaries, arterioles, and venules.

Whatever their origin, these cells ensheathe the fracture and differentiate into chondrocytes or osteoblasts. Low-oxygen tension, low pH, and movement favor the differentiation into chondrocytes; high-oxygen tension, high pH, and stability predispose to osteoblasts. Bone morphogenetic proteins (BMPs) and cytokines (IL-1, IL-6) are present during cartilage formation. This initial callus acts as an internal splint against bending and rotational deformation and, less effectively, against shearing and axial deformation. Because the stiffness of this callus in bending and torsion varies with the fourth power of the radius, its distribution around the fracture is important; peripheral distribution adds to rigidity. Clinically, the fracture becomes "sticky," and although some motion is detectable, the fracture is stable.

B. CARTILAGE FORMATION WITH SUBSEQUENT CALCIFICATION

Radiologic evidence of mineral formation signals the onset of this phase. Cartilage in callus is replaced by woven bone by a process analogous to the endochondral ossification seen in the fetus. The mechanism of mineralization is poorly understood but is thought to involve active transport of minerals and their precipitation from a supersaturated solution. Mineralization causes the chondrocytes themselves to degenerate and die. Capillary buds then invade the mineralized cartilage, bringing osteoblasts, which resorb part of the calcified cartilage and deposit coarse fibroid bone on its residuum. The proliferating cambium layer of the periosteum also lays down new bone on the exposed surface of the bone, if conditions are favorable.

The phase of mineralized callus leads to a state in which the fracture site is enveloped in a polymorphous mass of mineralized tissues consisting of calcified cartilage, woven bone made from cartilage, and woven bone formed directly.

C. CARTILAGE REMOVAL AND BONE FORMATION

The woven-bone mineralized callus has to be replaced by lamellar bone arranged in osteonal systems to allow the bone to resume its normal function. Before this stage of remodeling can start, it is necessary to consolidate the fracture site. The concept of consolidation is poorly defined but includes filling the gaps left by the previous phase between the ends of the bone; it is also called **gap-healing bone.** This bone has three major characteristics:

1. It forms only under conditions of mechanical stability;
2. It has the ability to replace fibrous or muscle tissue; and
3. It forms within the confines of the bone defect

Gap-healing bone is essentially coarse fibroid bone and, therefore, is not normal lamellar bone.

D. REMODELING

This final phase involves the replacement of woven bone by lamellar bone in various shapes and arrangements and is necessary to restore the bone to optimal function. This process involves the simultaneous meticulously coordinated removal of bone from one site and deposition in another.

Two lines of cells, osteoclasts and osteoblasts, are responsible for this process. Osteoclasts are derived from monocytes and are large multinucleated cells that remove bone. They are located on the resorption surfaces of the bone. Osteoblasts are mononuclear and are responsible for the accretion of bone.

Cartilage Healing

Articular cartilage consists of extracellular matrix (ECM) and chondrocytes. The ECM is formed by water (65% to 80%), collagen (95% type II) and proteoglycans (chondroitin sulfate and keratan sulfate). Collagen in the ECM provides form and tensile strength. Proteoglycans and water give the cartilage stiffness, resilience and endurance.

Chondrocytes are sparse in the adult cartilage, which is not a vascularized tissue. Their nutrition comes from the synovial fluid and depends on the health of the synovial membrane and adequate circulation of the fluid through the spongelike cartilage matrix. Motion of the joint is responsible for most of this circulation. A good part of the rationale behind rigid internal fixation of fractures is to allow early motion of the joints. The same argument can be made for early weight bearing of immobilized joints, which allows cyclical compression of the cartilage and circulation of the synovial fluid.

Rapidly applied forces to the articular cartilage prevent adequate fluid movement and load distribution leading to rupture of the ECM macromolecular framework and cell damage. Articular cartilage lesions are classified according to the type of damage and reparative response:

1. Injuries to the cartilage matrix and cells.
   Caused by acute or repetitive blunt trauma. Evidence of alterations in ECM (decrease in proteoglycans concentration, disruptions of the collagen fibril framework), without macroscopic evidence of damage. It has potential for repair.
2. Chondral fissures, flap tears, or chondral defects.
   Limited, short chondrocytic reparative response. Loss of segmental cartilage.
3. Osteochondral injuries.
   Hemorrhage, fibrin clot formation and inflammatory response. Fibrocartilage formation. Inferior mechanical properties.

Articular cartilage has limited reparative capacities because chondrocytes have a low baseline metabolic rate, a small cell-to-matrix ratio, and a restricted mode of nutrition. If the defect in the cartilage does not go through the calcified plate, the body attempts repair with hyaline cartilage. It will be, however, incomplete, except for the smallest defects. If the calcified plate is violated, the subchondral capillaries bring an inflammatory reaction, which fills the defect with granulation tissue and, eventually, fibrocartilage. The quality of this fibrocartilage can be improved by passive or active motion of the joint. Basic and clinical research has shown the potential of artificial matrices, growth factors, perichondrium, periosteum and transplanted chondrocytes and mesenchymal stem cells to stimulate the formation of cartilage in articular defects.

Tendon Healing

Tendons are specialized structures that allow muscles to concentrate or extend their action. The Achilles tendon, for example, concentrates the action of the bulky muscles of the calf over a small area where a large force needs to be applied for pushoff. Tendons consist of long bundles of collagen scattered with relatively inactive fibrocytes. These cells are nourished by the synovial fluid secreted by the one-cell-thick synovial membrane that covers the tendon (endotenon) and the parietal surface of the sheath (epitenon). The flexor tendons are covered by a richly vascularized adventitia (paratenon).

Muscle Healing

Human skeletal muscle is divided into fiber types depending on their metabolic activity and mechanical function. Type 1 fiber, known as **slow twitch, slow oxidative,** or **red,** muscle, has a slow speed of contraction and the greatest strength of contraction. It functions aerobically and, therefore, is fatigue-resistant. Type 2 fiber, known as **fast twitch** or **white** muscle, is subdivided into two types, according to metabolic activity level: fiber that functions by oxidative and glycolytic metabolism (type 2A) and fiber that is largely glycolytic (type 2B). Both subtypes of white fast-twitch muscles are fatigable but have high strength of contraction and high speed of contraction. Fiber type interconversion can occur, but this is generally believed to happen only under extreme conditions. It is generally conceded that the relative proportions of type 1 and type 2 fibers are defined genetically, with little capacity for change. Thus, sprinters are unlikely to become cross-country runners, and vice versa. Interconversion between type 2A and 2B fibers is much more likely, depending on the type of athletic training.

Traumatic injury to muscle can occur from a variety of mechanisms, including blunt trauma, laceration, or ischemia. Recovery occurs through a process of degeneration and regeneration, with new muscle cells arising from undifferentiated cells. Traumatic injuries include muscle laceration, muscle contusion (blunt injury), and strains resulting from excessive stretching. In addition to muscle regeneration, laceration repair requires reinnervation of denervated muscle areas. Muscle contusion frequently results in hematoma. The normal repair process includes an inflammatory reaction, formation of connective tissue, and muscle regeneration. Blunt trauma may result in myositis ossificans and may cause decreased function. Muscle strains go by a variety of names, including **muscle pull** and **muscle tear.** The failure frequently occurs at the myotendinous junction in experimental animals but may also be within the muscle itself rather than at the bone-tendon junction.

Of particular concern to the traumatologist is the effect of immobilization on muscle tissue. As with all tissues, immobilization and lack of activity result in atrophy. Loss of muscle weight initially occurs rapidly and then tends to stabilize, and loss of strength occurs simultaneously. Resistance to fatigue diminishes rapidly. These changes are minimized if immobilization occurs with some stretching of the muscle. Prevention of "fracture disease" after trauma requires an understanding of muscle physiologic principles.

Nerve Healing

Peripheral nerves have a distinct anatomic structure, with multiple nerve fibers combined to form a fascicle surrounded by perineurium. Multiple fascicles are surrounded by epineurium. Nerves fall into patterns of monofascicular, oligofascicular, and polyfascicular structures. The size and distribution of fascicles change as a function of length, reflecting greater or lesser nerve fibers in each fascicle. Around joints, fascicles typically tend to be multiple and small, perhaps to reduce injury from mechanical trauma. In addition, these nerves tend to have thicker epineurium near joints, with many small fascicles, and this may tend to protect the nerve from flexion and extension cycles. Nerve damage may occur through direct compression or stretching injuries. Ischemic damage from stretching may occur at elongation of 15%. Nerve injuries are now rated from 1 to 5 degrees. First-degree injury is the least severe and is equivalent to neurapraxia. The nerve (axon) is in continuity, and loss of function is reversible. Second-degree injury is equivalent to axonotmesis, with degeneration of the axon. The endoneurial sheath remains in continuity, however, and regeneration occurs by growth of the axon down its original endoneurial tube. Third-degree injury is the same as second-degree injury with the addition of loss of continuity of the endoneurial tube. The perineurium is preserved, however. Because of damage to the fascicle, some misdirection of regenerating axons may occur, and the extent of functional return depends on the extent of misdirection. Fourth-degree injuries preserve only the continuity of the nerve trunk but involve much more extensive degeneration of the fascicles. Despite the continuity of the nerve trunk,

this injury may require excision of the damaged segment, with reapproximation of the nerve ends to achieve a functional outcome. Fifth-degree injury involves complete loss of continuity of the nerve trunk. Surgical repair, obviously, is required to achieve restoration of function.

Functional recovery after nerve injury depends on a number of variables. The outcome is much more optimistic for children than adults, and the prognosis diminishes with age. Increasing distance from the nerve injury to the distal point of innervation reduces the likelihood of recovery. Other factors include the length of the damage to the nerve, the technical ability of the surgeon, and the length of time prior to repair.

Buckwalter JA. Articular cartilage injuries. Clin Orthop 2002; 402:21-37. [PMID: 14620787]

Jackson DW, Scheer MJ, Simon TM: Cartilage substitutes: Overview of basic science and treatment options. J Am Acad Orthop Surg 2001;9:37. [PMID: 11174162]

Browne JE, Branch TP: Surgical alternatives for treatment of articular cartilage lesions. J Am Acad Orthop Surg 2000;8:180. [PMID: 10874225]

Lee SK, Wolfe SW: Peripheral nerve injury and repair. J Am Acad Orthop Surg 2000;8:243. [PMID: 10951113]

Robinson LR: Role of neurophysiologic Evaluation in diagnosis. J Am Acad Orthop Surg 2000;8:190. [PMID: 10874226]

ORTHOPEDIC ASSESSMENT & MANAGEMENT OF POLYTRAUMA PATIENTS

A thorough understanding of the pathophysiology of trauma is essential for prompt diagnosis and timely treatment of musculoskeletal injuries. Sound therapeutic principles improve the overall outcome for the patient and optimize the utilization of limited health care resources.

Life-Threatening Conditions: The ABCs of Trauma Care

A systematic approach is required in all cases. The patient is assessed and treatment priorities are established according to the type of injury, stability of vital signs, and mechanism of injury. In a severely injured patient, treatment priorities are dictated by the patient's overall condition, with the first goal being to save life and preserve the major functions of the body. Assessment consists of four overlapping phases:

1. Primary survey (ABCDE)
2. Resuscitation
3. Secondary survey (head-to-toe evaluation and history) and
4. Definitive care

This process, identifies and treats life-threatening conditions, and can be remembered as follows:

Airway maintenance (with cervical spine protection);
Breathing and ventilation;
Circulation (with hemorrhage control);
Disability (neurologic status);
Exposure and environmental control (undress the patient but prevent hypothermia).

A brief overview of the treatment of polytrauma patients, with special emphasis on the orthopedic aspects, follows:

A. AIRWAY

Great care should be taken while assessing the airway. The cervical spine should be carefully protected at all times and not be hyperextended, hyperflexed, or rotated to obtain a patent airway. The airway should be rapidly assessed for signs of obstruction, foreign bodies and facial, mandibular, or tracheal/laryngeal fractures. A chin lift or jaw thrust maneuver should be used to establish an airway. A Glasgow Coma Scale of 8 or less is an indication for the placement of a definitive airway. The history of the trauma incident is essential because it provides immediate clues to associated injuries. A normal neurologic examination or cross-table lateral radiograph of the cervical spine, including the C7-T1 disk space, does not rule out cervical spine injuries; it only makes them less likely. Any patient with a blunt injury above the clavicle should be considered at risk for cervical spine injury).

B. BREATHING

The trauma surgeon should evaluate the patient's chest. Adequate ventilation requires not only airway patency but also adequate oxygenation and carbon dioxide elimination. Remember that the following four conditions, if present, must be addressed emergently:

1. Tension pneumothorax
2. Flail chest with pulmonary contusion
3. Open pneumothorax and
4. Massive hemothorax

C. CIRCULATION

Hemorrhage is the principal cause of postinjury deaths that are preventable. Postinjury hypotension is considered hypovolemic in origin until proved otherwise. Level of consciousness, skin color and pulses are simple to assess and reliably mirror the hemodynamic status of the patient, especially if recorded serially. Fractures of the femur or the pelvis can cause major blood loss, which can severely compromise the ultimate survival of the patient. (See sections on pelvic and femoral fracture.)The orthopaedic surgeon as a member of the trauma team should be alert to the possibility of extremity blood loss and communicate its estimate to the trauma team leader.

D. DISABILITY (NEUROLOGIC STATUS)

The Glasgow Coma Scale (see Chapter 13) should be used to assess neurologic status; it is quick, simple, and predictive of patient outcome. An even simpler way to monitor central neurologic status is to remember the mnemonic AVPU and check if the patient is

*A*lert and oriented,
or responds to *V*ocal stimuli,
or responds only to *P*ainful stimuli,
or is *U*nresponsive.

E. EXPOSURE AND ENVIRONMENTAL CONTROL

Recognition of lacerations, contusions, abrasions, swelling and deformity can only be accomplished in the completely disrobed patient. The safest way to achieve this is to cut off all clothing. This permits complete examination of the patient, prevents further displacement of fractures and minimizes the risk of overlooking significant problems. Hypothermia must be avoided, as cardiac function may be affected, especially when there is decreased blood volume. Sterile dressings should be applied to any wounds and wound exploration in the emergency department should be avoided to prevent further contamination.

F. CARE OF PATIENT BEFORE HOSPITALIZATION

The diagnosis and treatment of musculoskeletal injuries in polytrauma patients should be initiated in the field by the paramedics. Recognition and appropriate splinting of major fractures, adequate immobilization of the cervical spine, and proper handling of the injured patient are essential to prevent further damage to the neurovascular elements and limit hemorrhage. In many cases, proper care at this stage will prevent or limit shock as well as avoid catastrophic damage to the spinal cord.

The old saying "splint them where they lie" remains especially true when the exact nature and extent of the fractures remain obscure. As a general rule, the following measures should be taken:

1. The joints above and below the fracture should be immobilized.
2. Splints can be improvised with pillows, blankets, or clothing.
3. Immobilization does not need to be absolutely rigid.
4. Apply gentle in-line traction to realign the extremity in severe angulation.
5. Overt bleeding should be tamponaded with available dressings and firm pressure.
6. Tourniquets should be avoided, unless it is obvious that the patient's life is in danger.

Orthopedic Examination

A. HISTORY

Injury mechanism: an adequate assessment of the conditions in which the injury was sustained is crucial. Information from paramedics, patient relatives and bystanders should be recorded. Obtain the following information according to injury mechanism:

1. MVA: speed; direction (T bone, rollover etc.); patient location in the vehicle, impact location, postimpact location of the patient (if ejection, determine distance); internal and external damage to the vehicle; restraint use and type.
2. Falls: distance of the fall; landing position.
3. Crush: weight of the object, site of the injury, duration of weight application.
4. Explosion: blast magnitude; patient distance from the blast: primary blast injury (force of the blast wave); secondary blast injury (projectiles).
5. Vehicle-pedestrian: type of vehicle, site of collision, speed.

Environmental exposure, comorbidity, pre-hospital care and observations at the accident scene should be determined. Estimated bleeding, open wounds, deformity, motor and sensory function and delays in extrication or transport are recorded.

B. GENERAL EXAMINATION

The clinical orthopedic examination requires assessment of the axial skeleton, pelvis, and extremities. The extent of this examination depends on the patient's overall central neurologic status. Swelling, hematomas, and open wounds are assessed visually in the undressed patient. It is obligatory to palpate the entire spine, pelvis, and each joint. Examination soon after trauma may precede telltale swelling in joint or long bone injuries. In the unresponsive patient, only crepitation and false motion may be discerned. Patients with a better mental status, however, can provide feedback regarding pain resulting from palpation. The pelvis is examined by gentle compression of the iliac wings in a mediolateral, anterior-posterior direction and palpation of the pubis. However, if the patient is hemodynamically unstable, manipulation of the pelvis should be avoided in order to prevent increased bleeding. The AP pelvis x-ray must then be used to assess the pelvis as a potential source of shock.

C. NEUROLOGIC EXAMINATION

The neurologic examination of the extremities should be documented to the fullest extent possible, in light of the patient's mental status, as it is central to subsequent decision making. This examination includes delineation of sensory function in the major nerves and dermatomes in the upper and lower extremities. Perianal sensation is also important. Thus, in the upper extremity, dermatomes from C5–T1 and radial, ulnar, and median nerve function must be assessed.

D. MUSCLE EXAMINATION

Motor examination can be difficult because of pain or impaired mental status, but even in such cases, useful and relatively complete information can be obtained. In the upper extremity, the function of the deltoid, biceps, brachioradialis, extensor pollicis longus, flexor carpi radialis, and intrinsic muscles (first dorsal interosseus and opponens pollicis muscles) must be examined. A more complete examination is indicated if there is obvious trauma to this area. In the lower extremity, the motor supply to the extensor hallucis longus, tibialis anterior, peroneal muscles, gastrocnemius, and quadriceps muscles must be tested and graded. Muscle strength grading is desirable, but demonstration of a minimum of volitional control (even if withdrawal to painful stimuli) is important in verifying the presence of intact central sensory-motor integration.

Particularly important in the face of spinal cord injury or suspected injury are the reflexes of the anal "wink" and bulbocavernosus muscle. Other spinal reflexes (ie, of the biceps and triceps muscles, of the knee and ankle, and the Babinski reflex) are important in "fine-tuning" the neurologic examination. (These are discussed more fully in Chapter 5, "Disorders, Disease, & Injuries of the Spine.")

Imaging Studies

Radiologic assessment follows the same general hierarchy as the clinical assessment. The severely injured polytrauma patient requires plain films of the chest, abdomen, *and* pelvis to indicate sources of respiratory and circulatory compromise. The second level of examination requires the cervical spine cross-table lateral view. The information obtained from this film dictates treatment and the need for any further evaluation of the cervical spine. In the hemodynamically unstable patient, the AP pelvis film is sufficient to make immediate treatment decisions. Complementary pelvis films can be obtained later on.

Subsequent evaluation is dependent on clinical findings. Any long bone or joint with a laceration, hematoma, angulation, or swelling must undergo roentgenographic evaluation. Any long bone fracture requires complete evaluation of the joints proximal and distal to the fracture. At the minimum, two views of the extremities are needed, usually the anteroposterior and lateral views. Coordination of more sophisticated studies with other trauma specialties (eg, neurosurgery or urology) is necessary to allow cardiorespiratory monitoring of the patient while efficiently performing these studies. For example, magnetic resonance imaging (MRI) and computed tomographic (CT) scanning should be performed with the fewest changes of position possible that will also provide the necessary information for all surgical subspecialists.

"Clearing" the Cervical Spine

In the evaluation of the trauma patient, an important consideration is the status of the cervical spine. The cervical spine is easily injured because of the large mass of the head relative to the neck, especially in motor vehicle accidents involving rapid acceleration or deceleration. Consequently, the cervical spine can receive significant force and suffer injury. In the conscious and responsive patient, swelling or tenderness on physical examination of the cervical spine is readily apparent. In the unconscious patient, cervical spine injuries can go undetected, and a careful physical examination must be performed with heavy reliance upon radiographic evaluation.

The essential radiographs for evaluation of the cervical spine include anterior-posterior views, lateral views, and an open-mouth odontoid view. It is essential to be able to see to the top of T1. If this level is not visualized through these conventional views, then a "swimmer's view," which is a lateral cervical spine radiograph with the arm abducted and elevated, should be obtained.

After the cervical spine x-ray films have been reviewed, the ligamentous stability of the cervical spine can be further evaluated. Lateral cervical spine flexion and extension views can be analyzed to see if the lateral alignment of the anterior cervical spinal segments is correct. These can only be obtained in the alert and cooperative patient who can safely sit upright. These films are often delayed for a several-week period.

In the obtunded patient, CT and/or MRI scan is necessary to delineate further soft tissue injury. On the open-mouth view, the lateral masses of C1 should line up with the body of C2. The amount of total overhang of C1 over C2 should be less than 7 mm. On the lateral view, the anterior border of the bodies of the cervical segments should describe an arc. The distance from the basion to the posterior arch of C1 divided by the distance from the opisthion to the anterior arch of C1 should be less than 1 (Powers ratio) (Figure 3–1). A basion to odontoid tip distance above 10mm in children and 5 mm in adults indicates craniocervical dislocation, a potentially fatal injury. The posterior border of the anterior arc of C1 should be within 2–3 mm of the anterior border of C2. There should be no diastasis of the spinous processes, and the joints and facet joints should all be visible. If there is a change in orientation from one cervical spine level to another, then cervical fracture, jumped facets, or dislocation should be suspected. Suspected cervical spine fracture should be investigated with appropriate imaging, such as CT scan, to further delineate the injury pattern. Suspected cervical spine injuries should be treated with provisional stabilization using a cervical collar. Rotational subluxation should be managed with evaluation of soft tissues and reduction maneuvers. In the case of neurologic deficit, careful evaluation of the neurologic status is important, and immediate decompression-stabilization must be considered.

IMMEDIATE MANAGEMENT OF MUSCULOSKELETAL TRAUMA

The orthopedic injuries in the polytrauma patient are seldom truly emergency situations, except for those involving neural or vascular compromise.

For example, fracture-dislocation of the ankle or knee resulting in distal ischemia justifies immediate attempts at reduction to minimize the sequelae of ischemia. A more subtle situation requiring emergent treatment would be dislocation of the hip in which vascular com-

Figure 3–1. Powers ratio: a – anterior arch of atlas, b – basion, p – posterior arch of atlas, o – opisthion. The ratio of bp:oa should be approximately 0.77 in the normal population. Anterior occipito-atlantal dislocation is present when the Powers ratio is greater than 1.15.

promise of the femoral head may result. Arterial bleeding from an open fracture should be treated immediately with pressure to minimize blood loss. Other bone and joint injuries, although urgent, may be approached in a more deliberate manner.

Orthopedic management of traumatic injuries requires consideration of the entire individual as well as the entire extremity. It is short-sighted to treat only the area of injury revealed on radiograph, as the soft-tissue envelope around the bone is essential to fracture healing and the ultimate function of the patient. Repair of soft-tissue damage is clearly important in achieving satisfactory function after healing has occurred. A break in the skin is important, but the damage done to the entire extremity is more important than the extent of laceration.

Complications

From the orthopedist's viewpoint, the major complications associated with trauma are acute respiratory distress syndrome (ARDS), systemic inflammatory response syndrome (SIRS), fat embolism syndrome (FES), multisystem organ failure (MOF), thromboembolic disease, atelectasis, compartment syndrome, sepsis, and ectopic bone formation. The first five disorders involve pulmonary complications and must constantly be kept in mind in managing the polytrauma patient. The institution of early fixation of fractures with concomitant mobilization of the patient has helped to reduce the incidence of these four conditions significantly. They continue to be problems, however, and constant vigilance is necessary to prevent serious consequences. New research has begun to identify subsets of highly injured patients in whom some forms of early definitive fixation may accelerate the development of ARDS, SIRS, and MOF.

A. ACUTE RESPIRATORY DISTRESS SYNDROME

Acute respiratory distress syndrome (ARDS) can be a sequela of trauma with subsequent shock. Massive tissue injury activates the immunological system and releases inflammatory mediators, with subsequent disruption of the microvasculature of the pulmonary system. Some acute orthopaedic procedures have been shown to similarly activate the immune system. Pulmonary endothelial damage results, with decreased partial pressures of oxygen and arterial oxygen saturation and increased carbon dioxide levels. The onset is frequently within 24 hours after trauma and is revealed by hypoxemia, inflammatory reaction, and progressive decrease in arterial oxygen saturation if appropriate treatment is not instituted.

Fat embolism syndrome is a unique orthopedic manifestation of ARDS caused by the release of marrow fat into the circulation following fractures, particularly of the long bones. Pathologic examination of the lungs shows fat droplets, usually diffusely distributed throughout the pulmonary vasculature. This syndrome may also occur in nonfracture situations, as when the medullary canal of a long bone is pressurized during total knee replacement. Fat embolism syndrome occurs frequently as a subclinical occurrence that is insufficient to compromise the patient's pulmonary reserve, but in some cases it can result in severe pulmonary compromise and death.

The clinical diagnosis of ARDS is confirmed by a decrease in arterial PO_2, an increase in systemic PCO_2, infiltrates on chest radiograph, presence of petechiae, and mental confusion in a patient at risk. Relatively minor injuries can result in this syndrome in patients with limited pulmonary reserve. Treatment is directed toward minimizing hypoxemia with ventilatory support as needed. Prevention is enhanced by early mobilization of the patient, which often implies early fracture fixation.

B. ATELECTASIS

Atelectasis, or localized collapse of alveoli, is a frequent postoperative complication in elective patients and can be prominent in trauma patients because of the required immobilization. Significant hypoxemia can result, and the onset may be relatively rapid. This may be the source of postoperative fevers in the early recovery phase. Occasionally, radiograph examination, showing platelike collapse of areas of the lung, will confirm the diagnosis. By encouraging coughing and deep breathing, using incentive spirometry, and, in resistant cases, using respiratory therapy, rapid resolution can be expected.

C. PULMONARY EMBOLISM AND DEEP VENOUS THROMBOSIS

Although ARDS and atelectasis are seen in the early postoperative period, pulmonary embolism (PE) is uncommon sooner than 5 days after the onset of immobilization or bed rest. The trauma patient is at risk for PE, and the patient with spinal cord injury even more so. Population based studies have demonstrated recent trauma to be associated with a 13-fold increased risk of venous thromboembolism. Young multiple-trauma patients without prophylaxis have been shown to have a 1–2% incidence of fatal PE, which appears to decrease with a variety of prophylactic measures. Other groups of patients at risk include the elderly (>70 years), the obese, those with a history of prior venous thromboembolism, major surgery of the abdomen, pelvis or extremities, and fractures of the pelvis, hip or leg, and those with malignancy. Although it is uncommon, even a young (<30 years) healthy person can develop deep venous thrombosis (DVT) and be at risk for PE after a long car or airplane trip in which the legs are dependent. Oral contraceptive and smoking use may also increase the risk for a young healthy patient.

Geerts and colleagues examined the incidence of DVT and PE in trauma patients in a prospective series with venography. They found patients to be at significantly increased risk if they had suffered a pelvis or long bone fracture with greater than 5 days immobilization in bed, were obese, had a preexisting coagulopathy or an Injury Severity Score (ISS) greater than 8. Overall, they reported an incidence of 58% with 18% proximal DVT in patients without prophylaxis. The authors noted that fatal PE was the most common yet preventable form of death in the hospitalized trauma patient.

Patients at high risk for PE are those with DVT in the lower extremities, and pelvic veins. Clinically significant PE usually arise from the large veins proximal to the knee. Prevention of DVT in the venous system in this area reduces the risk of PE. Various strategies used to accomplish this include drug therapy with low-dose heparin, low-molecular-weight heparin, pentasaccharide, or sodium warfarin; and mechanical prophylaxis with intermittent pneumatic compression devices or inferior vena cava filters in the high risk patients with contraindications for pharmacologic prophylaxis.

Clinical diagnosis of DVT is unreliable. Definitive diagnosis is made with venography, duplex ultrasound scanning, impedance plethysmography, or CT or MRI venography. Prevention appears to be the best strategy as even routine surveillance screening in a trauma populations is cost-ineffective and does not appear to lower the overall rate of PE.

Pulmonary embolism is suspected in the orthopedic patient suffering an onset of tachypnea and dyspnea usually more than 5 days after an inciting event. The patient frequently reports chest pain and can often point to the painful area. Hemoptysis may also be present. On physical examination, tachycardia, cyanosis, and pleural friction rub can be noted.

Arterial blood gas studies demonstrate hypoxemia, although this is a nonspecific finding. Use of the d-dimer is unreliable in the early trauma patient but may be useful later in the recovery period. Definitive diagnosis is best made with pulmonary angiogram. Perfusion ventilation scanning is less invasive and may help determine whether there is a high or low probability of pulmonary embolus. Spiral CT is becoming useful in diagnosis of PE.

Treatment involves pulmonary support and heparin therapy. The natural history of treated PE is gradual lysis of the emboli, with the return of flow through the pulmonary arterial tree. The natural history of proximal DVT involves recanalization and arborization to bypass the clot. Patients may suffer from postphlebitic syndrome characterized by chronically painful swelling in the extremity.

D. COMPARTMENT SYNDROME

The term **compartment syndrome** refers to pathologic developments in a closed space in the body caused by buildup of pressure. Most commonly, such compartments are circumscribed by fascia and incorporate one or more bones. Pressure rises from edema or bleeding within the compartment, compromising circulation to the contents of the compartment over a period, and can result in necrosis of muscle and damage to nerves.

Compartment syndrome may result from a fracture; a soft-tissue injury; a vascular injury causing ischemia, necrosis, and edema; or from a burn. In an alcohol or drug user, it may be caused by external compression from immobilization that prevents normal postural changes. Failure to redistribute pressure through postural changes results in ischemia of the area under pressure because of collapse of capillaries.

The diagnosis of compartment syndrome must be considered in the postoperative or posttrauma patient who has pain out of proportion to that expected from the inciting injury. As the pain worsens, it can become totally unresponsive to narcotic medication. Epidural narcotics may mask the onset of compartment syndrome in the lower extremity.

The five P's (pulselessness, paresthesia, paresis, pain, and pressure) characteristic of compartment syndrome are helpful, but not diagnostic, for the experienced clinician. Pulses are poor indicators of compartment syndrome as they generally remain intact until late. Paresthesias occur only when the syndrome is significantly advanced. This points to the importance of careful documentation of sensory examination prior to the potential onset of compartment syndrome. Paresis, if present, is an unreliable finding. Subsequent to fracture or injury, pain is likely to induce guarding and thereby is also an unreliable finding. If normal muscle function is present, however, compartment syndrome is unlikely unless it is early. Pain with passive stretching of involved muscles is also a subjective finding and must be differentiated from pain arising from the original injury. To the experienced clinician, pain with passive stretching is a reliable clinical sign. Pressure is a key component of compartment syndrome, but palpation of a soft compartment does not rule out the diagnosis of compartment syndrome. Patients with equivocal clinical findings or those at high risk but without a reliable clinical examination (eg, those who are comatose, have psychiatric problems, or are under the influence of narcotics) should have compartmental pressure measurements. Intracompartmental pressure readings within 30 mm Hg or less of the diastolic blood pressure are indications for fasciotomy. Prior to fasciotomy, circular dressings including casts should be removed, and the patient should be observed for a short period for signs of improvement. Positive clinical findings may justify fasciotomy even despite normal pressures. Late fasciotomy may result in muscle damage or possible necrosis, with resulting risk of infection.

Although compartment syndrome can occur in almost any portion of the body, the two most common locations are the forearm and calf. In the forearm, an extensile volar incision to permit complete release, including the carpal tunnel distally and the lacertus fibrosus proximally, is necessary. Dorsally, a longitudinal incision is used. In the calf, two incisions are used to release the four compartments of the leg. The anterior and lateral compartments are decompressed using a longitudinal incision approximately over the anterior intermuscular septum. Posteromedially, a second incision is used to approach the superficial and deep posterior compartments. While single and limited incision approaches have been described, these may be unreliable and have a higher incidence of iatrogenic nerve injury in the trauma patients.

E. HETEROTOPIC BONE FORMATION

Clinically significant heterotopic ossification occurs as a consequence of trauma in perhaps 10% of cases and may cause pain or joint motion restriction even to the point of ankylosis. Trauma patients without head injuries frequently manifest heterotopic ossification on radiograph 1–2 months following trauma; if the ossification is clinically significant, resection may be indicated when the bone has matured as indicated by radiographs and bone scan. This can take up to 18 months to achieve.

Resection is accomplished by removing the entire piece of heterotopic bone. Selected patients may benefit from low-dose radiation (7 Gy) and oral indomethacin for 3–6 weeks. Further discussion of this topic can be found in Chapter 13, "Rehabilitation." Heterotopic bone is a much more common occurrence in patients with head injuries. This is believed to result from release of humeral modulators that have not yet been characterized.

Classification of Open Fractures

A. GUSTILO AND ANDERSON CLASSIFICATION

Gustilo and Anderson made a significant contribution to trauma care of long bones by introducing their classification of open fractures, which includes the degree of open or closed soft-tissue injury. Their system was initially designed for open tibial fractures; however, it has gone on to include all types of long bone fractures. This system uses three grades and divides the third most severe grade into three subtypes.

Grade I fracture is a low-energy injury with a wound less than 1 cm in length, often from an inside-out injury rather than an outside-in injury. These are generally simple transverse or short oblique fractures.

Grade II fracture involves a wound more than 1 cm long and significantly more injury, caused by more energy absorption during the production of the fracture. Grade II fractures usually display some comminution and have a minimal to moderate crushing component.

Grade III open fracture has extensive wounds more than 10 cm in length, significant fracture fragment comminution, and a great deal of soft-tissue damage. It is usually a high-energy injury. This type of injury results typically from high-velocity gunshots, close range shot-

gun blasts, motorcycle accidents, or injuries with contamination from outdoor sites such as with tornado disasters or farming accidents. Indeed, any open fracture resulting from a natural disaster, highly contaminated or comminuted, independent of wound size, is automatically classified as a grade III open fracture.

Grade III injuries are divided into subtypes A, B, and C. Grade IIIA fractures have extensive soft-tissue laceration with minimal periosteal stripping and have adequate bone coverage. These injuries include some gunshot injuries and segmental fractures and do not require major reconstructive surgery to provide skin coverage. Grade IIIB fractures, in contrast, have extensive soft-tissue injury with periosteal stripping and require a flap for coverage. Grade IIIC injuries involve vascular compromise requiring surgical repair or reconstruction to allow for reperfusion of the limb. The presence of an intact skin envelope may imply somewhat reduced severity of trauma. The soft-tissue and bony damage may be as severe for closed fractures, however, except for the lower risk of infection.

Severe soft-tissue and bony injuries, especially when open, raise the question of immediate amputation. This problem most frequently arises in the lower extremity between the knee and the ankle. The advent of microvascular surgery has reduced the absolute indication for amputation resulting from ischemia. Two years of reconstruction may be necessary to achieve a united tibia fracture without infection, and even then, function may be compromised by muscle or nerve damage. The patient may have also endured multiple operations, loss of work time, and the emotional trauma accompanying an injury of this magnitude. Prosthetic replacements, particularly in the trauma patient at the below-knee level, may well be a viable alternative to a poorly functioning, insensate lower extremity.

Early Total Care

The desirability of early total and appropriate orthopedic care in multiply injured patients has become well established. Benefits of timely and aggressive treatment include decreased rates of mortality, primarily due to reductions in ARDS and multisystem organ failure (MOF). In a classic study by Bone et al., 178 patients with femoral fractures were entered into an early fixation group (treatment within 24 hours) or a delayed fixation group (treatment after 48 hours). The incidence of pulmonary complications, such as ARDS, fat embolism, or pneumonia, was higher, the hospital stay was longer, and the intensive care unit requirements increased when the femoral fixation was delayed. Bone and collaborators did a follow-up retrospective, multicenter study of 676 patients who had an ISS (Injury Severity Score) greater than 18 and who had major pelvic or long-bone injuries treated under an early fixation protocol within 48 hours at one of six major US trauma centers. These results were compared with historical records of 906 patients from the American College of Surgeons Multiple Trauma Outcomes Study Database. The study, despite shortcomings in methodology, revealed a lower mortality rate for patients whose fractures were stabilized early.

In a study by Reynolds, Richards, and Spain, records of 424 consecutive trauma patients were reviewed. Of these, 105 had an ISS of 18 or greater. These patients did not receive definitive early long bone fixation. In general, femur fractures were stabilized on the day of admission if the patients were hemodynamically stable. These authors noticed that progressive surgical delays caused by decline in the patient's condition resulted in a significant increase in pulmonary complications for patients having an ISS less than 18. However, there was no relation between pulmonary complications and timing of femoral fixation when patients had an ISS of 18 or more. The authors concluded that the severity of injuries, not the timing of fracture fixation, tended to determine patient pulmonary outcome.

Damage Control Orthopaedics

Controversy exists, however, regarding the appropriate timing of orthopedic intervention for specific subsets of severely injured patients, particularly those with head injury or systemic hypotension. Long bone fracture fixation with reamed intramedullary rods, in particular, may cause intraoperative hypotension or an increased release of inflammatory mediators with deleterious results in specific patients.

The multiply injured patient's immunological system is stimulated or primed after trauma (first event). Subsequent resuscitation, hemorrhage, blood products, hypotension and surgery (second event), may produce an exaggerated systemic inflammatory response syndrome (SIRS), potentially leading to ARDS or MOF. Activated neutrophils are the principal effector of the inflammatory response, releasing active oxygen species, which damage the vascular endothelium. Bone marrow contents pushed to the systemic circulation during reaming and nailing can activate neutrophils leading to SIRS in polytrauma patients, particularly during the first 96 hours after trauma. Damage control Orthopaedics aims to decrease the additional surgical trauma through external fixation, and secondary definitive surgery. One study demonstrated that conversion of an external fixator to a reamed intramedullary nail is safe and effective if performed within 2 weeks.

Alternatives to modify the inflammatory response are currently under investigation. The potential advantage is to allow early total fracture care avoiding secondary surgeries.

Soft-Tissue Injuries & Traumatic Arthrotomies

Lacerations of the extremities can result in neural or vascular compromise to an extremity and may also cause traumatic arthrotomies. Compromise of the sterility of any joint requires surgical debridement of that joint. For many joints, arthroscopic irrigation and debridement will minimize trauma and improve the return to function. Other soft-tissue lacerations may require neural or vascular repair. Laceration of a tendon or muscle belly is often involved. Tendon repairs are frequently performed in the foot and the hand. All tendon lacerations of the hand, except for those of the palmaris longus, should be repaired. In the foot, extrinsic tendons are repaired to prevent late imbalance or loss of function. Muscle belly injuries generally require surgical debridement because their subfascial location makes simple irrigation difficult. Laceration involving only the muscle belly requires no surgical repair. Frequently, however, muscle belly laceration involves the continuation of the origin or the insertion tendon of the muscle. In this case, optimal function is obtained by reattaching the lacerated ends. Generally, they can be located by poking into the muscle with a forceps at the site of the blood clot on the surface of the cut end. The tendon portion has retracted and the muscle has expanded because of swelling, leaving a track with a blood clot inside.

In most cases, immediate treatment of open fractures and lacerations consists of surgical debridement. Prior to formal debridement, it is appropriate to splint fractures and cover open wounds with sterile dressings soaked in povidone-iodine. Antibiotic therapy is begun immediately, usually with a cephalosporin bactericidal antibiotic. Tetanus prophylaxis is administered if needed. Antibiotic therapy is continued based on the clinical course.

Irrigation and debridement are intended to convert a clean contaminated wound into a sterile wound. Copious irrigation, using an irrigating solution containing antibiotics, is effective in cleaning the wound. Debridement removes nonviable tissue. Generally, care should be taken to remove only tissue that is necrotic. Skin edges should be debrided, as should dead muscle, and the surface of any contaminated fat or fascia.

After debridement, bone surfaces and exposed tendons should be covered as well as possible with tissue to maintain moistness. Maintain soft tissue attachments to bone whenever possible. Fragments of bone, particularly cortical bone, without attachments, should be removed from the wound. Although the axiom "open fractures should be left open, closed fractures should be left closed" was suitable many years ago, experience has demonstrated that in certain cases minimal risk is assumed in closing the wound. It is acceptable practice, however, to leave any wound open. Grade I wounds may in some cases be closed completely, or the part that was opened to permit debridement may be closed, leaving the original débrided laceration open. This may close spontaneously. Grade II wounds may be treated in a similar fashion, with somewhat more risk. The possibility of gas gangrene must be entertained whenever such a wound is closed. Primary closure of Grade III wounds is rarely if ever done. Adequate closure to cover bone and other structures that may be damaged by desiccation, without completely closing the wound, may be attempted. Patients with massive wounds should be returned to the operating room in approximately 48 hours and then every 48 hours until the wound is completely clean and granulating. Smaller wounds that are left open may be closed safely at 3–5 days.

Flaps and Soft-Tissue Coverage for Open Trauma

Soft-tissue wounds in association with skeletal trauma (Gustilo grades I, II, and some IIIA wounds) can be treated by appropriate skeletal fixation, wound debridement, and limited skin grafts or rotation flaps to close the skin successfully. Larger wounds, however, require more aggressive surgical management. These wounds may be treated best by large regional soft-tissue flap reconstruction. Before the advent of microsurgery, the standard of care was pedicle flaps, such as chest wall flaps, applied to the arm for burn contractures around the elbow, cross-leg grafts for lower-extremity trauma, or groin flaps for soft-tissue trauma of the hand. With the advent of microsurgical techniques for skin, muscle, and fascia transplantation, the treatment of large soft-tissue trauma has changed. The classic study by Godina in *Plastic and Reconstructive Surgery* describes the results of immediate free flap reconstruction. Immediate free flap reconstruction is done within the first 48 h after trauma. The requirement for this procedure is radical debridement of the zone of injury, similar to the way one would resect a tumor. Using these techniques, there is little fibrosis of the bed and a fairly large soft-tissue defect for the viability of tissues with which to work and with which to place a free flap.

If radical debridement is not performed, then flap reconstruction should be delayed until soft tissues have healed at the margins, and there is no sign of infection. However, with large wounds, this often becomes a dilemma. Therefore, the use of free flaps gives an overall improved outcome by bringing a new source of vascularity to a compromised extremity, preventing infection and simultaneously providing soft-tissue coverage.

There are many sites that can be harvested for flaps. The most common and the hardiest flaps to use on a large scale include fasciocutaneous flaps from the latissimus dorsi, gracilis, serratus anterior, and rectus abdominis muscles. These are suitable for medium- to large-size wounds in a variety of locations. Additionally, there are a host of smaller tissue transfers designed for more specific uses that have some advantages in the matching of defect to donor and minimizing problems at the donor site. However, the flaps that have been listed are the mainstays of the reconstructive microsurgeon for the extremities.

A recent innovation in wound management is the Vacuum Assisted Closure Therapy (VAC). The VAC system exposes the wound bed to negative pressure in a closed system. The stretching stimulus is transformed into microchemical forces that promote wound healing through increased cell division and proliferation, angiogenesis stimulation, and local increase of growth factors. Also, edema fluid is removed from the extravascular space, eliminating the extrinsic cause of microcirculatory alteration and improving local blood supply. Although this device does not replace the need for surgical debridement, it may avoid the need for a free tissue transfer in patients with large traumatic wounds. Additional orthopaedic indications include the treatment of infected wounds after debridement, and fasciotomy wounds closure.

Gun-Shot Wounds

Optimum treatment of fractures caused by gun-shots relies upon an appreciation of the kinetic energy of injury, direction, caliber and, distance. This is particularly true with regard to soft-tissue injuries. Visual inspection alone at the time of initial evaluation is not always sufficient because it can underestimate the extent of damage. Gun-shot wounds to the musculoskeletal system result in complex soft-tissue lesions, fractures that are often comminuted, and related nerve, artery, and tendon involvement. Differences between high-velocity (>2000 feet/second) and low-velocity (<2000 feet/second) weapons and civilian and military settings for these wounds are also important. Additional characteristics are the efficiency of energy transfer, including deformation and fragmentation, kinetic energy, stability, profile of entrance, path through the body, and the biologic characteristics of the tissues. In general, kinetic energy (KE) associated with an injury is calculated by the formula

$$KE = \frac{M}{2} \times v^2$$

where *M* equals mass and *V* equals velocity. Thus velocity and missile mass are the determinants of resultant tissue damage. Velocity is more important than mass, doubling the velocity quadruples the kinetic energy. Shotgun injuries are different from single gun-shot wounds, because the weight of the shot causes an increase in the kinetic energy, resulting in a more severe injury. Additionally, shotgun shells have wadding that is made of plastic, felt, paper, or cord, between the powder and the shot charge, and this wadding can become embedded in the wound and be another important factor in wound management.

In gun-shot wounds and high-velocity missiles, shock waves, laceration and crushing, and cavitation result in tissue damage. Shock waves can produce injury in areas that are relatively distant from the direct path of the missile. Cavitation is an important mechanism of tissue damage in high-velocity injuries. The subatmospheric pressure in the cavity sucks contaminants in from both ends. Secondary missiles are the result of bone or bullet fragmentation, and can increase the extent of damage. Missile wound tracks close to a major vessel may be associated with occult vascular injury despite normal pulses. Doppler ultrasound is indicated when a vascular injury is suspected.

Low-velocity civilian gun-shot wounds and fractures are relatively simple to treat, because tissue damage is confined to the missile path, and local wound care, with or without antibiotic therapy, can effectively treat the injuries and decrease the incidence of wound sepsis and osteomyelitis. The use of immediate fixation by either internal or external fixator means is somewhat controversial. On the one hand, the danger of treatment of these open fractures with foreign material is a deterrent for immediate stabilization. However, in grossly unstable injuries, treatment that would be used for other open fractures appears to be reasonable in selected cases. The impact of gun-shot wounds in ballistic injuries can be significant. In a study by Brown in the *Journal of Orthopaedic Trauma*, a university-affiliated level-1 trauma center conducted a retrospective study through calendar year 1994 in which all patients admitted through the emergency department with a gun-shot wound for which the orthopedic surgery service was consulted were evaluated. These 284 patients were responsible for 24% of all orthopedic admissions, 33% of the average daily orthopedic census, and 14% of all the orthopedic surgery cases. Forty-five percent tested positive for alcohol and 65% for drugs. Eighty-seven percent of patients were male; only 4% of patients were privately insured. The authors concluded that during this 1-year study, gun-shot wound injuries required more orthopedic trauma resources than any other surgical areas. The majority of low-velocity gunshot wounds can be managed with local wound care and outpatient treatment. The wound should be left open for drainage. If the fracture requires surgical treatment, antibiotic prophylaxis is recommended. High velocity and shotgun fractures require surgical irrigation, appropriate debridement and at least 24 to 48 hours of IV antibiotics treatment.

Multiple Trauma Treatments—Strategies and Traumatic Scoring Systems

The surgeon who has to provide fracture care to patients who have multiple injuries will find that they fall into several categories. In the first are patients with multiple, isolated extremity injuries. In the second are patients with multiple orthopedic injuries who are otherwise medically stable. In a third category are patients with multiple orthopedic injuries and multisystem organ injuries.

Within these categories, orthopedic injuries are either life- or limb-threatening, emergent, urgent, or elective injuries in the timing of treatment. Timing of treatment is also related to the presence and severity of other injuries.

Several classification systems have been used to try to stratify these injuries and to determine severity. The

Table 3–1. Factors in evaluation of the mangled extremity severity score (MESS) variables.

	Points
A. Skeletal and soft-tissue injury	
Low energy (stab; simple fracture; "civilian" gunshot wound)	1
Medium energy (open or multiple fractures, dislocation)	2
High energy (close-range shotgun or "military" gunshot wound, crush injury)	3
Very high energy (above plus gross contamination, soft-tissue avulsion)	4
B. Limb ischemia[a]	
Pulse reduced or absent but perfusion normal	1
Pulseless; paresthesia, diminished capillary refilling	2
Cool, paralyzed, insensate, numb	3
C. Shock	
Systolic blood pressure almost more than 90 mm Hg	0
Hypotensive transiently	1
Persistent hypotension	2
D. Age	
<30 years	0
30–50 years	1
>50 years	2

[a]Score doubled for ischemia more than 6 hours.

Adapted and reproduced, with permission, from Johansen K et al: Objective criteria accurately predict amputation following lower extremity trauma. J Trauma 1990;30:369.

classification systems serve as a guide for both patient treatment and eventual outcomes. The Revised Trauma Score (RTS) was developed to help with patient triage. The scores for systolic blood pressure and respiratory rate are separated into five domains with each assigned a point value from 0 to 4. These scores are added to the Glasgow Coma Score to yield a Revised Trauma Score. In the United States, the American College of Surgeons' guidelines directs patients with an RTS of 11 or less to a designated trauma center.

The Abbreviated Injury Scale (AIS) divides injuries into nine body regions and stratifies the injuries from minor to fatal on a 6-point scale. These scores take into account life-threatening aspects of injuries, anticipated permanent impairment, treatment, and injury pattern.

The Injury Severity Score (ISS) is the sum of the squares of the highest AIS scores in the three most severely injured body regions, which are chosen from head and neck, chest, abdomen, extremities and pelvic girdle, and external. Multiple-trauma patients are defined as patients with ISS greater than or equal to 14. A good prognosis is associated with an ISS of less than 30, whereas an ISS greater than 60 is usually fatal.

Factors at the time of injury, which have a bearing on the decision to amputate, include status of the opposite leg, the time of limb ischemia, and the age of the patient. Many of these factors have been taken into account by Johansen and associates, who have defined a Mangled Extremity Severity Score (MESS). The MESS was previously used as a predictor of eventual amputation; however, recent studies have shown the MESS and other scoring systems to be inaccurate in predicting the functional outcome for mangled limb patients (Table 3–1).

Anglen JO: Wound irrigation in musculoskeletal injury. J Am Acad Orthop Surg 2001;9:219. [PMID: 11476531]

Bartlett CS: Ballistic and gunshot wounds: Effects on musculoskeletal tissues. J Am Acad Orthop Surg 2000;8:21. [PMID: 10666650]

Biffl WL, Smith WR, Moore EE, et al: Evolution of a multidisciplinary clinical pathway for the management of unstable patients with pelvic fractures. Ann Surg 2001;233:843. [PMID: 11407336]

Bone LB et al: Early vs delayed stabilization of femoral fracture. J Bone Joint Surg Am 1989;71A:336. [PMID: 2925704]

Bone LB et al: Mortality in multiple trauma patients with fractures. J Trauma 1994;37:262. [PMID: 8064927]

Bosse MJ et al: Adult respiratory distress syndrome, pneumonia, and mortality following thoracic injury and a femoral fracture treated either with intramedullary nailing with reaming or with a plate. A comparative study. J Bone Joint Surg Am 1997;79:799.

Bosse MJ, Mackenzie EJ, Kellam JF, et al: A prospective evaluation of the clinical utility of the lower-extremity injury-severity scores. J Bone Joint Surg AM. 2001;83-A(1):3–14.

Covey DC, Lurate RB, Hatton CT: Field hospital treatment of blast wounds of the musculoskeletal system during the Yugoslav civil war. J Orthop Trauma 2000;14: 278. [PMID: 10898201]

Dickson K et al: Outpatient management of low-velocity gunshot-induced fractures. Orthopedics 2001;24:951. [PMID: 11688773]

Dunham CM, Bosse MJ, Clancy TV et al: Practice management guidelines for the optimal timing of long-bone fracture stabilization in polytrauma patients: The EAST Practice Management Guidelines Work Group. J Trauma 2001;50(5):958.

Geerts W, Heit JA, Clagett GP et al. Prevention of venous thromboembolism. Chest 2001;119:132S. [PMID: 11157647]

Godina M: The tailored latissimus dorsi free flap. Plast Reconstr Surg 1987;80:304. [PMID: 3602183]

Gustilo RB, Anderson JT: Prevention of infection in the treatment of 1025 open fractures of long bones. J Bone Joint Surg Am 1976;58:453. [PMID: 773941]

Hammert WC, Minarchek J, Trzeciak MA: Free-flap reconstruction of traumatic lower extremity wounds. Am J Orthop 2000;29:22. [PMID: 11011776]

Hildebrand F, Giannoudis P, Krettek C, Pape HC. Damage control: extremities. Injury 2004;35:678. [PMID: 15203308]

Johansen K et al: Objective criteria accurately predict amputation following lower extremity trauma. J Trauma 1990;30:568. [PMID: 2342140]

MacKenzie EJ et al: Characterization of patients with high-energy lower extremity trauma. J Orthop Trauma 2000;14:455. [PMID: 11083607]

Mendelson SA et al: Early versus late femoral fracture stabilization in multiply injured pediatric patients with closed head injury. J Ped Orthop 2001;21:594. [PMID: 11521025]

Mullett H et al: Outcome of compartment syndrome following intramedullary nailing of tibial diaphyseal fractures. Injury 2001;32:411. [PMID: 11382428]

Nowotarski PJ, Turen CH, Brumback RJ, Scarbor JM. Conversion of external fixation to intramedullary nailing for fractures of the shaft of the femur in multiply injured patients. J Bone Joint Surg Am. 2000;82:781. [PMID: 10859097]

Perrier A et al: Performance of helical computed tomography in unselected outpatients with suspected pulmonary embolism. Ann Int Med 2001;135:88. [PMID: 11453707]

Pierce TD, Tomaino MM: Use of the pedicled latissimus muscle flap for upper-extremity reconstruction. J Am Acad Orthop Surg 2000;8:324. [PMID: 11029560]

Stannard JP et al: Mechanical prophylaxis against deep-vein thrombosis after pelvic and acetabular fractures. J Bone Joint Surg Am 2001;83-A:1047. [PMID: 11451974]

Van Belle A et al: Effectiveness of managing suspected pulmonary embolism using an algorithm combining clinical probability, D-dimer testing, and computed tomography. JAMA 2006; 295:172. [PMID: 16403929]

FAILURE OF FRACTURE HEALING

Fracture union is a gradual, continuous process where the mechanical integrity of a fractured bone is restored. The treating clinician needs measures of healing and definitions of failure that allows rational treatment decisions. Bone regeneration can occur by various histologic processes such as intramembranous, endochondral and/or osteonal remodeling. The speed of healing by periosteal callus depends on the extent of soft tissue disruption.

Generally, a fracture has united when there is radiographic evidence of bony bridging of the fracture on at least three cortices on orthogonal projections. Clinical criteria, such as absence of motion and resolution of pain at the fracture site, while helpful, are much less sensitive in confirming that a fracture has healed.

Many variables have an effect on the fracture healing process, including the fracture site, the blood supply, initial displacement of fracture fragments, whether the fracture is open or closed, the patient's age and nutritional status, and, possibly, medication use (eg, steroids, anticoagulants). In general, fractures will heal when the bone ends are in close apposition and the affected area has been adequately immobilized, has a good blood supply, is surrounded by a muscle envelope, and is not infected.

Nonunion of Fracture

Despite the best efforts and treatment, a certain percentage of fractures will fail to unite. The treatment of nonunited fractures has developed into a subspecialty area of orthopedic surgery. According to the Food and Drug Administration, **delayed union** of a long bone is defined as a fracture that has not gone on to full bony union after 6 months. Delayed union is represented by evident cessation of periosteal new bone formation before union has been achieved.

Nonunion is less well defined. Clearly, a fracture that fails to show progressive evidence of healing over a 4 to 6-month period can be considered a nonunion. One can immediately declare a fracture with a 2 inch bony defect, for example, a nonunion, as one knows that bony reconstitution will not occur spontaneously if this fracture is simply left immobilized.

Nonunion corresponds to scar formation in which the rate of endosteal and periosteal osteogenesis is zero or low and outweighed by bone resorption, with sclerosis of the medullary canal at the fracture surfaces. If the periosteum is active and there is no bridging despite new bone formation, the result is hypertropic nonunion. If no new bone formation is taking place, the morphology will be atrophic.

A. REASONS FOR NONUNION

There are many reasons why a fracture might not heal. The two most common reasons are lack of adequate blood supply at the fracture site and inadequate stabilization of the fracture. Other less common reasons include soft-tissue interposition at the fracture site, fractures stabilized in an unacceptable amount of distraction, metabolic abnormalities, and infection. Infection at the fracture site does not in and of itself preclude a fracture from healing, but it can be a contributing cause to the development of nonunion. Rosen has outlined the known causes of nonunion (Table 3–2).

The location of the fracture is also an important factor in healing. Certain areas of the skeleton are more prone to developing nonunion, even when appropriate treatment is rendered. The distal tibial diaphysis, scaphoid, and proximal diaphysis of the fifth metatarsal classically have a higher incidence of nonunion than other locations in the body. Fracture pattern also plays a role in the development of nonunion. Segmental fractures of long bones are much more prone to nonunion, as are fractures with large "butterfly" fragments, because of devascularization of the intermediary segment.

B. CLASSIFICATION OF NONUNIONS

Nonunions have been classified according to their radiologic characteristics. The most widely used classification is that developed by Weber and Cech, who classified nonunion of long bones as being either hypertrophic or atrophic. They utilized standard radiographs and strontium isotope studies to differentiate these two categories. **Hypertrophic nonunions** have viable bone ends, whereas **atrophic nonunions** have nonviable bone ends. This differentiation has importance both in prognosis and in determining appropriate treatment. They further subdivided hypertrophic nonunions into "elephant's foot type," "horse's foot type," and olig-

Table 3–2. Causes of nonunion.

1. Excessive motion: inadequate immobilization
2. Diastasis of fracture fragments
   a. Soft-tissue interposition
   b. Distraction from traction or internal fixation
   c. Malposition
   d. Loss of bone
3. Compromised blood supply
   a. Damage to nutrient vessels
   b. Stripping or injury to periosteum and muscle
   c. Free fragments; severe comminution
   d. Avascularity because of internal fixation devices
4. Infection
   a. Bone death (sequestrum)
   b. Osteolysis (gap)
   c. Loosening of implants (motion)
5. General: age, nutrition, steroids, anticoagulants, radiation, burns, predisposure to nonunion
6. Distraction from traction or internal fixation

Adapted and reproduced, with permission, from Rosen H: Treatment of nonunions: General principles. In: Chapman MW, (ed): *Operative Orthopedics*, 2nd ed. Lippincott, 1988.

otrophic nonunions (Figure 3–2). It is somewhat confusing as to what actually causes a viable hypertrophic nonunion to behave by laying down exuberant callus (elephant's foot type) versus no callus (oligotrophic type.) As a generalization, those nonunions with better blood supply and some degree of micromotion at the fracture site develop more callus, while those with either no motion, excess motion, or distraction and a less rich blood supply produce less callus.

C. COMPLICATIONS OF NONUNION

Grossly mobile hypertrophic or atrophic nonunions that are left untreated for an extended period often develop into a pseudarthrosis (false joint) (Figure 3–3). There is an actual synovial-lined capsule enveloping the bone ends. Synovial fluid is present in the cleft. As a joint now exists between the ununited bone ends, surgical intervention is the only treatment option available.

D. TREATMENT

Once nonunion has been established, the physician must establish treatment goals. The joints above and below the nonunion must be evaluated to determine their function and motion. The degree of shortening or deformity of the affected limb must also be determined. One must also determine the general health of the patient as well as the degree of functional impairment the patient is actually experiencing. This is especially important as some patients are actually asymptomatic and therefore do not warrant treatment. In the

Figure 3–2. Weber and Cech's subclassification of hypertrophic nonunions: elephant's foot (**A**); horse's foot (**B**); oligotrophic (**C**). (This can often resemble atrophic nonunion and is hard to distinguish.) (Reprinted, with permission, from Browner BD et al, eds: *Skeletal Trauma*, 2nd ed. WB Saunders, 1998.)

sick or elderly (>70 years), treatment must also be tailored, as these patients may not be able to safely tolerate surgical intervention.

1. Stimulation of osteogenesis by external forces— It is now known that several pathways exist to stimulate healing of nonunion. The pathways can be divided into the type of force required to stimulate osteogenesis. These inductive forces can be categorized as mechanical, electrical, and chemical and can be applied with varying success both operatively and nonoperatively.

a. Mechanical forces—Application of mechanical forces to achieve bony union has remained the most time-honored, well-tested method to date. Sarmiento has shown that the use of functional bracing incorporated with weight bearing can lead to union of documented tibial nonunions. His results for treating femoral nonunions were less successful using this method. Cyclic mechanical force of ambulation while the frac-

ture reduction is maintained with an external support is the presumed mechanism with which fracture healing is achieved without surgical intervention.

Mechanical forces can also be generated by surgical means. Mechanical stabilization of a long bone nonunion can be achieved either by placement of an intramedullary rod or compression plating. The rod works by providing mechanical stabilization of the fracture, hence allowing for cyclic axial loading of the limb without shearing forces caused by weight bearing. The compression plate provides stability as well as immediate rigid compression across the fracture fragments. These forms of treatment are often all that is necessary in elephant's foot type nonunions.

b. Electrical stimulation—Electrical fields have also been shown to stimulate the dormant chondrocytes and mesenchymal cells in the nonunion cleft to "turn on" and produce bone that results in healing. The mechanism of why this occurs has been postulated but to date is not well understood. Currently, most electrical bone growth stimu-

Figure 3–3. Fourteen-year-old distal humeral pseudarthrosis left untreated in an 89-year-old woman. All motion about the elbow is occurring through the pseudarthrosis, as the elbow ankylosed.

lators used are external devices that are incorporated in a cast or functional brace around the site of nonunion. Surgically implanted devices with internal coils wrapped into the nonunion site have also been used with somewhat equivocal success. Sharrard showed in a controlled double-blind study that application of an external pulsed electromagnetic field led to a statistically significant increase in healing of documented delayed tibial unions as compared with a control group. New interest in this field is now focusing on the use of nonpulsed electromagnetic fields and ultrasound. Nonunions being treated with adjuvant electrical fields are in fact being treated with mechanical forces as well, as these fractures are usually immobilized and weight bearing is often allowed on the affected limb.

c. Biological enhancement—Chemical modulators also play an important role in promoting nonunion healing. Application of autogenous cancellous bone graft (most frequently obtained from the iliac crest) is a potent stimulator of fracture healing. As a rigid nonunion will heal with autogenous bone grafting alone and no internal fixation, it is apparent that chemical modulators from the grafted cancellous bone are responsible for stimulating the healing response. There has been recent intense interest in determining the growth factors present in this cancellous bone responsible for "turning on" the healing process. Some surgeons have even reported success by obtaining bone marrow via a large-bore needle from the iliac crest and injecting this into the nonunion site. In the future, it is likely that the humoral modulator responsible will be isolated, synthesized in sufficient quantities by genetic engineering techniques, and simply injected into nonunion clefts to attain union.

d. Pathways of simulation—It is interesting to note that although three separate forces exist that can stimulate healing, it is unknown whether they act via a common pathway. As often happens in the body, these forces could actually work by different pathways so as to allow for some duplicity to help ensure that most fractures will heal.

2. Atrophic nonunions—Atrophic nonunions are not as easily treated as hypertrophic nonunions, and fewer treatment options are available. Electrical stimulation and nonoperative treatment methods have not been effective. The treatment most commonly utilized, and most successfully, is "freshening up" of the avascular bone ends, combined with rigid internal fixation and autogenous bone grafting. This same procedure is used in treating pseudarthroses.

The Ilizarov method has also shown great success in the treatment of complex hypertrophic and atrophic nonunions, sometimes in combination with autogenous bone grafting. This method allows not only for achievement of bony union but also for treatment of any accompanying deformity, segmental bone loss, or shortening that may be present.

Malunion of Fracture

A fracture that has healed with an unacceptable amount of angulation, rotation, or overriding that has resulted in shortening of the limb is defined as malunion. Shortening is better tolerated in the upper than the lower extremity, and angulatory deformities are better tolerated in bones such as the humerus than in the femur or tibia. Hence, no absolute guidelines can be given as to an acceptable versus an unacceptable malunion. Generally, shortening greater than 1 inch is poorly tolerated in the lower extremity. Smaller discrepancies, however, are well treated with just a shoe lift in most situations. When the degree of deformity is sufficient to cause pain (eg. caused by walking on the side of the foot secondary to varus malunion of the distal tibia) or impair normal function, then surgical correction of the malunion is indicated.

When correction of malunion is undertaken, proper preoperative planning is imperative. One must determine the true mechanical axis of the limb to determine the actual site of deformity. If an osteotomy is performed, the surgeon must decide whether to use a closing wedge (where a wedge of bone is removed) or an opening wedge (where a wedge of autogenous or allograft bone is added). This is important, as it will alter the limb length. If the limb is already short, the surgery should also include a limb-lengthening procedure. Proper fixation and often autogenous cancellous bone grafting should be incorporated to ensure that the osteotomy heals, for converting a malunion to a nonunion is only worsening an already bad situation. Special care must be paid to treatment of the soft tissues to prevent wound breakdown and infection.

Determination of the true plane of deformity is essential in planning for the surgical correction. Green and associates have shown in tibial malunions and nonunions that it is rare for the plane of deformity to be in the true sagittal or coronal plane. The true degree of deformity is therefore not fully appreciated on anterior to posterior and lateral radiographs, as the axis is usually in a plane somewhere between these. Thus, treatment of malunions can be appreciated as a difficult task that requires careful planning and execution to achieve anatomic results.

Ilizarov Method

The Ilizarov apparatus and the concepts of distraction osteogenesis have dramatically revolutionized the application of the principles of external fixation in the management of bony defects, nonunions, malunions, pseudarthroses, and osteomyelitis. Since its introduction in Kurgan, Siberia, in 1951 by Gavril A. Ilizarov, surgeons throughout the world have employed this method to pioneer modern limb salvaging and lengthening procedures. This method has numerous advantages, including immediate loading of the limb postoperatively and the use of healthy viable bone to replace devascularized bone in situ by corticotomy, localized transport, and osteogenesis. Accordingly, leg length discrepancy, deformity, nonunions, and infections may all be treated effectively.

The basic premise of the Ilizarov technique is that osteogenesis can occur at a specially controlled osteotomy site (referred to as a **corticotomy**), given the appropriate degree of retained vascularity, fixation, and quantified distraction. Ilizarov realized that healing and neogenesis both required a dynamic state, which could occur in either controlled distraction or compression. This dogma is a function of many principles that Ilizarov classified into three categories: biologic, clinical, and technical. Important biologic concepts include preservation of endosteal and periosteal blood supply via corticotomy and stable fixation. Ilizarov fixation prevents shearing forces but permits axial micromotion with postoperative weight bearing, which enhances bone formation. Distraction osteogenesis occurs at a rate of approximately 1 mm/day. Division of distraction into four equal increments appears to be more physiologically sound than one distraction per day, as used previously in lengthening procedures. At the termination of distraction, neutral fixation is required to allow maturation, calcification, and strengthening of the new bone. In essence, the technique fools the body into believing it is a child again, with the corticotomy site acting as a physis.

Clinical principles such as the geometry of the apparatus once it is constructed, adjustment of the rate of transport, and wound care directly affect the outcome of the procedure. The initial operation for the application of the apparatus is only one small part in the whole treatment scheme. The construct should be as safe and comfortable as possible because for an extended period of time. Pin tract infections are common and must be addressed aggressively with oral antibiotics and local pin care.

From a technical viewpoint, Ilizarov methodology relies on the use of an extremely rigid (in all planes except the axial loading plane), extremely versatile external fixator, employing K-wire fixation under tension. It is this "tension stress" phenomenon of gradually controlled distraction of bone ends at the corticotomy site that makes possible the limb lengthening or osteogenesis required in bone transport. Neogenesis of the accompanying soft tissues, including vessels, nerves, muscle, and skin, also occurs. Likewise, because of the dynamic nature of the apparatus, constant high loads of compression can be maintained across fracture sites to help stimulate fracture healing.

During distraction osteogenesis, the new tissues are aligned parallel to the distraction force vector. Accordingly, the surgeon has fine control over the direction of the regenerating bone. Ilizarov noted that tension stress neogenesis was similar to the natural conditions present in musculoskeletal growth. Mesenchymal cells fill the early distraction gap and soon differentiate into osteoblasts. A hyperemic state exists during distraction osteogenesis, with abundant neovascularization in the distraction gap. The overall blood flow to the affected limb is also increased up to 40%.

As noted earlier, the circular external fixator is attached to the limb using wires under tension. Two diameters of wires are used: 1.5 mm in small children and in upper extremities in adults, and 1.8 mm (twice as stiff in bending) in lower extremities in adults and adolescents. Beaded wires (olive wires) are utilized for bony transport, as well as to provide for rigidity of fixation, to prevent unwanted translation of the bone on the frame. An appropriately applied frame on the lower extremity should allow full weight bearing on the limb, irrespective of the extent of the bony defect present. In fact, Ilizarov felt that ambulation and the restoration of function to the limb were essential to achieve good bone regeneration and union. This cyclic axial loading of the affected limb is a crucial element of the Ilizarov method.

With the incorporation of hinges, plates, rods, and other elements, correction of a deformity can be accomplished in any plane. Hence, the apparatus has become an increasingly useful tool in the treatment of congenital, acquired, and posttraumatic limb deformities, as well as nonunion and malunion. What makes this treatment method unique is that all problems affecting a limb can be managed with the application of one apparatus. For instance, nonunion of the tibia with angulatory deformity and 5 cm of shortening can often be successfully treated with one operation. The surgery would entail application of the Ilizarov apparatus with either acute correction of the angulatory deformity or gradual correction via application of hinges. A corticotomy of the tibia is also performed at the time of surgery to proceed with distraction osteogenesis to restore the 5 cm of limb length. The nonunion is then compressed (once properly aligned) to achieve bony union. The lengthening of the limb is occurring at the same time that the nonunion is being compressed. Ilizarov also found that certain more rigid nonunions could actually heal in distraction. Therefore another treatment approach in the previous example would be primary gradual controlled distraction across the nonunion site for the purpose both of achieving bony union and restoring some of the limb length at the nonunion site. In essence, Ilizarov found that with few exceptions, healing could occur as long as a dynamic force, be it compression or distraction, was properly applied across a nonunion site. This dynamic force, when properly applied, causes the dormant mesenchymal cells in the nonunion gap to differentiate into functioning osteoblasts and allow for bone synthesis and resultant healing.

The Ilizarov method has revolutionized thinking about fracture healing and osteogenesis. It has greatly broadened the scope and indications for limb lengthening and has incorporated limb lengthening as a tool in both fracture and nonunion management. Ilizarov's introduction of the concept of distraction osteogenesis and the tension stress effect have changed Western thinking regarding limb lengthening and fracture healing. Close adherence to Ilizarov's principles makes it now possible to successfully treat a host of orthopedic conditions that previously were fraught with high morbidity rates and poor results. As experience broadens, application of the Ilizarov method will continue to grow.

Bhandari M et al: Reamed versus nonreamed intramedullary nailing of lower extremity long bone fractures: A systematic overview and meta-analysis. J Orthop Trauma 2000;14:2. [PMID: 10630795]

Einhorn TA, Lee CA: Bone regeneration: new findings and potential clinical applications. J Am Acad Orthop Surg 2001; 9:157. [PMID: 11421573]

Hak DJ, Lee SS, Goulet JA: Success of exchange reamed intramedullary nailing for femoral shaft nonunion or delayed union. J Orthop Trauma 2000;14:178. [PMID: 10791668]

Hupel TM et al: Effect of unreamed, limited reamed, and standard reamed intramedullary nailing on cortical bone porosity and new bone formation. J Orthop Trauma 2001;15:18. [PMID:11147683]

Ilizarov GA: The significance of the combination of optimal mechanical and biological factors in the regenerate process of transosseous synthesis. In: Abstracts of First International Symposium on Experimental, Theoretical, and Clinical Aspects of Transosseous Osteosynthesis Method Developed in Kniekot, Kurgan, USSR, September 20–23, 1983.

Ilizarov GA: Transosseous Osteosynthesis. Springer-Verlag, 1992.

Katsenis D et al: Treatment of malunion and nonunion at the site of an ankle fusion with the Ilizarov apparatus. J Bone Joint Surg Am 2005;87:302. [PMID: 15687151]

Lowenberg DW, Randall RL: The Ilizarov method. In: Braverman MH, Tawes RL (eds): Surgical Technology International II, 1993.

Marsh D. Concepts of fracture union, delayed union, and nonunion. Clin Orthop 1998;355S:S22. [PMID: 9917623]

Paley D, Maar DC: Ilizarov bone transport treatment for tibial defects. J Orthop Trauma 2000;14:76. [PMID: 10716377]

Weresh MJ et al: Failure of exchange reamed intramedullary nails for ununited femoral shaft fractures. J Orthop Trauma 2000; 14:335. [PMID: 11029556]

PRINCIPLES OF OPERATIVE FRACTURE FIXATION

Fractures occur when one or more types of stress, in excess of failure strength, are applied to bones. Fractures may occur from axial loading (tension, compression), bending, torsion (a twisting force), or shearing. All of these are observed at one time or another. It is frequently (but not always) helpful to recognize the type of failure in order to treat the fracture. Examples of these mechanisms are shown in Figure 3–4.

Biomaterials Used in Fracture Fixation

Operative fracture fixation requires strength and flexibility of the fixation materials. Two materials found to be useful in these regards are titanium alloy and stainless

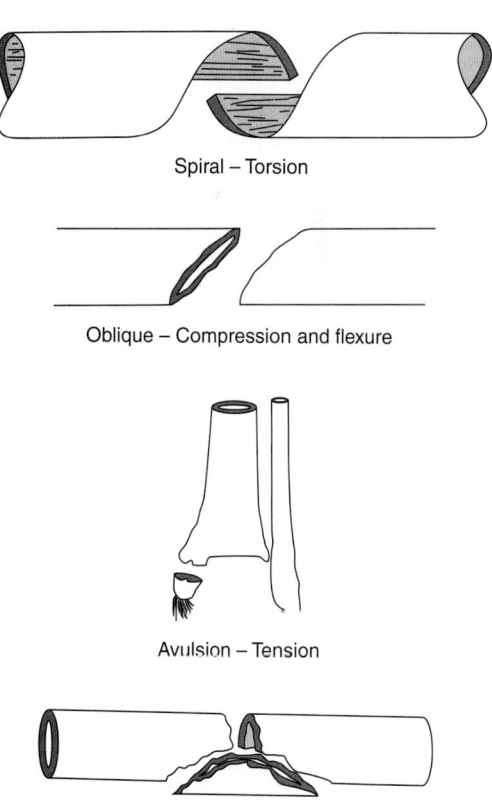

Spiral – Torsion

Oblique – Compression and flexure

Avulsion – Tension

Butterfly – Flexure

Figure 3–4. Mechanisms of failure of bones.

steel, both of which may be contoured to fit irregularities in bone surfaces at the time of surgery. They provide adequate strength and fatigue resistance to allow fracture healing to occur. The elastic modulus of titanium is half that of stainless steel, resulting in half the flexural rigidity in plates of equal size. Although it is recognized that more flexible devices decrease the disuse osteopenia underneath the plates, the clinical advantage of this difference has not been demonstrated. Other potential materials, including composites, cannot be contoured in the operative suite for particular applications.

Biomechanical Principles of Fracture Fixation

The principles of operative fracture fixation are demonstrated by several examples described here. These examples illustrate the importance of the location of a bone plate on a bone in relation to the loading applied to the bone and plate composite. They will demonstrate the bending stiffness of bone plates as a function of thickness and the load sharing that goes on between bone plates in bone. In addition, the effect of bending on the composite of an intramedullary rod and bone will be examined.

A. Bone Plate Thickness

One approach to solving the problem of bone plate fractures is to increase the thickness of the plate. If a bone plate is subjected to bending stress, the stress in the plate, assuming no loading is carried by the bone, can be calculated from the flexure formula: $s_{max} = Mc/I$, where M is the bending moment applied to the plate, c is one-half the thickness of the plate, and the area moment of inertia, I, is expressed by

$$\frac{bh^3}{12}$$

where h is the thickness of plate and b is the width of the plate. The maximum stress would then be equal to

$$s_{max} = \frac{6M}{bh^2}$$

because c is equal to one-half of h. Doubling the thickness decreases the stress to

$$\frac{6M}{4bh^2}$$

Thus, increasing the thickness of the plate by a factor of 2 reduces the stress by a factor of 4, meaning that the load would have to be four times higher before the failure stress would be reached. If one considers the area moment of inertia, I, to be proportional to the bending stiffness, then doubling the size of the plate would double h, which would mean that the plate is eight times

stiffer (but only four times stronger). Because the endurance limit of steel is approximately one-half the ultimate strength, four times higher cyclic loads can be tolerated without fear of failure caused by fatigue.

B. Titanium and Stainless Steel Rods

The second consideration is the difference in the stress carried by an intramedullary rod made of titanium alloy as compared with one constructed of stainless steel. Assume a tibia is a round bone with a hollow, round intramedullary canal 10 mm in diameter. The flexural rigidity is defined as the area moment of inertia times the elastic modulus. A higher flexural rigidity indicates a greater resistance to bending. The area moment of inertia of a thin tube is

$$p^3 r_{ave}^3 t$$

where r is the average radius and t is thickness. Assuming this equation holds for bone also, the ratio of the flexural rigidity of the intramedullary rod to the bone is expressed by the equation

$$\frac{E_m I_m}{E_b I_b} = \frac{r_m^3 t_m E_m}{r_b^3 t_b E_b}$$

The r_{ave} for the metal is 5 mm and for the bone 7.5 mm; t_m is 1 mm and t_b is 5 mm. The ratio E_m/E_b is approximately 10 for stainless steel and 5 for titanium alloy. Thus, the flexural rigidity ratio is

$$\frac{E_m I_m}{E_b I_b} = 0.60 \text{ for stainless steel}$$
$$= 0.30 \text{ for titanium alloy}$$

This indicates that the geometric contribution to stiffness of the construct is greater for bone than for metal. Thus, for a stainless steel rod, the bone and metal rod share the bending stress after healing in a 60:40 ratio, respectively, (75:25 for titanium alloy). It can be seen that the bone is much stiffer than titanium alloy or stainless steel alloy rods. The difference between the two metals is probably not significant for bone remodeling, but maximum strength of the bone would be attained by removal in either case.

C. Bone Plate

The placement of a plate on a bone has a significant bearing on its function. For example, on a curved bone such as the femur, which bows anteriorly, placement of the plate anteriorly tends to place the plate in tension and the posterior cortex of the femur in compression, owing to muscle action of the hamstrings and quadriceps. Conversely, placement of a plate posteriorly tends to cause the fracture to gap open anteriorly because of muscle action. This means that the bone in posterior placement is bearing none of the bending stress resulting from muscle forces and the bone plate has to resist all of this loading. When the bone plate is placed laterally, the axis of bending bisects the broad aspect of the plate, and thus the bone plate is much more able to tolerate the stress caused by muscle load. The plate, however, is susceptible to high stresses if abduction forces are applied to the femur or lower extremity. Thus, optimal placement of a bone plate is on the tension side of the bone, so that the bone will be placed in compressive loading as a result of muscle action. This stimulates healing and minimizes the stresses on the bone plate.

The conventional plate and screw system requires substantial bone exposure for access for open reduction and internal fixation. The surgeon-contoured plate is compressed onto the bone with screws resulting in anatomical reduction and absolute stability. The compressive forces acting on the bone-plate interface can compromise the blood supply and hence the healing process. The Low Contact Dynamic Compression (LCDC) plate was developed to reduce the bone-plate contact surface area.

The recently developed locking plates or internal fixators use a system where the screw head threads into the plate hole, thereby locking the plate just above the bone to minimize contact surface area and the resulting compressive forces. The locked screws in the plate also act as a second bone cortex and therefore self-tapping unicortical screws can be used. This achieves relative stability and therefore promotes callus formation at the fracture site. During fixation, the working length of the plate and screws should be kept in mind with the aim of increasing the working length of the plate and reducing the number of screws used.

D. EXTERNAL FIXATION

External fixation is an important treatment modality for musculoskeletal injuries. The basic principles are that pins are placed within the musculoskeletal system proximal and distal to the zone of injury. These pins are then placed on an external frame, a frame outside the confines of the bone and soft-tissue envelope to stabilize fractures. These devices can be useful as temporary treatment for musculoskeletal injuries, or as definitive treatment, depending on their location and the type of bone and soft-tissue trauma. In the upper extremity, they play a significant role in treating comminuted distal radius fractures by providing both provisional and definitive stabilization for healing as well as provisional treatment for grade III open fractures with segmental bone loss and large soft-tissue injuries in the forearm, elbow, and humerus.

For the pelvis, rapidly applied external fixation with compression for pelvic injuries can stabilize the pelvis, reduce blood loss, be of assistance in initial resuscitation, and provide definitive treatment of such injuries. In the lower extremity, external fixators are important in the treatment of tibia fractures, particularly open or commi-

nuted fractures, and in the treatment of open forefoot injuries and femur injuries with segmental defects. For femur and tibia fractures, external fixation may provide excellent initial or provisional stabilization, which can then be followed by intramedullary fixation for definitive care.

These specific uses of external fixation will be discussed in the individual sections on specific fractures.

Bone Substitutes Used in Fracture Fixation

A. AUTOGENOUS BONE GRAFTING

The gold standard for bone grafting material to stimulate bone growth is cancellous bone from the iliac crest. Obtaining bone graft is a process with potential morbidity, blood loss, infection, and, acute and/or chronic pain. Because of these possible problems, alternatives to autogenous bone grafting have been investigated.

B. OSTEOCONDUCTIVE GRAFT SUBSTITUTES

Hydroxyapatite and tricalcium phosphate, are inorganic structural bone graft substitutes that are primarily osteoconductive and do not stimulate bone formation. These materials can be injected into fracture sites to provide stabilization from compressive loads. A plethora of materials have come to market with variable degrees of clinical testing. The common denominator is that these are osteoconductive: They provide a scaffold for new bony ingrowth. They have been shown to be effective in well-vascularized areas such as the tibial plateau, distal radius and calcaneus.

C. DONOR BONE ALLOGRAFTS

The third alternative bone substitute is allograft derived from living or cadaveric donors. Femoral heads obtained at the time of hip replacement provide a source of living donor bone. Bone collected in the same fashion as transplant organs can also be made available for transplantation. It should be noted that all allograft bone is not the same. Immunogenicity, sterility, mechanical properties, and bone stimulation potential are all dependent on the treatment the bone receives from the time of collection until the time of implantation. The highest risk bone, because of occult viral and bacterial contamination, is that collected in a sterile manner from cadaveric donors and delivered in a sterile manner without further sterilization or processing. This bone also has the highest potential for containing bone growth factors and, therefore, the ability to stimulate new bone formation. Sterilization treatments, such as irradiation and ethylene oxide, are known to compromise these qualities to some extent, with ethylene oxide perhaps being worse than irradiation. Freeze-dried bone is convenient for storage at room temperature but must be sterilized secondarily with ethylene oxide. Because ethylene oxide is unable to penetrate to the depths of large pieces, secondary sterilization of large structural allografts is safer with radiation. The accepted dosage of gamma radiation is 2.5 mrad, but even this dose may not be sufficient to eradicate the human immunodeficiency virus.

D. OSTEO-INDUCTIVE AGENTS

Initially, bone substitutes consisted either of autogenous bone grafts, bone allografts, or material substitutes for bone growth such as hydroxyapatite. However, bone-derived protein extracts or bone morphogenic proteins (BMPs) have been identified as other important components of musculoskeletal repair for bone and cartilage growth. The identification of such specially purified BMPs, which had been shown to induce bone formation in a variety of ectopic and endogenous locations, has been coupled with recent advances in molecular biology and recombinant DNA techniques. Recombinant human bone morphogenic protein has been developed and has been undergoing human trials. These proteins can potentially be coupled with a collagen matrix and the addition of blood products from the patient to stimulate bone healing.

Demineralized bone matrix (DBM) is another osteo-inductive agent containing decalcified bone treated to reduce the potential for an immunogenic host reaction and transmissible infection. The resulting product is a biological scaffold with some remaining growth factors (BMPs). This has the potential to impart a greater osteoconductive effect than standard allograft, as the growth factors have not been exposed by demineralization in the latter.

Cobos JA, Lindsey RW, Gugala Z: The cylindrical titanium mesh cage for treatment of a long bone segmental defect: description of a new technique and report of two cases. J Orthop Trauma 2000;14:54. [PMID: 10630804]

El Maraghy AW et al: Influence of the number of cortices on the stiffness of plate fixation of diaphyseal fractures. J Orthop Trauma 2001;15:186. [PMID: 11265009]

Kurdy NG: Serology of abnormal fracture healing: The role of PII-INP, PICP, and BsALP. J Orthop Trauma 2000;14:48. [PMID: 10630803]

Laurencin C, Khan Y, El-Amin SF: Bone graft substitutes. Expert Rev Med Devices 2006;3:49. [PMID: 16359252]

MMWR 2002;51:207–210: Update: Allograft-associated bacterial infections—United States,2002. J Am Med Assoc 2002;287 (13):1642. [PMID: 11933914]

Radomisli TE et al: Weight-bearing alters the expression of collagen types I and II, BMP 2/4 and osteocalcin in the early stages of distraction osteogenesis. J Orthop Res 2001;19:1049. [PMID: 11781004]

Spinella-Jaegle S et al: Opposite effects of bone morphogenetic protein-2 and transforming growth factor-beta I on osteoblast differentiation. Bone 2001;29:323. [PMID: 11595614]

Wagner M: General principles for the clinical use of the LCP. Injury 2003 Nov;34 Suppl 2:B31-42. [PMID 14580984]

Zlotolow DA et al: The role of human bone morphogenetic proteins in spinal fusion. J Am Acad Orthop Surg 2000;8:3. [PMID: 10666648]

■ I. TRAUMA TO THE UPPER EXTREMITY

FRACTURES & DISLOCATIONS OF THE DISTAL AND MID-FOREARM

Anatomy & Biomechanical Principles

The articular surfaces of the radius, ulna, scaphoid, lunate and triquetral (in adduction) form the condyloid synovial joint of the wrist. The distal radius has three articular components (Figure 3–5): distally the scaphoid and lunate fossae, which allow articulation with the scaphoid and the lunate bones respectively; and the sigmoid notch, which allows articulation with the ulna medially. Between the scaphoid and the lunate fossa is a ridge that corresponds with the scapholunate interval. This entire surface is covered with articular cartilage. The radial styloid allows attachment of the brachioradialis tendon. Also, it is the origin of several important wrist ligaments, including the radial scapholunate and radial lunocapitate ligaments.

The third articular component of the distal radius is the sigmoid notch. This convex structure allows the radius to rotate around the distal ulna. The distal ulna itself has an ulnar styloid, which contains attachments to the triangular fibrocartilage complex, including the meniscus homolog, the volar and dorsal ulnar carpal ligaments, and the ulnar collateral ligament at the wrist. The concave elliptical distal radius is oriented in the sagittal plane with an average of 11 degrees of volar tilt. In the frontal plane, the average radial inclination is 23 degrees. Radial length is measured from the tip of the radial styloid to the ulnar articular surface and averages 13 mm.

In addition to the bony surfaces, the articular cartilage, joint capsule, and wrist ligaments, there are other soft tissues within the distal forearm and wrist. On the dorsal surface, six dorsal compartments contain wrist and digital extensor tendons (Figure 3–6). On the volar

Figure 3–5. Articular components of the distal radius. L = lunate articular surface; N = sigmoid notch; S = scaphoid articular surface. (Reproduced, with permission, from Green DP, Hotchkiss RN, Pederson WC, eds: *Operative Hand Surgery*, 4th ed. WB Saunders, 1999.)

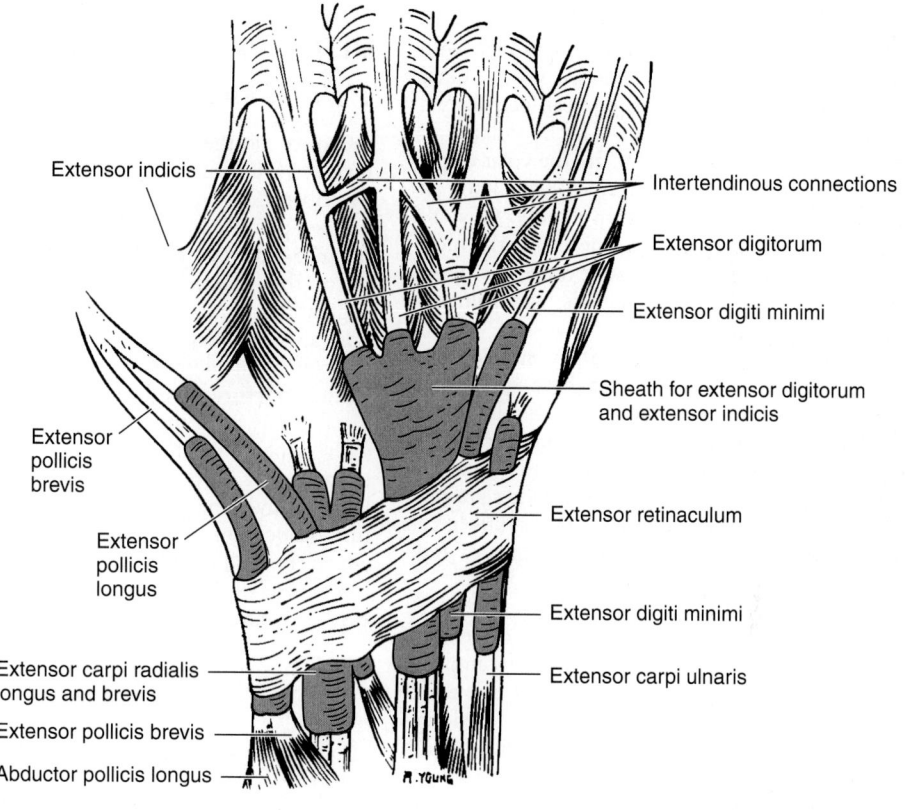

Extensor indicis

Intertendinous connections

Extensor digitorum

Extensor digiti minimi

Sheath for extensor digitorum and extensor indicis

Extensor pollicis brevis

Extensor pollicis longus

Extensor retinaculum

Extensor digiti minimi

Extensor carpi radialis longus and brevis

Extensor carpi ulnaris

Extensor pollicis brevis

Abductor pollicis longus

A. YOUNG

A

Tendon of palmaris longus

Tendon and sheath of flexor pollicis longus

Flexor retinaculum

Median nerve

Common flexor tendon sheath for flexor digitorum superficialis and profundus

Common sheath for abductor pollicis longus and extensor pollicis brevis

Ulnar artery and nerve

Tendon and sheath for flexor carpi radialis

Tendon and sheath for extensor carpi ulnaris

Tendon and sheath for extensor pollicis longus

Tendon and sheath for extensor digiti minimi

Common sheath for extensor carpi radialis longus and brevis

Common sheath for extensor digitorum and indicis

B

Figure 3–6. **A:** Dorsal section of the wrist, showing the six dorsal compartments of the extensor tendons. **B:** Cross section of the wrist, showing the tendons, arteries, and nerves. (Reproduced, with permission, from Jenkins DB: *Hollinshead's Functional Anatomy of the Limbs and Back,* 6th ed. WB Saunders, 1991.)

surface reside the contents of the carpal tunnel, with nine flexor tendons and the median nerve. On the ulnar surface, the flexor carpi ulnaris tendon can be palpated near its insertion on the pisiform. The boundaries of the ulnar tunnel, or Guyon's canal, are the volar carpal ligament and transverse carpal ligament, the hook of the hamate radially and the pisiform ulnarly. Guyon's canal contains the ulnar artery and nerve. In the most superficial soft tissue layer of the wrist reside the flexor carpi radialis layers, flexor carpi ulnaris, and palmaris longus.

The radius and the ulna structurally support the forearm. The distal radius and ulna have specialized articulations with the carpus and with each other. The shafts of the radius and ulna are approximately parallel. The ulnar shaft, however, remains fixed in its rotation at the ulnohumeral joint, and the radius rotates around the ulna in pronation and supination. The radius has a lateral bow that is crucial to the maintenance of full pronation and supination.

The interosseus membrane in the interosseous space connects the shafts of the radius and ulna. The central portion is thickened and has been shown to be important in force transmission between the radius and ulna. Origins of flexor and extensor muscles are located along the anterior and posterior surfaces of the radius, ulna, and interosseus membrane.

Berger RA: The anatomy of the ligaments of the wrist and distal radioulnar joints. Clin Orthop 2001;383:32. [PMID: 11210966]

Blazar PE et al: The effect of observer experience on magnetic resonance imaging interpretation and localization of triangular fibrocartilage complex lesions. J Hand Surg Am 2001;26: 742. [PMID: 11466652]

Cober SR, Trumble TE: Arthroscopic repair of triangular fibrocartilage complex injuries. Orthop Clin North Am 2001;32: 279. [PMID: 11331541]

Freeland AE, Geissler WB: The arthroscopic management of intraarticular distal radius fractures. Hand Surg 2000;5:93. [PMID:11301502]

Gupta R, Bozenthka DJ, Osterman AL: Wrist arthroscopy: Principles and clinical applications. J Am Acad Orthop Surg 2001; 9:200. [PMID: 11421577]

Lindau T, Adlercreutz C, Aspenberg P: Peripheral tears of the triangular fibrocartilage complex cause distal radioulnar joint instability after distal radial fractures. J Hand Surg Am 2000; 25:464. [PMID: 10811750]

McGinley JC et al: Mechanics of the antebrachial interosseous membrane: Response to shearing forces. J Hand Surg Am 2001;26:733. [PMID: 11466651]

Nakamura T et al: Origins and insertions of the triangular fibrocartilage complex: A histological study. J Hand Surg Br 2001; 26:446. [PMID: 11560427]

Poitevin LA: Anatomy and biomechanics of the interosseous membrane: Its importance in the longitudinal stability of the forearm. Hand Clin 2001;17:97. [PMID: 11280163]

DISTAL RADIUS & ULNA INJURIES

1. Distal Radius & Ulna Fracture

Fractures of the distal radius account for approximately 14% of all fractures. In 1814, Abraham Colles described distal radius fracture prior to the advent of radiographs. In his purely descriptive definition, the fracture most commonly involves the distal metaphysis of the radius. He described the resulting volar angulation, dorsal displacement, loss of radial inclination and resultant radial shortening as a "silver fork deformity." In contrast, the **Smith's fracture,** or **reverse Colles' fracture,** is a dorsally angulated fracture of the distal radius, with the hand and wrist displaced volarly with respect to the forearm. The fracture may be extraarticular, intraarticular, or a part of a fracture-dislocation involving the wrist. **Barton's fracture** is a fracture-dislocation with an intraarticular fracture in which the carpus and a rim of the distal radius are displaced together (Figure 3–7). The **Chauffeur's fracture** is a radial styloid fracture, described initially in

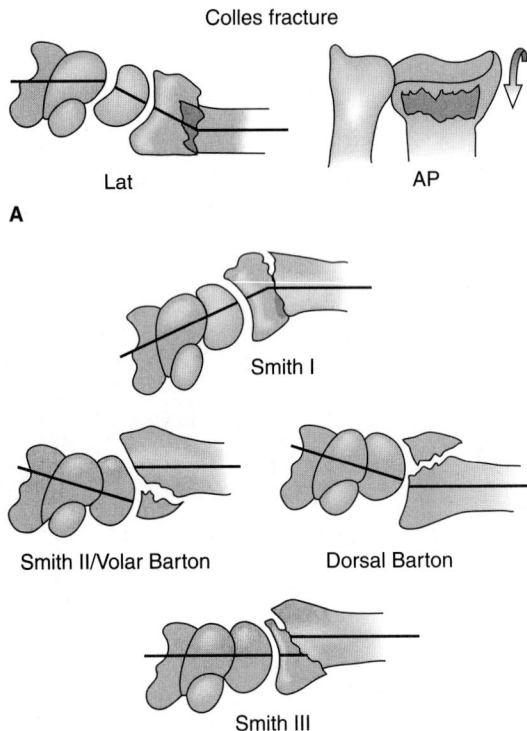

Figure 3–7. Schematic drawings of Colles fracture (**A**) and Smith and Barton fractures (**B**). (Reproduced, with permission, from Green DP, Hotchkiss RN, Pederson WC, eds: *Operative Hand Surgery,* 4th ed. WB Saunders, 1999.)

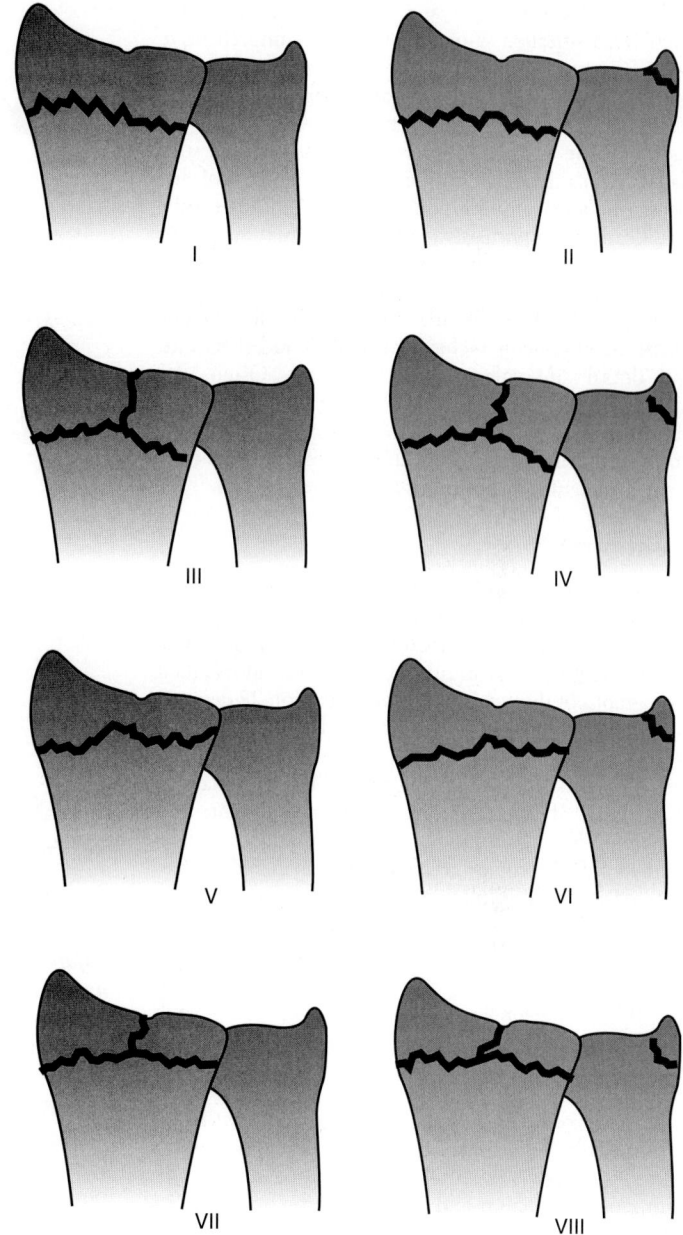

Figure 3–8. Classification of distal radius fractures according to Frykman. (Reproduced, with permission, from Green DP, Hotchkiss RN, Pederson WC, eds: *Operative Hand Surgery*, 4th ed. WB Saunders, 1999.)

car drivers operating automobiles, which required hand cranking to start. When the engine engaged, the crank would "kick back," and the Chauffeur's fracture would result.

Fracture Classification

In modern day fracture care, the emphasis has shifted from "named" fractures to anatomic descriptions of the injury.

No one fracture classification system is comprehensive in describing all important variables of distal radius fractures.

The Frykman classification categorizes fractures by the presence or absence of an ulnar styloid fracture and by whether fracture lines are extraarticular, intraarticular involving the radial carpal joint, intraarticular involving the distal radioulnar joint, or intraarticular involving both radiocarpal and distal radioulnar joints (Figure 3–8).

The AO classification and its derivative, the OTA fracture classification system are the most comprehensive systems currently used to classify distal radius fractures. Broadly, distal radius fractures are separated into three groups: extraarticular (type A), partial articular (type B), and complete articular (type C). Within these are sub-classifications that relate to the particular amount of displacement and comminution (Figure 3–9). These sub-classifications are primarily used for research.

Another useful classification that addresses intraarticular fractures is that popularized by Melone (Figure 3–10). The Melone classification describes four major fracture components including the shaft, radial styloid, and dorsal and volar medial fragments. Often, the lunate fossa is fractured into dorsal and volar components, with the scaphoid fossa a separate component. Four-part articular fractures can have varying degrees of displacement and comminution.

Treatment

Treatment of distal radius fractures should be influenced by fracture pattern and bone quality with a goal of restoring normal alignment and articular congruity. The normal alignment as measured in the AP and Lateral radiographs of the wrist are: radial inclination 22 degrees, volar tilt 11 degrees to 12 degrees and radial length 11 to 12 mm. Additional factors to consider are fracture displacement, intraarticular components, angulation, and degree of comminution; age of the patient; and functional level. Additional imaging techniques can be used to assess complex fracture patterns including CT scan for preoperative planning of intraarticular fractures; MRI to rule out injuries to the carpal ligaments or to the triangular fibrocartilage complex. Soft tissue injuries are commonly associated and should be carefully examined, including the triangular fibrocartilage complex (TFCC), lunotriquetral and scapholunate ligament.

A. Closed Procedures

1. Closed reduction with splinting and casting— Extraarticular distal radius fractures in certain individuals (classic Colles' fracture) can be treated successfully with closed reduction and splinting with conversion to a cast once swelling subsides. Radial length is generally not fully restored, nor is radial angulation with closed reduction techniques. Small amounts of radial shortening can lead to increased load in the lunate fossa, distal ulna, and triangular fibrocartilage. In most low-demand patients, however, this treatment can be successful, and functional wrist motion can be obtained. If shortening is significant, midcarpal instability may occur. Another potential problem is distal radioulnar joint arthrosis and ulnar carpal abutment, which may necessitate later reconstruction. In minimally displaced fractures, a rapid cast conversion to a supportive splint (2 or 3

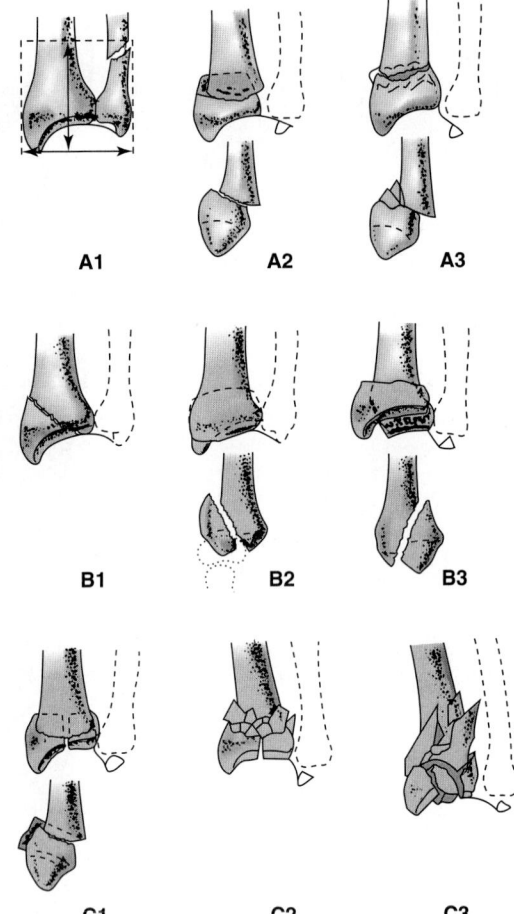

Figure 3–9. AO classification of distal radius fractures. **A:** Extraarticular metaphyseal fracture. Junction of the metaphysis and diaphysis is identified by the "square" or T method (greatest width on frontal plane of distal forearm; illustrated in **A1**). **A1:** Isolated fracture of distal ulna. **A2:** Simple radial fracture. **A3:** Radial fracture with metaphyseal impaction. **B:** intraarticular rim fracture (preserving the continuity of the epiphysis and metaphysis). **B1:** Fracture of radial styloid. **B2:** Dorsal rim fracture (dorsal Barton's fracture). **B3:** Volar rim fracture (reverse Barton's 5 Goyrand-Smith type 2, Letenneur). **C:** Complex intraarticular fracture (disrupting the continuity of the epiphysis and metaphysis). **C1:** Radiocarpal joint congruity preserved, metaphysis fractured. **C2:** Articular displacement. **C3:** Diaphyseal-metaphyseal involvement. It should be considered that injury of the distal radioulnar joint is possible in any of these fractures. (Reproduced, with permission, from Green DP, Hotchkiss RN, Pederson WC, eds: *Operative Hand Surgery,* 4th ed. WB Saunders, 1999.)

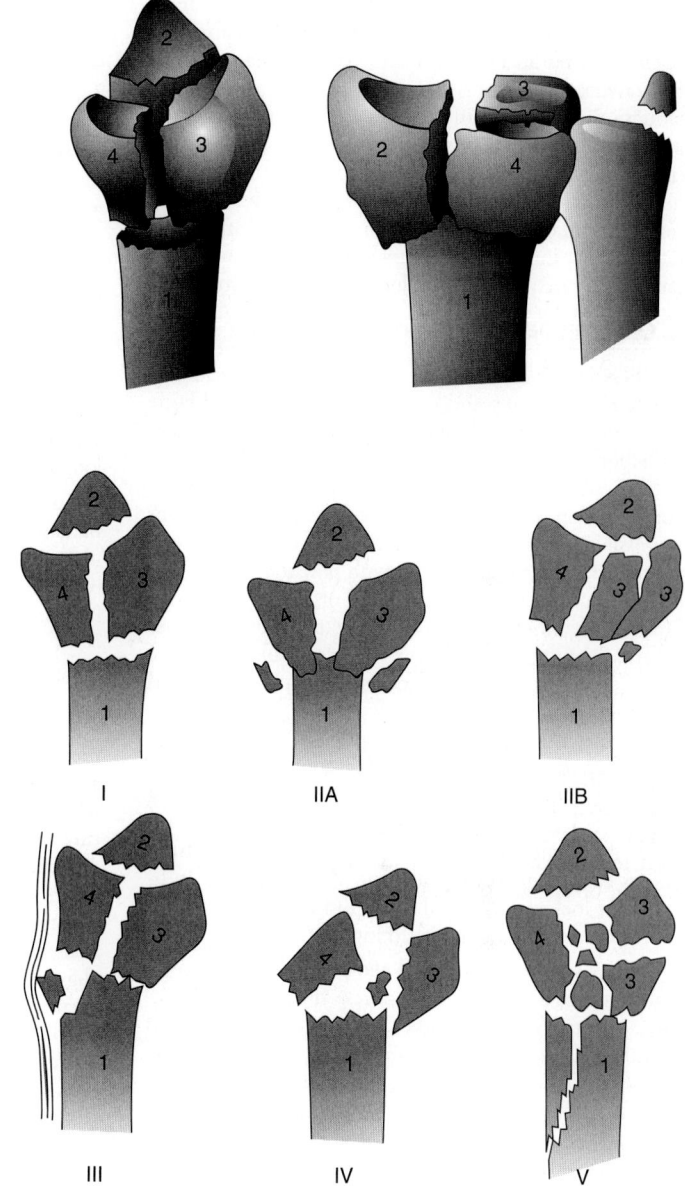

Figure 3–10. Intraarticular fracture classification of Melone. (Reproduced, with permission, from Green DP, Hotchkiss RN, Pederson WC, eds: *Operative Hand Surgery*, 4th ed. WB Saunders, 1999.)

weeks) and early mobilization can be safely done and may yield improved outcomes.

2. Percutaneous pin fixation—Percutaneous pins can be an effective adjunct to cast treatment or external fixation. The pins can hold large metaphyseal fragments in good position and prevent collapse or malalignment. In the **intrafocal pin technique,** the pin is placed in the fracture site itself. This can be an effective means of achieving anatomic alignment and preventing loss of reduction. The pins can be removed after 4 weeks but additional immobilization (cast or external fixation) should be used for 6 to 8

weeks. This technique requires good bone stock and additional stabilization using cast or external fixation. Loss of reduction is a potential complication in older patients. Also, granuloma formation around the pin can be seen.

3. External fixation—External fixation is an effective way to handle distal radius fractures. In particular, it provides more direct control of the overall length of the distal radius, and to some extent the inclination, compared with cast treatment. Use of indirect traction on fracture fragments, taking advantage of "ligamentotaxis" via the fixator pins, can be effective. There is the additional advantage of not devascularizing bony fragments and not creating a surgical wound. In cases of open fractures an external fixator can facilitate wound care. External fixation is effective in preventing loss of reduction and length in situations where there is comminution of bone. In intraarticular fractures, external fixation can be used but reductions are difficult to maintain without percutaneous pins or internal fixation. Complications are common however with external fixation including, pin tract infection, superficial radial nerve neuropathy, pin loosening, and stiffness.

B. OPEN REDUCTION AND INTERNAL FIXATION

1. Plate and screws—Plate and screws can be extremely effective in achieving and maintaining reduction. If bone fragments are large, it is also an effective way to maintain reduction. This technique has a tendency to fail, however, if there are multiple fragments and if there is sufficient comminution so that rigid internal fixation is difficult, or impossible, to achieve. Other drawbacks to this technique include creation of an incision, with potential subsequent scarring, and also the possibility of future hardware removal. Additionally, the operative technique involves soft-tissue stripping and potential devascularization of small fragments during the process of open reduction and internal fixation.

Recently, distal radius plates with fixed-angle screws have been devised specifically for comminuted distal radius fractures. These feature multiple small locking holes in a T configuration, allowing multiple screws for small fragment fixation. This highly stable construct allows early functional treatment. Recent studies indicate that locked plates and early postoperative range of motion may provide improved long-term results.

2. Arthroscopically assisted reduction—Arthroscopically assisted reduction can address the associated ligament injuries improving the final result, with limited scarring. A recent study reported that patients undergoing arthroscopically assisted procedures had a greater degree of supination, flexion, and extension than patients undergoing fluoroscopy-assisted fixation of intraarticular distal radius fractures.

C. TREATMENT DECISIONS

Besides fracture type and comminution, additional factors that modify treatment decisions include patient comorbidities, available resources for treatment and surgeon expertise. For a non-comminuted, non-displaced, methaphyseal distal radius fracture, nonoperative treatment with initial splint until the edema subsides and subsequent cast application is the appropriate treatment. In contrast, intraarticular comminuted fractures are difficult if not impossible to reduce and maintain without the addition of hardware. In presence of osteoporosis and intraarticular displacement, ORIF using a fixed angle device is probably the best option. When facing severe comminution, pinning and external fixator can be the most suitable treatment.

1. Extraarticular nondisplaced fractures—Extraarticular nondisplaced fractures can be treated with cast immobilization for 4-6 weeks, until fracture healing occurs, following by mobilization with an off the shelf brace.

2. Extraarticular displaced fractures—Closed reduction should be attempted on extraarticular displaced fractures. If radial length and volar tilt are restored, then a sugar tong splint or long arm cast can be effective in holding the reduction. If the reduction is not adequate by closed means then an external fixator (for ligamentotaxis) and percutaneous pins (to manipulate the fracture) may be necessary. Current trends toward plating via a volar approach with specialized locking plates may improve wrist motion and long-term outcomes even in extraarticular fractures.

3. Intraarticular fractures—The treatment of intraarticular fractures aims to restore the congruity of the articular surface and the anatomic axis of the distal radius in order to improve the outcome. Open reduction and internal fixation is the treatment of choice. For volar Barton's fractures, the treatment of choice is the volar buttress plate. The only contraindications to this treatment are cases with excessive comminution such that open reduction and internal fixation will fail to achieve a stable bony construct. In these situations, use of an external fixator as a distractor and neutralization device is generally indicated. Using a fluoroscopy unit to visualize the fracture will help ascertain that both articular alignment and overall radial length have been adequately restored with external fixation. Minor adjustments as necessary can be effectively done with adjunct percutaneous pins. These maneuvers may fail to achieve the appropriate articular alignment, particularly if some healing has already occurred or if the displacement is severe. In this case, open reduction and internal fixation should be performed. Justification for aggressive treatment of distal radius fractures in young patients (<60 years) comes from several studies. The goal should be articular step-off <2 mm, radial shortening <4 mm, dorsal tilt <15 degrees, volar tilt <20 degrees and loss of radial inclination <10 degrees. Arthroscopically assisted repair of distal radius fractures has been advocated. Intraarticular step-off and associated injuries such as triangular fibrocartilage, scapholunate, and lunotriquetral tears as well as osteochondral lesions can be accurately assessed. Some authors advocate bone grafting in the acute treatment of comminuted fractures.

2. Distal Radioulnar Joint Dislocation

The distal ulna transmits significant loads to the forearm through the distal ulna via the triangular fibrocartilage complex. Even minor disruptions of the precise anatomic relationships between the distal radius and ulna and ulnar carpus results in pain syndromes. The distal radioulnar joint (DRUJ) can be dislocated by a variety of mechanisms, including low- and high-energy trauma. These are associated with disruption of the ulnar soft-tissue triangular fibrocartilage complex, including the articular disk and associated ligaments. There should be a high index of suspicion in order to diagnose this lesion because radiographs that are not taken in the perfect lateral orientation will tend to look relatively normal. A displaced fracture at the ulnar styloid base indicates a high risk of distal radioulnar instability. In the presence of forearm and elbow fracture-dislocations, further evaluation of the radioulnar joint is mandatory.

Clinical Findings

The clinical examination is key, with identification of the distal radioulnar joint surface anatomy and clinical evaluation of the joint. The amount of stability should be carefully assessed and compared with that of the opposite wrist. The patient should position the wrist to reproduce the pain. With the hand pronated, the examiner tries to displace the ulnar head applying a dorsal to volar load 4 cm proximal to the DRUJ (piano key test). Little resistance to ballottement and volar movement of the ulna head corresponds to a positive "piano key test." Subluxation is much more common than anterior or posterior dislocation. Limitation of pronation and supination, or pain associated with such motion, would be expected in such a situation. Palpation of the sixth extensor compartment during resisted pronation is useful to identify any subluxation. The other common cause of distal radioulnar joint problems is rheumatoid arthritis.

Treatment

Dorsal dislocation, or subluxation, should be treated by reduction of the ulnar head into the sigmoid fossa and placement of the forearm in full supination. The arm should be immobilized in supination, which requires a long-arm cast or splint. Volar dislocation is relatively rare and is usually stable after reduction. If dorsal or volar dislocation or subluxation of the distal ulna cannot be reduced with manipulation in the outpatient setting, closed treatment can be attempted under anesthesia. If this fails, open reduction and soft-tissue reconstruction may be necessary. If this is performed, a retinacular flap may be used to transpose the extensor carpi ulnaris to a more dorsal position to stabilize the distal ulna, as has been described for Darrach reconstruction of the joint.

3. Malunion of Distal Radius

Malunion of the distal radius can have a variety of negative consequences. Alteration of the biomechanical function of the wrist may lead to weakness, limitation of motion, and midcarpal instability. Associated distal radioulnar joint arthrosis may be present, as well as ulnocarpal abutment. Also, rotational deformity is common with angulated malunions. CT of both wrists can be used to identify and measure malrotation preoperatively.

Treatment

The treatment of choice in such a situation, if conservative treatment fails, is reconstructive surgery. Fernandez has elegantly described the strategy. An osteotomy of the radius with iliac crest bone grafting and plate fixation is performed (Figure 3–11). The distal radioulnar joint

A   **B**

Figure 3–11. Wedge osteotomy of the distal radius with iliac crest bone graft and plate fixation. (Reproduced, with permission, from Green DP, Hotchkiss RN, Pederson WC, eds: *Operative Hand Surgery,* 4th ed. WB Saunders, 1999.)

Figure 3–12. Suave-Kapandji reconstruction of the distal radioulnar joint. (Reproduced, with permission, from Green DP, Hotchkiss RN, Pederson WC, eds: *Operative Hand Surgery,* 4th ed. WB Saunders, 1999.)

must be addressed and, depending upon the degree of subluxation or arthrosis, may require closed reduction, open reduction, or reconstruction using the Darrach or Sauve-Kapandji procedures (Figure 3–12). In this procedure, instead of distal ulnar resection as in the Darrach procedure, transverse segmental resection of the ulnar metaphysis is followed by creation of an arthrodesis of the distal ulna to the radius, using the resected bone as grafting material. Forearm rotation occurs through the ulnar metaphyseal pseudoarthrosis. Additionally, restoration of the radial length may be difficult with manipulation alone. Useful adjuncts to achieve restoration of appropriate length and orientation in severe malunion include use of laminar spreaders to distract the proximal and distal fragments of the radius after osteotomy. Alternatively, an external fixator may prove useful in helping to achieve appropriate length after osteotomy.

If the distal radius has settled into a position of shortening and significant angulatory deformity but the fracture is not yet fully healed, osteotomy for early or "nascent" malunion is justified. The advantage of taking down a nascent malunion is that the operation is technically simpler to perform, shortens the time of disability, and leads to better long-term results. Additionally, the distal radioulnar joint can be restored more reliably in these early reconstructions than when osteotomy is required for established malunion. The latter

often requires adjunctive distal radioulnar joint reconstruction with Darrach resection, Sauve-Kapandji, hemiresection, or matched resection arthroplasty.

Abboudi J, Culp RW: Treating fractures of the distal radius with arthroscopic assistance. Orthop Clin North Am 2001;32: 307. [PMID: 11331543]

Carter PB, Stuart PR: The Sauve-Kapandji procedure for post-traumatic disorders of the distal radio-ulnar joint. J Bone Joint Surg Br 2000;82:1013. [PMID: 11041592]

Chhabra A et al: Biomechanical efficacy of an internal fixator for treatment of distal radius fractures. Clin Orthop 2001;393: 318. [PMID: 11764365]

Jakob M, Rikli A, Regazzoni P: Fractures of the distal radius treated by internal fixation and early function. J Bone Joint Surg Br 2000;82-B:341. [PMID: 10813166]

Katz MA et al: Computed tomography scanning of intraarticular distal radius fractures: Does it influence treatment. J Hand Surg Am 2001;26:415. [PMID: 11418901]

Ladd AL, Pliam NB: The role of bone graft and alternatives in unstable distal radius fracture treatment. Orthop Clin North Am 2001;32:337. [PMID: 11331546]

Margaliot Z et al: A meta-analysis of outcomes of external fixation versus plate osteosynthesis for unstable distal radius fractures. J Hand Surg 2005;30:1185. [PMID: 16344176]

May MM, Lawton JN, Blazar PE. Ulnar styloid fractures associated with distal radius fractures: incidence and implications for distal radioulnar joint instability. J Hand Surg (Am). 2002; 27(6):965-71. [PMID: 12457345]

Mehta JA, Bain GI, Heptinstall RJ: Anatomical reduction of intraarticular fractures of the distal radius. J Bone Joint Surg Br 2000;82-B:79. [PMID: 10697319]

Orbay JL, Fernandez DL. Volar fixed-angle plate fixation for unstable distal radius fractures in the elderly patient. J Hand Surg [Am]. 2004 Jan;29(1):96-102. [PMID: 14751111]

Rogachefsky RA et al: Treatment of severely comminuted intraarticular fractures of the distal end of the radius by open reduction and combined internal and external fixation. J Bone Joint Surg Am 2001;83-A:509. [PMID: 11315779]

Schneeberger AG et al: Open reduction and plate fixation of displaced AO type C3 fractures of the distal radius: Restoration of articular congruity in eighteen cases. J Orthop Trauma 2001;15:350. [PMID: 11433140]

Viso R, Wegener EE, Freeland AE: Use of a closing wedge osteotomy to correct malunion of dorsally displaced extraarticular distal radius fractures. Orthopedics 2000;23:721. [PMID: 10917249]

DISLOCATION OF THE RADIOCARPAL JOINT

Dislocation of the radiocarpal joint is usually accompanied by significant carpal-ligamentous injury or fracture. Treatment of these injuries involves restoration of the bony architecture through immediate closed reduction, if possible, elective closed reduction, open reduction and internal fixation, or a combination of these procedures. Associated fractures, such as transscaphoid perilunate or distal radius fracture associated with carpal dislocation, should be treated with open reduction and internal fixation. Ligamentous repair should be performed at this time (see Chapter 10, Hand Surgery). Median nerve evaluation is mandatory, and surgical exploration indicated, if a dense neuropathy is present.

FOREARM SHAFT FRACTURES

In general, any fracture requires evaluation both clinically and radiographically of a joint above and joint below the fracture. It is not uncommon for fractures of the midshaft of the forearm to have significant consequences to either the wrist or elbow.

1. Isolated Fracture of the Ulna (Nightstick Fracture)

Nondisplaced or minimally displaced fractures of the ulnar shaft are fairly common and usually result from a direct blow.

Treatment

A variety of treatment options are possible for managing minimally displaced ulnar diaphyseal injuries. The time to union is about 3 months, with union achieved with cast immobilization and early mobilization of the wrist and elbow. Less stringent immobilization protocols have also resulted in satisfactory results. Sarmiento and Latta achieved excellent results using a functional brace for isolated ulnar fractures. After initial long arm cast fixation for immobilization until acute symptoms and swelling have subsided, cast removal is followed by Orthoplast sleeve or cast bracing with Velcro straps, with no limitation of pronation and supination. Some investigators report excellent results with minimal or no immobilization. In general, some sort of immobilization until pain subsides is preferable. With displaced fractures with angulation greater than 10 degrees or displacement greater than 50%, one must be extremely suspicious of an associated injury at the elbow or wrist. In isolated fractures of the ulna in the adult with displacement >50% or angulation >10 degrees (or both), open reduction and internal fixation is the treatment of choice. Current recommendations include fixation with a 3.5 mm dynamic or limited contact compression plate with six to eight cortices of fixation proximal and distal to the fracture. Intramedullary pinning seems to provide comparable results to plate fixation, but further studies are needed at this point.

2. Isolated Radial Shaft Fractures

A fracture anywhere along the length of the radius with or without associated ulnar fracture with injury to the distal radioulnar joint (DRUJ) is defined as a Galeazzi fracture. Injuries associated with the DRUJ include ulnar styloid fractures, radial shortening >5 mm, and DRUJ dislocation.

Treatment

Open reduction and internal fixation with plate fixation is recommended in adult patients to ensure a reasonable chance of restoration of the distal radioulnar joint. Hughston's series in 1957 had a 92% incidence of poor results with closed treatment. After open reduction and internal fixation of the radial shaft through a volar Henry approach using compression plating, the distal radioulnar joint should be carefully inspected. If it is unstable, pinning in a position of stability (usually full supination) is required. If it is frankly dislocated and cannot be reduced closed, and maintained by closed or percutaneous means, then open stabilization with repair of associated ligaments or removal of interposed soft tissue is mandatory.

3. Monteggia Fracture
Classification of Fractures

In 1814, Monteggia of Milan described an injury involving fracture of the proximal third of the ulna, with anterior dislocation of the radial head. This definition was extended by Bado to include the entire spectrum of these fractures with associated radial head dislocations, regardless of the direction of dislocation. They are classified in the following ways:

Type 1: Fracture of the ulnar diaphysis with anterior angulation and anterior dislocation of the radial head (60% of cases)

Type 2: Fracture of the ulnar diaphysis with posterior angulation or posterior or posterolateral dislocation of the radial head (15% of cases)

Type 3: Fracture of the ulnar metaphysis, with lateral or anterolateral dislocation of the radial head (20% of cases)

Type 4: Fracture of the ulna and radius at the proximal third, with anterior dislocation of the radial head (5% of cases).

Other authors have noted that type 3 fractures may be more common than type 2 fractures, but all agree that type 1 lesions are the most common.

Associated lesions include injury to the radial nerve; palsies of both the deep branch of the radial nerve and the posterior interosseous nerve have been described with Monteggia fractures. It is important to perform an adequate neurovascular examination at the time of evaluation. The index of suspicion must be high because radial head dislocation may be missed if appropriate radiographs are not obtained and scrutinized.

Treatment

Closed treatment is usually satisfactory for children, but open reduction and internal fixation is the treatment of choice for Monteggia lesions in an adult. Optimal results require early diagnosis, rigid internal fixation of the fractured ulna, complete reduction of the dislocated radial head, and immobilization for approximately 6 weeks to allow healing with sufficient stability. Internal fixation is best performed with a compression plate technique. The radial head can often be completely reduced by closed means once the ulnar fracture is reduced and rigidly fixed. If this is not possible, open reduction is required; attention should be paid to the relationship between the annular ligament, the lateral epicondyle, and the radial head. Entrapment of the soft tissues is the most common reason for inability to obtain concomitant closed radial head reduction at the time of open reduction and internal fixation of the ulna.

4. Fractures of Both the Radius & Ulna

Fractures of both the radius and ulna (both-bones fractures) usually result from high-energy injuries. These fractures are usually displaced because of the force required to produce such an injury. Careful neurovascular examination and adequate radiographs to show both the wrist and the elbow are mandatory.

Treatment

Treatment of choice for both-bones fractures is open reduction and internal fixation. The volar Henry approach should be used for radius repair, between the flexor carpi radialis and brachioradialis, with the ulna approached subcutaneously. Open reduction and internal fixation offers the best chance of restoring the normal positions of the radius and ulna, which is critical to forearm function and in particular pronation and supination. For fractures of the proximal half of the radius, the dorsal Thompson approach can be used; however, the risk of iatrogenic injury to the posterior interosseous nerve is increased. Technical points to be considered include minimal subperiosteal stripping only of the fracture site. The plates can be placed on top of the periosteum to preserve the blood supply as much as possible. A 3.5-mm dynamic compression plate or limited contact compression plate can be used for AO/ASIF compression plating. Bone grafting can be used for severely comminuted fractures with significant bone loss. Only the skin is closed so as not to cause compartment syndrome or Volkmann's contracture. Splinting of the affected extremity, as in all upper extremity surgery, is recommended, with early digital active and passive motion exercises.

Many authors recommend plate fixation for Gustilo type I, II, and IIIA open both-bones fractures. Use of an external fixator is a viable alternative, however, particularly if severe open wounds are present with skin and soft-tissue loss as in Gustilo type IIIB and IIIC injuries. Criteria for bone grafting include comminution involving more than one third the cortical circumference and comminution that compromises interfragmentary compression; however, the success of acute bone grafting has not been proved in long-term studies.

Catalano LW 3rd, Barron OA, Glickel SZ. Assessment of articular displacement of distal radius fractures. Clin Orthop 2004 Jun;423:79-84. [PMID: 15232430]

Chung KC, Spilson SV: The frequency and epidemiology of hand and forearm fractures in the United States. J Hand Surg Am 2001;26:908. [PMID: 11561245]

Dell'Oca AA et al: Treating forearm fractures using an internal fixator. Clin Orthop 2001;389:196. [PMID: 11501811]

Iqbal MJ, Abbas D: Distal radioulnar synostosis following K-wire fixation. Orthopedics 2001;24:61. [PMID: 11199355]

Qidwai SA: Treatment of diaphyseal forearm fractures in children by intramedullary Kirschner wires. J Trauma 2001;50:303. [PMID: 11242296]

Sarmiento A, et al: Isolated ulnar shaft fractures treated with functional braces. J Orthop Trauma. 1998;12:420. [PMID: 9715450]

Wei SY, et al: Diaphyseal forearm fractures treated with and without bone graft. J Trauma 1999;46:1045. [PMID: 10372622]

Ruch DS, Vallee J, Poehling GG, Smith BP, Kuzma GR. Arthroscopic reduction versus fluoroscopic reduction in the management of intraarticular distal radius fractures. Arthroscopy 2004;20:225. [PMID: 15007310]

INJURIES AROUND THE ELBOW

Anatomy & Biomechanical Principles

The elbow is one of the most confined articulations in humans. The trochlear notch covers almost 180° of the trochlea. The articular surface of the distal humerus is angulated 30° anteriorly, which is matched by a similar posterior angulation of the trochlear notch. Accessible surface structures at the elbow that can be inspected and palpated include the medial and lateral condyles and the olecranon. With the elbow in 90 degrees of flexion, these three palpable points form a triangle. Distally, the radial head can be palpated at the lateral aspect of the elbow joint, and the contour can be appreciated with pronation and supination. These bony landmarks are important when clinically assessing the elbow for fractures, dislocations, or effusions. Effusions can be discerned by swelling between the lateral epicondyle and the olecranon. On cross-section, the humerus is circular at the midshaft but flared and flattened at the distal end. Medial and lateral supracondylar columns diverge to increase the diameter of the distal humerus in the mediolateral plane. Each condyle contains an articulating portion for the radial head, or ulna, and nonarticulating epicondyles, which are terminal portions of the supracondylar ridges on which pronator-flexor muscles and supinator-extensor muscles originate. The three articulations at the elbow are the ulnotrochlear joint, the radiocapitellar joint, and the proximal radioulnar joint.

The radial head articulates with the capitellar portion of the lateral condyle. The articular surface of the medial condyle has prominent medial and lateral ridges that aid in stabilizing the articulation with the ulna. Anterior to these two condyles are the coronoid and radial fossa, which receive the coronoid process of the ulna and the radial head when the elbow goes into full flexion. The proximal ulna contains the olecranon process posteriorly, the coronoid process anteriorly, and the sigmoid, or semilunar notch, which articulates with the trochlea. The triceps has a broad tendinous insertion into the olecranon posteriorly; anteriorly, the brachialis inserts on the coronoid process and the tuberosity of the ulna. The radial head lines up in its lesser sigmoid, or radial notch, with the annular ligament surrounding it. Collateral ligaments make up the remainder of the soft-tissue structures of the elbow, with the most important portion being the anterior band of the medial or ulnar collateral ligament arising from the medial epicondyle and attaching to a small process on the medial surface of the coronoid. The lesser posterior portion of the medial collateral ligament attaches to the medial surface of the olecranon process. There is a similarly triangular fan-shaped lateral collateral ligament, whose origin is the lateral epicondyle inserting on the annular ligament of the radius. The ulnar nerve passes through the cubital tunnel at the medial column of the elbow and must be appropriately assessed following injury.

DISTAL HUMERUS FRACTURES

1. Intercondylar-T or -Y Fractures

Intercondylar humerus fractures are among the most challenging fractures treated by the orthopedic surgeon. The usual mechanism of injury is axial loading of the ulna in the trochlear groove. Studies have demonstrated increasing numbers of these injuries in the older (>60 years) population. It is critical to assess the integrity of the medial and lateral column for reconstructible bone fragments and the degree of comminution.

Classification

Jupiter and Mehne classified distal humerus fractures into intraarticular and extraarticular patterns. Intraarticular fractures are divided into the following types:

1. Single column: Divided into medial or lateral
2. Bicolumn: Divided into TT, TY, TH, lambda, or multiplane pattern
3. Capitellum fractures
4. Trochlea fractures

Extraarticular fractures are classified into intracapsular and extracapsular (Table 3–3).

Table 3–3. The Jupiter and Mehne classification of distal humerus fractures.

I. Intraarticular fracture
  A. Single-column fractures
    1. Medial
      a. High
      b. Low
    2. Lateral
      a. High
      b. Low
    3. Divergent
  B. Bicolumn fractures
    1. T pattern
      a. High
      b. Low
    2. Y pattern
    3. H pattern
    4. Lambda pattern
      a. Medial
      b. Lateral
    5. Multiplane pattern
  C. Capitellum fractures
  D. Trochlear fractures
II. Extraarticular intracapsular fractures
  A. Transcolumn fractures
    1. High
      a. Extension
      b. Flexion
      c. Abduction
      d. Adduction
    2. Low
      a. Extension
      b. Flexion
III. Extracapsular fractures
  A. Medial epicondyle
  B. Lateral epicondyle

Reproduced, with permission, from Browner BD et al, eds: *Skeletal Trauma,* 2nd ed. WB Saunders, 1998.

Treatment

Traditional treatment favored closed techniques because of the difficulty of fracture fixation for intercondylar fractures. Cast immobilization probably represents the worst of all possible worlds: inadequate reduction plus prolonged immobilization, leading to stiffness and ankylosis. Recent studies recommend open reduction, internal fixation (ORIF) in even the elderly (>70 years) population. Total elbow arthroplasty has similarly given good results in elderly patients with severely comminuted fractures involving osteoporotic bone. The goals of treating intraarticular distal humerus fractures include stable fixation with early motion.

Early operative methods consisted of pins and plaster or limited open reduction and internal fixation. With modern techniques, full ORIF is preferred for most fractures. Surgical exposure is through a transolecranon approach (ie, either transverse osteotomy or chevron osteotomy). A triceps-sparing, and a triceps-splitting posterior approach have also been described.

Intercondylar T fractures have two distinct components: the intraarticular intercondylar component and the supracondylar one. The intracondylar portion of the fracture can usually be secured surgically with provisional K-wire fixation, followed by definitive screw fixation. After intercondylar fracture, stabilization with restoration of either the medial or lateral column is required to complete the operative fixation. When possible, dual plate fixation can be used. The AO group recommends a posterolateral and a medially applied dynamic compression plate. The 90° plate configuration has been demonstrated to be the most stable construct. Locking compression plates are helpful for achieving stable fracture fixation in patients with osteoporosis and comminuted fractures.

In summary, intraarticular distal humerus fractures should in general be treated with (1) anatomic restoration of the articular surface with lag screw fixation of periarticular fragments (2) stable attachment of the metaphysis to the diaphysis with reconstruction or locking plates and (3) early range of motion.

2. Fracture of the Humeral Condyles

Both medial and lateral condyles can be disrupted. These fractures can correspond with the ossification centers of the distal humerus.

Lateral Condylar Fracture

Lateral column fractures are single-column injuries and are divided into "low" and "high." Low fractures have the lateral wall of the trochlea attached to the main mass of the humerus and are generally stable, whereas high fractures involve a majority of the trochlea and are unstable. "Low" and "high" correspond to Milch type I and II injuries, respectively. Stable internal fixation with early range of motion is generally recommended for displaced fractures.

Medial Condylar Fracture

Medial condyle fractures are similarly single-column injuries with low fractures (Milch type I) involving a portion of the trochlea, with preservation of the trochlear ridge and are generally stable. In high medial condyle fractures (Milch type II), the lateral trochlear ridge is included with the fracture portion.

Both fractures, if displaced, should be treated with ORIF and early range of motion.

3. Fracture of the Epicondyles

Although lateral epicondylar fractures are rare, medial epicondylar fractures are fairly common, especially among children or adolescents. They commonly present as avulsion fractures. Treatment depends on the amount of displacement. If displacement is minimal, then closed reduction is appropriate. A displaced fracture may require percutaneous pinning or open reduction. Elbow instability is not generally a problem; however, irritation of the ulnar nerve can result. Early motion seems to be important for restoration and ultimate function. If a displaced fracture results in ulnar symptoms or is itself symptomatic, the fragment can be excised at a later date.

OLECRANON FRACTURES

The olecranon is the most proximal posterior eminence of the ulna. It is on the dorsal subcutaneous border and contains broad attachments for the triceps posteriorly. Anteriorly, the olecranon forms the greater sigmoid (semilunar) notch of the ulna, which articulates with the trochlea. The ulnar nerve passes behind the medial epicondyle at the posterior medial aspect of the elbow and then pierces the volar forearm between the two flexor carpi ulnaris muscle heads.

Fracture of the olecranon commonly occur with a direct blow or as an avulsion injury with triceps contracture. The fractures generally are transverse or oblique in orientation and enter the semilunar notch.

Clinical Findings

Radiographic evaluation consists of a true lateral radiograph of the elbow, and classifications or descriptions generally analyze the fracture based on the percentage of articular surface involved in the fractured proximal fragment. This factor, the amount of comminution, the fracture angle, intraarticular step-off, and the degree of displacement, are all critical in evaluating the injury and selecting the appropriate treatment.

Treatment

Methods of treatment vary from closed treatment to ORIF. Nondisplaced fractures, or fractures with <2 mm displacement and an intact extensor mechanism, should be immobilized in a long arm cast with the elbow in 90 degrees of flexion.

Displaced transverse or short oblique fractures generally are best treated with ORIF. The optimal method for treating this fracture is tension banding with two longitudinal K-wires placed across the fracture site and stabilized with a figure-of-8 wire loop (Figure 3–13). More oblique fractures can be treated with interfragmentary screws with a neutralization plate. Wire protrusion and pain frequently result and may necessitate removal of the hardware.

If the articular surface is significantly comminuted, a low-profile, limited contact compression plate can be applied to the dorsal surface of the ulna. Selected comminuted fractures may be treated by selective bony excision or complete excision of the fragment followed by reattachment

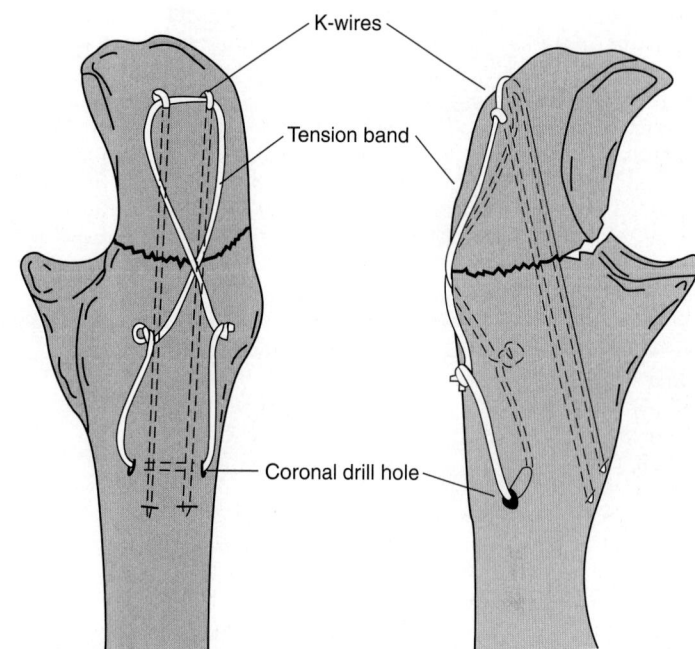

Figure 3–13. Tension band technique for fixation of olecranon fractures. (Reproduced, with permission, from Browner BD et al, eds: *Skeletal Trauma,* 2nd ed. WB Saunders, 1998.)

of the triceps. All these treatments generally can be accompanied with early protected range-of-motion exercises.

FRACTURE OF THE RADIAL HEAD

The incidence of fractures of the radial head is between 15% and 25% of elbow fractures. The radial head is seated in the lesser sigmoid notch and has contact axially with the capitellum of the distal humerus. The lateral portion contacts the ulna throughout forearm pronation and supination. Gripping or loading forces are transmitted through the interosseous membrane from the radius proximally to the ulnar distally. Load bearing occurs through the radial head.

Radial head fractures are generally caused by longitudinal loading from a fall on an outstretched hand; dislocation of the elbow is another cause.

Clinical Findings

One generally describes these fractures based on their location, percentage of articular involvement, and amount of displacement. Radiographs in the anteroposterior and lateral projections show the injury. The fat pad sign is usually present on the lateral projection (Figure 3–14).

Classification

Mason proposed a classification scheme for radial head fractures: Type I is a nondisplaced fracture; type II is a fracture that is displaced usually involving a single large frag-

ment; type III is a comminuted fracture and type IV is a fracture associated with an elbow dislocation (Figure 3–15).

Treatment

For type I fractures, nonoperative treatment with early motion can generally produce a good outcome.

The treatment of type II fractures is controversial. For fractures with near normal motion, <2 mm step-off and without associated injury, nonsurgical treatment is indicated.

Type II fractures with associated injuries that may compromise elbow stability or fractures with a mechanical block to full motion after injection of anesthetic into the elbow joint are indications for ORIF. Open reduction and internal fixation can be performed with pins, articular screws, or Herbert screws. Implants should be placed into the nonarticular safe zone to avoid impingement on the sigmoid fossa of the ulna. The safe zone corresponds to the lateral 100° arc with the forearm in neutral rotation.

The result of ORIF is less predictable when there is more than one fragment in Type II fractures, and limitation of forearm rotation not attributable to implant prominence can be expected.

Early excision with immediate motion is recommended for type III fractures with no associated elbow instability, coronoid fracture, wrist pain, or distal radio-ulnar joint injury. If any of these conditions exist, then current literature recommends placement of a metallic radial head prosthesis. The silastic implant has been associated with material failure and particulate synovitis that preclude permanent use

A

B

Figure 3–14. Positive fat pad sign on lateral radiograph of elbow. This finding indicates that fluid is in the elbow joint. In the acute setting, the fluid is blood, most commonly from a fracture.

of the implant. Replacement of the radial head becomes most important when there is evidence of soft-tissue disruption involving the interosseous membrane and the distal radioulnar ligaments. This can be determined through the clinical examination. Sometimes radiographic evidence will show proximal migration of the radius and carpus relative to the ulna if the radial head has not been replaced; this is called the Essex-Lopresti injury. Some authors suggest that replacement of the radial head should be considered in healthy, active patients even if the elbow and forearm are stable. Broberg and Morrey noticed a 92% incidence of arthrosis ten years after fracture-dislocation treatment without repair or replacement of the radial head.

1. Capitellar Fractures

Capitellar fractures frequently accompany and result from the same mechanism that causes radial head fractures. The medial collateral ligament, the interosseous ligament, and the distal radioulnar joint may also be injured. Various levels of injury, from cartilage damage to large osteochondral portions of the capitellum, can occur from impaction of the radius against the capitellum. Shearing forces can result in two different, more significant injuries: an osteochondral injury or complete fracture (type 1 or Hahn-Steinthal), an articular-cartilage-only injury (type 2 or Kocher-Lorenz), a comminuted fracture (type 3), or a fracture line extending into the trochlea (Hahn-Steinthal II). CT reconstructions are useful to further delineate the fracture and for surgical planning. Osteochondral pieces can be overlooked or confused with bone chips from radial head fractures.

Treatment

Today, anatomic reduction and early motion is the standard treatment for these injuries, whether obtained by open or closed means. Open reduction is performed through a lateral approach between the anconeus and extensor carpi ulnaris.

Type I

Type II

Type III

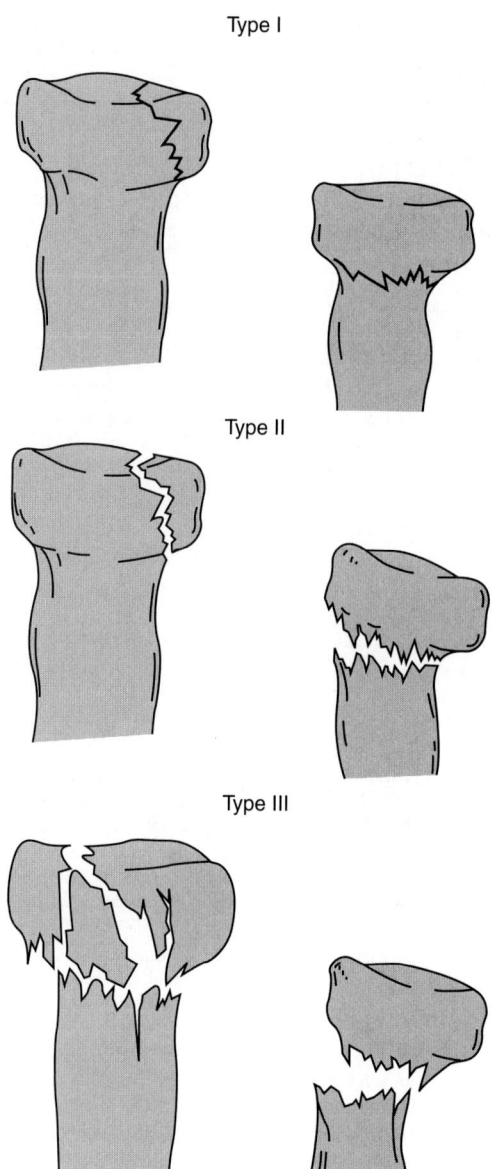

Figure 3–15. Mason classification of radial head fractures. (Reproduced, with permission, from Browner BD et al, eds: *Skeletal Trauma,* 2nd ed. WB Saunders, 1998.)

ELBOW DISLOCATION

Dislocations of the elbow occur when loads are placed on the structures about the elbow that exceed the intrinsic stability provided by the anatomic shape of the joint surfaces and soft-tissue constraints. These are potentially limb-threatening, as vascular compromise is

a possible sequela. Expeditious reduction of the elbow joint is the goal of treatment.

Although diagnosis of elbow dislocation can be made easily prior to the onset of swelling, the type of dislocation may not be obvious. Elbow dislocations are characterized, like all dislocations, according to direction of the distal bone. Thus, pure elbow dislocations are categorized as anterior, posterior, medial, or lateral, depending on the direction of displacement of the radius and ulna. Because two bones are present in the forearm, one more dislocation is possible, the divergent dislocation, but this is rare. This occurs when the radius and ulna are forced apart by the distal humerus. "Partial dislocations" also occur, in which the radial head or the ulna alone dislocate. The ulna has been observed to dislocate anteriorly or posteriorly. The radial head has more latitude and can dislocate laterally as well as in the anterior or posterior direction. Isolated radial head dislocation is rare; it is usually accompanied by an ulnar fracture (Monteggia fracture). When combinations of dislocations with concomitant fractures occur, treatment of the combined injury is usually dictated by the treated fracture. Adequate fracture care will usually cause secondary reduction of the dislocation.

Posterior Elbow Dislocations

Posterior dislocations are the most common type (80%) of elbow dislocations, resulting from an axial force applied to the extended elbow. Both collateral ligaments are disrupted, whether the dislocation is posteromedial or posterolateral.

Diagnosis is made by clinical examination and verified by radiograph to rule out associated fractures. The extremity is typically shortened and the elbow held slightly flexed.

Treatment is initiated after documenting the neurovascular examination. Anesthesia, either injected locally into the joint or administered intravenously is necessary. Traction on the extremity with correction of the medial or lateral displacement usually produces reduction with a "clunk." The elbow is put through a range of motion to ensure that reduction has been obtained and that there is no soft-tissue or bony mechanical blockage to motion. The elbow is generally splinted in flexion and pronation to maintain stability. Postreduction radiographs are necessary to rule out occult fracture.

Anterior Elbow Dislocations

Anterior dislocations are relatively rare. Soft-tissue damage is typically severe. Treatment is similar to that for posterior dislocations, except that the method of reduction is reversed.

Medial & Lateral Elbow Dislocations

The radius and ulna may be displaced medially or laterally. Some semblance of joint motion may be present with lateral dislocations, as the ulna may be displaced into the groove between the trochlea and the capitellum. The anteroposterior radiograph is diagnostic. Medial or lateral force is used, after attempting to distract the joint surfaces, to reduce these dislocations.

Isolated Ulnar Dislocations

Isolated ulnar dislocations occur when the humerus pivots around the radial head, causing the coronoid process to be displaced posterior to the humerus or the olecranon anterior to the humerus. The more common injury is posterior dislocation, which causes cubitus varus deformity of the forearm. Traction in extension and supination reduces the ulna.

General Treatment Procedures

A. EARLY TREATMENT

The elbow is tested for stability to varus and valgus stress and to pronation and supination. Stable dislocations are splinted for comfort at 90 degrees of flexion, and motion is instituted as soon as possible, generally within a few days. Maintenance of reduction is necessary, and radiographs should be taken periodically if any doubt exists. Immobilization does not guarantee maintenance of reduction. Unstable reductions are rare. Immobilization for longer periods may be necessary in these cases, as a stiff but stable elbow is preferable to an unstable elbow.

Uncomplicated elbow dislocations have a favorable long-term prognosis. A loss of extension of 5–10 degrees compared with the contralateral elbow can be expected following this injury. Posterolateral dislocation has been associated with persistent valgus instability in some patients, which is associated with a worse overall clinical result.

B. DELAYED TREATMENT

It would seem impossible for a patient not to seek immediate care for elbow dislocation. Treatment may be delayed, however, because of failure to seek medical attention, altered mental status, or missed diagnosis by the initial physician. Late reduction of elbow dislocations can be accomplished with closed techniques for up to several weeks from the time of injury. Dislocations left untreated for longer periods generally require open reduction techniques. Better function with less flexion contracture after open reduction of posterior dislocations is obtained by lengthening the triceps tendon.

C. ELBOW DISLOCATION AND CORONOID FRACTURE

An elbow dislocation and associated fracture of the coronoid process increases the risk of recurrent and chronic instability. The size of the coronoid fragment varies from a small marginal fragment (Reagan-Morrey Type I) to a larger fragment (Reagan-Morrey Type II), or includes the insertion of the anterior bundle of the medial collateral ligament (Reagan-Morrey Type III). The decision to fix a coronoid fracture should be made based on elbow stability. Even small rim fractures may require surgical fixation if instability is present after repair of associated fractures. Interfragmentary screws can be used to fix a large fragment. Otherwise a pullout technique can be used.

D. ELBOW DISLOCATION WITH RADIAL HEAD AND CORONOID FRACTURES

Denominated the terrible triad of the elbow, these injuries are difficult to treat and the reported results have been poor. The most common problems after these lesions are recurrent and chronic instability, stiffness, posttraumatic arthrosis, and pain. Appropriate treatment should include open reduction and internal fixation of the coronoid fracture and/or repair of the anterior capsule, ORIF or replacement of the radial head, and repair of the lateral ligament complex. Residual instability after treatment represents an indication for medial collateral ligament repair and/or application of a hinged external fixator.

Bailey CS et al: Outcome of plate fixation of olecranon fractures. J Orthop Trauma 2001;15:542. [PMID: 11733669]

Eygendaal D et al: Posterolateral dislocation of the elbow joint. J Bone Joint Surg Am 2000;82-A:555. [PMID: 10761945]

Hak DJ, Golladay GJ: Olecranon fractures: Treatment options. J Am Acad Orthop Surg 2000;8:266. [PMID: 10951115]

Mckee MD et al: Functional outcome following surgical treatment of intraarticular distal humeral fractures through a posterior approach. J Bone Joint Surg Am 2000;82-A:1701. [PMID: 11130643]

Paramasivan ON, Younge DA, Pant R: Treatment of nonunion around the olecranon fossa of the humerus by intramedullary locked nailing. J Bone Joint Surg Br 2000;82-B:332. [PMID: 10813164]

Popovic N, Rodriguez A, Lemaire R: Fracture of the radial head with associated elbow dislocation: Results of treatment using a floating radial head prosthesis. J Orthop Trauma 2000;14:171. [PMID: 10791667]

Pugh DMW et al: Standard surgical protocol to treat elbow dislocations with radial head and coronoid fractures. J Bone Joint Surg AM 2004;86:1122. [PMID: 15173283]

Sanchez-Sotelo J, Romanillos O, Garay EG: Results of acute excision of the radial head in elbow radial head fracture-dislocations. J Orthop Trauma 2000;14:354. [PMID: 10926244]

Wainwright AM, Williams JR, Carr AJ: Interobserver and intraobserver variation in classification systems for fractures of the distal humerus. J Bone Joint Surg Br 2000;82-B:636. [PMID: 10963156]

SHOULDER & ARM INJURIES

Anatomy & Biomechanical Principles

A. BONY ANATOMY

1. Humeral shaft—The humeral shaft extends from the level of the insertion of the pectoralis major muscle proximally to the supracondylar ridge distally. The upper portion of the shaft is cylindrical and then becomes more flattened in an anteroposterior direction as it proceeds distally. Medial and lateral intermuscular septae divide the arm into anterior and posterior compartments. In the anterior compartment reside the biceps brachii, coracobrachialis, and brachialis muscles, along with the neurovascular bundle coursing along the medial border of the biceps with the brachial artery and vein and the median, musculocutaneous, and ulnar nerves. In the posterior compartment reside the triceps brachii muscle and the radial nerve. Understanding the insertions of the muscle forces around the humerus helps explain the tendency for fractures to displace in predictable patterns, based on the influence of these muscles (Figure 3–16).

2. Shoulder girdle—The shoulder girdle is a complex arrangement of bony and soft-tissue structures. The shoulder has the largest range of motion of any major joint in the body. The glenoid cavity is a shallow socket, approximately one third the size of the humeral head. Stability of the joint depends on capsule, ligament, and muscle. A redundant capsule allows for motion; the rotator cuff controls the joint itself.

3. Proximal humerus—The proximal humerus contains the humeral head, lesser and greater tuberosities, bicipital groove, and proximal humeral shaft. The anatomic neck lies at the junction of the head and the tuberosities. The surgical neck lies below the greater and lesser tuberosities. The major blood supply to the humeral head is through the ascending branch of the anterior humeral circumflex artery, which penetrates the head at the bicipital groove and becomes the arcuate artery. Important structures that lie in the vicinity of the shoulder joint include the brachial plexus and axillary artery, which are anterior to the coracoid process of the scapula and humeral head. Nerves innervate muscles around the shoulder include the axillary, suprascapular, subscapular and musculocutaneous nerves. Fractures of the anatomic neck have a poor prognosis because of complete disruption of the blood supply to the head. Surgical neck fractures are common, and with these the blood supply to the head remains preserved. Within the bicipital groove lies the biceps tendon, which is covered by the transverse humeral ligament. The greater tuberosity provides attachment for the supraspinatus, infraspinatus, and teres minor muscles. The lesser tuberosity contains the attachment of the subscapularis muscle. The neck-shaft inclination angle measures an average of 145 degrees, and the humeral head is retroverted an average of 30 degrees. It is thought that the fusion of the three distinct ossification centers for the humeral head, greater and lesser tuberosities remains an area of weakness, and fractures occur in the areas corresponding to the epiphyseal scars. The acromion protects the superior aspect of the glenohumeral joint, provides origin for the deltoid muscles, and forms the lateral aspect of the acromioclavicular joint. The rotator cuff consists of four muscles: the subscapularis, supraspinatus,

A

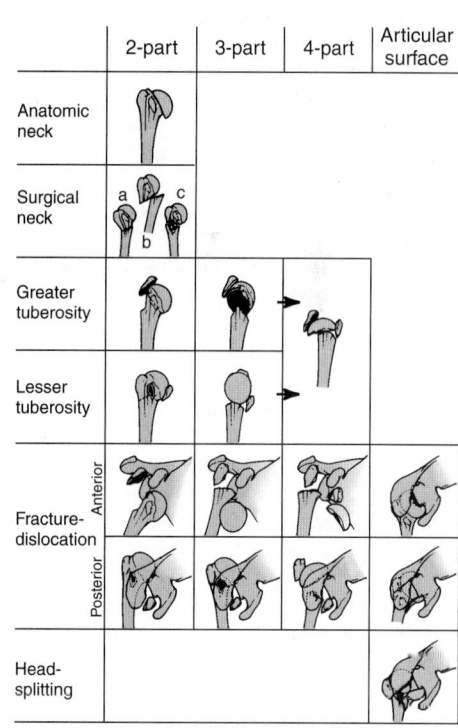

B

Figure 3–16. **A:** Muscle insertions on humerus and fracture displacement. **B:** Neer four-part classification of displaced fractures. (Reproduced, with permission, from Rockwood CA et al, eds: *Fractures in Adults,* 4th ed. Lippincott, 1996.)

infraspinatus, and teres minor muscles. The teres major is not a rotator cuff muscle. The cuff muscles serve as depressors of the humeral head to allow the deltoid to efficiently abduct the humerus. The infraspinatus and teres minor are external rotators, while the subscapularis is an internal rotator of the humerus. Two other important muscles in this region are the deltoid and the pectoralis major muscles. These muscles, along with the rotator cuff, cause predictable displacement of fractures around the proximal humerus. Additionally, injury to the rotator cuff, independent of injuries to the insertion of the tuberosities, may be encountered and need to be considered when evaluating the shoulder.

B. NERVE SUPPLY

Injuries to the nerves around the shoulders occur with fractures and dislocations. The brachial plexus and axillary artery can also be injured with anterior shoulder dislocations.

The most important evaluation consists of a neurovascular examination after injury around the arm and shoulder girdle. The radial nerve is commonly injured in humeral shaft fractures, particularly at the junction of the middle and distal third (Holstein-Lewis fracture). Careful evaluation of radial nerve sensory and motor function is critical. Evaluation should include sensation of the dorsal web space between the thumb and index finger, independent digital extension, and wrist extension.

Around the shoulder girdle, fractures of the proximal humerus and fracture-dislocations can on occasion result in axillary nerve and artery injuries. An axillary nerve injury from proximal humeral fracture or fracture-dislocation would result in paralysis of the deltoid muscle and anesthesia over the 'badge' region at the lateral proximal arm. Axillary artery injuries, although uncommon, generally result from fractures or fracture-dislocations in which a medial bone spike injures or penetrates the axillary artery. The index of suspicion is high if the arm, upon evaluation, shows significant color differences compared with the uninjured arm or has a bluish or cadaveric appearance. Pulses should be palpated and evaluated by Doppler studies; even if the pulse is present, if it is significantly different from the uninjured side, arterial injury should be suspected. Appropriate arterial studies should be obtained on an emergent basis or in the operating room. In late diagnosis, the outcome is determined by the neurological morbidity, even though the results of vascular reconstruction are good.

More subtle associated injuries involve the rotator cuff. This can generally be expected with fractures of the tuberosities, but it can also result from strictly soft-tissue injuries such as shoulder dislocations. Generally, rotator cuff avulsion is suspected when radiographs reveal no evidence of fracture but the patient is unable to actively externally rotate the shoulder against resistance. Evaluation of the integrity of the rotator cuff may be difficult in the acute setting, and special studies such as ultrasound, MRI, arthrogram or arthroscopy may be valuable in making this diagnosis.

HUMERAL SHAFT FRACTURE

Fractures of the shaft of the humerus usually result from a direct blow, a fall, an automobile injury, or a crushing injury. Missiles from firearms or shell fragments may pierce the arm and cause an open fracture. Other indirect means of injury, such as a fall on an outstretched upper extremity or violent muscle contracture, can cause midshaft fractures.

Classification

Fractures are classified according to whether they are open or closed and according to the level of the fracture in relation to the insertions of the pectoralis major and deltoid muscles. Characteristics of fracture and associated injury are also factors.

Clinical Findings

Clinical signs and symptoms include a shortened extremity with crepitus and pain at the diaphysis of the humerus. Confirmation should be obtained by radiographs in two planes. Both the shoulder and elbow joints should be thoroughly evaluated, clinically and radiographically, as should the neurovascular status.

Treatment

A. CLOSED TREATMENT

The recommended treatment in isolated diaphyseal humeral fractures involves closed methods. Nonoperative methods lead to good results with high union rates. Nonoperative methods include traction by hanging casts, coaptation splints, shoulder spica casts, Velcro bracing, cast humeral bracing, and skeletal traction. Cast bracing appears to be the most effective closed treatment.

1. Hanging cast—Treatment with a hanging cast involves placement of the arm in a Velcro cast with the elbow flexed to 90 degrees, with a sling fashioned over a loop placed on the radial aspect of the wrist. To correct angulation, loops may be placed on the dorsum or volar aspect of the wrist, and anterior or posterior angulation can be adjusted by the length of the sling or suspension apparatus. This treatment requires weekly radiographic evaluations; exercises both for shoulder and digital motion are helpful.

Patients with a large body habitus may develop more significant angulation at the time of healing with this technique, compared with slimmer patients. The vertical position must be maintained even at night. Spiral, comminuted, and oblique fractures have additional advantages of large fracture surfaces for ready healing. Transverse fractures may have more difficulty in healing. The musculature of the upper arm will accommodate 20 degrees of anterior angulation, 30 degrees of varus angulation and 3 cm of shortening without apparent deformity. One risk of this treatment is distraction of the fracture site and eventual nonunion.

2. Coaptation splint—A TU-shaped coaptation splint with cuff and collar is another method for treating humerus fractures. The more modern version of this is functional bracing, as popularized by Sarmiento. The sleeve is ready-made or custom-made from thermoplastic splinting materials and fixed with Velcro straps that can be adjusted to achieve the appropriate level of compression. Stand-alone slings or cuffs are used. Alternatively, a cast brace may be used with a hinge brace at the elbow with upper arm and forearm components. This can control flexion and protect against varus and valgus stresses as well as translational forces; it may be most useful for healing the more distal diaphyseal fractures.

3. Abduction humeral splinting and shoulder casting—Spica casting may be useful in certain unstable fractures, though it is a complex method of immobilization and requires close follow-up.

4. Skeletal traction—In special circumstances, skeletal traction has been used for humeral fractures. When treating other injuries, massive swelling, or open fractures requiring patient recumbency, skeletal traction may be indicated. Increasingly, however, multiple trauma patients are treated with aggressive internal fixation to allow early mobilization. The traction pin is inserted through the olecranon, going from a medial to lateral directions to avoid injury to the ulnar nerve. Differential traction on one side of a Steinmann pin bow or Kirschner wire bow can be used to achieve varus and valgus alignment; traction of the humerus longitudinally and flexion of the forearm and hand suspended overhead help to correct angulation. Positioning is checked with portable radiographs.

5. Sling and swathe—Elderly patients may be best treated by reducing fracture motion in a sling and stockinette body swathe for comfort. Aggressive maintenance of anatomic reduction is not a critical goal in this patient population; shoulder exercises should be initiated as early as possible to avoid shoulder contractures and adhesive capsulitis.

6. External fixation—External fixation is applicable to the humerus in the case of burns, gunshot wounds or severe comminuted open injuries with defects of skin, bone, or soft tissue. Other indications may include osteitis and infected non-union. Because of the soft-tissue envelope around the humerus, one uses external fixation only when other means of management are not applicable or appropriate. Half pins are generally inserted above

and below the fracture with access to the soft-tissue defect between the pins.

B. OPEN TREATMENT

Special circumstances may merit open reduction and internal fixation. Selected segmental fractures, inadequate closed reduction, "floating" elbow, bilateral humeral fractures, open fractures, multiple trauma, pathologic fractures, and trauma with associated vascular injuries requiring exploration may benefit from internal fixation. There are two general forms of internal fixation: (1) Compression plate and screw fixation using the AO techniques, with posterior, modified lateral and anterolateral surgical approaches. (2) Intramedullary nailing is especially useful in osteopenic bone, segmental and pathological fractures. In multiply injured patients, humeral stabilization, permitting mobilization, pulmonary toilet, and pain control, may be beneficial. The incidence of radial nerve palsy with acute fracture is about 16%; however, current literature does not recommend operative fixation and nerve exploration in these injuries.

FRACTURES & DISLOCATIONS AROUND THE SHOULDER

Classification

The classification of shoulder fractures and dislocations developed by Neer in 1970 is based on the work of Codman in 1934 and before that of Kocher in 1896. This comprehensive system considers the anatomy and biomechanical forces resulting in displacement of fracture fragments as they relate to diagnosis and treatment. Although useful, this system has been demonstrated to have significant interobserver variability. Fractures are classified by the number of parts that are displaced more than 1 cm or angulated more than 45 degrees. Displaced parts can include the anatomical neck, surgical neck, or tuberosities; other categories include fracture-dislocations and head-splitting injuries. The relationship of the humeral head to the displaced parts in the glenoid, as well as the blood supply, is also taken into consideration. The incidence of proximal humerus fractures has been estimated at 4–5% of all fractures. The likelihood of proximal humerus fractures increases in the older age groups (>65 years), especially with concomitant osteoporosis. The incidence of proximal humerus fractures was reported to be 105 per 100,000 people per year in 2002, while the mean patient age has increased from 73 in 1973 to 78 in 2002.

Clinical Findings

Clinical presentation is usually with pain, swelling, and ecchymosis.

Radiographic evaluation is a cornerstone for diagnosis and planning of treatment. The recommended series of radiographs is the so-called Neer trauma series, which consists of an (1) anterior-posterior view, (2) lateral view in the scapular plane, and (3) Velpeau modified axillary view. The lateral radiograph in the scapular plane is the tangential Y-view of the scapula. The combination of three of these views allows evaluation of the shoulder joint in three separate perpendicular planes. The axillary view is important for evaluating the glenoid articular surface and the relationship of the humeral head anteriorly and posteriorly. It can be obtained even in the traumatized patient, with gentle abduction of the arm, with the x-ray beam aimed toward the axilla and the plate placed above the patient's shoulder. On occasion, other studies, including CT scanning for detailing bony anatomy and MRI for detailing soft tissues such as the rotator cuff, may prove helpful.

Treatment

A. CLOSED TREATMENT

Approximately 85% of proximal humerus fractures are minimally displaced or nondisplaced and can be treated non-operatively with a sling for comfort and early motion exercises. The remaining 15% require supplemental techniques. The mainstay of closed treatment is initial immobilization and then early motion. Physical therapy or physician-directed exercises are essential and should be started at 7–10 days if possible. Monitoring of the exercises is important to prevent a program that is either too conservative (thus causing unnecessary contractures) or too aggressive (leading to displacement, with excessive pain and swelling).

B. SURGICAL TREATMENT

Techniques useful for the smaller percentage of fractures include closed reduction and percutaneous pinning, skeletal traction, and ORIF using a variety of techniques and implants. Good bone quality and simple fracture patterns are essential to make use of the minimal soft tissue dissection in the closed reduction and percutaneous pinning method. For severe fractures, especially four-part fractures or fracture-dislocations in elderly patients, primary prosthetic replacement of the injured humeral head is generally the treatment of choice due to the high risk of avascular necrosis of the humeral head. In younger patients ORIF may be possible even in comminuted fractures.

C. TWO-PART ANATOMIC NECK FRACTURES

Two-part anatomic neck fractures are rare. No single optimal method of management has been established. Closed reduction is difficult because controlling the articular fragment, which is usually rotated and angulated within the joint capsule, is difficult. The fragment can be preserved in a young (<40 years) patient with ORIF with pins or interfragmentary screws. It may be difficult to obtain adequate screw purchase without violating the articular surface. Additionally, the prognosis for head survival is poor because the blood supply is usually completely disrupted. In general, prosthetic hemiarthroplasty provides the most predictable result in the elderly (>75 years).

D. TWO-PART GREATER TUBEROSITY FRACTURES

Greater tuberosity fractures generally displace posteriorly and superiorly because of traction by the supraspinatus muscle. This is often associated with anterior glenohumeral dislocation. It is appropriate to attempt closed reduction, which may result in an acceptable position for the greater tuberosity. Neer has reported that displacement of the fragment by more than 1 cm is pathognomonic of a rotator cuff defect. The result of fracture healing in this position is subacromial impingement, with limitation of forward elevation and external rotation. In one series, patients with fractures that healed with more than 1 cm of displacement suffered permanent disability, whereas those with less than 0.5 cm of displacement did well. The group of patients in the midrange, 0.5–1 cm of displacement, had a 20% incidence of revision surgery for persistent pain. Open reduction and internal fixation is recommended if displacement is >5 mm with some references recommending ORIF with >3 mm displacement in the high-performance athlete as impingement symptoms may develop in these individuals. A variety of methods, including screws, pins, wires, and suture, can be used to repair the greater tuberosity. Nonabsorbable sutures can be used successfully; the rotator cuff defect can be repaired in a similar fashion. Treatment of this condition should be directed at rotator cuff repair as well as bony reconstruction. Percutaneous pinning tends to be inadequate for preventing re-displacement of greater tuberosity fractures. Despite these injuries being well recognized, there is a need for more studies to specifically evaluate the long-term outcome.

E. TWO-PART LESSER TUBEROSITY FRACTURES

If the displaced fragment (usually medially by subscapularis) is small, closed reduction of this rare injury is satisfactory. This fracture may be associated with posterior dislocation and may be treated by closed reduction in the acute setting. The position of immobilization in this case would be either neutral or slight external rotation. Larger fragments may require internal fixation.

F. TWO-PART SURGICAL NECK FRACTURES

In these conditions, both tuberosities remain attached to the head, and the rotator cuff in general remains intact. The diaphysis is often displaced anteromedially by the pull of the pectoralis major muscle. Reduction may be blocked by interposition of the periosteum, biceps tendon, or deltoid muscle, or by buttonholing of the shaft in the deltoid, pectoralis major, or fascial elements. One attempt at closed reduction is advisable; if this fails, operative intervention is recommended. If, on the other hand, the reduction is successful, percutaneous pinning under fluoroscopic control may be an excellent choice for the reducible but unstable fracture (Figure 3–17). If open reduction is required to remove displaced soft tissues, internal fixation can be accomplished by means of percutaneous pinning or intramedullary fixation in conjunction with a tension band wiring technique. In the past, an AO buttress plate has been used; however, complications including screw loosening (particularly in osteoporotic patients), retention of the plate, persistent varus, and interference with the blood supply have been reported. In the osteoporotic patient, wire or suture material for tension banding can be passed through the soft tissues and the rotator cuff, which may be superior to bone for fixation.

Another technique for internal fixation utilizes intramedullary devices such as Enders nails or Rush rods, which can be inserted through a limited deltoid-splitting incision. This may serve well to prevent displacement of the head in relation to the shaft; however, the control of rotational alignment is poor. For elderly (>75 years) or debilitated patients, this may be the best solution to achieve overall alignment with minimal surgical morbidity. Hardware removal is often necessary to treat resultant subacromial impingement. For complicated fractures, patients with osteoporotic bone, or other special circumstances, olecranon traction may be incorporated.

G. THREE-PART FRACTURES

Avascular necrosis in three-part fractures has been reported to be as high as 27%. Open reduction and internal fixation is the treatment of choice with the aim of achieving anatomic reduction and enough stability to allow early rehabilitation. The AO buttress plate has had

significant complications, including a high rate of avascular necrosis related in part to extension of soft-tissue displacement and dissection, superior placement of the plate with secondary impingement, loss of plate and screw fixation, malunion, and infections. Recent studies indicate that blade-plate devices tend to have stronger fixation than standard buttress plates. Other studies indicate that Ender nails combined with tension banding are good alternatives in osteoporotic bone. However, the properties of the locking compression plate (low stiffness and elasticity) have been shown to minimize peak stresses at the bone-implant interface. Screws, which lock into the plate, may decrease pullout in osteoporotic fractures. Finally, hemiarthroplasty should be considered in the elderly.

H. FOUR-PART FRACTURES

Open reduction and internal fixation of four-part fractures (as with three-part fractures) has generally produced unsatisfactorily high rates of complications such as avascular necrosis and malunion. Some authors recommend gentle open reduction and limited internal fixation in the active patient. In the less active or elderly (>75 years) patient, the accepted method of treatment is hemiarthroplasty, particularly because the avascular necrosis rate may be as high as 90% and the bone is usually osteoporotic. Appropriate prosthesis level and humeral retroversion, as well as the attachment of greater and lesser tuberosities, are critical in achieving a good result. Repair of any rotator cuff defects is necessary to prevent proximal migration of the humeral component as well as loss of rotator cuff power. With rehabilitation post-operatively, generally good pain relief can be expected, however function is usually limited.

I. FRACTURE-DISLOCATIONS

Fracture-dislocations require reduction of the humeral head, and their management is generally based on the fracture pattern. These injuries usually produce impression defects or head-splitting fractures, with concomi-

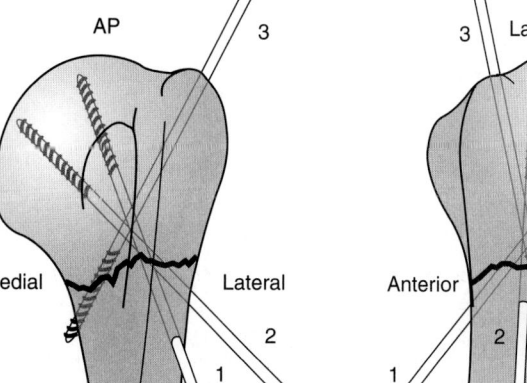

Figure 3–17. Pinning of the unstable surgical neck fracture. (Reproduced, with permission, from Fu FH, Smith WR, eds: Percutaneous pinning of proximal humerus fractures. Oper Tech Orthop 2001;11:235.)

tant posterior dislocation. Management is determined by the size of the impression defect and the time of persistent locked dislocation. Fractures of less than 20% will generally be stable with closed reduction and can be treated with immobilization in external rotation for 6 weeks to restore long-term stability. If the defect is 20–50%, however, transfer of the lesser tuberosity with the subscapularis tendon into the defect by open means is indicated. With impression fractures of greater than 50% or chronic dislocations, hemiarthroplasty may be the best treatment. If concomitant glenoid destruction is present, total shoulder arthroplasty may be required.

Complex Regional Pain Syndrome (CRPS)

This is defined as an abnormal reaction to injury characterized by pain, stiffness, vasomotor changes, swelling and osteoporosis of the affected limb. It is classified into 2 types: Type 1 (formerly reflex sympathetic dystrophy), and Type 2 (formerly causalgia). Type 1 is associated with pain out of proportion to the initial injury, hyperesthesia, restricted mobility and movement disorder, skin changes (color, texture and temperature), edema, patchy osteoporosis and spreading symptoms to become more diffuse. Type 2 includes the features of Type 1 with an identified nerve lesion. CRPS can be precipitated by trauma, infection, myocardial infarction, stroke, surgery, spinal cord disorders, and sometimes, without obvious cause. The pathophysiology is not fully understood but damage to the nervous control of the affected part has been speculated. There is an increased incidence in people aged 40–60. Early diagnosis is key to try to prevent chronic changes (muscle wasting and contractures) and can be made based on history and examination. Investigations include x-rays, bone scans, nerve conduction studies, and thermography. Primarily the cause, if identified, should be treated. Physical and occupational therapy, medications (tricyclic antidepressants, vasodilators and steroids) and sympathetic blockade (chemical or surgical) can be useful.

Clinically, reflex sympathetic dystrophy has three stages, which are not completely distinct from one another. During the first, or early, stage, a burning or aching pain may be present and may be increased by external stimuli; the pain is out of proportion to the severity of the injury and physical findings. The second stage generally develops at approximately 3 months and is characterized by significant edema, cold glossy skin, and joint limitations. Radiographs may reveal diffuse osteopenia. The third, or atrophic, stage is marked by progressive atrophy of skin and muscle and significant joint contractures.

Sudeck's atrophy is a radiographic term that is extended to a clinical condition. Spotty rarefaction is distinguished from generalized diffuse atrophy of bone and may occur 6–8 weeks after the onset of symptoms. **Shoulder-hand syndrome** is a variation of this phe-nomenon that often occurs with upper extremity disorders. Stiffness is characteristic, both at the shoulder and at the wrist and hand level.

Because the cause is unclear, the recommended treatment is an aggressive program of physical therapy modalities to help with soft-tissue sensitivity as well as prevention or treatment of joint contractures. Sympathetic blocks may be important. More recently, multi-disciplinary pain management services that incorporate counseling, evaluation of orthopedic musculoskeletal neurologic problems, and sympathetic blocks administered typically by anesthesiologists, have proved successful in helping to limit the time and extent of disability associated with these conditions. Progressive loading of the extremity and progressive resistance-type exercises can also be of benefit in the appropriate setting.

Blum J et al: Clinical performance of a new medullary humeral nail: Antegrade versus retrograde insertion. J Orthop Trauma 2001;15:342. [PMID:11433139]

Chapman JR et al: Randomized prospective study of humeral shaft fracture fixation: Intramedullary nails versus plates. J Orthop Trauma 2000;14:162. [PMID: 10791665]

Cox MA et al: Closed interlocking nailing of humeral shaft fractures with the Russell-Taylor nail. J Orthop Trauma 2000; 14:349. [PMID: 10926243]

Eberson CP et al: Contralateral intrathoracic displacement of the humeral head. J Bone Joint Surg Am 2000;82-A:105. [PMID: 10653090]

Helmy N, Hintermann B: New trends in the treatment of proximal humerus fractures. Clin Orthop 2006;442:100. [PMID: 16394747]

Hintermann B, Trouillier HH, Schafer D: Rigid internal fixation of fractures of the proximal humerus in older patients. J Bone Joint Surg Br 2000;82-B:1107. [PMID: 11132267]

McCormack RG et al: Fixation of fractures of the shaft of the humerus by dynamic compression plate or intramedullary nail. J Bone Joint Surg Br 2000;82-B:336. [PMID: 10813165]

Naranja RJ, Iannotti JP: Displaced three- and four-part proximal humerus fractures: Evaluation and management 2000;8:373. [PMID: 11104401]

Orthoteers: http//www.orthoteers.co.uk/Nrujp~ij33lm/Orthcrps.htm

Palvanen M, et al: Update on the epidemiology of proximal humerus fractures. Clin Orthop 2006;442:87. [PMID: 16394745]

Pickering RM, Crenshaw AH Jr, Zinar DM: Intramedullary nailing of humeral shaft fractures. Instr Course Lect 2002; 51:271–8. [PMID 12064112]

Ruch DS et al: Fixation of three-part proximal humeral fractures: A biomechanical evaluation. J Orthop Trauma 2000;14:36. [PMID: 10630801]

Sarmiento A et al: Functional bracing for the treatment of fractures of the humeral diaphysis. J Bone Joint Surg Am 2000;82: 478. [PMID: 10761938]

Steinmann SP, Moran EA: Axillary nerve injury: Diagnosis and treatment. J Am Acad Orthop Surg 2001;9:328. [PMID: 11575912]

Strothman D et al: Retrograde nailing of humeral shaft fractures: A biomechanical study of its effects on the strength of the distal humerus. J Orthop Trauma 2000;14:101. [PMID: 10716380]

II. TRAUMA TO THE LOWER EXTREMITY

FOOT & ANKLE INJURIES

The appropriate investigation of any foot injury requires obtaining, initially, a precise history of the mechanism of injury. A thorough physical examination will compare the injured extremity to the uninjured contralateral side (looking for ecchymosis, swelling, or deformity), palpating carefully all points of tenderness, stressing the different joints when indicated, and assessing the neurovascular status. Associated injuries and certain systemic disorders (particularly diabetes and peripheral vascular disease) should be identified. An appropriate radiographic evaluation is mandatory. Anteroposterior and lateral views are standard. Oblique and special views are requested according to clinical suspicion. Although some fracture patterns are still best delineated by conventional tomography, CT scanning with 3D rendering has recently proved to be valuable, especially for ankle and calcaneal fractures. Volume rendering helps demonstrate structures surrounding the fracture and shaded surface display is useful for obtaining disarticulated views in intraarticular fractures. Radionuclide imaging is helpful to identify occult injuries. MRI is gaining popularity and is particularly helpful in diagnosing soft-tissue damage to the tibialis posterior tendon or gastrocnemius muscle, osteochondral fractures, and avascular necrosis.

Anatomy & Biomechanical Principles

The foot is a complex, highly specialized structure that permits weight bearing in a smooth, energy-conserving pattern. The delicate balance between bones and soft tissues is necessary for optimal function. When planning treatment of an injured foot, both need to be addressed with equal rigor. High-energy injuries, such as crush injuries, generally have a poorer prognosis, even if the bones are anatomically reduced. Scarring of soft tissues, particularly specialized tissues like the heel fat pad or the plantar fascia, prevents normal function and is often painful.

Embryologically, the foot develops from proximal to distal into three functional segments: the tarsus, metatarsus, and phalanges. Anatomically, it is divided into the hindfoot (talus and calcaneus), the midfoot (navicular, cuboid, and three cuneiforms), and the forefoot (five metatarsals and 14 phalanges). Besides skin, vessels, and nerves, the soft tissues include extrinsic tendons, intrinsic musculotendinous units, a complex network of capsuloligamentous structures, and some uniquely specialized tissues such as fat pads.

The bones, ligaments and muscles of the foot actively maintain the integrity of the 3 arches of the foot. The 2 longitudinal arches aid in weight bearing and absorbing the forces during motion. The transverse arch helps with the movements of the foot.

Classically, the plantar aspect of the foot is divided into four layers, from superficial to deep. The first layer consists of the abductor hallucis, flexor digitorum brevis, and abductor digiti minimi. The second layer is made up of the tendons of the flexor hallucis longus and flexor digitorum longus, flexor digitorum accessorius, the quadratus plantae and lumbricales muscles. In the third layer are the flexor hallucis brevis, adductor hallucis, and flexor digiti minimi muscles. The peroneus longus and tibialis posterior tendons, as well as the unipennate plantar and bipennate dorsal interossei muscles, comprise the fourth and deepest layer.

These 28 bones, 57 articulations, and extrinsic and intrinsic soft tissues work harmoniously as a unit resembling functionally a ball and socket to allow walking, running, jumping, and accommodation of irregular surfaces with a minimal expense of energy.

Energy-effective gait requires optimal integration of all segments involved in locomotion, and proper coordination involves extremely complex pathways. Fluid motion minimizes energy expenditure, and a lot of the fine-tuning to attain this goal occurs in the foot. For example, the subtalar joint everts at heel strike, unlocking the midtarsal joint. Increasing the flexibility of the foot allows for better energy absorption and foot-to-ground accommodation. Conversely, the subtalar joint inverts at push-off, locking the midtarsal joint. This creates a rigid lever more mechanically advantageous for forward propulsion.

This superficial overview of the anatomy and biomechanical principles of the foot serves only to stress the complex relationship between bone and soft-tissue structures. Restoration of this relationship is often challenging, but is the goal of treatment of foot injuries.

FRACTURES COMMON TO ALL PARTS OF THE FOOT

1. Fatigue Fractures

Also known as **stress, march,** or **insufficiency** fractures, fatigue fractures occur when damage from cyclical loading of a bone overwhelms its physiologic repair capacity. Repetitive stress stimulates an attempt to strengthen areas of bone that are experiencing excessive stress. This process begins with resorption of bone to make room for the deposition of new stronger bone. Continued loading can lead to gross failure of the bone weakened by resorption.

This disorder is commonly seen in young active adults involved in vigorous and excessive exercise. A history of a single significant injury is usually lacking. Sites of fracture are most frequently the metatarsals and the calcaneus, but fatigue fractures can be found anywhere.

Clinical Findings

Incipient pain of varying intensity at rest is then accentuated by walking. Swelling and point tenderness are likely to be present. Depending on the stage of progress, radiographs may be normal or may show an incomplete or complete fracture line or only extracortical callus formation that can be mistaken for osteogenic sarcoma. Radionuclide imaging, CT and MRI can be helpful for occult fractures. Persistent unprotected weight bearing may cause arrest of bone healing and even displacement of the fracture fragment.

Treatment

Treatment is by protection in either a short leg cast, walking boot or a heavy stiff-soled shoe. Weight bearing is restricted until pain has subsided and restoration of bone continuity is confirmed radiographically, usually within 3–4 weeks.

2. Multiple High-Energy Injuries

Violent forces applied to the foot may cause more extensive damage than initially appreciated. Certain mechanisms of injury tend to produce specific patterns of lesions, and a high index of suspicion is necessary so as not to overlook some of the associated bony or ligamentous injuries.

Treatment

High-energy fractures are often open, and the basic principles of open fracture management should be applied. The objectives are to preserve circulation and sensation (particularly of the plantar region), maintain a plantigrade position of the foot, prevent or control infection, preserve plantar skin and fat pads, preserve gross motion of the different joints (both actively and passively), achieve bone union, and, ultimately, preserve fine motion. Fasciotomies of the severely injured foot may be necessary to avoid compartment syndromes and their serious sequelae.

Early stabilization of multiple fractures and dislocations will simplify wound management. This can be accomplished through external fixation or internal fixation with K-wires, plates, or screws. Early soft tissue coverage with local or free flaps is also beneficial.

3. Neuropathic Joint Injuries & Fractures

Fractures and other foot disorders often present in the patient with Charcot arthropathy. Neuropathic fractures are frequently seen with diabetes, tabes dorsalis,

syringomyelia, peripheral nerve injury or degeneration, leprosy, and other rare neurologic syndromes.

The potential for bone healing is normal if no other comorbidities exist. It has been found, however, that healing of fractures is often delayed in this patient group. Protection, rest, and elevation can result in union without deformity. Open reduction and internal fixation is sometimes necessary. Rarely, arthrodesis is indicated; however, the rate of nonunion is higher than for normal joints.

FOREFOOT FRACTURES & DISLOCATIONS

1. Metatarsal Fractures & Dislocations

Fracture of the metatarsals and dislocation of the tarsometatarsals are frequently caused by a direct crushing or indirect twisting injury to the forefoot. Besides osseous and articular injury, complicating soft tissue lesions are often present. With severe trauma, circulation may be compromised from injury to the dorsalis pedis artery, which passes between the first and second metatarsals.

Metatarsal Shaft Fractures

Undisplaced fractures of the metatarsal shafts cause only temporary disability, unless failure of bone healing occurs. Displacement is rarely significant when the first and fifth metatarsals are not involved because they act as internal splints.

These fractures can be treated with a hard-soled shoe with partial weight bearing, or, if pain is marked, a short leg walking cast.

For displaced fractures of the shaft, it is of paramount importance to correct angulation in the longitudinal axis of the shaft. Residual dorsal angulation causes prominence of the metatarsal head on the plantar surface. The concentrated local pressure may produce a painful skin callus. Residual plantar angulation of the first metatarsal will transfer weight to the heads of the second and third metatarsals. After reduction of angular deformity, a cast should be well molded to the plantar surface to minimize recurrence of deformity and support the transverse and longitudinal arches. If significant angulation or intraarticular displacement persists, open or closed reduction and internal fixation should be considered.

Metatarsal Neck & Head Fractures

Fractures of the metatarsal "neck" are close to the head but remain extraarticular. Dorsal angulation is common and should be reduced to avoid reactive skin callus formation from pressure on the plantar skin. Intraarticular fractures of the metatarsal heads are rare. Even when they heal in a displaced position, some remodeling occurs and the functional outcome is surprisingly good.

The indications for open reduction with or without internal fixation remain controversial.

Closed reduction of metatarsal fractures is best achieved by applying traction (Chinese finger traps) to the involved toes. Reduction is evaluated with intraoperative radiographs, and if judged unacceptable, ORIF with K-wires or plates and screws is indicated. Unstable reductions should also undergo percutaneous pinning under fluoroscopic imaging.

Tarsometatarsal (Lisfranc) Dislocations

The stability of the tarsometatarsal joint complex relies in part on strong ligamentous structures and in part on the bony architecture itself. The base of the second metatarsal is recessed proximally to the base of the other metatarsals in a cleft between the first and third cuneiforms, thus "locking" the joint. Injuries to this structure should alert the clinician to the possibility of other injuries along the entire tarsometatarsal complex.

The original injury, described by Napoleon's field surgeon Lisfranc, was attributed to a soldier falling from his horse with his foot trapped in the stirrup. The mechanism of the injury was an axial load acting on a hyper-plantarflexed foot. Three commonly occurring patterns of this injury are identified: total incongruity, partial incongruity, and divergent (Figure 3–18). The medial border of the second and fourth metatarsals should align with the medial borders of the middle cuneiform and the cuboid, respectively. Associated soft-tissue damage is almost always significant, with open wounds, vascular impairment, swelling, and blistering.

An attempt at closed reduction should be made as soon as possible; however, open reduction is often required. Gentle manipulation can be successful; however, residual instability is common. Postreduction radiographs are obtained, and if anatomic reduction is not obtained, then ORIF with K-wires on the lateral side of the foot to preserve mobility and screws on the medial side of the foot is indicated. The foot is then immobilized and elevated. Timing of hardware removal is controversial with some authors recommending 3 months and others recommending 6 months. Prognosis depends on maintenance of anatomical reduction. However, one study has reported that even in cases where anatomic reduction, normal walking patterns and excellent radiographic results were accomplished post tarsometatarsal fracture dislocation, subjective patient outcomes were less than satisfactory.

Some tarsometatarsal injuries present late (>3–4 weeks), when the healing process will prevent successful closed treatment. If displacement and deformity are significant, open reduction is indicated, but the patient should be advised to expect some residual joint stiffness. If displacement is minimal, it may be better to defer surgery and direct treatment toward functional

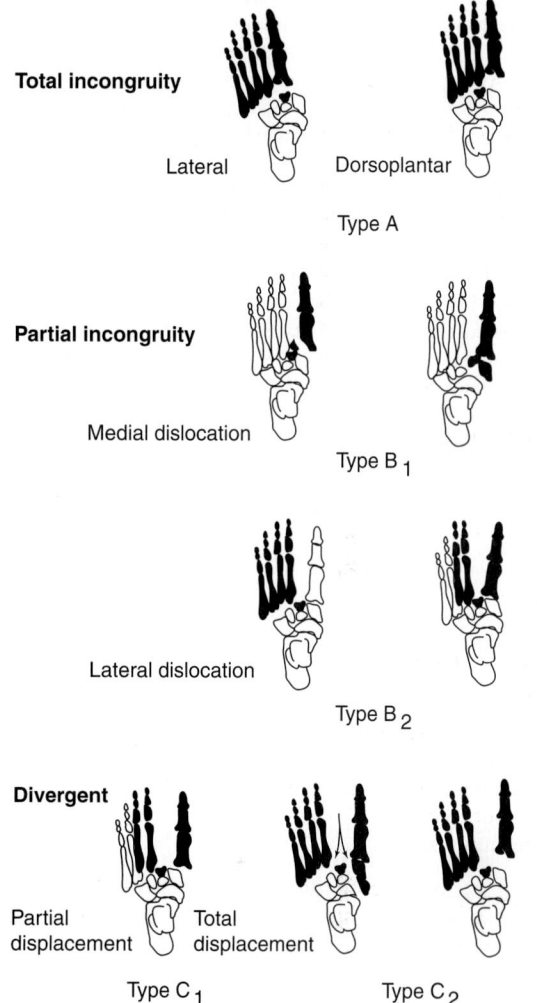

Figure 3–18. Classification of Lisfranc injuries. (Reproduced, with permission, from Coughlin MJ, Mann RA, eds: *Surgery of the Foot and Ankle*, 7th ed. WB Saunders, 1999.)

recovery. Reconstructive operations can be planned more suitably once residual disability is established.

Complications of this injury include chronic foot swelling, residual deformity making shoe fitting difficult, painful degenerative joint disease, and reflex sympathetic dystrophy. Arthrodesis should be considered for symptomatic post-traumatic arthritis.

Fracture of the Base of the Fifth Metatarsal

Three distinct patterns occur: (1) avulsion fracture of a variably sized portion of the tuberosity (styloid process) that may, on rare occasions, involve the joint between the cuboid and the fifth metatarsal; (2) acute Jones fracture involving the intermetatarsal joint(located at the metaphysial-diaphysial junction), and (3) transverse fracture of the proximal metatarsal diaphysis.

Avulsion fractures usually occur after adduction injury to the forefoot. The peroneus brevis muscle may pull and displace the fractured fragment proximally.

Symptomatic treatment is most often successful in a hard-soled shoe, and bony healing rarely fails to occur. Nonunions are rarely symptomatic but can be treated by internal fixation or fragment excision. In the rare event of a significant displaced intraarticular component, ORIF may be indicated.

Acute Jones fractures are best treated in a non-weight bearing cast for 6-8 weeks. Some authors recommend acute ORIF of Jones fractures in the high-performance athlete. Proximal diaphyseal fractures or "chronic Jones fractures" are most probably secondary to fatigue failure. Again, conservative treatment in a non-weight–bearing short leg cast for 6 weeks will usually bring healing of the fracture. Nonunions do occur (due to the poor inherent blood supply) and are often symptomatic. If there is no evidence of bone healing at 12 weeks, internal fixation and bone grafting are recommended.

2. Fractures & Dislocations of the Phalanges of the Toes

Fractures of the phalanges of the toes are most commonly caused by a direct force such as a crush injury. Spiral or oblique fractures of the shaft of the proximal phalanges of the lesser toes may occur as a result of an indirect twisting injury. The injury should be assessed in terms of deformity, soft tissue injury, neurovascular status and radiographically.

Treatment

Comminuted fracture of the proximal phalanx of the great toe, alone or in combination with fracture of the distal phalanx, is a disabling injury. Because wide displacement of fragments is not likely, correction of angulation and support by a splint usually suffices. A weight-bearing removable cast boot may be useful for relief of symptoms arising from associated soft-tissue injury. Spiral or oblique fracture of the proximal or middle phalanges of the lesser toes can be treated adequately by binding the involved toe to the adjacent uninjured toe (buddy taping). Comminuted fractures of the distal phalanx are treated as soft-tissue injuries.

Dislocation of the metatarsophalangeal joints and dislocation of the proximal interphalangeal joints usually can be reduced by closed manipulation. These dislocations are rarely isolated and usually occur in combination with other injuries to the forefoot.

3. Fracture of the Sesamoids of the Great Toe

Fractures of the sesamoid bones of the great toe are rare but may occur as a result of a crushing injury. These injuries must be differentiated from a bipartite sesamoid by comparing radiographs of the contralateral uninvolved foot.

Treatment

Undisplaced fractures require no treatment other than a hard-soled shoe or metatarsal bar. Displaced fractures may require immobilization in a walking boot or cast, with the toe strapped in flexion. Persistent delay of bone healing may cause disabling pain arising from arthritis of the articulation between the sesamoid and the head of the first metatarsal. If conservative modalities have been exhausted excision of the sesamoid may be necessary; however, this should be a last resort treatment.

Calder JD, Whitehouse SL, Saxby TS: Results of isolated LisFranc injuries and the effect of compensation claims. J Bone Joint Surg Br 2004;86:527. [PMID: 15174547]

Haapamaki V, Kiuru M, Koskinen S: Lisfranc fracture-dislocation in patients with multiple trauma: diagnosis with multidetector computed tomography. Foot Ankle Int 2004;25:614. [PMID: 15563381]

Kelly IP et al: Intramedullary screw fixation of Jones fractures. Foot Ankle Int 2001;22:585. [PMID: 11503985]

Kuo RS et al: Outcome after open reduction and internal fixation of Lisfranc joint injuries. J Bone Joint Surg Am 2000;82-A:1609. [PMID: 11097452]

Kura H et al: Mechanical behavior of the Lisfranc and dorsal cuneometatarsal ligaments: In vitro biomechanical study. J Orthop Trauma 2001;15:107. [PMID: 11232648]

Larson CM et al: Intramedullary screw fixation of Jones fractures: Analysis of failure. Am J Sports Med 2002;30:55. [PMID: 11798997]

Nunley JA: Fractures of the base of the fifth metatarsal: The Jones fracture. Orthop Clin North Am 2001;32:171. [PMID: 11465126]

Richter M et al: Fractures and fracture dislocations of the midfoot: Occurrence, causes and long-term results. Foot Ankle Int 2001;22:392. [PMID: 11428757]

Rosenberg GA, Sferra JJ: Treatment strategies for acute fractures and nonunions of the proximal fifth metatarsal. J Am Acad Orthop Surg 2000;8:332. [PMID: 11029561]

MIDFOOT FRACTURES & DISLOCATIONS

1. Navicular Fractures

Avulsion Fractures

Avulsion fractures of the tarsal navicular may occur as a result of severe midtarsal sprain and require neither reduction nor elaborate treatment. Avulsion fracture of the tuberosity near the insertion of the posterior tibialis tendon is uncommon and must be differentiated from a persistent ununited apophysis (accessory navicular) from the supernumerary sesamoid bone, or os tibiale externum. Dorsal lip avulsions also occur.

Body Fractures

Body fractures occur either centrally in a horizontal plane or, more rarely, in a vertical plane. They are occasionally characterized by impaction. Non-comminuted fractures with displacement of the dorsal fragment can be reduced. Closed manipulation by strong traction on the forefoot and simultaneous digital pressure over the displaced fragment can restore normal position. If a tendency to re-displace is apparent, this can be counteracted by temporary fixation with a percutaneously inserted Kirschner wire. Non-weight–bearing immobilization in a cast or splint is required for a minimum of 6 weeks. Comminuted and impacted fractures cannot be anatomically reduced in a closed manner. Where fragments involve >25% of the bone, ORIF may be required to prevent dorsal subluxation of the navicular fragment. Bone graft may be used for depressed areas. Some authorities offer a pessimistic prognosis for comminuted or impacted fractures. It is their contention that even though partial reduction has been achieved, posttraumatic arthritis supervenes, and that arthrodesis of the talonavicular and naviculocuneiform joints will be ultimately necessary to relieve painful symptoms.

Stress Fractures

The navicular is also a frequent site of fatigue fracture in runners. CT or radionuclide imaging is often necessary to make the diagnosis. Six weeks in a non-weight–bearing short leg cast is usually required for fracture healing.

2. Cuneiform & Cuboid Bone Fractures

Because of their relatively protected position in the midtarsus, isolated fractures of the cuboid and cuneiform bones are rarely encountered. Avulsion fractures occur as a component of severe midtarsal sprains. Extensive fractures usually occur in association with other injuries of the foot and often are caused by severe crushing. A "nutcracker" fracture is a compression fracture of the cuboid and, when associated with lateral column shortening, can be treated by lateral column lengthening, ORIF, and bone grafting.

1. Midtarsal Dislocations

Midtarsal dislocation through the naviculocuneiform and calcaneocuboid joints, or more proximally through the talonavicular and calcaneocuboid joints (Chopart's joint), may occur as a result of a twisting injury to the forefoot. Fractures of varying extent of adjacent bones are frequently associated.

When acute treatment is administered, closed reduction by traction on the forefoot and manipulation is generally effective. If reduction is unstable and displacement tends to recur upon release of traction, stabilization for 4 weeks by percutaneously inserted Kirschner wires is recommended.

HINDFOOT FRACTURES & DISLOCATIONS

1. Talus Fractures

Three fifths of the talus is covered with articular cartilage. The blood supply enters the neck area and is tenuous. Fractures and dislocations may disrupt this vascularization, causing delayed healing or avascular necrosis.

Major fractures of the talus commonly occur either through the body or the neck. Head fractures involve essentially a portion of the neck with extension into the head. Indirect injury is usually the cause of most fractures of the talus. Compression fracture or impaction of the tibial articular surface may be caused by the initial injury or may occur later in association with complicating avascular necrosis.

Fractures of the Neck of the Talus

The most common mechanism of talar neck fracture is hyperdorsiflexion with an axial load causing impingement between the talar neck and tibia. The most widely used classification is that of Hawkins:

Type 1: Nondisplaced vertical fracture

Type 2: Displaced fracture of the talar neck with subluxation or dislocation of the subtalar joint

Type 3: Displaced fracture of the talar neck with dislocation of the body of the talus from both the tibiotalar and subtalar joints

Type 4: Later, a type 4 fracture was described by Canale and Kelly to include rare variants which are essentially type 3 injuries with talonavicular subluxation or dislocation (Figure 3–19).

This classification is of prognostic value for avascular necrosis of the body: 0–13% for type 1 fractures, 25–50% for type 2 fractures, 80–100% for type 3 fractures, and 100% for type 4.

Less frequent complications of talar neck fractures include infection, delayed union or nonunion, malunion, and osteoarthritis of the tibiotalar and subtalar joints.

Treatment is aimed at minimizing the occurrence of these complications. Type 1 fractures are best treated with a non-weight–bearing below-knee cast for 2–3 months until clinical and radiologic signs of healing are present. Closed reduction is first attempted for type 2 fractures and, if this is successful in attaining anatomic

Figure 3–19. Hawkins classification of talar neck fractures. (Reproduced, with permission, from Coughlin MJ, Mann RA, eds: *Surgery of the Foot and Ankle,* 7th ed. WB Saunders, 1999.)

alignment, treatment is as for a type 1 fracture. In about 50% of cases, closed reduction is unsuccessful and open reduction and internal fixation with K-wires, pins, or screws is indicated. Closed reduction of types 3 and 4 fractures is almost never successful; ORIF is the rule. The postoperative regimen is the same as above. Progressive weight bearing will be allowed after fracture union if there is no avascular necrosis of the body. This can be determined on the anteroposterior radiograph of the ankle, taken out of the cast by the eighth week, if there is a subchondral lucency in the dome of the talus. This "Hawkins' sign" is possible only if the talar body is vascularized. The most sensitive method, however, appears to be MRI, which can, as early as 3 weeks, clearly define the extent of osteonecrosis in the body of the talus. When avascular necrosis is evident, revascularization can take up to 3 years. To avoid collapse of the talar dome during this process, partial weight bearing is recommended. One should also remember that there is not a direct correlation between avascular necrosis and permanently disabling symptoms.

Fractures of the Body of the Talus

Talus body fractures occur mainly due to shear and axial compression forces. The Hawkins classification describes 5 types of fracture:

    Type 1: Osteochondral fracture
    Type 2: Coronal, sagittal or horizontal fracture
    Type 3: Posterior process fracture
    Type 4: Lateral process fracture
    Type 5: Crush fracture of the body

Minimally displaced fractures of the talar body are not likely to cause disability if immobilization is continued until union is restored. If significant displacement occurs, the proximal fragment is apt to be dislocated from the subtalar and ankle joints. Associated fractures of the malleoli, talar neck and calcaneus occur frequently. Anterior-posterior, mortise, lateral and Broden (45 degrees internal oblique) views aid radiographic assessment of the injury and enable the quantification of articular surface involvement and displacement. CT is also used to assess comminution and associated fractures.

Reduction by closed manipulation is often difficult but is best achieved by traction and forced plantar flexion of the foot. Immobilization in a short leg cast, with the foot in plantar flexion for about 8 weeks, should be followed by further casting with the foot out of equinus until the fracture line has been obliterated and new bone is present on serial radiographs. Even though prompt adequate reduction is obtained by either closed manipulation or open reduction, extensive displacement of the proximal body fragments may be followed by avascular necrosis. If reduction is not anatomic, delayed healing of the fracture may follow, and posttraumatic arthritis is a likely sequela. If this occurs, arthrodesis of the ankle or subtalar joints may be necessary to relieve painful symptoms.

Osteochondral Fractures of the Talar Dome

These can occur with any type of injury to the ankle area, including sprains. A history of trauma is usual, but not always, present. Classically, lesions of the medial aspect of the talar dome are thicker, more extensive, and less likely to displace, whereas the lateral lesions are shallower, more wafer-like, and more prone to be displaced and symptomatic.

Initial radiograph evaluation often does not demonstrate these lesions. Presently, MRI is the best imaging modality for osteochondral talar lesions.

The Berndt and Harty classification is generally used:

Stage 1: Localized compression

Stage 2: Incomplete separation of the fragment

Stage 3: Completely detached but nondisplaced fragment

Stage 4: Completely detached, displaced fracture

A modified version of this classification to include MRI findings can help radiologists better classify these fractures.

Symptomatic stage 1, 2, and 3 lesions are usually initially treated conservatively with immobilization and restricted weight bearing. Healing is monitored radiographically with anterior-posterior and mortise views. Lesions that fail conservative treatment and all stage 4 lesions require surgical treatment. Reduction and pinning or fixation with screws and excision with or without drilling have been recommended. Arthroscopic management seems to give as good a result as arthrotomy, with fewer complications. Degenerative disease of the tibiotalar joint is a frequent long-term complication.

Compression fractures of the talar dome are rare injuries. They cannot be reduced by closed methods. If open reduction, with or without bone grafting, is elected, prolonged protection from weight bearing is the best means of preventing collapse of the healing area.

Other Talar Fractures

Other rare fractures include those of the lateral (snowboarders' fracture) or posterior process (Shepherd's fracture) or its lateral or medial tubercles. These fractures may be difficult to demonstrate. Special radiographs and radionuclide imaging can be very helpful.

Conservative treatment usually gives excellent results; however, consideration should be given to open reduction and fixation or fragment excision of displaced fractures and those involving the articular surface.

Subtalar Dislocation

Subtalar dislocation, also called **peritalar** dislocation, is the simultaneous dislocation of the talocalcaneal and talonavicular joints. Inversion injuries result in medial dislocations (85%), whereas eversion injuries result in lateral dislocations (15%). Anterior and posterior dislocations are rare.

Prompt gentle closed reduction is usually successful. Immobilization in a non-weight–bearing short leg cast for 6 weeks is usually satisfactory. Soft-tissue interposition, particularly of the posterior tibial tendon, may prevent closed reduction. Open reduction, with or without internal fixation, is then indicated.

Total Dislocation of the Talus

This injury usually results from high-energy trauma, and most are open dislocations. Despite adequate prompt reduction and thorough wound debridement, the complication rate is extremely high, including persistent infection and avascular necrosis. Talectomy and tibiocalcaneal fusion is a frequent final outcome.

2. Calcaneus Fractures

The calcaneus (os calcis) functions to provide support for body weight, maintains the lateral column of the foot and acts as a lever arm for the calf muscles. A fracture causing an impairment of any of the above functions will result in significant gait abnormalities. The most common mechanism of fracture is high-energy axial loading driving the talus downwards (e.g. a fall from a height). Ten percent of calcaneal fractures are associated with compression fractures of the thoracic or lumbar spine, and 5% are bilateral. Comminution and impaction are common features.

Clinical Findings

A. SYMPTOMS AND SIGNS

Pain is usually significant but may be masked by associated injuries. Swelling, deformity, and blistering of the skin occur frequently during the first 36 hours as a result of the severe damage to surrounding soft tissues. The heel pad in particular is a highly specialized fatty structure that acts as a hydraulic cushion. Major disruptions of the heel pad lead to persistent pain and deformity and can produce poor functional results in spite of adequate bony healing.

B. IMAGING STUDIES

Initial radiographs include three views: anteroposterior, lateral, and axial projection (Harris view). Disruption of Böhler's angle and the angle of Gissane can be determined from initial radiographs (Figure 3–20). Oblique

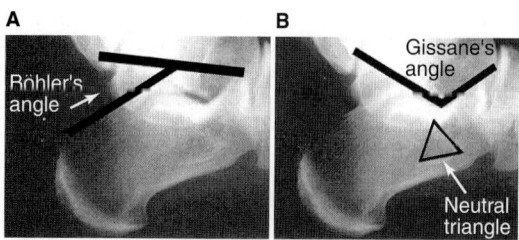

Figure 3–20. Böhler's angle (**A**) and Gissane's angle (**B**), indicating normal anatomic landmarks. (Reproduced, with permission, from Coughlin MJ, Mann RA, eds: *Surgery of the Foot and Ankle,* 7th ed. WB Saunders, 1999.)

or Broden's views are useful to demonstrate subtalar joint incongruity. CT scanning is the diagnostic tool of choice and will further delineate fracture patterns and occult injuries. Bone scanning may be useful to diagnose a stress fracture.

C. CLASSIFICATION

Various classifications have been advocated. Sanders has developed a classification system based upon coronal CT images (Figure 3–21). This classification has been found to be useful in both treatment and prognosis. Type I fractures are nondisplaced articular fractures. Type II fractures are two-part fractures of the posterior facet and are divided into A, B, and C based upon the location of the fracture line. Type III fractures are three-part fractures with a centrally depressed fragment, also divided into A, B, and C. Type IV fractures are four-part articular fractures with extensive comminution. To simplify classification, calcaneus fractures can be divided into intraarticular and extraarticular fractures. Intraarticular fractures occur frequently (75%), have a poorer prognosis, and are further subdivided into nondisplaced, tongue-type, joint depression and comminuted. Extraarticular fractures are rare (25%) and generally have a better prognosis.

Intraarticular Fractures

The subtalar joint is almost always involved, and occasionally the fracture line extends into the calcaneocuboid joint. Isolated fractures of the calcaneocuboid joint are rare.

A. TYPES OF FRACTURES

1. Nondisplaced fractures—These fractures are successfully treated by protection from weight bearing, for 4–8 weeks, until clinical and radiographic signs of healing are present.

2. Tongue-type fractures—This fracture pattern (Figure 3–22) involves the subtalar joint with a posterior extension in the transverse plane, creating a dorsal fragment.

3. Joint depression—This fracture pattern (Figure 3–23) creates a separate fragment of the posterior facet with joint incongruity.

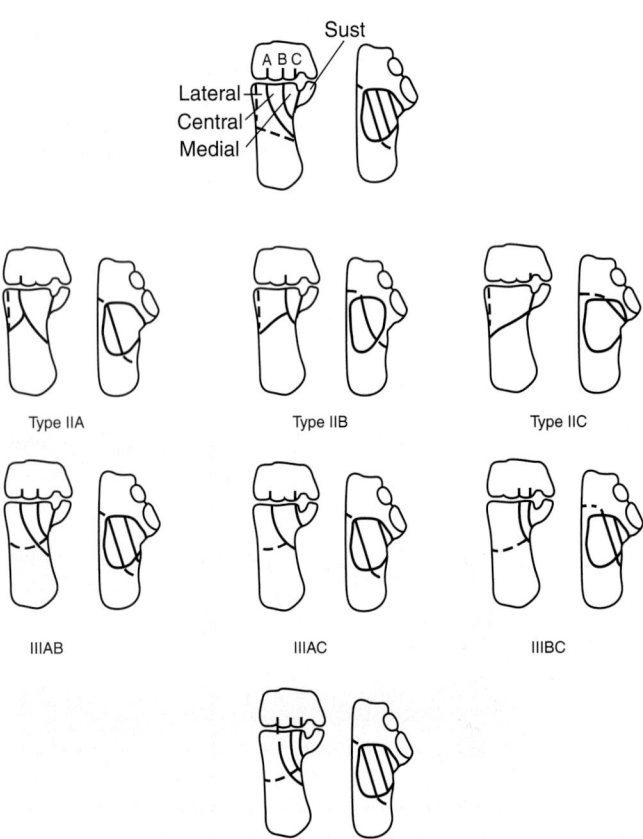

Figure 3–21. Sanders CT classification of calcaneus fractures. (Reproduced, with permission, from Coughlin MJ, Mann RA, eds: *Surgery of the Foot and Ankle,* 7th ed. WB Saunders, 1999.)

Figure 3–22. Tongue-type fracture of the calcaneus showing involvement of the subtalar joint.

4. Comminuted fractures—Some fracture patterns create such comminution and impaction that they defy classification. They all have in common significant soft tissue injury and subtalar joint incongruity.

B. TREATMENT

Treatment of displaced intraarticular fractures remains controversial. As already stated, the final outcome is much dependent on soft-tissue as well as bony healing. For the severely displaced fracture, the bursting nature of the injury may defy anatomic restoration.

Some surgeons still advise conservative treatment.

Other surgeons advocate early closed manipulation of displaced intraarticular fractures, to at least partially restore the external anatomic configuration of the heel region. Internal fixation with percutaneous pins may be performed. This is particularly successful for non-comminuted tongue-type fracture patterns. An axial pin is inserted in the tongue fragment, which is then disimpacted and reduced. The pin is then pushed further to stabilize the fracture (Essex-Lopresti technique). Open reduction and internal fixation with pins, screws, or plates, with or without bone grafting, has gained acceptance. The aim of ORIF is to restore Böhler's angle and improve heel alignment through stable fixation. A recent study has demonstrated a correlation between restoration of Böhlers angle and clinical outcome. Some authors advocate primary subtalar arthrodesis for severely comminuted fractures.

C. COMPLICATIONS

The most significant complication is posttraumatic degenerative arthritis. When only the subtalar joint is involved, talocalcaneal fusion is recommended. When the calcaneocuboid joint is also involved, triple arthrodesis should be performed. The rate of wound complications after ORIF has been reported to range from 0 to 12%. Other complications include compartment syndrome, neurovascular and tendon injury, heel pad pain and exostosis and, malunion. Compartment syndrome features in 10% of patients and should be excluded during the examination.

Extraarticular Fractures

Because posttraumatic joint disease is usually not a complication of these fractures, the final outcome is usually much better than that for intraarticular fractures. Fractures can affect any part of the bone.

A. TYPES OF FRACTURES

1. Fracture of the tuberosity—Isolated fractures of the calcaneal tuberosity are rare.

2. Horizontal fracture—These fractures may be limited to the superior portion of the region of the former apophysis (avulsion type) or extend toward the subtalar joint in the substance of the tuberosity (beak type). A pull from the Achilles tendon may displace the fragment proximally, and reduction may be indicated. If the fragment is big enough, the application of skeletal traction can reduce it to the plantar-flexed foot, and the pin is incorporated in a long leg cast with the knee flexed at 30 degrees. For smaller fragments or when closed reduction is unsuccessful, ORIF with screws, wires, or pullout sutures is indicated.

3. Vertical fracture—Vertical fracture occurs in the sagittal plane somewhat medially through the tuberosity. Because the minor medial fragment normally is not widely displaced, plaster immobilization is not required but may reduce pain. Limitation of weight bearing with crutches will also be helpful.

Figure 3–23. Joint depression-type fracture of the calcaneus. The posterior facet is separate fragment.

4. Non-articular fracture of the body—Comminuted fractures of the entire tuberosity, sparing the subtalar joint, are rare. Proximal displacement of the fragments may decrease the subtalar joint angle, but symptomatic degenerative arthritis is not an important sequela, even though some joint stiffness may persist permanently. Marked displacement may benefit from closed reduction to improve heel contour.

5. Fracture of the sustentaculum—A rare injury, fracture of the sustentaculum tali should be suspected in the patient with a history of eversion injury and pain below the medial malleolus, which is often accentuated by passive hyperextension of the great toe. Interposition of the flexor hallucis longus tendon may even prevent reduction. Conservative treatment is usually successful. In the rare instance of symptomatic nonunion, careful excision is indicated.

6. Fracture of the anterior process—Usually caused by forced inversion of the foot, it must be differentiated from midtarsal and ankle sprains. The firmly attached bifurcate ligament avulses a bony flake from the anterior process. Maximal tenderness and swelling occurs midway between the tip of the lateral malleolus and the base of the fifth metatarsal. A lateral oblique radiograph will demonstrate the fracture line.

Treatment is by a non-weight–bearing short leg cast in neutral position for 4 weeks.

7. Fracture of the medial process—This process gives origin to the abductor hallucis and part of the flexor digitorum brevis muscle and can be avulsed in eversion-abduction injuries. Conservative treatment with a well-molded short leg walking cast is usually successful.

B. COMPLICATIONS

Posttraumatic arthritis of the subtalar joint has already been mentioned as the most frequent complication of calcaneal fractures. Other complications include peroneal tendinitis, bone spurs, calcaneocuboid arthritis, and nerve entrapment syndromes (medial or lateral plantar branches and sural nerve, either from posttraumatic or postsurgical scarring).

Beals TC: Applications of ring fixators to complex foot and ankle trauma. Orthop Clin North Am 2001;32:205. [PMID: 11465130]

Berlet GC, Lee TH, Massa EG: Talar neck fractures. Orthop Clin North Am 2001;32:53. [PMID: 11465133]

Boon AJ et al: Snowboarder's talus fracture. Mechanism of injury. Am J Sports Med 2001;29:333. [PMID: 11394605]

Brunet JA: Calcaneal fractures in children. J Bone Joint Surgery Br 2000;82-B:211. [PMID: 10755428]

Fortin PT, Balazsy JE: Talus fractures: Evaluation and treatment. J Am Acad Orthop Surg 2001;9:114. [PMID: 11281635]

Harvey EJ et al: Morbidity associated with ORIF of intraarticular calcaneus fractures using a lateral approach. Foot Ankle Int 2001;22:868. [PMID: 11722137]

Juliano P, Nguyen HV: Fractures of the calcaneus. Orthop Clin North Am 2001;32:35. [PMID: 11465132]

Lim EV, Leung JP: Complications of intraarticular calcaneal fractures. Clin Orthop 2001;391:7. [PMID: 11603691]

Longino D, Buckley RE: Bone graft in the operative treatment of displaced intraarticular calcaneal fractures: Is it helpful? J Orthop Trauma 2001;15:280. [PMID: 11371794]

Rammelt S, Zwipp H: Calcaneus fractures: facts, controversies and recent developments. Injury 2004;35:443. [PMID 15081321]

ANKLE FRACTURES & DISLOCATIONS

Fractures and dislocations of the ankle are among the most common injuries treated by orthopedic surgeons. This injury is seen in all age groups, with a slightly different fracture pattern in children and adolescents than with adults. The ankle joint itself is limited to one plane of motion: plantarflexion and dorsiflexion in the sagittal plane. With incorporation of the motion of the subtalar joint (which allows for inversion and eversion in the coronal plane), the foot is able to move in a complex and varied arc in relationship to the leg.

Anatomy & Biomechanical Principles

The distal tibia and fibula are structures easily palpable because of their minimal soft-tissue coverage. The muscles, tendons, and neurovascular structures in the leg are generally grouped into anterior, lateral, and posterior compartments. In the distal leg, the compartments are predominantly tendinous, with little muscle being present. The tibia has a tubular diaphysis with wide flaring metaphyses both proximally and distally. The shape and size of the bone are markedly different in the proximal versus distal metaphysis. A cross-section of the midshaft tibia is approximately triangular, whereas a cross-section of the distal metaphysis is rounder and smaller in diameter. The inner and distal articular surfaces of the distal tibia and fibula form the ankle mortise (a uniplanar hinge joint). The ankle mortise serves as the "roof" over the talus. The articular portions of the lateral and medial malleoli serve as constraining buttresses to allow for controlled plantarflexion and dorsiflexion in the ankle mortise. This geometric configuration resists rotation of the talus in the ankle mortise. Further constraint and stability are provided by the interosseous membrane, the ankle capsule, the deltoid ligament medially and the lateral ligamentous complex (composed of the anterior talofibular, calcaneofibular, and posterior talofibular ligaments). The syndesmotic ligament connects the tibia to the fibula at the level of the tibial plafond. It allows for 1–2 mm of mortise widening, with ankle plantarflexion and dorsiflexion, accommodating the geometry of the talar dome. The bony architecture of the mortise also provides some constraint to posterior subluxation of the talus. This is provided by the cup-shaped tibial plafond and the slightly increased width of the talar dome anteriorly as compared with posteriorly.

The distal tibia also serves to absorb the compressive loads and stress placed on the ankle. The internal trabecular pattern of the bone helps transmit, diffuse, and resorb the compressive forces. Cross-sectional studies have shown that reduced activity and old age lead to resorption of cancellous bone, thereby decreasing the compressive resistance of the distal tibia.

Fracture-dislocations of the ankle are frequently referred to as **bimalleolar** (fractures of the medial and lateral malleoli) or **trimalleolar** (fractures of the medial, lateral, and posterior malleoli). Fracture of the lateral malleolus with complete rupture of the deltoid ligament (Dupuytren's fracture) or fracture of the medial malleolus with complete disruption of the syndesmosis and a proximal fibular shaft fracture (Maisonneuve's fracture) are also considered bimalleolar fractures on a functional basis.

Classification

The purpose of any classification scheme is to provide a means to better understand the extent of injury, describe an injury, and determine a treatment plan. Presently, the two most widely used classification schemes for describing ankle fractures are the Lauge-Hansen and Weber classifications.

In 1950, Lauge-Hansen described a classification system based on mechanism of injury that described over 95% of all ankle fractures (Figure 3–24). By stressing freshly amputated limbs in combinations of supination, pronation, adduction, abduction, and external rotation, he was able to describe nearly all fracture patterns. Pronation and supination refer to the position of the patient's foot at the instance of injury, while adduction, abduction, and external rotation refer to the vector of the force that is applied. Thus, four mechanisms of injury were described for ankle fractures: (1) supination adduction, (2) supination-external rotation, (3) pronation abduction, and (4) pronation-external rotation. Lauge-Hansen later added a fifth type of injury, the pronation dorsiflexion injury, in order to include a mechanism for tibial plafond fractures. This fifth type is caused by a compression-type injury.

The Weber classification is much simpler, and is based on the level at which the fibular fracture occurs.

Type A: Fracture in which the fibula is avulsed distal to the joint line. The syndesmotic ligament is

A	B	C
Supination-adduction stages I and II	Supination-external rotation stages I-IV	Pronation-abduction stages I-III	Pronation-external rotation stages I-IV

Figure 3–24. Comparison of Lauge-Hansen and Danis-Weber ankle classifications. (Reproduced, with permission, from Browner BD et al, eds: *Skeletal Trauma,* 2nd ed. WB Saunders, 1998.)

left intact, and the medial malleolus is either undamaged or is fractured in a shear-type pattern, with the fracture line angulating in a proximal-medial direction from the corner of the mortise.

Type B: Spiral fracture of the fibula beginning at the level of the joint line and extending in a proximal-posterior direction up the shaft of the fibula. Parts of the syndesmotic ligament complex can be torn, but the large interosseous ligament is usually left intact so that no widening of the distal tibiofibular articulation occurs. Complete syndesmotic disruptions, however can result from this fracture pattern.

The medial malleolus can either be left intact or sustain a transverse avulsion fracture. If the medial malleolus is left intact there can be a tear of the deltoid ligament. Avulsion fracture of the posterior lip of the tibia (posterior malleolus) can also occur.

Type C: Fracture of the fibula proximal to the syndesmotic ligament complex, with consequent disruption of the syndesmosis. Medial malleolar avulsion fracture or deltoid ligament rupture is also present. Posterior malleolar avulsion fracture can also occur. Figure 3–23 shows a comparison of the Weber and Lauge-Hansen schemes.

Many studies have stated that the above classification systems have failed to encompass all possible types of fracture. Furthermore, reproducibility is moderate and the fracture configuration is not predictive of prognosis. In fact, initial talar displacement and number of malleoli injured seem to be important for determining prognosis.

The AO classification system has better reproducibility as it is based on radiographic findings. However, it too cannot clearly separate fracture configurations to identify those that require surgical treatment.

Treatment

Four criteria should be met for the optimal treatment of ankle fractures: (1) dislocations and fractures should be reduced as soon as possible; (2) all joint surfaces must be precisely restored; (3) the fracture must be held in a reduced position during the period of bony healing, and (4) joint motion should be initiated as early as possible.

If these treatment goals are met, a good outcome can be expected, keeping in mind that disruption of the articular cartilage results in permanent damage.

Previous studies have demonstrated that the ankle has the thinnest articular cartilage but the highest ratio of joint congruence to articular cartilage thickness of any of the large joints. This suggests that loss in congruity of the ankle joint following fracture will be poorly tolerated and lead to posttraumatic arthritic changes. Thus, it is important to obtain anatomic reduction of the articular surfaces of the ankle after a fracture. A lat-

eral talar shift of as little as 1 mm will decrease surface contact at the tibiotalar joint by 40%.

Initial treatment of ankle fractures should include immediate closed reduction and splinting, with the joint held in the most normal position possible to prevent neurovascular compromise of the foot. An ankle joint should never be left in a dislocated position. If the fracture is open, the patient should be given appropriate intravenous antibiotics and taken to the operating room on an urgent basis for irrigation and debridement of the wound, fracture site, and ankle joint. The fracture should also be appropriately stabilized at this time.

With the advent of excellent results obtained from the techniques of open reduction and rigid internal fixation as developed by the AO group, the standard of care for displaced ankle fractures has become operative intervention. Exceptions to this rule are nondisplaced, isolated Weber type B lateral malleolar fractures (supination eversion stage 2), distal fibular avulsion fractures, fractures in nonambulatory (ie, paraplegic) patients, and fractures in patients for whom the surgical risks are greater than the consequences of non-anatomic reduction of the fracture. The isolated previously described lateral or medial malleolar fractures may be treated in a well-molded short leg walking cast for 6 weeks. Unstable ankle fractures treated by immobilization should be placed in a long leg cast with the knee flexed to prevent weight bearing on the involved limb. Most non-displaced medial malleolar fractures should be treated with internal fixation because of the risk of nonunion, when these fractures are treated non-operatively.

When performing ORIF of ankle fractures, several principles must be followed. It is important to gently handle the soft tissues about the ankle so as to minimize the risks of infection and wound-healing problems. In the treatment of bimalleolar and trimalleolar fractures, the lateral malleolus should usually be reduced and internally fixed first. This has two benefits: (1) it helps to correctly restore the original limb length, and (2) because of the strong ligamentous connections between the lateral malleolus and talus (anterior and posterior talofibular ligaments), initial fixation of the lateral malleolus will correctly position the talus in the mortise. If a long oblique fracture of the lateral malleolus is present, fixation can sometimes be adequately obtained with two interfragmentary screws. More commonly, however, further fixation, in the form of a neutralization plate and screws, is required.

When performing ORIF of the medial malleolus, it is important to remove any soft tissue or periosteum interposed in the fracture site. It is also preferable to fix the medial malleolus with either two cancellous-type screws or a screw and a K-wire to provide rotational control of the medial malleolar fragment.

The necessity for fixation of the posterior malleolar fragment is dependent on several factors. After the lateral and medial malleolar fractures have been internally fixed, ligamentotaxis often will anatomically reduce the posterior malleolar fragment. If this fragment represents less than 25% of the articular surface of the tibial plafond and there is less than 2 mm of displacement, internal fixation is not always required. If the fragment does not reduce on the intraoperative radiograph with ligamentotaxis, or if the fragment represents more than 25% of the articular surface, most authors agree that it should be internally fixed. Several methods have been described for this, utilizing either direct fixation posteriorly via the lateral or medial incisions, or a lag screw from anterior to posterior.

Following surgery, the limb is placed in a bulky sterile dressing with plaster splints from the ball of the foot to the proximal calf to allow for wound healing. The ankle is kept in neutral position to prevent equinus deformity. After the sutures are removed at 1–2 weeks, the surgeon must decide whether to begin early mobilization of the ankle joint. If the patient is reliable and stable fixation was achieved at the time of surgery, then early range of motion may be initiated, keeping the patient on crutches and not allowing weight bearing. If there is a question about patient reliability or stability of fixation, the limb can be placed in a short leg cast for added protection. Usually at 6 weeks all immobilization is discontinued and weight bearing is slowly advanced. Physical therapy often helps promote ankle motion, strengthening, and regained ankle proprioception.

Barrie J et al: Ankle fractures-Pathomechanics and classification. Blackburn foot and ankle hyperbook: http://www.blackburn-feet.org.uk/hyperbook/trauma/ankle_fractures/pathomechanics_and_classification.htm

Egol KA, Dolan R, Koval KJ: Functional outcome of surgery for fractures of the ankle. J Bone Joint Surg Br 2000;82-B:246. [PMID: 10755435]

Gehrmann RM et al: Athlete's ankle injuries: diagnosis and management. Am J Orthop 2005;34:551. [PMID: 16375063]

Hintermann B et al: Arthroscopic findings in acute fractures of the ankle. J Bone Joint Surg Br 2000;82-B:345. [PMID: 10813167]

Kay RM, Matthys GA: Pediatric ankle fractures: Evaluation and treatment. J Am Acad Orthop Surg 2001;9:268. [PMID: 11476537]

Obremskey WT et al: Change over time of SF-36 functional outcomes for operatively treated unstable ankle fractures. J Orthop Trauma 2002;15:30. [PMID: 11782630]

Pankovich AM: Acute indirect ankle injuries in the adult. J Orthop Trauma 2002;15:58. [PMID: 11782638]

Saltzman R, French BG, Mizel MS: Ankle fracture with syndesmotic injury: case controversies. J Orthop Trauma 2000; 14: 113. [PMID: 10716383]

Tabrizi P et al: Limited dorsiflexion predisposes to injuries of the ankle in children. J Bone Joint Surg Br 2000;82-B:1103. [PMID: 11132266]

Tornetta P: Competence of the deltoid ligament in bimalleolar ankle fractures after medial malleolar fixation. J Bone Joint Surg;82-A:843. [PMID: 10859104]

Tornetta P, Creevy W: Lag screw only fixation of the lateral malleolus. J Orthop Trauma 2001;15:119. [PMID: 11232650]

TIBIA & FIBULA INJURIES
Anatomy

The tibial diaphysis is straight and triangular in cross-section. Its anteromedial border and anterior crest are palpable throughout the entire length of the bone, and are useful landmarks for closed reduction techniques and cast molding with pressure relief, as are the palpable fibular head, distal third of the fibula, medial malleolus and patellar tendon. The distal half of the leg has more tendons and less muscle than the proximal half, and thus soft tissue coverage and blood supply of the distal tibia is more precarious than its proximal portion. The fibula transmits approximately one sixth of the axial load from the knee to the foot and the tibia five sixths.

From a surgical standpoint, the leg has been divided into four compartments. A compartment is defined by the unyielding boundaries, such as bone and fascia, enclosing a given content. The anterior compartment is limited medially by the tibia, posteriorly by the interosseous membrane, laterally by the fibula, and anteriorly by the crural fascia. It contains the tibialis anterior, extensor hallucis longus, extensor digitorum longus, and peroneus tertius muscles, as well as the anterior tibial artery and the deep branch of the peroneal nerve. It is responsible for ankle and toe extension. The lateral compartment contains the peroneus brevis and longus muscles responsible for ankle flexion and foot eversion and the superficial branch of the peroneal nerve. The superficial posterior compartment contains the gastrocnemius, soleus, plantaris, and popliteus muscles and the sural nerve. It is responsible for plantar flexion of the foot and ankle. The deep posterior compartment is enclosed by the tibia, the interosseous membrane, and the deep transverse fascia. It contains the tibialis posterior, flexor hallucis longus, and flexor digitorum longus muscles, and also the posterior tibial and peroneal arteries and the tibial nerve.

1. Tib-Fib Fractures

Fractures of the tibial or fibular diaphysis are the result of direct or indirect trauma, with some of these injuries being open fractures. A thorough assessment of the surrounding soft tissues is mandatory. One must remember that the size of the skin wound does not necessarily correlate with the amount of underlying soft tissue damage. A 1 cm skin laceration can be associated with an extensive muscle and periosteal injury, making the fracture a Gustilo grade 3 instead of 1, with a much poorer prognosis. Also, closed tibia fractures can be associated with significant soft tissue injury. Tscherne and Oestern in 1982 classified the soft tissue injury in ascending order of severity (grades 0 to 3):

Grade 0: soft-tissue damage is absent or negligible.

Grade 1: there is a superficial abrasion or contusion caused by fragment pressure from within.

Grade 2: a deep contaminated abrasion is present associated with localized skin or muscle contusion from direct trauma. Impending compartment syndrome is included in this category.

Grade 3: the skin is extensively contused or crushed and muscular damage may be severe. Also, subcutaneous avulsions, compartment syndrome and rupture of a major blood vessel associated with a closed fracture are additional criteria.

When the fracture is displaced, the clinical diagnosis is usually evident. All compartments should be palpated, and a thorough distal neurovascular examination should be recorded.

Radiographs in the anteroposterior and lateral projections are taken of the entire leg, including the knee and ankle joints. Oblique views are sometimes necessary. Fractures of the distal end of the tibia (pilon or plafond fractures) can be better visualized with CT scanning.

Fibula Diaphysis Fractures

Isolated fibula fractures can be associated with other injuries of the leg, such as fracture of the tibia or fracture-dislocation of the ankle joint. One should pay particular attention to the medial malleolus to rule out deltoid ligament rupture or medial malleolus fracture. Isolated fibula fracture can be the result of a direct or "tapping" mechanism; however, it can also coincide with syndesmosis disruption. If reduction of the mortise is congruent, radiographic follow-up needs to be careful to ensure maintenance of reduction.

Tibia Diaphyseal Fractures

Isolated fractures of the tibial diaphysis are usually the result of torsional stress. There is a tendency for the tibia to displace into varus angulation because of an intact fibula.

Fractures of both the tibia and fibula are more unstable, and displacement can recur after reduction. The fibular fracture usually heals independently of the reduction achieved. The same does not apply to the tibia. There is some controversy as to what is an acceptable reduction of a tibial shaft fracture in the adult. The following criteria are generally accepted: apposition of 50% or more of the diameter of the bone in both anteroposterior and lateral projections, no more than 5 degrees of varus or valgus angulation, 5 degrees of angulation in the anteroposterior plane, 10 degrees of rotation, and 1 cm of shortening. It is assumed that fracture healing in an unacceptable position (ie, malunion) will affect the mechanics of the knee or ankle joint and possibly lead to premature degenerative joint disease.

Acceptable reduction can be obtained in one of many ways, and this is another area of ongoing controversy: closed versus open treatment. The goal of any treatment is to allow the fracture to heal in an acceptable position with minimal negative effect on the surrounding tissues or joints. Closed reduction is obtained under general anesthesia if necessary, and the patient is immobilized in a long leg non-weight–bearing cast. Weekly radiographs for the first 4 weeks will help ensure that displacement does not occur. If it does, angulation can be corrected by "wedging" the cast. This involves dividing the plaster circumferentially and inserting wedges in the appropriate direction after corrective manipulation. At 6 weeks, some shaft fractures are stable enough to be put in a short leg weight-bearing cast, usually a patellar tendon-bearing cast or brace as recommended by Sarmiento. Protected weight bearing should be continued until clinical and radiologic healing is evident.

If acceptable and stable reduction cannot be obtained by closed means, other methods are required. Skeletal traction via a calcaneal transfixing pin is rarely used, although it is an acceptable short-term option in the polytraumatized patient. An external fixator with an outer frame is extremely useful for open fractures, as it provides rigid fixation and still allows access for wound care. This is still the initial treatment for some Gustilo type 3 injuries and in the hemodynamically unstable patient. A reamed intramedullary nail is the recommended treatment for most displaced closed and possibly Gustilo type 1-3a fractures. Intramedullary nails are introduced from a proximal starting point anterior to the tibial tubercle and across the fracture site under fluoroscopic control without opening the fracture site. Dynamic or static interlocking can be achieved with transfixing screws on both ends of the nail, and this maintains length and provides rotational control.

Open reduction and internal fixation with plates and screws using minimally invasive percutaneous plate osteosynthesis (MIPPO) techniques, avoids direct exposure of the fracture site and decreases soft-tissue dissection, devascularization of the bone, risk of infection, and delayed union. This technique is useful in periarticular fractures with diaphyseal extension.

Recent studies comparing tibia fractures treated with cast immobilization with those treated with intramedullary nailing indicate that the intramedullary nail group has a shorter time to healing, a better rate of healing, and an improved functional score. Disadvantages of operative treatment include infection, wound problems, and possible contractures. The advantages of closed treatment are early mobilization with or without weight bearing and a short hospital stay, with less risk of infection from the operative approach. Closed treatment does not preclude further surgical treatment. Disadvantages include residual deformity, knee or ankle joint stiffness, and more difficult wound care. Sound clinical judgment is needed in the decision-making process. An isolated closed tibial fracture in a compliant patient is a much different problem than the same tibial injury in a polytraumatized comatose patient.

Fracture of the Distal End of the Tibia

Also referred to as **pilon** or **plafond** fractures, these fractures involve the distal articular surface of the tibia at the tibiotalar joint. Ruedi and Allgower classified these injuries into I, II, and III based upon the amount of articular displacement and comminution, which represents a wide spectrum of injury (Figure 3–25).

As for any intraarticular fracture, the goal of treatment is to restore an anatomic articular surface. This can be difficult and sometimes impossible. Closed reduction

of displaced fractures is almost never successful and external fixation spanning the injury, with or without ORIF of the fibula can be initially performed. Once soft-tissue swelling subsides, minimally invasive open reduction and percutaneous techniques should be attempted. Bone graft can be added to metaphyseal defects to support the articular surface. When the fracture is so comminuted that internal fixation is impossible, an attempt at indirect reduction by ligamentotaxis should be done: ORIF of the fibular fracture to restore length, and closed reduction and external fixation of the tibia. This can usually restore normal contours and alignment of the distal leg and make an eventual tibiotalar fusion easier should disabling posttraumatic arthritis occur.

These fractures are notorious for associated soft-tissue damage. Swelling can be impressive, and prolonged

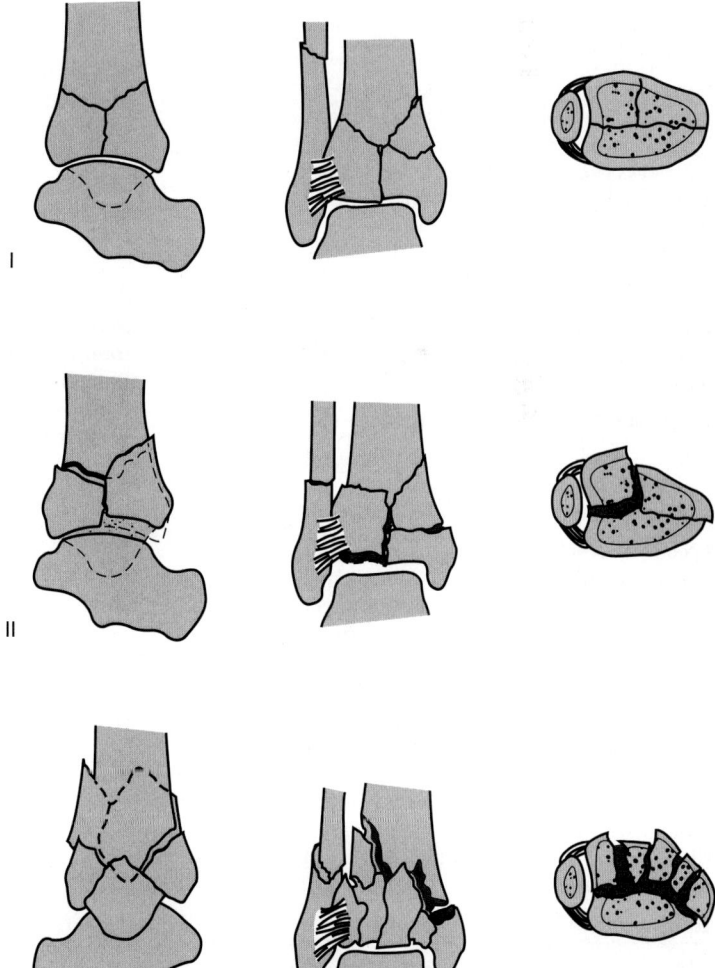

Figure 3–25. Ruedi and Allgower classification of Pilon fractures. (Reproduced, with permission, from Browner BD et al, eds: *Skeletal Trauma,* 2nd ed. WB Saunders, 1998.)

leg elevation is often necessary, especially to prevent surgical wound problems after open reduction. If open surgical treatment of the tibial pilon is planned, the surgery should be deferred until the soft tissue condition improves, usually 7 to 14 days, once the "wrinkle" sign appears. Surgical incisions through hemorrhagic blisters should be avoided. Healing is likely to be slow, and weight bearing should be carefully started only when radiologic evidence of bone healing is present.

Compartment Syndrome

Compartment syndrome is a frequent concern in tibia fractures and is caused by increased pressure in any of the four closed osteofascial spaces, compromising circulation and perfusion of the tissues within the involved compartment. Nerves and muscle tissue are particularly susceptible.

Fasciotomies are performed through a lateral and a medial incision in the skin and fascia of all four compartments. Compartment pressure measurements are taken after decompression to ensure adequate pressure reduction. Tissue debridement is kept to a minimum. The wounds are left open, sterilely dressed, and then treated by delayed primary closure or split-thickness skin grafting 5 days later. Delaying treatment of any compartment syndrome by more than 6–8 hours can lead to irreversible nerve and muscle damage.

Complications

Complications are common after tibia and fibula fractures and may be related to the nature of the injury itself or to its management.

A. Delayed Union or Nonunion

Because of its relatively poor soft-tissue coverage, the tibia, particularly its distal third, is prone to delayed union or nonunion. This occurs more frequently in high-energy, open, and segmental fractures. Pain and motion at the fracture are noted to be present more than 6 months after the injury. Radiographs show the persistence of the fracture line without bridging callus. Sclerosis and flaring of the bone ends characterize the hypertrophic nonunion, whereas osteopenia and thinning of the fragments are seen in atrophic nonunions. Early weight bearing is thought to stimulate bone healing. If nonunion develops in spite of this, rigid fixation (hypertrophic nonunion) or bone grafting (atrophic nonunion) may be required in order for the nonunion to heal. Electrical stimulation, ultrasound, and shock waves have limited efficacy but may achieve union in selected cases.

B. Malunion

Malunion may lead to premature degenerative joint disease. Corrective osteotomies may be required. When associated with shortening, multiple-plane correction and lengthening can be obtained after corticotomy and external fixation with Ilizarov-type devices, which allow progressive correction of the deformity.

C. Infection

Infection of the tibia following open fracture or surgical treatment remains the most severe complication, especially when associated with nonunion. Perioperative prophylactic antibiotic therapy and adequate debridement and irrigation of open fractures are not always successful in preventing this dreaded complication. Recently, the generous utilization of free muscle flaps to increase the local blood supply has significantly improved the overall results of treatment, although amputation is still occasionally required.

D. Complex Regional Pain Syndrome (Reflex Sympathetic Dystrophy)

Complex regional pain syndrome is a fortunately rare complication of unknown cause. It is characterized by pain out of proportion to the original injury. Swelling, pain, and vasomotor disturbances are the hallmarks of this syndrome. Gradual increase in weight bearing and early joint mobilization will minimize the occurrence of this complication. Chemical or surgical sympathetic blockade may be helpful for the more severe forms of this disease.

E. Other Complications

Posttraumatic arthritis is a frequent occurrence after pilon fractures or as a complication of tibial shaft malunion. Joint stiffness and ankylosis may occur after prolonged immobilization. Soft-tissue injuries, including those of nerve, vessels, or muscles, have been discussed in the compartment syndrome section. Sequelae may include dropfoot and claw toe deformities and may require further soft-tissue or bone procedures.

Blauth M et al: Surgical options for the treatment of severe tibial pilon fractures: A study of three techniques. J Orthop Trauma 2001;15:153. [PMID: 11265004]

Finkemeier CG et al: A prospective, randomized study of intramedullary nails inserted with and without reaming for the treatment of open and closed fractures of the tibial shaft. J Orthop Trauma 2000;14:187. [PMID: 10791670]

Gopal S et al: Fix and flap: The radical orthopaedic and plastic treatment of severe open fractures of the tibia. J Bone Joint Surg Br 2000;82-B:959. [PMID: 11041582]

Hernigou P, Cohen D: Proximal entry for intramedullary nailing of the tibia. J Bone Joint Surg Br 2000;82-B:33. [PMID: 10697311]

Keating JF et al: Reamed nailing of Gustilo grade-IIIB tibial fractures. J Bone Joint Surg Br 2000;82-B:1113. [PMID: 11132268]

Larsen LB, Madsen JE, Hoiness PR, Ovre S. Should insertion of intramedullary nails for tibial fractures be with or without reaming? A prospective, randomized study with 3.8 years' follow-up. J Orthop Trauma 2004;18(3):144-9. [PMID:15091267]

Lin J, Hou SM: Unreamed locked tight-fitting nailing for acute tibial fractures. J Orthop Trauma 2001;15:40. [PMID: 11132268]

Nassif JM et al: Effect of acute reamed versus unreamed intramedullary nailing on compartment pressure when treating closed tibial shaft fractures: A randomized prospective study. J Orthop Trauma 2000;14:554. [PMID: 11149501]

Tscherne H, Lobenhoffer P. A new classification of soft-tissue damage in open and closed fractures. Unfallheilkunde. 1982 Mar; 85(3):111–5.

Samuelson MA, McPherson EJ, Norris L: Anatomic assessment of the proper insertion site for a tibial intramedullary nail. J Orthop Trauma 2002;16:23. [PMID: 11782628]

Sarmiento A, Latta LL. 450 closed fractures of the distal third of the tibia treated with a functional brace. Clin Orthop. 2004 Nov;(428):261-71Thordarson DB: Complications after treatment of tibial pilon fractures: Prevention and management strategies. J Am Acad Orthop Surg 2000;8:253. [PMID: 10951114]

Vives MJ et al: Soft tissue injuries with the use of safe corridors for transfixion wire placement during external fixation of distal tibia fractures: An anatomic study. J Orthop Trauma 2001; 15:555. [PMID: 11733671]

Zelle BA et al: Treatment of distal tibia fractures without articular involvement: a systematic review of 1125 fractures. J Orthop Trauma 2006;20:76. [PMID: 16424818]

Ziran BH, Darowish M, Klatt BA, Agudelo JF, Smith WR. Intramedullary nailing in open tibia fractures: a comparison of two techniques. Int Orthop 2004;28(4):235-8. [PMID: 15160254]

INJURIES AROUND THE KNEE

Anatomy & Biomechanical Principles

The knee is a modified synovial hinge joint formed by three bones: the distal femur, the proximal tibia, and the patella. It is often divided into three compartments: medial, lateral, and patellofemoral.

The distal femoral diaphysis broadens into two curved condyles at the metaphyseal junction. Each condyle is convex and articulates distally with its corresponding tibial plateau. Their articular surfaces join anteriorly to articulate with the patella. Posteriorly, they remain separate to form the intercondylar notch. The lateral condyle is wider in the sagittal plane (preventing lateral patella displacement) and extends further proximally. The medial condyle is narrower but extends further distally. This difference in length of both condyles allows for the distance between both knees, when weight bearing, to be smaller than the distance between both hips. Both condylar surfaces form a horizontal plane parallel to the ground and create an anatomic angle (physiologic valgus position) of 5–7 degrees with the femoral shaft. Normally, the centers of the hip, knee, and ankle joints are all aligned to form a mechanical angle of 0 degrees. The supracondylar area of the femur is defined as the distal 9 cm. Fractures proximal to this are considered femoral shaft fractures and carry a different prognosis.

As for the distal femur, the proximal tibia widens proximally at the diaphyseal-metaphyseal junction to form the medial and lateral tibial plateaus (condyles). There is a 7–10 degrees slope from anterior to posterior of the tibial plateaus. The tibial eminence, with its medial and lateral spines, separates both compartments and is the attachment for the cruciate ligaments and the menisci. Distal to the joint itself, the tibia has two prominences: the tibial tubercle anteriorly, where the patellar tendon attaches, and Gerdy's tubercle anterolaterally, where the iliotibial band inserts. Posterolaterally, the under surface of the tibial condyle articulates with the fibular head to form the proximal tibiofibular joint.

The patella is the biggest sesamoid bone in the body. It lies within the substance of the quadriceps tendon. The distal third of the under surface is nonarticular and provides attachment for the patellar tendon. The proximal two thirds articulates with the anterior surface of the femoral condyles and is divided into medial and lateral facets by a longitudinal ridge. The area of contact at the patellofemoral joint varies according to the degree of knee flexion. On each side of the patella are the medial and lateral retinacular expansions formed by fibers of the vastus medialis and vastus lateralis muscles. These expansions bypass the patella to insert directly on the tibia. When intact, they can allow active knee extension even in the presence of a fractured patella. The blood supply to the patella is derived from anastomosis of the genicular vessels from the distal pole proximally. Avascular necrosis of a proximal fracture fragment is not uncommon.

The main plane of motion of the knee is flexion and extension, but physiologically, internal and external rotation, abduction and adduction (varus and valgus), and anterior and posterior translations also occur. The intrinsic bony configuration of the joint affords little stability. A complex soft-tissue network provides joint stability under physiologic loading. It includes passive stabilizers such as medial and lateral collateral ligaments, medial and lateral menisci, anterior and posterior cruciate ligaments, joint capsule, and active stabilizers such as the extensor mechanism, the popliteus muscle, and the hamstrings with their capsular expansions. All these soft tissue components work together in an extremely complex and finely tuned way to prevent excessive displacement of the joint surfaces throughout the full arc of motion under physiologic loading. When abnormal stresses that exceed the soft tissues' ability to resist them are transmitted across the joint, an infinite range of injuries can occur. These may be isolated or combined, partial or complete, and may or may not be associated with bony injuries. An accurate diagnosis, although sometimes difficult, is essential before the appropriate treatment can be decided upon.

LIGAMENTOUS INJURIES

As already stated, a wide spectrum of ligamentous injuries, from partial sprain of an isolated ligament to major soft-tissue disruption are seen in knee dislocations. Associated injuries to bone, cartilage, and menisci are common.

Knowledge of the mechanism of injury is of paramount importance, as certain injury patterns may be anticipated. Dashboard injuries may cause posterior translation of the tibia under the femur with posterior cruciate ligament damage. Hyperextension injuries, as seen in skiers, volleyball players, or basketball players, often involve the anterior cruciate ligament. Tackles at knee level in football often create a valgus flexion external rotation injury with damage to the medial collateral ligament, medial meniscus, and anterior cruciate ligament (The Terrible Triad). A good clinical examination is sometimes difficult, particularly in a young muscular athlete with a large lower extremity, but it is essential and will usually provide key diagnostic information.

Plain radiographs are of limited benefit. They will show fractures, bony avulsions at ligament attachment sites, or capsular avulsion signs such as the lateral capsular sign (Segond fracture), which is diagnostic of anterior cruciate ligament disruption (Figure 3–26).

Tomograms and contrast arthrograms have only limited indications because MRI has become so widely accepted. MRI is now by far the imaging tool of choice for ligamentous injuries of the knee, with an accuracy rate above 95%. Diagnostic arthroscopy is now reserved for cases when MRI is inconclusive or the surgeon is fairly sure that surgical treatment of a lesion will be necessary.

1. Medial (Tibial) Collateral Ligament Injury

This ligament normally resists valgus angulation at the knee joint. A history of abduction injury, often with a torsional component, is usually obtained. Examination reveals tenderness over the site of the lesion and often some knee effusion. When compared with the contralateral knee, valgus stressing with the knee flexed at 20–30 degrees will show exaggerated laxity at the joint line, signaling a complete tear. Stress radiographs can, on rare occasions, be useful in confirming the diagnosis.

Grade 1 and 2 sprains (incomplete) are treated with protective weight bearing in a hinged brace or cast to prevent further injury while healing progresses. Grade 3 sprains (complete) are rarely isolated. Known associated injuries, such as medial meniscus damage, anterior cruciate ligament tear, or lateral tibial plateau fractures, should be systematically ruled out. Most surgeons now favor conservative treatment of isolated grade 3 medial collateral ligament tears in a long leg hinged-knee brace for 4–6 weeks because surgical repair has not proved to provide any long-term benefit.

A

B

Figure 3–26. Lateral capsular sign, diagnostic of anterior cruciate ligament injury, as demonstrated by radiograph (**A**) and MRI studies (**B**).

2. Lateral (Fibular) Collateral Ligament Injury

This ligament originates from the lateral femoral condyle and inserts on the fibular head. It resists varus angulation at the knee joint. Isolated injuries are extremely rare. Most often, there is a combination of varying degrees of injury to the posterolateral corner, which includes the biceps tendon, posterolateral capsule, popliteus tendon, and iliotibial band. Injury to the peroneal nerve is not uncommon. Pain and tenderness are present over the lateral aspect of the knee, usually with some intraarticular effusion. In severe injuries, there is abnormal laxity on varus stressing compared with the other knee.

Radiographs often show avulsion of the fibular head. When this fragment is of sufficient size, internal fixation with a screw gives excellent results. Conservative management involves protected weight bearing in a long leg hinged-knee brace for 4–6 weeks. Most injuries require operative treatment, although conservative treatment may be indicated for the low-demand patient with mild laxity.

3. Anterior Cruciate Ligament Injury

This ligament originates at the posteromedial aspect of the lateral femoral condyle and inserts near the medial tibial spine. Because it is composed of at least two distinct fiber bundles, part of it remains taut throughout the normal flexion-extension arc of motion. It prevents anterior translation (gliding) of the tibia under the femoral condyles. Isolated injuries are frequent, especially with hyperextension mechanism, but associated medial collateral ligament, medial meniscus, posteromedial capsule, and even posterior cruciate ligament injuries are more common. When the tear is complete, it most often occurs within the substance of its fibers. Rarely, bony avulsion at the femoral or tibial attachment will be seen on plain radiograms.

Clinical Findings

The patient usually recalls the mechanism of injury, and classically feels a popping or snapping sensation in the knee. A moderate effusion usually accumulates during the first few hours is usually the rule. The only clinical finding in acute anterior cruciate ligament deficiency may be a positive Lachman's test, which is the anterior drawer test performed with 20–30 degrees of knee flexion. The classic drawer test, done with the knee flexed at 90 degrees and the foot resting on the table, is not as reliable. The injured knee should always be compared with the uninjured contralateral knee. In chronic anterior cruciate ligament deficiency, secondary restraints have stretched out and other clinical signs, such as the pivot shift and the active drawer sign, become more apparent.

Treatment

Treatment remains controversial despite the abundance of literature on this topic over the last 20 years. Most surgeons feel that surgical reconstruction affords the best long-term results. Non-operative treatment may have a role in the stable knee without signs of quadriceps wasting. When bony avulsions from the femur or tibia are present, surgical repair is indicated as bone-to-bone healing and good long-term results have been demonstrated.

Primary repair of the ligament stumps without reconstruction is likely to fail. The trend presently seems to reserve surgical reconstruction for young high-demand athletes. For others, conservative management with rehabilitation therapy and bracing can give satisfactory results. Those patients who remain unacceptably unstable after conservative treatment can still benefit from delayed reconstructive surgery. Favored techniques at the present include the arthroscopically assisted use of the middle third of the patellar tendon or harvest of an autogenous hamstrings graft.

4. Posterior Cruciate Ligament Injury

The posterior cruciate ligament is a broad thick ligament that extends from the lateral aspect of the medial femoral condyle posteriorly and inserts extraarticularly over the back of the tibial plateau approximately 1 cm below the joint line. It resists posterior translation (gliding) of the tibia under the femoral condyle. It usually ruptures after a posteriorly directed force on the proximal tibia as is sometimes seen in dashboard injuries. Posterior cruciate ligament ruptures can also occur as the end stage of severe hyperextension injuries.

Clinical Findings

The posterior drawer test will be positive, as will the sag test, showing posterior sagging of the tibia with the knee flexed to 90 degrees compared with the opposite side. As for the anterior cruciate ligament, the rupture may be at the bone-ligament junction or more often in the middle substance of the ligament.

Treatment

Reattachment of bony avulsions should restore functional competency of the ligament. Repair of the middle substance tear alone is of no value. Complex reconstructions have been described but remain of unproved value for non-athletic patients. Conservative treatment with rehabilitation (particularly of the extensor mechanism), and even bracing, of isolated posterior cruciate ligament injuries is currently recommended.

5. Meniscal Injury

The meniscus is a fibrocartilage that allows a more congruous fit between the convex femoral condyle and the flat tibial plateau. Both medial and lateral menisci are attached peripherally and have a central free border. They are wedge-shaped and thicker at the periphery. The medial meniscus is C-shaped and the lateral meniscus is O-shaped, with both anterior and posterior horns almost touching medially. They are vascularized only at their peripheral third. Tears involving that vascularized portion have a better repair potential. The menisci spread the load more uniformly on the underlying cartilage, thus minimizing point contact and wear. They are secondary knee stabilizers but are more important in the ligament-deficient knee.

Clinical Findings

Tears can be secondary to trauma or attrition. The medial meniscus is more often involved. Symptoms include pain, swelling, a popping sensation, and occasionally locking and giving way. Examination usually reveals nonspecific medial or lateral joint-line pain, and occasionally grinding or snapping can be felt with tibial torsion and the knee flexed to 90 degrees (McMurray's sign). Radiographs are of minimal value but may rule out other disorders; MRI has replaced contrast arthrography as the diagnostic tool of choice.

Treatment

Initial conservative management with immobilization, bracing, protective weight bearing, and exercises can give good results. Arthroscopic evaluation and treatment is recommended for recurrent or persistent locking, recurrent effusion, or disabling pain. If the tear is large enough and in the vascularized portion, repair should be attempted. For other tears, the affected area should be removed, leaving as much as possible of the healthy meniscus. Routine total meniscectomy has been abandoned because of the high incidence of subsequent arthritis.

6. Chondral & Osteochondral Injuries

The hyaline articular cartilage is avascular and has no intrinsic capability to repair superficial lacerations. Deep injuries involve the bone in the subchondral plate, and extrinsic repair occurs first with a fibrin clot replaced by granulation tissue, which is then transformed to fibrocartilage. Repetitive injury can cause abnormal motion with shearing stresses that can loosen chondral or osteochondral fragments. Compression injuries to the cartilage can lead to posttraumatic chondromalacia.

Clinical Findings

Chondral injuries usually give nonspecific symptoms that mimic meniscal injury. Plain radiographs will often reveal a loose body if the osteochondral fragment is big enough. Tunnel views and patellar tangential views can be helpful in visualizing fragments. Pure chondral fragments will only be seen with contrast arthrograms or MRI, both of which can easily miss the smaller fragments. Arthroscopy remains the most accurate diagnostic procedure.

Treatment

Treatment is controversial. The age of the patient, skeletal maturity and the presence of adequate subchondral bone all play an important part in guiding treatment.

Removal of the free fragment, debridement of the donor site, and drilling of the underlying subchondral bone to promote fibrin clot formation is the most accepted treatment. Rarely, an osteochondral fragment involving weight-bearing cartilage is large enough to warrant reduction and internal fixation.

7. Knee Dislocation

Traumatic dislocation of the knee is a rare injury that often results from high-energy trauma, but may occur from low energy injuries in the elderly. It is classified according to the direction of displacement of the tibia: anterior, posterior, lateral, medial, or rotatory. Complete dislocation can occur only after extensive tearing of the supporting ligaments and soft tissues. Injury to the neighboring neurovascular bundle is common and should be looked for systematically.

Treatment

Knee dislocations require prompt reduction. This is most easily accomplished in the emergency room by applying axial traction on the leg. Rarely, reduction can only be obtained under general anesthesia. The role of angiography is controversial. If pulses and ankle-brachial pressure index are normal, the limb is closely observed. Studies have shown that the isolated presence of abnormal foot pulses is not sensitive enough to detect a surgical vascular injury. Furthermore, one study demonstrated no vascular injury in any of their traumatic knee dislocations with initial normal vascular examination. Angiograms can be useful in the limb with obvious vascular injury, but should not delay treatment. Any vascular injury should be repaired as soon as possible. Ischemia of more than 4 hours implies a poor prognosis for salvage of a functional limb. Prophylactic fasciotomies should be performed at the time of vascular repair to prevent compartment syndrome caused by post-revascularization edema.

The timing of the treatment of the ligamentous damage is also controversial. Most authors now agree that surgical repair of all ligaments is indicated in relatively young (<50 years) active patients. Others still prefer closed management in a cast or braces. Whatever method is used, close follow-up is essential, especially at the beginning, to prevent subluxation, usually posteriorly. If subluxation occurs, the knee should be maintained in a reduced position using a femorotibial external fixator. After 6–8 weeks of immobilization, the knee is protected in a long leg brace and motion is started. Intensive quadriceps and hamstring rehabilitation is necessary to minimize functional loss. The need for a brace for strenuous activities may be permanent.

PROXIMAL TIBIA FRACTURES

1. Tibial Plateau Fractures

Proximal tibia fractures account for 1% of all fractures. There is a wide spectrum of fracture patterns that involve the medial tibial plateau (10–23%), the lateral tibial plateau (55–70%), or both (11–31%). These fractures occur through metaphyseal bone. Like all metaphyseal fractures, the spongiosa is impacted and once reduced, there can be a void with functional bone loss. These fractures usually result from axial loading, as seen in falls from a high place, combined most often with some varus and valgus forces. It is reported that at least 20% of unilateral tibial plateau fractures are associated with ligament rupture of the opposite compartment. The bone fails in compression and shear, with the ligament in tension. This is not easy to determine clinically,

because of pain and motion at the fracture site. A thorough neurovascular evaluation should be recorded.

Classification

Many different classification systems have been proposed, none with universal acceptance. The system most widely used today is the Schatzker classification; type I: split fracture of the lateral plateau, type II: split-depression of the lateral plateau, type III: depression of the lateral plateau, type IV: medial plateau fracture, type V: bicondylar fracture, and type VI: a fracture with metaphyseal-diaphyseal dissociation (Figure 3–27). Proper classification is based on quality radiographs, including oblique views if necessary. If fat is present in the knee aspirate and plain films fail to show any obvious fractures, occult injury needs to be ruled out. CT and more recently, MRI have all been used successfully for this purpose. MRI has also been useful to reduce inter-observer disparities in fracture classification, which in turn can affect management.

Treatment

The goal of treatment is to restore anatomic contours to the articular surface, to prevent posttraumatic degenerative joint disease, allow soft-tissue healing in optimal position, and prevent knee stiffness. Both closed and open treatment can achieve these goals. The choice will depend on multiple factors, including the patient's age and general medical condition, the degree of displacement and comminution of the fracture, associated local soft-tissue and bony injuries, local skin condition, residual knee stability, and fracture configuration.

Figure 3–27. Schatzker classification of tibial plateau fractures: **A** (type I: lateral split), **B** (type II: lateral split depression), **C** (type III: lateral depression), **D** (type IV: medial plateau), **E** (type V: bicondylar), **F** (type VI: bicondylar with separation of metaphysis from diaphysis). (Reproduced, with permission, from Rockwood CA et al, eds: *Fractures in Adults,* 4th ed. Lippincott, 1996.)

Closed treatment with a cast or fracture brace is appropriate for minimally displaced fractures with no ligament instability. Definite varus and valgus laxity at full extension is a poor prognostic sign for closed treatment. Articular step-off of 3 mm or less and condylar widening of 5 mm or less can be treated conservatively. Lateral or valgus tilt up to 5 degrees is well tolerated. Medial plateau fractures with any significant displacement should be surgically stabilized. Articular step-off >3 mm should be anatomically fixed. Bicondylar fractures with any medial displacement, valgus tilt >5 degrees or with significant articular step-off should be surgically stabilized. Range of motion is usually allowed after 6 weeks and weight bearing after 3 months. Noncomminuted fractures can undergo closed reduction with fluoroscopic imaging and percutaneous pinning with cannulated screws.

Recently, reduction of the articular fragment under arthroscopic visualization has become more popular, particularly for Schatzker type I, II, III, and IV injuries. The depressed fragment is elevated and bone graft packed underneath to prevent loss of reduction.

Open reduction and internal fixation with plates and screws remains the traditional approach of operative treatment. Reduction should be as anatomically precise as possible, and fixation should be solid enough to allow early mobilization. More recently, Minimally Invasive Plate Osteosynthesis (MIPO) and the Less Invasive Stabilization Systems (LISS) are being used in the treatment of these injuries. Bone defects should be grafted with either autograft, allograft or structural graft substitutes. Early range of motion is allowed according to the stability of the construct. Weight bearing is occasionally allowed at 6–8 weeks but more frequently after 12 weeks.

An external monolateral or ring fixator can be used for provisional and definitive treatment depending upon the clinical situation and experience of the surgical team.

Hybrid and ring external fixators have been found to be useful for bicondylar injuries with severe soft tissue trauma.

Bai B et al: Effect of articular step-off and meniscectomy on joint alignment and contact pressures for fractures of the lateral tibial plateau. J Orthop Trauma 2001;15:101. [PMID: 11232647]

Cain EL, Clancy WG: Treatment algorithm for osteochondral injuries of the knee. Clin Sports Med. 2001 Apr;20(2):321-42. [PMID 11398361]

Chen FS, Rokito AS, Pitman MI: Acute and chronic posterolateral rotatory instability of the knee. J Am Acad Orthop Surg 2000; 8:97. [PMID: 1075373]

Collinge CA, Sanders RW: Percutaneous plating in the lower extremity. J Am Acad Orthop Surg 2000;8:211. [PMID: 10951109]

Geller J et al: Tension wire position for hybrid external fixation of the proximal tibia. J Orthop Trauma 2000;14:502. [PMID: 11083613]

Griffin LY et al: Noncontact anterior cruciate ligament injuries: Risk factors and prevention strategies. J Am Acad Orthop Surg 2000;8:141. [PMID: 10874221]

Kumar A, Whittle AP: Treatment of complex (Schatzker type VI) fractures of the tibial plateau with circular wire external fixation: A retrospective case review. J Orthop Trauma 2000; 14:339. [PMID: 10926241]

Larsson S, Bauer TW: Use of injectable calcium phosphate cement for fracture fixation: a review. Clin Orthop 2002 Feb;(395): 23-32. [PMID 11937863]

Lonner JH, Dupuy DE, Siliski JM: Comparison of magnetic resonance imaging with operative findings in acute traumatic dislocations of the adult knee. J Orthop Trauma 2000;14:183. [PMID: 10791669]

Lundy DW, Johnson KD: "Floating knee" injuries: Ipsilateral fractures of the femur and tibia. J Am Acad Orthop Surg 2001; 9:238. [PMID: 11476533]

Stevens DG et al: The long-term functional outcome of operatively treated tibial plateau fractures. J Orthop Trauma 2001;15: 312. [PMID: 11433134]

Yacoubian SV et al: Impact of MRI on treatment plan and fracture classification of tibial plateau fractures. J Orthop Trauma 2002 Oct;16(9):632-7. [PMID 12368643]

Complications

Early complications include infection, deep vein thrombosis, compartment syndrome, loss of reduction, and hardware failure. Late complications include residual instability and posttraumatic degenerative joint disease that may require total knee replacement arthroplasty or arthrodesis.

2. Tibial Tuberosity Fracture

Tibial tuberosity fractures can occur with a violent quadriceps muscle contraction causing avulsion of the tibial tuberosity. When the fracture is complete, the extensor mechanism is disrupted and active knee extension is impossible.

Although conservative treatment of a nondisplaced avulsion fracture with a cylinder cast in extension for 6–8 weeks will allow it to heal, rigid fixation with percutaneous screws allows much earlier knee mobilization. Closed or open reduction and solid internal fixation is recommended for all fractures displaced by 5 mm or more.

3. Tibial Eminence (Spine) Fracture

A tibial eminence fracture occurs as an isolated injury or as part of the comminution of tibial plateau fractures. The isolated type of injury occurs mostly in the pediatric age group before physeal closure and is believed to be an avulsion fracture at the tibial attachment of the anterior cruciate ligament.

Myers has classified this lesion into three stages and has recommended open reduction for the displaced type 3 fractures. Type 1 and 2 fractures should be treated with a cylinder cast with the knee in extension for 4–6 weeks. When associated with other fractures of the tibial plateau, the tibial eminence fragment usually keeps its attachment to the anterior cruciate ligament, and anatomic reduction with rigid fixation should be obtained.

DISTAL FEMUR FRACTURES

These fractures involve the distal metaphysis and epiphysis of the femur. The incidence of distal femoral fractures has been estimated between 4 and 7% of all femoral fractures. It is important to distinguish between extraarticular (supracondylar) and intraarticular (condylar or intercondylar) fractures, and low energy fractures (usually in the elderly) and high energy fractures (young patient). The distal fragment is usually rotated into extension from traction by the gastrocnemius muscle. The distal end of the proximal fragment is apt to perforate the overlying quadriceps and may penetrate the suprapatellar pouch, causing hemarthrosis. The distal fragment may impinge on the popliteal neurovascular bundle, and an immediate thorough neurovascular examination is mandatory. Absence or marked decrease of pedal pulsations is an indication for immediate reduction. If this fails to restore adequate circulation, an arteriogram should be obtained immediately and the vascular lesion repaired as indicated. Injuries to the tibial or peroneal nerves are less frequent. Treatment should be aimed at restoring the mechanical axis, anatomic reduction of the articular surface and early knee range of motion.

A temporary spanning external fixation can be used to stabilize the fracture in polytrauma patients. Two pins can be rapidly allocated in the femoral shaft and two additional pins in the Tibial shaft. ORIF can be safely done in the first 2 weeks when the patient has been hemodynamically stabilized without increasing the risk of infection, provided that no infection at the pin sites has occurred. Complex Trauma of the Knee encompasses a distal supra or intercondylar femoral fracture combined with a proximal tibial fracture (floating knee); a supra or intercondylar femoral fracture with a second or third degree closed or open injury; or a complete knee dislocation and possible associated neurovascular injuries. Because of the complexity of injury and multidisciplinary team approach, this subset of patients is better treated in level 1 trauma centers.

1. Extraarticular Fractures

Most of these fractures, are best treated with internal fixation, which allows early mobilization of the patient and of the neighboring joints. Most fractures are best treated with fixed-angle plates, locking plates using MIPPO techniques, or retrograde intramedullary nailing. Skeletal traction treatment is reserved for patients for whom surgery is contraindicated and is fraught with all the previously mentioned complications that can accompany prolonged recumbency.

2. Intraarticular Fractures

As for any intraarticular fracture, maximal functional recovery of the knee joint requires anatomic reduction of the articular components and restitution of the mechanical axis. Closed reduction of displaced fragments is almost never successful. Displaced intraarticular fractures usually require open reduction and internal fixation with a variety of methods including Dynamic Compression Screws (DCS), AO buttress plating, LISS, with or without a percutaneous or minimally invasive plate osteosynthesis (MIPPO). For combined intercondylar and supracondylar fractures, or condylar fractures, the transarticular approach and retrograde plate osteosynthesis (TARPO) facilitates anatomic articular reconstruction and percutaneous plate insertion (Krettek et al., 1997).

3. Intercondylar Fracture

A comminuted fracture of the distal femoral epiphysis is classically described as a T or Y fracture, according to the configuration of the articular fragments. Displaced fractures are best treated by open reduction, to restore anatomic alignment of the articular surface, and by internal fixation using screws and condylar plates or screws. Even if the fracture heals in anatomic position, joint stiffness, pain, and posttraumatic arthritis are not uncommon outcomes.

4. Condylar Fracture

Isolated fractures of the lateral or medial femoral condyles are rare. They usually result from varus or valgus stress to the knee joint, and associated ligament injuries should be looked for systematically. Fractures of the posterior portion of one or the other condyle in the frontal plane can also be seen (Hoffa fracture)

Closed reduction of displaced fragments is rarely successful. Open reduction and internal fixation is usually indicated and requires anteroposterior lag screws. Associated ligamentous ruptures are repaired as needed. If fixation is solid, postoperative immobilization is kept at a minimum, and the patient can start moving the knee joint early. Weight bearing is usually allowed at 3 months when clinical and radiologic evidence of bone healing is present.

PATELLAR INJURIES

1. Transverse Patellar Fracture

Transverse fractures of the patella (Figure 3–28) are the result of an indirect force, usually with the knee in flexion. Fracture may be caused by sudden voluntary contraction of the quadriceps muscle or sudden forced flexion of the leg with the quadriceps contracted. The level of fracture is commonly in the middle. Associated tearing of the patellar retinacula depends upon the force of the initiating injury. The activity of the quadriceps muscle causes upward displacement of the proximal fragment, the magnitude of which depends on the extent of the retinacular tear.

Clinical Findings

Swelling of the anterior knee region is caused by hemarthrosis and hemorrhage into the soft tissues overlying the joint. If displacement is present, the defect in the patella can be palpated, and active extension of the knee is lost. A straight leg raise may be preserved if the retinacula is intact.

Treatment

Nondisplaced fractures can be treated with a walking cylinder cast or brace for 6–8 weeks followed by knee rehabilitation. Open reduction is indicated if the fragments are displaced >3 mm or if articular step-off is >2 mm. The fragments must be accurately repositioned to prevent early posttraumatic arthritis of the patellofemoral joint. If the minor fragment is small (no more than 1 cm in length) or severely comminuted, it may be excised and the quadriceps or patellar tendon (depending upon which pole of the patella is involved) sutured directly to the major fragment. Whenever possible, internal fixation of anatomically reduced fragments should be done, allowing early motion of the knee joint. This is best achieved by figure-of-eight tension banding over two longitudinal parallel K-wires.

Accurate reduction of the articular surface must be confirmed by lateral radiographs taken intraoperatively.

2. Comminuted Patellar Fracture

Comminuted fractures of the patella are usually caused by a direct force. Most often, little or no separation of the fragments occurs because the quadriceps retinaculum is not extensively torn. Severe injury may cause extensive destruction of the articular surface of both the patella and the opposing femur.

If comminution is not severe and displacement is insignificant, immobilization for 8 weeks in a cylinder extending from the groin to the supramalleolar region is sufficient.

Severe comminution can often be treated with ORIF with addition of a cerclage wire, but on rare occasions

Figure 3–28. Transverse fracture of the patella. (Reprinted from Campbells Operative Orthopaedics, 9/e, Vol. 3, Canale ST [ed], Copyright 1998, Mosby, with permission from Elsevier.)

excision of the patella and repair of the defect by imbrication of the quadriceps expansion is the only viable alternative. Excision of the patella can result in decreased strength, pain in the knee, and general restriction of activity. No matter what the treatment, high-energy injuries are frequently complicated by chondromalacia patella and patellofemoral arthritis.

3. Patellar Dislocation

Acute traumatic dislocation of the patella should be differentiated from episodic recurrent dislocation, as the latter condition is likely to be associated with occult organic lesions. When dislocation of the patella occurs alone, it may be caused by a direct force or activity of the quadriceps, and the direction of dislocation of the patella is almost always lateral. Spontaneous reduction is apt to occur if the knee joint is extended. If so, the clinical findings may consist merely of hemarthrosis and localized tenderness over the medial patellar retinaculum. Gross instability of the patella, which can be demonstrated by physical examination, indicates that injury to the soft tissues of the medial aspect of the knee has been extensive.

Reduction is maintained in a brace or cylinder cast with the knee in extension for 2–3 weeks. Isometric quadriceps exercises are encouraged. Physical therapy should be initiated to maximize the strength of the vastus medialis. Dynamic bracing may be helpful. Recurrent episodes require operative repair for effective treatment.

4. Tear of the Quadriceps Tendon

Tear of the quadriceps tendon occurs most often in patients over the age of 40. Apparent tears that represent avulsions from the patella occur in patients with renal osteodystrophy or hyperparathyroidism. Preexisting attritional disease of the tendon is apt to be present, and the causative injury may be minor. The tear commonly results from sudden deceleration, such as stumbling or slipping on a wet surface. A small flake of bone may be avulsed from the superior pole of the patella, or the tear may occur entirely through tendinous and muscular tissue.

Pain may be noted in the anterior knee region. Swelling is caused by hemarthrosis and extravasation of blood into the soft tissues. The patient is unable to extend the knee completely. Radiographs may show a bony avulsion from the superior pole of the patella.

Operative repair is recommended for complete tear. Postoperative immobilization should be encouraged in a walking cylinder cast or brace for 6 weeks, at which time knee mobilization is started.

5. Tear of the Patellar Tendon

The same mechanism that causes tears of the quadriceps tendon, transverse fracture of the patella, or avulsion of the tibial tuberosity may also cause the patellar ligament to tear. The characteristic finding is proximal displacement of the patella. A bony avulsion may be present adjacent to the lower pole of the patella if the tear takes place in the proximal patellar tendon.

Operative treatment is necessary for a complete tear. The ligament is resutured to the patella, and any tear in the quadriceps mechanism is repaired. The extremity should be immobilized for 6–8 weeks in a cylinder cast extending from the groin to the supramalleolar region. Guarded exercises may then be started

Jutson JJ, Zych GA: Treatment of comminuted intraarticular distal femur fractures with limited internal and external tensioned wire fixation. J Orthop Trauma 2000;14:405. [PMID: 1100141])

Meyer RW et al: Mechanical comparison of a distal femoral side plate and a retrograde intramedullary nail. J Orthop Trauma 2000 14;398. [PMID: 11001413]

Stahelin T, Hardegger F, Ward JC: Supracondylar osteotomy of the femur with use of compression. J Bone Joint Surg 2000; 82-A;712. [PMID: 10819282]

Woo SL et al: Healing and repair of ligament injuries in the knee. J Am Acad Orthop Surg 2000;8:364. [PMID: 11104400]

FEMORAL SHAFT FRACTURES

DIAPHYSEAL FRACTURES

Fracture of the shaft of the femur usually occurs as a result of severe trauma. Indirect force, especially torsional stress, is likely to cause spiral fractures that extend proximally or, more commonly, distally into the metaphyseal regions. Most are closed fractures; open fracture is often the result of compounding from within.

Clinical Findings

Extensive soft-tissue injury, bleeding, and shock are commonly present with diaphyseal fractures. The most significant features are severe pain in the thigh and deformity of the lower extremity. Hemorrhagic shock may be present, as multiple units of blood may be lost into the thigh, though only moderate swelling may be apparent. Careful radiographic examination in at least two planes is necessary to determine the exact site and configuration of the fracture pattern. The hip and knee should be examined and radiographs obtained to rule out associated injury. A femoral neck fracture may occur in association with a femur fracture and if overlooked can increase patient morbidity.

Injuries to the sciatic nerve and the superficial femoral artery and vein are uncommon but must be recognized promptly. Hemorrhagic shock and secondary anemia are the most important early complications. Later complications include those of prolonged recumbency, joint stiffness, malunion, nonunion, leg-length discrepancy, and infection.

Classification

No classification is universally accepted for fractures of the femoral diaphysis. Classically, the fracture is described according to its location, pattern, and comminution. Winquist has proposed a comminution classification that is now widely used.

Type 1: Fracture that involves no, or minimal, comminution at the fracture site, and does not affect stability after intramedullary nailing

Type 2: Fracture with comminution leaving at least 50% of the circumference of the two major fragments intact

Type 3: Fracture with comminution of 50–100% of the circumference of the major fragments. Nonlocked intramedullary nails do not afford stable fixation.

Type 4: Fracture with completely comminuted segmental pattern with no intrinsic stability

Treatment

Treatment depends upon the age and medical status of the patient as well as the site and configuration of the fracture.

A. CLOSED TREATMENT

This remains a treatment option for some skeletally immature patients. Depending on the age of the pediatric patient and the amount of initial displacement at the fracture site, treatment may consist of immediate immobilization in a hip spica cast, or skin or skeletal traction for 3–6 weeks, until the fracture is "sticky," and then spica casting.

Closed treatment of femoral shaft fractures in the adult is rarely indicated. Acceptable alignment may be difficult to maintain, and joint stiffness is frequent. Other rarer complications of prolonged recumbency, like pressure sores and deep vein thrombosis, can have disastrous consequences.

B. OPERATIVE TREATMENT

Most fractures in the middle third of the femur can be internally fixed by an intramedullary rod. Intramedullary fixation of femoral shaft fractures allows early mobilization of the patient (within 24–48 hour if the fracture fixation is stable), which is of particular benefit to the polytraumatized patient; more anatomic alignment; improved knee and hip function by decreasing the time spent in traction; and a marked decrease in the cost of hospitalization.

Although open nailing procedures have been described, intramedullary fixation is routinely performed closed.

In closed nailing, the fracture is reduced by closed manipulation on a fracture table under fluoroscopic control. An small incision is made proximal to the greater trochanter, and the nail is inserted through the piriformis fossa down into the intramedullary canal, after reaming to the appropriate size. The fracture site is not opened. Closed nailing decreases the chance of infection by decreasing the amount of soft-tissue dissection necessary and by limiting access to the fracture site to the medullary canal. It also does not disturb the periosteal circulation. Some authors feel that bone reamings at the fracture site further promote bone healing. Interlocking nails are the standard of treatment. Screws are inserted percutaneously through holes in both ends of the nail. Dynamic interlocking using screws at only one end of the nail, relies on interference friction of fracture fragments and muscle action to prevent rotation of the unlocked fragment. It allows axial compression at the fracture site. However, up to 10% of dynamic interlocking may undergo secondary rotation or shortening due to unseen fracture lines. Static interlocking (screws at both ends of the nail) provides rotational control and prevents

shortening of the bone at the fracture site; this is the recommended technique. Reamed interlocked nailing is recommended for most grade 1, 2, and 3a open fractures. When associated with extensive soft-tissue loss, as in grade 3b and 3c open fractures, temporary bony stability may be achieved with external fixation devices.

Complications of this procedure can arise from technical problems at the time of surgery (eg, choice of a rod that is too short or too narrow) and result in malalignment or shortening. Comminution of the fracture can occur during placement of the rod. Late bone fracture (weeks or months) can occur through interlocking screws, and severely comminuted fractures with weight bearing can suffer rod or screw breakage. Infection can occur after any open procedure but is uncommon with closed nailing. Occasionally, a painful bursa or heterotopic calcification may develop over the proximal end of the nail, causing discomfort when the patient sits or walks. The rod may be removed after healing is complete, usually at 12–16 months. The healing rate of femoral shaft fractures in general is high and approaches 100% after closed nailing techniques.

Other fixation devices are seldom used. Flexible intramedullary rods of the Ender type do not provide sufficient stability in the adult; however, they are routinely used in the pediatric population. Plates and screws require significant soft-tissue dissection and opening of the fracture hematoma and are usually reserved for special cases such as ipsilateral femoral neck and diaphyseal fractures. External fixation remains indicated in some open fractures. In polytrauma patients, initial external fixation may be indicated when early intramedullary nailing (first 24 hours after trauma), can be potentially hazardous due to hemodynamic instability, head or chest trauma. It has also recently gained acceptance as treatment for closed femoral shaft fractures in children to allow earlier mobilization and decreased hospital stays. The distal fragment pins should always be inserted with the knee in flexion to avoid quadriceps tenodesis that will prevent knee flexion. Superficial pin tract infection is common but rarely involves the bone. A course of oral antibiotics, proper pin care, and eventual pin removal, when the fracture is sufficiently healed, are usually all that are needed to control this problem.

SUBTROCHANTERIC FRACTURES

Subtrochanteric fractures occur below the level of the lesser trochanter and are usually the result of high-energy trauma in young to middle-aged adults. They are often comminuted, with distal or proximal extension toward the greater trochanter. Associated soft-tissue damage can be extensive.

The Russell and Taylor classification (Figure 3–29) is a treatment based classification system that incorpo-

A Type IA **B** Type 1B

C Type IIA **D** Type IIB

Figure 3–29. Russell and Taylor classification of subtrochanteric femur fractures. (Reproduced, with permission, from Browner BD et al, eds: *Skeletal Trauma,* 2nd ed. WB Saunders, 1998.)

rates involvement of the piriformis fossa. Type Ia Russell-Taylor fractures do not involve the piriformis fossa, with the lesser trochanter attached to the proximal fragment. These fractures may be treated with a first-generation intramedullary nail. Type Ib fractures do not involve the piriformis fossa; however, the lesser trochanter is detached from the proximal fragment. These fractures require a second-generation nail, with screw fixation into the head and neck. Type II fractures have fracture extension into the piriformis fossa and are best treated with a sliding hip screw or fixed angle plate. The patient usually presents with a swollen painful proximal thigh with or without shortening or malrotation. If the lesser trochanter is intact, the proximal fragment will tend to displace in flexion, external rotation, and abduction because of the unopposed pull of the iliopsoas and abductor muscles.

In the vast majority of cases, internal fixation (by closed or open methods) is now widely favored. Temporary skeletal traction will maintain femoral length until the definitive surgical procedure can be performed. A variety of devices are available.

Closed intramedullary interlocking nails have gained more popularity recently. Devices with cephalic proximal interlocking are available for those cases where conventional intertrochanteric proximal interlocking is contraindicated. Fixation can be obtained with first-generation intramedullary nails, "gamma nails," intramedullary hip screws, or with a variety of cephalomedullary nails or blades and long sideplates based upon the fracture pattern.

Postoperative activity depends on the adequacy of internal fixation. If fixation is solid, an agile cooperative patient can be out of bed within a few days after surgery and ambulating on crutches with toe-touch weight bearing on the affected side. The fracture is usually healed at 3–4 months, but delayed union and nonunion are not uncommon. Hardware failure in these cases are frequent. Repeat internal fixation with autogenous bone grafting is then the treatment of choice.

Brumback RJ, Virkus WW: Intramedullary nailing of the femur: Reamed versus nonreamed. J Am Acad Orthop Surg 2000; 8:83. [PMID: 10799093]

Dora C et al: Entry point soft tissue damage in antegrade femoral nailing: A cadaver study. J Orthop Trauma 2001;15:488. [PMID: 11602831]

Giannoudis PV et al: Nonunion of the femoral diaphysis. J Bone Joint Surg Br 2000;82-B:655. [PMID: 10963160]

Herscovici D et al: Treatment of femoral shaft fracture using unreamed interlocked nails. J Orthop Trauma 2000;14:10. [PMID: 10630796]

Nowotarski PJ et al: Conversion of external fixation to intramedullary nailing for fractures of the shaft of the femur in multiply injured patients. J Bone Joint Surg Am 2000;82-A:2000. [PMID: 1085909]

Ostrum RF et al: Prospective comparison of retrograde and antegrade femoral intramedullary nailing. J Orthop Trauma 2000; 14:496. [PMID: 11083612]

Patton JT et al: Late fracture of the hip after reamed intramedullary nailing of the femur. J Bone Joint Surg Br 2000;82-B:967. [PMID: 11041583]

Ricci WM et al: Angular malalignment after intramedullary nailing of femoral shaft fractures. J Orthop Trauma 2001;15:90. [PMID: 11232660]

Ricci WM et al: Retrograde versus antegrade nailing of femoral shaft fractures. J Orthop Trauma 2001;15:161. [PMID: 11265005]

Scalea TM, Boswell SA, Scott JD, Mitchell KA, Kramer ME, Pollak AN. External fixation as a bridge to intramedullary nailing for patients with multiple injuries and with femur fractures: damage control orthopedics. J Orthop Trauma. 2004 Sep;18(8 Suppl):S2-10; discussion S10-2. [PMID: 15472561]

Shepherd LE et al: Prospective randomized study of reamed versus undreamed femoral intramedullary nailing: An assessment of procedures. J Orthop Trauma 2001;15:28. [PMID: 11147684]

Tornetta P, Tiburzi D: Antegrade or retrograde reamed femoral nailing. J Bone Joint Surg Br 2000;82-B:652. [PMID: 10963159]

Tornetta P, Tiburzi D: Reamed versus nonreamed anterograde femoral nailing. J Orthop Trauma 2000;14:15. [PMID: 10630797]

HIP FRACTURES & DISLOCATIONS

Epidemiology & Social Costs

Hip fractures include intertrochanteric fractures and femoral neck fractures and constitute a major problem in the United States because of the disabling nature of these injuries. Ambulation is almost impossible in all fractures except femoral neck fractures until they have been treated surgically. These fractures primarily occur in older patients (>55 years), unable in many cases to care for themselves. The incidence of hip fractures sharply rises after menopause in women and the age of 70 in men. Fourteen billion dollars are spent yearly to take care of one million affected Americans. Of these, approximately a quarter regain pre-fracture function. Further, prompt and effective care is necessary to avoid the all too frequent occurrence of death in the elderly (>70 years) patient with a hip fracture (20–30% of patients in the first year after fracture). Thus, this injury justifies state-of-the-art care to minimize not only the societal cost but also the human suffering.

Anatomy & Biomechanical Principles

The hip joint is the articulation between the acetabulum and the femoral head. The trabecular pattern of the femoral head and neck, and that of the acetabulum, is oriented to optimally accept the forces crossing the joint. The total force across the joint is the vector sum of body weight and active muscle force. When the concept of lever arm is factored in, surprising forces across the hip joint are attained: 2.5 times body weight when standing on one leg, five times body weight when running, and 1.5 times body weight when lifting the leg from the supine position with the knee in extension. Using a cane in the opposite hand reduces the force to body weight when standing on that leg. For the same reasons, forces across the joint when the ipsilateral leg is kept in the air are significantly greater than when toe-touch weight bearing is allowed.

The hip capsule is a strong thick fibrous structure that attaches on the intertrochanteric line anteriorly and somewhat more proximally posteriorly. The intracapsular portion of the neck is not covered with periosteum, and fractures of the intracapsular part of the neck cannot heal with periosteal callus formation, only with endosteal union. Interposition of synovial fluid between fracture fragments, as in any joint, can delay or altogether prevent bony union.

The vascular supply of the femoral head is also of paramount importance. There are three main sources of vascular supply: (1) the retinacular vessels arising from the lateral femoral circumflex artery and the inferior metaphyseal artery and then running beneath the synovium along the neck, which they penetrate proximally both anteriorly and posteriorly; (2) the interosseous circulation crossing the marrow spaces from distal to proximal; and (3) unreliably, the ligamentum teres artery. Fractures of the femoral neck always disrupt the interosseous circulation; the femoral head then relies only on the retinacular arteries, which may also be disrupted or thrombosed. Secondary avascular necrosis of part or all of the femoral head can result. Union of a fracture can occur in the presence of an avascular fragment, but the incidence of nonunion is higher. Revascularization of the necrotic fragment occurs through the process of creeping substitution. Part of this process involves replacement of necrotic bony substrate with a "softer" granulation tissue and sets the stage for delayed segmental collapse.

Intertrochanteric fractures usually do not suffer this same fate. The capsule (and vessels) are still attached to the proximal fragment after fracture, and thus the blood supply remains patent.

1. Femoral Neck Fractures

Femoral neck fractures are intracapsular fractures. Because of the already mentioned unusual vascularization of the femoral head and neck, these fractures are at high risk of nonunion or avascular necrosis of the femoral head. The incidence of avascular necrosis increases with the amount of fracture displacement and the amount of time before the fracture is reduced.

Fractures of the femoral neck occur most commonly in patients over age 50. The involved extremity may be slightly shortened and externally rotated. Hip motion is painful, except in the rare cases of nondisplaced or impacted fractures, where pain may be evident only at the extremes of motion. Good quality anteroposterior and lateral radiographs are mandatory.

Classification

The Garden classification for acute fractures is the most widely used system:

Type 1: Valgus impaction of the femoral head

Type 2: Complete but nondisplaced

Type 3: Complete fracture, displaced less than 50%

Type 4: Complete fracture displaced greater than 50%

This classification is of prognostic value for the incidence of avascular necrosis: The higher the Garden number, the higher the incidence. The benefits of either skeletal or skin traction are unclear prior to definitive treatment. Traction may offer comfort in some patients but do not improve overall outcome.

Stable Femoral Neck Fractures

These include stress fractures and Garden type 1 fractures. Stress fractures may be difficult to diagnose. Physical examination, as well as the initial radiographs, may be normal. Repeat radiographs, radionuclide imaging, and MRI may be necessary to confirm the diagnosis. Reviews have shown that age, walking ability, and degree of impaction on the radiographs are important factors influencing fracture healing, and may guide the choice of treatment (conservative management versus internal fixation).

Toe-touch weight bearing (with crutches) until radiologic evidence of healing is usually successful for the compliant patient. Healing is usually complete in 3–6 months. Prophylactic internal fixation may be necessary and is indicated by failure of pain resolution with toe-touch weight bearing or by displacement.

The Garden type 1 fracture is impacted in valgus position and is usually stable. Impaction must be demonstrated on both anteroposterior and lateral views. The risk of displacement is nevertheless significant; most surgeons recommend internal fixation to maintain reduction and allow earlier ambulation and weight bearing. If surgery is contraindicated, closed treatment with toe-touch crutch ambulation and frequent radiographic follow-up until healing can be successful.

Unstable Femoral Neck Fractures

Although undisplaced, a Garden type 2 femoral neck fracture is unstable because displacement is probable under physiologic loading. Garden type 3 and 4 fractures are displaced and often comminuted. They can be life-threatening injuries, especially in elderly patients.

Treatment is directed toward preservation of life and restoration of hip function, with early mobilization. This is best attained by rigid internal fixation or primary arthroplasty as soon as the patient is medically prepared for surgery. Closed treatment in a spica cast is almost always bound to fail. Definitive treatment using skeletal traction requires prolonged recumbency with constant nursing care and is associated with numerous complications, including malunion, nonunion, pressure sores, deep vein thrombosis and pulmonary embolus, osteoporosis, and hypercalcemia, to name a few. If for some reason surgery is not possible, it is better to mobilize the patient as soon as pain permits. Subsequent nonunion can be treated at a later stage, electively. Surgical options are internal fixation or primary arthroplasty. In general, the younger the patient, the greater the effort is justified to save the femoral head.

Treatment

A. INTERNAL FIXATION

The goal of internal fixation is to preserve a viable femoral head fragment and provide the optimal setting for bony healing of the fracture while allowing the patient to be as mobile as possible. Because persistent displacement and motion at the fracture site may further jeopardize the femoral head blood supply, surgery should be performed as soon as possible. General or spinal anesthesia is used. The fracture is reduced under fluoroscopic imaging as anatomically accurately as possible. Gentle manipulation is usually sufficient. Rarely, open reduction may be necessary before fixation. Open reduction, if performed, should be approached anteriorly as this results in less disruption of blood supply than a posterior approach. Rigid internal fixation is obtained using multiple parallel partially threaded screws, a dynamic hip screw and plate, or a combination of both. The patient can usually be mobilized the following day, and weight bearing is allowed according to the stability of the construct.

B. PRIMARY ARTHROPLASTY

This procedure is indicated in the elderly patient for Garden type 4 fractures, in which avascular necrosis is highly probable, and for Garden type 3 fractures that cannot be satisfactorily reduced or for femoral heads with preexisting disease. The femoral head is sacrificed, but a definitive procedure is performed, whereas internal fixation of Garden type 4 fractures frequently fails and repeat surgery is required. When the acetabulum is undamaged, the most commonly accepted technique is hemiarthroplasty, using a femoral stem stabilized with methyl methacrylate or a surface that allows biologic fixation with bony ingrowth. If the hip joint itself is already damaged by preexisting disease, total hip replacement may be indicated. Primary head and neck resection (Girdlestone arthroplasty) may be rarely indicated in the presence of infection or local malignant growth.

Complications

The most common sequelae of femoral neck fractures are loss of reduction with or without hardware failure, nonunions or malunions, and avascular necrosis of the femoral head. This latter complication can appear as late as 2 years after injury. According to different series, the incidence of avascular necrosis for Garden type 1 fractures varies from 0 to 15%, for type 2 fractures 10–25%, for type 3 fractures 25–50%, and for type 4 fractures 50–100%. Secondary degenerative joint disease appears somewhat later. The most disabling complication, infection, is fortunately rare.

2. Trochanteric Fractures

Lesser Trochanter Fracture

Isolated fracture of the lesser trochanter is rare. When it occurs, it is the result of the avulsion force of the iliopsoas muscle. Rarely, a symptomatic nonunion may require fragment fixation or excision.

Greater Trochanter Fracture

Isolated fracture of the greater trochanter may be caused by direct injury or may occur indirectly as a result of the activity of the gluteus medius and gluteus minimus muscles. It occurs most commonly as a component of intertrochanteric fracture.

If displacement of the isolated fracture fragment is less than 1 cm and there is no tendency to further displacement (as determined by repeated radiographic examinations), treatment may be bed rest until acute pain subsides. As rapidly as symptoms permit, activity can increase gradually to protected weight bearing with crutches. Full weight bearing is permitted as soon as healing is apparent, usually in 6–8 weeks. If displacement is greater than 1 cm and increases on adduction of the thigh, extensive tearing of surrounding soft tissues may be assumed, and ORIF is indicated.

Intertrochanteric Fractures

By definition, these fractures usually occur along a line between the greater and the lesser trochanter. They typically occur at a later age than do femoral neck fractures. They are most often extracapsular and occur through cancellous bone. Bone healing within 8–12 weeks is the usual outcome, regardless of the treatment. Nonunion and avascular necrosis of the femoral head are not significant problems.

Clinically, the involved extremity is usually shortened and can be internally or externally rotated. The degree of displacement and comminution will determine the instability of the fracture. A wide spectrum of fracture patterns is possible, from the nondisplaced fissure fracture to the highly comminuted fracture with four major fragments (head and neck, greater trochanter, lesser trochanter, and femoral shaft). The Muller/AO system is useful in classifying intertrochanteric femur fractures and has gained more popularity in recent years (Figure 3–30).

The selection of definitive treatment depends upon the general condition of the patient and the fracture pattern. Rates of illness and death are lower when the fracture is internally fixed, allowing early mobilization. Operative treatment is indicated as soon as the patient is medically able to tolerate surgery. Overall mortality decreases if surgery can be performed within 48 hours. Initial treatment in the hospital should be by gentle skin traction to minimize pain and further displacement. Skeletal traction as the definitive treatment is rarely indicated and is fraught with complications such as pressure sores, deep vein thrombosis and pulmonary embolus, deterioration of mental status, and varus malunion. When surgery is contraindicated, it may be preferable to mobilize the patient as soon as pain permits and accept the eventual malunion or nonunion.

The great majority of these fractures are amenable to surgery. The goal is to obtain a fixation secure enough to allow early mobilization and provide an environment for sound fracture healing in a good position. Reduction of the fracture is usually accomplished by closed methods, using traction on the fracture table, and monitored using fluoroscopic imaging. Some surgeons do not attempt to anatomically reduce comminuted fractures but instead prefer to keep the distal fragment medially displaced, to enhance mechanical stability. Internal fixation is most widely obtained with a dynamic screw and sideplate. The screw can slide in the barrel of the sideplate, allowing the fracture to impact in a stable position. The patient can be taken out of bed the next day, and weight bearing with crutches or a walker is begun as soon as pain allows. The fracture usually heals in 6–12 weeks. Other devices used to treat intertrochanteric fractures include second-generation interlocked nails and prosthetic replacement. Recent results of series have shown more complications of fracture fixation with intramedullary techniques compared to the dynamic hip screw.

General complications include infection, hardware failure, loss of reduction, and irritation bursitis over the tip of the sliding screw.

3. Traumatic Dislocation of the Hip Joint

Traumatic dislocation of the hip joint may occur with or without fracture of the acetabulum or the proximal end of the femur. It is most common during the active years of life and is usually the result of high-energy trauma, unless there is preexisting disease of the femoral

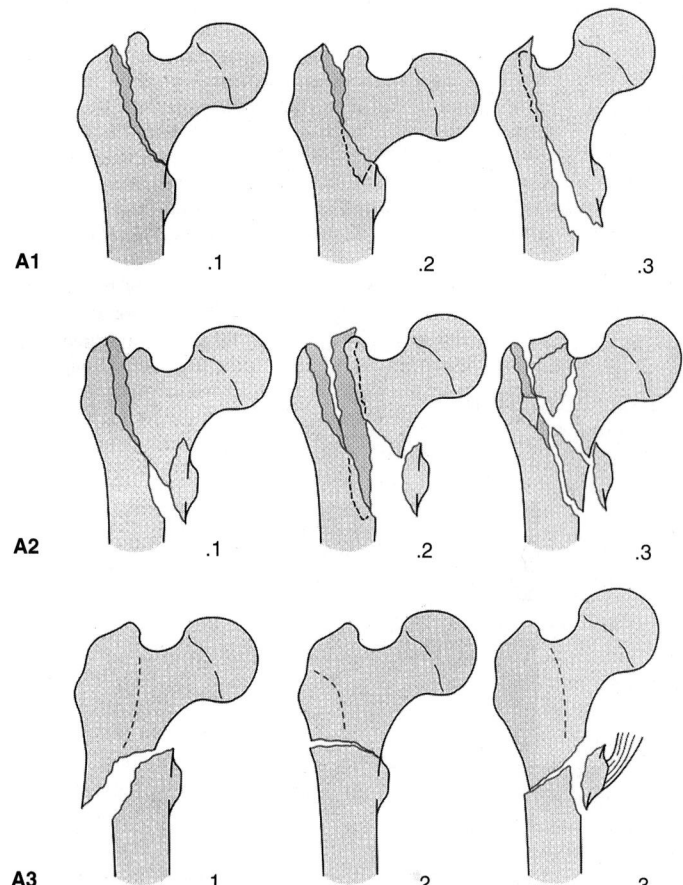

Figure 3–30. Muller/AO system for intertrochanteric femur fracture classification. (Reproduced, with permission, from Browner BD et al, eds: *Skeletal Trauma,* 2nd ed. WB Saunders, 1998.)

head, acetabulum, or neuromuscular system. The head of the femur cannot be completely displaced from the normal acetabulum, unless the ligamentum teres is ruptured or deficient because of some unrelated cause. Traumatic dislocations are classified according to the direction of displacement of the femoral head from the acetabulum.

Posterior Hip Dislocation

Usually, the head of the femur is dislocated posterior to the acetabulum when the thigh is flexed, for example, as may occur in a head-on automobile collision when the knee is driven violently against the dashboard. Posterior dislocation is also a complication of hip arthroplasty.

The significant clinical findings are shortening, adduction, and internal rotation of the extremity. Anteroposterior, lateral and, if fracture of the acetabulum is demonstrated, oblique radiographic projections

(Judet views) are required. Common associated injuries include fractures of the acetabulum or the femoral head or shaft and sciatic nerve injury. The head of the femur may be displaced through a tear in the posterior hip joint capsule. The short external rotator muscles of the femur are commonly lacerated. Fracture of the posterior margin of the acetabulum can create instability.

If the acetabulum is not fractured or if the fragment is small, reduction by closed manipulation is indicated. General anesthesia provides maximum muscle relaxation and allows gentle reduction. Reduction should be achieved as soon as possible, preferably within the first few hours after injury, as the incidence of avascular necrosis of the femoral head increases with time until reduction. The main feature of reduction is traction in the line of deformity followed by gentle flexion of the hip to 90 degrees with stabilization of the pelvis by an assistant. While manual traction is continued, the hip is gently rotated into internal and then external rotation to obtain reduction.

The stability of the reduction is evaluated clinically by ranging the extended hip in abduction and adduction and internal and external rotation. If stable, the same movements are repeated in 90 degrees of hip flexion. The point of redislocation is noted, the hip is reduced, and an anteroposterior radiograph of the pelvis is obtained. Soft tissue or bone fragment interposition will be manifested by widening of the joint space as compared to the contralateral side. Irreducible dislocations, open dislocations, and those that re-dislocate after reduction despite hip extension and external rotation (usually because of associated posterior wall fracture of the acetabulum) are indications for immediate open reduction and internal fixation if necessary. Most authors agree that a widened joint space on radiograph, despite a stable reduction, is also an indication for immediate arthrotomy. Others prefer obtaining a CT scan first, to further delineate the incarcerated fragments and associated injuries before surgery. Recently, hip arthroscopy has gained popularity, but it remains controversial.

Minor fragments of the posterior margin of the acetabulum may be disregarded, but larger displaced fragments are not usually successfully reduced by closed methods. Open reduction and internal fixation with screws or plates is indicated.

Postreduction treatment will vary according to the type of initial surgery. A strictly soft-tissue injury with a stable concentric reduction may be treated with light skin or skeletal traction for a few days to a week before exercises are begun. A motivated patient can then start crutch ambulation, progressing to full weight bearing at 6 weeks. An unstable reduction can be immobilized in a spica cast or abduction brace for 4–6 weeks. Securely fixed fractures are treated as soft-tissue injuries, but weight bearing is allowed when radiologic signs of bone healing are present. When fixation is tenuous, skeletal traction for 4–6 weeks or hip spica immobilization may be necessary.

Complications include infection, avascular necrosis of the femoral head, malunion, posttraumatic degenerative joint disease, recurrent dislocation, and sciatic nerve injury. Avascular necrosis occurs because of the disruption of the retinacular arteries providing blood to the femoral head. Its incidence increases with the duration of the dislocation. It can occur as late as 2 years after the injury. MRI studies enabling early diagnosis and protected weight bearing until revascularization has occurred are recommended. Sciatic nerve injury is present in 10–20% of patients with posterior hip dislocation. Although usually of the neurapraxia type, these lesions leave permanent sequelae in about 20% of cases. The rare patient who is neurologically intact before reduction but has a deficit after reduction should be explored surgically to see if the nerve has been entrapped in the joint. Associated injuries also, on rare occasions, include fracture of the femoral head. Small fragments or those involving the non-weight–bearing surface should be ignored if they do not disturb hip mechanics; otherwise they should be excised. Large fragments of the weight-bearing portion of the femoral head should be reduced and fixed if at all possible.

Anterior Hip Dislocation

Anterior dislocation of the hip is rare compared to its posterior counterpart. It usually occurs when the hip is extended and externally rotated at the time of impact. Associated fractures of the acetabulum and the femoral head or neck occur rarely. Usually, the femoral head remains lateral to the obturator externus muscle but can be found rarely beneath it (obturator dislocation) or under the iliopsoas muscle in contact with the superior pubic ramus (pubic dislocation).

The hip is classically flexed, abducted, and externally rotated. The femoral head is palpable anteriorly below the inguinal flexion crease. Anteroposterior and transpelvic lateral radiographic projections are usually diagnostic.

Closed reduction under general anesthesia is generally successful. Here also the surgeon must make sure of a concentric reduction comparing both hip joints on the postreduction anteroposterior radiograph. The patient starts mobilization within a few days when pain is tolerable. Active and passive hip motion, excluding external rotation, is encouraged, and the patient is usually fully weight bearing by 4–6 weeks. Skeletal traction or spica casting may rarely be useful for uncooperative patients.

4. Rehabilitation of Hip Fracture Patients

There has been an increased interest in the psychosocial outcome issues of patients with hip fractures. The goal of rehabilitation after hip injuries is to return the patient as rapidly as possible to the pre-injury functional level. Factors influencing rehabilitation potential include age, mental status, associated injuries, previous medical status, myocardial function, upper extremity strength, balance, and motivation.

For the rare patient treated conservatively, rehabilitation focuses early at preventing stiffness and weakness of the other extremities, and at eventually mobilizing the patient out of bed when pain is tolerable. Because the great majority of these injuries are now treated with internal fixation or prosthetic replacement, rehabilitation efforts are focused toward early range of motion, muscle strengthening, and weight bearing. Early full weight bearing as tolerated is encouraged for patients with prosthetic replacements, cemented or not, and for patients with stable fixation of an intertrochanteric fracture to allow compression of the fracture fragments.

Most authors now agree that the same applies for femoral neck fractures with stable internal fixation, although some still prefer partial weight bearing until radiologic evidence of bone healing is present to prevent hardware failure. When internal fixation does not provide stable fixation of the fracture fragments, supplemental protection may be added with a spica cast or brace However, it is highly undesirable in elderly patients. Otherwise, restricted range of motion or weight bearing may be allowed according to the surgeon's specifications.

Conn KS, Parker MJ: Undisplaced intracapsular hip fractures: results of internal fixation in 375 patients. Clin Orthop 2004 Apr;(421):249-54. [PMID 15123955]

Gotfried Y: Percutaneous compression plating of intertrochanteric hip fractures. J Orthop Trauma 2000;14:490. [PMID: 11083611]

Gruson et al: The relationship between admission hemoglobin level and outcome after hip fracture. J Orthop Trauma 2002; 15:39. [PMID: 11782632]

Jaglal S, Lakhani Z, Schatzker J: Reliability, validity and responsiveness of the lower extremity measure for patients with a hip fracture 2000; J Bone Joint Surg Am;82-A:955. [PMID: 10901310]

Kenny AM et al: Osteoporosis in older men and women. Conn Med 2003 Sep;67(8):481–6. [PMID: 14587128]

Parker MJ, Handoll HH, Bhargara A: Conservative versus operative treatment for hip fractures. Cochrane Database Syst Rev. 2000;(4):CD000337. [PMID 11034683]

Parker MJ, Handoll HH: Pre-operative traction for fractures of the proximal femur. Cochrane Database Syst Rev 2001;(3): CD000168. [PMID 11686954]

Parker MJ, Handoll HH: Gamma and other cephalocondylic intramedullary nails versus extramedullary implants for extracapsular hip fractures. Cochrane Database Syst Rev 2004;(1): CD000093. [PMID 14973946]

Rosen JE et al: Efficacy of preoperative skin traction in hip fracture patients: a prospective randomized study. J Orthop Trauma 2001;15:81. [PMID: 11232658]

Shah MR et al: Outcome after hip fracture in individuals ninety years of age and older. J Orthop Trauma 2001;15:34. [PMID: 11147685]

Tidermark J et al: Quality of life related to fracture displacement among elderly patients with femoral neck fractures treated with internal fixation. J Orthop Trauma 2002;15:34. [PMID: 11782631]

PELVIC FRACTURES & DISLOCATIONS

The innominate bones articulate with the sacrum through the sacroiliac joints and between themselves through the symphysis pubis. Upper body weight is transmitted across the hip joint to the lower limbs via the sciatic buttress and the acetabulum. The mechanism and severity of trauma will determine the pattern of injury. Osteoarticular structures and adjacent soft tissues will be involved to varying degrees depending upon the direction and magnitude of applied forces. Pelvic fractures are potentially life threatening with high mortality. A multidisciplinary team approach is necessary to reduce the likelihood of death and disability.

Mechanism of Injury

Four patterns of injury are responsible for pelvic fractures. Anteroposterior compression results in external rotation of the hemipelvis and rupture of the pelvic floor and anterior sacroiliac ligaments. Lateral compression creates compression fractures of the sacrum and disruption of the posterior sacroiliac ligament complex. The sacrospinous and sacrotuberous ligaments remain intact limiting the instability. In high energy lateral compression injuries, the contralateral hemipelvis can be pushed in external rotation, as seen in rollover or crush injuries. Combined external rotation-abduction is common in motorcycle accidents and the deforming forces are transmitted through the femur. The fourth pattern is a shear force vector resulting from fall from heights, where the grade of translational instability is variable.

Clinical Findings

Knowledge of the injury mechanism is of prime importance and should be assessed either by patient history or discussion with the prehospital provider. The physical examination includes inspection of the skin, perineum and rectum. Closed degloving injuries (Morel-Lavallée) should be properly identified. Palpation of the pelvic bony landmarks, including posterior palpation of the sacrum and sacroiliac joint, should be done. Rectovaginal examination is mandatory in all cases to identify open fractures. Bony spikes protruding through the mucosa contaminates the fracture hematoma. Anteroposterior and lateral iliac wing compression maneuvers to assess stability should be performed only once or avoided in hemodynamically unstable patients as excessive manipulation can increase bleeding. Associated injuries should also be systematically sought: lower urinary tract injuries, distal vascular status, and a thorough recorded neurologic examination.

An initial anteroposterior pelvic radiograph as per ATLS protocol is examined to evaluate the pelvic ring as a possible cause of shock. Following successful resuscitation, inlet and outlet views should be obtained. CT scan is essential to further define the fracture pattern Vascular and urologic imaging may also be required.

Open Pelvic Fractures

Open pelvic fractures account for 2–4% of all pelvic fractures. Because a higher energy is required to fracture the immature pelvic ring, the incidence of open pelvic fractures is increased among children. Motorcycle accidents are in part responsible for the increase in open pelvic fractures. Mortality has decreased from 50% in the 80s to 10–25%, probably because of the application of multidisciplinary protocols, including aggressive fracture management, selective fecal diversion and advances in critical care.

Treatment

Significant forces, either directly or indirectly through the lower extremities, are required to destabilize the pelvic ring. A systematic search for associated injuries is mandatory. Hemorrhage and shock are the primary causes of death due to pelvic fracture. The cornerstones of successful treatment include: identification of a significant pelvic injury; rapid resuscitation; hemorrhage control (using angiography or pelvic packing); assessment and treatment of associated injuries, and mechanical stabilization and in selected cases. In the hemodynamically unstable patient the ATLS® protocol should be followed. A pelvic binder or sheet can be used to stabilize the unstable pelvis temporarily. Antiseptic pressure dressings should be applied to bleeding sites. If there is continued hemodynamic instability after initial resuscitation (2 liters of IV fluids), a decision needs to be made in consultation with the trauma surgeon to perform pelvic packing with or without external fixation. If the patient's hemodynamic status stabilizes, the need for definitive versus temporizing mechanical fixation of the pelvis should be determined. This may involve anterior plating of the pubic symphysis, or the application of an external fixation device (pelvic clamp and /or anterior external fixator). Posterior fixation (either surgical or computed tomography guided percutaneous fixation) is usually deferred until a later time. When used to control pelvic fracture motion, the pelvic external fixator is a useful tool to manage volume depletion. It does not provide stable enough fixation to treat complex fractures or most unstable pelvic fractures. It usually resists stresses imposed by sitting but not those from weight bearing, and further internal fixation is often required at a later stage.

In open pelvic fractures, early surgical intervention using a multidisciplinary approach should be undertaken. Seventy-two percent of the open pelvic fractures are grade III open wounds, and should be appropriately treated. Swabs for microbiological examination followed by extensive irrigation and debridement are performed and repeated daily in an attempt to reduce the incidence of pelvic sepsis. Early selective faecal diversion in patients with perineal wounds can reduce sepsis and related mortality. The definitive method of stabilization of open pelvic fractures remains controversial. Internal fixation can be done when no gross contamination is present. Otherwise, external fixation is preferred when faecal or environmental contamination is present.

A. Associated Injuries

1. Hemorrhage—Bleeding associated with pelvic ring fractures usually comes from the small to medium-sized arteries and veins in the surrounding soft tissues and from the bone itself. After blunt trauma, the most common pelvic arteries injured are the superior gluteal artery, internal pudendal, obturator, and lateral sacral arteries. Occasionally, large vessels such as the femoral artery or the common iliac artery or vein are lacerated or torn. An arteriogram is diagnostic. Alternatively, contrast enhanced CT allows the early diagnosis of arterial bleeding. Arterial injuries causing significant bleeding occur only in about 10% of pelvic fractures, and surgery for repair or bypass is urgently required if there is distal ischemia.

2. Thrombosis—It is now well recognized that patients with pelvic fractures have a high incidence of thrombosis of the pelvic veins and, less frequently, of the femoral vein. Those treated with bed rest compound the risk of deep vein thrombosis and secondary pulmonary embolus. More trauma centers now use intermittent pneumatic compression after trauma and pharmacologic anticoagulation once the acute hemorrhagic phase has passed (24–48 hours). Severely traumatized patients with contraindications for pharmacological anticoagulation may benefit from temporary vena cava filters.

3. Neurologic injury—Neurologic injuries are common, with an overall incidence between 10% and 15% in pelvic fractures and are a common cause of disability following pelvic fracture. After unstable vertical shear sacral fractures the incidence rises to 50%. They involve either the roots (L5, S1) as they travel in or around the sacral foramen, or the peripheral nerve itself (sciatic, femoral, obturator, pudendal, or superior gluteal). Neurologic injury following closed or open reduction is not uncommon. Thus it is of paramount importance that a thorough neurologic examination be performed and recorded as soon as possible, searching for sensory or motor deficits in the distribution of all previously mentioned nerves. Peripheral nerve injuries have, overall, a better prognosis than root injuries. Partial nerve injuries also have a better outcome than complete ones. Most of the lesions are of the neurapraxia type, with favorable outcome. It is still accepted that nearly 10% have clinically significant permanent neurologic sequelae.

4. Urogenital injuries—Urogenital injuries are also common, especially in men. The incidence of bladder rupture and urethral disruption is estimated at 5–10% for each. These injuries should be suspected in the conscious patient who is unable to void or who has gross hematuria. Other signs include bloody urethral discharge, swelling or ecchymosis of the penis or perineum, or a high-riding or "floating" prostate on rectal examination. A retrograde urethrogram should be obtained before attempting to introduce a Foley catheter. If unremarkable, catheterization can be safely undertaken and a cystogram obtained later. When a partial or complete urethral disruption is diagnosed, a suprapubic cystostomy should be performed. Late sequelae are common and include urethral strictures, sexual dysfunction, and impotence.

1. Injuries to the Pelvic Ring

Pelvic ring fractures account for 3% of all fractures. There is an extremely wide spectrum between the innocuous avulsion fracture and the life-threatening severely unstable pelvic ring disruption. The choice between different treatment modalities revolves around one key issue: Is the fracture pattern stable or unstable?

From the anatomic standpoint, the posterior sacroiliac ligamentous complex is the single most important structure for pelvic stability. Injuries involving the pelvic ring in two or more sites create an unstable segment. The integrity of the posterior sacroiliac ligamentous complex will determine the degree of instability. Inlet and outlet views and CT scanning are necessary imaging techniques to make this determination. When intact, the hemipelvis will be rotationally unstable but vertically stable. When disrupted, the hemipelvis will be both rotationally and vertically unstable.

Classification & Treatment

Tile devised a dynamic classification system based on the mechanism of injury and residual instability (Table 3–4).

Type A: Fractures that involve the pelvic ring in only one place and are stable.

Type A1: Avulsion fractures of the pelvis, which usually occurs at muscle origins such as the anterosuperior iliac spine for the sartorius, anteroinferior iliac spine for the direct head of the rectus femoris, and ischial apophysis for the hamstring muscles. These fractures occur most often in the adolescent, and conservative treatment is usually sufficient. On rare occasions, symptomatic nonunion occurs, and this is best dealt with surgically.

Type A2: Stable fractures with minimal displacement. Isolated fractures of the iliac wing without intraarticular extension usually result from direct trauma. Even with significant displacement, bony healing is to be expected, and treatment is, therefore, symptomatic. On rare occasions, the soft tissue injury and accompanying hematoma may heal with significant heterotopic ossification.

Type A3: Obturator fractures. Isolated fractures of the pubic or ischial rami are usually minimally displaced. The posterior sacroiliac complex is intact, and the pelvis is stable. Treatment is symptomatic,

Table 3–4. The Tile classification of pelvic ring disruptions.

Type A: Stable, posterior arch intact
A1: Posterior arch intact, fracture of innominate bone (avulsion)
  A1.1 Iliac spine
  A1.2 Iliac crest
  A1.3 Ischial tuberosity
A2: Posterior arch intact, fracture of innominate bone (direct blow)
  A2.1 Iliac wing fractures
  A2.2 Unilateral fracture of anterior arch
  A2.3 Bifocal fracture of anterior arch
A3: Posterior arch intact, transverse fracture of sacrum caudal to S2
  A3.1 Sacrococcygeal dislocation
  A3.2 Sacrum undisplaced
  A3.3 Sacrum displaced
Type B: Incomplete disruption of posterior arch, partially stable, rotation
B1: External rotation instability, open-book injury, unilateral
  B1.1 Sacroiliac joint, anterior disruption
  B1.2 Sacral fracture
B2: Incomplete disruption of posterior arch, unilateral, internal rotation (lateral compression)
  B2.1 Anterior compression fracture, sacrum
  B2.2 Partial sacroiliac joint fracture, subluxation
  B2.3 Incomplete posterior iliac fracture
B3: Incomplete disruption of posterior arch, bilateral
  B3.1 Bilateral open-book
  B3.2 Open-book, lateral compression
  B3.3 Bilateral lateral compression
Type C: Complete disruption of posterior arch, unstable
C1: Complete disruption of posterior arch, unilateral
  C1.1 Fracture through ilium
  C1.2 Sacroiliac dislocation and/or fracture dislocation
  C1.3 Sacral fracture
C2: Bilateral injury, one side rotationally unstable, one side vertically unstable
C3: Bilateral injury, both sides completely unstable

with bed rest and analgesia, early ambulation, and weight bearing as tolerated.

Type B: Fractures that involve the pelvic ring in two or more sites. They create a segment that is rotationally unstable but vertically stable.

Type B1: Open-book fractures occur from anteroposterior compression. Unless the anterior separation of the pubic symphysis is severe (>6 cm), the posterior sacroiliac complex is usually intact and the pelvis relatively stable. Significant injury to perineal and urogenital structures is often present and should always be looked for. One should remember that fragment displacement at the time of injury might have been significantly more than what is apparent on radiograph. For minimally displaced symphysis injuries, only symptomatic treatment is needed. The same applies for the so-called straddle (four rami) fracture. For more displaced fracture-dislocations, reduction is done by lateral compression using the intact posterior sacroiliac complex as the hinge on which "the book is closed." Reduction can be maintained by external or internal fixation. "Closing the book" decreases the space available for hemorrhage. It also increases patient comfort, facilitates nursing care, and allows earlier mobilization, which is beneficial to the polytrauma patient.

Type B2 and B3: Lateral compression fractures. A lateral force applied to the pelvis causes inward displacement of the hemipelvis through the sacroiliac complex and the ipsilateral (B2) or, more often, contralateral pubic rami (B3, bucket-handle type). The degree of involvement of the posterior sacroiliac ligaments will determine the degree of instability. The posterior lesion may be impacted in its displaced portion, affording some relative stability. The hemipelvis is infolded, with overlapping of the symphysis. Major displacement requires manipulation under general anesthesia. This should be done soon after injury because disimpaction becomes difficult and hazardous after the first few days. Reduction can be maintained with external or internal fixation, or both. External fixation alone decreases pain and makes nursing care easier but is not strong enough for ambulation if the fracture is unstable posteriorly.

Type C: Fractures that are both rotationally and vertically unstable. They often result from a vertical shear mechanism, like a fall from a height. Anteriorly, the injury may fracture the pubic rami or disrupt the symphysis pubis. Posteriorly, the sacroiliac joint may be dislocated or there may be a fracture in the sacrum or in the ilium immediately adjacent to the sacroiliac joint, but there is always loss of the functional integrity of the posterior sacroiliac ligamentous complex. The hemipelvis is completely unstable. Three-dimensional displacement is possible, particularly proximal migration. Massive hemorrhage and injury to the lumbosacral nerve plexus are common. Indirect radiologic clues of pelvic instability should be looked for such as avulsion of the sciatic spine or fracture of the ipsilateral L5 transverse process. Reduction is relatively easy, with longitudinal skeletal traction through the distal femur or the proximal tibia. If chosen as definitive treatment, traction should be maintained for 8–12 weeks. Bony injuries heal quicker than ligamentous injuries. External fixation alone is insufficient to maintain reduction in highly unstable fractures, but

it may help control bleeding and eases nursing care. Open reduction and internal fixation is often required. The surgical technique is demanding, and there is a significant risk of complications. It is best left to experienced pelvic surgeons.

Complications

Long-term complications of unstable pelvic ring disruptions are more frequent and disabling than once thought. Of those patients with residual displacement of more than 1 cm, fewer than 30% are pain free at 5 years. Chronic low back pain and posterior sacroiliac pain is the most frequent long-term complaint, approaching 50% in some series. Nearly 5% of type C injuries are left with a leg length discrepancy of more than 2–5 cm. Residual gait abnormalities are present in 12–32% of cases. The overall nonunion rate is around 3%.

Clinically significant neurologic deficit is present in 6–10% of patients, but abnormal electromyographic findings are present in up to 46%. Long-term urologic complications include urethral strictures in 5–20% of cases and impotence in 5–30% of cases.

2. Fractures of the Acetabulum

The acetabulum results from the closure of the Y or triradiate cartilage and is covered with hyaline cartilage.

Fractures of the acetabulum occur through direct trauma on the trochanteric region or indirect axial loading through the lower limb. The position of the limb at the time of impact (rotation, flexion, abduction, or adduction) will determine the pattern of injury. Comminution is common.

Anatomy

The acetabulum appears to be contained within an arch. It is supported by the confluence of two columns and enhanced by two walls. The posterior column is the strongest one and where more space is available for fixation. It begins at the dense bone of the greater sciatic notch and extends distally through the center of the acetabulum to include the ischial spine and ischial tuberosity. The inner surface forms the posterior wall, and the anterior surface forms the posterior articular surface of the acetabulum. The anterior column extends from the iliac crest to the symphysis pubis. The anterior column rotates 90° just above the acetabulum as it descends. The medial part of the anterior column is the true pelvic brim. The quadrilateral plate is the medial structure preventing medial displacement of the hip, and is an independent structure between the two columns. The acetabular dome or weight-bearing area extends from the bone posterior to the anterior inferior iliac spine to the posterior column.

Classification

Letournel has classified acetabular fractures based on the involved column. Fractures may involve one or both columns in a simple or complex pattern.

Proper fracture classification requires good-quality radiographs. Two oblique views (Judet views) taken 45 degrees toward and away from the involved side complement the standard anteroposterior view of the pelvis. The obturator oblique view is obtained by elevating the fractured hip 45 degrees from the horizontal. This view shows the anterior column and the posterior lip of the acetabulum, and the iliac wing is perpendicular to its broad surface. In this view, the spur sign can be identified in 95% of cases of both-column fractures (Type C), and it corresponds to the area of the iliac wing above the acetabular roof. The Iliac oblique view is obtained by elevating the non-fractured hip 45°. This view best shows the posterior column, including the ischial spine, the anterior wall of the acetabulum, and the full expanse of the iliac wing. In addition, inlet and outlet pelvic views can be complimentary used if any doubt about pelvic ring compromise is present.

CT scanning gives further information on the fracture pattern, the presence of free intraarticular fragments, and the status of the femoral head and the rest of the pelvic ring.

Letournel has classified acetabular fractures into 10 different types: 5 simple patterns (one fracture line) and 5 complex patterns (the association of two or more simple patterns) (Figure 3–31). This is the most widely used classification system, as it allows the surgeon to choose the appropriate surgical approach.

Treatment

The goal of treatment is to attain a spherical congruency between the femoral head and the weight-bearing acetabular dome, and to maintain it until bones are healed. As with other pelvic fractures, acetabular fractures are frequently associated with abdominal, urogenital, and neurologic injuries, which should be systematically sought and treated. Significant bleeding can be present and should be addressed as soon as possible. Examination of the knee ligaments and vascular status of the extremities is mandatory. A careful neurologic

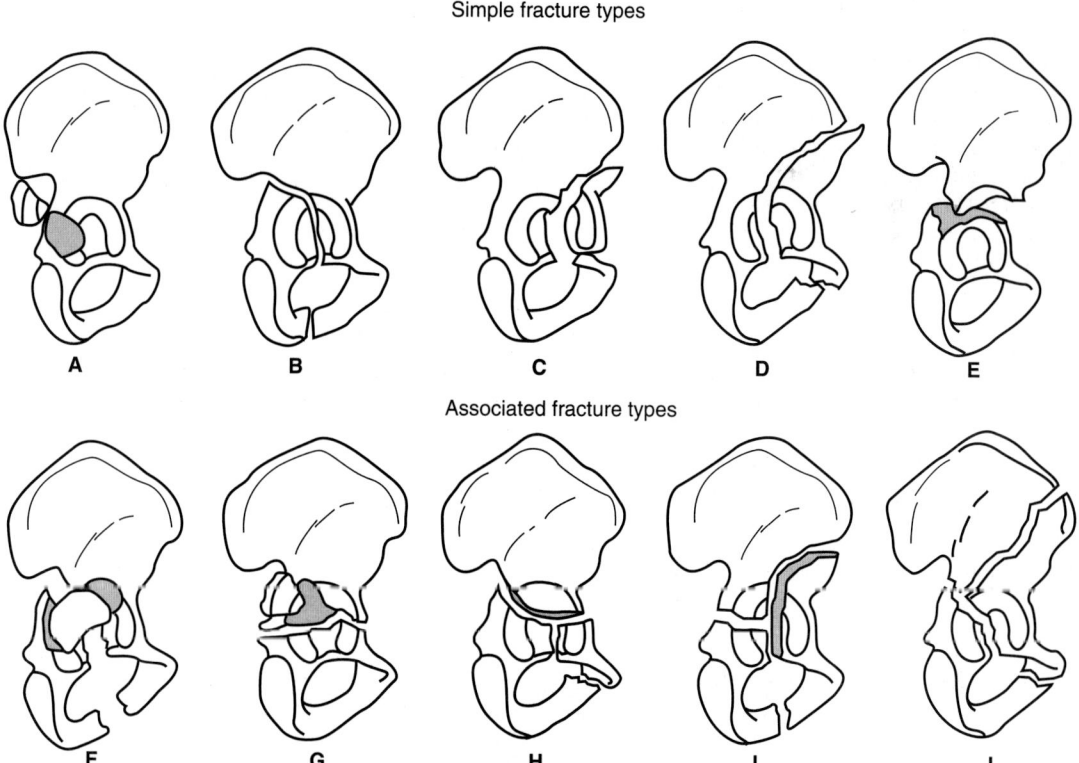

Figure 3–31. Letournel classification of acetabular fractures. (Reproduced, with permission, from Canale ST, ed: *Campbell's Operative Orthopaedics*, 9th ed. Lippincott, 1998.)

examination is necessary. Sciatic nerve compromise occurs in 20% of cases. The peroneal branch is often involved. Also, the tibial branch of the sciatic nerve, the femoral nerve, and the lateral femoral cutaneous nerve can be involved depending upon the fracture pattern and mechanism. Prophylaxis and surveillance for deep vein thrombosis (DVT) should be started soon after trauma. The reported incidence of DVT in patients with pelvic fractures has been as high as 60%.

The stabilized patient should be put in longitudinal skeletal traction through a distal femoral or proximal tibial pin pulling axially in neutral position. A trochanteric screw for lateral traction is contraindicated, as it will create a contaminated pin tract and thus preclude possible further surgical treatment. Postreduction radiographs are obtained. In general, a displaced acetabular fracture is rarely reduced adequately by closed methods. If the reduction is judged acceptable, traction is maintained for 6–8 weeks until bone healing is evident. Another 6–8 weeks is necessary before full weight bearing can be attempted. Surgical indications include intraarticular displacement of 2 mm or more, an incongruous hip reduction, marginal impaction >2 mm, or intraarticular debris. The choice of approach is of primary importance, and sometimes more than one approach will prove necessary. Acetabular surgery uses extensile approaches and sophisticated reduction and fixation techniques and is best performed by trained pelvic surgeons. Other surgical indications include free osteochondral fragments, femoral head fractures, irreducible dislocations, or unstable reductions.

Complications

Complications inherent to the injury include posttraumatic degenerative joint disease, heterotopic ossification, femoral head osteonecrosis, deep vein thrombosis, and other complications related to conservative treatment. Surgery is performed to prevent or delay osteoarthritis, but increases the possibility of complications such as infection, iatrogenic neurovascular injury, and increased heterotopic ossification. When the reduction is stable and fixation is solid, the patient can be mobilized after a few days with non-weight–bearing ambulation, and weight bearing may begin as early as 6 weeks. Most pelvic surgeons now routinely use postoperative prophylactic anticoagulation and heterotopic bone formation prophylaxis with irradiation or indomethacin, or both.

Bellabarba C, Ricci WM, Bolhofner BR: Distraction external fixation in lateral compression pelvic fractures. J Orthop Trauma 2000;14:475. [PMID: 11083609]

Carlson DA et al: Safe placement of S1 and S2 iliosacral screws: the vestibule concept. J Orthop Trauma 2000;14:264. [PMID: 10898199]

Ertel W et al: Control of Severe hemorrhage using C-clamp and pelvic packing in multiply injured patients with pelvic ring disruption. J Orthop Trauma 2001;15:468. [PMID: 11602828]

Grotz MRW, Allami MK, Harwood P, Pape HC, Kretekk C, Giannoudis PV. Open Pelvic Fractures: epidemiology, current concepts of management and outcome. Injury. 2005;1:1–13. [PMID: 15589906]

McCormick JP, Morgan SJ, Smith WR. Clinical effectiveness of the physical examination in diagnosis of posterior pelvic ring injuries. J Orthop Trauma. 2003 APR;17(4):257–61. [PMID: 12679685]

Routt ML, et al. Circumferential pelvic antishock sheeting: A temporary resuscitation aid. J Orthop Trauma 2002;15:45. [PMID: 11782633]

Saterbak AM et al: Clinical failure after posterior wall acetabular fractures: The influence of initial fracture patterns. J Orthop Trauma 2000;14:230. [PMID: 10898194]

Switzer JA, Nork SE, Routt ML: Comminuted fractures of the iliac wing. J Orthop Trauma 2000;14:270. [PMID: 10898200]

Tornetta P: Displaced acetabular fractures: Indications for operative and nonoperative management. J Am Acad Orthop Surg 2001;9:18. [PMID: 11174160]

Sports Medicine

4

Patrick J. McMahon, MD, & Lee D. Kaplan, MD

Introduction

Sports medicine developed in the 1970s as an orthopedic specialty focusing on competitive athletes. Today, sports medicine includes the overall care of athletes from many skill levels. Increasingly, care of recreational athletes has risen to that common for professional athletes. The initial focus of sports medicine on knee injuries now also includes other musculoskeletal injuries, including the shoulder, elbow, and ankle. In addition to the musculoskeletal system, emphasis is placed on the cardiovascular and pulmonary systems, and on training techniques, nutrition, and women's athletics. This wide range of care requires a multidisciplinary team of medical personnel, including athletic trainers, physical therapists, cardiologists, pulmonologists, orthopedic surgeons, and general practitioners.

■ KNEE INJURIES

Anatomy

The bones of the knee are the distal femur, the proximal tibia, and the patella. These bones depend on supporting ligaments, the joint capsule, and the menisci to provide stability for the joint.

A. MENISCI AND JOINT CAPSULE

The menisci, or semilunar cartilages, are C-shaped fibrocartilaginous disks in the knee that provide shock absorption, allow for increased congruency between joint surfaces, enhance joint stability, and aid in distribution of synovial fluid.

The medial and lateral menisci provide a concave surface with which the convex femoral condyles can articulate. If the menisci are not present, the convex femoral condyles articulate with the relatively flat tibial plateaus, and the joint surfaces are not congruent. This situation decreases the surface area of contact and increases the pressure on the articular cartilage of the

tibia and femur, which may lead to rapid deterioration of the joint surface. The medial meniscus is firmly attached to the joint capsule along its entire peripheral edge. The lateral meniscus is attached to the anterior and posterior capsule, but there is a region posterolaterally where it is not firmly attached (Figure 4–1). Therefore, the medial meniscus has less mobility than the lateral meniscus and is more susceptible to tearing when trapped between the femoral condyle and tibial plateau. The lateral meniscus is larger than the medial meniscus, and carries a greater share of the lateral compartment pressure than the medial meniscus carries for the medial compartment.

B. LIGAMENTS

Within the knee, the anterior cruciate ligament (ACL) travels from the medial border of the lateral femoral condyle to its insertion site anterolateral to the medial tibial spine. This ligament prevents anterior translation and rotation of the tibia on the femur (Figure 4–2). The posterior cruciate ligament (PCL) prevents posterior subluxation of the tibia on the femur. It runs from the lateral aspect of the medial femoral condyle to the posterior aspect of the tibia, just below the joint line (Figure 4–3). On the medial side, the medial collateral ligament has superficial and deep portions (Figure 4–4), which stabilize the knee to valgus stresses. The lateral collateral or fibular collateral ligament runs from the lateral femoral condyle to the head of the fibula. It is the main stabilizer against varus stress (Figure 4–5). The lateral collateral ligament is part of the posterolateral "complex" or "corner" of the knee that also resists external rotation. An important component is the popliteofibular ligament, present in 90% of knees, that runs from the tendon of the popliteus muscle to the styloid on the posterior fibular head.

History & Physical Examination

A. GENERAL APPROACH

The history of knee injury may be obtained by asking the patient the questions listed in Table 4–1. The physical examination begins with observation of the patient's gait. The uninjured knee is then examined as a

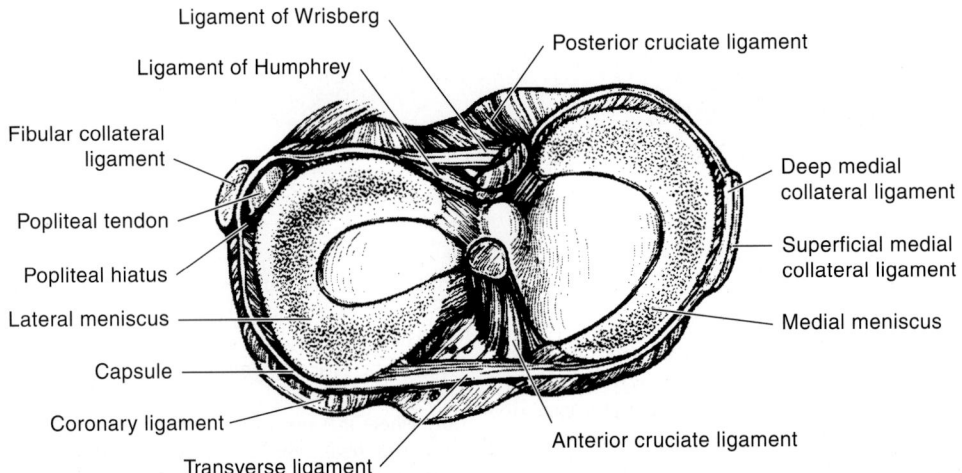

Figure 4–1. The medial and lateral menisci with their associated intermeniscal ligaments. *Note*: The lateral meniscus is not attached in the region of the popliteus tendon. (Reproduced, with permission, from Scott WN: *Ligament and Extensor Mechanism Injuries of the Knee: Diagnosis and Treatment.* Mosby-Year Book, 1991.)

Figure 4–2. Drawing of the anterior cruciate ligament with the knee in extension, showing the course of the ligament as it passes from the medial aspect of the lateral femoral condyle to the lateral portion of the medial tibial spine. (Reproduced, with permission, from Girgis FG et al: The cruciate ligaments of the knee joint: Anatomical, functional, and experimental analysis. Clin Orthop 1975;106:216.)

Figure 4–3. Drawing of the posterior cruciate ligament, showing the course of the ligament as it passes from the lateral aspect of the medial femoral condyle to the posterior surface of the tibia. (Adapted, with permission, from Girgis FG et al: The cruciate ligaments of the knee joint: Anatomical, functional, and experimental analysis. Clin Orthop 1975;106:216.)

Figure 4–4. Medial capsuloligamentous complex. (Reproduced, with permission, from Feagin JA Jr: *The Crucial Ligaments*. Churchill Livingstone, 1988.)

basis of comparison with the injured knee. Any swelling or effusion should be noted. A small effusion causes obliteration of the recesses on the medial and lateral aspects of the patellar tendon; with a larger effusion, diffuse swelling is present in the region of the suprapatellar pouch. Then, a fluid wave can be palpated on the sides of the patella. Active and then passive range of motion is tested carefully. The knee is palpated to define areas of localized tenderness. The joint lines are located at the level of the inferior pole of the patella when the knee is flexed to 90 degrees.

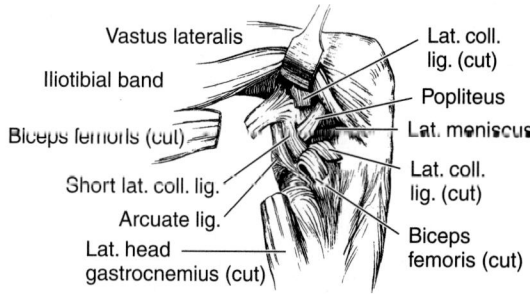

Figure 4–5. The lateral supporting structures of the knee. (Reproduced, with permission, from Rockwood CA Jr et al: *Fractures in Adults*, 2/e. New York Lippincott, 1984.)

Table 4–1. History of a knee injury.

Did an injury occur?	Yes: possible ligament tear or meniscus tear. No: overuse problem or degenerative condition.
Was it a noncontact injury?	Yes: often the ACL is the only ligament torn.
Was it a contact injury?	Yes: possible multiple ligament injuries, including ACL and MCL, ACL and LCL, ACL, PCL, and a collateral ligament.
Did the patient hear or feel a pop?	Yes: a pop often occurs with ACL tears.
How long did it take to swell up?	Within hours: often an ACL tear. Overnight: often a meniscus tear.
Does the knee lock?	Yes: often a meniscus tear flipping into and out of the joint.
Does it buckle (trick knee)?	Yes: not specific; may arise from quadriceps weakness, trapped meniscus, ligament instability, or patella dislocating.
Is climbing or descending stairs difficult?	Often patellofemoral problems.
Are cutting maneuvers difficult?	ACL tear.
Is squatting (deep knee bends) difficult?	Meniscus tear.
Is jumping difficult?	Patellar tendinitis.
Where does it hurt?	Medial joint line: medial meniscus tear or medial compartment arthritis. MCL: MCL sprain. Lateral joint line: lateral meniscus tear, injury, iliotibial band tendinitis, popliteus tendinitis.

ACL = anterior cruciate ligament; MCL = medial collateral ligament; LCL = lateral collateral ligament; PCL = posterior cruciate ligament.

B. Ligament Laxity Evaluation

To determine varus and valgus stability (Table 4–2), the patient's foot is held between the examiner's elbow and hip, with both hands free to palpate the joint (Figure 4–6). Stability should be determined at both full extension and 30 degrees of knee flexion. Grading of laxity is based on the amount of opening of the joint (grade 1, 0–5 mm; grade 2, 5–10 mm; and grade 3, 10–15 mm). Laxity in full extension to varus or valgus angulation is

Table 4–2. Anatomic correlation of clinical ligament instability examination of the knee.

Direction of Force	Position	Ligament Instability
Varus or valgus	Full extension	Posterior cruciate, posterior capsule
Varus	Flexion at 30 degrees	Lateral collateral ligament/complex
Valgus	Flexion at 30 degrees	Medial collateral ligament
Anterior	Flexion at 30 degrees neutral position (AP)	Anterior cruciate ligament
Anterior	Flexion at 90 degrees neutral internal or external rotation	Anterior cruciate ligament
Posterior	90 degrees (sag test)	Posterior cruciate ligament

AP = anteroposterior.

Figure 4–6. The collateral ligaments being tested in extension and 30 degrees of flexion with the foot held between the examiner's elbow and hip. (Reproduced, with permission, from Feagin JA Jr: *The Crucial Ligaments.* Churchill Livingstone, 1988.)

Figure 4–7. Lachman test. (Reproduced, with permission, from Feagin JA Jr: *The Crucial Ligaments.* Churchill Livingstone, 1988.)

an ominous sign that indicates disruption of key ligamentous structures. If significant valgus laxity is present in full extension, the posteromedial capsule and medial collateral ligament are torn. With varus laxity in full extension, the posterolateral capsular complex is torn, in addition to the lateral collateral ligament. With either varus or valgus laxity at full extension, anterior and posterior cruciate ligament tears are likely. At 30 degrees of flexion, the posterior capsule and cruciate ligaments are relaxed, and the medial and lateral collateral ligaments can best be isolated. Pain with varus or valgus stress is more suggestive of ligament damage than a meniscus tear.

1. The Lachman test—The Lachman test is the most sensitive test for ACL tears. It is done with the knee flexed at 20 degrees, stabilizing the distal femur with one hand and pulling forward on the proximal tibia with the other hand. (Figure 4–7). With an intact ligament, minimal translation of the tibia occurs and a firm end point is felt. With a torn ACL, more translation is noted, and the end point is soft or mushy. The hamstring muscles must be relaxed during this maneuver to prevent false-negative findings. Comparison of the injured and uninjured knees is essential.

2. Anterior drawer test—The anterior drawer test is done with the knee at 90 degrees of flexion and is not as sensitive as the Lachman test but serves as an adjunct in the evaluation of ACL instability (Figure 4–8). With the patient supine and the knee flexed to 90 degrees (hip flexed to approximately 45 degrees), the foot is restrained by sitting on it, and the exam-

iner's hands are placed around the proximal tibia. Then while the hamstrings are felt to relax and the tibia is pulled forward, the displacement and the endpoint are evaluated.

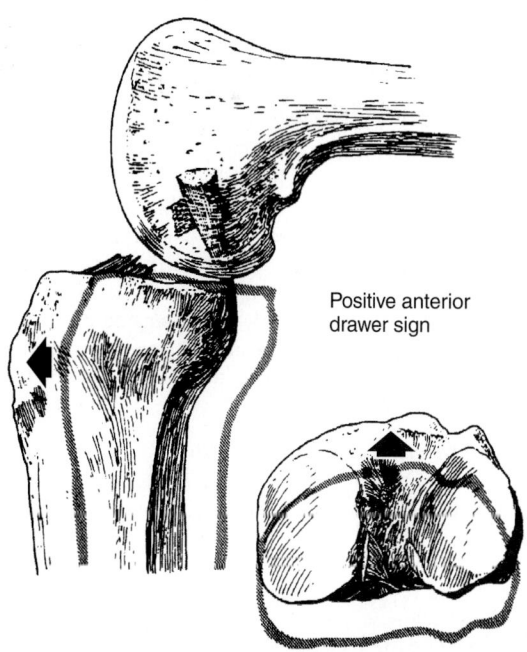

Positive anterior drawer sign

Figure 4–8. A positive anterior drawer test signifying a tear of the anterior cruciate ligament. (Reproduced, with permission, from Insall JN: *Surgery of the Knee.* Churchill Livingstone, 1984.)

Figure 4–9. The Losee pivot shift test. (Reproduced, with permission, from Scott WN: *Ligament and Extensor Mechanism Injuries of the Knee: Diagnosis and Treatment.* Mosby-Year Book, 1991.)

3. The Losee test—The pivot shift phenomenon demonstrates the instability associated with an ACL tear. Once demonstrated, it is often difficult to repeat because the patient may find this maneuver uncomfortable and will guard against having it done again. As described by Losee, a valgus and internal rotation force is applied to the tibia (Figure 4–9). Starting at 45 degrees of flexion, the lateral tibial plateau is reduced. Extending the knee causes the lateral plateau to subluxate anteriorly with a thud at approximately 20 degrees of flexion. It reduces quietly at full extension. Many other ways of doing this test are described, but the phenomenon and significance of the different tests are similar.

4. Posterior drawer test—The posterior drawer test evaluates the integrity of the PCL. It is performed with posterior pressure on the proximal tibia with the knee flexed at 90 degrees (Figure 4–10). Normally, the tibial plateau is anterior to the femoral condyles, and a step-off to the tibia is palpated when the thumb is slid down the femoral condyles. With a PCL injury, sagging of the tibial plateau may be appreciated, and no step-off is palpated (Figure 4–11). An associated contusion on the anterior tibia suggests a PCL injury.

5. The McMurray test—With the McMurray test, forced flexion and rotation of the knee elicits a clunk along the joint line if there is a meniscus injury (see Figure 4–12). Found in less than 10 percent of patients with a meniscus injury, joint line pain with the McMurray test is much more common.

Arthroscopic Examination

A. INDICATIONS FOR KNEE INJURIES

Indications for arthroscopic examination in the knee include the following:

1. acute hemarthrosis;
2. meniscus injuries;
3. loose bodies;
4. selected tibial plateau fractures;
5. patellar chondromalacia and/or malalignment;
6. chronic synovitis;
7. knee instability;
8. recurrent effusions; and
9. chondral and osteochondral fractures.

Today, a specific diagnosis of the type of knee injury can now usually be made with a history, physical examination, and appropriate imaging studies. With an examination under anesthesia and arthroscopic evaluation, a specific diagnosis can be confirmed, expanded, or revised, and treatment can be rendered as needed.

B. TECHNIQUE

Examination under anesthesia is very helpful in diagnosing ligament injuries and instability. It should be performed before the beginning of the procedure, before preparing and draping the extremity. For diagnostic arthroscopy, the knee joint is distended with irrigating fluid (usually saline or lactated Ringer's solution), which washes away blood and debris from the joint. A lateral portal, for the arthroscope, is placed approximately a thumb's breadth above the joint line and just lateral to the patellar tendon. The medial portal is placed at approximately the same level, but just medial to the patellar tendon for introducing arthroscopic tools such as a probe. One approach to the general inspection of the joint is to start in the suprapatellar pouch. Loose bodies and plicas are sought. The patellofemoral joint is then inspected and observed for tracking problems and cartilage damage. The lateral gutter and the popliteus tendon are examined by flexion and

Figure 4–10. The posterior drawer test is done in the same fashion as the anterior drawer test, except that the examiner exerts a posterior force. (Reproduced, with permission, from Scott WN: *Ligament and Extensor Mechanism Injuries of the Knee: Diagnosis and Treatment.* Mosby-Year Book, 1991.)

Figure 4–11. The posterior sag seen in posterior cruciate disruption. (Reproduced, with permission, from Scott WN: *Ligament and Extensor Mechanism Injuries of the Knee: Diagnosis and Treatment.* Mosby-Year Book, 1991.)

valgus stress to the leg, prior to entering the medial compartment. The medial meniscus is probed using a nerve hook through the medial portal. The intercondylar notch, including the ACL, is inspected. The lateral compartment is then examined in a similar manner. Documentation of findings and procedures performed is important and may be done by videotape, photo-

graphs, and diagrammatic sketches. With assessment of the pathologic changes, treatment can be initiated, such as debridement and repair of meniscus tears, removal of loose bodies, or ACL reconstruction.

Imaging & Other Studies

A. MAGNETIC RESONANCE IMAGING

MRI is a powerful technique for evaluation of the knee joint. Although the diagnosis is usually evident from the history and physical examination, MRI can be used to confirm the suspected injury. Other times, when a physical examination is not possible because of pain or the diagnosis remains elusive, MRI can aid in proper diagnosis. The specificity, sensitivity, and accuracy of MRI are greater than 90% for the medial and lateral menisci and the ACL and PCL. Therefore, MRI is often appropriate for ruling out the need for diagnostic arthroscopic examination. It is less helpful for the diagnosis of problems in knees with previous surgery.

B. IMAGING STUDIES

Roentgenographic examination of the knee is indicated in the evaluation of traumatic injury. In cases of minimal trauma, radiographs may not be needed if the

Figure 4–12. The McMurray test to produce click. (Reproduced, with permission, from American Academy of Orthopaedic Surgeons: *Athletic Training and Sports Medicine,* 2nd ed., 1991.)

injury proves to be self-limited. Arthrographic examination can be helpful in patients who are unable to undergo MRI because of claustrophobia, metal in the body that may be dislodged, or other contraindications.

C. LABORATORY TESTS

Laboratory tests may be helpful in ruling out nonmechanical disorders such as inflammatory arthritis as described in Chapter 7.

Chang CY et al: Imaging evaluation of meniscal injury of the knee joint: A comparative MR imaging and arthroscopic study. Clin Imaging 2004;28:372. [PMID: 15471672]

Luhmann SJ et al: Magnetic resonance imaging of the knee in children and adolescents. Its role in clinical decision-making. J Bone Joint Surg Am 2005;87-A:497. [PMID: 15741613]

Sanders TG, Miller MD: A systematic approach to magnetic resonance imaging interpretation of sports medicine injuries of the knee. Am J Sports Med 2005;33(1):131. [PMID: 15611010]

Scholten RJ et al. The accuracy of physical examination diagnostic tests for assessing meniscus lesions of the knee: A meta-analysis. J Fam Pract 2001,50:938. [PMID: 11711009]

MENISCUS INJURY

Meniscal injuries are the most common reason for arthroscopy of the knee. The medial meniscus is more frequently torn than the lateral meniscus because the medial meniscus is securely attached around the entire periphery of the joint capsule, whereas the lateral meniscus has a mobile area where it is not attached. Meniscus injury is rare in childhood, occurs in the late teens, and peaks in the third and fourth decades. After 50 years of age, meniscus tears are more often the result of arthritis than trauma.

Clinical Findings

Acute traumatic tears of the menisci are often caused by axial loading combined with rotation. Patients typically report pain and swelling. Patients with smaller tears may have a sensation of clicking or catching in the knee. Patients with larger tears in the meniscus may complain of locking of the knee as the meniscus displaces into the joint and/or femoral notch. Loss of knee motion with a block to extension may result from a large bucket-handle tear. In acute tears involving an associated ACL injury, the swelling may be more significant and acute. ACL injuries often involve a lateral meniscus tear as the lateral compartment of the knee subluxates forward, trapping the lateral meniscus between the femur and tibia.

Conversely, chronic or degenerative tears of the menisci often present in older patients (more than 40 years old) with the history of an insidious onset of pain and swelling with or without an acute increase superimposed. Often no identifiable history of trauma is obtained, or the inciting event may be quite minor, such as a bending or squatting motion.

The most important physical examination findings in the knee with a meniscus tear are joint line tenderness and an effusion. Other specialized tests include the McMurray, flexion McMurray, and Apley grind tests. The McMurray test is performed with the patient lying supine with the hip and knee flexed to approximately 90 degrees. While one hand holds the foot and twists it from external to internal rotation, the other hand holds the knee and applies compression (see Figure 4–12). A positive test is one that elicits a pop or click that can be felt by the examiner when the torn meniscus is trapped between the femoral condyle and tibial plateau. A variation of this test is the flexion McMurray, in which the knee is held as for the McMurray test. To test the medial meniscus, the foot is externally rotated and the knee maximally flexed. A positive test occurs when the patient experiences pain over the posteromedial joint line as the knee is gradually extended. The Apley grind test requires placing the patient prone with the knee flexed to 90 degrees. The examiner applies downward pressure to the sole of the foot while twisting the lower leg in external and internal rotation. A positive tests results in pain at either joint line.

In addition to the procedure just described, physical examination of the entire leg is essential. Assessing hip range of motion and irritability is useful, especially in children, because referred pain from the hip to the knee area is common. Examining for quadriceps atrophy and the presence of a knee effusion should also be done. Measurement of range of motion may reveal a loss of the normal knee extension. Assessing for tenderness of the femoral condyles, joint lines, tibial plateaus, and patellofemoral joint may give clues as to a possible osteochondral lesion, meniscus lesion, fracture, or chondrosis, respectively. Ligamentous testing, including varus and valgus stress testing at full extension and 30 degrees of flexion; Lachman; anterior drawer; and posterior drawer testing should be done to assess stability.

Tear Classification

Meniscal tears can be classified either by etiology or by their arthroscopic and MRI appearance. Etiologic classification divides tears into either acute tears (excessive force applied to an otherwise normal meniscus) or degenerative tears (normal force applied to a degenerative structure).

Classification should describe the tear location and its associated vascularity, morphology, and stability. Tear location is described by its location in the anteroposterior plane (anterior, middle, or posterior) and its circumferential location with respect to its vascularity. The common vascular zones include the most peripheral red/red zone near the meniscocapsular junction, the intermediate red/white zone, and the most central white/white zone. As tears occur more centrally, the vascularity decreases, as do the associated healing rates.

Tear morphology describes the orientation of the tear within the meniscus and includes vertical or horizontal longitudinal, radial (transverse), oblique, and complex (including degenerative) tears (Figure 4–13). Most acute tears in patients less than 40 years old involve vertical longitudinal or oblique tears, whereas complex and degenerative tears occur more commonly in patients more than 50 years old. Vertical longitudinal, or bucket-handle tears, can be complete or incomplete and usually start in the posterior horn and continue anteriorly a variable distance. Long tears can cause significant mobility of the torn meniscal fragment, allowing it to displace into the femoral notch and cause a locked knee (Figure 4–14). This more commonly occurs in the medial meniscus, possibly owing to its decreased mobility, which leads to increased sheer stresses. Oblique tears commonly occur at the junction of the middle and posterior thirds. They are often smaller tears, but the free edge of the tear can catch in the joint and cause symptoms of catching. Complex or degenerative tears occur in multiple planes, are often located in or near the posterior horns, and are more common in patients more than 50 years old with degenerative menisci. Horizontal longitudinal tears are often associated with meniscal cysts. They usually start at the inner margin of the meniscus and extend toward the meniscocapsular junction. They are thought to result from shear stresses and, when associated with meniscal cysts, they occur in the medial meniscus and cause localized swelling at the joint line.

Treatment & Prognosis

Small stable asymptomatic meniscus tears do not need to be treated surgically. Those causing persistent symptoms should be assessed with the arthroscope. Before the importance of the meniscus was understood and arthroscopy became available, the meniscus was often removed, even when normal. We now attempt to remove only the torn portion of the meniscus or repair the meniscus, if possible.

During arthroscopy, the meniscus should be visualized and palpated with a hooked probe. The inner two thirds of the meniscus is avascular and often requires resection when torn. A biting instrument is used to complete the resection of the torn portion of the meniscus, and the meniscus fragment is removed with a grasping instrument. Power shavers are used to smooth and contour the remaining meniscus to prevent further tearing from a jagged edge. Return to full function may be expected in 6–8 weeks.

Tears in the peripheral third of the meniscus, if small (less than 15 mm), may heal spontaneously because there is a blood supply in this portion of the adult meniscus. Larger tears need to be repaired. Patients who undergo meniscectomy at less than 40 years old are at risk of early osteoarthritis. These changes were first described by Fair-

Figure 4–13. Patterns of meniscal tears: bucket-handle, flap, horizontal cleavage, radial, degenerative, and double radial tear of a discoid meniscus. (Reproduced, with permission, from Scott WN: *Arthroscopy of the Knee.* WB Saunders, 1990.)

banks and include flattening of the femoral condyle, joint space narrowing, and osteophyte formation. Therefore, if a meniscus can be saved, it should be.

A. PARTIAL MENISCAL RESECTION

Partial meniscectomy has 90% good or excellent results in patients with normal knee stability and no degenerative changes. A major advantage over meniscus repair is a short recovery period, but results after partial meniscectomy are not as satisfactory when degenerative changes or knee ligament injuries are present. Also, results diminish over time; degenerative changes occur with follow-up beyond 10 years. Medial meniscus tears generally do better than lateral tears after partial resection, and an intact meniscal rim and normal articular cartilage surfaces are associated with a better prognosis.

B. MENISCUS REPAIR

Most surgeons attempt a meniscus repair rather than a partial meniscectomy in individuals less than 40 years old. Other commonly accepted criteria for meniscus repair include a complete vertical longitudinal tear greater than

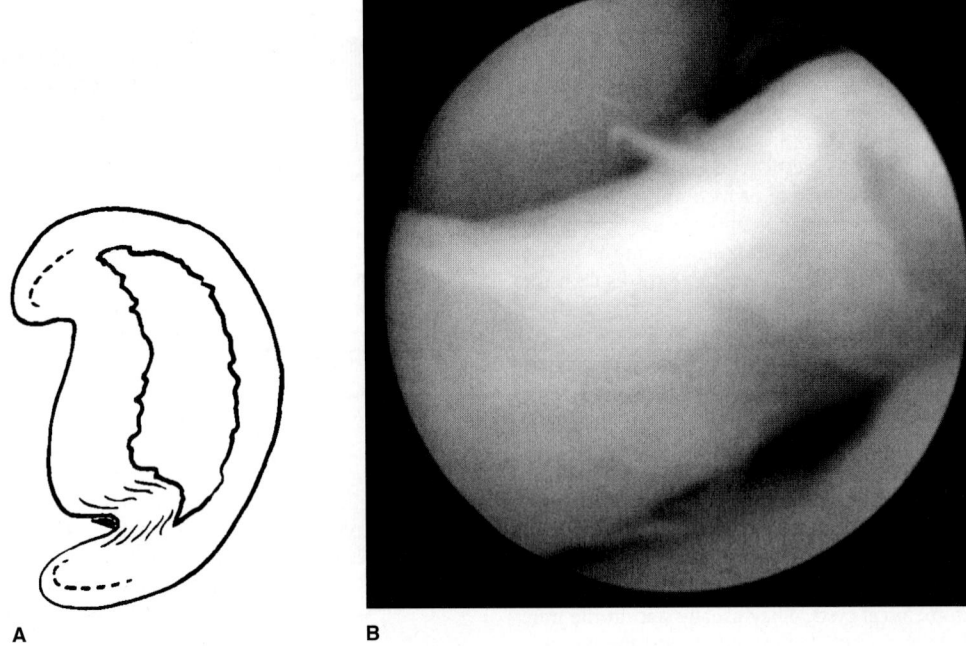

A   **B**

Figure 4–14. **A:** Diagram of a typical bucket-handle tear of the medial meniscus. **B:** Arthroscopic view of a bucket-handle fragment displaced into the intercondylar notch. (Reproduced, with permission, from McGinty JB: *Operative Arthroscopy.* Raven Press, 1991.)

15 mm in length, a tear within the peripheral 10–30% of the meniscus (ie, within 3–4 mm of the meniscocapsular junction), a peripheral tear that can be displaced toward the center of the plateau with a probe, the absence of secondary meniscus degeneration, and a tear in a patient undergoing concurrent ligament or articular cartilage repair.

Multiple factors affect the success of meniscus repair. Although no absolute age limit exists, patients younger than 40 years are thought to have a better chance for healing. Knees with associated ligamentous instability, particularly ACL instability, have inferior rates of meniscus healing because of abnormal meniscus stresses from tibiofemoral instability. The location of the tear and the time lapsed from injury to treatment are also important. Acute tears located in the peripheral red/red or red/white zone have better healing capability than chronic tears located in the red/white or white/white zones. Tears 5 mm or more from the periphery are considered avascular (white zone); those between 3 and 5 mm are variable in vascularity (red/white), and tears in the peripheral 3 mm are considered vascular (red). In areas with marginal vascularization, abrasion of the meniscocapsular junction or use of a fibrin clot may be used. It is thought that a vascular pannus forms from the abraded tissue, which aids in meniscus healing. Finally, the sta-

bility of the meniscus repair is a factor, with vertical mattress sutures generally considered the gold standard in meniscus repair.

Meniscus repair is successful in up to 90% of meniscus tears when done in conjunction with ACL reconstructions, as compared to approximately 50% in patients with stable ACLs who had meniscus repairs.

Types of repairs include the traditional open repair and arthroscopic repairs that can be dome with inside-out, outside-in, or all-inside techniques. Inside-out and outside-in repairs require a mini-incision and securing of the meniscus to the capsule with sutures. The all-inside technique has many device options, including both absorbable and nonabsorbable arrows, tacks, darts, and fasteners. Regardless of the type of repair chosen, adequate preparation of the tear site is required. The tear edges should be debrided or abraded with a shaver or rasp to stimulate bleeding. Restoration of biomechanical function is encouraged by anatomic apposition of the tear's edges to ensure good healing potential.

C. OPEN MENISCAL REPAIR

Open repair of meniscus tears has successful long-term results. The technique involves making a small incision through the subcutaneous tissue, capsule, and synovium to visualize the tear directly. Open repair is most useful in peripheral or meniscocapsular tears, often occurring in conjunction with open repair of a collateral ligament injury or a tibial plateau fracture. Follow-up studies of 10 years or longer show survival rates of repaired menisci of 80–90%, in part influenced by the peripheral nature of the tear and the associated hemarthrosis present in ligament tears or fracture repair cases.

D. ARTHROSCOPIC MENISCAL REPAIR

1. Inside-out meniscal repair—Arthroscopic inside-out meniscus repairs are performed using long needles introduced through cannula systems with attached absorbable or nonabsorbable sutures passed perpendicularly across the tear from inside the knee to a protected area outside the joint capsule. These sutures are able to obtain consistent perpendicular placement across the meniscus tear, which gives this method an advantage over other repair techniques. Improved suture placement is gained at the expense of possible neurovascular injury from passing the needle from inside the knee to outside the joint. This technique requires a posteromedial or posterolateral incision to protect the neurovascular structures and safely retrieve the exiting needles. Secondary to its ability to gain vertical mattress suture fixation, this technique remains the gold standard for many surgeons. Numerous retrospective and prospective studies using second-look arthroscopy or arthrography to evaluate healing of the meniscus repairs consistently show rates of 70–90% in isolated repairs and greater than 90% when done in conjunction with an ACL reconstruction. This technique is ideal for posterior and midposterior horn tears. There is difficulty in passing needles in mid- to anterior horn meniscus tears.

2. Outside-in meniscal repair—The arthroscopic outside-in repair was developed in part to decrease the neurovascular risk associated with the inside-out technique. The outside-in technique involves passing a needle from outside the joint, across the tear, and into the joint. Two options then exist for repair of the meniscus tear. One option is to retrieve the suture through an anterior portal, tie a knot outside the knee joint, and then bring the knot back in through the anterior portal placing the knot against the reduced meniscus body fragment. A second option is to use parallel needles and retrieve the suture through the second needle. This can be done using a suture relay. A knot is then tied outside the joint over the capsule. This method is useful for tears in the anterior horn or body of the menisci, but it does not work for tears in or near the posterior horn. Results of the outside-in technique using MRI, arthrography, or second-look arthroscopy to assess healing show complete or partial healing in between 74% and 87% of meniscus repairs that were successful. As expected, more

posterior horn tears and tears in unstable knees did worse.

3. All-inside meniscal repair—The popularity of the all-inside repairs has increased as numerous devices and techniques have been introduced in the last few years. Their popularity is due in part to the fact that they do not require accessory incisions thereby saving operative time, and they avoid more technical arthroscopic techniques required in other types of repairs. However, because of the speed of their introduction, their documented clinical effectiveness compared to more traditional techniques has lagged behind their use.

The initial devices introduced in the early 1990s included biodegradable meniscus arrows, meniscus darts, and simple suture devices such as the T-Fix (Acufex, Mansfield, MA). There was a good initial experience with these devices, particularly the meniscus arrows, which were the first to be introduced. Early studies showed success rates of 80% or higher at 1–2 year follow-ups. However, complications with these first-generation devices began to be reported and included retained fragments, foreign body reactions, inflammation, chronic effusions, and articular cartilage injuries. Additionally, mechanical testing of these first-generation devices showed pull-to-failure strengths closer to those of horizontal, not vertical, sutures.

Updated first-generation and second-generation devices were developed in response to these biomechanical strength concerns and to address the early complication rates. Implant design modifications included a change to smaller or rounded heads on the meniscus arrow and darts, polymer composition changes to decrease their resorption times, and the introduction of suture-based implants that did not require arthroscopic knot tying. Examples included contoured and headless arrow designs and suture based implants such as the FasT-Fix (Smith & Nephew, Endoscopy Div., Andover, MA) and RapidLoc (Mitek, Westwood, MA) devices.

It is difficult to compare studies for these updated first-generation devices or second-generation devices, but in general, studies can be classified into two groups: follow-up clinical studies on human implanted devices, and biomechanical cadaveric or animal studies. Secondary to their earlier introduction into clinical use, long-term follow-up studies are most prevalent for updated first-generation meniscus arrow devices. First reported in 1993, multiple studies show 60–90% clinical success rates using either second-look arthroscopy or clinical exam evaluations. Some were even comparable to traditional open suture techniques. Complications, including inflammatory reactions and articular cartilage damage, remain a concern for sutureless devices that may migrate from their original implanted meniscus tear position.

Biomechanical studies on second-generation devices are also published. A follow-up to the initial T-Fix device, the second-generation FasT-Fix suture device, shows superior results. Its biomechanical performance in load-to-failure, stiffness, and cyclic displacement tests has been equivalent to the gold standard of vertical mattress sutures. Other devices including other suture devices and the various meniscus arrows or screws have equivalent biomechanical performance to that of horizontal mattress sutures. It is generally believed that the superiority of vertical mattress over horizontal mattress sutures is derived from the ability of vertical mattress sutures to capture the strong circumferential fibers of the meniscus. Additionally, suture devices in general have a lower risk of loose body reactions because their fixation device is extracapsular. However, there is a learning curve associated with placement of suture devices that may cause their fixation strength to be suboptimal until the technique is mastered.

Caution should be exercised in interpreting biomechanical studies of meniscus repair devices. Virtually all larger studies involve porcine, bovine, or canine models secondary to increased cost and availability issues in obtaining human cadaveric menisci. Studies involving human menisci should also be evaluated for the source of their menisci because as older samples taken from arthritic total joint patients may not accurately reflect in vivo conditions. It is also not known if in vitro load to failure or cyclic loading testing is applicable to the in vivo stress environment.

In general, however, multidevice studies show that (1) vertical mattress sutures are superior to horizontal, (2) arrows and other nonsuture devices have 40–70% of the pull-to-failure strength and cyclic load displacement of vertical mattress sutures, and (3) sutures devices like the FasT-Fix have biomechanical profiles similar to vertical mattress sutures. What remains to be known, however, is the minimal strength that meniscus repair devices need to provide for meniscus healing to occur in vivo.

Repairable meniscus tears often occur with an ACL tear. Stabilizing the knee with ACL reconstruction protects the repaired meniscus from abnormal knee motion, which has a higher rate of success than if the knee is left unstable.

E. Meniscal Transplantation

An alternative to leaving the patient with a meniscus-deficient knee, and almost certain early osteoarthrosis, is meniscus transplantation. This technique yields satisfactory results in approximately two thirds of patients after a short-term follow-up. In the future, biologic scaffolds may enable menisci to be regenerated after meniscectomy.

Ahn JH, Wang JH, Yoo JC: Arthroscopic all-inside suture repair of medial meniscus lesion in anterior cruciate ligament—deficient knees: results of second-look arthroscopies in 39 cases. Arthroscopy 2004;20:936. [PMID: 15525926]

Englund M et al: Patient-relevant outcomes fourteen years after meniscectomy: Influence of the type of meniscus tear and size of resection. Rheumatology (Oxford) 2001,40:631. [PMID: 11426019]

McNicholas MJ et al: Total meniscectomy in adolescence: A thirty-year follow-up. J Bone Joint Surg 2000,82B:217. [PMID: 10755429]

Metcalf MH, Barrett GR: Prospective evaluation of 1485 meniscal tear patterns in patients with stable knees. Am J Sports Med 2004;32:675. [PMID: 15090384]

Rijk PC. Meniscal allograft transplantation—part I: Background, results, graft selection and preservation, and surgical considerations. Arthroscopy 2004;20:728. [PMID: 15483548]

Shelbourne KD, Dersam MD: Comparison of partial meniscectomy versus meniscus repair for bucket-handle lateral meniscus tears in anterior cruciate ligament reconstructed knees. Arthroscopy 2004;20:581. [PMID: 15241307]

Steenbrugge F, Verstraete K, Verdonk R. Magnetic resonance imaging of the surgically repaired meniscus: A 13-year follow-up study of 13 knees. Acta Orthop Scand 2004;75:323. [PMID: 15260425]

KNEE FRACTURE

Articular cartilage injuries of the knee are infrequent, and the examiner must have a high index of suspicion to detect them. Arthroscopy is very helpful with these injuries, especially pure articular cartilage injuries, where radiographs will be normal.

1. Osteochondral Lesions

Osteochondral Fracture

There is much confusion about the nomenclature and etiology of juvenile and adult osteochondral lesions (OCLs) of the knee. Initially, an inflammatory etiology for the condition was suggested. Further inquiry attributed the condition to an ossification abnormality. Still others thought that avascular necrosis might be responsible for the lesions. However, work in basic science, histopathology, and vascular studies did not support any of these etiologies as the cause of OCLs. The term *osteochondral injuries* was used to describe injuries ranging from acute osteochondral fractures to pure chondral injuries. Currently, OCLs are defined as potentially reversible idiopathic lesions of subchondral bone resulting in possible delamination or fragmentation with or without destruction of the overlying articular cartilage. OCLs are subdivided into juvenile and adult forms depending on the presence of an open distal femoral physes. In children, a combination of etiologies is now thought to be responsible for OCL lesions. For example, a stress fracture may develop in the subchondral bone of the distal femoral condyle. Such an injury may provoke further vascular compromise, which results in injury to the subchondral bone that was initially covered with normal articular cartilage. Loss of support from the subchondral bone may result in damage to the overlying articular cartilage. The vast majority of adult OCLs lesions are thought to have arisen from a persistent juvenile OCL lesion, although new lesions in adults are possible as well.

Both adult and juvenile lesions that do not heal have the potential for further sequelae including degenerative osteoarthritis. Juvenile lesions, defined as knees with an open physes, generally have a better prognosis than adult lesions. The classic location of an OCL is the posterolateral aspect of the medial femoral condyle, which accounts for 70–80% of all OCLs. Lateral condyle lesions are seen in 15–20% of patients, and patellar involvement ranges from 5% to 10%. The increased use of MRI and arthroscopy over the past decade may have resulted in greater recognition of OCL lesions.

Clinical Findings

A common presentation of a patient with an OCL is aching and activity-related anterior knee pain that is poorly localized. Pain may worsen with stair climbing or running. Patients with early or stable lesions usually do not complain of mechanical symptoms or knee instability. Mechanical symptoms are more common in patients with unstable or loose OCLs. Parents may note a limp in their child, and patients may complain of knee swelling with possible crepitus.

An antalgic gait may be observed as the patient. An effusion may be variably present, but generally crepitus or pain with range of motion is absent in patients with stable lesions. Tenderness with palpation of the femoral condyle may be observed with various degrees of knee flexion. Loss of range of motion or quadriceps atrophy may be noted in more long-standing cases.

Patients with unstable lesions may have crepitus and pain with range of motion, and an effusion is typically present in these patients. Involvement is bilateral in up to 25% of cases, so both knees should be evaluated regardless of symptoms. Initial evaluation should include anteroposterior, lateral, and tunnel views of both knees. The goal of plain radiographs is to exclude any bony pathology, evaluate the physes, and localize the lesion. Lesion location and an estimation of size can be determined as described by Cahill. MRI is frequently obtained once the diagnosis is confirmed on plain radiographs. MRI can give an estimation of the size of the lesion, the condition of the overlying cartilage and underlying subchondral bone, the extent of bony edema, the presence of a high signal zone beneath the fragment, and the presence of any loose bodies. There are four MRI criteria on T_2-weighted images: a line of high signal intensity at least 5 mm in length between the OCL and underlying bone, an area of increased homogeneous signal at least 5 mm in diameter beneath the lesion, a focal defect of 5 mm or more in the articular surface, and a high signal line traversing the subchondral plate into the lesion. A high signal line is the most common sign in patients found to have unstable lesions that are most likely to fail nonoperative treatment. Patient maturity and lesion size are also important predictors of failure of nonoperative treatment.

Equivocal prognostic value was found in the use of intravenous gadolinium in OCLs. Technetium bone scans were initially proposed to monitor the presence of healing. However, with MRI, that eliminates ionizing radiation and increased time required in bone scanning, it is not widely used.

Treatment & Prognosis

There is general agreement that initial nonoperative management should be pursued in the case of a child with open physes who presents with a stable OCL. The goal of nonoperative treatment is to obtain a healed lesion before physis closure so as to prevent early-onset osteoarthritis. Even if patients are within 6–12 months of physeal closure, a trial of nonoperative treatment is warranted.

As failure of the subchondral bone precedes failure of the overlying articular cartilage, most orthopedists recommend some sort of activity modification. Debate exists whether activity modification should include the use of cast or brace immobilization. The tenet of nonoperative treatment is to reduce the activity level where pain-free activities of daily living are possible. However, there is no optimal immobilization protocol available in the literature.

A general consensus is that patients should at least be non– or partial weight bearing with crutches for 3–6 weeks or until they are pain free. Repeat radiographs are obtained at approximately 6-week intervals. Physical therapy with full weight bearing may be initiated once patients are pain free. Physical therapy should focus on low-impact quadriceps and hamstring strengthening. If patients remain asymptomatic during this phase up to at least 3 months postdiagnosis, activity may be slowly advanced to higher impact activities such as running or jumping. Any recurrence of symptoms or pain or any progression of the OCL on plain radiographs should prompt repeat non–weight bearing and possible immobilization for a longer period. Obvious patient frustration and lack of compliance, especially in adolescents, is common, and a full discussion on the risks and benefits of nonoperative or operative treatment is required.

Operative treatment should be considered in the following instances: (1) detachment or instability of the fragment while the patient is under treatment, (2) persistence of symptoms despite nonoperative treatment in a compliant patient, (3) persistently elevated or worsening radiographic appearance (plain radiographs or MRI), (4) approaching or complete epiphyseal closure. Goals of operative treatment should include achievement of a stable osteochondral fragment that maintains joint congruity and allows early range of motion.

For stable lesions with an intact articular surface, arthroscopic drilling of the lesions is preferred. This creates channels for potential revascularization through the subchondral bone plate. Options include transarticular drilling versus transepiphyseal drilling. Multiple studies show radiographic healing and relief of symptoms in 80–90% of patients with open physes. This decreases to 50–75% in patients with closed physes.

Patients with flap lesions or partially unstable lesions should be managed depending on the status of the subchondral bone. Fibrous tissue between the lesion and subchondral bone should be debrided. If significant subchondral bone loss occurs, packing of autogenous bone graft in the crater prior to fragment reduction and fixation is advised. If significant subchondral bone remains attached to the fragment such that an anatomic fit into its donor site is possible, fixation should be attempted. Various fixation methods are described, including Herbert or cannulated screws and bioabsorbable screws or pins. Complication, however, is associated with these treatments.

Simple excision of the larger fragments shows poor results with more rapid progression of radiographic osteoarthritic changes. For lesions greater than 2 cm^2, drilling or microfracture methods that depend on replacement of the defect with fibrocartilage also show inferior results. These results tend to deteriorate with time with worsening radiographic changes. For these larger lesions, transplantation of autologous osteochondral plugs or autologous chondrocyte implantation was tried. Disadvantages of autologous osteochondral plugs or mosaicplasty include donor site morbidity and incongruent articular fit. Advantages include biologic fixation of autogenous material. Longer term results are now being published in patients less than 40 years old showing successful clinical results in up to 90% of patients. However, additional larger and longer term follow-up studies are needed.

Cepero S, Ullot R, Sastre S: Osteochondritis of the femoral condyles in children and adolescents: Our experience over the last 28 years. J Pediatr Orthop B 2005;14:24. [PMID: 15577303]

KNEE LIGAMENT INJURY

Knee injuries occur during both contact and noncontact athletic activities. Advances in the diagnosis and treatment of ligament injuries now allow athletes at all levels of ability to return to sports at their preinjury level of activity. The ligaments and menisci of the knee work in concert with one another, and frequently more than one structure is damaged when an acute injury occurs.

Ligament injuries are graded as follows: grade 1, stretching of the ligament with no detectable instability; grade 2, further stretching of the ligament with detectable instability, but with the fibers in continuity; and grade 3, complete disruption of the ligament.

Anatomy

Knee stability requires proper functioning of four ligaments. These ligaments include the ACL, the PCL, the medial collateral ligament (MCL), and the lateral collateral ligament (LCL). There are also several accessory or secondary stabilizers of the knee. Secondary stabilizers of the knee include the menisci, iliotibial band, and biceps femoris. These secondary stabilizers become more important when a primary stabilizer is injured.

The MCL is the primary static stabilizer against valgus stress at the knee. The MCL originates from the central sulcus of the medial epicondyle. The sulcus of the C-shaped medial epicondyle is located anterior and distal to the adductor tubercle. The MCL is made up of three main static medial stabilizers of the knee. This includes the superficial MCL, the posterior oblique ligament, and the deep capsular ligament.

The LCL is the primary static stabilizer against varus stress at the knee. The LCL originates from the lateral epicondyle. This is the most prominent point of the lateral femoral condyle. The LCL insertion is on the styloid process of the fibular head, which projects superiorly from the posterolateral fibular head. The LCL joins with the arcuate ligament, the popliteus muscle, and the lateral head of the gastrocnemius to form a lateral arcuate complex to control statically and dynamically varus angulation and external tibial torsion. The iliotibial band and biceps femoris also contribute to stability on the lateral aspect of the knee.

The ACL is the primary static stabilizer of the knee against anterior translation of the tibia with respect to the femur. The ACL originates from the posteromedial surface of the lateral femoral condyle in the intercondylar notch. The ACL inserts on the tibial plateau just medial to the anterior horn of the lateral meniscus, approximately 15 mm posterior to the anterior edge of the tibial articular surface. The blood supply to the ACL and PCL is the middle geniculate artery. Both the ACL and PCL are covered by a layer of synovium, making these ligaments intra-articular and extrasynovial.

The PCL is the primary static stabilizer of the knee against posterior translation of the tibia with respect to the femur. The PCL originates from the posterior aspect of the lateral surface of the medial femoral condyle in the intercondylar notch. The PCL inserts on the posterior aspect of the tibial plateau in a central depression just posterior to the articular surface. The insertion extends distally along the posterior aspect of the tibia for up to 1 cm in length. The PCL is a complex structure consisting of two major bands: the anterolateral and posteromedial bands. The anterolateral band is tight in flexion and loose in extension. The posteromedial band is loose in flexion and tight in extension. The cross-sectional area of the anterolateral band is twice as large as the posteromedial band. The meniscofemoral ligaments, the ligaments of Wrisberg and Humphrey, are the third component of the PCL. The meniscofemoral ligaments travel from the posterior horn of the lateral meniscus to the posteromedial femoral condyle.

Differential Diagnosis of Knee Instability

The differential diagnosis of acute or chronic knee instability can involve any of the knee ligaments and/or the structures of the posterolateral corner. There are often combinations of ligament injuries in addition to injuries of secondary stabilizing structures such as the menisci. The history and mechanism of injury are valuable information, if available. Similarly, the location of pain can help narrow the diagnosis. Clearly, however, a thorough physical examination helps distinguish which ligaments are injured. Additionally, imaging studies are often obtained to confirm clinical suspicions and to evaluate for occult injuries.

Brown JR, Trojian TH: Anterior and posterior cruciate ligament injuries. Prim Care 2004;31:925. [PMID: 15544828]

1. Medial Collateral Ligament Injuries

Clinical Findings

An MCL tear typically presents with medial knee pain after either a noncontact rotational injury or a direct valgus blow to the lateral knee. Instability may or may not be present, depending on the severity of the injury.

Symptoms (History)

How and when the patient was hurt are important parts of the history. Lower grade MCL injuries typically occur in a noncontact external rotational injury, whereas higher grade injuries generally involve lateral contact to the thigh or upper leg. Other important pieces of historical information include the location and presence of pain, instability, timing of swelling, and sensation of a pop or tear. Surprisingly, grade I and II injuries are often more painful than complete MCL rupture. Immediate swelling should make one suspicious of an associated cruciate ligament injury, fracture, and/or patellar dislocation. A prior history of knee injuries or instability should always be sought when evaluating a new knee injury.

Signs (Physical Examination)

MCL injuries are evaluated with a complete knee examination to evaluate for any other coexisting injuries.

This is especially true with ACL and PCL evaluation because an injury to either of these ligaments would significantly change the treatment. Given the frequency of coexisting patellar dislocations in MCL injuries, palpation of the patella and the medial parapatellar stabilizing ligaments should be performed in addition to patellar apprehension testing.

Medial joint line tenderness along the course of the MCL is typical at the location of the tear. Laxity to valgus stresses is assessed by the amount of medial joint space opening that occurs at 30 degrees of flexion. It is important to stress the knee at 30 degrees of flexion because with the knee in full extension, the posterior capsule and PCL stabilizes the knee to valgus stress. This stability to valgus stress in full extension could mislead the examiner to believe that the MCL is intact. Zero opening is considered normal, with 1–4 mm indicating a grade I injury; 5–9 mm indicating a grade II injury; and 10–15 mm indicating a complete or grade III injury. Additionally, grade I and II injuries typically have a firm endpoint, whereas a grade III injury tends to have a soft endpoint to valgus stress.

Imaging Studies

A. RADIOGRAPHS

A series of knee radiographs should be obtained in any patient with a suspected significant knee injury. Radiographs should be inspected for acute fracture, lateral capsular avulsion (the Segond fracture; see ACL imaging), loose bodies, Pellegrini-Stieda lesion (MCL calcification), and evidence of patellar dislocation. Stress radiographs should be obtained in patients prior to skeletal maturity to rule out an epiphyseal fracture.

B. MAGNETIC RESONANCE IMAGING

MRI is useful for confirming MCL injury and identifying the site of injury as well as the presence of meniscal and other injuries to the knee. Relative indications for an MRI include an uncertain ACL status despite multiple examinations, evaluation of a suspected meniscal tear, or preoperative evaluation for a planned MCL reconstruction or repair.

C. SPECIAL TESTS

An examination under anesthesia can be valuable when physical examination is unreliable because of the patient guarding the knee. Diagnostic arthroscopy can also be used to evaluate for coexistent pathology. MRI has largely replaced both of these diagnostic methods, however.

Treatment: Nonsurgical & Surgical

Treatment of an isolated MCL injury is generally nonoperative with protection against valgus stress and early motion. Grade I and grade II injuries can be placed in either a cast or a brace and bear weight as tolerated. Generally, knee motion is started within the first week or two, and full recovery is usually achieved more rapidly with early knee range of motion.

Grade III injuries are a bit more controversial. Several authors show increased instability in grade III tears treated nonsurgically, although most of these did not exclude knees with multiligamentous injuries. Comparison of isolated grade III MCL tears treated with surgical reconstruction versus nonsurgical management showed that the nonsurgical treatment group enjoyed better results in both subjective scoring and earlier return to activity.

The exception to the current trend of nonsurgical treatment of grade III injuries is in the setting of a multiligamentous knee injury. In this setting, particularly with a distal tibial avulsion of the MCL, nonsurgical treatment has not fared nearly as well as in isolated MCL injuries. MCL repair in the acute setting can include a primary repair, with shortening if needed, of the torn ligament. Similarly, avulsion fragments are treated with reduction and fixation in the acute setting. Primary repairs can be reinforced with autograft or allograft tissues if the remaining MCL is insufficient for a stand alone repair. Chronic reconstructions also often include autograft or allograft tissue reconstruction.

Traditionally, casting or operative treatment of MCL injuries significantly limited an early return to range-of-motion exercises. With the addition of functional bracing and early motion to a nonsurgical treatment protocol, motion and strengthening of the knee can occur at an early stage while the ligament is protected from valgus stress. As knee motion improves, isotonic strengthening exercises are introduced. As the strength of the extremity improves, the intensity of functional rehabilitation increases accordingly.

Complications

With nonsurgical treatment becoming the standard of care, complications associated with a MCL injury are decreasing. The main complication of nonsurgical therapy is residual valgus laxity or medial knee pain. Radiographs may show residual calcification of the MCL (Pellegrini-Stieda lesion). Potential surgical complications include arthrofibrosis, infection, damage to the saphenous nerve or vein, or recurrent valgus laxity.

Results/Return to Play

In general, good outcomes can be achieved with nonsurgical treatment and rehabilitation of isolated MCL injuries. Return to professional football after nonsurgical treatment of isolated MCL injuries is 98%.

Robinson JR et al: The posteromedial corner revisited. An anatomical description of the passive restraining structures of the medial aspect of the human knee. J Bone Joint Surg Br 2004; 86:674. [PMID: 15274262]

Woo SL, Vogrin TM, Abramowitch SD: Healing and repair of ligament injuries in the knee. J Am Acad Orthop Surg 2000; 8:364. [PMID: 11104400]

2. Lateral Collateral Ligament Injuries

Symptoms (History)

The most consistent symptom of an acute LCL injury is lateral knee pain. However, the symptoms of lateral and posterolateral instability are quite variable and depend on the severity of injury, patient activity level, overall limb alignment, and other associated knee injuries. For example, a sedentary individual with minimal laxity and overall valgus alignment typically has few if any symptoms. However, if LCL laxity is combined with overall varus alignment, hyperextension, and an increased activity level, symptoms are quite pronounced. These patients may complain of lateral joint line pain and a varus thrust of their leg with everyday activities. This is often described as the knee buckling into hyperextension with normal gait.

Signs (Physical Examination)

Patients with a LCL and/or posterolateral corner injury often also have additional ligamentous injuries to the knee. Therefore, a thorough knee examination should be performed to evaluate for coexistent knee pathology. Additionally, a careful neurovascular examination should be performed because the incidence of neurovascular injury, particularly peroneal nerve injury, is reported in 12–29% of posterolateral knee injuries.

The integrity of the LCL is assessed with a varus stress with the knee in full extension and 30 degrees of flexion. Baseline varus opening is widely variable and should be compared to the contralateral leg. The average baseline for varus opening is 7 degrees. Exam findings with an isolated LCL injury should include varus laxity at 30 degrees of flexion and no instability in full extension. This is because of the stabilizing effect that the intact cruciate ligaments provide in full extension.

Note that a significant posterolateral knee injury can be present without significant varus laxity. The most useful test to evaluate for posterolateral instability is the dial test, which is done by externally rotating each tibia and noting the angle subtended between the thigh and the foot. The dial test is performed at 30 degrees and 90 degrees of flexion with a significant difference being an angle 5 degrees or greater than the contralateral leg.

Imaging Studies

A. RADIOGRAPHS

A series of knee radiographs should be obtained in any patient with a suspected significant knee injury. Radiographs should be inspected for acute fractures, lateral capsular avulsion (Segond fracture; see ACL imaging), loose bodies, fibular head avulsions, and evidence of patellar dislocation. With chronic posterolateral instability, degenerative changes of the lateral compartment are often noted. Lateral joint space narrowing with osteophytes and subchondral sclerosis can be seen. Stress radiographs can help better quantify the amount of varus angulation present.

B. MAGNETIC RESONANCE IMAGING

MRI is often a useful adjunct for diagnosing posterolateral corner and LCL injuries in the severely injured knee. As mentioned earlier, this posterolateral injury can often go unnoticed during an initial evaluation, and MRI findings can refocus the examination to the posterolateral structures. Pain and guarding at the time of injury can often obscure posterolateral injury, and MRI can prove to be an extremely valuable adjunct in diagnosis.

C. SPECIAL TESTS/EXAMINATIONS

1. Reverse pivot shift test—This test involves starting with the knee flexed to 90 degrees. While the knee is extended, the leg is loaded axially with a valgus stress applied to the knee and the foot held in external rotation. A palpable shift is noted as the tibia reduces from its posteriorly subluxed position as the knee is extended.

2. External rotation recurvatum test—This test is performed with the patient supine and the hip and knee fully extended. The leg is lifted off the bed by the toes. Hyperextension, varus instability, and external rotation of the tibial tubercle occurs with adequate quadriceps relaxation in a patient with posterolateral instability.

3. Posterolateral drawer test—A standard posterior drawer test (see PCL physical examination) is performed with the tibia in internal rotation, neutral, and externally rotated positions. With posterolateral injury, the magnitude of the posterior drawer displacement is greatest with external tibial rotation.

4. Examination under anesthesia—An examination while the patient is relaxed under general anesthetic is extremely useful, particularly in the acute setting. If the patient with a multiligamentous knee injury is taken to the operating room, this is an excellent opportunity to examine the knee without guarding to improve the accuracy of the examination.

Treatment

A. NONSURGICAL

Isolated LCL ligament injuries, as noted earlier, are rare injuries. However, in the case of an isolated LCL ligament injury with grade II or less magnitude, a period of immobilization from 2 to 4 weeks followed by a quadriceps strengthening program usually yields good results. Grade III injuries often have better results with surgical treatment. The combination of delayed diagnosis along with an uncertain natural history of posterolateral instability make the treatment of these injuries a challenge.

B. SURGICAL

LCL and posterolateral ligaments, as already discussed, rarely occur in isolation. Therefore, other injuries must also be considered in the treatment plan of the multiligament knee injury. Ideally, the posterolateral and LCL injury is diagnosed in the acute setting. This allows the preferred surgical treatment of a primary repair of the injured structures with augmentation as needed. Primary repair is generally only feasible in the first few weeks following the knee injury.

The knee with chronic posterolateral instability often requires ligamentous reconstruction or advancement to reconstitute a static restraint to varus stresses. The key biomechanical concept of any lateral ligamentous reconstruction is that the isometric point of the LCL lies between the fibular head and the lateral epicondyle. Therefore, regardless of the graft material used to reconstruct the lateral ligamentous complex, a portion of the graft must pass between the lateral femoral epicondyle and the fibular head.

To improve the success rate of reconstruction of chronic lateral ligamentous instability, a proximal tibial valgus osteotomy may be performed to decrease the stress on the lateral structures of the knee.

Rehabilitation

The rehabilitation of the knee after posterolateral reconstructions or repairs is largely guided by associated injuries to the ACL or PCL. It is generally necessary, however, to limit weight bearing for at least 6 weeks and protect the lateral structures with a brace for at least 3 months.

Complications

The peroneal nerve runs just posterior to the fibular head. It is important to isolate the peroneal nerve prior to any lateral knee exposure to minimize the complication of a peroneal nerve injury.

Results

If injuries to the posterolateral corner of the knee are diagnosed and repaired acutely, the results are good for restoration of varus stability and return to play. Chronic posterolateral corner injury reconstructions also perform well when an isometric lateral reconstruction is achieved.

Jakob RP, Warner JP: Lateral and posterolateral instability of the knee. In *Orthopaedic Sports Medicine: Principles and Practice.* Eds. DeLee J, Drez D, Stanitski CL. Philadelphia: WB Saunders, 1994. [NLMID: 9411843]

Ross G et al: Evaluation and treatment of acute posterolateral corner/anterior cruciate ligament injuries of the knee. J Bone Joint Surg Am 2004;86 (Suppl 2):2. [PMID: 15691102]

Shahane SA, Ibbotson C, Strachan R et al: The popliteofibular ligament. An anatomical study of the posterolateral corner of the knee. J Bone Joint Surg Br 1999;81:636. [PMID: 10463736]

3. Anterior Cruciate Ligament Injuries

Symptoms (History)

The mechanism of injury should be elicited in any knee injury evaluation. This can guide the examination to additional structures that may also be injured. ACL injury can occur in a variety of ways; a few mechanisms predominate, however. The most common noncontact ACL injury mechanism involves a deceleration and rotational injury during running, cutting, or jumping activities. The most common contact injury involves either hyperextension and/or valgus forces to the knee by a direct blow.

ACL injury is often associated with a pop heard by the patient at the time of injury. This piece of history is not ACL specific, however. Upon return to competition, the patient often notices instability of the knee or describes the knee "giving out" with twisting activities. Substantial knee swelling secondary to a hemarthrosis typically occurs within the first 4 to 12 hours following the injury.

Signs (Physical Examination)

With the history obtained and a proper physical examination, an ACL tear should be able to be diagnosed without any additional tests. A complete examination of the knee should be performed to evaluate for any other associated injuries. The uninjured knee is examined first to familiarize the patient with the knee examination.

The Lachman test is the most useful test for anterior laxity of the knee. It is performed with the knee in 20–30 degrees of flexion as an anterior force is applied to the tibia while the other hand stabilizes the distal femur. The degree of anterior translation, as well as the presence and character of an endpoint, is assessed. The laxity is graded based on comparison to the uninjured contralateral knee. Grade 1 laxity is 1–5 mm of increased translation. Grade 2 laxity is 6–10 mm of

increased translation. Grade 3 laxity is more than 10 mm of translation as compared to the injured contralateral knee.

The anterior drawer test is another test to evaluate anterior tibial translation. This is performed with the knee in 90 degrees of flexion as an anterior force is applied to the tibia. This test is less sensitive than the Lachman test.

In the acute setting of an ACL tear, there is often a window where an accurate examination can occur before extensive knee swelling and guarding inhibit examination. Aspiration of a hemarthrosis can help decrease pain and improve the quality of the examination in the acute setting as well.

The pivot shift test is performed to test the rotational instability associated with an ACL tear. The test is based on the lateral tibial plateau subluxing anteriorly with extension and reduction of the lateral compartment with flexion. The most effective method of achieving this result is by flexing the knee with an axial load from full extension with valgus stress at the knee and internal rotation of the tibia. The reduction of the subluxation should occur at approximately 30 degrees of flexion. MCL injury and some meniscal tears may produce a false-negative test.

The pivot shift test is considered the most functional test to evaluate knee stability after ACL injury. An examination under anesthesia is also often useful in obtaining a more accurate pivot shift test. This can be useful in a patient with an unclear history of instability and an equivocal examination in the office.

Imaging Studies

Plain radiographs of the knee should be obtained to rule out fractures about the knee. The Segond fracture, as discussed earlier, is an avulsion of the anterolateral capsule of the tibia. Before skeletal maturity, an avulsion of the tibial insertion of the ACL can also be seen radiographically. Following radiographs, an MRI is the most useful examination for an evaluation of associated injuries. Although generally not needed for diagnosis of an ACL tear, MRI can diagnose an ACL tear with 95% or better accuracy. Bone bruises of the lateral femoral condyle and lateral tibial plateau are noted in up to 80% of ACL injuries.

Special Studies

Instrumented laxity evaluations can augment the physical examination and provide an objective baseline for future comparison. The most commonly used arthrometer, the KT-1000 (MEDmetric, San Diego, CA), uses a series of standard forces to measure anterior translation of the tibia with the knee in 20–30 degrees of flexion, similar to the Lachman test.

Treatment

A. NONSURGICAL

Rehabilitation following an isolated ACL injury should include an effort to regain knee motion and strengthen the muscles about the knee. Returning to activities that produce episodes of instability is discouraged. Once motion and strength are restored, a gradual return to activities can be attempted to determine the functional level that can be attained without instability.

Nonoperative management with rehabilitation after an ACL injury generally yields poor results in patients who return to competitive activities. Significant episodes of instability resulting in pain, swelling, and disability occur in approximately 80% of individuals that participate in sporting activities such as tennis, football and soccer. These episodes of instability are thought to place the menisci and articular cartilage of the knee at risk for further injury (Figure 4–15).

B. SURGICAL

The decision to reconstruct an ACL tear surgically is individualized and based on the patient's desire to return to competition, age, accompanying degenerative changes, and objective and subjective knee instability. For example, an active patient less than 40 years old with continued desire to compete in cutting and jumping sports with both objective and subjective knee instability may be best treated with surgical reconstruction. But an older patient with some degenerative arthritis of the knee and minimal desire for continued competitive athletics and no subjective instability would be much more suited to nonsurgical care.

Early in the history of ACL surgery, primary repairs of the ligament were found to do poorly. This gave way to ligament reconstruction using a variety of graft materials. Everything from synthetics to autograft and allograft tissues were used for reconstruction of the ACL. Over time, autograft bone-patellar tendon-bone, semi-tendinosus/gracilis hamstring autograft, and allograft bone-patellar tendon-bone constructs have proven to be the most commonly used grafts and are successful for ACL reconstructions.

The goal of ACL reconstruction is to reproduce the strength, location, and function of the intact ACL. Therefore, once a graft of adequate strength is selected,

Figure 4–15. Flow chart that summarizes the current management of acute anterior cruciate ligament injuries. (Reproduced, with permission, from Marzo JM, Warren RF: Results of nonoperative treatment of anterior cruciate ligament injury: Changing perspectives. Adv Orthop Surg 1991;15:59.)

the location of the graft is of utmost importance. The graft is generally passed through a bone tunnel in the tibia and a bone tunnel through the femur. The intraarticular placement of the tibial tunnel is generally in the center of the native ACL stump just in front of the PCL origin and just medial to the center of the notch in the coronal plane (Figures 4–16 and 4–17).

Once the graft is in place, the proper tension and fixation of the graft must occur to achieve a successful ACL reconstruction. Establishing proper tension in the graft is important. A lax ACL graft may not restore stability to the knee, and an overtightened graft may cause failure of the graft or limit knee range of motion. Fixation of the graft is achieved through a variety of measures. The most common method involves placing an interference screw up the bone tunnel that captures the graft in the tunnel. The graft can also be fixed via sutures tied over various devices located on the outer cortex of the tunnels.

Complications

Although ACL reconstruction often results in a successful outcome, several complications can occur. One of the most common is a loss of knee motion, which is minimized by obtaining and maintaining full knee extension immediately following surgery. Knee flexion exercises are

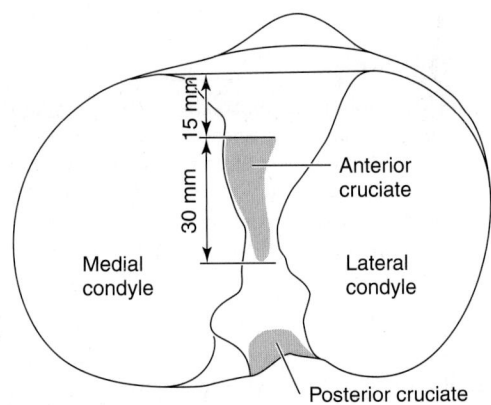

Figure 4–17. The upper surface of the tibial plateau to show average measurements and relations of the tibial attachments of the anterior cruciate ligament. (Reproduced, with permission, from Girgis FC et al: The cruciate ligaments of the knee joint: Anatomical, functional, and experimental analysis. Clin Orthop 1975;106:216.)

begun as soon as possible postoperatively with a goal of 90 degrees by 1 week after surgery. Additionally, patellar mobilization is performed in an attempt to minimize patellofemoral scarring. Another common complication of ACL reconstruction is anterior knee pain. The exact etiology of this pain is unclear; however, it is thought that patellar tendon autograft harvest may increase the incidence of patellofemoral pain. Less common complications (less than 1%) include patellar fracture, patellar tendon rupture, and quadriceps tendon rupture, depending on the graft harvest site.

Results/Return to Play

The goal of any rehabilitation protocol for an ACL reconstruction is to return the patient to the full desired level of activity in a short amount of time as possible while avoiding any complications or setbacks. Through improved surgical techniques and accelerated rehabilitation protocols, most studies show a 90% or better return to play and patient satisfaction. Patients generally are able to return between 4 and 6 months postoperatively, with some professional athletes returning successfully to competition in 3 months. Specific criteria for a return to sports vary from institution to institution with a combination of functional testing, subjective reporting, and clinical examination contributing to the decision. In general, the criteria for return to sports includes full range of motion, KT1000 testing within 2–3 mm of the uninjured knee, 85% or more of quadriceps strength and full hamstring strength, and functional testing within 85% of the contralateral leg.

Figure 4–16. Drawing of the medial surface of the right lateral femoral condyle showing the average measurements and body relations of the femoral attachment of the anterior cruciate ligament. (Reproduced, with permission, from Arnoczky SP: Anatomy of the anterior cruciate ligament. Clin Orthop 1983;172:19.)

Herrington L et al: Anterior cruciate ligament reconstruction, hamstring versus bone-patella tendon-bone grafts: A systematic literature review of outcome from surgery. Knee 2005;12:41. [PMID: 15664877]

Hewett TE, Myer GD, Ford KR: Reducing knee and anterior cruciate ligament injuries among female athletes: A systematic review of neuromuscular training interventions. J Knee Surg 2005;18:82. [PMID: 15742602]

Laxdal G et al: A prospective randomized comparison of bone-patellar tendon-bone and hamstring grafts for anterior cruciate ligament reconstruction. Arthroscopy 2005;21:34. [PMID: 15650664]

Marx RG et al: Beliefs and attitudes of members of the American Academy of Orthopaedic Surgeons regarding the treatment of anterior cruciate ligament injury. Arthroscopy 2003;19:762. [PMID: 12966385]

Seitz H et al: Anterior instability of the knee despite an intensive rehabilitation program. Clin Orthop 1996;328:159. [PMID: 8653950]

4. Posterior Cruciate Ligament Injuries

Symptoms (History)

When evaluating a patient for a PCL injury, it is important to obtain the mechanism of injury, the severity of the injury, and any potential associated injuries. In contrast to an ACL tear, it is rare for patients with PCL injuries to report hearing a pop or report any feelings of subjective instability. More commonly, patients complain of knee pain, swelling, and stiffness.

The presentation of a patient with a subacute or chronically injured PCL can range from asymptomatic to significant instability and pain. Patients with significant varus alignment or injury to the lateral structures of the knee often complain of feelings of instability and giving way. There are a few characteristic mechanisms of PCL injury that differ significantly from the mechanism of ACL injuries. One of the most common mechanisms of PCL injury is the so-called dashboard, injury during which the anterior tibia sustains a posteriorly directed force from the dashboard with the knee in 90 degrees of flexion. Sports injuries to the PCL result from an outside force or blow, in contrast to the typical deceleration twisting mechanism of an ACL injury. The most common methods of a sports PCL injury include a direct blow to the anterior tibia or via a fall onto the flexed knee with the foot in plantar flexion. The most common mechanism for isolated PCL injury in the athlete is a partial tear associated with hyperflexion of the knee. Additionally, significant knee multiligamentous injuries with PCL tears can be seen after a varus or valgus stress is applied to the hyperextended knee.

Signs (Physical Examination)

As with other ligamentous injuries, a thorough knee examination is necessary. Specific cues to injury to the PCL on initial inspection include abrasions or ecchymosis around the proximal anterior tibia and ecchymosis in the popliteal fossa. Assessment for meniscal damage and associated ligamentous injury should be performed. Evaluation of ACL laxity in the presence of an acute PCL injury is challenging because of the lack of a stable reference point to perform a Lachman or anterior drawer test.

Examination of the PCL in the acutely injured knee can be challenging. Despite increased awareness of the injury, many PCL injuries go undiagnosed in the acute setting. The most accurate clinical test of PCL integrity is the posterior drawer test. The knee is flexed to 90 degrees with the patient supine, and a posteriorly directed force is applied to the anterior tibia. The amount of posterior translation and the presence and character of the endpoint is noted. The extent of translation is assessed by noting the change in the distance of the step-off between the anteromedial tibial plateau and the medial femoral condyle. The tibial plateau is approximately 1 cm anterior to the medial femoral condyle on average. However, the contralateral knee must be examined to establish a baseline.

Another test for examination of the PCL is the posterior sag or Godfrey test. This test involves flexing the knee and hip and noting the posterior pull of gravity creating posterior "sag" of the tibia on the femur. An adjunct to this test involves watching for a reduction of this subluxation with active quadriceps contraction.

The reverse pivot shift is the analogue to the pivot shift in the evaluation of an ACL injury. This is performed by placing a valgus stress on the knee with the foot externally rotated. The knee is then extended from 90 degrees of flexion and a palpable reduction of the posterolateral tibial plateau is noted between 20 and 30 degrees of flexion.

It is extremely important to evaluate the posterolateral structures of the knee in the setting of a suspected PCL injury. Injury to the posterolateral structures is reported to occur in up to 60% of PCL injuries.

Imaging Studies

A. RADIOGRAPHS

Given the magnitude of the forces required to injure the PCL, plain radiographs of the knee are essential to evaluate for bony injuries, dislocation, or evidence of other associated injuries. Subtle posterior subluxation on the lateral radiograph may also indicate PCL injury. Stress posterior drawer radiographs and contralateral comparisons may also increase the sensitivity for detecting PCL injuries with plain radiographs. In the chronic setting of PCL injury, radiographs are useful to assess for patellofemoral and medial compartment degenerative changes that can occur over time.

B. Magnetic Resonance Imaging

Although plain films are necessary and useful in the evaluations of these injuries, MRI is the diagnostic study of choice for the knee with a presumed PCL injury. MRI is from 96% to 100% sensitive at diagnosing PCL tears. Equally or more importantly, MRI is extremely valuable in its ability to detect associated injuries. This is particularly important in diagnosing posterolateral corner injuries because these can often be missed on the initial clinical examination. In multiligamentous knee injuries, MRI can also be useful in assessing the ACL because clinical examination of the ACL is challenging in the setting of a complete PCL tear.

C. Special Studies

In the setting of a chronic isolated PCL tear, pain in the medial and patellofemoral compartments are generally evaluated with radiographs. If these are normal, some surgeons proceed with a bone scan to evaluate for increased uptake in these areas. Areas under increased stress demonstrate increased uptake on the bone scan before signs of advanced arthritis occur on radiographs. This subset of patients may benefit from a PCL reconstruction to decrease the stress and delay osteoarthritis.

Treatment

There is significant controversy in the treatment of isolated PCL injuries. Multiple factors must be evaluated in the decision to treat a complete PCL rupture. The patient's age, activity level, expectations, and associated injuries must be taken into account. The literature on operative versus nonsurgical treatment of these injuries can be difficult to interpret, and there is no long-term follow-up studies of randomized patient groups.

A. Nonsurgical

Rehabilitation of the PCL injured knee often largely depends on the associated injuries sustained by the knee. This is particularly true with the commonly associated posterolateral corner injury. Therefore, we focus on the rehabilitation of the isolated PCL injured knee. Regaining motion and strength are the two key objectives of a rehabilitation program. Obtaining full quadriceps strength is essential for achieving the optimal result with nonsurgical treatment. The initial treatment is aimed at keeping the tibia reduced under the femur and minimizing tension on the injured PCL. With partial injuries (grade I and II), the prognosis is quite good, and early motion with weight bearing is the usual course of therapy. In a complete PCL tear, most keep the knee immobilized in extension to protect the posterolateral structures. Early strengthening exercises focus on quadriceps strength with quadriceps sets, straight leg raises, and partial weight bearing in extension.

Overall, most patients benefit from nonsurgical treatment of a PCL tear. Despite objective findings of instability that are often noted on examination, most patients subjectively are satisfied with the function of the knee. Bracing is generally ineffective in controlling PCL laxity clinically.

The main subjective complaint with chronic PCL insufficiency, however, is pain rather than instability. A PCL deficient knee with posterior tibial subluxation places significantly increased stresses on the patellofemoral and medial compartments of the knee. In one series in which patients with PCL injuries were followed with serial radiographs, 60% of patients displayed some degenerative changes of the medial compartment.

B. Surgical

Surgical management of PCL injuries are broken down into avulsion fractures, isolated acute PCL injuries, multiligament injuries, and chronic PCL insufficiency. Avulsion fractures of the PCL are rare fractures. If nondisplaced, these injuries are treated nonsurgically. If significantly displaced, these fractures are generally treated with open reduction and internal fixation.

The majority of surgeons generally still treat isolated PCL injuries with nonsurgical care. However, nonoperative care of these injuries is not without consequences. Although subjective results in these patients are good in the short term, many continue to have objective instability and display degenerative arthritic changes over time. A follow up of PCL deficient knees at an average of 15 years after injury found 89% of patients with persistent pain and half with chronic effusions. All patients in this group showed degenerative changes when followed for 25 years. Therefore, given the risks of continued instability and the potential of an increased chance of arthritic changes, surgical reconstruction of the PCL is a reasonable choice.

Initially, surgical care of complete PCL tears consisted of a primary repair of midsubstance tears. The objective stability of these repairs was generally disappointing. Current reconstruction methods generally involve routing either autograft or allograft tendons through bone tunnels to reconstruct the PCL in an anatomic fashion. Although there are several different methods of reconstructing the PCL, the two main categories of PCL reconstruction consist of single- and double-bundle repairs. Classically, reconstructions of the PCL anatomically replicated the anterolateral bundle of the native PCL with a single-bundle reconstruction. As problems were noted with recurrence of posterior laxity in the postoperative period, a double-bundle technique was derived to reconstruct both the anterolateral and posteromedial bundles of the native PCL. The advantages of the double-bundle technique are thus far theoretical, and there is no long-term clinical follow-up demonstrating the superiority of a double-bundle reconstruction at this time.

The severe instability noted with PCL injuries associated with multiligamentous knee injuries make the argument for ligament reconstruction more compelling in this patient population. Many of the studies involving PCL reconstruction in these complex knee injuries have involved primary repair attempts. Although subjective results were generally good, residual excessive, objective laxity was very common following repairs. More recently ligament reconstructions with allograft and autograft have become the dominant method of PCL reconstruction in this challenging patient population.

Complications

The most common complication following PCL reconstruction is the return of objective posterior laxity on physical examination. This does not present as subjective laxity, however, and patient satisfaction remains high despite objective laxity. Acute PCL reconstructions in the setting of a multiligamentous knee repair/reconstruction can result in arthrofibrosis with extensive postoperative scarring.

Results/Return to Play

Even with nonsurgical management of a PCL injury, the prognosis for a functional recovery and return to competition is very good. A strong quadriceps muscle and extensor mechanism can significantly compensate for PCL laxity. Athletes should spend a minimum of 3 months in rehabilitation before attempting a return to competition. However, there is a subset of patients that experiences significant instability with a grade III PCL injury that does not allow a return to competition. This is a subset of patients that may benefit from PCL reconstruction.

However, the prognosis for a PCL tear associated with a multiligamentous knee injury is guarded with respect to return to play. Although prompt recognition of a multiligamentous injury and appropriately timed treatment, reconstruction, and rehabilitation is essential for optimal recovery, these injuries are such that a significant percentage of patients are not able to return to full competition.

Allen CR, Kaplan LD, Fluhme DJ et al: Posterior cruciate ligament injuries. Curr Opin Rheumatol 2002;14:142. [PMID: 11845019]

Fanelli GC, Edson CJ: Combined posterior cruciate ligament-posterolateral reconstructions with Achilles tendon allograft and biceps femoris tendon tenodesis: 2- to 10-year follow-up. Arthroscopy 2004;20:339. [PMID: 15067271]

5. Patella Dislocation

Dislocation of the patella is a potential cause of acute hemarthrosis and must be considered when evaluating a patient with an acute knee injury. The injury occurs when valgus force and external rotation of the tibia is applied to a flexed leg. It is most common in females in the second decade of life.

Clinical Findings

The patella almost always dislocates laterally. The patient may notice the patella sitting laterally or might say that the rest of the knee has shifted medially. It is unusual to see actual dislocation of the patella except at the time of injury. Reduction occurs when the knee is extended.

Examination demonstrates tenderness over the medial retinaculum and adductor tubercle, which is the origin of the medial patellofemoral ligament. The patient also has pain and apprehension when the patella is pushed laterally with the knee slightly bent. Radiographs, including an axial patellar view, should be obtained to determine whether there are osteochondral fractures. Often, a small fleck of bone is avulsed by the capsule on the medial aspect of the patella. This is not intraarticular and does not require removal. A displaced osteochondral fracture require excisions or internal fixation. Examination of the uninjured knee is recommended to determine whether there are predisposing factors for dislocation, such as patella alta, genu recurvatum, increased Q angle, and patellar hypermobility. Patella alta, or high-riding patella, is identified by measuring the length of the patellar tendon and dividing by the length of the patella. The upper limit of normal is 1.2. The Q angle is formed by a line through the patellar tendon intersecting a line from the anterior superior iliac spine in the center of the patella. A normal Q angle is approximately 10 degrees, with a range of approximately plus or minus 5 degrees. Patients with generalized hypermobility have increased extension of the knee, or genu recurvatum, which in effect gives them patella alta. They also often have hypermobility of all the capsular ligamentous structures, including the static stabilizers of the kneecap, giving them significant patellar hypermobility.

Treatment & Prognosis

A wide variety of treatment options are recommended for patellar dislocations, including immediate mobilization and strengthening exercises, immobilization in a cylinder cast for 6 weeks followed by rehabilitation, arthroscopy with or without retinacular repair, surgical repair of the torn retinaculum, or immediate patellar realignment.

Treatment is based on which predisposing factors are present. Little is lost by functional treatment, similar to the treatment of isolated medial collateral ligament sprains, which is often successful. If dislocation recurs, realignment may be performed. A long-term study showed that patients treated surgically for patellar malalignment problems had a higher incidence of osteoarthritis than those treated nonoperatively.

Atkin DM et al: Characteristics of patients with primary acute lateral patella dislocation and their recovery within the first 6 months of injury. Am J Sports Med 2000;28:472. [PMID: 10921637]

Bensahal H et al: The unstable patella in children. J Pediatr Orthop 2000,9:265. [PMID: 11143470]

Buchner M et al: Acute traumatic primary patellar dislocation: Long-term results comparing conservative and surgical treatment. Clin J Sport Med 2005;15:62. [PMID: 15782048]

KNEE TENDON INJURY

Ruptures of the quadriceps and patellar tendons usually result from a tremendous eccentric contraction of the quadriceps muscle, which may occur when an athlete stumbles and tries not to fall.

1. Rupture of the Quadriceps Tendon

Quadriceps tendon ruptures occur most frequently in patients older than 40 years. Biopsies of fresh rupture sites showed local degenerative changes already present, consistent with the theory that normal tendons do not rupture. Rarely, the injury occurs bilaterally, and it is often associated with gout, diabetes, or steroid use. When it does occur bilaterally with only a small amount of trauma, the diagnosis may be difficult to make because of the small amount of swelling or symptoms of injury.

The cardinal symptom is inability to extend the knee. When extension is attempted, a gap develops in the suprapatellar region. The patella rides at a slightly lower level, and the anterior border of the femoral condyles may be palpated.

Acute complete quadriceps tendon ruptures should be paired surgically. If left untreated, proximal migration and scarring of the quadriceps muscle occurs. Direct-end repair produces excellent results. Neutralizing the forces across the repair is difficult, and immobilization in extension is recommended. Repair of ruptures more than 2 weeks old may be difficult and may require quadriceps lengthening, muscle or tendon transfers, or a combination of these procedures.

Ilan DI et al: Quadriceps tendon rupture. J Am Acad Orthop Surg 2003;11:192. [PMID: 112828449]

Konrath GA et al: Outcomes following repair of quadriceps tendon ruptures. J Orthop Trauma 1998,12:273. [PMID: 9619463]

2. Rupture of the Patellar Tendon

Rupture of the patella tendon occurs more frequently in patients younger than 40 years. The patient cannot actively extend the knee, the patella is high riding, and a defect is palpable beneath the patella. Surgical repair is the treatment of choice. The tendon, along with the medial and lateral retinaculum, should be sewn end to end. A stress-relieving wire may be placed around the patella and through the tibial tubercle. The wire should be removed in 6–8 weeks. Chronic patellar tendon ruptures are very hard to treat. The quadriceps must be freed up from the femur and the patella pulled down to the proper location. The gracilis and semitendinosus tendons can be used to substitute for the patellar tendon.

The extensor mechanism may also be disrupted at the inferior pole of the patella where the patellar tendon originates. This usually occurs in a child between 8 and 12 years of age. The distal pole of the patella plus a large sleeve of articular cartilage is pulled off (Figure 4–18). This may be easily misdiagnosed if the fragment of bone is small. Reestablishment of an intact extensor mechanism is necessary. With displaced fractures, open reduction and internal fixation with tension band wiring are recommended.

KNEE PAIN

Pain in the knee region is a very common complaint of athletes. If there is no history of an acute injury, overuse is commonly the cause. The patient is often able to point to the area of pain. The history of activity must be obtained as well as overall evaluation of the extremities.

1. Anterior Knee Pain

Clinical Findings

A. SYMPTOMS AND SIGNS

Anterior knee pain is a common complaint and frequently bilateral. It is most common in females during the second decade of life. The patellofemoral joint is often the source of pain. Entities such as chondromalacia patella, patellofemoral arthralgia, and lateral patellofemoral compression syndrome are diagnostic considerations.

Patellar pain is often felt when going up or down hills or stairs, and there may be complaints of instability during walking, running, or other sports activities. These activities may create a joint reaction force of several times the body weight on the patella with each step. Swelling is seldom a complaint. If the pain is in one knee only, the patient may alter the way of climbing and descending stairs so that the affected leg is kept straight and each step leads with the same foot. This strategy significantly decreases the joint reaction force on the patellofemoral joint.

Many of these problems arise because the patel-lofemoral joint is semiconstrained, especially in the range of 0–20 degrees of flexion, and the constraint increases as flexion increases. The degree of constraint also depends on a number of other factors, including the angle of the sulcus of the femur, the presence or absence of patella alta, and the generalized ligamentous laxity of the patient. In addition, femoral anteversion and increased Q angle (Figure 4–19) may lead to increased instability of the patellofemoral joint. This lack of constraint may predispose the patella to frank dislocation, although subluxation is a much more common finding. The degree of congruity is anatomically variable and may lead to high-contact stresses caused by anatomic configuration and static and dynamic con-straints on the patella. Increased pressure may cause pain and patellofemoral osteoarthritis.

On physical examination of the patient with patel-lofemoral subluxation, minimal findings in relation to complaints may be present. Occasionally, crepitance, a crackling or clicking sound or feeling, is found with

A

B

Figure 4–18. Sleeve fracture of the patella. **A:** A small segment of the distal pole of the patella is avulsed with a relatively large portion of the articular surface. **B:** Lateral radiograph of the knee with a displaced sleeve fracture of the patella. Note that the small osseous portion of the displaced fragment is visible, but the cartilagi-nous portion is not seen. (Reproduced, with permission, from Rockwood CA Jr, ed: *Fractures in Children*, 3rd ed. Lippincott, 1991.)

Articular cartilage

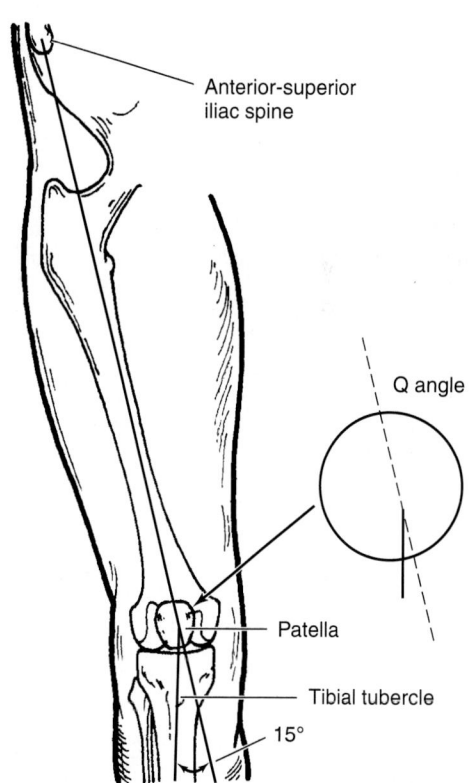

Anterior-superior iliac spine

Q angle

Patella

Tibial tubercle

15°

Figure 4–19. Q angle and valgus angulation. (Reproduced, with permission, from American Academy of Orthopaedic Surgeons: *Athletic Training and Sports Medicine*, 2nd ed. AAOS, 1991.)

flexion and extension. Quadriceps strength, tone, and bulk are usually reduced. Pain may be elicited at a particular angle of flexion by putting the knee through its range of motion with resistance. Subluxation may often be diagnosed with the apprehension sign, a rapid contraction of the quadriceps when the patella is passively moved laterally.

B. IMAGING STUDIES

Roentgenographic examination frequently shows a valgus angulation of the knee on anteroposterior views. Occasionally, patella alta may be identified on the lateral view, and tangential views of the patella at various knee flexion angles reveals a lack of contact of the medial facet of the patella with the medial facet of the trochlear groove of the femur. Lateral subluxation of the patellofemoral joint may also be observed.

This syndrome with a normal roentgenographic examination is frequently called chondromalacia patellae; with subluxation identified on radiograph, it is referred to as patellofemoral subluxation. A more accurate term would be patellofemoral arthralgia because patellofemoral subluxation was probably present prior to the onset of pain, and because chondromalacia patellae (softening of the patellar cartilage) is an arthroscopic or pathologic diagnosis. Patellofemoral arthralgia is a clinical diagnosis.

Treatment

A. CHONDROMALACIA PATELLAE

Initially, treatment is conservative, with the intent of improving quadriceps strength and stamina to stabilize the patellofemoral joint. Weight loss is prescribed to decrease the stress on the patellofemoral joint; reduction in loading the knee in the flexed position also accomplishes pressure reduction. Knee orthotics may be beneficial. When subluxation and fear of dislocation are major concerns, an orthotic that limits extension of the knee may be beneficial because the patella becomes inherently more stable with knee flexion. NSAIDs may be beneficial.

B. PATELLOFEMORAL ARTHRALGIA

Only when conservative treatment is exhausted should surgical treatment be considered. Alteration in the alignment of the patellofemoral joint may be beneficial in patellofemoral arthralgia. Lateral retinacular release followed by a period of conservative treatment is beneficial in some cases. Distal realignment may be necessary to achieve appropriate alignment and reduction in pain in those cases with an abnormality such as valgus knee or increased femoral anteversion.

C. PATELLOFEMORAL COMPRESSION SYNDROME

With lateral patellofemoral compression syndrome, there is tenderness along the lateral facet of the patella

or along the femoral condyle. Without cartilage damage, an effusion is rarely present. Treatment includes decreasing the activity level, including avoiding hills or step aerobics. Ice-massage, quadriceps and hamstring stretching, and short-arc quadriceps exercises against resistance are recommended to strengthen the vastus medialis obliquus muscle without aggravating the pain. Patellar supports or neoprene sleeves may also be helpful. Most patients respond to this regimen and gradually resume their activities. The role of releasing a contracted lateral patellofemoral retinaculum is controversial.

D. PATELLAR TENDINITIS

Patellar tendinitis, or jumper's knee, is seen in basketball and volleyball players. Tenderness along the tendon, usually at the inferior pole of the patella, is noted. Treatment with ice and avoiding jumping usually suffices. In refractory cases, debridement of mucinous degenerative material from the tendon may be successful.

Prognosis

The prognosis for jumper's knee is quite good. The condition is often persistent but self-limiting. The patient can always alleviate the symptoms by avoiding the activities that cause the problem.

Csintalan R et al: Gender effects on the biomechanical properties of the peripatellar retinaculum. Clin Orthop Rel Res 2002,(402):260. [PMID: 12218492]

Kettunen JA, Visuri T, Harilainen A et al: Primary cartilage lesions and outcome among subjects with patellofemoral pain syndrome. Knee Surg Sports Traumatol Arthrosc 2005;13:131. [PMID: 15756617]

Witvrouw E, Werner S, Mikkelsen C et al: Clinical classification of patellofemoral pain syndrome: Guidelines for non-operative treatment. Knee Surg Sports Traumatol Arthrosc 2005; 13:122. [PMID: 15703965]

2. Lateral Knee Pain

Lateral knee pain that is not located on the joint line may result from iliotibial band friction syndrome. This is a form of bursitis caused by rubbing of the iliotibial band against the lateral epicondyle. Tenderness over the lateral epicondyle at approximately 30 degrees of flexion when the knee is extended is indicative of this diagnosis. Runners and cyclists are commonly afflicted. Crossover gait or running on banked terrain is thought to be a causative factor.

Treatment involves decreasing the athlete's activities, ice-massage, stretching of the iliotibial tract, and use of a lateral wedge orthotic in those patients with heel varus. Running on flat terrain and changing the gait pattern may be helpful. In cyclists, lowering the seat height so the full extension of the knee is not reached and adjusting the pedals so the toes are not internally rotated should help. Steroid injections are infrequently needed, and release of the inflamed portion of the iliotibial band is seldom necessary. As for other overuse syndromes of the knee, the prognosis is good.

Gunter P, Schwellnus MP: Local corticosteroid injection in iliotibial band friction syndrome in runners: A randomised controlled trial. Br J Sports Med 2004;38:269; discussion 272. [PMID: 15155424]

■ ANKLE OR FOOT PAIN

Evaluation of foot and ankle injuries is described in Chapter 9. Injury specific to athletics includes chronic Achilles tendonitis, heel pain, plantar fasciitis and posterior tibial syndrome.

Clinical Findings

Achilles tendonitis, a frequent complaint in runners, may result from a contracted gastrocsoleus, or hyperpronation may cause overpulling of the medial insertion. Additionally, there may be a bony prominence on the superior-posterior aspect of the calcaneus, causing retrocalcaneal bursitis.

Heel pain is a common problem in runners and difficult to treat because of the uncertainty as to cause. Theories include painful heel spurs, bursitis, fat-pad atrophy, stress fracture, plantar fasciitis, or entrapment of the terminal branches of the posterior tibial nerve.

Many patients have pain localized in the posteromedial surface of the foot just distal to the attachment of the plantar fascia to the calcaneus (plantar fasciitis). This pain is often most severe on initially getting up in the morning and decreases as the day goes on.

Posterior tibial syndrome occurs in runners with hyperpronation. As the longitudinal arch flattens out, the posterior tibial musculotendinous unit elevates the flattened arch and has abnormal strain placed on it.

Treatment

Treatment depends on the cause of the injury, but it includes decreasing running activities, using a heel lift, and performing stretching exercises. If hyperpronation is thought to be the cause, an orthotic may be used. Steroid injections are not recommended because they could lead to weakening and subsequent rupture of the tendon.

Surgical intervention for chronic Achilles tendinitis or retrocalcaneal bursitis is seldom needed. This would be done to remove areas of fibrosis or calcium within the tendon and possibly some bone from the posterior

process of the calcaneus. The treatment for plantar fasciitis includes rest, ice-massage, and possibly antiinflammatory medications. A small shock-absorbing type of heel cup often is helpful, and a steroid injection may be given in recalcitrant cases. Acute rupture of the plantar fascia may occur. The pain is usually quite sharp and may cause significant disability for 6–12 weeks.

Hyperpronation may also cause fibular stress fractures. A semirigid orthosis may be recommended to decrease the amount and angular velocity of pronation. Using an orthosis while running actually increases the work of running, but if it decreases abnormal stresses in those who hyperpronate, it may be quite helpful.

Mizel MS et al: Evaluation and treatment of chronic ankle pain. Instr Course Lect 2004;53:311. [PMID: 15116624]
Shalabi A et al: Eccentric training of the gastrocnemius-soleus complex in chronic Achilles tendinopathy results in decreased tendon volume and intratendinous signal as evaluated by MRI. Am J Sports Med 2004;25:149. [PMID: 15244320]

■ OTHER INJURIES OF THE LOWER BODY

Many disorders seen while caring for athletes may be difficult to diagnose with certainty. The differential diagnosis must be carefully made to rule out more severe injuries. A period of rest followed by gradual return to activities is often the best treatment. During convalescence, application of ice packs, stretching exercises, and gradual strengthening of the injured limb facilitate return to sports activities.

OVERUSE SYNDROMES OF THE LOWER EXTREMITIES

Many athletes, such as runners, cyclists, aerobics enthusiasts, volleyball players, and basketball players, develop painful disorders of the lower extremities without an acute injury. History taking is very important, and the examiner should ask specific questions about the circumstances in which the discomfort occurs. In a runner, for example, the examiner should ask whether there was an increase in the distance run or a change in the running surface, at what point the pain was felt, and what home remedies were tried before the runner sought advice from a physician.

The physical examination should include not only the affected area, but also evaluation of the back, pelvis, leg lengths, genu varum or valgum, femoral and tibial torsion, and cavus or flatfoot deformities. The presence of hamstring and heel cord contracture should be determined, and the gait pattern should be observed. Running shoes should be inspected for wear patterns, which may be quite helpful.

1. Muscle Strains

Muscle strains of the lower extremity are frequent, and disabling muscle injuries, with strain of the distal muscle tendon junction, are the most common. Muscles may stretch to approximately 125% of their resting length before tearing. Strains are graded as mild, moderate, and severe, based on the degree of pain, spasm, and disability that the strain causes. A severe strain would be complete disruption of the muscle, with a palpable defect and balling up of the muscle proximally.

In spite of the frequency of muscle strains and the disability they produce, there is little scientific information on their pathologic basis. Muscles susceptible to more stretching are more susceptible to strains. In the lower extremity, the muscles most frequently injured are the hamstring, quadriceps, and gastrocnemius muscles. These muscles all cross two joints, and they may be unable to resist full stretching across both joints. The most powerful muscles are more likely to be strained, and strains are more common in so-called explosive-type athletics. Eccentric contraction (muscle contraction while the muscle is lengthening) is often thought to be causative in muscle strains.

Clinical Findings

The diagnosis is relatively easy. Often the athlete feels the muscle "grab" while he or she is accelerating. There is localized tenderness over the muscle and pain on stretching of the muscle. Because the two joint muscles are most frequently involved, the muscles should be stretched over both of the joints during examination.

Treatment & Prognosis

The treatment of muscle strains should begin with ice in the immediate postinjury period. Flexibility and strength should be regained prior to return to activity. This may take many months, and if the patient returns to activity too early, there may be a setback to the level of the original injury.

Strengthening of the muscles might make them less susceptible to being torn. It is commonly believed that flexibility helps prevent muscle strains, but there are conflicting reports regarding this idea, and it is still unproved.

Askling C, Karlsson J, Thorstensson A: Hamstring injury occurrence in elite soccer players after preseason strength training with eccentric overload. Scand J Med Sci Sports 2005;15:65. [PMID: 15679576]

Gabbe BJ, Finch CF, Bennell KL et al:. Risk factors for hamstring injuries in community level Australian football. Br J Sports Med 2005;39:106. [PMID: 15665208]

Levine WN et al: Intramuscular corticosteroid injection for hamstring injuries. A 13-year experience in the National Football League. Am J Sports Med 2000;28(3):297. [PMID: 10843118]

2. Shin Pain

Clinical Findings

A. SHIN SPLINTS

The term *shin splints* is widely used for shin pain, but it is not a diagnostic term. A more specific diagnosis should be made if possible. Shin splints are usually defined as pain associated with activity in the beginning of training after a relatively inactive period. The pain and tenderness are usually located over the anterior compartment and disappear in 1–2 weeks as the athlete becomes conditioned to the exercise. Care must be taken to differentiate shin splints from stress fractures of the tibia, which cause more localized pain and have many more potential complications if not cared for properly.

B. MEDIAL TIBIAL SYNDROME

Medial tibial syndrome is also seen in runners, occurring along the medial border of the distal tibia. After 3–4 weeks, some hypertrophy of the cortical bone and periosteal new bone formation may be seen on radiograph. It is thought to be either a periostitis or possibly an incomplete stress fracture. The pull of the tibialis posterior muscle from its origin on the tibia and posterior tibial tendinitis are also thought to be possible causes.

Treatment

Treatment for shin splints and medial tibial syndrome is rest and resumption of athletic activities in a graduated fashion.

3. Stress Fractures

Stress fractures may occur in the pelvis, femoral neck, tibia, navicular, and metatarsals. They are usually the result of a significant increase in training and activity. In the female athlete, poor nutrition, low bone density, and a history of menstrual disturbance are associated with a higher prevalence of stress fractures. The history is important in differentiating these injuries from infection or neoplasm, particularly when there is a finding on radiographs. Plain radiographs are normal at first. MRI or technetium bone scans are the best diagnostic tests. If symptoms persist for over a month, radiographs may become positive.

Treatment of stress fractures involves rest and avoidance of high-impact activities until healing occurs. This includes resolution of the tenderness and signs of fracture healing on plain radiographs. Continuous activity with stress fractures may lead to complete fractures. Patients must be made aware of this and all the complications that may develop with a complete fracture.

Armstrong DW III, Rue JP, Wilckens JH et al: Stress fracture injury in young military men and women. Bone 2004;35(3): 806. [PMID: 15336620]

Perron AD, Brady WJ, Keats TA: Principles of stress fracture management. The whys and hows of an increasingly common injury. Postgrad Med 2001;110:115.

4. Exertional Compartment Syndromes

Exertional compartment syndromes may result from muscle hypertrophy within the confining osseofascial compartment. As the muscles hypertrophy and the amount of edema within the compartment increases, the blood supply to the nerves and muscles within the involved compartment is diminished, and the pressure continues to increase.

The syndrome presents as recurrent claudication during exertional activity and is relieved by rest. After exercise, the findings of localized pain, pain on passive motion, and hypesthesia are indicative.

Treatment consists activity modification including gradual onset of training. If unsuccessful, compartment pressures may be measured while the patient is exercising on a treadmill, and if the pressures are elevated, surgical fasciotomy is usually effective.

Shah SN, Miller BS, Kuhn JE : Chronic exertional compartment syndrome. Am J Orthop 2004;33:335. [PMID: 15344575]

CONTUSIONS & AVULSIONS OF THE LOWER BODY

1. Contusion to the Quadriceps Muscle

Clinical Findings

A severe contusion to the quadriceps muscle (charley horse) is disabling and results in prolonged inactivity. It frequently occurs in football players. With significant bleeding into the muscle, there is inhibition of movement. Rarely, a compartment syndrome occurs.

Myositis ossificans may occur after these injuries. It may be apparent 2–4 weeks after the injury. Radiographically and histologically, myositis ossificans may be similar to osteogenic sarcoma; therefore, the history of contusion is very important. Radiographs should be obtained after such a contusion to minimize myositis ossificans being confused with cancer.

Treatment & Prognosis

Quadriceps contusions should be treated with elevation of the leg and the hip and knee flexed to tolerance to minimize bleeding. After a few days the knee can be moved with continuous passive motion or so-called drop-and-dangle gravity-assisted exercises. For the latter, the patient is seated on a table high enough to keep the feet off the floor. The patient then hooks the uninjured foot behind the ankle of the injured leg. The uninjured leg extends the knee of the injured leg, and gravity flexes the injured knee. Average length of disability for mild contusions is 2 weeks; for severe contusions, 3 weeks.

If heterotopic ossification is present, no specific treatment is recommended other than treatment for the contusion. Normal function may be obtained, but the recovery period is longer. Because early surgery may cause exacerbation of the heterotopic ossification, it should be avoided.

Cooper DE: Severe quadriceps muscle contusions in athletes. Am J Sports Med 2004;32:820. [PMID: 15090402]

Diaz JA, Fischer DA, Rettig AC et al: Severe quadriceps muscle contusions in athletes. A report of three cases. Am J Sports Med 2003;3:289. [PMID: 12642267]

CONTUSIONS ABOUT THE HIP AND PELVIS

Clinical Findings

Contusions about the pelvis and hip region may be very painful and disabling. Because of the subcutaneous location of the iliac crests and the greater trochanters, these regions are at risk in contact sports.

A contusion over the greater trochanter may cause persistent bursitis, tenderness directly over the greater trochanter, and increased pain with adduction of the leg. Females are more prone to trochanteric bursitis because of their broader pelvis.

A hip pointer is a very painful contusion over the iliac crest that occurs from many contact sports. It must be differentiated from an avulsion fracture in a child and a tear of the muscle aponeurosis in an adult. Profuse bleeding may occur and be very painful.

Treatment & Prognosis

For contusion over the greater trochanter, treatment consists of ice applications and decreased activities. Padding may be helpful to prevent recurrent injuries. The prognosis is good. For hip pointer injuries, initial treatment with ice is helpful. Protective pads are useful in preventing these injuries and returning the athlete to activities sooner.

AVULSION OF THE TIBIAL TUBERCLE

Clinical Findings

Tibial tubercle avulsions occur in adolescent athletes, most often in males between 14 and 16 years of age. They result from a powerful contraction of the quadriceps muscle against a fixed tibia, as in jumping, or with forced passive flexion of the knee against a powerful quadriceps contraction, as in an awkward landing at the end of a jump or fall. Avulsion of the tubercle may occur with either a sudden acceleration or deceleration of the knee extensor mechanism. The patellar tendon must pull hard enough to overcome the strength of the growth plate, the surrounding perichondrium, and the adjacent periosteum.

Swelling and tenderness are located over the proximal anterior tibia. A tense hemarthrosis may be present. A palpable defect in the anterior tibia is associated with a much-displaced avulsion. Proximal migration of the patella occurs, and the patella may seem to float off the anterior aspect of the femur. The knee is held flexed; with displaced fractures, the patient is unable actively to extend the knee.

Watson-Jones defined three types of avulsion fractures, which were subsequently refined as the following three types (Figure 4–20): type 1 fracture, in which the fracture line lies across the secondary center of ossification at the level of the posterior border of the patellar ligament; type 2 fracture, in which a separation breaks out at the primary and secondary ossification centers of epiphysis; and type 3 fracture, in which the separation propagates upward through the main portion of the proximal tibial epiphysis. The degree of displacement depends on the severity of injury to the surrounding soft-tissue moorings. A lateral radiograph with the tibia slightly internally rotated is the best view to see the fracture and the degree of displacement.

Differential Diagnosis

Osgood-Schlatter disease, or osteochondrosis of the tuberosity of the tibia, should not be confused with acute avulsion of the tibial tubercle. In the former, the patient is usually between 11 and 15 years of age and involved in athletics. Pain is located at the tibial tubercle, and it has usually been present intermittently over a period of several months. Walking on a flat surface is not difficult, but ascending or descending stairs causes difficulty. Radiograph examination shows slight separation of the tibial tubercle with new bone formation beneath it (Figure 4–21).

Treatment recommendations vary from decreasing the amount of running and jumping, but continuing participation in athletics, to cylinder cast immobilization for a short period of time. The long-term prognosis is excellent. Although symptoms are often present for 2 years, early short-term cast immobilization may shorten this period of discomfort to 9 months. In most children, casting is not necessary. Explaining the benign nature of the problem to both the patient and the parents, reassuring them that the long-term prognosis is good, and modifying activities usually allows continued

Figure 4–20. Classification of avulsion fractures of the tibial tubercle. Type 1 fracture (**left**) across the secondary ossification center at level with the posterior border of the inserting patellar ligament. Type 2 fracture (**center**) at the junction of the primary and secondary ossification centers of the proximal tibial epiphysis. Type 3 fracture (**right**) propagates upward across the primary ossification center of the proximal tibial epiphysis into the knee joint. This fracture is a variant of the Salter-Harris III separation and is analogous to the fracture of Tillaux at the ankle because the posterior portion of the physis of the proximal tibia is closing. (Reproduced, with permission, from Odgen JA et al: Fractures of the tibial tuberosity in adolescents. J Bone Joint Surg Am 1980;62:205.)

Patella alta

Osteo-
chondral
fragment

New bone
formation

Figure 4–21. Development of Osgood-Schlatter lesion. (**Left**) Avulsion of osteochondral fragment that includes surface cartilage and a portion of the secondary ossification center of the tibial tubercle. (**Right**) New bone fills in the gap between the avulsed osteochondral fragment and the tibial tubercle. (Reproduced, with permission, from Rockwood CA Jr (ed): *Fractures in Children*, 3rd ed. Lippincott, 1991.)

participation in athletics. Hamstring stretching and ice-massage ideally decrease symptoms during the time needed for maturation of the tibial tubercle. The pain goes away when the tubercle unites with the tibia. In a very small number of cases, chronic pain is present if the ossicle fails to unite. Painful ossicles in the adult are treated successfully with simple excision.

Treatment

Full function of the extensor mechanism is necessary, and therefore treatment of tibial tubercle avulsion fractures is aimed at this goal. If the fracture is minimally displaced, and the patient is able to extend the knee fully against gravity, nonoperative treatment is acceptable. A cylinder cast should be applied with the knee extended and worn for 4 weeks. Active range-of-motion and strengthening exercises should then commence. At 6 weeks, quadriceps exercises against resistance are initiated. For displaced fractures, open reduction and internal fixation are recommended, with screws if the piece or pieces are large enough. If rigid fixation of large fragments is obtained, early active flexion and passive extension may be initiated. If a tenuous repair is obtained, protection in a cast is advisable.

Prognosis

Because the injury occurs in children who are close to skeletal maturity, meaningful growth abnormalities at the proximal tibial physis do not occur. Return to activities is allowed after the athlete develops quadriceps mass and strength equal to the contralateral side.

AVULSIONS ABOUT THE PELVIS

Clinical Findings

In the skeletally immature athlete, the apophysis, or growth plate where the muscle attaches to bone, is the weak link in the bone-muscle-tendon unit. Therefore, just as the growth plate is prone to breaking in children's fractures, the bony origin of muscles may be pulled off. This most commonly occurs in athletes between 14 and 25 years of age. Comparison radiographs may be helpful to make sure the avulsion fracture is not just a normal anatomic variant. In the pelvis, this may occur at the iliac crest (abdominal muscles), anterior superior iliac spine (sartorius origin), anterior inferior iliac spine (rectus femoris origin), ischial tuberosity (hamstring origin), and lesser trochanter of the femur (iliopsoas insertion).

Treatment & Prognosis

Symptomatic care with a few days of rest followed by ambulation with crutches for approximately a month is recommended. It is usually 6–10 weeks before athletic activities may be resumed. Long-term athletic activity will probably not be affected. Open reduction and internal fixation do not show superior results, and therefore they are usually not warranted. Abundant calcification may occur in the ischial tuberosity region and may be the cause of chronic bursitis and pain. Excision of the exuberant callous should cure this problem. Another indication for surgery is a painful fibrous nonunion, which also may be cured with excision of the fragment.

Rossi F, Dragoni S: Acute avulsion fractures of the pelvis in adolescent competitive athletes: Prevalence, location and sports distribution of 203 cases collected. Skeletal Radiol 2001;30:127. [PMID: 11357449]

■ SHOULDER INJURIES

The shoulder is the third most commonly injured joint during athletic activities, after the knee and the ankle. Sports-related injuries of the shoulder may result from a direct traumatic event or repetitive overuse. Any activity that requires arm motion, particularly overhead arm motion such as throwing, may stress the soft tissues surrounding the glenohumeral joint to the point of injury. The shoulder is the most mobile joint in the body, partly as a result of minimal containment of the large humeral head by the shallow and smaller glenoid fossa. The trade-off for this mobility is less structural restraint to undesirable and potentially damaging movements. Thus, a fine balance must be struck to maintain full range of shoulder motion and normal glenohumeral joint stability.

Kim DH et al: Shoulder injuries in golf. Am J Sports Med 200432(5):1324. [PMID: 15262661]

Anatomy

A. THE BONY ARTICULATION OF THE GLENOHUMERAL JOINT

The glenohumeral joint is a modified ball-and-socket joint. The glenoid fossa is a shallow inverted, comma-shaped, articular surface one fourth the size of the humeral head. The articular surface of the humeral head is retroverted approximately 30 degrees relative to the transverse axis of the elbow. Because the scapula is oriented anterolaterally approximately 30 degrees on the thorax, relative to the coronal plane of the body, the face of the glenoid fossa matches the humeral head retroversion. The scapula rotates to direct the glenoid superiorly, inferiorly, medially, or laterally to accommodate changing humeral head positions. As a result, the humeral head is centered in the glenoid throughout most shoulder motions. When this centered position is disturbed, instability may result.

B. THE CLAVICLE AND ITS ARTICULATIONS

The clavicle articulates medially with the sternum at the sternoclavicular joint and laterally with the acromion of the scapula at the acromioclavicular joint. The clavicle rotates on its long axis and acts as a strut to stabilize the glenohumeral joint, serving as the only bone connecting the appendicular upper extremity to the axial skeleton.

C. THE GLENOHUMERAL JOINT CAPSULE, LIGAMENTS, AND LABRUM

The capsule of the glenohumeral joint may be the most lax of all the major joints, yet in certain positions it makes an important contribution to stability. The capsuloligamentous structures and the glenoid labrum share a common insertion. The anterior capsule is composed of the coracohumeral and superior glenohumeral ligaments, the middle glenohumeral ligament, and the inferior glenohumeral ligament (Figure 4–22). There is a variable relationship between the anterior capsuloligamentous structures and the labrum, such that certain anatomic variations may be associated with joint instability more often than others. For example, an anterosuperior sublabral hole is variably present within the glenohumeral joint, connecting with the subscapularis bursa that lies between the subscapularis tendon and the capsule.

The glenoid labrum not only acts as an attachment site for the capsuloligamentous structures but also as an extension of the articular cavity. Its presence deepens the glenoid socket by nearly 50%, and removal of the labrum decreases joint stability to shear stress. In this way, the triangular cross section of the labrum acts as a chock-block to help prevent subluxation.

D. THE SHOULDER MUSCULATURE

The muscles around the shoulder may be divided into three functional groups: glenohumeral, thoracohumeral, and those that cross both the shoulder and elbow.

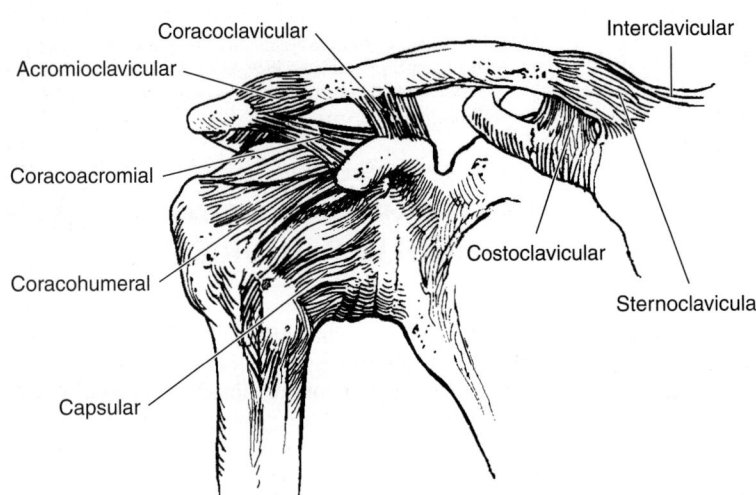

Figure 4–22. Ligaments about the shoulder girdle.

Glenohumeral Muscles

Four muscles compose the rotator cuff: the supraspinatus, subscapularis, infraspinatus, and teres minor. The supraspinatus has its origin on the posterosuperior scapula, superior to the scapular spine. It passes under the acromion, through the supraspinatus fossa, and inserts on the greater tuberosity with an extended attachment of fibrocartilage. The supraspinatus is active during the entire arc of scapular plane abduction; paralysis of the suprascapular nerve results in an approximately 50% loss of abduction torque. The infraspinatus and the teres minor muscles originate on the posterior scapula, inferior to the scapular spine, and insert on the posterior aspect of the greater tuberosity. Despite their origin below the scapular spine, their tendinous insertions are not separate from the supraspinatus tendon. These muscles function together to externally rotate and extend the humerus. Both account for approximately 80% of external rotation strength in the adducted position. The infraspinatus is more active with the arm at the side; the teres minor activates mainly with the shoulder in 90 degrees of elevation. The subscapularis muscle arises from the anterior scapula and is the only muscle to insert on the lesser tuberosity. The subscapularis is the sole anterior component of the rotator cuff and functions to rotate and flex the humerus internally. The tendinous insertion of the subscapularis is continuous with the anterior capsule so that both provide anterior glenohumeral stability.

The deltoid is the largest of the glenohumeral muscles. It covers the proximal humerus on a path from its tripennate origin at the clavicle, acromion, and scapular spine to its insertion midway on the humerus at the deltoid tubercle. Abduction of the joint results from activity of the anterior and middle portions. The anterior portion is also a forward flexor. The posterior portion does not abduct the joint but instead adducts and extends the humerus. The deltoid is active throughout the entire arc of glenohumeral abduction; paralysis of the axillary nerve results in a 50% loss of abduction torque. The deltoid muscle can fully abduct the glenohumeral joint with the supraspinatus muscle inactive.

The teres major muscle originates from the inferior angle of the scapula and inserts on the medial lip of the bicipital groove of the humerus, posterior to the insertion of the latissimus dorsi. The axillary nerve and the posterior humeral circumflex artery pass superior to it through the quadrilateral space also bordered by the teres minor, the triceps, and the humerus. It contracts with the latissimus dorsi muscle, and the two muscles function as a unit in humeral extension, internal rotation, and adduction.

Thoracohumeral Muscles

The pectoralis major and the latissimus dorsi muscles are powerful movers of the shoulder and hence contribute to the joint force that in turn usually stabilizes the glenohumeral joint. The pectoralis major muscle arises as a broad sheet of two distinct heads with the lowermost fibers of the sternal head inserting most proximally on the humerus.

Muscles that have origin on the thorax contribute to glenohumeral stability and may have roles in instability as well. When the shoulder is placed in horizontal abduction, similar to the apprehension position, the lowermost fibers of the sternal head of the pectoralis major muscle are stretched to an extreme. Because anterior instability also occurs from forcible horizontal abduction of the shoulder, the humeral head can be pulled out of the glenoid by passive tension in the pectoralis major and latissimus dorsi muscles.

Biceps Brachii Muscle

Both heads of the biceps brachii muscle have their origin on the scapula. The short head originates from the coracoid and with the coracobrachialis muscle forms the conjoined tendon. The long head of the biceps has its origin just superior to the articular margin of the glenoid from the posterosuperior labrum and the supraglenoid tubercle, and it is inside the synovial sheath of the glenohumeral joint. It traverses the glenohumeral joint, passing over the anterior aspect of the humeral head to the bicipital groove where it exits the joint under the transverse humeral ligament.

Its origin on the scapula and insertion of the radius leaves the long head of the biceps brachii muscle with potential for function at both the shoulder and the elbow. Its function at the elbow is well established to include both flexion and supination. Long considered a depressor of the humeral head, the role of the active biceps was questioned because electromyographic studies showed little or no activity of the biceps when elbow motion was controlled. This does not preclude a passive role or an active role associated with elbow motion because tension in the tendon may then contribute to glenohumeral joint stability.

E. THE NEUROVASCULAR SUPPLY

The axillary artery traverses the axilla, extending from the outer border of the first rib to the lower border of the teres minor muscle, forming the brachial artery. The axillary artery lies deep to the pectoralis muscle but is crossed in its midregion by the pectoralis minor tendon, just before the tendon inserts on the coracoid process. The axillary vein travels with the axillary artery, and branches of the axillary artery supply most of the shoulder girdle. The brachial plexus consists of the ventral rami of the fifth through eighth cervical nerves and the first thoracic nerve. This network of nerve fibers begins with the joining of the ventral rami proximally in the neck and continues anteriorly and distally, crossing into the axillary region obliquely underneath the clavicle at about the junction area of the distal one third and proximal two thirds. Clavicular fractures in this area have the potential of injuring the brachial plexus. The plexus then lies inferior to the coracoid process, where its cords form the peripheral nerves that continue down the arm. Muscles of the shoulder girdle are supplied by the nerves arising at all levels of the brachial plexus.

Eberly VC, McMahon PJ, Lee TQ: Variation in the glenoid origin of the anteroinferior glenohumeral capsulolabrum. Clin Orthop 2002;400,26. [PMID: 12072742]

Enad JG: Bifurcate origin of the long head of the biceps tendon. Arthroscopy 2004;20:1081. [PMID: 15592239]

Price MR et al: Determining the relationship of the axillary nerve to the shoulder joint capsule from an arthroscopic perspective. J Bone Joint Surg Am 2004;86-A:2135. [PMID: 15466721]

History & Physical Examination

A. GENERAL APPROACH

The history of shoulder complaints must include age, arm dominance, location, intensity, duration, temporal occurrence, aggravating and alleviating factors, radiation of discomfort, physical activity level, occupation, and the mechanism of injury. These responses, combined with the physical findings (Table 4–3) and imaging studies, can lead to accurate diagnosis of shoulder problems. Previous responses to treatment help to characterize their efficacy and establish a pattern of disease or injury progression. The physical examination begins with the patient undressing so both shoulders are fully exposed. Patients should be examined first in the standing position. The surface anatomy should be checked for asymmetry, atrophy, or external lesions. The supraspinatus and infraspinatus fossae are especially important to examine for atrophy. The area of pain should be pointed out by the patient prior to the physician manipulating the shoulder to avoid hurting the patient unnecessarily. A thorough neurovascular examination of the upper extremity should be performed.

B. SHOULDER RANGE OF MOTION

1. Types of movement—Many terms may be used to describe movements of the shoulder joint (Figure 4–23). Flexion occurs when the arm begins at the side and elevates in the sagittal plane of the body anteriorly. Extension occurs when the arm starts at the side and elevates in the sagittal plane of the body posteriorly. Adduction occurs when the arm moves toward the midline of the body, with abduction occurring as the arm moves away from the midline of the body. Internal rotation occurs when the arm rotates medially, inward toward the body, and external rotation occurs as the arm rotates laterally or outward from the body. Horizontal adduction occurs as the arm starts at 90 degrees of abduction and adducts forward and medially toward the center of the body, and horizontal abduction happens as the arm starts at 90 degrees of abduction and moves outward, away from the body. Elevation is the angle made between the thorax and arm, regardless if it is in the abduction plane, flexion plane, or in between.

2. Evaluation of movement—Range of motion of the injured shoulder should be compared with the opposite shoulder, along with the strength during abduction and rotation. This should be done both passively and actively. The shoulder should be inspected for any changes in synchrony, such as scapular winging, elevation of the scapula, muscle fasciculations indicating abnormal function, and any other irregular or asymmetric movements of the scapula. Information may be gained on loss of flexibility and instability resulting from muscle imbalance, fibrosis, and tendon, capsular, or ligament contractures. Loss of flexibility usually occurs in the capsular tissues of the glenohumeral joint. Sudden pain or clicking may indicate an intraarticular problem. Loss of motion in either internal or external rotation is suggestive of a chronic anterior or posterior dislocation, respectively.

3. Provocative tests—Specific tests are then performed that aid in making the correct diagnosis. The specific tests for instability, impingement syndrome, bicipital tendonitis, and superior capsulolabral/biceps anchor lesions are discussed later.

Imaging & Other Studies

Many varieties of radiologic views and projections are available to examine shoulder injuries. An initial radiographic evaluation of the shoulder should consist of an anteroposterior view of the glenohumeral joint in both internal and external rotation, and an axillary lateral. Additional plain radiographic views depend on the underlying pathology. MRI may be indicated in evaluation of rotator cuff disorders recalcitrant to conservative treatment. An MR arthrogram may be useful in detecting labral pathology. Traditional arthrography is rarely indicated because it is invasive and has little or no advantage over MRI. Ultrasonography is also useful in diagnosis of rotator cuff injury, but it is operator dependent. Electromyographic examination can be useful in identifying shoulder pain of cervical origin.

Arthroscopic Evaluation

A. INDICATIONS FOR ARTHROSCOPIC EVALUATION OF SHOULDER INJURIES

Indications for arthroscopic examination of the shoulder include the following:

Table 4–3. History and physical examination of the shoulder.

	History	Physical Examination
Cuff tendonitis	Pain over the lateral shoulder with overhead activity Night pain Mild weakness	Neer and Hawkin impingement signs Normal ROM Mild weakness Pain relieved with lidocaine injection into the subacromial space
Cuff tear	Pain over the lateral shoulder with overhead activity Night pain Weakness Loss of ROM	Neer and Hawkin impingement signs Loss of active ROM Weakness Pain relieved with lidocaine injection into the subacromial space
Instability	Joint "slips" out Pain and feelings of instability with shoulder abduction and external rotation (anterior instability only) Asymptomatic with the shoulder at rest	Apprehension of instability with shoulder abduction and external rotation (anterior instability only) Apprehension of instability with shoulder abduction and external rotation relieved by relocation test (if anterior instability only)
AC joint instability (separation)	History of fall onto the "point" of the shoulder Pain on top of the shoulder Pain with cross-body movements Bump at the AC joint	Tenderness at AC joint Deformity at AC joint: acromion displaced inferior to the distal clavicle Pain with cross-body movements Pain relieved with lidocaine injection into the AC joint
AC joint arthritis	Pain on top of the shoulder Pain with cross-body movements	Tenderness at AC joint Pain with cross-body movements Pain relieved with lidocaine injection into the AC joint
Stiffness	Decreased ROM Pain with shoulder at rest but worse at the limits of ROM	Decreased active and passive ROM Pain relieved with lidocaine injection into the glenohumeral joint
Arthritis	Decreased ROM Pain with shoulder at rest but worse with motion Crepitus with motion	Decreased active and passive ROM Crepitus with motion Pain relieved with lidocaine injection into the glenohumeral joint
Biceps tendonitis	Pain over the anterior shoulder with activity	Speed and Yerguson tests Tenderness at the bicipital groove Pain relieved with a lidocaine injection into the bicipital groove

AC = acromioclavicular; ROM = range of motion.

1. impingement syndrome including subacromial bursitis, rotator cuff tendonitis, and rotator cuff tears;
2. acromioclavicular joint osteoarthritis;
3. loose bodies;
4. chronic synovitis;
5. glenohumeral instability;
6. superior capsulolabral/biceps anchor lesions; and
7. adhesive capsulitis (frozen shoulder).

B. TECHNIQUE

With the patient either in the lateral decubitus or the beach chair position, the arthroscope is inserted into a posterior portal, medial and inferior to the posterolateral

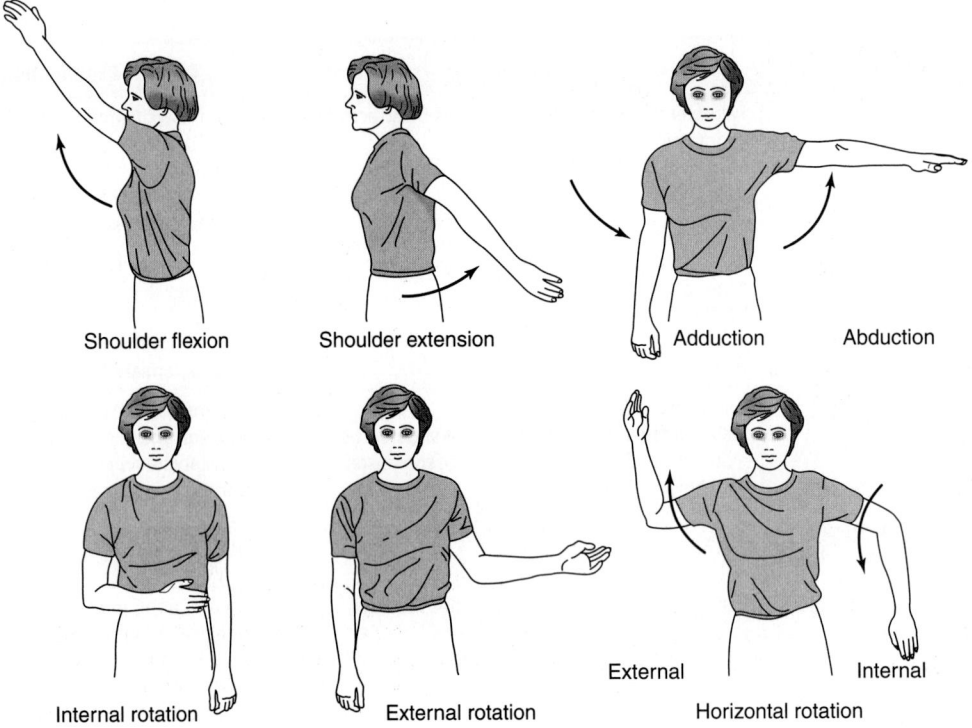

Figure 4–23. Description of shoulder motion.

corner of the acromion. With visualization of the gleno-humeral joint, an anterior portal immediately lateral to the coracoid allows additional inflow and entrance of additional instruments. Distal clavicle excision, removal of loose bodies, and capsular release of adhesive capsulitis can be performed. An additional anterior portal inferior to the first is required for instability repair with an arthroscopic technique. The arthroscope is then removed from the joint and placed into the subacromial bursa. Portals lateral to the acromion allow subacromial decompression and rotator cuff repair to be carried out with arthroscopic techniques.

C. STEPS IN EVALUATION

Examination of shoulder range of motion and stability with the patient under anesthesia is helpful in the diagnosis and treatment of shoulder injuries. This should be performed in the operating room prior to arthroscopy. The steps in arthroscopic examination should then include the following:

1. glenohumeral articular surfaces;
2. rotator cuff from inside the joint;
3. labrum including the biceps anchor;
4. anterior capsuloligamentous structures;
5. rotator cuff from the subacromial bursal space;
6. coracoacromial ligament;
7. acromion; and
8. acromioclavicular joint

Applegate GR et al: Chronic labral tears: Value of magnetic resonance arthrography in evaluating the glenoid labrum and labral-bicipital complex. Arthroscopy 2004;20:959. [PMID: 15525929]

Kaplan LD et al: Internal impingement: Findings on magnetic resonance imaging and arthroscopic evaluation. Arthroscopy 2004;20:701. [PMID: 15346111]

Lee DH et al: The double-density sign: A radiographic finding suggestive of an os acromiale. J Bone Joint Surg Am 2004;86-A:2666. [PMID: 15590851]

Lindauer KR et al: MR imaging appearance of 180–360 degrees labral tears of the shoulder. Skeletal Radiol 2005;34:74. [PMID: 15668822]

Magee T, Williams D, Mani N: Shoulder MR arthrography: Which patient group benefits most? AJR Am J Roentgenol 2004;183:969. [PMID: 15385288]

Middleton WD, Teefey SA, Yamaguchi K: Sonography of the rotator cuff: Analysis of interobserver variability. Am J Roentgenol 2004;183:1465. [PMID: 15505321]

Porcellini G et al: Arthroscopic treatment of calcifying tendinitis of the shoulder: Clinical and ultrasonographic follow-up findings at two to five years. J Shoulder Elbow Surg 2004;13:503. [PMID: 15383805]

Figure 4–24. The cycle of injury and reinjury resulting from rotator cuff impingement.

SHOULDER TENDON & MUSCLE INJURY

Rotator Cuff Tendon Injuries

Injury to the rotator cuff, a common cause of shoulder pain and disability, has a high prevalence during athletic activities. Injury of the rotator cuff may result in pain, weakness, and decreased range of motion. Symptoms are often worsened by activity, especially when the hand is positioned overhead. Night pain is also common, and many complain of awakening after rolling onto the affected shoulder. Although shoulder weakness and decreased range of motion usually result from a rotator cuff tendon tear, pain alone from subacromial bursitis or rotator cuff tendonitis may also be the cause. Each of these entities most often results from impingement syndrome.

Impingement Syndrome

Any prolonged repetitive overhead activity such as tennis, pitching, golf, or swimming may cause compromise of the space between the humeral head and the coracoacromial arch that includes the acromion, coracoacromial ligament, and the coracoid process. Impingement causes microtrauma to the rotator cuff, resulting in local inflammation, edema, cuff softening, pain, and poor function. These problems may even cause greater impingement, producing a continuous vicious cycle (Figure 4–24). This cycle may be precipitated by acute injury to the rotator cuff tendon itself. Blood supply to this tendon is precarious, thus decreasing its capacity for healing.

1. Subacromial Bursitis

Clinical Findings

Bursitis of the shoulder refers to the inflammation of the subacromial bursa. It has the mildest signs and symptoms of shoulder impingement. Pain is present with overhead activity, and there is usually no or mild pain with the arm at the side.

Active range of shoulder motion is limited by pain. No atrophy of the shoulder muscles is present, and manual muscle testing demonstrates mild weakness. Passively, when the internally rotated shoulder is moved into forward flexion, the patient experiences discomfort. This is called the Neer impingement sign (Figure 4–25). Injection of 10 mL of lidocaine into the subacromial space resolves the pain, and there is a dramatic increase in strength and range of motion with the Neer impingement test.

Radiographic views of the subacromial space, such as the supraspinatus outlet view, may show a spur on the undersurface of the acromion, causing narrowing of the subacromial space. Advances in imaging methods, such as ultrasonography and MRI, now aid in diagnosis of subacromial bursitis, rotator cuff tendonitis, and rotator cuff tendon tear (Figure 4–26).

Treatment & Prognosis

Treatment for impingement syndrome starts with conservative measures such as activity modification, physical therapy, and oral antiinflammatory medications. Activity modification is necessary to minimize overhead arm motion and effect a return to normal overhead throwing biomechanics. Modalities such as heat and cold, iontophoresis or phonophoresis, and microelectric nerve stimulation may also be helpful. Only with normal function of the rotator cuff tendons do glenohumeral mechanics improve and the impingement syndrome cease. If this treatment fails, a subacromial injection of corticosteroids may be helpful.

Surgical intervention is indicated only after failure of a prolonged conservative treatment program (a minimum of 3 months). If the subacromial space is narrow,

Figure 4–25. Evaluating for impingement of the supraspinatus tendon with the "empty can" test.

A   **B**

Figure 4–26. MRI demonstrating (**A**) normal shoulder anatomy and (**B**) cystic changes at the greater tuberosity with rotator cuff tear (*arrow*).

release of the coracoacromial ligament combined with shaving the undersurface of the acromion (known as acromioplasty or subacromial decompression) may result in relief of symptoms. This can be done with an arthroscopic technique to decrease postoperative discomfort and minimize the complication of deltoid muscle injuries.

Never has there been more controversy about this surgical procedure. It has been used since the 1930s to diminish symptoms associated with rotator cuff injury. The classic rationale for its efficacy is that any prolonged repetitive overhead activity, such as tennis, pitching, golf, or swimming, may cause compromise of the space between the humeral head and the coracoacromial arch, which includes the acromion, coracoacromial ligament, and the coracoid process. Known as impingement syndrome, microtrauma to the rotator cuff results in local inflammation, edema, cuff softening, pain, and poor function. These problems may even cause greater impingement, producing a continuous vicious cycle. This cycle may also be precipitated by acute injury to the rotator cuff tendon itself. Blood sup-

ply to this tendon is precarious, thus decreasing its capacity for healing. Removing subacromial spurs as well as increasing the size of the subacromial space may release pressure on the cuff tendons, ending the vicious cycle and allowing for healing.

Other rationales are proposed for the efficacy of subacromial decompression in treating rotator cuff injuries. The subacromial space, including the subacromial bursa and the subacromial periosteum, is richly innervated, primarily by branches of the suprascapular nerve. Subacromial decompression results in denervation of the subacromial space. Others have found increased inflammatory factors in the subacromial bursa of shoulders with rotator cuff injury that may normalize after subacromial decompression.

Rotator cuff pathology is associated with the shape and geometry of the acromion, especially if there is acromial encroachment onto the supraspinatus tendon. Bigliani and Morrison introduced a commonly used classification to describe the shape of the acromion in 1986. They found a higher incidence of rotator cuff tears in hooked (type III) acromions than in flat (type I) and curved (type

II) acromions. However, several studies show poor to moderate interobserver reliability of this classification, regardless if the clinicians used radiographs, MRI, or cadaveric scapulas to classify the acromions. Routine use of subacromial decompression in the treatment of rotator cuff tears is now questioned. A newer prospective, randomized study of rotator cuff repair found no statistical difference in outcome whether or not a subacromial decompression was done. To confuse matters even more, a study of nearly a hundred patients followed for nearly a decade found subacromial decompression may not prevent progression of impingement syndrome to a tear.

2. Rotator Cuff Tendonitis

Clinical Findings

Of the four rotator cuff muscles, the supraspinatus tendon is most often initially involved. Rotator cuff tendonitis also results from impingement syndrome and is characterized by pain with overhead activity. The patient may occasionally be awakened by pain at night. Active shoulder range of motion is limited by pain. Typically, no atrophy of the shoulder muscles is present and manual muscle testing demonstrates mild weakness. The Neer impingement sign is positive and the pain resolves with subacromial injection of lidocaine.

Treatment & Prognosis

Radiographic evaluation and treatment are similar to subacromial bursitis management. An exception is the athlete less than 40 years old with glenohumeral instability and secondary tendonitis. In this case, the instability should be treated first and the rotator cuff tendonitis then resolves.

3. Rotator Cuff Tendon Tear

Clinical Findings

A rotator cuff tendon tear is characterized by pain with overhead activity. However, the patient is often also awakened at night with pain. The athlete with a chronic rotator cuff tear may describe a gradual loss of strength. Pain may be persistent, occurring even with the arm at the side.

Active range of shoulder motion is limited, and if the tear is severe, there will be atrophy of the shoulder muscles. Manual muscle testing demonstrates weakness. The Neer impingement sign is positive, and the pain resolves with subacromial injection of lidocaine.

Treatment & Prognosis

Radiographic evaluation and treatment are similar to subacromial bursitis management. Unlike acute tears, chronic rotator cuff tears often present insidiously, with slow progression from subacromial bursitis to rotator cuff tendonitis and eventual tendon tear. Differentiating severe rotator cuff tendonitis from partial or small full-thickness chronic rotator cuff tears may be a difficult task.

Tears are most common at the humeral insertion site of the supraspinatus tendon, where stress is greatest with the joint in abduction. Tears may be partial thickness or involve the full thickness of the tendon. The size may be small (less than 1 cm), medium (1–3 cm), large (3–5 cm), or massive (more than 5 cm). Chronic rotator cuff tears may result partly from degeneration within the rotator cuff tendon. Poor vascularity and repetitive activity, especially in the athlete with a restricted subacromial space, may be contributing factors. A minor traumatic event may also cause a full-thickness tear in an athlete with mild or moderate tendon degeneration.

If the tear is small, a prolonged period of rest, lasting 4–9 months, may relieve symptoms. Range-of-motion exercises are also recommended, unless they cause significant discomfort. If this fails to control the symptoms, surgical repair of the tear is recommended. The thin degenerated tissue of a chronic rotator cuff tear makes surgical repair more difficult than repair of an acute tear. Surgical decompression of the subacromial space to remove spurs should also be considered.

Rehabilitation lasts from 6 months to a year with gradual exercise progression needed to restore normal, or near-normal function, and strength. This varies with the tear size repaired and type of surgery performed. Typically, immediately after the procedure, passive motion and isometric strengthening exercises start, along with elbow, hand, and grip strengthening exercises. At 6 weeks, the athlete may be able to begin low-intensity active strengthening exercises against gravity. The goals are to bring the athlete to normal strength with a functional, pain-free range of motion.

Although the lesion location and size are helpful in describing the rotator cuff tear, symptoms do not correlate with these factors alone. Both epidemiologic and imaging studies indicate a high incidence of partial-thickness rotator cuff tears at younger ages and a high incidence of full-thickness rotator cuff tears at older ages. Small full-thickness rotator cuff tears may be asymptomatic as long as the force couple of the anterior and posterior rotator cuff is preserved. Instead, a number of other factors influence the severity of symptoms, including acute/chronic nature of injury, patient age, activity level, humeral head superior migration, shoulder muscle strength, arthritis, pain tolerance, and workers' compensation status.

Partial-Thickness Rotator Cuff Tear

A partial articular sided tendon avulsion is much more common than a bursal side tear of the rotator cuff. As with other rotator cuff injuries, symptoms may resolve with appropriate physical therapy and analgesics. Yet some individuals with a partial-thickness tear have persistent or recurrent symptoms. If a conservative program of exercises and gradual return to activity does not lead to steady improvement, then further diagnostic evaluation with ultrasonography, MRI, or arthroscopy may be helpful. Arthroscopic debridement of the abnormal cuff may promote healing in athletes with partial-thickness posttraumatic tears. Following debridement, immediate resumption of range-of-motion and muscle-strengthening exercises begins. Typically, it requires 6–12 months for a throwing athlete to return to athletics following arthroscopic debridement of a partial-thickness rotator cuff tear.

Gartsman GM, O'Connor DP: Arthroscopic rotator cuff repair with and without arthroscopic subacromial decompression: A prospective, randomized study of one-year outcomes. J Shoulder Elbow Surg 2004;13:424. [PMID: 15220883]

Hyvonen P, Lohi S, Jalovaara P: Open acromioplasty does not prevent the progression of an impingement syndrome to a tear. Nine-year follow-up of 96 cases. J Bone Joint Surg Br 1998;80:813. [PMID: 9768891] See comment as well in J Bone Joint Surg Br 1999;82:743.

Klepps S et al: Prospective evaluation of the effect of rotator cuff integrity on the outcome of open rotator cuff repairs. Am J Sports Med 2004;32:1716. [PMID: 15494338]

Lam F, Mok D: Open repair of massive rotator cuff tears in patients aged sixty-five years or over: is it worthwhile? J Shoulder Elbow Surg 2004;13:517. [PMID: 15383807]

Millstein ES, Snyder SJ: Arthroscopic evaluation and management of rotator cuff tears. Orthop Clin North Am 2003;34:507. [PMID: 14984190]

O'Holleran JD et al: Determinants of patient satisfaction with outcome after rotator cuff surgery. J Bone Joint Surg Am 2005;87-A:121. [PMID: 15634822]

Rebuzzi E et al: Arthroscopic rotator cuff repair in patients older than 60 years. Arthroscopy 2005;21:48. [PMID: 15650666]

Romeo AA et al: Shoulder scoring scales for the evaluation of rotator cuff repair. Clin Orthop 2004;(427):107. [PMID: 15552145]

Sperling JW, Cofield RH, Schleck C: Rotator cuff repair in patients fifty years of age and younger. J Bone Joint Surg Am 2004;86-A:2212. [PMID: 15466730]

BICEPS TENDON INJURIES

1. Bicipital Tendinitis

Clinical Findings

The long head of the biceps muscle is an intraarticular structure deep in the rotator cuff tendon as it passes under the acromion to its insertion at the top of the glenoid. The same mechanism that initiates impingement syndrome symptoms in rotator cuff injuries may inflame the tendon of the biceps in its subacromial position, causing bicipital tendinitis. Tendinitis may also result from subluxation of the tendon out of its groove in the proximal humerus, which occurs with rupture of the transverse ligament. The symptoms of bicipital tendinitis, whether the result of impingement or tendon subluxation, are essentially the same. Pain is localized to the proximal humerus and shoulder joint, with resisted supination of the forearm aggravating the pain. Pain may also occur on manual testing of the elbow flexors and on palpation of the tendon itself. The Yergason test is used to test for instability of the long head of the biceps in its groove.

Treatment & Prognosis

If the tendinitis is associated with shoulder impingement, therapy aimed at treating the impingement syndrome relieves the bicipital tendinitis. If subluxation of the tendon within its groove is the cause of the irritation, conservative therapy includes NSAIDs and restriction of activities, followed by a slow resumption of activities after a period of rest. Strengthening of the muscles that assist the biceps in elbow flexion and forearm supination is also beneficial. Steroid injections into the sheath of the biceps tendon are helpful, but they may be hazardous if placed into the substance of the tendon because they promote tendon degeneration. Persistent symptoms may warrant tenodesis of the biceps tendon directly into the humerus. Recovery from this procedure is difficult, and it is doubtful if a competitive athlete could return to peak performance after such a procedure.

2. Biceps Tendon Rupture

Clinical Findings

The long head of the biceps tendon may rupture proximally, either from the supraglenoid tubercle of the scapula at the entrance of the bicipital groove proximally or at the exit of the tunnel at the musculotendinous junction. The muscle mass moves distally, producing a bulging appearance to the arm. Rupture of the long head of the biceps is predictive of a rotator cuff tear. Rupture of the biceps distally at its insertion involves both heads, and the muscle mass moves proximally. The mechanism is usually a forceful flexion of the arm and is more common in older athletes (greater than 50 years old) or with direct trauma. Microtears probably serve to render the tendon vulnerable to an acute tearing event. The degree of ecchymosis depends on the location of the tear, with avascular areas having less and the musculotendinous junction producing quite a noticeable amount of ecchymosis. Diagnosis is usually easily obvious because the deformity is evident.

Treatment & Prognosis

Surgical treatment of proximal ruptures, if indicated, is usually reserved for patients less than 40 years old. Open surgical repair leaves a long scar and usually does not completely restore the underlying anatomy. The coiled-up distal end of the tendon is usually found beneath the attachment of the pectoralis major. A correlation exists between proximal biceps tendon rupture and rotator cuff tears in middle-age and older athletes (more than 50 years old). Rupture of the distal biceps tendon often warrants surgical repair because of loss of forearm flexion and supination strength. In this case, the tendon is usually found approximately 5–6 cm above the elbow joint, and care must be taken to avoid damage to the lateral antebrachial cutaneous nerve.

Cope MR, Ali A, Bayliss NC: Biceps rupture in body builders: Three case reports of rupture of the long head of the biceps at the tendon-labrum junction. J Shoulder Elbow Surg 2004; 13:580. [PMID: 15383821]

Vidal AF, Drakos MC, Allen AA: Biceps tendon and triceps tendon injuries. Clin Sports Med 2004;23:707. [PMID: 15474231]

PECTORALIS MAJOR RUPTURE

Rupture of the pectoralis major tendon is an uncommon injury, usually occurring during bench press exercises in weight lifting caused by sudden unexpected muscle contraction during pulling or lifting. The athlete usually experiences sudden pain and develops local ecchymosis and swelling. As the swelling subsides, a sulcus and deformity may be visible, and the patient notices weakness of the arm in adduction and internal rotation. The rupture may be partial or complete, and nonoperative treatment usually results in satisfactory function for the activities of daily life. Surgery may be considered if the athlete wishes to return to heavy weight lifting.

Aarimaa V et al: Rupture of the pectoralis major muscle. Am J Sports Med 2004;32:1256. [PMID: 15262651]

GLENOHUMERAL JOINT INSTABILITY

To make the correct diagnosis, the glenohumeral joint must be tested for anterior, posterior, and inferior instability. Different classifications of glenohumeral joint instability are proposed, based on etiology, the direction of the instability, or on various combinations. TUBS is an acronym describing instability caused by a *t*raumatic event, which is *u*nidirectional, associated with a *B*ankart lesion, and often requires *s*urgical treatment. AMBRI refers to *a*traumatic, *m*ultidirectional instability that may be *b*ilateral and is best treated by *r*ehabilitation. In this classification, the etiology of multidirectional instability is thought to be enlargement of the capsule from genetic or microtraumatic origin.

The positive sulcus sign is used as the diagnostic hallmark for multidirectional instability, but we now know that the sulcus sign is sometimes found in asymptomatic shoulders of individuals with increased laxity. Laxity or joint play is a trait of body constitution that differs from one individual to another. Individuals may be loose or tight jointed. A shoulder is hyperlax if the examiner can easily subluxate the humeral head out of the glenoid in the anterior, posterior, and inferior directions without eliciting symptoms. Unfortunately, this makes classification of instability based on etiology, or direction alone, extremely difficult. Instead, classification is best based on the direction of instability that elicits symptoms and the presence or absence of hyperlaxity (Table 4–4).

Gerber C, Nyffeler RW: Classification of glenohumeral instability. Clin Orthop 2002;400:65. [PMID: 12072747]

Glenohumeral Joint Instability Evaluation

A. ANTERIOR INSTABILITY

The apprehension test is performed to assess anterior instability. The test applies an anterior directed force to the humeral head from the back with the arm in abduction and external rotation (Figure 4–27). A positive test results from the patient's apprehension that the joint will dislocate. This maneuver mimics the position of subluxation, or dislocation, and causes reflex guarding. Conversely, the relocation test is positive if relief is obtained by applying a posterior directed force to the humeral head (Figure 4–28).

B. POSTERIOR INSTABILITY

No single test has high sensitivity and specificity for posterior instability. The posterior apprehension test is performed by applying a posterior directed force to the forward flexed and internally rotated shoulder. To per-

Table 4–4. Classification of glenohumeral instability based on the direction of instability and the presence or absence of hyperlaxity.

Laxity \ Direction	UDI (Unidirectional Instability)	MDI (Multidirectional Instability)
Normal laxity	Very common 60%	Very rare 3%
Increased laxity	Common 30%	Rare 7%

Adapted, with permission, from Gerber C: Observations of the classification of instability. In Warner JJP et al eds: *Complex and Revision Problems in Shoulder Surgery.* Lippincott-Raven, 1997:9–18.

Figure 4–27. The apprehension test for anterior instability.

form the circumduction test, the patient is instructed to move the shoulder actively in a large circle starting from a flexed, internally rotated and cross-body position, then to forward flexion, then to an abducted and externally rotated position, and lastly to the arm at the side. The examiner stands behind the patient and palpates the posterior shoulder. If positive, the joint subluxes in the flexed, internally rotated, and cross-body position, and it reduces as the shoulder is moved. For the Jahnke test, a posteriorly directed force is applied to the forward flexed shoulder. The shoulder is then moved into the coronal plane as an anterior directed force is applied to the humeral head. A clunk occurs as the humeral head reduces from the subluxed position (Figure 4–29).

Figure 4–28. The relocation test is positive if relief is obtained by applying a posterior directed force to the humeral head.

C. INFERIOR INSTABILITY

The sulcus sign is used to evaluate laxity and inferior instability. The test is performed with the athlete in a sitting position with the arm at the side. A distraction force is applied longitudinally along the humerus. If positive, discomfort or apprehension of instability are experienced as the skin just distal to the lateral acromion hollows out (Figure 4–30).

A

B

Figure 4–29. The Jahnke test for posterior instability. **A:** A posterior directed force applied to the forward flexed shoulder (in the upper left column). **B:** The shoulder is then moved into the coronal plane as an anterior directed force is applied to the humeral head (in the lower left column). A clunk occurs as the humeral head reduces from the subluxed position. (Reprinted, with permission, from Hawkins RJ, Bokor DJ: Clinical evaluation of shoulder problems. In Rockwood CA et al (eds): *The Shoulder.* WB Saunders, 1998, p. 186.)

Figure 4–30. The sulcus test for inferior instability. (Reprinted, with permission, from Hawkins RJ, Bokor DJ: Clinical evaluation of shoulder problems. In Rockwood CA et al (eds): *The Shoulder*. WB Saunders, 1998, p. 189.)

1. Glenohumeral Dislocation

When the shoulder is forced beyond the limit of its normal range of motion, the articular surface of the humeral head may displace from the glenoid to varying degrees. The majority of glenohumeral dislocations, or subluxations, are in the anteroinferior direction.

Anterior Dislocation

A. CLINICAL FINDINGS

Anterior glenohumeral dislocation occurs from either an external rotation or abduction force on the humerus, a direct posterior blow to the proximal humerus, or a posterolateral blow on the shoulder large enough to displace the humeral head. The anterior capsule is either stretched or torn within its attachment to the anterior

glenoid. The head may be displaced into a subcoracoid, subglenoid, subclavicular, or intrathoracic position. Two major lesions are typically seen in patients with recurrent anterior dislocations (Figure 4–31). First is the Bankart lesion, an anterior capsular injury associated with a tear of the glenoid labrum off the anterior glenoid rim. The Bankart lesion may occur with fractures of the glenoid rim. Such fractures are often minimally displaced, and treatment is usually dictated by the joint instability. The second major lesion associated with recurrent anterior dislocations is the Hill-Sachs lesion, a compression fracture of the posterolateral articular surface of the humeral head. It is created by the sharp edge of the anterior glenoid as the humeral head dislocates over it. When large, both the Bankart and the Hill-Sachs lesions predispose to recurrent dislocations when the arm is placed in abduction and external rotation. If the glenoid rim fracture involves greater than 20% of the glenoid diameter, the joint becomes prone to instability and treatment with open reduction and internal fixation is indicated. If the fracture is old or the glenoid rim is worn to a similar level, corticocancellous bone grafting of the glenoid rim is indicated.

Other injuries associated with anterior dislocation may occur. These include avulsion of the greater tuberosity from the humerus, caused by traction from the rotator cuff, and injury to the axillary nerve, which may be stretched or torn. Permanent loss of axillary nerve function results in denervation of the deltoid muscle and loss of sensation over the proximal lateral aspect of the arm. Axillary nerve palsy may also occur during

ANATOMIC LESIONS

Figure 4–31. Anatomic lesions producing shoulder instability.

reduction of the dislocation, and therefore it should be tested both before and after reduction. The deltoid extension lag sign, described later in the section on axillary nerve injuries, may be the best way to assess function of this nerve. Lastly, the dead arm syndrome may occur after anterior joint instability. For example, a pitcher may report sudden inability to throw, with the arm going numb and becoming extremely weak after the ball release. The symptoms are transient, resolving within a few seconds to minutes.

Athletes who sustain a shoulder dislocation try to hold the injured extremity at the side, gripping the forearm with the opposite hand. Most athletes know their shoulder is dislocated, and they seek help immediately. On physical examination of an anterior dislocation, the examiner notes a space underneath the acromion where the humeral head should lie and a palpable anterior mass representing the humeral head in the anterior axilla.

B. TREATMENT AND PROGNOSIS

One must distinguish between acute and recurrent anterior glenohumeral dislocations because an acute dislocation sustains severe trauma with the increased probability of associated injuries. The recurrent dislocation may occur with minimal trauma, and reduction may be accomplished with much less effort. Anterior dislocations may be reduced by one of several techniques. Longitudinal traction may be exerted on the affected arm with external rotation, followed by internal rotation of the arm. Care must be taken to avoid direct pressure on the neurovascular structures. Another method is to have the patient lie face down on the table and tie or tape a bucket to the injured arm and slowly fill it with water. This allows the musculature around the shoulder to relax from the force of the weight and effects the spontaneous reduction.

Following reduction of an initial dislocation, the shoulder should be immobilized in internal rotation for 2–6 weeks. Healing generally takes at least 6 weeks. Before returning to athletics, the patient should have normal range of motion without pain, and normal strength in the shoulder. Emphasis must be placed on strengthening the rotator cuff muscles to compensate for the laxity of the ligamentous support. When weight training is begun, military press, fly exercises, a narrow grip while bench pressing, and deep shoulder dips must be excluded until considerable time elapses and complete healing is realized.

Recurrent dislocations should be treated with minimal immobilization until the pain subsides, followed by range-of-motion and muscle-strengthening exercises. Many restraining devices are available to help prevent recurrent dislocations during sporting activities, focusing on keeping the arm from going into abduction and external rotation. These orthotics may be effective, but because they limit the athlete's range of shoulder motion, their use is limited for certain competitive activities.

If an athlete has sustained multiple dislocations and is unresponsive to conservative treatment, surgical reconstruction of the shoulder joint may be indicated. There are a wide variety of procedures to correct the instability, with most involving repair of the labral defect and tightening of the anterior capsule and ligamentous structures through an anterior incision (Table 4–5).

For most surgical procedures, aggressive range-of-motion exercises do not start until at least 3 weeks postoperatively. The goal is to have full abduction and 90 degrees of external rotation. By 12 weeks, patients are often progressing well into their initial programs and may begin a variety of weight training exercises, avoiding exercises that strain the anterior capsule.

Posterior Dislocation

A. CLINICAL FINDINGS

Posterior glenohumeral dislocations result from the posterior capsule being torn, stretched, or disrupted from the posterior glenoid. A reverse Hill-Sachs lesion (Figure 4–31) may appear on the anterior articular surface of the humerus. With a posterior dislocation, the

Table 4–5. Repair of capsule and labrum back to the glenoid rim.

Bankart procedure
duToit procedure
Viek procedure
Eyre-Brook procedure
Moseley procedure
Muscle and capsule plication
Putti-Platt procedure
Symeonides procedure
Muscle and tendon sling procedures
Magnuson-Stack procedure
Bristow-Helfet-Latarjet procedure modifications
Boytchev procedure
Nicola procedure
Gallie-LeMesurier procedure
Boyd transfer of long head of biceps (for posterior dislocation)
Bone block
Eden-Hybbinette procedure
DeAnquin procedure (through a superior approach to the shoulder)
Osteotomies
Weber (humeral neck)
Saha (humeral shaft)

subscapularis, or its insertion on the lesser tuberosity, may be injured. Posterior dislocations are often difficult to diagnose because the patient may have a normal contour to the shoulder or the deltoid of a well-developed athlete may mask signs of a displaced humeral head. The patient holds the injured shoulder in internal rotation and the examiner cannot rotate it externally. Anteroposterior radiographs can be misleading, and axillary views must be obtained to diagnose a posterior dislocation.

B. TREATMENT AND PROGNOSIS

Applying traction in the line of the adducted humerus, with an anterior directed force to the humeral head, reduces a posterior dislocation. Anesthesia often helps decrease the trauma of reduction. Following reduction, the shoulder is immobilized for 2–6 weeks in external rotation and a small amount of abduction. Surgical treatment should be considered if these measures fail to provide the desired results.

Multidirectional Instability

A. CLINICAL FINDINGS

Some patients have instability in both the anterior and posterior directions, most often subluxation and not dislocation. This situation may result in a painful shoulder, especially if rotator cuff strength decreases. The pain is often primarily a result of rotator cuff inflammation, likely from attempts to stabilize the humeral head during activity.

B. TREATMENT AND PROGNOSIS

A rotator cuff strengthening program is often successful treatment.

Brophy RH, Marx RG: Osteoarthritis following shoulder instability. Clin Sports Med 2005;24:47. [PMID: 15636776]

Good CR, Macgillivray JD: Traumatic shoulder dislocation in the adolescent athlete: Advances in surgical treatment. Curr Opin Pediatr 2005;17:25. [PMID: 15659959]

Kim SH et al: Loss of chondrolabral containment of the glenohumeral joint in atraumatic posteroinferior multidirectional instability. J Bone Joint Surg Am 2005;87-A:92. [PMID: 15634818]

Kim SH et al: Painful jerk test: A predictor of success in nonoperative treatment of posteroinferior instability of the shoulder. Am J Sports Med 2004;32:1849. [PMID: 15572311]

Kirkley A et al: Prospective randomized clinical trial comparing the effectiveness of immediate arthroscopic stabilization versus immobilization and rehabilitation in first traumatic anterior dislocations of the shoulder: Long-term evaluation. Arthroscopy 2005;21:55. [PMID: 15701612]

Krishnan SG et al: A soft tissue attempt to stabilize the multiply operated glenohumeral joint with multidirectional instability. Clin Orthop 2004;(429):256. [PMID: 15577496]

GLENOID LABRUM INJURY

Clinical Findings

The glenoid labrum is a fibrocartilaginous rim around the glenoid fossa that deepens the socket and provides stability for the humeral head. It also is a connection for the surrounding capsuloligamentous structures. Glenoid labrum tears may occur from repetitive shoulder motion or acute trauma. In the athlete with repeated anterior subluxation of the shoulder, tears of the anteroinferior labrum may occur, leading to progressive instability.

Weight lifters may also develop glenoid labrum tears from repetitive bench pressing and overhead pressing. Weakness in the posterior rotator cuff may aggravate this condition. Tears of the glenoid labrum may also occur from acute trauma such as falling on an outstretched arm, but they are also seen in the leading shoulders of golfers and batters when they ground their clubs or bats.

Patients with glenoid labrum injuries may describe their pain as interrupting smooth functioning of the shoulder during their specific activity. On examination, they may have discomfort on forced external rotation at 90 degrees of abduction, with the pain typically not increasing as the arm goes into further abduction. Frequently, a labrum disruption may be felt as a pop or click on forced external rotation. The patient may also experience discomfort on forced horizontal adduction of the shoulder. Manual muscle testing may show associated weakness in the rotator cuff muscles. Diagnostic tests such as a CT scan and MRI following injection of contrast dye into the shoulder joint may allow early detection of glenoid labrum lesions.

Treatment & Prognosis

Range-of-motion exercises and gradual return to activity are often successful in relieving symptoms. However if nonoperative management fails, arthroscopic intervention may be indicated to debride a torn symptomatic labrum. During arthroscopy, care must be taken not to debride the inferior labrum because this may result in increased anterior shoulder instability, escalating the probability of anterior shoulder dislocation. Immediately following surgery, range-of-motion exercises and strengthening training begin. Usually within 2–3 weeks following surgery, the athlete may begin a throwing program. Baseball pitchers may be ready to throw 3 months postoperatively.

SLAP LESIONS

The use of shoulder arthroscopy in the diagnosis and treatment of shoulder disorders has led to increased awareness of superior labrum anterior posterior (SLAP) lesions. SLAP lesions involve the origin of the long head of the biceps brachii (biceps anchor) and the superior capsulolabral structures. A type I lesion has degeneration or fraying of the labrum without instability. Type II lesions are most common, accounting for more than 50% of patients with a SLAP lesion, and they involve detachment of the superior labrum from the glenoid. A type III lesion has a bucket-handle tear of the superior labrum with firm attachment of the remainder of the labrum. Type IV lesions also remain attached to the labrum, but they have an associated bucket-handle tear of the labrum that extends into the biceps tendon (Figure 4–32).

Types V through VII SLAP lesions were later added to this initial four-part classification. A type V lesion is an anterior-inferior Bankhart lesion that continues superiorly to include separation of the biceps tendon. A type VI lesion includes a biceps separation with an unstable flap tear of the labrum. Finally, a type VII is a superior labrum-biceps tendon separation that extends anteriorly beneath the middle glenohumeral ligament.

Figure 4–32. The five types of the SLAP lesion include fraying of the superior capsulolabrum (type 1), detachment of the superior capsulolabrum and the biceps anchor (type 2), bucket-handle tearing of the superior capsulolabrum (type 3), detachment of the superior capsulolabrum and tearing into the biceps anchor (type 4), and combinations of these (type 5).

Clinical Findings

Patients present with nonspecific shoulder pain associated with activity. A complicating factor in making the diagnosis is that the majority of SLAP lesions are associated with other shoulder pathology, such as rotator cuff tears, acromioclavicular joint pathology, and instability. Less than 28% of SLAP lesions are isolated.

No single test is both sensitive and specific for diagnosis of SLAP lesions. magnetic resonance arthrography (MRA) can be helpful. However, diagnostic arthroscopy remains the best means to diagnose SLAP lesions definitively. The active compression test may prove to be the most useful single provocative maneuver. The internally rotated shoulder is forward flexed to 90 degrees and then brought across the body in horizontal abduction of approximately 10 degrees. The test is positive if the patient has pain with resisted forward flexion that is relieved by external rotation of the shoulder.

Treatment

Treatment of SLAP lesions can be simplified by noting whether or not the lesion contributes to detachment of either the biceps anchor or the anterosuperior capsulolabrum. Lesions producing meaningful detachment of the anterior capsuloligamentous structures generally require repair of these structures back to the bony glenoid rim. Lesions producing significant defects extending into the biceps tendon may require biceps tenotomy, with or without tenodesis.

Holtby R, Razmjou H: Accuracy of the Speed's and Yergason's tests in detecting biceps pathology and SLAP lesions: comparison with arthroscopic findings. Arthroscopy 2004;20:231. [PMID: 15007311]

Musgrave DS, Rodosky MW: SLAP lesions: Current concepts. Am J Sports Med 2001;30:29. [PMID: 11198828]

Parentis MA, Mohr KJ, El-Attrache NS: Disorders of the superior labrum: Review and treatment guidelines. Clin Orthop 2002;400:77. [PMID: 12072748]

SHOULDER STIFFNESS

Clinical Findings

Often called adhesive capsulitis or frozen shoulder, shoulder stiffness is a painful condition characterized by significant restriction in both active and passive range of motion. The shoulder is characterized as being stiff when the articular surfaces are normal and the joint is stable, yet there is a restriction in range of motion. Stiffness may also result from pathologic connections between the articular surfaces, soft-tissue contracture, bursal adhesions, or a shortened muscle–tendon unit. Often of uncertain etiology, the restrictions of shoulder motion are global. That is, none of the shoulder planes of motion is spared.

Shoulder stiffness may be separated into idiopathic and posttraumatic etiologies. Idiopathic shoulder stiffness is most common in older individuals, especially women between 40 and 60 years of age. Other factors that predispose to idiopathic shoulder stiffness include cervical, cardiac, pulmonary, neoplastic, neurologic, and personality disorders. Patients with diabetes mellitus are also at a high risk of developing shoulder stiffness, with 10–35% of diabetics having restriction of shoulder motion. Diabetics who have been insulin dependent for many years have the greatest incidence and bilateral involvement. The pathophysiology of idiopathic shoulder stiffness remains uncertain, but the pathoanatomy is commonly limited to contracture of the glenohumeral capsule (Figure 4–33). Most prominently involved is the rotator interval that includes the coracohumeral ligament.

Although all patients can recall some traumatic event that preceded their shoulder stiffness, those with distinct trauma such as a prior fracture, rotator cuff tear, or surgical procedure have a posttraumatic etiology. Stiffness after shoulder surgery is typical and usually resolves with time and appropriate rehabilitation. But the shoulder should not be neglected after any surgery about the shoulder girdle. This includes axillary or cervical lymph node dissections, especially when combined with radiation therapy, cardiac catheterization in the axilla, coronary artery bypass grafting with sternotomy, and thoracotomy. All surgeons should be aware that these procedures may result in restricted shoulder motion.

The clinical presentation of idiopathic shoulder stiffness is classically described as having three phases. The first phase is the painful, freezing phase. The pain is typically achy, and sudden jolts or attempts at rapid motion exacerbate the chronic discomfort. The pain may begin at night, and shoulder motion becomes progressively limited. Patients often hold their arm at their side and in internal rotation with the forearm across the belly. They may also be treated for nonspecific shoulder pain with a sling in this position. This inflammatory phase often lasts between 2 and 9 months.

The second phase of progressive stiffness lasts between 3 and 12 months. Stiffness progresses to the point where shoulder motion is restricted in all planes. Essentially, the shoulder has undergone fibrous arthrodesis. Fortunately, pain progressively decreases from the initial inflammatory phase. With time, patients are able to use the shoulder with little or no pain, within the restricted range of motion, but attempts to exceed this range are accompanied by pain. The patient's symptoms then plateau. Unfortunately, this phase may be persistent with symptoms lasting for extended periods. In the resolution, or thawing phase, the shoulder slowly and progressively becomes more supple. It can be as short as a month but typically lasts 1–3 years.

Figure 4–33. Adhesive capsulitis of the shoulder. Note the small irregular joint capsule with addition of contrast material.

On clinical examination, there is loss of both active and passive range of shoulder motion. Often the first motion to be affected is internal rotation demonstrated by an inability to bring the arm up the back to the same level as the normal shoulder. Radiographic confirmation of adhesive capsulitis may be done by arthrography, which demonstrates marked reduction in the capacity of the joint. Often the affected shoulder does not take more than 2–3 mL of dye, although normal capacity is 12 mL.

Treatment & Prognosis

Treatment varies, but conservative modalities and progressive range-of-motion exercises seem effective. Range-of-motion exercises for external rotation and abduction help minimize the length of restriction in motion and dysfunction. Manipulation under anesthesia, long the mainstay of intervention, is being replaced by selective arthroscopic capsular release. Short-term results indicate a quicker return of motion. Whether treated with rehabilitation alone or with capsular release, a return of approximately 80% shoulder range of motion is usual.

Ide J, Takagi K: Early and long-term results of arthroscopic treatment for shoulder stiffness. J Shoulder Elbow Surg 2004; 13: 174. [PMID: 14997095]

Nicholson GP: Arthroscopic capsular release for stiff shoulders: Effect of etiology on outcomes. Arthroscopy 2003;19:40. [PMID: 12522401]

Wolf JM, Green A: Influence of comorbidity on self-assessment instrument scores of patients with idiopathic adhesive capsulitis. J Bone Joint Surg Am 2002;84-A:1167. [PMID: 12107317]

FRACTURES ABOUT THE SHOULDER

CLAVICULAR FRACTURE

The clavicle is one of the most commonly fractured bones in the body, with direct trauma being the usual cause in athletic events (Figure 4–34). Football, wrestling, and ice hockey are the sports most commonly involved in clavicular fractures, which is not surprising because all three are associated with high-speed contact between players.

Clinical Findings

Despite the proximity of vital structures, clavicular fractures that occur during athletic activities are rarely associated with neurovascular damage, and accompanying soft tissue disorders are uncommon. The patient usually gives a history of falling in the area of the shoulder or receiving a blow to the clavicle, experiencing immediate pain and inability to raise the arm. Radiography usually confirms the clinical impression and must show the entire clavicle, including the shoulder girdle, upper third of the humerus, and sternal end of the clavicle. Midclavicular fractures account for 80% of clavicular fractures, with distal fractures at 15% and proximal fractures at 5%. Most fractures of the shaft of the clavicle heal well. The potential for a rare but serious neurovascular complication, such as a tear of the subclavian artery or brachial plexus injury, must be kept in mind when evaluating and treating clavicular fractures, and a neurovascular examination on initial evaluation is very

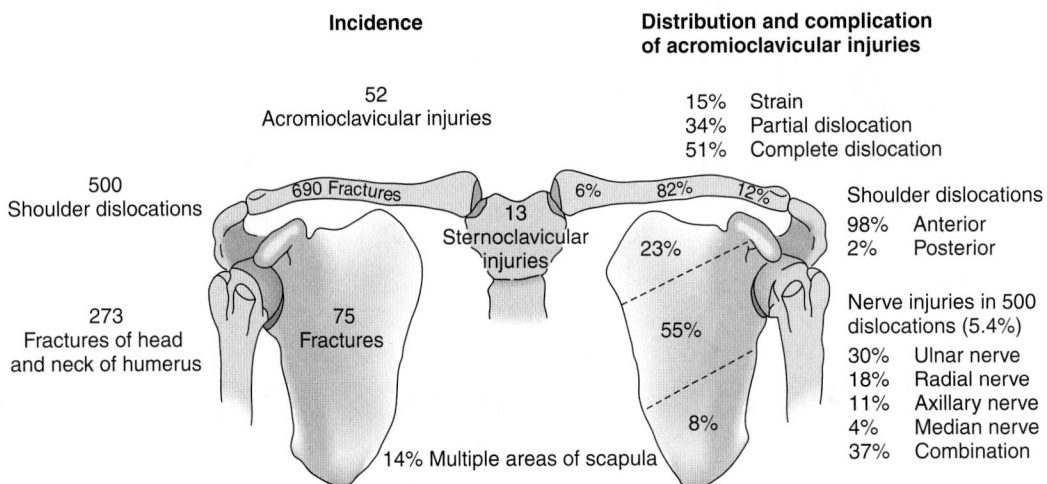

Figure 4–34. Analysis of 1603 shoulder girdle injuries, showing the frequency and location of fractures and dislocations.

important. Pulses in the distal part of the upper extremity, strength, and sensation must be carefully evaluated.

Because the clavicle is the single bone structure that fixes the shoulder girdle to the thorax, a fracture through the clavicle causes the shoulder to sag forward and downward. The pull of the sternocleidomastoid muscle may displace the proximal fragment superiorly. These forces tend to hinder the initial reduction and maintenance of reduction. In addition, distal fractures, which are more common in older age groups (more than 50 years old), may involve tears in the coracoclavicular ligament, which allows the proximal clavicle to ride up superiorly mimicking an acromioclavicular dislocation. Delayed union in this type of fracture is a much greater possibility than with other clavicular fractures.

Treatment & Prognosis

Mid and proximal clavicular fractures are usually treated with a short period of rest, and a sling may be used on the affected side to support the extremity. Immobilization is usually discontinued at 3–4 weeks, and once the clavicular fracture heals, range-of-motion and strengthening exercises should begin. Onset of exercises prior to healing may result in nonunion. Athletes should not be allowed to return to play until achieving their preinjury shoulder strength and range of motion. Generally, no special braces or pads are required when the athlete returns to play.

Grassi FS, Tajana MS, D'Angelo F: Management of midclavicular fractures: Comparison between nonoperative treatment and open intramedullary fixation in 80 patients. J Trauma 2001; 50:1096. [PMID: 11426125]

Robinson CM, Cairns DA: Primary nonoperative treatment of displaced lateral fractures of the clavicle. J Bone Joint Surg Am 2004;86-A:778. [PMID: 15069143]

Robinson CM, Court-Brown CM, McQueen MM et al: Estimating the risk of nonunion following nonoperative treatment of a clavicular fracture. J Bone Joint Surg Am 2004;86-A:1359. [PMID: 15252081]

PROXIMAL HUMERUS FRACTURE

Fractures of the proximal humerus, which represent approximately 4–5% of all fractures, are a relatively uncommon sports injury. They most often present in the early adolescent with open growth plates or in elderly (more than 70 years old) osteoporotic patients. When they do occur in the athlete, they are typically the result of a high-energy impact injury or are secondary to an underlying pathologic bone condition.

Clinical Findings

The proximal humerus consists of four major bony components: the humeral head, the greater tuberosity,

the lesser tuberosity and the humeral shaft. Fractures can occur between any or all of these regions, and they are traditionally defined by the location and displacement of the fracture fragments (see Figure 3–15). The patient with a proximal humerus fracture usually is able to report the mechanism of injury and complains of pain, swelling, and inability to use the shoulder. Physical examination often reveals loss of the normal contour of the shoulder, tenderness about the shoulder, ecchymosis that may extend down to the elbow, and crepitus on attempted range of motion. A thorough neurovascular exam is essential because brachial plexus and axillary nerve injuries are reported in association with proximal humerus fractures. Because the axillary nerve is the most commonly injured nerve in these cases, sensation to light touch and pinprick over the lateral aspect of the upper arm and deltoid muscle function must be tested. Accurate radiographic evaluation is necessary to confirm the type and severity of the fracture and is essential in determining the treatment plan. Necessary views include anteroposterior and lateral views in the plane of the scapula as well as an axillary view to rule out an associated glenohumeral dislocation.

Treatment & Prognosis

Most proximal humerus fractures are minimally displaced and can be treated nonoperatively with sling immobilization and early passive range of motion. However, an estimated 20% of these fractures should be treated operatively. Many factors contribute to this decision-making process, including fracture type and degree of displacement, bone quality, activity level, and associated injuries. Surgical options range from closed reduction and percutaneous pinning to open reduction with internal fixation to humeral head replacement.

For minimally displaced fractures, the prognosis is generally good. Loss of motion is the most common complication. It can take 12–18 months to attain the maximal result, so range-of-motion exercises should be continued for an extended period of time.

Fankhauser F et al: A new locking plate for unstable fractures of the proximal humerus. Clin Orthop 2005;430:176.

Iannotti JP, Ramsey ML, Williams GR et al: Nonprosthetic management of proximal humeral fractures. J Bone Joint Surg Am 2003;85:1578. [PMID: 15116630]

Robinson CM, Aderinto J: Posterior shoulder dislocations and fracture dislocations. J Bone Joint Surg Am 2005;87-A(3):639.

PROXIMAL HUMERAL EPIPHYSEAL FRACTURE

In skeletally immature athletes, epiphyseal fractures of the proximal humerus may occur. The separate growth centers of the articular surface, greater tuberosity, and lesser tuberosity coalesce at approximately 7 years of age, with the remaining growth plates closing at 20–22 years of age. Therefore, fracture separations may occur at any age until the growth plates close. Fortunately, fractures in this area usually do not arrest growth.

Injury can occur to the shoulder of the growing musculoskeletal system from overhead throwing sports. Proximal humerus pain, especially while throwing and associated with widening of the proximal humerus epiphysis, is termed *little league shoulder*. Although widening of the proximal humerus epiphysis can be an adaptive change to throwing, when painful it may represent an overuse fracture.

Dobbs MB et al: Severely displaced proximal humeral epiphyseal fractures. J Pediatr Orthop 2003;23:208. [PMID: 12604953]

Karatosun V et al: Treatment of displaced, proximal, humeral, epiphyseal fractures with a two-prong splint. J Orthop Trauma 2003;17:578. [PMID: 14504580]

ACROMIOCLAVICULAR JOINT INJURY

Clinical Findings

Acromioclavicular dislocations or subluxations, commonly referred to as separations, vary in severity depending on the extent of injury to the stabilizing ligaments and capsule. The typical mechanism of injury is a direct downward blow to the tip of the shoulder. Clinically, pain at the top of the shoulder over the acromioclavicular joint is the predominant symptom, with varying decreases in motion depending on the severity of the injury. The athlete who has sustained this type of injury typically leaves the field holding the arm close to the side.

When checking for instability of the acromioclavicular joint, the examiner should manipulate the midshaft of the clavicle, rather than the acromioclavicular joint, to rule out pain from contusion to the acromioclavicular area. For milder acromioclavicular injuries, the patient should put the hand of the affected arm on the opposite shoulder, and the examiner may then gently apply downward pressure at the patient's affected elbow, noting if this maneuver causes pain at the acromioclavicular joint.

Acromioclavicular joint injuries were initially divided into grades I through III (Figure 4–35). Grade I injuries are typically produced by a mild blow causing a partial tear of the acromioclavicular ligament. When the acromioclavicular ligament is completely torn, but the coracoclavicular ligament remains intact, a grade II injury that involves subluxation or partial displacement results. When the force of injury is severe enough to tear the coracoclavicular and acromioclavicular ligaments in addition to the capsule, a grade III injury occurs.

Three additional injuries were later added to the classification. In grade IV injuries, the clavicle is displaced posteriorly and buttonholed through the fascia of the trapezius muscle. Grade V injuries demonstrate

Figure 4–35. Grades of acromioclavicular joint separations.

severe inferior displacement of the glenohumeral joint, with the clavicle often 300% superior to the acromion. Lastly, in grade VI injuries, the distal end of the clavicle is locked inferior to the coracoid.

Acromioclavicular joint displacement is often obvious on physical examination, but it is best classified by radiography. An anteroposterior radiograph that is aimed 10 degrees cephalad allows visualization of the acromioclavicular joint. A radiograph of the entire upper thorax allows the vertical distance between the coracoid and the clavicle on both the involved and uninvolved sides to be compared. Anteroposterior radiographs with weights applied to the upper extremities are usually unnecessary. An axillary lateral radiograph is also essential for proper classification.

Treatment & Prognosis

Management of acromioclavicular joint injuries depends on their severity. Grade I and grade II injuries may be treated with a sling until discomfort dissipates, usually within 2–4 weeks. Next, a rehabilitation program starts, and normal range of motion and strength to the upper extremity begins to be restored. The treatment of grade III injuries or complete dislocations in athletes is controversial. Most feel that grade III injuries are best managed nonoperatively; others advocate operative treatment. Grade IV through VI injuries are best treated with open reduction and internal fixation along with reconstruction of the coracoclavicular ligament.

Nonsurgical treatment may either be a sling for comfort or an acromioclavicular sling to try to achieve reduction. The fit of the device must apply pressure to the distal clavicle sufficient to afford reduction, but not great enough to compromise the skin. Ice and other modalities are used for the acute acromioclavicular injury to reduce soreness and swelling. Pain is the limiting factor in beginning range-of-motion and isometric muscle strengthening exercises. It should be used as a guide for gradual initiation and escalation of these physical therapy regimes. Isotonic exercises may then follow because isometric exercises are more effective earlier when range of motion is limited.

Before resuming athletic activities, the patient must have full range of pain-free motion and no tenderness upon direct palpation of the acromioclavicular joint or pain when manual traction is applied. Athletes who do not require elevation of the arm, such as soccer or football players, tend to return to sports earlier than players who require overhead arm activity, such as tennis, baseball, and swimming athletes.

Fractures of the coracoid process are rare, usually seen in professional riflemen and skeet shooters, although they are also reported in baseball and tennis players. They are identified radiographically, and conservative treatment, including cessation of activity, usually results in uncomplicated healing after 6–8 weeks.

Dumonski M et al: Evaluation and management of acromioclavicular joint injuries. Am J Orthop 2004;33:526. [PMID: 15540856]

Su EP et al: Using suture anchors for coracoclavicular fixation in treatment of complete acromioclavicular separation. Am J Orthop 2004;33:256. [PMID: 15195920]

STERNOCLAVICULAR JOINT INJURY

In the skeletally mature adult athlete, injury to the sternoclavicular joint usually consists of the surrounding soft tissue and capsule tearing, leading to subluxation or dislocation. The mechanism of injury is either a blow to the point of the shoulder, which predisposes to anterior dislocation, or a direct blow to the clavicle or chest with the shoulder in extension, which predisposes to posterior dislocation. The injury may range from a symptomatic sprain to a complete sternoclavicular dislocation with disruption of the capsule and its restraining ligaments.

Anterior Dislocation

The most common type of sternoclavicular dislocation is anterior dislocation, which is recognized clinically by an anterior prominence of the proximal clavicle on the involved side. Radiographic documentation of an anterior sternoclavicular dislocation is difficult because of overlapping of the rib, sternum, and clavicle at the joint, but it may be confirmed by oblique views. A CT scan is usually very sensitive and should be done if radiographic appear normal but the diagnosis is suspected.

Although dislocation of the anterior sternoclavicular joint may cause considerable distress initially, the symptoms usually subside rapidly, with no loss of shoulder function. A variety of surgical and nonsurgical approaches are advocated, but most feel that surgery for anterior dislocations results in significant complications. Closed treatment modalities vary from a sling alone to attempted closed reduction, which may be successful initially but is difficult to maintain.

Posterior Dislocation

Posterior sternoclavicular dislocation is much less common but has more complications because of the potential for injury to the esophagus, great vessels, and trachea. Presenting symptoms range from mild to moderate pain in the sternoclavicular region to hoarseness, dysphagia, severe respiratory distress, and subcutaneous emphysema from tracheal injury.

In most instances, closed reduction of posterior dislocations, if performed early, are successful and stable. To effect reduction, a pillow is placed under the upper back of the supine patient and gentle traction is applied with the shoulder held in 90 degrees of abduction and at maximum extension (Figure 4–36). Rarely, closed reduction under general anesthesia or open reduction is required.

Figure 4–36. Method for reducing (**A**): anterior sternoclavicular dislocation and (**B**): posterior sternoclavicular dislocation.

After reduction, the patient is put in an immobilization splint, instructed to use ice and antiinflammatory agents. Once the joint heals sufficiently, usually within 2–3 weeks, range-of-motion exercises may begin. Elevation of the arm should not be attempted until 3 weeks after injury.

Medial Clavicular Epiphyseal Fracture

In athletes younger than 25 years, sternoclavicular injuries may not result in true dislocations but rather in fractures through the growth plate of the proximal clavicle. These clavicular epiphyseal fractures may appear clinically as dislocations, especially if some displacement is present, and they may be treated conservatively. Typically, these are not associated with growth deformities, and reduction of the fracture is not needed unless there is severe displacement. Symptomatic treatment for pain usually suffices. Sometimes an adolescent presents with an enlarging mass at the sternoclavicular joint and parents are worried about cancer. A careful history reveals trauma several weeks earlier, and the mass represents the callus of a healing clavicular epiphyseal fracture that can be demonstrated radiographically.

Battaglia TC et al: Interposition arthroplasty with bone-tendon allograft: A technique for treatment of the unstable sternoclavicular joint. J Orthop Trauma 2005;19:124. [PMID: 15677929]

SHOULDER NEUROVASCULAR INJURY

Brachial Plexus Injury

Brachial plexus injuries are typically caused by a fall on the shoulder as seen in acromioclavicular joint injuries. Most brachial plexus injuries do not involve motor loss and exhibit paresthesias, which resolve in a period of minutes to weeks, although some cases may persist for months or years. Early in the course of the injury, a transient slowing of conduction across the plexus or a mild prolongation of nerve latency possibly is seen. The "burner" or "stinger" is one of the most common brachial plexus injuries encountered in athletes. The key to diagnosis is short duration of upper extremity paresthesias and shoulder weakness, with pain-free range of motion of the cervical spine. Players may return to competition after shoulder strength and full pain-free range of motion returns.

Rarely, a severe injury occurs (eg, from motorcycle racing). Chronic injuries result in instability of the shoulder that may be treated with trapezius transfer. Arthrodesis is an alternative, initially or after failed muscle transfer.

Peripheral Nerve Injury

A. LONG THORACIC NERVE INJURY

Traction incidents may cause a long thoracic nerve palsy, with subsequent serratus anterior paralysis and winging of the scapula. Traction and blunt trauma may also cause injury to the spinal accessory nerve, another cause of winging of the scapula. These can be differentiated on physical examination by the position of the scapula. With serratus anterior palsy, the inferior portion of the scapula tends to go medially, whereas the opposite occurs with spinal accessory nerve palsy. Treatment is usually conservative, with return of function in weeks if the nerve is not divided.

Safran MR: Nerve injury about the shoulder in athletes, part 2: Long thoracic nerve, spinal accessory nerve, burners/stingers, thoracic outlet syndrome. Am J Sports Med 2004;32:1063. [PMID: 15150060]

B. SUPRASCAPULAR NERVE INJURY

Entrapment of the suprascapular nerve is often associated with activities such as weight lifting, baseball pitching, volleyball, and backpacking. Traction and repetitive shoulder use are the mechanisms of injury. Compression of the nerve may occur from entrapment at the anterior suprascapular notch of the scapula or at the level of the spinoglenoid notch. The latter occurs in volleyball players and baseball players likely caused by rapid overhead acceleration of the arm. Compression is associated with poorly localized pain and weakness in the posterolateral aspect of the shoulder girdle. This may be followed by atrophy of the supraspinatus or infraspinatus muscles. Eventually, there is weakness of forward flexion and external rotation of the shoulder. The diagnosis is confirmed by electromyography and nerve conduction studies.

Conservative therapy consists of rest, antiinflammatory medication, and physical therapy designed to increase muscular tone and strength. If this is unsuccessful, then surgical exploration is indicated, which may reveal hypertrophy of the transverse scapular ligament, anomalies of the suprascapular notch, and ganglion cysts. Results of surgery vary with the lesion discovered, but many patients return to full function postoperatively.

Safran MR: Nerve injury about the shoulder in athletes, part 1: Suprascapular nerve and axillary nerve. Am J Sports Med 2004; 32:803. [PMID: 15090401]

C. MUSCULOCUTANEOUS NERVE INJURY

The musculocutaneous nerve is susceptible to damage from direct frontal blows or surgical procedures. Injury is associated with numbness in the lateral forearm to the base of the thumb and weak to absent biceps muscle function. Most injuries seen in sports are transient and respond to conservative treatment in a matter of days to weeks.

Lo IK, Burkhart SS, Parten PM: Surgery about the coracoid: neurovascular structures at risk. Arthroscopy 2004;20:591. [PMID: 15241309]

D. AXILLARY NERVE INJURY

The usual mechanism of injury is trauma either by direct blow to the posterior aspect of the shoulder or following dislocation of the shoulder or fracture of the proximal humerus. Axillary nerve injury occurs in many sports, such as football, wrestling, gymnastics, mountain climbing, rugby, and baseball. The degree of injury to the nerve varies because the initial presentation may be mild weakness during elevation and abduction of the arm with or without numbness of the lateral arm. The deltoid extension lag sign is indicative of axillary nerve injury. To perform this test, the examiner elevates the arm into a position of near full extension and then releases the arm while asking the patient to hold the arm in this position. If there is complete deltoid paralysis, the arm drops. For partial nerve injuries, the magnitude of the angular drop, or lag, is an indicator of deltoid strength. Approximately 25% of all dislocated shoulder injuries are associated with axillary nerve traction injuries, which respond well to rest, physical therapy, and time. If recovery is not complete within 3–6 months, surgical intervention is recommended with exploration, utilizing neurolysis or grafting, or both, as necessary. Results of surgery are usually favorable, with sensory recovery occurring before motor recovery.

Hertel R et al: The deltoid extension lag sign for diagnosis and grading of axillary nerve palsy. J Shoulder Elbow Surg 1998; 7:97. [PMID: 9593085]

THORACIC OUTLET SYNDROME

The symptoms resulting from thoracic outlet compression may be neurologic, venous, or arterial. Obstruction of the subclavian vein may lead to stiffness, edema, and even thrombosis of the limb. Arterial obstruction may be the result of direct compression and manifests with pallor, coolness, and forearm claudication. Doppler examination reveals changes in arterial and venous flow. Electromyography and nerve conduction studies are also helpful in diagnosis.

Nonoperative treatment is recommended for less severe forms of this syndrome, and once the pain subsides, an exercise program to strengthen the pectoral girdle muscles is beneficial. Special exercises to strengthen the upper and lower trapezius, along with the erector spinae and serratus anterior muscles, yields good results. Correcting poor posture and an ongoing maintenance program are mandatory once improvement is reached. Progression of symptoms or failure of nonoperative treatment are indications for surgical exploration and correction of the pathologic factors encountered.

Degeorges R, Reynaud C, Becquemin JP: Thoracic outlet syndrome surgery: Long-term functional results. Ann Vasc Surg 2004;18:558. [PMID: 15534735]

ELBOW INJURIES

EPICONDYLITIS (TENNIS ELBOW)

Tennis elbow is the term given to many painful conditions about the elbow. An anatomic location may usually be found and specific diagnosis made.

Lateral Epicondylitis

Lateral tennis elbow involves the common tendon to the extensor muscles of the wrist and hand. Patients who perform repetitive wrist extension against resistance (such as the backhand stroke in tennis) are at risk. Their pain is usually chronic and more bothersome than disabling. Tenderness is located over the lateral humeral epicondyle, and pain is produced by extending the wrist against resistance. The tendon of the extensor carpi radialis brevis is identified as the most common site of the lesion. Other causes for lateral elbow pain should be considered, including radiocapitellar arthritis and posterior interosseous nerve compression. Radiographs only rarely reveal soft-tissue calcification near the lateral humeral epicondyle, and MRI is of questionable aid in making the diagnosis.

Treatment includes decreasing specific activities and using a tennis elbow band to distribute the tension of the muscular pull over a larger area, thereby decreasing the force per unit area. A lighter racquet, smaller grip on the racquet, and correcting backhand technique are also helpful. Exercises to strengthen the wrist extensor muscles should be included in the treatment plan. If this approach fails, an injection of local anesthetic and cortisone into the most tender region is often curative. Surgical treatment is needed in recalcitrant cases. Multiple procedures are described to take care of this malady. Commonplace in all procedures is release of the common extensor origin. Histologic studies of the afflicted tendon show degenerative changes with angiofibroblastic proliferation. These are thought to be similar to the pathologic changes of the torn rotator cuff, with diminished vascularity, an altered nutritional state, and tearing of the susceptible tendon.

Medial Epicondylitis

Medial epicondylitis involves the common flexor pronator origin. Treatment is similar to the management of lateral tennis elbow. Ulnar nerve compression at the elbow may occur in conjunction with medial tennis elbow. In approximately 60% of the cases treated surgically, ulnar nerve compression was present. The common flexor origin is an important medial stabilizer of the elbow, so if surgical treatment is indicated, the debrided tendon should be reattached rather than released from the medial epicondyle.

Ciccotti MC, Schwartz MA, Ciccotti MG: Diagnosis and treatment of medial epicondylitis of the elbow. Clin Sports Med 2004;23:693 [PMID: 15474230]

Jobe FW, Ciccotti MG: Lateral and medial epicondylitis of the elbow. J Am Acad Orthop Surg 1994;2:1. [PMID: 10708988]

ELBOW INSTABILITY

Rupture of the collateral ligaments of the elbow occurs most commonly from elbow dislocation. This can result from excessive valgus force, and initially the ulnar collateral ligament ruptures. Excessive posterolateral rotatory force may also result in rupture of the lateral ulnar collateral ligament. In either case, the elbow may dislocate, and typically the direction is posterior. Treatment after relocation and brief immobilization consists of active range-of-motion exercises. Recurrent instability is rare, and instead a small loss of elbow extension, usually less than 10 degrees, commonly results.

Valgus Instability

Valgus instability may result from overuse in overhead throwing sports, such as baseball, football, and javelin throwing. With acute medial collateral ligament rupture, a pop may be felt during a throw. Tenderness is present on the medial side of the elbow, usually just distal to the medial epicondyle. Instability can then be appreciated when a valgus force is applied to the elbow. This must be done with the elbow flexed 20 degrees because failure to unlock the olecranon from within the olecranon fossa in full extension creates a false sense of stability. Compari-

son to the contralateral side aids in making the correct diagnosis. If the ulnar collateral ligament was injured but remains intact, the valgus stress test may elicit pain but no instability. Then the so-called milking maneuver (Figure 4–37) also elicits pain along the medial side of the elbow. Eliciting pain while moving the elbow in flexion and extension with valgus stress during the milking maneuver may be the best test for diagnosing medial collateral ligament injuries in the elbow.

A stress radiograph may aid in making the diagnosis. An anteroposterior radiograph can be taken while the examiner performs the valgus stress test. Alternatively, gravity can be used to apply the valgus stress. For this, an anteroposterior radiograph of the elbow is taken with the shoulder externally rotated at 90 degrees with the elbow flexed at approximately 20 degrees. When instability is present, there will be a wider medial opening than on the contralateral normal side. MRI may also be useful, especially if an arthrogram is performed concurrently, because dye leaking through the ulnar collateral ligament is diagnostic of a rupture.

Surgical repair may be indicated in overhead throwing athletes who suffer an acute rupture of their ulnar collateral ligament and still want to continue to participate in their sport. Soccer players, basketball players, and other athletes participating in nonoverhead throwing may be treated with a program of early active range-of-motion exercises with expectation of full return to their sport. Chronic ulnar collateral ligament injuries resulting from overuse are best treated with rehabilitation, NSAIDs, and avoidance of throwing for as long as 3 months. Only those with residual pain and instability after participation in such a program should undergo reconstruction of the anterior band of the ulnar collateral ligament. In this surgery, pioneered by Dr. Frank

Figure 4–37. The valgus stress and milking maneuver tests for medial ulnar collateral ligament injury. (Reprinted, with permission, from Chen FS et al: Medial elbow problems in the overhead-throwing athlete. J Am Acad Orthop Surg 2001;9(2):102.)

Jobe, the palmaris longus tendon is woven through drill holes in the medial humeral epicondyle and olecranon. Nearly 70% of athletes are able to return to highly competitive throwing after such surgery.

Chen FS, Rokito AS, Jobe FW: Medial elbow problems in the overhead-throwing athlete. J Am Acad Orthop Surg 2001; 9(2):99.

O'Driscoll SW, Lawton RL, Smith AM: The "moving valgus stress test" for medial collateral ligament tears of the elbow. Am J Sports Med 2005;33:231. [PMID: 15701609]

Thompson WH et al: Ulnar collateral ligament reconstruction in athletes: Muscle-splitting approach without transposition of the ulnar nerve. J Shoulder Elbow Surg 2001;10:152. [PMID: 11307079]

Posterolateral Rotatory Instability

Posterolateral rotatory instability of the elbow may result from a fall on the outstretched upper extremity, surgery of the lateral side of the elbow, or chronic varus stress as may occur in long-term crutch walkers. The instability covers a spectrum of severity from mild subluxation to recurrent dislocation. Those with mild forms complain of intermittent symptoms on the lateral side of the elbow associated with supination of the forearm, such as pain, snapping, or catching. More severe symptoms include locking or sensations of elbow instability. To perform the posterolateral rotatory instability test, a valgus stress is applied to the supinated elbow with the patient supine and the upper extremity over the head (Figure 4–38). Subluxation of the radial head occurs with the elbow in extension and resolves when the elbow is flexed. This maneuver also reproduces the patient's symptoms. A lateral stress radio-graph, done with the elbow in extension as described for the posterolateral rotatory instability test, may also demonstrate the instability (see Figure 4–38). Treatment for acute cases consists of an elbow brace to hold the forearm in pronation and restricted terminal elbow extension for 6 weeks. Chronic cases are best treated with reconstruction of the lateral ulnar collateral ligament. Postoperatively the patient is put in the same brace as used for acute posterolateral rotatory instability for 6–12 weeks.

Olsen BS, Sojbjerg JO: The treatment of recurrent posterolateral instability of the elbow. J Bone Joint Surg Br 2003;85:342 [PMID: 12729105]

Sanchez-Sotelo J, Morrey BF, O'Driscoll SW: Ligamentous repair and reconstruction for posterolateral rotatory instability of the elbow. J Bone Joint Surg Br 2005;87:54. [PMID: 15686238]

OTHER ELBOW OVERUSE INJURIES

Posterior Elbow Impingement

Impingement may result from mechanical abutment of bone and soft tissues in the posterior elbow, which may or may not be associated with injury of the ulnar collateral ligament. Hyperextension injuries with an intact ulnar collateral ligament occur in gymnasts, football linemen, weight lifters, and others. The lesion is usually located in the center of the posterior elbow, and the pain is reproduced by forcible extension of the elbow. If there is insufficiency of the ulnar collateral ligament, as is often the case when there is posterior elbow impingement in overhead athletes, the lesion is posteromedial. In this case, the impingement is between the medial aspect of the olecranon and the lateral side of the medial

Figure 4–38. The posterolateral rotatory instability test reproduces the patient's symptoms.

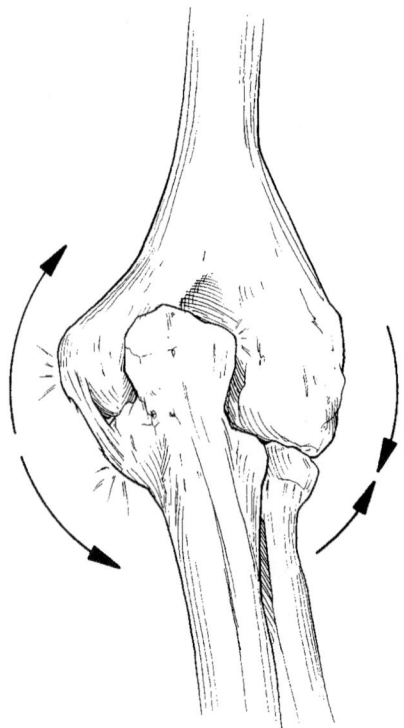

Figure 4–39. Mechanism of posteromedial impingement between the medial aspect of the olecranon and the lateral side of the medial wall of the olecranon fossa. (Reprinted, with permission, from Chen FS et al: Medial elbow problems in the overhead-throwing athlete. J Am Acad Orthop Surg 2001;9(2):105.)

wall of the olecranon fossa (Figure 4–39). Pain may be reproduced with the valgus stress test as described earlier for valgus instability, but the pain is posteromedial and medial. Radiographs may demonstrate osteophytes of the olecranon of the olecranon fossa.

As with most injuries caused by repetitive trauma, treatment begins with prevention. The number of innings pitched is probably the most important factor relating to injury. If symptoms persist, removal of osteophytes is successful treatment, providing no ulnar collateral ligament injury is present. Treatment of the valgus instability is also required for successful outcome.

Moskal MJ, Savoie FH III, Field LD: Arthroscopic treatment of posterior elbow impingement. Instr Course Lect 1999;48:399. [PMID: 10098066]

Fatigue Fracture of the Medial Epicondyle

In children, fatigue fractures of the medial epicondyle cause pain and swelling. This was blamed on throwing curve balls, but some studies show that a properly thrown

curve ball causes no more injuries than the traditional fastball. Prevention or minimization of damage involves several steps. First, it is important to maintain proper conditioning by continuing pitching practice in the off-season or beginning the baseball season in a slow progressive fashion. Second, pain and inflammation should be avoided, and if the elbow becomes painful, the athlete should stop throwing immediately. An accurate pitching count should be kept during a game, and a stopping point should be planned in advance. If the pitcher begins having pain or shows loss of control, pitching should be temporarily terminated, and treatment to decrease the swelling and inflammation should begin. No competitive throwing is allowed until full range-of-motion returns and no pain or tenderness is associated with throwing.

Osteochondritis Dissecans of the Capitellum

Osteochondritis dissecans of the capitellum usually affects pitchers older than 10 years (Figure 4–40). Changes in the radiocapitellar joint are very worrisome because of possible permanent loss of function. If fragmentation occurs, loose bodies may require excision.

Stubbs MJ, Field LD, Savoie FH: Osteochondritis dissecans of the elbow. Clin Sports Med 2001;20:1. [PMID: 11227698]

Figure 4–40. AP view of an elbow with osteochondritis dissecans of the capitellum.

SPINE INJURIES

CERVICAL SPINE INJURY

Cervical spine injuries in athletes are relatively infrequent, but the potential for serious injury to the nervous system exists. If spine injury is suspected, it is wise to be extremely cautious until a proper diagnosis can be made. This is the best way to prevent conversion of a repairable injury to a catastrophic outcome. Most often, a spine injury results from a collision, and sometimes it includes associated head injuries. The head and neck must be immobilized right away, and ease of breathing and level of consciousness ascertained immediately.

1. Brachial Plexus Neurapraxia

The most common cervical injury is pinching or stretching neurapraxia of the nerve root and brachial plexus. The injury is of short duration, and the patient has a full pain-free range of motion of the neck. These injuries are commonly called "stinger" or "burner" injuries. They result from lateral impact of the head and neck with simultaneous depression of the shoulder. This may cause stretching and pinching of the nerves of the brachial plexus, with burning pain, numbness, and tingling extending from the shoulder down into the hand and arms. Symptoms frequently involve the C5 and C6 root levels. Recovery is usually spontaneous within a few minutes after the acute episode.

Patients who demonstrate full muscle strength of the intrinsic muscles of the shoulder and upper extremity and have full pain-free range of motion of the cervical spine may return to their activities. If they have residual weakness or numbness, they should not be allowed to re-enter the game. Absence of neck pain should alert one to the possibility of a cervical spine injury, as neck pain is not part of the syndrome.

Persistence of paresthesia or weakness requires further evaluation before returning to play. This includes neurologic, electromyographic, and radiographic evaluation. The athlete should not participate in contact sports until full muscle strength is achieved and a repeat electromyogram shows evidence of axonal regeneration, usually at least 4–6 weeks.

Prevention of so-called stinger injuries is chiefly through correct head and neck techniques and strengthening of the neck musculature. Additionally, the use of cervical rolls may eliminate extremes of motion during impact.

2. Cervical Strain

Acute strains of the muscles of the neck are probably the most frequent cervical injuries in athletes. The word *strain* implies injury to a muscle, whereas a *sprain* is a ligamentous injury. A strain happens when a muscle tendon unit is overloaded or stretched. The clinical picture is common to all musculotendinous injuries. Motion of the neck becomes painful, reaching a peak after several hours or the next day. NSAIDs, heat, massage, and other modalities are beneficial.

3. Cervical Sprain

With cervical sprain, there is damage to the ligamentous and capsular structure connecting the facet joints and vertebra. It is often difficult to differentiate from a strain. There is limited motion and pain in the area of the injury and along the muscle groups overlying the area of the injury. Ligamentous disruption may be extensive enough to result in instability with associated neurologic involvement. Routine cervical spine radiographs are indicated. In those athletes with diminished motion as well as pain, stability of the cervical spine should be documented, which may be done with flexion and extension radiographs.

Treatment of a cervical sprain consists of immobilization, rest, support, and antiinflammatory therapy. Return to participation is permitted when motion and muscle strength normalize.

4. Cervical Spinal Cord Neurapraxia with Transient Tetraplegia

The phenomenon of cervical spinal cord neurapraxia with transient tetraplegia is a distinct clinical entity. Sensory changes include a burning pain, numbness, tingling, or loss of sensation. Motor changes include weakness or complete paralysis, which is usually transient, with complete recovery occurring in 10–15 minutes, although in some cases gradual resolution occurs over 36–48 hours. Complete motor function and full pain-free cervical motion returns. Routine radiographs of the cervical spine are negative for fractures or dislocations. Some radiographic findings include spinal stenosis, congenital fusions, cervical instability, and intervertebral disk disease. To determine whether cervical spinal stenosis is present, the anteroposterior diameter of the spinal canal is measured, and this figure is divided by the anteroposterior diameter of the vertebral body (Figure 4–11). If the ratio is less than 0.80, stenosis is present.

Athletes who have suffered transient tetraplegia are not known to be at any greater risk for permanent tetraplegia. Patients who have this syndrome and associated instability of the cervical spine or cervical disk disease should be precluded from further participation in contact sports. Those who have spinal stenosis alone should be treated on an individual basis.

More severe injuries, including fractures and dislocation of the cervical spine, may occur. Treatment of these

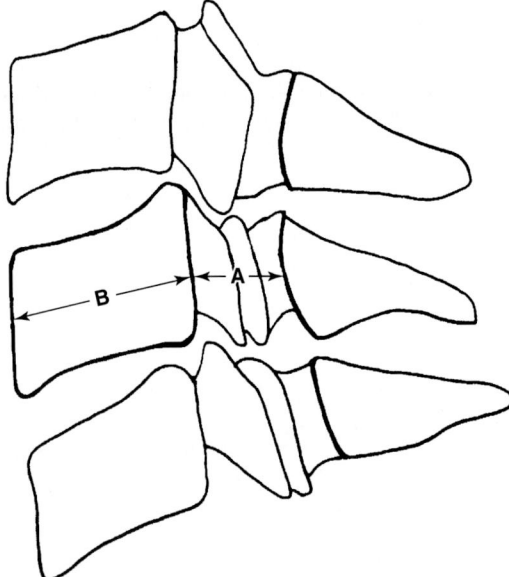

Figure 4–41. The ratio of the spinal canal to the vertebral body is the distance from the midpoint of the posterior aspect of the vertebral body to the nearest point on the corresponding spinolaminar line (**A**) divided by the anteroposterior width of the vertebral body (**B**). (Reproduced, with permission, from Torg JS et al: Neurapraxia of the cervical spinal cord with transient quadriplegia. J Bone Joint Surg Am 1986;68:1354.)

begins on the playing field, with immobilization of the spine. A face mask, if worn, may be cut off with bolt cutters. After thoroughly stabilizing the spine, the patient is moved to a spine board. Sandbags are used to immobilize the head and neck. The patient may then be transported to a local emergency room for further evaluation and treatment. Fractures and dislocations with or without permanent neurologic injury are treated like other spine injuries.

Torg JS et al. Cervical cord neurapraxia: Classification, pathomechanics, morbidity, and management guidelines. J Neurosurg 1997;87:843. [PMID: 9384393]

Torg JS et al: Neurapraxia of the cervical spinal cord with transient quadriplegia. J Bone Joint Surg Am 1986;68:1354. [PMID: 3782207]

LUMBAR SPINE INJURY

Clinical Findings

Spondylolysis is a disruption of the pars interarticularis, whereas spondylolisthesis involves anterior slippage of one vertebral body over the next. Spondylolysis is most often found at L5 and L4 but may occasionally be seen at L3 and L2. It is believed to result from repeated stress around the pars interarticularis during hyperextension of the lumbar spine. If continued hyperextension activity occurs, spondylolysis may become spondylolisthesis. Sports in which spondylolisthesis is commonly found include gymnastics, football, and weight lifting. Female teenage gymnasts, for example, often have back pain but normal early radiographs. Approximately 3–6 weeks later, a stress response may be seen around the pars interarticularis, with increased density developing. At this time, the bone scan is positive, indicating an impending stress fracture that will show up on plain radiographs in 2–4 weeks. A physician who is aware of which sports put stress on the pars interarticularis should consider a bone scan to rule out spondylolisthesis.

Treatment & Prognosis

The treatment of spondylolisthesis involves cessation of all aggravating sports and other actions producing spinal hyperextension. A certain percentage of these fractures heal spontaneously. Healing time for spondylolysis of the lumbar spine is usually approximately 6 months. If after that period of time no significant signs of healing are apparent, it is unlikely that spontaneous healing will take place. At this point, spinal fusion should be considered, or the patient should be willing to confine activities to less stressful pain-free sports.

Many patients with spondylolisthesis engage in high-level sporting activities without significant pain or neurologic deficit. Only a small percentage actually present for evaluation and care. Complete evaluation and treatment recommendations for spondylolisthesis and spondylolysis are found in the section on the spine.

Bono CM: Low-back pain in athletes. J Bone Joint Surg Am 2004;86-A:382. [PMID: 14960688]

Miller SF, Congeni J, Swanson K: Long-term functional and anatomical follow-up of early detected spondylolysis in young athletes. Am J Sports Med 2004;32:928. [PMID: 15150039]

Disorders, Diseases, & Injuries of the Spine

5

Serena S. Hu, MD, Clifford B. Tribus, MD, Bobby K-B Tay, MD, & Nitin N. Bhatia, MD

▋ OSTEOMYELITIS OF THE SPINE

Osteomyelitis of the spine comprises approximately 1% of all cases of pyogenic skeletal infections. Pathogenic organisms can infect the vertebra, the intervertebral disk, or the spinal canal through multiple mechanisms, including local spread from an adjacent infection or as a result of seeding from a noncontiguous source of infection either hematogenously or through the lymphatics. Bacteria can also be introduced directly to compromised tissues as a result of trauma, surgery, diskography, or intravenous or intradural catheterization. Although many organisms are implicated, the most frequently cultured organisms are *Staphylococcus aureus* and *Pseudomonas aeruginosa*. *Salmonella* should be strongly considered as a potential pathogen in patients with sickle cell disease. Infection with *Mycobacterium tuberculosis* is often seen in less developed countries and in prison populations. Spinal sepsis is most common in adolescents, the elderly (more than 60 years), intravenous drug abusers, patients with diabetes or renal failure, and patients who have undergone spinal surgery. Osteoporosis is also implicated as a predisposing factor secondary to increased blood flow. Eismont and Bohlman reported several risk factors for neurologic deterioration including patients with diabetes, rheumatoid arthritis, steroid use, age greater than 50 years, a cephalad level of infection, and infection with *S. aureus*. For additional information on osteomyelitis, see Chapter 8.

Clinical Findings

A. Symptoms and Signs

Patients with osteomyelitis of the spine may or may not present with symptoms relating to their spine. Pyogenic osteomyelitis is fundamentally different from tubercular osteomyelitis. In the latter, patients generally complain of indolent, chronic back pain. In pyogenic osteomyelitis, the symptoms of acute spontaneous back pain, fever, and weight loss are common but not always present. On physical examination, patients with diskitis or pyogenic osteomyelitis of the spine often exhibit significant percussion tenderness posteriorly over the affected vertebral segments. Paraspinal muscle spasm may be seen in more than 90% of patients. A history of fevers is found in less than 50% of affected patients. Neurologic involvement, fortunately, affects less than 10% of all patients with spinal infections. When the infection involves the cervical spine, patients may develop Horner syndrome, or dysphagia. Pyogenic osteomyelitis should be suspected in any patient who presents with back pain and a recent history of an acute systemic infection (eg, appendicitis, perinephritic abscess, pneumonia, genitourinary tract infection, or meningitis).

B. Laboratory Studies

The results of laboratory tests can be equivocal. The white cell count is elevated in only 42% of patients and often is normal. Both blood and spinal cultures may also be negative. Blood cultures are accurate in only 25% of cases, and closed biopsy techniques are diagnostic in only 70% of cases. The ESR rate is elevated in more than 90% of patients, and the C-reactive protein level (CRP) is also elevated at an earlier point in the infectious process. However, both of these tests are systemic indicators of inflammation and are relatively nonspecific. Thus, there is often a significant delay in diagnosis because many of the signs and symptoms of pyogenic vertebral osteomyelitis are subtle. Clearly, the diagnosis relies on having a high index of suspicion in at-risk patients as well as initiating the appropriate evaluation that will identify the organism and determine the extent of infection.

C. Imaging Studies

Radiographic signs of osteomyelitis typically lag behind symptomatic progression of the disease. MRI with vascular-based contrast enhancement (gadolinium) is the gold standard for early neurodiagnostic imaging. Radiographic findings may appear normal.

In pyogenic osteomyelitis, early radiographic changes may include loss of disk space height, erosion of the vertebral endplates, and vertebral destruction and collapse (Figure 5–1). In advanced cases, the vertebral bodies may become fused because of the inflammation and destruction of the intervertebral disk.

In tubercular osteomyelitis, radiographic studies typically demonstrate anterior vertebral body destruction with sparing of the intervertebral disk. Loss of bone stability in the cervical or thoracic spine may lead to kyphotic deformity and paralysis. Progression to solid fusion may occur but usually later than seen in pyogenic osteomyelitis.

Treatment

Early diagnosis and identification of the responsible organism is the cornerstone of treatment. Once the organism is confirmed by biopsy or blood culture, appropriate intravenous antibiotics should be initiated and continued for at least 6 weeks. Short-term bed rest for pain management is appropriate. Spinal column bracing is often necessary for pain relief, immobilization of the affected segments, and minimizing the progression of spinal deformity. Success of nonoperative treatment is linked to patient age younger than 60 years, immunocompetency, infection with *S. aureus,* and a decreasing erythrocyte sedimentation rate (ESR) with appropriate medical treatment. Indications for surgery other than tissue diagnosis include moderate to advanced destruction of the spine with instability, neurologic compromise, sequestrum formation, and failure to respond to intravenous antibiotics. Paraspinal abscesses may be managed conservatively with intravenous antibiotics unless the patient meets one of the surgical criteria just listed.

Pediatric diskitis often responds to spinal column bracing, immobilization, and rest. Although controversial, antibiotic therapy in the pediatric diskitis patient appears to improve nonoperative resolution of symptoms.

The incidence of epidural abscesses may be on the rise, associated with older patients and chronic illness. Epidural abscesses are best treated with early recognition, antibiotic therapy, and immediate surgical decompression. Preoperative paralysis and neurologic deterioration are poor prognostic factors of the disease. MRI is as sensitive as myelography with CT. For diagnostic purposes, MRI offers the advantage of being noninvasive and being able to delineate other disease entities, making it the imaging modality of choice.

For surgical candidates with osteomyelitis or diskitis, the treatment of choice consists of anterior surgical debridement and stabilization with an autogenous structural graft bone graft. Often posterior instrumentation and spinal fusion over the affected segments is necessary to prevent collapse of the anterior graft and to prevent late deformity. Foreign bodies, such as methylmethacrylate, are relatively contraindicated in spinal stabilization, although newer studies suggest that instrumentation can be safely used in an anterior column

A

B

Figure 5–1. Imaging studies in patients with osteomyelitis of the spine. **A:** Radiograph showing an epidural abscess and advanced collapse between L1 and L2. **B:** CT scan showing destruction of the vertebral body.

infection. Antibiotic-impregnated polymethylmethacrylate (PMMA) cement used as a temporary spacer may be useful in grossly contaminated sites. New minimally invasive surgical techniques that use laparoscopy and thoracoscopy appear to be an excellent alternative for operative management of spinal infections. These techniques employ similar surgical principles with expanding surgeon experience, although currently a thorough decompression of the spinal canal is not possible with the minimally invasive technique.

Dimar JR et al: Treatment of pyogenic vertebral osteomyelitis with anterior debridement and fusion followed by delayed posterior spinal fusion. Spine 2004;29:326; discussion 332. [PMID: 14752357]

Eismont FJ et al: Pyogenic and fungal vertebral osteomyelitis with paralysis. J Bone Joint Surg Am 1983;65:19. [PMID: 6849675]

Emery SE, Chan DP, Woodward HR: Treatment of hematogenous pyogenic vertebral osteomyelitis with anterior debridement and primary bone grafting. Spine 1989;14:284. [PMID: 2652335]

Fayazi AH et al: Preliminary results of staged anterior debridement and reconstruction using titanium mesh cages in the treatment of thoracolumbar vertebral osteomyelitis. Spine J 2004;4:388. [PMID: 15246297]

Frazier DD et al: Fungal infections of the spine. Report of eleven patients with long-term follow-up. J Bone Joint Surg Am 2001;83:560. [PMID: 11315785]

Gasbarrini AL, Bertoldi E, Mazzetti M et al: Clinical features, diagnostic and therapeutic approaches to haematogenous vertebral osteomyelitis. Eur Rev Med Pharmacol Sci 2005;9:53. [PMID: 15852519]

Hee HT et al: Better treatment of vertebral osteomyelitis using posterior stabilization and titanium mesh cages. J Spinal Disord Tech 2002;15:149. [PMID: 11927825]

Muckley T et al: The role of thoracoscopic spinal surgery in the management of pyogenic vertebral osteomyelitis. Spine 2004;29:E227. [PMID: 15167673]

Ogden AT, Kaiser MG: Single-stage debridement and instrumentation for pyogenic spinal infections. Neurosurg Focus 2004;17:E5.

Schuster JM et al: Use of structural allografts in spinal osteomyelitis: A review of 47 cases. J Neurosurg 2000;93(1 Suppl):8. [PMID: 10879752]

Tay BK, Deckey J, Hu SS: Spinal infections. J Am Acad Orthop Surg 2002;10:188. [PMID:12041940]

Weinstein MA, Eismont FJ: Infections of the spine in patients with human immunodeficiency virus. J Bone Joint Surg Am 2005; 87:604. [PMID: 15741629]

TUMORS OF THE SPINE

PRIMARY TUMORS OF THE SPINE

Primary tumors of the spine account for 0.04% of all tumors and 10% of all primary tumors of bone. The overwhelming majority of spinal tumors are metastatic. As with tumors elsewhere in the musculoskeletal system, primary lesions in the spine may be osteogenic, chondrogenic, fibrogenic, hematopoietic, neurogenic, or vascular. Generally, benign tumors typically occur in the younger age group (younger than 21 years), whereas up to 70% of malignant tumors are found in patients older than 21 years.

Principles of Diagnosis

A. HISTORY AND PHYSICAL EXAMINATION

If the presence of a spinal tumor is suspected, a thorough history and physical examination must be performed. Pain is the common presenting symptom. Persistent pain, especially at night, is the chief complaint in more than 80% of cases. The average time from onset of symptoms until diagnosis in patients with benign lesions is 19 months, whereas that in patients with metastatic disease is 4 months. The age of the patient is important in establishing the differential diagnosis (see Chapter 6). In adults, malignant lesions of bone occur twice as frequently as benign lesions. In children younger than 10 years, however, only 15–20% of tumors are malignant. Location within the spinal column also aids in establishing the diagnosis. Although 75% of tumors located in the vertebral bodies or pedicles are malignant, only 35% of those in the posterior elements are malignant.

On examination, the patient may complain of tenderness over the involved region of the spine. Although rare initially, radiculopathy secondary to nerve root compression may be the only finding. Signs and symptoms may mimic a herniated nucleus pulposus and may progress to localized weakness, sensory loss, and bowel or bladder dysfunction. Up to 70% of patients may develop motor weakness by the time the diagnosis is made. Pathologic fractures may present with acute onset of pain and paraparesis. Examination of the spine may reveal scoliosis, as occurs with osteomas or osteoblastomas, or it may reveal a painful kyphosis.

B. IMAGING STUDIES

The workup begins with high-quality plain radiographs, followed by CT scanning, radioisotope bone scanning, and MRI as necessary. The routine anteroposterior view may reveal the presence of the so-called winking owl sign, which is indicative of early pedicle destruction. As with other bony tumors, the more slowly expanding bony tumors of the spine are well circumscribed with reactive ossification. More aggressive lesions have a moth-eaten or erosive appearance. It is important to realize that radiographic evidence of bony destruction is not apparent until 30–50% of the trabecular bone is lost. Vertebral collapse with preservation of the disk space is a common finding.

Early on it is often difficult on plain radiographs to distinguish a neoplastic process from an infectious one. Technetium bone scans are an accurate and sensitive modality in detecting metastatic disease. False-positive results are acceptably low and usually a result of osteoarthritis. If the osteoblastic response is impaired, as in multiple myeloma or in highly lytic lesions, false-negative results may occur. However, with the advent of MRI, bone scanning is limited in its usefulness in staging of the tumor.

CT scanning with or without myelography is of great benefit in detecting and evaluating osseous lesions and dural impingement. CT scanning also allows an accurate assessment of the extent of bony destruction to help in preoperative planning. Evaluation of soft tissue and marrow has improved immensely with the advent of MRI. Tumor resolution is outstanding (Figure 5–2), and preoperative planning is greatly enhanced.

Arteriography enables the surgeon to evaluate the vascular supply to the tumor and the extent of vascular neogenesis. Highly vascular tumors, such as metastatic renal cell tumors, thyroid carcinoma, hemangiosarcoma, and aneurysmal bone cysts, are well visualized. Partial or complete embolization of highly vascular tumors may make operative resection significantly easier and safer. In addition, identification of feeder vessels in tumors in the lower thoracic spine may help identify possible vascular supply to the tumor from the artery of Adamkewitz. Inappropriate ligation of this major vessel may result in spinal cord ischemia and paralysis.

MRI is the study of choice in the diagnosis and evaluation of primary neoplasms of the spine. Its advantages include superior soft-tissue visualization, the availability of multiplanar images, and the ability to evaluate the extent of neural compression or infiltration.

C. BIOPSY

An open or closed percutaneous biopsy may be necessary for establishing the diagnosis. If the workup is consistent with a benign symptomatic tumor such as an osteoid osteoma, an excisional biopsy may be appropriate. When malignancy is suspected, needle biopsy should be performed prior to resection. Because the accuracy rate for needle biopsy is 75% or less, several specimens should be obtained. Open biopsy is necessary if aspiration is nondiagnostic.

D. SURGICAL TREATMENT

The surgical treatment of spinal tumors depends on (1) biologic tumor type, (2) location within spine, (3) percentage of vertebral involvement, (4) neurologic involvement, (5) potential for spine failure and instability, and (6) anticipated life expectancy of the patient.

Bauer HC: Controversies in the surgical management of skeletal metastases. J Bone Joint Surg Br 2005;87:608.

Bilsky MH et al: Operative management of metastatic and malignant primary subaxial cervical tumors. J Neurosurg Spine 2005;2:256. [PMID: 15796349]

Degen JW et al: CyberKnife stereotactic radiosurgical treatment of spinal tumors for pain control and quality of life. J Neurosurg Spine 2005;2:540. [PMID: 15945428]

Fisher CG et al: The surgical management of primary tumors of the spine: Initial results of an ongoing prospective cohort study. Spine 2005;30:1899. [PMID: 16103863]

A

B

Figure 5–2. Imaging studies in a patient with a hemangioendothelioma. **A:** CT scan showing the tumor invading the spinal canal. **B:** MRI of the thoracic spine, demonstrating tumor extension.

Flemming DJ et al: Primary tumors of the spine. Semin Musculoskelet Radiol 2000;4:299. Review. [PMID: 11371321]

Saad RS et al: Fine needle aspiration biopsy of vertebral lesions. Acta Cytol 2004;48:39. [PMID: 14969179]

Vialle R et al: Chondroblastoma of the lumbar spine. Report of two cases and review of the literature. J Neurosurg Spine 2005; 2:596. [PMID: 15945435]

Weinstein JN, McLain RF: Primary tumors of the spine. Spine 1987;12:843. [PMID: 3441830]

1. Benign Tumors

Benign primary tumors of the spine include osteoid osteoma, osteoblastoma, osteochondroma, aneurysmal bone cyst, hemangioma, eosinophilic granuloma, and giant cell tumor. For additional discussion of these tumors, see Chapter 6.

Osteoid Osteoma

Osteoid osteoma and osteoblastoma are osteoblastic lesions that are differentiated from each other by size. Lesions smaller than 2 cm are arbitrarily called osteoid osteomas, whereas tumors larger than 2 cm are called osteoblastomas. Osteoid osteoma affects males more frequently than females and is generally seen in patients between 10 and 20 years of age. This benign tumor is usually located in the posterior elements and most frequently involves the lumbar spine, followed by the cervical and then the thoracic spine.

The patient presents with a complaint of a progressive localized ache that may or may not have a radicular component but is usually relieved by the use of salicylates. Tenderness, muscle spasm, neurologic abnormalities, and even scoliosis may be present on examination. Torticollis may be associated with scoliosis of the cervical spine. Pelvic tilt may be seen in conjunction with lumbar spine scoliosis. Minimal correctability is seen with side bending. In the majority of cases, the tumor is located on the concave side of the curve.

Osteoid osteomas appear radiographically as a nidus surrounded by densely sclerotic bone. Tumors that grow close to the periosteum may cause a fusiform thickening of the overlying cortex secondary to hyperemia. Both the nidus and periosteal reaction can sometimes be seen on plain radiographs but are most easily delineated on the axial cuts of a CT scan. Although spontaneous resolution is reported in some cases, treatment of osteoid osteoma generally requires thorough local excision of the lesion because recurrence is likely. Spinal fusion is usually not indicated at the time of excision. In most cases, any scoliosis present preoperatively improves over the following 6–12 months. If the scoliosis is severe (more than 40 degrees) or the spine was rendered unstable by resection of the articular facets and pedicle, fusion should be considered.

Osteoblastoma

When osteoid osteomas grow larger than 2 cm, they are called osteoblastomas. Benign osteoblastomas account for fewer than 1% of all bone tumors. Although cases are rare, more than 40% of them involve the spine, and half of these spinal cases are associated with scoliosis. Osteoblastomas are more common in males than females and seen most frequently in patients younger than 30 years.

Patients generally complain of localized pain or scoliosis. Fifty-three percent of spinal osteoblastomas are found in the lumbar spine, and the rest are equally distributed in the thoracic and cervical spine.

Radiographic examination may reveal an expanded sclerotic cortex, although there are no classic characteristics. Rarely is the lesion lobulated. The posterior elements and pedicles are more frequently involved than the vertebral body. Vertebral involvement almost always occurs because of secondary expansion from the pedicle, and there may be an associated soft-tissue mass.

Curettage can offer a high rate of disease remission when the lesions are well contained within the vertebral bone. Wide excision of the lesion is always curative and may also provide reliable pain relief and resolution of the spinal deformity. However, marginal excision is safer, provides an excellent cure rate, and is the treatment of choice for these tumors. Even partial excision may offer symptom resolution if the nidus is removed. This can be aided by the use of adjuvant radiotherapy. The local recurrence rate can be up to 10% for some osteoblastomas, but malignant degeneration is a rare occurrence.

Osteochondroma

Osteochondromas result when metaplastic cartilage cells in the periosteum undergo progressive endochondral ossification. Multiple osteochondromatosis is the most common of all skeletal dysplasias, and approximately 7% of these patients have vertebral involvement. Spinal cord compression may occur and is the main indication for excision, which is almost always curative.

Aneurysmal Bone Cyst

Aneurysmal bone cysts result from an expansile hyperemic osteolytic process that erodes through bone. Approximately 80% of patients are younger than 20 years. An estimated 12–30% of these neoplasms occur in the spine, especially the lumbar areas. The tumor involves the posterior elements 60% of the time. Symptoms and signs include a rapid evolution of pain in the spine and radiculopathy. Radiographs reveal the presence of an osteolytic tumor with poor demarcation, peripheral ballooning, and cortical erosion with osseous septa within its substance. Like the chordoma but unlike most other tumors, the aneurysmal bone cyst may cross the intervertebral space. Scoliosis or kyphosis may be present.

The differential diagnosis includes giant cell tumors and cavernous hemangioma. Giant cell tumors usually occur in an older patient population and tend to involve the sacrum. A cavernous hemangioma is usually located in the vertebral body.

Appropriate treatment of aneurysmal bone cysts requires recognition that it may arise from or coexist with a preexisting neoplasm. For the isolated lesion, the treatment of choice is aggressive debulking. If the size and location of the tumor preclude complete surgical removal, incomplete curettage can be undertaken and usually eradicates the lesion. Bone grafting is often necessary. Spinal instrumentation, fusion, or both may be necessary, depending on the extent of the lesion.

Profound hemorrhage is a risk with primary surgical resection and may be controlled with preoperative embolization. Although aneurysmal bone cysts are sensitive to radiation, complications of irradiation-induced myelopathy and sarcoma are noted.

Hemangioma

Hemangiomas, common tumors of the vertebral column, arise from embryonic angioblastic tissue. They comprise approximately 7% of all benign tumors. They are much more common in females than in males and have a predilection for the lower thoracic and upper lumbar spine.

Hemangiomas are frequently asymptomatic. In some cases, they are found serendipitously on screening radiographs. In other cases, they are associated with a compression fracture, with the patient presenting with pain and neurologic symptoms. Radiographically, they present with classic vertebral striations resulting from the abnormally thickened bony trabeculae. CT scans easily delineate the lesion, and MRI shows high signal intensity on T_2-weighted images and low signal intensity on T_1-weighted images. If the patient presents with pain without neurologic deficit, low-dose irradiation is extremely effective in ameliorating the symptoms. If the patient shows signs of neurologic dysfunction, treatment should consist of anterior decompression, mass excision, and anterior fusion. Preoperative embolization of the feeding artery may facilitate surgical management.

Eosinophilic Granuloma (Langerhans Cell Histiocytosis)

Eosinophilic granuloma is a proliferative disorder of the Langerhans cells that is commonly seen in children younger than 10 years and rarely in adults. The disease has a male preponderance. Vertebral involvement is seen in 7–15% of cases and typically presents with a sudden onset of neck pain and torticollis.

Patients frequently present with localized pain. Spinal cord compression is a rare but reported event.

Eosinophilic granuloma can present with a spectrum of radiographic manifestations depending on the stage of the tumor. Early on, the tumor presents as a central lytic lesion with poorly defined margins. On plain radiographs, there is permeative bony destruction with a marked periosteal reaction. At this stage, the tumor is difficult to distinguish from a high-grade sarcoma such as Ewing sarcoma. Later in the evolution of the tumor, there is vertebral body collapse leading to a flattening of the vertebral bone between the adjacent intact disks. This phenomenon results in the classic "coin-on-end" appearance and "vertebra plana."

The differential diagnosis includes Ewing sarcoma and infection, and biopsy may be necessary to confirm the diagnosis.

Eosinophilic granuloma usually resolves spontaneously. If the patient suffers from disseminated Langerhans cell histiocytosis, chemotherapy may be appropriate. Local infiltration with corticosteroids is of some benefit. Low-dose irradiation (500–1000 rads) is used in cases associated with neurologic compromise. The use of anterior decompression and anterior fusion is the treatment of choice in patients with neurologic symptoms.

Giant Cell Tumor

Giant cell tumors comprise approximately 10% of all primary bone tumors. These tumors occur in people between 20 and 40 years of age with a slight female predominance (70.8%). Spinal involvement is seen in patients in the third and fourth decades of life. This tumor is locally aggressive and presents most commonly in the anterior vertebral structures. The presenting complaint is typically pain; however, as many as 50% of patients may present with neurologic deficits. Plain radiographs show a lytic lesion with matrix calcification and sclerosis. Aggressive surgical curettage or en bloc excision depending on the location and extent of tumor yield the best results. Because of the risk of sarcomatous transformation, radiation therapy should be reserved for patients with incomplete excision or local recurrence. There is a higher recurrence rate in those patients with soft-tissue extension, anterior and posterior tumor, and spinal canal involvement.

Bertram C, Madert J, Eggers C: Eosinophilic granuloma of the cervical spine. Spine 2002;27:1408. Review. [PMID: 12131737]

Brown CW et al: Treatment and outcome of vertebral Langerhans cell histiocytosis at the Children's Hospital of Eastern Ontario. Can J Surg 2005;48:230. [PMID: 16013628]

Fidler MW: Surgical treatment of giant cell tumours of the thoracic and lumbar spine: Report of nine patients. Eur Spine J 2001;10:69. [PMID: 11276839]

Garg S, Mehta S, Dormans JP: Modern surgical treatment of primary aneurysmal bone cyst of the spine in children and adolescents. J Pediatr Orthop 2005;25:387. [PMID: 15832161]

Kak VK et al: Solitary osteochondroma of the spine causing spinal cord compression. Clin Neurol Neurosurg 1985;87:135. [PMID: 4028590]

Ozaki T et al: Osteoid osteoma and osteoblastoma of the spine: experiences with 22 patients. Clin Orthop 2002;397:394. [PMID: 11953633]

Papagelopoulos PJ et al: Treatment of aneurysmal bone cysts of the pelvis and sacrum. J Bone Joint Surg Am 2001;83:1674. [PMID: 11701790]

Zileli M et al: Osteoid osteomas and osteoblastomas of the spine. Neurosurg Focus 2003;15:E5. Review. [PMID: 15323462]

2. Malignant Tumors

Primary malignant tumors of the spine are rare and carry a poor prognosis. Multiple myeloma is the most common. Osteosarcoma, Ewing sarcoma, chondrosarcoma, and chordoma occur much less frequently. For additional discussion of these tumors, see Chapter 6.

Solitary Plasmacytoma & Multiple Myeloma

Multiple myeloma and solitary plasmacytoma are B-cell lymphoproliferative diseases composed of abnormal aggregates of plasma cells. The neoplasm has a peak occurrence between 50 and 60 years of age with an equal sex distribution. Multiple myeloma is a multifocal plasma cell cancer of the osseous system whose neoplastic cells produce complete or incomplete immunoglobulins. The annual incidence of myeloma is approximately 2–3 per 100,000 among the general population. Genetic analysis of the tumor cells demonstrates abnormalities in band q32 of chromosome 14. The diagnosis is made on serum and urine evaluation for abnormal immunoglobulin levels. Serum protein electrophoresis shows increases in the levels of one of the immunoglobulin classes. The M-component is IgG in 55% of cases, IgA in 25% of cases, and rarely IgE, IgD, or IgM. Urine protein electrophoresis may detect the presence of immunoglobulin light chains called Bence Jones proteins in up to 99% of patients. In 60% of patients afflicted with multiple myeloma, both Bence Jones proteins and abnormal serum immunoglobulin levels are detected.

The initial treatment of myeloma consists of chemotherapy and irradiation. Chemotherapy is an effective means of controlling the advancement of the disease process but may increase the risk of secondary leukemia. The commonly employed agents include melphalan and prednisone. Newer agents such as gallium nitrate may attenuate the rate of skeletal bone loss from the disease and from steroid treatment. Radiation to affected osseous sites may reduce pain and prevent vertebral collapse, deformity, and neural compression. Patients with solitary plasmacytoma have a 5-year survival rate of 60%. In contrast, patients with multiple myeloma have only an 18% 5-year survival rate and a median survival of 24 months.

Osteosarcoma

Primary osteosarcoma is a malignant tumor of mesenchymal cells characterized by the direct formation of osteoid or bone by the tumor cells. It is the second most common primary neoplasm of bone behind myeloma. Most appear in persons younger than 20 years of age before epiphyseal closure. There is a slight male preponderance. In a series of patients with osteosarcoma, Barwick noted that 1–2% arose initially in the spine.

Patients with retinoblastoma (caused by a hereditary mutation in the q14 band of chromosome 13 that codes for a tumor suppressor gene) have a 500-fold greater risk of developing osteosarcoma. The overall consensus is that these tumors have a multifactorial origin involving genetic, constitutional, and environmental influences.

Radiographically, osteosarcomas present as mixed lytic and sclerotic lesions that cause cortical destruction and soft-tissue calcification. In advanced stages, vertebral collapse occurs from replacement of the structural elements of the spine with tumor. Traditional therapy involved limited tumor resection and radiotherapy. A more aggressive approach, as described by Sundaresan and Weinstein, with wide resection, combination chemotherapy, and local radiotherapy demonstrated promising early results. Secondary spinal osteosarcoma caused by malignant transformation of pagetoid or previously irradiated bone is extremely aggressive and associated with early metastasis. A 5-year survival rate of 17% is reported in cases involving pagetoid bone, and the prognosis is even poorer in cases involving irradiated bone.

Ewing Sarcoma

Ewing sarcoma is a malignant round cell tumor with a peak incidence in the second decade of life. The sarcoma was first described in 1921 by James Ewing, who called it an "endothelial myeloma." The neoplasm occurs twice as often in men as in women. Spinal involvement is seen in 3.5% of all Ewing sarcomas, and a large proportion of these arise in the sacrum.

Metastatic involvement of the spine is more common in the late stage of the disease. The vertebral body involvement seen on radiographs in patients with Ewing sarcoma can mimic the vertebra plana seen in patients with eosinophilic granuloma.

When the lesion is localized to the sacrum, the prognosis is worse because these particular lesions tend to be more aggressive and less responsive to chemotherapy and irradiation.

Chondrosarcoma

Chondrosarcoma is the third most common primary bone tumor behind myeloma and osteosarcoma. Although chondrosarcoma rarely affects the spine, it does so more often than osteosarcoma or Ewing sarcoma. The peak incidence of chondrosarcoma is in the fourth to sixth decade, with males affected four times more often than females. An estimated 6–10% of all chondrosarcomas arise in the spine.

Pain in the area of involvement is the first symptom. Fifty percent of patients have a palpable mass before being diagnosed. Approximately 4.5% have some form of neurologic deficit, varying from sensory deficits to frank paraplegia.

Radiographs show typical cortical destruction and paraspinal soft tissue calcification. MRI helps delineate the extent of soft-tissue and bony involvement.

Chondrosarcomas are radio resistant. Thus, the mainstay of treatment is wide excision. Survival is closely related to obtaining a clear surgical margin at the time of surgical excision. In the Mayo clinic series, 15 of 20 (75%) of the patients with chondrosarcoma died of local progression. Their 5-year survival rate was 21–55%, with a median survival of 6 years. High-dose irradiation therapy may have limited benefit for inoperable lesions.

Chordoma

A chordoma is a slow-growing tumor that arises from notochordal cells in the vertebral body. Physaliphorous cells, containing abundant vacuoles filled with glycogen and oxidative enzymes, are the distinctive cells of this neoplasm. Molecular analysis shows that chordoma cells express galectin-3, a carbohydrate binding protein that plays a role in cell differentiation, morphogenesis, and cancer biology. The neoplasm usually occurs in the fifth and sixth decades of life and afflicts men twice as often as women. Chordomas are found in the sacrum and coccyx in 55% of cases, in the basilar skull in 30%, and in the lumbar and cervical spine in 15%. The clinical course is indolent, and detection is often delayed until after metastasis occurs. Symptoms and signs include local pain, radiculopathy, and bowel or bladder dysfunction. Patients with cervicothoracic tumors can present with progressive dyspnea. Rectal examination can reveal a presacral mass.

After wide surgical resection, the local recurrence rate varies from 28–64%. Great care must be taken to prevent tumor spillage during resection because this can increase the local recurrence rate from 28% to 64%. Adjuvant radiation therapy is indicated when complete resection is not possible or when there is tumor spillage at the time of resection. Radiation therapy may allow an increased continuous disease-free survival. The 5-year survival rate in patients treated with irradiation alone is approximately 50%; that in patients treated with irradiation plus surgical resection is 71%. Virtually all patients eventually die from tumor recurrence.

Boriani S et al: Chondrosarcoma of the mobile spine: Report on 22 cases. Spine 2000;25:804. [PMID: 10751291]

Fourney DR, Gokaslan ZL: Current management of sacral chordoma. Neurosurg Focus 2003;15:E9. [PMID: 15350040]

Ilaslan H et al: Primary vertebral osteosarcoma: Imaging findings. Radiology 2004;230:697. Epub accessed January 28, 2004. [PMID: 14749514]

Lane JM et al: Kyphoplasty enhances function and structural alignment in multiple myeloma. Clin Orthop Relat Res 2004;426:49. [PMID: 15346051]

McLain RF, Weinstein JN: Solitary plasmacytomas of the spine: A review of 84 cases. J Spinal Dis 1989;2:69. [PMID: 2520065]

Ozaki T et al: Osteosarcoma of the spine: experience of the Cooperative Osteosarcoma Study Group. Cancer 2002;94:1069. [PMID: 11920477]

Papagelopoulos PJ et al: Chordoma of the spine: Clinicopathological features, diagnosis, and treatment. Orthopedics 2004;27:1256. [PMID: 15633956]

Sell M et al: Chordomas: A histological and immunohistochemical study of cases with and without recurrent tumors. Clin Neuropathol 2004;23:277. [PMID: 15584212]

Venkateswaran L et al: Primary Ewing tumor of the vertebrae: Clinical characteristics, prognostic factors, and outcome. Med Pediatr Oncol 2001;37:30. [PMID: 11466720]

Zeifang F et al: Long-term survival after surgical intervention for bone disease in multiple myeloma. Ann Oncol 2005;16:222. [PMID: 15668274]

METASTATIC DISEASE OF THE SPINE

Although the skeleton is the third most common site for metastatic disease, the spine, especially the thoracic spine, is the most frequently involved region of the skeleton. Approximately 70% of patients who die of cancer have evidence of vertebral metastasis on postmortem examination.

Lung, breast, prostate, renal, thyroid, and gastrointestinal carcinomas are all reported to metastasize to the spine, where lesions can lead to multilevel spinal instability and cord compression. Unfortunately, 30–50% of the bone must be destroyed before the metastatic involvement becomes evident on radiographs.

Many patients with spinal metastasis are asymptomatic. Symptoms, when they do occur, are typically a result of invasion of the tumor into the paravertebral soft tissues, compression of the spinal cord or nerve roots, or pathologic fracture and spinal instability. In these cases, patients frequently complain of severe, unrelenting back pain with or without neurologic sequelae. The pain typically wakes the patient up at night. The course may be rapid, leading to paraplegia or quadriplegia.

Technetium bone scanning reveals multiple sites of radioisotope uptake. MRI is the imaging study of choice to assess the extent of the tumor. Biopsy is necessary when the primary tumor is unknown and typically can be performed under CT guidance.

Most patients who do not develop progressive instability or neurologic compromise can be managed nonoperatively with systemic chemotherapy, local irradiation, and bracing.

Radiation therapy and chemotherapy protocols depend on the primary source of carcinoma. From 80% to 90% of patients suffering from spinal metastatic disease are reported to gain significant relief with radiation therapy. Irradiation can be started as early as 2 weeks after surgical decompression and fusion. Surgical intervention is warranted in patients who have severe pain and have failed to respond to conservative management. It is also indicated in patients who have significant neurologic dysfunction or spinal instability. Factors found to affect survival include preoperative neurologic status, anatomic site of primary

Figure 5–3. Radiograph showing metastasizing adeno-carcinoma of C4 and C5, treated with excision, methyl-methacrylate, and K-wire.

carcinoma, and number of vertebral bodies involved. Patients with a slower onset of neurologic compromise have a better prognosis for recovery of neurologic function than patients with acute onset of neurologic compromise. Stabilizing constructs can consist of bone, metal, or methylmethacrylate (Figure 5–3).

Alvarez L et al: Vertebroplasty in the treatment of vertebral tumors: Postprocedural outcome and quality of life. Eur Spine J 2003;12:356. Epub accessed March 22, 2003. [PMID: 12687441]

Barr JD et al: Percutaneous vertebroplasty for pain relief and spinal stabilization. Spine 2000;25:923. [PMID: 10767803]

Chataigner H, Onimus M: Surgery in spinal metastasis without spinal cord compression: Indications and strategy related to the risk of recurrence. Eur Spine J 2000;9:523. [PMID: 11189921]

Ghogawala Z, Mansfield FL, Borges LF: Spinal radiation before surgical decompression adversely affects outcomes of surgery for symptomatic metastatic spinal cord compression. Spine 2001;26:818. [PMID: 11295906]

Holman PJ et al: Surgical management of metastatic disease of the lumbar spine: experience with 139 patients. J Neurosurg Spine 2005;2:550.

Jeremic B: Single fraction external beam radiation therapy in the treatment of localized metastatic bone pain. A review. J Pain Symptom Manage 2001;22:1048. [PMID 11738168]

Manabe J et al: Surgical treatment of bone metastasis: Indications and outcomes. Int J Clin Oncol 2005;10:103. [PMID: 15864695]

North RB et al: Surgical management of spinal metastases: Analysis of prognostic factors during a 10-year experience. J Neurosurg Spine 2005;2:564. [PMID: 15945430]

Ryu S et al: Image-guided and intensity-modulated radiosurgery for patients with spinal metastasis. Cancer 2003;97:2013. [PMID: 12673732]

Togao O et al: Percutaneous vertebroplasty in the treatment of pain caused by metastatic tumor. Fukuoka Igaku Zasshi 2005; 96:93. [PMID: 15991606]

EXTRADURAL TUMORS

Extradural tumors include hemangiomas, lipomas, meningiomas, and lymphomas. Surgical management usually involves laminectomy and tumor excision. This is often all that is needed for symptomatic relief in these slow-growing tumors.

Loblaw DA et al: Systematic review of the diagnosis and management of malignant extradural spinal cord compression: The Cancer Care Ontario Practice Guidelines Initiative's Neuro-Oncology Disease Site Group. J Clin Oncol 2005;23:2028. [PMID: 15774794]

▮ INFLAMMATORY DISEASES OF THE SPINE

RHEUMATOID ARTHRITIS

Rheumatoid arthritis is the most common form of inflammatory arthritis. It affects 3% of women and 1% of men. The disease frequently affects the spine. The same inflammatory cells that destroy peripheral joints affect the synovium of apophyseal and uncovertebral joints, causing painful instability and neurologic compromise. Up to 71% of patients with rheumatoid arthritis show involvement of the cervical spine. The most common patterns of involvement are C1-C2 instability, basilar invagination, and subaxial subluxation. Sudden death associated with rheumatoid arthritis, most probably secondary to brain stem compression, is reported.

Clinical Findings

A. SYMPTOMS AND SIGNS

From 7% to 34% of patients present with neurologic problems. Documentation of neurologic function can be difficult because loss of joint mobility leads to general muscle weakness. Although many patients complain of nonspecific neck pain, atlantoaxial subluxation is the most common cause for pain in the upper neck, occiput, and forehead in patients with rheumatoid arthritis. Symptoms are aggravated by motion. Increasing compression of the spinal cord results in severe myelopathy with gait abnormalities, weakness, paresthesias, and loss of dexterity. Findings may also include Lhermitte sign (a tingling or electrical feeling that occurs in the arms, legs, or trunk when the neck is flexed), increased muscle tonus of the upper and lower extremities, and pathologic reflexes.

B. IMAGING STUDIES

Instability of the upper cervical spine is determined on lateral flexion-extension radiographs. An atlantodens interval (ADI) that exceeds 3.5 mm is abnormal. Subluxation with an atlasdens interval of 10–12 mm indicates disruption of all supporting ligaments of the atlantoaxial complex (transverse and alar ligaments). The spinal cord in this position is compressed between the dens and the posterior arch of C1. Although the ADI is an important measurement for traumatic instability of the C1-C2 complex, the posterior atlantodens interval (PADI) is more prognostic to assess neurologic compromise. The PADI is a direct measure of the space available for the spinal cord at the C1-C2 level. The PADI is measured from the posterior aspect of the odontoid process to the nearest posterior structure (the foramen magnum or the posterior ring of the atlas). If the space available for the spinal cord is less than 13 mm, the likelihood that the patient will develop myelopathy is extremely high.

Cranial settling is present in from 5% to 32% of patients. The odontoid process should not project more than 3 mm above the Chamberlain line, which is a line between the hard palate and the posterior rim of the foramen magnum. The tip of the dens should not project more than 4.5 mm above the McGregor line, which is a line connecting the posterior margin of the hard palate to the occiput. The Clark classification divides the axis into thirds in the sagittal plane. In severe cases of cranial settling, the anterior arch of C1 moves from station 1 (the upper third of C2) to station 3 (the lower third of C2). Neurologic compromise occurs as a result of impingement of the dens into the brainstem and the upper cervical spinal cord. The vertebral arteries can also become occluded as they course between the dens and the foramen magnum to enter the skull.

Lateral subluxation and posterior atlantoaxial instability are less frequent. From 10% to 20% of patients with rheumatoid arthritis present with subaxial subluxation. Erosion of the facet joints and narrowing of the disks leads to subtle anterior subluxations often found on several levels. This results in the characteristic so-called stepladder deformity that occurs most commonly at the C2-C3 and C3-C4 levels.

C. LABORATORY STUDIES

Rheumatoid factor is positive in up to 80% of patients. The ESR rate is elevated and the hemoglobin is decreased in the active phase of the disease.

After plain radiographs, which should include lateral flexion-extension views, MRI is the study of choice to evaluate the degree of neural compression and deformity.

Treatment

Indications for surgery are severe neck pain and increasing loss of neurologic function. Most commonly, a posterior arthrodesis between C1 and C2 is performed. A Gallie type or Brooks type of fusion can be done, or posterior transarticular screw fixation can be used. The latter obviates the need for postoperative halo immobilization. In cases of basilar invagination (cranial settling), extension of the fusion to the occiput is necessary. Preoperative halo traction is often required to reduce the subluxation or pull the odontoid process out of the foramen magnum. Often a suboccipital craniectomy is necessary to decompress the brainstem adequately. Good fixation can be obtained through the use of plate-screw and rod-screw constructs.

Alberstone CD, Benzel EC: Cervical spine complications in rheumatoid arthritis patients. Awareness is the key to averting serious consequences. Postgrad Med 2000;107:199. [PMID 10649674]

Boden SD et al: Rheumatoid arthritis of the cervical spine. A long-term analysis with predictors of paralysis and recovery. J Bone Joint Surg Am 1993;75:1282. [PMID: 8408150]

Christensson D, Saveland H, Rydholm U: Cervical spine surgery in rheumatoid arthritis. A Swedish nation-wide registration of 83 patients. Scand J Rheumatol 2000;29:314. [PMID: 11093598]

Clark CR, Goetz DD, Menezes AH: Arthrodesis of the cervical spine in rheumatoid arthritis. J Bone Joint Surg Am 1989; 71:381. [PMID: 2925711]

Faraj AA, Webb JK, Prince H: Surgical treatment for rheumatoid neck arthritis bilateral occipitospinal fusion with plate fixation. Acta Orthop Belg 2001;67:164. [PMID: 11383295]

Graziano GP, Hensinger R, Patel CK: The use of traction methods to correct severe cervical deformity in rheumatoid arthritis patients: A report of five cases. Spine 2001;26:1076. [PMID: 11337628]

Grob D: Posterior occipitocervical fusion in rheumatoid arthritis and other instabilities. J Orthop Sci 2000;5:82. [PMID: 10664444]

Haid RW Jr et al: C1-C2 transarticular screw fixation for atlanto-axial instability: A 6-year experience. Neurosurgery 2001; 49:65. [PMID: 11440461]

Kauppi MJ, Barcelos A, da Silva JA: Cervical complications of rheumatoid arthritis. Ann Rheum Dis 2005;64:355.

Matsunaga S, Ijiri K, Koga H: Results of a longer than 10-year follow-up of patients with rheumatoid arthritis treated by occipitocervical fusion. Spine 2000;25:1749. [PMID: 10888940]

Matsuyama Y et al: Long-term results of occipitothoracic fusion surgery in RA patients with destruction of the cervical spine. J Spinal Disord Tech 2005;18(Suppl):S101. [PMID: 15699794]

van Asselt KM et al: Outcome of cervical spine surgery in patients with rheumatoid arthritis. Ann Rheum Dis 2001;60:448. [PMID: 11302865]

ANKYLOSING SPONDYLITIS

Ankylosing spondylitis is a chronic seronegative inflammatory disease that affects the axial skeleton, especially the sacroiliac joints, hip joints, and spine. Extraskeletal involvement is found in the aorta, lung, and uvea. The incidence of ankylosing spondylitis is 0.5–1 per 1000 people. Although males are affected more frequently than females, mild courses of ankylosing spondylitis are more common in the latter. The disease usually has its onset during early adulthood. However, juvenile ankylosing spondylitis affects adolescents (younger than 16 years) and has a predisposition toward hip involvement. The HLA-B27 surface antigen is found in 88%–96% of patients, and investigators postulate that an endogenic component (ie, HLA-B27) and an exogenic component (eg, *Klebsiella* or *Chlamydia*) are responsible for triggering of the disease process. The ESR is elevated in up to 80% of the cases but does not accurately reflect disease activity. The serum creatine phosphokinase (CPK), however, is a good indicator of the severity of the disease process.

Clinical Findings

A. SYMPTOMS AND SIGNS

The onset is insidious, with early symptoms including pain in the buttocks, heels, and lower back. Patients complain typically of morning stiffness, the improvement of symptoms with activity during the day, and the return of symptoms in the evening. The earliest changes involve the sacroiliac joints and then extend upward into the spine. Spinal disease results in loss of motion and subsequent loss of lordosis in the cervical and lumbar spine. Synovitis in the early stages leads to progressive fibrosis and ankylosis of the joints during the reparative phase. Enthesitis occurs at the insertion of the annulus fibrosus on the vertebral body with eventual calcification that results in the characteristic "bamboo spine." The pain from the inflammatory process subsides after full ankylosis of the affected joints occurs.

Approximately 30% of patients develop uveitis, and 30% have chest tightness. Limited chest expansion indicates thoracic involvement. Fewer than 5% of patients have involvement of the aorta, characterized by dilation and possible conduction defects. In addition, patients may suffer from renal amyloidosis and pulmonary fibrosis.

B. IMAGING STUDIES

The earliest radiographic changes are visible in the sacroiliac joints. Symmetric bilateral widening of the joint space is followed by subchondral erosions and ankylosis. Bony changes in the spine affect the vertebral body. Changes include loss of the anterior concavity of the vertebral body, squaring of the vertebra, and marginal syndesmophyte formation, which give the spine the appearance of bamboo. Ankylosis of the apophyseal joints also develops. The disease generally starts in the lumbar spine and migrates cephalad to the cervical spine. Atlantoaxial instability is seen occasionally.

Treatment

The natural history of ankylosing spondylitis, with its slow progression over several decades, has to be considered in planning treatment. Initially, treatment consists of exercises and indomethacin. Approximately 10% of patients develop severe bony changes that eventually require surgical intervention. These changes characteristically include a fixed bony flexion deformity that limits their ambulatory potential. Hip disease should be addressed before correction of spinal deformities because correction of hip flexion deformities may allow significant compensation of the spinal kyphosis to allow adequate horizontal gaze.

Loss of lumbar lordosis can be treated by multilevel V-shaped osteotomies posteriorly (the Smith-Petersen procedure), by a decancellation procedure (the Heinig procedure) of L3 or L4, or by pedicle subtraction osteotomy based at L3 or L4. (Figure 5–4).

The spine is then fused in the corrected position. Utilization of modern fixation systems such as a pedicle screw system allows for early mobilization of the patient. Thorough preoperative assessment of the deformity and measuring of the chin-eyebrow-to-floor angle are helpful for the exact planning of the corrective osteotomy. Relative contraindications to surgery are poor general health and significant scarring of the major vessels, which may be injured when the spine is extended.

The cervical osteotomy is performed between C7 and T1. This approach avoids injury to the vertebral artery that usually enters the transverse foramen of C6. Although the procedure is usually performed under local anesthesia, the evolution of somatosensory and motor evoked potential monitoring of the spinal cord permits the use of general anesthesia. After removal of the poste-

Figure 5–4. Imaging studies in a patient with ankylosing spondylitis. **A:** Radiograph demonstrating flat back deformity, junctional kyphosis, and sagittal decompensation. **B:** Radiograph taken after a decancellation procedure of L3 and posterior fusion were performed to correct the alignment.

rior elements and neural decompression, the kyphotic deformity is corrected with gentle extension of the head. The head is held in the corrected position using internal fixation with plate-screw constructs or plate-rod constructs with adjunctive halo-vest immobilization.

Berven SH et al: Management of fixed sagittal plane deformity: Results of the transpedicular wedge resection osteotomy. Spine 2001;26:2036. [PMID: 11547205]

Braun J et al: Therapy of ankylosing spondylitis. Part II: Biological therapies in the spondyloarthritides. Scand J Rheumatol 2005;34:178. [PMID: 16134723]

Chen IH, Chien JT, Yu TC: Transpedicular wedge osteotomy for correction of thoracolumbar kyphosis in ankylosing spondylitis: Experience with 78 patients. Spine 2001;26:E354. [PMID: 11493864]

Danisa OA, Turner D, Richardson WJ: Surgical correction of lumbar kyphotic deformity: Posterior reduction "eggshell" osteotomy. J Neurosurg 2000;92(Suppl 1):50. [PMID: 10616058]

Kim KT et al: Clinical outcome results of pedicle subtraction osteotomy in ankylosing spondylitis with kyphotic deformity. Spine 2002;27:612. [PMID: 11884909]

Kubiak EN et al: Orthopaedic management of ankylosing spondylitis. J Am Acad Orthop Surg 2005;13:267.

Taggard DA, Traynelis VC: Management of cervical spinal fractures in ankylosing spondylitis with posterior fixation. Spine 2000;25:2035. [PMID: 10954633]

van der Linden S, van der Heijde D: Clinical aspects, outcome assessment, and management of ankylosing spondylitis and postenteric reactive arthritis. Curr Opin Rheumatol 2000; 12:263. Review. [PMID: 10910177]

DISEASES & DISORDERS OF THE CERVICAL SPINE

Principles of Diagnosis

In evaluating the cervical spine, the use of appropriate imaging studies is critical to a timely and precise diagnosis. Available imaging techniques include plain radiography, tomography, myelography, CT, CT with myelography, three-dimensional reconstruction CT, MRI, and scintigraphy. An understanding of the advantages and disadvantages of each technique is necessary for the proper selection of imaging studies and interpretation of results.

A. PLAIN RADIOGRAPHY

In evaluating the patient with neck pain, cervical spine radiographs are important in the initial search for a possible lesion. In the trauma setting, when a head or neck injury is suspected, radiographic studies must be carried out appropriately or a life-threatening lesion may be overlooked. The trauma series includes anteroposterior (AP), right oblique, left oblique, and open-mouth (odontoid) views in addition to an initial cross-table lateral view. When all five views are taken, sensitivity is 92%. Cervical spine precautions must be implemented throughout the radiographic evaluation (see Injuries of the Cervical Spine later in the chapter). In the absence of a history of trauma, the oblique and odontoid views are not always required.

The lateral view reveals the majority of traumatic lesions if performed correctly. Inadequate views can miss more than 20% of cervical spine injuries, however. All seven vertebrae should be clearly visible. Gentle traction on the upper extremities may be necessary to view C7. If this is unsuccessful, a swimmer's view may be necessary. Careful scrutiny of the prevertebral soft tissue, the anterior border of the vertebral bodies, the vertebral bodies themselves, the posterior border of the bodies, the spinal canal proper, and the posterior elements must be done.

The prevertebral region may reveal swelling consistent with a hematoma, and this may serve as the only clue to a traumatic lesion. The upper limits for the prevertebral space are 10 mm at C1; 5 mm at C2; 7 mm at

C3 and C4; and 20 mm at C5, C6, and C7. The contours of the cervical bony structures are regular, and subtle incongruities may indicate significant instability. Variations in normal cervical anatomy do exist, however, and a familiarity with them may prevent an overzealous workup. The ADI normally measures less than 3 mm in adults and less than 4 mm in children.

In reviewing the AP radiograph, careful assessment of the interspinous distance must be undertaken. Vertical widening at a given level greater than 1.5 times the level above and below indicates a hyperflexion injury with posterior instability or interlocking of the posterior facets. Traumatic tilting may also be noted in the AP plane while not appreciated on the lateral view.

Oblique views taken at 45 degrees allow visualization of the articulations of the facet joints. The open-mouth view permits evaluation of the odontoid process, the lateral masses, and the articulations of the lateral masses, and it also permits assessment of the distance between each lateral mass and the odontoid process. In atlantoaxial rotatory subluxation, the lateral mass of the atlas that is rotated forward is closer to the midline (medial offset); the opposite mass is farther away from the midline (lateral offset). Burst fractures of the C1 ring cause overhang of the C1 lateral masses on C2. A combined overhang exceeding 6.9 mm is highly correlated with insufficiency of the transverse ligament and C1-C2 sagittal instability.

This radiographic series is equally important in evaluating infants and children with suspected congenital or developmental defects and adults with insidious neck pain. Arthritic changes may be subtle or readily apparent with osteophytes, disk space narrowing, and facet sclerosis. Bone quality can also be assessed on plain radiographs.

B. COMPUTED TOMOGRAPHY

CT scans allow excellent visualization of the bony architecture and the paravertebral soft tissues of the cervical spine. The pedicles, laminae, spinous processes, and bony spinal canal can be examined with significantly better resolution when CT is used than when conventional radiographs are taken. CT with myelography or intrathecal contrast enhancement permits a visualization of the spinal canal contents.

CT is an appropriate modality for evaluating congenital variations and malformations, including spinal canal stenosis and spina bifida. Pars defects, atlantoaxial joint diseases, inflammatory changes, primary tumors, and metastatic carcinoma are well appreciated with CT. Although cervical disk disease is detectable when thin cuts and contrast enhancement are used with CT, it is better visualized with MRI.

In the trauma patient with questionable findings on plain radiographs, CT is integral in evaluating possible fractures or instability. Atrophy, deformity, and displacement of the spinal cord from acute or chronic injury are all appreciable with the use of intrathecal contrast. With the advent of MRI, however, CT is now reserved for the assessment of the bony architecture, which it does better than MRI.

Three-dimensional reconstruction of CT images gained wide clinical acceptance with the advancement of computer graphics. The reconstructions can be rotated in space to evaluate the anatomy from almost any perspective. This technique is valuable in the understanding of atlantoaxial rotatory subluxations or complex fractures of the spinal column.

C. MAGNETIC RESONANCE IMAGING

MRI permits axial, sagittal, coronal, or oblique plane analysis of the anatomy. It is routinely noninvasive, requiring contrast material in only selected cases.

MRI is the standard for assessing cervical spinal cord damage. Spinal cord tumors and trauma as well as central disk herniation can be easily visualized. In the preoperative evaluation of patients with spondylosis or disk herniation, MRI is the neuroimaging test of choice.

Intravenous paramagnetic agent gadolinium is commonly used to differentiate tissues receiving higher blood flow. This is helpful in the diagnosis of infection, tumor, and postsurgical scar.

D. SCINTIGRAPHY

Bone scans that employ technetium-99m phosphate permit assessment of physiologic processes within the musculoskeletal system. Metabolic, metastatic, and inflammatory abnormalities can be detected. Technetium-99m phosphate is incorporated into the hydroxyapatite in bone and reflects increased bone osteogenesis in a given region of bone. Early-phase imaging with technetium-99m gives blood flow information. Accordingly, subtle fractures, avascular necrosis, and osteomyelitis can be detected. Other radioisotopes used in scintigraphy include gallium-67 citrate, which labels serum proteins, and indium-111, which labels white blood cells. These labeling techniques are helpful in discerning areas of neoplasia or acute infection.

Daffner RH: Controversies in cervical spine imaging in trauma patients. Semin Musculoskelet Radiol 2005;9:105. [PMID: 15278699]

Holmes JF, Akkinepalli R: Computed tomography versus plain radiography to screen for cervical spine injury: a meta-analysis. J Trauma 2005;58:902. Review. [PMID: 15920400]

Larsson EM et al: Comparison of myelography, CT myelography and magnetic resonance imaging in cervical spondylosis and disk herniation. Pre- and postoperative findings. Acta Radiol 1989;30:233. [PMID: 2736175]

Mower WR et al: NEXUS Group. Use of plain radiography to screen for cervical spine injuries. Ann Emerg Med 2001;38:1. [PMID: 11423803]

Sanchez B et al: Cervical spine clearance in blunt trauma: Evaluation of a computed tomography-based protocol. J Trauma 2005;59:179.

Schuster R et al: Magnetic resonance imaging is not needed to clear cervical spines in blunt trauma patients with normal computed tomographic results and no motor deficits. Arch Surg 2005;140:762. [PMID: 16103286]

Taneichi H et al: Traumatically induced vertebral artery occlusion associated with cervical spine injuries: Prospective study using magnetic resonance angiography. Spine 2005;30:1955.

CONGENITAL MALFORMATIONS

The atlantooccipital region is a frequent location for abnormalities. Various combinations involving bone and nervous structures are possible. During embryologic development, 42 somites are formed from the paraxial mesoderm. The somites divide into sclerotomes, which form the vertebral bodies after separation into a caudal and cephalad portion. The middle portion builds the intervertebral disk. The second, third, and fourth somites fuse and become the occiput and posterior part of the foramen magnum. The fate of the first somite is unclear. The development of the neural tube progresses simultaneously with that of the cartilaginous skeleton.

Disturbances of embryologic development can result in incomplete development or absence of a tissue or part, as found in dysraphism, aplasia of the odontoid process, incomplete closure of the atlas, or absence of the atlas facet. Lack of segmentation results in atlantooccipital fusion, block vertebrae, and possible instability at adjacent cervical levels. A disturbance of neurologic development, alone or in combination with bony defects, can lead to basilar impression, Arnold-Chiari malformation, and syringomyelia, all of which manifest in myelopathy.

1. Os Odontoideum

Os odontoideum is an uncommon type of pseudarthrosis between the odontoid process and the body of the axis. It can cause significant atlantoaxial instability and myelopathy and can result in sudden death. The development of cervical myelopathy is thought to be a function of the amount of space available for the spinal cord. Because of the instability between C1 and C2, the spinal cord can become compressed against the anterior portion of the axis or the posterior ring of the atlas. In some cases, extrinsic compression of the vertebral arteries results in ischemic insult to the brain.

Clinical Findings

A. SYMPTOMS AND SIGNS

Patients with os odontoideum may be asymptomatic or may present with symptoms and signs that relate to atlantoaxial instability, such as ill-defined neck complaints or focal or diffuse neurologic deficits. A careful history may be needed to rule out trauma, although congenital os odontoideum may come to the attention of the surgeon secondary to a reported but inconsequential neck injury.

B. IMAGING STUDIES

The radiographic findings may be extremely subtle and difficult to distinguish. In the mature skeleton, os odontoideum appears as a radiographic lucency. In children younger than 5 years, however, an anomalous gap may be confused with a normal neural synchondrosis. Flexion-extension views must therefore be obtained to demonstrate motion between the odontoid process and the body of the axis. The ossicle in os odontoideum is either round or ovoid, with a smooth surface and uniform cortical thickness. It is usually approximately half the size of the normal odontoid process. In traumatic nonunion, the edge is irregular with a narrow gap. The fracture line may involve the body of C2 as well. An additional radiologic finding in os odontoideum is hypertrophy of the anterior ring of the atlas with a corresponding hypoplastic posterior ring. In flexion-extension views, the ossicle travels with the anterior ring of the atlas (Figure 5–5). In cases that are difficult to diagnose,

further studies include open-mouth views, tomograms, and CT reconstructions.

Treatment

Patients diagnosed with os odontoideum must be warned of the gravity of the situation because minimal trauma can be fatal. Patients with cervical myelopathy can be treated with traction, immobilization, or both, but they often require subsequent posterior fusion. Sometimes symptoms are reversible with or without intervention. Management of asymptomatic patients with instability is controversial. The benefits of surgical stabilization in an attempt to avoid potentially lethal injury from relatively minor trauma are counterbalanced by the possible complications of surgery.

If fusion is indicated, usually a posterior fusion of C1-C2 is adequate. Different fusion techniques are available. Most surgeons use the Gallie technique or the Brooks technique. The Gallie technique involves the use of a single block-shaped bone graft between the posterior ring of C1 and the spinous process of C2. A single sublaminar wire holds the graft in place. The Brooks technique uses from two to four sublaminar wires, and two bone grafts are wedged between the laminae of C1 and C2. The loss of motion between atlas and axis results in an overall decrease of 50% of cervical rotation. Use of transarticular

A **B**

Figure 5–5. Imaging studies in a patient with os odontoideum. **A:** Radiograph in flexion. The ossicle moves with the anterior ring of the atlas. **B:** Radiograph in extension.

screws or screw-rod constructs that purchase into the lateral masses of C1 and the pedicle of C2 are rigid enough to allow the patient to mobilize without a halo vest.

Dai L et al: Os odontoideum: Etiology, diagnosis, and management. Surg Neurol 2000;53:106. [PMID: 10713186]

Gluf WM, Brockmeyer DL: Atlantoaxial transarticular screw fixation: A review of surgical indications, fusion rate, complications, and lessons learned in 67 pediatric patients. J Neurosurg Spine 2005;2:164. [PMID: 15739528]

2. Klippel-Feil Syndrome

Klippel-Feil syndrome refers to an array of clinical disorders associated with congenital fusion of one or more cervical vertebrae. The fusion, which may be multilevel, results from a failure of the normal division of the cervical somites during the third through eighth weeks of embryogenesis. The cause of this failure is unknown. The syndrome was first described in 1912 by M. Klippel and A. Feil as a triad of clinical features: a short "web" neck, a low posterior hair line, and limited cervical neck motion. Interestingly, only 50% of patients with the syndrome that now bears the names of Klippel and Feil present with this classic triad.

Various conditions were subsequently seen in association with congenitally fused cervical vertebrae. These include scoliosis (seen in approximately 60% of cases), renal abnormalities (in 35%), deafness (in 30%), Sprengel deformity (in 30%), synkinesis or mirror movement (in 20%), congenital heart defects (in 14%), brainstem anomalies, congenital cervical stenosis, adrenal aplasia, ptosis, Duane contracture, lateral rectus palsy, facial nerve palsy, syndactyly, and upper extremity diffuse or focal hypoplasia.

Clinical Findings

A. SYMPTOMS AND SIGNS

Decreased range of motion is the most frequent finding in patients with cervical spine involvement. Involvement of only the lower cervical spine or fusion of fewer than three vertebrae results in minimal loss of motion, however. Patients may also be able to compensate at other cervical interspaces, masking any loss of motion.

Neck shortening is difficult to detect unless extreme. Webbing of the neck (pterygium colli), facial asymmetry, or torticollis is seen in fewer than 20% of patients. Webbing of the neck can nevertheless be dramatic, with underlying muscle involvement extending from the mastoid to the acromion. Sprengel deformity, which results from a failure of either or both scapulae to descend from their embryologic origin at C4, is seen in approximately 30% of patients. Sometimes an omovertebral bone bridges the cervical spine to the scapulae and limits the neck and shoulder motion.

Cervical spine symptoms in Klippel-Feil syndrome are related to the secondary hypermobility of the unfused vertebrae. Except for atlantoaxial joint involvement, resulting in a significant decrease in occipital rotation, the fused joints at a given level are asymptomatic. Because of the increased mechanical demands placed on the uninvolved joints, secondary osteoarthritis, disk degeneration, spinal stenosis, and instability may result at these levels. Neurologic sequelae, usually confined to the head, neck, and upper extremities, result from impingement of the cervical nerve roots. With progressive cervical instability, the spinal cord may become involved, leading to spasticity, weakness, hyperreflexia, and even quadriplegia or sudden death from minor trauma.

B. IMAGING STUDIES

Radiographic findings (Figure 5–6) of congenital cervical vertebral fusion are diagnostic of Klippel-Feil syndrome. This may present as synostosis of two vertebral bodies or as a multilevel fusion, as originally described in 1912. Other noteworthy findings are flattening of the involved vertebral bodies and the absence of disk spaces. Hypoplastic cervical disks in a child are often hard to appreciate radiographically. If suspected, flexion-extension views can be taken. CT scanning and MRI have improved the assessment of bony and nerve root involvement.

Spinal canal stenosis is not usually seen until adulthood. Although anterior spina bifida is infrequent, the posterior form is not. Enlargement of the foramen magnum with fixed hyperextension often accompanies the cervical spina bifida. Hemivertebrae are also noted.

Involvement of the upper thoracic spine can occur and may be the first sign of an undiagnosed cervical synostosis.

Because of the potential for multiorgan involvement in patients with Klippel-Feil syndrome, an electrocardiogram and renal ultrasound are also recommended.

Treatment

Treatment of the cervical spine abnormalities is limited. Multilevel involvement leads to hypermobility at uninvolved joints, so affected patients should be cautious in their activities. Prophylactic surgical stabilization is not routinely performed in asymptomatic patients because the risk-benefit ratio has not been well defined. In some cases, however, surgical fusion is performed.

Secondary osteoarthritis may be treated in the usual manner, including use of a cervical collar, traction, and antiinflammatory agents. Nerve root impingement requires careful evaluation before surgical decompression because more than one level may be involved and there may also be central abnormalities.

Figure 5–6. Imaging studies in a patient with Klippel-Feil syndrome and cervical myelopathy. **A:** Radiograph showing fusion of the atlas and the occiput and autofusion of the posterior elements of C3 and C4. **B:** CT scan demonstrates this as well. **C:** MRI demonstrating severe stenosis of the spinal canal. The odontoid process is above the level of the foramen magnum. **D:** Radiograph following posterior decompression and fusion between the occiput and C4.

Surgical correction of the aesthetic deformities is only moderately successful. Carefully selected candidates may benefit from soft tissue Z-plasty or tenotomies. This may improve the appearance of the patient but does not affect cervical motion.

Prognosis

Children with mild involvement can be expected to grow up to lead healthy, normal lives. Patients with more severe involvement can do comparably well if the associated conditions are successfully treated at an early age.

Herman MJ, Pizzutillo PD: Cervical spine disorders in children. Orthop Clin North Am 1999;30:457. Review. [PMID: 10393767]

Tracy MR, Dormans JP, Kusumi K: Klippel-Feil syndrome: Clinical features and current understanding of etiology. Clin Orthop 2004;424:183. [PMID: 15241163]

CERVICAL SPONDYLOSIS

Cervical spondylosis is defined as a generalized disease process affecting the entire cervical spine and related to chronic disk degeneration. In approximately 90% of men older than 50 years and 90% of women older than 60 years, degeneration of the cervical spine can be demonstrated by radiographs. Initial disk changes are followed by facet arthropathy, osteophyte formation, and ligamentous instability. Myelopathy, radiculopathy, or both may be seen secondarily. Cervical myelopathy is the most common form of spinal cord dysfunction in people older than 55 years. People older than 60 years are more likely to have multisegmental disease. The incidence of cervical myelopathy is twice as great in men as in women.

Pathophysiology

The relationship between the spinal cord and its bony arcade has been studied extensively. The first publication on the subject was written in the early 1800s and gave the first account of a "spondylotic bar," which was actually a thickened posterior longitudinal ligament protruding into the canal secondary to disk degeneration. Subsequent work revealed that disk degeneration and osteoarthritis could lead to spinal cord and nerve root impingement.

Acute traumatic disk herniation was distinguished from the chronic spondylotic process in the mid-1950s. Concurrently, anterior spinal artery impingement by the disk or osteophyte was proposed as part of the pathogenesis. As indicated in these studies, disk degeneration starts with tears in the posterolateral region of the annulus. The subsequent loss of water content and proteoglycans in the nucleus then leads to a decrease of disk height. The longitudinal ligaments degenerate and

form bony spurs at their insertion into the vertebral body. These so-called hard disks have to be distinguished from soft disks, which represent acute herniation of disk material into the spinal canal or into the neural foramen. The most frequently involved levels are the more mobile segments: C5-C6, C6-C7, and C4-C5. The converging of the cervical disk space may result in buckling of the ligamentum flavum, with further narrowing of the spinal canal. Segmental instability results in hypertrophic formation of osteophytes by the uncovertebral joint of Luschka and by the facet joints. These prominent spurs result in compression of both the exiting nerve roots and the spinal cord.

Further work revealed that the sagittal cervical canal diameter was appreciably smaller (3 mm on average) in the myelopathic spondylotic spine than in the normal spine. The anterior-posterior dimensions of the cervical spinal canal measure between 17 and 18 mm in normal individuals. Spinal canal stenosis is present when the canal diameter becomes less than 13 mm. With extension of the neck, both the spinal canal diameter and the neuroforaminal diameter decrease.

Clinical Findings

A. SYMPTOMS AND SIGNS

Headache may be the presenting symptom of cervical spondylosis. Usually, the headache is worse in the morning and improves throughout the day. It is commonly located in the occipital region and radiates toward the frontal area. Infrequently, patients complain of a painful, stiff neck. Signs include decreased range of motion, crepitus, or both. With more advanced cases, radicular or myelopathic symptoms may be present.

1. Cervical spondylotic radiculopathy—Cervical radiculopathy in spondylosis can be quite complex, with nerve root involvement seen at one or more levels and occurring either unilaterally or bilaterally. The onset may be acute, subacute, or chronic, and impingement on the nerve roots may be from either osteophytes or disk herniation. With radiculopathy, sensory involvement in the form of paresthesias or hyperesthesia is more common than motor or reflex changes. Several dermatomal levels may be involved, with radiation into the anterior chest and back. The chief complaint is radiation of pain into the interscapular area and into the arm. Typically, patients have proximal arm pain and distal paresthesias.

2. Cervical spondylotic myelopathy—Cervical myelopathy has a variable clinical presentation, given the complex pathogenic mechanisms involved. These include static or dynamic canal impingement, facet arthropathy, vascular ischemia, and the presence of spondylotic transverse bars. In addition, given its neuronal topography, the cord may be affected in dramatically different ways by relatively minor differences in anatomic regions of compression. The clinical course of myelopathy is usually progressive, leading to complete disability over a period of months to years with stepwise deteriorations in function.

Patients often present with paresthesias, dyskinesias, or weakness of the hand, the entire upper extremity, or the lower extremity. Deep aching pain of the extremity, broad-based gait, loss of balance, loss of hand dexterity, and general muscle wasting are found in patients with advanced myelopathy. Impotence is not uncommon in these patients.

Hyperextension injuries of the spondylotic cervical spine can precipitate a central cord syndrome in which motor and sensory involvement is typically greater in the upper extremities than the lower extremities. Recovery from this injury is usually incomplete. Complete quadriplegia can also occur if the preexisting stenosis is severe. In this setting, the 1-year mortality approaches 80%.

Deep tendon reflexes can be either hyporeflexic or hyperreflexic, with the former seen in anterior horn cell (upper extremity) involvement and the latter seen in corticospinal tract (lower extremity) involvement. Hyporeflexia is found at the level of compression; hyperreflexia occurs on the level below. Long-tract signs, such as the presence of the Hoffmann reflex or Babinski reflex, indicate an upper motor neuron lesion. Clonus is often present though asymmetric. Upper extremity involvement is often unilateral, whereas lower extremities are affected bilaterally. High cervical spondylosis (C3-C5) leads to complaints of numb and clumsy hands; myelopathy of the lower cervical spine (C5-C8) presents with spasticity and loss of proprioception in the legs.

Abdominal reflexes are usually intact, enabling the clinician to differentiate spondylosis from amyotrophic lateral sclerosis, in which reflexes are often absent. Multiple compressions of the spinal cord cause more severe deterioration functionally and electrophysiologically than a single-level compression does.

B. IMAGING STUDIES

Although spondylosis results from cervical spine degeneration, not every patient with radiographic evidence of cervical disk degeneration has symptoms. Furthermore, patients with all the radiographic stigmas of cervical spondylosis may be asymptomatic, and others with clinical evidence of myelopathy may show only modest radiographic changes. This paradox is explainable by canal size differences, with the smaller-diameter canal having less space to buffer the degenerative lesion.

The average AP diameter of the spinal canal measures 17 mm from C3 to C7. The space required by the spinal cord averages 10 mm. The dural diameter increases by 2–3 mm in extension. The smallest sagittal anteroposterior diameter is measured between an osteo-phyte on the inferior aspect of the vertebral body to the base of the spinous process of the next vertebra below. An absolute spinal canal stenosis exists with a sagittal diameter of less than 10 mm. The stenosis is relative if the diameter measures 10–13 mm.

Plain film findings also vary according to the stage of spondylosis at which they were taken. Radiographs may appear normal in early disk disease. Alternatively, they may show single or multilevel disk space narrowing with or without osteophytes. C5-C6 and C6-C7 are the two most commonly involved segments (Figure 5–7). Vertebral body sclerosis at the adjacent base plates may also be seen. Cortical erosion is uncommon and indicates an inflammatory process such as rheumatoid arthritis.

Oblique views permit evaluation of the facet joints and detection of osteophytosis and sclerosis. The superior facets undergo degeneration more frequently than their inferior counterparts. The superior joints may then subluxate posteriorly and erode into the lamina below. Inferior osteophytes, however, may prevent significant slippage. If instability seen on flexion-extension views is significant (greater than 3.5 mm when measured at the posteroinferior corner of the vertebral body), foraminal stenosis as well as vertebral artery impingement may result.

MRI permits visualization of the entire cervical canal and spinal cord by showing the spinal cord and nerve roots in two planes. The use of a contrast-enhanced CT scan is occasionally required in elderly (more than 60 years) patients with advanced degenerative bony changes of the cervical spine. Accurate identification of the location and extent of pathologic changes is necessary to determine the optimal approach for decompression. Selective nerve root blocks and electromyography may be useful to identify the level of involvement.

Differential Diagnosis

Inflammatory, neoplastic, and infectious conditions can mimic cervical spondylotic radiculopathy and myelopathy.

The cervical spine is affected in most rheumatoid arthritis patients. Atlantoaxial subluxation or subaxial instability can cause symptoms similar to those seen in degenerative cervical myelopathy. A primary tumor or metastatic disease can present with unremitting neck pain, often more intense at night. MRI can distinguish neoplastic conditions from degenerative disorders. Infections of the cervical spine occur in children and in elderly (more than 60 years) or immunocompromised individuals. Multiple sclerosis should be considered in the differential diagnosis. It occurs in younger patients but can present with similar motor signs. Pancoast tumors may invade the brachial plexus, resulting in upper extremity symptoms. Syringomyelia presents with tingling sensations plus motor weakness. A low protein concentration in the cerebrospinal fluid and characteristic changes on MRI are found. Disor-

A   B

Figure 5–7. Imaging studies in a patient with cervical spondylosis and chronic neck pain. **A:** Radiograph showing collapsed disk space between C5 and C6 and a large posterior osteophyte at the inferior endplate of C6. **B:** MRI showing collapsed disk spaces, a mild stenosis of the spinal canal, and effacement of the spinal cord by an osteophyte at C6.

ders of the shoulder, especially rotator cuff tendinitis, can imitate cervical radiculopathy. Compressive peripheral neuropathies, such as thoracic outlet syndrome, also have to be ruled out.

Treatment

Patients should be divided into three groups, according to the predominance of their symptoms: neck pain alone, radiculopathy, and myelopathy. The duration and progression of symptoms need to be considered in the planning of treatment. Several studies suggest that patients with cervical radiculopathy or myelopathy have better long-term results from surgery if symptoms are of short duration.

A. CONSERVATIVE TREATMENT

Initial management of patients with cervical spondylosis may involve a soft collar, antiinflammatory agents,

and physical therapy consisting of mild traction and the use of isometric strengthening and range-of-motion exercises. The soft cervical collar should be worn only briefly, until the acute symptoms subside. Analgesics are important in the acute phase, and muscle relaxants are helpful in breaking the cycle of muscle spasm and pain. Diazepam should be avoided because of its side effects as a clinical depressant. Epidural corticosteroid injections may be efficacious in patients with radicular pain. Trigger point injections are an empirical form of therapy that seems to work well in patients with chronic neck pain.

The value of cervical traction remains unclear. It is contraindicated in patients with cord compression, rheumatoid arthritis, infection, or osteoporosis. A careful screening of roentgenograms before treatment is mandatory. No evidence indicates that home traction is more effective than manual traction. Isometric strengthening exercises of the paravertebral musculature should be started after the acute symptoms resolve. The patient should be instructed to start a home exercise program early, to avoid long-term dependency on passive therapy modalities. Although ice, moist heat, ultrasound, and transcutaneous electrical nerve stimulation (TENS) are safe to use, there is no scientific proof of their efficacy.

B. SURGICAL TREATMENT

Surgical intervention should be considered if the patient does not respond to a conservative treatment protocol or shows evidence of deteriorating myelopathy or radiculopathy. The spinal cord can be effectively decompressed by either anterior, posterior, or combined approaches.

The anterior approach allows multilevel diskectomy, vertebrectomy, foraminotomy, and fusion with tricortical iliac crest bone grafts or strut grafts. Newer instrumentation techniques, such as cervical plates (Figure 5–8), alleviate the need for halo immobilization. However supplemental posterior fixation and fusion should be added if more than three vertebral levels are decompressed anteriorly. Posterior fixation minimizes the risk of anterior dislodgement of the graft even in the presence of solid anterior fixation. Anterior interbody fusion after decompression for a herniated cervical disk (Figure 5–9) has a high success rate.

Cervical disk replacement prostheses were also developed to provide a motion-sparing alternative to anterior cervical diskectomy and fusion. By maintaining existing motion or restoring motion to a diseased motion segment, these prostheses have the potential to decrease the rate of symptomatic adjacent segment degeneration. Currently, clinical trials approved by the Food and Drug Administration (FDA) are under way to assess the efficacy of these devices against the outcomes that can be obtained with anterior cervical diskectomy and fusion.

The number of involved levels may be important in deciding which of the surgical approaches to use. Patients with cervical myelopathy and involvement of more than three vertebral body levels may be best managed by a posterior approach. Multilevel laminectomy or laminoplasty shows excellent results. If laminectomies are performed, the facet joints and capsules should be preserved to minimize the chance of postlaminectomy deformity. Late swan-neck deformities after laminectomy can be avoided with simultaneous posterior fusion using lateral mass plates. Laminoplasty is advantageous in that the cervical spinal cord can be decompressed without the high risk of developing late deformity. In addition, the morbidity associated with instrumentation and fusion can be avoided.

Operative treatment in cases of cervical spondylotic radiculopathy and myelopathy must be individualized for every patient.

Prognosis

Cervical spondylosis is generally a progressive, chronic disease process. In a study of 205 patients with neck pain, Gore et al. found that many patients had decreased pain at the 10-year follow-up, but those with the most severe involvement did not improve. Conservative measures may retard the disease process in its early stages. If myelopathy or radiculopathy becomes clinically evident, surgical intervention is often necessary. For disease involving less than three vertebral levels, early anterior decompression and fusion improves the clinical outcome, particularly in the elderly (more than 60 years) individual who suffers from cervical myelopathy.

Belanger TA et al: Ossification of the posterior longitudinal ligament. Results of anterior cervical decompression and arthrodesis in sixty-one North American patients. J Bone Joint Surg Am 2005;87:610. [PMID: 15741630]

Chagas H et al: Cervical spondylotic myelopathy: 10 years of prospective outcome analysis of anterior decompression and fusion. Surg Neurol. 2005;64(Suppl 1):S1:30. [PMID: 15967227]

Edwards CC II et al: Cervical myelopathy. current diagnostic and treatment strategies. Spine J 2003;3:68. Review. [PMID: 14589250]

Edwards CC II, Heller JG, Murakami H: Corpectomy versus laminoplasty for multilevel cervical myelopathy: An independent matched cohort analysis. Spine 2002;27:1168. [PMID: 12045513]

Emery SE: Cervical spondylotic myelopathy: Diagnosis and treatment. J Am Acad Orthop Surg 2001;9:376. Review. [PMID: 11767723]

Epstein N: Anterior approaches to cervical spondylosis and ossification of the posterior longitudinal ligament: Review of operative technique and assessment of 65 multilevel circumferential procedures. Surg Neurol 2001;55:313. Review. [PMID: 11483184]

Heller JG et al: Laminoplasty versus laminectomy and fusion for multilevel cervical myelopathy: An independent matched cohort analysis. Spine 2001;26:1330. [PMID: 11426147]

Mehdorn HM, Fritsch MJ, Stiller RU: Treatment options and results in cervical myelopathy. Acta Neurochir Suppl 2005; 93:177. [PMID: 15986751]

Onari K et al: Long-term follow-up results of anterior interbody fusion applied for cervical myelopathy due to ossification of the posterior longitudinal ligament. Spine 2001;26:488. [PMID: 11242375]

Phillips FM, Garfin SR: Cervical disc replacement. Spine 2005; 30(Suppl 17):S27.

Takayama H et al: Proprioceptive recovery of patients with cervical myelopathy after surgical decompression. Spine 2005;30:1039.

Wada E et al: Subtotal corpectomy versus laminoplasty for multilevel cervical spondylotic myelopathy: A long-term follow-up study over 10 years. Spine 2001;26:1443. [PMID: 11458148]

Wang MY, Shah S, Green BA: Clinical outcomes following cervical laminoplasty for 204 patients with cervical spondylotic myelopathy. Surg Neurol 2004;62:487. [PMID: 15576110]

A

B

C

Figure 5–8. Imaging studies in a patient with cervical spondylotic myelopathy. **A:** Radiograph showing degenerative changes between C4 and C7. **B** and **C:** Radiographs taken after anterior vertebrectomy of C5 and C6, iliac crest strut graft, and anterior plate fixation.

A **B**

Figure 5–9. Imaging studies in a patient with cervical disk herniation. **A:** MRI showing herniation at C6-C7. **B:** Radiograph taken after anterior cervical fusion with a tricortical graft from the pelvis.

OSSIFICATION OF THE POSTERIOR LONGITUDINAL LIGAMENT

Ossification of the posterior longitudinal ligament (OPLL) is a relatively common cause of spinal canal stenosis and myelopathy in the Asian population. Its overall incidence is 2–3% in Japan, compared with 0.6% in Hawaii and 1.7% in Italy. Males are affected more often than females, and the peak age at onset of symptoms is the sixth decade. Although the cause of the disorder is unknown, it may be controlled by autosomal dominant inheritance because it is found in 26% of the parents and 29% of the siblings of affected patients. The disorder is associated with several rheumatic conditions, including diffuse idiopathic skeletal hyperostosis (DISH), spondylosis, and ankylosing spondylitis.

Clinical Findings

Almost all patients have only mild subjective complaints at the onset, although 10–15% of them complain of clumsiness and spastic gait. Nevertheless, minor trauma can lead to acute deterioration of symptoms and can result in quadriplegia. Spastic quadriparesis is the most common neurologic presentation.

Ossification of the posterior longitudinal ligament can easily be diagnosed on plain lateral radiographs. The levels most frequently involved are C4, C5, and C6. A segmental type of disorder is distinguished from the continuous, local, and mixed type on the basis of the distribution of lesions behind the vertebral bodies. CT scanning is helpful in assessing the thickness, lateral extension, and AP diameter of the ossified ligament. More than 95% of the ossification is localized in the cervical spine, although extension into the thoracic spine is reported to be a cause of persistent myelopathy following cervical decompression.

Enchondral ossification is mainly responsible for the formation of the ossified mass, which connects to the upper and lower margins of the vertebral bodies. In many cases, the ossified material is closely adherent to the underlying dura and makes excision quite hazardous. Compression of the spinal cord results in atrophy and necrosis in the gray matter and demyelinization of the white substance.

Treatment

Neurologic improvement with either conservative or surgical treatment is achieved in a significant proportion of patients. The patients with severe myelopathy require neural decompression by an anterior, posterior, or combined approach. Sophisticated posterior decompression techniques, such as the open-door laminoplasty, have yielded excellent long-term results for OPLL lesions that do not comprise more than 50% of the spinal canal cross-sectional area.

Belanger TA et al: Ossification of the posterior longitudinal ligament. Results of anterior cervical decompression and arthrodesis in sixty-one North American patients. J Bone Joint Surg Am 2005;87:610. [PMID: 15741630]

Chiba K et al: Multicenter study investigating the postoperative progression of ossification of the posterior longitudinal ligament in the cervical spine: A new computer-assisted measurement. J Neurosurg Spine 2005;3:17. [PMID: 16122017]

Epstein NE: Circumferential cervical surgery for ossification of the posterior longitudinal ligament: A multianalytic outcome study. Spine 2004;29:1340. [PMID: 15187635]

Kawaguchi Y et al: Progression of ossification of the posterior longitudinal ligament following en bloc cervical laminoplasty. J Bone Joint Surg Am 2001;83:1798. [PMID: 11741057]

Matsuoka T et al: Long-term results of the anterior floating method for cervical myelopathy caused by ossification of the posterior longitudinal ligament. Spine 2001;26:241. [PMID: 11224859]

Nakanishi K et al: Positive effect of posterior instrumentation after surgical posterior decompression for extensive cervicothoracic ossification of the posterior longitudinal ligament. Spine 2005;30:E382.

Ogawa Y et al: Long-term results of expansive open-door laminoplasty for ossification of the posterior longitudinal ligament of the cervical spine. J Neurosurg Spine 2004;1:168. [PMID: 15347002]

Takeshita K et al: Can laminoplasty maintain the cervical alignment even when the C2 lamina is contained? Spine 2005;30:1294.

■ DISEASES & DISORDERS OF THE LUMBAR SPINE

LOW BACK PAIN

Low back pain is a very common symptom in the general population. According to the Quebec Task Force on Spinal Disorders, more than 80% of the population experience some low back pain at some point in their life. The overall prevalence of low back pain in the United States is estimated to be approximately 18%. The annual incidence of low back pain is 15–20%. Males are affected as often as females, and the pain is usually self-limiting, with 50% of affected patients recovering by 2 weeks and 90% recovering by 6 weeks. Only 1% of the population in the United States is chronically disabled by back symptoms. If a patient stays off work for more than 2 years because of problems of the lower back, he or she is unlikely to return to work at all.

The socioeconomic impact of back problems is enormous. Over 14% of all new patient visits to physicians are for complaints of low back pain, and it is the most common reason for visits to the orthopedic surgeon. Costs are estimated to range from $20 billion to $50 billion annually, with 10% of the patients accounting for 85–90% of the costs. Investigators showed that patients with chronic low back pain tend to be dissatisfied with their vocation, viewing it as boring and repetitious. They also have an increased divorce rate, more problems with headaches and gastrointestinal ulcers, and a higher rate of alcoholism than the average population. The extensive use of the Minnesota Multiphasic Personality Inventory (MMPI) in the assessment of patients with chronic low back pain demonstrates an association among chronic pain, somatization, and hypochondriasis.

Etiology & Pathophysiology

The exact cause of symptoms is found in only 12–15% of patients. A thorough understanding of the lumbar anatomy and its function is important because lower back pain may originate from the disk, vertebral body, or posterior elements or may be unrelated to the spine. The earlier concept of a motor segment is now superseded by the concept of a functional spinal unit (FSU), or motion segment. The FSU consists of two adjacent vertebrae and the intervertebral disk. It forms a three-joint complex with the disk in front and two facet joints posteriorly. The motion segment involves joint capsules, ligaments, muscles, nerves, and vessels as well. Changes in one joint affect the other two. Disk degeneration leads to disk space narrowing, endplate sclerosis, abnormal stress on facet joints, and, ultimately, facet degeneration.

Significant emphasis is newly placed on the idea of the intervertebral disk as a pain generator. These axial pain syndromes of diskogenic origin are roughly categorized as internal disk disruption, degenerative disk disease, and disk degeneration as a sequela of segmental instability. The overriding principle is that the posterior portion of the annulus fibrosus is innervated by fibers of the sinuvertebral nerve that is a branch of the dorsal root ganglion. Irritation of the sinuvertebral nerve is thought to be responsible for axial back pain. In the rat, Suseki showed that these pain fibers are not innervated segmentally. Sensory information from the lumbar intervertebral disks is conducted to other spinal levels via the paravertebral sympathetic trunks. These data suggest that decompression of the nerve root at one level is unlikely to help with low back pain symptoms.

Principles of Diagnosis

A. HISTORY AND PHYSICAL EXAMINATION

A focused history and physical examination of the patient are crucial for the appropriate diagnosis and treatment. Typical initial questions include the following: What is the problem? Which areas are affected? How much does the pain interfere with sitting, standing, and walking? Were there previous episodes? If so, how long did they last? Are there bowel or bladder symptoms? The presence of bowel or bladder symptoms may indicate a cauda equina syndrome. Leg and buttock pain are usually indicative of nerve root irritation from a herniated disk or neuroforaminal stenosis, whereas axial low back pain is often mechanical. Drawing a diagram of the areas affected by pain may be of help, and a history of other medical problems may provide additional clues.

The physical examination is subjective and requires the patient's interpretation and cooperation. The diagnostic significance of range-of-motion measurements of the spine is questionable. Although a positive result in the straight leg–raising test is highly suggestive of nerve root irritation in a young patient, use of this test is less reliable in an older (more than 50 years) patient. In addition to noting a general impression of the patient and testing for sensory and motor deficits, the clinician should check the patient's response to local touch, axial loading, and simulated rotation and should record the presence of other nonorganic signs (Waddell signs). Patients with chronic low back pain demonstrate illness behavior and score high in nonorganic signs.

The pain is considered acute if it lasts less than 6 weeks and chronic if it lasts longer than 12 weeks. The most common cause is a lumbar strain after a lifting or twisting event or without known trauma. Patients usually present with localized pain in the lumbosacral area, in some cases with pain radiating into the buttocks. Palpation of the paraspinal muscles reveals spasms, and motion is limited. Results of the neurologic examination are normal, and the straight leg–raising test is negative. Sensation and reflexes are symmetric.

B. IMAGING STUDIES

1. Radiography—Radiographs are not necessary during the initial evaluation. If a patient's symptoms do not resolve, radiographs may be obtained. They are indicated in patients who are older than 50 years and have a history of trauma, cancer, weight loss, pain at rest, drug abuse, neurologic deficit, or fever. Radiographs may appear normal or demonstrate disk space narrowing, osteophyte formation, or localized instability on lateral flexion-extension views. No association is established between low back pain and the presence of disk space narrowing, transitional vertebrae, Schmorl nodes, the disk vacuum sign, claw spurs, lumbar lordosis, or spina bifida occulta. Routine flexion-extension views of the lumbar spine are not indicated and rarely demonstrate obvious segmental instability.

2. Other studies—If plain radiographs are unsuccessful in establishing the cause of the patient's problem and the patient does not respond to conservative therapy, additional imaging studies may be helpful.

MRI of the lumbar spine is noninvasive and excellent in assessing compromise of neural structures. For example, MRI with gadolinium enhances the imaging of intraspinal tissue and can help distinguish scar formation after previous surgery from new encroachment on neural structures by disk material. CT scanning, with and without enhancement by myelography, can be helpful if MRI studies are not possible or do not yield positive results. CT myelography is especially useful to assess patients who have had spinal instrumentation. If an infection of the spine is suspected, a gadolinium-enhanced MRI is an extremely sensitive and specific test for diskitis, spinal osteomyelitis, and epidural abscess.

Disk degeneration is common in adults with low back pain. Caution in interpreting the results of MRI and CT is necessary, however, because studies show that positive findings are seen in asymptomatic patients who undergo MRI or CT evaluation of the lumbar spine. When MRI was used to examine the lumbar spines of asymptomatic volunteers, disk herniation was found in 17% of those younger than 40 years, 22% of those between 40 and 59 years, and 36% of those older than 60 years. In the oldest group, 21% showed lumbar stenosis without symptoms. When CT was used to examine the lumbar spines of asymptomatic volunteers, disk herniation was found in 35.4% of the volunteers.

If disk degeneration is suspected to be the cause of lower back pain, a diskogram may be indicated. In this provocative test, dye is injected into the nucleus pulposus, and then a CT scan of the injected segment is taken. The pain response of the patient seems to be the most accurate indication that the injected disk might be responsible for the patient's pain. However, the use of provocative diskography in the evaluation of axial back pain continues to be controversial. The results are subjective and depend very much on the patient's psychological status at the time of the procedure. Diskography is more sensitive than MRI to assess internal disk disruption, although questions about the value of using diskography, facet blocks, and other invasive tests remain to be answered.

Principles of Treatment

Management of low back pain has to be tailored to the individual. The goal is early return to work. Most patients can simply modify their activities during the acute phase. If a serious pathologic condition is ruled out, a more aggressive approach is warranted because bed rest for more than 2 days has serious side effects: The body is in a catabolic state; 3% of muscle bulk is lost daily; 6% of bone is demineralized in 2 weeks; and restriction of social activities leads to illness behavior, depression, and loss of interest and motivation. Iatrogenic disability must be avoided. Patients with acute low back pain should avoid sitting and lifting. Mild analgesics and antiinflammatory agents are useful in the acute phase of the disease. Educational programs, aerobic endurance exercises, and abdominal conditioning also prove helpful.

No evidence indicates that the following treatment modalities are useful in the management of acute low back pain: TENS, interferential stimulation, traction, manipulation in the presence of radicular signs, acupuncture, biofeedback, narcotics for longer than 2 weeks, trigger point injections, and muscle relaxants.

Patients who have low back pain that persists for more than 3 months occasionally benefit from antidepressant medication. If narcotic analgesics are not needed and if surgery is ruled out, they may be candidates for a functional restoration program involving an interdisciplinary approach with physical therapists, occupational therapists, psychologists, and medical professionals. One study showed that 87% of program participants returned to work, whereas only 41% of control subjects did so.

A subgroup of patients who have persistent, disabling axial low back pain of diskogenic origin in the absence of other psychological or organic pathologies may benefit from complete diskectomy and interbody fusion. This can be performed through an anterior open or laparoscopic approach or via the posterior approach. Good to excellent outcomes are reported in up to 70–80% of patients.

Disk replacement surgery was first introduced in the early 1950s with variable results. As spinal fusion demonstrated itself to be a relatively efficacious procedure, spinal arthroplasty quickly lost its initial enthusiasm. However, as the limitations of spinal fusion became evident and technology improved to design better bearing surfaces, disk replacement is enjoying a resurgence in interest. The theoretical advantages, which include preserving or restoring motion after removal of the painful disk, preventing late adjacent segment degeneration, and improving function without the need for fusion, should be weighed against the possible complications. These include malpositioning of the prosthesis, extrusion of the device, failure of the polyethylene articulating surface, and osteolysis. Clinical outcomes of single-level lumbar total disk replacement are improved over single-level fusion in the first 6 months following surgery. However, the results are similar to fusion at 2-year follow-up. The SB-Charite III total disk replacement is the first device to be approved by the FDA for this application. Other comparable devices are currently under FDA-approved randomized, prospective clinical trials.

Other less invasive therapies for diskogenic axial back pain are also available. One of these, an intradiskal electrothermal therapy, attempts to thermally ablate the painful nerve fibers in the posterior annulus. The reported outcomes on this procedure are variable, and it is unclear whether the results are a significant improvement over the natural history of axial low back pain.

Blumenthal S et al: A prospective, randomized, multicenter Food and Drug Administration investigational device exemptions study of lumbar total disk replacement with the Charite artificial disc versus lumbar fusion: Part I. Evaluation of clinical outcomes. Spine 2005;30:1565. [PMID: 16025024]

Delamarter RB, Bae HW, Pradhan BB: Clinical results of ProDisc-II lumbar total disc replacement: Report from the United States clinical trial. Orthop Clin North Am 2005;36:301. [PMID: 15950690]

Derby R et al: The ability of pressure-controlled discography to predict surgical and nonsurgical outcomes. Spine 1999;24:364. [PMID: 10065521]

Fritzell P et al; Swedish Lumbar Spine Study Group, 2001 Volvo Award Winner in Clinical Studies: Lumbar fusion versus nonsurgical treatment for chronic low back pain: A multicenter randomized controlled trial from the Swedish Lumbar Spine Study Group. Spine 2001;26:2521. [PMID: 11725230]

Geisler FH et al: Neurological complications of lumbar artificial disc replacement and comparison of clinical results with those related to lumbar arthrodesis in the literature: Results of a multicenter, prospective, randomized investigational device exemption study of Charite intervertebral disc. Invited submission from the Joint Section Meeting on Disorders of the Spine and Peripheral Nerves, March 2004. J Neurosurg Spine 2004;1:143. [PMID: 15346999]

Humphreys SC et al: Comparison of posterior and transforaminal approaches to lumbar interbody fusion. Spine 2001;26:567. [PMID: 11242386]

McAfee PC et al: A prospective, randomized, multicenter Food and Drug Administration investigational device exemption study of lumbar total disc replacement with the CHARITE artificial disc versus lumbar fusion: Part II. Evaluation of radiographic outcomes and correlation of surgical technique accuracy with clinical outcomes. Spine 2005;30:1576. [PMID: 16025025]

Saal JA, Saal JS: Intradiscal electrothermal treatment for chronic discogenic low back pain: A prospective outcome study with minimum 1-year follow-up. Spine 2000;25:2622. [PMID: 11034647]

LUMBAR DISK HERNIATION

Symptomatic disk herniations are seen in all age groups but have their peak in patients between 35 and 45 years of age. Although smoking is a general risk factor for disk degeneration and herniation, occupational risk factors include sedentary work and motor vehicle driving. Sciatica, characterized by pain radiating down the leg in a dermatomal distribution, is the most common symptom and found in 40% of patients with disk herniation. Approximately 50% of patients recover within 1 month, and 96% function normally by 6 months. The rate of surgical treatment in the United States is three times higher than that in Sweden.

Pathophysiology

A disk herniation is usually preceded by degenerative changes inside the disk. Circumferential tears in the annulus progress to radial tears, and these in turn frequently cause internal disruption or frank herniation. Two pathologic patterns can be distinguished. In a contained disk protrusion, the annulus fibers are intact. In a noncontained disk herniation, the annulus is completely disrupted. Disk material can be subligamentous or sequestered as a free fragment. The pain accompanying disk herniation may be caused by direct pressure on the nerve root or may be induced by breakdown products from a degenerated nucleus pulposus or by an autoimmune reaction. Disk material is a direct source of chemically irritative substances such as phospholipase A2, prostaglandin E2, substance P, and lactic acid. Biochemical studies in operated disk fragments demonstrate an advanced aging process. The hydration of the disk changes from 90% during childhood to 70% by the sixth decade, and the ability of proteoglycans to aggregate decreases with advancing age.

Clinical Findings

A. SYMPTOMS AND SIGNS

The typical sciatica is commonly preceded by back pain for a period of days or weeks. This scenario suggests that a compression of nerve fibers in the outer layers of the annulus preceded the rupture of the disk material into the spinal canal and the advent of leg pain. A complete physical examination is necessary. Although the dominating symptom is pain, patients often present with scoliosis or a sciatic list. The mobility of the lumbar spine is diminished more in flexion than in extension. Coughing, sneezing, or a voluntary Valsalva maneuver commonly aggravates the radiating pain. Prolonged sitting also accentuates the pain.

In more than 90% of cases, lumbar disk herniations are localized at L4-L5 and L5-S1. Paracentral disk herniations typically affect the traversing nerve root at the affected level, whereas lateral and foraminal herniations affect the exiting nerve root at the affected level. Compression of the L4 nerve root, which leads to pain and numbness in the L4 dermatome, can occur in a central disk herniation at L3-L4 or in a lateral herniation at L4-L5. When the L4 nerve root is affected, there may be weakness of the quadriceps muscle, and the patella tendon reflex may be depressed or absent. Central or paracentral disk herniations at L4-L5 usually compromise the L5 nerve root, where they may cause numbness in the L5 dermatome and weakness of the foot and toe dorsiflexors. A disk herniation at L5-S1 usually compromises the S1 nerve root, causing numbness or pain in the S1 dermatome, weak plantarflexion of the foot, loss of the Achilles tendon reflex, or tingling in the nerve distribution.

The straight leg–raising test should be performed. The Lasègue sign (pain when the affected leg is elevated) is positive in 98% of patients with lumbar disk herniation, and the cross-Lasègue sign (pain radiating to the affected leg when the contralateral leg is elevated) is positive in 20%. This test is less accurate in older (more than 60 years) patients and in patients with chronic lumbar disk herniation. For lesions involving the L3 or L4 nerve root, the femoral nerve stretch test should be applied. The radicular pain is reproduced when the knee is flexed while the hip is slightly extended.

B. IMAGING STUDIES

MRI is the study of choice for diagnosis of a herniated disk (Figure 5–10). Because 28% of asymptomatic patients show a disk herniation on MRI, it is important to correlate the level of spinal involvement with the peripheral nerve deficit. CT scanning and myelography are less frequently used to confirm the diagnosis.

Differential Diagnosis

Radicular pain is typical and should be distinguished from referred pain, which commonly radiates from the lower back into the posterior thigh and ends at the knee level. The posterior spinal elements are frequently a source of this pain. Anterior thigh pain may indicate a retroperitoneal process, such as renal disease or a tumor of the uterus or bladder. Hip disorders, including trochanteric bursitis and coxarthrosis, must be ruled out. The presence of incontinence, perianal numbness, and bilateral leg pain associated with numbness suggests a cauda equina syndrome and requires immediate surgical attention. A primary tumor or metastatic disease involving the spine can present with radiculopathy, and symptoms and signs such as pain at night, a previous history of cancer, and loss of weight should raise the suspicion of the examiner.

Treatment

In cases of lumbar disk herniation, the goal of treatment is to return the patient to normal activities as quickly as possible. Unnecessary surgery should be avoided. In determining the proper treatment plan, a

Figure 5–10. MRI in a patient with disk herniation at L4-L5 and L5-S1. Both disks are markedly desiccated as compared with disks of the upper lumbar spine.

knowledge of the natural history of lumbar disk herniation is important. In a prospective study of 280 patients with lumbar disk herniations, Weber compared the outcome of a group treated conservatively with the outcome of a group treated with diskectomy. Although better results were seen in the surgically treated patients at 1-year follow-up, the groups showed nearly equal results in terms of function 4 and 10 years later. The study demonstrated a slight tendency to a more favorable outcome with surgery.

A. CONSERVATIVE TREATMENT

Two days of bed rest followed by a good physical therapy program will often lead to significant alleviation of symptoms within 2 or 3 weeks. Analgesics and nonsteroidal medication may also be included in the regimen. Chiropractic adjustments should be avoided in patients with documented disk herniation. Although the role of epidural corticosteroids is unclear, they seem to be successful in decreasing the acute sciatic pain.

B. SURGICAL TREATMENT

Approximately 10% of patients with lumbar disk herniation ultimately require surgery. Surgery is recommended if the sciatica is severe and disabling and tension signs are positive, if symptoms persist without improvement for longer than 1 month, or if findings on clinical examination and in diagnostic tests are consistent with nerve root compromise.

When a standard diskectomy is used, the overall success rate is 85%, and 95% of the patients with successful surgery return to work. Microdiskectomy minimizes the dissection and has an equally high success rate. Newer techniques using muscle-splitting approaches and small tubular retractors require even less soft-tissue violation than microdiskectomy. With this technique, only removal of the extruded part of the disk or of the free fragment is necessary. Postoperative discomfort is minimized and speed of recovery is maximized. Risks of surgery include dural tear, wrong-level exploration, hemorrhage, infection, and nerve deficit.

In cases of contained disk protrusion, percutaneous automated diskectomy or chemonucleolysis may be considered. Each of these approaches has a success rate of approximately 75%. When percutaneous diskectomy is used, a cannula is placed into the disk space under fluoroscopic control, a cutting instrument is fitted inside the cannula, and disk material is then cut and suctioned at the same time. Insertion of an optical device through an extra portal makes direct visualization of the disk possible. Although a multicenter analysis of percutaneous diskectomy showed that only 55% of patients returned to work following treatment, the success rate appears to be higher in the centers with the greatest experience.

Chemonucleolysis of herniated disks is used extensively in Europe. Chymopapain is injected into the nucleus of the contained herniated disk, and it degrades the nucleus pulposus enzymatically but leaves the annulus intact. This procedure fell into disfavor in the United States after a series of deaths occurred secondary to anaphylaxis. Other complications associated with the procedure include transverse myelitis, diskitis, seizures, and subarachnoid hemorrhage. Many of the previous bad results have been linked with poor patient selection or technical error.

Because experience with laser diskectomy is limited, this extradural approach must still be viewed as experimental. Thus far, its success rate is slightly lower than that of percutaneous diskectomy.

Atlas SJ et al: Long-term outcomes of surgical and nonsurgical management of sciatica secondary to a lumbar disc herniation: 10 year results from the Maine lumbar spine study. Spine 2005;30:927. [PMID: 15834338]

Burton AK, Tillotson KM, Cleary J: Single-blind randomised controlled trial of chemonucleolysis and manipulation in the treatment of symptomatic lumbar disc herniation. Eur Spine J 2000;9:202. [PMID: 10905437]

Choi JY, Choi YW, Sung KH: Anterior lumbar interbody fusion in patients with a previous discectomy: minimum 2-year follow-up. J Spinal Disord Tech 2005;18:347.

Dai LY et al: Recurrent lumbar disc herniation after discectomy: Outcome of repeat discectomy. Surg Neurol 2005;64:226.

Ito T, Takano Y, Yuasa N: Types of lumbar herniated disc and clinical course. Spine 2001;26:648. [PMID: 11246377]

Ng L, Chaudhary N, Sell P: The efficacy of corticosteroids in per-iradicular infiltration for chronic radicular pain: A randomized, double-blind, controlled trial. Spine 2005;30:857.

Nygaard OP, Kloster R, Solberg T: Duration of leg pain as a predictor of outcome after surgery for lumbar disc herniation: a prospective cohort study with 1-year follow up. J Neurosurg 2000;92(Suppl 2):131. [PMID: 10763681]

Park YK, Kim JH, Chung HS: Outcome analysis of patients after ligament-sparing microdiscectomy for lumbar disc herniation. Neurosurg Focus 2002;13:E4.

Riew KD et al: The effect of nerve-root injections on the need for operative treatment of lumbar radicular pain. A prospective, randomized, controlled, double-blind study. J Bone Joint Surg Am 2000;82:1589. [PMID: 11097449]

Yorimitsu E, Chiba K, Toyama Y et al: Long-term outcomes of standard discectomy for lumbar disc herniation: A follow-up study of more than 10 years. Spine 2001;26:652. [PMID: 11246379]

FACET SYNDROME

The facet joint is probably not a common source of pain. The term *facet syndrome* was introduced in 1933 by Ghormley, who thought a narrow disk space would lead to increased facet joint degeneration and serve as a potential source for sciatica. In the following decades, a distinction was made between radicular pain, which results from direct pressure on exiting nerve roots, and referred pain, which originates from the posterior spinal elements and the facet joints in particular.

Later research showed innervation of the facet joint by the medial branch of the posterior ramus of the spinal nerve. This nerve and its branches innervates the facet joints of a three-joint complex, making it virtually impossible to denervate a single joint by the injection of an agent at a single level.

The lumbar facet joints are biomechanically important. They absorb significant loads in extension and are a valuable part of the three-joint complex. Their role is to restrain excessive mobility of a spinal segment and to distribute axial loading over a broad area. In patients with symptomatic facet syndrome, biopsies have revealed cartilage changes that are similar to findings in chondromalacia patellae.

Clinical Findings

A. SYMPTOMS AND SIGNS

Although patients with facet syndrome tend to have problems localizing the exact source of their pain, they usually complain of low back pain that often increases on extension. The pain may radiate into the posterior thigh and commonly ends at the knee level. When patients wake up with low back pain, they frequently can alleviate the pain by changing position.

B. IMAGING STUDIES

Plain radiographs demonstrate a narrowed disk space. Oblique views of the lumbar spine may show osteophyte formation of the superior and inferior facet. A more accurate study is a CT scan, which allows axial cuts and demonstration of arthritic changes involving the facets.

Treatment

Conservative care with antiinflammatory medication, an external back support, and physical therapy should alleviate symptoms in most cases of facet syndrome. Intraarticular injections might be helpful as a diagnostic tool and buy time in these often difficult cases. The result of facet joint injections is unreliable, however. Medial branch ablation using a radiofrequency catheter shows some efficacy in the treatment of low back pain. However, better studies are necessary to assess accurately its overall efficacy in the management of this difficult problem. A low back fusion might be successful in extreme degenerative cases that failed to respond to conservative care, but the selection of fusion levels should not be based on the outcome of previous facet joint injections.

Jackson RP, Jacobs RR, Montesano PX: 1988 Volvo award in clinical sciences. Facet joint injection in low-back pain. A prospective statistical study. Spine 1988;13:966. [PMID: 2974632]

Oh WS, Shim JC: A randomized controlled trial of radiofrequency denervation of the ramus communicans nerve for chronic discogenic low back pain. Clin J Pain 2004;20:55. [PMID: 14668658]

Slipman CW et al: A critical review of the evidence for the use of zygapophysial injections and radiofrequency denervation in the treatment of low back pain. Spine J 2003;3:310. [PMID: 14589192]

van Wijk RM et al: Radiofrequency denervation of lumbar facet joints in the treatment of chronic low back pain: A randomized, double-blind, sham lesion-controlled trial. Clin J Pain 2005;21:335.

STENOSIS OF THE LUMBAR SPINE

Stenosis of the lumbar spine is a clinical entity responsible for a variety of complaints ranging from low back pain to lower-extremity dysfunction. The condition is defined as any developmental or acquired narrowing of the spinal canal, nerve root canals, or intervertebral foramina that results in compression of neural elements.

Pathophysiology

Some physiologic narrowing of the canal occurs with age. There are also normal variations in the cross-sectional areas and shapes of the lumbar spinal canal, with the narrowest area found between L2 and L4. The canal volume increases in flexion and decreases in extension. Narrowing of the spinal canal can further occur by bulging of the disk anteriorly, by buckling of the ligamentum flavum posteriorly, and by encroachment of the articular facets. Degeneration of the intervertebral disk causes increased stress on the facet joint and can lead to arthrosis and hypertrophy of facets and adjacent structures. This ultimately compromises the spinal canal. The decrease in canal volume occurs at such a slow and gradual pace that the neurologic structures in most patients accommodate to it, with the result that there may be surprisingly few neurologic symptoms even in patients with advanced degenerative stenosis.

The cause of pain experienced by patients with stenosis is perplexing and is attributed to mechanical, ischemic, inflammatory, and various other mechanisms. The simplest explanation, of course, is pure mechanical compression of cord and adjacent roots. The hourglass configuration and bulging of the dura as it is decompressed attests to the increased pressures within the stenotic canal. According to the neuroischemic explanation, the nerve fibers are nutritionally deprived by compression of the small nutrient vessels. Inflammatory conditions of the dura and exiting nerve roots are equally suspect. Common surgical findings are an adhesive arachnoiditis of the pia and the presence of friction neuritis, and these may constrict or tether the neural elements. The hypertrophic membranes also have reduced permeability and may obstruct the free flow of cerebrospinal fluid (CSF) from perfusing the root tissues. This can compromise the metabolism of nerve fibers because nearly 50% of their nutrients are derived from CSF.

According to a vascular and nutritional explanation for the onset of pseudoclaudication, the nerve fibers in the resting state diminish metabolic requirements that enable them to conduct sufficient impulses for minimal activity of the muscles. With increases in exertion, however, the metabolic requirements of the compromised nerve rise rapidly. The tension of root fixation and the reduced permeability to CSF hamper the delivery of necessary nutrients and the removal of noxious accumulations. The resulting relative neuroischemia renders the nerve more mechanosensitive, causing ectopic impulses to be conducted and to produce pain, paresthesias, and pseudoclaudication.

Gross morphologic changes include a compressed caudal sac, diffuse ligamentous and facet joint hypertrophy, disk space narrowing with or without concomitant protrusion, encroachment of the lamina, and occasional degenerative olisthesis. Microscopic changes include quantitative losses of neurons with numerous empty axons, various degrees of demyelinization, diffuse interstitial fibrosis with venous congestion, and coiled arterial "pigtails" on either side of the compressed lesion.

Classification

Spinal stenosis is classified as congenital or acquired. The congenital type is caused by developmental spinal anomalies that compromise the neural elements. This type is seen, for example, in patients with achondroplasia (Figure 5–11). The acquired type is more common and further divided into the degenerative, olistheticscoliotic, posttraumatic, and postoperative subtypes. Although the original shape of the spinal canal may be round, oval, or trefoil, the trefoil shape is most commonly associated with stenosis and may be a predisposing factor.

The location of stenosis can be central or lateral. In central stenosis, hypertrophied structures cause circumferential pressure of the spinal cord. Lateral stenosis is associated with narrowing of the foraminal canal, which is divided into three separate zones: the entrance zone, the middle zone, and the exit zone.

Clinical Findings

A. SYMPTOMS AND SIGNS

In degenerative spinal stenosis, which occurs primarily in elderly (more than 70 years) individuals and is seen more commonly in men than in women, the lower lumbar segments are affected the most severely. The

Figure 5–11. CT scan showing severe stenosis and typical trefoil shape of the lumbar spine in a patient with achondroplasia.

pattern of complaints varies among patients. In many cases, there is an insidious onset and slow progression of pain in the lower back, buttock, and thigh. The pain is generally diffuse rather than neurosegmental and is episodic. Nearly all patients report that their lower extremity pain is altered by changes in position. It generally occurs with standing or walking and is relieved by rest, lying, sitting, or adopting a position of flexion at the waist. In addition, patients may find it easier to walk uphill (when their trunk is flexed) than downhill (when their trunk is extended). They may also have greater walking tolerance pushing a shopping cart because they are able to ambulate in a more flexed position. These are the hallmarks of pseudoclaudication. Neurogenic and vascular claudication may be difficult to distinguish from each other. Thus, all patients should have their distal pulses examined as a part of the overall neurologic evaluation. Mistaken diagnoses are not uncommon.

In a study of 172 patients who had symptoms of claudication, were found on myelogram and CT to have lumbar stenosis, and were treated operatively, investigators found that 65% of the patients demonstrated objective weakness and 25% exhibited diminished deep tendon reflexes. Only 10% had positive results in the straight leg–raising test, indicating entrapment of a nerve root. Nine patients had peripheral vascular disease identified by ultrasound and arteriography, and six of these nine required additional vascular bypass surgery for persistent symptoms of lower extremity claudication.

B. Imaging Studies

Findings on plain radiographs include degenerative disk disease, osteoarthritis of the facets, spondylolisthesis, and narrowing of the interpedicular distance as seen on the AP view. Although myelography was commonly used in the past to evaluate spinal cord or root compression, it is an invasive procedure with possible side effects and no longer used routinely. CT scanning is commonly used to evaluate the spinal elements and allows for accurate measurement of the canal dimensions when combined with contrast enhancement. A dural sac with an anteroposterior diameter of less than 10 mm correlates with clinical findings of stenosis.

MRI is comparable to contrast-enhanced CT scanning in its ability to demonstrate spinal stenosis and is now the imaging modality of choice to assess the spinal canal and the neural structures. (Figure 5–12).

Differential Diagnosis

A complete physical examination is essential to exclude other causes of referred pain in the low back, such as retroperitoneal tumors, aortic aneurysms, peptic ulcer disease, renal lesions, and pathologic processes of the hips or pelvis.

Psychologic factors of low back pain often give rise to symptoms independent of spinal canal narrowing and can lead to confusing differential diagnoses. Depression is common in the elderly (more than 70 years), and prompt recognition and treatment of underlying depression as the cause of somatic complaints may result in marked diminution of symptoms.

Treatment

A. Conservative Treatment

Initial management of the patient with symptoms suggestive of spinal stenosis should consist of salicylates or nonsteroidal agents and an exercise program tailored to the patient's goals or lifestyle. Surprisingly, many patients show an appreciable response to this form of treatment. Narcotics may induce dependency and should be avoided. Epidural corticosteroid injections have a short-term success rate of 50% and a long-term success rate of 25%.

B. Surgical Treatment

If conservative methods fail, the patient's quality of life must be a key factor in deciding when to proceed with surgery. Decompressive laminectomy has a short-term success rate between 71% and 85%. Approximately 17% of older patients require reoperation for recurrent stenosis or instability. The disk should be preserved under any circumstances, to avoid postoperative instability. The best surgical results are seen in patients without coexisting morbid conditions (Figure 5–13).

Postoperative instability is reported in approximately 10–15% of patients treated. Preoperative risk factors for developing instability include disk space narrowing, osteoporosis, preexisting spondylolisthesis, and multilevel decompression. Late instability can occur when 50% of bilateral facets were resected, or when 100% of one facet joint was resected. In these cases, a prophylactic instrumented lateral fusion should be performed.

Atlas SJ et al: Long-term outcomes of surgical and nonsurgical management of lumbar spinal stenosis: 8 to 10 year results from the Maine lumbar spine study. Spine 2005;30:936. [PMID: 15834339]

Chang Y et al: The effect of surgical and nonsurgical treatment on longitudinal outcomes of lumbar spinal stenosis over 10 years. J Am Geriatr Soc 2005;53:785. [PMID: 15877553]

Galiano K et al: Long-term outcome of laminectomy for spinal stenosis in octogenarians. Spine 2005;30:332. [PMID: 15682015]

Ghiselli G et al: Adjacent segment degeneration in the lumbar spine. J Bone Joint Surg Am 2004;86:1497. [PMID: 15252099]

Ikuta K et al: Short-term results of microendoscopic posterior decompression for lumbar spinal stenosis. Technical note. J Neurosurg Spine 2005;2:624. [PMID: 15945442]

Knaub MA et al: Lumbar spinal stenosis: Indications for arthrodesis and spinal instrumentation. Instr Course Lect 2005;54: 313. [PMID: 15948459]

B

A

Figure 5–12. Imaging studies in a patient with degenerative stenosis of the lumbar spine. **A:** Radiograph showing degenerative spondylolisthesis between L4 and L5, as well as an old compression fracture of L3. **B:** MRI showing severe stenosis of the spinal canal at L4-L5, marked facet hypertrophy and ligamentous hypertrophy resulting in central canal stenosis, and lateral recess stenosis.

Kornblum MB et al: Degenerative lumbar spondylolisthesis with spinal stenosis: A prospective long-term study comparing fusion and pseudarthrosis. Spine 2004;29:726. [PMID: 15087793]

Lin SI, Lin RM: Disability and walking capacity in patients with lumbar spinal stenosis: Association with sensorimotor function, balance, and functional performance. J Orthop Sports Phys Ther 2005;35:220. [PMID: 15901123]

Palmer S, Turner R, Palmer R: Bilateral decompressive surgery in lumbar spinal stenosis associated with spondylolisthesis: Unilateral approach and use of a microscope and tubular retractor system. Neurosurg Focus 2002;13:E4. [PMID: 12296681]

Saint-Louis LA: Lumbar spinal stenosis assessment with computed tomography, magnetic resonance imaging, and myelography. Clin Orthop 2001;384:122. [PMID: 11249157]

Sengupta DK, Herkowitz HN: Lumbar spinal stenosis. Treatment strategies and indications for surgery. Orthop Clin North Am 2003;4:281. [PMID: 12914268]

Shapiro GS, Taira G, Boachie-Adjei O: Results of surgical treatment of adult idiopathic scoliosis with low back pain and spinal stenosis: A study of long-term clinical radiographic outcomes. Spine 2003;28:358. [PMID: 12590210]

Simotas AC: Nonoperative treatment for lumbar spinal stenosis. Clin Orthop 2001;384:153. [PMID: 11249160]

Truumees E: Spinal stenosis: Pathophysiology, clinical and radiologic classification. Instr Course Lect 2005;54:287. [PMID: 15948457]

Yuan PS, Booth RE Jr, Albert TJ: Nonsurgical and surgical management of lumbar spinal stenosis. Instr Course Lect 2005;54:303. [PMID: 15948458]

OSTEOPOROSIS AND VERTEBRAL COMPRESSION FRACTURES

Osteoporosis is characterized by a decline in overall bone mass in the axial and appendicular skeleton. The disease affects between 15 and 20 million people in the United States. Peak bone mass, attained between 16 and 25 years of age, slowly declines with age as the rate

A   B

Figure 5–13. Imaging studies in a patient with stenosis of the lumbar spine and leg pain. **A:** MRI showing stenosis at L3–L4. **B:** Radiograph taken after two-level laminectomy, which led to resolution of the preoperative leg pain.

of bone resorption exceeds that of bone formation. This phenomenon occurs in both men and women and is known as senile osteoporosis. Women are also susceptible to postmenopausal osteoporosis that occurs during the 15–20 years after the onset of menopause and is directly linked to estrogen deficiency. Environmental factors also play a role in accelerating the rate of skeletal bone loss. These include chronic calcium deficiency, smoking, excessive alcohol intake, hyperparathyroidism, and inactivity. Genetic influences may also play a role.

Vertebral compression fractures are one of the most frequent manifestations of osteoporosis in the elderly (more than 60 years). Over 700,000 vertebral compression fractures occur each year. Fortunately, the overwhelming majority of patients are asymptomatic.

Clinical Findings

Patients with symptomatic vertebral compression fractures typically complain of axial pain localized to the fractured level. Occasionally, the patient's family notices that the patient's back is becoming increasingly rounded and significant loss of height has occurred. This spinal deformity is known as the dowager's hump. In general, there is no neurologic dysfunction and no radiation of the pain in any dermatomal distribution. There is often no history of significant trauma or an inciting event.

Imaging

Plain radiographs and densitometric scans are the major imaging modalities in the assessment of osteoporotic bone and their pathologic counterparts (insufficiency fractures). Dual-energy x-ray absorptiometry (DXA) is the most useful of the densitometric imaging techniques because it carries a high degree of precision (0.5–2%) and subjects the patient to minimal amounts of radiation. It is also quite accurate for assessment of osteoporosis in both the axial and appendicular skeleton. Other imaging modalities include single-energy x-ray absorptiometry (SXA), quantitative computed tomography (QCT), and radiographic absorptiometry.

Posterior/anterior and lateral radiographs of the affected area of the spine are likely to reveal the location and severity of the osteoporotic fracture(s). In the thoracic spine, wedge compression fractures are most commonly encountered. In the lumbar spine, both compression and burst fractures can occur. Other imaging modalities include technetium bone scans and MRI scans. These studies should be reserved for the evaluation of fractures that remain symptomatic or progress after a course of conservative treatment. MRI is extremely useful in differentiating nonunited fractures from those that have healed and in differentiating osteoporotic fractures from those caused by malignancy.

Bone biopsy is indicated if a metabolic bone disease or a malignancy is suspected as the cause of the osteoporosis. The sample, typically retrieved from the anterior iliac crest, is examined using bone histomorphometry.

Treatment

Prevention still remains the best treatment for osteoporosis. Maximizing bone mineral density prior to the onset of bone loss and minimizing the bone loss that occurs is the optimal regimen to prevent the painful sequelae of the disease. In women, estrogen replacement therapy can be initiated if there is no history of breast cancer, thromboembolic disease, or endometrial disease. Routine gynecological examination is necessary once therapy is initiated. Calcitonin therapy can be used if estrogen therapy is contraindicated. Parathyroid hormone is currently under clinical trials for the treatment of osteoporosis. Early evidence suggests that it may help to increase skeletal bone mass significantly and may be useful as a first-line treatment for severe osteoporosis.

The bisphosphonates, etidronate and alendronate, prevent osteoclastic resorption of bone. They are the only FDA-approved compounds in widespread use that increase bone mineral density. However, the increase is relatively small.

The initial treatment of symptomatic vertebral compression fractures involves a trial of analgesic therapy and bracing for comfort. Evaluation and treatment for osteoporosis can be initiated if not done already. Conservative therapy should be attempted for at least 6–12 weeks or longer if the patient is improving.

Surgical Treatment

Patients who have fractures that cause neurologic deficits or significant spinal cord compression should be treated with anterior decompression and fusion fol-

lowed by posterior segmental instrumentation and fusion. The poor bone quality makes correction of deformity and maintenance of posterior constructs a challenging task.

Patients who have recalcitrant back pain from a nonunited vertebral compression fracture who have failed a course of conservative management can obtain excellent symptomatic relief from fracture stabilization through injection of PMMA bone cement into the fracture through a percutaneous technique. The two most popular procedures, vertebroplasty and kyphoplasty, are both safe and efficacious. In both techniques, a cannula is inserted intrapedicularly or extrapedicularly (lateral to the pedicle) into the anterior portion of the affected vertebral body, and acrylic cement is instilled into the fractured bone under fluoroscopic control. Once the cement cures, the fracture is immediately stabilized. In the kyphoplasty technique, a balloon is inflated in the vertebral body in an attempt to compress the existing bone, create a void for instillation of more viscous cement under lower pressure, and correct the wedge deformity. This technique has the theoretical advantage of allowing some deformity correction and preventing high-pressure-related extrusion of PMMA into the spinal canal.

The mechanism of pain relief achieved through vertebroplasty and kyphoplasty is unclear. Multiple mechanisms may play a role, including fracture stabilization, denervation of pain fibers by the heat generated during the cement curing process, and neurotoxicity of the PMMA monomer. In addition, longer follow-up has raised concerns over predisposing the adjacent segment to fracture by overstiffening the affected level. These concerns are currently under active investigation.

Coumans JV, Reinhardt MK, Lieberman IH: Kyphoplasty for vertebral compression fractures: 1-year clinical outcomes from a prospective study. J Neurosurg 2003;99(Suppl 1):44. [PMID: 12859058]

Diamond TH, Champion B, Clark WA: Management of acute osteoporotic vertebral fractures: A nonrandomized trial comparing percutaneous vertebroplasty with conservative therapy. Am J Med 2003;114:257. [PMID: 12681451]

Do HM et al: Prospective analysis of clinical outcomes after percutaneous vertebroplasty for painful osteoporotic vertebral body fractures. AJNR Am J Neuroradiol 2005;26:1623. [PMID: 16091504]

Grohs JG et al: Minimal invasive stabilization of osteoporotic vertebral fractures: A prospective nonrandomized comparison of vertebroplasty and balloon kyphoplasty. J Spinal Disord Tech 2005;18:238. [PMID: 15905767]

Guglielmi G et al: Percutaneous vertebroplasty: Indications, contraindications, technique, and complications. Acta Radiol 2000;46:256. [PMID: 15981722]

McGraw JK et al: Prospective evaluation of pain relief in 100 patients undergoing percutaneous vertebroplasty: results and follow-up. J Vasc Interv Radiol 2002;13:883. [PMID: 12354821]

Nussbaum DA, Gailloud P, Murphy K: A review of complications associated with vertebroplasty and kyphoplasty as reported to the Food and Drug Administration medical device related web site. J Vasc Interv Radiol 2004;15:1185. [PMID: 15525736]

Phillips FM et al: Minimally invasive treatments of osteoporotic vertebral compression fractures: Vertebroplasty and kyphoplasty. Instr Course Lect 2003;52:559. Review. [PMID: 12690882]

Steinmann J, Tingey CT, Cruz G et al: Biomechanical comparison of unipedicular versus bipedicular kyphoplasty. Spine 2005; 30:201. [PMID: 15644756]

Uppin AA et al: Occurrence of new vertebral body fracture after percutaneous vertebroplasty in patients with osteoporosis. Radiology 2003;226:119. [PMID: 12511679]

■ DEFORMITIES OF THE SPINE

SCOLIOSIS

Scoliosis is an abnormal curvature of the spine as viewed in the coronal plane. It is also generally associated with a rotational deformity, and it is the rotational component, manifested as a rib hump, prominent scapula, waist asymmetry, or lumbar fullness, that is most likely to call attention to the spinal curvature.

Etiology, Classification, & Pathophysiology

Scoliosis is classified according to its cause, with the most common causes summarized in Table 5–1. For example, if the curvature is secondary to a structural bony abnormality, it is described as congenital scoliosis. If it is caused by a neurologic disturbance or muscle disease (myopathy), it is described as neuromuscular scoliosis. If no cause can be determined, it is described as idiopathic scoliosis. The idiopathic type is the most common. Proposed etiologies for idiopathic scoliosis include abnormalities in melatonin, growth hormone or other hormones, platelet abnormalities, and posterior column abnormalities (ie, impaired proprioception and vibratory sensibility.

Particularly in idiopathic cases, scoliosis can also be classified according to the patient's age at onset. The age ranges for infantile, juvenile, adolescent, and adult scoliosis are shown in Table 5–1. Many surgeons consider juvenile scoliosis not to be a true separate entity, but rather a mix of late-presenting infantile scoliosis and early-developing adolescent scoliosis.

The curvature is named according to the side of the convexity, as well as the level of the apex, which is the most rotated vertebral body in the curve. For a cervical curve, the apex is at C1 through C6; for a cervicothoracic curve, C7 through T1; for a thoracic curve, T2

Table 5–1. Classification of scoliosis by cause.

I. Idiopathic scoliosis
  A. Infantile (under 3 years of age)
  B. Juvenile (from 3 to 10 years of age)
  C. Adolescent (from 10 years of age to skeletal maturity)
  D. Adult
II. Neuromuscular scoliosis
  A. Neuropathic
    1. Upper motor neuron
      a. Cerebral palsy
      b. Charcot-Marie-Tooth disease
      c. Syringomyelia
      d. Spinal cord trauma
    2. Lower motor neuron
      a. Poliomyelitis
      b. Spinal muscular atrophy
      c. Myelomeningocele
  B. Myopathic
    1. Arthrogryposis
    2. Muscular dystrophy
III. Congenital scoliosis
  A. Failure of formation
  B. Failure of segmentation
  C. Mixed failure of formation and segmentation
IV. Neurofibromatosis
V. Connective tissue scoliosis
  A. Marfan syndrome
  B. Ehlers-Danlos syndrome
VI. Osteochondrodystrophy
  A. Diastrophic dwarfism
  B. Mucopolysaccharidosis
  C. Spondyloepiphyseal dysplasia
  D. Multiple epiphyseal dysplasia
  E. Achondrodysplasia
VII. Metabolic scoliosis
VIII. Nonstructural scoliosis
  A. Postural, hysterical
  B. Secondary to nerve root irritation

Modified and reproduced, with permission, from Winter RB: Classification and terminology of scoliosis. In Lonstein JE et al, eds: *Moe's Textbook of Scoliosis and Other Spinal Deformities*, 3rd ed. WB Saunders, 1994.

through T11; for a thoracolumbar curve, T12 or L1; for a lumbar curve, L2 through L4; and for a lumbosacral curve, L5 or lower.

The most common types of curves in cases of idiopathic scoliosis are the right thoracic curve, followed by the double curve (right thoracic and left lumbar) and the right thoracolumbar curve. The primary curve or curves are considered structural. A secondary curve, known as a compensatory curve, permits the head to be centered over the pelvis. Compensatory curves are of lesser magnitude, more flexible, and less rotated; when they become less flexible and rotation is evident, it may be difficult to determine which curve is the primary one, and indeed they may be considered structural.

The natural history of spinal curvatures is affected by factors such as the magnitude of the curve, the age of the patient, and the underlying cause of the problem. With curve progression, the deformity can become severe, leading in some cases to a so-called razor-back deformity secondary to rib rotation. With thoracic curves measuring more than 60–90 degrees (depending on the chest anterior-posterior dimension), cardiopulmonary function can become compromised, and a secondary restrictive lung disease may result from the chest deformity. Curve progression is most common during continued skeletal growth; however, it is now evident that moderate curves of 40–50 degrees should be observed for progression in adulthood. Although the extent of progression in adulthood varies widely among patients, the average amount is 1 degree per year. Taking radiographs every 2–5 years appears to be satisfactory for adults who have idiopathic scoliosis without other clinical signs of progression. The likelihood of progression is greater in patients whose scoliosis is associated with conditions such as neurofibromatosis or connective tissue diseases, including Marfan syndrome and Ehlers-Danlos syndrome.

Principles of Diagnosis

A. HISTORY AND PHYSICAL EXAMINATION

In a patient with a spine deformity, the history should include the age when the deformity was first noted; the manner in which it was noted (by the patient or family member, by the pediatrician or other health professional during examination or school screening, etc.); the perinatal history; developmental milestones; other illnesses; and family history of scoliosis or other diseases that may affect the musculoskeletal system. Although the incidence of scoliosis in the general population is approximately 1%, the incidence is greater in the children of women with scoliosis and particularly in the daughters of these women. For this reason, the children of women with scoliosis should be screened repeatedly throughout their preadolescent and adolescent years. Idiopathic scoliosis of the adolescent type (see Table 5–1) is more common in females, whereas that of the infantile type is more common in males.

In children and adolescents, the curvature is generally not painful. If the patient complains of pain, appropriate diagnostic tests should be performed to determine whether the curvature is secondary to the presence of a bony or spinal tumor, herniated disk, or other abnormality.

The patient's skin, habitus, and back should be carefully inspected. The presence of café au lait spots, skin tags, or axillary freckles is suggestive of neurofibromatosis. The presence of hairy patches or dimples over the spine is suggestive of spinal dysraphism. Numerous clinical syndromes are associated with scoliosis (see Table 5–1), and some of these include unusual facies. Tall, long-limbed patients may have Marfan syndrome and should be examined for high-arched palate, cardiac murmur, and dislocated lenses. Dwarfs have a high incidence of spinal deformity, both kyphosis (see section on kyphosis) and scoliosis, as well as spinal instability.

In patients with scoliosis, the shoulders or pelvis may not be level, or waist asymmetry may be noted. Most commonly, these patients have scapular prominence, with rotational deformity and rib prominence. The rib hump, or the lumbar prominence of a lumbar curve, can be accentuated by having the patient lean forward from the waist, permitting the arms to hang down; the examiner then views the spine from above or below (Figure 5–14). The rib hump can be quantified by direct measurement of its height or by using a scoliometer, which permits measurement of angular deformity. Also important in the patient's examination is measurement of decompensation, if present. This can be deter-

Figure 5–14. The rotational deformity of scoliosis is manifested by a rib hump, which is accentuated by having the patient bend forward. (Reproduced, with permission, from Day LJ et al: Orthopedics. In Way LW, ed: *Current Surgical Diagnosis & Treatment,* 9th ed. Stamford: Appleton & Lange, 1991.)

Figure 5–15. Use of a plumb bob to measure coronal decompensation in a patient with scoliosis. (Reproduced, with permission, from McCarthy RE: Evaluation of the patient with deformity. In Weinstein SL, ed: *The Pediatric Spine*. Raven, 1994.)

mined by dropping a plumb bob from the prominence of the C7 spinous process and measuring where it falls with respect to the gluteal line (Figure 5–15).

Flexibility of the curve can be qualitatively assessed by having the patient bend in the direction that effects curve correction. The spinous processes within the curve as well as the rib hump can then be assessed for flexibility of the deformity.

B. NEUROLOGIC TESTS

Patients should demonstrate a normal gait and be able to walk on their toes and heels, unless other concomitant conditions are present. Motor and sensory testing of the lower extremities should be performed, and testing of the upper extremities should also be done if the curve pattern is atypical or if a neuromuscular condition is suspected. Reflexes should be tested, and the presence of asymmetry or a pathologic reflex (eg, clonus, a positive Babinski sign, or a positive Hoffmann sign) should be noted and suggest a nonidiopathic etiology.

An asymmetric abdominal reflex is the most common neurologic abnormality noted with an intracanal lesion, such as a syrinx, diastematomyelia, or spinal cord tumor. The abdominal reflex is assessed by gently scratching each of the four quadrants of the abdomen, just a few centimeters away from the umbilicus. The response is considered normal if the umbilicus moves slightly toward the direction scratched.

Abnormal neurologic test results are an indication for further workup, such as a spine MRI, particularly if the patient has an atypical curve (eg, a left thoracic curve) or a rapidly progressive spinal deformity.

C. IMAGING STUDIES

AP and lateral radiographs of the entire length of the spine should be taken, and this generally requires the use of an extra-long x-ray cassette. When the radiographs are taken, the patient should be in the standing position. If neuromuscular problems make it impossible for the patient to stand, however, radiographs can be taken with the patient sitting. Curves are measured using the Cobb method, as shown in Figure 5–16.

Views taken with the patient bending away from the concavity may be helpful or necessary, particularly if levels for fusion are being selected. These bend views allow for the assessment of the maximal correction of the curve. For curves measuring greater than 90 degrees or if the patient cannot perform the bending movement, traction films can be obtained by having two assistants exert longitudinal traction on the patient, either by grasping the legs and arms or via application of a head halter.

For severe curves (more than 90 degrees), the rotational deformity of the spine may distort the detail on an AP view. For this reason, a special Stagnara view should be obtained. The x-ray cassette is positioned parallel to the rib hump, and the x-ray beam is directed perpendicular to this to obtain an AP view of the spine, rather than of the patient (Figure 5–17).

For patients with abnormal results in the neurologic examination, atypical curve patterns, rapidly progressive curvatures, or congenital scoliosis, evaluation of the spinal canal is indicated. MRI or myelograms with CT scanning can be used. For young patients, sedation is often required. The radiologist should be advised to look for the following: a syrinx (a fluid-filled cyst within the spinal cord); a tethered cord (a fibrous band that is located distally and can prevent the normal cephalad migration of

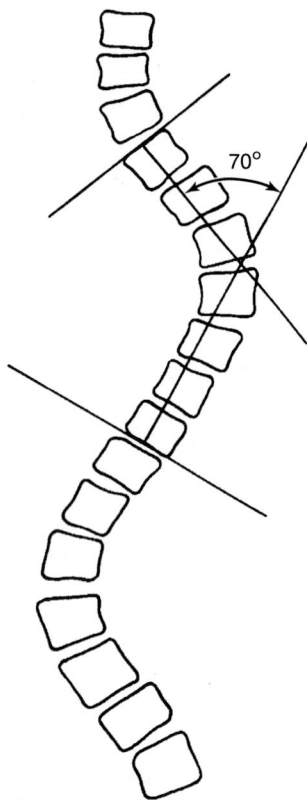

Figure 5–16. Use of the Cobb method to measure the scoliotic curve. First, lines are drawn along the end-plates of the upper and lower vertebrae that are maximally tilted into the concavity of the curve. Next, a perpendicular line is drawn to each of the earlier-drawn lines. The angle of intersection is the Cobb angle. (Reproduced, with permission, from Day LJ et al: Orthopedics. In Way LW, ed: *Current Surgical Diagnosis & Treatment*, 9th ed. Stamford: Appleton & Lange, 1991.)

the cord); a diastematomyelia (a bony or fibrous defect that divides the spinal cord and may cause a tether); or a diplomyelia (a reduplication of the spinal cord).

D. OTHER STUDIES

If the patient has a finding of intracanal abnormalities, particularly if surgical correction of the deformity is contemplated, neurosurgical evaluation may be indicated. In many cases, the release of a tethered cord or decompression of a syrinx can be performed prior to or at the same time as the scoliosis surgery.

Patients with curves greater than 60 degrees, those with respiratory complaints, and those with scoliosis resulting from a neuromuscular cause should undergo pulmonary function testing, particularly if surgery is being considered. In cases in which pulmonary function test values are less than 30% of predicted values based on the age, sex, and size of the patient, some clinicians recommend an aggressive approach with preoperative tracheostomy placement. We prefer, however, to caution patients about the possibility of tracheostomy placement if postoperative weaning from the respirator is prolonged, and we have rarely found tracheostomy to be necessary.

Principles of Treatment

Although general principles of treatment are discussed here, additional details about treatment of idiopathic scoliosis in adults, neuromuscular scoliosis, neurofibromatosis, and congenital scoliosis are given in subsequent sections of this chapter.

A. CONSERVATIVE TREATMENT

Mild curves (less than 20 degrees) can generally be managed conservatively. In most cases, curves less than 10 degrees require observation only, except in very young patients who have neuromuscular scoliosis and a high risk of progression in their collapsing-type curves.

Although some skeletally immature patients with curves greater than 20 degrees require bracing, others do not. If an adolescent has less than 2 years of skeletal growth remaining, has not demonstrated progression,

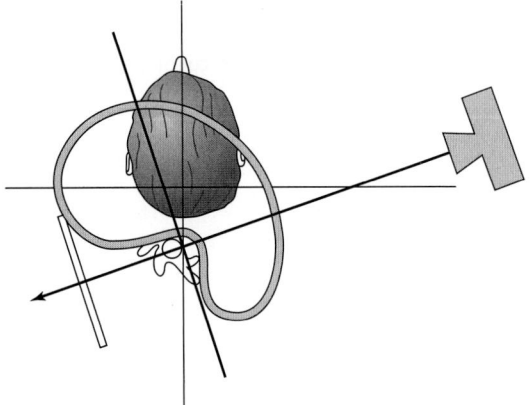

Figure 5–17. In cases of severe curvature, the x-ray beam and cassette are positioned as shown to obtain an anteroposterior view of the curve itself, rather than of the patient. This view is known as the Stagnara view. (Reproduced, with permission, from Lonstein JE: Patient evaluation. In Bradford DS et al, eds: *Moe's Textbook of Scoliosis and Other Spinal Deformities*, 2nd ed. WB Saunders, 1987.)

and has a curve that is still less than 30 degrees, the clinician may consider observation even at this point; however, considerations such as rotational deformity or a positive family history may suggest a more aggressive treatment for certain patients in this group. Any skeletally immature patient with a significant curve who shows progression of the curvature should be referred to an orthopedic surgeon with experience in treating scoliosis for possible brace treatment. Because the error of measurement of the Cobb angle is 3–5 degrees, progression of more than 5 degrees is considered significant.

Several types of braces are available for the treatment of scoliosis. The Milwaukee brace, which is also called the **cervical thoracolumbosacral orthosis,** can be used for nearly all curvatures, but its high profile makes it less desirable, particularly for a self-conscious adolescent. This brace (Figure 5–18) has a pelvic mold to which upright metal struts are attached. The struts are then joined to a neck ring. Corrective pads can be fastened to the metal struts, applying pressure to the rib at the apex of the convexity. If shoulder asymmetry is significant, a shoulder ring can be applied.

The thoracolumbosacral orthosis is a more cosmetically acceptable brace, but its use is limited to patients whose curves have an apex at T8 or below. The thoracolumbosacral orthosis is an external shell orthosis that is generally constructed of copolymer (largely polypropylene but with a small portion of polyethylene to prevent cracking). The shell is molded to the patient, and corrective pads are placed. One pad applies pressure at the apical rib, at the most prominent area. A second pad can be applied over the lumbar prominence if a double-curve pattern is present. If the patient shows significant decompensation to the left or right, a trochanteric extension can be included on that side to correct this tendency.

Because of the corrective forces being placed posteriorly, bracing may aggravate thoracic lordosis. For this reason, particular care should be made to place pads as laterally as possible. A decrease of normal thoracic kyphosis is common in idiopathic scoliosis and in fact contributes to the cardiovascular problems seen in patients because of the resultant decreased AP diameter of the thoracic cage.

For isolated lumbar curves, a lumbosacral orthosis can be used (Figure 5–19). Although the Boston brace is the most well-known type of lumbosacral orthosis, others are available. The various types of lumbosacral orthosis all use the corrective effect of flattening of lumbar lordosis to facilitate curve correction.

Although braces are designed to apply corrective forces to the spinal curvature and corrective effects are frequently noted on follow-up radiographs taken with the patient in the brace, braces do not afford long-term correction. Success may be achieved in preventing curve

Figure 5–18. The Milwaukee brace, which is also known as the cervical thoracolumbosacral orthosis (CTLSO), can be used to treat scoliosis.

progression during the growth period of the patient and improvement may even be noted, but the curvature generally returns to the preorthotic level of severity.

Unlike most braces, the Charleston night bending brace is worn only during the night. When this brace was used in the treatment of idiopathic scoliosis, with patients braced in maximal correction only at night, early results suggested that it was as effective as full-time brace wear; however, most of the patients had not yet achieved skeletal maturity.

Infants may require casting for management of severe curves. When the patients become large enough in size, a Milwaukee brace may be used.

Patients who are wearing braces for the treatment of scoliosis should be reexamined at intervals ranging from 4 to 6 months, depending on how close they are to their growth spurt. Some clinicians prefer that patients

Figure 5–19. The underarm brace, which is also known as the lumbosacral orthosis (LSO), can be used to treat lumbar scoliosis.

wear their braces during follow-up radiographs, but others prefer that the braces be removed on the day of the office visit and while radiographs are taken. Generally, it is felt that full-time brace wear (23 hours a day) is best, and some studies indicate that compliance with brace wear is correlated with the success of braces. Patients may be permitted to remove the brace during athletic activities. As children grow, corrective pads may not be applying force at the appropriate area, which should be checked clinically as well as with confirming radiographs where appropriate.

If an idiopathic curvature can be controlled with bracing, bracing should be continued until the end of skeletal growth. This progress can be assessed clinically by measuring the patient's height during each office visit as well as by following the patient's history (in female patients, for example, growth generally continues for approximately 2 years after menarche). Skeletal

growth can be assessed radiographically by evaluating the iliac apophysis (Risser sign, as shown in Figure 5–20) or by taking radiographs of the various physes in the wrist and comparing them with radiographs published in *Gruelich and Pyle's Radiographic Atlas of Skeletal Development of the Hand and Wrist.* Weaning from the brace can be begun as the patient nears the end of skeletal growth. Depending on the severity of the final curvature, follow-up radiographs may be necessary to assess the loss of correction. Some loss of correction should be expected; again, it is important not to anticipate permanent curve correction.

B. SURGICAL TREATMENT

Curves greater than 40 degrees are difficult to control with bracing because of the greater pressures that must be exerted to effect correction. Moreover, curves greater than 50 degrees are at risk for progression, even in adulthood. When conservative treatment is not possible, several options are available for surgical intervention.

Posterior fusion and Harrington rod instrumentation was historically used. This involves placing hooks on a ratcheted rod in distraction at the ends of the curve to be fused and then performing a fusion and bone grafting. Sublaminar wiring, because of the passage of each wire around the lamina and therefore into the spinal canal at each level, carries an

Figure 5–20. The Risser sign for skeletal maturity. The iliac apophysis first appears laterally and grows medially. Risser I is less than 25% ossification; Risser II is 50% ossification; Risser III is 75% ossification; Risser IV is completion of ossification; and Risser V denotes that the apophysis has fused with the iliac crest or complete skeletal maturity has occurred. (Reproduced, with permission, from McCarthy RE: Evaluation of the patient with deformity. In Weinstein SL, ed: *The Pediatric Spine.* Raven, 1994.)

increased risk of neurologic complications but gives better gradual and segmental control. The sublaminar wiring technique is generally reserved for neuromuscular scoliosis patients because of the need for better fixation in the generally osteoporotic bone, as well as for other patients who may have significant osteoporosis, such as older patients (more than 60 years).

Currently, variable hook-rod systems permit placement of hooks or screws at multiple selected sites

A **B**

Figure 5–21. Imaging studies in a patient with scoliosis. **A:** Radiograph showing preoperative curvature. **B:** Radiograph taken after treatment using Cotrel-Dubousset instrumentation.

along the deformity and the application of distraction or compression, as appropriate, to correct the curve (Figure 5–21). Detailed descriptions of the various instrumentation patterns are beyond the scope of this chapter, but the basic principle is to distract on the concavity of a curve and compress across the convexity. The patient's sagittal contours can also be corrected, if needed, by applying compression to decrease kyphosis or maintain lordosis and by applying distraction to increase kyphosis. The sagittal contours can also be improved by carefully bending the rod prior to insertion so that rotation of the rod converts the coronal curve to the sagittal kyphosis if desired. The systems use a concave and a convex rod. These two rods are usually cross-linked, and they provide rigid fixation so that postoperative brace wear is not needed for most young patients.

For more rigid curves, such as may be found in older patients (over 25 years), it may be necessary to perform an anterior release and fusion as well. With an anterior approach, the disk material can be removed completely, gaining additional mobility and correction and, because an anterior fusion is then performed as well, increasing the fusion rate through this region. Additional factors that may suggest the need for anterior release and fusion include rigid kyphosis, prior failed fusion, and the presence of severe spasticity, as found in some cases of neuromuscular scoliosis. When possible, the two operations are performed at the same surgical sitting, which appears to decrease the perioperative complications. Increasing use of pedicle screws throughout the lumbar and thoracic spine appears to decrease need for anterior release and fusion in many cases.

Some single curves, particularly thoracolumbar and lumbar curves, can be treated with an anterior approach rather than with a posterior approach if desired by the surgeon. In some cases, this can decrease the number of levels fused, which is particularly desirable in the lumbar spine. Screws are placed into the vertebral body on the convex side of the curve during the anterior fusion, connected to a rod, and compression is applied to gain correction (Figure 5–22). They are generally not used lower than the level of L4 because the common iliac vessels would then lie over them and face potential erosion.

Complications & Risks of Surgery

The incidence of complications in adolescent patients is quite low, although the complications outlined here should be discussed with the parent and child during obtaining of informed consent. The risk of major complications in adult scoliosis surgery is reported to be upward of 30%, with increased rates found in association with more complex cases, older patients, and patients with coexisting medical conditions.

A. NEUROLOGIC COMPROMISE

Among the risks faced by patients who undergo major spine fusion are paralysis and death. The incidence of paralysis, however, according to reports of the Scoliosis Research Society, is 0.4%, including both temporary and permanent deficits. Some of the neurologic risk appeared to be greater in the earlier days of using the variable hook-rod systems. These systems are powerful, and overcorrection and overdistraction can result. Because this is better understood today, the risk appears to have decreased.

B. CARDIOPULMONARY PROBLEMS

Cardiopulmonary complications are unusual in adolescents, but the incidence increases in older individuals. In patients with severe pulmonary disease or a history of cigarette smoking, prolonged intubation may be required. In older patients with a preexisting disease, the risk of cardiac ischemia is increased, particularly with long surgeries, significant blood loss, and controlled hypotension as might be induced by the anesthesia team. Controlled hypotension is used to minimize blood loss during many procedures but should be tailored to what can be tolerated by a given patient.

The risk of thromboembolic complications after spine surgery ranges from 0.5% to 50%. Many surgeons use antithromboembolic hose, sequential compression boots, or low-molecular-weight heparin during and after surgery. Pharmacologic anticoagulation poses the risk of postoperative bleeding into the surgical site, which can result in an epidural hematoma and compression of the neural elements and thus should be used with caution and only in high-risk patients. Although their efficacy is well documented with hip and knee arthroplasty, benefits are not yet demonstrated for spinal surgery patients.

C. INFECTION

Although perioperative antibiotics should and usually are given, patients undergoing spinal surgery are at risk for infection. We have found prior infection, smoking history, diabetes, staged anterior and posterior spinal fusion, and increasing age to result in increased risk for postoperative infection.

D. PSEUDARTHROSIS

Rarely occurring in the adolescent but seen occasionally in adults is pseudoarthrosis, or the failure of fusion. This can result in persistent pain or loss of curve correction. Although tomograms or bone scans are difficult to interpret because of the presence of metallic artifacts,

Figure 5-22. Illustration of the use of anterior instrumentation on a Thoracolumbar Scoliosis Curve.

they may help delineate suspicious areas. High suspicion for pseudarthrosis may necessitate reexploration and refusion, sometimes supplemented by anterior fusion. Instrumentation that is painful or broken may be an indication of pseudoarthrosis.

E. DECOMPENSATION

In cases of decompensation, the patient leans with the trunk shifted to one side. Decompensation, particularly in the coronal plane, can generally be attributed to overcorrection of the instrumented curves such that the flexibility of the compensatory curves is insufficient to allow righting of the patient.

F. FLAT BACK SYNDROME

Seen less frequently now that contoured rods are used, flat back syndrome can be a debilitating complication and reinforces the need to restore or maintain the normal sagittal contours of the spine. The distraction required to achieve curve correction by Harrington

rods, when applied across the lumbar spine, flattens the normal lumbar lordosis. This can also occur if the patient is positioned such that the spine is not adequately extended. Patients may need to hyperextend their hips to stand fully upright, or a hip-flexed, knee-flexed gait may be adopted. This is generally a late complication as patients lose their ability to compensate; affected patients note increasing back fatigue or pain and the inability to stand up straight. Surgical correction of flat back syndrome has a high rate of complications, although patient satisfaction is generally high.

G. LOW BACK PAIN

Lower distal levels of fusion appear to correlate with increasing risk of low back pain. This raises the concern of late degeneration below the spine fusion. If the clinician can attribute a patient's symptoms to a specific unfused level, extension of the fusion may be indicated.

Ascher M et al: Safety and efficacy of Isola instrumentation and arthrodesis for adolescent idiopathic scoliosis: Two- to 12-year follow-up. Spine 2004;29:2013. [PMID: 15371702]

Daneilsonn AJ, Nachemson AL: Back pain and function 22 years after brace treatment for adolescent idiopathic scoliosis: A case-control study—part I. Spine 2003;28:2078 [PMID: 14501917]

Daneilsson AJ, Nachemson AL: Back pain and function 23 years after fusion for adolescent idiopathic scoliosis: A case-control study—part II. Spine 2003;28:E373. [PMID: 14501939]

Danielsson AJ, Nachemson AL: Radiologic findings and curve progression 22 years after treatment for adolescent idiopathic scoliosis. Spine 2001;26:516. [PMID: 11242379]

Davids JR et al: Indications for magnetic resonance imaging in presumed adolescent idiopathic scoliosis. J Bone Joint Surg Am 2004;86:2187. [PMID: 15466727]

Dickson RA, Weinstein SL: Bracing (and screening)—Yes or no? J Bone Joint Surg Br 1999;80:193. [PMID: 10204919]

Gepstein R et al: Effectiveness of the Charleston bending brace in the treatment of single curve idiopathic scoliosis. J Pediatr Orthop 2002;22:84. [PMID: 11744860]

Gruelich W, Pyle S: *Radiographic Atlas of Skeletal Development of the Hand and Wrist.* Stanford University Press, 1959.

Lenke LG: Lenke classification system of adolescent idiopathic scoliosis: Treatment recommendations. Instr Course Lect 2005; 54:551. [PMID: 15948478]

Lenke LG et al: Radiographic results of arthrodesis with Cotrel-Dubousset instrumentation for the treatment of adolescent idiopathic scoliosis: A 5 to 10-year follow-up study. J Bone Joint Surg Am 1998;80:807. [PMID: 9655098]

Nachemson AL, Petersen P-E, and members of the Brace Study Group of the Scoliosis Research Society: Effectiveness of treatment with a brace in girls who have adolescent idiopathic scoliosis. J Bone Joint Surg Am 1995;77:815. [PMID: 7782353]

Parent S et al: Adolescent idiopathic scoliosis: Etiology, anatomy, natural history, and bracing. Instr Course Lect 2005;54:529. [PMID: 15948477]

Petersen L-E, Nachemson AL, and members of the Brace Study Group of the Scoliosis Research Society: Prediction of progression of the curve in girls who have adolescent idiopathic scoliosis of moderate severity. J Bone Joint Surg Am 1995;77:823. [PMID: 7782354]

Rowe DE et al: A meta-analysis of the efficacy of nonoperative treatments for idiopathic scoliosis. J Bone Joint Surg Am 1997;79:664. [PMID: 9160938]

1. Idiopathic Scoliosis in Adults

Indications for intervention in adults with scoliosis are pain and progression. Painful scoliosis can be treated with conservative measures, including antiinflammatory agents and physical therapy, in an approach similar to the treatment of low back pain without a deformity. Bracing of the curvature is rarely indicated because these patients have no skeletal growth remaining; however, a patient who cannot tolerate surgery for medical reasons may be braced as a salvage measure. In an otherwise reasonably healthy patient, if progression greater than 5 degrees can be documented or if symptoms are refractory to conservative measures, surgical correction may be indicated.

The same surgical principles apply to adults as younger patients. Adults are more likely to have rigid curves, which may require a combined anterior and posterior approach. Depending on the deformity and region of pain, fusion to the sacrum may be indicated. Patients with significant leg pain should have preoperative CT scanning or MRI to assess whether spinal stenosis accounts for the symptoms and warrants surgical decompression.

In adulthood, previously compensatory curves are often structural. It is important to consider the flexibility of all curves present in adult patients, including the fractional curve between L4 and the sacrum. (A fractional curve is one that does not cross the midline, such as that measured between a tilted L4 endplate and the horizontal and midline sacrum.) The preoperative bend films of all curves should be reviewed and the following question addressed: If correction of the major curve or curves is achieved as would be predicted by the curve flexibility, will the patient still be able to stand centered head over pelvis? If not, the clinician may need to consider fusing a lesser curve to balance the spine.

Another concern is the need to correct sagittal plane deformity, particularly kyphosis, or maintain normal sagittal contours.

Anterior release and fusion may be indicated prior to posterior instrumentation in some cases to permit the patient to stand upright with the head over the sacrum and the knees and hips straight. Before subjecting a patient to the significantly greater surgical risk of a combined anterior and posterior procedures, however, the surgeon should take into account issues such as spinal stenosis, hip disease, and pain from the patient's condition that may affect the patient's ability to stand fully upright.

For older patients, particularly women, osteoporosis may prevent optimal fixation of the instrumentation to the spine. Sublaminar wires, as previously mentioned, can improve the rigidity of the fixation because the multiple sites of attachment spread the load over more bony attachments. There is, however, a theoretical increase in risk of neurologic damage during surgery when this approach is used.

Use of iliac screws (Figure 5–23) should be considered for long fusions to the sacrum because it appears best at resisting flexion moments that are experienced at the lumbosacral junction. In complex and difficult cases such as the one discussed here, surgery should only be undertaken for relatively healthy patients who have failed to respond to nonoperative intervention and who have a clear under-

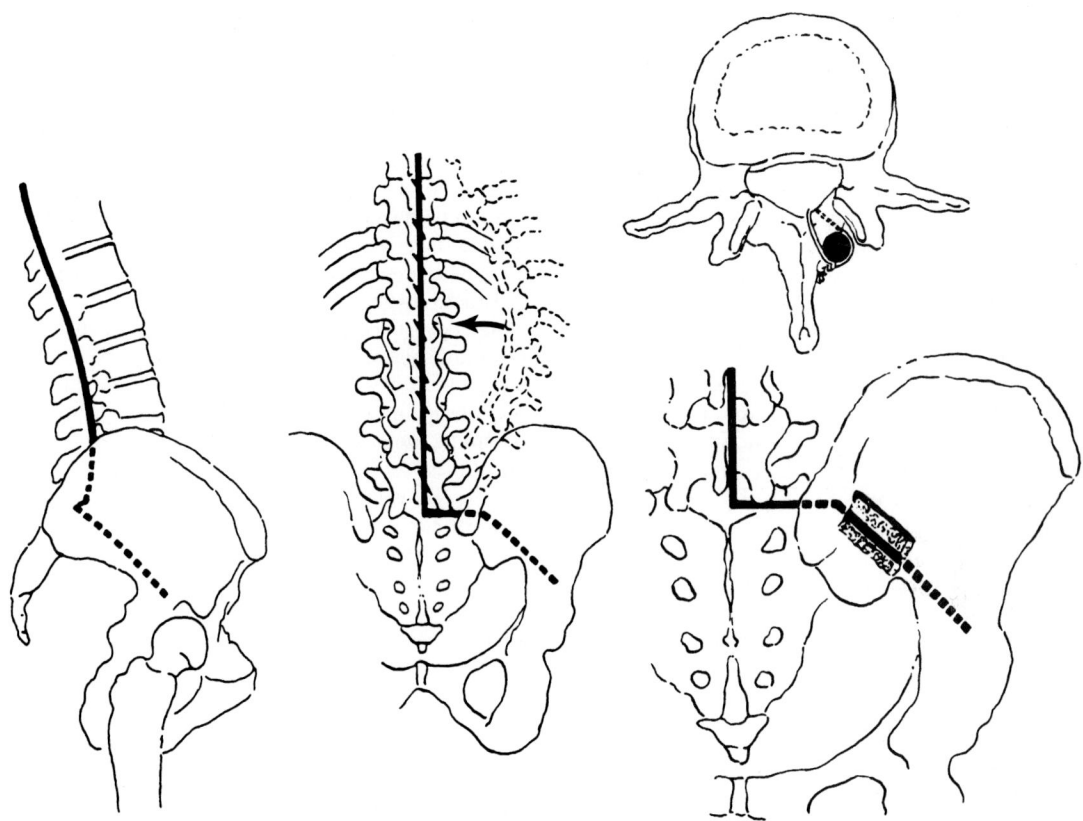

Figure 5–23. Use of the Galveston technique to obtain pelvic fixation. (Reproduced, with permission, from Shook JE, Lubicky JP: Paralytic spinal deformity. In Bridwell KH, DeWald RL, eds: *The Textbook of Spinal Surgery.* Lippincott, 1991.)

standing of the goals and the significant perioperative risks of surgery.

Postoperative care in the adult patient undergoing major reconstructive surgery requires detailed attention to the patient's systemic needs, much more so than is generally required by patients undergoing other orthopedic procedures. Those patients who require thoracotomy or thoracoabdominal approaches will have postoperative chest tubes and are at higher risk for pulmonary complications.

Fluid shifts can be significant after lengthy procedures, particularly those with large blood losses. Anterior approaches, although largely retroperitoneal, can lead to prolonged ileus, a problem compounded by the use of postoperative narcotics that all orthopedic patients require.

Bradford DS et al: Adult scoliosis: Surgical indications, operative management, complications, and outcomes. Spine 1999; 24(24):2617. [PMID: 10635525]

Connolly PJ et al: Adolescent idiopathic scoliosis. J Bone Joint Surg Am 1995;77A:1209. [PMID: 7642667]

Dickson JH et al: Results of operative treatment of idiopathic scoliosis in adults. J Bone Joint Surg Am 1995;77A:513. [PMID: 7713967]

Eck KR et al: Complications and results of long adult deformity fusions down to L4, L5 and the sacrum. Spine 2001;26(9): E182. [PMID: 11337635]

Grubb SA et al: Results of surgical treatment of painful adult scoliosis. Spine 1994;19(14):1619. [PMID: 7939999]

Kim YJ et al: Pseudoarthrosis in primary fusions for adult idiopathic scoliosis: Incidence, risk factors, and outcome analysis. Spine 2005;30(4):468. [PMID: 15706346]

Schwab F et al: Adult scoliosis: A health assessment analysis by SF-36. Spine 2003;28(6):603. [PMID: 12342769]

Schwab FJ et al: Adult scoliosis: A quantitative radiographic and clinical analysis. Spine 2002;27(4):387. [PMID: 11840105]

Weinstein SL et al: Health and function of patients with untreated idiopathic scoliosis: A 50 year natural history study. JAMA 2003;289(5):559. [PMID: 12578488]

2. Neuromuscular Scoliosis

Neuromuscular conditions frequently associated with scoliosis include muscular dystrophy, cerebral palsy, poliomyelitis, spinal cord tumor, spinal cord trauma, spinal muscular atrophy, Friedreich ataxia, syringomyelia, familial dysautonomia, and myelomeningocele (spina bifida). Spinal deformities tend to present early in life in patients with these conditions and often progress to severe deformities because of muscle weakness and the many years of ensuing growth. Although neuromuscular scoliosis can be subdivided into neurogenic and myogenic types (see Table 5–1), the principles of treatment for the two types are the same.

The assessment of patients should be detailed and include an evaluation of overall function, mental status, motor strength, ambulatory status, and sitting tolerance as well as a search for the presence of problems such as joint contractures, pelvic obliquity, and pressure sores. Joint contractures can lead to pelvic obliquity or can limit the patient's ambulatory or sitting ability. Pelvic obliquity or a dislocated hip can be primary and lead to scoliosis or can be secondary to the spinal deformity. The primary condition should be determined, and if corrected sufficiently early, may obviate or delay the need for further corrective surgery.

With neuromuscular scoliosis, as with idiopathic scoliosis, curvatures affecting the thoracic spine and therefore the chest cage can have adverse effects on the pulmonary system, which is already compromised in most neuromuscular scoliosis patients because of weakness of the respiratory musculature. Truncal imbalance or pelvic obliquity, or both, are often associated with neuromuscular scoliosis and can impair ambulatory ability or sitting balance in affected patients. Before treatment of neuromuscular scoliosis is undertaken, the goals should be understood by the clinician as well as the patient and family. In many cases, the conditions are progressive, and the long-term prognosis for the patient and the patient's curvature should be considered. Stabilization of a curvature clearly does not affect the disease process and therefore does not affect the life expectancy of the patient.

Studies show, however, that in patients with Duchenne-type muscular dystrophy, thoracic curvatures contribute in themselves to loss of pulmonary function, beyond that which would be experienced by the generalized loss of pulmonary function associated with the progressive weakness of the respiratory muscles. In patients with Duchenne-type muscular dystrophy, an increase of 10 degrees in thoracic scoliosis results in a loss of 4% of functional vital capacity.

The neuromuscular condition associated with scoliosis in each case should be well delineated and understood because the curvatures in neuromuscular scoliosis

have a higher likelihood of progression than those in idiopathic scoliosis, given the factors of muscle weakness, muscle imbalance, progression of disease, and the generally younger age at which the curves in patients with neuromuscular conditions are diagnosed. Particularly as pulmonary function is also progressively lost in many neuromuscular conditions, a more aggressive surgical approach is generally recommended, with intervention performed once the probable curve progression is established (by history, diagnosis, or degree of curvature) and preferably while the pulmonary function is still relatively good.

Unlike patients with idiopathic scoliosis, patients with neuromuscular scoliosis do not experience the active corrective effect of a brace. Instead, the brace functions as a shell of support, counteracting the effect of gravity on the collapsing spine. Bracing may adversely affect the breathing of these compromised patients but may slow progression in very young (less than 10 years) patients or while the course of the disease is being determined.

If surgery is recommended in cases of neuromuscular scoliosis, special concerns include whether the bone is osteoporotic, whether pelvic obliquity is present, and whether the patient has sitting balance. Osteoporotic bone often necessitates the use of sublaminar wiring, despite the theoretically increased neurologic risk associated with passage of the wire into the spinal canal. If pelvic obliquity exists or if the patient has poor sitting balance, fusion to the pelvis is advisable. This may be performed with the Galveston technique, in which the ends of a specially bent rod are placed between the inner and outer tables of the iliac wing. The proximal rod ends are then placed on either side of the spine after being bent to appropriate sagittal contours. The rods are subsequently attached to the spine with the sublaminar wires. Because of the collapsing nature of the spine in cases such as those described here, it is usually necessary to extend the fusion proximally to T3 or T4 to prevent kyphosis from developing above the fusion. Because sublaminar wires do not provide axial control, rigid proximal fixation, either hooks or screws, is recommended at the proximal end of the construct.

The perioperative management of neuromuscular scoliosis can be complex, and these patients often benefit from a multidisciplinary approach involving the orthopedic surgeon, pulmonologist, pediatrician, anesthesiologist, physical and occupational therapists, and additional specialists, depending on other system involvement. Patients with Duchenne-type muscular dystrophy, for example, may also develop cardiomyopathy. Those with Friedreich ataxia have a high incidence of cardiomyopathy and diabetes mellitus.

With aggressive medical and surgical management and a supportive family, the longevity and quality of life for patients with neuromuscular scoliosis can be optimized.

Benson ER et al: Results and morbidity in a consecutive series of patients undergoing spinal fusion for neuromuscular scoliosis. Spine 1998;23:2308. [PMID: 9820912]

Jones KB et al: Longitudinal parental perceptions of spinal fusion for neuromuscular spine deformity in patients with totally involved cerebral palsy. J Pediatr Orthop 2003;23:143. [PMID: 12604940]

Kannan S et al: Bleeding and coagulation changes during spinal fusion surgery: A comparison of neuromuscular and idiopathic scoliosis patients. Pediatr Crit Care Med 2002;3:364. [PMID: 12780956]

McCarthy RE: Management of neuromuscular scoliosis. Orthop Clin North Am 1999;30:435. [PMID: 10393765]

Miller F et al: Pulmonary function and scoliosis in Duchenne dystrophy. J Pediatr Orthop 1988;8:133. [PMID: 3350945]

Miller RG et al: The effect of spine fusion on respiratory function in Duchenne muscular dystrophy. Neurology 1991;41:38. [PMID: 1985293]

Olafsson Y et al: Brace treatment in neuromuscular spine deformity. J Pediatr Orthop 1999;19:376. [PMID: 10344323]

Yazici M et al: The safety and efficacy of Isola-Galveston instrumentation and arthrodesis in the treatment of neuromuscular spinal deformities. J Bone Joint Surg Am 2000;82:524. [PMID: 10761943]

3. Neurofibromatosis

Spinal deformity associated with neurofibromatosis poses some special considerations. Curvatures seen in affected patients may be of the idiopathic type or the dysplastic type. Curvatures of the first type exhibit the same curve patterns as seen in patients with idiopathic scoliosis and are most commonly right thoracic curves and may be managed in a similar manner. Curvatures of the second type can be much more malignant in behavior.

Dysplastic curves can be identified by evidence of dysplastic bone: penciling of the ribs or transverse processes, enlargement of the foramina, erosion of the vertebrae, and evidence of a shorter, more abrupt curve than that seen in idiopathic scoliosis. Dysplastic curves usually are associated with kyphosis, which also exists through a fairly short sharp segment. They may occur in the thoracic, thoracolumbar, or lumbar spine.

Dysplastic curves in patients with neurofibromatosis can progress rapidly and lead to severe deformity. Bony erosion can occur secondary to neurofibromas or to dural ectasia (expansions of the dural sac, which can account for enlargement of the foramina or erosion of the vertebrae). The short kyphotic curves and erosion of bone can in severe cases result in neurologic impairment, including paraplegia.

Surgery in patients with dysplastic curves is associated with a high incidence of pseudarthrosis. If surgery is indicated, it is usually recommended to perform both an anterior and a posterior fusion. This combined approach results in a satisfactory fusion rate of up to 80%. Because of the dysplastic bone stock, it may be necessary to use a combination of sublaminar wires, hooks, and screws. Preoperative MRI may be useful in assessing the extent of dural ectasia. Fusion levels are selected according to the end vertebra of the curvature. The end fusion level must lie centered over the middle of the sacrum, much like the selection for idiopathic scoliosis. Clearly, however, the fusion should not end above or below a dysplastic vertebra, although it would be rare for such a level not to be within the curve.

Akbarnia BA et al: Prevalence of scoliosis in neurofibromatosis. Spine 1992;17:S244. [PMID: 1523507]

Funasaki H et al: Pathophysiology of spinal deformities in neurofibromatosis: An analysis of 71 patients who had curves associated with dystrophic changes. J Bone Joint Surg Am 1994;76:692. [PMID: 8175817]

Vitale MG et al: Orthopaedic manifestations of neurofibromatosis in children: An update. Clin Orthop Relat Res 2002;401:107. [PMID: 12151887]

Winter RB et al: Spine deformity in neurofibromatosis. A review of one hundred and two patients. J Bone Joint Surg Am 1979;61A:677. [PMID 110813]

4. Congenital Scoliosis

Congenital scoliosis is caused by one of two types of structural bony abnormality (Figure 5–24). Type I is a failure of formation, such as that seen with hemivertebrae. Type II is a failure of segmentation, such as that seen with block vertebrae and that seen with unsegmented bars, where there is a tether to growth on one side of the spine. Mixed abnormalities are also found in patients with congenital scoliosis. Unilateral unsegmented bars with contralateral hemivertebrae have the greatest tendency for rapid progression and should be surgically fused as soon as the bony abnormality is evident. Unilateral unsegmented bars also tend to progress.

With respect to progression, hemivertebrae have a variable prognosis, depending on whether a contralateral hemivertebra is present that results in overall balance of the spine, whether multiple hemivertebrae are on one side of the spine, and how much growth potential is predicted for each endplate of the hemivertebra. Hemivertebrae at the cervicothoracic junction and the lumbosacral junction have a relatively poor prognosis because the spine above or below the abnormality cannot compensate. Hemivertebrae should be observed so as to delineate their growth potential and progression.

Bracing is ineffective in treating congenital scoliosis because the curves are inflexible. Bracing is sometimes used to prevent progression of the compensatory curve, however.

In patients with congenital scoliosis, the incidence of cardiac abnormalities is increased, as is the incidence of renal abnormalities (20–30%) and intracanal abnor-

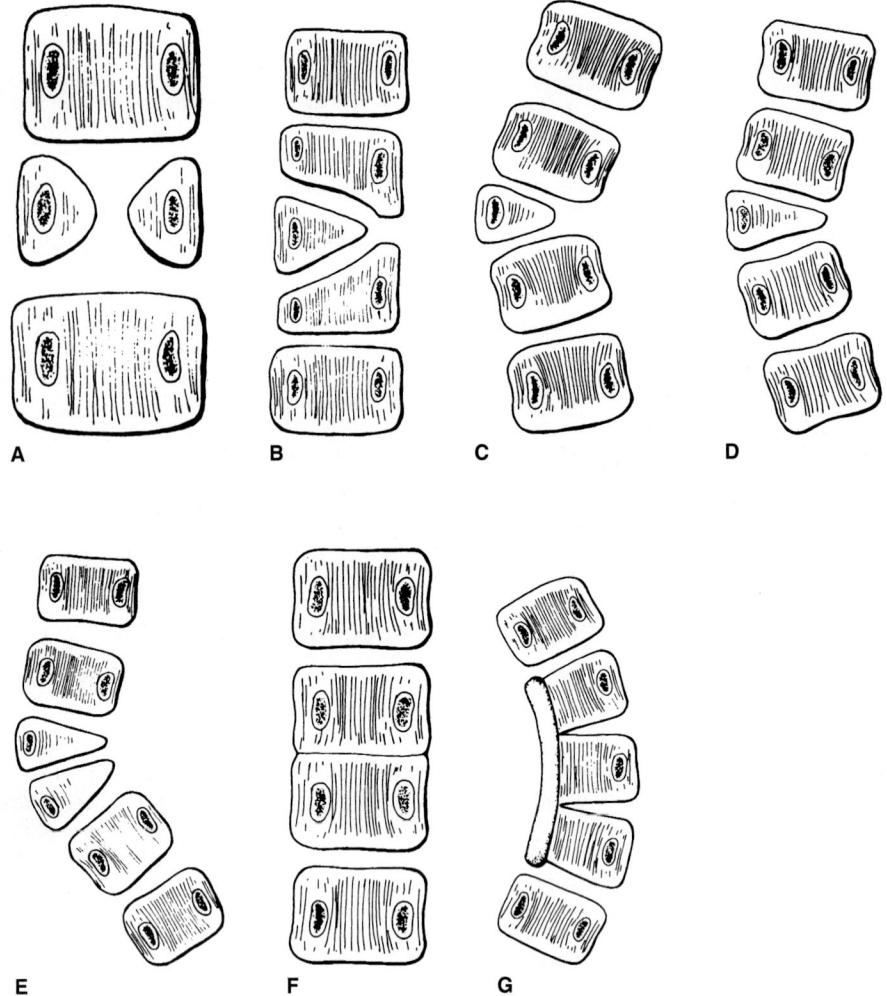

Figure 5–24. The major types of congenital scoliosis are failure of formation, as shown in diagrams A through E, and failure of segmentation, as shown in diagrams F and G. (Reproduced, with permission, from Hall JE: Congenital scoliosis. In Bradford DS, Hensinger RN, eds: *The Pediatric Spine.* Thieme, 1985.)

malities (10–50%). Abdominal ultrasound or other imaging tests should be used to rule out absent or abnormal kidneys. Intracanal abnormalities may include a syrinx (cyst within the cord), diastematomyelia or diplomyelia (division or reduplication of the cord, respectively), and tethered cord (presence of a tight filum terminale that does not permit the conus medullaris to migrate upward normally with growth).

If surgical intervention in patients with congenital scoliosis is indicated, several options are available. Fusion in situ is the simplest procedure. For very young (less than 10 years) patients, however, a posterior fusion

alone results in tethering of the posterior elements while the anterior elements continue to grow. This situation may lead to the crankshaft phenomenon, whereby the anterior growth in the spine results in a twisting deformity around the fused posterior elements. For this reason, combined anterior and posterior fusion is usually recommended for very young patients, halting growth circumferentially about the spine. (The crankshaft phenomenon can also occur in very young patients with noncongenital forms of scoliosis who were treated by posterior fusion. Age younger than 10 years, Risser stage 0 or 1, and the presence of an open triradiate cartilage are indicators of skeletal maturity at risk for development of crankshaft.)

In some cases of hemivertebra, hemiepiphysiodesis may be performed, arresting growth on the curve convexity but permitting continued growth on the curve concavity, with resultant gradual curve correction. This procedure has good results in selected patients but can be unpredictable with respect to the amount of actual correction that can be achieved.

In cases in which a hemivertebra is accompanied by significant coronal decompensation and compensatory growth would not be adequate to result in spinal balance, consideration can be given to hemivertebra excision via a combined anterior and posterior approach. Although this procedure is technically more demanding and has greater potential risks, it allows for better overall curve correction and improvement of coronal balance. Hemivertebra excision may be the preferred option in the lumbar spine or lumbosacral junction, where the neurologic risk is to the cauda equina rather than the spinal cord and where oblique takeoff of the vertebra above the hemivertebra can result in significant truncal decompensation.

Bradford DS: Partial epiphyseal arrest and supplemental fixation for progressive correction of congenital spinal deformity. J Bone Joint Surg Am 1982;64:610. [PMID: 7068703]

Bradford DS, Boachie-Adjei O: One-stage anterior and posterior hemivertebral resection and arthrodesis for congenital scoliosis. J Bone Joint Surg Am 1990;72:536. [PMID: 2324140]

Deviren V et al: Excision of hemivertebrae in the management of congenital scoliosis of the thoracic and thoracolumbar spine. J Bone Joint Surg Br 2001;83:496. [PMID: 11380117]

Holte DC et al: Excision of hemivertebrae and wedge resection in treatment of congenital scoliosis. J Bone Joint Surg Am 1995;77A:159. [PMID: 7844121]

Kim YJ, Otsuka NY, Flynn JM et al: Surgical treatment of congenital kyphosis. Spine 2001;26:2251. [PMID: 11598516]

Nakamura H, Matsuda H, Konishi S et al: Single-stage excision of hemivertebrae via the posterior approach alone for congenital spine deformity: Follow-up period longer than ten years. Spine 2002;27:110. [PMID: 11805647]

Prahinski JR, Polly DW Jr, McHale KA et al: Occult intraspinal anomalies in congenital scoliosis. J Pediatr Orthop 2000;20:59. [PMID: 10641690]

Thompson AG et al: Long term results of combined anterior and posterior convex epiphysiodesis for congenital scoliosis due to hemivertebrae. Spine 1995;20:1380. [PMID: 7676336]

KYPHOSIS

The normal sagittal contour of the spine includes cervical lordosis, thoracic kyphosis, and lumbar lordosis (Figure 5–25). Increases or decreases in any of these can be seen. If they are severe enough, they can cause disability, as discussed later in the cases of congenital kyphosis and Scheuermann kyphosis.

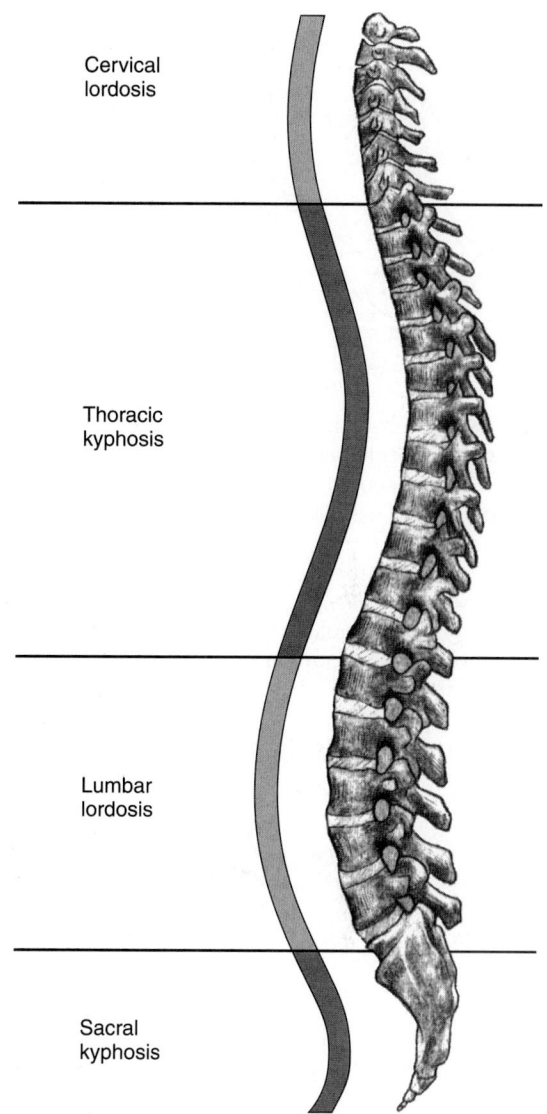

Figure 5–25. The normal sagittal contour of the spine. (Reproduced, with permission, from Bullough PG, Boachie-Adjei O: *Atlas of Spinal Diseases.* Gower, 1988.)

Cervical lordosis

Thoracic kyphosis

Lumbar lordosis

Sacral kyphosis

1. Congenital Kyphosis

As in congenital scoliosis (see previous discussion), congenital kyphosis can result from a failure of formation or a failure of segmentation. In congenital kyphosis, however, failures of formation have a much more dangerous clinical prognosis. These can lead to congenital or progressive "dislocation" of the spinal column (Figure 5–26) and paralysis if not treated appropriately. If

Canal in continuity   Step-off (dislocated spine)

Figure 5–26. Congenital kyphosis and congenital "dislocation" of the spinal column. (Reproduced, with permission, from Dubousset J: Congenital kyphosis. In Bradford DS, Hensinger RN, eds: *The Pediatric Spine.* Thieme, 1985.)

performed early enough, posterior fusion may be sufficient to prevent neurologic problems. Severe deficiencies, however, may require anterior and posterior fusion to achieve stability.

2. Scheuermann's Kyphosis

Normal thoracic kyphosis ranges from 25 to 45 degrees. Postural kyphosis can increase this curvature, but if no abnormalities are present, the curve is flexible and the posture can be easily corrected by the child. If endplate abnormalities are present and three or more vertebral bodies are wedged as seen on the lateral radiograph, the diagnosis of Scheuermann kyphosis can be made. Schmorl nodules, characterized by herniation of the disk material at the vertebral endplates, and increased thoracic kyphosis are also seen. Clinically, patients with this type of kyphosis have a curvature that is more abrupt than that observed in people with postural roundback, and this type is only partly correctable by forced extension. It can be demonstrated either by having the patient hyperextend or by taking a lateral radiograph with the patient lying over a pad at the apex of the kyphosis so the Cobb angle can be measured. Thoracic curves may cause pain and discomfort, although some report that pain is more commonly seen in thoracolumbar curves.

Bracing can be instituted if the kyphosis measures more than 45 or 55 degrees in a skeletally immature patient, particularly if the curvature is progressive or accompanied by pain. If lesser degrees of deformity are symptomatic, they can be treated with physical therapy exercises and observed for progression. Brace treatment requires the use of the Milwaukee brace, with two para-

spinal pads placed over the apical ribs posteriorly. Radiographs should be taken with the patient in the brace to confirm that adequate correction is being effected. The brace can be removed for sports and bathing but should otherwise be worn 23 hours a day. Repeat lateral radiographs should be taken at intervals of 4–6 months. If bracing is successful at controlling the curve, it should be continued until the patient nears skeletal maturity. Weaning should be performed slowly, so as to maintain correction. Although some correction may be lost, proper use of the Milwaukee brace can result in long-lasting improvement in many patients with kyphosis (which is not the case with brace treatment of adolescent idiopathic scoliosis).

Surgical treatment of kyphosis may be indicated if the curve magnitude increases despite bracing, if the patient has significant associated symptoms, or if the patient who is nearing skeletal maturity has a severe curvature. Posterior spinal fusion with a variable hook-rod system, such as the Cotrel-Dubousset system, is the treatment of choice in these cases. If the curve flexibility does not permit adequate correction as demonstrated on a hyperextension lateral radiograph, an anterior release and fusion prior to the posterior spinal fusion is indicated.

Reports describe the natural history of Scheuermann kyphosis, suggesting some functional limitations but little actual interference with lifestyle. The deformity can worsen over time. It appears clear, however, that many patients have their symptoms of back pain and deformity improved by surgery. Proper patient education and selection are essential for appropriate treatment of these patients.

Arlet V, Schlenzka D: Scheuermann's kyphosis: Surgical management. Eur Spine J 2005;14:817. [PMID: 15830215]

Lowe TG, Kasten MD: An analysis of sagittal curves and balance after Cotrel-Dubousset instrumentation for kyphosis secondary to Scheuermann's disease. Spine 1994;19:1680. [PMID: 7973960]

Murray PM et al: The natural history and long-term follow-up of Scheuermann's kyphosis. J Bone Joint Surg Am 1993;75:236. [PMID: 8423184]

MYELODYSPLASIA

Neural tube defects can result in complex spinal deformities secondary both to the neuromuscular collapsing nature of the spine and to the vertebral anomalies that can give rise to congenital kyphosis or congenital scoliosis. Myelomeningocele or meningocele is present at birth in a patient whose neural tube failed to close in utero. Sac closure is usually performed shortly after birth. In many cases, the affected infant also requires placement of a ventriculoperitoneal shunt because of hydrocephalus. The level of neurologic function usually corresponds to the level of the defect. For example, a low thoracic myelomeningocele patient has no lumbar nerve roots functioning and therefore no lower extremity function. An L4 myelomeningocele patient has a functioning tibialis anterior but no extensor hallucis and no gastrocnemius and usually no voluntary bowel and bladder control.

Neurologic function in patients with myelodysplasia is static and should not deteriorate with growth. Neurologic changes, especially during growth spurts, require evaluation for tethered cord, a common occurrence in affected children.

Orthopedic management includes maximizing the function of patients through the use of braces, ambulatory aids, wheelchairs, or surgery. The degree of spinal deformity is related to the neurologic level, with spinal collapse more likely in those with a higher neurologic level of involvement than in those with a lower level. The presence of bony abnormalities can affect this prognosis, of course.

As with many neuromuscular spinal deformities, curvatures may present early in life. If the clinician elects to treat a patient with bracing, it is important to remember that bracing in the presence of insensate skin can result in pressure sores if the brace is not adequately padded and the parents are not instructed regarding skin care.

In many cases, the curvature eventually requires surgical stabilization. Because of the magnitude and stiffness of the curvature as well as the absence of posterior elements, the preferred treatment is anterior and posterior fusion. Anterior instrumentation may improve rigidity of the surgical construct. In patients with myelodysplasia, fusion to the sacrum is invariably required because of pelvic obliquity or lack of sitting balance. Luque-Galveston instrumentation to the proximal thoracic spine is preferred, as with many neuromuscular deformities.

The lack of posterior elements in the myelodysplastic spine can lead to congenital kyphosis. Although kyphosis in these patients does not compromise neurologic function, it can lead to pressure sores over the prominent area. The treatment of choice for this problem is posterior kyphectomy and fusion.

Banit DM et al: Posterior spinal fusion in paralytic scoliosis and myelomeningocele. J Pediatr Orthop 2001;21:117. [PMID: 11176365].

Parsch D et al: Surgical management of paralytic scoliosis in myelomeningocele. J Pediatr Orthop 2001;10:10. [PMID: 11269805]

SPONDYLOLISTHESIS & SPONDYLOLYSIS

Spondylolisthesis is the slipping forward of one vertebra upon another. Spondylolysis is characterized by the presence of a bony defect at the pars interarticularis, which can result in spondylolisthesis.

The classification system most commonly used in spondylolisthesis was originated by Wiltse et al. in 1976 and subsequently modified by others. Type I, the dysplastic form of spondylolisthesis, is a congenital deficiency of the superior sacral facet, the inferior fifth lumbar facet, or both. Type II, the isthmic form, is caused by a defect in the pars interarticularis but can also be seen with an elongated pars. Types I and II are most commonly seen in younger (less than 15 years) patients and most likely to occur at the L5-S1 level. Type III, the degenerative form of spondylolisthesis, is seen in older patients and most frequently involves the L4-L5 level. Type IV, the traumatic form, is located other than at the pars. Type V, the pathologic form, is caused by conditions such as a neoplasm. The Wiltse classification of spondylolisthesis is shown in Figure 5–27.

Marchetti and Bartolozzi proposed a classification of spondylolisthesis that separates developmental and acquired types of spondylolisthesis. Developmental spondylolisthesis is divided into high dysplastic and

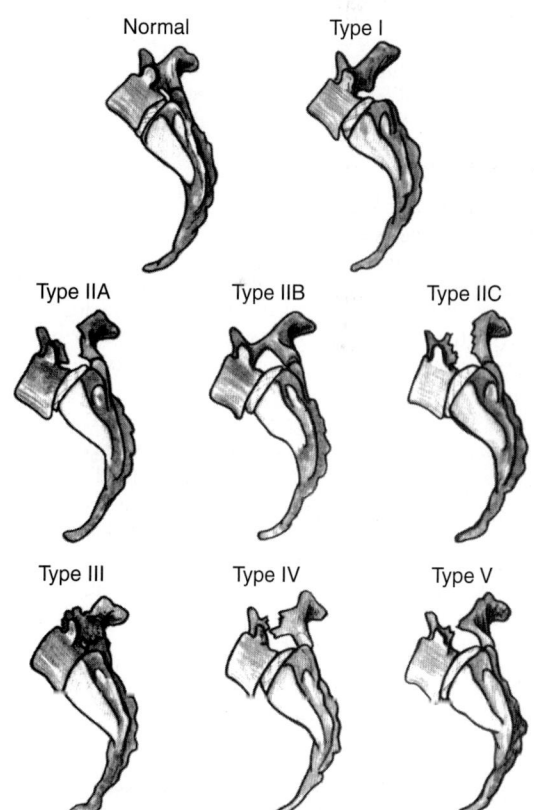

Figure 5–27. Classification of spondylolisthesis. (Reproduced, with permission, from Bradford DS, Hu SS: Spondylolysis and spondylolisthesis. In Weinstein SL, ed: *The Pediatric Spine.* New York: Raven, 1994.)

low dysplastic types, with each of these subdivided into those with lysis of the pars interarticularis or elongation of the pars interarticularis. Acquired types include degenerative, traumatic, postsurgical, and pathologic. A new classification based on clinical presentation and spinal morphology is now suggested for children and adolescents.

Bridwell KH, DeWal RL, eds: *The Textbook of Spinal Surgery,* 2nd ed. Lippincott-Raven, 1997.

Herman MJ, Pizzutillo PD: Spondylolysis and spondylolisthesis in the child and adolescent: A new classification. Clin Orthop 2005;434:46. [PMID: 15864031]

Marchetti PG, Bartolozzi P: Classification of spondylolisthesis as a guideline for treatment. In Wiltse LL et al: Classification of spondylolisthesis and spondylolysis. Clin Orthop 1976;117:23. [PMID: 11277669]

1. Isthmic Spondylolisthesis

The cause of isthmic spondylolisthesis may be developmental, with a congenital defect of dysplasia predisposing some individuals to spondylolysis. The overall incidence of spondylolysis is approximately 6%. The high incidence of spondylolysis in gymnasts, football players, weight lifters, and other athletes who place their lumbar spines in hyperextension suggests that repetitive injury may be a contributing mechanism. Biomechanical studies also suggest that the pars interarticularis is under the greatest stress in extension.

Clinical Findings

Spondylolysis and spondylolisthesis may be asymptomatic, or they may present with back pain and leg pain. Rarely, they present with radicular symptoms or bowel and bladder symptoms. Isthmic spondylolisthesis most commonly presents during the preadolescent growth spurt, between 10 and 15 years of age. The extent of slippage may not be correlated with the severity of pain. The L5 pars interarticularis defect, with resultant slippage of L5 forward on the sacrum, is most commonly seen.

In young patients, regardless of the extent of slippage, there may be tight hamstrings and a knee-bent, hips-flexed gait, the classic Phalen-Dickson sign. Careful palpation of the spine of the patient with spondylolisthesis may reveal a step-off secondary to the prominent spinous process of L5. With more severe slippage, the lumbosacral junction becomes more kyphotic and the trunk appears shortened, with the rib cage approaching the iliac crests (Figure 5–28).

Radiographic examination shows the defect on the lateral view, with the percentage of slippage measurable from this view. The Meyerding classification is most commonly used (Figure 5–29). Oblique radiographs demonstrate the "collar" or "broken neck" on the "Scottie dog" (Figure 5–30). If a unilateral defect is

Figure 5–28. Diagram showing how high-grade spondylolisthesis results in a short trunk, with the rib cage approaching the iliac crests. (Reproduced, with permission, from Bradford DS, Hu SS: Spondylolysis and spondylolisthesis. In Weinstein SL, ed: *The Pediatric Spine.* Raven, 1994.)

present, the contralateral pars or lamina may show sclerosis. If the history is suggestive of an early stress fracture and radiographic findings are negative, bone scans may be useful. CT scanning shows spondylolysis as an incomplete ring.

The slip angle, a measure of lumbosacral kyphosis, is useful in determining the likelihood of progression to higher grades of slippage in patients. A line is drawn along the posterior cortex of the sacrum, and the angle between its perpendicular and a line drawn along the inferior border of L5 is measured (Figure 5–31). If the slip angle is greater than 50 degrees, the likelihood of progression is high.

In patients with radicular symptoms or bowel or bladder impairment, CT scanning or MRI is essential if surgical intervention is considered.

Treatment

A. CONSERVATIVE TREATMENT

Low-grade spondylolisthesis (Meyerding grade I or II) can usually be managed with conservative measures, including restriction of the aggravating activity, bracing to reduce lumbar lordosis, and physical therapy. Patients with grade I slips who respond to conservative therapy may be permitted to resume all activities. For those with grade II slips who are improved with conservative treatment, it is usually recommended that they

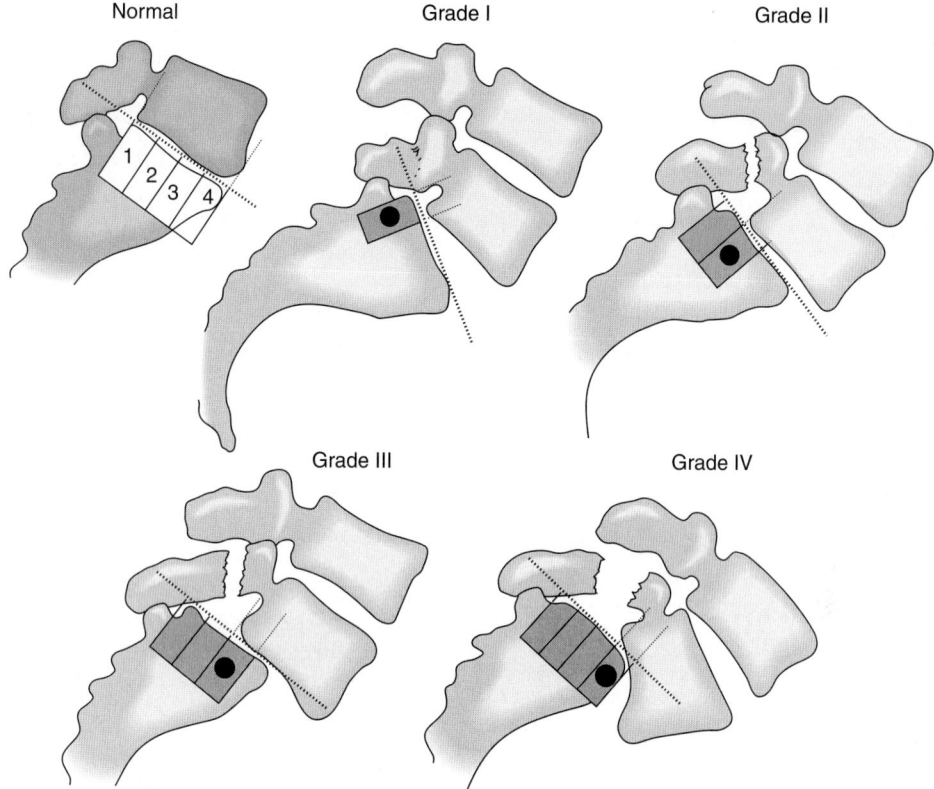

Figure 5–29. Meyerding classification of degree of slippage in spondylolisthesis. Grade I is 1–25% slippage; grade II is 26–50% slippage; grade III is 51–75% slippage; and grade IV is 76–100% slippage. (Reproduced, with permission, from Bradford DS, Hu SS: Spondylolysis and spondylolisthesis. In Weinstein SL, ed: *The Pediatric Spine.* Raven, 1994.)

refrain from activities that hyperextend the spine. Skeletally immature patients with grade III or higher slips are at significant risk for progression, and they are recommended for fusion.

B. SURGICAL TREATMENT:

1. Fusion and decompression—Fusion is indicated for patients who fail to respond to conservative measures, demonstrate progression, or have greater than 50% slippage and are skeletally immature. For most patients, fusion in situ is indicated. If slippage is less than 50%, fusion from L5 to S1 is sufficient. If slippage is greater than 50%, it is necessary to fuse from L4 to S1 to achieve a fusion bed that is under compression. Intertransverse fusion can result in fusion rates of 95% and good to excellent clinical outcomes in 75–100% of patients. This technique can be performed through two parallel paraspinal skin incisions. Alternatively, a midline skin incision with paraspinal fascial incisions, approximately two fingerbreadths off the midline, can be employed. The

sacrospinalis fibers can be split, and access to the transverse processes is obtained. The transverse processes, pars interarticularis, facet joint, and adjacent lamina are exposed and decorticated. Iliac crest bone graft is harvested and placed in corticocancellous strips over the fusion bed (Figure 5–32).

If neurologic findings such as numbness, leg pain, leg weakness, or bowel and bladder compromise are present, decompression may be needed. Central and foraminal stenosis can be evaluated with a CT scan or MRI. In many cases, fibrocartilaginous scarring at the site of the pars defect accounts for the compressive symptoms. Particularly for young (less than 18 years) patients, an isolated decompression without fusion is likely to result in slip progression, so decompression should be combined with fusion. Some reports indicate that signs of nerve root irritation, including hamstring tightness, resolve when fusion is used without surgical decompression. It may take up to 18 months for these signs to resolve after fusion alone.

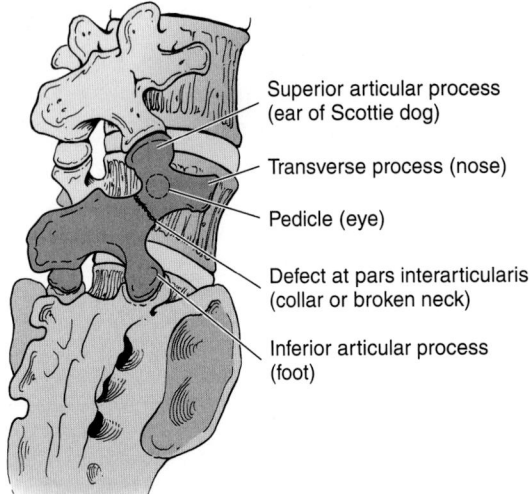

Figure 5–30. Diagram showing the "Scottie dog" (dark shaded area) seen on oblique radiographs of the lumbar spine in patients with spondylolisthesis.

Superior articular process (ear of Scottie dog)

Transverse process (nose)

Pedicle (eye)

Defect at pars interarticularis (collar or broken neck)

Inferior articular process (foot)

Bracing or casting may be indicated after fusion and may consist of the use of a lumbar corset, a thoracolumbar orthosis, or a thoracolumbosacral orthosis with leg extension or pantaloon spica cast, depending on the

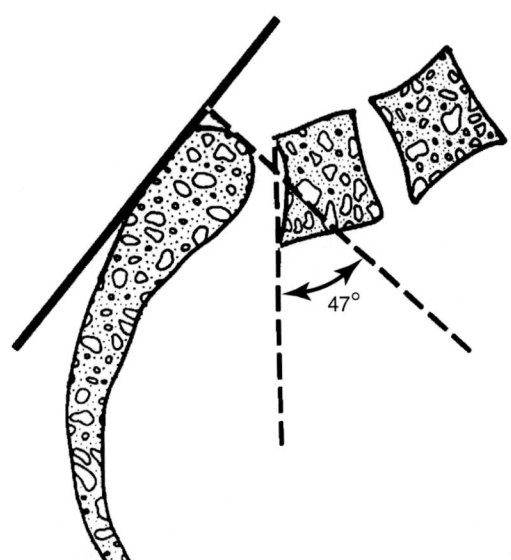

Figure 5–31. Measurement of the slip angle as a predictor of progression in spondylolisthesis. (Reproduced, with permission, from Bradford DS, Hu SS: Spondylolysis and spondylolisthesis. In Weinstein SL, ed: *The Pediatric Spine.* Raven, 1994.)

47°

Figure 5–32. Schematic diagram of fusion for spondylolisthesis, as described by Wiltse. (Reproduced, with permission, from Bradford DS, Hu SS: Spondylolysis and spondylolisthesis. In Weinstein SL, ed: *The Pediatric Spine.* Raven, 1994.)

preference of the surgeon. Once the patient's fusion is solid, full activities are permitted.

2. Pars repair—Pars repair may be indicated for young (less than 18 years) patients who have single-level or multiple-level L1-L4 pars defects without evidence of disk damage. Screw fixation or wiring of the transverse process to the spinous process (Figure 5–33) yields good results in appropriately selected patients.

3. Fibular strut graft—Bohlman and Cook described a technique for one-stage posterior decompression and interbody fusion for treatment of grade V spondylolisthesis (spondyloptosis). After wide decompression, a drill hole is prepared between the L5 and S1 nerve roots, passing through the sacrum to the L5 vertebral body that has slipped in front of the sacrum. The configuration is similar to that diagrammed in Figure 5–34 for anterior strut graft fusion. Autograft or allograft fibula is inserted and then countersunk to avoid dural impingement. Posterolateral fusion is also performed at this time.

4. Anterior fusion—Another option for achieving fusion is via an anterior transperitoneal or retroperitoneal approach. The surgeon can either perform disk space grafting with tricortical iliac crest or place a fibular graft through a drill hole from the L5 vertebral body to the sacrum (see Figure 5–34). For high-grade slips, anterior fusion places the graft in compression. Clearly, repeated neurologic assessments. It is less commonly used because of the availability of smaller pedicle screws. A posterolateral fusion can be performed after traction is completed or initially at the time of decompression. Anterior fusion may or may not be indicated,

Figure 5–33. Illustration of pars repair, which can be performed in younger patients with minimal slippage, particularly above L5. Wires are placed around the transverse process and wired around the spinous process. The pars defect itself must be cleared of fibrous tissue and then bone grafted. (Reproduced, with permission, from Bradford DS, Hu SS: Spondylolysis and spondylolisthesis. In Weinstein SL, ed: *The Pediatric Spine*. Raven, 1994.)

there are significant risks with the anterior approach, including the risk of vascular damage in male and female patients and the risk of retrograde ejaculation secondary to damage of the sympathetic nervous system in male patients. Because of these risks and because good results can generally be achieved with posterolateral fusion, anterior fusion is best reserved for patients with high-grade slippage or patients who have undergone unsuccessful posterior arthrodesis treatment.

5. Reduction—Reduction of high-grade spondylolisthesis remains controversial but may be considered in patients who have high-grade slippage and are unable to stand balanced with their head over the sacrum while keeping their knees straight. Reduction can improve the patient's overall trunk appearance, which is characterized by a short waist, transverse abdominal skin fold, and heart-shaped pelvis, all of which become more prominent with high grade spondylolisthesis. Improvement of the slip angle may prevent slip progression.

Although even fusion in situ of high-grade slips can lead to neurologic compromise and cauda equina syndrome, concern is raised over the neurologic risk with reduction techniques. Closed reduction using halopelvic or halo-femoral traction allows for gradual reduction while permitting the awake patient to have

Figure 5–34. Diagram showing the steps involved in an anterior strut grafting procedure for high-grade spondylolisthesis. This approach permits grafting of iliac crest or fibula from the L5 vertebra to the sacrum, with the graft being placed under compression. (Reproduced, with permission, from Bradford DS, Hu SS: Spondylolysis and spondylolisthesis. In Weinstein SL, ed: *The Pediatric Spine*. Raven, 1994.)

depending on the particular patient and on the reduction achieved.

Pedicle screw instrumentation can be used by experienced surgeons to distract and then posteriorly translate the slipped vertebra. Neurologic complications may occur but in most cases are temporary. Supplemental techniques, such as intrasacral rods with iliac buttressing, or iliac screws, appear to improve distal fixation as does performing an interbody fusion.

For severe slips, L5 vertebrectomy with reduction of L4 onto S1 is successfully performed. The technique shortens the spine and therefore theoretically poses less neurologic risk, but surgical manipulation of the nerve roots and posterior translation of L4 can result in neurologic compromise such as footdrop.

Complications

As noted earlier, neurologic compromise sometimes results even after fusion in situ. Particularly with decompression alone (which is rarely indicated) but also with high-grade slips even after fusion, progression of the slip can occur. This happens if there is pseudarthrosis (failure of fusion), but slippage can also occur postsurgically before the fusion becomes solid, or the fusion mass can bend if the forces across it are sufficiently great.

Incomplete pain relief is rare in adolescents but is sometimes a complaint of adults. The reasons for this are not entirely clear, but it is noted that secondary degenerative changes can occur either at the level of the spondylolisthesis or at the level above.

Frennered AK et al: Natural history of symptomatic isthmic low-grade spondylolisthesis in children and adolescents: A seven-year follow-up study. J Pediatr Orthop 1991;11:209. [PMID: 2010523]

Kakiuchi M: Repair of the defect in spondylolysis. J Bone Joint Surg Am 1997;79:818. [PMID: 9199377]

Labelle H et al: Spondylolisthesis, pelvic incidence, and spinopelvic balance: A correlation study. Spine 2004;29:2049. [PMID: 15371707]

Laursen M et al: Functional outcome after partial reduction and 360° fusion in grade III-V spondylolisthesis in adolescent and adult patients. J Spinal Dis 1999;12:300. [PMID: 10451045]

Minamide A et al: Transdiscal L5-S1 screws for the fixation of isthmic spondylolisthesis: A biomechanical evaluation. J Spinal Disord Tech 2003;16:114. [PMID: 12679668]

Ogilvie JW: Complications in spondylolisthesis surgery. Spine 2005;30:S97. [PMID: 15767893]

Petraco DM et al: An anatomic evaluation of L5 nerve stretch in spondylolisthesis reduction. Spine 1996;21:1133. [PMID: 8727186]

2. Degenerative Spondylolisthesis

Unlike isthmic spondylolisthesis, degenerative spondylolisthesis is found more commonly at the L4-L5 level, secondary to a number of factors. This level sees more stresses than other lumbar levels because the L5-S1 level is protected by the strong transverse-alar ligaments that run from the transverse process of L5 to the sacral ala and also because the lumbosacral junction usually lies below the iliac crest and is additionally protected from motion. Other lumbar levels have more motion segments above and below to disperse stress. With degeneration at the disk and facet joints occurring at a somewhat greater rate, narrowing of the disk can occur. Because of the configuration of the facet joints and the lumbar lordosis, this results in some slippage forward of the vertebral body upon the one below. Note that without surgical removal of the posterior elements, degenerative spondylolisthesis rarely reaches the severity seen in severe isthmic spondylolisthesis.

The narrowing at the disk level can lead to increased stresses at the facet joints, with resultant degenerative facet disease, including joint narrowing and hypertrophy of the facets. As this cycle continues, the hypertrophied facets and the redundant ligamentum flavum can result in spinal stenosis. The forward displacement of one vertebra upon the other can further narrow the canal.

Most patients with degenerative spondylolisthesis demonstrate symptoms of spinal stenosis with dysesthesias or leg pain. The spinal stenosis pattern of pain when walking beyond a well-defined distance (neurogenic claudication) is often present, relieved only by sitting down or bending over.

If degenerative spondylolisthesis is refractory to conservative measures (described earlier for isthmic spondylolisthesis), surgery may be indicated. Surgical intervention should consist of decompression. Fusion enhances surgical results after decompression for degenerative spondylolisthesis. Instrumentation such as pedicle screws may enhance fusion rates and prevent further slippage during the postdecompression period before the fusion consolidates.

Boden SD et al: Orientation of the lumbar facet joints: Association with degenerative disc disease. J Bone Joint Surg Am 1996;78:403. [PMID: 8613448]

Fischgrund JS et al: Degenerative lumbar spondylolisthesis with spinal stenosis: A prospective randomized study comparing decompressive laminectomy and arthrodesis with and without spinal instrumentation. Spine 1997; 22:2807. [PMID: 9431616]

Herkowitz HN: Spine update. Degenerative spondylolisthesis. Spine 1995;20:1084. [PMID: 7631240]

Kuntz KM, Snider RK, Weinstein JN et al: Cost-effectiveness of fusion with and without instrumentation for patients with degenerative spondylolisthesis and spinal stenosis. Spine 2000;25:1132. [PMID: 10788859]

Nork SE et al: Patient outcomes after decompression and instrumented posterior spinal fusion for degenerative spondylolisthesis. Spine 1999;24:561. [PMID: 10101820]

Sengupta DK, Herkowitz HN: Degenerative spondylolisthesis: Review of current trends and controversies. Spine 2005;30:S71. [PMID 15767890]

3. Thoracic Disk Disease

Disk herniation is found much less commonly in the thoracic spine than in the cervical and lumbar spine, presumably because of the decreased mobility seen in this region with the rib cage and sternum. Herniated thoracic disks account for 1–2% of operative disks, although the reported incidence in autopsy series is 7–15%.

Patients with thoracic disk disease may present with radicular symptoms at the level of involvement and complain of back or lower extremity pain, extremity weakness, numbness corresponding to the level of the disk herniation or below, and bowel or bladder dysfunction. They may demonstrate a spastic gait, with long-tract signs, if the disk is more central. Diagnosis is made by myelography, sometimes in conjunction with CT scanning or MRI.

In the absence of long-tract signs and paraparesis, conservative measures may include rest, antiinflammatory medications, and physical therapy, with a 70–80% success rate.

Surgical treatment is recommended for patients with signs of myelopathy, including paraparesis or hyperreflexia. Decompression is most safely performed via an anterior approach. The anterior extrapleural approach is advocated and yields good results.

When an anterior approach is used, 58–86% of patients show neurologic improvement and 72–87% experience pain relief. Neurologic deterioration is reported in up to 7% of patients who undergo surgery via an anterior or anterolateral approach and in 28–100% of patients who undergo posterior decompression. Posterior laminectomies are associated with a high rate of complications, including worsening neurologic function from manipulation of the cord and incomplete decompression of an inadequately visualized disk.

Bohlman H, Zdeblick T: Anterior excision of herniated thoracic discs. J Bone Joint Surg Am 1988;70:1038. [PMID: 3403572]

Brown CW et al: The natural history of thoracic disc herniation. Spine 1992;17:97. [PMID: 1631725]

Levi N, Gjerris F, Dons K: Thoracic disc herniation. Unilateral transpedicular approach in 35 consecutive patients. J Neurosurg Sci 1999;43:37. [PMID: 10494664]

Otani K et al: Thoracic disc herniation. Spine 1988;13:1262. [PMID: 3206285]

Regan JJ et al: A technical report on video-assisted thoracoscopy in thoracic spinal surgery. Spine 1995;20:831. [PMID: 7701398]

Vanichkachorn JS, Vaccaro AR: Thoracic disk disease: Diagnosis and treatment. J Am Acad Orthop Surg 2000;8:159. [PMID: 10874223]

Wood KB et al: Thoracic discography in healthy individuals. A controlled prospective study of magnetic resonance imaging and discography in asymptomatic and symptomatic individuals. Spine 1999;24:1548. [PMID: 10457574]

INJURIES OF THE CERVICAL SPINE

The cervical spine is the most mobile area of the spine, and as such it is prone to the greatest number of injuries. Injuries to the cervical spine and spinal cord are also potentially the most devastating and life altering of all injuries compatible with life. In the United States, approximately 10,000 spinal cord injuries occur each year. An estimated 80% of the victims are younger than 40 years, with the highest proportion of injuries reported in those between 15 and 35 years of age. Approximately 80% of all people who suffer from spinal column injuries are male. Falls account for 60% of injuries to the vertebral column in patients older than 75 years. In younger patients, 45% of injuries result from motor vehicle accidents, 20% from falls, 15% from sports injuries, 15% from acts of violence, and the remainder from other causes.

With the use of seat belts and air bags in motor vehicles and the advent of trauma centers and improved emergency service awareness of potential cervical injuries, fewer patients with cervical spine injuries are dying secondary to respiratory complications. The approach in treating these patients is early recognition of cervical spine injuries with rapid immobilization to prevent neurologic deterioration while the evaluation and treatment of associated injuries are carried out. After the patient is stabilized, the goals are restoration and maintenance of spinal alignment to provide stable weight bearing and facilitate rehabilitation.

Identification & Stabilization of Life-Threatening Injuries

Eighty-five percent of all neck injuries requiring medical evaluation are a result of a motor vehicle accident. Many of the affected patients are multiple-trauma victims and therefore may have more urgent life-threatening conditions. The ABCs of trauma are followed in order of priority, with *a*irway, *b*reathing (ventilation), and *c*irculation secured before further evaluation proceeds. Throughout the evaluation of other body systems, the cervical spine should be presumed injured and thus immobilized. Approximately 20% of patients with cervical trauma are hypotensive upon presentation. The hypotension is neurogenic in origin in approximately 70% of cases and related to hypovolemia in 30%. Concomitant bradycardia is suggestive of a neurogenic component. Another finding suggestive of cervical spine injury is an altered sensorium secondary to head trauma or lacerations and facial fractures. Appropriate diagnosis and fluid management are critical in the early hours of postinjury management. After all life-threatening injuries are identified and stabilized, the secondary evaluation, including an extremity examination and neurologic examination, can be safely carried out.

History & General Physical Examination

Details of the history of the injury should be obtained. If the patient is conscious, much of the information can be obtained directly. If not, family members or witnesses of the injury should be questioned. In the case of a motor vehicle accident, for example, pertinent questions include the following: Which part of the patient's body was the point of impact? Was the patient thrown from the car? Was there head trauma or a loss of consciousness? Were there any transient signs of paresis? Was the patient able to move any of his or her extremities at any time following the accident and before loss of function? What were the speeds of the involved motor vehicles? Was the patient restrained with a seat belt? Did an air bag deploy?

The history taken from the patient or family members should also include information about preexisting conditions such as epilepsy or seizures and about preexisting injuries. If the patient had any previous radiographic examinations, the radiographs might be useful for comparison.

It is helpful to question patients about what they are experiencing at the time of the examination. Are there areas of numbness, paresthesia, or pain? Can they move their extremities? The examiner should then proceed with the physical evaluation, beginning by observing the face and head of the patient for any areas of potential injury and attempting to determine the potential mechanism of injury. For instance, any lacerations or contusions to the forehead might indicate a hyperextension type injury. Observation should next include watching the extremities for any signs of motion. A genital examination should be performed because a sustained penile erection may be indicative of severe spinal cord injury. Then without moving the patient, palpation can be performed. Although palpation can be helpful in identifying potential levels of injury of the spine, it should not be used as the sole screening examination because false-negative results are possible.

Neurologic Evaluation

A meticulous neurologic examination should be performed following the history and general physical examination.

A. NEUROLOGIC TESTS

The neurologic evaluation should start with documentation of the function of the cranial nerves, working proximally to distally. Observation is particularly important in the unconscious patient. Spontaneous motion in an extremity may be a sole source of information regarding spinal cord function. Respiratory efforts made with intrathoracic musculature versus abdominal musculature are also significant. In the conscious patient who is able to follow commands, a motor examination should be fairly straightforward. Rectal and perirectal sensations should be documented because these may be the sole signs for distal spinal cord function.

An extensive sensory examination should also be performed with careful attention to dermatomal innervation. In the acute setting, it is useful to document sharp and dull sensations as well as proprioception. Sharp and dull sensations are carried via the lateral spinothalamic tract, whereas proprioception is carried through the posterior columns. Sharp and dull sensations are effectively tested with the sharp and blunt ends of a pen, and proprioception is tested by having the patient verify the position of the large toe and other joints as the examiner places them in dorsiflexion and plantarflexion. It proves helpful to make ink markings directly on the patient's skin to show the level of the dermatomal deficit, which decreases the chance for intraobserver or interobserver error over sequential examinations.

Reflexes should be checked bilaterally. In the upper extremity, the biceps reflex at the flexor side of the elbow evaluates the C5 nerve root, and the brachioradialis stretch reflex at the radial aspect of the forearm just proximal to the wrist checks the C6 nerve root. The triceps reflex is innervated by C7. In the lower extremity, the knee jerk reflex is innervated by L4, and the ankle jerk is innervated by S1.

The presence or absence of the four reflexes listed in Table 5–2 should be checked. The Babinski reflex (plan-

Table 5–2. Evaluation of reflexes in patients with injuries of the cervical spine.

Reflex	Root	Positive Response	Significance
Babinski	Upper motor neurons	Extension and spread of toes	Upper motor neuron lesion is present
Bulbocavernosus	S3 and S4	Contraction of anal sphincter	Spinal shock is over
Cremasteric	T12 and L1	Retraction of scrotal sac	Spinal shock is over
Anal wink	S2, S3, and S4	Contraction of anal sphincter	Spinal shock is over

tar reflex) is evaluated by firmly stroking the lateral plantar aspect of the foot distally and then medially over the metatarsal heads and then observing the toes. If the toes flex, the response is considered negative (normal). If the toes extend and spread, the response is considered positive (abnormal) and indicative of an upper motor neuron lesion. The bulbocavernosus reflex has its root in the S3 and S4 nerves and is evaluated by squeezing on the glans in a male patient or applying pressure to the clitoris in a female patient. This action should elicit a contraction of the anal sphincter. If a Foley catheter is in place, simply pulling on the Foley catheter can stimulate the anal sphincter contraction. The cremasteric reflex is evaluated by stroking the inner thigh and observing the scrotal sac, which should retract upward secondary to contraction of the cremasteric muscle. This function is innervated by T12 and L1. Finally, the anal wink, innervated by S2, S3, and S4, is elicited by stimulating the skin about the anal sphincter and eliciting a contraction.

The presence of spinal shock causes the absence of all reflexes and typically lasts up to 24 h after the injury. The bulbocavernosus reflex is the reflex that returns first (see Table 5–2), thus marking the end of spinal shock. This point has prognostic importance because recovery from a complete neurologic deficit that is still present at the end of spinal shock is extremely unlikely. A complete neurologic examination should be repeated over time as the patient is manipulated and treated.

B. ANATOMIC CONSIDERATIONS

The ability to interpret the results of a patient's neurologic examination appropriately depends on a thorough knowledge of the anatomy of the spinal cord and peripheral nerves.

Peripheral nerves are a combination of afferent fibers, which carry information from the periphery to the central nervous system, and efferent fibers, which carry information away from the central nervous system. As the peripheral nerve approaches the spinal cord, it becomes known as the spinal nerve. Proximal to the spinal cord, the fiber splits, with the afferent fibers becoming the dorsal root or sensory root and the efferent fibers becoming the ventral root. The afferent fibers are often regrouped in various plexuses that are located between the spinal cord and the periphery. This regrouping takes place before the fibers enter the dorsal root, therefore leading to significant overlap between the dorsal root and the respective dermatomes. The implications of this anatomic fact should be kept in mind by the clinician when performing a sensory examination. For example, a sectioned peripheral nerve is demonstrated by a highly specific sensory loss in that particular dermatome, whereas the clinical findings are more variable for a sectioned dorsal root.

The spinal cord is a caudal continuation of the brain, extending in an organized fashion from the foramen magnum at the base of the skull down to the proximal lumbar spine. The spinal cord has three primary functions: It provides a relay point for sensory information; it serves as a conduit for ascending sensory information and descending motor information; and it mediates body and limb movements because it contains both interneurons and motor neurons. Headed from caudal to rostral, the spinal cord is highly organized with a central butterfly-shaped area of gray matter and surrounding white matter.

The overall diameter of the spinal cord varies as a relative percentage of the spinal canal. The cord fills approximately 35% of the canal at the level of the atlas but increases to approximately 50% of the canal in the lower cervical spine. This variation results from the relative increasing and decreasing size of the spinal gray matter and spinal white matter. As the spinal roots become larger, as occurs at the base of the cervical spine, the size of the gray matter increases relative to the white matter, whereas the size of the white matter decreases linearly from cephalad to caudal.

The gray matter, so called because it appears gray on unstained cross sections, is divided into three zones: the dorsal horn, the intermediate zone, and the ventral horn. Made up predominantly of lower motor neurons, it is prominent in the cervical swellings and lumbar swellings, where axons concentrate before exiting to innervate the upper extremities and lower extremities, respectively.

The white matter derives its name from the fact that the axons in this area are myelinated, casting a white hue on unstained sections. White matter is functionally and anatomically divided into three bilaterally paired columns: the ventral columns, the lateral columns, and the dorsal columns.

The two major ascending systems that relay somatic sensory information are the dorsal columns and the anterolateral system. The ascending axon has its cell body located in the dorsal root ganglion before proceeding without synapsing through the dorsal horn at that level and then ascending along the dorsal column before synapsing at the approximate level of the medulla and crossing over to the contralateral side before proceeding to the cerebral cortex. The topography of the dorsal column is such that the sacrum and lower extremities are medial, with the trunk and cervical region being lateral. The anterolateral system carries pain and temperature sensorium. The afferent fibers have a cell body in the dorsal root ganglion and then synapse at that given level in the dorsal horn before crossing directly to the contralateral side and traveling up the spinothalamic tract.

Motor pathways originate in the cerebral cortex and travel distally to the contralateral side approximately at the level of the medulla and travel down the lateral corticospinal tract before synapsing with the lower motor neuron in the ventral horn of the gray matter. The topography of the corticospinal tract is such that the sacrum and legs lie lateral to the trunk and cervical axons. Thus, at the level of the cervical spine, the spinal cord contains both lower motor neurons traversing to the upper extremities and upper motor neurons being transmitted to the lower extremities. Therefore, injury in this area can give both upper and lower motor findings.

The anatomy of the reflex arc and especially its relationship to spinal shock should be kept in mind. The basic reflex circuitry is an afferent nerve coming from a stretch receptor through the dorsal horn of gray matter before synapsing with the lower motor neuron in the ventral horn of the gray matter, which sends a positive signal to the same muscle via an alpha motor neuron. This simple arc, however, is modulated by input from higher centers. If all descending influence is interrupted, such as would occur in a traumatic transection of the spinal cord, all reflexes are lost. This is also seen during spinal shock. If the local circuitry of the reflex arc is not disturbed, reflexes return at the end of spinal shock. The earliest reflex to return is the bulbocavernosus reflex, which typically returns within 24 hours of injury. Peripheral reflexes may take several months before they return.

C. RISK OF NEUROLOGIC DAMAGE

As mentioned earlier, the spinal cord varies in its diameter from cephalad to caudad. In the upper cervical spine, it occupies approximately a third of the spinal canal. In the lower cervical spine, it occupies approximately half of the canal. As inferred from this anatomy, the risk of neurologic damage from injury is greater in the lower cervical spine.

Cord compromise extends from two causes: mechanical destruction resulting directly from the trauma and vascular insufficiency. With vascular insufficiency, hypoxia and edema follow and result in further tissue damage. By approximately 6 hours after the trauma, axonal transport ends, and by 24 hours, cord necrosis begins.

D. CLASSIFICATION OF NEUROLOGIC STATUS

1. Intact—Approximately 60% of injuries to the cervical spine result in no neurologic sequelae. In most of these cases, the injuries are in the upper cervical spine, where the ratio of the spinal cord to the spinal canal is smaller. It is obviously critical to identify unstable injuries of the cervical spine in the intact patient because the evolution of neurologic deficits is both potentially catastrophic and preventable.

2. Nerve root injuries—Eight cervical nerve roots correspond to the seven cervical vertebral bodies. Each of the first seven nerve roots exits above its respective body (the C1 nerve exiting above the C1 vertebral body, the C2 nerve exiting above the C2 body, and so

forth), whereas the C8 nerve root exits through the foramen between the C7 and T1 vertebral bodies. Nerve root injuries can happen either in isolation or in conjunction with more severe spinal cord injuries. Injury to the nerve root alone may result from a compression or fracture of the lateral bone mass and thus impingement on the neural foramen. The clinical findings of a root injury would be those of a lower motor neuron lesion. If the nerve root is still intact and the ongoing pressure to the root is removed, the prognosis for recovery of nerve root function is good.

3. Incomplete versus complete neurologic injury—In the acute setting, any evidence of neurologic function distal to the level of injury is significant and defines the lesion as being incomplete rather than complete. As Lucas and Ducker reported in a prospective study published in 1979, "The less the injury, the greater the recovery," and "partial lesions partially recover, whereas complete lesions do not."

According to the Frankel system, which is the most widely used system for classifying sensory and motor deficits in patients with spinal cord lesions, there are five categories of injury: (A) sensory function absent, motor function absent (complete injury); (B) sensation present, motor absent; (C) sensation present, motor active but not useful; (D) sensation present, motor active and useful; and (E) normal sensory function, normal motor function.

In the acutely injured spinal cord patient, the documentation of sacral nerve root function by testing perianal sensation, rectal tone, and flexion of the great toe is critically important. Intact sacral function may be the only sign of an at least partially functioning spinal cord. In contrast, the absence of sacral function may be the only finding on physical examination in patients with an injury to the conus medullaris or cauda equina at the distal spinal column. Because these patients can move their lower extremities, a cursory examination might easily miss these significant deficits.

E. CLINICAL FEATURES OF SPINAL CORD SYNDROMES

Combining the findings on examination with knowledge of the cross-sectional anatomy of the spinal cord allows the examiner to identify specific injury patterns (Figure 5–35).

1. Central cord syndrome—The most common of the incomplete cord syndromes is the central cord syndrome, which occurs most frequently in elderly (more than 65 years) people with underlying degenerative spondylosis but can also be found in younger people who have had a severe hyperextension injury with or without evidence of a fracture. Central cord syndrome is defined by the American Spinal Injury Association (ASIA) as a clinical presentation characterized by "dissociation in degree of motor weakness with lower limbs

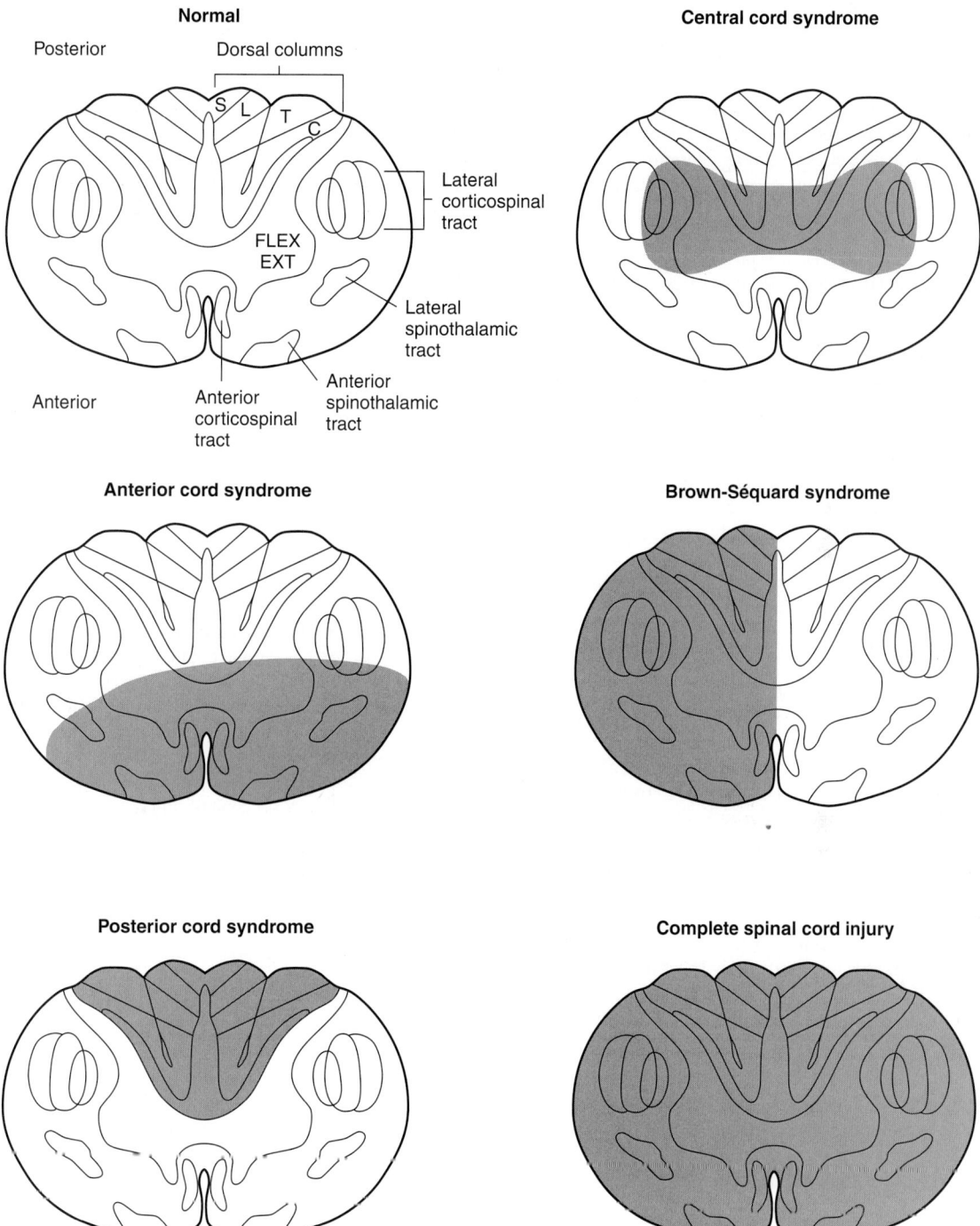

Figure 5–35. Diagrams illustrating cross-sectional views of the normal and injured spinal cord. The diagram of the normal spinal column shows the segmental arrangement (S = sacral, L = lumbar, T = thoracic, and C = cervical) and the area of flexors and extensors (FLEX and EXT). Central cord syndrome, anterior cord syndrome, Brown-Séquard syndrome, and posterior cord syndrome are incomplete injuries, with affected areas shaded. In complete spinal cord injury, all areas are affected.

stronger than upper limbs and sacral sensory sparing." The syndrome typically occurs following a hyperextension injury and is thought to be caused by an expanding hematoma or edema forming in the central aspect of the spinal cord. Central cord syndrome can be quite variable in presentation and in recovery. A mild presentation may consist of a slight burning sensation in the upper extremities, whereas a severe central cord syndrome includes motor impairment in both the upper and lower extremities, bladder dysfunction, and a variable sensory deficit below the level of injury. The pattern of clinical presentation is directly related to the cross-sectional anatomy of the spinal cord. Because the lower extremity and sacral tracts of the spinothalamic and corticospinal tracts are lateral, these areas are often spared in central cord syndrome. In cases in which they are involved, they are the areas whose function returns first. The upper extremity deficit is caused by a lesion in the gray matter, and the damage here is largely irreversible.

From 50% to 75% of patients with central cord lesions show some neurologic improvement, but the amount of improvement varies considerably among patients. The usual order in which motor function recovery occurs is as follows: return of lower extremity strength, return of bladder function, return of upper extremity strength, and return of intrinsic function of the hand.

2. Anterior cord syndrome—The patient with an anterior cord syndrome typically presents with immediate paralysis and loss of pain and temperature sensation. Both the spinothalamic and corticospinal tracts are located in the anterior aspect of the spinal cord and therefore involved. With the dorsal columns preserved, the patient still has intact proprioception and vibratory sense as well as intact sensation to deep pressure. This clinical presentation is the most common in the younger (less than 35 years) trauma victim. The mechanism of injury is typically a flexion injury to the cervical spine. It is usually associated with an identifiable lesion of the cervical spine, most commonly a vertebral body burst fracture or a herniated disk. Return of useful motor function is reported in only 10–16% of patients with anterior cord syndrome. The prognosis is slightly improved, however, if evidence of spinothalamic tract function is present early.

3. Brown-Séquard syndrome—Patients with this syndrome have a motor weakness on the ipsilateral side of the lesion and a sensory deficit on the contralateral side caused by a functional hemisection of the spinal cord. For example, a cervical lesion on the right side of the spinal cord disrupts the ipsilateral corticospinal tract, which is the tract that carries motor function to the right side of the body distal to the level of the lesion. The right spinothalamic tract is also disrupted. This tract carries pain and temperature fibers from the contralateral side of the body distal to the level of injury. Position sense and vibratory

sense, which are carried in the posterior column, have not yet crossed the midline; therefore, these sensory functions are disrupted on the ipsilateral side of the injury.

Brown-Séquard syndrome may result from a closed rotational injury such as a fracture-dislocation or may result from a penetrating trauma such as a stab wound. The prognosis in cases resulting from a closed injury is quite favorable, with 90% of patients regaining function of the bowel and bladder as well as the ability to walk.

4. Posterior cord syndrome—The posterior cord syndrome is the least common of the incomplete syndromes and typically a result of an extension type injury. Its clinical presentation is one of loss of position and vibratory sense below the level of injury secondary to disruption of the dorsal columns. With these deficits as isolated findings, the prognosis for recovery of ambulation and function of the bowel and bladder is excellent.

5. Complete spinal cord injury—A complete neurologic deficit is characterized by a total absence of sensation and voluntary motor function caudal to the level of spinal cord injury in the absence of spinal shock. Initial evaluation must rule out any evidence of sacral sparing and the presence of a bulbocavernosus reflex. In the absence of sacral sparing and with the return of the bulbocavernosus reflex, which typically occurs within 24 hours, the spinal cord injury is termed complete and there is virtually no likelihood of functional spinal cord recovery. Affected patients may gain some root function about the level of the injury—a phenomenon called root escape because this damage to nerve roots is a peripheral nerve injury. Although the presence of root escape should not be taken as a potential return of spinal cord function, it can significantly improve the patient's rehabilitation efforts because vital function of the upper extremities may be regained.

Imaging Studies

A. RADIOGRAPHY

1. Screening radiograph—A lateral radiograph of the cervical spine may be the only screening tool obtained upon initial radiographic evaluation of the multiple-trauma patient. This radiograph must be carefully reviewed. Should a patient present with a complete neurologic injury or a densely affected incomplete neurologic injury indicating a traumatically malaligned cervical spine, closed reduction of the cervical spine should be urgently attempted with axial traction through Gardner-Wells tongs. Once the patient is fully evaluated and life-threatening injuries are stabilized, secondary diagnostic studies can then be undertaken. If the patient is fully alert, has full pain-free rotational range of motion, no palpable tenderness, and no other injuries, the cervical spine can be cleared on clinical grounds.

2. Subsequent plain radiographs—Full radiographic evaluation of the cervical spine with plain radiographs includes lateral, AP, open-mouth (odontoid), right oblique, and left oblique views. The lateral radiograph, if adequate, visualized approximately 85% of significant cervical spine injuries. It must display the base of the skull with all seven cervical vertebrae, as well as the proximal half of the T1 vertebral body. If the C7-T1 junction is not visualized, a repeat radiograph should be done with axial traction on the upper extremities caudally to attempt to visualize the C7-T1 junction. If this is unsuccessful, a swimmer's view, which is a transthoracic lateral with the patient's arm fully abducted, should be taken. If this plain radiograph is not satisfactory and if suspicion of injury is still high, a CT scan must be obtained.

When evaluating a lateral cervical spine radiograph, the clinician should first evaluate the bony anatomy. Four lines or curves should be kept in mind (Figure 5–36). The anterior spinal line and the posterior spinal line are imaginary lines drawn from the anterior cortex and posterior cortex, respectively, of the cervical vertebral body from C2 all the way down to T1. The spinal laminar curve is an imaginary line drawn from the posterior aspect of the foramen magnum connecting the anterior cortex of each successive spinous process. These three lines (labeled A, B, and C in Figure 5–36) should have a gentle, continuous lordotic curve with no areas of acute angulation. The fourth line (labeled D in Figure 5–36) is known as the basilar line of Wackenheim, and it is drawn along the posterior surface of the clivus and should thus be tangent to the posterior cortex of the tip of the odontoid process. After the clinician examines the radiograph in terms of these four lines or curves, he or she should look at the individual vertebral bodies to see if there is loss of height of any of them or if a rotational deformity is present with alterations in the alignment of the facets.

The evaluation of soft tissues can also prove valuable diagnostically. Prevertebral soft tissues have an upper limit of normal width beyond which a prevertebral hematoma indicative of vertebral injury can be suspected. The upper ends of normal are 11 mm at C1, 6 mm at C2, 7 mm at C3, and 8 mm at C4. The measurements below C4 become more variable and therefore less reliable clinically.

The AP view of the cervical spine is at first a confusing projection to those who are unfamiliar with cervical anatomy, yet careful attention to bony detail in the AP view can be of significant diagnostic aid in picking up subtle injuries. The bony and soft-tissue anatomy seen on the AP projection should be symmetric. The spinous processes should be equally spaced because a single level of increased intraspinous process distance suggests posterior instability. Abrupt malalignment of the spinous processes suggests a rotatory injury such as a unilateral facet dislocation. After checking for these problems, the

Figure 5–36. Diagram illustrating normal lines and curves in the bony anatomy of the cervical spine. The anterior spinal line (line A), the posterior spinal line (line B), and the spinal laminar curve (line C) should have a gentle, continuous lordotic curve. The basilar line of Wackenheim (line D) is drawn along the posterior surface of the clivus and should thus be tangent to the posterior cortex of the tip of the odontoid process. (Reproduced, with permission, from El-Khoury GY, Kathol MH: Radiographic evaluation of cervical spine trauma. Semin Spine Surg 1991;3:3.)

clinician should inspect the lateral masses. The facet joints are typically angled away from the vertical and therefore not clearly seen on the AP projection. If, however, the facet joint can be seen at a particular level, this is indicative of a fracture through the lateral masses and a rotational malalignment of the facet.

The open-mouth (odontoid) view is the projection most useful for looking at C1-C2 anatomy. It permits visualization of both the dens in the AP plane, and the lateral masses of C1 on C2.

The right and left oblique views can be taken of the cervical spine with the patient in the supine position. These views are useful as confirmatory studies in ruling in or out lateral mass injuries.

3. Stress radiographs—Two techniques are used in obtaining cervical stress radiographs. The first is to apply axial distraction to the cervical spine through a halo or traction device and obtain a lateral radiograph. This technique should be carefully performed in the presence of a physician and only after gross instabilities of the cervical spine are ruled out. Serial lateral radiographs are taken as weight is sequentially added, reaching an amount equivalent to approximately a third of body weight or 30 kg, depending on the level of suspected injury. Occult instability can be inferred by noting an interspace angulation of at least 11 degrees or an interspace separation of at least 1.7 mm (Figure 5–37).

The second technique, which should only be performed in a fully alert and cooperative patient, is used to obtain flexion-extension lateral radiographs that are helpful in the diagnosis of late instability. The technique is to have the patient flex the head forward as far as possible while a lateral radiograph is taken and then to have the patient put the head in full extension while another radiograph is taken. Findings presumptive of instability are facet subluxation, forward subluxation of 3.5 cm of one vertebral body on the next, and interbody angulation of greater than 11 degrees.

A   B

Figure 5–37. **A:** Diagram illustrating an increase of the C2-C3 interdisk space in a patient with type IIA traumatic spondylolisthesis. **B:** Radiograph demonstrating an increased space. (Reproduced, with permission, from Levine AM, Rhyne AL: Traumatic spondylolisthesis of the axis. Semin Spine Surg 1991;3:47.)

B. COMPUTED TOMOGRAPHY

CT scanning is the most useful means for definitive delineation of bony fracture anatomy. Its advantages are its ready availability and its ability to be performed with a minimal amount of patient manipulation. CT scans provide excellent axial detail, and if the sections are taken with close enough cuts, the computer can reconstruct images in sagittal, coronal, or oblique planes. CT scans can now even be reformatted into a three-dimensional construct for excellent visualization of the bony anatomy.

C. MAGNETIC RESONANCE IMAGING

MRI is the most effective way to evaluate the soft-tissue component of cervical trauma. The major advantage of MRI is that it can visualize occult disk herniation, hematoma, or edema about the spinal cord, as well as ligamentous injury. Current disadvantages are that MRI is disrupted by metallic objects, so these should be removed from the area of examination, and it also requires a prolonged amount of time to perform, therefore making close monitoring of the acutely ill patient difficult.

Diagnostic Checklist of Spinal Instability

The concept of spinal stability is central to the understanding and treatment of cervical spine injuries. In a broad sense, patients with injuries that are deemed unstable require surgical intervention, whereas those deemed to have stable injury patterns can be treated nonoperatively. Spinal injuries, however, are not readily divided into unstable and stable injuries, and in actuality they fall along a spectrum of spinal instability.

White and Panjabi's diagnostic checklist of spinal instability (Table 5–3) has nine categories, each of which

is assigned a point value. If a total of 5 points is present in a given patient, the injury is deemed unstable.

Holdsworth's two-column theory of spine stability, as well as Denis's three-column theory, proposed for application to the thoracolumbar spine, are also applied to the cervical spine in an attempt to better predict stability in the neck.

General Principles of Managing Acute Injuries of the Cervical Spine

Management of acute cervical spine injury is predicated on two principles: protection of the uninjured spinal cord and prevention of further damage to the injured spinal cord. This is accomplished by following spine precaution principles from the very onset of medical care, starting at the accident scene. The cervical spine should be considered injured until proven otherwise and securely immobilized before the patient is transported to a medical center. The equipment for initial immobilization should not be removed until the definitive means of immobilization can be put in place or the cervical spine is cleared of injury. Use of a spinal board, with the patient's head taped to the board and held between two sandbags, is the most secure form of immobilization readily available in the field. This technique can be supplemented by a Philadelphia collar. When the medical center is reached, if a definitive cervical spine injury is identified and deemed unstable, skeletal traction for immobilization, reduction, or both may be applied. Gardner-Wells traction is easily applied and adequate for axial traction. Halo traction affords the added advantage of four-point fixation and thus controlled traction in three planes. Halo traction can also be easily converted at a later time to halo-vest immobilization.

Table 5–3. White and Panjabi's diagnostic checklist of spinal instability.

Checklist Category	Description	Point Value[a]
1	Disruption of the anterior elements, with greater than 25% loss of height	2
2	Disruption of the posterior elements	2
3	Sagittal plane translation of greater than 3.5 mm or greater than 20% of the antero-posterior diameter of the vertebral body	2
4	Intervertebral sagittal rotation of greater than 11 degrees	2
5	Intervertebral distance of greater than 1.7 mm on a stretch test	2
6	Evidence of cord damage	2
7	Evidence of root damage	1
8	Acute intervertebral disk space narrowing	1
9	Anticipated abnormally large stress	1

[a]If a total of 5 points is present in a given patient, the injury is deemed unstable.

Modified and reproduced, with permission, from White AA III, Panjabi MM: Update on the evaluation of instability of the lower cervical spine. Instr Course Lect 1987;36:513.

Among the various agents that show potential benefits in laboratory studies of models of spinal cord injury are corticosteroids, opiate receptor antagonists (such as naloxone or thyrotropin-releasing hormone), and diuretics (such as mannitol). The National Acute Spinal Cord Injury Studies (NASCIS) II and III reported neurologic improvement with steroid treatment given within 8 hours of injury. Those treated within 3 hours did best; those treated between hours 3 and 8 only did better by extending to 48 hours of treatment. Criticism of the NASCIS studies called to question the validity of the conclusions, and many professional organizations downgraded their enthusiasm for the use of methylprednisolone in the patient with the acutely injured spinal cord. However, many hospitals still use the protocol in blunt trauma cord injuries if the medicine can be administered within 3 hours of the injury. The recommended dosage of methylprednisolone in an acute setting is 30 mg/kg given as a bolus and followed by 5.4 mg/kg/h for 24 hours. However, some thought should be given to its use because, for example, the Congress of Neurological Surgeons stated that steroid therapy "should only be undertaken with the knowledge that the evidence suggesting harmful side effects is more consistent than any suggestion of clinical benefit."

Bracken MB et al: Administration of methylprednisolone for 24 or 48 hours or tirilazad mesylate for 48 hours in the treatment of acute spinal cord injury; Results of the Third National Acute Spinal Cord Injury Randomized Control Trial. JAMA 1997;277:1597.

Denis F: The three-column spine and its significance in the classification of acute thoracolumbar spinal injuries. Spine 1983; 8:817.

Nesathurai S: Steroids and spinal cord injury: revisiting the NASCIS 2 and NASCIS 3 trials. J Trauma 1998;45(6):1088.

White AA III, Panjabi MM: Update on the evaluation of instability of the lower cervical spine. Instr Course Lect 1987;36:513.

INJURIES OF THE UPPER CERVICAL SPINE

With the exception of occipitoatlantal dissociation, traumatic injuries to the upper cervical spine are less frequently associated with significant neurologic injury than are traumatic injuries to the lower cervical spine. This is secondary to the fact that the spinal cord occupies only a third of the upper spinal canal versus a half of the lower spinal canal.

Occipitoatlantal Dissociation

Occipitoatlantal dissociation is a disruption of the cranial vertebral junction, and it implies a subluxation or complete dislocation of the occipitoatlantal facets. This injury is typically fatal, yet the clinician must be aware of it because unrecognized occipitoatlantal dissociation may

have catastrophic results. The mechanism of dissociation is poorly understood, but it most likely results from either a severe flexion or distraction type of injury. Anterior translation of the skull on the vertebral column is a common presentation and most likely a hyperflexion injury. Bucholz, however, presented the pathologic anatomic findings of fatal occipitoatlantal dissociation and proposed a mechanism of hyperextension with resultant distractive force applied across the craniovertebral junction.

When the dissociation is a frank dislocation, the findings are clear on a lateral radiograph. When the dissociation is a subluxation, however, findings may be more subtle. In normal individuals, the distance between the tip of the dens and the basion (the anterior aspect of the foramen magnum) should be no greater than 1.0 cm, and the previously described Wackenheim line should run from the base of the basion tangentially to the tip of the dens. If the dens penetrates this line, anterior translation of the cranium is implied. Calculation of the Powers ratio can also be helpful in securing the diagnosis. Powers and his colleagues described a ratio of two lines (Figure 5–38), the first of which runs from the tip of the basion to the midpoint of the posterior lamina of the atlas (line BC) and the second of which runs from the anterior arch of C1 to the opisthion (line AO). When the ratio of BC to AO is greater than 1:1, anterior occipitoatlantal dissocia-

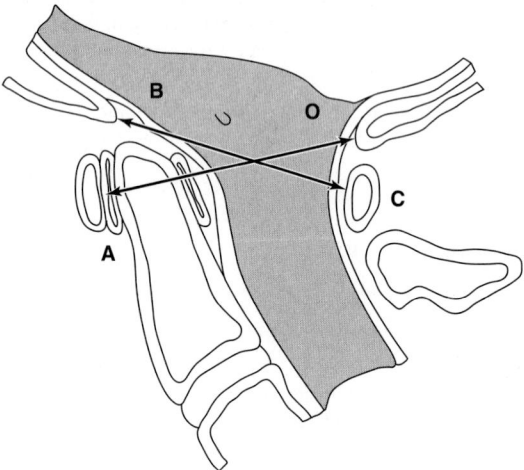

Figure 5–38. Diagram showing lines used in the calculation of the Powers ratio, which is helpful in diagnosing occipitoatlantal dissociation. The distance between the basion (point B) and the posterior arch (point C) is divided by the distance between the anterior arch of C1 (point A) and the opisthion (point O). The normal ratio of BC to AO is 1:1. A ratio of greater than 1 suggests the head is dislocated anteriorly on the spine.

tion is present. Other radiographic signs include marked soft-tissue swelling and the presence of avulsion fractures at the occipitovertebral junction.

Early recognition and surgical stabilization are the mainstays of treatment in cases of occipitoatlantal dissociation.

Fractures of Vertebra C1 (Atlas Fractures)

The mechanism of injury in the fracture of the atlas is most typically axial compression with or without extension force, and the anatomic findings of the fracture are indicative of the specifics of the force and the position of the head at the time of impact. In 1920, Jefferson presented his classic description of the four-part fracture of the atlas following an axial injury. This fracture is a burst type that occurs secondary to the occipital condyles being driven into the interior portions of the ring of the atlas and driving the lateral masses outward, resulting in a two-part fracture of the anterior ring of the atlas as well as a two-part fracture of the posterior ring. More common than the classic four-part atlas fracture, however, are the two-part and three-part fractures. Isolated anterior arch fractures are the least common, and they are typically associated with fractures of the dens, whereas the more common posterior arch fracture is typically the result of a hyperextension injury.

A fracture of the atlas is typically diagnosed on plain radiographs. Findings may be subtle on the lateral cervical spine radiograph. The open-mouth (odontoid) view may show asymmetry of the lateral masses of C1 on C2 with overhang (Figure 5–39). A bilateral overhang totaling more than 6.9 mm is presumptive evidence of a disruption to the transverse ligament and suggests potential late instability. Presumptive evidence for transverse ligament disruption can also be seen on the lateral radiograph if the ADI is greater than 4 mm.

The treatment for fractures of the atlas as isolated injuries is typically nonoperative (Figure 5–40). If there are signs of transverse ligament disruption, halo traction is indicated with later transfer to halo-vest immobilization for a total of 3–4 months. Immediate halo-vest application is indicated in cases involving a moderately displaced fracture with lateral mass overhang up to 5 mm, although collar immobilization is preferred in cases involving a minimally displaced fracture of the atlas. At completion of bony union, flexion-extension views should be obtained to rule out any evidence of late instability. If late instability is present and the bony elements were allowed to heal, a limited C1-C2 fusion can address the instability. If a nonunion is present or if the posterior arch remains disrupted, an occiput to C2 fusion is necessary to control the late instability.

Dislocations & Subluxations of Vertebrae C1 & C2

A. ATLANTOAXIAL ROTATORY SUBLUXATION

Atlantoaxial rotatory subluxation is most common in children and may be associated with minimal trauma or even occur spontaneously. Although some patients are asymptomatic, others present with neck pain or torticollis (a position in which the head is tilted toward one side and rotated toward the other). Inasmuch as the mechanism of injury is often unclear, the propensity for the C1-C2 location is based on anatomic factors. In approximately 50% of cases, cervical spine rotation occurs at the C1-C2 junction, where the facet joints are more horizontal and less inherently stable in rotation.

The diagnosis of atlantoaxial rotatory subluxation is typically suspected on the basis of radiographs taken in several views. The odontoid view may show displacement of the lateral masses with respect to the dens; a lateral view may show an increased ADI; and the AP view may show a lateral shift of the spinous process of C1 on C2. CT scanning can be used to confirm the diagnosis, and a dynamic CT scan with full attempted right and left rotation can demonstrate a fixed deformity.

There are four types of atlantoaxial rotatory subluxations. In type I, the ADI is less than 3 mm, which suggests the transverse ligament is still intact. In type II, the interval is 3–5 mm, which suggests the transverse ligament is not structurally intact. In type III, the interval exceeds 5 mm, which is indicative of disruption of the transverse ligament as well as secondary stabilization of the alar ligament. In type IV, there is a complete posterior dislocation of the atlas on the axis, a finding typi-

Figure 5–39. Open-mouth (odontoid) radiographic view demonstrating asymmetry of the lateral masses of C1 on C2 with overhang in a patient with a Jefferson fracture. (Reproduced, with permission, from El-Khoury GY, Kathol MH: Radiographic evaluation of cervical spine trauma. Semin Spine Surg 1991:3:3.)

B

A

Figure 5–40. Imaging studies in a patient who was in a motor vehicle accident and sustained a distractive extension injury to his cervical spine and a three-part fracture of his atlas (a Jefferson fracture). **A:** Lateral radiographic view showing a fracture of the posterior arch. **B:** Axial section of a CT scan further delineating the fracture anatomy. This injury was deemed stable and treated nonoperatively in a halo vest.

cally associated with a hypoplastic odontoid process such as that seen in several forms of mucopolysaccharidosis (eg, the Morquio syndrome).

Treatment of atlantoaxial subluxation is typically conservative, consisting of traction followed by immobilization. Approximately 90% of patients respond to this treatment regimen. There is a high incidence of recurrence, however. For patients who do not respond to conservative measures and for patients with recurrent problems, C1-C2 arthrodesis may be required to control the deformity.

B. DISRUPTION OF THE TRANSVERSE LIGAMENT

The transverse ligament and secondarily the alar ligament are the main constraints to anterior displacement of C1 on C2. It was previously presumed that because anterior subluxation of C1 on C2 typically involves a fracture through the dens, the transverse ligament is in fact stronger than the bony elements of the dens. Fielding and his colleagues, however, showed that experimentally this was

not the case, yet clinically the higher association of anterior dislocation of dens fractures still holds true.

The mechanism of disruption is typically a flexion injury, and the diagnosis is made on lateral radiographs. The ADI should not exceed 3 mm in the adult. If the interval is 4 mm or larger and the dens is intact, a rupture of the transverse ligament is presumed.

High-resolution CT scan can be used to categorize this injury into two types. Type 1 is a disruption in the substance of the transverse ligament, whereas type 2 involves an avulsion fracture of the insertion of the transverse ligament on the lateral mass of C1. Type 1 injuries predictably fail conservative treatment and should be managed with a C1-C2 arthrodesis. A trial of nonoperative care in type 2 injuries using a rigid cervical orthosis may be a reasonable alternative. A 74% success rate can be anticipated, with surgery reserved for patients who fail nonoperative care, showing persistent instability after 12 weeks in mobilization.

C. FRACTURE OF THE ODONTOID PROCESS

Fracture of the odontoid process is typically associated with high-velocity trauma, and the mechanism of injury is flexion in most cases. Depending on the fracture pattern, extension may be the predominant force in a smaller subset of cases. Associated injuries, particularly fractures of the ring of the atlas, should be ruled out. Neurologic involvement is relatively rare with odontoid fractures. In a study of 60 patients with acute fractures of the odontoid process, Anderson and D'Alonzo reported that 15 had some neurologic deficit on presentation, but only 5 of the 15 had major neurologic involvement, and only 2 of this group of 5 remained quadriparetic at follow-up.

Odontoid fractures may be suspected on the basis of clinical presentation and confirmed on plain radiographs, although spasm and overlying shadows can obscure the diagnosis. CT scan with sagittal and coronal reconstruction is the most sensitive study to diagnose these injuries. CT scan with axial sectioning alone may miss the horizontal fracture line typical of these injuries; thus, the reconstructions are necessary.

Both the risk of nonunion with delayed instability and the method of treating odontoid fracture depends on the classification of the fracture. Reported rates of nonunion range from 20% to 63%. According to the classification system proposed in 1974 by Anderson and D'Alonzo, there are three types of fracture of the odontoid process (Figure 5–41).

Type I is a fracture through the tip of the odontoid process. In this configuration, the blood supply is maintained through the base of the odontoid process and through the attachment of the alar transverse ligaments. The mechanical stability of this fracture pattern is left intact. Symptomatic care and immobilization are the treatment of choice.

Type II, the most common type, is a fracture through the base of the odontoid process at its junction with the body of the axis. In this configuration, soft-tissue attachments to the fracture fragment cause distraction at the fracture site. Because the amount of cancellous bone available for opposition is limited, a high nonunion rate is expected, particularly if displacement is significant or the patient is older (more than 60 years). In this case, primary surgical treatment may be indicated. Anterior screw fixation of the odontoid process is now the treatment of choice for most type 2 odontoid fractures. Although it is technically demanding, it does allow for the maintenance of motion at C1-C2 (Figure 5–42).

Type III is a fracture through the body of the axis. The blood supply is maintained through soft-tissue attachments, and abundant cancellous bone opposition at the fracture site facilitates a high rate of union. The treatment, therefore, is conservative, consisting of halo traction or halo-vest immobilization until bony union occurs.

Figure 5–41. Diagram showing the three types of fractures of the odontoid process.

D. HANGMAN'S FRACTURE (TRAUMATIC SPONDYLOLISTHESIS OF VERTEBRA C2)

Hangman's fracture occurs when a fracture line passes through the neural arch of the axis. The anatomy of the axis is such that the superior facets are anterior and the inferior facets are posterior, thus concentrating stress through the neural arch. Because of the high ratio of spinal canal size to spinal cord size at this level, neurologic damage associated with hangman's fracture should be unusual. However, in his postmortem studies, Bucholz reported that traumatic spondylolisthesis was second only to occipitoatlantal dislocations in cervical injuries leading to fatalities.

According to the scheme proposed by Levine and Rhyne, hangman's fractures can be classified on the basis of anatomic factors and the presumed mechanism of injury. Treatment depends on the type of fracture. Imaging studies in a patient with hangman's fracture are shown in Figure 5–43.

Type I is typically caused by hyperextension with or without additional axial load. There is no angulation of the deformity, and the fracture fragments are separated by less than 3 mm. Treatment should consist of immobilization in a cervical collar or halo vest until union occurs, which is typically 12 weeks.

A

B   C

Figure 5–42. Imaging studies in a patient with a type II odontoid fracture nonunion. **A:** Open-mouth radiographic view showing the fracture line at the base of the odontoid process. **B:** Sagittal reconstruction using CT scanning to better delineate the fracture anatomy. **C:** Radiograph taken after the patient underwent anterior placement of two odontoid screws under fluoroscopic control using a cannulated screw system.

B

A

Figure 5–43. Imaging studies in a patient who was in a motor vehicle accident and sustained a hangman's fracture, or traumatic spondylolisthesis of C2. **A:** Lateral radiographic view, which is largely unremarkable. **B:** Sagittal reconstruction using CT scanning to better delineate the fracture site at the base of the posterior elements. The patient was treated nonoperatively.

Type II is thought to be caused by hyperextension and axial load with a secondary flexion component leading to displacement of the fracture. Reduction of the anterior angulation in this type of fracture is necessary and typically obtained by traction therapy and then followed by placement of a halo vest until union occurs. An atypical type II hangman's fracture is described. This fracture occurs through the posterior aspect of the vertebral body, potentially resulting in cord compromise as the anterior aspect of the vertebral body flexes forward. A higher likelihood of neurologic injury with this atypical pattern is seen, and halo-vest immobilization is recommended.

Type IIA has the same fracture pattern as type II but with a component of distraction that also occurred at the time of injury and led to disruption of the C2-C3 disk space, rendering this injury inherently unstable. Traction should be avoided in cases of type IIA fracture because it exacerbates the injury. Treatment should consist of immediate halo-vest application, with the patient's head positioned in slight extension to afford a reduction.

Type III includes a fracture through the neural arch, a facet dislocation, and a disruption of the C2-C3 disk space that renders the injury highly unstable. Treatment generally consists of early closed reduction of the

facet dislocation and application of a halo vest to maintain the reduction. If the reduction cannot be obtained in a closed fashion or cannot be maintained conservatively, treatment with open reduction of the dislocation and anterior or posterior fusion is indicated.

Anderson LD, D'Alonzo RT: Fractures of the odontoid process of the axis. J Bone Joint Surg Am 1974;56:1663.

Govender S et al: Fractures of the odontoid process. J Bone Joint Surg Br 2000;82(8):1143. [PMID: 11132275]

Powers B et al: Traumatic anterior atlanto-occipital dislocation. Neurosurgery 1979;4:12.

Vieweg U, Schultheiss R: A review of halo vest treatment of upper cervical spine injuries. Arch Orthop Trauma Surg 2001; 121(1–2):50. [PMID: 21034862]

Ziai WC, Hurlbert RJ: A six year review of odontoid fractures: The emerging role of surgical intervention. Can J Neurol Sci 2000;27(4):297. [PMID: 11097519]

INJURIES OF THE LOWER CERVICAL SPINE

As stated earlier, fractures and dislocations of the lower cervical spine have a greater frequency of catastrophic neurologic involvement because of the decreased ratio of spinal canal to spinal cord in the lower levels. Treatment of affected patients again relies on early recognition of the injury, recognition of inherent stability or instability of the injury pattern, and institution of appropriate definitive care.

In 1982, Allen and colleagues developed a classification system for closed indirect fractures and dislocations of the lower cervical spine. After reviewing numerous cases previously described by other authors as well as 165 of their own cases, they grouped the injuries into six categories, based on the position of the cervical spine at the time of impact and on the dominant mode of failure. The six categories were compressive flexion, vertical compression, distractive flexion, compressive extension, distractive extension, and lateral flexion. Of these, the distractive flexion injuries were the most common, followed by the compressive extension injuries and the compressive flexion injuries. Some of the categories were further divided into stages, as described next.

Compressive Flexion Injury

There are five stages of compressive flexion injuries, which are labeled compression flexion stage (CFS) I through V (Figure 5–44). CFS I shows a slight blunting and rounding to the anterior superior vertebral margin, without any evidence of posterior ligamentous damage. CFS II shows some additional loss of height of the anterior vertebral body, again sparing the posterior elements. CFS III has an additional fracture line passing from the anterior surface of the vertebral body through to the inferior subchondral plate, with minimal displacement. CFS IV has less than 3 mm of displacement of the inferior posterior vertebral fragment into the neural canal. CFS V has severe displacement of the inferior posterior fragment into the canal, with widening of the spinous processes posteriorly, indicative of three-column disruption.

Within the compressive flexion category are two types of fractures, more commonly referred to as the **compression fracture** and the **teardrop fracture.** Most compression fractures without disruption of the posterior elements are thought to be stable, so no surgical intervention is required. The more severe compression fracture injuries, however, can result in displacement of bone into the spinal canal, and if a neurologic injury is present, these require anterior decompression and stabilization. All patients should be carefully checked with flexion-extension views at the completion of their treatment to rule out any evidence of late instability.

Vertical Compression Injury

Vertical compression spinal (VCS) injuries occur secondary to axial loading and are divided into three stages. VCS I consists of an endplate central fracture with no evidence of ligamentous failure. VCS II is a fracture of both vertebral endplates, again with only minimal displacement. VCS III is the more commonly termed **burst fracture** with a spectrum of fragmentation of the vertebral body, with or without posterior element disruption.

The treatment for VCS injuries is typically nonoperative. Traction is applied to obtain and maintain alignment, and bony union is generally complete after 3 months of halo-vest immobilization. Flexion-extension views should be obtained at the completion of healing because a posterior ligamentous injury can result in late instability.

Distractive Flexion Injury

The category of distractive flexion spinal (DFS) injury was the most common injury category reported by Allen and colleagues, and it includes both unilateral and bilateral facet subluxation and dislocation. There are four stages of DFS injury. DFS I, termed a **flexion sprain,** is characterized by subluxation of the facet joint, with possible interspinous process widening. This injury has subtle radiographic findings and may easily be missed during initial evaluation and therefore result in late symptomatic instability (Figure 5–45). DFS II is a unilateral facet dislocation, the diagnosis of which can be confirmed on plain radiographs. The lateral radiograph would reveal an anterior subluxation of one vertebra of approximately 25% of vertebral body width at the affected level. The facet itself may be perched or fully dislocated. DFS III is a bilateral facet dislocation with approximately 50% anterior dislocation at the affected level. DFS IV, which is also termed a **floating vertebra,** is a bilateral facet dislocation with displacement of a full vertebral width.

Treatment of DFS injuries depends on the severity of the injury. Achievement of anatomic alignment and spinal stability yields the best results. Patients with unilateral facet dislocation should be treated with closed reduction in the acute phase, followed by immobilization. If closed reduction is not possible, open reduction and fusion are indicated (Figure 5–46). Bilateral facet dislocations are associated with a higher incidence of both neurologic injury and instability. Treatment consisting of closed reduction and immobilization is feasible, but because it results in a high percentage of late instability, which eventually requires posterior fusion, the use of early posterior fusion is indicated.

Another fracture pattern that should be included in the discussion on flexion injuries is the clay shoveler's fracture, which is a fracture of the spinous process, typically at level C6, C7, or T1. This is an avulsion injury that generally occurs in flexion by the counteractive forces of the muscular attachments. As an isolated injury, it is considered stable and usually treated nonoperatively.

Figure 5–44. Radiographs showing the five stages of compressive flexion injury. **A** shows CFS I. **B** shows CFS II. **C** shows CFS III. **D** shows CFS IV. **E** shows CFS V. (Reproduced, with permission, from Allen BL et al: A mechanistic classification of closed, indirect fractures and dislocations of the lower cervical spine. Spine 1982;7:1.)

A

B

Figure 5–45. Imaging studies in a patient with a distractive flexion injury of the cervical spine. **A:** This lateral radiographic view demonstrates anterior subluxation of C5 on C6. **B:** The follow-up radiograph shows progression of the subluxation. The patient was treated with a posterior spinal fusion of C5-C6.

Compressive Extension Injury

The category of compressive extension (CES) injury was the second most common injury category reported by Allen and colleagues. It is divided into five stages. CES I is a fracture of the vertebral arch unilaterally, with or without displacement, and CES II is a bilateral fracture. CES III and CES IV were not encountered in the series reported by Allen and colleagues but are theoretic interpolations between CES II and CES V. CES III is a bilateral fracture of the vertebral arch articular processes, lamina, or pedicle without vertebral displacement, whereas CES IV is the same fracture pattern but with moderate vertebral body displacement. Three patients in the Allen series had CES V injuries, which were bilateral vertebral arch fractures with 100% anterior displacement.

Treatment of CES injuries is related to the three-column theory. Stabilization with a posterior, anterior, or combined approach is indicated if there is significant disruption of the middle column or of two of the three columns.

Distractive Extension Injury

Distractive extension (DES) injuries are typically soft-tissue lesions and divided into two stages. DES I is a disruption of the anterior ligamentous complex or, rarely, a nondisplaced fracture of the vertebral body. Radiographs may appear entirely normal. One clue to the diagnosis is widening of the disk space, which is sometimes present. DES II is a disruption of the posterior soft-tissue complex, which can allow posterior displacement of the upper vertebral body into the spinal canal. This lesion is often reduced at the time of lateral radiographs and may show only subtle or no changes on routine radiographs. When neurologic involvement is present, it is most commonly a central cord syndrome, and provided that no coexisting compression lesions are present, some neurologic recovery is expected.

A   **B**

Figure 5–46. Imaging studies in a man who fell from a height and suffered a C6-C7 fracture-dislocation with a perched facet but remained neurologically intact. **A:** Lateral radiographic view demonstrating the fracture-dislocation at C6-C7. **B:** MRI demonstrating the anterior subluxation of C6 on C7, with the intervertebral disk retropulsed behind the C6 vertebral body. The patient was treated with an anterior diskectomy, reduction, and fusion.

The DES injury is usually stable and does not require surgical intervention. Late flexion-extension views, however, are indicated to rule out any evidence of late instability.

Lateral Flexion Injury

Allen and colleagues included the injuries of five patients in the category of lateral flexion (LFS) injury. This category is further divided into two stages. LFS I is an asymmetric compression fracture of the vertebral body and ipsilateral posterior arch, with no displacement in the coronal plane. LFS II has a similar fracture pattern but with displacement in the coronal plane, which suggests ligamentous disruption on the tension side of the injury. This mechanism can lead to brachial plexus injuries of varying degrees on the distracted side.

Because of the rarity of LFS injuries, treatment protocols are not well established. Surgical stabilization should be considered if late instability is expected or if there is a neurologic deficit.

Treatment Decisions

Ultimately the treating physician must decide on a treatment plan. The Allen classification, although quite useful to describe an injury, is a mechanistic system that is challenging to apply to the individual patient to assess operative indications. The decision whether to operate is based on a spectrum of spinal stability and neurologic compromise. A patient with a three-column injury, continued neurologic compression, and neurologic symptoms has a clear operative indication either through an anterior, posterior, or combined approach. A fully neurologically intact patient with a one-column

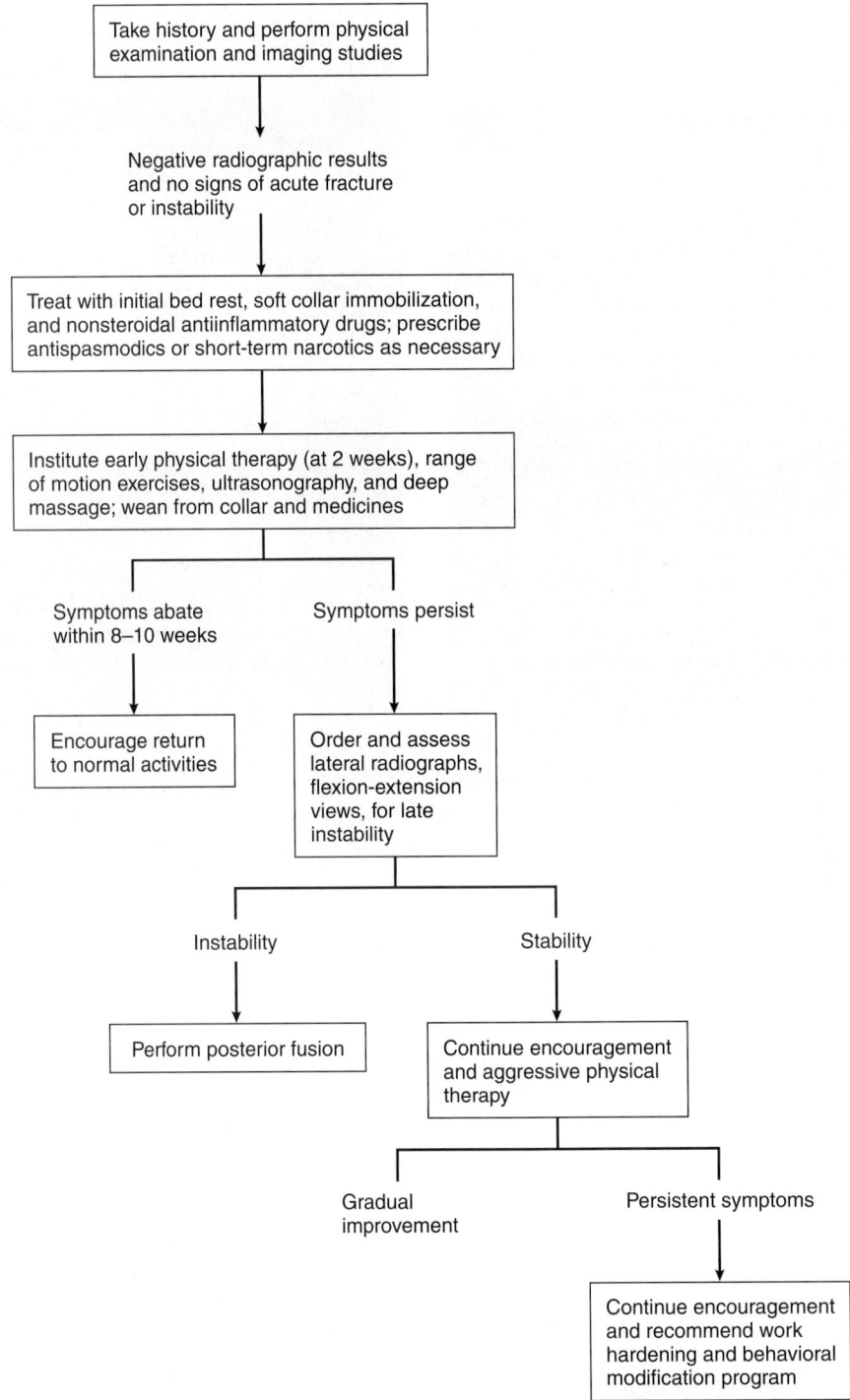

Figure 5–47. Algorithm for management of patients with cervical strain.

injury generally does fine in a brace. Patients with injury patterns in between must be treated on a case-by-case basis.

Cervical Strains & Sprains (Whiplash Injury)

Cervical strains and sprains, which are commonly referred to as a whiplash injury when associated with motor vehicle accidents, can produce a protracted and confusing clinical picture. Pain is typically the one unifying feature, yet there may be numerous other complaints, including local tenderness, decreased range of motion, headaches that are typically occipital, blurred or double vision, dysphagia, hoarseness, jaw pain, difficulty with balance, and even vertigo. It is often difficult for the physician to correlate radiographic findings, diagnostic test results, and other objective findings with the subjective complaints of the patient. The constellation of symptoms is fairly uniform, however, and should certainly not be discounted, and many investigators propose an anatomic basis for the clinical complaints. McNabb proposed that paresthesias in the ulnar distribution may be secondary to spasm of the scalenus muscle, and certainly symptoms such as hoarseness and dysphagia can be related to retropharyngeal hematoma. The cervical zygapophysial joint and facet capsule are implicated as a source for chronic pain after whiplash injury.

Figure 5–47 presents an algorithm for management of cervical strain. Radiographs should be taken because the amount of neck trauma that the patient has sustained may be significant. Radiographic findings, however, may be subtle or entirely negative. Cervical lordosis may be reversed, indicating spasm. Subtle signs of instability may also be present, and these can be further delineated on flexion-extension views if symptoms persist. The prevertebral soft-tissue window should be within normal limits to rule out any prevertebral hematoma.

Once the stability of the spine is ensured, the care of the cervical sprain or whiplash injury should be symptomatic. Initial rest, bed rest if necessary, and soft collar immobilization are indicated, along with the use of antiinflammatory medications. Early mobilization with progressive range of motion and weaning from external supports should be encouraged, however. Frequent reassurance is often necessary because the symptoms may be long lasting.

Approximately 42% of patients have persistent symptoms beyond 1 year, with approximately a third having persistent symptoms beyond 2 years. Most patients who do improve do so within the first 2 months. Factors associated with a poor prognosis include the presence of occipital headaches, interscapular pain, or reversal of cervical lordosis. Women have a worse prognosis than men, and hyperextension injuries are thought to have a worse prognosis than hyperflexion injuries.

Hartling L et al: Prognostic value of the Quebec classification of whiplash associated disorders. Spine 2001;26(1):36. [PMID: 11148643]

McNabb I: The "whiplash syndrome." Orthop Clin North Am 1971;2:389.

Siegmund GP et al: Mechanical evidence of facet capsule injury during whiplash—A cadaveric study using combined shear, compression, and extension loading. Spine 2001;26(19):2095. [PMID: 11698885]

Yoganandan N et al: Whiplash injury determination with conventional spine imaging and cryomicrotomy. Spine 2001;26(22):2443. [PMID: 11707708]

Musculoskeletal Oncology

R. Lor Randall, MD, and Bang H. Hoang, MD

Tumors of the musculoskeletal system are an extremely heterogeneous group of neoplasms consisting of well over 200 benign types of neoplasms and approximately 90 malignant conditions. The relative incidence of benign to malignant disease is 200:1. The tumors uniformly arise from embryonic mesoderm and are categorized according to their differentiated or adult histology. Current classification schemes are essentially descriptive. Each histologic type of tumor expresses individual, distinct behaviors with great variation between tumor types. Benign disease, by definition, behaves in a nonaggressive fashion with little tendency to recur locally or to metastasize. Malignant tumors or sarcomas, such as osteosarcoma and synovial cell sarcoma, are capable of invasive, locally destructive growth with a tendency to recur and to metastasize.

Neoplastic processes arise in tissues of mesenchymal origin far less frequently than those of ectodermal and endodermal origin. In 2004, soft-tissue and bone sarcomas had an annual incidence in the United States of more than 8600 and 2400 new cases, respectively. When compared with the overall cancer mortality of 563,000 cases per year in 2004, sarcomas are a small fraction of the problem. However, although a relatively uncommon form of cancer, these mesenchymal tumors behave in an aggressive fashion with reported current mortality rates in some series greater than 50%. According to the National Cancer Institute's Surveillance, Epidemiology, and End Results (SEER) program, approximately 8600 new soft-tissue sarcomas developed in the United States in 2004 with over 3600 sarcoma-related deaths. The associated morbidity is much higher. These tumors inflict a tremendous emotional and financial toll on individuals and society alike. Furthermore, sarcomas are more common in older patients, with 15% percent affecting patients younger than 15 years and 40% percent affecting persons older than 55 years. Accordingly, as the population ages, as it is doing at a rapid rate, the incidence of these tumors will increase.

ETIOLOGY OF MUSCULOSKELETAL TUMORS

Tumorigenesis is a complex multiple-step process by which healthy tissue progressively transforms from a normal phenotype into an abnormal colony of proliferating cells. During this process, cells acquire genetic abnormalities in oncogenes, tumor suppressor genes, and other genes that directly or indirectly control proliferation. Such a process may progress beyond the controlled state of benign disease to become a dedifferentiated, aggressive, and immortal phenotype by genomic instability. It is this instability that allows the cell to progress to fulminant malignancy. DNA regulation and, correspondingly, integrity is ultimately lost and a cancer is born.

To appreciate how bone or soft-tissue tumors develop, one must have a basic understanding of the cell cycle during which cell division occurs. The cell cycle is divided into four distinct phases: G1 (gap 1), S (DNA synthesis), G2 (gap 2), and M (mitosis). DNA synthesis occurs during the S phase, with chromosomal separation and cell division occurring in the M phase. The majority of cell growth takes place during G1. The mature state for mesenchymal tissues is normally in a resting, nonproliferative phase designated G0. It is the factors that affect the exit of the cell from G0, with entrance into G1, that is the hallmark of neoplastic disease.

Control of the cell cycle is a function of numerous regulatory proteins and checkpoints. The checkpoints allow for the monitoring and correction in the genetic sequence. The proteins are encoded by two basic gene types: oncogenes (stimulatory) and tumor suppressor genes (inhibitory). The retinoblastoma (Rb) protein and its phosphorylation state are critically important in regulating cell cycle progression (from G1 to S phase). Therefore, the activation state of Rb is a highly regulated cellular event. In addition, multiple cyclins and cyclin-dependent kinases are being studied actively to elucidate their role in regulation of the cell cycle.

Oncogenes, encoding a variety of growth factors, promote progression of the cell through G1, effecting a mitogenic signal. Suppressor genes, such as wild-type *TP53*, act to arrest the cell cycle. Specifically, *TP53* acts to stop the cell cycle at the G1/S border as a final attempt to abort proliferation. Other suppressor genes work earlier to keep reproduction at bay. A complex array of molecules can serve as either an induction or suppressor function. When this pathway is not orchestrated properly, a given cell obtains the potential for limited or even immortal proliferation. A normal cell progresses through a preneoplastic state on its way to becoming neoplastic via the accumulation of mutations. A critical step during tumor progression is the loss of suppressor gene function, which occurs by a variety of defects, including deletions, translocations, promoter silencing, loss of heterozygosity, point mutations, microsatellite changes, and telomeric associations. The degree to which the daughter cells dedifferentiate into a malignant phenotype is a function of the amount of genomic instability that arises with each subsequent mitosis. Mutation begets mutation as the checkpoints and regulatory machinery continually fail to repair the genetic code.

Factors that influence these mechanisms include both inheritable genetic conditions (eg, Li-Fraumeni syndrome, retinoblastoma) or environmental factors. It is well established that oncogenic viruses, radiation, and chemical carcinogens can affect these processes, ultimately compromising genomic stability.

The neoplastic process may arrest in the so-called benign state, with further genomic instability curtailed, or it can almost progress to a sarcomatous state. For example, if the cell type of origin is a lipocyte, then a lipoma or liposarcoma may develop. Furthermore, a liposarcoma can progress in its dedifferentiation such that its phenotype, as a high-grade lesion, minimally reflects its lipocytic origin. This possibility does not imply, however, that all benign lesions are necessarily at risk for malignant degeneration. It is not a surgical indication to remove a lipoma because of concern over developing a liposarcoma.

Although a plethora of molecular markers are being studied, understanding the details of genomic instability and subsequent tumor formation is lacking. The initiation of the neoplastic process and subsequent disease progression is a complex multistep process in gene expression and deregulation. There is no single pathway by which all neoplasms arise; instead, multiple genetic targets are altered in a variety of sequences with the common result of cellular proliferation that is tumorigenesis.

EVALUATION & STAGING OF TUMORS

History & Physical Examination

When evaluating a new patient with a possible tumor, the workup must commence with a thorough history and physical examination. Prior to ordering any diagnostic studies, particular questions must be answered, and the physical characteristics of the mass in question must be assessed. This procedure prevents unnecessary tests and better enables the physician to determine which tests will be most helpful in diagnosing the condition as well as facilitating therapeutic interventions if needed.

The clinical history is of paramount importance (Table 6–1). The age of the patient permits the generation of a list of potential diagnoses (Table 6–2), which,

Table 6–1. Questions that must be asked in the workup of a possible tumor.

1. **The patient's age.** Certain tumors are relatively specific to particular age groups.
2. **Duration of complaint.** Benign lesions generally have been present for an extended period (years). Malignant tumors usually have been noticed for only weeks to months.
3. **Rate of growth.** A rapidly growing mass, as in weeks to months, is more likely to be malignant. Growth may be difficult to assess by the patient if it is deep seated, as can be the case with bone. Deep lesions may be much larger than the patient thought ("tip-of-the-iceberg" phenomenon).
4. **Pain associated with the mass.** Benign processes are usually asymptomatic. Osteochondromas (see text) may cause secondary symptoms because of encroachment on surrounding structures. Malignant lesions may cause pain.
5. **History of trauma.** With a history of penetrating trauma, one must rule out osteomyelitis. With a history of blunt trauma, healing fracture must be entertained.
6. **Personal or family history of cancer.** Adults with a history of prostate, renal, lung, breast, or thyroid tumors are at risk for developing metastatic bone disease. Children with neuroblastoma are prone to bony metastases. Patients with retinoblastoma are at an increased risk for osteosarcoma. Secondary osteosarcomas and other malignancies can result from treatment of other childhood cancers. Family history of conditions such as Li-Fraumeni syndrome must raise suspicion of any bone lesion. Furthermore, certain benign bone tumors can run in families (eg, hereditary multiple exostoses; see text).
7. **Systemic signs or symptoms.** Generally there should be no significant findings on the review of systems with benign tumors. Fevers, chills, night sweats, malaise, change in appetite, weight loss, and so on, should alert the physician that an infectious or neoplastic process may be involved.

Table 6–2. Distribution of bone tumors by age (years).

Type of Tumor	0	10	20	30	40	50	60	70	80
Benign bone tumors									
Osteoid osteoma	X	X	X	X					
Osteoblastoma		X	X	X					
Osteofibrous dysplasia	X	X							
Enchondroma		X	X	X	X	X			
Periosteal chondroma		X	X	X	X	X			
Osteochondroma		X	X	X	X	X			
Chondroblastoma		X	X	X					
Chondromyxoid fibroma		X	X	X					
Fibrous cortical defect	X	X	X	X	X	X			
Nonossifying fibroma	X	X	X	X	X	X			
Fibrous dysplasia	X	X	X	X	X	X			
Solitary bone cyst	X	X							
Aneurysmal bone cyst		X	X						
Epidermoid cyst			X	X	X				
Giant cell tumor			X	X	X	X			
Hemangioma		X	X	X	X	X			
Malignant bone tumors									
Classic osteosarcoma		X	X	X					
Hemorrhagic osteosarcoma		X	X	X					
Parosteal osteosarcoma		X	X	X					
Periosteal osteosarcoma		X	X						
Secondary osteosarcoma						X	X	X	X
Low-grade intramedullary osteosarcoma		X	X	X	X	X			
Irradiation-induced osteosarcoma			X	X	X	X	X	X	X
Multicentric osteosarcoma		X	X						
Primary chondrosarcoma				X	X	X	X		
Secondary chondrosarcoma				X	X	X	X		
Clear cell chondrosarcoma			X	X	X	X			
Dedifferentiated chondrosarcoma						X	X	X	
Mesenchymal chondrosarcoma			X	X					
Ewing sarcoma	X	X	X						
Lymphoma			X	X	X	X			
Multiple myeloma				X	X	X	X	X	X
Solitary plasmacytoma				X	X	X			
Fibrosarcoma		X	X	X	X	X	X		
Malignant fibrous histiocytoma		X	X	X	X	X	X	X	X
Adamantinoma		X	X	X	X				
Vascular sarcoma		X	X	X	X	X	X		
Chordoma				X	X	X	X	X	X
Metastatic carcinoma			X	X	X	X	X	X	X

300

Table 6–3. Aspects of physical exam that should be documented when evaluating a patient with a mass.[a]

---

1. **Skin color**
2. **Warmth**
3. **Location**
4. **Swelling.** Swelling, in addition to the primary mass effect, may reflect a more aggressive process.
5. **Neurovascular exam.** Changes may reflect a more aggressive process.
6. **Joint range of motion** of all joints in proximity to the region in question, above and below.
7. **Size.** A mass greater than 5 cm should raise the suspicion of malignancy.
8. **Tenderness.** Tenderness may reflect a more rapidly growing process.
9. **Firmness.** Malignant tumors tend to be firmer on examination than benign processes. This applies more to soft-tissue tumors than osseous ones.
10. **Lymph nodes.** Certain sarcomas (eg, rhabdomyosarcoma, synovial sarcoma, epithelioid, and clear cell sarcomas) all have increased rates of lymph node involvement.

---

[a]*Note:* These findings assume the absence of trauma.

when combined with the history and a few additional studies, should permit establishing a diagnosis. The duration of symptoms, rate of growth, the presence of pain, and a history of trauma can help elucidate the diagnosis. A careful past medical history, family history, and review of systems must not be overlooked either.

A thorough physical exam is also critical (Table 6–3). The clinician must assess the location and size of the mass, the quality of the overlying skin, the presence of warmth, any associated swelling, the presence of tenderness, and the firmness of the lesion. Range of motion of all joints in proximity to the tumor, above and below, must be recorded as well as a complete neurovascular exam. An assessment of the related lymph node chains as well as an examination for an enlarged liver or spleen should be performed.

The clinician must also consider pseudotumors in addition to true neoplastic conditions. A history of trauma suggests a possible stress fracture or myositis ossificans as a diagnosis. The history of stress-related physical activity and the exact timing of symptom presentation and variations of symptoms with the passage of time are important considerations in establishing a differential diagnosis.

Imaging Studies

A. RADIOGRAPHY

Initial evaluation should begin with plain radiography. In every patient with a suspected tumor, orthogonal antero-

posterior (AP) and lateral views of the affected area should be taken. This includes soft-tissue masses as well. In many cases, radiographic examination is diagnostic, and no further imaging studies are indicated. However, in the case of a more aggressive process, the diagnosis may be determined on the plain radiographs but further evaluation with advanced studies is usually indicated to determine the extent of local soft-tissue involvement as well as to assess the extent of disseminated disease (staging).

The initial radiographic images must be scrutinized. For bone lesions, the location within the bone (eg, epiphyseal, metaphyseal, or diaphyseal) facilitates the diagnosis. Epiphyseal tumors are usually benign. The more malignant primary sarcomas, such as osteosarcoma, are typically seen in a metaphyseal location; however, round cell tumors, such as Ewing sarcoma, multiple myeloma, and lymphomas, are usually medullary diaphyseal lesions. A tumor arising from the surface of a long bone may be a benign lesion, such as an osteochondroma, or it may be a low-grade sarcoma, such as a parosteal osteosarcoma.

Terms such as *geographic, well circumscribed, permeative,* and are used to describe the appearance of radiographic abnormalities. Geographic or well circumscribed implies that the lesion has a distinct boundary and is sharply marginated, suggesting a benign tumor (Figure 6–1). A poorly defined, infiltrative process is described as permeative or moth eaten and reflects a more aggressive process such as a malignancy (Figure 6–2), although aggressive but benign processes can have this radio-

Figure 6–1. Radiograph of an enchondroma of the second metacarpal. Notice its geographic appearance.

Figure 6–2. Radiograph of a proximal fibular osteosarcoma demonstrating the destructive, permeative nature of malignant bone tumors.

graphic quality as well (Figure 6–3). An exception to this rule is multiple myeloma, which frequently demonstrates a punched-out, well-demarcated appearance but in multiple locations.

With a careful history, physical, and appropriate radiographs, the physician can reach a working diagnosis of the lesion. Although benign and malignant tumors can mimic each other, some tumors can be ruled out on the basis of the history, the age of the patient, the location of the tumor (in which bone and where in the bone), and the radiographic appearance of the tumor, as shown in Tables 6–1 through 6–6. For example, a 20-year-old man with a 3-month history of pain in the knee is found to have an epiphyseal lesion in the distal femur. The lesion has a benign geographic appearance. If the tumor is benign, the criteria of the patient's age (see Table 6–2) eliminates only solitary bone cyst and osteofibrous dysplasia, but all other benign tumors remain possibilities. If the tumor is malignant, it is likely to be an osteosarcoma (various types), Ewing sarcoma, fibrosarcoma, vascular sarcoma, or, possibly, chondrosarcoma, according to the age criterion. The most common site for bone tumors is about

the knee, especially the distal femur. The likely benign tumors are giant cell tumor, nonossifying fibroma, chondroma, osteochondroma, and chondroblastoma. The likely malignant tumors in this age group are osteosarcoma, Ewing sarcoma, fibrosarcoma, and, possibly, chondrosarcoma. Most malignant tumors are metaphyseal. Based on location in the bone (Table 6–4), the most likely benign tumors are chondroblastoma and giant cell tumor. Most malignant tumors are metaphyseal. The geographic appearance implies a benign radiographic appearance. Thus, the working diagnosis would be chondroblastoma or, possibly, giant cell tumor if the lesion were benign, whereas it would be osteosarcoma or chondrosarcoma if the lesion were malignant, which is less likely. In this age group, metastatic disease is very unlikely, but low-grade infection may mimic a tumor, particularly if the patient is immunocompromised, as can be determined from the patient's history. Table 6–5 indicates the most useful studies for further workup.

B. ISOTOPE BONE SCANNING

Technetium-99 radioisotope scans are used to assess the degree of osteoblastic activity of a given lesion

Figure 6–3. Radiograph of a giant cell tumor of the thumb. This is a typical moth-eaten appearance.

(Figure 6–4). In general, they are quite sensitive, with a few exceptions, for active lesions of bone. Accordingly, technetium-99 scans are excellent screening tools for remote lesions (staging). The best indication for a bone scan is suspected multiple bony lesions, such as those commonly seen in metastatic carcinomas and lymphomas of bone. Isotope bone scanning is far simpler to perform, less expensive, and requires less total body irradiation than skeletal surveys. It is common practice to use serial isotope scans to follow patients with suspected metastatic disease and at the same time evaluate the effectiveness of their systemic therapy program.

Isotope scanning is also used in the staging process of a primary sarcoma such as an osteosarcoma to make sure the patient does not have an asymptomatic remote skeletal lesion. Technetium-99 scans are also useful in distinguishing blastic lesions of bone. Given that the study reflects metabolic activity, an enostosis (bone island) would not demonstrate significant increased activity compared with a blastic prostate metastasis. Inflammatory disease and trauma also show increased activity. It is important to note, however, that multiple myeloma and metastatic squamous cell carcinoma may not demonstrate technetium uptake (ie, a false-negative result). Skeletal surveys are preferable for screening for additional sites of involvement in such cases.

C. COMPUTED TOMOGRAPHY AND MAGNETIC RESONANCE IMAGING

Computed tomography (CT) remains a standard imaging procedure for use in well-selected clinical situations. Perhaps the best indication for CT is for smaller lesions that involve cortical structures of bone or spine (Figure 6–5). In such cases, CT is superior to MRI because the resolution of cortical bone using MRI is inferior. CT scan of the lung is the modality of choice for evaluating patients with sarcoma for possible lung metastases. Abdominal CT scan is invaluable in surveying for a primary tumor in patients who present with bone metastases. For tumors involving the pelvis and sacrum, CT can help elucidate the extent of bone involvement (Figure 6–6). In cases involving a soft-tissue lesion, MRI is far superior to CT unless there is a heavily calcified process.

MRI is the imaging modality of choice for evaluating bone marrow involvement as well as noncalcific soft-tissue lesions. The two most commonly used MRI sequences are the T_1-weighted and T_2-weighted spin echo (Figure 6–7). MRI can also demonstrate the normal anatomy of soft structures, including nerves and vessels, thereby nearly eliminating the need for arteriography and myelograms. Dynamic-enhanced MRI, with its ability to estimate tumor blood flow by examining the rate of contrast uptake and clearance, may

serve as a predictor of clinical outcome or tumor response to chemotherapy.

Laboratory Studies

A. BIOPSY

The biopsy should usually be the final staging procedure. Although the biopsy can distort the imaging studies, such as MRI, pathologic evaluation and interpretation may require information provided by the prior workup. Complications relating to the biopsy are not infrequent. Accordingly, careful preoperative planning is imperative. The imaging studies aid the surgeon in selecting the best site for a tissue diagnosis. In most cases, the best diagnostic tissue is found at the periphery of the tumor, where it interfaces with normal tissue. For example, in the case of a malignant bone tumor, soft-tissue invasion is usually evident outside the bone, and this area can be sampled without violating cortical bone and thus without causing a fracture at the biopsy site. If a medullary specimen is needed, a small round or oval hole should be cut to decrease the chance of fracture. If the medullary specimen is malignant, the cortical hole should be plugged with bone wax or bone cement to reduce soft-tissue contamination following the procedure.

Obtaining an adequate specimen is critical. A frozen section determines if viable and adequate tissue were obtained. A few experienced tumor centers may make a definitive diagnosis based on a frozen section, allowing the surgeon to proceed with definitive operative treatment of the tumor. However, freezing artifact can cause overinterpretation of the material, so an aggressive resection should always be deferred until the permanent analysis is complete. Additional studies beyond conventional light microscopy, such as immunocytochemistries and cytogenetics, may also be necessary.

The placement of the biopsy site is a major consideration. If the surgeon is inexperienced and not familiar with surgical oncologic principles, a serious contamination of a vital structure such as the popliteal artery or sciatic nerve may occur. Such an error might necessitate an amputation instead of a limb-sparing procedure. To avoid this problem in the case of a suspected malignant condition, the surgeon who performs the biopsy should be the same surgeon who will perform the definitive operative procedure.

Transverse incisions should be avoided because removing the entire biopsy site with the widely resected subjacent tumor mass is difficult. Adequate hemostasis is mandatory to avoid formation of a contaminating hematoma. A drain may be helpful but frequently is unnecessary. If a drain is used, it must be placed in line with the incision.

Table 6–4. Skeletal distribution of bone tumors, ranked from most common (1) to less common (5) sites.

Type of Tumor	Femur	Tibia	Foot or Ankle	Humerus	Radius	Ulna	Hand or Wrist	Scapula	Clavicle	Rib	Vertebra	Sacrum	Pelvis	Skull	Face
Benign bone tumors															
Osteoid osteoma	1	2		4			5				3				
Osteoblastoma	3	4		5							1				2
Osteofibrous dysplasia		1													
Chondroma	2		4	3		5	1								
Osteochondroma	1	3		2				5					4		
Chondroblastoma	1	3		2				5					4		
Chondromyxoid fibroma	3	1	2		5								4		
Fibrous cortical defect	2	1		3	4				5						
Nonossifying fibroma	2	1		3	4				5						
Solitary bone cyst	2	3		1		5							4		
Aneurysmal bone cyst	1	2		4							3		5		
Giant cell tumor	1	2		5	3							4			
Hemangioma	3	4		5							2			1	
Malignant bone tumors															
Classic osteosarcoma	1	2		3									4		
Hemorrhagic osteosarcoma	1	2		3							5		4		
Parosteal osteosarcoma	1	2		3		4									

	1	2	3	4	5	6	7	8	9	10	11	12
Periosteal osteosarcoma	1		3		4					1		4
Secondary osteosarcoma	2	5	3		5						4	
Low-grade intramedullary osteosarcoma	1	2								2		
Irradiation-induced osteosarcoma	1		2	4			3	5				
Primary chondrosarcoma	1		4			3	5		3	2		
Secondary chondrosarcoma	2		3	4			5		1			
Dedifferentiated chondrosarcoma	1		3	4		5			2			
Mesenchymal chondrosarcoma	5					3	2		1			4
Ewing sarcoma	1		3	5		4			2			
Lymphoma	1		4			5	3		2			
Myeloma	4		5			2	1		3			
Fibrosarcoma	1	2	4						3		5	
Malignant fibrous histiocytoma	1	3	5						2	4		
Adamantinoma	3	1		4	2							
Vascular sarcoma	3	4	3			5	1		2			
Chordoma						3	3	1		2		
Metastatic carcinoma	2		5			4	1		3			

Table 6-5. Bone tumors: imaging characteristics, location in a long bone, and beneficial studies, ranked from most common or most beneficial (1) to less common or less beneficial (3).

Type of Tumor	Imaging Characteristics			Location in a Long Bone					Beneficial Studies				
	Geographic	Moth Eaten	Permeative	Epiphyseal	Meta-physeal	Metadi-aphyseal	Diaphyseal	Surface	Plain Radiograph	CT Scan	MRI	Isotope Bone Scan	Blood Studies
Benign bone tumors													
Osteoid osteoma	1				1	2	3		1	2		3	
Osteoblastoma	2	1			2	1	3		1	2		3	
Osteofibrous dysplasia		1				2	1		1	2		3	
Chondroma	1				3	1	2		1	2		3	
Osteochondroma	1				2			1	1	2			
Chondroblastoma	1	2		1	2				1	2			
Chondromyxoid fibroma	1	2			1	2			1	2		3	
Fibrous cortical defect	1				1	2			1				
Nonossifying fibroma	1	2			1	2			1	2			
Solitary bone cyst	1				1	2	3		1				
Aneurysmal bone cyst	3	2	1		1	2		3	1	2	3		
Giant cell tumor	3	1	2	1	2				1	2			3
Hemangioma	2	1			3	1	2		1	2			
Malignant bone tumors													
Classic osteosarcoma	3	1	2		1	2	3		1	2	2	3	
Hemorrhagic osteosarcoma		1	2		1	2			1	2	2		3
Parosteal osteosarcoma	2	1			2	3		1	2	1			

	C1	C2	C3	C4	C5	C6	C7	C8	C9	C10	C11	C12
Periosteal osteosarcoma	2			3	2	3	1	2	1	1		
Secondary osteosarcoma	1	2		1	2	3		2	1	3	3	
Low-grade intramedullary osteosarcoma	1			1	2	3		1	2		3	
Irradiation-induced osteosarcoma	1	2		1	2	3		1	1	2	3	
Primary chondrosarcoma	2		3	1	2			2	1	3		
Secondary chondrosarcoma	2			2	3		1	2	1			
Dedifferentiated chondrosarcoma	1	2		1	2	3		2	3	1		
Mesenchymal chondrosarcoma	1	2		1	2			2	3			
Ewing sarcoma	2	1		1	2	3		2		1	3	
Lymphoma	2	1		3	1	2		3		1	2	
Myeloma	1	2		1	3	2		1			3	2
Fibrosarcoma	1	2		1	2	3		2		1		
Malignant fibrous histiocytoma	1	2		1	2	3		2		1		
Adamantinoma	2			3	2	1		1	2	3		
Vascular sarcoma	2	3		1	2	3		1		2	3	
Chordoma	2				1	2		3	2	1		
Metastatic carcinoma	3	2		1	2	3		2	3		1	

Table 6–6. Distribution of soft-tissue tumors by age (years).

Type of Tumor	0	10	20	30	40	50	60	70	80
Benign soft-tissue tumors									
Desmoid tumor		█	█	█	█				
Intramuscular lipoma			█	█	█	█	█		
Spindle-cell lipoma					█	█	█		
Angiolipoma			█	█					
Diffuse lipomatosis		█	█	█					
Benign lipoblastoma	█	█	█						
Hibernoma			█	█					
Capillary hemangioma	█								
Cavernous hemangioma		█	█	█					
Arteriovenous hemangioma		█	█						
Epithelioid hemangioma			█	█					
Pyogenic granuloma		█	█	█	█	█	█		
Lymphangioma		█	█	█					
Glomus tumor			█	█					
Benign hemangiopericytoma			█	█					
Neurilemoma			█	█					
Solitary neurofibroma			█	█					
Neurofibromatosis		█	█	█					
Intramuscular myxoma					█	█	█	█	█
Malignant soft-tissue tumors									
Pleomorphic MFH						█	█		
Myxoid MFH						█	█		
Giant cell MFH						█	█		
Angiomatoid MFH			█	█					
Dermatofibrosarcoma protuberans			█	█	█				
Fibrosarcoma				█	█				
Leiomyosarcoma					█	█			
Well-differentiated liposarcoma					█	█	█		
Myxoid liposarcoma					█	█	█		
Round cell and pleomorphic liposarcoma					█	█	█		
Embryonal rhabdomyosarcoma	█	█							
Alveolar rhabdomyosarcoma		█	█						
Pleomorphic rhabdomyosarcoma					█	█	█	█	█
Synovial sarcoma		█	█						
Solitary malignant schwannoma				█	█	█	█	█	█
Multiple malignant schwannoma				█	█	█	█	█	█
Angiosarcoma				█	█	█	█	█	█
Alveolar soft part sarcoma		█	█						
Epithelioid sarcoma			█	█					
Clear cell sarcoma			█	█					

MFH = malignant fibrous histiocytoma.

Figure 6–4. Technetium-99 scan demonstrating extensive osteoblastic activity in a patient with metastatic adenocarcinoma.

Figure 6–5. CT scan of an osteoblastoma arising from the right pedicle of a lumbar vertebral body.

Needle biopsies, either core or fine needle, can be used by experienced tumor centers, especially for lesions that are easily diagnosed, such as metastatic carcinomas or round cell tumors. Because the subtype of sarcoma is proving to be very important, architecture of the tumor is generally needed, which requires a core biopsy rather than a fine-needle aspirate. Core biopsies also allow the surgeon to sample various areas of the tumor to avoid sampling error in a heterogeneous tumor. In the case of a deep pelvic lesion or a spinal lesion, a CT-guided nee-

Figure 6–6. Pelvic CT demonstrating the bony destruction of the sacrum caused by a giant cell tumor.

A   **B**

Figure 6–7. Synovial sarcoma involving the popliteal fossa. (**A**) T_1 weighted. (**B**) T_2 weighted.

dle biopsy is ideal because it avoids excessive multicompartmental contamination.

In general, excisional biopsies are discouraged unless the lesion is particularly small (less than 2–3 cm) or in an area where a cuff of healthy uninvolved tissue of at least 1 cm can be removed as well. This technique ideally avoids a second procedure to remove the entire biopsy site if the lesion turns out to be malignant.

B. CULTURES AND SPECIAL STUDIES

The damage of biopsy specimens after retrieval can make it impossible to perform special studies such as immunohistochemistry, cytogenetics, flow cytometry, and electron microscopy. For this reason, the biopsy surgeon should consult with the pathologist before specimens are retrieved and handled. Furthermore, many current studies require fresh tissue (no formalin). It is also a good habit to obtain cultures for bacterial culture (anaerobic and aerobic) as well as fungal and acid-fast bacteria if clinical suspicion warrants.

Molecular diagnostics is on the verge of revolutionizing sarcoma diagnostics. Specific translocations were found in a variety of tumors (Table 6–7). Furthermore, therapeutics are beginning to be designed against specific molecular

defects in malignancies. Gastrointestinal stromal tumor (GIST), a malignant mesenchymal tumor arising from the gastrointestinal (GI) tract, omentum, and mesentery, overexpresses a mutant form of c-*kit*. The *KIT* gene encodes a tyrosine kinase receptor for the growth factor named stem cell factor or mast cell growth factor. Therapy directed against c-*kit* is having an early and remarkable effect on the previously difficult treatment of malignancy. Similar pathways are being elicited in other sarcomas.

Staging Systems

After the appropriate studies are completed, staging begins. *Staging* refers to an assessment of the grade of the tumor and the extent to which the disease has spread. There are several staging systems, but all have the purpose of helping the physician plan a logical treatment program and establish a prognosis for the patient. The two major systems are discussed here.

A. SYSTEM OF THE AMERICAN JOINT COMMITTEE ON CANCER

The American Joint Committee on Cancer (AJCC) system (5th edition) is used by most surgical oncologists

Table 6–7. Common translocations seen in sarcomas.

Ewing/primitive neuroectodermal tumor: t(11;22) (q24; q12), (t21; 22) (q22; q12), (t7; 22) (p22; q12)
Myxoid chondrosarcoma: t(9; 22) (q22; q12)
Myxoid & round cell liposarcoma: t(12; 16) (q12; p11)
Synovial sarcoma: t(X; 18) (p11; q11)
Alveolar rhabdomyosarcoma: t(2; 13) (q35; q14), t(1; 13) (p36; q14)
Alveolar soft parts sarcoma: t(X; 17) (p11.2; q25)
Desmoplastic small round cell tumor: t(11; 22) (p13; q12)
Congenital fibrosarcoma: t(12; 15)

---

when dealing with soft-tissue sarcomas. It classifies sarcomas according to their histologic grade (low or high), depth (superficial or deep), and size (with large tumors more than 5 cm in greatest dimension). Adverse prognostic factors include large tumor size, deep location within the extremity, and high histologic grade.

B. SYSTEM OF THE AMERICAN MUSCULOSKELETAL TUMOR SOCIETY (ENNEKING SYSTEM)

Orthopedic oncologists generally prefer the Enneking system, which addresses the unique problems related to sarcomas of the extremities and applies to tumors of the bone as well as those of soft tissue. The Enneking system has a 3-point scale for classifying tumors as stage I, II, or III on the basis of their histologic and biologic appearance and their likelihood of metastasizing to regional lymph nodes or distant sites such as the lung. Stage I refers to low-grade sarcomas with less than 25% chance of metastasis. Stage II refers to high-grade sarcomas with more than 25% chance of metastasis. Stage III is for either low-grade or high-grade tumors that have metastasized to a distant site, such as a lymph node, lung, or other distant organ system.

The Enneking system further classifies tumors on the basis of whether they are intracompartmental (type A) or extracompartmental (type B). Type A tumors are constrained by anatomic boundaries such as muscle fascial planes and stand a better chance for local control of tumor growth with surgical removal than type B tumors do. A lesion contained in a single muscle belly or a bone lesion that has not broken out into the surrounding soft tissue would be classified as a type A tumor. A lesion in the popliteal space, axilla, pelvis, or midportion of the hand or foot would be classified as a type B tumor. Although compartmentalization of a tumor is an important concept, studies show that the size of the tumor rather than whether it is contained within a compartment is more prognostic. Larger tumors, greater than 5 cm, are prognostically unfavorable.

A low-grade fibrosarcoma located inside the fascial plane of the biceps muscle and having no evidence of metastasis would be classified as a stage IA tumor. A typical malignant osteosarcoma of the distal femur with breakthrough into the surrounding muscle as determined by MRI would be classified as a stage IIB lesion. If CT scanning revealed metastatic involvement of the lung, the osteosarcoma would then be classified as a stage IIIB lesion.

Enneking WF: A system of staging musculoskeletal neoplasms. Clin Orthop 1985;204:9.

Mankin HJ et al: The hazards of the biopsy, revisited. J Bone Joint Surg Am 1996;78:656. [PMID 8642021]

Miettinen M et al: Gastrointestinal stromal tumors—Definition, clinical, histological, immunohistochemical, and molecular genetic features and differential diagnosis. Virchows Arch 2001;438(1):1. [PMID: 11688571]

Moley JF et al: Soft-tissue sarcomas. Surg Clin North Am 2000; 80(2):687. [PMID: 10836012]

Oliveira AM et al: Grading in soft tissue tumors: Principles and problems. Skeletal Radiol 2001;30(10):543. [PMID: 11685477]

Reddick WE et al: Dynamic MR imaging (DEMRI) of microcirculation in bone sarcoma. J Magn Reson Imaging 1999;10(3): 277. [PMID: 10508287]

Simon MA et al: Diagnostic strategy for bone & soft tissue tumors. J Bone Joint Surg Am 1993;75:622. [PMID: 8478392]

Skrzynski MC et al: Diagnostic accuracy and charge savings of outpatient care needle biopsy compared with open biopsy of musculoskeletal tumors. J Bone Joint Surg Am 1996;78:644. [PMID: 8642019]

Zahm SH et al: The epidemiology of soft tissue sarcoma. Semin Oncol 1997;24(5):504. [PMID: 9344316]

■ DIAGNOSIS & TREATMENT OF TUMORS

BENIGN BONE TUMORS

Benign bone tumors have certain characteristics that favor their diagnosis over malignant conditions. If the condition is benign, the patient is frequently asymptomatic, and the radiograph usually shows a well-defined geographic lesion with sclerotic reactive margins that suggest a long-standing process associated with slow growth potential. In contrast, if the condition is malignant, the patient usually complains of pain, and the radiograph commonly shows a more permeative lesion with lytic destruction and poorly defined margins that suggest rapid progression. In many cases, further studies such as MRI or bone isotope studies are not necessary for a typical benign tumor, such as fibrous dysplasia, enchondroma, or nonossifying fibroma. A system of staging exists for benign bone tumors. Stage 1 lesions are considered latent. They generally are asymptomatic but not always. Although they can progress, they usually resolve. Initially, these lesions should be observed. Stage 2 lesions are considered active. They tend not to resolve spontaneously and are less well demarcated than stage 1 lesions. They frequently require surgical intervention with aggressive treatment. Recurrence is not infrequent. Stage 3, or aggressive lesions, demonstrate extensive destruction. Treatment often requires wide en bloc resection.

The more common types of benign bone tumor seen by the practicing orthopedic surgeon are discussed in this section.

Benign Osteoid-Forming Tumors

A. OSTEOID OSTEOMA

The most common benign osteoid-forming tumor is the osteoid osteoma, accounting for 10% of all benign bone tumors. It is more common in males than in females, with a peak incidence in the second decade of life. The proximal femur is the most common site. Dull aching pain is the most frequent symptom. Symptoms are relieved with nonsteroidal antiinflammatory drugs (NSAIDs) secondary to a high concentration of prostaglandins in the nidus. Osteoid osteoma may have a unique pathogenic nerve supply as well, a unique finding among bone tumors.

The characteristic radiographic feature of the osteoid osteoma is the central lytic nidus that measures up to 1 cm in diameter. In the common cortical lesion (Figure 6–8), an extensive reactive sclerosis is evident, creating a fusiform bulge on the bone surface. However, if the nidus is more centrally located in metaphyseal bone, less sclerosis is seen and the radiographic appearance is less diagnostic. If the nidus is close to a joint or actually in the joint, as in the case of a femoral neck lesion, inflammatory synovitis results and suggests the diagnosis of a pyarthrosis or rheumatoid disease. Technetium bone scans are invariably positive. A CT scan is helpful to better anatomically locate the lesion in preoperative planning.

In the spine, the typical location for an osteoid osteoma is in the posterior elements, such as the lamina or pedicle. The lumbar spine is most commonly involved; the dorsal spine is the second most commonly involved. A secondary scoliosis may develop, with the convexity toward the lesion. Furthermore, if the nidus is in proximity to a nerve root, root irritation can develop. In the lumbar spine, this pain can present as sciatica and suggest the diagnosis of a herniated disk.

Previously, some investigators believed that the osteoid osteoma was an inflammatory process such as a Brodie abscess, which has a similar clinical and radiographic appearance. Currently, it is accepted that osteoid osteoma is a true osteoid-forming neoplasm and absent of lymphocytes or plasma cells. Histologically, the nidus shows aggressive but benign woven bone formation, with large numbers of osteoblasts and osteoclasts in a vascular fibrous stroma. No chondroid areas are seen.

Most cases of osteoid osteoma are stage 1 lesions and can be treated symptomatically with aspirin or NSAIDs. If the patient fails such treatment, surgical intervention is warranted. If surgery is undertaken, the entire symptomatic nidus must be eradicated. Removal of a large amount of the surrounding sclerotic bone should be avoided because it can severely weaken the bone and may result in a pathologic fracture. If the lesion is in cortical bone, adequate exposure is required so the surgeon can visualize the bulging cortex. Intralesional resection via the so-called burr-down technique is generally preferred over en bloc resection. The nidus can be identified visually by the hyperemic pink color in the reactive bone adjacent to it. Simple curettage of the nidus followed by high-speed burring to advance the margin another 2–3 mm is all that is necessary. If the lesion is not visible on the surface, as in the case of a medullary lesion, radiographic markers should be placed intraoperatively prior to placing the round cortical window. CT-guided radiofrequency ablation (RFA) is reported as an effective, less invasive method of treating osteoid osteoma. This method employs probes with high-frequency alternating current to induce ionic agitation and frictional heat to cause tumor necrosis. RFA is used extensively as a less invasive treatment modality with similar success rate as surgical excision.

B. OSTEOBLASTOMA

Osteoblastoma is a large osteoid osteoma that demonstrates a propensity for the posterior elements of the spine. The tumors are found more commonly in males than in females and occur in the same age group as osteoid osteomas. Osteoblastomas are less common than osteoid osteomas, accounting for 1% of all bone tumors. A few can be found in the metaphyses of long bone (raising suspicion about a possible osteosarcoma), and a few can be seen in the ankle and wrist areas. These lesions are usually stage 1–2 lesions.

Radiographically, the osteoblastoma has a more lytic and destructive appearance than the osteoid osteoma. Its nidus, which is greater than 1–2 cm, has a less sclerotic reactive bone at the periphery and may take on the appearance of an aneurysmal bone cyst. Histologically, the nidus of the osteoblastoma is nearly identical to that

Figure 6–8. Radiograph (**A**), isotope bone scan (**B**), CT scan (**C**), and photomicrograph (**D**) of an osteoid osteoma in the femur of a 19-year-old man.

of the osteoid osteoma and shows excessive osteoblastic activity and osteoid formation with numerous giant cells in a vascular fibrous stroma.

In the spine area, the effects of osteoblastoma are similar to those of osteoid osteoma, with pressure on nerve roots causing pain down the leg or arm (Figure 6–9). In the thoracic area, a large lesion could result in cord compromise.

In patients with osteoblastomas, treatment usually consists of a vigorous curettage of the lesion, which may require a bone graft if instability results. Radiofre-

quency ablation may also prove useful in the management of this lesion.

C. OSTEOFIBROUS DYSPLASIA

Osteofibrous dysplasia is a rare condition that is seen almost exclusively in the tibia of children younger than 10 years. It is more common in boys than in girls and usually asymptomatic. It commonly affects the diaphysis and results in anterior cortical bowing. Osteofibrous dysplasia can occur in the fibula and even more rarely can be seen bilaterally. It is most likely a hamartoma-

Figure 6–9. Radiograph of osteoblastoma in the pedicle area of the C3 vertebra of a 14-year-old boy.

tous process and tends to involute spontaneously with skeletal maturity.

In osteofibrous dysplasia (Figure 6–10), the lytic changes seen in the anterior tibial cortex surrounded by sclerotic margins, thus creating a soap-bubbly appearance similar to the radiographic picture of both fibrous dysplasia and adamantinoma. Histologically, the lytic lesion shows a benign trabecular alphabet-soup pattern in a fibrous stroma. The histologic findings are similar to those in fibrous dysplasia, although the lesions of fibrous dysplasia lack the prominent surface layer of osteoblasts seen in osteofibrous dysplasia. These lesions are stage 1–2.

In a report of experience with 35 cases of osteofibrous dysplasia, investigators indicated that early attempts at curettage and grafting of the lesions resulted in a high failure rate because of recurrence. For this reason, they suggested waiting until patients reach the age of 15 years and their disease arrests spontaneously before proceeding with a definitive debridement and bone grafting.

Benign Chondroid-Forming Tumors

A. ENCHONDROMA

Enchondroma refers to a centrally located chondroma of bone. These tumors are relatively common lesions, accounting for greater than 10% of benign bone tumors. In 50% of cases, the tumor is found in the small tubular bone of the hands and feet. It arises in growing bones as a hamartomatous process but is frequently asymptomatic and may avoid detection until the patient reaches adulthood, at which time the lesion may be discovered in association with a pathologic fracture or as an incidental finding on a routine radiographic examination.

Radiographs of enchondromas show geographic lysis with sharp margination and central calcification (Figure 6–11). In the case of an enchondroma of the hand, the cortex is frequently thinned out with slight dilation. In contrast, with involvement of the large long bones, the lesion is centrally located with minimal evidence of cortical erosion or dilatation. Enchondromas are either stage 1 or 2 lesions.

Figure 6–10. Radiograph of osteofibrous dysplasia in the tibia of an 8-year-old boy.

Figure 6–11. Radiograph of an enchondroma of the proximal phalanx of the ring finger.

Multiple enchondromatosis, or Ollier disease (Figure 6–12), is a rare nonfamilial dysplasia typically seen on half of the body and appears similar to fibrous dysplasia. This condition can be quite extensive, with significant involvement of metaphyseal areas resulting in bowing and shortening of the long bones. Such dramatic changes are rarely seen in cases of a solitary enchondroma. In patients with Maffucci syndrome, enchondromatosis is seen in association with multiple soft-tissue hemangiomas.

A large solitary enchondroma in a large bone converts to a low-grade chondrosarcoma in fewer than 5% of cases, and the conversion takes place during adulthood. A solitary enchondroma on the hand rarely converts to a chondrosarcoma. A secondary chondrosarcoma in enchondromatosis can arise in up to 20% of cases and may be related to inactivation of particular tumor suppressor genes.

There is no need to treat an asymptomatic patient with a solitary enchondroma of the hand or foot. If the patient has a pathologic fracture, it is best to allow the fracture to heal and then at a later date to perform a simple curettage and bone grafting procedure, which usually results in good function and a low chance of recurrence. Patients with Ollier or Maffucci disease must be followed carefully because of the increased risk of malignant degeneration.

B. PERIOSTEAL CHONDROMA

A benign chondroma seen on the surface of a bone is called a periosteal chondroma. Patients usually have more than one lesion, and the most common location is on the proximal humeral metaphysis. Radiographically, the lesions appear to lie on the cortical surface and appear to saucerize the underlying cortex (Figure 6–13). These

lesions are stage 1–2. Periosteal chondromas can grow to a sizable mass, but anything larger than 4 cm suggests a peripheral primary chondrosarcoma.

Management of periosteal chondromas generally consists of observing the lesion at intervals to make sure it does not continue growing as the patient reaches adulthood. In cases in which simple local resection without bone graft is indicated, the procedure is associated with a low recurrence rate.

C. OSTEOCHONDROMA

The nonossifying fibroma of bone is the most common benign tumor of bone, and the solitary osteochondroma is the second most common. Like the enchondroma, the osteochondroma is a developmental, or hamartomatous, process that arises from a defect in the outer edge of the growth plate on the metaphyseal side and results in an exostosis that always points away from the joint of origin as the lesion moves away from the growth plate during the growing years.

Figure 6–12. Radiograph of Ollier disease of the upper and lower extremities.

Figure 6–13. Radiograph of a periosteal chondroma of the distal femur.

The bony base of an osteochondroma is in direct communication with the medullary canal of the bone from which it arises. These lesions can be either pedunculated, as is commonly seen around the knee, or sessile, as is typically seen in the proximal humerus. There must be an associated cartilaginous cap on the bony base to make the diagnosis of osteochondroma (Figure 6–14). This cap has the histologic features of a normal growth plate during the growing years. However, osteochondroma growth plate activity subsides at the same time as the activity in the larger plate from which the osteochondroma arose.

A familial form of osteochondroma, called hereditary multiple exostosis (HME), is an autosomal-dominant disorder that is one tenth as common as solitary osteochondroma. Three genetic loci are associated with HME involving the tumor suppressor *EXT* genes (*EXT1, EXT2,* and *EXT3*). This condition can vary from quite mild to extensive involvement with symmetric limb shortening. Forearm involvement can be quite deforming. The metaphyseal portions of long bones are deformed

and widened (Figures 6–15 and 6–16). The histologic findings in multiple exostoses are similar to those in solitary osteochondroma.

Conversion of solitary osteochondroma to chondrosarcoma occurs only during adulthood. The overall rate of conversion for all types of solitary lesions is quite rare. In HME, there is approximately a 1% chance of malignant conversion to secondary chondrosarcoma in the cartilaginous cap, especially in the larger, more proximal lesions.

Osteochondromas are stage 1 lesions. Most children and adults with a solitary osteochondroma are asymptomatic and therefore do not require surgical treatment. In some cases, the lesion may be palpable and irritating. Surgical removal is appropriate in these cases to address the symptoms only and not as a prophylaxis for chondrosarcomatous degeneration. In HME, symptomatic lesions are addressed surgically as needed. Corrective osteotomy is occasionally required because of angulatory deformity in the lower extremity. If a previously quiescent lesion begins to enlarge, in adults with either a solitary osteochondroma or with multiple exostoses, it

Figure 6–14. Radiograph of an osteochondroma of the distal femur.

Figure 6–15. Radiograph of multiple exostoses of both hips.

should be removed. The surgical margin should be wide enough to include the entire cartilaginous cap because this is where malignant degeneration can occur.

D. CHONDROBLASTOMA

The term *chondroblastoma* suggests a benign cartilage-forming tumor, but in fact this epiphyseal lesion of childhood has a histologic appearance that is more typical of the benign metaphyseal-epiphyseal giant cell tumor of young adulthood. The chondroblastoma is approximately one fifth as common as the giant cell tumor. It differs from other bone tumors in that it is almost always associated with epiphyseal or apophyseal bone. The majority of cases arise in the second decade of life. Males are affected more often than females. The most common location is the outer portion of the proximal humeral epiphysis, but other common locations are the distal femoral and proximal tibial epiphyseal areas. Because of its proximity to a joint, chondroblastoma can present with a symptomatic joint effusion.

In cases of chondroblastoma, the radiograph demonstrates a lytic tumor with a sharp sclerotic margin and central stippled or flocculated calcification occurring in the chondroid portion of the tumor (Figure 6–17). As the growth plate closes, the tumor can expand gradually into the metaphyseal area, and it sometimes becomes quite aneurysmal, as in the case of a giant cell tumor. The chondroblastoma has the histologic appearance of a giant cell tumor, with numerous macrophages seen usually in areas of hemorrhage. The stromal cells of the chondroblastoma are polyhedral, like those of a giant cell tumor, but with associated halos that give the chondroblastoma a so-called chicken-wire appearance. Although chondroid metaplasia in the chondroblastoma is not easy to find, it must be present to firmly establish the diagnosis. Most chondroblastomas are stage 2 lesions, but some can be stage 3.

The spontaneous conversion of chondroblastoma to a malignant tumor is extremely rare. However, as with the case of giant cell tumors, conversion to sarcoma can occur following radiation treatment. Even though the chondroblastoma is considered benign, it is reported to metastasize to the lung on rare occasions. Nevertheless, it carries an excellent prognosis.

Treatment for chondroblastoma consists of aggressive intralesional resection with curettage; bone graft or bone cement (polymethyl methacrylate) may be used to reconstruct the defect. It is our experience that this suffices, with local recurrence less than 10%. Some authors, however, recommend more aggressive marginal or wide resection.

E. CHONDROMYXOID FIBROMA

The chondromyxoid fibroma, a very rare tumor, generally affects males in the second or third decade of life. The most common location of the tumor is the proximal tibial metaphysis, followed by the distal femur and the first ray of the foot. The tumor is slow growing and accompanied by mild pain symptoms.

Figure 6–16. Radiograph of multiple exostoses in the knee.

Figure 6–17. Radiograph of a chondroblastoma in the proximal humeral epiphysis of a 15-year-old boy.

Radiographs of chondromyxoid fibroma show a lytic tumor with sharp sclerotic margins and a pseudoloculated pattern resembling that of a bone cyst. The tumor is eccentrically located in metaphyseal bone with a slightly dilated and thinned-out cortex similar to that shown in Figure 6–18. Histologic findings include a strange but specific mixture of fibrous, myxomatous, and chondroid tissues, which could mistakenly suggest the diagnosis of a chondrosarcoma. The findings also commonly include giant cells, which may suggest the diagnosis of a chondroblastoma seen in epiphyseal bone. This stage 2 lesion is quite active locally, especially in children. With simple curettage and bone grafting, the recurrence rate can approach 25%. Aggressive marginal excision should be performed. The conversion of chondromyxoid fibroma to chondrosarcoma is extremely rare.

Benign Fibrous Tumors of Bone

A. FIBROUS CORTICAL DEFECT

Fibrous cortical defects, or cortical desmoids, are small hamartomatous fibromas seen almost exclusively in the metaphyseal areas of the lower extremities of growing children. They can be multiple, and as many as 25% of normal children demonstrate these asymptomatic lesions at 5 years of age. The lesions tend to disappear as the result of bone remodeling before skeletal maturity. If excessive stress is placed across the lesions, they can become symptomatic and can also cause findings of increased activity on an isotope bone scan.

In the case of fibrous cortical defects, microscopic studies show benign-appearing fibroblasts with an occasional area of histiocytes, foam cells, and benign giant cells. The radiographic appearance is so characteristic of this entity

(Figure 6–19) that a biopsy is usually not necessary. These are stage 1 lesions and can generally be observed.

B. NONOSSIFYING FIBROMA

Just as the osteoblastoma is considered a larger or more extensive form of osteoid osteoma, the nonossifying fibroma is considered a larger form of the fibrous cortical defect. It is typically seen in the lower extremity of children. Because of its size, it may not entirely resolve by skeletal maturity and can persist into adult life. If the lesion is quite large, approaching 50% of the diameter of the bone, pathologic fracture may ensue. The fracture-healing process may facilitate resolution of the lesions. Careful consideration to fracture prophylaxis should be reserved for large lesions only in children older than 10 years. Nonossifying fibromas are stage 1 lesions, and neither they nor fibrous cortical defects require biopsy because their radiographic appearance is so characteristic.

With nonossifying fibroma, multiple lesions may take on the appearance of fibrous dysplasia and can be associated with café au lait skin defects. Large lesions in the

Figure 6–18. Radiograph of a chondromyxoid fibroma in the proximal tibia of an 11-year-old boy.

Figure 6–19. Radiograph of a metaphyseal fibrous defect in a 15-year-old boy.

proximal tibia can assume the appearance of a chondromyxoid fibroma (Figure 6–20). The lesions have a well-defined sclerotic margin and a pseudomultiloculated lytic center that gives them a soap-bubbly radiographic appearance. Histologically, they appear identical to fibrous cortical defects and are characterized by benign fibrous tissue speckled with areas of histiocytes, foam cells, and giant cells. As the lesion involutes in adulthood and the number of giant cells and histiocytes diminishes, large areas of cholesterol deposits become evident, which may suggest the diagnosis of a xanthofibroma or xanthoma of bone. Nonossifying fibromas are clearly separated from fibrous dysplasia by the absence of the metaplastic osteoid formation in the fibrous stroma.

C. FIBROUS DYSPLASIA

Fibrous dysplasia can present in a variety of ways: monostotic, polyostotic, and with or without associated syndromes (Figure 6–21). Most cases are diagnosed within the first three decades and have a distinct female predilection. The monostotic presentation is more common than polyostotic. This condition is a dysplastic anomaly of bone-forming mesenchymal tissue with an inability to produce mature lamellar bone. Accordingly, the bone is arrested in the woven state with a resultant proliferation of spindle cell fibroblasts. In the polyostotic form, it tends to involve one side of the body rather than bilaterally. Nevertheless, it can involve any bone of the body. The most common location is the proximal femur, where it results in the so-called shepherd's crook deformity. Other areas frequently involved include the tibia, pelvis, humerus, radius, and ribs.

In addition to bony involvement, patients can demonstrate café au lait skin pigmentation. These patches usually have a rough border, in contrast to the smooth border of those seen in neurofibromatosis. Patients with fibrous dysplasia may have associated endocrine problems. For example, 5% of patients with the polyostotic form of fibrous dysplasia also exhibit precocious puberty

(McCune-Albright syndrome). Other associated endocrine abnormalities include hyperthyroidism, acromegaly, Cushing disease, and hypophosphatemic osteomalacia. Polyostotic fibrous dysplasia with soft-tissue myxomas is known as Mazabrand syndrome. Fibrous dysplasia can also involve the skull and jaw bones, mimicking ossifying fibroma of jaw bone.

In fibrous dysplasia, microscopic findings include an alphabet-soup pattern of metaplastic woven bone scattered through a benign fibrous tissue stroma. This woven stroma has an absence of osteoblastic rimming. Foam cells, giant cells, and cholesterol deposits can be seen. Large cystic areas and even areas of cartilage formation are commonly present.

The molecular basis for fibrous dysplasia is associated with mutations affecting the alpha subunit of G protein. These mutations affect cells of the osteoblastic lineage, resulting in decreased differentiation and increased proliferation. These mutations cause constitutive elevation of cAMP in fibrous dysplasia and thus alter cAMP target genes such *c-fos, c-jun,* IL-6, and IL-11.

Figure 6–20. Radiograph of a nonossifying fibroma of the distal tibia.

Figure 6–21. Radiograph of polyostotic fibrous dysplasia of the pelvis.

Fibrous dysplasia tends to be active during the growing years and then burns out in adult life. Fewer than 1% of lesions convert to osteosarcoma, fibrosarcoma, or even chondrosarcoma. If conversion does occur, it almost always happens during adulthood. Generally, this disease is either stage 1 or 2.

In pediatric patients with active disease, curettage and grafting should be avoided because of high recurrence rates. The goals in treating pediatric patients should be the prevention and treatment of deformity, especially in the lower extremity. Most cases should become quiescent with skeletal maturity. If not, the best surgical treatment in adults consists of rigid fixation with an intramedullary implant with strut grafting as needed. The best surgical treatment in adults consists of the use of long autogenous fibular struts combined with autogenous cancellous bone graft. This treatment has a higher success rate in the adult group than in the pediatric group. Medical management with bisphosphonates is of benefit in some cases. Irradiation is contraindicated because it may lead to irradiation-induced sarcoma at a later date.

Cystic Lesions of Bone

A. SIMPLE BONE CYST

Simple bone cysts are a common pseudotumor of bone and the most frequent cause of pathologic fractures in children. Bone cysts typically affect patients between 5 and 15 years of age and occur more often in boys than in girls (2:1) with an incidence of 1 per 10,000 children per year. They are found in the proximal humerus in 50% of cases and in the upper femur in 25%. Patients are asymptomatic until a pathologic fracture occurs. Fractures seem to arise from the central metaphyseal side of an epiphyseal or apophyseal growth plate. The cystic process continues to grow away from the physis. When it remains in contact with the physis it is termed "active." When it separates it is termed "inactive."

Radiographs typically show a solitary cyst that is centrally located in the metaphyseal area and has marked thinning of the adjacent cortical bone and a pseudoloculated appearance (Figure 6–22). The bone cyst is filled with a clear serous fluid, and there is increased pressure during the active phase. The fact that this pressure gradually decreases as the cyst becomes inactive suggests a hydrodynamic mechanism.

The cyst cavity, lined with a fibrinous membrane that contains giant cells, foam cells, and a slight osteoid formation, is similar to the fibrous tissues seen in other fibrous bone lesions, including fibrous dysplasia. The periosteal covering in the area of a cyst is normal, and thus the pathologic fractures heal normally and in most cases do not require surgery. Unfortunately, the cyst usually persists after fracture union and requires further treatment. Bone-resorbing factors, such as matrix metalloproteinases, prostaglandins, IL-1, IL-6, tumor necrosis factor alpha (TNF), and oxygen free radicals, are demonstrated in the cyst fluid. Elevated nitrate and nitrite levels are also noted to be higher in the cyst fluid than in serum.

Before the mid-1970s, the standard treatment for a solitary bone cyst was aggressive curettage or even resection followed by bone grafting. In patients with active disease, the recurrence rate was 30–50%, and repeated grafting was frequently necessary. In patients with inactive disease, particularly those older than 15 years, the surgical results were much better and the recurrence rate was lower. Unicameral bone cysts are generally considered

Figure 6–22. Radiograph of a solitary bone cyst on the proximal humerus of a 13-year-old boy.

stage 1 lesions, but occasionally they may be stage 2. Currently, treatment is a function of location. In weight-bearing bones, such as the proximal femur, lesions should be treated aggressively. Initial management usually involves aspiration/injection with either bone marrow or corticosteroid. The injections are carried out with bone biopsy needles and are repeated three to five times at intervals of 2–3 months, depending on the radiographic response. The best results are when the patient is between 5 and 15 years of age, at which time the disease is active and macrophage activity is greatest in the cyst lining. Curettage and bone grafting may also be an effective modality. Demineralized bone matrix injected in combination with autogenous bone marrow shows encouraging results, with an approximately 20% recurrence rate and low morbidity.

Physicians should note that sarcomas can take on the radiographic appearance of a solitary bone cyst. For this reason, if needle aspiration does not reveal cystic fluid or if it is impossible to inject contrast material and obtain radiologic confirmation of the diagnosis, an open biopsy is indicated to rule out a sarcoma.

B. ANEURYSMAL BONE CYST

Aneurysmal bone cyst is a hemorrhagic lesion with many characteristics of a giant cell tumor but occurs only half as frequently. Although 75% of the cases of aneurysmal bone cyst occur in patients 10–20 years old, giant cell tumor is rare in patients younger than 20 years of age. Both aneurysmal bone cyst and giant cell tumor are more common in females than in males. The femur is the most frequently affected site, followed by the tibia, pelvis, and spine. In the spine, two thirds of aneurysmal bone cysts arise from posterior elements and one third arise from the vertebral body, whereas most giant cell tumors arise from the vertebral body.

Initially, the aneurysmal bone cyst appears on radiograph as an aggressive osteolytic lesion with extensive permeative cortical destruction that gives the impression of a malignant process such as Ewing sarcoma or hemorrhagic osteosarcoma. Next, a large aneurysmal bulge occurs outside the bone, with a thin reactive shell of bone forming at the outer edge. Less soap-bubbly pseudoseptation is seen in an aneurysmal bone cyst than in a solitary cyst (Figure 6–23).

At the time of biopsy, the aneurysmal bone lesion demonstrates large hemorrhagic cysts, but bleeding is modest. The hemorrhagic cysts are broken up by thick spongy fibrous septa that histologically contain great numbers of large giant cells and have thin osteoid seams. Even if a few mitotic figures are seen, the diagnosis of a benign lesion can remain. A carefully placed biopsy with multiple samples is needed to rule out other well-known skeletal tumors that may demonstrate an aneurysmal component. These include giant cell tumor, chondromyxoid fibroma, and malignant hemorrhagic osteo-

Figure 6–23. Radiograph of an aneurysmal bone cyst on the proximal femur of a 5-year-old boy.

sarcoma. Some authors believe there is no such entity as the aneurysmal bone cyst and that it is merely a morphologic variant of some other underlying neoplastic process. Like the solitary bone cyst, this cyst may have a hydraulic pressure origin that is secondary to hemorrhage and could be traumatically induced. However, abnormal cytogenetic findings were noted in aneurysmal bone cysts, which may suggest a distinct cellular pathogenetic etiology. Specifically, a t(16,17) translocation resulting in a CDH11-USP6 fusion gene product is frequently observed in aneurysmal bone cyst. Aneurysmal bone cyst is either a stage 2 or 3 lesion and frequently symptomatic.

If an aneurysmal cyst is left untreated, it may involute spontaneously, during which time it develops a heavy shell of reactive bone at the periphery. This involutional process can be hastened by surgical curettage and bone grafting. Radiation is no longer recommended. Another option for treating extremely large lesions is repeated embolization to reduce the rate of hemorrhagic expansion.

C. EPIDERMOID CYST

The least common bone cyst is the epidermoid bone cyst. This lesion is found either in the distal phalanx or in the skull. No other bone is affected. In the case of the phalanx, the cyst is usually the result of nail bed epithelium being driven into the subjacent distal phalanx by a crushing blow. The ectopic squamous epithelium produces a keratinized cavity that is filled with clear fluid and creates a surface erosion with a sclerotic reactive base (Figure 6–24). The bulbous cyst seen at the fingertip transilluminates with flashlight examination. Other conditions that might have a similar appearance are the glomus tumor and the enchondroma. The epidermoid cyst is treated with a simple curettage and, in some cases, a bone graft.

Figure 6–24. Radiograph of an epidermoid cyst in the distal phalanx.

Giant Cell Tumor of Bone

Numerous types of tumors contain giant cells but are not true benign giant cell tumors. Most of the variants are seen in children and include aneurysmal bone cyst, chondroblastoma, simple bone cyst, osteoid osteoma, and osteoblastoma. The giant cell–rich osteosarcoma is the most malignant of the variants, and it is sometimes difficult to distinguish from an aggressive benign giant cell tumor. The giant cell reparative granuloma is a benign variant seen in jaw bones or hand bones and has more spindle cells than a classic giant cell tumor. The brown tumor of hyperparathyroidism is a nonneoplastic variant seen in both primary and secondary hyperparathyroidism. Only after all of the variant conditions are excluded can the diagnosis of benign giant cell tumor be made. Giant cell tumor of bone is now associated with overexpression of osteoprotegerin ligand (OPGL), an important stimulator of osteoclast differentiation, suggesting overactivity of osteoclast in the etiology of this neoplasm.

Between 5% and 10% of all benign bone tumors are true giant cell tumors, occurring most frequently in the third decade of life. They are more frequently found in females than in males. In approximately half of the cases, the tumor is found about the knee. The next most common locations are the distal radius and sacrum. The tumor is usually painful for several months prior to diagnosis and can cause a pathologic fracture. It can also cause a painful effusion because of its juxtaposition to a major joint. Giant cell tumors may present as either stage 2 or stage 3 disease and less frequently as stage 1. On radiograph, the lesion appears lytic in nature and is located in the epiphyseal-metaphyseal end of a long bone (Figure 6–25). The lesion grows toward the joint surface and frequently comes into contact with articular cartilage but rarely breaks into the joint.

Like the chondroblastoma, the benign giant cell tumor has a 1–2% chance of metastasizing to the lung. Recurrent tumors have a 6% chance. Accordingly, pulmonary staging is an importantcomponent in the initial evaluation and follow-up of giant cell tumor of bone. The prognosis for survival with this complication is favorable, and the tumors may resolve spontaneously. The benign giant cell tumor can later convert to a malignant condition such as an osteosarcoma or malignant fibrous histiocytoma. It is generally believed that this is secondary to treatment. A conversion rate of 15–20% is reported in patients who were treated previously with more than 3000 cGy of radiation, with conversion occurring 3 or more years after treatment. The conversion rate in patients who do not receive radiation therapy is less than 5%. This finding has come into question with newer radiation therapy modalities.

Until recent years, the standard treatment for giant cell tumor was curettage and bone grafting. The recurrence

Figure 6–25. Radiograph of a giant cell tumor on the proximal tibia of a 22-year-old woman.

rate with this treatment was reported as up to more than 50%. Follow-up treatment consisted of an aggressive resection of the recurrent lesion and reconstruction with a large osteoarticular allograft, endoprosthesis, or an excisional arthrodesis. Currently, most surgeons elect an aggressive curettage, followed by high-speed burring and adjuvant phenol, hydrogen peroxide, or liquid nitrogen and by the subsequent packing of the defect with bone cement. With this new approach, the recurrence rate is between 10% and 25%. When giant cell tumor infrequently involves an expendable bone such as the proximal fibula or ilium, it should be primarily resected. En bloc resection continues to be used to treat multiple recurrent tumors, intensive soft-tissue involvement, or massively destructive cases. Embolization may also prove palliative or curative in unresectable cases. For advanced, multiply recurrent, or aggressive metastatic cases, investigators are developing experimental medical protocols. Close follow-up for locally recurrent disease and pulmonary involvement is critical. Surveillance should include a plain chest radiograph every 6–12 months for the first 2–3 years at least.

Hemangioma

Hemangioma of bone is a hamartomatous process that occurs more frequently in females than in males. It is most commonly found in vertebral bodies (Figure 6–26). It is found only rarely in the diaphysis of long bone. Hemangiomas of bone can be associated with hemangiomas of soft tissue. The spinal lesion is usually discovered as an incidental radiographic finding and demonstrates a characteristic vertically oriented honeycombed or moth-eaten appearance. On rare occasions, a lesion can cause cord compression that may require surgical resection. In such cases, preoperative angiography is critical in evaluating the vascular blood supply to the spinal cord. Alternatively an attempt at arterial embolization may prove successful and is less aggressive.

Gorham disease, characterized by massive osteolysis in children or young adults, is usually associated with the presence of benign cavernous hemangiomas or lymphangiomas of bone. This strange condition usually affects a particular area (such as the spine or the hip) but can involve multiple bones of that area and tends to resolve spontaneously.

Figure 6–26. Radiograph of a hemangioma of the tibia in a 14-year-old boy.

Baruffi MR et al: Aneurysmal bone cyst with chromosomal changes involving 7q and 16p. Cancer Genet Cytogenet 2001;129(2): 177. [PMID: 11566352]

Bottner F et al: Cyclooxygenase-2 inhibitor for pain management in osteoid osteoma. Clin Orthop 2001;393:258. [PMID: 11764357]

Boutou-Bredaki S et al: Prognosis of giant cell tumor of bone. Histopathological analysis of 15 cases and review of the literature. Adv Clin Path 2001;5(3):71. [PMID: 11753878]

Bovee JV et al: Malignant progression in multiple enchondromatosis (Ollier's disease): An autopsy-based molecular genetic study. Hum Pathol 2000;31(10):1299. [PMID: 11070122]

Cantwell CP et al: Current trends in treatment of osteoid osteoma with an emphasis on radiofrequency ablation. Eur Radiol 2004;14(4):607. [PMID: 14663625]

Cheung P et al: Etiological point mutations in the hereditary multiple exostoses gene EXT1: A functional analysis of heparan sulfate polymerase activity. Am J Hum Genet 2001;69(1):55. [PMID: 11391482]

Flemming DJ et al: Primary tumors of the spine. Semin Musculoskelet Radiol 2000;4(3):299. [PMID: 11371321]

Gallazzi MB et al: Percutaneous radio-frequency ablation of osteoid osteoma: Technique and preliminary results. Radiol Med (Torino) 2001;102(5-6):329. [PMID: 11779979]

Kivioja A et al: Chondrosarcoma in a family with multiple hereditary exostoses. J Bone Joint Surg Br 2000;82(2):261. [PMID: 10755438]

Komiya S et al: Increased concentrations of nitrate and nitrite in the cyst fluid suggesting increased nitric oxide synthesis in solitary bone cysts. J Orthop Res 2000;18(2):281. [PMID: 10815830]

Lindner NJ et al: Percutaneous radiofrequency ablation in osteoid osteoma. J Bone Joint Surg Br 2001;83(3):391. [PMID: 11341426]

Maki M et al: Comparative study of fibrous dysplasia and osteofibrous dysplasia: Histopathological, immunohistochemical, argyrophilic nucleolar organizer region and DNA ploidy analysis. Pathol Int 2001;51(8):603. [PMID: 11564214]

Marie PJ: Cellular and molecular basis of fibrous dysplasia. Histol Histopathol 2001;16(3):981. [PMID: 11510989]

Nakase T et al: Involvement of BMP-2 signaling in a cartilage cap in osteochondroma. J Orthop Res 2001;19(6):1085. [PMID: 11781009]

Oliveira AM et al: USP6 (Tre2) fusion oncogenes in aneurysmal bone cyst. Cancer Res 2004;64(6):1920. [PMID: 15026324]

Ramappa AJ et al: Chondroblastoma of bone. J Bone Joint Surg Am 2000;82-A(8):1140. [PMID: 10954104]

Randall RL et al: Aggressive aneurysmal bone cyst of the proximal humerus. Clin Orthop 2000;(370):212. [PMID: 10660716]

Robinson P et al: Periosteal chondroid tumors: Radiologic evaluation with pathologic correlation. Am J Roentgenol 2001; 177(5):1183. [PMID: 11641198]

Rougraff BT et al: Treatment of active unicameral bone cysts with percutaneous injection of demineralized bone matrix and autogenous bone marrow. J Bone Joint Surg Am 2002;84-A(6):921. [PMID: 12063325]

Safar A et al: Recurrent anomalies of 6q25 in chondromyxoid fibroma. Hum Pathol 2000;31(3):306. [PMID: 10746672]

Soder S et al: Cell biology and matrix biochemistry of chondromyxoid fibroma. Am J Clin Pathol 2001;116(2):271. [PMID: 11488075]

Yanagawa T et al: The natural history of disappearing bone tumours and tumour-like conditions. Clin Radiol 2001;56(11): 877. [PMID: 11603890]

MALIGNANT BONE TUMORS

Osteoid-Forming Sarcomas

Aside form multiple myeloma, osteosarcoma of bone is the most common primary malignant tumor of bone, constituting 20% of all primary malignancies of bone. In the United States, between 500 and 1000 new cases are diagnosed each year. The global incidence is felt to be between 1 and 3 per million people annually. There are currently many subtypes of osteoid-forming sarcomas, ranging from the extremely low-grade variants, such as the parosteal osteosarcoma, to the extremely high-grade variants, such as osteosarcoma secondary to Paget disease.

The molecular pathobiology of osteosarcoma is a subject of intense investigation. Several gene families were investigated as potential biomarkers of disease progression. Among these are genes involved in angiogenesis (eg, vascular endothelial growth factor, or VEGF), growth factors and their receptors (eg, transforming growth factor-beta, Wnt receptor LRP5, *HER2*), cytoskeletal protein (eg, ezrin), and cellular senescent protein (ie, telomerase).

This discussion begins with the more common, central form of sarcoma that is seen in children and known as classic osteosarcoma.

A. CLASSIC OSTEOSARCOMA

The classic form of osteosarcoma is typically seen in patients in their second or third decade, with a peak in the adolescent growth spurt. It occurs more frequently in males than in females and is found in the metaphyseal

areas of long bones, with 50% of lesions seen about the knee joint (Figures 6–27 and 6–28). The distal femur is the most common site, followed by the proximal tibia and then the proximal humerus. It is rare to see osteosarcoma in small bones of the feet or hands or in the spine. When seen in the foot, it occur in the larger bones of the hindfoot. The prognosis is more favorable for a tumor in a small bone than for one in a large bone.

Most patients with classic osteosarcoma have symptoms of pain before a tumor mass is noticeable. A mass near a major joint may exist for several weeks or even as long as 4 months before a diagnosis is made. Dilated veins may be seen in the overlying skin. The radiographic findings include permeated lytic destruction of metaphyseal bone, with eventual cortical breakthrough into the subperiosteal space and subsequent formation of the Codman triangle at the diaphyseal end of the tumor. As the tumor continues to push its way into the extracortical soft tissue, a typical sunburst pattern neoplastic bone may be seen outside the involved bone.

In less than 2–25% of cases, an additional lesion may be found at a higher level in the femur. Such a so-called

Figure 6–27. Osteosarcoma of the distal femur of a 15-year-old female patient. Notice the sunburst appearance.

Figure 6–28. Gross surgical specimen from Figure 6–27. Notice the sharp upper medullary margin located about the same level as the extracortical mass. The tumor has not invaded the growth plate.

skip lesion may portend a worse probability of survival and should be considered a true metastatic focus (stage III [Enneking], stage IV [AJCC]). Approximately 50% of osteosarcomas are of the more typical osteoblastic type, followed by chondroblastic, with a small percentage of them fibroblastic. Whether the subtype portends a better or worse prognosis is controversial. Confounding variables such as multidrug resistance (*p*-glycoprotein expression) may be differentially expressed in different subtypes. *P*-glycoprotein overexpression itself bears a substantial relationship to clinical outcome.

Staging of osteosarcoma must include an MRI of the involved extremity (Figure 6–29). This technique offers excellent contrast of the extracortical portion of the tumor and at the same time gives good intramedullary contrast of the high-signal tumor next to a low-signal fatty marrow. The periphery of the tumor can readily be appreciated and represents the most anaplastic and rapidly growing part of the tumor. This region is the best tissue for a biopsy because it is easy to reach, soft enough for a diagnostic fro-

zen section, and representative of the most aggressive portion of the tumor. Furthermore, the MRI provides the necessary anatomic data to determine the level of transection through the femur for a safe margin and to determine whether a limb-sparing procedure is feasible.

Before the advent of adjuvant multidrug chemotherapy, the treatment for osteosarcoma was radical amputation. Eighty percent of these patients proceeded to die from disseminated pulmonary disease. Today, with the combination of chemotherapy and surgical treatment, the prognosis for 5-year survival approaches 70%.

The drugs commonly used today include high-dose methotrexate, doxorubicin, cisplatin, and ifosfamide. They are administered intravenously in cyclic intervals of 3–4 weeks for approximately 11–15 weeks prior to surgery. Surveillance imaging studies are performed during this period to assess possible reduction in tumor volume. Tumor necrosis secondary to neoadjuvant chemotherapy, determined at the time of tumor resection, is an important prognostic factor. Patients with greater than 90% tumor necrosis have a significantly improved 5-year survival rate, approaching 85%. Approximately half

Figure 6–29. Fat-subtraction (STIR [short tau inversion recovery]) MRI of a femoral osteosarcoma.

of patients demonstrate this response to current chemotherapy regimens. Furthermore, the postoperative drug regimen can be adjusted based on this evaluation.

In extremity osteosarcoma, limb-sparing surgery, with wide resection of the tumor, is the standard approach. Amputation is reserved for the exceptional or recurrent case. In less than 10% of cases, amputation is performed at a level approximately 5 cm above the upper pole of the tumor. Limb salvage techniques continue to evolve with reconstruction options including large prostheses, structural allografts, and composites reconstructions. Endoprosthetics are composed of modular components in various lengths, linked together with taper fittings (Figures 6–30 and 6–31). The intramedullary stems are of various diameters and lengths and usually cemented. The immediate functional results are excellent, with minimal early compli-

A   **B**

Figure 6–30. **A:** Two examples of distal femoral replacement systems. **B:** Modularity of system allows different-size intercalary body segments.

its pathogenesis. The *p53* suppressor genes have an increased mutation rate in osteosarcoma. However, wild-type *TP53* and *MDM2* assays in and of themselves are not of prognostic value. Loss of heterozygosity of the *Rb* gene is a predictive feature of osteosarcoma. The *F33* isoform also demonstrates a strong correlation with osteosarcoma disease progression. *ErbB-2* (*HER-2/neu*), a protooncogene and transforming growth factor-beta, isoform 3 expression is also correlated with a worse prognosis in osteosarcoma patients. Controversy surrounds the significance of cytoplasmic versus membranous staining in *HER-2/*neu expression as relates to prognosis in osteosarcoma.

B. HEMORRHAGIC OR TELANGIECTATIC OSTEOSARCOMA

Telangiectatic osteosarcoma, an extremely lytic and destructive variant of classic osteosarcoma, is seen in the same age group and location. Its radiographic appearance is similar to that of an aneurysmal bone cyst, thereby making the diagnosis difficult (Figure 6–32). The pathologic specimen is hemorrhagic, with micro-

Figure 6–31. Lateral radiograph of distal femoral replacement system in skeletally immature patient. Expansion with larger intercalary body is possible.

cations. However, subsequent loosening at 5–10 years occurs in as many as 15–30% of cases. Another limb-sparing procedure consists of the use of an osteoarticular allograft alone or in combination with a prosthesis. The major drawback with large bone allografts is a 10–15% chance of infection, nonunion, or stress fracture, especially in the immunosuppressed patient receiving chemotherapy. The use of an excisional arthrodesis was more popular in the past but is rarely elected today because patients have better function with a mobile joint.

Prior to the introduction of chemotherapy, the finding of a pulmonary metastasis portended a very poor prognosis. Today, however, in larger tumor centers where aggressive surgical approaches with multiple thoracotomies and continued chemotherapy are used, the 5-year survival rate is approximately 30%.

Molecular oncologic evaluation of osteosarcoma specimens is beginning to elucidate factors involved in

Figure 6–32. Radiograph of hemorrhagic osteosarcoma in a 6-year-old girl.

scopic evaluation demonstrating the presence of malignant-appearing stromal cells with giant cells.

Because hemorrhagic osteosarcoma is a high-grade, purely lytic tumor, the incidence of pathologic fracture in the early course of the disease is high. If significant contamination of the adjacent neurovascular structures results, a pathologic fracture may necessitate amputation rather than limb salvage (Figure 6–33). This situation must be carefully evaluated with a preoperative MRI. Accordingly, in cases with significant risk for fracture during the preoperative treatment regiment, it may be appropriate to immobilize the involved extremity or proceed with limb-sparing surgery earlier than usual. Prior to the advent of aggressive multidrug chemotherapy, the prognosis for patients with hemorrhagic osteosarcoma was extremely poor. At present, however, it is the same as the prognosis for patients who have classic osteosarcoma and is treated with similar protocols.

C. Parosteal Osteosarcoma

Parosteal osteosarcoma is a low-grade variant arising in an exophytic pattern from the cortical surface of bone. There is no medullary involvement. It is low-grade with a 5-year survival rate in excess of 90% and a 10-year survival rate of 80%. It accounts for 3–4% of all osteosarcomas.

The tumor is composed of a spindle-cell fibroblastic component with well-developed bone trabeculae. There also may be areas of cartilage present. Osteoblasts are well differentiated, and few mitotic figures are present.

Parosteal osteosarcoma is more common in females than in males and affects a slightly older age group than classic osteosarcoma (see Table 6–2). It is a slow-growing tumor with minimal symptoms initially. It is metaphyseal in origin, with the vast majority of cases involving the posterior aspect of the distal femur (Figure 6–34).

Because the parosteal osteosarcoma is low grade, it does not respond well to either chemotherapy or radiation therapy. Therefore, the only treatment is wide surgical resection. This usually requires distal femoral removal, but in smaller cases side resection of the posterior cortex and tumor only may be feasible, sparing the knee joint. Nevertheless, a negative tumor margin is imperative. Otherwise, recurrence is likely. Recurrence may occur as late as 5–10 years because of the tumor's slow growth.

On occasion, low-grade parosteal osteosarcoma can dedifferentiate into a high-grade sarcoma. Such a lesion carries a similar prognosis to classic osteosarcoma.

D. Periosteal Osteosarcoma

Periosteal osteosarcoma is another surface osteosarcoma of low to intermediate grade. This lesion represents less than 2% of all osteosarcomas. It arises beneath the periosteum, elevating it and inducing vigorous neoosteogenesis with a predominant chondroblastic differentiation. It is slightly more common in females, with a peak incidence in the

Figure 6–33. Clinical photograph of patient that sustained a pathologic fracture through a distal femur osteosarcoma contaminating the neurovascular structures precluding limb salvage.

B

A

Figure 6–34. Radiograph (**A**) and CT scan (**B**) of a parosteal osteosarcoma of the distal femur in a 21-year-old woman.

second decade of life. It almost exclusively arises in the long bone. The lesion can mimic an aneurysmal bone cyst or periosteal chondroma radiographically (Figure 6–35).

Because of its low to intermediate grade, periosteal osteosarcoma is generally not treated with chemotherapy but may be in more advanced cases. Wide surgical resection is the modality of choice. Because periosteal osteosarcoma is a low-grade tumor, it carries a better prognosis than the classic osteosarcoma. Approximately 25% of patients succumb to metastatic disease within 2–3 years. The surgical treatment is usually a limb-sparing procedure, and because the tumor is more diaphyseal in location, the adjacent joints may often be spared.

E. Secondary Osteosarcoma

Osteosarcoma can arise from benign disease through a process that may involve a second mutation and usually occurs at a later age (see Table 6–2). Among the benign conditions that can result in secondary osteosarcoma are Paget disease, osteoblastoma, fibrous dysplasia, benign giant cell tumor, bone infarction, and chronic osteomyelitis.

The classic example of a secondary osteosarcoma is seen in a small percentage of patients with Paget disease. Pagetic osteosarcomas, which represent approximately 3% of all osteosarcomas, are the most common osteosarcomas in the older (more than 65 years) age group. The most frequent location for pagetic osteosarcoma is the humerus, followed next by the pelvis and femur. The typical patient has a long history (15–25 years) of dull, aching pain associated with the inflammation of Paget disease before a new acute pain arises in an area of recent lytic destruction and the diagnosis of pagetic osteosarcoma is established (Figure 6–36). The prognosis for patients with pagetic osteosarcoma is extremely poor (5-year survival rate of approximately 8%). Because of the older age group involved, chemotherapy is usually not an option secondary to intolerance.

F. Low-Grade Intramedullary Osteosarcoma

Another rare and low-grade osseofibrous variant of osteosarcoma is the central or intramedullary form. Although this variant has a microscopic appearance similar to that of the parosteal osteosarcoma, it is usually located in metaphyseal bone about the knee joint in adults between 15 and 65 years of age. Males and females are equally affected. Radiographically, intramedullary osteosarcoma creates a sclerotic density in metaphyseal bone (Figure 6–37). Like the parosteal osteosarcoma, the low-grade intramedullary osteosar-

Figure 6–35. Radiograph of a periosteal osteosarcoma of the distal tibia in a 15-year-old boy.

coma carries an excellent prognosis and can be treated with local surgery alone.

G. IRRADIATION-INDUCED OSTEOSARCOMA

Radiation-induced osteosarcoma may arise after any form of significant radiation exposure (in excess of 30 Gy) (Figure 6–38). Onset is usually delayed an average of 15 years (range: 3–55). Other irradiation-induced sarcomas, besides the osteosarcoma type, include irradiation-induced fibrosarcoma and malignant fibrohistiocytoma. All of these secondary sarcomas are invariably high grade and carry a poor prognosis for survival, with a very high rate of metastasis.

H. MULTICENTRIC OSTEOSARCOMA

Multicentric osteosarcoma has two clinical presentations: (1) synchronous, occurring in childhood and adolescents, and (2) metachronous, occurring in adults. The synchronous type is a high-grade sclerosing intramedullary type, which is lethal. The adult form is less aggressive, with a lower histologic appearance, but prognosis remains grim (Figure 6–39).

I. SOFT-TISSUE OSTEOSARCOMA

Osteosarcoma can occur in muscle tissue outside bone and accounts for approximately 4% of all osteosarcomas (Figure 6–40). Soft-tissue osteosarcoma is rarely seen in patients younger than 40 years. The number of cases is equal in males and females, and the tumor is usually seen in large muscle groups of the pelvis and thigh areas.

Soft-tissue osteosarcoma must be differentiated from the more common myositis ossificans. Although soft-tissue osteosarcoma shows heavy mineralization in the central area (see Figure 6–40), myositis ossificans has a zonal pattern of ossification, with the mature dense ossification concentrating at the periphery of the lesion.

The treatment of the soft-tissue form of osteosarcoma is the same as for the high-grade osseous form and includes a wide resection and adjuvant chemotherapy. The prognosis is worse with the soft-tissue form of osteosarcoma, with a high rate of chemotherapy resistance.

Figure 6–36. Radiograph of a pagetic osteosarcoma of the tibia.

A

Figure 6–37. Radiograph (A) and CT scan (B) of a low-grade intramedullary osteosarcoma in the distal femur of a 65-year-old man.

Chondroid-Forming Sarcomas

Chondroid-forming sarcomas are a heterogenous group of neoplasms consisting of a cartilage-based histology. A cornerstone to the diagnosis of chondrosarcoma is the absence of osteoid formation. If any osteoid is present with a malignant stroma, the tumor is considered an osteosarcoma with chondroblastic features. It is important to make the distinction because chondrosarcomas behave differently from osteosarcomas. However, this can be a difficult task. The surgeon must consider the age of the patient and carefully assess the radiographic and histologic features to confirm the diagnosis.

A. PRIMARY OR CENTRAL CONVENTIONAL CHONDROSARCOMA

The typical primary chondrosarcoma is a low-grade tumor seen in adults between 30 and 60 years of age. The tumor is found more frequently in men than in women. Minimal symptoms of pain may occur over a period of several years before a radiograph is obtained. The pelvis and femur are the most common locations, followed by the rib cage, proximal humerus, scapula, and upper tibia. Primary chondrosarcoma is extremely rare in small bones, including the hand and foot. The metaphysis is the most common location in a long bone; however, a diaphyseal location is not unusual.

Figure 6–38. Radiograph of irradiation-induced osteosarcoma of the peritrochanteric area in a 35-year-old woman.

Figure 6–39. Isotope bone scan of multicentric osteosarcoma in an 8-year-old girl.

Approximately 85% of central chondrosarcomas are low-grade lesions with a typical matrix calcification that can be described as flocculated. The high-grade lesions are rare, and radiographically they lose their typical lobulated and calcific pattern and take on the appearance of a more permeative high-grade tumor, such as a malignant fibrous histiocytoma. At the same time, histologically the high-grade chondrosarcomas lose their chondroid matrix pattern, which is replaced with that of a more aggressive spindle-cell tumor.

The radiologic feature that clearly separates this lesion from a benign enchondroma is the permeative lysis seen in the surrounding cortex (Figure 6–41). Because of the weakened cortex, the patient usually complains of local pain not experienced with an enchondroma. Because most chondrosarcomas are low grade, they do not respond well to adjuvant irradiation or chemotherapy. Therefore, aggressive surgical management is imperative. However, optimal surgical management is controversial. Although wide en bloc

resection is ideal from a margin standpoint, it can often produce considerable morbidity. On the contrary, aggressive intralesional resection (curettage) and margin expansion with an adjuvant therapy (eg, phenol or liquid nitrogen) can reduce morbidity and may provide equal local control. In fact, some authors found that for grade 1 chondrosarcoma the margin of resection is not significant in terms of local recurrence or disease progression.

In general, the prognosis for low-grade central chondrosarcoma is very good, with a low rate of pulmonary metastasis if the primary lesion is widely resected. Nevertheless, recurrences can occur late, even over 15 years later. For any intermediate- or high-grade chondrosarcoma, wide, en bloc resection is mandatory (Figure 6–42).

B. SECONDARY CHONDROSARCOMA

The vast majority of secondary chondrosarcomas arise from osteochondromas in patients afflicted with HME.

Figure 6–40. Radiograph of a soft-tissue osteosarcoma in the calf area of a 67-year-old man.

Figure 6–41. Radiograph of a low-grade primary chondrosarcoma in the distal femur of an 83-year-old man.

Patients with solitary osteochondromas do not generally form secondary chondrosarcomas in their lesions, making prophylactic removal unnecessary and unwarranted unless the solitary lesion is otherwise symptomatic. Even in patients with HME, the rate of malignant degeneration is less than 1% and generally does not occur in patients prior to skeletal maturity. However, patients with secondary chondrosarcoma tend to be younger than those with primary chondrosarcomas (see Table 6–2). The lesions tend to be slow growing with minimal to mild symptoms. The most common site is the pelvis, followed by the proximal femur, proximal humerus, and ribs. Plain radiographs demonstrate a flocculated calcific pattern (Figure 6–43). Anything thicker than 1–2 cm should raise suspicion of a secondary chondrosarcoma. The overall prognosis for patients with secondary or peripheral chondrosarcoma is even better than that for patients with primary or central chondrosarcoma. Surgical removal, without violation of the cartilage cap, is the only effective treatment modality.

C. DEDIFFERENTIATED CHONDROSARCOMA

Dedifferentiated chondrosarcoma is the most malignant variant of chondrosarcoma, accounting for between 5% and 10% of all chondrosarcomas. It is heralded by the transformation of areas of conventional chondrosarcoma into malignant fibrous histiocytoma or osteosarcoma. Histologically, it is characterized by two distinct but neighboring areas of low- to intermediate-grade malignant chondroid tumor and heterogenous high-grade sarcoma. Dedifferentiated chondrosarcoma occurs in older patients, usually between 50 and 70 years of age. It is found in the same areas affected by central primary chondrosarcomas, including the pelvis, femur, and proximal humerus (Figure 6–44). Radiographs show areas of rarefaction within the tumor with cortical attenuation. Pathologic fracture is not uncommon.

The prognosis in dedifferentiated chondrosarcoma is bleak, with the majority of patients developing and dying of metastatic disease within 1 year (historically, 1-year survival rate approached 10%). Chemotherapy and radiation therapy are less effective than in a malignant fibrous histiocytoma or osteosarcoma that arose de novo. Surgical resection remains the mainstay of treatment, with adjuvant modalities employed in younger patients.

D. CLEAR CELL CHONDROSARCOMA

Clear cell chondrosarcoma is a rare low-grade variant of chondrosarcoma. Clear cell lesions occur more often in males than in females and are usually seen in patients between 20 and 50 years of age. The vast majority of lesions are found in the femoral head (Figure 6–45). The radiographic appearance is one of a lytic tumor with sharp margination and a central matrix calcification, creating the appearance of a chondroblastoma. Although microscopic examination reveals the presence of some giant cells, as seen in a chondroblastoma, areas of low-grade chondrosarcoma are also evident in which no giant cells are seen. Even on gross examination, the clear cell chondrosarcoma does not look like a chondrosarcoma, which explains why it is frequently mistaken for a chondroblastoma in younger adult patients. The tumor cells have abundant glycogen, giving them their characteristic clear cell phenotype. Although no significant genetic alteration is found in clear cell chondrosarcoma, newer findings show that alkaline phosphatase activity may correlate with prognosis.

The treatment for clear cell chondrosarcoma is a wide excision and reconstruction. The prognosis with this type of treatment is good. In contrast, when lesions are mistaken for chondroblastomas and treatment consists of a simple curettage and bone grafting, the prognosis is poor and the recurrence rate is high.

Figure 6–42. Preoperative radiograph of a large central chondrosarcoma in the proximal humerus of a 52-year-old woman (**A**), placement of a Neer prosthesis (**B**), and postoperative radiograph (**C**).

Figure 6–43. CT scan of a secondary peripheral chondrosarcoma in the ilium of a 56-year-old man with multiple exostoses.

E. MESENCHYMAL CHONDROSARCOMA

Another rare variant of chondrosarcoma is the mesenchymal chondrosarcoma. It is a highly cellular tumor composed of primitive mesenchymal cells with foci of cartilage differentiation. This tumor involves the soft tissue in a third of cases, occurs more frequently in females than in males, and is seen in young adults (see Table 6–2). The jaw is the most common location, followed by the spine and ribs, with very few cases noted in long bones.

Mesenchymal chondrosarcoma is a high-grade tumor with histologic features of low-grade chondrosarcoma. Heavily calcified areas, mixed with areas of malignant round cells, may give it the appearance of Ewing sarcoma or hemangiopericytoma.

Treatment consists of resection, with a wide margin if possible, and adjuvant chemotherapy and radiation therapy. Despite aggressive treatment, the prognosis is very poor, with a high incidence of pulmonary metastasis.

Round Cell Sarcomas

This so-called group of tumors is composed of distinct tumors that, other than their similar microscopic appearance using hematoxylin-eosin stain, are quite different. They behave and are treated in a variety of ways, given that each arises from a different cell type.

A. THE EWING FAMILY OF TUMORS

1. Ewing sarcoma—Ewing sarcoma is a well-known clinical entity originally described by James Ewing as a diffuse endothelioma of bone. Since the time of his description, many theories have evolved regarding the

tumor's true histogenesis. Based on electron microscopic and immunohistochemical findings, experts currently believe the tumor represents an undifferentiated member of the family of neural tumors distinct from neuroblastoma. Cytogenetic studies identified a chromosomal abnormality with a reciprocal translocation in chromosomes 11 and 22 seen in 90% of cases. This translocation is also seen in primitive neuroectodermal tumor (PNET) and Askin tumors. The breakpoints were cloned, and it is now known that the Ewing sarcoma and *FLI1* genes are involved. The Ewing sarcoma gene encodes a homologous sequence to the RNA binding site in RNA polymerase II. The FLI product is a transcription factor. Accordingly, in the resultant fusion protein, the *FLI1* transcription factor is placed under control of the Ewing sarcoma promoter. Two other translocations are also described in Ewing/PNET: t(21:22) and t(7:22).

In 90% of cases, Ewing sarcoma is found in patients between 5 and 25 years of age. If the patient is younger

Figure 6–44. Radiograph of dedifferentiated chondrosarcoma in the distal femur of a 73-year-old woman.

Figure 6–45. Radiograph of clear cell chondrosarcoma of the femoral head in a 25-year-old man.

than 5 years, the most likely diagnosis is metastatic neuroblastoma. Males are affected more frequently than females and carry a worse prognosis. The pelvis is the most common location, followed by the femur, tibia, humerus, and scapula. However, because Ewing sarcoma is a myelogenous tumor, it can be found in any bone in the body.

Ewing sarcoma appears radiographically as a central lytic tumor of the diaphyseal-metaphyseal bone. It creates extensive permeative destruction of cortical bone, and as it breaks through under the periosteum, it takes on a typical onionskin, multilaminated appearance. Another radiographic feature is the reactive hair-on-end appearance created by bone forming along the periosteal vessels that run perpendicularly between the cortex and the elevated periosteum (Figure 6–46).

Ewing sarcoma can frequently masquerade as osteomyelitis because it is a high-grade lesion with resultant areas of necrosis, liquefaction may occur that may be mistaken for pus. Furthermore, patients frequently present with systemic symptoms of low-grade intermittent fever, elevated white cell count, and erythrocyte sedimentation rate (ESR).

Microscopically, small roundlike cells predominate in densely packed sheets. Formation of pseudorosettes may also be seen (in less than 20%). The rosette-like patterns are more frequently seen in PNET.

Ewing sarcoma is an aggressive malignancy with a high local recurrence and metastatic rate. Patients with locally resectable disease treated with multidrug chemotherapy have a 5-year survival rate of approximately 70%. Unfortunately, 15–25% of patients present with nonlocalized disease. For the patient who presents with advanced, metastatic disease, the 5-year survival rate is 30%. Resection of lung metastasis, if possible, does improve survival.

Ewing sarcoma is a radiosensitive tumor. Historically, this was a modality of choice employing 45–50 Gy over 5 weeks to treat local disease. Because of the not insignificant risk of secondary sarcomas, surgery was investigated as the primary modality for local control. If the margins are contaminated, local irradiation must still be used postoperatively. However, prospective well-controlled studies do not yet clearly establish that surgery significantly improves survival without radiation.

2. Primitive neuroectodermal tumor—PNET is the less common relative to Ewing sarcoma. Like Ewing, this tumor demonstrates expression of neural markers by immunocytochemistry. PNET also exhibits the t(11:22) translocation with the resulting EWS/FI1-fusion protein. In fact, because of such similarities, it is generally agreed that PNET and Ewing represent ends of a spectrum of disease.

By strict criteria, PNET is a rare tumor, representing approximately 10% of Ewing-like tumors. The demographics are identical to those of Ewing-like tumors. Treatment of PNET is similar to that of Ewing; however, the survival rate is slightly less. Accordingly, some authors feel it should be distinguished from Ewing.

Figure 6–46. Radiograph of periosteal response in Ewing sarcoma of the femur in a 15-year-old boy.

B. LYMPHOMA

Lymphoblastic tumors are considered systemic neoplasms of the lymphatic organs, including the bone marrow, and they account for 7% of all malignant bone tumors. They can be roughly divided into Hodgkin lymphomas and non-Hodgkin lymphomas, both of which can affect bone. Of the two groups, the lymphomas associated with Hodgkin disease carry a much better prognosis. When they are found in bone, they tend to be localized and have a considerable blastic response, especially when involving the vertebra.

There are two main types of non-Hodgkin lymphomas. The type emphasized in this section is the primary lymphoma of bone, in which a localized lytic destruction occurs in a single bone, and the results of staging studies (including an isotope bone scan, a CT scan of the chest and abdomen, and marrow aspiration) all prove negative for other areas of involvement. The other type is the more generalized or systemic form of lymphoma, in which many lymphoid organs are involved, including the lymph nodes, liver, spleen, and bone. The prognosis is better for an isolated primary lymphoma of bone, but years later involvement may become generalized or systemic and carry a worse prognosis. This is similar to the case with plasma cell tumors, in which the findings in a patient can change from that of a solitary plasmacytoma with an excellent prognosis to that of the multiple myeloma form of the disease with a poor prognosis.

Primary lymphoma of bone, which was formerly called reticulum cell sarcoma of bone, accounts for approximately half of all lymphomas. To meet the criteria of being a primary bone lymphoma, there must be a 4–6-month interval from the onset of skeletal manifestations to the development of systemic disease. It occurs more frequently in males than in females, is usually found in patients older than 25 years, and affects the spine or pelvis in more than 50% of the cases. In the extremities, the femur is the most commonly involved area, followed next by the humerus and the tibia. Multiple skeletal involvement occurs in 10–40% of cases.

Radiographic findings in primary lymphoma include extensive lytic permeation of cortical bone, with minimal sclerotic response in diaphyseal, metaphyseal, and epiphyseal locations (Figure 6–47). MRI studies demonstrate that the actual marrow involvement is frequently more extensive than the cortical disruption seen on simple radiographs suggests.

The most common histologic types of lymphoma of bone are the large cell or mixed small and large cell types. The cells tend to demonstrate little cytoplasmic structure. However, the nuclear pattern shows indented and folded nuclear patterns and a prominent pink-staining nucleolus, which may help to distinguish it histologically from Ewing sarcoma. Immunohistochemical staining is often necessary to differentiate Ewing sarcoma from the B-cell and T-cell subtypes of lymphoma. In the case of lymphomas, the glycogen stain is usually negative, but the reticulum stain is often positive.

In primary lymphoma of bone, as in Ewing sarcoma, multidrug chemotherapy has greatly improved the 5-year survival rate, which now is approximately 70% for patients with either of these tumors. Like Ewing sarcoma, primary lymphoma of bone is highly sensitive to local irradiation. If the primary lymphoma is localized, a wide resection and limb-salvage reconstruction may be carried out, thereby avoiding the need for local irradiation and possibly effect a cure. However, if the involvement is more extensive, as is commonly the case, it is necessary to use intralesional techniques such as cemented intramedullary nails or a long-stem prosthesis and subsequently use whole bone irradiation, similar to the management of metastatic carcinoma with pathologic fractures. In cases of exten-

Figure 6–47. Radiograph of a lymphoma in the proximal humerus of a 64-year-old woman.

sive systemic involvement, bone marrow transplantation can be used.

C. PLASMA CELL TUMOR

A bone tumor composed of malignant monoclonal plasma cells is referred to as a myeloma or plasmacytoma. It is rare for a patient to have a solitary myeloma or plasmacytoma. Tumors are almost always found on multiple bony sites, in which case the term *multiple myeloma* is used.

1. Myeloma—Multiple myeloma, which is the most common primary tumor of bone, accounts for 45% of all malignant bone tumors. It is the second most common hematopoietic malignancy. An estimated 90% of cases are in patients older than 40 years. It accounts for 1% of all malignancies in Caucasians and 2% in African Americans.

The disease is characterized by a triad of osteolytic punched-out lesions (multifocal) (Figure 6–48) neoplastic proliferation of atypical plasma cells and a monoclonal gammopathy. Diagnostic criteria are established for myeloma. Major criteria include plasmacytosis on biopsy of a lesion, marrow plasmacytosis, and an abnormal serum protein electrophoresis and light (Bence Jones) proteinuria. It causes bony destruction similar to that caused by lymphomas, with most lesions occurring in the trunk, hip, and shoulder areas. Many advances were made in the biology of myeloma in the last decade. The observation that myeloma cells enhance osteoclasts formation (through osteoprotegerin/RANKL [receptor activator of nuclear factor κ] pathway) forms the basis for new treatment paradigms aimed at inhibiting RANKL and thereby decreasing osteolysis. A naturally occurring inhibitor of the Wnt signaling pathway called Dkk-1 is secreted by myeloma cells and promotes osteolysis.

Lesions are rarely found distal to the knee or elbow. Approximately 3% of patients with myeloma have a sclerotic form of the disease, which appears to carry a better prognosis and is associated with peripheral neuropathy. The serum protein electrophoresis shows an elevated monoclonal immunoglobulin on either the a or y spike. Bence Jones proteinuria is secondary to light-chain immunoglobulin spillover. Occasionally, electrophoresis of a urine sample yields positive results, whereas that of a serum sample yields negative results. In aggressive forms of myeloma, the extensive bone breakdown causes hypercalcemia, which can lead to a semicomatose state and over a long period results in nephrocalcinosis. Renal damage also results from protein plugging of the renal tubules and renal failure.

A marrow aspirate usually demonstrates the abnormal plasma cells. These cells show an eccentrically placed nucleus in a well-structured eosinophilic cytoplasm. Although normal B-cell–derived plasma cells

Figure 6–48. Radiograph of multiple myeloma in the femoral shaft of a 72-year-old man.

produce antibodies, the abnormal B-cell–derived plasma cells produce immunoglobulin that is ineffective, which helps explain the increased infection rate in patients with myelomas. Patients may also demonstrate extraosseous infiltrates, with the majority seen in the upper airway and oral cavity. Amyloidosis may be seen concurrently in 10–15% of cases. A quarter of these have extensive cardiac involvement. In such cases the median survival is 4 months.

Plain radiographs show myeloma lesions to be sharply demarcated lytic lesions with minimal periostitis. Pathologic fixation is frequent. Bone scans have a high false-negative rate thought to be caused by almost exclusive osteoclast activity.

Less than 2% of myeloma cases demonstrate the POEMS syndrome (*p*olyneuropathy, *o*rganomegaly, *e*ndocrinopathy, *M*-component spike, *s*kin changes, *s*cleroses of bone).

Although treatment and prognosis have improved, myeloma remains a fatal disease, with more than 90% of patients dying within 2–3 years. Chemotherapy such as melphalan and cortisone may induce a transient remission in 50–70% of cases.

Local treatment of myeloma is similar to that of metastatic disease, with cemented intramedullary nails and prosthetic devices used after an intralesional debridement. The amount of bleeding at the surgical site is usually extensive, similar to that encountered with surgery for metastatic renal cell carcinoma and certain thyroid metastases. After surgery, the entire bone should be irradiated with 5500 cGy. Spinal lesions should be handled just like metastatic tumors, as discussed in a later section.

2. Solitary myeloma—Solitary lesions are rare (Figure 6–49). By definition, there must be no marrow involvement. Seventy-five percent of these cases have an entirely normal serum protein electrophoresis (SPEP) and urine protein electrophoresis (UPEP). The remaining 25% may have mild abnormalities. Vertebral involvement is the most common site. Patients also tend to be younger (less than 50 years). Unfortunately, 70% of these solitary cases develop multiple myeloma within 3 years. Until this happens, the treatment is only local, with a wide resection if possible or intralesional debridement and reconstruction followed by radiation therapy.

Figure 6–49. Radiograph of a solitary plasmacytoma in the proximal femur of a 46-year-old man.

Fibrous Sarcomas of Bone

Malignant fibrous tumors of bone are clinically similar to the osteosarcoma, but they affect an older (more than 20 years) age group of patients and show a complete absence of tumor osteoid formation. The two major tumors in this category are the fibrosarcoma and the malignant fibrous histiocytoma.

A. Fibrosarcoma of Bone

Fibrosarcoma of bone is a malignant spindle-cell tumor seen in an older patient population with a peak incidence in the fourth decade. It is 10 times less frequent than osteosarcoma but tends to involve similar locations. The most common site of fibrosarcoma is the distal femur, followed next in order by the proximal tibia, pelvis, proximal femur, and proximal humerus. It is rarely seen in the spine, hand, or foot.

On radiograph, fibrosarcomas appear to be almost purely osteolytic and permeative, similar to lymphomas. For this reason, they are painful and can lead to a pathologic fracture. Microscopically, myofibroblastic differentiation with osteoid formation or histiocytes permits distinction from fibroblastic osteosarcoma and malignant fibrous histiocytoma (MFH) of bone. The low-grade form is characterized by malignant-appearing fibroblasts that form a large amount of collagen fiber, giving the appearance of an aggressive desmoplastic fibroma. The high-grade form is characterized by a more anaplastic fibroblast with a higher index of mitotic activity and less collagen fiber formation. It is common to see a basket-woven or storiform pattern in the microscopic picture.

The prognosis and treatment are directly related to the histologic grade of the tumor. Low-grade fibrosarcoma has a better prognosis than osteosarcoma does, but it must be treated by means of an aggressive and wide resection to avoid local recurrence. Because the low-grade form has a low mitotic index, adjuvant chemotherapy and radiation therapy are of little help. High-grade fibrosarcoma has a prognosis and a rate of metastasis that are similar to those of osteosarcoma, and it is usually treated in a similar manner with a combination of surgery and, if the patient is young enough to tolerate the systemic toxicity, adjuvant chemotherapy.

B. Malignant Fibrous Histiocytoma of Bone

Prior to 1970, MFH was rarely diagnosed in bone but was commonly found in soft tissue. Now MFH is more common in bone than fibrosarcoma, but the two types of tumor run a similar clinical course. MFH of bone is seen in middle-age and older (see Table 6–2) adults, is more common in males than in females, and affects the same bony sites as the fibrosarcoma and osteosarcoma.

MFH is a purely lytic tumor that shows aggressive permeation of metaphyseal-diaphyseal bone, similar to the findings in lymphoma (Figure 6–50). Lytic destruction is diffuse, with no evidence of a periosteal response to blastic repair. Microscopic analysis of MFH usually shows the tumor to be high grade and have highly anaplastic fibroblasts mixed with malignant histiocytes and a few giant cells in a typical storiform pattern.

Because MFH is closely related to the high-grade fibrosarcoma, it carries a poor prognosis, with high rates of local recurrence and metastasis. The treatment program is therefore similar to that for high-grade fibrosarcoma and osteosarcoma, and it includes an aggressive wide resection and the use of adjuvant chemotherapy.

Adamantinoma of Bone

Adamantinomas account for only 0.33% of all malignant bone tumors; occur with equal frequency in males and females, usually during the second and third decades of life; are found in the tibia in 90% of cases; and are usually diaphyseal in location, frequently starting in the anterior cortex. The cause of adamantinoma remains unknown, although angioblastic synovial cells and epithelial cells were considered in the past. Newer investigations, including immunohistochemistry and electron microscopic studies, lend support to the hypothesis of an epithelial origin, which goes along with the histologic appearance of a basal cell carcinoma and might explain the common site of origin subcutaneously in the anterior tibial cortex. The name *adamantinoma* was given to the tibial lesion because its histologic appearance is similar to that of the adamantinoma of jaw bone (ameloblastoma), but the two entities have no other relationship clinically.

In patients with adamantinoma, the radiograph shows a benign tumor with a lytic central core that is surrounded by reactive sclerotic bone that typically bulges the anterior cortex and thus takes on the appearance of either fibrous dysplasia or osteofibrous dysplasia (Figure 6–51). One consideration in the differential

A   **B**

Figure 6–50. Radiograph (**A**) and T$_1$-weighted MRI (**B**) of malignant fibrous histiocytoma in the distal femur of a 50-year-old woman.

Figure 6–51. Adamantinoma of the tibia. Initial anteroposterior radiograph (**A**), lateral radiograph (**B**), bone scan (**C**), MRI (**D**). *Continued.*

341

E

F

G

H

Figure 6–51. (Continued) Immediate postoperative after resection with intercalary allograft reconstruction and vascularized fibula transport anteroposterior radiograph (**E**), lateral radiograph 3 years postoperative (**F**), anteroposterior radiograph (**G**), lateral radiograph (**H**). *Continued.*

I   J   K

Figure 6–51. (Continued) **I–K:** Clinical photos 3 years postoperative.

diagnosis is that osteofibrous dysplasia is painless, whereas pain is a frequent symptom in adamantinoma. Another is that fibrous lesions of bone stop growing at bone maturity, whereas the adamantinoma continues on into adult life, at which point a biopsy of the progressive lytic portion of the disease should be performed. There have been cases of osteofibrous dysplasia combined with small areas of adamantinoma scattered in the benign osseofibrous tissue. Adamantinoma is also occasionally found in both the tibia and fibula, so the physician should look for multiple sites.

Microscopic findings include nests or cords of epithelial or angioid tissue growing in a fibrous tissue stroma, which can give adamantinoma the appearance of a low-grade angiosarcoma or a metastatic carcinoma.

Adamantinoma grows extremely slowly, over many years, but on occasion metastasizes to regional lymph nodes and the lung. For this reason, it should be treated by a wide resection, which in most cases is a segmental diaphyseal resection followed by an allograft reconstruction over an intramedullary nail. Because of the low-grade nature of this tumor, adjuvant irradiation or chemotherapy is rarely indicated. Even if pulmonary metastases occur, they can be resected, and there is a fairly good prognosis for survival.

Vascular Sarcomas of Bone

Vascular sarcomas are relatively rare. They include the hemangioendothelioma, angiosarcoma, and hemangiopericytoma of bone. The terms *hemangioendothelioma* and *angiosarcoma* are frequently used synonymously; however, the first term refers to a low-grade tumor, and the second term usually suggests a higher grade lesion with a poorer prognosis. The vascular sarcomas have two different cell-line origins: endothelial cells for the hemangioendotheliomas, in contrast to hemangiopericytes for the hemangiopericytomas.

A. HEMANGIOENDOTHELIOMA

The hemangioendothelioma, which is more common in males than in females, is seen in a wide range of ages between the second and seventh decades. The femur, pelvis, spine, and ribs are the usual sites of origin, and the diaphyses and metaphyses of the long bones are also involved. One third of cases are multicentric, usually in the same bone or limb.

Radiographically, the lesion appears lytic, with surrounding sclerotic bone. The more anaplastic the disease process is, the less reactive bone is. The clinical picture varies widely, depending on the histologic grade of the tumor. The low-grade lesions look like benign hemangiomas, are slow growing, and carry an excellent prognosis. The high-grade lesions are fast-growing lytic lesions with a poor prognosis.

Treatment depends on the histologic grade. The low-grade lesions do well with simple curettement and bone graft, but the high-grade lesions require a more aggressive wide resection and reconstruction. Adjuvant chemotherapy and radiation therapy can be considered for high-grade lesions, especially in patients with multifocal disease.

B. HEMANGIOPERICYTOMA

The hemangiopericytoma is an extremely rare form of vascular sarcoma that also has a wide spectrum of clinical presentations, depending on the histologic grading. This tumor is the malignant counterpart of the glomus tumor, discussed later in the section on soft-tissue tumors. The hemangiopericytoma is a round cell tumor located outside the endothelial membrane of the vascular channel. This can be demonstrated clearly by a silver staining of the reticulum fibers lying between the inner endothelial cells and the outer hemangiopericytes.

Chordomas

Chordoma of bone is rare and accounts for 4% of malignant bone tumors. It takes its origin from the primitive notochord and has the clinical appearance of a chondrosarcoma. Chordomas affect males more frequently than females and are seen in patients between 30 and 80 years of age. Although 50% of the tumors are sacrococcygeal in origin, 37% arise in the sphenoccipital area, and the remainder arise from vertebral bodies of the cervical or lumbar spine. The cranial lesions are seen in a younger age group and carry a poor prognosis because of the dangerous location next to the brain, where surgical removal is difficult.

On radiograph, the chordoma appears as a centrally located lytic process that has minimal sclerotic response at the periphery and may show slight matrix calcification, as in a chondrosarcoma. If the sacrum is involved, the lesion is seen usually in the lower three sacral segments and presents as an extracortical lobulated mass both in front and behind the sacrum. Because of the slow tumor growth, pain may not occur early, but constipation can be an early symptom that results from pressure on the rectum. Because the true anatomic borders are not readily defined by routine radiography, it is best to image this tumor with CT or MRI (Figure 6–52). Microscopically, nests or cords of cells, sprinkled in a sea of mucinous tissue, give an appearance similar to low-grade chondrosarcoma. In most cases, large vacuolated cells appear like a signet ring and are referred to as physaliferous cells.

Treatment for the sacral lesions is an aggressive wide resection, which can be difficult because of excessive bleeding. Significant neurogenic bowel and bladder deficits can result. At the present time, it is common to use adjuvant radiation therapy to help reduce the chance of postoperative recurrence. Newer studies recommend using up to 5000 cGy preoperatively, followed with a boost of 1500 cGy postoperatively. If the surgeon is successful in obtaining clean margins, the local recurrence rate is approximately 30%. With contaminated margins, the recurrence rate climbs to 65%. Recurrence 10–15 years following surgery is common. Because of the low-grade characteristics of the chordoma, it is rare to see a pulmonary metastasis, even after a local recurrence following an inadequate local surgical resection.

Anthouli-Anagnostopoulou FA et al: Juxtacortical osteosarcoma. A distinct malignant bone neoplasm. Adv Clin Path 2004(3):127. [PMID: 11080792]

Bacci G et al: Neoadjuvant chemotherapy for osteosarcoma of the extremity: Long-term results of the Rizzoli's 4th protocol. Eur J Cancer 2001;37(16):2030. [PMID: 11597381]

Bacci G et al: Histologic response of high-grade nonmetastatic osteosarcoma of the extremity to chemotherapy. Clin Orthop 2001;(386):186. [PMID: 11347833]

Bacci G et al: Telangiectatic osteosarcoma of the extremity: Neoadjuvant chemotherapy in 24 cases. Acta Orthop Scand 2001; 72(2):167. [PMID: 11372948]

Barrille-Nion S et al: Advances in biology and therapy of multiple myeloma. Hematology (Am Soc Hematol Educ Program) 2003;248–278. Review. [PMID: 14633785]

Berend KR et al: Adjuvant chemotherapy for osteosarcoma may not increase survival after neoadjuvant chemotherapy and surgical resection. J Surg Oncol 2001;78(3):162. [PMID: 11745799]

Bruns J et al: Chondrosarcoma of bone: An oncological and functional follow-up study. Ann Oncol 2001;12(6):859. [PMID: 11484965]

Crapanzano JP et al: Chordoma: A cytologic study with histologic and radiologic correlation. Cancer 2001;25;93(1):40. [PMID: 11241265]

Ewing J: Diffuse endothelioma of bone. Proc NY Pathol Soc 1921; 21:17.

Gokgoz N et al: Comparison of p53 mutations in patients with localized osteosarcoma and metastatic osteosarcoma. Cancer 2001;92:2181. [PMID: 11596036]

Gorlick R et al: Expression of HER2/erbB-2 correlates with survival in osteosarcoma. J Clin Oncol 1999;17(9):2781. [PMID: 10561353]

Hoang BH et al: Expression of LDL receptor-related protein 5 (LRP5) as a novel marker for disease progression in high-grade osteosarcoma. Int J Cancer 2004;109(1):106. [PMID: 14735475]

Hoang MP et al: Mesenchymal chondrosarcoma: A small cell neoplasm with polyphenotypic differentiation. Int J Surg Pathol 2000;8(4):291. [PMID: 11494006]

Kanamori M et al: Extra copies of chromosomes 7, 8, 12, 19, and 21 are recurrent in adamantinoma. J Mol Diagn 2001;3(1): 16. [PMID: 11227067]

Kaste SC et al: Thallium bone imaging as an indicator of response and outcome in nonmetastatic primary extremity osteosarcoma. Pediatr Radiol 2001;31(4):251. [PMID: 11321742]

Figure 6–52. Sacral chordoma in middle-age woman: T₂ sagittal image (**A**), T₂ transverse image (**B**).

Kaya M et al: Vascular endothelial growth factor expression in untreated osteosarcoma is predictive of pulmonary metastasis and poor prognosis. Clin Cancer Res 2000;6(2):572. [PMID: 10690541]

Khanna C et al: The membrane-cytoskeleton linker ezrin is necessary for osteosarcoma metastasis. Nat Med 2004;10(2):182. [PMID: 14704791]

Kilpatrick SE et al: Clinicopathologic analysis of HER-2/neu immunoexpression among various histologic subtypes and grades of ostesosarcoma. Mod Pathol 2001;14(12):1277. [PMID: 11743051]

Kloen P et al: Expression of transforming growth factor-beta (TGF-beta) isoforms in osteosarcomas: TGF-beta3 is related to disease progression. Cancer 1997;80(12):2230. [PMID: 9404699]

Lewis VO et al: Parosteal osteosarcoma of the posterior aspect of the distal part of the femur. Oncological and functional results following a new resection technique. J Bone Joint Surg Am 2000;82-A(8):1083. [PMID: 10954096]

Maitra A et al: Aberrant expression of tumor suppressor proteins in the Ewing family of tumors. Arch Pathol Lab Med 2001; 125(9):1207. [PMID: 11520274]

Mandahl N et al: Cytogenetic aberrations and their prognostic impact in chondrosarcoma. Genes Chromosomes Cancer 2002; 33(2):188. [PMID: 11793445]

Oberlin O et al: Study of the French Society of Paediatric Oncology (EW88 study). Br J Cancer 2001;85(11):1646. [PMID: 11742482]

Ogose A et al: Elevation of serum alkaline phosphatase in clear cell chondrosarcoma of bone. Anticancer Res 2001;21(1B):649. [PMID: 11299821]

Park YK et al: Overexpression of p53 and absent genetic mutation in clear cell chondrosarcoma. Int J Oncol 2001;19(2):353. [PMID: 11445851]

Pring ME et al: Chondrosarcoma of the pelvis. A review of sixty-four cases. J Bone Joint Surg Am 2001;83-A(11):1630. [PMID: 11701784]

Reddick WE et al: Dynamic MR imaging (DEMRI) of microcirculation in bone sarcoma. J Magn Reson Imaging 1999; 10(3):277. [PMID: 10508287]

Rizzo M et al: Chondrosarcoma of bone: Analysis of 108 cases and evaluation for predictors of outcome. Clin Orthop 2001; (391):224. [PMID: 11603673]

Roland Durr H et al: Multiple myeloma: Surgery of the spine: Retrospective analysis of 27 patients. Spine 2002;27(3):320. [PMID: 11805699]

Scully SP et al: Pathologic fracture in osteosarcoma: Prognostic importance and treatment implications. J Bone Joint Surg Am 2002;84-A(1):49. [PMID: 11792779]

Sluga M et al: The role of surgery and resection margins in the treatment of Ewing's sarcoma. Clin Orthop 2001;(392):394. [PMID: 11716413]

Smith SE et al: Primary musculoskeletal tumors of fibrous origin. Semin Musculoskelet Radiol 2000;4(1):73. [PMID: 11061693]

Tallini G et al: Correlation between clinicopathological features and karyotype in 100 cartilaginous and chordoid tumours. A report from the Chromosomes and Morphology (CHAMP) Collaborative Study Group. J Pathol 2002;196(2):194. [PMID: 11793371]

Tian E et al: The role of the Wnt-signaling antagonist DKK1 in the development of osteolytic lesions in multiple myeloma. N Engl J Med 2003;349(26):2483. [PMID: 14695408]

Weisstein JS et al: Detection of c-fos expression in benign and malignant musculoskeletal lesions. J Orthop Res 2001;19(3):339. [PMID: 11398843]

Zhou H et al: Her-2/neu staining in osteosarcoma: Association with increased risk of metastasis. Sarcoma 2001;5(S1):9.

BENIGN SOFT-TISSUE TUMORS

Soft tissue can be defined as nonepithelial, extraskeletal mesenchymal exclusive of the reticuloendothelial system and glia. This definition would include fat, fibrous tissue, muscle, and the relating neurovascular structures.

Benign soft-tissue tumors, by definition, represent a differentiated neoplastic process with a limited capacity for autonomous growth. They generally demonstrate a marginal capacity to invade locally with infrequent local recurrence. Because of the extensive numbers of benign soft-tissue tumors, discussion is limited here to the more common entities.

Lipomas

The lipoma is by far the most common soft-tissue tumor and has a large number of variants. Some examples include the superficial subcutaneous lipoma; the intramuscular lipoma; the spindle-cell lipoma; the angiolipoma; the benign lipoblastoma; and the lipomas of tendon sheaths, nerves, synovium, periosteum, and the lumbosacral area.

A. SUPERFICIAL SUBCUTANEOUS LIPOMA

The most frequently seen type of lipoma is the superficial subcutaneous type, which can be solitary or multiple. Subcutaneous lipomas occur with equal frequency in men and women and seem to arise spontaneously during the fifth and sixth decade of life. The most common locations are the back, shoulder, and neck.

On palpation this tumor is soft and ballotable. Although it is found more commonly in obese patients, the size of the lipoma does not correlate with the weight of the patient. Lipomas do not reduce in volume with weight loss. They generally grow to a limited size and sarcomatous degeneration does not occur. Surgical treatment is usually cosmetic in nature, and the recurrence rate is less than 5%.

B. INTRAMUSCULAR LIPOMA

The deep intramuscular lipoma is seen in adults between 30 and 60 years of age, affects men more frequently than women, and is commonly found in the large muscles of the extremities. The lesions are slow growing and painless. The intramuscular lipoma has a characteristic radiolucency that contrasts with the surrounding muscle (Figure 6–53). On MRI this tumor demonstrates a uniform high-signal image on the T_1-weighted spin-echo sequence. On gross examination, the tumor can appear quite infiltrative in surrounding muscle and has a faint yellow color on sectioning. Histologic studies show that the intramuscular lipoma, like the subcutaneous lipoma, is composed of benign lipocytes with small pyknotic nuclei that are difficult to see on the surface of the large fat-laden cell. When samples are taken for biopsy purposes, the pathologist must take care to rule out a low-grade, well-differentiated liposarcoma that can coexist with a benign lipoma. On rare occasions, a lipoma can have chondroid or osseous hamartomatous elements that have caused it to be classified as a mesenchymoma in the past. In other cases, evidence of hemorrhage or necrosis can be found in a lipoma and creates low-signal changes on the MRI that are similar to the changes seen in liposarcoma.

A marginal surgical excision is indicated for treatment of intramuscular lipoma. Local recurrence rates of 15–60% are reported.

C. SPINDLE-CELL LIPOMA

The spindle-cell lipoma is seen typically in the posterior neck and shoulder area in men between 45 and 64 years

A   B

Figure 6–53. Radiograph (**A**) and coronal view T$_1$-weighted MRI (**B**) of an intramuscular lipoma in the quadriceps muscle of a 72-year-old man.

of age. On gross examination, the spindle-cell lipoma has the appearance of an ordinary lipoma but with areas of gray-white gelatinous foci streaking through it. Microscopic examination of these areas reveals the presence of benign fibroblasts. Thus, with imaging studies, dense areas are scattered throughout the normal radiolucent areas of a lipoma. On MRI, findings generally consist of a low-signal streaking through the typical high-signal pattern of a benign lipoma.

The treatment for this lesion is a simple marginal resection. The chance for local recurrence is minimal.

D. Angiolipoma

The angiolipoma (Figure 6–54) is a subcutaneous lesion seen in young (see Table 6–6) adults, usually on the forearm. Multiple lesions are frequently present and usually painful because of their vascularity. Grossly, the lobular lipoma demonstrates vascular channels.

Treatment of angiolipoma consists of marginal excision.

E. Diffuse Lipomatosis

An extremely rare variant of the lipoma is diffuse lipomatosis, characterized by the presence of multiple superficial and deep lipomas that involve one entire extremity or the trunk and usually have their onset during the first 2 years of life. Histologically, an individual lesion in a patient with diffuse lipomatosis looks no different from a typical solitary lipoma. An involved limb may become massive in size, sometimes making it impossible to remove the fatty tumors surgically. If this is the case, amputation may be indicated.

F. Lumbosacral Lipoma

The lumbosacral lipoma occurs in the lumbosacral area posterior to a spina bifida defect. It is frequently associated with both intradural and extradural lipomas and

A

B

Figure 6–54. Radiograph (**A**) and T$_1$-weighted MRI (**B**) of a soft-tissue angiolipoma in the volar aspect of the forearm of a 27-year-old woman.

thus can result in neurologic deficits. Although lumbosacral lipoma is generally considered a pediatric tumor, it can be seen in adults (Figure 6–55).

Surgical treatment consists of a marginal resection of the entire lipoma, including the portion arising from the vertebral canal and lumbosacral roots.

G. BENIGN LIPOBLASTOMA AND DIFFUSE LIPOBLASTOMATOSIS

The benign and diffuse types of lipoma are seen in the extremities of infants. The lesions, solitary or multiple, can be superficial or deep in muscle tissue. They demonstrate cellular immaturity, with lipoblasts similar to the myxoid form of liposarcoma. Even with the cellular aggressiveness of the lesions, the prognosis is excellent following simple surgical resection.

H. HIBERNOMA

Hibernoma, a rare lipoma usually seen in young (see Table 6–6) adults, commonly occurs in the scapular and interscapular regions, is painless and slow growing, and ranges between 10 and 15 cm in diameter. The hibernoma is composed of finely granular or vacuolated cells characteristic of brown fat and contains a considerable amount of glycogen. The treat-

ment is marginal surgical resection with a low potential for recurrence.

Benign Vascular Tumors

Benign vascular proliferative tumors are the second most common benign tumor after lipomas. Three types of vascular tumors are discussed here: hemangiomas, lymphangiomas, and glomus tumors.

Like lipomas, angiomas occur in a wide variety of clinical conditions seen more often in females than in males. The most common type of angioma is the hemangioma, which can be a superficial cutaneous lesions or a deep and intramuscular one. The lymphatic counterpart of the hemangioma is known as the lymphangioma or hygroma. In most cases, the lesion is solitary or localized. If it is extensive and involves an entire limb, the term *angiomatosis* is used. Because most hemangiomas and lymphangiomas are congenital, the term *hamartomatous* or *arteriovenous malformation* is applied in their classification. Hemangiomas and lymphangiomas arise from developmental dysplasias of the endothelial tube, whereas glomus tumors and heman-

Figure 6–55. T$_1$-weighted MRI of a lumbosacral lipoma.

giocytomas arise from hemangiopericytes, which are cells that lie outside the endothelial tube. Most vascular anomalies arise sporadically, but some familial, autosomal-dominant inheritance patterns are also described. Genetic analysis of these families identified specific gene mutations supporting the genomic role in the regulation of angiogenesis.

A. HEMANGIOMA

Hemangiomas are the most frequently seen tumors of childhood and account for 7% of all benign tumors.

1. Solitary capillary hemangioma—The most common type of hemangioma is the solitary capillary type, which appears as an elevated red to purple cutaneous lesion on the head or neck. The lesion occurs during the first few weeks after birth, grows rapidly over a period of several months, and regresses over a 7-year period in 75–90% of cases.

Because of the spontaneous regression, no treatment is needed in most cases. In the past, treatment consisted of cryosurgery, sclerotherapy, or irradiation, but frequently this treatment was worse than the disease itself. Today, lasers are used with good preliminary results. This may prove to be the treatment of choice in selected cases.

2. Cavernous hemangioma—The cavernous hemangioma is larger and less common than the capillary hemangioma. The enlarged vascular spaces of the cavernous lesion give it the appearance of a cluster of purple grapes. It lies deep in the extremity, with common involvement of muscles and even the synovial membrane of the joints.

Imaging may be characteristic (Figure 6–56). In some patients with deep intramuscular forms of hemangioma, the skin shows no abnormalities and no phleboliths are apparent on radiograph. With MRI, deep intramuscular hemangiomas can be easily detected by the characteristic mixed-signal serpiginous pattern seen in the T_1-weighted image.

The muscle lesions are usually asymptomatic until intralesional hemorrhage occurs either spontaneously or after a minor injury. The pain symptoms are usually short lived but recur infrequently. In some patients, the pain is more severe and associated with muscle contracture and joint deformity. These patients may require surgical resection of the scarred-down lesion to allow for better joint function and to reduce the pain. In rare cases of multiple hemangiomas involving the entire limb, amputation may be indicated. Vascular embolization of the feeder vessels can be attempted but may lead to a significant compartment syndrome, with severe contractures or with loss of muscle strength and limitation of joint movement.

A   B   C

Figure 6–56. Clinical appearance (**A**) and radiographic appearance (**B**) of a cavernous hemangioma in the foot of one patient, and T_1-weighted and T_2-weighted MRIs (**C**) of a cavernous hemangioma in the foot of another patient.

3. Arteriovenous hemangioma—The arteriovenous hemangioma is seen in young patients (see Table 6–6) usually in the head, neck, or lower extremity. It is associated with significant arteriovenous shunting in the tumor, which creates increased perfusion. This results in increased local temperature, pain, and continuous thrill or bruit over the mass. In the extremity, it also results in an overgrowth of the limb.

If shunting is excessive, surgical removal of the hemangioma may be necessary to prevent increased pulse pressure from leading to high-output heart failure. Arteriograms are helpful in determining the degree of shunting prior to treatment. Embolization or surgical ligation of feeder vessels is frequently not a successful form of treatment.

4. Epithelioid hemangioma (Kimura disease)—This cutaneous hemangioma is found on the head or neck in women between 20 and 40 years old. It is associated with inflammatory changes and eosinophilia, and it sometime ulcerates. Its name is derived from the epithelial appearance of the endothelia-lined capillary structures.

5. Pyogenic granuloma—The pyogenic granuloma is a polypoid capillary hemangioma that affects the skin or mucosal surfaces of males and females in all age groups. It may be associated with trauma and is found about the mouth, gingivae, or fingers. The lesions have a purple-red color, bleed easily, and ulcerate.

B. Lymphangioma

The lymphangioma is nothing more than an angioma composed of lymphatic endothelial tubes filled with lymphatic fluid, rather than being filled with blood, as the hemangioma is. Lymphangiomas can be localized, which occurs with the cystic hygroma, and they are usually seen about the head, neck, or axilla of young boys and girls (see Table 6–6). As with hemangiomas, the larger lymphomas are cavernous lesions seen in older patients with deeper involvement. In both lymphangioma and hemangioma, because of increased regional perfusion, bony overgrowth can occur (Figure 6–57).

C. Glomus Tumor

The glomus tumor arises from the hemangiopericyte, which is a cell seen at the periphery of the capillary vascular network and normally involved with the regulation of blood flow through the capillary system. Microscopic examination of the tumor reveals large vascular spaces surrounded by a homogeneous field of round epithelioid hemangiopericytes, with no evidence of mitotic activity.

The glomus tumor is a pink lesion that measures less than 1 cm in diameter. It represents 1.6% of all soft-tissue tumors and occurs with equal frequency in men and women, usually between 20 and 40 years of age. Although the tumor is found most commonly in the subungual area of a digit, where it is readily visible, it

Figure 6–57. Radiograph of a lymphangioma in the forearm and hand of a 23-year-old woman.

also occurs subcutaneously on the hand, wrist, forearm, or foot, where it may be invisible and thus difficult to diagnose until localized lancinating pain leads to a surgical exploration. After the lesion is surgically removed, the pain subsides, and recurrence is unlikely.

Extraabdominal Desmoid Tumors (Aggressive Fibromatosis)

In comparison with the infantile fibrous lesions mentioned earlier, the desmoid tumor is seen in older children and young adults up through 40 years of age. Whereas abdominal desmoids are seen in the abdominal wall of women following pregnancy, the extraabdominal desmoids usually occur in men and are more common in proximal areas about the shoulder and buttock, followed next by the posterior thigh, popliteal area, arm, and fore-

Figure 6–58. T_1-weighted MRI of a desmoid tumor in the gluteal area of a 45-year-old woman.

arm. In most cases, it presents as a solitary tumor. Multicentric involvement is seen at times, however, and can be associated with Gardner syndrome, which is characterized by polyposis of the large bowel and by craniofacial osteomas. In patients with familial adenomatous polyposis (FAP), an inherited disease caused by mutations in the *APC* gene, desmoids are a significant source of morbidity and mortality. The *APC* gene, located on chromosome 5, encodes for a 300-kDa protein, in which a germline mutation is an early event in tumor formation.

Desmoids are deep-seated tumors that arise from muscle fascial planes and infiltrate extensively into adjacent muscle tissue, tendons, joint capsules, and even bone. Compared with malignant fibrosarcomas, desmoids are poorly marginated and thus difficult to resect surgically. Desmoids can engulf surrounding vessels and nerves, whereas fibrosarcomas usually push these structures aside. A desmoid may cause local pain and grow quite rapidly, suggesting a malignant tumor. The desmoid tends to grow more longitudinally along muscle planes to a considerable size, frequently resulting in restricted joint motion about the shoulder, hip, or knee. Because the local aggressiveness of desmoids is so similar to that of malignant fibrosarcomas or malignant fibrous histiocytomas, some experts believe the desmoid may be a low-grade fibrosarcoma that has lost its potential to metastasize; however, molecular analyses may suggest otherwise.

On gross examination, a desmoid tumor is firm and heavily collagenized. Microscopically, it has a low mitotic index, similar to that of a plantar or palmar fibromatosis. Radiographically, a desmoid is noncalcified and appears dense in comparison with normal muscle. It is easily seen in soft window CT scanning. More exact presurgical imaging can be obtained with MRI (Figure 6–58). As with an abdominal desmoid, an extraabdominal desmoid physical injury may play a role in the activation of a preexisting oncogene located in the damaged fibroblast.

Desmoids are usually treated surgically with an aggressive wide resection similar to that used in treating a primary sarcoma. Even following a clean resection of the desmoid, the recurrence rate may approach 50%. For this reason, it is common to administer 50 Gy of radiation to the surgical site starting 2 weeks postoperatively. With radiation therapy, the recurrence rate decreases to 15%. In rare cases an amputation may be necessary after multiple recurrences. A few cases of spontaneous involution of desmoid tumors are reported after 40 years of age.

Based on clinical and experimental evidence, estrogen may play a role in the development of desmoid tumors. Accordingly, agents such as tamoxifen are being used in some centers because of their antiestrogen effects. NSAIDs were also implemented in attempts to treat aggressive cases. In selected patients with progressive disease, low-dose vinblastine and methotrexate chemotherapy may be used.

Benign Tumors of Peripheral Nerves

Benign tumors of peripheral nerve sheaths are common and take their origin from Schwann cells, which normally produces myelin and collagen fiber.

A. NEURILEMOMA

The neurilemoma (neurinoma or benign schwannoma) is the least common of the benign tumors of peripheral nerve sheaths. It usually affects individuals between 20 and 50 years of age and occurs with equal frequency in men and women. It has a predilection for spinal roots and for superficial nerves on the flexor surfaces of both upper and lower extremities. In most cases, the lesion is solitary, but multiple lesions are occasionally seen in Recklinghausen disease. The neurinoma is slow growing and rarely causes pain or a neurologic deficit.

Unlike the neurofibroma, which has a fusiform appearance, the neurilemoma is round (Figure 6–59). Micro-

Figure 6–59. T_1-weighted MRI of a neurilemoma of the ulnar nerve in a 69-year-old man.

scopic studies reveal the presence of a characteristic Verocay body, which consists of palisading Schwann cells and is found in the fibrotic Antoni A substance of the tumor. Other areas reveal a more mucinous Antoni B substance. Neurilemomas may occur in an axial fashion involving spinal roots, often presenting as a dumbbell-shaped extradural defect (Figure 6–60). In comparison with the less restricted peripheral lesions, the nerve root lesions are more apt to cause pain associated with neurologic deficiency because of their bony constriction.

In some cases, simple excision of the neurilemoma is clinically indicated, which often can be performed without serious damage to the nerve. If the patient is asymptomatic, observation is appropriate because there is little chance for malignant degeneration.

B. Solitary Neurofibroma

The solitary neurofibroma is a fusiform fibrotic tumor arising centrally from a smaller peripheral nerve (Figure 6–61). The tumor is seen with equal frequency in men and women, usually between 20 and 30 years of age. It is 10 times more common than the multiple form seen

Figure 6–61. Photographic appearance of a solitary neurofibroma.

in Recklinghausen disease, is usually smaller, and carries less chance of malignant degeneration. Microscopic examination of the solitary neurofibroma shows interlacing bundles of elongated spindle cells with benign-appearing nuclei and occasionally with areas resembling the Antoni A tissue seen in the neurilemoma.

Treatment of the solitary neurofibroma consists of simple excision.

C. Neurofibromatosis (Recklinghausen Disease)

Recklinghausen disease is a familial dysplasia, inherited as an autosomal-dominant trait, with an incidence of approximately 1 in every 3000 live births. The disease usually begins during the first few years of life with the emergence of small café au lait spots. Over time, these lesions grow in number and size. Unlike the lesions seen in fibrous dysplasia, the lesions in Recklinghausen disease do not have rough edges. If a patient has more than six lesions that have smooth edges and are greater than 1.5 cm in diameter, the diagnosis of Recklinghausen disease is certain.

Later in life, the patient develops multiple neurofibromas, each of which appears as a soft cutaneous nodule (Figure 6–62). This pedunculated skin lesion, which is called fibroma molluscum, can be large and pendulous. More pathognomonic of the disease is the plexiform neurofibroma, which appears in larger nerves and can involve an entire extremity (see Figure 6–62). When the overlying skin of an extremity is loose and hyperpigmented, the condition is called elephantiasis neuromatosa, or "elephant man syndrome." (It is now thought that John Merrick, the so-called elephant man, was actually affected by Proteus syndrome.) Among the bony changes seen in Recklinghausen disease are angular scoliosis, spinal meningocele, scalloping of the vertebra, pseudarthrosis of the tibia, and osteolytic lesions in bone.

Figure 6–60. Myelogram of a neurilemoma in the cervical spine.

Figure 6–62. Cutaneous manifestations of neurofibromatosis.

A major threat to the patient's life is that a malignant schwannoma will develop from one of the large and deep neurofibromas. This occurs at a later age in 3–5% of patients.

Intramuscular Myxomas

The intramuscular myxoma is a rare tumor seen in patients older than 40 years and affecting the large muscles about the thighs, shoulders, buttocks, and arms. It is a slow-growing well-marginated tumor that has the gelatinous physical quality of a ganglion cyst or myxoid liposarcoma. The intramuscular myxoma causes no pain and can grow to greater than 15 cm in diameter. Although it appears radiolucent on CT scan, MRI demonstrates an intermediate signal on the T_1-weighted image and an extremely high signal on the T_2-weighted image. Multiple myxomas are associated with polyostotic fibrous dysplasia.

The intramuscular myxoma can be resected marginally. After this procedure, the recurrence rate is extremely low.

Azzarelli A et al: Low-dose chemotherapy with methotrexate and vinblastine for patients with advanced aggressive fibromatosis. Cancer 2001;92(5):1259. [PMID: 11571741]

Bertario L et al: Genotype and phenotype factors as determinants of desmoid tumors in patients with familial adenomatous polyposis. Int J Cancer 2001;95(2):102. [PMID: 11241320]

Chun YS et al: Lipoblastoma. J Pediatr Surg 2001;36(6):905. [PMID: 11381423]

Kang HJ et al: Schwannomas of the upper extremity. J Hand Surg [Br] 2000;25(6):604. [PMID: 11106529]

Richards KA et al: The pulsed dye laser for cutaneous vascular and nonvascular lesions. Semin Cutan Med Surg 2000;19(4):276. [PMID: 11149608]

Shields CJ et al: Desmoid tumours. Eur J Surg Oncol 2001; 27(8): 701. [PMID: 11735163]

Sorensen SA et al: Long-term follow-up of von Recklinghausen neurofibromatosis: Survival and malignant neoplasms. N Engl J Med 1986;314:1010. [PMID: 3083258]

Vikkula M et al: Molecular genetics of vascular malformations. Matrix Biol 2001;20(5-6):327. [PMID: 11566267]

MALIGNANT SOFT-TISSUE TUMORS

Sarcomas are capable of invasive, locally destructive growth with a tendency to recur and to metastasize. All sarcomas do not behave the same, however. Some sarcomas, such as dermatofibrosarcoma protuberans, rarely metastasize. Malignant fibrous histiocytoma, in contrast, does so with alacrity.

A. Fibrohistiocytic Tumors

Until recently, MFH was the most common soft-tissue sarcomas seen in adults (Figure 6–63). Strangely, although more frequently encountered than other adult soft-tissue sarcomas, the cell type(s) of origin remain unclear. Current debate is centered on whether MFH is a distinct entity or a diverse group of sarcomas that on histologic evaluation appear similar. The latest World Health Organization classification for sarcomas no longer includes MFH as a distinct entity. The current nomenclature for the majority of MFH is undifferentiated pleomorphic sarcoma.

1. Storiform pleomorphic—Storiform pleomorphic is the most common subtype of MFH. It occurs more frequently in men than in women, primarily affecting individuals between 50 and 70 years of age. Usually it is a deep lesion found in the large muscles about the thigh, hip, and retroperitoneal areas. The tumor may be asymptomatic.

On gross examination, the tumor appears multinodular and may demonstrate several separate satellite lesions in the same muscle belly, especially at the superior and interior poles. It may be necrotic and ranges in color from dirty gray to a reddish tan. Microscopy demonstrates that it is composed of malignant fibroblasts mixed with anaplastic and pleomorphic histiocytes.

The prognosis and treatment vary, depending on the size and location of the tumor. The overall local recurrence potential is 45%, with a 40% incidence of metastasis to the lung and with a 10% incidence of regional lymph node involvement. Tumors smaller than 5 cm in diameter and found in a subcutaneous location in the distal body parts carry a good prognosis, with a 5-year survival rate of 80%, whereas tumors that are 5 cm or more in diameter and located deep in a more proximal

Figure 6–63. Clinical appearance (**A**), T$_1$-weighted MRI (**B**), T$_2$-weighted MRI (**C**), and resected surgical specimen (**D**) of a large pleomorphic malignant fibrous histiocytoma in the posterior thigh of a 55-year-old man.

muscle group carry a poor prognosis, with a 5-year survival rate of only 55%.

Although the treatment depends on the clinical situation, it generally consists of an aggressive wide resection after careful preoperative staging, including an MRI of the primary and CT scan of the chest. Amputation is rare, with limb salvage possible in the majority of cases.

The use of adjuvant radiation therapy is important in reducing the local recurrence rate. Most clinicians administer 55 Gy to a wide area, followed by a boost to 65 Gy aimed at the surgical site. An attempt is made to leave a longitudinal strip of tissue out of the field of radiation to reduce the chance of postirradiation edema distal to the treatment site. Some centers advocate preoperative and postoperative radiation with 50 Gy given before resection and approximately 15 Gy postoperatively. Some institutions employ preoperative radiation exclusively. Local recurrence rates are generally between 5% and 25%.

The use of adjuvant chemotherapy is more controversial. Because limited data suggest that chemotherapy results in a significant improvement in survival and because most patients are older individuals who cannot tolerate the high-dose protocols, medical oncologists are divided on whether to advocate the use of chemotherapeutic agents in the treatment of MFH.

2. Myxoid—The myxoid type is the second most common type of MFH and is seen in the same age group of patients and the same locations as the pleomorphic type. On gross examination, myxoid MFH has a multinodular and translucent or gelatinous appearance similar to the appearance of a myxoid liposarcoma or a benign myxoma of muscle. Because of its gelatinous nature, myxoid MFH has a greater chance for local contamination and thus has a higher local recurrence rate than pleomorphic MFH. However, the metastasis rate in cases of myxoid MFH is approximately 25%.

3. Giant cell—The giant cell type of MFH also affects older patients and is seen in large muscle groups, but it is hemorrhagic and carries a 50% chance of pulmonary metastasis.

4. Inflammatory—The inflammatory type of MFH affects the older age groups, is more common in the retroperitoneal areas, and has a 50% metastasis rate.

B. DERMATOFIBROSARCOMA PROTUBERANS

Dermatofibrosarcoma protuberans, a low- to intermediate-grade fibrohistiocytic tumor, is unique because of its nodular cutaneous location. It is seen more commonly in males than females and occurs in young or middle-age (20–40 years) adults. It is typically located about the trunk and proximal extremities. Antecedent trauma is recorded in 10–20% of cases. Dermatofibrosarcoma protuberans begins as a painless subcutaneous nodule or nodules and slowly develops into an elevated multinodular plaque (Figure 6–64). Microscopic examination of the lesion reveals the same storiform or basket-weave pattern of a benign or malignant fibrous histiocytoma but with a very low mitotic index. The pattern tends to infiltrate extensively into surrounding subcutaneous fat and skin, which accounts for the high local recurrence rate, sometimes reported to approach 50%.

Characteristic cytogenetic abnormalities are described with characteristic features such as reciprocal t(17;22)(q22;q13) or, more commonly, supernumerary ring chromosomes containing sequences from chromosomes 17 and 22.

Surgical treatment, consisting of an aggressive resection, is associated with a lower recurrence rate of 20%. Because of the low mitotic index, radiation therapy is not usually indicated, and the chance of pulmonary metastasis is only 1%.

C. FIBROSARCOMA

Fifty years ago, fibrosarcoma was considered the most common of the soft-tissue sarcomas, secondary to imprecise pathologic classification of MFH, certain liposarcomas, rhabdomyosarcoma, leiomyosarcomas, and malignant

Figure 6–64. Clinical appearance of dermatofibrosarcoma protuberans on the bottom of the heel of a 30-year-old man.

peripheral nerve sheath tumors. Currently, fibrosarcoma is considered one of the least common soft-tissue sarcomas. The diagnosis is reserved for those tumors in which the histology demonstrates a uniform fasciculated growth pattern of spindle cells (malignant fibroblasts). It is clinically similar to MFH, occurs with nearly equal frequency in men and women, is found in patients between 30 and 55 years of age, is sometimes slow growing and painless, and tends to affect deep fascial structures of muscle about the knee and thigh, followed next by the forearm and leg.

On gross examination, fibrosarcoma appears as a firm and lobulated lesion that has a yellowish white to tan color. The lesion may demonstrate a few calcific or osseous deposits on radiographic exam. Microscopy reveals spindle, uniformly shaped fibroblasts that have varying degrees of mitotic activity. Fibrosarcomas contain no malignant histiocytes.

The treatment and prognosis depend on the grade of tumor in a particular patient. Low-grade fibrosarcoma is nearly the same tumor as a benign desmoid tumor and has an extremely low rate of metastasis. However, high-grade fibrosarcoma requires an aggressive wide surgical resection, along with radiation therapy, and has a pulmonary metastasis rate of 50–60%. Lymph node involvement is rare. The use of chemotherapy is considered controversial in patients with fibrosarcoma, as it is in patients with MFH.

D. LIPOSARCOMAS

Liposarcoma is the second most common soft-tissue sarcoma after MFH. Like MFH, liposarcoma is a tumor of older (40–60 years) patients and can be large and deep seated. Four types of liposarcoma are discussed in the following sections. The well-differentiated type and the myxoid type are associated with a low chance for lung metastasis, whereas the round cell and the pleomorphic types tend to behave more aggressively.

1. Well-differentiated liposarcoma—This very low grade tumor affects individuals who are 40–60 years of age and occurs more frequently in men than in women. It grows extremely slowly and reaches a large size without causing pain. The deep-seated tumor is found in the retroperitoneum, buttock, or thigh. In some cases of well-differentiated liposarcoma, findings include inflammation and sclerosis.

On gross examination, this tumor has a fatty lobulated appearance similar to a benign lipoma. Even under the microscope, many large areas of the tumor appear benign. However, with proper sampling, the pathologist will find a few areas of lipoblast activity to suggest the diagnosis of a liposarcoma. MRI findings are sometimes difficult to distinguish from a large deep lipoma (Figure 6–65).

In cases of well-differentiated liposarcoma, a conservative wide resection is performed to avoid local recurrence. Adjuvant radiation therapy is not helpful, and chemo-

Figure 6–65. T₁-weighted MRI of a well-differentiated liposarcoma in the thigh of a 63-year-old man.

therapy is never used. The chance of metastatic disease is very low, and the prognosis for survival is excellent.

2. Myxoid liposarcoma—Myxoid liposarcoma is the most common fat sarcoma, accounting for 40–50% of all liposarcomas. The myxoid type is low to intermediate grade and seen in older patients (see Table 6–6). The clinical presentation is similar to the well-differentiated liposarcoma.

Gross examination of a myxoid liposarcoma reveals a lobulated pattern with some areas that appear similar to those of a lipoma but with other myxomatous areas. Microscopic examination shows myxoid tissue with areas of signet ring lipoblasts. It is common to find a delicate pattern of capillaries running through the myxoid areas. MRI frequently demonstrates a heterogeneous high- and low-signal pattern typical of myxoid liposarcoma but not present in cases of benign lipoma (Figure 6–66).

Characteristic translocations are also seen in myxoid liposarcoma. The predominant type is t(12;16)(q13;p11); however, t(12;22)(q13;q12) is also described.

Multifocal myxoid liposarcoma is also described. Consideration for additional advanced axial imaging should be entertained with this histologic subtype.

Although myxoid liposarcoma carries a very good prognosis, the tumor should be removed with wide margins, and adjuvant radiation therapy should be given. Chemotherapy is not indicated.

3. Round cell and pleomorphic liposarcoma—These high-grade liposarcomas are seen in the same locations and age group as the well-differentiated and myxoid subtypes. But unlike the latter, the round cell and pleomorphic types are fast-growing tumors that may be painful.

In cases of round cell or pleomorphic liposarcoma, the lesion does not have a fatty appearance on gross examination but instead looks more like an MFH or a fibrosarcoma. Moreover, on MRI, the lesion appears more like an MFH, with a low-signal pattern in the T₁-weighted image and a high-signal pattern in the T₂-weighted image. Microscopically, the round cell type of liposarcoma shows areas of uniformly shaped round cells similar to those found in Ewing sarcoma or lymphoma and also shows areas of myxoid tissue. In the pleomorphic type of liposarcoma, large and bizarre giant cells occur similar to those found in the pleomorphic type of MFH and rhabdomyosarcoma.

In round cell and pleomorphic liposarcoma, there is an early and high rate of pulmonary metastasis. Accordingly, the prognosis for survival is poor. Thus, the treatment should include aggressive resection, adjuvant radiation therapy as necessary, and chemotherapy in selected patients.

E. RHABDOMYOSARCOMAS

Rhabdomyosarcomas account for 20% of all soft-tissue sarcomas. The embryonal and alveolar types of rhabdo-

Figure 6–66. Sagittal view T₁-weighted MRI of a myxoid liposarcoma in the thigh of a 32-year-old man.

myosarcoma affect pediatric patients, and the rarer pleomorphic type affects adults.

1. Embryonal rhabdomyosarcoma—The embryonal type is seen in patients from birth to 15 years of age and encountered more frequently in boys than in girls. It is most common in the head and neck area. The so-called botryoid form is seen as a cluster of grapes under mucous membranes in the vagina, bladder, or retroperitoneal area. Histologically, it is a round cell tumor like Ewing sarcoma, but some rhabdomyoblasts with cross striations are present in a few areas.

Embryonal rhabdomyosarcoma is treated with local surgical resection plus preoperative and postoperative chemotherapy consisting of vincristine, dactinomycin, cyclophosphamide, and doxorubicin given in cyclic courses during a 2-year span. If the surgical margins are contaminated, local radiation therapy is used. With this program, the 5-year survival rate is 80%. Prior to the advent of chemotherapy, it was only 10%.

2. Alveolar rhabdomyosarcoma—This type of rhabdomyosarcoma affects individuals between 10 and 25 years of age and is found more commonly in males than in females. Besides affecting the head and neck, it can be seen in the extremities, especially the thigh and calf. Microscopic examination of the lesion reveals a typical alveolar pattern of round cells, with fewer rhabdomyoblasts seen in this type of rhabdomyosarcoma than in the embryonal type. This type of rhabdomyosarcoma is associated with the fusion genes *PAX3-FKHR* and *PAX7-FKHR*. Although not definitive, the presence of the translocation t(2;13)/*PAX3-FKHR* may be an adverse prognostic factor, with molecular screening being implemented in the future. Currently, the treatment is the same as for the embryonal type, but the prognosis is a bit worse.

3. Pleomorphic rhabdomyosarcoma—In the 1940s, pleomorphic rhabdomyosarcoma was a popular histologic diagnosis and MFH was a rare one. Based on today's criteria, most of the old cases classified as pleomorphic rhabdomyosarcoma would now be classified as MFH. Currently, the pleomorphic type of rhabdomyosarcoma is the rarest type.

Pleomorphic rhabdomyosarcoma is a high-grade tumor that affects middle-age and older adults and is seen most commonly in the large muscle groups of the proximal extremities, usually the lower extremities. Microscopic examination of the tumor reveals large atypical giant cells, along with racket- or tadpole-shaped malignant rhabdomyoblasts that stain positive for glycogen, actin, and myosin. The tumor carries a poor prognosis and is associated with a high rate of metastasis to the lung. The treatment for pleomorphic rhabdomyosarcoma is similar to that for MFH and consists of a wide local resection and adjuvant radiation therapy. Chemotherapy is rarely indicated.

F. LEIOMYOSARCOMA

Leiomyosarcoma is a very rare soft-tissue tumor whose cell type of origin is smooth muscle. It is seen in the middle-age (see Table 6–6) adult and is much more common in women than in men. Its usual locations, in order of frequency, are retroperitoneal, intraabdominal, cutaneous, and subcutaneous. In some cases, the lesion has a venous wall origin and is found in the vena cava or large vessels of the leg. On microscopic examination, leiomyosarcoma can demonstrate a palisading, orderly fascicular pattern similar to a malignant schwannoma. A specific immunohistochemical staining for actin may be helpful in the differential diagnosis.

The prognosis and the treatment for leiomyosarcoma are similar to those for fibrosarcoma. However, leiomyosarcomas of venous wall origin have a worse prognosis because they are difficult to resect and have a high rate of pulmonary metastasis.

G. SYNOVIAL SARCOMAS

Synovial sarcoma (Figure 6–67) is the fourth most common soft-tissue sarcoma. It is seen in young adults between 15 and 35 years of age and affects males slightly more than females. The name of this tumor suggests a synovial cell origin, but only 10% of synovial sarcomas are found in a major joint. Nevertheless, they frequently arise from juxtaarticular structures, especially around the knee, and they can also arise from tendon sheaths, bursal sacs, fascial planes, and deep muscles. Synovial sarcomas can be seen about the shoulder, arm, elbow, and wrist and are the most common soft-tissue sarcoma in the foot.

Synovial sarcomas initially grow slowly and cause pain in approximately half of the affected patients. The tumors may appear after an injury, and because dystrophic calcification or even heterotopic bone formation is seen in half of the cases, the tumors are assumed to be a benign process for 2–4 years before a diagnostic biopsy is performed.

Microscopic examination of the tumor shows a typical biphasic pattern composed of epithelium-like cells that form nests, clefts, or tubular structures surrounded by malignant fibroblastic spindle cells. The epithelium-like cells produce a mucinous material that suggests a synovial cell origin, although this origin is unlikely. A monophasic form of synovial sarcoma is described and reported to consist of a dominant fibroblastic or epithelial cell pattern. If the lesion shows no biphasic component, however, it is difficult to confirm the diagnosis of synovial sarcoma.

Molecular characterization of this tumor reveals a particular translocation, t(X;18), representing the fusion of *SYT* (at 18q11) with either *SSX1* or *SSX2* (both at Xp11). Both *SYT* and *SSX* appear to be transcription regulation factors whose fusion product is seen in the majority of synovial sarcomas.

A

B

Figure 6–67. Radiograph (**A**) and microscopic appearance (**B**) of a synovial sarcoma in the shoulder of a 20-year-old woman.

Despite the slow growth of synovial sarcoma, the 5-year and 10-year survival rates are only 50% and 25%, respectively. In cases in which the tumors are heavily calcified, the 5-year survival rate is 80%. Because of the poor prognosis, the treatment plan should include aggressive wide resection, along with both radiation therapy and chemotherapy. Lymph node involvement is seen in 20% of affected patients and may require a surgical excision followed by local radiation therapy.

H. MALIGNANT PERIPHERAL NERVE SHEATH TUMOR

A malignant peripheral nerve sheath tumor can arise from a preexisting benign solitary neurofibroma but more frequently arises from the multiple lesions of neurofibromatosis type 1. In both cases, the tumor mass is usually larger than 5 cm in diameter and may arise from a large deep neurogenic structure such as the sciatic nerve (Figure 6–68) or one of the spinal roots. Smaller nerves, even cutaneous branches, however, can give rise to these sarcomas.

Malignant degeneration from a solitary neurofibroma usually occurs after 40 years of age with a 5-year survival rate of 75%. In contrast, patients whose schwannoma arose from the lesions of neurofibromatosis type 1 are generally younger and have a 5-year survival rate of 30%. Surgical treatment consists of a wide resection if possible. Adjuvant radiation and chemotherapy are used in selected cases.

I. MALIGNANT VASCULAR TUMORS

l. Kaposi sarcoma—Of the malignant vascular tumors, Kaposi sarcoma is the most common with four specific subtypes: (1) chronic, (2) lymphadenopathic, (3) transplant associated, (4) AIDS related. It is found directly beneath the skin, generally in the lower extremity of adults, is seen more often in men than in women, and is endemic in central Africa. The cutaneous lesions seen frequently in the foot and ankle area are purplish in color and are nodular (Figure 6–69). Microscopic examination of Kaposi sar-

A

B

Figure 6–68. Clinical appearance of a café au lait defect in the skin overlying a malignant schwannoma in the buttock area of a 42-year-old man (**A**), and gross appearance of the tumor in resected sciatic nerve (**B**).

Figure 6–69. Clinical appearance of Kaposi sarcoma of the foot.

coma shows an aggressive vascular pattern with rare mitosis. However, over a period of many years, the tumor progresses into a full-blown angiosarcoma or fibrosarcoma. It is associated with AIDS and other immunosuppressive disorders and is also seen with lymphomas and multiple myeloma. Although the behavior of Kaposi sarcoma is a function of the immunologic status of the patient and other variables, the overall mortality rate is 10–20%.

2. Angiosarcoma—Soft-tissue angiosarcoma is rare, accounting for less than 1% of all sarcomas. Although angiosarcomas are usually cutaneous lesions and tend to affect men more than women, they sometimes take the form of a deep tumor, and they are typically seen in the upper extremities of women who have chronic lymphedema following radical breast surgery and radiation therapy. Histologic examination of angiosarcoma shows anaplastic endothelial cells surrounded by reticulum fiber. Prognosis for the older patient is poor. Smaller lesions in younger (less than 50 years) patients have a distinctively better outcome. The treatment is wide resection, sometimes with radiation therapy.

3. Hemangiopericytoma—This rare perivascular tumor arises from pericytes. Pericytes are highly arborized perivascular cells that line capillaries and venules. The lesion, which affects male and female adults with equal frequency, is usually found deep in muscle bellies and generally located in the thigh or retroperitoneal area of the pelvis. Microscopic examination of the malignant hemangiopericytoma reveals tightly packed cells with round nuclei with moderate amounts of cytoplasm with poorly defined borders. The bifurcating sinusoidal vessels have a typical staghorn appearance. Cytogenetic analysis reveals multiple chromosome translocations including t(12;19) and t(13;22). Treatment consists of a wide surgical resection, followed by local radiation therapy. Some authors recommend preoperative embolization or afferent vessel ligation (or both) intraoperatively.

MISCELLANEOUS SOFT-TISSUE SARCOMAS

The remaining soft-tissue sarcomas are rare and only a brief description of their clinical patterns is summarized.

A. SOFT-TISSUE CHONDROSARCOMA

There are three types of soft-tissue chondrosarcomas.

1. Myxoid chondrosarcoma—The myxoid chondrosarcoma is sometimes referred to as a chordoid sarcoma because it looks like a chordoma. It is a slow-growing tumor seen in adults, usually in deep structure of the leg. It has a myxoid appearance, does not calcify, and is low grade. Like the chordoma, the myxoid chondrosarcoma responds only to surgical removal.

2. Mesenchymal chondrosarcoma—This tumor affects individuals between 15 and 40 years of age, is found deep in the lower extremity and neck areas, is fast growing, and carries a poor prognosis because of the high risk of pulmonary metastasis. Calcification may be seen on radiograph, and microscopic examination reveals round cells scattered in a chondroid matrix. Treatment consists of a wide resection in conjunction with chemotherapy and radiation therapy.

3. Synovial chondrosarcoma—The conversion of a synovial chondromatosis to a malignant synovial chondrosarcoma is an extremely rare phenomenon. It can occur with lesions of the hip or knee region in older (more than 60 years) adults.

B. EWING SARCOMA

Extraskeletal Ewing sarcoma can be found in individuals between 10 and 30 years of age and is usually located in the paravertebral area, thorax, or deep muscle area of the lower extremity. It is a fast-growing tumor with minimal pain symptoms. It carries the same prognosis as its counterpart in bone and is treated with the same combination of surgery, chemotherapy, and radiation therapy.

C. ALVEOLAR SOFT PART SARCOMA

This round cell sarcoma affects more females than males, is usually found in patients between 15 and 35 years of age, and arises in the deep muscle tissue of the lower extremity, usually the thigh. Alveolar soft part sarcoma is a slow-growing tumor but carries a poor prognosis because of early pulmonary metastasis. The tumor has increased vascularity and is thought to originate from a neurogenic stem cell. It derives its name from its alveolar pattern, which is seen on microscopic examination and can cause this tumor to be mistaken for an alveolar form of rhabdomyosarcoma. A cytogenetic, unbalanced abnormality, t(x;17)(p11.2;q25), is described. Treatment of alveolar soft part sarcoma consists of a wide surgical resection plus radiation therapy and chemotherapy.

D. EPITHELIOID SARCOMA

Although this superficial skin lesion is seen most commonly in the palm of the hand, it can also be found on the dorsum of the forearm or on the plantar aspect of the foot. It is a slow-growing tumor that affects patients between 20 and 30 years of age, causes minimal pain symptoms, and is associated with ulceration.

Because epithelioid sarcoma has a whitish color that under the microscope demonstrates cords of epithelium-like cells, it can be mistaken for a synovial sarcoma. Moreover, because of its firm multilobulated presentation, the epithelioid sarcoma may be mistaken for a plantar of palmar fibromatosis (Figure 6–70).

Epithelioid sarcoma spreads as a lumpy nodularity along tendon sheaths or fascial planes and frequently involves local lymph nodes. Local surgical resection is followed by a high local recurrence rate, and a late pulmonary metastasis is common. For this reason, early treatment should consist of an aggressive wide surgical resection.

E. CLEAR CELL SARCOMA

The clear cell sarcoma is thought to be a deep, noncutaneous variant of the well-known cutaneous melanoma. It is extremely rare, affects women more often than men, and commonly occurs between 20 and 40 years of age. It arises in tendon sheaths and fascial planes, most frequently in the foot and ankle but also in the knee and arm. Clear cell sarcoma starts slowly as a painless lump and has a high potential to spread to local lymph nodes. The lesion in many cases demonstrates evidence of melanin and melanosomes and may be of neural crest origin. The microscopic clear cell appearance can cause this sarcoma to be confused with epithelioid sarcoma and synovial sarcoma.

The prognosis is poor because of a high rate of pulmonary metastasis. This tumor may spread via lymphatics as well. Treatment consists of early aggressive wide resection and may include chemotherapy and local radiation therapy.

Figure 6–70. Clinical appearance of epithelioid sarcoma on the plantar aspect of the foot of a 36-year-old man.

Ahmad SA et al: Extraosseous osteosarcoma: Response to treatment and long-term outcome. J Clin Oncol 2002;20(2):521. [PMID: 11786582]

Anderson J et al: Detection of the PAX3-FKHR fusion gene in paediatric rhabdomyosarcoma: A reproducible predictor of outcome? Br J Cancer 2001;85(6):831. [PMID: 11556833]

Antonescu CR et al: Monoclonality of multifocal myxoid liposarcoma: Confirmation by analysis of TLS-CHOP or EWS-CHOP rearrangements. Clin Cancer Res 2000;6:2788. [PMID: 10914725]

Bowne WB et al: Dermatofibrosarcoma protuberans: A clinicopathologic analysis of patients treated and followed at a single institution. Cancer 2000;88(12):2711. [PMID: 10870053]

Cormier JN et al: Concurrent ifosfamide-based chemotherapy and irradiation. Analysis of treatment-related toxicity in 43 patients with sarcoma. Cancer 2001;92(6):1550. [PMID: 11745234]

Dei Tos AP: Liposarcoma: New entities and evolving concepts. Ann Diagn Pathol 2000;4(4):252. [PMID: 10982304]

dos Santos NR et al: Molecular mechanisms underlying human synovial sarcoma development. Genes Chromosomes Cancer 2001;30(1):1. [PMID: 11107170]

Gibbs J et al: Malignant fibrous histiocytoma: An institutional review. Cancer Invest 2001;19(1):23. [PMID: 11291552]

Hayes-Jordan AA et al: Nonrhabdomyosarcoma soft tissue sarcomas in children: Is age at diagnosis an important variable? J Pediatr Surg 2000;35(6):948; discussion 953. [PMID: 10873042]

Ladanyi M: Fusions of the SYT and SSX genes in synovial sarcoma. Oncogene 2001;20(40):5755. [PMID: 11607825]

Meis-Kindblom JM et al: Cytogenetic and molecular genetic analyses of liposarcoma and its soft tissue simulators: Recognition of new variants and differential diagnosis. Virchows Arch 2001; 439(2):141. [PMID: 11561754]

Nishio J et al: Supernumerary ring chromosomes in dermatofibrosarcoma protuberans may contain sequences from 8q11.2-qter and 17q21-qter: A combined cytogenetic and comparative genomic hybridization study. Cancer Genet Cytogenet 2001; 129(2):102. [PMID: 11566338]

Orvieto E et al: Myxoid and round cell liposarcoma: A spectrum of myxoid adipocytic neoplasia. Semin Diagn Pathol 2001; 18:267. [PMID: 11757867]

Spillane AJ et al: Synovial sarcoma: A clinicopathologic, staging, and prognostic assessment. J Clin Oncol 200015;18(22):3794. [PMID: 11078492]

■ MANAGEMENT OF CARCINOMA METASTASIZED TO BONE

Incidence & Natural History of Metastases

A. COMMON METASTATIC CARCINOMAS AND AREAS OF SKELETAL INVOLVEMENT

Metastatic involvement of the musculoskeletal system is one of the most significant clinical issues facing orthopedic oncologists. The number of patients with metastasis to the skeletal system from a carcinoma is 15 times greater than the number of patients with primary bone tumors of all types. Approximately a third of all diagnosed adenocarcinomas include skeletal metastases, resulting in approximately 300,000 cases per year. Furthermore, 70% of patients with advanced terminal carcinoma demonstrate bone metastases at autopsy. The carcinomas that commonly metastasize to bone are prostate, breast, kidney, thyroid, and lung carcinomas. One study showed that nearly 90% of patients with these types of carcinoma had bone metastases. Among the carcinomas that less commonly metastasize to bone are cancers of the skin, oral cavity, esophagus, cervix, stomach, and colon.

The spine is the most frequent area of bone metastasis. Other common skeletal sites include the pelvis, femur, rib, proximal humerus, and skull, in that order. Metastatic lesions are rarely found distal to the elbow or knee. If lesions are found in these areas, the lung is the most common source. Solitary bone lesions comprise only approximately 10% of cases of bone metastasis.

B. CLINICAL COURSE OF METASTASES

The mechanism of metastases is accounted for in a modified "seed/soil" theorem. Less then 1 in 10,000 neoplastic cells that escape into the circulation from the primary site are able to set up a metastatic focus, a complex multistep process by which the cell must first break free. This is a function of *degradative* enzymes such as collagenases, hydrolases, cathepsin D, and proteases. Once the cell invades the vascular channel, it circulates through the body. It is theorized that the cell is protected by a fibrin platelet clot. However, clinical trials with heparin do not show a significant change in metastatic outcome. Local factors such as integrins are instrumental in attracting the circulating metastatic cell to a particular remote tissue site. Once within the new tissue, the metastatic cell releases factors such as tumor angiogenesis factor, inducing neovascularization, which in turn facilitates growth of the metastatic focus.

Patients with advanced metastatic disease frequently experience dysfunction of their hematopoietic and calcium homeostases systems. Patients may develop a normochromic, normocytic anemia with leukocytosis. In response to the anemia, the increased production of immature cells is noted on the peripheral blood smear. This is termed the *leukoerythroblastic reaction.* Hypercalcemia may result in up to 30% of cases with extensive metastases. This is most frequently seen in myeloma, breast cancer, and non–small cell lung cancer.

Blastic metastases are frequently painless and associated with a lower incidence of pathologic fracture because the bone is not as severely weakened (Figures 6–71 and 6–72). Not all tumors that metastasize from the prostate to the bone are blastic. The lytic variants are painful and can cause pathologic fractures.

Most tumors that metastasize from the breast to the bone are blastic, but some demonstrate mixtures

Figure 6–71. Radiograph of a blastic carcinoma that metastasized from the prostate to the pelvis in an 85-year-old man.

of blastic and lytic areas in the same bone. By taking serial radiographs and noting the appearance of bone metastases, it is possible to follow the progress of treatment consisting of systemic therapy with hormones or chemotherapeutic agents plus local radiation therapy. A favorable response may show a gradual conversion from a lytic to a blastic appearance as the pain decreases.

Bone destruction in lytic lesions is a response by native osteoclasts to the tumor. Neovascularity is common. Among the tumors that are characteristic for this hemorrhagic response are thyroid carcinomas (Figure 6–73), renal cell (Figure 6–74), and multiple myeloma. Before a surgical intervention, it is beneficial to perform a prophylactic embolization of the area to reduce perioperative bleeding. If a lesion is unexpectedly found to be aneurysmal at the time of surgical exploration, it is best to debulk the friable tumor mass rapidly down to normal bone and then pack the area until it can be stabilized with bone cement.

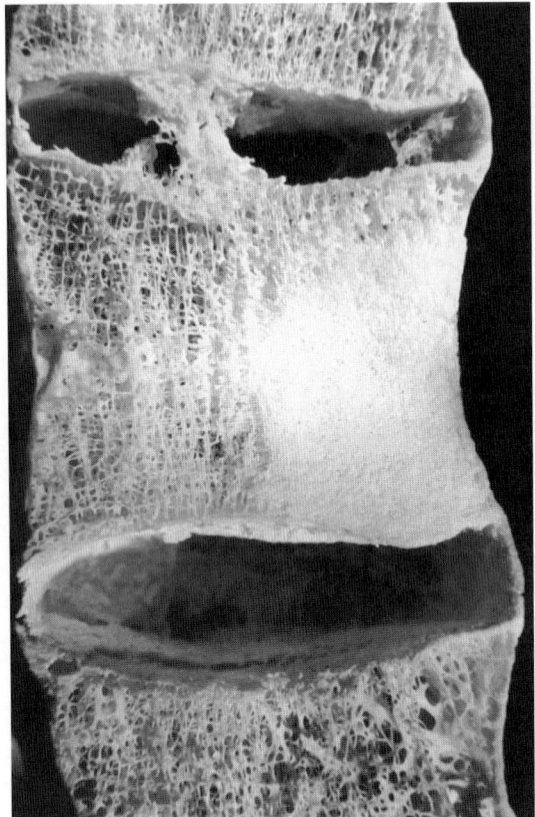

Figure 6–72. Skeletal specimen of a blastic carcinoma that metastasized from the prostate to the lumbar spine.

Diagnosis

A. GENERAL APPROACH

A methodical approach is mandatory in the workup of a patient with presumed metastatic disease to bone to locate the primary tumor. A thorough biopsy and physical examination must be completed prior to laboratory and radiographic analysis. Eight percent of patients may have their primary carcinoma detected on physical exam. Laboratory analysis should include complete blood count, ESR, renal and liver panels, alkaline phosphate, and serum protein electrophoresis.

Radiographic examination should follow with a plain chest radiograph and radiographs of known involved bones. Approximately 45% of primaries are detected in the lung on the chest radiograph. The workup should also include a staging bone scan. If this is negative, myeloma should be suspected. Furthermore, a lesion at a more convenient biopsy site may be found. Bone scan is also more sensitive than plain radiographs in detecting early lesions. CT scans of the chest, abdomen, and pelvis

should be performed. Lung CT can detect up to 15% of primaries missed on the plain radiograph.

These studies in conjunction with a well-planned biopsy detect the majority of cases. Routine radiographic screening studies in search of early metastatic disease are not very helpful (Figure 6–75). Lytic changes become evident on routine radiographs only when cortical destruction approaches 30–50% (Figure 6–76).

Treatment & Prognosis

A. NONSURGICAL TREATMENT

Nonsurgical management of metastatic carcinoma to bone includes observation, radiation treatment, and hormonal/cytotoxic chemotherapy. Radiation is reserved for palliative management. Each patient must be carefully evaluated as a candidate for radiation therapy. The histologic type of disease, extent of disease, prognosis, marrow reserve, and overall constitution must be assessed.

After sustaining a pathologic fracture secondary to metastatic carcinoma, the average survival time is 19 months. Each histologic type has varying lengths of survival (prostate, 29 months; breast, 23 months; renal, 12 months; lung, 4 months). Furthermore, each type of carcinoma exhibits varying radiosensitivity. Prostate and lymphoreticular types demonstrate excellent sensitivity. Breast is intermediate, and renal and gastrointestinal are poor. When used, appropriately 90% of patients gain at least minimal relief, with up to two thirds obtaining complete relief. Seventy percent of patients who are ambulatory retain this function after radiation therapy to the lower extremities. Systemic radioisotopes may also be used. Strontium-89 mimics calcium distribution in the body and shows promise in clinical applications.

When a patient has sustained a true pathologic fixation (rather than an impending lesion) surgical stabilization is usually indicated with subsequent radiation therapy. Because of poor bone quality, augmentation of fixation with bone cement may be necessary.

Hormonal therapy has an important role in the management of metastatic breast and prostate cancer. Fortunately, these agents are easy to administer and have few side effects.

For breast cancer, medical hormonal manipulation can be done by use of antiestrogens, progestins, luteinizing hormone-releasing hormone, or adrenal-suppressing agents. Tamoxifen is effective in 30% of all breast cancer cases but increases to 50–75% of cases when the tumor is known to be estrogen receptor, progesterone receptor positive. Surgical ablation (oophorectomy) may also have a role in certain cases.

For prostate cancer, reduction in testosterone levels via bilateral orchiectomy or administration of estrogens or antiandrogens may produce dramatic results in cer-

A

B

Figure 6–73. Clinical appearance (**A**) and radiographic appearance (**B**) of aneurysmal lesions in a case of carcinoma that metastasized from the thyroid to the hand.

tain cases. Estrogens are no longer used as a first agent because of the risk of cardiovascular complication.

Cytotoxic chemotherapy is used in adenocarcinoma treatment quite extensively. In older (more than 60 years) patients with advanced disease, however, the side effects of the drugs may be too severe.

B. SURGICAL TREATMENT

The goals for surgical intervention in the patient with metastatic carcinoma to bone are relief of pain; prevention of impending pathologic fixations; stabilization of true fixations; enhancement of mobility, function, and quality of life; and perhaps improvement of survival. It is generally agreed that a patient must have a life expectancy of at least 6 weeks to warrant operative intervention. Special considerations to surgical management include noting that bone quality is attenuated and healing will be delayed if even possible. Cancer patients, irrespective of their age, may have increased difficulty protecting their fixation device/ prothesis secondary to systemic debilitation. Accordingly, rigid fixation, with polymethylmethacrylate (PMMA) augmentation as needed, is mandatory.

1. Hip—Seventy-five percent of all surgery for cancer that has metastasized to bone is performed in the hip area (Figure 6–77). Prior to 1970, surgeons attempted to stabilize these fractures with conventional hip nails

Figure 6–74. Radiograph of a metastatic hypernephroma in the ilium.

A   **B**

Figure 6–75. Radiograph (**A**) and gross appearance (**B**) of bone in a case of carcinoma that metastasized from the lung to the spine.

Figure 6–76. Radiograph of the spine of a 45-year-old woman whose cancer had metastasized from the breast.

Figure 6–77. Radiograph of the pathologic fractures of both hips in a 55-year-old man with lung carcinoma.

or Austin Moore prostheses, but results were poor because of deficient local bone stock. After 1970, with the advent of bone cement as an adjuvant form of therapy, these same devices could be used, with improved results in most cases, along with local radiation therapy starting 2 weeks after the surgery. This technique allowed for early ambulation with less pain. However, as time passed and survival times increased, more failures were noted after 1–2 years with the hip nail and cement technique. For this reason, most surgeons currently use a cemented bipolar hemiarthroplasty for the femoral neck fractures and a longer stem calcar replacement hemiarthroplasty for the intertrochanteric fractures. Before these procedures are performed, it is wise to evaluate the entire shaft of the femur and the supraacetabular area for other lytic lesions that might require a longer stem femoral component for the shaft or a modified cemented acetabular component with a total hip replacement for acetabular lesions.

In many cases, the diagnosis of metastasis to the proximal femur is made before a fracture occurs. In these cases, it is the responsibility of the orthopedic surgeon to decide whether the patient should receive some form of internal stabilization prior to radiation therapy. A CT scan of the involved area helps make this decision. Criteria for the performance of a prophylactic stabilization procedure include the following: (1) 50% cortical lysis, (2) a femoral lesion greater than 2.5 cm in diameter, (3) an avulsion fracture of the lesser trochanter, and (4) persistent pain in the hip area 4 weeks following the completion of radiation therapy. These criteria are not perfect, however, and large errors arise in estimation of the load-bearing capacity of the bone.

2. Supraacetabular area—In the case of a small supraacetabular lesion with intact cortical bone, a

A

Figure 6–78. Preoperative (**A**) and postoperative (**B**) radiographs of the pelvis of a 73-year-old woman whose cancer had metastasized from the breast.

B

cemented cup with a total hip system is generally most appropriate. Augmentation of the fully cemented reconstruction with threaded Steinmann pins or similar anchoring screws may be necessary in advanced cases (Figure 6–78). The principles of treatment are always the same, irrespective of the extent of disease: aggressive intralesional curettage of the area back to healthy bone, followed by the placement of large (4.76 mm) threaded Steinmann pins into the sacroiliac area. The pins are placed with an initial foundation batch of cement, leaving them exposed for a second batch of cement, on top of which the cup is placed. A routine femoral component is then cemented.

3. Femoral shaft—Diaphyseal lesions that affect the femur but spare the peritrochanteric area are best handled with some form of intramedullary nail (Figure 6–79). Fixation of the entire femur, including the peritrochanteric area, with a reconstruction type nail is preferable in the event the disease progresses within the bone. Current intramedullary fixation devices often do not need cement augmentation. However, in cases of severe bone deficiency, PMMA introduction, either directly into the defect or indirectly at the nail insertion site, is preferable.

4. Humerus—The principle for the management of metastatic disease to the humerus is no different from that for the femur. In the case of diaphyseal lesions,

A   B

Figure 6–79. Preoperative (**A**) and postoperative (**B**) radiographs of the midshaft of the femur of a patient whose treatment involved fixation with a cemented intramedullary nail.

surgeons either use a conventional intramedullary rod or they plate the lesion. PMMA may be used with either technique.

In the case of the proximal humerus involving a large amount of the humeral head and neck, it is frequently necessary to cement a long-stem prosthesis (Figure 6–80). Just as with the proximal femur, in the proximal humerus there is no need to widely resect the tumor, and the rotator cuff is usually left intact.

5. Spine—In most cases of metastasis to the spine, the patient's pain can be managed adequately with local radiation therapy and medication. However, in cases of mechanical collapse associated with bony protrusion into the vertebral canal and cord compromise, surgical decompression and stabilization are frequently indicated. In the past, most of these prob-lems were treated with posterior decompression by laminectomy alone. The results were poor because the spine was further destabilized, which resulted in increased kyphosis and anterior cord compression. With advances in the area of spinal instrumentation, the treatment shifted toward a more aggressive anterior decompression and stabilization if the patient's general condition allows. Even in cases in which the patient's general health does not tolerate the larger anterior approach, a less aggressive alternative might include posterior decompression supplemented by posterior spinal fixation.

The midthoracic spine is the most common area for paraplegia secondary to metastasis because of the narrow vertebral canal at this level of the spine. The ideal surgical approach to the problem in a patient with a reasonable prognosis consists of an anterior thoracotomy and anterior decompression by verte-

A   **B**

Figure 6–80. Preoperative (**A**) and postoperative (**B**) radiographs of the proximal humerus of a patient whose treatment involved the use of a cemented long-stem Neer prosthesis.

Figure 6–81. Preoperative T_1-weighted MRI (**A**) and postoperative radiograph (**B**) of the spine of a patient whose treatment involved use of posterior rods and sublaminal wires for stabilization.

brectomy, followed by anterior stabilization. As an alternative approach in a patient with a worse prognosis and a circumferential cord compression, a posterior decompression stabilization can be considered (Figure 6–81).

The second most common site for cord compression is the thoracolumbar region. The anterior reconstruction is the same in the thoracolumbar area as in the midthoracic area. A posterior stabilization may be advisable, especially in cases in which the prognosis is good.

The cervical spine is the least likely area for surgical treatment, mainly because the vertebral canal is wide at this level and cord compromise is uncommon. If surgery is needed, an ideal reconstruction is an anterior decompression and stabilization.

Radiation therapy is required postoperatively with all of these reconstructions. The use of bone graft is therefore undesirable because of inhibited osteoblastic healing.

Beauchamp CP: Errors and pitfalls in the diagnosis and treatment of metastatic bone disease. Orthop Clin North Am 2000; 31(4):675. [PMID: 11043105]

Hipp JA et al: Predicting pathologic fracture risk in the management of metastatic bone defects. Clin Orthop 1995;312:120. [PMID: 7634597]

Hortobagyi GN et al: Efficacy of pamidronate in reducing skeletal complications in patients with breast cancer and lytic bone metastases. N Engl J Med 1996;24:1785. [PMID: 8965890]

Mirels H: Metastatic disease in long bones. A proposed scoring system for diagnosing impending pathologic fractures. Clin Orthop 1989;(249):256. [PMID: 2684463]

Mundy GR: Mechanisms of bone metastasis. Cancer 1997;80S: 1546. [PMID: 9362421]

Rougraff BT et al: Skeletal metastases of unknown origin: A prospective study of a diagnostic strategy. J Bone Joint Surg AM 1993;75:1276. [PMID: 8408149]

Wedin R: Surgical treatment for pathologic fracture. Acta Orthop Scand Suppl 2001;72(302):2p. [PMID: 11582636]

Wedin R et al: Surgical treatment for skeletal breast cancer metastases: A population-based study of 641 patients. Cancer 2001;92(2):257. [PMID: 11466677]

DIFFERENTIAL DIAGNOSIS OF PSEUDOTUMOROUS CONDITIONS

In addition to benign, malignant, and metastatic neoplasms, a group of pseudotumors masquerade as bone and soft-tissue tumors. These lesions actually appear with greater frequency than either primary bone or soft-tissue tumors.

Stress-Reactive Lesions

The most common pseudotumors are those related to either bone or soft-tissue injury.

A. STRESS FRACTURE OF BONE

Stress fractures are common in young (less than 30 years) athletic individuals and can produce radiographic features that might suggest the diagnosis of a bone-forming sarcoma or Ewing sarcoma. It is important to obtain a careful history from patients regarding their physical activity both at work and at play. There will be no history of a single injury if the bone symptoms are caused by repetitive impact loading stress such as occurs with working out for cross-country running. The stress fracture usually occurs several weeks after a sudden increase of physical activity for which the patient is not properly conditioned. This is a common situation in the military, particularly during initial training.

Stress fractures are commonly located in the metaphyseal-diaphyseal areas of long weight-bearing bones. Early radiographs frequently appear normal before periosteal new bone begins to form. The most sensitive early diagnostic tool is a bone scan, which can appear hot or abnormal in the case of stress fractures, neoplasms, and infections. The MRI is sensitive to early fluid shifts in the periosteum overlying a stress fracture, but it is also sensitive to neoplastic and infectious conditions. One of the best methods to help rule out tumors and infection is to simply stop all physical stress to the injured bone for a period of 4 weeks. In patients with stress fracture, the pain should resolve spontaneously during this period, and a follow-up radiograph taken after this period reveals a typical fusiform circumferential periosteal callous formation. In patients with a tumor or infection, the pain persists, and the radiographic signs of permeative osteolysis predominate, in which case a biopsy and culture are indicated.

At times, the clinical picture of a stress fracture is confused by the preexistence of a benign stress raiser, such as a nonossifying fibroma or fibrous cortical defect (Figure 6–82).

In older patients, especially in postmenopausal women, stress fractures can occur with minimal physi-

A

B

C

Figure 6–82. Radiograph (**A**), isotope bone scan (**B**), and T_1-weighted MRI (**C**) of the proximal tibia in a 16-year-old boy with a stress fracture.

cal activity. The circumstances under which the fracture occurred might not come out in a routine history. A common location of osteoporotic stress fractures is in the sacrum (Figure 6–83).

A

B

C

Figure 6–83. T$_1$-weighted MRI (**A**), isotope bone scan (**B**), and CT scan (**C**) of the sacrum in a 71-year-old woman with stress fracture.

B. Myositis Ossificans

Another common stress-reactive pseudotumor seen in the extremity is myositis ossificans, which occurs most frequently in the lower extremity in young men. The

quadriceps muscle is commonly involved because of direct blows or tearing injury to this muscle. The pseudotumor mass may not arise for several months after the injury and may not be related to a specific injury. In older (more than 40 years), more sedentary patients, there may be no history of stress injury.

Early radiographs may not reveal soft-tissue calcification. With maturation, ossification occurs in the traumatized muscle fascial planes, which may suggest the diagnosis of a synovial sarcoma or other calcifying sarcoma. If the myositis pseudotumor is attached to the subjacent bone, it can mimic a parosteal osteosarcoma (Figure 6–84).

Infectious Diseases

Bacterial, viral, tuberculous, or fungal infections of the bone or soft tissue can frequently mimic a neoplastic process. This is particularly the case with infections that are not highly virulent, do not create systemic symptoms or a febrile response, and do not cause a large alteration in acute-phase reactant laboratory work. If a tender mass is present on examination and a bone or soft-tissue tumor is suggested by imaging studies, a biopsy may be indicated and should include a tissue culture to make the correct diagnosis. Inflammatory pseudotumors can be seen in any age group but are more common in children and frequently affect the lower extremity.

A. Bacterial Infection

Bacterial infections of bone can take on the appearance of a round cell tumor such as Ewing sarcoma in children or lymphoma in adults (Figure 6–85). In contrast, tuberculous and fungal infections are less inflammatory and thus have more localized, well-marginated lesions that take on the imaging appearance of a benign tumor.

B. Tuberculous or Fungal Infection

A tuberculous or fungal infection of the spine or extremity can present as a pseudotumor in children or young adults, especially in Asian or Mexican patients (Figure 6–86). The incidence of tuberculous and fungal infections, which are low-grade infections that typically have an insidious onset, is also increased in patients with AIDS.

C. Caffey Disease

Caffey disease can mimic a neoplastic process. It is an idiopathic form of periostitis that is seen in infants younger than 6 months and affects the extremities, shoulder girdle, and mandible (Figure 6–87). It may have a viral origin and is currently much rarer than it was 30 years ago. The bony changes are osteoblastic and could suggest the diagnosis of an osteosarcoma, which is rare in infants. Caffey disease is self-

A

B

Figure 6–84. Radiograph (**A**) and gross appearance of a resected specimen (**B**) of myositis ossificans in the adductor muscles of a 12-year-old girl.

limiting and usually clears spontaneously without disability.

Metabolic Disorders

A. BROWN TUMOR
OF PRIMARY HYPERPARATHYROIDISM

Brown tumor is the most common metabolic disorder that mimics a neoplastic process in bone. The lytic giant cell lesions occur symmetrically in metaphyseal-epiphyseal bone as the result of increased parathyroid hormone production by a solitary parathyroid adenoma, by hyperplastic parathyroid glands, or by a solitary parathyroid carcinoma. Brown tumors occur three times more often in females than in males and are usually seen between 15 and 70 years of age. They are most common in the ends of the long bone, followed next in frequency in the pelvis, long bone diaphysis, maxillary bone, cranium, rib, and hand. Brown tumors are rarely seen in the spine. Symptoms of pain are related to the local bone destruction, but widespread pain may result from generalized osteomalacia. The hyperparathyroid condition can lead to weight loss, psychologic disorders, gastrointestinal disorders, renal stones, polyuria, and polydipsia.

The radiographic features of the brown tumor in bone include a round lytic area that may be multicentric and may suggest the diagnosis of metastatic carcinoma, multiple myeloma, or histiocytic lymphoma (Figure 6–88). In the case of a solitary lesion, it may suggest the diagnosis of a nonossifying fibroma, fibrous dysplasia, giant cell tumor, or aneurysmal bone cyst. At the time of biopsy, the brown tumor has the reddish brown appearance of a giant cell tumor. Microscopically, it looks like a giant cell tumor except that the background stromal cells are more fibroblastic and the bone trabeculae demonstrates abnormally thick and poorly mineralized osteoid seams. Because of the marked similarity between the brown tumor and the giant cell tumor, clinicians should routinely order an analysis of serum calcium, phosphorus, and alkaline phosphatase levels in all patients with bone lesions that produce giant cells.

In patients with brown tumors, the treatment consists of removing the source of the excessive parathyroid hormone. After this, the bony defects usually heal spontaneously. Bone grafting is rarely required. Although the secondary hyperparathyroidism seen in renal failure patients does not usually develop into brown tumors, it does produce pseudotumor-

Figure 6–85. Radiograph of acute osteomyelitis caused by *Staphylococcus aureus* in the proximal humerus of a 13-year-old boy.

ous calcification in soft tissue, a condition similar to tumoral calcinosis, which is discussed later in this section.

B. PAGET DISEASE

Paget disease is frequently included in discussions of metabolic bone disorders, although the demonstration of cytoplasmic and nuclear inclusion bodies in osteoclasts of pagetic bone similar to paramyxovirus infections may suggest a viral origin. Most clinicians are familiar with the late changes in Paget disease, which include the bowing of long bones and the finding of dense blastic changes on radiographic examination. However, many are unfamiliar with the early lytic phase of Paget disease when the radiographic findings are more suggestive of metastatic carcinoma, histiocytic lymphoma, primary sarcoma, or even primary hyperparathyroidism (Figure 6–89).

C. GAUCHER DISEASE

Gaucher disease is a rare familial disorder in which accumulation of glucocerebroside causes enlargement of the liver, spleen, and marrow tissues. The marrow infiltration in children and young adults causes a gradual loss of bone that can mimic a neoplastic condition. The most common areas involved include the distal femur, tibia, humerus, vertebral column, skull, and mandible. Isolated focal destructive changed with endosteal scalloping and moth-eaten patterns may suggest the diagnosis of metastatic disease, myelomatosis, primary sarcoma, or fibrous dysplasia (Figure 6–90).

Hemorrhagic Conditions

A. PSEUDOTUMOR OF HEMOPHILIA

A hematoma in the soft tissue or bone under the periosteum may be difficult to distinguish from a tumor.

Figure 6–86. Radiograph of tuberculous osteomyelitis in the proximal tibia of a 10-year-old girl.

Figure 6–87. Preoperative (**A**) and postoperative (**B**) radiographs of Caffey disease in the upper extremity and shoulder of a 5-month-old infant.

Hematoma formation is frequently precipitated by some form of trauma, and the bones most commonly involved are the femur, pelvis, tibia, and small bones of the hand. It is rare to see multiple lesions. The bony lesions can be central or eccentric. The finding of lytic destruction fol- lowed by sclerotic reaction at the periphery may mimic the radiographic picture of an aneurysmal bone cyst or a giant cell tumor. In the hand bones, the osseous pseudo- tumors take on the appearance of a giant cell reparative granuloma or an osteoblastoma. The subperiosteal lesions

Figure 6–88. Radiograph (**A**) and photomicrograph (**B**) of a brown tumor of hyperparathyroidism in the proxi- mal humerus of a 40-year-old woman.

A   **B**

Figure 6–89. Early and late radiographs of Paget disease of the tibia, taken when the male patient was 45 years of age (**A**) and when he was 65 years of age (**B**).

bulge into the surrounding soft tissue and show reactive periosteal new bone formation and subjacent cortical erosion that may mimic Ewing sarcoma or hemorrhagic osteosarcoma (Figure 6–91).

B. Intramuscular Hematoma

Another hemorrhagic disorder that can produce a pseudotumor of soft tissue is the intramuscular hematoma. It is similar to the soft-tissue pseudotumor of hemophilia but without a bleeding abnormality. Intramuscular hematomas are almost always related to blunt trauma, but they occasionally result from a traction injury that may subsequently produce myositis ossificans. There may be no superficial signs of bruising in the overlying skin, and sometimes the hematoma grows in size at a later date, even as long as several years after the initial injury. The radiographic examination is of little help because no calcification or bony abnormality is evident. The MRI is the best imaging study, but unfortunately, the appearance of an intramuscular hematoma on MRI can mimic that of a deep soft-tissue sarcoma such as a malignant fibrous histiocytoma (Figure 6–92).

Ectopic Calcification

Ectopic calcification in soft tissue has many causes, most of which are related to chronic degenerative disorders in collagenous structures such as tendons or ligaments about a joint. However, in cases in which the

dystrophic calcification is associated with a soft-tissue mass, the clinician must rule out the diagnosis of a soft-tissue sarcoma such as synovial sarcoma.

A. Tumoral Calcinosis

Tumoral calcinosis, seen about the hip, shoulder, and elbow, is characterized by extensive calcium phosphate deposition in a benign fibrous mass. It is an idiopathic condition that affects patients between 10 and 30 years of age and occurs more frequently in males than in females. Multiple lesions occur, and the lesions cause minimal pain and tenderness.

In cases of tumoral calcinosis, the extensive central fluffy calcification might suggest the diagnosis of a synovial sarcoma, soft-tissue chondrosarcoma, or tuberculosis (Figure 6–93). At biopsy, a chalky white paste exudes from a spongelike fibrous mass. Microscopic findings include extensive amorphous calcium phosphate deposits in a fibrous stroma speckled with macro-

Figure 6–90. Radiograph of a pathologic fracture secondary to Gaucher disease involving the distal femur in a 29-year-old man.

A   **B**

Figure 6–91. Anteroposterior (**A**) and lateral (**B**) radiographs of a pseudotumor of hemophilia in the distal femur of a 14-year-old boy.

phages and inflammatory cells. If the pseudotumor is not completely removed, a recurrence is very likely.

A similar condition is seen in patients with renal osteodystrophy with secondary hyperparathyroidism, and the mechanism for the deposition in this case is a high level of calcium phosphorus production.

B. COMPARTMENT SYNDROME

The ischemic calcification and even ossification that occur in traumatic compartment syndromes in the lower extremity can often mimic a tumor. The initial injury is usually a crushing type that causes increased compartment pressure from muscle swelling. This pressure eventually leads to ischemic necrosis of the compartment muscle, which several years later becomes calcific or even ossified. Because the muscle appears firm and calcified on radiographic examination, the clinician may not relate the finding to an old injury and may suspect a calcifying sarcoma such as synovial sarcoma. The most common place for this pseudotumor is in one of the

Figure 6–92. Axial view T$_2$-weighted MRI of a hematoma in the quadriceps muscles of a 46-year-old man.

A

B

Figure 6–93. Radiograph (**A**) and T₁-weighted MRI (**B**) of tumoral calcinosis in the hip of a 54-year-old woman.

muscle compartments of the leg, and it causes stiffness and muscle weakness at the ankle and foot area (Figure 6–94). This process can mimic soft-tissue calcifications secondary to a neoplastic process (Figure 6–95).

Dysplastic Disorders

Many developmental or dysplastic conditions can create bony abnormalities, which, on radiographic examination, can mimic a bone tumor. These are usually focal defects in enchondral bone formation that result from a failure to remodel primary woven bone forming at the metaphyseal end of the physis.

A. OSTEOMA

Osteoma commonly occurs in the skull or maxilla and is composed of dense unorganized woven bone seen just beneath the cortex. There is no lytic component in or around the dense bone, and no symptoms are associated with the presence of osteomas. Because the lesions are commonly seen in the metaphyseal areas about the

knee, the clinician may become concerned about the diagnosis of an early osteosarcoma. However, the lack of periosteal response and minimal uptake on an isotope bone scan help rule out sarcoma (Figure 6–96). In such cases, there should be no concern about future problems from the lesion, and usually no intervention is necessary.

B. BONE ISLAND

The bone island is an even more sharply marginated dysplastic process than the osteoma. It is most commonly located in the pelvis. It can mimic a blastic metastatic lesion in patients with prostate cancer. However, with a bone island, as with an osteoma, the bone scan shows minimal and very focal activity, and the CT scan and MRI show no reaction in the surrounding

Figure 6–94. Radiograph of an old compartment syndrome in the flexor hallucis longus.

Figure 6–95. Radiograph of calcification in synovial sarcoma of the leg.

marrow. Figure 6–97 shows the findings of a bone island through the pelvis of a 35-year-old man.

Bone Infarcts

The two types of bone infarcts that can mimic bone tumors are the metaphyseal type and the epiphyseal type. They can be idiopathic in origin or secondary to increased alcohol consumption or corticosteroid use.

A. METAPHYSEAL BONE INFARCT

The most common bone infarct is in the metaphyseal region, which is typically seen about the knee, hip, and shoulder in adults. Radiographically, the infarct can mimic a low-grade cartilaginous tumor such as an

enchondroma. An infarct presents with a sclerotic honeycombed pattern (Figure 6–98), whereas a cartilaginous lesion presents with central flocculated calcification (Figure 6–99).

B. EPIPHYSEAL BONE INFARCT

Although epiphyseal bone infarcts have the same etiology as those in the metaphysis, these are most commonly found in the femoral condyles and the proximal femoral and humeral epiphyses. In these locations, the lytic change seen in the epiphyseal bone can mimic a chondroblastoma. The differential diagnosis can be difficult before the appearance of a crescent sign or other radiographic signs of subchondral collapse that usually rule out the chondroblastoma (Figure 6–100).

A

B

Figure 6–96. Radiograph (**A**) and T$_2$-weighted MRI (**B**) of a dysplastic process in the distal femur of a 64-year-old woman.

A

vis, maxilla, vertebral body (vertebra plana), clavicle, and scapula, listed in the order of frequency. Besides affecting flat bones, it can arise in the diaphysis of long bones, followed next by the metaphysis, and it is least common in the epiphysis.

Eosinophilic granuloma can be extremely permeative and destructive, especially in long bones (Figure 6–101) and vertebrae (Figure 6–102), thereby mimicking a more aggressive process, such as Ewing sarcoma, metastatic neuroblastoma, or osteomyelitis. It can also produce a so-called onionskin periostitis of the type seen in Ewing sarcoma. The lesion has a more aggressive pattern in younger children and later becomes more focal and granulomatous. Microscopic findings include large pale-staining histiocytes speckled with small bright-staining eosinophils and an occasional giant cell.

A

B

Figure 6–97. CT scan (**A**) and T$_2$-weighted MRI (**B**) of a bone island through the pelvis of a 35-year-old man.

Histiocytic Disorders

A. Langerhans Cell Histiocytosis

Sometimes inappropriately called histiocytosis X, Langerhans cell histiocytosis can present in a variety of ways. Previously considered distinct diseases, including eosinophilic granuloma, Hand-Schüller-Christian disease, and Letterer-Siwe disease, they are now considered part of the same spectrum of histiocytosis presentation. Of these, the localized granulomatous form, which is called eosinophilic granuloma or Langerhans cell granulomatosis, is the one that mimics a tumor radiographically. Eosinophilic granuloma is seen twice as often in boys as in girls and commonly occurs between 5 and 15 years of age. It is usually monostotic but in 10% of cases involves two or three separate areas. It is a histiocytic process of unknown cause but may have a viral origin. It causes local inflammatory pain and may result in low-grade fever associated with an elevated sedimentation rate. Although the most common location of eosinophilic granuloma is the skull, it is also seen in the rib, pel-

B

Figure 6–98. Radiograph (**A**) and T$_1$-weighted MRI (**B**) of a metaphyseal infarct in the distal femur of a 52-year-old woman.

Figure 6–99. Radiograph of a large enchondroma in the distal femur.

Figure 6–100. Radiograph of an epiphyseal infarct in the femoral condyle of a 45-year-old woman.

Figure 6–101. Radiograph of an eosinophilic granuloma of the humerus in a 12-year-old boy.

Eosinophilic granulomas tend to involute spontaneously without treatment, and therefore treatment should be conservative. Simple curettement and corticosteroid injections are beneficial. In difficult areas such as the spine or pelvis, low-dose radiation treatment (10 Gy) can be considered. In more disseminated cases that do not respond to simple treatment, low-dose chemotherapy is appropriate.

B. PIGMENTED VILLONODULAR SYNOVITIS

Although this form of synovitis can mimic a histiocytic tumor, it is thought to be a nonneoplastic condition involving histiocytic proliferation. It occurs in the subsynovial tissue about major joints of the lower extremity in patients between 20 and 40 years of age. The knee joint is the most common site of involvement, followed next by the hip, ankle, and foot. Involvement of the upper extremity is rare.

The histopathology of pigmented villonodular synovitis is similar to that of a giant cell tumor of the tendon

Figure 6–103. T$_1$-weighted MRI of pigmented villonodular synovitis in the popliteal space of a 50-year-old man.

Figure 6–102. Radiograph of an eosinophilic granuloma in the body of the C3 vertebra in a 5-year-old girl.

sheath, which presents with soft-tissue tumors about the ankle and on the fingers of the hand. The usual situation involves spontaneous swelling of one knee secondary to synovial hypertrophy. The swelling can grow gradually to a massive amount and be associated with intermittent hemarthroses. The inflamed synovium can cause juxtaarticular erosion into bone at the point of attachment of the joint capsule, as is seen in any chronic proliferative synovitis, including hemophilia and coccidioidomycosis.

In fewer than 10% of cases, pigmented villonodular synovitis is more localized and presents as a focal soft-tissue mass high in the suprapatellar pouch or in the popliteal space, and no generalized swelling of the knee occurs. In these cases, the mass can mimic a soft-tissue sarcoma such as a synovial sarcoma (Figure 6–103). Cortical erosion with secondary bony changes can also be appreciated frequently (Figure 6–104).

Figure 6–104. Laminagram of pigmented villonodular synovitis in the proximal tibia of a young man.

Mankin HJ et al: Gaucher disease. New approaches to an ancient disease. J Bone Joint Surg Am 2001;83-A(5):748. [PMID: 11379747]

Roodman GD: Studies in Paget's disease and their relevance to oncology. Semin Oncol 2001;28(4 Suppl 11):15. [PMID: 11544571]

Shidham V et al: Evaluation of crystals in formalin-fixed, paraffin-embedded tissue sections for the differential diagnosis of pseudogout, gout, and tumoral calcinosis. Mod Pathol 2001; 14(8):806. [PMID: 11504841]

Zelger B: Langerhans cell histiocytosis: A reactive or neoplastic disorder? Med Pediatr Oncol 2001;37(6):543. [PMID: 11745894]

Adult Reconstructive Surgery

7

Robert S. Namba, MD, Harry B. Skinner, MD, PhD, & Ranjan Gupta, MD

Adult reconstructive surgery in orthopedics has rapidly evolved over the past 30 years. Prior to the successful development of so-called low-friction arthroplasty of the hip in the late 1960s, reconstructive options for the hip and the knee were limited. Reconstructive procedures with high success rates are now available for a variety of disorders, from marked degenerative hip disease to rotator cuff tears of the shoulder. Research done in the last 30 years has increased the understanding of major joint function and contributed to the success of reconstructive surgical procedures in almost all cases, and there is now a tremendous demand for these procedures. In 1997, total knee arthroplasty and total hip arthroplasty procedures numbered 338,000 and 289,000, respectively, the result of their great success in returning patients to active lifestyles. Millions of Americans are now benefiting from these procedures for extended periods. Because their cumulative procedure failure rate is approximately 1% per year, 10 years after their operation, patients have approximately a 90% chance of still having a successful, well-functioning joint replacement.

Statistics from American Academy of Orthopedic Surgeons: *Arthroplasty and Total Joint Replacement Procedures in the United States 1990 to 1997.* http://www.aaos.org/wordhtml/press/arthropl.htm

■ ARTHRITIS & RELATED CONDITIONS

Evaluation of Arthritis

To treat arthritic conditions of the joints appropriately, an understanding of the disease process is essential. This begins with accurate diagnosis and a history of the progression of the disease, so that the future progression can be predicted and appropriate decisions regarding treatment can be made. The physician must evaluate the possibility of traumatic, inflammatory, developmental, idiopathic, and metabolic causes of the arthritis (Table 7–1).

Evaluation of the history, physical examination, and laboratory data is helpful in arriving at a diagnosis.

A. History

Clearly the history is important in defining the disease process. The time course, including duration and behavior of symptoms since onset, is a key factor. Gradual rather than acute onset implies a nontraumatic cause. Swelling in the joints is an important sign, as is the distribution of joints if more than one is involved. The degree of interference with activities indicates the seriousness of the disorder.

The presence and extent of pain are valuable pieces of information. Constant pain, night and day, implies infection, cancer, or a functional disorder. Pain only with activity such as walking, standing, or running suggests joint loading. Pain that awakens the patient is considered severe and requires evaluation. Location helps distinguish referred pain from joint pain.

Knowledge of the age distribution of the various arthritic disorders can be very helpful to the student in diagnosing the disease. A hip disorder in the patient under age 40 is unlikely to be OA unless a predisposing condition is present, such as trauma. A more likely diagnosis is osteonecrosis. Similarly, a chronic condition of the knee in the 45-year-old man is likely to be a degenerative meniscus tear, unless the patient had a meniscectomy in his early 20s. This concept can be extended to all age groups for the common disorders of the hip and knee (Figures 7–1 and 7–2). Further, a history of one of these disorders at an earlier age predisposes a patient to earlier osteoarthrosis.

Hip pain is felt typically in the groin or in the lateral aspect of the hip or anterior thigh but seldom in the buttock. Pain arising from the spine may be appreciated in the buttock and less often in the groin and anterior thigh. Acetabular pain or femoral head pain is frequently felt in the groin. Proximal femur pain is usually appreciated in the anteroproximal thigh.

Knee pain is frequently anterior (patellofemoral), medial (medial compartment), or lateral (lateral compartment). It may also be poorly localized by the patient. Pain in the back of the knee may result from a popliteal cyst (Baker cyst) or a torn meniscus. A swol-

Table 7–1. Causes of arthritic conditions.

Traumatic causes	Traumatic arthritis, osteonecrosis (posttraumatic)
Inflammatory causes	Infectious arthritis, gout, pseudogout, rheumatoid arthritis, systemic lupus erythematosus, ankylosing spondylitis, juvenile rheumatoid arthritis, Reiter syndrome
Developmental causes	Developmental dysplasia of the hip, hemophilic arthritis, following slipped capital fermoral epiphysis, following Legg-Calvé-Perthes disease
Idiopathic causes	Osteoarthritis, osteonecrosis
Metabolic causes	Gout, calcium pyrophosphate deposition disease, ochronosis, Gaucher disease

Figure 7–2. The age distribution of knee disorders is given schematically as a function of age. Blount's ds = tibia vara; P-F ds = patellofemoral arthralgia; and OA = osteoarthrosis. Meniscal tears can be either medial or lateral and are traumatic in the younger age group and degenerative in the older age group. Osteoarthrosis shows an earlier onset with the knee than with the hip because there is an incidence of medial gonarthrosis in the 40s and 50s caused by medial meniscectomy in the late teens and early 20s.

len knee may be painful because of pressure. Pain with any motion may indicate a septic joint or possibly a gouty joint. Arthritic pain in the elbow and shoulder is less clearly defined by patients, and in such cases the physical examination is important. Shoulder pain may be caused by cervical, cardiac, or even diaphragmatic disorders.

B. Physical Examination

1. Hip—The physical examination of the hip is important to verify that the reported pain arises from the hip joint and to determine the severity of the pain. It is also useful to document range of motion (ROM), gait, leg-length discrepancy, and muscle weakness. Pain arising from the hip is typically elicited at the extremes of

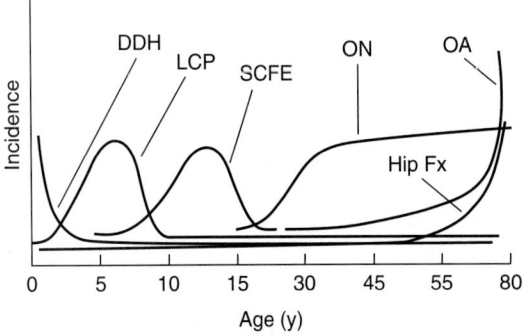

Figure 7–1. The age distribution of hip disorders is given in a schematic representation. DDH = developmental dysplasia of the hip; LCP = Legg-Calvé-Perthes disease; SCFE = slipped capital femoral epiphysis; ON = osteonecrosis; OA = osteoarthrosis; and Hip Fx = hip fracture.

ROM. Active straight leg raising or resisted straight leg raising may produce pain (Figure 7–3). Log rolling (internal and external rotation of the hip in extension) usually elicits hip pain if pain is severe. Frequently, internal rotation of the hip in flexion is limited; this condition is one of the first signs of osteoarthritis (OA) of the hip. Abduction of the hip against gravity loads the hip and may produce hip pain of arthritis, but does not do so if pain in the buttock or thigh is referred from the spine. Increased loading may be achieved by applying resistance to abduction. In the young (under age 40) patient with groin pain, provocative maneuvers can be used to diagnose labral tears. Flexion of the hip with external rotation (ER) and abduction (ABD) is followed by extension, adduction (ADD), and internal rotation (IR). Clicking or catching is observed in patients with anterior labral tears. Posterior tears of the labrum are identified by moving the hip from extension, ABD, and ER to flexion, ADD, and IR.

The ROM in flexion, extension (flexion contracture), ABD, ADD, and IR and ER is measured. Decreased IR is an early finding in OA.

2. Knee—The physical examination of the knee localizes the pain to the knee and to the specific involved compartment. ROM of the hip should be evaluated to rule out referred hip pain. Ligamentous stability is discerned in the mediolateral and anteroposterior (AP) planes (see Chapter 4). Instability is not common in osteoarthritis but is often seen in rheumatoid arthritis.

Figure 7–3. Resisted straight leg–raising test. The examiner asks the patient to actively raise the straight leg to approximately 30 degrees. This produces hip pain in severe arthritis. If no pain is produced, the examiner applies pressure to the thigh, which the patient resists. This increased joint loading uncovers mild to moderate hip pain.

Alignment of the knee (varus or valgus) while standing is measured. Varus and valgus alignment increase the odds of progression of OA fourfold and fivefold, respectively, in 18 months. ROM of the knee is measured, and any flexion contracture or extensor lag is noted. Flexion contracture is an inability to come to full extension passively, whereas an extensor lag indicates an inability to extend the knee actively as far as it will extend passively. The contracture is common in advanced OA, whereas the lag is generally a quadriceps muscle or tendon problem. The medial and lateral compartments are loaded during flexion and extension with varus and valgus stress, respectively, to elicit pain arising from arthritis in each compartment. The patellofemoral joint may be assessed for pain and bone-on-bone crepitation by flexion and extension with pressure on the patella. The presence of fluid, synovitis, and erythema is also important.

3. Shoulder—After the cervical spine is ruled out as the source of pain, examination of the shoulder begins with visual inspection for obvious asymmetry of bone and muscle contours. Palpation of muscle tone and of the clavicle, as well as the acromioclavicular and sternoclavicular joints, follows. Tenderness over the anterolateral humeral head is often found with rotator cuff disorders. Tendinitis of the long head of the biceps is easily demonstrated by palpation of the tendon over the anteromedial humeral head. Active ROM is then assessed in flexion and abduction. External rotation is reproducibly measured by keeping the elbow on the waist and rotating the hand away from the body. Internal rotation is best recorded by measuring how high the thumb can be positioned along the spine. Most individuals can position the thumb to the midthoracic area (eg, T6 or T7). When internal rotation is limited, the thumb may only

be elevated to L5. If active ROM is at all limited, passive ROM should be assessed. Strength of the upper extremity muscle is then evaluated along with sensation and deep tendon reflexes. Decreased strength in external rotation with the elbow at the side indicates significant rotator cuff weakness. Provocative tests can help evaluate the cause of pain, particularly with instability. The apprehension test is positive, indicating anterior instability, when abduction, extension, and external rotation of the shoulder elicit anxiety or discomfort. Impingement signs are present with rotator cuff disorders and produce pain with passive flexion or internal rotation of the flexed and adducted arm.

4. Elbow—Inspection of the elbow includes measurement of the "carrying angle," the normal 5–7 degree angle of valgus inclination between the humerus and forearm. Scars and obvious deformities are noted, as well as swelling or masses. Bony prominences are palpated, including the mediolateral epicondyles, radial head, and olecranon. Active and passive motion is recorded for both flexion and extension and pronation and supination. Tenderness over the lateral epicondyle exacerbated by resisted wrist dorsiflexion is often seen in lateral epicondylitis (tennis elbow). Tenderness over the medial epicondyle with pain elicited by resisted wrist flexion is seen in medial epicondylitis. Limitation of flexion and extension is seen with arthritis and posttraumatic stiffness.

C. IMAGING STUDIES

Radiologic data, synovial fluid analysis, and blood testing may be beneficial in confirming the diagnosis of arthritis. The most fundamental radiographic data can be provided by a plain radiograph with a minimum of two views. Evaluation of joint pain includes ruling out fracture, joint space narrowing, osteophyte formation, or osteopenia. Views of the hip include a modified AP view of the pelvis (which clips the iliac wings to show the proximal femora) and a lateral view of the affected hip (either "frog," an AP view with the hip externally rotated and abducted, or a true lateral view). Views of the knee should include a 10 degrees down-angled beam posteroanterior radiograph of the bent knee (30–45 degrees of flexion) taken while the patient is standing, a lateral view, and a tangential patellar view (Merchant view, 45 degrees of flexion) (Table 7–2). Views of the shoulder should include AP, axillary, and lateral views of the scapula. Supraspinatus outlet views may be helpful in revealing acromial bone spurs, which produce impingement. The elbow usually can be visualized with AP and lateral radiographs.

D. LABORATORY FINDINGS

Basic blood testing should include a complete blood count and sedimentation rate. These are indicated in a suspected septic process or in the evaluation of a painful

Table 7–2. Radiographic findings in arthritis.

Disease State	Findings in Hip or Knee
Osteoarthritis	Joint space narrowing, subchondral sclerosis, osteophytes, subchondral cysts Hip: Superior or medial narrowing Knee: Early narrowing on Rosenberg views; flattening of femoral condyles
Rheumatoid arthritis or sytemic lupus erythematosus	Uniform joint narrowing, erosion near joint capsule
Ankylosing spondylitis	Osteopenia, osteophytes, ankylosis of sacroiliac joints
Gout	Tophi, erosions
Calcium pyrophosphate deposition disease	Calcification of menisci and hyaline cartilage
Osteonecrosis	Crescent sign, spotty calcification
Gaucher disease	Erlenmeyer flask appearance, distal femora
Neuropathic joint	Four *Ds*: destruction, debris, dislocation, densification (sclerosis, hypertrophy)
Hemophilic arthropathy	Epiphyseal widening, sclerosis, cysts, joint space narrowing

joint replacement. A normal white cell count may be helpful in the diagnosis of gout, especially in an inflamed joint other than the first metatarsophalangeal joint.

Synovial fluid analysis is indicated at any time to rule out infection, and it may also be quite helpful in the diagnosis of other arthritides. Table 8–4 shows the significance of yellow and clear synovial fluid. Aspiration of synovial fluid may reveal hemorrhagic fluid. If this is the result of a traumatic tap, it should be so noted and the fluid should be sent for analysis. If the fluid is grossly hemorrhagic, several diagnoses must be entertained, including hemophilia, neuropathic arthropathy, pigmented villonodular synovitis, hemangioma, or trauma. A finding of fat floating on the bloody fluid in the setting of a traumatic injury suggests the presence of an intraarticular fracture.

The combined history, physical examination, and appropriate laboratory studies should narrow the diagnoses to a relative few, if not the definitive one. It is helpful to consider diagnoses in categories, which, despite some overlap, provide a framework for further workup. Many of these arthritic conditions are described in the following pages.

Sharma L et al: The role of knee alignment in disease progression and functional decline in knee osteoarthritis. JAMA 2001; 286:188.

Solomon DH et al: Does this patient have a torn meniscus or ligament of the knee? Value of physical exam of the knee. JAMA 2001;286:1610.

1. Noninflammatory Arthritis

The term **osteoarthritis** is a misnomer, because inflammation is not the primary pathologic process observed in this form of articular joint disruption. More accurately described as degenerative joint disease, the disease represents a final common pathway of injury to articular cartilage. Although the true nature and cause of OA are unclear, radiographic findings and gross and microscopic pathologic features are fairly typical in most cases.

Categorization of primary and secondary forms of OA, although still useful, are blurred. A designation of primary or idiopathic OA was made when no identifiable predisposing conditions could be recognized. OA is considered secondary when an underlying cause such as trauma, previous deformity, or systemic disorder exists. Although many cases of hip OA were considered idiopathic when the end-stage changes were observed, careful analysis indicated predisposing conditions such as slipped capital femoral epiphysis and mild forms of acetabular dysplasia in many cases.

The joints most commonly involved include the hip; knee; distal interphalangeal, proximal interphalangeal, and first carpometacarpal joints of the hand; and cervical, thoracic, and lumbar spine.

Primary Osteoarthritis

A. Epidemiologic Features

OA is a widespread joint disorder in the United States, significantly affecting approximately 40 million people. Though autopsy studies show degenerative changes of weight-bearing joints in 90% of people older than 40 years, clinical symptoms are usually not present. The prevalence and severity of OA increase with age.

When all ages are considered, men and women are equally affected. Younger than 45 years, the disease is more prevalent in men; older than 55 years, women are more commonly afflicted. The pattern of joint involvement commonly includes the joints of the hands and knees in women and the hip joints in men.

The incidence of hip OA is higher in European and American white males than in Chinese, South African blacks, and East Indian persons. Primary hip OA in Japanese persons is rare, but secondary OA is common because of developmental dysplasia of the hip.

Evidence indicates that some distinct forms of OA may be inherited as a dominant trait with a mendelian pattern. These include a primary generalized OA in which Heberden nodes and Bouchard nodes are a prominent feature, and symmetric and uniform loss of articular cartilage of the knee and hip joints is evident. Other types of inherited OA include familial chondrocalcinosis (with deposition of calcium pyrophosphate dihydrate crystals in cartilage), Stickler syndrome (characterized by vitreoretinal degeneration), hydroxyapatite deposition disease, and multiple epiphyseal dysplasias. Certain inherited forms are caused by mutations in the gene for cartilage-specific type II procollagen.

B. PATHOLOGIC FEATURES

Early features of OA include focal swelling and softening of the cartilage matrix. Mild loss of metachromatic staining ability represents loss of proteoglycans in the extracellular matrix. Surface irregularities in the form of fibrillation occur. Diffuse hypercellularity of the chondrocytes can be seen. The tidemark, an interface plane between hyaline cartilage and the zone of calcified cartilage, is thin and wavy early in OA.

Later features of OA include progressive loss of proteoglycans manifesting as reduction in safranin-O staining. Fibrillations in the surface deepen into fissures and later into deeper clefts. Chondrocyte cloning is seen and also reduplication of the tidemark, with discontinuous parallel lines indicating progression of calcification of the basal portion of the articular cartilage. Regions of eburnated bone represent complete loss of cartilage.

New bone formation occurs in a subchondral location as well as at margins of the articular cartilage. Areas of rarefaction of bone below eburnation are represented by "cysts" on radiographs and on gross inspection.

C. LABORATORY FINDINGS

Specific diagnostic tests for OA are currently not available. Routine blood tests, urinalysis, and even synovial fluid analysis do not provide useful information, except for exclusion of inflammatory or infectious arthritis. Experimental work on identification of markers of cartilage degradation in OA may provide diagnostic tests in the future. These include sensitive and specific assays for synovial fluid cytokines, proteinases and their inhibitors, matrix components and their fragments, serum antibodies to cartilage collagen, and identification of proteoglycan subpopulations.

D. IMAGING STUDIES

Typical radiographic features indicate late pathologic changes in OA. Specifically, narrowing of the joint space, subchondral sclerosis, bony cysts, and marginal osteophytes are seen. End-stage disease is complicated by bony erosions, subluxation, loose bodies, and deformity.

Heberden nodes are commonly seen in primary OA, represented by bony and cartilaginous enlargement of the distal interphalangeal joints of the fingers. Similar enlargements of the proximal interphalangeal joints of the fingers are called **Bouchard nodes.**

Secondary Osteoarthritis

The term **secondary osteoarthritis** is applied when an underlying recognizable local or systemic factor exists. These include conditions leading to joint deformity or destruction of cartilage, followed by signs and symptoms typically seen with primary OA. Examples of preexisting conditions leading to secondary osteoarthritic changes in joints include acute and chronic trauma, Legg-Calvé-Perthes disease, developmental dysplasia of the hip, rheumatoid arthritis, bleeding dyscrasias, achondroplasia, infection, crystal deposition disease, neuropathic disorders, overuse of intraarticular steroids, and multiple epiphyseal dysplasias. Radiographic features of secondary OA reflect the underlying pathologic changes plus the changes resulting from the primary OA.

Bjell A: Cartilage matrix in hereditary pyrophosphate arthropathy. J Rheumatol 1981;8:959.

Hoaglund FT, Steinbach LS: Primary osteoarthritis of the hip: Etiology and epidemiology. J Am Acad Orthop Surg 2001;9(5):320.

Kellgren JH et al: Genetic factors in generalized osteoarthrosis. Ann Rheum Dis 1963;22:237.

Knowlton RG et al: Genetic linkage analysis of hereditary arthroophthalmopathy and the type II procollagen gene. Am J Hum Genet 1989;65:681.

Lawrence RC et al: Estimates of the prevalence of arthritis and selected musculoskeletal disorders in the United States. Arthritis Rheum 1999;42(2):396.

Lowman EW: Osteoarthritis. JAMA 1955;157:487.

Marcos JC et al: Idiopathic familial chondrocalcinosis due to apatite crystal deposition. Am J Med 1981;71:557.

Mukhopadhaya B, Barooah B: Osteoarthritis of hip in Indians. Indian J Orthop 1975;1:55.

Palotie A et al: Predisposition to familial osteoarthrosis linked to type II collagen gene. Lancet 1989;1:924.

Reginato AJ: Articular chondrocalcinosis in the Chiloé islanders. Arthritis Rheum 1976;19:396.

Solomon L et al: Rheumatic disorders in the southern African Negro. S Afr Med J 1975;49:1737.

Spranger J: The epiphyseal dysplasias. Clin Orthop 1975;114:46.

Stickler GB et al: Hereditary progressive arthro-ophthalmopathy. Mayo Clin Proc 1965;40:433.

2. Inflammatory Arthritis

Rheumatoid Arthritis

A chronic systemic inflammatory disorder, rheumatoid arthritis (RA) is a crippling disease affecting approximately 1% of the population in the United States. Although similar synovial histopathologic and joint abnormalities are identifiable in all patients, the articular and systemic manifestations, outcomes, and differences in genetic makeup and serologic findings vary widely in individual patients. The cause is unknown, although the disease probably occurs in response to a pathogenic agent in a genetically predisposed host. Possible triggering factors include bacterial, mycoplasmal, or viral infections, as well as endogenous antigens in the form of rheumatoid factor, collagens, and mucopolysaccharides.

Joint involvement is typically symmetric, affecting the wrist, metacarpal, phalangeal, proximal, interphalangeal elbow, shoulder, cervical spine, hip, knee, and ankle joints. The distal interphalangeal joints are typically spared. Extraarticular manifestations include vasculitis, pericarditis, skin nodules, pulmonary fibrosis, pneumonitis, and scleritis. The triad of arthritis, lymphadenopathy, and splenomegaly, known as **Felty syndrome,** is associated with anemia, thrombocytopenia, and neutropenia.

A. EPIDEMIOLOGIC FEATURES

RA occurs two to four times more often in women than men. The disease occurs in all age groups, but increases in incidence with advancing age, with a peak between the fourth and sixth decades.

Evidence for a genetic basis is provided by the association of RA with a certain haplotype of class II gene products of the major histocompatibility complex. Seventy-five percent of patients with RA carry circulating rheumatoid factors, which are autoantibodies against portions of the IgG antibody. In rheumatoid factor–positive patients, there is a high incidence of HLA-DR4, except in black patients. Only a minority of individuals with HLA-DR4 develop RA, however. (See Chapter 13, especially Tables 13–5 and 13–6.)

B. PATHOLOGIC FEATURES

Early rheumatoid synovitis consists of a local inflammatory response with accumulation of mononuclear cells. The antigen-presenting cell (macrophage) activates T lymphocytes, resulting in cytokine production, B-cell proliferation, and antibody formation. Chronic inflammation results in formation of a pannus, a thickened synovium filled with activated T and B lymphocytes and plasma cells, as well as fibroblastic and macrophagic types of synovial cells. Joint destruction begins with exposed bone at the margins of articular cartilage denuded of hyaline cartilage. Eventually, the cartilage itself is destroyed by inflammatory byproducts of the pannus. The synovial fluid, in contrast to the mononuclear cell infiltrate seen in the synovial membrane, has neutrophils forming 75–85% of the cells.

Rheumatoid factors are antibodies specific to antigens on the Fc fragment of IgG. The antibodies include IgM, IgG, IgA, and IgE classes, but the IgM rheumatoid factor is typically measured. Rheumatoid factor may be a triggering factor for RA and may contribute to the chronic nature of the disease. Rheumatoid factor is also frequently found in patients with other inflammatory diseases, however, as well as in 1–5% of normal patients.

C. LABORATORY FINDINGS

No specific laboratory test exists for RA, but a series of test results help in the diagnosis. A high titer of rheumatoid factor (more than 1:160) is the most significant diagnostic finding. Anemia is moderate, and leukocyte counts are normal or mildly elevated. Acute-phase reactants reflect the degree of inflammation nonspecifically and are often elevated in RA. These include the erythrocyte sedimentation rate (ESR) and levels of C-reactive protein and serum immune complexes. Antinuclear antibodies are often positive in patients with severe RA (up to 37% in one study) but are not specific for the disease.

D. IMAGING STUDIES

Early radiographic changes in RA include swelling of the small peripheral joints and marginal bony erosions. Joint space narrowing occurs later and is uniform, unlike the focal narrowing seen in OA. Regional osteoporosis occurs, unlike the sclerosis seen in OA. Advanced changes include bone resorption, deformity, dislocation, and fragmentation of affected joints. Protrusio acetabuli may be seen in the hips, and ulnar subluxation is common in the metacarpophalangeal joints.

Lipsky PE et al: The role of cytokines in the pathogeneis of rheumatoid arthritis. Springer Semin Immunopathol 1989;11: 123. [PMID: 2479111]

Saulsbury FT: Prevalence of IgM, IgA, and IgG rheumatoid factors in juvenile rheumatoid arthritis. Clin Exp Rheumatol 1990; 8:513. [PMID: 2261713]

Sutton B et al: The structure and origin of rheumatoid factors. Immunol Today 2001;21:177.

Winchester RG: Genetic aspects of rheumatoid arthritis. Springer Semin Immunopathol 1981;4:89.

Zvaifler NJ: Etiology and pathogenesis of rheumatoid arthritis. In McCarty DJ, ed: *Arthritis and Allied Conditions.* Lea & Febiger, 1989.

Ankylosing Spondylitis

A seronegative (negative rheumatoid factor) inflammatory arthritis, ankylosing spondylitis consists of bilateral sacroiliitis with or without associated spondylitis and uveitis. An insidious disease, the diagnosis is often delayed because of vagueness of the early symptom of low back pain. Diagnostic clinical criteria include low back pain, limited lumbar spine motion, decreased chest expansion, and sacroiliitis.

Joint involvement is primarily axial, including all portions of the spine, sacroiliac joint, and hip joints. Extraskeletal involvement includes dilation of the aorta, anterior uveitis, and restrictive lung disease secondary to restriction of thoracic cage mobility.

A. Epidemiologic Features

The association of HLA-B27 and ankylosing spondylitis is strong, with 90% of patients testing positive for this haplotype; however, only 2% of HLA-B27-positive patients develop ankylosing spondylitis. First-degree family members of a patient who has ankylosing spondylitis and is positive for HLA-B27 have a 20% risk of developing the disease. Clinical and experimental evidence shows that *Klebsiella* infection may be a triggering factor for arthritis in patients positive for HLA-B27.

B. Laboratory Findings

During the active phase of the disease, the ESR is increased. Testing for rheumatoid factor and antinuclear antibodies is negative.

C. Imaging Studies

Early in the course of ankylosing spondylitis, the sacroiliac joints may be widened, reflecting bony erosions of the iliac side of the joint. Later, the inflamed cartilage is replaced by ossification, resulting in ankylosis of the bilateral sacroiliac joints. Vertebrae of the thoracolumbar spine are squared off, with bridging syndesmophytes, forming a so-called bamboo spine. Ankylosis of peripheral joints may be seen. MRI may provide sensitive and specific radiographic evidence of sacroiliitis.

Ebringer RW et al: Sequential studies in ankylosing spondylitis: Association of *Klebsiella pneumoniae* with active disease. Ann Rheum Dis 1978;37:146.

Geczy AF et al: A factor in *Klebsiella* filtrates specifically modifies an HLA-B27 associated cell-surface component. Nature 1980; 283:782.

Luong AA, Salonen DC: Imaging of the seronegative spondyloarthropathies. Curr Rheumatol Rep 2000;2(4):288.

Moll JMH, Wright V: New York clinical criteria for ankylosing spondylitis: A statistical evaluation. Ann Rheum Dis 1973; 32:354.

Van der Linden S et al: The risk of developing ankylosing spondylitis in HLA-B27 positive individuals: A family and population study. Br J Rheum 1983;22(Suppl):18.

Psoriatic Arthritis

A seronegative inflammatory arthritis associated with psoriasis, psoriatic arthritis was long considered a variant of RA. The discovery of rheumatoid factor led to the division of inflammatory arthritides into seropositive and seronegative diseases, separating psoriatic arthritis from RA.

Although psoriatic arthritis is characterized by a relatively benign course in most patients, up to 20% develop severe joint involvement. The distal interphalangeal joints of the fingers are commonly affected, but several patterns of peripheral arthritis exist, including an asymmetric oligoarthritis, a symmetric polyarthritis (similar to RA), arthritis mutilans (a destructive, deforming type of arthritis), and a spondyloarthropathy (similar to ankylosing spondylitis, with sacroiliac joint involvement).

In addition to the dry erythematous papular skin lesions, nail changes are found. These include pitting, grooves, subungual hyperkeratosis, and destruction.

A. Epidemiologic Features

A third of patients with psoriasis have arthritis, with joint symptoms delayed as long as 20 years after onset of skin lesions. Both sexes are affected equally.

B. Laboratory Findings

There are no specific laboratory tests for psoriatic arthritis. Nonspecific inflammatory markers may be elevated, including the ESR. Rheumatoid factor is usually negative but is present in up to 10% of patients.

C. Imaging Studies

Coexistence of erosive changes and bone formation is seen in peripheral joints, with absence of periarticular osteoporosis. Gross destruction of phalangeal joints (so-called pencil-in-cup appearance) and lysis of terminal phalanges are seen. Bilateral sacroiliac joint ankylosis and syndesmophytes of the spine are seen, as in ankylosing spondylitis.

Gladman DD et al: HLA antigens in psoriatic arthritis. J Rheum 1986;13:586.

Hohler T, Marker-Hermann E: Psoriatic arthritis: Clinical aspects, genetics, and the role of T cells. Curr Opin Rheumatol 2001;13(4):273.

Mader R, Gladman D: Psoriatic arthritis: Making the diagnosis and treating early. J Musculoskel Med 1993;10:18.

Juvenile Rheumatoid Arthritis

Juvenile rheumatoid arthritis (JRA) is an inflammatory arthritic syndrome with a variety of symptoms. Early diagnosis is often difficult. Criteria for JRA include distinction of mode of onset as systemic, polyarticular, or pauciarticular. Systemic onset (also known as **Still disease**) occurs in 20% of patients and is characterized by high fever, rash, lymphadenopathy, splenomegaly, carditis, and varying degrees of arthritis. Polyarticular onset occurs in 30–40% of patiemnts and is notable for fewer systemic symptoms, low-grade fever, and synovitis of four or more joints. Pauciarticular onset develops in 40–50% of patients and involves one to four joints; there are no systemic signs, but there is an increased incidence of iridocyclitis. Iridocyclitis is an insidious complication that requires early ophthalmologic slit-lamp evaluation, if JRA is suspected, to prevent blindness.

A. EPIDEMIOLOGIC FEATURES

The two peak ages of onset are between 1 and 3 years and between 8 and 12 years. Females are affected twice as often as males.

B. LABORATORY FINDINGS

Leukocytosis up to 30,000/mL is seen with systemic-onset JRA, with mild elevations in polyarticular-onset disease and normal values in pauciarticular-onset disease. White blood cell counts in synovial fluid range from 150 to 50,000/mL. The ESR rate is elevated, as are other acute-phase reactants.

Rheumatoid factor is typically negative in JRA. As many as 50% of patients have positive antinuclear antibodies, a finding correlated with iridocyclitis and pauciarticular-onset disease.

C. IMAGING STUDIES

Soft-tissue swelling and premature closure of physes may be seen early, as well as juxtaarticular osteopenia. Erosive changes are seen late and resemble those of RA.

Falcini F, Cimaz R: Juvenile rheumatoid arthritis. Curr Opin Rheumatol 2000;12(5):415.

Schaller JG: The association of antinuclear antibodies with the chronic iridocyclitis of juvenile rheumatoid arthritis. Arthritis Rheum 1974;17:409.

Systemic Lupus Erythematosus

Systemic lupus erythematosus (SLE) is a chronic inflammatory disease that may affect multiple organ systems. It is an autoimmune disorder in which autoantibodies are formed. The large variety of clinical appearances and laboratory findings may mimic many disorders. The diagnosis is based on the presence of 4 of the following 11 criteria: (1) malar rash; (2) discoid rash; (3) photosensitivity; (4) oral ulcers; (5) arthritis; (6) serositis; (7) renal disorders (proteinuria or casts); (8) neurologic disorders (seizures or psychosis); (9) hematologic disorders (hemolytic anemia, leukopenia, lymphopenia, thrombocytopenia); (10) immunologic disorders (positive lupus erythematosus [LE] cell preparation, anti-DNA antibody, anti-Sm antibody, false-positive serologic test for syphilis); and (11) abnormal titer of antinuclear antibody.

A. EPIDEMIOLOGIC FEATURES

Females are affected eight times as often as males. An increased risk for SLE is noted for Asians and Polynesians over whites in Hawaii. Black females are also associated with an increased risk over white females. Genetic susceptibility is demonstrated with increased frequency (5%) among relatives of patients with the disease. An inherited complement deficiency is inferred from the absence, or near absence, of individual complement components, the most common being C2.

B. LABORATORY FINDINGS

Antinuclear antibody determination is the most helpful screening test for SLE. The LE cell preparation was the first immunologic test for SLE, but it is laborious, insensitive, and difficult to interpret. In patients with untreated active disease, 98% have positive antinuclear antibody tests. The higher the titer of antinuclear antibodies, the more likely is the diagnosis of SLE or related rheumatic syndrome. A low value for the antinuclear antibody test is 1:320; values greater than 1:5120 are considered high.

If antinuclear antibody levels are positive, more specific tests may be performed, including testing for anti-DNA antibodies, antibodies to extractable nuclear antigens, and complement levels. High titers of antibodies to double-stranded DNA are highly suggestive for SLE. Low complement levels (C3, C4, and total hemolytic complement levels) are found in the disease but are also seen in related illnesses.

Anemia, leukopenia, and thrombocytopenia are seen, as well as elevations in the ESR. Renal function tests and muscle and liver enzyme tests are often abnormal, reflecting multiple organ system involvement.

C. IMAGING STUDIES

The radiographic features of arthritis in SLE are similar to those of RA. Much of the joint pain may be related to osteonecrosis, particularly of the femoral and humeral heads.

Agnello V: Association of systemic lupus erythematosus and systemic lupus erythematosus-like syndromes with hereditary and acquired complement deficient states. Arthritis Rheum 1978;21:S146.

Block SR et al: Immunologic observations on 9 sets of twins either concordant or discordant for systemic lupus erythematosus. Arthritis Rheum 1976;19:545.

Kaine JL, Kahl LE: Which laboratory tests are useful in diagnosing SLE? J Musculoskel Med 1992;9:15.

Serdula MK, Rhoads GG: Frequency of systemic lupus erythematosus in different ethnic groups in Hawaii. Arthritis Rheum 1979;22:328.

Tan EM et al: Revised criteria for classification of systemic lupus erythematosus: ARA subcommittee. Arthritis Rheum 1982; 25:1271.

Arthritis Associated with Inflammatory Bowel Disease

Peripheral arthritis and spondylitis are associated with ulcerative colitis and Crohn disease. Joint involvement is typically monarticular or oligoarticular and often parallels the activity of the bowel disease. The arthritis, frequently migratory, is self-limiting in most cases, with only 10% of patients having chronic arthritis. The joints most commonly affected are the knees, hips, and ankles, in order of prevalence. Spondylitis associated with inflammatory bowel disease occurs in two forms. One is very similar to ankylosing spondylitis, including the increased incidence of the HLA-B27 haplotype. The other form has no identifiable genetic predisposition.

A. EPIDEMIOLOGIC FEATURES

Up to 25% of patients with inflammatory bowel disease develop arthritis. There is no difference between the sexes in incidence.

B. LABORATORY FINDINGS

There is no specific diagnostic test. Synovial fluid analysis reveals an inflammatory process, with leukocyte counts of 4000–50,000/mL.

C. IMAGING STUDIES

Peripheral arthritis is nonerosive, with juxtaarticular osteopenia and joint space narrowing. Spondylitis associated with inflammatory bowel disease resembles ankylosing spondylitis.

Enlow RW et al: The spondylitis of inflammatory bowel disease. Arthritis Rheum 1980;23:1359.

Morris RI et al: HLA-B27, a useful discriminator in the arthropathy of inflammatory bowel disease. N Engl J Med 1974; 290:1117.

Wollheim FA: Enteropathic arthritis: How do the joints talk with the gut? Curr Opin Rheumatol 2001:13(4):305.

Reiter Syndrome

The classic triad of conjunctivitis, urethritis, and peripheral arthritis is known as **Reiter syndrome.** **Reactive arthritis** is becoming accepted as a more precise term because the initiating condition may be enteritis as well as a sexually transmitted disease. The peripheral arthritis is polyarticular and asymmetric, with knees, ankles, and foot joints most commonly affected.

A. EPIDEMIOLOGIC FEATURES

Nongonococcal urethritis caused by *Chlamydia* accounts for the precipitating event in approximately 20% of cases. Patients who test positive for HLA-B27 are predisposed to developing arthritis after contracting nongonococcal urethritis. A reactive arthritis following enteric infection with *Salmonella, Shigella, Yersinia,* and *Campylobacter* is also noted. For enteric infections with *Shigella,* the risk of developing arthritis in individuals positive for HLA-B27 is close to 20%.

B. LABORATORY FINDINGS

There are no specific diagnostic tests for Reiter syndrome. Anemia, leukocytosis, and thrombocytosis occur, and the ESR is often elevated.

C. IMAGING STUDIES

The radiographic features of Reiter syndrome are similar to those of ankylosing spondylitis, with calcifications of ligamentous insertions and ankylosing of joints. The sacroiliitis is unilateral, unlike in ankylosing spondylitis.

Bradshaw CS et al: Etiologies of nongonococcal urethritis, bacteria, viruses, and the association with orogenital exposure. J Infect Dis 2006;193:366. [PMID: 16388480]

Caelin A, Fries JF: An "experimental" epidemic of Reiter's syndrome revisited: Follow-up evidence on genetic and environmental factors. Ann Intern Med 1976;85:563.

Ford DK: Reiter's syndrome: Reactive arthritis. In McCarty DJ, ed: *Arthritis and Allied Conditions.* Lea and Febiger, 1989.

Grayston JT, Wan SP: New knowledge of chlamydiae and the diseases they cause. J Infect Dis 1975;132:87.

3. Metabolic Arthropathy

Gout

Deposition of monosodium urate crystals in the joints produces gout. Although most patients with gout have hyperuricemia, few patients with hyperuricemia develop gout. The causes of hyperuricemia include disorders resulting in overproduction or undersecretion of uric acid or a combination of these two abnormalities. Examples of uric acid overproduction include enzymatic mutations, leukemias, hemoglobinopathies, and excessive purine intake.

The first attack involves sudden onset of painful arthritis, most often in the first metatarsophalangeal joint, but also in the ankle, knee, wrist, finger, and elbow. The intensity of the pain is comparable to that from a septic joint, and differentiation is necessary because the treatment is different. Coexistence of a septic joint is unusual but possible. Rapid resolution with colchicine or indomethacin is seen. Chronic gouty arthritis is notable for tophaceous deposits, joint deformity, constant pain, and swelling. Definitive diagnosis is made upon demonstration of intracellular monosodium urate crystals in synovial cell leukocytes.

A. EPIDEMIOLOGIC FEATURES

Primary gout has hereditary features, with a familial incidence of 6–18%. It is likely that the serum urate concentration is controlled by multiple genes.

B. LABORATORY FINDINGS

The key diagnostic test is detection of monosodium urate crystals in white blood cells in synovial fluid. Negative birefringence of the needle-shaped crystals is seen by their yellow coloration on polarized light microscopy.

Hyperuricemia is usually seen, but up to a fourth of gout patients may have normal uric acid levels. Uric acid levels are elevated when they exceed 7 mg/dL. An elevated white blood cell count and sedimentation rate can be seen in acute gout, and thus these tests cannot be used to differentiate between the two processes. Aspirates should be sent for culture to rule out coexisting infection.

C. IMAGING STUDIES

Tophi may be seen when they are calcified. Soft-tissue swelling is seen, as well as erosions. Chronic changes consist of extensive bone loss, joint narrowing, and joint deformity.

Abubaker MY et al: The management of gout. N Engl J Med 1996;334:445.

Agudelo CA, Wise CM: Gout: Diagnosis, pathogenesis, and clinical manifestations. Curr Opin Rheumatol 2001;13(3):234.

Emmerson BT: Coexistence of acute gout and septic arthritis. Arthritis Rheum 2000;43:S189.

Kelley WN et al: Gout and related disorders of purine metabolism. In Kelly WN et al, eds: *Textbook of Rheumatology.* WB Saunders, 1989.

Levinson DJ: Clinical gout and the pathogenesis of hyperuricemia. In McCarty DJ, ed: *Arthritis and Allied Conditions.* Lea & Febiger, 1989.

Calcium Pyrophosphate Crystal Deposition Disease

Calcium pyrophosphate crystal deposition disease, a goutlike syndrome, is also known as pseudogout or chondrocalcinosis. Crystals of calcium pyrophosphate dihydrate are deposited in a joint, most commonly the knee and not the first metatarsophalangeal joint, as in gout. The diagnosis is made by demonstration of the crystals in tissue or synovial fluid and by the presence of characteristic radiographic findings.

Aging and trauma are associated with this disorder, as well as conditions such as hyperparathyroidism, gout, hemochromatosis, hypophosphatasia, and hypothyroidism.

A. EPIDEMIOLOGIC FEATURES

Hereditary forms of calcium pyrophosphate dihydrate deposition disease are reported, with transmission as an autosomal trait. Idiopathic cases were not rigorously examined for genetic factors or association with other diseases.

B. PATHOLOGIC FEATURES

Calcification of multiple joint structures occurs, including hyaline cartilage and capsules, with heaviest deposi-

tion in fibrocartilaginous structures such as the menisci. The crystals are more difficult to see than urate crystals but have weak positive birefringence.

C. IMAGING STUDIES

Calcification of menisci and hyaline cartilage is seen as punctate or linear radiodensities, which delineate these normally radiolucent structures. Bursas, ligaments, and tendons may have calcifications as well. Bony signs include subchondral cyst formation, signs of carpal instability, sacroiliac joint erosions with vacuum phenomenon, and crowning of the odontoid process.

Kohn NN et al: The significance of calcium phosphate crystals in the synovial fluid of arthritis patients: The "pseudogout syndrome." II. Identification of crystals. Ann Intern Med 1982;56:738.

McCarty DJ et al: The significance of calcium phosphate crystals in the synovial fluid of arthritis patients: The "pseudogout syndrome." I. Clinical aspects. Ann Intern Med 1962;56:711.

Resnick D: Rheumatoid arthritis and pseudorheumatoid arthritis in calcium pyrophosphate dihydrate crystal deposition disease. Radiology 1981;140:615.

Rosenthal AK: Calcium crystal-associated arthritides. Curr Opin Rheumatol 1998;10(3):273.

Ochronosis

A hereditary deficiency in the enzyme homogentisic acid oxidase is present in the disease known as **alkaptonuria.** The presence of unmetabolized homogentisic acid results in a brownish black color of the urine (thus the name of the disease). The term **ochronosis** describes the clinical condition of homogentisic acid deposited in connective tissues, manifested by bluish black pigmentation of the skin, ear, and sclera, and in cartilage.

The diagnosis is made when the triad of dark urine, degenerative arthritis, and abnormal pigmentation is present. Freshly passed urine is normal in color but turns dark when oxidized. Spondylosis is common, with knee, shoulder, and hip joint involvement also seen.

A. EPIDEMIOLOGIC FEATURES

Transmission of alkaptonuria is by a recessive autosomal gene.

B. IMAGING STUDIES

Spondylosis is seen, with calcification of intervertebral disks with few osteophytes. Joint involvement is similar in appearance to that of OA, except for protrusio acetabuli.

Schumacher HR, Holdsworth DE: Ochronotic arthropathy: Clinicopathologic studies. Semin Arthritis Rheum 1977;6:207.

4. Osteochondroses

Osteonecrosis of the Femoral Head

A variety of conditions and diseases are associated with femoral head osteonecrosis, but the pathogenesis is unknown in most cases. Direct injury to the blood supply of the femoral head is implicated in traumatic causes of avascular necrosis such as subcapital femoral neck fracture and dislocation of the hip. The disorder is bilateral in more than 60% of cases and affects other bones in approximately 15% of cases. The leading nontraumatic causes of osteonecrosis of the femoral head include alcoholism, idiopathic causes, and systemic steroid treatment. The mechanism by which steroids cause osteonecrosis may be by adipogenesis because the effects may be reduced, at least in an animal model, by using lovastatin.

Other associated conditions include hemoglobinopathies, Gaucher disease, caisson disease, hyperlipidemia tobacco use, hypercoagulable states, irradiation, and diseases of bone marrow infiltration such as leukemia and lymphoma.

A. PATHOLOGIC FEATURES

Regardless of underlying causes, the early lesions in femoral head osteonecrosis include necrosis of marrow and trabecular bone, usually in a wedge-shaped area in the region of the anterolateral superior femoral head. The overlying articular cartilage is largely unaffected because it is normally avascular, obtaining nutrition from the synovial fluid. The deep calcified layer of cartilage, however, does derive nutrition from epiphyseal vessels and also undergoes necrosis. Histologically, necrotic marrow and absence of osteocytes in lacunae are seen.

Leukocytes and mononuclear cells collect around necrotic and fibrovascular tissue and eventually replace necrotic marrow. Osteoclasts resorb dead trabeculae, and osteoblasts then attempt to repair the damaged tissue; during attempted repair, the necrotic trabeculae are susceptible to fatigue fracture. Grossly, a subchondral fracture forms, with deformation of overlying hyaline cartilage. With time, fragmentation of articular cartilage ensues, resulting in degenerative arthritis.

B. IMAGING STUDIES

Ficat created a classification based on the plain radiographic appearance of femoral head osteonecrosis in progressive stages. Stage I represents normal or minimal changes (mild osteopenia or sclerotic regions) in an asymptomatic hip. In stage II, subchondral sclerosis and osteopenia are evident, often in a well-demarcated wedge in the anterolateral femoral head seen best with radiographs taken with the patient in the frog-leg position from the lateral views. Stage III is heralded by collapse of subchondral bone, known as the crescent sign, and is pathognomonic for femoral head osteonecrosis.

Femoral head flattening is often seen, but the joint space is preserved. Stage IV consists of advanced degenerative arthritic changes, with loss of joint space and bony changes in the acetabulum.

A newer classification system, devised by Steinberg, is popular and based on extent of head involvement as determined by MRI. This system, called the University of Pennsylvania system, has seven stages from normal (stage 0) to stage VI in which advanced degenerative changes are evident. Stages I to V are divided into three subcategories of mild, moderate, and severe. Stage III of the Steinberg system corresponds to stage III of the Ficat system.

Cui Q et al: The Otto Aufranc Award: Lovastatin prevents steroid-induced adipogenesis and osteonecrosis. Clin Orthop 1997; 344:8.

Ficat RP: Idiopathic bone necrosis of the femoral head: Early diagnosis and treatment. J Bone Joint Surg Br 1985;67:3.

Lavernia CJ et al: Osteonecrosis of the femoral head. J Am Acad Orthop Surg 1999;7:250.

Steinberg ME et al: A quantitative system for staging avascular necrosis. J Bone Joint Surg 1995;77B:34.

5. Other Disorders Associated with Arthritis

Hemophilia

Hemophilia A is a heritable bleeding disorder produced by deficiency of factor VIII. Hemophilia B is a disease caused by lack of clotting factor IX. Both hemophilia A (classic hemophilia) and hemophilia B (Christmas disease) are sex-linked recessive disorders, although 30% of patients may have no family history of the disease. Hemophilic arthropathy primarily involves the knee joint, with the elbow and ankle joints affected less frequently.

A. PATHOLOGIC FEATURES

Recurrent hemarthrosis produces deposits of hemosiderin and synovitis. In the acute phase, hypertrophy of synovium occurs, causing a higher risk of repeated bleeding. A pannus may form, as in RA, with underlying cartilage destruction. With time, synovial fibrosis occurs, resulting in joint stiffness.

B. IMAGING STUDIES

Soft-tissue swelling, seen early, is associated with hemarthroses. Later stages include widening of epiphyseal regions caused by overgrowth from increased vascularity. Skeletal changes are manifested as subchondral sclerosis and cyst formation early, with later loss of cartilage and secondary osteophyte formation. Squaring of the patella is seen, possibly resulting from overgrowth.

Luck JV, Kasper CK: Surgical management of advanced hemophilic arthropathy. Clin Orthop 1989;242:60.

Gaucher Disease

A rare familial disorder, Gaucher disease is an inborn error of metabolism caused by a deficiency of the lysosomal hydrolase enzyme β-glucocerebrosidase. Accumulation of glucosylceramidase in phagocytic cells of the reticuloendothelial cells occurs, including the liver, spleen, lymph nodes, and bone marrow.

The femur is the most commonly affected bone, but the vertebrae, ribs, sternum, and flat bones of the pelvis may also be affected. The manifestations of skeletal disease are the result of mechanical effects of infiltration of the abnormal cells, leading to erosion of cortices and interference with the normal vascular supply. Expansion of bone and areas of osteolysis predispose affected bones to pathologic fracture, and vascular interruption leads to avascular necrosis of the femoral hip.

A. Epidemiologic Features

Inherited in an autosomal recessive manner, Gaucher disease is the most common inherited disorder of lipid metabolism. The disease is especially common in the Ashkenazi Jewish community.

B. Pathologic Features

Histologic examination of involved reticuloendothelial tissues demonstrates foam cells, which are large lipid-laden macrophages.

C. Imaging Studies

Early stages of skeletal involvement in Gaucher disease include diffuse osteoporosis and medullary expansion. The distal femur may expand to form a characteristic Erlenmeyer flask deformity. Localized erosions and sclerotic areas are seen. Osteonecrosis may be seen in the femoral head, humeral head, and distal femur. Secondary degenerative changes follow collapse of necrotic articular bone.

Amstutz HC, Carey EJ: Skeletal manifestations and treatment of Gaucher's disease. J Bone Joint Surg Am 1966;48:670.

Goldblatt J et al: The orthopaedic aspects of Gaucher's disease. Clin Orthop 1978;137:208.

Hip Labral Tears

The hip has a cartilaginous extension of the bony acetabulum called the labrum that deepens the acetabulum and stabilizes the hip. Labral tears were newly rediscovered as a source of pain and a cause of osteoarthrosis, partially because of the relative ease of evaluating their presence and subsequently treating them. Arthroscopy can be used to remove the torn labrum, similar to torn menisci.

A. Pathologic Features

The normal labrum is triangular in shape and variable in size from 1 to 10 mm in length. The pathologic labrum is classified into types A and B, depending on whether the labrum is traumatic (triangular: A) or degenerative (thick and rounded: B) and three stages: (1) intrasubstance degeneration, (2) partial tear, and (3) complete tear.

B. Imaging Studies

MRI arthrography is the test of choice for suspected labral tears. Contrast is seen going into the tear, which is frequently in the weight-bearing area of the acetabulum. CT arthrography and MRI are not as sensitive.

Plotz GM et al: Magnetic resonance arthrography of the acetabular labrum. J Bone Joint Surg Br 2000;82:426.

■ MEDICAL MANAGEMENT

Nonsteroidal Antiinflammatory Drugs

The use of nonsteroidal antiinflammatory drugs (NSAIDs) in the management of OA is widespread but controversial. Because only minimal inflammatory changes are present in joints with OA, the use of acetaminophen is advocated as a first-line drug. In a short-term study of patients treated for OA, acetaminophen (4000 mg/d) was found to be as effective as ibuprofen (2400 mg/d).

The therapeutic effect of NSAIDs can be dramatic in the osteoarthritic patient, even with severe disease. The main problems with routine NSAID therapy are the gastrointestinal (GI) and renal complications and the inhibition of normal platelet function. Thus, alternative therapies should be carefully considered, and therapy should be closely monitored. Current NSAIDs work by altering prostaglandin synthesis through nonspecific inhibition of both cyclooxygenase isoforms 1 (COX-1) and 2 (COX-2). COX-1 inhibition can have deleterious effects on hemostasis and the GI tract.

Patients treated with NSAIDs have a three times greater relative risk of developing GI complications than nonusers. In one study, NSAIDs were associated with acute hospital admissions of 30% of elderly patients. Patients at high risk for developing ulcers with use of NSAIDs are those with any of the following characteristics: age older than 65 years, history of prior ulcer disease, use of multiple dose or high-dose NSAIDs, or use of concomitant corticosteroids. The antiprostaglandin effects of NSAIDs can reduce renal blood flow, leading to acute and chronic renal insufficiency. Patients at risk for acute renal insufficiency because of NSAIDs are elderly patients, those with atherosclerotic cardiovascular disease, and those with preexisting renal impairment. The platelet effects of these drugs are variable, depending on the NSAID half-life, on whether the NSAID inhibits thromboxane A, and on whether that inhibition is reversible. Aspirin, for example, is permanent for the life of the platelet. Many patients report increased bruising as a result of taking these drugs.

Table 7–3 compares the toxicities of currently available NSAIDs. Because the effects are not caused solely by the inhibitory effects on prostaglandin synthesis, the various chemical origins of these drugs may lead to slightly different clinical effects in different patients.

The chemical families of these drugs are noted in Table 7–4 with their half-lives and their dosing frequency. Dosing frequency is important because patient compliance with use of these drugs goes up with less frequent dosing, such as daily or twice daily.

Much anticipated is the development of COX-2-selective NSAIDs, which are now available. Most of the side effects attributable to NSAIDs are caused by inhibition of COX-1, an isoform that is normally present ("constitutive") in renal and GI tissues. COX-2-selective NSAIDs inhibit the isoenzyme that develops

("inducible") as a response to inflammation. By selectively inhibiting COX-2, the efficacy of NSAIDs is retained with much less side effects.

Although COX-2-selective NSAIDs are purportedly safe, they are not without side effects. Celecoxib did not exhibit statistically significant decreased rates of complicated upper GI events in a randomized controlled trial. Rofecoxib was shown to decrease complicated upper GI events significantly compared with conventional NSAIDs, but the rate of myocardial infarction was increased, possibly related to loss of the antiplatelet effect normally present in NSAIDs.

The choice of an appropriate NSAID should be based on the following factors: clotting problems, compliance of the patient, GI symptom history, renal function, drug cost, and the effect on the patient with previously used NSAIDs. Patients taking warfarin would probably be better treated with a drug having no platelet effect that is COX-2-specific. Patients with a poor response to one type of NSAID may benefit from a trial with one from another chemical family. A patient with a history of poor drug compliance with other medications would benefit from daily dosing, whereas a patient

Table 7–3. Toxicity profiles of currently available NSAIDs.

Generic Name	Proprietary Name	Gastrointestinal Toxicity	Renal Toxicity	Platelet Effects (d)[a]	Other Toxicity[b]
Diclofenac	Voltaren	Moderate	Moderate	1	Hepatitis
Etodolac	Lodine	Low[c]	Moderate	NA	—
Indomethacin	Indocin	High	Moderate	1	Headache
Nabumetone	Relafen	Low[c]	Moderate	NA	Hepatitis
Sulindac	Clinoril	Moderate	Low	1	Dermatitis
Tolmetin	Tolectin	Moderate	Moderate	2	—
Meclofenamate	Meclomen	Moderate	Moderate	1	Diarrhea
Piroxicam	Feldene	Moderate	Moderate	14	—
Fenoprofen	Nalfon	Moderate	Moderate	1	—
Flurbiprofen	Ansaid	Moderate	Moderate	1	—
Ibuprofen	Motrin	Moderate	Moderate	1	—
Ketoprofen	Orudis	Moderate	Moderate	2	—
Naproxen	Naprosyn	Moderate	Moderate	4	—
Oxaprozin	Daypro	Moderate	Moderate	NA	—
Ketorolacq	Toradol	High	Moderate	1	—
Salicylsalicylic acid[d]	Disalcid	None	None	None	—
Sodium salicylate[d]	—	None	None	None	—
Aspirin	—	High	Moderate	10	Tinnitus
Diflunisal[e]	Dolobid	Low	Low	None	—
Celecoxib	Celebrex	Low	Low	None	Sulfa allergies

[a]Average time to normal platelet function after discontinuation of drug.
[b]Other NSAIDs may have similar toxicity, but the effects are more prevalent with these agents.
[c]Simultaneous efficacy comparisons in inflammatory disease not available.
[d]No prostaglandin inhibition.
[e]Weak prostaglandin inhibitor.
NA = data not available.

Table 7–4. Dosage data of currently available NSAIDs.

Generic Name	Proprietary Name	Largest Unit Dose (mg)	Half-Life (h)	Dosing Frequency[a]	Family
Diclofenac	Voltaren	75	2	bid	Acetic acid
Etodolac	Lodine	300	6	qid	Acetic acid
Indomethacin	Indocin	50	4	tid	Acetic acid
Nabumetone	Relafen	500	20–30	2 qd	Acetic acid
Sulindac	Clinoril	200	8–14	bid	Acetic acid
Tolmetin	Tolectin	400	1–2	tid	Acetic acid
Meclofenamate	Meclomen	100	2	tid	Fenamates
Piroxicam	Feldene	20	30–86	qd	Oxicams
Fenoprofen	Nalfon	600	2–3	qid	Proprionates
Flurbiprofen	Ansaid	100	6	tid	Proprionates
Ibuprofen	Motrin	800	2	qid	Proprionates
Ketoprofen	Orudis	75	3	tid	Proprionates
Naproxen	Naprosyn	500	14	bid	Proprionates
Oxaprozin	Daypro	600	40–50	2 qd	Proprionates
Ketorolac	Toradol	10	5	qid	Pyrrolo-pyrrole
Salicylsalicylic acid	Disalcid	750	1	qid	Salicylates
Sodium salicylate	—	650	0.5	q4h	Salicylates
Aspirin	—	325	0.25	2q4h	Salicylates
Diffunisal	Dolobid	500	10	bid	Salicylates
Celecoxib	Celebrex	200	11	bid	Sulfonamide

[a]Dosage required for treatment of inflammation.

bid = twice a day; qd = each day; q4h = every 4 hours; qid = four times a day; tid = three times a day.

already taking another drug three times daily would probably find three-times-daily dosing more convenient. Obviously, a patient with renal disease should be treated with a drug having not only low renal toxicity, but also probably a short half-life to minimize the accumulation of the drug in the body because of lack of renal excretion. The COX-2-selective NSAIDs will not eliminate the need for the other drugs. The vast majority of patients tolerate the side effects of the older drugs, and the risk-benefit ratio for these drugs is quite favorable, especially for short courses of treatment.

The advent of the COX-2-specific NSAIDs adds to their safety as analgesics for acute pain because the COX-2 inhibitors block the pain, fever, and inflammatory response while not affecting clotting. Thus, their use in the perioperative setting is significantly increased.

Surgical intervention is generally indicated for patients who have failed conservative therapy with NSAIDs. For patients who are not surgical candidates, a long-term regimen of narcotic medication may be considered.

Batchlor EE, Paulus HE: Principles of drug therapy. In Moskowitz RW et al, eds: *Osteoarthritis: Diagnosis and Medical Surgical Management.* WB Saunders, 1993.

Berger RG: Nonsteroidal anti-inflammatory drugs: Making the right choice. J Am Acad Orthop Surg 1994;2:255.

Bombardier C et al: Comparison of upper gastrointestinal toxicity of rofecoxib and naproxen in patients with rheumatoid arthritis. VIGOR Study Group. N Engl J Med 2000;343(21):1520.

Bradley JD et al: Comparison of an anti-inflammatory dose of ibuprofen, an analgesic dose of ibuprofen, and acetaminophen in the treatment of patients with osteoarthritis of the knee. N Engl J Med 1991;325:87.

Gabriel SE et al: Risk for serious gastrointestinal complications related to use of nonsteroidal anti-inflammatory drugs. Ann Intern Med 1991;115:787.

Hochberg MC et al: Guidelines for the medical management of osteoarthritis: I. Osteoarthritis of the hip. Arthritis Rheum 1995;38:1535.

Hochberg MC et al: Guidelines for the medical management of osteoarthritis: II. Osteoarthritis of the knee. Arthritis Rheum 1995;38:1541.

Hosie J et al: Meloxicam in osteoarthritis: A 6-month, double-blind comparison with diclofenac sodium. Br J Rheumatol 1996;35(Suppl 1):39.

Silverstein FE et al: Gastrointestinal toxicity with celecoxib vs nonsteroidal anti-inflammatory drugs for osteoarthritis and rheumatoid arthritis: The CLASS study: A randomized controlled trial. Celecoxib long term arthritis safety study. JAMA 2000;284(10):1247.

Simon LS et al: Preliminary study of the safety and efficacy of SC-58635, a novel cyclooxygenase 2 inhibitor: Efficacy and safety in two placebo-controlled trials in OA and rheumatoid arthritis, and studies of gastrointestinal and platelet effects. Arthritis Rheum 1998;41:1591.

Disease-Modifying Agents in Rheumatoid Arthritis

Three new disease-modifying antirheumatic drugs (DMARDs) are now available for the medical treatment of rheumatoid arthritis. Although the experience of these new agents is limited, the mechanisms of their actions may guide orthopedic surgeons with respect to their potential effect on the surgical procedures. Etanercept is an artificially bioengineered molecule that binds to the receptor of TNF (tumor necrosis factor), preventing activation of the inflammatory cascade. Infliximab is a chimeric antibody that also targets TNF. Both of these drugs probably have little effect on healing and most likely can be continued up to any surgical procedure. Leflunomide inhibits an enzyme, decreasing levels of pyrimidine nucleotides, inhibiting clonal expansion of T cells in RA. This DMARD should probably be discontinued 1 week prior to surgery, similar to methotrexate.

Kremer JM: Rational use of new and existing disease-modifying agents in rheumatoid arthritis. Ann Intern Med 2001;134:695.

OTHER THERAPIES

Nutritional Supplements

The nutritional supplements glucosamine sulfate and chondroitin sulfate are popular as nonprescription products for arthritis therapy. This popularity arises from the concept that these products may serve as substrate for the reparative processes in cartilage. Glucosamine sulfate is found as an intermediate product in mucopolysaccharide synthesis, and an elevated urinary excretion is seen in patients with OA and RA. Oral administration of glucosamine sulfate was compared with analgesic doses of ibuprofen in a 4-week trial in patients with OA of the knee. Ibuprofen was found to provide pain relief more quickly, but the response rates were similar at 4 weeks.

Chondroitin sulfate is another glycosaminoglycan present in articular cartilage; its oral administration in one study resulted in no change in serum levels. In another study, patients with OA of the hip and knee used fewer NSAIDs when given chondroitin sulfate compared with a placebo control group. Although glucosamine sulfate and chondroitin sulfate are unproven therapies at this time, their use may provide safe and effective symptomatic relief in some patients with OA. Newer reports indicate improved symptoms of OA with oral glucosamine and chondroitin sulfate, but the mechanisms of action are unknown.

Brief AA et al: Use of glucosamine and chondroitin sulfate in the management of osteoarthritis. J Am Acad Orthop Surg 2001;9:71.

Houpt JB et al: Effect of glucosamine hydrochloride (GHCl) in the treatment of pain of osteoarthritis of the knee. J Rheumatol 1998;25(Suppl 52):8.

Hughes RA, Carr AJ: A randomized double-blind placebo-controlled trail of glucosamine to control pain in osteoarthritis of the knee. Arthritis Rheum 2000;43(Suppl 9):S384.

Leffter CT et al: Glucosamine, chondroitin, and manganese ascorbate for degenerative joint disease of the knee or low back: A randomized, double-blind, placebo-controlled pilot study. Mil Med 1999;164(2):85.

Mazieres B et al: Chondroitin sulfate in the treatment of gonarthrosis and coxarthrosis. Five-month results of a multicenter double-blind controlled prospective study using placebo. Rev Rhum Mal Osteoartic 1992;59:466.

McAlindon TE et al: Glucosamine and chondroitin for treatment of osteoarthritis: A systemic quality assessment and meta-analysis. JAMA 2000;283:1469.

Muller-Fabender H et al: Glucosamine sulfate compared to ibuprofen in osteoarthritis of the knee. Osteoarthritis Cartilage 1994;2:61.

Reginster JY et al: Long term effects of glucosamine sulphate on osteoarthritis progression: A randomized, placebo-controlled clinical trial. Lancet 2001;357:251.

Rindone JP et al: Randomized, controlled trial of glucosamine for treating osteoarthritis of the knee. West J Med 2000;172(2):91.

Injections

One of the mainstays of the treatment of osteoarthrosis and RA is the cortisone injection, which can be used for joints, bursae, and trigger points. Generally, shoulders, elbows, wrists, finger joints, knees, ankles, and joints of the foot can be given in the office without radiographic control. Hips and some joints of the foot and hand are best done with radiographic control to ensure location of the injection. The injections can be therapeutic with steroids or diagnostic with local anesthetic. For example, differentiation between the amount of a patient's pain coming from the back and the proportion coming from the hip can be ascertained with a lidocaine injection into the hip. This reliably informs the patient as to the realistic expectations of pain relief after a hip replacement. Similarly, an ankle injection predicts pain relief after ankle fusion. Intraarticular administration of hyaluronic acid is now available for treatment of OA of the knee with products of different molecular weight. The treatment protocols for these drugs call for weekly injections for 3–5 weeks to obtain a therapeutic effect.

Hyaluronic acid is a long-chain polysaccharide responsible for the viscoelastic properties of synovial joint fluid. In pathologic states, such as OA and RA, both the concentration and molecular size of hyaluronic acid is diminished. In animal experimental models, evidence indicates that hyaluronic injections may retard progression of OA. Serial injections of hyaluronic acid in patients with osteoarthritic knees are reported to reduce pain for up to 10 months, but the mechanism of action is unknown.

Because of the short half-life of hyaluronic acid, it is unlikely that the injections significantly boost lubrication of arthritic joints. Rather than being a disease-modifying therapy, the injectable hyaluronic acid products should be considered long-acting pain-relieving drugs.

Adams ME et al: The role of viscosupplementation with hylan G-F 20 (Synvisc) in the treatment of osteoarthritis of the knee: A Canadian multicenter trial comparing hylan G-F 20 alone, hylan G-F 20 with nonsteroidal anti-inflammatory drugs (NSAIDs) and NSAIDs alone. Osteoarthritis Cartilage 1995;3(4):213.

Altman RD, Moskowitz R: Intraarticular sodium hyaluronate (Hyalgan) in the treatment of patients with osteoarthritis of the knee: A randomized clinical trial. Hyalgan Study Group. J Rheumatol 1998;25(11):2203.

Marshall KW et al: Amelioration of disease severity by intraarticular hylan therapy in bilateral canine osteoarthritis. J Orthop Res 2000;18(3):416.

Watterson JR, Esdaile JM: Viscosupplementation: Therapeutic mechanisms and clinical potential in osteoarthritis of the knee. J Am Acad Orthop Surg 2000;8:277.

Orthotic Treatment

The use of orthotics can ameliorate the symptoms of osteoarthrosis in the knee, the ankle, and possibly the elbow, but other joints are not really amenable to this treatment. The medial compartment of the knee is more commonly affected than the lateral, leading to, or resulting from varus deformity. Thus, this disorder lends itself to orthotic treatment to remove the deformity. Heel wedges and valgus braces can be helpful in relieving the pain and improving the ambulatory function of patients with medial gonarthrosis. Similarly, orthotics to control varus and valgus forces at the ankle can be very helpful for ankle arthrosis.

Draper ERC et al: Improvement of function after valgus bracing of the knee. J Bone Joint Surg Br 2000;82:1001.

Pollo FE: Bracing and heel wedging for unicompartmental osteoarthritis of the knee. Am J Knee Surg 1998;11:47.

SURGICAL MANAGEMENT

PROCEDURES FOR JOINT PRESERVATION

A joint can potentially deteriorate for the following reasons: (1) trauma, which may distort the joint so abnormal loads are applied; (2) hemophilia, which forces the joint to dispose of blood on multiple occasions, causing synovitis; (3) rheumatoid arthritis, which causes a proliferation of the synovium, which may destroy the hyaline joint cartilage; and (4) osteonecrosis, which may result in fatigue fractures and collapse of the joint, with subsequent incongruity or (5) rotator cuff tear, leading possibly to cuff arthropathy. Certain procedures can slow progression of the deterioration and prolong the useful service of the joint. These include synovectomy, core decompression, osteotomy, and rotator cuff repair.

Rotator Cuff Repair

Chronic rotator cuff tears of the shoulder can lead to a degenerative condition called **cuff arthropathy.** The rotator cuff functions to counter the upward shear force on the articular cartilage exerted by the unopposed deltoid musculature. By repairing a torn rotator cuff, kinematic balance can be restored, preventing degeneration of the glenohumeral joint. Rotator cuff tears are repaired by mobilizing the rotator cuff and debriding the degenerated margins. These freshened edges are then sutured into bone at their insertion to restore function of the rotator cuff muscles. Removal of acromial spurs and excision of the coracoacromial ligament are also performed at the time of repair.

Synovectomy

Synovectomy is a treatment that may prolong the life of the hyaline joint surface through removal of proliferative synovitis, which damages cartilage. Synovectomy is indicated for chronic but not acute synovitis. Chronic synovitis is a clinical entity characterized by proliferation of the synovium and may be monarticular, as in pigmented villonodular synovitis, or polyarticular, as in RA or hemophilia. The term **synovitis** is relatively nonspecific, and the disorder is usually the result of a reaction to joint irritation.

A. INDICATIONS AND CONTRAINDICATIONS

The most common indication for synovectomy is RA, but the procedure may be beneficial in many other conditions, such as synovial osteochondromatosis, pigmented villonodular synovitis, and hemophilia, and occasionally following chronic or acute infection.

More specific indications for synovectomy include the following conditions:

1. synovitis with disease limited to the synovial membrane with little or no involvement of the other structures of the joint;

2. recurrent hemarthroses in conditions such as pigmented villonodular synovitis or hemophilia;

3. imminent destruction of the joint by lysosomal enzymes derived from white blood cells that may be liberated from infection; and

4. failure of an adequate trial of conservative management.

Contraindications include reduced ROM, significant degenerative arthrosis of the involved joint or other joint, or cartilage involvement.

B. TECHNIQUE

Synovectomy is most commonly performed on the knee and also often on the elbow, ankle, and wrist. Three main techniques are available: open synovectomy, synovectomy with use of the arthroscope, and radiation synovectomy.

1. Open synovectomy—Open synovectomy is becoming less common because of pain that causes difficulty in obtaining full motion following surgery. Continuous passive motion may be beneficial in these cases. Open synovectomy may be necessary in cases of pigmented villonodular synovitis or synovial osteochondromatosis, although these diseases may also be treated by arthroscopy, which permits noninvasive complete removal of the synovium in many cases.

2. Synovectomy with use of arthroscope—Synovectomy with use of the arthroscope may be tedious, especially in large joints such as the knee, because complete treatment requires removal of the entire synovium in many cases.

A study of pigmented villonodular synovitis of the knee treated by total and partial arthroscopic synovectomy demonstrated that total synovectomy resulted in a low recurrence rate, whereas partial synovectomy resulted in symptomatic and functional improvement but a fairly high recurrence rate. Arthroscopic synovectomy was recommended only for localized lesions.

3. Radiation synovectomy—Radiation synovectomy is a technique that is becoming much more popular. It is used in knee joints affected by RA. An injection of dysprosium-165-ferric hydroxide macroaggregates is given and leads to improvement in a significant percentage of patients. Proliferation of synovium decreases following this procedure, and there is less pain, blood loss, and expense than with more invasive procedures.

A similar technique is used in the knee joint in hemophiliacs. Phosphorus-32 chromic phosphate colloid is used and can be given on an outpatient basis. This is a safer technique for health care personnel, who have less contact with the blood of the hemophiliac patients, many of whom have become HIV positive through contaminated blood factor replacement.

Cartilage Transplant Techniques

Defects of hyaline cartilage were long considered permanent injuries, and the irrevocable sequelae were gradual deterioration of the architecture of the tissue. The treatment of cartilaginous diseases and injuries was limited by the slow and poorly understood metabolism of articular chondrocytes. Current development of cartilage repair procedures pertain only to focal defects of full-thickness cartilage loss. Such injuries occur typically in young (less than 40 years) patients during athletic activities or in patients with osteochondritis dissecans.

Because cartilaginous tissues are avascular, prior surgical treatment consisted of chondroplasty, where underlying subchondral bone was either drilled, burred, or microfractured to produce bleeding and an inflammatory response. Although multiple growth factors may be released with bleeding, the ensuing repair tissue is essentially fibrous scar tissue with inferior load-bearing capabilities compared with hyaline articular cartilage. As a result, the repair tissue eventually degrades, leaving the defect little better than if left alone.

Much enthusiasm followed the procedure described by Brittberg and colleagues, in which viable articular chondrocytes are harvested from a patient with a focal cartilaginous defect and cultured in a laboratory. The population of chondrocytes is expanded and placed back in the patient at the site of the cartilage injury. The cells are held in place with a flap of periosteum sutured to surrounding healthy cartilage. Although encouraging early clinical results were reported with this method, similar results are shown using only the flap of periosteum. Further, the procedure using cells failed to demonstrate reconstitution of normal hyaline cartilage in a canine model experiment.

Another method of dealing with focal defects of cartilage includes transplantation of small plugs of mature cartilage and bone. Small cylinders of cartilage and bone are removed from non–weight-bearing portions of cartilage and transplanted into focal femoral defects. Although encouraging short-term results are reported, whether the reconstructed cartilage endures remains to be seen.

In contrast, OA is a more prevalent affliction of cartilage, affecting more than 40 million patients in the United States. The early pathologic observations of OA indicate structural degradation of the superficial layers of the cartilage architecture. Meaningful spontaneous repair of injuries limited to cartilage are not observed clinically, but a variety of experimental evidence suggests a latent ability to effect some degree of healing after injury and possibly in OA. These suppositions include observation of increased DNA synthesis and proteoglycan synthesis in chondrocytes during intermediate stages of OA. The procedures just described for cartilage repair do not apply for osteoarthritic involvement of any significant portions of a joint.

Brittberg M et al: Treatment of deep cartilage defects in the knee with autologous chondrocyte implantation. N Engl J Med 1994;331:889.

Hangody L et al: Mosaicplasty for the treatment of articular defects of the knee and ankle. Clin Orthop 2001;391(Suppl):S328.

Rodrigo JJ et al: Improvement of full-thickness chondral defect healing in the human knee after debridement and microfracture using continuous passive motion. Am J Knee Surg 1994;7:109.

Core Decompression with or without Structural Bone Grafting

A. INDICATIONS AND CONTRAINDICATIONS

Core decompression with or without bone grafting is a surgical treatment primarily used for the femoral head because the hip is the joint most commonly affected by osteonecrosis. The knee and the shoulder may also be affected. Osteonecrosis results from loss of blood supply to the bone and is associated with a variety of conditions. Under repetitive stress, microfractures occur, are not repaired, and eventually lead to collapse of the necrotic bone and disruption of the joint surface.

The treatment of osteonecrosis is controversial because the outcome is frequently unsatisfactory. Spontaneous repair of the osteonecrotic lesion may occur but is an exception to the usual natural history of osteonecrosis. Core decompression, core decompression with electrical stimulation and bone grafting, and core decompression with structural bone grafting are considered acceptable forms of treatment for this disorder. Another treatment involves use of a free vascularized fibula transplant after core decompression.

B. TECHNIQUE

The goal of core decompression is to alleviate hypertension in the bone caused by obstructed venous egress from the affected area. The theory is that drilling a hole in an involved bony area diminishes pressure and permits the ingrowth of new blood vessels, which allow repair of the avascular bone and prevent joint destruction. Corticocancellous bone grafting is considered an alternative to simple core decompression because some evidence indicates this would place the femoral head at less risk of collapse in the postoperative period before new bone formation can occur. Core decompression or structural bone grafting is indicated in early osteonecrosis prior to collapse of the femoral head (Ficat stage I or II).

Core decompression is usually performed on the hip but may also be done on the knee or the shoulder. A lateral approach is used for the hip, and a pin is placed into the osteonecrotic area under fluoroscopic control. A reamer or core device is then passed over the pin to achieve decompression, and a sample of bone may be obtained for pathologic analysis. If structural bone grafting is to be performed, the graft may be placed over the pin (allograft or autograft fibula). Again, placement is performed under direct radiograph control.

The results of core decompression are mixed, possible as a result of poor technique, lack of standardization of staging, and factors causing the osteonecrosis. The major complication of the procedure in the hip is torsional failure resulting from the stress concentration site in the lateral aspect of the cortex. Reports of structural bone grafting by some investigators are highly favorable, with a high percentage of asymptomatic hips showing no evidence of progression of necrosis or collapse. One series reported a relatively high rate of postoperative or intraoperative fracture (4 of 31 cases).

Osteotomy

Osteotomy should be considered part of the armamentarium of the orthopedic surgeon in the treatment of biomechanical disorders of the knee and the hip. Osteotomy of the hip for OA is less frequently performed than osteotomy of the knee. Abnormal distribution of load may be alleviated by osteotomy. Femoral head coverage may be improved with osteotomy of the pelvis, orientation of the femoral head may be improved with osteotomy of the proximal femur, and realignment of the load on the medial and lateral condyles of the tibia may be improved with osteotomy of the femur and the tibia. The most common procedure is high tibial osteotomy, sometimes referred to as **Coventry osteotomy,** which corrects varus deformity of the knee by removal of a wedge of bone from the lateral side of the tibia. Other osteotomies are performed for residual deformity for fracture. These are tailored to the particular problem presented by the patient. Either intraarticular (ie, condylar osteotomy of the medial compartment [Figure 7–4]) or extraarticular osteotomies can be done to correct deformity.

A. HIGH TIBIAL OSTEOTOMY

Alleviation of abnormal stress through high tibial osteotomy prevents osteoarthrosis or, alternatively, reduces pain caused by unicompartmental gonarthrosis. The procedure is indicated in relatively young (less than 55 years) patients who have unicompartmental degeneration with relative sparing of the patellofemoral joint. The knee should have a good ROM, preferably with no flexion contracture. The knee must be stable, with no demonstrated medial or lateral subluxation. The ideal patients are younger than 65 years, not obese, and wish to continue an active lifestyle, including activities such as skiing or tennis. These activities are contraindicated in total joint replacement or unicompartmental replacement. Evaluation of the uninvolved compartment (either medial or lateral) may be accomplished by arthroscopy or with a technetium bone scan. A cold scan of the uninvolved compartment indicates relative normalcy. The normal anatomic axis of 5–7 degrees (angle between the shaft of the femur and the shaft of the tibia) on the standing AP film must usually be overcorrected to 10 degrees. High tibial osteotomy is usually indicated for patients with medial gonarthrosis, although it can be performed in patients with a valgus angulation of less than 12 degrees. If the angle is outside of this range, the patient may be a candidate for distal femoral supracondylar osteotomy. A high tibial osteotomy that results in a joint line that is not parallel to the ground indicates that the osteotomy should probably be performed through the distal femur.

A **B**

Figure 7–4. An intraarticular osteotomy can be of benefit in tibial plateau fractures. **A:** Preoperative radiograph of an intracondylar fracture of the tibial plateau. **B:** Postoperative view after osteotomy of the medial tibial condyle.

Proximal tibial osteotomy is performed through a lateral hockey-stick incision or a straight lateral incision. Exposure of the lateral, anterior, and posterior aspects of the tibia is made, and a closing wedge osteotomy is performed. The proximal portion of this osteotomy is made parallel to the joint surface under image intensifier control (Figure 7–5). With the help of guide pins, the appropriate distal cut is made, as determined from preoperative standing radiographs, to provide the necessary correction, which in the average case is approximately 1 mm per degree of correction as measured on the lateral cortex. This technique should only be used to double-check previous calculations, however. Resection of the fibular head or the proximal tibiofibular joint allows correction of the valgus angle. Fixation can reliably be obtained with staples, and other commercial fixation devices are available. Care must be taken to avoid damage to the peroneal nerve. Other problems that may be encountered include fracture of the proximal fragment or avascular necrosis of this fragment, which may occur if care is not exercised in performing the procedure.

The results of high tibial osteotomy are not as predictable as unicompartmental knee replacement or total knee replacement. Although pain is relieved in a high percentage of patients, this relief deteriorates over time. Clinical reports indicate that approximately 65–85% of patients have a good result after 5 years. Results of series vary because of the differences in patient population, surgical technique, and preexisting pathologic factors. The procedure should be considered in a patient who wants to maintain a more active lifestyle and would be willing to accept the possibility of some pain or loss of pain relief over time.

Lateral gonarthrosis from genu valgum is a relatively frequent result of lateral tibial plateau fractures, although RA, rickets, and renal osteodystrophy may also produce this disorder. There has been limited success in using varus tibial osteotomy in treating genu valgum because the procedure frequently produces a joint line that is not parallel to the ground, resulting in medial subluxation of the femur. Several reports of distal femoral osteotomy for genu valgum demonstrated this is a viable alternative for treating painful lateral gonarthrosis.

Figure 7–5. High tibial osteotomy, showing staples holding the osteotomy in place.

B. Osteotomy of the Hip

Certain unusual conditions of the hip can be treated with osteotomy to prevent or retard coxarthrosis. These include osteochondritis dissecans and other traumatic conditions that produce localized damage to the surface of the hip. Various biomechanical theories are proposed regarding the benefit of osteotomy of the pelvis and hip in decreasing the load on the hip. Although the theoretical arguments may be correct, in practical terms the two reasons for performing this procedure are (1) a normal viable cartilage surface is moved to the weight-bearing area where previously there was degenerated, thinned articular cartilage; and (2) the biomechanical loads on the joints that cause pain are reduced. These can be reduced either through alteration of moment arms for muscles or, alternatively, by releasing or weakening the muscles. Significantly lengthening or shortening a muscle reduces the force it can apply across a joint. In hip disorders, disease on one side of the hip joint cannot be addressed by an operation on the other side. For example, although it is tempting to use femo-

ral osteotomy to treat acetabular dysplasia, only temporary relief may be obtained.

1. Treatment for acetabular dysplasia—Acetabular dysplasia may be defined by the center edge angle. The normal center edge angle is 25–45 degrees; an angle of less than 20 degrees is definitely considered dysplastic (Figure 7–6). The anterior center edge angle can also demonstrate an acetabulum that is too open anteriorly; an angle of 17–20 degrees is considered the lower limit on the false profile view. In individuals with a mature skeleton, limited pelvic osteotomies such as the Salter innominate or shelf procedure are not appropriate. These measurements are probably best considered in a three-dimensional view with CT.

To improve coverage and hip biomechanics significantly, an acetabular-reorienting procedure that also permits medialization is ideal. The Wagner spherical osteotomy permits complete redirection of the acetabulum but does not permit medialization and is technically demanding. A triple osteotomy is useful in positioning the acetabulum but causes severe pelvic instability. The periacetabular osteotomy described by Ganz permits acetabular redirection and medialization but preserves the posterior column, minimizing instability.

2. Treatment of femoral disorders—Osteotomy of the femur can safely and reliably be performed in the intertrochanteric region, with the expectation of union. Osteotomy of the femoral neck is likely to compromise the blood supply to the femoral head. Intertrochanteric

Figure 7–6. Anteroposterior pelvis film demonstrating the center edge angle.

osteotomies of the femur of various types are described. The goal of osteotomy is removal of degenerated articular cartilage from the weight-bearing dome and replacement of it with more viable cartilage. This procedure may involve any of the three degrees of freedom: varus and valgus angle, internal and external rotation, and flexion and extension. It is necessary when planning these procedures to be sure the osteotomy will provide an adequate ROM for the patient. These osteotomies have usefulness in very specific cases for osteoarthrosis, but their usefulness for osteonecrosis is extremely limited in the United States.

Bonfiglio M, Voke EM: Aseptic necrosis of the femoral head and nonunion of the femoral neck: Effect of treatment by drilling and bone-grafting (Phemister technique). J Bone Joint Surg Am 1968;50:48.

Buckley PD et al: Structural bone-grafting for early atraumatic avascular necrosis of the femoral head. J Bone Joint Surg Am 1991;73:1357.

Coventry MB: Osteotomy about the knee for degenerative and rheumatoid arthritis: Indications, operative technique, and results. J Bone Joint Surg Am 1973;55:23.

Crockarell JR et al: The anterior center-edge angle: A cadaver study. J Bone Joint Surg Br 2000:82.532.

Edgerton BC et al: Distal femoral varus osteotomy for painful genu valgum: A five-to-11-year follow-up study. Clin Orthop 1993; 288:263.

Fairbank AC et al: Long-term results of core decompression for ischaemic necrosis of the femoral head. J Bone Joint Surg Br 1995;77:42.

Haddad FS et al: CT evaluation of periacetabular osteotomies. J Bone Joint Surg Br 2000:82;526.

Mont MA et al: Core decompression versus nonoperative management for osteonecrosis of the hip. Clin Orthop 1996;324:169.

Morita S et al: Long-term results of valgus-extension femoral osteotomy for advanced osteoarthritis of the hip. J Bone Joint Surg Br 2000:82;824.

Ogilvie-Harris DJ et al: Pigmented villonodular synovitis of the knee: The results of total arthroscopic synovectomy, partial arthroscopic synovectomy, and arthroscopic local excision. J Bone Joint Surg Am 1992;74:119.

Ohashi H et al: Factors influencing the outcome of Chiari pelvic osteotomy: A long-term follow-up. J Bone Joint Surg Br 2000: 82;517.

Shoji H, Insall J: High tibial osteotomy for osteoarthritis of the knee with valgus deformity. J Bone Joint Surg Am 1973;55:963.

Sledge CB et al: Synovectomy of the rheumatoid knee using intraarticular injection of Dysprosium-165-ferric hydroxide macroaggregates. J Bone Joint Surg Am 1987;69:970.

Urbaniak JR, Harvey EJ: Revascularization of the femoral head in osteonecrosis. J Am Acad Orthop Surg 1998;6(1):44.

JOINT SALVAGE PROCEDURES

1. Arthrodesis

Arthrodesis is the creation of a bony union across a joint. The creation of a fibrous union across a joint

with no motion is ankylosis. With bony union across a joint, motion of one bone on another is eliminated, relieving pain caused by arthritis. Although ankylosis may prevent observable motion, micromotion may be associated with significant pain. Ankylosis or arthrodesis may occur spontaneously, as in infection or ankylosing spondylitis, or may be surgically produced. The functional results of spontaneous arthrodesis are not ideal because the patient typically holds the joint in the position that causes minimum pain, which frequently is an inappropriate angle for function. Although surgical arthrodesis can be created in almost any joint, including the spine, the most common joints fused are the ankle, knee, shoulder, and hip. The technique used in any of the joints follows the same general pattern. The articular surfaces are denuded of remaining hyaline cartilage and then placed together in the optimal position of function after shaping to achieve maximum contact between the two opposing surfaces. Bone grafting is frequently used, and some form of fixation, either internal (plates, rods, or screws) or external (external fixators or a cast), is used to immobilize the arthrodesis site in the optimal position (Table 7–5). After adequate healing, the rehabilitation process is begun. Multiple techniques of arthrodesis are described for each joint.

Ankle Arthrodesis

The orthopedic community generally considers arthrodesis of the tibiotalar joint to be a good operation for treatment of tibiotalar arthrosis. A well-done ankle arthrodesis results in freedom from pain and nearly normal walking ability. Perhaps the main reason that the ankle arthrodesis is regarded so highly, however, is that other options, such as total ankle replacement, are less viable.

The indications for ankle arthrodesis are as follows:

1. degenerative arthrosis;
2. rheumatoid arthritis;
3. posttraumatic arthritis;
4. avascular necrosis of the talus;
5. neurologic disease resulting in an unstable ankle; and
6. neuropathic ankle joint.

The relative contraindications include degenerative joint disease in the subtalar and midtarsal joints.

The ankle arthrodesis can be performed through an anterior, lateral, or medial approach, and even posterior approaches are described. Arthroscopic techniques are now employed. The most common techniques are probably external fixation or internal screw fixation to achieve compression. Preparation of the ankle for arthrodesis is performed as mentioned earlier. Positioning of the ankle is important, with the talus in a neutral position or at an angle of 5 degrees of dorsiflexion. The midtarsal joints have a greater ROM in plantar flexion than in dorsiflex-

Table 7–5. Optimal position of joints after arthrodesis.

Joint	Angle	Length	Other Consideration
Ankle	0° dorsiflexion 0–5° valgus of hindfoot 5–10° external rotation	Slight shortening	Talus displaced posteriorly.
Knee	15° flexion 5–8° flexion	Slight shortening	—
Shoulder	20–30° flexion 20–40° abduction (lateral border of scapula) 25–40° internal rotation	—	Patient's hand should be able to touch the head and face.
Hip	25° flexion 0–5° abduction (measured between the shaft and a line through the ischia) 0–5° external rotation	Slight shortening	Do *not* destroy abductor mechanism.

ion, resulting in a more flexible foot. The talus is also displaced slightly posteriorly to make it easier for the patient to roll the foot over at the completion of the stance phase. A varus position is to be avoided because this restricts mobility at the midtarsal joints.

Kitaoka HB, Patzer GL: Arthrodesis for the treatment of arthrosis of the ankle and osteonecrosis of the talus. J Bone Joint Surg 1998;80:370.

Scranton PE: An overview of ankle arthrodesis. Clin Orthop 1991;268:96.

Knee Arthrodesis

Knee arthrodesis is seldom done for primary problems and generally done as the last resort for other problems. Indications for the procedure include infection, such as tuberculosis, neuropathic joint secondary to syphilis or diabetes, and loss of quadriceps function. The latter is a relative indication for arthrodesis because joint mobility can be maintained without quadriceps function, and joint stability can be obtained through the use of orthosis, which locks the joint in the fully extended position but can be unlocked for sitting. Although knee arthrodesis is usually successful and provides pain-free weight bearing, it is associated with other problems, especially in tall people. Sitting in airplanes, movie theaters, and even automobiles may be difficult. The most common indication for knee arthrodesis at the present time is failed total knee arthroplasty, usually because of infection. In a patient who wishes to maintain an active lifestyle, such as hunting on rough ground or performing manual labor, a knee arthrodesis is a viable alternative. The relative contraindications include bilateral disease or a problem such as an above-knee amputation of the other leg. In such a case, it would be extremely difficult for a person to arise from a chair with an arthrodesis on the contralateral side.

The technique of arthrodesis varies with the problem being treated. After infection, particularly when it is asso-

ciated with total knee replacement, bone loss is often moderate to severe. Cancellous bone from the distal femur and proximal tibia may be nearly nonexistent, and external fixation may be necessary to obtain adequate immobilization for arthrodesis. For less severe cases, intramedullary rod fixation may be indicated, particularly if the infection is under control. Similarly, use of double plates at 90 degrees is a viable method of immobilization. Frequently, iliac crest bone grafting is necessary to stimulate healing. Although bone loss often makes it necessary to shorten the extremity, some shortening (2–3 cm) is desirable to prevent a circumduction gait after fusion. The knee should be positioned at 10–15 degrees of flexion and at the normal valgus alignment of 5–8 degrees, if possible.

Donley BG et al: Arthrodesis of the knee with an intramedullary nail. J Bone Joint Surg Am 1991;73:907.

Nichols SJ et al: Arthrodesis with dual plates after failed total knee arthroplasty. J Bone Joint Surg Am 1991;73:1020.

Papilion JD et al: Arthroscopic assisted arthrodesis of the knee. Arthroscopy 1991;7:237.

Elbow Arthrodesis

Elbow arthrodesis is an uncommon procedure. Loss of elbow motion may be particularly disabling. Thus, the indications for arthrodesis are few, and few are performed because fusion causes severe functional limitations. To perform activities of daily living, a flexion arc of 100 degrees from 30 degrees of extension to 130 degrees of flexion is required. A range of 100 degrees for pronation and supination is also required. Painful arthrosis in a patient who is willing to accept the trade-off between stability and loss of motion is the indication for arthrodesis. Infectious processes, such as tuberculosis or fungus, are also indications for arthrodesis.

Several techniques are described, but the relative rarity of the operation prevents recommendation of one particular method. One report recommends screw fixation. Resection of the radial head may be necessary to allow for pronation and supination. The position of fusion is 90 degrees.

Irvine GB, Gregg PJ: A method of elbow arthrodesis: Brief report. J Bone Joint Surg Br 1989;71:145.

Morrey BF et al: A biomechanical study of normal elbow motion. J Bone Joint Surg Am 1981;62:872.

Shoulder Arthrodesis

Paralysis of the deltoid muscle and sepsis after an arthroplasty are possible indications for shoulder arthrodesis. Obtaining fusion may be a relatively difficult process because of the very long lever arm on the shoulder joint. This is accentuated by the position of fusion, which places the arm in abduction. Before the advent of comprehensive internal fixation devices, intraarticular and extraarticular arthrodeses were performed to provide a reasonable probability of obtaining fusion.

The AO technique (Arbeitsgemeinschaft für Osteosynthesefragen technique) is the most promising because it provides rigid internal fixation and the potential for immobilization without postoperative external immobilization. The patient is placed in the lateral decubitus position. The incision is made over the spine of the scapula, over the acromion, and down the lateral aspect of the humerus. The surface of the glenohumeral joint and the undersurface of the acromion are cleaned of residual cartilage and cortical bone to provide as much contact as possible with the arm in the appropriate position (see Table 7–5). A broad bone plate or pelvic reconstruction plate is then used to fix the humerus to the scapula. The bone plate is fixed to the spine of the scapula and the shaft of the humerus and bent into the appropriate position. Additional fixation may be obtained by placing another plate posteriorly. Bone grafting may be necessary for defects. Rigid fixation must be obtained. After surgery, a soft dressing is used until pain is controlled. A shoulder spica cast is preferred for immobilization by some surgeons. Exercises are begun to gently obtain scapular motion if no cast is used.

A modification of the AO technique that uses an external fixator to neutralize forces on interfragmentary screws has good results. Functional results are varied and depend on the position of fusion. Overhead work or work with the arm abducted is not possible. Excessive internal and external rotation must be avoided.

Johnson CA et al: External fixation shoulder arthrodesis. Clin Orthop 1986;211:219.

Muller ME et al: *Manual of Internal Fixation.* Berlin: Springer-Verlag, 1970.

Richards RR et al: Shoulder arthrodesis using a pelvic-reconstruction plate. J Bone Joint Surg Am 1988;70;416.

Riggins RS: Shoulder fusion without external fixation: A preliminary report. J Bone Joint Surg Am 1976;58:1007.

Hip Arthrodesis

Arthrodesis of the hip, as of other joints, produces a relatively pain-free stable joint that allows the patient to perform heavy labor. The disadvantage of hip arthrodesis in a young person who performs heavy labor is that over a period of time, degenerative disk disease of the lumbar spine and degenerative arthrosis of the ipsilateral knee frequently occur, even with optimal position of the arthrodesis. In fact, an indication for converting a hip fusion to a total hip arthroplasty is incapacitating back or knee pain.

The most obvious indication for arthrodesis of the hip is tuberculosis. Chronic osteomyelitis is a relative indication. Contraindications to arthrodesis include limited motion of the ipsilateral knee or degenerative arthrosis of the ipsilateral knee, as well as significant degenerative lumbar spine disease and arthrosis of the contralateral hip. Perhaps the biggest problem in performing a hip arthrodesis in a patient with adequate indications is obtaining agreement from the patient. Because joint replacement offers mobility, early rehabilitation, and a less extensive operation, patients are reluctant to consider the potential problems of hip arthrodesis. This is particularly true when total hip arthroplasty is performed in professional athletes, permitting some of them to continue in sports. Because of these factors, hip arthrodesis is now a relatively uncommon operation.

Multiple techniques are described for performing hip arthrodesis. Truly rigid fixation is difficult to achieve, and cast immobilization after surgery is usually needed. During the fusion procedure, care should be taken to preserve the abductors, so future reconstructive procedures may be performed if desired. The crucial aspect of the operation is fusing the hip in the appropriate position. The optimal position is slight flexion (25 degrees) from the normal position of the pelvis and spine, slight external rotation (5 degrees), and neutral abduction and adduction. Previously, the hip was placed in abduction, producing a very abnormal gait with additional stress on the lumbar spine. A position of neutral to slight abduction minimizes this problem because the body's center of gravity when the patient is in a one-legged stance is moved closer to the foot. Too much flexion makes both walking and lying in bed difficult, and too little flexion makes sitting difficult. Too much external rotation forces the knee joint to move in a plane oblique from that defined by the collateral and cruciate ligaments.

Blasier RB, Holmes JR: Intraoperative positioning for arthrodesis of the hip with the double bean bag technique. J Bone Joint Surg Am 1990;72:766.

Callaghan JJ et al: Hip arthrodesis: A long-term follow-up. J Bone Joint Surg Am 1984;67:1328.

2. Resection Arthroplasty

Resection arthroplasty, or excisional arthroplasty, is a procedure that is applied primarily to the hip, the elbow, and, more recently, the knee. Resection arthroplasty, or a modification called **fascial arthroplasty,** was a procedure used in the elbow for many years. Resection arthroplasty of the hip is also called **Girdlestone pseudoarthrosis** and dates back to 1923. Resection arthroplasty of the knee is a relatively new procedure that is used when infection compromises total knee replacement. Similarly, Girdlestone pseudoarthrosis is performed with increasing frequency as an intervening, sometimes permanent treatment for infection following total hip arthroplasty.

Hip Arthroplasty

Resection arthroplasty of the hip produces a relatively pain-free joint with reasonably good motion. It is indicated as a primary procedure when ankylosis causes the hip to be placed in an unsuitable position; such patients would otherwise be at high risk for dislocation or infection with a total hip arthroplasty. Spinal cord injury, head injury, and, perhaps, severe Parkinson disease would be diagnoses that might warrant primary resection arthroplasty. Disadvantages of the procedure result from lack of mechanical continuity between the femur and the pelvis; this causes an abnormal gait and the need for support with a cane or other device, and shortening occurs with each step. Patients who previously had infection following total hip replacement usually have the most stable hip joints because dense scar tissue has formed. The procedure can be very helpful in reambulating wheelchair-bound patients in whom peroneal care is very difficult.

For infection compromising total hip replacement, resection arthroplasty is accomplished by removing all of the cement, the prosthesis, any necrotic bone, and the soft tissue. In primary resection arthroplasty, the procedure is more of a reconstructive procedure in which the femoral head and neck are removed flush with the intertrochanteric line and the capsule is reconstructed to help provide some stability of the hip. Traction with a pin in the tibia is frequently used for variable periods to maintain leg length.

Knee Arthroplasty

Resection arthroplasty of the knee has a much less satisfactory functional result. After removal of an infected knee prosthesis, there is usually significant bone loss and the knee is quite unstable. Bracing improves the condition only modestly, and the patient still requires crutches or a walker to ambulate.

Elbow Arthroplasty

Resection arthroplasty or fascial arthroplasty of the elbow is one means of managing ankylosis after trauma or infection. Resection arthroplasty may be performed for failure of total elbow arthroplasty resulting from sepsis. Resection arthroplasty in the patient with RA should be discouraged because one of the problems associated with the procedure is instability. The rheumatoid patient frequently depends on the upper extremity to ambulate with walking aids. Interpositional arthroplasty, using fascia or split-thickness skin grafts, was thought to reduce resorption of bone, but the additional benefit of the interpositional tissue is doubtful. Although resection arthroplasty frequently relieves pain, instability is a major problem, and bracing is required in most cases. With the availability of elbow arthroplasty, this procedure is rarely performed.

Milgram JW, Rana NA: Resection arthroplasty for septic arthritis of the hip in ambulatory and nonambulatory adult patients. Clin Orthop 1991;272:181.

Thornhill TS et al: Alternatives to arthrodesis for failed total knee arthroplasty. Clin Orthop 1982;170:131.

JOINT REPLACEMENT PROCEDURES

1. Hemiarthroplasty

Hemiarthroplasty is the replacement of only one side of a diarthrodial joint. The procedure is indicated for displaced fractures of the femoral neck or four-part fractures of the humeral head, but there are other indications in adult reconstructive surgery. In both the shoulder and the hip, osteonecrosis may result in collapse of the humeral or femoral articulating surface, with sparing of the glenoid or acetabulum. In the hip, nonunion of the femoral neck after open reduction and internal fixation may also be an indication for endoprosthetic replacement. In either joint, pathologic fracture or tumor may be an indication. Contraindications include active infection, RA, and possibly the patient's age. Endoprosthetic replacement in a young individual is certain to result, with time, in destruction of the articular surface of the acetabulum. This may, however, take many years, and the patient may have a serviceable joint in the intervening period.

The choice of prosthesis depends on factors such as life expectancy, cost, and physiologic demand. For the shoulder, a cemented prosthesis should probably be modular to permit conversion to total shoulder replacement at a later date without removal of the stem, should that become necessary. Similar concerns for the hip apply. The femoral head can be replaced with a unipolar or bipolar prosthesis. The bipolar prosthesis allows motion to occur between the acetabulum and the prosthesis, as well as between the prosthesis and the articulating surface of the metal femoral head. This articulation is metal or ceramic on plastic and certain to produce debris from wear that may be detrimental to the durability of the hip prosthesis. Selection of a monopolar prosthesis, however, must not compromise conversion of the hemiarthroplasty to a total hip arthroplasty, should this become necessary.

The operative technique is quite similar to that of total joint replacement for each joint. The main difference in the hip is that the capsule is usually repaired after hemiarthroplasty. A posterolateral approach is most commonly used in the hip, although an anterolateral approach may be preferred in a patient with associated mental problems that may limit postoperative cooperation. If the posterolateral approach is used in such patients, a knee immobilizer may be necessary to prevent hip flexion that might lead to dislocation.

2. Total Joint Arthroplasty

Joint replacement surgery became a viable treatment for arthritic afflictions of joints when the low-friction hip arthroplasty was developed by Sir John Charnley in the 1960s. This procedure consisted of the articulation of a metal femoral head on an ultrahigh-molecular-weight polyethylene (UHMWPE) acetabular component, with both components fixed in place with acrylic cement (polymethylmethacrylate [PMMA]). The long-term results are quite satisfactory, and the concept is now applied to other joints with variable success. The knee replacement, shoulder replacement, and elbow replacement have evolved to the point that satisfactory results are routine when the indications for surgery are appropriate. Other arthroplasties, such as the ankle, wrist, and first metatarsophalangeal joint, are less successful. In fairness, the application of technology to these joints is not at the level applied to other joints. Success of all arthroplasties depends on the skill of the surgeon, the surgeon's understanding of the basic biomechanics underlying the joint function, the design of the prosthesis, and the technical equipment used to insert the prosthesis.

The design of the prosthesis is an evolutionary process that depends on laboratory and clinical experience. Hip replacement surgery, performed often, is highly successful. Less frequently performed arthroplasties, such as elbow replacement, are associated with less clinical and laboratory experience.

Total Hip Arthroplasty

The original Charnley total hip arthroplasty was a stainless steel femoral prosthesis with a small collar, a rectangular cross section, and a 22-mm femoral head. The acetabular component was a UHMWPE cup (Figure 7–7). Both components were cemented into place with acrylic bone cement. Since then, an entire industry

has evolved to produce new designs for hip components, including different head sizes (22, 25, 25.4, 28, 32, and 35 mm); different femoral component lengths (ranging from 110 mm to 160 mm for standard prostheses); different cross sections (square, round, oval, I-beam); a porous coating for bone ingrowth attachment; and metal backing for the acetabulum (cemented or porous coated). The two generic designs that evolved from experience with bone attachment technique are the porous ingrowth and cement fixation prostheses.

A. INDICATIONS

The indications for hip arthroplasty are incapacitating arthritis of the hip combined with appropriate physical and roentgenographic findings. The historical data that justify consideration of hip replacement surgery include pain requiring medication stronger than aspirin, inability to walk more than a few blocks without stopping, pain following activity, pain that wakes the patient at night, difficulty with shoes and socks or foot care such as cutting nails, and difficulty in climbing stairs. It is good practice to use a clinical rating score to evaluate these historical data (Table 7–6).

Figure 7–7. Radiograph of a Charnley arthroplasty.

Table 7–6. Harris hip evaluation (modified).

I. Pain (44 possible)
  A. None or ignores it 44
  B. Slight, occasional, no compromise in activities 40
  C. Mild pain, no effect on average activities, rarely moderate pain; with unusual activity may take aspirin 30
  D. Moderate pain, tolerable, but makes concessions to pain; some limitation of ordinary activity or work;
     may require occasional pain medicine stronger than aspirin 20
  E. Marked pain, serious limitation of activities 10
  F. Totally disabled, crippled, pain in bed, bedridden. 0
II. Function (47 possible)
  A. Gait (33 possible)
    1. Limp
      a. None 11
      b. Slight 8
      c. Moderate 5
      d. Severe 0
    2. Support
      a. None 11
      b. Cane for long walks 7
      c. Cane most of the time. 5
      d. One crutch. 3
      e. Two canes 2
      f. Two crutches 0
      g. Not able to walk (specify reason). 0
    3. Distance walked
      a. Unlimited 11
      b. Six blocks 8
      c. Two or three blocks 5
      d. Indoors only 2
      e. Bed and chair 0
  B. Activities (14 possible)
    1. Stairs
      a. Normally without using a railing 4
      b. Normally using a railing 2
      c. In any manner 1
      d. Unable to do stairs 0
    2. Shoes and socks
      a. With ease 4
      b. With difficulty. 2
      c. Unable. 0
    3. Sitting
      a. Comfortably in ordinary chair 1 hour. 5
      b. On a high chair for one-half hour 3
      c. Unable to sit comfortably in any chair. 0
      4. Enter public transportation. 1

  C. Range of Motion   R   L
    Flexion   _____ _____
    Flexion contracture   _____ _____
    Abduction   _____ _____
    Adduction   _____ _____
    External rotation   _____ _____
    Internal rotation   _____ _____
  D. Location of pain
    Groin   _____ _____
    Thigh   _____ _____
    Buttock   _____ _____

Physical examination typically demonstrates a limited ROM, pain at extremes of motion, a positive Trendelenburg test, a limp, and groin or anterior thigh pain with active straight leg raising.

Radiographs demonstrate loss of joint space and other findings consistent with the cause of the disorder. Noteworthy features requiring special considerations for surgery are dysplasia of the acetabulum, protrusio acetabuli, and proximal femoral deformity or the presence of metal implants from previous operations.

After consideration of the lifestyle requirements of the patient, the surgeon may suggest this procedure as a means of alleviating pain, which is the main indication for hip replacement surgery. Other reconstructive procedures should be considered, including arthrodesis, osteotomy, and hemiarthroplasty. When selecting a procedure, one should consider the patient's goals in terms of work and leisure activity. A young person who performs heavy labor and has unilateral traumatic arthritis may be best served by arthrodesis. A 50-year-old bank executive who does not ski, play tennis, or ride horses but does swim and bicycle will probably have best results with hip arthroplasty.

A choice must be made between cemented and uncemented arthroplasty, with the uncemented acetabular component nearly universally indicated. Its advantages include a consistently pain-free result, long-lasting fixation, and modularity to permit latitude in selecting head size and acetabular polyethylene component offset designs. Its disadvantages include the need for metal backing of the polyethylene liner, which may increase wear, and the possibility of dissociation of the plastic component from the metal. A cemented acetabular component manufactured from UHMWPE is usually reserved for an individual with a life expectancy of 10 years or less. The indications for an uncemented femoral component vary with the surgeon but usually depend on the age of the patient, with younger patients most likely to benefit from the porous-coated prosthesis.

B. SURGICAL TECHNIQUE

Certain aspects of hip replacement surgery apply to all arthroplasty techniques, including cement technique and bone surface preparation.

1. Posterolateral approach—The most common approach for total hip arthroplasty is the posterolateral approach. After administration of anesthesia and placement of a thromboembolic stocking and intermittent compression stocking on the unaffected limb, the patient is rolled into the lateral decubitus position, with the affected side superior. Draping should leave the entire leg free and extending above the iliac crest. Kidney rests are used to support the pelvis at the pubis and the sacrum, and bony prominences should be protected. The incision is outlined on the skin before the skin is completely covered with an adhesive drape. By flexing the hip to 45 degrees, the incision can be made in line with the femur from approximately 10 cm proximal to the tip of the trochanter to 10 cm distal to the tip of the trochanter.

Alternatively, with the hip in the extended position, the incision is made from 10 cm distal to the tip of the trochanter extending proximally along the line of the trochanter and then curving posteriorly at approximately a 45-degree angle for another 10 cm. The incision is deepened to show the fascia lata and the gluteus maximus. An incision is made in the fascia lata directly lateral and extended proximally into the gluteus maximus, which is split in line with its fibers. A Charnley retractor is placed, and fat overlying the external rotators is removed. After putting the femur into internal rotation, the external rotators (piriformis, gemelli, obturator internus, and quadratus femoris) are tagged with sutures for reattachment and removed from their attachments at the trochanter. The gluteus minimus is separated from the capsule and preserved and protected, and a capsulectomy is performed. Alternatively, portions of the posterior capsule can be reflected for later reattachment. If the patient is not paralyzed with nondepolarizing muscle relaxant agents, excision of the capsule with electrocautery signals whether the sciatic nerve is particularly closely applied to the posterior of the acetabulum. The sciatic nerve must be identified and protected throughout the procedure if there is electrical transmission. Internal rotation of the flexed hip dislocates the hip, and the femoral head is delivered into the operative field. Using an appropriate template, the femoral head is resected with an oscillating saw. The femur is then externally rotated, and Taylor retractors are placed anteriorly and posteriorly to permit visualization of the acetabulum. The acetabulum is medialized if appropriate when medial osteophytes are present. Anterior osteophytes, if present, are removed under direct visualization. Reaming of the acetabulum is performed until a good bed of bleeding subchondral bone is obtained; progressive reamers are usually used. At this point, techniques diverge based on whether a cemented or an uncemented cup is used.

If a cemented cup is used, multiple holes with a diameter of $1/4$–$3/8$ inch are drilled in the acetabulum to provide firm cement interdigitation. One of the commercially available techniques that prevents bottoming out of the acetabular cup should be used, so the medial cement mantle will be adequate. The position of the cup is determined with trials, using the native acetabulum for guidance and radiograph if there is any concern about positioning. The cup is cemented into place after the acetabular bone is prepared with pulsatile lavage, epinephrine-soaked sponges, and pressurization of the cement.

If an uncemented cup is used, reaming progresses to a diameter 1–2 mm smaller than the actual size of the cup to be implanted. The cup is impacted into place, ensuring appropriate positioning. Fixation is achieved with screws or pegs, as specified by the manufacturer. A trial plastic component is inserted, and attention is returned to the femur.

The hip is internally rotated, flexed to approximately 80 degrees, and adducted, so the cut femoral neck is presented to the surgeon. Homan retractors may be used to help elevate the amputated femoral neck into the wound. A box chisel is then used to remove the femoral neck laterally. The canal is broached with a curet to provide an indication of the direction of the intramedullary canal. The femoral canal is then broached with increasing sizes of broaches, until all weak cancellous bone is removed. The prosthesis size is determined, and a cement restrictor is placed 2 cm distal to the final position of the stem tip. The canal is prepared for cementing with pulsatile lavage, medullary canal brushing, and sponges soaked with hydrogen peroxide or epinephrine. The cement is prepared and centrifuged or vacuum mixed and inserted into the femoral canal with a cement gun. The cement is pressurized, and the prosthesis is inserted into appropriate anteversion (approximately 10 degrees) and held in position until the cement cures. When the appropriate broach, as indicated by preoperative templating, is reached, a trial femoral prosthesis is inserted, the neck length is checked, and the prosthesis is reduced into position. Range of motion is tested at 90 degrees of flexion and should be stable to 40–45 degrees of internal rotation. External rotation to 40 degrees in the fully extended position must be obtained without impingement on the femoral neck posteriorly. Proper myofascial tension is assessed by telescoping the hip at 45 degrees (approximately 3 or 4 mm). Proper leg length is usually achieved when the rectus femoris tightness (flexion of the knee with the hip extended) is similar to prior to surgery. A further check on leg lengths can be made by comparing the center of the femoral head preoperatively with the proximal tip of the trochanter to trochanter-prosthesis center distance with the prosthesis in place. Measuring devices are designed to measure leg lengths, but up to a centimeter of discrepancy can still occur. An extended lip on the UHMWPE component may provide additional stability but may form a fulcrum on which the head may be levered out. The prosthesis trial is removed, and the permanent polyethylene component is put into place in the acetabular metallic shell. The femoral canal is then prepared for cementing.

After the cement hardens, a trial femoral head is used to put the hip through a second ROM. The optimal neck length is selected, and the appropriate prosthetic component is impacted into place. When combining modular components held together with a Morse-type taper, the manufacturers' components should not be mixed. It is mandatory that the surfaces be clean and dry. The bore in the femoral head is placed on the trunnion and twisted and impacted into place with several sharp blows. The acetabulum is cleaned of debris, the femoral head is reduced, and the wound is closed. The external rotators are reattached with sutures placed through bone while the hip is in external rotation and abduction. The fascia is closed with interrupted sutures.

The design and insertion technique of the uncemented femoral components are quite variable and therefore are not described here.

Abbreviated mini incisions for the posterolateral approach to the hip are described. These generally use a small portion of the routine incision but are carefully placed to optimize visualization of the hip.

2. Lateral approach—The lateral approach to the hip is performed with a trochanteric osteotomy after the fascia of the tensor fascia lata and gluteus maximus are entered. The patient may be in the supine position with a bump under the hip or in the lateral position. Prior to osteotomy, the trochanter is mobilized, and the trochanteric osteotomy is performed with an osteotome or a Gigli saw. The gluteus minimus is peeled off the capsule as the trochanter is mobilized proximally. After capsulectomy, the femoral head is dislocated anteriorly. The procedure is essentially identical from this point on until the trochanter is reattached. Various modifications of trochanteric osteotomy techniques are described. The abductor mechanism is extremely important in preserving the stability of the hip as well as the gait. Thus, extreme care must be taken to reattach the trochanter when the procedure is completed, so reliable union is achieved. Even in the best of hands, approximately 1 in 20 trochanters fails to unite, although the number of people who have disability or pain from a fibrous union is much lower. If wires are used to reattach the trochanter, they should be biocompatible with the prosthetic component, and a minimum of three should be used to achieve adequate fixation.

3. Anterolateral approach (Watson-Jones approach)—The interval between the gluteus medius muscle and the tensor fascia lata is utilized proximally to gain access to the femoral neck and hip joint. The patient is in the supine position, with a bump under the buttock. The skin incision follows the shaft of the femur distally and curves slightly anteriorly proximally. The fascia is incised in line with the skin incision and proximally splits the interval between the tensor fascia lata and the gluteus medius. The tensor fascia lata is then retracted anteriorly, and the gluteus medius is retracted superiorly and laterally. Because the fibers of the gluteus medius and minimus tend to run anteriorly, particularly in the osteoarthritic hip with destruction and shortening, these fibers must be released to provide access to the hip joint. The hip is externally rotated. The anterior capsule is incised, and the hip joint can then be dislocated. Osteotomy of the femoral neck proceeds at the appropriate level. Capsulotomy is performed, retractors are placed to provide acetabular exposure, and hip replacement is performed. The femur during this procedure is externally rotated. Care must be taken in exposing the acetabulum to prevent damage to the femoral nerve and femoral muscles.

4. Other approaches—Other approaches are used for hip replacement, some of which are successful according to the skill of the individual surgeon. Some approaches, including the direct lateral approach, may be fraught with problems such as abductor weakness after surgery, and the result may be disappointing to the patient as well as the surgeon.

C. IMPLANTS

The two basic types of total hip replacement are cemented and uncemented. The bearing surfaces for both are the same, either cobalt chromium alloy or ceramic (alumina or zirconia), articulating with a UHMWPE bearing surface. The femoral stem replacement may be cobalt chromium or titanium alloy, either of which is also used for the metal backing of the acetabulum. Cobalt chromium alloy is associated with much less stress on the bone–cement interface because of its higher modulus; this prolongs fixation. The femoral component should be designed to provide intrinsic torsional stability without having sharp edges that would create stress concentration sites in the bone cement. A matte surface should be created to allow some mechanical interlocking with the cement, although currently this is controversial, and some surgeons recommend a polished surface. Adequate offset is necessary to restore the mechanical advantage of the abductors.

The choice of material for the femoral head is a trade-off between cost and theoretical advantages. The harder, wettable surface of ceramic heads theoretically results in less production of debris from wear and longer service of the hip replacement without loosening, but the cost is two to three times that of an equivalent-sized cobalt chromium (Co/Cr) head. Thus, in most individuals undergoing total hip arthroplasty, a Co/Cr head is probably optimal. In younger patients, the increased cost of a ceramic head may be warranted. Femoral heads are available now in 22-, 26-, 28-, and 32-mm sizes. One clinical investigation of total hip replacements showed that 26- and 28-mm heads are associated with the least amount of linear and volumetric wear. A head of 22 mm may be necessary for patients with smaller acetabular sockets to provide adequate thickness of the polyethylene bearing surface. A minimum of 6 mm, preferably 8 mm or more, is suggested to lower the contact stress on the polyethylene and thereby reduce wear.

New bearing surfaces for the articulation of the hip joint are becoming popular. The possibilities include ceramic on ceramic, Co/Cr on Co/Cr, and ceramic or Co/Cr on radiation cross-linked polyethylene. The impetus for this change is the possibility of lower wear debris. These articulation couples require long-term follow-up to determine if they will live up to their promise.

No evidence justifies use of a metal backing on the cemented acetabular component. Other design considerations to avoid are deep grooves that might evolve into cracks in the PMMA. The surface must be rough enough to allow the cup to bond to the cement through mechanical interlock.

Uncemented acetabular components have a spherical outer surface with at least one hole to permit the surgeon to determine if the prosthesis is fully impacted into place. The shell should have a minimum of 3 mm of metal to reduce the risk of fatigue failure. Cobalt chromium alloy or titanium alloy appears to be equally efficacious. The inner surface should lock the polyethylene in some fashion to reliably limit rotation and dissociation. The inner surface should be the mate of the polyethylene outer surface to reduce the chance of cold flow of the plastic as well as wear from relative motion. Recommended materials are listed in Table 7–7.

Table 7–7. Preferred materials for total hip replacement.

Component	Material	Alternative Material
Uncemented femoral component	Titanium alloy	Cobalt chromium alloy
Cemented femoral component	Cobalt chromium alloy (forged)	Cast cobalt chromium alloy, titanium alloy
Femoral head	Cobalt chromium alloy	Zirconia, alumina
Cemented acetabulum bearing surface	Ultrahigh-molecular-weight polyethylene component (no metal backing)	—
Uncemented acetabulum bearing surface	Ultrahigh-molecular-weight polyethylene component	—
Acetabulum ingrowth surface	Titanium alloy, cobalt chromium alloy	—

Design considerations for the uncemented femoral component are unclear at present. Use of porous coating, hydroxyapatite, or tricalcium phosphate coating is driven by manufacturing concerns and prosthesis strength requirements rather than an understanding of the biologic principles of hip replacement. Two design factors are important: (1) If a prosthesis is excessively stiff in relation to the bone to which it is attached, proximal osteopenia may result from "stress shielding" or "stress bypassing" of the bone; and (2) stiffer prostheses also seem to be associated with more pain in the thigh. Therefore, strategies to reduce stiffness seem appropriate. Both of these factors are addressed by using titanium alloy as opposed to cobalt chromium alloy, but other factors may surface to affect this choice. Creating slots or grooves to reduce the torsional and bending stiffness also seems to be effective in reducing stiffness and resulting thigh pain.

D. COMPLICATIONS

Any major surgery is associated with a certain incidence of complications, which is certainly true for total hip arthroplasty. The surgeon must recognize these complications in a timely manner and treat them appropriately. The most common complications include deep venous thrombosis (DVT), fracture or perforation of the femoral shaft, infection, instability (dislocation), heterotopic bone formation, and nerve palsies.

1. Deep venous thrombosis—Although some morbidity results from DVT, the real risk is pulmonary embolism, which is occasionally fatal. The incidence of DVT is high, but the incidence of fatal pulmonary emboli fortunately is low, in the range of 0.3%. The high incidence of DVT during hip replacement surgery is related to femoral vein damage from manipulation or retraction, intraoperative or postoperative venous stasis caused by immobility and limb swelling, and a hypercoagulable state directly resulting from the surgical trauma to the patient. Certain factors are recognized as predisposing the patient to higher risk for DVT, including a prior history of pulmonary embolus, estrogen treatment, preexisting cancer, older (more than 60 years) age of the patient, and length of the operative procedure, one factor that is under the surgeon's control.

Pharmacologic and mechanical measures are used to reduce the risk of DVT. Some surgeons prefer surveillance through clinical or laboratory tests such as duplex scanning, venograms, and fibrinogen scans, followed by anticoagulation therapy in patients with clot formation. The National Institutes of Health Consensus Conference concluded that mechanical measures such as intermittent pneumatic compression provide adequate prophylaxis for patients who are mobilized quickly, whereas anticoagulation therapy is recommended for those expected to undergo prolonged bed rest. Pharmacologic prophylaxis includes sodium warfarin, subcutaneous heparin, and aspirin. The efficacy of subcutaneous minidose heparin and aspirin is controversial. The first low-molecular-weight heparin (enoxaparin) is administered subcutaneously and was approved by the Food and Drug Administration (FDA) for prophylaxis in total hip arthroplasty patients. This drug offers the benefit of twice-daily administration without the need for coagulation monitoring. Its indications were extended to total knee replacement prophylaxis. Other similar low-molecular-weight heparin products are now available and may permit single daily dosing. These include such products as dalteparin sodium and tinzaparin sodium. These drugs offer higher factor Xa inhibition in relation to factor IIa inhibition than unfractionated heparin, which prevents clotting without affecting the activated partial thromboplastin time (PTT). Other chemotherapeutic agents include fondaparinux, a pentasaccharide that is a factor Xa inhibitor, also given by injection once daily. On the horizon are oral thrombin (IIa) inhibitors that may be more convenient for outpatient use.

Because DVT can lead to a catastrophic outcome, preventative measures are indicated starting in the presurgical area. The patient should wear an antiembolic stocking on the unaffected extremity, and both extremities can be treated with intermittent pneumatic compression during the operative procedure. Following surgery, a low-molecular-weight heparin (enoxaparin or dalteparin) is the treatment of choice. Patients who develop pulmonary embolus should receive routine treatment with heparin followed by warfarin.

2. Nerve palsies—Three degrees of nerve injury are recognized. In order of increasing severity, these are neurapraxia, in which conduction is disrupted; axonotmesis, in which the neuron is affected but not the myelin sheath; and neurotmesis, in which the nerve is completely disrupted, as in laceration. In total hip arthroplasty, the most common injuries are neurapraxia and axonotmesis. Neurotmesis is unlikely to occur, except when severe scar tissue predisposes the nerve to laceration. Early nerve recovery (days to weeks) indicates neurapraxia; while longer recovery (months) indicates axonotmesis.

Nerve palsies after total hip arthroplasty are relatively infrequent, but the incidence increases as the complexity of the surgical procedure increases. The sciatic nerve is most commonly involved, with the peroneal division of the sciatic nerve at the greatest risk (80% of cases). The femoral nerve is involved less frequently. An early study indicated an overall prevalence of 1.7%, with total hip arthroplasty for congenital hip dysplasia having a rate of 5.2% and for osteoarthrosis 1%, but a subsequent review suggested that the overall rate of palsy was reduced to approximately 1%. Revision surgery was associated with a rate of 3.2%. The type of injury most likely to produce nerve palsy is stretching or compression, although other mechanisms, such as ischemia, intraneural hemorrhage, dislocation of the femoral component, and cement extrusion, are also suggested as causes.

Nerve injury may be prevented by identifying high-risk cases, protecting the sciatic nerve from compression, and evaluating the sciatic nerve for possible stretching before the wound is closed. Stretching the sciatic nerve by as little as 2 cm increases the risk of palsy significantly. Palpation of the sciatic nerve for tautness with the hip and knee extended and with the hip flexed and knee extended (straight leg–raising test) indicates whether there is danger of stretching the sciatic nerve. Shortening the femoral neck is one means of addressing this problem. If any doubt exists about whether stretching occurred, the patient should be placed in the hospital bed following operation with the hip extended and the knee flexed to relieve tension of the nerve, until the patient is awake and function of the nerve can be monitored.

Management of nerve palsy is generally conservative, with observation when the nerve is known to be in continuity and not stretched. Electromyograms and nerve conduction studies may be helpful but may not show changes until 3 weeks after injury. Recovery of some motor function in the hospital heralds a good prognosis, and if complete return is to occur, it does so by 21 months, according to one study.

3. Vascular complications—Significant vascular complications are reported to occur in approximately 0.25% of total hip replacements. These may be caused by placement of retractors and acetabular screws and by damage to atherosclerotic vessels. Early recognition is important in these injuries.

4. Fracture or perforation—The typical fracture associated with total hip arthroplasty involves the femoral shaft, but other fractures do occur. Fatigue fractures of structures such as the pubic ramus may occur following increased activity after hip replacement relieves pain. The intraoperative problem of fracture or perforation of the femur is relatively uncommon in primary arthroplasty. Perforation may occur in disorders such as sickle cell anemia and osteopetrosis or following previous internal fixation. These conditions may have resulted in sclerotic bone, which may direct the broach astray. Perforations are relatively easily managed by extending the prosthesis past the area of perforation. This distance is generally considered to be two femoral diameters for a perforation with a cemented arthroplasty, but longer distances may be necessary with unce-

mented arthroplasties, depending on the size of the perforation. An alternative is to use a structural allograft held in place with cerclage wires. In either case, cancellous bone grafting is prudent to facilitate healing.

After total hip arthroplasty, the stress state of the bone is definitely changed, and there is a stress concentration area at the tip of the prosthesis. Fractures in the periprosthetic area are relatively common. These fractures are classified as type A, involving the greater or lesser trochanter; type B1, B2, B3, around or just below the stem, with the stem well fixed (B1), stem loose (B2), or poor bone stock in the proximal femur (B3); or type C, well below the stem. Type A fractures are treated nonoperatively unless the cause is osteolysis, which may predispose the femur to more serious injury. Type B and C fractures are generally treated surgically. Revision is usually the treatment of choice if the prosthesis demonstrates loosening on plain radiographs. Bone grafting is generally necessary with bone deficiencies, and bicortical onlay grafting techniques may be necessary with poor bone stock. Open reduction and internal fixation may be indicated if the prosthesis is tight (types B1 and C), but generous bone grafting and careful observation are necessary to ensure healing. Fracture fixation devices applied in the vicinity of the femoral component may be tenuous, and these devices must not compromise the integrity of the cement mantle or prosthesis.

5. Dislocation following total hip arthroplasty— The incidence of dislocation following total hip arthroplasty varies somewhat from series to series, but ranges from 1% to 8% and averages 2–2.5%. Several factors are associated with higher rates of dislocation, including female sex of the patient and nonunion of the trochanteric osteotomy, revision surgery, and use of the posterior approach. Dislocation after revision surgery in one series was 10% after the first revision and 26.7% after two or more revisions. An ununited trochanter after revision was associated with a 25% rate of dislocation.

Factors important in preventing dislocation are proper placement of components, adjustment of myofascial tension, component design, and patient compliance. Variables found to have no effect on the dislocation rate include the ROM of the hip and the femoral head size. A 32-mm head has a theoretic advantage over a 22-mm head because a neck of the same diameter would impinge earlier with a 22-mm head. At the time of surgery, the myofascial tension is tested by traction on the femur. Displacement of 1 cm or more suggests an increased probability of dislocation after surgery.

The risk of dislocation after total hip arthroplasty diminishes as time passes without dislocation. A first dislocation often occurs within 6 weeks following surgery and is frequently a result of patient noncompliance with postsurgical guidelines. For a first dislocation, closed reduction is used, and careful assessment of the cause of dislocation should be made. If component position appears to be adequate, bracing for 3 months is recommended, along with careful explanation of hip dislocation precautions to the patient. Alternatively, removal of the acetabular component with replacement by a bipolar into the reamed acetabulum may be the best salvage procedure. Recurrent dislocation should be examined carefully for cause, with radiographs taken to evaluate the abduction and anteversion of the cup as well as the anteversion of the femoral head (Figure 7–8). Examination under fluoroscopy may reveal impingements, and push-and-pull films may reveal inadequate myofascial tension.

After careful evaluation of the cause(s) of dislocation, surgical correction may be undertaken. Possible solutions include reorienting the offset lip of the acetabulum, changing the anteversion or abduction of the acetabulum, changing the anteversion of the femoral component, or advancing the trochanter to tighten the muscle envelope. Failure of these methods may require

Figure 7–8. Approximate determination of the abduction-adduction angle and angle of anteversion of the cup. Exact measurement requires careful control of the direction of the x-ray beam.

the use of a constrained acetabulum to prevent dislocation. This treatment should be considered a last resort because the reduced ROM resulting from the design of these cups can predispose the patient to dislocation as a result of levering out of the cup from neck impingement. Long-term bracing is a possible solution for recurrent dislocation in a patient with limited goals for activity. Recurrent dislocation causes significant anxiety, which encourages patients to seek surgical correction. The recurrence rate in such patients is as high as 20% after surgical correction.

6. Leg-length discrepancy—During hip replacement surgery, an attempt is made to maintain the preoperative length of the affected leg, so it is as long as the unaffected leg. This goal, however, is sometimes incompatible with (and therefore subservient to) myofascial tension in the ligamentously lax individual or may be a potential cause of damage to nerve or vascular structures. Hence, most surgeons advise their patients that the leg may be longer or shorter than normal after operation.

7. Trochanteric nonunion—The rate of trochanteric nonunion after a primary total hip arthroplasty is approximately 5%. The percentage of patients who develop symptoms from this complication is smaller. Usually, migration of less than 1 cm is not associated with functional symptoms or pain.

The rate of nonunion after revision surgery is much higher, as much as 40%, particularly if there has been nonunion following the primary procedure. Diminished function, as evidenced by weakness in abduction and a limp that cannot be compensated for with a cane, is an indication for an attempt at reattachment of the trochanter. The surfaces should be freshened and rigidly fixed together; bone grafting may be necessary. Subperiosteal release of the iliac wing muscles may be necessary to allow the trochanter to be reattached to the femur.

Pain after trochanteric nonunion may be the result of a painful pseudoarthrosis or, alternatively, to fixation wires that may form a painful bursa.

8. Heterotopic ossification—The incidence of significant heterotopic ossification after total hip arthroplasty is 5% or 10%, although it is present to a lesser degree in perhaps 80% of patients. Definite risk factors include previous heterotopic ossification, ankylosing spondylitis, diffuse idiopathic skeletal hyperostosis or spinal ostosis (Forestier disease), unlimited hip motion preoperatively, head injury, and male sex of the patient. Other possible risk factors include trochanteric osteotomy, interoperative fracture, bone grafting, or localized muscle damage or hematoma.

Heterotopic bone is classified by either the Brooker or the Mayo classification (Table 7–8). Patients identified as being at risk for heterotopic ossification should undergo prophylactic treatment, careful surgical treat-

Table 7–8. Heterotopic bone classification systems.

Stage	Mayo Classification	Brooker Classification
I	5 mm or less	Islands of bone
II	< 50% bridging laterally	Bone spurs 1 cm or greater gap
III	> 50% bridging laterally	Bone spurs less than 1 cm
IV	Apparent ankylosis	Apparent ankylosis

Reprinted, with permission, from Brooker AF et al: Ectopic ossification following total hip replacement. J Bone Joint Surg Am 1973; 55:1629; and Morrey BF, Adams RA, Cabanela ME: Comparison of heterotopic bone after anterolateral, transtrochanteric, and posterior approaches for total hip arthroplasty. Clin Orthop 1984;188:160.

ment, wound drainage, and irrigation of the wound prior to closing. In patients at risk, low-dose radiation, 6–8 cGy in the first 3 days after surgery, prevents grade 3 or 4 heterotopic ossification. Indomethacin is effective, although it may be poorly tolerated by some patients. Early studies indicate that the bone inhibition is a COX-1 function, suggesting that COX-2 inhibitors may not prevent heterotopic bone. Diphosphonates are not effective in prevention of heterotopic ossification and should not be used. Indomethacin may not be optimal for prophylaxis in uncemented total hip arthroplasty because ingrowth may be retarded. Irradiation may cause problems if ingrowth components are not appropriately shielded.

If heterotopic ossification causes symptoms (pain, decreased ROM), surgical excision may be considered after the ossification is fully mature. Irradiation and NSAIDs are recommended postoperatively to prevent recurrence.

9. Infection—Prevention of infection after total hip arthroplasty is important because of the grave consequences. Frequently, the only way to treat an infected total hip arthroplasty is to remove the components and control the infection with antibiotics. Reinsertion of the components is then required 1.5–6 months later.

An innovation in the treatment of infected total hips and knees is the prosthetic antibiotic-loaded acrylic cement (PROSTALAC) technique. The prostheses are removed, sterilized, and reinserted as press-fit components with a layer of antibiotic-impregnated bone cement covering all surfaces except the bearing surface. This procedure is performed at the initial meticulous debridement, to provide a spacer for subsequent, definitive joint replacement.

Prevention is much more desirable than subsequent treatment of infection. Total joint arthroplasty implants are such large foreign bodies that all reasonable prophylactic measures should be employed. Laminar flow and ultraviolet lights are used in operating rooms to reduce the number of viable particles per volume of air in the room. Because bacteria are shed from people, keeping the number of people in an operating room to a minimum and reducing the exposed skin area may be beneficial. Antimicrobial therapy may be the single most important prophylaxis against infection. Good surgical technique and minimal operating times also contribute to lowering of infection rates. Infections occurring 6 weeks to 3 months after surgery probably originate from intraoperative contamination. Careful surveillance in this period for signs of infection, including pain, elevated white blood cell count, fever, and wound drainage, allows for early identification of deep wound infection, and early debridement is then indicated to eradicate the infection. Similarly, large hematomas should be debrided because they may cause chronic drainage and constitute a culture media for infectious agents. One report indicates that prophylactic antibiotics given in the period before and immediately after significant dental procedures may be beneficial in preventing hematogenous infection of total joints, despite recent recommendations that routine prophylaxis 2 years after joint arthroplasty is not necessary.

Amoxicillin, 3 g taken 1 hour before and 1.5 g taken 6 hours after a dental procedure, is recommended to reduce the risk of hematogenous infection. For penicillin-allergic patients, erythromycin, 1 g before and 500 mg after the procedure, is recommended.

Barrack RL, Harris WH: The value of aspiration of the hip joint before revision total hip arthroplasty. J Bone Joint Surg Am 1993;75:66.

Callaghan JJ et al: Charnley total hip arthroplasty with cement: Minimum twenty-five year follow-up. J Bone Joint Surg Am 2000;82:487.

Coventry MB: Late dislocations in patients with Charnley total hip arthroplasty. J Bone Joint Surg Am 1985;67:832.

Daly P, Morrey BF: Operative correction of an unstable total hip arthroplasty. J Bone Joint Surg Am 1992;74:1334.

DeHart MM and Riley LH: Nerve injuries in total hip arthroplasty. J Am Acad Orthop Surg 1999;7:101.

Dorr LD et al: Total hip arthroplasty with use of the Metasul metal-on-metal articulation: Four to seven year results. J Bone Joint Surg Am 2000;82:789.

Harris WH: Traumatic arthritis of the hip after dislocation and acetabular fractures: Treatment by mold arthroplasty. J Bone Joint Surg Am 1969;51:737.

Harris WH, Barrack RL: Contemporary algorithms for evaluation of the painful total hip replacement. Orthop Rev 1993;22:531.

Huddleston HD: An accurate method for measuring leg length and hip offset in hip arthroplasty. Orthopedics 1997;20:331.

Khan MAA et al: Dislocation following total hip arthroplasty. J Bone Joint Surg Br 1981;63:214.

Lester DK, Helm M: Mini-incision posterior approach for hip arthroplasty. Orthop Traumatol 2001;4:245.

Lewinnek GE et al: Dislocations after total hip replacement arthroplasties. J Bone Joint Surg Am 1970;60:217.

Markolf KL et al: Mechanical stability of the greater trochanter following osteotomy and reattachment by wiring. Clin Orthop 1979;141:111.

McDonald DJ, Fitzgerald RH Jr: Two-stage reconstruction of a total hip arthroplasty because of infection. J Bone Joint Surg Am 1989;71:828.

Mont MA et al: Total hip replacement without cement for noninflammatory osteoarthrosis in patients who are less than forty-five years old. J Bone Joint Surg Am 1993;75:740.

Ritter MA: A treatment plan for the dislocated total hip arthroplasty: Treatment with an above-knee hip spica cast. Clin Orthop 1980;153:153.

Schmalzried TP et al: Update on nerve palsy associated with total hip replacement. Clin Orthop 1997;344:188.

Waldman BJ et al: Total knee arthroplasty infections associated with dental procedures. Clin Orthop 1997;343:164.

Revision Total Hip Arthroplasty

The clinical success of revision total hip arthroplasty (THA) procedures historically was greatly inferior to the results of primary hip arthroplasty procedures. Loosening rates from 13% to 44% of cemented femoral revision procedures were reported at follow-ups of less than 5 years.

Improved techniques of cementing femoral stems led to improved results with cemented femoral revision. Pressurization of cement delivered, in a doughy stage, with a cement gun; pulsatile lavage; and an intramedullary plug permitted reproducible creation of adequate cement mantles. Only 14% of revised cemented femoral components were loose radiographically in one series after an average of 6 years. Other series indicate a revision rate of approximately 10% at 10 years, which is much improved from earlier series but inferior to those obtained with primary cemented stems.

Estok DMD II, Harris WH: Long-term results of cemented femoral revision surgery using second-generation techniques: An average 11.7 years follow-up evaluation. Clin Orthop 1994;299:190.

Katz RP et al: Cemented revision total hip arthroplasty using contemporary techniques: A minimum ten-year follow-up study. J Arthroplasty 1994;9:103.

Kavanagh BF et al: Revision total hip arthroplasty. J Bone Joint Surg 1985;67:517.

Pellicci PM et al: Revision total hip arthroplasty. Clin Orthop 1982;170:34.

Rubash HE, Harris WH: Revision of nonseptic, loose, cemented femoral components using modern cementing techniques. J Arthroplasty 1988;3:241.

Cementless reconstructions of failed femoral components were developed in response to the early high rates of failure with cemented revision procedures. However, early cementless revision series were generally unsuccessful, with failure rates of 4–10% at follow-ups less than 4 years. The use of proximally porous coated stems with inadequate stabilization, in the setting of deficient femoral bone stock, led to unreliable bone ingrowth fixation. Encouraging reports were obtained with modular proximally coated stems, such as the S-ROM (Johnson and Johnson, Raynham, MA) prosthesis, and extensively porous coated stems, such as the AML and Solution (Depuy, Warsaw, IN). Re-revision rates from 1.5% to 6% were achieved with use of these types of cementless femoral component at follow-ups from 5 to 8.4 years.

Gustilo RB, Pasternak HS: Revision total hip arthroplasty with titanium ingrowth prosthesis and bone grafting for failed cemented femoral component loosening. Clin Orthop 1988;235:111.

Harris WH et al: Results of cementless revisions of total hip arthroplasties using the Harris-Galante prosthesis. Clin Orthop 1988;235:120.

Hedley AK et al: Revision of failed total hip arthroplasties with uncemented porous-coated anatomic components. Clin Orthop 1988;235:75.

Lawrence JM et al: Revision total hip arthroplasty: Long term results with cement. Orthop Clin North Am 1993;24:635.

McCarthy JC et al: Revision of the deficient femur with a modular femoral component. Orthop Trans 1993;17:966.

Paprosky WG et al: Cementless femoral revision in the presence of severe proximal bone loss using diaphyseal fixation. Orthop Trans 1993;17:965.

In the situation where inadequate femoral bone stock exists, the use of allograft bone is advocated. For extended loss of proximal femoral bone stock, cementing a smooth tapered femoral stem in a bed of impacted particulate allogenic bone produces promising short-term clinical results. When deficiency of proximal bone stock is severe, use of structural femoral allografts may be required, and short-term reports suggest good clinical results.

Gie GA et al: Impacted cancellous allografts and cement for revision total hip replacement. J Bone Joint Surg 1993;75:14.

Gross AE et al: Proximal femoral allografts for reconstruction of bone stock in revision arthroplasty of the hip. Clin Orthop 1995;319:151.

Similar to early experience with cemented revisions of the femoral component, acetabular revision with cement was generally unsuccessful. Because of the difficulty of interdigitating cement into a sclerotic and often deficient acetabular bone stock, failure rates of loosening were reported from 53% to 93% at follow-ups from only 2–4.5 years.

Kavanagh BF et al: Charnley total hip arthroplasty with cement: Fifteen-year results. J Bone Joint Surg 1985;71:1496.

Snorrason F, Karrholm J: Early loosening of revision hip arthroplasty: A roentgen stereophotogrammetric analysis. J Arthroplasty 1990;5:217.

The introduction of cementless porous-coated acetabular implants for revision of failed cemented cups greatly facilitated early clinical results. Large hemispherical cementless acetabular implants can accommodate most bone defects encountered after removal of failed cemented cups. Where an adequate press-fit cannot be obtained, adjuvant fixation of the implant with screws or spikes can provide adequate stability to permit bone ingrowth fixation. Re-revision rates are reported from 0% to 1.6% with follow-up of 2–4 years.

Engh CA et al: Results of cementless revision for failed cemented total hip arthroplasty. Clin Orthop 1988;235:91.

Harris WH et al: Results of cementless revision of total hip arthroplasties using the Harris-Galante prosthesis. Clin Orthop 1988;235:120.

Hedley AK et al: Revision of failed total hip arthroplasties with uncemented porous-coated anatomic components. Clin Orthop 1988;235:75.

Padgett DE et al: Revision of the acetabular component without cement after total hip arthroplasty: Three- to six-year follow-up. J Bone Joint Surg 1993;75A:663.

Where inadequate bone stock of the acetabulum precludes reconstructions with conventional hemispherical implants, structural allografts fixed to the pelvis with screws can provide acceptable middle-term results. Other alternatives include the use of eccentric shaped cementless implants and cemented reconstructions with particulate allografting and antiprotrusio cages.

Berry DJ, Muller M: Revision arthroplasty using an antiprotrusio cage for massive acetabular bone deficiency. J Bone Joint Surg 1992;74:711.

Garbuz D et al: Revision of the acetabular component of a total hip arthroplasty with a massive structural allograft. J Bone Joint Surg 1996;78:693.

Peters CL, Curtain M, Samuelson KM: Acetabular revision with the Burch-Schnieder antiprotrusio cage and cancellous allograft bone. J Arthroplasty 1995;10:307.

Sutherland CJ: Early experience with eccentric acetabular components in revision total hip arthroplasty. Am J Orthop 1996;25:284.

Total Knee Arthroplasty

A. INDICATIONS

As with other joints, the primary indication for total knee arthroplasty is pain. Absolute contraindications to total knee arthroplasty include active sepsis, absence of an extensor mechanism, and neuropathic joint. Relative contraindications include a patient's young (less than 40 years) age, heavy demand for activity, or a patient's unreliability.

When both hips and knees are involved with painful arthritis, the joint causing the most discomfort should be replaced first. If hips and knees are equally painful, hip arthroplasty should precede knee arthroplasty. Rehabilitation following total hip arthroplasty is easier and less affected by a painful knee than vice versa. Additionally, motion of the hip joint greatly facilitates surgery for the knee.

B. IMPLANTS

Early designs of total knee arthroplasty were developed in Europe and may be categorized as constrained or resurfacing. Constrained devices consisted of fixed hinges, and resurfacing devices relied on ligaments for stability. Constrained devices predictably loosened, although they were used primarily in severe bone or ligamentous deficiency states. Early resurfacing implants were flat, roller pin–shaped implants or unicondylar devices that replaced only the medial or lateral compartment. Early knee replacements did not resurface the patellofemoral joints.

Contemporary total knee replacements represent a convergence of two major designs developed in the United States during the early 1970s: the total condylar and the duopatellar prostheses. The total condylar prosthesis had a femoral component made of Co/Cr and an all-polyethylene tibial component with a central peg. Excision of the posterior cruciate ligament was required because the entire surface of the tibial plateau was resurfaced. The patellar component was a dome-shaped polyethylene implant. All components were fixed with acrylic cement.

The Duocondylar knee replacement was the forerunner of the duopatellar prosthesis and did not resurface the patellofemoral joint. Extension of the anterior flange of the Co/Cr femoral component provided an articulation surface for an all-polyethylene dome-shaped patellar component. The tibial component was originally designed with separate medial and lateral runners, allowing preservation of the central insertion of the posterior cruciate ligament. Later, the two components were joined together, but a cutout was made posteriorly to permit retention of the posterior cruciate ligament.

Retention of the posterior cruciate ligament permitted increased flexion over that with the total condylar design because the normal femoral rollback during knee flexion was retained. Shifting of the center of rotation posteriorly during knee flexion greatly improves the lever arm of the quadriceps mechanism. The ability to climb stairs was superior when the cruciate ligament was retained. Central to the design of a cruciate-retaining prosthesis is avoidance of excessive constraint by the tibial surface to permit rollback.

To overcome limitations in flexion and stair-climbing function, the total condylar prosthesis was modified with a cam mechanism (posterior-stabilized condylar prosthesis). The central cam design permits substitution of the function of the posterior cruciate ligament, providing a mechanical recreation of femoral rollback.

The differences in ROM and stair-climbing function achieved with cruciate-retaining and posterior-stabilized knee replacements are now considered negligible. Arguments in favor of the posterior-stabilized implant include technical ease in reconstructing severely deformed knees and less shear force at the articular bearing because sliding is reduced. The arguments in favor of cruciate-retaining designs are reduction of bone–cement interface forces because of less constraint, improved stability in flexion, less removal of bone from the intercondylar region, and absence of patellofemoral impingement syndrome (formed by scar tissue in the intercondylar recess of the posterior stabilized femoral component).

Problems with high-contact, stress-inducing fatigue wear of the polyethylene surfaces stimulated a new design concept in knee replacement. This design uses a polyethylene component that can move in relation to the tibial base plate. Thus, the surface of polyethylene in contact with the femoral component can be made to be more conforming because it can change positions during flexion and extension of the knee. Two types have evolved: the rotating platform, which only allows rotation of the polyethylene around an axis approximating the axis of the tibia, and variations on the "meniscal bearing" knee. In this design, the individual medial and lateral poly components can rotate (tibial axis) and translate (AP direction), or the entire poly plateau can rotate and translate in the AP direction. The latter concept seems to better address the biomechanical aspects of the knee, but results are early or limited on all designs.

C. SURGICAL TECHNIQUE

Total knee replacement surgery is greatly facilitated by use of a thigh tourniquet. Following exsanguination of the lower limb with an elastic wrap, the tourniquet is inflated to 250–300 mm Hg. An anterior midline skin incision is made, followed most commonly by a deep medial parapatellar approach. The lateral flap containing the patella is everted to allow exposure of the tibiofemoral joint. Remnants of menisci and anterior cruciate ligament are excised, with careful release of contracted soft-tissue structures as needed.

Instrumentation systems guide the surgeon to create bone cuts with a saw that match the prosthetic fixation surface and reproduce anatomic alignment of the knee joint. Typically, in the coronal plane, the tibial plateau is cut horizontally to be at a right angle with the shaft of the tibia. The distal femur is usually cut at 5–7 degrees of valgus from the shaft of the femur. Such bone cuts provide a neutral mechanical alignment in the coronal plane so a line can be drawn from the center of the femoral head, through the middle of the knee joint, and through the center of the ankle joint. In the sagittal plane, the femoral cut is at right angles to the femoral shaft, but the tibial cut is made with 3–5 degrees of posterior slope. Slight external rotation of the femoral component allows symmetric tension of collateral ligaments during knee flexion and facilitates tracking of the patellar component.

Retention or sacrifice of the posterior cruciate ligament depends on the design of the implant used. When the cruciate ligament is sacrificed, bone from the intercondylar notch is removed to accommodate the box that houses the cam mechanism.

When the patellar surface is replaced, a saw is used to create a flat surface with symmetric bone thickness. Inadequate resection predisposes to subluxation because excessive extensor mechanism length is used, and the lateral ligamentous structures are relatively tightened. Many patellar components are 10 mm thick; thus, adequate resection must be almost 10 mm, within the limits of the anatomy of the patella. At least 10 mm and preferably 15 mm of patella (AP thickness) should remain. Patellar tracking is assessed by using trial components and ranging the knee from full extension to full flexion. In knees with valgus deformity, it is common to have lateral subluxation of the patella. In such cases, a careful lateral retinacular release that preserves the superior lateral geniculate vessels is performed. Positioning the patellar implant slightly medially on the patellar bone surface also improves tracking.

After appropriate trials are used to confirm accurate sizes of the components as well as ligamentous stability, cementing is performed. Careful cleansing of the bone surfaces with pulsatile lavage facilitates interdigitation of doughy-stage methylmethacrylate cement. The prosthetic components must be seated in the correct orientation, and excess acrylic cement must be removed. Before closure of the knee, it is prudent to lavage fragments of bone and cement and release the tourniquet to obtain hemostasis. At surgery, little bleeding is seen in the flexed knee. Thus, many surgeons close the wound and maintain the knee in flexion for periods up to 24 hours to decrease blood loss.

D. CLINICAL RESULTS

Long-term results of contemporary cemented total knee arthroplasty designs are excellent. Survivorship of the total condylar prosthesis is calculated to be 90–95% at 15 years. Excellent functional results of posterior stabilized total knee replacements are also reported, with a 12-year survival rate of 94% for functional prostheses. Similarly, excellent function and only a 1% rate of loosening of the tibial or femoral component was reported with a cruciate ligament–retaining knee replacement when followed up at 10–14 years.

E. COMPLICATIONS

Complications are infrequent with total knee arthroplasty but include many of the same problems encountered with total hip arthroplasty. Additional problems arise from wound healing, fracture, extensor mechanism problems, and stiffness of the knee.

1. Deep vein thrombosis—DVT is common following knee arthroplasty, occurring in more than 50% of patients in one study. Further, 10–15% of patients develop DVT in the contralateral leg after unilateral knee arthroplasty. The use of the tourniquet during surgery does not have a clear detrimental effect on thrombus formation. The incidence of pulmonary embolism is lower than that reported in hip arthroplasty. This may be caused by the greater propensity to form calf thrombi after total knee arthroplasty; these thrombi may be less likely to cause emboli than thigh thrombi. Antithrombotic prophylactic measures include use of pulsatile compression stockings and administration of warfarin or low-molecular-weight heparin.

2. Wound problems—Wound problems can arise from incision-related issues and from patient-related risk factors. The skin incision should optimally be midline and longitudinal, and the skin should have minimal undermining. Preexisting skin incisions should be used when possible. Because wound healing is crucial to the success of the procedure, preoperative plastic surgery consultation may be beneficial if multiple scars, burns, or previous irradiation to the skin are present. Patient-related risk factors include chronic corticosteroid use, obesity, malnutrition, tobacco use, diabetes, and hypovolemia.

Treatment of wound problems depends on the type of problem. Drainage of serous material that does not clear in 5–7 days is an indication for open debridement. Hematoma formation (without drainage) is treated nonoperatively unless there are signs of impending skin necrosis or compromise of ROM. Small areas of superficial necrosis at the wound edge are treated with routine local wound care. Full-thickness soft-tissue necrosis places the joint space at high risk of infection and must be treated aggressively. Debridement with flap closure is frequently required. The medial gastrocnemius flap is useful because the tissue necrosis is frequently medial.

Prevention of wound problems through careful planning, gentle handling of soft tissues, and patient education to minimize risk factors is preferable to subsequent treatment of the problems.

3. Nerve palsy—Nerve palsies are a rare complication of total knee arthroplasty. The peroneal nerve is believed to be at increased risk for injury from surgery performed on valgus knees with flexion contractures or other significant deformity, ischemia from stretching small vessels in the surrounding soft tissue, and compression resulting from a tight dressing or splint. The risk is reported to be approximately 0.6%.

4. Femoral fracture—Notching of the anterior femoral cortex may predispose to distal femoral fracture. A technical error, notching can be prevented by careful femoral sizing before use of the anterior distal femur cutting block and by avoidance of posterior displacement or extension of the cutting block. Use of an intramedullary stem extension is advised if notching occurs. Fracture of the medial or lateral condyle may occur, particularly in patients with poor bone stock, such as those with RA or osteoporosis or in patients with cruciate-sacrificing femoral components. Large intercondylar boxes in these prostheses can cause weakening of the distal femur. Prevention is the rule, facilitated by vigilance during exposure of a stiff knee. Useful techniques to avoid avulsion include a V turndown quadriceps-plasty, quadriceps "snip," tibial tubercle osteotomy, and placement of a Steinmann pin in the tubercle to prevent excessive traction on the patellar tendon. Treatment of the disruption is similar to the treatment in a normal knee. The patellar tendon is attached to bone, and the repair is protected with a wire around the patella and the tibial tubercle, holding the patella at the correct length from the tibial tubercle.

Patellar complications include maltracking, loosening of the patellar component, fractures, and impingement. The patellofemoral forces are among the highest anywhere in the body, and avoidance of intraoperative technical errors may minimize patellar complications. Patellar tracking should be assessed intraoperatively during flexion and extension of the prosthetic knee. Lateral patellar subluxation or dislocation may be caused by internal rotation of the femoral or tibial component, as well as a tight lateral patellar retinaculum. Careful release of the lateral patellar retinaculum may correct maltracking. Subluxation can predispose to patellar component loosening, as can abnormal stress caused by uneven patellar bone resection. Excessive bone resection and avascularity, caused by damage to the superior lateral geniculate artery during lateral release, can predispose to fractures. When using a posterior stabilized prosthesis, maintaining the inferior pole of the patella within 10–30 mm of the joint line may prevent impingement syndrome, which is characterized by pain or clicking when peripatellar synovial scar tissue impinges against the intercondylar box of the femoral component during flexion and extension.

In some studies, patellar complications are the cause for as many as half of the knee revisions performed. For this reason, some surgeons do not resurface the patella when the appearance is relatively normal. Because most patellofemoral replacement problems are attributed to technical errors, inferior prosthetic design, and excessive loads, replacement will probably become more prevalent as these problems are resolved.

5. Extensor mechanism complications—Many extensor mechanism problems can be prevented by careful surgical technique because many of these arise from technical problems, such as quadriceps (or patellar) tendon rupture, patellofemoral instability, and patella fracture.

Intraoperative rupture of the patellar or quadriceps tendon at the time of arthroplasty can be repaired, but a repair complicates the postoperative ROM regimen, at least to some extent. The incidence ranges from 0.2% to 2.5%.

6. Knee stiffness—Knee stiffness is a common problem in the early postoperative period. Methods to reduce stiffness include physical therapy (active or active-assisted ROM) and continuous passive motion (CPM). The CPM machine moves the knee through a preset passive ROM This modality is generally accepted and even liked by patients but does not affect the final ROM or reduce hospital stay. An acceptable ROM is 90–95 degrees of flexion with less than 10 degrees of flexion contracture, but the activities of daily living, such as getting out of a chair or climbing stairs, should be painless. Postoperative stiffness should generally subside by 6–8 weeks after surgery, and improvement in ROM should occur for 1 year with most gain in the first 3 months. The preoperative ROM is an important indicator of the ROM to be expected postoperatively.

Prevention of significant flexion contracture at the time of surgery and in the early postoperative period is important because improvement with manipulation is unrewarding. Manipulation with or without steroid injection can be beneficial in the first 3 months. Arthroscopic debridement may be necessary after intraarticular fibrosis occurs. Decreases in ROM after initial gains should alert the surgeon to possible infection, reflex sympathetic dystrophy, or mechanical problems, such as loose components or interposed soft tissue.

Ayers DC et al: Common complications of total knee arthroplasty. J Bone Joint Surg Am 1997;79:278.

Barrack RL, Wolfe MW: Patellar resurfacing in total knee arthroplasty. J Am Acad Orthop Surg 2000;8:75.

Callaghan JJ et al: Cemented rotating-platform total knee replacement: A nine to twelve year follow-up study. J Bone Joint Surg Am 2000;82:705.

Callaghan JJ et al: Mobile-bearing knee replacement: Concepts and results. J Bone Joint Surg 2000;82:1020.

Figgi HF et al: The influence of tibial-patellofemoral location on function of the knee in patients with the posterior stabilized condylar knee prosthesis. J Bone Joint Surg Am 1986;68:1035.

Hahn SB et al: A modified Thompson quadricepsplasty for stiff knee. J Bone Joint Surg Br 2000;82:992.

Rinonapoli E et al: Long-term results and survivorship analysis of 89 total condylar knee prostheses. J Arthroplasty 1992;7:241.

Scuderi GR et al: Survivorship of cemented knee replacements. J Bone Joint Surg Br 1989;71:798.

Ververeli PA et al: Continuous passive motion after total knee arthroplasty: Analysis of cost and benefits. Clin Orthop 1995;321:208.

Total Shoulder Arthroplasty

A. INDICATIONS

The primary indication for shoulder arthroplasty is severe pain that was treated unsuccessfully with nonsurgical management. The underlying causes for the loss of articular cartilage and the incongruent osseous surfaces of the glenohumeral joint are usually OA, RA, posttraumatic arthritis, and dislocation arthropathy. The functional status of the soft tissues is vitally important because they provide a significant component of the joint stabilizing force through the concavity-compression mechanism. Techniques for replacement of the glenoid remains controversial based on the glenoid wear pattern. Newer reports suggest that asymmetric loading with excessive or repetitive overhead activities may eventually lead to posterior glenoid erosion. Most surgeons currently still recommend that glenoid replacement may be performed if and only if the rotator cuff is intact or reparable at the time of surgery. Although still controversial, a shoulder hemiarthroplasty is performed for patients with rotator cuff arthropathy and osteonecrosis. In this subset of patients, a surface replacement arthroplasty is an option to preserve bone stock. For patients with rotator cuff arthropathy or severe glenohumeral arthritis with an irreparable rotator cuff, a "reverse" or "inverted" shoulder prosthesis was reintroduced to improve function. With this design, the socket is placed in the humerus and the ball is placed in the glenoid with hopes of resisting glenohumeral subluxation. There is currently not enough follow-up data available to determine the efficacy of these devices. If RA has caused profound bony erosion of the glenoid medially to the level of the coracoid process, hemiarthroplasty may be the only viable option because the glenoid may not be able to support a prosthetic component. Contraindications to shoulder arthroplasty include active sepsis, neuropathic arthropathy, and the absence of a functional deltoid.

B. SURGICAL TECHNIQUE

A deltopectoral surgical approach is performed, with careful retraction of the conjoined tendon medially to avoid injury to the musculocutaneous nerve. Although some suggest releasing the subscapularis tendon 1 cm lateral to its humeral insertion because it may facilitate later repair, most currently recommend detaching the subscapularis directly off the humeral insertion. Attachment of the subscapularis to the edge of the humeral osteotomy lengthens the muscle-tendon unit so a coronal Z-plasty is not required to improve external rotation of the glenohumeral joint. Palpation of the axillary nerve medially along the inferior border of the subscapularis is recommended to avoid injury to this vital nerve. A capsulotomy is then performed from the humeral attachment, and the humeral head is delivered out of the wound, with extension and external rotation of the arm. The humeral head is carefully resected to protect the rotator cuff insertion, and the humeral component is placed in 30–35 degrees of retroversion. Preparation of the humeral intramedullary canal is followed by insertion of a trial stemmed humeral component. After the appropriate thickness of the humeral head and stem is determined, the trial humeral head component is removed, and the stem is left in place to tamponade the intramedullary bleeding and to provide strength to the humerus during glenoid preparation. Posterior displacement of the proximal humerus is performed using a humeral head retractor, such as a Fukuda retractor, for exposure of the glenoid vault. Minimal bone is removed from the glenoid bone with a motorized burr to preserve cortical bone for support of the glenoid component. Long-term follow-up studies show that both bone grafting of deficient glenoid bone and building up defects with cement are not routinely recommended. With posterior glenoid wear, bone is removed form the glenoid anteriorly to match the posterior aspect of the glenoid. A keel or drill holes for peg insertion are made for cemented applications. To date, the FDA has not approved any noncemented glenoid components. There are glenoid components with trabecular metal for bony ingrowth that are currently in clinical trials. The humeral component is then implanted with or without cement, depending on surgeon preference and quality of bone stock. The closure must include a robust repair of the subscapularis tendon so that physical therapy may be initiated in the immediate postoperative period.

C. IMPLANTS

Early total shoulder arthroplasties were designed with constrained articulations between the humeral and glenoid components. Predictably, glenoid loosening and implant failures were commonplace, leading to development of unconstrained designs. Currently, nonconstrained resurfacing devices are primarily used with stemmed metal humeral components. Options include modular head and neck assemblies as well as a porous coating for cementless implantation. Although most commonly used glenoid components are made of high-density polyethylene, some designs of metal backing with porous coating and screw fixation for cementless applications are being explored.

D. CLINICAL RESULTS

Shoulder arthroplasty has made significant progress, similar to the advances in hip and knee arthroplasty. The current so-called third-generation prosthetic designs incorporate variable offset and inclination, anatomic humeral heads, precision instruments, and variable glenoid curvature in their designs. Pain relief is reliably

achieved with shoulder arthroplasty in more than 90–95% of patients. Pain relief obtained from hemiarthroplasties is equivalent to total shoulder replacement in selected patients younger than 50 years. As would be expected, shoulder arthroplasty performed in a high-volume hospital or high-volume surgeons are more likely to have a better outcome than their counterparts who perform the surgery infrequently.

Functional results are variable, however, depending largely on the underlying cause. A ROM three quarters to four fifths of normal can be expected in patients treated for OA or osteonecrosis. For RA, one half to two thirds of normal motion is usually obtained. For patients with cuff tear arthropathy, the ROM achieved may be only one third to one half of normal. Furthermore, the results for either hemiarthroplasty or total shoulder arthroplasty for patients younger than 50 years show higher failure rates. As such, alternative solutions in these younger patients may be explored.

The major complication associated with total shoulder arthroplasty involves loosening of the glenoid component; instability and late rotator cuff tears are next in frequency. Less common complications are humeral component loosening, sepsis, nerve injury, and humeral fractures. The incidence of shoulder arthroplasty infection is less than 0.5% and usually attributed to the abundant blood supply and surrounding musculature of the joint.

Radiolucent lines were observed around the glenoid component in 30–90% of cases in most published series, but the rate of definite and probable radiographic loosening is between 0% and 11%. Despite this, the revision rate for glenoid loosening is approximately 6% at 12 years. A higher failure rate caused by glenoid component loosening is associated with deficiency of the rotator cuff. Superior migration of the humeral articulation leads to eccentric loading and a rocking-horse effect on the glenoid component and loosening. Most surgeons currently perform hemiarthroplasty for rotator cuff tear arthropathy. In certain cases of cuff tear arthropathy or of significant medial glenoid erosion, a large-diameter humeral head or bipolar hemiarthroplasty may be used to lateralize the joint center, thereby facilitating the mechanical advantage of the deltoid. Alternatively, the so-called reverse or inverted shoulder prosthesis is being offered at certain centers for rotator cuff arthropathy, but it should be entertained in only select patients.

Baumgarten KM et al: Glenoid resurfacing in shoulder arthroplasty: Indications and contraindications. Instr Course Lect 2004;53:3.

Gupta R, Lee TQ: Positional-dependent changes in glenohumeral joint contact pressure and force: Possible biomechanical etiology of posterior glenoid wear. J Shoulder Elbow Surg 2005;14:S105.

Harman M et al: Initial glenoid component fixation in "reverse" total shoulder arthroplasty: A biomechanical evaluation. J Shoulder Elbow Surg 2004;14:S162.

Jain N et al: The relationship between surgeon and hospital volume and outcomes for shoulder arthroplasty. J Bone Joint Surg Am 2004; 86-A:496.

Levy O et al: Copeland surface replacement arthroplasty of the shoulder in rheumatoid arthritis. J Bone Joint Surg Am 2004;86-A:512.

Lyman S et al: The association between hospital volume and total shoulder arthroplasty outcomes. Clin Orthop 2005;432:132.

Sperling J et al: Minimum fifteen-year follow-up of Neer hemiarthroplasty and total shoulder arthroplasty in patients aged fifty years or younger. J Shoulder Elbow Surg 2004;13:604.

Total Elbow Arthroplasty

A. Indications

Although total elbow arthroplasty (TEA) may be an appropriate method of restoring joint function and stability, its primary goal is pain relief. With increased surgical experience, improvement of prosthetic designs, and evolving biomechanical knowledge, the indications for TEA have broadened to include the following, in order of frequency:

1. rheumatoid arthritis (RA);
2. posttraumatic arthritis;
3. juvenile rheumatoid arthritis (JRA);
4. distal humeral nonunions and severe comminuted distal humeral fractures, especially in the elderly; and
5. primary OA.

The severity of the disease and the choice of prosthesis in all of these situations are critical to the final outcome. TEA achieves its best results in individuals who do not tax the functional design of the prosthesis and who do not expect to use their upper limb beyond the level of basic daily functional activities such as combing hair, eating, and drinking. Active sepsis is an absolute contraindication to total elbow arthroplasty. Relative contraindications for TEA include previously open wound associated with trauma around the elbow, a previous infection of the elbow associated with prior TEA, arthrodesis, paralysis of the biceps or triceps, severe joint capsule contracture, and poor patient compliance. Lifting limitations after TEA remain 2.25 kg for repetitive lifting and 4.5 kg for single-episode lifting. Because most devices have higher failure rates approximately 10 years after implantation, alternative therapeutic interventions such as interpositional arthroplasty should be considered for younger (less than 60 years) patients. Thus, patient selection, compliance, and age become critical factors in determining the successful long-term outcome of prosthetic elbows.

B. Surgical Technique

Attention to the soft tissue, including the triceps insertion, collateral ligaments, and the ulnar nerve, is of vital importance when performing a TEA. Although the direct posterior approach is routinely recommended, especially early in the surgeon's learning curve, failures in TEA are attributed to this approach. After the flap of triceps muscle is turned down, the tissue may be devascularized and lead to overlying skin necrosis and weakness of the triceps muscle. If this approach is used, careful reattachment of the triceps insertion to the ulna is mandatory.

Because maintenance of the collateral ligaments is of vital importance when a nonconstrained device is used, the Kocher posterolateral approach allows preservation of the ulnar collateral ligament. This ligament provides the major restraint against valgus forces in the flexed elbow, and so it must be preserved when a nonconstrained device is used. The surgical plane is between the anconeus and extensor carpi ulnaris muscles distally and proximally between the triceps and brachioradialis muscles.

The Bryan posteromedial approach is routinely used for implantation of semiconstrained devices. The surgical plane is between the medial triceps and forearm flexors proximally and between the flexor carpi ulnaris and flexor carpi radialis distally. This approach allows direct visualization of the ulnar nerve and facilitates transposition of the nerve. Great care should be taken when encountering Sharpey fibers during elevation of the triceps from its olecranon insertion to prevent discontinuity with the forearm fascia. Release of the medial collateral ligament is required to proceed with implantation.

C. Implants

Early TEA designs included constrained devices, which predictably failed because of early aseptic loosening. In response to these failures, devices with less constraint and those permitting more normal elbow kinematics were developed. The two currently available types of elbow implants include resurfacing nonconstrained devices and semiconstrained devices. The most popular semiconstrained devices are the Coonrad Morrey, Pritchard-Walker, and GSB III (Geschwend-Scheier-Bahler III) prostheses. These implants have a linked hinge that provides stability but less constraint than early designs. The sloppy fit of these hinges permits varus, valgus, and rotatory forces to the implant and fixation to be dissipated. The inherent stability of these designs permits application in cases of soft-tissue and bony insufficiency, but theoretically there is increased risk of loosening. Excision of the radial head is also recommended during implantation of semiconstrained total elbow arthroplasties. Nonconstrained devices are widely used outside the United States, and the most popular devices are the Souter-Strathclyde, Roper-Tuke, and the Kudo implants. These nonconstrained implants permit restoration of the center of rotation of the ulnotrochlear joint with a metal-on-polyethylene articulation. The humeral and ulnar components are not linked, minimizing stresses to the fixation of these components. Because these implants lack intrinsic stability, they should not be used in cases of ligamentous instability or deficiency of supporting bone.

D. CLINICAL RESULTS

Ten-year follow-up studies for TEA are currently only available for two semiconstrained linked devices—the Coonrad-Morrey and the GSB III designs—as well as for three nonconstrained devices: the Kudo, the Souter-Strathclyde, and the Roper-Tuke designs. Most of the experience using resurfacing devices in the United States was with the capitellocondylar design. Although no consistent 10-year studies exist for the capitellocondylar device, supporters of these implants report functional outcome of TEAs with nonconstrained devices comparable to those with semiconstrained device. Nevertheless, most of the reported past experiences suggest that high complication rates, particularly joint subluxations and dislocations, are associated with the use of these devices. The currently available 10-year long-term studies, as well as previous intermediate follow-up results, seem to suggest that the better semiconstrained designs may be associated with smaller numbers of revisions and aseptic loosening and greater success in maintaining pain relief and joint stability compared with the best nonconstrained devices.

Although previous radial head resection and synovectomy does not increase the rate of revision surgery for the subsequent elbow arthroplasty, this prior procedure did increase the complication rate when the elbow arthroplasty was performed. Newer data support the use of interpositional arthroplasty for younger patients because a semiconstrained arthroplasty remains a viable option at a later date. Although not as effective for pain relief, debridement arthroplasty and ulnohumeral arthroplasty are also options in active, younger high-demand patients who are not ready to accept the limitations of an elbow prosthesis.

Common complications encountered following TEA include aseptic loosening and joint instability, ulnar neuropathy, and infections. Ulnar neuropathies do not tend to require additional procedures, usually manifesting as paraesthesias and rarely showing signs of motor weakness. Many cases resolve or ameliorate over time. Many patients with RA already have preoperative evidence of ulnar neuropathy and the TEA did not contribute significantly to postoperative ulnar nerve dysfunction. Aseptic loosening of the cement–stem interface, polyethylene bushing wear (in semiconstrained devices), metallosis, and infections are major reasons for reoperation. For these patients that require revision procedures for aseptic loosening, the use of a longer stem prosthesis may be required. Alternatively, impaction grafting into the distal humerus or proximal

ulna may be an option. These remain extremely challenging procedures with significant morbidity and often require multiple subsequent procedures. Infections are the most serious complications among these indications and have the potential to develop further into devastating local and systemic complications.

Blaine TA et al: Total elbow arthroplasty after interposition arthroplasty for elbow arthritis. J Bone Joint Surg Am 2005;87-A:286.

Chafik D, Lee TQ, Gupta R: Total elbow arthroplasty: Current indications, factors affecting outcomes, and follow-up results. Am J Orthop 2004;33:496.

Kelly EW et al: Five- to thirteen-year follow-up of the GSB III total elbow arthroplasty. J Shoulder Elbow Surg 2004;13:434.

Loebenberg MI et al: Impaction grafting in revision total elbow arthroplasty. J Bone Joint Surg Am 2005;87-A:99.

Malone AA et al: Successful outcome of the Souter-Strathclyde elbow arthroplasty. J Shoulder Elbow Surg 2004;13:548.

Sarris I et al: Ulnohumeral arthroplasty: Results in primary degenerative arthritis of the elbow. Clin Orthop 2004;420:190.

Wada T et al: Debridement arthroplasty for primary osteoarthritis of the elbow. J Bone Joint Surg Am 2005;87-A:95.

Whaley A et al: Total elbow arthroplasty after previous resection of the radial head and synovectomy. J Bone Joint Surg Br 2005;87:47.

Total Ankle Arthroplasty

The total ankle arthroplasty was under development for many years as a result of the success with total joint replacement of the knee and the hip. Initial designs met with modest short-term success and caused almost an abandonment of the procedure because of the comparison to ankle arthrodesis. The longevity of present total ankle joint replacements is somewhat erratic for a variety of reasons. The articular surface that must be replaced is unlike any other joint, and thus, experience cannot be carried directly from the knee or the hip to the ankle. Joint loads and requirements are less well characterized, and surgical technique is less well developed and, therefore, less reliable. For these reasons, total ankle replacement remains a developmental procedure indicated for patients with low activity demand and the need for ankle motion.

Encouraging early reports with newer designs of total ankle arthroplasty have emerged and are being closely observed. Results with the Scandinavian total ankle replacement (STAR) prosthesis in short-term follow-up are promising. Total ankle replacement is desirable because of the drawbacks of ankle arthrodesis, which include a significant pseudoarthrosis rate of 10–20%, despite extended cast immobilization to achieve arthrodesis. Furthermore, extended arthrodesis results in osteopenia and diminished motion in the subtalar and midtarsal joints. The additional stress on these joints from the ankle arthrodesis predisposes them to degenerative changes over the long term, as is seen frequently above and below the arthrodesis in other joints such as the cervical spine, the lumbar spine, and the hip.

Kitaoka HB, Patzer GL: Clinical results of the Mayo total ankle arthroplasty. J Bone Joint Surg 1996;78:1658.

Pyevich MT et al: Total ankle arthroplasty: A unique design. Two to twelve-year follow-up. J Bone Joint Surg 1998;80:1410.

Evaluation of Painful Total Joint Arthroplasty

A certain degree of adaptation and accommodation is possible in the normal joint, allowing it to last for a lifetime in most persons. After replacement of a diseased joint by a metal-and-plastic artificial joint, no remodeling or accommodation is possible. Loosening of the interface between bone and prosthesis is possible and, indeed, may be inevitable. In addition, during and subsequent to the implantation process, bacteria may find their way into a prosthetic joint, causing pain or loosening. Implantation of a new joint markedly alters the stress state in the bone, particularly with uncemented prostheses, and a certain amount of pain may result. The presence of the new joint is likely to alleviate pain markedly, and the patient's activity level may increase, resulting in bone remodeling around the prosthesis or at a remote site or even fatigue fractures. All of these problems may result in a painful arthroplasty. Evaluation is complicated by the presence of the artificial joint, which introduces several new variables when compared with a normal arthritic joint. The same process of evaluation is used as with an arthritic joint; a history is obtained, physical examination is performed, and laboratory data are obtained.

A. History

Referred pain from other sources must be ruled out, particularly with the shoulder and the hip, where referred pain from the lumbar and cervical spine may confuse the picture. A history of pain radiating into the shoulder with motion of the neck, for example, may be helpful in this process. Pain related to activity of the affected joint, as compared with pain all the time, is an important fact, with constant pain or night pain suggesting chronic infection. Pain in the hip or knee that occurs with the first few steps but then improves is likely to be caused by loosening of the prosthesis. This pain probably arises from a fibrous membrane between the prosthesis and bone, which, with weight bearing, compresses and provides better contact, thereby lessening the pain. A history of swelling, redness, fevers, or chills must be obtained.

B. Physical Examination

The same tests are performed as for an arthritic joint to evaluate the location, magnitude, and severity of pain.

C. Workup

1. Laboratory findings—Laboratory data may be helpful. The ESR (more than 35–40 mm/h) or C-reactive protein (more than 0.7) points toward an infected arthroplasty; with the knee, a lower rate does not rule out infected arthroplasty. A complete blood count is sometimes also helpful in demonstrating an elevated white blood cell count.

2. Arthrographic evaluation—Arthrographic evaluation may be helpful by showing dye penetration into the cement–bone interface, prosthesis–bone interface, or prosthesis–cement interface. The most important aspect of arthrographic evaluation is the fluid obtained for culture. Arthrographic evaluation is mainly indicated when infection is suspected because there is a risk of contaminating the joint as well as the possibility of obtaining false-positive and false-negative cultures. Another important aspect of arthrographic evaluation is the pain response to injection of lidocaine into the joint. Alleviation of essentially all pain when weight bearing is attempted after injection localizes the problem to the affected joint.

Bone scans have little value immediately after surgery. Significant bone remodeling is present, which continues for several months. Bone scans may not be helpful until 6 months to 1 year after surgery. At that point, increased uptake indicates bone remodeling and loosening of the prosthesis.

3. Indium-labeled white blood cell scan—This nuclear medicine study uses the patient's polymorphonuclear leukocytes, which are labeled with radioactive indium and injected back into the patient. It may be quite beneficial in localizing acute infectious processes but is frequently not helpful in the evaluation of chronic infection.

4. Plain radiographs—Roentgenographic examination is the single most useful test in the evaluation of nonseptic loosening. Important signs are radiolucent lines adjacent to the prosthesis or cement, particularly if they are 2 mm or greater or are becoming enlarged on serial radiographs (Figure 7–9). Fracture of the cement and change in position of the component are indications of loosening.

Treatment of Infected Total Joint Arthroplasty

Definitive evidence of a septic total joint arthroplasty forecasts a poor prognosis for the patient. The infectious process is either acute or chronic, and the infection is either gram negative or gram positive. The components are either tightly fixed to bone, or one or more of the components is loose. In acute infection with tightly fixed components, most surgeons debride the

Figure 7–9. Radiograph of radiolucent lines around an acetabular component.

joint without removing the components and treat the infection locally and with systemic antibiotic therapy. A chronically infected or loose prosthesis is usually treated with removal of the prosthesis, local wound care, and systemic antimicrobial therapy. Therapy for an acutely infected, firmly fixed prosthesis varies according to surgeon preference.

There is general concurrence that thorough debridement of the joint, synovectomy, removal of necrotic material, and copious irrigation are necessary at the time of debridement. Because of the potential presence of glycocalyx, surfaces of the prosthesis available for inspection are scrubbed with Dakin solution, which dissolves the glycocalyx. Removable components are removed, and the undersurfaces are cleaned with Dakin solution. New polyethylene components are inserted if available; if this is not possible, the old polyethylene prothesis is scrubbed with Dakin solution and reinserted. To prevent superinfection, the wound must be tightly closed. To help eradicate the existing infection,

however, irrigation and drainage must be continued. One suitable method is that described by Jergesen and Jawetz, in which small volumes of antibiotic solution are instilled into the joint twice a day, the joint is sealed off for 3 hours, followed by 9 hours of suction (Figure 7–10). This protocol begins 24 hours after surgery, during which time suction drainage is maintained. The instillation-suction system is maintained for 10 days. At the end of the course of irrigation and instillation, a culture is aspirated from the joint after one antibiotic instillation. This system can also be used for osteomyelitis and routine joint infections. Antibiotics are continued for an appropriate period of time (usually 6 weeks) after the tubes are withdrawn.

In cases of loose prostheses, little alternative is available except to remove the prosthesis. A similar system of instillation and suction is then used, using the same protocol. If reimplantation is likely after infected total knee prosthesis, an antibiotic cement block is used to separate the bone ends and maintain a potential joint space. An alternative to the cement block is the PROSTALAC system as described earlier. This technique has the benefit of maintaining quadriceps length and elasticity. In patients in whom reimplantation is planned, the ESR is followed monthly until it is normal without antibiotic therapy. In patients with RA or other disorders in which the rate may be elevated, 6 months is an appropriate time to wait for possible recrudescence of the infection. At this point, either an aspiration arthrogram or a Craig needle biopsy is used to obtain specimens for culture. If these are negative, reimplantation surgery is planned.

Figure 7–10. Schematic diagram of the Jergesen system of instillation of antibiotics. The antibiotics can be varied depending on the susceptibility of the infecting bacteria (fungus). The amount instilled is approximately 5 mL per tube plus the dead space from the valve to the joint.

Orthopedic Infections

Scott C. Wilson, MD, & Harry B. Skinner, MD, PhD

■ OVERVIEW

Introduction

Musculoskeletal infections are common; they can affect all parts of the musculoskeletal system; and they can be dangerous and even life threatening. Much has been learned in the last 20 years to treat a wide range of musculoskeletal infections effectively. Often a team including orthopedic surgeons, plastic surgeons, infectious disease specialists, as well as internists, nutritionists, and therapists, must collaborate to orchestrate the multidisciplinary care that may be required to treat these patients optimally. This chapter summarizes the pathogenesis, diagnosis, and treatment of infections relevant to orthopedics. The management of osteomyelitis, septic arthritis, and soft tissue infections is discussed and highlighted with clinical examples.

Because this subject is so important, other chapters in this book include discussions of special aspects of infection. Chapter 3 (Musculoskeletal Trauma Surgery) discusses appropriate management of open fractures, traumatic arthrotomies, and gunshot wounds to minimize the risk of infection. Chapter 5 (Disorders, Diseases, & Injuries of the Spine) describes the clinical identification and management of osteomyelitis of the spine, diskitis, and epidural abscess. Chapter 7 (Adult Reconstructive Surgery) outlines the care of patients with prosthetic joint infections. Chapter 9 (Foot & Ankle Surgery) carefully details the management of diabetic foot ulcers and infections. Chapter 10 (Hand Surgery) discusses the treatment of paronychia, felons, chronic hand infections, human bites, and web space abscesses. Chapter 11 (Pediatric Orthopedic Surgery) reviews acute hematogenous osteomyelitis, septic arthritis especially of the hip joint, puncture wounds of the foot, skeletal tuberculosis, and spinal diskitis.

Pathogenesis

A. GENERAL

All clinical infections must be thought of in terms of the attacking microbes and the host's defenses. Infections are more likely to occur if the organisms are more virulent and if the inoculum is larger. Bacteria can gain entry into the body from direct penetrating trauma, by hematogenous spread from adjacent or remote sites of infection, or during surgical exposures. This wide spectrum of clinical possibilities ranges from fight bites to seeding from bacterial endocarditis to intraoperative breaks in sterile technique.

In acute osteomyelitis in children, the metaphysis is commonly involved. It is thought that the end vessels of the nutrient artery empty into much larger sinusoidal veins, causing a slow and turbulent flow of blood at this junction. These conditions predispose bacteria to migrate through adjacent gaps in the endothelium and adhere to the matrix. Also, low oxygen tension in this region may compromise phagocytic activity of white blood cells. Thrombosis caused by infection results in a region of avascular necrosis that may lead to abscess formation. As pus accumulates and pressurizes, it can track through the cortex via the haversian system and Volkmann canals to collect beneath the periosteum. Subperiosteal abscesses may stimulate the formation of a periosteal involucrum. Once out of the cortex, pus can also track through soft tissues to the surface of the skin, forming a draining sinus.

The physis and joint capsule act as barriers to the flow of pus. However, secondary septic arthritis may occur if the infection begins in a region of bone within the confines of a joint capsule. Thus, the hip joint is particularly susceptible to secondary infection arising from a spreading osteomyelitis of the femoral head or neck. Additionally, pus may track through the transphyseal vessels found in infants up to 6 months of age, causing secondary septic arthritis.

In hematogenous septic arthritis, the synovial membrane lacks a basement membrane, facilitating the ingress of hematogenous bacteria into the joint space and resulting in an acute inflammatory reaction. The synovium becomes hyperemic and produces increased amounts of synovial fluid. Acute white blood cells infiltrate the joint space and the synovium hypertrophies. The cartilage may be eroded by the proteolytic enzymes released during phagocytosis. Cytokines and other inductive molecules produced by the leukocytes and synovial tissue recruit a further inflammatory response, which can eventually destroy all articular surfaces. Concurrent bone erosion usually begins in the periarticular folds of synovium at the junction of synovium and cartilage. Arthritis is the end result of articular bone and cartilage loss caused by joint sepsis.

B. ORGANISMS

Although the musculoskeletal system may be infected by any infectious agent, the great majority of infections are bacterial. *Staphylococcus aureus, Streptococcus,* and *Haemophilus influenzae* are the most common causes of acute hematogenous osteomyelitis in children. The most common causes of septic arthritis are *Neisseria gonorrhoeae, S. aureus,* and group A *Streptococcus.* Septic arthritis is less often caused by gram-negative organisms, including *Escherichia coli, Pseudomonas aeruginosa, Klebsiella, Enterobacter, Serratia, Proteus,* and *Salmonella.* Uncommon bacterial organisms include *Borrelia burgdorferi* (Lyme disease), *Mycobacterium tuberculosis, Brucella,* and the anaerobes *Clostridium* and *Bacteroides.* Unusual organisms that may preferentially infect immunocompromised patients include fungi (*Blastomyces, Cryptococcus, Histoplasma, Sporotrichum,* and *Coccidioidomycoses*) and atypical mycobacteria (*kansasii, avium-intracellulare, fortuitum, triviale,* and *scrofulaceum*). The increase in the immunocompromised population because of iatrogenic causes (eg, transplantation of organs) and other diseases (eg, AIDS and rheumatoid arthritis) has increased the spectrum of bacteria that can cause musculoskeletal infection. Some evidence even suggests that Paget disease is the manifestation of a slow virus infection of bone.

Table 8–1 lists common conditions associated with specific bacterial species. Antibiotic resistance is conferred in these circumstances by spontaneous mutation, transduction of resistance genes via plasmids, and conjugation.

Ahmed S, Ayoub EM: Poststreptococcal reactive arthritis. Pediatr Infect Dis J 2001;20:1081. [PMID: 11734716]

Bezwada HP et al: Haemophilus influenza infection complicating a total knee arthroplasty. Clin Orthop 2002;402:202.

Brook I: Joint and bone infections due to anaerobic bacteria in children. Pediatr Rehabil 2002;5:11. [PMID: 12396847]

Dubost JJ et al: No changes in the distribution of organisms responsible for septic arthritis over a 20 year period. Ann Rheum Dis 2002;61:267. [PMID: 11830437]

Franz JK, Krause A: Lyme disease (Lyme borreliosis). Best Pract Res Clin Rheumatol 2003;17:241. [PMID: 12787524]

Geyik MF et al: Musculoskeletal involvement of brucellosis in different age groups: A study of 195 cases. Swiss Med Wkly 2002;132;98. [PMID: 11971204]

Gonzalez TB et al: Acute bacterial arthritis caused by group C streptococci. Semin Arthritis Rheum 2001;31:43. [PMID: 11503138]

McCarthy JJ et al: Musculoskeletal infections in children: Basic treatment principles and recent advancements. Instr Course Lect 2005;54:515. [PMID: 15948476]

Table 8–1. Bacterial species associated with common conditions.

Organism	Common Occurrence
Staphylococcus aureus	Most common organism in osteomyelitis, acute hematogenous osteomyelitis (90%), and infected metal implants.
Group B strep	Infants < 1 year old
Haemophilus influenzae	Children 1–16 years old
Pseudomonas aeruginosa	Nosocomial, puncture wound through shoe
Pasteurella multocida	Animal bite
Eikenella corrodens	Human bite
Salmonella	Sickle cell disease
Anaerobes	Diabetic ulcers, fight bites
Candida albicans	Immunocompromised
Aspergillus	Immunocompromised
Atypical mycobacteria	Immunocompromised
Escherichia coli	Neonatal
Neisseria gonorrhoeae	Septic arthritis in young sexually active adult

McLemore MM, Stapleton FB: Atypical septic arthritis due to *Neisseria meningitides.* J Tenn Med Assoc 1984;77:149.

Press J et al: Leukocyte count in the synovial fluid of children with culture-proven brucellar arthritis. Clin Rheumatol 2002; 21:191. [PMID: 12111621]

Shirtliff ME, Mader JT: Acute septic arthritis. Clin Microbiol Rev 2002;15:527. [PMID: 12364368]

Tachi M et al: Pathophysiology and treatment of streptococcal toxic shock syndrome. Scan J Plast Reconstr Surg 2002;36: 305. [PMID: 12477090]

Weinstein MA, Eismont FJ: Infections of the spine in patients with human immunodeficiency virus. J Bone Joint Surg Am 2005; 87:604. [PMID: 15741629]

C. HOST FACTORS

Any host with compromised immunity and wound healing or with an implanted synthetic or allograft material has an increased risk for musculoskeletal infection. Nonspecific factors include the skin as a mechanical barrier. Local host factors include the adequacy of the vascular supply and the presence of tissue injury. Systemic host factors that compromise immunocompetence include nutritional wasting; comorbid diseases such as diabetes mellitus, chronic renal and liver disease, cancer, AIDS, and autoimmune connective tissue diseases; and usage of immunosuppressing medications such as corticosteroids, methotrexate, or tumor necrosis factor inhibitors.

Patients with chronic renal and liver disease, diabetes, cancer, AIDS, autoimmune connective tissue disease, and nutritional wasting and those on immunosuppressive medications are particularly susceptible to infection.

Nutritional depletion with negative nitrogen balance, weight loss, and tissue wasting can easily develop in patients with severe musculoskeletal injuries, as well as in patients who suffer from cancer, gastrointestinal malabsorption syndromes, and other chronic medical conditions. The signs of gross long-standing malnutrition, including profound weight loss, pitting edema, and intercostal wasting, are easily identified, but the signs of acute malnutrition are less apparent and often go undetected. A patient with a major fracture has a 20–25% increase in energy expenditure, and one with multiple trauma or infection has a 30–55% increase. Liver and skeletal muscle glycogen stores can be depleted within 12 hours during severe stress. Even with adequate stores of fat, visceral and skeletal muscle protein may not be spared because fat is not a readily available energy source during severe stress. Therefore, patients who are malnourished have significantly higher infection rates after surgery than patients who have normal nutritional status. Table 8–2 outlines methods to detect malnutrition.

D. FOREIGN MATERIAL

Experimental studies indicate that all biomaterials commonly used for total joint arthroplasty increase the incidence of *S. aureus* infections. In contrast, biomaterials appear to have no effect on *E. coli* and *S. epidermidis* infections except when polymethylmethacrylate is used, in which case the incidence rises markedly.

Adherence of bacteria to the surface of implants is promoted by a polysaccharide biofilm called glycocalyx that acts as a barrier against host defense mechanisms and antibiotics. In addition, this film makes culture of organisms difficult, even with the use of special techniques.

Mixing antibiotics such as vancomycin and gentamicin to methacrylate cement can lower the risk of infection from cemented metal joint replacements, presumably by killing surface bacteria before they can produce glycocalyx.

Implantation of small amounts of allograft bone and connective tissue may slightly increase the risk of postoperative infection, but massive osteoarticular allografts can dramatically elevate the risk (8–12%). Fresh and fresh-frozen allograft bone and soft tissue harvested and processed into implants in an aseptic manner are implicated in clostridium infections because of problems with not detecting contaminated donors and not sterilizing the tissue for spores. In 2001, approximately 875,000 of these implants were used in the United States, with a rate of infection with properly selected donors and treated tissues of much less than 0.1%

Table 8–2. Tests to measure nutritional depletion.

Serology	
Albumin	< 3.5 g/dL
Prealbumin	< 10 mg/dL
Total lymphocyte count	< 1500/µL
Transferrin	< 150 mg/dL
Other	
Anergy panel	Nonreactive
Weight loss	> 4.5 kg
Arm circumference	< 80% standard

Synthetic suture materials such as nylon and polyglycolic acid are less likely to facilitate wound infection than natural suture materials such as silk and cotton. In this regard, monofilaments are superior to braided sutures in preventing infection, and resorbable materials are superior to nonresorbable materials. Therefore synthetic resorbable monofilaments are preferred in wounds that are potentially susceptible to infection.

Archibald LK et al: Update: Allograft-associated bacterial infections—United States, 2002. MMWR Morb Mortal Wkly Rep 2002;51:207. [PMID: 11922189]

Kainer MA et al: Clostridium infections associated with musculoskeletal-tissue allografts. N Engl J Med 2004;350:2564. [PMID: 15201413]

Mankin HJ, Hornicek FJ, Raskin KA: Infection in massive bone allografts. Clin Orthop 2005;432:210. [PMID: 15738824]

Menovsky T et al: Skin closure in carpal tunnel surgery: A prospective comparative study between nylon, polyglactin 910 and stainless steel sutures. Hand Surg 2004;9:35. [PMID: 15368623]

Prophylaxis

A. GENERAL

Transmission of bacterial and viral infections can easily occur in the clinic and hospital setting because health care workers are often in direct contact with patients. The risk of transmission can be reduced by using universal precautions, including hand washing before and after all patient or body fluid contact, and wearing gloves, masks, eye protection, and gowns when in contact with patients with known infections. Proper disposal of patients' waste, dressing materials, and surgical drains should be mandatory. Blades and needles (which should not be recapped) must be disposed of in a dedicated sharps box. Inpatients with easily transmitted infections or infections caused by bacteria resistant to certain antibiotics should be isolated in private rooms, and movement of these patients should be limited to reduce possible contact with other patients or health care workers.

B. ANTIBIOTICS

The administration of prophylactic antibiotics immediately before surgery and intraoperatively for cases lasting longer than 3–4 hours is now a uniformly accepted standard of practice. Generally a first-generation cephalosporin is used. Vancomycin, clindamycin, or ciprofloxacin are useful alternatives if the patient has a cephalosporin allergy or an anaphylactic response to penicillin that indicates a potential cross-reactivity. Although the consensus opinion suggests that antibiotic prophylaxis should be administered approximately a half hour prior to skin incision, this may not allow adequate tissue levels to be obtained for some antibiotics in the area of interest. The administration of preoperative antibiotics should be withheld when intraoperative bacterial cultures are to be obtained because they inhibit the in vitro growth of the cultured bacteria and reduce the ability to identify the causative organism(s).

C. OPERATING ROOM STERILITY

Sterile technique in the operating room is extremely important. The operative site is thoroughly prepped with a variety of topical antiseptics including isopropyl alcohol, chlorhexidine soaps, and iodine-based scrubs and paints. Sterile drapes effectively isolate the operative site from the rest of the patient, and sterile gowns and gloves isolate the surgeons and assistants from the patient. Surgeons may use double gloves, space suits, adherent plastic drapes, pulsatile lavage, and laminar flow operating rooms or rooms with ultraviolet lights as additional techniques that may lower the risk of intraoperative contamination, which is approximately 1% for clean, elective orthopedic cases. Breaks in sterile technique should be dealt with immediately and aggressively even if the operative site has to be reprepped and redraped and the surgeons have to regown and reglove.

D. EXPOSURE TO BLOOD-BORNE PATHOGENS

Health care workers may be accidentally exposed to infection when poked by a needle or sharp wire, cut by a knife or a sharp bone fracture edge, or splashed in the eye. The primary concern is the possible transmission of hepatitis B virus (HBV), hepatitis C virus (HCV), and human immunodeficiency virus (HIV). The estimated risk of acquiring an infection by accidental blood transmission is 6–30% for HBV, 1.8% for HCV, and 0.3% for HIV. Logically, larger inoculations confer an increased risk of infection. If exposure with a potentially infected source occurs, the worker must wash the contact area with disinfectant and immediately report to the occupational health center to document the exposure. The viral status is determined in the exposed worker and the source patient by obtaining serologic tests for HBV, HCV, and HIV. HIV testing requires

the source's informed written consent. (Rapid plasma reagent [RPR] for syphilis should also be checked.)

The threat of health care workers acquiring hepatitis B is now dramatically reduced because many health care institutions require their employees to be immunized against HBV. Immunization status is confirmed if the concentration of hepatitis B serum antibody (anti-HBV) is equal to 10 mIU/mL. However, if the worker is unvaccinated or a nonresponder to the vaccine and the source is known to be positive for hepatitis B, the worker should receive hepatitis B immunoglobulin (HBIG) and a series of hepatitis B vaccinations.

Currently there is no vaccination against HCV and no recommended prophylactic therapy for workers exposed to HCV. However, new drugs are being developed to treat active HCV infections and effective prophylaxis may soon be developed. If the source is known to have HIV, the worker should immediately begin a 28-day course of double or triple antiretroviral therapy.

Workers with any viral exposures should be subsequently monitored with serologic tests for HIV, HBV, and HCV at 6 weeks, 3 months, 6 months, and 1 year after exposure. These guidelines are frequently updated, and specific treatment recommendations should be discussed with the institution's occupational health specialist (Table 8–3).

Clarke MT et al: Contamination of primary total hip replacements in standard and ultra-clean operating theaters detected by the polymerase chain reaction. Acta Orthop Scand 2004;75:544. [PMID: 15513484]

Gillespie WJ, Walenkamp G: Antibiotic prophylaxis for surgery for proximal femoral and other closed long bone fractures. Cochrane Database Syst Rev 2001;1:CD000244. [PMID: 11279687]

Owers KL, James E, Bannister GC: Source of bacterial shedding in laminar flow theatres. J Hosp Infect 2004;58:230. [PMID: 15501339]

Tai CC et al: Antibiotic prophylaxis in surgery of the intervertebral disc. A comparison between gentamicin and cefuroxime. J Bone Joint Surg Br 2002;84:1036. [PMID: 12358368]

Diagnosis

A. RADIOLOGIC WORKUP

1. Plain films—Plain radiographs are useful in establishing a diagnosis of osteomyelitis or chronic septic arthritis. Initially plain radiographs do not show any bony changes in early osteomyelitis. After 7–10 days, an area of osteopenia may appear, heralding cancellous bone destruction. As the infection progresses, a periosteal reaction may be seen, and focal areas of cancellous and cortical bone destruction may become apparent. Chronic osteomyelitis is identified by more extensive bone destruction and the appearance of a reactive rim of bone called the involucrum, which envelops a scle-

Table 8–3. Testing and treatment of exposed persons, assuming source tests positive and exposed person tests negative.

Virus	Seroconversion (percutaneous exposure)[a]	Serologic Test of Exposed Person	Prophylaxis	Efficacy of Rx
Hepatitis B	6–30%	Virus antibody-positive	None, immunity intact	
		Virus antibody-negative	Hepatitis B immunoglobulin	90%
			Hepatitis B vaccination series	
			None[b]	
Hepatitis C	1.8% (0–7%)		Antiretroviral drugs for 4 weeks	81%
HIV	0.3%[c]		Two- or three-drug regimen[d]	

[a]Larger inoculations from increased exposure confer higher risk of seroconversion.
[b]Patient may benefit from early treatment if symptoms develop.
[c]0.09% risk of seroconversion from mucosal exposure.
[d]Three drugs recommended if large exposure or source has AIDS.
Adapted, with permission, from Updated U.S. Public Health Service guidelines for the management of occupational exposures to HBV, HCV and HIV and recommendations for postexposure prophylaxis. MMWR 50(RR11):1–42, 2001. And from Guidelines for using retroviral agents among HIV infected adults and adolescents. Recommendations of the Panel on Clinical Practices for Treatment of HIV. MMWR 51(RR–7):1, 2002.

rotic focus of necrotic bone called the sequestrum. The sequestrum is often radiodense compared with the adjacent involucrum.

Plain radiographs are usually normal in early septic arthritis. Only later in the disease do radiographs show cartilage loss and periarticular bone erosion. These radiographic features are not specific for infection and may be present in other arthropathies such as rheumatoid arthritis (RA) and pigmented villonodular synovitis.

Soft-tissue infections are virtually invisible on plain radiographs except for an occasional suggestion of soft-tissue swelling. The striking exception is encountered with air-producing infections causing "gas gangrene." Air in the soft tissues is quite clearly identifiable on plain radiographs as discrete radiolucent areas, analogous to bowel gas in a plain radiograph of the abdomen. Figure 8–1 is a radiograph of air in the calf of a patient with a life-threatening clostridial infection.

2. Ultrasound—Ultrasound is useful at identifying a joint effusion and particularly beneficial in the evaluation of pediatric patients with suspected infections of the hip joint. Ultrasound may also aid in the identification and aspiration of soft-tissue abscesses.

3. Radionuclide imaging—Radionuclide imaging is not routinely necessary to diagnose acute osteomyelitis and is often falsely negative in acute septic arthritis. This imaging modality is very sensitive but nonspecific in identifying bone disease. Commonly, infection cannot be distinguished from neoplasm, infarction, trauma, gout, stress fracture, postsurgical changes, adjacent soft-tissue infection, neurotrophic joints (Charcot joint), or arthritis. However, in equivocal cases, radio-

nuclide imaging may help identify an infectious process before an invasive procedure is performed.

The most common imaging agents are technetium-99m and indium-111. Technetium-99m is administered intravenously. An early-phase scan is performed in 10–15 minutes. At this time most of the radioisotope is in equilibrium with the extracellular compartment and accumulates in areas of increased blood flow, such as areas associated with cellulitis. The late-phase scan is performed in 3 hours, and the radioisotope is localized to the skeleton in both the organic matrix and the mineral phase of the bone.

Imaging with indium-111 requires collection of 80–90 mL of venous blood, separation of the leukocytes in the sample, and labeling the leukocytes with indium-111 in vitro. The indium-labeled leukocytes are then returned to the patient's bloodstream intravenously, and scanning is done 18–24 hours later. One study found a sensitivity of 91% and a specificity of 62% for detecting osteomyelitis for indium-111 white cell scans.

Imaging with technetium-99m methylene diphosphonate is a highly sensitive technique and useful in cases of suspected acute hematogenous osteomyelitis. In an extensive study of 280 children, the sensitivity of technetium-99m imaging in accurately detecting acute osteomyelitis was 89%, the specificity was 94%, and the overall accuracy was 92%. All soft-tissue infections were correctly identified by this technique, and 37 studies were positive for septic arthritis, although 8 were falsely positive.

Although radionuclide imaging can be sensitive for chronic musculoskeletal infections, it is often nonspecific, and false-positive results may hinder diagnosis.

Figure 8–1. Plain radiograph of the knee, showing air in the soft tissues of the calf and thigh arising from a necrotizing clostridial infection.

Radionuclide imaging often cannot distinguish a chronic infection from aseptic loosening in patients with painful prosthetic joint replacements, and it is rarely necessary in establishing a diagnosis of septic arthritis.

4. Computed tomography—Computed tomography (CT) with sagittal and coronal reformatting is particularly useful in identifying sequestra in cases of chronic osteomyelitis. Routinely discrete sequestra are isolated from the viable bone and are more radiodense than the surrounding involucrum. Also, sagittal and coronal reformatting can be very useful in further assessing the mechanical integrity of the bone and in determining the extent of fracture healing even in the presence of metal fixation hardware. CT can show expansion of a joint capsule and any evidence of bony destruction but is not specific for septic arthritis.

5. Magnetic resonance imaging—Magnetic resonance imaging (MRI) with T_2 and inversion recovery sequencing offers unparalleled visualization of bone marrow and soft-tissue inflammation associated with infection. Intravenous (IV) gadolinium concentrates in areas of increased vascularity and enhances regions of inflammation. Fluid collections are identified as dark signal voids where the gadolinium cannot penetrate because of the absence of vascular ingress. Thus, contrast MRI facilitates the identification of fluid collections within bones, joint spaces, and soft tissues that may represent abscesses and septic effusions.

Acute inflammation in bone and soft tissues is nonspecific. Acute inflammatory arthropathies may reveal synovial and adjacent soft-tissue inflammation, effusion, and periarticular bone inflammation, especially at the synovial-cartilage junction. These findings may be identical with acute septic arthritis, gout, or other inflammatory arthropathies including neuropathic Charcot joints. Pigmented villonodular synovitis may have many of the same features, although it can often be distinguished by areas of decreased signal uptake on T_2 images that represent areas of hemosiderin deposition.

As infection progresses in a joint, eroded cartilage and subchondral bone can be seen along with hypertrophic synovium and pronounced effusion. Periarticular erosion usually precedes erosion along weight-bearing surfaces. These changes are accompanied by generalized inflammation in the adjacent bone marrow and soft tissues, including bursas and tendon sheaths. Formation of abscesses, synovial cysts, and sinus tracts are particularly well visualized.

Keat A: Reactive arthritis or post-infective arthritis? Best Pract Res Clin Rheumatol 2002;16:507. [PMID: 12406424]

Palestro CJ et al: Osteomyelitis: diagnosis with (99m) Tc-labeled antigranulocyte antibodies compared with diagnosis with (111)In-labeled leukocytes—Initial experience. Radiology 2002;223:758. [PMID: 12034946]

Roddy E, Jones AC: Reactive arthritis associated with genital tract group A streptococcal infection. J Infect 2002;45:208. [PMID: 12387782]

Sigal LH: Update on reactive arthritis. Bull Rheum Dis 2001;50:1. [PMID: 12386943]

B. IDENTIFICATION OF PATHOGENS

Whenever possible, antibiotic therapy must be delayed until deep cultures of the infection site are obtained. It is imperative to take appropriate cultures prior to antibiotic administration because antibiotics can often inhibit bacterial growth in vitro. If the cultures fail to grow, the clinician must choose antibiotics empirically. However well informed the clinician may be, the selection of empirical antibiotics is a matter of guesswork, and treatment failure is more likely.

Deep cultures must be obtained percutaneously or intraoperatively using strict sterile technique. The overlying skin must be prepped with antiseptic to decrease the concentration of skin flora that might contaminate the culture sample. In addition to swabs of purulent fluid, bone and soft-tissue samples of the infected site should also be obtained. Additional tissue should be sent for histologic analysis because an acute suppurative infection can be distinguished from a chronic granulomatous infection, and an infection can be distinguished from an unsuspected neoplasm.

Superficial swabs of skin ulcers and draining sinus tracts usually identify colonizing bacteria rather than the pathogenic bacteria that must be eradicated. Therefore, the practice of obtaining superficial cultures of deep-seated infections should be avoided. Also, it is important to employ appropriate techniques for anaerobic cultures because these organisms can be difficult to isolate and may be responsible for a considerable amount of osteomyelitis. This is particularly true for diabetic patients with infected foot ulcers who have a high risk for mixed aerobic/anaerobic infections.

A Gram stain of the culture samples is not diagnostic by itself but may help identify the organism. Therefore, the preliminary information gained from a Gram stain should be used to confirm clinical suspicions such as a staphylococcal osteomyelitis (positive cocci in clusters) or a gonococcal septic arthritis (gram-negative cocci in pairs). Blood cultures should also be obtained in patients who present with acute symptoms of bacteremia, such as fever, chills, and sweats.

Joint aspiration is usually necessary to identify the organisms responsible for septic arthritis, although blood cultures may also be helpful in acute cases. The synovial fluid from an infected joint is opaque, light yellow or light gray, and nonviscous. Cell analysis often reveals a white blood count (WBC) of more than 100,000 and more than 90% polymorphonuclear (PMN) leukocytes (Table 8–4). Similarly, for infected prosthetic knee joints, cell counts and PMN leukocyte percentages were higher, with an average of 18,900/mL and 92% neutrophils compared to 300/mL and 7% neutrophils for joints with aseptic loosening. Iatrogenic contamination of a sterile joint space may occur if the arthrocentesis needle passes through an overlying soft-tissue infection. Therefore, erythematous skin or indurated soft tissue should be avoided when choosing a site for arthrocentesis.

C. HISTOLOGY

Pathologic examination of a tissue sample can help determine the presence of an infection, characterize the type and time frame of the infection histologically, identify the causative organism, and occasionally distinguish an infection from an unsuspected neoplasm.

During revision arthroplasty, samples of periprosthetic tissue may be submitted for frozen section analysis. If less than 5 PMN leukocytes occur per high-powered field, there is a low probability of residual infection. Extensive debridement and prosthetic removal should be considered rather than reimplantation of revision components if there are greater than 10 PMN leukocytes per high-powered field.

Histologic study can distinguish between acute inflammatory responses characterized by the presence of PMN leukocytes and chronic inflammatory responses characterized by plasma cells and lymphocytes. Granulomatous

Table 8–4. Analysis of synovial fluid.

Analysis	Normal Results	Noninflammatory Effusion	Inflammatory Effusion	Septic Effusion
Gross Exam				
Volume	1–4 mL	Increased	Increased	Increased
Clarity	Transparent	Transparent	Transparent	Opaque
Color	Clear/pale yellow	Yellow	Yellow/white	Yellow/white/gray
Viscosity	High	High	Low	Low
Mucin clotting	Good	Good/fair	Fair/poor	Poor
Microscopic Exam				
Leukocytes	< 300	< 2000	2000–80,000	> 80,000
Neutrophils	< 25%	< 25%	25–75%	> 75%
Bacterial smear	Negative	Negative	Negative	Positive
Serum				
Glucose ratio	0.8–1.0	0.8–1.0	0.5–0.8	< 0.5
Protein g/dL	< 3	< 3	≤ 8	≤ 8
Culture	Negative	Negative	Negative	Positive

Normal synovial fluid is clear and viscous. Inflammation causes synovial fluid to become more cloudy as the concentration of white cells increases. Traditionally, newsprint can be read through a vial of noninfectious transudate but not through a vial of infectious exudate. The synovial fluid/serum glucose ratio will decrease and the synovial protein concentration will increase. Besides a positive bacterial smear the most helpful indicators of infection are a white blood cell count greater than 50,000 and a percentage of polymorphonuclear leukocytes exceeding 75%. Many acute bacterial infections will generate a white cell count of greater than 100,000 and > 90% PMNs.

responses with central caseation help establish the diagnosis of *Mycobacterium tuberculosis.* Noncaseating granulomas can occur with fungal and atypical mycobacterial infections.

Occasionally, the inciting organisms can be identified as well. For example, budding yeast forms of *Blastomyces dermatitidis* can be visualized with special stains or by using immunohistochemical markers. This is particularly important because mycobacterial and fungal organisms are slow growing in vitro, and they may take 3–6 weeks to identify in culture. Also, histologic analysis can distinguish an infection from an unsuspected tumor such as squamous cell carcinoma arising within a chronic infection or a tumor that radiographically may mimic an infection such as eosinophilic granuloma, Ewing sarcoma, and lymphoma of bone.

Lu TS et al: Concurrent acute gouty and gonococcal arthritis. Lancet Infect Dis 2002;2:313. [PMID: 12062998]

Trampuz A et al: Synovial fluid leukocyte count and differential for the diagnosis of prosthetic knee infection. Am J Med 2004; 117:556. [PMID: 15465503]

Treatment

A. ANTIBIOTICS

1. Selection and use—Whenever possible, antibiotics should be chosen based on the antibiotic sensitivities of the specific organisms that were cultured from the infection site. Consultation with infectious disease experts is prudent for unusual or resistant organisms or if a lengthy course of therapy is anticipated. Because patterns of bacterial resistance to antibiotics vary from region to region, these experts work closely with local clinical laboratories to establish locally specific bacterial sensitivity profiles. Also, infectious disease experts are often more closely attuned to the latest clinical research regarding antibiotic treatment of musculoskeletal infections (information that is not usually encountered in the primary orthopedic literature) and the continually changing patterns of bacterial resistance. For example, *Staphylococcus epidermidis* is becoming increasingly resistant to methicillin, and certain strains of enterococci and *S. aureus* are resistant to vancomycin. Resistance to second- and third-generation cephalosporins is emerging in some gram-negative bacilli, and penicillin resistance is increasing in *Bacteroides* and *Clostridium* species. Even if an organism is sensitive to a given antibiotic, addition of a second antibiotic may be necessary to lessen the risk of treatment failure because of the development of antibiotic resistance.

Antibiotic therapy is usually continued for 6 weeks for patients with septic arthritis or osteomyelitis. In acute pediatric infections caused by sensitive organisms, a shorter course of therapy may be sufficient. In patients with multiple medical problems, retained orthopedic hardware, or persistent open wounds, a longer course of therapy may be required.

Erythrocyte sedimentation rates (ESRs) and C-reactive protein (CRP) levels should be serially checked weekly or semiweekly to monitor the success of treatment. Quantitative CRP levels usually decrease before ESR levels in adequately treated infections. A patient with persistently elevated ESR and CRP levels toward the end of planned antibiotic treatment may have an incompletely treated infection. Persistence of the infection may be caused by the retention of orthopedic hardware, the incomplete debridement of necrotic tissue, the immunocompromised status of the host, or the development of antibiotic resistance by the causative bacteria. Ideally, surgical reexploration should be performed on these patients and tissue samples should be recultured after the patient is off antibiotics to determine if additional treatment is required.

Occasionally, antibiotics must be given for palliation rather than cure. Chronic suppressive antibiotic therapy may be appropriate in selected patients with severe immunocompromise, those who are not surgical candidates, or those with stable joint prostheses infected by sensitive organisms. Close monitoring of these patients is necessary to detect possible antibiotic resistance.

For example, an 80-year-old woman with a history of a revision total hip arthroplasty 10 years previously underwent a Girdlestone arthroplasty 5 years ago to treat septic loosening of the prosthesis. All components were removed, the bones debrided, and antibiotic beads were placed in the acetabulum (Figure 8–2). During this time, a severe hematologic bleeding disorder was diagnosed that prohibited further surgery. Her lateral hip incision healed incompletely, and she developed a mature deep sinus that tracked down to the cut end of the femur. The antibiotic beads could not be retrieved through this opening. She also developed a new sinus tract in her medial thigh. These wounds were treated with daily absorptive alginate dressings, and occasionally she had debridement of the sinus tracts in clinic to prevent them from closing. When the sinus tracts closed, the undrained pus rapidly created a pressurized abscess that resulted in a prompt increase in local inflammation, bacteremia, and acute febrile illness. Her infection was suppressed using culture-specific oral antibiotics for staphylococcal and enterococcal bacteria. Over the past 5 years she has lived with her infection and controlled her pain with oral narcotics. She is able to stand to transfer and walk short distances with a walker.

2. Intravenous route of administration—Use of a peripheral intravenous central catheter (PICC) line is now the standard IV access for extended antibiotic

Figure 8–2. Anteroposterior pelvic radiograph depicting the Girdlestone arthroplasty and retained antibiotic beads in the left hip area and a painless malunion of a subcapital fracture of the right hip.

therapy. PICC lines can be inserted by qualified nursing personnel in an outpatient setting, and the placement of the line can be confirmed by a chest radiograph. Specialized personnel in the radiology department can also place PICC lines using ultrasound to identify suitable veins and fluoroscopy to ensure appropriate catheter placement with the tip of the catheter in the superior vena cava. A subclavian central line such as a Hickman catheter is used as a backup if peripheral access cannot be established. These catheters are generally placed in an operating room setting with the patient heavily sedated or under general anesthesia.

Most home health agencies are expert in managing PICC lines and administering antibiotics to patients in a home setting. Portable computerized IV pumps with replaceable drug cartridges are often used to automate the delivery of antibiotics throughout a 24-hour period.

3. Methicillin-resistant *Staphylococcus aureus/epidermidis*—Methicillin-resistant *Staphylococcus aureus* (MRSA) is the most common resistant bacteria encountered in orthopedic practice. *S. epidermidis* is rapidly becoming a concern as isolates start to demonstrate methicillin resistance. This is particularly important because one study showed the methicillin-resistant *Staphylococcus epidermidis* (MRSE) rate on routine screening for total joint replacement was 55% of samples that grew *S. epidermidis*. A 6-week course of vancomycin (1 g IV every 12 hours) is the current standard treatment for MRSA. However, this drug has relatively poor bone penetration, and it requires close monitoring because, rarely, it can be the cause of nephrotoxicity and ototoxicity. Establishing therapeutic drug levels by adjusting the dose and interval of treatment should be performed

based on drug peak and trough levels. Generally, if the peak level is too high, the dose has to be lowered; and if the trough is too high, the interval between doses has to be lengthened. Dosing has to be adjusted in patients with renal insufficiency based on creatinine clearance, and one daily dose or one dose every other day is not uncommon in this setting. Toxicity is more likely to occur if the trough level remains above the acceptable range. Many infectious disease experts treat MRSA with a two-drug regimen, often adding rifampin to vancomycin. There are reports of vancomycin-resistant MRSA. Newer antibiotics such as linezolid (Zyvox) are now being introduced for MRSA and can be administered orally.

B. SURGERY

1. Septic arthritis—Complete surgical evacuation of a purulent effusion offers the best protection against cartilage destruction in patients with acute infectious pyarthrosis. The greatest risk of cartilage damage comes from proteolytic enzymes produced by the recruited polymorphonuclear leukocytes rather than from direct action of the bacteria. Although serial needle aspirations may accomplish this goal in the acute setting, surgical drainage, irrigation, and drain tube placement are more efficient and better tolerated by the patient. Whenever technically possible arthroscopy is preferred, especially when dealing with septic arthritis of the knee joint. Limited open arthrotomy may also be used because the synovium need not be extensively debrided in acute infections.

In chronic septic arthritis, a pannus of hypertrophic synovium forms that must be surgically debrided to ensure successful treatment. Debridement debulks the bacterial load and decreases the production of inflammatory agents that destroy cartilage.

2. Osteomyelitis—Successful treatment of bone and soft-tissue infections requires the surgical removal of all nonviable tissue and foreign debris. Necrotic tissue shelters bacteria from access by white blood cells and from therapeutic concentrations of antibiotics. In acute open fractures, all devitalized soft tissue and all free bony fragments that are completely denuded of periosteum must be removed from the wound. Although buckshot and isolated bullets do not need to be removed from gunshot victims, thorough exploration of the bullet wounds is necessary to remove any embedded bullet wadding and clothing fragments. In chronic osteomyelitis, the sequestrum must be completely removed, although the involucrum should be left in place. Involucrum is viable reactive tissue that has a generous vascular supply and contributes to the mechanical stability of the bone.

Skin, subcutaneous fat, and muscle should be sharply debrided until they bleed freely. The appearance of viable cancellous bone is easily discerned by the presence of bleeding trabecular surfaces. It is more difficult to tell the viability of cortical bone because of its normally sparse vascularity. Biologic dyes such as fluorescein and isosulfan blue and flow Doppler examination are used intraoperatively to estimate the vascularity of cortical bone. However, visual inspection for punctate bleeding remains the simplest and most popular method of determining the viability of cortical bone. The so-called paprika sign should be apparent after water-cooled high-speed burring of all exposed cortical surfaces to ensure that all dead bone tissue was removed (Figure 8–3).

Infections occasionally are so severe or are located in such unforgiving anatomic locations that amputation is the best method of curing the infection surgically. For example, a 60-year-old man with insulin-dependent diabetes and extensive peripheral vascular disease developed a rapidly worsening heel infection that exposed his calcaneus (Figure 8–4). During physical examination, a cotton swab could easily probe exposed cancellous bone of the calcaneus and subtalar joint. A subtotal calcanectomy with free flap coverage after peripheral arterial bypass would have been necessary for any chance of infection control and limb salvage. The patient elected to proceed with a recommended below-knee amputation.

3. Implantable antibiotics—An excellent method to supplement the IV administration of systemic antibiotics is to implant local antibiotics into the wound using polymethylmethacrylate bone cement as a carrier. Antibiotic "spacers" and "beads" have the added advantage of provisionally filling dead spaces so that bacteria-rich fluids do not accumulate and thwart the host's defenses. Intraoperatively, methacrylate powder is thoroughly mixed with powdered antibiotics and then made into a dough by adding the liquid methacrylate monomer. The antibiotic dough can be fashioned into a string of beads using gauge-5 wire or number 5 nonabsorbable suture (Figure 8–5). Antibiotic-laden cement spacers can be molded into a disk shape like a hockey puck for the knee joint after removal of a total knee prosthesis. Also cement spacers can be molded into the shape of a femoral head and secured to the femur using a rush rod placed in the femur. Alternatively, hip and knee joint prostheses made of antibiotic bone cement are now commercially available. Palacos cement has superior

Figure 8–3. Intraoperative photograph of the so-called paprika sign, representing punctate bleeding from the endosteal surface of a tibia that has just undergone aggressive debridement with a high-speed burr.

Figure 8–4. Calcaneus ulcer with exposed bone and blackened eschar.

antibiotic elution characteristics when compared with other bone cements. Vancomycin and tobramycin are commonly used in combination to treat presumed staphylococcal infections. A standard recipe in a patient without renal insufficiency is to mix one full bag of Palacos with 2 g of vancomycin and 3.6 g of tobramycin. Scoring the surface of a spacer and using numerous small beads rather than a few large beads increases the overall surface area of the antibiotic cement implant, enhances the elution of the antibiotics, and results in higher local concentrations of antibiotics. Initially the local serum concentrations may be as much as 100 times the minimal inhibitory concentration for *Staphy-lococcus*. After 3 weeks the antibiotic concentrations drop below the minimal inhibitory concentration. Although spacers and beads are left in place indefinitely, it is a good practice to remove them after the infection is treated to ensure that the cement does not act as a foreign body and precipitate a new infection.

4. Soft-tissue and bone reconstruction—Assuming musculoskeletal infections were treated comprehensively with antibiotics and debridement, bone reconstruction can proceed in a standard fashion. Total joints can be reimplanted, and structural bone defects can be filled with bone graft. Intercalary long bone defects can

Figure 8–5. Two strings of antibiotic beads were molded onto a number 5 braided nonabsorbable suture with the knotted ends incorporated into the outermost beads.

be spanned with bone transport techniques, vascularized structural bone autotransplants supported by external fixators, or even structural allografts secured with intramedullary rods.

Expeditious soft-tissue coverage is the first reconstructive priority in the contemporary management of acute open fractures. Rotation, pedicled, or free flaps are used to accomplish wound closure. Early flap reconstruction also ensures a good vascular supply to the injured area that promotes bone healing and resistance to local infection. If definitive bone fixation must be delayed until after complete debridement and soft-tissue coverage is accomplished, provisional stabilization of the bone can be achieved with orthotics, skeletal traction, or external fixation.

An acute infection occasionally develops after orthopedic fixation of a fracture. Assuming good soft-tissue coverage of the fracture area, the patient is treated with antibiotics, and the implanted hardware is left in place until the fracture heals. Once biologic union of the fracture is achieved, surgical debridement of the wound and removal of the fixation hardware can be performed without having to be concerned about a mechanically unstable bone. Alternatively, debridement of dead bone and removal of hardware with the placement of an external fixator can provide stabilization until the infection is under control. Bone graft for small defects or bone transport for segmental defects can successfully achieve union.

C. ADJUNCTIVE THERAPIES

1. Local wound care—Newer alginate dressing materials are more absorbent and may be left in place for 24 hours. Saline wet-to-dry dressings can be used for initial mechanical debridement of wounds that contain necrotic material and must be changed every 6 hours. Antiseptic solutions such as hydrogen peroxide, povidone-iodine, isopropyl alcohol, and sodium hypochlorite (Dakin solution, 5% NaClO) are now used only for the first few days until the bacterial load is reduced and necrotic tissue is debrided. Extended use of these caustic agents inhibits fibrogenesis. Instead, petroleum gel or topical antibiotic cream are placed on the wounds to keep the tissues from desiccating and to promote fibroblast growth.

Treatment of open wounds is now transformed using a new method that employs a sealed sponge dressing to which a negative pressure is applied using a portable pump (Figure 8–6). An open-cell sponge is cut to fit the shape of the wound and secured by an airtight plastic dressing (see Figure 8–12D and E). The sponge is connected to a vacuum pump by way of a plastic tube. When the pump is activated, a partial vacuum is generated within the wound. The porous sponge partially collapses, causing contraction of the walls of the wound. All drainage fluids are sucked out through the sponge and tubing and collected in a container located

Figure 8–6. Portable wound suction pump (also known as a wound *vacuum-assisted closure* device, or VAC). Note the tubing that runs from the pump to a black sponge placed in a patient's ischial decubitus.

in the pump unit. The wound is kept quite clean, and the dressing is changed every 2–3 days. The units are portable and can be serviced by visiting nurses in an outpatient setting.

2. Hyperbaric oxygen—Hyperbaric oxygen (HBO) therapy is used to treat a variety of orthopedic disorders. Specialized diving chambers developed for medical purposes expose patients to 100% oxygen at 2 or more atmospheres of pressure. During an HBO treatment, superphysiologic concentrations of oxygen from the lungs are dissolved into the serum. These high serum oxygen levels stimulate neoangiogenesis, sustain hypoxic tissues, support the activity of phagocytic white blood cells, and inhibit infections caused by anaerobic bacteria. It does not cause oxygen to be absorbed from the skin or wound surface, and it does not revitalize tissue that is already necrotic. Therefore, an adequate vascular inflow to the wound is necessary for HBO to work. When appropriately indicated, HBO can be a useful adjunct to good medical and surgical wound management.

Acute problems that can be helped by HBO include severe crush injury, compromised muscle flaps, and necrotizing fasciitis. Each of these conditions is characterized by soft tissues that have become acutely hypoxic and are at risk for infection. So-called acute HBO protocols usually require higher pressures (2.4–3 atm) and more frequent sessions (two to three times a day) for several days. To be effective, an acute HBO treatment protocol must be started as soon as possible after the injury because a 48-hour delay in initiating HBO can render it ineffective.

Chronic wounds that can be helped by HBO are primarily related to chronic ischemic ulcers that are not caused by peripheral vascular disease, venous stasis disease, or pressure necrosis. Diabetic foot ulcers in particular may benefit from HBO protocols with a reduction in risk for major amputation. The older literature includes uncontrolled studies that expound the use of treating chronic osteomyelitis with HBO. However, newer reconstruction techniques, including free flaps for soft-tissue coverage and bone transport for bone defect restoration, have empowered the surgeon to perform more comprehensive debridement and more aggressive wound closure. Better surgical management results in better cure rates for chronic osteomyelitis.

3. Nutritional support—Patients with severe infections and large wounds have increased nutritional and caloric needs. Nutritional depletion can be measured using the following tests: albumin, prealbumin, total protein, total lymphocyte count, and anergy panel (see Table 8–2). Dietary supplementation to restore normal healing in a compromised host may be accomplished using enteral tube feedings or parenteral infusions.

Antony SJ, Diaz-Vasquez E, Stratton C: Clinical experience with linezolid in the treatment of resistant gram-positive infections. J Natl Med Assoc 2001;93:386. [PMID: 11688919]

Centers for Disease Control and Prevention: Vancomycin-resistant *Staphylococcus aureus*—Pennsylvania, 2002. JAMA 2002;288: 2116.

Connolly LP et al: Acute hematogenous osteomyelitis of children: Assessment of skeletal scintigraphy-based diagnosis in the era of MRI. J Nucl Med 2002;43:1310. [PMID: 12368368]

Gristina AG et al: The glycocalyx, biofilm, microbes, and resistant infection. Semin Arthroplasty 1994;5:160. [PMID: 10155159]

Hanssen AD, Spangehl MJ: Practical applications of antibiotic-loaded bone cement for treatment of infected total joint replacements. Clin Orthop 2004;427:79. [PMID: 15552141]

Herscovici D Jr et al: Vacuum-assisted wound closure (VAC therapy) for the management of patients with high-energy soft tissue injuries. J Orthop Trauma 2003;17:683. [PMID: 14600567]

Hiramatsu K: Vancomycin-resistant *Staphylococcus aureus*: A new model of antibiotic resistance. Lancet Infect Dis 2001;1:147. [PMID: 11871491]

Jenson JE et al: Nutrition in orthopaedic surgery. J Bone Joint Surg Am 1982;64:1263. [PMID: 7142234]

Jones S et al: Cephalosporins for prophylaxis in operative repair of femoral fractures. Levels in serum, muscle, and hematoma. J Bone Joint Surg Am 1985;67:921. [PMID: 4019541]

Kartsonis N et al: Efficacy of caspofungin in the treatment of esophageal candidiasis resistant to fluconazole. J Acquir Immune Defic Syndr 2002;31:183. [PMID: 12394797]

Ledermann HP et al: Pedal abscesses in patients suspected of having pedal osteomyelitis: Analysis with MR imaging. Radiology 2002;224:649. [PMID: 12202694]

Mazza A: Ceftriaxone as short-term antibiotic prophylaxis in orthopedic surgery: A cost-benefit analysis involving 808 patients. J Chemother 2000;12(Suppl 3):29. [PMID: 11432680]

Mohanty SS, Kay PR: Infection in total joint replacements: Why do we screen MRSA when MRSE is the problem? J Bone Joint Surg Br 2004;86:266. [PMID: 15046444]

Neut D et al: Biomaterial-associated infection of gentamicin-loaded PMMA beads in orthopaedic revision surgery. J Antimicrob Chemother 2001;47:885. [PMID: 11389124]

Perea S, Patterson TF: Antifungal resistance in pathogenic fungi. Clin Infect Dis 2002;35:1073. [PMID: 12384841]

Petty W et al: The influence of skeletal implants on the incidence of infection: Experiments in a canine model. J Bone Joint Surg Am 1985;67:1236. [PMID: 3802846]

Roeckl-Wiedmann I, Bennett M, Kranke P: Systematic review of hyperbaric oxygen in the management of chronic wounds. Br J Surg 2005;92:24. [PMID: 15635604]

Schmidt AH, Swiontkowski MF: Pathophysiology of infections after internal fixation of fractures. J Am Acad Orthop Surg 2000;8:285. [PMID: 11029556]

Segreti J: Efficacy of current agents used in the treatment of Gram-positive infections and the consequences of resistance. Clin Microbiol Infect 2005;11(Suppl 3):29. [PMID: 15811022]

Shirtliff ME, Mader JT: Acute septic arthritis. Clin Microbiol Rev 2002;15:527. [PMID: 12364368]

Stewart PS, Costerton JW: Antibiotic resistance of bacteria in biofilms. Lancet 2001;358:135. [PMID: 11463434]

Stott NS: Review article: Paediatric bone and joint infection. J Ortho Surg (Hong Kong) 2001;9:83. [PMID: 12468850]

Stratton RJ et al: Malnutrition in hospital outpatients and inpatients: Prevalence, concurrent validity and ease of use of the "malnutrition universal screening tool" ("MUST") for adults. Br J Nutr 2004;92:799. [PMID: 15533269]

Stumpe KD et al: FDG positron emission tomography for differentiation of degenerative and infectious endplate abnormalities in the lumbar spine detected on MR imaging. AJR Am J Roentgenol 2002;179:1151. [PMID: 12388490]

Tarkowski A et al: Current status of pathogenetic mechanisms in staphylococcal arthritis. FEMS Microbiol Lett 2002;217:125. [PMID 12480095]

Tomas MB et al: The diabetic foot. Br J Radiol 2000;73:443. [PMID: 10844873]

Turpin S, Lambert R: Role of scintigraphy in musculoskeletal and spinal infections. Radiol Clin North Am 2001;39:169. [PMID: 11316353]

van de Belt H: Infection of orthopedic implants and the use of antibiotic-loaded bone cements. A review. Acta Orthop Scand 2001;72:557. [PMID: 11817870]

Vandecasteele SJ et al: New insights in the pathogenesis of foreign body infections with coagulase negative staphylococci. Acta Clin Belg 2000;55:148. [PMID: 10981322]

Webb LX: New techniques in wound management: Vacuum-assisted wound closure. J Am Acad Orthop Surg 2002;10:303. [PMID: 12374481]

Zhuang H et al: Exclusion of chronic osteomyelitis with F-18 fluorodeoxyglucose positron emission tomographic imaging. Clin Nucl Med 2000;25:281. [PMID: 10750968]

Zhuang H et al: Persistent non-specific FDG uptake on PET imaging following hip arthroplasty. Eur J Nucl Med Mol Imaging 2002;29:1328. [PMID: 12271415]

■ OSTEOMYELITIS

Classification Systems

Several classification systems are used to describe osteomyelitis. The traditional system divides bone infections according to the duration of symptoms: acute, subacute, and chronic (Table 8–5). Acute osteomyelitis is identified within 7–14 days of onset. Acute infections are most frequently associated with hematogenous seeding of bones in children. However, adults may also develop acute hematogenous infections, especially around implanted metal prostheses and fixation hardware. The duration of subacute osteomyelitis is between several weeks and several months. Chronic osteomyelitis is a bone infection that is present for at least several months. It is associated with an epicenter of bone necrosis called a sequestrum that is generally encased in vascular reactive bone called an involucrum.

Another system, developed by Waldvogel, categorizes bone infections based on etiology and chronicity: hematogenous, contiguous spread (with or without concomitant vascular disease), and chronic (see Table 8–5). Hematogenous and contiguous spreading infections may be acute, although the latter is associated with trauma or preexisting localized soft-tissue infections such as diabetic foot ulcers. Compromise in soft-tissue vascular supply may inhibit the immunological response to an infection. Therefore, Waldvogel created this subcategory to acknowledge the increased difficulty in treating infections in hosts with compromised vascularity.

Cierny and Mader developed a staging system for osteomyelitis that is classified by the anatomic extent of the infection and by the physiologic status of the host rather than by chronicity or etiology (see Table 8–5 and Box 8–1). The four stages are characterized by the pattern of bony involvement of the infection in order of increasing complexity: stage 1—medullary only, stage 2—superficial cortex only, stage 3—localized medullary and cortical, and stage 4—diffuse medullary and cortical (see Box 8–1). The latter two categories are best distinguished by the presence or absence of mechanical compromise of the involved bone. Localized infections have not created an unsta-

Table 8–5. Classification systems for osteomyelitis.

Traditional system

Type	Time of onset
Acute	≤ 2 weeks
Subacute	Weeks to months
Chronic	≥ 3 months

Waldvogel system
Hematogenous
Arising from contiguous infection
   No vascular disease
Vascular disease present
Chronic

Cierny-Mader system
Anatomic extent of infection
1. Medullary only (acute hematogenous)
2. Superficial cortex (contiguous spread or soft tissue trauma)
3. Localized (cortical and medullary, mechanically stable)
4. Diffuse (cortical and medullary, mechanically unstable)
5. Subtype by host's physiologic status

A	Healthy
Bs	Compromised because of systemic factors
Bl	Compromised because of local factors
Bls	Compromised because of both local and systemic factors
C	Treatment worse than the disease

ble bone. However, diffuse infections have sufficiently weakened the bone that surgical stabilization of the bone is necessary.

Host factors that mitigate healing are subcategorized into three groups: A—healthy host, B—compromised host, and C—"incurable" host (the treatments necessary to cure the disease are worse than living with the symptoms of the disease itself). A good example is an ambulatory diabetic smoker with peripheral vascular disease who has a stage 3 infection in a mechanically stable femur. Appropriate local wound care and suppressive antibiotic therapy may indeed be preferable to extensive surgical debridement that would risk destabilizing the bone, worsening a nonhealing soft-tissue wound, and increasing the risk of an above-knee amputation.

Systemic factors that compromise the host include diabetes mellitus, immunosuppression (eg, corticosteroid or cyclosporin usage), immune disease (eg, AIDS), malnutrition (often associated with alcohol or IV drug abuse), renal or hepatic failure, chronic hypoxia, and extremes of age. Local factors include peripheral vascular disease, venous stasis disease, chronic lymphedema, extensive soft-tissue scarring, radiation fibrosis, arteritis, diabetic dysvascularity of small vessels, neuropathy, and tobacco use.

BOX 8-1. THE CIERNEY AND MADER STAGING SYSTEM.

A   Stage 1

B   Stage 2

C   Stage 3

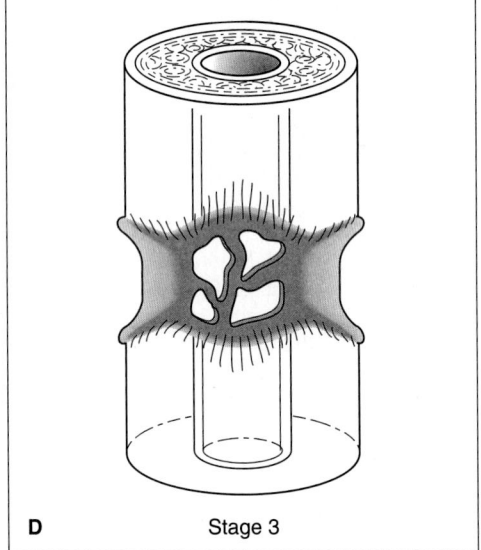

D   Stage 3

The Cierny and Mader staging system for osteomyelitis is classified by the anatomic extent of the infection and by the physiologic status of the host rather than by chronicity or etiology. The four stages are characterized by the pattern of bony involvement of the infection in order of increasing complexity: stage 1—medullary only, stage 2—superficial cortex only, stage 3—localized medullary and cortical, and stage 4—diffuse medullary and cortical.

Belzunegui J et al: Musculoskeletal infections in intravenous drug addicts: Report of 34 cases with analysis of the microbiological aspects and pathogenic mechanisms. Clin Exp Rheumatol 2000;18:383. [PMID: 10895378]

Casado E et al: Musculoskeletal manifestations in patients positive for human immunodeficiency virus: Correlation with CD4 count. J Rheumatol 2001;28:802. [PMID: 11327254]

Gilad J et al: Polymicrobial polyarticular septic arthritis: A rare clinical entity. Scand J Infect Dis 2001;33:381.

Lazzarini L, Mader JT, and Calhoun JH: Osteomyelitis of long bones. J Bone Joint Surg Am 2004;86:2305. [PMID: 15466746]

ACUTE OSTEOMYELITIS

1. Acute Hematogenous Osteomyelitis

Acute hematogenous osteomyelitis (AHO) is most frequently encountered in the metaphysis of long bones in children. Clinically, patients have the signs and symptoms of an acute inflammation. Pain is usually localized, although it may radiate to adjacent regions of the body. For example, if a child complains of knee pain, the hip joint must be thoroughly evaluated for the possibility of septic arthritis. If a bone in the leg is infected, the child may limp or stop walking altogether. Children may also demonstrate guarding of an infected arm, refusing to use it and holding it to their side. Exam usually reveals local tenderness and occasionally limited motion of an adjacent joint, but swelling and redness are less frequent. Systemic signs of fever and chills may be present, and infants may be irritable or lethargic and uninterested in eating.

Serology characteristically shows dramatic elevations in the CRP and the ESR. The WBC is usually elevated, and a left shift may be apparent. Peripheral blood cultures grow the offending organism in up to half of acutely infected children.

Plain radiographs taken early in the course of disease are usually negative. After a week or two, radiographs may reveal a radiolucent lesion and periosteal elevation. Reactive sclerosis is absent because it is encountered only in chronic bone infections. Technetium bone scan shows increased activity on soft tissue and delayed bone images. CT may show a radiolucent area in cancellous bone and signs of periosteal elevation. MRI shows early inflammation of bone marrow with inflammation of the periosteum and adjacent soft tissues as the infection progresses. In later stages abscess formation may be seen as a signal void on gadolinium contrast images.

The clinical and radiologic appearance of AHO may be similar to inflammatory neoplasms such as acute lymphocytic leukemia, Ewing sarcoma, and Langerhans cell histiocytosis (also known as eosinophilic granuloma). Therefore, a biopsy may be required to distinguish an infection from a tumor.

Standard evaluation of a patient with suspected AHO includes a needle or open biopsy to obtain tissue for culture *and* histology and subsequent initiation of empirical antibiotics. If an abscess is identified, thorough irrigation and local debridement through a small cortical window should be performed. Once the culture results and sensitivities are obtained, the final antibiotic regimen may be selected. Six weeks of antibiotic therapy are usually indicated. In pediatric patients with sensitive staphylococcal infections, 2 weeks of parenteral antibiotics may be followed by 4 weeks of oral antibiotic therapy. Close clinical follow-up is necessary to ensure that the patient's inflammatory symptoms are resolving. Serial ESR and CRP should return to normal within the treatment period.

If the patient does not improve, temporary discontinuation of antibiotics may be necessary prior to performing a surgical exploration to culture the infected site. Often antibiotics, even those to which the bacteria are resistant, may suppress the bacteria enough that they will not grow in culture. Although a 2-week waiting period off antibiotics, which is customary for cases of chronic osteomyelitis, may not be tolerated by patients with acute osteomyelitis, even waiting for several days may increase the culture yield. This further highlights the potential problems of beginning an empirical regimen using inappropriate antibiotics and then having difficulty obtaining productive cultures. Either a delay in treatment occurs or the patient has to be placed on several antibiotics to cover all possible organisms.

In patients with stable prosthetic joints who acquire an acute hematogenous infection because of a sensitive organism, thorough soft-tissue debridement, exchange of the polyethylene liner or temporary substitution of the polyethylene with a molded antibiotic spacer, and 6 weeks of IV antibiotic therapy confer a salvage rate approaching 50%.

Clinical Example

A 13-year-old girl complained of acute knee pain beginning 7 days earlier when arising from sleep. Her pain worsened to the point where she had to stay at home from school because she could not walk. On exam her thigh was tender, and her hip and knee motion severely restricted because of pain, but there was no knee effusion. Her temperature was 38.2°C (100.9°F). The serum white blood cell count was 17,000 with a left shift, and the ESR was four times normal. Plain films of the femur were normal. An MRI of the thigh showed significant inflammation of the marrow and adjacent soft tissues on T_2-weighted images (Figure 8–7A). Intraoperatively the midfemur was exposed, a hole was drilled in the femur, and a collection of pus was aspirated from the marrow cavity (Figure 8–7B). Irrigation was performed through the drill hole and the wound closed over a drain. *Staphylococcus aureus* was cultured, and the patient was successfully treated with 6 weeks of IV antibiotics.

A **B**

Figure 8–7. **A:** T$_2$-weighted MRI of the thigh, showing marrow edema in the femur and surrounding musculature. **B:** Aspiration of the medullary cavity of the femur produces 10 mL of pus in the syringe.

2. Acute Osteomyelitis Caused by Puncture Wound

Acute osteomyelitis must be considered in the evaluation of a patient who has suffered a deep puncture wound. The feet and hands are the most frequent sites of these injuries. The soft tissue wound may appear insignificant. It may be difficult to detect a foreign body made of wood or plastic on plain radiography, and wound exploration for a foreign body in a clinic setting is frequently unrewarding. Refer to Chapter 9 (Foot & Ankle Surgery) and Chapter 10 (Hand Surgery) for further information.

Clinical Example

An 11-year-old boy punctured his foot when he stepped on a sharp object. Initial radiographs of the foot showed no evidence of a foreign body (Figure 8–8A). In retrospect, a small puncture wound can be visualized in the middistal diaphysis. He was initially treated with a limited irrigation and debridement in the emergency depart-

ment and discharged on oral antistaphylococcal antibiotics. Two weeks later. the arch of his foot became swollen and drainage emanated from the puncture wound (Figure 8–8B). He was admitted to the hospital and placed empirically on triple IV antibiotics. Superficial swabs of the wound grew *Pseudomonas.*

A technetium bone scan identified a significant uptake of radiotracer in the distal aspect of the first metatarsal compared with the opposite normal foot (Figure 8–8C). New radiographs of the foot depicted a circular region of osteolysis with a slight elevation of the adjacent periosteum (Figure 8–8D). The patient underwent a thorough irrigation and debridement in the operating room. No foreign body was identified. Deep cultures of the wound revealed *Mycobacterium fortuitum,* a rapidly growing mycobacteria other than tuberculosis (MOTT). He clinically improved within several days of beginning oral clarithromycin and continued this treatment for 9 months.

This case illustrates the need to obtain accurate wound cultures in order to choose appropriate antibiotic therapy. Superficial cultures often reveal skin con-

A

B

C

D

Figure 8–8. **A:** Initial plain radiograph of the first metatarsal. **B:** Preoperative view of the puncture wound. **C:** Bone phase of a technetium bone scan of the feet. **D:** Follow-up radiograph of the first metatarsal taken 2 weeks after Figure 8–8A.

441

taminants that are not representative of the organisms actually causing the infection. When infections do not respond to routine empirical antibiotic therapy, it is always important to consider surgical exploration to obtain deep cultures of the wound for mycobacterium and fungal organisms as well as for aerobic and anaerobic organisms.

Agrawal A et al: Cryptococcal arthritis in an immunocompetent host. J S C Med Assoc 2000;96:297. [PMID: 10933007]

Babhulkar SS, Pande SK: Unusual manifestations of osteoarticular tuberculosis. Clin Orthop 2002;398:114. [PMID: 11964639]

Blumberg HM, Leonard MK Jr, Jasmer RM: Update on the treatment of tuberculosis and latent tuberculosis infection. JAMA 2005;293:2776. [PMID: 15941808]

Caspofungin: New preparation. A last resort for invasive aspergillosis. Prescrire Int 2002;11:142. [PMID: 12378745]

Centers for Disease Control and Prevention: Trends in Tuberculosis—United States, 2004. MMWR Morb Mortal Wkly Rep 2005;54:149. [PMID: 15772584]

Dhillon MS et al: Tuberculosis of the sternoclavicular joints. Acta Orthop Scand 2001;72:514. [PMID: 11728080]

Hansen BL, Andersen K: Fungal arthritis. A review. Scan J Rheumatol 1995;24:248. [PMID: 7481591]

Nolan CM, Goldberg SV: Treatment of isoniazid-resistant tuberculosis with isoniazid, rifampin, ethambutol and pyrazinamide for 6 months. Int J Tuberc Lung Dis 2002;6:952. [PMID: 12475140]

Silber JS et al: Insidious destruction of the hip by *Mycobacterium tuberculosis* and why early diagnosis is critical. J Arthroplasty 2000;15:392. [PMID: 10794239]

SUBACUTE OSTEOMYELITIS

Subacute infections are often associated with pediatric patients. These infections are usually caused by organisms of low virulence and associated with muted symptoms. Ultimately, the infection appears to reach a stalemate with the host's defenses and does not progress. Subacute osteomyelitis shares some of the radiographic characteristics of both acute and chronic infections. Like acute osteomyelitis, regions of osteolysis and periosteal elevation may be present. Like chronic osteomyelitis, a circumferential zone of reactive sclerotic bone may be visualized. When subacute osteomyelitis affects the diaphysis of a long bone, it may be particularly difficult to distinguish from Langerhans cell histiocytosis (also known as eosinophilic granuloma) or Ewing sarcoma.

Clinical Example

A 14-year-old boy presented with a 2-month history of left ankle pain and swelling that occurred when he jumped off a farm trailer. His symptoms persisted, although some improvement was reported. He denied any fever, chills, or night sweats and could walk without assistance. On exam he was still tender and focally erythe-matous over the anterior region of the ankle. His WBC was normal and the ESR was only slightly elevated.

Anteroposterior (AP) and lateral radiographs of the tibia show mixed areas of radiodensity and radiolucency in the metaphysis and a slightly raised periosteum (Figures 8–9A and B). Axial T_2-weighted MRI shows marrow edema and periosteal elevation—identified as the outer dark ring just superficial to the cortex. A halo of inflammation surrounds the raised periosteum (Figure 8–9C). Coronal T_2-weighted MRI shows the periosteal elevation along the metadiaphysis and the marrow edema extending as far proximally as the midtibia (Figure 8–9D). During open surgical biopsy, purulent material was encountered within the metaphysis but not along the periosteal surface or in the ankle joint. Thorough irrigation and debridement of the area was performed with primary closure of the incision over a drain. The patient was subsequently cured of his subacute nonresistant *S. aureus* infection with 6 weeks of IV nafcillin.

Lazzarini L, Lipsky BA, Mader JT: Antibiotic treatment of osteomyelitis: What have we learned from 30 years of clinical trials? Int J Infect Dis 2005;9:127. [PMID: 15840453]

Mader JT et al: Antibiotic therapy for musculoskeletal infections. Instr Course Lect 2002;51:539. [PMID: 12064145]

Vinod MB et al: Duration of antibiotics in children with osteomyelitis and septic arthritis. J Paediatr Child Health 2002;38:363. [PMID: 12173997]

CHRONIC OSTEOMYELITIS

Chronic osteomyelitis is the result of untreated acute or subacute osteomyelitis. It can occur hematogenously, iatrogenically, or as a result of penetrating trauma. Chronic infections are often associated with orthopaedic metal implants used to replace joints, fuse spine segments, or fix fractures. Direct intraoperative inoculation or subsequent hematogenous seeding of metal or dead bone surfaces may provide a haven for the bacteria, protecting them from white blood cells and effective concentrations of antibiotics. Therefore, removal of the metal and dead bone are necessary in addition to appropriate antibiotics to eradicate chronic osteomyelitis.

Surgical debridement of necrotic bone for infection control is akin to curettage of a benign bone tumor. A study validating the Cierny-Mader classification system substaging A and B was reported. Debridements were wide marginal or intralesional.

Clinical Example

A 62-year-old man sustained a closed femur fracture when he fell from a ladder 40 years ago. His fracture was fixed with an intramedullary rod that was subsequently removed after the fracture healed. Unfortunately, the patient's leg became infected postoperatively

Figure 8–9. **A:** Anteroposterior radiograph of the distal tibia. **B:** Lateral radiograph of the distal tibia. Notice focal region of osteopenia immediately above the growth plate. **C:** Axial T$_2$-weighted MRI of both tibias in the region of the distal metaphysis shows marrow edema and periosteal elevation and inflammation on the affected left side. **D:** Coronal T$_2$-weighted MRI of both tibias shows extensive marrow edema and periosteal inflammation ascending to the midtibia on the affected side.

and a draining sinus tract developed adjacent to the fracture site. He subsequently had several local debridements when oral antibiotics would not resolve his symptoms. He enjoyed extended asymptomatic intervals of up to 14 years between successive debridements. For the last 4 years he had an intermittently draining sinus tract and occasional bouts of pain relieved with brief courses of oral ciprofloxacin.

At the time of presentation he had had a fever of 38.5°C (101.3°F) and increasing leg pain and swelling for 1 week. Once the sinus tract opened up and began to drain pus, he defervesced and his leg symptoms modestly improved, although it was still difficult for him to walk. On physical examination the sinus tract was probed with a cotton swab, which easily reached the surface of the femur. Serologic exam yielded these results: CRP, 7.5 (0.5 is normal); ESR, 38 (0–15 mm Hg is normal), and WBC, 7.9 (5–10 k is normal). A sensitive *S. aureus* was cultured.

Radiographs depict an irregularly expanded callus of sclerotic bone at the prior fracture site (Figure 8–10A). An indium-labeled WBC scan was focally positive (Figure 8–10B). CT showed small free fragments of bone not connected to the main shaft (Figure 8–10C). The main fragment was further outlined using computer-generated sagittal reconstructions and was thought to be a sequestrum (Figure 8–10D). A T_1-weighted fat saturation MRI with gadolinium contrast further characterized the infected area outlining the relatively small area of focal inflammation (Figure 8–10E).

Curettage of the femur produced a 3.5-cm sequestrum (Figure 8–10F). A water-cooled high-speed burr was used to debride the adjacent cortical bone extensively until it bled freely. A string of antibiotic beads were made on a number 5 nonabsorbable braided suture using 2 g of vancomycin powder, 3 g of tobramycin powder, and one bag of polymethylmethacrylate bone cement (see Figure 8–5). The beads were counted and snugly placed into the cavity in a way that they could easily be retrieved later (Figure 8–10G). The adjacent soft tissues were curetted to remove necrotic material, but the sinus tract was not closed or excised. Operative cultures grew sensitive *S. aureus* and a 6-week course of IV nafcillin (2 g every 4 hours) was begun as an outpatient. A visiting nurse administered the antibiotic through a PICC line using a programmable computerized pump.

Three weeks later, the beads were removed and a mixture of posterior iliac crest bone graft, demineralized bone matrix, and allograft cancellous bone chips were placed into the cavity (Figure 8–10H). Further cultures of the wound were sterile. At the conclusion of his antibiotic therapy, the patient's ESR and CRP had returned to normal values, his sinus tract had completely healed, and he was asymptomatic.

OSTEOMYELITIS CAUSED BY OPEN FRACTURES

Osteomyelitis caused by trauma may present acutely or chronically. In acute cases the signs of infection may be masked by the local open wound and may be delayed by the use of empirical antibiotics and surgical debridement that is not complete. Similar bone changes can be seen on radiographic imaging even in the presence of fractures and fixation hardware. Open wounds where the bone is exposed must undergo comprehensive irrigation and debridement in the operating room. Foreign material, including road dirt, clothing, and bullet shell wadding, must be completely removed, and all necrotic areas of the soft tissues must be excised. If a fracture is present, all fracture fragments completely stripped of their blood supply must also be removed. Viable bone fragments where the periosteum is still attached may be left in the wound but must be carefully monitored. Pulsatile lavage using at least 6 L of saline, with or without antibiotics, is a proven adjunct to sharp surgical debridement. In cases of large soft-tissue defects, early flap coverage is ideal to prevent ongoing contamination of deep tissues and to provide a robust blood supply to the injured area for enhanced antibiotic delivery. Serial debridements every 48 hours may be necessary to establish the viability of injured tissues and to ensure that complete removal of all devitalized tissue is accomplished. In cases where soft-tissue coverage must be delayed, a wound vacuum-assisted closure (VAC) device is an ideal way to manage the wound. This system is easy to apply and only needs to be changed every 2–3 days. Because the pump is portable and the wound is sealed and dry, patient acceptance is high. For these reasons, the wound VAC system has largely replaced open continuous irrigation systems that are more labor intensive to maintain and less well tolerated by the patient.

Fractures can heal even in the presence of a soft-tissue or bone infection. If an acute infection is present in an open wound where a fracture was fixed with a rod or plate, it must be determined if the soft and bony tissues are viable. If they are viable, the fixation hardware should be left in place until the fracture heals. If tissue is necrotic, redebridement to remove all areas of necrosis must first be performed, even if the fixation hardware has to be replaced. If there is a large defect in the bone after comprehensive debridement, the bone should be held to length with an external fixator until the infection is resolved. Placement of temporary antibiotic beads may help provide local antibiotic delivery and eliminate the dead space. Then reconstruction with autograft, vascularized bone graft, or bone transport may be performed.

Chronic osteomyelitis caused by open trauma may often be associated with a healed fracture and an open wound where the bone or fixation hardware may be

Figure 8–10. **A:** Lateral radiograph of the femur. **B:** Indium-labeled white blood count bone scan. **C:** Axial CT scan of the infected area. **D:** Computer-reformatted CT with sagittal image of the femur. *Continued.*

Figure 8–10. (Continued) **E:** An axial T$_1$-weighted fat-saturated MRI with gadolinium contrast. **F:** Sequestrum. **G:** Beads placed in the operative wound. **H:** Ingredients used to bone graft the bone defect (clockwise from bottom: allograft cancellous bone chips, demineralized bone matrix, autograft iliac crest bone).

exposed. The hardware must be removed, and the site of infection must be treated like any chronic osteomyelitis with thorough bone debridement, use of local antibiotic beads, and systemic IV antibiotics. Once the infection is controlled, bone grafting or other reconstruction of the defect may take place, often in association with a local or free flap to reconstruct the soft tissue defect.

Antibiotic therapy for osteomyelitis remains controversial. Antibiotic therapy specific for the offending organism is obvious, but which of several potential agents to use is less clear. Further, use of more than one antibiotics is more effective, according to some studies. Another issue is the length and route of therapy; 6 weeks is the usual empirical recommendation but is not supported by a strong body of literature. With the expense and inconvenience to the patient of IV antibiotics, the length of therapy takes on significant importance. Oral antibiotic therapy could be less burdensome to the

patient and the health system, and it was used for pediatric patients in several studies for the final 4 weeks of therapy. Despite years of clinical trials, these questions in the treatment of osteomyelitis remain unanswered.

Clinical Example

A 42-year-old woman sustained an open fracture of the proximal third of her tibia. She underwent debridement and fracture fixation with a 10-hole plate. The fracture healed after 6 months but remained painful and began to drain purulent material from three sinus tracts (Figure 8–11A). A lateral radiograph shows the tibia before and after plate removal and debridement using a water-cooled high-speed burr (Figures 8–11B and C). The tibia was then packed with a string of antibiotic beads and primarily closed. Half way through the 6-week course of IV antibiotic therapy the beads were removed

(Figure 8–11D) and the defect bone grafted. Graft incorporation occurred over the next 3 months, at which point unrestricted ambulation was permitted.

SQUAMOUS CELL CARCINOMA ARISING FROM A CHRONIC OSTEOMYELITIS

Squamous cell carcinoma may arise in the chronically infected granulation tissue that is adjacent to a chroni-

cally infected bone. This rare complication can occur in areas of burn scars, chronic pressure ulcers, and ostomies, as well as at sites of chronic draining osteomyelitis. The patient usually has had stable chronic osteomyelitis for an average of approximately 20 years, although the latent period can be as little as 18 months. The tumor can be difficult to distinguish visually from the granulation tissue. The focus of carcinoma appears to be an exuberance of proliferative, lobulated, and friable

Figure 8–11. **A:** Leg with draining sinus tracts. **B:** Preoperative radiograph showing fracture fixation plate. **C:** Postoperative radiograph showing extent of bony debridement. **D:** Second surgical exposure of clean tibia and the antibiotic beads that were removed.

"granulation tissue." A recent and progressive worsening of the soft-tissue defect in an otherwise stable case of chronic osteomyelitis is a clue that carcinoma has developed. Liberal sampling of the wound can easily be done in a clinic setting with a disposable skin punch biopsy trephine that dermatologists use for skin biopsies. Histologic examination of the biopsy specimens enables the pathologist to distinguish readily between squamous cell carcinoma and chronic granulation.

Staging studies, including contrast CT scan of the chest, abdomen, and pelvis; technetium total body bone scan; and PET scan, are used to detect other sites of disease. PET is particularly helpful in detecting regional and systemic lymphatic spread of the tumor. Wide surgical excision of the primary site and any positive lymph nodes are necessary to render the patient surgically free of disease. Adjunctive radiotherapy for local control and chemotherapy for systemic control are used in conjunction with surgical excision in most cases.

Clinical Example

A 49-year-old man presented with a 30-year history of ischial decubitus ulcers and rectal fistulas. He had spinal meningitis during infancy resulting in severe paraparesis, hypoesthesia, and incontinence of bowel and bladder. Despite a long series of local debridement procedures, muscle flaps, and skin grafts; his buttock region remained open to some degree during this entire time. More recently, he was concerned about a reactivation of his ischial osteomyelitis. On physical exam, a 15-cm region of friable spongelike neogranulation was identified adjacent to a scarred ulcer overlying the ischium (Figure 8–12A). Plain films suggested chronic reactive changes in the ischium caused by infection and prior surgery. Punch biopsies of the concerning area of neogranulation revealed squamous cell carcinoma. CT of the chest abdomen and pelvis were negative except for enlarged inguinal lymph nodes. The patient underwent a permanent diverting colostomy and inguinal and retroperitoneal lymph node dissection. All lymph nodes were negative. The tumor subsequently was radically excised, including a partial excision of the ischium (Figures 8–12B and C). A wound VAC was used for local wound care (Figures 8–12D and E). Eight weeks later, the wound edges had retracted, and normal healthy granulation tissue covered the bony defect (Figure 8–12F). The area was subsequently covered with skin graft to achieve complete healing.

Copcu E et al: Thirty-one cases of Marjolin's ulcer. Clin Exp Dermatol 2003;28:138. [PMID: 12653697]

Gonzalez MH, Weinzweig N: Muscle flaps in the treatment of osteomyelitis of the lower extremity. J Trauma 2005;58:1019. [PMID: 15920418]

Kuokkanen HO et al: Radical excision and reconstruction of chronic osteomyelitis with microvascular muscle flaps. Orthopedics 2002;25:137. [PMID: 11871378]

Moroni A et al: State of the art review: Techniques to avoid pin loosening and infection in external fixation. J Orthop Trauma 2002;16:189. [PMID: 11880783]

Strauss MB, Bryant B: Hyperbaric oxygen. Orthopedics 2002;25:303. [PMID: 11918035]

Thio D et al: Malignant change after 18 months in a lower limb ulcer: Acute Marjolin's revisited. Br J Plast Surg 2003;56:825. [PMID: 14615262]

■ SEPTIC ARTHRITIS

Diagnosis

There is no formal classification system for septic arthritis. Most joint infections are acute rather than chronic, monoarticular rather than polyarticular, and they arise from a hematogenous source of organisms rather than by direct inoculation or extension from an adjacent infection. The most important clinical question that often arises is whether the patient's inflamed joint is caused by an infection or a noninfectious inflammatory process. Inflammatory arthropathies are numerous, and patients often require systemic medical treatment to control the joint symptoms. They are often categorized as seropositive (for rheumatoid factor) or seronegative. Common conditions include crystal arthropathies (gout and pseudogout) and autoimmune disorders with joint involvement (RA, systemic lupus erythematosus, and inflammatory bowel disease). Finally, arthropathy from osteoarthritis and avascular necrosis may present with inflammatory symptoms and mimic an indolent infection.

Diagnosis of septic arthritis depends much more on arthrocentesis for synovial fluid analysis (see Table 8–4) and culture than it does on radiologic imaging. Early plain radiographs are usually normal. Ultrasound is better at diagnosing increased fluid within a joint space but is not specific as to the cause. Many of the radiographic features of bone scan, CT, and MRI are nonspecific and leave the diagnosis of septic arthritis in question.

ACUTE SEPTIC ARTHRITIS

Hematogenous septic arthritis commonly affects patients with compromised immunologic defense mechanisms. The underlying source of infection can frequently be determined, and blood cultures are positive in approximately half of patients. Patients at risk include those with specific immune deficiencies from HIV or chemotherapy; those with chronic disease, including RA, gout, renal failure, and sickle cell disease; and IV drug abusers. Patients with known arthropathy from other causes are also at increased risk for superimposed infections. Patients rou-

Figure 8–12. **A:** Photograph of chronic ulcerative wound with neogranulation tissue laterally. **B:** Wound and tumor bed after wide excision of the carcinoma. **C:** Tumor/wound specimen, 18 cm in diameter. **D:** Wound vacuum-assisted closure (VAC) sponge being measured over wound. **E:** Wound VAC sponge in place, partially contacting wound. **F:** Eight weeks after wound VAC and antibiotic therapy. Bed ready for skin grafting.

tinely complain of severe pain with passive motion of the affected joint. Rest pain, guarding, swelling, erythema, and heat become more pronounced as the infection progresses. Fever and chills are not sensitive indicators of septic arthritis.

The most common joint affected by hematogenous septic arthritis is the knee. The hip, ankle, wrist, shoulder, and elbow follow in frequency of involvement. The differential diagnosis includes Charcot joint, gout, pseudogout, RA, and other inflammatory arthropathies. The diagnosis is tentatively made on joint fluid analysis (see Table 8–4).

Although infections often spread from joints to affect adjacent metaphyseal bone, tumors seldom do except at the sacroiliac joint. Surgical decompression and irrigation of all large joints is preferred to serial needle aspirations. In the acute setting, arthroscopy is ideal for culturing synovial tissue, thoroughly irrigating the joint space, and for placement of an indwelling drainage tube.

Clinical Example

A 53-year-old woman with RA and a painful left hip presented with a 3-week history of rapidly worsening groin pain, slight fever, and lethargy. Degenerative narrowing of the hip joint is seen on a prior AP radiograph (Figure 8–13A). Although the patient's WBC was normal, the hematocrit was only 18! Her groin was extremely tender, and any motion of the hip joint elicited excruciating pain. The patient was admitted to the hospital directly from the clinic. A bone scan showed intense activity in the region of the hip (Figure 8–13B). A CT of the pelvis outlines a loculated soft-tissue mass anterior to the femoral head displacing the femoral artery and vein medially (Figure 8–13C). Using CT guidance, the region was aspirated, and a pigtail catheter was inserted to drain the abscess cavity. MRI with T_1 fat-saturated sequences and gadolinium contrast further characterized the infection, revealing significant inflammation in the femoral head and an effusion of the hip joint (Figure 8–13D). A plain radiograph at that time showed a dramatic collapse of the femoral head (Figure 8–13E). A Girdlestone arthroplasty was performed, and the remainder of the femoral head was submitted for histologic analysis (Figure 8–13F). An antibiotic spacer was orthotopically placed to stabilize the femur, and the wound was closed over drains (Figure 8–13G). A 6-week course of IV antibiotics was given. Afterward, the hip was surgically reexamined, and no evidence of persistent infection was seen grossly or by frozen section analysis. At that time a total hip prosthesis was successfully implanted.

CHRONIC SEPTIC ARTHRITIS

Unlike acute septic arthritis, which is intensely painful, chronic septic arthritis presents with indolent joint symptoms that are often muted by oral or intraarticular injections of antiinflammatory medications and may be attributed to coexistent chronic joint arthritis. Immunocompromised patients are susceptible to less virulent and slower growing organisms such as atypical mycobacteria and fungus. These organisms may solicit a subdued chronic inflammatory response that generates less pain and joint effusion, resulting in a delay in diagnosis.

Clinical Example

A 52-year-old man with AIDS on retroviral therapy presented with a 4-month history of arthritic pain and effusion in his knee and a 1-week history of an enlarging painful mass on the medial aspect of his knee (Figure 8–14A). One year earlier he was diagnosed with a large popliteal abscess in the same leg caused by *S. epidermidis* that was successfully treated with surgical drainage and 6 weeks of IV antibiotics. Exam revealed focal swelling, warmth, erythema, and restricted motion because of pain. During arthrotomy, the medial swelling was found to communicate directly with the knee joint. Intraoperative findings included a large quantity of pus, extensive erosion of cartilage, and chronic proliferative synovial tissue (Figure 8–14B). After irrigation and debridement, the wound was primarily closed over drainage catheters. Cultures grew *Candida albicans,* and the patient was treated with fluconazole (Diflucan).

Even though this patient's symptoms appeared acute, he actually had chronic septic arthritis that likely began 4 months previously when he began having arthritic pain. Because he was immunocompromised, his inflammatory symptoms were muted, causing a delay in clinical presentation. Unusual pathogens are a hallmark of immunocompromised patients. Therefore, it is essential to acquire mycobacterial and fungal cultures in addition to aerobic and anaerobic bacterial cultures. Unless the cause of immunosuppression is known, a comprehensive diagnostic survey must be undertaken to identify the underlying causes, including cancer, severe malnutrition, immune disorders, and chronic viral infection.

Aubry A et al: Sixty cases of *Mycobacterium marinum* infection: Clinical features, treatment, and antibiotic susceptibility of the causative isolates. Arch Intern Med 2002;162:1746. [PMID: 12153378]

Biviji AA et al: Musculoskeletal manifestations of human immuno-deficiency virus infection. J Am Acad Orthop Surg 2002;10: 312. [PMID: 12374482]

Le Dantec C et al: Occurrence of mycobacteria in water treatment lines and in water distribution systems. Appl Environ Microbiol 2002;68:5318. [PMID: 12406720]

Laine M, Luukkainen R, Toivanen A: Sindbis viruses and other alpha viruses as a cause of human arthritic disease. J Intern Med 2004;256:457. [PMID: 15554947]

Figure 8–13. **A:** Initial anteroposterior radiograph of hip joint with narrowed cartilage caused by rheumatoid arthritis. **B:** Technetium bone scan shows intense activity in region of left hip. **C:** CT scan shows loculated soft-tissue mass anterior to the femoral head displacing the femoral artery and vein medially. **D:** T_1-weighted fat-saturated MRI with gadolinium contrast shows intense inflammation around hip joint and in acetabulum and femoral head. A retroperitoneal abscess is depicted in the enlarged iliopsoas muscle by a dark central area of signal void surrounded by a halo of bright inflammation. *Continued.*

F

E

G

Figure 8–13. (Continued) **E:** Preoperative plain radiograph showing extensive collapse of the weight bearing portion of the femoral head. **F:** Surgical specimen showing flattened femoral head (upper portion). Note the cut surface of the neck (lower right). **G:** Radiograph of an antibiotic spacer molded around a rush rod that was implanted in the femoral canal.

Mylonas AD et al: Natural history of Ross River virus-induced epidemic polyarthritis. Med J Aust 2002;177:356. [PMID: 12358577]

Stahl HD et al: Detection of multiple viral DNA species in synovial tissue and fluid of patients with early arthritis. Ann Rheum Dis 2000;59:342. [PMID: 10784515]

SEPTIC ARTHRITIS CAUSED BY ADJACENT INFECTION

Contiguous spread of infection to a joint most commonly occurs in pediatric patients with AHO or in adults with chronic wounds such as ischial decubiti and diabetic foot ulcers. Chronic soft-tissue and bone infections may extend into joints in adults as well. Of particular concern is occurrence in patients who are immunocompromised or insensate.

Clinical Example

A 28-year-old man with paraplegia and a long-standing history of sacral and ischial decubiti presented with a 2-week history of fevers, anemia, and increased spasticity of the lower extremities. Two large fist-sized decubiti, one over the sacrum and one over the right ischium, were observed (Figure 8–15A). The underlying bone was easily palpated at the base of both of these ulcers. Further examination with a probing finger revealed a deep sinus that tracked to the posterior aspect of the femoral head. Plain films revealed a chronically dislocated hip with cephalad migration of the femur and concomitant destruction of the ilium (Figure 8–15B). Axial CT scan showed air within and surrounding the dislocated femoral head (Figure 8–15C). MRI with inversion recovery sequenc-

A

Figure 8–14. A: A large focal erythematous soft-tissue swelling and a longitudinal scar from prior surgical drainage of a popliteal abscess are seen along the medial aspect of the knee. **B:** With the patella everted to the left, the articular surfaces of the femur are seen at the top and the hypertrophic synovium is seen below. Note the complete loss of cartilage on the medial femoral condyle to the right.

B

ing depicted extensive inflammation of the femur, the ilium, and the surrounding gluteal musculature (Figure 8–15D). An extensive surgical debridement of the acetabulum and removal of the proximal femur was performed through the lateral ulcer. A wound VAC was placed on both ulcers, and culture-specific antibiotics were administered. The patient refused a hip disarticulation with an anterior thigh flap that would close both ischial and sacral decubiti, and he was subsequently treated with chronic oral antibiotic suppression and daily wound packing.

Goergens ED et al: Acute osteomyelitis and septic arthritis in children. J Pediatr Child Health 2005;41:59. [PMID: 15670227]

Li SF et al: Laboratory tests in adults with monoarticular arthritis: Can they rule out a septic joint? Acad Emerg Med 2004; 11:276. [PMID: 15001408]

Salter RB, Bell RS, Keeley FW: The protective effect of continuous passive motion on living articular cartilage in acute septic arthritis. Clin Orthop 1981;159:223. [PMID: 7285461]

Shirtliff ME, Mader JT: Acute septic arthritis. Clin Microbiol Rev 2002;15:527. [PMID: 12364368]

Swan A, Amer H, Dieppe P: The value of synovial fluid analysis in the diagnosis of joint disease: A literature survey. Ann Rheum Dis 2002;61:493. [PMID: 12006320]

Yu KH et al: Concomitant septic and gouty arthritis—An analysis of 30 cases. Rheumatology (Oxford) 2003;42:1062. [PMID: 12730521]

■ SOFT-TISSUE INFECTIONS

CELLULITIS

Skin infections are common, and it is important to distinguish cellulitis from noninfectious rashes and from deeper infections that have a component of cellulitis, such as osteomyelitis, septic arthritis, myositis, and necrotizing fasciitis. Stasis dermatitis may visually mimic cellulitis. Patients often present with a rash over areas of increased peripheral edema.

Figure 8–15. A: Large sacral and right ischial ulcer. **B:** Anteroposterior radiograph of the pelvis. **C:** CT scan of pelvis. **D:** MRI with inversion recovery sequence of the pelvis.

Unlike patients with cellulitis, these patients do not have a fever or elevated WBC.

Clinical Example

A 43-year-old man fell 3 weeks ago, injuring his leg. He presented with progressively worsening pain and swelling in his thigh. On examination, cellulitis of the anterior and lateral thigh was manifested by erythema, diffuse and tense swelling with shiny skin, and dramatic pain with knee flexion and tenderness with light palpation (Figure 8–16A). No swelling or erythema of the calf or foot was noted, and distal pulses and sensation were intact. Plain radiographs of the femur were

A **B**

Figure 8–16. **A:** Cellulitis and diffuse thigh swelling. **B:** Axial T₂-weighted MRI of the thigh.

normal. Doppler ultrasound ruled out a deep venous thrombosis but identified diffuse swelling of the muscle compartment. A T₂-weighted MRI depicted characteristic expansion of the subcutaneous tissues with feathery streaks of increased water content circumferentially. It also revealed an underlying fluid collection within the vastus lateralis and intermedius (Figure 8–16B). Surgical inspection of this fluid revealed pus from an underlying myositis. An intramuscular hematoma from nonpenetrating trauma to the thigh had become hematogenously seeded with *S. aureus.* The infection caused an expanding abscess with myositis and superficial cellulitis. Culture acquisition, serial irrigation and debridement with open packing, and antibiotic therapy were started. Delayed primary closure and 6 weeks of culture-sensitive IV antibiotics cured the patient's infection. It should be noted in this case that the cellulitis was manifested after the leg began to swell, indicating clinically that the cellulitis was a secondary finding. In this circumstance a search for an underlying cause was necessary to understand the source of infection.

PYOMYOSITIS

Pyomyositis is usually caused by hematogenous spread of bacteria rather than direct inoculation via penetrating trauma. Usually there is very limited muscle necrosis, and a very vascular fibrous reactive capsule contains the abscess. Open exploration with copious irrigation, limited debridement, and primary wound closure over a surgical drain is the surgical treatment of choice. Evaluation for contiguous spread to bone or joint must be performed. Aspiration for culture and insertion of a pigtail catheter for drainage can be done with ultrasound or CT guidance.

Clinical Example

A 6-year-old boy presented with a 2-week history of a posterior thigh mass. Focal tenderness and swelling were present, but no erythema was noted (Figure 8–17A). Further inspection revealed numerous insect bites around his ankle and leg that had become open pustules because of vigorous scratching. A T₁-weighted fat-saturated MRI with gadolinium clearly characterized a fluid collection represented by a black signal void (Figure 8–17B). A halo of increased signal uptake along the rim of the fluid collection represents intense localized inflammation. The patient underwent surgical exploration, and pus was easily expressed from the thigh. The wound was debrided, irrigated, and a surgical drainage tube was placed. The wound was primarily closed. Staining revealed gram-positive cocci in clusters, and cultures grew a sensitive *S. aureus.* IV antibiotics were initiated, and the patient's symptoms rapidly improved. A week later he was discharged to home with 5 weeks of oral antibiotics that cured his infection.

BURSITIS

A bursa occasionally becomes infected by hematogenous spread or because of open trauma to the overlying skin. The patient complains of pain and stiffness and possibly a fever. A tender, inflamed bursal region is seen clinically with significant erythema and swelling. Because these findings may also occur in acute exacerbations of rheumatism and flare-ups of gout, the patient must be carefully questioned regarding a possible history of these diagnoses. For example, aspiration of a soft, inflamed olecranon tophus may yield fluid that is strikingly similar to pus. Gram stain and polarized microscopy are necessary to identify negatively birefringent crystals.

A   B

Figure 8–17. **A:** Prone patient with focal swelling of the posterior region of the midthigh. Note the insect bites scarring the skin. **B:** T_1-weighted MRI with gadolinium contrast showing dark signal void in center of abscess.

If infectious bursitis is identified within the first several days, an oral course of antibiotics may successfully treat the infection. If skin erythema spreads and the bursa fills with fluid, the patient must be admitted to the hospital to aspirate and culture the bursal fluid and to begin empirical IV antibiotics. If the infection does not begin to resolve clinically within 48 hours, surgical bursectomy and primary closure of the wound over a drain should be performed.

Clinical Example

An 18-year-old woman skinned her knee on the gym floor during a game of basketball 1 week prior to presentation. She was noted on exam to have a dramatically painful, swollen, and erythematous prepatellar region with only slight loss of knee motion. A small central eschar, indicative of a floor burn, was observed (Figures 8–18A and B). Gram stain of the aspirate from the prepatellar bursa revealed gram-positive cocci in clusters. Despite 2 days of IV antistaphylococcal antibiotic therapy, the inflammation worsened. A complete bursectomy was performed (Figure 8–18C). A layer of normal appearing fatty tissue was left to cover the surface of the patella (Figure 8–18D), and the wound was closed over a surgical drain. The inflammation quickly improved within 3 days, and the patient was sent home with 3 weeks of culture-specific antibiotics.

NECROTIZING FASCIITIS

Necrotizing fasciitis is a rare but extremely aggressive, life-threatening soft-tissue infection of the subcutaneous and fascial tissues often encountered in diabetic patients. The muscle tissues are generally spared. Clinical examination of the skin reveals streaking erythema and sometimes small blisters, arising in the region of an incidental puncture wound. Local induration is always found, and occasionally subcutaneous crepitation caused by gas in the soft tissues is encountered. Air in the soft tissues can usually be seen on plain radiographs in gas-producing clostridial infections (see Figure 8–1). Serial exams are necessary to track the leading edge of the infection, which rapidly progresses in the direction of venous drainage. Emergent surgical debridement of devitalized tissues (sometimes necessitating amputation) along with antibiotics and intensive care treatment for hypotension are required to prevent death.

Clinical Example

A 38-year-old woman with a history of insulin-dependent diabetes mellitus sustained a penetrating trauma to the dorsum of her wrist while using scissors. Two days later she presented to the emergency room with a very painful arm and an infected stab wound that was draining serous fluid, an erythematous rash that extended from the wound to her elbow, and an increase of her forearm circumference of 6 cm compared with the other arm. She had a temperature of 38.6°C (101.5°F), a serum WBC of 22,000 with a left shift, and normal plain radiographs of the forearm.

The patient was admitted to the hospital and started empirically on a ticarcillin with clavulanate potassium (Timentin) and gentamicin. After 24 hours, however, the arm pain progressively worsened, and the rash advanced above the elbow (Figure 8–19A). MRI showed significant soft-tissue edema in the subcutaneous tissues but not in the muscle compartments (Fig-

Figure 8–18. A: Anterior view of acute prepatellar bursitis. Notice small dark eschar. **B:** Lateral view of swollen prepatellar bursa. **C:** Bursa sectioned sagittally. Note the white-appearing rind of reactive fibrosis surrounding the central cavity. **D:** Intraoperative view of knee after bursectomy. Notice that the adipose tissue covering periosteum of patella was retained.

ures 8–19B and C). Concerned about an uncontrolled necrotizing fasciitis, surgical exploration was emergently performed. Although most of the skin and all of the muscle tissues were viable, necrosis of the subcutaneous tissues and fascia was extensive (Figures 8–19D and E). All necrotic tissue was sharply excised. The necrotic tissue could easily be distinguished because it was friable to palpation. Normal-appearing tissue was

firmer, and a finger could not easily dissect the plane between the subcutaneous tissue and the fascia. The wound was copiously irrigated with a pulsatile lavage device and packed open with moist gauze dressings secured with sterile rubber bands and staples in a shoelace fashion (Figure 8–19F). Gram-positive cocci in chains were identified intraoperatively, and the antibiotics were switched to oxacillin and clindamycin.

Figure 8–19. **A:** A small draining puncture wound is noted at the middorsum of the hand, and an extensive erythematous rash covers the forearm. **B:** Axial MRI inversion recovery sequence showing circumferential subcutaneous inflammation. **C:** Sagittal MRI inversion recovery sequence showing subcutaneous inflammation but absence of inflammation in muscle tissue. **D:** Dorsal forearm incision revealing extensive subcutaneous necrosis. **E:** Necrosis in subcutaneous tissues but not in muscle tissue. **F:** Open packing of wound with saline-dampened gauze sponges secured with staples and sterile rubber bands in a shoelace fashion. *Continued.*

G   H

Figure 8–19. (Continued) **G:** Appearance of viable wound after 1 week of serial debridements, antibiotics, and hyperbaric oxygen treatments. **H:** Delayed primary closure with interrupted retention sutures.

Hyperbaric oxygen treatments using an acute protocol of 2.4 atm for 90 minutes three times daily was begun, and daily surgical debridements were performed for 3 days (Figure 8–19G). Some skin died and was debrided. The patient's infection cleared, and the wound was left to heal by delayed primary closure with use of split-thickness skin grafts where necessary (Figure 8–19H).

Tiu A et al: Necrotizing fasciitis: Analysis of 48 cases in South Auckland, New Zealand. ANZ J Surg 2005;75:32. [PMID: 15740513]

Foot & Ankle Surgery

Jeffrey A. Mann, MD, Loretta B. Chou, MD, & Steven D. K. Ross, MD

BIOMECHANIC PRINCIPLES OF THE FOOT & ANKLE

The following is a limited discussion of the biomechanic principles governing the foot and ankle during the gait cycle. The physician must have a clear understanding of these principles to evaluate problems affecting the foot and ankle accurately. Once normal biomechanic function is understood, anatomic and functional abnormalities are more easily detected.

Gait

Gait is the orderly progression of the body through space while expending as little energy as possible. As the body moves through a gait cycle, forces are generated actively, by action of the body's muscles, and passively, by the effects of gravity on the body. To accommodate these forces, the foot is flexible at the time of heel strike, when it must absorb the impact of the body against the ground, and rigid at the time of toe-off, when it must assist in moving the body forward. The magnitude of the forces on the foot increases significantly as the speed of gait increases. For example, when an individual is walking, the initial force with which the foot meets the ground is approximately 80% of body weight, whereas when an individual is jogging, it is approximately 160%. The peak force against the foot during walking is approximately 110% of body weight, whereas for jogging it is approximately 240%. This marked increase probably contributes to some of the injuries seen in runners.

The Walking Cycle

The walking cycle is discussed more extensively in Chapter 1, but pertinent aspects relating to the foot are discussed here (Figure 9–1).

Observation of the patient while walking may give the clinician insight into the cause of a gait anomaly (Figure 9–2). For example, equinus deformity resulting from spasticity or contracture may cause the toe to make initial contact with the ground rather than the heel. At 7% of the gait cycle, the foot is usually flat on the ground, but spasticity or tightness of the Achilles tendon causes this to be delayed. At 12% of the cycle,

the opposite foot toes off and the swing phase begins. Heel rise of the standing foot begins at 34% of the cycle as the swinging leg passes the standing limb. Heel rise may be premature in spasticity or prolonged in weakness of the gastrocsoleus muscle. Heel strike of the opposite foot occurs at 50% of the cycle, ending the period of single-limb support; this may occur sooner if there is weakness of the contralateral calf muscle. Toe-off of the opposite foot occurs at 62% of the cycle, at the beginning of the swing phase. These markers of the gait cycle should be kept in mind when observing gait, so pathologic conditions may be identified.

Motions of the Foot & Ankle

The names for various motions about the foot and ankle may be confusing and used incorrectly. The motions that occur at the ankle joint are dorsiflexion and plantar flexion. The motions of the heel medially and laterally, which occur at the subtalar joint, are inversion (varus) and eversion (valgus), respectively. The motion occurring at the transverse tarsal joint (talonavicular and calcaneocuboid) is adduction, which is movement toward the midline, and abduction, which is movement away from the midline.

Supination and *pronation* are terms for two different combinations of movements, but unfortunately these terms are sometimes used in the literature interchangeably. *Pronation* refers to dorsiflexion of the ankle joint, eversion of the subtalar joint, and abduction of the transverse tarsal joint. *Supination* is the opposite; namely, plantar flexion of the ankle joint, inversion of the subtalar joint, and adduction of the transverse tarsal joint.

The nomenclature may also be confusing when such terms as *forefoot varus* and *forefoot valgus* are used (Figure 9–3). Forefoot varus or valgus is an anatomic deformity that is observed when the hindfoot is placed in neutral position. Neutral position is achieved when the calcaneus is aligned with the long axis of the tibia and the head of the talus is covered with the navicular bone. Forefoot varus deformity is present when the lateral aspect of the forefoot is in greater plantar flexion than the medial aspect. With a flexible deformity, the foot lies flat on the floor during stance, but with a fixed deformity, excessive weight is borne on the lateral side of the foot. As a result,

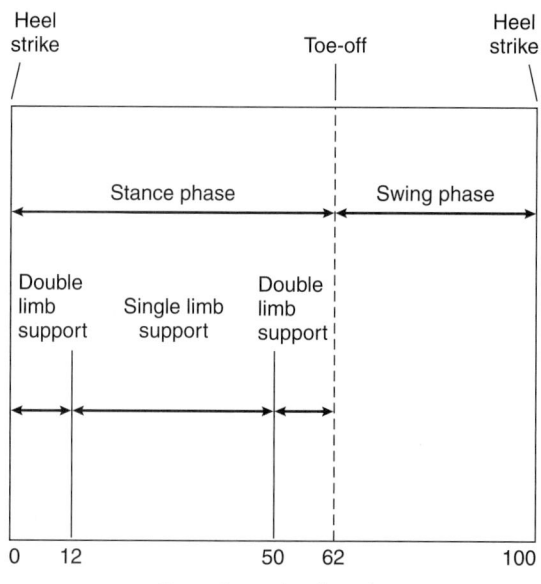

Figure 9–1. Phases of the walking cycle. Stance phase constitutes approximately 62% and swing phase 38% of the cycle. (Reproduced, with permission, from Mann RA, Coughlin MJ: *The Video Textbook of Foot and Ankle Surgery.* Medical Video Productions, 1991.)

as the weight passes onto the forefoot region, the calcaneus goes into valgus position, and this may result in lateral impingement of the calcaneus against the fibula if severe. In forefoot valgus deformity, the medial side of the foot has greater plantar flexion than the lateral side and results in excessive weight bearing by the first metatarsal head. To accommodate for this deformity, the calcaneus assumes a varus position, which may result in a feeling of instability at the ankle joint.

Mechanisms of the Foot during Weight Bearing

As mentioned previously, the normal foot is flexible at the time of heel strike to absorb the impact of striking the ground. As a result, the subtalar joint literally collapses into a position of valgus, causing internal rotation of the tibia and resulting distally in unlocking of the transverse tarsal (talonavicular and calcaneocuboid) joint. Thus, the forefoot is more flexible. The only muscle group that is functioning about the foot and ankle during heel strike is the anterior compartment muscle group, which helps control the initial rapid plantar flexion following heel strike by an eccentric or lengthening contraction. The flexibility of the foot is greatest at approximately 7% of the cycle, and a series of changes is then initiated. With the foot fixed to

the ground, the body passes over the foot, which lifts the heel up and forces the metatarsophalangeal joints into extension. As this occurs, the foot is converted into a rigid lever that supports the body at the time of toe-off. The mechanisms that bring about conversion of the foot from a flexible to a rigid structure are (1) the tightening of the plantar aponeurosis, the windlass mechanism, (2) the progressive external rotation of the lower extremity, which begins at the pelvis and is passed distally across the ankle joint into the subtalar joint, and (3) the stabilization of the transverse tarsal joint, which results from the progressive inversion of the subtalar joint.

Joints About the Foot & Ankle

A. ANKLE JOINT

The ankle joint consists of the articulation of the talus with the tibia and fibula, with a range of motion (ROM) of 15 degrees of dorsiflexion and 55 degrees of plantar flexion. There is also a small amount of motion in the transverse plane, approximately 15 degrees. The anterior compartment muscles of the leg, the tibialis anterior and the toe extensors, control the amount of plantar flexion of the ankle joint at the time of heel ground contact to 10% stance. In addition, these muscles provide dorsiflexion of the ankle joint during swing phase. If this muscle group does not function, a footslap is observed at the time of heel strike, and a dropfoot occurs during swing phase. The greatest force across the ankle joint during walking is calculated to be approximately 4.5 times body weight; this force is present at 40% of the walking cycle.

B. SUBTALAR JOINT

The subtalar joint is the articulation between the talus and the calcaneus. The primary joint surface is the

Figure 9–2. Events of the walking cycle. (Reproduced, with permission, from Mann RA, Coughlin MJ: *The Video Textbook of Foot and Ankle Surgery.* Medical Video Productions, 1991.)

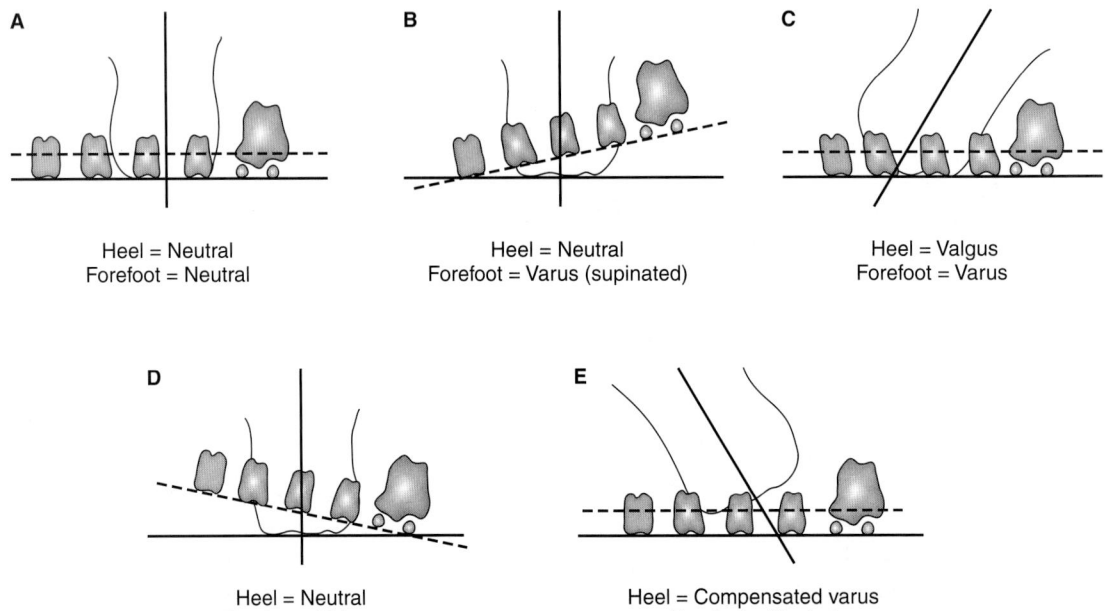

Figure 9–3. Biomechanics of foot posture. **A:** Normal alignment: forefoot perpendicular to heel. **B:** Forefoot varus (uncompensated): lateral aspect of forefoot plantar flexed in relation to medial aspect. **C:** Forefoot varus (compensated): With the forefoot flat on the floor, the heel assumes a valgus position. **D:** Forefoot valgus (uncompensated): medial aspect of forefoot plantar flexed in relation to lateral aspect. **E:** Forefoot valgus (compensated): With the forefoot flat on the floor, the heel assumes a varus position. (Reproduced, with permission, from Mann RA, Coughlin MJ: *The Video Textbook of Foot and Ankle Surgery.* Medical Video Productions, 1991.)

posterior facet, with much smaller middle and anterior facets. The motion of this joint is inversion of approximately 30 degrees and eversion of approximately 10 degrees. The tibialis posterior causes inversion and the peroneus brevis eversion at the subtalar joint. At the time of initial ground contact, eversion is a passive mechanism and occurs because of the shape of the articulations and their ligamentous support. Inversion occurs both actively and passively at the time of toe-off. Active control is achieved by the gastrocsoleus and posterior tibial muscles, and passive inversion occurs by the action of the plantar aponeurosis, the external rotation of the lower extremity, and the oblique metatarsal break.

C. TALONAVICULAR JOINT AND CALCANEOCUBOID JOINT

The talonavicular and calcaneocuboid joints functionally act as a unit known as the *transverse tarsal joint.* Motion at the transverse tarsal joint is approximately 10 degrees of abduction and approximately 15 degrees of adduction. The head of the talus is firmly seated into the navicular at the time of toe-off, adding stability to the foot. The stability of the transverse tarsal joint is controlled by the position of the subtalar joint. When the subtalar joint is in an inverted position, the axes of these two joints are nonparallel, giving rise to increased stability of the hindfoot. When the calcaneus is in an everted position at the time of heel strike, these joints are parallel to one another, thereby giving rise to increased flexibility of these joints (Figure 9–4). The clinical implication is that when carrying out a subtalar arthrodesis, placement of the subtalar joint into a varus position locks the transverse tarsal joint, causing increased stiffness of the forefoot and, frequently, discomfort. When the hindfoot is everted into a position of 5–7 degrees of valgus, the flexibility of the transverse tarsal joint is maintained. This allows the forefoot to be more supple and makes ambulation easier.

D. METATARSOPHALANGEAL JOINTS

The motion at the metatarsophalangeal joints is between 50 and 70 degrees of dorsiflexion (extension) and 15 and 25 degrees of plantar flexion (flexion). The role of the metatarsophalangeal joints during gait is discussed in the section on deformities of the first toe.

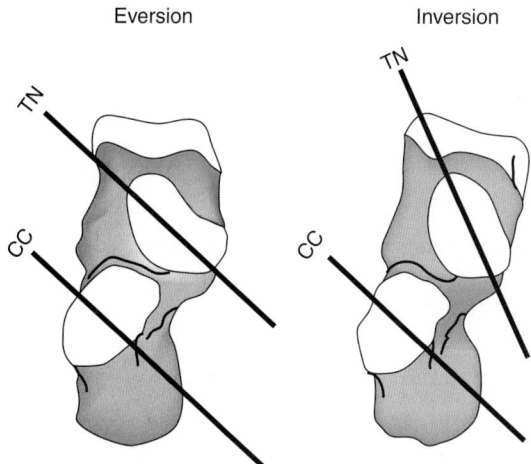

Figure 9–4. The function of the transverse tarsal joint as described by Elftman demonstrates that when the calcaneus is in eversion, the resultant axes of the talonavicular and calcaneocuboid joints are parallel or congruent. When the subtalar joint is in an inverted position, the axes are incongruent, giving increased stability to the midfoot. (Reproduced, with permission, from Mann RA, Coughlin MJ: *The Video Textbook of Foot and Ankle Surgery.* Medical Video Productions, 1991.)

E. THE PLANTAR APONEUROSIS

Although the plantar aponeurosis is not an articulation per se, it probably plays the predominant role in the overall stability of the foot. The plantar aponeurosis arises from the tubercle of the calcaneus and passes distally to insert into the base of each proximal phalanx (Figure 9–5). As the metatarsophalangeal joints pass into dorsiflexion in the last half of the stance phase, the rigidity of the plantar aponeurosis forces the metatarsal heads into a plantarward direction, which raises the longitudinal arch. This is known as a windlass mechanism. It also increases the effect that a tensile force in the tendo Achilles has on the tensile force in the plantar fascia. The now-rigid foot provides support to the body for the push-off phase of gait. Secondarily, this mechanism also helps bring about inversion of the subtalar joint.

F. GAIT ABNORMALITIES

The following is a brief description of the more common gait abnormalities.

1. Dropfoot gait—Patients with dropfoot gait lack ankle dorsiflexion, resulting in plantar flexion at the ankle joint. When walking, these patients adopt a steppage-type gait. This gait pattern is manifested by increased flexion of the hip and knee to enable the swinging leg to clear the ground. If this compensatory mechanism does not occur, the patient may catch the toes on the ground and fall.

2. Equinus gait—In an equinus gait pattern, the ankle joint is fixed in plantar flexion throughout the entire gait cycle. This situation may result from a stroke or head injury, trauma to the lower extremity, or a congenital deformity, and it often is associated with tightness of the posterior capsule. This gait pattern is characterized by forefoot floor contact (no heel contact). The anterior loading of the foot results in a back knee thrust, which may, over a long period of time, result in a hyperextension deformity of the knee. A weak quadriceps muscle may accentuate this problem.

3. Cavus deformity—A cavus deformity is an excessive elevation of the longitudinal arch. A moderate decrease in the ROM of the foot usually accompanies this deformity. In addition, the hindfoot is often in a varus posture and the forefoot in valgus posture. This is most frequently observed in Charcot-Marie-Tooth disease but may also be seen in poliomyelitis and occasionally as a late result of calf compartment syndrome. The deformity significantly diminishes the overall surface available for weight bearing in these patients. Clawing of the toes may further reduce contact with the ground. Thus, the gait pattern in these patients is altered, with increased pressure on the heel at initial ground contact, followed by increased pressure along the lateral side of the foot and underneath the first metatarsal head as the gait cycle progresses.

4. Pes planus deformity—Usually, the patient with a pes planus deformity demonstrates just the opposite of cavus deformity; the foot is too flexible. At the time of initial ground contact, there is excessive valgus of the hindfoot and in severe cases breaking down of the longitudinal arch with an associated abduction of the forefoot. This results in an increased weight-bearing surface and often easy fatigability because of the lack of adequate support of the longitudinal arch.

Carlson RE, Fleming LL, Hutton WC: The biomechanical relationship between the tendoachilles, plantar fascia and metatarsophalangeal joint dorsiflexion angle. Foot Ankle Int 2000;21:18–25. [PMID: 10710257]

Hunt AE, Smith RM, Torode M: Extrinsic muscle activity, foot motion and ankle joint moments during the stance phase of walking. Foot Ankle Int 2001;22:31–41. [PMID: 11206820]

Mann RA: Biomechanics of the foot and ankle. In Mann RA, Coughlin MJ, eds: *Surgery of the Foot and Ankle.* Mosby-Year Book, 1993.

Nester CJ, Findlow AF, Bowder P et al: Transverse plane motion at the ankle joint. Foot Ankle Int 2003;24:164. [PMID: 12627625]

Saunders JB, Inman VT, Eberhart HD: The major determinants in normal and pathologic gait. J Bone Joint Surg Am 1953;35:543. [PMID: 13069544]

Figure 9–5. Windlass mechanism. **A:** The plantar aponeurosis, which arises from the tubercle of the calcaneus, divides and inserts into the base of each of the proximal phalanges. **B:** Dorsiflexion of the metatarsophalangeal joints wraps the plantar aponeurosis around the metatarsal head, depressing the metatarsal heads and elevating the longitudinal arch. (Reproduced, with permission, from Mann RA, Coughlin MJ: *The Video Textbook of Foot and Ankle Surgery.* Medical Video Productions, 1991.)

DEFORMITIES OF THE FIRST TOE

Biomechanic Principles

The first metatarsophalangeal joint functions mainly as a weight-bearing structure and stabilizer of the medial aspect of the longitudinal arch. The static stability of the first metatarsophalangeal joint is provided by the collateral ligaments and the strong plantar plate, which consists of the plantar aponeurosis and the joint capsule. Added dynamic stability is provided by the abductor hallucis and adductor hallucis muscles, which insert along the medial and lateral sides of the metatarsal head, respectively. No muscle inserts into the metatarsal head per se, and therefore it is suspended in a sling of muscles and tendons. This allows the metatarsal head to be pushed in a medial or lateral direction, depending on the deviation of the proximal phalanx.

As previously discussed, the plantar aponeurosis forces the metatarsal heads into plantar flexion during the last third of the stance phase of the walking cycle. As a result, pressure that is present under the metatarsal heads is transferred to the toes, especially the hallux (see Figure 9–5). If this windlass mechanism for the hallux is lost as occurs in a bunion deformity, pressure is no longer transferred to the toes but remains beneath the metatarsal heads. Metatarsalgia results from this transfer of load, especially beneath the lesser metatarsal heads. The second metatarsal frequently bears the load because the weight-bearing ability of the first metatarsal is disrupted.

Any type of surgical procedure that disrupts this mechanism may result in the development of transfer lesions as well. This problem can be seen after the Keller arthroplasty, in which the base of the proximal phalanx is removed, or after prosthetic replacement of the first metatarsal joint. Metatarsal osteotomy with excessive shortening (more than 5–7 mm) or dorsiflexion of the first metatarsal may also cause this problem.

Normal Anatomy

The first metatarsophalangeal joint consists of the articulating surfaces of the metatarsal head and the base of the proximal phalanx. On the plantar aspect of the foot beneath the metatarsal head are the two sesamoid bones, which are embedded in the dual tendons of the flexor hallucis brevis and lie on either side of the crista. Medially and laterally, the collateral ligaments stabilize the metatarsophalangeal joint, and toward the plantar surface, they blend with the adductor and abductor hallucis tendons along the lateral and medial sides of the joint. Further toward the plantar surface, the sesamoids are stabilized by the firm attachment of the encapsulating plantar aponeurosis, which inserts into the base of the proximal phalanx. Plantar to the sesamoids passes the flexor hallucis longus tendon. Dorsally, the extensor hallucis longus tendon is stabilized by a medial and lateral hood mechanism similar to that present in the hand, and the extensor digitorum brevis muscle inserts into the proximal phalanx along the lateral aspect of the joint. Normal motion of the metatarsophalangeal joint consists of dorsiflexion and plantar flexion.

Hallux Valgus

The most common deformity of the metatarsophalangeal joint is hallux valgus or the so-called bunion deformity, which results from the lateral deviation of the proximal phalanx and the resultant medially directed pressure exerted against the metatarsal head. The medial eminence becomes prominent as the proximal phalanx drifts into a valgus position. Attenuation of the medial joint capsule and contracture of the lateral joint capsule occur. As the metatarsal head is pushed medially, the sesamoids, which are firmly anchored by the adductor hallucis tendon and transverse metatarsal ligament, slowly erode the crista. Eventually the sesamoids subluxate from underneath the first metatarsal, with the fibular sesamoid lying in the first web space. The extensor hallucis longus and flexor hallucis longus, which insert into the base of the distal phalanx, also deviate in a lateralward direction and contribute to the progressive hallux valgus deformity. As the deformity becomes more severe, both the extrinsic and intrinsic muscles lie lateral to the longitudinal axis of the first metatarsophalangeal joint, thereby further enhancing the deformity. As the deformity progresses, pronation of the great toe occurs. Attenuation of the weakest portion of the capsule (the dorsomedial aspect) allows the abductor hallucis tendon to slide beneath the metatarsal head and rotate the proximal phalanx into a position of pronation. More rapid progression of the deformity may occur in a small percentage of patients whose first metatarsocuneiform joint demonstrates a significant degree of instability.

Etiology of Hallux Valgus Deformity

Hallux valgus deformity occurs in women approximately 10 times more frequently than in men. The incidence is also significantly higher in persons who wear shoes than in those who do not. The conclusion can therefore be made that a major contributing cause of hallux valgus deformity is wearing tight pointed-toed shoes that women often wear. Other factors that may contribute to hallux valgus are congenital deformity or predisposition, severe flatfoot deformity, chronic tightness of the Achilles tendon, spasticity, hypermobility of the first metatarsocuneiform joint, and systemic disease such as rheumatoid arthritis (RA).

Clinical Findings

A. History

The clinical evaluation of hallux valgus deformity begins with a careful history to obtain the chief complaint, which may be primarily medial eminence pain, plantar first metatarsal or lesser metatarsal head pain, impingement upon the second toe, resultant deformities of the lesser toes, or the inability to wear certain shoes. The examiner should ask about factors that seem to aggravate the discomfort, the patient's occupation and level of athletic endeavors, and what type of shoe is most commonly worn.

B. Physical Examination

The physical examination starts with the patient in a standing position to observe the degree of deformity of the great toe and lesser toes. The overall posture of the foot is noted. The patient's gait is observed, looking for evidence of abnormal ground contact or early heel rise, which would indicate possible tightness of the Achilles tendon. In the seated position, the ROM of the ankle, subtalar, transverse tarsal, and metatarsophalangeal joints is noted. The neurovascular status of the foot is carefully assessed, noting venous stasis changes. Doppler studies are obtained if there is any question regarding the circulatory status of the foot. The plantar aspect of the foot is examined for abnormal callus formation, particularly beneath the metatarsal head and along the medial aspect of the great toe.

The motion of the first metatarsophalangeal joint is carefully observed in its deformed position and after the toe is carefully brought back toward normal alignment. Restriction of motion gives the clinician insight into the degree of surgical correction that can be obtained at the joint without impairing motion of the joint. The first metatarsocuneiform joint is examined for hypermobility by moving it in a dorsomedial and plantolateral direction.

C. Imaging Studies

The radiographic evaluation consists of weight-bearing anteroposterior, lateral, and oblique radiographs. From these radiographs, the following measurements are made:

1. The hallux valgus angle is the angle created by the intersection of the lines that longitudinally bisect the proximal phalanx and first metatarsal. A normal angle is less than 15 degrees (Figure 9–6A).
2. The intermetatarsal angle is defined as the angle created by the intersection of the lines bisecting the first and second metatarsal shafts. This angle should be less than 9 degrees.
3. The distal metatarsal articular angle measures the relationship of the distal articulating surface of the first metatarsal to the long axis of the metatarsal. Normally there is less than 10 degrees of lateral deviation (Figure 9–6B).
4. A determination is made as to whether or not the first metatarsophalangeal joint is congruent or incongruent. A congruent joint is one in which no lateral subluxation of the proximal phalanx occurs on the metatarsal head; an incongruent joint is one in which lateral subluxation of the proximal phalanx on the metatarsal head does occur (Figure 9–7).
5. The shape of the metatarsocuneiform joint is observed, looking for evidence of excessive medial deviation of this articulation. This observation alerts the examiner to the fact that hypermobility may be present.
6. The presence of arthrosis of the metatarsophalangeal joint is evaluated, as characterized by narrowing or osteophyte formation about the joint.
7. The size of the medial eminence is measured by a line drawn down the medial aspect of the first metatarsal shaft.
8. The presence of a hallux valgus interphalangeus is characterized by lateral deviation of the proximal or distal phalanx, or both, in relation to a line drawn across the base of the proximal phalanx. Normal is considered up to approximately 10 degrees of lateral deviation.

Treatment

A. Nonoperative Treatment

The patient should be encouraged to wear shoes of adequate size and shape. This simple form of management may relieve most symptoms.

A variety of pads are available to address symptoms that occur because of the bunion deformity. Pads may be placed in the first web space or over the median eminence to help take pressure off a painful median eminence. Pads are also available that can be placed underneath the metatarsal heads to take pressure off painful calluses or sesamoids.

If after adequate conservative management the patient continues to have discomfort, surgical intervention may be considered. Surgery is not performed for cosmetic reasons or to allow patients to wear fashionable shoes, but rather to correct a symptomatic structural deformity.

Juvenile hallux valgus deformity presents a significant problem in management, but as a general rule, conservative management should be continued until

A

B

Figure 9–6. Radiologic evaluation. **A:** Hallux valgus (HV) and intermetatarsal (IM) angles. **B:** Distal metatarsal articular angle (DMAA = 27). (Reproduced, with permission, from Mann RA, Coughlin MJ: *The Video Textbook of Foot and Ankle Surgery.* Medical Video Productions, 1991.)

growth is completed, after which surgery may be considered. Extra care must be taken into consideration in the juvenile population where cosmetic appearance may play a greater role in the patient's or parents' desire for surgery.

Hallux valgus surgery is generally contraindicated in high-performance athletes or dancers until they are no longer able to perform at the level necessary to continue in their vocation or avocation. Premature surgery in these individuals may diminish their special abilities.

B. Surgical Treatment

1. Algorithm for surgical treatment—If surgery is being considered, the patient's chief complaint, the physical findings, and the radiographic measurements must be correlated to enable the surgeon to select the best procedure. No single procedure succeeds for all

hallux valgus deformities, and careful preoperative planning is essential.

The following factors need to be considered in the decision-making process:

1. patient's chief complaint;

2. physical findings;

3. degree of hallux valgus and intermetatarsal angle;

4. distal metatarsal articular angle;

5. congruency or incongruency of the metatarsophalangeal joint;

6. presence of arthrosis of the joint;

7. degree of pronation of the hallux;

8. age of the patient;

9. circulatory status; and

10. patient expectations for outcome of operation.

Figure 9–7. **Left:** Congruent joint. **Right:** Incongruent joint. (Reproduced, with permission, from Mann RA, Coughlin MJ: *The Video Textbook of Foot and Ankle Surgery.* Medical Video Productions, 1991.)

The algorithm in Figure 9–8 divides hallux valgus deformities into three main groups: those with a congruent joint, those with an incongruent joint, and those associated with degenerative joint disease. The algorithm lists the operative procedure that may best correct the deformity within each classification. Although no one scheme is all inclusive, this algorithm is helpful in organizing the treatment plan.

In using this algorithm, the first question to ask is if the deformity is congruent or incongruent. A congruent metatarsophalangeal joint implies that the goal is mainly treatment of an enlarged medial eminence, and little or no correction of the stable metatarsophalangeal is required. For the congruent joint, a chevron procedure or Akin procedure with removal of the medial eminence usually results in satisfactory correction.

If the deformity is incongruent to the degree that the proximal phalanx is subluxed laterally on the metatarsal head, a procedure that moves the proximal phalanx back onto the metatarsal head is required. The procedure of choice depends on the severity of the deformity (see Figure 9–8).

If the first metatarsocuneiform joint is hypermobile, the distal soft-tissue procedure with a metatarsocuneiform arthrodesis should be considered. Generally, in the patient with severe hallux valgus deformity, greater than 45–50 degree hallux valgus angle, and degenerative joint disease, arthrodesis of the joint is indicated. If routine hallux valgus repair is attempted in the patient with advanced arthrosis, stiffness of the metatarsophalangeal joint frequently results. Use of a prosthetic replacement, as a general rule, does not produce a satisfactory long-term result, particularly in active individuals.

2. Surgical procedures—

a. Distal soft-tissue procedure—The distal soft-tissue procedure was previously referred to as the McBride procedure, which was first modified by DuVries and subsequently modified further and given its current designation. The procedure is indicated for mild hallux valgus deformity, usually with an intermetatarsal angle of less than 12–13 degrees and a hallux valgus deformity of less than 30 degrees. Within this range of deformity, a satisfactory outcome can usually be anticipated from this procedure.

Figure 9–8. Algorithm for hallux valgus deformities. STP = soft-tissue procedure; M-C = metatarsocuneiform; MPJ = metatarsal phalangeal joint. (Redrawn, with permission, from Mann RA, Coughlin MJ: *The Video Textbook of Foot and Ankle Surgery.* Medical Video Productions, 1991.)

The procedure requires releasing the soft-tissue contracture on the lateral side of the metatarsophalangeal joint, including the lateral joint capsule, the adductor hallucis tendon, and the transverse metatarsal ligament (Figure 9–9). On the medial side of the metatarsophalangeal joint, the medial eminence is removed 2–3 mm medial to the sagittal sulcus and in line with the medial aspect of the metatarsal shaft. The capsule on the medial side of the joint is plicated to hold the toe in correct alignment. Postoperatively, the patient is maintained in a firm compression dressing, which is changed on a weekly basis for 8 weeks. During this period, the patient is permitted to ambulate in a postoperative shoe.

The most common complication consists of recurrence of the deformity, usually because the deformity was too severe to be corrected by the procedure. In these cases, a metatarsal osteotomy added to the distal soft-tissue procedure completes the correction.

Hallux varus deformity is a medial deviation of the proximal phalanx on the metatarsal head, a complication that may occur in approximately 5–7% of cases. This deformity is usually a result of excessive excision of the medial eminence or fibular sesamoidectomy, which causes joint instability. Occasionally, the medial joint capsule is overplicated or the lateral joint capsule fails to attain adequate strength. Mild hallux varus deformity, up to 7–10 degrees, usually is of no clinical significance unless the joint is also hyperextended.

Figure 9–9. Distal soft-tissue procedure. **A:** The adductor tendon inserts into the lateral aspect of the fibular sesamoid and into the base of the proximal phalanx. **B:** The adductor tendon was removed from its insertion into the lateral side of the fibular sesamoid and base of the proximal phalanx. **C:** The transverse metatarsal ligament is passed from the second metatarsal into the fibular sesamoid. **D:** The transverse metatarsal ligament was transected. **E:** The three contracted structures on the lateral side of the metatarsophalangeal joint were released. **F:** The medial capsular incision begins 2–3 mm proximal to the base of the proximal phalanx, and a flap of tissue measuring 3–8 mm is removed. **G:** The medial eminence is exposed by creating a flap of capsule that is based proximally and plantarward. **H:** The medial eminence is removed in line with the medial aspect of the first metatarsal. **I:** The postoperative dressings are critical. Note that the metatarsal heads are firmly bound with the gauze, and the great toe is rotated so as to keep the sesamoids realigned beneath the metatarsal head. This necessitates dressing the right great toe in a counterclockwise direction and the left great toe in a clockwise direction when one is standing at the foot of the bed. (Reproduced, with permission, from Mann RA, Coughlin MJ: *The Video Textbook of Foot and Ankle Surgery.* Medical Video Productions, 1991.)

b. Distal soft-tissue procedure with proximal metatarsal osteotomy—Addition of the proximal metatarsal osteotomy to the distal soft-tissue procedure significantly expands the capability of this procedure to correct hallux valgus deformity. If the intermetatarsal angle exceeds 13 degrees, the degree of deformity between the first and second metatarsal prevents adequate correction of alignment of the metatarsophalangeal joint with the distal soft-tissue procedure alone. Realignment of the fixed bony deformity present between the first and second metatarsals permits the combined procedure to be used for deformities with up to 50 degrees of hallux valgus and a 25-degree intermetatarsal angle.

In carrying out this operative procedure, the distal soft-tissue procedure is performed as described earlier. The metatarsal osteotomy is carried out through a third incision, which is centered over the dorsal aspect of the base of the metatarsal shaft. The most commonly used osteotomy is a crescentic-shaped osteotomy whose concavity is directed proximally (Figure 9–10). This enables the surgeon to rotate the metatarsal head laterally as the metatarsocuneiform joint is pushed in a medialward direction. This usually results in approximately 2–3 mm of lateral displacement of the osteotomy site. Stabilization is carried out with a screw, which passes from distal to proximal. Other types of osteotomies are used to realign the first metatarsal, including oblique, chevron-shaped, and closing-wedge osteotomies.

Postoperatively, the treatment is the same as for the distal soft-tissue procedure, with 8 weeks of dressing changes and immobilization in a postoperative shoe. As a general rule, cast immobilization is not necessary.

The long-term postoperative results following the distal soft-tissue procedure with proximal osteotomy result in greater than 90% patient satisfaction. The addition of the osteotomy does create an increased risk of complications, but is reported to be uniformly low. Dorsiflexion of the osteotomy site may occur but is usually not of clinical significance. Nonunion of the osteotomy may develop in 1% of cases. Excessive lateral displacement of the metatarsal head can result in hallux varus deformity, which is more resistant to treatment than when osteotomy is not included.

c. Chevron osteotomy—The chevron osteotomy is usually indicated for hallux valgus deformity of less than 30 degrees, with an intermetatarsal angle of less than 12 degrees. The distal metatarsal articular angle should not be more than 12 degrees, or complete correction will not be obtained. The operative procedure is based on lateral translation of the metatarsal head, along with plication of the medial joint capsule. The joint is approached surgically through a medial incision, the capsule opened, and the medial eminence removed. A chevron-shaped cut with the apex based distally is carried out and translated laterally approxi-

Figure 9–10. The osteotomy site is reduced by pushing the proximal fragment medially with a small freer while pushing the metatarsal head laterally. This locks the lateral side of the osteotomy site so the internal fixation can be inserted. (Reproduced, with permission, from Mann RA, Coughlin MJ: *The Video Textbook of Foot and Ankle Surgery.* Medical Video Productions, 1991.)

mately 3–4 mm. The medial bony prominence created by the shift of the metatarsal head is excised and the medial joint capsule plicated. The osteotomy site is fixed with a pin or a screw (Figure 9–11).

Postoperatively, the foot is firmly bandaged for 6–8 weeks, and the patient is permitted to ambulate in a postoperative shoe. If a pin was used for fixation, it is removed after 4 weeks.

Uniformly good results, short and long term, are reported following a chevron procedure. In addition, more than 10-year follow-up showed consistent improvement with time. There was no difference between patients younger and older than 50 years; patients had equally positive outcomes. If it is used to correct a deformity that is too severe, the outcome may be unsuccessful. The most serious complication, occurring in 1–2% of cases, is avascular necrosis of the metatarsal head, which is probably the result of extensive stripping of the soft tissue surrounding the head. As with any type of osteotomy, the distal fragment is capable of migrating either too far laterally or medially, giving rise either to hallux varus deformity or recurrent hallux valgus deformity. Occasionally, arthrofibrosis of the joint is noted, resulting in significant joint stiffness.

A

B

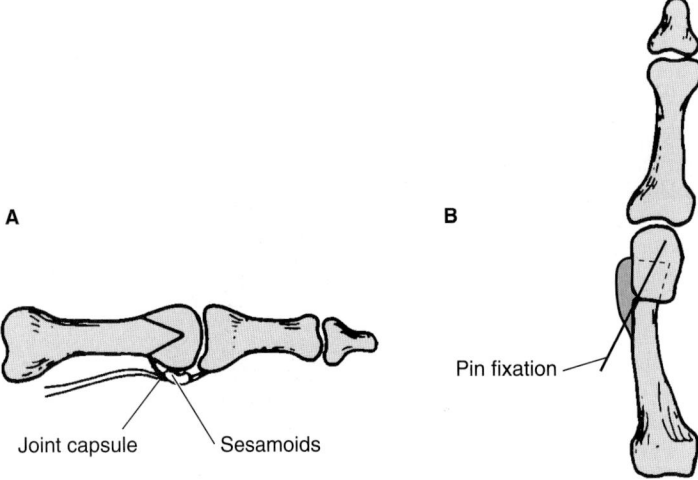

Joint capsule   Sesamoids

Pin fixation

Figure 9–11. Chevron procedure.
A: The apex of the chevron osteotomy
starts in the center of the metatarsal
head and is brought proximally. The
plantar aspect of the line of the osteotomy should be proximal to the
joint capsule, thereby avoiding the
sesamoid bones. **B:** The osteotomy
site is displaced laterally 20–30% of
the width of the shaft. (Reproduced,
with permission, from Mann RA, Coughlin
MJ: *The Video Textbook of Foot and Ankle
Surgery.* Medical Video Productions, 1991.)

d. Akin procedure—The Akin procedure consists of
a medial closing-wedge osteotomy at the base of the
proximal phalanx. This procedure is used along with
simple excision of the median eminence or with a chevron procedure to correct a hallux valgus deformity with
a congruent joint. The Akin procedure is indicated for
a hallux valgus deformity of less than 25 degrees, with
an intermetatarsal angle of 12 degrees or less.

The operative procedure consists of a medial approach
to the base of the proximal phalanx and the median eminence. After removing the median eminence in line with
the metatarsal, a wedge of bone is removed from the
medial aspect of the proximal phalanx. The osteotomy is
closed down and stabilized internally with sutures or
wires, or externally with a Kirschner wire (K-wire). Dressings are applied for 6–8 weeks postoperatively.

e. Keller procedure—The Keller procedure is reserved
for the older, less active patient, in a patient prone to skin
problems, or in the case of an arthritic joint. This procedure is contraindicated in an active person.

The procedure consists of removal of the base of the
proximal phalanx, which decompresses the metatarsophalangeal joint, and excision of the medial eminence. An
attempt is made to reapproximate the intrinsic muscles
that were detached by placing them into the remaining
stump of bone (Figure 9–12). As a rule, a longitudinal pin
is used to stabilize the operative site for approximately 4
weeks. Postoperatively, the patient is permitted to ambulate in a postoperative shoe, and dressings are changed for
approximately 6 weeks.

Results in the older (more than 65 years) patient with
low functional demand are satisfactory. If the procedure
is used in a younger patient, a certain degree of instability and loss of weight bearing by the first metatarsophalangeal joint occurs because the base of the proximal

phalanx was removed. There is significant loss of foot
function, and a transfer lesion may develop beneath the
second metatarsal head because the great toe no longer
carries adequate weight. The metatarsophalangeal joint
often becomes cocked upward and into varus.

f. Arthrodesis of the first metatarsophalangeal joint—
Arthrodesis of the first metatarsophalangeal joint is indicated in the patient with hallux valgus who also has
advanced degenerative arthrosis of the joint, or as a salvage
procedure following a previously failed surgical attempt to
realign the metatarsophalangeal joint. The procedure is
also indicated in the patient with advanced hallux valgus
deformity that cannot be corrected by the previously
described procedures. Hallux valgus deformity in which
the proximal phalanx is subluxed more than 50% of the
metatarsal head or one with a significant degree of stiffness about the metatarsophalangeal joint should be considered for fusion.

The arthrodesis is carried out by creating two flat
surfaces or a ball-and-socket type of configuration.
The arthrodesis site is stabilized with an interfragmentary screw and plate or Steinmann pins if the bone
stock is poor. The position of the arthrodesis is critical. The joint should be placed in 15–20 degrees of
valgus and 10–15 degrees of dorsiflexion in relation to
the ground or the plantar aspect of the foot. In relation to the first metatarsal shaft, which is inclined
plantarward approximately 15 degrees, it should be in
approximately 30 degrees of dorsiflexion (Figure 9–
13). Any pronation that is present must also be corrected at the same time.

The patient must wear a postoperative shoe until
arthrodesis occurs in 10–12 weeks. The unreliable
patient should be treated in a short leg walking cast
until fusion occurs.

Figure 9–12. Keller procedure. **A:** The medial eminence is removed in line with the medial aspect of the metatarsal shaft. The proximal third of the proximal phalanx is removed. **B:** An attempt is made to reapproximate the plantar and medial capsular structures to the remaining base of the proximal phalanx. (Reproduced, with permission, from Mann RA, Coughlin MJ: *The Video Textbook of Foot and Ankle Surgery.* Medical Video Productions, 1991.)

The main complication associated with arthrodesis of the first metatarsophalangeal joint is malposition. If the toe is not placed into adequate dorsiflexion or valgus, excessive stress occurs against the interphalangeal joint, which may result in a painful arthritic condition of the joint. The fusion rate is approximately 95%. Occasionally, the degree of valgus and dorsiflexion is correct but the toe is left in a pronated position, which results in pressure along the medial side of the interphalangeal joint and possible discomfort.

The patient's gait following arthrodesis of the first metatarsophalangeal joint in proper alignment is most satisfactory. These patients are able to roll over the fusion site and have little or no difficulty carrying out everyday activities. Squatting is the only activity that is difficult because the toe must be in full dorsiflexion when this activity is carried out. Patients are able to return to most types of athletic activities, although at a somewhat slower pace.

Hallux Rigidus

A. GENERAL CONSIDERATIONS

Hallux rigidus or first metatarsophalangeal joint arthritis is a relatively common problem, often affecting people at a much younger age than arthritis of other joints. Hallux rigidus is seen in patients from their 30s onward. The reason why arthritis of this joint is seen in younger patients is unclear but may be associated with an unrecognized chondral injury to the metatarsal head. It is also associated with hallux valgus interphalangeus, bilateral involvement in those with a family history, and female gender. Hallux rigidus is not associated with elevatus, first ray hypermobility, a long first metatarsal, Achilles tightness, abnormal foot posture, symptomatic hallux valgus, adolescent onset, shoe wear, or occupation.

Figure 9–13. Arthrodesis of the first metatarsophalangeal joint. **A:** The joint is placed into approximately 15 degrees of valgus. **B:** The joint is placed into approximately 10–15 degrees of dorsiflexion in relation to the floor, which is approximately 25–30 degrees of dorsiflexion in relation to the first metatarsal shaft. (Reproduced, with permission, from Mann RA, Coughlin MJ: *The Video Textbook of Foot and Ankle Surgery.* Medical Video Productions, 1991.)

B. CLINICAL FINDINGS

Patients present with complaints of joint stiffness and pain with dorsiflexion of the joint. The symptoms are worse with increased physical activities. Patients also complain of a painful dorsal prominence over the metatarsal neck that makes shoe wear uncomfortable. Radiographs show varying degrees of joint space narrowing and, invariably, a large osteophyte on the dorsal aspect of the metatarsal neck.

C. CONSERVATIVE TREATMENT

Conservative treatment consists of nonsteroidal anti-inflammatories (NSAIDs) and wearing a stiff-soled shoe with a deep toe box. In older (more than 60 years), sedentary patients, these measures are usually adequate. In more active individuals, however, surgical treatment is usually indicated.

D. SURGICAL TREATMENT

Several surgical treatment methods are available for treating hallux rigidus. Resection of the dorsal bone spur, known as cheilectomy, is efficacious and the least intrusive surgical option. Approximately 25% of the dorsal aspect of the metatarsal head is removed along with the bone spur, and a thorough synovectomy of the joint is performed. Postoperatively, patients regain up to 50% of their dorsiflexion and have improvement of their total motion. More than 90% of patients have improvement of pain and increased physical abilities. This procedure is less likely to have a favorable outcome on joints with advanced arthritis.

A resection arthroplasty (Keller procedure) can be used on older, less active patients, but has a high rate of complications, as previously discussed. Prosthetic replacement of the arthritic first metatarsophalangeal joint can be used in older, lower demand patients but has high rates of failure in younger, more active individuals.

First metatarsophalangeal joint arthrodesis provides predictable pain relief and longevity for advanced arthritis. The drawback is that of lost motion at the joint. However, patients can remain quite active with a first metatarsophalangeal joint fusion as described previously.

Sesamoid Disorders

A. GENERAL CONSIDERATIONS

The two sesamoid bones on the plantar aspect of the first metatarsophalangeal joint can become painful for a variety of reasons. Fractures, osteonecrosis, arthritis, and subluxation can affect these small bones. Often they can become painful for no clear reason, a condition referred to as sesamoiditis.

B. CLINICAL FINDINGS

The patient with a painful sesamoid complains of discomfort on the plantar aspect of the foot, directly under the affected bone. The pain is worse with weight-bearing activities. The history may be significant for a trauma to the toe causing a fracture, but most commonly, the pain has an insidious onset.

C. PHYSICAL EXAMINATION

The painful sesamoid is determined by direct palpation. Postural abnormalities of the foot that may be contributing to the condition are evaluated. For example, hallux valgus deformity may cause a subluxation of the sesamoid from its normal articulation with the plantar aspect of the metatarsal head, causing pain.

D. RADIOGRAPHIC FINDINGS

Radiographs of the foot are taken, including a skyline or sesamoid view, which is a tangential view of the sesamoid metatarsal head articulation. Abnormalities may be seen, such as subluxation of the sesamoids in the case of hallux valgus, fragmentation as seen in osteonecrosis, or joint space narrowing as seen in the case of arthritis. Displaced fractures are easy to determine, but nondisplaced fractures may be difficult to distinguish from a bipartite sesamoid that is a normal finding. A bone scan may be helpful in the case of normal radiographs to diagnose osteonecrosis or sesamoiditis.

E. TREATMENT

If an acute injury has occurred and radiographs are consistent with a fracture of the sesamoid, a short leg walking cast is placed. If symptoms came on gradually, a stiff-soled shoe is used, with a soft pad placed just proximal to the sesamoids to take the pressure off the involved area. Usually the majority of symptoms resolve in a matter of weeks, although some degree of discomfort may persist for several months. If 6–12 months of conservative treatment does not relieved the symptoms, the affected sesamoid can be removed, which relieves the pain.

Coughlin MJ, Shurnas PS: Hallux rigidus: Demographics, etiology, and radiographic assessment. Foot Ankle Int 2003;24:731. [PMID: 14524514]

Coughlin MJ, Shurnas PS: Hallux rigidus: Grading and long-term results of operative treatment. J Bone Joint Surg Am 2005;85:2072. [PMID: 14630834]

Machacek F, Easley ME, Gruber F et al: Salvage of the failed Keller resection arthroplasty. J Bone Joint Surg 2005;87A(Suppl):86. [PMID: 15743850]

Schneider W, Aigner N, Pinggera O et al: Chevron osteotomy in hallux valgus. Ten-year results of 112 cases. J Bone Joint Surg 2004;86B:1016. [PMID: 15446530]

Veri JP, Pirani SP, Claridge R: Crescentic proximal metatarsal osteotomy for moderate to severe hallux valgus: A mean 12.2 year follow-up study. Foot Ankle Int 2001;22:817. [PMID: 11642533]

DEFORMITIES OF THE LESSER TOES

The most common problems involving the four lesser toes include mallet toe, hammer toe, clawtoe, and hard and soft corns. More proximally, at the metatarsophalangeal joint, subluxation or dislocation of the joint may occur. All of these conditions alter the shape of the foot and at times make wearing shoes difficult. Furthermore, in the patient with an insensitive foot, ulcerations may form over the bony prominences of these deformities.

The most common cause of clawtoe, hammer toe, and mallet toe deformities are the long-term use of tightly fitting shoe wear. These deformities may also result from intrinsic or extrinsic factors, including inflammatory arthritis, trauma, congenital abnormalities, or neuromuscular disorders. Additional predisposing factors are a wide foot or an abnormally long second ray and occasionally postural abnormalities of the foot. Identifying the etiology is important to help treat the deformity properly.

Anatomy & Pathophysiologic Findings

The metatarsophalangeal joint is stabilized on the plantar aspect by a consolidation of the plantar capsule and plantar aponeurosis (plantar plate) and medially and laterally by the collateral ligaments. Plantar flexion of the metatarsophalangeal joint is affected by the intrinsic muscles, the interossei, and lumbricals, whose lines of action pass plantarward to the axis of the metatarsophalangeal joint. The flexor digitorum brevis and flexor digitorum longus muscles produce plantar flexion of the proximal interphalangeal and distal interphalangeal joints, respectively. On the dorsal aspect of the joint, the extensor digitorum longus and brevis tendons and the extensor hood or sling constitute the extensor mechanism. This mechanism causes dorsiflexion of the metatarsophalangeal joint and can cause extension of the distal interphalangeal and proximal interphalangeal joints if the proximal phalanx is in a neutral or plantarflexed position. When the metatarsophalangeal joint is hyperextended, the ability of the extensor hood to extend the distal interphalangeal and proximal interphalangeal joints is significantly diminished. Chronic hyperextension of the metatarsophalangeal joint eventually leads to fixed flexion deformities at the interphalangeal joints. As a general rule, a fixed deformity is significantly more bothersome to the patient than a flexible deformity.

1. Mallet Toe Deformity

A mallet toe is a flexion deformity of the distal interphalangeal joint. It may be a fixed or flexible deformity. In general, the deformity involves the second toe, usually because of its excessive length in relation to the adjacent toes.

Clinical Findings

A. SYMPTOMS AND SIGNS

A mallet toe tends to cause pain over the dorsal aspect of the distal interphalangeal joint or occasionally at the tip of the toe from striking the ground. This may result in a callus or, in cases associated with neuropathy, an ulceration. Occasionally, the nail itself is deformed if the pressure was chronic.

The initial physical examination is carried out with the patient standing to evaluate the severity of the deformity and ascertain whether deformities are present in other toes. The interphalangeal joint is then carefully palpated to determine whether the deformity is fixed or flexible. If the distal interphalangeal joint is flexible, plantar flexion of the ankle permits the joint to be straightened out completely. As the ankle joint is brought into dorsiflexion, however, the deformity recurs. In the case of a fixed deformity, ankle motion does not affect the deformity.

B. IMAGING STUDIES

Radiographic evaluation confirms the clinical findings of the flexion deformity of the distal interphalangeal joint.

Treatment

A. CONSERVATIVE MANAGEMENT

The patient should be encouraged to obtain a shoe with a wide enough toe box to accommodate the deformed toe. An extra-depth shoe may be necessary if the deformity is too severe. If the main complaint is pain under the tip of the toe, a small pad can be placed underneath the toe to keep it from striking the ground, or lamb's wool can be wrapped around the toe.

B. SURGICAL TREATMENT

Surgical treatment of a flexible mallet toe deformity requires release of the flexor digitorum longus tendon, which is carried out under local anesthesia by incising the tendon on the plantar aspect of the toe at the level of the middle phalanx. This usually results in resolution of the problem.

A fixed mallet toe deformity requires a condylectomy, which is carried out through an elliptical incision made over the dorsal aspect of the distal interphalangeal joint. Along with the ellipse of skin, the extensor tendon is excised, the collateral ligaments released, and the distal portion of the middle phalanx removed. The distal phalanx is reduced and held in place either with a 0.045-in. K-wire for 4 weeks or with Telfa bolsters (Figure 9–14).

Good results may be expected following this procedure. The most common complication occurs because a contracture of the flexor digitorum longus tendon was not appreciated prior to surgery or because insufficient bone was removed from the middle phalanx to decompress the deformity adequately.

2. Hammer Toe Deformity

A hammer toe deformity is a plantar flexion deformity of the proximal interphalangeal joint, which may either be fixed or flexible. It is frequently associated with varying degrees of hyperextension of the metatarsophalangeal joint. A flexion deformity of the distal interphalangeal joint usually accompanies a hammer toe, but an extension deformity is occasionally observed.

Clinical Findings

A. Symptoms and Signs

Clinical evaluation is similar to that of a mallet toe deformity, with care taken to distinguish between a fixed or flexible deformity. Also, the metatarsophalangeal joints of each toe are evaluated for hyperextension deformities. Callus formation or even an ulcer may be present over the extensor surface of the proximal interphalangeal joint. Metatarsophalangeal joint correction may be necessary to alleviate the hammer toe. Similarly, a significant hallux valgus deformity that is impinging on the second toe may require treatment to make room for correction of the hammer toe.

B. Imaging Studies

Radiographs help in the evaluation of proximal interphalangeal flexion deformity, hyperextension deformity at the metatarsophalangeal joint, and hallux valgus deformity. It is critical that all joints be assessed when hammer toe correction is being considered.

Treatment

A. Conservative Management

The conservative management of hammer toe deformities is foremost that of proper shoe wear, as previously emphasized. In addition, toe sleeves are available that pad the painful callus.

Conservative management becomes more difficult if a significant fixed deformity is present, particularly if it is associated with extension of the metatarsophalangeal joint or a significant hallux valgus deformity.

B. Surgical Treatment

Surgical decision making regarding the hammer toe hinges on whether (1) the deformity is fixed or flexible, (2) any deformity of the metatarsophalangeal joint needs to be corrected concomitantly, and (3) a space must be created for the toe by correcting the hallux valgus deformity.

1. Flexible hammer toe deformity—A flexible hammer toe deformity is corrected with the Girdlestone flexor tendon transfer. In this procedure, the long flexor tendon is harvested from the plantar aspect of the foot, brought up on either side of the extensor hood mechanism, and sutured into the extensor hood with the toe held in approximately 5 degrees of plantar flexion and the ankle in plantar flexion (Figure 9–15). This causes the long flexor tendon to act as an extensor of the interphalangeal joints and a flexor of the metatarsophalangeal joint, thereby correcting the deformity. A soft

A   **B**

Figure 9–14. Mallet toe repair. **A:** Resection of condyles of the middle phalanx. **B:** Intramedullary K-wire fixation. (Reproduced, with permission, from Mann RA, Coughlin MJ: *The Video Textbook of Foot and Ankle Surgery.* Medical Video Productions, 1991.)

Figure 9–15. Flexor tendon transfer for flexible hammer toe deformity. **A:** Lateral view of lesser toe. **B:** The long flexor is detached from its insertion and delivered through the proximal plantar wound. It is split longitudinally along the median raphe. **C:** Each limb is transferred dorsally on either side of the proximal phalanx and secured on the dorsal aspect. **D:** Dorsal view after tendon transfer. **E:** Cross section showing flexor digitorum longus tendon in sheath. (Reproduced, with permission, from Mann RA, Coughlin MJ: *The Video Textbook of Foot and Ankle Surgery.* Medical Video Productions, 1991.)

dressing is applied and a postoperative shoe is worn for 4 weeks, after which ambulation is allowed.

2. Fixed hammer toe deformity—The DuVries proximal phalangeal condylectomy is used for the fixed deformity. This procedure, which is identical to that described for treatment of the mallet toe deformity, involves the proximal interphalangeal joint instead of the distal interphalangeal joint (Figure 9–16). Clinical results show a majority of patients were satisfied and a low risk of recurrence of deformity.

3. Complications—The main complication observed with either procedure is inadequate correction of the deformity, usually because of failure to appreciate a contracture of the flexor digitorum longus tendon at the time of surgery.

A

B

Figure 9–16. Fixed hammer toe repair. **A:** Resection of the head of the proximal phalanx. **B:** Intramedullary K-wire fixation. (Reproduced, with permission, from Mann RA, Coughlin MJ: *The Video Textbook of Foot and Ankle Surgery.* Medical Video Productions, 1991.)

3. Clawtoe Deformity

Clawtoe deformity involves both the metatarsophalangeal and interphalangeal joints and may be flexible or fixed. Clawtoe deformity can be disabling, particularly in the patient with a neuromuscular disorder. This deformity is characterized by marked dorsiflexion of the metatarsophalangeal joint, which results in pain secondary to chafing over the interphalangeal joints against the shoe and pain beneath the metatarsal heads because the metatarsal heads are forced into plantar flexion. In contrast to hammer toe or mallet toe deformities, which usually involve a single toe, clawtoe deformity usually involves all of the lesser toes. An associated deformity of the great toe may occur as well.

Clinical Findings

A. SYMPTOMS AND SIGNS

The clinical evaluation is similar to that described for the previous lesser toe deformities. The metatarsal heads are palpated because the fat pad may be displaced distally and the skin beneath the metatarsal heads may be atrophic. Callosities may be present on the extensor surface of the proximal interphalangeal joints and on the plantar aspect of the metatarsophalangeal joints.

B. IMAGING STUDIES

Radiographs demonstrate the deformity, which is present at the metatarsophalangeal and interphalangeal joints. The posture of the entire foot needs to be evaluated, looking for the presence of a cavus-type foot deformity,

characterized by increased dorsiflexion pitch of the calcaneus and increased plantar flexion of the first metatarsal.

Treatment

A. CONSERVATIVE MANAGEMENT

An extra-depth shoe reduces the pressure on the lesser toes, and arch supports placed under the metatarsal head area may relieve the pain. Flexible mild deformities can be treated with shoe inserts placed immediately proximal to the metatarsophalangeal joints. These can have the effect of balancing the extensors and flexors of the toes.

B. SURGICAL TREATMENT

The type of operative intervention depends upon the nature of the deformity. Flexible deformities can be treated with the Girdlestone flexor tendon transfer. In addition, however, the extensor tendons usually must be lengthened to permit correction of the metatarsophalangeal joints to neutral plantar flexion.

A concomitant fixed contracture of the proximal interphalangeal joint requires a DuVries proximal phalangeal condylectomy as well as the Girdlestone tendon transfer procedure. Furthermore, release of the dorsal capsule, collateral ligaments, and extensor tendon is performed at the metatarsophalangeal joint. Postoperative management for the patient with clawtoe deformity is the same as discussed earlier for hammer toe deformity.

Following this surgical procedure no active motion of the toes occurs. The toes are usually well aligned in a plantigrade position. The marked deformity of the proximal interphalangeal joints is relieved so they no longer strike the top of the shoe. The main problems that can occur after surgery are (1) failure to correct a fixed hammer toe deformity adequately by use of the tendon transfer and (2) failure to release the fixed deformity adequately at the metatarsophalangeal joint, resulting in recurrence of the deformity.

4. Hard Corn & Soft Corn (Clavus Durum & Clavus Mollum)

A corn is a keratotic lesion that forms over a bony prominence on the lesser toes because of excessive pressure on the skin. A hard corn occurs most commonly over the dorsal and lateral aspect of the fifth toe, usually over the lateral condyle of the proximal phalanx. A soft corn represents a keratotic lesion in a web space and is so named because maceration results from moisture between the toes. The soft corn may occur anywhere along the toe where a bony excrescence is present and frequently occurs in the fourth web space between the base of the proximal phalanx of the fourth toe and the medial condyle of the head of the proximal phalanx of the fifth toe. At times, an ulceration may occur because of the extent of the maceration.

Treatment

A. CONSERVATIVE MANAGEMENT

The main objective of conservative management is reducing pressure on the bony prominences. Footwear with a large toe box can relieve this pressure. Debridement or shaving of the lesion reduces pain. The procedure can frequently be carried out by younger patients without assistance but becomes increasingly difficult in older individuals because of decreasing flexibility and poor eyesight. Skin compromise, especially in the diabetic patient, must be avoided. At times, soft pads or lamb's wool can be placed around the toe to minimize pressure on the involved area, but the patient must wear a shoe with an adequate toe box to accommodate such modalities.

B. SURGICAL TREATMENT

1. Surgical treatment of the hard corn—The hard corn, over the fifth toe, is managed surgically by removing the distal portion of the proximal phalanx and occasionally the dorsolateral aspect of the proximal portion of the middle phalanx. The longitudinal incision is made over the dorsal aspect so the scar will not chafe against the shoe. The extensor tendon is split, the collateral ligaments cut, and the condyle exposed. With a bone cutter, the distal portion of the proximal phalanx is generously removed and the edges smoothed with a rongeur. Following closure, a compression dressing is applied for several days. The toe is taped to the adjacent fourth toe for 8 weeks. Long-term results show a high level of patient satisfaction and a low recurrence rate. Removal of excessive bone is the major complication, which causes the small toe to become too floppy, creating a nuisance for the patient.

2. Surgical treatment for the soft corn—Soft corns are treated surgically by making an incision over the lesion and using a small rongeur to remove the underlying bony excrescence. This is a simple procedure and almost invariably results in satisfactory resolution of the problem.

3. Syndactyly—Because the soft corn is caused by pressure on the skin, removal of the skin between the toes can resolve the problem. Syndactyly is a procedure by which the skin is removed between the fourth and fifth toes and the two toes are sutured together to eliminate the problem of a soft corn in the web space. Although the soft corn can usually be managed with a condylectomy, as described earlier, occasionally a great deal of maceration or ulceration precludes treating it only with a condylectomy. In these cases, syndactyly is indicated. Occasionally, a floppy fifth toe from previous surgery can be stabilized by syndactyly.

5. Subluxation & Dislocation of the Metatarsophalangeal Joint

Dorsal subluxation or dislocation of the metatarsophalangeal joint occurs because of weakening of the supporting plantar capsule and collateral ligament structures, which maintain the stability of the metatarsophalangeal joint. Secondary changes such as hammer toe may occur in the toe itself. Pain usually occurs either beneath the metatarsophalangeal joint or over the dorsal aspect of the toe as it strikes the top of the shoe.

Etiologic Findings

The most common cause of a subluxed or dislocated joint is probably a progressive hallux valgus deformity pressing against the second toe. Over time, subluxation and eventual dislocation of the second metatarsophalangeal joint can occur.

A nonspecific synovitis, isolated to the metatarsophalangeal joint and usually involving the second metatarsophalangeal joint, is the next most common cause. The clinical picture is one of generalized swelling about the metatarsophalangeal joint that subsides over a period of 3–6 months, followed by progressive subluxation and eventual dislocation of the joint. Occasionally, subluxation or dislocation of the metatarsophalangeal joint may result from trauma.

Arthritic conditions such as rheumatoid or psoriatic arthritis can cause subluxation or dislocation at multiple joints. Advanced neuromuscular disorders may cause severe subluxation of the metatarsophalangeal joint, but dislocation is unusual.

A variant of this condition results from attenuation of collateral ligaments on one side of the metatarsophalangeal joint. The cause may be idiopathic but occasionally may follow a steroid injection into the area. The metatarsophalangeal joint, instead of subluxing in a dorsalward direction, deviates medially or occasionally laterally, crossing over the adjacent toe. This again is most common in the second metatarsophalangeal joint. When the toe deviates in a medialward direction and crosses over the great toe, the patient may have difficulty wearing shoes.

Clinical Findings

A. SYMPTOMS AND SIGNS

Patients complain of pain on the dorsal and plantar aspects of the affected joint. They may note swelling as well and complain of an associated hammer toe or lateral deviation of the toe if present. The degree of deformity is evaluated with the patient in a standing and sitting position. The affected metatarsophalangeal joint is palpated for active synovitis, flexibility of the joint, and degree of subluxation.

The dorsal-plantar stability of the joint is evaluated by holding the proximal phalanx between the examiner's fingers and moving it dorsally and plantarward, similar to a Lachman test of the knee. If a significant hallux valgus deformity is associated with crossover of the second toe on the first toe, the hallux valgus requires evaluation.

B. IMAGING STUDIES

The radiographs of the foot reveal the extent of the subluxation or dislocation. The severity of the hallux valgus is evaluated, and changes about the articular surface of the joint are observed. In RA, multiple joint involvement is noted.

Treatment

A. CONSERVATIVE MANAGEMENT

Conservative management consists of using a shoe with a wide enough toe box to accommodate the deformity and prescribing a well-molded, soft orthotic device to relieve pressure on the metatarsal head. Unfortunately, this may raise the forefoot, causing impingement on the toe box area of the shoe and some discomfort. A series of cortisone injections into the affected joint may be performed. No more than three injections are given, and at least 1 month is allowed between injections. If the patient cannot be accommodated adequately with these modalities, surgical intervention may be indicated. A significant hallux valgus deformity indicates the need for correction to make a space for second toe correction. Failure to treat both problems results in recurrence.

B. SURGICAL TREATMENT

The subluxed metatarsophalangeal joint with a flexible hammer toe is treated by releasing the dorsal contracture of the extensor tendons and joint capsule, followed by a Girdlestone flexor tendon transfer, as previously described. This technique usually brings the toe into better alignment, although the patient loses some selective voluntary control of the toe, which is usually not of any significance. If a fixed hammer toe is present, a proximal phalanx condylectomy is added to the procedure.

The more severe complete dorsal dislocation of the metatarsophalangeal joint is a difficult surgical problem. In the past it was treated by an aggressive release of the dorsal joint capsule and collateral ligaments and a synovectomy of the metatarsophalangeal joint. The distal third of the metatarsal head is removed to decompress the joint. Accompanying hammer toe procedures are performed to correct the invariably present fixed hammer toe.

A longitudinal K-wire stabilizes the correction for 2 weeks. After pin removal, motion is started at the metatarsophalangeal joint. This procedure results in significant joint stiffness and possible resubluxation of the joint.

An osteotomy of the metatarsal neck is now used to treat dislocated or advanced subluxation of the metatarsophalangeal joint. An oblique osteotomy is performed, starting at the metatarsal neck and aimed proximally at a shallow angle to the metatarsal shaft, creating a long osteotomy site. Once the osteotomy is complete, the metatarsal head is allowed to slide proximally to the appropriate level that will allow the joint to assume a reduced position.

The amount of shortening is usually between 4.0 mm and 6.0 mm. The osteotomy is fixed with a single 2.5-mm or smaller diameter cortical screw. Accompanying hammer toe procedures are then performed if necessary. Good short-term results are noted with this procedure without the complication of joint stiffness as occurs with the previously described procedures. Common complications include plantar penetrating hardware and floating-toe deformity (extension contracture of the metatarsophalangeal joint causing the toe not to touch the ground).

Repair of the medially or laterally dislocated metatarsophalangeal joint can be a technically difficult problem. Satisfactory correction can be achieved with one of two techniques. A soft-tissue release of the joint capsule can be performed on the side to which the toe deviates, allowing realignment of the toe. Alternatively, a closing-wedge osteotomy at the base of the proximal phalanx can also achieve good realignment of the toe. Severe deformities can be corrected with an oblique metatarsal neck osteotomy, previously described for treatment of dorsally subluxated metatarsophalangeal joints. The technique is identical, although some soft-tissue balancing may need to be added to the procedure.

Coughlin MJ: Lesser toe abnormalities. Instr Course Lect 2003; 52:421. [PMID: 12690869]

Coughlin MJ, Kennedy MP: Operative repair of fourth and fifth toe corns. Foot Ankle Int 2003;24:147. [PMID: 12627623]

Dhukaram V, Hossain S, Sampath J et al: Correction of hammer toe with an extended release of the metatarsophalangeal joint. J Bone Joint Surg Br 2003;84:986. [PMID: 12358391]

Migues A, Slullitel G, Bilbao F et al: Floating-toe deformity as a complication of the Weil osteotomy. Foot Ankle Int 2004; 25:609. [PMID: 15563380]

Trnka HJ, Gebhard C, Muhlbauer M et al: The Weil osteotomy for treatment of dislocated lesser metatarsophalangeal joints: Good outcome in 21 patients with 42 osteotomies. Acta Orthop Scand 2002;73:190. [PMID: 12079018]

REGIONAL ANESTHESIA FOR FOOT & ANKLE DISORDERS

Regional anesthesia is becoming more commonly used because many foot and ankle procedures are performed in the outpatient setting. Most procedures below the ankle can be performed without general anesthesia, eliminating the hazards of central nervous system depression. Pain develops gradually as the anesthesia wears off, and the analgesic requirements of the patient are thereby reduced significantly. Efficacy, safety, and high patient satisfaction are demonstrated.

Digital Block

A. INDICATIONS

Digital block is suitable for procedures used in the toes, such as treatment of nail disorders, correction of hammer toe or mallet toe, tendon releases, and some meta-tarsophalangeal joint procedures.

B. TECHNIQUE

Short- and longer-term anesthesia is provided by digital block using a 1:1 mixture of 1% lidocaine hydrochloride and 0.25% bupivacaine. A short 25-gauge needle is used to inject approximately 1.5 mL on either side of the toe within the subcutaneous layer between the skin and deeper fascia. The needle is then passed toward the plantar aspect of the toe to anesthetize the digital nerves. Both sides of the toe should be anesthetized. Anesthesia should be administered before the operative site is prepared to allow approximately 15 minutes necessary for the block to take effect before starting a procedure.

Ankle Block

A. INDICATIONS

Ankle block anesthesia is commonly used for operations on the forefoot and midfoot, such as bunion procedures, neuroma excision, metatarsal osteotomies, and tarsometatarsal fusions. If more than one lesser toe procedure is being performed, an ankle block is preferred to multiple digital blocks. Ankle block anesthesia is not recommended for hindfoot or ankle procedures, such as hindfoot fusions or ankle arthroscopy.

B. TECHNIQUE

The successful ankle block must anesthetize the posterior tibial nerve, superficial branch of the deep peroneal nerve, sural nerve, saphenous nerve, and superficial peroneal nerve. The posterior tibial nerve requires a larger 3-cm, 22- or 25-gauge needle and approximately 7–10 mL of a 1:1 mixture of 1% lidocaine hydrochloride and 0.25% bupivacaine. The landmark for the posterior tibial nerve behind the malleolus is approximately two finger breadths proximal to the tip of the malleolus and along the medial border of the Achilles tendon (Figure 9–17). The needle is inserted perpendicular to the shaft of the tibia until the posterior cortex of the tibia is palpated with the tip of the needle. The needle is then withdrawn approximately 2 mm. Approximately 5 mL of anesthetic agent is injected into this area after aspiration is done to confirm that the needle is not in a vessel.

To anesthetize the deep peroneal nerve, the site of the injection is located by palpating the extensor hallucis and extensor digitorum longus tendons at the level of the navicular. The deep peroneal nerve lies just lateral to the dorsalis pedis artery. The 25-gauge needle is inserted and advanced to bone and then withdrawn 1–2 mm, aspiration is attempted, and approximately 5 mL of anesthetic is injected.

The saphenous nerve is identified one to two finger breadths proximal to the tip of the medial malleolus and just posterior to the saphenous vein. A 25-gauge needle is inserted and 5 mL of anesthetic injected.

The sural nerve is blocked approximately 1–1.5 cm distal to the tip of the lateral malleolus and can often be palpated in the subcutaneous fat. A 25-gauge needle is inserted and approximately 5 mL of anesthetic injected.

The superficial peroneal nerve branches are blocked starting two finger breadths proximal and anterior to the tip of the lateral malleolus, and the injection is carried out below the subcutaneous veins but above the long extensor tendons in a ring-type block. Approximately 5 mL of anesthetic agent is used. The anesthesia for ankle block takes effect within 15–20 minutes.

Popliteal Block

A. INDICATIONS

The popliteal block is used for major foot or ankle procedures. These include ankle arthrodesis, hindfoot arthrodesis, calcaneal osteotomy, tarsometatarsal arthrodesis, posterior tibial tendon reconstruction, and surgical treatment of calcaneal or ankle fractures. The popliteal block can be placed by the anesthesiologist or surgeon, and it can be used with general anesthesia, sedation, or as the sole anesthetic technique.

B. TECHNIQUE

The patient is placed in the lateral decubitus position with a pillow between the knees. The landmarks of the popliteal fossa are identified, using the horizontal popliteal skin crease that divides the fossa into superior and inferior quadrants (Figure 9–18). Approximately 7–8 cm superior to the popliteal skin crease and 1 cm lateral to the midline is where the common peroneal branch separates from the tibial branch of the sciatic nerve. A nerve stimulator is set at 3 mA to assist in locating the nerve. When a twitch is found, the stimulator is decreased until there is loss of twitch at 0.8 to 1.0 mA (Figure 9–19). Following aspiration, 30 mL of 0.5% bupivacaine with 1:200,000 epinephrine are slowly injected. The saphenous nerve can be infiltrated with 3–5 mL of 0.5% bupivacaine proximal to the ankle.

Delgado-Martinez AD, Marchal-Escalona JM: Supramalleolar ankle block anesthesia and ankle tourniquet for foot surgery. Foot Ankle Int 2001;22:836. [PMID: 11642537]

Jarrett GJ, Rongstad KM, Snyder M: Popliteal nerve block by surgeon in the lateral decubitus position. Foot Ankle Int 2004;25:37. [PMID: 14768963]

Provenzano DA, Viscusi ER, Adams SB Jr et al: Safety and efficacy of the popliteal fossa nerve block when utilized for foot and ankle surgery. Foot Ankle Int 2002;23:394. [PMID: 12043982]

METATARSALGIA

Metatarsalgia is a general term for pain arising from the metatarsal head region. The center of pressure during nor-

Figure 9–17. Anesthetic technique for ankle block. H: extensor hallucis longus tendon; T: tibialis anterior tendon; TP: tibialis posterior tendon. (Reproduced, with permission, from Delgado-Martinez AD, Marchal-Escalona JM: Supramalleolar ankle block anesthesia and ankle tourniquet for foot surgery. Foot Ankle Int 2001.)

mal gait is initially applied to the heel and progresses along the plantar aspect of the foot. For more than 50% of the stance time, the pressure is concentrated beneath the metatarsal head area. This extended period of pressure can cause bothersome pain. A precise diagnosis is necessary in metatarsalgia to direct treatment toward the specific cause.

Etiologic Findings

Metatarsalgia encompasses a broad spectrum of conditions with various causes arising out of the anatomic structures in the area. It may be associated with abnormalities of the metatarsal head subluxation or dislocation of the metatarsophalangeal joints, systemic diseases, dermatologic lesions, soft-tissue disorders, or iatrogenic causes. Table 9–1 lists the various causes of metatarsalgia and the differential diagnoses that should be considered in evaluating these patients.

Clinical Findings

A. SYMPTOMS AND SIGNS

The clinical evaluation begins with a careful history directed toward delineating the precise location of the pain. The physical examination of the foot and lower extremity begins with the patient standing. Any deformities of the toes are noted, such as clawing of the toes, a long second ray, or swelling around any of the joints. The patient should be evaluated for a postural problem of the foot, such as a flat foot or cavus foot. The plantar aspect of the foot is carefully evaluated for evidence of callus formation. The metatarsal heads are palpated individually to assess for generalized plantar fat pad atrophy, a prominent fibular condyle, synovitis, or possibly a transfer lesion beneath a metatarsal head resulting from previous forefoot surgery.

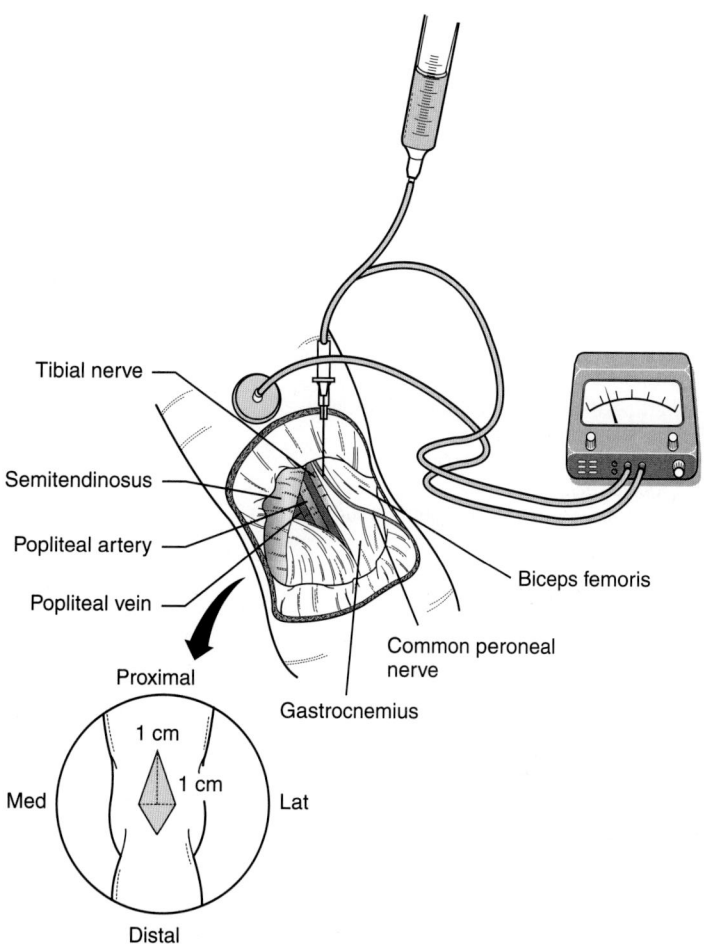

Tibial nerve

Semitendinosus

Popliteal artery

Popliteal vein

Biceps femoris

Common peroneal nerve

Gastrocnemius

Proximal

1 cm

1 cm

Med

Lat

Distal

Figure 9–18. Anesthetic technique. The popliteal block is performed with the needle tip inserted 7–8 cm above the popliteal crease and 1 cm lateral to the midline. (Reproduced, with permission, from Rongstad KM, Mann RA, Prieskorn D et al: Popliteal sciatic nerve block for postoperative analgesia. Foot Ankle Int 1996.)

Popliteal fascia

Semitendinosus

Semimembranosus

Popliteal artery and vein

Tibial nerve

Common peroneal nerve

Sciatic nerve

Biceps femoris

Femur

Figure 9–19. Anesthetic technique for the popliteal block. The needle tip is positioned to localize the sciatic nerve, and aspiration ensures no vascular penetration. (Reproduced, with permission, from Rongstad KM, Mann RA, Prieskorn D et al: Popliteal sciatic nerve block for postoperative analgesia. Foot Ankle Int 1996.)

Table 9–1. Causes of metatarsalgia.

Bone causes
   Prominent fibular condyle of the metatarsal head
   Long metatarsal
   Morton foot
   Hypermobile first ray
   Posttraumatic malalignment of metatarsals
   Abnormal foot posture such as forefoot varus or valgus,
      cavus foot, or equinus deformity
   Systemic disease, rheumatoid arthritis, psoriatic arthritis
Dermatologic lesions
   Wart, seed corn, hyperkeratosis of the skin
Soft tissue disorders
   Atrophy of the plantar fat pad
   Sequelae of a crush injury
   Plantar scars secondary to trauma or surgery
Metatarsophalangeal joint disorders
   Subluxed or dislocated joint
   Freiberg infraction
   Nonspecific synovitis
Iatrogenic causes
   Residuals of metatarsal surgery
   Transfer lesion due to previous surgery
   Hallux valgus surgery (eg, shortening or dorsiflexion of
      the metatarsal)

B. IMAGING STUDIES

The radiographic evaluation includes weight-bearing anteroposterior, lateral, and oblique views of the foot. Occasionally, the so-called skyline view of the metatarsal heads (obtained with the metatarsophalangeal joints in dorsiflexion) is helpful to evaluate their overall alignment, particularly in cases resulting from previous surgery, by demonstrating the height of the metatarsal heads. MRI can be useful in the diagnosis of metatarsalgia, such as distinguishing among a neuroma, cyst, bursa, or synovitis.

Treatment

A. CONSERVATIVE MANAGEMENT

Conservative management is directed at relieving the pressure beneath the area of maximum pain. Initially, the patient must obtain a shoe of appropriate style and adequate size to allow an orthotic device to be inserted. A lace-type shoe with a soft sole material and an adequate toe box is appropriate. High-heeled shoes, loafers, or tight shoes are inappropriate because they have decreased volume for the foot and may cause increased pressure against the involved area. As a general rule, the softer the orthotic device, the more comfortable the patient. A hard acrylic orthotic device is not particularly comfortable for the patient and should usually be avoided.

B. SURGICAL TREATMENT

The surgical management of metatarsalgia depends on the cause and is discussed in different sections of this chapter. In general, pain from a bony prominence can be relieved by a partial ostectomy or osteotomy, dermatologic lesions such as warts can often be burned off with liquid nitrogen or excised, or pain caused by a subluxated metatarsophalangeal joint can be corrected with tendon transfer. The outcome depends on the severity of the problem and the type of surgical intervention required to correct it.

KERATOTIC DISORDERS OF THE PLANTAR SKIN

Friction and pressure over bony prominences, particularly on the plantar skin, can often result in callus formation. Modest callus formation is normal, but more extensive callus formation, particularly on the plantar aspect of the foot, may become symptomatic and occasionally quite disabling.

Etiologic Findings

Many of the intractable plantar keratoses arise from the bony abnormalities presented in Table 9–1.

Clinical Findings

A. SYMPTOMS AND SIGNS

A careful history of the problem is extremely important, especially if the patient has had multiple surgical procedures. The patient's activities, type of shoes that exacerbate or relieve the pain, how often the lesion needs to be trimmed, and the type of orthotic devices used are all important. The physical examination, however, is the most important single factor in the diagnosis of intractable plantar keratoses. First, the overall posture of the foot needs to be evaluated to determine whether the condition is the result of a postural abnormality. Specifically, a rigid plantar-flexed first metatarsal could cause a diffuse callus beneath the first metatarsal head, or a hypermobile first ray that fails to support the medial forefoot may result in generalized callus formation beneath the lesser metatarsal heads. Varus posture of the forefoot (the lateral aspect of the foot in greater plantar flexion than the medial aspect) may result in callus formation beneath the fifth metatarsal head.

The nature of the callus itself is important because it helps determine the cause of the problem. A well-localized lesion beneath the metatarsal head is often caused by a prominent fibular condyle on the second or third metatarsal. A diffuse callus is usually associated with a long metatarsal. The callus may have arisen after trauma or surgery in which an adjacent metatarsal was dorsiflexed, thereby increasing the weight-bearing load of the metatarsal. A callus on the bottom of the foot must be differentiated from a plantar wart, which can occasionally mimic a plantar callosity. Shaving the lesion reveals bleeding from end arteries in a plantar wart, whereas a keratotic lesion consists only of hyperkeratotic tissue.

B. IMAGING STUDIES

Routine weight-bearing radiographs of the foot are performed and correlated with the clinical findings in evaluation of these patients.

Treatment

A. CONSERVATIVE MANAGEMENT

A wide, soft lace-up shoe is recommended, often with the addition of a soft metatarsal support. The orthotic device usually consists of a soft pad (Figure 9–20). It is

A

B

Figure 9–20. **A:** A metatarsal pad may help redistribute weight bearing and relieve symptoms. **B:** A soft insole may be added to help absorb pressure and allow transfer of the metatarsal pad from one shoe to another. (Reproduced, with permission, from Mann RA, Coughlin MJ: *The Video Textbook of Foot and Ankle Surgery.* Medical Video Productions, 1991.)

usually not necessary for an orthotic device to be fabricated early in the treatment of metatarsalgia because the less expensive, commercially available pads are sufficient in most cases.

B. SURGICAL TREATMENT

The surgical management of metatarsalgia depends on the cause of the condition. The following causes of intractable plantar keratoses may respond to surgical intervention.

Localized intractable plantar keratosis beneath a metatarsal head is usually caused by a prominent fibular condyle. It occurs most frequently underneath the second metatarsal but may also be found underneath the third and fourth metatarsals. Surgical treatment is accomplished through a dorsal hockey stick incision over the metatarsophalangeal joint. The toe is plantar flexed to allow removal of 30% of the plantar condyle of the metatarsal head, thereby removing the sharp bony prominence (Figure 9–21). This procedure results in predictable pain relief of the affected toe, although 5–10% of patients develop a transfer lesion beneath the adjacent metatarsal head.

A diffuse callus beneath the second metatarsal that is the result of a dorsiflexed or hypermobile first metatarsal can be treated with dorsiflexion osteotomy done at the base of the second metatarsal. If the lesion is the result of an excessively long metatarsal, it may be shortened to the level of a line drawn between the adjacent metatarsal

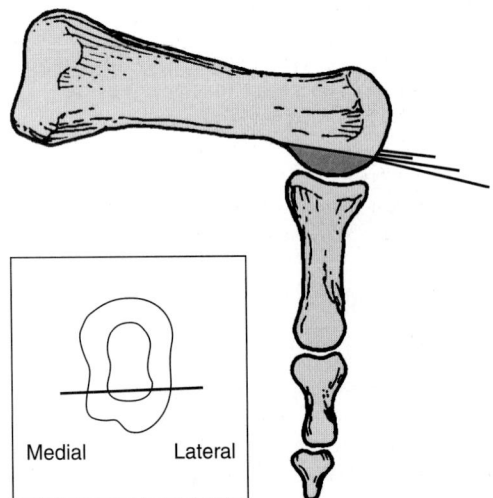

Figure 9–21. A plantar condylectomy is performed with resection of one fourth to one third of the plantar surface of the metatarsal head. (Reproduced, with permission, from Mann RA, Coughlin MJ: *The Video Textbook of Foot and Ankle Surgery.* Medical Video Productions, 1991.)

heads, thereby reestablishing a smooth metatarsal pattern. If the callus is a result of a dislocated metatarsophalangeal joint, the joint must be surgically reduced, using one of the techniques previously described, to alleviate the chronic downward pressure against the metatarsal head. All of these surgical procedures to eliminate a callus are fairly successful, although the possibility of a transfer lesion developing is approximately 5–10%.

Occasionally, a well-localized callus is present beneath the tibial sesamoid, which can be treated surgically by shaving the plantar third of the sesamoid. This alleviates the callus in almost all cases, with the only significant complication being caused by inadvertent disruption of the plantar medial cutaneous nerve during the surgical approach to the sesamoid.

Bunionettes are caused by prominence of the fifth metatarsal head and may lead to metatarsalgia. A diffuse callus beneath the fifth metatarsal head can be treated with a midshaft metatarsal osteotomy to bring it out of its plantar-flexed position, which usually alleviates the condition. It is unusual for a transfer lesion to occur beneath the fourth metatarsal head.

At times, the fifth metatarsal head is too prominent on the lateral aspect of the foot rather than the plantar aspect. In these cases, a chevron osteotomy of the fifth metatarsal head, displacing it in a medialward direction, alleviates the condition (Figure 9–22), sometimes with slight loss of motion of the metatarsophalangeal joint.

A subhallux sesamoid can cause a small callus beneath the interphalangeal joint of the great toe and be quite bothersome to the patient. Surgical excision of the sesamoid is indicated, with good results and little or no disability.

Mann RA, DuVries HL: Intractable plantar keratosis. Orthop Clin North Am 1973;4:67.

Mann RA, Mann JA: Keratotic disorders of the plantar skin. AAOS Instr Course Lect 2004;53:287. [PMID: 15116622]

Yu JS, Tanner JR: Considerations in metatarsalgia and midfoot pain: An MR imaging perspective. Semin Musculoskelet Radiol 2002;6:91. [PMID: 12077699]

DIABETIC FOOT

Approximately 22 million people in the United States are diabetic, and foot problems are the most common cause for hospitalization, accounting for 20% of all inpatient days in this population. More than half of all nontraumatic amputations are performed on diabetics. One report showed a 68% incidence of foot disorders in a large diabetic clinic, and the cost of care of these problems approaches $100 million per year. Treatment of the diabetic, who presents with foot problems, can be complex and require a team approach, involving the primary care physician, vascular surgeon, orthopedic surgeon, infectious disease specialist, orthotist, diabetic

A

B

Figure 9–22. **A:** Lateral view of chevron fifth metatarsal osteotomy. **B:** Diagram following completion of this procedure. (Reproduced, with permission, from Mann RA, Coughlin MJ: *The Video Textbook of Foot and Ankle Surgery.* Medical Video Productions, 1991.)

nurse specialist, and, whenever possible, the patient's family members.

Pathophysiologic Findings

Diabetes is a metabolic disorder that involves all the organ systems. Those of primary interest to the orthopedist are integumentary with the risk of ulceration, neurological with the loss of protective sensation, vascular with diminished perfusion, and immunologic with limited ability to fight infection. The most frequent problem faced by the diabetic is breakdown of the skin of the foot (Figure 9–23). The cause of foot ulcers is multifactorial but stems from diminished sensation resulting from neuropathic disease. Unappreciated local stresses are placed on the skin externally by poorly fitting shoes and internally by skeletal deformity. Autonomic neuropathy causes dry skin and cracks in the dermis, which may become portals of entry for infection. Reactive hyperemia, which normally helps clear infections, is blunted by autonomic neuropathy. Motor neuropathy affects the intrinsic muscles of the foot and may lead to clawtoe deformities with metatarsal heads and proximal interphalangeal joints becoming prominent and predisposed to ulcerations. (Figure 9–24). Hyperglycemia can impair wound healing strength as well as damage vascular endothelium, which is a precur-

sor to atherosclerosis and leads to diminished extremity blood flow and limited healing potential. Elevated blood glucose levels over a long period also leads to glycation of the body's proteins and is commonly measured by the hemoglobin A1c. Glucose covalently binds to lycine in proteins in a reversible process. It is believed that the addition of glucose molecules changes the flexibility of tissues, especially fibrous tissue, making tissues such as skin less able to handle shear stresses. The neuropathy in diabetics is caused by the loss of myelinated and unmyelinated nerve fibers. Other factors that affect healing in diabetics include nutritional deficiencies, diminished microcirculation, and lowered resistance to infection.

History

When a diabetic patient presents to an orthopedist, the four areas of impact are ulcers and their prevention, amputations, Charcot arthropathy, and toenail abnormalities. With an infected foot ulceration, it is essential to obtain a history that will help delineate why the ulcer occurred and how to optimize the patient's healing potential. A past history of foot surgery is sought, previous or current antibiotic usage is detailed, and any recent trauma to the foot is noted. A history is taken about the severity of the patient's diabetes, including

Figure 9–23. Ulceration over the dorsolateral aspect of the fifth toe as the result of pressure from a shoe. (Reproduced, with permission, from Mann RA, Coughlin MJ: *The Video Textbook of Foot and Ankle Surgery.* Medical Video Productions, 1991.)

how long ago the diabetes was diagnosed, whether the patient is taking insulin, the recent level of control, what other organ systems are involved, and the degree of neuropathy present in the patient's feet.

Clinical Findings

A. GENERAL EXAMINATION

Examination of the diabetic patient should begin with inspection of the shoe for internal and external wear patterns. The leg and foot are inspected for overall appearance of the skin, hair growth, perfusion, pulses, and color.

B. FOOT EXAMINATION

Any bony prominences are recognized as areas of potential skin breakdown. The most common prominences are located at the apex of deformities. Neurologic examination should test for the presence of protective sensation, as defined by the patient's ability to feel the 10-g Semmes-Weinstein monofilament as well as motor function. Ulcers should be carefully documented and evaluated for evidence of infection in the adjacent soft tissues. Wounds should be measured for length, width, and depth as well as documenting their location. Open wounds should be probed with a sterile cotton swab or other appropriate instrument to evaluate the extent of involvement of deeper structures, such as tendons, joints, and bone. A positive probe-to-bone test usually indicates the presence of osteomyelitis.

C. VASCULAR FINDINGS

Vascular evaluation is essential to ensure that the patient has adequate perfusion to allow healing. The patients with palpable pedal pulses and normal capillary filling have adequate blood supply and usually do not require further vascular evaluation. For those patients with less perfusion, one method of assessing the overall potential for healing of foot lesions is the ischemic index, obtained by dividing the blood pressure measurement in the brachial artery by that in the dorsalis pedis and posterior tibial arteries, as measured by Doppler ultrasound with a calf cuff. If the index is 0.45 or greater, there is a 90% chance that a foot ulcer will heal. Lower indexes are an indication for a vascular surgery consultation. It must be kept in mind, however, that falsely elevated values of blood pressure in the foot may result from calcification of major blood vessels. Thus, apparent vascular insufficiency in the light of an adequate ischemic index also warrants a vascular surgery consultation. A laser Doppler study can also be beneficial in assessing local skin perfusion. This information can be used to help predict the patient's response to surgical intervention.

D. IMAGING STUDIES

Radiographic studies should include weight-bearing radiographs of both feet and ankles as indicated. Plain radiographs can help identify bony prominences that predispose the patient to ulcer formation, and osteomyelitis or changes consistent with a neuropathic foot may be identified. Early Charcot (neuropathic) joint changes may be difficult to differentiate from osteomyelitis. The

Figure 9–24. Clawtoe deformity involves hammer toe deformity associated with dorsiflexion of metatarsophalangeal joint. (Reproduced, with permission, from Mann RA, Coughlin MJ: *Surgery of the Foot and Ankle,* 6th ed. Mosby-Year Book, 1993.)

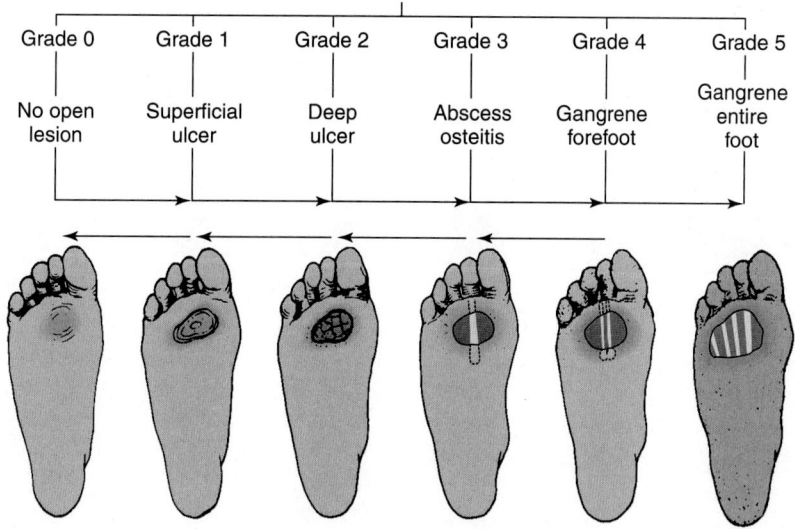

Figure 9–25. The original Rancho Los Amigos classification by Wagner and Meggitt presented the first widely referenced classification of diabetic foot lesions. Two concepts included in this classification are now in need of revision, in light of further experience. The first is the concept that all lesions of the diabetic foot from grade 1 ulcers to grade 5 gangrene occur along a natural continuum. Although this may often be true for the grade 1 ulcer, which progresses to the grade 3 lesion of osteomyelitis, this is not the case with grades 4 and 5. Grades 4 and 5 are vascular lesions or descriptions of the vascular status of the foot and not necessarily related to the progression of the lesser grades. The ischemic lesions of grades 4 and 5 may exist separately from the lesser grades or coincide with any of them, including a forefoot that is otherwise grade 1 (ie, a superficial lesion). Vascular pathologic changes can and should be graded also, but there is not necessarily a relationship between the depth of ulcerative lesions (ie, grades 0, 1, 2, and 3) and the dysvascularity of the foot (ie, grades 4 and 5). Moreover, the grade 5 foot is truly no longer a foot problem but belongs in the domain of salvage of the proximal portion of the leg. The second concept that needs to be refined is that there are not necessarily pathways backward and forward from each grade of lesion (eg, grade 4 feet [partial gangrene] cannot be reversed to grade 3). (Reproduced, with permission, from Brodsky JW: The diabetic foot. In Mann RA, Coughlin MJ, eds: *Surgery of the Foot and Ankle,* 6th ed. Mosby-Year Book, 1993.)

four D's of neuropathic joints are helpful in delineating more advanced cases: debris, destruction, dislocation, and densification.

The presence of bony infection may be delineated on serial radiographs as progressive osteolysis, realizing that changes on plain films are late findings and suggesting the infection was present for weeks. A technetium bone scan is sensitive in detecting early osteomyelitis but quite nonspecific. MRI can demonstrate bone and soft-tissue changes, such as edema or the extent of an abscess cavity, and can be helpful in distinguishing Charcot changes from osteomyelitis.

Classification & Treatment of Diabetic Foot Ulcers

The Rancho Los Amigos Hospital classification of diabetic foot ulcers (Figure 9–25) is based on the depth of tissue affected and extent of the foot involved. Treatment choice depends on the grade of ulcer (Figure 9–26). Table 9–2 shows treatment based on classification of foot ulcers.

As a general rule in treating infections of the foot, a balance must be struck between salvage of tissue and foot function. A healed amputation at a more proximal level is

A   **B**

Figure 9–26. Comparison of grade 1 (**A**) and grade 2 (**B**) ulcers (new depth and ischemia classification). Note the exposed deep tissues of the grade 2 ulcer. (Reproduced, with permission, from Brodsky JW: The diabetic foot. In Mann RA, Coughlin MJ, eds: *Surgery of the Foot and Ankle,* 6th ed. Mosby-Year Book, 1993.)

Table 9–2. Classification and treatment of diabetic foot ulcers.

Grade	Classification	Treatment
0	Foot is "at risk" for developing ulcer. Skin remains intact, but underlying bone deformity places foot at risk for skin breakdown.	Proper footwear plus other preventive measures such as patient education and surgical correction as described in text.
1	Lesion affects skin only	Outpatient dressing changes or total contact cast. Antibiotics usually not necessary.
2	Deep lesions that involve underlying tendons, bones, or ligaments (Figure 9–25).	Surgical debridement and hospitalization for aggressive wound care and intravenous antibiotics. Goal is conversion to grade 1 ulcer.
3	Abscess or osteomyelitis present as complication of ulcer.	Emergency surgery for drainage of acute infection. Wound often left open, with dressing changes performed until definitive closure or amputation is done at a later date.
4	Gangrene is present in the toes or forefoot.	Appropriate amputation.
5	Entire foot is gangrenous.	Appropriate amputation.

more advantageous to the patient than leaving a marginally viable area of the foot that requires constant wound care.

Large wounds heal slowly with the risk of secondary infection, and if possible, they should not be left to heal by secondary intention. Split-thickness skin grafts, especially on the sole of the foot or over an amputation site, are prone to breakdown.

A. SURGICAL TREATMENT FOR RELIEVING BONY PROMINENCES

As previously stated, a major goal of treatment in the ulcerated or at-risk foot is to relieve bony prominences that cause pressure on the skin. Treatment consists of measures to relieve the pressure. Many appropriate measures are available to relieve pressure on the skin from the outside. Examples include extradepth shoes for clawtoes and accommodative foot orthoses with metatarsal pads to relieve pressure under a prominent metatarsal head. If these measures fail or are inappropriate, the pressure should be relieved from the inside by correcting the bony deformity. These prominences are located at several common sites.

The hallux may have a prominence beneath the metatarsal head, on the plantar-medial aspect of the interphalangeal joint, or over the median eminence secondary to a bunion deformity (Figure 9–27). A prominence caused by the medial sesamoid can be relieved by complete or partial removal of the sesamoid. If this does not relieve the prominence adequately, a dorsiflexion osteotomy or resection of the metatarsal head can be performed. Ulcers found over the plantarmedial aspect of the interphalangeal joint can often be relieved by simple excision of the prominent medial condyles or by resection of the

Figure 9–27. Four procedures for recalcitrant ulceration over the condyles of the Interphalangeal joint of the hallux. **A:** Reduction of the condyles of the joint. **B:** Resection of the interphalangeal joint. **C:** Modified Keller procedure (resection of the base of the proximal phalanx). **D:** Dorsiflexion osteotomy of the base of the proximal phalanx. **E:** K-wire fixation of dorsiflexion osteotomy. (Reproduced, with permission, from Brodsky JW: The diabetic foot. In Mann RA, Coughlin MJ, eds: *Surgery of the Foot and Ankle,* 6th ed. Mosby-Year Book, 1993.)

entire joint. A prominence over the median eminence can be addressed with a routine bunion procedure.

The diabetic patient is subject to clawtoe deformities resulting from motor neuropathy, causing prominences under the metatarsal heads and over the dorsum of the proximal interphalangeal joints. Depending on the severity, treatment varies from reduction of the metatarsophalangeal joints and proximal interphalangeal arthroplasties to resection of the metatarsal heads and interphalangeal fusions.

A collapsed longitudinal arch from Charcot changes causes the classic rocker-bottom foot with prominences along the plantar and medial aspects of the midfoot. This can be addressed with a simple exostectomy for a mild deformity, or an appropriate osteotomy and arthrodesis for a more complex deformity.

B. TREATMENT OF OSTEOMYELITIS

Osteomyelitis is a common complication present in a grade 3 diabetic foot ulcer. The infection is seldom eradicated without surgical debridement of the bone. Frequently, more radical treatment than simple exostectomy is required. For example, infection of a proximal phalanx is usually treated by resection of the phalanx. Osteomyelitis of the metatarsal may require ray amputation if more than just the head is involved. If multiple metatarsals are infected, a transmetatarsal amputation is often the best treatment with the reminder to always consider lengthening the tendo Achilles to decrease load on the residual forefoot.

Osteomyelitis of the midfoot is a complication of a collapsed Charcot foot. The treatment options for such an infection include wide local debridement with exostectomy or a more proximal amputation. Similarly, osteomyelitis of the calcaneus can be treated with a partial calcanectomy or a more proximal amputation.

Treatment of ulcers should make sense. A patient with a superficial wound with good blood supply, minimal infection, and protective sensation would be treated with topical wound care, a shoe to accommodate the dressing, and limited activity to control swelling. A patient with an infected deep wound with osteomyelitis and nonreconstructable dysvascularity would probably be best served with early amputation. Of course, each patient is unique and deserves an evaluation of all organ systems to develop an appropriate treatment plan.

Wound dressings should try to mimic skin. They should try to provide a healing environment that is bacteria free, warm, moist, strain free, nontoxic, and well oxygenated. There is nothing that will provide all of these. Dressings should be chosen based on the needs of the wound, possibly needing infection control and debridement in the initial phases but later only requiring protection and absorption of wound drainage. The gold standard for treating plantar ulcers is a total contact or healing cast. This protective cast provides wound protection, edema control, and a moist environment, and it decreases plantar loading to the ulcer. When the wound is draining, the cast does require frequent changing or the odor can be intolerable.

Biological wound healing products that provide wound healing factors can be helpful in the patient with marginal healing potential. Larger wounds, especially those with considerable drainage, can benefit from vacuum-assisted closure where a constant negative suction pressure is applied to a sealed wound, thereby decreasing its size and pulling away wound drainage.

A small number of patients who are marginal wound healers benefit from hyperbaric oxygen treatment. When placed at 2 atm of pure oxygen, the serum becomes supersaturated and benefits some patients who receive serial treatments.

C. CHARCOT FOOT

A Charcot joint is also referred to as a neuropathic, neurotrophic, or neuroarthropathic joint. Diabetes is by far the leading cause of Charcot joints. A Charcot foot is characterized by destruction of joint surfaces, fractures often accompanied by dislocations of one or more joints in a patient with an inappropriate pain response (Figure 9–28). The requirements are an active patient who has neuropathy and adequate blood supply. The pathophysiology is not fully understood, but there are two theories. The neurotraumatic theory claims that cumulative mechanical strains in a patient with inadequate sensory protection leads to stress fractures that are progressive because the patient does not have adequate sensory feedback to limit his or her activity. The neurovascular theory suggests there is a neurally initiated vascular reflex that leads to juxtaarticular osteopenia weakening the bone in this area while glycation of the joint capsule causes stiffness. These factors when combined with mechanical stress can lead to the fracture dislocations commonly seen.

Eichenholtz defined three stages in Charcot arthropathy. Stage 1 is the acute inflammatory phase where there is swelling, redness, and increased warmth. Radiographs likely show fractures and dislocations and the involved area is unstable. The concern in this stage is to rule out infection. If the patient is neuropathic with good blood supply and has an acute, red, hot, swollen foot without an ulcer or a history of an ulcer in that area, it is probably Charcot arthropathy and not infection. Hematogenous osteomyelitis is very rare; infections in the foot are usually introduced locally through the skin. Stage 2 is the subacute phase where there are signs of healing, less swelling, warmth, and radiographic signs of new bone formation. Stage 3 is the chronic phase with consolidation and resolution of inflammation. Typical locations include the midfoot with the creation of the rocker-bottom foot deformity as the arch collapses, the hindfoot, and the ankle with the risk of collapse into varus or valgus that can lead to ulceration.

Figure 9–28. A, B: The classic rocker-bottom Charcot foot, with collapse and then reversal of the longitudinal arch. **C:** Loss of the normal calcaneal pitch, or angle relative to the floor, in patients with Charcot collapse of the arch. This leads to a mechanical disadvantage for the Achilles tendon. (Reproduced, with permission, from Brodsky JW: The diabetic foot. In Mann RA, Coughlin MJ, eds: *Surgery of the Foot and Ankle,* 6th ed. Mosby-Year Book, 1993.)

1. Principles of treatment—There are several important principles to follow in the treatment of Charcot joints. The primary goal is to limit joint destruction and preserve a stable plantigrade foot that protects the soft tissues and prevents ulceration.

2. Treatment of acute phase—For a patient who presents in the acute phase of Charcot joint, the initial treatment should be immobilization and elevation of the foot. This can best be achieved with a non–weight-bearing total contact cast for those patients who can be placed in a plantigrade position. The skin must be checked at weekly intervals initially to look for breakdown. Surgery is rarely attempted on the acute Charcot foot, unless necessitated by the inability to obtain a stable plantigrade position. Even in those patients who require acute stabilization to obtain a plantigrade foot, it is best to allow the swelling and inflammation to diminish by offloading and immobilization prior to surgical intervention. Once the acute phase subsides and the fractures heal, immobilization can be accomplished by means of an ankle-foot orthosis (AFO) or other appropriate removable support. Custom-made shoes can then be fitted to accommodate for the bony prominences.

3. Treatment of subacute phase—In this phase the foot has stabilized, and there is no ongoing bony destruction. Operations address the bony prominences that were created by Charcot destruction and collapse. Simple removal of a prominence is often all that is required, and, sometimes, fusion of one or several joints is necessary. One of the most common foot deformities is a collapsed arch and rocker-bottom deformity from subluxation of multiple joints in the midfoot. An exostectomy of the prominent bones on the plantar aspect of the midfoot usually is sufficient. Alternatively, an osteotomy and arthrodesis of the midfoot can be performed to realign the foot and reconstitute the arch in cases where a simple exostectomy is inadequate (Figure 9–29). This procedure has a high complication rate and an extended time to achieve union. In the case of Charcot involvement of the ankle joint, the goal is a stable and plantigrade foot, which often requires arthrodesis. Retrograde intramedullary nailing is successful in achieving union but also has significant complication rates.

Figure 9–29. **A:** Patient with advanced midfoot Charcot deformity and soft-tissue breakdown over an extruded medial cuneiform. **B:** Limited arthrodesis with internal fixation and iliac grafting to relieve pressure on soft tissue and reestablish weight bearing of the first ray. (Reproduced, with permission, from Brodsky JW: The diabetic foot. In Mann RA, Coughlin MJ, eds: *Surgery of the Foot and Ankle,* 6th ed. Mosby-Year Book, 1993.)

Andros G: Diagnostic and therapeutic arterial interventions in the ulcerated diabetic foot. Diabetes Metab Res Rev 2004;20 (Suppl 1):S29. [PMID: 15150810]

Brem H, Sheehan P, Boulton AJ: Protocol for the treatment of diabetic foot ulcers. Am J Surg 2004;187(5)(Suppl 1):S1. [PMID: 15147985]

Eldor R et al: New and experimental approaches to treatment of diabetic foot ulcers: A comprehensive review of emerging treatment strategies. Diabet Med 2004;21:1161. [PMID: 15498081]

Gil H, Morrison WB: MR imaging of diabetic foot infection. Semin Musculoskelet Radiol 2004;8(3):189. [PMID: 15478022]

Lipsky B: Medical treatment of diabetic foot infections. Clin Infect Dis 2004;39:S104. [PMID: 15306988]

Perry JE et al: The use of running shoes to reduce plantar pressures in patients who have diabetes. J Bone Joint Surg 1995;778: 1819. [PMID: 8550649]

Pinzur M: Surgical versus accommodative treatment for Charcot arthropathy of the midfoot. Foot Ankle Int 2004;25(8):545. [PMID: 15363375]

Pinzur MS, Kelikian A: Charcot ankle fusion with a retrograde locked intramedullary nail. Foot Ankle Int 1997;18:699. [PMID: 9391814]

Wagner FW Jr: A classification and treatment program for diabetic, neuropathic, and dysvascular foot problems. Instr Course Lect 1979;28:143.

DISORDERS OF THE TOENAILS

Toenail problems in younger (less than 20 years) patients usually involve trauma, such as stubbing the toe or, more frequently, improper nail care, which can contribute to ingrown toenails. This is usually the result of tearing off a toenail, which leaves the nail too short and predisposes it to become ingrown.

Toenail problems in the older age group are more varied, including an incurvating nail, a thickened hypertrophied nail associated with a chronic fungal infection, an ingrown nail resulting from improper nail cutting, and on rare occasions a subungual exostosis.

Etiologic Findings

The anatomy of the toenail is demonstrated in Figure 9–30. The nail unit consists of four components: the proximal nail fold, the nail matrix, the nail bed, and the hyponychium. The area in which most of the problems occur is the lateral or medial nail groove, where an ingrown nail occurs at the level of the nail bed or hyponychium.

Clinical Findings

A. SYMPTOMS AND SIGNS

The history of most nail problems is not complex and usually quickly defines the nature of the problem.

1. Infection of the toenails—Infection of the toenails usually begins slowly, with erythema and swelling along the margin of the nail, followed by increasing pain and drainage, and finally the development of granulation tissue, usually in response to the foreign body reaction of the nail itself.

2. Mycotic nail—In the case of the mycotic (fungal) nail, there is usually a long, slow history of development of deformation of the nail, often with medial or lateral deviation of the nail, marked hypertrophy, and increased pain when wearing shoes. At times, an incurvated nail condition develops in which one or both edges of the nail slowly curve inward, resulting in pinching of the nail plate. This may cause a localized infection, or just the sheer pressure of the nail against the skin may be the cause of the pain. Medical therapy is based on direct microscopy (KOH [potassium hydroxide]) and culture studies.

3. Subungual exostosis—The patient who develops subungual exostosis usually notes pain evolving beneath the toenail over a long period. Erosion of the nail from below occurs because of the pressure of the exostosis against the nail itself. The patient often does not seek help until there is actual breakdown of the tissue, giving rise to a rather ugly-appearing lesion that seems much more ominous than the condition itself.

B. IMAGING STUDIES

Radiographs are necessary when evaluating a toenail problem for subungual exostosis, which is clearly seen with a lateral view. In patients with long-standing infected ingrown toenails, a radiograph can be important to rule out underlying osteomyelitis.

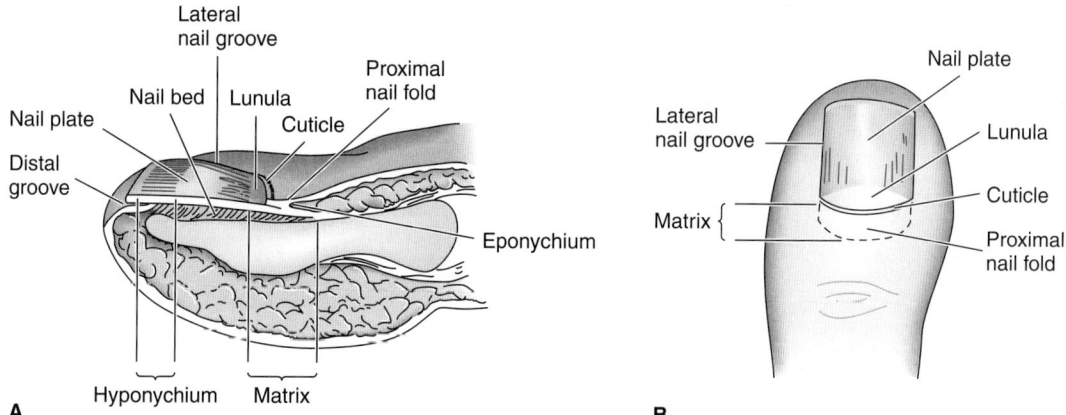

Figure 9–30. **A:** Cross section of the toe demonstrates the components of the toenail and supporting structures. **B:** The proximal nail is covered by the proximal nail fold and cuticle. The lunula is the main germinal area. (Reproduced, with permission, from Mann RA, Coughlin MJ: *The Video Textbook of Foot and Ankle Surgery.* Medical Video Productions, 1991.)

Treatment

A. CONSERVATIVE MANAGEMENT

1. Chronic ingrown toenail—For the chronic ingrown toenail, the margin of the nail is removed to relieve the pressure of the nail against the skin. This procedure, along with local care and occasionally systemic antibiotics, usually permits the condition to resolve. It is important, however, to explain to the patient the necessity of permitting the nail to grow out over the ungual labia, to depress it and prevent the ingrown nail from recurring.

2. Chronic onychophosis of the nail—Chronic onychophosis of the nail must be kept debrided. If an ingrown nail occurs, the margins must be trimmed to relieve the pressure against the skin.

3. Subungual exostosis—Subungual exostosis that is symptomatic is treated by excision.

B. SURGICAL TREATMENT

1. Ingrown toenail—The surgical management of the recurrent ingrown toenail consists of the Winograd procedure, in which the medial or lateral margin of the offending nail plate is removed along with the underlying nail matrix. The nail matrix is removed as thoroughly as possible to prevent the possible growth of a nail horn, which occurs in approximately 5% of cases. The nail matrix can be removed by sharp dissection or ablated with a laser or treated with phenol to kill the nail matrix.

2. Chronic infection—If chronic infections has caused severe distortion of the nail, the nail and the nail bed can be removed in their entirety. This usually results in a horny base where the nail existed, often a satisfactory outcome. The terminal Syme amputation can be carried out to eliminate the nail and matrix completely (Figure 9–31). Although results are usually satisfactory, some patients do not like the appearance of the toe or absence of the toenail because of its somewhat bulbous appearance. The terminal Syme procedure can be carried out under digital block in most patients. An elliptical incision is made over the distal end of the toe, removing the nail and its matrix in their entirety. The distal portion of the distal phalanx is removed and the edges smoothed, thus shortening the toe. The tip of the toe is defatted and loosely sutured. In this manner, the nail is completely removed and soft tissue covers the area of the former nail bed. The only significant complication associated with this procedure is the regrowth of some nail matrix beneath the healed flap, which results in an inclusion cyst that must be drained and the residual nail matrix excised.

3. Subungual exostosis—Surgical management of subungual exostosis requires lifting the nail, identification of the exostosis, and complete removal of the exostosis and its stalk. The dissection must be carefully carried out and the entire exostosis removed to prevent recurrence. The nail bed is repaired to cover the defect.

Baran R, Dawber RPR: *Diseases of the Nails and Their Management.* Blackwell Scientific Publications, 1984.

Coughlin MJ: Toenail abnormalities. In Mann RA, Coughlin MJ, eds: *Surgery of the Foot and Ankle.* Mosby-Year Book, 1993.

Mann RA, Coughlin MJ: Toenail abnormalities. In Mann RA, Coughlin MJ, eds: *The Video Textbook of Foot and Ankle Surgery.* Video Medical Productions, 1990.

Mayeaux EJ: Nail disorders. Prim Care 2000;27:333. [PMID: 10815047]

Rounding C, Hulm S: Surgical treatments for ingrowing toenails. Cochrane Database Syst Rev 2000;(2):CD001541. [PMID: 10796808]

Summerbell RC, Cooper E, Bunn U et al: Onychomycosis: A critical study of techniques and criteria for confirming the etiologic significance of nondermatophytes. Med Mycol 2005;43:39. [PMID: 15712607]

A   **B**   **C**

Figure 9–31. Syme amputation of toenail. **A:** Elliptical or rectangular incision is centered over the nail bed and matrix. **B:** The distal half of the distal phalanx is resected. **C:** Excess skin is resected, and skin edges are approximated. (Reproduced, with permission, from Mann RA, Coughlin MJ: *The Video Textbook of Foot and Ankle Surgery.* Medical Video Productions, 1991.)

NEUROLOGIC DISORDERS OF THE FOOT

1. Interdigital Neuroma (Morton Neuroma)

An interdigital neuroma is a painful affliction involving the plantar aspect of the forefoot. It usually involves the third interspace and is characterized by a well-localized area of pain on the plantar aspect of the foot that radiates into the web space. The symptoms are usually aggravated by ambulation and relieved by rest. As a rule, wearing a tight-fitting shoe aggravates the pain, and walking barefoot often relieves it.

Etiologic Findings

The precise cause of interdigital neuroma is not determined. It occurs in women approximately 10 times more frequently than men, and, as a result, high-fashion shoe wear is implicated. Several studies demonstrate that the changes in the nerve appear to occur just distal to the transverse metatarsal ligament. This finding has given rise to the hypothesis that the neuroma results from the constant traction of the nerve against the ligament as the toes are brought into a dorsiflexed position, a theory that explains the higher incidence in women wearing high-heeled shoes. Although this condition is called **interdigital neuroma,** it is not a true neuroma. The pathologic changes involve actual degeneration of the nerve fibers associated with deposition of amorphous eosinophilic material that is felt to be consistent with an entrapment neuropathy (Figure 9–32).

Clinical Findings

A. SYMPTOMS AND SIGNS

Patients with an interspace neuroma usually present with a complaint of localized pain in the metatarsal head region that is increased by walking and relieved by rest and by removing the shoe. Palpation of the involved interspace produces sharp pain that often radiates into the toes. There can be a palpable mass, and squeezing the forefoot, thereby narrowing the intermetatarsal space while compressing the mass, often reproduces the patient's symptoms. If this maneuver produces a snapping sensation, it is referred to as a Mulder click. The third interspace is more frequently involved than the second, and it is extremely rare to have involvement of the first or fourth web space. Pain over the metatarsophalangeal joint itself is caused by disease involving the metatarsophalangeal joint, and pain in the interspace must be distinguished from pain associated with pathology in the metatarsophalangeal joint. The differential diagnosis of metatarsalgia includes avascular necrosis (Freiberg disease), synovitis caused by mechanical insta-

Figure 9–32. An interdigital neuroma impingement occurs beneath the intermetatarsal ligament. (Reproduced, with permission, from Mann RA, Coughlin MJ: *The Video Textbook of Foot and Ankle Surgery.* Medical Video Productions, 1991.)

bility, synovial cysts, or even referred pain from tarsal tunnel compression or lumbar disk disease.

B. IMAGING STUDIES

Radiographs are not helpful in the diagnosis of an interdigital neuroma but may reveal pathology at the metatarsophalangeal joint as the cause of the patient's symptoms. There are several reports regarding the use of ultrasound to evaluate the presence of nerve enlargement, but this is very user dependent. MRI can be used effectively but is rarely necessary.

Treatment

A. CONSERVATIVE MANAGEMENT

Conservative management begins with wearing a wider soft-soled shoe to accommodate the foot without mediolateral compression and lowering the heel. A soft metatarsal support is placed in the shoe proximal to the area of the neuroma, thereby spreading the metatarsal heads and lifting them. Approximately a third of patients respond to this treatment. Steroid injection into the web space can be helpful in resolving the symptoms but is not without the hazard of local fat atrophy, which can lead to diminished padding under the metatarsal heads or local skin thinning and discoloration.

B. SURGICAL TREATMENT

Surgical excision of the nerve is indicated if conservative treatment fails. A dorsal incision is made in the midline of the involved web space and carried down to the transverse metatarsal ligament, which is cut. The nerve is noted to lie just beneath the transverse metatarsal ligament. A quite thickened nerve is reassuring evidence that the correct diagnosis was made; however, a nerve of normal thickness should still be removed if the clinical diagnosis of neuroma was made from other evidence. The nerve is delivered into the interspace by plantar pressure and freed up distally and proximally, transected proximal to the metatarsal head, and then dissected out distally, where it is cut just past its bifurcation. Care is taken not to disrupt the surrounding fatty tissue or intrinsic muscles. A compression dressing is used for 3 weeks after routine wound closure, and ambulation is permitted in a postoperative shoe. Decreased sensation in the toes on either side of the web space is expected postoperatively. Approximately 80% of patients are totally satisfied with the results of the procedure; 20% obtain little or no relief. The precise cause of this failure rate is a bit of an enigma. Obviously in some patients, the diagnosis was made incorrectly, and the metatarsophalangeal joint was actually involved.

C. RECURRENT NEUROMA

A recurrent neuroma is indeed a true surgical bulb neuroma that resulted following the transection of the common digital nerve on the plantar aspect of the foot. True neuritic symptoms occur in some cases in which transection was not proximal enough or the nerve became adherent and trapped beneath the metatarsal head. Careful percussion of the plantar aspect to elicit the Tinel sign can frequently localize the cut end of the nerve (bulb neuroma). If the severed nerve can be clinically well localized, reexploration for the neuroma is carried out either through a dorsal or plantar approach. The neuroma is identified and transected to a more proximal level or implanted into muscle, and symptoms are relieved in 60–70% of patients.

2. Tarsal Tunnel Syndrome

Tarsal tunnel syndrome is a compressive or traction neuropathy of the posterior tibial nerve as it passes behind the medial malleolus. The tarsal tunnel is formed by the fibroosseous tunnel resulting from the flexor retinaculum as it wraps around the posterior aspect of the medial malleolus (Figure 9–33). Tarsal tunnel syndrome causes poorly localized dysesthesias on the plantar aspect of the foot. The symptom complex is often aggravated by activity and relieved by rest. Some patients complain mainly of nocturnal dysesthesias.

Etiologic Findings

Tarsal tunnel syndrome may arise from a space-occupying lesion within the tarsal tunnel (eg, a ganglion, synovial cyst, or lipoma) or distally against one of the two terminal branches: the medial or lateral plantar nerve. It occasionally follows severe trauma to the lower extrem-

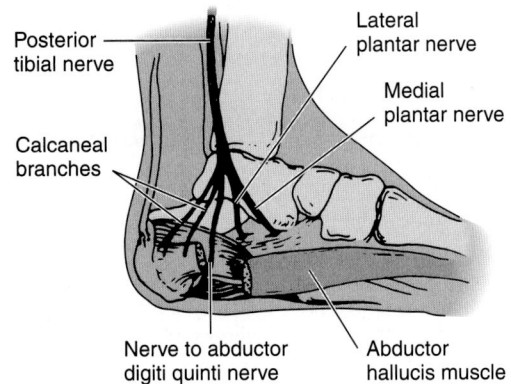

Figure 9–33. Posterior tibial nerve and major branches. (Reproduced, with permission, from Mann RA, Coughlin MJ: *The Video Textbook of Foot and Ankle Surgery.* Medical Video Productions, 1991.)

ity, probably because of edema or scarring. Other causes are severe venous varicosities, tenosynovitis, or a tumor within the nerve. Traction neuropathy can occur in those patients who have an excessively valgus hindfoot position, especially those that are unstable. As the patient walks, the posterior tibial nerve is subjected to stretching as it courses around the convex side of the deformity. In more than half of the cases, however, the precise cause cannot be determined.

Clinical Findings

A. SYMPTOMS AND SIGNS

The diagnosis is entertained after obtaining a history of paresthesias or burning in the posterior tibial nerve distribution. Careful evaluation of the patient in the standing and sitting positions is necessary to check posture and increased fullness, thickening, or swelling in the involved tarsal tunnel area. Careful percussion may elicit a Tinel sign over the posterior tibial nerve in the tarsal tunnel or distally along the divisions of the posterior tibial nerve (the medial calcaneal nerve and medial and lateral plantar nerves). Muscle weakness is usually not observed, but loss of sensation and two-point discrimination may be occasionally detected.

Electrodiagnostic studies should be carried out to help confirm the diagnosis of tarsal tunnel syndrome. Nerve conduction velocities along the medial plantar nerve to the abductor hallucis muscle (latency less than 6.2 ms) and of the lateral plantar nerve to the abductor digiti quinti (latency usually less than 7 ms) should be within 1 ms of each other, otherwise indicating nerve compression in the tarsal tunnel. Motor-evoked potentials that demonstrate a decreased amplitude and increased duration are also indicative of tarsal tunnel syndrome. The most accurate study for tarsal tunnel syndrome appears to be sensory nerve conduction velocity, although this is also the least reproducible study.

The definitive diagnosis of tarsal tunnel syndrome should be based on (1) the clinical history of ill-defined burning, tingling pain in the plantar aspect of the foot, (2) positive physical findings of Tinel sign along the course of the nerve, and (3) electrodiagnostic studies. If all three factors are not positive, the diagnosis of tarsal tunnel syndrome should be suspect. MRI may be quite useful in demonstrating the presence of a space-occupying lesion.

Treatment

A. CONSERVATIVE MANAGEMENT

The tarsal tunnel syndrome should be managed with NSAIDs and an occasional steroid injection into the tarsal tunnel area. Aspiration and injection of a cyst or ganglion may be attempted but is rarely successful. Immobilization in a polypropylene AFO may also be useful, especially in the patient with unstable valgus.

B. SURGICAL TREATMENT

Surgical intervention can be considered if conservative management fails. Approximately 75% of patients operated on for tarsal tunnel syndrome are satisfied with the result. The other 25% may continue to have varying degrees of discomfort. The surgical release uses an incision behind the medial malleolus that is carried distally to about the level of the talonavicular joint. The investing retinaculum is exposed and released. The posterior tibial nerve is identified proximal to the tarsal tunnel area and carefully traced distally behind the medial malleolus. The division into its three terminal branches is identified. Because the medial calcaneal branch passes from the posterior aspect of the lateral plantar nerve, the dissection should be carried out along its dorsal aspect. There may be one or more medial calcaneal branches. The medial plantar nerve should be traced distally until it passes through the fibroosseous tunnel in the abductor hallucis muscle. The lateral plantar nerve should be traced behind the abductor hallucis muscle until it passes toward the lateral aspect of the foot. A preoperative Tinel sign distal to the tarsal tunnel area requires that the area be carefully explored to determine whether there is a ganglion or cyst within the tendon sheath as a cause of the tarsal tunnel syndrome.

Postoperatively, a compression dressing is applied and weight bearing is prohibited for 3 weeks, before progressive ambulation is permitted.

The results following tarsal tunnel release depend on the pathology found at the time of surgery. Removal of a space-occupying lesion usually relieves all of the symptoms. Involvement of a single nerve branch, such as the medial or lateral plantar nerve, also portends good results after surgery. If more diffuse pain is felt throughout the foot before surgery and no definite constriction on the nerve is found at exploration, only one half to two thirds of patients can be expected to experience pain relief. Patients with traction neuropathy caused by the unstable valgus foot are treated by correction of the instability, usually with arthrodesis, and not with soft tissue tarsal tunnel release.

3. Traumatic Neuromas About the Foot

A traumatic neuroma about the foot presents a difficult problem in management because footwear can cause constant irritation of the neuroma. The most frequent cause of traumatic neuroma in the foot is previous surgery. Despite caution in making incisions about the foot, many lesser and occasionally major nerve trunks can be injured. The dorsal aspect of the foot is most frequently involved (Figure 9–34).

Clinical Findings

The clinical evaluation begins with a careful history of the problem and an evaluation of the area involved to determine the precise location of the neuroma, which is essential for proper treatment. Rarely is any type of electrodiagnostic study indicated, and radiographs are not usually necessary.

Figure 9–34. **A:** Common area of traumatic nerve entrapment. **B:** Frequent incisions that may lead to entrapment of dorsal sensory nerves. (Reproduced, with permission, from Mann RA, Coughlin MJ: *The Video Textbook of Foot and Ankle Surgery.* Medical Video Productions, 1991.)

Treatment

A. CONSERVATIVE MANAGEMENT

Attempts to relieve pressure on the neuroma with a large shoe or a carefully designed pad may be of benefit. A cortisone injection into the area occasionally may help, particularly when a small nerve is involved. Surgical intervention is indicated if conservative measures fail.

B. SURGICAL TREATMENT

Careful planning must be undertaken prior to the excision of a traumatic neuroma. The exact location of the neuroma and the area of sensitivity proximal to it must be determined. The incision must be made as precisely as possible to identify the neuroma and trace the nerve proximally into an area that would not be affected by pressure from shoes and boots. The neuroma is excised, leaving enough nerve to bring the cut end into an area of minimal pressure. The cut end is buried into an excavation in bone, if possible, or beneath a muscle such as the extensor digitorum brevis muscle. When carrying out a resection of the sural nerve, it is important, particularly in an individual who wears heavy work boots, that the end of the nerve is brought proximally enough so the top of the boot will not press on the nerve, resulting in continued symptoms.

The results following resection of a traumatic neuroma are quite variable. Initial relief from removing the traumatic neuroma is routine, but unless the nerve is buried where it will not be exposed to pressure, the symptoms may recur in time. It is therefore preferable to bury the end of the nerve into bone, if possible. Resection of most neuromas accentuate a sensory deficit, which is usually not a significant clinical problem.

4. Entrapment of the Superficial Branch of the Deep Peroneal Nerve

Osteophyte formation at the talonavicular or metatarsocuneiform joint may entrap the superficial branch of the deep peroneal nerve as it passes beneath the extensor retinaculum. Patient complaints are of dysesthesias on the foot or difficulty in wearing shoes, depending on the location of the entrapment.

The superficial branch of the deep peroneal nerve passes onto the dorsum of the foot between the extensor hallucis longus and extensor digitorum longus tendons. It continues beneath the extensor retinaculum, coursing along the dorsal surface of the talus and navicular and more distally across the metatarsocuneiform joints. Osteophyte formation at any point along the course of the nerve may cause sufficient pressure against the nerve to cause an entrapment problem.

Clinical Findings

A. SYMPTOMS AND SIGNS

The clinical evaluation begins with a careful history regarding the patient's complaint of dysesthesias over the dorsum of the foot. The physical examination demonstrates tingling along the course of the superficial branch of the deep peroneal nerve, which radiates into the first web space. Often the precise location of the nerve entrapment can be identified by careful palpation and by rolling the nerve across the involved bony prominence.

B. IMAGING STUDIES

Radiographs usually reveal the offending osteophytes, often along the area of the talonavicular or metatarsocuneiform joints. Placing a radiographic marker at the area of maximum tenderness can help identify the offending bony prominence.

Treatment

A. CONSERVATIVE MANAGEMENT

Conservative management consists of attempting to keep the pressure off the involved area, either by padding the tongue of the shoe or by trying to create a pad that will not put pressure directly on the nerve. If these measures fail, decompression of the nerve usually brings about satisfactory resolution of the condition.

B. SURGICAL TREATMENT

Depending on the area of entrapment (talonavicular or metatarsocuneiform), a slightly curved incision is made and carried down through the retinaculum to expose the nerve. Great caution must be taken during the approach so the nerve is not inadvertently damaged. The nerve is carefully lifted off of its bed, exposing the osteophytes, which are removed with a rongeur. The bone surfaces are coated with bone wax prior to laying the nerve back on its bed. After wound closure in layers, the foot is immobilized for approximately 3 weeks in a postoperative shoe.

The results following release of the superficial portion of the deep peroneal nerve are usually satisfactory. Because the nerve itself usually is not damaged by the entrapment, a favorable outcome is expected.

Bailie DS, Kelikian AS: Tarsal tunnel syndrome: Diagnosis, surgical technique, and functional outcome. Foot Ankle Int 1998; 2:65. [PMID: 9498577]

Beskin JL: Nerve entrapment syndromes of the foot and ankle. J Am Acad Orthop Surg 1997;5:261. [PMID: 10795062]

Coughlin M et al: Concurrent interdigital neuroma and MTP joint instability: Long-term results of treatment. Foot Ankle Int 2002;23:1018. [PMID: 12449407]

Okafor B, Shergill G, Angel J: Treatment of Morton's neuroma by neurolysis. Foot Ankle Int 1997;5:284. [PMID: 9167928]

Stamatis ED, Myerson MS: Treatment of recurrence of symptoms after excision of an interdigital neuroma. J Bone Joint Surg Br 2004;86:48. [PMID: 14765865]

RHEUMATOID FOOT

The foot is involved in 90% of patients with long-standing RA, and the involvement is almost always bilateral. The forefoot is most commonly involved, and these joints are often the first joints to be affected, but deterioration of the subtalar joint is noted in approximately 35% of patients and of the ankle joint in approximately 30%.

Etiologic Findings

The changes in the forefoot are caused by chronic synovitis, which destroys the supporting structures about the metatarsophalangeal joints. The joint capsules are distended and the ligaments destroyed. When these structures no longer function to provide stability for the joint, progressive dorsal subluxation and eventual dislocation of the metatarsophalangeal joints occur. As the metatarsophalangeal joints progress from subluxation to dislocation, the plantar fat pad is drawn distally, and the base of the proximal phalanx eventually comes to rest on the metatarsal head. Thus, the metatarsals are forced into a position of plantar flexion, which results in significant callus formation beneath the metatarsal heads. The changes at the metatarsophalangeal joints result in imbalance of the intrinsic muscles, and severe hammer toe and clawtoe deformities usually result.

Significant midfoot and hindfoot pathology is also found in patients with RA. A severely flattened longitudinal arch can result from long-standing subtalar joint involvement with subluxation. Pain with less severe deformity is present in isolated talonavicular involvement of the midfoot.

Clinical Findings

A. SYMPTOMS AND SIGNS

The clinical evaluation of the rheumatoid patient begins with a careful history of the disease and the medications the patient is taking and an attempt to ascertain whether the disease process is currently in an active or a quiescent stage. It is important to obtain some indication of the patient's wound-healing capacity in the foot or elsewhere in the body.

The vascular status of the foot and quality of the skin is noted. The feet are assessed with the patient standing, which often demonstrates marked deformities of multiple joints or localized involvement of only one or two joints. The patient is then seated and a careful evaluation of all the joints about the foot and ankle is carried out to determine precisely the degree to which they are affected. Careful palpation of the metatarsophalangeal joints often demonstrates the degree of the synovial activity as well as the degree of stability of the joints. The plantar aspect of the foot is inspected for the callus formation and past or present ulcerations. Flattening of the longitudinal arch and any hindfoot valgus are evaluated with a careful assessment of joint stability to determine the risk of deformity progression.

B. IMAGING STUDIES

Radiographs help assess the number of joints involved and the degree of involvement. Bilateral involvement is frequently asymmetric. Standing radiographs are beneficial in assessing the effect of joint stability on the severity of deformity.

Treatment

A. CONSERVATIVE MANAGEMENT

Conservative management includes medical management, carried out by the patient's rheumatologist. The patient with sufficient deformity should wear an extra-depth shoe with a soft accommodative liner to reduce pressure on the metatarsal heads and the toes, which may be severely contracted dorsally. Frequently, the patient is quite comfortable in this shoe and does not require further treatment. With significant hindfoot involvement, an AFO may be required to help relieve pain by providing adequate stabilization.

B. SURGICAL TREATMENT

The main goal of surgical management of the forefoot is to create a stable foot that will alleviate the pain beneath the metatarsal head region (Figure 9–35). Arthrodesis of the first metatarsophalangeal joint is the procedure most commonly used, with the joint placed in approximately 15 degrees of dorsiflexion in relation to the floor and approximately 15 degrees of valgus position. The lesser metatarsophalangeal joints are corrected by release of the soft-tissue contracture and resection arthroplasty. The metatarsal heads are excised to decompress the metatarsophalangeal joints, and the fat pad is brought back down onto the plantar aspect of the foot by realigning and securing the plantar plates of the joints under the residual metatarsals. The hammer toes can be corrected by closed osteoclasis, which often results in satisfactory realignment. Open hammer toe procedures are also very effective in correcting residual deformities. The toes and metatarsophalangeal joint area are stabilized with longitudinal K-wires postoperatively for approximately 4 weeks.

The results of this rheumatoid forefoot repair are most gratifying in that approximately 90% of patients are satisfied with the results. There are few complica-

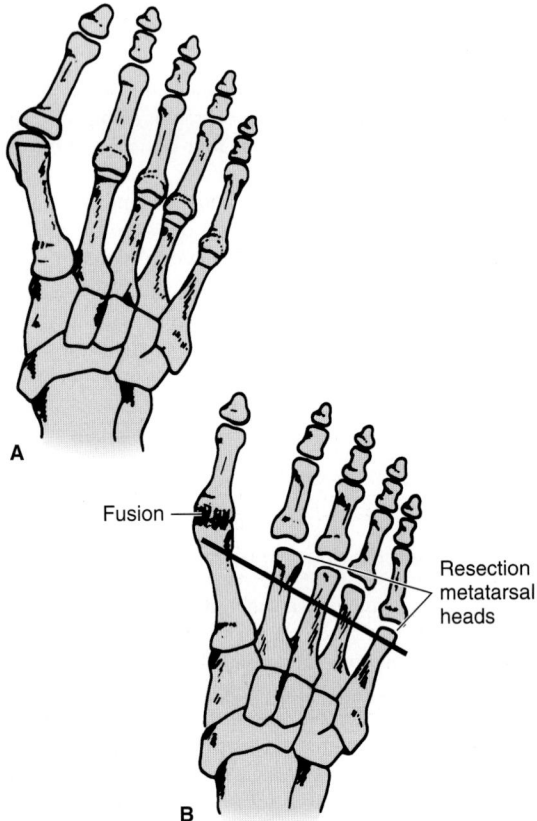

A

Fusion —

Resection
metatarsal
heads

B

Figure 9–35. **A:** Resection of metatarsal heads.
B: Symmetric resection of metatarsal heads minimizes
recurrence of intractable plantar keratoses. (Reproduced, with permission, from Mann RA, Coughlin MJ: *The
Video Textbook of Foot and Ankle Surgery.* Medical Video Productions, 1991.)

tions, although the blood supply to the toes is always of
concern because the procedure is extensive. Occasionally, wound healing is delayed, particularly if the
patient is taking high dosages of corticosteroids or the
antimetabolite drugs.

Hindfoot and ankle disease is usually managed
medically unless there is instability and progressive
deformity. Orthotic support or bracing can be beneficial, but if the deformity is increasing and the
patient's thin skin cannot tolerate further pressure,
surgical stabilization with arthrodesis is necessary. If
only a single joint is involved with the rheumatoid
process, a less extensive procedure is carried out. For
isolated talonavicular RA with no significant deformity of the arch, an isolated talonavicular fusion is
adequate. If significant deformity is present because

of subtalar joint subluxation, a triple arthrodesis is
required. Ankle joint involvement is treated with
ankle joint fusion or total ankle arthroplasty. The
details of the surgical procedures are described elsewhere in this chapter.

Cracchiolo A III: Surgery for rheumatoid disease. Part I. Foot
   abnormalities in rheumatoid arthritis. Instr Course Lect
   1984;33:386. [PMID: 6400419]

James D et al: Orthopaedic intervention in early rheumatoid arthritis. Occurrence and predictive factors in an inception
   cohort of 1064 patients followed for 5 years. Rheumatology
   2004;43:369. [PMID: 14722346]

Kavlak Y et al: Outcome of orthoses intervention in the rheumatoid
   foot. Foot Ankle Int 2003;24(6):494. [PMID: 12854671]

Mann RA, Schakel ME: Surgical correction of rheumatoid forefoot deformities. Foot Ankle Int 1995;16:1. [PMID:
   7697146]

McGarvey SR, Johnson KA: Keller arthroplasty in combination
   with resection arthroplasty of the lesser metatarsophalangeal
   joints in rheumatoid arthritis. Foot Ankle 1988;9:75.
   [PMID: 3224902]

Ostendorf B et al: Diagnostic value of magnetic resonance imaging
   of the forefeet in early rheumatoid arthritis when findings on
   imaging of the metacarpophalangeal joints of the hands remain normal. Arthritis Rheum 2004;50(7):2094. [PMID:
   15248206]

HEEL PAIN

Heel pain can be caused by several distinct entities.
When evaluating the patient for heel pain, the clinician
must attempt to define as precisely as possible the location and hence the cause of the pain.

Table 9–3 presents the causes of heel pain, which are
quite variable and need to be carefully defined, so the
proper treatment can be chosen.

Table 9–3. Causes of heel pain.

Causes of plantar heel pain
Plantar fascitis
Atrophy of heel pad
Posttraumatic (eg, calcaneal fracture)
Enlarged calcaneal spur
Neurologic conditions such as tarsal tunnel syndrome or entrapment of nerve to abductor digiti quinti
Degenerative disk disease with radiation toward heel
Systemic disease (eg, Reiter syndrome, psoriatic arthritis)
Acute tear of plantar fascia
Calcaneal apophysitis
Causes of posterior heel pain
Retrocalcaneal bursitis
Achilles tendinitis
Haglund deformity
Degeneration of Achilles tendon insertion

Clinical Findings

A. SYMPTOMS AND SIGNS

The clinical evaluation begins with a careful history of the onset and location of the pain. The patient's activities and types of footwear that aggravate and relieve the pain are discussed. Specific inquiry regarding radiation of pain proximally in the lower extremity may suggest lumbar disk disease as the cause. Patients active in sports should be questioned regarding significant changes in their level of activity because heel pain often is the result of increased stress on the foot. The cause of the patient's heel pain can usually be determined by palpating the area of maximum tenderness.

Plantar fasciitis, the most common cause of plantar heel pain, usually has an area of maximum tenderness along the plantar medial aspect of the heel, which corresponds to the origin of the plantar fascia at the medial calcaneal tuberosity. In most cases the pain is most severe with the first steps upon arising. The pain is usually aggravated by dorsiflexion of the toes, the so-called windlass stretch, because this applies more tension on the damaged plantar fascia.

Achilles tendonitis/tendinosis typically occurs at one of two discrete sites: at the calcaneal insertion or centered 3–4 cm proximal to the insertion. Insertional Achilles tendinitis/tendinosis is characterized by pain and swelling that is increased by activity. There is usually tenderness in the posterior midline with local increased warmth. Noninsertional Achilles tendinitis/tendinosis is usually associated with a thickened tendon and often quite severe pain to palpation of the thickened area in the midportion of the tendon. Both of these are more degenerative than true inflammatory processes and more properly referred to as tendinosis.

Heel pain can also be caused by inflammation of the retrocalcaneal bursa, which sits between the tendo Achilles and the posterior calcaneus and is often associated with the Haglund heel deformity.

Tarsal tunnel syndrome with involvement of the medial calcaneal branches should be investigated by careful percussion of the posterior tibial nerve. Evidence of degenerative disk disease requires careful testing of motor function and sensation more proximally in the calf.

B. IMAGING STUDIES

Radiographs may demonstrate calcaneal spur formation or calcification at either the insertion of the Achilles tendon or the origin of the plantar fascia. Alternatively, the posterosuperior aspect of the calcaneus may be too prominent and protrude into the Achilles tendon, a condition known as Haglund disease or Haglund deformity, with the symptoms coming from the inflamed retrocalcaneal bursa. A bone scan sometimes reveals increased activity diffusely about the calcaneus, as may be seen in systemic diseases such as Reiter syndrome or a discrete area of uptake as in a stress fracture. MRI scan may help delineate the degree of the Achilles tendon degeneration present in cases of Achilles tendinosis and can help identify rupture of the tendon if this is in question.

Treatment

A. CONSERVATIVE MANAGEMENT

The conservative management of heel pain depends on the specific cause. Because many causes are related to abnormal stress on the foot, the basic principles involve reducing the stress on the involved area. Activity modification, footwear with a softer, more resilient heel, and use of a soft orthotic device under the longitudinal arch to relieve some of the pressure on the region of pain can be helpful. NSAIDs are often useful as is physical therapy to teach stretching exercises of the Achilles tendon and plantar fascia. Plantar fasciitis is treated initially with stretching exercises, soft cushioned heel shoes, NSAIDS if they are tolerated, and avoidance of strong toe-off activities such as running and jumping. The use of a night splint to help keep the Achilles tendon and plantar fascia stretched often relieves the acute pain patients experience when they first get up in the morning. Patients refractory to treatment may benefit from a steroid injection into the plantar fascia origin, although there is a risk of plantar fascia rupture. Cast immobilization also benefits these refractory patients.

In general, the treatment of heel pain is often prolonged, requiring a great deal of patience on the part of the physician and patient. It is important to explain to the patient the nature of the problem and the fact that it is often a chronic condition requiring many months to resolve.

Achilles tendinosis is treated with stretching exercises, activity modification, NSAIDS, and a heel lift. If these modalities are inadequate, bracing or casting provides more strain relief to the damaged tissue.

B. SURGICAL TREATMENT

Patients with plantar fasciitis, in whom symptoms cannot be controlled after 9–12 months of conservative management, may become candidates for surgery. The options include orthotripsy or surgical release of the medial half of the plantar fascial origin. With surgical release, the success rate is approximately 75%. Caution must be exercised with the approach to the medial side of the heel to avoid damage to the medial calcaneal branch of the posterior tibial nerve. Disruption of this nerve causes an area of heel numbness and possibly a troublesome neuroma along the medial side of the heel. An endoscopic approach for plantar fascia release is described in patients who do not have a plantar heel spur that requires removal. Orthotripsy, although less invasive, still has conflicting literature about its effectiveness.

Surgical treatment of Achilles tendinosis is offered if 6–9 months of conservative measures do not help eliminate symptoms. Insertional Achilles tendinosis is treated with debridement of degenerative tendon and excision of bone spurs with repair of the Achilles insertion. If a Haglund deformity is present, it is also resected. Noninsertional Achilles tendinosis is treated with debridement of the degenerative tendon. In either case, if the majority of the tendon is nonviable, it must be repaired, often requiring a graft such as the flexor hallucis longus tendon.

Baxter DE, Pfeffer GB: Treatment of chronic heel pain by surgical release of the first branch of the lateral plantar nerve. Clin Orthop 1992;279:229. [PMID: 1600660]

Boyle RA, Slater GL: Endoscopic plantar fascia release: A case series. Foot Ankle Int 2003;24:176. [PMID: 12627628]

Erdimir A Piazza SJ: Changes in foot loading following plantar fasciotomy: A computer modeling study. J Biomech Eng 2004;126:237. [PMID: 15179854]

Jerosch J et al: Indication, surgical technique and results of endoscopic fascial release in plantar fasciitis (E FRPF). Knee Surg Sports Traumatol Arthrosc 2004;12:471. [PMID: 15088083]

Ogden J et al: Plantar fasciopathy and orthotripsy: The effect of prior cortisone injection. Foot Ankle Int 2005;26:231. [PMID: 15666426]

Williams SK, Brage M: Heel pain-plantar fasciitis and Achilles enthesopathy. Clin Sports Med 2004;23:123. [PMID: 15062587]

Zhu F et al: Chronic plantar fasciitis: Acute changes in the heel after extracorporeal high-energy shock wave therapy—Observations at MR imaging. Radiology 2005;234:206. [PMID: 15564391]

ARTHRODESIS ABOUT THE FOOT & ANKLE

General Considerations

A. GOALS OF ARTHRODESIS

Arthrodesis is surgical fixation of a joint to obtain fusion of the joint surfaces. Arthrodesis about the foot and ankle can be effective in achieving the following goals:

1. elimination of joint pain;
2. correction of deformity;
3. stabilization of the foot or ankle when adequate muscle function or ligamentous support is lacking, as in residual poliomyelitis or the acquired flat foot caused by peritalar instability; and
4. restoration of function by salvaging a situation in which no reasonable reconstructive procedure is available, as in fusion of the first metatarsophalangeal joint after failed hallux valgus repair.

B. PRINCIPLES OF ARTHRODESIS

An arthrodesis about the foot and ankle requires adherence to these general principles:

1. To be effective, the arthrodesis must produce a plantigrade foot.
2. Broad, cancellous bony surfaces must be placed into apposition.
3. The arthrodesis site should be stabilized with rigid internal fixation, preferably with interfragmentary compression.
4. When correcting malalignment of the foot, it is imperative that the hindfoot be placed into 5–7 degrees of valgus and the forefoot in neutral position with regard to abduction, adduction, pronation, and supination.
5. The surgical approaches should be carried out in such a way as to minimize the risk of damage to the nerves.

C. EFFECTS OF ARTHRODESIS ON JOINT MOTION

Following ankle arthrodesis, residual dorsiflexion and plantar flexion movement occurs within the subtalar and transverse tarsal joints, and additional, compensatory motion may develop over time. Arthritic changes in these joints may become symptomatic following ankle arthrodesis, and in time, extension of the fusion may be required.

The subtalar joint and transverse tarsal joints must be viewed as a joint complex similar to the universal joint of a car. Movement in these joints is interrelated. After subtalar arthrodesis, inversion and eversion is lost, but transverse tarsal joint motion is minimally affected. Arthrodesis of the talonavicular joint, however, eliminates most of the subtalar joint motion because rotation must occur around the head of the talus for subtalar motion to occur.

A triple arthrodesis eliminates the subtalar and transverse tarsal joint motion, causing increased stress on the ankle joint and the midtarsal joints distal to the fusion site. A small percentage of patients develop degenerative changes in the ankle joint following triple arthrodesis. It is imperative, therefore, to evaluate the ankle joint carefully prior to carrying out a triple arthrodesis.

Arthrodesis of the tarsometatarsal joints does not significantly affect motion of the foot and ankle, but a certain degree of stiffness is noted through the midtarsal area following this fusion. Fusion of the first metatarsophalangeal joint places added stress on the interphalangeal joint of the great toe, particularly with poor alignment. Although up to 40% of patients may develop degenerative changes in this joint, they are rarely of clinical significance.

D. DISADVANTAGES OF ARTHRODESIS

Although arthrodesis is an effective reconstructive tool, the resulting loss of motion places increased stress on the surrounding joints, making them more prone to developing arthritis or worsening preexisting degenerative changes. Thus, correction of a problem without arthrodesis is preferable whenever possible, such as with an osteotomy, tendon transfer, or both.

Ankle Fusion

A. INDICATIONS

The main indications for ankle arthrodesis are the following:

1. arthrosis of the ankle joint usually secondary to a previous ankle fracture, although primary arthrosis does occur;

2. arthritis secondary to rheumatoid disease; and

3. instability with malalignment of the ankle joint as the result of an epiphyseal injury or previous fracture.

B. TECHNIQUE

The surgical approach preferred by the authors is a transfibular approach (Figure 9–36). The incision begins along the fibula, approximately 10 cm proximal to the tip of the fibula, and is carried distally along the shaft of the fibula and then curves toward the base of the fourth

Figure 9–36. Technique for ankle arthrodesis. Skin incision is placed between superficial peroneal nerve and sural nerve. (Reproduced, with permission, from Mann RA, Coughlin MJ: *The Video Textbook of Foot and Ankle Surgery.* Medical Video Productions, 1991.)

Sural nerve

Incision

Superficial peroneal nerve

Resected area

Figure 9–37. The fibula is excised approximately 2–2.5 cm proximal to the ankle joint, and the distal portion of the tibia is cut, producing a flat cut perpendicular to the long axis of the tibia. (Reproduced, with permission, from Mann RA, Coughlin MJ: *The Video Textbook of Foot and Ankle Surgery.* Medical Video Productions, 1991.)

metatarsal. In this way, the incision avoids the sural nerve posteriorly and the superficial peroneal nerve dorsally. The flaps created are full thickness, to lessen the possibility of wound-healing problems. The dissection is carried across the anterior aspect of the ankle joint, to the medial malleolus and along the lateral aspect of the neck of the talus. Posteriorly, the fibula and the posterior aspect of the ankle joint are exposed; distally, the subtalar joint and sinus tarsi area are exposed. The fibula is removed approximately 2 cm proximal to the joint, after which the residual cartilage and subchondral bone are removed from the distal tibia (Figure 9–37). This cut should be made as perpendicular as possible to the long axis of the tibia and should extend to the medial malleolus but not through it. The foot is placed into a plantigrade position and a cut made in the dome of the talus parallel to the cut in the tibia, thereby creating two flat surfaces and correcting any malalignment. At this point, the ankle should be aligned in neutral position, insofar as dorsiflexion and plantar flexion are concerned, and at approximately 5 degrees of valgus. The degree of rotation should be equal to that of the opposite extremity, which is usually 5–10 degrees of external rotation. If the two joint surfaces do not easily oppose each other, it is because the medial malleolus is too long, and the malleolus should be exposed through a dorsomedial incision and the distal centimeter removed.

The two flat surfaces should now be in total apposition, with little or no pressure being exerted. Temporary fixation is obtained by inserting two 0.062 K-wires. Interfragmentary compression is gained with at least two 6.5-mm cancellous screws. These screws should be placed to gain adequate interfragmentary compression (Figure 9–38). Following insertion of the screws, there should be rigid fixation of the arthrodesis site. Because

Sinus tarsi

Figure 9–38. Diagram demonstrating placement of the 6.5-mm screws across the arthrodesis site. (Reproduced, with permission, from Mann RA, Coughlin MJ: *The Video Textbook of Foot and Ankle Surgery.* Medical Video Productions, 1991.)

the joint surfaces are fully opposed, there is no room for bone grafting. In the immediate postoperative period, a firm compression dressing incorporating plaster splints is applied. After swelling is decreased, a short leg cast is applied and weight bearing is not allowed for 6 weeks. Weight bearing is then allowed with the short leg cast in place for another 6 weeks. Arthrodesis generally occurs following 12 weeks of immobilization.

C. COMPLICATIONS

Nonunion of the ankle joint, although uncommon, does occur. Using the surgical technique described earlier, a fusion rate of 90% can be anticipated. If nonunion occurs, bone grafting and further internal fixation may be required.

Malalignment of the ankle joint with the foot in too much internal rotation is poorly tolerated and often requires revision surgery. Excessive plantar flexion causes a back knee thrust and eventually some knee discomfort; excessive dorsiflexion causes increased stress on the heel (which can usually be treated with adequate padding); varus deformity may cause subtalar joint instability; excessive valgus causes stress on the medial aspect of the knee joint. It is extremely important not to place any pin or screw across the subtalar joint for fear of damaging the posterior facet, which may lead to arthrosis.

D. SPECIAL CONSIDERATIONS

Avascular necrosis of the talus requires excision and tibiocalcaneal fusion or a fusion that bypasses the necrotic bone. Bone grafting may also be necessary when attempting to carry out a fusion after a severely comminuted pilon fracture because there are often defects that affect stability because of the previous crushing of cancellous bone.

Total Ankle Arthroplasty

Total ankle arthroplasty is an alternative to ankle arthrodesis for painful arthrosis of the ankle joint. Advantages include maintenance of some ankle joint motion with a more normal gait and thus less stress on adjacent joints. Unfortunately, the procedure is technically difficult with a steep learning curve, there is a higher complication rate than arthrodesis, and the long-term survival rate is unknown. The intermediate-term survival rate of the Agility total ankle reported by Saltzman suggests the outcome is durable in selected patients. Several other prostheses, including the STAR and the HINTEGRA, used primarily in Europe, have reported promising early results. The long-term results are necessary before widespread use is advocated.

Subtalar Arthrodesis

A. INDICATIONS

The main indications for subtalar arthrodesis are the following:

1. arthrosis of the subtalar joint, usually following a calcaneal fracture, but occasionally for primary arthrosis of the joint;

2. varus or valgus deformity secondary to RA;

3. varus deformity secondary to residual clubfoot or possibly following compartment syndrome;

4. unstable subtalar joint secondary to poliomyelitis, a neuromuscular disorder, or tendon dysfunction, such as posterior tibial tendon dysfunction; and

5. symptomatic talocalcaneal coalition without secondary changes in the talonavicular or calcaneocuboid joints.

B. TECHNIQUE

The incision for subtalar arthrodesis begins at the tip of the fibula and is carried distally toward the base of the fourth metatarsal. As the incision is deepened, the sural nerve or one of its branches should be carefully noted and retracted. Small twigs of nerve may be present that unfortunately may be cut and give rise to a painful neuroma. The sinus tarsi area is exposed by reflecting the extensor digitorum brevis muscle distally. The use of a lamina spreader in the subtalar joint enhances the exposure.

The articular cartilage is removed from the joint surfaces, which include the middle and posterior facets. The bony joint surfaces are then deeply feathered or scaled using a small osteotome. These cuts through the subchondral bone greatly enhance the possibility of fusion. The area around the floor of the sinus tarsi and anterior process region can be carefully shaved to obtain local bone graft for the fusion.

The alignment of the subtalar joint is critical. It must be aligned into approximately 5–7 degrees of valgus position, producing a supple transverse tarsal joint. If it is placed in varus position, the foot is stiff and the patient must walk on the side of the foot.

Rigid fixation of the subtalar joint is achieved by using a 7-mm cannulated interfragmentary screw starting at the posterior tip of the calcaneus and passing into the body or neck of the talus. The guide pin is first placed up into the posterior facet, the subtalar joint is then manipulated into proper alignment, and the guide pin is passed into the talus. The alignment of the screw is verified on radiograph, and the screw is inserted.

Following adequate internal fixation, the local bone graft is packed into the sinus tarsi area. Additional bone may be obtained from the area of the medial malleolus, the proximal tibia, or occasionally the iliac crest, although the latter site significantly adds to the morbidity of the procedure.

Postoperatively, a firm compression dressing incorporating plaster splints is applied. A short leg cast is applied, and weight bearing is not allowed for 6 weeks. The cast is changed, and weight bearing is allowed for another 6 weeks. Twelve weeks of immobilization generally achieves an arthrodesis.

C. COMPLICATIONS

Nonunion of the subtalar joint is uncommon, although it can occur. Careful surgical technique and heavy scaling of the joint surfaces can help prevent this complication. If nonunion occurs, bone grafting and added fixation are required to attempt to achieve a solid union.

Misalignment of the subtalar joint may also be a complication. An excessive valgus deformity following subtalar fusion may result in impingement laterally against the fibula or peroneal tendons. It also causes excessive stress along the medial aspect of the midfoot and occasionally the knee joint. A varus deformity of the subtalar joint imparts rigidity to the transverse tarsal joint, resulting in stiffness of the forefoot. This also increases pressure along the lateral aspect of the foot, particularly in the area of the base of the fifth metatarsal.

D. SPECIAL CONSIDERATIONS

The patient with RA or posttraumatic complications may have lateral subluxation of the calcaneus in relation to the talus, which usually requires CT scanning for identification. The calcaneus must be displaced medially during surgery to align it with the lateral aspect of the talus and place it under the tibia in a proper weight-bearing position. If the calcaneus is fused with significant lateral deviation, the abnormal alignment places added stress on the ankle and midfoot region.

Special attention to the peroneal tendons is necessary when a subtalar arthrodesis is done to correct an old calcaneal fracture. Protrusion of the lateral wall of the body of the calcaneus from the healed fracture results in impingement on the peroneal tendons beneath the fibula. This protrusion must be carefully excised when the subtalar fusion is carried out, so the lateral aspect of the talus and calcaneus are in line. Further, the peroneal tendon sheath should be dissected subperiosteally off the calcaneus to provide tendon sheath and protect the peroneal tendons from the raw, bony surface of the calcaneus.

Occasionally a bone block distraction arthrodesis of the subtalar joint is performed in cases of severe deformity after a calcaneus fracture. If the talus assumes a horizontal position because of flattening of Böhler's angle, it can cause limited ankle joint dorsiflexion. Placing a tricortical block of iliac crest into the posterior facet of the subtalar joint helps improve the overall alignment of the hind foot and regain ankle joint dorsiflexion.

Talonavicular Arthrodesis

A. INDICATIONS

Talonavicular arthrodesis is indicated in the following conditions:

1. posttraumatic injury, RA, or primary arthrosis;
2. unstable talonavicular joint secondary to rupture of the posterior tibial tendon and the peritalar ligaments and RA; and
3. double or triple arthrodesis of the hindfoot.

B. TECHNIQUE

The talonavicular joint is approached through a medial or dorsomedial incision that starts in the region of the naviculocuneiform joint and extends to the neck of the talus. The soft tissues are stripped from around the joint and the articular cartilage removed with a curet or curved osteotome. Distraction of the joint by placing a towel clip into the navicular often facilitates exposure and debridement of the joint. Correct alignment of the talonavicular joint is extremely critical because this fusion essentially eliminates motion in the subtalar joint. The fusion position of the subtalar joint is 3–5 degrees of valgus with the forefoot in a plantigrade position (Figure 9–39). After the foot is properly aligned to correspond to the opposite foot, fixation of the joint is carried out. Proper alignment of this joint is particularly critical when treating the laterally subluxed talonavicular joint in the patient with a ruptured posterior tibial tendon. The internal fixation is carried out by using interfragmentary compression with a single large screw (6.5 mm), two smaller screws (4.0 mm), or multiple staples.

Figure 9–39. Talonavicular fusion. **A:** Changes that occur in the talonavicular joint with a flatfoot deformity. Note that the head of the talus deviates medially as the forefoot deviates laterally into abduction. **B:** The forefoot was brought into adduction so the navicular is once again centered over the head of the talus. (Reproduced, with permission, from Mann RA, Coughlin MJ: *The Video Textbook of Foot and Ankle Surgery.* Medical Video Productions, 1991.)

Postoperatively the patient is immobilized in a non–weight-bearing cast for 6 weeks followed by a weight-bearing cast for an additional 6 weeks.

The talonavicular joint has a relatively high incidence of nonunion, which is probably the result of the difficulty in exposing the joint. If the joint is also approached medially to gain additional exposure, the surfaces can be well scaled, and the fusion rate should approach 90%.

C. COMPLICATIONS

Complications of nonunion and misalignment are similar to those discussed for subtalar joint fusion.

D. SPECIAL CONSIDERATIONS

An isolated talonavicular joint fusion usually produces a satisfactory result, particularly in relatively sedentary patients older than 50 years. In younger, more active individuals with no other affliction (eg, RA), consider-

ation should be given to including the calcaneocuboid joint at the same time to obtain a more stable transverse tarsal joint and enhance the fusion of the talonavicular joint through added stability.

Double Arthrodesis (Calcaneocuboid & Talonavicular Joints)

A. INDICATIONS

Double arthrodesis today is a procedure that provides the same degree of stability to the foot as a triple arthrodesis (Figure 9–40). By locking the transverse tarsal joint (calcaneocuboid and talonavicular), further subtalar motion is prevented because these three joints function together. This procedure is also indicated in the younger, active patient in whom an isolated talonavicular fusion is contemplated because it gives added stability to the foot.

Figure 9–40. Double arthrodesis consisting of a talonavicular and calcaneocuboid fusion. (Reproduced, with permission, from Mann RA, Coughlin MJ: *The Video Textbook of Foot and Ankle Surgery.* Medical Video Productions, 1991.)

Indications for double arthrodesis are as follows:

1. arthrosis of the talonavicular and calcaneocuboid joints (eg, following trauma);
2. unstable talonavicular and calcaneocuboid joint following rupture of the posterior tibial tendon or neuromuscular disease when a flexible subtalar joint is present; and
3. arthrosis of the talonavicular joint or calcaneocuboid joint in an active individual, usually younger than 50 years of age, to give the midfoot a greater degree of stability.

B. TECHNIQUE

The talonavicular joint is approached through a medial or dorsomedial incision, as previously described, and the calcaneocuboid joint is approached through the same incision along the lateral side of the foot as described for subtalar fusion. Once these joints are exposed, the joint surfaces are denuded of articular cartilage and the subchondral bone heavily feathered.

The alignment when carrying out a double arthrodesis is extremely critical because once this fusion is achieved, the subtalar joint or the transverse tarsal joint no longer move. Therefore, the foot must be placed into a plantigrade position prior to the fixation of the arthrodesis site. The desired position is 5 degrees of valgus of the calcaneus, neutral abduction and adduction of the transverse tarsal joint, and correction of any forefoot varus that is present. This alignment creates a plantigrade foot. The fixation of the talonavicular joint is done first with the insertion of a screw (6.5 mm) or screws (4 mm) or possibly the use of multiple staples. The calcaneocuboid joint is then fixed the same way. Postoperative care is the same as for other foot fusions.

C. COMPLICATIONS

Complications of nonunion and malalignment are similar to those discussed for subtalar joint fusion.

Triple Arthrodesis

The triple arthrodesis is a fusion of the talonavicular, calcaneocuboid, and subtalar joints (Figure 9–41). In the past, it was the procedure of choice for all hindfoot problems, before isolated fusions became more accepted. Now, this procedure is still commonly used when limited fusions are inadequate.

A. INDICATIONS

Indications for triple arthrodesis are as follows:

1. arthrosis secondary to trauma involving the subtalar, talonavicular, or calcaneocuboid joints;
2. arthrosis or instability of the talonavicular or calcaneocuboid joints in association with a fixed deformity of the subtalar joint;
3. instability of the foot secondary to posterior tibial tendon dysfunction with a fixed subtalar joint that cannot be realigned by a double arthrodesis;
4. unstable hindfoot secondary to poliomyelitis, nerve injury, or RA;
5. symptomatic, unresectable calcaneonavicular bar; and
6. malalignment of the hindfoot secondary to trauma such as a crush injury or compartment syndrome.

B. TECHNIQUE

The triple arthrodesis is carried out as previously described for subtalar fusion and talonavicular fusion. The foot is fixed after manipulation back into a plantigrade position (3–5 degrees of valgus of the subtalar joint), neutral position as far as abduction and adduction of the transverse tarsal joint, and correction of forefoot varus. Postoperative care is the same as for subtalar fusion.

C. COMPLICATIONS

The main complication is failure of fusion of one of the joints, which is uncommon, because the successful

Figure 9–41. Diagram of a triple arthrodesis. (Reproduced, with permission, from Mann RA, Coughlin MJ: *The Video Textbook of Foot and Ankle Surgery.* Medical Video Productions, 1991.)

fusion rate exceeds 90%. The talonavicular joint is most likely to have nonunion. Malalignment of the foot or forefoot may require revision and technically is a difficult procedure. The sural nerve may become entrapped or disrupted through the lateral approach.

Tarsometatarsal Arthrodesis

Arthrodesis in the tarsometatarsal area may involve a single tarsometatarsal joint, usually the first joint, or multiple joints. The fusion mass not infrequently extends proximally to include the intertarsal bones and sometimes even the naviculocuneiform joints. A careful determination of the involved joints is important when considering a tarsometatarsal fusion for a patient with posttraumatic disorders. At times, in addition to the plain radiograph, a CT scan and bone scan may be necessary to help define the involved area precisely.

A. INDICATIONS

The indications for a tarsometatarsal fusion are as follows:

1. hypermobility of the first metatarsocuneiform joint associated with a hallux valgus deformity in a small percentage of patients with a bunion deformity;

2. arthrosis involving one or more of the tarsometatarsal joints either resulting from trauma or as a primary disease process; and

3. arthrosis associated with a deformity resulting from an old Lisfranc fracture-dislocation.

B. TECHNIQUE

The surgical approach to the first metatarsocuneiform joint is through a dorsomedial longitudinal incision to expose the joint. If multiple joints are involved, the second incision is centered over the second metatarsal, through which the lateral side of the first and all of the second and third metatarsocuneiform joints can be adequately viewed (Figure 9–42). The incision must be sufficiently long to permit adequate exposure of the joints and must be extended proximally if the naviculocuneiform joints are going to be fused as well. Cautious dissection is necessary because there are numerous superficial nerves as well as the neurovascular bundle (dorsalis pedis and superficial branch of the deep peroneal nerve) passing over the area of the second metatarsocuneiform joint in this approach. If the fourth and fifth metatarsocuboid joints are to be fused, a third longitudinal incision is made over this area to enable adequate exposure. The articular cartilage is carefully removed from the tarsometatarsal and intertarsal joints, depending on the extent of the fusion mass. The bones are heavily feathered to create a good environment for healing. If a deformity is present (usually an abduction deformity of the foot or possibly dorsiflexion), it should be corrected.

Figure 9–42. Longitudinal incisions used for a tarsometatarsal arthrodesis. (Reproduced, with permission, from Mann RA, Coughlin MJ: *The Video Textbook of Foot and Ankle Surgery.* Medical Video Productions, 1991.)

The first metatarsocuneiform joint is aligned and fixed using 4-mm cancellous screws or a dorsomedial plate. Interfragmentary longitudinal compression of the other joints is obtained to prevent possible nonunion. The screw pattern found to be most useful for the first metatarsocuneiform joint is one brought from the dorsal aspect of the cuneiform directed distally, and a second screw from the dorsal aspect of the metatarsal base directed proximally, crossing the metatarsocuneiform joint. Care must be taken to also correct any dorsiflexion or abduction deformity that is present.

Postoperatively, the joint is placed in a short leg, non–weight-bearing cast for 6 weeks, and then in a weight-bearing cast for another 6 weeks.

C. COMPLICATIONS

The possibility of nonunion exists, but with interfragmentary compression the risk is minimized. If nonunion occurs, bone grafting may be required as well as improved internal fixation. When multiple tarsometatarsal joints are fused, a moderate amount of swelling and tension is placed against the incisions. It is critical postoperatively to use a compression dressing to minimize the risk of swelling and prevent possible wound sloughing. If sloughing occurs, it must be treated appropriately, and, occasionally, skin grafting is required.

A tarsometatarsal fusion involving multiple joints may cause a plantar callus because one of the metatarsals was placed in a position of too much plantar flexion. Osteotomy at the base of the metatarsal may be necessary to realign the metatarsal.

Staples should be avoided as a means of internal fixation of the tarsometatarsal joints because they have a tendency to cause dorsiflexion of the metatarsals, which could result in transfer pressure problems under the uninvolved metatarsal heads.

First Metatarsophalangeal Joint Arthrodesis

See the discussion of hallux valgus at the beginning of the chapter.

Interphalangeal Joint Arthrodesis (Hallux Arthrodesis)

A. INDICATIONS

Interphalangeal joint arthrodesis is usually indicated for the following problems:

1. arthrosis, usually secondary to trauma or occasionally following a first metatarsophalangeal joint arthrodesis; and

2. stabilization of the interphalangeal joint when carrying out a transfer of the extensor hallucis longus into the neck of the first metatarsal (first toe Jones procedure).

B. TECHNIQUE

The interphalangeal joint is approached through a dorsal transverse incision centered over the joint. An ellipse of skin is usually removed, exposing the ends of the involved joints. Using a small power saw, the end of the distal portion of the proximal phalanx and the proximal portion of the distal phalanx are removed, placing the distal phalanx into approximately 5–7 degrees of plantar flexion and 3–4 degrees of valgus position. Internal fixation is achieved by using a longitudinal screw (4 mm) or crossed K-wires, or both. A postoperative shoe is used, with weight bearing allowed but avoiding the toe-off phase of gait until fusion occurs, usually in 8 weeks.

C. COMPLICATIONS

Nonunion of interphalangeal joint fusion is uncommon. If it does occur, it often is asymptomatic and does not require treatment. If it is symptomatic, usually the fusion needs to be revised because the area is too small for adequate bone grafting.

Buchner M, Sabo D: Ankle fusion attributable to posttraumatic arthrosis: A long-term followup of 48 patients. Clin Orthop 2003;406:155. [PMID: 12579015]

Buck P et al: The optimum position of arthrodesis of the ankle. J Bone Joint Surg Am 1987;69:1052. [PMID: 3654697]

Clain MR, Baxter DE: Simultaneous calcanealcuboid and talonavicular fusion: Long term follow up study. J Bone Joint Surg Am 1994;76:133. [PMID: 8300657]

Harper MC: Talonavicular arthrodesis for the acquired flat foot in the adult. Clin Orthop 1999;365:65. [PMID: 10627687]

Hintermann B et al: The HINTEGRA ankle: rationale and short-term results of 122 consecutive ankles. Clin Orthop 2004;424:57. [PMID: 15241144]

Knecht S et al: The Agility Total Ankle Arthroplasty J Bone Joint Surg AM 2004;86:1161. [PMID: 15173288]

Kofoed H: Scandinavian Total Ankle Replacement (STAR). Clin Orthop 2004;424:73. [PMID: 15241146]

Kofoed H, Sorensen TS: Ankle arthroplasty for rheumatoid arthritis and osteoarthritis. J Bone Joint Surg Br 1998;80;328. [PMID: 9728697]

Komenda GA et al: Results of arthrodesis of the tarsometatarsal joints after traumatic injury. J Bone Joint Surg 1996; 78:1665. [PMID: 8934480]

Mann RA, Beaman DN, Horton GA: Isolated subtalar arthrodesis. Foot Ankle Int 1998;19:511. [PMID: 9728697]

Rosenfeld FF, Budgen SA, Saxby TS: Triple arthrodesis: Is bone grafting necessary? The results of 100 consecutive cases. J Bone Joint Surg Br 2005;87:175. [PMID: 15736738]

Robinson JF, Murphy GA: Arthrodesis as salvage for calcaneal malunions. Foot Ankle Clin 2002;7:107. [PMID: 12380384]

Winson IG, Robinson DE, Allen PE: Arthroscopic ankle arthrodesis. J Bone Joint Surg Br 2005;87:343. [PMID: 15773643]

CONGENITAL FLATFOOT

Congenital flatfoot is the term used to describe a flatfoot present since birth. The condition may not be apparent during the early years of life but is usually identified toward the end of the first or during the second decade. The typical asymptomatic flexible flatfoot is probably a normal variant of the longitudinal arch. This deformity must be differentiated from the symptomatic flexible or more rigid flatfoot, which usually becomes symptomatic in the early teen years and is often caused by a tarsal coalition. These individuals have a fairly flexible foot until adolescence, when the foot often becomes somewhat more rigid and symptomatic.

The patient with a tarsal coalition frequently presents with a peroneal spastic flatfoot, usually around the age of 10–12 years. The theory is that the foot is locked in a valgus position by the peroneal muscle spasm that is trying to immobilize the painful peritalar joints. A tarsal coalition is the union of two or more tarsal bones, usually occurring between the calcaneus and the navicular or between the talus and the calcaneus. This process is a congenital failure of segmentation between the bones of the hindfoot. Coalitions are usually not symptomatic until adolescence, with symptoms brought on by increasing stiffness of the hindfoot as the cartilaginous coalition begins to ossify. Flatfoot associated with an accessory navicular bone usually becomes symptomatic in the early to mid teenage years and may be unilateral or bilateral. Residual congenital deformity from conditions such as clubfoot or congenital vertical talus are present from birth and discussed in Chapter 11, Pediatric Orthopedic Surgery.

The patient with generalized dysplasia, such as Marfan syndrome or Ehlers-Danlos syndrome, may present with flatfoot. A generalized ligamentous laxity is present from the time of birth, and the diagnosis is usually already known.

Clinical Findings

A. SYMPTOMS AND SIGNS

The clinical evaluation begins with the patient in a standing position. In all cases of congenital flatfoot, the longitudinal arch flattens when the patient is standing. In the case of tarsal coalition with peroneal spastic flatfoot, the calcaneus is in a severe fixed valgus position. A tarsal coalition or an accessory navicular may be unilateral, as well as the residuals of a congenital deformity such as clubfoot or congenital vertical talus. The symptomatic and asymptomatic flexible flatfoot and the generalized dysplasias are present bilaterally.

The physical examination of these patients is extremely important. The asymptomatic flexible flatfoot usually demonstrates a satisfactory ROM and no contracture of the Achilles tendon. The symptomatic flexible flatfoot, however, almost invariably demonstrates an equinus contracture. To test adequately for tightness of the Achilles tendon, the head of the talus is covered with the navicular, after which the foot is brought up into dorsiflexion with the knee extended. If the foot is brought into dorsiflexion, permitting lateral subluxation of the talonavicular joint, the examiner often is fooled into thinking that dorsiflexion is adequate when indeed it is not.

The patient with tarsal coalition usually demonstrates restricted hindfoot motion secondary to peroneal spasm and to the cartilaginous or bony bar. The peroneal tendons can actually be felt to be bow strung behind the fibula, not permitting any passive or active inversion of the subtalar joint to occur. On occasion, clonus can be elicited. As a rule, stressing of these joints causes the patient increased discomfort. In flatfoot associated with an accessory navicular, pain is present over the prominence. Frequently, stressing of the posterior tibial tendon aggravates the condition. The patient with residual congenital deformity often demonstrates a certain degree of stiffness of the foot and, not infrequently, varying degrees of deformity of the remainder of the foot. The patient with generalized dysplasia demonstrates marked hypermobility of all the joints, with no contractures whatsoever.

B. IMAGING STUDIES

The radiographic evaluation is useful in differentiating the various types of flatfoot. In almost all cases, the lateral view shows a lack of normal dorsiflexion pitch of the calcaneus, which is approximately 20 degrees or more. In symptomatic flexible flatfoot, the calcaneus may even be in a mild degree of equinus position. On the lateral radiograph, a line drawn through the long axis of the talus and first metatarsal demonstrates an angle of more than 30 degrees in severe flatfoot, 15–30 degrees in moderate flatfoot, and 0–15 degrees in mild flatfoot (Figure 9–43).

The calcaneonavicular coalition is best observed on an oblique radiograph and identified as a bridge from

Normal 0°

Mild 15°

Severe 30°

Figure 9–43. Measurement of flatfoot deformity by using the lateral talometatarsal angle: 0 degrees, normal; 1–15 degrees, mild; 16–30 degrees, moderate; greater than 30 degrees, severe. (Reproduced, with permission, from Bordelon RL: Correction of hyper mobile flatfoot in children by molded insert. Foot Ankle 1980;1:143.)

Figure 9–44. Oblique view of the foot at 45-degree angle demonstrating calcaneonavicular coalition. (Reproduced, with permission, from Mann RA, Coughlin MJ: *Surgery of the Foot and Ankle,* 6th ed. St. Louis: Mosby-Year Book, 1993.)

Figure 9–45. CT scan demonstrating osseous coalition on one side (left) and fibrous coalition on the other (right). (Reproduced, with permission, from Mann RA, Coughlin MJ, eds: *Surgery of the Foot and Ankle,* 6th ed. Mosby-Year Book, 1993.)

the anterior process of the calcaneus to the inferior lateral aspect of the navicular (Figure 9–44). The subtalar or talocalcaneal bar is best demonstrated on a CT scan taken in the coronal plane (Figure 9–45). Flatfoot associated with an accessory navicular demonstrates the accessory bone along the medial side of the navicular, but occasionally a medial oblique view is necessary to outline the size of the fragment (Figure 9–46). In a patient with a residual congenital deformity, such as a clubfoot or congenital vertical talus, the changes about the foot are often sufficient to make the diagnosis fairly

obvious. The patient with generalized dysplasia often demonstrates complete collapse of the longitudinal arch.

Treatment

A. CONSERVATIVE MANAGEMENT

Conservative management is undertaken for congenital flatfoot deformities. A longitudinal arch support may benefit the patient but is usually not necessary for the

Figure 9–46. Large accessory navicular. **A:** Preoperatively, a cartilaginous plate is loose and painful. **B:** One year postoperatively. (Reproduced, with permission, from Mann RA, Coughlin MJ, eds: *Surgery of the Foot and Ankle,* 6th ed. St. Louis: Mosby-Year Book, 1993.)

A

B

asymptomatic flexible flatfoot. For symptomatic flexible flatfoot, a semirigid longitudinal arch support and Achilles stretching exercises may be of some benefit.

The tarsal coalition can be treated conservatively with a short leg walking cast, followed by a polypropylene AFO or a University of California Biomechanics Laboratory (UCBL) insert. If adequate pain relief is achieved, further treatment is not necessary. Flatfoot with an accessory navicular may respond to modification of the shoe to relieve some of the pressure from the involved area. Occasionally, the use of a longitudinal arch support relieves the pressure.

Residual flatfoot resulting from congenital problems can be treated with an AFO or UCBL insert if symptomatic. The patient with generalized dysplasia usually does not require any treatment at all.

B. SURGICAL MANAGEMENT

Surgical procedures are never appropriate for asymptomatic flatfoot. Symptomatic flexible or semiflexible flatfoot occasionally is treated surgically, particularly if equinus contracture is observed after 5 or 6 years of age. A significant equinus contracture may benefit from lengthening of the Achilles tendon. A lateral column lengthening procedure, such as an Evans calcaneal osteotomy, is indicated in cases of symptomatic flexible flatfoot that fail conservative management. This procedure helps correct heel valgus and forefoot abduction and should be done as late into growth as possible to avoid disturbing open growth centers. A triple arthrodesis should only rarely be carried out because it leaves a young patient with a very stiff foot.

A tarsal coalition that does not respond to conservative management may require resection. The surgical approach to the calcaneonavicular bar is identical to that of the subtalar joint. The bar is carefully outlined and then resected in its entirety. Talocalcaneal coalitions are resectable throughout the adolescent years, if less than 20% of the posterior facet of the subtalar joint is involved or if the coalition is confined only to the middle facet. More extensive involvement of the subtalar joint in an adolescent or any bar in an adult patient is an indication for subtalar arthrodesis. The approach is through a medial incision centered over the middle facet, and caution is taken to carefully reflect the tendons and posterior tibial nerve. The extent of the coalition is identified, and it is resected to expose the area of normal-appearing articular cartilage. Bone wax is applied to the edges or a free fat graft is inserted to prevent reformation of the bar. Flatfoot associated with an accessory navicular may require excision of the accessory navicular and plication of the posterior tibial tendon (Kidner procedure). This fairly successful operation is usually carried out during the late adolescent years.

Residual congenital deformity or generalized dysplasias usually do not require surgical management. In severe cases, a triple arthrodesis is indicated after the foot has matured.

Coleman S: *Complex Foot Deformities in Children*. Lea and Febiger, 1983.

Frischhut B et al: Foot deformities in adolescents and young adults with spina bifida. J Pediatr Orthop B 2000;9:161. [PMID: 10904902]

Giannini S et al: Operative treatment of flatfoot with talocalcaneal coalition. Clin Orthop 2003;411:178. [PMID: 12782874]

Gonzalez P, Kumar SJ: Calcaneonavicular coalition treated by resection and interposition of the extensor digitorum brevis muscle. J Bone Joint Surg 1990;72:71. [PMID: 2104855]

Varner KE, Michelson JD: Tarsal coalition in adults. Foot Ankle Int 2000;21:669. [PMID: 10966365]

ACQUIRED FLATFOOT DEFORMITY

Acquired flatfoot deformity is a condition affecting a foot that at one time had a normal functioning longitudinal arch. Over time, the arch progressively flattens, often causing the foot to become symptomatic. This deformity is different from congenital flatfoot deformity, present since birth. Acquired flatfoot deformity in the adult may be caused by the following conditions:

1. posterior tibial tendon dysfunction;
2. arthrosis of the tarsometatarsal joints, which may be primary or secondary to a previous Lisfranc fracture or dislocation;
3. Charcot changes in the midfoot resulting from a peripheral neuropathy; or
4. talonavicular collapse resulting from trauma or RA.

Acquired flatfoot deformities are complex deformities that affect different areas of the midfoot and hindfoot. The deformities may include dorsal subluxation of the talonavicular joint and tarsometatarsal joints, abduction of the forefoot, valgus deformity of the hindfoot, or all three. The extent of the deformity varies widely and is usually progressive. Depending on the etiology, acquired flatfoot deformity may affect a patient bilaterally.

Clinical Findings

A. SYMPTOMS AND SIGNS

A careful history is important to help distinguish among differing causes of acquired flatfoot deformity. Usually, no specific traumatic event is recalled by the patient who presents with dysfunction of the posterior tibial tendon. In approximately half of patients with tarsometatarsal joint arthrosis, a Lisfranc fracture-dislocation has occurred, whereas the other half has primary arthrosis. The patient with Charcot foot usually gives a relevant history of the cause of the peripheral neuropathy, such as diabetes. The patient with collapse of the talonavicular joint gives a history of prior trauma to the talus or navicular or has RA, which causes disruption of the spring ligament complex.

The physical examination begins by observing the foot with the patient standing, observing for unilateral or bilateral flattening of the longitudinal arch. Varying degrees of abduction of the forefoot and hindfoot valgus should also be evaluated.

The patient with posterior tibial tendon dysfunction demonstrates little or no active inversion strength. Usually, the posterior tibial tendon is thick and swollen and there is increased warmth and pain to palpation over the tendon sheath. When the patient is asked to stand on tiptoe, the involved calcaneus remains in valgus position rather than inverting, as normally occurs. When the patient is viewed from the posterior aspect, more toes are visible laterally on the involved foot than the uninvolved foot, commonly known as the "too many toes sign."

Arthrosis of the tarsometatarsal joints creates a deformity of abduction of the forefoot with varying degrees of dorsiflexion, giving rise to a rather prominent medial cuneiform. Not infrequently, palpable osteophytes are present on the dorsal and plantar aspect of the tarsometatarsal joints.

A Charcot foot presents with varying degrees of swelling and deformity. In the early stages, the foot demonstrates generalized swelling and increased warmth, with loss of sensation in a stocking-glove distribution. Deformity may vary from a mild flat foot to a severe rocker-bottom deformity. It is important to palpate for bony prominences on the medial and plantar aspects of the foot that make it at risk for ulcerations.

In the patient with RA, most of the changes occur within the talonavicular joint. In this case, the head of the talus is often palpable on the plantar medial aspect of the foot. When the subtalar joint is more involved, a fixed hindfoot valgus deformity is usually present as well.

The posttraumatic deformity may vary, depending on precisely which joints are involved. If trauma led to a collapse of the navicular, the longitudinal arch is flattened with little forefoot abduction, and the head of the talus is often palpable on the plantar medial aspect of the foot. There is usually little or no motion in the hindfoot and midfoot joints.

B. IMAGING STUDIES

Radiographs usually differentiate the cause of the problem. In the patient with posterior tibial tendon dysfunction, there is sagging of the talonavicular joint and abduction of the navicular on the head of the talus. The patient with tarsometatarsal joint arthrosis demonstrates typical degenerative changes at the affected joints, along with varying degrees of lateral and dorsal

subluxation of the joints. Patients with Charcot foot demonstrate characteristic changes seen in a neuropathic joint, including dramatic bone destruction and joint dislocations (Figure 9–47). The patient with RA demonstrates the typical destructive changes observed with this disease process, with joint space narrowing but little osteophyte formation.

Treatment

A. CONSERVATIVE MANAGEMENT

Conservative management is aimed at providing support to the longitudinal arch and ankle with a polypropylene AFO. The orthosis must be shaped to accommodate any prominences that might be present. Unfortunately, these prominences present the potential for skin breakdown, particularly in the neuropathic foot. A rocker-bottom-type shoe with an adequate toe box is sometimes indicated to give the patient a smoother gait pattern.

B. SURGICAL TREATMENT

The surgical management of these various conditions is specific for each problem. Posterior tibial tendon dysfunction with a satisfactory ROM of the joints of the hindfoot and midfoot can be treated with reconstruction of the posterior tibial tendon, using a flexor digitorum longus tendon transfer. A calcaneal osteotomy is performed as well, if a significant valgus deformity of the heel is present. Alternatively, a lateral column lengthening, consisting of a calcaneal-cuboid distraction arthrodesis, can be used to correct a flexible flat foot with significant abduction of the forefoot. When a fixed deformity is present in the hindfoot or forefoot, a triple arthrodesis is indicated.

The patient with Charcot foot is treated in a short leg cast until the acute process subsides, after which a polypropylene AFO is used. Occasionally, a bony prom-

Figure 9–47. Charcot midfoot changes resulting in joint dislocations and a rocker-bottom deformity of the foot.

inence that continues to cause skin breakdown may be excised to permit the patient to use an AFO. In extreme rocker-bottom deformities, midfoot correction with an osteotomy may be required. The rheumatoid patient usually requires stabilization of the involved area with an isolated talonavicular fusion if little deformity is present, or a triple arthrodesis if there is a hindfoot or midfoot deformity.

The posttraumatic foot with involvement of the talonavicular joint requires a triple arthrodesis. The fusion may need to be extended distally to include the naviculocuneiform joints if arthrosis is present at these joints.

The patient with arthrosis of the tarsometatarsal joints responds well to surgical management by realigning the foot and carrying out arthrodesis of the involved joints.

Castro MD: Arthrodesis of the navicular. Foot Ankle Clin 2004;9(1):73. [PMID: 15062215]

Guyton GP et al: Flexor digitorum longus transfer and medial displacement calcaneal osteotomy for posterior tibial tendon dysfunction: A middle-term clinical follow-up. Foot Ankle Int 2001;22:627. [PMID: 11527022]

Mann RA, Thompson FM: Rupture of the posterior tibial tendon causing flatfoot: Surgical treatment. J Bone Joint Surg Am 1985;67:556. [PMID: 3980501]

Thomas RL et al: Preliminary results comparing two methods of lateral column lengthening. Foot Ankle Int 2001;22:107. [PMID: 11249219]

Trepman E et al. Current topics review: Charcot neuroarthropathy of the foot and ankle. Foot Ankle Int 2005;26(1):46. [PMID: 15680119]

Trnka HJ: Dysfunction of the tendon of tibialis posterior. J Bone Joint Surg Br 2004;86(7):939. [PMID: 15446514]

CAVUS FOOT

Cavus foot deformity is characterized by an abnormal elevation of the longitudinal arch, with resulting decrease in the plantar weight-bearing area and stress concentrated on the metatarsal heads. The condition may be aggravated by clawing of the toes, further reducing the forefoot weight-bearing area. Generalized stiffness of the joints is common, causing the patient to avoid prolonged use of the foot.

Etiologic Findings

The various causes of cavus foot deformity include the following:

1. anterior horn cell disease, such as poliomyelitis, diastematomyelia, and spinal cord tumor;
2. nerve disorders, such as Charcot-Marie-Tooth disease and spinal dysraphism;
3. muscular diseases, such as muscular dystrophy;
4. long tract and central diseases, such as Friedreich ataxia and cerebral palsy;

5. idiopathic conditions, such as residual clubfoot, arthrogryposis, and cavus foot of undetermined cause; and
6. posttraumatic disorders following injuries, such as compartment syndrome or crush injury.

Anatomy

Cavus foot deformity is extremely variable in its presentation, from mild to extremely severe degree of cavus. The types of deformities can be classified based on the localizing of the area of deformity:

1. Posterior cavus deformity—This deformity mainly involves the calcaneus, which has a dorsiflexion pitch angle of greater than 40 degrees measured on a weight-bearing lateral radiograph. Normally, the dorsiflexion pitch to the calcaneus is approximately 20 degrees. Some degree of varus deformity of the heel is usually present as well.

2. Anterior cavus deformity—In anterior cavus deformity, there is a forefoot equinus deformity with the hindfoot in a neutral position. The anterior cavus may be localized, mainly involving the first and second metatarsal, or it may be more global, with the entire forefoot in a position of plantar flexion. Some degree of adduction of the forefoot is usually present.

3. Combined cavus deformity—In a combined cavus deformity, which is the most severe, there are both anterior and posterior components.

Clinical Findings

A. SYMPTOMS AND SIGNS

A careful history regarding the onset of the condition and progression is important. A detailed family history should also be obtained because idiopathic cavus deformity does tend to run in families. Progression of deformity should be ascertained, particularly in the adolescent, because it may indicate a spinal cord abnormality or neoplasm. Activity level and ambulation should also be carefully evaluated as markers of progression of neural or muscular disease.

The degree of deformity of the foot must be examined with the patient in a standing position. This also reveals any evidence of atrophy of the calf muscles, as seen in Charcot-Marie-Tooth disease, clubfoot, or arthrogryposis. The active and passive ROM of the joints of the foot and ankle should be carefully measured. The muscle strength of each muscle must be carefully evaluated, especially if considering a tendon transfer. The degree of deformity and flexibility of the rearfoot, forefoot, metatarsophalangeal joints, and lesser toes must be ascertained. The presence of a tight plantar fascia should also be noted. The lateral ankle ligaments must be evaluated for integrity because they often become stretched out with long-standing varus heel deformity.

B. IMAGING STUDIES

Weight-bearing radiographs of the foot and ankle are obtained to help classify the type of cavus deformity and formulate a treatment plan. Any degree of arthrosis or varus tilting of the talus in the ankle mortise is also evaluated.

Treatment

A. CONSERVATIVE MANAGEMENT

Conservative care is tailored to the severity of the cavus deformity. Mild deformities may only require a softer-soled shoe. Significant clawing of the lesser toes may require an extra-depth shoe. A custom-made Plastazote

liner with a built-in arch support helps decrease the stress on the metatarsal heads. A significant motor deficit may require an AFO to stabilize the ankle. Most cases of cavus foot can be managed with conservative modalities.

B. SURGICAL TREATMENT

Surgical treatment for the cavus foot is aimed at correcting the site of the deformity. The most frequent pattern consists of plantar flexion of the first metatarsal, contracture of the plantar fascia, and varus deformity of the calcaneus. These problems respond to release of the plantar fascia, dorsiflexion osteotomy of the first and perhaps second metatarsal, and lateral closing-wedge osteotomy (Dwyer procedure) of the calcaneus to correct the varus deformity. Fusion of the joints is avoided to maintain as much flexibility of the foot as possible (Figure 9–48).

Figure 9–48. Technique for correction of cavus foot. **A:** For first metatarsal osteotomy, a dorsally based wedge of bone was removed approximately 1 cm distal to the metatarsocuneiform joint. The plantar fascia was released. Dorsiflexion of the osteotomy site helps correct the cavus deformity by flattening the arch. **B:** Heel varus is corrected by a closing-wedge calcaneus osteotomy. (Reproduced, with permission, from Mann RA, Coughlin MJ: *The Video Textbook of Foot and Ankle Surgery.* Medical Video Productions, 1991.)

A more severe deformity involving dorsiflexion of the calcaneus can be treated with sliding osteotomy of the calcaneus (Samilson procedure), correcting any varus deformity with a lateral closing-wedge osteotomy and releasing the plantar fascia (Figure 9–49). Forefoot deformity is treated with osteotomy of the first and sometimes second metatarsal. In some patients, transfer of the peroneus longus tendon into the brevis and lengthening of the posterior tibial tendon provides dynamic muscle balance for the foot.

Severe deformities not amenable to procedures that retain joint motion require triple arthrodesis. A Siffert beak-type triple arthrodesis corrects the deformity because the navicular is mortised under the head of the talus to help reduce the elevation of the longitudinal arch (Figure 9–50). A first metatarsal osteotomy may need to be added to the procedure as well.

The lesser toes may have either fixed or flexible clawtoe deformities. Flexible deformity often responds to release of the extensor tendons and a Girdlestone flexor tendon transfer. If a fixed deformity is present, a DuVries phalangeal condylectomy corrects the hammer

Figure 9–50. A diagram of a beak-type triple arthrodesis. This mortises the navicular underneath a portion of the head of the talus to allow rotation of the distal portion of the foot, permitting flattening of the longitudinal arch and correction of the cavus deformity. (Reproduced, with permission, from Mann RA, Coughlin MJ: *The Video Textbook of Foot and Ankle Surgery*. Medical Video Productions, 1991.)

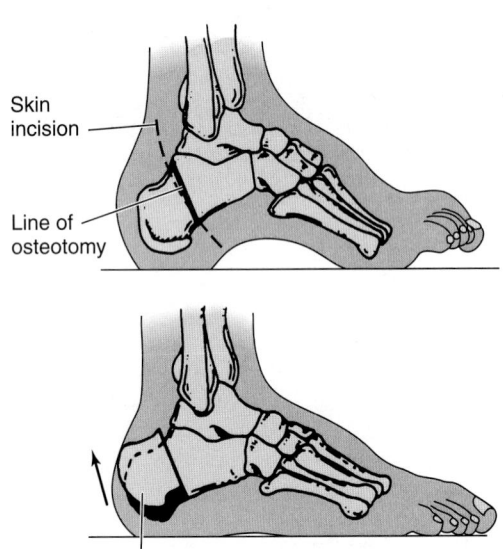

Skin incision

Line of osteotomy

Dorsal displacement of posterior calcaneus

Figure 9–49. Techniques of calcaneal osteotomy. In the treatment of pes cavus, the osteotomy permits the calcaneus to be moved into a more dorsal position and, if necessary, to be closed laterally to correct heel varus. (Reproduced, with permission, from Mann RA, Coughlin MJ: *The Video Textbook of Foot and Ankle Surgery*. Medical Video Productions, 1991.)

toe, followed by extensor tendon release and the Girdlestone procedure.

Hyperextension of the first metatarsophalangeal joint is corrected by interphalangeal arthrodesis of the hallux and transfer of the extensor hallucis longus tendon into the neck of the first metatarsal (Jones procedure) (Figure 9–51).

Breusch SJ et al. Function after correction of a clawed great toe by a modified Robert Jones transfer. J Bone Joint Surg (Br) 2000:82-B:250. [PMID: 10755436]

Giannini S et al. Surgical treatment of adult idiopathic cavus foot with plantar fasciotomy, naviculocuneiform arthrodesis, and cuboid osteotomy. A review of thirty-nine cases. J Bone Joint Surg Am. 2002;84-A Suppl 2:62. [PMID: 12479341]

Siffert RS del Torto U "Beak" triple arthrodesis for severe cavus deformity. Clin Orthop Relat Res 1983;181:64. [PMID: 6641068]

Sammarco GJ, Taylor R Cavovarus foot Treated with combined calcaneus and metatarsal osteotomies. Foot Ankle Int 2001; 22:19. [PMID: 11206819]

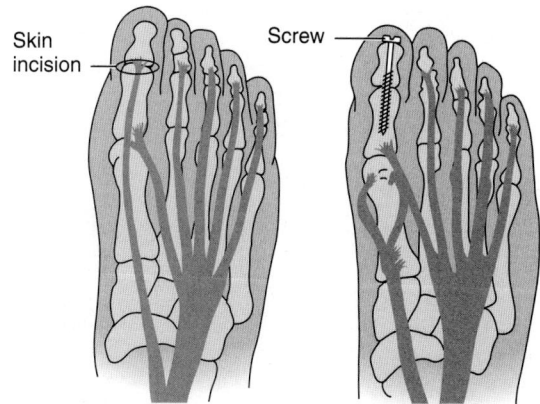

Figure 9–51. Diagram of the first toe Jones procedure. This procedure moves the pull of the extensor hallucis longus tendon from the great toe into the neck of the metatarsal. An interphalangeal arthrodesis of the hallux is carried out. (Reproduced, with permission, from Mann RA, Coughlin MJ, eds: *Surgery of the Foot and Ankle.* Mosby-Year Book, 1993.)

ORTHOTIC DEVICES FOR THE FOOT & ANKLE

Orthotic devices are used to redistribute stresses on the foot as it makes contact with the ground and to accommodate for abnormal function of defective muscles or ligaments. This is achieved by controlling the posture of the foot and padding certain areas to relieve pressure and provide increased comfort for the foot. Orthoses are also used to limit motion in arthritic joints, making them less painful. The orthotic device may be attached to the sole of the shoe, may be inserted inside the shoe as an insole, may cup the foot (UCBL insert), or may extend across the ankle to hold the entire foot and ankle in place (AFO).

Orthotic Shoe Sole Devices

A variety of heel and sole corrections are available to accommodate foot postural abnormalities. A medial or lateral heel or sole wedge (or a combination of both) can help control excessive pronation or supination from weak tendons, ligamentous instability, or fixed deformities. A wide heel is used to increase the stability of the subtalar joint. A rocker sole helps stabilize the forefoot in the case of a fracture or arthritis and also aids a patient with an ankle fusion to allow a more normal gait pattern.

Orthotic Insole Devices

Insole orthotic devices can be used for flexible deformities to alter the posture of the foot and for fixed deformi-

ties to redistribute stress. The simplest device is a soft liner for a shoe or boot made out of a high-density foam material. Other simple orthoses include a soft felt pad to relieve pressure on the metatarsal heads or a combination of materials to produce a more rigid support to help control a forefoot deformity such as forefoot varus or valgus deformity. Orthotic devices take up space in the shoe, and the patient may need a larger or deeper shoe.

University of California Biomechanics Laboratory Insert

The principle of the UCBL insert is to correct a foot deformity such as flatfoot by stabilizing the calcaneus in neutral position and molding the orthosis to block abduction of the forefoot. Posting along the medial aspect may compensate for forefoot varus. In theory, this orthotic device is excellent for controlling the rearfoot and forefoot, but two caveats apply to the use of this device. The first is that the foot must be flexible because correction of a rigid deformity is impossible. The second is that a bony prominence can chafe against the polypropylene material, resulting in pain or skin breakdown over the prominence.

Ankle-Foot Orthosis

An AFO is a molded polypropylene device that passes along the posterior aspect of the calf and then onto the plantar aspect of the foot to the metatarsal heads. Alterations are made in a variety of ways to accommodate the patient's problem (Figure 9–52). Ankle problems such as arthrosis or dorsiflexion weakness require adequate rigidity to eliminate ankle joint motion. An orthosis for a subtalar joint problem should have enough flexibility to provide ankle joint motion but must be rigid enough to immobilize the subtalar joint. When the problem involves the transverse tarsal joint, the AFO can be fabricated to permit some ankle joint motion but maintain immobilization of the transverse tarsal joint area, usually by blocking abduction of the forefoot. When managing tarsometatarsal arthritis, the footpiece is carried to the tips of the toes. Again, a significant fixed bony deformity results in pressure points, making fitting of the device difficult. If the patient has loss of sensation, careful construction and padding are essential to minimize the risk of ulcers forming over a bony prominence. In cases of marked instability or discomfort, an anterior shell can be added to the AFO, and the brace is extended proximally to create a patellar tendon bearing surface.

Double Upright Orthosis

The double upright orthosis with a hinged ankle may be used when individuals require stability but are engaged in physically demanding activities. The double upright orthosis is somewhat more cumbersome than the AFO

A   **B**

Figure 9–52. Types of ankle-foot orthoses (AFOs). **A:** A standard AFO with a trim-line cut to maximum stability of the ankle joint. If the trim line is cut more posteriorly, there would be some give at the ankle joint. **B:** An anterior shell was added to the AFO to increase the stability of the foot and ankle within the brace. (Reproduced, with permission, from Mann RA, Coughlin MJ, eds: *Surgery of the Foot and Ankle,* 6th. ed. Mosby-Year Book, 1993.)

but provides rigid immobilization. The hinge mechanism of the ankle joint may be changed, depending on the nature of the patient's problem. The ankle joint can be free, which allows dorsiflexion and plantar flexion to occur, or it can be fixed to prevent plantar flexion past 90 degrees. This brace can be modified with a spring load to provide dorsiflexion for the patient with dropfoot resulting from paralysis but should not be used for the patient with spasticity because it may accentuate the spasticity.

Prescriptions for Orthotic Devices

The following are typical prescriptions for orthotic devices.

A. METATARSALGIA OR ATROPHY OF PLANTAR FAT PAD

1. Treatment—A full-length well-molded orthosis for metatarsal arch support is used to relieve pressure under the metatarsal heads. Soft insole material should be used.

2. Explanation—In the treatment of metatarsalgia or atrophy of the plantar fat pad, a full-length orthosis is needed that is molded to the plantar aspect of the foot and built up just proximal to the metatarsal heads to relieve pressure on them. The material should be soft to provide extra cushioning for the foot.

B. RUPTURED POSTERIOR TIBIAL TENDON WITH MODERATELY SEVERE FLEXIBLE FLATFOOT DEFORMITY

1. Treatment—AFO with trim-line cut to permit 30% ankle joint motion is molded to reestablish the longitudinal arch and built up on the lateral aspect of the footpiece to block abduction of the forefoot.

2. Explanation—With a moderately advanced flexible flatfoot deformity, an in-shoe orthotic device alone does not provide sufficient support; the AFO is needed to provide adequate stability. Some ankle joint motion is included, which makes ambulation more comfortable for the patient. The longitudinal arch is molded to support the foot in a plantigrade position, and the lateral aspect of the AFO is built up to prevent the forefoot from moving into an abducted position. By blocking abduction, the amount of pressure needed beneath the longitudinal arch to prevent it from collapsing is decreased.

C. POSTERIOR TIBIAL TENDON INSUFFICIENCY WITH MILD FLATFOOT DEFORMITY AND 5 DEGREES OF FOREFOOT VARUS DEFORMITY

1. Treatment—Use a well-molded longitudinal arch support, with a 5-degree varus post and a 3-degree medial heel lift.

2. Explanation—Insufficiency of the posterior tibial tendon that has not produced a significant foot deformity can be treated with a well-molded longitudinal arch support. The 5-degree varus forefoot post compensates for the fixed forefoot varus, and the 3-degree heel lift likewise helps tilt the hindfoot from valgus deformity closer to neutral position.

D. DROPFOOT SECONDARY TO PERONEAL NERVE INJURY

1. Treatment—An AFO with a full footpiece is molded to the longitudinal arch.

2. Explanation—A dropfoot secondary to a peroneal nerve injury responds well to an AFO with a full footpiece. The footpiece supports the toes so they do not drop and makes it easier for the patient to put on shoes.

E. DIABETIC NEUROPATHY WITH CLAWFOOT DEFORMITY

1. Treatment—An extra-depth shoe with a molded Plastazote liner is backed with a Pelite material.

2. Explanation—The patient with clawfoot deformity requires a shoe that has extra height in the toe box. The extra-depth shoe provides enough room for the toes, so they do not chafe against the top of the shoe. The molded Plastazote liner is an excellent means of providing full contact to the plantar aspect of the foot. Plastazote has a tendency to bottom out, as it were, and by backing the material with a Pelite liner or some comparable material, the life expectancy of the Plastazote is extended significantly.

Bordelon RL: Orthotics, shoes, and braces. Orthop Clin North Am 1989;20:751. [PMID: 2797761]

Major RE et al: A new structural concept in moulded fixed ankle foot orthoses and comparison of the bending stiffness of four constructions. Prosthet Orthot Int 2004;28:44. [PMID: 15171577]

Pfeffer G et al: Comparison of custom and prefabricated orthoses in the initial treatment of proximal plantar fasciitis. Foot Ankle Int 1999;20:214. [PMID: 10229276]

Pinzur M: Surgical versus accommodative treatment for Charcot arthropathy of the midfoot. Foot Ankle Int 2004;25:545. [PMID: 15363375]

Raikin SM et al: Biomechanical evaluation of the ability of casts and braces to immobilize the ankle and hindfoot. Foot Ankle Int 2001;22:214. [PMID: 11310863]

LIGAMENTOUS INJURIES ABOUT THE ANKLE JOINT

Ankle ligament injuries represent the most common musculoskeletal injury; therefore, accurate assessment and treatment of these injuries are important. The lateral collateral ligament complex is most commonly injured, but damage to other important structures around the ankle joint should not be overlooked, as discussed in this section.

Functional Anatomy

The lateral collateral ligament structure of the ankle consists of three distinct ligamentous bands: the anterior and posterior talofibular ligaments (ATFL and PTFL) and the calcaneal fibular ligament (CFL).

When the ankle joint is in plantar flexion, the ATFL is positioned in line with the fibula and therefore placed under stress with an inversion injury and will be damaged. Conversely, when the ankle joint is in dorsiflexion, the CFL is positioned in line with the long axis of the fibula and is therefore subject to injury. If the applied stress is severe, both the ATFL and the CFL may be torn, no matter the position of the ankle joint. The syndesmosis ligament complex tethers the tibia and fibula together and is injured by an external rotational force to the foot. The deltoid ligament is the sole medial stabilizer of the ankle joint. An isolated deltoid ligament injury can occur with an eversion or external rotation force on the foot. The deltoid ligament can also sustain injury in conjunction with a syndesmosis ligament injury, with lateral ankle sprains, or with a concomitant fibula fracture (known as a Maisonneuve fracture).

Clinical Findings

A. CLASSIFICATION

Lateral collateral ankle ligament injuries are divided into three degrees of severity. A grade I sprain is confined to the ATFL and demonstrates no instability. A grade II sprain involves injury to both the ATFL and CFL, with mild laxity of one or both ligaments. A grade III sprain involves injury and significant laxity of both the ATFL and CFL.

B. SYMPTOMS AND SIGNS

A past history of injuries of the ankle and problems with chronic ankle ligament instability should be ascertained. A careful physical examination is important to evaluate the degree of involvement of each ligament and to rule out injury to any adjacent bony or soft-tissue structures. The ATFL, PTFL, CFL, and syndesmosis ligaments are palpated for tenderness. To rule out fractures, pain should be elicited in the area of the distal fibula, the anterior process of the calcaneus, the lateral process of the talus, and at the base of the fifth metatarsal. Other areas where an injury must be ruled out include the subtalar joint and the peroneal tendon sheath.

A patient with significant medial joint pain with or without lateral ligament pain should be evaluated for an injury to the deltoid ligament complex, the posterior tibial tendon, and the medial talar dome. Assessment of ankle ligament stability requires clinical and radiographic stress examinations. To perform an anterior drawer maneuver, which tests stability of the ATFL, the ankle is placed in 30 degrees of equinus, and the ankle is pulled in an anterior and slightly internally rotated direction (Figure 9–53). A feeling of subluxation is present if a significant ligament injury has occurred. A talar tilt maneuver is performed by placing an inversion stress on the heel. With the foot in plantar flexion, this tests the stability of the ATFL. With the foot in neutral or dorsiflexion, a talar tilt maneuver tests the stability of the CFL. If clinical instability is suggested by either maneuver, radiographic confirmation can be performed, with comparison to the unaffected ankle.

Deltoid ligament insufficiency may cause a feeling of instability and giving way, affecting the medial aspect of the ankle joint. Stress examination is performed by pulling the foot laterally and into valgus while stabilizing the distal tibia.

Injury to the syndesmosis ligament complex is suspected if the region between the distal anterior tibia and fibula is tender to palpation. If extensive swelling is present more than 2 cm proximal to the ankle joint, syndesmosis rupture is a strong possibility. Pain elicited by squeezing the tibia and fibula together in the midcalf is diagnostic of a syndesmosis ligament tear. A syndesmosis ligament injury is also suspected if external rotation of the foot is painful or if lateral translation of the talus in the ankle mortice occurs with direct lateral force on the foot.

C. IMAGING STUDIES

Standard anteroposterior, lateral, and oblique radiographs of the ankle should be obtained to rule out a fracture of the fibula, talus, or calcaneus. If ligament laxity is suggested on clinical examination, stress radiographs should be obtained. An anteroposterior view is taken while a talar tilt maneuver is performed, and a lateral view is taken while an anterior drawer maneuver is performed. More than 10 degrees of tilt and more than 5–7 mm of anterior drawer are considered abnormal.

If a syndesmosis ligament injury is suspected, careful attention must be paid to the joint spaces to rule out

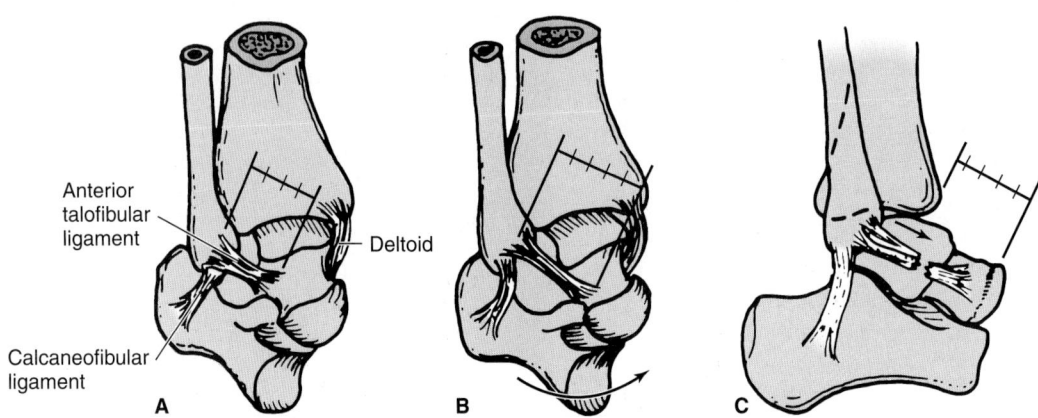

Figure 9–53. Mechanics of carrying out a stress test of the lateral ankle ligaments. **A:** Normal anatomic alignment, which demonstrates the checkrein effect of the anterior talofibular ligament on the talus. **B:** The stress test for the calcaneofibular ligament is carried out by firmly inverting the calcaneus. **C:** The anterior talofibular ligament is tested by placing the ankle joint in neutral position and applying an anterior pull with slight medial rotation. (Reproduced, with permission, from Mann RA, Coughlin MJ, eds: *Surgery of the Foot and Ankle,* 6th. ed. Mosby-Year Book, 1993.)

widening of the ankle mortise. If instability is suspected, a stress radiograph is performed by externally rotating the foot with the tibia held still.

MRI or CT scan may be helpful in some instances if there is a high index of suspicion for an accompanying injury. Osteochondral injuries to the talus should be ruled out with an MRI scan. If a talus or calcaneus fracture is suspected, either MRI or CT scan may be of benefit.

Treatment

A. CONSERVATIVE MANAGEMENT

Acute grade I ligament tears are treated with a lateral stabilizing ankle brace, ice, and avoidance of painful activities. Immediate full weight-bearing is allowed, as are non–weight-bearing physical activities, such as bicycling and swimming. The brace can be discontinued in 1 month.

Grade II ligament tears are treated with protected weight bearing and a lateral stabilizing ankle brace. The patient can begin non–weight-bearing exercise (stationary bicycle) after 7 days, along with peroneal strengthening exercises. Weight-bearing exercise (jogging) may resume after 2–4 weeks.

In a grade III ligament tear, the ankle is immobilized with a removable walking cast for 3–4 weeks. This is followed by a period of physical therapy consisting of range-of-motion (ROM) exercises, peroneal strengthening, and proprioception training using a biomechanical ankle platform system (BAPS) board.

Treatment of isolated deltoid ligament sprains depends on the severity of the injury and is similar to lateral ligament injuries. Mild injuries can be treated with immediate mobilization and rapid return to activity, whereas more severe injuries should be casted for 3–4 weeks.

Syndesmosis ligament tears, if mild, can be treated with weight bearing in a cast or brace and close follow-up to assess for widening of the ankle joint mortise. If the interosseous membrane is damaged, as evidenced by massive swelling of the leg proximal to the ankle joint, treatment depends on the radiographic appearance of the ankle. If the mortise has not widened, the patient is kept on a non–weight-bearing regime in a cast for 6 weeks, with close radiographic follow-up. If initial or follow radiographs show a widened mortise, the patient requires surgical repair of the syndesmosis ligaments with temporary screw placement until the ligaments heal.

B. SURGICAL TREATMENT

The surgical treatment of an acute ligamentous injury is indicated only for the occasional elite athlete. Most ligamentous injuries, even grade III sprains, heal sufficiently with no significant disability if properly treated, as just described. However, even less severe ankle sprains may cause chronic pain or functional instability if left untreated.

The indication for a lateral ligament reconstruction is functional ligament instability. A patient with ligament instability complains of recurrent sprains that occur with sports activities or even with activities of daily living, despite 4–6 months of physical therapy and use of a lateral stabilizing brace. A patient with functional ligament instability also complains of difficulty walking on uneven ground. This history must be found in conjunction with physical examination findings of ligament instability.

Although many lateral ankle reconstruction procedures are described for chronic lateral ankle ligament instability, a Broström repair is generally the procedure of choice. The Broström procedure is a soft-tissue ligamentous repair in which the ATFL and CFL are plicated and reattached to their anatomic positions (Figure 9–54). The repair is reinforced by bringing up a portion of the inferior extensor retinaculum. The Broström procedure is highly effective and has lower morbidity than other procedures that harvest the peroneus brevis tendon. In patients who have severe and long-standing laxity or have failed a Broström repair, revision surgery with an allograft or autograft tendon is indicated.

Chronic lateral ankle pain following an ankle sprain may be caused by a previously undiagnosed condition rather than chronic ankle instability. The differential diagnosis for chronic ankle pain is similar to that following an acute injury and also includes subtalar joint instability, subtalar joint chondral damage or synovitis, and dislocating or torn peroneal tendons. Impingement of scar tissue in the lateral gutter between the talus and fibula may also cause chronic lateral ankle pain. In addition to a careful physical examination, an MRI or CT scan may be helpful for distinguishing among these possible causes of pain.

Surgical treatment may help relieve symptoms of chronic lateral ankle pain, once an accurate diagnosis is made. Chondral or osteochondral fractures involving the ankle or subtalar joints can be treated with arthroscopic or open debridement or pinning. Subtalar joint instability is addressed with a Broström procedure. A fracture of the anterior or lateral process of the talus is either removed if it is small or fixed if it is a large fragment. Tears or dislocations of the peroneal tendons are repaired or stabilized. Scar tissue in the lateral gutter can be treated with arthroscopic debridement.

Chronic instability of the deltoid ligament or syndesmosis ligament is uncommon but can occur after an untreated injury. Diagnosis of either condition is made with stress radiographs. Treatment usually requires a free tendon graft to reconstruct the damaged ligament, with the addition of internal fixation for chronic syndesmosis tears.

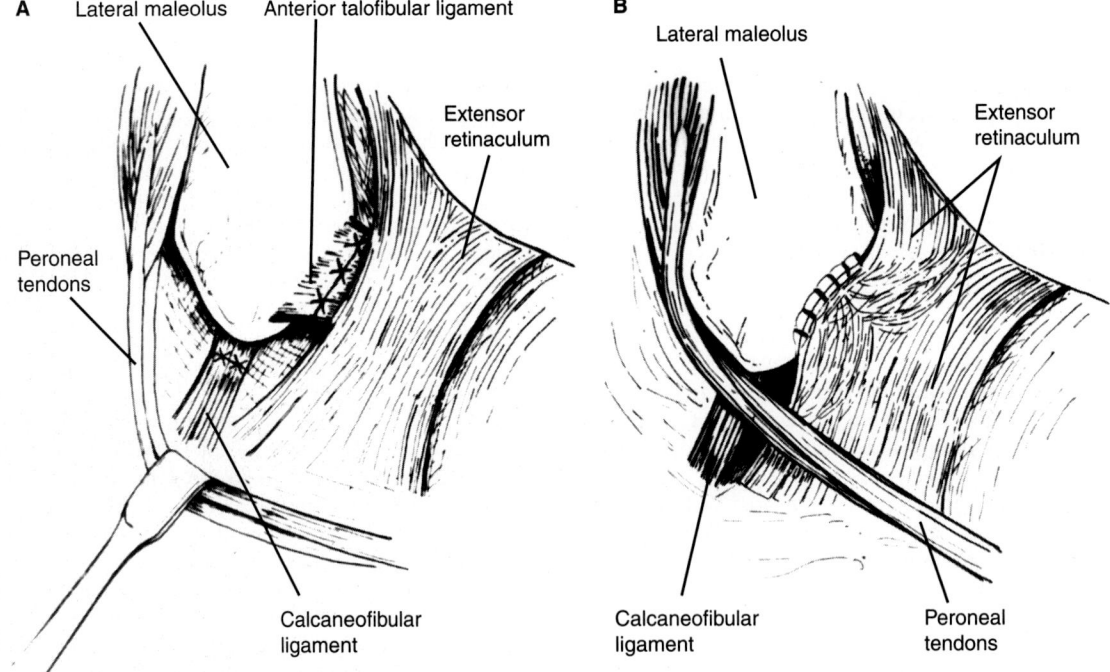

A Lateral maleolus   Anterior talofibular ligament   **B** Lateral maleolus

Extensor retinaculum   Extensor retinaculum

Peroneal tendons

Calcaneofibular ligament   Calcaneofibular ligament   Peroneal tendons

Figure 9–54. Modified Broström anatomic reconstruction. **A:** Imbrication of anterior talofibular and calcaneofibular ligaments. **B:** Imbrication of inferior extensor retinaculum to reinforce the repair. (Reproduced, with permission, from Coughlin MJ, Mann RA, eds: *Surgery of the Foot and Ankle,* 7th ed. Mosby, 1999. Modified from Renstrom PA, Trevino S, eds: *Operative Techniques in Sports Medicine,* Vol. 2. WB Saunders, 1994.)

Coughlin MJ et al: Comprehensive reconstruction of the lateral ankle for chronic instability using a free gracilis graft. Foot Ankle Int 2004;25:231. [PMID: 15132931]

DiGiovanni BF et al: Acute ankle injury and chronic lateral instability in the athlete. Clin Sports Med 2004;23:1. [PMID: 15062581]

Hintermann B et al: Medial ankle instability: An exploratory, prospective study of fifty-two cases. Am J Sports Med 2004; 32:183.

Hoiness P, Stromsoe K: Tricortical versus quadricortical syndesmosis fixation in ankle fractures: A prospective, randomized study comparing two methods of syndesmosis fixation. J Orthop Trauma 2004;18:331. [PMID: 15213497]

Krips R et al: Long-term outcome of anatomical reconstruction versus tenodesis for the treatment of chronic anterolateral instability of the ankle joint: A multicenter study. Foot Ankle Int 2001;22:415. [PMID: 11428761]

Messer TM et al: Outcome of the modified Broström procedure for chronic lateral ankle instability using suture anchors. Foot Ankle Int 2000;21:996. [PMID: 11139039]

Pijnenburg ACM et al: Treatment of ruptures of the lateral ankle ligaments: A meta-analysis. J Bone Joint Surg Am 2000; 82:761. [PMID: 10859095]

ARTHROSCOPIC EXAMINATION OF THE FOOT & ANKLE

Arthroscopy is an important tool for use in diagnosis and treatment of foot and ankle disorders. With developments in instrumentation, more ankle joint conditions can be treated arthroscopically. Arthroscopy of the subtalar joint is also now an accepted method for diagnosing and treating some subtalar joint abnormalities.

Advantages of Ankle Arthroscopy over Ankle Arthrotomy

Arthroscopy of the ankle joint offers distinct advantages over open exploration of the ankle. The entire joint can be visualized using the arthroscope, including the lateral and medial gutters and the posterior aspect of the joint. Dynamic studies can be performed to stress ligaments or identify areas of soft-tissue or bony impingement. Furthermore, the low morbidity of arthroscopy allows rapid rehabilitation.

Table 9–4. Proven indications for ankle arthroscopy.

Loose body removal
Irrigation and debridement for infection
Shaving of small osteophytes
Debridement of localized general synovitis
Debridement of osteochondral fractures
Debridement of osteochondritis dissecans lesions
Debridement of soft-tissue impingement

Indications

Table 9–4 lists the indications for ankle joint arthroscopy. In addition, arthroscopic examination can be used as a diagnostic tool in some instances when the precise cause of ankle pain remains in question.

A. THERAPEUTIC INDICATIONS

1. Loose bodies—Intraarticular loose bodies are generally easy to identify and remove arthroscopically. These bony or cartilaginous fragments may occur as a result of a single incident or repetitive trauma, or they may represent a fragment of an osteochondritis dissecans lesion. They cause pain or locking symptoms of the ankle and are diagnosed on plain radiographs, CT, or MRI scan.

2. Ankle joint infection—Arthroscopic irrigation, drainage, and synovectomy is an excellent method of treating ankle joint infections.

3. Synovitis—Synovitis may be present as a result of inflammatory arthritis (RA) or neoplastic diseases (pigmented villonodular synovitis), following trauma, or for unknown reasons (idiopathic). Whether the synovitis is localized or diffuse, arthroscopic debridement of inflamed synovium often relieves symptoms. Synovectomy is more easily and thoroughly performed arthroscopically.

4. Osteophyte formation—Repetitive trauma or early osteoarthritis can lead to osteophyte formation on the anterior lip of the tibia and the neck of the talus. These lesions can cause pain and limited ankle joint dorsiflexion and can be removed arthroscopically with a high-speed burr.

5. Other lesions within the joint—Chondral or osteochondral lesions, whether caused by trauma or osteochondritis dissecans, can be treated arthroscopically. This may involve debridement of loose cartilage flaps, drilling of subchondral bone, or pinning of large osteochondral fragments.

Patients who present with ankle pain over the anterolateral joint line and a history of a severe ankle sprain or recurrent sprains may have impingement of scar tissue in the lateral gutter between the talus and fibula. This entity responds well to arthroscopic debridement of scar tissue from the lateral gutter.

6. Ankle arthrodesis—Techniques for arthroscopically assisted ankle arthrodesis are well detailed, and several published studies discuss this method. The technique causes less morbidity and allows a shorter time to fusion than open methods of ankle fusion. But this is a technically demanding procedure and cannot be used to correct any joint deformity.

7. Ankle arthritis—Arthroscopic debridement of the arthritic ankle joint is not beneficial for generalized arthritis but may help for localized degenerative changes accompanied by early osteophyte formation.

8. Ankle fractures—Arthroscopically assisted fixation of ankle fractures is described and potentially allows for more accurate realignment of the joint surfaces and identification of chondral lesions that might otherwise be missed. However, the use of arthroscopy in the treatment of most routine ankle fractures is probably not indicated.

B. DIAGNOSTIC INDICATIONS

Ankle arthroscopy can be a valuable diagnostic tool when the cause of symptoms remains unclear (Table 9–5). Chronic ankle pain or swelling that remains refractory to conservative measures and was not diagnosed by conventional imaging studies may warrant arthroscopic exploration to help make a diagnosis. Chondral damage or inflamed synovium are examples of symptomatic lesions that may not be demonstrated on imaging studies, including MRI. Patients with episodes of locking, stiffness, or instability for which a cause cannot be found may be aided by diagnostic ankle arthroscopy. Loose bodies, cartilage flaps, or arthrofibrosis may be contributing to such symptoms, all of which can be treated arthroscopically (see Table 9–5).

Table 9–5. Refractory conditions diagnosed by arthroscopy.

Chondromalacia
Synovitis
Locking of the joint
Chronic stiffness
Instability
Loose bodies
Cartilage flaps
Arthrofibrosis

Technique of Ankle Arthroscopy

The patient is placed supine on the operating table with the foot positioned to allow access from all directions. This can be achieved with the foot placed off the edge of the bed or with the thigh held flexed in a well-padded thigh holder (Figure 9–55). General or spinal anesthesia is necessary for full relaxation of the extremity.

The use of distraction greatly enhances arthroscopic procedures, providing better views of the structures of the joint and allowing tools to be introduced into the joint. Noninvasive distractors with padded straps over the foot and heel are most commonly used (see Figure 9–55) Invasive distractors require placement of pins or screws through the tibia proximally and the calcaneus or talus distally. Stronger distraction forces can be obtained in this manner, but the morbidity is higher when using an invasive distractor.

Most ankle arthroscopies are performed using two anterior portals: anterolateral and anteromedial (Figure 9–56). A posterolateral portal may be helpful for use as outflow or to access the posterior aspect of the joint. Thorough knowledge of the anatomy of the tendons, nerves, and vessels is essential to prevent damage to any of these structures with portal placement. The anterolateral portal is placed just lateral to the tendon of the peroneus tertius muscle, taking care to avoid branches of the superficial peroneal nerve. The anteromedial portal is placed just medial to the anterior tibial tendon, taking care to avoid the saphenous nerve and vein. The

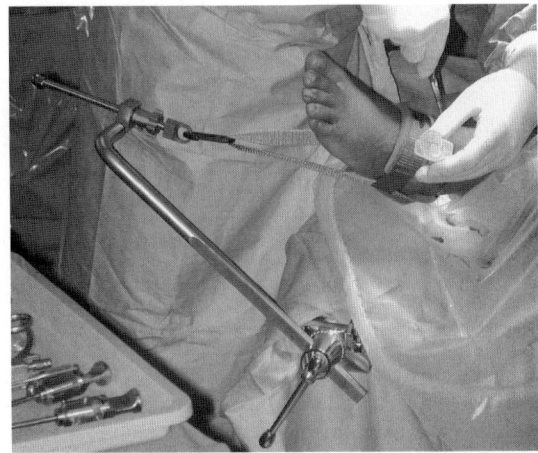

Figure 9–55. Soft strap type of distractor used during ankle arthroscopy.

posterolateral portal is placed just lateral to the Achilles tendon, to avoid damage to the sural nerve.

Initially, the entire joint is explored systematically, to ensure that abnormalities are not overlooked. The cartilaginous surfaces of the talus and tibia are thoroughly examined for osteochondral defects, unstable cartilage flaps, and areas of softening. The medial and lateral gutters are explored, paying special attention to tibiotalar

Figure 9–56. **A:** The anterior portals used for ankle arthroscopy are illustrated. The anterocentral portal is not used. **B:** The posterolateral portal is the only posterior portal utilized for ankle arthroscopy. (Reproduced, with permission, from Ferkel RD: Arthroscopy of the ankle and foot. In Mann RA, Coughlin MJ, eds: *Surgery of the Foot and Ankle,* 6th ed. Mosby-Year Book, 1993.)

and talofibular articulations. The synovium is inspected for inflammation. Ligamentous structures are identified, specifically the deltoid and talofibular ligaments, which are observed closely for signs of laxity while varus and valgus forces are applied. Loose bodies are carefully searched for, especially in the anterior and posterior recesses of the joint. The presence of osteophytes on the distal tibia and talar neck is also evaluated.

After a thorough diagnostic examination, surgical procedures are performed. These include synovial biopsy or synovial resection, removal of loose bodies, debridement of abnormal cartilaginous surfaces with subchondral drilling, and removal of bone spurs.

Postoperatively, a compression dressing is applied with a posterior splint for 5 to 7 days to allow the portals to heal. Weight bearing is then progressed as tolerated, and activities are advanced to normal.

Complications

Although several complications are reported, the most common is nerve damage in the form of hypesthesias or neuroma formation associated with portal placement. Postoperative joint infection, draining sinuses, arterial or tendon damage, and infections at the sites of distraction pins are all described but are very uncommon complications of ankle arthroscopy.

Subtalar Joint Arthroscopy

The subtalar joint is technically challenging for arthroscopy, given its complex shape and the difficulty distracting the joint. Subtalar joint arthroscopy is indicated for several conditions involving the subtalar joint. Talocalcaneal interosseous ligament tears, chondral lesions, synovitis, and focal degenerative changes may respond to arthroscopic debridement of the subtalar joint.

For subtalar joint arthroscopy, the patient can either be placed supine with a bump under the ipsilateral hip or in the lateral decubitus position. Two portals are used over the anterolateral subtalar joint, approximately 1.5 cm apart. The anterior and lateral portions of the posterior facet and the interosseous ligament can be visualized from these portals. A third portal is placed posterolaterally, for outflow and for visualization of the posterior aspect of the joint. The references here provide additional details about the technique of subtalar joint arthroscopy.

Frey C et al: Arthroscopic evaluation of the subtalar joint: Does sinus tarsi syndrome exist? Foot Ankle Int 1999;20:185. [PMID: 10195298]

Henderson I, La Valette D: Ankle impingement: Combined anterior and posterior impingement syndrome of the ankle. Foot Ankle Int 2004;25:632. [PMID: 15563385]

Kim SH, Ha KI: Arthroscopic treatment for impingement of the anterolateral soft tissues of the ankle. J Bone Joint Surg Br 2000;82-B;1019. [PMID: 11041593]

Okuda R et al: Arthroscopic findings in chronic lateral ankle instability: Do focal chondral lesions influence the results of ligament reconstruction? Am J Sports Med 2005;33:35. [PMID: 15610997]

Philbin TM et al: Arthroscopy for athletic foot and ankle injuries. Clin Sports Med 2004;23:35. [PMID: 15062583]

Schimmer RC et al: The role of ankle arthroscopy in the treatment strategies of osteochondritis dissecans lesions of the talus. Foot Ankle Int 2001;22:895. [PMID: 11722142]

Stroud CC: Arthroscopic arthrodesis of the ankle, subtalar, and first metatarsophalangeal joint. Foot Ankle Clin 2002;7:135. [PMID: 12380386]

Thordarson DB et al: The role of ankle arthroscopy on the surgical management of ankle fractures. Foot Ankle Int 2001;22:123. [PMID: 11249221]

■ TENDON INJURIES

Tendon injuries about the foot and ankle are common causes of disability because large forces are acting on these tendons in a repetitive fashion during walking, running, and athletic activities. The tendons cross the ankle joint at an acute angle, which further predisposes them to injury. Injury to tendons may be caused by acute trauma, such as in Achilles tendon ruptures, or may be caused by chronic strain, such as posterior tibial tendon dysfunction.

ACHILLES TENDON INJURIES

Achilles tendon abnormalities are extremely common, especially among active men and women between 30 and 50 years of age. The primary disorders are Achilles tendinitis, either insertional or noninsertional, and Achilles tendon ruptures. Achilles tendinitis was previously discussed in the section on heel pain.

1. Achilles Tendon Rupture

Pathogenesis

The mechanism of injury is usually mechanical overload from an eccentric contraction of the gastrocsoleus muscle complex. This occurs as a sudden, forceful dorsiflexion of the foot as the gastrocsoleus is contracted. The tear usually occurs 3–6 cm proximal to the insertion of the Achilles tendon, at the site of its poorest blood supply (Figure 9–57). At times, a history of intermittent pain in the tendon is elicited, suggestive of a prior tendinitis. The typical patient is between 30 and 50 years of age and a recreational athlete. These factors suggest that insufficient conditioning of the musculotendon unit plays a role in many injuries. The most common sports activities leading to Achilles tendon ruptures are basketball, racket sports, soccer, and softball.

A

B

Figure 9–57. Examples of acute Achilles tendon ruptures. **A:** Complete rupture with minimal fraying of the tendon. **B:** Achilles tendon rupture with marked fraying of the tendon. (Reproduced, with permission, from Plattner P, Mann RA: Disorders of tendons. In Mann RA, Coughlin MJ, eds: *Surgery of the Foot and Ankle,* 6th ed. Mosby-Year Book, 1993.)

Clinical Findings

A. SYMPTOMS AND SIGNS

The patient describes sudden pain in the calf after attempting a pushing-off movement, often accompanied by an audible pop. Immediate weakness is noted in the affected leg. On physical examination, a palpable defect is often present in the tendon. Ankle plantar flexion is markedly weak compared with the unaffected side. A positive Thompson test, diagnostic of complete Achilles tendon rupture, is performed with the patient prone and the affected knee bent 90 degrees. Squeezing the calf causes plantar flexion of the foot if the Achilles tendon is intact or partially torn but not if there is complete rupture of the tendon.

B. IMAGING STUDIES

Plain radiographs are not helpful in diagnosing Achilles tendon tear, unless there is an avulsion off the calcaneus with a fragment of bone, an uncommon condition. MRI is extremely sensitive in diagnosing this disorder and in determining if some tendon remains in continuity (Figure 9–58). However, MRI is rarely needed because physical exam is usually diagnostic of Achilles tendon rupture.

Treatment

Methods for treating Achilles tendon rupture include primary repair, using open or percutaneous techniques, or cast immobilization. Surgical repair is recommended for active individuals, in the case of a rerupture, or if the injury is older than 2 weeks.

Cast treatment for Achilles tendon ruptures is recommended for more sedentary individuals, patients who are at increased risk of developing wound prob-

lems, or high-risk surgical patients. The primary risk of cast immobilization is a higher chance of rerupture. For the vast majority of patients, either treatment method results in a good outcome.

Figure 9–58. MRI of Achilles tendon rupture.

A. Nonsurgical Treatment

Once an acute rupture is diagnosed, the patient should be placed in a gravity equinus cast. A below-knee cast is adequate in a reliable patient. If there is a question of whether the tendon edges are properly apposed in the cast, an MRI scan be done, although this is not routine. After 4 weeks, the cast is changed, with correction of approximately half of the previous equinus. Over the next 4 weeks, the patient is brought down to neutral with serial casts. Once at neutral, the patient is given a removable walking cast for 4 weeks. Supervised strengthening activities then begin.

B. Surgical Treatment

The surgical approach is on the medial side of the Achilles tendon sheath. The frayed edges of the tendon are debrided. The foot is positioned in equinus position equal to the resting equinus of the opposite ankle. Two heavy nonabsorbable sutures are woven through 3–4 cm of each tendon edge using a Bunnell or Kessler stitch (Figure 9–59). The repair can be reinforced with lighter, absorbable sutures at the site of the tear. If the plantaris tendon is intact, it can be harvested and used to reinforce the repair.

Postoperatively, a hard cast is used for 3 weeks, followed by a removable cast with adjustable ankle motion. Over the next 2–3 weeks, the joint should be gradually brought out of equinus. Weight bearing is then allowed, and ROM exercises are begun. The cast is discontinued at 6–8 weeks, and supervised strengthening exercises are performed.

The primary risk of surgical repair is wound healing problems, which occur in approximately 5% of patients. A percutaneous method of Achilles tendon repair is listed in the references.

C. Treatment of Chronic Ruptures or Reruptures

Chronic Achilles tendon ruptures, more than 6 weeks old, or reruptures of previously treated injuries can be challenging reconstruction problems because of retraction and degeneration of the tendon ends. A number of different procedures are described to address this problem, including a variety of synthetic and interpositional grafts (Figure 9–60).

Small defects can be bridged by turning down a strip of gastrocnemius fascia, which is sutured into the distal tendon stump. Larger defects can be treated by using a V-Y lengthening of the gastrocnemius aponeurosis. If the deficit is too large for V-Y lengthening, transfer of the flexor hallucis longus tendon can be performed. The tendon of the flexor hallucis longus is transected distally in the foot, and the distal segment is tenodesed to the flexor digitorum longus to maintain flexion of the great toe. The proximal tendon is secured to the calcaneus

Figure 9–59. Suture techniques used to reapproximate the ruptured Achilles tendon. (Reproduced, with permission, from Mann RA, Coughlin MJ, eds: *Surgery of the Foot and Ankle,* 6th ed. Mosby-Year Book, 1993.)

through a drill hole or by using an absorbable anchor or screw. A central slip of the Achilles tendon is advanced to bridge the gap, and then the repair is reinforced by securing it to the flexor hallucis (Figure 9–61).

The postoperative course for these procedures includes 6 weeks of non–weight bearing and a total of 3 months protection in a cast.

POSTERIOR TIBIAL TENDON INJURIES

This topic is covered in the section on acquired flatfoot deformities.

PERONEAL TENDON INJURIES

Peroneal tendon injuries fall into the categories of peroneal tendonitis, peroneal tendon tears, and peroneal tendon subluxation or dislocation.

1. Peroneal Tendonitis

Pathogenesis

Inflammation of the peroneal tendons may be caused by acute trauma, inflammatory arthropathy conditions, or repetitive motion. Traumatic events that may induce tendonitis include a direct blow to the posterolateral ankle, a fracture of the calcaneus or fibula, or a severe inversion sprain of the ankle. Most tendonitis is caused by repetitive motion injury from recurrent rubbing of the peroneal tendons on the distal end of the fibula. Often there is an abnormal bony contour of the distal

Figure 9–60. Various methods of reconstruction for untreated Achilles tendon ruptures. **A:** Repair using fascial strip from proximal gastrocsoleus complex. *a:* Distally based fascial strip is passed transversely through proximal tendon fragment. *b:* The strip is woven across the gap. *c:* Enlarged diagram of *b*. **B:** Repair using peroneus brevis tendon. The peroneus brevis is isolated and detached from its insertion into the fifth metatarsal. *a:* A transverse drill hole is placed in the calcaneus. *b:* The peroneus brevis is transferred through the drill hole. *c:* The tendon is sutured to itself and to the Achilles tendon proximally and distally. (**A:** Reproduced, with permission, from Bosworth DM: Repair of defects in the tendo achillis. J Bone Joint Surg Am 1956;38:111. **B:** Reproduced, with permission, from Plattner P, Mann RA: Disorders of tendons. In Mann RA, Coughlin MJ, eds: *Surgery of the Foot and Ankle,* 6th ed. Mosby-Year Book, 1993.)

fibula or the peroneal tubercle. Tendonitis of the peroneus longus may be associated with abnormality of the os peroneum, a small sesamoid bone located in the tendon where it curves around the lateral border of the cuboid.

Clinical Findings

A. SYMPTOMS AND SIGNS

The patient complains of pain over the lateral aspect of the ankle, made worse with activity, and improved with

Figure 9–61. Delayed repair of ruptured Achilles tendon using flexor digitorum longus (FDL) transfer. **A:** Operative technique demonstrating incisions. **B:** Tenodesis of the FDL stump to the flexor hallucis longus (FHL). **C:** Flexor digitorum longus pulled through drill hole in calcaneus. **D:** Augmentation of spanned gap by turndown of fascial strip from gastrocsoleus complex. (Reproduced, with permission, from Plattner P, Mann RA: Disorders of tendons. In Mann RA, Coughlin, MF, eds: *Surgery of the Foot and Ankle,* 6th ed. Mosby-Year Book, 1993.)

rest and NSAIDs. The onset may be insidious, or it may be associated with an acute injury. Physical examination usually demonstrates pain located along the course of the peroneal tendons. Pain and weakness is noted with resisted eversion of the foot.

B. IMAGING STUDIES

An MRI scan may help distinguish between tendonitis and a tendon tear, although small tears may not be identified on an MRI.

Treatment

A. NONSURGICAL

If symptoms are mild, the recommended treatment includes NSAIDs, activity modification, and an ankle brace. Four to 6 weeks of cast immobilization is used for more advanced symptoms or for patients who do not respond to initial treatment. Occasionally, a diagnostic injection with bupivacaine is given into the tendon sheath.

B. Surgical

Operative intervention is recommended for patients who fail conservative treatment. The tendon sheath is explored, inflamed synovium is removed, and the tendons are carefully explored to look for tears or degenerative lesions. Postoperatively, early ROM is encouraged.

2. Peroneal Tendon Tears

Pathogenesis

The majority of peroneal tendon tears are attritional in nature, caused by mechanical irritation within the fibular groove. The peroneus longus tendon, which lies posterior, places pressure on the brevis tendon. Also, a sharp lateral edge of the fibula may predispose to a longitudinal split of the tendons. Laxity of the tendon sheath and subluxation of the tendons out of the fibular groove may contribute to tears as well. Acute tears of the peroneal tendons may occur with a sudden, severe stress to the ankle, but usually there is some degree of preexisting degeneration within the tendon.

Clinical Findings

Clinical presentation is similar to that of peroneal tendonitis, but with a more acute onset of pain and swelling along the tendon sheath.

Treatment

A. Nonsurgical

Initial treatment is similar to that of peroneal tendonitis, but it is less likely to result in resolution of symptoms if a tear is present.

B. Surgical

Surgical repair of a peroneal tendon tear is indicated when nonoperative treatment fails to relieve symptoms. At surgery, both tendons are carefully examined, the fibula is explored for sharp edges, and the tendon sheath is evaluated for laxity. Small areas of the tendon that demonstrate significant degeneration are removed. The remainder of the tendon is repaired with nylon or polypropylene suture. Postoperatively, the ankle is immobilized for 4 weeks; then weight bearing and gentle ROM is allowed.

3. Peroneal Tendon Subluxation and Dislocation

Pathogenesis

Peroneal tendon dislocation is caused by a sudden forceful dorsiflexion motion of the ankle combined with a simultaneous strong contraction of the peroneal musculature. This mechanism injures the superior peroneal retinaculum, which holds the peroneal tendons in place along the posterior border of the distal fibula. The retinaculum is either stripped off the fibular periosteum or avulsed with a small piece of fibular cortex. This permits the creation of a false pouch and laxity of the retinaculum, allowing the peroneal tendons to dislocate anteriorly. If this condition goes unrecognized, either the tendons remain dislocated, or they relocate with the propensity for recurrent subluxation or dislocation.

Clinical Findings

A. Symptoms and Signs

The patient usually recalls an acute episode of trauma and frequently the sensation of the tendon dislocating. Pain and swelling is localized to the peroneal tendon sheath around the tip of the fibula. With recurrent subluxation or dislocation, the tendons are felt to pop out of place. On examination, resisted eversion of the ankle elicits pain and may cause the tendons to subluxate. Unfortunately, many acute peroneal tendon dislocations go unrecognized as lateral ankle sprains.

B. Imaging Studies

Radiographs may show a small piece of bone lateral to the distal fibula, indicative of avulsion of the retinaculum. MRI scan usually details the injury well if careful attention is paid to this area.

Treatment

A. Nonsurgical

Treatment of acute peroneal tendon dislocations consists of casting in plantarflexion and inversion for 4 weeks, followed by a walking cast for an additional 2 weeks. Cast treatment has at least a 50% failure rate. Once a tendon is chronically dislocated or recurrently subluxates, only surgical treatment will keep it in position.

B. Surgical

Surgical repair is recommended for an athletic individual following an acute dislocation of the peroneal tendons. It is also recommended for patients with recurrent dislocation if their physical activities are significantly restricted. The procedure consists of repairing the superior peroneal retinaculum to the fibula, either through drill holes or with suture anchors. In the case of attenuated retinaculum caused by chronic dislocations, the repair can be reinforced with a strip of Achilles or by rerouting the calcaneofibular ligament over the tendons. At the time of surgical repair, the tendons are inspected for tears and the contour of the posterior fibular groove is evaluated. If a shallow groove is noted, a bony procedure to deepen the groove is necessary to prevent recurrent dislocations. Postoperatively, the patient is immobilized in a cast for 6 weeks.

ANTERIOR TIBIAL TENDON RUPTURE

Pathogenesis

Rupture of the anterior tibial tendon occurs infrequently, and most often in patients older than 60. The mechanism is either chronic rubbing against the inferior edge of the extensor retinaculum or rubbing against an exostosis at the first metatarsocuneiform joint. The rupture usually occurs at the distal 2–3 cm of tendon. Nondegenerative traumatic ruptures of the anterior tibial tendon are rare.

Clinical Findings

A. SYMPTOMS AND SIGNS

Patients with a degenerative rupture present with complaints of pain and swelling over the anterior ankle. They sense the foot slapping down, or they may be catching their toes on the ground when they walk. Patients frequently present after the symptoms have been bothersome for several months. Physical exam is notable for weakness of ankle dorsiflexion, often with a palpable mass over the anterior ankle joint.

B. Imaging Studies

If the diagnosis is in doubt, MRI scan can accurately determine if the tendon is ruptured.

Treatment

A. NONSURGICAL

In the case of a less active patient, nonsurgical treatment appears to give equal functional results to surgical repair. Cast immobilization is followed by long-term use of an AFO.

B. SURGICAL

Acute tendon rupture in an active individual should be surgically repaired. Chronic ruptures that are symptomatic usually require reconstruction using an extensor tendon graft or tendon transfer because the distal stump is usually too degenerated to perform a primary repair.

Brandes CB, Smith RW: Characterization of patients with primary peroneus longus tendinopathy: A review of twenty-two cases. Foot Ankle Int 2000;21:462. [PMID: 10884103]

Haji A et al: Percutaneous versus open tendo Achilles repair. Foot Ankle Int 2004;25:215. [PMID: 15132928]

Jaakkola JI et al: Early ankle motion after triple bundle technique repair vs casting for acute Achilles tendon rupture. Foot Ankle Int 2001;22:979. [PMID: 11783925]

Tan V et al: Superior peroneal retinaculoplasty: A surgical technique for peroneal subluxation. Clin Orthop 2003;410:320. [PMID: 12771847]

van der Linden-van der Zwaag HM et al: Results of surgical versus non-surgical treatment of Achilles tendon rupture. Int Orthop 2004;28:370. [PMID: 15241626]

Wong MW, Ng VW: Modified flexor hallucis longus transfer for Achilles insertional rupture in elderly patients. Clin Orthop 2005;431:201. [PMID: 15685076]

OSTEOCHONDRAL LESIONS OF THE TALUS

Osteochondral lesions of the talus (OLTs) are defects of cartilage and subchondral bone in the talar dome. More sophisticated imaging techniques allow for precise diagnosis of OLTs, and advanced arthroscopic and open methods are available to treat this difficult problem.

Pathogenesis

OLTs, also known as osteochondritis dissecans lesions, are generally located in one of two areas on the talar dome: either posteromedial or anterolateral. The more common posteromedial lesions are usually deeper lesions involving subchondral bone. Their origin is thought to involve ischemia, often with an episode of trauma exacerbating the underlying condition. Anterolateral lesions are a result of a single traumatic episode or repetitive trauma from lateral ankle sprains. These lesions tend to be purely cartilaginous.

Clinical Findings

A. SYMPTOMS AND SIGNS

Patients usually present with several months of ankle pain following a routine ankle sprain. Sometimes they recount a history of recurrent sprains to the ankle. The pain is usually located over the anterior aspect of the ankle on the side of the lesion, but it may be diffuse. Occasionally, there is a sensation of locking in the ankle when a loose flap of cartilage is present. A high index of suspicion is necessary because OLTs can be misdiagnosed as a chronic ankle sprain, as discussed in the section on ligamentous injuries about the ankle joint.

B. IMAGING STUDIES

Radiographs are often normal in OLTs. MRI scan is the imaging procedure of choice for determining the size, location, and extent of bony or cartilaginous involvement (Figure 9–62).

Figure 9–62. MRI scan of extensive osteochondral lesion of the talus.

Treatment

A. NONSURGICAL

A 6-week trial of cast immobilization is warranted if the MRI scan shows no evidence of a displaced bone or cartilage fragment.

B. SURGICAL

The surgical treatment method depends on the type of lesion. Acutely displaced lesions can be reduced and pinned with an absorbable pin by either open or arthroscopic methods. Purely cartilaginous lesions are curetted to a stable rim and drilled to stimulate vascular ingrowth and fibrocartilage formation. OLTs with significant bony involvement require bone grafting in addition to drilling and curettage. A medial malleolar osteotomy is required to access a posteromedial lesion. If a bony lesion has intact overlying cartilage, drilling and bone grafting can be performed under radiographic guidance through the talus, thereby sparing the overlying cartilage. Postoperatively, patients are kept non–weight bearing for 4 weeks, but early ROM is encouraged.

New techniques were developed for larger lesions or ones that fail curettage and drilling. Osteochondral autograft or allograft plugs can be used to replace bone and cartilage defects. Autograft plugs are generally harvested from the ipsilateral knee. Intermediate-term follow-up data shows good results in most patients following this technique. Autologous chondrocyte implantation is also used to a limited extent for OLTs.

Barnes CJ, Ferkel RD: Arthroscopic debridement and drilling of osteochondral lesions of the talus. Foot Ankle Clin 2003; 8:243. [PMID: 12911239]

Hangody L: The mosaicplasty technique for osteochondral lesions of the talus. Foot Ankle Clin 2003;8:259. [PMID: 12911240]

Hunt SA Sherman O: Arthroscopic treatment of osteochondral lesions of the talus with correlation of outcome scoring systems. Arthroscopy 2003;19:360. [PMID: 12671618]

Petersen L et al: Autologous chondrocyte transplantation of the ankle. Foot Ankle Clin 2003;8:291. [PMID: 12911242]

Robinson DE et al: Arthroscopic treatment of osteochondral lesions of the talus. J Bone Joint Surg Br 2003;85:989. [PMID: 14516033]

Takao M et al: Arthroscopic drilling with debridement of remaining cartilage for osteochondral lesions of the talar dome in unstable ankles. Am J Sports Med 2004;32:332. [PMID: 14977656]

Hand Surgery

10

Michael S. Bednar, MD, & Terry R. Light, MD

Function of the Hand

The hand is a vital part of the human body, allowing humans to directly interact with their environment. The functional capabilities of the hand are many because the hand is ultimately an end organ of the human mind. The hand's enormous capacity for adaptability allowed primitive humans to make stone tools and modern humans to pilot complex aircraft.

The human hand is capable of prehension, which involves approaching an object, grasping it, modulating and maintaining grasp, and ultimately releasing the object. When a power grasp is used, the object is pushed by the flexed fingers against the palm while the thumb metacarpal and proximal phalanx stabilize the object. When an object is held with a precision pinch pattern, the object is secured between the pulp of the thumb distal phalanx and the index finger or index and middle fingers.

The hand can touch objects or other human beings while sensing temperature, vibration, and texture. This quality of tactile gnosis is sophisticated enough to allow blind individuals to read the pattern of small elevations that distinguish one Braille letter from another. The hand is also an instrument of communication, whether by making a gesture, playing a musical instrument, drawing, writing, or typing.

General Considerations in Treatment of Hand Disorders

Treatment of hand disorders requires an understanding of normal anatomy and its common variations. Treatment usually attempts to restore the normal anatomy, but when that is not possible, the goal should be restoration of maximal function. The appearance of the hand is vital because the hand is usually uncovered and exposed to the scrutiny of others. Imperfections are often a source of embarrassment. Effective treatment requires a mature balancing of the need for optimal function and normal appearance of the hand. Complex reconstruction that restores prehension but results in a hideous appearance of the hand are ineffective if the patient is so reluctant to expose the hand that he or she avoids using it. Conversely, a functionless stiff finger leading to awkward motion of an otherwise supple hand may cause the patient more embarrassment than amputation.

DIAGNOSIS OF DISORDERS OF THE HAND

History

When a patient seeks evaluation of a hand disorder, the physician should ask many general questions as well as questions specific to hand function and injury. The chief complaint as perceived by the patient should be summarized in one or two sentences. The patient's hand dominance, age, gender, and occupation should be noted, as well as any hobbies that require hand dexterity or strength. The approximate date of onset of symptoms should be recorded. If injury is the cause of discomfort, the exact date and mechanism of injury should be noted and whether the injury occurred at the workplace. The patient should be questioned about prior treatment and his or her perception of its effectiveness.

Complaints should then be further detailed, such as the nature of pain (sharp, aching, dull, or burning), whether night symptoms are present, and whether the pain is worse upon awakening in the morning or after a full day of work. The patient should be asked whether symptoms include numbness or tingling. Specific motor difficulties, such as difficulty in writing or unscrewing jar tops, should be noted. If the patient complains principally of unilateral symptoms, the examiner should ask whether similar symptoms are occurring on the opposite side. Finally, because the hand is an exposed area of the body, the impact of altered appearance should be discussed.

The medical history should include any prior hand injuries and any systemic diseases such as rheumatoid arthritis (RA) or other inflammatory arthropathies, diabetes, other endocrine disorders, renal disease, or vascular disease. Women of childbearing age should be questioned about recent pregnancies. A careful history suggests the correct diagnosis in approximately 90% of patients with hand problems.

535

Figure 10–1. Normal cascade of digital flexion posture. When the wrist is in slight extension and the fingers are at rest, there is progressively less flexion from the little finger to the index finger. (Reproduced, with permission, from Carter PR: *Common Hand Injuries and Infections.* WB Saunders, 1983.)

Examination of the Hand

A. GENERAL EXAMINATION

Examination of the hand should begin with observation. Vascular condition can be assessed by noting the color of the fingers. Some hint of nerve function can be obtained by observing pseudomotor function as revealed by sweatiness or dryness of the finger pulps. The extent and timing of injury is suggested by the degree of swelling and ecchymosis. The posture of the digits and the wrist may signal tendon or bone disruption. Normally, a cascade of increased digital flexion is noted when ulnar digits are observed next to radial digits (Figure 10–1).

A diagram of the hand is often helpful in documenting the abnormality. Laceration sites, previous scars, ampu-

tated fingers, and subjective areas of decreased sensation can be noted on the diagram.

Next, the hand, wrist, and forearm are gently palpated. The temperature and moisture of the fingers should be noted. When the skin is blanched in the paronychial region, circulation should return within 3 seconds. Areas of tenderness on palpation are carefully noted.

B. RANGE OF MOTION

The passive and active range of motion (ROM) of the shoulder, elbow, forearm, wrist, and hand are evaluated. The normal ROM of the wrist and fingers is indicated in Table 10–1. In documenting ROM, active extension should be to the left and active flexion to the right. When the range of passive extension and flexion is different from that of active motion, the passive ROM values are noted in parentheses next to the corresponding active ROM values. The ROM of a stiff proximal interphalangeal joint could thus be recorded as 20/70 (15/80), indicating an arc of active motion from 20 to 70 degrees and a passive arc of motion from 15 to 80 degrees.

C. MUSCLE FUNCTION

The integrity of individual muscles should be documented. The flexor digitorum profundus to each finger is tested by stabilizing the middle phalanx and asking the patient to flex the distal interphalangeal joint (Figure 10–2). The flexor digitorum superficialis of each finger is tested by keeping all fingers except the one to be tested in full extension. The patient is then asked to flex the finger being evaluated at the proximal interphalangeal joint (Figure 10–3). The function of the flexor

Table 10–1. Normal range of motion in joints of arm and hand.

Elbow: Extension and flexion 0°/135°
Forearm: Supination and pronation 90°/90°
Wrist: Flexion and extension 80°/70°
      Radial deviation and ulnar deviation 20°/30°
Finger
  MP: Extension and flexion 0°/90°
  PIP: Extension and flexion 0°/110°
  DIP: Extension and flexion 0°/65°
Thumb
  CMC: Extension and flexion 50°/50°
    Abduction and adduction 70°/0°
   MP: Extension and flexion—variable, up to 0°/90°
   IP: Extension and flexion—variable, up to 0°/90°

MP = metacarpal phalangeal; PIP = proximal interphalangeal; DIP = distal interphalangeal; CMC = carpometacarpal; IP = interphalangeal.

Figure 10–2. Testing of flexor digitorum profundus integrity. If the distal interphalangeal joint can be actively flexed while the proximal interphalangeal joint is stabilized, the profundus tendon is not severed. (Reproduced, with permission, from American Society for Surgery of the Hand: *The Hand: Examination and Diagnosis,* 2nd ed. Churchill Livingstone, 1983.)

pollicis longus is tested by asking the patient to flex the interphalangeal joint of the thumb.

The function of the extrinsic extensors is tested by asking the patient to extend the metacarpophalangeal joints of the fingers. If the examiner simply asks the patient to open the hand, the proximal and distal interphalangeal joints may be extended by contraction of the interosseous muscles, which may mislead the examiner to conclude that digital extension is normal. Interosseous muscle function is screened by asking the patient to

abduct the fingers. The examiner assesses the strength of muscle force while palpating the contraction of the hypothenar and the first dorsal interosseous muscles.

D. SENSORY FUNCTION

Examination of sensory function requires evaluation of the integrity of the median, ulnar, and radial nerves as well as the component proper digital nerves to each side of each finger. Each of the major nerves has an autogenous sensory zone, an area of the hand supplied predominantly by that nerve (Figure 10–4). The autogenous zone of the median nerve is the pulp of the index finger, whereas the ulnar nerve provides sensory fibers from the pulp of the little finger. The skin on the dorsum of the first web space is innervated by the superficial branch of the radial nerve.

1. Two-point discrimination—The integrity of each digital nerve may be evaluated using either a blunt-tipped caliper or an unfolded paper clip to test two-point discrimination. The two points of the testing instrument are held apart at a measured distance. The examiner alternates between touching the skin with one or two

Figure 10–3. Testing of flexor digitorum superficialis integrity. If the proximal interphalangeal joint can be actively flexed while the adjacent fingers are held completely extended, the sublimis tendon is not severed. (Reproduced, with permission, from American Society for Surgery of the Hand: *The Hand: Examination and Diagnosis,* 2nd ed. Churchill Livingstone, 1983.)

Figure 10–4. Sensory distribution in the hand. Light shading = ulnar nerve; medium shading = radial nerve; darkest shading = median nerve. (Reproduced, with permission, from Way LW, ed: *Current Surgical Diagnosis & Treatment,* 10th ed. Appleton & Lange, 1994.)

points. The points may be either touched (static two-point discrimination) or longitudinally moved (moving two-point discrimination) against the skin on either the radial or ulnar side of the finger. The points should be pressed against the finger until the skin just begins to blanch. The two-point discrimination value is the smallest distance between the two points that the patient can correctly detect in two out of three trials. Because of the increased sensory cues provided by movement, moving two-point discrimination has a value less than or equal to static two-point discrimination. Static two-point discrimination is normal if the distance is less than 7 mm, impaired if 7–14, and absent if 15 mm or greater.

E. MOTOR FUNCTION

Examination of motor function may be organized by considering groups of muscles within specific nerve domains (Table 10–2). Proximally, the median nerve innervates the pronator teres, flexor carpi radialis, palmaris longus, and flexor digitorum superficialis muscles. The anterior interosseous nerve branch of the median nerve innervates the flexor digitorum profundus of the index and middle fingers, flexor pollicis longus, and pronator quadratus muscles. The motor branch of the median to the thenar musculature innervates the opponens pollicis, abductor pollicis brevis, and superficial portion of the flexor pollicis brevis. The index- and long-finger lumbricals are innervated by median motor fibers running with the sensory nerve branches of the median nerve to the index and middle fingers.

Table 10–2. Innervation of the hand and forearm.

Median nerve
  Proximal median nerve: pronator teres, flexor carpi radialis, flexor digitorum superficialis
  Anterior interosseous nerve: flexor pollicis longus, index and middle flexor digitorum profundus, pronator quadratus
  Distal median nerve: index and middle lumbrical, opponens pollicis, abductor pollicis brevis, flexor pollicis brevis
Ulnar nerve
  Proximal ulnar nerve: flexor carpi ulnaris, ring and small flexor digitorum profundus
  Distal ulnar nerve: flexor digiti minimi, abductor digiti minimi, opponens digiti minimi, volar and dorsal interossei, flexor pollicis brevis, adductor pollicis, ring and small lumbricals
Radial nerve: brachioradialis, extensor carpi radialis longus, supinator, anconeus
Posterior interosseous nerve: extensor carpi radialis brevis, extensor digitorum communis, extensor indicis proprius, extensor digiti minimi, extensor carpi ulnaris, abductor pollicis longus, extensor pollicis longus, extensor pollicis brevis

The ulnar nerve innervates the flexor carpi ulnaris and flexor digitorum profundus of the ring and little fingers proximally. Within the hand, the ulnar nerve innervates the hypothenar musculature, flexor digiti quinti, and abductor digiti quinti. The deep motor branch of the ulnar nerve innervates the dorsal and palmar interosseous muscles, lumbricals to the ring and little fingers, deep portion of the flexor pollicis brevis, and adductor pollicis muscles.

The radial nerve innervates the triceps, brachioradialis, extensor carpi radialis longus and brevis, supinator, and anconeus muscles. The posterior interosseous division of the radial nerve then distally innervates the extensor digitorum communis, extensor indicis proprius, extensor digiti minimi, extensor carpi ulnaris, abductor pollicis longus, and extensor pollicis longus and brevis.

Muscle strength should be graded according to the British muscle grading system based on a scale of 0 to 5, with 5/5 being normal strength, 4/5 less than normal strength but with ability to resist a fair amount of resistance, 3/5 resistance against gravity, 2/5 resistance with gravity eliminated, and 1/5 only a trace or flicker of contraction without significant motion.

Diagnostic Studies

A number of studies may be helpful in establishing the proper diagnosis in a patient with hand or wrist pain. The choice of technique should be based on a careful history and physical examination.

A. IMAGING STUDIES

In most instances, radiographic evaluation includes anteroposterior and lateral films. The importance of obtaining a true lateral radiograph of the finger and wrist cannot be overemphasized because many disorders, particularly interphalangeal joint subluxation and carpal instability, are not evident on oblique views. Oblique views may be useful in defining phalangeal fracture patterns. Tangential views are useful in assessing a carpometacarpal boss. The carpal tunnel view may allow visualization of a fracture of the hook of the hamate.

Stress views allow assessment of ligamentous stability. This is particularly useful in the evaluation of collateral ligament stability of the thumb metacarpophalangeal joint.

Ligamentous stability of the wrist may also be evaluated by radial and ulnar deviation views and by clenched-fist grip views. Grip views and ulnar deviation views may demonstrate a gap between the scaphoid and the lunate that is not apparent on simple anteroposterior and lateral studies.

B. ELECTRODIAGNOSTIC STUDIES

Electrodiagnostic studies include both nerve conduction studies and electromyography. Nerve conduction studies measure both motor (proximal to distal) and sensory (distal to proximal) conduction. Electromyography allows evaluation of muscle function.

C. COMPUTED TOMOGRAPHY SCAN

A CT scan allows excellent visualization of the distal radioulnar joint. The relationship of the distal ulna to the sigmoid notch should be viewed in pronation, neutral, and supination. CT scanning may be helpful in evaluating displacement as well as healing of scaphoid fractures.

D. MAGNETIC RESONANCE IMAGING

MRI provides direct visualization of soft-tissue structures. The integrity of the transverse carpal ligament may be evaluated, which is particularly helpful in patients with persistent symptoms following carpal tunnel release. Evaluation of tumors and avascular necrosis is also facilitated by MRI. MRI scans also allow visualization of many triangular fibrocartilage complex and intercarpal ligament tears.

E. BONE SCAN

The technetium-99 MDP bone scan is a useful physiologic test in the evaluation of unexplained hand or wrist pain. This test can rule out bone involvement and can be used to localize inflammatory processes for further study with CT or MRI scans (Figure 10–5).

F. WRIST ARTHROSCOPY

Arthroscopic examination of the wrist allows for direct visualization of articular surfaces, wrist ligaments, and the triangular fibrocartilage complex. The effect of stress maneuvers on intercarpal kinematics may be directly observed. Wrist arthroscopy is particularly helpful in the debridement or repair of the triangular fibrocartilage complex tears. Partial tears of either the scapholunate or lunotriquetral ligaments may be debrided. Intraarticular fracture of the distal radius may be anatomically aligned and pinned under direct observation.

Bernstein MA, Nagle DJ, Martinez A et al: A comparison of combined arthroscopic triangular fibrocartilage complex debridement and arthroscopic wafer distal ulna resection versus arthroscopic triangular fibrocartilage complex debridement and ulnar shortening osteotomy for ulnocarpal abutment syndrome. Arthroscopy 2004;20:392. [PMID: 15067279]

Cerezal L, del Pinal F, Abascal F et al: Imaging findings in ulnar-sided wrist impaction syndromes. Radiographics. 2002;22:105. [PMID: 11796902]

Kocharian A, Adkins MC, Amrami KK et al: Wrist: improved MR imaging with optimized transmit-receive coil design. Radiology 2002;223:870. [PMID: 12034961]

Morley J, Bidwell J, Bransby-Zachary M: A comparison of the findings of wrist arthroscopy and magnetic resonance imaging in the investigation of wrist pain. J Hand Surg 2001; 26B:544. [PMID: 11884109]

Potter HG, Weiland AJ: Magnetic resonance imaging of triangular fibrocartilage complex lesions. J Hand Surg [Am] 2002;27(2): 363. [PMID: 11901408]

Slutsky DJ: Wrist arthroscopy through a volar radial portal. Arthroscopy 2002;18:624. [PMID: 12098124]

SPECIAL TREATMENT PROCEDURES FOR HAND DISORDERS

1. Replantation

Replantation is the reattachment of a body part that was totally severed from the body, without any residual soft-

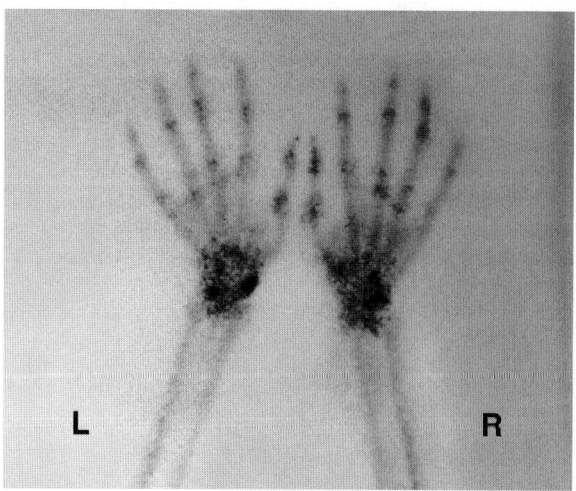

A

B

Figure 10–5. Radiograph (**A**) and bone scan (**B**) demonstrating increased activity in the region of the scaphoid in a woman with a symptomatic cyst.

tissue continuity. Revascularization is the reconstruction of damaged blood vessels to prevent an attached but ischemic body part from becoming necrotic.

Initial Care of Patient

Effective treatment of the patient and the ischemic or detached body part requires appropriate initial care and prompt referral to a surgeon at a center capable of mobilizing resources for early surgical care. The initial treating physician should place the amputated part in a sponge soaked with either normal saline or Ringer's lactate solution. The wrapped part should then be placed into a plastic bag, which is sealed and immersed in an ice-water solution. Under no circumstances should the amputated part be placed directly into ice water or exposed to dry ice.

A tourniquet is usually not required to control bleeding. A compressive dressing should be applied to the amputation stump. No attempt should be made to ligate bleeding vessels because it might compromise subsequent neurovascular repair. If the amputated part is not cooled, ischemia is poorly tolerated and successful revascularization is unlikely after 6 hours. Cooled parts may be replanted up to 12 hours after injury.

Indications & Contraindications

Replantation is indicated for severed thumbs or multiple digits, transmetacarpal hand amputations, wrist- or distal forearm-level amputations, and amputations of almost any body part in a child. In more proximal levels of amputation, only sharp or moderately avulsed parts can be considered for replantation. The more proximal the amputation, the greater the amount of ischemic muscle mass and the more urgent the need for revascularization.

Contraindications to replantation include severely crushed or mangled parts; multilevel amputation; amputations in patients with arteriosclerotic vessels; amputations in patients with other serious injuries or diseases; and amputations with prolonged warm ischemic times, particularly at proximal levels.

In adults, replantation of a single finger proximal to the insertion of the flexor digitorum superficialis is usually contraindicated because of the likelihood of stiffness. Limited tendon function in these replanted fingers is caused by simultaneous zone 2 flexor digitorum superficialis and profundus tendon disruption, phalangeal fracture, and extensor tendon disruption. Replantation at this level may be considered in children or for aesthetic reasons.

Surgical Procedure

The preferred method of anesthesia is axillary block because this technique provides a sympathetic block resulting in vasodilation. The surgical sequence of replantation begins with a wide surgical exposure that allows identification and isolation of arteries, veins, and nerves. The soft tissue is then meticulously debrided. The bone is shortened and securely internally fixed with sufficient stability to allow institution of early postoperative motion.

The extensor tendons are repaired first and then the flexor tendons. Anastomosis of one or preferably two arteries is then performed, followed by repair of the nerves and anastomosis of the veins. Two veins should be repaired for each artery repaired. Skin should be closed loosely, with care taken to approximate soft tissue over repaired vessels and nerves.

In replantations proximal to the distal forearm, fasciotomies of all muscle compartments should be performed at the time of replantation. The patient should be returned to the operating room in 48–72 hours, so the wound may be reevaluated and any additional necrotic tissue debrided.

Postoperative Care

Postoperatively, the hand is protected in an elevated, loose, bulky dressing. Anticoagulation should be given in the perioperative period to diminish the likelihood of anastomosis thrombosis. Low-molecular-weight dextran for 5–7 days and aspirin are among the recommended regimens. Some patients, particularly children, may require sedation to decrease early postoperative arterial spasm. Vasospastic agents such as nicotine, caffeine, theophylline, and theobromine should be restricted for the first few weeks after replantation or revascularization. The patient should be placed on a broad-spectrum antibiotic for 5–7 days. Clinical monitoring of the replanted or revascularized part may be supplemented with a pulse oximeter, laser Doppler, or temperature probe.

In those replanted or revascularized parts that show impending failure by change in color, capillary refill, or tissue turgor, the dressing should be loosened. Hand position should be changed to relieve pressure on the part. Patients may be given a heparin bolus of 3000–5000 U. The patient must be kept well hydrated and the room warm. If no improvement is seen after 4–6 hours, the patient may be returned to the operating room for exploration of the anastomoses. Vascular revision is most successful when carried out within 48 hours of injury.

Technical problems involving vascular anastomoses are most often caused by thrombosis, an ill-placed suture occluding the lumen, poor proximal flow secondary to spasm, or undetected intimal vessel damage. If vascular damage is found, a larger segment of the vessel should be resected and a vein graft interposed. If failure appears secondary to poor venous outflow, the intermittent application of leeches (*Hirudo* species) for 1–5 days may provide transient venous drainage while adequate venous drainage is reestablished.

Prognosis

Approximately 85% of replanted parts remain viable. Sensory recovery with two-point discrimination of 10 mm or less occurs in approximately 50% of adults. Patients with viable replanted or revascularized parts often complain of cold intolerance during the first 2 or 3 years after replantation. ROM in replanted digits largely depends on the level of injury and averages approximately half of the normal side.

In most children, normal sensation is regained after digital replantation, and the epiphyseal plates remains open and achieves approximately 80% of normal longitudinal growth. Although the functional results are more promising in children, the viability rate is lower in children because of the greater technical demands of the small vessel anastomoses and the greater sympathetic tone.

Because nerves transected in the proximal arm must regenerate over the considerable length of the limb, only limited motor return is seen in the forearm and hand in proximal limb replantations in adults. One potential benefit of a proximal upper limb replantation may be converting a traumatic above-elbow amputation to an assistive limb with elbow control. Replantation may provide dramatic restoration of hand function when the level of initial amputation is either in the distal forearm or at the wrist level (Figure 10–6).

2. Amputation

The purpose of amputation is to preserve maximal function consistent with bone loss and to achieve an aesthetically acceptable appearance. Priority should be given to preserving functional length, minimizing scar and joint contractures, and preventing the development of symptomatic neuromas.

Phalangeal Amputation

Digital amputation may be carried out through a phalanx or an interphalangeal joint. If the amputation is through the proximal or distal interphalangeal joint, the distal articular surface is reshaped to remove the palmar condylar prominences. If the normal insertion of a tendon was amputated, the tendon should be pulled distally, severed proximally, and allowed to retract. The flexor and extensor tendons should never be sewn over the amputation bone end to provide soft-tissue coverage. Nerves should be identified, gently drawn distally, and transected proximally to prevent the development of a neuroma adherent to the skin scar. If possible, the thick well-padded skin of the palmar surface of the finger should be used to cover the amputation stump. A nontender, shortened, well-padded digit is preferable to a poorly covered, slightly longer, tender digit.

A   B   C

Figure 10–6. Replantation of hand. Intraoperative view (**A**). Following operation, flexion (**B**) and extension (**C**) are restored.

Ray Resection

Amputations through the proximal portion of the proximal phalanx or at the metacarpophalangeal joint of the index or little finger may leave an unsightly bony prominence on the border of the palm, and amputations at a similar level in the middle or ring finger may create an awkward interdigital gap that allows small objects to fall through the palm. Ray resection of a digit's phalanges and metacarpal may be employed to close traumatic wounds, remove dysfunctional or dysesthetic digits, or treat malignant tumors. The aesthetic and functional advantages of ray resection must be balanced against the loss of palmar breadth and, hence, diminution of grip strength.

Index-ray resection creates a normal-appearing web between the middle finger and the thumb. Similarly, resection of the little-finger metacarpal leaves a smooth ulnar contour. Little-finger ray resection is contraindicated in patients who prefer maximal grip strength over cosmesis. Resection of the middle- or ring-finger ray should be accompanied by either soft-tissue coaptation or metacarpal transposition. Resection of the middle ray through the proximal metacarpal metaphysis allows transposition of the corresponding distal portion of the index ray to the middle-ray position (Figure 10–7). Ring-finger ray resection may be closed by either osteotomizing the little-finger metacarpal and moving it to the ring-finger base or by pulling the little finger radialward across the hamate by tight repair of the deep transverse intermetacarpal ligament between the middle and little fingers.

Adani R, Marcoccio I, Castagnetti C et al: Long-term results of replantation for complete ring avulsion amputations. Ann Plast Surg 2003;51:564. [PMID: 14646649]

Melikyan EY, Beg MS, Woodbridge S et al: The functional results of ray amputation. J Hand Surg 2003;8:47. [PMID: 12923934]

Nuzumlali E, Orhun E, Ozturk K et al: Results of ray resection and amputation for ring avulsion injuries at the proximal interphalangeal joint. J Hand Surg 2003B;28:578. [PMID: 14599832]

Wilhelmi BJ, Lee WP, Pagensteert GI et al: Replantation in the mutilated hand. Hand Clin 2003;19:89. [PMID: 12683449]

Yu JC, Shieh SJ, Lee JW et al: Secondary procedures following digital replantation and revascularisation. J Plast Surg 2003B;56:125. [PMID: 12791355]

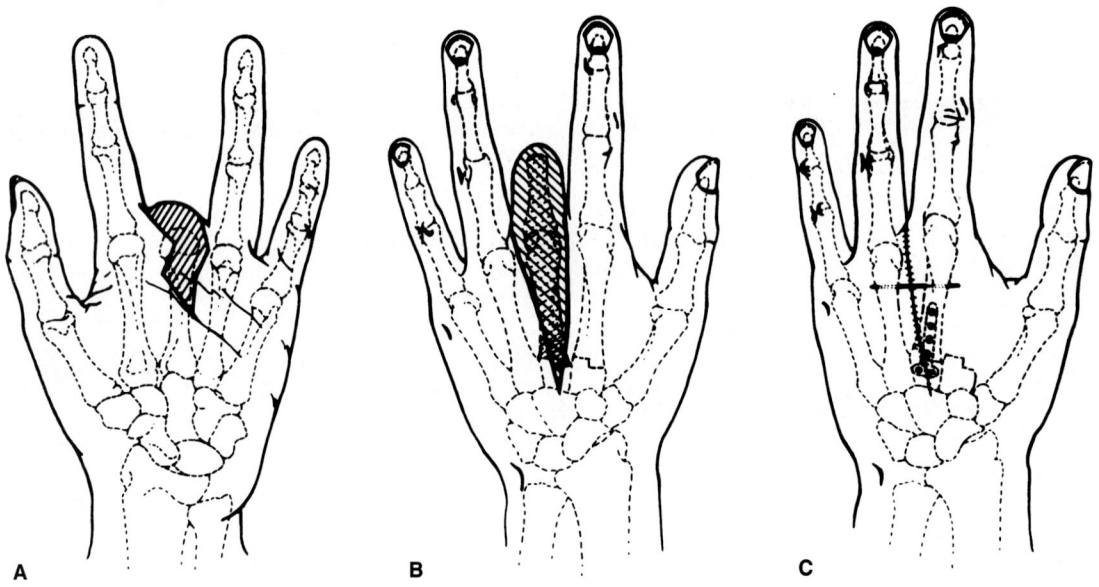

Figure 10–7. Middle-ray resection and index-ray transposition. **A:** Converging chevron incisions reduce palmar skin and soft-tissue redundancy. **B:** Corresponding step-cut osteotomies are fashioned in both the index and middle metacarpal proximal metaphyses. **C:** The transposed index finger is fixed to the middle finger with a plate and further stabilized with K-wire into the ring-finger metacarpal. (Reproduced, with permission, from Chapman MW, ed: *Operative Orthopaedics,* Vol. 2, 3/e, 2001.)

■ DISORDERS OF THE MUSCULATURE OF THE HAND

Anatomy

Control of digital posture requires a complex balance of extrinsic and intrinsic muscle forces. Extrinsic muscles have their origin outside of the hand and their insertion on the hand or carpus, whereas intrinsic muscles have both origin and insertion within the hand. Extrinsic muscles are either flexors or extensors, and intrinsic muscles contribute to both digital flexion and extension.

A. EXTRINSIC EXTENSOR MUSCLES

The extrinsic extensors run through six different fibro-osseous retinacular compartments at the wrist level (Figure 10–8A). The first (most radial) compartment contains the abductor pollicis longus and the extensor pollicis brevis. The abductor pollicis longus inserts at the base of the thumb metacarpal and radially abducts the thumb, whereas the extensor pollicis brevis inserts on the dorsum of the proximal aspect of the proximal phalanx of the thumb and actively extends the metacarpophalangeal joint of the thumb.

The second extensor compartment contains the extensor carpi radialis longus and the extensor carpi radialis brevis. The extensor carpi radialis longus, inserting on the index metacarpal, dorsiflexes and radially deviates the wrist, and the extensor carpi radialis brevis, inserting into the base of the middle metacarpal, provides balanced wrist dorsiflexion.

The third compartment contains the extensor pollicis longus, which runs longitudinally down the forearm through the third compartment and turns abruptly radialward about Lister tubercle, a dorsal prominence on the distal radius. Because its insertion is on the distal phalanx, the extensor pollicis longus provides forceful extension of the thumb interphalangeal joint. The oblique course of the extensor pollicis longus tendon provides a significant adduction component to the pull of the extensor pollicis longus.

The fourth extensor compartment contains the extensor indicis proprius and the extensor digitorum communis, whereas the fifth compartment contains the extensor digiti quinti. These three muscles each have a role in digital extension at the metacarpophalangeal, proximal interphalangeal, and distal interphalangeal joints of the fingers. The principal bony insertion of the extrinsic digital extensors is on the dorsal proximal aspect of the middle phalanx. Metacarpophalangeal joint extension is provided by extrinsic extensor force

transmitted through the sagittal bands. Distal interphalangeal joint extension is achieved through the conjoined lateral bands that are composed of tendinous slips from the extrinsic and intrinsic tendons.

The extensor indicis proprius inserts on the index finger ulnar to the extensor digitorum communis. The extensor digitorum communis inserts on the index, middle, ring, and, in some cases, little fingers. The extensor digiti quinti tendon inserts on the little finger ulnar to the extensor digitorum communis insertion.

The extensor carpi ulnaris tendon runs through the sixth compartment and inserts at the base of the little-finger metacarpal. It provides wrist extension and ulnar deviation.

The extensor digitorum communis tendons of the middle, ring, and little fingers are tethered together by juncturae tendinum over the dorsum of the hand proximal to the metacarpophalangeal joint (Figure 10–8B). The extensor indicis proprius tendon may be recognized at the wrist level as possessing the most distal muscle belly of any of the digital extensor tendons.

The digital extensor tendons are stabilized over the midline of the metacarpophalangeal joint by their attachment to sagittal band fibers (Figure 10–9). The sagittal band fibers insert onto the volar proximal phalanx and onto the lateral borders of the volar plate. The sagittal band fibers form a sling that allows proximal extrinsic extensor tension to be transmitted to the proximal phalanx, permitting metacarpophalangeal joint extension without a tendinous insertion onto the proximal phalanx. By holding the extrinsic extensor tendon balanced over the prominence of the metacarpal head, the sagittal bands normally keep the extrinsic extensor as far as possible away from the center of rotation of the metacarpophalangeal joint, thereby giving it the greatest mechanical efficiency. With rupture or attenuation of the sagittal band fibers, the extrinsic extensor tendon sublux to the ulnar side of the metacarpal head.

B. EXTRINSIC FLEXOR MUSCLES

The extrinsic finger flexors are the flexor digitorum profundus and the flexor digitorum superficialis. The flexor digitorum profundus inserts on the proximal volar aspect of the distal phalanx, flexing the distal interphalangeal joint as well as the proximal interphalangeal and metacarpophalangeal joints. The flexor digitorum superficialis acts as a flexor of the proximal interphalangeal and metacarpophalangeal joints. It lies palmar to the flexor digitorum profundus tendon in the palm, splits at the level of the metacarpophalangeal joint, and passes dorsal to the flexor digitorum profundus tendon before reattaching or inserting into the middle phalanx. Although the extrinsic flexors provide metacarpophalangeal joint flexion, this occurs only

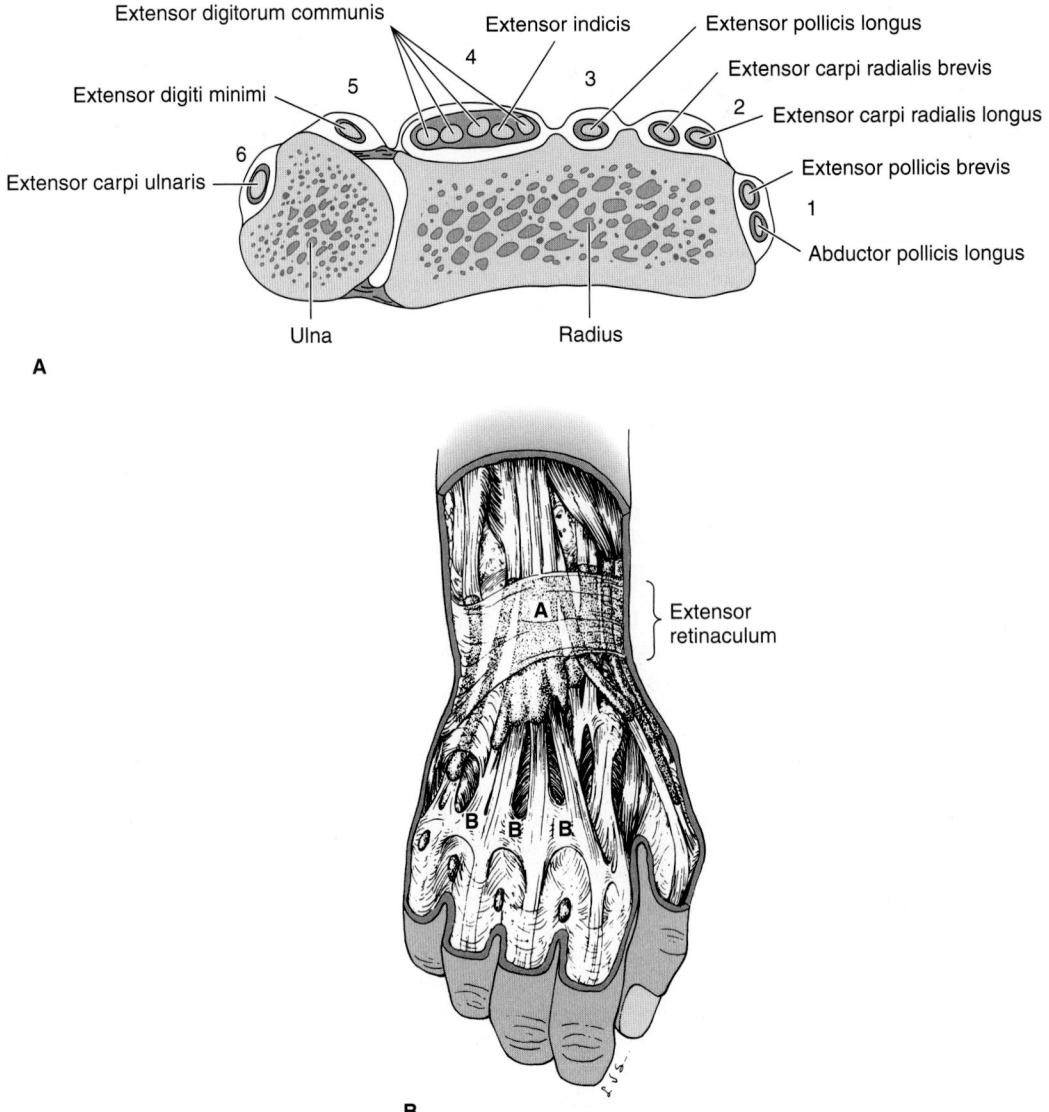

Extensor digitorum communis
Extensor indicis
Extensor pollicis longus
Extensor digiti minimi
Extensor carpi radialis brevis
Extensor carpi radialis longus
Extensor carpi ulnaris
Extensor pollicis brevis
Abductor pollicis longus
Ulna
Radius
A

Extensor retinaculum
B

Figure 10–8. The six dorsal compartments of the wrist. **A:** Cross-section of pronated right wrist viewed from distal to proximal. (Reproduced, with permission, from Reckling FW et al: *Orthopaedic Anatomy and Surgical Approaches.* Mosby-Year Book, 1990.) **B:** Dorsal view. A = extensor retinaculum over the compartments; B = juncturae tendinum (conexus intertendineus). (Reproduced, with permission, from Way LW, ed: *Current Surgical Diagnosis & Treatment,* 10th ed. Appleton & Lange, 1994.)

after most of their excursion is expended flexing the interphalangeal joints.

C. INTRINSIC MUSCLES

The intrinsic muscles that control finger posture are the dorsal and palmar interossei, lumbricals, and hypothenar muscles. These muscles are responsible for primary flexion, abduction, and adduction of the metacarpophalangeal joints and primary extension of the proximal interphalangeal and distal interphalangeal joints.

The index metacarpal is abducted by the first dorsal interosseous muscle and adducted by the first palmar interosseous muscle. The middle finger is radially abducted by the second dorsal interosseous muscle and ulnarly

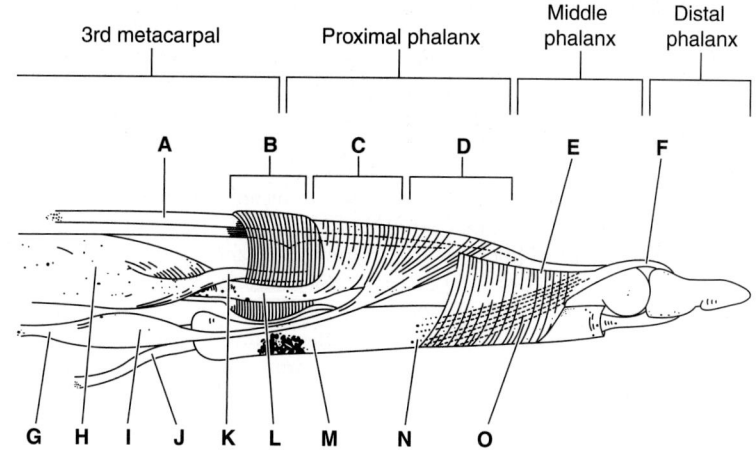

A. Common extensor tendon
B. Sagittal bands
C. Transverse fibers of the interossei
D. Oblique fibers of the interossei
E. Lateral conjoined tendon
F. Terminal tendon
G. Flexor digitorum profundus tendon
H. Interosseous muscle (second dorsal) deep head
I. Lumbrical muscle
J. Tendon of flexor digitorum superficialis
K. Medial tendon, superficial head of second dorsal interosseous
L. Lateral tendon of deep head of second dorsal interosseous
M. Fibrous flexor pulley
N. Oblique retinacular ligament
O. Transverse retinacular ligament
P. Medial interosseous band
Q. Central slip of the common extensor
R. Lateral slip of the common extensor
S. Triangular ligament

Figure 10–9. Extensor hood mechanism. The dorsal hood apparatus provides points of insertion of both extrinsic extensors and intrinsic muscles of the hand. (Modified and reproduced, with permission, from Way LW, ed: *Current Surgical Diagnosis & Treatment,* 10th ed. Appleton & Lange, 1994.)

abducted by the third dorsal interosseous muscle. The ring finger is adducted by the second volar interosseous muscle and abducted by the fourth dorsal interosseous muscle. The little finger is adducted by the third volar interosseous muscle and abducted by the abductor digiti quinti muscle.

The first, second, and fourth dorsal interossei have both superficial and deep muscle bellies, with the superficial belly giving rise to a tendon of insertion on the proximal phalanx tubercle. The deep muscle belly inserts into the hood of the dorsal aponeurosis and thus contributes to metacarpophalangeal joint flexion and proximal and distal interphalangeal joint extension. The third dorsal interosseous usually has a single muscle belly, which inserts into the dorsal hood apparatus. The insertion of the volar interosseous muscles is also into the hood apparatus (see Figure 10–9).

All interosseous muscles course palmar to the axis of motion of the metacarpophalangeal joint and dorsal to the transverse intermetacarpal ligament. Their tendinous insertions are into the lateral band fibers, which pass dorsal to the axis of motion of the proximal and distal interphalangeal joints. When the metacarpophalangeal joint is flexed, the interossei are less effective in extending the interphalangeal joints than when the metacarpophalangeal joint is in extension or slight flexion.

The four lumbrical muscles insert into the radial lateral band of the dorsal hood aponeurosis of each finger. The lumbricals originate from the flexor digitorum profundus tendons of the corresponding finger. Their course is more volar than that of the dorsal or palmar interosseous muscles because they lie palmar to the transverse intermetacarpal ligament. The lumbrical muscles modulate flexor and extensor digital tone and may have a role in digital proprioception. Contraction of the profundus muscle belly draws the profundus tendon proximally and shifts the lumbrical origin proximally, thereby increasing tension on the dorsal hood fibers that extend the proximal and distal interphalangeal joints. Contraction of the lumbrical muscle draws the proximal profundus distally and reduces tension on the flexor digitorum profundus at the distal interphalangeal joint, so that distal interphalangeal joint extension is facilitated.

The abductor digiti quinti, like the first, second, and fourth interossei, has two tendons of insertion. One of these tendons inserts directly onto the bone of the abductor tubercle along the ulnar aspect of the little finger proximal phalanx, and the other insertion is into the dorsal hood apparatus. The flexor digiti quinti inserts onto the ulnar tubercle at the base of the proximal phalanx but does not insert into the dorsal hood apparatus. The primary function of the flexor digiti quinti is flexion of the metacarpophalangeal joint.

D. Dorsal Hood Apparatus

The dorsal hood apparatus, frequently referred to as the extensor mechanism, is the confluence of intrinsic and extrinsic tendon insertions on the dorsal aspect of the finger (see Figure 10–9). Through dorsal hood attachments, the extrinsic extensor muscles extend the metacarpophalangeal joint, the intrinsic muscles flex the metacarpophalangeal joint, and both the intrinsic and extrinsic muscles extend the proximal and distal interphalangeal joints.

Extension of the metacarpophalangeal joint is achieved through the action of the extrinsic extensor tendons pulling through the sagittal band sling mechanism, which lifts up the proximal phalanx. Flexion of the metacarpophalangeal joint is achieved both by the tendinous insertion of the intrinsics on the proximal phalanx and by a similar sling effect created by oblique fibers of the intrinsic mechanism blending into the hood, which flexes the metacarpophalangeal joint. Additionally, the flexor digitorum profundus and superficialis secondarily flex the metacarpophalangeal joint.

Extension of the proximal interphalangeal joint is achieved through the action of the central slip, which is the bony insertion of the extrinsic digital extensors on the middle phalanx. In addition, the intrinsic muscles contribute to proximal interphalangeal joint extension through medial slips from the lateral band, which run centrally to insert on the proximal dorsal aspect of the middle phalanx as part of the central slip.

Distal interphalangeal joint extension is achieved through both intrinsic and extrinsic forces pulling through the radial and ulnar conjoined lateral bands, which merge to form the terminal tendon insertion. The intrinsic contribution to the conjoined lateral band is through its insertion into the lateral band. The extrinsic contribution to distal interphalangeal joint extension occurs through lateral slip fibers that diverge from the central slip over the dorsum of the proximal phalanx and join the lateral band to form the conjoined lateral band. The conjoined lateral bands from the radial and ulnar side converge distally as the terminal tendon inserting on the distal phalanx.

DISRUPTION OF EXTENSOR MUSCLE INSERTIONS

1. Sagittal Band Disruption

Anatomy & Clinical Findings

The sagittal band fibers transmitting extrinsic extensor power may be disrupted by laceration or, more often, may become attenuated because of underlying synovitis of the metacarpophalangeal joint, as occurs in RA. When the sagittal band fibers along either the radial or ulnar aspect of the dorsal hood become attenuated, the extensor tendon may sublux into the valley between the adjacent metacarpal heads. Because the subluxed extrinsic extensors are mechanically less effective at extending the metacarpophalangeal joint, full active extension of this joint may be lost. This phenomenon occurs commonly in RA. It also may result from tearing of the sagittal band fibers with torquing activity such as occurs in the middle finger with pitching a baseball.

Treatment

An acute tear of the radial sagittal band may be treated by splinting. If this is ineffective, surgical repair may be indicated. Chronic injuries are treated by releasing the ulnar sagittal band and recentralizing the extensor tendon by placing a strip of the tendon around the radial collateral ligament.

2. Boutonnière Deformity

Anatomy & Clinical Findings

When the central slip is disrupted by laceration or closed rupture or elongated by synovitis of the proximal interphalangeal joint, the direct bony insertion of the extrinsic extensors on the middle phalanx is lost. When the insertion of the medial slips from the lateral band is also lost, active proximal interphalangeal joint extension is lacking. The finger is rapidly drawn into a position of proximal interphalangeal joint flexion as the unopposed motion of the flexor digitorum sublimis and profundus draws the finger into flexion (Figure 10–10). The lateral bands migrate apart as the finger is flexed and are drawn into a progressively more palmar position, eventually coming to lie palmar to the axis of flexion of the joint. In the subluxed position, the lateral bands become a deforming force contributing to the tendency of the finger to flex at the proximal interphalangeal joint.

With central slip disruption, the force normally transmitted through the central slip to the middle phalanx from both extrinsic extensor and intrinsic muscles bypasses the proximal interphalangeal joint and is refocused on the distal interphalangeal joint, amplifying the force of extension of this joint and hyperextending it. Because the distal interphalangeal joint is relatively resistant to active flexion, contraction of the flexor digitorum profundus muscle primarily flexes the proximal interphalangeal joint and is relatively ineffective in flexing the distal interphalangeal joint, unless the proximal interphalangeal joint is supported in maximal extension. The digit rapidly assumes the boutonnière deformity posture of proximal interphalangeal joint flexion and distal interphalangeal joint hyperextension.

Treatment

Because the proximal interphalangeal joint is at the center of the complex balance of the intrinsic and extrinsic forces, restoration of proper balance and tension on the central slip may be technically difficult. When the central slip is acutely lacerated, it should be directly repaired and the joint pinned in full extension for 3–6 weeks to protect the integrity of the repair. Closed ruptures of the central slip, if diagnosed acutely, should be treated with

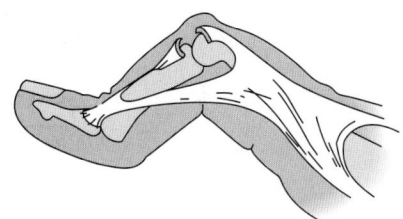

Figure 10–10. Boutonnière deformity caused by loss of active proximal interphalangeal extension secondary to loss of the central slip insertion on the proximal dorsal middle phalanx. (Reproduced, with permission, from Way LW, ed: *Current Surgical Diagnosis & Treatment*, 10th ed. Appleton & Lange, 1994.)

6 weeks of splinting of the proximal interphalangeal joint in full extension. When diagnosis is delayed even a few weeks, a fixed flexion contracture of the proximal interphalangeal joint is usual.

Surgical treatment of closed rupture of the central slip in a finger that develops a fixed flexion contracture is frequently disappointing because the surgical procedure must both release the contracture on the palmar aspect of the joint and augment proximal interphalangeal joint extension on the dorsal aspect. A better strategy employs prolonged splinting to diminish the extent of the fixed proximal interphalangeal joint flexion contracture. Among the variety of splints available for this, the Capener splint and the Joint Jack splint are particularly useful. Serial casting of the finger with a circumferential digital cast that is changed every few days may also be helpful in bringing the proximal interphalangeal joint into extension. During the period of splinting, the patient should be instructed to carry out active flexion of the distal interphalangeal joint, with the middle phalanx supported in extension. Care should be taken to assure that splints and casts allow distal interphalangeal joint flexion. Once full proximal interphalangeal joint extension is achieved, splinting should be continued full time for an additional 6–12 weeks. In many instances, this achieves sufficient tightening of the central slip to permit satisfactory active proximal interphalangeal joint extension.

If active extension cannot be restored with prolonged splinting, several operative interventions may be considered. The first, a Fowler type of tenotomy, obliquely divides the dorsal hood apparatus over the middle phalanx, proximal to the terminal tendon insertion. This diminishes distal interphalangeal joint hyperextension and may improve active proximal interphalangeal joint extension by refocusing intrinsic and extrinsic forces at the more proximal joint.

Alternatively, other surgical techniques attempt to more directly augment proximal interphalangeal joint extension, either by shortening the central slip or by mobilizing portions of one or both lateral bands. Although such techniques may increase active extension of the joint, they often do so at the loss of full proximal interphalangeal joint flexion.

3. Mallet Finger

Anatomy & Clinical Findings

The mallet finger deformity is characterized by a loss of full active distal interphalangeal joint extension with full passive ROM evident. The mallet finger reflects the loss of normal extensor force transmission via the terminal tendon insertion onto the distal phalanx. The unopposed flexor digitorum profundus pulls the distal joint into flexion (Figure 10–11). The usual mechanism of injury involves sudden passive flexion of the actively extended distal interphalangeal joint. Disruption of the terminal tendon may be entirely confined to the tendon or may involve an avulsed fracture fragment from the dorsal lip of the distal phalanx proximal articular surface.

Because the avulsed fragment includes the terminal tendon insertion, the clinical appearance of soft tissue and bony mallet fingers is similar. The distal joint rests in flexion, a posture that cannot be actively changed. Full passive extension of the distal interphalangeal joint is possible.

Treatment

A radiograph should be obtained to determine whether a fracture is present and, if the dorsal fragment is large, whether the distal phalanx is subluxed palmarward. If the joint is congruent, splinting is recommended even if a small articular surface fracture site gap persists. The distal interphalangeal joint should be splinted in extension continuously for 8 weeks, and the finger may then be tested. If residual drooping of the distal joint is noted, an additional 2–4 weeks of splinting is required.

Kalainov DM et al: Non-surgical treatment of closed mallet finger fractures. J Hand Surg Am 2005;30:580. [PMID: 15925171]

Figure 10–11. Mallet finger deformity is secondary to loss of terminal tendon insertion on the distal phalanx. (Reproduced, with permission, from Way LW, ed: *Current Surgical Diagnosis & Treatment,* 10th ed. Appleton & Lange, 1994.)

Figure 10–12. Intrinsic plus position.

INTRINSIC PLUS & INTRINSIC MINUS POSITIONS

Together, the interossei and lumbricals flex the metacarpophalangeal joints and extend the proximal and distal interphalangeal joints. Hence, the posture of the hand in which the metacarpophalangeal joints are flexed and the proximal and distal interphalangeal joints are extended is known as the intrinsic plus position (Figure 10–12). This is an ideal position for splinting the hand because the collateral ligaments of the metacarpophalangeal and interphalangeal joint are taut, and because it is also ideal for immobilization of most hand injuries, it is termed the *position of safety* or *position of advantage.*

The normal excursion of the intrinsic muscles is sufficient to allow simultaneous passive positioning of the metacarpophalangeal joints in extension while the proximal and distal interphalangeal joints are flexed. This posture, known as the intrinsic minus position, requires full excursion of the relaxed intrinsic muscles (see Figure 10–12, Figure 10–13). When the intrinsic muscles are paralyzed, the hand tends to assume the intrinsic minus posture, sometimes referred to as a clawhand. Although the extrinsic extensors have fibers that can provide proximal and distal interphalangeal joint extension in the hand with competent intrinsic muscles, in the intrinsic minus hand their excursion is expended in unopposed metacarpophalangeal joint hyperextension. Thus, the hand devoid of intrinsic power is unable to achieve active extension of the proximal and distal interphalangeal joints, unless the metacarpophalangeal joint is flexed by other means.

Figure 10–13. Intrinsic minus position secondary to low median and ulnar nerve palsies.

Treatment

Surgical correction of the intrinsic minus hand must either prevent passive hyperextension of the metacarpophalangeal joint or restore active control of metacarpophalangeal joint flexion. This may be achieved either by tenodesis or capsulodesis across the metacarpophalangeal joint or by an active tendon transfer. Once metacarpophalangeal joint hyperextension is prevented, the extrinsic extensors usually can effectively open the hand by extending the proximal and distal interphalangeal joints. If active proximal interphalangeal joint extension is not possible through the extrinsic extensors when the metacarpophalangeal joint is flexed, then tendon transfer for metacarpophalangeal joint flexion should be inserted into the digital lateral bands. This augments proximal interphalangeal joint extension and provides metacarpophalangeal joint flexion.

INTRINSIC MUSCLE TIGHTNESS
Anatomy & Clinical Findings

When the lumbricals and interossei become contracted and overly tight, the limitation of their excursion does not permit full simultaneous metacarpophalangeal joint extension and interphalangeal joint flexion. The intrinsic tightness test was originally described by Finochietto and later by Bunnell (Figure 10–14). It is accomplished by first determining that the metacarpophalangeal and interphalangeal joints each have a full range of passive joint motion in a reduced position. The metacarpophalangeal joint is then passively held in an extended position while the examiner attempts to flex the proximal and distal inter-

Figure 10–14. Intrinsic tightness test is performed by flexing the proximal interphalangeal joint with the metaphalangeal joint extended and flexed. Tightness to proximal interphalangeal flexion occurs with the metaphalangeal joint extended. (Reproduced, with permission, from Green DP, ed: *Operative Hand Surgery*, 2nd ed. Churchill Livingstone, 1988.)

phalangeal joints passively. If full passive flexion of the proximal and distal interphalangeal joints is not possible in this position, the intrinsic muscles are deemed tight.

Causes of intrinsic muscle tightness include conditions as diverse as RA, neurologic dysfunction secondary to closed head injury, and crush injury of the hand.

Treatment

Surgical treatment of intrinsic tightness may be carried out as an isolated procedure or in combination with metacarpophalangeal joint reconstruction. The intrinsic force is diminished either by intrinsic muscle tenotomy or by resection of a triangular segment of one or both lateral bands. The intrinsic tightness test may be used intraoperatively to judge the adequacy of intrinsic muscle release.

SWAN-NECK DEFORMITY

Anatomy & Clinical Findings

Swan-neck deformity is characterized by hyperextension of the proximal interphalangeal joint and flexion of the distal interphalangeal joint (Figure 10–15). The pathophysiology of swan-neck deformity involves either primary or secondary stretching or disruption of the volar plate's restraint on proximal interphalangeal joint hyperextension. Synovitis of the proximal interphalangeal joint secondary in patients with RA may distend the joint and thus render the volar plate ineffective in preventing proximal interphalangeal joint hyperextension. Overly forceful intrinsic muscle contraction (as occurs with an intrinsic plus deformity) transmits an abnormally high force through the central slip, hyperextending the proximal interphalangeal joint. When the proximal interphalangeal joint is hyperextended, the dorsal hood apparatus is relatively ineffective in extending the distal interphalangeal joint, allowing the distal interphalangeal joint to fall into flexion.

In some fingers, a fixed extension contracture or ankylosis of the proximal interphalangeal joint may occur as a consequence of swan-neck deformity. In other fingers, the proximal interphalangeal joint remains supple but the finger is locked in a hyperextended posture.

Treatment

Surgical treatment of swan-neck deformity secondary to intrinsic tightness requires diminishing intrinsic muscle force, usually through resection of a triangle of the proximal lateral band and dorsal hood. A new checkrein to proximal interphalangeal joint extension is created, either through tenodesis of one slip of the flexor digitorum superficialis or tenodesis in which one of the lateral bands is rerouted volar to the center of rotation of the proximal interphalangeal joint, recreating the sagittal oblique retinacular ligament.

Figure 10–15. Swan-neck deformity. (Reproduced, with permission, from American Society for Surgery of the Hand: *The Hand: Examination and Diagnosis,* 2nd ed. Churchill Livingstone, 1983.)

Bruner S, Wittemann M, Jester A et al: Dynamic splinting after extensor tendon repair in zones V to VII. J Hand Surg. 2003B;28:224. [PMID: 12809652]

■ DISORDERS OF THE TENDONS OF THE HAND

FLEXOR TENDON INJURY

Anatomy

The extrinsic flexors of the finger consist of the flexor digitorum profundus and the flexor digitorum superficialis. The flexor digitorum profundus originates from the proximal ulna and the interosseous membrane. In the forearm, it divides into two muscle groups: the most radial component supplying the index finger and the ulnar component supplying the middle, ring, and little fingers. The flexor digitorum profundus and the flexor pollicis longus muscles form the deep compartment of the volar forearm. As the flexor digitorum profundus and flexor pollicis longus tendons travel through the carpal tunnel, they occupy the floor of the carpal tunnel.

The tenosynovial sheath of the flexor pollicis longus is continuous with the radial bursa; the tenosynovial sheath to the little finger is continuous with the ulnar digital bursa. In some patients, these two bursae communicate, allowing a so-called horseshoe abscess to spread between the thumb and little finger if infection occurs in the flexor tendon sheath of either one of these digits.

The lumbricals originate from the radial side of the index, middle, ring, and little fingers in the palm. The profundus tendon passes through the bifurcation of the flexor digitorum superficialis before inserting into the proximal palmar base of the distal phalanx. The innervation of the flexor digitorum profundus of the index and middle fingers is through the anterior interosseous branch of the median nerve, whereas the profundus of the ring and little fingers is innervated by the ulnar nerve. The flexor digitorum profundus provides digital flexion at both the proximal and distal interphalangeal joints.

The flexor digitorum superficialis has two heads: The radial head originates from the proximal shaft of the radius, and the humeral ulnar head originates from the medial humeral epicondyle and coronoid process of the ulna. Each digit has a corresponding independent superficialis muscle. As the superficialis tendons pass through the carpal tunnel, the tendons of the middle and ring fingers are more superficial and central than those of the index and little fingers. In the proximal aspect of the finger, the flexor digitorum superficialis tendon bifurcates around the flexor digitorum profundus at the beginning of the A2 pulley. The flexor digitorum superficialis tendon slips then reunite distally at the Camper chiasm, with approximately half of the fibers staying on the ipsilateral side and half crossing to the contralateral side of the finger. The tendon then inserts via radial and ulnar slips into the proximal metaphysis of the middle phalanx. The entire flexor digitorum superficialis muscle receives innervation from the median nerve. The primary function of the superficialis is digital flexion at the proximal interphalangeal joint.

The flexor pollicis longus originates from two heads: The radial head takes origin from the proximal radius and interosseous membrane, and an accessory head originates from the coronoid process of the ulna and from the medial epicondyle of the humerus. In the palm, the flexor pollicis longus tendon transverses between the abductor pollicis brevis and the flexor pollicis brevis. The flexor pollicis longus inserts into the proximal base of the thumb distal phalanx and is innervated by the anterior interosseous branch of the median nerve. The flexor pollicis longus flexes both the interphalangeal and metacarpophalangeal joints of the thumb.

As the flexor tendons pass distal to the metacarpal neck, they enter the fibroosseous tunnel, or digital flexor sheath. The fibroosseous tunnel extends distally to the proximal aspect of the distal phalanx. The tendinous sheath consists of annular pulleys, which provide mechanical stability, and cruciate pulleys, which provide flexibility (Figure 10–16). The first, third, and fifth annular pulleys (A1, A3, and A5) are located over the metacarpophalangeal, proximal interphalangeal, and distal interphalangeal joints, respectively, and the second and fourth pulleys (A2 and A4) are situated over the middle portion of the proximal and middle phalanges. The A2 and A4 pulleys are the most essential in maintaining the mechanical advantage of the flexor tendons.

The tenosynovium that lines the fibroosseous tunnel supplies both nutrition and lubrication to the poorly vascularized flexor tendons. Proximal to the sheath, the tendons are well vascularized by the peritenon. Within the sheath, tendon vascularity is supplied via the vincula system: the vinculum longus and brevis.

Following injury, the flexor tendon heals through both extrinsic and intrinsic mechanisms. Extrinsic tendon healing occurs via cells brought to the site of repair by ingrowth of capillaries and fibroblasts; formation of adhesions follows at the repair site. Intrinsic healing occurs from tenocyte within the tendon. The goal of flexor tendon repair and postoperative care is to encourage both intrinsic and extrinsic healing without the formation of thick adhesions, which would limit tendon excursion and ultimately result in restricted motion of the finger.

Clinical Findings

The time since injury as well as the mechanism of injury (sharp open injury versus closed avulsion injury) should be noted in the history.

A. NORMAL CASCADE OF FINGERS

The resting posture of the fingers should be observed. Disruption of the normal cascade of increasing flexion in the relaxed fingers as one moves from the index finger to the little finger should arouse suspicion of tendon disruption (Figure 10–17).

B. NORMAL TENODESIS PHENOMENON

Tendon integrity may also be evaluated by taking advantage of the normal tenodesis positioning of the

Figure 10–16. Annular (A) and cruciate (C) pulley locations.

Figure 10–17. If the index finger remains extended when the hand is at rest, its flexor tendons are severed.

digits, which occurs as the wrist is passively brought through a ROM. Normally, as the wrist is dorsiflexed, the digital extensors relax and the finger flexors become taut, passively flexing the fingers in the normal cascade pattern. When the muscles of the proximal forearm are squeezed, the fingers normally flex involuntarily.

C. TESTING OF INDIVIDUAL TENDONS

Isolated testing of the superficialis and profundus tendons is employed to determine the integrity of each tendon (see Figures 10–2 and 10–3). Because the flexor digitorum superficialis of the little finger is not independent of the ring finger in many individuals, either because of cross connections between the two tendons or because of congenital absence of the tendon, it may be impossible from clinical examination to detect injury to the flexor digitorum superficialis tendon of the little finger. The strength of flexion should be noted as each of the tendons is tested. If the patient is able to flex the finger but experiences pain with flexion and is unable to generate full power against resistance, a partial flexor tendon injury should be suspected.

Treatment

Functional outcomes are equivalent if the repair is done the day of injury (primary repair) or within the first 7–10 days after the injury (delayed primary repair).

Because repair requires proper visualization of both ends of the tendon, the wound may need to be electively extended. The tendon ends must be gently retrieved because trauma to the flexor tendon sheath creates adverse scarring. Tendons should not be grasped along their tenosynovial surfaces. The A2 and A4 pulleys should be preserved. A maximum of 1 cm may be debrided from the tendon ends without compromising eventual digital extension. A core suture of either 3-0 or 4-0 braided synthetic material is secured to coapt tendon ends (Figure 10–18).

The flexor tendon repair is strengthened by employing four strands of suture across the repair site rather than two. A running 6-0 nylon epitendinous suture completes the tendon repair. The role of flexor tendon sheath repair remains controversial.

Because the results and complications of flexor tendon repair vary by level of injury, five zones of injury are defined (Figure 10–19). Zone I extends from the insertion of the profundus on the distal phalanx to the insertion of the flexor digitorum superficialis on the middle phalanx. The tendon may be directly repaired if the distal stump is large enough, or it may be reinserted to bone. Care must be taken not to advance the tendon more than 1 cm.

Zone II, which extends from the proximal portion of the A1 pulley to the insertion of the superficialis tendon, is the most problematic region of injury because it contains both the profundus and superficialis tendons in a relatively avascular region. Care must be taken to preserve the vincular blood supply. When both the superficialis and profundus tendons are divided, it is preferable to repair both tendons because greater digital independence of motion may be achieved with a somewhat lower risk of tendon rupture during the rehabilitation period. Repair of the superficialis tendon as well as the profundus tendon also diminishes the likelihood of proximal interphalangeal joint hyperextension deformity.

Zone III injuries are located between the proximal edge of the A1 pulley and the distal edge of the transverse carpal ligament.

In zone IV injuries, the area beneath the transverse carpal ligament, a step-cut release and repair of the transverse carpal ligament should be performed to prevent flexor tendon bowstringing.

Zone I and II injuries of the thumb are handled similarly to those of analogous finger zones. In zone III of the thumb, it is difficult to access the flexor pollicis longus tendon as it passes through the thenar musculature. Options for treatment of injuries at this level include either primary tendon grafting or step-cut lengthening of the tendon in the forearm, so the repair is distal to the obscuring thenar muscles.

Improved results of flexor tendon surgery in recent years are substantially because of the evolution of postoperative therapy programs. Immobilization of the fin-

Figure 10–18. Kessler sutures and other types of sutures for flexor tendon repair. (Reproduced, with permission, from Green DP, ed: *Operative Hand Surgery*, 2nd ed. Churchill Livingstone, 1988.)

ger after tendon repair is appropriate only in very young or otherwise uncooperative patients. Following flexor tendon injury, the wrist should be immobilized at approximately 30 degrees of flexion, the metacarpophalangeal joints at approximately 45 degrees of flexion, and the interphalangeal joints at 0–15 degrees of flexion. A program of passive ROM exercises should be initiated that decreases the adhesions at the repair site and enhances intrinsic tendon repair. Passive motion may be achieved either through rubber band splinting to flex the finger passively or by having the patient move the finger passively. At 4–6 weeks following repair, active flexion and extension exercises are allowed as splinting is discontinued. At 6–8 weeks, passive extension exercises and isolated blocking is encouraged. After 8 weeks, the patient may begin flexion against resistance.

When a four-strand repair is performed, active assisted motion is begun within the first 2 weeks. In this program, the wrist is extended and the fingers are passively flexed. The patient is then asked to flex the fingers actively to hold this position.

With four-strand techniques for flexor tendon repair, active motion can begin earlier than with a two-strand repair. In properly motivated and cooperative patients, an active hold program is begun during the first week. The therapist passively brings the hand into flexion and the patient is asked to maintain the position.

Flexor Tendon Avulsion Injuries

The flexor tendon may be avulsed from its bony insertion, usually by forced extension of the finger while the finger is simultaneously actively flexed. An estimated 75% of flexor digitorum profundus avulsion injuries involve the ring finger. Such injuries commonly occur in football or rugby, when the athlete grabs an opponent's jersey and a finger is involuntarily extended as the opponent attempts to elude tackle.

Flexor digitorum profundus avulsion injuries may be classified according to the level of profundus tendon retraction. In type 1 injuries, the tendon retracts proximally from the sheath into the palm. Repair of these

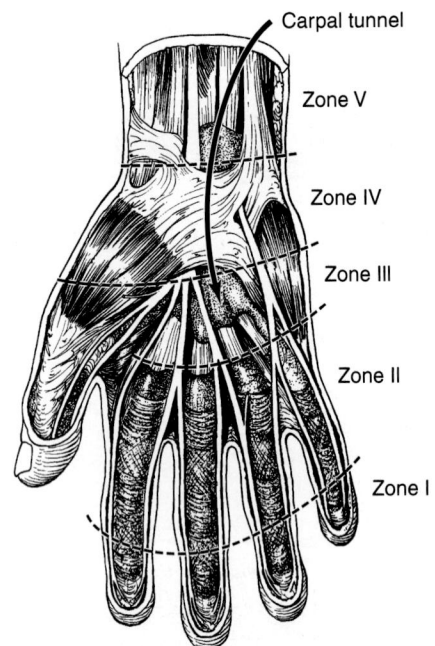

Carpal tunnel

Zone V

Zone IV

Zone III

Zone II

Zone I

Figure 10–19. Flexor tendon injury zones. (Modified and reproduced, with permission, from Way LW, ed: *Current Surgical Diagnosis & Treatment*, 10th ed. Stamford: Appleton & Lange, 1994.)

injuries should be performed within 10 days to avoid myostatic contracture, which will limit the ability to bring the tendon to its normal insertion without undue tension. In type 2 injuries, the tendon retracts to the level of the proximal interphalangeal joint. A small bony avulsion fragment may be seen on a lateral radiograph of the finger in these injuries. The tendon may be reinserted into the distal phalanx up to 6 weeks after injury. Type 3 injuries involve an osseous distal phalangeal avulsion fragment that is so large, it blocks retraction of the flexor digitorum profundus proximal to the A4 pulley. These injuries also may be repaired up to 6 weeks after injury. Missed or neglected profundus avulsion injuries, if symptomatic, may be treated by staged tendon reconstruction, distal interphalangeal joint arthrodesis, or tenodesis.

Moiemen NS, Elliot D: Primary flexor tendon repair in zone 1. J Hand Surg Br 2000;25:78. [PMID: 10763731]

Flexor Tendon Reconstruction

Direct repair of a disrupted flexor tendon is not possible if there is loss of the tendon substance, long-standing myostatic contracture, or unresolved soft-tissue defects. If the flexor digitorum superficialis tendon is intact with a full active range of proximal interphalangeal joint motion, arthrodesis or tenodesis of the distal interphalangeal joint may be elected, creating a so-called superficialis finger. If the patient requires active motion at the distal interphalangeal joint, tendon grafting is necessary. Tendon grafting is usually indicated when neither flexor digitorum superficialis nor flexor digitorum profundus tendons can be repaired.

Primary tendon grafting may be performed when there is satisfactory skin coverage, full passive range of metacarpophalangeal and interphalangeal joint motion, an intact annular pulley system, minimal scarring in the sheath, adequate digital circulation, and at least one intact digital nerve. Possible donor tendon sources include the palmaris longus, plantaris, or toe extensor tendons. The palmaris longus and plantaris tendons are absent in a significant minority of individuals.

A. SURGICAL PROCEDURE

The donor tendon graft is secured into the distal phalanx. The tendon graft is threaded beneath the flexor tendon sheath pulleys. The proximal attachment of the donor tendon to the profundus motor is performed either with a tendon weave or an end-to-end repair.

Establishing appropriate tension on the tendon graft is critical. If insufficient tension is placed on the tendon graft, a lumbrical plus deformity occurs. With this condition, as the patient pulls the proximal portion of the profundus tendon proximally, the lumbrical is placed under tension, and all of this tension is transmitted to the dorsal hood apparatus rather than to the flexor tendon graft. As a result, as the patient attempts to flex the finger, the finger paradoxically extends both the proximal and distal interphalangeal joints.

If the tendon graft tension is too tight, full extension is impossible. The results of primary tendon grafting are inferior to primary repair in similar circumstances.

Primary tendon repair is contraindicated if the fibroosseous sheath is extensively scarred or if critical pulleys are absent. Restoration of flexion in such situations requires a staged tendon reconstruction. In stage 1, the tendon remnants are excised from the sheath and joint contractures are released. At a minimum, the A2 and A4 pulleys are reconstructed using a flexor tendon remnant, a tendon graft, or a strip of the wrist extensor retinaculum. A silicone rod similar in size to the anticipated tendon graft is secured to the distal phalanx and threaded through the sheath. Early passive ROM stimulates the development of a pseudosheath surrounding the silicone tendon rod.

The second stage of the procedure occurs at least 3 months after the initial procedure. Full digital passive ROM and soft-tissue equilibrium must be achieved before the second stage is undertaken. The silicone tendon rod is replaced with a tendon graft. The donor tendon is secured to the distal phalanx and to the donor motor in a manner similar to primary tendon grafting.

B. COMPLICATIONS

1. Adhesions—The most common complication following flexor tendon surgery is formation of adhesions, which may occur in spite of an appropriate therapy program. Following flexor tendon repair or graft tenolysis should be considered when active flexion is restricted, despite a normal passive ROM, in a wound that has reached soft-tissue equilibrium (usually at least 3 months since repair or reconstruction), in a motivated patient.

Ideally, tenolysis should be performed under local anesthesia with intravenous sedation. Elevation of skin flaps allows wide exposure of the sheath. Care is taken to preserve the annular pulleys while adhesions are released between the tendon and the sheath and between the tendon and the phalanges. Evaluation of the adequacy of lysis may be obtained by asking the patient under local anesthesia to flex the finger actively. If regional or general anesthesia is employed, the tendon must be identified at a more proximal level and traction applied to the tendon at this level to confirm the improvement in joint motion.

Active ROM exercise is begun within the first 24 hours after surgery. Electrical stimulation of the proximal muscle belly may facilitate early motion.

2. Tendon repair rupture—The second major postoperative complication of flexor tendon repair is rupture of the repair. When the rupture is promptly diagnosed, a second repair should be attempted because success rates approach those of uncomplicated primary repair. If rupture is not promptly diagnosed, the ruptured tendon ends must be resected, and either free tendon grafting or staged tendon reconstruction is necessary to restore active flexion.

3. Failure of staged reconstruction—If staged reconstruction fails, arthrodesis or amputation of the digit may be considered, particularly when neurovascular compromise occurs.

Beredjiklian PK: Biologic aspects of flexor tendon laceration and repair. J Bone Joint Surg Am 2003;85:539. [PMID: 12637445]

Beris AE et al: Two-stage flexor tendon reconstruction in zone II using a silicone rod and a pedicled intrasynovial graft. J Hand Surg Am 2003;28:652. [PMID: 12877856]

Slade JF et al: Zone II tendon repairs augmented with autogenous dorsal tendon graft: A biomechanical analysis. J Hand Surg Am 2001;26:813. [PMID: 11561232]

TENOSYNOVITIS

Tenosynovitis may develop about any of the extrinsic flexor or extensor tendons, either throughout their course or, more commonly, at points of constraint by fibrous pulleys or retinacular sheaths.

1. de Quervain Tenosynovitis

Clinical Findings

The abductor pollicis longus and extensor pollicis brevis tendons may become inflamed beneath the retinacular pulley at the radial styloid region. Symptoms are provoked by lifting activity in which the thumb is adducted and flexed while the hand is ulnarly deviated. Activities such as inflating a blood pressure cuff, picking up an infant out of a crib, or lifting a heavy frying pan off the stove may provoke pain along the radial aspect of the wrist.

Physical examination reveals tenderness directly over the first extensor compartment. A provocative maneuver, the Finkelstein test, is helpful in diagnosing this disorder (Figure 10–20).

Treatment

Initial treatment includes either splinting or steroid injection. Immobilization limits extensor pollicis brevis tendon excursion using a forearm-based thumb spica splint, which prevents both wrist deviation and thumb carpometacarpal and metacarpophalangeal motion while allowing interphalangeal joint motion. Steroid injection into the first extensor compartment along the course of the extensor pollicis brevis may diminish swelling and pain.

If de Quervain tenosynovitis is unresponsive to conservative care, surgical release of the overlying retinacu-

Figure 10–20. Finkelstein maneuver. The patient's thumb is enclosed in the palm. The wrist is then abruptly deviated ulnarward by the examiner. In a positive test, pain is produced on the radial border of the wrist. (Reproduced, with permission, from Lister G: *The Hand: Diagnosis and Indications,* 3rd ed. Churchill Livingstone, 1993.)

lum may be elected. Because most patients with symptomatic disease have more than one abductor pollicis longus slip, the extensor pollicis brevis tendon must be identified and decompressed. In some cases, the first extensor compartment is divided by a septum, creating two separate tendon sheaths. In such cases, the more dorsal component sheaths must be opened to allow unconstrained extensor pollicis brevis tendon gliding.

Extreme caution must be exercised in carrying out the skin incision and subcutaneous dissection in this region because injury to the sensory branch of the radial nerve as it runs over the first compartment is a troublesome complication that may overshadow any benefit from tendon decompression.

2. Flexor Tenosynovitis (Trigger Finger & Trigger Thumb)

Clinical Findings

Flexor tenosynovitis or tenovaginitis is characterized by pain and tenderness in the palm at the proximal edge of the digital A1 pulley (Figure 10–21). Patients frequently

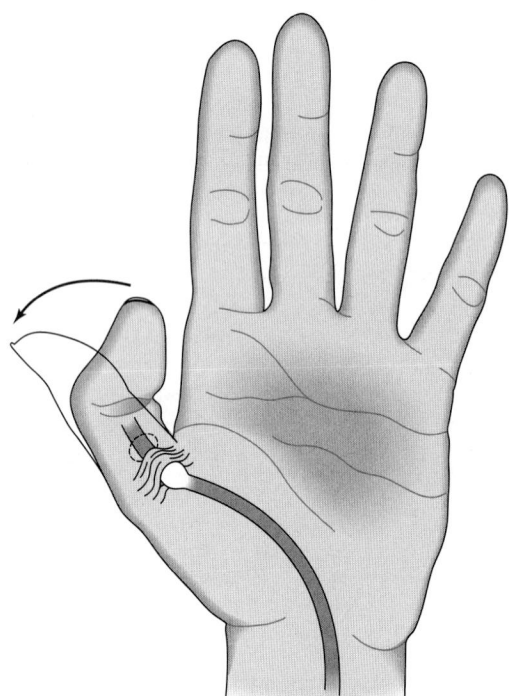

Figure 10–21. Trigger thumb. (Reproduced, with permission, from American Society for Surgery of the Hand: *The Hand: Examination and Diagnosis,* 2nd ed. Churchill Livingstone, 1983.)

note catching or triggering of the affected finger or thumb after forceful flexion. In more severe cases, the opposite hand must be used to force the finger or thumb passively into extension. In the most severe cases, the finger becomes locked in a flexed position. Triggering is often more pronounced in the morning than later in the day. Stenosing tenosynovitis is more common in diabetic patients than in nondiabetic patients. When multiple digits are involved, the possibility of diabetes should be considered.

Treatment

Most triggering digits may be successfully treated by long-acting steroid injection into the flexor sheath. To inject a trigger finger, the needle is inserted at the proximal palmar crease for the index finger and the distal palmar crease for the middle, ring, and small fingers. The needle enters the flexor tendon and pressure is applied to the plunger. The needle is slowly backed out until the needle is between the tendon and the tendon sheath, discerned by loss of plunger resistance. One milliliter of a combination of a short-acting anesthetic and steroid are given. The injection may be repeated if symptoms recur after an initially positive response to injection.

Surgical release of the A1 pulley is curative in digits refractory to steroid injection. Release is accomplished by directly exposing the pulley and incising its transversely oriented fibers longitudinally. The fibers of the A2 pulley must be spared to preserve effective digital flexion. Percutaneous release of the A1 pulley may be accomplished with a needle on the middle and ring fingers, especially if they actively lock. In patients with RA, the entire annular pulley system should be preserved to prevent further ulnar drift of the fingers. Triggering in these patients is treated by tenosynovectomy and excision of one slip of the flexor digitorum superficialis.

3. Flexor Carpi Radialis Tenosynovitis

Clinical Findings

Flexor carpi radialis tenosynovitis is characterized by pain with wrist motion, particularly active wrist flexion or passive wrist dorsiflexion. Marked tenderness is elicited on palpation of the skin overlying the tendon, particularly over the trapezium.

Treatment

Conservative care includes splinting the wrist in flexion and administration of oral antiinflammatory medication. If these measures are ineffective, a long-acting steroid may be injected about the tendon at the trapezial level.

Surgical decompression of the flexor carpi radialis is considered if conservative measures are ineffective. Decompression unroofs the tendon sheath in the distal forearm and across the wrist. The fibroosseous sheath is further decompressed by resection of the palmar ulnar ridge of the trapezium overlying the tendon.

Finsen V, Hagen S: Surgery for trigger finger. Hand Surg 2003; 8:201. [PMID: 15002098]

Hwang M et al: Referred pain pattern of the abductor pollicis longus muscle. Am J Phys Med Rehabil 2005;84:593. [PMID: 16034228]

Ragoowansi R, Acornley A, Khoo CT: Percutaneous trigger finger release: The "lift-cut" technique. Br J Plast Surg 2005;58:817. [PMID: 15936736]

Wilhelmi BJ et al: Trigger finger release with hand surface landmark ratios: An anatomic and clinical study. Plast Reconstr Surg 2001;108(4):908. [PMID: 11547146]

Zingas C et al: Injection accuracy and clinical relief of de Quervain's tendinitis. J Hand Surg Am 1998;22:89.

■ VASCULAR DISORDERS OF THE HAND

Anatomy

The blood supply to the hand is predominantly through the ulnar and radial arteries. The ulnar artery is larger than the radial artery and provides the primary arterial contribution to the hand. In most hands, the ulnar artery supplies the superficial palmar arch, which provides the principal blood supply to the common and proper digital arteries. The radial artery enters the hand by passing deep to the tendons of the first dorsal compartment across the anatomic snuffbox, dives palmarward between the bases of the first and second metacarpals, and forms the deep palmar arch. The median artery, a remnant of the embryologic vascular supply to the developing upper limb, contributes to the superficial palmar arch in 10% of patients.

The superficial palmar arch is located distal to the deep palmar arch. The arterial arch is complete, with total communication between the radial and ulnar arteries in 34% of hands and incomplete communication in 20%. The remaining hands have limited communication between the ulnar and radial arteries in varied configurations. The deep palmar arch runs alongside the motor branch of the ulnar nerve as it travels transversely just palmar to the proximal metacarpal shafts. The princeps pollicis artery is derived from the deep palmar arch in 98% of patients. The deep palmar arch also supplies the deep metacarpal arterial branches, which provide secondary blood flow to the digital arteries.

Clinical Findings

Patients with vascular insufficiency frequently complain of cold intolerance. When color changes occur, paleness or whiteness of the fingers is more suggestive of loss of inflow, whereas redness or bluish discoloration suggests inadequate venous return. Ulcerations of the tips of the fingers may denote ischemia.

The duration of vascular symptoms should be noted. If the abnormality is congenital in origin, changes in symptoms over time should be documented. The occupational history should record whether the patient uses vibrating tools or is subjected to repetitive blunt hand trauma during work. Occupations requiring outdoor work in all seasons (construction) or in a cold environment indoors (butchering) are noted. A history of trauma may suggest arterial or periarterial damage. Any sports activities that involve repeated trauma to the hand should be recorded; golfers, baseball catchers, and handball players are particularly at risk of closed vascular injury. Exposure to vasoconstrictive drugs, and particularly tobacco, should be noted. Other evidence of vascular disease should be sought, as well as diseases with vascular effects such as scleroderma or diabetes. Pulses are palpated, noting thrills or bruits.

A. ALLEN TEST

The Allen test allows assessment of the extent of connection between the radial and ulnar arteries through the palmar arches. The examiner compresses both the radial and ulnar arteries at the wrist and then asks the patient to flex and extend the fingers repetitively. After the hand blanches, pressure is released from the radial artery while compression is maintained on the ulnar artery. The examiner observes how long it takes for each of the fingers to regain its pink color. The initial step is repeated with both vessels compressed, and the ulnar artery occlusion is then released while pressure is maintained on the radial artery. Again, examination of the reperfusion of the fingers reveals which digits are primarily supplied through the ulnar artery. In this fashion, the extent of interconnections between the radial and ulnar arteries may be assessed.

B. DIAGNOSTIC STUDIES

Noninvasive vascular diagnostic studies include Doppler scans, which detect the presence of flow; plethysmography, which determines the pulse volume difference between brachial and digital arteries; and cold stress testing, a technique that evaluates the effect of cold on arterial spasm. Invasive diagnostic procedures include arteriography, digital subtraction arteriography, and early-phase radionuclide scans.

ARTERIAL OCCLUSION

1. Arterial Trauma

Clinical Findings

Partial or complete division of an artery may occur as the result of lacerations, acute injection trauma, or cannulation injuries. Hemorrhage from arterial disruption should initially be treated with direct pressure. Total arterial division must be repaired if distal vascularity is inadequate. Partial arterial injuries may bleed profusely because the lacerated vessel ends are tethered to one another and are unable to retract, constrict, and occlude further flow. Partial arterial injury may require resection with or without reconstruction to prevent the formation of aneurysms or arteriovenous fistulas. Injection injury may produce either spasm or occlusion.

Treatment

The primary objective in treating arterial injuries is the restoration of adequate distal blood flow. Attempts may be made to remove distal clots with Fogarty catheters. If this is unsuccessful, clot-dissolving agents such as urokinase, local or systemic vasodilators, and stellate ganglion blocks may be employed to diminish vascular spasm. Care must be taken when using multiple agents to ensure they do not interfere with one another. For instance, use of urokinase after an axillary block may produce axillary artery hemorrhage, thereby compounding the problem.

2. Thrombosis

Clinical Findings

The ulnar artery is the most common site of upper extremity arterial thrombosis. This entity, also known as ulnar hammer syndrome hypothenar hammer syndrome, is most often the result of repetitive trauma to the hypothenar area of the hand. Patients may complain of a tender pulsatile mass on the ulnar side of the palm. In some instances, presenting symptoms reflect a low ulnar nerve palsy secondary to compression of the ulnar nerve by the aneurysm at the level of the Guyon canal. Distal vascular insufficiency may be evident in the ring and little fingers.

Treatment

If evaluation demonstrates that all the fingers are well perfused by the radial artery alone, excision of the segment of the ulnar artery containing the aneurysm or thrombosed segment and ligation of the vessel ends is curative. Simple division of the vessel may confer a modest sympathectomy effect to the residual ulnar artery because sympathetic fibers surrounding the ulnar artery are disrupted at the time of vessel division. If, however, digital perfusion is inadequate after a vessel segment is resected and the tourniquet deflated, a segmental vein graft is required to reconstitute the ulnar artery.

3. Aneurysm

A distinction should be made between true and false aneurysms. In a true aneurysm, all layers of the arterial wall are involved. These aneurysms are usually caused by blunt trauma but may also be secondary to degeneration or infection. False aneurysms are characterized by partial wall involvement, with periarterial tissues forming a false wall lined by endothelium. False aneurysms are most common following penetrating trauma, such as stab wounds.

Both true and false aneurysms should be treated with resection. As discussed in the section about ulnar hammer syndrome, the necessity of vascular reconstruction is dictated by the adequacy of distal perfusion after tourniquet release.

VASOSPASTIC CONDITIONS

Clinical Findings

Raynaud phenomenon, Raynaud disease, and Raynaud syndrome are often confused. Raynaud phenomenon is a condition in which pallor of the digits occurs with or without cyanosis on exposure to cold. Raynaud disease (primary Raynaud) is present when Raynaud phenomenon occurs without another associated or causative disease. Raynaud disease most commonly occurs in young (less than 40 years) women and is often bilateral, without demonstrable peripheral arterial occlusion. In severe cases, patients may develop gangrene or atrophic changes limited to the distal digital skin. Raynaud syndrome (secondary Raynaud) occurs when Raynaud phenomenon is associated with another disease, such as connective tissue disorders (systemic lupus erythematosus), neurologic disorders, arterial occlusive disorders, or blood dyscrasias.

Treatment

All patients with Raynaud phenomenon experience cyclic episodes of digital pallor alternating with episodes of cyanosis and hyperemia. Treatment includes protection of the hands from cold by the use of gloves or mittens. Patients should be strongly encouraged to cease all cigarette or cigar smoking. Drug treatment attempts to diminish occlusive phenomena. Alpha-receptor blocking agents, nitroglycerin ointment, nifedipine, and other calcium channel blockers are effective in decreasing spasm. Digital artery sympathectomy, the surgical stripping of the periarterial tissue of the common digital artery over a short segment at the distal palmar level, may improve circulation to ischemic digits.

Balogh B et al: Adventitial stripping of the radial and ulnar arteries in Raynaud's disease. J Hand Surg Am 2002;27:1073.

Ruch DS et al: Arterial reconstruction for radial artery occlusion. J Hand Surg [Am] 2000;25:282. [PMID: 10722820]

Ruch DS et al: Periarterial sympathectomy in scleroderma patients: Intermediate-term follow-up. J Hand Surg [Am] 2002;27(2): 258. [PMID: 11901385]

■ DISORDERS OF THE NERVES OF THE HAND

PERIPHERAL NERVE INJURY

Anatomy

Peripheral nerves consist of a mixture of myelinated and unmyelinated axons. Motor, sensory, and sympathetic fibers often travel together in a single nerve. Axons are grouped in bundles termed *fascicles,* which are surrounded by perineurium. The fine connective tissue between axons within a fascicle is called *endoneurium.* Fascicles are held together as a nerve by the epineurium. Nerves are considered monofascicular, oligofascicular, or polyfascicular, depending on the number of fascicles. The relationship between fascicles changes along the longitudinal course of the nerve. The degree of fascicular change decreases distally. The mesoneurium, which is the connective tissue surrounding the epineurium, facilitates longitudinal gliding of the nerve.

After a nerve is injured, a number of changes occur. The somatosensory cortex reorganizes so the area represented by the injured nerve diminishes. The cell body of the lacerated axon increases in size. The production of materials for repair of the cytoskeleton is increased, and the production of neurotransmitters decreases. At the proximal segment of the injured axon, further proximal degeneration occurs based on the severity of the injury. In the axon distal to the laceration, Schwann cells phagocytose the axon, allowing the surrounding myelin tube to collapse.

Within 24 hours of injury, axonal sprouting occurs from the proximal stump. Multiple axons in a fascicle form a regenerating unit. The number of axons in the unit decreases with time. Longitudinal growth of the regenerating nerve depends on the ability of the axons to adhere to trophic factors in the basal lamina of the Schwann cell. Changes also occur at the distal end of the nerve. At the motor endplate, the muscle fibers atrophy. The sensitivity and number of acetylcholine receptors increases as their location expands from pits to the entire length of the muscle fiber. If the muscle fiber is reinnervated, both old and new motor endplates become active. The recovery of strength is greatest after primary nerve repair, less vigorous after repair with nerve grafting, and weakest after direct implantation of the nerve end into muscle. Muscle reinnervation occurs only if the axon reaches the muscle within a year. In contrast, sensory receptors may be effectively reinnervated years after injury.

Nerve injures are classified into three types. (1) Neurapraxia is a conduction block that occurs without axonal disruption. Recovery is usually complete within days to a few months. (2) Axonotmesis describes an injury in which axonal disruption occurs, with the endoneurial tube remaining in continuity. The intact endoneurial tube provides the regenerating sprouting axons with a well-defined path to the end organs. Because axonal growth occurs at approximately 1 mm/day, recovery is good but slow. (3) Neurotmesis refers to transection of the nerve. Unless the nerve is repaired, the regenerating axons cannot find a suitable path and recovery does not occur. The frustrated sprouting axons form a neuroma at the distal end of the proximal segment of the lacerated nerve.

Diagnostic Studies

Preoperative and postoperative assessment of motor and sensory function include quantitative measurement of pinch and grip strength, static and moving two-point discrimination, and vibration and pressure measurements. Two-point discrimination reflects innervation density, whereas vibration and pressure measurements gauges innervation threshold.

Treatment

Nerve repair should be carried out with magnification and microsurgical technique. A tension-free repair provides the ideal environment for nerve regeneration. Tension at the repair site may be diminished by advancement of the nerve (ie, anterior transposition of the ulnar nerve for proximal forearm ulnar nerve laceration) or by limitation of joint motion. If a tension-free repair is impossible, nerve grafting is necessary to bridge the defect in the nerve. Frequently used donor nerves include the sural nerve, the anterior branch of the medial antebrachial cutaneous nerve, and the lateral antebrachial cutaneous nerve.

Primary repair is preferred to nerve grafting because the latter procedure requires two sites of nerve coaptation. Epineurial repair is usually performed under magnification, using 8-0 or 9-0 suture (Figure 10–22A). When a particular fascicular group (eg, motor branch of the median nerve) is recognized as mediating a specific function, it may be repaired separately (Figure 10–22B). Postoperative therapy may include motor and sensory reeducation to maximize the clinical result.

Primary nerve repair is indicated after a sharp nerve division occurs. After avulsion injuries, repair even by nerve grafting cannot be performed until the proximal and distal extent of injury is known. When closed nerve injury occurs, sensory and motor function is closely monitored. If no recovery is seen within 3 months, electrodiagnostic studies are carried out. If no electrical evidence of recovery is documented, the nerve is explored, and neurolysis, secondary nerve repair, or nerve grafting is accomplished.

A. Epineurial repair   **B.** Group fascicular repair

Figure 10–22. **A:** Schematic diagram of epineurial repair technique. **B:** Group fascicular repair technique. (Reproduced, with permission, from Mackinnon SE, Dellon AL: *Surgery of the Peripheral Nerve.* Thieme, 1988.)

COMPRESSIVE NEUROPATHIES

Compressive neuropathies are a group of nerve injuries that have common pathophysiology factors and occur at predictable sites of normal anatomic constraint. Nerve dysfunction is the result of neural ischemia in the compressed segment. Symptoms may resolve after release of the anatomic structures producing pressure on the nerve, particularly when compression is neither severe nor long standing.

1. Median Neuropathy

Carpal Tunnel Syndrome

A. ANATOMY

Compression of the median nerve within the carpal tunnel is the most common upper extremity compressive neuropathy. The carpal tunnel is that space along the palmar aspect of the wrist anatomically bounded by the scaphoid tubercle and the trapezium radially, the hook of the hamate and the pisiform ulnarly, the capitate dorsally, and the transverse carpal ligament palmarly (Figure 10–23).

B. CLINICAL FINDINGS

Carpal tunnel syndrome is often idiopathic. It is associated with pregnancy, amyloidosis, flexor tenosynovitis, overuse phenomenon, acute or chronic inflammatory conditions, traumatic disorders of the wrist, endocrine disorders (diabetes mellitus and hypothyroidism), and tumors within the carpal tunnel.

Differential diagnosis includes compression of the median nerve or cervical roots in other anatomic locations. Diabetic neuropathy may produce symptoms similar to those of carpal tunnel syndrome, and patients with diabetic neuropathy may develop concomitant carpal tunnel syndrome.

1. Symptoms and signs—Most patients complain of numbness in the thumb and index and middle fingers, though many note that the entire hand feels numb. Pain rarely prevents the affected individual from falling asleep but characteristically awakens the patient from sleep after a number of hours. After a period of moving the fingers, most patients are able to return to sleep. Many patients complain of finger stiffness upon arising in the morning.

Discomfort or numbness, or both, may be incited by activities in which the wrist is held in a flexed position for a sustained period of time (eg, holding a steering wheel, telephone receiver, book, or newspaper). Discomfort and pain may radiate from the hand up the arm to the shoulder or neck. The patient may complain of clumsiness when trying to perform tasks such as unscrewing a jar top and may experience difficulty in holding on to a glass or cup securely.

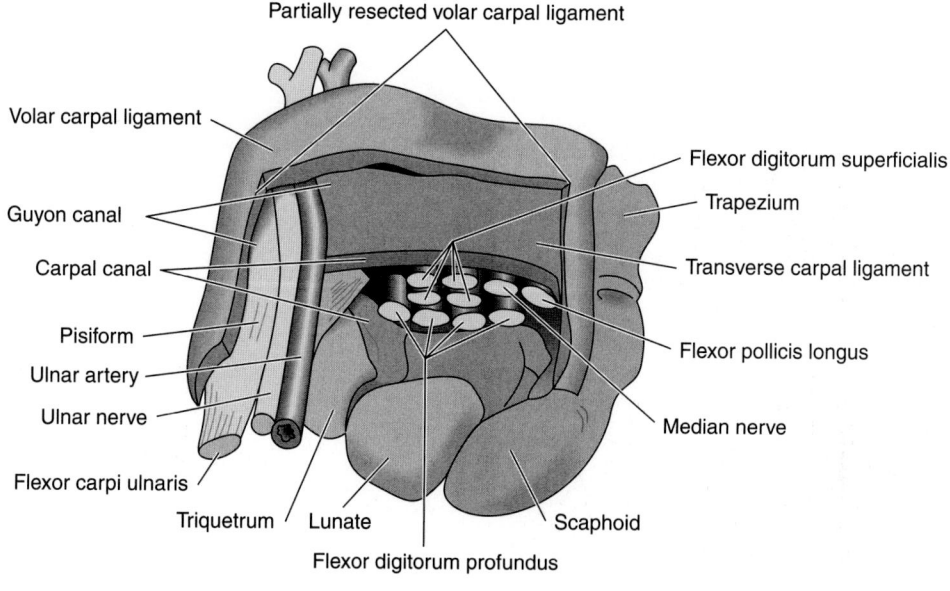

Partially resected volar carpal ligament

Volar carpal ligament

Guyon canal

Carpal canal

Pisiform

Ulnar artery

Ulnar nerve

Flexor carpi ulnaris

Triquetrum   Lunate

Flexor digitorum profundus

Flexor digitorum superficialis

Trapezium

Transverse carpal ligament

Flexor pollicis longus

Median nerve

Scaphoid

Dorsal

Figure 10–23. The Guyon canal and carpal tunnel and contents. (Cross section of supinated right wrist, viewed from proximal to distal.) Note the relationship between the transverse carpal ligament and the volar carpal ligament (partially resected). (Reproduced, with permission, from Reckling FW, Reckling JB, Mohn MP: *Orthopaedic Anatomy and Surgical Approaches.* Mosby-Year Book, 1990.)

Atrophy of muscles innervated by the median nerve is visible in severe long-standing cases but is uncommon in most cases of recent onset. Weakness of the abductor pollicis brevis muscle may be detected by careful manual muscle testing.

2. Provocative tests—Three provocative tests, the Phalen maneuver, the Tinel sign, and the wrist compression test, are helpful in establishing the diagnosis of carpal tunnel syndrome.

a. Tinel sign—The Tinel sign is elicited by percussing the skin over the median nerve just proximal to the carpal tunnel; when it is positive, the patient complains of an electric or tingling sensation radiating into the thumb, index, middle, or ring fingers.

b. Phalen maneuver—The Phalen wrist flexion sign, or Phalen maneuver, is usually positive in patients with carpal tunnel syndrome and is thought by many to be even more diagnostic than the Tinel sign. When this maneuver is performed, the elbow should be maintained in extension while the wrist is passively flexed (Figure 10–24). The time is then measured from initiation of wrist flexion to onset of symptoms; onset within 60 seconds is considered supportive of the diagnosis of carpal tunnel syndrome. Both the time to onset and the location of paresthesias should be recorded.

c. Wrist compression test—pressure over the median nerve proximal to the wrist provoke symptoms within 30 seconds. The test is confirmatory to other physical signs of median nerve compression.

3. Two-point discrimination test—Two-point discrimination is often diminished in the finger pulps of patients with carpal tunnel syndrome. Sensation in the radial aspect of the palm should be normal, however, because the palmar cutaneous branch of the median nerve does not pass through the carpal tunnel.

4. Imaging studies—The diagnostic evaluation may include a radiograph of the wrist, including a carpal tunnel view.

5. Electrodiagnostic studies—Nerve conduction velocities and electromyography help localize nerve compression to the wrist and evaluate residual neural and motor integrity. Nerve conduction velocity (NCV) and electromyogram (EMG) studies are indicated for patients who have failed conservative care and are considered candidates for surgery. A motor distal latency greater than 3.5–4.0 ms is the best indicator of carpal tunnel syndrome.

C. TREATMENT

1. Conservative measures—Because the pressure within the carpal tunnel increases if the wrist is held in sus-

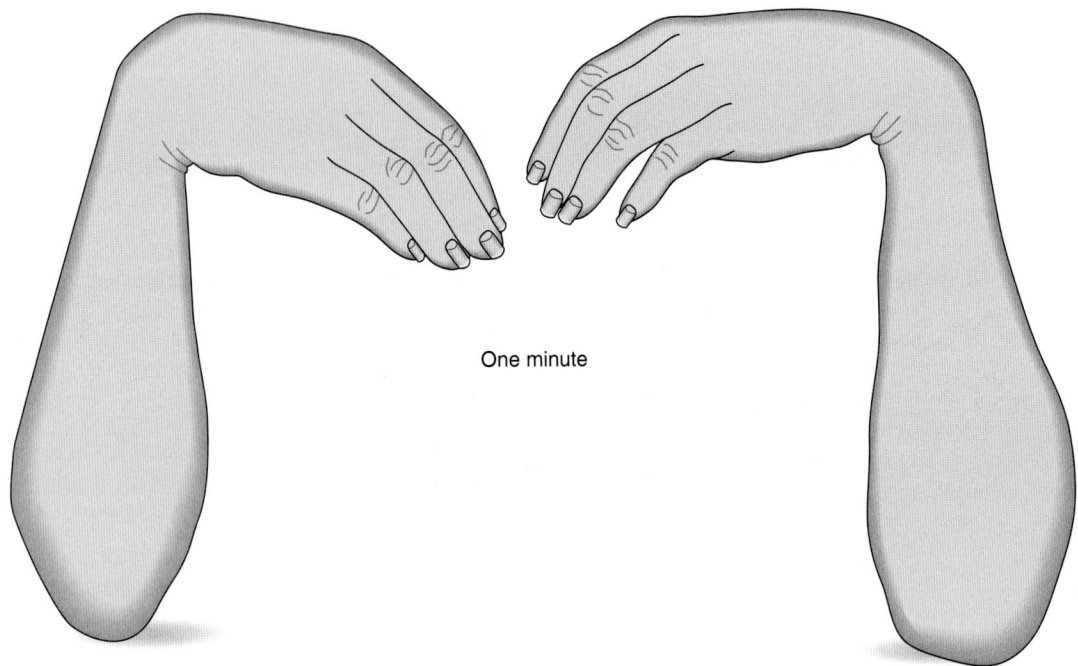

One minute

Figure 10–24. Phalen maneuver. (Reproduced, with permission, from American Society for Surgery of the Hand: *The Hand: Examination and Diagnosis,* 2nd ed. Churchill Livingstone, 1983.)

tained flexion (usual sleep posture) or sustained extension, the initial treatment of carpal tunnel syndrome should include a splint that maintains the wrist in a neutral position at night. Clinical improvement with this simple measure adds further support to the diagnosis of carpal tunnel syndrome. Activities that provoke symptoms may be modified with simple measures such as adjustment of keyboard height and rotation of repetitive job activities.

Injection of steroids into the carpal tunnel often decreases the inflammatory response around the flexor tendons and diminishes symptoms. To inject the carpal tunnel, a 25-gauge 1.5-inch needle is placed at the palmar wrist crease just ulnar to the palmaris longus tendon. If the palmaris longus is absent, a line along the radial border of the ring finger is drawn to the wrist crease. Before placing the needle, patients are told they may experience an electric shock sensation in the fingers. If this sensation occurs, the needle may be in the median nerve, and the injection should not be given. The needle is withdrawn and placed a few millimeters ulnar. When inserting the needle, first the skin is punctured, then a pop is felt as the needle passes through the transverse carpal ligament. A mixture of a short-acting anesthetic and steroid is injected. Transient relief of symptoms after injection suggests a greater likelihood of a favorable result after surgical decompression.

2. Surgical treatment—Patients unresponsive to conservative measures may benefit from surgical division of the transverse carpal ligament. This division may be accomplished through either direct open exposure or through an endoscopic approach. The open incision is made in the palm over the transverse carpal ligament, staying ulnar to the axis of the palmaris longus, along the longitudinal axis of the radial border of the ring finger. This incision avoids injury to the palmar cutaneous branch of the median nerve. After incising the palmar fascia longitudinally, the transverse carpal ligament is identified and sectioned longitudinally under direct observation. Endoscopic division of the transverse carpal ligament avoids a potentially tender palmar incision with either a single wrist portal proximal to the palm or with a combined proximal portal and short midpalmar portal along the axis of the open incision. Although some studies noted an earlier return to work activities after endoscopic release, the incidence of iatrogenic nerve and tendon injuries and late recurrence of symptoms form incomplete ligament division may be higher with endoscopic release than with open release. Both types of procedures are effective ways of treating carpal tunnel syndrome. The decision of which technique to use is based on the surgeon's experience. Endoscopic carpal tunnel release should not be used for treatment of recurrent carpal tunnel syndrome.

Patients are encouraged to actively move their fingers from the first postoperative day. Wrist motion is begun within the first week. Incisional tenderness often prevents patients from fully using their hands and returning to unrestricted work for the first 4–8 weeks. If patients have difficulty with hand function 3–4 weeks after surgery, a therapy program is prescribed consisting of desensitization, ROM, and strengthening.

Pronator Syndrome

A. Anatomy

The median nerve may be compressed in the proximal forearm by one or more of the following structures: ligament of Struthers, lacertus fibrosus, pronator teres muscle, or proximal fibrous arch on the undersurface of the flexor digitorum superficialis muscle.

B. Clinical Findings

Patients with pronator syndrome complain of pain that is usually more severe in the volar forearm than in the wrist or hand. Pain usually increases with activity. Complaints of numbness in the thumb, index, middle, and ring fingers may initially suggest the possibility of carpal tunnel syndrome. Night symptoms, however, are unusual in cases of isolated pronator syndrome.

Examination may reveal sensory and motor deficits similar to those seen in carpal tunnel syndrome, but significant differences may be detected on careful evaluation. Dysesthesia may include the distribution of the palmar cutaneous nerve. The Tinel sign is positive at the forearm level rather than at the wrist. The Phalen maneuver does not provoke symptoms. Patients may experience pain with resistance to contraction of the pronator teres or flexor digitorum superficialis muscles tested by resistance to forearm pronation or to isolated flexion of the proximal interphalangeal joints of the long and ring fingers.

C. Treatment

Evaluation of symptomatic patients should include electrodiagnostic studies if a 6-week course of immobilization fails to effect improvement. Surgical treatment requires generous decompression of all potentially constricting sites.

Anterior Interosseous Syndrome

A. Anatomy

The anterior interosseous nerve branch divides from the median nerve 4–6 cm below the elbow. This branch of the nerve innervates the flexor pollicis longus, flexor digitorum profundus of the index and middle fingers, and pronator quadratus muscles. The anterior interosseous nerve may be compressed by the deep head of the pronator teres, the ori-gin of the flexor digitorum superficialis, a palmaris profundus, or the flexor carpi radialis. In addition, accessory muscles connecting the flexor digitorum superficialis to the flexor digitorum profundus proximally and Gantzer muscle (the accessory head of the flexor pollicis longus) may impinge on the anterior interosseous nerve.

B. Clinical Findings

Patients affected with anterior interosseous nerve syndrome complain of inability to flex either the thumb interphalangeal joint or the index-finger distal interphalangeal joint. In contrast to those with pronator syndrome, these patients do not complain of numbness or pain.

C. Treatment

Surgical decompression of the anterior interosseous nerve may be indicated when the syndrome does not spontaneously improve. All potentially compressing structures must be exposed and released.

2. Ulnar Neuropathy

Cubital Tunnel Syndrome

A. Anatomy

The ulnar nerve is most commonly compressed at the cubital tunnel, along the medial side of the elbow. Compression may occur between the ulnar and humeral origins of the flexor carpi ulnaris or at the proximal border of the cubital tunnel because the nerve is tethered anteriorly with elbow flexion (Figure 10–25).

B. Clinical Findings

Patients affected with cubital tunnel syndrome most often complain of paresthesia and numbness involving the ring and little fingers. Because symptoms may be aggravated or provoked by sustained elbow flexion, patients may complain of increased symptoms while talking on the telephone. Many patients complain of being awakened at night by the symptoms, most often when sleeping with the elbows flexed. Patients whose exam demonstrates weakness of muscles innervated by the ulnar nerve may note clumsiness and lack of dexterity.

1. Provocative tests—

a. Tinel sign—A positive Tinel sign is noted when percussion over the ulnar nerve at the elbow provokes paresthesias along the ulnar forearm and hand. The nerve may be noted to sublux over the medial epicondyle as the arm is brought into flexion.

b. Motor strength—Motor strength should be assessed both in intrinsic muscles innervated by the ulnar nerve (first dorsal interosseous muscle) and in extrinsic muscles innervated by the ulnar nerve (flexor digitorum profundus of the little finger).

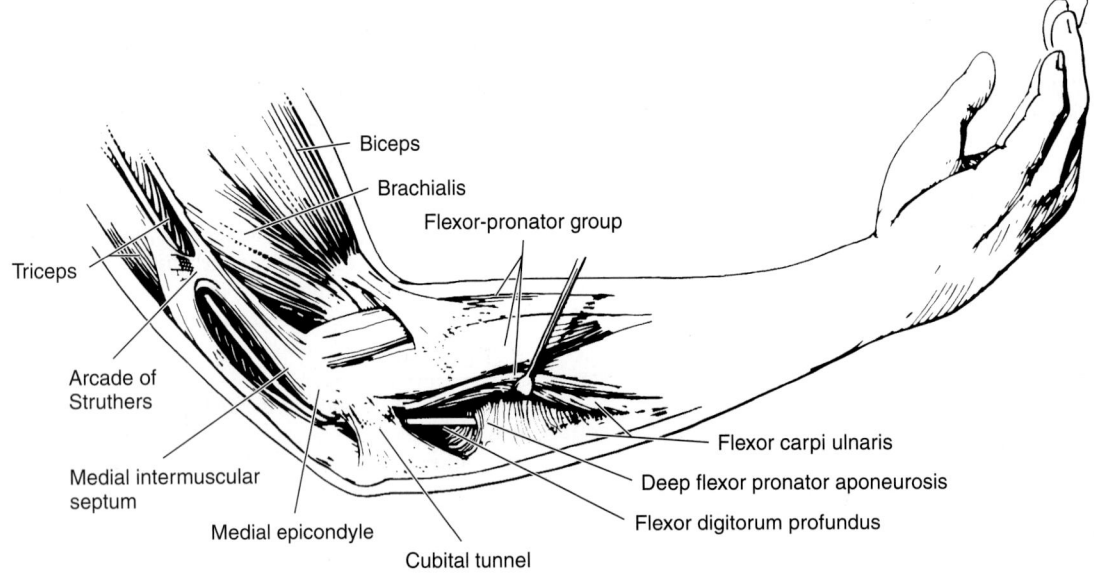

Figure 10–25. Points of constriction of the ulnar nerve at the elbow. (From Amadio PC: Anatomic basis for a technique of ulnar nerve transposition. Surg Radiol Anat 1986;8:155; used, with permission, from Mayo Foundation.)

c. Froment sign—With weakness of the ulnar nerve innervated adductor pollicis muscle, a positive Froment sign may be observed. As the patient tries to hold a piece of paper placed between the thumb and the index finger, the thumb interphalangeal joint flexes in an attempt to substitute flexor pollicis longus activity for inadequate adductor pollicis strength.

d. Elbow flexion test—The ulnar nerve may be rendered symptomatic by fully flexing the elbow with the wrist in the neutral position. The elbow flexion test, a provocative maneuver, is considered positive if paresthesia is elicited in the ring and little fingers within 60 seconds. The location of the paresthesia and the time between initiation of elbow flexion and the onset of symptoms should be recorded.

C. Treatment

1. Conservative treatment—Conservative treatment may include the use of an elbow pad to protect the nerve from trauma or a splint holding the elbow at approximately 45 degrees of flexion. The splint may be worn continuously or at night only, depending on the frequency and intensity of symptoms.

2. Surgical treatment—Electrodiagnostic studies should be obtained if conservative treatment does not alleviate the symptoms, particularly if motor weakness is evident. The reliability of nerve conduction studies at the elbow

depends on the ability of the electromyographer to measure the length of the ulnar nerve accurately.

Numerous procedures are described to relieve ulnar nerve compression at the elbow. These include simple decompression of the ulnar nerve within the cubital tunnel or decompression with anterior transposition of the nerve subcutaneously, intramuscularly, or submuscularly into the flexor pronator mass. When the nerve is transposed, great care must be taken to excise the medial intermuscular septum proximally and to release the aponeurosis between the humeral and ulnar origins of the flexor carpi ulnaris distally, to avoid creating a new area of impingement.

An alternative surgical strategy involves decompression of the nerve and medial epicondylectomy. This technique removes the prominence against which the ulnar nerve is tethered with elbow flexion. After surgery, initial rehabilitation focuses on regaining elbow ROM. Strengthening begins at 4–6 weeks, and the patient is usually able to return to unrestricted work at 8–12 weeks.

Ulnar Tunnel Syndrome

A. Anatomy

The ulnar nerve passes from the forearm into the hand through the Guyon canal (see Figure 10–23). The anatomic borders of the Guyon canal are the pisiform and pisohamate ligament ulnarly, the hook of the hamate and insertion of the transverse carpal ligament radially, and the volar carpal ligament forming the roof of the tunnel.

B. CLINICAL FINDINGS

Examination should document ulnar nerve sensory and motor integrity. In contrast to the findings in cubital tunnel syndrome, the Tinel sign is positive at the wrist rather than at the elbow. Extrinsic motor function is normal. The region of compression should be delineated by electrodiagnostic studies. In some cases MRI studies demonstrate a space-occupying lesion such as a ganglion compressing the nerve within the Guyon canal.

C. TREATMENT

When splinting is ineffective, surgical decompression should be considered. When symptoms exist in tandem with carpal tunnel syndrome, release of the transverse carpal ligament favorably alters the shape and size of the Guyon canal. Postoperative care is the same as following carpal tunnel release.

3. Radial Neuropathy
Radial Tunnel Syndrome
A. ANATOMY

The radial nerve may be rendered symptomatic if compressed in the region of the radial tunnel. Points of impingement along the radial tunnel, located at the level of the proximal radius, include fibers spanning the radiocapitellar joint, the radial recurrent vessels, the extensor carpi radialis brevis, the tendinous origin of the supinator (arcade of Frohse), and the point at which the nerve emerges from beneath the distal edge of the supinator.

B. CLINICAL FINDINGS

Because radial tunnel syndrome often occurs in combination with lateral epicondylitis, the two diagnoses are frequently confused. Patients with radial tunnel syndrome experience pain over the midportion of the mobile wad (brachioradialis, extensor carpi radialis longus, and extensor carpi radialis brevis muscles), whereas the pain experienced by patients with lateral epicondylitis is located at or just distal to the lateral epicondyle. Patients with radial tunnel syndrome experience pain when simultaneously extending the wrist and fingers while the long finger is passively flexed by the examiner (positive long-finger extension test). Patients with radial tunnel syndrome often also experience pain with resisted forearm supination.

C. TREATMENT

Conservative treatment of radial tunnel syndrome includes measures to avoid forceful extension of the wrist and fingers. The wrist is splinted in dorsiflexion while the forearm is immobilized in supination. Persistent symptoms in spite of splinting may be treated by surgical decompression of the radial nerve. Concomitant lateral epicondylitis should be treated surgically at the same time that the radial nerve is decompressed.

Posterior Interosseous Nerve Syndrome
A. ANATOMY

The radial nerve splits into the posterior interosseous nerve and the superficial sensory branch of the radial nerve after passing anteriorly to the radiocapitellar joint. The posterior interosseous nerve then passes beneath the origin of the extensor carpi radialis brevis, radial recurrent artery, and arcade of Frohse. The posterior interosseous nerve is most commonly entrapped at the proximal edge of the supinator, although entrapment may also occur at either the middle or the distal edge of the supinator muscle.

B. CLINICAL FINDINGS

In contrast to radial tunnel syndrome, patients with posterior interosseous nerve syndrome experience extrinsic extensor weakness. Pain may be less than that of patients with radial tunnel syndrome.

Paralysis may be either partial or complete. Because the brachioradialis, extensor carpi radialis longus, supinator, and often extensor carpi radialis brevis are innervated by the radial nerve proximal to the posterior interosseous nerve branch, these muscles are spared. Digital extension at the metacarpophalangeal joint is the principal deficit from loss of extensor digitorum communis, extensor indicis proprius, and extensor digit quinti function.

The differential diagnosis in a patient with spontaneous loss of digital extension should include the possibility of multiple tendon ruptures in addition to possible radial neuropathy, particularly in patients with RA. The tenodesis effect, in which the fingers extend as the wrist is passively flexed, is preserved in posterior interosseous nerve syndrome but absent if the extensor tendons are ruptured.

C. TREATMENT

Treatment of posterior interosseous nerve syndrome requires thorough decompression of the nerve. If motor recovery does not occur, tendon transfers restore digital extension.

4. Thoracic Outlet Syndrome
Anatomy

The brachial plexus exits the base of the neck and upper thorax through the thoracic outlet. Anatomic boundaries of the outlet are the scalenus anterior muscle anteriorly, the scalenus medius muscle posteriorly, and the first rib inferiorly. Thoracic outlet syndrome, usually resulting from irritation of the C8- and T1-derived nerves, may be caused by a cervical rib, a fiber spanning from a rudimentary cervical rib, tendinous bands from the scalenus anterior to the medius muscles, or hypertrophic clavicle fracture callus. Poor posture with slumping shoulders or prolonged military brace position are each implicated as a contributing factor.

Clinical Findings

The symptoms of thoracic outlet syndrome are often vague. Symptoms may include pain in the C8-T1 dermatome, with a variable degree of intrinsic muscle weakness. Patients may experience vascular symptoms if the axillary artery is simultaneously being compressed in the thoracic outlet region.

A. PROVOCATIVE TESTS

1. Elevated stress test—Physical examination of the patient with suspected thoracic outlet syndrome should include an elevated stress test, in which the patient's shoulders are kept extended and the arm is externally rotated 90 degrees at the shoulder. The patient is then asked to open and close the hands with the arms elevated for 3 minutes. Reproduction of symptoms is suggestive of thoracic outlet syndrome.

2. Other tests—The Adson sign and the Wright test may be helpful in detecting vascular compression. In a positive Adson test, the radial pulse is obliterated when the arm is dependent and the head is turned to the affected side. In the Wright test, the pulse is obliterated when the shoulder is abducted, externally rotated, and the head is turned away from the involved shoulder. In addition, this maneuver should reproduce the patient's symptoms. Physical examination should document C8-T1 sensation and intrinsic muscle strength.

B. DIAGNOSTIC STUDIES

Workup of the symptomatic patient should include radiographs of the cervical spine to rule out a cervical rib, electrodiagnostic studies to assess the function of the lower nerve roots, and Doppler studies of the arm in varied positions to assess compression of the axillary artery.

Treatment

Initial treatment includes postural exercises. Patients who are unresponsive to conservative treatment or have demonstrable weakness may benefit from surgi-

cal resection of a cervical rib, resection of the first rib, or scalenotomy.

5. Cervical Root Compression

Clinical Findings

Cervical spine root compression may result in complaints of hand pain or weakness. It is useful to inquire routinely about pain or limitation of motion of the cervical spine. If the patient was involved in an accident involving sudden neck flexion and extension, this should be noted. Cervical root compression may occur from a herniated cervical disk, cervical spondylosis, intervertebral foraminal osteophytes, or, rarely, a cervical cord tumor.

Patients with cervical root compression most often complain of pain in a radicular rather than a peripheral nerve distribution. In spite of symptoms involving the hand, most patients, when carefully questioned, are able to distinguish pain that begins in the neck and radiates to the hand from pain that begins in the hand and radiates proximally to the neck. Pain may be exacerbated with neck motion (flexion and extension, lateral bending, or rotation), coughing, or sneezing.

A. SPURLING TEST

Physical examination of the patient with cervical radiculopathy frequently demonstrates either a decreased range of neck motion or pain with neck motion. Symptoms may be reproduced with axial compression on the patient's head (positive Spurling test). Detailed sensory and motor examination may reveal deficits in the domain of one or more roots.

B. DOUBLE-CRUSH SYNDROME

The occasional simultaneous presentation of cervical radiculopathy with peripheral entrapment neuropathy is termed the *double-crush syndrome*. Whether compression at one level renders a nerve more vulnerable to compressive forces at a second level or whether such cases simply represent two common entities in the same extremity remains the subject of debate.

Treatment

If a nerve is compressed at more than one location, the more symptomatic area is usually treated first. If both areas are equally symptomatic, the simpler of the two operations is chosen.

Lindley SG, Kleinert JM: Prevalence of anatomic variations encountered in elective carpal tunnel release. J Hand Surg Am 2003;28:849. [PMID: 14507518]

Morgenlander JC et al: Surgical treatment of carpal tunnel syndrome in patients with peripheral neuropathy. Neurology 1997;49:1159. [PMID: 9339710]

Naidu SH et al: Median nerve function in patients undergoing carpal tunnel release: Pre- and post-op nerve conductions. Electromyogr Clin Neurophysiol 2003;43:393. [PMID: 14626718]

Trumble TE et al: Single-portal endoscopic carpal tunnel release compared with open release: A prospective, randomized trial. J Bone Joint Surg Am 2002;84:1107. [PMID: 12107308]

Upton AR, McComas AJ: The double crush in nerve entrapment syndromes. Lancet 1973;2:359. [PMID: 4124532]

■ DISORDERS OF THE FASCIA OF THE HAND

DUPUYTREN DISEASE

Dupuytren disease is characterized by a nodular thickening on the palmar surface of the hand affecting the preexisting palmar fascia (Figure 10–26). It is a progressive condition, resulting from pathologic changes mediated by the myofibroblast. Dupuytren disease occurs most commonly in patients between 40 and 60 years of age. It is observed more often in men, in whom it appears earlier and is often more aggressive. Flexion contractures most frequently occur at the metacarpophalangeal joints but may also tether the proximal interphalangeal joint and, less commonly, the distal interphalangeal joint. The little and ring fingers and the thumb index web are the most commonly involved areas. Ectopic deposits may occur in the dorsum of the proximal interphalangeal joint (knuckle pads), the dorsum of the penis (Peyronie disease), and the plantar fascia of the foot (Ledderhose disease).

Epidemiologic Factors

A number of predisposing factors are identified. The disease most commonly appears in patients of northern European ancestry and is occasionally encountered in Asians; it is rarer in other racial groups. Dupuytren disease is associated with epilepsy medications taken for seizure disorders and with alcoholism, smoking, and diabetes. The relationship of work and trauma to the development of the disease remains controversial. The most aggressive disease occurs in patients who have a family history of disease and in those who have onset of disease prior to 40 years of age. More severely involved patients may have extensive bilateral involvement and ectopic deposits on the dorsum of the hands and the feet. Although these patients often undergo surgery at an early age, both extension and recurrence of the disease is common.

Figure 10–26. Dupuytren contracture. (Reproduced, with permission, from American Society for Surgery of the Hand: *The Hand: Examination and Diagnosis,* 2nd ed. Churchill Livingstone, 1983.)

Anatomy

Dupuytren contracture distorts the anatomy of the palmar fascia. Flexion contractures of the metacarpophalangeal joint are caused by pathologic contracture of pretendinous bands at a superficial level. Contracture of the natatory ligaments produces web space contractures and scissoring of the fingers. The transverse fibers of the palmar aponeurosis remain uninvolved, except at the base of the thumb. In the fingers, the superficial volar fascia, lateral digital sheath, spiral band, and Grayson ligaments may contract alone or in combination to produce flexion contracture of the proximal interphalangeal joint. When a spiral band contracts, the digital nerve is often displaced palmarly to the band from proximal lateral to distal central in the region of the proximal phalanx.

Treatment

Nonsurgical treatment is ineffective in reversing or halting Dupuytren disease. The primary indication for surgery is a fixed contracture of more than 30 degrees at the metacarpophalangeal or any degree of flexion contracture at the proximal interphalangeal joint.

Surgical exposure may be achieved through either transverse or longitudinal skin incisions. A transverse incision across the distal palmar skin crease is useful when extensive palmar involvement is anticipated. Transverse incisions are usually sutured; if there is excessive tension, the wound may be left open to heal by secondary intention. When longitudinal exposure of the finger is needed, Brunner zigzag incisions are useful. An alternative is a longitudinal incision that is modified for closure by a series of Z-plasty flap transpositions.

The goal of surgical release is to achieve a regional fasciectomy or subtotal palmar fasciectomy that allows maximal untethered joint motion. A local fasciotomy may occasionally be elected in older, more debilitated patients with severe joint contractures.

Severe or recurrent proximal interphalangeal joint disease may occasionally be best treated with a salvage procedure, usually proximal interphalangeal joint arthrodesis. Amputation may be considered when profound stiffness or neurovascular compromise is present in patients with recurrent disease.

Complications

The most common postoperative complication is hematoma, which may expand and compromise skin flaps and act as a nidus for infection. To diminish the possibility of postoperative hematoma, the tourniquet should be released and meticulous hemostasis obtained prior to wound closure. Tight skin closure should be avoided. If limited flap necrosis occurs, the affected regions should be treated by open dressing changes. If skin loss is extensive, skin graft application may be necessary to gain early wound closure.

Joint stiffness may occur, particularly after extensive surgical release of the long-standing fixed proximal interphalangeal joint. Extensive therapy is often necessary, consisting of both active and passive exercises and splinting.

Mild sympathetically mediated pain (reflex sympathetic dystrophy) is not uncommon. For patients who have a more severe form, hospitalization with elevation, sympathetic blocking agents, oral steroids, and intensive therapy may be necessary.

Prognosis

Contracture correction is usually maintained at the metacarpophalangeal joints. Recurrence is more common at the proximal interphalangeal joint, particularly when the extent of preoperative proximal interphalangeal joint contracture was more than 60 degrees. Long-term postoperative night splinting may diminish the extent of residual digital flexion contracture.

Forsman M et al: Dupuytren's contracture; increased cellularity—Proliferation, is there equality? Scand J Surg 2005;94:71. [PMID: 15865122]

Godtfredsen NS et al: A prospective study linked both alcohol and tobacco to Dupuytren's disease. J Clin Epidemiol 2004;57:858. [PMID: 15485739]

Ketchum LD, Donahue TK: The injection of nodules of Dupuytren's disease with triamcinolone acetonide. J Hand Surg Am 2000;25:1157. [PMID: 11119679]

McFarlane RM: On the origin and spread of Dupuytren's disease. J Hand Surg [Am] 2002;27(3):385. [PMID: 12015711]

■ COMPARTMENT SYNDROMES

Compartment syndromes are a group of conditions that result from increased pressure within a limited anatomic space, acutely compromising the microcirculation and threatening the viability of the tissue within that space.

Recurrent or chronic compartment syndrome results from increased pressure within the compartment with a specific activity, most commonly in athletes during exercise. Symptoms of muscle weakness may be severe enough to stop the exercise activity in spite of the patient being asymptomatic between recurrences.

The Volkmann ischemic contracture is the result of an acute compartment syndrome in which fibrous tissue has replaced dead muscle. Because nerve injury is not always associated with this condition, sensation and intrinsic muscle function may be normal distal to the involved compartment. Because there is often no associated nerve injury, no sensory deficit or loss of motor function may be detected in the nerve domain distal to the involved compartment.

Etiologic Factors

The most common causes of compartment syndrome are fractures, soft-tissue crush injuries, arterial injuries either caused by localized hemorrhage or postischemic swelling, drug overdose with prolonged limb compression, and burn injuries. In most cases, fractures are closed or, if open, are grade 1 injuries, with only limited disruption of the compartmental soft-tissue envelopes.

The pathophysiology of compartment syndrome is a consequence of closure of small vessels. Increased compartment pressure increases the pressure on the walls of arterioles within the compartment. Increased local pressure also occludes small veins, resulting in venous hypertension within the compartment. The arteriovenous gradient in the region of the pressurized tissue becomes insufficient to allow tissue perfusion. Because the elevated pressure within the compartment is not high enough to occlude major arteries completely as they pass through the compartment, distal pulses usually remain strong in spite of increasing tissue ischemia in the affected soft-tissue compartment.

Clinical Findings

The diagnosis of compartment syndrome is established predominantly on clinical findings. The clinician must have a high index of suspicion whenever a closed compartment has the potential for bleeding or swelling. Compartment syndromes are characterized by pain out of proportion to the initial injury. Pain is often persistent, progressive, and unrelieved by immobilization. Pain may be accentuated by passive stretching of involved muscles. Diminished sensation may be noted in the distribution of the nerve whose compartment is being compressed. This phenomenon is believed to be secondary to nerve ischemia. A third sign is weakness and paralysis of muscles within the compartment. A fourth sign is tenseness of the compartment on palpation. Of the preceding signs and symptoms, pain with passive muscle stretching is the most sensitive in detecting compartment syndrome.

If the diagnosis of compartment syndrome is in question, the clinician is obligated to ascertain the pressure within the potential affected compartments. Various methods are available, including a portable hand-held pressure monitor or a simple modification of a mercury manometer connected to tubing and a three-way stopcock. Although the exact pressure threshold for requiring fasciotomy is controversial, fasciotomy should be strongly considered whenever the compartment pressure is greater than 30 mm Hg in the forearm. Pressure measurements of the compartments of the hand

are difficult to interpret. The decision to perform a fasciotomy of the hand or finger is based solely on clinical judgment.

Treatment

Once the diagnosis of compartment syndrome is established, fasciotomy of the involved compartment should be performed as soon as possible because elevation of compartment pressure of more than 30 mm Hg for more than 8 hours is associated with irreversible tissue death. Prophylactic fasciotomy should also be considered in patients in whom ischemia is present for more than 4 hours. All patients undergoing forearm or arm replantation should have a fasciotomy performed at the time of the initial surgical procedure.

The volar compartment of the forearm is the upper extremity compartment most often requiring release (Figure 10–27A). The skin incision should extend from the elbow to the carpal tunnel. The preferred skin incision extends from the medial side of the biceps and swings ulnarly toward the medial epicondyle. Care must be taken to incise the lacertus fibrosus at the elbow

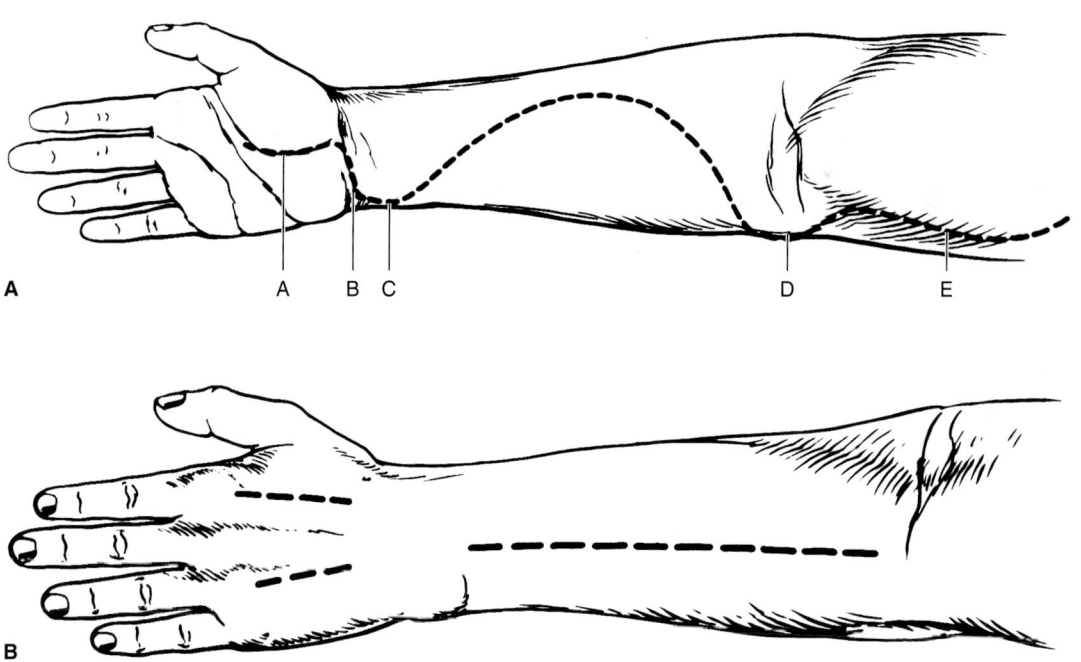

Figure 10–27. **A:** Various skin incisions used for performing a volar arm fasciotomy. **B:** To decompress the dorsal and mobile wad compartments, straight incisions are preferred because fewer veins are damaged. (Reproduced, with permission, from Green DP, ed: *Operative Hand Surgery*, 2nd ed. Churchill Livingstone, 1988.)

level. The incision may be extended in a radial direction to allow decompression of the mobile wad. In the distal half of the forearm, the incision runs along the ulnar border. The flap is designed to allow coverage of the median nerve in the distal forearm when the wounds are left open at the conclusion of the procedure. The incision is extended obliquely across the wrist to provide exposure of the carpal tunnel in the proximal palm.

An epimysiotomy of the individual superficial and deep compartment muscle bellies should be performed as needed. Care should be taken to ensure that the deep compartment musculature (the flexor pollicis longus and flexor digitorum profundus muscles) is completely decompressed. The skin incision should be partially closed over the median nerve in the hand and distal forearm. The proximal wound over muscle should be left open. The patient should be returned to the operating room within 48 hours for reevaluation. At the second surgery, dressings are changed and secondary debridement is accomplished if nonviable muscle remains. In some instances, it is possible to close the wound secondarily; in most cases, split-thickness skin grafting of the residual skin defect is a safer alternative. Decompression of the dorsal forearm when necessary may be accomplished with a dorsal longitudinal incision (Figure 10–27B).

In the hand, the connections between compartments are limited; therefore, each compartment should be released individually. This may be accomplished by two longitudinal dorsal incisions over the index and ring metacarpals. Through these incisions, each of the interosseous compartments can be entered on both the radial and ulnar sides of each metacarpal. Separate volar incisions are needed when decompression of the thenar and hypothenar compartments is necessary on the palm of the hand.

In the finger, fasciotomy may be required for treatment of either severe trauma or snakebite injuries. Because compartment pressures in the finger are impossible to measure accurately, the indications for finger fasciotomy are based on the degree of swelling. Midaxial incisions along the ulnar side of the index, middle, and ring fingers and the radial side of the little finger and thumb allow satisfactory digital decompression. Care is taken to retract the neurovascular bundle palmarward, and the fascia between the neurovascular bundle and the flexor tendon sheath are then incised. Digital wounds are left open postoperatively, and wound closure is achieved either secondarily or with a split-thickness skin graft.

Botte MJ, Keenan MA, Gelberman RH: Volkmann's ischemic contracture of the upper extremity. Hand Clin 1998;14:483. [PMID: 9742427]

Dente CJ et al: A review of upper extremity fasciotomies in a level I trauma center. Am Surg 2002;70:188. [PMID: 15663051]

Hovius SE, Ultee J: Volkmann's ischemic contracture. Prevention and treatment. Hand Clin 2000;16:647. [PMID: 11117054]

Ultee J, Hovius SE: Functional results after treatment of Volkmann's ischemic contracture: A long-term followup study. Clin Orthop 2005;431:42. [PMID: 15685054]

■ FRACTURES & DISLOCATIONS OF THE HAND

FRACTURES & DISLOCATIONS OF THE METACARPALS & PHALANGES

Fractures of the metacarpals and phalanges account for approximately 10% of all fractures. More than half of all hand fractures are work related. Fractures of the border digits, thumb, and little finger are most common. The most commonly fractured bone is the distal phalanx, accounting for 45–50% of all hand fractures.

Clinical Findings

Description of a phalangeal or metacarpal fracture should include notation of the bone involved, the location within the bone (base, shaft, or neck), and whether the fracture is open or closed. Further determination should be made as to whether the fracture is displaced or nondisplaced, if it has an intraarticular component, and whether rotational or angular deformity is present.

Because rotational malalignment of a metacarpal or phalangeal fracture is difficult to evaluate from a radiograph, physical examination is essential. The patient is asked to flex actively the fingers individually and together. Nail rotation, finger orientation, and overlapping of the fingers is assessed. Associated vascular, nerve, and tendon injuries, as well as the adequacy of soft-tissue coverage, also should be evaluated.

Treatment

Treatment of metacarpal and phalangeal fractures requires accurate diagnosis, reduction, sufficient immobilization to maintain the fracture reduction, with early motion of the uninvolved fingers to prevent stiffness. Immobilization should usually place the hand in an intrinsic plus, or safe, position to avoid secondary joint contracture (see Figure 10–12). Immobilization should rarely exceed 3 weeks for phalangeal fractures or 4 weeks for metacarpal fractures. Because radiologic union usually lags behind clinical union in the hand, initiation of digital motion should not be delayed until radiologic union is visible. Prolonged immobilization increases the likelihood of residual stiffness.

The fixation required to maintain fracture reduction depends on the fracture characteristics. Stable fractures may be treated by either buddy taping the affected finger to an adjacent finger and allowing early motion or with a brief period of splint immobilization. Repeat radiographs at 7–10 days document maintenance of fracture reduction. Initially displaced unstable fractures that require closed reduction to achieve proper alignment require external immobilization with a cast or splint.

When external immobilization is impossible or unlikely to maintain fracture reduction, internal fixation is required. Internal fixation techniques useful in the management of hand fractures include Kirschner (K)-wire fixation, interosseous wiring, tension band wiring, interfragmentary screw fixation, or fixation with plates and screws. K-wire fixation is versatile but lacks the rigidity of other techniques. Additional stability may be achieved by combining K-wire fixation with tension band wires. Interfragmentary screws provide ideal fixation for long oblique fractures, in which the obliquity of the fracture is more than two times the diameter of the fractured bone. Plates and screws in the hand are particularly helpful in open metacarpal fractures with bone loss. When segmental bone loss occurs, initial treatment includes debridement of an associated open wound and maintenance of skeletal length with either internal or external fixation. After the soft-tissue coverage is established, bony graft reconstruction may be coupled with definitive internal fixation.

1. Physeal Fractures

Approximately a third of all fractures of the immature skeleton involve the epiphysis. Salter-Harris physeal fractures are divided into five types. Type 1 fractures, which shear through the growth plate without extension into the epiphysis or metaphysis, may be effectively treated with simple immobilization. Type 2 fractures, in which a metaphyseal fracture fragment is attached to the epiphysis, can usually be reduced in a closed fashion and immobilized with a splint. One of the more common type 2 fractures is the so-called extraoctave fracture at the base of the proximal phalanx of the little finger, caused by forceful ulnar deviation of the finger. Reduction may be accomplished by metacarpophalangeal joint flexion and little-finger radial deviation. Type 3 and 4 fractures are intraarticular injuries. When displaced, these fractures require open reduction to achieve restoration of the articular surface and physis. Type 5 fractures are uncommon in the phalanges, occurring most often in the finger metacarpals as a result of axial compression. Type 5 crush injuries to the growth plate may provoke either partial or complete fusion of the physis and thereby result in late angular deformity or digital shortening.

2. Distal Phalanx Fractures

Distal phalangeal fractures occur most often in the middle finger and the thumb. These fractures usually result from a crushing injury, such as occurs with a misdirected hammer striking a thumb holding a nail or a protruding middle-finger distal phalanx caught in a closing door.

Precise reduction of distal phalangeal fracture fragments is not required in closed injuries, unless the articular surface is involved. Treatment consists of splinting the bone and distal interphalangeal joint for protection and pain relief. While the distal interphalangeal joint is splinted, motion should be encouraged at the metacarpophalangeal and proximal interphalangeal joints. Splint protection may be discontinued at 3 weeks.

Nail matrix injuries are often associated with open distal phalanx fractures. Proper treatment of these fractures requires removal of the nail, irrigation of the fracture and nail bed, and nail bed repair with fine absorbable sutures. Fracture reduction is usually accomplished by nail matrix repair and replacement of the nail. In rare cases, pin fixation of markedly displaced distal phalanx fractures may be required. After nail bed repair, either the original nail, a nail prosthesis, a piece of aluminum suture package, or a piece of gauze should be interposed between the nail roof and the nail bed to prevent synechia (adhesion) formation.

Displaced open distal phalangeal epiphyseal injuries are most often caused by flexion of the distal phalanx with the apex at the dorsal physis. The nail is often avulsed dorsal to the eponychia. Treatment requires nail removal, irrigation, reduction of the fracture, and nail bed repair. Failure to appreciate the open nature of a displaced type 1 fracture of the distal phalanx may result in osteomyelitis with growth arrest of the distal phalanx.

3. Proximal & Middle Phalanx Fractures

Angulation of fractures of the proximal and middle phalanges reflects the tendon forces inserting on the bone. The middle phalanx has an extensor force transmitted to it by the central slip attaching dorsally and proximally. The terminal extensor tendon inserts dorsally and distally into the terminal phalanx, providing a secondary dorsiflexion force. The flexor digitorum superficialis inserts volarly over the middle three fifths of the middle phalanx. Therefore, middle phalanx fractures that occur proximal to the flexor digitorum superficialis insertion angulate with the fracture apex dorsally; fractures that occur distal to the superficialis insertion angulate with the apex palmarly. Proximal phalangeal fractures tend to angulate with the apex palmarly because of the force of lateral bands that pass palmarward to the axis of the metacarpophalangeal joint and dorsalward to the axis of the proximal interphalangeal joint.

Adhesions involving the flexor or extensor tendons are a major complication of proximal and middle phalangeal fractures. Fracture displacement increases the likelihood of tendon adherence and limitation of joint motion. Malunion or malrotation of the fractures may require secondary correction.

Early appropriate treatment of these fractures attempts to prevent complications. In a stable nondisplaced or impacted fracture, only temporary splint protection is required, followed by dynamic splinting such as buddy taping to an adjacent finger. Radiographic follow-up is needed to document maintenance of the reduction. Patients who require closed reduction and immobilization should have the forearm, wrist, and injured digits as well as an adjacent digit immobilized in a plaster cast or gutter splint.

4. Metacarpal Fractures

Metacarpal Head Fractures

Intraarticular fractures of the metacarpal head require open reduction and internal fixation if more than 20–30% of the joint surface is involved. Realigned articular fracture fragments may be held in place with either a K-wire or small screw. Fractures with marked comminution of the metacarpal head distal to the ligament origin may not be amenable to precise internal fixation and may be treated with early mobilization with distraction traction.

Metacarpal Neck Fractures

Metacarpal neck fractures are most frequent in the little finger, although they may occur in any metacarpal. Metacarpal neck fractures result from a direct blow, either delivered to the hand or by the hand striking a solid object (animate or inanimate). Comminution of the volar cortex results in collapse deformity with apex dorsal angulation (Figure 10–28). Greater residual fracture angulation may be accepted in the ring and little fingers because the greater mobility in the ulnar carpometacarpal joints allows greater compensatory motion. The flexion and extension arc is 15 degrees in the ring-finger carpometacarpal joint and 30 degrees in the little finger.

Fracture site angulation of more than 10 degrees should not be accepted in the index and middle fingers. Fractures of the ring and little fingers with initial angulation of less than 15 degrees should be immobilized in a gutter splint for 10–14 days. When angulation is 15–40 degrees, reduction should be accomplished before an ulnar gutter splint immobilization is employed for 3

Figure 10–28. Boxer's fracture. If the angulation in a metacarpal neck fracture is severe, clawing may result when the patient attempts to extend the finger. This is a good clinical test to supplement the evaluation of the severity of the angulation as seen radiographically. (Reproduced, with permission, from Rockwood CA Jr et al, ed: *Fractures in Adults,* 3rd ed. Lippincott, 1991.)

weeks. With angulation of more than 40 degrees, extensor lag may be noted at the proximal interphalangeal joint, and the patient may complain of a "marble" in the palm when making a fist. If closed reduction cannot be maintained, internal fixation may be employed.

Metacarpal Shaft Fractures

Metacarpal shaft fractures result from a direct blow or crushing injury. Dorsal angulation of the fracture fragments is secondary to the interosseous muscle forces. The closer the fracture is to the carpometacarpal joints, the greater the lever arm and, hence, the less angulation can be tolerated. Less shortening occurs in isolated fractures of the middle and ring metacarpals than in the index or little fingers because the deep intermetacarpal ligaments of two adjacent rays tether the fractured metacarpal distally. Isolated metacarpal fractures may be treated with cast or splint immobilization for 4–6 weeks. Displaced metacarpal shaft fractures may be fixed percutaneously with a longitudinal pin or by percutaneously pinning the fractured metacarpal to an adjacent metacarpal. Skeletal fixation is essential if metacarpal rotational deformity cannot be corrected with closed means because modest metacarpal malrotation results in substantial digital overlap. Dorsal angulation of more than 10 degrees in index and middle metacarpals and more than 20 degrees in ring and little metacarpals, shortening of more than 3 mm, or multiple displaced metacarpal fractures should be treated with operative intervention. Long spiral fractures may be effectively fixed with multiple screws, and transverse fractures are usually most securely fixed with dorsally applied plates. When two or more metacarpals are simultaneously fractured, the splinting effect of the intact adjacent metacarpals is lost. Secure fixation with screws or plates should be employed in at least one of the multiple injured metacarpals.

5. Joint Injuries

Distal Interphalangeal Joint

The most common intraarticular fracture of the distal interphalangeal joint is a bony mallet finger, in which a portion of the articular surface is avulsed by the extensor tendon. Most bony mallet injuries can be treated with splinting in extension for 6 weeks. Indications for fixation of these fractures are controversial. Internal fixation should be considered in fractures that include articular surface loss greater than 30% and subluxation of the joint.

Dislocation of the distal interphalangeal joint is uncommon without an associated fracture. Closed reduction with temporary splint protection allows early mobilization to begin within 7–10 days.

Condylar Fractures

Condylar fractures may occur in either the proximal or middle phalanges. These fractures are most often athletic injuries. Anteroposterior, lateral, and oblique radiographs are necessary to identify the fracture fragments. If the injury is inadequately appreciated, angulation of the finger and joint incongruity may lead to stiffness, deformity and early degenerative arthritis. Displaced fracture should be openly reduced and internally fixed if the condylar fracture is displaced by more than 2 mm. If both condyles are fractured, they must be precisely secured together and then secured to the phalangeal shaft. The collateral ligament insertion to the condyle must be preserved because it is the only blood supply to the fragment. Permanent stiffness may be anticipated in complex condylar fractures.

Proximal Interphalangeal Joint Dislocation & Fracture-Dislocation

Dorsal dislocations of the proximal interphalangeal joint are more common than palmar or lateral dislocations. Dorsal dislocations may be separated into three types (Figure 10–29). In type 1 dislocations, a hyperextension injury avulses the volar plate from the base of the middle phalanx, and the collateral ligaments partially split from the middle phalanx and the joint surface remain intact. Type 2 dislocations are dorsal dislocations similar to type 1 injuries, except that a larger portion of the collateral ligament is torn. In type 3 injuries, dorsal dislocation occurs with proximal retraction of the middle phalanx. A portion of the middle phalangeal palmar base may be sheared away. Stable fracture-dislocations are associated with fractures in which less than 40% of the middle phalanx base is fractured. Unstable fracture-dislocations have more than 40% bone fracture involvement and are associated with complete loss of collateral ligament stability.

Treatment of proximal interphalangeal joint dislocations depends on the dislocation type. Stable type 1 and 2 injuries should be treated by closed reduction and immobilization in a dorsal splint in 30 degrees of flexion for 1–2 weeks. After reduction and splinting, a radiograph should document the reduction. While in the splint, patients are encouraged to flex the proximal interphalangeal joint actively. After 2–3 weeks, the splint is removed. The finger may be buddy taped to an adjacent finger during sports for the next month.

Unstable fracture-dislocations should be treated with closed reduction. Considerable flexion (more than 75 degrees) may be necessary to achieve reduction. Again,

Figure 10–29. Various dorsal dislocations of the proximal interphalangeal joint. **A:** Type 1 (hyperextension). The volar plate is avulsed, and an incomplete longitudinal split occurs in the collateral ligaments. The articular surfaces maintain congruous contact. **B:** Type 2 (dorsal dislocation). There is complete rupture of the volar plate and a complete split in the collateral ligaments, with the middle phalanx resting on the dorsum of the proximal phalanx. The proximal and middle phalanges lie in almost parallel alignment. **C:** Type 3 (fracture-dislocation). The insertion of the volar plate, including a portion of the volar base of the middle phalanx, is disrupted. The major portion of the collateral ligaments remains with the volar plate and flexor sheath. A major articular defect may be present.

radiographs must document congruent joint reduction. An extension block splint allows active proximal interphalangeal joint flexion while constraining extension. The splint is straightened by 10-degree increments each week until approximately 6 weeks after reduction, when splinting may be discontinued. If closed reduction cannot be achieved, open reduction is required. When a single large palmar articular fragment is present, internal fixation may be attempted. If the fracture is comminuted, however, either volar plate arthroplasty or an axial traction technique that allows early controlled passive joint motion is necessary.

Radial lateral proximal interphalangeal dislocation is six times more common than ulnar lateral interphalangeal dislocation. These dislocations are associated with avulsion of the volar plate, extensor mechanism, or a portion of the phalangeal base. After the joint is reduced, the residual joint stability should be assessed by observing the active ROM. Stable fracture-dislocations are immobilized at 5–10 degrees of flexion for 3 weeks, and then active ROM activities are allowed.

Palmar proximal interphalangeal dislocations are unusual. The condyle of the proximal phalanx may buttonhole between the central slip and the lateral bands. Closed reduction may be attempted by applying traction to the fingers after flexing both the metacarpophalangeal and proximal interphalangeal joints. If closed reduction is successful, the digit should be splinted in extension for 3–6 weeks to allow healing of the extensor rent. If closed reduction is unsuccessful, open reduction is necessary to free the condyle from the rent in the extensor mechanism.

Metacarpophalangeal Joint

Dorsal metacarpophalangeal dislocations most commonly involve either the index or little finger. The volar plate is ruptured proximally from the metacarpal by hyperextension injury. If the joint is subluxed and the volar plate has not yet become interposed in the joint, closed reduction may be achieved by flexion of the joint. Traction across the subluxated metacarpophalangeal joint can transform a reducible joint into an irreducible, dislocated joint. Once the joint dislocates, the volar plate becomes interposed between the dislocated articular surfaces. This injury, termed *complex* or *irreducible,* requires open reduction to extract the volar plate from between the articular surfaces (Figure 10–30). Open reduction may be accomplished through either a palmar or dorsal approach. If the palmar approach is used, care should be taken to avoid injury to the radial digital nerve of the index finger or the ulnar digital nerve of the small finger. The A1 pulley is incised to release the tension of the flexor tendons on the volar plate. If the dorsal approach is used, the volar plate is incised longitudinally to facilitate reduction.

Figure 10–30. Complex dislocation of the metacarpophalangeal joint. In the upper lateral diagram, the palmar plate is locked between the head of the metacarpal and the base of the proximal phalanx. In the lower diagram, an anterior view, the head of the metacarpal can be seen trapped between the flexor digitorum profundus on one aspect and the lumbrical on the other. (Reproduced, with permission, from Lister G: *The Hand: Diagnosis and Indications,* 3rd ed. Churchill Livingstone, 1993.)

Postoperatively, the metacarpophalangeal joint is immobilized in approximately 30 degrees of flexion for 3–5 days. Splinting that allows active motion is maintained for 3 weeks.

Although lateral dislocations of the metacarpophalangeal joint are rare, isolated radial collateral ligament ruptures may occur. These injuries should also be immobilized in approximately 30 degrees of flexion for 3 weeks. The fingers should be protected from ulnar stress for an additional 3 weeks. Unstable index- and middle-finger radial collateral ligament tears may be surgically repaired.

Finger Carpometacarpal Joints

Sprains and fracture-dislocations may involve any of the carpometacarpal joints. Sprains of the index- and middle-finger carpometacarpal joints may occur with palmar flexion and torsion. If tenderness is localized to the carpometacarpal joint and careful radiographs fail to demonstrate fracture, a sprain may be diagnosed.

Treatment of acute sprain injuries consists of 3–6 weeks of immobilization. If localized pain persists, steroid injection may be considered. Chronic pain at the index middle trapezoid capitate joint may be treated with either carpal boss excision or arthrodesis of the carponmetacarpal joint. Carpometacarpal fracture-dislocations of the ring and little fingers are usually secondary to direct or longitudinal blows. Dorsal dislocations are more common than volar dislocations. Oblique views with partial pronation and supination may be required to visualize the carpometacarpal joint clearly. Closed reduction may be achieved with longitudinal distraction. The reduction may be maintained by percutaneous K-wire fixation. When fracture-dislocation of the little-finger metacarpal articular surface shears off a fragment of the hamate, displacement of the metacarpal shaft is likely. Because of forces of the extensor carpi ulnaris and the hypothenar muscles, the metacarpal shaft tends to displace proximally and angulate palmarly. Longitudinal traction and percutaneous K-wire fixation of the ring- and little-finger metacarpals stabilize these fractures. Open reduction is necessary for an irreducible dislocation or for chronic fracture-dislocations. If the patient develops degenerative arthritis of the hamate metacarpal joint, arthrodesis of the ring- or small-finger carpometacarpal joint (or both) is well tolerated.

Thumb Metacarpophalangeal Joint

The most common injury to the metacarpophalangeal joint is sprain of the ulnar collateral ligament of the thumb (gamekeeper's thumb, skier's thumb). This injury occurs when the thumb is forced into radial deviation, stressing the ulnar collateral ligament. When the ulnar collateral ligament tears from its phalangeal insertion, the adductor aponeurosis may become interposed between the retracted ligament, preventing healing of the ligament to the proximal phalanx with closed treatment (Stener lesion). Evaluation of the integrity of the ligament may be made by radially stressing the flexed metacarpophalangeal joint under local anesthesia. Radial deviation that is more than 30 degrees from that of the opposite thumb is diagnostic of a totally disrupted, incompetent ligament.

Closed treatment of a partial ligament tear may be accomplished with a thumb spica splint for 3–4 weeks. Complete disruption of the ligament requires surgical exploration and reattachment to the bone. Avulsion of the ulnar collateral ligament may also occur with a bony fragment. If the fragment is greater than 15% of the articular surface or if the avulsed fragment is displaced more than 5 mm, open repair of the ligament is recommended.

Chronic symptomatic ulnar collateral ligament injuries may be repaired if the residual ligament is of sufficient quality. Supplementation of the repair with either tendon transfer or tendon grafting may be useful. In patients who develop traumatic arthritis or if ligament reconstruction is not deemed feasible, arthrodesis of the metacarpophalangeal joint is preferred.

Thumb Carpometacarpal Joint

Four patterns of thumb metacarpal fracture are most commonly encountered.

A. BENNETT FRACTURE

Bennett fracture is an intraarticular fracture in which the small volar radial fragment of the metacarpal articular surface remains attached to the anterior oblique ligament, and the remainder of the metacarpal articular surface and shaft is displaced proximally, radially, and into adduction in response to the force of the adductor pollicis and abductor pollicis longus muscles insertion on the metacarpal (Figure 10–31). Acute Bennett fractures may often be reduced by traction and pressure on the proximal metacarpal, with slight pronation. The reduction may then be stabilized by percutaneous pin fixation through the metacarpal shaft into either the fragment or the trapezium. If satisfactory reduction cannot be achieved by closed means, open reduction and internal fixation is required.

B. ROLANDO FRACTURE

The Rolando fracture is a comminuted T or Y intraarticular fracture of the base of the thumb metacarpal. When large fragments are present, open reduction and internal fixation is possible. When the joint is highly comminuted, cast immobilization, traction, or limited open reduction and internal fixation with cast immobilization may be employed.

Abductor pollicis longus

Figure 10–31. Bennett fracture. The first metacarpal shaft is displaced by the pull of the muscle. (Reproduced, with permission, from American Society for Surgery of the Hand: *The Hand: Examination and Diagnosis*, 2nd ed. Churchill Livingstone, 1983.)

C. EXTRAARTICULAR FRACTURE

Extraarticular fractures are less likely to develop traumatic arthritis than intraarticular fractures. Because of the mobility of the carpometacarpal joint of the thumb, up to 30 degrees of angulation can be accepted without functional loss.

D. EPIPHYSEAL FRACTURE

Epiphyseal fractures of the thumb metacarpal are treated in a fashion similar to other Salter-Harris fractures.

Freeland AE, Lineaweaver WC, Lindley SG: Fracture fixation in the mutilated hand. Hand Clin 2003;19:51.

Kiefhaber TR, Stern PJ: Fractures dislocations of the proximal interphalangeal joint. J Hand Surg Am 1998;23:368.

Page SM, Stern PJ: Complications and range of motion following plate fixation of metacarpal and phalangeal fractures. J Hand Surg Am 1998;23:827.

WRIST INJURIES

Scaphoid Injuries

The scaphoid is the most commonly fractured bone in the carpus. Anatomically, the scaphoid may be divided into proximal, middle, and distal thirds. The middle third is termed the *waist.* The scaphoid tubercle forms a distal volar prominence. Because the scaphoid articulates with four carpal bones and the radius, most of its surface is composed of articular cartilage, leaving little room for vascular perforation. Therefore, the vascular supply to the scaphoid comes through a narrow nonarticular region in the waist. Most of the blood supply to the scaphoid enters distally. In approximately a third of fractures at the waist level, there is diminished flow to the proximal pole, which may result in ischemic necrosis of the proximal pole of the scaphoid. Almost 100% of proximal pole fractures develop ischemic or aseptic necrosis.

Middle third fractures account for approximately 70% of scaphoid fractures, proximal pole fractures for 20%, and distal pole fractures for the rest.

Cast immobilization is recommended in the treatment of all nondisplaced scaphoid fractures, defined as fractures with less than 2 mm of displacement and no fracture site angulation. On average, middle third fractures heal in 6–12 weeks, distal third fractures in 4–8 weeks, and proximal third fractures in 12–20 weeks. When initial radiographs demonstrate fracture displacement, open reduction and internal fixation is required to prevent malunion. Internal fixation is accomplished with either smooth K-wires or a buried compression screw. Because of the time to union in scaphoid fractures, some surgeons recommend primary fixation of these fractures even when nondisplaced. Newer studies demonstrate that percutaneous fixation of nondisplaced waist fractures decreases or eliminates the period of cast immobilization.

Delayed union may be treated with either prolonged casting or open reduction, curettage, and bone grafting. Nondisplaced ununited fractures may be treated by percutaneous screw fixation. If fracture site angulation or collapse is present, a cortical cancellous volar graft is employed to correct the deformity. The graft must be stabilized with either a buried compression screw or K-wires. If the proximal pole is avascular and no radiocarpal arthritis is present, revascularization of the scaphoid with a vascularized bone graft from the dorsal radius should be performed.

Once degenerative arthritis is evident at the radiocarpal joint, salvage procedures include proximal row carpectomy, scaphoid excision and midcarpal arthrodesis, or total wrist arthrodesis.

Lunate & Perilunate Dislocations

Lunate and perilunate dislocations are the result of a powerful force causing disruption of the ligamentous support about the lunate. The mechanism of these injuries is usually dorsiflexion, ulnar deviation, and intercarpal supination. Mayfield defined four stages of disruption. Stage 1 injuries demonstrate disruptions of the scapholunate ligament. Stage 2 injuries also include tears of the ligaments dorsal to the lunate. In stage 3 injuries, the arc of disruption extends across the lunotriquetral ligament. Stage 4 injuries have total disruption of the entire lunate ligamentous support. The sequence of injuries is paralleled by a progression of clinical entities from scapholunate dissociation to perilunate dislocation to lunate dislocation.

When the entire carpus except the lunate dislocates and the lunate remains normally seated in the lunate fossa of the radius, the abnormality is termed *perilunate dislocation* (Figure 10–32). When the relationship between the carpus and the radius is maintained but the lunate is dislocated palmarward into the carpal tunnel, the condition is termed *lunate dislocation.* Both lunate and perilunate dislocations imply disruption of ligamentous connections between the scaphoid and the lunate, between the capitate and the lunate, and between the lunate and the triquetrum. Although the lunate is bound to the scaphoid by the scapholunate ligament and to the triquetrum through the lunotriquetral ligament, the interval between the lunate and the capitate, known as the space of Poirier, lacks direct ligamentous connection.

A variant of perilunate dislocation is transscaphoid perilunate dislocation. With this injury, the arc of disruption passes through the scaphoid rather than the scapholunate ligament. The disruption then passes between the proximal scaphoid and the capitate, between the capitate and the lunate, and between the lunate and the triquetrum.

Intercarpal ligamentous disruptions heal if the normally connected bones are maintained in an anatomic

A   **B**

Figure 10–32. Perilunate dislocation: Anteroposterior view (**A**); lateral view (**B**).

relationship. Intercarpal dislocations should be reduced initially in a closed fashion. Reduction is usually achieved by longitudinal traction and direct pressure on the dislocated carpal bone or bones. Occasionally, anatomic alignment of the carpus can be achieved and maintained with closed reduction and cast application. In most instances, however, open reduction, pin fixation, and direct ligamentous repair is necessary to secure anatomic reduction. Surgical treatment of perilunate and lunate dislocations often requires both palmar and dorsal approaches. Through the dorsal approach, intercarpal alignment is visualized, adjusted, and stabilized. The palmar approach is employed to release the median nerve at the carpal tunnel and to repair the rent in the space of Poirier.

Kienböck Disease

Kienböck disease results from ischemic necrosis of the lunate. The cause of the condition is the subject of extensive debate. The condition is more common in patients with a negative ulnar variance, in which the

ulna is shorter than the radius. It is unclear whether the relatively shorter ulna alters and increases the force transmitted to the lunate through the lunate fossa of the radius or whether the altered stress causes the lunate to be shaped in a more triangular and less cuboid or trapezoidal configuration.

Kienböck disease may be classified based on the extent of collapse (Figure 10–33). Stage I disease demonstrates a linear compression fracture but an otherwise normal-appearing architecture and density. MRI studies show poor vascularity of the lunate in stage I (Figure 10–34). In stage II disease, the density is abnormal on plain films. By stage III, lunate collapse is present. Stage III disease is subdivided into stage IIIA, in which the lunate is collapsed but carpal height remains normal, and stage IIIB, in which the lunate is collapsed and carpal height is also abnormal. In stage IV wrists, extensive osteoarthritic changes are present.

The current recommendations for the treatment of Kienböck disease include radial shortening osteotomy for ulnar-negative or neutral variance when no carpal collapse is present. If the patient initially demonstrates a

Stage I   Stage II

Stage III   Stage IV

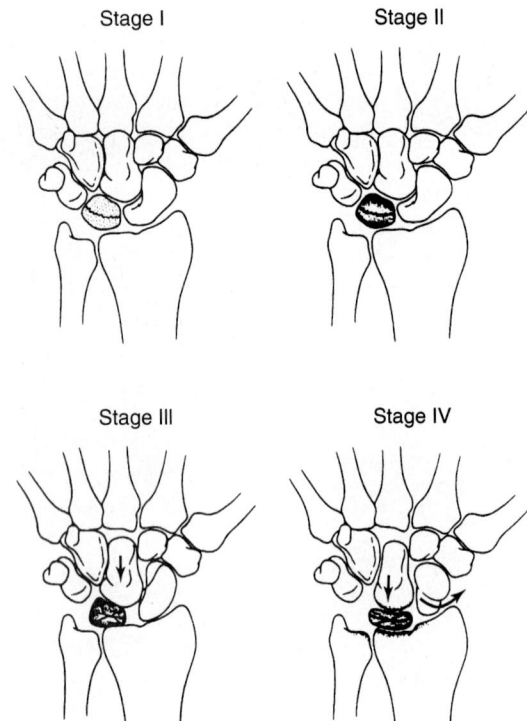

Figure 10–33. Staging of Kienböck disease (after Lichtman). Stage I: Routine radiographs (posteroanterior, lateral) are normal, but tomography may show a linear fracture, usually transverse through the body of the lunate. MRI confirms avascular changes. Stage II: Bone density increase (sclerosis) and a fracture line are usually evident on the posteroanterior radiograph. Posteroanterior and lateral tomograms demonstrate sclerosis, cystic changes, and often a clear fracture. There is no collapse deformity. Stage III: Advanced bone density changes are present, with fragmentation, cystic resorption, and collapse. The diagnosis is evident from posteroanterior radiograph. Tomograms (posteroanterior and lateral) show the degree of lunate infractionation and amount of fracture displacement. Proximal migration of the capitate is present, and there is mild to moderate rotary alignment of the scaphoid. Stage IV: Perilunate arthritic changes are present, with complete collapse and fragmentation of the lunate. Carpal instability is evident, with scaphoid malalignment and capitate displacement into the lunate space. (Reproduced, with permission, from Rockwood CA Jr et al, eds: *Fractures in Adults,* 3rd ed. Lippincott, 1991.)

positive ulnar variance, recommendations include either a capitate shortening osteotomy or an intercarpal arthrodesis of the scaphoid, trapezium, and trapezoid. A new technique restores the anatomic height of the lunate with a vascularized bone graft and additional cancellous bone. In stage IIIB and IV wrists, consideration is given to either proximal row carpectomy or wrist arthrodesis. Silicone replacement of the lunate is no longer advised for Kienböck disease.

Carpal Instability

To evaluate the orientation of the carpus properly, true anteroposterior and lateral radiographs are required. The anteroposterior view should be obtained with the forearm positioned in neutral rotation to allow a precise standardized evaluation of the relationship between the distal radius and the distal ulna. When the ulna is shorter than the radius, the term *negative ulnar variance* is used, and when the ulna extends further distally than the radius, the term *positive ulnar variance* is used.

The anteroposterior radiograph should demonstrate the close relationship of the scaphoid and the lunate. Normally, the ossified portions of these two bones are separated by their abutting respective articular cartilage shells, creating a radiographic gap of 3 mm or less. In an adult a gap of more than 3 mm is considered abnormal and indicates separation of these two bones secondary to ligamentous disruption. When the scapholunate gap is abnormally wide on a standard radiograph, the abnormality is referred to as static scapholunate dissociation (Figure 10–35). When the standard anteroposterior radiograph is normal but an anteroposterior radio-

Figure 10–34. MRI showing Kienböck disease.

Figure 10–35. Anteroposterior view of static scapholunate dissociation.

graph taken with the fingers squeezing tightly to form a fist reveals an abnormal gap, the condition is referred to as dynamic scapholunate dissociation.

The lateral radiograph should be obtained with the wrist in a neutral position, neither flexed nor extended. The lateral radiograph is often overlooked because of the projected superimposition of shadows. This normal overlapping allows measurement of a number of angles between bones. Normally, the middle metacarpal, capitate, lunate, and radius are collinear. The long axis of the radius is readily defined. Establishing the relationship of the scaphoid to the radius requires defining a line drawn along the most palmar portions of the distal and proximal poles of the scaphoid. The axes of the radius and the scaphoid intersect, forming the radioscaphoid angle (Figure 10–36). This angle is usually between 40 and 60 degrees. When the angle is greater than 60 degrees, the scaphoid is abnormally flexed.

The orientation of the lunate viewed on the lateral radiograph is derived by first establishing a line between the most distal palmar and dorsal lips of the lunate. A second line is then drawn perpendicular to the first line, establishing the axis of the lunate. The angle between the radial and lunate axes (radiolunate angle) is normally less than 15 degrees.

The orientation of the lunate seen on the lateral radiograph normally reflects a ligamentous balancing of the influences of the adjacent scaphoid and triquetrum. The scaphoid tends to tether the lunate into flexion through the scapholunate ligament, whereas the triquetrum tends to tether the lunate into extension (dorsi-

flexion) through the lunotriquetral ligament. When the scapholunate ligament is disrupted, the scaphoid tends to flex excessively, and the lunate, under the unopposed influence of the triquetrum, dorsiflexes (dorsal intercalated segment instability [DISI]) (Figure 10–37). When the lunotriquetral ligament is disrupted, the lunate, under the unopposed influence of the scaphoid, is flexed

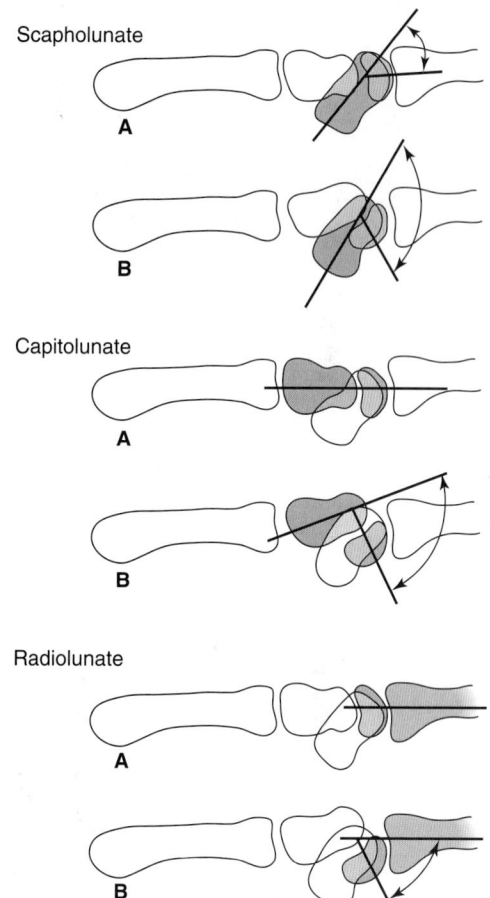

Scapholunate

Capitolunate

Radiolunate

Figure 10–36. Carpal angle measurements are of considerable aid in identifying carpal instability patterns. A = normal angle; B = abnormal angle seen in dorsiflexion instability. The capitolunate angle should theoretically be 0 degrees with the wrist in neutral position, but the range of normal probably extends to as much as 15 degrees. The scapholunate angle may be the most helpful; an angle of greater than 80 degrees is definite evidence of dorsiflexion instability. The radiolunate angle is abnormal if it exceeds 15 degrees. (Reproduced, with permission, from Green DP, ed: *Operative Hand Surgery,* 2nd ed. Churchill Livingstone, 1988.)

Figure 10–37. Lateral radiograph of dorsal intercalated segment instability.

(volar intercalated segment instability [VISI]). The optimal treatment for DISI is currently an area of intense interest. Acute ligamentous disruption is usually treated with direct ligamentous reapproximation and repair. When ligamentous repair is not possible and articular surfaces are free of degenerative change, ligamentous reconstruction, dorsal capsular ligamentodesis, or intercarpal fusions may be considered.

Degenerative arthritis occurs in wrists subjected over time to loads applied to noncongruently articulating carpal bones. The scapholunate advanced collapse (SLAC) wrist pattern describes the evolution of degenerative arthritis resulting from disruption of the scapholunate ligament (Figure 10–38). The earliest evidence of degenerative change is seen at the radioscaphoid joint, and, with time, degenerative change progresses to include the capitate lunate articulation. When radioscaphoid change is present but the articular surface of the capitate retains its normal articular cartilage, proximal row carpectomy (removal of the scaphoid, lunate, and triquetrum) allows preservation of wrist motion as the capitate head shifts proximally to articulate within the lunate fossa of the distal radius. When degenerative change is present at the capitate lunate portion of the midcarpal joints in addition to radioscaphoid change, the scaphoid may be excised and intercarpal fusion of the capitate, lunate, triquetrum, and hamate is accomplished. This selective intercarpal fusion procedure provides motion through the residual radiolunate articulation. The ultimate salvage procedure, complete wrist fusion, provides reliable pain relief while permanently sacrificing wrist motion.

Distal Radioulnar Joint

The distal radioulnar joint (DRUJ) is composed of two joints. The proximal and distal articulations of the ulna and radius allow forearm rotation. The ulna also articulates with the ulnar carpus through the triangular fibrocartilage complex (TFCC). Approximately 20% of the load from the hand to the forearm passes through the ulnocarpal joint. Problems at the DRUJ are related to one or both of these joints.

When the ulnar variance is positive, the patient may develop an ulnocarpal impaction syndrome. This often presents with pain on the ulnar side of the wrist, particularly with ulnar deviation. Radiographs may demonstrate degenerative changes of the distal ulna and ulnar lunate. Treatment consists of shortening the ulna, accomplished by removing 2–3 mm of the ulnar head (wafer procedure) either by open method, by arthroscope, or by an ulnar-shortening osteotomy, performed in the diaphyseal ulna, and fixed with a plate and screws. After the wafer procedure, patients often complain of ulnar pain for a prolonged (3–6 month) period. Approximately 50% of patients who have an ulnar shortening osteotomy require plate removal after osteotomy healing.

Figure 10–38. Scapholunate advanced collapse pattern.

Another source of ulnar-sided wrist pain is a tear of the TFCC. Tears are divided into degenerative and traumatic types. Degenerative tears are usually related to ulnocarpal impaction. Traumatic tears usually occur after a twisting injury of the wrist. Central tears and tears near the attachment of the TFCC to the radius are usually treated with an arthroscopic debridement. Tears in the well-vascularized periphery of the TFCC are treated with either arthroscopic or open repair. After repair, patients are maintained in a long arm cast for 6 weeks to allow fibrocartilage healing.

Arthritis between the distal radius and ulna can be caused by traumatic, degenerative, or inflammatory arthritis. Treatment consists of hemiresection or complete excision of the ulnar head (Darrach procedure). An alternative treatment, the Suave-Kapandji procedure, fuses the DRUJ and creates a pseudarthrosis of the distal ulna. This is particularly useful in the presence of ulnar translocation of the carpus.

Instability of the DRUJ is difficult to treat. Instability is usually the result of trauma, but it may occur after an excessive distal ulna resection. Treatment requires detection and correction of any degree of malunions in the radius or ulna. A number of soft-tissue operations are designed to stabilize the distal ulna, all with varying degrees of success.

Adams BD, Berger RA: An anatomic reconstruction of the distal radioulnar ligaments for posttraumatic distal radioulnar joint instability. J Hand Surg [Am] 2002;27(2):243. [PMID: 11901383]

Aldridge JM III, Mallon WJ: Hook of the hamate fractures in competitive golfers: Results of treatment by excision of the fractured hook of the hamate. Orthopedics 2003;26:717. [PMID: 12875568]

Berger RA: The anatomy of the ligaments of the wrist and distal radioulnar joints. Clin Orthop 2001;(383):32. Review. [PMID: 11210966]

Cohen MS, Kozin SH: Degenerative arthritis of the wrist: Proximal row carpectomy versus scaphoid excision and four-corner arthrodesis. J Hand Surg [Am] 2001;26:94. [PMID: 11172374]

Gelberman RH et al: Ulnar variance with Kienböck's disease. J Bone Joint Surg Am 1975;57:674. [PMID: 1150712]

Rettig ME et al: Open reduction and internal fixation of acute displaced scaphoid waist fractures. J Hand Surg [Am] 2001;26(2):271. [PMID: 11279573]

Shin AY et al: Treatment of isolated injuries of the lunotriquetral ligament. A comparison of arthrodesis, ligament reconstruction and ligament repair. J Bone Joint Surg Br 2001;83(7):1023. [PMID: 11603516]

Shin AY, Bishop AT: Pedicled vascularized bone grafts for disorders of the carpus: Scaphoid nonunion and Kienböck's disease. J Am Acad Orthop Surg 2002;10:210. [PMID: 12041942]

Slade JF III et al: Percutaneous internal fixation of selected scaphoid nonunions with an arthroscopically assisted dorsal approach. J Bone Joint Surg Am 2003;85:20. [PMID: 14652390]

Steinmann SP et al: Use of the 1,2 intercompartmental supraretinacular artery as a vascularized pedicle bone graft for difficult scaphoid nonunion. J Hand Surg [Am] 2002;27(3):391. [PMID: 12015712]

Szabo RM et al: Dorsal intercarpal ligament capsulodesis for chronic, static scapholunate dissociation: Clinical results. J Hand Surg Am 2002;27A:978. [PMID: 12457347]

■ FINGERTIP INJURIES

SOFT-TISSUE INJURIES

Because of the importance of the fingertip in providing a contact surface for sensate prehension, injuries to the fingertip may result in troublesome disability. The pulp of the fingertip is normally covered by tough, highly innervated skin, anchored to the phalanx by fibrous septa. The dorsum of the fingertip is composed of the nail and nail bed.

Treatment

The goals in treatment of fingertip injuries are to provide adequate sensation, minimal tenderness, satisfactory appearance, and full joint motion. Preservation of length should be balanced with the other goals.

The choice of treatment depends on the size and location of the defect. The mechanism of injury (sharp, crushing, or avulsion), the presence of exposed bone, and the angle of soft-tissue loss are considered in planning treatment.

A. OPEN WOUND CARE

The simplest treatment is open wound care, which is indicated in most injuries in children and in defects of 1 cm^2 or less in adults. The wound is thoroughly cleansed. Bone is shortened so it is covered by soft tissue and the length of the bone is the same as the length of the nail bed. Dressings are changed until the wound is healed. The disadvantages of the open method are the possibility of stump tenderness and prolonged healing time. Advantages include the ability to initiate movement immediately and to thus preserve full digital motion.

B. COMPOSITE GRAFTING

Replacement of the amputated part as a composite graft (skin and subcutaneous tissue) is indicated in children and selected adults with sharp distal amputations. When successful, this treatment gives the best appearance. The disadvantage, the unpredictable viability of the part, may result in recovery delayed by failure and secondary procedures.

C. MICROVASCULAR REPLANTATION

Microvascular replantation is possible in selected sharp amputations distal to the distal interphalangeal joint. Disadvantages include the expense of complex surgery and the time lost from work.

D. PRIMARY SHORTENING AND CLOSURE

Primary bone shortening and closure is indicated when more than 50% of the distal phalanx is lost or the nail matrix is irreparably damaged. This one-stage procedure allows for immediate mobilization. In performing the procedure, the end of the distal phalanx bone should be trimmed to provide a tension-free soft-tissue closure. The nail bed should be trimmed as far proximal as the bone. If the nail bed is pulled over the end of the shortened bone, a hook-shaped nail results. Neurectomy of digital nerves under traction allows the nerve ends to retract into soft tissue proximal to the ultimate scar.

E. SKIN GRAFTING

Skin grafting may also be employed to obtain closure if no bone is exposed. Split-thickness grafts may be placed on a less well vascularized bed. Split-thickness grafts contract more than full-thickness grafts. As the graft shrinks, the area of sensory loss also shrinks. The appearance and durability of scar tissue may be less than ideal, however.

Full-thickness skin grafts provide more durable coverage and better appearance. Care should be taken to match the pigmentation of the skin at the donor and recipient sites. The ulnar border of the hand provides an ideal donor source. Full-thickness grafts require a better vascularized bed to assure survival.

F. SKIN FLAPS

Local advancement skin flaps are useful in the treatment of fingertip injuries.

1. V-Y advancement skin flaps—V-Y advancement skin flaps may advance palmar tissue or unite two lateral skin flaps. These skin flaps are helpful in the management of transverse or dorsal oblique amputations in which soft-tissue tip coverage is needed and further skeletal shortening deemed undesirable. Complete separation of the vertical septa between the skin and the bone is required to mobilize skin flaps for advancement. The septa between the flap and the proximal skin must then be divided. Traction on the flap helps differentiate the septa from vessels and nerves.

2. Moberg palmar advancement flap—Defects of up to 1.5 cm on the thumb may be covered by a palmar advancement flap, first described by Moberg. Bilateral midlateral incisions dorsal to the neurovascular bundles of the thumb allow mobilization of the flap from the flexor tendon sheath. The flap may be maximally advanced by flexion of the thumb interphalangeal joint. When additional coverage is required, the skin of the flap may be transversely divided at the metacarpophalangeal crease while the neurovascular bundles are preserved, the distal portion of the flap may be advanced further, and a skin graft may be placed between the dis-

tal flap and the proximal flap. Disadvantages of this flap include the possibility of interphalangeal joint flexion contracture and the potential for dorsal tip necrosis if dorsal vascular branches to the digit are injured.

3. Regional skin flaps—Regional skin flaps are considered when fingertip skin is lost but nail and bone are preserved.

a. Cross-finger flap—The cross-finger flap is the most commonly used distant flap. Skin is elevated from the dorsum of the adjacent finger, with care taken not to incise the extensor paratenon. The skin is then rotated palmarward and sewn to the palmar defect of the involved finger. The donor region on the donor finger is skin grafted. The transposed flap is divided from the donor finger after 2 weeks. Joint stiffness is a potential complication in both the donor and recipient digits. The creation of a defect on a normal digit is another disadvantage.

b. Thenar flap—The thenar flap may be used in children and young (less than 25 years) adults in whom the potential for joint stiffness is less. More subcutaneous fat is transferred with a thenar flap than with a cross-finger flap. Thenar skin flaps usually result in good matching of color and texture with the pulp.

◼ NAIL BED INJURIES

Clinical Findings

Nail bed injuries, often neglected, should be carefully attended to because the nail enhances sensibility, provides protection and fine manipulation of the finger, and gives the finger a normal appearance. The nail bed may be injured by subungual hematoma, nail matrix laceration, avulsion of the nail matrix from the nail fold, or complete loss of the nail matrix.

Treatment

When a subungual hematoma involves more than 50% of the subungual area, the nail should be removed and the nail bed laceration repaired with fine absorbable suture. Either the nail is replaced or a dressing is placed under the nail fold to prevent synechia formation with resultant splitting of the nail. Nail bed defects are treated with split-thickness nail bed grafts taken from either an adjacent uninjured fingernail or a toenail.

When nail bed injuries occur with an open distal phalangeal fracture, pin fixation of the fracture may be considered because it stabilizes the nail bed repair.

Caution is required in the treatment of nail bed injuries in children, who often suffer injury from having a fingertip slammed in a door. The nail often lies dorsal to the nail fold, and a small subungual hematoma is noted. If a radiograph is obtained, usually a physeal fracture of the distal phalanx is observed. Because the nail bed laceration communicates with the physeal fracture, this injury represents an open fracture and must be treated appropriately. The nail should be removed and the fracture site irrigated. An interposed portion of the nail bed often must be extracted from between the fragments of the physeal fracture. If the fracture is unstable, pin fixation facilitates nail bed repair. Failure to appreciate the open nature of this pediatric injury may result in osteomyelitis and physeal arrest of the distal phalanx.

Heistein JB, Cook PA: Factors affecting composite graft survival in digital tip amputations. Ann Plast Surg 2003;50:299. [PMID: 12800909]

■ THERMAL INJURY

ACUTE BURN INJURY

Degree of Injury

A. First-Degree Burns

Burns are characterized by the depth of skin injury. First-degree burns involve only the epidermis. Patients usually present with swollen red areas, and care is symptomatic.

B. Second-Degree Burns

Second-degree burns involve both the epidermis and the superficial portion of the dermis. These burns may be identified by skin blistering and blanching of the skin when pressure is applied. Second-degree burns are subdivided into superficial and deep burns. Superficial second-degree burns are treated with topical antibiotics such as silver sulfadiazine. The extremity is elevated and the hand splinted in the intrinsic plus position. With the wrist in 30 degrees of extension, the metacarpophalangeal joint is flexed and the interphalangeal joints are extended. The thumb should be maintained in an abducted position to prevent contracture of the first web space. The patient should begin a vigorous therapy program emphasizing active ROM as soon as it is tolerated. Compression garments may deduce swelling and scar hypertrophy after reepithelialization.

In deep second-degree burns, excision of the remaining portion of the skin and application of a skin graft does not produce long-term results superior to those achieved with spontaneous healing. Therefore, the treatment of deep second-degree burns should be similar to that of superficial second-degree burns.

C. Third-Degree Burns

Third-degree burns involve the entire epidermis, dermis, and a portion of the subcutaneous region. These burns result in waxy dry regions often having a nontender central area, caused by burning of the neural tissue. Third-degree burns should be treated with excision within the first 3–7 days and a split-thickness skin graft applied to the involved areas.

D. Fourth-Degree Burns

In addition to involvement of the skin, fourth-degree burns involve deep tissues, including muscle, tendon, and bone. Often, the only effective treatment for these burns is amputation of the involved part, with appropriate soft-tissue coverage of the residual stump.

Complications

A. Neurovascular Complications

The neurovascular status of the burned hand should be carefully monitored. Massive swelling necessitates release of compartments of the hand and forearm. Digital releases are best performed by longitudinal releases along the ulnar border of the index, middle, and ring fingers and along the radial border of the thumb and little finger. Longitudinal incisions on the dorsal hand allow decompression of interosseous muscle compartments. Incisions are made along the medial and lateral aspects of the arm and forearm.

B. Late Complications

1. Joint contractures—Joint contractures are the most common complications of upper extremity burns. At the elbow, these are most often flexion contractures. Treatment consists of soft-tissue release and either skin grafting of open regions or rotation of local skin flaps. Elbow motion may also be limited by the development of heterotopic ossifications. Excision of the ossification may be successful if delayed until the area of ossification has matured, often 1.5–2 years after the burn injury. Because the area of most intense heterotopic ossification is posteromedially, care must be taken to define and protect the ulnar nerve during elbow release surgery.

2. Wrist and hand contractures—Wrist contracture may tether the hand into either a flexed or extended position, depending on the region of the burn. In the fingers, burns usually involve the thin skin on the dorsum of the finger, often disrupting the central slip insertion onto the middle phalanx. The loss of active proximal interphalangeal joint extension combined with dorsal hand burns may result in development of a clawlike deformity, with flexion contractures of the proximal interphalangeal joints and hyperextension contracture at the metacarpophalangeal joint.

Treatment of metacarpophalangeal joint extension contracture usually requires release of the dorsal scar, addition of a dorsal skin graft, and dorsal metatarsophalangeal joint capsular release. Proximal interphalangeal flexion contractures may also occur secondary to scarred volar skin. In such cases, soft tissue release may be accomplished with either Z-plasty flap transposition or by palmar scar excision and full-thickness skin graft application. The most predictable treatment of severe proximal interphalangeal joint contracture in the burn patient is arthrodesis of the proximal interphalangeal joint.

Adduction contracture, the most common thumb deformity in the burned hand, may be difficult to resolve fully. The extent of release required depends on the degree of contracture. A modest adduction contracture may be effectively treated with Z-plasty of the thenar skin to regain adequate abduction in the first web space. With more severe contracture, release of the adductor pollicis from its origin or at its insertion and release of the first dorsal interosseous muscle origin from the thumb metacarpal may be required. If web space skin coverage is inadequate after muscle release, full-thickness skin grafting or local or distant skin flaps may be needed.

Ideally, first web space contracture should be avoided by carefully maintaining the first web space during the initial phases of burn treatment. When the extent of web space burn is severe and the normal first web cannot be maintained with dressings, an external fixator should be placed, spanning the thumb and index-finger metacarpals.

ELECTRICAL BURNS

The extent of injury in electrical burns is proportional to the amount of current that passes through the involved portion of the body. The Ohm law states that the amount of current is equal to the voltage divided by the resistance. Therefore, for a given voltage, those structures that have a lower resistance conduct a greater amount of current. The relative resistance of structures in the arm from least resistance to greatest resistance is as follows: nerve, vessel, muscle, skin, tendon, fat, and bone. Alternating current is more injurious than direct current. Because of its frequency, alternating current produces muscle tetany in the finger flexors, which may prevent the patient from releasing the grasped current source. The duration of contact plays a direct role in the severity of injury because a longer contact period results in more electrical energy passing through the body.

Clinical Findings

The greatest current density occurs at the entrance and exit wounds, usually apparent as charred areas that are blackened and surrounded by a gray-white zone, an area of tissue necrosis in which the tissue is still intact but will die. These areas are surrounded by a red zone, in which there is a variable extent of vessel thrombosis, coagulation, and necrosis.

High-voltage, or arc, burns produce a greater thermal than electric injury. Arc burns may extend across flexor surfaces from the hand to the wrist or from the forearm to the arm. Arc burns are usually associated with a high temperature of 3000–5000°C.

It is difficult to assess precisely the extent of tissue necrosis in burn wounds at the time of initial presentation. All burn patients should be examined for fractures, particularly cervical spine fractures, because electrical burn patients were possibly thrown a distance by the current. The possibility of either compartment syndrome or concomitant peripheral nerve injury must also be considered. Patients should be admitted to an intensive care unit and monitored for cardiac arrhythmia, renal failure, sepsis, secondary hemorrhage, and neurologic complications to the brain, spinal cord, or peripheral nerves.

Treatment

Treatment for upper extremity burns consists of initially debriding clearly nonviable tissue. The decision to carry out fasciotomy and nerve decompression should be guided by examination. A second debridement is performed 48–72 hours later, for tissue in the gray-white zones. Debridement should be continued every 48–72 hours until a stable wound is achieved. The extent of necrosis often appears to increase with each successive debridement. This phenomenon reflects both an underestimation of the extent of initial injury and progressive vascular thrombosis. After all necrotic tissue is debrided, reconstruction is accomplished with either local or distant skin flaps or amputation.

CHEMICAL BURNS

The severity of chemical burns is directly proportional to the concentration and penetrability of the offending agent, the duration of skin exposure, and the mechanism of contact. Tissue destruction continues until either the chemical combines with tissue or the agent is neutralized by an applied secondary agent or washed from the skin surface. The mainstay of treatment of chemical burns of the skin is irrigation with water.

Two notable exceptions are burns resulting from hydrofluoric acid and from white phosphorous. Because hydrofluoric acid cannot be removed with water, calcium gluconate 10%, either applied to the skin as a gel or injected subcutaneously, is required to neutralize the acid. Patients with hydrofluoride burns experience severe pain seemingly out of proportion to the injury. White phosphorus burns, also refractory to water irrigation, are treated with 1% copper sulfate solution.

Iatrogenic chemical burns may occur with extravasation of chemotherapeutic agents administered intravenously. Chemotherapeutic agents are classified as vesicants, which include doxorubicin and vincristine and have a high probability of causing skin necrosis, and nonvesicants, which include cyclophosphamide. Management of both types of injury requires early surgical debridement of the region of extravasation. Secondary wound coverage may be obtained by either split-thickness skin grafting or skin flap coverage.

COLD INJURY (FROSTBITE)

Clinical Findings

Frostbite occurs as the result of cellular injury when the cell membrane is punctured by ice crystals formed in the extracellular space. With the formation of ice crystals, osmotic gradients develop, leading to cell dehydration and electrolyte disturbances. Patients may develop severe vasoconstriction as a result of increased sympathetic tone. Vessel endothelial injury may cause thrombosis. With capillary endothelial damage, leakage occurs into the extracellular space, resulting in hemoconcentration and sludging within the capillary system.

Frostbite injuries may be classified as either superficial or deep. Superficial frostbite involves only the skin and usually heals spontaneously, whereas deep frostbite damages both the skin and subcutaneous structures (Figure 10–39). As with burn injuries, the depth of the area of necrosis is difficult to determine initially.

Treatment

The initial treatment of frostbite consists of rewarming the part and providing pain relief. The core body temperature should be restored and the frozen extremity rapidly rewarmed in a water bath at 38–42°C. Because rapid rewarming induces considerable pain, it should be delayed until adequate analgesia can be administered. After rewarming, treatment should include elevation of the hand, local wound care, and dressing changes. Frequent whirlpool debridement and active ROM exercises should be instituted. The role of anticoagulants and sympathectomy in increasing blood flow is controversial.

Long-Term Sequelae

Long-term sequelae depend on the extent of initial injury. Adult patients may develop osteoarthritis of the

Figure 10–39. Radiograph of deformities of the fingers of the left hand in a 12-year-old girl caused by frostbite incurred at 2 years of age. Note destruction of epiphyses of middle and distal phalanges of all fingers and deformity of epiphysis of proximal phalanx of little finger. Osseous changes in right hand were similar.

interphalangeal joints. Skeletally immature patients may develop epiphyseal destruction, with digital shortening, nail dysplasia, and joint destruction. Severe injuries may produce intrinsic muscle atrophy or vasospastic syndrome secondary to increased sympathetic tone. Vasospasm may lead to severe pain, coldness, or edema of the finger; trophic changes leading to decreased nail or hair growth; or Raynaud phenomenon. In severe injuries, mummification of nonviable portions of the fingers may become apparent. Amputation or surgical debridement of these mummified parts should usually be delayed 60–90 days, unless local infection develops. This delay allows maximal reepithelialization beneath the nonviable tissue.

Woo SH, Seul JH: Optimizing the correction of severe postburn hand deformities by using aggressive contracture releases and fasciocutaneous free-tissue transfers. Plast Reconstr Surg 2001;107(1):1. [PMID: 11176593]

■ HIGH-PRESSURE INJECTION INJURY

Injection machinery used in industry may create pressures of 3000–10,000 psi. The amount of pressure reflects both the design of the nozzle aperture and the distance between the nozzle and the finger. Virtually all patients who sustain injuries with pressures of over 7000 psi require amputation.

Clinical Findings

Injection injuries usually puncture the palmar digital pulp, track to the flexor tendon sheath, and fill the tendon sheath with the injected material. These injuries have a poor prognosis. Injections into the palm have a somewhat better prognosis because the site of the material is unconfined by fascial planes. Prognostic factors include the time interval from injury to treatment, as well as the amount and type of material injected. Whereas paint injection may cause more necrosis of the finger, grease injection more often leads to fibrosis of the finger. The amputation rate for paint injection injuries is approximately 60%; the rate for grease injection injuries is 20%.

The examiner must be wary of an innocuous-appearing entrance wound at the time of presentation. Initial pain may be modest but increases with time as more distal swelling and early necrosis occur.

Treatment

The effectiveness of corticosteroids administered every 6 hours remains controversial in the treatment of injection injuries. Patients should be operatively treated soon after the injury occurs. Thorough debridement of all injected material is easier when the injected material is pigmented. Nonpigmented materials such as kerosene or turpentine are considerably more difficult to remove thoroughly. The hand should be splinted in the safe position. Sympathetic blocks may be helpful in managing pain. Repeat debridement should be done if there is doubt about the adequacy of the initial procedure.

Although injection injuries may appear simple, these severe injuries compromise function and result in amputation. The seriousness of these injuries should be recognized at the time of presentation.

Christodoulou L et al: Functional outcome of high-pressure injection injuries of the hand. J Trauma 2001;50:717. [PMID: 11303170]

Gutowski KA et al: High-pressure hand injuries caused by dry cleaning solvents: Case reports, review of the literature, and treatment guidelines. Plast Reconstr Surg 2003;111:174. [PMID: 12496578]

Luber KT, Rehm JP, Freeland AE: High-pressure injection injuries of the hand. Orthopedics 2005;28:129. [PMID: 15751366]

■ INFECTIONS OF THE HAND

Felon

A felon is an abscess of the pulp space of the distal phalanx. Vertical septa between the skin and the bone create small closed compartments within the pulp space. Infection in this region produces localized erythema, swelling, and throbbing pain.

Treatment of these infections requires incision and drainage, with release of the vertical septa to decompress the pulp space completely (Figure 10–40). A drain is placed in the wound, the hand is elevated, and intravenous antibiotics are administered.

Paronychia

Paronychia is the most common digital infection. The paronychia is the gutter along both the radial and ulnar borders of the fingernail. The eponychium is the roof of the nail over the nail lunula. Paronychial infections may be classified as acute or chronic.

A. Acute Infection

Acute infections are most often caused by *Staphylococcus aureus.* These infections begin as a localized cellulitis, with erythema around the nail. Untreated, this cellulitis may progress to an abscess at the nail margin.

Treatment of early infection includes warm soaks and oral antibiotics. Once an abscess forms, incision and drainage is required. To debride the region adequately, either an incision is made in the abscess and the abscess packed, or a portion of the lateral nail is removed and the abscess decompressed.

B. Chronic Infection

Chronic paronychial infections are most often caused by *Candida* species. These occur commonly in patients who work with their hands in water, such as bartenders or dishwashers. Patients may have repeated episodes of acute infection in addition to chronic infection.

Treatment of chronic infection may be accomplished by eponychial marsupialization, excision of a segment of the eponychia without incision of the nail roof. Simultaneous nail removal may increase the effectiveness of marsupialization.

Web Space Abscess

Web space abscesses most often occur after palmar puncture wounds. The infection spreads from the palm along the path of least resistance to the dorsal web space. Treatment requires dorsal and palmar incision, drain placement, open wound care, and appropriate antibiotic coverage.

Figure 10–40. Incisions for drainage of felons. **A:** Unilateral longitudinal approach that should be used for most felons. It is generally made on the ulnar side of the finger, unless it is the little finger, to preserve sensation. **B:** The hockey stick, or J, incision should be reserved for extensive or severe abscess or felon. **C:** The incision must decompress the longitudinal septa but should not go through and through. **D:** The felon that points volarly may be decompressed through a longitudinal midline incision, which is preferable because of less risk to sensory nerves. A transverse incision may also be made, but there is risk of damage to the digital nerves. (Courtesy of HB Skinner, ©copyright 2002.)

Flexor Suppurative Tenosynovitis

Kanavel described four cardinal signs of acute suppurative tenosynovitis: (1) pain on passive digital extension; (2) flexed position of the digit; (3) symmetric swelling of the digit, which may include the palm; and (4) tenderness with palpation along the flexor tendon sheath. Acute suppurative tenosynovitis of the flexor pollicis longus sheath may extend into the thenar space. Likewise, infections in the flexor sheath of the little finger may extend into the ulnar bursa. In some patients, coalescence between the radial and ulnar bursas may allow infection to track in a horseshoe pattern, extending from the thumb to the little finger.

Treatment of acute suppurative tenosynovitis requires incision, irrigation, and drainage. Although an extensive midlateral incision may be used, limited incisions are preferred. Short incisions over the proximal (metacarpophalangeal joint region) and distal (distal interphalangeal region) margins of the flexor tendon sheath allow thorough sheath irrigation (Figure 10–41). The sheath is opened distally and a small tube (16-gauge catheter or number 8 pediatric feeding tube) is inserted. A drain is

Figure 10–41. Drainage and closed irrigation for flexor sheath infection. The antibiotic solution drips in through the distal catheter and drains out through the proximal one. (Reproduced, with permission, from Way LW, ed: *Current Surgical Diagnosis and Treatment*, 10th ed. Appleton & Lange, 1994.)

placed in the flexor sheath through the proximal wound. Irrigation of the finger is performed with 5 mL of saline injected every 2 hours. Intravenous antibiotics are administered, and the hand is elevated.

Two days after surgery the dressing is changed. Swelling should be significantly decreased. The catheter is removed, and the patient is encouraged to begin active ROM exercises.

Bite Injuries

Although bite wounds may initially appear harmless, a bite may inoculate deep tissues with virulent organisms.

A. CAT AND DOG BITES

Because the small puncture wounds of cat bites are more likely to be disregarded than the large tearing wounds of dog bites, late sequelae are more common after cat bites. Cat and dog bites frequently harbor *Pasteurella multocida*, an organism best treated with ampicillin, penicillin, or a first-generation cephalosporin. Acute animal bites may be treated with incision and drainage and an initial course of intravenous antibiotics in the emergency room followed by oral antibiotics.

B. HUMAN BITES

Most human bite wounds result from a fist striking a tooth, which readily penetrates the skin, subcutaneous tissue, extensor tendon, and capsule of the metacarpophalangeal joint (Figure 10–42). Human bites often contain *Eikenella corrodens*, an organism best treated with penicillin or ampicillin. Human bite wounds should be excised and drained, and intravenous antibiotic therapy instituted. Arthrotomy of the metacarpophalangeal joint and irrigation is necessary if this injury is suspected.

C. SPIDER BITES

Although most spider bites are innocuous, the bite of a brown recluse spider requires early wide excision to control the locally injected toxin.

Infection Caused by Unusual Organisms

A. ATYPICAL MYCOBACTERIAL INFECTION

Mycobacterium marinum infection may present as a chronically inflamed finger that was punctured by the spine or a fin of a saltwater fish. Successful culture of the organism is difficult but is most likely at a temperature of 30–32°C. Antitubercular drug therapy is effective in treating and eradicating these infections.

B. GRAM-NEGATIVE INFECTION

Because of the risk of a gram-negative infection following mutilating farm injuries or injuries with possible

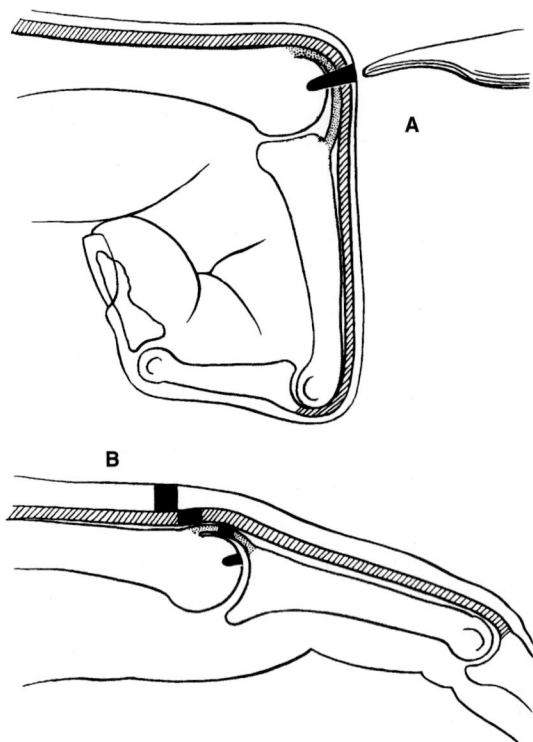

Figure 10–42. Human bite wound of metacarpophalangeal joint. **A:** The tooth pierces the clenched fist of the attacker, penetrating skin, tendon, joint capsule, and metacarpal head. **B:** When the finger is extended by swelling and at surgery, the four puncture wounds do not correspond. (Reproduced, with permission, from Lister G: *The Hand: Diagnosis and Indications*, 3rd ed. Churchill Livingstone, 1993.)

fecal contamination, these patients should be treated with broad-spectrum antibiotics.

C. ANAEROBIC INFECTION

When *Clostridium perfringens* infection occurs after hand injury, immediate wide fasciotomy and intravenous penicillin should be instituted. Hyperbaric oxygen therapy may be helpful. If infection cannot be adequately controlled, amputation may be necessary to avoid death.

The possibility of *Clostridium tetani* contamination must be remembered with any puncture wound. Initial evaluation of all patients with penetrating wounds must include questioning about tetanus inoculation. If inoculation is not up to date, antitoxin should be administered.

D. GONORRHEA

A patient who presents with an isolated septic joint or tenosynovitis without a history of puncture wound may have a hematogenous gonorrheal infection. Treatment consists of culturing the involved organism on the appropriate media and treatment with penicillin or tetracycline.

E. NECROTIZING FASCIITIS

The causative agent in necrotizing fasciitis is most commonly hemolytic *Staphylococcus*. Treatment consists of wide surgical debridement to the fascia and appropriate antibiotics.

F. HERPETIC WHITLOW

Herpes simplex infections may involve the fingertips. They are most common in medical or dental personnel who care for the oral tracheal area and are also seen in small children. It may be difficult to distinguish herpetic lesions from acute bacterial infections of the fingers. Close examination reveals the presence of groups (crops) of vesicles, with surrounding erythema. Aspiration of a vesicle yields clear fluid. Serial viral titers confirm the diagnosis. Unlike bacterial infections, herpetic whitlow should not be incised but simply treated with splinting and elevation.

Connor RW, Kimbrough RC, Dabezies MJ: Hand Infections in patients with diabetes. Orthopedics 2001;24:1057. [PMID: 11727802]

Huish SB et al: Pyoderma gangrenosum of the hand: A case series and review of the literature. J Hand Surg 2001;26A:679. [PMID: 11466644.]

Karanas YL, Bogdan MA, Chang J: Community acquired methicillin-resistant *Staphylococcus aureus* hand infections: Case reports and clinical implications. J Hand Surg Am 2000;25:760. [PMID: 1093220]

Perron AD, Miller MD, Brady WJ: Orthopedic pitfalls in the ED: Fight bites. Am J Emerg Med 2002;20:114. [PMID: 11880877]

■ ARTHRITIS OF THE HAND

OSTEOARTHRITIS

Osteoarthritis is a slowly progressive polyarticular disorder of unknown cause, predominantly affecting the hands and large weight-bearing joints. Clinically, osteoarthritis is characterized by pain, deformity, and limitation of motion. Focal erosions, articular cartilage space loss, subchondral sclerosis, cyst formation, and peripheral joint osteophytes are evident on radiographic examination.

Epidemiologic Factors

The disease occurs commonly in older individuals, with approximately 80–90% of adults older than 75 years showing radiographic evidence of osteoarthritis. The strongest predictors of developing osteoarthritis of the hand are female gender, increasing age, and positive family history.

The most frequently involved joints in the hand are the distal interphalangeal joints, carpometacarpal joint of the thumb (Figure 10–43), and proximal interphalangeal joints. The bony enlargements commonly seen in the osteoarthritic distal interphalangeal joint are referred to as Heberden nodes, whereas osteoarthritic enlargements at the proximal interphalangeal joint are known as Bouchard nodes.

Secondary osteoarthritis may develop in the hand as the result of trauma, avascular necrosis, prior inflammatory arthritis, or metabolic disorders.

Figure 10–43. Osteoarthritis of the carpometacarpal joint of the thumb.

Clinical Findings

Patients with osteoarthritis of the hand often complain of activity-induced or work-related pain. Most patients experience periods of exacerbation and remission. Functional limitations result from pain, weakness, loss of motion, and deformity. Tenderness and enlargement of the distal and proximal interphalangeal joints are noted on examination. Axial compression of the thumb trapeziometacarpal with a circumduction motion (grind test) reproduces pain. As the disease progresses, radial subluxation of the thumb metacarpal on the trapezium may develop, leading to adduction deformity of the metacarpal.

Treatment

Nonoperative treatment includes oral nonsteroidal anti-inflammatory medication (NSAIDs), long-acting intraarticular steroid injection, and splint immobilization.

The primary indication for surgery is pain unresponsive to oral medication and splinting. Distal interphalangeal joint arthrodesis relieves pain, corrects deformity, and resolves joint instability. Because the severely arthritic distal interphalangeal joint is often stiff, the additional loss of motion occasioned by arthrodesis is usually well tolerated. The distal interphalangeal joint is fused in 10–15 degrees of flexion, a position in which the fingernail is parallel with the axis of the middle phalanx.

At the proximal interphalangeal joint, pain is the primary indication for surgery. Implant arthroplasty may be helpful in relieving pain and retaining motion in the ring and little fingers. The motion attained from implant arthroplasty is less in the proximal interphalangeal joints than in the metacarpophalangeal joints. Implant arthroplasty is usually avoided in the index- or middle-finger proximal interphalangeal joint because of residual instability to lateral or key pinch.

Arthrodesis effectively relieves pain at the proximal interphalangeal joint and provides pinch stability. The ideal position of arthrodesis varies from the radial to the ulnar digits. The index-finger proximal interphalangeal joint is usually fused at 40 degrees of flexion, the middle finger at 45 degrees, the ring finger at 50 degrees, and the little finger at 55 degrees.

At the trapeziometacarpal joint, conservative treatment includes a hand-based thumb spica splint with the interphalangeal joint left free, cortisone injections, and NSAIDs. Many patients with advanced degenerative changes on radiograph obtain good pain relief with conservative therapy.

The primary indication for surgery is persistent pain. Trapezium resection arthroplasty relieves pain at the trapeziometacarpal joint and allows retention of full metacarpal base motion. Either the distal half of the tra-

pezium or the entire trapezium may be resected. A tendon interposition is created using either the flexor carpi radialis or a slip of the abductor pollicis longus. The tendon may be threaded through a drill hole in the articular surface of the thumb metacarpal to suspend the thumb. The remaining tendon is rolled into a so-called anchovy and placed in the space of the excised trapezium. This reconstruction prevents impingement of the metacarpal on the scaphoid. After surgery, the thumb is immobilized in a cast or splint for 6 weeks.

Arthrodesis of the thumb carpometacarpal joint is an alternative to trapeziectomy. With the joint fused, patients are unable to lay their hand flat on a table. However, pain relief is excellent, and it may be the procedure of choice for a young laborer.

RHEUMATOID ARTHRITIS

RA is a chronic inflammatory disease of unknown cause. The combined effect of tenosynovitis and synovitis on joints and periarticular tissues results in progressive joint destruction and deformity. RA affects 0.3–1.5% of the population. Women are two to three times more commonly affected than men.

Clinical Findings

Evaluation of the hand affected by RA requires care. The goal is to determine which of the patient's many problems—pain, weakness, or mechanical dysfunction—is most problematic. Evaluation detects tendon rupture, adherence, or triggering as well as nerve compression symptoms. The most common nerve compression syndromes involve compression of the median nerve at the wrist and compression of the radial nerve at the elbow. The appearance of rheumatoid nodules and ulnar drift deformity at the metacarpophalangeal joint may be disturbing aesthetically. Rheumatoid nodules, occurring in 20–25% of patients with RA, are not treated unless associated with erosion, pain, or infection.

Treatment

The shoulder, elbow, forearm, wrist, and hand should be examined individually. The goal of surgical reconstruction is restoration of a functional upper extremity, not just a functional hand. Indications for surgical intervention include relieving pain, slowing the progression of disease, improving function, and improving appearance.

Surgical treatment may be classified as either preventive or corrective. Preventive options include tenosynovectomy and synovectomy. Corrective procedures include tendon transfers, nerve decompression, soft-tissue reconstruction, and arthrodesis.

Synovectomy is considered in patients who have pauciarticular persistent synovitis while under good medical control. Contraindications to synovectomy include rapidly progressive disease, multiple joint involvement, and underlying joint destruction.

A. ELBOW RECONSTRUCTION

Synovitis of the elbow joint may cause pain, joint destruction, and radial nerve compression. Nodules or bursas are common over the olecranon. Surgical treatment of the rheumatoid elbow includes radial head excision and synovectomy. As the disease progresses, consideration may be given to total elbow arthroplasty.

B. WRIST RECONSTRUCTION

RA frequently involves the wrist and occurs in a predictable pattern. On the radial side of the wrist, the radioscaphocapitate and the radiolunototriquetral ligaments are attenuated, permitting rotatory displacement of the scaphoid. Scapholunate dissociation is followed by radiocarpal collapse.

On the ulnar side of the wrist, the ulnar carpal ligaments become attenuated, allowing the carpus to drift radially as the carpus translates ulnarward. Attenuation of the distal radioulnar joint allows the head of the ulna to displace dorsally, producing caput-ulnae syndrome. The extensor carpi ulnaris tendon displaces volarly. These changes lead to supination of the carpus on the radius, ulnar translocation of the carpus, and a concomitant radialward displacement of the metacarpals (Figure 10–44). The carpus may also dislocate volarly beneath the radius.

Surgical treatment consists of extensor tenosynovectomy, with transposition of the dorsal retinaculum over the wrist joint to reinforce the capsule, and wrist synovectomy. The extensor carpi ulnaris tendon can be relocated from a volar to a dorsal position.

Figure 10–44. Radialward displacement of the metacarpals in rheumatoid arthritis.

If pain is present over the distal ulna or if rupture of the little- or ring-finger extensor tendon results from a sharp prominence of the distal ulna, then resection of the distal ulna is performed. Fusion of the rheumatoid wrist provides stability and may increase function. Either a total wrist arthrodesis or a radiolunate arthrodesis may be elected, depending on the extent of midcarpal joint involvement.

C. HAND RECONSTRUCTION

Triggering of the digits is a common problem caused by flexor tenosynovitis. The A1 pulley should not be incised in the treatment of rheumatoid trigger digits. Loss of the A1 pulley increases the tendency of the fingers to drift ulnarward. Instead, tenosynovectomy and excision of the ulnar slip of the sublimis tendon should be considered.

If flexor tendon rupture occurs, treatment may include tendon transfer, bridge grafting, or joint fusion. The flexor tendon that most commonly ruptures is the flexor pollicis longus because it rubs over an osteophyte on the volar aspect of the scaphotrapezial joint (Mannerfelt lesion). Extensor tendon ruptures are caused by attrition of the common extensor tendon of the ring and little fingers over the distal ulna (Vaughn-Johnson syndrome).

Treatment of the arthritic hand depends on the joints involved. The distal interphalangeal joint is usually best treated by arthrodesis. At the proximal interphalangeal joint, synovectomy may be performed if synovitis is isolated to the proximal interphalangeal joint without multiple joint involvement. Alternatives for the more involved joint are arthroplasty or arthrodesis.

At the metacarpophalangeal joint, inflammation of the synovium may cause the extensor mechanism to sublux ulnarly because of attenuation of the radial sagittal band. The mechanism may be relocated to improve function of the joint. For isolated joints without significant destruction, synovectomy may be performed. With more severe joint destruction, resection implant arthroplasty is required (Figure 10–45). Subluxation and ulnar drift alone are not absolute indications for arthroplasty if satisfactory function of the hand remains. Arthroplasty does not increase the ROM of the metaphalangeal joints, but it changes its arc. Because most patients have severe flexion and ulnar deviation of the joints, arthroplasty provides a more functional ROM, especially for grasping large objects. Because the implants fracture with extensive use, silicone arthroplasty is indicated only in the low-demand hand and is therefore better suited to rheumatoid than osteoarthritic patients.

1. Boutonnière deformity—In addition to arthritis, various finger deformities occur related to soft-tissue damage. At the proximal interphalangeal joints, the most common is boutonnière deformity. Because of proximal interphalangeal joint synovitis, the central slip is either elongated or ruptured, which allows the proximal interphalangeal joint to flex and the lateral bands to

A   **B**

Figure 10–45. **A:** Preoperative view of metacarpophalangeal joint in rheumatoid arthritis. **B:** Following resection arthroplasty.

sublux volarly. As the lateral bands migrate below the proximal interphalangeal joint axis, they become active proximal interphalangeal flexors rather than extensors. In addition to increasing the proximal interphalangeal joint deformity, the relative shortening of the extensor mechanism leads to distal interphalangeal joint hyperextension. Treatment of mild boutonnière deformities, which are passively correctable, consists of synovectomy and splinting. Lateral band reconstruction may be considered to relocate the bands dorsal to the axis of rotation. Alternatively, tenotomy of the terminal slip may be done to allow relaxation of the extensor mechanism and prevent hyperextension of the distal interphalangeal joint. Once moderate deformity of the proximal interphalangeal joint occurs (30- to 40-degree flexion deformity, with a flexible joint and preservation of the joint space), consideration may be given to reconstruction of the central slip as well as lateral band reconstruction and terminal tendon tenotomy. In the final stage of boutonnière deformity, the joint deformity becomes fixed, and the best form of treatment is arthroplasty or fusion.

2. Swan-neck deformity—Swan-neck deformities consist of hyperextension at the proximal interphalangeal joint and flexion at the distal interphalangeal joint. The mechanism of swan-neck deformity is terminal tendon rupture or attenuation, with secondary hyperextension of the proximal interphalangeal joint resulting from overpulling of the central slip or proximal interphalangeal joint hyperextension caused by laxity of the volar plate, rupture of the flexor digitorum superficialis, or intrinsic tightness. The most common of these mechanisms is intrinsic tightness secondary to metacarpophalangeal joint synovitis.

Swan-neck deformities are divided into four stages. In stage 1, the joints are supple in all positions. Treatment consists of splinting, distal interphalangeal joint fusion, or soft-tissue reconstruction to limit proximal interphalangeal joint hyperextension. In stage 2, proximal interphalangeal flexion is limited because of intrinsic tightness. Intrinsic release with or without reconstruction of the metacarpophalangeal joint may be of benefit. In stage 3, proximal interphalangeal joint motion is limited in all positions, yet the joint is still preserved. Mobilization of the lateral bands may help relieve this deformity. Finally, in stage 4, the proximal interphalangeal joint is arthritic. Either proximal interphalangeal arthrodesis or arthroplasty should be considered for stage 4 joint destruction.

3. Synovitic metacarpophalangeal joint deformity— The metacarpophalangeal joints subluxes volarly and ulnarly in RA. This deformity results from synovial invasion of the collateral ligaments with secondary laxity, volar and ulnar forces that are normally present on the joint, augmentation of these forces by radial deviation of the wrist, attenuation of the radial sagittal band (allowing ulnar subluxation of the extensor tendon), and contracture of the intrinsic muscles. Treatment of the synovitic metacarpophalangeal joint consists of medical management and splinting. When the joint space is preserved, surgical synovectomy may provide symptomatic relief. Once moderate joint destruction or volar subluxation and ulnar deviation occurs, the decision about surgery is based on the function of the hand. When the patient is still able to use the hand for activities of daily living, splinting and other assistive aids are provided. Once loss of function is noted, metacarpophalangeal arthroplasty is considered. In performing metacarpophalangeal arthroplasty, the wrist deformity should first be corrected, and all soft-tissue releases required to relieve the subluxing forces should be performed. The radial collateral ligament of the index finger should be reconstructed, and the extensor tendon should be relocated. Postoperatively, extensive splinting and therapy are required to hold the hand in proper position. Therapy utilizes an outrigger splint holding the wrist in dorsiflexion and the metaphalangeal joints in full extension and neutral radial-ulnar alignment. The splint is worn full time for 6 weeks and part time for 3 months. The patient wears a resting pan splint at night for 1 year.

D. THUMB RECONSTRUCTION

Three patterns of rheumatoid thumb deformities are defined. In type 1 deformity, the metacarpophalangeal joint is flexed while the interphalangeal joint is hyperextended and the thumb metacarpal is secondarily abducted. In type 2 and 3 deformities, carpometacarpal subluxation leads to metacarpal adduction. In type 2 deformities, interphalangeal joint hyperextension develops with metacarpophalangeal flexion, and in type 3 deformities, the metacarpophalangeal joint is hyperextended and the interphalangeal joint is flexed. Type 2 deformities are unusual. Type 1 deformities are usually initiated by synovitis of the metacarpophalangeal joint, leading to attenuation of the extensor pollicis brevis tendon, intrinsic muscle tightness, and ulnar and volar displacement of the extensor pollicis longus.

Treatment is based on the degree of progression. In type 1 deformities, if the metacarpophalangeal and inter-

phalangeal joints are passively correctable, synovectomy and extensor reconstruction may be performed. If the metacarpophalangeal joint flexion deformity is fixed, arthrodesis or arthroplasty of the joint is considered. When fixed metacarpophalangeal flexion and interphalangeal extension deformities are present simultaneously, the interphalangeal joint is fused and the metacarpophalangeal joint is replaced with an arthroplasty or also undergoes arthrodesis.

Type 3 deformities are analogous to swan-neck deformities of the fingers. The carpometacarpal joint disease allows dorsal and radial subluxation of the joint, with secondary adduction contraction of the metacarpal and hyperextension of the metacarpophalangeal joint. Treatment with minimal metacarpophalangeal deformity (stage 1) or passively correctable metacarpophalangeal deformity (stage 2) consists of splinting and carpometacarpal arthroplasty or fusion. Once the metacarpophalangeal deformity becomes fixed (stage 3), first web release and carpometacarpal arthroplasty are required.

E. SURGICAL PRIORITIES

When multilevel deformity is present, consideration should be given to combined procedures. If wrist and metacarpophalangeal deformities are both present, the wrist should be fused prior to or simultaneously with metacarpophalangeal joint reconstruction. When both metacarpophalangeal and proximal interphalangeal joint deformities are present, motion-preserving procedures such as arthroplasty should be carried out at the metacarpophalangeal joint. Treatment of concomitant proximal interphalangeal joint involvement depends on the stage of deformity. Mild to moderate proximal interphalangeal joint deformities can either be ignored or treated by closed manipulation and pin fixation. With severe deformity, arthrodesis of the proximal interphalangeal joint should be performed.

In all cases, attempts should be made to perform multiple procedures under a single anesthetic. These patients often require numerous operations for multiple joints of the upper and lower extremities, and surgical and rehabilitation time must be used judiciously.

Other Inflammatory Arthritides

Other inflammatory conditions related to RA may affect the hand, producing joint destruction and deformity.

A. JUVENILE RHEUMATOID ARTHRITIS

In juvenile rheumatoid arthritis (JRA), early epiphyseal closure occurs as a result of synovitis and increased periarticular blood flow. Narrowing of phalangeal and metacarpal medullary canals makes implant arthroplasty difficult. The metacarpophalangeal joints may deviate radially rather than ulnarly.

B. ARTHRITIS MUTILANS

In arthritis mutilans, axial shortening because of marked bone loss occurs while the soft-tissue envelope is preserved. Early joint fusion is required to avoid progressive bone loss.

C. SYSTEMIC LUPUS ERYTHEMATOSUS

Systemic lupus erythematosus (SLE) affects periarticular soft tissue, resulting in joint laxity with secondary dysfunction. Synovitis is minimal in lupus, and therefore the articular cartilage is preserved. Soft-tissue reconstruction is ineffective, and joint fusions are preferable to restore stability and function. The exception to this is the metacarpophalangeal joints, where implant arthroplasty may be appropriate, even though normal articular cartilage is sacrificed.

D. PSORIATIC ARTHRITIS

Psoriatic arthritis presents deformities similar to that of RA. The hand has a marked tendency to become stiff. In psoriatic arthritis, the metacarpophalangeal joints become stiff in extension, whereas in RA, these joints tend to become stiff in flexion.

Davis TR, Brady O, Dias JJ: Excision of the trapezium for osteoarthritis of the trapeziometacarpal joint: A study of the benefit of ligament reconstruction or tendon interposition. J Hand Surg Am 2004;29:1069. [PMID: 15576217]

Day CS et al: Basal joint osteoarthritis of the thumb: A prospective trial of steroid injection and splinting J Hand Surg Am 2004;29:247. [PMID: 15043897]

Fulton DB, Stern PJ: Trapeziometacarpal arthrodesis in primary osteoarthritis: A minimum two-year follow-up study. J Hand Surg Am 2001;26:109. [PMID: 11172376.]

Jain A et al: Influence of steroids and methotrexate on wound complications after elective rheumatoid hand and wrist surgery. J Hand Surg Am 2002;27:449. [PMID: 12015719]

■ HAND TUMORS

Nearly all mass lesions in the hand or wrist are benign conditions. Foreign body granulomas, epidermoid inclusion cysts, and neuromas are usually related to prior trauma. Ganglions and fibroxanthomas arise adjacent to joints or tendon sheaths.

Ganglion

Ganglions are the most common soft-tissue tumors of the hand and wrist. They are cystic structures filled with a mucinous fluid but without a synovial or epithelial lining. In most cases, a stalk can be identified communicating between the cyst and an adjacent joint or

tendon sheath. The most common locations for ganglions are the wrist, digital flexor sheath, and distal interphalangeal joint (Figure 10–46).

A. DORSAL WRIST GANGLION

Dorsal wrist ganglions arise from the dorsal capsule of the scapholunate joint. Small firm dorsal ganglions may be barely palpable but highly symptomatic, whereas large ganglions are often soft and only mildly symptomatic. Aspiration and steroid injection may provide transient symptomatic relief, but recurrence is frequent. Symptomatic lesions can be surgically excised, with expectation of cure if care is taken to excise the stalk of the lesion with a capsular base from the lesion's origin. Because these lesions arise from the dorsal portion of the scapholunate ligament, care must be taken to preserve the ligament's integrity to avoid an iatrogenic scapholunate dissociation.

B. PALMAR WRIST GANGLION

Palmar wrist ganglions present as swellings on the palmar radial aspect of the wrist, adjacent to the radial artery. These lesions arise from either the palmar radios-

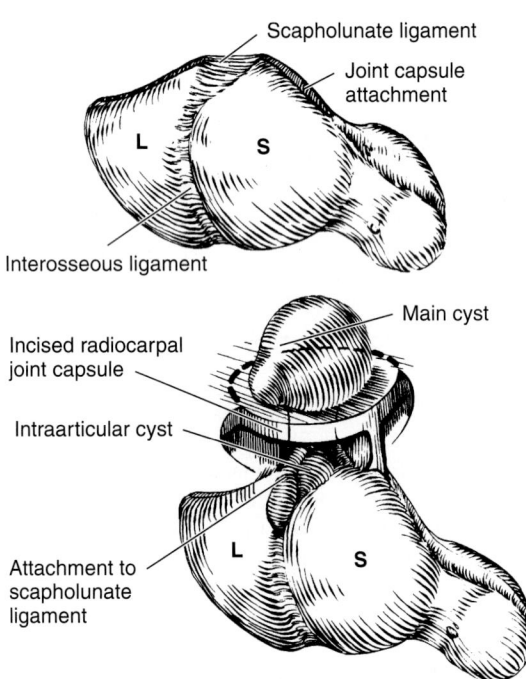

Figure 10–46. The ganglion and scapholunate attachments are isolated from the remaining uninvolved joint capsule (not shown). (Reproduced, with permission, from Green DP, ed: *Operative Hand Surgery*, 2nd ed. Churchill Livingstone, 1988.)

caphoid or palmar scaphotrapezial joint. Surgical resection of the palmar radial ganglion requires mobilization and protection of the adjacent radial artery.

C. Flexor Sheath Ganglion

Flexor sheath ganglions present as firm mass lesions over the palmar aspect of the flexor sheath. The mass is usually between 3 and 8 mm in diameter and often so firm that it is presumed to be a bone exostosis. Treatment of symptomatic lesions is accomplished with aspiration or excision.

D. Mucous Cyst

Mucous cysts are ganglions arising from the distal interphalangeal joint. The neck of the ganglion arises either the radial or ulnar side of the extensor terminal tendon. Surgical excision requires debridement of the joint osteophyte. If the skin is thinned, a local rotation flap is required for soft-tissue coverage after excision.

E. Fibroxanthoma

Fibroxanthomas are also known as giant cell tumors of tendon sheath or tendon sheath xanthomas. These slowly enlarging, firm lesions are usually painless, often arising from an interphalangeal joint. They lesion are usually fixed to deep tissues, more often on the palmar aspect of the hand or finger. Surgical resection requires delineation of adjacent nerves that may be displaced, compressed, or encircled by a fibroxanthoma.

F. Epidermoid Inclusion Cyst

Epidermoid inclusion cysts are usually the result of previous trauma, such as a puncture wound, stab wound, or laceration. Epidermal cells become embedded in the subcutaneous tissue, gradually into an enlarging pearlike mass. Eventually, the mass becomes noticeable, particularly when it is located over the palmar aspect of the pulp. Surgical treatment is excision of the mass without rupture.

G. Foreign Bodies

Foreign bodies may act as a nidus, inciting the development of a surrounding granuloma. This situation may be associated with a local inflammatory reaction or frank infection. Treatment consists of excision.

H. Neuromas

Neuromas, the bulbous enlargement of the distal end of a severed nerve, are a normal response to nerve transection. Neuromas are inevitable in all amputations of the hand. If the neuroma enlargement of the distal end of the proximal segment of the transected nerve is in an area of palmar pulp contact, the lesion may be highly symptomatic. Treatment alternatives include neuroma revision or transposition of the neuroma to a location away from contact stress.

◼ CONGENITAL DIFFERENCES

Congenital hand differences occur in approximately 1 in 1500 live births. The term *differences* is favored over the traditional terms *abnormality, anomaly,* or *malformation.* Many congenital hand differences are part of a well-delineated association or syndrome. The abnormality may suggest that other regions of the body or organ systems be evaluated. When an infant is seen with bilateral total absence of the radius and normal or very mildly hypoplastic thumbs, the possibility of thrombocytopenia with absent radius (TAR) syndrome should be considered and a platelet count obtained. Radial absence may also be associated with the VATER association, children with abnormalities that may include *v*ertebral, *a*nal, *t*racheal, *e*sophageal, and *r*enal defects.

A number of frequently encountered conditions such as cleft hand are inherited as autosomal-dominant traits. The expertise of an experienced geneticist is invaluable in providing counsel to families considering additional children and to patients wishing to know the likelihood that their offspring would be affected by the disorder.

The two most commonly encountered conditions are syndactyly and polydactyly. In white populations, syndactyly is more common, and in African American populations, polydactyly is the most commonly encountered congenital hand anomaly.

Syndactyly

Syndactyly, the webbing together of digits, is simple if soft tissue alone is involved and complex if bone or nails are joined (Figure 10–47). Surgical release of syndactyly requires the use of local flaps to create a floor for the interdigital web space and to partially surface the adjacent sides of the separated digits. Residual defects along

Figure 10–47. Bilateral complex syndactyly of the ring and little fingers.

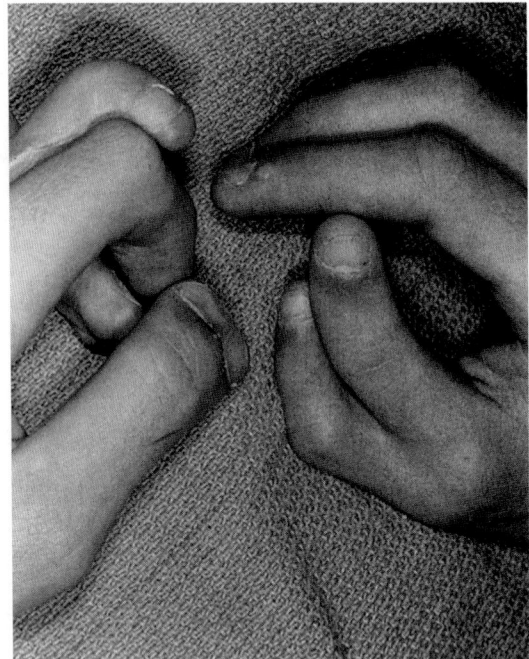

Figure 10–48. Thumb polydactyly.

the sides of the separated fingers are covered with full-thickness skin grafts. Surgery is indicated when the webbing occurs distal to the usual point of separation of the fingers and the webbing prohibits full use of the fingers. Surgery is usually performed at 6–12 months of age.

Polydactyly

Radial polydactyly is usually manifest as thumb duplication. When two thumbs are present in the same hand, they are rarely both normal in size, alignment, and mobility (Figure 10–48). The more ulnar thumb component is usually better developed than the more radial thumb component. The level of bifurcation varies from a wide distal phalanx with two nails, to two digits each possessing a metacarpal and a proximal and distal phalanx. In the most common form of thumb duplication, a single broad metacarpal supports two proximal phalanges, each of which support a distal phalanx. Optimal reconstruction requires merging of elements of both component digits. Usually the ulnar thumb is maintained. If the duplication occurs at the metacarpophalangeal joint, the radial collateral ligament is preserved with the metacarpal and attached to the proximal phalanx of the ulnar thumb. Surgery is usually performed at 6–12 months of age. Ulnar polydactyly, frequent in black children, may usually be treated by simple excision.

Partial or Absent Structures

Absence or partial deficiency of the radius results in inadequate support of the hand and carpus. The unsupported hand angulates radially. Stretching of contracted radial soft-tissue structures is accomplished through repeat manipulation, casting, splinting, or distraction lengthening. The hand is then surgically reoriented onto the end of the ulna by a centralization procedure.

Mild hypoplasia of the thumb is treated by release of the first web space, metacarpophalangeal joint collateral reconstruction and opponensplasty tendon transfer. More sever hypoplasia or absence of the thumb may be treated by pollicization of the index finger. This procedure shifts the index finger to the thumb position and repositions the index-finger extrinsic extensor tendons as well as the dorsal and palmar interosseous tendons to provide balanced control of the shifted digit.

McCarroll HR: Congenital anomalies: A 25-year overview. J Hand Surg Am 2000;25:1007. [PMID: 11119659]

Giele H et al: The incidence and epidemiology of congenital upper limb anomalies: A total population study. J Hand Surg Am 2001;26:628. [PMID: 11466636]

Pediatric Orthopedic Surgery

11

George T. Rab, MD

The scope of pediatric orthopedics ranges from congenital anomalies to injuries in the adolescent. The pathophysiologic manifestations of many of these disorders differ from analogous adult problems because of the added dimension of growth. The physician's relationship with the pediatric patient generally occurs in the context of a protective family environment, in contrast to the more independent relationship the physician may form with an adult. The natural tendency for children to be active and the remarkable regenerative processes of the immature skeleton frequently make formal rehabilitation unnecessary following surgery or serious injury.

Guidelines for Pediatric Orthopedics

The following rules may be helpful when applying general orthopedic principles to the child:

1. A growing bone normally tends to remodel itself toward the adult configuration. This process occurs faster in younger children and in deformities near the ends of bone. Remodeling is faster when deformity is in the plane of motion of the nearest joint.
2. Skeletal deformities worsen as abnormal growth continues (eg, following permanent damage to the growth plate), especially near rapidly growing areas such as the knee. This characteristic is exaggerated in younger children.
3. Children tolerate long-term immobilization better than adults and tend to recover soft-tissue mobility spontaneously following most injuries.
4. Fracture healing is usually more rapid and predictable in the actively growing skeleton than in the adult skeleton.
5. Joint surfaces in children are generally more tolerant of irregularity than those of the adult. Although degenerative arthritic changes may follow childhood injury, there is often an asymptomatic interval of many decades before the process becomes clinically evident.
6. Many so-called deformities, such as metatarsus adductus, internal tibial torsion, and genu valgum (knock-knee), are actually physiologic variations that correct spontaneously with growth. Thus, the clinician must distinguish between conditions that need no treatment and those requiring early intervention.

GROWTH DISORDERS

General skeletal growth is discussed in detail in Chapter 1.

1. Limb-Length Inequality

Limb-length inequality may reflect either a congenital deficiency or any of a wide variety of acquired conditions (Table 11–1). Upper extremities of unequal length are usually only of cosmetic interest and can easily be compensated for by modifying clothing. In the lower extremities, however, length discrepancies may be severe enough—greater than 1 inch (2.5 cm)—to limit function and require treatment. Lesser discrepancies can be managed with a shoe lift.

Treatment

A. CALCULATION OF LIMB LENGTH AT MATURITY

Clinical management of limb-length inequality in pediatric patients should include calculation of projected lengths at maturity. Several mathematical methods, based on skeletal age, gender, and normal growth rates, are available. The following general rule can be used to estimate the extent of future growth: The average growth rates of the distal femur and proximal tibia are 10–12 mm/year and 5–6 mm/year, respectively, with growth continuing until bone age 14 in females and 16 in males.

B. SURGICAL TREATMENT

1. Epiphysiodesis—The simplest surgical procedure to treat pediatric bone-length discrepancies is epiphysiodesis (surgical closure of the growth plate). In the longer limb, it involves curetting or drilling the physis or inserting small bone grafts across the medial and lateral edges of the plate. Epiphysiodesis is usually performed at the distal femoral physis, proximal tibial physis, or both, because they are rapidly growing and easily accessible surgically. The remaining open physes in the limb allow for continued growth but at a slower rate. The exact timing of epiphysiodesis is crucial to attaining equal limb lengths at skeletal maturity. Timing is calculated by the same method used to predict ultimate adult leg length. The effectiveness of epiphysiodesis requires that bone still be growing and that accurate

Table 11–1. Causes of limb-length inequality.

Infectious causes
    Osteomyelitis
    Septic arthritis
Neoplastic causes
    Arteriovenous malformations
    Hemangioma
Neuromuscular causes
    Cerebral palsy
    Isolated limb paralysis
    Poliomyelitis
Traumatic causes
    Malunion of long bones
    Physeal injury
Other causes
    Avascular necrosis of femoral head (and physis)
    Congenital amputations
    Legg-Calvé-Perthes disease

---

data be collected on this growth for several years (ie, scanograms for leg-length measurement, skeletal age).

2. Femoral shortening—If a child reaches the age when bone growth is insufficient to make epiphysiodesis practical, the long leg may be shortened at skeletal maturity by femoral shortening. This may be performed as an open procedure by removing a segment of femur and fixing the bone with a plate and screws. It may also be done as a closed procedure, using an intramedullary femoral rod introduced through a buttock incision for fixation. A cylindrical segment of femur is cut out of the bone using intramedullary saws, and the bone is pushed aside to allow the femur to shorten over the rod. The excised bone segment eventually resorbs.

3. Other techniques—Leg-length inequalities projected to be 6 cm or more generally do not respond well to the previously described treatments, which in these cases may lead to unacceptably short stature or limb segments. Although some discrepancies are so severe that amputation of the foot and prosthetic fitting are required, techniques of bone lengthening are successful in treating these children (see Chapter 1).

Anderson M et al: Growth and predictions of growth in the lower extremities. J Bone Joint Surg Am 1963;45:1.

Birch JG, Samchukov ML: Use of the Ilizarov method to correct lower limb deformities in children and adolescents. J Am Acad Orthop Surg 2004;12:144. [PMID: 15161167]

Little DG et al: A simple calculation for the timing of epiphysiodesis. J Pediatr Orthop 1996;16:173.

Moseley CF: Assessment and prediction in leg-length discrepancy. Instr Course Lect 1989;38:325.

Surdam JW, Morris CD, DeWeese JD et al: Leg length inequality and epiphysiodesis: Review of 96 cases. J Pediatr Orthop 2003;23:381. [PMID: 12724605]

2. Dwarfism & Other Disorders of Growth

Orthopedic disorders (achondroplasia, multiple epiphyseal dysplasia) or other syndromes (Down syndrome, Marfan syndrome) often accompany dwarfism. The classification of skeletal syndromes and dysplasias is undergoing rapid change as knowledge is gained using molecular, biologic, and genetic techniques. A detailed review is outside the scope of this text; Table 11–2 lists

Table 11–2. Orthopedic involvement in selected syndromes and dwarfing conditions.

Achondroplasia
    Short limbs; genu varum; exaggerated lumbar lordosis; spinal stenosis; ligamentous laxity
Apert syndrome
    Foot deformities; hand and foot polydactyly
Arthrogyposis
    Severe joint stiffness, contractures, and dislocations; resistant clubfoot
Cleidocranial dysplasia
    Absent clavicles; coxa vara
Diastrophic dysplasia
    Severe clubfoot; joint dislocations; joint stiffness; cervical kyphosis; scoliosis
Down syndrome
    Cervical (C1–C2) instability; hip dislocation; ankle valgus; ligamentous laxity
Enchondromatosis
    Asymmetric multiple enchondromas in long bones; limb-length inequality; angulation of long bones
Fibrous dysplasia
    Multiple fibrous lesions in bone; limb bowing or shortening; occasional endocrine disorders
Larsen syndrome
    Hip, knee, and radial head dislocations; severe cervical kyphosis and instability; scoliosis
Marfan syndrome
    Scoliosis
Metaphyseal chondrodysplasia
    Moderate dwarfing; genu varum; ligamentous laxity; cervical instability
Multiple epiphyseal dysplasia
    Mild dwarfism; joint surface deformities with premature osteoarthritis; angular limb deformities
Multiple hereditary exostoses
    Mild dwarfing; osteochondroma (external enlargements) at all long bone ends
Osteogenesis imperfecta
    Bone fragility and multiple fractures; bowing of bones; scoliosis; mild to moderate dwarfing
Spondyloepiphyseal dysplasia
    Severe dwarfing; coxa vara; genu valgum; scoliosis; odontoid hypoplasia, instability, and deformity

---

some of these conditions and the major orthopedic problems associated with them.

INFECTIOUS PROCESSES

1. Hematogenous Osteomyelitis

Osteomyelitis, an infection of bone tissue, usually occurs in the marrow cavity but sometimes affects the cortex as well. In children, it is most commonly the result of hematogenous spread, frequently following an upper respiratory infection or partially treated distant infection. Direct inoculation of bacteria into an open fracture or penetrating wound can also lead to infection and may resemble other serious bacterial infections in children (Table 11–3).

Clinical Findings

Acute bacterial hematogenous osteomyelitis usually occurs in the metaphysis following sludging of bacteria-laden blood in the venous sinusoids. The majority of cases are caused by *Staphylococcus aureus*. As the infection progresses, edema fluid and infected purulent tissue invade the porous cortex and elevate the periosteum, which is highly resistant to infection because of its extreme vascularity. The pressure of the pus beneath the richly innervated periosteum causes localized pain. Eventually, if the infection is untreated, the periosteum itself ruptures, and infected tissue spills into the surrounding soft tissue or ruptures the skin (Figure 11–1).

Table 11–3. Common pathogens in pediatric bone and joint infections.

Osteomyelitis
   Group A *Streptococcus*
   Salmonella (with sickle cell)
   Staphylococcus aureus
Septic joint
   Escherichia coli (neonatal)
   Group A *Streptococcus*
   Haemophilus influenzae (age 6–24 months) in non-HIB
      immunized patients
   Neisseria gonorrhoeae (adolescent)
   Pneumococcus
   Proteus (neonatal)
   Staphylococcus aureus
   Streptococcus fecalis (neonatal)
Soft-tissue Infection
   Escherichia coli (neonatal)
   Group A *Streptococcus*
   Proteus
   Pseudomonas
   Staphylococcus aureus
   Streptococcus fecalis (neonatal)

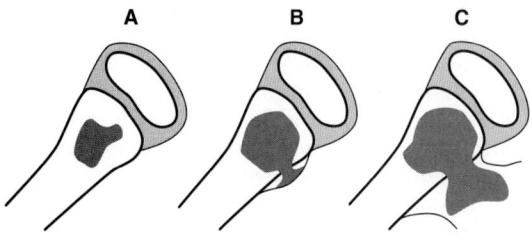

Figure 11–1. Hematogenous osteomyelitis in children. Cellulitic phase (**A**) can exude through the cortex, raising periosteum (**B**). Late rupture into soft tissues (**C**) is rare, unless infection is untreated.

The accumulated purulence in the marrow cavity and under the periosteum creates an efficient avascular culture medium in the cortex between them. This dead cortex is called sequestrum, and, if it is large, surgical removal may be required to control the infection.

The elevated periosteum responds to infection by producing a shell of periosteal new bone called involucrum, which provides some stability to the infected bone and rarely becomes infected itself.

Pain and tenderness at the infection site are universal signs, limping is common, and frequently the child is irritable. Fever and leukocytosis are common but not universal, and the erythrocyte sedimentation rate (ESR) is almost always elevated, usually to 50 mm/hour or more. C-reactive protein (CRP) is elevated. Clinical examination is usually sufficient to make the diagnosis; occasionally bone scans or MRI may be required to help localize lesions. Although the diagnosis is usually clear, osteomyelitis should be suspected if a child has bone pain in the absence of other systemic signs but has recently received antibiotic treatment for other conditions.

Treatment

A. EARLY TREATMENT

Treatment depends on the duration of symptoms and findings on radiograph. If the infection is detected early, no visible radiograph changes usually are apparent except for soft-tissue swelling. In that case, intravenous and, later, oral antibiotics may resolve the infection. Aspiration of the metaphysis should be done for culture before beginning antibiotic therapy. Up to 30–40% of cultures may be negative despite other clear evidence of bacterial infection; in that case, empirical treatment (usually with antistaphylococcal antibiotics) is appropriate.

B. TREATMENT FOR ADVANCED INFECTION

In advanced cases, lytic defects or osteoporosis may be present, and periosteal reaction may be visible on radiograph; such cases require open drainage and debridement of the infected metaphysis. Treatment must be continued until there is no evidence of residual infection because bacteria can survive in bone tissue that is not well perfused with antibiotic. In such cases, a 3-month prolonged regimen of oral antibiotics minimizes the possibility of chronic osteomyelitis.

Hamdy RC et al: Subacute hematogenous osteomyelitis: Are biopsy and surgery always necessary? J Pediatr Orthop 1996; 16:220.

Scott RJ et al: Acute osteomyelitis in children: A review of 116 cases. J Pediatr Orthop 1990;5:649.

2. Septic Joint

Septic arthritis in children, like osteomyelitis, usually is hematogenous in origin. The bacterial complications are similar to those seen in bone infections (see Table 11–3). Septic joints frequently follow upper respiratory infections; they may be delayed in onset by a week or more and may present in an attenuated form when a previous infection was partially treated.

Clinical Findings

The classic septic joint in a child presents a dramatic picture: The joint is splinted by muscle spasm, and motion of even a few degrees causes extreme pain. There may be effusion, but findings may be less striking if antibiotics were used in the recent past. During this acute inflammatory phase, children are more comfortable if the involved joint is immobilized.

Although white blood cell counts and the ESR are usually elevated, the definitive diagnosis of septic joint requires aspiration and synovial fluid analysis. Sterile aspiration does not harm the joint and should be done immediately when the diagnosis is suspected. Aspiration of deep joints such as the hip may require radiographic control.

Synovial white blood cell counts range from 50,000/μL (in nonpyogenic infections such as *Neisseria gonorrhoeae*) to over 250,000/μL (*S. aureus*). This white cell response, with the concomitant high level of lysosomal enzyme release, is most destructive of articular cartilage in septic joints. Although synovial fluid cultures give definitive guidance for therapy, antibiotic treatment can initially be based on results of Gram staining. In addition, immunochemical tests may offer rapid identification of certain pathogens.

Treatment

Treatment always includes drainage of the joint. In easily accessible joints, such as the finger or knee, certain low-grade infections may respond well to repeated aspi-

rations. In most cases, however, surgical drainage by arthrotomy or arthroscopy is preferable.

Antibiotics easily cross the synovial membrane and are continued until the joint inflammation is resolved, usually for at least 3 weeks. Intravenous administration is used initially but may often be followed by oral medication once the temperature, sedimentation rate, and leukocyte count return to normal.

Darville T, Jacobs RF: Management of acute hematogenous osteomyelitis in children. Pediatr Infect Dis J 2004;23:255. [PMID: 15014303]

Kim HKW et al: A shortened course of parenteral antibiotic therapy in the management of acute septic arthritis of the hip. J Pediatr Orthop 2000;20:44. [PMID: 10641687]

3. Septic Hip

Septic hip is one of the true surgical emergencies in pediatric orthopedics. It must be differentiated from transient synovitis of the hip, which is a benign condition (see the section on transient synovitis of the hip).

Because of the unique structure and blood supply of this joint (Figure 11–2), purulence within the joint cap-

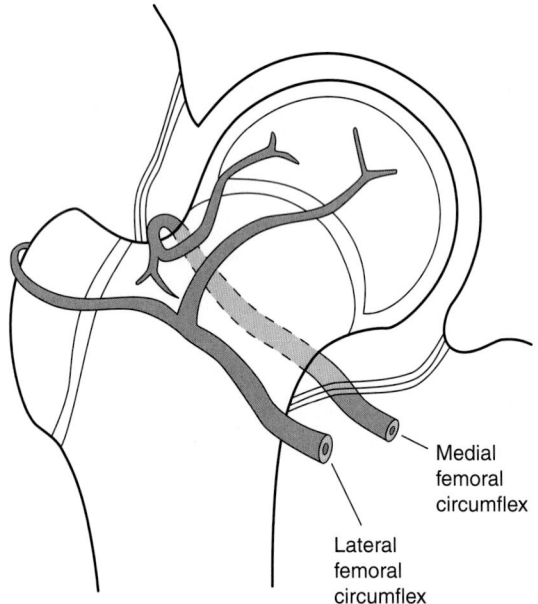

Figure 11–2. The blood supply of the proximal femur is unusual because the capsule interferes with the direct routing of blood vessels. The epiphyseal vessels emerge distal to the capsule and course up the surface of the femoral neck, rendering them susceptible to injury, thrombosis, or blockage by increased intraarticular pressure.

Medial femoral circumflex

Lateral femoral circumflex

sule can cause thrombosis of epiphyseal vessels and necrosis of the proximal femoral epiphysis. Neglected septic hips may subluxate or dislocate because of effusion and laxity caused by hyperemia. For these reasons, septic hip (or osteomyelitis of the proximal femur) always requires surgical drainage. Delay of even 4–6 hours may compromise the vascularity of the hip. An anterior approach is preferred to reduce the risk of vascular injury and subluxation.

Septic hip in a growing child is also a special orthopedic case because the femoral neck (which is intraarticular) is actually the anatomic metaphysis of the proximal femur. It is thus susceptible to hematogenous osteomyelitis, which may rupture into the hip joint and cause sepsis.

A common clinical problem is the differentiation between septic and hip and transient synovitis of the hip. Juvenile arthritis may occasionally be included in the differential. Table 11–4 highlights differences in the conditions.

Kocher MS, Mandiga R, Zurakowski D et al: Validation of a clinical prediction rule for the differentiation between septic arthritis and transient synovitis of the hip in children. J Bone Joint Surg Am 2004;86-A:1629. [PMID: 15292409]

4. Puncture Wounds of the Foot

Sneakers and tennis shoes offer little protection from nail punctures of the plantar surface of the foot. The penetrating nail may carry *Pseudomonas* bacteria (which contaminates the soles of tennis shoes) into the plantar fascia, although one series found *S. aureus* or Group A *Streptococcus* to be most common.

The symptoms of infection include redness, swelling, and pain that persist longer than 1 week. Surgical incision and drainage of the abscess and foreign body excision, when present (approximately one sixth of cases), are usually curative. Interestingly, prophylactic use of antibiotics does not seem to lessen the chance of developing late abscess. Late presentation is a marker for deep infection.

Eidelman M et al: Plantar puncture wounds in children: Analysis of 80 hospitalized patients and late sequelae. Isr Med Assoc J 2003;5:268. [PMID: 14509132]

5. Skeletal Tuberculosis

As in the adult, *Mycobacteria* organisms may invade the pediatric skeleton by hematogenous spread to bone or synovium while the initial pulmonary infection goes undetected. The most common sites of invasion are the hip and spine. Tuberculosis should be considered, and skin tests performed, in children suffering from chronic atypical musculoskeletal infections, particularly if the child is immunosuppressed.

Clinical Findings

Hip involvement is characterized by a chronic limp associated with a flexion contracture. In addition, muscle atrophy of the thigh may be striking. Radiographic examination discloses osteoporosis, joint narrowing, and irregular erosions.

Spine involvement may include paraspinal abscess (best visualized by CT scan or MRI), vertebral destruction, or kyphosis, which may be severe and lead to paralysis.

Treatment

Treatment of skeletal tuberculosis consists of combination chemotherapy, with surgical debridement in resistant cases. Occasionally, surgical fusion of joints or spine may be required.

Teo HE, Peh WC: Skeletal tuberculosis in children. Pediatr Radiol 2004;34:853. [PMID: 15278319]

Table 11–4. Clinical differential diagnosis of inflammatory hip conditions.

	Septic Hip	Transient Synovitis of Hip	Juvenile Arthritis of Hip
Pain	Severe	Moderate–severe	Moderate
Gait	Cannot walk	Limp or cannot walk	Limp
Fever	Common	No	No or low grade
Radiograph	Negative	Negative	Joint narrowing
WBC	Elevated	Normal	Normal–elevated
Aspirate	Turbid; 5000–250,000 WBC; bacteria present	Normal	25,000–50,000 WBC with monocytes
Treatment	Urgent surgical drainage; antibiotics	Symptomatic	Salicylates, rest, physical therapy

WBC = white blood cells.

6. Diskitis in Children

Diskitis is a low-grade inflammatory process involving the intervertebral disk, usually in the lumbar spine. It affects children at any age, although it is most frequent between 2 and 6 years of age. The disorder is caused by hematogenous bacterial seeding, with the most common cultures growing *S. aureus* from the disk aspirate. The classic presentation in a toddler is refusal to walk; pain is not a prominent symptom in this age group. Older children (up to early teen years) may have either back or abdominal pain.

Clinical Findings

Small children may have limitation of passive hyperextension of the spine (in the prone position) with no other findings. Older children have splinting of the paraspinous muscles and pain with percussion. The ESR may be normal or elevated; those patients with an elevated ESR are more likely to have bacterial growth if cultures are done. Aspirate cultures may be negative in up to 40% of patients. Radiographs at first are normal but eventually demonstrate disk space narrowing with sclerosis of adjoining endplates, best visualized on spot lateral views. Bone scan is positive in those children with negative radiographs.

Treatment

Management depends on the severity of clinical findings because a large number of diskitis patients have self-limited disease and improve spontaneously. Children with sepsis or elevated ESR may benefit from disk aspiration and culture. Less ill children are usually treated with empirical antistaphylococcal oral antibiotics for 6 weeks. Pantaloon spica cast may occasionally be required for symptom relief. Long-term outcome is universally favorable, although occasional spontaneous fusion of the disk space occurs.

Early SD, Kay RM, Tolo VT: Childhood diskitis. J Am Acad Orthop Surg 2003;11:413. [PMID: 14686826]

METABOLIC DISORDERS

1. Rickets & Rickets-Like Conditions

Nutritional rickets is a dietary deficiency of vitamin D that interferes with skeletal ossification. In the United States, vitamin supplementation of food and milk has virtually eliminated the dietary form of rickets. Numerous rickets-like metabolic conditions persist with orthopedic consequences, however.

Renal Osteodystrophy

Renal osteodystrophy, a disorder of calcium, phosphorus, vitamin D, and parathyroid function in children with chronic renal disease, has potentially serious skeletal manifestations. In transplantation patients, the condition can be aggravated by chronic illness and antimetabolite or steroid usage.

Osteoporosis, leading to compression fractures of the spine, is a common complication. Delayed healing of fractures is also common. Inadequate metaphyseal ossification during skeletal growth results in wide, irregular cartilaginous growth plates, which tend to slip slowly, sometimes producing grotesque hip, knee, and ankle deformities. Such deformities are usually best treated only after transplantation or other improvement in renal status. Occasionally, severe functional disabilities may require osteotomy to correct deformity before renal transplantation. Healing may be delayed, however, and the condition may recur.

Hypophosphatemic Rickets

Hypophosphatemic rickets (vitamin D–resistant rickets) is an dominant X-linked condition in which vitamin D production and metabolism are normal but renal tubular loss of phosphate interferes with skeletal ossification. The major manifestations are a mild-to-moderate decrease in stature and bowing of the lower extremities.

The medical history usually discloses a parent or sibling with short stature and bowlegs. In addition, serum phosphorus is reduced, and serum calcium is normal. Radiographic examination discloses characteristic widening of growth plates, funnel-like beaking of the metaphyses, and curvature of the femoral and tibial shafts, which are normally straight (Figure 11–3).

Medical treatment with megadoses of vitamin D and phosphorus supplementation may not be curative. Functionally disabling deformities can be corrected by multiple-level osteotomies, which usually require bilateral surgery. Because postosteotomy healing is delayed and recurrence of deformity is common until maturity, surgery should be postponed until adolescence, if possible.

Saland JM: Osseous complications of pediatric transplantation. Pediatr Transplant 2004;8:400. [PMID: 15265169]

Santos F et al: Alterations of the growth plate in chronic renal failure. Pediatr Nephrol 2004;20:330. [PMID: 15549411]

HIP DISORDERS

1. Transient Synovitis of the Hip

Transient synovitis of the hip is a benign, nontraumatic, self-limited disorder that mimics septic hip in clinical presentation. The physician confronting this condition must exclude septic hip, which is a surgical emergency.

Although the cause of transient synovitis is unclear, evidence suggests it is associated with immune responses to viral or bacterial antigens, mediated through the synovial membrane. Synovial fluid rapidly accumulates under pressure in the hip joint, and there may be severe pain from capsular distension. The fluid is resorbed within 3–7 days, with no long-term sequelae.

Figure 11–3. Hypophosphatemic rickets. Radiographs demonstrate bowing of long bones and flared, irregular physes (see text).

Clinical Findings

As with septic hip, upper respiratory tract infections often precede transient synovitis by a few days to 2 weeks. The hip contains excess synovial fluid and is held in flexion, abduction, and external rotation because this is the joint's position of maximum capacity. The joint may be sore and resistant to movement, but subluxation does not occur. Usually, the patient allows careful passive movement.

Radiographs reveal only capsular swelling, and effusion may be detected on ultrasound. Leukocytosis is absent, and ESR and CRP are not elevated.

Although experienced physicians frequently suspect transient synovitis based only on clinical examination, aspiration of the hip following confirmation of needle position by radiograph is the safest approach. Synovial fluid does not show elevation of the white blood cell count, and bacterial cultures are negative.

Treatment

Treatment of transient synovitis includes simple analgesics and splintage, usually by bed rest, until symptoms resolve.

The early stages of Legg-Calvé-Perthes disease (see section on Legg-Calvé-Perthes disease) may include a synovitic stage that, until the development of characteristic radiograph findings, is indistinguishable from transient synovitis. No evidence indicates that transient synovitis leads to Legg-Calvé-Perthes disease itself. Typically, the pain is less severe than in transient synovitis, the children are a bit older (older than 4–5 years), and there is no history of recent illness.

Luhmann SJ et al: Differentiation between septic arthritis and transient synovitis of the hip in children with clinical prediction algorithms. J Bone Joint Surg Am 2004;86:956. [PMID: 15118038]

2. Developmental Dysplasia of the Hip

Developmental dysplasia of the hip is one of the most serious problems in pediatric orthopedics. The neonatal hip is a relatively unstable joint because the muscle is undeveloped, the soft cartilaginous surfaces are easily deformed, and the ligaments are lax. Exaggerated positioning in acute flexion and adduction in utero may occur, especially in breech presentation. This situation may cause excess stretching of the posterior hip capsule, which renders the joint unstable after delivery. Laxity may reflect family history or the presence of maternal relaxin hormone in the fetal circulatory system.

This relative instability may lead to asymptomatic subluxation (partial displacement) or dislocation (complete displacement) of the hip joint. Displacement of the femoral head in the infant is proximal (posterior and superior) because of the pull of the gluteal and hip flexor muscles. In the subluxated hip, asymmetric pressure causes progressive flattening of the posterior and superior acetabular rim and medial femoral head (*dysplasia* is the term to describe these structural deviations from normal).

In the completely dislocated hip, dysplasia also occurs because normal joint development requires concentric motion with normally mated joint surfaces. The shallow, deformed dysplastic joint surfaces predispose to further mechanical instability and the inexorable progression of undetected, and therefore untreated, developmental dysplasia of the hip.

Developmental dysplasia of the hip (DDH) occurs in approximately 1 in 1000 live births in whites, is less common in blacks, and may be more common in certain ethnic groups such as North American Indians. In all groups, this disorder is more likely if certain risk factors are present, such as positive family history, ligamentous laxity, breech presentation (and, by association, cesarean delivery), female gender, large fetal size, and first-born status. Dislocations may be bilateral but are more often unilateral and on the left side.

Clinical Findings

Reversal of dysplasia and subsequent normal hip development depend on early detection of DDH. Early detection is made more challenging by lack of a definitive test or finding on examination. Moreover, because this disorder is painless, there are no symptoms in the infant. Detection of bilateral dislocations may be particularly difficult.

Radiographs are usually not useful in newborn infants because the femoral head is composed of radiolucent cartilage. Ultrasound examination is helpful, but false-positive results are common before 8–10 weeks of age. The test is expensive, and interpretation requires comprehensive training. Thus, the best test for this disorder is careful physical examination at birth, repeated at each well-infant check until the child is walking normally. A high index of suspicion is mandatory, especially if risk factors are present.

A. TESTS FOR DYSPLASIA

Several examination maneuvers require a quiet, relaxed infant and commonly produce false-negative findings. Although it is imperative to detect subluxated or dislocated hips, it is also helpful to identify the very lax (unstable) but still located hip. This type of joint may either dislocate later or exhibit subtle dysplasia during growth that can cause premature osteoarthritis.

1. Asymmetric skin folds—A dislocated hip displaces proximally, causing the leg to be marginally shorter. This occasionally leads to the accordion phenomenon, with wrinkling of thigh skin folds. The most significant fold is between the genitals and gluteus maximus region. This test is not very reliable, frequently producing false-positive and false-negative results (Figure 11–4A).

2. Galeazzi test—With the child lying on a flat surface, flex the hips and knees so the heels rest flat on the table, just distal to the buttock (Figure 11–4B). A dislocated hip is signaled by relative shortening of the thigh compared with the normal leg, as shown by the difference in knee height level. This test is almost always useless in children younger than 1 year and is negative if dislocation is bilateral.

3. Passive hip abduction—The flexed hips are gently abducted as far as possible (Figure 11–4C). If one or both hips are dislocated, the femoral head (the pivot point during abduction) is posterior, causing relative tightness of the adductor muscles. Asymmetric abduction or limited abduction (usually less than 70 degrees from the midline) is a positive finding. When the hip is lax (dislocatable but not dislocated), the abduction test is normal despite the presence of subluxation or dislocation.

4. Barlow test—A provocative test that picks up an unstable but located hip, the Barlow test is unsuitable for

Figure 11–4. Clinical examination of developmental dislocation of the hip. In all pictures, the child's left hip is the abnormal side. **A:** Asymmetric skin folds. **B:** Galeazzi test. **C:** Limitation of abduction. **D, E, F:** Ortolani and Barlow tests (see text).

a dislocated hip. The flexed calf and knee are gently grasped in the hand, with the thumb at the lesser trochanter and fingers at the greater trochanter (knee flexion relaxes the hamstrings). The hip is adducted slightly and gently pushed posteriorly and laterally with the palm (Figure 11–4D, F). Detection of so-called pistoning, or the sensation of the femoral head subluxating over the posterior rim of the acetabulum, is a positive finding.

5. Ortolani test—This test detects hips that are already dislocated. The flexed limb is grasped as in the Barlow test. The hip is abducted while the femur is gently lifted with the fingers at the greater trochanter (Figure 11–4D, E). In a positive test, there is a sensation of the hip reducing back into the acetabulum. Reduction is felt but not heard: The old concept of a so-called hip click is incorrect. The Ortolani test may be negative at 2–3 months of age, even when the hip is dislocated, because of the development of soft-tissue contracture.

B. Imaging Studies

In the infant, diagnosis is made by physical examination alone, and radiographs are generally unnecessary. Dysplasia, instability, and dislocation may appear on ultrasound studies, which can allow visualization of hip contour and stability before ossification is present. Sonography is a dynamic examination that requires an experienced interpreter, and there can be false positives prior to 6–10 weeks of age. Radiographs may be used at any age, but the absence of ossified structures renders them inaccurate in the newborn. After 4–6 months, when the ossific nucleus appears in the femoral head, radiographs are more helpful. Because much of the skeleton is cartilaginous at this age, certain lines and angles may be drawn on radiographs to allow estimates of geometric parameters (Figure 11–5). These may suggest evidence of acetabular dysplasia (a more vertical slope of the acetabular roof, measured as the acetabular index); femoral dysplasia (small or absent ossification center in the femoral head); or lateral superior displacement of the femoral head.

Increased femoral anteversion (external rotation of the femoral head and neck) is often present in DDH but not visible. Increased anteversion may be seen as an increase in relative femoral neck valgus in the older child.

C. Detection of Dysplasia in the Older Child

As the infant grows older, many diagnostic maneuvers that are positive in a young infant become negative because soft-tissue changes accommodate the displaced structures. Thus, the Ortolani and Barlow signs can be negative, even in the face of grossly abnormal hip development, making detection particularly difficult (especially between 4 and 15 months of age). The first signs of developmental dysplasia may then not be recognized until the child begins to walk and demonstrates a waddling gait with excessive lumbar lordosis. Radiographs at this age are diagnostic.

Treatment

Treatment of DDH should be initiated as soon as the diagnosis is suspected. Early treatment is generally successful, whereas a delay in treatment may result in permanent dysplastic changes. Exact treatment depends on patient age at presentation and degree of involvement. Regardless of age, treatment may fail, and the physician may need to institute a more complex treatment plan. The current recommendations described next.

A. Age 0–6 Months

A dislocated hip at this age may spontaneously reduce over 2–3 weeks if the hip is held in a position of flexion. This is best accomplished with the Pavlik harness (Figure 11–6), a canvas device that holds the hips flexed at 100 degrees and prevents adduction but does not limit

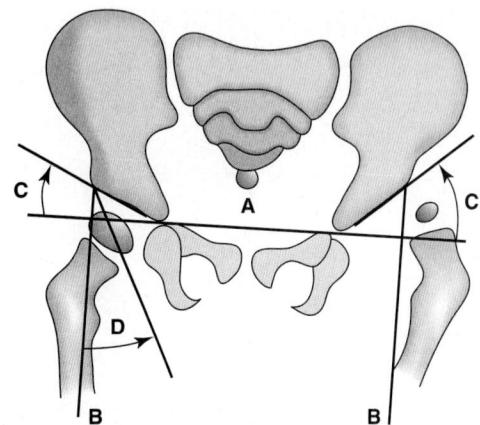

Figure 11–5. Lines drawn for measurement in developmental dysplasia of the hip. In the figure, the patient's left hip (on the right of the figure) is the subluxated one. **A:** Hilgenreiner line is a horizontal line of the pelvis, drawn between the triradiate cartilages. The proximal femoral ossification center should be below this line. **B:** Perkins line is a vertical line (perpendicular to Hilgenreiner line) drawn down from the lateral edge of the acetabulum. The femoral head ossification center, as well as the medial beak of the proximal metaphysis, should fall medial to this line. **C:** The acetabular index is the angle between Hilgenreiner line and a line joining the acetabular center (triradiate) with the acetabular edge as it intersects Perkins line. It measures acetabular depth and should be below 30 degrees by 1 year of age and below 25 degrees by 2 years of age. **D:** The center-edge angle is the angle between Perkins line and a line joining the lateral edge of the acetabulum with the center of the femoral head. It is a measure of lateral subluxation that becomes smaller as the hip subluxates laterally. Normal is 20 degrees or greater.

further flexion. Movement in the harness is beneficial for the joint and helps achieve gradual spontaneous reduction and stabilization of the hip. The Pavlik harness presents a low risk of avascular necrosis (see section on avascular necrosis of the hip). This treatment should not be continued beyond 3–4 weeks if there is no improvement. The failure rate of the Pavlik harness is approximately 10%, necessitating more invasive treatment, such as closed or open reduction.

B. Age 6–15 Months (Before Walking)

Gentle manipulative reduction of the dislocation under a general anesthetic and maintenance of a located position for 2–3 months in a spica cast usually stabilizes the joint. Even after the hip is stable, any residual dysplasia

Figure 11–6. The Pavlik harness, a device used for treatment of hip dislocation, subluxation, and dysplasia.

must be treated by bracing or surgery. In the past, prereduction skin traction was thought to reduce the risk of avascular necrosis. It is now believed that adequate hip flexion and limited abduction in the spica cast is the most important safety factor, and most surgeons no longer use traction.

C. AGE 15 MONTHS TO 2 YEARS

In toddlers or young children in whom closed reduction failed, open reduction of the hip is required. Severe flattening of the acetabulum with distortion of the normal spherical femoral head shape is found on opening the hip. The limbus (acetabular rim) may be flattened and inverted, and the ligamentum teres is always hypertrophic. Fibrofatty tissue occupying the center of the acetabulum must be removed. Femoral shortening osteotomy may be required at the time of open reduction to reduce soft-tissue tension and minimize the risk of avascular necrosis. After reduction, the position is maintained by capsular repair (capsulorrhaphy) and a cast, until stability is achieved. Prolonged bracing or surgery is often

required to resolve the residual dysplasia that accompanies untreated dysplasia in this group of children.

D. AGE OLDER THAN 2 YEARS

Significant residual dysplasia is present in children with DDH who are untreated at this age. Dysplasia may also persist despite successful reduction performed by any method at an earlier age. The dysplasia may be accompanied by a limp, and radiographs show a high acetabular index (more vertical acetabular roof), increased valgus of the femoral neck, and subluxation of the femoral head.

Surgical correction of dysplasia creates a stable mechanical environment that permits remodeling to a more normal joint during growth. Treatment requires bony procedures, either on the acetabular or femoral sides of the joint, or on both sides. Acetabular procedures, such as the Salter or Pemberton osteotomies, improve the acetabular index and increase the mechanical stability of the joint.

Femoral osteotomy corrects the anteversion and femoral neck valgus that characterize femoral dysplasia. The exact selection of osteotomy site may be based on maximum radiographic dysplasia or on the individual surgeon's preference. All of the osteotomies require that the femoral head be spherical and the hip joint concentrically reduced before an attempt can be made to correct the dysplasia. In general, the osteotomy should address the site of dysplasia, that is, acetabular dysplasia is not ideally treated with femoral osteotomy. Nevertheless, femoral osteotomy, if performed before 4 years of age, stimulates a dysplastic shallow acetabulum to remodel into a more normal shape. This occurs because the femoral osteotomy renders the hip joint more stable, thus allowing the normal mechanisms of growth to take over. Similarly, patients exhibit a progressive decrease in femoral dysplasia following successful acetabular osteotomy.

1. Salter osteotomy—Salter osteotomy is a surgical procedure to redirect the acetabulum in DDH (Figure 11–7). Animal models demonstrate that residual hip dysplasia is accompanied by acetabular malrotation and deficiency in the anterolateral acetabular rim. Salter osteotomy corrects this deficiency by rotating the acetabular region anteriorly and laterally.

The procedure is indicated in children 18 months to 10 years of age in whom concentric reduction of the hip was achieved. It is used to correct moderate acetabular dysplasia and can improve the acetabular index by 15 degrees. It may also be used to stabilize the hip at the time of open reduction. The pelvis above the hip joint is exposed subperiosteally. A transverse cut is made, using a wire saw, from the sciatic notch to the anteroinferior iliac spine, and the entire distal fragment (including the acetabulum) is spun on the pivot points

Figure 11–7. Salter innominate osteotomy, used for managing acetabular dysplasia. After a transverse cut is made above the acetabulum (**A**), the acetabular fragment is rotated forward and outward (**B**) to improve acetabular coverage.

of the notch and the pubic symphysis. This redirects the entire dysplastic acetabulum to a more horizontal stable position. A bone graft and pins hold the osteotomy open until it heals. A spica cast is used for 6 weeks to protect the graft during healing.

Salter osteotomy requires a second operation to remove the fixation pins. Because the geometric reorientation afforded is limited, there may be residual dysplasia. In addition, failure to achieve a concentric reduction before pelvic osteotomy usually renders the procedure ineffective.

2. Pemberton osteotomy—Indications for the Pemberton osteotomy (Figure 11–8) are similar to those of the Salter osteotomy, and frequently one or the other is selected according to the surgeon's experience or preference. The Pemberton procedure is particularly suited for correction of the long stretched-out dysplastic acetabulum because it reduces the capacity of an overly spacious acetabulum. This is done by cutting above the acetabular roof, down to the flexible triradiate cartilage (the growth plate of the center of the acetabulum). The roof fragment is then pried down to a more horizontal position and held in place by wedging a bone graft into the resulting defect. The fold thus produced in the center of the acetabulum may cause temporary stiffness. In younger children, this quickly remodels, but it is the major reason many surgeons do not perform this procedure on children older than 7–8 years.

Like the Salter procedure, Pemberton osteotomy requires concentric reduction before it is performed. For the Pemberton osteotomy, the pelvis is exposed above the joint. Under radiographic guidance, a curved osteotome is used to cut the pelvic bone from the acetabular roof down to the triradiate cartilage (the central growth plate of the acetabulum). The flexible cartilage allows the fragment to be hinged down over the femoral head, producing a more horizontal acetabular roof. A bone graft from the upper ilium wedges into the osteotomy site to maintain correction, and a spica cast is used until healing, which takes approximately 6 weeks.

Rarely, early extrusion or graft collapse occurs, and transient stiffness may be seen in older children. Because there is no internal fixation, a second procedure is unnecessary.

3. Femoral osteotomy—Femoral osteotomy (Figure 11–9) may be used to correct severe increased femoral anteversion or coxa valga (a high neck-shaft angle), conditions that are sometimes seen in residual DDH.

Figure 11–8. Pemberton pericapsular iliac osteotomy. An osteotomy cut is made above the acetabulum down to the flexible triradiate cartilage (**A**). The fragment is pried down to improve acetabular coverage and held with a bone graft (**B**).

Figure 11–9. Femoral osteotomy is performed at the intertrochanteric level and fixed with a plate and screws.

The procedure is particularly indicated when radiographs taken with the hip in abduction and external rotation show improvement in the overall congruency of the hip. Redirection of an anteverted proximal femur in valgus angulation stimulates spontaneous improvement in dysplastic acetabula in children younger than 4 years.

Femoral osteotomy is performed using a lateral approach, with the cut made across the intertrochanteric region of the femur. This site is chosen both because it is distal to the blood supply of the femoral head and because the cancellous bone heals easily. A metal bladeplate is placed in the proximal (femoral neck) fragment, usually after positioning with a provisional guidewire. The femoral neck fragment is rotated into a more horizontal position (varus) and is then internally rotated to correct excessive anteversion. The exact degree of correction is determined by preoperative radiograph positioning to achieve maximum congruence and correction of radiographic dysplasia. The plate portion is then clamped to the shaft of the bone and fixed with screws. A spica cast is usually used to supplement fixation.

After healing (6 weeks), the patient may resume walking. A Trendelenburg limp is common for 1–2 years after femoral osteotomy because of the geometric distortion of the relationship between the joint and insertion of the abductor muscles. This resolves as the femur remodels with growth and does not present a long-term problem.

Avascular Necrosis of the Hip

If a reduction maneuver for DDH was forceful or if there is tension in the soft tissues around the hip, the resulting compression of the joint may cause transient blockage of the blood supply to the femoral head. The subsequent death of the ossific nucleus and proximal growth plate of the femur (avascular necrosis) is a complication of treatment rather than of the disorder itself. A well-recognized cause of avascular necrosis is exaggerated forced abduction in the spica cast used after closed or open reduction. Avascular necrosis may be mild (involving a small fraction of the ossific nucleus), in which case it may go undetected and be of little significance. At the other extreme, avascular necrosis may lead to complete femoral head death and loss of future growth at the proximal physis. As it revascularizes, a dead femoral head may deform significantly, subluxate further, and require abduction bracing or osteotomy. Thus, it can cause leg-length inequality or early osteoarthritis of the hip. The best treatment for avascular necrosis is prevention.

Lehmann HP, Hinton R, Morello P et al: Developmental dysplasia of the hip practice guideline: Technical report. Committee on Quality Improvement, and Subcommittee on Developmental Dysplasia of the Hip. Pediatrics 2000;105(4):E57. [PMID: 10742378]

Weinstein SL, Mubarak SJ, Wenger DR: Developmental hip dysplasia and dislocation: Part II. Instr Course Lect 2004; 53:531. [PMID: 15116642]

3. Legg-Calvé-Perthes Disease

Legg-Calvé-Perthes disease (LCP, Perthes disease) is a serious but self-limited pediatric hip disorder. Although its cause is unknown, the disease is thought to be related to avascular necrosis of the hip. It affects children between 4 and 10 years of age and is somewhat more common in boys. Children with the disease are often small for their age and have retarded bone age. The disease is generally unilateral. If it is bilateral, other conditions, such as Gaucher disease or multiple epiphyseal dysplasia, must be considered. Newer investigations suggest that some cases of LCP might be related to a variety of transient or permanent hypercoagulation states. This research is not yet been confirmed in multiple centers. Surprisingly, trauma is not considered a causative factor in LCP.

Although early radiographs may be negative, they eventually show fragmentation, irregularity, and collapse of part or all of the femoral head ossification center (Figure 11–10). The few pathologic specimens that were examined suggest that multiple rather than single episodes of avascular necrosis occur over a period of months. Early bone scans may show a filling defect corresponding to areas of necrosis, and MRI is typical of avascular necrosis. The disease has a characteristic course (see Figure 11–10). Initially, the avascular episodes are silent and the child is asymptomatic. As the disease progresses, the necrotic femoral epiphysis is revascularized. Osteoclasts remove dead bone while osteoblasts simultaneously lay down new bone on the dead trabeculae (a process known as creeping substitution). During this phase, the femoral head is mechanically weak. Fragmentation and collapse of the bony structure may then occur, causing geometric flattening and deformity of the ossific nucleus and femoral head. The newly replaced bone takes the shape of the collapsed head.

At this point, continued growth may allow gradual remodeling and improvement of the femoral head shape until maturity. The symptomatic collapse phase rarely exceeds 1–1.5 years, but full revascularization and remodeling may continue silently for several years thereafter.

Clinical Findings and Classification

A. SYMPTOMS AND SIGNS

The clinical presentation of LCP in a child 4–10 years of age is usually a painless limp. If pain is present, it may be mild and referred to the thigh or knee. Physical examination discloses atrophy of the thigh on the affected side and, usually, limited hip motion. The typical patient has a flexion contracture of 0–30 degrees,

Figure 11–10. Legg-Calvé-Perthes disease. **A:** Central necrotic fragment with collapse. **B:** Same patient after healing and partial remodeling.

loss of abduction compared with the opposite side (in severe cases, no abduction beyond 0 degrees), and loss of internal rotation of the hip.

B. IMAGING STUDIES

Radiographs may be negative at first, probably because the initial softening of the femoral head is sufficient to cause symptoms but insufficient to change the radiographic appearance of the femoral head. The eventual characteristic collapse of portions of the femoral head is diagnostic of the disease, however.

The exact extent of necrosis, which is usually estimated in fourths of the head using the Catterall classification (Figure 11–11), is helpful in determining whom to treat. It may require additional radiographs.

An alternative radiograph classification uses the lateral third of the femoral epiphysis (the so-called lateral pillar). Collapse of this structure suggests a poor prognosis for late deformity, whereas maintenance of pillar height correlates with good long-term results. Partial collapse suggests an intermediate prognosis. The difficulty with all classification systems is their reproducibility and the need to delay until the collapse phase before the exact extent of involvement is clear.

There is little value in bone scans or MRI in the clinical management of LCP.

Treatment Options

A. NO TREATMENT

Children with bone age less than 5 years and children who exhibit relatively minor involvement (less than half of the femoral head) rarely need treatment. In these children, so much of the femoral head is cartilage, and therefore unaffected by necrosis, that mechanical collapse does not markedly decrease sphericity. Also, younger children have tremendous remodeling potential, and minor collapse can be outgrown before maturity. Older children who exhibit some radiograph changes but have excellent range of motion (ROM) may require only observation and serial reexamination.

B. NONOPERATIVE AND OPERATIVE TREATMENT

The issues surrounding selection of patients with LCP who need treatment are as highly controversial as the treatment itself. Most experts agree that children who maintain excellent motion (particularly abduction greater than 30 degrees in the absence of flexion contracture) may not require intervention. In children older than 4–5 years with significant collapse or progressive loss of abduction, treatment is frequently recommended.

	AP	Frog-leg lateral
I		
II		
III		
IV		

Figure 11–11. The Catterall classification is used to determine probable course and prognosis of Legg-Calvé-Perthes disease. It is based on progressive involvement of approximate fourths of the femoral head.

No evidence indicates that use of crutches or relief of weight bearing has any effect on femoral head collapse in this disease. For those children requiring it, however, treatment should minimize the effects of collapse and subluxation that often occur when the femoral head deforms. This is best achieved by abduction of the hip until subluxation resolves. The molding action of the acetabular shape is thought to help improve the contour of the collapsing femoral head. Abduction can be accomplished nonoperatively by holding the legs in abduction (Petrie) casts or using an ambulatory brace (Figure 11–12).

Operative procedures are advocated by some and include varus femoral osteotomy and Salter osteotomy, which were adapted from hip dysplasia treatment to control the subluxation seen in some cases of LCP. Healing usually occurs within 18 months.

Despite many studies, there is still no consensus for the best method of treatment; some patients do well without treatment, whereas others have a poor

Figure 11–12. Abduction bracing is one method used for ambulatory treatment of Legg-Calvé-Perthes disease.

result after aggressive treatment. Prognosis can often be predicted from the knowledge of certain factors (Table 11–5).

Balasa VV, Gruppo RA, Glueck CJ et al: Legg-Calve-Perthes disease and thrombophilia. J Bone Joint Surg Am 2004;86-A:264. [PMID: 15590848]

Herring JA, Kim HT, Browne R: Legg-Calve-Perthes disease. Part II: Prospective multicenter study of the effect of treatment on outcome. J Bone Joint Surg Am 2004;86-A:2121. [PMID: 15466720]

Table 11–5. Factors in long-term prognosis for patients with Legg-Calvé-Perthes disease.

Relative Prognosis	Good	Poor
Age at diagnosis	< 5 years	> 8–9 years
Hip motion[a]	Maintained (abduction > 30°)	Stiff (abduction < 15°)
Extent of involvement	< 50% of femoral head	> 50% or total femoral head
Radiograph features	Little or no subluxation	Subluxation, lateral calcification

[a]During first year of treatment.

4. Slipped Capital Femoral Epiphysis

Slipped capital femoral epiphysis is an adolescent hip disorder characterized by displacement of the femoral head on the femoral neck. Displacement changes the geometry of the upper end of the femur and hinders hip function (Figure 11–13). This disorder is one of the main causes of premature osteoarthritis in young adults.

Slipped capital femoral epiphysis usually affects both male and female adolescents 11–13 years of age. In 30% of patients, the condition is bilateral, although both legs are not always affected simultaneously. The typical patient is overweight—often markedly so—and is in either late prepuberty or early puberty. Rarely, the patient is tall, asthenic, and rapidly growing.

This disorder occurs at a time when the cartilage physis of the proximal femur is thickening rapidly under the influence of growth hormone. The vigorous secretion of sex hormone has not yet begun, however, so the mechanical effect of sex hormones on closure and stabilization of the growth plate is absent. This combination of thick growth plate cartilage (weaker than bone and subject to shear), lack of sexual maturity (which would stabilize the physis), mechanical stress (caused by obesity), and the peculiar anatomic mechanics of the hip joint renders the growth plate susceptible to slippage.

The direction of the slip is always posterior and often medial, and the mechanical bases of chronic and acute disorders are the same. In chronic slipped capital femoral epiphysis, the most common form (90% of patients), the femoral head slips insidiously at the growth plate over the course of several months. In the acute form, the femoral head is suddenly displaced, a condition that can be superimposed on chronic changes. Displacement may occur during normal activity or following minor trauma.

Because slipped capital femoral epiphysis is a progressive disorder and the prognosis depends on the severity of the slippage, early detection and prompt treatment are imperative.

Clinical Findings

A. SYMPTOMS AND SIGNS

The onset of chronic slipped capital femoral epiphysis is usually insidious, with a history of a painful limp for 1 to several months prior. The pain is characteristically aching and located in the thigh or knee rather than the hip. This referred pain to the knee is responsible for many misdiagnoses. Patients may be seen for knee pain and dismissed as normal after a negative knee examination and radiographs. A high index of suspicion is required to detect slipped capital femoral epiphysis in the obese limping adolescent complaining of knee pain. The change in hip ROM is usually diagnostic. Loss of abduction and internal rotation of the hip are evident, although these may be difficult to identify in the grossly overweight child. There is almost always a characteristic obligatory external rotation of the hip when it is flexed because of the distorted hip anatomy caused by the disorder. The femoral head is posterior to its normal position, so the flexed hip must externally rotate to keep the head within the acetabulum.

Acute slipped capital femoral epiphysis is accompanied by severe pain and limping, which may render the patient immobile. The onset is sudden, following little or no trauma, and examination discloses a painful, guarded, restricted range of hip motion. An acute slip is analogous to an epiphyseal fracture. In its unstable form, the patient is unable to bear weight, and there is a high rate of avascular necrosis. In its stable form, the sudden increase in displacement is painful, but limited weight bearing is possible and the risk of avascular necrosis appears to be lower.

B. IMAGING STUDIES

Slipped capital femoral epiphysis can be difficult to detect on standard anteroposterior (AP) radiographs (Figure 11–14). A frog-leg lateral view is the best for detecting mild forms because slippage is always poste-

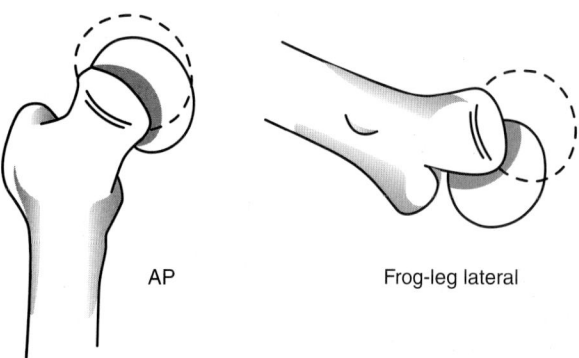

AP   Frog-leg lateral

Figure 11–13. Anteroposterior (AP) and frog-leg views of a slipped epiphysis. The dotted lines show the normal position of the femoral head.

A

B

Figure 11–14. Radiograph diagnosis of left slipped capital femoral epiphysis. **A:** Anteroposterior film shows subtle medial displacement of left epiphysis, best appreciated by drawing a line (Klein line) along the lateral side of the normal and abnormal femoral neck. The slipped epiphysis does not protrude lateral to this line. **B:** Frog-leg lateral radiograph clearly demonstrates posterior displacement.

rior. A radiograph also shows changes suggesting acute or chronic forms, information that may be critical to management of the disorder.

Establishing the severity of slippage is important in determining treatment and prognosis. Severity is estimated by the percentage of femoral neck left exposed. Slippage of less than 25% of neck width is mild; 25–50% is moderate; and more than 50% is severe.

Treatment

Slipped capital femoral epiphysis is usually a progressive disease that requires prompt surgical treatment. Because the changes in the chronic form occur so slowly, it is impossible to manipulate the femoral head into a better position. Treatment consists of fixing the slip in its current position and preventing progression. This is done by inserting one or more screws or pins across the growth plate, regardless of the severity of the slip (pinning in situ).

Following surgery, aching rapidly resolves, and during the remaining 2–3 years of skeletal growth, the extent of remodeling of the distorted proximal femur may be considerable, leading to an improved ROM.

Acute slips, if unstable, may be gently reduced before fixation, but the risk of further damage to the tenuous blood supply of the proximal femur and subsequent avascular necrosis is always significant. For this reason, many surgeons accept the position of an acute slip and pin it in situ.

In some cases, high-grade slipped capital femoral epiphysis does not remodel sufficiently with growth, despite treatment. In these cases, a residual, chronically painful limp is present, requiring correction by proximal femoral osteotomy. The osteotomy site may be at the level of the slip, which is mechanically effective but relatively risky for the blood supply. Alternatively, osteotomy can be performed at the trochanteric level; this is a safer procedure for correction of the functional deformity but does not resolve the exact anatomic deformity.

Complications

A. CHONDROLYSIS

In addition to the problems of impingement of the anterior metaphyseal prominence, which can impede motion, some patients with slipped capital femoral epiphysis develop chondrolysis, a poorly understood degeneration of the hip articular cartilage. It may be painful and may progress to severe joint narrowing and degenerative changes within 6 months.

During chondrolysis, cartilage is replaced by fibrous tissue, the joint capsule thickens and contracts, and joint motion is lost. Typically, the joint stiffens in flexion, abduction, and external rotation. Radiographs disclose joint narrowing, irregularity, and subchondral sclerosis, as well as regional osteoporosis from disuse.

Chondrolysis can result from iatrogenic malposition (permanent penetration) of pins or screws used for fixation of slipped capital femoral epiphysis. Although brief penetrations during surgery are probably common and cause no complications, unrecognized permanent pin penetration is disastrous. Chondrolysis also appears without obvious penetration and occasionally is detected in patients before treatment begins.

Chondrolysis is treated by nonsteroidal antiinflammatory medications (NSAIDs), aggressive physical therapy and ROM exercises, and observation. Capsular release is sometimes useful in resistant cases. Approximately half of patients eventually recover satisfactory painless motion. The other half may require hip fusion for symptomatic relief.

B. AVASCULAR NECROSIS

Patients with an acutely slipped capital femoral epiphysis can develop avascular necrosis of the femoral head (see section on developmental dysplasia of the hip). Because such patients are teenagers, the prognosis is poor, although some patients with partial head involvement regain a painless hip after a 1–2 years of symptoms. Some patients with painless but abnormal ROM may be treatable by intertrochanteric osteotomy to reorient the arc of motion. Long-term pain following avascular necrosis is treated by hip fusion.

C. PROGNOSIS

A slipped epiphysis is a major cause of early osteoarthritis. In general, the higher the degree of slip, the earlier the degenerative changes begin. In fact, a statistical increase in degenerative arthritis is evident even in the radiographically normal hip of patients with a contralateral slipped epiphysis. This suggests that subclinical bilateral involvement is more common than recognized.

Loder RT, Greenfield ML: Clinical characteristics of children with atypical and idiopathic slipped capital femoral epiphysis: Description of the age-weight test and implications for further diagnostic investigation. J Pediatr Orthop 2001;21:481. [PMID: 11433161]

Perron AD, Miller MD, Brady WJ: Orthopedic pitfalls in the ED: Slipped capital femoral epiphysis. Am J Emerg Med 2002;20:484. [PMID: 12216050]

Tokmakova KP, Stanton RP, Mason DE: Factors influencing the development of osteonecrosis in patients treated for slipped capital femoral epiphysis. J Bone Joint Surg Am 2003;85-A:798. [PMID: 12728027]

FOOT DISORDERS

1. Metatarsus Adductus

Metatarsus adductus (metatarsus varus) is the most common foot deformity in the newborn infant, occurring in 5 in 1000 live births, frequently bilaterally. Although it is usually isolated, several apparently unrelated deformities (such as DDH) are statistically more likely to occur in the presence of this disorder. The cause is unknown but might be related to so-called uterine packing.

Clinical Findings

The hallmark of metatarsus adductus is medial deviation of the forefoot, with the apex of the deformity at the midtarsal region. The hindfoot is normal. A deep skin crease frequently is evident at the medial border of the foot, suggesting the deformity has been present for some time. The adducted forefoot usually can be passively corrected to a neutral position but occasionally is fairly rigid. When the examining physician places a hand on the forefoot so as to hide it, the ankle has full movement.

Treatment

Metatarsus adductus tends to be self-correcting. Even severe cases generally resolve by 12–18 months of age without treatment. Nevertheless, many orthopedists use passive stretching to reassure parents the child is being treated. Indeed, some evidence indicates that passive correction and serial plaster casting can speed resolution of the disorder. Recurrence after brief casting is frequent in young children, however, and treatment for metatarsus adductus is usually not recommended.

2. Congenital Clubfoot

Congenital clubfoot (equinovarus foot; talipes equinovarus) is a severe fixed deformity of the foot (Figure 11–15). It is characterized by fixed ankle plantar flexion

Midfoot adducted and supinated

Ankle plantarflexed

Heel inverted and internally rotated

Figure 11–15. Clinical appearance of congenital right clubfoot.

(equinus), inversion and axial internal rotation of the subtalar (talocalcaneal) joint (varus), and medial subluxation of the talonavicular and calcaneocuboid joints (adductus). Severe cavus may be present, with a medial and plantar midfoot crease. Whether unilateral or bilateral, the deformity is more common in males, although when it occurs in females, it tends to be more severe.

The incidence in the newborn population is 1 in 1000, with increased risk for families in which even distant members have the deformity. There is considerable evidence that clubfoot is an inherited trait, but the disorder appears to reflect polygenetic expression, and exact inheritance patterns are unclear. Although most are isolated deformities and considered idiopathic, clubfoot may frequently be present in association with a wide variety of syndromes that affect the musculoskeletal system.

Clinical Findings

A. SYMPTOMS AND SIGNS

Clinical diagnosis of clubfoot is uncomplicated. Because it is a rigid deformity, clubfoot cannot be passively corrected the way metatarsus adductus can. Frequently, the foot is so severely internally rotated and inverted that the sole faces superiorly. Occasionally, the plantar flexion of the ankle is not obvious because the posterior tip of the calcaneus is small, high, and difficult to palpate. Clubfoot is always associated with a permanent decrease in calf circumference related to fibrosis of the calf musculature. This may not be obvious at birth but becomes more apparent after the child begins to walk.

Special attention should be paid to the presence of spine deformity, caudal dimpling, or midline spinal hairy patches, all of which may imply a neurogenic component. Thus, the examining physician should carefully search for features of other deformities or syndromes.

B. IMAGING STUDIES

Increasingly, clubfoot is suspected from prenatal ultrasound examination. Radiographs are rarely of value in the initial clubfoot evaluation because the bones of the foot are minimally ossified at birth. Radiographs become more important if the physician is considering surgical intervention or if the child has reached walking age, and radiographs can quantify the completeness of correction achieved by casting or surgery.

The typical radiographic findings of incompletely treated clubfoot include the following features:

1. presence of hindfoot plantar flexion;
2. lack of the normal angular relationship between the talus and calcaneus (so-called parallelism of talus and calcaneus); and

3. residual medial subluxation or displacement of the navicular on the talus and the cuboid on the calcaneus (Figure 11–16).

Treatment

A. CONSERVATIVE TREATMENT

Clubfoot always requires treatment, which should begin at birth. The initial approach is passive manipulation and positioning to the corrected position. In the United States, the majority of orthopedists use serial manipulation and casting, usually at 1-week intervals in the first month of life, and at 1- to 2-week intervals thereafter. In other parts of the world, strapping (with adhesive tape) or splinting with a variety of braces are popular methods (in addition to serial casting) for maintaining the manipulated correction. When casting is performed, there is agreement that specific techniques are more likely to be successful (Ponseti method). Even when the deformity responds to casting, there is usually sufficient Achilles tightness that a heel cord lengthening needs to be done at 4 weeks or later to facilitate cast correction.

The combination of careful casting and limited release allows most clubfeet to be corrected adequately, and long-term bracing for a year or more maintains the correction until the child is walking well. When satisfactory correction is not obtained, more extensive surgery is necessary. Although nonoperative treatment may be conceptually similar to training a bonsai tree, in that the joints are carefully held in a corrected position during growth, the analogy is limited. In clubfoot, the ligaments and joint capsules are severely contracted and thickened and, unlike supple tree limbs, may not stretch despite carefully executed manipulation and casting. In addition, the manipulation that encourages tension in these shortened ligaments may produce damaging compressive forces on delicate cartilaginous anlages of future tarsal bones. For these reasons, many surgeons limit nonoperative treatment to 12 weeks and then reassess the degree of correction attained. If clinical and radio-

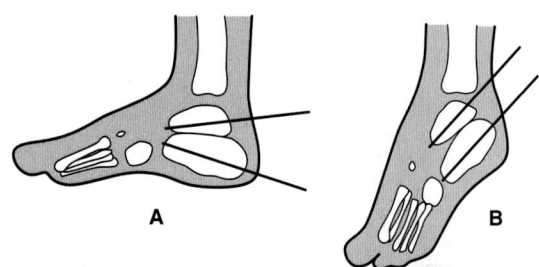

Figure 11–16. Diagrammatic appearance of radiograph in clubfoot. **A:** Normal foot. **B:** Clubfoot.

Figure 11–17. Cincinnati incision used for surgical correction of clubfoot.

logic evidence indicates significant correction, casting continues. Otherwise, surgery is required. Failure of nonoperative treatment is common, particularly in girls (where the deformity is often more severe) and in bilateral cases.

B. Surgical Treatment

Surgical correction of all clubfoot deformities is generally performed in one stage. At times, the casting corrects most of the midfoot deformity, and simple posterior release (ankle capsulotomy and Achilles tendon lengthening) are all that is required. Frequently, the surgeon must consider correction of the entire group of deformities through a comprehensive, extensive surgical approach.

One common approach uses the so-called Cincinnati incision, which extends from the navicular bone medially, around the superior portion of the heel, to the cuboid bone laterally (Figure 11–17). During surgery, the medial posterior tibial neurovascular bundle must be identified and protected. The tendons of the posterior tibialis, flexor digitorum longus, flexor hallucis longus, and Achilles tendon are Z-lengthened. The capsules of the talonavicular joint, subtalar (talocalcaneal) joint, and posterior ankle joint are released to allow repositioning of the bones of the hindfoot and midfoot. The navicular is usually subluxated medially on the head of the talus and must be repositioned onto its normal location. The calcaneus is both inverted and internally rotated on the talus. This is corrected by manually derotating the subtalar joint and tilting the calcaneus back into a neutral position. These corrections are usually held in place after reduction by inserting small K-wires, which are removed after 4–6 weeks.

The ankle is repositioned by dorsiflexion to neutral prior to repair of the lengthened Achilles tendon. Postoperative casting allows the gaping capsule to reform with the bones of the clubfoot in their appropriate, corrected position.

C. Complications

Early complications of clubfoot surgery are rare, but the rate of recurrence within 3 years is 5–10%. Mild recurrence of deformity is fairly common, and even when deformity is permanently corrected, the foot always remains smaller and stiffer than normal and calf circumference is reduced. Families must be informed of this possibility early in treatment so they have realistic expectations about the outcome.

If surgical release is too aggressive, overcorrection with late heel valgus and an overlengthened heel cord can occur. There is broad agreement that a slightly underreleased clubfoot is much more functional that an overreleased one, and the trend to less surgery and more conservative treatment is currently strong.

Dobbs MB, Morcuende JA, Gurnett CA et al: Treatment of idiopathic clubfoot: An historical review. Iowa Orthop J 2000;20:59. [PMID: 10934626]

Herzenberg JE, Radler C, Bor N: Ponseti versus traditional methods of casting for idiopathic clubfoot. J Pediatr Orthop 2002;22:517. [PMID: 12131451]

3. Calcaneovalgus Foot

Calcaneovalgus foot is generally considered a uterine-packing problem in which the foot is markedly dorsiflexed at birth so the dorsum of the foot sits against the anterior surface of the tibia (Figure 11–18). The hind-

A   **B**

Figure 11–18. Calcaneovalgus foot as it appears in relaxed position (**A**) and maximally plantar flexed (**B**).

foot is usually in moderate eversion (valgus) as well. Although some flexibility is present with the deformity, there is resistance to full motion, and most cases do not allow ankle plantar flexion beyond a right angle.

Despite its dramatic appearance, calcaneovalgus foot corrects spontaneously within 2–3 months. Although some orthopedists brace or apply serial casts and many recommend stretching exercises, all true calcaneovalgus feet resolve without treatment.

Congenital Vertical Talus

Calcaneovalgus foot must be differentiated from a much rarer condition known as congenital vertical talus (congenital rocker-bottom foot, congenital complex pes valgus). In this deformity, although the foot appears to lie against the anterior tibia, the hindfoot is actually plantar flexed because of contracture of the posterior calf muscles. To accommodate plantarflexion of the hindfoot and dorsiflexion of the forefoot, the midfoot joints (talonavicular and calcaneocuboid joints) must subluxate or dislocate dorsally.

Congenital vertical talus often accompanies genetic disorders, syndromes such as arthrogryposis, or neuromuscular disorders such as spina bifida. It is occasionally found in otherwise normal infants, however. Treatment is usually surgical, and casting does not resolve the disorder.

4. Cavus Foot

Cavus foot is a foot with an abnormally high arch. Although it is difficult to ascribe a particular threshold of arching beyond which treatment is necessary, most deformities are dramatic enough to make diagnosis straightforward (Figure 11–19).

Cavus foot frequently accompanies hindfoot varus deformity (cavovarus foot), and there may be clawing of the toes and demonstrable weakness of ankle or foot muscles. In addition, calluses beneath the metatarsal heads and heel skin are common.

Clinical Findings

One of the most common symptoms of cavus foot is anterior ankle pain, sometimes associated with toe walking. This paradoxical situation occurs because of the pathologic anatomy of the cavus foot. The forefoot is severely plantar flexed on the hindfoot, requiring marked ankle dorsiflexion to compensate. When the cavus becomes too severe, ankle dorsiflexion is blocked, leading to anterior ankle impingement and pain. The inability to dorsiflex further compromises forefoot clearance, and, eventually, only the metatarsals can contact the floor. This can be misinterpreted as ankle plantarflexion contracture, leading to unnecessary (and possibly harmful) heel cord release.

Figure 11–19. Cavus foot: clinical appearance and radiographic appearance.

The cause of cavus foot is usually muscle imbalance in a growing foot. Thus, cavus is rarely found in early childhood but is fairly frequent after 8–10 years of age. Although intrinsic muscle weakness is a major cause of cavus foot, weakness of the peroneal or anterior tibialis muscles is also implicated. Cavus foot is rarely found in the absence of an underlying neuromuscular condition.

Cavus foot is a marker for neuromuscular disease. Diagnosis requires a thorough search for the underlying cause and may require neurologic consultation, spinal MRI, and electromyographic (EMG) studies. Table 11–6 lists common neuromuscular causes of cavus foot.

Treatment

Conservative treatment of cavus foot includes accommodation by shoe modifications or inserts. These modalities

Table 11–6. Common neuromuscular causes of cavus foot.

Cerebral palsy
Charcot-Marie-Tooth disease
Compartment syndrome
Diastematomyelia
Friedrich ataxia
Muscular dystrophy
Spinal cord tumor
Spinal dysraphism (spina bifida)

---

do not actually correct the condition; severe deformity requires surgical correction by tendon transfers to restore muscle balance, by midfoot osteotomy to correct bony deformity, or by triple arthrodesis (hindfoot fusion in a corrected position).

Schwend RM, Drennan JC: Cavus foot deformity in children. J Am Acad Orthop Surg 2003;11:201. [PMID: 12828450]

5. Pes Planus (Flatfoot)

Flatfoot refers to loss of the normal longitudinal arch of the medial foot. Many cases of flatfoot are inherited, and a careful family history may uncover other persons with the condition. The foot is usually flexible, so the arch appears when the foot is not bearing weight. Hindfoot valgus (heel eversion) is often present. In severe cases, flatfoot may be painful, but this aspect of the deformity is often overemphasized.

Clinical Findings

Physical determination of the flexibility of the flatfoot requires careful examination. Subtalar motion is usually normal. In feet that exhibit a flat arch and valgus heel while standing, examination from the posterior aspect frequently discloses a normal arch and varus heel by muscle action when the patient stands on tiptoe. If these signs of a flexible flatfoot are not present, alternative diagnoses such as tarsal coalition (see section on tarsal coalition) should be considered. The physician should also look for painful plantar calluses.

Standing radiographs disclose loss of the normal medial longitudinal arch and may show mild lateral subluxation of the talonavicular joint as well. In severe chronic cases, degenerative talonavicular spurring may be present.

Treatment

Symptomatic treatment (shoe modifications, arch supports, and plantar inserts) is appropriate because no long-term treatment can alter the anatomic features of

the disorder. Posterior tibial advancement, subtalar joint elevation or fusion, and elongation osteotomy of the lateral calcaneal neck may not provide reproducible, predictable resolution of the problem.

6. Tarsal Coalition

Tarsal coalition is a congenital connection between two or more tarsal bones. Coalitions may be fibrous, cartilaginous, or bony. Coalitions usually occur between two bones and are cartilaginous in early life but eventually ossify (or nearly ossify) as the foot matures. Frequently bilateral, coalitions often follow an autosomal-dominant inheritance pattern.

The most common sites for tarsal coalition are between the calcaneus and the navicular laterally (Figure 11–20) and between the talus and the calcaneus medially.

Clinical Findings

Symptoms of tarsal coalition may include foot pain and stiffness as the lesion begins to ossify during early adolescence. The resulting stiffness and abnormal intertarsal movement patterns in the hindfoot lead to progressive loss of subtalar motion and fixed valgus (eversion) of the heel. Tarsal coalition is often called peroneal spastic flatfoot because the peroneals appear to be protectively overactive. As the lesion matures, pain may diminish but stiffness increases, and the abnormal valgus posture persists.

This diagnosis should be suspected in adolescents with foot pain, valgus heel, and decreased subtalar motion. Lateral anteroposterior and oblique radiographs of the foot confirm the diagnosis of calcaneonavicular coalition, but special subtalar radiographs (Harris views), CT scan, or MRI may be necessary to delineate medial talocalcaneal lesions.

Figure 11–20. Calcaneonavicular tarsal coalition is best seen on oblique radiograph projection.

Treatment

Not all coalitions require treatment. The decision to initiate treatment depends on the severity of pain, stiffness, and fixed valgus. Conservative treatment consists of casting to reduce pain and peroneal spasm. If this fails, the coalition can be surgically resected and the resultant space filled with autologous fat or muscle to prevent recurrence. In late or neglected cases with pain or deformity, hindfoot fusion by triple arthrodesis is effective treatment for both symptoms.

Harris EJ, Vanore JV, Thomas JL et al: Clinical Practice Guideline Pediatric Flatfoot Panel. Diagnosis and treatment of pediatric flatfoot. J Foot Ankle Surg 2004;43:341. [PMID: 15605048]

7. Toe Deformities

Toe deformities occur as isolated conditions, in association with similar hand deformities, and as part of other syndromes. The more commonly found deformities are presented here, with mention of associated hand problems.

Simple Syndactyly

Simple syndactyly, a connection of two or more toes, is the most common toe deformity. The webbing is complete, or a proximal fraction of the web is absent. This disorder demonstrates a strongly familial inheritance pattern and causes no symptoms. It is rarely treated in the foot. In the hand, however, surgical separation is required to restore normal finger function.

Acrosyndactyly

Acrosyndactyly is joining of the tip of two or more toes distally with an open web. It is most commonly seen in conjunction with oligohydramnios, congenital soft-tissue constriction bands, and congenital amputations (Streeter dysplasia).

In the hand, acrosyndactyly interferes with independent finger function and should be treated surgically (usually at approximately 6–12 months of age). In the foot, it is usually asymptomatic and may be left untreated.

Polydactyly

Polydactyly is the presence of more than five digits on either the hands or the feet. It is frequently hereditary and often bilateral. Duplication of the thumbs may mirror duplication of the great toes, and both generally require surgical treatment. Both preaxial (duplication of medial toes and radial digits) and postaxial polydactyly (duplication of the lateral toes or ulnar digits) often accompany genetic syndromes and should prompt the physician to look for other symptoms.

8. Constriction Bands (Amniotic Bands)

During gestation, protein-laden amniotic material can condense around limb segments. These amniotic bands may indent delicate embryonic tissues, causing constriction rings or even necrosis and resorption of the distal segment (congenital amputation). Constriction bands may be isolated or associated with Streeter dysplasia. The syndactyly of Streeter dysplasia differs from simple syndactyly in that the distal, rather than proximal, web is obliterated (acrosyndactyly). It is thought to be an acquired, rather than hereditary, condition, caused by shearing of the delicate tips of the embryonic digits, followed by conjoined healing of distal digits.

Constriction bands may be very deep and circumferential and occasionally must be released surgically by Z-plasty immediately after birth to avoid postnatal necrosis. Usually, only half of the circumference of a band is released at one time, to protect any remaining blood supply in the other half. Reports of successful one-stage resection and Z-plasty of constriction bands suggest that the remaining blood supply is probably subfascial and interosseous.

9. Adolescent Bunions (Hallux Valgus)

Although bunion (prominence of the medial metatarsophalangeal joint of the great toe) is rare in children, this troublesome deformity often requires treatment. It is frequently hereditary, usually seen in early adolescence, and almost always found in conjunction with a wide forefoot caused by varus (medial deviation) of the first metatarsal shaft (metatarsus primus varus). The wide forefoot allows severe lateral deviation of the great toe (hallux valgus), causing the prominent base of the great toe to rub against the inside of the shoe and create a painful bunion (Figure 11–21).

Although conservative measures may relieve discomfort, many adolescent bunions are progressive and require surgical management. Surgery must address each aspect of the deformity. The surgeon must trim the bunion, correct the varus angulation of the first metatarsal by osteotomy, and centralize and balance the hallux valgus by lengthening the adductor hallucis muscle. There is a fairly high incidence of recurrence of the deformity following surgery.

Johnson AE et al: Treatment of adolescent hallux valgus with the first metatarsal double osteotomy: The Denver experience. J Pediatr Orthop 2004;24:358. [PMID: 15205615]

TORSIONAL & ANGULAR DEFORMITIES OF THE KNEE & LEG

Torsional (rotational) and angular deformities are a major source of referrals to pediatric orthopedic surgeons (Figure 11–22). Most of these patients are young

Figure 11–21. Adolescent bunion (hallux valgus) is generally accompanied by a wide forefoot with splaying of the first metatarsal (metatarsus primus varus).

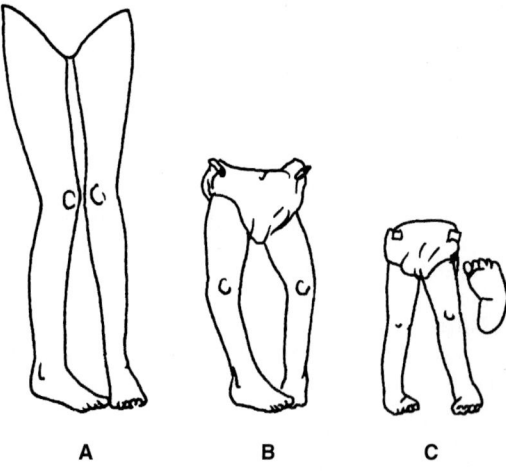

Figure 11–22. The major causes of clinical in-toeing include increased femoral anteversion (**A**), internal tibial torsion (**B**), and metatarsus adductus (**C**).

(less than 5 years) and have internal rotational deformities resulting in a so-called pigeon-toed gait.

The internal rotation, which can occur at the level of the thigh, leg (shin), or foot, is a cosmetic problem. Little evidence indicates that any of the so-called torsional deformities are harmful to the child or cause significant disability in the adult. Angular deformities (usually varus or valgus at the knee) are also usually benign, although careful evaluation and workup, including radiograph or other imaging modalities, occasionally disclose conditions requiring treatment. Nevertheless, most torsional and angular deformities are physiologic variations of normal anatomy, and they correct spontaneously over time.

Increased Femoral Anteversion

The normal femoral neck does not lie exactly in the frontal (coronal) plane but rather projects anteriorly from the plane at an angle called the angle of anteversion (Figure 11–23). Infants have anteversion of as much as 40 degrees, but this angle gradually reduces with growth, so normal adult femurs exhibit anteversion of 15 degrees. In some children, this gradual regression is slow or incomplete, causing the child to have excessive anteversion compared with an average child of the same age. This excessive anteversion produces a relative increase in internal femoral rotation.

The clinical manifestation of this increased internal rotation and decreased external rotation of the hip is in-toeing during walking.

Observation of the walking child discloses internal rotation of the entire femur by the medial position of the patella. Although parents may consider this pigeon-toed gait unsightly, increased femoral anteversion is a normal variant that has no effect on function.

Increased femoral anteversion gradually decreases, with improvement in in-toeing, until 9 years of age. Subsequently, persistent in-toeing in the adult becomes more likely. Increased femoral anteversion requires no treatment.

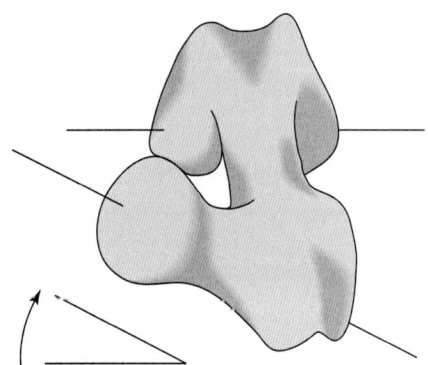

Figure 11–23. The angle of anteversion describes the inclination of the femoral neck forward of (anterior to) the frontal plane.

Internal Tibial Torsion

Some infants are born with a relatively dramatic internal twisting (torsion) of the tibia that makes the foot and ankle appear markedly rotated inward, relative to the axis of the knee. This internal tibial torsion is usually bilateral, frequently familial, and inevitably a normal variant in the wide torsional range seen in infants.

Internal tibial torsion can be clinically measured by comparing the bimalleolar axis (imaginary line connecting the medial and lateral malleoli of the ankle) with the frontal plane of the knee as determined by the position of the patella.

Torsion of 30–40 degrees is not uncommon in the newborn. When the child starts to walk, torsion can cause significant in-toeing, which, in turn, causes excessive tripping.

With growth, internal tibial torsion spontaneously resolves, and normal foot position and walking eventually occur. Some children improve by 24 months of age but may require up to 4 years for full resolution of the torsion. Internal tibial torsion requires no treatment. There is no scientific evidence that braces or shoe modifications alter the natural correction of the deformity.

Metatarsus Adductus

Metatarsus adductus may cause apparent in-toeing in the young child, leading to its inclusion as a torsional deformity. It is described in the previous section on the foot (Table 11–7).

Staheli LT et al: Lower extremity rotational problems in children. Normal values to guide management. J Bone Joint Surg AM 1985;67:39.

Bowlegs, Knock-Knee, & Genu Varum

Many infants have bilateral symmetric bowing of the legs, which may persist in the first 1–2 years of walking before developing into an exaggerated knock-kneed condition. The knock-knee is most dramatic at 3–6 years of age when it is known as physiologic genu valgum. At this time, the anatomic angle may be as high as 15 degrees of valgus. The genu valgum then gradually remodels spontaneously to the adult average value of 5–7 degrees of valgus.

Bowing of the legs in infants and excessive valgus of the knees in children 6 years of age are normal phenomena that require no treatment, although parents may have to be reassured that the condition is benign. The rare case of bowing that persists beyond 3 years of age may require further evaluation or treatment. Following are disorders that cause bowing.

A. INTERNAL TIBIAL TORSION

Internal tibial torsion may masquerade as bowing when the child walks with the feet forward and the knees rotated externally rather than internally. As the laterally facing knees flex, they give the appearance of bowlegs. Careful physical examination discloses internal tibial torsion, which spontaneously resolves by 4 years of age. As the torsion corrects, the apparent bowlegs disappear.

B. BLOUNT DISEASE

Also known as tibia vara, Blount disease is a poorly understood loss of medial tibial physeal growth that causes progressive bowing of the leg (Figure 11–24). It may occur as early as 3 years of age and can be bilateral or unilateral. If unilateral, the condition may be suspected earlier because it is obvious by comparison with the other leg. Excessive loading of the knee by early walking in heavy children with physiologic bowing of the legs may contribute to the development of Blount disease, but this is not proven. It occurs in all racial groups but is particularly common in blacks and Hispanic children.

Diagnosis of Blount disease is based on radiographic evidence of decreased medial tibial physeal growth. Later, the medial articular surface is distorted and the medial physis fuses. This allows progressive angular deformity to develop as the lateral growth plate continues elongating while the medial side is tethered.

Mild cases of Blount disease may improve spontaneously. Although some orthopedists recommend bracing to assist the process, there is no consensus that this is necessary or effective.

Table 11–7. In-toeing summary.

	Metatarsus Adductus	Internal Tibial Torsion	Internal Femoral Torsion (Increased Femoral Anteversion)
Age at resolution	12 months	3–4 years	9–10 years
Leg position	Femur and tibia normal	Patella forward; foot/ankle internally rotated	Patella internally rotated
Hip examination	Normal	Normal	Internal rotation exceeds external rotation

Figure 11–24. The Langenskiöld diagrammatic classification of radiographic changes in Blount disease (infantile tibia vara). The higher grades are associated with permanent closure of the medial tibial physis, which leads to progressive varus and internal rotation deformity with growth.

Severe or progressive cases of Blount disease require surgical correction by tibial osteotomy to regain the normal physiologic valgus angle of the knee. Surgery reduces the physiologic load on the medial tibial plateau and may allow normal growth. Slight overcorrection of the bowing often ensures load reduction, and the resulting valgus slowly resolves as the child grows.

Surgical treatment early in life is now popular, and many orthopedists recommend osteotomy after 3–4 years of age if radiographic changes are present. In early cases, surgical correction may cause reversal of the radiographic findings. Once physeal bridging occurs, however, there is no alternative to repeated surgical correction of angular deformity and leg-length inequality until growth ceases at maturity. Controlled studies of the issues involved in treatment of Blount disease by bracing and surgery are not available.

C. Rickets

Metabolic disorders of calcium intake can decrease the rate of calcification and ossification of physeal cartilage, causing the development of softer bones, so to speak, that are prone to bowing. Vitamin and calcium dietary supplements have virtually eliminated nutritional rickets in the United States. Hypophosphatemic rickets was discussed earlier in the section on metabolic bone disease.

Accadbled F, Laville JM, Harper L: One-step treatment for evolved Blount's disease: Four cases and review of the literature. J Pediatr Orthop 2003;23:747. [PMID: 14581778]

Ferrick MR, Birch JG, Albright M: Correction of non-Blount's angular knee deformity by permanent hemiepiphysiodesis. J Pediatr Orthop 2004;24:397. [PMID: 15205622]

Fraser RK et al: Medial physeal stapling for primary and secondary genu valgum in late childhood and adolescence. J Bone Joint Surg BR 1995;77:733.

Heath CH, Staheli LT: Normal limits of knee angle in white children—genu varum and genu valgum. J Pediatr Orthop 1993;13:259.

Langenskild A, Riska EB: Tibia vara (osteochondrosis deformans tibiae): A survey of seventy-one cases. J Bone Joint Surg Am 1964;46:1405.

Tibial Bowing & Pseudarthrosis

The tibia has a propensity to exhibit congenital angular deformities (bowing of the tibial shaft), which, although rare, are significant. The direction of the bowing is important in both diagnosis and prognosis and usually detectable at birth. Bowing direction is described by the apex of the bow, not the direction of displacement of the distal part (Figure 11–25).

A. Congenital Posteromedial Bowing of Tibia

Congenital posteromedial bowing of the tibia is a unilateral birth deformity of the distal fourth of the tibia. The apex of the bow is posteromedial, and often a skin dimple is present over the area. Because of the angle of

A   **B**

Figure 11–25. The major types of tibial bowing. **A:** Posteromedial bowing. The angulation spontaneously corrects, but with limb-length inequality. **B:** Anterolateral bowing. This disorder eventually progresses to spontaneous tibial fracture with resistant pseudarthrosis (see text).

bowing (often approximately 50 degrees) and the proximity to the ankle joint, the clinical appearance often mimics calcaneovalgus foot. The spatial position of the ankle joint, however, not the foot itself, is responsible for the deformity. Radiographs of posteromedial bowing disclose the curvature of the distal tibia, often with sclerosis in the underlying section of bone.

Despite its dramatic appearance, posteromedial tibial bowing corrects spontaneously in all cases. Some authors recommend casting to bring the dorsiflexed foot down to plantigrade position, but because the actual deformity is not related to the foot, this advice is not logical: Patients who are never casted resolve as quickly as those who are.

The tibial curvature remodels enough by 3 years of age that the limb appears cosmetically straight, although some bowing may be evident on radiograph for 5–8 years. All patients with posteromedial bowing are left with a leg-length discrepancy. At maturity, the involved limb is relatively as much shorter than the longer limb as it was at birth. Therefore, although the angular deformity needs no treatment, long-term follow-up and treatment of limb inequality is necessary in all cases.

Pseudarthrosis of Tibia

B. Congenital Anterolateral Bowing of Tibia and Congenital Pseudoarthrosis of the Tibia

Congenital anterolateral bowing of the tibia and congenital pseudoarthrosis of the tibia represent the other extreme of tibial bowing. For reasons not understood, anterolateral bowing in the distal third of the tibia and fibula is associated with inevitable progressive sclerosis and atrophy of the tibial shaft underlying the deformity. The ultimate fate of this atrophic abnormal bone is spontaneous fracture, which does not heal as readily as most fractures in children do (ie, pseudoarthrosis). Some children with this condition are born with a tibial fracture, whereas others simply have anterolateral bowing and sclerosis at birth, with fractures occurring up to 8–10 years of age. In approximately 30% of cases, coexisting neurofibromatosis is present.

All children with variations of this disorder require treatment. Because the prognosis is worse for those whose fracture occurs at a younger age, treatment methods vary. If anterolateral bowing is present but fracture has not occurred, protective bracing might be indicated. The fracture may heal in children whose first fracture occurs at 8 years or older, using prolonged casting or surgical bone grafting (with or without internal fixation).

Bone grafting in children whose fracture occurs before 3 years of age almost always fails, although repeated attempts to graft show some success.

The dismal results with conventional treatment of congenital pseudarthrosis of the tibia in younger patients prompted some surgeons to try innovative treatments. Electrical stimulation, free microvascular transfer of the fibula, and Ilizarov transport of normal bone to the defect are all reported to improve the success of treatment. So much surgery may be required to achieve a functional result, however, that many patients eventually undergo amputation to achieve rapid return to the normal functional activities of childhood.

Johnston CE: Congenital pseudarthrosis of the tibia: Results of technical variations in the Charnley-Williams procedure. J Bone Joint Surg Am 2002;84:1799. [PMID: 12377911]

Kim HW, Weinstein SL: Intramedullary fixation and bone grafting for congenital pseudarthrosis of the tibia. Clin Orthop 2002;405:250. [PMID: 12461381]

Morrissey RT: Congenital pseudarthrosis of the tibia: Factors that affect results. Clin Orthop 1982;166:21.

Ohnishi I et al: Treatment of congenital pseudarthrosis of the tibia: A multicenter study in Japan. J Pediatr Orthop 2005;25:219. [PMID: 15718906]

Tudisco C et al: Functional results at the end of skeletal growth in 30 patients affected by congenital pseudarthrosis of the tibia. J Pediatr Orthop B; 2000,9:94.

KNEE DISORDERS

1. Discoid Meniscus

The normal menisci of the knee are semilunar in shape and wedge shaped in cross section. They deepen the flat tibial articular surface to allow cupping of the rounded femoral condyles. The medial meniscus is longer and narrower than the lateral meniscus.

Rarely, the lateral meniscus remains congenitally round (or discoid) instead of acquiring its normal semilunar shape (Figure 11–26). This reduces its cupping function and may cause some instability of either the lateral compartment of the knee or hypermobility of the lateral meniscus itself.

A   **B**

Figure 11–26. **A:** Normal lateral meniscus. **B:** Discoid lateral meniscus, which may cause clicking, effusion, or pain.

Clinical Findings

The classic physical finding of discoid meniscus is loud clicking over the lateral meniscus during flexion and extension of the knee. This clicking is usually painless but may be accompanied by aching or effusion. Physical exam may demonstrate an extension block. Discoid meniscus may be suspected on radiograph by widening of the lateral knee compartment, a subtle increase in subchondral sclerosis laterally, and convexity of the lateral tibial articular surface. Confirmation is attained on arthrography or MRI. The abnormal mechanical function of discoid lateral meniscus makes it susceptible to tears, particularly in children older than 10 years.

Treatment

In the past, symptomatic discoid menisci were treated by total lateral meniscectomy, but the resultant late degenerative knee changes dictate a far more conservative course. Current practice is to avoid treatment unless symptoms are significant and disabling. If treatment is required, the safest approach appears to be arthroscopic removal of the central portion of the discoid shape, thus sculpting the lateral meniscus into a roughly semilunar form.

Ahn JH et al: Discoid lateral meniscus in children: Clinical manifestations and morphology. J Pediatr Orthop 2001;21:812. [PMID: 11675561]

Kelly BT, Green DW: Discoid lateral meniscus in children. Current Opin Pediatr 2002;14:54. [PMID: 11880735]

Washington ER III et al: Discoid lateral meniscus in children. Long-term follow-up after excision. J Bone Joint Surg AM 1995;77:1357. [PMID: 7673286]

2. Chondromalacia and Internal Derangements of the Knee

Patellar chondromalacia and patellar subluxation are common in active adolescents, particularly in females who have small patellas and a slight exaggeration of knee valgus and quadriceps (Q) angle. Meniscal and ligament injuries are managed as in the adult, although these injuries are not as common in children.

A somewhat more conservative approach to suspect internal knee derangements is warranted in most children. The diagnostic accuracy of both physical exam and complex imaging studies (such as MRI) is surprisingly low in children. False-positive MRIs are particularly typical in children.

These disorders are described in Chapter 3, Musculoskeletal Trauma Surgery, and Chapter 4, Sports Medicine.

3. Osteochondritis Dissecans

Osteochondritis dissecans is a poorly understood disorder usually of the distal femoral condyle ossification center, although other joints (talus, elbow) can be affected. A portion of the joint surface softens, shears, or separates through the articular cartilage and underlying bone (Figure 11–27). This disorder is common, but not exclusive, in children 8–14 years of age; however, it is an infrequent problem in the adult.

The disease appears to be caused by a combination of two factors: (1) mechanical shearing or injury from activity and (2) femoral condyle susceptibility (fragility) resulting from immature ossification of the femoral condyle (which can be quite irregular in children). The importance of each factor depends on age. Athletic trauma seems more important in older children and adults, whereas in younger children, ossification defects render the femoral condyle more susceptible to minor repetitive injury.

Clinical Findings

A. SYMPTOMS AND SIGNS

Symptoms and physical findings can be highly variable. Younger children may have an asymptomatic radiographic abnormality of condylar fragmentation or may simply have a vague aching after strenuous activity. Older children and adults may have pain, effusion, and locking or catching if the affected fragment actually separates and becomes a loose body in the knee joint.

B. IMAGING STUDIES

Plain radiographs show an irregular fragment of the surface that is usually sclerotic but may be osteopenic, and is usually on the lateral side of the medial condyle. It is often necessary to obtain tangential views of the condyle such as notch views. Occasionally, the defect is visible only on lateral projection. Contralateral comparison views should

A   **B**   **C**

Figure 11–27. Various forms of the osteochondritis dissecans lesion found in children. **A:** Defect in ossification center without cartilage defect. **B:** Lesion with a hinged flap. **C:** Complete separation of bone and cartilage, which can lead to loose body in the knee joint.

always be obtained. So-called ossification defects that mimic osteochondritis dissecans may be normal ossification fronts, seen to be bilateral and symmetric.

In children older than 11–12 years, MRI or arthrography is used to determine whether the underlying bone alone is involved or whether there is an actual separation of overlying cartilage. Although these studies are helpful in refining treatment strategy in this age group, they are seldom useful in younger children.

Treatment

Young children with asymptomatic osteochondritis dissecans need not be treated because most of these lesions heal spontaneously. In preadolescents with symptoms or with large lesions seen on radiographs, simple immobilization with either a knee immobilizer or cylinder cast for 6 weeks frequently heals the defect and eliminates symptoms.

Sometimes immobilization is not effective, though. If the lesion is large and accompanied by cartilage separation or displacement, or if the skeleton has reached maturity, treatment may be the same as in the adult. This includes arthroscopic debridement and stabilization of the loose fragment using pins for internal fixation. Excision is less likely to result in a good result. The presence of open physes may necessitate modifications of standard adult techniques.

Hefti F et al: Osteochondritis dissecans: A multicenter study of the European Pediatric Orthopedic Society. J Pediatr Orthop B 1999;8:231.

Letts M, Davidson D, Ahmer A: Osteochondritis of the talus in children. J Pediatr Orthop 2003;23:617. [PMID: 12960624]

Wright RW et al: Osteochondritis of the knee: Long-term results of the excision of the fragment. Clin Orthop 2004;424:239. [PMID: 15241178]

4. Ligament & Epiphyseal Injury

Children who have not reached skeletal maturity have far fewer major ligament injuries of the knee than do older children and adults. Smaller children tend to participate in lower impact activities and sports, and their lack of muscle bulk (which increases during adolescence) limits body acceleration and the force of collision. In addition, ligaments are relatively strong in the immature skeleton compared with bone or cartilaginous physes. Therefore, physeal fractures and bony avulsions of ligament attachments are more likely than traumatic ruptures of the ligaments themselves.

Residual instability may occur in the child's knee after varus or valgus injury. In the adult, such instability is considered clinical evidence of ligament injury. In children, however, the physis rather than the ligament may be the site of failure. Instability can be caused by a physeal fracture that hinges open rather than the joint opening (Figure 11–28). It is usually clinically obvious

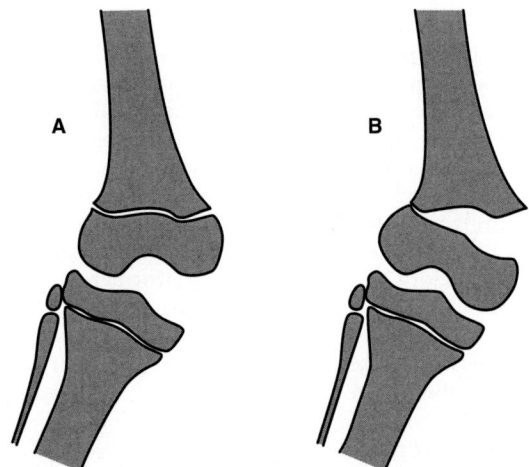

Figure 11–28. Stress radiograph of the unstable knee in an immature patient may reveal ligament rupture (**A**) or separation of the femoral physis (**B**).

that fracture is present, although stress radiographs may help in questionable cases.

Major intraarticular disruptions of the knee joint (meniscal tear or cruciate ligament injury) are rare in children. Detection may be delayed because symptoms may be less severe than in the adult and their presence not given as much weight in the differential diagnosis. Meniscus injury, particularly when peripheral, may lend itself to arthroscopic repair because of the excellent blood supply in children. Anterior cruciate rupture can be difficult to manage surgically in children because the anatomic sites of the tibial or femoral physes limit the options for reattachment. With the exception of cruciate injuries, most childhood knee ligament injuries are treatable by 2–4 weeks of splinting and return to function, as tolerated by pain. Physical therapy is rarely necessary in children younger than 15 years. A review of the major signs, symptoms, diagnostic procedures, and treatment options can be found in Chapter 4, Sports Medicine.

Not all effusions in the knee are traumatic, particularly in younger children. Because children at play are always suffering minor injuries, a history of injury may be inaccurate. The physician must remember to consider septic arthritis and pauciarticular juvenile rheumatoid arthritis in the differential diagnosis of effusion.

Beasley LS, Chudik SC: Anterior cruciate ligament injury in children: Update of current treatment options. Curr Opin Pediatr 2003;15:45. [PMID: 12544271]

Luhmann SJ: Acute traumatic knee effusions in children and adolescents. J Pediatr Orthop 2003;23:199. [PMID: 12649021]

OSGOOD-SCHLATTER DISEASE

The proximal tibial physis contains a transverse component that contributes to longitudinal growth and an anterior tongue that contains the attachment of the patellar tendon. In preadolescent and adolescent children (usually boys), the distal tip of this tongue may undergo fragmentation from chronic tensile stress, and enlargement from the resultant hyperemic response, which is known as Osgood-Schlatter disease. As the tibial tubercle becomes increasingly prominent, a painful bursa can form over it.

Clinical Findings

Symptoms vary from mild aching at the tubercle to severe pain with patellar function and exaggerated bursal tenderness. Radiographs of the lateral proximal tibia show the characteristic fragmentation (Figure 11–29).

Treatment

Treatment is symptomatic, including analgesics, knee pads to avert direct pressure, quadriceps stretching, avoidance of sports activities, and brief casting or splinting for painful cases. The disorder resolves spontaneously when the physis closes at skeletal maturity. No evidence indicates that physical activity within the limits of pain is harmful to the child with Osgood-Schlatter disease.

Figure 11–29. Osgood-Schlatter disease. The radiographs would show characteristic fragmentation of the tibial tubercle apophysis, similar to diagram.

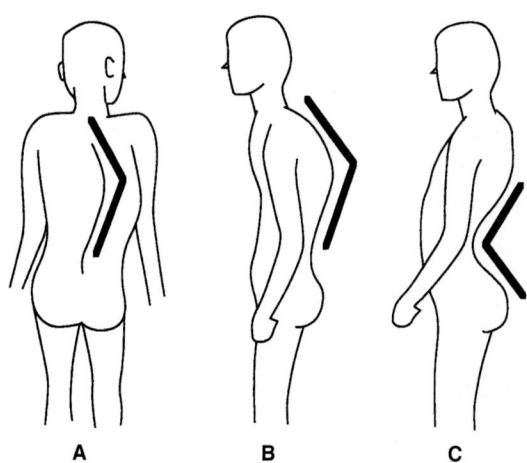

A   **B**   **C**

Figure 11–30. Definitions of spinal deformities. **A:** Scoliosis. **B:** Kyphosis. **C:** Lordosis. Frequently, a combination of deformities occur in individual patients (ie, kyphoscoliosis).

Krause BL et al: Natural history of Osgood-Schlatter disease. J Pediatr Orthop 1990;10:65.

SPINAL CURVATURE

Spinal curvature may occur in any age group and present with variable findings. Curvatures may be idiopathic, congenital, or accompany a wide variety of neuromuscular disorders, tumors, and infections. Curvatures may be small and nonprogressive or may worsen and require aggressive treatment. Sometimes, spinal curvature is the first clue to important underlying disease. Figure 11–30 shows the different types of spinal deformities.

Types of Curvatures

A. SCOLIOSIS

Scoliosis is a lateral spinal curvature in the frontal plane, best appreciated by physical examination from the patient's back and by anteroposterior radiographs. Curvatures, which may be single or multiple, are described by the direction of their convexity. In a flexible spine, the presence of a single (more rigid) curvature can lead to physiologic compensatory curvatures in the opposite direction, above and below the primary curvature. True scoliosis always includes a rotational component that may not be fully appreciated on radiograph and generally includes a lordotic component as well (see section on lordosis). Surprisingly, lateral curvature is often undetected externally. The rotation of vertebrae that accompanies scoliosis is the physical feature that allows clinical detection.

B. Kyphosis

Kyphosis is a forward (flexed) curvature of the spine in the sagittal plane, best appreciated from the side and by lateral radiographs. If kyphosis is acutely angular, a posterior prominence called a gibbus may be evident in the sagittal plane.

C. Lordosis

Lordosis is a hyperextension deformity of the spine, most common in the lumbar spine but also often accompanying scoliosis. Lumbar lordosis may be secondary to flexion contracture of the hip.

Detection of Curvature

Although spinal curvatures may be detected first during routine radiograph, most lesions are best diagnosed by physical examination. Spinal examination should proceed according to the following specific protocol:

1. Place the patient in the standing position (Figure 11–31).
2. Check the level of the pelvis and look for obvious asymmetry of the rib, scapula, neck, and shoulder height (leg-length inequality can cause apparent scoliosis, which disappears when the short leg is elevated on blocks).
3. Level the pelvis by seating the child on a firm surface if the pelvis cannot be leveled while standing. This is the case in children with hip contracture from neuromuscular disease.
4. Have the child bend forward, carefully noting any asymmetric prominence of the lumbar paraspinous muscle, rib cage, or scapula, which suggests the rotational portion of scoliosis. The magnitude of

asymmetry corresponds to the severity of the curvature, with convexity of the curvature directed toward the most prominent side.

5. From the side, check for prominence of the spine that might indicate kyphosis, both in the upright and forward-bending position.
6. Perform a careful neurological exam, including upper extremity reflexes and abdominal reflexes in addition to thorough lower extremity neurological examination.
7. Use radiographs to assess type, severity, and location of the curvature and to look for underlying lesions. Because primary scoliosis and kyphosis curvatures are always stiffer than uninvolved spine segments, bending radiographs may reveal which curvatures are "structural" and which are more flexible compensations (secondary curvature). The Cobb method is usually used to measure curvatures (Figure 11–32). The degree of tilt between the most affected vertebral end plates describes curvature magnitude.

Scoliosis

A. Idiopathic Scoliosis

Idiopathic scoliosis has no apparent underlying cause. It is most common in early adolescent girls, although it can be found in either gender at any age. Adolescent idiopathic scoliosis typically is a convex curvature to the right in the thoracic portion of the spine (right thoracic curvature pattern). Patients with atypical curvature patterns and idiopathic curvature in younger children may require more extensive testing (eg, EMG, MRI) before the cause can be definitively designated idiopathic.

Many idiopathic curvatures progress in magnitude with growth and continue to do so until skeletal maturity. Therefore, the clinician must determine if the curvature is progressing and if the spine is still growing. Radiographs document progression, and observations of the ossification pattern of the iliac crest apophysis (Risser sign) are used to estimate skeletal maturity. This ossification pattern begins laterally at puberty and spreads medially across the ilium, capping and fusing with the bone at maturity.

Growing children with progressive curvatures should be treated. A variety of spinal braces is available to treat progression of idiopathic scoliosis. Children who mature with curvatures smaller than 35–40 degrees generally have no symptoms and no progression in adulthood. If a curvature progresses despite adequate bracing, surgery is the treatment of choice. Some curvatures are too rigid to brace effectively and can only be observed if they are relatively small. If curve magnitude exceeds 40 degrees, bracing is generally ineffective and surgical correction is the treatment of choice.

Figure 11–31. Examination of the spine for deformity is best carried out by observing for asymmetry and deformity as the patient bends forward (see text).

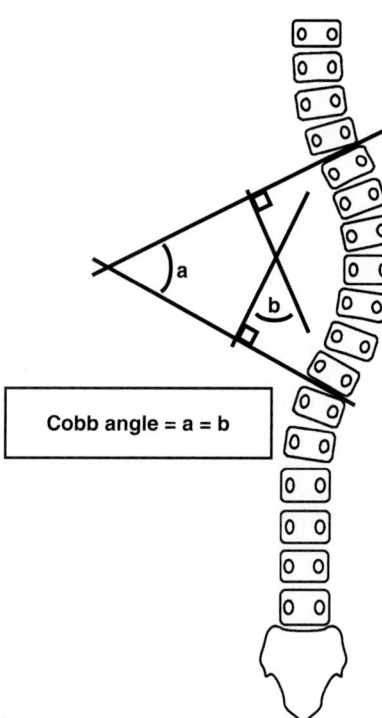

Figure 11–32. The Cobb method of measurement is commonly used to assess spinal curvature. It measures the angle between the far (top and bottom) endplates of the most inclined vertebrae. To allow the measurement lines to fit on the radiograph, lines at 90-degree angles to the endplates are often drawn, and their relative angles measured. Geometrically, these angles are the same.

Surgery for scoliosis corrects the deformity using metal rods that can be configured to push, pull, distract, or compress portions of the spine with curvature. The involved spinal segments are then fused together using iliac or allograft bone. Typically, a posterior fusion of the laminas and facets is sufficient for many cases of idiopathic scoliosis. Severe cases may also require anterior fusion through the thorax or retroperitoneal space.

B. Congenital Scoliosis

Congenital scoliosis is caused by malformations of vertebral shape. It does not refer to the age of the patient: Newborns can have idiopathic scoliosis, despite being born with spinal curvatures. Congenital vertebral malformations generally occur in early embryonic life (before 7 weeks) and are thought to represent errors in formation or segmentation of the spinal segments that originate from primitive mesenchymal condensations of embryonic cells (Figure 11–33).

Curvatures can originate when vertebral parts fail to form (eg, hemivertebrae, wedge vertebrae, butterfly vertebrae) or when embryonic somites fail to segment properly into individual vertebrae (eg, block vertebrae, unilateral unsegmented bar). Because of the embryonic timing of this process, children with congenital scoliosis frequently have abnormalities of other organ systems that form during the same embryonic period (eg, cardiac and renal systems).

Diagnosis of congenital scoliosis must be followed by a careful cardiac examination and by ultrasound or intravenous pyelography evaluation of the kidneys. Although neural tube damage is relatively rare, careful imaging of the spinal canal (MRI, EMG) may be required, especially if surgery is contemplated.

Congenital scoliosis may encompass one or many deformed vertebrae, and different types of vertebral abnormalities are often seen in the same patient. Sometimes, two deforming vertebrae cancel each other out, as it were, and no curvature is visible. For this reason, prediction of progression of the scoliosis depends on serial radiographs. If progression occurs, bracing is usually the first treatment, although surgery is indicated if progression is not halted by external means. Curvatures caused by unilateral unsegmented bars have such a strong tendency to progress that they should be treated by surgery as soon as they are detected.

C. Neuromuscular Scoliosis

Neuromuscular scoliosis includes a diverse group of curvature patterns that occur in association with various neuromuscular diseases. The cause varies with the disease. For example, scoliosis in children with cerebral palsy is usually caused by a combination of spasticity (overactivity of muscle) and weakness. Scoliosis in children with muscular dystrophy is the result of severe progressive muscle weakness that eliminates the paraspinous stability of the spinal column. Scoliosis in infants with spina

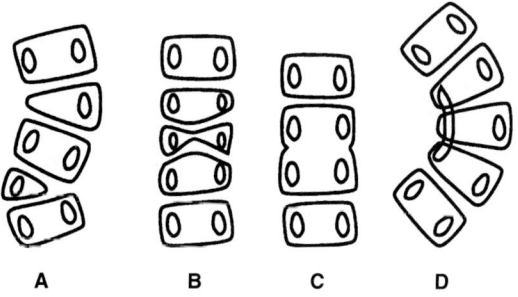

A   B   C   D

Figure 11–33. Vertebral anomalies of congenital scoliosis. **A:** Hemivertebra. **B:** Butterfly vertebra. **C:** Block vertebra. **D:** Unilateral unsegmented bar.

bifida (myelomeningocele) is frequently congenital (see previous discussion), related to loss of posterior elements, or associated with the development of a syrinx (central cystic fluid collection) in the spinal cord, a process similar to hydrocephalus.

Patients with neuromuscular scoliosis often develop curvatures at an early age, when surgical treatment is either impossible or would result in severe stunting of spinal growth. It is common to treat such children by daytime bracing, despite the fact that bracing alone is rarely sufficient to eliminate progression or the need for later surgery. In such cases, some surgeons feel that bracing may slow progression enough to allow additional skeletal growth, and spinal correction and fusion is postponed until puberty.

D. OTHER SCOLIOSES

Childhood scoliosis can be associated with benign tumors of the spine, usually osteoid osteoma and osteoblastoma. Treatment of the tumor is usually curative, although long-standing lesions may require fusion as well.

Neurofibromatosis is associated with both scoliosis and kyphosis and characteristically leads to short high-grade curvatures requiring surgical treatment.

Dobbs MB et al: Prevalence of neural axis abnormalities in patients with infantile idiopathic scoliosis. J Bone Joint Surg Am 2002; 84:2230. [PMID: 12473713]

Kyphosis

Kyphosis may be congenital, traumatic, or acquired. Some patients with kyphosis need no treatment, whereas others require immediate surgical attention.

A. POSTURAL KYPHOSIS (POSTURAL ROUNDBACK)

Postural kyphosis, a variation of normal posture, is a cosmetic problem. There is no associated underlying disease, and the spine is flexible and capable of hyperextension. Although it may be worrisome to parents, little scientific evidence indicates that it requires, or responds to, treatment.

B. SCHEUERMANN KYPHOSIS

Scheuermann kyphosis is a disorder of growth of the vertebral end plates that affects adolescents, particularly boys, and produces a progressive rigid forward curvature of the thoracic spine. Less commonly, it involves the lumbar spine, causing decreased lumbar lordosis (relative kyphosis). It is often moderately painful. Radiographs show wedging of vertebral bodies, irregularity of the endplates with radiographic lucent pits known as Schmorl nodules, and kyphosis (Figure 11–34).

Figure 11–34. Scheuermann kyphosis is characterized by vertebral wedging, endplate changes, and kyphosis.

Lumbar Scheuermann kyphosis responds to symptomatic treatment with nonnarcotic pain medications or a supportive lumbar corset. Thoracic involvement with pain or kyphosis of 15–20 degrees greater than normal can be managed with a Milwaukee brace. Brace treatment is usually effective in controlling pain and producing structural correction of the kyphosis. It can sometimes be used at night only so it will not have to be worn during school hours.

Scheuermann disease is the exception to the general rule that spinal bracing must be done during the growth phase to improve deformity. Patients as old as 18 years of age show improvement with the Milwaukee brace. Severe cases (40 degrees excessive kyphosis) may require surgical correction by spinal instrumentation and fusion.

C. CONGENITAL KYPHOSIS

Congenital kyphosis is a rare but important group of diseases, which, like congenital scoliosis, may be caused by failure of formation of vertebrae (hemivertebrae) or failure of embryonic segmentation (anterior unsegmented bar). In most cases, the lesion tends to cause uneven growth, so kyphosis gradually increases as the spine elongates. This can produce bowstringing of the spinal cord over the kyphotic prominence and eventually cause paraplegia. For this reason, any progressive congenital kyphosis must be fused to prevent neurologic complications, regardless of the child's age.

D. TRAUMATIC KYPHOSIS

Traumatic kyphosis is a traumatic compression of vertebrae that may lead to either cosmetic or symptomatic kyphosis. This may be prevented by early surgical stabilization of high-grade unstable traumatic spinal injuries.

E. INFECTIOUS KYPHOSIS

Infectious kyphosis refers to septic destruction of vertebral bodies, which can lead to severe kyphosis. In particular, tuberculous vertebral osteomyelitis can produce soft-tissue abscess, high-grade kyphosis, a sharp gibbus, and paraplegia. Bacterial infection can mimic this, although dramatic deformities are far more unusual.

Treatment includes chemotherapy, surgical debridement and drainage, decompression of the spinal cord, and spinal fusion to prevent further deformity.

Treatment

A. BRACING

Bracing can be used to slow progression of spinal curvatures, prevent progression, or improve underlying structural deformities. Many different types of braces are available, each with its own advocates and specific applications (Figure 11–35). When the goal is to provide postural support, slow progression, or postpone (but not prevent) surgery, a polypropylene body jacket, or so-called clamshell brace, may suffice for waking or sitting hours.

Long-term braces designed to arrest progression must be custom molded for the patient, with pads placed to exert appropriate pressure to reduce deformity. Depending on the anatomic level of the curvature, they may be positioned under the arm or may extend to the neck (Milwaukee brace). This type of brace is usually worn 24 hours a day.

All braces must be modified or replaced to accommodate growth. In general, bracing is only effective with flexible curvatures in growing children.

B. SURGICAL TREATMENT

Surgical intervention is indicated for curvatures that progress despite adequate conservative treatment (usually bracing). It is also required when spinal compression is imminent (tuberculous kyphosis, congenital kyphosis) or when a curvature is so severe that bracing is impossible and future progression likely.

Figure 11–35. Two popular brace styles used for the treatment of spinal deformity are the Milwaukee brace (**A**) and the low-profile (Boston-type) brace (**B**).

1. Surgical stages—Surgery involves two separate stages: correction and stabilization. After posterior exposure of the spine, correction is achieved with a variety of mechanical internal fixation devices. These are usually rods with hooks, screws, wires, or other mechanisms to distract, compress, or bend spinal segments. Correction is rarely complete because mechanical and safety considerations limit the force that can be applied. Once correction is obtained, the cortex of spine is removed and bone graft is placed over the raw bone. Subsequently, solid fusion occurs within 6 months, permanently stabilizing the spine (Figure 11–36).

2. Treatment of severe curvatures—For small curvatures, posterior instrumentation and fusion are sufficient. Some large idiopathic curves and neuromuscular curves require anterior release and bone grafting to render enough acute flexibility for curvature correction and enough late stability for dependable fusion. Occasionally, fusion may fail, causing a pseudarthrosis that may be painful or may allow progression of a previously corrected curvature. In this case, fusion must be repeated.

Lonstein JE: Adolescent idiopathic scoliosis: Screening and diagnosis. Instr Course Lect 1989;38:105. [PMID: 2649563]

Danielsson AJ, Nachemson AL: Radiologic findings and curve progression 22 years after treatment for adolescent idiopathic scoliosis: Comparison of brace and surgical treatment with

A   **B**

Figure 11–36. Treatment of a scoliotic curve by instrumentation and fusion. Preoperative view (**A**) and postoperative view (**B**).

matching control group of straight individuals. Spine 2001; 26:516. [PMID: 11242379]

Weinstein SL, Ponseti IV: Curve progression in idiopathic scoliosis. J Bone Joint Surg Am 1983;65:455. [PMID: 6833318]

NEUROMUSCULAR DISORDERS

Because muscle weakness or imbalance changes the underlying structure of a growing skeleton, neuromuscular diseases of children often require orthopedic evaluation. Treatment may be required to reverse skeletal deformity and contracture or to effect functional improvement.

Many childhood neuromuscular diseases require coordinating the services of the pediatrician, neurologist, physiatrist, therapist, educator, social worker, nurse, and parent.

1. Cerebral Palsy

Cerebral palsy is a static encephalopathy in a growing child. Although it is often birth related, the term also includes childhood head injury, stroke, metabolic brain conditions, and degenerative neurologic conditions.

The challenges to physicians evaluating cerebral palsy are making an accurate diagnosis and detecting correctable conditions. It is essential that functional evaluation of the child's condition take into account the need for education, communication, socialization, and mobility.

Types of Cerebral Palsy

The hallmark of most cases of cerebral palsy is alteration in motor tone (spasticity or dystonia). Spasticity is increased tone associated with stretching of muscle; dystonia is present without changing muscle length. Diagnosis of spasticity can be direct (increased tone, increased deep tendon reflexes, clasp-knife rigidity, and clonus) or inferred (shortening of muscles, contractures of joints, joint dislocations, and scoliosis). Dystonia can be confused with spasticity, but it does not generally lead to contractures.

A. HEMIPLEGIA

Hemiplegia is spasticity involving only one side of the body. Most hemiplegia involves the pyramidal tract, especially at the cerebral cortex. It may be mild or severe and typically is more pronounced in the distal skeleton (hand and foot-ankle). Hemiplegia is usually caused by congenital loss of portions of the parietal, contralateral cerebral cortex. This loss may reflect vascular insufficiency, trauma, or porencephalic cysts.

Many patients with hemiplegia have normal development and intelligence. Children with hemiplegia frequently walk at a normal age, although sometimes with marked posturing of the involved side. Right hemiplegia (left cerebral cortex) may involve the Broca area and thus cause speech deficits. Because sensory and motor cortex areas are contiguous, hemiplegia is strongly associated with abnormalities of sensation and proprioception in the affected limbs. This may prove more disabling than the spasticity because a child may not appreciate an insensate limb as part of overall body image.

B. DIPLEGIA

Diplegia, or diplegic cerebral palsy, is an encephalopathy usually associated with prematurity. It is characterized by relatively symmetric involvement of the lower extremities and lesser involvement of the upper extremities. Prematurity is often accompanied by intracerebral hemorrhage and periventricular leukomalacia, which lead to edema and necrosis in the region of the trigone. This involvement of the pyramidal tract and associated basal ganglia is the main cause of diplegia.

Most diplegic children exhibit mixed patterns of spasticity with a variety of less obvious neurologic symptoms, including ataxia, rigidity, and athetosis (dystonia). Many have normal intelligence (if the cortex is spared) but may suffer developmental delays caused by damage to associative fibers in the brain. Although they may initially be hypotonic ("floppy"), most diplegic patients develop high tone (dystonic rigidity) and spasticity by 12–18 months of age.

Diplegia, usually more severe in the lower extremities, is relatively symmetric. Many children with diplegia eventually walk, exhibiting a crouching gait characterized by flexed, internally rotated hips, flexed knees, and plantar-flexed ankles.

C. QUADRIPLEGIA

Quadriplegia (total body involvement) often occurs in children who suffer birth asphyxia, metabolic encephalopathy, or encephalitis. Severe spasticity, seizures, mental retardation, joint contractures, and scoliosis are typical but not always individually present in this type of cerebral palsy. Children with quadriplegia are particularly susceptible to spontaneous hip dislocations (because of hip muscle imbalance) and high-grade scoliosis. Both of these conditions interfere with sitting and may require surgery. Most quadriplegic patients require wheelchair assistance and do not walk.

D. MIXED NEUROLOGIC INVOLVEMENT

Mixed neurologic involvement of extrapyramidal portions of the brain can cause athetosis, dystonia, ballismus, and ataxia. Many children with cerebral palsy exhibit subtle signs of some of these disorders, in addition to spasticity. In some children, one of these signs may predominate, but spasticity is absent. In general, prognosis varies with the anatomy of involvement.

Treatment

Before treating cerebral palsy, specific goals should be set for the patient. Although many important goals are not orthopedic, the surgeon may help the patient achieve them. Increased mobility, for instance, may facilitate achieving a variety of nonorthopedic goals. Especially urgent are the patient's ability to communicate, move independently, and socialize. Orthopedic treatment may improve sitting position in the wheelchair or improve walking by releasing muscles or joints.

Many children benefit from physical or occupational therapy during the first few years of life. Although the exact role of such therapy in cerebral palsy remains undefined, therapists often help parents and children deal more effectively with the complex problems presented by the disease. Therapists also help parents and children set optimistic and realistic goals for the future.

Bracing or surgery may be required to control effects of spasticity on individual joints and to decrease spasticity, correct dislocation or contracture, or control scoliosis. Surgery is ineffective in the case of extrapyramidal neurologic symptoms. A variety of nonorthopedic treatments are also used for cerebral palsy. Selective dorsal rhizotomy, a neurosurgical procedure to cut a portion of the posterior roots of the lumbar spinal cord, may reduce spasticity in selected patients by interrupting the reflex arc. Botulinum toxin injection (or phenol injection) into the motor endplate region of a muscle temporarily interrupts the nerve supply, relaxing a spastic muscle for several months and allowing therapy or other evaluation. Oral baclofen can reduce overall spasticity. Intrathecal baclofen, delivered by a subcutaneous pump,

may offer relaxation of troublesome lower extremity muscle tension in both dystonic and spastic patients.

Hip subluxation is common in quadriplegia, and pelvic radiographs in young quadriplegic patients are needed to detect early, reversible involvement. Subluxation may be treated in children younger than 3–4 years by adductor muscle release, which improves abduction. Rarely, the anterior obturator nerve (which innervates the adductor longus muscle) is resected to weaken the adductors. In older children, bony reconstruction by varus-derotation osteotomy and acetabular reorientation or supplementation may be necessary to correct the bone malformation that results from the force of spastic muscles on the growing skeleton. Children who develop hip subluxation often develop scoliosis as well (see section on scoliosis).

A. ADDUCTOR RELEASE

Adductor release may be done as an open procedure (usually by myotomy or transverse sectioning of the adductor longus and a portion of the adductor brevis) or by percutaneous adductor tenotomy (section of the tendon origin of the adductor longus at the pelvis). The exact technique and amount of release is dictated by the severity of contracture and other factors. When done for hip subluxation, adductor release is most effective before 3–4 years of age. It should be sufficient to allow hip abduction of 70–80 degrees on the operating table. When frank subluxation is present, some surgeons perform an anterior obturator neurectomy in addition to the adductor myotomy. This open procedure removes a segment of the obturator nerve that supplies the released adductor longus muscle, so the muscle remains loose after spontaneously reattaching after surgery.

Obturator neurectomy must be used carefully because it can cause excessive weakening of the adductors and, subsequently, late hip abduction contracture. After each of these procedures, the patient is casted in abduction for 3–4 weeks to allow muscle healing in the new elongated position.

Dynamic spasticity or joint contracture (the result of chronic spasticity) can interfere with walking in children with hemiplegia or diplegia. This may be treated by bracing involved joints in a functional position or by surgical lengthening of the muscle–tendon unit. Such muscle releases can be done by complete tenotomy, tendon Z-lengthening (common at the Achilles tendon), or lengthening of the aponeurosis of a muscle, which is often done for the iliopsoas or hamstrings (Figure 11–37).

It is convenient to combine multiple procedures for children with cerebral palsy. For example, a typical hemiplegic with a tiptoe (equinus) gait may benefit from lengthening the Achillis tendon to make the foot plantargrade. A typical diplegic patient with a crouching gait may benefit from hip flexor, hamstring, and Achilles tendon lengthenings performed bilaterally during a single operation. The exact timing and extent of surgery

Figure 11–37. Schematic representation of surgical options for muscle release or lengthening in cerebral palsy. **A:** Myotomy; **B:** tenotomy; **C:** aponeurotomy.

are controversial among experts in cerebral palsy. Three-dimensional computerized gait analysis, performed in motion laboratories, can guide the surgeon.

B. MUSCLE RELEASE FOR DYNAMIC DEFORMITY

Muscle releases for dynamic deformity may be done in several ways, depending on the specific muscle, the presence of contracture, and the surgeon's preference. The goal is to weaken spastic muscles to reduce their abnormal influence while not lengthening them so much that the opposite deformity occurs. The more common procedures are described here.

1. Achilles tendon lengthening—Achilles tendon lengthening is usually done by Z-lengthening of the distal tendon. Cuts for Z-lengthening can be either open or percutaneous. The ankle is carefully dorsiflexed just beyond neutral to allow the tendon fibers to slide into an elongated position. The surgeon must avoid overlengthening (a matter of judgment) because an excessively weakened gastrocnemius-soleus group hinders walking and can actually encourage a deeper crouching gait.

2. Gastrocnemius lengthening—Gastrocnemius lengthening is required in patients whose gastrocnemius is considerably more spastic than the soleus. In such cases, ankle dorsiflexion is limited and ankle clonus occurs when the knee is extended, but free dorsiflexion occurs when the knee is flexed. In such patients, the gastrocnemius alone may be released by approaching the musculotendinous junction in the calf and sectioning the aponeurosis or by release of the insertion of the gastrocnemius where it attaches to the soleus and Achilles tendon. This effectively recesses the muscle, selectively weakening it while retaining soleus strength for pushoff during walking.

3. Hamstring lengthening—Hamstring lengthening is indicated when the hamstrings are tight (limited straight-leg raising) and knee flexion is persistent during the stance phase of gait (crouching gait). Usually, the distal medial and lateral hamstrings are released, but procedures vary widely among surgeons. On the medial side, the gracilis and semitendinosus tendons are usually Z-lengthened or tenotomized (transversely released). The semimembranosus is lengthened by transverse incision of its aponeurosis, which allows the interior muscle fibers to stretch and lengthen. Laterally, both heads of the biceps femoris can be managed by aponeurotic lengthening as well. The procedure must be done carefully to avoid cutting or stretching the sciatic or peroneal nerves. The leg is splinted or casted in extension for 3–4 weeks to allow soft-tissue healing.

4. Iliopsoas lengthening—The hip flexors (psoas and iliacus) may be released at the insertion of the conjoined tendon into the lesser trochanter, usually done in sitters also undergoing adductor release for spastic hip subluxation. If the child is walking and less weakening of hip flexion is desired, the psoas tendon alone can be sectioned at the level of the pelvic brim, retaining the iliacus portion of the muscle for strength.

DeLuca PA: The musculoskeletal management of children with cerebral palsy. Pediatr Clin North Am 1996;43:1135.

2. Myelomeningocele (Spina Bifida)

Myelomeningocele is a complex birth defect affecting the spinal cord and central nervous system. Although the cause is not fully understood, there is a hereditary component. Lack of maternal folic acid is identified as a causative factor in an estimated 50–70% of cases.

Embryologic Defect

The basic embryologic defect is a failure of complete tubulation and dorsal closure of the embryonic neural tube and placode, including incomplete closure of the skin over the spinal cord, resulting from lack of induction. In its mildest form, this spinal dysraphism consists of a simple spina bifida occulta or isolated meningocele (protrusion of spinal membranes, but not nerve, outside of the spinal canal, without neurologic deficit). The more severe varieties include herniation of membranes and nervous tissue through large dorsal bony and skin defects at birth and hydrocephalus with cerebral malformations (Figure 11–38).

Myelomeningocele can occur at any spinal level but usually is seen between levels T12 and S2. Because neural tissue fails to form properly, the child is paraplegic and insensate below the level of the dysraphism. The clinical determination of neurologic level is most easily accomplished by describing the last muscles contracting under active voluntary motor control (Table 11–8). This may

Figure 11–38. Spina bifida (myelomeningocele). The sac includes dysplastic spinal cord and membrane elements, and it must be surgically closed in the first days of life. Hydrocephalus and congenital scoliosis are commonly associated.

be difficult because of anatomic variability, the age of the child, and other central nervous system involvement.

Treatment of Orthopedic Problems

Orthopedic problems associated with myelomeningocele include clubfoot or congenital vertical talus, torsional deformities of the legs, contractures, hip dislocations, and scoliosis. The lack of sensation may allow extensive pressure sores to develop, or painless fractures may go undetected by patients. The health defects of children with spina bifida, in addition to their paralysis, usually include nonmusculoskeletal organ system problems such as hydrocephalus or Arnold-Chiari malformation (brain), syrinx formation or tethering (spinal cord), and neurogenic bladder or hydronephrosis (renal system). Early in life, most of these are more important than the orthopedic manifestations, and a team approach is needed to decide when and how best to coordinate management. The most pressing needs of the infant born with spina bifida are usually neural defect closure and ventricular shunting.

Orthopedic management depends on the deformities and the long-term mobility goals for the child. The level of paralysis often is helpful in determining whether the child will ultimately be able to walk (L5 or S1 function usually required) or will require a wheelchair (because of function only proximal to L4 or L5). Foot deformities such as clubfoot or congenital vertical talus usually require surgery. If foot deformities recur or progress, tethered cord should be suspected.

Spina bifida is theoretically a static neurologic disease, but many children exhibit a drifting deterioration

of neurologic function as they grow; progression of foot deformities, especially during growth spurts, suggests tethering (and therefore stretching) of the cord. Hip dislocations, although dramatic on radiograph, frequently require no treatment; they are painless and tend to occur in children with neurologic involvement at L2 to L4, which precludes long-term walking.

A young child with scoliosis may require bracing until the thorax is long enough for spinal fusion. Scoliosis surgery is complicated by absent posterior neural arches. Some scoliosis seen with spina bifida is congenital (see section on scoliosis). If rapidly progressive scoliosis occurs, the physician should suspect a neurologic cause such as syrinx. Because of chronic exposure to latex materials in contact with mucous membranes and internal tissues (shunts, catheters), children with spina bifida are exceedingly susceptible to latex allergy, which can be fatal. Steps to limit latex exposure are essential in this population and must be observed by medical personnel working with them.

Bunch WH: Myelomeningocele: Part I. General concepts. Instr Course Lect 1976;xxv:61–64.

CDC (Centers for Disease Control and Prevention): Spina bifida and anencephaly before and after folic acid mandate—United States, 1995–1996 and 1999–2000. MMWR Morb Mortal Wkly Rep 2004;53:362. [PMID: 15129193]

Mazur JM, Menelaus MB: Neurologic status of spina bifida patients and the orthopedic surgeon. Clin Orthop 1991;264:54.

Oakshott P, Hunt GM: Long-term outcome in open spina bifida. Br J Gen Pract 2003;53:632. [PMID: 14601340]

Wehby MC et al: Occult tight filum terminale syndrome: Results of surgical untethering. Pediatr Neurosurg 2004;40:51. [PMID: 15292632]

Table 11–8. Muscle function at neurologic levels in myelomeningocoele (spina bifida).

Neurologic Level	Functions	Muscles Active
T12	Hip flexion (weak)	Iliopsoas (weak)
L1	Hip flexion	Iliopsoas
L2	Hip adduction (weak)	Adductor longus, brevis (weak)
L3	Hip adduction	Adductors
	Knee extension (weak)	Quadriceps (weak)
L4	Knee extension	Quadriceps
	Ankle dorsiflexion	Anterior tibialis (variable)
L5	Knee flexion	Medial hamstring
	Hip abduction	Tensor fascia lata
S1	Knee flexion	All hamstrings
	Ankle plantar flexion	Gastrocnemius-soleus
S2	Toe flexion	Flexor digitorum longus

3. Muscular Dystrophy

Duchenne muscular dystrophy is an X-linked disorder that presents orthopedic features in boys 6–9 years of age. The disorder is one of progressive muscle weakness, usually first involving more proximal muscles of the limb girdles. Pseudohypertrophy caused by replacement of gastrocnemius muscles (or other muscles) with fat is a classic finding, as is Gower sign (an inability to rise from the floor without using the hands to walk up the body and legs). As the muscles weaken, imbalance can cause fixed flexion contractures of the hip, knee, and ankle plantar flexors, which limits walking ability. Because weakness eventually forces patients into a wheelchair, a decision to brace or correct these contractures surgically depends on estimates of remaining strength and likely duration of ambulation after treatment. Most often, progressive foot deformities (usually equinovarus) require muscle release and correction (including bracing) because use of the wheelchair also requires relatively well-positioned feet.

As weakness progresses, the child requires an electric wheelchair for mobility. At this point, scoliosis begins to appear and is usually relentlessly progressive. Attempts to control the scoliosis of muscular dystrophy by wheelchair inserts and braces are ineffective. Early surgery (before cardiorespiratory status deteriorates) is often the best answer. Chapter 13, Rehabilitation, provides more information.

4. Myotonic Dystrophy

Myotonic dystrophy is a genetic muscle disease whose name reflects the hallmark of the disease: myotonic EMG potentials. The disease is often associated with mild-to-moderate retardation, obesity, and foot deformities. Initial diagnosis is made by identifying the characteristic myotonic face (weak perioral muscles with a distinctive pyramidal mouth), confirmed by EMG. Myotonic dystrophy worsens with each succeeding generation; genetic markers are available for diagnosis.

The most frequent foot deformity is equinovarus, often with weakness of the anterior tibialis and overactivity of the posterior tibialis. Surgery is often required, and recurrence requiring additional surgery is common. Surgical treatment of myotonic dystrophy foot deformities includes joint release (for passive correction of the deformity) and muscle transfers (for rebalancing muscle forces).

5. Spinal Muscular Atrophy

This heterogeneous group of disorders includes static and degenerative lesions of the anterior horn cell population in the spinal cord. These disorders all involve muscle weakness caused by a lower motor neuron lesion, that is, flaccid paralysis. Sensation is intact, and the major goals are mobility (with electric wheelchair), adaptive devices to aid in daily living (eg, feeding devices), and control of scoliosis, which is similar to management of scoliosis in advanced muscular dystrophy (see section on muscular dystrophy).

Green NE: The orthopaedic care of children with muscular dystrophy. Instr Course Lect 1987;36:267.

Voisin V, de la Porte S: Therapeutic strategies for Duchenne and Becker dystrophies. Int Rev Cytol 2004;240:1. [PMID: 15548414]

6. Arthrogryposis (Arthrogryposis Multiplex Congenita)

Arthrogryposis is not a disease per se but rather a symptom complex that includes joint contractures or dislocations, rigid skeletal deformities (especially clubfoot), shiny skin with decreased wrinkling and subcutaneous tissue, weakness, and muscle wasting. Although many factors contribute to arthrogryposis, the common link among the symptoms appears to be decreased fetal movement during a critical period in limb development. This can be caused by neurologic lesions (congenital absence of anterior horn cells, Werdnig-Hoffman spinal muscular atrophy, myelomeningocele), myopathic lesions (myotonic dystrophy, congenital myopathies), various syndromes (Moebius syndrome), or physical restriction associated with oligohydramnios.

Arthrogrypotic infants frequently have extension or flexion contractures of knees and elbows, dislocated hips, and severe clubfeet. The contractures may partially resolve with passive ROM therapy in the first 6–12 months of life; however, they must be released surgically after that if they interfere with walking or arm use. Hip dislocations may not limit function and often are not treated. Clubfeet require surgery, which is often of limited success; multiple operations are frequently necessary. Arthrogrypotic children are generally highly resourceful in achieving mobility, and they care for themselves completely independently, despite seemingly overwhelming skeletal problems.

TUMORS

Skeletal neoplasms, particularly benign ones, are fairly common in children. Common benign bone lesions of childhood include osteochondroma, osteoid osteoma, unicameral (simple) bone cysts, chondroblastoma, hemangioma, histiocytosis X (eosinophilic granuloma), and fibrous dysplasia. Malignant tumors, which are usually seen after 10 years of age, include Ewing sarcoma and osteosarcoma. Certain systemic diseases can be manifested in childhood as apparent bone tumors (hyperparathyroidism, renal disease, leukemia). Chapter 6 offers a detailed discussion of bone tumors.

AMPUTATIONS

Congenital Amputations & Absence of Segments

Congenital absence of limb segments at birth can occur sporadically, as part of a syndrome (Streeter dysplasia) or as a result of mutagens (eg, thalidomide). Absence may be terminal (eg, congenital below-knee amputation) or intercalary (eg, congenital shortening or absence of the humerus).

Although congenital amputations can be dramatic in appearance, the missing limb is not part of the child's body image. Thus, the child has a natural instinct to be mobile. Children with severe limb deficiencies at birth are almost always able to be completely independent and functional. They accept prostheses quite readily but only if the device truly improves their efficiency. For example, nearly all congenital above-elbow amputees reject artificial limbs, opting for function over appearance. Parents may harbor strong feelings of guilt over the child's condition, so the psychological issues associated with the condition are more those of the adults than the child.

It is not unusual for congenital amputations to require conversion to a level more easily fitted with a prosthesis. For example, fibular hemimelia (severe shortening of the tibia with absent fibula and foot deformity) sometimes can be most effectively treated by removing the foot and converting the limb to an ankle disarticulation level. This facilitates prosthetic fitting and simplifies management of the leg-length discrepancy, thus permitting normal function.

Boostra AM et al: Children with congenital deficiencies or acquired amputations of the lower limbs: Functional aspects. Prosthet Orthot Int 2000;24:19. [PMID: 10855435]

Ephraim PL et al: Epidemiology of limb loss and congenital limb deficiency: A review of the literature. Arch Phys Med Rehabil 2003;84:747. [PMID: 12736892]

Fixsen JA: Major lower limb congenital shortening: A mini review. J Pediatr Orthop B 2003;12:1. [PMID: 12488764]

Krebs DE, Fishman S: Characteristics of the child amputee population. J Pediatr Orthop 1984;4:8. [PMID: 6693574]

Rijnders LJ et al: Lower limb deficient children in the Netherlands: Epidemiological aspects. Prosthet Orthot Int 2000;24:13. [PMID: 10855434]

Traumatic Amputation

In contrast to the congenital amputee, the child with a traumatic amputation is particularly likely to be male, adolescent, rebellious, and troubled. Although pediatric traumatic amputations are often caused by inadvertent incidents, many result from high-risk behavior. These factors must be taken into account when dealing with the psychological issues of the patient and family; social, as well as medical, intervention is often appropriate.

The orthopedic management of traumatic amputees is modified in children by the presence of growth plates and the remarkable healing and rehabilitation powers of children. This must be considered during surgical completion of amputations because injury to the physis may cause severe shortening or angulation of a stump, rendering the amputation far less satisfactory than a similar amputation in the adult. The child amputee rarely has vascular problems, however, and the use of split-thickness skin grafting may allow preservation of length that would be impossible in most adults.

Overgrowth of Amputation Stump

Amputations through the long bones of children exhibit the unique phenomenon of terminal overgrowth. Eventually, the distal end of the stump may develop a long, thin, sometimes painful bony prominence. Overgrowth is not physeal in origin (ie, closure of the physis by epiphysiodesis does not eliminate its formation), and it appears to be related to aggressive bone formation associated with the periosteal membrane.

Although overgrowth can occur in any bone, it is most troublesome in the tibia, fibula, and humerus. When symptomatic, overgrowth is treated by resecting the spike of bone (revision of the amputation), but the process does continue, and recurrence is common. Some pediatric amputees require two or more surgical revisions during growth. Overgrowth ceases at skeletal maturity. Various attempts at capping the overgrowing bone end (using foreign materials or free epiphyseal grafts) have met with inconsistent success.

Tenholder M et al: Surgical management of juvenile amputation overgrowth with a synthetic cap. J Pediatr Orthop 2004;24:218. [PMID: 15076611]

FRACTURES

Common Pediatric Fracture Patterns

Many fractures in children are similar to their counterparts in adults. However, the added factor of growth contributes to the unique issues of fracture care in children. Pediatric bone is softer and more easily broken than adult cortical bone. Thus, the amount of energy required to produce a fracture is less in the child, even as soft-tissue injury is frequently less severe in the child than in the adult. In addition, the periosteal membrane in children is far thicker and more osteogenic than in adults. The periosteum is so leathery in immature humans that it frequently holds bone ends together, contributing greatly to stability and ease of manipulative reduction. The excellent osteogenic potential of pediatric periosteum permits rapid, aggressive fracture healing, so nonunions are extremely rare in children.

Figure 11–39. Softer bone in children can lead to unique fracture behavior (in addition to the fracture patterns seen in adults). **A:** Greenstick fracture; **B:** torus fracture; **C:** plastic deformation.

Figure 11–40. Remodeling of bone after fracture is most rapid when it is in the plane of a nearby joint. Schematically, if the joint is thought of as a hinge, the fracture above (in the plane of the hinge) is likely to remodel faster than the fracture below the hinge (out of plane).

Less brittle pediatric bone is subject to fracture patterns unique to children (Figure 11–39). A greenstick fracture is a transverse crack that retains its continuity, just as a small moist twig breaks without actually snapping apart.

A torus fracture is a small buckle or impaction of one cortex with a slight bend on the opposite cortex. Plastic deformation is a change in the natural shape of a bone without a detectable fracture line.

Remodeling (gradual correction in alignment or size of a fractured bone back to normal) is generally far more rapid in children than in adults. Remodeling of angular deformities is particularly rapid when the deformity is in the same plane of motion as the nearest joint (Figure 11–40) or when the deformity is near a rapidly growing physis. Remodeling of rotational deformities is less reliable. Overgrowth is a singular feature of remodeling that occurs in certain fractures of the long bones, particularly the femur. It is a product of physeal stimulation by the hyperemic response to fracture and healing and may increase the length of a bone by 2 cm or more over the course of a year.

The combination of low-energy injury, rapid bone healing, and dependable remodeling of angular deformity makes it possible to treat many pediatric fractures by simple closed reduction (often incomplete) and casting. Surgical management of children's fractures is rarely required. The surgeon may accept a less-than-perfect reduction if the fracture is known to remodel into satisfactory alignment.

1. Epiphyseal Fracture

The cartilage physeal plates are a region of low strength relative to the surrounding bone and are susceptible to fracture in the child. They are analogous to a scratch on a pane of glass, in which concentrated force facilitates damage. Once injury occurs, the physis usually is able to recover and resume growth. But if an offset occurs in the physeal substance, bone may grow across it (from epiphyseal bone to metaphyseal bone), forming a bridge that anchors further growth and leads to either progressive shortening or a worsening angulation (Figure 11–41).

Figure 11–41. Progressive angular deformity can occur if there is asymmetric closure of the physis after fracture.

Because physes are near joints and physeal fractures are common, children may suffer injuries to joint surfaces that require careful surgical repair and realignment. Thus, open reduction is more likely in fractures involving physes and joints than in other pediatric fractures.

Most physeal fractures propagate through the weakest region of the cartilage. Physeal cartilage begins in a dense resting zone on the epiphyseal side, and chondrocytes gradually multiply, elongate, and arrange into longitudinal columns that produce longitudinal growth. Hypertrophic, balloonlike chondrocyte columns then undergo cell death, and the remaining cell walls are calcified and eventually ossify to form metaphyseal bone.

The weakest spot is usually the interface between hypertrophic dying columns of cells and the stiff calcified cell walls beneath them; this area is highly susceptible to shearing forces. Fortunately, the region also represents the boundary between the process of epiphyseal elongation (supported by the epiphyseal blood supply) and metaphyseal ossification (supported by the metaphyseal blood supply). Thus, physeal fractures do not often damage the growth potential of the physis because they do not interrupt its critical blood supply.

Although physeal fractures can occur in a wide variety of configurations, certain patterns are seen frequently enough that a descriptive classification aids in understanding physeal injury (Figure 11–42). Fractures

Figure 11–42. The Salter-Harris classification of physeal fractures is widely used to describe such injuries. With some exceptions, the potential for problems with growth arrest is greater in the higher numbered patterns.

that either cross the joint or result in spatial malalignment of portions of the physis have the worst prognosis.

Physeal fractures heal rapidly, usually within 4 weeks. Careful monitoring is required to detect early posttraumatic closure of the growth plate. Occasionally, an epiphyseal–metaphyseal bony bridge forms and tethers growth. If this growth is minor, surgical removal of the bridge (epiphyseal bar resection) may successfully restore physeal growth. Otherwise, the procedures for evaluation and treatment of limb-length inequality should be followed (see section 1. Limb-length inequality).

Salter RB, Harris WR: Injuries involving the growth plate. J Bone Joint Surg Am 1963;45:587.

2. Upper Extremity Fractures

Clavicle Fracture

Clavicle fractures are among the most common injuries in children. They are usually closed and may be treated with a simple sling. Healing occurs rapidly with abundant callus, which leaves a lump that may concern parents. This enlargement remodels over several years of growth.

An extremely rare condition, atraumatic congenital pseudarthrosis of the clavicle, can mimic the radiographic appearance of fracture. It may be right sided or bilateral, with little or no pain and no history of trauma. Treatment is generally unnecessary.

Proximal Humerus Fracture

Proximal humerus fractures are usually epiphyseal injuries (usually Salter-Harris type II injuries) that may progress into significant varus angulation (medial deviation). Fortunately, the proximal humerus is a rapidly growing physis and shoulder motion is full in all planes, so remodeling is rapid. These fractures generally require only a sling or shoulder immobilization for 3–4 weeks, without reduction. Rarely, fractures with extreme angulation (more than 90 degrees) may require surgical reduction and fixation.

Elbow Region Fracture

Most elbow region fractures are indirect injuries caused by a fall on the outstretched hand. Both diagnosis and treatment can be difficult in this serious group of injuries. Epiphyseal ossification is incomplete in the group that is susceptible to falls (2–10 years of age), making radiographs difficult to interpret (Figure 11–43). Swelling, if severe, can block venous or arterial structures and lead to forearm compartment syndromes. Reductions are often unstable, and operative intervention may be required. Most surgeons immobilize pediatric elbow fractures for 4 weeks after treatment. The most important fractures are listed next.

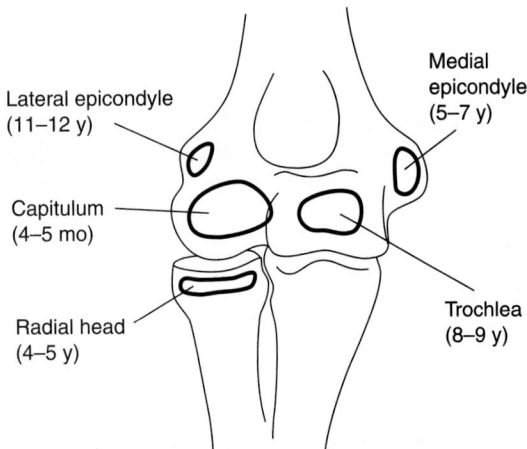

Figure 11–43. Ages of appearance of ossification centers. The ossification centers of the elbow region emerge at different ages as indicated and can complicate the interpretation of radiographs. It is often advisable to obtain comparison radiographs of the opposite elbow if injury is suspected.

A. SUPRACONDYLAR FRACTURE OF HUMERUS

Supracondylar fracture of the humerus occurs at the metaphyseal bone, proximal to the elbow joint, and does not involve the growth plate (Figure 11–44). Displacement may be severe, and nerve injury, usually caused by stretching, is common. If swelling is marked, there may be interruption of the blood supply; it is not uncommon for such a distal extremity to lack a pulse.

The most appropriate treatment is rapid anatomic reduction under general anesthesia. Because the reduction is highly unstable, many surgeons prefer to fix the fracture after reduction with percutaneous wires. Once the fracture is reduced, the swelling recedes rapidly and the pulse returns. On rare occasions, the surgeon must perform vascular or nerve exploration or repair.

Some displaced supracondylar humerus fractures are incompletely reduced or lose position because of fracture instability after apparently adequate initial reduction. These progress to a characteristic malunion with an apex-lateral angular deformity of the elbow (known as cubitus varus or so-called gunstock deformity). Although cosmetically unsightly, cubitus varus rarely has any significant functional consequences. If desired, it may be corrected by valgus osteotomy at the old fracture site.

B. LATERAL CONDYLE FRACTURE

The lateral condyle fracture is an oblique shearing fracture of the lateral portion of the joint surface that occurs when the radial head drives into the capitulum of the humerus during a fall. The lack of significant ossification may obscure the fracture or give the false appearance of a benign Salter-Harris II fracture pattern, but most lateral condyle fractures are highly unstable Salter-Harris IV fractures (Figure 11–45). Because both the joint surface and the physis are displaced, they usually require open reduction and fixation using pins.

C. RADIAL NECK FRACTURE

Fracture of the radial neck is similar to a lateral condyle fracture. The radial neck just distal to the joint may angulate up to 70–80 degrees, although lesser angulation is more common (Figure 11–46). It is important to determine the location of the radial head despite traumatic angulation of the radial neck. Surprisingly, angulation of 45 degrees or less usually remodels spontaneously and requires only symptomatic treatment that permits early return to activity. Larger degrees of angulation can often respond to closed manipulation.

D. FOREARM FRACTURE

Forearm fractures are a common result of falls. If they involve both bones, one bone may be completely displaced while the other only bends or suffers a greenstick fracture. In children, most forearm fractures that involve both bones can be treated successfully by closed reduction and casting; minor angular malalignment can easily be tolerated if rotational alignment of the bone ends is accurate. In addition, the ends of fractured bones often overlap. This is not necessarily of concern if alignment is satisfactory because side-to-side bone healing and remodeling are rapid in children.

E. MONTEGGIA FRACTURE

Monteggia fracture is fracture of the ulna only, with the radius remaining intact. Because two-bone systems generally must fail in two spots if they break at all, the radial head dislocates from the capitulum. In such cases, reduction must include the elbow component. As with other pediatric forearm fractures, closed reduction is usually successful, although some Monteggia fractures require open reduction. The physician should be alert to the possibility of Monteggia fracture because the fracture can lead to chronic loss of elbow motion if it is not properly reduced.

In children, Galeazzi fracture of the radius, in which the distal radioulnar joint is dislocated, is far less common than the analogous Monteggia fracture.

F. TORUS FRACTURE OF RADIUS

Torus fracture of the radius is a minor buckle of the dorsal cortex of the distal radius, usually 1–2 cm proximal to the distal radial physis. It occurs after a minor fall on the hand. Many torus fractures are mistaken for wrist sprains because they are stable and not as painful

A   **B**

Figure 11–44. Displaced supracondylar fracture of the humerus. Injury film (**A**); after closed reduction and internal fixation using percutaneous pins (**B**).

as unstable fractures. They heal uneventfully in 3–4 weeks, with excellent long-term results.

Laumay F et al: Lateral humeral condyle fractures in children: A comparison of two approaches to treatment. J Pediatr Orthop 2004;24:385. [PMID: 15205620]

Mirsky EC et al: Lateral condyle fractures in children: Evaluation of classification and treatment. J Orthop Trauma 1997;11:117. [PMID: 9057147]

Wattenbarger JM, Gerardi J, Johnston CE: Late open reduction internal fixation of lateral condyle fractures. J Pediatr Orthop 2002;22:394. [PMID: 11961463]

Metacarpal & Phalangeal Fractures

Fractures of the metacarpals and phalanges commonly occur from crush injuries in children (eg, catching a hand or finger in a door) and are generally quite stable because the periosteum remains intact. Rarely severely angulated or rotationally malaligned, they can usually be managed by immobilization for 2–3 weeks.

3. Lower Extremity Fractures

Pelvic Fracture

Pelvic fractures in children are usually seen in conjunction with major blunt trauma. Gross displacement is fairly uncommon and usually can be treated symptomatically because the intact periosteum stabilizes the large flat bones. The patient should be carefully evaluated for intraabdominal and other injuries. Properly treated pelvic fractures in an immature skeleton resolve satisfactorily.

Adolescents exhibit a special type of avulsion fracture of apophyses because aggressive pulling of muscles during sports can detach an apophysis from its parent bone. These avulsion fractures are sometimes called transitional fractures because the physes are in transition within 2 years of skeletal maturity. During this time, relatively weak cartilage physes may not be strong enough to withstand the pull of growing muscles sud-

Figure 11–45. Lateral condyle fracture of the humerus (**A**) can easily be mistaken for a relatively simple Salter-Harris type II injury, which carries a good prognosis (**B**). In reality, however, it is almost always a Salter-Harris type IV injury, with a fracture pattern crossing both the joint surface and the physis (**C**); unless it is not displaced, it requires open reduction.

denly grown powerful under the influence of hormones. Transitional avulsion fractures may occur at the iliac crest (abdominal muscles), lesser trochanter of the femur (iliopsoas muscle), or ischial tuberosity (hamstring muscle). Transitional fractures of the pelvis and femur are treated symptomatically. Although these frac-

tures do not require reduction, they may heal with a significant bump that requires excision later.

Tsirikos AI et al: Transepiphyseal fracture-dislocation of the femoral neck: A case report and review of the literature. J Orthop Trauma 2003;17:648. [PMID: 14574194]

Figure 11–46. Fracture of the radial neck may angulate greatly yet still remodel spontaneously in the younger child.

Hip Fracture

Pediatric hip fractures are rare but may be serious because trauma to this area may produce significant injury. As in the adult, the fracture pattern may disrupt the blood supply of the proximal femoral head and lead to avascular necrosis of the proximal femoral epiphysis, femoral neck, or both. In older children, this can be a devastating complication; it is treated like LCP but may result in such severe collapse that hip fusion is required.

Femoral neck fractures in children are highly unstable and treated by reduction and internal fixation. The mechanical fixation may be imperfect because the surgeon must avoid injury to the proximal femoral physis. For this reason, a spica cast (body and legs) is generally used as well.

Odent T et al: Traumatic dislocation of the hip with separation of the capital epiphysis: 5 adolescent patients with 3–9 years of follow-up. Acta Orthop Scand 2003;74:49. [PMID: 12635793]

Femoral Shaft Fracture

Fractures of the femoral shaft are common injuries caused by falls as well as bicycle and motor vehicle accidents. In young children, they may be the result of child abuse. Although most are closed injuries, blood loss can be significant because of bleeding into the soft tissues of the thigh. Nerve injury is rare, and the fact that the fracture is surrounded by richly nourished muscle ensures rapid solid union (usually within 6 weeks).

Longitudinal muscle pull and spasm cause femoral shaft fractures to shorten and angulate. Initial treatment requires longitudinal traction (skin traction in younger children, skeletal traction in older children) to restore length and alignment. At this point, treatment largely depends on the patient's age.

Femur fractures in children 2–10 years of age have a strong tendency to exhibit overgrowth of 1–2.5 cm because of fracture hyperemia. In this age group, therefore, it may be desirable to use a cast and allow some shortening to occur. Rapid remodeling of the bone makes perfect reduction unnecessary. Most surgeons apply a spica cast immediately or within the first week.

Femoral overgrowth following fracture becomes unlikely in children older than 10 years. In these older children, the bone either must be kept to anatomic length by traction for 3–4 weeks (until sufficient callus has formed to stabilize length) or treated by intramedullary nails or other operative measures, as in the adult. Currently, flexible intramedullary nails are popular because they do not require reaming prior to insertion, and they are less likely to disrupt the precarious blood supply of the proximal femur. There is now a tendency at many centers to fix femur fractures using flexible nails in children 6 years and older.

After healing or cast removal, the child may begin walking. Limping is common in the first month after fracture because the hip girdle musculature regains its strength only slowly. No physical therapy is required, however, because normal walking permits spontaneous recovery, and long-term results of pediatric femur fractures are excellent.

Epiphyseal Separation

Epiphyseal separations (fracture) of the distal femoral physis are usually Salter-Harris type I or II injuries. All are caused by significant trauma, and injury to the growth mechanism of the plate is common. As many as 50% of cases exhibit subsequent growth arrest. Major neurovascular injury can occur, as with knee dislocations. Displaced epiphyseal separations require gentle reduction under general anesthesia. Some are so unstable, however, that they require percutaneous pin fixation for several weeks until the fracture is sticky, as it were, or healed enough so displacement does not occur. If physeal closure occurs, the treatment depends on age and remaining growth potential. (See discussion of limb-length inequality.)

Tibial Eminence Injury

The tibial eminence (spine), located entirely on the proximal tibial epiphysis, is the site of attachment of the anterior cruciate ligament. Twisting injuries of the knee can shear off the eminence and may displace it within the joint. Usually, the fragment reduces with full

Figure 11–47. Tibial eminence fracture usually includes an anterior cruciate avulsion component. It can be treated nonoperatively if the fragment reduces with extension of the knee.

extension of the knee, but open reduction can be performed if necessary. Casting in extension is used for 6 weeks, until the bone heals (Figure 11–47). Unlike many other pediatric fractures, tibial eminence injuries often lead to mild long-term knee symptoms, especially during athletic activities.

Tibial Tubercle Avulsion Fracture

Tibial tubercle avulsion fractures are most often seen in adolescent males (13–14 years of age) who suffer sports-related injuries. The anterior tongue of the proximal tibial epiphysis is the site of attachment of the patellar tendon. During strenuous jumping, as in basketball, the tongue may avulse and displace. Sometimes the fracture extends into the joint and across the tibial joint surface. Tibial tubercle avulsions are transitional fractures in that they occur immediately before physeal closure and are not seen in younger children. Nearly all these fractures require open reduction and internal fixation, although the surgeon need not take the usual precautions when operating near the physis because maturity follows too rapidly to permit deformity.

Proximal Tibial Metaphyseal Fracture

Proximal tibial metaphyseal fractures are usually undisplaced or minimally displaced. In the absence of fibular overgrowth (Figure 11–48), they can exhibit trou-

blesome late angular deformity (valgus) caused by tibial overgrowth after fracture. The phenomenon is most pronounced at the age of maximum physiologic valgus (3–6 years). Over a number of years, the valgus has a tendency to remodel, so the best approach is observation.

Tibial Shaft Fracture

Tibial shaft fractures, which are usually accompanied by fibula fractures, generally result from major trauma. An exception is the nondisplaced, isolated spiral tibial fracture often seen after minor trauma in children just learning to walk (toddler's fracture). In the pediatric population, open tibia fractures are fairly common. As

Figure 11–48. Even when not displaced, fracture of the proximal tibial metaphysis can stimulate the tibial physis and cause progressive valgus deformity, especially in patients younger than 6 years. Long-term observation indicates that slow remodeling eventually occurs.

in the adult, injury to neurovascular structures and compartment syndromes are major risks (see Chapter 3, Musculoskeletal Trauma Surgery). Open fractures of the tibia and fibula require surgical debridement, but because skin loss is less likely than in the adult, they can often be managed the same way as closed fractures, following lavage.

Most tibial fractures in children can be adequately aligned and immobilized in above-knee casts. Rare, unstable cases, some open fractures, or fractures in older children also may require external fixation or other devices to maintain reduction and alignment. As in the adult, pediatric tibia fractures are relatively slow to heal, frequently requiring 10–12 weeks; nonunion is rare, however.

Ankle Fracture & Distal Tibial Fracture

Ankle fractures and distal tibial fractures in younger children are often either metaphyseal or Salter-Harris type II distal tibial physeal injuries that heal rapidly. These fractures have very little tendency to suffer growth arrest or other serious consequences (Figure 11–49). In children 8–11 years of age, inversion injuries can push off the medial malleolus, causing an oblique Salter-Harris type IV fracture that disrupts both the joint and the growth plate. These fractures generally require open reduction for accurate realignment of the physis and articular surface. Subsequent growth arrest can cause a medial physeal bridge and produce a progressive varus deformity of the distal tibial articular surface as the lateral physis continues untethered elongation. If this occurs, either epiphyseal bar resection or corrective tibial osteotomy should be considered.

Figure 11–50. The triplane (**A**) and juvenile Tillaux (**B**) fractures are variations of ankle fracture that occur in the adolescent shortly before physeal closure. Because they involve the joint surface, such fractures may require open reduction.

The distal tibia is the site of several distinct transitional fracture patterns. These physeal injuries occur only at the end of growth, shortly before complete distal tibial physeal closure at maturity. The distal physis begins early closure medially, with gradual lateral closure over the next year. The exact fracture pattern depends on how much of the plate is still open and on the force applied (ie, mechanism of injury). When just the medial physis is closed, a triplane fracture (ie, sagittal, transverse, and frontal) of the distal tibia occurs (Figure 11–50). This fracture contains a complex of fracture lines and crosses the growth plate. Triplane fractures usually require open reduction, although minimally displaced injuries can be managed nonoperatively. CT scans may be necessary to define the exact fracture configuration for accurate treatment.

In slightly older patients, when only a small anterolateral segment of the physis remains open, this anterolateral fragment can be avulsed by fibers of the distal tibiofibular syndesmosis (juvenile Tillaux fracture). This is a Salter-Harris type III fracture involving the articular surface and frequently requires open reduction to restore perfect joint anatomy.

Figure 11–49. Simple fracture of the distal tibia (and fibula) at the ankle is usually a Salter-Harris type II pattern in patients younger than 10 years.

Spiegel PG et al: Epiphyseal fractures of the distal ends of the tibia and fibula: A retrospective study of two hundred and thirty-seven cases in children. J Bone Joint Surg Am 1978; 60:1046.

Figure 11–51. The presence of multiple fractures of various ages as well as unexplained long-bone fracture in a young child should suggest the diagnosis of child abuse.

INJURIES RELATED TO CHILD ABUSE

Child abuse crosses all socioeconomic boundaries and takes many forms. The musculoskeletal system is frequently the site of abuse-related injuries, but findings may be subtle or misleading. The most critical issue to consider in suspected abuse is whether the history can explain the injury adequately and believably.

The classic radiographic picture of abuse is the presence of multiple healing fractures of various ages; in the absence of a bone fragility syndrome, the diagnosis may thus be obvious (Figure 11–51). Soft-tissue injuries were found in 92% of children suspected of having been physically abused, with ecchymosis as the most common finding, increasing in incidence with age. Long bones (femur or humerus) are the bones most commonly fractured during child abuse. These fractures are transverse or oblique shaft injuries, a common pattern that is not by itself diagnostic. The history is often one of a minor fall or a limb "catching" in the side of the crib. But studies of fractures in young children disclosed that injury mechanisms of this type are almost never the cause of serious skeletal injury, and the dichotomy between story and findings is highly suggestive of abuse. A good rule of thumb is to consider any long bone fracture in a child younger than 3 years as abuse until proved otherwise.

The orthopedic management of abuse fractures is rarely complex, and simple closed methods usually suffice. Nearly all such fractures carry an excellent prognosis and heal or remodel rapidly. It is the detection of the abuse, and its subsequent social management, that are the main determinant of outcome.

McMahon P et al: Soft-tissue injury as an indication of child abuse. J Bone Joint Surg AM 1995;77:1179.

Oral R, Blum KL, Johnson C: Fractures in young children: Are physicians in the emergency department and orthopedic clinics adequately screening for possible abuse? Pediatr Emerg Care 2003;19:148. [PMID: 12813297]

Amputations

12

Douglas G. Smith, MD

Amputations are performed to remove extremities that are severely diseased, injured, or no longer functional. Although medical advances in antibiotics, trauma care, vascular surgery, and the treatment of neoplasms have improved the prospects for limb salvage, in many cases prolonged attempts to save a limb that should be amputated lead to excessive morbidity or even death. To counsel a patient regarding amputation versus limb salvage adequately, the physician must provide sufficient information about the surgical and rehabilitative steps involved with each procedure and must also appraise the probable outcome for function realistically with each alternative. Attempting to salvage a limb is not always in the best interest of the patient.

The decision to amputate is an emotional process for the patient, the patient's family, and the surgeon. The value of taking a positive approach to amputation cannot be overemphasized. It is not a failure and should never be viewed as such. The amputation is a reconstructive procedure designed to help the patient create a new interface with the world and to resume his or her life. The residual limb must be surgically constructed with care to maintain muscle balance, transfer weight loads appropriately, and assume its new role of replacing the original limb.

For patients to achieve maximal function of the residual limb, they also need a clear understanding of what to expect for an early postoperative prosthetic fitting, a rehabilitation program, and for long-term medical and prosthetic needs. For these discussions, the team approach to meeting the patient's needs can be especially rewarding. Nurses, prosthetists, physical and occupational therapists, and amputee support groups can be invaluable in providing the physical, psychologic, emotional, and educational support needed in returning patients to a full and active life. Many new amputees state that a peer visitor program was one of the most helpful events during their hospitalization and rehabilitation. The Amputee Coalition of America, a not-for-profit organization, supports this peer visitor training and can help locate programs that are available throughout the country.

SPECIAL CONSIDERATIONS IN THE TREATMENT OF PEDIATRIC PATIENTS

In infants and children, amputations are frequently associated with congenital limb deficiencies, trauma, and tumors. Congenital limb deficiencies are commonly described using the Birch revision of the Frantz and O'Rahilly classification system. Amelia is the complete absence of a limb; hemimelia is the absence of a major portion of a limb; and phocomelia is the attachment of the terminal limb at or near the trunk. Hemimelias can be further classified as terminal or intercalary. A terminal hemimelia is a complete transverse deficit at the end of the limb. An intercalary hemimelia is an internal segmental deficit with variable distal formation. In discussions of limb deficiencies, preaxial refers to the radial or tibial side of a limb, and postaxial refers to the ulnar or fibular side. The International Organization for Standardization (ISO) published a recommended classification for limb deficiencies in 1989 based on standard anatomic and radiologic characteristics and terminology. Although the ISO intentionally avoided the use of the terminology in the Frantz and O'Rahilly system, the older system is widely used, and the definitions and unusual language must still be understood by those caring for children with limb deficiency.

Reamputation of a congenital upper limb deficiency is rarely indicated, and even rudimentary appendages can often be functionally useful. In the lower limb, however, the ability to bear weight and the relative equality of leg lengths are mandatory for maximal function. Reamputation may be indicated in proximal femoral focal deficiency and congenital absence of the fibula or tibia to produce a more functional residual limb and improve prosthetic placement.

In the growing child, proportional change occurs in residual limb length from childhood to adulthood—an important concept to keep in mind when determining the surgical approach. A diaphyseal amputation in an infant or young child removes one of the epiphyseal growth centers, and the involved bone therefore does not keep proportional growth with the rest of the body. What initially appears to be a long transfemoral amputation in a small child can turn out to be a short and troublesome residual limb when the child reaches skeletal maturity. All attempts should be made to save the distal-most epiphysis by disarticulation. If this is not technically possible, the greatest amount of bone length should be saved.

Terminal overgrowth occurs in 8–12% of pediatric patients who had a surgical amputation. The growth of appositional bone at the transected end of a long bone exceeds the growth of the surrounding soft tissues. If left untreated, the appositional bone can penetrate through the skin (Figure 12–1). Terminal overgrowth of the transected bone does not occur as a result of the normal growth from the proximal physis pushing the distal end of the bone through the soft tissues, nor does it occur in limb disarticulations. Terminal overgrowth occurs most commonly in the humerus, fibula, tibia, and femur, in that order. Although numerous surgical procedures are used to manage this problem, the best approach consists of stump revision with adequate bone resection or autogenous osteochondral stump capping as originally described by Marquardt (Figure 12–2). If the stump-capping procedure is done at the time of original amputation, the graft material can be obtained from part of the amputated limb, such as the distal tibia, talus, or calcaneus. If a procedure is done later, the graft material can be obtained from the posterior iliac crest. Although techniques with nonautologous material are used, significant complications are reported. A report of using a modified Ertl osteomyoplasty to prevent terminal overgrowth in childhood limb deficiencies was not successful.

Figure 12–2. Stump-capping procedure. The bone end was split longitudinally and the osteochondral graft fixed temporarily with K-wires.

In a growing child, the fitting of a prosthesis can be challenging and requires frequent adjustments. Specialty pediatric amputee clinics can ease this process, provide family support, and make care more cost effective. The timing of prosthetic fitting should be initiated to coincide closely with normal motor skill development.

Prosthetic fitting for the upper limb should begin near the time the child gains sitting balance, usually around 4–6 months of age. A passive terminal device with blunt rounded edges is used initially. Active cable control and a voluntary opening terminal device are added when the child exhibits initiative in placing objects in the terminal device, usually in the second year of life. Myoelectric devices are usually not prescribed until the child masters traditional body-powered devices. The physical demand placed on prosthetic devices by children can often exceed the durability of current myoelectric designs, so maintenance and repair costs must be considered. The decision to prescribe a myoelectric device for a child is individual and depends on many factors, including the physical characteristics of the residual limb, the desires of the child, the training available, the proximity of prosthetic facilities for fitting and maintenance, and issues about funding.

Prosthetic fitting for the lower limb commonly begins when the child develops the ability to crawl and pull to a standing position, which is usually at 8–12 months. A child with a Syme amputation or a transtibial amputation generally adapts to a prosthesis with surprising ease, and although formal gait training is not required, educational efforts are focused on teaching

Figure 12–1. Terminal overgrowth of the transected bone in a pediatric amputee.

the parents about the prosthesis. For a child with a transfemoral amputation, control of a knee unit should not be expected immediately. The knee unit should be eliminated or locked in extension until the child is ambulating well and demonstrates proficient use of the prosthesis. The initial gait pattern used by a child with a transfemoral amputation is not a normal heel strike, midstance, toe-off gait pattern but is instead a more circumducted gait pattern with a prolonged foot flat phase. Formal gait training is seldom warranted until the child reaches 5 or 6 years of age. Attempts to force gait training too early can be frustrating for all involved. When pediatric patients are allowed to develop their own gait patterns as they grow and gain improved motor coordination, they are surprisingly adept at discovering the most efficient gait pattern without formal training.

Bernd L et al: The autologous stump plasty: Treatment for bony overgrowth in juvenile amputees. J Bone Joint Surg Br 1991; 73:203. [PMID: 2005139]

Birch JG et al: Syme amputation for the treatment of fibular deficiency. An evaluation of long-term physical and psychological functional status. J Bone Joint Surg Am 1999;81(11):1511. [PMID: 10565642]

Drvaric DM, Kruger LM: Modified Ertl osteomyoplasty for terminal overgrowth in childhood limb deficiencies. J Pediatr Orthop 2001;21(3):392. [PMID 1137827]

Fixsen JA: Major lower limb congenital shortening: A mini review. J Pediatr Orthop B 2003;12:1. [PMID: 124887464]

Greene WG, Cary JM: Partial foot amputation in children: A comparison of the several types with the Syme's amputation. J Bone Joint Surg Am 1982;64:438. [PMID: 7061561]

International Organization for Standardization: ISO 8548-1: Prosthetics and orthotics—Limb deficiencies, Part 1: Method of describing limb deficiencies present at birth. International Organization for Standardization, 1989.

Pfeil J et al: The stump-capping procedure to prevent or treat terminal osseous overgrowth. Prosthet Orthot Int 1991;15:96.

Weber M: Neurovascular calcaneo-cutaneus pedicle graft for stump capping in congenital pseudarthrosis of the tibia: Preliminary report of a new technique. J Pediatr Orthop B 2002;11(1): 47. [PMID: 11866081]

GENERAL PRINCIPLES OF AMPUTATION

Epidemiology

Epidemiologic data on the incidence of amputation in the United States from 1993 to 2001 show the number of lower extremity amputations increased 14% from 99,522 to 113,379, and the average hospital charge for this procedure increased 38% from $24,332 to $33,562. Nearly two thirds of amputations are performed in individuals with diabetes, even though people with diabetes represent only 6% of the population.

Preoperative Evaluation & Decision Making

The decision to amputate a limb and the choice of amputation level can be difficult and are often subject to differences in opinion. Advances in the treatment of infection, peripheral vascular disease, replantation, and limb salvage complicate the decision-making process. The goals are to optimize a patient's function and reduce the level of morbidity.

A. VASCULAR DISEASE AND DIABETES

Ischemia resulting from peripheral vascular disease remains the most frequent reason for amputation in the United States. Nearly two thirds of patients with ischemia also have diabetes. The preoperative assessment of these patients includes a physical examination and an evaluation of perfusion, nutrition, and immunocompetence. Preoperative screening tests can be helpful, but no single test is 100% accurate in predicting successful healing. Clinical judgment based on experience in examining and following many patients with vascular disease and diabetes is still the most important factor in preoperative assessment.

1. Doppler ultrasound studies—The most readily available objective measurement of limb blood flow and perfusion is by Doppler ultrasound. Arterial wall calcification increases the pressure needed to compress the vessels of patients with vascular disease, and this often gives an artificially elevated reading. Low-pressure levels are indicative of poor perfusion, but normal and high levels can be confusing because of vessel wall calcification and are not predictive of normal perfusion or of wound healing. Digital vessels are not usually calcified, and blood pressure levels in the toes appear to be more predictive of healing than do those in the ankles.

2. Transcutaneous oxygen tension measurements— Tests to measure transcutaneous partial pressure of oxygen (PO_2) are noninvasive and becoming more readily available in many vascular laboratories. These tests use a special temperature-controlled oxygen electrode to measure the PO_2 diffusing through the skin. The ultimate reading is based on several factors: the delivery of oxygen to the tissue, the utilization of oxygen by the tissue, and the diffusion of oxygen through the tissue and skin. Caution in interpreting the transcutaneous PO_2 measurements during acute cellulitis or edema is warranted because the presence of either of these disorders can increase oxygen utilization and decrease oxygen diffusion, thereby resulting in lower measurements of PO_2. Paradoxical measurements are also reported on the plantar skin of the foot. In spite of these limitations, transcutaneous PO_2 and transcutaneous partial pressure of carbon dioxide (PCO_2) are both statistically accurate in predicting amputation healing, but this does not rule out false-negative results.

3. Xenon studies—Xenon-133 (^{133}Xe) skin clearance studies are used successfully to predict healing of amputations, but the preparation of the mixture containing xenon-133 gas and saline solution and the administration of the test are time consuming, highly technician dependent, and expensive. A small amount of the xenon and saline solution is injected intradermally at various sites, and the rate of washout is monitored by gamma camera. Xenon-133 is almost never used today and is primarily of historical interest.

4. Fluorescence studies—Skin fluorescence studies use intravenous injection of fluorescein dye and subjective observation or digital fluorometers to assess skin blood flow and correlate this with the likelihood of successful wound healing. The technique is not commonly used, and studies to assess its accuracy yielded conflicting results.

5. Arteriography—Arteriography is not helpful in predicting successful healing of amputations, and this invasive test is probably not indicated solely for the purpose of selecting the proper level of amputation. Arteriography is indicated if the patient is truly a candidate for arterial reconstruction or angioplasty.

6. Nutrition and immunocompetence studies—Both nutrition and immunocompetence correlate directly with amputation wound healing. Many laboratory tests are available to assess nutrition and immunocompetence, but some are quite expensive. Screening tests for albumin level and total lymphocyte count are readily available and inexpensive. Several studies show increased healing of amputations in patients who have vascular disorders but have a serum albumin level of at least 3 g/dL and a total lymphocyte count exceeding 1500/mL. Nutritional screening is recommended to allow for nutritional improvement preoperatively and to help determine whether a higher level of amputation is needed.

7. Other issues—Activity level, ambulatory potential, cognitive skills, and overall medical condition must be evaluated to determine if the distal-most level of amputation is really appropriate for the patient.

For patients who are likely to remain ambulatory, the goals are to achieve healing at the distal-most level that can be fit with a prosthesis and to make successful rehabilitation possible. Newer studies of patients with vascular insufficiency and diabetes demonstrate that successful wound healing can be achieved in 70–80% of these patients at the transtibial or more distal amputation level. This is in sharp contrast to 25 years ago, when because of a fear of wound failure, surgeons elected to perform 80% of all lower extremity amputations at the transfemoral level.

For nonambulatory patients, the goals are not simply to obtain wound healing but also to minimize complications, improve sitting balance, and facilitate position transfers. Occasionally, a more proximal amputation

more successfully meets these goals. For example, a bedridden patient with a knee flexion contracture might be better served with a knee disarticulation than a transtibial amputation, even if the biologic factors are present to heal the more distal amputation. Preoperative assessment of the patient's potential ability to use a prosthesis, the patient's specific needs for maintaining independent transfers, and the best weight distribution for seating can help in making wise decisions concerning the appropriate level of amputation and the most successful type of postoperative rehabilitation program.

Some nonambulatory patients do benefit from a partial foot amputation, or even transtibial amputation with prosthetic fitting, not with the goal of walking but to use that leg as a standing pivot for independent transfers. In these cases, prosthetic fitting is justified.

B. TRAUMA

As vascular reconstruction techniques improved, more attempts to salvage limbs were initially made, often with the result that multiple surgical procedures were subsequently required. In many cases, amputation was ultimately performed after a substantial investment of time, money, and emotional energy. Current studies offer guidelines for immediate or early amputation and show the value of amputation not only in saving lives but also in preventing the emotional, marital, and financial disasters that can follow unwise and desperate limb salvage attempts. Although several scoring systems for mangled limbs are published, none can perfectly predict when an amputation should be performed. These scores can help in the decision-making process, but good clinical experience and judgment are still required.

The absolute indication for amputation in trauma remains an ischemic limb with unreconstructable vascular injury. Massively crushed muscle and ischemic tissue release myoglobin and cell toxins, which can lead to renal failure, adult respiratory distress syndrome, and even death. In two groups of high-risk patients (multiply injured patients and elderly patients with a mangled extremity), limb salvage, even though technically possible, can become life-threatening and generally should be avoided. In all patients, the decision about whether to undertake immediate or early amputation of a mangled limb must also depend on whether it is an upper extremity or lower extremity.

An upper extremity can function with minimal or protective sensation, and even a severely compromised arm can serve as an assistive limb. An assistive upper extremity often functions better than the currently available prosthetic replacements. The decision of salvage versus amputation in the upper limb should be based on the chance of maintaining some useful function, even if that function is limited.

In the lower extremity, weight bearing is mandatory. A lower limb functions poorly without sensation, and an assistive limb is not useful. A salvaged lower limb often functions worse than a modern prosthetic replacement unless the limb can tolerate full weight bearing, is relatively pain free, has enough sensation to provide protective feedback, and has durable skin and soft-tissue coverage that does not break down whenever walking is attempted. The decision to salvage a mangled lower extremity should be based on providing a limb that can tolerate the demands of walking.

C. FROSTBITE

Exposure to cold temperatures can directly damage the tissue and cause a related vascular impairment from endothelial vessel injury and increased sympathetic tone. If the foot or hand is wet or directly exposed to the wind, cold injury can result even in temperatures above freezing. The immediate treatment involves restoring the core body temperature and then rewarming the injured body part in a water bath at a temperature of 40–44°C for 20–30 minutes. Rewarming can be painful, and the patient often requires opiate analgesia. After rewarming, the involved part should be kept dry, blisters left intact, and dry gauze dressings used. The goals are to keep the injured extremity clean and dry and to prevent maceration, especially between the digits.

The temptation to perform early amputation should be avoided because the amount of recovery can be dramatic. As the extremity recovers from frostbite, a zone of mummification (dry gangrene) develops distally, and a zone of intermediate tissue injury forms just proximal to this. Even at the time of clear demarcation, the tissue just proximal to the zone of mummification continues to heal from the cold insult, and although the outward appearance is often pink and healthy, this tissue is not totally normal. Delaying amputation can improve the chance of primary wound healing. It is not unusual to wait 2–6 months for definitive surgery. In spite of having mummified tissue, infection is rare if the tissue is kept clean and dry.

D. TUMORS

Patients with musculoskeletal neoplasms face new choices in treatment with the development of limb salvage techniques and adjuvant chemotherapy and radiation therapy. If an amputation is chosen, the amputation incisions must be carefully planned to achieve the appropriate surgical margin.

Surgical margins (Figure 12–3) are characterized by the relationship of the surgical incision to the lesion, to the inflammatory zone surrounding the lesion, and to the anatomic compartment in which the lesion is located. The four types of margins are the intralesional margin, in which the surgical incision enters the lesion; the marginal margin, in which the incision enters the inflammatory zone but not the lesion; the wide margin, in which the incision enters the same anatomic compartment as the lesion but is outside of the inflammatory zone; and the radical margin, in which the incision remains outside of the involved anatomic compartment. Biopsy incisions and amputation incisions must be planned with careful consideration as to the tumor margin required.

Newer studies continue to evaluate the complex issues and outcomes of amputation versus limb-sparing procedures for patients with extremity sarcomas. Studies still suggest that functional outcomes in terms of kinesiologic parameters are comparable with either limb salvage or amputation. Both treatment groups report quality of life problems involving employment, health insurance, social isolation, and poor self-esteem. Overall survival remains comparable with either treatment. In some tumors, amputation may achieve better local disease control. These results confirm that the decision about treatment must be made on an individual basis, according to the specific lifestyle and needs of the patient.

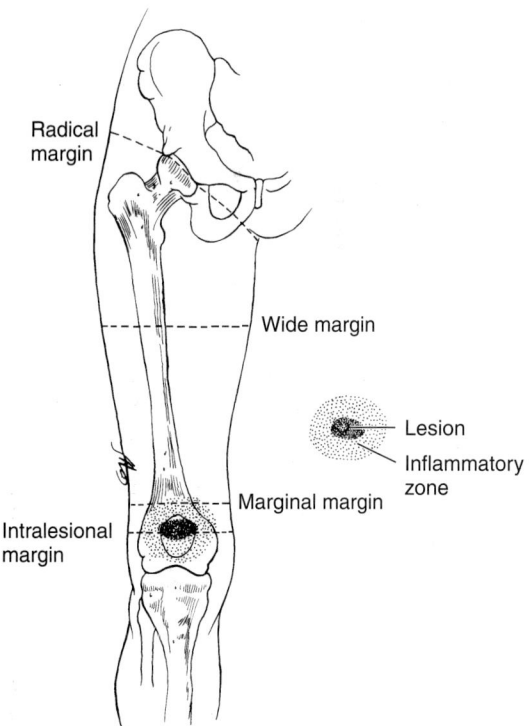

Figure 12–3. Surgical margins in tumors of the extremity.

Surgical Definitions & Techniques

Terminology for amputation level now uses an accepted international nomenclature. *Transtibial* should be used instead of below knee, and *transfemoral* instead of above knee. In the upper extremity, the terms *transradial* and *transhumeral* replace the older terms below elbow and above elbow.

Careful surgical techniques, especially in soft-tissue handling, are more critical to wound healing and functional outcome in amputation procedures than in many other surgical procedures. The tissues are often traumatized or poorly vascularized, and the risk of wound failure is high, particularly if close attention is not paid to soft-tissue technique. Flaps should be kept thick, avoiding unnecessary dissection between the skin and subcutaneous, fascial, and muscle planes. In adults, periosteum should not be stripped proximal to the level of transection. In children, however, removing 0.5 cm of the distal periosteum may help prevent terminal overgrowth. The rounding of all bone edges and the beveling of prominences are necessary for optimal prosthetic use.

Muscle loses its contractile function when the skeletal attachments are divided during amputation. Stabilizing the distal insertion of muscle can improve residual limb function by preventing muscle atrophy, providing counterbalance to the deforming forces resulting from amputation, and providing stable padding over the end of the bone. Myodesis is the direct suturing of muscle or tendon to the bone or the periosteum. Myodesis techniques are most effective in stabilizing strong muscles needed to counteract strong antagonistic muscle forces, such as in cases involving transfemoral or transhumeral amputation and in cases involving knee or elbow disarticulation. Myoplasty involves the suturing of muscle to muscle over the end of the bone. The distal stabilization of the muscle is more secure with myodesis than with myoplasty. Care must be taken to prevent a mobile sling of muscle over the distal end of the bone, which usually results in a painful bursa.

The transection of nerves always results in neuroma formation, but all neuromas are not symptomatic. Historical attempts to diminish symptomatic neuromas include clean transection, ligation, crushing, cauterization, capping, perineural closure, and end-loop anastomosis. No technique is more effective than careful and meticulous isolation, retraction, and clean transection of the nerve. This allows the cut end to retract into the soft tissues, away from the scar, pulsating vessels, and prosthetic pressure points. Ligation of a nerve is still indicated to control bleeding from the blood vessels contained within larger nerves, such as the sciatic.

Split-thickness skin grafts are generally discouraged except as a means to save a knee or elbow joint that has a stable bone and good muscle coverage. Skin grafts do best with adequate soft-tissue support and are least durable when closely adherent to bone. New prosthetic interfaces, such as silicone-based liners, can help reduce the shear at the interface and improve durability in skin-grafted residual limbs.

An open amputation is occasionally necessary to control a severe ascending infection. The term *guillotine amputation* should be avoided because it gives the impression that the limb is transected at one level through skin, muscle, and bone. Open amputations need to be performed with careful planning and forethought as to how the amputation will eventually be closed. The surgical plan must obviously consider adequate debridement of tissue necrosis and drainage of infection but must also consider the surgical flaps and tissue needed for a functional closure of the amputation to allow prosthetic fitting.

The problem of ascending infection is seen, for example, in a diabetic patient with a severe infection of the foot and cellulitis extending upward to the calf. The open amputation removes the source of infection, provides adequate drainage, and allows the acute cellulitis to resolve. After resolution, a definitive amputation and closure can be done safely. In the case of a diabetic foot infection, an open ankle disarticulation is simple, relatively bloodless, and preserves the posterior calf flap for a definitive transtibial amputation. Occasionally, it is necessary to make a longitudinal incision to drain the posterior tibial, anterior tibial, or peroneal tendon sheaths, in which case care should be taken not to violate the posterior flap of the definitive amputation. This approach often prevents having open, transected muscle bellies that can retract and become edematous—a problem that commonly occurs if an open calf-level amputation was initially performed and one that can make the definitive amputation difficult. In more severe infections or in cases in which the level of the definitive amputation will clearly be transfemoral, an open knee disarticulation has the same advantages as the open ankle disarticulation.

Postoperative Care

A. POSTOPERATIVE CARE AND PLANNING

The terminal amputation allows the unique opportunity to manipulate the physical environment of the wound during healing. A variety of methods are described, including rigid dressings, soft dressings, controlled environment chambers, air splints, and skin traction. The use of a rigid dressing controls edema, protects the limb from trauma, decreases postoperative pain, and allows early mobilization and rehabilitation.

The use of an immediate postoperative prosthesis, or IPOP (Figure 12–4), is effective in decreasing the time to limb maturation and the time to definitive prosthetic fitting. In most cases involving a lower limb amputation,

Figure 12–4. Immediate postoperative prosthetic cast for transtibial amputation.

the surgeon has the patient start with partial weight bearing if the wound appears stable after the first cast change, which usually takes place between the fifth and tenth day after surgery. Immediate postoperative weight bearing can be initiated safely in selected patients, usually young patients in whom an amputation was performed following a traumatic injury and above the zone of injury. Rigid dressings and the IPOP need to be applied carefully, but their application is easily learned and well within the scope of interested physicians. For upper extremity amputations, an IPOP can be applied immediately. Early training with an IPOP is believed to increase the long-term acceptance and use of a prosthesis. Chapter 13 offers a detailed discussion of rehabilitation.

To counsel patients adequately , some insight into the typical surgical and postoperative course can be helpful. Many patients require inpatient hospital care for 5–8 days after a transtibial amputation. Epidural or patient-controlled analgesia is usually required for pain control. Assistance with basic mobility and emotional support are also necessary. Antibiotics can minimize the risk of infection. The cast applied at the end of the surgical procedure is changed about postoperative day 5. If the wound healing is adequate, a new cast with a foot attachment is applied, and the patient can begin ambulating with approximately 30 lb of weight on the amputated extremity. Transtibial amputees are discharged to home or a nursing facility typically 5 or 8 days after sur-

gery. Outpatient visits are scheduled weekly to change the cast, which frequently becomes loose as edema lessens, and to monitor wound healing and allow suture removal. Active and active-assisted knee range of motion (ROM) is performed between each cast. On average, approximately six casts are applied on a weekly basis until the wound heals, edema resolves, wrinkles return to the skin, and the patient is ready for prosthetic fitting. The cast and the prosthetic foot attachment are applied and aligned by either the surgeon or the prosthetist. New prefabricated, removable postoperative prosthetic systems are alternatives to the traditional casting techniques. Unfortunately, comparison trails versus traditional techniques have not been done.

Close interaction between the patient, the physical therapist, and the prosthetist is required in the first 12–18 months. The socket made for the first prosthesis must allow modifications as the residual limb continues to change shape during this time. Volume changes and mismatch between the shape of the socket and the evolving shape of the residual limb are treated with amputation socks and by adding pads to the socket or socket liner. Pads are usually needed in the region that contacts the anteromedial and anterolateral tibial flares, and posteriorly, in the popliteal region. Even with careful modifications, the prosthetic socket must be changed two or three times in the first 18 months. Because of these frequent prosthetic modifications, encouraging the patient to work with a prosthetic provider who is located close to the patient's residence can help tremendously in this rehabilitation phase. Many patients have an immediate desire to have the most advanced and high-tech components in their first prosthesis. But often these components are designed for higher activity levels than are typically achieved in the rehabilitation phase and are too rigid. Discussing how the prosthesis will evolve and be upgraded as the patient's activity increases can ease this process. A new prosthesis is typically required around month 18; the old components often can be turned into a shower leg.

B. Prevention and Treatment of Complications

1. Failure of the wound to heal properly—Problems with wound healing, especially in diabetic and ischemic limbs, occur as the result of insufficient blood supply, infection, or errors in surgical technique. Healing failure rates are difficult to interpret because they depend so much on the level of amputation selected. Low failure rates can be achieved by doing amputations at an extremely proximal level in the majority of cases, but this sacrifices the rehabilitation potential of many patients because the ability to ambulate decreases dramatically with a transfemoral amputation. Wound healing failure that necessitates reamputation at a more proximal level occurs in approximately 5–10% of cases at centers specializing in amputee treatment.

Most surgeons prefer open wound care if the wound gap is less than 1 cm wide and prefer revision surgery if the gap is wider. If the surgical edema has resolved and some atrophy has already occurred, a wedge excision of all nonviable tissue can be performed and still allow primary closure without any tension at the original level. If it is not possible to oppose the viable tissue gently without tension, bone shortening or reamputation at a more proximal level should be performed.

In patients with small local areas of wound-healing failure, successful treatment with rigid dressings and an IPOP is reported. The wounds are debrided weekly and packed open, and the IPOP is applied to allow some weight bearing. The stimulation of weight bearing can increase local circulation, decrease edema, and promote wound healing.

2. Infection—Infection without widespread tissue necrosis or flap failure may be seen after surgery, especially if active distal infection was present at the time of the definitive amputation or if the amputation was done near the zone of a traumatic injury. Hematomas can also predispose a wound to infection. In cases involving infection or hematomas, the wound must be opened, drained, and debrided. If the wound is allowed to remain open for an extended time, the flaps retract and become edematous, which makes delayed closure difficult or impossible without shortening the bone. One solution, which can be instituted after thorough debridement and irrigation, is to close only the central one third to one half of the amputation wound and to use open packing for the medial and lateral corners (Figure 12–5). This method provides coverage of the bone but also allows adequate drainage and open wound management for the edges. If the original problem was truly infection and not tissue failure, the open portions of the wound heal secondarily, and the result is still a residual limb suitable for prosthetic fitting.

3. Phantom sensation—Phantom sensation is the feeling that all or a part of the amputated limb is still present. This sensation is felt by nearly everyone who undergoes surgical amputation, but it is not always bothersome. Phantom sensation usually diminishes over time, and telescoping (the sensation that the phantom foot or hand has moved proximally toward the stump) commonly occurs.

4. Pain and phantom pain—Phantom pain is defined as a bothersome, painful, or burning sensation in the part of the limb that is missing. Although from 80% to 90% of patients with acquired amputation experience some episodes of phantom pain, the episodes are often infrequent and brief. The dreaded problem of unrelenting phantom pain fortunately occurs only in a much smaller minority of patients. Surgical intervention for this problem is not very successful.

Figure 12–5. Partial closure of the infected transtibial amputation.

Local physical measures, including massage, cold packs, exercise, neuromuscular stimulation by external electrical currents, acupuncture, and regional sympathectomy, may under given circumstances have a place in therapy when the pain is intractable. A technique that has gained some acceptance and success is the use of transcutaneous electrical nerve stimulation (TENS), incorporated either into a prosthesis or used as an isolated unit. The TENS system can be worn by the amputee at night and even during the day with the battery pack attached to the belt or inside a pocket. We use this TENS system with moderate short-term success, but it is rare to see a patient who continues to use a TENS system for more than a year.

Pharmacologic treatment shows some success with several oral agents including gabapentin, amitriptyline, carbamazepine, phenytoin, and mexiletine. Medications can decrease the frequency of phantom pain episodes and decrease the intensity of these episodes. The appropriate use of an intravenous lidocaine challenge is predictive of a favorable response to oral mexiletine. Unfortunately, no indicators are good at predicting who will respond to treatment with gabapentin, amitriptyline, carbamazepine, or phenytoin . Psychological support can be beneficial, particularly when personality problems seem to accentuate the occurrence of pain. The individual needs patience and reassurance that the discomfort will improve with time, especially when a supportive social environment is present.

The sensations described by patients with phantom pain may be similar to the symptoms of reflex sympathetic dystrophy after an injury. Reflex sympathetic dystrophy can occur in amputated limbs and should be treated aggressively if present. Although rare, pain unrelated to the amputation can easily be overlooked. The differential diagnosis includes radicular nerve pain from proximal entrapment or disk herniation, arthritis of proximal joints, ischemic pain, and referred visceral pain.

Research has progressed in the prevention of phantom limb pain. Several authors document that the use of perioperative epidural anesthesia or intraneural anesthesia can block the acute pain associated with amputation surgery and decrease the opiate requirements in the immediate postoperative period. They also suggest that perioperative analgesia can prevent or decrease the later incidence of phantom pain, although this is difficult to document. The literature unfortunately is not conclusive on whether preemptive measures can truly reduce the frequency or severity of phantom limb pain. Some reports dispute the claims that preemptive analgesia reduces the frequency of phantom limb problems. A randomized trial by Lambert and colleagues found that perioperative epidural block started 24 hours before amputation is not superior to infusion of local anesthetic via a perineural catheter in preventing phantom pain but does give better relief in the immediate postoperative period.

5. Edema—Postoperative edema is common in patients who have undergone amputation. Rigid dressings can help reduce this problem. If soft dressings are used, they should be combined with stump wrapping to control edema, especially if the patient is a prosthetic candidate. The ideal shape of a residual limb is cylindrical, not conical. One common mistake is wrapping the stump too tightly at the proximal end, which can lead to congestion and worsening edema and also cause the residual limb to become shaped like a dumbbell. Another common mistake is not wrapping transfemoral amputations in a waist-high soft spica cast that includes the groin. If wrapped incorrectly, the limb has a narrow, conical shape, and a large adductor roll develops. Because of the difficulty in wrapping the transfemoral amputation with elastic bandages, shrinker socks with a waist belt are frequently used as a safer alternative for the transfemoral level.

Stump edema syndrome is a condition commonly caused by proximal constriction and characterized by edema, pain, blood in the skin, and increased pigmentation. The syndrome usually responds to temporary removal of the prosthesis, elevation of the residual limb, and compression.

6. Joint contractures—Joint contractures usually develop between the time of amputation and prosthetic fitting. Contractures that exist preoperatively can seldom be corrected postoperatively.

In transfemoral amputees, the deforming forces are flexion and abduction. Adductor and hamstring stabilization can oppose the deforming forces. During the postoperative period, patients should avoid propping up the residual limb on a pillow and should begin active and passive motion exercises early, including lying prone to stretch the hip.

In transtibial amputees, knee flexion contractures greater than 15 degrees can cause major prosthetic problems and failure. Long leg rigid dressings, early postoperative prosthetic fitting, quadriceps-strengthening exercises, and hamstring stretching can prevent this complication. Because contractures in below-knee amputees can seldom be corrected, their prevention is paramount.

In the upper extremity amputee, shoulder and elbow flexion contractures often follow amputation, especially with short residual limbs. Efforts should be directed at prevention, with aggressive physical therapy beginning soon after surgery.

7. Dermatologic problems—Good general hygiene includes keeping the residual limb and prosthetic socket clean, rinsed well to remove all soap residual, and thoroughly dry. Patients should avoid the application of foreign materials and be encouraged not to shave a residual lower limb. Shaving seems to increase the problems with ingrown hairs and folliculitis.

Reactive hyperemia is the early onset of redness and tenderness after amputation. It is usually related to pressure and resolves spontaneously.

Epidermoid cysts commonly occur at the prosthetic socket brim, especially posteriorly. These cysts are difficult to treat and commonly recur, even after excision. The best initial approach is to modify the socket and relieve pressure over the cyst. Warm heat, often with a warm tea bag; topical agents; and oral antibiotics can be required as local treatment.

Verrucous hyperplasia is a wartlike overgrowth of skin that can occur on the distal end of the residual limb. It is caused by a lack of distal contact and failure to remove normal keratin. The disorder is characterized by a thick mass of keratin, sometimes accompanied by fissuring, oozing, and infection. The infection should be addressed first, and then the limb should be soaked and treated with salicylic acid paste to soften the keratin. Topical hydrocortisone is occasionally helpful in resistant cases. Prosthetic modifications to improve distal contact must be made to prevent recurrences. Because the distal limb is often tender and prosthetic modifications are uncomfortable, an aggressive preventive approach is warranted.

Contact dermatitis sometimes occurs in amputees and can be confused with infection. The primary irritation type of dermatitis is caused by contact with acids, bases, or caustics and frequently results from failure to rinse detergents and soaps from prosthetic socks. Patients should be instructed to use mild soap and to rinse extremely well. Allergic contact dermatitis is commonly caused by the nickel and chrome in metal, antioxidants in rubber, carbon in neoprene, chromium salts used to treat leather, and unpolymerized epoxy and polyester resins in plastic laminated sockets. After infection is ruled out and contact dermatitis is confirmed, treatment begins and consists of removal of the irritant and use of soaks, corticosteroid creams, and compression with elastic wraps or shrinkers.

Superficial skin infections are common in amputees. Folliculitis occurs in hairy areas, often soon after the patient starts to wear a prosthesis. Pustules develop in the eccrine sweat glands surrounding the hair follicles, and this problem is often worse if the patient shaves. Hidradenitis, which occurs in apocrine glands in the groin and axilla, tends to be chronic and responds poorly to treatment. Socket modification to relieve any pressure in these areas can be helpful. Candidiasis and other dermatophytoses present with scaly, itchy skin, often with vesicles at the border and clearing centrally. Dermatophytoses are diagnosed with a potassium hydroxide preparation and treated with topical antifungal agents.

C. LENGTHENING OF RESIDUAL LIMBS

The ultimate function of an amputation depends on both the length of the bone and the quality of the soft-tissue envelope for the residual limb. Ilizarov techniques of distraction osteogenesis are applied to lengthen the tibia or ulna in amputees. Bone lengthening can be successful, but often issues of soft-tissue coverage remain. Although great success is described in a small series of congenital short transradial amputations, another author describes the pending necrosis of the skin over the tip of the lengthened ulna. Nonadherent, mobile soft tissue that can pad the distal end of the bone is vitally important to successful prosthetic fitting. Microsurgical techniques are also applied to use free tissue transfer to supply this type of coverage over bone in select patients, most often in trauma or tumor surgery. By using these techniques, the gracilis or latissimus dorsi muscle can be transferred to the end of the residual limb and covered with skin graft. The transposed tissues do not have sensation, and the bulk of the flap can lead to tremendous volume changes over the first 2 years. Lack of sensation and volume issues do complicate prosthetic fitting and function. These extraordinary techniques are probably best reserved for very select and unique circumstances.

D. PRESCRIPTION OF PROSTHETIC LIMBS

For lower limb prostheses, the major advances include the development of new lightweight structural materials (see Chapter 1), the incorporation of elastic response ("energy-storing") designs, the use of computer-assisted design and computer-assisted manufacturing technology in sockets, and microprocessor control of the prosthetic knee joint. For upper limb use, new electronic technology has increased the success and durability of myoelectric prostheses. The surgeon who prescribes prosthetic limbs should have a basic understanding of the general features available to match optimally the components with the patient's specific needs.

A good prosthetic prescription specifies the socket type, suspension, shank construction, specific joints, and terminal device. The socket can be a hard socket with no or minimal interface, or it can incorporate a liner. For the transfemoral amputee, a wide variety of socket shapes are available and range from the traditional quadrilateral design to the newer narrow mediolateral design. The prosthesis is suspended from the body by straps, belts, socket contour, liners that roll on the limb and then lock to the socket, suction, friction, or physiologic muscle control.

Shank construction can be either exoskeletal or endoskeletal. The older exoskeletal type has a rigid outer shell that is hollow in the center. The endoskeletal type has a central pylon or pipe surrounded by a soft and lightweight cosmetic foam cover. In the past, exoskeletal systems were more durable; however, as materials technology has improved, so has the durability and cosmetic appearance of endoskeletal systems. The endoskeletal systems also allow more adjustment and fine tuning of alignment and are now considered structurally as durable as the older exoskeletal designs. However, the cosmetic and foam covers for the endoskeletal systems are not as durable as an exoskeletal shell. Exoskeletal systems are rarely prescribed, except for very active patients without easy access to prosthetic services or for those involved in activities that would stain, tear, or destroy the endoskeletal cover. As the public's impression of disability has evolved, many active patients now decide not to cover the prosthesis and often take pride in the high-tech look of the titanium or carbon fiber components incorporated in an endoskeletal prosthesis.

A large variety of elbow, wrist, knee, and ankle joints are now available, as well as numerous terminal devices, including hands, hooks, feet, and special adaptive equipment for sports and work. The choice of an appropriate terminal device is extremely important. For an upper extremity amputee, there is no sensation in the prosthesis, and the critical feedback of touch and proprioception is missing. Initially, a hook may be a better choice than a prosthetic hand because vision must substitute for upper extremity proprioception, and a prosthetic hand blocks vision and makes dexterous use of the terminal device difficult and clumsy. In each case, the prosthetic prescription must be individualized to ensure the most efficient system for a particular patient.

Nearly all prosthetic sockets are fabricated by forming a thermoplastic or laminate socket over a plaster mold. An exact mold of the residual limb does not make a good socket for a prosthesis. The original mold must be modified to relieve the socket over areas that cannot tolerate pressure and to indent the socket over areas that can. Test sockets of clear plastic are commonly made to visualize the blanching of the skin at troublesome areas. automated fabrication of mobility aids (AFMA) technology uses computer-assisted design and manufacturing to aid the prosthetist by digitizing the residual limb, adding the standard modifications usually applied to a mold, and allowing additional fine manipulation of the shape on the computer screen. The computer can direct the carving of the mold or fabrication of the socket. AFMA technology can decrease the time needed for the fabrication of prostheses and increase the time available for the evaluation and training of patients. The best use of AFMA is to allow fabrication of multiple sockets for one patient during the fitting process. By using computer modifications, refinements are added in each iteration, ultimately to optimize the fit and comfort of the final socket. Before AFMA, this technique was not cost effective.

Myoelectric components are exciting but should generally not be prescribed for patients until they master traditional body-powered devices and their residual limb volume is stable. Myoelectric devices are used most successfully by patients with a midlength transradial amputation. Although a long below-elbow limb has better rotation, it is less able to contain the electronics. The need for myoelectric devices is greater in patients with a more proximal upper extremity amputation, but the weight and slow speed of the myoelectric components is a deterrent for their use. Hybrid devices utilizing body power and myoelectric components can be effective. Muscles stabilized by myodesis or myoplasty techniques seem to generate a better signal for myoelectric use.

Microprocessor control systems are applied to the knee units for transfemoral amputees. The microprocessor control alters the resistance of the knee unit to flexion or extension appropriately by sensing the position and velocity of the shank relative to the thigh. The current microprocessor-controlled knee units still do not provide power for active knee extension that would assist in rising from the sitting position or in providing power to the amputee's gait and rise up stairs. The new microprocessor-controlled so-called intelligent knee units do offer superior control when walking at varied speeds, descending ramps and stairs, and walking on uneven surfaces. Patients report improved confidence and a decrease in the tendency for the knee unit to buckle. One transfemoral amputee credits this new technology for his survival by allowing him to descend 70 stories in the World Trade Center at a normal pace during the terrorist attacks.

Attal N, Rouaud J, Brasseur L et al: Systemic lidocaine in pain due to peripheral nerve injury and predictors of response. Neurology 2004;62(2):218. [PMID: 14745057]

Bone M, Critchley P, Buggy DJ: Gabapentin in postamputation phantom limb pain: A randomized, double-blind, placebo-controlled, cross-over study. Reg Anesth Pain Med 2002;2 7(5):481. [PMID: 12373695]

Bosse MJ et al: A prospective evaluation of the clinical utility of the lower-extremity injury-severity scores. J Bone Joint Surg Am 2001;83-A(1):3. [PMID: 11205855]

Boyko EJ et al: A prospective study of risk factors for diabetic foot ulcer. The Seattle Diabetic Foot Study. Diabetes Care 1999; 22(7):1036. [PMID: 10388963]

Brooks B et al: TBI or not TBI: That is the question. Is it better to measure toe pressure than ankle pressure in diabetic patients? Diabet Med 2001;18(7):528. [PMID: 11553180]

Burgess EM et al: *The Management of Lower-Extremity Amputations*. Publication TR 10-6. U.S. Government Printing Office, 1969.

Carter SA, Tate RB: The value of toe pulse waves in determination of risks for limb amputation and death in patients with peripheral arterial disease and skin ulcers or gangrene. J Vasc Surg 2001;33(4):708. [PMID: 11296321]

Ehde DM et al: Chronic phantom sensations, phantom pain, residual limb pain, and other regional pain after lower limb amputation. Arch Phys Med Rehabil 2000;81(8):1039. [PMID: 10943752]

Lambert AW et al: Randomized prospective study comparing preoperative epidural and intraoperative perineural analgesia for the prevention of postoperative stump and phantom limb pain following major amputation. Reg Anesth Pain Med 2001;26(4):316. [PMID: 11464349]

Lane JM et al: Rehabilitation for limb salvage patients: Kinesiological parameters and psychological assessment. Cancer 2001;92 (Suppl 4):1013. [PMID: 11519028]

Marks LJ, Michael JW: Science, medicine, and the future: Artificial limbs. BMJ 2001;323(7315):732. [PMID: 11576982]

Mayfield JA et al: Trends in lower limb amputation in the Veterans Health Administration, 1989–1998. J Rehabil Res Dev 2000;37(1):23. [PMID: 10847569]

Melzack R: Phantom limbs. Sci Am 1992;266:120. [PMID: 1566028]

Mertens P, Lammens J: Short amputation stump lengthening with the Ilizarov method: Risks versus benefits. Acta Orthop Belg 2001;67(3):274. [PMID: 11486691]

Misuri A et al: Predictive value of transcutaneous oximetry for selection of the amputation level. J Cardiovasc Surg (Torino) 2000;41(1):83. [PMID: 10836229]

Nikolajsen L et al: Phantom limb pain. Curr Rev Pain 2000;4(2):166. [PMID: 10998730]

Nikolajsen L et al: Randomized trial of epidural bupivacaine and morphine in prevention of stump and phantom pain in lower limb amputation. Lancet 1997;350:1353.

Peabody TD et al: Evaluation and staging of musculoskeletal neoplasms. J Bone Joint Surg Am 1998;80(8):1204. [PMID: 9730132]

Reiber GE, Ledoux W: Epidemiology of foot ulcers and amputations in the diabetic foot: Evidence for prevention. In Williams R et al (eds): *The Evidence Base for Diabetes Care.* Wiley, 2002.

Siddle L: The challenge and management of phantom limb pain after amputation. Br J Nurs 2004;13(11):664. [PMID: 15218432]

Smith DG, Burgess EM: The use of CAD/CAM technology in prosthetics and orthotics—Current clinical models and a view to the future. J Rehabil Res Dev 2001;38(3):327. [PMID: 11440264]

Smith DG, McFarland LV, Sangeorzan BJ et al: Postoperative dressing and management strategies for transtibial amputations: A critical review. J Rehabil Res Dev 2003;40(3):213. Review. [PMID: 14582525]

Soucacos PN: Indications and selection for digital amputation and replantation. J Hand Surg [Br] 2001;26(6):572. Review. [PMID: 11884116]

Stojadinovic A et al: Amputation for recurrent soft tissue sarcoma of the extremity: Indications and outcome. Ann Surg Oncol 2001;8(6):509. [PMID: 11456050]

Waters RL et al: The energy cost of walking of amputees: Influence of level of amputation. J Bone Joint Surg AM 1976; 58:42. [PMID: 1249111]

■ TYPES OF AMPUTATION

UPPER EXTREMITY AMPUTATIONS & DISARTICULATIONS

Hand Amputation

Although microsurgical replantation techniques have reduced the incidence of hand amputations, for many patients replantation is still not feasible or results in failure. There is considerable controversy about the best treatment for any given hand injury, and the optimal treatment takes into consideration the injured patient's occupation, hobbies, skills, and hand of dominance. The hand is a highly visible and important part of body image. Many patients with partial hand amputations can benefit tremendously from using a cosmetic partial hand prosthesis.

A. FINGERTIP AMPUTATION

Fingertip injuries occur frequently, and fingertip amputation is the most common type of amputation. The treatment of choice usually depends on the geometry of the defect and whether or not bone is exposed. Although a large variety of local flap procedures are used to cover defects of different shapes and sizes, there is also a growing understanding that allowing secondary healing of fingertip injuries is the treatment least prone to complications in adults as well as in children. Even if bone is exposed, simply rongeuring back the exposed bone

proximal to the soft-tissue defect and allowing secondary healing can give excellent results. The amount of the bone that can be removed is limited because at least a third of the distal phalanx must be left intact to prevent a hook deformity of the nail.

Two problems frequently result from fingertip amputations: cold intolerance and hypersensitivity. Overall, regardless of which treatment is chosen, approximately 30–50% of patients experience these problems. One criticism of the many local flap procedures used to obtain coverage and primary wound healing is that all of them involve incising and advancing uninjured tissue, which extends the area of scarring and damages the fine branches of the digital nerves. Newer studies suggest that the incidence of cold intolerance and hypersensitivity may be lower with secondary healing than with skin grafts or local flaps.

B. THUMB AMPUTATION

The thumb, with its unique range of motion, plays the major role in all three prehensile activities of the hand: palmar grip, side-to-side pinch, and tip-to-tip pinch. Amputation of the thumb can result in the loss of virtually all hand function. Thumb amputations can involve (1) the distal third of the thumb (ie, distal to the interphalangeal joint), (2) the middle third of the thumb (ie, from the metacarpophalangeal joint to the interphalangeal joint), or (3) the proximal third of the thumb.

Thumb amputation of the distal third allows the patient to retain a tremendous amount of thumb function. Cold intolerance and hypersensitivity are frequent problems, as noted in the previous discussion of fingertip amputations. Treatment of distal third injuries should allow secondary healing of the thumb or should use relatively uncomplicated techniques for coverage.

Thumb amputation in the middle third is more complicated. The issues here are length, stability, and sensate skin coverage. More aggressive procedures may well be warranted and may consist of cross-finger flaps, volar advancement flaps, neurovascular island flaps from the dorsal index finger (radial nerve) or volar middle finger (median nerve), bone lengthening, or web space deepening.

Thumb amputation in the proximal third has a devastating impact on hand function. Local reconstruction for this degree of loss is not generally successful. Pollicization of another digit, a toe-to-hand transfer, or other complicated surgical techniques may be indicated to restore function.

C. DIGIT AMPUTATION

Isolated amputation of a lesser digit can cause a variety of functional and cosmetic problems. Digit amputations distal to the insertion of the sublimis flexor tendon retain active flexor tendon activity and maintain useful metacarpophalangeal joint flexion. The long flexor tendon should not be sewn to the extensor tendon because it limits the excursion of both tendons and definitely limits the function of the remaining digits.

Amputations proximal to the sublimis tendon insertion retain approximately 45 degrees of proximal phalanx flexion at the metacarpophalangeal joint through the action of the intrinsic muscles. This is usually enough to keep small objects from falling through the defect and to allow the residual finger to participate to some degree in grip. If the patient uses a cosmetic finger prosthesis and wears a ring to cover the proximal edge of the prosthesis, the amputation is almost unnoticeable.

The index finger participates principally in side-to-side and tip-to-tip pinch with the thumb. After an amputation of the index finger at the metacarpophalangeal joint, the middle finger assumes this important role. The residual second metacarpal can interfere with side-to-side pinch between the thumb and the middle finger, however. Converting this amputation to a ray amputation often can improve function and cosmesis, but the drawback is that it also narrows the width of the palm and can decrease grip and torque strength significantly. Surgical decisions must be individualized, but the second metacarpal should probably be retained if the patient uses hand tools extensively, as does a carpenter or machinist.

Amputation of the middle or ring finger at the metacarpophalangeal joint can make it difficult for the patient to hold small objects because they tend to fall through the defect. Full ray resection can narrow the central defect and occasionally improve function, but narrowing the palm can decrease grip and torque strength.

Amputation of the small finger at the metacarpophalangeal joint is often cosmetically unacceptable because of the abrupt and noticeable change in contour of the hand. Although converting a fifth digital amputation to a ray amputation by including the metacarpal can improve cosmesis, it also narrows the width of the palm and can decrease grip and torque strength. Surgical decisions must be based on individual factors and concerns.

D. CARPUS AMPUTATION

Amputations through the carpus are generally discouraged. Most surgeons believe the result to have no real advantages over a wrist disarticulation or transradial amputation. There are isolated reports of patients valuing the little bit of wrist flexion and extension that allows them to hold objects against their body and to stabilize objects for two-handed grasp. The flexor and extensor carpi radialis and ulnaris tendons must be reattached to provide this limited motion. The prosthetic options are less standard and generally considered to be less functional than the traditional transradial designs.

Carpus amputations should probably be considered in bilateral cases. Although rare, more patients sustaining tissue loss from ischemia are seen in the intensive care unit after prolonged resuscitations and the use of vasopressors. Without the vasopressors, these patients would die. Unfortunately, part of the body's response to these lifesaving medications can be to shunt blood flow from the distal extremities, resulting in demarcation and dry gangrene in the hands and feet. Just as in frostbite, if infection is not present, it is worthwhile to delay any surgical intervention and allow adequate time for tissue demarcation and recovery. Partial hand amputation is occasionally necessary, and if required, the carpus level should be considered.

Wrist Disarticulation

Wrist disarticulation continues to be controversial. Proponents frequently argue that it has two advantages over the shorter transradial amputation: It retains the distal radioulnar joint, which preserves more forearm rotation, and it retains the distal radial flare, which dramatically improves prosthetic suspension. Volar and dorsal fish-mouth incisions are usually best, and removal of the radial and ulnar styloids can prevent painful pressure points. Tenodesis of the major forearm motors stabilizes the muscle units and thereby improves physiologic and myoelectric performance.

Opponents of wrist disarticulation argue that prosthetic substitution after this procedure is slightly more complicated than it is after a standard transradial amputation. The prosthetic socket is more difficult to fabricate because of the bone contours. Conventional wrist units add too much length to the prosthetic arm after wrist disarticulation and therefore cannot be used. The terminal device for a wrist disarticulation also needs to be modified because of length. Myoelectric prostheses are difficult to fit because there is less space to conceal the electronics and power supply.

In spite of these prosthetic concerns, wrist disarticulation patients are often excellent upper extremity prosthetic users. Some patients with an unsatisfactory hand can gain improved function by undergoing a wrist disarticulation and using a standard prosthesis. This decision must be individualized and based on contributory factors such as severity of tissue loss, pain, functional requirements, and the patient's body image.

Transradial Amputation

The transradial amputation is extremely functional, and successful prosthetic rehabilitation and sustained use are achieved in 70–80% of patients who undergo amputation at this level. Forearm rotation and strength are proportional to the length retained. Surgical incisions are best with equal volar and dorsal flaps. A myodesis should be performed to prevent a painful bursa, facilitate physiologic muscular suspension, and allow for myoelectric prosthetic use. An extremely short transradial residual limb requires the use of a Muenster-type socket, which molds up around the humeral condyles for added suspension. Occasionally, side hinges and a humeral cuff are required to achieve suspension of the prosthesis. Both of these types of suspension preserve elbow flexion and extension but limit rotation.

The value of preserving the elbow joint cannot be overemphasized. Skin grafts and even composite grafts should be considered to retain the tremendous functional benefit of an elbow with some active motion. Even a limited range of elbow motion can be useful, and an ingeniously designed, geared step-up elbow hinge can convert a limited active range of elbow motion to an improved prosthetic ROM. Although body-powered prostheses are extremely functional at the transradial level of amputation, this level is also the most successful level at which to use myoelectric devices.

Krukenberg Amputation

The Krukenberg kineplastic operation transforms the transradial amputation stump into radial and ulnar digits that are capable of strong prehension and have excellent manipulative ability because of retained sensation on the "fingers" of the forearm. The operation should not be performed as a primary amputation.

The Krukenberg amputation can be performed as a secondary procedure in a transradial amputee who has a residual limb of at least 10 cm from the tip of the olecranon, an elbow flexion contracture of less than 70 degrees, and good psychological preparation and acceptance. In this case, the amputee can become completely independent in daily activities because of the retained sensory ability of the pincers as well as the quality of the grasping mechanism (Figure 12–6). The Krukenberg amputation traditionally was indicated for blind patients with bilateral below-elbow amputations, but it also may be indicated at least unilaterally in bilateral below-elbow amputees who are able to see and in those who have limited access to prosthetic facilities.

A conventional prosthesis can be worn over the Krukenberg forearm, and myoelectric devices can be adapted to use the forearm motion. The major disadvantage is the appearance of the arm, which many people consider grotesque and do not accept. As society continues to become more understanding and accepting of disabled individuals, concerns about appearance may diminish. Intensive preoperative preparation and counseling are mandatory.

Elbow Disarticulation

Elbow disarticulation can be a satisfactory amputation level and has the advantage of retaining the condylar flare

Figure 12–6. A patient with bilateral Krukenberg hands demonstrates bimanual dexterity in sharpening a pencil. (Reproduced, with permission, from Garst RJ: The Krukenberg hand. J Bone Joint Surg Br 1991;73:385.)

to improve prosthetic suspension and allow for the transfer of humeral rotation to the prosthesis. The longer lever arm improves strength. The disadvantage is in the design of the prosthetic elbow hinge. An outside hinge is bulky and hard on clothing, whereas the conventional elbow unit provides a disproportionately long upper arm and short forearm. Whether the advantages of the elbow disarticulation outweigh the disadvantages remains controversial. Surgically, volar and dorsal flaps work best, and myodesis of the biceps and triceps tendons are needed to preserve the distal muscle attachments.

Transhumeral Amputation

When transhumeral amputation is performed, efforts should be made to retain as much as possible of the bone length that has suitable soft-tissue coverage. Even if only the humeral head remains and no functional length is salvageable, an improved shoulder contour and cosmetic appearance results. Myodesis helps preserve biceps and triceps strength, prosthetic control, and myoelectric signals. In most cases of transhumeral amputation, an immediate postoperative prosthesis and rigid dressings can be used successfully. Physical therapy should focus on proximal joint and muscle function. Because the terminal prosthetic device is usually controlled by active shoulder girdle motion, early prosthetic use and therapy can prevent contracture and maintain strength.

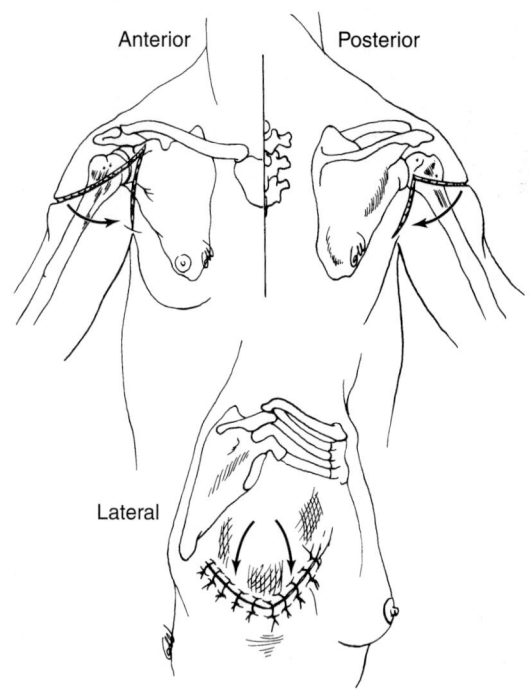

Figure 12–7. Shoulder disarticulation.

transhumeral amputation because of brachial plexus injury—one group without shoulder arthrodesis and one group with it—found a somewhat better return-to-work rate in the group without shoulder arthrodesis. Prosthetic expectations in these patients should be limited because prosthetic fitting adds weight to a dysfunctional shoulder girdle, often defeating one of the original goals of the amputation.

Shoulder Disarticulation & Scapulothoracic (Forequarter) Amputation

The performance of shoulder disarticulation (Figure 12–7) or scapulothoracic amputation (Figure 12–8) is rare. When either operation is performed, it is usually in cases of cancer or severe trauma. Either operation results in a loss of the normal shoulder contour and causes the patient difficulty because clothing does not fit well. Saving the humeral head, if possible, can improve the contour of a shoulder disarticulation tremendously. The scapulothoracic amputation, usually performed for proximal tumors, removes the arm, scapula, and clavicle. Dissection often extends into the neck and into the thorax.

Elaborate myoelectric prostheses are available for patients but are expensive, heavy, and require intensive maintenance. Body-powered prostheses are also heavy,

Prosthetic suspension traditionally was incorporated in the body-powered harness, which can be somewhat uncomfortable. Among the alternative techniques are humeral angulation osteotomy (rarely used), socket-suction suspension, and the newer elastomeric roll on locking liners. Many prosthetic options are available for the transhumeral amputee. One option is a prosthesis that is totally body powered. Another is a hybrid prosthesis that uses myoelectric control of one component (either the terminal device or the elbow device) and body-powered control of the other. The transhumeral prosthesis is heavy, often considered slow, and requires much mental concentration to use effectively. These issues lead many unilateral transhumeral amputees to choose not to wear a prosthesis at all or to wear only a lightweight cosmetic prosthesis for special occasions.

Transhumeral amputation is sometimes elected to manage a dysfunctional arm following a severe brachial plexus injury. The advantages of amputation are that it unloads the weight from the shoulder and scapulothoracic joints and eliminates the problem of having a paralyzed arm that gets in the way and hinders body function. The decision to undertake shoulder arthrodesis in combination with transhumeral amputation is controversial and should be made on an individualized basis. Investigators who compared two groups of patients with

Figure 12–8. Forequarter amputation.

hard to suspend comfortably, and difficult to use. Most patients request prosthetic help for improved cosmesis and fitting of clothes. Often a simple soft mold to fill out the shoulder meets these expectations and is an alternative to a full-arm cosmetic prosthesis.

Postural Abnormalities after High Upper Extremity Amputation

Normally, the weight of the arm and the muscle activity associated with shoulder and arm function keep the shoulders appropriately level. Unilateral hypertrophy of an upper limb, including the shoulder girdle, occurs in certain occupations and is also seen in some sports. Some people are born with a degree of asymmetry of their shoulders, which is a relatively minor postural abnormality and does not require special clothing.

When the arm is removed and the clavicle and scapula remain, the muscles elevating the shoulder girdle are unopposed by both the weight of the arm and those muscles that pass across the shoulder and tend to depress the shoulder and arm. The consequence of this imbalance is an upward elevation described as "hiking" of the shoulder girdle. This high shoulder tends to accentuate the cosmetic loss, even when the individual is wearing a cosmetic shoulder filler or a cosmetic limb. Abnormal shoulder elevation can be countered by corrective exercises beginning as soon as they can be tolerated after the amputation. The wearing of a prosthesis with its dependent weight also diminishes shoulder hike. In most circumstances, the shoulder girdle elevation is inevitable; however, its degree can be minimized by appropriate physical measures.

Removal of the entire upper limb in the growing skeleton can result in a scoliosis of the spine. Muscular imbalance is considered to be the cause of the deformity. It may be seen to a slighter degree in the adult but is primarily confined to the growing skeleton. The combined postural deformity of upper dorsal spine scoliosis and elevation of the shoulder girdle produces asymmetry of the head and neck on the trunk, with the head appearing to be placed asymmetrically as the person stands.

In general, no corrective splinting or orthotic device can successfully counteract the postural changes associated with shoulder-level amputation. Neck and shoulder-girdle exercises offer the most effective prophylaxis and treatment. The postural deficits are particularly evident with forequarter amputation. Soft, light polyurethane cosmetic restoration, either as part of a cosmetic prosthesis or separately used with the empty sleeve, counters to some degree the unsightly upper body contour.

Hand Transplantation

Hand transplantation and the suppression of rejections is now technically possible. Approximately 25 documented cases of hand transplantation have been performed with varying degrees of success. The potential benefits for the amputee are certainly many, but they must be balanced against the real risks. In general, skin, muscle, and bone marrow appear to reject earlier and more aggressively than bone, cartilage, or tendon. Preventing this rejection is an ongoing and lasting issue, with real consequences for the individual's health and life expectancy. The current immunosuppressive drugs needed to prevent rejection of a composite hand transplant include toxic side effects, opportunistic infections, and increase in malignancies.

Also, the real psychological impact following hand and other organ transplantation should not be underestimated. One study examining the issues 5 years following heart transplant showed a significant increase in emotional issues such as irritability, depression, and low self-esteem. Even for a patient with no preexisting psychological issues, living with a hand transplantation, which remains constantly in view, may not be easy.

Baumeister S, Kleist C, Dohler B et al: Risks of allogeneic hand transplantation. Microsurgery 2004;24(2):98. Review. [PMID: 15038013]

Crandall RC, Tomhave W: Pediatric unilateral below-elbow amputees: Retrospective analysis of 34 patients given multiple prosthetic options. J Pediatr Orthop 2002;22(3):380. [PMID: 11961460]

Goel A et al: Replantation and amputation of digits: User analysis. Am J Phys Med Rehabil 1995;74(2):134. [PMID: 7710728]

Hatrick NC, Tonkin MA: Hand transplantation: A current perspective. ANZ J Surg 2001;71(4):245. [PMID: 11354126]

Martin C, Gonzalez del Pino J: Controversies in the treatment of fingertip amputations. Conservative versus surgical reconstruction. Clin Orthop 1998;(353):63. [PMID: 9728160]

Neusel E et al: Results of humeral stump angulation osteotomy. Arch Orthop Trauma Surg 1997;116:263. [PMID: 9177800]

Peimer CA et al: Hand function following single ray amputation. J Hand Surg [Am] 1999;24(6):1245. [PMID: 10584948]

Schatz RL, Rosenwasser MP: Krukenberg kineplasty: A case study. J Hand Ther 2002;15(3):260. [PMID: 12206329]

Waikakul S, Sakkarnkosol S, Vanadurongwan V et al: Results of 1018 digital replantations in 552 patients. Injury 2000;31(1):33. [PMID: 10716048]

Wilkinson MC et al: Brachial plexus injury: When to amputate? Injury 1993;24(9):603. [PMID: 8288380]

LOWER EXTREMITY AMPUTATIONS & DISARTICULATIONS

Foot Amputation

A. Toe Amputation

Toe amputations can be performed with side-to-side or plantar-to-dorsal flaps to use the best available soft tissue. The bone should be shortened to a level that allows adequate soft-tissue closure without tension.

In great toe amputations, if the entire proximal phalanx is removed, the sesamoids can retract and expose the keel-shaped plantar surface of the first metatarsal to weight bearing. This often leads to high local pressure, callous formation, or ulceration. The sesamoids can be stabilized in position for weight bearing by leaving the base of the proximal phalanx intact or by performing tenodesis of the flexor hallucis brevis tendon.

An isolated amputation of the second toe commonly results in severe hallux valgus deformity of first toe (Figure 12–9). This situation may be prevented by amputation of the second ray or by fusion of the first metatarsal and phalanx. In the shorter toe amputations at the metatarsophalangeal joint level, transferring the extensor tendon to the capsule may help elevate the metatarsal head and maintain an even distribution for weight bearing. Prosthetic replacement is not required after toe amputations.

B. RAY AMPUTATION

A ray amputation removes the toe and all or some of the corresponding metatarsal. Isolated ray amputations can be durable. Multiple ray amputations, however, especially in patients with vascular disease, can narrow the foot excessively. This increases the amount of weight that must be borne by the remaining metatarsal heads and can lead to new areas of increased pressure, callous formation, and ulceration. Surgically, it is often difficult

Figure 12–10. Fifth ray amputation for fifth metatarsal head ulcer.

to achieve primary closure of ray amputation wounds because more skin is usually required than is readily apparent. Instead of closing these wounds under tension, it is usually advisable to leave them open and allow for secondary healing.

The fifth ray amputation is the most useful of all the ray amputations. Plantar and lateral ulcers around the fifth metatarsal head often lead to exposed bone and osteomyelitis. A fifth ray amputation allows the entire ulcer to be excised and the wound to be closed primarily (Figure 12–10). In general, for more extensive involvement of the foot, a transverse amputation at the transmetatarsal level is more durable. Prosthetic requirements after ray amputations include extra-depth shoes with custom-molded insoles. The insole should include a metatarsal pad that loads the shafts of the metatarsal and unloads some of the pressure at the metatarsal heads.

C. MIDFOOT AMPUTATION

The transmetatarsal and Lisfranc amputations are reliable and durable. The Lisfranc amputation is actually a disarticulation just proximal to the metatarsals where the cuneiform and cuboid bones are retained. Surgically, a healthy, durable soft-tissue envelope is more important than a specific anatomic level of amputation, so the length of bone to be removed should be based on the ability to perform soft-tissue closure without tension. A long plantar flap is preferable, but equal dorsal

Figure 12–9. Severe hallux valgus deformity occurring after isolated second toe amputation.

and plantar flaps work well, especially for transmetatarsal amputation in the treatment of metatarsal head ulcers (Figure 12–11).

Muscle balance around the foot should be carefully evaluated preoperatively, with specific attention to tightness of the heel cord and strength of the anterior tibial, posterior tibial, and peroneal muscles. Midfoot amputations significantly shorten the lever arm of the foot, so lengthening of the Achilles tendon should be done if necessary. Tibial or peroneal muscle insertions should be reattached if they are released during bone resection. For example, if the base of the fifth metatarsal is resected, the peroneus brevis tendon should be reinserted into the cuboid bone. In patients with vascular disease, this can be performed with a minimal amount of dissection to prevent further compromise of the tissues.

Postoperative casting prevents deformities, controls edema, and speeds rehabilitation. Prosthetic requirements can vary widely. During the first year following amputation, many patients benefit from the use of an ankle-foot orthosis (AFO) with a long footplate and a toe filler. To prevent an equinus deformity from developing, patients should be advised to wear the orthosis except when taking a bath or shower. Later, the use of a simple toe filler combined with a stiff-soled shoe may be adequate. Cosmetic partial foot prostheses are also available.

D. Hindfoot Amputation

A Chopart amputation removes the forefoot and midfoot and saves only the talus and calcaneus. Rebalancing procedures are required to prevent equinus and varus deformities. Achilles tenotomy, transfer of the anterior tibial or extensor digitorum tendons, and postoperative casting are all usually necessary. Although tendon transfer to the talus was previously recommended, transfer to the calcaneus is now done to minimize varus positioning. Beveling the inferior, anterior surface of the calcaneus can remove a potential bone pressure point.

Two other types of hindfoot amputations are the Boyd and the Pirogoff amputations. The Boyd procedure consists of a talectomy and calcaneal-tibial arthrodesis after forward translation of the calcaneus. The Pirogoff procedure consists of a talectomy with calcaneal-tibial arthrodesis after the vertical transection of the calcaneus through the midbody and a forward rotation of the posterior process of the calcaneus under the tibia. These two types of hindfoot amputations are done mostly in children to preserve length and growth centers, prevent heel pad migration, and improve socket suspension.

Studies in which various procedures in children are compared showed that a hindfoot amputation results in better function than a Syme amputation (see section on Syme amputation) in cases in which the hindfoot is balanced and no equinus deformity has developed.

The hindfoot prosthesis requires more secure stabilization than a midfoot prosthesis to keep the heel from pistoning during gait. An anterior shell can be added to an ankle-foot prosthesis, or a posterior opening socket prosthesis can be used.

E. Partial Calcanectomy

Partial calcanectomy, which consists of excising the posterior process of the calcaneus (Figure 12–12), should be considered an amputation of the back of the foot. In selected patients with large heel ulcerations or calcaneal osteomyelitis, partial calcanectomy can be a functional alternative to transtibial amputation. The removal of the entire posterior process of the calcaneus allows for fairly large soft-tissue defects to be closed primarily. Patients must have adequate vascular perfusion and nutritional competence for wound healing to occur. As with other amputations, partial calcanectomy creates a functional and cosmetic deformity. Use of an ankle-foot prosthesis with a cushion heel is usually required to replace the missing heel and prevent further skin ulceration.

Figure 12–11. Transmetatarsal amputation with Achilles tendon lengthening.

Figure 12–12. Partial calcanectomy.

Syme Amputation

In the Syme amputation, the surgeon removes the calcaneus and talus while carefully dissecting on bone to preserve the heel skin and fat pad to cover the distal tibia (Figure 12–13). The surgeon must also remove and contour the malleoli, but whether this should be done during the initial operation or 6–8 weeks later remains controversial. Proponents of the two-stage procedure argue that it can improve healing in patients with vascular disease. Opponents point out that it delays rehabilitation because the patient cannot bear weight until after the second stage of the operation. One series supports the use of the one-stage procedure, even in the presence of vascular disease or diabetes. A late complication of the Syme amputation is the posterior and medial migration of the fat pad. One of these surgical procedures can be done to stabilize the fat pad: tenodesis of the Achilles tendon to the posterior margin of the tibia through drill holes; transfer of the anterior tibial and extensor digitorum tendons to the anterior aspect of the fat pad; or removal of the cartilage and subchondral bone to allow scarring of the fat pad to bone, with or without pin fixation. Careful postoperative casting can also help keep

the fat pad centered under the tibia during healing. The Syme amputation is one of the most difficult amputations to perform in terms of surgical technique and achievement of primary healing and heel pad stability.

Syme amputation should be designed to allow end bearing. Retaining the smooth, broad surface of the distal tibia and the heel pad allows direct transfer of weight from the end of the residual limb to the prosthesis. A transtibial or transfemoral amputation does not allow this direct transfer of weight. Because of the ability to end-bear, the amputee can occasionally ambulate without a prosthesis in emergency situations or for bathroom activities.

The Syme prosthesis is wider at the ankle level than is a transtibial prosthesis, and this cosmetic problem can be bothersome to some patients. The surgical narrowing of the malleolar flare and the use of new materials in the prosthesis, however, can improve the appearance of the final prosthesis. Moreover, patients can now benefit from energy-storing technology provided by the newly designed lower profile elastic response feet. Sockets do not need the high contour of a patellar-tendon bearing design because of the end-bearing quality of the residual limb. The socket can be windowed either posteriorly or medially if the limb is bulbous, or a flexible socket

Figure 12–13. Syme amputation with tenodesis of the Achilles tendon to the distal tibia.

within a rigid frame design can be used if the limb is less bulbous. Because of the tibial flare, the socket used following Syme amputation is usually self-suspending.

Transtibial Amputation

Transtibial amputation is the most commonly performed major limb amputation. The long posterior flap technique (Figure 12–14) is now standard, and good results can be expected even in the majority of patients with vascular disease. Anterior and posterior flaps, sagittal flaps, and skewed flaps can be helpful in specific patients.

Efforts should be made to preserve as much bone length as possible between the tibial tubercle and the junction of the middle and distal thirds of the tibia, based on the available healthy soft tissues. Amputations in the distal third of the tibia should be avoided because they result in poor soft-tissue padding and are more difficult to fit comfortably with a prosthesis. The goal is a cylindrically shaped residual limb with muscle stabilization, distal tibial padding, and a nontender and nonadherent scar (Figure 12–15). The transtibial amputation is especially well suited to rigid dressings and immediate postoperative prosthetic management.

Distal tibiofibular synostosis (Ertl procedure) should be considered for the treatment of a wide trauma-induced

Figure 12–15. Bilateral transtibial amputations that emphasize the benefits of the long posterior flap technique. The right limb, amputated by using equal anterior and posterior flaps, is conically shaped and atrophic. The left limb, amputated by using the long posterior flap technique, is cylindrical and well padded. (Reproduced, with permission, from Smith DG, Burgess EM, Zettl JH: Fitting and Training the Bilateral Lower-Limb Amputee, in Bowker JH, Michael JW (eds): *Atlas of Limb Prosthetics Surgical, Prosthetic, and Rehabilitation Principles.* Rosemont, IL, American Academy of Orthopaedic Surgeons, 2002, pp 599–622.)

diastasis to improve stabilization of the bone and soft tissue. The procedure is less often indicated in the treatment of patients with vascular disease. The synostosis is developed to create a broad bone mass terminally to improve the distal end-bearing property of the limb and minimize motion between the tibia and fibula. Although there is renewed interest in these techniques, true comparison of patients with osteomyoplastic techniques versus standard techniques has not been done.

A wide variety of prosthetic designs are available for the transtibial amputee. Sockets can be designed to incorporate a liner, which offers the advantages of increased comfort and accommodation of minor changes in residual limb volume. Disadvantages include increased perspiration and a less sanitary, less comfortable feeling in hot humid weather. Hard sockets are designed to have cotton or wool stump socks of an appropriate ply or thickness as the interface between the leg and the socket. Hard sockets are easier to clean and more durable than the liners are.

The Icelandic-Swedish-New York (ISNY) socket refers to the use of a more flexible socket material that is supported by a rigid frame. The flexible socket changes shape to accommodate underlying muscle contraction. This socket style can also be useful for limbs that are scarred or difficult to fit. Open-ended sockets with side joints and a thigh corset are not used much today except by patients who wore them successfully in the

Figure 12–14. Transtibial amputation with long posterior flap technique.

past and by patients with limited access to prosthetic care. The patellar tendon-bearing shape is most commonly used for the transtibial amputee. In spite of its name, the majority of the weight is borne on the medial tibial flare and laterally on the interosseus space, whereas the rest of the weight is borne on the patellar tendon area. Even the new so-called total-contact transtibial socket, which is designed to have increased contact on all areas of the residual limb, preferentially loads the tibial flare and patellar tendon regions.

Numerous types of suspension devices are available for the transtibial prosthesis. The simplest and most common is a suprapatellar strap, which wraps above the femoral condyles and patella. Sockets can be designed to incorporate a supracondylar mold or wedge to grip above the femoral condyles, but this higher profile is bulkier and less cosmetic when the patient is sitting. A waist belt and fork strap are helpful for the patient who has a very short transtibial residual limb because these devices decrease pistoning in the socket; they are also helpful for the patient whose activities require extremely secure suspension. If the patient has a limb with poor soft tissue or has intrinsic knee pain, side hinges and a thigh corset can help unload the lower leg and transfer some of the weight to the thigh.

External suspension sleeves made of latex or neoprene are still used quite frequently. Latex is more cosmetic but less durable and can be constricting. Neoprene is more durable and not as constricting but sometimes causes contact dermatitis. The newest suspension uses an elastomeric or silicone-based liner that is rolled on over the residual leg and offers an intimate friction fit. A small metal post on the distal end of the liner then locks into a catch in the prosthetic socket to suspend the socket securely to the liner. Many patients who use these elastomeric locking liners like the secure suspension and feeling of improved control of the prosthesis. The liners have the disadvantages of being less durable and requiring frequent replacement. These elastomeric locking liners can be expensive. Although elastomeric locking liners were originally touted as preventing skin problems; rashes, skin irritation, and skin breakdown remain a frequent complaint even with this new technology, however. Approximately a third of amputees cannot tolerate the forces generated at the distal part of the amputation with liners using the metal post or pin lock system. New techniques were designed to attach the elastomeric liner to the socket with vacuum pumps, clips on the side of the liner, or sealing liners and one-way socket valves to maintain a suction between the liner and the socket. Suspension must be individualized, and no system is yet proven acceptable to all amputees.

Many different designs for prosthetic feet are now available, ranging from the original solid ankle cushion heel (SACH) foot to the newer elastic response technology with a variety of keel, ankle, and pylon designs.

Cost and function can vary widely, and care should be used in prescribing an appropriate prosthetic foot for an individual patient. A common error is to prescribe a foot that is either too stiff or does not get to feel flat quickly enough for an individual patient, especially in the first 12–18 months after an amputation.

Knee Disarticulation

Disarticulation through the knee joint (Figure 12–16) is indicated in ambulatory patients when a below-knee amputation is not possible but suitable soft tissue is present for a knee disarticulation. These circumstances are most commonly found in cases involving traumatic injuries. In patients with vascular disease, the blood supply is such that if a knee disarticulation would heal, a short transtibial amputation would usually heal as well. The knee disarticulation is indicated in patients who have vascular problems and are nonambulatory, especially if knee flexion contractures or spasticity are present. Although sagittal flaps or the traditional long posterior flap can be used to take advantage of the best available soft-tissue coverage, newer literature supports use of the posterior flap technique when possible. The patella is retained and the patellar tendon sutured to the cruciate stumps to stabilize the quadriceps muscle complex. The biceps tendons can also be stabilized to the

Figure 12–16. Knee disarticulation.

patellar tendon. A short section of gastrocnemius muscle can be sutured to the anterior capsule to pad the distal end. Although many techniques are described to trim the condyles of the femur, trimming is rarely necessary, and radical trimming can decrease some of the advantages of the knee disarticulation.

For ambulatory patients, the advantages of a knee disarticulation over a transfemoral amputation include improved socket suspension by contouring above the femoral condyles, the added strength of a longer lever arm, the retained muscle balance of the thigh, and, most important, the end-bearing potential to transfer weight directly to the prosthesis. In the past, the objections to a bulky prosthesis and asymmetric knee-joint level led many surgeons to abandon the practice of performing knee disarticulations. New materials allow a less bulky prosthesis to be fabricated, and the four-bar linkage knee unit, which can fold under the socket, improves the appearance of the prosthesis when the patient is sitting. The four-bar linkage knee remains the prosthetic knee of choice for a knee disarticulation. It is low profile, has excellent stability, and can incorporate a hydraulic unit for control during the swing phase of gait in patients who can walk at different cadences.

For nonambulatory patients, a knee disarticulation eliminates the problem of knee flexion contractures, provides a balanced thigh to decrease hip contractures, and provides a long lever arm for good sitting support and transfers.

The Gritti-Stokes amputation is not recommended. In this operation, the patella is advanced distally and fused by arthrodesis to the distal femur, theoretically to allow direct weight bearing. The concept behind this operation is flawed because even in normal kneeling, the weight is borne on the pretibial and patellar tendon areas and not on the patella. The added length and the asymmetry of the knee joints complicate prosthetic fitting.

Transcondylar amputation can be performed, but the end-bearing comfort and improved suspension of a transcondylar amputation appear to be diminished when compared with the true knee disarticulation.

Transfemoral Amputation

Transfemoral amputation is usually performed with equal anterior and posterior fish-mouth flaps. Atypical flaps can and should be used to save all possible femoral length in cases of trauma because the amount of function is directly proportional to the length of the residual limb.

Muscle stabilization is more important in the transfemoral amputation than in any other major limb amputation. The major deforming force is into abduction and flexion. Myodesis of the adductor muscles through drill holes in the femur can counteract the abductors, prevent a difficult adductor tissue roll in the groin, and improve

prosthetic control (Figure 12–17). Without muscle stabilization, the femur commonly migrates laterally through the soft-tissue envelope to a subcutaneous location. Newer transfemoral socket designs attempt to better control the position of the femur, but they are not as effective as muscle stabilization. Even in nonambulatory patients, muscle stabilization is helpful in creating a more durable, padded residual limb by preventing migration of the femur.

An IPOP and rigid dressings are more difficult to apply and keep positioned after a transfemoral amputation than after more distal amputations. IPOP techniques do offer the advantages of early rehabilitation and control of edema and pain, and these techniques are preferred if the expertise to use them is available. The major complaints of patients with the transfemoral IPOP are the weight of the cast and the discomfort when sitting. In many cases, only a soft compressive dressing alone is used, and in these patients, the dressing should be carried proximally around the waist as a spica to better suspend the dressing and to include the medial thigh and prevent the development of an adductor roll of tissue. Proper postoperative positioning and therapy are essential to prevent hip flexion contractures.

Figure 12–17. Transfemoral amputation with adductor myodesis.

The limb should be positioned flat on the bed, rather than elevated on a pillow, and hip extension exercises and prone positioning should be started early.

Suspension of the prosthesis is more complicated in transfemoral amputations than in more distal amputations because of the short residual limb, the lack of bony contours, and the increased weight of the prosthesis. The transfemoral amputation prosthesis can be suspended by suction, Silesian bandage, hip-joint and pelvic band, or by the newer elastomeric locking liners.

Traditional socket-suction suspension works when the skin forms an airtight seal against the socket. Air is forced distally through a small one-way valve when the prosthesis is donned and with each step during gait, thus maintaining negative pressure distally in the socket. No prosthetic sock or other liner is used between the hard socket and the limb because air leaks out around the sock and prevents suction from developing. Donning a socket-suction prosthesis requires skill and exertion, and patients must have good coordination, upper extremity function, and balance to perform this task. Socket-suction systems work well for average-to-long transfemoral residual limbs that have adequate soft tissues and stable shape and volume. It is usually comfortable and the most cosmetically acceptable method of socket suspension.

A Silesian bandage is a flexible strap that attaches laterally to the prosthesis, wraps back around the waist and over the contralateral iliac crest, and then comes forward to attach to the anterior proximal socket (Figure 12–18). It provides good suspension and added rotational control of the prosthesis. A Silesian bandage is commonly used to augment suction suspension for patients who have shorter-length limbs or for patients whose activities require more secure suspension than suction alone can offer.

As with the transtibial prosthesis, the newer elastomeric locking liners can provide excellent suspension and control. An elastomeric or silicone-based liner is rolled onto the leg similar to the way a condom is applied. This liner has an intimate fit with the residual limb and avoids pistoning and rotational forces. A small metal post at the distal end of the liner locks down into a catch at the bottom of the prosthetic socket to create a secure mechanical suspension. A small button must be pushed to disengage the lock and release the prosthesis. Many amputees express an improved sense of security and improved proprioception with these systems. The disadvantages continue to be the added cost, the need to replace the liners as they tear, and, rarely, developing a contact dermatitis. As discussed with transtibial amputees, approximately a third of amputees cannot tolerate the forces generated at the distal part of the amputation with liners using the metal post or pin lock system. For these patients, new methods to attach the liner to the socket must be explored.

Figure 12–18. Silesian band suspension of a transfemoral prosthesis.

The hip joint and pelvic band provides extremely secure suspension and control, but the band is bulky, the least cosmetically acceptable method of suspension, and the least comfortable, especially when the patient is sitting. The pelvic band, made of metal or plastic, is thicker than a Silesian bandage. The pelvic band runs from the hip hinge, around the waist, between the contralateral iliac crest and trochanter, and back to the hip hinge. The hinge is located laterally, just anterior to the trochanter, over the anatomic axis of the hip joint. Hip joint and pelvic band suspension is indicated for very short transfemoral limbs, geriatric patients who cannot don a suction suspension, and obese patients who cannot get adequate control with suction, silicone suspension sleeves, or Silesian band suspension.

Socket design for the transfemoral amputation has changed. The traditional quadrilateral socket has a narrow anteroposterior diameter to keep the ischium positioned back and up on top of the posterior brim of the socket for weight bearing. The anterior wall of the socket is 5–7 cm higher than the posterior wall to hold the leg back on the ischial seat. Anterior pain is a frequent complaint and should be addressed by modification of the prosthetic socket in a small local area such as over the anterior superior iliac spine. If the entire anterior wall is lowered or relieved, the ischium slips inside the socket and totally alters the load transfer and pressure areas. Even though the lateral wall is contoured to hold the femur in adduction, the overall dimensions of the quadrilateral socket are not anatomic and provide poor femoral stability in the coronal plane.

Narrow mediolateral transfemoral socket designs attempt to solve the problems of a traditional quadrilateral socket by contouring the posterior wall to set the ischium down inside the socket, not up on the brim. Weight is transferred through the gluteal muscle mass and lateral thigh instead of the ischium, which eliminates the need for anterior pressure from a high anterior wall. Attention is then focused on a narrow mediolateral contour to better hold the femur in adduction and minimize the relative motion between the limb and the socket. The normal shape and normal alignment (NSNA) socket and the contoured adducted trochanteric-controlled alignment method (CAT-CAM) socket are two of the narrow mediolateral designs available.

A socket made of flexible material with a rigid frame can also be used. The flexible material allows socket wall expansion with underlying muscle contraction. A flexible socket can be made in either the traditional quadrilateral or narrow mediolateral shapes. Advantages of this type of socket include improved comfort in walking and sitting and possibly improved muscular efficiency. One drawback is that the flexible material is less durable, and cracks can result in the loss of suction suspension and skin irritation.

Prosthetic knee joints are available in many designs to address specific patient needs. The traditional standard was the single-axis constant-friction knee. The constant-friction knee is simple, durable, lightweight, and inexpensive. The friction can be set at only one level to optimize function at one cadence, and patients have difficulty when walking at different speeds.

Outside hinges were the old standard for the knee disarticulation patient, to better approximate the center of motion of the knee. Outside hinges are cosmetically poor but still available for patients who used them successfully in the past and remain satisfied with them. For new patients, other types of knee units are used.

The term *stance control knee* has replaced the term *safety knee*. It refers to a knee unit that has weight-activated friction to increase stability and resistance to buckling as more of the amputee's body weight is applied. This unit is particularly useful for patients who are older, feel less secure, and have a very short residual limb, weak hip extensors, or hip flexion contractures.

A polycentric knee provides a changing center of rotation that is located more posteriorly than other knee joints. The posterior center of rotation offers more stability during stance and the first few degrees of flexion than other knee units do. The four-bar knee is one of many polycentric knee units available.

A hydraulic or pneumatic unit can be added to most knee joints to provide superior control of the prosthesis in swing phase by using fluid hydraulics to vary the resistance according to the speed of gait. This option is useful in active amputees who walk and run at different speeds.

The variable-friction knee unit can be a less expensive way to accommodate patients who walk at different speeds. This knee changes the friction according to the degree of flexion in the knee unit and leads to an improvement in the swing phase of walking. Although a variable-friction knee is less costly and requires less maintenance than a hydraulic unit, it is not as effective in allowing the amputee to walk at different cadences.

A manual locking option can also be added to most knee units to lock the knee in full extension. Locking is helpful if the patient is blind, feels less secure, has a very short residual limb, or is a bilateral amputee.

As mentioned previously, microprocessor-controlled so-called intelligent knee units incorporate the latest technology to provide superior control of the swing and stance characteristics or the knee and respond to the amputee's speed, cadence, and accelerations. Technology has not yet advanced enough for knee units to replace the tremendous motor power lost when an amputation is done above the knee.

Specifically designed prostheses known as *stubbies* are initially recommended for bilateral knee disarticulation or transfemoral amputees, regardless of age, who have lost both legs simultaneously but are candidates for ambulation. Stubbies consist of prosthetic sockets mounted directly over rocker-bottom platforms that serve as feet. The rocker-bottom platforms have a long posterior extension to prevent the patient from falling backward, and they have a shortened anterior process that allows smooth rollover into the push-off phase of gait. These prostheses look as if the foot were positioned backward. The use of stubbies results in a lowering of the center of gravity, and the rocker bottom provides a broad base of support that teaches trunk balance, provides stability, and allows the patient to build confidence during standing and ambulation. As the patient's confidence and skills improve, periodic lengthening of the stubbies is permitted until the height becomes nearly compatible with full-length prostheses, at which time the transition is attempted. Many patients reject full-length prostheses and prefer the stability and balance afforded by the stubbies.

Hip Disarticulation

Hip disarticulation (Figure 12–19) is rarely performed. Surgically, the traditional racket-shaped incision with

Lateral
(rotation 90°)

Figure 12–19. Hip disarticulation.

an anterior apex is used in patients with vascular problems and in trauma-injured patients when possible. In tumor surgery, creative flaps based on the uninvolved anatomic compartments must be designed.

Prosthetic replacement can be successful in healthy young patients who required hip disarticulation because of trauma or cancer but is generally not indicated for patients with vascular disease. The standard prosthesis is the Canadian hip disarticulation prosthesis. The socket contains the involved hemipelvis and suspends over the iliac crests. Although the hip joint and other endoskeletal components are made of lightweight materials in an effort to keep the weight to a minimum, the prosthesis is still heavy and difficult to manipulate. Ambulation with the prosthesis usually requires more energy than it would take to ambulate with crutches and a swing-through gait. For this reason, many ambulatory patients use crutches and no prosthesis. The advantage of the prosthesis is that it does allow freer use of the upper extremities.

Hemipelvectomy

Although a hemipelvectomy (Figure 12–20) is even less frequently required than a hip disarticulation, it is some-

times indicated for trauma injuries or cancer involving the pelvis. Use of a prosthesis after this procedure is extremely rare because the body weight must be transferred onto the sacrum and thorax. Special considerations for seating are usually required after hemipelvectomy.

Prosthetic Prescription following Amputation at or Above the Knee

To be considered a candidate for a high anatomic level prosthesis (knee disarticulation and higher), a patient must be able to transfer independently, rise from sitting to standing independently, and ambulate using one leg and a swing-through gait over a distance of 100 feet on the parallel bars or with a walker. Although these requirements seem extreme, they are necessary for the successful use of this heavy and complicated prosthesis. The use of a transtibial prosthesis can make it easier to transfer and to ambulate. But a current transfemoral prosthesis can make it much more difficult to rise from sitting to standing because the powerful motor force required to extend the knee is not present. High-level prosthetic devices can actually increase the energy required for walking compared with one-leg swing-through gait. Unfortunately, without the ability to meet the activity demands unas-

Figure 12–20. Hemipelvectomy.

sisted, a prosthesis acts as an anchor to decrease overall independence. We use these same activity requirements as a functional test before prescribing a prosthesis for all transfemoral, hip disarticulation, and hemipelvectomy amputees.

Percutaneous Direct Skeletal Attachment of Artificial Limbs

The benefits of attaching prosthetic limbs through the skin, directly to the skeleton, was envisioned for nearly 100 years. Documentation of temporary external fixation for fractures dates to Malgaigne in 1845. During and just after World War II, independent attempts were made in Germany and the United States to attach a transtibial prosthesis directly to the tibia. Four humans were fit in May 1946 by Drummer, a general surgeon in Pinneberg, Germany. The two major hurdles continue to be the bone–implant interface, and the skin–implant interface. Breakthrough work by Branemark in Gothenburg, Sweden, advanced the use of titanium and improved design implants that led to over 30 years of successful dental and maxillofacial reconstruction with prosthetic devices directly connected to the bone of the mouth and face.

The skin of the extremities posed a larger challenge to the cutaneous–implant interface. Improvements in implant design and surgical technique, however, made it possible to implant and fit thumb, forearm, and transfemoral amputees successfully. Approximately 60 amputees have undergone surgical implantation and prosthetic fitting in Sweden, the United Kingdom, and Australia.

The early results confirm the potential promise of major improvements in attachment, proprioception, and function of osseointegrated prosthetic limbs compared with socket-style prostheses. Much work remains to be accomplished, however, especially in the skin–implant interface. A tremendous improvement in the bone–implant interface led to results that far outdistance historical attempts at directly attaching artificial limbs to the skeleton. Without true cutaneous–implant integration that provides a durable and biologic barrier, however, the risk of bacterial migration causing infection and loosening continues. It is fantastic to see this dream continue and advance.

Smith DG, Michael JW, Bowker JH: *Atlas of Amputations and Limb Deficiencies: Surgical, Prosthetic, and Rehabilitation Principles,* 3rd ed. American Academy of Orthopaedic Surgeons, 2004.

Bowker JH et al: North American experience with knee disarticulation with use of a posterior myofasciocutaneous flap. Healing rate and functional results in seventy-seven patients. J Bone Joint Surg Am 2000;82-A(11):1571. [PMID: 11097446]

Branemark R et al: Osseointegration in skeletal reconstruction and rehabilitation: A review. J Rehabil Res Dev 2001;38(2):175. Review. No abstract available. [PMID: 11392650]

Gaine WJ, McCreath SW: Syme's amputation revisited: A review of 46 cases. J Bone Joint Surg Br 1996;78:461.

Gottschalk F et al: Does socket configuration influence the position of the femur in above-knee amputation? J Prosthet Orthot 1989;2:94.

Kock HJ, Friederichs J, Ouchmaev A et al: Long-term results of through-knee amputation with dorsal musculocutaneous flap in patients with end-stage arterial occlusive disease. World J Surg 2004;28(8):801. Epub accessed August 3, 2004. [PMID: 15457362]

Pinzur MS, Bowker JH, Smith DG et al: Amputation surgery in peripheral vascular disease. Instr Course Lect 1999;48:687. [PMID: 10098097]

Unruh T et al: Hip disarticulation: An eleven-year experience. Arch Surg 1990;125:791.

Rehabilitation

Mary Ann E. Keenan, MD, & Samir Mehta, MD

GENERAL PRINCIPLES OF REHABILITATION

In the past, rehabilitation was regarded as aftercare, but today, rehabilitation is recognized as an important part of the acute-care program. Physicians, therapists, and other health care workers in the field of orthopedics are involved in rehabilitation programs for a variety of patients, including those with congenital or acquired musculoskeletal problems (eg, bone deformities, arthritis, or fractures) as well as those with neurologic trauma or diseases that affect limb function (eg, spinal cord injury [SCI], stroke, or poliomyelitis). Rehabilitation in these patients frequently involves correcting limb deformities, increasing muscle strength, maximizing motor control, training individuals to make the most effective use of residual function, and providing adaptive equipment.

The most successful model for rehabilitation addresses the physical, emotional, and other needs of the patient and is based on a team approach. Among those frequently included in the team are physicians and nurses from various medical specialties, physical and occupational therapists, speech therapists, psychologists, orthotists, and social workers as well as the patient and members of the patient's family. The shared goal of team members is to prevent barriers to rehabilitation by (1) diagnosing accurately all current problems in the patient, (2) treating the problems adequately, (3) establishing adequate nutrition, (4) monitoring the patient for any complications that might impede progress in recovery, (5) mobilizing the patient as soon as possible, and (6) restoring function or helping the patient adjust to an altered lifestyle.

Management of Common Problems in Rehabilitation

Inadequate nutrition, decubitus ulcers, urinary tract infections, impaired bladder control, spasticity, contractures, acquired musculoskeletal deformities, muscle weakness, and physiologic deconditioning are common complications that can obstruct rehabilitation efforts and cause further loss of function in an already compromised patient. Because these problems are costly in both human and financial terms, every effort should be made to prevent them.

A. INADEQUATE NUTRITION

Good nutritional status is the basis for avoiding many of the previously listed complications. In trauma patients, the nutritional requirements are markedly increased from the normal maintenance requirement of 30 kcal/kg/day. Most trauma patients have been receiving intravenous fluids with minimal nutritional benefit and so arrive at the rehabilitation center in various degrees of malnutrition. Patients with chronic illnesses commonly have poor appetites. Physically handicapped people expend much of their energy performing simple activities of daily living (ADLs) and may also have difficulty in obtaining and preparing adequate amounts of food. Yet another form of poor nutrition that should be noted is obesity. Inactivity leads to diminished calorie need, but boredom may result in increased consumption.

B. DECUBITUS ULCERS (PRESSURE SORES)

The combination of poor nutritional status, lack of sensation at pressure points of the body, and decreased ability to move can cause decubitus ulcers (Figure 13–1) and greatly add to the length and cost of the patient's hospital stay. The ulcer is a potential source of sepsis in an already compromised individual and often requires that a flap graft be rotated to cover the defect. After a sacral flap is rotated, the patient must remain in a prone position until the graft heals. This significantly hampers the patient's participation in a rehabilitation program because mobility and ability to interact with others are hindered. Prevention is the best treatment. The clinical rule of protecting the patient's skin is to change position every 2 hours. No cushion can completely prevent decubitus ulcers.

C. URINARY TRACT INFECTIONS AND IMPAIRED BLADDER CONTROL

Urinary tract infections are a common source of sepsis and prolonged illness. An indwelling catheter is the most frequent source of contamination. In an acutely ill or multiply injured patient, an indwelling catheter may be necessary for medical reasons but should be removed as soon as possible. Urinary incontinence is not sufficient reason for continued use of an indwelling catheter. In male patients, incontinence can be managed

Figure 13–1. Patient with contractures and a decubitus ulcer over the greater trochanter of the femur.

with a carefully applied condom catheter. Care must be taken to inspect the penis frequently for signs of skin maceration or pressure. In female patients, diapering and frequent linen changes are necessary.

Restoring bladder function to achieve adequate reflex voiding or a balanced bladder may require the use of an intermittent catheterization program. In a balanced bladder, the volume of residual urine should not exceed a third of the volume of voided urine. In general, an intermittent catheterization program is initiated if the residual volume is greater than 100 mL or if the voided volume exceeds 400 mL. The patient is catheterized every 4 hours initially and then every 6 hours for 24 hours. Then the patient is reassessed. Good records are necessary throughout the program.

D. MUSCLE WEAKNESS AND PHYSIOLOGIC DECONDITIONING

During sustained exercise, the metabolism is mainly aerobic. The principal fuels for aerobic metabolism are carbohydrates and fats. In aerobic oxidation, the substrates are oxidized through a series of enzymatic reactions that lead to the production of adenosine triphosphate (ATP) for muscular contraction. A physical conditioning program can increase the aerobic capacity by improving cardiac output, increasing hemoglobin levels, enhancing the capacity of cells to extract oxygen from the blood, and increasing the muscle mass by hypertrophy.

Prolonged immobilization of extremities, bed rest, and inactivity lead to pronounced muscle wasting and physiologic deconditioning in a short period of time. Because disabled patients generally expend more energy than normal individuals in performing the routine

ADLs, they must be mobilized as quickly as possible to prevent unnecessary physiologic decline. They should also be placed on a daily exercise program to maximize muscle strength and aerobic capacity.

E. SPASTICITY

Patients with spasticity exhibit an excessive response to the quick stretch of a muscle, which leads to hyperactive deep tendon reflexes and clonus. Spasticity must be managed aggressively to prevent permanent deformities and joint contractures.

1. Spasmolytic drugs—Drugs can be of some assistance in controlling spasticity associated with upper motor neuron diseases. Drugs are used when spasticity affects multiple large muscle groups in the body and when the spasticity is not severe.

Baclofen (Lioresal) can inhibit both polysynaptic and monosynaptic reflexes at the spinal cord level. It does, however, depress general central nervous system function. Use of oral baclofen is avoided in traumatic brain-injured patients when possible because it may cause sedation and impede cognitive recovery. Patients with attention deficits or memory disorders may be compromised by antispastic agents, such as baclofen, diazepam, and clonidine, that have sedating properties. The drug tizanidine (Zanaflex) affects the central nervous system less than other agents and may be useful. Even a drug such as dantrolene sodium, which acts peripherally, may also cause drowsiness.

Baclofen pump technology has an advantage over oral drug therapy because of the small concentrations it introduces intrathecally. The small intrathecal doses control spasticity effectively while minimizing central side effects. The pump is placed in a subcutaneous pocket in the abdominal wall. A catheter is routed subcutaneously from the intrathecal space to the pump. The pump can be refilled by injection into the reservoir chamber. The dosage and rate of administration can be easily adjusted by using a laptop computer that sends radio signals to the pump.

Dantrolene (Dantrium), another drug that can be used to control spasticity, is the drug of choice for treating clonus. Dantrolene produces relaxation by directly affecting the contractile response of skeletal muscle at a site beyond the myoneural junction. It causes dissociation of the excitation–contraction coupling probably by interfering with the release of calcium from the sarcoplasmic reticulum. Although it does not affect the central nervous system directly, it does cause drowsiness, dizziness, and generalized weakness, which may interfere with the patient's overall function. Use of dantrolene for the control of spasticity is indicated in upper motor neuron diseases, such as SCI, cerebral palsy, stroke, or multiple sclerosis. The most serious problem encountered with the use of dantrolene is hepatotoxicity. The risk appears greatest in females, in patients older than 35 years, and in patients taking other medications. When using dantrolene, the lowest effective dose should be used, and liver enzyme functions should be monitored closely. If no effect is noted after 45 days of use, the drug should be stopped.

2. Casts—Casting temporarily reduces muscle tone and is frequently used to correct a contracture. The cast is changed weekly until the problem is corrected. If a cast must be used for a prolonged period, the patient should be placed on anticoagulant therapy to prevent deep venous thrombosis.

3. Splints—Anterior and posterior clamshell splints can be used to control joint position and still allow for active and passive range of motion (ROM) of the joints in therapy. A splint applied to only one side of an extremity is not sufficient to control excessive spasticity and may result in skin breakdown from motion of the extremity against the splint. A splint can also obscure an early contracture.

4. Nerve-blocking agents—Anesthetic and phenol nerve blocks are often combined with a casting or splinting program.

Anesthetic nerve blocks are commonly used to eliminate muscle tone temporarily. They can be used diagnostically to evaluate what portion of a deformity is dynamic (occurring because of muscle spasticity) and what portion is secondary to myostatic contracture. The block can give an advanced indication of the likely results of surgical neurectomy or tendon lengthening. Repeated blocks of local anesthetics give a carryover effect to decrease muscle tone.

When muscle spasticity requires control for an extended period of time but the patient still has potential for spontaneous improvement, a phenol nerve block may be indicated. Phenol exerts two actions on the nerves. The first is a short-term effect, similar to the effect produced by a local anesthetic and directly proportional to the thickness of the nerve fibers. The second is a long-term effect that results from protein denaturation. Although this leads to wallerian degeneration of the axons, experimental studies in animals showed that the nerves regenerate with time. In patients, the direct injection of a nerve with a 3–5% solution of phenol after surgical exposure gives relief of spasticity for up to 6 months. Mixed nerves containing sensory fibers should not be injected because it could cause unwanted sensory loss or painful dysesthesia. Reduction of spasticity for up to 3 months can also be achieved by the percutaneous injection of muscle motor points with an aqueous solution of phenol after localization using a needle and nerve stimulator (Figure 13–2).

a. Botulinum toxin—Ordinarily, an action potential propagating down to a motor nerve to the neuro-

Figure 13–2. Use of a Teflon-coated needle and nerve stimulator to locate the motor points of spastic forearm muscles for phenol injection.

muscular junction triggers the release of acetylcholine (ACh) into the synaptic space. The released ACh causes depolarization of muscle membrane. Botulinum toxin type A is a protein produced by *Clostridium botulinum* that attaches to the presynaptic nerve terminal and inhibits the release of ACh at the neuromuscular junction. Botulinum toxin is injected directly into a spastic muscle. Clinical benefit lasts 3–5 months. Current practice is not to administer a total of more than 400 U in a single treatment session to avoid excessive weakness or paralysis. This upper limit of 400 U may be reached rather quickly when injecting a few large muscles. A delay of 3–7 days between injection of botulinum toxin A and the onset of clinical effect is typical. The patient does not see effects immediately, and usually a follow-up visit is arranged to check the result. Because botulinum toxin is the most potent biologic toxin known, and the cost is relatively high, the smallest possible dose should be used to achieve results. Most studies report side effects in 20–30% of patients per treatment cycle. The incidence of adverse effects varies based on the dosage used (ie, the higher the dose, the more frequent the adverse effects); however, the incidence of complications is not related to the total dose of botulinum toxin used. Local pain at the injection site is the most commonly reported side effect. Other adverse effects (eg, local hematoma, generalized fatigue, lethargy, dizziness, flulike syndrome, pain in neighboring muscles) are also reported.

5. Surgical procedures—If muscle spasticity is permanent and no change in muscle tone is anticipated, definitive procedures such as dorsal rhizotomy, peripheral neurectomy, tendon lengthening or release, and tendon transfer should be considered.

Figure 13–3. Upper extremity contractures in a patient with untreated spasticity.

F. Joint Contractures

Inactivity and uncontrolled spasticity often lead to joint contractures (Figure 13–3), which are difficult to correct and greatly extend the needed rehabilitation program. Contractures may cause difficulties in positioning an individual in a bed or chair or problems in using orthotic devices. They can also cause difficulties with hygiene and skin care and increase the risk of decubitus ulcers. Shoe wear may be rendered impossible secondary to foot deformities.

Muscle weakness is accentuated by contractures and malalignment, which cause the muscle to function at a mechanical disadvantage. Sitting and standing balance are compromised when contractural deformities displace the location of the center of gravity relative to the base of support. Functional use of the extremities is severely limited by lack of adequate joint motion. Joint contractures may require surgical release, which could further decrease function in an already compromised individual. Moreover, in children, joint contractures can lead to structural changes in the skeleton. Muscle growth lags behind skeletal growth, and this discrepancy in growth rates can cause increasing deformity with time.

To prevent contractures, exercises to maintain ROM must be performed several times daily. The patient, family members, therapists, and nursing personnel should all participate in this task.

Splinting can help maintain joints in a functional position when motor control is lacking. Splints should be removed regularly to inspect the skin condition and reassess their efficacy in maintaining the desired position.

Treatment of established contractures can be time consuming and expensive. In general, if a contracture is present for less than 3 months, it may be amenable to nonsurgical methods of correction such as serial casting or electrical stimulation of the antagonist muscles. Excessive muscle tone must be treated aggressively if present because it will only accentuate the tendency to form contractures. An anesthetic nerve block can be given to eliminate excessive tone temporarily and provide analgesia prior to manipulation of the joint and application of a cast. Each week, the cast is removed, a nerve block is given, and a new cast is applied. When the desired limb position is obtained, a holding cast is used to maintain the position for an additional week. The cast can then be bivalved and made into anterior and posterior clamshell splints, which can be removed for ROM or other activities. Another useful technique is the application of a dropout cast (Figure 13–4), which allows for further correction of the contracture while preventing the original deformity from recurring.

When contractural deformities are long standing and fixed, surgical release is indicated. Tendons, ligaments, and joint capsules are all involved. If the deformity is severe, complete correction at the time of surgery may be impossible. Neurovascular structures must be protected from excessive traction. Serial casts or dropout casts may be necessary following surgery to gain the desired limb position.

G. Other Acquired Musculoskeletal Deformities

Paralysis or weakness of trunk muscles can lead to scoliotic deformities of the spine. These deformities can impair respiratory function and tend to cause balance problems when the patient walks and sits. External support in the form of bracing or seating modifications can eliminate or minimize this tendency.

Figure 13–4. An elbow dropout cast used to increase elbow extension while preventing flexion.

Disuse and lack of muscle tone lead to osteoporosis, which in turn predisposes patients to fractures. The fractures should be treated aggressively and in a manner that maximizes function rather than prolonging immobilization.

Peripheral nerve palsy can result from pressure secondary to decreased mobility in patients confined to a bed or chair. Pressure can also result from braces, splints, and casts, and these require careful monitoring. In those patients who form heterotopic ossification, the new bone formation and the accompanying inflammation may impinge on peripheral nerves, thereby causing nerve palsy.

Evaluation of Impairment

A. NERVES

Many disabilities requiring rehabilitation result from diseases affecting the nervous system. The location and the extent of the primary lesion determine not only the degree of paralysis but also the extent to which motor control is impaired and spasticity is present. In injuries or diseases of the peripheral nerves, the damage is confined to the lower motor neurons. Normal motor control is preserved, spasticity is absent, and the magnitude of disability depends on the extent of paralysis and weakness (paresis). In pathologic conditions of the brain or spinal cord, the upper motor neurons are affected, which not only causes muscular weakness but also impairs motor control.

Motor activity can be considered as a hierarchic system of voluntary and involuntary neurologic mechanisms.

1. Voluntary muscle activity—Two types of voluntary muscle activity are clinically identifiable: selective and patterned movements. The highest level of motor activity, selective movement, depends on the integrity of the cerebral cortex. Selective movement is the ability to flex or extend one joint preferentially without initiating a mass flexor or extensor motion at other joints of the limb. Patterned movement (synergy) at a joint refers to the ability to move one joint by invoking a mass flexion or extension synergy involving movement at other joints of the limb. Patients with central nervous system disorders may have voluntary patterned movement but lack selective movement. Because most patients have mixtures of selective and patterned movement at different joints, however, the strength of each type of activity must be assessed at each joint. Patterned flexion and extension movements of the lower limb can provide sufficient motor control for ambulation, but patterned motion does not provide sufficient fine control for upper extremity function.

2. Involuntary muscle activity—Spasticity relates to two types of involuntary muscle activity: clonic and tonic responses. Each type depends on the sensitivity of the muscle spindle to the rate of stretch. If a muscle is quickly extended above the threshold of the velocity-sensitive receptors of the spindle, a phasic response may be elicited. If spasticity is severe, sudden stretch may trigger clonus, which consists of repeated bursts of phasic activity at 6–8 cycles per second. The phasic stretch response has practical clinical significance. For example, if an ankle equinus deformity is present and spasticity is severe, clonus of the triceps surae may be triggered in the stance phase each time the patient takes a step. A rigid ankle-foot orthosis (AFO) that blocks ankle motion and prevents the triceps surae from stretching may inhibit clonus, enabling the foot to be held in a neutral position. An articulated or flexible AFO that allows the ankle to move and the triceps surae to stretch may not prevent clonus from being elicited and may be less effective.

If the muscle is stretched slowly below the threshold of the velocity components of the spindle, a phasic response is not triggered, but the spindle is still capable of detecting changes in length that may generate a tonic response consisting of continuous muscle hypertonus. The tonic muscle activity during slow stretch is called **clasp-knife resistance.** This tonic activity is also of practical significance. Even if the ankle is slowly dorsiflexed for a prolonged time, hypertonus may persist in the triceps surae and restrict normal motion. Consequently, it may be necessary to differentiate spasticity from myostatic contracture by performing peripheral nerve blocks.

Patients with injury involving the brainstem may exhibit severe hypertonus that is continuously present and is called either **decorticate rigidity** or **decerebrate rigidity,** depending on the posture of the limbs. In decerebrate posturing, the patient's arms are held tightly flexed while the legs are held in extension. In decorticate posturing, both the upper and lower extremities are in rigid extension. Patients with severe muscular rigidity are at extreme risk of developing contractural deformities.

When a spastic patient is sitting or standing, labyrinthine activation increases tone in the extensor muscles of the lower extremity and also increases upper limb flexion. Consequently, patients who are examined for spasticity should be evaluated in the upright rather than supine position, to elicit the maximal stretch response. Conversely, patients who are examined for maximal ROM should be evaluated in the supine position, to minimize muscle tone and enable maximal joint range. The limb posture of patients also influences the intensity of reflex and voluntary activity.

3. Sensory perception—The final steps of sensory integration occur in the cerebral cortex, where basic sensory data are integrated into the more complex sensory phenomena. When central nervous system injury involves the cerebral cortex, the patient responds to basic modalities of touch and pain. Responses to tests of more complex aspects of sensation (such as shape, texture, and proprioception) and two-point discrimination may be impaired, however. These simple tests quickly determine the patient's ability to interpret basic sensory information. Patients with absent proprioception across the major lower joints have balance abnormalities or are unable to walk. Most patients do not routinely use an affected hand unless proprioception is intact. Patients without lesions of the cerebral cortex can generally discriminate between two points less than 10 mm apart applied simultaneously to the fingers.

B. MUSCLES

Manual muscle testing is often useful for evaluating an individual's ability to perform functional tasks and also documents progress made in the rehabilitation program. Several systems are currently used, but all are based on the grading system introduced by Robert Lovett in 1932. The evaluation is subjective, but the use of gravity resistance provides a measure of objective standardization (Table 13–1). A normal muscle grade as determined by manual testing does not always imply normal strength. A significant amount of weakness (a 25–30% loss of strength) must be present to be detected by this method.

C. GAIT

1. Normal gait—Normal gait is the combination of postures and muscle activities that produce forward motion with minimal energy expenditure (Figure 13–5).

   a. Swing phase—The swing phase (Figures 13–5 and 13–6) is divided into three equal periods: initial swing, midswing, and terminal swing. During the three-part phase, the pelvis rotates from backward to forward and the hip flexes 20–30 degrees. The knee flexes to 60 degrees initially and then extends in preparation for

Table 13–1. Muscle strength.

Grade	Strength	Description
0	Absent	Muscle does not contract.
1	Trace	Muscle contracts, but no motion is generated.
2	Poor	Muscle contraction produces movement, but muscle cannot function against gravity.
3	Fair	Muscle functions against gravity.
4	Good	Muscle can overcome some outside resistance as well as gravity.
5	Normal	Muscle can overcome resistance to motion.

contact with the ground. The knee flexion is largely responsible for the foot clearing the ground during swing. Knee flexion occurs as the result of the forward momentum of the limb swinging and not as a result of hamstring contraction. The ankle joint initially plantarflexes 10 degrees and then assumes a neutral position during terminal swing so that the heel normally contacts the floor first.

The hip flexor muscles provide the power for advancing the limb and are active during the initial two thirds of the swing phase. The ankle dorsiflexors become active during the latter two thirds of the phase to ensure foot clearance as the knee begins to extend. The hamstring muscles decelerate the forward motion of the thigh during the terminal period of the swing phase.

   b. Stance phase—The stance phase (Figures 13–5 and 13–7) accounts for 60% of the gait cycle and can be divided into five distinct activities: initial contact, the loading response, midstance, terminal stance, and preswing. At initial ground contact, the ankle is in neutral position, the knee is extended, and the hip is flexed. The hip extensor muscles contract to stabilize the hip because the body's mass is behind the hip joint. During the loading response, the knee flexes to 15 degrees, and the ankle plantarflexes to absorb the downward force and conserve energy by minimizing the up-and-down movement of the body's center of gravity. As the knee flexes and the stance leg accepts the weight of the body, the quadriceps muscle becomes active to stabilize the knee. In midstance, the knee is extended, and the ankle is in a neutral position. As the body's mass moves forward of the ankle joint, the calf muscles become active to stabilize the ankle and allow the heel to rise from the floor. In terminal stance, the heel leaves the floor, and the knee begins to flex as momentum carries the body forward. In the final portion of terminal stance, as the body rolls forward over the forefoot, the toes dorsiflex at the metatarsophalangeal joints. During preswing, the knee is flexed to 35 degrees and the ankle plantarflexes to 20 degrees. Because the opposite extremity is also in contact with the floor, the preswing is called the time of double-limb support.

Throughout the stance phase, the hip gradually extends and the pelvis rotates backward. During the first portion of the stance phase, the ankle dorsiflexors and hamstring muscles remain active. During the loading response and early midstance, the gluteus and quadriceps muscles become active to provide hip and knee stability. In midstance, the gastrocnemius and soleus muscles become active to stabilize the ankle joint and control the forward advancement of the tibia. This allows the heel to rise from the floor and the body weight to roll forward over the forefoot.

2. Abnormal gait—The study of movement (kinesiology) provides many important tools for evaluating patients with gait abnormalities. Among the areas of study are

	SWING 40%			STANCE 60%				
	Initial swing	Mid-swing	Terminal swing	Initial contact	Loading response	Mid-stance	Terminal stance	Pre-swing
TRUNK	Erect neutral	Erect neutral	Erect neutral	Erect neutral	Erect neutral	Erect neutral	Erect neutral	Erect neutral
PELVIS	Level: backward rotation 5°	Level: neutral rotation	Level: forward rotation 5°	Level: maintains forward rotation	Level: less forward rotation	Level: neutral rotation	Level: backward rotation 5°	Level: backward rotation 5°
HIP	Flexion 20° Neutral rotation abduction adduction	Flexion 20°–30° Neutral rotation abduction adduction	Flexion 30° Neutral rotation abduction adduction	Flexion 30° Neutral rotation abduction adduction	Flexion 30° Neutral rotation abduction adduction	Extending to neutral Neutral rotation abduction adduction	Apparent hyperext 10° Neutral rotation abduction adduction	Neutral extension Neutral rotation abduction adduction
KNEE	Flexion 60°	Flexion 60°–30°	Extension to 0°	Full extension	Flexion 15°	Extending to neutral	Full extension	Flexion 35°
ANKLE	Plantar flexion 10°	Neutral	Neutral	Neutral heel first	Plantar flexion 15°	From plantar flexion to 10° dorsiflexion	Neutral with tibia stable and heel off prior to initial contact opposite foot	Plantar flexion 20°
TOES	Neutral	Neutral	Neutral	Neutral	Neutral	Neutral	Neutral IP extended MP	Neutral IP extended MP

Figure 13–5. The normal gait cycle. (Reproduced, with permission, from American Academy of Orthopaedic Surgeons: Home study syllabus. In Heckman JD, ed: *Orthopaedic Knowledge Update*, I. American Academy of Orthopaedic Surgeons, 1984.)

stride analysis, motion analysis (kinematics), force analysis (kinetics), and muscle activity analysis.

Three of the many specialized tools used in these studies are dynamic electromyography, force plate studies, and motion analysis. Dynamic electromyography, which records the electrical activity in multiple muscles simultaneously during functional activities, elucidates the patterns of motor control in both the upper and the lower extremities and helps in the management of spasticity and gait abnormalities. Force plate studies, which measure ground reaction forces and the fluctuations of the center of pressure, can be used to analyze gait problems and quantify balance reactions in impaired patients. Motion analysis uses multiple cameras located at different positions around the room. The cameras detect sensors placed on the patient and create a three-dimensional model of the patient moving through space.

Muscle strength can be accurately measured using torque, which can be correlated with joint position. Joint stiffness can also be assessed by measuring torque while moving the joint through a passive arc of motion. Joint powers can be calculated by multiplying joint moment times angular velocity.

Figure 13–6. Swing phase of gait. (Reproduced, with permission, from American Academy of Orthopaedic Surgeons: Home study syllabus. In Heckman JD, ed: *Orthopaedic Knowledge Update*, I. American Academy of Orthopaedic Surgeons, 1984.)

Measurement of velocity, stride length, cadence, and single- and double-limb support times can be combined with dynamic electromyography, force plate studies, and joint goniometric recordings to present a complete analysis of gait dysfunction. These studies can also be used to assess the influence of surgery, orthotic corrections, or prosthetic design on gait characteristics.

D. OXYGEN CONSUMPTION AND AEROBIC CAPACITY

Perhaps the most important measurement for understanding the difficulties faced by disabled people comes from oxygen consumption studies. Oxygen consumption indicates the energy required to perform an activity. Measuring an individual's maximal aerobic capacity is the single best indicator of the level of physical fitness.

1. Effects of disease and aging on energy expenditure—Cardiorespiratory disease, anemia, muscle atrophy, and any other condition that restricts oxygen uptake causes a decrease in the maximal aerobic capacity. Even in a healthy person, 3 weeks of bed rest decreases maximal aerobic capacity by up to 30%.

During normal walking, the rate of energy expenditure by adults varies from approximately 30% to 45% of the maximal aerobic capacity, with the higher percentage used in people over 60. Because of the decline in maximal aerobic capacity with age, an older person is more susceptible than a person under 50–60 years of age to the penalties of a gait disability.

2. Effects of exercise on energy expenditure—When exercise is performed at less than 50% of an individual's maximal aerobic capacity, the exercise can be continued for prolonged periods because the ATP needed for muscle contraction is provided by aerobic pathways. Anaerobic pathways of ATP production, which do not use oxygen, increasingly come into play when exercise is performed at work rates exceeding approximately 50% of maximal aerobic capacity. The amount of energy that can be delivered by anaerobic metabolism is limited, and fatigue ensues because of the accumulation of lactate in the muscle. Consequently, the normal ADLs and working that must be performed throughout an 8-hour day, including walking, are performed below anaerobic threshold.

3. Effects of musculoskeletal impairment on energy expenditure—Gait abnormalities that interfere with efficient, coordinated limb movement can increase energy demand. Some affected patients respond to this increased demand by working harder, which increases the output of physiologic energy and is reflected in the higher-than-normal heart rate and oxygen consumption rate. Rather than increasing the rate of energy expenditure, however, most patients slow their gait velocity in an effort to keep the power requirement from exceeding normal limits.

Figure 13–7. Stance phase of gait. (Reproduced, with permission, from American Academy of Orthopaedic Surgeons: Home study syllabus. In Heckman JD, ed: *Orthopaedic Knowledge Update*, I. American Academy of Orthopaedic Surgeons, 1984.)

Among amputees, patients progressively walk slower at increasingly more proximal amputation levels. Younger patients with traumatic or congenital amputations walk faster than older dysvascular amputees because of their greater maximal aerobic capacity. Patients with limited joint movement or with arthritis and painful joints also reduce their gait velocity. The heart rate and energy expenditure rate do not exceed normal in any of these groups of patients if crutches are not required.

Patients requiring crutches and exerting considerable force to support the body often have high heart rates and energy expenditure rates. A swing-through, crutch-assisted gait in a paraplegic or a patient who has a fracture and is unable to bear weight on one leg requires strenuous physical exertion, which is why few paraplegics use swing-through gait and why older patients with fractures can ambulate for only short distances. Even patients who use a reciprocal gait pattern, such as patients with low lumbar paraplegia resulting from SCI or myelodysplasia, use their arms for considerable exertion. Consequently, these types of patients may also be restricted ambulators in the community.

Patients with hip and knee flexion deformities caused by fixed or dynamic contractures require increasing muscle effort not only to walk but also to maintain an upright posture because the center of gravity during stance passes farther away from the axis of rotation of the joint. The fact that knee flexion greater than 30 degrees significantly increases the energy expenditure rate even in otherwise normal persons points to the importance of preventing and correcting contractures.

Children who have cerebral palsy and diplegia and who walk in a crouch gait may have energy expenditure rates that are above the anaerobic threshold. This is why these children are restricted ambulators who frequently discontinue walking when they mature and their maximal aerobic capacities decrease.

Use of Orthoses

Orthotic (brace) prescription plays a vital role in rehabilitation. The physician must understand the functional needs of the patient and provide the orthotist with an exact prescription that specifies the materials, type of joints, joint position, and ROM. Brace prescriptions should not be left to the discretion of the patient and orthotist.

A temporary orthosis may be used in an early stage of illness until a definitive, custom-fitted orthosis is fabricated. Definitive orthoses for the lower extremity are the below-knee ankle-foot orthosis (AFO) and the above-knee knee-ankle-foot orthosis (KAFO).

The bichannel adjustable ankle-locking (BiCAAL) type of AFO is commonly applied as the first orthosis following stroke, head trauma, spinal injury, or other condition that causes extensive muscle imbalance about the foot and ankle (Figure 13–8). A rigid ankle is useful in controlling plantarflexion spasticity, stabilizing the ankle in a flaccid limb, and correcting a dynamic varus deformity (inversion of the foot). The adjustable ankle joint mechanism enables the clinician to determine the optimal ankle position in the acute period following onset of illness when the neurologic picture and orthotic requirement are changing. Once neurologic recovery stabilizes, a plastic (polypropylene) orthosis often becomes the treatment of choice (Figure 13–9).

The use of plastic materials in lower extremity orthotics is now widespread. Orthoses fabricated from plastics are lighter, more comfortable, and more attractive. A plastic AFO can be rigid or can be flexible, allowing motion at the ankle. Polypropylene is presently the most practical plastic material. Skillful fitting is critical because of the close skin and bone contact.

A. Ankle-Foot Orthosis

1. Types—Of several currently available orthoses classified as limited-motion ankle joint orthoses, two are commonly used: the conventional metal, double-upright, single-adjustable ankle joint with dorsiflexion spring assist (Klenzak) and the molded plastic posterior shells made

Figure 13–8. The bichannel adjustable ankle-locking (BiCAAL) type of ankle-foot orthosis.

Figure 13–9. The molded polypropylene ankle-foot orthosis.

from 116-inch polypropylene. The use of plastic materials makes the latter design preferable for most patients. When a greater restriction of ankle motion is desired, rigidity can be attained in several ways: by using a thicker sheet of polypropylene, by extending the lateral trim lines farther anteriorly at the ankle to serve as side struts, by adding an anterior shell to the posterior shell and totally enveloping the ankle, or by stiffening the posterior shell with the use of carbon fiber or lamination techniques. The trim lines may be reinforced with metal or additional layers of plastic. The foot plate of the orthosis extends just proximal to the metatarsal heads. Total circumferential orthoses combining anterior and posterior shells require exceptionally careful fitting to avoid excessive skin pressure over bony prominences. They are not recommended for routine use.

Insertion of a polypropylene orthosis inside a shoe generally requires a shoe size that is a half size larger and wider than that previously worn by the patient. To eliminate the need to purchase two pairs of shoes of different sizes, an inlay can be inserted in the shoe of the sound limb to prevent excessive looseness once a shoe is

fitted on the polypropylene side. The ankle position of the polypropylene orthosis should be assessed with the patient wearing his or her shoe with the normal heel height.

2. Indications—The primary requirement for orthotic support is that all joints must be passively capable of being positioned in adequate alignment. An orthosis cannot correct a fixed bony deformity or fixed joint contracture.

a. Inadequate dorsiflexion for foot clearance during swing—An AFO is indicated for inadequate toe clearance (footdrop) during the midswing phase of gait. This problem may result from inadequate ankle dorsiflexion caused by weakness of the dorsiflexors or by the inability of dorsiflexors to overcome spasticity of the triceps surae. A lightweight, flexible polypropylene orthosis is indicated if inadequate dorsiflexion is the only problem at the ankle. A flexible orthosis can also be used for a mild swing-phase varus deformity (foot inversion). A rigid orthosis is needed in patients who have excessive plantarflexion resulting from severe spasticity and in patients who initiate a strong extensor pattern activity prior to heel strike.

b. Inadequate dorsiflexion for initial contact—A patient with inadequate dorsiflexion from any cause contacts the ground with the forefoot or with the foot flat and the tibia extended backward. This problem is commonly combined with varus deformity, and weight bearing is on the lateral edge of the foot. The results are a backward thrust to the limb, which decreases forward momentum and produces excessive hyperextension forces on the knee, which leads to knee instability in the patient who is a functional walker. A rigid AFO in the neutral position provides heel strike for the patient who has full-knee extension and allows the tibia to rotate forward during stance.

c. Medial-lateral subtalar instability during stance—Varus deformity is more common than valgus deformity. The patient walks on the lateral border of the foot and is hesitant to accept weight on the leg. A rigid orthosis can correct the varus deformity unless spasticity is severe. To correct a mild varus deformity, a limited ankle orthosis may be used. No orthosis is effective in controlling the severe spastic varus deformity.

d. Inadequate tibial stability during stance—Some patients have inadequate strength or control of the plantarflexors for maintenance of normal tibial position and alignment during stance. Early after midstance, this problem is manifested by excessive dorsiflexion and accompanying knee flexion. Whether or not the limb collapses during weight bearing depends on the amount of quadriceps muscle control and strength. Patients with sufficient proprioception learn to compensate by locking the knee in hyperextension as the foot contacts the floor, which keeps the knee from buckling. A rigid orthosis that prevents both dorsiflexion and plantarflexion is indicated to provide vertical tibial alignment during midstance. Its use prevents tibial collapse forward during terminal stance as a substitution for adequate calf control.

A knee extension thrust, caused by inadequate calf control as described earlier, may result also from severe plantarflexion tone or fixed equinus deformity resulting from contracture. At foot strike, the forefoot strikes the floor first, resulting in a knee extension or hyperextension thrust. A rigid AFO with a plantarflexion block prevents the development of knee instability and pain.

A T-strap (a leather T-shaped strap attached to the brace at the ankle and applied around the ankle to hold the foot from either an inverted or everted position) is usually not desirable for correction of severe varus deformity in patients fitted with metal orthoses. If a T-strap is applied with sufficient force to provide significant control to prevent foot twisting, it usually causes excessive pressure over the lateral malleolus in the patient with severe spasticity. This problem can be treated better by the use of a split anterior tibial tendon transfer or by the addition of a lateral wedge and flare to the shoe of the nonsurgical candidate.

B. KNEE-ANKLE-FOOT ORTHOSIS

A KAFO may be used if quadriceps muscle weakness or hamstring muscle spasticity is present. A knee immobilizer may be used as a training aid before having a KAFO fabricated. A KAFO is more difficult to don than a below-knee brace, and most patients with a central nervous system disease such as stroke or cerebral palsy have difficulty walking with a KAFO. Consequently, if hamstring spasticity rather than quadriceps spasticity necessitates external support to align the knee in extension, it is preferable to perform hamstring tenotomy or tendon lengthening, thereby eliminating the need for knee support.

Most patients with lower extremity quadriceps paresis resulting from SCI lack sufficient proprioception to walk with a free-knee mechanism (unlocked knee joint mechanism).

When a KAFO is prescribed for quadriceps paresis, it is necessary to determine if the knee will be locked while walking or if it will be freely movable to allow knee flexion in swing. When a KAFO is prescribed because of knee instability or because of varus or valgus instability, a polycentric joint (a joint in which the center of rotation moves following the anatomic instantaneous center of rotation) permits flexion extension movement but blocks medial and lateral angulation. A posterior stop added to the knee mechanism prevents excessive hyperextension.

If proprioception is intact, as is the case with poliomyelitis, even patients with considerable quadriceps weakness may be able to walk with an unlocked knee using an offset knee joint. This is accomplished by careful orthotic alignment. The center of rotation of the orthosis is positioned anterior to the center of rotation of the knee. As long as the patient can fully extend the knee in the swing stage preparatory to limb loading, the resulting movement caused by vertical loading acts to extend the knee against the posterior stop, thereby locking the knee in extension. This requires at least fair (grade 3) hip flexor strength (see Table 13–1) to provide sufficient forward momentum of the leg to position the knee in full extension.

The substitution of plastic components, such as a pretibial shell, has led to significantly improved fit and reduced weight in KAFOs.

Esquenazi A. Evaluation and management of spastic gait in patients with traumatic brain injury. J Head Trauma Rehabil 2004; 19(2):109. [PMID: 15247822]

Hebela N, Smith DG, Keenan MA: What's new in orthopaedic rehabilitation. J Bone Joint Surg Am 2004;86-A(11):2577. [PMID: 15523043]

Hsu JD: Rancho Los Amigos Medical Center. A unique orthopaedic resource and teaching institution. Clin Orthop 2000; 374:125. [PMID: 10818973]

Kaelin DL, Oh TH, Lim PA et al: Rehabilitation of orthopedic and rheumatologic disorders. 4. Musculoskeletal disorders. Arch Phys Med Rehabil 2000;81(3 Suppl 1):S73. [PMID: 10721764]

Pearson OR, Busse ME, van Deursen RW et al: Quantification of walking mobility in neurological disorders. QJM 2004;97(8): 463. [PMID: 15256604]

Schmalz T, Blumentritt S, Jarasch R: Energy expenditure and biomechanical characteristics of lower limb amputee gait: The influence of prosthetic alignment and different prosthetic components. Gait Posture 2002;16(3):255. [PMID: 12443950]

Ulkar B, Yavuzer G, Guner R et al: Energy expenditure of the paraplegic gait: Comparison between different walking aids and normal subjects. Int J Rehabil Res 2003;26(3):213. [PMID: 14501573]

SPINAL CORD INJURY

Trauma to the spinal cord causes dysfunction of the cord, with nonprogressive loss of sensory and motor function distal to the point of injury. Approximately 400,000 people have spinal cord damage in the United States, and the incidence rate is estimated to be 10,000 per year. The leading causes of SCI are motor vehicle accidents, gunshot wounds, falls, sports (especially diving) injuries, and water injuries.

Patients are generally categorized into three groups. The first consists predominantly of younger individuals who sustained their injury from a motor vehicle collision or other high-energy traumatic accident. The second consists of individuals over 50 years of age with cervical spinal stenosis caused by congenital narrowing or spondylosis. Patients in this second group often sustained their injury from minor trauma and commonly have no vertebral fracture. The third group consists of people with gunshot wounds, which are now the leading cause of spinal injury in many urban centers in the United States. With the benefits of an organized program of medical care, the life expectancy of survivors of SCI is now approaching the normal level.

Terminology

A. TETRAPLEGIA

The term *tetraplegia* (preferred to *quadriplegia*) refers to loss or impairment of motor or sensory function (or both) in the cervical segments of the spinal cord with resulting impairment of function in the arms, trunk, legs, and pelvic organs.

B. PARAPLEGIA

Paraplegia refers to loss or impairment of motor or sensory function (or both) in the thoracic, lumbar, or sacral segments of the spinal cord. Arm function is intact but, depending on the level of the cord injured, impairment in the trunk, legs, and pelvic organs may be present.

C. COMPLETE INJURY

The term *complete injury* refers to an injury with no spared motor or sensory function in the lowest sacral segments.

D. INCOMPLETE INJURY

Incomplete injury refers to an injury with partial preservation of sensory or motor function (or both) below the neurologic level and includes the lowest sacral segments.

Neurologic Impairment & Recovery

A. NEUROLOGIC EXAMINATION

The neurologic examination is critical to the classification and treatment of spinal injuries because it determines the patient's potential level of recovery. The neurologic level of the lesion refers to the highest neural segment having normal motor and sensory function. Patients are further subdivided according to whether they have complete or incomplete spinal cord function. This is determined by the absence or presence of motor or sensory function in the most distal part of the spinal cord innervating the sacral nerves. The presence of sacral nerve function is critical because patients with incomplete injuries have the potential to recover normal neurologic function over a time span of up to 2 years even if paralysis is initially complete.

1. Spinal shock—The diagnosis of complete SCI cannot be made until the period of spinal shock is over, as evidenced by the return of the bulbocavernosus reflex. To elicit this reflex, the clinician examines the patient's rectum digitally, feeling for contraction of the anal sphincter while squeezing the glans penis or clitoris. The concept of spinal shock is important and can be understood on the basis of the monosynaptic stretch reflex. At a given neural segment of the spinal cord, afferent sensory fibers enter the spinal cord and anastomose with the anterior motor neurons at the same level. If trauma to the spinal cord causes complete injury, reflex activity at the site of injury will not return because the reflex arc is permanently interrupted. When spinal shock disappears, however, reflex activity does return in the distal segments below the level of injury. In a patient with complete SCI, spinal shock may last for as little as several hours or as long as several months. Patients with complete SCI who have recovered from spinal shock have a negligible chance for any useful motor return.

2. Sacral reflexes—The presence or absence of sacral function determines the completeness of the injury. Sacral motor function is assessed by testing contraction of the external anal sphincter (graded as present or absent). Sacral sensation is tested at the anal mucocutaneous junction. Additionally, testing of the external anal sphincter is performed by assessing perceived deep sensation as present or absent when the examiner's finger is inserted.

B. SPINAL CORD SYNDROMES

1. Anterior cord syndrome—Anterior cord syndrome commonly results from direct contusion to the anterior cord by bone fragments or from damage to the anterior spinal artery. Depending on the extent of cord involvement, only posterior column function (proprioception and light touch) may be present. The ability to respond to pain (tested by discriminating sharp and dull) and to light touch (tested with a wisp of cotton) signifies that the entire posterior half of the cord has some intact function and thus offers a better prognosis for motor recovery. If there is no recovery of motor function and pain sensation 4 weeks after injury, the prognosis for significant motor return is poor.

2. Central cord syndrome—Central cord syndrome can be understood on the basis of the spinal cord anatomy. The gray matter in the spinal cord contains nerve cell bodies and is surrounded by white matter consisting primarily of ascending and descending myelinated tracts. The central gray matter has a higher metabolic requirement and is therefore more susceptible to the effects of trauma and ischemia. Central cord syndrome often results from a minor injury such as a fall in an older patient with cervical spinal canal stenosis. The overall prognosis for patients with central cord syndrome is variable. Most patients are able to walk despite severe paralysis of the upper extremity.

3. Brown-Séquard syndrome—Brown-Séquard syndrome is caused by a complete hemisection of the spinal cord, resulting in a greater ipsilateral proprioceptive motor loss and a greater contralateral loss of pain and temperature sensation. Affected patients have an excellent prognosis and can usually ambulate.

4. Mixed syndrome—Mixed syndrome is characterized by a diffuse involvement of the entire spinal cord. Affected patients have a good prognosis for recovery. As with all incomplete SCI syndromes, early motor recovery is the best prognostic indicator.

Management

A. ACUTE MANAGEMENT

Most patients with spinal cord injuries have associated injuries. In this setting, assessment and treatment of airway, respiration, and circulation takes precedence. The patient is best treated initially in the supine position.

Airway management in the setting of SCI, with or without a cervical spine injury, is complex and difficult. The cervical spine must be maintained in neutral alignment at all times. Clearing of oral secretions and/or debris is essential to maintain airway patency and to prevent aspiration. Failure to intubate emergently when indicated because of concerns regarding the instability of the patient's cervical spine is a potential pitfall.

Hypotension may be hemorrhagic and/or neurogenic in acute SCI. Because of the vital sign confusion in acute SCI and the high incidence of associated injuries, a diligent search for occult sources of hemorrhage must be made. The most common causes of occult hemorrhage are chest, intraabdominal, or retroperitoneal injuries and pelvic or long bone fractures. Appropriate investigations, including radiography or CT scanning, are required.

Once occult sources of hemorrhage are excluded, initial treatment of neurogenic shock focuses on fluid resuscitation. Judicious fluid replacement with isotonic crystalloid solution to a maximum of 2 liters is the initial treatment of choice.

Associated head injury occurs in approximately 25% of SCI patients. A careful neurologic assessment for associated head injury is compulsory. The presence of amnesia, external signs of head injury or basilar skull fracture, focal neurologic deficits, associated alcohol intoxication or drug abuse, and a history of loss of consciousness mandates a thorough evaluation for intracranial injury, starting with noncontrast head CT scanning.

Ileus is common. Placement of a nasogastric tube is essential. Aspiration pneumonitis is a serious complication in the SCI patient with compromised respiratory function. Antiemetics should be used aggressively.

The National Acute Spinal Cord Injury Studies (NASCIS) II and III, a Cochrane review of all randomized clinical trials and other published reports, verified significant improvement in motor function and sensation in patients with complete or incomplete spinal cord injuries who were treated with high doses of methylprednisolone within 8 hours of injury. The current recommendation is to treat all SCI patients within 3 hours of injury with the following steroid protocol: methylprednisolone 30 mg/kg bolus over 15 minutes and an infusion of methylprednisolone at 5.4 mg/kg/hour for 23 hours beginning 45 minutes after the bolus.

The NASCIS III study evaluated methylprednisolone 5.4 mg/kg/hour for 24 or 48 hours versus tirilazad 2.5 mg/kg every 6 hours for 48 hours. (Tirilazad is a potent lipid preoxidation inhibitor. High doses of steroids or tirilazad are thought to minimize the secondary effects of acute SCI.) All patients received a 30 mg/kg bolus of methylprednisolone intravenously. The study found that in patients treated earlier than 3 hours after injury, the administration of methylprednisolone for 24 hours was best. In patients treated 3–8 hours after injury, the use of methylprednisolone for 48 hours was best. Tirilazad was equivalent to methylprednisolone for 24 hours.

The use of high-dose methylprednisolone in nonpenetrating acute SCI is the standard of care in North America. However, the validity of these results came into question on the basis of statistical analysis, randomization, and clinical endpoints. The risks of steroid therapy are not inconsequential. An increased incidence of infection and avascular necrosis is documented. Nevertheless, most physicians practice the administration of high-dose steroids within 3 hours of injury for all acute SCI patients.

Two studies addressed the administration of GM-1 ganglioside following acute SCI. The available medical evidence does not support a significant clinical benefit. It is recommended as a treatment option after the administration of methylprednisolone.

B. LOWER EXTREMITIES

Prevention of contractures and maintenance of ROM are important in all patients with SCI and should begin immediately following the injury. Teaching the patient to sleep in the prone position is the most effective means of preventing hip and knee flexion contractures. Passive stretching of the hamstring muscles with the knee extended is initiated to prevent shortening of these muscles secondary to spasticity. For patients to be able to dress the lower parts of their body independently, they must be able to flex the lumbar spine and hip 120 degrees with the knee extended.

Patients with extensive paralysis of the lower extremity need strength in both arms to manipulate crutches and bring the body to a standing position. Patients who lack at least fair (grade 3) strength in their quadriceps muscles (see Table 13–1) require KAFOs to stabilize the knee and also require the knee to be locked in extension while walking. Patients who have bilateral KAFOs commonly use a swing-through, crutch-assisted gait rather than a reciprocal gait. Because strenuous upper extremity exertion is required and the rate of energy expenditure is extremely high when crutches are used, nearly all patients prefer to use a wheelchair. In contrast, patients who have fair (grade 3) or greater strength in their hip flexors and knee extensors are able to walk with unlocked (free) knees and only require AFOs to stabilize their feet and ankles. These patients also usually require crutches because of absent or impaired hip extensor and adductor muscles, but they are able to achieve a reciprocal gait pattern and can walk for a limited duration outside the home. Most of them prefer a wheelchair when they must ambulate over long distances.

Because most ambulatory patients with SCI have impaired hip extensor support, they learn to hyperextend the lumbar spine so the center of gravity of the trunk is posterior to the hip joint in the stance phase of gait. This prevents forward collapse and decreases the demand on the arms during crutch use. Spine stabilization procedures that decrease the flexibility of the lower lumbar spine or reduce the amount of lordosis deprive the patient of an important gait maneuver.

C. UPPER BODY AND EXTREMITIES

1. C4 level function—Patients with cervical lesions above C4 may have impairment of respiratory function, depending on the extent of injury, and may require a tracheostomy and mechanical ventilatory assistance.

Phrenic nerve stimulation via implanted surgical electrodes enables patients to use their own diaphragm and ventilate without mechanical assistance if the cause of their diaphragm paralysis is upper motor neuron injury. With training, these patients should be able to achieve a vital capacity that is 50–60% of normal using only the diaphragm.

Patients with high tetraplegia can use chin or tongue controls to operate an electric wheelchair with attached respiratory equipment. Mouth sticks that are lightweight rods attached to a dental bite plate enable patients to perform desktop skills, operate push-button equipment, and pursue vocational and recreational activities.

2. C5 level function—At the C5 level, the key muscles are the deltoid and biceps muscles, which are used for shoulder abduction and elbow flexion. If these muscles are weak, the patient benefits from mobile arm supports attached to a wheelchair that are balanced to exert a vertical force to counteract gravity. This enables the patient with poor muscle strength to feed independently and perform other functional tasks with the hands. A ratchet wrist-hand orthosis (WHO) with a fixed wrist joint and a passively closing mechanism attached to the thumb and fingers enables the patient to grasp objects between the thumb and fingers.

Surgery can further enhance upper extremity function. The goals of surgery are to provide active elbow and wrist extension and to restore the ability to pinch the thumb against the index finger (key pinch or lateral pinch). Transferring the posterior deltoid to the triceps muscle provides active elbow extension. Transferring the brachioradialis to the extensor carpi radialis brevis provides active wrist extension. Attaching the flexor pollicis longus tendon to the distal radius and fusing the interphalangeal joint of the thumb provides for key pinch by tenodesis when the wrist is extended.

3. C6 level function—At the C6 level, the key muscles are the wrist extensors, which enable the patient to propel a wheelchair manually, transfer from one position to another, and even live independently.

If wrist extensor strength is poor, an orthosis is indicated. A WHO with a free wrist joint and a rubber-band extensor-assist mechanism enables the patient to complete wrist extension. A wrist-driven WHO with a flexor hinge mechanism that causes the metacarpophalangeal joint to flex when the wrist is extended enables the patient to grasp actively between the fingers and thumb. Some patients develop a natural tenodesis of their thumb and finger flexor muscles because of myostatic contracture or spasticity, and this tenodesis enables them to grasp without an orthosis.

Most patients with good wrist extensor strength are able to operate a manual wheelchair but may require an electric wheelchair for long distances. These patients may also be able to transfer independently if they have no elbow flexion contractures and they can lock their elbows passively in extension while transferring.

The goals of surgery in the C6 patient are the restoration of lateral pinch and active grasp. Lateral pinch can be restored either by tenodesis of the thumb flexor or by transfer of the brachioradialis to the flexor pollicis longus. Active grasp can be restored by transfer of the pronator teres to the flexor digitorum profundus.

4. C7 level function—At the C7 level, the key muscle is the triceps. All patients with intact triceps function should be able to transfer and live independently if no other complications are present. Despite their ability to extend the fingers, these patients may also require a WHO with a flexor hinge mechanism.

The goals of surgery in the C7 tetraplegic patient are active thumb flexion for pinch, active finger flexion for grasp, and hand opening by extensor tenodesis. Transfer of the brachioradialis to the flexor pollicis longus provides active pinch. Transfer of the pronator teres to the flexor digitorum profundus allows for active finger flexion and grasp. If the finger extensors are weak, tenodesis of these tendons to the radius provides hand opening with wrist flexion.

5. C8 level function—At the C8 level, the key muscles are the finger and thumb flexors, which enable a gross grasp. The functioning flexor pollicis longus enables patients to obtain lateral pinch between the thumb and the side of the index finger. Intrinsic muscle function is lacking, and clawing of the fingers is usually present. A capsulodesis of the metacarpophalangeal joints corrects the clawing and improves hand function. Active intrinsic function can be gained by splitting the superficial finger flexor tendon of the ring finger into four slips and transferring these tendons to the lumbrical insertions of each finger.

D. Skin

Maintaining skin integrity is crucial to spinal injury care. From the moment the patient enters the emergency room, preventive measures are instituted to avoid skin breakdown even while critical diagnostic procedures and lifesaving measures are performed. Only 4 hours of continuous pressure on the sacrum is sufficient to cause full-thickness skin necrosis. Turning the patient from side to back to side every 2 hours avoids skin ulceration, a problem that greatly prolongs the cost and length of rehabilitation. Following the simple procedures outlined here usually obviates the need for flotation devices, Stryker frames, cyclically rotating beds, and similar equipment.

Once the patient is allowed to sit, a progressive program to increase the time of sitting tolerance is undertaken. Paraplegics with normal upper extremity function are taught to perform raises automatically in the wheelchair and decompress the skin for approximately 15 seconds every 15 minutes. Tetraplegics who are unable to perform raises can lean to either side or lean forward for 1-minute intervals every hour to achieve decompression. Those patients unable to perform decompressive maneuvers require assistance from another person or may use an electric wheelchair with a powered recliner that enables them to assume a supine posture every hour.

All patients must be taught to inspect their skin at least twice a day, when dressing and undressing. Mirrors attached to a rod enable paraplegics to examine their skin over the sacrum and ischia independently. Tetraplegics usually require assistance with skin inspection.

If there is evidence of chronic skin inflammation over bony prominences or if redness persists 30 minutes after removal of pressure, action must be taken to avoid incipient pressure necrosis. Pressure transducers placed under the bony prominences determine if pressure exceeds acceptable levels. Up to 40 mm Hg is well tolerated by most patients. If pressures exceed this amount, a custom-fitted foam cushion with appropriate cutouts is prescribed.

Development of any open areas in the skin over the ischia or sacrum, even superficial areas, is an indication to discontinue sitting temporarily. The patient must remain in a prone or side-lying position to avoid pressure until the lesion is healed. Failure to take aggressive steps to eliminate pressure and allow healing leads to chronic inflammation, scarring, and a loss of elasticity, creating a vicious cycle that further increases susceptibility to pressure necrosis.

Excessive hip and knee flexor spasticity that prevents patients from assuming the prone position or lying supine and requires them constantly to assume a side-lying posture when in bed can lead to excessive pressure over the greater trochanters. Flexor spasticity or contracture that prevents continuous turning should be corrected medically prior to development of pressure sores and must be performed before skin flap placement. Failure to correct flexion deformities inevitably decreases the likelihood of successful skin closure. Surgical tenotomy and myotomy of hip and knee flexors is the most effective surgical method for correcting the problem when nonoperative measures fail. Neurosurgical procedures such as myelotomy or rhizotomy are usually less effective and run the risk of interfering with reflex bladder emptying and penile erections.

In the neglected patient with a full-thickness pressure sore, surgery is necessary. The initial phase consists of debridement of all infected soft tissue and bone as well as treatment of spasticity and contractures that may have predisposed the patient to pressure sores. Once all wounds have a clean granulating base and the patient is able to remain prone 24 hours a day, he or she becomes a candidate for a rotational flap. The gluteus maximus, the tensor fasciae latae, and other types of musculocutaneous flaps give the surgeon a superior and reliable method of providing skin coverage. Sitting tolerance must be carefully reestablished following flap surgery. Because most pressure sores in patients with chronic SCI are the result of failure to relieve pressure by appropriate measures, patient education is the key element of a successful rehabilitation outcome.

Ischial or trochanteric pressure sores commonly lead to septic arthritis of the hip. In such cases, femoral head and neck resection is required. In the paraplegic with an intact hip joint, the passive weight of the limbs cantilevered about the posterior thigh exerts an upward force on the pelvis, which decompresses the ischia. Consequently, approximately 30% of the body weight is supported on the thigh. Femoral head and neck resection disrupts the bony leg of the femur to the pelvis and results in a greater concentration of pressure on the ischia, thereby increasing the chance of recurrence even after successful flap closure.

Pressure sores affecting the ankle commonly occur over the heel or malleolus. After initial debridement, wound healing can nearly always be obtained by placing the patient in a short leg cast that protects the wound from any external pressure. The cast is changed every 1 or 2 weeks until healing occurs. Rotational flaps are rarely needed.

E. BLADDER FUNCTION

Intermittent catheterization is the factor most responsible for the nearly normal life span of patients with spinal cord injuries. In this group, urinary tract infection is no longer the leading cause of death. Most patients who have intact sacral reflex activity following complete injury are able to obtain reflex bladder emptying. Some patients with complete SCI are able to trigger reflex bladder emptying by tapping the suprapubic area, stroking the thighs, or using the Credé method (applying external pressure on the bladder to induce emptying) or the Valsalva maneuver (forcibly exhaling against the closed glottis). These patients require an external condom catheter for men or diapering for women. Patients with nonreflex bladders void by the application of pressure on the bladder by the Valsalva maneuver or Credé method. Not all so-called reflex bladders empty reflexively, and some, despite reflex emptying, have an excessive amount of residual urine. Anticholinergic medications to decrease bladder neck spasm of the smooth muscle of the internal sphincter or spasmolytic medications to decrease tone in the striated muscle of the external sphincter may improve bladder emptying. Some patients require surgical sphincterotomy.

Bladder diversion using an ileal conduit as a primary means of achieving bladder drainage is contraindicated. This procedure leads to a chronic acid–base imbalance, osteoporosis, and, ultimately, renal failure from secondary infection. The suprapubic catheter also is to be avoided as a means of primary treatment for the same reasons that permanent indwelling catheters are contraindicated. The constant presence of an indwelling catheter leads to bladder constriction and increases the risks of renal calculi, infection, and death from renal failure. For male patients, the external condom catheter is the treatment of choice. For female patients, padding or diapering is the preferred treatment, although some women prefer an indwelling catheter despite the risks of a shortened life span.

F. SEXUAL FUNCTION

Women with or without intact reflex activity can perform coitus and deliver normal children. Approximately 90% of men with complete SCI and sacral reflex activity can be expected to have reflex erections. Most of these men are able to perform coitus; however, fewer than half can ejaculate. Sacral sparing plays a great role in prognosticating sexual potential in the male patient. Those able to distinguish pain (discrimination of sharp and dull) are usually able to achieve psychogenic erections.

G. AUTONOMIC DYSREFLEXIA

Splanchnic outflow conveying sympathetic fibers to the lower body exits at the T8 region. Patients with lesions above T8 are prone to autonomic dysreflexia. They are subject to bouts of hypertension that may be heralded by dizziness, sweating, and headaches. A plugged catheter is the most common precipitating cause of dysreflexia. The catheter should be carefully checked and the bladder irrigated. Other frequent causes of dysreflexia include calculi or infections in any portion of the urinary system, fecal impaction, and pressure sores. If the patient's blood pressure does not lower in response to treatment of the causative agent, management with antihypertensive medication is begun.

Recovery

The *International Standards for Neurological and Functional Classification of Spinal Cord Injury,* published by the American Spinal Injury Association (ASIA) and the International Medical Society of Paraplegia (IMSOP), represent the most reliable instrument for assessing neurologic status in SCI. These standards provide a quantitative measure of sensory and motor function.

Neurologic recovery is assessed by determining the change in ASIA Motor Score (AMS) between successive neurologic examinations. The AMS is the sum of strength grades for each of the 10 key muscles tested bilaterally that represent neurologic segments from C5 to T1 and L2 to S1. In a neurologically intact individual, the total possible AMS is 100 points.

The most important prognostic indicator of recovery is completeness of injury using the sacral-sparing definition. Using completeness and level of injury (tetraplegia or paraplegia), patients are divided into four groups: complete tetraplegia, incomplete tetraplegia, complete paraplegia, and incomplete paraplegia. The rate of motor recovery in all groups declines rapidly in the first 6 months following injury with minimal further changes after this time (Figure 13–10).

A. COMPLETE PARAPLEGIA

Patients with paraplegia that remains complete 1 month after injury have a 96% chance of remaining complete. Thirty-eight percent of those with injuries at or below T9 recover some lower extremity function. No patients with a neurologic level above T9 regain volitional lower extremity motor function. Only 5% of muscles with a strength of 0/5 at 1 month recover to 3/5 or greater strength 1 year after injury. Furthermore, only 5% of individuals become independent community ambulators at 1 year.

B. INCOMPLETE PARAPLEGIA

Motor recovery is better in individuals with incomplete injuries. Between 1 month and 1 year after injury, the

Figure 13–10. Recovery rates of ASIA Motor Score for persons with incomplete and complete paraplegia and tetraplegia. (Reproduced from Waters RL et al: Functional and neurological recovery following acute SCI. J Spinal Cord Med 1998;21:195.)

AMS increases by an average of 12 points regardless of the level of injury. Additionally, these patients have a 76% chance of becoming community ambulators.

C. COMPLETE TETRAPLEGIA

Ninety percent of individuals with complete tetraplegia 1 month after injury remain complete. Among the 10% who undergo late conversion to incomplete status, lower extremity motor recovery is minimal and inadequate for ambulation. Recovery of AMS points is independent of neurologic level. Waters and colleagues reported that with the exception of the triceps muscle, all upper extremity muscles with grade of at least 1/5 1 month after injury recover to at least 3/5 1 year following injury.

D. INCOMPLETE TETRAPLEGIA

In patients with incomplete tetraplegia, motor recovery of upper and lower extremity muscles occurs concurrently. Nearly all muscles with at least 1/5 strength 1 month after injury recover to at least 3/5 1 year postinjury. Forty-six percent of the patients examined by Waters and colleagues attained independent community ambulation status 1 year after injury. The number of individuals with incomplete tetraplegia who can attain independent community ambulation is less than for individuals with incomplete paraplegia and comparable lower extremity function. This is because upper extremity function may be insufficient to allow crutch-assisted ambulation in the former group, whereas those with incomplete paraplegia have normal upper extremity strength.

Taken as a whole, a minority of individuals with SCI can ambulate independently after injury. The proportion of patients who can ambulate does, however, vary with the level and completeness of the injury. The lower extremity motor score (LEMS), which is the sum of the strength grades of the bilateral key lower extremity muscles, can be used to predict successful ambulation (Table 13–2). The motor groups are as follows: L2, hip flexors (iliopsoas); L3, knee extensors (quadriceps); L4, ankle

Table 13–2. Community ambulators at 1 year postinjury.

ASIA Lower Extremity Motor Score[a] (at 30 days postinjury)	Complete Paraplegia (%)	Incomplete Paraplegia (%)	Incomplete Tetraplegia (%)
0	< 1	33	0
1–9	45	70	2
10–19		100	63
20 or greater		100	100
Total	5	76	46

[a]Score based upon five key muscles.
Total possible 50 points for both lower extremities for normals.
Reprinted, with permission, from Waters RL et al: Functional and neurological recovery following acute SCI. J Spinal Cord Med 1998;21:195.

dorsiflexors (tibialis anterior); L5, long toe extensors (extensor hallucis longus); and S1, ankle plantarflexors (gastrocnemius, soleus). In an individual with no deficit, the total possible LEMS is 50 points. The LEMS at 30 days is used to predict the chance of successful ambulation in incomplete tetraplegics, incomplete paraplegics, and complete paraplegics. All individuals with a LEMS of at least 20 and an incomplete injury are expected to be community ambulators 1 year after injury.

American Spinal Injury Association, International Medical Society of Paraplegia: *International Standards for Neurological Classification of Spinal Cord Injury* (revised). American Spinal Injury Association, 2000.

Banovac K et al: Prevention of heterotopic ossification after spinal cord injury with indomethacin. Spinal Cord 2001;39:370. [PMID: 11464310]

Bracken MB: Methylprednisolone and acute spinal cord injury: An update of the randomized evidence. Spine 2001;26(Suppl 24):S47. [PMID: 11805609]

Bracken MB, Holford TR: Neurological and functional status 1 year after acute spinal cord injury: Estimates of functional recovery in National Acute Spinal Cord Injury Study II from results modeled in National Acute Spinal Cord Injury Study III. J Neurosurg Spine 2002;96(3):259. [PMID: 11990832]

Burns AS, Ditunno JF: Establishing prognosis and maximizing functional outcomes after spinal cord injury: A review of current and future directions in rehabilitation management. Spine 2001;26:S137. [PMID: 11805621]

Hebela N, Smith DG, Keenan MA: What's new in orthopaedic rehabilitation. J Bone Joint Surg Am 2004;86-A(11):2577. [PMID: 15523043]

Hurlbert RJ: Methylprednisolone for acute spinal cord injury: An inappropriate standard of care. J Neurosurg Spine 2000; 93(1):1. [PMID: 10879751]

Keith MW, Hoyen H: Indications and future directions for upper limb neuroprostheses in tetraplegic patients: A review. Hand Clin 2002;18(3):519, viii. [PMID: 12474601]

Kirshblum SC, O'Connor KC: Levels of spinal cord injury and predictors of neurologic recovery. Phys Med Rehabil Clin North Am 2000;11(1):1, vii. [PMID: 10680155]

Lee TT, Green BA: Advances in the management of acute spinal cord injury. Orthop Clin North Am 2002;33(2):311. [PMID: 12389277]

Little JW et al: Neurologic recovery and neurologic decline after spinal cord injury. Phys Med Rehabil Clin North Am 2000; 11(1):73. [PMID: 10680159]

Macciocchi SN, Bowman B, Coker J et al: Effect of co-morbid traumatic brain injury on functional outcome of persons with spinal cord injuries. Am J Phys Med Rehabil 2004;83(1):22. [PMID: 14709971]

McKinley WO, Seel RT, Gadi RK et al: Nontraumatic vs. traumatic spinal cord injury: A rehabilitation outcome comparison. Am J Phys Med Rehabil 2001;80(9):693. [PMID: 11523972]

Nockels RP: Nonoperative management of acute spinal cord injury. Spine 2001;26(24 Suppl):S31. [PMID: 11805606]

Pollard ME, Apple DF: Factors associated with improved neurologic outcomes in patients with incomplete tetraplegia. Spine 2003;28:33. [PMID: 12544952]

Salisbury SK, Choy NL, Nitz J: Shoulder pain, range of motion, and functional motor skills after acute tetraplegia. Arch Phys Med Rehabil 2003;84:1480. [PMID: 14586915]

Van der Putten JJ et al: Factors affecting functional outcome in patients with nontraumatic spinal cord lesions after inpatient rehabilitation. Neurorehabil Neural Repair 2001;15:99. [PMID: 11811258]

von Wild KR: New development of functional neurorehabilitation in neurosurgery. Acta Neurochir Suppl (Wien) 2003;87:43. [PMID: 14518522]

Waters RL, Sie IH: Spinal cord injuries from gunshot wounds to the spine. Clin Orthop 2003;408:120. [PMID: 12616048]

STROKE

Stroke (cerebrovascular accident or brain attack) occurs when thrombosis, embolism, or hemorrhage interrupts cerebral oxygenation and causes the death of neurons in the brain. This leads to deficits in cognition and in motor and sensory function.

In the United States, where cerebrovascular accidents are the leading cause of hemiplegia in adults and the third leading cause of death, 2 million people have permanent neurologic deficits from stroke. The annual incidence of stroke is 1 in 1000, with cerebral thrombosis causing nearly three fourths of the cases. More than half of stroke victims survive and have an average life expectancy of approximately 6 years. Most survivors have the potential for significant function and useful lives if they receive the benefits of rehabilitation.

Neurologic Impairment & Recovery

Infarction of the cerebral cortex in the region of the brain supplied by the middle cerebral artery (MCA) or one of its branches is most commonly responsible for stroke. Although the middle cerebral artery supplies the area of the cerebral cortex responsible for hand function, the anterior cerebral artery supplies the area responsible for lower extremity motion (Figure 13–11). The typical clinical picture following middle cerebral artery stroke is contralateral hemianesthesia (decreased sensation), homonymous hemianopia (visual field deficit), and spastic hemiplegia with more paralysis in the upper extremity than in the lower extremity. Because hand function requires relatively precise motor control, even for activities with assistive equipment, the prognosis for the functional use of the hand and arm is considerably worse than for the leg. Return of even gross motor control in the lower extremity may be sufficient for walking.

Infarction in the region of the anterior cerebral artery causes paralysis and sensory loss of the opposite lower limb and to a lesser degree the arm. Patients who have cerebral arteriosclerosis and suffer repeated bilateral infarctions are likely to have severe cognitive impairment that limits their general ability to function even when motor function is good.

Middle cerebral artery

Anterior cerebral artery

Posterior cerebral artery

Figure 13–11. Cerebral artery circulation.

After stroke, motor recovery follows a fairly typical pattern. The size of the lesion and the amount of collateral circulation determine the amount of permanent damage. Most recovery occurs within 6 months, although functional improvement may continue as the patient receives further sensorimotor reeducation and learns to cope with disability.

Initially after a stroke, the limbs are completely flaccid. Over the next few weeks, muscle tone and spasticity gradually increase in the adductor muscles of the shoulder and in the flexor muscles of the elbow, wrist, and fingers. Spasticity also develops in the lower extremity muscles. Most commonly, there is an extensor pattern of spasticity in the leg, characterized by hip adduction, knee extension, and equinovarus deformities of the foot and ankle (Figure 13–12). In some cases, however, a flexion pattern of spasticity occurs, characterized by hip and knee flexion.

Whether the patient recovers the ability to move one joint independently of the others (selective movement) depends on the extent of the cerebral cortical damage. Dependence on the more neurologically primitive patterned movement (synergy) decreases as selective control improves. The extent to which motor impairment restricts function varies in the upper and lower extremities. Patterned movement is not functional in the upper extremity, but it may be useful in the lower extremity,

where the patient uses the flexion synergy to advance the limb forward and the mass extension synergy for limb stability during standing.

The final processes in sensory perception occur in the cerebral cortex, where basic sensory information is integrated to complex sensory phenomena such as vision, proprioception, and perception of spatial relationships, shape, and texture. Patients with severe parietal dysfunction and sensory loss may lack sufficient perception of space and awareness of the involved segment of their body to ambulate. Patients with severe perceptual loss may lack balance to sit, stand, or walk. A visual field deficit further interferes with limb use and may cause patients to be unaware of their own limbs.

Management

A. ACUTE MANAGEMENT

Medical intervention in the treatment of a stroke is most effective when initiated within 3 hours from the onset of symptoms. However, pharmacologic intervention may play a role, although limited, if administered within 24 hours of onset.

1. Thrombolytics

a. Tissue plasminogen activator (t-PA) (also known as recombinant t-PA or recombinant tissue-type plasminogen activator [rt-PA])—The efficacy of intravenous t-PA was established in two randomized double-blind placebo-controlled studies published in combination by the National Institute of Neurological Disorders and Stroke (NINDS). At 3 months after stroke, approximately 12% more patients in the t-PA group experienced a cure of symptoms relative to those who did not receive

Figure 13–12. Equinovarus deformities of the feet in a patient with spasticity.

it. The risk of intracerebral hemorrhage in the t-PA group was 6% (50% of which were fatal), compared to 0.6% in the placebo group. Despite the differences in hemorrhage rates, there were no differences in mortality (17% in the t-PA group versus 21% in the placebo group).

Key points about the administration of thrombolytic agents include the following:

1. They must be administered within 3 hours of symptom onset. Patients who wake up with symptoms or those who cannot describe accurately the time of their symptom onset are timed to when they were last known to be well.

2. An imaging study of the head (CT scan or MRI) must be performed prior to treatment to rule out hemorrhage as a cause of symptoms.

3. Blood pressure should be lower than 185 systolic and 110 diastolic. Agents such as labetalol may be used to lower the blood pressure for the purposes of treatment.

4. Blood must be tested for platelet count (should be over 100,000); international normalized ratio (INR) (many recommend under 1.6); partial thromboplastin time (PTT) (many recommend less than 40); and glucose (should be 50–400).

b. Prourokinase (also known as recombinant prourokinase, or r-pro-UK)—This intraarterial therapy requires the involvement of a skilled interventionist. The time window is 6 hours from symptom onset. In addition, and in contrast to the NINDS t-PA study, patients with a CT scan showing over a third involvement of the MCA territory as seen on CT scan are not eligible for treatment. The absolute percentage increase in patients with slight or no disability at 3 months was 15% in the prourokinase group compared with the placebo group. The hemorrhage rate in the prourokinase group was 10% versus 2% in subjects who received placebo. No difference was noted, however, in mortality (25% in the prourokinase group versus 27% in the placebo group).

This therapy may be especially useful for patients who arrive later than 3 hours from symptom onset and who have less than a third involvement of the MCA territory on initial scan.

2. Antiplatelet agents

a. Aspirin—The Chinese Acute Stroke Trial (CAST) and the International Stroke Trial (IST) are two large studies evaluating the use of aspirin (160–300 mg/d) within 48 hours of ischemic stroke symptom onset. Compared to no treatment, there was approximately a 1% absolute reduction in stroke and death in the first few weeks. At further time points (eg, 6 months), there was a similar absolute reduction of approximately 1% in death or dependence.

b. Abciximab—An ongoing phase III study of the efficacy of abciximab (ReoPro) in acute stroke is being conducted. A phase II study of 400 patients found an 8% absolute reduction in poor outcomes at 3 months ($P < 0.05$). Symptomatic intracranial hemorrhage occurred in 3.6% of patients on abciximab and in 1.0% of patients on placebo.

3. Anticoagulants

a. Warfarin—No studies have evaluated use of warfarin for the acute treatment of stroke.

b. Heparin and heparinoids—At this time, only one randomized trial showed benefit for heparins or heparinoids in acute ischemic stroke. In that study, no benefit was seen at 10 days or 3 months, only at 6 months. Other large studies failed to find benefit of heparin or heparinoids, either intravenous or subcutaneous, at 3 months. An exploratory post hoc analysis of one intravenous low molecular randomized study suggested benefit in patients with severe large vessel (eg, carotid) atherosclerosis; however, the authors conclude that these findings need to be properly evaluated in a prospective randomized trial.

4. Neuroprotectants—Various classes of neuroprotectants were tested and include calcium channel antagonists, potassium channel openers, glutamate antagonists, antiadhesion molecules, N-methyl-D-aspartate (NMDA) receptor antagonists and modulators, α-amino-3-hydroxy-5-methylisoxazole-4-propionic acid (AMPA) receptor antagonists, membrane stabilizers, growth factors, and glycine site antagonists. At this time, no neuroprotectant shows efficacy in the treatment of acute stroke.

B. Lower Extremities

1. Hemiplegia—To walk independently, the hemiplegic patient requires intact balance reactions, hip flexion to advance the limb, and stability of the limb for standing. If a patient meets these criteria and has acceptable cognition, the orthopedic surgeon can restore ambulation in most cases by prescribing an appropriate lower extremity orthosis and an upper extremity assistive device such as a cane. Surgery to rebalance the muscle forces in the leg can greatly enhance ambulation.

Except for the correction of severe contractures in nonambulatory patients, surgical procedures should be delayed for at least 6 months to allow spontaneous neurologic recovery to occur and the patient to learn how to cope with the disability. After this time, surgery may safely be performed to improve usage in the functional limb.

In the nonfunctional limb, surgery may be performed to relieve pain or correct severe hip and knee flexion contractures caused by spasticity. Most severe contractural deformities in the nonfunctional limb, however, are the result of an ineffective program of daily passive ROM, splinting, and limb positioning.

Most hemiplegics with motor impairment have hip abductor and extensor weakness. A quad cane (cane with four feet to provide more stability) or a hemi-walker is prescribed to provide better balance. Because of paralysis in the upper extremity, the hemiplegic patient is unable to use a conventional walker.

2. Limb scissoring—Scissoring of the legs caused by overactive hip adductor muscles is a common problem. This gives the patient an extremely narrow base of support while standing and causes balance problems. When no fixed contracture of the hip adductor muscles is present, transection of the anterior branches of the obturator nerve denervates the adductors and allows the patient to stand with a broader base of support. If a contracture of the adductors occurs, surgical release of the adductor longus, adductor brevis, and gracilis muscles should be performed (Figure 13–13).

3. Stiff-knee gait—Patients with a stiff-knee gait are unable to flex the knee during the swing phase of gait. The deformity is a dynamic one meaning that it only occurs during walking. Passive knee motion is not restricted, and the patient does not have difficulty sitting. Usually the knee is maintained in extension throughout the gait cycle. Toe drag, which is likely in the early swing phase, may cause the patient to trip. Thus, balance and stability are also affected. The limb appears to be functionally longer. Circumduction of the involved limb, hiking of the pelvis, or contralateral limb vaulting may occur as compensatory maneuvers.

A gait study with dynamic electromyography (EMG) should be done preoperatively to document the activity of the individual muscles of the quadriceps. Dyssynergic activity is commonly seen in the rectus femoris from pre-swing through terminal swing throughout the gait cycle. Abnormal activity is also common in the vastus interme-dius, vastus medialis, and vastus lateralis muscles. If knee flexion is improved with a block of the femoral nerve or with botulinum toxin injection of the quadriceps, the rationale for surgical intervention is strengthened. Any equinus deformity of the foot should be corrected prior to evaluation of a stiff-knee gait because equinus causes a knee extension force during stance. Because the amount of knee flexion during swing is directly related to the speed of walking, the patient should be able to ambulate with a reasonable velocity to benefit from surgery. Hip flexion strength is also needed for a good result because the forward momentum of the leg normally provides the inertial force to flex the knee. In the past a selective release of the rectus femoris or rectus and vastus interme-dius was done to remove their inhibition of knee flexion. On average, a 15-degree improvement in peak knee flex-ion was seen after surgery. Transfer of the rectus femoris to a hamstring tendon not only removes it as a deform-ing muscle force; it also converts the rectus into a correc-tive flexion force. This procedure provides improved

Figure 13–13. Release of the hip adductor tendons and neurectomy of the anterior branches of the obturator nerve to correct the problem of limb scissoring. (Illustration by Anthony C. Berlet. Reproduced, with permission, from Keenan MAE et al: *Manual of Orthopaedic Surgery for Spasticity.* Raven, 1993.)

knee flexion over selective release. When any of the vasti muscles are involved, they can be selectively lengthened at their myotendinous junction (Figure 13–14) and knee flexion improves.

4. Knee flexion deformity—A knee flexion deformity increases the physical demand on the quadriceps muscle, which must continually fire to hold the patient upright. Knee flexion often leads to knee instability and causes falls. It is most often caused by spasticity of the ham-string muscles. A KAFO can be used to hold the knee in extension on a temporary basis as a training aid in physi-cal therapy. Such an orthosis, however, is difficult for the stroke patient to don and wear for permanent usage.

Surgical correction of the knee flexion deformity is the most desirable treatment. Hamstring tenotomy (Figure 13–15) eliminates the dynamic component of the deformity and generally results in a 50% correction of the contracture at the time of surgery. The residual joint contracture is then corrected by serial casting done weekly after surgery. Hamstring function posterior to the knee joint is not necessary for ambulation. In fact, ambulation may only be feasible in patients with knee flexion deformities of greater than 30 degrees if a ham-string release is done.

5. Equinus or equinovarus foot deformity—Surgical correction of an equinus deformity is indicated when the foot cannot be maintained in the neutral position with the heel in firm contact with the sole of the shoe in a well-fitted, rigid AFO. Despite a wide variety of surgical methods designed to decrease the triceps surae spasticity, none is more effective than Achilles tendon

Figure 13–14. Selective lengthening of the rectus femoris tendon to correct a stiff-knee gait abnormality.

lengthening. In this procedure, triple hemisection tenotomy is performed via three stab incisions, with the most distal cut based medially to alleviate varus pull of the soleus muscle (Figure 13–16).

An anesthetic block of the posterior tibial nerve can be a valuable tool in preoperative assessment of the patient with equinus deformity because it demonstrates the potential benefits of Achilles tendon lengthening if the deformity is a result of increased muscle tone. Surgical release of the flexor digitorum longus and brevis tendons at the base of each toe (Figure 13–17) is done prophylactically at the time of Achilles tendon lengthening because increased ankle dorsiflexion fol-

lowing heel cord tenotomy increases tension on the long toe flexor and commonly leads to excessive toe flexion (toe curling). The flexor hallucis longus and flexor digitorum longus tendons can be transferred to

Figure 13–15. Distal release of the hamstring tendons to correct a knee flexion contracture. (Illustration by Anthony C. Berlet. Reproduced, with permission, from Keenan MAE et al: *Manual of Orthopaedic Surgery for Spasticity*. Raven, 1993.)

Figure 13–16. Hoke triple hemisection Achilles tendon lengthening to correct an equinus foot deformity. (Illustration by Anthony C. Berlet. Reproduced, with permission, from Keenan MAE et al: *Manual of Orthopaedic Surgery for Spasticity*. Raven, 1993.)

the os calcis to provide additional support to the weakened calf muscles.

Surgical correction of varus deformity is indicated when the problem is not corrected by a well-fitted orthosis. It is also indicated to enable the patient to walk without an orthosis when varus deformity is the only significant problem. The tibialis anterior, tibialis posterior, extensor hallucis longus, flexor hallucis longus, flexor digitorum, and soleus pass medial to the axis of the subtalar joint and are potentially responsible for varus deformity. EMG studies demonstrate that the peroneus longus and peroneus brevis are generally inactive, and the tibialis posterior is also usually inactive or minimally active.

The tibialis anterior is the key muscle responsible for varus deformity, and in most patients, this can be confirmed by visual examination or palpation while the patient walks. A procedure known as the split anterior tibial tendon transfer (Figure 13–18) diverts the inverting deforming force of the tibialis anterior to a corrective force. In this procedure, half of the tendon is transferred laterally to the os cuboideum. When the extensor hallucis longus muscle is overactive, it can be transferred to the middorsum of the foot as well.

Treatment of equinovarus deformity consists of simultaneously performing the Achilles tendon lengthening procedure and the split anterior tibial tendon transfer. At surgery, the tibialis anterior is secured and held suffi-

Figure 13–18. Split anterior tibial tendon transfer to correct a spastic varus foot deformity. (Illustration by Anthony C. Berlet. Reproduced, with permission, from Keenan MAE et al: *Manual of Orthopaedic Surgery for Spasticity.* Raven, 1993.)

ciently taut to maintain the foot in a neutral position. After healing, 70% of patients are able to walk without an orthosis.

C. UPPER EXTREMITIES

1. Spasticity—The first objective in treating the spastic upper extremity is to prevent contracture. Severe deformities at the shoulder, elbow, and wrist are seen in the neglected or noncompliant patient. Assistive equipment can be used to position the upper extremity, to aid in prevention of contractures, and to support the shoulder. Positioning extends spastic muscles but does not subject them to sudden postural changes that trigger the stretch reflex and aggravate spasticity. Brief periods should be scheduled when the upper extremity is not suspended and time can be devoted to ROM therapy and hygiene.

Most hemiplegics do not use their hand unless some selective motion is present at the fingers or thumb. Thumb opposition begins with opposition of the thumb to the side of the index finger (lateral or key pinch) and proceeds by circumduction to oppose each fingertip. In most stroke patients with selective thumb–finger extension, proximal muscle function is comparatively intact. Hence, orthotic stabilization of proximal joints is rarely necessary in the patient with a functional hand.

Figure 13–17. Release of the flexor digitorum longus and brevis tendons to correct the problem of toe curling. (Illustration by Anthony C. Berlet. Reproduced, with permission, from Keenan MAE et al: *Manual of Orthopaedic Surgery for Spasticity.* Raven, 1993.)

Figure 13–19. Technetium bone scan showing the periarticular increase in activity characteristic of reflex sympathetic dystrophy.

An overhead suspension sling attached to the wheelchair is used for patients with adductor or internal rotator spasticity of the shoulder. An alternative is an arm trough attached to the wheelchair.

It is usually not possible to maintain the wrist in neutral position with a WHO when wrist flexion spasticity is severe or when the wrist is flaccid. With minimal to moderate spasticity, either a volar or dorsal splint can be used. The splint should not extend to the fingers if the finger flexor spasticity is severe because slight motion and sensory contact of the fingers or palm may elicit the stretch reflex or grasp response, causing the fingers to jack-knife out of the splint.

2. Shoulder or arm pain—The hemiplegic shoulder deserves special attention because it is a common source of pain. A variety of different factors contribute to the painful shoulder: reflex sympathetic dystrophy, inferior subluxation, spasticity with internal rotation contracture, adhesive capsulitis, and degenerative changes about the shoulder. If early ROM exercises are performed and the extremity is properly positioned with a sling to reduce subluxation, severe or chronic pain at the shoulder can usually be prevented or minimized.

The classic clinical signs of reflex sympathetic dystrophy (swelling and skin changes) may not be apparent in the hemiplegic patient. If the patient complains that the arm is painful and no cause is apparent, a technetium bone scan assists in establishing the diagnosis (Figure 13–19). Treatment should be instituted immediately, and the patient should be given positive psychological reinforcement. The use of narcotics must be avoided. Treatment options include the use of medications such as corticosteroids, amitriptyline, or gabapentin (Neurontin), physical therapy, or nerve blocks (stellate ganglion blocks, brachial plexus blocks, or Bier IV regional blocks). Each of these techniques is successful with some patients; however, none is reliable for all patients.

3. Shoulder contracture—Contracture of the shoulder can cause pain, hygiene problems in the axilla, and difficulty in dressing and positioning. Shoulder adduction and internal rotation are caused by spasticity and myostatic contracture of four muscles: the pectoralis major, the subscapularis, the latissimus dorsi, and the teres major.

When the deformity is not fixed, lengthening of the pectoralis major, latissimus, and teres major at their myotendinous junction provides satisfactory correction of the deformity. In a nonfunctional extremity, surgical release of all four muscles (Figure 13–20) is usually necessary to resolve the deformity. Release of the subscapularis muscle is performed without violating the glenohumeral joint capsule. The joint capsule should not be opened because instability or intraarticular adhesions may result. A

Figure 13–20. Release of the pectoralis major, subscapularis, latissimus dorsi, and teres major to correct an internal rotation and adduction contracture of the shoulder. (Illustration by Anthony C. Berlet. Reproduced, with permission, from Keenan MAE et al: *Manual of Orthopaedic Surgery for Spasticity.* Raven, 1993.)

Z-plasty of the axilla may be needed if the skin is contracted. After the wound heals, an aggressive mobilization program is instituted. Gentle ROM exercises are employed to correct any remaining contracture. Careful positioning of the limb in abduction and external rotation is necessary for several months to prevent recurrence.

4. Elbow flexion contracture—Persistent spasticity of the elbow flexors causes a myostatic contracture and flexion deformity of the elbow. Frequent accompanying problems include skin maceration, breakdown of the antecubital space, and compression neuropathy of the ulnar nerve.

Surgical release of the contracted muscles and gradual extension of the elbow corrects the deformity and decreases the ulnar nerve compression. The brachioradialis muscle and biceps tendon are transected. The brachialis muscle is fractionally lengthened at its myotendinous junction by transecting the tendinous fibers on the anterior surface of the muscle while leaving the underlying muscle intact (Figure 13–21). Complete release of the brachialis muscle is not performed unless a severe contracture was present for several years. An anterior capsulectomy is not needed and should be avoided because of the associated increased stiffness and intraarticular adhesions that occur postoperatively. Anterior transposition of the ulnar nerve may be necessary to further improve ulnar nerve function.

Approximately 50% correction of the deformity can be expected at surgery without causing excessive tension on the contracted neurovascular structures. Serial casts or dropout casts can be used to obtain further correction over the ensuing weeks.

Figure 13–22. The superficialis-to-profundus tendon transfer to correct a severe clenched-fist deformity in a nonfunctional hand. (Illustration by Anthony C. Berlet. Reproduced, with permission, from Keenan MAE et al: *Manual of Orthopaedic Surgery for Spasticity.* Raven, 1993.)

5. Clenched-fist deformity—A spastic clenched-fist deformity in a nonfunctional hand causes palmar skin breakdown and hygiene problems. Recurrent infections of the fingernail beds are also common.

Adequate flexor tendon lengthening to correct the deformity cannot be attained by fractional or myotendinous lengthening without causing discontinuity at the musculotendinous junction. Transection of the flexor tendons is not recommended because any remaining extensor muscle tone may result in an unopposed hyperextension deformity of the wrist and digits. The recommended procedure is a superficialis-to-profundus tendon transfer (Figure 13–22), which provides sufficient flexor tendon lengthening with preservation of a passive tether to prevent a hyperextension deformity. The wrist deformity is corrected by release of the wrist flexors. A wrist arthrodesis is done to maintain the hand in a neutral position and to eliminate the need for a permanent splint. Because intrinsic muscle spasticity is always present in conjunction with severe spasticity of the extrinsic flexors, a neurectomy of the motor branches of the ulnar nerve in the Guyon canal should be routinely performed along with the superficialis-to-profundus tendon transfer to prevent the postsurgical development of an intrinsic plus deformity.

After surgery, the wrist and digits are immobilized for 4 weeks in a short arm cast extended to the fingertips.

Botte MJ, Bruffey JD, Copp SN et al: Surgical reconstruction of acquired spastic foot and ankle deformity. Foot Ankle Clin 2000;5(2):381. [PMID: 11232236]

Fuller DA, Keenan MA, Esquenazi A et al: The impact of instrumented gait analysis on surgical planning: Treatment of spastic equinovarus deformity of the foot and ankle. Foot Ankle Int 2002;23(8):738. [PMID: 12199388]

Figure 13–21. Surgery of the brachioradialis muscle, biceps tendon, and brachialis muscle to correct an elbow flexion contracture in a nonfunctional arm. (Illustration by Anthony C. Berlet. Reproduced, with permission, from Keenan MAE et al: *Manual of Orthopaedic Surgery for Spasticity.* Raven, 1993.)

Gardner MJ, Ong BC, Liporace F et al: Orthopedic issues after cerebrovascular accident. Am J Orthop 2002;31(10):559. [PMID: 12405561]

Keenan MA, Fuller DA, Whyte J et al: The influence of dynamic polyelectromyography in formulating a surgical plan in treatment of spastic elbow flexion deformity. Arch Phys Med Rehabil 2003;84(2):291. [PMID: 12601663]

Keenan MA, Mehta S: Neuro-orthopedic management of shoulder deformity and dysfunction in brain-injured patients: A novel approach. J Head Trauma Rehabil 2004;19(2):143. [PMID: 15247824]

Mayer NH: Choosing upper limb muscles for focal intervention after traumatic brain injury. J Head Trauma Rehabil 2004;19(2):119. [PMID: 15247823]

Pollock A, Baer G, Pomeroy V et al: Physiotherapy treatment approaches for the recovery of postural control and lower limb function following stroke. Cochrane Database Syst Rev 2003;2:CD001920. [PMID: 12804415]

Vuagnat H, Chantraine A: Shoulder pain in hemiplegia revisited: Contribution of functional electrical stimulation and other therapies. J Rehabil Med 2003;35:49. [PMID: 12691333]

GERIATRIC ORTHOPEDICS

General Principles

A major challenge facing society is the aging of the population. By 2020, 52 million Americans will be older than 65 years. By 2040, 68 million people will be older than 65 years. Both the absolute numbers and proportion of elderly people is increasing dramatically. People are living longer and have higher expectations for a good quality of life. Despite this trend, proportionally less disability occurs among the elderly now than in the past.

Although the passage of time, chronological age, is the convenient measure used, it is not necessarily the most precise marker of aging. A more sensitive marker would be to consider the person's functional age, but this is often difficult to define and measure. Age 65 is generally considered the beginning of old age.

The young elderly are those individuals 65 to 75 years of age. These people are usually functionally intact. They have isolated orthopedic problems, such as mild osteoporosis, osteoarthrosis, overuse injuries (sports), and occasionally cancer.

The frail very elderly are those persons older than 80 years. These people tend to have multiple musculoskeletal impairments such as advanced osteoporosis, generalized muscle weakness, multiple organ diseases, and dementia.

1. Disability

The leading causes of death in the elderly are heart disease, malignant neoplasms, and cerebrovascular disease. The overall leading causes of disability in the elderly are cancer, heart disease, dementia, and musculoskeletal disorders. The leading causes of disease-related disability before death are arthritis, hypertension, hearing impairment, heart disease, and orthopedic conditions. Despite the increasing incidence of disability with aging, only 5% of Americans live in nursing homes.

When evaluating the elderly, five functional domains of disability need to be considered:

1. *Physical ADLs* include activities such as bathing, dressing, eating, and walking.

2. *Instrumental ADLs* are home management tasks such as shopping, meal preparation, money management, using the telephone, and performing light housework.

3. *Cognitive functioning* is particularly important in the elderly. Dementia is one of the four leading causes of disability in the elderly and a principal reason for institutionalization.

4. *Affective function* is important. Secondary depressions are common in the elderly, and suicide is a more frequent cause of death in the elderly than in the young.

5. *Social functioning* is less of a problem. Only 1% of the elderly rate their social interactions as inadequate.

Disability in basic ADLs is common among community-dwelling older persons, with prevalence rates ranging from 7% in those 65 to 74 years of age to 24% in those 85 years of age or older. Restricted activity, defined as staying in bed for at least half a day and/or cutting down on usual activities because of an illness, injury, or other problem, is common among community-living older persons, regardless of risk for disability, and it is usually attributable to several concurrent health-related problems. Although disability in older persons is often thought to be progressive or permanent, previous research shows it is a dynamic process, with individuals moving in and out of states of disability. To set realistic goals and plan for appropriate care, disabled older persons, along with their families and clinicians, need accurate information about the likelihood and time course of recovery. Prevention of functional decline and disability includes not only management of acute episodes of disability and promotion of recovery, but also ongoing evaluation and management of key risk factors for disability and use of preventive interventions. The high likelihood of recurrent disability among older persons suggests that those who recently recovered from an episode of disability are an important target population for preventive interventions. Although some interventions designed to prevent recurrent disability may be disease specific (eg, anticoagulation after embolic stroke), others may be broadly applicable regardless of the specific precipitant of disability (eg, exercise-based programs).

2. Challenges for the Orthopedic Surgeon

When working with the elderly, the orthopedic surgeon becomes a member of a multidisciplinary team. The people making up this team include internists, geriatricians, rehabilitation specialists, psychiatrists, psychologists, social workers, nutritionists, skin care specialists, physical and occupational therapists, and the so-called young elderly children of the patient. Osteoporosis, fractures, arthritis, foot disorders, stroke, and amputations are the most frequent causes of musculoskeletal impairment.

3. Osteoporosis

Osteoporosis is an age-related disorder characterized by decreased bone mass and increased fracture risk in the absence of other recognizable causes of bone loss. Osteoporosis can occur either as a primary disorder or secondary to other diseases.

A. PRIMARY OSTEOPOROSIS

Primary osteoporosis, the most common form of the disease, occurs in people from 51 to 65 years of age with a female-to-male ratio of 6:1. Primary osteoporosis can be further subdivided into two types. Type I, postmenopausal osteoporosis, results from decreased circulating levels of estrogen. It is seen in postmenopausal women and affects the majority of persons older than 70 years. Bone loss is rapid. There is swift trabecular bone loss up to 8% per year. Type I osteoporosis causes primarily trabecular bone loss with only 0.5% cortical bone loss per year. Fractures occur in locations of trabecular bone loss such as the distal radius and vertebrae. The cause of primary osteoporosis is a changing hormonal milieu.

Type II, senile osteoporosis, is a consequence of aging. It causes a more global bone loss affecting cortical and cancellous bone such as in the femoral neck. Type II osteoporosis is seen in persons older than 70 years. The female-to-male ratio is 2:1. The bone loss occurs in both the trabecular and cortical bone and averages 0.3–0.5% per year. Fractures occurring as the result of type II osteoporosis typically involve the hip, pelvis, humerus, tibia, and vertebral bodies. The causes of senile osteoporosis are those seen with aging and include calcium deficiency, decreased vitamin D, and increased parathormone activity.

B. SECONDARY OSTEOPOROSIS

Secondary osteoporosis results from a variety of causes. The most common are chronic or prolonged corticosteroid use and endocrine disorders. The endocrine disorders associated with osteoporosis are hyperthyroidism; hyperparathyroidism; diabetes, Cushing disease, and euplastic disorders.

Prevention Strategies

Restoration of bone is difficult. It is therefore imperative to maximize peak bone mass during skeletal growth and then to maintain it during maturity. This requires adequate dietary calcium and vitamin D intake. The recommended amounts for adults are 1200 mg/day of calcium and 400 mg of vitamin D. For postmenopausal women, 1500 mg/day of calcium is recommended. Impact exercise is effective in maintaining bone mass. It is also important to avoid those factors that promote osteoporosis such as the use of tobacco products and excessive alcohol consumption.

Diagnosis

Osteoporosis is a clinical diagnosis often made following a fracture. Radiographic findings include osteopenia (seen with more than 30% mineral loss); loss of horizontal trabeculae in vertebral bodies; thoracic wedge fractures; lumbar spine endplate fractures; stress fractures of the pelvis; and fractures of humerus, wrist, hip, supracondylar femur, tibial plateau. Quantification of bone mass is done for confirmation and follow-up. Dual-energy x-ray absorptiometry (DEXA) is used to quantify bone mass. The following criteria for diagnosis are based on the DEXA scan:

Normal: within 1 standard deviation (SD) of young adult reference

Osteopenia: between 1.0 and 2.4 SD below reference

Osteoporosis: 2.5 or more SD below reference

Severe osteoporosis: 2.5 plus one or more fragility fractures

Treatment

Calcium alone does not prevent bone loss during the early postmenopausal period, but adequate daily calcium replacement is helpful. In late menopause (more than 6 years), calcium replacement does reduce bone loss. Weight-bearing exercise is also useful in maintaining bone mass.

Newer treatments using bisphosphonates show promise in treating osteoporosis. The bisphosphonates are a class of compounds similar to pyrophosphate that are readily adsorbed by bone mineral surfaces. Once bound, they inhibit the bone absorption activity of osteoclasts. Two bisphosphonates currently are available for clinical use: alendronate sodium (Fosamax) and risedronate sodium (Actonel).

Only approximately a third of women in the United States diagnosed with osteoporosis during the 1990s were offered treatment for the condition. Fewer than 2% of the women 60 years and older were diagnosed with osteoporosis, but the rate increased from 1.2% in 1993 to 2.7% in 1997. Overall, 36% of women diagnosed with osteoporosis were prescribed calcium, vitamin D, or drugs to treat the disease, but this also increased, from 20% in 1993 to 55% in 1997.

Exercise

The ability to walk safely is vital for independent living. Both strength and endurance determine the capacity for independent movement. Muscle strength is associated with the capacity to perform ADLs. A reduction in strength with age is attributed to these factors:

1. a loss of muscle mass because of smaller and fewer fibers;
2. a loss of motor neurons (anterior horn cells);
3. changes in muscle architecture;
4. a defect in the excitation-contraction mechanism; and
5. psychosocial changes leading to reduced capacity to activate motor units.

Strength training can lead to major functional improvements in the elderly. The plasticity of the motor system to adapt to a training load appears to be maintained into the 10th decade of life. Strength training has no effect on the central determinants of aerobic capacity such as maximum heart rate, blood pressure hemoglobin concentration, and blood volume.

Aerobic exercise does lead to increased endurance and functional capacity. Endurance is the time a person can maintain either a static force or a power level involving a combination of concentric or eccentric muscular contractions. The stress that exercise imposes on a person and the tolerance or endurance for that exercise intensity depends on how much energy is needed to perform the task in relation to the person's maximal capacity. With training, activities become easier to perform. The person has increased endurance for submaximal exercise. Improvements in movement can lower the energy cost of an activity.

4. Arthritis

Osteoarthritis is very prevalent in the elderly. Total joint arthroplasty has dramatically improved the mobility and quality of life for the elderly. A variety of studies confirm the appropriateness and effectiveness of both total hip and total knee arthroplasty in the elderly with low complication rates. The elderly patient is more likely to require the use of an upper extremity assistive device for ambulation following joint replacement.

5. Fractures

A. GENERAL CONSIDERATIONS

One of the most compelling reasons to determine the etiology of a fracture and provide appropriate treatment is that a previous low-energy fracture is among the strongest risk factors for new fractures. Specifically, patients with a low-energy fracture of the wrist, hip, proximal humerus, or ankle have nearly a two- to fourfold greater risk for future fractures than individuals who have never experienced a fracture. Furthermore, up to half of patients with a prior vertebral fracture experience additional vertebral fractures within 3 years, many within the first year. Indeed, compared to individuals with no history of fracture, a patient with a prior vertebral fracture has nearly a fivefold increased risk of future vertebral fractures and up to a sixfold increased risk of hip and other nonvertebral fractures. Taken together, these data indicate that patients with a history of any type of prior fracture have a two- to sixfold increased risk of subsequent fractures compared to those without a previous fracture.

These findings emphasize that optimal care of fragility fracture patients includes not only management of the presenting fracture, but also evaluation, diagnosis, and treatment of the underlying cause(s) of the fracture, including low bone density or other medical conditions. In this regard, supplementation with calcium and vitamin D lowers fracture risk in the elderly. In addition, several pharmacologic agents reduce the risk of future fracture by as much as 50% in patients with existing fractures. Nonpharmacologic interventions, such as fall prevention programs and individually tailored exercise programs, reduce falls among the elderly, which may decrease the incidence of fractures. In addition, trochanteric padding dramatically reduces hip fractures among those at highest risk. Thus, initiating interventions soon after a fragility fracture occurs may significantly reduce the incidence and severity of subsequent fractures.

In the elderly, fractures result from low-energy injuries. Falls in the home most frequently result in fractures of the hip, distal radius, pelvis, proximal humerus, and ribs. Approximately 90% of fractures of the pelvis, hip, and forearm result from a fall. Only 3–5% of falls result in fractures.

Many of the risk factors for fracture are also risk factors for falls. Risk factors can be divided into categories. Risk factors associated with aspects of aging include primary osteoporosis, impaired vision or balance; gait abnormalities; and loss of muscle and fat padding the bones. Environmental risk factors consist of uneven surfaces; slippery surfaces; obstacles such as throw rugs, pets, and steps; poor lighting; and lack of railings or other supports for balance. Fall prevention programs include home safety measures such as the installation of safety bars in the bathtub and shower, elimination of heavily waxed floors and slippery rugs, and the use of rubber sole shoes with low wide heels that provide more stability.

Genetic factors are seen in both gender and race. Women sustain more fractures than men. Whites have more fractures than African Americans. Illnesses commonly associated with fractures include stroke, syncope, hypotension, secondary osteoporosis, Parkinson disease, dementia, and paraparesis. The use of medications such as benzodiazepines, tricyclic antidepressants, antipsychotics, corticosteroids, and barbiturates are connected with fractures. Lifestyle factors include exercise, nutrition, alcohol or other substance abuse, immobilization, and shoe style.

Other factors contribute to the risk of traumatic fractures occurring in falls. The first is the orientation of the fall. A fall that happens while standing still or walking very slowly imparts little or no forward momentum so the point of impact is near the hip. Gait velocity slows with aging, putting the hip more at risk of injury in a fall. Protective responses during a fall decrease with age. Local shock absorbers, muscle and fat, that surround the bone decrease with age. Bone strength is less secondary to the osteoporosis associated with aging.

B. Hip Fractures

Fractures of the hip are classified by location and severity. The basic considerations are whether the fracture occurs in the intracapsular or extracapsular area and the stability of the fracture pattern. Intracapsular fractures occur along the neck of the femur. When they are displaced, the blood supply to the femoral head is likely disrupted, which increases the possibility of osteonecrosis.

Treatment of hip fractures is operative whenever possible. The nonoperative treatment of hip fractures is very occasionally chosen for patients at high medical risk. It is sometimes recommended for demented nonambulatory patients. The nonoperative treatment of a hip fracture involves months of bed rest and sometimes traction. It requires excellent nursing care to avoid decubitus ulcers and respiratory dysfunction. Fracture malunion, limb-length inequality, pain, and higher mortality rates are common with nonoperative care. The chances for eventual ambulation are only 55% compared with 76% for patients treated operatively.

The basic principles of treatment of hip fractures are well established. Nondisplaced fractures of the femoral neck are usually treated with multiple pins or screws. Displaced fractures of the femoral neck are usually treated with a hemiarthroplasty because of the high incidence of avascular necrosis. Stable intertrochanteric fractures are generally treated with a sliding screw and side plate system. Unstable intertrochanteric fractures may require additional measures to gain adequate medial support. In very osteoporotic bone, it may be necessary to add methyl methacrylate bone cement to gain sufficient fixation and stability. When a patient is known to have severe arthritis, a primary total hip arthroplasty may be performed.

The postoperative rehabilitation of the elderly patient is critical to a successful outcome. Non–weight-bearing ambulation is extremely difficult and more often impossible for elderly patients. Every effort should be made in the operative treatment to gain enough stability of the fracture to allow weight bearing as tolerated. The patient should be mobilized on the first or second day after surgery to prevent the many complications of immobility. Pain management is important to allow mobilization, but oversedation of the elderly patient needs to be avoided. When a prosthesis was inserted, dislocation must be avoided. The elderly patient may not remember the precautions. Use of elevated chairs and toilet seats helps avoid the excessive hip flexion associated with posterior dislocation. A knee immobilizer splint while in bed prevents knee flexion that in turn results in flexion of the hip. It is prudent occasionally to place the patient in a hip brace, which limits flexion and adduction while soft-tissue healing occurs.

C. Fractures of the Pelvis

A common pelvic classification is based on whether or not the ring of the pelvis is disrupted because this indicates the amount of energy involved with the initial trauma. A fracture that does not disrupt the pelvic ring such as a pubic ramus fracture is a low-energy injury. Formerly, pelvic fractures were associated with high-energy trauma, were displaced, and occurred in patients less than 40 years old. With the aging of America, now more than 50% of fractures occur in those older than 60 years, with a preponderance occurring in women. The majority of pelvis fractures in the elderly are low-energy injuries and can be treated nonoperatively with analgesia and bed rest. Early mobilization is desirable to prevent the complications of immobility. Full weight bearing is allowed. A walker or other assistive device is useful to decrease pain and increase stability during walking. Stool softeners are often helpful. Fractures of the coccyx and sacrum are treated in a similar manner.

D. Fractures of the Distal Femur

The management of distal femur fractures in the elderly patients must be individualized. Advanced age in itself is not a contraindication to surgery. The objects of surgical treatment of the distal femur are anatomic reduction and stable fixation. In the presence of severe osteopenia, stable fixation is difficult. The addition of methyl methacrylate or long-stem knee replacement can help with stability. Occasionally, a postoperative cast brace is needed to supplement the internal fixation.

E. Fractures of the Forearm

Most fractures of the distal radius (Colles fracture) can be treated by closed reduction and casting. Significant loss of radial height and dorsal comminution can occur in osteoporotic bone even after lower energy injuries. In this situation, most surgeons would agree that external fixation and bone grafting of the fracture are warranted to obtain and maintain a more anatomic reduction. Early ROM exercises for both the shoulder and the fingers should be encouraged to avoid stiffness.

F. FRACTURES OF THE PROXIMAL HUMERUS

Fractures of the proximal humerus account for 4–5% of all fractures and occur most commonly in the elderly. Humeral fractures in the elderly are minimally displaced 80% of the time. In these cases, sling immobilization is used to control pain. Pendulum exercises are begun early to prevent excessive stiffness in the shoulder. Limited external rotation of the shoulder predisposes to a future spiral fracture of the humerus during dressing. In unstable and markedly displaced fractures of the humeral head, a hemiarthroplasty can be considered. If coexisting severe osteoarthritis of the glenohumeral joint is present, a total shoulder arthroplasty can be considered.

6. Stroke

Stroke is a common cause of disability in the elderly. This topic was covered in detail earlier in this chapter.

7. Foot Disorders

The foot tends to widen with age as the transverse arch support weakens and abnormal bony alignments of the foot become common. Surgical reconstruction of foot deformities may be contraindicated in the frail elderly patient, particularly because of peripheral vascular disease. Nonoperative treatment consists of active and passive ROM exercises of the foot to maximize flexibility. Strengthening exercises of the lower extremity can be useful to improve the overall gait pattern. The patient should try to optimize body weight to eliminate excessive forces on the foot. Functional orthoses of a semirigid material with little or no posting may improve the foot position and provide symptomatic relief. Accommodative orthoses of a soft material may also be used. These soft orthoses are designed to control foot posture and eliminate areas of pressure, but they are not intended to correct the foot position. Orthoses are used in combination with soft extra-depth shoes that provide more clearance for deformities of the toes. Flat shoes are helpful for forefoot deformities because they prevent the foot sliding forward in the shoe. A shoe with a low heel is desirable for patients with a severe pronation deformity because the Achilles tendon is commonly tight. Placing the heel cord on stretch only increases the pronation forces on the foot.

8. Amputation

The majority of amputations done in a civilian population are of the lower extremity. Most amputations are done in the sixth decade of life or later, so this is largely a problem of the elderly. The issues associated with amputation are discussed in Chapter 12.

Chao EY, Inoue N, Koo TK et al: Biomechanical considerations of fracture treatment and bone quality maintenance in elderly patients and patients with osteoporosis. Clin Orthop 2004; (425):12. [PMID: 15292783]

Gehlbach SH et al: Recognition of osteoporosis by primary care physicians. Am J Public Health 2002;92:271. [PMID: 11818304]

Gill TM, Allore HG, Holford TR et al: Hospitalization, restricted activity, and the development of disability among older persons. JAMA 2004;292(17):2115. [PMID: 15523072]

Hardy SE, Gill TM: Factors associated with recovery of independence among newly disabled older persons. Arch Intern Med 2005;165(1):106. [PMID: 15642885]

Hooven F, Gehlbach SH, Pekow P et al: Follow-up treatment for osteoporosis after fracture. Osteoporos Int 2005;16:296–301. [PMID: 15221208]

Lorich DG, Geller DS, Nielson JH: Osteoporotic pertrochanteric hip fractures: Management and current controversies. Instr Course Lect 2004;53:441. [PMID: 15116633]

Phillips FM: Minimally invasive treatments of osteoporotic vertebral compression fractures. Spine 2003;28(Suppl 15):S45. [PMID: 12897474]

Stromsoe K: Fracture fixation problems in osteoporosis. Injury 2004;35(2):107. [PMID: 14736465]

Tosi LL, Kyle RF: Fragility fractures: The fall and decline of bone health. Commentary on "Interventions to improve osteoporosis treatment following hip fracture" by Gardner et al. J Bone Joint Surg Am 2005;87-A(1):1. [PMID: 15634807]

BRAIN INJURY

Brain injury resulting from trauma to the head is a leading cause of death and disability. Head injury is at least twice as common in males as in females and occurs most often in people 15–24 years of age. Approximately half of the injuries result from motor vehicle accidents. In the United States, 410,000 new cases of traumatic brain injury can be expected each year, with each case presenting a challenge to the team of health care providers involved in providing emergency treatment and long-term management.

Neurologic Impairment & Recovery

The Glasgow Coma Score (Table 13–3) is frequently used to evaluate eye opening, motor response, and verbal response of patients with impaired consciousness. Analysis of scores from patients in several countries sheds light on the chances for survival and neurologic recovery. According to the data, approximately 50% of patients with impaired consciousness survived.

Table 13–3. The Glasgow Coma Score.

Response	Description	Numerical Value
Eye opening	Spontaneous response	4
	Response to speech	3
	Response to pain	2
	No response	1
Motor response	Obeying response	6
	Localized response	5
	Withdrawal	4
	Abnormal flexion	3
	Extension	2
	No response	1
Verbal response	Oriented conversation	5
	Confused conversation	4
	Inappropriate words	3
	Incomprehensible sounds	2
	No response	1

Adapted, with permission, from: Teasdale G, Jennett B: Assessment of coma and impaired consciousness. A practical scale. Lancet 1974;2:81.

Six months after injury, moderate or good neurologic recovery was seen in 82% of patients with initial (24-hour) Glasgow scores of 11 or higher, 68% of patients with initial scores of 8–10, 34% with initial scores of 5–7, and 7% with initial scores of 3 or 4. Age was an important factor related to neurologic outcome, with 62% of patients younger than 20 years and 46% of patients between 20 and 29 years of age showing moderate or good recovery.

The incidence of good recovery declines not only with advancing age but also with advancing duration of coma. Patients recovering from coma within the first 2 weeks of injury have a 70% chance of good recovery. The recovery rate drops to 39% in the third week and to 17% in the fourth week. Decerebrate or decorticate posturing indicates a brainstem injury and is indicative of a poor prognosis.

Management

The rehabilitation process has three distinct phases: the acute injury period, the subacute period of neurologic recovery, and the residual period of functional adaptation. Health care workers from a variety of disciplines are involved in each phase.

A. PHASES OF PATIENT CARE AND REHABILITATION

1. Acute injury phase—The initial phase of rehabilitation begins as soon as the patient reaches the acute-care hospital. Brain injury is frequently the result of a high-velocity accident. Diagnosis is problematic because multiple injuries are common, resuscitation and other lifesaving efforts make a complete examination difficult, and the patient who is comatose or disoriented cannot assist in the history or physical examination.

Under the circumstances, three important principles should be followed. The first is to make an accurate diagnosis based on a thorough examination. Fractures or dislocations are missed in 11% of patients, and peripheral nerve injuries are missed in 34%. The second is to assume that the patient will make a good neurologic recovery. Basic treatment principles should not be waived on the erroneous assumption that the patient will not survive. The third principle is to anticipate uncontrolled limb motion and lack of patient cooperation. The patient often goes through a period of agitation as neurologic recovery progresses. Traction and external fixation devices are best avoided for extremity injuries. Open reduction and internal fixation of fractures and dislocations diminishes complications, requires less nursing care, allows for earlier mobilization, and results in fewer residual deformities.

2. Subacute phase of neurologic recovery—During the subacute phase, when the patient is generally in a rehabilitation facility, spontaneous neurologic recovery occurs. During this recovery period, which may last from 12 to 18 months, spasticity is frequently present, and heterotopic ossification may develop. Management is aimed at preventing limb deformities, maintaining a functional arc of motion in the joints, and meeting both the physical and the psychological needs of the patient.

3. Residual phase or period of functional adaptation—When neurologic recovery reaches a plateau, the third phase of rehabilitation begins. Medical and surgical management is aimed at correction of residual limb deformities and excision of heterotopic ossification while specialists from various disciplines continue moving toward the goals planned for the individual patient.

B. THE TEAM APPROACH TO PATIENT CARE AND REHABILITATION

Members of the rehabilitation team are involved in setting short-term goals, which are meant to be accomplished by the time of discharge from the rehabilitation program, and long-term goals, which will take an extended period of time to achieve. The identification of needs and the setting of goals are performed independently by health care workers from each discipline.

The team members then meet to discuss their goals and draw up a coordinated plan.

1. Medical management—General medical goals are usually straightforward. Because most patients with traumatic brain injuries are younger persons, chronic premorbid illnesses are uncommon. Prevention and treatment of infections are important goals, especially while shunts, tubes, and catheters are in place. If seizures are present, controlling them without causing sedation is vital.

In patients with decreased ROM in a joint, the cause of the problem should be explored. Possible causes include increased muscle tone, pain, myostatic contracture, periarticular heterotopic ossification, an undetected fracture or dislocation, and lack of patient cooperation secondary to diminished cognition. Peripheral nerve blocks with local anesthetics are useful in distinguishing between severe spasticity and fixed contractures.

Phenol blocks or botulinum toxin injections are used to decrease spasticity only during the period of potential neurologic recovery. The rationale for phenol injection is that by the time the nerve regenerates, the patient will have recovered more control of the affected muscle.

The technique for administering the phenol block depends on the anatomic accessibility and composition of the nerve; the direct injection of a peripheral nerve gives the most complete and long-lasting block. If a peripheral nerve has a large sensory component, however, direct injection is not recommended because loss of sensation is undesirable and some patients may develop painful hyperesthesia. In some cases, it is necessary to dissect surgically the individual motor branches of a nerve that runs to a muscle and inject each branch separately. In other cases, the motor points of the muscles can be localized using a needle electrode and nerve stimulator and then injected. Motor point injections do not completely relieve spasticity but can be helpful in reducing muscle tone. The duration of motor point blocks is approximately 2 months, and the blocks can be repeated as necessary.

Botulinum toxin is injected directly into the muscle belly. The onset of action is delayed but lasts for approximately 3 months. The injections can be repeated as needed and do not result in any scarring of the muscle. The limitation of botulinum toxin is the total dose tolerated at a given time and its high cost relative to phenol.

2. Nursing care—Nursing goals concentrate on basic bodily needs such as nutrition, hygiene, and handling of secretions. Removal of tubes at the earliest possible time is a desirable goal.

Tracheostomy tubes are commonly used in patients with brain injury. General principles of care include changing an uncuffed tube as soon as possible to prevent pressure necrosis of the trachea, adding mist if necessary to provide moisture to the artificial airway, establishing suctioning procedures to prevent trauma and infection, and eliminating the dressing once the tracheostomy incision is healed because the dressing can be a source of infection. The size of the tube is gradually reduced, and the tube is then plugged to tolerance. When continual plugging is tolerated for 3 consecutive days, the tube can be removed.

Feeding tubes are also commonly used. If oral feeding is not anticipated in the near future, a percutaneous endoscopic gastrostomy tube is recommended. If oral feeding is anticipated soon, a nasogastric tube is inserted, cleaned daily, and changed once a week. Instituting and carrying out an oral feeding program requires the combined efforts of the nursing and physical therapy staffs. Head and trunk control are necessary to provide alignment of swallowing structures. The presence of a cough reflex indicates some measure of laryngeal control and the ability to clear the airway. The presence of a swallowing reflex indicates inherent coordination of swallowing structures. The gag reflex, although protective, is not necessary for functional swallowing. Oral feeding should be started with thickened liquids and pureed foods, which provide more oral stimulus and allow time to initiate swallowing. Thin liquids are more easily aspirated.

The ability to inhibit voiding is generally a cognitive function. Restoring continence in the brain-injured patient requires a consistent routine with repeated instructions and positive feedback. Bowel programs should be initiated as soon as the patient begins taking nourishment via the gastrointestinal tract. Again, a consistent routine is most successful.

3. Cognitive and neuropsychological management—The return of cognitive abilities follows the same sequence of stages that normal cognitive development follows, with each new level of cognitive function stemming from the previous level. Table 13–4 shows the eight levels. Cognitive and behavioral management focuses on providing stimulation for patients with a level II or III response; providing structure for patients with a level IV, V, or VI response; and encouraging community activities for patients with a level VII or VIII response.

Memory loss and diminished cognitive function are frequently the most pervasive limitations to overall function. Cognitive retraining is an essential part of the rehabilitation process at every stage. As cognition increases and the patient becomes more aware of the injury, he or she also becomes increasingly aware of the possible consequences of the injury and requires counseling and psychological support.

4. Speech therapy—After traumatic brain injury, patients may have temporary or permanent physical handicaps that prevent them from communicating effectively. In communicating with nonverbal patients, a variety of methods and devices can be used, ranging from yes-and-no signals to communication boards and electronic devices. Patients need to acquire at least a minimal level of attentional, memory, and organiza-

Table 13–4. Cognitive function.

Level	Description
I	No response
II	Generalized response
III	Localized response
IV	Confused, agitated response
V	Confused, inappropriate response
VI	Confused, appropriate response
VII	Automatic, appropriate response
VIII	Purposeful, appropriate response

Adapted from Malkmus D et al: *Rehabilitation of the Head-Injured Adult. Comprehensive Cognitive Management.* Professional Staff Association of Rancho Los Amigos Hospital, Inc: Downey, CA. 1980.

tional skills to facilitate use of such communication devices. In verbal patients, language disorders may be present because of an underlying cognitive disruption following head trauma. The most frequent residual language disorders are those seen in the areas of work retrieval and auditory processing. Language therapy in patients with these long-term disorders should be directed toward reorganization of the cognitive process.

5. Physical therapy—Areas of concern in physical therapy include patient positioning, mobility, and performance of daily activities. Making it possible for bedridden patients to sit can significantly improve the quality of life and greatly enhance the opportunities to interact with other people. In some patients, casts or orthotic devices may be required to maintain the desired limb positions. Aggressive joint ROM exercises are necessary to prevent contractures.

Among the factors that influence whether a patient can walk are limb stability, motor control, good balance reactions, and adequate proprioception. Equipment and devices to aid in movement (canes, walkers, wheelchairs, etc.) should always be of the least complex design to accomplish the goal and should be chosen on the basis of the individual patient's cognitive and physical level of function.

In developing appropriate exercises and activities for a patient, the physical therapist should consider factors such as the joint ROM, muscle tone, motor control, and cognitive functions of the patient. Even the confused and agitated patient may respond to simple, familiar functional activities such as washing the face and brushing the teeth. Patients with higher cognitive function should be encouraged to carry out hygiene, grooming, dressing, and feeding activities.

6. Surgical management of residual musculoskeletal problems—After neurologic recovery stabilizes, surgical procedures may be indicated to correct residual limb deformities and to excise heterotopic ossification.

a. Correction of limb deformities in the lower extremities—In functional lower limbs, surgery is most often directed at correcting the equinovarus deformity of the foot (see Figure 13–12). The procedures needed for correction of the deformity are determined by clinical evaluation combined with laboratory assessment using dynamic polyelectromyography (poly-EMG). Commonly several procedures are done simultaneously: lengthening of the Achilles tendon (see Figure 13–16), release of the flexor digitorum longus, flexor hallucis longus and flexor brevis tendons (see Figure 13–17), a split anterior tibial tendon transfer (see Figure 13–18), and transfer of the flexor digitorum longus tendon to the heel. The object of surgery is to provide a plantigrade foot for standing and walking, and the surgery is highly successful in this goal. Seventy percent of patients are able to ambulate without a brace after surgery.

A stiff-knee gait is a common deformity that causes the patient to hike the pelvis and circumduct the leg for clearance of the foot during the swing phase of walking. Inappropriate activity in the quadriceps muscle at this time prevents knee flexion. If the vasti muscles of the quadriceps muscle are firing out of phase, the affected head or heads can be lengthened surgically (see Figure 13–14) to allow knee flexion while retaining quadriceps function. Transfer of the rectus femoris muscle to the sartorius or gracilis muscle provides active knee flexion during swing.

In nonfunctional lower limbs, surgery commonly consists of releasing contractures of the hips and knees.

b. Correction of limb deformities in the upper extremities—In functional upper limbs, surgery is frequently needed to correct problems of the wrist, fingers, and thumbs. If active hand opening is restricted by flexor spasticity, lengthening of the extrinsic finger flexors (Figure 13–23) weakens the overactive flexors and improves hand function while preserving the ability of the patient to grasp objects. In cases in which spastic thenar muscles cause thumb-in-palm deformity, a procedure consisting of proximal release of the thenar muscles (Figure 13–24) corrects the problem while preserving function of the thumb. In some patients, adequate placement of the hand for functional activities is impaired by elbow spasticity, although triceps function is generally normal. In these patients, lengthening the elbow flexors (Figure 13–25) enhances the ability to extend the elbow smoothly while preserving active flexion.

In nonfunctional upper limbs, common procedures consist of releasing various contractures and performing neurectomies to eliminate muscle spasticity. The problems of shoulder contracture, elbow contracture, and clenched-fist deformity are discussed in the section on

Figure 13–25. Lengthening of the elbow flexors to correct flexor spasticity and improve movement of the elbow. (Illustration by Anthony C. Berlet. Reproduced, with permission, from Keenan MAE et al: *Manual of Orthopaedic Surgery for Spasticity*. Raven, 1993.)

Figure 13–23. Lengthening of the extrinsic finger flexors to correct the problem of flexor spasticity and improve hand function while preserving the ability to grasp objects. (Illustration by Anthony C. Berlet. Reproduced, with permission, from Keenan MAE et al: *Manual of Orthopaedic Surgery for Spasticity*. Raven, 1993.)

stroke (see previous discussion), and the surgical procedures used in their treatment are shown in Figures 13–20, 13–21, and 13–22.

c. Excision of heterotopic ossification—Surgical measures for treatment of this problem are discussed later in this chapter.

Figure 13–24. Proximal release of the thenar muscles to correct a thumb-in-palm deformity while preserving function of the thumb. (Illustration by Anthony C. Berlet. Reproduced, with permission, from Keenan MAE et al: *Manual of Orthopaedic Surgery for Spasticity*. Raven, 1993.)

d. Occupational therapy and social services—Before patients are released from the hospital or rehabilitation facility, both they and their families must be informed about social service agencies, support groups, and special programs that can be of help. Social adjustment and the resumption of occupational pursuits and leisure activities depend on the recovery of mental factors first, personality status second, and physical factors third. Physical factors are more responsive to rehabilitation than are mental, personality, or social factors. Mental impairment, however, interferes the most with independence in ADLs.

7. Inpatient rehabilitation—Changes in the rules governing inpatient rehabilitation hospitals and units, particularly the implementation of the new prospective payment system for inpatient rehabilitation facilities by the Centers for Medicare & Medicaid Services (CMS), complicate the admission of patients with rehabilitation goals to an inpatient setting.

Physicians generally agree on the circumstances that justify a medical or surgical patient's hospitalization. In addition, in some cases an admission to a rehabilitation hospital or to the rehabilitation service of a short-term hospital can be justified on essentially the same medical or surgical grounds. In other cases, however, a patient's medical or surgical needs alone may not warrant inpatient hospital care, but hospitalization may nevertheless be necessary because of the patient's need for rehabilitative services.

Patients needing rehabilitative services require a hospital level of care if they need a relatively intense rehabilitation program that requires a multidisciplinary coordinated team approach to upgrade their ability to function (eg, patients with traumatic brain injury or SCI after corrective extremity surgery). Two basic requirements must be met for inpatient hospital stays for rehabilitation care to be covered:

1. The services must be reasonable and necessary (in terms of efficacy, duration, frequency, and amount) for the treatment of the patient's condition; and

2. It must be reasonable and necessary to furnish the care on an inpatient hospital basis, rather than in a less intensive facility such as a skilled nursing facility (SNF), or on an outpatient basis.

To meet the requirements just cited, the following basic components must be met:

1. Close medical supervision by a physician with specialized training or experience in rehabilitation;

2. The patient requires the 24-hour availability of a registered nurse with specialized training or experience in rehabilitation;

3. The general threshold for establishing the need for inpatient hospital rehabilitation services is that the patient must require and receive at least 3 hours a day of physical and/or occupational therapy; and

4. A multidisciplinary team (usually includes at minimum a physician, rehabilitation nurse, and one therapist).

Banovac K, Sherman AL, Estores IM et al: Prevention and treatment of heterotopic ossification after spinal cord injury. J Spinal Cord Med 2004;27(4):376. [PMID: 15484668]

Botte MJ, Bruffey JD, Copp SN et al: Surgical reconstruction of acquired spastic foot and ankle deformity. Foot Ankle Clin 2000;5(2):381. [PMID: 11232236]

Dahners LE, Mullis BH: Effects of nonsteroidal anti-inflammatory drugs on bone formation and soft-tissue healing. J Am Acad Orthop Surg 2004;12(3):139. [PMID: 15161166]

Esquenazi A et al: Dynamic polyelectromyography, neurolysis, and chemodenervation with botulinum toxin A for assessment and treatment of gait dysfunction. Adv Neurol 2001;87:321. [PMID: 11347237]

Gardner MJ, Ong BC, Liporace F et al: Orthopedic issues after cerebrovascular accident. Am J Orthop 2002;31(10):559. [PMID: 12405561]

van Kuijk AA, Geurts AC, van Kuppevelt HJ: Neurogenic heterotopic ossification in spinal cord injury. Spinal Cord 2002; 40(7):313. [PMID: 12080459]

HETEROTOPIC OSSIFICATION

Heterotopic ossification is commonly detected 2 months after traumatic brain injury or SCI and is characterized by increasing pain and decreasing ROM about a joint. The problem affects adults but is virtually unheard of in children. Although the cause of heterotopic ossification is unknown, a genetic predisposition is suspected. Unidentified humoral factors that enhance osteogenesis are demonstrated in the sera of patients with brain injury. Other contributing factors include soft-tissue trauma and spasticity.

Clinical Findings

Clinically significant heterotopic ossification is seen in 20% of adults with traumatic brain injuries or spinal cord injuries and may affect one joint or multiple joints. The overall rate of joint ankylosis is 16%. In affected patients, the bone forms in association with spastic muscles, and the alkaline phosphatase level is elevated. Bone scans may aid in early diagnosis, and the diagnosis is most commonly confirmed by radiographs.

In 27% of patients with heterotopic ossification, shoulder involvement is found inferomedial to the glenohumeral joint. Although ankylosis of the joint in these cases is unusual, motion may be sufficiently restricted to require surgical resection. Elbow involvement is seen in 26% of patients with heterotopic ossification and in 89% of those who suffered a fracture or dislocation about the elbow. When ossification forms posterior to the elbow joint, pressure neuritis of the ulnar nerve is common. Anterior transposition of the ulnar nerve is frequently required to prevent entrapment, and this procedure also facilitates later bone resection. Joint ankylosis is a common complication in patients with elbow involvement. Hip involvement is seen in 44% of patients who form ectopic bone. Bilateral hip involvement and joint ankylosis are common in these patients. Heterotopic ossification in the knee joint is less common but significantly impedes both flexion and extension of the joint.

Management

A. EARLY MEASURES

Aggressive treatment of spasticity is necessary because this problem appears to play an etiologic role in mechanically stimulating bone formation. To eliminate spasticity in the muscle groups adjacent to the bone formation, phenol blocks are administered. To prevent the deposition of calcium crystals in the collagen matrix of the periarticular connective tissue, etidronate disodium (Didronel) is used. When the heterotopic bone is detected very early, the use of intravenous etidronate sodium, 300 mg for 3 days, followed by oral therapy is very effective. The recommended dosage is 20 mg/kg/day orally in a single dose, and the drug should be taken on an empty stomach for proper absorption. Antiinflammatory medications are also used to control the intense inflammatory reaction that occurs during the formation of heterotopic bone. The most commonly documented medication is indomethacin, 75–150 mg daily, but in theory, other medications are equally effective. Physical therapy is aimed at providing gentle ROM to the joint to prevent ankylosis. Forceful joint manipulation is not advised because it can cause fractures or soft-tissue damage with contracture formation.

B. Definitive Treatment

Surgical excision is the definitive treatment for heterotopic ossification. To prevent recurrence of the problem, excision should be delayed until the heterotopic bone is fully mature. A true bone cortex should be visible radiographically. The serum alkaline phosphatase level does not need to be normal. If the patient has voluntary motion about the joint, surgical excision predictably results in an increased ROM. Following surgery, a single dose of radiation therapy (800 rads) and oral etidronate therapy for 6 weeks is used to prevent recurrence. Physical therapy is continued after surgery.

Banovac K, Sherman AL, Estores IM et al: Prevention and treatment of heterotopic ossification after spinal cord injury. J Spinal Cord Med 2004;27(4):376. [PMID: 15484668]

Burd TA et al: Indomethacin compared with localized irradiation for the prevention of heterotopic ossification following surgical treatment of acetabular fractures. J Bone Joint Surg Am 2001;83-A:1783. [PMID: 11741055]

Dahners LE, Mullis BH: Effects of nonsteroidal anti-inflammatory drugs on bone formation and soft-tissue healing. J Am Acad Orthop Surg 2004;12(3):139. [PMID: 15161166]

Kaplan FS, Glaser DL, Hebela N et al: Heterotopic ossification. J Am Acad Orthop Surg 2004;12(2):116. [PMID: 15089085]

van Kuijk AA, Geurts AC, van Kuppevelt HJ: Neurogenic heterotopic ossification in spinal cord injury. Spinal Cord 2002; 40(7):313. [PMID: 12080459]

Viola RW, Hastings H II: Treatment of ectopic ossification about the elbow. Clin Orthop 2000;(370):65. [PMID: 10660703]

RHEUMATOID ARTHRITIS

Rheumatoid arthritis (RA) is a systemic disease that affects connective tissue and results in chronic inflammatory synovitis. The cause of the disease remains unknown. An infectious agent, perhaps viral, is suspected to be the initiating factor. A genetic predisposition may also be a factor.

Immune mechanisms are involved, as evidenced by the presence of large numbers of lymphocytes in the synovial tissue and by the presence of rheumatoid factor (IgM antibodies) in the serum and synovial fluid of 80% of patients. The antigen-antibody reactions activate the complement system and attract neutrophils to the joint fluid. The immune complexes are then phagocytized, and lysosomal enzymes are released into the synovial fluid. These enzymes and the inflammatory synovial pannus are in part responsible for the destruction of articular cartilage and periarticular structures. Tendons are also directly invaded by the inflammatory synovium and may attenuate and rupture. Ligaments and joint capsules become weakened by the chronic inflammatory process and may become stretched by repeated joint effusions (Figure 13–26).

The erosion of articular cartilage is greatly enhanced by the superimposition of mechanical derangements on a joint weakened by chronic inflammation and enzy-

Figure 13–26. Chronic synovitis of the joints and extensor tendons in a patient with rheumatoid arthritis.

matic deterioration. Osteoporosis results from the hyperemia of inflammation. Disuse of limbs secondary to pain, weakened muscle action, and mechanical derangements enhances the osteoporosis.

Clinical Findings

RA affects synovial joints, bones, muscles, fasciae, ligaments, and tendons. Because it is a systemic disease, it can also affect internal organs. The diagnosis is made primarily on clinical grounds and supported by radiographic and laboratory data (Table 13–5). RA is two or three times more common in women than men. The disease is seen in some children but has increasing prevalence with increasing age up to the seventh decade. Rheumatic complaints are responsible for the largest share of chronic disability in the United States.

The clinical course of RA is variable with respect to the extent and intensity of the disease. The time course of the disease, measured in months and years, is progressive. Several factors affect the course of disease and are associated with a poor prognosis. These factors include insidious onset, symmetric disease, presence of rheumatoid factor in the serum, and presence of rheumatoid nodules, which occur in patients with rheumatoid factor. In patients under 40 years of age, with RA, females have a worse prognosis than males. Eosinophilia of 5% or greater is associated with an increased incidence of vasculitis, pleuropericarditis, pulmonary fibrosis, and subcutaneous nodules.

The multisystem nature of RA and its variable clinical pattern make it difficult to devise a precise system for describing the overall functional ability of the patient. The most commonly employed scale is the functional classification devised by the American Rheumatism Association (Table 13–6).

Table 13–5. American Rheumatism Association criteria for diagnosing and categorizing rheumatoid arthritis.

Category	Description
Classic rheumatoid arthritis	Presence of 7 of the following findings: (1) morning stiffness,[a] (2) pain on motion of 1 joint[a] (3) swelling of 1 joint[a] (4) swelling of an additional joint[a] (5) symmetric swelling of joints, (6) presence of subcutaneous nodules, (7) presence of rheumatoid factor in the serum, (8) poor results in the mucin clot test of synovial fluid, (9) characteristic roentgenographic changes, (10) characteristic histopathologic findings in the synovial fluid, and (11) characteristic histopathologic findings in nodule biopsies.
Definite rheumatoid arthritis	Presence of 5 of the above findings.
Probable rheumatoid arthritis	Presence of 3 of the above findings.

[a]Finding must be present for at least 6 weeks.

Management

A. THE TEAM APPROACH TO PATIENT CARE AND TREATMENT

Optimal management requires an interdisciplinary team approach involving many specialists, including a liaison nurse, rheumatologist, orthopedic surgeon, physical therapist, occupational therapist, psychologist, and social worker. The patient and members of his or her family are also important members of the team. Because the disease is an ongoing and progressive process, the goal of management is to prevent deformities and maintain function for the patient over a lifetime.

1. Nursing care and patient education—The liaison nurse functions as the coordinator of the team. The nurse provides the critical link between the inpatient medical and surgical management of the disease and the continuation of treatment in the outpatient environment.

Much of the responsibility for patient education in the daily care of the disease rests with the nurse, who explains the techniques for protecting joints; advises patients about the need to perform exercises for maintaining joint ROM and optimizing failing muscle strength; cautions patients that exercising too vigorously can damage weakened joints and ligaments; and

reminds patients that because the disease tends to decrease their physical activity, they will need regular periods of rest during the day and good nutrition to maximize their general health and to prevent obesity.

2. Medical and surgical management—The rheumatologist is commonly the team leader and in charge of medical management, which is directed toward the control of synovitis, the relief of pain, and the prevention or treatment of other organ involvement by the disease. The medications used for treatment include aspirin, nonsteroidal antiinflammatory drugs (NSAIDs), corticosteroids, immunosuppressive drugs, and suppressive agents. A local injection of corticosteroids can be useful in controlling an acute inflammatory process in a specific joint. Corticosteroids can also be used systemically but are generally avoided because of undesirable side effects. Agents that produce suppression or remission of arthritis inclumde gold salts, antimalarial drugs, and penicillamine. Immunosuppressive drugs or total lymphoid irradiation can also be used to suppress immune reactions. The most important measure to treat RA successfully is the use of disease-modifying antirheumatic drug (DMARDs), which can retard or prevent disease progression and, thus, joint destruction and subsequent loss of function. Until the full action of DMARDs takes effect, antiinflammatory or analgesic medications may be required as bridging therapy to reduce pain and swelling. DMARDs can be classified into xenobiotic and biologic agents. Methotrexate (MTX) and sulfasalazine (SSZ) are the most active xenobiotic compounds in terms of frequency of remissions and time to onset of action and provide the best risk-benefit ratios. MTX alone or in combination with other agents is now the standard of care for moderate-to-severe RA.

Table 13–6. American Rheumatism Association classification of function in patients with rheumatoid arthritis.

Class	Description
I	Complete function; able to perform usual duties without handicap.
II	Adequate function for normal activities, despite handicap of pain or limited range of motion in one or more joints.
III	Limited function; able to perform few or none of the duties of usual occupation or self-care.
IV	Largely or wholly incapacitated; bedridden or confined to a wheelchair; able to perform little or no self-care.

The recognition of TNF-α and IL-1 as central proinflammatory cytokines led to the development of biologic agents that block these cytokines or their effects. The first such biologics were the TNF blockers etanercept and infliximab. These agents are expensive. Consensus statements do not recommend their use until at least one xenobiotic DMARD, usually MTX, was administered without sufficient success. A new addition to the biologics is anakinra (interleukin-1 receptor antagonist [IL-1RA]). IL-1RA occupies the IL-1 receptor without triggering it and prevents receptor binding of IL-1.

The orthopedic surgeon should be involved early in the course of the patient's disease and not merely be called on when medical management fails to be effective. A knowledge of biomechanics, gait dynamics, and energy requirements can be useful in preserving function for the patient. The orthopedist can often recommend orthotic supports, walking aids, and shoe wear that minimize unwanted stress on joints and maximize strength.

In selected situations, early surgical intervention may prevent excessive deterioration of joint structure and function. Synovectomy is effective in preventing tendon rupture in the hand, whereas arthroscopic synovectomy of the knee and shoulder show promise for preventing joint destruction. Fusion of an unstable cervical spine can prevent the disastrous effect of a SCI.

Most surgical procedures are reconstructive. Because relief of pain is the most consistent result of reconstructive surgery, pain is the primary indication for surgery. Restoration of motion and function and the correction of deformity are additional indications for surgical intervention but are more difficult goals to achieve. Preoperative assessment is a painstaking process. In addition to performing a physical examination and reviewing radiographic findings, the surgeon must attempt to elicit sufficient information from the patient, family, and therapists to ascertain which deformities are causing the greatest functional losses. The patient can only tolerate a finite number of surgical procedures, and these must be carefully staged to obtain the maximal result.

For further discussion of medical and surgical treatment, see the section Management Approaches Based on the Area of Disease Involvement.

3. Physical therapy—The physical therapist uses modalities such as heat and ultrasound to decrease joint stiffness and relieve pain. An exercise program is essential for preserving the functional abilities of the patient. The exercise should gently put all joints through their full arc of motion to maintain this range.

Patients with joint effusions and synovitis automatically assume positions that minimize intraarticular pressure and therefore minimize pain. These positions are usually not optimal for function and can result in flex-

ion deformities. An abnormal position may be reversible if discovered early. Daily joint ROM exercises are central to preventing unwanted contractures.

Muscles weakened by the concomitant myopathy need strengthening but are susceptible to damage from overuse or from an excessively vigorous exercise program. Orthotics may be indicated to support weakened ligaments and provide a means of joint protection and support for functional activities such as walking. Upper extremity walking aids may be useful to give the patients additional support. These aids often require modification to meet the specific needs of the individual. Forearm troughs allow the patient to use the entire arm for support when the hands and wrists are weak or deformed. They are also useful for protecting the hands from excessive stress. A rolling walker, which does not require the patient to lift the walker for advancement, may be useful in patients with limited strength.

4. Occupational therapy—The occupational therapist evaluates and instructs the patient in modified techniques for performing ADLs, such as grooming, dressing, and meal preparation. Because of the weakness and deformities imposed by the arthritis, adaptive equipment and alternative methods are commonly needed. Modifications in clothing, such as larger fasteners for ease of manipulation, Velcro strips at seams or on shoes, and front openings, can all facilitate dressing. Upper extremity splints can be used to provide joint protection and stabilization and to prevent further deformity from occurring. The splints must be lightweight and easily donned by the patient.

5. Psychological counseling—It is not uncommon for patients or their family members to have feelings of anxiety, denial, anger, or depression. The psychologist provides assistance in dealing with these feelings and coping with alterations in lifestyle and self-image. Comprehensive care involves an understanding of how patients respond to weakness, fatigue, altered physical appearance, progressive disability, diminished independence, and the financial burdens of chronic illness. Coping skills are needed to deal with these problems as well as with pain, which becomes an everyday occurrence and may interfere with both intellectual and emotional functioning.

6. Social services—A variety of modifications in lifestyle accompany chronic illness with RA. Occupational changes may be necessary, or the patient may no longer be able to work at all. Additional assistance may be needed in the home for housework and the preparation of meals. In more advanced stages, the patient may require help for personal care. Transportation needs become more complex, and the patient finds it increasingly difficult to leave the home. The social worker becomes an invaluable team member in helping families with the numerous practical arrangements required for everyday existence and for locating financial aid to help defray the mounting costs.

B. MANAGEMENT APPROACHES BASED ON THE AREA OF DISEASE INVOLVEMENT

Orthopedic surgery is frequently necessary for patients with RA affecting the cervical spine or extremities.

1. Cervical spine—Depending on the study and diagnostic criteria, involvement of the cervical spine is found in anywhere from 6.4% to 90% of patients with RA. Three forms of cervical spine involvement are seen.

The first and most common form is atlantoaxial instability (Figure 13–27), which results from erosion of the transverse and alar ligaments. These ligaments normally function to maintain the odontoid process of the axis within the anterior third of the atlas ring, where the two bones articulate with each other. Disruption of the transverse and alar ligaments results in excessive motion between C1 and C2. Forward flexion of the head causes anterior subluxation of the atlas on the axis and possible impingement of the spinal cord or occlusion of the vertebral arteries. This is best seen in lateral flexion and extension radiographs of the cervical spine.

The second form of cervical spine involvement is subaxial instability (Figure 13–28), which may lead to subluxation of two or more cervical vertebrae below the level of C2. If subluxation is severe or its appearance is sudden, it can exert sufficient pressure on the spinal cord to cause permanent quadriparesis. If subluxation occurs slowly over a long time, however, as commonly happens, the spinal cord is able to adapt to the pressure, so that a severe degree of deformity occurs before clinical symptoms appear.

Figure 13–28. Radiograph of the cervical spine, showing multiple levels of subaxial instability in a patient with rheumatoid arthritis.

The third and least common form of cervical spine involvement is superior migration of the odontoid process of C2 resulting from severe degrees of bone erosion. This form of involvement is reported in from 3.8% to 15% of patients with RA. As the dens migrates proximally, radiographic detail is lost because of the overlapping of bony structures. CT scanning is most useful in elucidating the exact nature of the involvement and can show rotational instability caused by asymmetric bone erosions (Figure 13–29).

Orthotic supports are useful in controlling the patient's symptoms. Posterior cervical fusion is indicated when the spinal cord is at risk of damage. The most common level of fusion is C1 to C2, supplemented by wire fixation. If the subluxation is irreducible or if severe osteoporosis is present, fusion to the occiput may be necessary. Occasionally, it is useful to supplement the bone graft with polymethyl methacrylate fixation.

In patients with severe erosive disease of the cervical spine and proximal migration of the odontoid

Figure 13–27. Tomogram of the upper cervical spine, showing atlantoaxial instability in a patient with rheumatoid arthritis.

Figure 13–29. CT scan showing rotational instability of C1 on C2 in a patient with advanced psoriatic arthritis.

process, a rotational deviation of the larynx may occur, making intubation impossible except with the use of a flexible fiber optic scope (Figure 13–30). Because cervical spine disease often presents difficulties in endotracheal intubation at the time of surgery, the stability of the cervical spine should be assessed preoperatively in all patients with RA. Lateral flexion-extension radiographs taken within 1 year of surgery are sufficient to detect significant instability problems. Use of the flexible fiber optic bronchoscope for such problems is valuable. Among the indications for fiber optic intubation in patients with arthritis are an unstable cervical spine on flexion and extension; limited mobility of the cervical spine; and impaired motion of the temporomandibular joints, with or without associated micrognathia.

Figure 13–30. *Left*: Diagram showing the normal relationship of the trachea and larynx. The insert shows the view seen through the fiber optic bronchoscope. *Right*: Diagram showing the triple-plane rotational deviation of the larynx noted secondary to cervical spine disease in inflammatory arthritis. (Illustrations by Ted Bloodhart. Reproduced, with permission, from Keenan MA et al: Acquired laryngeal deviation associated with cervical spine disease in erosive polyarticular arthritis. Anesthesiology 1983;58:441.)

2. Lower extremities

a. Hips—Total joint replacement has vastly improved the quality of life for patients with RA. Special problems exist in this group of patients, however, and must be considered before total hip arthroplasty is performed. Because osteoporosis is pronounced, fracture can occur easily during surgery. Protrusio acetabuli, another common problem, may require bone grafting. The risk of infection is increased in this population, and wound healing may also be delayed, especially if the patient has been taking systemic corticosteroids. In patients under the 60 years, excess femoral anteversion may be present and distort the anatomy. Moreover, the small size of the bone may require a special prosthesis. Despite these problems, total joint arthroplasty remains the treatment of choice for the arthritic hip.

b. Knees—Knee pain is common and may be the result of a valgus deformity of the hindfoot, which places excessive stress on the knee proximally. Mild medial knee pain can be relieved with the use of an AFO to correct the valgus deformity. Knee pain may also be caused by the presence of a joint effusion, which increases the intraarticular pressure and thereby increases the pain. When patients attempt to minimize pain by placing the knee in 30 degrees of flexion, this encourages the formation of flexion contractures.

Arthroscopic evaluation of the rheumatoid knee demonstrates the importance of the meniscus in the degeneration of the knee. The synovium directly invades the body of the meniscus and tears it. The mechanical derangement resulting from the torn meniscus then causes rapid deterioration of the articular surfaces, which were rendered abnormal by the action of enzymes. Synovectomy of the joint line and partial meniscectomy are easily accomplished under arthroscopic control and may have a role in preventing articular damage in the rheumatoid knee.

Total knee arthroplasty is effective in restoring knee alignment and motion and relieving pain. When a valgus deformity is present, serial releases of the soft tissue should be performed to realign the limb prior to cutting the bone for insertion of the prosthetic components. The lateral retinaculum, popliteal tendon, proximal iliotibial band, posterolateral capsule, and lateral collateral ligament can be released in this sequence to provide soft-tissue balance. A flexion deformity is corrected at the time of arthroplasty by releasing the posterior capsule from the femur or by removing additional bone from the distal femur in severe cases.

c. Feet—Forefoot involvement is common in RA. Clawtoe deformities with plantar subluxation of the metatarsal heads result in painful callosities on the plantar surface of the forefoot. These problems are usually accompanied by a hallux valgus deformity. Skin ulcerations may form over bony prominences. Forefoot pain prevents the patient from transferring body weight over the foot during terminal stance, which results in an awkward gait with a shortened step length. Extra-depth shoes with wide toe boxes and molded pressure-relieving inserts may be sufficient to relieve pain and improve gait. When the deformities are marked, resection of the metatarsal heads in conjunction with arthroplasty or fusion of the metatarsophalangeal joint of the great toe is indicated.

Hindfoot involvement is also common and results in a planovalgus or pronation deformity. A longitudinal arch support or similar shoe insert is not sufficient to hold the hindfoot in alignment. When the deformity is supple, an AFO with a well-molded arch support can control the position of the heel and subtalar joint during gait. This also reduces the valgus thrust on the knee joint. If the deformity is fixed, a triple arthrodesis aligns the hindfoot.

3. Upper extremities

a. Shoulders—In patients with RA, shoulder involvement is common but is generally insidious in onset or episodic in nature. Because the pain is not constant early in the course of the disease, shoulder involvement is often not appreciated until a significant amount of destruction occurs. The shoulders must be examined regularly to detect early loss of motion and function.

Arthroscopy provides a useful tool in examining the shoulder and assessing the integrity of the glenoid labrum, rotator cuff, and biceps tendon. Arthroscopy can also be used to perform synovectomy of the shoulder joint.

Normally, the glenohumeral joint has more motion than any other joint. This motion is rotation, and it is facilitated by the shallow shape of the glenoid labrum. The rotator cuff muscles, which are central to the normal functioning of the shoulder, provide stability to the humeral head and also provide rotation. If the rotator cuff ruptures, the humeral head rides upward and is subjected to abnormal muscle forces as the patient attempts to compensate for the loss of motion. This results in the rapid deterioration of the glenohumeral joint. Normally, the anterior portion of the deltoid muscle provides forward elevation of the humerus. This is the position of function and the most common arc of motion for activities involving the upper extremity. The tendon of the long head of the biceps muscle serves to stabilize the humeral head against riding upward and also to reduce subacromial impingement. Whenever surgery of the shoulder is performed, it is important to preserve the deltoid muscle fibers and their attachments as well as the intraarticular portion of the biceps tendon.

The subacromial bursa is often involved with the inflammatory response of RA and may become thickened. The inflammatory process may cause a decrease in nutrition of the rotator cuff tendons and lead to attrition of the tendons with or without rupture of the rotator cuff. Subacromial bursitis can be treated by local injection of a corticosteroid preparation. When the inflammation subsided, the patient is begun on a program of gentle ROM exercises.

Repair of a ruptured rotator cuff is often possible and should be performed. If the rupture is detected early, excessive damage to the glenohumeral joint can be avoided. If extensive joint damage is already present, repair or reconstruction of the rotator cuff is done at the time of prosthetic arthroplasty of the glenohumeral joint. Preoperative radiographic evaluation should include axillary radiographs to assess the glenoid alignment. The glenoid labrum is often eroded asymmetrically, and the prosthetic component must be accurately aligned to ensure optimal function and to minimize the abnormal forces that might lead to prosthetic loosening. In patients with total shoulder replacement, pain is effectively alleviated. Shoulder function depends on the integrity of the soft tissues and on muscle function. Resurfacing of the glenoid should be reserved for those patients with an intact rotator cuff. If the rotator cuff is destroyed, humeral hemiarthroplasty is the preferred surgical treatment. A careful postoperative therapy program is essential for maximizing shoulder function.

b. Elbows—The elbow joint consists of three separate articulations: radiocapitellar, ulnotrochlear, and radioulnar. These articulations allow the hand to rotate 180 degrees around the longitudinal axis of the forearm. The function of the hand depends on being placed in space as necessary for use. The elbow is the most important joint for positioning the hand. Unlike the shoulder or wrist, if the elbow is fused, the functional loss is great. The goal of treatment is to maintain a painless arc of motion.

Olecranon bursitis is common in patients with RA. The usual treatment consists of aspirating the bursa and injecting a corticosteroid preparation. Rarely, chronic bursitis develops and requires surgical excision of the bursa.

Subcutaneous rheumatoid nodules are common along the extensor surface of the ulna. The nodules are often sensitive to pressure when the arm is resting on any surface, and they may interfere with the use of forearm troughs on walking aids. If they are bothersome, the nodules should be excised surgically. The patient should be advised, however, that nodules can recur.

Radiocapitellar arthritis is often the predominant feature of elbow involvement and can cause marked pain and a decrease in motion. The pain is most pronounced with pronation and supination of the forearm.

When the joint destruction is severe, prosthetic arthroplasty is indicated. Elbow prostheses fall into two basic categories: semiconstrained and unconstrained. An unconstrained design is less likely to loosen. The shoulder should be evaluated carefully prior to prosthetic elbow arthroplasty. A patient with limited shoulder motion exerts greater forces on the elbow in an effort to compensate for the decrease in shoulder function.

c. Wrists and hands—In patients with RA, evaluating the wrist and hand deformities and developing a

rational treatment plan can be a complex task for the surgeon. Many joints, tendons, and ligaments are involved in a linked system of structure and function. Treatment can be divided into three categories: nonsurgical treatment, preventive surgery, and reconstructive or salvage surgery. Nonoperative treatment consists of resting inflamed joints; exercising joints for short periods of time but frequently and gently to maintain motion; using resting or dynamic splints to alleviate pain and prevent deformity; and judiciously using local corticosteroid injections for control of synovitis.

(1) Tendons—Dorsal tenosynovitis is common. It is of significance because it often results in rupture of the extensor tendons either from attrition or from direct invasion of the inflamed synovial tissue into the tendon substance. Tenosynovectomy should be performed in patients whose synovitis has persisted for 4–6 months despite medical treatment. Recurrence of the synovitis is rare following synovectomy, and the procedure prevents extensor tendon rupture.

Rupture of an extensor tendon can result from attenuation of the tendon caused by chronic inflammation, friction against abnormal bony surfaces, ischemia secondary to interference with the normal circulation to the tendon, or direct invasion of the tendon by synovium. The most common tendons to rupture, listed in order of frequency, are the extensors of the fifth finger, the extensors of the ring finger, and the long extensor of the thumb (the extensor pollicis longus). Surgical repair by tendon transfer is more successful when fewer tendons are involved. Therefore, prompt diagnosis and treatment are essential for a successful outcome. For a single tendon rupture in the fifth and ring fingers, a side-to-side repair using the adjacent extensor tendon is advised. The tendon of the index finger extensor can be transferred to repair a rupture of the thumb extensor tendon or a rupture of two finger tendons. For more complex ruptures, tendon transfer from the wrist extensors or from the superficial flexor muscles of the fingers may restore function.

Synovitis in the flexor tendon sheaths is characterized by crepitation that is palpable in the palm during finger flexion and extension. Triggering of the fingers may result from the inflamed synovial tissue catching on the flexor pulleys with motion. Carpal tunnel syndrome may also occur as a result of swelling within the carpal canal, which causes pressure on the median nerve. Early treatment consists of local corticosteroid injection to reduce the inflammation, application of a splint, and medical management of the underlying synovitis. Persistent synovitis may require carpal tunnel release and synovectomy. Rupture of the flexor tendons is rare.

(2) Wrist joints—The wrist joint is a frequent site of synovitis and may begin to show radial deviation and volar subluxation. The radioulnar joint is commonly inflamed and painful. Early treatment consists of splinting for support and medical control of the synovitis. Dorsal synovectomy of the extensor compartments is indicated when medications do not control the synovitis adequately. Dorsal synovectomy prevents rupture of the extensor tendons. Radial deviation of the carpus can be corrected by transfer of the extensor carpi radialis longus tendon to the extensor carpi ulnaris.

When the wrist becomes unstable, several choices of surgical treatment are available. If the deformity is mild, bone stock can be preserved and motion maintained by a limited carpal fusion. The lunate and scaphoid bones are fused to the distal radius to prevent further displacement of the carpus. The distal ulna can be fused to the distal radius to provide a platform to support the wrist. A segment of the ulna is removed just proximal to the fusion to allow for pronation and supination of the forearm. If the intercarpal joints are severely affected by the arthritis, the base of the capitate bone can be removed and a tendon spacer inserted to preserve motion at the intercarpal row.

Another option is to perform a prosthetic arthroplasty of the wrist. More bone stock is removed with this procedure, but revision is still possible in the event of fracture of the prosthesis. Several designs of total joint prosthesis are available for the wrist.

Fusion of the wrist joint provides a stable pain-free joint and remains a reasonable surgical choice for selected patients. Because fusion may interfere with personal hygiene tasks, it is advisable to avoid fusing both wrist joints.

(3) Metacarpophalangeal and carpometacarpal joints—Finger and wrist deformities commonly occur together in a collapsing zigzag pattern. The wrist deviates in a radial direction, and the fingers then drift ulnarward at the metacarpophalangeal joint level. When both deformities are present, the wrist must be realigned prior to correcting the finger deformities, or the ulnar deviation of the fingers recurs.

Ulnar deviation and volar subluxation of the fingers at the metacarpophalangeal joint level are common. With ulnar deviation, the extensor tendons move into the valleys between the metacarpal heads. This condition can be confused with extensor tendon rupture. If the joint surfaces are preserved, function can be improved by a synovectomy, soft-tissue release of the volar capsule, and realignment of the extensor tendons. If the joint surfaces are destroyed, then a total wrist arthroplasty can be considered. If the joints are unstable because of ligament loss, it may be necessary to reconstruct the radial collateral ligament using a portion of the volar plate to provide a stable pinch. Tightness of the intrinsic tendons commonly occurs in conjunction with the subluxation of the metacarpophalangeal joints. To correct this problem, a release of the intrinsic tendons is performed along with the arthroplasty. Dynamic splinting of the fingers, which maintains alignment while allowing motion, is used continuously for 6 weeks following surgery and then for an additional 6 weeks at night.

Flexion of the metacarpophalangeal joint with extension of the interphalangeal joint in the thumb is the equivalent of a boutonnière deformity. The reverse deformity can also be seen, with extension of the metacarpophalangeal joint and flexion of the interphalangeal joint. An adduction deformity of the metacarpal bone places increased stress on the metacarpophalangeal joint and produces lateral instability and hyperextension. Adduction of the thumb occurs when the carpometacarpal joint shifts radially. Derangements of the carpometacarpal joint can be treated by fusion or by arthroplasty. Interposition arthroplasty is desirable to maintain motion and can be performed using a Silastic spacer or soft tissue.

(4) Interphalangeal joints—Continued synovitis gradually attenuates the capsular and ligamentous structures and results in tendon imbalance. In the fingers, this will be seen as either a flexion or an extension deformity.

Flexion deformity results from rupture or attenuation of the central slip of the extensor mechanism, with gradual volar displacement of the lateral bands. As the lateral bands shift in the volar direction, a hyperextension deformity of the distal interphalangeal joint results. This flexion malalignment, called a **boutonnière,** or **buttonhole, deformity,** interferes with the ability to grasp large objects but does not usually impede the pinch function used for picking up small items. Interposition arthroplasty using a Silastic spacer gives unpredictable results. Fusion of the interphalangeal joints gives dependable results when the boutonnière deformity is fixed. In the index and long fingers, stability for pinch is required for good function and is more important than a large arc of motion. In the ring and small fingers, motion is more important for a functional grasp. When arthroplasty is considered, the ring and fifth fingers are usually selected.

Hyperextension deformities, or swan-neck deformities, can be either primary or secondary. Primary deformities are caused by stretching of the volar plate from synovitis or rupture of the flexor digitorum superficialis tendon. Secondary deformities are characterized by flexion of the metacarpophalangeal joints, with tightness of the intrinsic muscles proximally and presence of a mallet deformity distally. This hyperextension deformity interferes with picking up small objects but does not cause much difficulty with grasping larger objects. If the deformity is treated early and is secondary to intrinsic muscle tightness, a release of the intrinsic tendons corrects the imbalance. If the deformity is seen late and is rigid, joint fusion or arthroplasty is indicated.

Derangements of the distal interphalangeal joints are either mallet deformities secondary to rupture of the extensor tendon or lateral deformities from loss of capsular and ligamentous support. When the deformities interfere with function, fusion of the joint is indicated.

Abboud JA, Beredjiklian PK, Bozentka DJ: Metacarpophalangeal joint arthroplasty in rheumatoid arthritis. J Am Acad Orthop Surg 2003;11(3):184. [PMID: 12828448]

Belt EA et al: Outcome of ankle arthrodesis performed by dowel technique in patients with rheumatic disease. Foot Ankle Int 2001;22:666.

Berger RA et al: Long-term follow-up of the Miller-Galante total knee replacement. Clin Orthop 2001;388:56. [PMID: 11451133]

Chen AL, Joseph TN, Zuckerman JD: Rheumatoid arthritis of the shoulder. J Am Acad Orthop Surg 2003;11(1):12. [PMID: 12699368]

Dionne RA et al: Analgesia and COX-2 inhibition. Clin Exp Rheumatol 2001;19:S63. [PMID: 11695255]

Gordon P et al: A 10-year prospective followup of patients with rheumatoid arthritis 1986–96. J Rheumatol 2001;28:2409. [PMID: 11708411]

Johnstone BR: Proximal interphalangeal joint surface replacement arthroplasty. Hand Surg 2001;6:1. [PMID: 11677661]

Kauffman JI, Chen AL, Stuchin S et al: Surgical management of the rheumatoid elbow. J Am Acad Orthop Surg 2003;11(2):100. [PMID: 12670136]

King JA, Tomaino MM: Surgical treatment of the rheumatoid thumb. Hand Clin 2001;17:275. [PMID: 11478050]

Nelissen RG: The impact of total joint replacement in rheumatoid arthritis. Best Pract Res Clin Rheumatol 2003;17(5):831. [PMID: 12915160]

Shen FH, Samartzis D, Jenis LG et al: Rheumatoid arthritis: Evaluation and surgical management of the cervical spine. Spine J 2004;4(6):689. [PMID: 15541704]

POLIOMYELITIS

Poliomyelitis is caused by an enterovirus that attacks the anterior horn cells of the spinal cord. Infection can lead to a variety of clinical findings, ranging from minor symptoms to paralysis. The last major epidemics in the United States occurred during the early 1950s. Because of effective immunization programs, acute poliomyelitis has now become rare in the United States and other developed nations of the world. Nevertheless, orthopedic surgeons today are frequently called on to treat patients with postpoliomyelitis syndrome.

Classification

Four stages of poliomyelitis are recognized.

A. ACUTE POLIOMYELITIS

All of the anterior horn cells are attacked during the acute stage, which accounts for the diffuse and severe paralysis seen with the initial infection. The anterior horn cells control the skeletal muscle cells of the trunk and limbs.

Clinically, the infection is characterized by the sudden onset of paralysis and the presence of fever and acute muscle pain, often accompanied by stiff neck. Paralysis of the respiratory muscles is life-threatening in the acute stage. When the shoulder muscles are involved, respiratory compromise should be suspected because of the close proximity of the anterior horn cells controlling each in the spinal cord. Mechanical support of ventilation may be required.

A variable number of anterior horn cells survive the initial infection. The treatment in the acute stage of the disease consists of providing the needed respiratory support, decreasing muscle pain, and performing regular ROM exercises to prevent the formation of joint contractures.

B. SUBACUTE POLIOMYELITIS

Anterior horn cell survival, axon sprouting, and muscle hypertrophy occur in the subacute phase and provide three mechanisms for regaining strength. An average of 47% (range of 12–94%) of the anterior horn cells in the spinal cord survive the initial attack. Because cell survival occurs in a random fashion, the distribution of paralysis is variable and depends on which anterior horn cells were destroyed. Each anterior horn cell innervates a group of muscle cells. When a group of muscle cells is orphaned, as it were, by the death of the anterior horn cell that supports it, a nearby nerve cell can sprout additional axons and adopt some of the orphaned cells. By means of this process, a motor unit (defined as a nerve cell and the muscle cells it innervates) can expand greatly. Moreover, muscle cells in the unit enlarge, and this hypertrophy provides additional strength for the patient.

C. RESIDUAL POLIOMYELITIS

It is only after 16–24 months following onset that the ultimate extent of poliomyelitis can be determined and procedures to restore lost function and provide structural stability can be instituted.

D. POSTPOLIOMYELITIS SYNDROME

Patients who had acute poliomyelitis during childhood often complain of increased muscle weakness 30–40 years later. This weakness is not a result of infectious spread of the earlier disease but, rather, is caused by the overuse of muscles that were originally affected, whether or not they were known to have been affected at the onset of the disease. Studies show that a muscle must lose from 30% to 40% of its strength for weakness to be detected using manual muscle testing. Studies of gait also demonstrate that the ADLs require more muscle strength and stamina than were previously appreciated. The traditional program, which encouraged patients to work harder to regain strength and was based on the concept of "no pain, no gain," proved detrimental because it encouraged chronic overuse of muscles and resulted in further deterioration of function.

The diagnosis of postpoliomyelitis syndrome is based on a history of poliomyelitis; a pattern of increased muscle weakness that is random and does not follow any nerve root or peripheral nerve distribution; and the presence of additional symptoms such as muscle pain, severe fatigue, muscle cramping or fasciculations, joint pain or instability, sleep apnea, intolerance to cold, and depression. No pathognomonic tests for the syndrome are currently available. Electromyography can demonstrate the presence of large motor units resulting from the previous axon sprouting. This finding is supportive but not diagnostic of poliomyelitis.

Management

A. Acute Poliomyelitis

When the shoulder muscles are involved, respiratory compromise should be suspected, and mechanical support of ventilation should be instituted. Other measures are aimed at decreasing muscle pain and preventing complications. Regular ROM exercises prevent the formation of joint contractures.

B. Subacute Poliomyelitis

During the subacute stage, which may last as long as 24 months, the emphasis is on preventing deformities and preserving function. Splints and braces are often helpful for maintaining joint position and supplementing function.

C. Residual Poliomyelitis

Patients with compromised function of the diaphragm can be taught glossopharyngeal breathing. This method, in which air is swallowed into the lungs, provides sufficient air exchange for the patient to perform light activities in the sitting position. Mechanical support of ventilation may still need to be continued while the patient sleeps. It is during the residual stage that orthopedic surgery is commonly performed to restore lost function and provide structural stability. If the patient is still growing, it is important to prevent the formation of skeletal deformities that result from muscle imbalance. Before any surgery that requires general anesthesia or significant sedation is performed, the vital capacity should be assessed to determine the patient's need for respiratory support.

D. Postpoliomyelitis Syndrome

Treatment is directed at preserving current muscle strength and preventing further weakness from occurring. Generally, strength cannot be restored in a muscle that was weakened by poliomyelitis. Some gain in strength can be seen, however, when chronic overuse is corrected.

General management strategies consist of modifying lifestyle to prevent chronic overuse of weak muscles; instituting a limited exercise program that incorporates frequent rest periods to prevent disuse atrophy and weakness; providing lightweight orthotic support of the limbs to protect joints and substitute for muscle function; and performing orthopedic surgery to correct limb or trunk deformities.

Specific management strategies depend on the areas of disease involvement.

1. Spine—Back pain is a common complaint and usually results from postural strain caused by excessive lumbar extension in patients who have weak or paralyzed hip extensor muscles. Neck pain, like back pain, is a common complaint associated with slowly increasing weakness. Both complaints can be treated by the use of external supports. Patient education is imperative because many patients are reluctant to don braces again, after having passed decades without using them. Patients should be instructed in methods to relieve excess strain on the neck muscles and prevent further deterioration. Tilting the seat of a chair 10 degrees backward is often sufficient to relieve the fatigue of the posterior cervical muscles from supporting the head.

Paralysis of the cervical spine musculature can result in the inability to maintain the head erect and can interfere with the performance of a vast number of functions, including ambulation. Surgical fusion of the cervical spine corrects the problem.

Scoliosis is common in patients with muscle imbalance caused by paralysis. The condition is particularly pronounced in patients with leg-length discrepancies. External supports can be used to hold the spine in position, but these often interfere with respiration if the patient depends on the use of accessory muscles for breathing. Posterior spinal fusion may be needed to control the spine adequately. After fusion is performed, prolonged immobilization must be avoided. Segmental spine fixation may be helpful.

2. Lower extremities—Full ROM of the hip and knee joints is needed for function. Contractures should be corrected when possible to permit more effective bracing. In iliotibial band contractures, which are common deformities, the hip assumes a position of flexion, external rotation, and abduction; the knee assumes a valgus alignment; and the tibia is externally rotated on the femur. Release or lengthening of the iliotibial band corrects the deformity.

A patient with flailing lower extremities can stand using crutches and a KAFO with the knees locked in extension and the ankles in slight dorsiflexion by hyperextending the hips and using the strong anterior hip capsule for support. Flexion contractures of the hips or knees prevent this alignment. If trunk support and upper extremity strength are adequate, the patient could ambulate with a swing-through gait for short distances. This gait has high energy demands. With time, the posterior knee joint capsule becomes stretched, and the knee develops a recurvatum deformity that is painful and can lead to arthritic degeneration of the knee. A KAFO protects the knee and provides improved stability for walking. If there is fair (grade 3) strength in the hip flexor muscles (see Table 13–1) and passive full-knee extension, then the knee joints can be left unlocked for walking. In this case, a posteriorly offset knee joint is used to stabilize the knee, and ankle dorsiflexion is limited to minus 3 degrees of neutral dorsiflexion to provide a hyperextension moment to the knee for stability. Thus, at stance phase, the net ankle plantarflexion locks the knee in hyperextension, restrained by posterior capsular static structures.

Quadriceps muscle strength is not essential for ambulation. A strong gluteus maximus and good calf strength can substitute by keeping the knee locked in extension. If the calf strength is inadequate to control the forward motion of the tibia in mid to late stance, an AFO is needed. It is not necessary to fix the ankle in mild plantarflexion to provide knee stability, and such a position could cause a recurvatum deformity in any case. An equinus position of the foot inhibits forward momentum and limits step length by preventing body weight from rolling over the forefoot prior to contact of the contralateral extremity with the ground. When good hamstring function is present, the biceps femoris and the semitendinosus can be transferred anteriorly to the quadriceps tendon to provide dynamic knee stability.

Muscle imbalances in the foot can lead to deformity. When muscle imbalances exist, tendon releases or transfers should be considered prior to the development of fixed deformities.

Equinus contracture of the ankle is a common problem and results in genu recurvatum. Accommodating the equinus posture by using an elevated heel places excessive stress on the calf muscles to control the leg. A surgical procedure to lengthen the Achilles tendon is frequently needed to correct the equinus contracture of the ankle and to permit adequate bracing.

A cavus foot deformity causes forefoot equinus, which also limits bracing. If no fixed bony abnormalities are present, then release of the plantar fascia is sufficient to correct the deformity. If the cavus deformity is caused by bony abnormalities, then a closing wedge osteotomy is needed. A triple arthrodesis of the hindfoot can also be used to correct deformities and provide a stable base of support.

The long-standing muscle imbalances, patterns of muscle substitution, and resulting joint and ligament strains often lead to degenerative arthritis. Total joint replacement can be performed, but several special considerations are needed. In patients with postpoliomyelitis syndrome, osteoporosis is common because of prolonged lack of muscle action on the bone. Joint contractures

must be corrected at the time of surgery to prevent excessive forces on the prosthetic components because these forces might lead to loosening of the prosthesis. Weak muscles must be supported with the appropriate orthoses after surgery. The rehabilitation program is lengthy because it takes an extended period to regain joint motion and muscle function. Continuous passive motion devices and frequent joint ROM must be used to gain joint mobility after surgery. Because the hip joint is difficult to brace, there must be at least fair (grade 3) strength (see Table 13–1) in the hip extensors, abductors, and flexors to provide stability to the hip after surgery. Surgery can be expected to weaken the surrounding muscles, which must be taken into account before total hip arthroplasty is undertaken to prevent chronic dislocation.

3. Upper extremities

a. Shoulders—The shoulder is important for placing the hand in the desired position for use. The shoulder totally depends on muscle strength for active mobility. In patients who use a wheelchair, weak muscles about the shoulder can be made more functional with the use of mobile arm supports on the wheelchair. These supports allow the patient a greater arc of motion with less muscle strength. Shoulder stability is more important in the ambulatory patient who requires upper extremity aids. A glenohumeral fusion may be helpful if the patient has sufficient strength in the scapulothoracic muscles. When the shoulder is fused, scapulothoracic motion is maintained, allowing use of the extremity for tabletop activities. Glenohumeral fusion does restrict the ability of the patient to position the hand for bathroom hygiene, so it is undesirable to perform the procedure on both shoulders.

Preservation of shoulder strength should be a priority of treatment. Rotator cuff tears are a common problem in postpolio patients. Surgical repair of the torn rotator cuff should be done when possible. In large tears that cannot be repaired, arthroscopic debridement offers significant relief of pain. Shoulder weakness is found in 95% of patients with postpoliomyelitis syndrome and correlates closely with the amount of lower extremity weakness present. Patients with weak legs use their arms to push up from a chair and pull themselves up stairs. They also lean heavily on upper extremity aids while walking. It is therefore important to remove as many unnecessary strains from the shoulders as possible with the use of elevated seats, motorized lift chairs, elevators or motorized stair chair glides, and optimal lower extremity bracing. In minimally ambulatory or nonambulatory patients, an electric wheelchair or motorized scooter should be prescribed to prevent excessive strain on the shoulder muscles caused by propelling a manual wheelchair.

b. Elbows—The elbow requires sufficient flexor strength to lift an object against gravity for function. A mobile arm support can maximize the effectiveness of the muscle strength for the patient. Tendon transfers, such as those involving the deltoid and biceps muscles, may also be useful in restoring active flexion.

c. Wrists and hands—Opponens paralysis is common in the hand and results in a 50% loss of hand function. A splint used during the acute and recovery phases is useful in preventing an adduction contracture. Opponens function can be restored by tendon transfer. The most common muscle transferred is the flexor digitorum superficialis of the ring finger.

Paralysis of the intrinsic muscles of the hand interferes with function. A lumbrical bar orthosis prevents hyperextension of the metacarpophalangeal joints and allows the long extensors to extend the fingers and open the hand. Surgical capsulodesis to limit metacarpophalangeal joint extension accomplishes the same result.

Paralysis of the finger flexors and extensors can be overcome with the use of a flexor hinge orthosis if wrist extensor function is present. Tendon transfers can provide the same result, allowing the tenodesis effect to provide grasp and pinch functions.

Bruno RL: Paralytic vs. "nonparalytic" polio: Distinction without a difference? Am J Phys Med Rehabil 2000;79(1):4. [PMID: 10678596]

Chasens ER, Umlauf MG: Post-polio syndrome. Am J Nurs 2000;100(12):60. [PMID: 11202787]

Dhillon MS, Sandhu HS: Surgical options in the management of residual foot problems in poliomyelitis. Foot Ankle Clin 2000;5(2):327. [PMID: 11232234]

Gandevia SC, Allen GM, Middleton J: Post-polio syndrome: Assessments, pathophysiology and progression. Disabil Rehabil 2000;22(1-2):38. [PMID: 10661756]

Giori NJ, Lewallen DG: Total knee arthroplasty in limbs affected by poliomyelitis. J Bone Joint Surg Am 2002; 84-A(7):1157. [PMID: 12107315]

Klein MG et al: Changes in strength over time among polio survivors. Arch Phys Med Rehabil 2000;81:1059. [PMID: 10943755]

Klein MG et al: The relationship between lower extremity strength and shoulder overuse symptoms: A model based on polio survivors. Arch Phys Med Rehabil 2000;81:789. [PMID: 10857526]

Sunnerhagen KS, Grimby G: Muscular effects in late polio. Acta Physiol Scand 2001;171(3):335. [PMID: 11412146]

CEREBRAL PALSY
(Static Encephalopathy)

Cerebral palsy is a nonprogressive and nonhereditary disorder of impaired motor function. The onset may be prenatal, perinatal, or postnatal. An exact cause is not always known, but the impairment is sometimes associated with prematurity, perinatal hypoxia, cerebral trauma, or neonatal jaundice. In the United States, more than 500,000 people are affected by cerebral palsy. The degree of neurologic impairment is severe in a third of patients and mild in approximately a sixth.

Classification

Because of the diversity of neurologic findings seen in patients with cerebral palsy, a classification system is essential. The disease can be classified by the types of movement disorder and by the patterns of neurologic deficit.

A. TYPES OF MOVEMENT DISORDER

Three types of disorder are seen.

1. Spastic disorders—These are characterized by the presence of clonus and hyperactive deep tendon reflexes. Patients with spastic movement can be helped by orthopedic intervention.

2. Dyskinetic disorders—Among the conditions classified as dyskinetic disorders are athetosis, ballismus, chorea, dystonia, and ataxia. For practical purposes, these conditions are grouped together because they are not amenable to surgical correction.

3. Mixed disorders—These usually consist of a combination of spasticity and athetosis with total body involvmement.

B. PATTERNS OF NEUROLOGIC INVOLVEMENT

1. Monoplegia—With single-limb involvement, the disorder is usually spastic in nature. Because monoplegia is rare, it is advisable to test the patient before making the diagnosis. The stress of performing an activity such as running at a fast pace often uncovers spasticity in another limb.

2. Hemiplegia—Spasticity affects the upper and lower extremities ipsilaterally. Equinovarus posturing is common in the lower extremity. The upper extremity is usually held with the elbow, wrist, and fingers flexed and the thumb adducted. The major problem interfering with upper extremity function, however, is a loss of proprioception and stereognosis. Surgery for the upper extremity is aimed at making the hand assistive and at improving cosmesis. An arm that is involuntarily held in severe flexion while the patient walks can present a major social disadvantage for the patient.

3. Paraplegia—In paraplegia, neurologic deficits involve only the lower extremities. Because paraplegia is rare in patients with spastic cerebral palsy, the existence of a high spinal cord lesion that could also be responsible for the neurologic findings must be ruled out. Bladder problems coexist with spastic paralysis that affects the lower extremities and is secondary to spinal cord damage.

4. Diplegia—Spastic diplegia, seen in 50–60% of cerebral palsy patients in the United States, is the most common neurologic pattern. It is characterized by major involvement in both lower extremities with only minor incoordination in the upper extremities. Findings in the lower extremities include marked spasticity, particularly about the hips, hyperactive deep tendon reflexes, and a positive Babinski sign. The hips are commonly held in a position of flexion, adduction, and internal rotation secondary to the spasticity. The knees are in the valgus position and may have excessive external rotation of the tibia. The ankles are held in the equinus position, with a valgus attitude of the feet. Speech and intellectual functions are usually normal or only slightly impaired. Esotropia and visual perception problems are common.

5. Total body involvement—Sometimes referred to as quadriplegia, total body involvement is characterized by impairments affecting all four extremities, the head, and the trunk. Sensory deficits are typical, and speech and swallowing are commonly impaired. The most serious deficit is often the inability to communicate with others. Although mental retardation is found in approximately 45% of patients, intelligence is often masked by communication dysfunction. Ambulation is not usually a goal because the equilibrium reactions of affected patients are severely impaired or absent. Sitting may require braces or adaptive supportive devices. Scoliosis, contractures, and dislocated hips are common orthopedic problems and may interfere with sitting.

Management

Because cerebral palsy in children is discussed elsewhere (see Chapter 11), the following discussion concentrates on the needs of the adult with cerebral palsy.

A. Special Considerations in Adult Patients

1. Musculoskeletal problems—Long-standing deformities may be rigid. Bony deformities are common and may preclude surgery for soft-tissue rebalancing unless concomitant osteotomies are done. In comparison with the young patient, the adult patient has a greater body mass to support and therefore has increased energy demands. Spastic muscles are weak and frequently further compromised by the chronic overuse of muscles to compensate for contractural deformities.

2. Mobility—The patient who can sit independently has good balance and may propel a wheelchair. It may be easier to propel the wheelchair backward, using the feet to push. A self-propped sitter may require some external support to remain erect, whereas a propped sitter needs a straight spine and flexible hips to remain erect with support.

Ambulation can be divided into four categories: community ambulation, household ambulation, physiologic ambulation (exercise), and wheelchair ambulation. A patient categorized as a community ambulator is able to maneuver independently and safely around obstacles normally encountered in the community. Orthotics or upper extremity walking aids may be required. A household ambulator is able to walk independently for short distances but requires assistance to negotiate obstacles such as stairs or curbs and requires a wheelchair for long distances. A physiologic ambulator is someone who is capable of walking for short distances with assistance or walks as a means of exercise but finds it impractical to walk for normal activities. The energy requirements for walking determine the category to which a patient belongs and also determine the types of equipment that are recommended. It is unreasonable to expect patients to expend all their energy in merely transporting themselves from one location to another.

B. Treatment of Patients with Lower Extremity Problems

1. Hips—An adduction and internal rotation deformity of the hip is sometimes seen during ambulation. Release of the hip adductor tendons (see Figure 13–13) may be needed to correct this tendency.

A crouch gait and lumbar lordosis are evidence of hip flexion deformity. In patients with cerebral palsy, gait studies with dynamic poly-EMG demonstrated dysphasic activity of the iliopsoas, which is the main hip flexor muscle. Gait studies with poly-EMG should be undertaken to evaluate the activity of the iliopsoas and pectineus and to aid in surgical decision making. If release of the iliopsoas is indicated, the tendon is cut distally and allowed to retract proximally to the point where it reattaches to the anterior hip capsule (Figure 13–31). Release of the pectineus muscle is often also necessary.

Figure 13–31. Release of the iliopsoas tendon from its insertion on the lesser trochanter of the femur to correct a hip flexion deformity. (Illustration by Anthony C. Berlet. Reproduced, with permission, from Keenan MAE et al: *Manual of Orthopaedic Surgery for Spasticity.* Raven, 1993.)

2. Knees—Correction of a knee flexion deformity in a patient with a crouch gait may be necessary. Attention should first be paid to the hip deformity. Weakness of the gastrocnemius and soleus muscles and inability to maintain the position of the tibia may also contribute to a crouch posture and should be considered prior to performing any knee surgery. Gait electromyograms are useful in determining which muscles are responsible for the abnormal posture. Release of the offending hamstring tendons (see Figure 13–15) or hamstring lengthening may be useful.

3. Feet—Equinus posturing of the ankle is common. If no fixed contracture is present, an AFO controls the position of the foot. If the deformity is the result of an equinus contracture, Achilles tendon lengthening (see Figure 13–16) should be performed to bring the foot to a neutral position. The foot should be held in a short leg walking cast for 6 weeks following surgery. An AFO is then used to maintain the position of the foot and support the tibia during walking.

Equinovarus posturing of the ankle is also common. Although the anterior tibial muscle is the primary varus force in patients with stroke or traumatic brain injuries, it is equally likely that the posterior tibial muscle may be causing equinovarus posturing in patients with cerebral palsy. Therefore, in order to find the cause and make the correct decision concerning surgery, it is important to make dynamic EMG recordings while the patient walks.

If the anterior tibial muscle is overactive, Achilles tendon lengthening should be accompanied by a split anterior tibial tendon transfer (see Figure 13–18). If the posterior tibial muscle is overactive, it is advisable to lengthen the posterior tendon. If the EMG studies show that the posterior tibial muscle is active only during the swing phase of gait, it may be more logical to transfer the posterior tendon through the interosseous membrane to the dorsum of the foot, rather than performing a split anterior tibial tendon transfer. After surgery is performed, a short leg cast that allows weight bearing is worn for 6 weeks, and the leg is then supported with an AFO. If hallux valgus subsequently develops, management consists of correcting the subtalar deformity and realigning the first digital ray.

A pes cavus deformity of the foot is occasionally seen in patients with spasticity of the intrinsic muscles. If the problem is detected early, it can be corrected by plantar fasciotomy and release of the flexor origins from the os calcis. If the problem is detected late and a concomitant bony deformity is present, a wedge osteotomy of the midtarsal bones should be performed.

C. Treatment of Patients with Upper Extremity Problems

Function of the upper extremities depends on a variety of factors, including cognition, intact sensation, and the ability to place the hand in space. The amount of spasticity present also affects the ability to control movement of the arm and hand. Surgery can influence hand placement and modify spasticity, but a successful outcome requires the ability to cooperate with postoperative therapy programs. Mental impairment, motion disorders, and poor sensation are relative contraindications to surgery in the functional arm and hand.

1. The functional upper extremity—In patients with problems involving the functional hand, treatment begins with careful clinical evaluation of motor and sensory deficits. Dynamic EMG is extremely useful in determining which muscles should be lengthened or transferred to improve function. The least severely involved hands exhibit a minor degree of spasticity in the flexor carpi ulnaris and a resulting mild flexion deformity of the wrist. In this case, all that is required to improve hand function and position is surgical lengthening of the flexor carpi ulnaris tendon.

In some patients, release of objects from the hand is a problem. In this case, the synergistic action of the finger extensors and wrist flexors causes difficulty with finger extension when the wrist is extended. This resembles the tenodesis effect seen in paralytic hands, but the mechanism is a dynamic one. Selective lengthening of the overactive finger flexors (see Figure 13–23) improves hand function.

Transfer of a wrist flexor to a wrist extensor should be done with caution. Often a patient flexes the wrist to adjust the dynamic balance between the finger flexors and extensors. Holding the wrist in extension can rob the patient of this important method of compensation.

The thumb-in-palm deformity is treated by proximal release of the thenar muscles (see Figure 13–24) and lengthening of the flexor pollicis longus tendon. Distal release of the thenar muscles is not recommended because it may cause a hyperextension deformity of the metacarpophalangeal joint of the thumb.

2. The nonfunctional upper extremity—Surgery may be indicated in the nonfunctional upper extremity to prevent skin breakdown, to improve hygiene or cosmesis, or to make dressing easier. The problems of shoulder contracture and elbow contracture are discussed in the section on stroke, and the surgical procedures used in their treatment are shown in Figures 13–20 and 13–21. Patients who have a flexed wrist with flexed fingers and a thumb-in-palm deformity should be treated because severe wrist flexion can cause median nerve compression against the proximal edge of the transverse carpal ligament. An arthrodesis of the wrist in neutral position, combined with a superficialis-to-profundus tendon transfer (see Figure 13–22), reliably corrects the wrist deformity and also improves skin care. Management of the thumb deformity consists of lengthening the flexor pollicis longus tendon, fusing the interphalangeal joint, and performing a proximal release of the thenar muscles (see Figure 13–24).

D. TREATMENT OF PATIENTS WITH TOTAL BODY INVOLVEMENT

Patients with total body involvement are rarely functional ambulators, although they may transfer from one position to another either independently or with assistance. They frequently have a combination of spasticity and motion disorders such as athetosis, and they spend most of their time in a chair. Flexible hips and a straight spine are needed for functional sitting.

Occasionally, knee flexion deformities require distal hamstring release or lengthening to allow for greater flexibility in positioning the patient. Rigid extension contractures of the knee are sometimes seen and interfere with sitting tolerance. Lengthening of the quadriceps tendon (Figure 13–32) allows the knee to flex.

Foot deformities in the spastic patient are extremely common and require treatment to allow shoe wear and to prevent skin breakdown. Sitting balance is improved when the feet can be positioned on the leg support of a wheelchair.

Figure 13–32. The dV-Y incision (*top*) and lengthening (*bottom*) of the quadriceps tendon to correct a rigid extension contracture of the knee and allow improved sitting. (Illustration by Anthony C. Berlet. Reproduced, with permission, from Keenan MAE et al: *Manual of Orthopaedic Surgery for Spasticity.* Raven, 1993.)

The spine is of major concern in patients with total body involvement because scoliosis is common. Adaptive seating or orthotics are useful in supporting the spine and helping the patient maintain an erect posture while seated. Spinal fusion with instrumentation is indicated for treatment of progressive scoliosis. Obliquity of the pelvis greatly interferes with sitting. When this problem is present, fusion should include the sacrum.

Buckon CE, Thomas SS, Piatt JH Jr et al: Selective dorsal rhizotomy versus orthopedic surgery: A multidimensional assessment of outcome efficacy. Arch Phys Med Rehabil 2004; 85(3):457. [PMID: 15031833]

Johnston TE, Finson RL, McCarthy JJ et al: Use of functional electrical stimulation to augment traditional orthopaedic surgery in children with cerebral palsy. J Pediatr Orthop 2004;24(3):283. [PMID: 15105724]

Koman LA: Cerebral palsy: Past, present, and future. J South Orthop Assoc 2002;11(2):93. [PMID: 12741589]

Moran CG, Tourret LJ: Recent advances: Orthopaedics. BMJ 2001; 322(7291):902. [PMID: 11302907]

Pfister AA, Roberts AG, Taylor HM et al: Spasticity in adults living in a developmental center. Arch Phys Med Rehabil 2003; 84(12):1808. [PMID: 14669188]

Sussman MD, Aiona MD: Treatment of spastic diplegia in patients with cerebral palsy. J Pediatr Orthop B 2004;13(2):S1. [PMID: 15076595]

Tilton AH: Management of spasticity in children with cerebral palsy. Semin Pediatr Neurol 2004;11(1):58. [PMID: 15132254]

Wren TA, Rethlefsen S, Kay RM: Prevalence of specific gait abnormalities in children with cerebral palsy: Influence of cerebral palsy subtype, age, and previous surgery. J Pediatr Orthop 2005;25(1):79. [PMID: 15614065]

NEUROMUSCULAR DISORDERS

The neuromuscular disorders represent a diverse group of chronic diseases characterized by the progressive degeneration of skeletal musculature, which results in weakness, atrophy, joint contractures, and increasing disability. These disorders are best classified as motor unit diseases because the primary abnormality may involve the motor neuron, the neuromuscular junction, or the muscle fiber. Two broad categories are considered. Myopathies are diseases of the muscle fibers. Neuropathies are disorders in which muscle degeneration is seen secondary to lower motor neuron disease. Most of the neuromuscular disorders are hereditary (Table 13–7), although point mutations may result in spontaneous cases. Early diagnosis is important not only for initiation of appropriate therapy but also for genetic counseling. Treatment programs are aimed at symptomatic and supportive care. Appropriate orthopedic intervention can significantly increase the functional capacity of patients with neuromuscular disorders.

Table 13–7. Classification of the more commonly encountered neuromuscular disorders.

Disorder	Inherited	Creatine Phosphokinase Level	Electromyographic Pattern	Nerve Conduction	Biopsy Pattern
Muscular dystrophies					
Duchenne (pseudohypertrophic) type	Yes	Markedly elevated	Myopathic	Normal	Myopathic
Facioscapulohumeral type	Yes	Normal or elevated	Myopathic	Normal	Myopathic
Limb-girdle type	Yes	Elevated	Myopathic	Normal	Myopathic
Spinal muscular atrophy					
Werdnig-Hoffmann and Kugelberg-Welander types	Yes	Normal or slightly elevated	Neuropathic	Normal	Neuropathic
Hereditary motor and sensory neuropathies					
Type I (Charcot-Marie-Tooth disease)	Yes	Normal	Neuropathic	Markedly decreased	Neuropathic
Type II	Yes	Normal	Neuropathic	Decreased or normal	Neuropathic
Type III	Yes	Normal	Neuropathic	Decreased	Neuropathic
Type IV	Yes	Normal	Neuropathic		Neuropathic
Type V	Yes	Normal	Neuropathic	Normal	Neuropathic
Myopathies					
Central core, nemaline, mini-core, mitochondrial, myo-tubular, and other types	Often	Often normal	Normal or mildly myopathic	Usually normal	Myopathic
Poliomyelitis	No		Neuropathic	Normal	Neuropathic
Guillain-Barré syndrome	No	Normal	Neuropathic	Slow in acute phase	Neuropathic
Polymyositis	No	Normal or elevated	Myopathic	Normal	Myopathic
Myotonic diseases	Usually	Usually normal	Diagnostic	Normal	
Myasthenia gravis	Sometimes		Diagnostic		

Data compiled by Irene Gilgoff, MD, Rancho Los Amigos Medical Center, Downey, CA.

Diagnosis

A. HISTORY AND PHYSICAL EXAMINATION

A careful genetic history is important. The clinical history and physical examination delineates the onset and pattern of muscle involvement. Neuropathies generally present with distal involvement. Muscle fasciculation and spasticity are common, and muscle atrophy is in excess of the weakness. Myopathies usually display weakness of the proximal limb musculature initially. Fasciculations and spasticity are not seen. The weakness is more pronounced than the atrophy. Disorders of neuromuscular transmission, such as myasthenia gravis, present with fatigue and ptosis.

B. MUSCLE ENZYME STUDIES

Serum levels of muscle enzymes are elevated in myopathies but normal in neuropathies. The enzymes studied include creatine phosphokinase (CPK), lactate dehydrogenase (LDH), aldolase, aspartate aminotransferase (AST, SGOT), and alanine aminotransferase (ALT, SGPT). CPK levels are the most elevated in the Duchenne type of muscular dystrophy and less elevated in the more slowly progressive disease forms. In Duchenne-type muscular dystrophy, the highest enzyme levels are seen at birth and during the first few years of life, before the disease is clinically apparent. As the disease progresses and the muscle mass deteriorates, the enzyme levels decrease.

C. ELECTROMYOGRAPHY AND NERVE CONDUCTION STUDIES

EMG and nerve conduction studies differentiate between primary muscle diseases and neuropathies (see Table 13–7). EMG is useful in differentiating among muscle diseases, peripheral nerve disorders, and anterior horn cell abnormalities. A myopathic pattern on EMG is characterized by (1) increased frequency, (2) decreased duration, and (3) decreased amplitude of action potentials. In addition, increased insertional activity, short polyphasic potentials, and a retained interference pattern are evident. A neuropathic pattern on EMG is characterized by the opposite constellation of findings: (1) decreased frequency, (2) increased duration, and (3) increased amplitude of action potentials. In addition, frequent fibrillation potentials, a group polyphasic potential, and a decreased interference pattern can be seen. In myasthenia gravis and the myotonic diseases, the patterns on EMG are diagnostic. In myasthenia gravis, the fatigue phenomenon is exhibited. In myotonia, the EMG is characterized by positive waves and trains of potentials that fire at high frequency and then wax and wane until they slowly disappear.

D. MUSCLE BIOPSY

To gain the maximal amount of information from muscle biopsy, the clinician should choose a muscle that has mild to moderate involvement and was not recently traumatized by electrodes during EMG. Muscle biopsy can be used to differentiate myopathy, neuropathy, and inflammatory myopathy. The biopsy, however, cannot be used to determine prognosis. Histochemical staining further distinguishes the congenital forms of myopathy.

Histologically, myopathies are characterized by muscle fiber necrosis, fatty degeneration, proliferation of the connective tissue, and an increased number of nuclei, some of which have migrated from their normal peripheral position to the center of the muscle fiber.

Neuropathies display small, angulated muscle fibers. Bundles of atrophic fibers are intermingled with bundles of normal fibers. There is no increase in the amount of connective tissue.

Biopsy findings in polymyositis include prominent collections of inflammatory cells, edema of the tissues, perivasculitis, and segmental necrosis with a mixed pattern of fiber degeneration and regeneration.

Dietz FR, Mathews KD: Update on the genetic bases of disorders with orthopaedic manifestations. J Bone Joint Surg AM 1996;78:1583. [PMID: 88765869]

Esquenazi A et al: Dynamic polyelectromyography, neurolysis, and chemodenervation with Botulinum toxin A for assessment and treatment of gait dysfunction. In Ruzicka E et al, eds: *Advances in Neurology: Gait Disorders,* Vol. 87. Lippincott Williams & Wilkins, 2001.

Roberts A, Evans GA: Orthopedic aspects of neuromuscular disorders in children. Curr Opin Pediatr 1993;5:379.

1. Duchenne-Type Muscular Dystrophy

Duchenne-type muscular dystrophy, which is also called **pseudohypertrophic muscular dystrophy,** is a progressive disease that affects males. It is inherited in an X-linked recessive manner and has its onset in early childhood. Generally, affected children have a normal birth and developmental history. But by the time they reach 3–5 years of age, sufficient muscle mass has been lost to impair function.

Clinical Findings

Early signs of disease include pseudohypertrophy of the calf, which is the result of the increase in connective tissue; planovalgus deformity of the feet, which is secondary to heel cord contracture; and proximal muscle weakness. Muscle weakness in the hips may be exhibited by the Gower sign, in which the patient uses the arms to support the trunk while attempting to rise from the floor. Other signs are hesitance when climbing stairs, acceleration during the final stage of sitting, and shoulder weakness.

Weakness and contractures prevent independent ambulation in approximately 45% of patients by 9 years of age and in the remainder by 12 years of age. It is common for patients to have difficulty first in rising from the floor, next in ascending the stairs, and then in walking. Cardiac involvement is seen in 80% of patients. Findings generally include posterobasal fibrosis of the ventricle and electrocardiographic changes. In patients with a decreased level of activity, clinical evidence of cardiomyopathy may not be obvious. Pulmonary problems are common in the advanced stages of the disease and are found during periodic evaluations of pulmonary function. Mental retardation, noted in 30–50% of patients, is present from birth and not progressive.

Management

Efforts are made to keep patients ambulating for as many years as possible to prevent the complications of obesity, osteoporosis, and scoliosis. The hip flexors, tensor fasciae latae, and triceps surae develop ambulation-limiting contractures. With progressive weakness and contractures, the base of support decreases and the patient cannot use normal mechanisms to maintain upright balance. The patient walks with a wide-based gait, hips flexed and abducted, knees flexed, and the feet in equinus and varus position. Lumbar lordosis becomes exaggerated to compensate for the hip flexion contractures and weak hip extensor musculature.

Equinus contractures of the Achilles tendon occur early and are caused by the muscle imbalance between the calf and pretibial muscles. Initially, this problem can be managed by heel cord stretching exercises and night splints. A KAFO may be needed to control foot position and substitute for weak quadriceps muscles. Stretching exercises and pronation can be employed to treat early hip flexion contractures.

Surgical intervention is directed toward the release of ambulation-limiting contractures. Early postoperative mobilization is important to prevent further muscle weakness. Anesthetic risks are increased in these patients because of their limited pulmonary reserve and because the incidence of malignant hyperthermia is higher than normal in patients with muscle disease.

The triceps surae and tibialis posterior are the strongest muscles in the lower extremity of the patient with muscular dystrophy. These muscles are responsible for equinus and varus deformities. Management that consists of releasing the contracted tensor fasciae latae, lengthening the Achilles tendon, and transferring the tibialis posterior muscle anteriorly is indicated and prolongs walking for approximately 3 years. Postoperative bracing is required.

Scoliosis is common in nonambulatory patients confined to a wheelchair. Adaptive seating devices that hold the pelvis level and the spine erect are useful in preventing deformity. Alternatively, a rigid plastic spinal torso orthosis may be used for support. When external support is not effective, scoliosis develops rapidly. Spinal fusion is occasionally indicated. Blood loss during surgery is high, and the incidence of pseudarthrosis is increased. Postoperative immobilization is to be avoided; therefore, segmental spinal stabilization is often the preferred technique of internal stabilization.

Fractures in patients with myopathies occur secondary to osteoporosis from the inactivity and the loss of muscle tension. No abnormalities of bone mineralization are present. The incidence of fracture increases with the severity of the disease. Most fractures are metaphyseal in location, show little displacement, cause minimal pain, and heal in the expected time without complication.

Bentley G et al: The treatment of scoliosis in muscular dystrophy using modified Luque and Harrington-Luque instrumentation. J Bone Joint Surg Br 2001;83:22. [PMID: 11245532]

Biggar WD, Klamut HJ, Demacio PC et al: Duchenne muscular dystrophy: Current knowledge, treatment, and future prospects. Clin Orthop 2002;401:88. [PMID: 12151886]

Do T: Orthopedic management of the muscular dystrophies. Curr Opin Pediatr 2002;14(1):50. [PMID: 11880734]

Sussman M: Duchenne muscular dystrophy. J Am Acad Orthop Surg 2002;10(2):138. [PMID: 11929208]

Yamashita T et al: Prediction of progression of spinal deformity in Duchenne muscular dystrophy: A preliminary report. Spine 2001;26:E223. [PMID: 11389405]

2. Spinal Muscular Atrophy

Spinal muscular atrophy is a neuropathic disorder in which fewer anterior horn cells are present in the spinal cord congenitally. The severe infantile form of the disease is called **Werdnig-Hoffmann paralysis.** The disorder is inherited in an autosomal-recessive pattern.

Approximately 20% of patients with spinal muscular atrophy are ambulatory, and 1% are totally dependent. Fractures are common in these patients and occur secondary to decreased mobility and function.

The goal of orthopedic intervention is to prevent collapse of the spine and contractures. Orthotic support is often needed to stabilize the spine. In the nonambulatory patient, adaptive seating devices or orthotics may be used. If collapse of the spine occurs, spinal fusion is indicated.

Bentley G et al: The treatment of scoliosis in muscular dystrophy using modified Luque and Harrington-Luque instrumentation. J Bone Joint Surg Br 2001;83:22. [PMID: 11245532]

Frugier T, Nicole S, Cifuentes-Diaz C et al: The molecular bases of spinal muscular atrophy. Curr Opin Genet Dev 2002;12(3):294. [PMID: 12076672]

Hopf CG, Eysel P: One-stage versus two-stage spinal fusion in neuromuscular scolioses. J Pediatr Orthop B 2000;9(4):234. [PMID: 11143465]

Iannaccone ST, Burghes A: Spinal muscular atrophies. Adv Neurol 2002;88:83. [PMID: 11908238]

Iannaccone ST, Smith SA, Simard LR: Spinal muscular atrophy. Curr Neurol Neurosci Rep 2004;4(1):74. [PMID: 14683633]

Nicole S, Diaz CC, Frugier T et al: Spinal muscular atrophy: Recent advances and future prospects. Muscle Nerve 2002;26(1):4. [PMID: 12115944]

Noordeen MH et al: Blood loss in Duchenne muscular dystrophy: Vascular smooth muscle dysfunction? J Pediatr Orthop B 2001;8:212. [PMID: 10399127]

3. Charcot-Marie-Tooth Disease

Charcot-Marie-Tooth disease is the most common of the hereditary degenerative myopathies. It is generally inherited in an autosomal-dominant pattern. EMG studies show a neuropathic pattern, and the nerve conduction velocity of the involved nerves is markedly decreased. Muscle enzyme levels are normal. Clinical onset of the disease is between 5 and 15 years of age.

The peroneal muscles are affected early in the course of the disease. For this reason, Charcot-Marie-Tooth disease is sometimes referred to as **progressive peroneal muscular atrophy.** The intrinsic muscles of the feet and hands are affected later. Patients usually present with progressive clawtoe and cavus deformities of the feet. In the skeletally immature patient, release of the plantar fascia is done to correct the cavus deformity. This is often combined with transfer of the extensor digitorum longus tendon to the neck of the metatarsal and fusion of the proximal interphalangeal joints of the toes to correct the clawtoe deformities. If the tibialis posterior muscle is active during swing phase, it can be transferred through the interosseous membrane to the lateral cuneiform bone. Triple arthrodesis is often necessary in the adult to correct the deformity.

The intrinsic minus hand deformity causes difficulty in grasping objects. An orthosis with a lumbrical bar to hold the metacarpophalangeal joints flexed improves hand use. A capsulodesis of the volar portion of the metacarpophalangeal joints accomplishes the same objective. To restore active intrinsic muscle function in the hand, the flexor digitorum superficialis tendon of the ring finger can be divided into four slips and transferred through the lumbrical passages to the proximal phalanx.

Aktas S, Sussman MD: The radiological analysis of pes cavus deformity in Charcot Marie Tooth disease. J Pediatr Orthop B 2000;9:137. [PMID: 10868366]

Borg K, Ericson-Gripenstedt U: Muscle biopsy abnormalities differ between Charcot-Marie-Tooth type 1 and 2: Reflect different pathophysiology? Exerc Sport Sci Rev 2002;30:4.

Guyton GP, Mann RA: The pathogenesis and surgical management of foot deformity in Charcot-Marie-Tooth disease. Foot Ankle Clin 2000;5(2):317. [PMID: 11232233]

Olney B: Treatment of the cavus foot. Deformity in the pediatric patient with Charcot-Marie-Tooth. Foot Ankle Clin 2000;5(2): 305. [PMID: 11232232]

Smith AG: Charcot-Marie-Tooth disease. Arch Neurol 2001;58: 1014. [PMID: 11405820]

Schwend RM, Drennan JC: Cavus foot deformity in children. J Am Acad Orthop Surg 2003;11(3):201. [PMID: 12828450]

PARKINSON DISEASE

A. Epidemiology

Parkinson disease (PD) is a progressive neurodegenerative disorder associated with a loss of dopaminergic nigrostriatal neurons. PD is recognized as one of the most common neurological disorders, affecting approximately 1% of individuals older than 60 years. The incidence and prevalence of PD increase with age. The average age of onset is approximately 60 years. Onset in persons younger than 40 years is relatively uncommon.

B. Pathophysiology

The major neuropathologic findings in PD are a loss of pigmented dopaminergic neurons in the substantia nigra and the presence of Lewy bodies. The loss of dopaminergic neurons occurs most prominently in the ventral lateral substantia nigra. Approximately 60–80% of dopaminergic neurons are lost before clinical symptoms of PD emerge.

C. History

Onset of PD is typically asymmetric, with the most common initial finding being an asymmetric resting tremor in an upper extremity. Approximately 20% of patients first experience clumsiness in one hand. Over time, patients notice symptoms related to progressive bradykinesia, rigidity, and gait difficulty. The initial symptoms of PD may be nonspecific and include fatigue and depression.

D. Physical Examination

The three cardinal signs of PD are resting tremor, rigidity, and bradykinesia. Of these cardinal features, two of three are required to make the clinical diagnosis. Postural instability is the fourth cardinal sign, but it emerges late in the disease, usually after 8 years or more.

E. Medical Care

The goal of medical management of PD is to provide control of signs and symptoms for as long as possible while minimizing adverse effects. Medications (eg, levodopa) usually provide good symptomatic control for 4–6 years. After this, disability progresses despite best medical management, and many patients develop long-term motor complications including fluctuations and dyskinesia. Additional causes of disability in late disease include postural instability (balance difficulty) and dementia.

F. Neurosurgical Care

When medical management is exhausted, neurosurgical interventions include deep brain stimulation, thalamotomy, pallidotomy, and fetal cell transplantation.

G. Orthopedic Care

Treatment of orthopedic problems in patients with PD can be problematic and include failure of fixation or prosthetic dislocation. Despite successful pain relief, the functional results of total joint arthroplasty in patients with Parkinson disease are poor, especially in patients older than 65 years, and complications are more frequent. Success in terms of pain relief and no further need for intervention can be obtained with appropriate medical management of the PD after orthopedic intervention.

Gauggel S, Rieger M, Feghoff TA: Inhibition of ongoing responses in patients with Parkinson's disease. J Neurol Neurosurg Psychiatry 2004;75(4):539. [PMID: 15026491]

Tabamo RE, Fernandez HH, Friedman JH et al: Spinal surgery for severe scoliosis in Parkinson's disease. Med Health R I 2000;83(4):114. [PMID: 10821012]

Weber M, Cabanela ME, Sim FH et al: Total hip replacement in patients with Parkinson's disease. Int Orthop 2002;26(2):66. [PMID: 12078878]

BURNS

More than 2 million people sustain burns of sufficient severity each year in the United States to require medical attention. Of these, 50,000 individuals remain hospitalized for more than 2 months, attesting to the serious nature of their injuries.

Thermal burns affect the skin most directly but can also involve the underlying muscles, tendons, joints, and bones. Scar contractures cause the greatest limitation to later function and the greatest deformity. Rehabilitation efforts ideally should begin when the patient first enters the hospital, immediately following acute resuscitation and continuing through the reconstruction process.

Classification

Burn wounds are traditionally classified as first, second, or third degree, depending on the depth of the damage. Currently, it is thought to be more useful to simply divide burns into two categories: partial thickness (involving part of the dermis) and full thickness (involving the entire dermis).

First-degree burns damage only the epidermis. They cause erythema, minor edema, and pain. The skin surface remains intact, and healing occurs uneventfully in 5–10 days, without residual scar formation.

Second-degree burns involve the epidermis and a variable amount of the underlying corium. The depth of damage to the corium determines the outcome of healing. In the more superficial second-degree burns, blister formation is prominent and occurs secondary to the osmotic gradient formed by particles in the vesicle fluid. Superficial second-degree burns heal in 10–14 days, with minimal scarring. Deep dermal burns are characterized by either a reddish appearance or by the presence of a white tissue that is barely perceptible and adheres to the underlying viable dermis. These wounds may advance to a full-thickness loss if infection occurs. They heal with a fragile epithelial covering. Healing occurs over 25–30 days, and dense scar formation is common.

Third-degree burns are full-thickness injuries that damage the epidermis and the entire corium. Because of the loss of pain receptors, which are normally found within the corium, pain is absent. The burns have a thick leathery surface of dead tissue.

Management

A. TECHNIQUES FOR MAINTAINING FUNCTIONAL POSITION

Burn scars contract and become rigid, so it is critical to maintain the head, trunk, and extremities in a functional position. Contractures, if allowed to form, severely limit later function. The location of the burns determines which techniques are useful in preventing deformity.

To prevent deformities of the neck and jaw in patients with burns of the neck or upper torso, molded splints should be applied early to maintain the head and neck in a neutral position or in slight extension. Patients with burns in the shoulder region are at risk for contractures characterized by a protracted scapula with an adducted arm. Placing a roll between the scapulae and providing support with a firm mattress help prevent scapula protraction. To keep the arms abducted 75–80 degrees and the shoulder flexed 20–30 degrees, axillary foam pads are used and can be held in position with a figure-of-8 wrapping, which maintain the glenohumeral joint in a functional position. Untreated contractures not only limit limb motion but also can result in joint subluxation from extremes in positioning.

When the burns involve the torso, the goal is to maintain a straight spine in the face of contracting scar tissue. Burns involving only one side of the trunk sometimes result in scoliosis. This should be corrected by scar excision and splinting. If left uncorrected, the scoliosis becomes structural, with resultant bony changes. Burns in the groin area tend to cause flexion and adduction contractures of the hip. To prevent this, the patient should be positioned with the hips extended and in 15–20 degrees of abduction. If the patient is lying on a soft mattress, mild flexion deformities of the hips may be masked. Daily pronation is useful in maintaining the extension range of the hips.

Regardless of the location of burn wounds on the extremities, the knees and elbows tend to develop flexion contractures. Custom-molded thermoplastic splints can be applied over dressings or skin grafts to maintain the extremities in extension. The splints should be removable to allow for daily wound care. Burns in the ankle area result in equinus contractures with inversion of the foot. Splints can be used here also to maintain the foot in a neutral position, but care must be taken to ensure the splint is holding the foot adequately and not merely obscuring a deformity. Custom-molded splints applied to the anterior and posterior surfaces in a clamshell fashion are more effective in maintaining the desired position. They also assist in the control of edema and can be removed for wound care and motion exercises. Burns on the dorsum of the foot cause hyperextension deformities of the toes. Early grafting and toe traction are useful.

Burns of the hands present special problems. Scar contracture results in a flexion deformity of the wrist and a clawhand position similar to that seen with loss of the intrinsic musculature. The hand should be splinted with the wrist in neutral or in a slightly extended position. The metacarpophalangeal joints should be flexed 60–75 degrees and the interphalangeal joints extended. The thumb should be held with the metacarpal in abduction and flexion, the metacarpophalangeal joint in mild flexion, and the interphalangeal joint in the extended position.

B. SKELETAL TRACTION AND EXTERNAL SUSPENSION

In patients with circumferential burns on an extremity, the use of skeletal traction or external fixators and suspension is efficacious and has several advantages. It permits access to all surfaces, elevates the limb to decrease edema, and maintains the extremity in the desired position while allowing joint motion. Traction can be used to correct contractures. In addition, traction still allows for daily hydrotherapy. Generally, traction is only employed for a 2-week period because longer use may result in a pin tract infection with formation of sequestra.

Special splints are fabricated for use in the hand. The traction frame is secured proximally with a pin inserted through the distal radius. Pins are also placed through the distal phalanges of the fingers and thumb by drilling through the nail bed from the dorsal to the volar surface. Traction is applied to the fingers in the desired direction by attaching rubber bands from the distal pins to the outrigger frame. The frame can be modified for use in the foot to apply traction to the toes. In this case, the traction frame is secured proximally with a pin inserted through the calcaneus.

C. PRESSURE DRESSINGS

Consistent pressure of 25 torr applied evenly aids in the prevention of hypertrophic scar formation and contracture. Elastic wraps applied over splints are used early after the injury and following grafting because they can be adjusted for changes in the amount of edema present. Later, when the amount of swelling shows little fluctuation, custom elastic garments are employed. Pressure must be continued for as long as the scar tissue is biologically active. When the skin is soft and flat and returns to normal color, the pressure can be discontinued. Pressure dressings should be employed for a minimum of 6 months and may be necessary for as long as a year. The daily application of lanolin relieves the dryness of grafted skin or substitutes for the loss of sebaceous gland secretions in deep burns.

D. MOBILIZATION

Early motion is desirable for burned and uninvolved extremities. Splints should be removed frequently to allow for ROM exercises. If the patient is being treated with skeletal traction, motion exercises can be performed on the extremities. If the patient is receiving hydrotherapy for the burn wounds, the motion exercises are facilitated with the extremities supported in the fluid environment.

Patients with burns of the lower extremities can begin to stand or walk before skin grafts are performed, provided the legs are wrapped with elastic supports to control edema. Ambulation should be resumed after skin grafting as soon as the grafts are stable. Early mobilization not only preserves joint motion but also decreases the incidence of sequelae such as osteoporosis, physiologic deconditioning, muscle atrophy, and heterotopic ossification.

E. TREATMENT OF SPECIAL PROBLEMS

1. Fractures—If fractures occurred at the time of the burn, they can be treated with the use of skeletal traction or external supports such as splints. Diagnosis may be delayed if the fractures do not result in any obvious deformity. If fractures occur secondary to disuse osteoporosis, they are usually minimally displaced and heal uneventfully. Pathologic fractures are less common with early mobilization.

2. Osteomyelitis—Osteomyelitis is not a common complication, despite the high incidence of sepsis associated with burns. Prolonged exposure of bone sometimes results in the formation of a tangential sequestrum in the devitalized cortex. Exposed bone surfaces can be drilled to promote the formation of a granulation tissue bed for skin grafting without an increased risk of infection. The prolonged use of pins for skeletal traction causes infection in 5% of patients who require traction. The use of threaded traction pins minimizes the motion of the pin in the bone. Pins should be removed as soon as possible.

3. Exposed joints—Children and adolescents with exposed joint surfaces may retain some function after healing, but adults often develop joint ankylosis or deformities that require arthrodesis at a later date. To maintain the joint in the desired position, traction can be used. The joint should be irrigated with hypochlorite solution daily and debrided as necessary. The exposed bone surfaces can be drilled to promote the formation of granulation tissue. When the bed of tissue covers the joint, skin grafting is performed.

4. Heterotopic ossification—Periarticular bone formation is seen in 2–3% of patients with severe burns. Although the cause is unknown, predisposing factors include full-thickness burns involving more than 30% of the body surface, prolonged immobilization, and superimposed trauma. The location of the heterotopic bone is not determined by the distribution of the burns. Ossification can occur in any of the major joints. In adults, the elbow is the joint most frequently affected; the hip is rarely affected. In children, the hip and elbow are common sites; the shoulder is an uncommon site.

Heterotopic bone can continue to form as long as open granulating wounds are present. If joint ankylosis does not occur, the ossification gradually diminishes after the burns heal. In children, it may disappear completely. If joint ankylosis occurs, surgical resection is indicated and usually restores a functional arc of motion, particularly when the heterotopic bone is in a single plane and the articular surface is not violated. When the heterotopic bone is present in multiple planes, the problem may recur after resection. Early mobilization of patients with burns decreases the incidence and severity of heterotopic ossification.

Edgar D, Brereton M: Rehabilitation after burn injury. BMJ 2004;329(7461):343. [PMID: 15297346]

Goldberg DP et al: Reconstruction of the burned foot. Clin Plast Surg 2000;27:145. [PMID: 10665363]

James J: The treatment of severe burns of head, hands and feet. Trop Doct 2001;31:178. [PMID: 11444349]

Luce EA: The acute and subacute management of the burned hand. Clin Plast Surg 2000;27:49. [PMID: 10665355]

Prakash V, Bajaj SP: A new concept for the treatment of postburn contracture of the elbow. Ann Plast Surg 2000;45:339. [PMID: 10987541]

Silverberg R et al: Gait variables of patients after lower extremity burn injuries. J Burn Care Rehabil 2000;21:259. [PMID: 10850909]

Tilley W et al: Rehabilitation of the burned upper extremity. Hand Clin 2000;16:303. [PMID: 10791175]

Index

Note: Page numbers in **boldface** type indicate a major discussion. Page numbers followed by *b* indicate boxed material; page numbers followed by *f* indicate figures; and page numbers followed by *t* indicate tables.